UNIT VI
Psychosocial Basis for Nursing Practice

UNIT VII
Physiological Basis for Nursing Practice

NINTH EDITION

FUNDAMENTALS OF NURSING

Patricia A. Potter, RN, MSN, PhD, FAAN
Director of Research
Patient Care Services
Barnes-Jewish Hospital
St. Louis, Missouri

Anne Griffin Perry, RN, MSN, EdD, FAAN
Professor Emerita
School of Nursing
Southern Illinois University Edwardsville
Edwardsville, Illinois

Patricia A. Stockert, RN, BSN, MS, PhD
President, College of Nursing
Saint Francis Medical Center College of Nursing
Peoria, Illinois

Amy M. Hall, RN, BSN, MS, PhD, CNE
Chair and White Family Endowed Professor of Nursing
Dunigan Family Department of Nursing and Health Sciences
University of Evansville
Evansville, Indiana

SECTION EDITOR:
Wendy R. Ostendorf, RN, MS, EdD, CNE
Professor of Nursing
Neumann University
Aston, Pennsylvania

ELSEVIER

ELSEVIER

3251 Riverport Lane
St. Louis, Missouri 63043

FUNDAMENTALS OF NURSING, NINTH EDITION ISBN: 978-0-323-32740-4

Notices

Knowledge and best practice in this field are constantly changing. As new research and experience broaden our understanding, changes in research methods, professional practices, or medical treatment may become necessary.

Practitioners and researchers must always rely on their own experience and knowledge in evaluating and using any information, methods, compounds, or experiments described herein. In using such information or methods they should be mindful of their own safety and the safety of others, including parties for whom they have a professional responsibility.

With respect to any drug or pharmaceutical products identified, readers are advised to check the most current information provided (i) on procedures featured or (ii) by the manufacturer of each product to be administered, to verify the recommended dose or formula, the method and duration of administration, and contraindications. It is the responsibility of practitioners, relying on their own experience and knowledge of their patients, to make diagnoses, to determine dosages and the best treatment for each individual patient, and to take all appropriate safety precautions.

To the fullest extent of the law, neither the Publisher nor the authors, contributors, or editors, assume any liability for any injury and/or damage to persons or property as a matter of products liability, negligence or otherwise, or from any use or operation of any methods, products, instructions, or ideas contained in the material herein.

Previous editions copyrighted 2013, 2009, 2005, 2001, 1997, 1993, 1989, and 1985.

International Standard Book Number: 978-0-323-32740-4

Executive Content Strategist: Tamara Myers
Content Development Manager: Jean Sims Fornango
Senior Content Development Specialist: Tina Kaemmerer
Publishing Services Manager: Jeff Patterson
Senior Project Manager: Jodi M. Willard
Design Direction: Maggie Reid

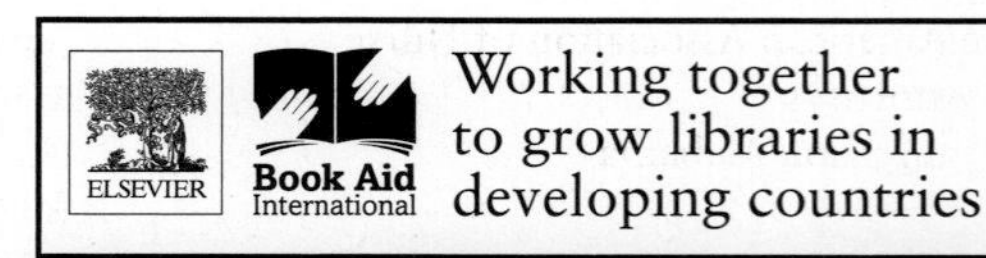

Printed in Canada

Last digit is the print number: 9 8 7 6 5 4 3

CONTRIBUTORS

Michelle Aebersold, PhD, RN
Clinical Associate Professor
Director—Clinical Learning Center
School of Nursing
University of Michigan
Ann Arbor, Michigan

Katherine N. Ayzengart, MSN, RN
Associate Faculty
Nursing
MiraCosta College
Oceanside, California

Brenda Battle, RN, BSN, MBA
Vice President, Care Delivery Innovation, Urban Health Initiative and Chief Diversity and Inclusion Officer
University of Chicago Medicine and Biological Sciences
Chicago, Illinois

Janice C. Colwell, RN, MS, CWOCN, FAAN
Advanced Practice Nurse
Surgery
University of Chicago Medicine
Chicago, Illinois

Maureen F. Cooney, DNP, FNP-BC
Adjunct Associate Professor of Nursing
FNP Program
Lienhard School of Nursing
College of Health Professions
Pace University
Pleasantville, New York;
Nurse Practitioner
Pain Medicine
Westchester Medical Center
Valhalla, New York

Cheryl A. Crowe, RN, MS
Assistant Professor
Saint Francis Medical Center College of Nursing
Peoria, Illinois

Alice E. Dupler, JD, APRN-ANP, Esq.
Associate Professor
School of Nursing & Human Physiology
Gonzaga University
Spokane, Washington;
Corresponding Secretary
Executive Board of Directors
The American Association of Nurse Attorneys
Birmingham, Alabama

Margaret Ecker, RN, MS
Director of Nursing Quality (Retired)
Kaiser Permanente Los Angeles Medical Center
Los Angeles, California

Antoinette Falker, DNP, RN, CMSRN, CBN, GCNS-BC
Adjunct Faculty
Nursing Department
Webster University
Webster Groves, Missouri;
Clinical Nurse Specialist
Trauma, Geriatric Trauma, Acute Care Surgery, Bariatric Services
Barnes-Jewish Hospital
St. Louis, Missouri

Jane Fellows, MSN, CWOCN
Wound/Ostomy CNS
Advanced Clinical Practice
Duke University Health System
Durham, North Carolina

Linda Felver, PhD, RN
Associate Professor
School of Nursing
Oregon Health & Science University
Portland, Oregon

Susan Fetzer, RN, GSWN, MSN, MBA, PhD
Associate Professor
College of Health and Human Services
University of New Hampshire
Durham, New Hampshire

Victoria N. Folse, PhD, APN, PMHCNS-BC, LCPC
Director and Professor
Caroline F. Rupert Endowed Chair of Nursing
School of Nursing
Illinois Wesleyan University
Bloomington, Illinois

Kay E. Gaehle, PhD, MSN, BSN
Associate Professor
School of Nursing, Primary Care Department
Southern Illinois University Edwardsville
Edwardsville, Illinois

Lorri A. Graham, RN
Assistant Professor
Nursing
Saint Francis Medical Center College of Nursing
Peoria, Illinois

Tara Hulsey, PhD, RN, CNE, FAAN
Dean and E. Jane Martin Professor
School of Nursing
West Virginia University
Morgantown, West Virginia

Noël Kerr, PhD, RN, CMSRN
Assistant Professor
School of Nursing
Illinois Wesleyan University
Bloomington, Illinois

Mary Koithan, PhD, RN, CNS-BC, FAAN
Anne Furrow Professor and Associate Dean, Professional and Community Engagement
College of Nursing
University of Arizona
Tucson, Arizona

Gayle L. Kruse, RN, ACHPN, GCNS-BC
APN Instructor
Graduate Department
Saint Anthony College of Nursing
Rockford, Illinois

Jerrilee LaMar, PhD, RN, CNE
Associate Professor of Nursing
Dunigan Family Department of Nursing and Health Sciences
University of Evansville
Evansville, Indiana

Kathryn Lever, MSN, WHNP-BC
Associate Professor of Nursing
College of Education and Health Sciences
University of Evansville
Evansville, Indiana

Erin H. McCalley, RN, BSN, MS, CCRN, CCNS
Clinical Nurse Specialist
Nursing Education and Practice
Stanford Health Care
Stanford, California

Emily L. McClung, MSN, RN, PhD(c)
Nursing Instructor
Hiram College
Hiram, Ohio

Judith A. McCutchan, RN, ASN, BSN, MSN, PhD
Adjunct Nursing Faculty
Dunigan Family Department of Nursing and Health Sciences
University of Evansville
Evansville, Indiana

Patricia A. O'Connor, RN, MSN, CNE
Assistant Professor
College of Nursing
Saint Francis Medical Center College of Nursing
Peoria, Illinois

Jill Parsons, PhD, RN
Associate Professor of Nursing
MacMurray College
Jacksonville, Illinois

Beverly J. Reynolds, RN, EdD, CNE
Professor
Graduate Program
Saint Francis Medical Center College of Nursing
Peoria, Illinois

Kristine Rose, BSN, MSN
Assistant Professor
Nursing Education
Saint Francis Medical Center College of Nursing
Peoria, Illinois

Patsy L. Ruchala, DNSc, RN
Professor and Director
Orvis School of Nursing
University of Nevada, Reno
Reno, Nevada

Matthew R. Sorenson, PhD, APN, ANP-C
Associate Professor/Associate Director
School of Nursing
DePaul University
Chicago, Illinois;
Clinical Scholar
Physical Medicine and Rehabilitation
Northwestern University Feinberg School of Medicine
Chicago, Illinois

Donna L. Thompson, MSN, CRNP, FNP-BC, CCCN-AP
Continence Nurse Practitioner
Division of Urogynecology
University of Pennsylvania Medical Center
Philadelphia, Pennsylvania;
Continence Nurse Practitioner
Urology Health Specialist
Drexel Hill, Pennsylvania;
Continence Consultant/Owner
Continence Solutions, LLC
Media, Pennsylvania

Jelena Todic, MSW, LCSW
Doctoral Student
Social Work
University of Texas at Austin
Austin, Texas

CONTRIBUTORS TO PREVIOUS EDITIONS

Jeanette Adams, PhD, MSN, APRN, CRNI
Paulette M. Archer, RN, EdD
Myra. A. Aud, PhD, RN
Marjorie Baier, PhD, RN
Sylvia K. Baird, RN, BSN, MM
Karen Balakas, PhD, RN, CNE
Lois Bentler-Lampe, RN, MS
Janice Boundy, RN, PhD
Anna Brock, PhD, MSN, MEd, BSN
Sheryl Buckner, RN-BC, MS, CNE
Jeri Burger, PhD, RN
Linda Cason, MSN, RN-BC, NE-BC, CNRN
Pamela L. Cherry, RN, BSN, MSN, DNSc
Rhonda W. Comrie, PhD, RN, CNE, AE-C
Eileen Costantinou, MSN, RN
Ruth M. Curchoe, RN, MSN, CIC
Marinetta DeMoss, RN, MSN
Christine R. Durbin, PhD, JD, RN
Martha Keene Elkin, RN, MS, IBCLC
Leah W. Frederick, MS, RN CIC
Mimi Hirshberg, RN, MSN
Steve Kilkus, RN, MSN
Judith Ann Kilpatrick, RN, DNSc
Lori Klingman, MSN, RN
Karen Korem, RN-BC, MA
Anahid Kulwicki, RN, DNS, FAAN
Joyce Larson, PhD, MS, RN
Kristine M. L'Ecuyer, RN, MSN, CCNS
Ruth Ludwick, BSN, MSN, PhD, RNC
Annette G. Lueckenotte, MS, RN, BC, GNP, GCNS
Frank Lyerla, PhD, RN
Deborah Marshall, MSN
Barbara Maxwell, RN, BSN, MS, MSN, CNS
Elaine K. Neel, RN, BSN, MSN
Wendy Ostendorf, BSN, MS, EdD
Dula Pacquiao, BSN, MA, EdD
Nancy C. Panthofer, RN, MSN
Elaine U. Polan, RNC, BSN, MS
Debbie Sanazaro, RN, MSN, GNP
Marilyn Schallom, RN, MSN, CCRN, CCNS
Carrie Sona, RN, MSN, CCRN, ACNS, CCNS
Marshelle Thobaben, RN, MS, PHN, APNP, FNP
Ann B. Tritak, EdD, MA, BSN, RN
Janis Waite, RN, MSN, EdD
Mary Ann Wehmer, RN, MSN, CNOR
Pamela Becker Weilitz, RN, MSN(R), BC, ANP, M-SCNS
Joan Domigan Wentz, BSN, MSN
Katherine West, BSN, MSEd, CIC
Terry L. Wood, PhD, RN, CNE
Rita Wunderlich, PhD, RN
Valerie Yancey, PhD, RN

REVIEWERS

Colleen Andreoni, DNP, FNP-BC, ANP-BC, CEN
Assistant Professor and Department Chair
Health Promotion & Risk Reduction
Marcella Niehoff School of Nursing
Loyola University Chicago
Chicago, Illinois

Suzanne L. Bailey, PMHCNS-BC, CNE
Associate Professor of Nursing
University of Evansville
Evansville, Indiana

Lisa Boggs, BSN, RN
ER Staff Nurse
Mercy Hospital
Lebanon, Missouri;
Teaching Assistant
Sinclair School of Nursing
University of Missouri—Columbia
Columbia, Missouri

Leigh Ann Bonney, PhD, RN, CCRN
Assistant Professor
College of Nursing
Saint Francis Medical Center College of Nursing
Peoria, Illinois

Anna M. Bruch, RN, MSN
Nursing Professor
Illinois Valley Community College
Oglesby, Illinois

Jeanie Burt, MSN, MA, CNE
Carr College of Nursing
Harding University
Searcy, Arkansas

Pat Callard, DNP, RN, CNL, CNE
Assistant Professor of Nursing
College of Graduate Nursing;
Director
Interprofessional Education, Phase II
Pomona, California

Susan M.S. Carlson, MS, RN, APRN-BC, NPP
Associate Professor
Monroe Community College
Rochester, New York

Tracy Colburn, MSN, RN, C-EFM
Assistant Professor of Nursing
Lewis and Clark Community College
Godfrey, Illinois

Barbara Coles, PhD(c), RN-BC
Registered Nurse
James A. Haley VA Hospital
University of South Florida
Tampa, Florida

Dorothy Diaz, MSN, RN-BC
Caregiver Support Coordinator
James A. Haley VA Hospital
Tampa, Florida

Holly J. Diesel, PhD, RN
Associate Professor
Goldfarb School of Nursing
Barnes-Jewish College
St. Louis, Missouri

Dawna Egelhoff, MSN, RN
Associate Professor
Lewis and Clark Community College
Godfrey, Illinois

Amber Essman, MSN, APRN, FNP-BC, CNE
Assistant Professor
Chamberlain College of Nursing
Columbus, Ohio

Margie L. Francisco, EdD, MSN
Nursing Professor
Illinois Valley Community College
Oglesby, Illinois

Linda Garner, PhD, RN, CHES
Assistant Professor
Department of Nursing
Southeast Missouri State University
Cape Girardeau, Missouri

Amy S. Hamlin, PhD, MSN, FNP-BC, APN
Professor of Nursing
Austin Peay State University
Clarksville, Tennessee

Nicole M. Heimgartner, RN, MSN, COI
Associate Professor of Nursing
Kettering College
Kettering, Ohio

Mary Ann Jessee, MSN, RN
Assistant Professor
School of Nursing
Vanderbilt University
Nashville, Tennessee

Kathleen C. Jones, MSN, RN, CNS
Associate Professor of Nursing
Walters State Community College
Morristown, Tennessee

Lori L. Kelley, RN, MSN, MBA
Associate Professor of Nursing
Aquinas College
Nashville, Tennessee

Shari Kist, PhD, RN, CNE
Assistant Professor
Goldfarb School of Nursing
Barnes-Jewish College
St. Louis, Missouri

Laura Szopo Martin, MSN, RN, CNE
Professor
College of Southern Nevada
Las Vegas, Nevada

Angela McConachie, DNP, FNP-C
Instructor
Goldfarb School of Nursing
Barnes-Jewish College
St. Louis, Missouri

Tammy McConnell, MSN, APRN, FNP-BC
Associate Professor of Nursing
Admission and Progression Coordinator
Clinical Coordinator
Greenville Technical College
Greenville, South Carolina

Janis Longfield McMillan, RN, MSN, CNE
Nursing Faculty
Coconino Community College
Flagstaff, Arizona

Pamela S. Merida, MSN, RN
Assistant Professor, Nursing
St. Elizabeth School of Nursing
Lafayette, Indiana

Jeanie Mitchel, RN, MSN, MA
Nursing Professor
South Suburban College
South Holland, Illinois

Katrin Moskowitz, BSN, MSN, FNP
Family Nurse Practitioner
Bristol Hospital Multispecialty Group
Bristol, Connecticut

Cindy Mulder, RNC, MS, MSN, WHNP-BC, FNP-BC
Instructor
The University of South Dakota
Vermillion, South Dakota

Cathlin Buckingham Poronsky, PhD, APRN, FNP-BC
Assistant Professor
Director of the Family Nurse Practitioner Program
Marcella Niehoff School of Nursing
Loyola University Chicago
Chicago, Illinois

Beth Hogan Quigley, MSN, RN, CRNP
Family and Community Health Department Advanced Senior Lecturer
University of Pennsylvania School of Nursing
Philadelphia, Pennsylvania

Cherie R. Rebar, PhD, MBA, RN, FNP, COI
Director, Division of Nursing
Chair, Prelicensure Nursing Programs
Professor
Kettering College
Kettering, Ohio

Anita K. Reed, MSN, RN
Department Chair
Adult and Community Health Practice
St. Elizabeth School of Nursing
Saint Joseph's College
Lafayette, Indiana

Rhonda J. Reed, MSN, RN, CRRN
Learning Resource Center Director—Technology Coordinator
Indiana State University
Terre Haute, Indiana

Carol A. Rueter, RN, PhD(c)
Bereavement Coordinator/Clinical Instructor
James A. Haley VA Hospital
University of South Florida
Tampa, Florida

Susan Parnell Scholtz, RN, PhD
Associate Professor of Nursing
Moravian College
Bethlehem, Pennsylvania

Gale P. Sewell, PhD(c), MSN, RN, CNE
Associate Professor
University of Northwestern
St. Paul, Minneapolis

Cynthia M. Sheppard, RN, MSN, APN-BC
Assistant Professor of Nursing
Schoolcraft College
Livonia, Michigan

Elaine R. Shingleton, RN, MSN, OCN
Service Unit Manager, Oncology/Infusion
The Permanente Medical Group
Walnut Creek, California

Crystal D. Slaughter, DNP, APN, ACNS-BC
Assistant Professor
College of Nursing
Saint Francis Medical Center College of Nursing
Peoria, Illinois

Mindy Stayner, RN, MSN, PhD
Professor
Northwest State Community College
Archbold, Ohio

Laura M. Streeter
Coordinator, Clinical Simulation Learning Center
University of Missouri—Columbia
Columbia, Missouri

Estella J. Wetzel, MSN, APRN, FNP-C
Family Nurse Practitioner
Integrated Care
Scioto Paint Valley Mental Health Clinic
Chillicothe, Ohio;
Clark State Community College
Springfield, Ohio

Laura M. Willis, MSN, RN, FNP
Assistant Professor
Coordinator of Service Learning
Kettering College
Kettering, Ohio

Lea Wood, MSN, BSN-RN
Coordinator, Clinical Simulation Learning Center
University of Missouri—Columbia
Columbia, Missouri

Damien Zsiros, MSN, RN, CNE, CRNP
The Pennsylvania State University
Lemont Furnace, Pennsylvania

I have been incredibly fortunate to have a career that has allowed me to develop long-lasting friendships with amazing professional nurses. I dedicate this book to one of those amazing nurses, Coreen Vlodarchyk. She is the consummate nurse and leader who has allowed me to pursue a different direction in my career, offering her enthusiastic and unfettered support.

Patricia A. Potter

To all nursing faculty and professional nurses who work each day to advance clinical nursing. Your commitment to nursing education and nursing practice inspires us all to be the guardians of the discipline. I also want to acknowledge all the reviewers and contributors to this text. A great thank you goes out to my coauthors. Together we challenge, encourage, and support one another to produce the best textbook.

I also want to thank my family for their loving support. A special thank you to my grandchildren, Cora Elizabeth Bryan, Amalie Mary Bryan, Shepherd Charles Bryan, and Noelle Anne Bryan, who always tell it like it is.

Anne Griffin Perry

To my husband, Drake, and daughters, Sara and Kelsey. Thank you for your love and patience as I have spent time writing, reviewing, and editing for this edition of Fundamentals. Your support has made this endeavor possible for me! And to all the nurses and nursing faculty, especially the faculty at Saint Francis Medical Center College of Nursing. Thank you for all your hard work, caring, compassion, and presence as you work with patients and nursing students on a daily basis. Your commitment to nursing and nursing education is the foundation that makes nurses the most trusted professionals!

Patricia A. Stockert

To Debbie, Suzanne, Melissa, Donna, Joan, Cindy, Jerrilee, Theresa, and Kathy. Your never-ending enthusiasm for helping to shape the nurses of our future inspire me all the time. I value your friendship and support. To Patti, Anne, and Pat for your friendship, support, and quest for excellence. And to Greg, the love of my life, for supporting and encouraging me to spread my wings and grow both personally and professionally.

Amy M. Hall

STUDENT PREFACE

Fundamentals of Nursing provides you with all of the fundamental nursing concepts and skills you will need as a beginning nurse in a visually appealing, easy-to-use format. We know how busy you are and how precious your time is. As you begin your nursing education, it is very important that you have a resource that includes all the information you need to prepare for lectures, classroom activities, clinical assignments, and exams—and nothing more. We've written this text to meet all of those needs. This book was designed to help you succeed in this course and prepare you for more advanced study. In addition to the readable writing style and abundance of full-color photographs and drawings, we've incorporated numerous features to help you study and learn. We have made it easy for you to pull out important content. **Check out the following special learning aids:**

32

Medication Administration

OBJECTIVES

- Discuss nursing roles and responsibilities in medication administration.
- Describe the physiological mechanisms of medication action.
- Differentiate among different types of medication actions.
- Discuss developmental factors that influence pharmacokinetics.
- Discuss factors that influence medication actions.
- Discuss methods used to educate patients about prescribed medications.
- Compare and contrast the roles of the health care provider, pharmacist, and nurse in medication administration.
- Implement nursing actions to prevent medication errors.
- Describe factors to consider when choosing routes of medication administration.
- Calculate prescribed medication doses correctly.
- Discuss factors to include in assessing a patient's needs for and response to medication therapy.
- Identify the six rights of medication administration and apply them in clinical settings.
- Correctly and safely prepare and administer medications.

KEY TERMS

Absorption, p. 611
Adverse effects, p. 613
Anaphylactic reactions, p. 613
Biological half-life, p. 614
Biotransformation, p. 612
Buccal, p. 615
Detoxify, p. 612
Idiosyncratic reaction, p. 613
Infusions, p. 614
Injection, p. 611
Instillation, p. 617
Intraarticular, p. 616
Intracardiac, p. 616
Intradermal (ID), p. 615
Intramuscular (IM), p. 615
Intraocular, p. 617
Intravenous (IV), p. 615
Irrigations, p. 618
Medication allergy, p. 613
Medication error, p. 624
Medication interaction, p. 613
Medication reconciliation, p. 625
Metric system, p. 617
Nurse Practice Acts (NPAs), p. 610
Ophthalmic, p. 638
Parenteral administration, p. 615
Peak, p. 614
Pharmacokinetics, p. 611
Polypharmacy, p. 633
Prescriptions, p. 623
Pressurized metered-dose inhalers (pMDIs), p. 638
Side effects, p. 613
Solution, p. 618
Subcutaneous, p. 615
Sublingual, p. 615
Synergistic effect, p. 613
Therapeutic effect, p. 613
Toxic effects, p. 613
Transdermal disk, p. 616
Trough, p. 614
Verbal order, p. 621
Z-track method, p. 650

MEDIA RESOURCES

http://evolve.elsevier.com/Potter/fundamentals/

- Review Questions
- Video Clips
- Concept Map Creator
- Case Study with Questions
- Skills Performance Checklists
- Audio Glossary
- Calculations Tutorial
- Content Updates

Patients with health problems use a variety of strategies to restore or maintain their health. One strategy they often use is medication, a substance used in the diagnosis, treatment, cure, relief, or prevention of health problems. No matter where patients receive health care (i.e., hospitals, clinics, or home), nurses play an essential role in preparing, administering, and evaluating the effects of medications. Family members, friends, or home care personnel often administer medications when patients cannot administer them themselves at home. In all settings nurses are responsible for evaluating the effects of medications on the patient's ongoing health status, teaching him or her about medications and side effects, encouraging adherence to the medication regimen, and evaluating the patient's and family caregiver's ability to administer medications.

SCIENTIFIC KNOWLEDGE BASE

Because medication administration and evaluation are a critical part of nursing practice, nurses need to understand the actions and effects of all medications taken by their patients. Administering medications safely requires an understanding of legal aspects of health care,

609

Learning Objectives begin each chapter to help you focus on the key information that follows.

Key Terms are listed at the beginning of each chapter and are boldfaced in the text. Page numbers help you quickly find where each term is defined.

Evolve Resources sections detail what electronic resources are available to you for every chapter.

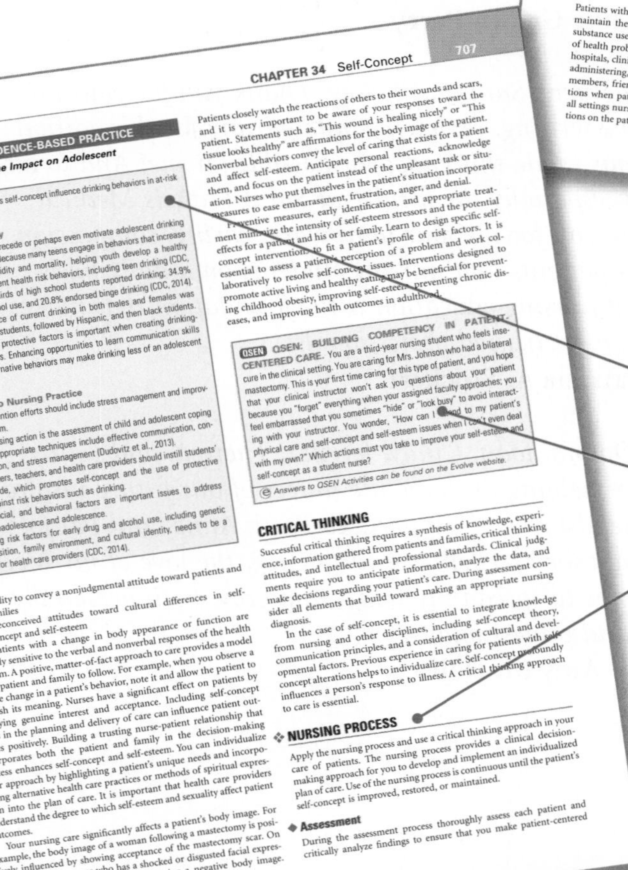

CHAPTER 34 Self-Concept 707

BOX 34-4 EVIDENCE-BASED PRACTICE

Self-Concept and the Impact on Adolescent Drinking Behaviors

PICO Question: How does self-concept influence drinking behaviors in at-risk adolescents?

Evidence Summary

Low self-concept may precede or perhaps even motivate adolescent drinking (Dudovitz et al., 2013). Because many teens engage in behaviors that increase the potential for morbidity and mortality, helping youth develop a healthy self-concept may prevent health risk behaviors, including teen drinking (CDC, 2014). In 2013 two thirds of high school students reported drinking; 34.9% reported current alcohol use, and 20.8% endorsed binge drinking (CDC, 2014). Overall the prevalence of current drinking in both males and females was higher among white students, followed by Hispanic, and then black students. Identifying risk and protective factors is important when creating drinking-prevention programs. Enhancing opportunities to learn communication skills and engage in alternative behaviors may make drinking less of an adolescent risk behavior.

Application to Nursing Practice

- Drinking-prevention efforts should include stress management and improving self-esteem.
- A priority nursing action is the assessment of child and adolescent coping strategies. Appropriate techniques include effective communication, conflict resolution, and stress management (Dudovitz et al., 2013).
- Families, peers, teachers, and health care providers should instill students' cultural pride, which promotes self-concept and the use of protective factors against risk behaviors such as drinking.
- Family, social, and behavioral factors are important issues to address during preadolescence and adolescence.
- Identifying risk factors for early drug and alcohol use, including genetic predisposition, family environment, and cultural identity, needs to be a priority for health care providers (CDC, 2014).

- Ability to convey a nonjudgmental attitude toward patients and families
- Preconceived attitudes toward cultural differences in self-concept and self-esteem

Some patients with a change in body appearance or function are extremely sensitive to the verbal and nonverbal responses of the health care team. A positive, matter-of-fact approach to care provides a model for the patient and family to follow. For example, when you observe a positive change in a patient's behavior, note it and allow the patient to establish its meaning. Nurses have a significant effect on patients by conveying genuine interest and acceptance. Including self-concept issues in the planning and delivery of care can influence patient outcomes positively. Building a trusting nurse-patient relationship that incorporates both the patient and family in the decision-making process enhances self-concept and self-esteem. You can individualize your approach by highlighting a patient's unique needs and incorporating alternative health care practices or methods of spiritual expression into the plan of care. It is important that health care providers understand the degree to which self-esteem and sexuality affect patient outcomes.

Your nursing care significantly affects a patient's body image. For example, the body image of a woman following a mastectomy is positively influenced by showing acceptance of the mastectomy scar. On the other hand, a nurse who has a shocked or disgusted facial expression contributes to the woman developing a negative body image. Patients closely watch the reactions of others to their wounds and scars, and it is very important to be aware of your responses toward the patient. Statements such as, "This wound is healing nicely" or "This tissue looks healthy" are affirmations for the body image of the patient. Nonverbal behaviors convey the level of caring that exists for a patient and affect self-esteem. Anticipate personal reactions, acknowledge them, and focus on the patient instead of the unpleasant task or situation. Nurses who put themselves in the patient's situation incorporate measures to ease embarrassment, frustration, anger, and denial.

Preventive measures, early identification, and appropriate treatment minimize the intensity of self-esteem stressors and the potential effects for a patient and his or her family. Learn to design specific self-concept interventions to fit a patient's profile of risk factors. It is essential to assess a patient's perception of a problem and work collaboratively to resolve self-concept issues. Interventions designed to promote active living and healthy eating may be beneficial for preventing childhood obesity, improving self-esteem, preventing chronic diseases, and improving health outcomes in adulthood.

QSEN: BUILDING COMPETENCY IN PATIENT-CENTERED CARE. You are a third-year nursing student who feels insecure in the clinical setting. You are caring for Mrs. Johnson who had a bilateral mastectomy. This is your first time caring for this type of patient, and you hope that your clinical instructor won't ask you questions about your patient because you "forget" everything when your assigned faculty approaches; you feel embarrassed that you sometimes "hide" or "look busy" to avoid interacting with your instructor. You wonder, "How can I attend to my patient's physical care and self-concept and self-esteem issues when I can't even deal with my own?" Which actions must you take to improve your self-esteem and self-concept as a student nurse?

Answers to QSEN Activities can be found on the Evolve website.

CRITICAL THINKING

Successful critical thinking requires a synthesis of knowledge, experience, information gathered from patients and families, critical thinking attitudes, and intellectual and professional standards. Clinical judgments require you to anticipate information, analyze the data, and make decisions regarding your patient's care. During assessment consider all elements that build toward making an appropriate nursing diagnosis.

In the case of self-concept, it is essential to integrate knowledge from nursing and other disciplines, including self-concept theory, communication principles, and a consideration of cultural and developmental factors. Previous experience in caring for patients with self-concept alterations helps to individualize care. Self-concept profoundly influences a person's response to illness. A critical thinking approach to care is essential.

NURSING PROCESS

Apply the nursing process and use a critical thinking approach in your care of patients. The nursing process provides a clinical decision-making approach for you to develop and implement an individualized plan of care. Use of the nursing process is continuous until the patient's self-concept is improved, restored, or maintained.

Assessment

During the assessment process thoroughly assess each patient and critically analyze findings to ensure that you make patient-centered

Evidence-Based Practice boxes summarize the results of a research study and indicate how that research can be applied to nursing practice.

Building Competency scenario boxes focus on one of the six QSEN key competencies and provide a short case study and question.

The 5-step **Nursing Process** provides a consistent framework for presentation of content in clinical chapters.

Cultural Aspects of Care boxes prepare you to care for patients of diverse populations.

Focus on Older Adults boxes prepare you to address the special needs of older adults.

Patient Teaching boxes emphasize important information to teach patients.

Nursing Assessment Questions boxes help you learn how to properly pose assessment questions when you interview patients.

The unique **Critical Thinking Model** clearly shows how critical thinking is to be applied during steps of the nursing process to help you provide the best care for your patients.

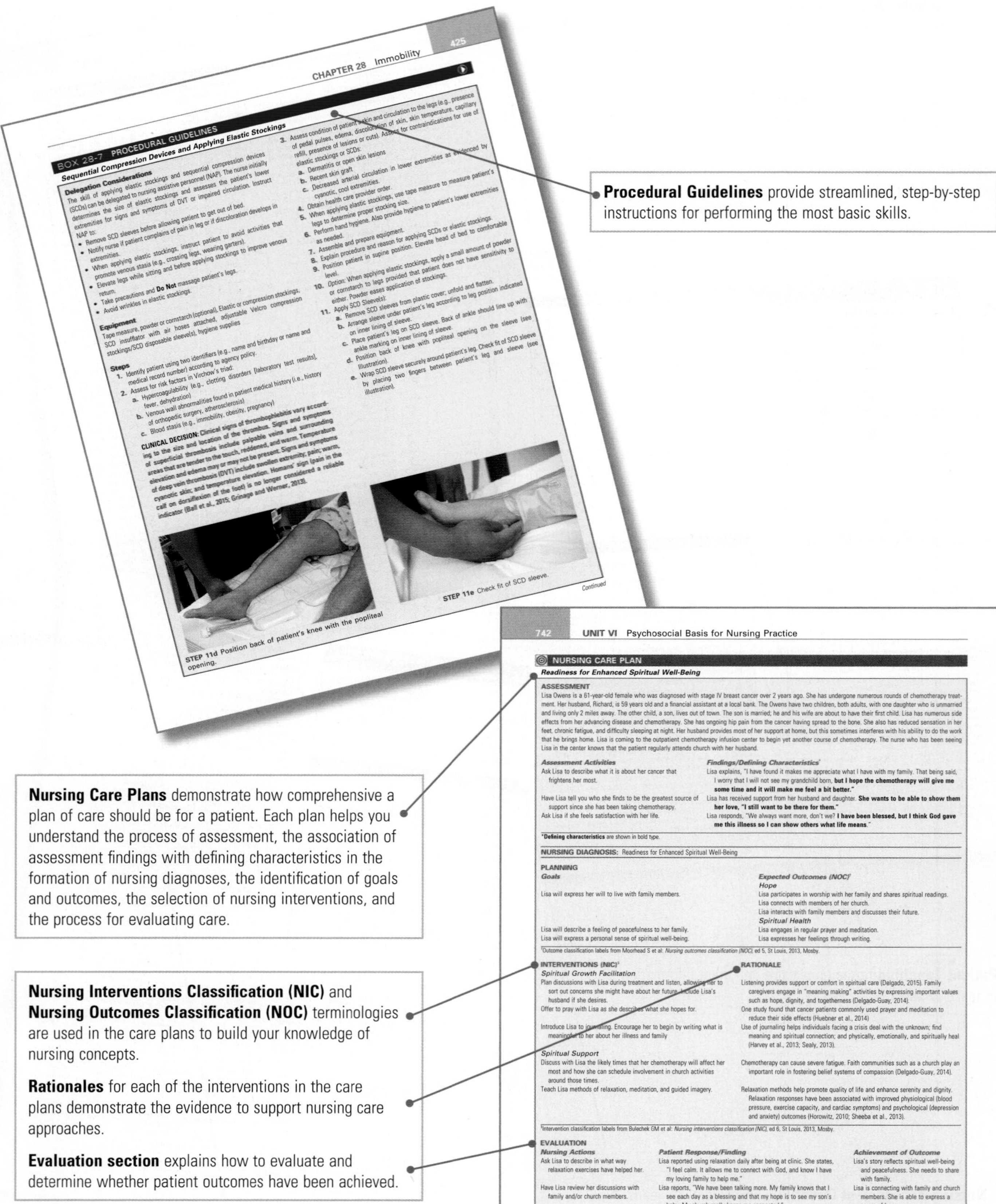

Procedural Guidelines provide streamlined, step-by-step instructions for performing the most basic skills.

Nursing Care Plans demonstrate how comprehensive a plan of care should be for a patient. Each plan helps you understand the process of assessment, the association of assessment findings with defining characteristics in the formation of nursing diagnoses, the identification of goals and outcomes, the selection of nursing interventions, and the process for evaluating care.

Nursing Interventions Classification (NIC) and **Nursing Outcomes Classification (NOC)** terminologies are used in the care plans to build your knowledge of nursing concepts.

Rationales for each of the interventions in the care plans demonstrate the evidence to support nursing care approaches.

Evaluation section explains how to evaluate and determine whether patient outcomes have been achieved.

Concept Maps help you see the connections between your patient's medical problems and your plan of care.

Nursing Skills are presented in a clear, two-column format that includes Steps and Rationales to help you learn how and why a skill is performed. Each skill begins with a **Safety Guidelines** section that will help you focus on safe and effective skill performance.

Delegation Considerations guide you in delegating tasks to assistive personnel.

Equipment lists show specific items needed for each skill.

Video Icons indicate video clips associated with specific skills that are available on the free Evolve Student Resources website.

Clinical Decisions alert you to important information within a skill to consider to ensure safe and effective patient care.

Clear, close-up **photos** and **illustrations** show you how to perform important skill procedures.

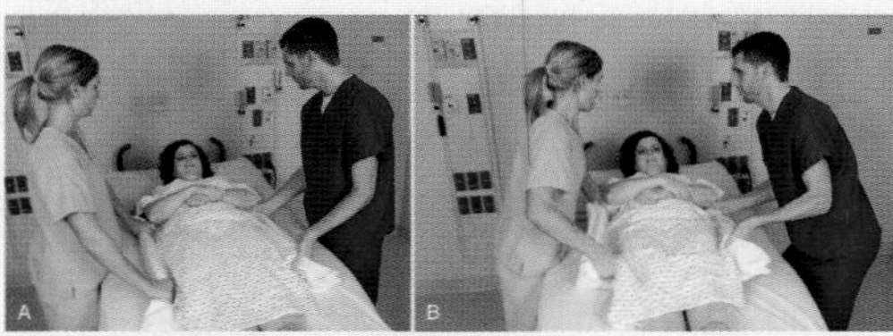

STEP 1b(6) A and B, Moving immobile patient up in bed with drawsheet.

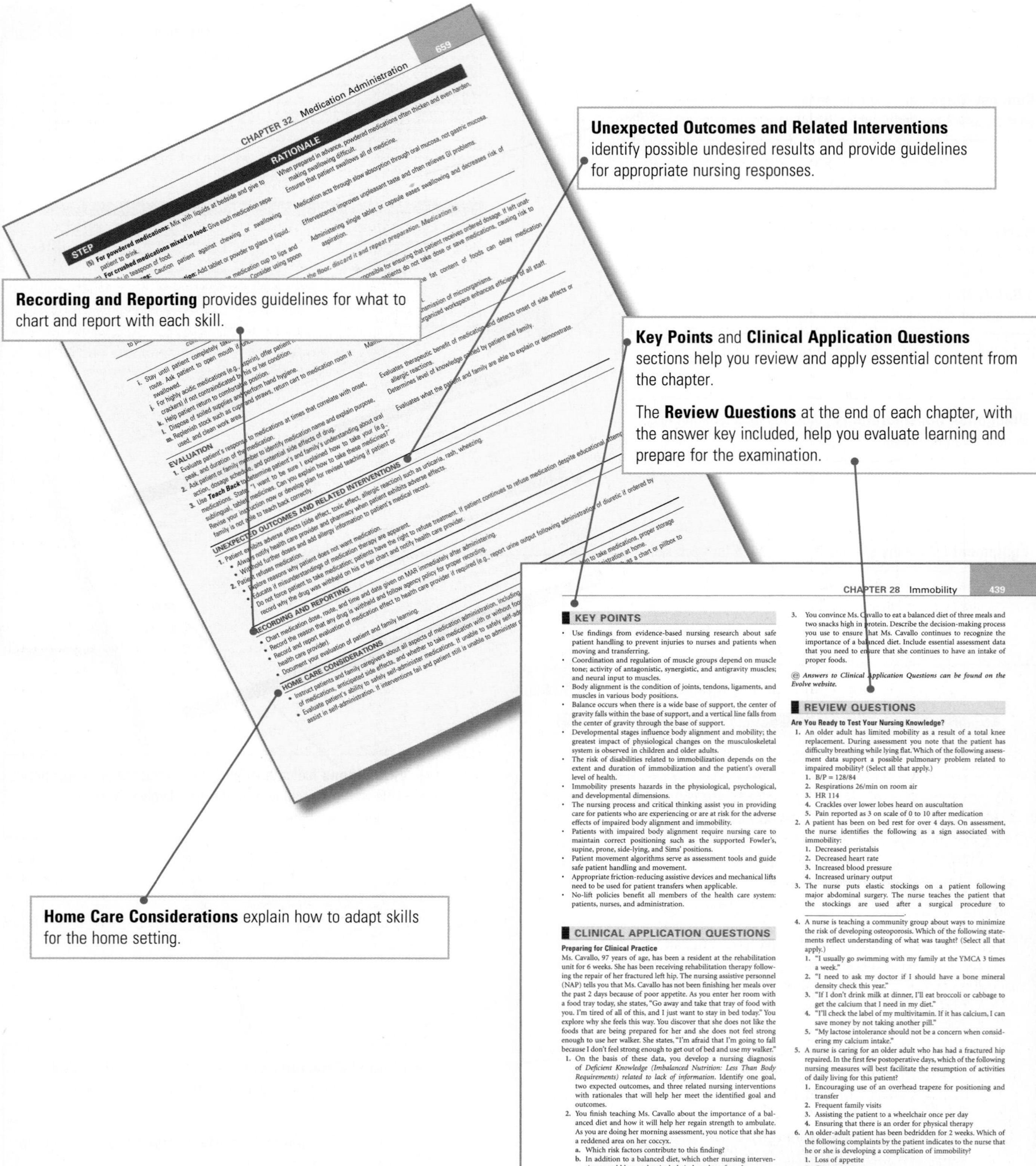

Unexpected Outcomes and Related Interventions identify possible undesired results and provide guidelines for appropriate nursing responses.

Recording and Reporting provides guidelines for what to chart and report with each skill.

Key Points and **Clinical Application Questions** sections help you review and apply essential content from the chapter.

The **Review Questions** at the end of each chapter, with the answer key included, help you evaluate learning and prepare for the examination.

Home Care Considerations explain how to adapt skills for the home setting.

CHAPTER 28 Immobility 439

KEY POINTS

- Use findings from evidence-based nursing research about safe patient handling to prevent injuries to nurses and patients when moving and transferring.
- Coordination and regulation of muscle groups depend on muscle tone; activity of antagonistic, synergistic, and antigravity muscles; and neural input to muscles.
- Body alignment is the condition of joints, tendons, ligaments, and muscles in various body positions.
- Balance occurs when there is a wide base of support, the center of gravity falls within the base of support, and a vertical line falls from the center of gravity through the base of support.
- Developmental stages influence body alignment and mobility; the greatest impact of physiological changes on the musculoskeletal system is observed in children and older adults.
- The risk of disabilities related to immobilization depends on the extent and duration of immobilization and the patient's overall level of health.
- Immobility presents hazards in the physiological, psychological, and developmental dimensions.
- The nursing process and critical thinking assist you in providing care for patients who are experiencing or are at risk for the adverse effects of impaired body alignment and immobility.
- Patients with impaired body alignment require nursing care to maintain correct positioning such as the supported Fowler's, supine, prone, side-lying, and Sims' positions.
- Patient movement algorithms serve as assessment tools and guide safe patient handling and movement.
- Appropriate friction-reducing assistive devices and mechanical lifts need to be used for patient transfers when applicable.
- No-lift policies benefit all members of the health care system: patients, nurses, and administration.

CLINICAL APPLICATION QUESTIONS

Preparing for Clinical Practice

Ms. Cavallo, 97 years of age, has been a resident at the rehabilitation unit for 6 weeks. She has been receiving rehabilitation therapy following the repair of her fractured left hip. The nursing assistive personnel (NAP) tells you that Ms. Cavallo has not been finishing her meals over the past 2 days because of poor appetite. As you enter her room with a food tray today, she states, "Go away and take that tray of food with you. I'm tired of all of this, and I just want to stay in bed today." You explore why she feels this way. You discover that she does not like the foods that are being prepared for her and she does not feel strong enough to use her walker. She states, "I'm afraid that I'm going to fall because I don't feel strong enough to get out of bed and use my walker."

1. On the basis of these data, you develop a nursing diagnosis of *Deficient Knowledge (Imbalanced Nutrition: Less Than Body Requirements) related to lack of information*. Identify one goal, two expected outcomes, and three related nursing interventions with rationales that will help her meet the identified goal and outcomes.
2. You finish teaching Ms. Cavallo about the importance of a balanced diet and how it will help her regain strength to ambulate. As you are doing her morning assessment, you notice that she has a reddened area on her coccyx.
   a. Which risk factors contribute to this finding?
   b. In addition to a balanced diet, which other nursing interventions would be good to include in her plan of care?
3. You convince Ms. Cavallo to eat a balanced diet of three meals and two snacks high in protein. Describe the decision-making process you use to ensure that Ms. Cavallo continues to recognize the importance of a balanced diet. Include essential assessment data that you need to ensure that she continues to have an intake of proper foods.

Answers to Clinical Application Questions can be found on the Evolve website.

REVIEW QUESTIONS

Are You Ready to Test Your Nursing Knowledge?

1. An older adult has limited mobility as a result of a total knee replacement. During assessment you note that the patient has difficulty breathing while lying flat. Which of the following assessment data support a possible pulmonary problem related to impaired mobility? (Select all that apply.)
   1. B/P = 128/84
   2. Respirations 26/min on room air
   3. HR 114
   4. Crackles over lower lobes heard on auscultation
   5. Pain reported as 3 on scale of 0 to 10 after medication
2. A patient has been on bed rest for over 4 days. On assessment, the nurse identifies the following as a sign associated with immobility:
   1. Decreased peristalsis
   2. Decreased heart rate
   3. Increased blood pressure
   4. Increased urinary output
3. The nurse puts elastic stockings on a patient following major abdominal surgery. The nurse teaches the patient that the stockings are used after a surgical procedure to ________.
4. A nurse is teaching a community group about ways to minimize the risk of developing osteoporosis. Which of the following statements reflect understanding of what was taught? (Select all that apply.)
   1. "I usually go swimming with my family at the YMCA 3 times a week."
   2. "I need to ask my doctor if I should have a bone mineral density check this year."
   3. "If I don't drink milk at dinner, I'll eat broccoli or cabbage to get the calcium that I need in my diet."
   4. "I'll check the label of my multivitamin. If it has calcium, I can save money by not taking another pill."
   5. "My lactose intolerance should not be a concern when considering my calcium intake."
5. A nurse is caring for an older adult who has had a fractured hip repaired. In the first few postoperative days, which of the following nursing measures will best facilitate the resumption of activities of daily living for this patient?
   1. Encouraging use of an overhead trapeze for positioning and transfer
   2. Frequent family visits
   3. Assisting the patient to a wheelchair once per day
   4. Ensuring that there is an order for physical therapy
6. An older-adult patient has been bedridden for 2 weeks. Which of the following complaints by the patient indicates to the nurse that he or she is developing a complication of immobility?
   1. Loss of appetite
   2. Gum soreness

PREFACE TO THE INSTRUCTOR

The nursing profession is always responding to dynamic change and continual challenges. Today nurses need a broad knowledge base from which to provide care. More important, nurses require the ability to know how to apply best evidence in practice to ensure the best outcomes for their patients. The role of the nurse includes assuming the lead in preserving nursing practice and demonstrating its contribution to the health care of our nation. Nurses of tomorrow, therefore, need to become critical thinkers, patient advocates, clinical decision makers, and patient educators within a broad spectrum of care services.

The ninth edition of ***Fundamentals of Nursing*** was revised to prepare today's students for the challenges of tomorrow. This textbook is designed for beginning students in all types of professional nursing programs. The comprehensive coverage provides fundamental nursing concepts, skills, and techniques of nursing practice and a firm foundation for more advanced areas of study.

Fundamentals of Nursing provides a contemporary approach to nursing practice, discussing the entire scope of primary, acute, and restorative care. This new edition continues to address a number of key current practice issues, including an emphasis on patient-centered care and evidence-based practice. Evidence-based practice is one of the most important initiatives in health care today. The increased focus on applying current evidence in skills and patient care plans helps students understand how the latest research findings should guide their clinical decision making.

KEY FEATURES

We have carefully developed this ninth edition with the student in mind. We have designed this text to welcome the new student to nursing, communicate our own love for the profession, and promote learning and understanding. Key features of the text include the following:

- Students will appreciate the **clear, engaging writing style.** The narrative actually addresses the reader, making this textbook more of an active instructional tool than a passive reference. Students will find that even complex technical and theoretical concepts are presented in a language that is easy to understand.
- **Comprehensive** coverage and readability of all fundamental nursing content.
- The **attractive, functional design** will appeal to today's visual learner. The clear, readable type and bold headings make the content easy to read and follow. Each special element is consistently color-keyed so students can readily identify important information.
- Hundreds of **large, clear, full-color photographs and drawings** reinforce and clarify key concepts and techniques.
- The **nursing process** format provides a consistent organizational framework for clinical chapters.
- **Learning aids** help students identify, review, and apply important content in each chapter and include Objectives, Key Terms, Key Points, Clinical Application Questions, and Review Questions.
- **Evolve Resources** lists at the beginning of every chapter detail the electronic resources available for the student.
- **Health promotion and acute and continuing care** are covered to address today's practice in various settings.
- A **health promotion/wellness** thread is used consistently throughout the text.
- **Cultural awareness**, care of the **older adult,** and **patient teaching** are stressed throughout chapter narratives and are highlighted in special boxes.
- **Procedural Guidelines** boxes provide more streamlined, step-by-step instructions for performing very basic skills.
- **Concept Maps** in each clinical chapter show you the association between multiple nursing diagnoses for a patient with a selected medical diagnosis and the relationship between nursing interventions.
- **Nursing Care Plans** guide students on how to conduct an assessment and analyze the defining characteristics that indicate nursing diagnoses. The plans include NIC and NOC classifications to familiarize students with this important nomenclature. The evaluation sections of the plans show students how to evaluate and then determine the outcomes of care.
- A **critical thinking model provides a framework** for all clinical chapters and show how elements of critical thinking, including knowledge, critical thinking attitudes, intellectual and professional standards, and experience are integrated throughout the nursing process for making clinical decisions.
- **More than 50 nursing skills** are presented in a clear, two-column format with steps and supporting rationales that are often supported with current, evidence-based research.
- **Delegation Considerations** guide when it is appropriate to delegate tasks to assistive personnel.
- **Unexpected Outcomes and Related Interventions** are highlighted within nursing skills to help students anticipate and appropriately respond to possible problems faced while performing skills.
- **Video Icons** indicate video clips associated with specific skills that are available online in the Evolve Student Resources.
- **Printed endpapers** on the inside back cover help students locate specific assets in the book, including Skills, Procedural Guidelines, Nursing Care Plans, and Concept Maps.

NEW TO THIS EDITION

- Information related to the **Quality and Safety Education for Nurses** (**QSEN**) initiative is highlighted by headings that coordinate with the key competencies. Building Competency scenarios in each chapter incorporate one of the six key competencies in QSEN. Answers to these activities can be found online in the Evolve Student Resources.
- The latest **NANDA 2015-2017** diagnoses are included for up-to-date content.
- **A new skill** covers Fall Prevention in Health Care Settings.
- **Review Questions** have been updated in each chapter, with a minimum of four alternate-item type questions. Answers are provided with questions and rationales on Evolve.
- **Evidence-Based Practice** boxes in each chapter have been updated to reflect current research topics and trends.
- Both ***Healthy People 2020*** and The Joint Commission's **2016 National Patient Safety Goals** are covered in this new edition, promoting the importance of current research.
- **Chapter 28: Immobility** and **Chapter 39: Activity and Exercise** have been completely reorganized to reduce redundancy, improve clarity, and increase the clinical focus of both chapters.
- **Chapter 9: Cultural Awareness** has been completely rewritten and revised to better address this topic for fundamentals students.

LEARNING SUPPLEMENTS FOR STUDENTS

- The **Evolve Student Resources** are available online at http://evolve.elsevier.com/Potter/fundamentals/ and include the following valuable learning aids organized by chapter:
  - Chapter Review Questions from the book in an interactive format! Includes hundreds of questions to prepare for examinations.
  - Answers and rationales to Chapter Review Questions
  - Answers and rationales to Clinical Application Questions
  - Answers and rationales to Building Competency scenario questions
  - Video clips to highlight common skills and procedural guidelines
  - Concept Map Creator (included in each clinical chapter)
  - Conceptual Care Map (included in each clinical chapter)
  - Case Study with Questions
  - Audio Glossary
  - Fluids & Electrolytes Tutorial
  - Calculation Tutorial
  - Printable versions of Chapter Key Points
  - Interactive Skills Performance Checklists (included for each skill in the text)
- A thorough ***Study Guide*** by Geralyn Ochs provides an ideal supplement to help students understand and apply the content of the text. Each chapter includes multiple sections:
  - Preliminary Reading includes a chapter assignment from the text.
  - Comprehensive Understanding provides a variety of activities to reinforce the topics and main ideas from the text.
  - Review Questions are NCLEX®-style multiple-choice questions that require students to provide rationales for their answers. Answers and rationales are provided in the answer key.
  - Clinical chapters include an Application of Critical Thinking Synthesis Model that expands the case study from the chapter's Care Plan and asks students to develop a step in the synthesis model based on the nurse and patient in the scenario. This helps students learn to apply both content learned and the critical thinking synthesis model.
- The handy ***Clinical Companion: Just the Facts*** complements, rather than abbreviates, the textbook. Content is presented in a tabular, list, and outline format that equips your students with a concise, portable guide to all the facts and figures they'll need to know in their early clinical experiences.
- **Virtual Clinical Excursions** is an exciting workbook and CD-ROM experience that brings learning to life in a virtual hospital setting. The workbook guides students as they care for patients, providing ongoing challenges and learning opportunities. Each lesson in *Virtual Clinical Excursions* complements the textbook content and provides an environment for students to practice what they are learning. This CD/workbook is available separately or packaged at a special price with the textbook.

TEACHING SUPPLEMENTS FOR INSTRUCTORS

The **Evolve Instructor Resources** (available online at http://evolve.elsevier.com/Potter/fundamentals) are a comprehensive collection of the most important tools instructors need, including the following:

- **TEACH for Nurses** ties together every chapter resource you need for the most effective class presentations, with sections dedicated to objectives, teaching focus, nursing curriculum standards (including QSEN, BSN Essentials, and Concepts), instructor chapter resources, student chapter resources, answers to chapter questions, and an in-class case study discussion. Teaching Strategies include relations between the textbook content and discussion items. Examples of student activities, online activities, new health promotion-focused activities, and large group activities are provided for more "hands-on" learning.
- The **Test Bank** contains 1500 questions with text page references and answers coded for NCLEX Client Needs category, nursing process, and cognitive level. Each question was involved in an instructor piloting process to ensure the best possible exam for students. The ExamView software allows instructors to create new tests; edit, add, and delete test questions; sort questions by NCLEX category, cognitive level, nursing process step, and question type; and administer/grade online tests.
- Completely revised **PowerPoint Presentations** include more than 1500 slides for use in lectures. Art is included within the slides, and progressive case studies include discussion questions and answers.
- The **Image Collection** contains more than 1150 illustrations from the text for use in lectures.
- **Simulation Learning System** is an online toolkit that helps instructors and facilitators effectively incorporate medium- to high-fidelity simulation into their nursing curriculum. Detailed patient scenarios promote and enhance the clinical decision-making skills of students at all levels. The system provides detailed instructions for preparation and implementation of the simulation experience, debriefing questions that encourage critical thinking, and learning resources to reinforce student comprehension. Each scenario in *Simulation Learning System* complements the textbook content and helps bridge the gap between lectures and clinicals. This system provides the perfect environment for students to practice what they are learning in the text for a true-to-life, hands-on learning experience.

MULTIMEDIA SUPPLEMENTS FOR INSTRUCTORS AND STUDENTS

- **Nursing Skills Online 3.0** contains 18 modules rich with animations, videos, interactive activities, and exercises to help students prepare for their clinical lab experience. The instructionally designed lessons focus on topics that are difficult to master and pose a high risk to the patient if done incorrectly. Lesson quizzes allow students to check their learning curve and review as needed, and the module exams feed out to an instructor grade book. Modules cover Airway Management, Blood Therapy, Bowel Elimination/Ostomy Care, Chest Tubes, Enteral Nutrition, Infection Control, Injections, IV Fluid Administration, IV Fluid Therapy Management, IV Medication Administration, Nonparenteral Medication Administration, Safe Medication Administration, Safety, Specimen Collection, Urinary Catheterization, Vascular Access, Vital Signs, and Wound Care. Available alone or packaged with the text.
- **Mosby's Nursing Video Skills: Basic, Intermediate, Advanced, 4th edition** provides 126 skills with overview information covering skill purpose, safety, and delegation guides; equipment lists; preparation procedures; procedure videos with printable step-by-step guidelines; appropriate follow-up care; documentation guidelines; and interactive review questions. Available online, as a student DVD set, or as a networkable DVD set for the institution.

ACKNOWLEDGMENTS

The ninth edition of *Fundamentals of Nursing* is one that we believe continues to prepare the student nurse to be able to practice in the challenging health care environment. Collaboration on this project allows us to be creative, visionary, and thoughtful as to students' learning needs. Each edition is a new adventure for all of us on the author team as we try to create the very best textbook for beginning nurses. Each of us wishes to acknowledge the professionalism, support, and commitment to detail from the following individuals:

- The editorial and production professionals at Mosby/Elsevier, including:
    - Tamara Myers, Executive Content Strategist, for her vision, organization, professionalism, energy, and support in assisting us to develop a text that offers a state-of-the-art approach to the design, organization, and presentation of *Fundamentals of Nursing.* Her skill is in motivating and supporting a writing team so it can be creative and innovative while retaining the characteristics of a high-quality textbook.
    - Jean Sims Fornango, Content Development Manager for *Fundamentals of Nursing*, for her professionalism and commitment to excellence. Her editorial and publishing skills provide a vision for organizing and developing the manuscript while ensuring that all pieces of the book and ancillary materials are creative, stimulating, and state-of-the-art. She, like the rest of the team, goes the extra mile sharing her energy and spirit.
    - Tina Kaemmerer as our Senior Content Development Specialist for *Fundamentals of Nursing.* She is dedicated to keeping the writing team organized and focused, performing considerable behind-the-scenes work for ensuring accuracy and consistency in how we present content within the textbook. She has limitless energy and is always willing to go the extra mile.
    - Jodi Willard, Senior Project Manager, consistently performs miracles. She is an amazing and accomplished production editor who applies patience, humor, and attention to detail. It is an honor to work with Jodi because of her professionalism and ability to coordinate the multiple aspects of completing a well-designed finished product.
- StoryTrack, St. Louis, Missouri, for their excellent photography.
- Maryville University, who allowed us to use the new Myrtle E. and Earl E. Walker Hall for the new photographs.
- To our contributors and clinician and educator reviewers, who share their expertise and knowledge about nursing practice and the trends within health care today, helping us to create informative, accurate, and current information. Their contributions allow us to develop a text that embodies high standards for professional nursing practice through the printed word.
- And special recognition to our professional colleagues at Barnes-Jewish Hospital, Southern Illinois University—Edwardsville, Saint Francis Medical Center College of Nursing, and the University of Evansville.

We believe that *Fundamentals of Nursing*, now in its ninth edition, is a textbook that informs and helps to shape the standards for excellence in nursing practice. Nursing excellence belongs to all of us, and we are happy to have the opportunity to continue the work we love.

Patricia A. Potter
Anne Griffin Perry
Patricia A. Stockert
Amy M. Hall

CONTENTS

Any updates to this textbook can be found in the Content Updates folder on Evolve at http://evolve.elsevier.com/Potter/fundamentals/.

1

Nursing Today

OBJECTIVES

- Discuss the development of professional nursing roles.
- Describe educational programs available for professional registered nurse (RN) education.
- Describe the roles and career opportunities for nurses.
- Discuss the influence of social, historical, political, and economic changes on nursing practices.

KEY TERMS

Advanced practice registered nurse (APRN), p. 4
American Nurses Association (ANA), p. 2
Caregiver, p. 3
Certified nurse-midwife (CNM), p. 4
Certified registered nurse anesthetist (CRNA), p. 4
Clinical nurse specialist (CNS), p. 4
Code of ethics, p. 3
Continuing education, p. 10
Genomics, p. 9
In-service education, p. 10
International Council of Nurses (ICN), p. 2
Nurse administrator, p. 5
Nurse educator, p. 4
Nurse practitioner (NP), p. 4
Nurse researcher, p. 5
Nursing, p. 2
Patient advocate, p. 3
Professional organization, p. 10
Quality and Safety Education for Nurses (QSEN), p. 7
Registered nurse (RN), p. 9

MEDIA RESOURCES

http://evolve.elsevier.com/Potter/fundamentals/

- Review Questions
- Case Study with Questions
- Audio Glossary
- Content Updates

Nursing is an art and a science. As a professional nurse you will learn to deliver care artfully with compassion, caring, and respect for each patient's dignity and personhood. As a science, nursing practice is based on a body of knowledge that is continually changing with new discoveries and innovations. When you integrate the art and science of nursing into your practice, the quality of care you provide to your patients is at a level of excellence that benefits patients and their families.

NURSING AS A PROFESSION

A variety of career opportunities are available in nursing, including clinical practice, education, research, management, administration, and even entrepreneurship. As a student it is important for you to understand the scope of professional nursing practice and how nursing influences the lives of your patients, their families, and their communities.

The patient is the center of your practice. Your patient includes individuals, families, and/or communities. Patients have a wide variety of health care needs, knowledge, experiences, vulnerabilities, and expectations; but this is what makes nursing both challenging and rewarding. Making a difference in your patients' lives is fulfilling (e.g., helping a dying patient find relief from pain, helping a young mother learn parenting skills, and finding ways for older adults to remain independent in their homes). Nursing offers personal and professional rewards every day. This chapter presents a contemporary view of the evolution of nursing and nursing practice and the historical, practical, social, and political influences on the discipline of nursing.

Nursing is not simply a collection of specific skills, and you are not simply a person trained to perform specific tasks. Nursing is a profession. No one factor absolutely differentiates a job from a profession, but the difference is important in terms of how you practice. To act professionally you administer quality patient-centered care in a safe, prudent, and knowledgeable manner. You are responsible and accountable to yourself, your patients, and your peers.

Health care advocacy groups recognize the importance of the role quality professional nursing has on the nations' health care. One such program is the Robert Wood Johnson Foundation (RWJF) *Future of Nursing: Campaign for Action* (RWJF, 2014a). This program is a multifaceted campaign to transform health care through nursing, and it is a response to the Institute of Medicine (IOM) publication on *The Future of Nursing* (IOM, 2010). Together these initiatives prepare a professional workforce to meet health promotion, illness prevention, and complex care needs of the population in a changing health care system.

Science and Art of Nursing Practice

Because nursing is both an art and a science, nursing practice requires a blend of the most current knowledge and practice standards with an insightful and compassionate approach to patient care. Your patients' health care needs are multidimensional and constantly changing. Thus your care will reflect the needs and values of society and professional standards of care and performance, meet the needs of each patient, and integrate evidence-based findings to provide the highest level of care.

Nursing has a specific body of knowledge; however, it is essential that you socialize within the profession and practice to fully

BOX 1-1 Benner: From Novice to Expert

- **Novice:** Beginning nursing student or any nurse entering a situation in which there is no previous level of experience (e.g., an experienced operating room nurse chooses to now practice in home health). The learner learns via a specific set of rules or procedures, which are usually stepwise and linear.
- **Advanced Beginner:** A nurse who has had some level of experience with the situation. This experience may only be observational in nature, but the nurse is able to identify meaningful aspects or principles of nursing care.
- **Competent:** A nurse who has been in the same clinical position for 2 to 3 years. This nurse understands the organization and specific care required by the type of patients (e.g., surgical, oncology, or orthopedic patients). He or she is a competent practitioner who is able to anticipate nursing care and establish long-range goals. In this phase the nurse has usually had experience with all types of psychomotor skills required by this specific group of patients.
- **Proficient:** A nurse with more than 2 to 3 years of experience in the same clinical position. This nurse perceives a patient's clinical situation as a whole, is able to assess an entire situation, and can readily transfer knowledge gained from multiple previous experiences to a situation. This nurse focuses on managing care as opposed to managing and performing skills.
- **Expert:** A nurse with diverse experience who has an intuitive grasp of an existing or potential clinical problem. This nurse is able to zero in on the problem and focus on multiple dimensions of the situation. He or she is skilled at identifying both patient-centered problems and problems related to the health care system or perhaps the needs of the novice nurse.

Data from Benner P: *From novice to expert: excellence and power in clinical nursing practice,* Menlo Park, CA, 1984, Addison-Wesley.

BOX 1-2 ANA Standards of Nursing Practice

1. **Assessment:** The registered nurse collects comprehensive data pertinent to the patient's health and/or the situation.
2. **Diagnosis:** The registered nurse analyzes the assessment data to determine the diagnoses or issues.
3. **Outcomes Identification:** The registered nurse identifies expected outcomes for a plan individualized to the patient or the situation.
4. **Planning:** The registered nurse develops a plan that prescribes strategies and alternatives to attain expected outcomes.
5. **Implementation:** The registered nurse implements the identified plan.
   - 5a. **Coordination of Care:** The registered nurse coordinates care delivery.
   - 5b. **Health Teaching and Health Promotion:** The registered nurse uses strategies to promote health and a safe environment.
   - 5c. **Consultation:** The graduate level–prepared specialty nurse or advanced practice registered nurse provides consultation to influence the identified plan, enhance the abilities of others, and effect change.
   - 5d. **Prescriptive Authority and Treatment:** The advanced practice registered nurse uses prescriptive authority, procedures, referrals, treatment, and therapies in accordance with state and federal laws and regulations.
6. **Evaluation:** The registered nurse evaluates progress toward attainment of outcomes.

understand and apply this knowledge and develop professional expertise. Clinical expertise takes time and commitment. According to Benner (1984), an expert nurse passes through five levels of proficiency when acquiring and developing generalist or specialized nursing skills (Box 1-1).

Expert clinical nursing practice is a commitment to the application of knowledge, ethics, aesthetics, and clinical experience. Your ability to interpret clinical situations and make complex decisions is the foundation for your nursing care and the basis for the advancement of nursing practice and the development of nursing science (Benner, 1984; Benner et al., 1997, 2010). Critical thinking skills are essential to nursing (see Chapter 15). When providing nursing care, you need to make clinical judgments and decisions about your patients' health care needs based on knowledge, experience, critical-thinking attitudes, and standards of care. Use critical thinking skills and reflections to help you gain and interpret scientific knowledge, integrate knowledge from clinical experiences, and become a lifelong learner (Benner et al., 2010).

Use the competencies of critical thinking in your practice. This includes integrating knowledge from the basic sciences and nursing, applying knowledge from past and present experiences, applying critical thinking attitudes to a clinical situation, and implementing intellectual and professional standards. When you provide well–thought out care with compassion and caring, you provide each patient the best of the science and art of nursing care (see Chapter 7).

Scope and Standards of Practice

When giving care, it is essential to provide a specified service according to standards of practice and to follow a code of ethics (ANA, 2015). Professional practice includes knowledge from social and behavioral sciences, biological and physiological sciences, and nursing theories. In addition, nursing practice incorporates ethical and social values, professional autonomy, and a sense of commitment and community (ANA, 2010b). The following definition from the American Nurses Association (ANA) illustrates the consistent commitment of nurses to provide care that promotes the well-being of their patients and communities (ANA, 2010a). Nursing is *the protection, promotion, and optimization of health and abilities; prevention of illness and injury; alleviation of suffering through the diagnosis and treatment of human response; and advocacy in the care of individuals, families, communities, and populations* (ANA, 2010b). The International Council of Nurses (ICN, 2014) has another definition: *Nursing encompasses autonomous and collaborative care of individuals of all ages, families, groups, and communities, sick or well, and in all settings. Nursing includes the promotion of health; prevention of illness; and the care of ill, disabled, and dying people. Advocacy, promotion of a safe environment, research, participation in shaping health policy and in patient and health systems management, and education are also key nursing roles.* Both of these definitions support the prominence and importance that nursing holds in providing safe, patient-centered health care to the global community.

Since 1960 the ANA has defined the scope of nursing and developed Standards of Practice and Standards of Professional Performance (ANA, 2010b). It is important that you know and apply these standards in your practice (Box 1-2). Most schools of nursing and practice settings have published copies of the scope and standards of nursing practice. The scope and standards of practice guide nurses to make significant and visible contributions that improve the health and well-being of all individuals, communities, and populations (ANA, 2010b).

Standards of Practice. The Standards of Practice describe a competent level of nursing care. The levels of care are demonstrated by a critical thinking model known as the nursing process: assessment,

BOX 1-3 ANA Standards of Professional Performance

1. **Ethics:** The registered nurse practices ethically.
2. **Education:** The registered nurse attains knowledge and competency that reflects current nursing practice.
3. **Evidence-Based Practice and Research:** The registered nurse integrates evidence and research findings into practice.
4. **Quality of Practice:** The registered nurse contributes to quality nursing practice.
5. **Communication:** The registered nurse communicates effectively in all areas of practice.
6. **Leadership:** The registered nurse demonstrates leadership in the professional practice setting and the profession.
7. **Collaboration:** The registered nurse collaborates with health care consumer, family, and others in the conduct of nursing practice.
8. **Professional Practice Evaluation:** The registered nurse evaluates her or his own nursing practice in relation to professional practice standards and guidelines, relevant statutes, rules, and regulations.
9. **Resources:** The registered nurse uses appropriate resources to plan and provide nursing services that are safe, effective, and financially responsible.
10. **Environmental Health:** The registered nurse practices in an environmentally safe and healthy manner.

diagnosis, outcomes identification and planning, implementation, and evaluation (ANA, 2010b). The nursing process is the foundation of clinical decision making and includes all significant actions taken by nurses in providing care to patients (see Unit III).

Standards of Professional Performance. The ANA Standards of Professional Performance (Box 1-3) describe a competent level of behavior in the professional role (ANA, 2010b). The standards provide a method to assure patients that they are receiving high-quality care, that the nurses must know exactly what is necessary to provide nursing care, and that measures are in place to determine whether nursing care meets the standards.

Code of Ethics. The code of ethics is the philosophical ideals of right and wrong that define the principles you will use to provide care to your patients. It is important for you to also incorporate your own values and ethics into your practice. As you incorporate these values, you explore what type of nurse you will be and how you will function within the discipline (ANA, 2015). Ask yourself how your ethics, values, and practice compare with established standards. The ANA has a number of publications that address ethics and human rights in nursing. *The Code of Ethics for Nurses With Interpretive Statements* is a guide for carrying out nursing responsibilities that provide quality nursing care; it also outlines the ethical obligations of the profession (ANA, 2015). Chapter 22 provides a review of the nursing code of ethics and ethical principles for everyday practice.

Professional Responsibilities and Roles

You are responsible for obtaining and maintaining specific knowledge and skills for a variety of professional roles and responsibilities. Nurses provide care and comfort for patients in all health care settings. Nurses' concern for meeting their patient's needs remains the same whether care focuses on health promotion and illness prevention, disease and symptom management, family support, or end-of-life care.

Autonomy and Accountability. Autonomy is an essential element of professional nursing that involves the initiation of independent nursing interventions without medical orders. Although the nursing profession regulates accountability through nursing audits and standards of practice, you also need to develop a commitment to personal professional accountability. For example, you independently implement coughing and deep-breathing exercises for a patient who recently had surgery. As you continue to care for this patient, a complication arises. You note that the patient has a fever and the surgical wound has a yellow-green discharge. You collaborate with other health professionals to develop the best treatment plan for this patient's surgical wound infection. With increased autonomy comes greater responsibility and accountability. Accountability means that you are responsible professionally and legally for the type and quality of nursing care provided. You must remain current and competent in nursing and scientific knowledge and technical skills.

Caregiver. As a caregiver you help patients maintain and regain health, manage disease and symptoms, and attain a maximal level of function and independence through the healing process. You provide healing through psychomotor and interpersonal skills. Healing involves more than achieving improved physical well-being. You need to meet all health care needs of a patient by providing measures to restore a patient's emotional, spiritual, and social well-being. As a caregiver you help patients and families set realistic goals and meet them.

Advocate. As a patient advocate you protect your patient's human and legal rights and provide assistance in asserting these rights if the need arises. As an advocate you act on behalf of your patient and secure your patient's health care rights (Emrich et al., 2013). For example, you provide additional information to help a patient decide whether or not to accept a treatment, or you find an interpreter to help family members communicate their concerns. You sometimes need to defend patients' rights to make health care decisions in a general way by speaking out against policies or actions that put patients in danger or conflict with their rights (Wilson et al., 2013).

Educator. As an educator you explain concepts and facts about health, describe the reason for routine care activities, demonstrate procedures such as self-care activities, reinforce learning or patient behavior, and evaluate the patient's progress in learning. Some of your patient teaching is unplanned and informal. For example, during a casual conversation you respond to questions about the reason for an intravenous infusion, a health issue such as smoking cessation, or necessary lifestyle changes. Other teaching activities are planned and more formal such as when you teach your patient how to self-administer insulin injections. Always use teaching methods that match your patient's capabilities and needs and incorporate other resources such as the family in teaching plans (see Chapter 25).

Communicator. Your effectiveness as a communicator is central to the nurse-patient relationship. It allows you to know your patients, including their strengths, weaknesses, and needs. Communication is essential for all nursing roles and activities. You will routinely communicate with patients and families, other nurses and health care professionals, resource people, and the community. Without clear communication it is impossible to advocate for your patients or to give comfort and emotional support, give care effectively, make decisions with patients and families, protect patients from threats to well-being, coordinate and manage patient care, assist patients in rehabilitation, or provide patient education (Emrich et al., 2013). Quality communication is a critical factor in meeting the needs of individuals, families, and communities (see Chapter 24).

Manager. Today's health care environment is fast paced and complex. Nurse managers need to establish an environment for collaborative patient-centered care to provide safe, quality care with positive patient outcomes. A manager coordinates the activities of members of the nursing staff in delivering nursing care and has personnel, policy, and budgetary responsibility for a specific nursing unit or agency. A manager uses appropriate leadership styles to create a nursing environment for patients and staff that reflects the mission and values of the health care organization (see Chapter 21).

Career Development

Innovations in health care, expanding health care systems and practice settings, and the increasing needs of patients have created new nursing roles. Today the majority of nurses practice in hospital settings, followed by community-based care, ambulatory care, and nursing homes/extended care settings.

Nursing provides an opportunity for you to commit to lifelong learning and career development. Because of increasing educational opportunities for nurses, the growth of nursing as a profession, and a greater concern for job enrichment, the nursing profession offers different career opportunities. Your career path is limitless. You will probably switch career roles more than once. Take advantage of the different clinical practice and professional opportunities. Examples of these career opportunities include advanced practice registered nurses (APRNs), nurse researchers, nurse risk managers, quality improvement nurses, consultants, and even business owners.

Provider of Care. Most nurses provide direct patient care in an acute care setting. However, as changes in health care services and reimbursement continue, there will be an increase in the direct care activities provided in the home care setting and an increased need for community-based health promotion activities.

Educate your patients and families how to maintain their health and implement self-care activities. While collaborating with other health care team members, focus your care on returning a patient to his or her home at an optimal functional status.

In the hospital you may choose to practice in a medical-surgical setting or concentrate on a specific area of specialty practice such as pediatrics, critical care, or emergency care. Most specialty care areas require some experience as a medical-surgical nurse and additional continuing or in-service education. Many intensive care unit and emergency department nurses are required to have certification in advanced cardiac life support and critical care, emergency nursing, or trauma nursing.

Advanced Practice Registered Nurses. The advanced practice registered nurse (APRN) is the most independently functioning nurse. An APRN has advanced education in pathophysiology, pharmacology, and physical assessment and certification and expertise in a specialized area of practice (AACN, 2011). There are four core roles for the APRN: clinical nurse specialist (CNS), certified nurse practitioner (CNP), certified nurse midwife (CNM), and certified RN anesthetist (CRNA). The educational preparation for the four roles is in at least one of the following six populations: adult-gerontology, pediatrics, neonatology, women's health/gender related, family/individual across the life span, and psychiatric mental health. APRNs function

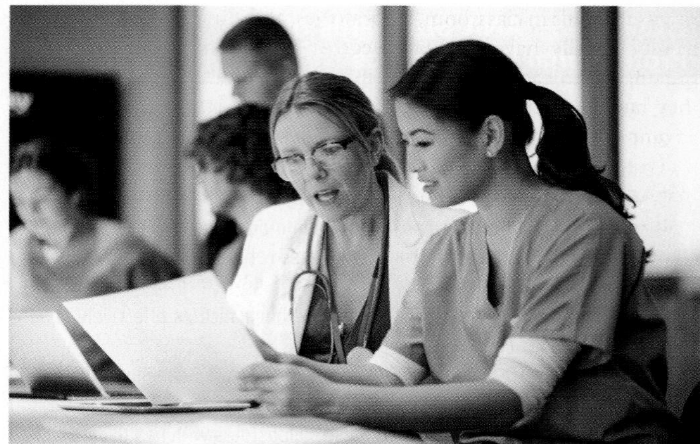

FIGURE 1-1 Nurse specialist consults on a difficult patient case. (iStock.com/Sturti.)

as clinicians, educators, case managers, consultants, and researchers within their area of practice to plan or improve the quality of nursing care for patients and families.

Clinical Nurse Specialist. A clinical nurse specialist (CNS) is an APRN who is an expert clinician in a specialized area of practice (Figure 1-1). The specialty may be identified by a population (e.g., geriatrics), a setting (e.g., critical care), a disease specialty (e.g., diabetes), a type of care (e.g., rehabilitation), or a type of problem (e.g., pain) (National CNS Competency Task Force, 2010). Some examples of CNS practice settings include community, acute care, restorative, and palliative.

Nurse Practitioner. A nurse practitioner (NP) is an APRN who provides health care to a group of patients, usually in an outpatient, ambulatory care, or community-based setting. NPs provide care for patients with complex problems and a more holistic approach than physicians. The NP provides comprehensive care, directly managing the nursing and medical care of patients who are healthy or who have chronic conditions. An NP establishes a collaborative provider-patient relationship and works with a specific group of patients or with patients of all ages and health care needs.

Certified Nurse-Midwife. A certified nurse-midwife (CNM) is an APRN who is also educated in midwifery and is certified by the American College of Nurse-Midwives. The practice of nurse-midwifery involves providing independent care for women during normal pregnancy, labor, and delivery and care for the newborn. It includes some gynecological services such as routine Papanicolaou (Pap) smears, family planning, and treatment for minor vaginal infections.

Certified Registered Nurse Anesthetist. A certified registered nurse anesthetist (CRNA) is an APRN with advanced education from a nurse anesthesia–accredited program. Before applying to a nurse anesthesia program, a nurse must have at least 1 year of critical care or emergency experience. Nurse anesthetists provide surgical anesthesia under the guidance and supervision of an anesthesiologist who is a physician with advanced knowledge of surgical anesthesia.

Nurse Educator. A nurse educator works primarily in schools of nursing, staff development departments of health care agencies, and patient education departments. Nurse educators need experience in clinical practice to provide them with practical skills and theoretical knowledge. A faculty member in a nursing program educates students to become professional nurses. Nursing faculty members are responsible for teaching current nursing practice; trends; theory; and necessary skills in classroom, laboratories, and clinical settings. Nursing faculty usually have graduate degrees such as a master's degree in nursing or an earned doctorate in nursing or related field. Generally they have a specific clinical, administrative, or research specialty and advanced clinical experience.

Nurse educators in staff development departments of health care institutions provide educational programs for nurses within their institution. These programs include orientation of new personnel, critical care nursing courses, assisting with clinical skill competency, safety training, and instruction about new equipment or procedures. These nursing educators often participate in the development of nursing policies and procedures.

The primary focus of the nurse educator in a patient education department of an agency such as a wound treatment clinic is to teach and coach patients and their families how to self-manage their illness or disability and make positive choices or change their behaviors to promote their health. These nurse educators are usually specialized and hold a certification such as a certified diabetes educator (CDE) or an ostomy care nurse and see only a specific population of patients.

Nurse Administrator. A nurse administrator manages patient care and the delivery of specific nursing services within a health care agency. Nursing administration begins with positions such as clinical care coordinators. Experience and additional education sometimes lead to a middle-management position such as nurse manager of a specific patient care area or house supervisor or to an upper-management position such as an associate director or director of nursing services.

Nurse manager positions usually require at least a baccalaureate degree in nursing, and director and nurse executive positions generally require a master's degree. Chief nurse executive and vice president positions in large health care organizations often require preparation at the doctoral level. Nurse administrators often have advanced degrees such as a master's degree in nursing administration, hospital administration (MHA), public health (MPH), or an MBA.

In today's health care organizations directors have responsibility for more than one nursing unit. They often manage a particular service or product line such as medicine or cardiology. Vice presidents of nursing or chief nurse executives often have responsibilities for all clinical functions within the hospital. This may include all ancillary personnel who provide and support patient care services. The nurse administrator needs to be skilled in business and management and understand all aspects of nursing and patient care. Functions of administrators include budgeting, staffing, strategic planning of programs and services, employee evaluation, and employee development.

Nurse Researcher. The nurse researcher conducts evidence-based practice and research to improve nursing care and further define and expand the scope of nursing practice (see Chapter 5). She or he often works in an academic setting, hospital, or independent professional or community service agency. The preferred educational requirement is a doctoral degree, with at least a master's degree in nursing.

Nursing Shortage

There is an ongoing shortage of qualified RNs to fill vacant positions (AACN, 2014; IOM, 2010). This shortage affects all aspects of nursing, including patient care, administration, and nursing education; but it also represents challenges and opportunities for the profession (Tanner and Bellack, 2010). Many health care dollars are invested in strategies aimed at recruiting and retaining a well-educated, critically thinking, motivated, and dedicated nursing workforce (Benner et al., 2010). There is a direct link between direct care by an RN and positive patient outcomes, reduced complication rates, and a more rapid return of the patient to an optimal functional status (Aiken, 2010, 2013a,b).

Professional nursing organizations predict that the number of nurses will continue to diminish (AACN, 2011; Aiken, 2010, 2013a). With fewer available nurses, it is important for you to learn to use your patient contact time efficiently and professionally. Time management, therapeutic communication, patient education, and compassionate implementation of bedside skills are just a few of the essential skills you need. It is important for your patients to leave the health care setting with a positive image of nursing and a feeling that they received quality care. Your patients should never feel rushed. They need to feel that they are important and are involved in decisions and that their needs are met. If a certain aspect of patient care requires 15 minutes of contact, it takes you the same time to deliver organized and compassionate care as it does if you rushed through your nursing care.

HISTORICAL INFLUENCES

Nurses have responded and always will respond to the needs of their patients. In times of war they responded by meeting the needs of the wounded in combat zones and military hospitals in the United States and abroad. When communities face health care crises such as disease outbreaks or insufficient health care resources, nurses establish community-based immunization and screening programs, treatment clinics, and health promotion activities. Our patients are most vulnerable when they are injured, sick, or dying.

Today nurses are active in determining best practices in a variety of areas such as skin care management, pain control, nutritional management, and care of individuals across the life span. Nurse researchers are leaders in expanding knowledge in nursing and other health care disciplines. Their work provides evidence for practice to ensure that nurses have the best available evidence to support their practices (see Chapter 5).

Knowledge of the history of the nursing profession increases your ability to understand the social and intellectual origins of the discipline. Although it is not practical to describe all of the historical aspects of professional nursing, some of the more significant nursing leaders and milestones are described in the following paragraphs.

Florence Nightingale

In *Notes on Nursing: What It Is and What It Is Not,* Florence Nightingale established the first nursing philosophy based on health maintenance and restoration (Nightingale, 1860). She saw the role of nursing as having "charge of somebody's health" based on the knowledge of "how to put the body in such a state to be free of disease or to recover from disease" (Nightingale, 1860). During the same year she developed the first organized program for training nurses, the Nightingale Training School for Nurses at St. Thomas' Hospital in London.

Nightingale was the first practicing nurse epidemiologist. Her statistical analyses connected poor sanitation with cholera and dysentery. She volunteered during the Crimean War in 1853 and traveled the battlefield hospitals at night carrying her lamp; thus she was known as the "lady with the lamp." The sanitary, nutrition, and basic facilities in the battlefield hospitals were poor at best. Eventually she was tasked with organizing and improving the quality of sanitation facilities. As a result, the mortality rate at the Barracks Hospital in Scutari, Turkey, was reduced from 42.7% to 2.2% in 6 months (Donahue, 2011).

The Civil War to the Beginning of the Twentieth Century

The Civil War (1860 to 1865) stimulated the growth of nursing in the United States. Clara Barton, founder of the American Red Cross, tended soldiers on the battlefields, cleansing their wounds, meeting their basic needs, and comforting them in death. Mother Bickerdyke organized ambulance services and walked abandoned battlefields at night, looking for wounded soldiers. Harriet Tubman was active in the Underground Railroad movement and helped to lead over 300 slaves to freedom (Donahue, 2011). The first professionally trained African-American nurse was Mary Mahoney. She was concerned with the effect culture had on health care, and as a noted nursing leader she brought forth an awareness of cultural diversity and respect for the individual, regardless of background, race, color, or religion.

Nursing in hospitals expanded in the late nineteenth century. However, nursing in the community did not increase significantly until 1893, when Lillian Wald and Mary Brewster opened the Henry Street Settlement, which focused on the health needs of poor people who lived in tenements in New York City (Donahue, 2011).

Twentieth Century

In the early twentieth century a movement toward developing a scientific, research-based defined body of nursing knowledge and practice evolved. Nurses began to assume expanded and advanced practice roles. Mary Adelaide Nutting, who became the first nursing professor at Columbia Teacher's College in 1906, was instrumental in moving nursing education into universities (Donahue, 2011).

As nursing education developed, nursing practice also expanded, and the Army and Navy Nurse Corps were established. By the 1920s nursing specialization began. Graduate nurse-midwifery programs began; in the last half of the century specialty-nursing organizations were created.

Twenty-First Century

Today the profession faces multiple challenges. Nurses and nurse educators are revising nursing practice and school curricula to meet the ever-changing needs of society, including an aging population, bioterrorism, emerging infections, and disaster management. Advances in technology and informatics (see Chapter 26), the high acuity level of care of hospitalized patients, and early discharge from health care institutions require nurses in all settings to have a strong and current knowledge base from which to practice.

Nursing organizations and the RWJF are currently involved in programs to support nursing scholars, decrease the nursing shortage, and improve the health of the nation's population (RWJF, 2014a,b). Nursing is taking a leadership role in developing standards and policies to address the needs of the population now and in the future.

CONTEMPORARY INFLUENCES

Multiple external forces affect nursing, including the need for nurses' self-care, the Affordable Care Act (ACA) and rising health care costs, demographic changes of the population, human rights, and increasing numbers of medically underserved.

Importance of Nurses' Self-Care

You cannot give fully engaged, compassionate care to others when you feel depleted or do not feel cared for yourself. Nurses experience grief and loss too. Many times, even before a nurse has a chance to recover from an emotionally draining situation, he or she encounters another difficult human story. Nurses in acute care settings often witness prolonged, concentrated suffering on a daily basis, leading to feelings of frustration, anger, guilt, sadness, or anxiety. Nursing students report feeling initially hesitant and uncomfortable with their first encounters with a dying patient and identify feelings of sadness, anxiety, and discomfort.

Frequent, intense, or prolonged exposure to grief and loss places nurses at risk for developing compassion fatigue. *Compassion fatigue* is a term used to describe a state of burnout and secondary traumatic stress (Potter et al., 2013a). It occurs without warning and often results from giving high levels of energy and compassion over a prolonged period to those who are suffering, often without experiencing improved patient outcomes (Potter et al., 2010). Secondary traumatic stress is the trauma that health care providers experience when witnessing and caring for others suffering trauma. Examples include an oncology nurse who cares for patients undergoing surgery and chemotherapy over the long term for their cancer or a spouse who witnesses his wife deteriorating over the years from Alzheimer's disease.

Burnout is the condition that occurs when perceived demands outweigh perceived resources (Potter et al., 2013a). It is a state of physical and mental exhaustion that often affects health care providers because of the nature of their work environment. Over time, giving of oneself in often intense caring environments sometimes results in emotional exhaustion, leaving a nurse feeling irritable, restless, and unable to focus and engage with patients (Potter et al., 2013b). This often occurs in situations in which there is a lack of social support, organizational pressures influencing staffing, and the inability of the nurse to practice self-care. Compassion fatigue typically results in feelings of hopelessness, a decrease in the ability to take pleasure from previously enjoyable activities, a state of hypervigilance, and anxiety.

Compassion fatigue impacts the health and wellness of nurses and the quality of care provided to patients. Nurses experience changes in job performance and in their personal lives, increased demands, and a desire to leave the profession or their specialty. In addition, these factors affect an agency's ability to maintain a caring, competent staff and patient satisfaction.

When health care agencies develop interventions to help nurses manage compassion fatigue, nurse retention and job satisfaction rates improve. Agency-based programs that provide opportunities to validate the caregiver's experiences and an opportunity to talk about the challenges of the type of care nurses give are basic interventions to begin to manage these factors and their implication for professional nursing care. More complex interventions include specific programs that teach nurses how to more effectively cope with the challenges of care to offset the stress related to the care (Potter et al., 2010).

When a nurse experiences ongoing stressful patient relationships, he or she often disengages (Slatten et al., 2011). This disengagement can also occur when perceived stress comes from nurse-physician or nurse-nurse relationships. It is not uncommon for nurses who are experiencing compassion fatigue to become angry or cynical and have difficulty relating with patients and co-workers (Young et al., 2011).

Compassion fatigue may contribute to what is described as *lateral violence.* Health care providers do not always voice concerns about patients and actively avoid conflict in clinical settings (Lyndon et al., 2011). However, lateral violence sometimes occurs in nurse-nurse interactions and includes behaviors such as withholding information, making snide remarks, and demonstrating nonverbal expressions of disapproval such as raising eyebrows or making faces. New graduates and nurses new to a unit are most likely to face problems with lateral or horizontal violence (Lachman, 2014).

All nurses require resiliency skills to better manage the stressors that contribute to compassion fatigue and lateral violence. Skills such as managing stress and conflict, building connections with colleagues to share difficult stories, and self-care are helpful in dealing with difficult situations and contribute to safe and effective care (Mahon and Nicotera, 2011).

However, interventions in the health care agency alone are not enough. Nurses need to be self-aware, allowing them to identify their own vulnerability to secondary traumatic stress and burnout (see Chapter 38). Participating in health promotion activities is also effective in identifying and managing the stressors that lead to compassion fatigue. Chapter 6 provides a guide to identify effective interventions that help nurses identify and manage health-related risk factors from prolonged caregiver stress.

The Affordable Care Act and Rising Health Care Costs

The ACA affects how health care is paid for and delivered (see Chapter 2). There will be greater emphasis on health promotion, disease prevention, and illness management in the future. The ACA impacts how and where nursing care is provided. More nursing services will be in community-based care settings. As a result, more nurses will be needed to practice in community care centers, schools, and senior centers. This will require nurses to be better able to assess for resources, identify service gaps, and help patients adapt to safely return to their community.

Skyrocketing health care costs present challenges to the nursing profession, consumer, and health care delivery system. As a nurse you are responsible for providing patients with the best-quality care in an efficient and economically sound manner. The challenge is to use health care and patient resources wisely. Chapter 2 summarizes reasons for the rise in health care costs and its implications for nursing

Demographic Changes

The U.S. Census Bureau (2014) continues to predict a continuing rise in the population, with an increase in the population over 65. This change alone requires expanded health care resources. To effectively meet all the health care needs of the expanding and aging population, changes need to occur as to how care is provided, especially in the areas of outpatient-, community-, and home-based services (see Chapters 2 and 3). The population is still shifting from rural areas to urban centers, and more people are living with chronic and long-term illness (RWJF, 2014b).

Medically Underserved

Unemployment, underemployment and low-paying jobs, mental illness, homelessness, and rising health care costs all contribute to increases in the medically underserved population. Caring for this population is a global issue; the social, political, and economic factors of a country affect both access to care and resources to provide and pay for these services (Huicho et al., 2010). In addition, the number of underserved patients who require home-based palliative care services is increasing. This is a group of patients whose physical status does not improve and health care needs increase. As a result, the cost for home-based care continues to rise, to the point that some patients opt out of all palliative services because of costs (Fernandes et al., 2010).

TRENDS IN NURSING

Nursing is a dynamic profession that grows and evolves as society and lifestyles change, as health care priorities and technologies change, and as nurses themselves change. The current philosophies and definitions of nursing have a holistic focus, which addresses the needs of the whole person in all dimensions, in health and illness, and in interaction with the family and community. In addition, there continues to be an increasing awareness for patient safety in all care settings.

Evidence-Based Practice

Today the general public is more informed about their health care needs, the cost of health care, and the incidence of medical errors within health care institutions. Your practice needs to be based on current evidence, not just according to your education and experiences and the policies and procedures of health care facilities (see Chapter 5). Health care organizations can show their commitment to each health care stakeholder (e.g., patients, insurance companies, and governmental agencies) to reduce health care errors and improve patient safety by implementing evidence-based practices (National Quality Forum, 2010). In addition, many hospitals are achieving Magnet Recognition, which recognizes excellence in nursing practice (ANCC, 2014). A component of excellence in practice is quality of care, which is achieved by implementing evidenced-based practice (see Chapter 2).

Quality and Safety Education for Nurses

The RWJF sponsored the **Quality and Safety Education for Nurses (QSEN)** initiative to respond to reports about safety and quality patient care by the IOM (Barton et al., 2009). QSEN addresses the challenge to prepare nurses with the competencies needed to continuously improve the quality of care in their work environments (Table 1-1). The QSEN initiative encompasses the competencies of patient-centered care, teamwork and collaboration, evidence-based practice, quality improvement, safety, and informatics (Cronenwett et al., 2007). For each competency there are targeted knowledge, skills, and attitudes (KSAs). The KSAs are elements that are integrated in a nursing prelicensure program (Jarzemsky et al., 2010). As you gain experience in clinical practice, you will encounter situations in which your education helps you to make a difference in improving patient care (Box 1-4).

Whether that difference in care is to provide evidence for implementing care at the bedside, identifying a safety issue, or reviewing patient data to identify trends in outcomes, each of these situations requires competence in patient-centered care, safety, or informatics. Although it is not within the scope of this textbook to present the QSEN initiative in its entirety, subsequent clinical chapters will provide you an opportunity to address how to build competencies in one or more of these areas.

> QSEN **QSEN: BUILDING COMPETENCY IN PATIENT-CENTERED CARE** You are caring for Kitty, a 10-year-old with severe delayed development. Kitty, an only child, lives with her parents and goes to a school that is able to meet her needs. Her mom gives her seizure medicine each day, and her seizures are well controlled. Kitty has very little independent function. She needs assistance with all of her activities of daily living (e.g., bathing, toileting, eating, and hygiene). Up to now Kitty's parents are able to provide all of her care and meet her needs. As Kitty gets older and bigger, it will be difficult for her mom and dad to provide this care. They want to keep Kitty in her current school as long as possible. They are looking at in-home physical care assistance and anticipate needing to make decisions about Kitty's home care within the next 2 years. After thinking about this scenario, which questions do you need to ask to determine how best to guide the family to establish a comprehensive home care team? How would you help Kitty's parents ask these questions when they interview home care services?
>
> *Answers to QSEN Activities can be found on the Evolve website.*

TABLE 1-1 Quality and Safety Education for Nurses

Competency	Definition with Examples
Patient-Centered Care	Recognize the patient or designee as the source of control and full partner in providing compassionate and coordinated care based on respect for patient's preferences, values, and needs. Examples: Involve family and friends in care. Elicit patient values and preferences. Provide care with respect for diversity of the human experience.
Teamwork and Collaboration	Function effectively within nursing and interprofessional teams, fostering open communication, mutual respect, and shared decision making to achieve quality patient care. Examples: Recognize the contributions of other health team members and patient's family members. Discuss effective strategies for communicating and resolving conflict. Participate in designing methods to support effective teamwork.
Evidence-Based Practice	Integrate best current evidence with clinical expertise and patient/family preferences and values for delivery of optimal health care. Examples: Demonstrate knowledge of basic scientific methods. Appreciate strengths and weaknesses of scientific bases for practice. Appreciate the importance of regularly reading relevant journals.
Quality Improvement	Use data to monitor the outcomes of care processes and use improvement methods to design and test changes to continuously improve the quality and safety of health care systems. Examples: Use tools such as flow charts and diagrams to make process of care explicit. Appreciate how unwanted variation in outcomes affects care. Identify gaps between local and best practices.
Safety	Minimize risk of harm to patients and providers through both system effectiveness and individual performance. Examples: Examine human factors and basic safety design principles and commonly used unsafe practices. Value own role in preventing errors.
Informatics	Use information and technology to communicate, manage knowledge, mitigate error, and support decision making. Examples: Navigate an electronic health record. Protect confidentiality of protected health information in electronic health records.

Adapted from Cronenwett L et al: Quality and safety education for nurses, *Nurs Outlook* 57:122, 2007.

BOX 1-4 EVIDENCE-BASED PRACTICE

Safety Competencies and Patient-Centered Care

PICO Question: Do teaching strategies targeted at interprofessional communication develop competencies in teamwork and collaboration in new graduates?

Evidence Summary

Patient care needs are increasingly complex, and this trend is expected to continue well into the future. The American Association of Colleges of Nursing (AACN) (AACN, 2008) endorsed a new set of guidelines that parallel the QSEN competencies to direct the preparation of baccalaureate nurses to provide safe, high-quality patient care (Barton et al., 2009). Health professions education must prepare all students for "deliberately working together" toward a safer and better health care system. Collaboration and teamwork are essential competencies in delivering safe, effective patient-centered care (Headrick et al., 2012).

Students need more than classroom and clinical experiences to understand the intricacies of effective teamwork and collaboration. Institution of QSEN content into schools' curricula enables students to practice teamwork and collaboration in safe, clinical simulations (Barnsteiner et al., 2013). For teamwork and collaboration to be successful, there must be strong and clear communication between and among all health care professions. Adverse events, omission of care, and confusion are serious events in today's health care environments.

An academic/clinical partnership provides consistent class and clinical environments for students to safely incorporate teamwork and collaboration early in the clinical practicum (Didion et al., 2013). Inaccurate communication among health care providers leads to serious events (Barnsteiner et al., 2013). Teaching effective communication strategies across the disciplines is an effective method to help bridge this gap (Robinson et al., 2010).

Application to Nursing Practice

- Communicate with clarity and precision when designing multidisciplinary plans of care (Robinson et al., 2010).
- Create a safety huddle so all health care staff are aware of the clinical objectives (Didion et al., 2013).
- Set up communication simulations to increase caregiver's knowledge about the expertise of other health care disciplines (Headrick et al., 2012; Didion et al., 2013).
- Recognize that electronic communication may be quick but in some situations may not be effective (Robinson et al., 2010). When patient care issues are at stake, a focused, well-organized interdisciplinary meeting is more effective than a series of "round-robin" e-mails (Robinson et al., 2010).
- It usually takes the same amount of time to communicate and collaborate ineffectively as it does to do it effectively.

Impact of Emerging Technologies

Many emerging technologies have the potential to rapidly change nursing practice. Some of these help nurses use noninvasive, more accurate assessment tools; implement evidence-based practices; collect and trend patient outcome data; and use clinical decision support systems. The electronic health record (EHR) offers an efficient method to record and manage patient health care information (see Chapter 26). In addition, computerized physician/provider order entry (CPOE) is a key patient safety initiative (Houston, 2014).

Three skills sets are needed to respond to these emerging technologies (Houston, 2013). First, you need to use technology to facilitate mobility, communication, and relationships. Telehealth and telemedicine functions, video conferencing, and simulations provide opportunities for nurses, health care professionals, and patients and families to communicate about specific health care issues. Second, you need to develop an expertise to acquire and distribute knowledge. Evidence-based practice, clinical decision support systems, and case-based reasoning are all methods to increase information acquisition and distribution. Last, you need to understand and use genomics. Effective use of genomic information in a confidential, ethical, and culturally appropriate manner helps health care providers and patients make informed care decisions (Houston, 2013).

Genomics

Genetics is the study of inheritance, or the way traits are passed down from one generation to another. Genes carry the instructions for making proteins, which in turn direct the activities of cells and functions of the body that influence traits such as hair and eye color. Genomics is a newer term that describes the study of all the genes in a person and interactions of these genes with one another and with that person's environment (CDC, 2015). Using genomic information allows health care providers to determine how genomic changes contribute to patient conditions and influence treatment decisions (Miaskowski and Aouizerat, 2012). For example, when a family member has colon cancer before the age of 50, it is likely that other family members are at risk for developing this cancer. Knowing this information is important for family members who will need a colonoscopy before the age of 50 and repeat colonoscopies more often than the patient who is not at risk. In this case nurses are essential in identifying the patients' risk factors through assessment and counseling patients about what this genomic finding means to them personally and to their family.

Public Perception of Nursing

Nursing is a pivotal health care profession. As frontline health care providers, nurses practice in all health care settings and constitute the largest number of health care professionals. They are essential to providing skilled, specialized, knowledgeable care; improving the health status of the public; and ensuring safe, effective quality care (ANA, 2010b).

Consumers of health care are more informed than ever; with the Internet consumers have access to more health care and treatment information. For example, *Hospital Compare* is a consumer-oriented website that allows people to select multiple hospitals and directly compare performance measure information on specific diseases such as health attack, heart failure, pneumonia, and surgery (CMS, 2014). This information can help consumers make informed decisions about health care.

Consumers can also access *Hospital Consumer Assessment of Healthcare Providers Systems* (HCAHPS) to obtain information about patients' perspectives on hospital care. Although many hospitals collect information on patient satisfaction, HCAHPS helps consumers obtain valid comparisons about patient perspectives across all hospitals. This information is intended to allow consumers to make "apples to apples" comparisons to support their choice (HCAHPS, 2015).

Publications such as *To Err Is Human* (IOM, 2000) describe strategies for government, health care providers, industry, and consumers to reduce preventable medical errors. When you care for patients, realize how your approach to care influences public opinion. Always act in a competent professional manner.

Impact of Nursing on Politics and Health Policy

Political power or influence is known as the ability to influence or persuade an individual holding a government office to exert the power of that office to affect a desired outcome. Nurses' involvement in politics is receiving greater emphasis in nursing curricula, professional organizations, and health care settings. Professional nursing organizations and state nursing boards employ lobbyists to urge state legislatures and the U.S. Congress to improve the quality of health care (Mason et al., 2012).

The ANA works for the improvement of health standards and the availability of health care services for all people, fosters high standards of nursing, stimulates and promotes the professional development of nurses, and advances their economic and general welfare. The ANA's purposes are unrestricted by considerations of nationality, race, creed, lifestyle, color, gender, or age.

Nurses are active in social policy and political arenas. Nurses and their professional organizations lobby for health care legislation to meet the needs of patients, particularly the medically underserved. For example, nurses in communities provide home visits to newborns of high-risk mothers (e.g., adolescent, poorly educated, or medically underserved). These visits result in fewer emergency department visits, fewer newborn infections, fewer developmental delays, and reduced infant mortality (Mason et al., 2012).

You can influence policy decisions at all governmental levels. One way to get involved is by participating in local and national efforts (Mason et al., 2012). This effort is critical to exerting nurses' influence early in the political process. When nurses become serious students of social needs, activists in influencing policy to meet those needs, and generous contributors of time and money to nursing organizations and to candidates working for universal good health care, the future is bright indeed (Mason et al., 2012).

PROFESSIONAL REGISTERED NURSE EDUCATION

Nursing requires a significant amount of formal education. The issues of standardization of nursing education and entry into practice remain a major controversy. Most nurses agree that nursing education is important to practice and that education needs to respond to changes in health care created by scientific and technological advances. Various education preparations are available for an individual intending to be an RN. In addition, graduate nurse education and continuing and in-service education are available for practicing nurses.

Currently in the United States the most frequent way to become a registered nurse (RN) is through completion of either an associate or baccalaureate degree program. Graduates of both programs are eligible to take the National Council Licensure Examination for Registered Nurses (NCLEX-RN®) to become RNs in the state in which they will practice.

The associate degree program in the United States is a 2-year program that is usually offered by a university or community college. This program focuses on the basic sciences and theoretical and clinical courses related to the practice of nursing.

The baccalaureate degree program usually includes 4 years of study in a college or university. It focuses on the basic sciences; theoretical and clinical courses; and courses in the social sciences, arts, and humanities to support nursing theory. In Canada the degree of Bachelor of Science in Nursing (BScN) or Bachelor in Nursing (BN) is equivalent to the degree of Bachelor of Science in Nursing (BSN) in the United States. The *Essentials of Baccalaureate Education for Professional Nursing* (AACN, 2008) delineates essential knowledge, practice and values, attitudes, personal qualities, and professional behavior for the baccalaureate-prepared nurse and guides faculty on the structure and evaluation of the curriculum. Standards published by nursing program accrediting organizations typically specify core competencies for the professional nurse that should be in the nursing curriculum. In addition, one of the IOM recommendations is that 80% of nurses be prepared with a baccalaureate in nursing by 2020 (IOM, 2010) (see Chapter 2). Thus nurses with associate degrees often return to school to earn their baccalaureate degree.

Graduate Education

After obtaining a baccalaureate degree in nursing, you can pursue graduate education leading to a master's or doctoral degree in any number of graduate fields, including nursing. A nurse completing a graduate program can receive a master's degree in nursing. The graduate degree provides the advanced clinician with strong skills in nursing science and theory. Graduate education emphasizes advance knowledge in the basic sciences and research-based clinical practice. A master's degree in nursing is important for the roles of nurse educator and nurse administrator, and it is required for an APRN.

Doctoral Preparation. Professional doctoral programs in nursing (DSN or DNSc) prepare graduates to apply research findings to clinical nursing. Other doctoral programs prepare nurses for more rigorous research and theory development and award the research-oriented Doctor of Philosophy (PhD) in nursing. Recently the AACN recommended the Doctor of Nursing Practice (DNP) as the terminal practice degree and required preparation for all APRNs. The DNP is a practice-focused doctorate. It provides skills in obtaining expanded knowledge through the formulation and interpretations of evidence-based practice (Chism, 2010).

The need for nurses with doctoral degrees is increasing. Expanding clinical roles and continuing demand for well-educated nursing faculty, nurse administrators, and APRNs in the clinical settings and new areas of nursing specialties such as nursing informatics are just a few reasons for increasing the number of doctoral-prepared nurses.

Continuing and In-Service Education

Nursing is a knowledge-based profession, and technological expertise and clinical decision making are qualities that our health care consumers demand and expect. Continuing education programs help nurses maintain current nursing skills, gain new knowledge and theory, and obtain new skills reflecting the changes in the health care delivery system (Hale et al., 2010). **Continuing education** involves formal, organized educational programs offered by universities, hospitals, state nurses associations, professional nursing organizations, and educational and health care institutions. An example is a program on caring for older adults with dementia offered by a university or a program on safe medication practices offered by a hospital. Continuing education updates your knowledge about the latest research and practice developments, helps you to specialize in a particular area of practice, and teaches you new skills and techniques (Hale et al., 2010). In some states continuing education is required for RNs to keep their licenses.

In-service education programs are instruction or training provided by a health care agency or institution. An in-service program is held in the institution and is designed to increase the knowledge, skills, and competencies of nurses and other health care professionals employed by the institution. Often in-service programs are focused on new technologies such as how to correctly use the newest safety syringes. Many in-service programs are designed to fulfill required competencies of an organization. For example, a hospital might offer an in-service program on safe principles for administering chemotherapy or a program on cultural sensitivity.

NURSING PRACTICE

You will have an opportunity to practice in a variety of settings, in many roles within those settings, and with caregivers in other related health professions. The ANA standards of practice, standards of performance, and code of ethics for nurses are part of the public recognition of the significance of nursing practice to health care and implications for nursing practice regarding trends in health care. State and provincial nurse practice acts (NPAs) establish specific legal regulations for practice, and professional organizations establish standards of practice as criteria for nursing care.

Nurse Practice Acts

In the United States the State Boards of Nursing oversee NPAs. NPAs regulate the scope of nursing practice and protect public health, safety, and welfare. This protection includes shielding the public from unqualified and unsafe nurses. Although each state defines for itself the scope of nursing practice, most have similar NPAs. The definition of nursing practice published by the ANA is representative of the scope of nursing practice as defined in most states. However, in the last decade many states have revised their NPAs to reflect the growing autonomy of nursing and the expanded roles of nurses in practice. For example, NPAs expanded their scope to include minimum education requirements, required certifications, and practice guidelines for APRNs such as nurse practitioners and certified RN anesthetists. The expansion of scope of practice includes skills unique to the advanced practice role (e.g., advanced assessment, prescriptive authority for certain medications and diagnostic procedures, and some invasive procedures).

Licensure and Certification

Licensure. In the United States all boards of nursing require RN candidates to pass the NCLEX-RN®. Regardless of educational preparation, the examination for RN licensure is exactly the same in every state in the United States. This provides a standardized minimum knowledge base for nurses. Other requirements for licensure such as criminal background checks vary from state to state.

Certification. Beyond the NCLEX-RN®, the nurse may choose to work toward certification in a specific area of nursing practice. Minimum practice requirements are set, based on the certification the nurse seeks. National nursing organizations such as the ANA have many types of certification to enhance your career such as certification in medical surgical or geriatric nursing. After passing the initial examination, you maintain your certification by ongoing continuing education and clinical or administrative practice.

PROFESSIONAL NURSING ORGANIZATIONS

A **professional organization** deals with issues of concern to those practicing in the profession. In addition to the educational organizations previously discussed, a variety of specialty organizations exist. For example, some organizations focus on specific areas such as critical care, advanced practice, maternal-child nursing, and nursing research. These organizations seek to improve the standards of practice, expand nursing roles, and foster the welfare of nurses within the specialty areas. In addition, professional organizations present educational programs and publish journals.

As a student you have the opportunity to take part in organizations such as the National Student Nurses Association (NSNA) in the United States and the Canadian Student Nurses Association (CSNA) in Canada. These organizations consider issues of importance to nursing students such as career development and preparation for licensing. The NSNA often cooperates in activities and programs with the professional organizations.

KEY POINTS

- Nursing responds to the health care needs of society, which are influenced by economic, social, and cultural variables of a specific era.

- Changes in society such as increased technology, new demographic patterns, consumerism, health promotion, and the women's and human rights movements lead to changes in nursing.
- Nursing definitions reflect changes in the practice of nursing and help bring about changes by identifying the domain of nursing practice and guiding research, practice, and education.
- Nursing standards provide the guidelines for implementing and evaluating nursing care.
- Professional nursing organizations deal with issues of concern to specialist groups within the nursing profession.
- Nurses are becoming more politically sophisticated and, as a result, are able to increase the influence of nursing on health care policy and practice.

CLINICAL APPLICATION QUESTIONS

Preparing for Clinical Practice

1. You are on the patient safety committee at your hospital. Your assignment is to identify two sources related to safety. One resource must relate to the individual nurse, and the second must relate to the practice and work environment. Identify the ANA website and use this site to identify the resources.
2. Mrs. Langman is in the hospital recovering from hip replacement surgery. Her surgery involved insertion of a new type of hip replacement prosthesis and newer postsurgical care. The advanced practice registered nurse (APRN) is preparing her discharge medication and rehabilitation prescriptions. The staff nurse is preparing to transfer Mrs. Langman to a rehabilitation facility. The nurse educator is conducting bedside rounds to explain the new prosthesis and related postoperative care.
   a. Discuss the roles of the staff nurse, APRN, and nurse educator.
   b. What is the educational preparation for each role?

Answers to Clinical Application Questions can be found on the Evolve website.

REVIEW QUESTIONS

Are You Ready to Test Your Nursing Knowledge?

1. You are preparing a presentation for your classmates regarding the clinical care coordination conference for a patient with terminal cancer. As part of the preparation you have your classmates read the Nursing Code of Ethics for Professional Registered Nurses. Your instructor asks the class why this document is important. Which of the following statements best describes this code?
   1. Improves self–health care
   2. Protects the patient's confidentiality
   3. Ensures identical care to all patients
   4. Defines the principles of right and wrong to provide patient care
2. An 18-year-old woman is in the emergency department with fever and cough. The nurse obtains her vital signs, listens to her lung and heart sounds, determines her level of comfort, and collects blood and sputum samples for analysis. Which standard of practice is performed?
   1. Diagnosis
   2. Evaluation
   3. Assessment
   4. Implementation
3. A patient in the emergency department has developed wheezing and shortness of breath. The nurse gives the ordered medicated nebulizer treatment now and in 4 hours. Which standard of practice is performed?
   1. Planning
   2. Evaluation
   3. Assessment
   4. Implementation
4. A nurse is caring for a patient with end-stage lung disease. The patient wants to go home on oxygen and be comfortable. The family wants the patient to have a new surgical procedure. The nurse explains the risk and benefits of the surgery to the family and discusses the patient's wishes with them. The nurse is acting as the patient's:
   1. Educator.
   2. Advocate.
   3. Caregiver.
   4. Case manager.
5. The nurse spends time with the patient and family reviewing the dressing change procedure for the patient's wound. The patient's spouse demonstrates how to change the dressing. The nurse is acting in which professional role?
   1. Educator
   2. Advocate
   3. Caregiver
   4. Case manager
6. The examination for registered nurse (RN) licensure is exactly the same in every state in the United States. This examination:
   1. Guarantees safe nursing care for all patients.
   2. Ensures standard nursing care for all patients.
   3. Ensures that honest and ethical care is provided.
   4. Provides a minimal standard of knowledge for an RN in practice.
7. Contemporary nursing requires that the nurse has knowledge and skills for a variety of professional roles and responsibilities. Which of the following are examples? (Select all that apply.)
   1. Caregiver
   2. Autonomy and accountability
   3. Patient advocate
   4. Health promotion
   5. Lobbyist
8. Match the advanced practice nurse specialty with the statement about the role.

1. Clinical nurse specialist	a. Provides independent care, including pregnancy and gynecological services
2. Nurse anesthetist	b. Expert clinician in a specialized area of practice such as adult diabetes care
3. Nurse practitioner	c. Provides comprehensive care, usually in a primary care setting, directly managing the medical care of patients who are healthy or have chronic conditions
4. Nurse-midwife	d. Provides care and services under the supervision of an anesthesiologist

9. Health care reform will bring changes in the emphasis of care. Which of the following models is expected from health care reform?

1. Moving from an acute illness to a health promotion, illness prevention model
2. Moving from an illness prevention to a health promotion model
3. Moving from an acute illness to a disease management model
4. Moving from a chronic care to an illness prevention model

10. A nurse meets with the registered dietitian and physical therapist to develop a plan of care that focuses on improving nutrition and mobility for a patient. This is an example of which Quality and Safety in the Education of Nurses (QSEN) competency?
    1. Patient-centered care
    2. Safety
    3. Teamwork and collaboration
    4. Informatics
11. A critical care nurse is using a computerized decision support system to correctly position her ventilated patients to reduce pneumonia caused by accumulated respiratory secretions. This is an example of which Quality and Safety in the Education of Nurses (QSEN) competency?
    1. Patient-centered care
    2. Safety
    3. Teamwork and collaboration
    4. Informatics
12. How does knowledge of genomics affect patient treatment decisions?
13. The nurses on an acute care medical floor notice an increase in pressure ulcer formation in their patients. A nurse consultant decides to compare two types of treatment. The first is the procedure currently used to assess for pressure ulcer risk. The second uses a new assessment instrument to identify at-risk patients. Given this information, the nurse consultant exemplifies which career?
    1. Clinical nurse specialist
    2. Nurse administrator
    3. Nurse educator
    4. Nurse researcher
14. Nurses in an acute care hospital are attending a unit-based education program to learn how to use a new pressure-relieving device for patients at risk for pressure ulcers. This is which type of education?
    1. Continuing education
    2. Graduate education
    3. In-service education
    4. Professional Registered Nurse Education
15. Which of the following Internet resources can help consumers compare quality care measures? (Select all that apply.)
    1. WebMD
    2. Hospital Compare
    3. Magnet Recognition Program
    4. Hospital Consumer Assessment of Healthcare
    5. The American Hospital Association's webpage.

Answers: 1. 4; **2.** 3; **3.** 4; **4.** 2; **5.** 1; **6.** 4; **7.** 1, 2, 3, 4; **8.** 1b, 2d, 3c, 4a; **9.** 1; **10.** 3; **11.** 4; **12.** See Evolve; **13.** 4; **14.** 3; **15.** 2, 4.

Rationales for Review Questions can be found on the Evolve website.

REFERENCES

Aiken LH: Economics of nursing, *Policy Politics Nurs* 9(93):73, 2010.

Aiken LH: The impact of research on staffing: an interview with Linda Aiken, Part 1, *Nurs Econ* 31(5):216, 2013a.

Aiken LH: The impact of research on staffing: an interview with Linda Aiken, Part 2, *Nurs Econ* 31(5):216, 2013b.

American Association of Colleges of Nursing (AACN): *Essentials of baccalaureate education for professional nursing*, Washington, DC, 2008, The Association.

American Association of Colleges of Nursing (AACN): *Essentials of master's education for advanced practice nursing*, Washington, DC, 2011, The Association.

American Association of Colleges of Nursing (AACN): *Nursing shortage, news release*, Washington, DC, 2014, The Association. http://www.aacn.nche.edu/media-relations/fact-sheets/nursing-shortage. Accessed May 2015.

American Nurses Association (ANA): *Nursing's social policy statement: the essence of the profession*, Silver Spring, MD, 2010a, American Nurses Publishing.

American Nurses Association (ANA): *Nursing: scope and standards of practice*, ed 2, Silver Spring, MD, 2010b, The Association.

American Nurses Association (ANA): *Guide to the code of ethics for nurses: interpretation and application*, Silver Spring, MD, 2015, The Association.

American Nurses' Credentialing Center (ANCC): *Magnet Recognition Program Model*, 2014, http://www.nursecredentialing.org/Magnet/ProgramOverview/New-Magnet-Model. Accessed May 2015.

Benner P: *From novice to expert: excellence and power in clinical nursing practice*, Menlo Park, CA, 1984, Addison-Wesley.

Benner P, et al: The social fabric of nursing knowledge, *Am J Nurs* 97(7):16, 1997.

Benner P, et al: *Educating nurses: a call for radical transformation*, Stanford, CA, 2010, Carnegie Foundation for the Advancement of Teaching.

Centers for Disease Control and Prevention (CDC): *Genomics and health frequently asked questions*, 2015, http://www.cdc.gov/genomics/public/faq.htm. Accessed May 2015.

Centers for Medicare & Medicaid Services (CMS): *Hospital compare*, Updated December 2014, http://www.cms.gov/Medicare/Quality-Initiatives-Patient-Assessment-Instruments/hospital QualityInits/HospitalCompare.html. Accessed May 2015.

Chism LA: *The doctor of nursing practice: a guidebook for role development and professionals' issues*, Sudbury, MA, 2010, Jones & Bartlett Publishers.

Cronenwett L, et al: Quality and safety education for nurses, *Nurs Outlook* 57:122, 2007.

Donahue MP: *Nursing: the finest art—an illustrated history*, ed 3, St Louis, 2011, Mosby.

Fernandes R, et al: Home-based palliative care services for underserved populations, *J Palliat Med* 13(4):413, 2010.

Hale MA, et al: Continuing education needs of nurses in a voluntary continuing nursing education state, *J Cont Educ Nurs* 41(3):107, 2010.

Hospital Consumer Assessment of Healthcare Providers and Systems (HCAHPS): *CAHPS Survey®*, April 2015 update, http://www.hcahpsonline.org/home.aspx. Accessed May 2015.

Houston C: The impact of emerging technology on nurse care: warp speed ahead, *Online J Issues Nurs* 18(2):1, 2013.

Houston C: Technology in the health care workplace: benefits, limitations, and challenges. In Houston CJ, editor: *Professional issues in nursing: challenges and opportunities*, ed 3, Philadelphia, 2014, Lippincott Williams & Wilkins.

Huicho L, et al: Increasing access to health workers in underserved areas: a conceptual framework for measuring results, *Bull World Health Organ* 88:357, 2010.

Institute of Medicine (IOM): *To err is human*, Washington, DC, 2000, The Institute.

Institute of Medicine (IOM): *The future of nursing: leading change, advancing health*, Washington DC, 2010, National Academies Press.

International Council of Nurses (ICN): *ICN definition of nursing*, 2014, http://icn.ch/definition.htm. Accessed May 2015.

Jarzemsky P, et al: Incorporating quality and safety education for nurses' competencies in simulation scenario design, *Nurse Educ* 35(2):90, 2010.

Lachman VD: Ethical issues in the disruptive behaviors of incivility, bullying, and horizontal/lateral violence, *Medsurg Nurs* 23(1):56, 2014.

Mahon NM, Nicotera AM: Nursing and conflict communication: avoidance as a preferred strategy, *Nurs Adm Q* 35(2):152, 2011.

Mason DJ, et al: *Policy & politics in nursing and health care*, ed 6, Philadelphia, 2012, Saunders.

National CNS Competency Task Force, Core Competencies, National Association of Clinical Nurse Specialists: *Core competencies*, Philadelphia, 2010, The Association.

National Quality Forum (NQF): *Safe practices for better healthcare—2010 update: a consensus report*, Washington, DC, 2010, NQF. http://www.qualityforum.org/Publications/2010/04/

Safe_Practices_for_Better_Healthcare_–_2010_Update.aspx. Accessed May 2015.

Nightingale F: *Notes on nursing: what it is and what it is not*, London, 1860, Harrison and Sons.

Robert Wood Johnson Foundation (RWJF). *Future of nursing: campaign for action is chalking up successes that will improve patient care*, 2014a, http://www.rwjf.org/en/library/articles-and-news/2014/06/campaign-for-action-is-chalking-up-successes-that-will-improve-p.html. Accessed May 2015.

Robert Wood Johnson Foundation (RWJF). *More newly licensed nurse practitioners choosing to work in primary care, federal study finds*, RWJF, Human Capital Blog, June 10, 2014b, http://www.rwjf.org/en/culture-of-health/2014/06/more_newly_licensed.html. Accessed May 2015.

Tanner CA, Bellack JP: Our faculty for the future, *J Nurs Educ* 49(3):123, 2010.

US Census Bureau, Population Division: *2014 National population projections*, 2014, http://www.census.gov/population/projections/data/national/2014.html. Accessed May 2015.

RESEARCH REFERENCES

Barnsteiner J, et al: Diffusing QSEN competencies across schools of nursing: The AACN/RWIF faculty development institutes, *J Prof Nurs* 29:68, 2013.

Barton AJ, et al: A national Delphi to determine developmental progression of quality and safety competencies in nursing education, *Nurs Outlook* 57(6):313, 2009.

Didion J, et al: Academic/clinical partnership and collaboration in quality, safety, and education for nurse education, *J Prof Nurs* 29:88, 2013.

Emrich IA, et al: Clinical ethics and patient advocacy: the power of communication in health care, *HEC Forum* 26:111, 2013.

Headrick LA, et al: Results of an effort to integrate quality and safety into nursing school curricula and foster joint learning, *Health Aff* 31(2):2669, 2012.

Lyndon A, et al: Effective physician-nurse communication: a patient safety essential for labor and delivery, *Am J Obstet Gynecol* 205(2):91, 2011.

Miaskowski C, Aouizerat BE: Biomarkers: symptoms, survivorship, and quality of life, *Semin Oncol Nurs* 28(2):129, 2012.

Potter PA, et al: Compassion fatigue and burnout: prevalence among oncology nurses, *Clin J Oncol Nurs* 14(5):E56, 2010.

Potter PA, et al: Developing a systemic program for compassion fatigue, *Nurs Adm Q* 37(4):326, 2013a.

Potter PA, et al: Evaluation of a compassion fatigue resilience program for oncology nurses, *Oncol Nurs Forum* 40(2):180, 2013b.

Robinson FP, et al: Perceptions of effective and ineffective nurse-physician communication in hospitals, *Nurs Forum* 45(3):206, 2010.

Slatten LA, et al: Compassion fatigue and burnout: what managers should know, *Health Care Manag (Frederick)* 30(4):325, 2011.

Wilson F, et al: Autonomy and choice in palliative care: time for a new model?, *J Adv Nurs* 70(5):1020, 2013.

Young J, et al: Compassion satisfaction, burnout, and secondary traumatic stress in heart and vascular nurses, *Crit Care Nurs Q* 34(3):227, 2011.

2

The Health Care Delivery System

OBJECTIVES

- Explain the structure of the United States health system.
- Compare the various methods for financing health care.
- Discuss the types of settings that provide various health care services.
- Discuss the role of nurses in different health care delivery settings.
- Explain the impact of quality and safety initiatives on delivery of health care.
- Discuss the implications that changes in the health care system have on nursing.
- Discuss opportunities for nursing within the changing health care delivery system.
- Explain the relationship between evidence-based practice and performance improvement.
- Describe the components of a quality improvement program.

KEY TERMS

Acute care, p. 18
Adult day care centers, p. 22
Assisted living, p. 21
Capitation, p. 15
Diagnosis-related groups (DRGs), p. 15
Discharge planning, p. 19
Extended care facility, p. 20
Globalization, p. 26
Home care, p. 20
Hospice, p. 22
Integrated delivery networks (IDNs), p. 17
Managed care, p. 15
Medicaid, p. 15
Medicare, p. 15
Minimum Data Set (MDS), p. 21
Nursing informatics, p. 25
Nursing-sensitive outcomes, p. 25
Patient-centered care, p. 24
Pay for performance, p. 24
Performance improvement (PI), p. 27
Primary health care, p. 17
Professional standards review organizations (PSROs), p. 15
Prospective payment system (PPS), p. 15
Quality improvement (QI), p. 27
Rehabilitation, p. 20
Resource utilization groups (RUGs), p. 15
Respite care, p. 22
Restorative care, p. 20
Skilled nursing facility, p. 20
Utilization review (UR) committees, p. 15
Vulnerable populations, p. 26
Work redesign, p. 18

MEDIA RESOURCES

http://evolve.elsevier.com/Potter/fundamentals/
- Review Questions
- Case Study with Questions
- Audio Glossary
- Content Updates

The U.S. health care system is complex and constantly changing. A broad variety of services are available from different disciplines of health professionals, but gaining access to services is often very difficult for those with limited health care insurance. Uninsured patients present a challenge to health care and nursing because they are more likely to skip or delay treatment for acute and chronic illnesses and die prematurely (Kovner and Knickman, 2011). The continuing development of new technologies and medications, which shortens length of stay (LOS), also causes health care costs to increase. Thus health care institutions are managing health care more as businesses than as service organizations. Challenges to health care leaders today include reducing health care costs while maintaining high-quality care for patients, improving access and coverage for more people, and encouraging healthy behaviors (Kovner and Knickman, 2011). Health care providers are discharging patients sooner from hospitals, resulting in more patients needing nursing homes or home care. Often families provide care for their loved ones in the home setting. As a nurse you face major challenges to prevent gaps in health care across health care settings so individuals remain healthy and well within their own homes and communities.

Nursing is a caring discipline. Values of the nursing profession are rooted in helping people to regain, maintain, or improve health; prevent illness; and find comfort and dignity. The health care system of the new millennium is less service oriented and more business oriented because of cost-saving initiatives, which often causes tension between the caring and business aspects of health care (Kovner and Knickman, 2011). The Institute of Medicine (IOM) calls for a health care delivery system that is safe, effective, patient centered, timely, efficient, and equitable (IOM, 2001). The National Priorities Partnership is a group of 52 organizations from a variety of health care disciplines that have joined together to work toward transforming health care with the aims of healthy people and healthy communities and better and affordable care (National Priorities Partnership, 2014). The group set the following national priorities:

- Work with communities to promote wide use of best practices to enable healthy living and well-being.
- Promote the most effective prevention, treatment, and intervention practices for the leading causes of mortality, starting with cardiovascular disease.
- Ensure person- and family-centered care.
- Make care safer.
- Promote effective communication and care coordination.
- Make quality care affordable for people, families, employers, and governments.

The IOM (2011) put forth a vision for a transformed health care delivery system. The health care system of the future makes quality care accessible to all populations, focuses on wellness and disease prevention, improves health outcomes, and provides compassionate care across the life span. Transformations in health care are changing the practice of nursing. Nursing continues to lead the way in change and retain values for patient care while meeting the challenges of new roles and responsibilities. These changes challenge nurses to provide evidence-based, compassionate care and continue in the role as patient advocate (Singleton, 2010). According to the IOM report (IOM, 2011), nurses need to be transformed by:

- Practicing to the full extent of their education and training.
- Achieving higher levels of education and training through an improved education system that provides seamless progression.
- Becoming full partners with physicians and other health care providers in redesigning the health care system.
- Improving data collection and information infrastructure for effective workforce planning and policy making.

HEALTH CARE REGULATION AND REFORM

Through most of the twentieth century, few incentives existed for controlling health care costs. Insurers or third-party payers paid for whatever the health care providers ordered for a patient's care and treatment. As health care costs continued to rise out of control, regulatory and competitive approaches had to control health care spending. The federal government, the biggest consumer of health care, which paid for **Medicare** and **Medicaid**, created **professional standards review organizations (PSROs)** to review the quality, quantity, and cost of hospital care. Medicare-qualified hospitals had physician-supervised **utilization review (UR) committees** to review the admissions and identify and eliminate overuse of diagnostic and treatment services ordered by physicians caring for patients on Medicare.

One of the most significant factors that influenced payment for health care was the **prospective payment system (PPS)**. Established by Congress in 1983, the PPS eliminated cost-based reimbursement. Hospitals serving patients who received Medicare benefits were no longer able to charge whatever a patient's care cost. Instead the PPS grouped inpatient hospital services for Medicare patients into **diagnosis-related groups (DRGs)**. Each group has a fixed reimbursement amount with adjustments based on case severity, rural/urban/regional costs, and teaching costs. Hospitals receive a set dollar amount for each patient based on the assigned DRG, regardless of the patient's LOS or use of services. Most health care providers (e.g., health care networks or managed care organizations) now receive capitated payments. **Capitation** means that the providers receive a fixed amount per patient or enrollee of a health care plan (Sultz and Young, 2014). Capitation aims to build a payment plan for select diagnoses or surgical procedures that consists of the best standards of care at the lowest cost.

Capitation and prospective payment influence the way health care providers deliver care in all types of settings. Many now use DRGs in the rehabilitation setting and **resource utilization groups (RUGs)** in long-term care. In all settings health care providers try to manage costs so the organizations remain profitable. For example, when patients are hospitalized for lengthy periods, hospitals have to absorb the portion of costs that are not reimbursed. This simply adds more pressure to ensure that patients are managed effectively and discharged as soon as is reasonably possible. Thus hospitals started to increase discharge planning activities, and hospital lengths of stay began to shorten. Because patients are discharged home as soon as possible, home care agencies now provide complex technological care, including mechanical ventilation and long-term parenteral nutrition.

Managed care describes health care systems in which a provider or health care system receives a predetermined capitated payment for each patient enrolled in the program. In this case the managed care organization assumes financial risk in addition to providing patient care. The focus of care of the organization shifts from individual illness care to prevention, early intervention, and outpatient care. If people stay healthy, the cost of medical care declines. Systems of managed care focus on containing or reducing costs, increasing patient satisfaction, and improving the health or functional status of individuals (Sultz and Young, 2014). Table 2-1 summarizes the most common types of health care insurance plans.

In 2011 the National Quality Forum (NQF) revised and defined a list of 29 "Never Events" that are devastating and preventable. The "Never Events" are organized in seven categories: surgical, product or device, patient protection, care management, environmental, radiological, and critical. The Joint Commission (TJC) labels "Never Events" as sentinel events and requires a root cause analysis following the event. Many states now require mandatory reporting of these events when they occur (AHRQ PSNet, 2012). In 2007 Medicare ruled that it would no longer pay for medical costs associated with these errors. In the current culture of patient safety and quality, health care organizations are implementing processes to eliminate "Never Events."

Major health care reform came in 2010 with the signing into law of the Patient Protection and Affordable Care Act (PPACA) (Public Law No. 111-148). Health care reform of this magnitude has not occurred in the United States since the 1960s when Medicare and Medicaid were signed into law. It is predicted that implementing the proposed changes with PPACA will be a lengthy process and will change the current health care system (Kovner and Knickman, 2011). The PPACA focused on the major goals of increasing access to health care services for all, reducing health care costs, and improving health care quality. Examples of key provisions in the law include (Kovner and Knickman, 2011; Sultz and Young, 2014):

- All individuals are required to have some form of health insurance by 2014 or pay a penalty through the tax code.
- Public program eligibility, including state Medicaid and Children's Health Insurance, is expanded. Primary care physician payments for Medicaid services increased to equal Medicare payments.
- States will create health insurance exchanges whereby individuals and small business owners can purchase more affordable health insurance. The exchanges will also provide individuals and small employers with consumer information to aid them in making decisions regarding alternative health insurance policies.
- Insurance regulations that prevent private insurance companies from denying insurance coverage for any reason and from charging higher premiums based on health status and gender will be implemented.

TABLE 2-1 Examples of Health Care Plans

Type	Definition	Characteristics
Managed care organization (MCO)	Provides comprehensive preventive and treatment services to a specific group of voluntarily enrolled people. Structures include a variety of models.	Focuses health maintenance, primary care. All care is provided by a primary care physician. Referral is needed for access to specialist and hospitalization. May use capitated payments.
Preferred provider organization (PPO)	Type of managed care plan that limits an enrollee's choice to a list of "preferred" hospitals, physicians, and providers. An enrollee pays more out-of-pocket expenses for using a provider not on the list.	Contractual agreement exists between a set of providers and one or more purchasers (self-insured employers or insurance plans). Comprehensive health services are at a discount to companies under contract. Focus is on health maintenance.
Medicare	A federally administrated program by the Commonwealth Fund or the Centers for Medicare and Medicaid Services (CMS); a funded national health insurance program in the United States for people 65 years and older. Part A provides basic protection for medical, surgical, and psychiatric care costs based on diagnosis-related groups (DRGs); also provides limited skilled nursing facility care, hospice, and home health care. Part B is a voluntary medical insurance; covers physician, certain other specified health professional services, and certain outpatient services. Part C is a managed care provision that provides a choice of three insurance plans. Part D is a voluntary Prescription Drug Improvement (Sultz and Young, 2014).	Payment for plan is deducted from monthly individual Social Security check. Covers services of nurse practitioners. Does not pay full cost of certain services such as skilled nursing facilities. Supplemental insurance is encouraged.
Medicaid	Federally funded, state-operated program that provides: (1) health insurance to low-income families; (2) health assistance to low-income people with long-term care (LTC) disabilities; and (3) supplemental coverage and LTC assistance to older adults and Medicare beneficiaries in nursing homes. Individual states determine eligibility and benefits.	Finances a large portion of care for poor children, their parents, pregnant women, and disabled very poor adults. Reimburses for nurse-midwifery and other advanced practice nurses (varies by state). Reimburses nursing home funding.
Private insurance	Traditional fee-for-service plan. Payment is computed after patient receives services on basis of number of services used.	Policies are typically expensive. Most policies have deductibles that patients have to meet before insurance pays.
Long-Term Care (LTC) insurance	Supplemental insurance for coverage of LTC services. Policies provide a set amount of dollars for an unlimited time or for as little as 2 years.	Very expensive. Often has a minimum waiting period for eligibility; payment for skilled nursing, intermediate, or custodial care and home care.
State Children's Health Insurance Program (SCHIP)	Federally funded, state-operated program to provide health coverage for uninsured children. Individual states determine participation eligibility and benefits.	Covers children not poor enough for Medicaid.

- A financial penalty will be assessed to employers of more than 50 employees if they do not offer health insurance coverage to employees.
- Adult children up to the age of 26, regardless of student status, are allowed to be covered under their parents' health insurance plan.

EMPHASIS ON POPULATION WELLNESS

The United States health care delivery system faces many issues such as rising costs, increased access to services, a growing population, and improved quality of health outcomes. As a result, the emphasis of the health care industry today is shifting from managing illness to managing health of a community and the environment.

The Health Services Pyramid developed by the Core Functions Project serves as a model for improving the health care of U.S. citizens (Figure 2-1). The pyramid shows that population-based health care services provide the basis for preventive services. These services include primary, secondary, and tertiary health care. Achievements in the lower tiers of the pyramid contribute to the improvement of health care delivered by the higher tiers. Health care in the United States is moving toward practices that emphasize managing health rather than managing illness. This emphasis on wellness and health of populations and the environment enhances quality of life (Stanhope and Lancaster, 2012). The premise is that in the long term health promotion reduces health care costs. A wellness perspective focuses on the health of populations and the communities in which they live rather than just on finding a cure for an individual's disease. Life expectancy for Americans is 78.7 years, which has shown a steady increase in the past century. Along with increased life expectancy, adult deaths related to coronary heart disease and stroke continue a long-term decreasing trend, and there is a decreasing trend in deaths of children since 1900 (Murphy et al., 2013). The reduction in mortality rates has been credited to advancements in sanitation and prevention of infectious diseases (e.g., water, sewage, immunization, and crowded living conditions); patient teaching (e.g., dietary habits, decrease in tobacco use, and blood pressure control); and injury prevention programs (e.g., seat belt restraints, child seats, and helmet laws).

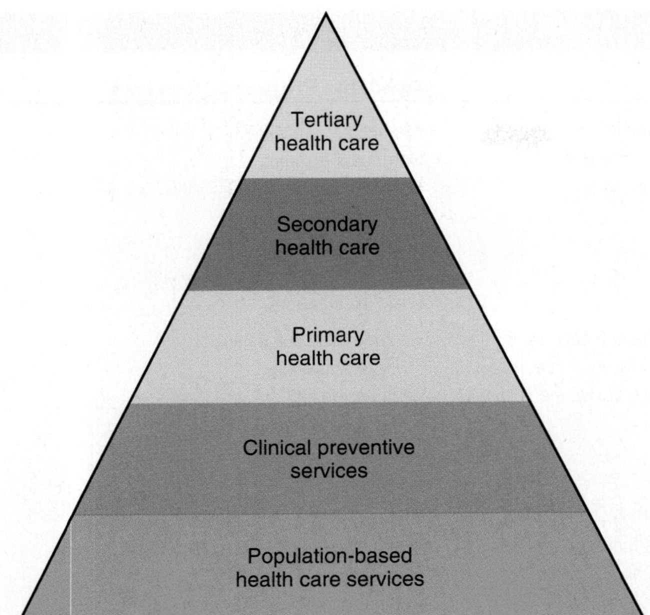

FIGURE 2-1 Health services pyramid. US Public Health Service: *The core functions project,* Washington, DC, 1994/update 2000, Office of Disease Prevention and Health Promotion. (From Stanhope M, Lancaster J: *Public health nursing: population-centered health care in the community, revised reprint,* ed 8, St Louis, 2014, Mosby.)

BOX 2-1 Examples of Health Care Services

Primary Care (Health Promotion)
- Prenatal and well-baby care
- Nutrition counseling
- Family planning
- Exercise, yoga, and mediation classes

Preventive Care
- Blood pressure and cancer screenings
- Immunizations
- Mental health counseling and crisis prevention
- Community legislation (e.g., seat belts, air bags, bike helmets, no texting while driving)

Secondary Acute Care
- Emergency care
- Acute medical-surgical care
- Radiological procedures for acute problems (e.g., x-rays, computed tomography [CT] scans)

Tertiary Care
- Intensive care
- Subacute care

Restorative Care
- Cardiovascular and pulmonary rehabilitation
- Orthopedic rehabilitation
- Sports medicine
- Spinal cord injury programs
- Home care

Continuing Care
- Assisted living
- Psychiatric and older adult day care

HEALTH CARE SETTINGS AND SERVICES

Currently the U.S. health care system has five levels of care for which health care providers offer services: disease prevention; health promotion; and primary, secondary, and tertiary health care. The health care settings within which the levels of care are provided include preventive, primary, secondary, tertiary, restorative, and continuing care settings (Box 2-1). Larger health care systems have **integrated delivery networks (IDNs)** that include a network of facilities, providers, and services organized to deliver a continuum of care to a population of patients at a capitated cost in a particular setting. An integrated system reduces duplication of services across levels or settings of care to ensure that patients receive care in the most appropriate settings.

Changes unique to each setting of care have developed because of health care reform. For example, many health care providers now place greater emphasis on wellness, directing more resources toward primary and preventive care services. Nurses are especially important as patient advocates in maintaining continuity of care throughout the levels of care. They have the opportunity to provide leadership to communities and health care systems. The ability to find strategies that better address patient needs at all levels of care is critical to improving the health care delivery system.

Health care agencies seek accreditation and certification as a way to demonstrate quality and safety in the delivery of care and to evaluate the performance of the organization based on established standards. Accreditation is earned by the entire organization; specific programs or services within an organization earn certifications (TJC, 2013). TJC accredits health care organizations across the continuum of care, including hospitals and ambulatory care, long-term care, home care, and behavioral health agencies. Other accrediting agencies have a specific focus such as the Commission on Accreditation of Rehabilitation Facilities (CARF) and the Community Health Accrediting Program (CHAP). Disease-specific certifications are available in most chronic diseases. Accreditation and certification survey processes help organizations identify problems and develop solutions to improve the safety and quality of delivered care and services.

Preventive and Primary Health Care

Primary health care focuses on improved health outcomes for an entire population. It includes primary care and health education, proper nutrition, maternal/child health care, family planning, immunizations, and control of diseases. Primary health care requires collaboration among health professionals, health care leaders, and community members. This collaboration needs to focus on improving health care equity, making health care systems person centered, developing reliable and accountable health care leaders, and promoting and protecting the health of communities (WHO, 2015). In settings in which patients receive preventive and primary care such as schools, physician's offices, occupational health clinics, community health centers, and nursing centers, health promotion is a major theme (Table 2-2). Health promotion programs lower the overall costs of health care by reducing the incidence of disease, minimizing complications, and thus reducing the need to use more expensive health care resources. In contrast, preventive care is more disease oriented and focused on reducing and controlling risk factors for disease through activities such as immunization and occupational health programs. Chapter 3 provides a more comprehensive discussion of primary health care in the community.

TABLE 2-2 Preventive and Primary Care Services

Type of Service	Purpose	Available Programs/Services
School health	These are comprehensive programs that include health promotion principles throughout a school curriculum. They emphasize program management, interdisciplinary collaboration, and community health principles.	Positive life skills Nutritional planning Health screening Physical fitness Counseling Communicable disease prevention Crisis intervention
Occupational health	This is a comprehensive program designed for health promotion and accident or illness prevention in the workplace setting. It aims to increase worker productivity, decrease absenteeism, and reduce use of expensive medical care	Environmental surveillance Physical assessment Health screening Health education Communicable disease control Counseling
Physicians' offices	They provide primary health care (diagnosis and treatment). Many focus on health promotion practices. Nurse practitioners often partner with a physician in managing a patient population (e.g., diabetes, arthritis).	Routine physical examination Health screening Diagnostics Treatment of acute and chronic ailments
Nurse-managed clinics	These clinics provide nursing services with a focus on health promotion and education, chronic disease assessment management, and support for self-care and caregivers.	Day care Health risk appraisal Wellness counseling Employment readiness Acute and chronic care management
Block and parish nursing	Nurses living within a neighborhood provide services to older patients or those unable to leave their homes. It fills in gaps not available in traditional health care system.	Running errands Transportation Respite care Homemaker aides Spiritual health
Community health centers	These are outpatient clinics that provide primary care to a specific patient population (e.g., well-baby, mental health, diabetes) that lives in a specific community. They are often associated with a hospital, medical school, church, or other community organization.	Physical assessment Health screening Disease management Health education Counseling

Secondary and Tertiary Care

In secondary and tertiary care the diagnosis and treatment of illnesses are traditionally the most common services. With managed care, these services are now delivered in primary care settings. For example, many surgeons now perform simple surgeries in office surgical suites. Disease management is the most common and expensive service of the health care delivery system. Chronic illness causes disability, decreased quality of life, and increased health care costs (CDC, 2015). Often patients with chronic illnesses need care from a specialist, leading to increased health care costs.

People who do not have health care insurance often wait longer before presenting for treatment; thus they are usually sicker and need more health care. As a result, secondary and tertiary care (also called acute care) are more costly. Young adults turning 19 years of age are in danger of being uninsured because of the inability to attend college, instability with financial independence, and challenges finding employment with health care benefits (Kirzinger et al., 2013). With the passage of the PPACA in 2010, the number of young adults with either private health insurance coverage or employer-sponsored health insurance has increased (Kirzinger et al., 2013). People in this age-group are also less likely to see a doctor on a regular basis and follow up on a problem if they do not have health insurance. With the arrival of more advanced technology and managed care, physicians now perform simple surgeries in office surgical suites instead of in the hospital. Cost to the patient is lower in the office because the general overhead cost of the facility is lower.

Hospitals. Hospital emergency departments, urgent care centers, critical care units, and inpatient medical-surgical units provide secondary and tertiary levels of care. Quality, safe care is the focus of most acute care organizations, and patient satisfaction with the health care services provided is important. Patient satisfaction becomes a priority in a busy, stressful location such as the inpatient nursing unit. Patients expect to receive courteous and respectful treatment, and they want to be involved in daily care decisions. As a nurse you play a key role in bringing respect and dignity to a patient. Acute care nurses need to be responsive to learning patient needs and expectations early to form effective partnerships that ultimately enhance the level of nursing care given.

Because of managed care, the number of days patients can expect to be hospitalized is limited based on their DRGs on admission. Therefore you need to use resources efficiently to help patients successfully recover and return home. To contain costs, many hospitals have redesigned nursing units. Because of work redesign, more services are available on nursing units, thus minimizing the need to transfer and transport patients across multiple diagnostic and treatment areas.

Hospitalized patients are acutely ill and need comprehensive and specialized tertiary health care. The services provided by hospitals vary considerably. Some small rural hospitals offer only limited emergency and diagnostic services and general inpatient services. In comparison, large urban medical centers offer comprehensive, up-to-date diagnostic services, trauma and emergency care, surgical intervention, intensive care units (ICUs), inpatient services, and rehabilitation facilities. Larger hospitals also offer professional staff from a variety of specialties such as social service, respiratory therapy, physical and occupational therapy, and speech therapy. The focus in hospitals is to provide the highest quality of care possible so patients are discharged early but safely to home or another health care facility that will adequately manage remaining health care needs.

Discharge planning begins the moment a patient is admitted to a health care facility. You play an important role in **discharge planning** in the hospital, where continuity of care is important. To achieve continuity of care, use critical thinking skills and apply the nursing process (see Unit III). To anticipate and identify a patient's needs, work with all members of the interdisciplinary health care team. They take the lead to develop a plan of care that moves a patient from the hospital to another level of health care such as the patient's home or a nursing home. Discharge planning is a centralized, coordinated, interdisciplinary process that ensures that a patient has a plan for continuing care after leaving a health care agency.

Because patients leave hospitals as soon as their physical conditions allow, they often have continuing health care needs when they go home or to another facility. For example, a surgical patient requires wound care at home after surgery. A patient who has had a stroke requires ambulation training. Patients and families worry about how they will care for unmet needs and manage over the long term. Help by anticipating and identifying patients' continuing needs before the actual time of discharge and by coordinating health care team members in achieving an appropriate discharge plan.

Some patients are more in need of discharge planning because of the risks they present (e.g., patients with limited financial resources, limited family support, and long-term disabilities or chronic illness). However, any patient who is being discharged from a health care facility with remaining functional limitations or who has to follow certain restrictions or therapies for recovery needs discharge planning. All caregivers who care for a patient with a specific health problem participate in discharge planning. The process is truly interdisciplinary. For example, patients with diabetes visiting a diabetes management center require the group effort of a diabetes nurse educator, dietitian, and physician to ensure that they return home with the right information to manage their condition. A patient who has experienced a stroke will not be discharged from a hospital until the team has established plans with physical and occupational therapists to begin a program of rehabilitation.

Effective discharge planning often requires referrals to various health care disciplines. In many agencies a health care provider's order is necessary for a referral, especially when planning specific therapies (e.g., physical therapy). It is best to have patients and families participate in referral processes so they are involved early in any necessary decision making. Some tips on making the referral process successful include the following:

- Make a referral as soon as possible.
- Provide the care provider receiving the referral as much information about the patient as possible. This avoids duplication of effort and exclusion of important information.
- Involve the patient and family caregiver in the referral process, including selecting the necessary referral. Explain the service that the referral will provide, the reason for the referral, and what to expect from the services of the referral.
- Determine what the care provider receiving the referral recommends for the patient's care and include this in the treatment plan as soon as possible.

Provide information about community resources available to improve the long-term outcomes of patients with limitations. Discharge planning depends on comprehensive patient and family education (see Chapter 25). Patients and family caregivers need to know what to do when they get home, how to do it, and for what to observe when problems develop. Patients require the following instruction before they leave health care facilities:

- Safe and effective administration of medications
- Safe and proper use of medical equipment
- Instruction in potential food-drug interactions and counseling on nutrition and modified diets
- Rehabilitation techniques to support adaptation to and/or functional independence in the environment
- Access to available and appropriate community resources
- When and how to obtain further treatment
- The patient's and family's responsibilities in the patient's ongoing health care needs and the knowledge and skills needed to carry out those responsibilities
- When to notify their health care provider for changes in functioning or new symptoms

Intensive Care. An ICU or critical care unit is a hospital unit in which patients receive close monitoring and intensive medical care. ICUs have advanced technologies such as computerized cardiac monitors and mechanical ventilators. Although many of these devices are on regular nursing units, patients hospitalized within ICUs are monitored and maintained on multiple devices. Nursing and medical staff have special knowledge about critical care principles and techniques. An ICU is the most expensive health care delivery site because each nurse usually cares for only one or two patients at a time and because of all the treatments and procedures the patients in the ICU require.

Psychiatric Facilities. Patients who suffer emotional and behavioral problems such as depression, violent behavior, and eating disorders often require special counseling and treatment in psychiatric facilities. Located in hospitals, independent outpatient clinics, or private mental health hospitals, psychiatric facilities offer inpatient and outpatient services, depending on the seriousness of the problem. Patients enter these facilities voluntarily or involuntarily. Hospitalization involves relatively short stays with the purpose of stabilizing patients before transfer to outpatient treatment centers. Patients with psychiatric problems receive a comprehensive interdisciplinary treatment plan that involves them and their families. Medicine, nursing, social work, and activity therapy work together to develop a plan of care that enables patients to return to functional states within the community. At discharge from inpatient facilities, patients usually receive a referral for follow-up care at clinics or with counselors.

Rural Hospitals. Access to health care in rural areas has been a serious problem. Most rural hospitals have experienced a severe shortage of primary care providers. Many have closed because of economic failure. In 1989 the Omnibus Budget Reconciliation Act (OBRA) directed the U.S. Department of Health and Human Services (USDHHS) to create a new health care organization, the rural primary care hospital (RPCH). The Balanced Budget Act of 1997 changed the designation for rural hospitals to Critical Access Hospital (CAH) if certain criteria were met (DHHS CMS, 2012). A CAH is located in a rural area and provides 24-hour emergency care, with no more than 25 inpatient beds for providing temporary care for 96 hours or less to acutely ill or injured patients needing stabilization before transfer to a larger, better-equipped facility. Basic radiological and laboratory services are also available. Physicians, nurse practitioners, or physician assistants staff a CAH.

With health care reform, more big-city health care systems are branching out and establishing connections or merging with rural hospitals. The rural hospitals provide a referral base to the larger tertiary care medical centers. With the development of advanced technologies such as telemedicine, rural hospitals have increased access to specialist consultations. Nurses who work in rural hospitals or clinics require competence in physical assessment, clinical decision making, and emergency care. Having a culture of evidence-based practice (EBP) is important in rural hospitals so nurses practice using the best evidence to achieve optimal patient outcomes and an environment of quality and safety (Newhouse and Morlock, 2011). Advanced practice nurses (e.g., nurse practitioners and clinical nurse specialists) use medical protocols and establish collaborative agreements with staff physicians to ensure that they provide safe, evidence-based care.

Restorative Care

Patients recovering from an acute or chronic illness or disability often require additional services to return to their previous level of function or reach a new level of function limited by their illness or disability. The goals of restorative care are to help individuals regain maximal functional status and enhance quality of life through promotion of independence and self-care. With the emphasis on early discharge from hospitals, patients usually require some level of restorative care. For example, some patients require ongoing wound care and activity and exercise management until they have recovered enough following surgery to independently resume normal activities of daily living.

The intensity of care has increased in restorative care settings because patients leave hospitals earlier. The restorative health care team is an interdisciplinary group of health professionals and includes a patient and family or significant others. In restorative settings nurses recognize that success depends on effective and early collaboration with patients and their families. Patients and families require a clear understanding of goals for physical recovery, the rationale for any physical limitations, and the purpose and potential risks associated with therapies. Patients and families are more likely to follow treatment plans and achieve optimal functioning when they are involved in restorative care.

Home Care. Home care is the provision of medically related professional and paraprofessional services and equipment to patients and families in their homes for health maintenance, education, illness prevention, diagnosis and treatment of disease, palliation, and rehabilitation. Nursing is one service that most patients use in home care. However, home care also includes medical and social services; physical, occupational, speech, and respiratory therapy; and nutritional therapy. A home care service also coordinates the access to and delivery of home health equipment, or durable medical equipment, which is a medical product adapted for home use.

Health promotion and education are traditionally the primary objectives of home care, yet at present most patients receive home care because they need nursing care. Examples of home nursing care include monitoring vital signs; assessment; administering parenteral or enteral nutrition, medications, and intravenous (IV) or blood therapy; and wound or respiratory care. The focus is on patient and family independence. Nurses address recovery and stabilization of illness in the home and identify problems related to lifestyle, safety, environment, family dynamics, and health care practices.

Approved home care agencies usually receive reimbursement for services from the government (such as Medicare and Medicaid in the United States), private insurance, and private pay. The government has strict regulations that govern reimbursement for home care services. An agency cannot simply charge whatever it wants for a service and expect to receive full reimbursement. Government programs set the cost of reimbursement for most professional services.

Nurses in home care provide individualized care. They have a caseload and help patients adapt to permanent or temporary physical limitations so they are able to assume a more normal daily home routine. Home care requires a strong knowledge base in many areas such as family dynamics (see Chapter 10), cultural practices (see Chapter 9), spiritual values (see Chapter 36), and communication principles (see Chapter 24).

Rehabilitation. Rehabilitation restores a person to the fullest physical, mental, social, vocational, and economic potential possible. Patients require rehabilitation after a physical or mental illness, injury, or chemical addiction. Specialized rehabilitation services such as cardiovascular, neurological, musculoskeletal, pulmonary, and mental health rehabilitation programs help patients and families adjust to necessary changes in lifestyle and learn to function with the limitations of their disease. Drug rehabilitation centers help patients become free from drug dependence and return to the community.

Rehabilitation services include physical, occupational, and speech therapy and social services. Ideally rehabilitation begins the moment a patient enters a health care setting for treatment. For example, some orthopedic programs now have patients perform physical therapy exercises before major joint repair to enhance their recovery after surgery. Initially rehabilitation usually focuses on preventing complications related to an illness or injury. As the condition stabilizes, it helps to maximize a patient's functioning and level of independence.

Rehabilitation occurs in many health care settings, including special rehabilitation agencies, outpatient settings, and the home. Frequently patients needing long-term rehabilitation (e.g., patients who have had strokes and spinal cord injuries) have severe disabilities affecting their ability to carry out the activities of daily living. When rehabilitation services occur in outpatient settings, patients receive treatment at specified times during the week but live at home the rest of the time. Health care providers use rehabilitation strategies specific to the home environment. Nurses and other members of the health care team visit homes and help patients and families learn to adapt to illness or injury.

Extended Care Facilities. An extended care facility provides intermediate medical, nursing, or custodial care for patients recovering from acute illness or those with chronic illnesses or disabilities. Extended care facilities include intermediate care and skilled nursing facilities. Some include long-term care and assisted-living facilities. At one point extended care facilities primarily cared for older adults. However, because hospitals discharge their patients sooner, there is a greater need for intermediate care settings for patients of all ages. For example, health care providers transfer a young patient who has experienced a traumatic brain injury resulting from a car accident to an extended care facility for rehabilitative or supportive care until discharge to the home becomes a safe option.

An intermediate care or skilled nursing facility offers skilled care from a licensed nursing staff. This often includes administration of IV fluids, wound care, long-term ventilator management, and physical rehabilitation. Patients receive extensive supportive care until they are able to move back into the community or into residential care. Extended care facilities provide around-the-clock nursing coverage. Nurses who work in a skilled nursing facility need nursing expertise similar to that of nurses working in acute care inpatient settings, along with a background in gerontological nursing principles (see Chapter 14).

Continuing Care

Continuing care describes a variety of health, personal, and social services provided over a prolonged period. These services are for people who are disabled, who were never functionally independent, or who suffer a terminal disease. The need for continuing health care services is growing in the United States. People are living longer, and many of those with continuing health care needs have no immediate family members to care for them. A decline in the number of children families choose to have, the aging of care providers, and the increasing rates of divorce and remarriage complicate this problem. Continuing care is available within institutional settings (e.g., nursing centers or nursing homes, group homes, and retirement communities), communities (e.g., adult day care and senior centers), or the home (e.g., home care, home-delivered meals, and hospice) (Meiner, 2011).

Nursing Centers or Facilities. The language of long-term care is confusing and constantly changing. The nursing home has been the dominant setting for long-term care (Meiner, 2011). With the 1987 OBRA, *nursing facility* became the term for nursing homes and other facilities that provided long-term care. Now *nursing center* is the most appropriate term. A nursing center typically provides 24-hour intermediate and custodial care such as nursing, rehabilitation, dietary, recreational, social, and religious services for residents of any age with chronic or debilitating illnesses. In some cases patients stay in nursing centers for room, food, and laundry services only. The majority of people living in nursing centers are older adults. A nursing center is a resident's temporary or permanent home, with surroundings made as homelike as possible (Sorrentino and Remmert, 2012). The philosophy of care is to provide a planned, systematic, and interdisciplinary approach to nursing care to help residents reach and maintain their highest level of function.

The nursing center industry is one of the most highly regulated industries in the United States. These regulations raised the standard of services that nursing centers are required to provide (Box 2-2). One regulatory area that deserves special mention is that of resident rights. Nursing facilities have to recognize residents as active participants and decision makers in their care and life in institutional settings (Meiner, 2011). This also means that family members are active partners in planning residents' care.

Interdisciplinary functional assessment of residents is the cornerstone of clinical practice within nursing centers (Meiner, 2011). Government regulations require that staff comprehensively assess each resident and make care planning decisions within a prescribed period. A resident's functional ability (e.g., ability to perform activities of daily living) and long-term physical and psychosocial well-being are the focus. Staff must complete the Resident Assessment Instrument (RAI) on all residents. The RAI consists of the **Minimum Data Set (MDS)** (Box 2-3), Resident Assessment Protocols, and utilization guidelines of each state. The collected information provides a national database for nursing facilities so policy makers will better understand the health care needs of the long-term care population. The MDS is a rich resource for nurses in determining the best interventions to support the health care needs of this growing population.

Assisted Living. Assisted living is one of the fastest growing industries within the United States. There are approximately 31,000 assisted-living facilities that house more than 971,000 people in the United States (NCAL, 2014). **Assisted living** offers an attractive long-term care setting with an environment more like home and greater resident autonomy. Residents require some assistance with activities of daily living but remain relatively independent within a partially protective setting. A group of residents live together, but each resident has his or her own room and shares dining and social activity areas. Usually people keep all of their personal possessions in their residences. Facilities range from hotel-like buildings with hundreds of units to modest group homes that house a handful of seniors. Assisted living provides independence, security, and privacy all at the same time (Touhy and Jett, 2012). These facilities promote physical and psychosocial health (Figure 2-2). Services in an assisted-living facility include laundry, assistance with meals and personal care, 24-hour oversight, and housekeeping (NCAL, 2014). Some facilities provide assistance with medication administration. Nursing care services are not always directly available, although home care nurses can visit patients in

BOX 2-2 Major Regulatory Requirements Defined by the 1987 Omnibus Budget Reconciliation Act

- Resident rights
- Admission, transfer, and discharge rights
- Resident behavior and facility practices
- Quality of life
- Resident assessment
- Quality of care
- Nursing services
- Dietary services
- Physician services
- Specialized rehabilitative services
- Dental services
- Pharmacy services
- Infection control
- Physical environment
- Administration

From Health Care Financing Administration, Department of Health and Human Services: *Requirements for states and long-term care facilities,* 42 CFR 483 Subpart B (483.1-75), 2014, http://www.gpo.gov/fdsys/pkg/CFR-2011-title42-vol5/pdf/CFR-2011-title42-vol5-part483.pdf. Accessed July 9, 2015.

BOX 2-3 Minimum Data Set and Examples of Resident Assessment Protocols

Minimum Data Set

- Resident's background
- Cognitive, communication/hearing, and vision patterns
- Physical functioning and structural problems
- Mood, behavior, and activity patterns
- Psychosocial well-being
- Bowel and bladder continence
- Health conditions
- Disease diagnoses
- Oral/nutritional and dental status
- Skin condition
- Medication use
- Special treatments and procedures

Resident Assessment Protocols (Examples)

- Delirium
- Falls
- Pressure ulcers
- Psychotropic drug use

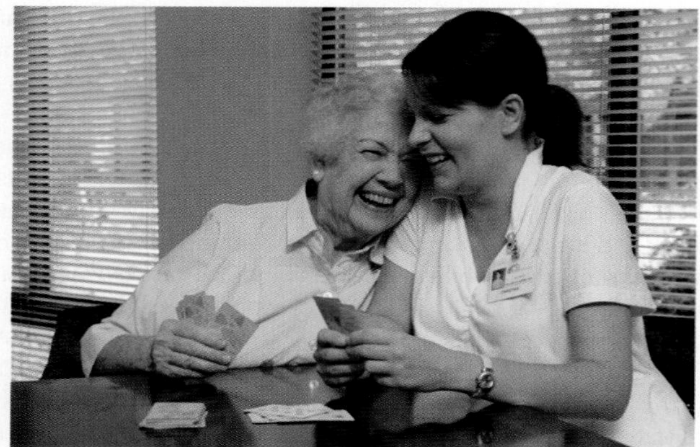

FIGURE 2-2 Providing nursing services in assisted-living facilities promotes physical and psychosocial health.

assisted-living facilities. Unfortunately most residents of assisted-living facilities pay privately. The national median monthly fee is $3500 for a private unit (NCAL, 2014). With no government fee caps and little regulation, assisted living is not always an option for individuals with limited financial resources.

Respite Care. The need to care for family members within the home creates great physical and emotional problems for family caregivers, especially if the people for whom they care have either physical or cognitive limitations. A family caregiver not only has the responsibility for providing care to a loved one, but usually needs to maintain a full-time job, raise a family, and manage the routines of daily living as well. Respite care is a service that provides short-term relief or "time off" for people providing home care to an individual who is ill, disabled, or frail (Meiner, 2011). Respite care is offered in the home, a day care setting, or a health care institution that provides overnight care. The family caregiver is able to leave the home for errands or some social time while a responsible person stays in the home to care for the loved one. There are few formal respite care programs in the United States because of cost. Currently Medicare does not cover respite care, and Medicaid has strict requirements for services and eligibility (Sultz and Young, 2014).

Adult Day Care Centers. Adult day care centers provide a variety of health and social services to specific patient populations who live alone or with family in the community. Services offered during the day allow family members to maintain their lifestyles and employment and still provide home care for their relatives (Meiner, 2011). Day care centers are associated with a hospital or nursing home or exist as independent centers. Frequently the patients need continuous health care services (e.g., physical therapy or counseling) while their families or support people work. The centers usually operate 5 days per week during typical business hours and usually charge on a daily basis. Adult day care centers allow patients to retain more independence by living at home, thus potentially reducing the costs of health care by avoiding or delaying an older adult's admission to a nursing center. Nurses working in day care centers provide continuity between care delivered in the home and the center. For example, nurses ensure that patients continue to take prescribed medication and administer specific treatments. Knowledge of community needs and resources is essential in providing adequate patient support (Touhy and Jett, 2012).

Hospice. A hospice is a system of family-centered care that allows patients to live with comfort, independence, and dignity while easing the pains of terminal illness. The focus of hospice care is palliative care, not curative treatment (see Chapters 37 and 44). Hospice care can be provided in the patient's home, an inpatient hospice unit or a free-standing hospice home. The interdisciplinary team in the hospice works continuously with a patient's health care provider to develop and maintain a patient-directed individualized plan of care. Many hospice programs provide respite care, which is important in maintaining the health of the primary caregiver and family.

Care Coordination

A problem that many patients face in today's complex health care delivery system is lack of coordination of care and services. Health care reform has stimulated the development of two models focused on coordinating medical care for patients and families. The first, accountable care organizations (ACOs) were developed to coordinate medical care by primary care and specialty physicians, hospitals, and other health care providers, with the goal of providing high-quality coordinated care (Colpas, 2013). An ACO strives to ensure that patients receive the right care at the right time, without duplication of services or incidence of medical errors (CMS, 2012). In an ACO, all health care providers are accountable for the quality and cost of care delivered to patients. Nurses are a key part of the ACO, acting as leaders and care coordinators (Amara et al., 2013).

The second model of care developed to improve coordination of care is the patient-centered medical home (PCMH). The goal of a PCMH is to make care for patients more efficient, effective, continuous, comprehensive, patient centered, and coordinated (Kovner and Knickman, 2011; NCQA, 2014). The PCMH uses technology, teamwork, and effective communication with patients to make care culturally sensitive and accessible, gather clinical data, promote patient participation in decision-making, and monitor patient outcomes (NCQA, 2014). The primary care health provider functions as the "hub" of the PCMH (Sultz and Young, 2014). Reports indicate that patients in a PCMH have increased access to care and that the PCMH helps to decrease disparities for lower-income patients (NCQA, 2014).

ISSUES AND CHANGES IN HEALTH CARE DELIVERY

The climate in health care today influences both health care professionals and consumers. Because those who provide patient care are the most qualified to make changes in the health care delivery system, you need to participate fully and effectively within all aspects of health care. As you face issues of how to maintain health care quality while reducing costs, you need to acquire the knowledge, skills, and values necessary to practice competently and effectively. It is also more important than ever to collaborate with other health care professionals to design new approaches for patient care delivery.

Nursing Shortage

There are more than 3.1 million nurses in the United States, making nursing the largest health care profession in the country (American Association of Colleges of Nursing [AACN], 2011). Although nearly 57% of the nurses work in medical-surgical hospitals, they are involved in delivering health care at all levels, including primary and preventive care (AACN, 2011). In spite of the large number of practicing nurses, a critical shortage of nurses is projected in the United States. It is expected that this shortage will worsen with increased need for health care services by the aging baby-boomer generation (AACN, 2014). The U.S. Department of Labor (2013) lists nursing as one of the top job growth professions through 2022, predicting that by 2022 there will be 1.05 million job openings for nurses. The age of the nursing workforce is increasing, with over 55% of the workforce over the age of 50 years (AACN, 2014). One factor contributing to the shortage is the slow growth in nursing school enrollments, often because of nursing faculty shortages, space limitations, and clinical site availability (AACN, 2014).

Competency

The Pew Health Professions Commission, a national and interdisciplinary group of health care leaders, recommended 21 competencies for health care professionals in the twenty-first century (Pew Health Professions Commission, 1998). The competencies emphasize the importance of public service, caring for the health of communities, and developing ethically responsible behaviors. In addressing the continued challenge facing the health care system, the IOM (2001) identified five interrelated competencies that are essential for all health care workers in the twenty-first century (Box 2-4). Shifting the emphasis on prevention and management places increased importance on the competencies of care management and coordination, patient education, public health, and transitional care (IOM, 2011). The IOM also identified 10 important rules of performance for a health care system to follow to better meet patient needs (Box 2-5) (IOM, 2003).

The health care practitioner competencies are an excellent tool for measuring how well a nurse practices nursing and serve as a guide for the development of a professional nursing career. A consumer of health care expects that the standards of nursing care and practice in any health care setting are appropriate, safe, and effective. Health care organizations ensure quality care by establishing policies, procedures, and protocols that are evidence based and follow national accrediting standards. Your responsibility is to follow policies and procedures and know the most current practice standards. Ongoing competency is your responsibility. You are also responsible for obtaining necessary continuing education, following an established code of ethics, and earning certifications in specialty areas.

BOX 2-4 Institute of Medicine Competencies for the Twenty-First Century

Provide Patient-Centered Care
- Recognize and respect differences in patients' values, preferences, and needs.
- Relieve pain and suffering.
- Coordinate continuous care.
- Effectively communicate with and educate patients.
- Share decision making and management.
- Advocate for disease prevention and health promotion.

Work in Interdisciplinary Teams
- Cooperate, collaborate, and communicate.
- Integrate care to ensure that it is continuous and reliable.

Use Evidence-Based Practice
- Integrate best research with clinical practice and patient values.
- Participate in research activities as possible.

Apply Quality Improvement
- Identify errors and hazards in care.
- Practice using basic safety design principles.
- Measure quality in relation to structure, process, and outcomes.
- Design and test interventions to change processes.

Use Informatics
- Use information technology to communicate, manage knowledge, reduce error, and support decision-making.

Adapted from Institute of Medicine (IOM): *Crossing the quality chasm: a new health system for the 21st century,* Washington DC, 2001, National Academies Press; and Institute of Medicine: *Health professions education: a bridge to quality,* Washington, DC, 2003, National Academies Press.

Quality and Safety in Health Care

Nursing plays an important role in quality and safety in health care (Box 2-6). Quality health care is the "degree to which health services for individuals and populations increase the likelihood of desired health outcomes and are consistent with current professional knowledge" (IOM, 2001). Safety is a critical part of quality health care. The

BOX 2-5 Ten Rules of Performance in a Redesigned Health Care System

1. Care is based on continuous healing relationships.
2. Care is individualized based on patient needs and values.
3. The patient is the source of control, participating in shared decision making.
4. Knowledge is shared, and information flows freely.
5. Decision making is evidence based, with care based on the best available scientific knowledge.
6. Safety is a system property and focused on reducing errors.
7. Transparency is necessary through sharing information with patients and families.
8. Patient needs are anticipated through planning.
9. Waste is continuously decreased.
10. Cooperation and communication among clinicians are priorities.

Adapted from Institute of Medicine (IOM): *Crossing the quality chasm: a new health system for the 21st century,* Washington DC, 2001, National Academies Press; and Institute of Medicine: *Health professions education: a bridge to quality,* Washington, DC, 2003, National Academies Press.

BOX 2-6 EVIDENCE-BASED PRACTICE

End-of-Shift Reporting Practices and Patient Satisfaction

PICO Question: Does the practice of bedside shift-to-shift report versus traditional report improve patient satisfaction in hospitalized adults?

Evidence Summary

Shift-to-shift report is an important nursing activity that allows nurses to share information about patients so nursing care can be delivered safely and competently. Historically shift-to-shift report occurred at the nurses' station or in a conference room and did not include patients (Radtke, 2013). In efforts to improve nursing communication, nursing report has moved to the bedside and includes the patient. Bedside shift report or hand-off allows patients to receive information about their care and ask questions (Dempsey et al., 2014). Patient satisfaction with nurse-patient communication is a key factor in patient satisfaction surveys. Bedside shift report is recognized by patients as an activity that enhances nurse-patient communication and involves the patient in decision making related to his or her care (Cairns et al., 2013; Dempsey et al., 2014; Radtke, 2013). Improvement of nurse-patient communication has a direct effect on improving patient satisfaction (Dempsey et al., 2014).

Application to Nursing Practice
- Use a standardized report to ensure that all pertinent patient information is communicated to the next shift nurse.
- Respond to all patient questions during bedside shift report.
- Use bedside shift report as a time to provide information to patients related to discharge (Dempsey et al., 2014).
- Encourage patients to participate in making decisions related to their care.

NQF (2014) endorsed performance measures to improve health care transparency related to safety and quality; ensure that health care is safer; ensure accountability of health care providers; and generate information to help individuals make informed health care decisions. Examples of NQF practices include hand hygiene, teamwork, training, influenza prevention, central line–associated bloodstream infection prevention, catheter-associated urinary tract infection prevention, pressure ulcer prevention, fall prevention, and medication reconciliation (NQF, 2010). Health care providers define the quality of their services by measuring health care outcomes that show how a patient's health status has changed. Examples of outcomes that are monitored are readmission rates for patients who have had surgery, functional health status of patients after discharge (e.g., ability and time frame for returning to work), and the rate of infection after surgery. You play an important role in gathering and analyzing quality outcome data.

Pay for performance programs and public reporting of hospital quality data are designed to promote quality, effective, and safe patient care by physicians and health care organizations. These programs are quality improvement strategies that reward excellence through financial incentives to motivate change to achieve measurable improvements. Nurses play an important role in helping hospitals meet measures for quality, efficiency, and patient satisfaction. You are often the health care provider who ensures that performance measures occur. Some health care organizations use balanced scorecards to report data on their key performance indicators. These scorecards are reported publicly so health care consumers can use the information when choosing health care services.

More and more health care institutions are focused on improving processes as a way to improve quality and safety. Many use strategies such as Six Sigma, Lean Six Sigma, or Value Stream Analysis. Six Sigma is a data-driven approach to process improvement that reduces variation in process. For example, a nursing unit sets up a project to collect data on the process of administering the first dose of an ordered chemotherapy. The audit reveals delays in getting the drug from the pharmacy to the nursing unit. Using Six Sigma, the collected data are analyzed, and unnecessary steps in the process are identified. On the basis of this analysis the process is streamlined to decrease time from ordering to administration. Lean Six Sigma and value stream analysis are two other methods that focus on improvement of processes through studying each step of a process to determine if the step adds value and reduces the time, costs, and resources of the health care organization (Carey, 2010). The aim of both is to eliminate unnecessary, non–value-added costly steps to reduce waste.

Health plans throughout the United States rely on the Healthcare Effectiveness Data and Information Set (HEDIS) as a quality measure. The National Committee for Quality Assurance (NCQA) created HEDIS to collect various data to measure the quality of care and services provided by different health plans. It is the database of choice for the Centers for Medicare and Medicaid Services (CMS). HEDIS compares how well health plans perform on measures across eight domains of care in the key areas of quality and effectiveness of care, access to care, and patient satisfaction with the health plan and doctors (NCQA, 2015). For accreditation purposes TJC requires health care organizations to determine how well an organization meets patient needs and expectations. Organizations are using outcomes such as patient satisfaction to redesign how they manage and deliver care in hopes of improving quality in the long term.

Patient Satisfaction. Every major health care organization measures certain aspects of patient satisfaction. The Hospital Consumer of Assessment of Healthcare Providers and Systems (HCAHPS) is a standardized survey developed to measure patient perceptions of their hospital experience (HCAHPS, 2013). HCAHPS was developed by the CMS and the Agency for Healthcare Research and Quality (AHRQ) as a way for hospitals to collect and report data publicly for comparison purposes. The survey is administered to a randomly selected sample of adults who were discharged from a hospital between 48 hours and 6 weeks ago. The telephone survey asks patients questions about communication with nurses and physicians, responsiveness of hospital staff, pain management, communication about medications, discharge planning, cleanliness and quietness of the environment, overall satisfaction, and willingness to recommend the hospital (HCAHPS, 2013).

Patient- and family-centered health care is an approach to health care delivery that builds relationships among the health care provider, patients, and families. This approach leads to improved outcomes and greater patient and family satisfaction (IPFCC, 2010). Identifying patient and family expectations, knowledge, preferences, cultural beliefs, and values is an important part of patient-centered care (IPFCC, 2010; QSEN, 2014). Concepts of **patient-centered care** include respect and dignity, sharing of information, participation in care and care decisions, and collaboration (IPFCC, 2010). By learning early what a patient expects with regard to information, comfort, and availability of family and friends, you are able to better plan care. Ask about a patient's expectations when a patient first enters a health care setting, while care continues, and when the patient is discharged. Research often helps explain the relationship between patient expectations and patient satisfaction. Enhancing relationships through nursing actions such as asking about patient expectations, explaining care, being caring and compassionate, involving patients in care, and providing timely care improves patient satisfaction (Jeffs et al., 2013; Reck, 2013). A Patient and Family Advisory Council is one strategy that is effective in obtaining patient and family feedback to develop patient- and family-centered care (IPFCC, 2010).

> **QSEN QSEN: BUILDING COMPETENCY IN PATIENT-CENTERED CARE** Nathan, a new graduate nurse, is assigned to care for a patient of the Muslim faith who had surgery yesterday for cancer. The patient tells Nathan that his pain is an 8 on the 0 to 10 pain scale. Identify strategies that Nathan can use to meet his patient's expectations.
>
> *Answers to QSEN Activities can be found on the Evolve website.*

Magnet Recognition Program

The American Nurses Credentialing Center (ANCC) established the Magnet Recognition Program to recognize health care organizations that achieve excellence in nursing practice (ANCC, 2014b). In the United States approximately 7% of health care organizations have achieved Magnet status (ANCC, 2013). Health care organizations that apply for Magnet status must demonstrate quality patient care, nursing excellence, and innovations in professional practice. The professional work environment needs to allow nurses to practice with a sense of empowerment and autonomy to deliver quality nursing care. The revised Magnet model has five components affected by global issues that are challenging nursing today (ANCC, 2014a). The five components are Transformational Leadership; Structural Empowerment; Exemplary Professional Practice; New Knowledge, Innovation, and Improvements; and Empirical Quality Results (Box 2-7). Institutions achieve Magnet status through an appraisal process that requires them to present evidence showing achievement of the 14 forces of magnetism. Magnet status requires nurses to collect data on specific nursing-sensitive quality indicators or outcomes and compare their outcomes against a national, state, or regional database to demonstrate quality of care.

BOX 2-7 Model and Forces of Magnetism

Magnet Model Components	Forces of Magnetism
Transformational Leadership—A vision for the future and the systems and resources to achieve the vision are created by nursing leaders.	• Quality of Nursing Leadership • Management Style
Structural Empowerment—Structures and processes provide an innovative environment in which staff are developed and empowered and professional practice flourishes.	• Organizational Structure • Personnel Policies and Programs • Community and the Health Organization • Image of Nursing • Professional Development
Exemplary Professional Practice—Strong professional practice is established, and accomplishments of the practice are demonstrated.	• Professional Models of Care • Consultation and Resources • Autonomy • Nurses As Teachers • Interdisciplinary Relationships
New Knowledge, Innovations, and Improvements—Contributions are made to the profession in the form of new models of care, use of existing knowledge, generation of new knowledge, and contributions to the science of nursing.	• Quality Improvement
Empirical Quality Outcomes—Focus is on structure and processes and demonstration of positive clinical, workforce, and patient and organizational outcomes.	• Quality of Care

Adapted from American Nurses Credentialing Center (ANCC): *Magnet program overview,* 2014b, http://www.nursecredentialing.org/Magnet/ProgramOverview. July 1, 2015.

Nursing-Sensitive Outcomes. Nursing-sensitive outcomes are patient outcomes and nursing workforce characteristics that are directly related to nursing care such as changes in patients' symptom experiences, functional status, safety, psychological distress, registered nurse (RN) job satisfaction, total nursing hours per patient day, and costs. As a nurse you assume accountability and responsibility for achieving and accepting the consequences of these outcomes. The American Nurses Association developed the National Database of Nursing Quality Indicators (NDNQI) to measure and evaluate nursing-sensitive outcomes with the purpose of improving patient safety and quality care (NDNQI, 2015) (Box 2-8). The NDNQI reports quarterly results on nursing outcomes at the nursing unit level. This provides a database for individual hospitals to compare their performance against nursing performance nationally. The evaluation of patient outcomes and nursing workforce characteristics remains important to nursing and the health care delivery system. Chapter 5 describes approaches for measuring outcomes.

Because of the importance of nursing-sensitive outcomes, AHRQ funded several nursing research studies that looked at the relationship of nurse staffing levels to adverse patient outcomes. These studies found a connection between higher levels of staffing by registered nurses (RNs) in hospitals and fewer negative patient outcomes. For example, the incidence of hospital-acquired pneumonia was highly sensitive to RN staffing levels (AHRQ/USDHHS, 2008). Adding just 30 minutes of RN staffing per patient day greatly reduced the incidence of pneumonia in patients following surgery. These studies also found that increased levels of nurse staffing positively impacted nurse satisfaction. Future studies will examine how nurses' workloads affect patient safety and how their working conditions affect medication safety. Measuring and monitoring nursing-sensitive outcomes reveal the interventions that improve patients' outcomes. Nurses and health care facilities use nursing-sensitive outcomes to improve nurses' workloads, enhance patient safety, and develop sound policies related to nursing practice and health care.

BOX 2-8 Nursing Quality Indicators

- Patient falls/falls with injuries
- Falls in ambulatory settings
- Pressure ulcers—hospital acquired, unit acquired
- Pressure ulcer incidence rates from electronic health record (EHR)
- Skill mix (registered nurse [RN], licensed practical nurse [LPN], unlicensed assistive personnel [UAP])—hospital units, emergency department (ED), perioperative and perinatal units
- Nursing hours per patient day
- Nursing care hours in ED, perioperative and perinatal units
- RN surveys on job satisfaction and practice environment scale
- RN education and certification
- Pain assessment intervention/reassessment cycle
- Hospital readmission rates
- Physical/sexual assault
- Physical restraints
- Nurse turnover
- Hospital-acquired infections of ventilator-associated pneumonia and events, central line–associated bloodstream infection, catheter-associated urinary tract infection

Data from National Database of Nursing Quality Indicators (NDNQI): *Turn nursing quality insights into improved patient experiences,* 2015. http://pressganey.com/ourSolutions/performance-and-advanced-analytics/clinical-business-performance/nursing-quality-ndnqi. Accessed July 1, 2015.

Nursing Informatics and Technological Advancements

Quality and Safety Education for Nurses (QSEN) identified informatics as a competency for nurses (QSEN, 2014). Nursing informatics "uses information and technology to communicate, manage knowledge, mitigate error, and support decision-making" (QSEN, 2014). Data are individually distinct pieces of reality. Examples of data that nurses collect and use to deliver safe patient care include a patient's blood pressure or the measurement of a patient's wound. Nurses gain or use *information* when they organize, structure, or interpret data. You use information when looking at trends in a patient's blood pressure readings over the past 24 hours or when evaluating the changes in the size of a wound over the past 3 weeks. Knowledge develops when you combine and identify relationships between different pieces of information. For example, you know that diet plays an important role in blood pressure control and wound healing. You use this knowledge to teach patients at risk for developing high blood pressure to limit their salt intake and to teach patients who have wounds the importance of eating a well-rounded diet that includes adequate protein, vitamins, and minerals. Knowledge and skills in informatics also provides the ability to access quality electronic sources of health care information to plan and coordinate patient care (QSEN, 2014). The focus of nursing informatics is not on the technology or the computer; rather, its focus is on the organization, analysis, and dissemination of information

(ANA, 2008). Chapter 26 provides a thorough review of how nursing informatics improves the way nurses provide health care through use of the electronic health record.

Advances in technology are constantly evolving. People work, play, and view the world much differently because of these advances. Technological advancements influence where and how you provide care to patients and help you deliver evidence-based care (Simpson, 2012). Sophisticated equipment such as electronic IV infusion devices, cardiac telemetry (a device that monitors a patient's heart rate wherever the patient is on a nursing unit), and computerized medication dispensation systems (see Chapter 32) are just a few examples that have changed health care. In many ways technology makes your work easier, but it does not replace nursing judgment. For example, it is your responsibility when managing a patient's IV therapy to monitor the infusion to be sure that it infuses on time and without complications. An electronic infusion device provides a constant rate of infusion, but you need to be sure that you calculate the rate correctly. The device sets off an alarm if the infusion slows, making it important for you to respond to the alarm and troubleshoot the problem. Technology does not replace your critical eye and clinical judgment. Challenges arise when technologies create inefficient delivery systems or uses or need repairs.

Telemedicine or telehealth is an emerging technology that is used to improve patient outcomes. In telemedicine electronic medical records and video teleconferencing are used by health care providers and nurses to provide care from a remote location (Mullen-Fortino et al., 2012). Vital signs and other types of physiological assessment findings are transmitted to monitor patient status (Radhakrishanan and Jacelon, 2012). Patient and family education and building of the patient's self-care abilities are other interventions used in telehealth or telemedicine. Telehealth has been found to be an effective tool in promoting self-care in patients with heart failure (Radhakrishanan and Jacelon, 2012) and improved survival rates in patients in ICUs (Mullen-Fortino et al., 2012).

Technology also affects the way we communicate with others. Personal computers, cell phones, and tablets allow us to communicate and share information or data with others in a variety of formats around the world. People expect accurate information to be delivered to them as it develops. Managing communication, information, and data is challenging in health care. Health care agencies use data to measure their outcomes and improve patient care. Accrediting bodies, insurance companies, and Medicare/Medicaid all require collection and reporting of accurate data. Furthermore, you need accurate, up-to-date information to make the best decisions about patient care. Therefore it is crucial that you help health care agencies develop an effective way to manage the collection, interpretation, and distribution of information.

Nurses need to play a role in evaluating and implementing new technological advances. You use technology and informatics to improve the effectiveness of nursing care, enhance safety, and improve patient outcomes. Most important, it is essential for you to remember that the focus of nursing care is not the machine or the technology; it is the patient. Therefore you need to constantly attend to and connect with your patients and ensure that their dignity and rights are preserved at all levels of care.

Globalization of Health Care

Globalization, the increasing connectedness of the world's economy, culture, and technology, is one of the forces reshaping the health care delivery system (Oulton, 2012). Advances in communication, primarily through the Internet, allow nurses, patients, and other health care providers to talk with others worldwide about health care issues. Improved communication, easier air travel, and easing of trade restrictions are making it easier for people to engage in "health tourism." Health tourism is the travel to other nations to seek out health care.

Many problems affect the health status of people around the world. For example, poverty is still deadlier than any disease and is the most frequent reason for death in the world today. It increases the disparities in health care services among vulnerable populations (Finkelman and Kenner, 2010). Nations and communities that experience poverty have limited access to vaccines, clean water, and standard medical care. The growth of urbanization also currently is affecting global health. As cities become more densely populated, problems with pollution, noise, crowding, inadequate water, improper waste disposal, and other environmental hazards become more apparent. Children, women, and older adults are **vulnerable populations** most threatened by urbanization. Nurses work toward improving the health of all populations (Finkelman and Kenner, 2010). Although globalization of trade, travel, and culture improves the availability of health care services, the spread of communicable diseases such as Ebola, tuberculosis, and severe acute respiratory syndrome has become more common. Finally, the results of global environmental changes and disasters affect health. Changes in climate and natural disasters threaten food supplies and often allow infectious diseases to spread more rapidly.

You need to understand how worldwide communication and globalization of health care influence nursing practice. Health care consumers demand quality and service and have become more knowledgeable. They often have searched the Internet about their health concerns and medical conditions. They also use the Internet to select their health care providers. As a result of globalization, health care providers have to make their services more accessible. Because of advances in communication, nurses and other health care providers practice across state and national boundaries. In response to the nursing shortage in the early 2000s, health care institutions recruited nurses from around the world to work in the United States. This was an effort to continue to provide quality, safe patient care. This trend is expected to continue to fill vacant nursing positions. The migration of nurses from their home countries to other countries often leaves the home country with insufficient resources to meet their own health needs (Nichols et al., 2010). The hiring of nurses from other nations has required American hospitals to better understand and work with nurses from different cultures and with different needs.

As a leader in health care, remain aware of what is happening in your community, nation, and around the world. The International Council of Nurses (ICN), based in Switzerland, represents nursing worldwide. The mission of the ICN is to represent nursing worldwide, advancing the professions and influencing health policy. It does this by enhancing the health of individuals, populations, and societies (ICN, 2015). The goals of ICN are to bring nursing together, advance the nursing profession, and influence health policy worldwide (ICN, 2015). The unique focus of nursing on caring helps nurses address the issues presented by globalization. Nurses and the nursing profession are able to help overcome these issues by working together to improve nursing education throughout the world, retaining nurses and recruiting people to be nurses, and being advocates for changes that will improve the delivery of health care. Be prepared for future health care issues. Globalization has influenced many other industries. As a leader, nursing has to take control and be proactive in developing solutions before someone outside of nursing takes control.

QUALITY AND PERFORMANCE IMPROVEMENT

Every health care organization gathers data on a number of health outcome measures as a way to gauge and improve its quality of care.

This is the focus of outcomes management. Examples of quality data include fall rates, number of medication errors, incidence of pressure ulcers, and infection rates. Health care organizations actively promote efforts for improving patient care and outcomes, particularly with respect to reducing medical errors and enhancing patient safety. Quality data are the outcome of both quality improvement (QI) and performance improvement (PI) initiatives. **Quality improvement (QI)** is an approach to the continuous study and improvement of the processes of providing health care services to meet the needs of patients and others and inform health care policy. The QI program of an institution focuses on improvement of health care–related processes (e.g., medication delivery or fall prevention). Performance measurement analyzes what an institution does and how well it does it. In **performance improvement (PI)** an organization analyzes and evaluates current performance and uses the results to develop focused improvement actions. PI activities are typically clinical projects conceived in response to identified clinical problems and designed to use research findings to improve clinical practice (Melnyk and Fineout-Overholt, 2014).

QI data inform you about how processes work within an organization and thus offer information about how to make EBP changes (see Chapter 5). When implementing a research project, EBP and QI can inform opportunities for research. Rapid-cycle improvements measured through QI often identify gaps in evidence. Similarly EBP literature reviews often identify gaps in scientific evidence. When implementing a QI project, you consider information from research and EBP that aims to improve or better understand practice, thus helping to identify worthy processes to evaluate. Here is an example of how the three processes can merge to improve nursing practice. A nursing unit has an increase in the number of patient falls over the last several months. QI data identifies the type of patients who fall, time of day of falls, and possible precipitating factors (e.g., efforts to reach the bathroom, multiple medications, or patient confusion). A thorough analysis of QI data then leads clinicians to conduct a literature review and implement the best evidence available to prevent patient falls for the type of patients on the unit. Once the staff apply the evidence in a fall-prevention protocol, they implement the protocol (in this case, focusing efforts on care approaches during evening hours) and evaluate its results. Recurrent problems with falls lead staff to conduct a research study specific to the problem.

Quality Improvement Programs

A well-organized QI program focuses on processes or systems that contribute to patient, staff, or system outcomes. A systematic approach ensures that all employees support a continuous QI philosophy. An organizational culture in which all staff members understand their responsibility toward maintaining and improving quality is essential. Typically in health care many individuals are involved in single processes of care. For example, medication delivery involves the nurse who prepares and administers the drugs, the health care provider who prescribes medications, the pharmacist who prepares the dosage, the secretary who communicates about new orders, and the transporter who delivers medications. All members of the health care team collaborate together in QI activities. As a member of the nursing team, you participate in recognizing trends in practice, identifying when recurrent problems develop, and initiating opportunities to improve the quality of care.

The QI process begins at the staff level, where problems are defined by the staff. This requires staff members to know the practice standards or guidelines that define quality. Unit QI committees review activities or services considered to be most important in providing quality care to patients. To identify the greatest opportunity for improving quality, the committees consider activities that are high-volume (greater than 50% of the activity of a unit), high-risk (potential for trauma or death), and problem areas (potential for patient, staff, or institution). TJC's annual National Patient Safety Goals provide another focus for QI committees to explore and identify problem areas (TJC, 2015). Sometimes the problem is presented to a committee in the form of a sentinel event (i.e., an unexpected occurrence involving death or serious physical or psychological injury). Once a committee defines the problem, it applies a formal model for exploring and resolving quality concerns. There are many models for QI and PI. One model is the PDSA cycle:

Plan—Review available data to understand existing practice conditions or problems to identify the need for change.

Do—Select an intervention on the basis of the data reviewed and implement the change.

Study—Study (evaluate) the results of the change.

Act—If the process change is successful with positive outcomes, act on the practices by incorporating them into daily unit performance.

Six Sigma or Lean is another QI model. In this model organizations carefully evaluate processes to reduce costs, enhance quality and revenue, and improve teamwork while using the talents of existing employees and the fewest resources. In a lean organization all employees are responsible and accountable for integrating QI methodologies and tools into daily work (DelliFraine et al., 2014; Kimsey, 2010).

Some organizations use a QI model called rapid-cycle improvement or rapid-improvement event (RIE). RIEs are very intense, usually week-long events, in which a group gets together to evaluate a problem with the intent of making radical changes to current processes (Kimsey, 2010). Changes are made within a very short time. The effects of the changes are measured quickly, results are evaluated, and further changes are made when necessary. An RIE is appropriate to use when a serious problem exists that greatly affects patient safety and needs to be solved quickly (DelliFraine et al., 2014).

Once a QI committee makes a practice change, it is important to communicate results to staff in all appropriate organizational departments. Practice changes will likely not last when QI committees fail to report findings and results of interventions. Regular discussions of QI activities through staff meetings, newsletters, and memos are good communication strategies. Often a QI study reveals information that prompts organization-wide change. An organization is responsible for responding to the problem with the appropriate resources. Revision of policies and procedures, modification of standards of care, and implementation of new support services are examples of ways an organization responds.

THE FUTURE OF HEALTH CARE

Any discussion of the health care delivery system must begin with the issue of change. Change is often threatening, but it also opens up opportunities for improvement. The ultimate issue in designing and delivering health care is ensuring the health and welfare of the population. Health care in the United States and around the world is not perfect. Often patients are uninsured or underinsured and do not have access to necessary services. However, health care organizations are trying to become better prepared to deal with the challenges. Increasingly they are changing how they provide their services, reducing unnecessary costs, improving access to care, and trying to provide high-quality patient care. Professional nursing is an important player in the future of health care delivery. The solutions necessary to improve the quality of health care depend largely on the active participation of nurses.

KEY POINTS

- Increasing costs and decreasing reimbursement are forcing health care institutions to deliver care more efficiently without sacrificing quality.
- The Medicare prospective reimbursement system is based on payment calculated on the basis of DRG assignment.
- Levels of health care describe the range of services and settings in which health care is available to patients in all stages of health and illness.
- Health promotion occurs in home, work, and community settings.
- Nurses are facing the challenge of keeping populations healthy and well within their own homes and communities.
- Successful community-based health programs involve building relationships with the community and incorporating cultural and environmental factors.
- Hospitalized patients are acutely ill, requiring better coordination of services before discharge.
- The goal of rehabilitation is to allow individuals to return to a level of normal or near-normal function after a physical or mental illness, injury, or chemical dependency.
- Home care agencies provide a wide variety of health care services with an emphasis on patient and family independence.
- Discharge planning begins at admission to a health care facility and helps in the transition of a patient's care from one environment to another.
- Health care organizations are evaluated on the basis of outcomes such as prevention of complications, patients' functional outcomes, and patient satisfaction.
- Nurses need to remain knowledgeable and proactive about issues in the health care delivery system to provide quality patient care and positively affect health.
- Providing patient- and family-centered care is a key component to patient satisfaction.
- A thorough analysis of QI data leads clinicians to understand work processes and the need to change practice.

CLINICAL APPLICATION QUESTIONS

Preparing for Clinical Practice

Community Hospital is a 400-bed urban hospital, one of six hospitals in a health care system. The nursing department of the hospital is applying to the American Nurses Credentialing Center for Magnet status. Nursing units are working on a number of projects to prepare for the Magnet application process.

1. You are a staff nurse on a medical-surgical floor at the hospital. The unit is trying to improve its culture in patient safety. How would you go about helping to improve the culture of safety on the unit?
2. Discuss four strategies that the nursing unit can use to deliver patient- and family-centered care.
3. You are asked by a newly hired nurse what the nursing-sensitive outcomes mean and why it is important that the unit measure the outcomes. What is your response?

ⓔ *Answers to Clinical Application Questions can be found on the Evolve website.*

REVIEW QUESTIONS

Are You Ready to Test Your Nursing Knowledge?

1. A community center is presenting a nurse-led program on the Patient Protection and Affordable Care Act. Which statement made by a participant indicates a need for further teaching?
   1. "My small company will now have to offer the 75 employees health insurance or pay a penalty."
   2. "As long as my son is a full-time student in college, I will be able to keep him on my health insurance until he is 26 years old."
   3. "I signed up for the state health insurance exchange before the designated deadline to make sure I had health insurance."
   4. "Since I have now been diagnosed with diabetes, my health insurance plan cannot charge me higher premiums."
2. Which activity performed by a nurse is related to maintaining competency in nursing practice?
   1. Asking another nurse about how to change the settings on a medication pump
   2. Regularly attending unit staff meetings
   3. Participating as a member of the professional nursing council
   4. Attending a review course in preparation for a certification examination
3. A patient tells a nurse that she is enrolled in a preferred provider organization (PPO) but does not understand what this is. What is the nurse's best explanation of a PPO?
   1. This health plan is for people who cannot afford their own health insurance.
   2. This health plan is operated by the government to provide health care to older adults.
   3. This health plan gives you a list of physicians and hospitals from which you can choose.
   4. This is a fee-for-service plan in which you can choose any physician or hospital.
4. Which of the following are examples of a nurse participating in primary care activities? (Select all that apply.)
   1. Providing prenatal teaching on nutrition to a pregnant woman during the first trimester
   2. Assessing the nutritional status of older adults who come to the community center for lunch
   3. Working with patients in a cardiac rehabilitation program
   4. Providing home wound care to a patient
   5. Teaching a class to parents at the local grade school about the importance of immunizations
5. Nurses on a nursing unit are discussing the processes that led up to a near-miss error on the clinical unit. They are outlining strategies that will prevent this in the future. This is an example of nurses working on what issue in the health care system?
   1. Patient safety
   2. Evidence-based practice
   3. Patient satisfaction
   4. Maintenance of competency
6. Which of the following statements is true regarding Magnet status recognition for a hospital?
   1. Nursing is run by a Magnet manager who makes decisions for the nursing units.
   2. Nurses in Magnet hospitals make all of the decisions on the clinical units.
   3. Magnet is a term that is used to describe hospitals that are able to hire the nurses they need.
   4. Magnet is a special designation for hospitals that achieve excellence in nursing practice.
7. A group of staff nurses notice an increased incidence of medication errors on their unit. After further investigation it is determined that the nurses are not consistently identifying the patient

correctly. A change is needed quickly. What type of quality improvement method would be most appropriate?
1. PDSA
2. Six Sigma
3. Rapid-improvement event (RIE)
4. A randomized controlled trial

8. Which of the following are characteristics of managed care systems? (Select all that apply.)
1. Provider receives a predetermined payment for each patient in the program.
2. Payment is based on a set fee for each service provided.
3. System includes a voluntary prescription drug program for an additional cost.
4. System tries to reduce costs while keeping patients healthy.
5. Focus of care is on prevention and early intervention.

9. Which of the following nursing activities is provided in a secondary health care environment?
1. Conducting blood pressure screenings for older adults at the Senior Center
2. Teaching a clinic patient with chronic obstructive pulmonary disease purse-lipped breathing techniques
3. Changing the postoperative dressing for a patient on a medical-surgical unit
4. Doing endotracheal suctioning for a patient on a ventilator in the medical intensive care unit

10. A nurse is using the Plan-Do-Study-Act (PDSA) strategy to do a quality improvement project to decrease patient falls on a nursing unit. Place the steps in the correct sequence for PDSA.
1. Bedside change of shift report is piloted on two medical-surgical units.
2. Patient satisfaction levels after implementation of the bedside report are compared to patient satisfaction levels before the change.
3. The nursing council develops a strategy for bedside change of shift report.
4. After modifications are made in the shift report elements, bedside shift report is implemented on all nursing units.

11. The nursing staff is developing a quality program. Which of the following are nursing-sensitive indicators from the National Database of Nursing Quality Indicators (NDNQI) that the nurses can use to measure patient safety and quality for the unit? (Select all that apply.)
1. Use of physical restraints
2. Pain assessment, intervention, and reassessment
3. Patient satisfaction with food preparation
4. Registered nurse (RN) education and certification
5. Number of outpatient surgical cases per year

12. A nurse is providing restorative care to a patient following an extended hospitalization for an acute illness. Which of the following is an appropriate goal for restorative care?
1. Patient will be able to walk 200 feet without shortness of breath.
2. Wound will heal without signs of infection.
3. Patient will express concerns related to return to home.
4. Patient will identify strategies to improve sleep habits.

13. A nurse is presenting information to a management class of nursing students on the topic of financial reimbursement for achievement of established, measurable patient outcomes. The nurse is presenting information to the class on which topic?
1. Prospective payment system
2. Pay for performance
3. Capitation payment system
4. Managed care systems

14. A nurse is using data collected from the unit to monitor the incidence of falls after the unit implemented a new fall protocol. The nurse is working in which area?
1. Quality improvement (QI)
2. Health care patient system
3. Nursing informatics
4. Computerized nursing network

15. The nurses on a medical unit have seen an increase in the number of pressure ulcers that develop in their patients. They decide to initiate a quality improvement project using the Plan-Do-Study-Act (PDSA) model. Which of the following is an example of "Do" from that model?
1. Implementing the new skin care protocol on all medicine units
2. Reviewing the data collected on patients cared for using the protocol
3. Reviewing the quality improvement reports on the six patients who developed ulcers over the last 3 months
4. Based on findings from patients who developed ulcers, implementing an evidence-based skin care protocol

Answers: 1. 2; **2.** 4; **3.** 3; **4.** 1, 2, 5; **5.** 1; **6.** 4; **7.** 3; **8.** 1, 4, 5; **9.** 3, 4; **10.** 3, 1, 2, 4; **11.** 1, 2, 4; **12.** 1; **13.** 2; **14.** 1; **15.** 4.

Rationales for Review Questions can be found on the Evolve website.

REFERENCES

Agency for Healthcare Research and Quality Patient Safety Network (AHRQ PSNet): *Patient safety primer: never events*, 2012. http://psnet.ahrq.gov/printviewPrimer.aspx?primerID=3. Accessed July 1, 2015.

Amara S, et al: Nursing's role in ACOs, *Nurs Manage* October:20, 2013.

American Association of Colleges of Nursing (AACN): *Nursing fact sheet*, 2011. http://www.aacn.nche.edu/media-relations/fact-sheets/nursing-fact-sheet. Accessed July 1, 2015.

American Association of Colleges of Nursing (AACN): *Nursing shortage fact sheet*, 2014. http://www.aacn.nche.edu/media-relations/NrsgShortageFS.pdf. Accessed July 1, 2015.

American Nurses Association (ANA): *Nursing informatics scope and standards of practice*, Silver Springs, Md, 2008, The Association.

American Nurses Credentialing Center (ANCC): *Growth of the program*, 2013. http://www.nursecredentialing.org/Magnet/ProgramOverview/HistoryoftheMagnetProgram/GrowthoftheProgram. Accessed May 8, 2014.

American Nurses Credentialing Center (ANCC): *Magnet Recognition Program Model*, 2014a, http://www.nursecredentialing.org/Magnet/ProgramOverview/New-Magnet-Model. Accessed July 1, 2015.

American Nurses Credentialing Center (ANCC): *Magnet program overview*, 2014b. http://www.nursecredentialing.org/Magnet/ProgramOverview. Accessed July 1, 2015.

Carey B: *Comparing and blending ISO9000 and lean six sigma*, 2010. http://www.isixsigma.com/community/awards-and-standards/comparing-and-blending-iso9000-and-lean-six-sigma. Accessed July 1, 2015.

Centers for Disease Control and Prevention (CDC): *Chronic disease overview*, 2015. http://www.cdc.gov/chronicdisease/overview/index.htm. Accessed July 1, 2015.

Centers for Medicare and Medicaid Services (CMS): *Accountable care organizations (ACO)*, 2012. http://www.cms.gov/Medicare/Medicare-Fee-for-Service-Payment/ACO/index.html?redirect=/ACO/. Accessed July 1, 2015.

Colpas P: Accountable care organizations help to coordinate care, *Health Manag Technol* 34(7):6, 2013.

Department of Health and Human Services Center for Medicare and Medicaid Services (DHHS CMS): *Critical Access Hospitals*, 2012. http://www.cms.gov/Outreach-and-Education/Medicare-Learning

-Network-MLN/MLNProducts/downloads/CritAccessHospfctsht.pdf. Accessed July 1, 2015.

Finkelman A, Kenner C: *Professional nursing concepts: competencies for quality leadership*, Sudbury, MA, 2010, Jones & Bartlett.

HCAHPS: *Fact sheet (CAHPS hospital survey, August 2013)*, 2013. http://www.hcahpsonline.org/files/August_2013_HCAHPS_Fact_Sheet3.pdf. Accessed July 1, 2015.

Institute for Patient and Family Centered Care [IPFCC]: *FAQ*, 2010. http://www.ipfcc.org/faq.html. Accessed July 1, 2015.

Institute of Medicine (IOM): *Crossing the quality chasm: a new health system for the 21st century*, Washington DC, 2001, National Academies Press.

Institute of Medicine (IOM): *Health professions education: a bridge to quality*, Washington, DC, 2003, National Academies Press.

Institute of Medicine (IOM): *The future of nursing: leading change, advancing health*, Washington DC, 2011, National Academies Press.

International Council of Nurses [ICN]: *Our mission, strategic intent, core values, and priorities*, 2015. http://www.icn.ch/who-we-are/our-mission-strategic-intent-core-values-and-priorities/. Accessed July 1, 2015.

Kimsey DB: Lean methodology in health care, *AORN J* 92(1):53, 2010.

Kirzinger WK et al.: Trends in insurance coverage and source of private coverage among young adults aged 10-25: United States, 2008-2012, *NCSH Data Brief*, No. 137, December 2013. http://www.cdc.gov/nchs/data/databriefs/db137.pdf. Accessed July 10, 2015.

Kovner AR Knickman JR: The current U.S. healthcare system. In Kovner AR, Knickman JR, editors: *Jonas & Kovner's Health care delivery in the United States*, ed 10, New York, 2011, Springer.

Meiner SE: *Gerontologic nursing*, ed 4, St Louis, 2011, Mosby.

Melnyk BM, Fineout-Overholt E: *Evidence-based practice in nursing and health care: a guide to best practice*, ed 3, Philadelphia, 2014, Lippincott Williams & Wilkins.

Murphy SL, et al: *National vital statistics: deaths: final data for 2010*, 2013. http://www.cdc.gov/nchs/data/nvsr/nvsr61/nvsr61_04.pdf. Accessed July 1, 2015.

National Center for Assisted Living [NCAL]: *Assisted living community profile*, 2014. http://www.ahcancal.org/ncal/resources/Pages/ALFacilityProfile.aspx. Accessed July 1, 2015.

National Committee for Quality Assurance (NCQA): *The future of patient-centered medical homes: foundation for a better medical system*, 2014. http://www.ncqa.org/Portals/0/Public%20Policy/2014%20Comment%20Letters/The_Future_of_PCMH.pdf. Accessed July 1, 2015.

National Committee for Quality Assurance [NCQA]: *HEDIS and performance measurement*, 2015. http://www.ncqa.org/HEDISQualityMeasurement.aspx. Accessed July 1, 2015.

National Database of Nursing Quality Indicators (NDNQI): *Turn Nursing Quality Insights into Improved Patient Experiences*, 2015. http://pressganey.com/ourSolutions/performance-and-advanced-analytics/clinical-business-performance/nursing-quality-ndnqi. Accessed July 1, 2015.

National Priorities Partnership: *National priorities partnership and the national quality strategy*, 2014. https://www.qualityforum.org/Setting_Priorities/NPP/Input_into_the_National_Quality_Strategy.aspx. Accessed July 1, 2015.

National Quality Forum [NQF]: *Safe practices for better healthcare—2010 update: a consensus report*, Washington, DC, 2010, National Quality Forum.

National Quality Forum [NQF]: *Committee guide to NQF's measure endorsement process*, Washington, DC, 2014, National Quality Forum.

Oulton J: Nursing in the international community: a broader view of nursing issues. In Mason DJ, et al: *Policy and politics in nursing and health care*, ed 6, St Louis, 2012, Saunders.

Pew Health Professions Commission, The Fourth Report of the Pew Health Professions Commission: *Recreating health professional practice for a new century*, 1998, The Commission.

Quality and Safety Education for Nurses (QSEN): *Pre-licensure KSAs*, 2014. http://qsen.org/competencies/pre-licensure-ksas/. Accessed July 1, 2015.

Simpson RL: Technology enables value-based nursing care, *Nurse Admin Q* 36(1):85, 2012.

Singleton KA: Lead, follow, and get in the way: the medical-surgical nurse's role in health care reform, *Medsurg Nurs* 19(1):5, 2010.

Sorrentino SA, Remmert LN: *Mosby's textbook for nursing assistants*, ed 8, St Louis, 2012, Mosby.

Stanhope M, Lancaster J: *Public health nursing population-centered health care in the community*, ed 8, St Louis, 2012, Mosby.

Sultz HA, Young KM: *Health care USA: understanding its organization and delivery*, ed 7, Sudbury, 2014, Jones & Bartlett.

The Joint Commission (TJC): *Accreditation guide for hospitals*, 2013. http://www.jointcommission.org/assets/1/6/Accreditation_Guide_Hospitals_2011.pdf. Accessed July 1, 2015.

The Joint Commission (TJC): *2014 National Patient Safety Goals (NPGs)*, 2015, TJC. http://www.jointcommission.org/standards_information/npsgs.aspx. Accessed July 1, 2015.

Touhy TA, Jett K: *Ebersole & Hess' Toward healthy aging: human needs and nursing response*, ed 8, St Louis, 2012, Mosby.

US Department of Labor: *Economic news release: 2013 Occupations with the largest projected number of job openings due to growth and replacement needs, 2012 and projected 2022*, 2013. http://www.bls.gov/news.release/ecopro.t08.htm. Accessed July 1, 2015.

World Health Organization [WHO]: *Primary health care*, 2015. http://www.who.int/topics/primary_health_care/en/. Accessed July 1, 2015.

RESEARCH REFERENCES

Agency for Health Care Research and Quality, U.S. Department of Health and Human Services (AHRQ/USDHHS): *Patient safety and quality: an evidence-based handbook for nurses,* AHRQ Pub No 08-0043, Rockville, MD, 2008, AHRQ/USDHHS.

Cairns LL, et al: Utilizing bedside shift report to improve the effectiveness of shift handoff, *J Nurs Admin* 43(3):160, 2013.

DelliFraine JL, et al: The use of Six Sigma in health care management: are we using it to its full potential, *Q Manage Health Care* 23: 240, 2014.

Dempsey C, et al: Improving the patient experience: real-world strategies for engaging nurses, *J Nurs Admin* 44(3):142, 2014.

Jeffs L, et al: Quality nursing care and opportunities for improvement: insights from patients and family members, *J Nurs Care Qual* 28(10):76, 2013.

Mullen-Fortino M, et al: Bedside nurses' perceptions of intensive care unit telemedicine, *Am J Crit Care* 21(1):24, 2012.

Newhouse RP, Morlock L: Rural hospital nursing: results of a national survey of nurse executives, *J Nurse Admin* 41(3):129, 2011.

Nichols BL, et al: An integrative review of global nursing workforce: issues, *Annu Rev Nurs Res* 28:113, 2010.

Radhakrishanan K, Jacelon C: Impact of telehealth on patient self-management of heart failure: a review of the literature, *J Cardiovasc Nurs* 27(1):33, 2012.

Radtke K: Improving patient satisfaction with nurse communication using bedside shift report, *Clin Nurse Spec* 27(1):19, 2013.

Reck DL: Can and should nurses be aware of patients' expectations for their nursing care? *Nurs Admin Q* 37(2):109, 2013.

3

Community-Based Nursing Practice

OBJECTIVES

- Explain the relationship between public health and community health nursing.
- Differentiate community health nursing from community-based nursing.
- Discuss the role of the community health nurse.
- Discuss the role of the nurse in community-based practice.
- Identify characteristics of patients from vulnerable populations that influence the community-based nurse's approach to care.
- Describe the competencies important for success in community-based nursing practice.
- Describe elements of a community assessment.

KEY TERMS

Community-based nursing, p. 33
Community health nursing, p. 33
Health disparities, p. 33
Incident rates, p. 32
Population, p. 33
Public health nursing, p. 33
Social determinants of health, p. 32
Vulnerable populations, p. 34

MEDIA RESOURCES

http://evolve.elsevier.com/Potter/fundamentals/

- Review Questions
- Case Study with Questions
- Audio Glossary
- Content Updates

Community-based care focuses on health promotion, disease prevention, and restorative care. Because patients are often discharged quickly from acute care settings, there is a growing need to provide health care delivery services where people live, work, socialize, and learn. One way to achieve this goal is through a community-based health care model. Community-based health care is a collaborative, evidence-based model designed to meet the health care needs of a community (Olson et al., 2011). A healthy community includes elements that maintain a high quality of life and productivity. For example, safety and access to health care services are elements that enable people to function productively in their community (U.S. Department of Health and Human Services [USDHHS], 2015). As more community health care partnerships develop, nurses are in a strategic position to play an important role in health care delivery and improve the health of the community.

The focus of health promotion and disease prevention continues to be essential for the holistic practice of professional nursing. The history of nursing documents the roles of nurses in establishing and meeting the public health needs of their patients. Within community health settings, nurses are leaders in assessing, diagnosing, planning, implementing, and evaluating the types of public and community health services needed. Community health nursing and community-based nursing are components of a health care delivery system that improve the health of the general public.

COMMUNITY-BASED HEALTH CARE

It is important to understand the focus of community-based health care. Community-based health care is a model of care that reaches everyone in a community (including the poor and underinsured), focuses on primary rather than institutional or acute care, and provides knowledge about health and health promotion and models of care to the community. Community-based health care occurs outside traditional health care institutions such as hospitals. It provides services to individuals and families within the community for acute and chronic conditions (Stanhope and Lancaster, 2014).

Today the challenges in community-based health care are numerous. Political policy and the Affordable Care Act (ACA); social determinants of health, increases in health disparities, and economics all influence public health problems and subsequent health care services. Some of these problems include a lack of adequate health insurance, chronic illnesses such as heart disease and diabetes, an increase in sexually transmitted infections, and underimmunization of infants and children (USDHHS, 2015). More than ever before, the health care system must commit to reform and bring attention and health care services to all communities.

Achieving Healthy Populations and Communities

The USDHHS Public Health Service designed a program to improve the overall health status of people living in this country. The *Healthy People Initiative* was created to establish ongoing health care goals (see Chapter 6). The 2020 document strives to ensure that *Healthy People 2020* is relevant to diverse public health needs and seizes opportunities to achieve its goals. Since its inception, *Healthy People* has become a broad-based, public engagement initiative with thousands of citizens helping to shape it at every step along the way. The overall goals of *Healthy People 2020* are to increase life expectancy and quality of life and eliminate health disparities through improved delivery of health care services (USDHHS, 2015).

Improved delivery of health care occurs through assessment of health care needs of individuals, families, and communities; development and implementation of public health policies; and improved access to care. For example, assessment includes systematic data collection on the population, monitoring the health status of the population, and accessing available information about the health of the community (Stanhope and Lancaster, 2014). A comprehensive community assessment sometimes leads to community health programs such as adolescent smoking prevention, sex education, and proper nutrition. Some examples of assessment include gathering information on **incident rates** such as identifying and reporting new infections or diseases, determining adolescent pregnancy rates, and reporting the number of motor vehicle accidents caused by teenage drivers.

Health professionals provide leadership in developing public policies to support the health of the population (Stanhope and Lancaster, 2014). Strong policies are driven by community assessment. For example, assessing the level of lead poisoning in young children often leads to a lead cleanup program to reduce the incidence of lead poisoning. Identifying evidence-based practices to help more people manage chronic illnesses in the home and the community addresses the needs of nurses and their patients (Kirkpatrick et al., 2012) (Box 3-1).

Improved access to care ensures that essential community-wide health services are available and accessible to the entire community (Stanhope and Lancaster, 2014). Community development, social capital, and capacity are essential in establishing community-wide health promotion and health maintenance activities. As a result the community is empowered to be part of the health care agenda (Piper, 2011). Examples include prenatal care programs and programs focusing on disease prevention, health protection, and health promotion. The five-level health services pyramid is an example of how to provide community-based services within existing health care services in a community. In this population-focused health care services model, the goals of disease prevention, health protection, and health promotion provide a foundation for primary, secondary, and tertiary health care services (see Figure 2-1 on p. 17).

A rural community does not always have a hospital to meet the acute care needs of its citizens. However, a community assessment might reveal which services are available to meet the needs of expectant mothers, reduce teenage smoking, or provide nutritional support for older adults. In addition, this same community assessment identifies the health care gaps for a specific community. Community-based programs provide these services and are effective in improving the health of the community. In other situations a community has the resources for providing childhood immunizations, flu vaccines, and primary preventive care services and is able to focus on child developmental problems and child safety.

Public health services aim at achieving a healthy environment for all individuals. Health care providers apply these principles for individuals, families, and the communities in which they live. Nursing plays a role in all levels of the health services pyramid. By using public health principles you are better able to understand the types of environments in which patients live and the types of interventions necessary to help keep them healthy.

BOX 3-1 EVIDENCE-BASED PRACTICE

Promoting Informed Decision Making in a Community Setting

PICO Question: Do community centers that provide informed decision making for prostate cancer screening (PCS) have better outcomes than those centers that do not provide informed decision making?

Evidence Summary

Often a community health center is the first, if not only, health care resource for some of the population. Social determinants of health, health disparities, and inequalities in health care all contribute to a population's level of health. Cultural beliefs, experiences with health care services, and health literacy all impact how patients access health care and make health care decisions (Chan et al., 2011). Translating research evidence and creating an evidence-based community nursing practice also impact health care outcomes (Kirkpatrick et al., 2012).

Health promotion and related health screenings are essential in maintaining an individual and community level of health. Health practices related to PCS are often lacking in ethnically diverse communities. For example, both Hispanic and African-American men tend to have lower participation in PCS when compared with Caucasian men (Chan et al., 2011; Gash & McIntosh, 2013). This most likely happens for many reasons, such as limited knowledge about PCS, poor access to health care, and mistrust of the health care system. Lower participation in PCS often leads to a diagnosis of cancer at a later, more aggressive stage and poorer health outcomes in these populations (Gash & McIntosh, 2013).

Chan et al. (2011) found that community centers that provide culturally appropriate information related to PCS improves knowledge and promotes more active involvement in decision making about PCS screening activities. Including the spouse or significant other in educational interventions may be especially helpful because men's decision making about health screening and their coping patterns often includes family or friends (Gash & McIntosh, 2013). Thus patients who seek health care at community centers that provide gender neutral, culturally appropriate, and targeted education regarding decision making about PCS may experience better health outcomes when compared with community centers that do not provide this type of educational interventions.

Application to Nursing Practice

- Help increase patients knowledge about appropriate screening practices.
- Reinforce patients' decision-making rights.
- Understand the social and cultural dynamics of the community.
- Use community resources and leadership to develop culturally appropriate educational interventions (Chan et al., 2011).
- Include spouses and significant others in educational sessions when appropriate to enhance patients' involvement in their decision making about health screenings (Gash & McIntosh, 2013).

Social Determinants of Health

Our health is also determined in part by access to social and economic opportunities; the resources and support systems available in our homes, neighborhoods, and communities; the quality of our schooling; the safety of our workplaces; the cleanliness of our water, food, and air; and the nature of our social interactions and relationships.

Health starts in our homes, schools, workplaces, neighborhoods, and communities. We know that taking care of ourselves by eating well and staying active, not smoking, getting the recommended immunizations and screening tests, and seeing a doctor when we are sick all influence our health. However there are also social determinants of health. **Social determinants of health** are factors that contribute to a person's current state of health. These factors may be biological, socioeconomic, psychosocial, behavioral, or social in nature. Scientists generally recognize five determinants of health: biology and genetics (sex and age), individual behavior (such as alcohol, injection drug use, unprotected sex, and smoking), social environment (such as discrimination, income, and gender), physical environment (where a person lives or crowding conditions), and health services (such as access to quality health care and having health insurance) (CDC, 2014b). Whether these factors affect a single family or the community, they impact the overall health and wellness of that community.

Health Disparities

Health disparities negatively affect groups of people who have systematically experienced social or economic obstacles to health. These obstacles stem from characteristics historically linked to discrimination or exclusion such as race or ethnicity, religion, socioeconomic status, gender, mental health, sexual orientation, or geographic location. Other characteristics include cognitive, sensory, or physical disability.

Health disparities are preventable differences in the burden of disease, injury, violence, or opportunities to achieve optimal health that are experienced by socially disadvantaged populations. Populations can be defined by factors such as race or ethnicity, gender, education or income, disability, geographic location (e.g., rural or urban), or sexual orientation. Health disparities are inequitable and are directly related to the historical and current unequal distribution of social, political, economic, and environmental resources. They result from multiple factors, including poverty, environmental threats, inadequate access to health care, individual and behavioral factors, and educational inequalities (CDC, 2014a).

COMMUNITY HEALTH NURSING

Frequently the terms *community health nursing* and *public health nursing* are used interchangeably, although they are different. A **public health nursing** focus requires understanding the needs of a **population** or a collection of individuals who have one or more personal or environmental characteristics in common (Stanhope and Lancaster, 2014). Examples of populations include high-risk infants, older adults, or an ethnic group such as Native Americans. A public health nurse understands factors that influence health promotion and health maintenance, the trends and patterns influencing the incidence of disease within populations, environmental factors contributing to health and illness, and the political processes used to affect public policy. For example, a nurse uses data on increased incidence of playground injuries to lobby for a policy to use shock-absorbing material rather than concrete for new public playgrounds.

Public health nursing requires preparation at the basic entry level and sometimes requires a baccalaureate degree in nursing that includes educational preparation and clinical practice in public health nursing. A specialist in public health has a graduate level education with a focus in the public health sciences (American Nurses Association [ANA], 2013).

Community health nursing is nursing practice in the community, with the primary focus on the health care of individuals, families, and groups within the community. The goal is to preserve, protect, promote, or maintain health (Stanhope and Lancaster, 2014). The emphasis of such nursing care is to improve the quality of health and life within that community. In addition, the community health nurse provides direct care services to subpopulations within a community. These subpopulations often have a clinical focus in which the nurse has expertise. For example, a case manager follows older adults recovering from stroke and sees the need for community rehabilitation services, or a nurse practitioner gives immunizations to patients with the objective of managing communicable disease within the community. By focusing on subpopulations, a community health nurse cares for the community as a whole and considers an individual or family as only one member of a group at risk.

Competence as a community health nurse requires the ability to use interventions that include the broad social and political context of the community (Stanhope and Lancaster, 2014). The educational requirements for entry-level nurses practicing in community health nursing roles are not as clear as those for public health nurses. Not all hiring agencies require an advanced degree. However, nurses with a graduate degree in nursing who practice in community settings are considered community health nurse specialists, regardless of their public health experience (Stanhope and Lancaster, 2014).

Nursing Practice in Community Health

Community health nursing practice requires a unique set of skills and knowledge. In the health care delivery system nurses who become experts in community health practice usually have advanced nursing degrees, yet the baccalaureate-prepared nurse generalist is also able to formulate and apply population-focused assessments and interventions. The expert community health nurse understands the needs of a population or community through experience with individual families, which includes working through their social and health care issues. In this context, critical thinking involves applying knowledge of public health principles, community health nursing, family theory, and communication in finding the best approaches to partner with families.

Successful community health nursing practice involves building relationships with the community and being responsive to changes within the community. For example, when there is an increase in the incidence of grandparents assuming child care responsibilities, a community health nurse becomes an active part of a community by establishing an educational program in cooperation with local schools to assist and support grandparents in this caregiving role. The nurse knows the community members, along with their needs and resources, and then works in collaboration with community leaders to establish effective health promotion and disease prevention programs. This requires working with highly resistant systems (e.g., welfare system) and trying to encourage them to be more responsive to the needs of a population. Skills of patient advocacy, communicating people's concerns, and designing new systems in cooperation with existing systems help to make community nursing practice effective.

COMMUNITY-BASED NURSING

Community-based nursing care takes place in community settings such as a home or clinic, where nurses focus on the needs of an individual or family. It involves the safety needs and acute and chronic care of individuals and families, enhances their capacity for self-care, and promotes autonomy in decision making (Stanhope and Lancaster, 2014). It requires critical thinking and decision making for the individual patient and family—assessing health status, diagnosing health problems, planning care, implementing interventions, and evaluating outcomes of care. Because nurses provide direct care services where patients live, work, and play, it is important that they place the perspectives of the community members first and foremost when planning care (Jackson et al., 2012).

Community-based nursing centers function as the first level of contact between members of a community and the health care delivery system (Figure 3-1). Ideally health care services are provided near where patients live. This approach helps to reduce the cost of health care for the patient and the stress associated with the financial burdens of care. In addition, these centers offer direct access to nurses and patient-centered health services and readily incorporate the patient and the patient's family or friends into a plan of care. Community-based nursing centers often care for the most vulnerable of the population (Olson et al., 2011).

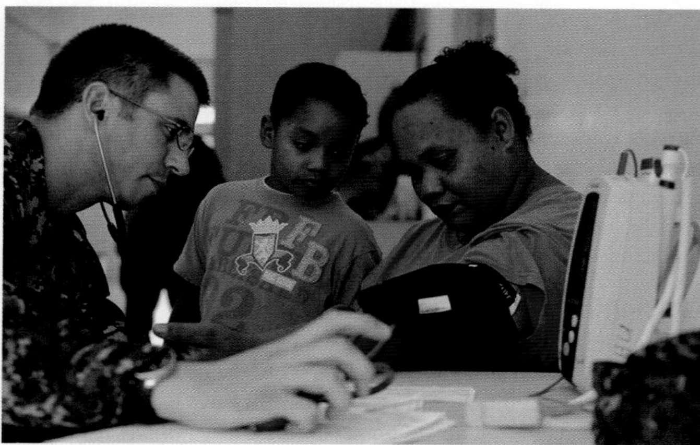

FIGURE 3-1 Patient and family receiving care in a community-based care center. (Courtesy Mass Communication Specialist 2nd Class Daniel Viramontes.)

With the individual and family as the patients, the context of community-based nursing is family-centered care within the community. This focus requires a strong knowledge base in family theory (see Chapter 10), principles of communication (see Chapter 24), group dynamics, and cultural diversity (see Chapter 9). Nurses partner with their patients and families to enable them to ultimately assume responsibility for their health care decisions.

Vulnerable Populations

In a community setting nurses care for patients from diverse cultures and backgrounds and with various health conditions. However, changes in the health care delivery system have made high-risk groups the principal patients. For example, you are not likely to visit low-risk mothers and babies. Instead, you are more likely to visit adolescent mothers or mothers with drug addiction. **Vulnerable populations** are groups of patients who are more likely to develop health problems as a result of excess health risks, who are limited in access to health care services, or who depend on others for care. Individuals living in poverty, older adults, people who are homeless, immigrant populations, individuals in abusive relationships, substance abusers, and people with severe mental illnesses are examples of vulnerable populations. These vulnerabilities are often associated with the individual's/community's social determinants of health or individual health disparities.

Public and community health nursing and primary care providers share health care responsibility for health promotion, screening, and early detection and disease prevention for vulnerable populations. These patients have intense health care needs that are unmet or ignored or require more care than can be provided in outpatient or hospital settings. Individuals and their families who are vulnerable often belong to more than one of these groups. In addition, health care vulnerability affects all age-groups (Sebastian, 2014).

Patients who are vulnerable often come from varied cultures, have different beliefs and values, face language and literacy barriers, and have few sources of social support. Their special needs will be a challenge for you as you care for increasingly complex acute and chronic health conditions.

To provide competent care for vulnerable populations, you need to assess these patients accurately (Box 3-2). In addition, you need to evaluate and understand a patient's and family's cultural beliefs, values, and practices to determine their specific needs and the interventions that will be most successful in improving their state of health (see Chapter 9). It is important not to judge or evaluate your patient's beliefs and values about health in terms of your own culture, beliefs, and values. Communication and caring practices are critical in learning a patient's perceptions of his or her problems and then planning health care strategies that will be meaningful, culturally appropriate, and successful.

BOX 3-2 Guidelines for Assessing Members of Vulnerable Population Groups

Setting the Stage

- Create a comfortable, nonthreatening environment.
- Obtain information about a patient's culture so you understand the practices, beliefs, and values that affect the patient's health care.
- If the patient speaks a different language, use a professional interpreter and observe nonverbal behavior to complete a culturally competent assessment (Chapter 9).
- Be sensitive to the fact that patients often have priorities other than their health care (e.g., financial, legal, or social issues). Help them with these concerns before beginning a health assessment. If a patient needs financial assistance, consult a social worker. If there are legal issues, provide the patient with a resource. Do not attempt to provide financial or legal advice yourself.

Nursing History of an Individual or Family

- Because you often have only one opportunity to conduct a nursing history, you need to obtain an organized history of all of essential information to help an individual or family during that visit.
- Collect data on a comprehensive form that focuses on the specific needs of the vulnerable population with whom you work. However, be flexible so as not to overlook important health information. For example, when with an adolescent mother, obtain a nutritional history on both the mother and baby. Be aware of the developmental needs of the adolescent mom and listen to her social needs as well.
- Identify both developmental and health care needs. Remember, the goal is to collect enough information to provide family-centered care.
- Identify any risks to the patient's immune system. This is especially important for vulnerable patients who are homeless and sleep in shelters.

Physical Examination and Home Assessment

- Complete as thorough a physical and/or home assessment as possible. However, only collect data that are relevant to providing care to the patient and family.
- Be alert for signs of physical or substance abuse (e.g., inadequately clothed to hide bruising, underweight, runny nose).
- When assessing a patient's home, observe: Is there adequate water and plumbing? What is the status of the utilities? Are foods and perishables stored properly? Are there signs of insects or vermin? Is the paint peeling? Are the windows and doors adequate? Are there water stains on the ceiling, evidence of a leaky roof? What is the temperature? Is it comfortable? What does the outside environment look like: Are there vacant houses/lots nearby? Is there a busy intersection? What is the crime level?

Modified from Stanhope M, Lancaster J: *Foundations of nursing in the community: community oriented practice*, ed 4, St Louis, 2014, Mosby.

Barriers to access and use of services often lead to adverse health outcomes for vulnerable populations (Jackson and Saltman, 2011; Rew et al., 2009). Because of these poorer outcomes, vulnerable populations have shorter life spans and higher morbidity rates. Members of vulnerable groups frequently have multiple risks, which make them more sensitive to the cumulative effects of individual risk factors. It is essential for community-based nurses to assess members of vulnerable populations by taking into account the multiple stressors that affect their patients' lives. It is also important to learn patients' strengths and resources for coping with stressors. Complete assessment of vulnerable populations enables a community-based nurse to design interventions within the context of the patient's community (Sebastian, 2014).

Immigrant Population. Researchers predict a continued increase in immigrant population (Camarota, 2012). This continued growth creates many social and health care needs. Immigrant populations face multiple diverse health issues that cities, counties, and states need to address. These health care needs pose significant legal and policy issues. For some immigrants access to health care is limited because of language barriers and lack of benefits, resources, and transportation. Immigrant populations often have higher rates of hypertension, diabetes mellitus, and infectious diseases; decreased outcomes of care; and shorter life expectancies (Stanhope and Lancaster, 2014).

Frequently the immigrant population practices nontraditional healing practices (see Chapter 9). Although many of these healing practices are effective and complement traditional therapies, it is important that you know and understand your patient's health beliefs about these healing practices.

Certain immigrant populations left their homes as a result of oppression, war, or natural disaster (e.g., Afghans, Bosnians, and Somalis). Be sensitive to these physical and psychological stressors and consequences and identify the appropriate resources to help understand your patients and their health care needs (Stanhope and Lancaster, 2014).

Effects of Poverty and Homelessness. People who live in poverty are more likely to have more health disparities because they often live in hazardous environments, work at high-risk jobs, eat less nutritious diets, have multiple stressors in their lives, have poor or unavailable transportation, and are at risk for homelessness.

Patients who are homeless have even fewer resources than the poor. They are often jobless, do not have the advantage of a permanent shelter, and must continually cope with finding food and a place to sleep at night. Chronic health problems tend to worsen because of poor nutrition and the inability to store nutritional foods. In addition, people who are homeless usually walk the streets and neighborhoods to seek shelter, leading to an imbalance of rest and activity (Jackson et al., 2012).

Patients Who Are Abused. Physical, emotional, and sexual abuse and neglect are major public health problems affecting older adults, women, and children. Risk factors for abusive relationships include mental health problems, substance abuse, socioeconomic stressors, and dysfunctional family relationships (Landenburger and Campbell, 2014). For some, risk factors may not be present. When dealing with patients at risk for or who have suffered abuse, it is important to provide protection. Interview a patient you suspect is abused at a time when the patient has privacy and the individual suspected of being the abuser is not present. Patients who are abused may fear retribution if they discuss their problems with a health care provider. Most states have abuse hot lines that nurses and other health care providers must notify when they identify an individual as being at risk.

Patients with Mental Illness. When a patient has a severe mental illness such as schizophrenia or bipolar disorder, you need to explore multiple health and socioeconomic problems. Many patients with severe mental illnesses are homeless or live in poverty. Others lack the ability to remain employed or even to care for themselves on a daily basis (Prochaska et al., 2012). Patients who have a mental illness often require medication therapy, counseling, housing, and vocational assistance. In addition, they are at a greater risk for abuse and assault.

Patients with mental illnesses are no longer routinely hospitalized in long-term psychiatric institutions. Instead resources are offered within the community. Although comprehensive service networks are in every community, many patients still go untreated. Many are left with fewer and more fragmented services, with little skill in surviving and functioning within the community (Happell and Cleary, 2012).

Older Adults. With the increasing older-adult population, simultaneous increases in the number of patients suffering from chronic diseases and a greater demand for health care services are seen. Take time to understand what health means to an older adult and which assessment findings to expect; view health promotion in the older adult within a broad context (see Chapter 14). Help older adults and their families understand which steps they need to take to maintain their health and improve their level of function (Piper, 2011). Design appropriate community-based interventions that provide an opportunity to improve the lifestyle and quality of life of older adults (Table 3-1).

Competency in Community-Based Nursing

A nurse in community-based practice needs a variety of skills and talents to be successful. In addition to assisting patients with their health care needs and developing relationships within the community, the community-based nurse needs skills in health promotion and disease prevention. The nurse uses the nursing process and critical thinking (see Unit III) to ensure individualized nursing care for specific patients and their families. Students' clinical practice in a community-based care setting will probably be in partnership with a community nurse.

Caregiver. First and foremost is the role of caregiver (see Chapter 1). In the community setting you manage and care for the health of patients and families in the community. Use a critical thinking approach to apply the nursing process (see Unit III) and ensure appropriate, individualized nursing care for specific patients and their families.

Historically well-baby and child care were integral to community nursing practices. Because of changes in the health care delivery system, changing economics, homelessness, and the medically underinsured, community child care services are increasing. Community nurses are undertaking more complex and expanded child health services for increasingly diverse client populations (Borrow et al., 2011).

In addition, you individualize care within the context of a patient's community so long-term success is more likely. Together with the patient and family you develop a caring partnership to recognize actual and potential health care needs and identify needed community resources. As a caregiver, you also help build a healthy community, which is one that is safe and includes elements to enable people to achieve and maintain a high quality of life and function.

> **QSEN QSEN: BUILDING COMPETENCY IN SAFETY** Jan Carrel is a 30-year-old single woman who has multiple sclerosis (MS). She owns a condo and is an executive for a car rental firm. Her MS has progressed to the point that she needs ambulatory assistive devices. Depending on her level of mobility, these devices range from a walker to a motorized chair; and the amount of assistance Jan requires changes during the week. She is able to stand to transfer to the toilet or to her handicapped-accessible vehicle or to reach items in the kitchen. However, because of her muscle weakness, her activity intolerance, and imbalance, she cannot stand for long periods of time. Both she and her doctor have requested a home safety assessment. What information do you need to begin this assessment?
>
> *Answers to QSEN Activities can be found on the Evolve website.*

TABLE 3-1 Major Health Problems in Older Adults and Community-Based Nursing Roles and Interventions

Problem	Community-Based Nursing Roles and Interventions
Hypertension	Monitor blood pressure and weight; educate about nutrition and antihypertensive drugs; teach stress management techniques; promote a good balance between rest and activity; establish blood pressure screening programs; assess patient's current lifestyle and promote lifestyle changes; promote dietary modifications by using techniques such as a diet diary.
Cancer	Obtain health history; promote monthly breast self-examinations and annual Papanicolaou (Pap) smears and mammograms for older women; promote regular physical examinations; encourage smokers to stop smoking; correct misconceptions about processes of aging; provide emotional support and quality of care during diagnostic and treatment procedures.
Arthritis	Educate adult about management of activities, correct body mechanics, availability of mechanical appliances, and adequate rest; promote stress management; counsel and assist the family to improve communication, role negotiation, and use of community resources; help adult avoid the false hope and expense of arthritis fraud.
Visual impairment (e.g., loss of visual acuity, eyelid disorders, opacity of the lens)	Provide support in a well-lighted, glare-free environment; use printed aids with large, well-spaced letters; help adult clean eyeglasses; help make arrangements for vision examinations and obtain necessary prostheses; teach adult to be cautious of false advertisements.
Hearing impairment (e.g., presbycusis)	Speak with clarity at a moderate volume and pace and face audience when performing health teaching; help make arrangements for hearing examination and obtain necessary prostheses; teach adult to be cautious of false advertisements.
Cognitive impairment	Provide complete assessment; correct underlying causes of disease (if possible); provide for a protective environment; promote activities that reinforce reality; help with personal hygiene, nutrition, and hydration; provide emotional support to the family; recommend applicable community resources such as adult day care, home care aides, and homemaker services.
Alzheimer's disease	Maintain high-level functioning, protection, and safety; encourage human dignity; demonstrate to the primary family caregiver techniques to dress, feed, and toilet adult; provide frequent encouragement and emotional support to caregiver; act as an advocate for patient when dealing with respite care and support groups; protect the patient's rights; provide support to maintain family members' physical and mental health; maintain family stability; recommend financial services if needed.
Dental problems	Perform oral assessment and refer to dentist as necessary; emphasize regular brushing and flossing, proper nutrition, and dental examinations; encourage patients with dentures to wear and take care of them; calm fears about dentist; help provide access to financial services (if necessary) and dental care facilities.
Substance and alcohol abuse	Get drug use history; educate adult about safe storage, risks for drug, drug-drug, drug-alcohol, and drug-food interactions; give general information about drug (e.g., drug name, purpose, side effects, dosage); instruct adult about presorting techniques (using small containers with one dose of drug that are labeled with specific times to take drug). Counsel adults about substance abuse; promote stress management to avoid need for drugs or alcohol and arrange for and monitor detoxification if appropriate.
Sexually transmitted infections	Perform a full sexual risk assessment and bring awareness regarding risk factors and susceptibility to human immunodeficiency virus/acquired immunodeficiency syndrome (HIV/AIDS). Educate about safe sexual practices such as abstinence, use of condoms and refer as necessary for HIV testing.

Data from Stanhope M, and Lancaster J: *Foundations of nursing in the community: community-oriented practice,* ed 4, St Louis, 2014, Mosby; Goodman C et al: Activity promotion for community-dwelling older people: a survey of the contribution of primary care nurses, *Br J Community Nurs* 16(1):12, 2011; Baym-Williams J, Salyer J: Factors influencing the health-related lifestyles of community-dwelling older adults, *Home Health Care Nurse* (28)115–121, 2010; Jacobson SA: HIV/AIDS interventions in an aging US population, *Health Soc Work*: 2(36):149, 2011.

Case Manager. In community-based practice case management is an important competency (see Chapter 2). It is the ability to establish an appropriate plan of care based on assessment of patients and families and to coordinate needed resources and services for a patient's well-being across a continuum of care. Generally a community-based case manager assumes responsibility for the case management of multiple patients. The greatest challenge is coordinating the activities of multiple providers and payers in different settings throughout a patient's continuum of care. An effective case manager eventually learns the obstacles, limits, and even the opportunities that exist within the community that influence the ability to find solutions for patients' health care needs.

Change Agent. A community-based nurse is also a change agent. This involves identifying and implementing new and more effective approaches to problems. You act as a change agent within a family system or as a mediator for problems within a patient's community. You identify any number of problems (e.g., quality of community child care services, availability of older-adult day care services, or the status of neighborhood violence). As a change agent you empower individuals and their families to creatively solve problems or become instrumental in creating change within a health care agency. For example, if your patient has difficulty keeping regular health care visits, you determine why. Maybe the health clinic is too far and difficult to reach, or perhaps the hours of service are incompatible with a patient's transportation resources. You work with the patient to solve the problem and help identify an alternative site such as a nursing clinic that is closer and has more convenient hours.

To effect change you gather and analyze facts before you implement the program. This requires you to be very familiar with the community itself. Many communities resist change, preferring to provide services in the established manner. Before analyzing facts, it is often necessary to manage conflict among the health care providers, clarify their roles, and clearly identify the needs of the patients. If the community has a history of poor problem solving, you will have to focus on developing problem-solving capabilities (Stanhope and Lancaster, 2014).

Patient Advocate. Patient advocacy is more important today in community-based practice because of the confusion surrounding access to health care services. Your patients often need someone to help them walk through the system and identify where to go for services, how to reach individuals with the appropriate authority, which services to request, and how to follow through with the information they receive. It is important to provide the information necessary for patients to make informed decisions in choosing and using services appropriately. In addition, it is important for you to support and at times defend your patients' decisions.

Collaborator. In community-based nursing practice you need to be competent in working not only with individuals and their families but also with other related health care disciplines. Collaboration, or working in a combined effort with all those involved in care delivery, is necessary to develop a mutually acceptable plan that will achieve common goals (Stanhope and Lancaster, 2014). For example, when your patient is discharged home with terminal cancer, you collaborate with hospice staff, social workers, and pastoral care to initiate a plan to support end-of-life care for the patient in the home and support the family. For collaboration to be effective, you need mutual trust and respect for each professional's roles, abilities, and contributions.

Counselor. Knowing community resources is a critical factor in becoming an effective patient counselor. A counselor helps patients identify and clarify health problems and choose appropriate courses of action to solve those problems. For example, in employee assistance programs or women's shelters, a major amount of nurse-patient interaction is through counseling. As a counselor you are responsible for providing information; listening objectively; and being supportive, caring, and trustworthy. You do not make decisions but rather help your patients reach decisions that are best for them (Stanhope and Lancaster, 2014). Patients and families often require assistance in first identifying and clarifying health problems. For example, a patient who repeatedly reports a problem in following a prescribed diet is actually unable to afford nutritious foods or has family members who do not support good eating habits. You need to discuss with your patient factors that block or aid problem resolution, identify a range of solutions, and then discuss which solutions are most likely to be successful. You also encourage your patient to make decisions and express your confidence in the choice the patient makes.

Educator. In a community-based setting you work with single individuals and groups of patients. Establishing relationships with community service organizations offers educational support to a wide range of patient groups. Prenatal classes, infant care, child safety, and cancer screening are just some of the health education programs provided in a community practice setting.

When the goal is to help your patients assume responsibility for their own health care, your role as an educator takes on greater importance (Stanhope and Lancaster, 2014). Patients and families need to gain skills and knowledge to care for themselves. Assess your patient's learning needs and readiness to learn within the context of the individual, the systems with which the individual interacts (e.g., family, business, and school), and the resources available for support. Adapt your teaching skills so you can instruct a patient within the home setting and make the learning process meaningful. In this practice setting you have the opportunity to follow patients over time. Planning for return demonstration of skills, using follow-up phone calls, and referring to community support and self-help groups give you an opportunity to provide continuity of instruction and reinforce important instructional topics and learned behaviors (see Chapter 25).

Epidemiologist. As a community-based nurse, you also apply principles of epidemiology. Your contacts with families, community groups such as schools and industries, and health care agencies place you in a unique position to initiate epidemiological activities. As an epidemiologist, you are involved in case finding, health teaching, and tracking incident rates of an illness. For example, a cafeteria worker in the local high school is diagnosed with active tuberculosis (TB). As a community health nurse, you help find new TB exposures or active disease within the worker's home, employment network, and community.

Nurse epidemiologists are responsible for community surveillance for risk factors (e.g., tracking incidence of elevated lead levels in children and identifying increased fetal and infant mortality rates, increases in adolescent pregnancy, presence of infectious and communicable diseases, and outbreaks of head lice). Nurse epidemiologists protect the level of health of the community, develop sensitivity to changes in the health status of the community, and help identify the cause of these changes.

COMMUNITY ASSESSMENT

When practicing in a community setting, you need to learn how to assess the community at large, especially in community health nursing. Community assessment is the systematic data collection on the population, monitoring the health status of the population, and making information available about the health of the community (Stanhope and Lancaster, 2014). This is the environment in which patients live and work. Without an adequate understanding of that environment, any effort to promote a patient's health and bring about necessary change is unlikely to be successful. The community has three components: structure or locale, the people, and the social systems. To develop a complete community assessment, take a careful look at each of the three components to identify needs for health policy, health programs, and needed health services (Box 3-3).

When assessing the structure or locale, you travel around the neighborhood or community and observe its design, the location of services, and the locations where residents meet. You obtain the demographics of the population by accessing statistics on the community from a local public health department or public library. You acquire information about existing social systems such as schools or health care facilities by visiting various sites and learning about their services.

Once you have a good understanding of the community, you can perform all individual patient assessments against that background. For example, when assessing a patient's home for safety, you consider the following: does the patient have secure locks on doors? Are windows secure and intact? Is lighting along walkways and entryways operational? As you conduct a patient assessment, it is important to know the level of community violence and the resources available when help is necessary. Always assess an individual in the context of the community.

CHANGING PATIENTS' HEALTH

In community-based practice nurses care for patients from diverse backgrounds and in diverse settings. It is relatively easy over time to become familiar with the available resources within a particular community practice setting. Likewise, with practice you learn how to identify the unique needs of individual patients. Similarly, nurses bring together the resources necessary to improve a patient's continuity of care. When you collaborate with your patients and their health care providers, you help to reduce duplication of health care services.

BOX 3-3 Community Assessment

Structure
- Name of community or neighborhood
- Geographical boundaries
- Emergency services
- Water and sanitation
- Housing
- Economic status (e.g., average household income, number of residents on public assistance)
- Transportation

Population
- Age distribution
- Sex distribution
- Growth trends
- Density
- Education level
- Predominant ethnic groups
- Predominant religious groups

Social System
- Education system
- Government
- Communication system
- Welfare system
- Volunteer programs
- Health system

For example, when caring for a patient with a healing wound, it is important to coordinate wound care services and help the patient and family locate cost-effective dressing materials.

However, the challenge is promoting and protecting a patient's health within the context of the community using an evidence-based practice approach when possible. For example, can nurses help men in an ethnic community change their decision-making processes regarding prostate cancer screening (Chan et al., 2011; Gash & McIntosh, 2013; see Box 3-1)? Kirkpatrick et al. (2012) investigated the effect of an evidence-based approach used by community health nurses to develop strategies to support patients with chronic obstructive pulmonary disease (COPD) in the community setting. Patients improved their self-care practices, managed panic attacks, and improved their medication compliance in this study.

Perhaps the most important theme to consider is how well you understand your patients' lives. This begins by establishing strong, caring relationships with patients and their families (see Chapter 7). As you gain experience and are accepted by a patient's family, you are able to advise, counsel, and teach effectively and understand what truly makes a patient unique. The day-to-day activities of family life are the variables that influence how you will adapt nursing interventions. The time of day a patient goes to work, the availability of the spouse and patient's parents to provide child care, and the family values that shape views about health are just a few examples of the many factors you will consider in community-based practice. Once you acquire a picture of a patient's life, you then design interventions to promote health and prevent disease within the community-based practice setting.

KEY POINTS

- Principles of public health nursing practice focus on helping individuals and communities achieve and maintain a healthy living environment.
- Essential public health functions include community assessment, policy development, and access to resources.
- When population-based health care services are effective, there is a greater likelihood that higher levels of services will contribute efficiently to health improvement of the population.
- A community health nurse cares for a community as a whole and assesses individuals or families within the context of the community.
- Successful community health nursing practice involves building relationships with a community and being responsive to changes within the community.
- A community-based nurse's competence is based on decision making at the level of the individual patient.
- The special needs of vulnerable populations are a challenge that nurses face in caring for these patients' increasingly complex acute and chronic health conditions.
- A community-based nurse is competent as a caregiver, collaborator, educator, counselor, change agent, patient advocate, case manager, and epidemiologist.

CLINICAL APPLICATION QUESTIONS

Preparing for Clinical Practice

You are managing community care for Katie, age 17, who has cerebral palsy and is severely disabled. Because of the impact of this adolescent's disability, you are also providing care to her mother, Monica, age 50, who is a single parent. Monica has cardiac disease, and all three of her siblings died in their late 50s. She is not able to work and is on public health insurance; Katie is covered through her state insurance program. Katie attends special education programs through the school district, and she will remain eligible for this education until she is 21.

Katie's two siblings, Josh (22) and Marilyn (19), both have cardiac disease and follow strict health promotion activities, which include diet and exercise. Both are in college and currently live at home. Monica is encouraging them to live in their own apartment when they graduate and have a job.

1. Identify some of the social determinants of health for this family. Use the following reference to assist you: Centers for Disease Control and Prevention (CDC): *Social Determinants of Health, Definitions,* 2014b, http://www.cdc.gov/socialdeterminants/Definitions.html.
2. Which resources do you need to identify for the family?
3. How would you help the family begin to envision the new family structure as Josh and Marilyn move out of the home?

ⓔ ***Answers to Clinical Application Questions can be found on the Evolve website.***

REVIEW QUESTIONS

Are You Ready to Test Your Nursing Knowledge?

1. A community nurse in a diverse community is working with health care professionals to provide prenatal care for underemployed and underinsured South African women. Which overall goal of *Healthy People 2020* does this represent?
   1. Assess the health care needs of individuals, families, or communities.
   2. Develop and implement public health policies and improve access to care.

3. Gather information on incident rates of certain diseases and social problems.
4. Increase life expectancy and quality of life and to eliminate health disparities.

2. Using *Healthy People 2020* as a guide, which of the following would improve delivery of care to a community? (Select all that apply.)
   1. Community assessment
   2. Implementation of public health policies
   3. Home safety assessment
   4. Increased access to care
   5. Determining rates of specific illnesses
3. A nursing student in the last semester of a baccalaureate nursing program is beginning the community health practicum and will be working in a clinic with a focus on asthma and allergies. What is the primary focus of the community health nurse in this clinic setting? (Select all that apply.)
   1. Decrease the incidence of asthma attacks in the community
   2. Increase patients' ability to self-manage their asthma
   3. Treat acute asthma attack in the hospital
   4. Provide asthma education programs for the teachers in the local schools
   5. Provide scheduled immunizations to people who come to the clinic
4. The nurse caring for a Bosnian community identifies that the children are undervaccinated and the community is unaware of resources. The nurse assesses the community and determines that there is a health clinic within a 5-mile radius. The nurse meets with the community leaders and explains the need for immunizations, the location of the clinic, and the process of accessing health care resources. Which of the following practices is the nurse providing? (Select all that apply.)
   1. Providing community resources for the children
   2. Teaching the community about health promotion and illness prevention
   3. Promoting autonomy in decision-making about health practices
   4. Improving the health care of the community's children
   5. Participating in professional development activities to maintain nursing competency
5. Vulnerable populations of patients are those who are more likely to develop health problems as a result of:
   1. Chronic diseases, homelessness, and poverty
   2. Poverty and limits in access to health care services
   3. Lack of transportation, dependence on others for care, and homelessness
   4. Excess risks, limits in access to health care services, and dependency on others for care
6. Which of the following are major public health problems commonly affecting older adults? (Select all that apply.)
   1. Substance abuse
   2. Confusional states
   3. Financial limitations
   4. Communicable diseases
   5. Acute and chronic physical illnesses
7. Some nurses are collecting data to determine how many adolescents attempt suicide in a community. This is an example of what type of community assessment data?
8. Many older homes in a neighborhood are undergoing a lot of restoration. Lead paint was used. The community clinic in the neighborhood is initiating a lead screening program. This activity is based on which social determinant of health?
9. Following a community assessment that focused on adolescent health behaviors, a nurse determines that a large number of adolescents smoke and designs a smoking cessation program at the youth community center. This is an example of which nursing role:
   1. Educator
   2. Counselor
   3. Collaborator
   4. Case manager
10. A nurse in a community health clinic noticed an increase in the number of positive tuberculosis (TB) skin tests from students in a local high school during the most recent academic year. After comparing these numbers to the previous years, 10% increase in positive tests was found. The nurse contacts the school nurse and the director of the health department. Together they begin to expand their assessment to all students and employees of the school district. The community nurse was acting in which nursing role(s)? (Select all that apply.)
    1. Epidemiologist
    2. Counselor
    3. Collaborator
    4. Case manager
    5. Caregiver
11. A nursing student is giving a presentation to a group of other nursing students about the needs of patients with mental illnesses in the community. The nursing professor needs to clarify the student's presentation when the student states:
    1. "Many patients with mental illness do not have a permanent home."
    2. "Unemployment is a common problem experienced by people with a mental illness."
    3. "The majority of patients with mental illnesses live in long-term care settings."
    4. "Patients with mental illnesses are often at a higher risk for abuse and assault."
12. The nurse in a new community-based clinic is requested to complete a community assessment. Order the steps for completing this assessment.
    1. Structure or locale
    2. Social systems
    3. Population
13. On the basis of an assessment, the nurse identifies an increase in the immigrant population group in the community. How would the nurse determine the health needs of this population? (Select all that apply.)
    1. Identify what the immigrant population views as the two most important health needs.
    2. Apply information from *Healthy People 2020*.
    3. Determine how the population uses available health care resources.
    4. Determine which health care agencies will accept immigrant populations.
    5. Identify perceived barriers for health care.
14. A patient is worried about her 76-year-old grandmother who is in very good health and wants to live at home. The patient's concerns are related to her grandmother's safety. The neighborhood does not have a lot of crime. Using this scenario, which of the following are the most relevant to assess for safety?
    1. Crime rate, locks, lighting, neighborhood traffic
    2. Lighting, locks, clutter, medications
    3. Crime rate, medications, support system, clutter
    4. Locks, lighting, neighborhood traffic, crime rate

15. The public health nurse is working with the county health department on a task force to fully integrate the goals of *Healthy People 2020*. In the immigrant community most of the population does not have a primary care provider, nor do they participate in health promotion activities; the unemployment rate in the community is 25%. How does the nurse determine which goals need to be included or updated? (Select all that apply.)
    1. Assess the health care resources within the community.
    2. Assess the existing health care programs offered by the county health department.
    3. Compare existing resources and programs with *Healthy People 2020* goals.
    4. Initiate new programs to meet *Healthy People 2020* goals.
    5. Implement educational sessions in the schools to focus on nutritional needs of the children.

Answers: 1. 4; **2.** 1, 2, 4, 5; **3.** 1, 2, 4; **4.** 1, 2, 4; **5.** 4; **6.** 1, 2, 3, 5; **7.** Incident rates; **8.** Physical environment; **9.** 2; **10.** 1, 3; **11.** 3; **12.** 1, 3, 2; **13.** 1, 2, 3, 5; **14.** 2; **15.** 1, 2, 3.

Rationales for Review Questions can be found on the Evolve website.

REFERENCES

American Nurses Association: *Standards of public health nursing practice*, ed 2, Washington, DC, 2013, The Association.

Camarota S: Immigrants in the United States: a profile of America's foreign born population, *Center for Immigration Studies*, 2012, http://cis.org/2012-profile-of-americas-foreign-born-population.

Centers for Disease Control and Prevention (CDC): *Adolescent and school health, health disparities*, 2014a, http://www.cdc.gov/healthyyouth/disparities/.

Centers for Disease Control and Prevention (CDC): *Social determinants of health, definitions*, 2014b, http://www.cdc.gov/socialdeterminants/Definitions.html.

Happell B, Cleary M: Promoting health and preventing illness: promoting mental health in community nursing practice, *Contemp Nurse* 41(1):88, 2012.

Jackson D, Saltman D: Recognising the impact of social exclusion: the need for advocacy and activism in health care, *Contemp Nurse* 40(1):57, 2011.

Jackson D, et al: Family and community health nursing: challenges and moving forward, *Contemp Nurse* 43(1):141, 2012.

Landenburger KM, Campbell JC: Violence and human abuse. In Stanhope M, Lancaster J, editors: *Foundations of nursing in the community: community-oriented practice*, ed 4, St Louis, 2014, Mosby.

Olson KI, et al: Cornerstones of public health nursing, *Public Health Nurs* 28(3):249, 2011.

Piper M: Community empowerment for health visiting and other public health nursing, *Community Pract* 84(8):28, 2011.

Prochaska T, et al: *Public health for an aging society*, Baltimore, MD, 2012, John Hopkins University Press.

Sebastian JG: Vulnerability and vulnerable populations: an overview. In Stanhope M, Lancaster J, editors: *Foundations of nursing in the community: community-oriented practice*, ed 4, St Louis, 2014, Mosby.

Stanhope M, Lancaster J: *Foundations of nursing in the community: community-oriented practice*, ed 4, St Louis, 2014, Mosby.

US Department of Health and Human Services [USDHHS]: *Public Health Service: Healthy People 2020: a systematic approach to health improvement*, Washington, DC, 2015 update, US Government Printing Office. http://www.healthypeople.gov/2020/topicsobjectives2020/default.

RESEARCH REFERENCES

Borrow S, et al: Community-based child health nurses: an exploration of current practice, *Contemp Nurse* 40(1):71, 2011.

Chan ECY, et al: A community-based intervention to promote informed decision making for prostate cancer screening among Hispanic American men changed knowledge and role preferences: a cluster RCT, *Patient Educ Couns* 84(2):e44, 2011.

Gash J, McIntosh GV: Gender matters: health beliefs of women as a predictor of participation in prostate cancer screening among African American men, *Diversity Equality Health Care* 10(1):23, 2013.

Kirkpatrick P, et al: Research to support evidence-based practice in COPD community nursing, *Br J Community Nurs* 17(10):486, 2012.

Rew L, et al: Development of a dynamic model to guide health disparities research, *Nurs Outlook* 57(3):132, 2009.

4

Theoretical Foundations of Nursing Practice

OBJECTIVES

- Explain the influence of nursing theory on a nurse's approach to practice.
- Describe types of nursing theories.
- Describe the relationship among nursing theory, the nursing process, and patient needs.
- Review selected nursing theories.
- Review selected shared theories from other disciplines.
- Describe theory-based nursing practice.

KEY TERMS

Assumptions, p. 42
Conceptual framework, p. 42
Concepts, p. 42
Content, p. 45
Descriptive theories, p. 44
Domain, p. 42
Environment/situation, p. 43
Feedback, p. 45
Grand theories, p. 44
Health, p. 42
Input, p. 45
Middle-range theories, p. 44
Nursing, p. 43
Nursing metaparadigm, p. 42
Nursing theory, p. 41
Output, p. 45
Paradigm, p. 42
Person, p. 42
Phenomenon, p. 42
Practice theories, p. 44
Prescriptive theories, p. 44
Shared theory, p. 45
Theory, p. 41

MEDIA RESOURCES

http://evolve.elsevier.com/Potter/fundamentals/

- Review Questions
- Case Study with Questions
- Audio Glossary
- Content Updates

Providing patient-centered nursing care is an expectation for all nurses. As you progress through your nursing classes, you will learn to apply knowledge from nursing; social, physical and biobehavioral sciences; ethics; and health policy. Theory-based nursing practice helps you to design and implement nursing interventions that address individual and family responses to health problems. Some nurses find nursing theory difficult to understand or appreciate. However, as your knowledge about theories improves, you will find that they help to describe, explain, predict, and/or prescribe nursing care measures. Common questions nurses have about theory include: What is theory? How are nursing theories created? Why is theory important to the nursing profession? This chapter answers these questions and will help you understand how to use theory in your nursing practice.

Imagine that you are building a house. You need to complete the foundation before you start building the walls. Without a strong foundation, the house will not stand. Such is the case with nursing practice. Theory serves as the foundation for the art and science of nursing. Nurses use theory every day but are not always aware of it. For example, when a nurse ensures that a patient's room is free of clutter, excess noise, and soiled linens, she or he is using Florence Nightingale's environmental theory to promote healing and comfort. When encouraging a patient to set goals for his recovery, a nurse is using Imogene King's theory of goal attainment. A nurse uses Dorothea Orem's self-care deficit theory when feeding or bathing a patient until the patient is able to do this independently. Even though the term *theory* may sound intimidating, you will find that it is a standard part of everyday nursing practice.

The scientific work used to develop theories expands the scientific knowledge of the profession. Theories offer well-grounded rationales for how and why nurses perform specific interventions and for predicting patient behaviors and outcomes. Expertise in nursing is a result of knowledge and clinical experience. Nursing knowledge improves nursing practice by connecting theory and research. Theory, research, and practice are bound together in a continuous interactive relationship (Figure 4-1). Nurses develop theories to explain the relationship among variables by testing the theory through research and applying it in practice. Throughout this process new information often comes to light that indicates the need to revise a theory, and the cycle repeats (McEwen and Wills, 2014). Throughout your nursing career you need to reflect and learn from your experiences to grow professionally and use well-developed theories as a basis for your approach to patient care.

THEORY

What is theory? A **theory** helps explain an event by defining ideas or concepts, explaining relationships among the concepts, and predicting outcomes (McEwen and Wills, 2014). In the case of nursing, theories are designed to explain a phenomenon such as self-care or caring.

A **nursing theory** conceptualizes an aspect of nursing to describe, explain, predict, or prescribe nursing care (Meleis, 2012). Theories

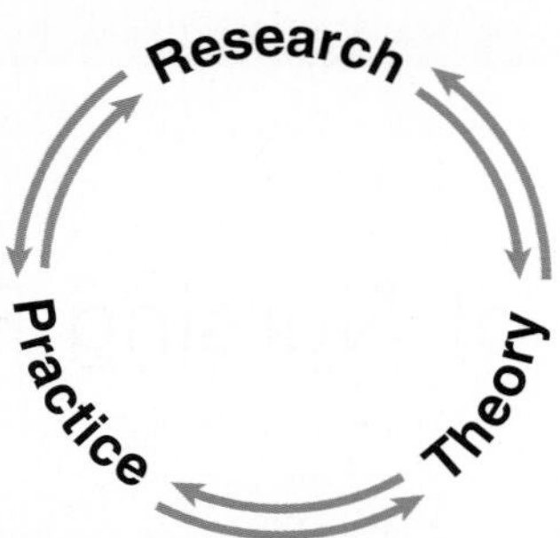

FIGURE 4-1 Cyclical relationship among theory, research, and practice. (Adapted from McEwen M, Wills EM: *Theoretical basis for nursing,* ed 4, Philadelphia, 2014, Wolters Kluwer Health.)

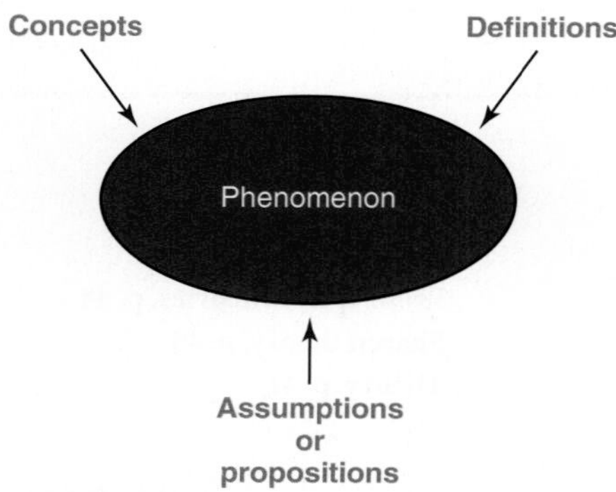

FIGURE 4-2 Components of a nursing theory.

offer a perspective for assessing your patients' situations. They also help you organize, analyze, and interpret data. For example, if you use Orem's theory in practice, you assess and interpret data to determine patients' self-care needs, deficits, and abilities in the management of their disease. Orem's theory then guides your development of patient-centered nursing interventions.

Nursing is both a science and an art. The *science* of nursing is based on data obtained from current research, whereas the *art* of nursing stems from a nurse's experience and the unique caring relationship that a nurse develops with a patient (McEwen and Wills, 2014). A nursing theory helps to identify the focus, means, and goals of practice. Nursing theories enhance communication and accountability for patient care (Meleis, 2012).

Components of a Theory

A theory contains a set of concepts, definitions, and assumptions or propositions that explain a phenomenon. It explains how these elements are uniquely related in the phenomenon (Figure 4-2). These components provide a foundation of knowledge for nurses to direct and deliver caring nursing practices. Researchers test theories, and as a result they gain a clearer perspective and understanding of all parts of a phenomenon.

Phenomenon. Nursing theories focus on the phenomena of nursing and nursing care. A **phenomenon** is the term, description, or label given to describe an idea or responses about an event, a situation, a process, a group of events, or a group of situations (Meleis, 2012). Phenomena may be temporary or permanent. Examples of phenomena of nursing include caring, self-care, and patient responses to stress.

Concepts. A theory also consists of interrelated concepts that help describe or label phenomena. "Concepts are the words or phrases that identify, define, and establish structure and boundaries for ideas generated about a particular phenomenon" (Johnson and Webber, 2014, p. 18). Think of **concepts** as ideas and mental images. They can be abstract such as emotions or concrete such as physical objects (McEwen and Wills, 2014). For example, in Watson's transpersonal theory of caring (see Chapter 7), concepts include meeting human needs and instilling faith-hope (Watson, 2010). Theories use concepts to communicate meaning.

Definitions. Theorists use definitions to communicate the general meaning of the concepts of a theory. Definitions may be *theoretical/conceptual* or *operational.* Theoretical or conceptual definitions simply define a particular concept, much like what can be found in a dictionary, based on the theorist's perspective (Meleis, 2012; McEwen and Wills, 2014). Operational definitions state how concepts are measured (Johnson and Webber, 2014). For example, a nursing concept *conceptually* defines pain as physical discomfort and *operationally* as a patient reporting a score of three or above on a pain scale of zero to ten.

Assumptions. **Assumptions** are the "taken-for-granted" statements that explain the nature of the concepts, definitions, purpose, relationships, and structure of a theory. Assumptions are accepted as *truths* and are based on values and beliefs (Masters, 2015; Meleis, 2012). For example, Watson's transpersonal caring theory has the assumption that a conscious intention to care promotes healing and wholeness (Watson, 2010).

The Domain of Nursing

The **domain** is the perspective or territory of a profession or discipline (Meleis, 2012). It provides the subject, central concepts, values and beliefs, phenomena of interest, and central problems of a discipline. The domain of nursing provides both a practical and theoretical aspect of the discipline. It is the knowledge of nursing practice and nursing history, nursing theory, education, and research. The domain of nursing gives nurses a comprehensive perspective that allows you to identify and treat patients' health care needs in all health care settings.

A **paradigm** is a pattern of beliefs used to describe the domain of a discipline. It links the concepts, theories, beliefs, values, and assumptions accepted and applied by the discipline (McEwen and Wills, 2014). Often used synonymously with paradigm is the term **conceptual framework.** A conceptual framework provides a way to organize major concepts and visualize the relationship among phenomena. Different frameworks provide alternative ways to view the subject matter of a discipline and represent the perspective of the author. For example, the grand theorists all address similar concepts in their respective theories, but each theorist defines and describes the concepts in a different way on the basis of the theorist's own ideas and experiences (Fawcett and DeSanto-Mayeda, 2013).

The **nursing metaparadigm** allows nurses to understand and explain what nursing *is,* what nursing *does,* and *why* nurses do what they do (Fawcett and DeSanto-Mayeda, 2013). The nursing metaparadigm includes the four concepts of person (or human beings), health, environment/situation, and nursing. **Person** is the recipient of nursing care, including individual patients, groups, cultures, families, and communities. The person is central to the nursing care you provide. Because each person's needs are often complex, it is important to provide individualized patient-centered care. **Health** has different meanings for each patient, the clinical setting, and the health care profession (see Chapter 6). It is a state of being that people define in relation to their own values, personality, and lifestyle. It is dynamic and continuously changing. Your challenge as a nurse is to provide the best possible care based on a patient's level of health and health care needs at the time of care delivery.

Environment/situation includes all possible conditions affecting patients and the settings where they go for their health care. There is a continuous interaction between a patient and the environment. This interaction has positive and negative effects on a person's level of health and health care needs. Factors in the home, school, workplace, or community all influence the level of these needs. For example, an adolescent girl with type 1 diabetes needs to adapt her treatment plan to adjust for physical activities of school, the demands of a part-time job, and the timing of social events such as her prom.

Nursing is the "… protection, promotion, and optimization of health and abilities, prevention of illness and injury, alleviation of suffering through the diagnosis and treatment of human response, and advocacy in the care of individuals, families, communities, and populations" (ANA, 2014). The scope of nursing is broad. For example, a nurse does not medically diagnose a patient's health condition as heart failure. However, he or she assesses a patient's response to the decrease in activity tolerance as a result of the disease and develops *nursing diagnoses* of fatigue, activity intolerance, and ineffective coping (see Chapter 17). From these nursing diagnoses the nurse creates a patient-centered plan of care for each of the patient's health problems (see Chapter 18). Use critical thinking skills to integrate knowledge, experience, attitudes, and standards into the individualized plan of care for each of your patients (see Chapter 15).

Evolution of Nursing Theory. How are theories created? Nursing theories often build on the works of prior theories. Florence Nightingale is generally regarded as the first nursing theorist; her theory was founded on her belief that nursing could improve a patient's environment to facilitate recovery and prevent complications. In the Nightingale era nurses were trained to observe each patient's condition and report changes to the doctor, thus beginning the status of nursing as subservient to the physician—a sign of the Victorian era in which Nightingale lived (Warelow, 2013).

With the twentieth century approaching, nursing began to transition from a vocation to a profession, which prompted American nurses to standardize nursing education in diploma programs and encouraged more nurses to seek academic degrees. The first national gathering of nurses occurred at the World's Fair in Chicago in 1893, and the first edition of the *American Journal of Nursing* (AJN) was published in 1900 (Alligood, 2014). The "curriculum era" of nursing spanned the 1900s to the 1940s. During this period nursing education expanded beyond basic anatomy and physiology courses to include courses in the social sciences, pharmacology, and "nursing arts" that addressed nursing actions, skills, and procedures (Alligood, 2014).

The "research era" encompassed the 1950s, '60s, and '70s, during which nurses became increasingly involved in conducting studies and sharing their findings. However, the earliest research studies had a psycho-social, anthropological, or educational focus. Nurses studied their own attitudes, their relationships with other disciplines, and their functions in work and political settings. In the early years, nursing research did not explore clinical questions based on the medical model of research because the discipline was attempting to show its uniqueness from medicine. At this same time the "graduate education era" began, and early versions of nursing theories were developed that offered more structure to nursing research. The renowned theorists of this time period included Johnson, King, Levine, Neuman, Orem, Rogers, and Roy (Alligood, 2014).

The *theory* era, which included the 1980s and 1990s, significantly contributed to knowledge development, and the nursing metaparadigm was proposed by Fawcett. This era resulted in the publication of several nursing journals, the development of nursing conferences, and the offering of more doctoral programs in nursing (Alligood, 2014).

The twenty-first century is considered the era of *theory utilization.* Today nurses strive to provide evidence-based practice (EBP), which stems from theory, research, and experience. The focus of EBP is safe, comprehensive, individualized, quality health care (see Chapter 5). The original *grand* theories served as springboards for the development of the more modern *middle-range* theories, which, through testing in research studies, provided "evidence" for EBP and promoted the translation of research into practice. Theory use is congruent with current national goals for quality health care (Alligood, 2014).

Historical eras of knowledge development in nursing are represented in Table 4-1. Nursing theories have changed over time in response to changes in society and the world. The environment of war was a primary factor in developing Nightingale's theory. At the other end of the nursing spectrum Rogers' vision of aerospace nursing was developed during the 1980s when the advent of the space shuttle program made the concept of space travel a possible reality for everyone (Warelow, 2013).

TABLE 4-1 Historical Eras of Knowledge Development in Nursing

Historical Areas	Major Question	Emphasis	Outcomes	Emerging Goal
Curriculum era: 1900 to the 1940s	What curriculum content should student nurses study?	Courses taught in nursing programs	Standardized curricula for diploma programs	Specialized knowledge and higher education
Research era: 1950 to the 1970s	What is focus for nursing research?	Role for nurses and what to research	Problem studies and studies of nurses	Theory-based studies for unified knowledge
Graduate education era: 1950 to the 1970s	What knowledge is needed for nursing practice?	Carving out an advanced role and basis for nursing pracice	Nurses have an important role in quality health care	Focus graduate education on knowledge development
Theory era: 1980 to the 1990s	How do these frameworks guide research and practice?	The many ways to think about nursing	Nursing theoretical works clearly focus on the patient	Guide nursing research and practice
Theory utilization era: twenty-first century	Which new theories are needed as evidence for quality care?	Nursing theory as a guide for research, practice, education, and administration	Middle-range theories are from quanititative or qualitative approaches	Nursing frameworks as the knowledge (evidence) for quality care

From Alligood MR: *Nursing theory: utilization and application,* ed 5, St Louis, 2014, Mosby.

BOX 4-1 Goals of Theoretical Nursing Models

- Identify domain and goals of nursing.
- Provide knowledge to improve nursing administration, practice, education, and research.
- Guide research to expand the knowledge base of nursing.
- Identify research techniques and tools used to validate nursing interventions.
- Develop curriculum plans for nursing education.
- Establish criteria for measuring quality of nursing care, education, and research.
- Guide development of a nursing care delivery system.
- Provide systematic structure and rationale for nursing activities.

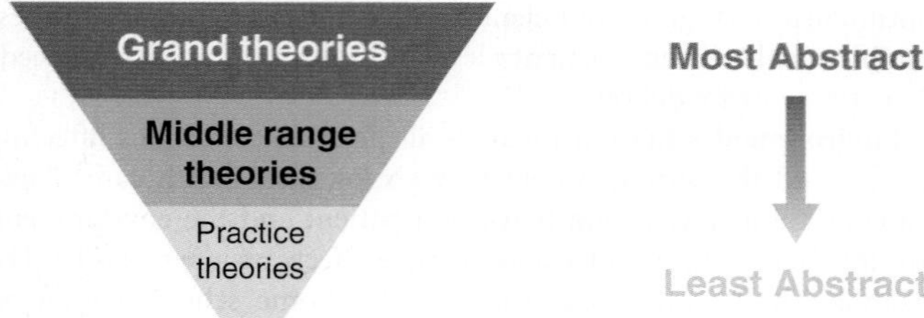

FIGURE 4-3 Correlation of theory category with level of abstraction. (Adapted from McEwen M, Wills EM: *Theoretical basis for nursing,* ed 4, Philadelphia, 2014, Wolters Kluwer Health.)

Theorists developed their theories from their own experiences in nursing education and nursing practice and from knowledge gained from the disciplines of philosophy, sociology, psychology, and anthropology. Many nursing theorists revise their theories over time to remain current with health care changes. Such evolution shows that theories are not stagnant; rather they are dynamic and responsive to the changing environment in which we live (Warelow, 2013).

Types of Theory

The unique theories of a discipline help to distinguish the discipline from other professions. Before the development of nursing theories, nursing was considered to be a task-oriented occupation that functioned under the direction of the medical profession (McEwen and Wills, 2014). "The primary use of theory is to provide insights about nursing practice situations and guide research" and to provide a guideline or explanation of why nurses do what they do (Meleis, 2012, p. 35). Theories have different purposes and are sometimes classified by levels of abstraction (grand versus middle-range versus practice theories) or the goals of the theory (descriptive or prescriptive). For example, a descriptive theory describes a phenomenon such as grief or caring and also identifies conditions or factors that predict a phenomenon. A prescriptive theory details nursing interventions for a specific phenomenon and the expected outcome of the care. Box 4-1 summarizes goals of theoretical nursing models.

Grand theories are abstract, broad in scope, and complex; therefore they require further clarification through research so they can be applied to nursing practice. A grand theory does not provide guidance for *specific* nursing interventions; but it provides the structural framework for general, global ideas about nursing. Grand theories intend to answer the question, "What is nursing" and focus on the *whole* of nursing rather than on a *specific* type of nursing. The grand theorists developed their works based on their own experiences and the time in which they were living, which helps to explain why there is so much variation among the theories. Grand theories address the nursing metaparadigm components of person, nursing, health, and environment.

Middle-range theories are more limited in scope and less abstract. They address a specific phenomenon and reflect practice (administration, clinical, or teaching). A middle-range theory tends to focus on a concept found in a specific field of nursing such as uncertainty, incontinence, social support, quality of life, and caring rather than reflect on a wide variety of nursing care situations as the grand theories do (Meleis, 2012). For example, Kolcaba's theory of comfort encourages nurses to meet patients' needs for comfort in physical, psychospiritual, environmental, and sociocultural realms (Krinsky et al, 2014). Like many middle-range theories, Kolcaba's theory was based on the works of a grand theorist—in this case, Nightingale. Middle-range theories are also sometimes developed from research, nursing practice, or the theories of other disciplines (McEwen and Wills, 2014; Meleis, 2012).

Practice theories, also known as situation-specific theories, bring theory to the bedside. Narrow in scope and focus, these theories guide the nursing care of a *specific* patient population at a *specific* time (Meleis, 2012). An example of a practice theory is a pain-management protocol for patients recovering from cardiac surgery. "Practice theories have had the benefit of trial and error through clinical practice" and are often easier to understand and apply than the grand and middle-range theories (Warelow, 2013, p. 41). Figure 4-3 demonstrates the level of abstraction for each of the grand, middle-range, and practice theory categories.

Descriptive theories are the first level of theory development. They describe phenomena and identify circumstances in which the phenomena occur (Meleis, 2012). For example, theories of growth and development describe the maturation processes of an individual at various ages (see Chapter 11). Descriptive theories do not direct specific nursing activities or attempt to produce change but rather help to explain patient assessments.

Prescriptive theories address nursing interventions for a phenomenon, guide practice change, and predict the consequences. Nurses use prescriptive theories to anticipate the outcomes of nursing interventions (McEwen and Wills, 2014).

Theory-Based Nursing Practice

Why is theory important to the nursing profession? Nursing knowledge is derived from basic and nursing sciences, experience, aesthetics, nurses' attitudes, and standards of practice. As nursing continues to grow as a practice-oriented profession, new knowledge is needed to prescribe specific interventions to improve patient outcomes. Nursing theories and related concepts continue to evolve. Florence Nightingale spoke with firm conviction about the "nature of nursing as a profession that requires knowledge distinct from medical knowledge" (Nightingale, 1860). The overall goal of nursing knowledge is to explain the practice of nursing as different and distinct from the practice of medicine, psychology, and other health care disciplines. Theory generates nursing knowledge for use in practice, thus supporting EBP (see Chapter 5). The integration of theory into practice leads to coordinated care delivery and therefore serves as the basis for nursing (McEwen and Wills, 2014).

The nursing process is used in clinical settings to determine individual patient needs (see Unit III). Although the nursing process is central to nursing, it is not a theory. It provides a systematic process for the delivery of nursing care, not the knowledge component of the discipline. However, nurses use theory to provide direction in how to *use* the nursing process. For example, the theory of caring influences what nurses need to assess, how to determine patient needs, how to

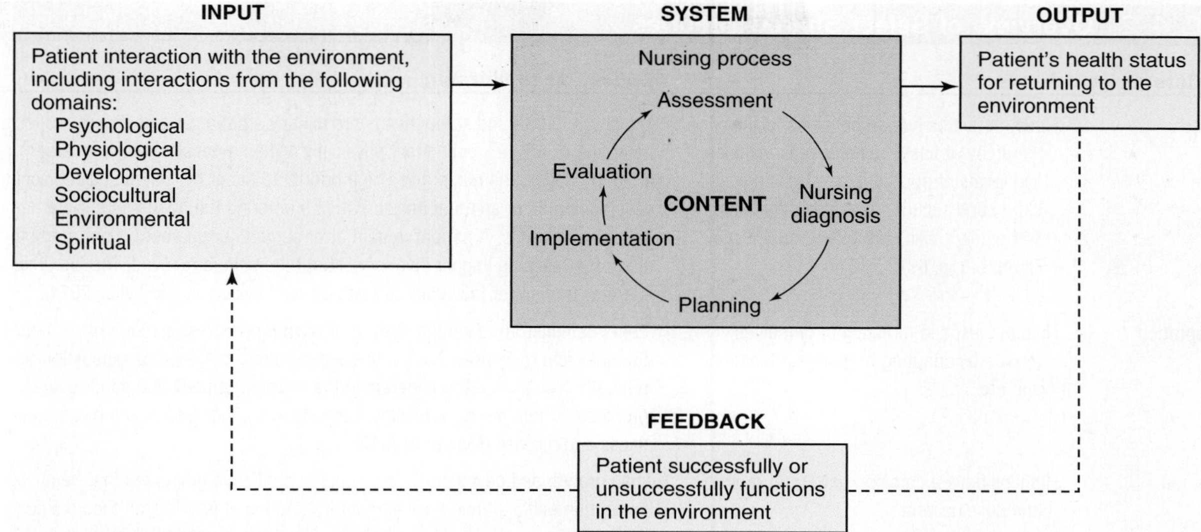

FIGURE 4-4 Providing nursing services in assisted-living facilities promotes physical and psychosocial health.

plan care, how to select individualized nursing interventions, and how to evaluate patient outcomes.

SHARED THEORIES

To practice in today's health care systems, nurses need a strong scientific knowledge base from nursing and other disciplines such as the biomedical, sociological, and behavioral sciences. Also known as a *borrowed* or *interdisciplinary* theory, a **shared theory** explains a phenomenon specific to the discipline that developed the theory (McEwen and Wills, 2014). For example, Piaget's theory of cognitive development helps to explain how children think, reason, and perceive the world (see Chapter 11). Knowledge and use of this theory help pediatric nurses design appropriate therapeutic play interventions for ill toddlers or school-age children. Knowles's adult learning theory helps a nurse plan and provide appropriate discharge teaching for a patient who is recovering from surgery. Several nursing theories are based on systems theory, and the nursing process is also a system (Figure 4-4). Like all systems, the nursing process has a specific purpose or goal (see Unit III). The goal of the nursing process is to organize and deliver patient-centered care. As a system the nursing process has the following components: input, output, feedback, and content. **Input** for the nursing process is the data or information that comes from a patient's assessment. **Output** is the end product of a system; and in the case of the nursing process it is whether the patient's health status improves, declines, or remains stable as a result of nursing care.

Feedback serves to inform a system about how it functions. For example, in the nursing process the outcomes reflect the patient's responses to nursing interventions. The outcomes are part of the feedback system to refine the plan of care. Other forms of feedback in the nursing process include responses from family members and consultation from other health care professionals.

The **content** is the product and information obtained from the system. For example, patients with impaired bed mobility have common skin care needs and interventions (e.g., hygiene and scheduled positioning changes) that are very successful in reducing the risk for pressure ulcers. Table 4-2 provides an overview of additional select shared theories that are often used in nursing practice.

SELECT NURSING THEORIES

Definitions and theories of nursing can help you understand the practice of nursing. The following sections describe select theories and their concepts. See Table 4-3 for a review of additional grand and middle-range nursing theories.

Nightingale's Environmental Theory

Known as the founder of modern nursing, Florence Nightingale is credited with developing the first nursing theory. The focus of Nightingale's grand theory is a patient's environment, which Nightingale believed nurses should manipulate (e.g., ventilation, light, decreased noise, hygiene, nutrition) so nature is able to restore a patient to health (McEwen and Wills, 2014). Through observation and data collection, she linked the patient's health status with environmental factors and initiated improved hygiene and sanitary conditions during the Crimean War. Nightingale taught and used the nursing process, noting that "vital observation [assessment] ... is not for the sake of piling up miscellaneous information or curious facts, but for the sake of saving life and increasing health and comfort" (Nightingale, 1860).

Peplau's Interpersonal Theory

Hildegard Peplau is considered to be the mother of psychiatric nursing; the focus of her middle-range theory includes interpersonal relations among a nurse, a patient, and a patient's family and developing the nurse-patient relationship (McEwen and Wills, 2014). According to Peplau, nurses help patients reduce anxiety by converting it into constructive actions (McEwen and Wills, 2014). They develop therapeutic relationships with patients that are respectful, empathetic, and nonjudgmental (Senn, 2013). The following phases characterize the nurse-patient interpersonal relationship: preorientation (data gathering), orientation (defining issue), working phase (therapeutic activity), and resolution (termination of relationship). In developing a nurse-patient relationship, the nurse serves as a resource person, counselor, and surrogate. For example, when a patient seeks help, the nurse and patient first discuss the nature of any problems, and the nurse explains the services available. As the nurse-patient relationship develops, the nurse and patient mutually define the problems and potential solutions.

TABLE 4-2 Overview of Select Shared Theories

Theory Categories	Focus	Application to Nursing
Human needs	Need motivates human behavior. Maslow's hierarchy of basic human needs includes five levels of priority (e.g., physiological, safety and security, love and belonging, self-esteem, and self-actualization) (see Figure 6-3, p. 68.).	Basic physiological and safety needs are usually a patient's first priority, especially when he or she is severely dependent physically. When a patient has no emergent physical or safety needs, the nurse gives high priority to his or her psychological, sociocultural, developmental, or spiritual needs. Patients entering the health care system generally have unmet needs. A patient in pain after surgery (basic need) is not ready for discharge teaching (higher level need) until the pain is relieved. The hierarchy of needs is a way to plan for individualized patient care (McEwen and Wills, 2014).
Stress/adaptation	Humans respond to actual or perceived threats by adapting to maintain function and life.	Patients demonstrate a similar pattern of reacting to stress through physiological and psychological responses. Failure to adapt to stress can lead to exhaustion and decline in health. Nurses need to understand the reaction of body and mind to stress and intervene to help patients develop methods of coping/adapting to prevent or manage illness and disease (Master's, 2015).
Developmental	Humans have a common pattern of growth and development.	Human growth and development are orderly, predictive processes that begin with conception and continue through death. Varieties of well-tested theories describe and predict behavior and development at various phases of the life continuum (McEwen and Wills, 2014).
Biomedical	Theory explains causes of disease; principles related to physiology.	Nurses must have knowledge of theories from the fields of biology, medicine, public health, physiology, and pharmacology to provide holistic patient care, promote health, and prevent illness (McEwen and Wills, 2014).
Psychosocial	Theory explains and/or predicts human responses within the physiological, psychological, sociocultural, developmental, and spiritual domains	Nursing is a diverse discipline that strives to meet holistic needs of patients. Chapter 9 discusses models for understanding cultural diversity and implementing care to meet the diverse needs of the patient. Chapter 10 describes family theory and how to meet the needs of the family when the family is the patient or the caregiver. Chapter 37 discusses several models of grieving and demonstrates how to help patients through loss, death, and grief.
Educational	Theory explains the teaching-learning process by examining behavioral, cognitive, and adult learning principles.	Nurses provide education to patients, families, community groups, and members of the health care team. A basic understanding of various teaching-learning theories is critical for this aspect of the professional nursing role (Butts and Rich, 2015).
Leadership/ management	Theory promotes organization, change, power/empowerment, motivation, conflict management, and decision-making.	Nurses often assume leadership positions in the health care realm and as such are expected to effectively manage individuals and groups to promote change and improve quality care and outcomes (McEwen and Wills, 2014).

TABLE 4-3 Overview of Select Grand and Middle-Range Nursing Theories

Theory Category	Theorist	Focus	Application
Grand theory	Henderson	Principles and practice of nursing	Nurses assist patients with 14 activities (breathing, eating/drinking, elimination, movement/positioning, sleep/rest, clothing, body temperature, hygiene, safety, communication/socialization/play, practice of faith, learning) until patients can meet these needs for themselves; or they help patients have a peaceful death (Butts and Rich, 2015; McEwen and Wills, 2014).
	Johnson	Behavioral system	Nurses perceive patients as being more important than their disease; a patient is viewed as a collection of subsystems that form an overall behavioral system focused on meeting basic drives of achievement, affiliation, aggression/protection, dependence, elimination, ingestion, sex, and restoration. The goal of nursing is to help the patient attain/maintain balance, function, and stability in each of the subsystems (Butts and Rich, 2015).
	Neuman	Systems	Nurses view a patient (physical, psychological, sociocultural, developmental, and spiritual) as being an open system that is in constant energy exchange with both internal and external environments. Nurses help a patient/client (individual, group, family, or community) cope with intrapersonal, interpersonal, and extra-personal *stressors* that can break through the patient's line of defense and cause illness. The role of nursing is to stabilize a patient or situation, and the focus is on *wellness* and *prevention* of disease (McEwen and Wills, 2014).

TABLE 4-3 Overview of Select Grand and Middle-Range Nursing Theories—cont'd

Theory Category	Theorist	Focus	Application
	Abdellah	Patient-centered care	Nurses address 21 "nursing problems" to meet patients' physical, psychological, and social needs and should strive to *know* each patient. Nurses use knowledge constructed from previous experiences to determine a general plan of care and then personalizes the plan to the patient to provide *patient-centered care.* A nurse should involve a patient's family in the plan of care (McEwen and Wills, 2014).
	Levine	Conservation	Nurses promote *balance* between nursing interventions and patient participation to help patients *conserve energy* needed for healing; *conserve structural integrity* by limiting the extent of tissue involvement/damage; *conserve personal integrity* by involving them in their care decisions; and *conserve social integrity* by facilitating patient interactions with family and loved ones (Johnson and Webber, 2014).
	King	Goal attainment	Nurses view a patient as a unique personal system that is constantly interacting/transacting with other systems (e.g., nurse, family, friends); nurses help patients become active participants in their care by working *with* them to establish goals for attaining, restoring, or maintaining health (Johnson and Webber, 2014; McEwen and Wills, 2014).
	Roy	Adaptation	Nurses help a patient cope with or adapt to changes in physiological, self-concept, role function, and interdependence domains (Masters, 2015).
	Erickson-Tomlin-Swain	Modeling/role modeling	Nurses understand a patient's *model of the world* or world view (e.g., how the patient thinks, acts, feels, communicates) and help a patient use internal and external resources to make appropriate changes *(role modeling)* to attain optimal health (McEwen and Wills, 2014).
	Watson	Caring	Nurses understand that caring is a fundamental component of professional nursing practice and is based on 10 *carative factors* (see Chapter 7). The purpose of nursing is to understand the interrelationship among health, illness, and human behavior rather than focus on the disease-cure model. Caring occurs when a nurse and patient engage in a *transpersonal relationship* that facilitates the patient's ability for self-healing (Johnson and Webber, 2014).
	Rogers/Parse/Newman	Unitary beings/human becoming/expanding consciousness	Nurses view a patient as a unique, dynamic energy field in constant energy exchange with the environment; nursing care focuses on helping a patient use his or her *own* potential to identify and alter personal rhythms/patterns (e.g., eating, breathing, sleeping, communicating, touching) to promote and maintain health. Nurses understand that patients are responsible for their own health and that health stems from how patients live their lives in accordance with their own values; the nurse's role is to be truly *present* with the patient and accepting of his or her view of reality while providing guidance to the patient in making health-related choices in accordance with his or her belief system (Johnson and Webber, 2014; McEwen and Wills, 2014).
Middle-range theory	Benner	Skill acquisition	Nurses progress through five stages of skill acquisition: novice, advanced beginner, competent, proficient, and expert (Butts and Rich, 2015).
	Kolcaba	Comfort	Nurses facilitate health-seeking behaviors in patients by striving to relieve physical, emotional, social, environmental, and/or spiritual distress (McEwen and Wills, 2014).
	Pender	Health promotion	Nurses understand that a patient's personal characteristics, experiences, and beliefs affect his or her motivation for adopting healthy behaviors (see Chapter 6) (McEwen and Wills, 2014).
	American Association of Critical-Care Nurses	Synergy	Matching nurse competencies to patient needs in the critical care environment improves patient outcomes (McEwen and Wills, 2014).
	Mishel	Uncertainty in illness	Nurses facilitate patient coping and adaptation by performing interventions aimed at helping patients process and find meaning related to their illness (Adelstein et al., 2014).
	Eakes, Burke, and Hainsworth	Chronic sorrow	Nurses understand that the disparity between *desired* and *actual* reality often leads to continuous cycles of grief. For example, chronic sorrow sometimes occurs in parents of children with disabilities or in individuals diagnosed with a chronic illness (Vitale and Falco, 2014).

When the patient's original needs are resolved, new needs sometimes emerge. This middle-range theory is useful in establishing effective nurse-patient communication when obtaining a nursing history, providing patient education, or counseling patients and their families (see Chapter 24).

Orem's Self-Care Deficit Nursing Theory

Dorothea Orem's theory is commonly used in nursing practice (Alligood, 2014). When applying this grand theory, a nurse continually assesses a patient's ability to perform self-care and intervenes as needed to ensure that the patients meets physical, psychological, sociological, and developmental needs. According to Orem, people who participate in self-care activities are more likely to improve their health outcomes (Rustøen et al., 2014). Nursing care becomes necessary when patients are unable to fulfill biological, psychological, developmental, or social needs. Nurses continually assess and determine why patients are unable to meet these needs, identify goals to help them, intervene to help them perform self-care, and evaluate how much self-care they are able to perform. For example, a patient may need a nurse to bathe or feed him or her while acutely ill; but as his or her condition improves, the nurse encourages the patient to begin doing these activities independently.

Leininger's Culture Care Theory

As early as the 1950s Madeleine Leininger recognized the need to focus on culture in nursing as she predicted that nursing and health care would become more global. She blended her background in anthropology with nursing to form her middle-range theory of cultural care diversity and universality (Alligood, 2014). Human caring varies among cultures in its expressions, processes, and patterns. Social structure factors such as a patient's politics, culture, and traditions are significant forces affecting care and influencing the patient's health and illness patterns. Think about the diversity of patients and their nursing care needs (see Chapter 9). The major concept of Leininger's theory is cultural diversity, and the goal of nursing care is to provide a patient with culturally specific nursing care (Alligood, 2014). To provide care to patients of unique cultures, nurses safely integrate their cultural traditions, values, and beliefs into a plan of care. Leininger's theory recognizes the importance of culture and its influence on everything that involves a patient, including health beliefs, the role of family and community, and dietary practices (Alligood, 2014). For example, some cultures believe that the leader of the community needs to be present during health care decisions. As a result, a health care team needs to reschedule when rounds occur to include the community leader. In addition, symptom expression also differs among cultures. A person with an Irish background might be stoic and not complain about pain, whereas a person from a Middle Eastern culture might be very vocal about pain. In both cases a nurse needs to skillfully incorporate the patient's cultural practices in assessing his or her level of pain (e.g., is the pain getting worse or remaining the same?).

QSEN QSEN: BUILDING COMPETENCY IN PATIENT-CENTERED CARE You are caring for a patient from India who is visiting family in the United States. On entering this patient's room, you notice that he has not eaten any of the food on his tray. When you ask if he wasn't hungry, he replies, "I am very hungry, but I cannot eat this food." How could you use *Leininger's culture care theory* to respond to this patient?

Answers to QSEN Activities can be found on the Evolve website.

LINK BETWEEN THEORY AND KNOWLEDGE DEVELOPMENT IN NURSING

Nursing has its own body of knowledge that is both theoretical and experiential. You acquire theoretical knowledge through "reading, observing, or discussing" concepts (Alligood, 2014, p. 123). Theoretical knowledge stimulates thinking and creates a broad understanding of nursing science and practice. Experiential, or clinical, knowledge, often called the *art* of nursing, is formed from nurses' clinical experience. Both types of knowledge are needed to provide safe, comprehensive nursing care.

Nursing theories guide nursing practice (McEwen and Wills, 2014). When using theory-based nursing practice, you apply the principles of a theory in delivering nursing interventions. Grand theories help shape and define your practice; middle-range theories continue to advance nursing knowledge through nursing research; and practice theories help you provide specific care for individuals and groups of diverse populations and situations (Im and Chang, 2012).

Relationship Between Nursing Theory and Nursing Research

Research validates, refutes, supports, and/or modifies theory; and theory stimulates nurse scientists to explore significant issues in nursing practice, leading to the improvement of nursing care (McEwen and Wills, 2014; Meleis, 2012). The relationship between nursing theory and nursing research builds the scientific knowledge base of nursing, which is then applied to practice. Nurses better understand the appropriate use of a theory to improve patient care as more research is conducted. The relationships between the components of a theory often help identify research questions and determine the overall design of a study. For example, nurse researchers used Peplau's interpersonal theory as the framework for a study about standardized shift report as a means of improving nurse-to-nurse communication. The results showed improved patient satisfaction with nursing care (Radtke, 2013).

Sometimes research is used to develop new theories (Meleis, 2012). *Theory-generating* research uses logic to explore relationships among phenomena (McEwen and Wills, 2014). In theory-generating research an investigator makes observations (*without* any preconceived ideas) to view a phenomenon in a new way. Middle-range theories are often developed in this manner. For example, the middle-range theory of chronic sorrow stemmed from a researcher's initial observations of cyclic periods of sadness in parents of children with intellectual or developmental disabilities (Vitale and Falco, 2014).

Theory-testing research determines how accurately a theory describes a nursing phenomenon. Testing develops the evidence for describing or predicting patient outcomes. A researcher has *some* preconceived idea as to how patients describe or respond to a phenomenon and generates research questions or hypotheses to test the assumptions of the theory. No one study tests *all* components of a theory; researchers test the theory through a variety of research activities. For example, nurse researchers studied Kolcaba's middle-range nursing theory of comfort in relation to the pain and discomfort experienced by patients with heart disease. The researchers explored the specific intervention of "quiet time" as a comfort measure in this patient population (Krinsky et al, 2014).

Theory-generating or theory-testing research refines the knowledge base of nursing. As a result, nurses incorporate research-based interventions into theory-based practice (Box 4-2). As research activities continue, not only does the knowledge and science of nursing increase, but patients receive high-quality evidence-based nursing practice (see Chapter 5). As an art, nursing relies on knowledge gained from practice and reflection on past experiences. The "expert nurse" translates both the art and science of nursing into the realm of *creative caring,* which takes the extra step of individualizing care to the specific needs of each patient. For example, a nurse provides creative caring when arranging for a hospitalized patient to visit with a beloved pet or finding a way to honor a patient's wish to die at home.

As you progress in your nursing education and practice, you will use theory in a variety of ways. Keep in mind that these theories are not only applicable to patient care but are also useful in communicating with other members of the health care team. Theory is the

BOX 4-2 EVIDENCE-BASED PRACTICE

Theory-Based Practice in the Management of Patients with Cancer

PICO Question: In patients with cancer (P), how does application of Mishel's uncertainty in illness theory (I) compared to no specific theory application (C) influence physical and psychological coping abilities (O)?

Evidence Summary

Patients with cancer experience many stressors, including pain, side effects of treatment, and an uncertain future. Patients perceive this uncertainty as either a danger or an opportunity. Coping and adaptation to illness depends on reducing the uncertainty in the situation or accepting it as a sign of hope (Adelstein et al., 2014). According to Mishel's theory, people with serious illness improve their coping skills and their quality of life by helping patients "think" about their disease in a way that allows them to find meaning in their illness. This helps patients adapt to their disease and improve their quality of life. Mishel's theory provides a framework for nursing interventions to improve psychological and behavioral outcomes, especially when illness and treatment become very complex, inconsistent, random, and unpredictable (Germino et al., 2013). Although Mishel's uncertainty in illness theory can be applied to any patient experiencing a serious illness, it has been used in several research studies with patients who have cancer. For example, nursing interventions based on this theory have been found to reduce feelings of uncertainty and significantly improve coping strategies to manage uncertainty, self-efficacy, and sexual dysfunction in women with breast cancer (Germino et al., 2013; Kim et al, 2012). Research also supports the use of this theory to enhance adaptation and coping; reduce physical, psychosocial, and spiritual challenges; and achieve positive personal growth in patients who received stem cell transplants as a result of blood cancers (Adelstein, Anderson, and Taylor, 2014). Finally, nursing actions based on Mishel's theory reduced anxiety and preserved quality of life in patients with incurable brain cancer (Cahill et al., 2012).

Application to Nursing Practice

- Promote meaning-making in patients with cancer or other serious illnesses.
- Help patients find meaning in their illness to improve their ability to adapt and cope.
- Implement nursing actions that reduce anxiety and preserve quality of life to balance the uncertainty that occurs when the disease is not curable.
- Recognize that a patient's sense of uncertainty often changes over the course of an illness and its treatment.

foundation of nursing; it defines our unique profession and sets it apart from other disciplines. Theory provides a basis for research and practice and serves as a guide in providing safe, comprehensive, individualized care, which is the hallmark of nursing.

KEY POINTS

- A nursing theory conceptualizes an aspect of nursing to describe, explain, predict, and/or prescribe nursing care.
- Grand theories provide complex structural frameworks for broad, abstract ideas.
- Middle-range theories address specific phenomena or concepts and reflect practice. Thus they are more limited in scope and less abstract.
- Practice or situation-specific theories bring theory to the bedside by focusing on specific types of patients in specific situations.
- The metaparadigm of nursing identifies four concepts of interest to the profession: the person, health, environment/situation, and nursing. These four components are essential to the development of nursing theory.
- Theory generates nursing knowledge used in practice. Nurses use the nursing process to apply the theory or knowledge. The integration of theory and nursing process is the basis for professional nursing.
- Theory-generating research discovers and describes relationships without imposing preconceived notions (e.g., hypotheses) of what the phenomenon under study means.
- Theory-testing research determines how accurately a theory describes nursing phenomena.

CLINICAL APPLICATION QUESTIONS

Preparing for Clinical Practice

1. Your nursing class is debating the issue of the usefulness of grand theories in current practice. Make a case for the applicability of grand theories in modern nursing and describe how nurses can use the original nursing theory—Nightingale's environmental theory—in the following settings:
   a. Critical Care Unit
   b. Emergency Department (ED)
   c. Home Health
2. You are providing care to a patient with chronic obstructive pulmonary disease (COPD) who has been readmitted 3 times within the past month for difficulty breathing. Explain how you would apply Peplau's interpersonal theory to help this patient prevent complications and promote self-management of his disease.
3. For the same patient described previously, how would you apply Orem's self-care deficit theory to help the patient? Compare and contrast the use of Peplau's and Orem's theories for this patient.

ⓔ ***Answers to Clinical Application Questions can be found on the Evolve website.***

REVIEW QUESTIONS

Are You Ready to Test Your Nursing Knowledge?

1. The components of the nursing metaparadigm include:
   1. Person, health, environment, and theory
   2. Health, theory, concepts, and environment
   3. Nurses, physicians, health, and patient needs
   4. Person, health, environment, and nursing
2. Theory is essential to nursing practice because it: (Select all that apply.)
   1. Contributes to nursing knowledge.
   2. Predicts patient behaviors in situations.
   3. Provides a means of assessing patient vital signs.
   4. Guides nursing practice.
   5. Formulates health care legislation.
   6. Explains relationships between concepts.
3. A nurse ensures that each patient's room is clean; well ventilated; and free from clutter, excessive noise, and extremes in temperature. Which theorist's work is the nurse practicing in this example?
   1. Henderson
   2. Orem
   3. King
   4. Nightingale

4. The nurse is caring for a patient admitted to the neurological unit with the diagnosis of a stroke and right-sided weakness. The nurse assumes responsibility for bathing and feeding the patient until the patient is able to begin performing these activities. The nurse in this situation is applying the theory developed by:
1. Neuman.
2. Orem.
3. Roy.
4. Peplau.

5. Match the following types of theory with the appropriate description.

1. Middle-range theory	**a.** Very abstract; attempts to describe nursing in a global context
2. Shared theory	**b.** Specific to a particular situation; brings theory to the bedside
3. Grand theory	**c.** Applies theory from other disciplines to nursing practice
4. Practice theory	**d.** Addresses a specific phenomenon and reflects practice

6. Match the following descriptions to the appropriate grand theorist.

1. King	**a.** Based on the theory that focuses on ***wellness*** and ***prevention*** of disease
2. Henderson	**b.** Based on the belief that people who participate in self-care activities are more likely to improve their health outcomes
3. Orem	**c.** Based on 14 activities, the belief that the nurse should assist patients with meeting needs until they are able to do so independently
4. Neuman	**d.** Based on the belief that nurses should work with patients to develop goals for care

7. Match the following description to the appropriate middle-range theory.

1. Benner's Skill Acquisition	**a.** The nurse strives to relieve patients' distress.
2. AACN's Synergy Model	**b.** The nurse progresses through five stages of expertise.
3. Mishel's Uncertainty in Illness	**c.** The nurse helps the patient to process and find meaning related to his or her illness.
4. Kolcaba's Theory of Comfort	**d.** Matching nurse competencies to patient needs can improve patient outcomes.

8. Which of the following statements related to theory-based nursing practice are correct? (Select all that apply.)
1. Nursing theory differentiates nursing from other disciplines.
2. Nursing theories are standardized and do not change over time.
3. Integrating theory into practice promotes coordinated care delivery.
4. Nursing knowledge is generated by theory.
5. The theory of nursing process is used in planning patient care.
6. Evidence-based practice results from theory-testing research.

9. A nurse is caring for a patient who recently lost a leg in a motor vehicle accident. The nurse best assists the patient to cope with this situation by applying which of the following theories?
1. Roy
2. Levine
3. Watson
4. Johnson

10. Using Maslow's hierarchy of needs, identify the priority for a patient who is experiencing chest pain and difficulty breathing.
1. Self-actualization
2. Air, water, and nutrition
3. Safety
4. Esteem and self-esteem needs

11. Which of the following categories of shared theories would be most appropriate for a patient who is grieving the loss of a spouse?
1. Biomedical
2. Leadership
3. Psychosocial
4. Developmental

12. While working in a rehabilitation facility, it is important to obtain nursing histories and develop a therapeutic nurse-patient relationship. List in correct order the phases of Peplau's theory as applied in this setting. The nurse:
1. Ensures that the patient has access to appropriate community resources for long-term care.
2. Collaborates with the patient to identify specific patient needs.
3. Collects essential information from the patient's health record.
4. Works with the patient to develop a plan for resolving patient issues.

13. Nurses have developed theories in response to: (Select all that apply.)
1. Changes in health care.
2. Prior nursing theories.
3. Changes in nursing practice.
4. Research findings.
5. Government regulations.
6. Theories from other disciplines.
7. Physician opinions.

14. Which of the following types of theory influence the "evidence" in current "evidence-based practice (EBP)"?
1. Grand theory
2. Middle-range theory
3. Practice theory
4. Shared theory

15. A nurse is preparing to begin intravenous fluid therapy for a patient. Which category of theory would be most helpful to the nurse at this time?
1. Grand theory
2. Middle-range theory
3. Practice theory
4. Shared theory

Answers: 1. 4; **2.** 1, 2, 4, 6; **3.** 4; **4.** 2; **5.** 1d, 2c, 3a, 4b; **6.** 1d, 2c, 3b, 4a; **7.** 1b, 2d, 3c, 4a; **8.** 1, 3, 4, 6; **9.** 1; **10.** 2; **11.** 3; **12.** 3, 2, 4, 1; **13.** 1, 2, 3, 4, 6; **14.** 2; **15.** 3.

Ⓔ ***Rationales for Review Questions can be found on the Evolve website.***

REFERENCES

Alligood MR: *Nursing theory utilization & application*, ed 5, St Louis, 2014, Mosby.

American Nurses Association (ANA): *What is nursing?* ©2014, American Nurses Association. http://www.nursingworld.org/EspeciallyForYou/What-is-Nursing. Accessed July 4, 2015.

Butts JB, Rich KL: *Philosophies and theories for advanced nursing practice*, ed 2, Burlington, MA, 2015, Jones & Bartlett Learning.

Fawcett J, DeSanto-Mayeda S: *Contemporary nursing knowledge: analysis and evaluation of nursing models and theories*, ed 3, Philadelphia, 2013, FA Davis.

Im E, Chang SJ: Current trends in nursing theories, *J Nurs Sch* 44(2):156, 2012.

Johnson BM, Webber PB: *An introduction to theory and reasoning in nursing*, ed 4, Philadelphia, PA, 2014, Lippincott Williams & Wilkins.

Masters K: *Nursing theories: a framework for professional practice*, ed 2, Burlington, MA, 2015, Jones & Bartlett Learning.

McEwen M, Wills EM: *Theoretical basis for nursing*, ed 4, Philadelphia, PA, 2014, Lippincott Williams & Wilkins.

Meleis AI: *Theoretical nursing: development & progress*, ed 5, Philadelphia, PA, 2012, Lippincott Williams & Wilkins.

Nightingale F: *Notes on nursing: what it is and what it is not*, London, 1860, Harrison & Sons.

Senn JF: Peplau's theory of interpersonal relations: application in emergency and rural nursing, *Nurs Sci Q* 26(1):31, 2013.

Vitale SA, Falco C: Children born prematurely: risk of parental chronic sorrow, *J Pediatric Nurs* 29:248, 2014.

Warelow PJ: Changing philosophies: a paradigmatic nursing shift from Nightingale, *Aust J Adv Nurs* 31(1):36, 2013.

Watson J: Caring science and the next decade of holistic healing: transforming self and system from the inside out, *Am Holistic Nurses Assoc* 30(2):14, 2010.

RESEARCH REFERENCES

Adelstein KE, et al: Importance of meaning-making for patients undergoing hematopoietic stem cell transplantation, *Oncol Nurs Forum* 42(2):E172, 2014.

Cahill J, et al: Brain tumor symptoms as antecedents to uncertainty: an integrative review, *J Nurs Sch* 44(2):145, 2012.

Germino BB, et al: Outcomes of an uncertainty management intervention in younger African-American and Caucasian breast cancer survivors, *Oncol Nurs Forum* 40(1):82, 2013.

Kim SH, et al: Symptoms and uncertainty in breast cancer survivors in Korea: differences by treatment trajectory, *J Clin Nurs* 21:1014, 2012.

Krinsky R, et al: A practical application of Katharine Kolcaba's comfort theory to cardiac patients, *Appl Nurs Res* 27:147, 2014.

Radtke K: Improving patient satisfaction with nursing communication using bedside shift report, *Clin Nurse Spec* 27(1):19, 2013.

Rustøen T, et al: A randomized clinical trial of the efficacy of a self-care intervention to improve cancer pain management, *Cancer Nurs* 37(1):34, 2014.

5

Evidence-Based Practice

OBJECTIVES

- Discuss the benefits of evidence-based practice.
- Describe the steps of evidence-based practice.
- Develop a PICOT question.
- Explain the levels of evidence available in the literature.
- Discuss ways to apply evidence in practice.
- Explain how nursing research improves nursing practice.
- Discuss the steps of the research process.
- Discuss priorities for nursing research.
- Explain the relationship between evidence-based practice and performance improvement.

KEY TERMS

Bias, p. 58
Clinical guidelines, p. 55
Confidentiality, p. 61
Empirical data, p. 58
Evaluation research, p. 60
Evidence-based practice (EBP), p. 52
Experimental study, p. 59
Generalizability, p. 58
Hypotheses, p. 56
Inductive reasoning, p. 60
Informed consent, p. 61
Nursing research, p. 58
Peer-reviewed, p. 55
Performance improvement (PI), p. 57
PICOT question, p. 54
Qualitative nursing research, p. 60
Quantitative nursing research, p. 59
Reliability, p. 58
Research process, p. 60
Scientific method, p. 58
Validity, p. 58
Variables, p. 56

MEDIA RESOURCES

http://evolve.elsevier.com/Potter/fundamentals/

- Review Questions
- Case Study with Questions
- Audio Glossary
- Content Updates

Rick is a registered nurse (RN) on a general surgical unit. Since he started working there 5 years ago, standard nursing care includes significant patient education, administration of pain medications, and promoting a quiet environment to manage anxiety and pain for patients after surgery. Rick notices that many patients are experiencing higher levels of anxiety and pain, which is interfering with their recovery and delaying their discharge. Rick raises the question with other RNs in the department, "What if we had our patients listen to music after they have surgery? Is it possible that music will help better manage our patients' anxiety and pain?"

Most nurses like Rick practice nursing according to what they learn in nursing school, their experiences in practice, and the policies and procedures of their health care agency. This approach to practice does not guarantee that nursing practice is always based on up-to-date scientific information. Sometimes it is based on tradition and not on current evidence. If Rick went to the scientific literature for articles about how listening music affects postsurgical pain and anxiety, he would find some studies that show having patients listen to music following surgery sometimes helps them recover more quickly. The evidence from research and the opinions of nursing experts provide a basis for Rick and his colleagues to make evidence-based changes to their care of patients following surgery. The use of evidence in practice enables clinicians like Rick to provide the highest quality of care to their patients and families.

THE NEED FOR EVIDENCE-BASED PRACTICE

Quality and cost issues drive the direction of the current health care environment (Garner et al., 2013). As a professional nurse you are accountable and responsible for providing the best nursing care possible. People are more informed about their own health and the incidence of medical errors within health care institutions across the country. Evidence-based care improves quality, safety, patient outcomes, and nurse satisfaction while reducing costs (Melnyk and Fineout-Overholt, 2014). Thus implementing **evidence-based practice (EBP)** helps you make effective, timely, and appropriate clinical decisions in response to the broad political, professional, and societal forces present in today's health care environment (Peterson et al., 2014).

Nurses make important clinical decisions when caring for patients (e.g., what to assess in a patient and which interventions are best to use). It is important to translate best evidence into best practices at a patient's bedside. For example, changing how patients' pain is managed after surgery is one way that Rick uses evidence at the bedside (see previous case study). EBP is a problem-solving approach to clinical practice that integrates the conscientious use of best evidence in combination with a clinician's expertise and patient preferences and values in making decisions about patient care (Figure 5-1) (Melnyk and Fineout-Overholt, 2014). Today EBP is an expectation of all health care institutions and professional nurses (Peterson et al., 2014).

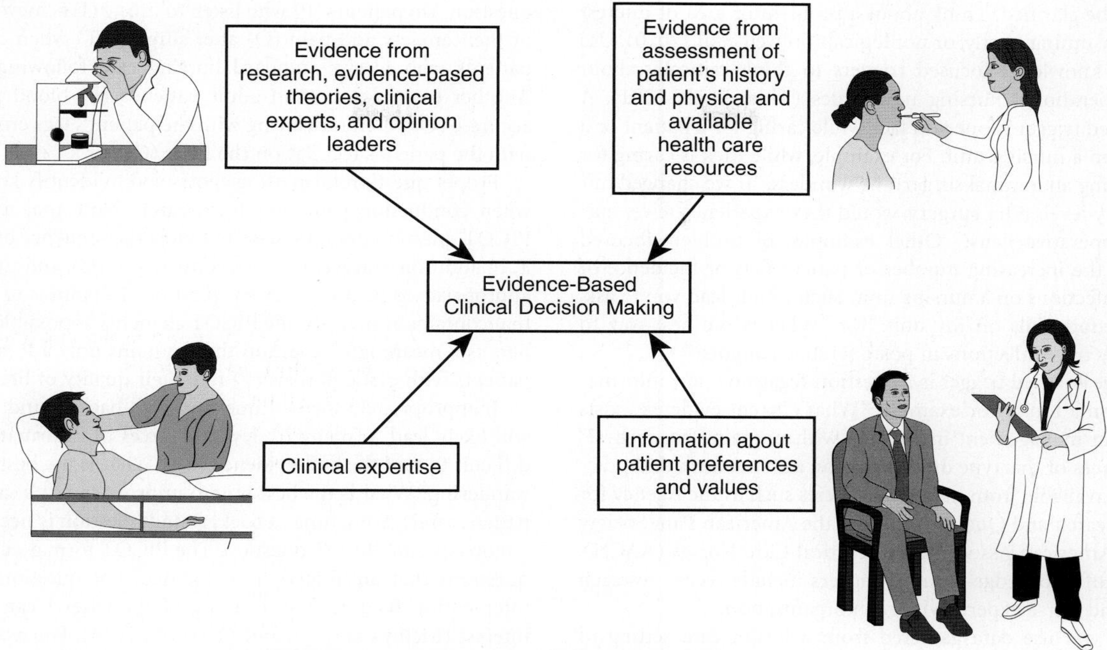

FIGURE 5-1 Model for evidence-based clinical decision making.

There are many sources of evidence. A good textbook incorporates evidence into the information, practice guidelines, and procedures it includes. Articles from nursing and health care literature are available on almost any topic involving nursing practice in either journals or on the Internet. Although the scientific basis of nursing practice has grown, some nursing care practices do not have adequate research to guide practice decisions. The challenge is to obtain the very best, most relevant, current, and accurate information at the right time, when you need it for patient care.

The best information is evidence that comes from well-designed, systematically conducted research studies, mostly found in scientific journals. Unfortunately much of that evidence never reaches the bedside. Nurses in practice settings, unlike in educational settings, do not always have easy access to databases for scientific literature. Instead they often care for patients on the basis of tradition or convenience (Flynn-Makic et al., 2014). Other sources of evidence come from quality improvement and risk management data; international, national, and local standards of care; infection control data; benchmarking, retrospective, or concurrent chart reviews; and clinicians' expertise. It is important to rely more on research evidence rather than solely on evidence that is not research based. When you face a clinical problem, always ask yourself where you can find the best evidence to help you find the best solution in caring for patients.

Even when you use the best evidence available, application and outcomes will differ on the basis of your patient's values, preferences, concerns, and/or expectations (Sherwood and Zomorodi, 2014). As a nurse you develop critical thinking skills to determine whether evidence is relevant and appropriate to your patients and to a clinical situation. For example, a single research article suggests that using medical clowns is an effective intervention for reducing fear and anxiety in children (Tener et al., 2012). However, if your patient is afraid of clowns, you will need to search for a better evidence-based therapy that he or she will accept. Using your clinical expertise and considering patient values and preferences ensures that you apply the evidence available in practice both safely and appropriately.

Steps of Evidence-Based Practice

EBP is a systematic, problem-solving process that facilitates achievement of best practices. Consistently following a step-by-step approach ensures that you obtain the strongest available evidence to apply in patient care. There are seven steps of EBP, which are numbered from zero to six (Melnyk and Fineout-Overholt, 2014):

0. Cultivate a spirit of inquiry.
1. Ask a clinical question in PICOT format.
2. Search for the most relevant and best evidence.
3. Critically appraise the evidence you gather.
4. Integrate all evidence with your clinical expertise and patient preferences and values.
5. Evaluate the outcomes of practice decisions or changes using evidence.
6. Share the outcomes of EBP changes with others.

Cultivate a Spirit of Inquiry. Changes in health care are often made slowly because of multiple barriers that often prevent the implementation of EBP. Gaps between what is known to improve patient care and what we actually do when caring for patients sometimes lead to inappropriate or unnecessary care (Holmes et al., 2012). When your care is not evidence based, your patients will sometimes experience poor outcomes. To be an effective change agent and foster optimal patient care, you need to have a never-ending spirit of inquiry. Constantly questioning current clinical practices and believing in the value of EBP leads to the consistent use of EBP in clinical nursing practice. You need to gain knowledge and skills associated with EBP and maintain a commitment to provide the best care possible to your patients and their families. In addition, health care agencies need to adopt a culture that supports EBP (e.g., through staff-led practice councils and journal clubs) and provide essential resources and tools to promote evidence-based care (Melnyk and Fineout-Overholt, 2014).

Ask a Clinical Question. Always think about your practice when caring for patients. Question what does not make sense to you and what needs to be clarified. Think about a problem or area of interest that is time consuming, costly, or not logical (Stilwell et al., 2010). Use problem- and knowledge-focused triggers to think critically about clinical and operational nursing unit issues (Titler et al., 2001). A problem-focused trigger is one you face while caring for a patient or a trend you see on a nursing unit. For example, while Rick is caring for patients following abdominal surgery, he wonders, "If we changed our patients' activity levels after surgery, would they experience fewer episodes of postoperative ileus?" Other examples of problem-focused trends include the increasing number of patient falls or incidence of urinary tract infections on a nursing unit. Such trends lead you to ask, "How can I reduce falls on my unit?" or "What is the best way to prevent urinary tract infections in postoperative patients?"

A knowledge-focused trigger is a question regarding new information available on a topic. For example, "What current evidence exists to improve pain management in patients with migraine headaches?" Important sources of this type of information are standards and practice guidelines available from national agencies such as the Agency for Healthcare Research and Quality (AHRQ), the American Pain Society (APS), or the American Association of Critical Care Nurses (AACN). Other sources of knowledge-focused triggers include recent research publications and nurse experts within an organization.

Sometimes you use data gathered from a health care setting to examine clinical trends when developing clinical questions. For example, most hospitals keep monthly records on key quality of care or performance indicators such as medication errors or infection rates. All magnet-designated hospitals maintain the National Database of Nursing Quality Improvement (NDNQI) (see Chapter 2). The database includes information on falls, falls with injuries, pressure ulcer incidence, and nurse satisfaction. You use quality and risk-management data to help you understand the nature or severity of problems that then allow you to form practice questions. The questions you ask eventually lead you to the evidence for an answer. When you ask a question and then go to the scientific literature, you don't want to read 100 articles to find the handful that are most helpful. You want to be able to read the best four-to-six articles that specifically address your practice question. Melnyk and Fineout-Overholt (2014) suggest using a PICOT format to state your question. Box 5-1 summarizes the five elements of a **PICOT question**. The more focused your question is, the easier it becomes to search for evidence in the scientific literature. For example, Rick is a member of the evidence-based council committee of his unit. The nurses on the committee develop the following PICOT question: Do patients (P) who listen to music (I) achieve better control of their anxiety and pain (O) after surgery (T) when compared with patients who receive standard nursing care following surgery (C)? Another example is: Is an adult patient's (P) blood pressure more accurate (O) when measuring with the patient's legs crossed (I) versus *with* the patient's feet flat on the floor (C)?

Proper question formatting allows you to identify key words to use when conducting your literature search. Note that a well-designed PICOT question does not have to follow the sequence of P, I, C, O, and T. In addition, intervention (I), comparison (C), and time (T) are not appropriate to be used in every question. The aim is to ask a question that contains as many of the PICOT elements as possible. For example, here is a meaningful question that contains only a P and O: How do patients with cystic fibrosis (P) rate their quality of life (O)?

Inappropriately formed questions are background questions that will likely lead to many irrelevant sources of information, making it difficult to find the best evidence (e.g., What is the best way to reduce wandering? What is the best way to improve family's satisfaction with patient care?). Sometimes a background question is needed to identify a more specific PICOT question. The PICOT format allows you to ask questions that are intervention focused. For questions that are not intervention focused, the meaning of the letter I can be an area of interest (Melnyk and Fineout-Overholt, 2014). For example, What is the difference in retention (O) of new nursing graduates (P) who go through a nurse residency program (I) versus those who do not (C) *2* years post hire date (T)?

The questions you ask using a PICOT format help to identify knowledge gaps within a clinical situation. Asking well–thought out questions allows you to identify evidence needed to guide clinical practice. Remember: do not be satisfied with clinical routines. Always question and use critical thinking to consider better ways to provide patient care.

BOX 5-1 Developing a PICOT Question

P = Patient population of interest

Identify patients by age, gender, ethnicity, and disease or health problem.

I = Intervention of interest

Which intervention is worthwhile to use in practice (e.g., a treatment, diagnostic test, prognostic factor)?

C = Comparison of interest

What is the usual standard of care or current intervention used now in practice?

O = Outcome

What result do you wish to achieve or observe as a result of an intervention (e.g., change in patient behavior, physical finding, or patient perception)?

T = Time

What amount of time is needed for an intervention to achieve an outcome (e.g., the amount of time needed to change quality of life or patient behavior)?

QSEN QSEN: BUILDING COMPETENCY IN EVIDENCE-BASED PRACTICE While attending a professional nursing conference about the care of surgical patients, Rick hears a report about common nursing practices that are not supported by research. One practice is the size or gauge of an intravenous (IV) needle that nurses need to use when infusing packed red blood cells (PRBCs). Traditionally nurses were taught that it is necessary to insert the largest IV needle possible and to use at least a 20-gauge IV needle when administering PRBCs to minimize destruction of the blood. However, current evidence indicates that PRBCs are not damaged by small IV needles. Rather it is high pressure during PRBC administration that damages blood cells. The evidence presented at the conference indicated that it is safe and effective to use IV needles as small as 22 gauge in adults and 24 gauge in infants and toddlers when administering PRBCs. Using this information, develop a PICOT question that Rick could use to further investigate this intervention. Identify each part of the PICOT question.

ⓔ *Answers to QSEN Activities can be found on the Evolve website.*

Collect the Best Evidence. Once you have a clear and concise PICOT question, you are ready to search for evidence. A variety of sources will provide the evidence needed to answer your question such as agency policy and procedure manuals, quality improvement data, existing clinical practice guidelines, and journal articles. Do not hesitate to ask for help to find appropriate evidence. Key resources include nursing faculty, librarians, advanced practice nurses, staff educators, risk managers, and infection control nurses.

When using scientific literature for evidence, seek the assistance of a medical librarian who knows the various online databases that are

TABLE 5-1 Searchable Scientific Literature Databases and Sources

Databases	Sources
AHRQ	Agency for Healthcare Research and Quality; includes clinical guidelines and evidence summaries http://www.ahrq.gov
CINAHL	Cumulative Index of Nursing and Allied Health Literature; includes studies in nursing, allied health, and biomedicine http://www.cinahl.com
MEDLINE	Includes studies in medicine, nursing, dentistry, psychiatry, veterinary medicine, and allied health http://www.ncbi.nim.nih.gov
EMBASE	Biomedical and pharmaceutical studies http://www.embase.com
PsycINFO	Psychology and related health care disciplines http://www.apa.org/psycinfo/
Cochrane Database of Systematic Reviews	Full text of regularly updated systematic reviews prepared by the Cochrane Collaboration; includes completed reviews and protocols http://www.cochrane.org/reviews
National Guidelines Clearinghouse	Repository for structured abstracts (summaries) about clinical guidelines and their development; also includes condensed version of guideline for viewing http://www.guideline.gov
PubMed	Health science library at the National Library of Medicine; offers free access to journal articles http://www.nlm.nih.gov
World Views on Evidence-Based Nursing	Electronic journal containing articles that provide a synthesis of research and an annotated bibliography for selected references

available to you (Table 5-1). The databases contain large collections of published scientific studies, including peer-reviewed research. A **peer-reviewed** article is reviewed for accuracy, validity, and rigor and approved for publication by experts before it is published. MEDLINE and the Cumulative Index of Nursing and Allied Health Literature (CINAHL) are among the best-known online databases to search for scientific knowledge in health care (Melnyk and Fineout-Overholt, 2014). Some databases are available through vendors at a cost, some are free of charge, and some offer both options. Students typically have access to an institutional subscription through a vendor purchased by their school. One of the more common vendors is OVID, which offers several different databases. Databases are also available on the Internet free of charge. The Cochrane Database of Systematic Reviews is a valuable source of high-quality evidence. It includes the full text of regularly updated systematic reviews and protocols for reviews currently under way. Collaborative review groups prepare and maintain the reviews. The protocols provide the background, objectives, and methods for reviews in progress (Melnyk and Fineout-Overholt, 2014).

The National Guidelines Clearinghouse (NGC) is a database supported by the AHRQ. It contains **clinical guidelines**, which are systematically developed statements about a plan of care for a specific set of clinical circumstances involving a specific patient population. Examples of clinical guidelines on NGC include care of children and adolescents with type 1 diabetes and practice guidelines for the treatment of adults

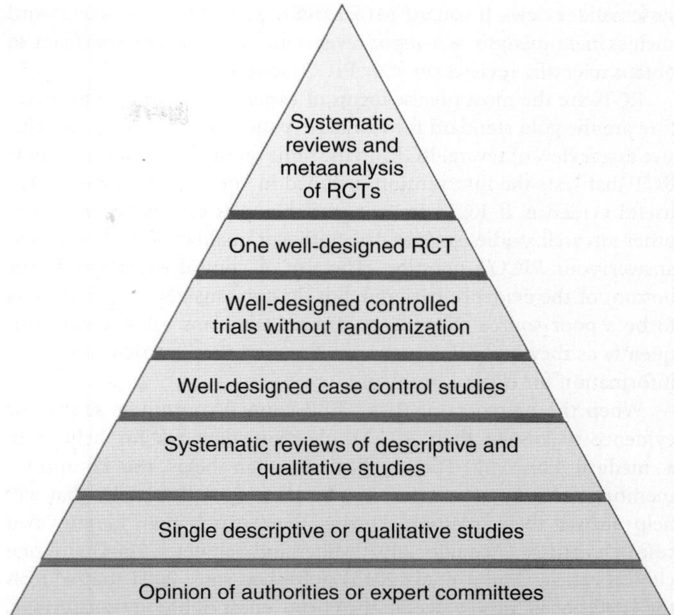

FIGURE 5-2 Hierarchy of evidence. *RCT,* Randomized controlled trial. (Data from Guyatt G, Rennie D: User's guide to the medical literature, Chicago, 2002, American Medical Association; Harris RP et al: Current methods of the US Prevention Services Task Force: a review of the process, *Am J Prev Med* 20:21, 2001; Melnyk BM, Fineout-Overholt E: *Evidence-based practice in nursing and healthcare: a guide to best practice,* ed 3, Philadelphia, 2014, Lippincott Williams & Wilkins.)

with low back pain. The NGC is invaluable when developing a plan of care for a patient (see Chapter 18).

Seek the help of a librarian to identify the appropriate databases and key words that will provide the best evidence to answer your PICOT question. When conducting a search, you need to enter and manipulate different key words until you get the combination of terms that provides the best articles that will help answer your question. It usually takes several searches before you find the most appropriate articles. The key words you select often have one meaning to one author and a very different meaning to another. Be patient and persistent and keep trying different words and different combinations of words until you find the evidence you need.

Figure 5-2 represents the hierarchy of available evidence. The level of rigor or amount of confidence you can have in the findings of a study decreases as you move down the pyramid. At this point in your nursing career, you cannot be an expert on all aspects of the types of studies conducted. But you can learn enough about the types of studies to help you know which ones have the best scientific evidence. At the top of the pyramid are systematic reviews or meta-analyses, which are state-of-the-art summaries from an individual researcher or panel of experts. Meta-analyses and systematic reviews are the perfect answers to PICOT questions because they rigorously summarize current evidence.

During either a meta-analysis or a systematic review, a researcher asks a PICOT question, reviews the highest level of evidence available (e.g., randomized controlled trials [RCTs]), summarizes what is currently known about the topic, and reports if current evidence supports a change in practice or if further study is needed. The main difference is that in a meta-analysis the researcher uses statistics to show the effect of an intervention on an outcome. In a systematic review no statistics are used to draw conclusions about the evidence. In the Cochrane Library all entries include information on meta-analyses and systematic reviews. If you use MEDLINE or CINAHL, enter a text word such as *meta-analysis, systematic reviews,* or *evidence-based medicine* to obtain scientific reviews on your PICOT question.

RCTs are the most precise forms of experimental study and therefore are the gold standard for research. A single RCT is not as conclusive as a review of several RCTs on the same question. However, a single RCT that tests the intervention included in your question yields very useful evidence. If RCTs are not available, you can use results from other research studies such as descriptive or qualitative studies to help answer your PICOT question. The use of clinical experts is at the bottom of the evidence pyramid, but do not consider clinical experts to be a poor source of evidence. Expert clinicians use evidence frequently as they build their own practice, and they are rich sources of information for clinical problems.

When the members of Rick's EBP council committee search for evidence to answer their PICOT question, they ask for help from a medical librarian. The medical librarian helps the committee members learn how to choose key terms to identify articles that will help answer their question. During their search they identify two research articles (Acquillo, 2007; Miller and Schlueter, 2004) and one clinical article (Makic et al., 2013) published since 2004 that address the effects of IV needle size on the effectiveness of blood transfusions. Other articles they found about this question were published in the 1980s and 1990s.

Critically Appraise the Evidence. Perhaps the most difficult step in the EBP process is critiquing or analyzing the available evidence. Critiquing evidence involves evaluating it, which includes determining the value, feasibility, and usefulness of evidence for making a practice change (ONS, n.d.). When critiquing evidence, first evaluate the scientific merit and clinical applicability of the findings of each study. Then with a group of studies and expert opinion determine which findings have a strong enough basis for use in practice. After critiquing the evidence you will be able to answer the following questions. Do the articles offer evidence to explain or answer my PICOT question? Do the articles show support for the reliability and validity of the evidence? Can I use the evidence in practice?

It takes time to develop skills needed to critique the evidence like an expert. When you read an article, do not put it down and walk away because of the statistics and technical language. Know the elements of an article and use a careful approach when reviewing each one. Evidence-based articles include the following elements:

- *Abstract.* An abstract is a brief summary that quickly tells you if the article is research or clinically based. An abstract summarizes the purpose of the article. It also includes the major themes or findings and the implications for nursing practice.
- *Introduction.* The introduction contains more information about the purpose of the article. There is usually brief supporting evidence as to why the topic is important. Together the abstract and introduction help you decide if you want to continue to read the entire article. You will know if the topic of the article is similar to your PICOT question or related closely enough to provide useful information. If you decide that an article will most likely help answer your question, continue to read the next elements of the article.
- *Literature review or background.* A good author offers a detailed background of the level of science or clinical information about the topic. The literature review offers an argument about what led the author to conduct a study or report on a clinical topic. This section of an article is very valuable. Even if the article itself does not address your PICOT question the way you desire, the literature review may lead you to other more useful articles. After reading a literature review, you should have a good idea of how past research led to the researcher's question. For example, a study designed to test an educational intervention for older-adult family caregivers reviews literature that describes characteristics of caregivers, the type of factors influencing caregivers' ability to cope with stressors of caregiving, and previous educational interventions used with families.
- *Manuscript narrative.* The "middle section" or narrative of an article differs according to the type of evidence-based article it is (Melnyk and Fineout-Overholt, 2014). A clinical article describes a clinical topic, which often includes a description of a patient population, the nature of a certain disease or health alteration, how patients are affected, and the appropriate nursing therapies. An author sometimes writes a clinical article to explain how to use a therapy or new technology. A research article contains several subsections within the narrative, including the following:
  - *Purpose statement:* Explains the focus or intent of a study. It includes research questions or **hypotheses**—predictions made about the relationship or difference among study **variables** (concepts, characteristics, or traits that vary within or among subjects). An example of a research question is: Does music therapy reduce a patient's pain and anxiety?
  - *Methods or design:* Explains how a research study was organized and conducted to answer the research question or test the hypothesis. This section explains the type of study that was conducted (e.g., RCT, case control study, or qualitative study) and the amount of subjects or people who participated in the study. In health care research, subjects often include patients, family members, or health care staff. The methods section is sometimes confusing because it explains details about how the researcher designed the study to obtain the most accurate results possible. Use your faculty member as a resource to help interpret this section.
  - *Results or conclusions:* Clinical and research articles have a summary section. In a clinical article the author explains the clinical implications for the topic presented. In a research article the author details the results of the study and explains whether a hypothesis is supported or how a research question is answered. This section includes a statistical analysis if it is a quantitative research study. A qualitative study summarizes the descriptive themes and ideas that arise from the researcher's analysis of data. Do not let the statistical analysis in an article overwhelm you. Read carefully and ask these questions: Does the researcher describe the results? Were the results significant? A good author also discusses limitations to a study in this section. The information on limitations is valuable in helping you decide if you want to use the evidence with your patients. Have a faculty member or an expert nurse help you interpret statistical results.
  - *Clinical implications:* A research article includes a section that explains if the findings from the study have clinical implications. The researcher explains how to apply findings in a practice setting for the type of subjects studied.

After Rick's EBP council critiques each article for their PICOT question, they combine the findings from the three articles he found about the IV needle gauge needed to safely administer a blood transfusion. They use critical thinking to consider the settings where the studies were performed, the scientific rigor of the evidence, the number of patients involved, and how well the evidence answers their PICOT question. They also consider the evidence in light of surgical patients' typical concerns and preferences. As nurses, the committee judges whether to use the evidence for patients who usually are admitted on the surgical unit. Patients frequently have complex medical histories and patterns of responses (Melnyk and Fineout-Overholt, 2014). Ethically it is important for the committee to consider evidence that will benefit patients and do no harm. They need to decide if the evidence is relevant, is easily applicable in this setting of practice, and has the potential for improving patient outcomes.

Integrate the Evidence. If you decide that the evidence is strong and applicable to your patients and clinical situation, you begin to identify how to incorporate it into practice. Your first step is simply to apply the research in your plan of care for a patient (see Chapter 18). Use the evidence you find as a rationale for an intervention you plan to try. For instance, you learned about an approach to bathe older adults who are confused and decide to use the technique during your next clinical assignment. If you find that the bathing technique is successful with your own assigned patients, you may begin to work with a group of other students or nurses to revise the policy and procedure for bathing patients or develop a new clinical protocol.

The literature that Rick's committee found reveals that using a 22-gauge IV needle may be safe and effective when administering a blood transfusion. However, they only found two research articles, both of which used small sample sizes (Acquillo, 2007; Miller and Schlueter, 2004). Because this is not enough evidence to support a practice change at this time, the committee members meet with their colleagues on the hospital-wide nursing practice committee to recommend further investigation into this practice issue. The nursing practice committee decides to consult with advanced practice nurses on the IV therapy team to search for professional guidelines that address the IV needle size needed when infusing blood.

Evidence is integrated in a variety of ways through teaching tools, clinical practice guidelines, policies and procedures, and new assessment or documentation tools. Depending on the amount of change needed to apply evidence in practice, it becomes necessary to involve a number of staff from a given nursing unit. It is important to consider the setting where you want to apply the evidence. Is there support from all staff? Does the practice change fit with the scope of practice in the clinical setting? Are resources (time, secretarial support, and staff) available to make a change? When evidence is not strong enough to apply in practice, your next option is to conduct a pilot study to investigate your PICOT question. A pilot study is a small-scale research study or one that includes a quality or performance improvement (PI) project.

Evaluate the Practice Decision or Change. After applying evidence in your practice, your next step is to evaluate the outcome. How does the intervention work? How effective was the clinical decision for your patient or practice setting? Sometimes your evaluation is as simple as determining if the expected outcomes you set for an intervention are met (see Chapters 18 and 20). For example, after the use of a transparent IV dressing, does the IV dislodge, or does the patient develop the complication of phlebitis? When using a new approach to preoperative teaching, do patients learn what to expect after surgery?

When an EBP change occurs on a larger scale, an evaluation is more formal. For example, evidence showing factors that contribute to pressure ulcers lead a nursing unit to adopt a new skin care protocol. To evaluate the protocol, nurses track the incidence of pressure ulcers over a course of time (e.g., 6 months to a year). In addition, they collect data to describe patients who develop ulcers and those who do not. This comparative information is valuable in determining the effects of the protocol and whether modifications are necessary.

When evaluating an EBP change, determine if the change was effective, if modifications in the change are needed, or if the change needs to be discontinued. Events or results that you do not expect may occur. For example, a hospital that implements a new method of cleaning IV line puncture sites discovers an increased rate of IV line infections and reevaluates the new cleaning method to determine why infections have increased. If the hospital does not evaluate this change in practice, more patients will develop IV site infections. Never implement a practice change without evaluating its effects.

In Rick's case nurses from the EBP committee of the unit, the hospital-wide nursing practice committee, and the IV therapy team decide to collect data to determine how many patients on surgical units require a blood transfusion and how many require multiple IV sticks to start at least a 20-gauge IV needle. After completing chart reviews, the nurses discover that patients who need blood transfusions and who require multiple IV sticks to start a 20-gauge or larger IV tend to be elderly and experience an increase in complications associated with their IV sites. Since the evidence does not provide a clear answer to their PICOT question, the nurses decide to present this information during the hospital grand rounds to gather more expert opinions from physicians and continue researching this issue. The physicians decide to join the nurses. They work together to conduct a pilot study evaluating the efficacy of using 22-gauge IV needles for blood transfusions in adults who cannot have larger IVs started.

Share the Outcomes with Others. After implementing an EBP change, it is important to communicate the results. If you implement an evidence-based intervention with one patient, you and the patient determine the effectiveness of that intervention. When a practice change occurs on a nursing unit level, the first group to discuss the outcomes of the change is often the clinical staff on that unit. To enhance professional development and promote positive patient outcomes beyond the unit level, share the results with various groups of nurses or other care providers such as the nursing practice council or the research council. Clinicians enjoy and appreciate seeing the results of a practice change. In addition, the practice change will more likely be sustainable and remain in place when staff are able to see the benefits of an EBP change.

As a professional nurse it is critical to contribute to the growing knowledge of nursing practice. Nurses often communicate the outcomes of EBP changes at professional conferences and meetings. Being involved in professional organizations allows them to present EBP changes in scientific abstracts, poster presentations, or even podium presentations.

After completing the pilot study, Rick presents the outcomes to the nursing research committee at his hospital. The chief nursing officer hears Rick's presentation and encourages him to submit an abstract about his study to a national professional nursing conference. Rick submits his abstract for consideration as a poster presentation at the annual Midwest Nursing Research Society conference, and it is accepted. During the conference Rick tells other nurses about the findings of this study and is contacted after the conference by several nurses who are interested in studying this problem further.

NURSING RESEARCH

After completing a thorough review and critique of the scientific literature, you might not have enough strong evidence to make a practice change. Instead you may find a gap in knowledge that makes your PICOT question go unanswered. When this happens, the best way to answer your PICOT question is to conduct a research study. At this time in your career you will not be conducting research. However, you may observe more senior nurses performing research within the hospital. It is important for you to understand the process of nursing research and how it generates new knowledge.

Nursing research improves the health and welfare of people (NINR, n.d.). **Nursing research** is a way to identify new knowledge, improve professional education and practice, and use nursing and health care resources effectively. Research means to search again or to examine carefully. It is a systematic process that asks and answers questions to generate knowledge. The knowledge provides a scientific basis for nursing practice and validates the effectiveness of nursing interventions. Nursing research improves professional education and practice and helps nurses use resources effectively (e.g., how to best use human resources by determining the best practice mix of nurses and unlicensed assistive personnel on a nursing unit). The scientific knowledge base of nursing continues to grow today, thus furnishing evidence that nurses can use to provide safe and effective patient care. Many professional and specialty nursing organizations support the conduct of research for advancing nursing science.

An example of how research can expand our practice can be seen in the work of Dr. Norma Metheny who has spent many years asking questions about how to prevent the aspiration of tube feeding in patients who receive feeding through nasogastric tubes (Metheny et al., 1988, 1989, 1990, 1994, 2000, 2007, 2010, and 2012; Metheny, 2006; Metheny and Meert, 2014). Through her program of research she has identified factors that increase the risk for aspiration and approaches to use in determining tube feeding placement. Dr. Metheny's findings are incorporated into this textbook and have changed the way nurses administer tube feedings to patients. Through research Dr. Metheny has contributed to the scientific body of knowledge that has saved patients' lives and helped to prevent the serious complication of pulmonary aspiration.

Outcomes Research

In today's health care delivery system it is more important than ever to understand the results of health care practices. Outcomes research helps patients, health care providers, and those in health care policy make informed decisions on the basis of current evidence (PCORI, 2015). Outcomes research typically focuses on the benefits, risks, costs, and holistic effects of a treatment on patients. For example, researchers are conducting outcomes research when they study the effects of managing Parkinson disease in patients using videoconferencing and telemedicine to increase access to health care.

Care delivery outcomes are the observable or measurable effects of health care interventions (Melnyk and Fineout-Overholt, 2014). Similar to the expected outcomes you develop in a plan of care (see Chapter 18), a care-delivery outcome focuses on the recipients of service (e.g., patient, family, or community) and not the providers (e.g., nurse or physician). For example, an outcome of a diabetes education program is that patients are able to self-administer insulin, not the nurses' success in instructing patients newly diagnosed with diabetes.

A problem in outcomes research is the clear definition or selection of measurable outcomes. Components of an outcome include the outcome itself, how it is observed (the indicator), its critical characteristics (how it is measured), and its range of parameters (Melnyk and Fineout-Overholt, 2014). For example, health care settings commonly measure the outcome of patient satisfaction when they introduce new services (e.g., new care delivery model or outpatient clinic). The outcome is patient satisfaction, observed through patients' responses to a patient satisfaction instrument, including characteristics such as nursing care, physician care, support services, and the environment. Patients complete the instrument, responding to a scale (parameter) designed to measure their degree of satisfaction (e.g., scale of 1 to 5). The combined score on the instrument yields a measure of patient satisfaction, an outcome that the facility can track over time.

Nurse-sensitive indicators are outcomes that are sensitive to nursing practice (Press Gainey Associates, 2015) (see Box 2-8). Although it is important to research the effects of nursing care on nurse-sensitive indicators, some researchers choose outcomes that do not measure a direct effect of nursing care such as length of stay, mortality, quality of life, and patient satisfaction. Researchers need to select appropriate outcomes to measure when designing their studies. For example, if a nurse researcher intends to measure the success of a nurse-initiated protocol to manage blood glucose levels in patients who are critically ill, the researcher will not likely measure mortality because it is too broad and susceptible to many factors outside of the control of the nurse-initiated protocol (e.g., the selection of medical therapies, the patients' acuity of illness). Instead the nurse researcher will have a better idea of the effects of the protocol by measuring the outcome of patients' blood glucose ranges. He or she obtains the blood glucose level of patients placed on the protocol and compares them to a desired range that represents good blood glucose control.

Scientific Method

The **scientific method** is the foundation of research and the most reliable and objective of all methods of gaining knowledge. This method is an advanced, objective means of acquiring and testing knowledge. Aspects of the method guide you in applying evidence gained from research in practice and conducting future research. When using research evidence to change practice, you need to understand the process that a researcher uses to guide a study. For example, when Rick's committee considered if blood transfusions could be infused safely with smaller-gauge IV needles, they needed to know if this had been tested on patients similar to the ones admitted on their unit and the outcomes or results of the studies. Otherwise the evidence might not be relevant to patients on Rick's unit. The scientific method is a systematic, step-by-step process. When completed correctly, you know that the study supports the **validity**, **reliability**, and **generalizability** of the data. Thus you can safely apply the findings of this study to similar subjects in a different study.

Researchers use the scientific method to understand, explain, predict, or control a nursing phenomenon (Polit and Beck, 2011). Systematic, orderly procedures reduce the possibility for error. Although this possibility always exists, the scientific method minimizes the chance that **bias** or opinion by a researcher will influence the results of research and thus the knowledge gained. Scientific research includes the following characteristics:

- The research identifies the problem area or area of interest to study.
- The steps of planning and conducting a research study are systematic and orderly.
- Researchers try to control external factors that are not being studied but can influence a relationship between the phenomena they are studying. For example, if a nurse is studying the relationship between diet and heart disease, he or she controls other characteristics among subjects such as stress or smoking history because they are risk factors for heart disease. Patients on an experimental diet and those on a regular diet would both need to have similar levels of stress and smoking histories to test the true effect of the diet.
- Researchers gather **empirical data** through the use of observations and assessments and use the data to discover new knowledge.
- The goal is to apply the knowledge gained from a study to a broader group of patients.

Nursing and the Scientific Approach

In the past much of the information used in nursing practice was borrowed from other disciplines such as biology, physiology, and psychology. Often nurses applied this information to their practice without testing it. For example, nurses use several methods to help patients sleep. Interventions such as giving a patient a back rub, making sure that the bed is clean and comfortable, and preparing the environment by dimming the lights are nursing measures that are used frequently and in general are logical, commonsense approaches. However, when these measures are considered in greater depth, questions arise about their applications. For example, are they the best methods to promote sleep? Do different patients in different situations require other interventions to promote sleep?

Research allows you to study nursing questions and problems in greater depth within the context of nursing. Nurses who do not use an evidence-based approach to practice often rely solely on personal experience or the advice of nursing experts. These nurses do not question if there is an intervention that produces better outcomes. When an intervention is not successful, nurses who do not use EBP will usually use an approach practiced by a colleague or try a different sequence of accepted measures. Even if an intervention discovered with this trial-and-error approach is effective for one or more patients, it is not always appropriate for patients in other settings. Nursing interventions must be tested through research to determine the measures that work best with specific patients.

Nursing research addresses issues important to the discipline of nursing. Some of these issues relate to the profession itself, education of nurses, patient and family needs, and issues within the health care delivery system. Once research is completed, it is important to disseminate or communicate the findings. One method of dissemination is through publication of the findings in professional journals. Nursing research uses many methods to study clinical problems (Box 5-2). There are two broad approaches to research: quantitative and qualitative methods.

Quantitative Research. Quantitative nursing research is the study of nursing phenomena that offers precise measurement and quantification. Two examples of quantitative research are (1) a study dealing with a new pain therapy quantitatively measures participants' pain severity, and (2) a study testing different forms of surgical dressings measures the extent of wound healing. Quantitative research is the precise, systematic, objective examination of specific concepts. It focuses on numerical data, statistical analysis, and controls to eliminate bias in findings (Polit and Beck, 2011). Although there are many quantitative methods, the following sections briefly describe experimental, nonexperimental, survey, and evaluation research.

Experimental Research. An RCT is a true experimental study that tightly controls conditions to eliminate bias with the goal of generalizing the results of the study to similar groups of subjects. Researchers test an intervention (e.g., new drug, therapy, or education method) against the usual standard of care (Box 5-3). They randomly assign subjects to either a control or a treatment group. All subjects in an RCT have an equal chance to be in either group. The treatment group receives the experimental intervention, and the control group receives the usual standard of care. The researchers measure both groups for the same outcomes to see if there is a difference. When an RCT is completed, the researcher hopes to know if the intervention leads to better outcomes than the standard of care.

Controlled trials without randomization are studies that test interventions, but researchers have not randomized the subjects into control or treatment groups. Thus there is bias in how the study is conducted. Some findings are distorted because of how the study was designed. A researcher wants to be as certain as possible when testing an intervention that the intervention is the reason for the desired outcomes. In a nonrandomized controlled trial the way in which subjects fall into the control or treatment group sometimes influences the results. This suggests that the intervention tested was not the only factor affecting the results of the study. Careful critique allows you to determine if bias

BOX 5-2 Types of Research

- **Historical research:** Studies designed to establish facts and relationships concerning past events. Example: Study examining the societal factors that led to the acceptance of advanced practice nurses by patients.
- **Exploratory research:** Initial study designed to develop or refine the dimensions of phenomena (facts or events) or to develop or refine a hypothesis about the relationships among phenomena. Example: Pilot study testing the benefits of a new exercise program for older adults with dementia.
- **Evaluation research:** Study that tests how well a program, practice, or policy is working. Example: Study measuring the outcomes of an informational campaign designed to improve parents' ability to follow immunization schedules for their children.
- **Descriptive research:** Study that measures characteristics of people, situations, or groups and the frequency with which certain events or characteristics occur. Example: Study to examine RNs' biases toward caring for obese patients.
- **Experimental research:** Study in which the investigator controls the study variable and randomly assigns subjects to different conditions to test the variable. Example: RCT comparing chlorhexidine with Betadine in reducing the incidence of IV-site phlebitis.
- **Correlational research:** Study that explores the interrelationships among variables of interest without any active intervention by the researcher. Example: Study examining the relationship between RNs' educational levels and their satisfaction in the nursing role.

RNs, Registered nurses; *RCT,* randomized controlled trial; *IV,* intravenous.

BOX 5-3 Example of a Randomized Controlled Trial

- **Research question:** Will an educational program for patients at risk for diabetes compared with a traditional educational pamphlet improve patient's blood glucose level and weight control?
- **Subjects:** 130 adult patients with risk factors for diabetes who visit a local medicine clinic
- **Randomization:** Patients are randomly assigned to one of two groups using a random-numbers table.
- **Treatment group:** 65 patients attend an 8-hour class on diabetes prevention, with group discussion, lecture, and interactive computer program use.
- **Control group:** 65 patients receive a printed pamphlet outlining risks for diabetes and health promotion strategies.
- **Outcome measure:** Both groups have blood glucose levels and weight measured before receiving education and every month for 3 months after receiving education.
- **Analysis:** Statistical tests comparing the blood glucose levels and weight for the two groups will demonstrate if the treatment group shows significant improvements in blood glucose levels and weight as predicted.

was present in a study and what effect, if any, the bias had on the results of the study.

Although RCTs investigate cause and effect and are excellent for testing drug therapies or medical treatments, this approach is not always the best for testing nursing interventions. The nature of nursing care causes nurse researchers to ask questions that are not always answered best by an RCT. For example, nurses help patients with problems such as knowledge deficits and symptom management. When researchers attempt to plan an RCT, it is often realized that ethical issues will develop if the control group does not receive the new therapeutic intervention. Also, learning to understand how patients experience health problems cannot always be addressed through an RCT. Therefore nonexperimental descriptive studies are often used in nursing research.

Nonexperimental Research. Nonexperimental descriptive studies describe, explain, or predict phenomena. Two examples include a study examining factors that lead to an adolescent's decision to smoke cigarettes and a study determining factors that lead patients with dementia to fall in a hospital setting.

A case control study is one in which researchers study one group of subjects with a certain condition (e.g., asthma) at the same time as another group of subjects who do not have the condition. A case control study determines if there is an association between one or more predictor variables and the condition (Melnyk and Fineout-Overholt, 2014). For example, is there an association between predictor variables such as family history or environmental exposure to dust and the incidence of asthma? Often a case control study is conducted retrospectively, or after the fact. Researchers look back in time and review available data about their two groups of subjects to understand which variables explain the condition. These studies involve a small number of subjects, creating a risk of bias. Sometimes the subjects in the two groups differ on certain other variables (e.g., amount of stress or history of contact allergies) that also influence the incidence of the condition, more so than the variables being studied. Correlational studies describe the relationship between two variables (e.g., the age of the adolescents and if the adolescents smoke). The researcher determines if the two variables are correlated or associated with one another and to what extent.

Many times researchers use findings from descriptive studies to develop studies that test interventions. For example, if the researcher determines that adolescents 15 years old and older tend to smoke, he or she might later test if participation in a program about smoking for older adolescents is effective in helping adolescents stop smoking.

Surveys. Surveys are common in quantitative research. They obtain information regarding the frequency, distribution, and interrelation of variables among subjects in the study (Polit and Beck, 2011). An example is a survey designed to measure nurses' perceptions of physicians' willingness to collaborate in practice. Surveys obtain information about practices, perceptions, education, experience, opinions, and other characteristics of people. The most basic function of a survey is description. Surveys gather a large amount of data to describe the population and the topic of study. It is important in survey research that the population sampled is large enough to keep sampling error at a minimum.

Evaluation Research. Evaluation research is a form of quantitative research that determines how well a program, practice, procedure, or policy is working (Polit and Beck, 2011). An example is outcomes research. Evaluation research determines why a program or some components of the program are successful or unsuccessful. When programs are unsuccessful, evaluation research identifies problems with the program and opportunities for change or barriers to program implementation.

Qualitative Research. Qualitative nursing research is the study of phenomena that are difficult to quantify or categorize such as patients' perceptions of illness or quality of life. This research method describes information obtained in a nonnumeric form (e.g., data in the form of transcribed written transcripts from a series of interviews). Qualitative researchers aim to understand patients' experiences with health problems and the contexts in which the experiences occur. Patients have the opportunity to tell their stories and share their experiences in these studies. The findings are in depth because patients are usually very descriptive in what they choose to share. Examples of qualitative studies include "patient's perceptions of nurses' caring in a palliative care unit," and "the perceptions of stress by family members of critically ill patients."

Qualitative research involves inductive reasoning to develop generalizations or theories from specific observations or interviews (Polit and Beck, 2011). For example, a nurse extensively interviews cancer survivors and then summarizes the common themes from all of the interviews to inductively determine the characteristics of cancer survivors' quality of life. Qualitative research involves the discovery and understanding of important behavioral characteristics or phenomena. An example is a qualitative research study conducted by Nixon and Narayanasamy (2010) that described the spiritual needs of patients with brain tumors and how well nurses support these needs.

There are a number of different qualitative research methods, including ethnography, phenomenology, and grounded theory. Each is based on a different philosophical or methodological view of how to collect, summarize, and analyze qualitative data.

RESEARCH PROCESS

The research process is an orderly series of steps that allow a researcher to move from asking the research question to finding the answer. Usually the answer to the initial research question leads to new questions and other areas of study. The research process builds knowledge for use in other similar situations. For example, a nurse researcher wants to seek knowledge about the best way to provide psychosocial support for patients with breast cancer. The research process ultimately provides knowledge that nurses from a variety of settings will use to provide evidence-based nursing care. Table 5-2 summarizes steps of the research process. Initially the researcher identifies an area of inquiry (identifying a problem), which often results from clinical practice. For example, a nurse notices that many surgical patients experience nausea after colon surgery. While speaking with a researcher at a professional nursing conference, the nurse decides to conduct a pilot study on the nursing unit to determine if chewing peppermint gum following colon surgery prevents patients from having nausea and reduces the incidence of postoperative ileus. The nurse reviews the relevant literature to determine what is known about chewing peppermint gum and its effect on bowel mobility and nausea following abdominal surgery. The nurse notes that, although many patients report problems with nausea and return of bowel function, there is limited research on the effects of chewing gum on these two outcomes.

Following identification of the problem and review of the literature, the nurse forms a research team who designs a study with the help of a nurse researcher. The research team includes nurses, gastrointestinal surgeons, and a statistician. The study sample includes all patients who are having elective colon resections. Subjects are excluded if they need to have surgery because of an emergency situation. After obtaining approval from the hospital institutional review board, the research team places each subject into one of the two groups (experimental or control) on the basis of random assignment. The control group receives standard postoperative care. The experimental or treatment group

TABLE 5-2 Comparison of Steps of the Nursing Process with the Research Process

Nursing Process	Research Process
Assessment	Identify area of interest or clinical problem. • Review literature. • Formulate theoretical framework. • Reflect on personal practice and/or discuss clinical issues with experts to better define the problem.
Diagnosis	Develop research question(s)/hypotheses.
Planning	Determine how study will be conducted: • Select research design/methodology. • Identify plan to recruit sample, taking into consideration population, number, and assignment to groups. • Identify study variables: specific interventions (independent variable) and outcomes (dependent variables). • Select data collection methods. • Select approach for measuring outcomes: questionnaires, surveys, physiological measures, interviews, observations. • Formulate plan to analyze data: statistical methods to answer research questions/hypotheses.
Implementation	Conduct the study: • Obtain necessary approvals. • Recruit and enroll subjects. • Implement the study protocol/collect data.
Evaluation	Analyze results of the study: • Continually analyze study methodology. Is study consistently carried out? Are all investigators following study protocol? • Interpret demographics of study population. • Analyze data to answer each research question/hypothesis. • Interpret results, including conclusions, limitations. Use of the findings: • Formulate recommendations for further research. • Determine implications for nursing. • Disseminate the findings: presentations, publications, need for further study, how to apply findings in practice.

receives standard postoperative care, and they chew gum for 5 minutes 3 times a day. Subjects have a 50-50 chance of being in each group. The research team selects appropriate instruments to measure postoperative nausea and decides to use patient assessment data to determine when nurses first hear bowel sounds and when patients first pass flatus and have their first bowel movement after surgery.

Before conducting any study with human subjects, a researcher obtains approvals from the human subjects committee or institutional review board (IRB) of an agency. An IRB includes scientists and laypeople who review all studies conducted in the institution to ensure that ethical principles, including the rights of human subjects, are followed. **Informed consent** means that research subjects (1) are given full and complete information about the purpose of a study, procedures, data collection, potential harm and benefits, and alternative methods of treatment; (2) are capable of fully understanding the research and the implications of participation; (3) have the power of free choice to voluntarily consent or decline participation in the research; and (4) understand how the researcher maintains confidentiality or anonymity. **Confidentiality** guarantees that any information a subject provides will not be reported in any manner that identifies the subject and will not be accessible to people outside the research team.

Once the study begins, the nurses on the unit collect data as indicated in the study protocol. The team analyzes the data from the nausea instrument and the chart review about bowel function from the two groups studied. With the help of the statistician, analysis of the results determines whether patients who chewed peppermint gum experienced less nausea and a quicker return of bowel function than the patients who had standard nursing care. The results from this study may advance postoperative nursing care.

Researchers always need to consider study limitations. Limitations are factors that affect study findings such as a small sample of subjects, a unique setting where the study was conducted, or the failure of the study to include representative cultural groups or age-groups. The research team conducted a pilot study because little data were available about the benefits of chewing gum following abdominal surgery. The sample size only included 20 patients in each group, and it was challenging to collect all the data from the patient charts because of inconsistencies in documentation. Therefore the results of the study have limited generalizability to other patients who are experiencing abdominal surgery. These limitations help the team decide how to refine or adapt the study for further investigation in the future.

A researcher also addresses the implications for nursing practice. This ultimately helps fellow researchers, clinicians, educators, and administrators know how to apply findings from a study in practice. At the end of the chewing gum study, the research team recommends that patients who have elective colon resections be offered the opportunity to chew peppermint gum following surgery. The surgeons on the unit agreed to the change in practice. The team decides to conduct another study to investigate this intervention with patients who have other types of abdominal surgeries to enhance the generalizability of the results. In addition, the team suggests ways to effectively introduce the use of chewing gum into other surgical units following surgery.

THE RELATIONSHIP BETWEEN EBP, RESEARCH, AND QUALITY IMPROVEMENT

EBP, research, and quality improvement (QI) are closely interrelated (Figure 5-3; see Chapter 2). All three processes require you to use the best evidence to provide the highest quality of patient care. As a nurse you are professionally accountable to know the differences and which process to select when facing clinical problems or when you desire to improve patient care. Although you will use all of these in nursing practice, it is important to know the similarities and differences among them (Table 5-3). When implementing an EBP project, it is important to first review evidence from appropriate research and QI data. This information helps you better understand the extent of a problem in practice and within your organization. QI data inform you about how processes work within an organization and thus offer information about how to make EBP changes. EBP and QI sometimes provide opportunities for research.

The following is an example of how the three processes merge to improve nursing practice:

A nursing unit is experiencing a decrease in patient satisfaction with pain management over the last several months. QI data identify factors associated with pain management (e.g., the types of pain medications typically ordered, patient reports of pain relief following administration of pain medications). A thorough analysis of QI data leads a unit-based quality council team of nurses to conduct a literature review and implement the best evidence available to improve their pain-management protocol for the type of patients on the unit. The staff implement the revised protocol and evaluate its results. Despite the implementation of the revised pain-management protocol, patient satisfaction data continue to be lower than desired. Thus staff decide to conduct a research study to further investigate this clinical problem and improve patient care.

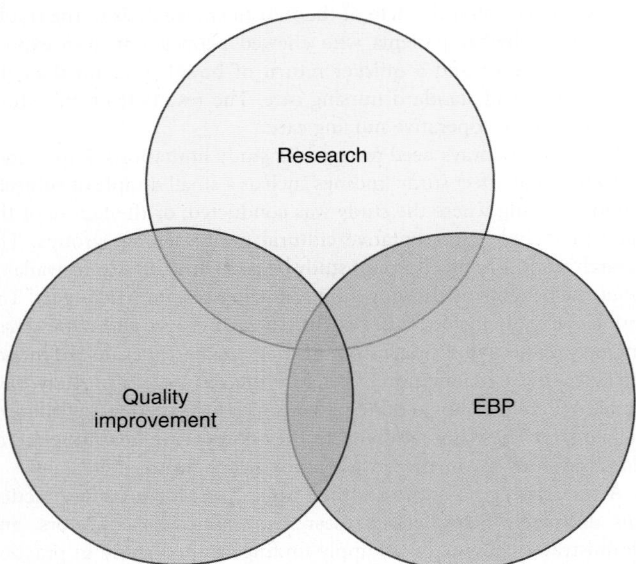

FIGURE 5-3 The overlapping relationship among research, evidence-based practice, and quality improvement. *EBP,* Evidence-based practice.

KEY POINTS

- A challenge in EBP is to obtain the very best and most relevant, accurate, and current information at the right time, when you need it for patient care.
- Using your clinical expertise and considering patients' values and preferences ensures that you will apply the evidence in practice both safely and appropriately.
- The steps of EBP provide a systematic approach to rational clinical decision making.
- A focused PICOT question allows you to search for evidence in the scientific literature.
- The hierarchy of available evidence offers a guide to the types of literature or information that offer the best scientific evidence.
- An RCT is the highest level of experimental research.
- Expert clinicians are a rich source of evidence because they use it frequently to build their own practice and solve clinical problems.
- The critique or evaluation of evidence includes determining the value, feasibility, and usefulness of evidence for making a practice change.
- After critiquing all articles for a PICOT question, synthesize or combine the findings to consider the scientific rigor of the evidence and whether it has application in practice.
- When you decide to apply evidence, consider the setting and whether there is support from staff and available resources.
- Research is a systematic process that asks and answers questions that generate knowledge, which provides a scientific basis for nursing practice.
- Outcomes research is designed to assess and document the effectiveness of health care services and interventions.

TABLE 5-3 Similarities and Differences Among Evidence-Based Practice, Research, and Quality Improvement

	Evidence-Based Practice	Research	Quality Improvement
Purpose	Use of information from research, professional experts, personal experience, and patient preferences to determine safe and effective nursing care with the goal of improving patient care and outcomes	Systematic inquiry answers questions, solves problems, and contributes to the generalizable knowledge base of nursing; it may or may not improve patient care.	Improves local work processes to improve patient outcomes and efficiency of health systems; results usually not generalizable
Focus	Implementation of evidence already known into practice	Evidence is generated to find answers for questions that are not known about nursing practice.	Measures effects of practice and/or practice change on specific patient population
Data sources	Multiple research studies, expert opinion, personal experience, patients	Subjects or participants have predefined characteristics that include or exclude them from the study; researcher collects and analyzes data from subjects.	Data from patient records or patients who are in a specific area such as on a patient care unit or admitted to a particular hospital
Who conducts the activity?	Practicing nurses and possibly other members of the health care team	Researchers who may or may not be employed by the health care agency and usually are not a part of the clinical health care team conduct it.	Employees of a health care agency such as nurses, physicians, pharmacists
Is activity part of regular clinical practice?	Yes	No	Yes
Is IRB approval needed?	Sometimes	Yes	Sometimes
Funding sources	Internal, from health care agency	Funding is usually external such as a grant.	Internal, from health care agency

IRB, Institutional review board.

- Nursing research involves two broad approaches for conducting studies: quantitative and qualitative methods.
- Although EBP, research, and QI are closely related, they are separate processes.
- When posed with a clinical problem, you need to use the appropriate approach.

CLINICAL APPLICATION QUESTIONS

Preparing for Clinical Practice

The nursing staff on Rick's surgical unit have been reviewing their patients' medical records and have seen a steady increase in the incidence of catheter-acquired urinary tract infections (CAUTIs) in patients over the last 3 months. The staff agrees to look into the current practice guidelines about the prevention of CAUTIs and determine if a change in practice is indicated.

1. What is an appropriate PICOT question for this group to ask? Identify each part of the PICOT question.
2. The nurses on Rick's unit conduct a literature search and gather research articles about the PICOT question. Which step of the evidence-based practice (EBP) process do they need to implement next? Describe what the nurses will do during this step.
3. The staff on the surgical unit implemented a new protocol 4 months ago for patients who have catheters after surgery. The staff need to determine if this practice change has been effective. Identify one outcome the nurses could measure to determine the effectiveness of this change. Describe one method they could use to measure this outcome.

ⓔ *Answers to Clinical Application Questions can be found on the Evolve website.*

REVIEW QUESTIONS

Are You Ready to Test Your Nursing Knowledge?

1. A nurse researcher studies the effectiveness of a new program designed to educate parents to promote the immunization of children. The nurse divides the parents randomly into two groups. One group receives the typical educational program and the other group receives the new program. This is an example of which type of study?
   1. Historical
   2. Qualitative
   3. Correlational
   4. Experimental
2. A nurse who works on a pediatric unit asks, "I wonder if children who interact with therapy dogs have reduced anxiety when they are in the hospital." In this example of a PICOT question, which of the following is the O?
   1. Children
   2. Therapy dogs
   3. The pediatric unit
   4. Anxiety
3. A nurse researcher wants to know which factors are associated with a person's decision to exercise. The nurse distributes a survey to people who recently joined an exercise wellness program and analyzes the data to determine which factors and characteristics are most significantly linked to the decision to start exercising. Which type of a research study is this?
   1. Qualitative
   2. Descriptive
   3. Correlational
   4. Randomized controlled trial
4. A group of nurses have identified that the elderly patients on their unit have a high incidence of pressure ulcers after they have a stroke. During a unit meeting they discuss different interventions that they think may reduce the development of pressure ulcers. What is the nurses' next step to investigate this clinical problem further?
   1. Conduct a literature review
   2. Share the findings with others
   3. Conduct a statistical analysis
   4. Create a well-defined PICOT question
5. Arrange the following steps of evidence-based practice (EBP) in the appropriate order.
   1. Integrate the evidence.
   2. Ask the burning clinical question.
   3. Create a spirit of inquiry.
   4. Evaluate the practice decision or change.
   5. Share the results with others.
   6. Critically evaluate the evidence you gather.
   7. Collect the most relevant and best evidence.
6. When recruiting subjects to participate in a study about the effects of an educational program to help patients at home take their medications as ordered, the researcher tells the subjects that their names will not be used and no one but the research team will have access to their information and responses. This is an example of:
   1. Bias.
   2. Anonymity.
   3. Confidentiality.
   4. Informed consent.
7. Nurses in a community clinic have seen an increase in the numbers of obese children. The nurses who care for children are discussing ways to reduce childhood obesity. One nurse asks a colleague, "I wonder what the most effective ways are to help school-age children maintain a healthy weight?" This question is an example of a/an:
   1. Hypothesis.
   2. PICOT question.
   3. Problem-focused trigger.
   4. Knowledge-focused trigger.
8. The nurses on a medical unit have seen an increase in the number of medication errors on their unit. They decide to evaluate the medication administration process on the basis of data gained from chart reviews and direct observation of nurses administering medications. Which process are the nurses using?
   1. Evidence-based practice
   2. Research
   3. Quality improvement
   4. Problem identification
9. A nursing student is preparing to read the methods section of a research article. Which type of information will the student expect to find in this section? (Select all that apply.)
   1. How the researcher conducted the study
   2. A description about how to use the findings of the study
   3. The number and type of subjects who participated in the study
   4. Summaries of other research articles that support the need for this study
   5. Implications for future research studies
10. A group of nurses on the research council of a local hospital are measuring nursing-sensitive outcomes. Which of the following is a nursing-sensitive outcome that the nurses need to consider measuring? (Select all that apply.)

1. Frequency of low blood sugar episodes in children at a local school
2. Number of patients who develop a urinary tract infection from a Foley catheter
3. Number of patients who fall and experience subsequent injury on the evening shift
4. Number of sexually active adolescent girls who attend the community-based clinic for birth control
5. Patient-reported quality of life following coronary artery bypass graft surgery and cardiac rehabilitation

11. Which of the following statements about evidence-based practice (EBP) made by a nursing student would require the nursing professor to correct the student's understanding?
1. "In evidence-based practice the patients are the subjects."
2. "It is important to talk with experts and patients when making an evidence-based decision."
3. "A nurse wanting to investigate the evidence to solve a problem starts by forming a PICOT question."
4. "It is important to ask a librarian for help when searching for literature to help you answer your PICOT question."

12. A nurse is reading a research article. The nurse just finished reading a brief summary of the research study that included the purpose of the study and its implications for nursing practice. Which part of the article did the nurse just read?
1. Abstract
2. Analysis
3. Discussion
4. Literature review

13. A researcher is studying the effectiveness of an individualized evidence-based teaching plan on young women's intention to wear sunscreen to prevent skin cancer. In this study which of the following research terms best describes the individualized evidence-based teaching plan?
1. Sample
2. Intervention
3. Survey
4. Results

14. A nurse researcher wants to conduct historical research. Which of the following ideas for a study could the nurses conduct? (Select all that apply.)
1. Determining the effect of unemployment on emergency room usage
2. Understanding how Clara Barton shaped nursing in America
3. Evaluating the effect of the Vietnam War on nursing leadership and practice
4. Analyzing the evolution of nursing and patient care during recent disasters
5. Investigating barriers to exercise in women who have become mothers in the past year

15. A nurse researcher is collecting data following approval from the institutional review board (IRB). In which part of the research process is this nurse?
1. Analyzing the data
2. Designing the study
3. Conducting the study
4. Identifying the problem

Answers: **1.** 4; **2.** 4; **3.** 3; **4.** 4; **5.** 3, 2, 7, 6, 1, 4, 5; **6.** 3; **7.** 3 ; **8.** 3; **9.** 1, 3; **10.** 2, 3; **11.** 1; **12.** 1; **13.** 2; **14.** 2, 3, 4; **15.** 3.

Rationales for Review Questions can be found on the Evolve website.

REFERENCES

Flynn-Makic MB, et al: Examining the evidence to guide practice: challenging practice habits, *Crit Care Nurse* 34(2):28, 2014.

Holmes B, et al: Translating evidence into practice: the role of health research funders, *Implementation Sci* 7(39), 2012. http://www.implementationscience.com/content/7/1/39. Accessed July 6, 2015.

Makic MBF, et al: Putting evidence into nursing practice: four traditional practices not supported by the evidence, *Crit Care Nurse* 33(2):28, 2013.

Melnyk BM, Fineout-Overholt E: *Evidence-based practice in nursing and healthcare: a guide to best practice*, ed 3, Philadelphia, 2014, Lippincott Williams & Wilkins.

National Institute of Nursing Research (NINR): *The National Institute of Nursing Research*, n.d., http://www.ninr.nih.gov/. Accessed July 6, 2015.

Oncology Nursing Society (ONS): *Putting evidence into practice*, n.d., https://www.ons.org/practice-resources/pep/evaluation-process. Accessed July 6, 2015.

Patient-Centered Outcomes Research Institute (PCORI): *PCORI*, 2015, http://www.pcori.org/ Accessed July 6, 2015.

Peterson M, et al: Choosing the best evidence to guide clinical practice: application of AACN levels of evidence, *Crit Care Nurse* 34(2):58, 2014.

Polit DF, Beck CT: *Nursing research: generating and assessing evidence for nursing practice*, ed 9, Philadelphia, 2011, Lippincott Williams & Wilkins.

Press Gainey Associates: *Nursing quality*, 2015, NDNQI. http://pressganey.com/ourSolutions/performance-and-advanced-analytics/clinical-business-performance/nursing-quality-ndnqi. Accessed July 6, 2015.

Sherwood G, Zomorodi M: A new mindset for quality and safety: the QSEN competencies redefine nurses' roles in practice, *Nephrol Nurs J* 41(1):2014.

Stilwell SB, et al: Asking the clinical question: a key step in evidence-based practice, *Am J Nurs* 110(3):58, 2010.

RESEARCH REFERENCES

Acquillo G: Blood transfusion flow rate, *J Vasc Access* 12(4):225, 2007.

Garner S, et al: Reducing ineffective practice: challenges in identifying low-value health care using Cochrane systematic reviews, *J Health Serv Res Policy* 18(1):6, 2013.

Metheny N, et al: Measures to test placement of nasogastric and nasointestinal feeding tubers: a review, *Nurs Res* 37:324, 1988.

Metheny N, et al: Effectiveness of pH measurement in predicting feeding tube placement, *Nurs Res* 38(5):262, 1989.

Metheny N, et al: Effectiveness of the auscultatory method in predicting feeding tube location, *Nurs Res* 39(5):262, 1990.

Metheny N, et al: Visual characteristics of aspirates from feeding tubes as a method for predicting tube location, *Nurs Res* 43:282, 1994.

Metheny N, et al: Development of a reliable and valid bedside test for bilirubin and its utilization for improving prediction of feeding tube location, *Nurs Res* 49(6):202, 2000.

Metheny N: Preventing respiratory complications of tube feedings: evidence-based practice, *Am J Crit Care* 15(4):360, 2006.

Metheny NA, et al: Complications related to feeding tube placement, *Curr Opin Gastroenterol* 23(2):178, 2007.

Metheny NA, et al: Effectiveness of an aspiration risk-reduction protocol, *Nurs Res* 59(1):18, 2010.

Metheny NA, et al: Blind insertion of feeding tubes in intensive care units: a national survey, *Am J Crit Care* 21(5):352, 2012.

Metheny NA, Meert KL: Effectiveness of an electromagnetic feeding tube placement device in detecting inadvertent respiratory placement, *Am J Crit Care* 23(3):240, 2014.

Miller MA, Schlueter AJ: Transfusions via hand-held syringes and small-gauge needles as risk factors for hyperkalemia, *Transfusion* 44(3):373, 2004.

Nixon A, Narayanasamy A: The spiritual needs of neuro-oncology patients from patients' perspective, *J Clin Nurs* 19(15–16):2259, 2010.

Tener D, et al: The use of medical clowns as a psychological distress buffer during anogenital examination of sexually abused children, *J Loss Trauma* 17(1):12, 2012.

Titler MG, et al: The Iowa model of evidence-based practice to promote quality care, *Crit Care Clin North Am* 13(4):497, 2001.

6

Health and Wellness

OBJECTIVES

- List the four general *Healthy People 2020* public health goals for Americans.
- Discuss the definition of health.
- Discuss the health belief, health promotion, basic human needs, and holistic health models to understand the relationship between patients' attitudes toward health and health practices.
- Describe variables influencing health beliefs and practices.
- Describe health promotion, wellness, and illness prevention activities.
- Discuss the three levels of preventive care.
- Describe four types of risk factors affecting health.
- Discuss risk-factor modification and changing health behaviors.
- Describe variables influencing illness behavior.
- Describe the effect of illness on patients and families.
- Discuss a nurse's role in health and illness.

KEY TERMS

Active strategies of health promotion, p. 71
Acute illness, p. 74
Chronic illness, p. 74
Health, p. 66
Health behavior change, p. 73
Health behaviors, p. 66
Health belief model, p. 66
Health promotion, p. 70
Holistic health model, p. 68
Illness, p. 73
Illness behavior, p. 74
Illness prevention, p. 70
Passive strategies of health promotion, p. 71
Primary prevention, p. 71
Risk factor, p. 72
Secondary prevention, p. 71
Tertiary prevention, p. 72
Wellness, p. 70

MEDIA RESOURCES

http://evolve.elsevier.com/Potter/fundamentals/
- Review Questions
- Case Study with Questions
- Audio Glossary
- Content Updates

In the past most individuals and societies viewed good health, or wellness, as the opposite or absence of disease. This simple attitude ignores the states of health that exist between disease and good health. Health is a multidimensional concept and is viewed from a broader perspective. An assessment of a patient's state of health is an important aspect of nursing.

Models of health offer a perspective to understand the relationships among the concepts of health, wellness, and illness. Nurses are in a unique position to help patients achieve and maintain optimal levels of health. They need to understand the challenges of today's health care system and embrace the opportunities to promote health and wellness and prevent illness. In an era of rising costs and advanced technology, nurses are a vital link to the improved health of individuals and society. Through assessment and knowledge of patients, nurses identify actual and potential risk factors that predispose an individual or a group to illness. In addition, a nurse uses risk factor modification strategies to promote health and wellness and prevent illness.

Different attitudes cause people to react in different ways to illness or the illness of a family member; this reaction is *illness behavior.* Nurses who understand how patients react to illness can minimize its effects and help them and their families maintain or return to the highest level of functioning.

HEALTHY PEOPLE DOCUMENTS

Healthy People provides evidence-based, 10-year national objectives for promoting health and preventing disease. In 1979 an influential document, *Healthy People: the Surgeon General's Report on Health Promotion and Disease Prevention,* was published; it introduced a goal for improving the health of Americans by 1990. The report outlined priority objectives for preventive services, health protection, and health promotion that addressed improvements in health status, risk reduction, public and professional awareness of prevention, health services and protective measures, surveillance, and evaluation. The report served as a framework for the 1990s as the United States increased the focus on health promotion and disease prevention instead of illness care. The strategy required is a cooperative effort by government, voluntary and professional organizations, businesses, and individuals. Widely cited by popular media, in professional journals, and at health conferences, it has inspired health promotion programs throughout the country.

Healthy People 2000: National Health Promotion and Disease Prevention Objectives, published in 1990, identified health improvement goals and objectives to be reached by the year 2000 (U.S. Department of Health and Human Services [USDHHS, Public Health Service], 1990). *Healthy People 2010,* published in 2000, served as a road map for improving the health of all people in the United States for the first decade of the twenty-first century (USDHHS, 2000). This edition emphasized the link between individual and community health and the premise that the health of communities determines the overall health status of the nation. *Healthy People 2020* was approved in December 2010. Healthy People 2020 promotes a society in which all people live long, healthy lives. There are four overarching goals: (1) attain high-quality, longer lives free of preventable disease, disability, injury, and premature death; (2) achieve health equity, eliminate disparities, and improve the health of all groups; (3) create social and physical environments that promote good health for all; and (4) promote quality of life, healthy development, and healthy behaviors across all life stages (USDHHS, n.d.).

DEFINITION OF HEALTH

Defining health is difficult. The World Health Organization (WHO) defines **health** as a "state of complete physical, mental, and social well-being, not merely the absence of disease or infirmity" (WHO, 1947). Many aspects of health need to be considered. Health is a state of being that people define in relation to their own values, personality, and lifestyle. Each person has a personal concept of health. Pender and colleagues (2015) define health as the actualization of inherent and acquired human potential through goal-directed behavior, competent self-care, and satisfying relationships with others while adjustments are made as needed to maintain structural integrity and harmony with the environment.

Individuals' views of health vary among different cultural orientations (Pender et al., 2015). Pender (1996) explains that "all people free of disease are not equally healthy." Views of health have broadened to include not only physical well-being, but also mental, social, and spiritual well-being and a focus on health at the family and community levels.

To help patients identify and reach health goals, nurses discover and use information about their concepts of health. Pender et al. (2015) suggest that for many people conditions of life rather than pathological states define health. Life conditions can have positive or negative effects on health long before an illness is evident (Pender et al., 2015). Life conditions include socioeconomic variables such as environment, diet, lifestyle practices or choices, and many other physiological and psychological variables.

Health and illness are defined according to individual perception. Health often includes conditions previously considered to be illness. For example, a person with epilepsy who has learned to control seizures with medication and who functions at home and work or a person fully recovered from a stroke with limited paralysis and living independently may no longer consider himself or herself ill. A nurse needs to consider the total person and the environment in which the person lives to individualize nursing care and enhance meaningfulness of the patient's future health status.

MODELS OF HEALTH AND ILLNESS

A model is a theoretical way of understanding a concept or idea. Models represent different ways of approaching complex issues. Because health and illness are complex concepts, models explain the relationships between these concepts and a patient's attitudes toward health and **health behaviors**.

Health beliefs are a person's ideas, convictions, and attitudes about health and illness. They may be based on factual information or misinformation, common sense or myths, or reality or false expectations. Because health beliefs usually influence health behavior, they can positively or negatively affect a patient's level of health. Positive health behaviors are activities related to maintaining, attaining, or regaining good health and preventing illness. Common positive health behaviors include immunizations, proper sleep patterns, adequate exercise, stress management, and nutrition. Negative health behaviors include practices actually or potentially harmful to health such as smoking, drug or alcohol abuse, poor diet, and refusal to take necessary medications.

Nurses developed the following health models to understand patients' attitudes and values about health and illness and to provide effective health care. These nursing models allow you to understand and predict patients' health behavior, including how they use health services and adhere to recommended therapy. Positive health models focus on the individual's strengths, resiliencies, resources, potential, and capabilities rather than on disease or pathology (Pender et al., 2015).

Health Belief Model

Rosenstoch's (1974) and Becker and Maiman's (1975) **health belief model** (Figure 6-1) addresses the relationship between a person's beliefs and behaviors. The health belief model helps you understand factors influencing patients' perceptions, beliefs, and behavior to plan care that will most effectively help patients maintain or restore health and prevent illness.

The first component of this model involves an individual's perception of susceptibility to an illness. For example, a patient needs to recognize the familial link for coronary artery disease. After this link is recognized, particularly when one parent and two siblings have died in their fourth decade from myocardial infarction, the patient may perceive the personal risk of heart disease.

The second component is an individual's perception of the seriousness of the illness. This perception is influenced and modified by demographic and sociopsychological variables, perceived threats of the illness, and cues to action (e.g., mass media campaigns and advice from family, friends, and medical professionals). For example, a patient may not perceive his heart disease to be serious, which may affect the way he takes care of himself.

The third component is the likelihood that a person will take preventive action. This component results from a person's perception of the benefits of and barriers to taking action. Preventive actions include lifestyle changes, increased adherence to medical therapies, or a search for medical advice or treatment. A patient's perception of susceptibility to disease and his or her perception of the seriousness of an illness help to determine the likelihood that the patient will or will not partake in healthy behaviors.

Health Promotion Model

The health promotion model (HPM) proposed by Pender (1982; revised, 1996) was designed to be a "complementary counterpart to models of health protection" (Figure 6-2). It defines health as a positive, dynamic state, not merely the absence of disease (Pender et al., 2015). Health promotion is directed at increasing a patient's level of well-being. The HPM describes the multidimensional nature of people as they interact within their environment to pursue health (Pender, 1996; Pender et al., 2015). The model focuses on the following three areas: (1) individual characteristics and experiences; (2) behavior-specific knowledge and affect; and (3) behavioral outcomes, in which the patient commits to or changes a behavior. The HPM notes that each person has unique personal characteristics and experiences that affect subsequent actions. The set of variables for behavioral-specific knowledge and affect have important motivational significance. These variables can be modified through nursing actions. Health-promoting

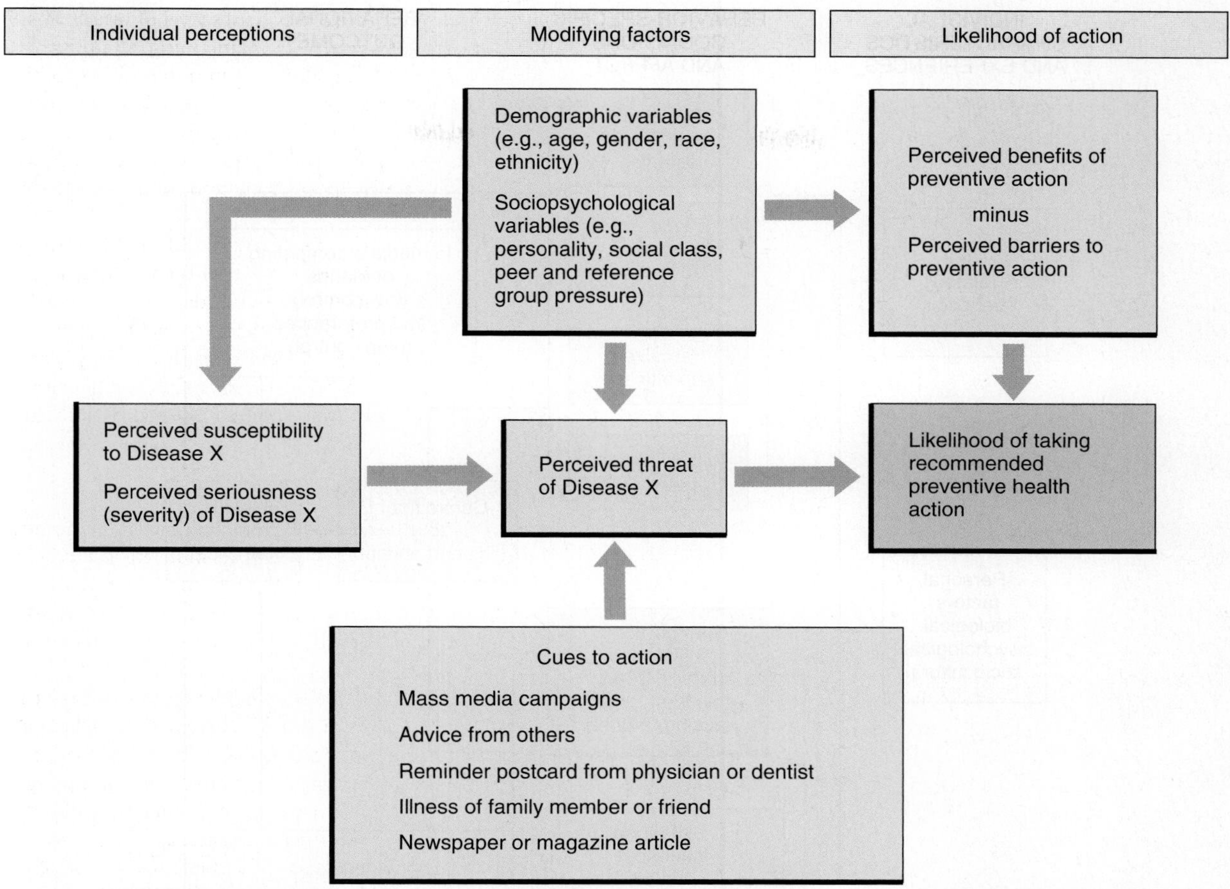

FIGURE 6-1 Health belief model. (Data from Becker M, Maiman L: Sociobehavioral determinants of compliance with health and medical care recommendations, *Med Care* 13[1]:10, 1975.)

behavior is the desired behavioral outcome and the end point in the HPM. Health-promoting behaviors result in improved health, enhanced functional ability, and better quality of life at all stages of development (Pender et al., 2015) (Box 6-1).

Maslow's Hierarchy of Needs

Basic human needs are elements that are necessary for human survival and health (e.g., food, water, safety, and love). Although each person has unique needs, all people share the basic human needs, and the extent to which people meet their basic needs is a major factor in determining their level of health.

Maslow's hierarchy of needs is a model that nurses use to understand the interrelationships of basic human needs (Figure 6-3). According to this model, certain human needs are more basic than others (i.e., some needs must be met before other needs [e.g., fulfilling the physiological needs before the needs of love and belonging]). Self-actualization is the highest expression of one's individual potential and allows for continual self-discovery. Maslow's model takes into account individual experiences, which are always unique to that individual (Touhy and Jett, 2012).

The hierarchy of needs model provides a basis for nurses to care for patients of all ages in all health settings. However, when applying the model, the focus of care is on a patient's needs rather than on strict adherence to the hierarchy. It is unrealistic to always expect a patient's

BOX 6-1 FOCUS ON OLDER ADULTS

Health Promotion

- Promote healthy lifestyles by encouraging regular physical activity tailored to the individual's ability, accepting responsibility for one's own health, using stress-management strategies, focusing on self-care abilities, improving self-efficacy, and practicing relaxation exercises (Pascucci et al., 2012; Pender et al., 2015).
- Consider an older adult's social environment and strengthen social support to promote health and provide access to resources (Touhy and Jett, 2012).
- Injury prevention is a key strategy to promote and improve health (Touhy and Jett, 2012).
- Promote community-based exercise programs to decrease social isolation and increase independence (Wallace et al., 2014).
- Factors that have been reported to affect older adults' willingness to engage in health promotion activities may include socioeconomic factors, beliefs and attitudes of patients and providers, encouragement by a health care professional, specific motivation based on efficacy beliefs, access to resources, age, number of chronic illnesses, mental and physical health, marital status, ability for self-care, gender, education, and support system presence (Byam-Williams and Salyer, 2010; Pascucci et al., 2012).
- Encourage frequent healthy meals that are well balanced and contain fruits, vegetables, and dairy (Pascucci et al., 2012).

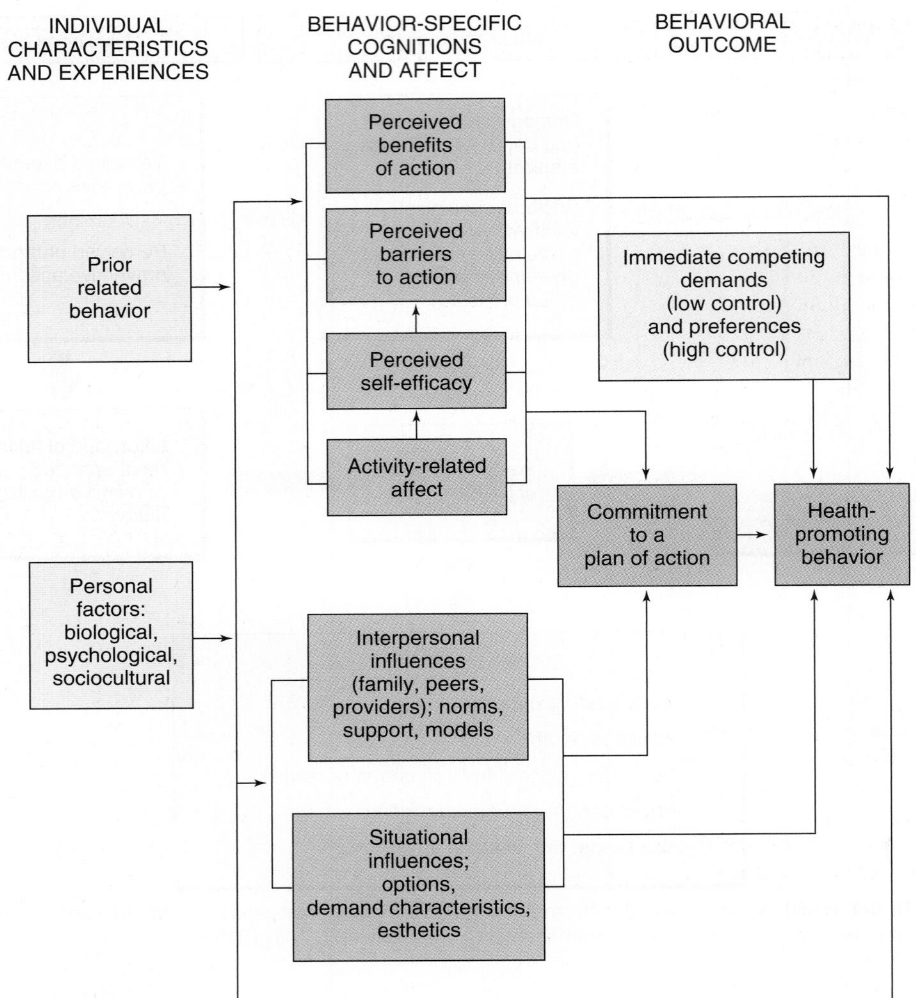

FIGURE 6-2 Health promotion model (revised). (Redrawn from Maslow AH, Frager RD (Editor), Fadiman J (Editor): *Motivation and personality,* ed 3. ©1987. Reprinted with permission of Ann Kaplan.)

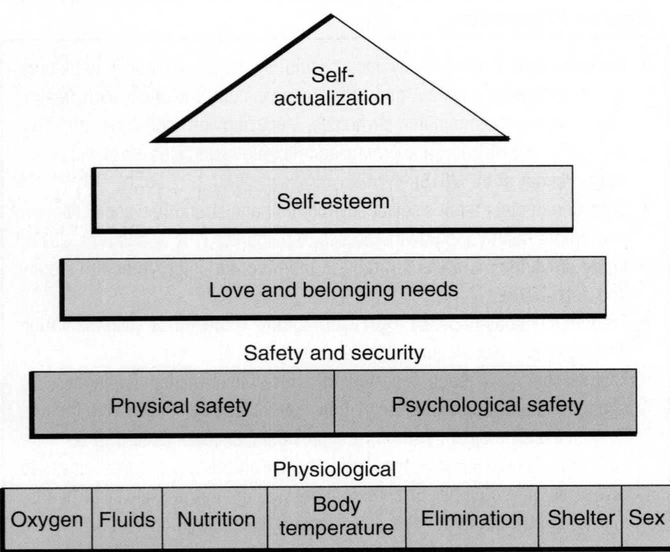

FIGURE 6-3 Maslow's hierarchy of needs. (Redrawn from Maslow AH: *Motivation and personality,* ed 3, Upper Saddle River, NJ, 1970, Prentice Hall.)

basic needs to occur in the fixed hierarchical order. In all cases an emergent physiological need takes precedence over a higher-level need. In other situations a psychological or physical safety need takes priority. For example, in a house fire, fear of injury and death takes priority over self-esteem issues. Although it would seem that a patient who has just had surgery might have the strongest need for pain control in the psychosocial area, if the patient just had a mastectomy, her main need may be in the areas of love, belonging, and self-esteem. It is important not to assume the patient's needs just because other patients reacted in a certain way. Maslow's hierarchy can be very useful when applied to each patient individually. To provide the most effective care, you need to understand the relationships of different needs and the factors that determine the priorities for each patient.

Holistic Health Models

Health care has begun to take a more holistic view of health by considering emotional and spiritual well-being and other dimensions of an individual to be important aspects of physical wellness. The **holistic health model** of nursing attempts to create conditions that promote a patient's optimal level of health. In this model nurses using the nursing process consider patients to be the ultimate experts concerning their own health and respect patients' subjective experience as relevant in maintaining health or assisting in healing. In the holistic health model patients are involved in their healing process, thereby assuming some responsibility for health maintenance (Edelman and Mandle, 2014).

Nurses using the holistic nursing model recognize the natural healing abilities of the body and incorporate complementary and alternative interventions such as meditation, music therapy, reminiscence, relaxation therapy, therapeutic touch, and guided imagery because they are effective, economical, noninvasive, nonpharmacological complements to traditional medical care (see Chapter 33). These holistic strategies, which can be used in all stages of health and illness, are integral in the expanding role of nursing.

Nurses use holistic therapies either alone or in conjunction with conventional medicine. For example, they use reminiscence in the geriatric population to help relieve anxiety for a patient dealing with memory loss or for a cancer patient dealing with the difficult side effects of chemotherapy. Music therapy in the operating room creates a soothing environment. Relaxation therapy is frequently useful to distract a patient during a painful procedure such as a dressing change. Breathing exercises are commonly taught to help patients deal with the pain associated with labor and delivery.

VARIABLES INFLUENCING HEALTH AND HEALTH BELIEFS AND PRACTICES

Many variables influence a patient's health beliefs and practices. Internal and external variables influence how a person thinks and acts. As previously stated, health beliefs usually influence health behavior or health practices and likewise positively or negatively affect a patient's level of health. Therefore understanding the effects of these variables allows you to plan and deliver individualized care.

Internal Variables

Internal variables include a person's developmental stage, intellectual background, perception of functioning, and emotional and spiritual factors.

Developmental Stage. A person's thought and behavior patterns change throughout life. A nurse considers a patient's level of growth and development when using his or her health beliefs and practices as a basis for planning care (see Chapter 11). The concept of illness for a child, adolescent, or adult depends on the individual's developmental stage. Fear and anxiety are common among ill children, especially if thoughts about illness, hospitalization, or procedures are based on lack of information or lack of clarity of information. Emotional development may also influence personal beliefs about health-related matters. For example, you use different techniques for teaching about contraception to an adolescent than you use for an adult. Knowledge of the stages of growth and development helps predict a patient's response to the present illness or the threat of future illness. Adapt the planning of nursing care to developmental expectations and to the patient's abilities to participate in self-care.

Intellectual Background. A person's beliefs about health are shaped in part by the person's knowledge, lack of knowledge, or incorrect information about body functions and illnesses, educational background, traditions, and past experiences. These variables influence how a patient thinks about health. In addition, cognitive abilities shape the *way* a person thinks, including the ability to understand factors involved in illness and apply knowledge of health and illness to personal health practices. Cognitive abilities also relate to a person's developmental stage. A nurse considers intellectual background so these variables can be incorporated into communication and instructional approaches (Edelman and Mandle, 2014).

Perception of Functioning. The way people perceive their physical functioning affects health beliefs and practices. When you assess a patient's level of health, gather subjective data about the way the patient perceives physical functioning such as level of fatigue, shortness of breath, or pain. Then obtain objective data about actual functioning such as blood pressure, height measurements, and lung sound assessment. This information allows you to more successfully plan and implement individualized approaches, such as self-care and mobility.

Emotional Factors. The patient's degree of stress, depression, or fear can influence health beliefs and practices. The manner in which a person handles stress throughout each phase of life influences the way he or she reacts to illness. A person who generally is very calm may have little emotional response during illness, whereas another individual may be unable to cope emotionally with the threat of illness and may overreact or deny the presence of symptoms and not take therapeutic action (see Chapter 38).

Spiritual Factors. Spirituality is reflected in how a person lives his or her life, including the values and beliefs exercised, the relationships established with family and friends, and the ability to find hope and meaning in life. Spirituality serves as an integrating theme in people's lives (see Chapter 36). Religious practices are one way that people exercise spirituality. Some religions restrict the use of certain forms of medical treatment. For example, persons of the Jehovah Witness faith do not receive blood transfusions. You need to understand patients' spiritual dimensions to involve patients effectively in nursing care.

External Variables

External variables influencing a person's health beliefs and practices include family practices, psychosocial and socioeconomic factors, and cultural background.

Family Practices. The way that patients' families use health care services generally affects their health practices. Their perceptions of the seriousness of diseases and their history of preventive care behaviors (or lack of them) influence how patients think about health. For example, if a young woman's mother never had annual gynecological examinations or Papanicolaou (Pap) smears, it is unlikely that the daughter will have annual Pap smears.

Psychosocial and Socioeconomic Factors. Socioeconomic and psychosocial factors increase the risk for illness and influence the way that a person defines and reacts to illness. Psychosocial variables include the stability of the person's marital or intimate relationship, lifestyle habits, and occupational environment. A person generally seeks approval and support from social networks (neighbors, peers, and co-workers), and this desire for approval and support affects health beliefs and practices.

Socioeconomic variables partly determine how the health care system provides medical care. The organization of the health care system determines how patients obtain care, the treatment method, cost to patients, and potential reimbursement to the health care agency or patients.

Economic variables often affect a patient's level of health by increasing the risk for disease and influencing how or at what point the patient enters the health care system. A person's compliance with a treatment designed to maintain or improve health is also affected by economic

BOX 6-2 CULTURAL ASPECTS OF CARE

Cultural Health Beliefs

The cultural backgrounds of patients shape their views of health, how to treat and prevent illness, and what constitutes good care (Narayan, 2010; Purnell, 2013). Two common beliefs of health exist: the individual, family, or community is able to influence its own health; or the individual has little control over his or her health because health is a gift from a higher being or power (Purnell, 2013). Health beliefs often vary within a cultural group; therefore it is important to assess the health beliefs of each patient and not stereotype a patient based on cultural background (Kersey-Matusiak, 2012). Cultural health beliefs influence individuals' responses to health and illness such as eye contact, response to pain and pain management, use of touch, perception and treatment of mental illness, and sick role behaviors (Narayan, 2010; Purnell, 2013). Other examples of cultural beliefs that affect health care practices include yin/yang balance, hot-and-cold foods, influence of humors, the importance of hexes, and spirits and soul loss (Giger, 2013). Recognizing a patient's health beliefs helps the nurse provide culturally competent nursing care that considers the physical, psychological, social, emotional, and spiritual needs of each patient. Nurses need to use culturally appropriate resources and be able to provide evidence-based cultural practices (Douglas et al., 2011).

Implications for Patient-Centered Care

- Be aware of the effect of culture on a patient's view and understanding of illness.
- Understand a patient's traditions, values, and beliefs and how these dimensions may affect health, wellness, and illness.
- Do not stereotype patients based on their culture and do not assume that they will adopt all cultural beliefs and practices (Kersey-Matusiak, 2012).
- When teaching patients about their illness and treatment regimens, you need to understand that unique cultural perceptions exist regarding the cause of an illness and its treatment.
- Use a trained interpreter if possible when a patient and family do not speak English to avoid misinterpretation of information (Purnell, 2013).
- Be aware of your own cultural background and recognize prejudices that lead to stereotyping and discrimination (Purnell, 2013).

BOX 6-3 EVIDENCE-BASED PRACTICE

Health Promotion Strategies

PICO Question: For individuals in the community, do psychosocial strategies effectively promote health and assist individuals with lifestyle changes?

Evidence Summary

Nurses use a variety of psychosocial strategies to improve health promotion in individuals. Research shows that some are more effective than others. One growing strategy is faith community nursing (FCN). FCN is a specialized area of nursing in which parish nurses focus on the goals of holistic health promotion (Dandridge, 2014). A wide variety of health promotion programs are presented by the parish nurses in their faith communities. Further research is needed on the outcomes of these FCN programs (Dandridge, 2014).

Face-to-face communication is another psychosocial strategy. Motivational interviewing (MI) is a face-to-face communication strategy that nurses use to assess an individual's readiness for change (Droppa and Lee, 2014). Through engaging individuals in communication, nurses who use MI are better able to understand their patients' motivation, help their patients work through resistance to change, empower the individual, and help support his or her self-efficacy (Droppa and Lee, 2014). MI techniques help move the individual through established targets in their health promotion journey. Han and Yan (2014) also found that face-to-face communication is effective in improving physical activity in individuals.

Application to Nursing Practice

- Use face-to-face dialogues when possible to encourage individuals regarding health promotion and lifestyle changes (Han and Yan, 2014).
- Provide support to individuals as they work on lifestyle changes (Hornsten et al., 2014).
- Determine if the individual has access to FCN—sponsored health promotion programs (Dandridge, 2014).
- Use motivational interview techniques to determine an individual's concerns and motivation for change (Droppa and Lee, 2014).

status. A person who has high utility bills, cares for a large family, and has a low income tends to give a higher priority to food and shelter than to costly drugs or treatment or expensive foods for special diets. Some patients decide to take medications every other day rather than every day as prescribed to save money, which greatly affects the effectiveness of the medications.

Cultural Background. Cultural background influences beliefs, values, and customs. It influences the approach to the health care systems, personal health practices, and the nurse-patient relationship. Cultural background also influences an individual's beliefs about causes of illness and remedies or practices to restore health (Box 6-2). If you are not aware of your own cultural patterns of behavior and language, you will have difficulty recognizing and understanding your patient's behaviors and beliefs. You will also probably have difficulty interacting with patients. As with family and socioeconomic variables, you need to incorporate cultural variables into a patient's care plan (see Chapter 9).

HEALTH PROMOTION, WELLNESS, AND ILLNESS PREVENTION

Currently, health care is more focused on health promotion, wellness, and illness prevention. In addition, changes in health care cost and insurance coverage have motivated people to seek ways to improve health, decrease incidence of disease and disability, and minimize the results of disease or disability.

The concepts of health promotion, wellness, and illness prevention are closely related and in practice overlap to some extent. All are focused on the future; the difference among them involves motivations and goals. **Health promotion** activities such as routine exercise and good nutrition help patients maintain or enhance their present levels of health. They motivate people to act positively to reach more stable levels of health. **Wellness** education teaches people how to care for themselves in a healthy way and includes topics such as physical awareness, stress management, and self-responsibility. Wellness strategies help people achieve new understanding and control of their lives. **Illness prevention** activities such as immunization programs protect patients from actual or potential threats to health. They motivate people to avoid a decline in health or functional levels.

Nurses emphasize health promotion activities, wellness-enhancing strategies, and illness-prevention activities as important forms of health care because they help patients maintain and improve health. The goal of a total health program is to improve a patient's level of well-being in all dimensions, not just physical health. Total health programs are based on the belief that many factors can affect a person's level of health (Box 6-3).

Examples of the health topics and objectives as defined by *Healthy People 2020* include physical activity, adolescent health, tobacco use, substance abuse, sexually transmitted diseases, mental health and

TABLE 6-1 Three Levels of Prevention

PRIMARY PREVENTION		SECONDARY PREVENTION		TERTIARY PREVENTION
Health Promotion	**Specific Protection**	**Early Diagnosis and Prompt Treatment**	**Disability Limitations**	**Restoration and Rehabilitation**
Health education Good standard of nutrition adjusted to developmental phases of life Attention to personality development Provision of adequate housing and recreation and agreeable working conditions Marriage counseling and sex education Genetic screening Periodic selective examinations	Use of specific immunizations Attention to personal hygiene Use of environmental sanitation Protection against occupational hazards Protection from accidents Use of specific nutrients Protection from carcinogens Avoidance of allergens	Case-finding measures: individual and mass screening activities Selective examinations to cure and prevent disease process, prevent spread of communicable disease, prevent complications and sequelae, and shorten period of disability	Adequate treatment to arrest disease process and prevent further complications and sequelae Provision of facilities to limit disability and prevent death	Provision of hospital and community facilities for retraining and education to maximize use of remaining capacities Education of public and industry to use rehabilitated persons to fullest possible extent Selective placement Work therapy in hospitals Use of sheltered colony

Data from Leavell H, Clark AE: *Preventive medicine for the doctors in his community,* ed 3, New York, 1965, McGraw-Hill; and modified from Edelman CL, Mandle CL: *Health promotion throughout the life span,* ed 7, St Louis, 2014, Mosby.

mental disorders, injury and violence prevention, environmental health, immunization and infectious disease, and access to health care (USDHHS, 2015). A complete list of topics and objectives is available on the *Healthy People* website (www.healthypeople.gov). These objectives and topics show the importance of health promotion, wellness, and illness prevention and encourage all to participate in the improvement of health.

Individual practices such as poor eating habits and little or no exercise influence health. Physical stressors such as a poor living environment, work stress, exposure to air pollutants, and an unsafe environment also affect health. Hereditary and psychological stressors such as emotional, intellectual, social, developmental, and spiritual factors influence one's level of health. Total health programs are directed at individuals' changing their lifestyles by developing more health-oriented habits.

Other programs are aimed at specific health care problems. For example, support groups help people with human immunodeficiency virus (HIV) infection. Exercise programs encourage participants to exercise regularly to reduce their risk of cardiac disease. Stress-reduction programs teach participants to cope with stressors and reduce their risks for multiple illnesses such as infections, gastrointestinal disease, and cardiac disease.

Some health promotion, wellness education, and illness prevention programs are operated by health care agencies; others are operated independently. Many businesses have on-site health promotion activities for employees. Likewise, colleges and community centers offer health promotion and illness prevention programs. Some nurses actively participate in these programs, providing direct care, and others act as consultants or refer patients to them. The goal of these activities is to improve a patient's level of health through preventive health services, environmental protection, and health education.

Health care professionals who work in the field of health promotion use proactive attempts to prevent illness or disease. Health promotion activities are passive or active. With **passive strategies of health promotion**, individuals gain from the activities of others without acting themselves. The fluoridation of municipal drinking water and the fortification of homogenized milk with vitamin D are examples of passive health promotion strategies. With **active strategies of health promotion**, individuals adopt specific health programs. Weight-reduction and smoking-cessation programs require patients to be actively involved in measures to improve their present and future levels of wellness while decreasing the risk of disease.

Health promotion is a process of helping people improve their health to reach an optimal state of physical, mental, and social well-being (WHO, 2009). An individual takes responsibility for health and wellness by making appropriate lifestyle choices. Lifestyle choices are important because they affect a person's quality of life and well-being. Making positive lifestyle choices and avoiding negative lifestyle choices also play a role in preventing illness. In addition to improving quality of life, preventing illness has an economic impact because it decreases health care costs.

Levels of Preventive Care

Nursing care oriented to health promotion, wellness, and illness prevention is described in terms of health activities on primary, secondary, and tertiary levels (Table 6-1).

Primary Prevention. **Primary prevention** is true prevention; it precedes disease or dysfunction and is applied to patients considered physically and emotionally healthy. Primary prevention aimed at health promotion includes health education programs, immunizations, nutritional programs, and physical fitness activities. It includes all health promotion efforts and wellness education activities that focus on maintaining or improving the general health of individuals, families, and communities (Edelman and Mandle, 2014). Primary prevention includes specific protection such as immunization for influenza and hearing protection in occupational settings.

Secondary Prevention. **Secondary prevention** focuses on individuals who are experiencing health problems or illnesses and are at risk for developing complications or worsening conditions. Activities are directed at diagnosis and prompt intervention, thereby reducing severity and enabling the patient to return to a normal level of health as early as possible (Edelman and Mandle, 2014). A large portion of nursing care related to secondary prevention is delivered in homes, hospitals, or skilled nursing facilities. It includes screening techniques and treating early stages of disease to limit disability by averting or delaying the consequences of advanced disease. Screening activities also become a key opportunity for health teaching as a primary prevention intervention (Edelman and Mandle, 2014).

Tertiary Prevention. Tertiary prevention occurs when a defect or disability is permanent and irreversible. It involves minimizing the effects of long-term disease or disability by interventions directed at preventing complications and deterioration (Edelman and Mandle, 2014). Activities are directed at rehabilitation rather than diagnosis and treatment. For example, a patient with a spinal cord injury undergoes rehabilitation to learn how to use a wheelchair and perform ADLs independently. Care at this level helps patients achieve as high a level of functioning as possible, despite the limitations caused by illness or impairment.

RISK FACTORS

A risk factor is any situation, habit, or other variable such as social, environmental, physiological, psychological, developmental, intellectual, or spiritual that increases the vulnerability of an individual or group to an illness or accident. An example would be risk factors for falls, such as impaired gait, reduced vision, and lower extremity weakness. Risk factors and behaviors, risk factor modification, and behavior modification are integral components of health promotion, wellness, and illness prevention. Nurses in all areas of practice have opportunities to reduce patients' risk factors to promote health and decrease risks of illness or injury.

The presence of risk factors does not mean that a disease will develop, but risk factors increase the chances that the individual will experience a particular disease or dysfunction. Nurses and other health care professionals are concerned with risk factors, sometimes called *health hazards,* for several reasons. Risk factors play a major role in how a nurse identifies a patient's health status. They also often influence health beliefs and practices if a person is aware of their presence. Risk factors are often placed in the following interrelated categories: genetic and physiological factors, age, physical environment, and lifestyle.

Genetic and Physiological Factors

Physiological risk factors involve the physical functioning of the body. Certain physical conditions such as being overweight place increased stress on physiological systems (e.g., the circulatory system), increasing susceptibility to illness. Heredity, or genetic predisposition to specific illness, is a major physical risk factor. For example, a person with a family history of diabetes mellitus is at risk for developing the disease later in life. Other documented genetic risk factors include family histories of cancer, heart disease, kidney disease, or mental illness.

Age

Age affects a person's susceptibility to certain illnesses and conditions. For example, premature infants and neonates are more susceptible to infections. As a person ages, the risk of heart disease and many types of cancers increases. Age risk factors are often closely associated with other risk factors such as family history and personal habits. Nurses need to educate their patients about the importance of regularly scheduled checkups for their age-group. Various professional organizations and federal agencies develop and update recommendations for health screenings, immunizations, and counseling. Access to scientific evidence, recommendations for clinical prevention services, and information on how to incorporate recommended preventive services into practice can be found at http://www.ahrq.gov/professionals/prevention-chronic-care/index.html.

Environment

Where we live and the condition of that area (its air, water, and soil) determine how we live, what we eat, the disease agents to which we are exposed, our state of health, and our ability to adapt. The physical environment in which a person works or lives can increase the likelihood that certain illnesses will occur. For example, some kinds of cancer and other diseases are more likely to develop when industrial workers are exposed to certain chemicals or when people live near toxic waste disposal sites. Nursing assessments extend from the individual to the family and the community in which they live focusing on the short term effects of exposure and the potential for long-term effects (Edelman and Mandle, 2014).

Lifestyle

Many activities, habits, and practices involve risk factors. Lifestyle practices and behaviors have positive or negative effects on health. Those with potential negative effects are risk factors. Some habits are risk factors for specific diseases. For example, excessive sunbathing increases the risk of skin cancer; smoking increases the risk of lung diseases, including cancer; and a poor diet and being overweight increase the risk of cardiovascular disease. Because patients often take risks, there is an increased emphasis for nurses to provide preventive care. Lifestyle choices lead to health problems that cause a huge impact on the economics of the health care system. Therefore it is important to understand the effect of lifestyle behaviors on health status. Nurses educate their patients and the public on wellness-promoting lifestyle behaviors.

Stress is a lifestyle risk factor if it is severe or prolonged or if the person is unable to cope with life events adequately. Stress threatens both mental health (emotional stress) and physical well-being (physiological stress). Both play a part in the development of an illness and affect a person's ability to adapt to potential changes associated with the illness and survive a life-threatening illness. Stress also interferes with patients adopting health promotion activities and the ability to implement needed lifestyle modifications. Some emotional stressors result from life events such as divorce, pregnancy, death of a spouse or family member, and financial instabilities. For example, job-related stressors overtax a person's cognitive skills and decision-making ability, leading to "mental overload" or "burnout" (see Chapters 1 and 38). Stress also threatens physical well-being and is associated with illnesses such as heart disease, cancer, and gastrointestinal disorders (Pender et al., 2015). Always review life stressors as part of a patient's comprehensive risk factor analysis.

The goal of risk factor identification is to help patients visualize the areas in their life that they can modify, control, or even eliminate to promote wellness and prevent illness. You can use a variety of available health risk appraisal forms to estimate a person's specific health threats based on the presence of various risk factors (Edelman and Mandle, 2014). Link the health risk appraisal tool with educational programs and other community resources if a patient needs to make lifestyle changes and reduce health risks (Pender et al., 2015).

RISK-FACTOR MODIFICATION AND CHANGING HEALTH BEHAVIORS

Identifying risk factors is the first step in health promotion, wellness education, and illness prevention. Discuss health hazards with a patient following a comprehensive nursing assessment, then help the patient decide if he or she wants to maintain or improve his or her health status by taking risk-reduction actions (Edelman and Mandle, 2014). Risk-factor modification, health promotion, illness prevention activities, or any program that attempts to change unhealthy lifestyle behaviors is a wellness strategy. Emphasize wellness strategies that teach patients to care for themselves in a healthier way because they have the

TABLE 6-2 Stages of Health Behavior Change

Stage	Definition	Nursing Implications
Precontemplation	Not intending to make changes within the next 6 months	Patient is not interested in information about the behavior and may be defensive when confronted with it.
Contemplation	Considering a change within the next 6 months	Ambivalence may be present, but patients will more likely accept information since they are developing more belief in the value of change.
Preparation	Making small changes in preparation for a change in the next month	Patient believes that advantages outweigh disadvantages of behavior change; needs assistance in planning for the change.
Action	Actively engaged in strategies to change behavior; lasts up to 6 months	Previous habits may prevent taking action relating to new behaviors; identify barriers and facilitators of change.
Maintenance stage	Sustained change over time; begins 6 months after action has started and continues indefinitely	Changes need to be integrated into the patient's lifestyle.

Data from Prochaska JO, DiClemente CC: Stages of change in the modification of problem behaviors, *Prog Behav Modif* 28:184, 1992; and Conn VS: A staged-based approach to helping people change health behaviors, *Clin Nurs Spec* 8(4):187, 1994.

ability to increase their quality of life and decrease the potential high costs of unmanaged health problems.

Some attempts to change are aimed at the cessation of a health-damaging behavior (e.g., tobacco use or alcohol misuse) or the adoption of a healthy behavior (e.g., healthy diet or exercise) (Pender et al., 2015). It is difficult to change negative health behavior, especially when the behavior is ingrained in a person's lifestyle patterns. The importance of nurses using a health promotion model to identify risky behaviors and implement the change process cannot be overemphasized because it is the nurse who spends the greatest amount of time in direct contact with patients. In addition, leading causes of death continue to relate to health behaviors that require a change, and nurses are able to motivate and facilitate important health behavior change when working with individuals, families, and communities (Edelman and Mandle, 2014).

Understanding the process of changing behaviors will help you support difficult **health behavior changes** in patients. It is believed that change involves movement through a series of stages. DiClemente and Prochaska (1998) describe the stages of change in the transtheoretical model of change (Table 6-2). These stages range from no intention to change (precontemplation), considering a change within the next 6 months (contemplation), making small changes (preparation), and actively engaging in strategies to change behavior (action) to maintaining a changed behavior (maintenance stage). As individuals attempt a change in behavior, relapse followed by recycling through the stages frequently occurs. When relapse occurs, a person will return to the contemplation or precontemplation stage before attempting the change again. Relapse is a learning process, and people can apply the lessons learned from relapse to their next attempt to change. It is important to understand what happens at the various stages of the change process to time the implementation of interventions (wellness strategies) adequately and provide appropriate assistance at each stage.

Once an individual identifies a stage of change, the change process facilitates movement through the stages. To be most effective, you choose nursing interventions that match the stage of change (DiClemente and Prochaska, 1998). Most behavior-change programs are designed for (and have a chance of success when) people are ready to take action regarding their health behavior problems. Only a minority of people are actually in this action stage (Prochaska, 1991). Changes are maintained over time only if they are integrated into an individual's overall lifestyle (Box 6-4). Maintaining healthy lifestyles can prevent hospitalizations and potentially lower the cost of health care.

BOX 6-4 PATIENT TEACHING

Lifestyle Changes

Objective

- Patient will reduce health risks related to poor lifestyle habits (e.g., high-fat diet, sedentary lifestyle) through behavior change.

Teaching Strategies

- Practice active listening and ask the patient how he or she prefers to learn.
- Begin with determining information that the patient knows regarding health risks related to poor lifestyle.
- Ask which barriers the patient perceives with the planned lifestyle change.
- Help the patient establish goals for change.
- In collaboration with the patient, establish time lines for modification of eating and exercise lifestyle habits.
- Reinforce the process of change.
- Use written resources at an appropriate reading level (Ward-Smith, 2012).
- Ensure education materials are culturally appropriate (Douglas et al., 2011).
- Include family members to support the lifestyle change.

Evaluation

- Ask the patient to repeat back the teaching on reducing risks and lifestyle changes (Ward-Smith, 2012).
- Have the patient maintain an exercise and eating calendar to track adherence and provide positive reinforcement.
- Ask the patient to discuss success with lifestyle changes such as minutes spent in activity or actual number of fruits and vegetables eaten.

ILLNESS

Illness is a state in which a person's physical, emotional, intellectual, social, developmental, or spiritual functioning is diminished or impaired. Cancer is a disease process, but one patient with leukemia who is responding to treatment may continue to function as usual, whereas another patient with breast cancer who is preparing for surgery may be affected in dimensions other than the physical. Therefore illness is not synonymous with disease. Although nurses need to be familiar with different types of diseases and their treatments, they often are concerned more with illness, which may include disease but also includes the effects on functioning and well-being in all dimensions.

QSEN QSEN: BUILDING COMPETENCY IN SAFETY Sandy, a registered nurse, works in the Health Center of the local university. This spring, the university had 25 cases of measles break out among the college students. The measles outbreak was a part of a larger outbreak of measles in colleges and universities across the country. Sandy plans to use the health belief model to develop a risk reduction program. On the basis of this model, which strategies does Sandy need to consider?

Answers to QSEN Activities can be found on the Evolve website.

Acute and Chronic Illness

Acute and chronic illnesses are two general classifications of illness used in this chapter and throughout this text. Both acute and chronic illnesses have the potential to be life threatening. An **acute illness** is usually reversible, has a short duration, and is often severe. The symptoms appear abruptly, are intense, and often subside after a relatively short period. An acute illness may affect functioning in any dimension. A **chronic illness** persists, usually longer than 6 months, is irreversible, and affects functioning in one or more systems. Patients often fluctuate between maximal functioning and serious health relapses that may be life threatening. A person with a chronic illness is similar to a person with a disability in that both have varying degrees of functional limitations that result from either a pathological process or an injury (Larsen, 2013a). In addition, the social surroundings and physical environment in which an individual lives frequently affect the abilities, motivation, and psychological maintenance of the person.

Chronic illnesses and disabilities remain a leading health problem in North America for older adults and children. Issues of coping and living with a chronic illness can be complex and overwhelming. The Centers for Disease Control and Prevention report that in 2012 about half of the adults in the United States had at least one chronic disease or health problem (CDC, 2015). Many chronic illnesses are related to four modifiable health behaviors: physical inactivity, poor nutrition, use of tobacco, and excessive alcohol consumption (CDC, 2015). A major role for nursing is to provide patient education aimed at helping patients manage their illness or disability. The goal of managing a chronic illness is to reduce the occurrence or improve the tolerance of symptoms. By enhancing wellness, nurses improve the quality of life for patients living with chronic illnesses or disabilities.

Patients with chronic diseases and their families continually adjust and adapt to their illnesses. How an individual perceives an illness influences the type of coping responses. In response to a chronic illness, an individual develops an illness career. The illness career is flexible and changes in response to changes in health, interactions with health professionals, psychological changes related to grief, and stress related to the illness (Larsen, 2013b).

Illness Behavior

People who are ill generally act in a way that medical sociologists call **illness behavior**. It involves how people monitor their bodies, define and interpret their symptoms, take remedial actions, and use the resources in the health care system (Mechanic, 1995). Personal history, social situations, social norms, and past experiences affect illness behaviors (Larsen, 2013b). How people react to illness varies widely; illness behavior displayed in sickness is often used to manage life adversities (Mechanic, 1995). In other words, if people perceive themselves to be ill, illness behaviors become coping mechanisms. For example, illness behavior results in a patient being released from roles, social expectations, or responsibilities. A homemaker views the "flu" as either an added stressor or a temporary release from child care and household responsibilities.

Variables Influencing Illness and Illness Behavior

Internal and external variables influence both health and health behavior and illness and illness behavior. The influences of these variables and a patient's illness behavior often affect the likelihood of seeking health care, adherence to therapy, and health outcomes. Plan individualized care based on an understanding of these variables and behaviors to help patients cope with their illness at various stages. The goal is to promote optimal functioning in all dimensions throughout an illness.

Internal Variables. Internal variables such as patient perceptions of symptoms and the nature of the illness influence patient behavior. If patients believe that the symptoms of their illnesses disrupt their normal routine, they are more likely to seek health care assistance than if they do not perceive the symptoms to be disruptive. Patients are also more likely to seek assistance if they believe the symptoms are serious or life threatening. Persons awakened by crushing chest pains in the middle of the night generally view this symptom as potentially serious and life threatening, and they will probably be motivated to seek assistance. However, such a perception can also have the opposite effect. Individuals may fear serious illness, react by denying it, and not seek medical assistance.

The nature of the illness, either acute or chronic, also affects a patient's illness behavior. Patients with acute illnesses are likely to seek health care and comply readily with therapy. On the other hand, a patient with a chronic illness in which symptoms are not cured but only partially relieved may not be motivated to adhere to the therapy plan. Some patients who are chronically ill become less actively involved in their care, experience greater frustration, and adhere less readily to care. Because nurses generally spend more time than other health care professionals with chronically ill patients, they are in the unique position of being able to help these patients overcome problems related to illness behavior. A patient's coping skills and his or her locus of control (the degree to which people believe they control what happens to them) are other internal variables that affect the way the patient behaves when ill (see Chapter 38).

External Variables. External variables influencing a patient's illness behavior include the visibility of symptoms, social group, cultural background, economic variables, accessibility of the health care system, and social support. The visibility of the symptoms of an illness affects body image and illness behavior. A patient with a visible symptom is often more likely to seek assistance than a patient with no visible symptoms.

Patients' social groups either assist in recognizing the threat of illness or support the denial of potential illness. Families, friends, and co-workers all potentially influence patients' illness behavior. Patients often react positively to social support while practicing positive health behaviors. A person's cultural background teaches the person how to be healthy, how to recognize illness, and how to be ill. The effects of disease and its interpretation vary according to cultural circumstances. For example, ethnic differences influence decisions about health care and the use of diagnostic and health care services. Dietary practices and cultural beliefs contribute to illness and disease maintenance (Giger, 2013).

Economic variables influence the way a patient reacts to illness. Because of economic constraints, some patients delay treatment and in many cases continue to carry out daily activities. Patients' access to the health care system is closely related to economic factors. The health care system is a socioeconomic system that patients enter, interact within, and exit. For many patients entry into the system is complex or confusing, and some patients seek nonemergency medical care in an emergency department because they do not know how otherwise to obtain health services or do not have access to care. The physical proximity of patients to a health care agency often influences how soon they enter the system after deciding to seek care.

Impact of Illness on the Patient and Family

Illness is never an isolated life event. The patient and family deal with changes resulting from illness and treatment. Each patient responds uniquely to illness, requiring you to individualize nursing interventions. The patient and family commonly experience behavioral and emotional changes and changes in roles, body image and self-concept, and family dynamics.

Behavioral and Emotional Changes. People react differently to illness or the threat of illness. Individual behavioral and emotional reactions depend on the nature of an illness, a patient's attitude toward it, the reaction of others to it, and the variables of illness behavior.

Short-term, non–life-threatening illnesses evoke few behavioral changes in the functioning of a patient or family. For example, a father who has a cold lacks the energy and patience to spend time in family activities. He becomes irritable and prefers not to interact with his family. This is a behavioral change, but the change is subtle and does not last long. Some may even consider such a change a normal response to illness.

Severe illness, particularly one that is life threatening, leads to more extensive emotional and behavioral changes such as anxiety, shock, denial, anger, and withdrawal. These are common responses to the stress of illness. You can develop interventions to help a patient and family cope with and adapt to this stress when the stressor itself usually cannot be changed.

Impact on Body Image. Body image is the subjective concept of physical appearance (see Chapter 34). Some illnesses result in changes in physical appearance. Patients' and families' reactions differ and usually depend on the type of changes (e.g., loss of a limb or an organ), their adaptive capacity, the rate at which changes take place, and the support services available.

When a change in body image such as that which results from a leg amputation occurs, the patient generally adjusts in the following phases: shock, withdrawal, acknowledgment, acceptance, and rehabilitation. Initially the patient is in shock because of the change or impending change. He or she depersonalizes the change and talks about it as though it were happening to someone else. As the patient and family recognize the reality of the change, they become anxious and often withdraw, refusing to discuss it. Withdrawal is an adaptive coping mechanism that helps the patient adjust. As a patient and family acknowledge the change, they move through a period of grieving (see Chapter 37). At the end of the acknowledgment phase, they accept the loss. During rehabilitation the patient is ready to learn how to adapt to the change in body image through use of prosthesis or changing lifestyles and goals.

Impact on Self-Concept. Self-concept is a mental self-image of strengths and weaknesses in all aspects of personality. Self-concept depends in part on body image and roles but also includes other aspects of psychology and spirituality (see Chapters 34 and 36). The effect of illness on the self-concepts of patients and family members is usually more complex and less readily observed than role changes.

Self-concept is important in relationships with other family members. For example, a patient whose self-concept changes because of illness may no longer meet family expectations, leading to tension or conflict. As a result, family members change their interactions with the patient. In the course of providing care, you observe changes in the patient's self-concept (or in the self-concepts of family members) and develop a care plan to help them adjust to the changes resulting from the illness.

Impact on Family Roles. People have many roles in life such as wage earner, decision maker, professional, child, sibling, or parent. When an illness occurs, parents and children try to adapt to the major changes that result. Role reversal is common (see Chapter 10). If a parent of an adult becomes ill and cannot carry out usual activities, the adult child often assumes many of the parent's responsibilities and in essence becomes a parent to the parent. Such a reversal of the usual situation sometimes leads to stress, conflicting responsibilities for the adult child, or direct conflict over decision making.

Such a change may be subtle and short term or drastic and long term. An individual and family generally adjust more easily to subtle, short-term changes. In most cases they know that the role change is temporary and will not require a prolonged adjustment. However, long-term changes require an adjustment process similar to the grief process (see Chapter 37). The patient and family often require specific counseling and guidance to help them cope with role changes.

Impact on Family Dynamics. As a result of the effects of illness on the patient and family, family dynamics often change. Family dynamics are the processes by which the family functions, makes decisions, gives support to individual members, and copes with everyday changes and challenges. When a parent in a family becomes ill, family activities and decision making often come to a halt as the other family members wait for the illness to pass, or the family members delay action because they are reluctant to assume the ill person's roles or responsibilities. This often creates tension or anxiety in the family. Role reversal is also common. If a parent of an adult becomes ill and is unable to carry out usual activities, the adult child often becomes the family caregiver and assumes many of the parent responsibilities. Such reversal leads to conflict responsibilities for the adult child and often direct conflict over decision making. The nurse views the whole family as a patient under stress, planning care to help the family regain the maximal level of functioning and well-being (see Chapter 10).

CARING FOR YOURSELF

To be able to provide competent, quality and safe care, nurses need to take care of themselves to ensure they remain healthy. Nurses are particularly susceptible to the development of compassion fatigue, which is a combination of secondary traumatic stress (STS) and burnout (BO) (see Chapter 1). Secondary traumatic stress develops as a result of the relationships that nurses develop with their patients and families, whereas BO stems from conflicts or nurse job dissatisfaction within the work setting (Boyle, 2011; Potter et al., 2013a). Compassion fatigue frequently affects a nurse's health, often leading to a decline in health, changes in sleep and eating patterns, emotional exhaustion, irritability, restlessness, impaired ability to focus and engage with patients, feelings of hopelessness, inability to take pleasure from activities, and anxiety (Potter et al., 2013a). In the workplace the effects of compassion fatigue are often manifested by diminished performance, reduced ability to feel empathy, depersonalization of the patient, poor judgment, chronic absenteeism, high turnover rates, and conflict between nurses (Jenkins and Warren, 2012). It is important for nurses to engage in personal and professional strategies to help combat compassion fatigue and promote resiliency.

Personal strategies focus on health-promoting behaviors and healthy lifestyle choices. In an effort to combat STS and BO, you need to eat a nutritious diet, get adequate sleep regularly, engage in regular exercise and relaxation activities, establish a good work-family balance, and engage in regular nonwork activities (Beck, 2011). Other strategies that can help you prevent or deal with STS and BO include developing coping skills, allowing personal time for grieving the loss of patients, and focusing on one's own spiritual health (Beck, 2011). Another strategy is to find a mentor or experienced nurse who understands the stress of the job and is able to help you identify coping strategies (Lombardo and Eyre, 2011).

An increasing number of health care institutions and organizations are offering educational programs for the nursing staff that are designed to help decrease compassion fatigue and increase resiliency (Flarity et al., 2013; Jenkins and Warren, 2012). These programs educate nurses about compassion fatigue and its negative effects and provide resources and tools for nurses to use to prevent or cope with STS and BO (Potter et al., 2013b). Participating in debriefing sessions or a compassion fatigue support group allows nurses to identify stressors and work as a group to develop healthy coping strategies (Beck, 2011; Boyle, 2011). Health care organizations need to also provide resources for nurses such as a mental health professional to provide assistance in managing STS and BO (Beck, 2011). It is important that organizations provide nurses with the education and resources needed to care for themselves.

KEY POINTS

- Health and wellness are not merely the absence of disease and illness.
- A person's state of health, wellness, or illness depends on individual values, personality, and lifestyle.
- Multiple models of health in which persons are active participants explain relationships among health beliefs, health behaviors, health promotion, and individual well-being.
- Health beliefs, practices, and illness behaviors are influenced by internal and external variables, and you need to consider them when planning care.
- Health promotion activities help maintain or enhance health, whereas wellness education teaches patients how to care for themselves.
- Illness prevention activities protect against health threats and thus maintain an optimal level of health.
- Nursing incorporates health promotion activities, wellness education, and illness prevention activities rather than simply treating illness.
- The three levels of preventive care are primary, secondary, and tertiary.
- Risk factors threaten health, influence health practices, and are important considerations in illness prevention activities.
- Improvement in health usually involves a change in health behaviors.
- The transtheoretical model of change describes a series of changes through which patients progress for successful behavior change rather than simply assuming that all patients are in an action stage.
- Illness has many effects on a patient and family, including changes in behavior and emotions, family roles and dynamics, body image, and self-concept.
- Using personal and professional strategies that focus on caring for self can help to decrease or prevent compassion fatigue.

CLINICAL APPLICATION QUESTIONS

Preparing for Clinical Practice

Ms. Thom, age 46, works as an RN in the intensive care unit at a large busy medical center. Over the last three years she has gained 30 lbs and quit attending the fitness classes at the local recreation center. Her co-workers keep trying to get her to come back to fitness class, but she says that she is too tired after work and just wants to go home. She has smoked for 15 years, but says that she is trying to cut back on the number of cigarettes each day because she watched her mother die from emphysema. She has picked up some literature from Employee Health on smoking cessation. She was recently diagnosed with hypertension.

1. Using the health belief model, identify the modifying factors impacting Ms. Thom's likelihood of taking a preventive health action.
2. Which primary intervention activities are important for Ms. Thom?
3. Using the transtheoretical model of change, in which stage is Ms. Thom most likely related to her smoking? Explain your answer.

ⓔ *Answers to Clinical Application Questions can be found on the Evolve website.*

REVIEW QUESTIONS

Are You Ready to Test Your Nursing Knowledge?

1. A nurse is presenting a program to workers in a factory covering safety topics, including the wearing of hearing protectors when workers are in the factory. Which level of prevention is the nurse practicing?
   1. Primary prevention
   2. Secondary prevention
   3. Tertiary prevention
   4. Quaternary prevention
2. A patient had surgery for a total knee replacement a week ago and is currently participating in daily physical rehabilitation sessions at the surgeon's office. In what level of prevention is the patient participating?
   1. Primary prevention
   2. Secondary prevention
   3. Tertiary prevention
   4. Quaternary prevention
3. Based on the transtheoretical model of change, what is the most appropriate response to a patient who states: "Me, stop smoking? I've been smoking since I was 16!"
   1. "That's fine. Some people who smoke live a long life."
   2. "OK. I want you to decrease the number of cigarettes you smoke by one each day, and I'll see you in 1 month."
   3. "I understand. Can you think of the greatest reason why stopping smoking would be challenging for you?"
   4. "I'd like you to attend a smoking cessation class this week and use nicotine replacement patches as directed."
4. A patient comes to the local health clinic and states: "I've noticed how many people are out walking in my neighborhood. Is walking good for you?" What is the best response to help the patient through the stages of change for exercise?
   1. "Walking is OK. I really think running is better."
   2. "Yes, walking is great exercise. Do you think you could go for a 5-minute walk next week?"
   3. "Yes, I want you to begin walking. Walk for 30 minutes every day and start to eat more fruits and vegetables."

4. "They probably aren't walking fast enough or far enough. You need to spend at least 45 minutes if you are going to do any good."

5. A male patient has been laid off from his construction job and has many unpaid bills. He is going through a divorce from his marriage of 15 years and has been seeing his pastor to help him through this difficult time. He does not have a primary health care provider because he has never really been sick and his parents never took him to a physician when he was a child. Which external variables influence the patient's health practices? (Select all that apply.)
   1. Difficulty paying his bills
   2. Seeing his pastor as a means of support
   3. Age of patient (46 years)
   4. Stress from the divorce and the loss of a job
   5. Family practice of not routinely seeing a health care provider

6. A nurse is conducting a home visit with an older-adult couple. While in the home the nurse weighs each individual and reviews the 3-day food diary with them. She also checks their blood pressure and encourages them to increase their fluids and activity levels to help with their voiced concern about constipation. The nurse is addressing which level of need according to Maslow?
   1. Physiological
   2. Safety and security
   3. Love and belonging
   4. Self-actualization

7. When taking care of patients, a nurse routinely asks if they take any vitamins or herbal medications, encourages family members to bring in music that the patient likes to help the patient relax, and frequently prays with her patients if that is important to them. The nurse is practicing which model?
   1. Holistic
   2. Health belief
   3. Transtheoretical
   4. Health promotion

8. Using the Transtheoretical Model of Change, order the steps that a patient goes through to make a lifestyle change related to physical activity.
   1. The individual recognizes that he is out of shape when his daughter asks him to walk with her after school.
   2. Eight months after beginning walking, the individual participates with his wife in a local 5K race.
   3. The individual becomes angry when the physician tells him that he needs to increase his activity to lose 30 lbs.
   4. The individual walks 2 to 3 miles, 5 nights a week, with his wife.
   5. The individual visits the local running store to purchase walking shoes and obtain advice on a walking plan.

9. Which statement made by a nurse shows that the nurse is engaging in an activity to help cope with secondary traumatic stress and burnout?
   1. "I don't need time for lunch since I am not very hungry."
   2. "I am enjoying my quilting group that meets each week at my church."
   3. "I am going to drop my gym membership because I don't have time to go."
   4. "I don't know any of the other nurses who met today to discuss hospital-wide problems with nurse satisfaction."

10. Which of the following are symptoms of secondary traumatic stress and burnout that commonly affect nurses? (Select all that apply.)
   1. Regular participation in a book club
   2. Lack of interest in exercise
   3. Difficulty falling asleep
   4. Lack of desire to go to work
   5. Anxiety while working

11. After a class on Pender's health promotion model, students make the following statements. Which statement does the faculty member need to clarify?
   1. "The desired outcome of the model is health-promoting behavior."
   2. "Perceived self-efficacy is not related to the model."
   3. "The individual has unique characteristics and experiences that affect his or her actions."
   4. "Patients need to commit to a plan of action before they adopt a health-promoting behavior."

12. A patient registered at the local fitness center and purchased a pair of exercise shoes. The patient is in what stage of behavioral change?
   1. Precontemplation
   2. Contemplation
   3. Preparation
   4. Action

13. As part of a faith community nursing program in her church, a nurse is developing a health promotion program on breast self-examination for the women's group. Which statement made by one of the participants is related to the individual's perception of susceptibility to an illness?
   1. "I have a door hanging tag in my bathroom to remind me to do my breast self-examination monthly."
   2. "Since my mother had breast cancer, I know that I am at increased risk for developing breast cancer."
   3. "Since I am only 25 years of age, the risk of breast cancer for me is very low."
   4. "I participate every year in our local walk/run to raise money for breast cancer research."

14. The nurse assesses the following risk factors for coronary artery disease (CAD) in a female patient. Which factors are classified as genetic and physiological? (Select all that apply.)
   1. Sedentary lifestyle
   2. Mother died from CAD at age 48
   3. History of hypertension
   4. Eats diet high in sodium
   5. Elevated cholesterol level

15. Which activity shows a nurse engaged in primary prevention?
   1. A home health care nurse visits a patient's home to change a wound dressing.
   2. A nurse is assessing risk factors of a patient in the emergency department admitted with chest pain.
   3. A school health nurse provides a program to the first-year students on healthy eating.
   4. A nurse schedules a patient who had a myocardial infarction for cardiac rehabilitation sessions weekly.

Answers: 1. 1; **2.** 3; **3.** 3; **4.** 2; **5.** 1, 5; **6.** 1; **7.** 1; **8.** 3, 1, 5, 4, 2; **9.** 2; **10.** 2, 3, 4, 5; **11.** 2; **12.** 3; **13.** 2; **14.** 2, 3, 5; **15.** 3.

Rationales for Review Questions can be found on the Evolve website.

REFERENCES

Becker M, Maiman L: Sociobehavioral determinants of compliance with health and medical care recommendations, *Med Care* 13(1):10, 1975.

Boyle DA: Countering compassion fatigue: a requisite nursing agenda, *Online J Issues Nurs* 16(1):1, 2011.

Centers for Disease Control and Prevention [CDC]: *Chronic diseases and health promotion*, 2015, http://www.cdc.gov/chronicdisease/overview/index.htm. Accessed June 21, 2015.

DiClemente C, Prochaska J: Toward a comprehensive transtheoretical model of change. In Miller WR, Healther N, editors: *Treating addictive behaviors*, New York, 1998, Plenum Press.

Douglas MK, et al: Standards of practice for culturally competent nursing care, 2011 update, *J Transcult Nurs* 22(4):317, 2011.

Edelman CL, Mandle CL: *Health promotion throughout the life span*, ed 8, St Louis, 2014, Mosby.

Giger JN: *Transcultural nursing: assessment and intervention*, ed 6, St Louis, 2013, Mosby.

Kersey-Matusiak G: Culturally competent care: are we there yet?, *Nursing* 43(4):49, 2012.

Larsen PD: Chronicity. In Lubkin IM, Larsen PD, editors: *Chronic illness: impact and intervention*, ed 8, Boston, 2013a, Jones & Bartlett.

Larsen PD: The illness experience. In Lubkin IM, Larsen PD, editors: *Chronic illness: impact and intervention*, ed 8, Boston, 2013b, Jones & Bartlett.

Lombardo B, Eyre C: Compassion fatigue: a nurse's primer, *Online J Issues Nurs* 16(1):1, 2011.

Mechanic D: Sociological dimensions of illness behavior, *Soc Sci Med* 41(9):1207, 1995.

Narayan MC: Culture's effects on pain assessment and management, *Am J Nurs* 110(4):38, 2010.

Pender NJ: *Health promotion and nursing practice*, Norwalk, Conn, 1982, Appleton-Century-Crofts.

Pender NJ: *Health promotion and nursing practice*, ed 3, Stamford, Conn, 1996, Appleton & Lange.

Pender NJ, et al: *Health promotion in nursing practice*, ed 7, Upper Saddle River, NJ, 2015, Prentice Hall.

Prochaska JO: Assessing how people change, *Cancer* 67(3 Suppl):805, 1991.

Purnell LD: *Transcultural health care: a culturally competent approach*, ed 4, Philadelphia, 2013, FA Davis.

Rosenstoch I: Historical origin of the health belief model, *Health Educ Monogr* 2:334, 1974.

Touhy TA, Jett K: *Ebersole and Hess' Toward healthy aging: human needs and nursing response*, ed 8, St Louis, 2012, Mosby.

US Department of Health and Human Services [USDHHS], Public Health Service: *Healthy People 2000: national health promotion and disease prevention objectives*, Washington, DC, 1990, US Government Printing Office.

US Department of Health and Human Services [USDHHS]: *Healthy People 2010: understanding and improving health*, ed 2, Washington, DC, 2000, US Government Printing Office.

US Department of Health and Human Services [USDHHS]: *Healthy People 2020 Framework*, n.d., www.healthypeople.gov/sites/default/files/HP2020Framework.pdf. Accessed June 21, 2015.

US Department of Health and Human Services [USDHHS]: *HealthyPeople.gov: About Healthy People*, 2015, http://www.healthypeople.gov/2020/default.aspx. Accessed June 21, 2015.

Ward-Smith P: Health literacy, *Urol Nurs* 32(3):168, 2012.

World Health Organization Interim Commission [WHO]: *Chronicle of WHO*, Geneva, 1947, The Organization.

World Health Organization [WHO]: *Milestones in health promotion: statement from global conferences*, Geneva, Switzerland, 2009, WHO Press.

RESEARCH REFERENCES

Beck CT: Secondary traumatic stress in nurses: a systematic review, *Arch Psychiatr Nurs* 25:2011.

Byam-Williams J, Salyer J: Factors influencing the health-related lifestyle of community-dwelling older adults, *Home Healthc Nurse* 28(2):115, 2010.

Dandridge R: Faith community/parish nurse literature, *J Christ Nurs* 31(2):100, 2014.

Droppa M, Lee H: Motivational interviewing: a journey to improve health, *Nursing* 44(3):40, 2014.

Flarity K, et al: The effectiveness of an education program on preventing and treating compassion fatigue in emergency nurses, *Adv Emerg Nurs J* 35(3):247, 2013.

Han Y, Yan J: The effect of face-to-face-interventions in promoting physical activity, *Am J Nurs* 114(4):23, 2014.

Hornsten A, et al: Strategies in health promoting dialogues—primary nurses' perspectives—a qualitative study, *Scand J Caring Sci* 28:235, 2014.

Jenkins B, Warren NA: Concept analysis: compassion fatigue and effects upon critical care nurses, *Crit Care Nurs Q* 35(4):388, 2012.

Pascucci MA, et al: Health promotion for the oldest of the old people, *Nurs Older People* 24(3):22, 2012.

Potter P, et al: Developing a systematic program for compassion fatigue, *Nurse Admin Q* 37(4):326, 2013a.

Potter P, et al: Evaluation of a compassion fatigue resiliency program for oncology nurses, *Oncol Nurs Forum* 40(2):180, 2013b.

Wallace R, et al: Effects of a 12-week community exercise programme on older people, *Nurs Older People* 26(1):20, 2014.

7

Caring in Nursing Practice

OBJECTIVES

- Discuss the role that caring plays in building the nurse-patient relationship.
- Compare and contrast theories on caring.
- Discuss the evidence that exists about patients' perceptions of caring.
- Explain how an ethic of care influences nurses' decision making.
- Describe ways to express caring through presence and touch.
- Describe the therapeutic benefit of listening to patients.
- Explain the relationship between knowing a patient and clinical decision making.
- Discuss the relationship of compassion to caring.
- Describe the significance of caring as part of the nurses' personal philosophy of nursing.

KEY TERMS

Caring, p. 80
Comforting, p. 84
Compassion, p. 80
Ethic of care, p. 83
Presence, p. 84
Transcultural, p. 80
Transformative, p. 81

MEDIA RESOURCES

http://evolve.elsevier.com/Potter/fundamentals/

- Review Questions
- Case Study with Questions
- Audio Glossary
- Content Updates

Caring is central to nursing practice, but it is even more important in today's hectic, high-tech health care environment. The demands, pressure, and time constraints in the health care environment leave little room for caring practice, which results in nurses and other health professionals becoming dissatisfied with their jobs and cold and indifferent to patient needs (Watson, 2009; 2010). Increasing use of technological advances for rapid diagnosis and treatment often causes nurses and other health care providers to perceive the patient relationship as less important. However, it is important to preserve a relationship-centered approach to patient care for all aspects of nursing, whether the care focuses on pain management, teaching self-care, or basic hygiene measures (Winsett and Hauck, 2011). Technological advances become dangerous without a context of skillful and compassionate care. Despite these challenges in health care, more professional organizations are stressing the importance of caring in health care and keeping the nurse engaged at the patient's bedside (RWJF, 2014). *Nursing's Agenda for the Future* (ANA, 2002) states that "Nursing is the pivotal health care profession highly valued for its specialized knowledge, skill, and caring in improving the health status of the individual, family, and the community." The American Organization of Nurse Executives (AONE, 2015) describes caring and knowledge as the core of nursing, with caring being a key component of what a nurse brings to a patient experience (Figure 7-1).

It is time to value and embrace caring practices and expert knowledge that are the heart of competent nursing practice (Benner et al., 2010). When you engage patients in a caring and compassionate manner, you learn that the therapeutic gain in caring makes enormous contributions to the health and well-being of your patients.

Have you ever been ill or experienced a problem requiring health care intervention? Think about that experience. Then consider the following two scenarios and select the situation that you believe most successfully demonstrates a sense of caring.

A nurse enters a patient's room, greets the patient warmly while touching him or her lightly on the shoulder, makes eye contact, sits down for a few minutes and asks about the patient's thoughts and concerns, listens to the patient's story, looks at the intravenous (IV) solution hanging in the room, briefly examines the patient, and then checks the vital sign summary on the bedside computer screen before leaving the room.

A second nurse enters the patient's room, looks at the IV solution hanging in the room, checks the vital sign summary sheet on the bedside computer screen, and acknowledges the patient but never sits down or touches him or her. The nurse makes eye contact from above while the patient is lying in bed. He or she asks a few brief questions about the patient's symptoms and leaves.

There is little doubt that the first scenario presents the nurse in specific acts of caring. The nurse's calm presence, parallel eye contact, attention to the patient's concerns, and physical closeness all express a patient-centered, comforting approach. In contrast, the second scenario is task-oriented and expresses a sense of indifference to patient concerns. Both of these scenarios take approximately the same amount of time but leave very different patient perceptions. It is important to remember that, during times of illness or when a person seeks the professional guidance of a nurse, caring is essential in helping the individual reach positive outcomes.

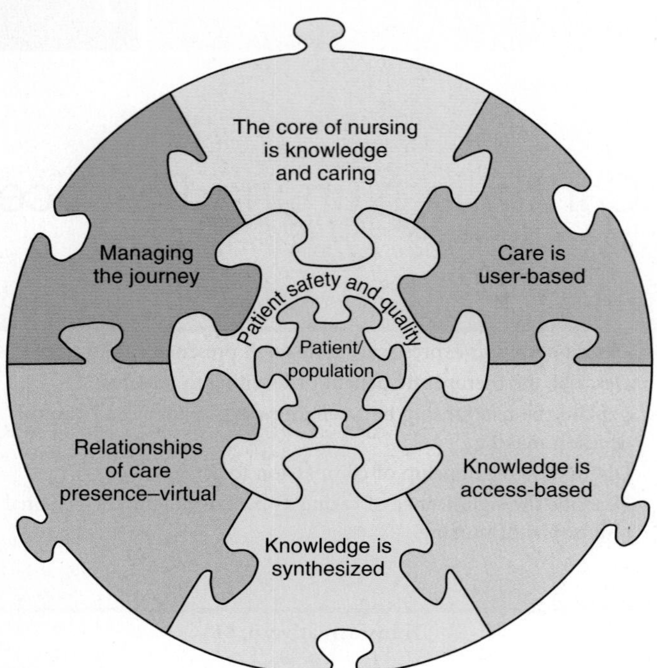

FIGURE 7-1 AONE guiding principles for the role of the nurse in future patient care delivery. (Copyright© 2015 by the American Organization of Nurse Executives [AONE]. All rights reserved.)

THEORETICAL VIEWS ON CARING

Caring is a universal phenomenon influencing the ways in which people think, feel, and behave in relation to one another. Since Florence Nightingale, nurses have studied caring from a variety of philosophical and ethical perspectives. A number of nursing scholars have developed theories on caring because of its importance to nursing practice. This chapter does not detail all of the theories of caring, but it is designed to help you understand how caring is at the heart of a nurse's ability to work with all patients in a respectful and therapeutic way.

Caring Is Primary

Benner offers nurses a rich, holistic understanding of nursing practice and caring through the interpretation of expert nurses' stories. After listening to nurses' stories and analyzing their meaning, she described the essence of excellent nursing practice, which is caring. The stories revealed the nurses' behaviors and decisions that expressed caring. Caring means that people, events, projects, and things matter to people (Benner and Wrubel, 1989; Benner et al., 2010). It is a word for being connected.

Caring determines what matters to a person. It underlies a wide range of interactions, from parental love to friendship, from caring for one's work to caring for one's pet, to caring for and about one's patients (Burtson and Stichler, 2010). Benner and Wrubel (1989) note: "Caring creates possibility." Personal concern for another person, an event, or a thing provides motivation and direction for people to care. Through caring, nurses help patients recover in the face of illness, give meaning to their illness, and maintain or reestablish connection. Understanding how to provide humanistic caring and compassion begins early in nursing education and continues to mature through experiential practice (Gallagher-Lepak and Kubsch, 2009).

Patients are not all the same. Each person brings a unique background of experiences, values, and cultural perspectives to a health care encounter. Caring is always specific and relational for each nurse-patient encounter. As nurses acquire more experience, they typically learn that caring helps them focus on the patients for whom they care. Caring facilitates a nurse's ability to know a patient, allowing the nurse to recognize a patient's problems and find and implement individualized solutions on the basis of the patient's unique needs, which is one of the primary objectives of using the nursing process.

Illness is a human experience. It impacts an individual's independent function, and the associated treatments disrupt a patient's lifestyle and social and family interactions. Expert nurses understand the differences among health, illness, and disease. Develop a caring relationship with your patients and listen to their stories to fully understand the meaning and impact of their condition. This information and understanding helps you provide individualized patient-centered care.

Leininger's Transcultural Caring

From a transcultural perspective, Madeleine Leininger (1991) describes the concept of care as the essence and central, unifying, and dominant domain that distinguishes nursing from other health disciplines (see Chapter 4). Care is an essential human need, necessary for the health and survival of all individuals. Care, unlike cure, helps an individual or group improve a human condition. Acts of caring refer to nurturing and skillful activities, processes, and decisions to assist people in ways that are empathetic, compassionate, and supportive. An act of caring depends on the needs, problems, and values of the patient. Leininger's studies of numerous cultures around the world found that care helps protect, develop, nurture, and provide survival to people. It is needed for people of all cultures to recover from illness and to maintain healthy life practices.

Leininger (1991) stresses how important it is for nurses to understand cultural caring behaviors. Even though human caring is a universal phenomenon, the expressions, processes, and patterns of caring vary among people of different cultures (Box 7-1). Caring is very personal; thus its expression differs for each patient. For caring to be effective, nurses need to learn culturally specific behaviors and words that reflect human caring in different cultures to identify and meet the needs of all patients (see Chapter 9). As nurses we care for patients from certain "subcultures" that have very unique needs (e.g., the chronically ill, physically disabled, developmentally challenged, foster children, the homeless). When caring for your patients, you must remember that a difference in culture does not always mean that a person is from a different country.

Watson's Transpersonal Caring

Caring is a central focus of nursing and it is integral to maintain the ethical and philosophical roots of the profession (Watson 2008; Lusk and Fater, 2013). Patients and their families expect a high quality of human interaction from nurses; however, unfortunately many conversations between patients and their nurses are very brief and disconnected. Many are not really "conversations," but rather simply the nurse reporting information to the patient and family. Watson's theory of caring is a holistic model for nursing that suggests that a conscious intention to care promotes healing and wholeness (Watson, 2008, 2010). It integrates the human caring processes with healing environments, incorporating the life-generating and life-receiving processes of human caring and healing for nurses and their patients (WCSI, 2014). The theory describes a consciousness that allows nurses to raise new questions about what it means to be a nurse, to be ill, and to be caring and healing. The transpersonal caring theory rejects the disease orientation to health care and *places care before cure* (Watson, 2008). When the nurse focuses on transpersonal caring, he or she looks for deeper sources of inner healing to protect, enhance, and preserve a person's dignity, humanity, wholeness, and inner harmony (see also Chapter 4).

In Watson's view caring becomes almost spiritual. It preserves human dignity in the technological, cure-dominated health care system (Watson, 2009). Creating caring-healing environments in the current high-tech health care system is crucial to establishing and maintaining the nurse-patient relationship (Jackson, 2012). In Watson's model the emphasis is on the nurse-patient relationship. The focus is on carative behaviors and the nurse-patient caring relationship (Table 7-1). A nurse communicates caring-healing to a patient through the nurse's consciousness. This takes place during a single caring moment between nurse and patient when a connection forms. The model is **transformative** because the relationship influences both the nurse and the patient for better or for worse (Watson, 2008, 2010). Caring-healing consciousness promotes healing. Application of Watson's caring model in practice enhances nurses' caring practices (Box 7-2).

BOX 7-1 CULTURAL ASPECTS OF CARE

Nurse Caring Behaviors

Caring includes knowing a patient's cultural values and beliefs. Although the need for human caring is universal, its application is influenced by cultural norms. As a result, expectations may change across cultures (Kelley et al., 2013; Suliman et al., 2009). For example, providing time for family presence is often more valuable than a nursing presence. Using touch to convey caring sometimes crosses cultural norms. Sometimes a gender-congruent caregiver or the patient's family needs to provide caring touch. When listening to a patient, remember that some cultures view eye contact as disrespectful.

Implications for Patient-Centered Care

- Know the patient's beliefs and attitudes regarding health care and caring practices.
- Know the patient's cultural practices regarding end-of-life care. In some cultures it is considered insensitive to tell the patient that he or she is dying (Maroon, 2012).
- Determine if a member of the patient's family or cultural group is the best resource to guide the use of caring practices such as providing presence or touching (Lusk and Fater, 2013).
- Know the patient's cultural practices regarding the removal of life support (Maroon, 2012).
- Know the patient's cultural practices regarding care of the body after death.

Swanson's Theory of Caring

Kristen Swanson (1991) studied patients and professional caregivers in an effort to develop a theory of caring for nursing practice. This theory of caring was developed from three perinatal studies involving interviews with women who miscarried, parents and health care professionals in a newborn intensive care unit, and socially at-risk mothers who received long-term public health intervention (Swanson, 1999). After analyzing the stories and descriptions of the three groups, Swanson developed a theory of caring, which includes five caring processes (Table 7-2). Swanson (1991) defines caring as a nurturing way of relating to an individual (i.e., when one feels a personal sense of commitment and responsibility). The theory provides direction for how to develop useful and effective caring strategies appropriate for multiple age-group and health care settings (Andershed and Olsson, 2009). It supports the claim that caring is a central nursing phenomenon but not necessarily unique to nursing practice.

Summary of Theoretical Views

Nursing caring theories have common themes. Duffy et al. (2007) identify these commonalities as human interaction or communication, mutuality, appreciating the uniqueness of individuals, and improving

TABLE 7-1 Watson's 10 Carative Factors (Watson, 2008)

Carative Factor	Example in Practice
Forming a human-altruistic value system	Use loving kindness to extend yourself. Use self-disclosure appropriately to promote a therapeutic alliance with your patient (e.g., share a personal experience in common with your patient such as a childrearing experience, an illness, or an experience with a parent who needs assistance).
Instilling faith-hope	Provide a connection with the patient that offers purpose and direction when trying to find the meaning of an illness.
Cultivating a sensitivity to one's self and to others	Learn to accept yourself and others for their full potential. A caring nurse matures into becoming a self-actualized nurse.
Developing a helping, trusting, human caring relationship	Learn to develop and sustain helping, trusting, authentic caring relationships through effective communication with your patients.
Promoting and expressing positive and negative feelings	Support and accept your patients' feelings. In connecting with your patients you show a willingness to take risks in sharing in the relationship.
Using creative problem-solving, caring processes	Apply the nursing process in systematic, scientific problem-solving decision making in providing patient-centered care.
Promoting transpersonal teaching-learning	Learn together while educating the patient to acquire self-care skills. The patient assumes responsibility for learning.
Providing for a supportive, protective, and/or corrective mental, physical, societal, and spiritual environment	Create a healing environment at all levels, physical and nonphysical. This promotes wholeness, beauty, comfort, dignity, and peace.
Meeting human needs	Help patients with basic needs with an intentional care and caring consciousness.
Allowing for existential-phenomenological-spiritual forces	Allow spiritual forces to provide a better understanding of yourself and your patient.

BOX 7-2 EVIDENCE-BASED PRACTICE

Enhancing Caring

PICO Question: Do patient satisfaction scores among hospitalized adult patients improve when carative nursing practices are used?

Evidence Summary

Patient satisfaction is an important indicator for the quality of health care received. Caring practices facilitate healing and improve patient satisfaction with nursing care (Palese et al., 2011; Zolnierek, 2014). Caring behaviors were integrated into a nursing care model in multiple European hospitals; and researchers wanted to determine if (1) there were any correlations between caring and patient satisfaction; (2) there were any differences across countries; and (3) did caring behaviors affect patient satisfaction. Caring behaviors, especially those of connectedness, presence, and respect, highly correlated with patient satisfaction; and there were no differences across countries. Nurses' knowledge and skill level were expectations of care and did not correlate with patient satisfaction scores (Palese et al., 2011). Carative nursing practices improve and solidify the nurse-patient relationship and contribute to patient-centered care and patient satisfaction measures (Dobrina et al., 2014; Lusk and Fater, 2013).

Application to Nursing Practice

- Use caring nursing practices to design a wholistic approach for individualized patient-centered care (Maroon, 2012).
- Use caring practices of listening, presence, and connectedness to partner with the patient and family through their illness. Use these practices with humility, love, kindness, and compassion (Dobrina et al., 2014).
- Knowing the patient enables a nurse to partner with a patient and family to obtain vital health care information, understand the patient's expectation and fears, and identify health care priorities. Knowing the patient is continuous, and the nurse must use every patient interaction to "know" the patient better (Kelley et al., 2013; Zolinierek, 2014).
- Being with and doing for a patient are components of presence, whether it is a dedicated one-on-one interaction during a nursing shift or quietly sitting with a patient (Drenkard, 2008; Yagasaki and Komatsu, 2013). Presence often helps elicit important health care information from a patient and reduces patient fears and anxiety.

TABLE 7-2 Swanson's Theory of Caring (Swanson, 1991)

Caring Process	Definitions	Subdimensions
Knowing	Striving to understand an event as it has meaning in the life of the other	Avoiding assumptions Centering on the one cared for Assessing thoroughly Seeking clues to clarify the event Engaging the self or both
Being with	Being emotionally present to the other	Being there Conveying ability Sharing feelings Not burdening
Doing for	Doing for the other as he or she would do for self if it were at all possible	Comforting Anticipating Performing skillfully Protecting Preserving dignity
Enabling	Facilitating the other's passage through life transitions (e.g., birth, death) and unfamiliar events	Informing/explaining Supporting/allowing Focusing Generating alternatives Validating/giving feedback
Maintaining belief	Sustaining faith in the other's capacity to get through an event or transition and face a future with meaning	Believing in/holding in esteem Maintaining a hope-filled attitude Offering realistic optimism "Going the distance"

the welfare of patients and their families. Caring is highly relational. A nurse and patient enter into a relationship that is much more than one person simply "doing tasks for" another. There is a mutual give-and-take that develops as nurse and patient begin to know and care for one another (Jackson, 2012; Parcells and Locsin, 2011). Caring theories are valuable when assessing patient perceptions of being cared for in a multicultural environment (Suliman et al., 2009). Frank (1998) described a personal situation when he was suffering from cancer: "What I wanted when I was ill was a mutual relationship of *people* who were also clinician and patient." It was important for Frank to be seen as one of two fellow human beings, not the dependent patient being cared for by the expert technical clinician.

Caring seems highly invisible at times when a nurse and patient enter a relationship of respect, concern, and support. A nurse's empathy and compassion become a natural part of every patient encounter. However, when caring is absent, it becomes very obvious. For example, if a nurse shows disinterest or chooses to avoid a patient's request for help, his or her inaction quickly conveys an uncaring attitude. Benner and Wrubel (1989) relate the story of a clinical nurse specialist who learned from a patient what caring is all about: "I felt that I was teaching him a lot, but actually he taught me. One day he said to me (probably after I had delivered some well-meaning technical information about his disease), 'You're doing an OK job, but I can tell that every time you walk in that door you're walking out.'" In this nurse's story the patient perceived that the nurse was simply going through the motions of teaching and showed little caring toward the patient. Patients quickly know when nurses fail to relate to them.

As you practice caring, your patient will sense your commitment and willingness to enter into a relationship that allows you to understand his or her experience of illness. In a study of patients receiving oral chemotherapy, patients noted that it was essential for nurses to develop a partnership and connect with them, to be attentive, and be proactive in providing committed patient support (Yagasaki and Komatsu, 2013). Thus the nurse becomes a coach and partner rather than a detached provider of care.

One aspect of caring is enabling, when a nurse and patient work together to identify alternatives in approaches to care and resources. Consider a nurse working with a patient recently diagnosed with diabetes mellitus who must learn how to administer daily insulin injections. The nurse enables the patient by providing instruction in a manner that allows the patient to successfully modify lifestyle to incorporate diabetes self-management strategies such as medication administration, exercise, and changes in diet.

Another common theme of caring is to understand the context of a person's life and illness. It is difficult to show caring for another

TABLE 7-3 Comparison of Research Studies Exploring Nurse Caring Behaviors (As Perceived by Patients)

Surgical Patient Satisfaction As an Outcome of Nurses' Caring Behaviors: a Descriptive and Correlational Study in Six European Countries (Palese et al., 2011)	Information Needed to Support Knowing the Patient (Kelley et al., 2013)	The Need for a Nursing Presence in Oral Chemotherapy (Yagasaki and Komatsu, 2013)
Caring behaviors and patient satisfaction are intertwined. Major caring factors associated with patient satisfaction follow. Connecting (connectedness) with patients and their families allows them to tell their health care story. Being present (presence) shows time, interest, and caring. Respecting the patient's values, beliefs, and health care choices further solidifies the nurse patient relationship. Although nurses' knowledge and skill level is an expectation of patient-centered care, it alone does not impact patient satisfaction.	Knowing the patient is an essential element of caring nursing practice. How the nurse obtains the information needed to support knowing the patient is crucial in establishing and maintaining caring practice. Displaying compassion and patience is important. Developing patient-nurse trust and responsiveness to the patient is critical to collecting clinical and personal information so the nurse can better know and understand the patient's health care story and expectations for care, identify and correct for missing information, and design individualized care.	Nursing presence contributes to knowing the patient. Illness and treatments often cause major changes in a patient's lifestyle. Nursing presence for patients receiving oral chemotherapy is as important as identifying those patients at risk for nonadherence. It is the nursing presence that provides emotional and knowledge-based support for patients who are new to or receiving additional oral chemotherapy.

individual without gaining an understanding of who the person is and his or her perception of the illness. Exploring the following questions with your patients helps you understand their perceptions of illness: How was your illness first recognized? How do you feel about the illness? How does your illness affect your daily life practices? Knowing the context of a patient's illness helps you choose and individualize interventions that will actually help the patient. This approach is more successful than simply selecting interventions on the basis of your patient's symptoms or disease process.

PATIENTS' PERCEPTIONS OF CARING

Theories of caring provide an excellent beginning to understanding the behaviors and processes that characterize caring. Researchers have explored nurse caring behaviors as perceived by patients (Table 7-3). Their findings emphasize what patients expect from their caregivers and thus provide useful guidelines for your practice. Patients continue to value nurses' effectiveness in performing tasks; but clearly patients value the affective dimension of nursing care. When we talk about the art and science of nursing, caring is a significant part of the art of nursing.

The study of patients' perceptions is important because health care is placing greater emphasis on patient satisfaction (see Chapter 2). Health care consumers can search online for specific information about health care agencies with regard to their ratings by patients in various areas of performance. The Caring Assessment Tool (CAT) was developed to measure caring from a patient's perspective (Duffy et al., 2007). This tool and other caring assessments help you, as a beginning professional, to appreciate the type of behaviors that hospitalized patients identify as caring. When patients sense that health care providers are sensitive, sympathetic, compassionate, and interested in them as people, they usually become active partners in the plan of care (Gallagher-Lepak and Kubsch, 2009). Suliman et al. (2009) studied the impact of Watson's caring theory as an assessment framework in a multicultural environment. Patients in the study indicated that they did not perceive any cultural bias when they perceived nurses to be caring. As institutions strive to improve patient satisfaction, creating an environment of caring is a necessary and worthwhile goal. Patient satisfaction with nursing care is an important factor in a patient's decision to return to a specific health care facility.

As you begin clinical practice, consider how patients perceive caring and the best approaches to provide care. Behaviors associated with caring offer an excellent starting point. It is also important to determine an individual patient's perceptions and unique expectations. Frequently patients and nurses differ in their perceptions of caring. For that reason focus on building a relationship that allows you to learn what is important to your patients (Gallagher-Lepak and Kubsch, 2009). For example, your patient is fearful of having an intravenous catheter inserted, and you are still a novice at catheter insertion. Instead of giving a lengthy description of the procedure to relieve anxiety, you decide that the patient will benefit more if you obtain assistance from a skilled staff member. Knowing your patients helps you select caring approaches that are most appropriate to their needs.

ETHIC OF CARE

Caring is a moral imperative, not a commodity to be bought and sold. Caring for other human beings protects, enhances, and preserves human dignity. It is a professional, ethical covenant that nursing has with its public (Watson, 2010). Caring science provides a disciplinary foundation from which you deliver patient-centered care. Chapter 22 explores the importance of ethics in professional nursing. The term *ethic* refers to the ideals of right and wrong behavior. In any patient encounter a nurse needs to know what behavior is ethically appropriate. An ethic of care is unique so professional nurses do not make professional decisions based solely on intellectual or analytical principles. Instead, an ethic of care places caring at the center of decision making. For example, which resources should be used to care for an indigent patient? Is it caring to place a terminally ill patient on a ventilator or a disabled relative in a long-term care facility?

An **ethic of care** is concerned with relationships between people and with a nurse's character and attitude toward others. Nurses who function from an ethic of care are sensitive to unequal relationships that lead to an abuse of one person's power over another—intentional or otherwise. In health care settings patients and families are often on unequal footing with professionals because of a patient's illness, lack of information, regression caused by pain and suffering, and unfamiliar circumstances. An ethic of care places the nurse as the patient's advocate, solving ethical dilemmas by attending to relationships and giving priority to each patient's unique personhood.

CARING IN NURSING PRACTICE

It is impossible to prescribe ways that guarantee whether or when a nurse becomes a caring professional. Experts disagree as to whether caring is teachable or more fundamentally a way of being in the world. For those who find caring a normal part of their lives, it is a product of their culture, values, experiences, and relationships with others. People who do not experience care in their lives often find it difficult to act in caring ways. As you deal with health and illness in your practice, you grow in your ability to care and develop caring behaviors. We learn from our patients. Our patients tell us that a simple touch, a simple phrase (e.g., "I'm here") or a promise to remain at the bedside represent caring and compassion (Engle, 2010).

Caring is one of those human behaviors that we can give and receive. As a nurse it is important to assess both your caring needs and your caring behaviors. Recognize the importance of nurses' self-care (see Chapters 1 and 6). You cannot give fully engaged, compassionate care when you feel depleted or uncared for. Take time to recognize stressors and reach out to colleagues and family and friends for help in coping with these stressors. Use caring behaviors to reach out to your colleagues and care for them as well (Jackson, 2012). Whether you are giving or receiving care, the value of caring in your nursing practice benefits your patients, your colleagues, and your health care agency.

Providing Presence

In today's high-tech health care environment in which patients are discharged quickly from hospitals, nursing practice and patient satisfaction improves when "nursing presence" is part of the health care culture (Yagasaki and Komatsu, 2013). Providing **presence** is a person-to-person encounter conveying a closeness and sense of caring. Presence involves "being there" and "being with." "Being there" is not only a physical presence; it also includes communication and understanding. Nursing presence is the connectedness between the nurse and the patient (Kostovich, 2012).

Presence is an interpersonal process that is characterized by sensitivity, wholism, intimacy, vulnerability, and adaptation to unique circumstances. It results in improved mental well-being for nurses and patients and improved physical well-being in patients (Finfgeld-Connett, 2008). The interpersonal relationship of "being there" depends on the fact that a nurse is attentive to the patient. Presence translates into an actual caring art that affects the healing and well-being of both the nurse and patient. Nurses use presence in conjunction with other nursing interventions such as establishing the nurse-patient relationship, providing comfort measures, providing patient education, and listening (Kostovich, 2012). The outcomes of nursing presence include alleviating suffering, decreasing a sense of isolation and vulnerability, and personal growth (Lai and Lee, 2012). This type of presence is something you offer to each patient in achieving patient care goals.

"Being with" is also interpersonal. A nurse gives of himself or herself, which means being available and at a patient's disposal. If a patient accepts a nurse, the patient will invite the nurse to see, share, and touch his or her vulnerability and suffering. One's human presence never leaves one unaffected (Watson, 2010). The nurse then enters the patient's world. In this presence the patient is able to put words to feelings and understand himself or herself in a way that leads to identifying solutions, seeing new directions, and making choices.

When a nurse establishes presence, eye contact, body language, voice tone, listening, and a positive and encouraging attitude act together to create openness and understanding. Establishing presence enhances a nurse's ability to learn from patients, including their hopes, dreams, need for support, and expectations of care. Learning from a patient strengthens a nurse's ability to provide adequate and appropriate nursing care (Dobrina et al., 2014).

It is especially important to establish presence and caring when patients are experiencing stressful events or situations. Awaiting a physician's report of test results, preparing for an unfamiliar procedure, and planning for a return home after serious illness are just a few examples of events in the course of a person's illness that can create unpredictability and dependency on care providers. A nurse's presence and caring help to calm anxiety and fear related to stressful situations. Giving reassurance and thorough explanations about a procedure, remaining at the patient's side, and coaching the patient through the experience all convey a presence that is invaluable to a patient's well-being.

Touch

Patients face situations that are embarrassing, frightening, and painful. Whatever the feeling or symptom, they look to nurses to provide comfort. The use of touch is one **comforting** approach that reaches out to patients to communicate concern and support (Busch et al., 2012).

Touch is relational and leads to a connection between nurse and patient. It involves contact and noncontact touch. Contact touch involves obvious skin-to-skin contact, whereas noncontact touch refers to eye contact. It is difficult to separate the two. Both in turn are providing a connectedness between a patient and nurse (Palese et al., 2011; Jackson, 2012). Before implementing touch be aware of your patient's cultural practices and past experiences. For some people a simple touch on the arm may be perceived as invasive, and for victims of abuse a simple touch may be perceived as a threat.

Nurses use task-oriented touch when performing a task or procedure. The skillful and gentle performance of a nursing procedure conveys security and a sense of competence. An expert nurse learns that any procedure is more effective when it is explained and administered carefully and in consideration of any patient concern. For example, if a patient is anxious about having a procedure such as the insertion of a nasogastric tube, offer comfort through a full explanation of the procedure and what the patient will feel. Then perform the procedure safely, skillfully, and successfully. This is done as you prepare the supplies, position the patient, and gently manipulate and insert the nasogastric tube. Throughout a procedure talk quietly with the patient to provide reassurance and support.

Caring touch is a form of nonverbal communication, which successfully influences a patient's comfort and security, enhances self-esteem, increases confidence of the caregivers, and improves mental well-being (Gillespie et al., 2012). You express this in the way you hold a patient's hand, give a back massage, gently position a patient, or participate in a conversation. When using a caring touch, you connect with the patient physically and emotionally.

Protective touch is a form of touch that protects a nurse and/or patient (Fredriksson, 1999). The patient views it either positively or negatively. The most obvious form of protective touch is preventing an accident (e.g., holding and bracing the patient to avoid a fall). Protective touch can also protect a nurse emotionally. A nurse withdraws or distances herself or himself from a patient when he or she is unable to tolerate suffering or needs to escape from a situation that is causing tension. When used in this way, protective touch elicits negative feelings in a patient (Fredriksson, 1999).

Because touch conveys many messages, use it with discretion. Touch itself is a concern when crossing cultural boundaries of either the patient or the nurse (Benner et al., 2010). Patients generally permit task-orientated touch because most individuals give nurses and physicians a license to enter their personal space to provide care (see Box 7-1). Know and understand if patients accept touch and how they interpret your intentions.

Listening

Caring involves an interpersonal interaction that is much more than two people simply talking back and forth (Bunkers, 2010). Listening is a critical component of nursing care and is necessary for meaningful interactions with patients. It is a planned and deliberate act in which the listener is present and engages the patient in a nonjudgmental and accepting manner. It includes "taking in" what a patient says, interpreting and understanding what the patient is saying, and then giving back that understanding to the patient. Listening to the meaning of what a patient says helps create a mutual relationship. True listening leads to knowing and responding to what really matters to the patient and family.

When an individual becomes ill, he or she usually has a story to tell about the meaning of the illness. Any critical or chronic illness affects all of a patient's life choices and decisions, and sometimes the individual's identity. Being able to tell that story helps the patient break the distress of illness. Thus a story needs a listener. Frank (1998) described his own feelings during his experience with cancer: "I needed a [health care professional's] gift of listening in order to make my suffering a relationship between *us,* instead of an iron cage around *me.*" He needed to be able to express what he needed when he was ill. The personal concerns that are part of a patient's illness story determine what is at stake for the patient. Caring through listening enables you to become a participant in the patient's life.

To listen effectively you need to silence yourself and listen with openness (Fredriksson, 1999). Fredriksson describes silencing one's mouth and also the mind. It is important to remain intentionally silent and concentrate on what the patient has to say. Give patients your full, focused attention as they tell their stories.

When an ill person chooses to tell his or her story, it involves reaching out to another human being. Telling the story implies a relationship that develops only if the clinician exchanges his or her stories as well. Frank (1998) argues that professionals do not routinely take seriously their own need to be known as part of a clinical relationship. Yet, unless the professional acknowledges this need, there is no reciprocal relationship, only an interaction. There is pressure on a clinician to know as much as possible about a patient, but it isolates the clinician from the patient. By contrast, in knowing and being known, each supports the other.

Through active listening you begin to truly know your patients and what is important to them (Bunkers, 2010). Learning to listen to a patient is sometimes difficult. It is easy to become distracted by tasks at hand, colleagues shouting instructions, or other patients waiting to have their needs met. However, the time you take to listen effectively is worthwhile, in both the information gained and the strengthening of the nurse-patient relationship. Listening involves paying attention to the individual's words and tone of voice and entering his or her frame of reference (see Chapter 24). By observing the expressions and body language of the patient, you find cues to help the patient explore ways to achieve greater peace.

Knowing the Patient

Knowing the patient is a complex process with a temporal nature that occurs within the context of the nurse-patient relationship (Zolnierek, 2014). It is an essential element of nursing practice and is linked to patient satisfaction and successful outcomes of care (Kelley et al., 2013). One of the five caring processes described by Swanson (1991) is knowing the patient. Knowing the patient comprises both a nurse's understanding of a specific patient and his or her subsequent selection of interventions. It is essential when providing patient-centered care. Knowing emerges from a caring relationship between a nurse and a patient, in which the nurse engages in a continuous assessment, striving to understand and interpret the patient's needs across all dimensions (Kelley et al., 2013).

Two elements that facilitate knowing are continuity of care and clinical expertise. When patient care is fragmented, knowing the patient declines, and patient-centered care is compromised (Zolinierek, 2014). Knowing develops over time as a nurse learns the clinical conditions within a specialty and the behaviors and physiological responses of patients. Intimate knowing helps the nurse respond to what really matters to the patient. To know a patient means that a nurse avoids assumptions, focuses on the patient, and engages in a caring relationship with the patient that reveals information and cues that facilitate critical thinking and clinical judgments (see Chapter 15). Knowing the patient is at the core of the clinical decision-making process.

Factors that contribute to knowing the patient include time, continuity of care, teamwork of the nursing staff, trust, and experience. Barriers to knowing the patient are often related to the organizational structure of the organization and economic constraints. Organizational changes often result in decreasing the amount of time that registered nurses are able to spend with their patients, which in turn affects the nurse-patient relationships. Decreased length of stay also reduces the interactions' between nurses and their patients (Zolnierek, 2014).

Consequences of not knowing the patient are many. For example, in the acute care setting, not knowing the patient contributes to risk for falls and actual falls. Patients and their families don't understand the complexities of treatment and their participation in care (Kelley et al., 2013). Finally, patients do not adequately understand their discharge guidelines and may administer their home medications or treatments incorrectly. A caring nurse-patient relationship helps you to better know the patient as a unique individual and choose the most appropriate and efficacious nursing therapies (WCSI, 2014).

A caring relationship coupled with your growing knowledge and experience provides a rich source of meaning when changes in a patient's clinical status occur. Expert nurses develop the ability to detect changes in patients' conditions almost effortlessly (Benner et al., 2010). Clinical decision making, perhaps the most important responsibility of a professional nurse, involves various aspects of knowing the patient: responses to therapies, routines and habits, coping resources, physical capacities and endurance, and body typology and characteristics. Experienced nurses know additional facts about their patients such as their experiences, behaviors, feelings, and perceptions (Benner et al., 2010). You will achieve improved patient satisfaction and patient health outcomes when you make clinical decisions accurately in the context of knowing a patient well (Zolnierek, 2014). When you base care on knowing a patient, the patient perceives care as personalized, comforting, supportive, and healing.

The most important thing for a beginning nurse to recognize is that knowing a patient is more than simply gathering data about the patient's clinical signs and condition. Success in knowing the patient lies in the relationship you establish. To know a patient is to enter into a caring, social process that also includes interaction with members of the health care team, which results in a deep nurse-patient relationship whereby the patient comes to feel known by the nurse (Kelley et al., 2013).

QSEN QSEN: BUILDING COMPETENCY IN PATIENT-CENTERED CARE Knowing the patient and family helps you gain information about their health status, relationships, and fears. Knowing as much as possible about your patient helps you plan safe, effective patient-centered care. Read the following case study and determine factors related to planning and implementing patient-centered care for a patient who is preparing for discharge from a hospital.

Mrs. Martinez is 72 and lives in a mother-in-law suite in the home of her son and daughter-in-law. When she was a child she lived in a multigenerational home. She and her family believe that it is important to invite the grandparents to live in one of the children's home and, if necessary, care for them. Mrs. Martinez has three sons, and they are married with children. All the family members and Mrs. Martinez believed that it was best to have her living with one of her sons vs. sharing time with all the sons.

There are two grandchildren who are grown and out of the home. Mrs. Martinez's son and daughter-in-law have full-time jobs and are out of the house from 8:00 AM to 6:00 PM each day.

Each summer each of her sons and their family visit Mrs. Martinez while the son with whom she lives, his wife, and their two grown children and their families go on vacations. During the holidays Mrs. Martinez's sons, their families, and all the grandchildren spend the holidays together.

Presently she is independent. She takes medication for high blood pressure and an irregular heartbeat. At times these medications make her "light-headed." She also has occasional dizziness from a middle ear problem when she changes position too fast. She is afraid that, if she shared this information with her doctor, he'd think that she'd fall and say she must give up her activities. She equates this with losing her independence.

Given the information about her living situation, current level of independence, and symptoms of light-headedness and dizziness, how can you continue to provide patient-centered care?

Answers to QSEN Activities can be found on the Evolve website.

Spiritual Caring

An individual achieves spiritual health after finding a balance between his or her own life values, goals, and belief systems and those of others (see Chapter 36). An individual's beliefs and expectations affect his or her own physical well-being.

Research shows that nurses who develop spiritual caring practices early in their career development are able to identify methods to incorporate these practices into routine care and do not perceive variables such as a lack of sufficient time or patient census as barriers (Ronaldson et al., 2012). Establishing a caring relationship with a patient involves interconnectedness between the nurse and the patient. This interconnectedness is why Watson (2008, 2010) describes the caring relationship in a spiritual sense. Spirituality offers a sense of connectedness: intrapersonally (connected with oneself), interpersonally (connected with others and the environment), and transpersonally (connected with the unseen, God, or a higher power). In a caring relationship the patient and the nurse come to know one another so both move toward a healing relationship by (Watson, 2010; WCSI, 2014):

- Mobilizing hope for the patient and the nurse.
- Finding an interpretation or understanding of illness, symptoms, or emotions that is acceptable to the patient.
- Assisting the patient in using social, emotional, or spiritual resources.
- Recognizing that caring relationships connect us human to human, spirit to spirit.

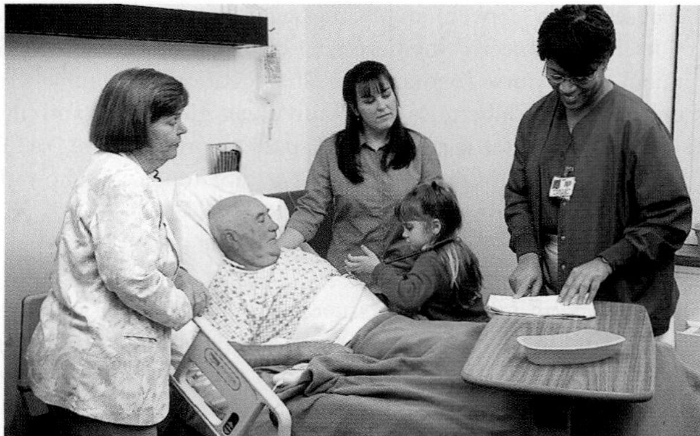

FIGURE 7-2 Nurse discusses patient's health care needs with the family.

Relieving Symptoms and Suffering

Relieving symptoms such as pain and nausea and suffering is more than giving pain medications, repositioning the patient, cleaning a wound, or providing end-of-life care. The relief of symptoms and suffering encompasses caring nursing actions that give a patient comfort, dignity, respect, and peace and provide necessary comfort and support measures to the family or significant others (Maroon, 2012). Ensuring that the patient care environment is clean and pleasant and includes personal items makes the physical environment a place that soothes and heals the mind, body, and spirit (Gallagher-Lepak and Kubsch, 2009). This is a responsibility of a professional nurse and not a task automatically delegated to nursing assistive personnel. Always be aware of your patient's environment, assess symptoms thoroughly, and take the necessary steps to make the environment comfortable.

Through skillful and accurate assessment of a patient's level and type of pain or other symptoms, you are able to design patient-centered care to improve the patient's level of comfort. There are multiple interventions for pain relief (see Chapter 44) and approaches for relieving nausea or fatigue. However, knowing about the patient and the meaning of his or her symptoms guides your care. Often conveying a quiet caring presence, touching a patient, or listening helps you to assess and understand the meaning of your patient's discomfort. The caring presence helps you and your patient design goals for symptom relief.

Human suffering is multifaceted, affecting a patient physically, emotionally, socially, and spiritually. It also affects a patient's family and friends. You may find yourself working with a young family whose newborn baby has multiple developmental challenges. Their emotional suffering encompasses anger, guilt, fear, or grief. You cannot fix it, but you can provide comfort through a listening, nonjudgmental caring presence. Patients and their families are comforted by a caring listener.

Family Care

People live in their worlds in an involved way. Each person experiences life through relationships with others. Thus caring for an individual cannot occur in isolation from that person's family. As a nurse it is important to know the family almost as thoroughly as you know a patient (Maroon, 2012). The family is an important resource (Figure 7-2). Success with nursing interventions often depends on their willingness to share information about the patient, their acceptance and understanding of therapies, whether the interventions fit with their daily practices, and whether they support and deliver the therapies recommended.

BOX 7-3 Nurse Caring Behaviors as Perceived by Families

- Providing honest, clear, and accurate information
- Listening to patient and family concerns, complaints, fears
- Advocating for patient's care preferences and end-of-life decisions
- Asking permission before doing something to a patient
- Providing comfort (e.g., offering warm blanket, rubbing a patient's back)
- Reading patient passages from religious texts, favorite book, cards, or mail
- Providing for and maintaining patient privacy
- Informing the patient about the types of nursing services and the people who may enter the personal care area
- Assuring the patient that nursing services will be available
- Helping patients do as much for themselves as possible
- Teaching the family how to keep the relative physically comfortable

Data from Maroon, AM: Ethical palliative family nursing care: a new concept of caring for patients and families, *JONA's Healthc Law Ethics Regul* 14(4):115, 2012; Lusk JM, Fater K: A concept analysis of patient-centered care, *Nurs Forum* 48(2):89, 2013.

Families of patients with cancer perceived many nurse caring behaviors to be most helpful (Box 7-3). It is critical that a nurse ensures the patient's well-being and safety and helps the family members to be active participants (AONE, 2015). Although specific to families of patients with cancer, these behaviors offer useful guidelines for developing a caring relationship with all families. Begin a relationship by learning who makes up the patient's family and their roles in the patient's life. Showing a family that you care for and are concerned about the patient creates an openness that then enables a relationship to form with a family. Caring for the family takes into consideration the context of the patient's illness and the stress it imposes on all members (see Chapter 10).

THE CHALLENGE OF CARING

Assisting individuals during a time of need is the reason many enter nursing. When you are able to affirm yourself as a caring individual, your life achieves a meaning and purpose (Benner et al., 2010). Caring is a motivating force for people to become nurses, and it becomes a source of satisfaction when nurses know that they have made a difference in their patients' lives.

Today's health care system presents many challenges for the nurse to provide a caring patient-centered plan of care (Lusk and Fater, 2013). Nurses are often torn between the human caring model and the task-oriented biomedical model and institutional demands that consume their practice (Winsett and Hauck, 2011). They have increasingly less time to spend with patients, making it much harder to know who they are. A reliance on technology and cost-effective health care strategies and efforts to standardize and refine work processes all undermine the nature of caring. Too often patients become just a number, with their real needs either overlooked or ignored.

The American Nurses Association (ANA), National League for Nursing (NLN), American Organization of Nurse Executives (AONE), and American Association of Colleges of Nursing (AACN) recommend strategies to reverse the current nursing shortage. A number of these strategies have potential for creating work environments that enable nurses to demonstrate more caring behaviors. In addition, the Robert Wood Johnson Foundation's "Future of Nursing: Campaign for Action" is identifying methods to improve both patient care and satisfaction and nurse job satisfaction. This campaign is focusing on increasing the amount of time nurses actually spend with their patients and families. Environmental factors promote a more artful nursing and caring presence that further enhances patient-centered care. Strategies include greater emphasis on improving the work environment to facilitate more nurse-patient interaction, improving nurse staffing, providing nurses with autonomy over their practice, and promoting increased educational requirements and opportunities (RWJF, 2014).

If health care is to make a positive difference in their lives, patients cannot be treated like machines or robots. Instead health care must become more wholistic and humanistic. Nurses play an important role in making caring an integral part of health care delivery. This begins by making it a part of the philosophy and environment in the workplace. Incorporating caring concepts into standards of nursing practice establishes the guidelines for professional conduct. Finally, during day-to-day practice with patients and families, nurses need to be committed to caring and willing to establish the relationships necessary for personal, competent, compassionate, and meaningful nursing care. "Consistent with the wisdom and vision of Nightingale, nursing is a lifetime journey of caring and healing, seeking to understand and preserve the wholeness of human existence and to offer compassionate, informed knowledgeable human caring …" (Watson, 2009).

KEY POINTS

- Caring is the heart of a nurse's ability to work with people in a respectful and therapeutic way.
- Caring is specific and relational for each nurse-patient encounter.
- For caring to achieve cure, nurses need to learn the culturally specific behaviors and words that reflect human caring in different cultures.
- Because illness is the human experience of loss or dysfunction, any treatment or intervention given without consideration of its meaning to the individual is likely to be worthless.
- Caring involves a mutual give-and-take that develops as nurse and patient begin to know and care for one another.
- Presence involves a person-to-person encounter that conveys closeness and a sense of caring that involves "being there" and "being with" patients.
- Research shows that touch, both contact and noncontact, includes task-orientated touch, caring touch, and protective touch.
- The skillful and gentle performance of a nursing procedure conveys security and a sense of competence in the nurse.
- Listening is not only "taking in" what a patient says; it also includes interpreting and understanding what the patient is saying and giving back that understanding.
- Knowing the patient is at the core of the process that nurses use to make clinical decisions.

CLINICAL APPLICATION QUESTIONS

Preparing for Clinical Practice

1. Mrs. Lowe is a 52-year-old patient being treated for lymphoma (cancer of the lymph nodes) that occurred 6 years after a lung transplant. Mrs. Lowe is discouraged about her current health status and has a lot of what she describes as muscle pain. The unit where Mrs. Lowe is receiving care has a number of very sick patients and is short staffed.
   a. You enter her room to do a morning assessment and find Mrs. Lowe crying. How are you going to use caring practices to help her, knowing that your day has just begun and you have many nursing interventions to complete?

b. When you listen to Mrs. Lowe, she explains that her muscle pain is very bothersome and it was worse when she was alone. Both you and Mrs. Lowe determine that an injection for her pain would be beneficial. In what way can you show caring in the way you administer the injection to Mrs. Lowe?
c. Mrs. Lowe's day is getting better. She seems more comfortable and is crying less. You find that your day is more controlled. What else can you do for Mrs. Lowe?

2. During your next clinical practicum, select a patient to talk with for at least 15 to 20 minutes. Ask the patient to tell you about his or her illness. Review the skills of listening in this chapter and in Chapter 24. Immediately after your discussion, reflect on the discussion with the patient and determine if you have enough information about him or her to answer the following questions:
   a. What do you believe the patient was trying to tell you about his or her illness?
   b. Why was it important for the patient to share his or her story?
   c. What did you do that made it easy or difficult for the patient to talk with you? What did you do well? What could you have done better?
   d. Would you rate yourself a good listener? How can you listen better?

ⓔ ***Answers to Clinical Application Questions can be found on the Evolve website.***

REVIEW QUESTIONS

Are You Ready to Test Your Nursing Knowledge?

1. A nurse hears a colleague tell a nursing student that she never touches a patient unless she is performing a procedure or doing an assessment. The nurse tells the student that from a caring perspective:
   1. She does not touch the patients either.
   2. Touch is a type of verbal communication.
   3. Touch is only used when a patient is in pain.
   4. Touch forms a connection between nurse and patient.
2. Of the five caring processes described by Swanson, which describes "knowing the patient?"
   1. Anticipating the patient's cultural preferences
   2. Determining the patient's physician preference
   3. Establishing an understanding of a specific patient
   4. Gathering task-oriented information during assessment
3. A Muslim woman enters the clinic to have a woman's health examination for the first time. Which nursing behavior applies Swanson's caring process of "knowing the patient?"
   1. Sharing feelings about the importance of having regular woman's health examinations
   2. Gaining an understanding of what a woman's health examination means to the patient
   3. Recognizing that the patient is modest; and obtaining gender-congruent caregiver
   4. Explaining the risk factors for cervical cancer
4. **Fill-in-the-Blank.** Swanson's caring process of ______ is demonstrated by a nurse helping a new mother through the birthing experience.
5. A patient is fearful of upcoming surgery and a possible cancer diagnosis. He discusses his love for the Bible with his nurse, who recommends a favorite Bible verse. Another nurse tells the patient's nurse that there is no place in nursing for spiritual caring. The patient's nurse replies:
   1. "You're correct; spiritual care should be left to a pastoral care professional."
   2. "You're correct; religion is a personal decision."
   3. "Nurses should explain their own religious beliefs to patients."
   4. "Spiritual, mind, and body connections can affect health."
6. Which of the following is a strategy for creating work environments that enable nurses to demonstrate more caring behaviors? (Select all that apply.)
   1. Decreasing the number of consecutive shifts of the nursing staff
   2. Increasing salary and vacation benefits of the nursing staff
   3. Increasing the number of nurses who work each shift to decrease the nurse-patient ratio
   4. Encouraging increased input concerning nursing functions from health care providers
   5. Providing nursing staff an opportunity to discuss practice changes they can implement to enhance opportunities for patient caring
7. When a nurse helps a patient find the meaning of cancer by supporting beliefs about life, this is an example of:
   1. Instilling hope and faith.
   2. Forming a human-altruistic value system.
   3. Cultural caring.
   4. Being with.
8. An example of a nurse caring behavior that families of acutely ill patients perceive as important to patients' well-being is:
   1. Making health care decisions for patients.
   2. Having family members provide a patient's total personal hygiene.
   3. Injecting the nurse's perceptions about the level of care provided.
   4. Asking permission before performing a procedure on a patient.
9. A nurse demonstrated caring by helping family members to: (Select all that apply.)
   1. Become active participants in care.
   2. Remove themselves from personal care.
   3. Make health care decisions for the patient.
   4. Have uninterrupted time for family and patient to be together.
   5. Have opportunities for the family to discuss their concerns.
10. Listening is not only "taking in" what a patient says, but it also includes:
    1. Incorporating the views of the physician.
    2. Correcting any errors in the patient's understanding.
    3. Injecting the nurse's personal views and statements.
    4. Interpreting and understanding what the patient means.
11. A nurse is caring for an older adult who needs to enter an assisted-living facility following discharge from the hospital. Which of the following is an example of listening that displays caring?
    1. The nurse encourages the patient to talk about his concerns while reviewing the computer screen in the room.
    2. The nurse sits at the patient's bedside, listens as he relays his fear of never seeing his home again, and then asks if he wants anything to eat.
    3. The nurse listens to the patient's story while sitting on the side of the bed and then summarizes the story.
    4. The nurse listens to the patient talk about his fears of not returning home and then tells him to think positively.
12. Presence involves a person-to-person encounter that:
    1. Enables patients to care for self.
    2. Provides personal care to a patient.
    3. Conveys a closeness and a sense of caring.
    4. Describes being in close contact with a patient.

13. A nurse enters a patient's room, arranges the supplies for a Foley catheter insertion, and explains the procedure to the patient. She tells the patient what to expect; just before inserting the catheter, she tells the patient to relax and that, once the catheter is in place, she will not feel the bladder pressure. The nurse then proceeds to skillfully insert the Foley catheter. This is an example of what type of touch?
    1. Caring touch
    2. Protective touch
    3. Task-oriented touch
    4. Interpersonal touch
14. A hospice nurse sits at the bedside of a male patient in the final stages of cancer. He and his parents made the decision that he would move home and they would help him in the final stages of his disease. The family participates in his care, but lately the nurse has increased the amount of time she spends with the family. Whenever she enters the room or approaches the patient to give care, she touches his shoulder and tells him that she is present. This is an example of what type of touch?
    1. Caring touch
    2. Protective touch
    3. Task-oriented touch
    4. Interpersonal touch
15. Match the following caring behaviors with their definitions.

1. Knowing	a. Sustaining faith in one's capacity to get through a situation
2. Being with	b. Striving to understand an event as meaning for another person
3. Doing for	c. Being emotionally there for another person
4. Maintaining belief	d. Providing for another as he or she would do for themselves

Answers: 1. 4; **2.** 3; **3.** 2; **4.** Enabling; **5.** 4; **6.** 3, 5; **7.** 1; **8.** 4; **9.** 1, 4, 5; **10.** 4; **11.** 3; **12.** 3; **13.** 3; **14.** 1; **15.** 1b, 2c, 3d, 4a.

Rationales for Review Questions can be found on the Evolve website.

REFERENCES

American Nurses Association [ANA]: *Nursing's agenda for the future: a call to the nation,* 2002, http://infoassist.panpha.org/docushare/dsweb/Get/Document-1884/PP-2002-APR-Nsgagenda.pdf. Accessed February 2015.

American Organization of Nurse Executives [AONE]: *Guiding principles for the role of the nurse in future health care delivery toolkit,* 2015, http://www.aone.org/resources/leadership%20tools/guideprinciples.shtml. Accessed February 2015.

Benner P, Wrubel J: *The primacy of caring: stress and coping in health and illness,* Menlo Park, CA, 1989, Addison Wesley.

Benner P, et al: *Educating nurses: a call for radical transformation,* Stanford, CA, 2010, Carnegie Foundation for the Advancement of Teaching.

Bunkers SS: The power and possibility in listening, *Nurs Sci Q* 23(1):22, 2010.

Burtson L, Stichler JF: Nursing work environment and nurse caring: relationship among motivational factors, *J Adv Nurs* 66(8):1819, 2010.

Busch M, et al: The implementation and evaluation of therapeutic touch in burn patients: and instructive experiences of conducting a scientific study within a non-academic nursing setting, *Patient Educ Couns* 89(3):439, 2012.

Drenkard KN: Integrating human caring science into a professional nursing practice model, *Crit Care Nurs Clin North Am* 20:402, 2008.

Engle M: *I'm here: compassionate communication in patient care,* Orlando, FL, 2010, Phillips Press.

Frank AW: Just listening: narrative and deep illness, *Fam Syst Health* 16(3):197, 1998.

Gallagher-Lepak S, Kubsch S: Transpersonal caring: a nursing practice guideline, *Holist Nurs Pract* 23(3):171, 2009.

Jackson C: The interface of caring, self-care, and technology in nursing education and practice, *Holist Nurs Pract* 26(2):69, 2012.

Leininger MM: *Culture care diversity and universality: a theory of nursing,* Pub No 15-2402, New York, 1991, National League for Nursing Press.

Maroon AM: Ethical palliative family nursing care: a new concept of caring for patients and families, *JONAS Healthc Law Ethics Regul* 14(4):115, 2012.

Robert Wood Johnson Foundation (RWJF). *Future of nursing: campaign for action is chalking up successes that will improve patient care,* 2014, http://www.rwjf.org/en/about-rwjf/newsroom/newsroom-content/2014/06/campaign-for-action-is-chalking-up-successes-that-will-improve-p.html. Accessed February 2015.

Watson Caring Science Institute (WCSI) and International Caritas Consortium: *Caring science theory and research,* 2014, http://watsoncaringscience.org/about-us/caring-science-definitions-processes-theory/. Accessed February 2015.

Watson J: *The philosophy and science of caring,* Boulder, 2008, University Press of Colorado.

Watson J: Caring science and human caring theory: transforming personal and professional practices of nursing and health care, *J Health Human Serv Adm* 31(4):466, 2009.

Watson J: Caring science and the next decade of holistic healing: transforming self and system from the inside out, *Am Holist Nurses Assoc* 30(2):14, 2010.

RESEARCH REFERENCES

Andershed B, Olsson K: Review of research related to Kristen Swanson's middle-range theory of caring, *Scand J Caring Sci* 23:598, 2009.

Duffy JR, et al: Dimensions of caring: psychometric evaluation of the caring assessment tool, *Adv Nurs Sci* 30(3):235, 2007.

Dobrina R, et al: An overview of hospice and palliative care nursing models and theories, *Int J Palliat Nurs* 20(2):75, 2014.

Finfgeld-Connett D: Qualitative comparison and synthesis of nursing presence and caring, *Int J Nurs Terminol Classif* 19(3):111, 2008.

Fredriksson L: Modes of relating in a caring conversation: a research synthesis on presence, touch, and listening, *J Adv Nurs* 30(5):1167, 1999.

Gillespie GL, et al: Caring in pediatric emergency nursing, *Res Theory Nurs Pract* 26(3):216, 2012.

Kelley T, et al: Information needed to support knowing the patient, *Adv Nurs Sci* 36(4):351, 2013.

Kostovich CT: Development and psychometric assessment of the presence in nursing scale, *Nurs Sci Q* 25(2):167, 2012.

Lai HL, Lee LH: Effects of music intervention with nursing presence and recorded music on psycho-physiological indices of cancer patient caregivers, *J Clin Nurs* 21(5):745, 2012.

Lusk JM, Fater K: A concept analysis of patient-centered care, *Nurs Forum* 48(2):89, 2013.

Palese A, et al: Surgical patient satisfaction as an outcome of nurses' caring behaviors: a descriptive and correlational study in six European countries, *J Nurs Scholarsh* 43(4):341, 2011.

Parcells DA, Locsin RC: Development and psychometric testing of the technological competency as caring in nursing instrument, *Int J Human Caring* 15(4):8, 2011.

Ronaldson S, et al: Spirituality and spiritual caring: nurses' perspectives and practice in palliative and acute care environments, *J Clin Nurs* 21(15):2126, 2012.

Suliman WA, et al: Applying Watson's nursing theory to assess patient perceptions of being cared for in a multicultural environment, *J Nurs Res* 17(4):293, 2009.

Swanson KM: Empirical development of a middle-range theory of caring, *Nurs Res* 40(3):161, 1991.

Swanson KM: Effects of caring, measurement, and time on miscarriage impact and women's well being, *Nurs Res* 48(6):288, 1999.

Winsett RP, Hauck S: Implementing relationship-based care, *J Nurs Adm* 41(6):285, 2011.

Yagasaki K, Komatsu H: The need for a nursing presence in oral chemotherapy, *Clin J Oncol Nurs* 17(5):512, 2013.

Zolnierek CD: An integrative review of knowing the patient, *J Nurs Scholarsh* 46(1):3, 2014.

8

Caring for the Cancer Survivor

OBJECTIVES

- Discuss the concept of cancer survivorship.
- Describe the influence of cancer survivorship on patients' quality of life.
- Discuss the effects that cancer has on the family.
- Explain the nursing implications related to cancer survivorship.
- Discuss the essential components of survivorship care.

KEY TERMS

Biological response modifiers (biotherapy), p. 90
Cancer-related fatigue (CRF), p. 92
Cancer survivorship, p. 90
Chemotherapy, p. 90
Chemotherapy-induced peripheral neurotoxicity, (CIPN), p. 91
Chemotherapy-related cognitive impairment (CRCI), p. 92
Hormone therapy, p. 90
Neuropathy, p. 91
Oncology, p. 97
Paresthesias, p. 91
Posttraumatic stress disorder (PTSD), p. 92
Radiation therapy, p. 90

MEDIA RESOURCES

http://evolve.elsevier.com/Potter/fundamentals/

- Review Questions
- Case Study with Questions
- Audio Glossary
- Content Updates

Currently there are 14.5 million adult and childhood cancer survivors in the United States; the number of survivors will continue to grow since more than 1.7 million new cases of cancer are diagnosed each year (American Cancer Society [ACS], 2014a; National Cancer Institute [NCI], 2015). Most cancer survivors (64%) were diagnosed initially 5 or more years ago; 50% of cancer survivors are 70 years of age or older (ACS, 2014a; NCI, 2015).

It is estimated that by January 2024 there will be 19 million cancer survivors in the United States (ACS, 2014a). Increased detection at the early stage of disease and improvements in all modes of treatment through research increase a prolonged life such that cancer diagnosis equates to cure for some and for others cancer is a managed chronic illness. The major forms of cancer therapy—surgery, immunotherapy, **chemotherapy**, **hormone therapy**, **biological response modifiers (biotherapy)**, and **radiation therapy**—often create unwanted long-term effects on tissues and organ systems that impair a person's health and quality of life (QOL) in many ways (Institute of Medicine [IOM], 2006).

There are many stages of the cancer continuum (Figure 8-1). Children and adolescents who receive aggressive chemotherapy and radiation are at greatest risk for developing secondary malignancies, sometimes related to the initial treatment received for the primary cancer. Adult cancer survivors may also experience new malignancies related to prior treatment but also may be genetically predisposed to recurrent tumors. With continued focus on cancer treatment going beyond acute treatment, health care providers are improving care needed for all long-term cancer survivors. Thus cancer survivorship has enormous implications for the way these individuals monitor and manage their health throughout their lives. As a nurse you will care for these patients when they seek care for their cancer and other medical conditions.

Cancer survivorship begins at the time of cancer diagnosis, includes treatment, and extends to the rest of the person's life (National Coalition for Cancer Survivorship [NCCS], 2015). Family members and friends are also survivors because they experience the effects that cancer has on their loved ones. Cancer is a life-changing event. Although progress is being made, evidence shows that many cancer survivors do not receive adequate follow-up care during the period following first diagnosis and initial treatment and before the development of a recurrence of the initial cancer or death (IOM, 2006). Following treatment, contact with a cancer care provider often stops, and survivors' needs go unnoticed or untreated. Improvements have occurred in follow-up treatment for some cancer survivors, but many long-term survivors suffer unnecessarily and die from delayed second cancer diagnoses or treatment-related chronic disease.

Nurses have the responsibility to better understand the needs of cancer survivors and provide the most current evidence-based approaches for managing late and long-term effects of cancer and cancer treatment. Although progress in early detection is improving in the underserved, more work is needed. Being able to provide comprehensive care to a cancer survivor begins with recognizing the effects of cancer and its treatment and learning about the survivor's own meaning of health.

THE EFFECTS OF CANCER ON QUALITY OF LIFE

As people live longer after diagnosis and treatment for cancer, it becomes important to understand the types of distress that many

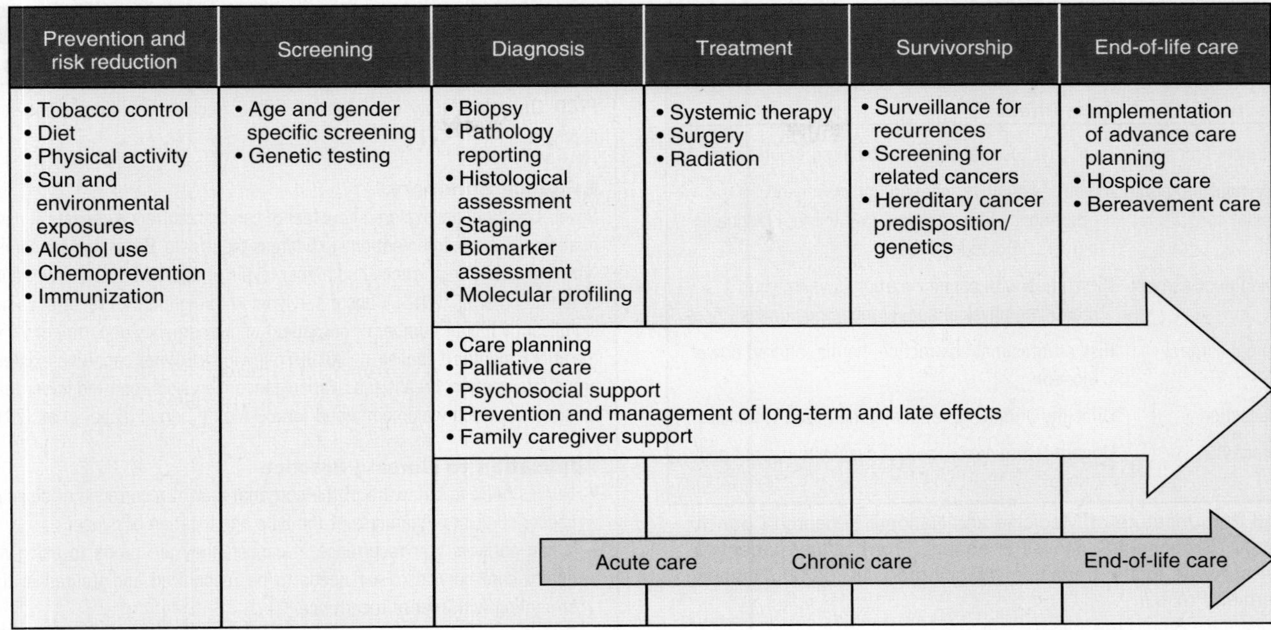

FIGURE 8-1 Domains of the cancer care continuum. (From Laura Levit et al, editors: Committee on Improving the Quality of Cancer Care: *Addressing the challenges of an aging population;* Board on Health Care Services, Institute of Medicine: *Delivering high-quality care: charting a new course for a system in crisis,* Washington, D.C., 2013, National Academies Press.)

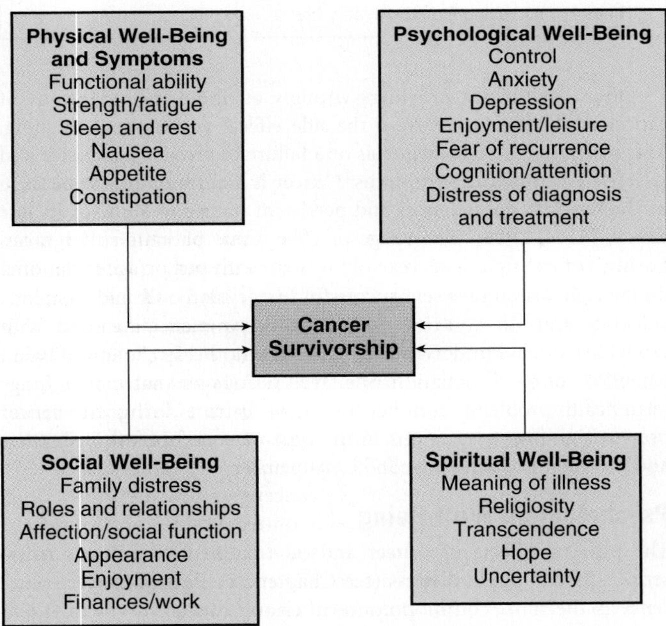

FIGURE 8-2 Dimensions of quality of life affected by cancer. (From Ferrell B: Introduction to cancer survivorship strategies for success: survivorship education for quality cancer care, Pasadena, CA, 2006, City of Hope National Medical Center.)

survivors experience and how it affects their QOL (Figure 8-2). QOL in cancer survivorship means having a balance between the experience of increased dependence while seeking both independence and interdependence. Of course there are always exceptions in regard to the level of distress that survivors face. For some, cancer becomes an experience of self-reflection and an enhanced sense of what life is about. Regardless of each survivor's journey with cancer, having cancer affects each person's physical, psychological, social, and spiritual well-being.

Physical Well-Being and Symptoms

Cancer survivors are at increased risk for cancer (either a recurrence of the cancer for which they were treated or a second cancer) and for a wide range of treatment-related problems (IOM, 2006). The increased risk for developing a second cancer is the result of cancer treatment, genetic factors, other susceptibility, or an interaction between treatment and susceptibility (ACS, 2014a). The risk for treatment-related problems is associated with the complexity of the cancer itself (e.g., type of tumor and stage of disease); the type, variety, and intensity of treatments used (e.g., chemotherapy and radiation combined); and the age and underlying health status of the patient.

A number of tissues and body systems are impaired as a result of cancer and its treatment (Table 8-1). Late effects of chemotherapy and/or radiation include osteoporosis, heart failure, diabetes, amenorrhea in women, sterility in men and women, impaired gastrointestinal motility, abnormal liver function, impaired immune function, **paresthesias**, hearing loss, and problems with thinking and memory (IOM, 2006).

Chemotherapy-induced peripheral neurotoxicity (CIPN) refers to peripheral nerve damage resulting from the effects of certain chemotherapeutic agents (Park et al., 2013). Damage to large sensory nerves causes feelings of numbness and tingling in the hands and feet. Motor function may also be affected, but usually to a lesser degree than sensory function. Permanent chronic **neuropathy** occurs in 58% of patients with CIPN, resulting in increased falls and other motor and sensory dysfunction (Gewandter et al., 2013).

Certain conditions resolve over time, but tissue damage causes some symptoms to persist indefinitely, especially when patients receive high-dose chemotherapy. Health care professionals do not always recognize these conditions as delayed problems. Often conditions such as osteoporosis, hearing loss, or change in memory are instead considered to be age related. It is common for patients with cancer to have multiple symptoms, and more attention is being given to the existence

TABLE 8-1 Examples of Late Effects of Surgery Among Adult Cancer Survivors

Procedure	Late Effect
Any surgical procedure	Pain, psychosocial distress, impaired wound healing
Surgery involving brain or spinal cord	Impaired cognitive function, motor sensory alterations, altered vision, swallowing, language, bowel and bladder control
Head and neck surgery	Difficulties with communication, swallowing, breathing, physical appearance/body image
Abdominal surgery	Risk of intestinal obstruction, hernia, altered bowel function
Lung resection	Difficulty breathing, fatigue, generalized weakness
Prostatectomy	Urinary incontinence, sexual dysfunction, poor body image

Modified from Institute of Medicine and National Research Council, Hewitt M, Greenfield S, Stovall E, editors: From cancer patient to cancer survivor: lost in transition, Washington, DC, 2006, National Academies Press.

of symptom clusters. A symptom cluster is a group of several related and coexisting symptoms such as pain-insomnia-fatigue or pain-depression-fatigue (Nguyen et al., 2011; Oh et al., 2012). Researchers are trying to better understand symptom clusters, their effects on patients, and whether clusters require a different treatment approach than current symptom management.

Cancer-related fatigue (CRF) and associated sleep disturbances are among the most frequent and distressing complaints of people with cancer. The symptoms often last many months after chemotherapy and radiation. The fatigue affects patients physically, psychologically, and socially and limits their ability to function and socialize in enjoyable activities (Borneman et al., 2012).The National Comprehensive Cancer Network (NCCN) *Clinical Practice Guidelines* (2014) for CRF treatment includes interventions for controlling fatigue through routine physical exercise, rest (such as taking an entire day off), development of good sleep habits, eating a balanced diet, and counseling for depression that often accompanies CRF.

Chemotherapy-related cognitive impairment (CRCI) is consistently associated with people who receive systemic chemotherapy. In addition to chemotherapy, radiation, hormone therapy, and the use of tranquilizers may also contribute to cognitive impairment in survivors (Rey et al., 2012) Breast cancer survivors report having difficulty with short-term memory, focusing, working, reading with comprehension, and driving (Myers, 2012).

A 44-year-old woman reported the following when asked if chemotherapy was responsible for memory deterioration … . "Yes absolutely. I mean I was forgetful before but not to the degree I am now. I would have had some vague memory of someone saying something, but now I really just don't remember. It doesn't ring any bells. It's just a complete blank." (Mitchell and Turton, 2011).

Suggested positive coping strategies include writing things down, focusing on one task at a time, allowing others to help with activities requiring focus, reading simpler texts, using audiobooks, and giving oneself permission to make mistakes (Potrata et al., 2010). There is no way to predict if a person will have CRCI or the degree of cognitive change. Some people who experience this symptom have difficulty working and processing information, which affects daily functioning and the quality of their work and social life.

BOX 8-1 EVIDENCE-BASED PRACTICE

Fear of Cancer Recurrence Among Cancer Survivors

PICO Question: How does fear of cancer recurrence affect adult cancer survivors?

Evidence Summary

Several researchers explored how fear of cancer recurrence impacts survivors' health care use or interventions to address their fears. Breast cancer survivors with high fear of recurrence had higher levels of depression and lower quality of life (Koch et al., 2014). Cancer survivors with high fear of recurrence had a significantly higher number of outpatient and emergency department visits in the prior 6 months (Lebel et al., 2013). Following a 6-week cognitive-existential group intervention, breast and ovarian cancer survivors reported lower fear of recurrence, which was maintained for a 3-month period (Lebel et al., 2014).

Application to Nursing Practice

- Nurses need to be aware of the potential fear of recurrence of disease in cancer survivors regardless of the type and location of cancer.
- When patients fear recurrence of cancer, they are prone to using more health care services. Fear needs to be recognized and treated in those struggling with fear of recurrence.
- Cognitive-based therapies (exploration of relationships among a person's thoughts, feelings, and behaviors) show promise in helping cancer survivors deal with fear of recurrent disease and maintain an improved perspective.
- Further research needs to be done to clearly identify additional interventions and screening tools to identify fear of recurrence.

Often health care providers wrongly attribute the symptoms of cancer or the symptoms from the side effects of treatment to aging. This often leads to late diagnosis or a failure to provide aggressive and effective treatment of symptoms. Cancer is a chronic disease because of the serious consequences and persistent nature of some of its late effects (IOM, 2006). The range of effects that patients suffer varies greatly. For example, a 46-year-old woman with early-stage melanoma on the right arm underwent successful surgery and only had an inconspicuous scar. In contrast, a 52-year-old woman diagnosed with Hodgkin's disease underwent intensive chemotherapy followed by an extended course of radiation. She faced serious and substantial long-term health problems from her treatment. Patients living with cancer present significant variations in the type of conditions they develop and the length of time the conditions persist.

Psychological Well-Being

The physical effects of cancer and its treatment sometimes cause serious psychological distress (see Chapter 38). Fear of cancer recurrence is the most common concern among cancer survivors (Koch et al., 2014, Ness et al., 2013; Simard et al., 2013). Cancer diagnosis and time since diagnosis impact prevalence and severity of fears (Ness et al., 2013). Being younger and considering oneself as a tumor patient increase the likelihood of moderate-to-high fear of recurrence in long-term breast cancer survivors (Koch et al, 2014) (Box 8-1).

Another common psychological problem for survivors is **posttraumatic stress disorder (PTSD)**. PTSD is a psychiatric disorder characterized by an acute emotional response to a traumatic event or situation. When incidence of PTSD-like symptoms is measured, rates range from 20% in patients with early-stage cancer to 80% in those with recurrent cancer (NCI, 2014b). Grief, intrusive thoughts about the disease, nightmares, relational difficulties, or fear may present in these people. Being unmarried or less educated or having a lower income and less social and emotional support increases the risk for PTSD in adult survivors (Stuber et al., 2010). In young adults with cancer, higher rates of PTSD appear in those who are unemployed or not in school, had surgical treatment for cancer, currently receive treatment, and have a diagnosis of a cancer type with a 90% to 100% survival rate (Kwak et al., 2013). In these young adults PTSD symptoms observed as early as 6 months following the diagnosis remained stable for 12 months.

The following description is an example of a cancer survivor's response to the stressors of cancer treatment:

> The first question I asked my radiation oncologist after completing treatment for non-metastatic breast and ovarian cancer was: "When can I go back to my job?" He said, "Considering the work you do, I would think that 8 weeks of rest and recovery is the minimum." I left the clinic excited that my treatments were over and I could get on with my life. Eight weeks later I woke up tired after sleepless nights. I was bald and had peripheral neuropathy in my hands and feet that was crippling, and the drug I was taking made me feel like I had arthritis all over my body. Where was my energy and soft blond hair? Why couldn't I think straight? There is no way I could do my job like this. I felt like I was drowning (Bush, 2009, p. 395).

The disabling effects of chronic cancer symptoms disrupt family and personal relationships, impair individuals' work performance, and often isolate survivors from normal social activities. Such changes in lifestyle create serious implications for a survivor's psychological well-being. When cancer changes a patient's body image or alters sexual function, the survivor frequently experiences significant anxiety and depression in interpersonal relationships. In the case of breast cancer survivors, studies show that poorer self-ratings of QOL are associated with poor body image, coping strategies, and a lack of social support (IOM, 2006).

The NCCN guidelines (NCCN, 2014) suggest a variety of nonpharmacological interventions to treat anxiety and depression in cancer survivors. Therapies include education, routine exercise, adequate sleep, supportive therapy or cognitive behavioral intervention, and reassurance that anxiety and depression are commonly seen in cancer survivors. Pharmacological intervention may also be warranted based on individual survivor response. Patients who use problem-oriented, active, and emotionally expressive coping processes also manage stress well (see Chapter 38). Survivors who have social and emotional support systems and maintain open communication with their treatment providers will also likely have less psychological distress.

Social Well-Being

Cancer affects any age-group (Figure 8-3). The developmental effects of cancer are perhaps best seen in the social impact that occurs across the life span. For adolescents and young adults, cancer seriously alters social skills, sexual development, body image, and the ability to think about and plan for the future (see Chapter 12). Adults (ages 30 to 59) who have cancer experience significant changes in their families. Once a member of the family is diagnosed with cancer, every family member's role, plans, and abilities change. The healthy spouse often takes on added job responsibilities to provide additional income for the family. A spouse, sibling, grandparent, or child often assumes caregiving responsibilities for the patient.

Adult patients who experience changes in sexuality, intimacy, and fertility see their marriages affected, often resulting in divorce. Impaired fertility is a concern since chemotherapy and radiation may be gonadotoxic (Kort et al., 2014). Infertility or subfertility may be present following cancer treatment. Male cancer survivors may also face erectile dysfunction; female survivors may face premature menopause or

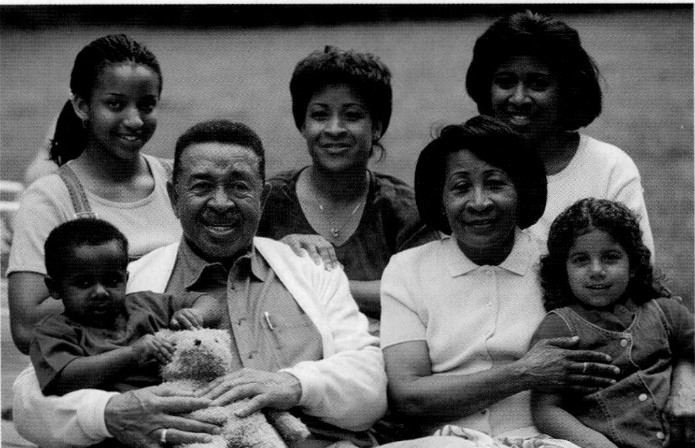

FIGURE 8-3 A family representing young and old. Each member could be a cancer survivor.

changes in vaginal tissue, impacting sexual intercourse. All of these reproductive challenges may impact sexual health between cancer survivor and spouse. The potential fertility issues secondary to chemotherapy and radiation impact family planning. To cope with these issues, pretreatment discussions regarding potential effect of treatment on sexual relations and fertility are essential (Harden et al., 2013; Kort et al., 2014; NCCN, 2014; Rossen et al., 2012). Guidelines from NCCN (2014) suggest cryopreservation of ova or sperm pretreatment to address fertility concerns.

A history of cancer significantly affects employment opportunities and has affected the ability of survivors to obtain and retain health and life insurance in the past. However, changes in the availability and affordability of health insurance resulting from the Patient Protection and Affordable Care Act of 2010 has made insurance more attainable for cancer survivors (NCCS, 2012a). There are now many options for health insurance. Cancer survivors should obtain comprehensive health coverage that will pay for all of their basic health care needs such as hospital and doctor care, lab tests, medical equipment, and prescription drugs. Beginning in 2014, most people are required to have comprehensive health coverage that includes a defined set of essential health benefits that provide minimum essential coverage (NCCS, 2012b).

Often a survivor experiences health-related work limitations that require a reduced work schedule or a complete change in employment. Between 64% and 84% of cancer survivors who worked before their diagnosis return to work (Steiner et al., 2010). The most common problems reported by survivors who return to work are physical effort, heavy lifting, stooping, concentration, and keeping up with the work pace. Factors that affect a return to work include cancer site, prognosis, type of treatment, socioeconomic status, and characteristics of the work to be done. The economic burden of cancer is enormous. If a survivor's illness affects his or her ability to work, less income goes to the individual and family. The problems are even greater for low-income survivors if they are underinsured. The ACS (2014b) offers excellent tips on returning to work after cancer treatment: http://www.cancer.org/treatment/survivorshipduringandaftertreatment/stayingactive/workingduringandaftertreatment/returning-to-work-after-cancer-treatment.

Older adults face many social concerns as a result of cancer. The disease causes some survivors to retire prematurely or decrease work hours, thus decreasing income. The older adult faces a fixed income and the limitations of Medicare reimbursement. Many older adults have moved to retirement residences in other states and find themselves isolated from the social support of their families. Older adults also face a high level of disability as a result of cancer and cancer treatment and report a higher incidence of limitations in activities of daily living than older adults without cancer (IOM, 2006). As a result, many older cancer survivors require ongoing caregiving support either from family members or professional caregivers.

Spiritual Well-Being

Cancer challenges a person's spiritual well-being (see Chapter 36). Key features of spiritual well-being include a harmonious interconnectedness, creative energy, and a faith in a higher power or life force. Cancer and its treatment create physical and psychological changes that cause survivors to question, "Why me?" and wonder if perhaps their disease is a form of punishment. Cancer survivors who participate in religious activities and report belief in God experience increased emotional function and coping (Holt et al., 2011; Schreiber, 2011). Relationships with a God, a higher power, nature, family, or community are critical for survivors. Cancer threatens relationships because it makes it difficult for survivors to maintain a connection and a sense of belonging. It isolates survivors from meaningful interaction and support, which then threatens their ability to maintain hope. Long-term treatment, cancer recurrence, and the lingering side effects of treatment create a level of uncertainty for survivors.

CANCER AND FAMILIES

A survivor's family takes different forms: the traditional nuclear family, extended family, single-parent family, close friends, and blended families (see Chapter 10). Once cancer affects a member of the family, it affects all other members as well. Although the research is from 2006, a summary of issues affecting families of patients with cancer still holds true (Lewis, 2006):

- Family members are substantially distressed when a member has cancer.
- Family members do not know, understand, or respond supportively to the expressed thoughts, feelings, and behavior of other family members about the cancer.
- Families try to cope with both the impact of the cancer and tension in the family caused or worsened by the cancer.
- Family members struggle to maintain their core functions when one of them is a long-term survivor.

Usually a member of the family becomes the patient's caregiver. Family caregiving is a stressful experience, depending on the relationship between patient and caregiver and the nature and extent of the patient's disease. Members of the "sandwich generation" (i.e., caregivers who are 30 to 50 years old) are often caught in the middle of caring for their own immediate family and a parent with cancer. The demands are many, from providing ongoing encouragement and support and assisting with household chores to providing hands-on physical care (e.g., bathing, assisting with toileting, or changing a dressing) when cancer is advanced. Caregiving also involves the psychological demands of communicating, problem solving, and decision making; social demands of remaining active in the community and work; and economic demands of meeting financial obligations.

Families struggle to maintain core functions when one of their members is a cancer survivor. Core family functions include maintaining an emotionally and physically safe environment, interpreting and reducing the threat of stressful events (including the cancer) for family members, and nurturing and supporting the development of individual family members (Lewis, 2006). In childrearing families, this means providing an attentive parenting environment for children and information and support to children when their sense of well-being becomes threatened. Spouses often do not know what to do to support the survivor, and they struggle with how to help. In the end family functions become fragmented, and family members develop an uncertainty about their roles.

IMPLICATIONS FOR NURSING

Cancer survivorship creates many implications for nurses who help survivors plan for optimal lifelong health. Nurses are in a strong position to take the lead in improving public health efforts to manage the long-term consequences of cancer. Improvement is also necessary in the education of nurses and survivors about the phenomenon of survivorship. This section addresses approaches to incorporate cancer survivorship into your nursing practice.

Survivor Assessment

Knowing that there are many cancer survivors in the health care system, consider how to assess patients who report a history of cancer. It is important to assess a cancer survivor's needs as a standard part of your practice. When you are collecting a nursing history (see Chapters 16 and 31), have patients tell you their stories through a narrative. A narrative makes it possible to know people through their stories (i.e., the narratives they tell) and provides contextual detail and person-revealing characteristics that make them individuals (Hall and Powell, 2011). As you explore the patient's history of cancer and the treatment received in the past, ask questions such as, "How did that come about?" vs. why or yes/no questions. Let the patient take you on a journey explaining his or her condition. You might ask, "Tell me how your disease most affects you right now," or "What are the biggest problems that you're having from cancer?" or "What can I do to help you at this point?" A narrative approach elicits stories that will illustrate the social context of events and implicitly provide answers to questions of feeling and meaning (Hall and Powell, 2011). Show a caring approach so patients know that their stories are accepted.

Be aware that some patients do not always report that they have had cancer. Thus, when a patient tells you that he or she has had surgery, ask if it was cancer related. When a patient reveals a history of chemotherapy, radiation, biotherapy, or hormone therapy, refer to resources to help you understand how these therapies typically affect patients in both the short and long term. Then extend your assessment to determine if these treatment effects exist for your patient. Consider not only the effects of the cancer and its treatment (such as potential symptoms) but how it will affect any other medical condition. For example, if a patient also has heart disease, how will cancer-related fatigue affect this individual?

As of 2015 all accredited cancer centers must meet new standards of the American College of Surgeons Commission on Cancer (2012). Standard 2.3 includes risk assessment and genetic counseling for people at risk for familial or hereditary cancers. Genetic testing provides early detection and improved outcomes in appropriate patients and their family members. This should also be included in patient assessments.

Symptom management is an ongoing problem for many cancer survivors. If cancer is their primary diagnosis, it will be natural for you to explore any presenting symptoms. Be sure to learn specifically how symptoms are affecting the patient. For example, is pain also causing fatigue, or is a neuropathy causing the patient to walk with an abnormal gait? If cancer is secondary, you do not want important symptoms to go unrecognized. Ask the patient, "Since your diagnosis of and treatment for cancer, which physical changes or symptoms have you had?" "Tell me how these changes affect you now?" You explore each symptom that a patient identifies to gain a complete picture of his or her health

TABLE 8-2 Examples of Assessment Questions for Cancer Survivors

Category	Examples of Questions
Symptoms	• Tell me about the symptoms you're having from your cancer treatment. • Describe any pain or discomfort in the area where you had surgery or radiation; discomfort, pain, or unusual sensations in your hands or feet; weakness in your legs or arms; or problems moving around. • Describe for me the fatigue, sleeplessness, or shortness of breath you're feeling. • Sometimes people believe that they are starting to have problems after chemotherapy such as paying attention, remembering things, or finding words. Have you noticed any changes like these?
Psychosocial problems	• How distressed are you feeling at this point on a scale of 0 to 10, with 10 being the worst distress that you could imagine? • Tell me how you think your family is handling your cancer? • What do you see in your family members' responses to your cancer that concerns you?
Sexuality problems	• If you have had sexual changes, which strategies have you tried to make things better? Have these strategies worked? • Would you be open to a health care provider who knows how to help you? • Since your cancer, do you see yourself differently as a person?

status (Table 8-2). Some patients are reluctant to report or discuss their symptoms. Be patient and, once you identify a symptom, explore the extent to which the symptom is currently affecting the patient.

Because you know that cancer affects a patient's QOL in many ways, be sure to explore the patient's psychological, social, and spiritual needs and resources. Sometimes you will not be able to conduct a thorough assessment when you perform an initial nursing history. If this is the case, incorporate your assessment into your ongoing patient care. Observe your patient's interactions with family members and friends. When you are administering care to patients, talk about their daily lives and determine the extent to which cancer has changed their lifestyle.

One area that is often difficult for nurses to assess well is a patient's sexuality. Sexuality is more than simply the physical ability to perform a sex act or conceive a child. It also includes a person's self-concept and body image (see Chapter 34), sexual response (e.g., interest and satisfaction), and sexual roles and relationships (see Chapter 35). Surgery for many cancers is disfiguring, and chemotherapy and radiation often alter a patient's sexual response (e.g., prostate, breast, and gynecological cancers). Cancer therapies have the potential to cause fatigue, apathy, nausea, vomiting, malaise, and sleep disturbances, all of which interfere with a patient's sexual function. It is important to simply realize that cancer often influences the patient's sexuality. It helps to develop a comfort level in acknowledging with patients that sexual changes are common at any age level. Ask a patient, "Since your diagnosis of and treatment for cancer, has your ability or interest in sexual activity changed? If so, how?" Patients will appreciate your sensitivity and interest in their well-being. When they begin to discuss their sexuality, be familiar with the expert resources in your institution (e.g., psychologist or social worker) available for patient referral.

Patient Education

When you care for a cancer patient, it is important to understand whether the patient administers most of his or her own self-care or if support is required from a family caregiver. This is essential to provide the most appropriate patient education, both in the form of content and in your teaching approach. Schumacher et al. (2006) developed a conceptual model, the transactional model of cancer family caregiving skill, which describes the relationship among cancer patients and family caregivers in the performance of family caregiving skills (Figure 8-4). The model offers a perspective on caregivers and cancer survivors both as individuals and as a team. Family caregiving skill is the ability to respond effectively and smoothly to the demands of an illness and pattern of care using multiple caregiving processes. Illness demands of cancer include dealing with symptoms, responding to illness behaviors (e.g., role changes, avoiding interaction), modifying activities for an illness situation, nutritional support, interpersonal care, use of community resources, managing acute illness episodes, and implementing treatments. The patient and caregiver follow a continuum of three patterns of care: the self-caregiving pattern (patients are mostly independent with caregivers in a standby role), the collaborative care pattern (patients and caregivers share care activities and respond together to illness demands), and the family caregiving pattern (patients are unable to perform independently and require extensive caregiver involvement) (Schumacher et al., 2006).

A patient's and caregiver's response to a caregiving demand involves performing caregiving processes (e.g., monitoring [observing for problems], interpreting [identifying the problem], making decisions and adjustments, accessing resources, and providing hands-on care). In terms of providing hands-on care, family caregivers often provide complex nursing procedures in the home such as managing intravenous infusions or irrigating wounds. Knowledge about caregiving or self-care, previous experience, and emotions influence the way caregivers and survivors respond and acquire caregiving processes. Schumacher's model is a helpful resource for you to apply when initially assessing the patient and caregiver condition, identifying their learning needs, and recognizing the type of information to teach. Learn where the patient and caregiver are along the caregiving continuum and determine the information needed to support them in meeting caregiving demands and performing caregiving processes. Frequently this means that any education will involve both the patient and family caregiver together, unless the relationship is strained and the patient chooses not to involve the caregiver.

It is a nurse's responsibility to educate cancer survivors and their families about the effects of cancer and cancer treatment. This means that, when you care for a cancer survivor, you need to understand the nature of the patient's particular disease and know the short- and long-term effects of each therapy. When designing education that promotes self-management in caregiving, plan activities on the basis of the family caregiver's and cancer survivor's perceived disease-related problems and help them problem solve and gain the self-efficacy or confidence to deal with these problems. The online publication, *Facing Forward: Life After Cancer Treatment* (NCI, 2014a) provides information about follow-up medical care and managing physical, social, work, and intimacy concerns. Available in both English and Spanish, it is a valuable resource for cancer survivors to guide a forward perspective in managing life challenges. Patient education helps survivors assume healthier lifestyle behaviors that will give them control of aspects of their health and improve outcomes from cancer and chronic illness.

When caring for patients with an initial diagnosis of cancer, reinforce their health care provider's explanations of the risks related to their cancer and treatment, what they need to self-monitor (e.g.,

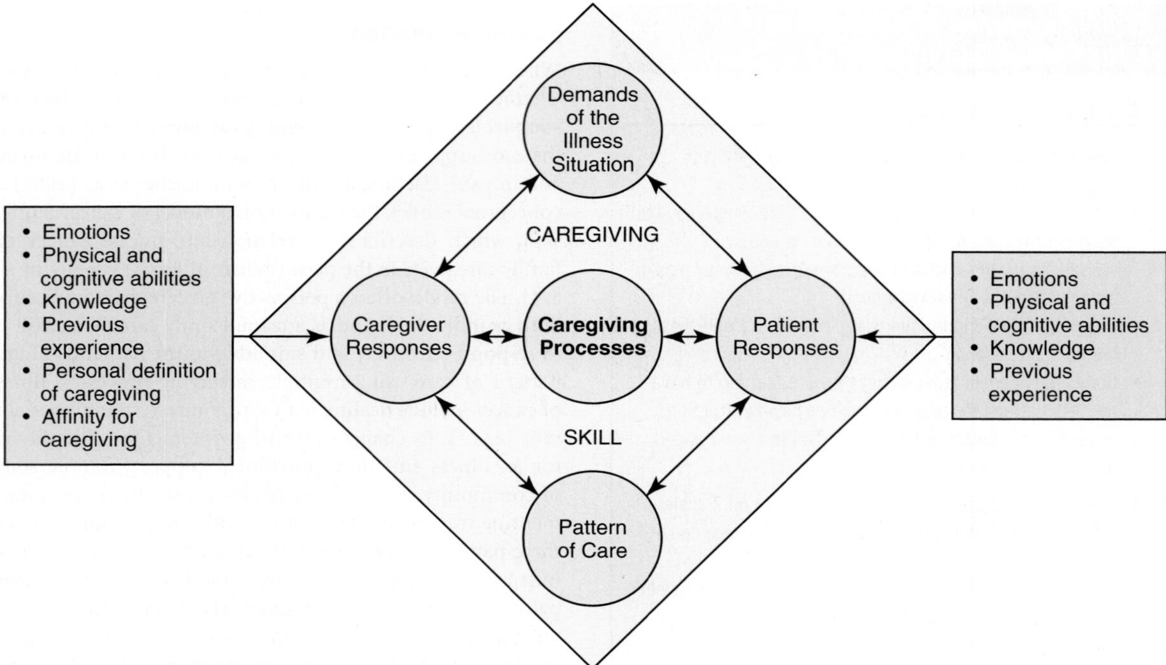

FIGURE 8-4 Transactional model of cancer family caregiving skill. (From Schumacher KL et al: A transactional model of family caregiving skill, *Adv Nurs Sci* 29(3):271, 2006.)

appetite, weight, and effects of fatigue), and what to discuss with health care providers in the future. If you teach patients and their family caregivers about the potential for treatment effects such as pain, neuropathy, or cognitive change, they are more likely to report their symptoms. It allows them to know which signs or changes to anticipate and monitor. Survivors need to learn how to manage problems related to persistent symptoms. For example, survivors with neuropathy need to learn how to protect the hands and feet, prevent falls, and avoid accidental burns.

Because survivors have an increased risk for developing a second cancer and/or chronic illness, it is important to educate them about lifestyle behaviors and the importance of participating in ongoing cancer screening and early detection practices. Lifelong cancer screening provides the opportunity to identify new cancers in early stages. Female cancer survivors who have a history of nonmetastatic cancer are more likely to participate in mammography and pelvic/Papanicolaou screening than women with no cancer history (Schumacher et al., 2012). This may be related to fear of cancer recurrence and a health care provider's recommendation for follow-up screening in cancer survivors. Many survivors become interested in learning more about dietary supplements and nutritional complementary therapies to manage disease symptoms (IOM, 2006). Scientific evidence shows that several health promotion areas are of interest to cancer survivors (i.e., smoking cessation, physical activity, diet and nutrition) (see Chapter 45), and the use of complementary and alternative medicine (see Chapter 33). Teach patients useful strategies to promote their health.

Providing Resources

Numerous organizations provide resources to cancer survivors. However, many survivors do not receive timely and appropriate referrals to them. As a nurse you will find that many people (e.g., friends, neighbors, and family members) come to you for advice about health care before they actually become a patient. It is important to know that cancer-related hospital and ambulatory care are not standardized. For example, when a patient with cancer is hospitalized, the availability of ancillary services for long-term care varies by care setting. Hospital-based oncologists are usually in larger hospitals and not in smaller ones. An NCI-designated cancer center offers the most comprehensive and up-to-date clinical care. NCI-designated centers also conduct important clinical trials to investigate the most current cancer therapies. Your role is to tell patients about the different resources available so they are able to make informed choices about their care. Refer patients to the NCI website (http://www.cancer.gov/). It contains a current list of NCI-designated comprehensive cancer centers.

A wealth of cancer-related community support services is available to survivors through voluntary organizations such as the ACS (www.cancer.org) and the NCCS (http://www.canceradvocacy.org). Most offer their services at no cost. Many supportive services offer call centers and Internet-based information and discussion boards in addition to direct-service delivery (IOM, 2006). Health care professionals are not consistent in referring patients to these valuable services. In addition, although community-based services help most survivors, there are gaps in service provision for assistance with transportation, home care, child care, and financial assistance. Become knowledgeable about the services within your community.

COMPONENTS OF SURVIVORSHIP CARE

Once primary cancer treatment ends, health care professionals need to develop an organized plan for survivorship care. This does not always occur because of inadequacies in the health care system, including a health care provider not assuming responsibility for coordinating care, fragmentation of care between specialists and general practitioners, and a lack of guidance about how survivors can improve their health outcomes (IOM, 2006). Patients with cancer often do not receive noncancer care (e.g., care for diabetes or heart conditions) when their cancer diagnosis shifts attention away from care that is routine but necessary. The IOM (2006) recommends four essential components of

BOX 8-2 A Survivorship Care Plan

On discharge from cancer treatment, every patient and his or her primary health care provider should receive a record of all care received from the oncologist. The patient and health care provider should also receive a follow-up plan incorporating available evidence-based standards of care.

Care Summary

- Diagnostic tests performed and results
- Tumor characteristics (e.g., site, stage, and grade)
- Dates when treatment started and stopped
- Surgery, chemotherapy, radiotherapy, transplant, hormone therapy, or gene therapy provided, including the specific agents used
- Psychosocial, nutritional, and other supportive services provided
- Full contact information for treating institutions and key providers
- Identification of a key point of contact and coordinator of care

Follow-Up Plan

- Need for ongoing treatment and clinic follow-up plan
- Description of recommended cancer screening and other periodic testing/examinations
- Information about possible late and long-term effects of treatment and symptoms of such effects
- Information about possible signs of recurrence and second tumors and follow-up tests
- Recommendations for healthy behaviors (e.g., nutrition, sun screen use, exercise, no smoking)
- Information about genetic counseling and testing as appropriate
- Referrals to specific follow-up care providers
- A listing of cancer-related resources and information

Data from American Society of Clinical Oncology: *New ASCO survivorship care plan template is simpler, faster for healthcare providers*, October 14, 2014, http://www.asco.org/advocacy/new-asco-survivorship-care-plan-template-simpler-faster-healthcare-providers.

survivorship care: (1) prevention and detection of new cancers and recurrent cancer; (2) surveillance for cancer spread, recurrence, or second cancers; (3) intervention for consequences of cancer and its treatment (e.g., medical problems, symptoms, and psychological distress); and (4) coordination between specialists and primary care providers.

Survivorship Care Plan

To meet the health care needs of cancer survivors, it is essential for a "survivorship care plan" to be written by the principal provider who coordinates the patient's **oncology** treatment (Box 8-2) (IOM, 2006). The care plan contains important information about the patient's treatment, the need for future check-ups and cancer tests, the potential long-term late effects of the treatment, and ideas for improving the patient's health (ASCO, 2015). When a survivor is released from an oncologist, the internist and other health care providers provide and coordinate care on the basis of knowledge of prior cancer history and treatment. On the basis of Standard 3.3 of the American College of Surgeons Commission on Cancer (2012), by 2015 fully accredited cancer centers must develop and disseminate a comprehensive patient specific follow-up survivorship care plan for all patients when they complete treatment. Some patients receive care at cancer centers without this type of resource and may not have a survivorship care plan.

The IOM (2006) also recommends that health insurance plans cover care outlined in a survivorship care plan. Survivor plans are not always developed, and health insurance companies do not routinely cover this type of care. Ideally you review a survivorship care plan with a patient when he or she is formally discharged from a treatment program. The plan then becomes a guide for any future cancer or cancer-related care. Health care providers use the plan as a guide for patient education and screening for secondary cancers. Survivors use it to raise questions with health care providers to prompt appropriate care during follow-up visits.

QSEN QSEN: BUILDING COMPETENCY IN PATIENT-CENTERED CARE Mrs. Henry is a 45-year-old patient who received treatment for breast cancer at an outpatient clinic. Her cancer treatments ended 1 year ago. This is the first time she is coming to the primary health provider for a physical examination. As the nurse, you ask her to bring a copy of her survivorship care plan with her to the appointment. Mrs. Henry says that she does not have one. She said her oncologist has told her to follow up with her care with her primary health provider. What is the best response to Mrs. Henry? Which nursing assessments need to be done before her first appointment at the physical examination?

Answers to QSEN Activities can be found on the Evolve website.

Barriers to develop and implement survivorship care plans (SCPs) focus on financial and human resource costs (Stricker and O'Brien, 2014). Average reimbursement of patient visits for assessment and discussion of an SCP is 55% of the billed amount. Some private insurance companies reimbursed an average of 38% for the visit while Medicare/Medicaid averages 59% of the bill (Rosales et al., 2014). No reimbursement exists for the development costs of an SCP.

Cancer organizations such as the Lance Armstrong Foundation (http://www.livestrong.org/), the Association of Cancer Online Resources (ACOR) (http://www.acor.org) and the NCCS (http://www.canceradvocacy.org/toolbox/) provide Internet guides for the development of survivorship care plans. Many NCI-designated cancer centers and pediatric cancer centers provide survivorship care planning (NCI, 2014a). Many survivors do not receive care at NCI-designated cancer centers and are discharged with no survivor plan. Thus nurses and other health care providers need to become more vigilant in recognizing cancer survivors and attempting to link them with the support and resources they require. Nurses make a difference when they consider the long-term issues that cancer survivors face after their time of diagnosis and in contributing to solutions to manage or relieve cancer-associated health problems. A strong interprofessional approach that includes nurses, oncology specialists, dietitians, social workers, pastoral care, and rehabilitation professionals is necessary. Together an interprofessional team provides a plan of care that addresses treatment-related problems and future health risks and offers a wellness focus to give patients a sense of hope as he or she enters the survivor experience.

KEY POINTS

- Nurses care for cancer survivors when they seek care for their cancer and other medical conditions.
- Cancer survivors may have serious health problems related to their treatments.
- How well a survivor adapts to the cancer experience psychologically depends on predisposing factors, the person's current psychological status, the extent of his or her disease, and the presence of disruptive signs and symptoms.
- The disabling effects of chronic cancer symptoms disrupt family and personal relationships, impair individuals' work performance, and often isolate survivors from normal social activities.

- Adults who have cancer experience significant changes within their families, including a change in each member's role.
- Relationships among cancer survivors and family members become difficult to maintain because family members often do not know, understand, or have the skills or confidence to support the survivor's reactions to cancer.
- Because survivors are at an increased risk for developing a second cancer and/or chronic illness, it is important to educate them about lifestyle behaviors that will improve the quality of their lives.
- Fear of recurrence is a common concern of cancer survivors and should be addressed to determine if it exists and if intervention is needed.
- Once a patient's primary cancer treatment ends, health care professionals should develop an organized plan for survivorship care.
- Ideally you review a survivorship care plan with a patient when he or she is formally discharged from a treatment program, and it becomes a guide for any future cancer or cancer-related care.

CLINICAL APPLICATION QUESTIONS

Preparing for Clinical Practice

1. Do you have a friend or family member who has cancer and is willing to talk about it? If so, ask the individual to tell you what the experience has been like and what he or she would recommend to help you provide better care for survivors.
2. Ms. Ritter is a 32-year-old woman who visits the medical outpatient clinic to discuss her treatment options for breast cancer. She is married and has one child, a daughter, who is 6 years old. She and her husband hoped to have another child in the near future but now wonder if that will be possible. She shares with the nursing staff her concerns about the future and how cancer will affect her and her family. Identify two follow-up care plan components that would be important when considering Ms. Ritter's role as a wife and parent.
3. Ms. Ritter tells her nurse, "This chemotherapy has made me feel so tired, and there are many nights when I can't sleep very well. I'm looking forward to this ending." What is an appropriate response the nurse might give Ms. Ritter?

ⓔ *Answers to Clinical Application Questions can be found on the Evolve website.*

REVIEW QUESTIONS

Are You Ready to Test Your Nursing Knowledge?

1. Cancer survivors are at risk for treatment-related problems. Which of the patients listed here has the greatest risk for developing such problems?
   1. An 80-year-old woman undergoing surgery for removal of a basal cell carcinoma on the face
   2. A 71-year-old man getting high-dose chemotherapy/radiation for advanced-stage lymphoma
   3. A 26-year-old man receiving chemotherapy for testicular cancer that is localized to the testicle
   4. A 48-year-old woman receiving radiation for Hodgkin's disease that involves lymph nodes extending above and below the diaphragm
2. A 34-year-old patient who is a 5-year survivor of Hodgkin's disease continues to have symptoms related to chemotherapy treatment. The patient is a computer expert and enjoys Internet discussion groups. Which of the following is the best resource a nurse can recommend to help the patient access a survivorship care plan?
   1. Association of Cancer Online Resources (ACOR)
   2. National Coalition for Cancer Survivorship
   3. American Cancer Society (ACS)
   4. National Cancer Institute (NCI)
3. A nurse reviews the medical record of a 40-year-old patient newly admitted to the medical nursing unit for evaluation of diabetes. While reviewing the medical history, the nurse notices that the patient had bladder surgery 3 years ago. Which of the following assessment questions is most appropriate for the nurse to ask to determine if the patient is a cancer survivor?
   1. Determining if the patient had additional surgeries recently
   2. Assessing the patient's medication history
   3. Determining if the surgery was cancer related
   4. Assessing if the patient's parents had cancer
4. A nurse working in a gynecological oncology clinic knows that it is important to recognize that cancer survivors may have impaired sexual function. Which of the following statements is most appropriate to determine if sexual impairment is a problem?
   1. "I'm embarrassed to ask you this, but is your sex life OK?"
   2. "Treatment for cervical cancer may change sexual relations. Describe concerns you have about this.
   3. "You're probably too tired to have intercourse with your husband, right?"
   4. "Did the doctor tell you that you can still have sex while you are being treated?"
5. A 20-year-old man who has been diagnosed with testicular cancer is about to begin treatment, including intense chemotherapy, radiation, and surgery. He says to the nurse, "I'm scared that I'll never be able to be a father." The most appropriate response by the nurse is:
   1. "You're young. You'll beat this cancer and have a long and happy life."
   2. "Tell me what you mean about your fear of never being a father."
   3. "Cancer treatment has really improved, and more people are surviving it."
   4. "Your doctor is really good and has a high cure rate. He'll take care of you. "
6. Symptoms of chemotherapy-related cognitive impairment (CRCI) may include difficulty: (Select all that apply.)
   1. Driving a car.
   2. Sleeping 6 to 8 hours at night.
   3. Reading with comprehension.
   4. Walking with a steady gait.
   5. Focusing on balancing a checkbook.
   6. Eating a balanced diet.
7. A support group of cancer survivors is discussing cancer-related fatigue (CRF). The survivor most likely to gain relief from CRF is the survivor who does which of the following? (Select all that apply.)
   1. Takes naps during the day and evening
   2. Drinks energy drinks daily
   3. Exercises at least every other day
   4. Eats a balanced diet
   5. Joins a cancer support group
8. A patient has received multiple chemotherapy regimens and a course of radiation for colon cancer. He performs his own hygiene but needs assistance from his wife to move about safely in the

home because of ongoing fatigue and weakness. His wife helps him dress when he becomes excessively tired. This caregiving skill pattern is best described as which of the following?
1. The self-caregiving pattern
2. The collaborative care pattern
3. The family caregiving pattern
4. The team caregiving pattern

9. A 50-year-old patient who has completed systemic chemotherapy and radiation for breast cancer tells you that she is having difficulty remembering things and paying attention to a television show for over 5 minutes. Interventions that may help the patient include: (Select all that apply.)
1. Stop reading any nonessential materials.
2. Identify a trusted support person to help with banking and bill payment.
3. Rest as much as possible and do not exercise.
4. Try listening to a book on tape and see if that helps understanding.
5. Eat as much protein and as many vitamin K—enriched foods as possible.
6. Write appointments on your calendar and keep a list to organize what you are to do.

10. A nurse in an oncology outpatient clinic has been seeing a woman and her husband since the woman was diagnosed with breast cancer. Sometimes the husband appears supportive, asking questions about his wife's care. At other times the husband seems easily distracted and uninterested. The nurse decides to reassess the psychosocial condition of the patient and her husband. Which of the following questions best elicits needed psychosocial information?
1. "In what way does the pain you have affect you on a daily basis?"
2. "Describe what you eat in a typical day."
3. "Tell me how you think you and your husband are dealing with your cancer."
4. "Are the two of you having any relational difficulties because of your cancer?"

11. A child in remission for leukemia and her mother come to the pediatrician's office for a routine physical examination. The nurse asks the child whether she is having continued symptoms. Her mom says, "I don't know why you want all of this information about her cancer treatment. The leukemia is gone." The best response from the nurse in support of the child and mother would be:
1. "The doctor likes to keep the records complete on all of her patients."
2. "Just because she is in remission does not mean that it will stay that way."
3. "Children sometimes have delayed effects from treatment; we need this information to plan her care properly."
4. "I understand your concern. If you don't want to provide the information, sign this release form."

12. A 60-year-old breast cancer survivor was told by her physician that she is experiencing late effects of chemotherapy and chest radiation. Which of the following are known late effects of cancer treatment? (Select all that apply.)
1. Impaired immune function
2. Heart failure
3. Osteoporosis
4. Loss of sense of smell
5. Abnormal liver function

13. A 45-year-old patient who has recurrent cancer is having nightmares and obsessive thoughts about the disease, is unable to focus on anything else, and has a breakdown in relationships with her family. These symptoms are associated with:
1. Chemotherapy-related cognitive impairment (CRCI).
2. Cancer-related fatigue (CRF).
3. Family dysfunction caused by cancer.
4. Posttraumatic stress disorder (PTSD).

14. Survivorship care plans should include information to provide future caregivers with important information about the treatment a patient with cancer has received. The most important entries in a well-written survivorship care plan include: (Select all that apply.)
1. Type of tumor and dates of diagnosis.
2. Screening tests that are appropriate for future use.
3. Type of chemotherapy or radiation treatment used and length of dose.
4. Typical side effects the patient experienced immediately after a dose of chemotherapy was given.
5. Lifestyle recommendations for diet and exercise.

15. Caring for a patient with cancer is unique because of the effects of the disease and associated treatment. An understanding of a patient's symptom experience is critical and best revealed by a nurse asking which of the following questions? (Select all that apply.)
1. "What symptoms do you think you're having as a result of your cancer?"
2. "Describe how the symptoms affect you in your daily life."
3. "Let's discuss your pain. Tell me how it affects you."
4. "Describe how your family provides care for your symptoms."

Answers: 1. 2; **2.** 1; **3.** 3; **4.** 2; **5.** 2; **6.** 1, 3, 5; **7.** 3, 4; **8.** 2; **9.** 2, 4, 6; **10.** 3; **11.** 3; **12.** 1, 2, 3, 5; **13.** 4; **14.** 1, 2, 3, 5; **15.** 1, 2, 3.

Rationales for Review Questions can be found on the Evolve website.

REFERENCES

American Cancer Society (ACS): *Cancer Treatment and Survivorship Facts & Figures 2014–2015*, Atlanta, 2014a, American Cancer Society. http://www.cancer.org/acs/groups/content/@research/documents/document/acspc-042801.pdf. Accessed June 24, 2015.

American Cancer Society (ACS): *Returning to work after cancer treatment*, 2014b, http://www.cancer.org/treatment/survivorshipduringandaftertreatment/stayingactive/workingduringandaftertreatment/returning-to-work-after-cancer-treatment. Accessed June 24, 2015.

American College of Surgeons Commission on Cancer: *Cancer program standards 2012: ensuring patient-centered care manual,* V 1.2.1 Chicago, IL, 2012. https://www.facs.org/quality-programs/cancer/coc/standards. Accessed June 24, 2015.

American Society of Clinical Oncology (ASCO): *ASCO Cancer treatment summaries and survivorship care plans,* 2015, http://www.cancer.net/survivorship/follow-care-after-cancer-treatment/asco-cancer-treatment-summaries-and-survivorship-care-plans. Accessed June 24, 2015.

Bush N: Post-traumatic stress disorder related to the cancer experience, *Oncol Nurs Forum* 36(4):395, 2009.

Hall JM, Powell J: Understanding the person through narrative, *Nurs Res Pract*, 2011, Article ID 293837. http://dx.doi.org/10.1155/2011/293837. Accessed June 24, 2015.

Institute of Medicine (IOM) and National Research Council, et al, editors: *From cancer patient to cancer survivor: lost in transition*, Washington, DC, 2006, National Academies Press.

Kort J, et al: Fertility issues in cancer survivorship, *CA Cancer J Clin* 64(2):118, 2014.

National Cancer Institute (NCI): *Cancer trends progress report—2011/2012 Update*, Bethesda, MD, 2015, NIH, DHHS. http://progressreport.cancer.gov/. Accessed June 24, 2015.

National Cancer Institute (NCI): *Facing forward: life after cancer treatment*, NIH#14-2424, Bethesda, MD, 2014a, DHHS, Last revised May 2014. Available at: https://pubs.cancer.gov/ncipl/detail.aspx?prodid=p119. Accessed June 24, 2015.

National Cancer Institute (NCI): *Post-traumatic stress disorder*, 2014b, http://cancer.gov/cancertopics/pdq/supportivecare/post-traumatic-stress/health professional. Accessed August 30, 2014.

National Coalition for Cancer Survivorship (NCCS): *Cancer survivorship*, 2015, NCCS, Available at www.canceradvocacy.org. Accessed June 24, 2015.

National Coalition for Cancer Survivorship (NCCS): *Comprehensive Cancer Care Improvement Act*, 2012a. Available at http://www.canceradvocacy.org/cancer-policy/cccia/. Accessed June 24, 2015.

National Coalition for Cancer Survivorship (NCCS): *What cancer survivors need to know about health insurance*, 2012b. Available at http://www.canceradvocacy.org/wp-content/uploads/2013/01/Health-Insurance.pdf Accessed June 28, 2015.

National Comprehensive Cancer Network (NCCN): *NCCN Clinical practice guidelines in oncology: survivorship*, Version 2, 2014, https://www.nccn.org/. Accessed June 24, 2015.

Park SB, et al: Chemotherapy-induced peripheral neurotoxicity: a critical analysis, *CA Cancer J Clin* 63(6):419, 2013.

Stricker C, O'Brien M: Implementing the commission on cancer standards for survivorship care plans, *Clin J Oncol Nurs* 18(Suppl 15):22, 2014.

RESEARCH REFERENCES

Borneman T, et al: A qualitative analysis of cancer related fatigue in ambulatory oncology, *Clin J Oncol Nurs* 16(1):10, 2012.

Gewandter JS, et al: Falls and functional impairments in cancer survivors with chemotherapy-induced peripheral neuropathy (CIPN): a University of Rochester CCOP study, *Support Care Cancer* 21(7):205, 2013.

Harden J, et al: Survivorship after prostate cancer treatment: spouses quality of life at 36 months, *Oncol Nurs Forum* 40(6):567, 2013.

Holt C, et al: Role of religious involvement and spirituality in functioning among African Americans with cancer: testing a mediational model, *J Behav Med* 34:437, 2011.

Koch L, et al: Fear of recurrence in long-term breast cancer survivors-still an issue, *Psychooncology* 23:547, 2014.

Kwak M, et al: Prevalence and predictors of post-traumatic stress symptoms in adolescent and young adult cancer survivors: a 1-year follow-up study, *Psychooncology* 22(8):1798, 2013.

Lebel S, et al: Does fear of cancer recurrence predict cancer survivors' health care use?, *Support Care Cancer* 21(3):901, 2013.

Lebel S, et al: Addressing fear of cancer recurrence among women with cancer: a feasibility and preliminary outcome study, *J Cancer Surviv* 8(3):485, 2014.

Lewis FM: The effects of cancer survivorship on families and caregivers: more research is needed on long-term survivors, *Am J Nurs* 106(3):20, 2006.

Mitchell T, Turton P: "Chemobrain": concentration and memory effects in people receiving chemotherapy—a descriptive phenomenological study, *Eur J Cancer Care (Engl)* 20:539, 2011.

Myers J: Chemotherapy-related cognitive impairment: the breast cancer experience, *Oncol Nurs Forum* 39(1):E31, 2012.

Ness S, et al: Concerns across the survivorship trajectory: results from a survey of cancer survivors, *Oncol Nurs Forum* 40(1):35, 2013.

Nguyen J, et al: A literature review of symptom clusters in patients with breast cancer, *Expert Rev Pharmacoecon Outcomes Res* 11(5):533, 2011.

Oh H, et al: The identification of multiple symptom clusters and their effects on functional performance in cancer patients, *J Clin Nurs* 21:19, 2012.

Potrata B, et al: "Live a sieve": an exploratory study on cognitive impairments in patients with multiple myeloma, *Eur J Cancer Care (Engl)* 19:721, 2010.

Rey D, et al: Self-reported cognitive impairment after breast cancer treatment in young women from the ELIPPSE40 cohort, *Breast J* 5:406, 2012.

Rosales A, et al: Comprehensive survivorship care with cost and revenue analysis, *J Oncol Pract* 10(2):e81, 2014.

Rossen P, et al: Sexuality and body image in long-term survivors of testicular cancer, *Eur J Cancer* 48:571, 2012.

Schreiber J: Image of God: effect on coping and psychospiritual outcomes in early breast cancer survivors, *Oncol Nurs Forum* 38(3):293, 2011.

Schumacher KL, et al: A transactional model of cancer family caregiving skill, *ANS Adv Nurs Sci* 29(3):271, 2006.

Schumacher JR, et al: Cancer screening of long-term cancer survivors, *J Am Board Fam Med* 25(4):460, 2012.

Simard S, et al: Fear of cancer recurrence in adult cancer survivors: a systematic review of quantitative studies, *J Cancer Surviv* 7(3):300, 2013.

Steiner JF, et al: Returning to work after cancer: quantitative studies and prototypical narratives, *Psychooncology* 9(2):115, 2010.

Stuber ML, et al: Prevalence and predictors of posttraumatic stress disorder in adult survivors of childhood cancer, *Pediatrics* 125(5):e1124, 2010.

9

Cultural Awareness

OBJECTIVES

- Describe cultural influences on health and illness.
- Explain how the many facets of culture affect a health care provider's ability to provide culturally congruent care.
- Describe health disparities and social determinants of health.
- Describe steps toward developing cultural competence.
- Describe the relationship between cultural competence and patient-centered care.
- Use cultural assessment to plan culturally competent care.
- Discuss research findings applicable to culturally competent care.
- Discuss research finding applicable to equity-focused quality improvement.

KEY TERMS

Core measures, p. 111
Cultural assessment, p. 106
Cultural competency, p. 103
Culturally congruent care, p. 103
Culture, p. 102
Explanatory model, p. 107
Health care disparities, p. 102
Health disparity, p. 101
Intersectionality, p. 102
Linguistic competence, p. 108
Marginalized groups, p. 102
Oppression, p. 102
Social determinants of health, p. 102
Transcultural nursing, p. 103
World view, p. 105

MEDIA RESOURCES

http://evolve.elsevier.com/Potter/fundamentals/
- Review Questions
- Case Study with Questions
- Audio Glossary
- Content Updates

In the United States many individuals face greater obstacles to good health on the basis of one or more of the following factors: racial or ethnic group; religion; socioeconomic status; gender; age; mental health; cognitive, sensory, or physical disability; sexual orientation or gender identity; geographic location; or other characteristics historically linked to discrimination or exclusion (U.S. Department of Health and Human Services [USDHHS], 2015). The concept of culture comprises all of these factors. Research findings reveal differences in rates of cancer, diabetes, infant mortality, organ transplantation, and many other health conditions because of cultural factors. For example, African-Americans have the highest mortality rate of any racial and ethnic group for all cancers combined, contributing in part to a lower life expectancy for both African-American men and women (Office of Minority Health [OMH], 2013a). Asian Americans generally have lower cancer rates than the non-Hispanic white population, but they also have the highest incidence rates of liver cancer for both sexes compared with Hispanic, non-Hispanic Whites, or non-Hispanic Blacks (OMH, 2013b). Hispanic youths ages 2 to 19 are more likely to be overweight or obese than the non-Hispanic White or Black youths of the same age, which places them at a greater risk of developing a number of chronic diseases such as type 2 diabetes, high blood pressure, and asthma (Leadership for Healthy Communities, 2014).

Discrimination based on the cultural factors of sexual orientation and gender identity contributes to health and health care inequities. Gay, lesbian, and bisexual young people have a significantly increased risk for depression, anxiety, and substance use disorders and are four times as likely as their straight peers to make suicide attempts that require medical attention (Hollenbach et al., 2014). Transgender individuals are more likely to postpone medical care because of lack of insurance and encounters with discrimination than people who do not identify as transgender (Hollenbach et al., 2014).

The cultural differences in infant mortality are also alarming. In American Indian and Alaska Native populations, the infant mortality rate is 60% higher than in non-Hispanic Whites (OMH, 2014). In 2008 the infant mortality rate for African-American infants was more than twice the rate for non-Hispanic white infants. Disparities in infant mortality remain even when comparing groups of similar socioeconomic status. For example, the infant mortality rate among children born to college-educated African-American women is significantly higher than among babies born to white women who are similarly educated (Kaiser Family Foundation, 2008).

HEALTH DISPARITIES

Healthy People 2020 defines a **health disparity** as "a particular type of health difference that is closely linked with social, economic, and/or environmental disadvantage" (USDHHS, 2015). The word *parity* means "equality." Health *dis*parity is literally an inequality or difference (i.e., a gap) between the health status of a disadvantaged group such as people with low incomes and wealth and an advantaged group such as people with high incomes and wealth. Members of the disadvantaged group bear a burden of disease, injury, and violence that is out of proportion to the size of the group (CDC, 2013). Although Americans' health overall has improved during the past few decades, the health of members of marginalized groups has actually declined (CDC, 2013).

So what causes health disparities? People in **marginalized groups** are more likely to have poor health outcomes and die at an earlier age because of a complex interaction between individual genetics and behaviors; public and health policy; community and environmental factors; and quality of health care (United Health Foundation, 2014). Many organizations have developed different models incorporating **social determinants of health** to explain the complexity of these interactions (McGovern et al., 2014). According to the World Health Organization (2013), social determinants of health are "the conditions in which people are born, grow, live, work and age...shaped by the distribution of money, power and resources at global, national, and local levels." Income and wealth, family and household structure, social support, education, occupation, discrimination, neighborhood conditions, and social institutions are some examples of social determinants of health (McGovern et al., 2014).

Health Disparities and Health Care

Health disparities are the differences among populations in the incidence, prevalence, and outcomes of health conditions, diseases, and related complications. On the other hand, **health care disparities** are differences among populations in the availability, accessibility, and quality of health care services (e.g., screening, diagnostic, treatment, management and rehabilitation) aimed at prevention, treatment, and management of diseases and their complications.

Poor access to health care is one social determinant of health that contributes to health disparities. Access to primary care is an important indicator of broader access to health care services. A patient who regularly visits a primary care provider is more likely to receive adequate preventive care than a patient who lacks such access. The 2013 National Healthcare Disparities Report (AHRQ, 2013a) revealed that African-Americans, Asians, and Hispanics are less likely than non-Hispanic Whites to see a primary care provider regularly.

A similar disparity in access to care exists in other disadvantaged groups. Less care is available or accessible to people in low- and middle-income groups compared with people in high-income groups. Uninsured people ages 0 to 64 are less likely to have a regular primary care provider than those with private or public insurance (AHRQ, 2013a). Research suggests that some subgroups of the LGBT community have more chronic health conditions and a higher prevalence and earlier onset of disabilities than heterosexuals (Ranji et al., 2015).

In addition to the poor access to health care, a large body of research shows that health care systems and health care providers can contribute significantly to the problem of health disparities. More than a decade ago, reports by the Institute of Medicine (IOM, 2001, 2010) defined quality health care as care that is safe, effective, patient centered, timely, efficient, and equitable or without variation in outcomes as determined by stratified outcomes data. Although the U.S. health care system has improved in most of these areas since the IOM reports were published, the focus on equity has lagged behind (Mutha et al., 2012). Inadequate resources, poor patient-provider communication, a lack of culturally competent care, fragmented delivery of care, and inadequate access to language services all compromise patient outcomes (NQF, 2012). As a result, many disparities in health care and health outcomes remain.

Disparities in access to care, quality of care, preventive health, health education, and available resources to enable self-management when patients are outside of the health care setting contribute to poor population health. Health disparities are also very costly. Recent analysis estimates that 30% of direct medical costs for Blacks, Hispanics, and Asian Americans are excess because of health inequities and that overall the economy loses an estimated $309 billion per year because of the direct and indirect costs of disparities (Kaiser Family Foundation, 2012).

Addressing Health Care Disparities

The United States is a complex multicultural society. By the year 2050 the percentage of racial and ethnic minority groups in the United States is expected to climb to 50%. According to the Administration on Aging (2014), the population age 65 years and over increased from 35.9 million in 2003 to 44.7 million in 2013 (a 24.7% increase) and is projected to more than double to 98 million in 2060. The American Community Survey reports that the number of people in poverty increased to about 48.8 million or 15.9%, with African-Americans, Hispanics, and Native Americans having the highest national poverty rates (U.S. Census Bureau, 2013). According to the 2003 *National Adult Assessment of Literacy* (NAAL), only 12% of U.S. adults are proficient in obtaining, processing, and understanding basic health information and services needed to make appropriate health decisions (NCES, 2006). In addition, more than ever before, individuals are openly expressing their religious views, sexual orientation, and gender identities. All of these factors contribute to the complexities of delivering health care in the United States. Thus nurses, other health care providers, and health care organizations need to consider which skills, knowledge, attitudes, and policies can help them deliver the best care to all patients.

The Joint Commission (TJC), the National Quality Forum (NQF), and the National Commission on Quality Assurance (NCQA) are a few of the influential organizations that have responded to these complexities by implementing new standards focused on cultural competency, health literacy, and patient- and family-centered care. These standards recognize that valuing each patient's unique needs improves the overall safety and quality of care and helps to eliminate health disparities.

CULTURE

Culture is associated with norms, values, and traditions passed down through generations. It also has been perceived to be the same as ethnicity, race, nationality, and language (Kleinman and Benson, 2006). A more contemporary view of culture acknowledges its many other facets such as gender, sexual orientation, location, class, and immigration status. This more dynamic perspective recognizes that we all belong simultaneously to multiple social groups within changing social and political contexts, a framework often referred to as **intersectionality** (Box 9-1). According to this framework our memberships in social groups are not neutral. **Oppression** is a formal and informal system of advantages and disadvantages tied to our membership in social groups, such as those at work, at school, and in families (Adams et al., 2007). It impacts an individual's access to resources such as health care, housing, education, employment, and legal services. Whether we live in a disadvantaged community or a community with access to social power and resources, we are all affected by the system of oppression. Understanding the dynamics of oppression that operate on various levels while simultaneously affecting you and your patients helps you engage in the process of becoming more culturally competent.

The many categories that comprise culture are not isolated from each other—they stand alone, interact and are interdependent and mutually reinforcing. Although both groups and individuals within cultural groups may share commonalties in their experiences of oppression(s), there are also differences in these experiences. Including oppression in our definition of culture helps us recognize the profound effect it has on the individual and group experiences of all of us.

BOX 9-1 Key Concepts of Intersectionality

Intersectionality refers to the notion that intersecting categories such as race, ethnicity, gender, socioeconomic status, sexual orientation, and other axes of identity contribute to systemic injustice and social inequality (Cho et al., 2013).

- Social inequality: Groups have unequal access to resources, services, and positions.
- Overinclusion and underinclusion: Many groups have been overlooked in research and the design of interventions. For example, much of what is currently known about racial and ethnic disparities is drawn from national information sources and combines both sexes, despite the large body of evidence of sex and gender differences in the prevalence of health conditions and the use of health services (James et al., 2009).
- Marginalization: Groups are left out (e.g., limited access or exclusion from facets of the society such as political system, labor market, positions of power).
- Social location: One's place in society is based on membership in a social group (e.g., gender, race, class, sexual orientation) that determines access to resources. Social location is not based on biology but on the meaning that society constructs and gives to one's social group.
- Matrix of domination: Instead of thinking about race, gender, immigration status, class, and other axes of identity as descriptive categories only, it is important to understand them within the context of the larger system of power and privilege that permeates society.

Adapted from Murphy Y et al: Incorporating intersectionality in social work practice, research, policy, and education, Washington, DC, 2009, NASW Press.

To better understand this more dynamic and complex way of thinking about culture, consider this example. As a nurse think about how a 27-year-old homeless woman with diabetes, an 85-year-old African-American retired nurse from rural Alabama, a 32-year-old Latina lesbian executive in San Francisco who is Catholic, and an undocumented immigrant woman from Eastern Europe who has a 3-year-old child with a developmental disability experience their womanhood. How may their experiences compare to the experiences of others as they live in America? How do their experiences compare with regard to using a health care system, managing their diabetes, or perceiving the presence or absence of opportunities to live a happy, safe, and productive life? How could age affect their perspective? How would these answers change if one looked at their lives 15 or 35 years ago? How would the experiences change if these individuals were men or transgender? These scenarios are likely to draw a wide range of responses.

Understanding culture requires you to adopt an intersectional perspective like the one in the example. This allows you to consider the multitude of different experiences of your patients so that you can provide effective, evidence-based, culturally competent care.

Culturally Congruent Care

Leininger (2002) defines **transcultural nursing** as a comparative study of cultures to understand their similarities (culture that is universal) and the differences among them (culture that is specific to particular groups). The goal of transcultural nursing is to provide **culturally congruent care**, or care that fits a person's life patterns, values, and system of meaning. Patterns and meaning are generated by people themselves rather than from predetermined criteria. For example, rather than instructing all patients to always take their medications at the same set times during a day, you learn their lifestyle patterns, eating habits, sleep habits, and beliefs about medications and then try to plan a dosage schedule that fits each patient's needs. Culturally congruent care is sometimes different from the values and meanings of the professional health care system. Discovering patients' cultural values, beliefs, and practices as they relate to nursing and health care requires you to assume the role of learner and to partner with your patients and their families to determine what is needed to provide meaningful and beneficial nursing care (Leininger and McFarland, 2002). Effective nursing care integrates the cultural values and beliefs of individuals, families, and communities with the perspectives of a multidisciplinary team of health care providers.

When you provide culturally congruent care, you bridge cultural gaps to provide meaningful and supportive care for all patients. For example, during nursing school you are assigned to care for a female patient who observes Muslim beliefs. You notice the woman's discomfort with several of the male health care providers. You wonder if this discomfort is related to your patient's religious beliefs. While preparing for clinical, you learn that Muslims differ in their adherence to tradition but that modesty is the "overarching Islamic ethic" pertaining to interaction between the sexes (Rabin, 2010). Thus you say to the patient, "I know that for many of our Muslim patients, modesty is very important. Is there some way I can make you more comfortable?" You do not assume that the information will automatically apply to this patient. Instead you combine your knowledge about a cultural group with an attitude of helpfulness and flexibility to provide quality, patient-centered, culturally congruent care.

Meaning of Disease and Illness

Culture affects social determinants of health and how an individual defines the meaning of illness. It also provides the context in which a person interacts with family members, peers, community members, and institutions (e.g., educational, religious, media, health care, legal). Culture and life experiences shape a person's world view about health, illness, and health care.

To provide culturally congruent care, you need to understand the difference between disease and illness. Illness is the way that individuals and families react to disease, whereas disease is a malfunctioning of biological or psychological processes. People tend to react differently to diseases on the basis of their unique cultural perspective. Most health care providers in the United States are primarily educated to treat disease, whereas most individuals seek health care because of their experience with illness. In addition, there is a lack of cultural diversity among health care providers (OMH, 2013c). This often frustrates patients and providers, fostering a lack of trust, lack of adherence, and poor health outcomes. Providing safe, quality care to all patients means taking into consideration both disease and illness.

CULTURAL COMPETENCY

Cultural competency is defined by the National Institutes of Health (2015) as the enabling of health care providers to deliver services that are respectful of and responsive to the health beliefs, practices, and cultural and linguistic needs of diverse patients. Developing cultural competency allows systems, agencies, and groups of professionals to function effectively to understand the needs of groups accessing health information and health care and thus help eliminate health care disparities and ultimately health disparities (NIH, 2015). It is a developmental process that evolves over time. Both individuals and organizations are at various levels of awareness, knowledge, and skills that affect their ability to effectively function in a multicultural context (National Center for Cultural Competence [NCCC], n.d.). According to the NCCC framework, culturally competent organizations:

- Value diversity
- Conduct a cultural self-assessment
- Manage the dynamics of difference
- Institutionalize cultural knowledge
- Adapt to diversity

A culturally competent organization integrates these principles and capabilities into all aspects of the organization (e.g., policy making, administration, service delivery) and systematically involves consumers, key stakeholders, and communities.

In 2000 the Office of Minority Health (OMH) developed the Culturally and Linguistically Appropriate Standards (CLAS). In 2013, after 10 years of successful implementation, the OMH updated the standards to reflect the tremendous growth in the field and the increasing diversity of the nation (Box 9-2). The enhanced national CLAS are intended to advance health equity, improve quality, and help eliminate health care disparities by establishing a blueprint to help individuals and health care organizations implement culturally and linguistically appropriate services (OMH, 2013c).

In its early stages, the field of cultural competency primarily focused on the cultural barriers between health care providers educated in Western health care practices and immigrants arriving from non-Western parts of the world. The early pioneers in cross-cultural medicine outlined a set of universal skills that are still applicable for helping health care providers work effectively with patients from any culture (Berlin and Fowkes, 1982; Kleinman, 1980; Leininger, 2002). These skills include:

1. Respecting a patient's health beliefs as valid and understanding the effect of his or her beliefs on health care delivery
2. Shifting a model of understanding a patient's experience from a disease happening in his or her organ systems to that of an illness occurring in the context of culture (biopsychosocial context)
3. Ability to elicit a patient's explanation of an illness and its causes (patient's explanatory model)
4. Ability to explain to a patient in understandable terms the health care provider's perspective on the illness and its perceived causes
5. Being able to negotiate a mutually agreeable, safe, and effective treatment plan

Expanding the original focus on interpersonal skills, many of the current approaches to cultural competency now also focus on: (1) all marginalized groups and not just immigrants; (2) prejudice, stereotyping, and social determinants of health; and (3) the health system, communities, and institutions (Saha et al., 2008).

You broaden your understanding of the world by learning about other people's world views, which determines how people perceive others, how they interact and relate to reality, and how they process information (Walker et al., 2010). Cultural competency is dynamic and developmental, thus taking time to evolve as a new nurse. A variety of models for acquiring cultural competency exist. One model suggests that nurses see themselves as *becoming* rather than being culturally competent (Campinha-Bacote, 2007) because cultural competency is developmental. Campinha-Bacote's model of cultural competency (2002) has five interrelated components:

- **Cultural awareness:** An in-depth self-examination of one's own background, recognizing biases, prejudices, and assumptions about other people

BOX 9-2 National Standards for Culturally and Linguistically Appropriate Services (CLAS) in Health and Health Care

The National CLAS Standards are intended to advance health equity, improve quality, and help eliminate health care disparities by establishing a blueprint for health and health care organizations to:

Principal Standard

1. Provide effective, equitable, understandable, and respectful quality care and services that are responsive to diverse cultural health beliefs and practices, preferred languages, health literacy, and other communication needs.

Governance, Leadership, and Workforce

2. Advance and sustain organizational governance and leadership that promotes CLAS and health equity through policy, practices, and allocated resources.
3. Recruit, promote, and support a culturally and linguistically diverse governance, leadership, and workforce that are responsive to the population in the service area.
4. Educate and train governance, leadership, and workforce in culturally and linguistically appropriate policies and practices on an ongoing basis.

Communication and Language Assistance

5. Offer language assistance to individuals who have limited English proficiency and/or other communication needs, at no cost to them, to facilitate timely access to all health care and services.
6. Inform all individuals of the availability of language assistance services clearly and in their preferred language, verbally and in writing.
7. Ensure the competence of individuals providing language assistance, recognizing that the use of untrained individuals and/or minors as interpreters should be avoided.
8. Provide easy-to-understand print and multimedia materials and signage in the languages commonly used by the populations in the service area.

Engagement, Continuous Improvement, and Accountability

9. Establish culturally and linguistically appropriate goals, policies, and management accountability, and infuse them throughout the organization's planning and operations.
10. Conduct ongoing assessments of the organization's CLAS-related activities and integrate CLAS-related measures into assessment measurement and continuous quality improvement activities.
11. Collect and maintain accurate and reliable demographic data to monitor and evaluate the impact of CLAS on health equity and outcomes and to inform service delivery.
12. Conduct regular assessments of community health assets and needs and use the results to plan and implement services that respond to the cultural and linguistic diversity of populations in the service area.
13. Partner with the community to design, implement, and evaluate policies, practices, and services to ensure cultural and linguistic appropriateness.
14. Create conflict- and grievance-resolution processes that are culturally and linguistically appropriate to identify, prevent, and resolve conflicts or complaints.
15. Communicate the organization's progress in implementing and sustaining CLAS to all stakeholders, constituents, and the general public.

From the United States Department of Health and Human Services (USDHHS): *National standards for culturally and linguistically appropriate services (CLAS) in health and health care,* Washington, D.C., 2013. USDHHS Office of Minority Health.

- **Cultural knowledge:** Sufficient comparative knowledge of diverse groups, including the values, health beliefs, care practices, world view, and bicultural ecology commonly found within each group
- **Cultural skills:** Ability to assess social, cultural, and biophysical factors that influence patient treatment and care
- **Cultural encounters:** Cross-cultural interactions that provide opportunities to learn about other cultures and develop effective intercultural communication
- **Cultural desire:** The motivation and commitment to caring that moves an individual to learn from others, accept the role as a learner, be open to and accepting of cultural differences, and build on cultural similarities.

Blanchet and Pepin (2015) have recently described the processes involved in the development of cultural competence among registered nurses and undergraduate student nurses. Clinical experience and interactions with patients and fellow clinicians help to build cultural competency. The researchers describe three dimensions of cultural competence:

- Building a relationship with the other
- Working outside the usual practice framework
- Reinventing practice in action

When you compare features of the models and the universal skills associated with cultural competence, a central theme is being able to know patients through their eyes and learning their stories. Failing to understand a person's world view may result in your being very impersonal and detached from the individual, and unique, lively individuals become static objects of your assessment. You do not form the important relationship that is needed to provide patient-centered care. You may be tempted to categorize people according to simplistic differences if you approach understanding all patients in the same way (Kumagai and Lypson, 2009). By describing people only in terms of how they differ from the majority, you unintentionally reinforce the dominant culture and lose the details of each individual's character and behavior. As a nurse you are responsible for assessing patients' health issues within their world view. For example, are their issues simply the effects of their illness, or are they associated with underlying societal conditions (Grace and Willis, 2012) such as poverty, lack of transportation, or an unsafe neighborhood?

Patient-Centered Care

Two landmark reports from the Institute of Medicine (IOM)—*Crossing the Quality Chasm* (IOM, 2001) and *Unequal Treatment* (Smedley et al., 2003)—highlight the importance of patient-centered care and cultural competence. *Crossing the Quality Chasm* identifies patient-centered care as one of six "aims" for high quality health care, and *Unequal Treatment* stresses the importance of developing cultural competence among health care providers to eliminate racial/ethnic health care disparities (Box 9-3). The differences between cultural competence and patient-centered care are not always clear. However, Beach and colleagues (2006) succinctly summarize the differences and similarities between these two concepts:

> Both patient-centeredness and cultural competence aim to improve health care quality, but each emphasizes different aspects of quality. The primary goal of the patient-centeredness movement has been to provide individualized care and restore an emphasis on personal relationships. It aims to elevate quality for all patients. Alternatively, the primary aim of the cultural competence movement has been to increase health equity and reduce disparities by concentrating on people of color and other disadvantaged populations (p. vii).

BOX 9-3 Patient-Centered Care for LGBT Patients

- Create a welcoming environment that is inclusive of LGBT patients. A health care organization should have a prominently posted nondiscrimination policy or patient bill of rights that explicitly mentions sexual orientation and gender identity. Any displayed art and health materials should include images and topics relevant to LGBT patients.
- Health care organizations should create or designate unisex or single-stall restrooms because patients whose appearance may not conform to traditional gender expressions may feel less comfortable using traditional male- and female-designated restrooms.
- Ensure that visitation policies are fair and implemented in a nondiscriminatory manner. Any denial of access should have a clear medical explanation.
- Avoid assumptions about sexual orientation and gender identity, remembering that any patient can be LGBT, regardless of his or her age, appearance, and other axis of identification.
- Include LGBT-inclusive language on forms and assessments to facilitate disclosure, knowing that disclosure is a choice impacted by many factors. For example, provide options such as "partnered" under relationship status. For parents, use parent/guardian, instead of mother/father.
- Use neutral and inclusive language when talking with patients (e.g., partner or significant other), listening and reflecting patient's choice. Remember that some LGBT patients are also legally married.

Data from Gay and Lesbian Medical Association (GLMA): *Guidelines for care of lesbian, gay, bisexual, and transgender patients,* 2006, http://www.clark.wa.gov/public-health/hiv/documents/GLMA%20Welcoming.pdf. Accessed August 2015.

Campinha-Bacote (2011) views cultural competency as an expansion of patient-centered care. More specifically, cultural competence can be seen as a necessary set of skills for nurses to attain in order to render effective patient-centered care. It is important for nurses to see themselves as becoming culturally competent. Your ability to exercise cultural competence by applying the components of Campinha-Bacote's (2002) model of cultural competency will allow you to deliver patient centered care.

Cultural Awareness. Curiosity about other ways of being in the world is an important attitude for cultural competence; however, it is also important for you to understand the forces that influence your own world view. Everyone holds biases about human behavior. A bias is a predisposition to see people or things in a certain light, either positive or negative. Becoming more self-aware of your biases and attitudes about human behavior is the first step in providing patient-centered care. You should spend time reflecting on what you learned, formally and informally, throughout your life about health, illness (physical and mental), health care system, gender roles, sexual orientation, race, ability, age, family, and many other issues as a part of your commitment to becoming a culturally competent nurse. It is helpful to think about cultural competence as a lifelong process of learning about others and also about yourself.

Cultural Knowledge—World Views. Historical and social realities shape an individual's or group's **world view**, which determines how people perceive others, how they interact and relate to reality, and how they process information (Walker et al., 2010). World view refers to "the way people tend to look out upon the world or their universe to form a picture or value stance about life or the world around them" (Leininger, 2006). The cycle of socialization is the lifetime process of interacting with family, peers, communities, organizations, media, and institutions through which we develop our world view (Figure 9-1). As a nurse it is important that you advocate for patients by gaining knowledge about their world view. When you assess a patient's cultural background and needs, you take into account each patient's world view, then you plan and provide nursing care in partnership with each patient to ensure that it is safe, effective, and culturally sensitive (McFarland and Eipperle, 2008).

In any intercultural encounter there is an insider perspective (emic world view) and an outsider perspective (etic world view). For example, a Korean woman requests seaweed soup for her first meal after giving birth. This request puzzles her nurse. The nurse has an insider's view of professional postpartum care but is an outsider to the Korean culture. As such, the nurse is not aware of the significance of the meal to the patient. Conversely the Korean patient has an outsider's view of American professional postpartum care and assumes that seaweed soup is available in the hospital because, according to her cultural beliefs, the soup cleanses the blood and promotes healing and lactation (Edelstein, 2011).

It is easy for nurses to stereotype various cultural groups after reading general information about ethnic practices and beliefs (Kleinman, 2013). Avoid stereotypes or unwarranted generalizations about any particular group that prevents an accurate assessment of an individual's unique characteristics and world view. Instead approach each person individually and ask questions to gain a better understanding of his or her perspective and needs.

Health care has its own culture of hierarchies, power dynamics, values, beliefs, and practices. Research supports the idea that group membership such as membership in a professional group shapes one's world view (Sue, 2006). Most health care providers educated in Western traditions are immersed in the culture of science and biomedicine through their course work and professional experience. Consequently they often have a world view that differs from that of their patients (Kleinman, 2013). As a nurse it is best to see every patient encounter as being cross-cultural.

Even when a patient and health care provider are similar in age or have the same gender or ethnicity, two different perspectives are present each time they interact. When patients access the health care system, they want to: (1) see their health care provider, and (2) feel better. In return the health care providers expect patients to: (1) make and keep appointments; (2) give a medication history; (3) give informed consent; (4) follow (discharge) instructions; (5) read, understand, and use health education materials; (6) correctly complete insurance forms; (7) pay their bills; and (8) go home and manage their care by taking their medication the right way, eating the right foods, and stopping/starting/changing a variety of behaviors (AMA, 2007). This list shows how complex each patient interaction is even before the interaction begins. The complexity increases as you consider the interactive effect between a health care provider's and patient's multiple social group identities and unique life experiences.

Nurses, patients, and all other health care providers bring each of their world views into the care process. The Iceberg Analogy (Figure 9-2) is a tool that helps you to visualize the visible and invisible aspects of your world view and recognize that the same applies to your patients. Just as most of an iceberg lies beneath the surface of the water, most aspects of a person's world view lie outside of his or her awareness and are invisible to those around the person. For example, a young female patient who has willingly agreed to be admitted to the hospital for a serious medical condition requiring surgery may refuse the surgery for religious reasons. In the patient's view she came to the hospital for help to eliminate the pain and infection from her illness. At the same time she believes that she needs to seek God's will for a decision that entails removing a body part. The patient's health care provider assumes that the patient is in the hospital to receive care for a serious illness and is willing to accept any and all treatments to cure the illness. The patient's deeply held religious beliefs about removing a body part are not obvious by assessing for a religious preference. Thus you would need to conduct a comprehensive **cultural assessment** (Box 9-4) to understand the patient's world view, including how her religious values affected her willingness to receive care. These deeply held values reside underneath the iceberg. The observed behavior (in this case, coming to the hospital) is a visible sign of a person's world view, but the beliefs, attitudes, knowledge, and experiences that guide the behavior are not visible to others; they lie under the surface. Conflict arises when health care providers interpret the behaviors of patients through their own world view lens instead of trying to uncover the world view that guides this behavior.

Because of differences in age, gender, political preferences, class, religion, or other variables, cultural values frequently differ within a

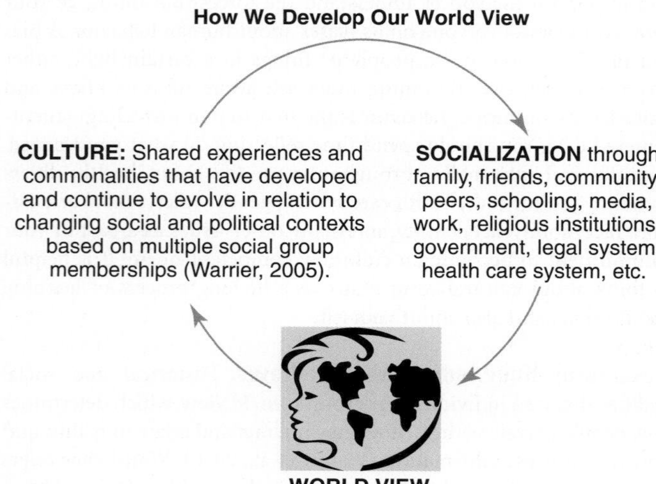

FIGURE 9-1 How we develop our world view. (Copyright © 2011 Barnes-Jewish Hospital Center for Diversity and Cultural Competence.)

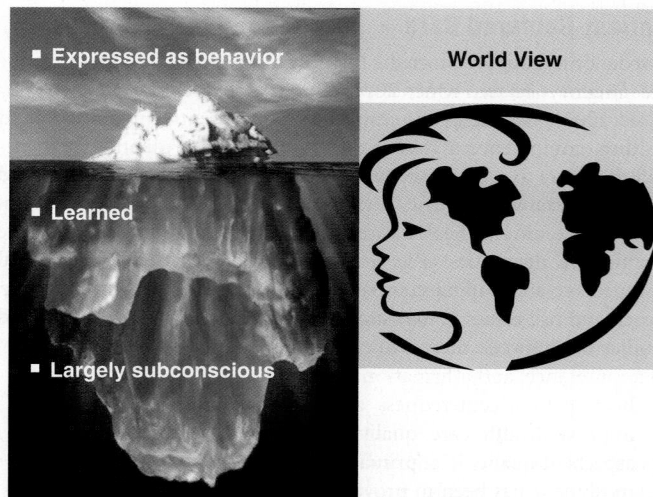

FIGURE 9-2 Both nurse and patient act in accordance with their own world views. This model has been adapted from Campinha-Bacote et al. (2005) Iceberg Analogy. It incorporates the Kleinman (1980) explanatory model. (Copyright © 2011 Barnes-Jewish Hospital Center for Diversity and Cultural Competence.)

BOX 9-4 Nursing Assessment Questions

Open-Ended
- What do you think caused your illness?
- How do you want us to help you with your problem?
- Tell me how your beliefs affect your views on medical treatment choices and your willingness to receive care.

Focused
- Did you have this problem before?
- Is there someone with whom you want us to talk about your care?

Contrast
- How different is this problem from the one you had previously?
- What is the difference between what we are doing and what you think we should be doing for you?

Ethnohistory
- What is your ethnic background or ancestry?
- For patients who are first- or second-generation immigrants:
  - How long have you/your parents resided in this country?
  - Tell me why you/your family left your homeland.
  - How different is your life here from back home?

Sexual Orientation and Gender Identity
- What is your legal name?
- How do you prefer to be addressed?
- What is your preferred pronoun? (he, she, they, or something else)
- What is your gender?
- Are your current sexual partners men, women, or both?
- In the past have your sexual partners been men, women, or both?
- What is your current relationship status?

Social Organization
- Who lives with you?
- Whom do you consider members of your family?
- Where do other members of your family live?
- Who makes the decisions for you or your family?
- To whom do you go outside of your family for support?
- What expectations do you have of your family members and support people? Are there different expectations for family members and support people of different ages and genders?

Socioeconomic Status
- What is your main source of income?
- If employed: What do you do for a living?

Bicultural Ecology and Health Risks
- What caused your problem?
- How does this problem affect or how has it affected your life and your family?
- How do you treat this problem at home?
- What other problems do you have?

Language and Communication
- What language(s) do you speak at home?
- What language(s) do you use to read and write?
- How should we address you or what should we call you?
- Which kinds of communication upset or offend you?

Caring Beliefs and Practices
- What do you do to keep yourself well?
- What do you do to show someone you care?
- How do you take care of sick family members?
- Which caregivers do you seek when you are sick?
- How different is what we do from what your family does for you when you are sick?

single social group such as a family or a group of nurses. For patients, family members, and members of the health care team alike, culture is a process through which ordinary activities such as greeting another person or selecting a doctor take on an emotional tone and moral meaning beyond that which appears on the surface (Kleinman, 2013). Think about the complexity of culture and world views. Realize the need to develop your assessment skills and cultural interventions that will allow you to successfully negotiate the various world views present in encounters with patients and families (and frequently other team members). Most important, remember that the core of this negotiation is compassionate care. Perhaps it may be helpful to think about these encounters as gift exchanges between individuals whose relationship to one another really matters (Kleinman, 2013). During these encounters participants not only exchange information but also acknowledgment, presence, and affirmation (Kleinman, 2013).

Skills and Interventions. You need to develop assessment skills and be able to provide culturally congruent interventions to become culturally competent. To provide patient-centered culturally competent care, you must know how to collect relevant cultural data about a patient's presenting health problem(s) and how to then use it (Campinha-Bacote, 2011). Critical to success is your ability to conduct a systematic cultural assessment, communicate effectively), and have the skills to successfully manage world view differences with others.

Cultural Assessment. The goal of a cultural assessment is to obtain accurate information from a patient that allows you to formulate a mutually acceptable and culturally relevant plan of care for each health problem of a patient (Campinha-Bacote, 2011). Nurses need skills to perform a systematic cultural assessment of individuals, groups, and communities as to their cultural beliefs, values, and practices. Numerous models and assessment tools exist to facilitate cultural assessment, including Leininger's Sunrise Model (2002), Giger and Davidhizar's Transcultural Assessment Model (2002), and the Purnell Model for Cultural Competence (Purnell, 2002). Regardless of which one you select, using a cultural assessment model will help you focus on the information that is most relevant to your patient's problems. It will also help you better understand the complex factors that influence your patient's cultural world view. You need to assess and interpret a patient's perspective during your assessment. Use open-ended, focused, and contrasted questions. Encourage your patients to describe the values, beliefs, and practices that are significant to their care. Culturally oriented questions are by nature broad and require learning more about the patient's personal narratives (see Box 9-4).

One effective approach to assessment is to ask questions that will help you understand a patient's **explanatory model**—his or her views about health and illness and its treatment. There are five questions in most explanatory models: etiology, time and mode of onset of symptoms, pathophysiology, course of illness (including severity and type of sick role), and treatment for an illness episode. Understanding a patient's perceptions of these concepts and the relationship among them helps you provide patient-centered care that combines a patient's values and beliefs with your perspectives. Using a cultural model during your assessment (such as the one in Figure 9-3 that integrates Kleinman's explanatory model with the previously discussed Iceberg Analogy) will help you develop open-ended questions that effectively reveal your patient's views on illness (Kleinman and Benson, 2006). Table 9-1 summarizes and contrasts a patient's explanatory model of illness with the biomedical explanatory model of illness (Lynch and Medin, 2006).

In contrast to standard approaches for health assessment, cultural assessment is intrusive and may take more time to conduct because it requires building a trusting relationship between participants. Miscommunication commonly occurs in intercultural transactions. This occurs because of differences in verbal communication between participants and differences in interpreting one another's behaviors.

TABLE 9-1 Explanatory Model Comparison

Patient's Explanatory Model	Biomedical Explanatory Model
What do you call your problem? What name does it have?	Etiology
What do you think has caused your problem? Why do you think it started when it did?	Time and mode of onset
What do you think your sickness does to you? How does this illness work inside your body?	Pathophysiology
What will happen to you? What do you fear most about your sickness? What are the chief problems your sickness has caused for you?	Course of illness (including symptom severity and trajectory: acute, chronic, impaired)
How should your sickness be treated?	Recommended treatment

Adapted from Lynch E, Medin D: Explanatory models of illness: study of within-culture variation, *Cogn Psychol* 53(4):285, 2006.

You can use transcultural communication skills to better understand a patient's behavior and to behave in a culturally congruent way. Effective communication is a critical skill in providing quality and safe care.

A number of authors have developed mnemonic cultural assessment and planning tools. Mnemonics, or memory aids, offer you a different option that makes it easier to perform assessments and communicate effectively with patients about their plan of care (Box 9-5). They help you remember the steps of each communication technique. For example, if you use the LEARN mnemonic, your first step is to ***l***isten to the patient's explanation or story of the presenting problem. Then you ***e***xplain your perception of the patient's problem, whether it is physiological, psychological, or cultural. Then you ***a***cknowledge the similarities and differences between the two perceptions. It is important to recognize differences but build on the similarities (Campinha-Bacote, 2011). The fourth step involves ***r***ecommendations that require you to involve the patient and family when appropriate. The last step is to then ***n***egotiate a mutually agreeable, culturally oriented, patient-centered plan. Remember, cultural assessment and care planning requires a level of negotiation. Leininger (2006) describes cultural care negotiation as assistive, accommodating, facilitative, or enabling creative provider care actions or decisions that help people with different backgrounds adapt to or negotiate with others for culturally congruent care.

Linguistic Competence. Linguistic competence is the ability of an organization and its staff to communicate effectively and convey information in a manner that is easily understood by diverse audiences. These audiences include people of limited English proficiency, those who have low literacy skills or are not literate, individuals with disabilities, and those who are deaf or hard of hearing. Linguistic competency requires organizational resources (e.g., instructional resources designed at a 6th-grade reading level or lower, interpreters) and providers who are able to respond effectively to the health and mental health literacy needs of the populations served. One important service that health care organizations must provide is an interpretive service.

Most health care providers and virtually all health care organizations nationwide are subject to federal civil rights laws. These laws outline requirements for the provision of language access services.

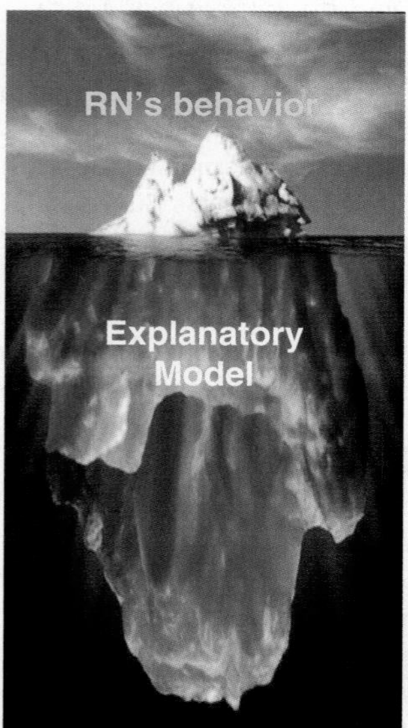

1. What do you call the problem? What name does it have?
2. What do you think has caused the problem?
3. Why do you think it started when it did?
4. What does your sickness do to you? How does it work?
5. How severe is it? Will it last a long or short time?
6. What do you fear most about this sickness?
7. What are the chief problems your sickness has caused for you?
8. What type of treatment do you think you should receive? What are the most important results you hope to receive from the treatment?

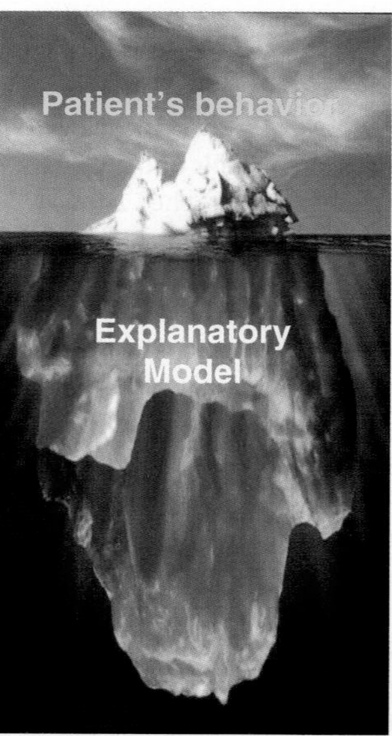

FIGURE 9-3 Cultural Model that integrates Kleinman's explanatory model with the Iceberg Analogy. (Copyright © 2011 Barnes-Jewish Hospital Center for Diversity and Cultural Competence.)

BOX 9-5 Communication Techniques Using Mnemonics

Communication Technique	Process
LEARN	
Berlin EA, Fowkes WC Jr: A teaching framework for cross-cultural health care, *West J Med* 139(6):934, 1982.	*L*isten with empathy and understanding to patient's perception of problem. *E*xplain your perceptions of the problem (physiological, psychological, spiritual, and/or cultural). *A*cknowledge and discuss cultural differences and similarities between you and your patient. *R*ecommend treatment (involving patient). *N*egotiate agreement (incorporate selected aspects of patient's culture into patient-centered plan).
RESPECT	
Bigby JA, editor: *Cross-cultural medicine,* Philadelphia, 2003, American College of Physicians, p. 20.	*R*apport • Connect on a social level. • Seek the patient's point of view. • Consciously attempt to suspend judgment. • Recognize and avoid making assumptions. *E*mpathy • Remember that the patient has come to you for help. • Seek out and understand the patient's rationale for his or her behaviors or illness. • Verbally acknowledge and legitimize the patient's feelings. *S*upport • Ask about and try to understand barriers to care and adherence. • Help the patient overcome barriers by providing resources. • Involve family members if appropriate. • Reassure the patient that you are and will be available to help. *P*artnership • Be flexible with regard to issues of control. • Negotiate roles when necessary. • Stress that you will be working together to address medical problems. *E*xplanations • Check often for understanding. • Use verbal clarification techniques. *C*ultural Competence • Respect the patient and his or her culture and beliefs. • Understand that the patient's view of you may be influenced by stereotypes. • Be aware of your own biases and preconceptions. • Know your limitations in addressing medical issues across cultures. • Understand your personal style and recognize when it may not be working with a given patient. *T*rust • Self-disclosure may be difficult for some patients. • Do not assume trust; instead take necessary time and consciously work to earn trust.
ETHNIC	
Levin S, Like, R, Gottlieb J: *ETHNIC: a framework for culturally competent clinical practice.* New Brunswick, NJ, 2000, Department of Family Medicine, UMDNJ-Robert Wood Johnson Medical School.	*Explanation*—Patient explains his or her perception of problem, or you ask what most concerns the patient. *Treatment*—Which types of treatments have the patient tried for the problem? *Healers*—Has the patient sought advice from alternative health practitioners? *Negotiate*—Try to find an option that is mutually acceptable. *Intervention*—Agree on an appropriate intervention, which may incorporate alternate treatments. *Collaboration*—Include patient, family members, and other health care professionals, healers, and community resources.
C-LARA	
C-LARA was developed by the organization Love Makes a Family; *C* (check your pulse) addition has been contributed by the organization Nonviolent Peaceforce.	*Calm* yourself down. Take a deep breath. Check your pulse. *Listen* to the patient's and family's perspective. *Affirm:* Express connection with something that was shared: a feeling, perspective, principle. *Respond:* To what was said. Answer the question. *Add:* Share additional information for the patient and family to consider. In this step you can educate.

They also help ensure meaningful access to health care for people with limited English proficiency (LEP) and offer effective communication services for those who are deaf or hard-of-hearing (TJC, 2013). As a nurse, it is critical for you to know that these laws require health care organizations to do the following:

- Provide language assistance services free of charge at all points of contact to all patients who speak limited English or are deaf
- Notify patients, both verbally and in writing, of their right to receive language-assistance services

- Take steps to provide auxiliary aids and services, including qualified interpreters, note takers, computer-aided transcription services, and written materials
- Ensure that interpreters are competent in medical terminology and understand issues of confidentiality and impartiality

Do not use a patient's family members to interpret for you or other health care providers. Cultural dynamics, lack of interpreting skills, low health literacy, and bias could lead to inaccurate interpretation. Box 9-6 provides guidelines for effectively working with an interpreter.

Health Literacy. The concept of linguistic competence encompasses both health literacy and limited English proficiency. Choosing a healthy lifestyle, knowing how to seek medical care, and taking advantage of preventive health care measures requires people to understand and use health information. Health literacy is the ability to obtain, process, and understand health information needed to make informed health decisions (Office of Disease Prevention and Health Promotion, n.d.). Studies show that health literacy has direct effects on health outcomes, linking poor health outcomes to limited health literacy (Berkman et al., 2011; Cho et al., 2008; DeWalt et al., 2004). More specifically, lower health literacy has been associated with higher risk of mortality for seniors, poorer ability to demonstrate taking medications appropriately, poorer ability to interpret labels and health messages, and poorer overall health status among seniors (Berkman et al., 2011). Approximately nine out of ten people in the United States experience challenges in using health care information (NCES, 2006). Patients who are especially vulnerable are the elderly (age 65+), immigrants, people with low incomes, people who do not have a high-school diploma or GED, and people with chronic mental and/or physical health conditions (AMA, 2007).

Commonly used measures of health literacy include literacy measures such as the Rapid Estimate of Adult Literacy in Medicine (REALM), which is a word recognition test; and the Test of Functional Health Literacy in Adults (TOFHLA), which measures reading skills and numeracy. No gold-standard instrument is currently available to assess adequately the more global concept of health literacy, including the interactions of reading ability, numeracy, and oral literacy (Berkman et al., 2011). However, researchers are beginning to develop instruments more specifically for health literacy (e.g., Newest Vital Sign, Diabetes Numeracy Test) that are framed in specific health contexts and assess condition-related skills (Berkman et al., 2011). Interestingly, in a study involving patients in the Veterans Administration (VA) system, the single question, "How confident are you filling out medical forms for yourself", showed a high correlation with being able to detect inadequate health literacy (Chew et al., 2008).

Teach Back. Evidence suggests that health care providers who attend to both health literacy and cultural differences help reduce medical errors and improve adherence, patient-provider-family communication, and outcomes of care at both individual and population levels (Lie et al., 2012). Clear communication is essential for effective delivery of quality and safe health care, but most patients experience significant challenges when communicating with their health care providers. The Teach Back method is an intervention that helps you to confirm that you have explained what a patient needs to know in a manner that the patient understands. The Teach Back technique is an ongoing process of asking patients for feedback through explanation or demonstration and presenting information in a new way until you feel confident that you communicated clearly and that your patient has a full understanding of the information presented (Figure 9-4) (see Chapter 25). You also use Teach Back to help you identify explanations and communication strategies that your patients most commonly understand (AHRQ, 2013b).

When using the Teach Back technique, do not ask a patient, "Do you understand?" or "Do you have any questions?" Instead ask open-ended questions to verify his or her understanding. You can ask the question in the following ways.

- "I've given you a lot of information to remember. Please explain it back to me so I can be sure that I gave you the information you need to take good care of yourself."

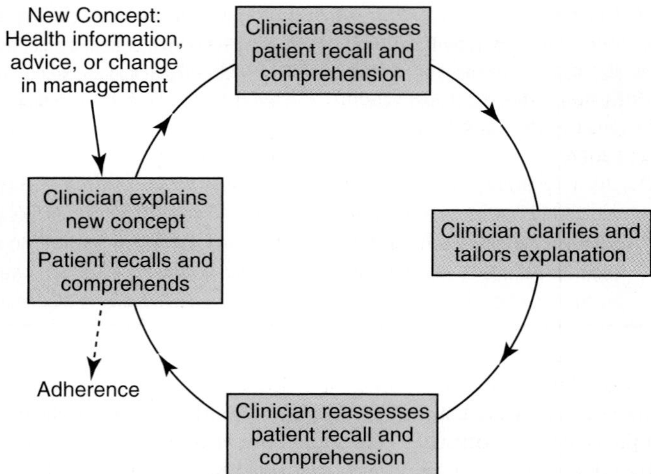

FIGURE 9-4 Using Teach Back technique to close the loop. (From the U.S. Health Resources and Services Administration.)

BOX 9-6 Working with Interpreters

If a patient needs an interpreter, do not ask the patient's family members and friends or other health care providers not trained as medical interpreters to help with communication. Instead request a medically trained interpreter. The interpreter could be available in person or via technology such as speakerphone or video. During each encounter:

- Introduce yourself to the interpreter and briefly describe the purpose of the meeting.
- Determine the interpreter's qualifications.
- Make sure that the interpreter can speak the patient's dialect or has an appropriate level of certification in case of American Sign Language (ASL).
- Consider the possible impact of differences in educational and socioeconomic status between the patient and the interpreter.
- Make sure that both the patient and interpreter are compatible and that both understand the expectations of the interpreter role.
- Introduce the interpreter to the patient.
- Do not expect the interpreter to interpret your statements word for word. Although the interpreter must ensure that everything that was said is interpreted, he or she may need to use more or fewer words to convey the meaning of your conversation with a patient.
- If you sense that the interpretation is not going well, stop and address the situation directly with the interpreter.
- Pace your speech by using short sentences but do not break your sentences. Allow time for the patient's response to be interpreted.
- Direct your questions to the patient. Look at the patient instead of at the interpreter.
- Ask the patient for feedback and clarification at regular intervals.
- Observe the patient's nonverbal and verbal behaviors.
- Thank both patient and interpreter.

- "What will you tell your wife (or husband/partner/child) about the changes we made to your medications today?"
- "We've gone over a lot of information today about how you might change your diet, and I want to make sure that I explained everything clearly. In your own words, please review what we talked about. How will you make it work at home?"

It is important to understand that Teach Back is not intended to test a patient but rather to confirm the clarity of your communication (AHRQ, 2013b). Many patients are embarrassed by their inability to sort out health information or instructions. By regarding Teach Back as a test of your communication skills, you take responsibility for the success or failure of the interaction and create a shame-free environment for your patients.

Helpful hints to consider when trying the Teach Back method follow.

- *Plan your approach.* Think about how you will ask your patient to teach back in a shame-free way. Keep in mind that some situations are not appropriate for Teach Back (AHRQ, 2013b).
- *Use handouts, pictures,* and *models* to reinforce your teaching (AHRQ, 2013b).
- *Clarify.* If a patient cannot remember or accurately repeat your instructions, clarify your information and allow him or her to teach it back again. Do this until the patient is able to teach back in his or her own words without parroting back what you said (AHRQ, 2013b). Understand Teach Back as a process of "closing the loop" (see Figure 9-4).
- *Practice.* Although it takes time to get used to Teach Back, studies show that it doesn't take longer to perform once it becomes a part of your routine (AHRQ, 2013b).

Cultural Encounters. A cultural encounter is an intervention that involves a nurse directly interacting with patients from culturally diverse backgrounds (Campinha-Bacote, 2011). The use of a caring, therapeutic, and culturally congruent relationship will lessen the likelihood of conflict when you engage in such encounters. A cultural encounter enables new forms of community and collective identity between you and your patients. Campinha-Bacote (2011) describes two goals of a cultural encounter: (1) to generate a wide variety of responses and to send and receive both verbal and nonverbal communication accurately and appropriately, and (2) to continuously interact with patients from culturally diverse backgrounds in order to validate, refine, or modify existing values, beliefs, and practices and to develop cultural desire, awareness, skill, and knowledge. The challenge is being able to show compassion, especially if cross-cultural conflict develops. However, conflict gives you an excellent opportunity for developing compassion and sharing one's suffering to achieve better health outcomes for your patients. A patient-centered and culturally competent encounter must be viewed as a "win-and-lose" situation for a patient and a "win-and-lose" situation for a nurse. Such an encounter effectively resolves cultural conflict by avoiding a "win-or-lose" situation for either the patient or nurse and instead results in a "win-lose/win-lose" situation in which the values of both the patient and nurse are respected (Campinha-Bacote, 2011).

Cultural Desire. It is easy to avoid cultural encounters with patients. Time, our personal discomfort in communicating with others who are "different," and a focus on physical care priorities are just some of the factors that may limit encounters with patients. Cultural desire is the motivation of a health care professional to "want to"—not "have to"—engage in the process of becoming culturally competent (Campinha-Bacote, 2011). It involves a natural inclination to engage in the cultural competence process that is characterized by passion, commitment, and caring. An ethically responsible professional nurse must embrace the importance of cultural competency and apply principles in daily patient encounters.

Within health care organizations today, more changes are occurring to integrate cultural competence principles into everyday organizational processes and practices. Health care regulatory agencies, national think tanks, and government agencies expect health care organizations to incorporate cultural competence into policies and practices to ensure effective communication, patient safety and quality, and patient-centered care. Examples of such organizational policies and practices include:

- Instituting a requirement for all staff to be trained in cultural competence.
- Embedding a broad description of family in written policies.
- Expanding visitation policies and practices to include a patient's preferences.
- Requiring nursing staff to conduct and document a cultural assessment on all patients within the clinical documentation system.
- Ensuring that people who are deaf or speak limited English have access to an interpreter.
- Embedding health literacy principles in written and verbal communication.
- Collecting race, ethnicity, and language information from patients on admission and stratifying outcomes data by these and other demographic indicators to identify disparities in care.
- Using stratified outcomes data to improve the health of populations.

CORE MEASURES

The Joint Commission (TJC) and the Centers for Medicare and Medicaid Services (CMS) are two of the many regulatory bodies that hold health care providers accountable for considering patients' unique cultural perspectives to provide safe and quality care. To improve health outcomes, TJC and the CMS developed a set of evidence-based, scientifically researched standards of care called *core measures* (TJC, 2013). The **core measures** are key quality indicators that help health care institutions improve performance, increase accountability, and reduce costs. All of the core measures such as screening for depression and controlling high blood pressure are consistent with national health priorities. They represent clinical conditions such as heart failure, acute myocardial infarction, pneumonia, and surgical-site infections. Following these standards of care on a nationwide scale is expected to reduce mortality, complications, and inpatient readmissions (Chassin et al., 2010; VanSuch et al., 2006).

In addition, core measures are intended to reduce health disparities. According to the 2013 National Health Care Disparities Report, Blacks and Hispanics received worse care than Whites for about 40% of quality measures; American Indians and Alaska Natives received worse care than Whites for about 30% of core measures; Asians received worse care than Whites for about 25% of core measures; poor people received worse care than high-income people for about 60% of core measures (AHRQ, 2013a).

Although most disparities in quality are significantly worse for some populations compared to White patients, there are some improvements in these outcomes as more and more effort is focused on addressing these disparities. Box 9-7 provides an example of a successful equity-focused QI effort and an evidence-based process for conducting equity-focused QI. The 2013 National Health Care Disparities Report identified that the number of disparities that are getting smaller

BOX 9-7 EVIDENCE-BASED PRACTICE

Equity-Focused Quality Improvement

PICO Question: What is the most effective quality improvement (QI) process that nurses can use to eliminate disparities in patient outcomes on their unit?

Evidence Summary

Health care disparities persist and indicate a clear inequity in care quality on the basis of race, ethnicity, sexual orientation, socioeconomic status, and other accesses of social identity. However, evidence for QI interventions that successfully decreased disparities is limited because of many challenges in developing, implementing, and studying QI with vulnerable populations or in under-resourced settings (Lion and Raphael, 2015). In addition, general QI interventions designed to improve overall quality (as opposed to targeting the specific needs of the population experiencing disparities) may not improve disparities and in some cases may increase them if there is greater uptake or effectiveness of the intervention among the population with better outcomes at baseline (Lion and Raphael, 2015). Designing equity-centered QI efforts is key to eliminating health care disparities.

In a recent study the investigators used an information technology (IT) surveillance for identifying and tracking patients overdue for colorectal cancer (CRC) screening to reduce socioeconomic disparities in their screening (Berkowitz et al., 2015). CRC is the third leading cause of cancer mortality for men and women and can be effectively prevented through different screening strategies (Berkowitz et al., 2015). The investigators implemented this effort in 18 primary care practice sites, including four community health centers within a practice-based research network in and around Boston. After the investigators discovered that CRC screening completion was lower for patients who had not finished high school than for patients who did, they contacted identified patients via letter or a telephone call. In addition, high-risk patients received patient navigation. The intervention resulted in a 3% increase in CRC screening overall and modestly reduced screening disparity among those with a lower level of educational attainment. Although the investigators achieved only a modest reduction in disparities, the intervention demonstrated overall screening improvement from a population health standpoint (Paluri, 2015). This study serves as an example that equity-centered QI efforts can address quality and equity.

Finding Answers, a national program office of the Robert Wood Johnson Foundation (RWJF), has been researching strategies and interventions to eliminate disparities in health outcomes. After conducting 12 systematic literature reviews and funding 33 innovative research projects, Finding Answers recommended a road map for organizations looking to implement equity-focused QI efforts and eliminate disparities in health outcomes (Clarke et al., n.d.).

Application to Nursing Practice

Emerging evidence-based strategies can help health care organizations working to reduce disparities in health outcomes. The road map offers a comprehensive approach to achieving equity. Use the following six steps described in *A Roadmap and Best Practices for Organizations to Reduce Racial and Ethnic Disparities in Health Care* (Chin et al., 2012) to implement equity-focused QI in your practice:

1. *Recognize disparities and commit to reducing them.* The Affordable Care Act makes the collection of a health care organization's performance data stratified by race, ethnicity, and language (REL) a priority. Cultural competency will improve your ability to assess for patient disparities.
2. *Implement a basic quality improvement structure and process.* An ongoing process is needed for a health care organization to build interventions. Nursing staff play a role in identifying opportunities to improve practice approaches for vulnerable patient groups.
3. *Make equity an integral component of quality improvement efforts.* It is necessary for health care organizations to think about the needs of vulnerable patients served as they design interventions to improve patient care.
4. *Design the intervention(s).* Interventions should be designed using evidence-based strategies; however, they must be tailored to fit the patient population and the context. They should target one or more of the appropriate levels of influence (i.e., the patient, provider, microsystem, organization, community, or policy).
5. *Implement, evaluate, and adjust the intervention(s).* Organizations should start by implementing a change on a small scale (pilot testing), learning from each test, and refining the intervention through performance improvement cycles (e.g., plan, do, study, and act) (PDSA) (see Chapter 5). This process will help organizations prepare for implementation on a larger scale
6. *Sustain the intervention(s).* Any change in practices must be continuously evaluated to ensure that recommended interventions are maintained.

exceeded the number that are getting larger for Blacks, Hispanics, Asians, and individuals with lower socioeconomic status (AHRQ, 2013a).

Nurses and other health care providers need to be familiar with how policies and institutional forces enable or inhibit their ability to provide culturally competent, patient-centered, high-quality, safe care to all patients. When policies impede the delivery of effective care, you and your colleagues must advocate for policy change.

QSEN QSEN: BUILDING COMPETENCY IN QUALITY IMPROVEMENT You are a nurse on a cardiology floor. Some of your patients have been readmitted to the hospital within 30 days of discharge with the same predischarge diagnosis. You don't know why some patients are readmitted at a rate that seems higher than other patients. How might you identify patients with the highest readmission rate? What are some steps you could take to determine the patient's ability to self-manage post-discharge?

Answers to QSEN Activities can be found on the Evolve website.

KEY POINTS

- Disparities in the access to quality of health care, preventive health, and health education contribute to poor population health.
- Health care systems and providers contribute to the problem of health disparities as a result of inadequate resources, poor patient-provider communication, lack of culturally competent care, fragmented delivery of care, and inadequate access to language services.
- Culturally competent health care providers and organizations can contribute to elimination of health disparities.
- Current evidence shows that addressing limited health literacy and cultural differences often reduces medical errors and improves adherence, patient-provider-family communication, and outcomes of care.
- Cultural desire involves a natural inclination to engage in the cultural competence process that is characterized by passion, commitment, and caring.
- A person's culture and life experiences shape his or her world view about health, illness, and health care.

- An effective approach to patient assessment is to use a patient's explanatory model instead of a traditional biomedical model to reveal your patient's views on illness
- Becoming culturally competent is an ongoing long-term process for a health care provider.

CLINICAL APPLICATION QUESTIONS

Preparing for Clinical Practice

Ms. Jackson is a 44-year-old overweight woman who was diagnosed with diabetes 2 years ago and is now insulin dependent. In 2012 the company she worked for downsized, and Ms. Jackson lost her job. As a result she was unable to pay her mortgage and became homeless. Since then she has been staying with various family members and friends because she has not been able to afford her own apartment. She has been working as an office temp from time to time but has not been able to find full-time work. She arrived at the emergency department (ED) with a blood sugar of 322 (normal range is 80 to 120) and a hemoglobin A1C of 11% (normal is approximately 5%).

Sam is a 23-year-old nursing student assigned to care for Ms. Jackson. After Sam reads Ms. Jackson's chart, she notices that she has come to the ED on several occasions over the past 6 months with the same issue. She also notices that health care providers who took care of Ms. Jackson during the previous visits documented that she verbalized an understanding of how to manage her diabetes but has been nonadherent with her treatment plan.

After Sam conducts a cultural assessment using an explanatory model with questions, she learns that Ms. Jackson fears that she will eventually die because her mother died of diabetes. She also learns that Ms. Jackson cannot get her medications filled because she doesn't have health insurance. After obtaining this information, Sam consults with a social worker, who tells Sam about a community health center within eight blocks of the place where Ms. Jackson is currently living. This health center has a diabetes management program and can offer ongoing support to Ms. Jackson. Sam spends time with Ms. Jackson explaining that people do not die from diabetes if they manage it effectively. Sam also discusses with Ms. Jackson some realistic ways to manage her diabetes given her challenging circumstances. In addition, she escorts Ms. Jackson to the social worker's office so they can discuss possible housing and unemployment resources. Sam realizes that there is an opportunity for her to learn more about the social determinants of health that affect Ms. Jackson's ability to manage her care. She also realizes that by gaining skills in cultural competence she will be more confident in providing culturally competent care to her patients.

1. List some of the social determinants of health that Sam most likely discovered while conducting a cultural assessment with Ms. Jackson.
2. On the basis of a cultural assessment, Sam discovers that Ms. Jackson believes that she may die. Select the C-LARA communication mnemonic listed in this chapter and plot a discussion that might help Ms. Jackson understand that diabetes is a manageable chronic illness that does not have to result in death.
3. Ms. Jackson is discharged and returns to the ED several months later because she is having difficulty managing her diabetes again. You are assigned to care for her. How will her weight, history of nonadherence, and past visits to the ED possibly affect your treatment? How could these factors trigger biases and assumptions that will get in the way of providing quality care? How could self-awareness help you reduce the effect of bias on the quality of care you provide?

Answers to Clinical Application Questions can be found on the Evolve website.

REVIEW QUESTIONS

Are You Ready to Test Your Nursing Knowledge?

1. A nurse enters the examination room of the emergency clinic and meets a 29-year-old patient who missed her last two follow-up appointments. The nurse notes from the medical record that the patient has high blood pressure that the doctor has been trying to help her manage. The patient just spoke with her doctor who left the room frustrated because the patient has not been taking her medication as prescribed. The patient confronts the nurse, saying, "I'm tired of being treated this way; no one cares. I need to find another doctor!" Using the C-LARA mnemonic, match the nurse's response to the correct letter of the mnemonic.
   1. C ____
   2. L ____
   3. A ____
   4. R ____
   5. A ____

   a. The nurse acknowledges that it is absolutely reasonable for patients to expect that their health care providers care about their situations and that it is disappointing when they have experiences that make them feel like they do not.
   b. The nurse uses a relaxation technique before responding to the patient's concerns. Calm yourself. Take a deep breath. Check your pulse.
   c. The nurse says, "I want to help you. I can do that better if you tell me what's making it difficult for you to come to your appointments and take your medicine each day."
   d. The nurse maintains eye contact and allows the patient to discuss her perspective while remaining attentively quiet.
   e. The nurse explains, "One thing I want you to understand is that your blood pressure medicine will only work if you take the same amount each day. Your follow-up appointments are important so we can get this blood pressure under control. Let me get a social worker who can help you figure out these transportation issues or see if he can find a doctor closer to your house."
2. Which of the following are considered social determinants of health? (Select all that apply.)
   1. Lack of primary health care providers in a zip code
   2. Poor-quality public school education that prevents a person from developing adequate reading skills
   3. Lack of affordable health insurance
   4. Employment opportunities that do not provide paid vacation or sick leave
   5. The number of times a person exercises during a week
   6. Neighborhood safety that prevents a person from walking around the block or socializing with neighbors outside of his or her home
3. Which of the following changes can help create a more inclusive environment for lesbian, gay, bisexual, and transgender (LGBT) patients? (Select all that apply.)
   1. Explicitly including sexual orientation and gender identity into nondiscrimination policies
   2. Displaying art that reflects LGBT community
   3. Modifying health care forms to provide opportunities for gender identity and sexual orientation disclosure
   4. Not asking patients about their gender identity and sexual orientation to avoid making them uncomfortable
   5. Ensuring access to unisex or single-stall bathrooms

4. Which of the following are examples of problems with the health care system that contribute to health disparities? (Select all that apply.)
   1. A health care provider assumes that the patient missed two appointments because the patient does not care about his or her health and does not inquire about the reasons for missed visits.
   2. The discharge nurse at a hospital uses Teach Back with a patient to ensure that she has communicated the discharge instructions clearly.
   3. A community hospital lacks an adequate staff of social workers who are able to ensure patients' access to resources they need to take care of their health.
   4. A hospital discharges a patient without ensuring that the patient has a primary care provider and has made a follow-up appointment.
   5. A nurse uses a family member as an interpreter to explain the patient's medications.
   6. The hospital conducts quality improvement without stratifying data by race, ethnicity, language, socioeconomic status, sexual orientation, and other axes of social group identities.
5. Match each letter of the RESPECT mnemonic with a statement that describes the concept the letter represents.
   1. R. ____
   2. E. ____
   3. S. ____
   4. P. ____
   5. E. ____
   6. C. ____
   7. T. ____

   a. Ask about and try to understand barriers to care and adherence, and then offer resources to help the patient overcome them, involving family members if appropriate, and reassuring the patient that you are and will be available to help.
   b. Patients may have different reasons for not disclosing important information. Earn a patient's confidence through actions and attitude that demonstrate respect, compassion, and your interest in partnership.
   c. Work closely together with the patient by being flexible with regard to issues of control, negotiating roles when necessary, and stressing that you will be working together to mutually address medical problems.
   d. Provide explanations for the process and your action, checking often for understanding and using verbal clarification techniques such as Teach Back.
   e. Approach each encounter thinking about cultural competence and how you can demonstrate respect for the patient and his or her culture and beliefs.
   f. Approach the encounter with empathy, remembering that the patient has come to you for help. Seek out and understand the patient's rationale for his or her behaviors or illness, verbally acknowledging and legitimizing his or her feelings.
   g. Connect on a social level, seeking the patient's point of view; consciously attempt to suspend judgment; and avoid making assumptions.
6. A patient is admitted through the emergency department (ED) after a serious car accident. The nurse assesses the patient and quickly learns that he speaks little English. Spanish is his primary language. The nurse speaks some Spanish. Which interventions would be appropriate at this time? (Select all that apply.)
   1. The nurse requests a professional interpreter.
   2. Since this is an emergent situation, the nurse will interpret and identify the patient's priority needs.
   3. The nurse determines the interpreter's qualifications and makes sure that the interpreter can speak the patient's dialect.
   4. The nurse uses short sentences to explain the treatments provided in the ED.
   5. The nurse directs questions to the patient by looking at the patient instead of at the interpreter.
7. A new nurse is caring for a hospitalized obese patient who is homeless. This is the first time the patient has been admitted to the hospital, and the patient is scheduled for surgery. Which of the following is a universal skill that will help the nurse work effectively with this patient?
   1. The nurse shifts her focus to understanding the patient by asking her, "Describe for me the course of your illness."
   2. The nurse tells the patient, "Your choices of foods and unwillingness to exercise are adding to your health problems."
   3. The nurse asks the patient, "Tell me about the main problems you have had with your health from not having a home."
   4. The nurse explains, "Because you have obesity, it is important to know the effects it has on wound healing because of reduced tissue perfusion."
8. Which statement made by a new graduate nurse about the teach-back technique requires intervention and further instruction by the nurse's preceptor?
   1. "After teaching a patient how to use an inhaler, I need to use the Teach Back technique to test my patient's understanding."
   2. "The Teach Back technique is an ongoing process of asking patients for feedback."
   3. "Using Teach Back will help me identify explanations and communication strategies that my patients will most commonly understand."
   4. "Using pictures, drawings, and models can enhance the effectiveness of the Teach Back technique."
9. In the United States, there has never been a president of Asian or Hispanic culture. This is an example of:
   1. Social inequality
   2. Marginalization
   3. Under inclusion
   4. Social location
10. A nurse has worked in a home health agency for a number of years. She goes to visit a patient who has diabetes and who lives in a public housing facility. This is the first time the nurse has cared for the patient. The patient has four other family members who live with her in the one-bedroom apartment. Which of the following, based on Campinha-Bacote's (2002) model of cultural competency, is an example of cultural awareness?
    1. The nurse begins a discussion with the patient by asking, "Tell me about your family members who live with you?"
    2. The nurse asks, "What do you believe is needed to make you feel better?"
    3. The nurse silently reflects about how her biases regarding poverty can influence how she assesses the patient.
    4. The nurse uses a therapeutic and caring approach to how she interacts with the patient.
11. Match the following definitions with the key terms related to intersectionality.
    1. Under inclusion
    2. Social inequality
    3. Social location

    a. Groups have unequal access to resources, services, and positions.
    b. A group has been overlooked in research and the design of interventions.
    c. One's place in society is based on membership in a social group that determines access to resources.

12. A nurse is preparing to perform a cultural assessment of a patient. Which of the following questions is an example of a contrast question?
    1. Tell me about your ethnic background.
    2. Have you had this problem in the past?
    3. Where do other members of your family live?
    4. How different is this problem from the one you had previously?
13. How can a nurse work on developing cultural awareness? (Select all that apply.)
    1. Reflect on his or her past learning about health, illness, race, gender, and sexual orientation
    2. Develop greater self-knowledge about personal biases
    3. Recognize consciously the multiple factors that influence his or her own world view
    4. Engage in an in-depth self-examination of his or her own background
    5. Learn as many facts as possible about an ethnic group
14. During an encounter with an elderly patient, the nurse recognizes that a thorough cultural assessment is necessary because the patient has recently come to the United States from Russia and has never been hospitalized before. The nurse wants to discuss cultural similarities between herself and the patient. Which step of the LEARN mnemonic is this?
    1. Listen
    2. Explain
    3. Acknowledge
    4. Recommend treatment
    5. Negotiate agreement
15. When you care for a patient who does not speak English, it is necessary to call on a professional interpreter. Which of the following are proper principles for working with interpreters? (Select all that apply.)
    1. Expect the interpreter to interpret your statements word-for-word so there is no misunderstanding by the patient.
    2. If you feel an interpretation is not correct, stop and address the situation directly with the interpreter.
    3. Pace a conversation so there is time for the patient's response to be interpreted.
    4. Direct your questions to the interpreter.
    5. Ask the patient for feedback and clarification at regular intervals.

Answers: 1. 1b, 2d, 3a, 4c, 5e; **2.** 1, 2, 3, 4, 6; **3.** 1, 2, 3, 5; **4.** 1, 3, 4, 5, 6; **5.** 1g, 2f, 3a, 4c, 5d, 6e, 7b; **6.** 1, 3, 4, 5; **7.** 3; **8.** 1; **9.** 2; **10.** 3; **11.** 1b, 2a, 3c; **12.** 4; **13.** 1, 2, 3, 4; **14.** 3; **15.** 2, 3, 5.

ⓔ ***Rationales for Review Questions can be found on the Evolve website.***

REFERENCES

Adams M, et al: *Teaching for diversity and social justice*, ed 2, New York, 2007, Routledge.

Administration on Aging: *Profile of Older Americans: future growth,* 2014, http://www.aoa.acl.gov/Aging_Statistics/Profile/2014/4.aspx. Accessed July 13, 2015.

Agency for Healthcare Research and Quality (AHRQ): *2013 National Healthcare Disparities Report,* 2013a, http://www.ahrq.gov/research/findings/nhqrdr/nhdr12/index.html. Accessed May, 2014.

Agency for Healthcare Research and Quality (AHRQ): *Health literacy universal precautions toolkit,* 2013b, http://www.ahrq.gov/professionals/quality-patient-safety/quality-resources/tools/literacy-toolkit/index.html. Accessed April 5, 2015.

American Medical Association (AMA): *Health literacy and patient safety: help patients understand*, Chicago, 2007, American Medical Association Foundation.

Beach MC, et al: The role and relationship of cultural competence and patient-centeredness in health care quality, Commonwealth Fund Publication No. 960, *Medicine* 82(2):193, 2006.

Berlin EA, Fowkes WC Jr: A teaching framework for cross-cultural health care, *West J Med* 139(6):934, 1982.

Campinha-Bacote J: The process of cultural competence in the delivery of healthcare services: a model of care, *J Transcult Nurs* 13(3):181, 2002.

Campinha-Bacote J: *The process of cultural competence in the delivery of healthcare services: the journey continues*, ed 5, Cincinnati, OH, 2007, Transcultural C.A.R.E. Associates.

Campinha-Bacote J: Delivering patient-centered care in the midst of a cultural conflict: the role of cultural competence, *Online J Issues Nurs* 16(2):5, 2011.

Centers for Disease Control and Prevention (CDC): Health disparities and inequalities report—United States, 2013, *MMWR Suppl* 62(3):1, 2013.

Chassin MR, et al: Accountability measures—using measurement to promote quality improvement, *N Engl J Med* 363(7):6838, 2010.

Chin MH, et al: A Roadmap and Best Practices for Organizations to Reduce Racial and Ethnic Disparities in Health Care, *J Gen Int Med* 27(8):992–1000, 2012.

Cho S, et al: Toward a field of intersectionality studies: theory, applications, and praxis, *Signs (Chic)* 38(4):785, 2013.

Edelstein S: *Food, cuisine and cultural competency for culinary, hospitality and healthcare professionals*, Sudbury, MA, 2011, Jones & Bartlett.

Giger JN, Davidhizar RD: The Giger and Davidhizar transcultural assessment model, *J Transcult Nurs* 13(3):185, 2002.

Grace P, Willis D: Nursing responsibilities and social justice: an analysis in support of disciplinary goals, *Nurs Outlook* 60(4):198, 2012.

Hollenbach AD, et al: *Implementing curricular and institutional climate changes to improve health care for individuals who are LGBT, gender nonconforming, or born with DSD: a resource for medical educators*, Washington, 2014, Association of American Medical Colleges.

Institute of Medicine (IOM): *Crossing the quality chasm: a new health system for the 21st century*, Washington DC, 2001, National Academy of Sciences, National Academies Press.

Institute of Medicine (IOM): *Future directions for the National Healthcare Quality and Disparities Reports*, Washington DC, 2010, National Academy of Sciences, National Academies Press.

James C, et al: *Putting women's health care disparities on the map: examining racial and ethnic disparities at the state level*, Menlo Park, CA, 2009, Kaiser Family Foundation. http://kff.org/disparities-policy/report/putting-womens-health-care-disparities-on-the/. Accessed July 13, 2015.

Kaiser Family Foundation (KFF): *Eliminating racial/ethnic disparities in health care: what are the options?* 2008, http://kff.org/disparities-policy/issue-brief/eliminating-racialethnic-disparities-in-health-care-what/. Accessed April 5, 2015.

Kaiser Family Foundation: *Disparities in health and health care: five key questions and answers,* November 2012, http://kff.org/disparities-policy/issue-brief/disparities-in-health-and-health-care-five-key-questions-and-answers/. Accessed July 8, 2015.

Kleinman A: *Patients and healers in the context of culture*, Berkeley, 1980, University of California Press.

Kleinman A: From illness as culture to caregiving as moral experience, *N Engl J Med* 368(15):1376, 2013.

Kleinman A, Benson P: Anthropology in the clinic: the problem of cultural competency and how to fix it, *PLoS Med* 3(10):e294, 2006.

Kumagai A, Lypson M: Beyond cultural competence: critical consciousness, social justice, and multicultural education, *Acad Med* 84(6):782, 2009.

Leadership for Healthy Communities: *Overweight and obesity among Latino Youths*, Princeton, NJ, 2014, The Robert Wood Johnson Foundation. http://www.rwjf.org/en/library/research/2014/05/overweight-and-obesity-among-latino-youths.html. Accessed July 18, 2015.

Leininger MM: Culture care theory: a major contribution to advance transcultural nursing knowledge and practices, *J Transcult Nurs* 13(3):189, 2002.

Leininger MM: Cultural care diversity and universality theory and evolution of the ethnonursing method. In Leininger MM, McFarland MR, editors: *Culture care diversity and universality: worldwide nursing theory*, ed 2, Sudbury, MA, 2006, Jones & Bartlett Learning, p 1.

Leininger MM, McFarland MR: *Transcultural nursing: concepts, theories, research and practice*, ed 3, New York, 2002, McGraw-Hill.

Lie D, et al: What do health literacy and cultural competence have in common? Calling for a collaborative health professional pedagogy, *J Health Commun* 17:13, 2012.

Lion KC, Raphael JL: Partnering health disparities research with quality improvement science in pediatrics, *Pediatrics* 135(2):354, 2015.

Lynch E, Medin D: Explanatory models of illness: a study of within-culture variation, *Cogn Psychol* 53(4):285, 2006. [Epub April 18, 2006].

McFarland MR, Eipperle MK: Culture care theory: a proposed practice theory guide for nurse practitioners in primary care settings, *Contemp Nurse* 28(1–2):48, 2008.

McGovern L, et al: *The relative contribution of multiple determinants to health outcomes*, 2014, Robert Wood Johnson Foundation, Health Policy Brief. http://www.rwjf.org/content/dam/farm/articles/articles/2014/rwjf415185. Accessed April 5, 2015.

Mutha S, et al: *Bringing equity into quality improvement: an overview and opportunities ahead*, San Francisco, 2012, Center for the Health Professions at the University of California. http://futurehealth.ucsf.edu/Public/Publications-and-Resources/Content.aspx?topic=Bringing_Equity_Into_QI_1. Accessed July 13, 2015.

National Center for Cultural Competence (NCCC): *The cultural competence and linguistic competence policy assessment (CLCPA)*, Washington, DC, n.d., Georgetown University Center for Child and Human Development. http://www.clcpa.info/. Accessed April 5, 2015.

National Center for Education Statistics (NCES): *The health literacy of America's adults: results from the 2003 National Assessment of Adult Literacy*, Washington, DC, 2006, US Department of Education. http://nces.ed.gov/pubsearch/pubsinfo.asp?pubid=2006483. Accessed April 5, 2015.

National Institutes of Health (NIH): *Cultural competency*, 2015. http://www.nih.gov/clearcommunication/culturalcompetency.htm. Accessed July 13, 2015.

National Quality Forum (NQF): *Healthcare disparities and cultural competence consensus standards: technical report*, 2012, http://www.qualityforum.org/Publications/2012/09/Healthcare_Disparities_and_Cultural_Competency_Consensus_Standards_Technical_Report.aspx. Accessed July 21, 2015.

Office of Disease Prevention and Health Promotion: *Quick Guide to Health Literacy: Fact Sheet- Health Literacy and Health Outcomes*, n.d. Available at http://www.health.gov/communication/literacy/quickguide/factsliteracy.htm. Accessed July 18, 2015.

Office of Minority Health (OMH), US Department of Health and Human Services (USDHHH): *Cancer and African Americans*, 2013a, http://minorityhealth.hhs.gov/omh/browse.aspx?lvl=4&lvlid=16. Accessed July 8, 2015.

Office of Minority Health (OMH), US Department of Health and Human Services (USDHHH): *Chronic liver disease and Asian Americans/Pacific Islanders*, 2013b, http://minorityhealth.hhs.gov/omh/browse.aspx?lvl=4&lvlid=47. Accessed July 8, 2015.

Office of Minority Health (OMH), US Department of Health and Human Services (USDHHH): *Think cultural health: CLAS and continuing education*, 2013c, https://www.thinkculturalhealth.hhs.gov/index.asp. Accessed July 8, 2015.

Office of Minority Health (OMH), US Department of Health and Human Services (USDHHH): *Infant Mortality Disparities Fact Sheet*, 2014, http://minorityhealth.hhs.gov/omh/content.aspx?ID=6907&lvl=3&lvlID=8. Accessed July 8, 2015.

Paluri R: Capsule commentary on Berkowitz et al, Building equity improvement into quality improvement: reducing socioeconomic disparities in colorectal cancer screening as part of population health management, *J Gen Intern Med* 30(7):1001, 2015.

Purnell L: The Purnell model for cultural competence, *J Transcult Nurs* 13(3):193, 2002.

Rabin RC: *Respecting Muslim patient's needs*, 2010, New York Times, http://www.nytimes.com/2010/11/01/health/01patients.html?_r=0. Accessed December 29, 2013.

Ranji U, et al: *Health and access to care and coverage for lesbian, gay, bisexual, and transgender individuals in the U.S.: The Henry J Kaiser Family Foundation Disparities Policy*, April 23, 2015, http://kff.org/disparities-policy/issue-brief/health-and-access-to-care-and-coverage-for-lesbian-gay-bisexual-and-transgender-individuals-in-the-u-s/ Accessed July 13, 2015.

Saha S, et al: Patient centeredness, cultural competence, and healthcare quality, *J Natl Med Assoc* 100(11):1275, 2008.

Smedley B, et al: *Unequal treatment: confronting racial and ethnic disparities in health care*, Washington, DC, 2003, National Academies Press.

Sue DW: *Multicultural social work practice*, Ken, NJ, 2006, John Wiley & Sons.

The Joint Commission (TJC): *Core measure sets*, Chicago, 2013, TJC. http://www.jointcommission.org/core_measure_sets.aspx. Accessed April 5, 2015.

United Health Foundation: *America's health rankings: United States overview*, 2014 edition results, 2014, http://cdnfiles.americashealthrankings.org/SiteFiles/Reports/Americas%20Health%20Rankings%202014%20Edition.pdf. Accessed April 5, 2015.

US Census Bureau: *The American community survey, 2008-2012*, 2013, http://www.census.gov/acs/www/. Accessed August 15, 2015.

US Department of Health and Human Services (USDHHS): *Healthy people 2020: health disparities*, 2015, http://www.healthypeople.gov/2020/about/foundation-health-measures/Disparities. Accessed July 18, 2015.

VanSuch M, et al: Effect of discharge instructions on readmission of hospitalized patients with heart failure: do all of the Joint Commission on Accreditation of Healthcare Organization's heart failure core measures reflect better care? *Qual Saf Health Care* 15(6):414, 2006.

World Health Organization (WHO): *Social determinants of health*, Commission on Social Determinants of Health, 2005-2008, 2013, http://www.who.int/social_determinants/thecommission/finalreport/key_concepts/en/index.html. Accessed April 5, 2015.

RESEARCH REFERENCES

Berkman ND, et al: *Health literacy interventions and outcomes: an updated systematic review*, Evidence Report/Technology Assessment No. 199. (Prepared by RTI International–University of North Carolina Evidence-based Practice Center under contract No. 290-2007-10056-I.) AHRQ Publication Number 11-E006, Rockville, MD, 2011, Agency for Healthcare Research and Quality.

Berkowitz SA, et al: Building equity improvement into quality improvement: reducing socioeconomic disparities in colorectal cancer screening as part of population health management, *J Gen Intern Med* 30(7):942, 2015.

Blanchet G, Pepin J: A constructivist theoretical proposition of cultural competence development in nursing, *Nurse Educ Today* 2015. pii: S0260-6917(15)00247-6. [Epub ahead of print].

Chew LD, et al: Validation of screening questions for limited health literacy in a large VA outpatient population, *J Gen Intern Med* 23(5):561–566, 2008.

Cho YI, et al: Effects of health literacy on health status and health service utilization amongst the elderly, *Soc Sci Med* 66(8):1809–1816, 2008.

Clarke AR, et al: *A roadmap to reduce racial and ethnic disparities in health care*, n.d., Robert Wood Johnson Foundation.

DeWalt DA, et al: Literacy and health outcomes: a systematic review of the literature, *J Gen Int Med* 19(12):1228–1239, 2004.

Walker RL, et al: Ethnic group differences in reasons for living and the moderating role of cultural worldview, *Cultur Divers Ethnic Minor Psychol* 16(3):372, 2010.

10

Caring for Families

OBJECTIVES

- Discuss current trends in the American family.
- Discuss how the term *family* reflects family diversity.
- Explain how the relationship between family structure and patterns of functioning affects the health of individuals within the family and the family as a whole.
- Discuss common family forms and their health implications.
- Discuss the role of families and family members as caregivers.
- Discuss factors that promote or impede family health.
- Compare family as context to family as patient and explain the way these perspectives influence nursing practice.
- Use the nursing process to provide for the health care needs of the family.

KEY TERMS

Family, p. 117
Family as context, p. 123
Family as patient, p. 123
Family as system, p. 123
Family caregiving, p. 127
Family forms, p. 118
Hardiness, p. 122
Resiliency, p. 122

MEDIA RESOURCES

http://evolve.elsevier.com/Potter/fundamentals/

- Review Questions
- Case Study with Questions
- Audio Glossary
- Content Updates

THE FAMILY

The family is a central institution in society; however, the concept, structure, and functioning of the family unit continue to change over time. Families face many challenges, including the effects of health and illness, childbearing and childrearing, changes in family structure and dynamics, and caring for older parents. Family characteristics or attributes such as durability, resiliency, and diversity help families adapt to these challenges.

Family durability is a system of support and structure within a family that extends beyond the walls of the household. For example, the parents may remarry, or the children may leave home as adults, but in the end the "family" transcends long periods and inevitable lifestyle changes.

Family resiliency is the ability of a family to cope with expected and unexpected stressors. The family's ability to adapt to role and structural changes, developmental milestones, and crises shows resilience. For example, a family is resilient when the wage earner loses a job and another member of the family takes on that role. The family survives and thrives as a result of the challenges they encounter from stressors.

Family diversity is the uniqueness of each family unit. For example, some families experience marriage for the first time and then have children in later life. Another family includes parents with young children and grandparents living in the home. Every person within a family unit has specific needs, strengths, and important developmental considerations.

As you care for patients and their families, you are responsible for understanding family dynamics, which include the family makeup (configuration), structure, function, problem-solving, and coping capacity. Use this knowledge to build on a patient's and family's strengths and resources (Duhamel, 2010). The rapidly changing health care delivery system promotes early discharge of patients back to the community. Living as a family in the midst of an illness is challenging; family functions, communications, and roles are altered (Arestedt et al., 2013). The goal of family-centered nursing care is to address the comprehensive health care needs of the family as a unit; and to advocate, promote, support, and provide for the well-being and health of the patient and individual family members (Martin et al., 2013; Brazil et al., 2012; Popejoy, 2011).

Concept of Family

The term family brings to mind a visual image of adults and children living together in a satisfying, harmonious manner (Figure 10-1). For some this term has the opposite image. Families represent more than a set of individuals, and a family is more than a sum of its individual members (Kaakinen et al., 2014). Families are as diverse as the individuals who compose them. Patients have deeply ingrained values about their families that deserve respect.

The specific relationships among patient, families, and health care providers are at the center of patient and family care. Unfortunately these relationships are often defined and shaped by the beliefs of health care providers (Bell, 2013), and not the needs of the patient and family caregiver. As a nurse, you need to assess for and understand how your patients define their families and how they perceive the general state of member relationships. Think of a **family** as a set of relationships that a patient identifies as family or as a network of individuals who influence one another's lives, whether or not there are actual biological or legal ties.

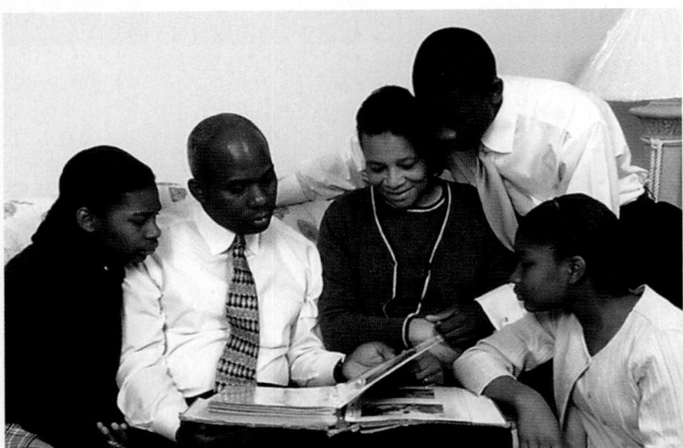

FIGURE 10-1 Family celebrations and traditions strengthen the role of the family.

BOX 10-1 Family Forms

Nuclear Family
The nuclear family consists of a married couple (and perhaps one or more children).

Extended Family
The extended family includes relatives (aunts, uncles, grandparents, and cousins) in addition to the nuclear family.

Single-Parent Family
The single-parent family is formed when one parent leaves the nuclear family because of death, divorce, or desertion or when a single person decides to have or adopt a child.

Blended Family
The blended family is formed when parents bring unrelated children from prior adoptive or foster parenting relationships into a new, joint living situation.

Alternative Family
Relationships include multi-adult households, "skip-generation" families (grandparents caring for grandchildren), communal groups with children, "nonfamilies" (adults living alone), and cohabitating partners.

Definition: What Is a Family?

Defining family initially appears to be a simple undertaking. However, different definitions result in heated debates among social scientists and legislators. The definition of family is significant and affects who is included on health insurance policies, who has access to children's school records, who files joint tax returns, and who is eligible for sick-leave benefits or public assistance programs. The family is defined biologically, legally, or as a social network with personally constructed ties and ideologies. For some patients, family includes only people related by marriage, birth, or adoption. To others, aunts, uncles, close friends, cohabitating people, and even pets are family. Understand that families take many forms and have diverse cultural and ethnic orientations. No two families are alike; each has its own strengths, weaknesses, resources, and challenges. You must care for both the family and the patient. Effective nursing administrators have a clear vision that caring for families is crucial to the mission of the health care facility and the health of the nation (Bell, 2014).

FAMILY FORMS AND CURRENT TRENDS

Family forms are patterns of people considered by family members to be included in a family (Box 10-1). Although all families have some things in common, each family form has unique problems and strengths. Remain open about who makes up a family so you do not overlook potential resources and concerns.

Although the institution of the family remains strong, the family itself is changing. In some situations people are marrying later, women are delaying childbirth, and couples are choosing to have fewer children or none at all. The number of people living alone is expanding rapidly and represents approximately 25% of all households (U.S. Bureau of the Census, 2011). Between 2006 and 2010, the Centers for Disease Control and Prevention reported the probability of a first marriage lasting at least 10 years as 68% for women and 70% for men and the probability of a first marriage surviving 20 years as 52% for women and 56% for men (Copen et al., 2012). A number of divorced adults remarry. Remarriage often results in a blended family with a complex set of relationships among all members

Marital roles are also more complex as families increasingly comprise two wage earners. The majority of women work outside the home, and about 60% of mothers are in the workforce (U.S. Bureau of the Census, 2011). Balancing employment and family life creates a variety of challenges in terms of child care and household work for both parents.

The number of single-parent families appears to be stabilizing. Forty-one percent of children are living with mothers who have never married; many of these children are a result of an adolescent pregnancy. Although mothers head most single-parent families, father-only families are on the rise (U.S. Bureau of the Census, 2011).

Adolescent pregnancy is an ever-increasing concern. The majority of adolescent mothers continue to live with their families. A teenage pregnancy has long-term consequences for the mother. For example, adolescent mothers frequently quit high school and have inadequate job skills and limited health care resources. The overwhelming task of being a parent while still being a teenager often severely stresses family relationships and resources. In addition, there is an increased risk for subsequent adolescent pregnancy, inability to obtain quality job skills, and poor lifestyles (Harper et al., 2010). Stressors are also placed on teenage fathers when their partner becomes pregnant. Teenage fathers usually have poorer support systems and fewer resources to teach them how to parent. In addition, adolescent fathers report early adverse family relationships such as exposure to domestic violence and parental separation or divorce and lack positive fathering role models (Biello et al., 2010). As a result, both adolescent parents often struggle with the normal tasks of development and identity but must accept a parenting role that they are not ready for physically, emotionally, socially, and/or financially.

Many homosexual couples define their relationship in family terms. Approximately half of all gay male couples live together compared to three fourths of lesbian couples. Same-sex couples are more open about their sexual preferences and more vocal about their legal rights. Some homosexual families include children, through adoption or artificial insemination or from prior relationships (Reczek and Umberson, 2012).

The fastest-growing age-group in America is 65 years of age and over. For the first time in history the average American has more living parents than children, and children are more likely to have living

BOX 10-2 FOCUS ON OLDER ADULTS

Family Caregiver Concerns

- Assess a family for the existence of caregivers who provide daily or respite care for older-adult family members. For example, determine the caregiving roles for members of the family (e.g., providing additional financial support, designating someone to obtain groceries and medications, providing hands-on physical care).
- Assess for caregiver burden such as tension in relationships between family caregivers and care recipients, changes in level of health of caregivers, changes in mood, and anxiety and depression (Tamayo et al., 2010).
- Assess caregivers' spiritual well-being. Many older adults use spirituality and religion to cope with life changes and maintain psychological well-being (Kim et al., 2011).
- Later-life families have a different social network than younger families because friends and same-generation family members often have died or been ill themselves. Look for social support within the community and through church affiliation (Tamayo et al., 2010).
- Take time to provide and reinforce individualized caregiver instruction. Teach caregivers the importance of presence, hope, and sharing with loved one and other family caregivers (Dobrina et al., 2014).

grandparents and even great-grandparents. This "graying" of America continues to affect the family life cycle, particularly the "sandwich generation"—composed of the children of older adults (see section on restorative care). These individuals, who are usually in the middle years, have to meet their own needs along with those of their children and their aging parents. This balance of needs often occurs at the expense of their own well-being and resources.

Family caregivers also require support from professional health professionals (Touhy and Jett, 2014). These caregivers frequently provide more than 20 hours of care per week, and this care is integrated into current family and work obligations (Touhy and Jett, 2014). Caring for a frail or chronically ill relative is an ongoing process in which families must continue to redefine their relationships and roles (Arestedt et al., 2013). It is not uncommon for spouses in their 60s and 70s to be the major caregivers for one another, and these caregivers have unique concerns (Box 10-2).

More grandparents are raising their grandchildren (U.S. Bureau of the Census, 2011). This new parenting responsibility is the result of a number of societal factors: military deployment, unemployment, adolescent pregnancy and substance abuse; and divorce rate resulting in single parenthood. Most grandparents resume a parenting role for their grandchildren as a consequence of legal intervention when parents are unfit or renounce their parental obligations (Touhy and Jett, 2014).

Families face many challenges, including changing structures and roles in the changing economic status of society. In addition, social scientists identify five further trends as threats or concerns facing families: (1) changing economic status (e.g., declining family income and lack of access to health care), (2) homelessness, (3) domestic violence, (4) the presence of acute or chronic illnesses or trauma, and (5) end-of-life care (Kim et al., 2011; Martin et al, 2013).

Changing Economic Status

For some families, making ends meet is a daily concern because of their declining economic status. Economics affects families at the lower end of the economic scale, and single-parent families are especially vulnerable. As a result, many families have inadequate health insurance coverage. Because of recent economic trends, adult children are often faced with moving back home after college because they cannot find employment or in some cases lose their jobs.

The number of American children living below the poverty level continues to rise. There are 16.4 million children living below the poverty level; and approximately 8 million children are uninsured (Children's Defense Fund [CDF], 2014). Although the Affordable Care Act (ACA) aims to improve access to affordable health insurance, the challenge to access appropriate health care continues (USDHHS, 2014). When caring for these families, be sensitive to their need for independence and help them obtain appropriate financial and health care resources. For example, help a family by providing information about resources within the community to obtain assistance with energy bills, dental and health care, and school supplies.

Homelessness

Homelessness is a major public health issue. According to public health organizations, absolute homelessness describes people without physical shelter who sleep outdoors, in vehicles, in abandoned buildings, or in other places not intended for human habitation. Relative homelessness describes those who have a physical shelter but one that does not meet the standards of health and safety (National Coalition for the Homeless, 2014).

The fastest growing section of the homeless population is families with children. This includes complete nuclear families and single-parent families. It is expected that 3.5 million people are homeless and 1.35 million are families with children. Poverty, mental and physical illness, and lack of affordable housing are primary causes of homelessness (National Coalition for the Homeless, 2014). Homelessness severely affects the functioning, health, and well-being of the family and its members (CDF, 2014). Children of homeless families are often in fair or poor health and have higher rates of asthma, ear infections, stomach problems, and mental illness (see Chapter 3). As a result, usually the only access to health care for these children is through an emergency department.

Children who are homeless face difficulties such as meeting residency requirements for public schools, inability to obtain previous enrollment records, and enrolling in and attending school. As a result, they are more likely to drop out of school and become unemployable (National Coalition for the Homeless, 2014). Homeless families and their children are at serious risk for developing long-term health, psychological, and socioeconomic problems. For example, children are frequently under immunized and at risk for childhood illnesses; they may fall behind in school and are at risk of dropping out; or they can develop risky behaviors (CDF, 2014).

Domestic Violence

Domestic violence includes not only intimate-partner relationships of spousal, live-in partners, and dating relationships, but also familial, elder, and child abuse. Abuse includes emotional, physical, and sexual abuse, which occurs across all social classes (Futures without Violence, 2014).

Factors associated with family violence are complex and include stress, poverty, social isolation, psychopathology, and learned family behavior. Other factors such as alcohol and drug abuse, pregnancy, sexual orientation, and mental illness increase the incidence of abuse within a family (Futures without Violence, 2014). Although abuse sometimes ends when one leaves a specific family environment, negative long-term physical and emotional consequences often linger. One of the consequences includes moving from one abusive situation to another. For example, an adolescent girl sees marriage as a way to leave her parents' abusive home and in turn marries a person who continues the abuse in her marriage.

IMPACT OF ILLNESS AND INJURY

Any acute or chronic illness influences an entire family economically, emotionally, socially, and functionally and affects a family's decision-making and coping resources. Hospitalization of a family member is stressful for the whole family. Hospital environments are foreign, physicians and nurses are strangers, the medical language is difficult to understand or interpret, and family members are separated from one another.

Acute/Chronic Illness

During an acute illness such as a trauma, myocardial infarction, or surgery, family members are often left in waiting rooms to receive information about their loved one. Communication among family members may be misdirected from fear and worry. Sometimes previous family conflicts rise to the surface, whereas others are suppressed. When implementing a patient-centered care model, patients' family members and surrogate decision makers must become active partners in decision making and care. Involving family during bedside handover from one care provider to another, for example, provides an opportunity to involve the patient and family in discussing the present and long-term plan of care (Tobiano et al., 2012). When possible, patients and family caregivers want to participate in shared decision making about treatment and ongoing disease/symptom management (Brazil et al., 2012). Incorporating a patient's and family's cultural beliefs, values, and communication patterns is essential to provide individualized patient/family-centered care (Campinha-Bacote, 2011).

Chronic illnesses are a global health problem and present continuous challenges for families. Frequently family patterns and interactions, social activities, work and household schedules, economic resources, and other family needs and functions must be reorganized around the chronic illness or disability. Despite the stressors, families want to accept and manage the illness and strive to gain a balance in family life (Arestedt et al., 2013). Astute nursing care involves the patient and family in preventing and/or managing medical crises, controlling symptoms, learning how to provide specific therapies, adjusting to changes over the course of the illness, avoiding isolation, obtaining community resources, and helping the family with conflict resolution (Arestedt et al., 2013; O'Shea et al., 2014).

Trauma

Trauma is sudden, unplanned, and sometimes life-threatening. Family members often struggle to cope with the challenges of a severe life-threatening event, which can include the stressors associated with a family member hospitalized in an intensive care environment, anxiety, depression, economic burden, and the impact of the trauma on family functioning and decision making (McDaniel and Allen, 2012). The powerlessness that family members experience makes them very vulnerable and less able to make important decisions about the health of the family. In caring for family members, advocate for the patient and family and answer their questions honestly (Grant and Ferrell, 2012). When you do not know the answer, find someone who does. Provide realistic assurance; giving false hope breaks the nurse-patient trust and also affects how the family can adjust to "bad news." When a patient who has experienced trauma is hospitalized, take time to make sure that the family is comfortable. You can bring them something to eat or drink, give them a blanket, or encourage them to get a meal. Sometimes telling a family that you will stay with their loved one while they are gone is all they need to feel comfortable in leaving.

End-of-Life Care

You will encounter many families with a terminally ill member. Although people equate terminal illness with cancer, many diseases have terminal aspects (e.g., heart failure, pulmonary and renal diseases, and neuromuscular diseases). Although some family members may be prepared for their loved one's death, their need for information, support, assurance, and presence is great (see Chapter 37). Use presence to refine a therapeutic relationship with a patient and family (see Chapter 7). Also use presence and therapeutic communication to enhance family members' relationships with one another and to promote shared decision making (Dobrina et al., 2014). The more you know about your patient's family, how they interact with one another, their strengths, and their weaknesses, the better. Each family approaches and copes with end-of-life decisions differently. Encourage the patient and family to make decisions about care (e.g., pain control or preferred nonpharmacologic comfort measures) and specific therapies. Help the family set up home care if they desire and obtain hospice and other appropriate resources, including grief support (Brazil et al., 2012). Provide information about the dying process and make sure family members know what to do at the time of death. If you are present at the time of death, be sensitive to the family's needs (e.g., provide for privacy and allow sufficient time for saying good-byes).

APPROACHES TO FAMILY NURSING: AN OVERVIEW

Understanding family developmental stages and attributes enables you to provide nursing care to a patient, the family as a whole, and individuals within the family structure. These theoretical perspectives and their concepts provide the foundation for family assessment and interventions.

Developmental Stages

Families, like individuals, change and grow over time. Although they are far from identical to one another, they tend to go through common stages. Each developmental stage has its own challenges, needs, and resources and includes tasks that need to be completed before the family is able to successfully move on to the next stage. Societal changes and an aging population have caused changes in the stages and transitions in the family life cycle. For example, adult children are not leaving the nest as predictably or as early as in the past, and many are returning home. In addition, more people are living into their 80s and 90s. Sixty-five is now considered the "backside of middle age," and the length of the midlife stage in the family life cycle has increased, as has the later stage in family life.

McGoldrick and Carter based their 1985 classic model of family life stages on expansion, contraction, and realignment of family relationships that support the entry, exit, and development of the members (Kaakinen et al., 2014). This model describes the emotional aspects of lifestyle transition and the changes and tasks necessary for the family to proceed developmentally (Table 10-1). Use this model to promote family behaviors to achieve essential tasks and help families prepare for later transitions (e.g., preparing for a new baby or adjusting to dealing with chronic illness) (see Chapter 13).

Attributes of Families

It is important to assess for and understand how family attributes affect the care of a family. Families have a structure and a way of functioning. Structure and function are closely related and continually interact with one another and impact family health.

TABLE 10-1 **Stages of the Family Life Cycle**

Family Life-Cycle Stage	Emotional Process of Transition: Key Principles	Changes in Family Status Required to Proceed Developmentally
Unattached young adult	Accepting parent-offspring separation	Differentiating self in relation to family of origin Developing intimate peer relationships Establishing self in work
Joining of families through marriage: newly married couple	Committing to new system	Forming marital system Realigning relationships with extended families and friends to include spouse
Family with young children	Accepting new generation of members into system	Adjusting marital system to make space for children Taking on parental roles Realigning relationships with extended family to include parenting and grandparenting roles
Family with adolescents	Increasing flexibility of family boundaries to include children's independence	Shifting parent-child relationships to permit adolescents to move into and out of system Refocusing on midlife material and career issues Beginning shift toward concerns for older generation
Family with young adults	Launching children and moving on Accepting multitude of exits from and entries into family system	Adjusting to reduction in family size Developing adult-to-adult relationships between grown children and their parents Realigning relationships to include in-laws and grandchildren Dealing with disabilities and death of parents (grandparents)
Family without children	Maintaining flexibility	Refocusing on career issues and new career opportunities Refocusing on partner and marriage issues Redefining recreational activities
Family in later life	Accepting shifting of generational roles	Maintaining own or couple functioning and interests in the face of physiological decline; exploring new familial and social role options Making room in system for wisdom and experience of older adults; supporting older generations without overfunctioning for them Dealing with retirement Dealing with loss of spouse, siblings, and other peers and preparation for own death; a life review, in which one reviews life experiences and decisions

From Duvall EM, Miller BC: Marriage and family development, ed 6, Boston, 2005, Allyn & Bacon. Printed and electronically reproduced by permission of Pearson Education, Upper Saddle River, NJ.

Structure. Structure is based on the ongoing membership of the family and the pattern of relationships, which are often numerous and complex. Each family has a unique structure and way of functioning. For example, a family member may have a relationship with a spouse, child, employer, and work colleagues. Each of these relationships has different demands, roles, and expectations. The multiple relationships and their expectations are often sources for personal and family stress (see Chapter 38).

Although the definitions of structure vary, you can assess family structure by asking the following questions: "Who is included in your family?" "Who performs which tasks (e.g., cooking, managing finances, caring for parent)?" and "Who makes which decisions?" Structure either enhances or detracts from a family's ability to respond to the expected and unexpected stressors of daily life. Structures that are too rigid or flexible sometimes threaten family functioning. Rigid structures specifically dictate who accomplishes different tasks and also limit the number of people outside the immediate family allowed to assume these tasks. For example, in a rigid family structure, the mother is the only acceptable person to provide emotional support for the children and/or to perform all of the household chores. The husband is the only acceptable person to provide financial support, maintain the vehicles, do the yard work, and/or make all of the home repairs. A change in the health status of the person responsible for a task places a burden on a rigid family because no other person is available, willing, or considered acceptable to assume that task. An extremely flexible structure also presents problems for the family. There is sometimes an absence of stability that would otherwise lead to automatic action during a crisis or rapid change.

Function. Family functioning is what a family does. Specific functional aspects include the way a family reproduces, interacts to socialize its young, cooperates to meet economic needs, and relates to the larger society. Family functioning also focuses on the processes used by the family to achieve its goals. Some processes include communication among family members, goal setting, conflict resolution, caregiving, nurturing, and use of internal and external resources. Traditional reproductive, sexual, economic, and educational goals that were once universal family goals no longer apply to all families. For example, a married couple who decides not to have children still consider themselves a family. Another example includes a blended family whose spouses bring school-age children into the new marriage. However, the spouses decide not to comingle their finances and have separate educational goals for their minor children. As a result, this family does not have the traditional economic patterns of a nuclear family.

Families achieve goals more successfully when communication is clear and direct. Clear communication enhances problem solving and conflict resolution, and it facilitates coping with life-changing or life-threatening stressors. Another process to facilitate goal achievement includes the ability to nurture and promote growth. For example, some families have a specific celebration for a good report card, a job well done, or specific milestones. They also nurture by helping children know right and wrong. In this situation a family might have a specific form of discipline such as "time out" or taking away privileges, and the children know why the discipline is given. Thus when a situation occurs, the child is disciplined and learns not to behave like that again.

Families need to have multiple resources available. For example, a social network is an excellent resource. Social relationships such as friends or churches within the community are important for family celebrations but also act as buffers, particularly during times of stress, and reduce a family's vulnerability.

Family and Health. When assessing a family, it is important to use a guide such as the family health system (FHS) approach to identify all of their needs. The FHS is a holistic model that guides the assessment and care for families (Anderson, 2000; Anderson and Friedemann, 2010). It includes five realms/processes of family life: interactive, developmental, coping, integrity, and health. The FHS approach is one method for family assessment to determine areas of concern and strengths, which helps you develop a plan of care with outcomes and specific family nursing interventions. As with all systems, the FHS has both unspoken and spoken goals, which vary according to the stage in the family life cycle, family values, and individual concerns of the family members. When working with families, the goal of care is to improve family health or well-being, assist in family management of illness conditions or transitions, and achieve health outcomes related to the family areas of concern.

Many factors influence the health of a family (e.g., its relative position in society, economic resources, and geographical boundaries). Although American families exist within the same culture, they live in very different ways as a result of race, values, social class, and ethnicity. In some minority groups multiple generations of single-parent families live together in one home. Class and ethnicity produce differences in the access of families to the resources and rewards of society. This access creates differences in family life, most significantly in different life chances for its members.

Distribution of wealth greatly affects the capacity to maintain health. Low educational preparation, poverty, and decreased social support compound one another, magnifying their effect on sickness in the family and the amount of sickness in the family. Economic stability increases a family's access to adequate health care, creates more opportunity for education, increases good nutrition, and decreases stress (CDF, 2014; National Coalition for the Homeless, 2014).

The family is the primary social context in which health promotion and disease prevention take place. A family's beliefs, values, and practices strongly influence health-promoting behaviors of its members. In turn the health status of each individual influences how a family unit functions and its ability to achieve goals. When a family satisfactorily functions to meet its goals, its members tend to feel positive about themselves and their family. Conversely, when they do not meet goals, families view themselves as ineffective (Epley et al., 2010).

Some families do not place a high value on good health. In fact, some families accept harmful practices. In some cases a family member gives mixed messages about health. For example, a parent chooses to smoke while telling children that smoking is bad for them. Family environment is crucial because health behavior reinforced in early life has a strong influence on later health practices. In addition, the family environment is a crucial factor in an individual's adjustment to a crisis. Although relationships are strained when confronted with illness, research indicates that, when family members receive support from health care professionals, they have the potential to adapt to the stressors and develop coping mechanisms (Arestedt et al., 2013).

Attributes of Healthy Families. The family is a dynamic unit; it is exposed to threats, strengths, changes, and challenges. Some families are crisis proof, whereas others are crisis prone. The crisis-proof, or effective, family is able to combine the need for stability with the need for growth and change. This type of family has a flexible structure that allows adaptable performance of tasks and acceptance of help from outside the family system. The structure is flexible enough to allow adaptability but not so flexible that the family lacks cohesiveness and a sense of stability. The effective family has control over the environment and influences the immediate environment of home, neighborhood, and school. The ineffective, or crisis-prone family lacks or believes it lacks control over its environments.

Hardiness and resiliency are factors that moderate a family's stress. Family hardiness is the internal strengths and durability of the family unit. A sense of control over the outcome of life, a view of change as beneficial and growth producing, and an active rather than passive orientation in adapting to stressful events characterize family hardiness (McCubbin et al., 1996). Resiliency helps to evaluate healthy responses when individuals and families experience stressful events. Resources and techniques that a family or individuals within the family use to maintain a balance or level of health aid in understanding a family's level of resiliency.

Genetic Factors. Genetic factors reflect a family's heredity or genetic susceptibility to diseases that may or may not result in actual development of a disease. The scope of genomics in nursing care is broad and encompasses risk assessment, risk management, counseling and treatment options, and treatment decisions (Calzone et al., 2012). Clinical applications of genetic and genomic knowledge for nurses have implications for care of people, families, communities, and populations across the life span (Calzone et al., 2013).

In certain families identification of genetic factors and genetic counseling help family members decide whether or not to test for the presence of a disease and/or to have children (Calzone et al., 2013; Kirk, 2013). Some families choose not to have children, whereas others choose not to know genetic risks and have children; other families choose to know the risk and then determine whether or not to have children. Some of these diseases (e.g., heart or kidney disease) are manageable. With genetic risks for certain cancers such as certain breast cancers, a woman may choose prophylactic bilateral mastectomies to reduce the risk for developing the disease. Families with genetic neurological diseases such as Huntington's disease may choose not to have children. When families know of these risks, they have the opportunity to make informed decisions about their lifestyle and health behaviors, are more vigilant about recognizing changes in their health, and in some cases seek medical intervention earlier (Kirk, 2013).

FAMILY NURSING

To provide compassion and caring for your patients and their families, you need a scientific knowledge base in family theory and knowledge in family nursing. A focus on the family is necessary to safely discharge patients back to the family or community settings. The members of the family may need to assume the role of primary caregiver. Family caregivers have unique nursing and caregiving needs. They often need to understand the disease process and outcomes and learn how to provide nursing skills, but too often they feel abandoned by the health care system (Plank et al., 2012). When a life-changing illness occurs, the family has to make major adjustments to care for a family member. Often the psychological, social, and health care needs of the caregiver go unmet (Tamayo et al., 2010).

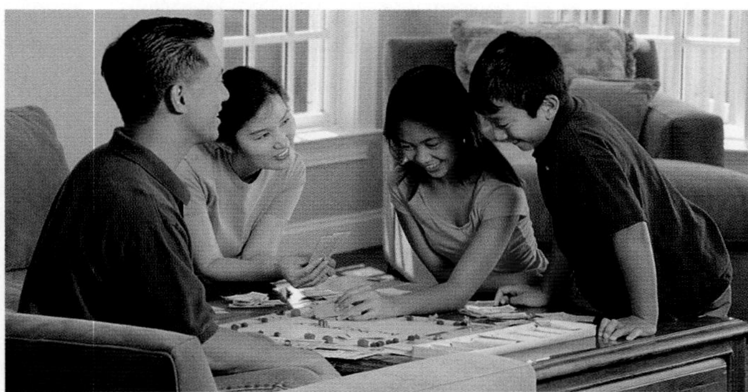

FIGURE 10-2 Family recreational activities strengthen family functioning. (Courtesy Bill Branson, National Cancer Institute.)

Family nursing is based on the assumption that all people, regardless of age, are members of some type of family form such as the traditional nuclear family or an alternate family (Figure 10-2). The goal of family nursing is to help a family and its individual members reach and maintain maximum health throughout and beyond the illness experience. Family nursing is the focus of the future across all practice settings and is important in all health care environments.

There are different approaches for family nursing practice. For the purposes of this chapter, family nursing practice has three levels of approaches: (1) **family as context**; (2) **family as patient**; and (3) the newest model, called **family as system**. Family as system includes both relational and transactional concepts. All approaches recognize that patient-centered care for one member influences all members and affects family functioning. Families are continually changing. As a result, the need for family support changes over time, and it is important for you to understand that the family is more complex than simply a combination of individual members.

Family As Context

When you view a family as context, the primary focus is on the health and development of an individual member existing within a specific environment (i.e., the patient's family). Although the focus is on an individual's health status, assess how much the family provides the individual's basic needs. These needs vary, depending on the individual's developmental level and situation. Because families provide more than just material essentials, you also need to consider their ability to help patients meet psychological needs.

Family As Patient

When you view a family as patient, the family processes and relationships (e.g., parenting or family caregiving) are the primary focuses of nursing care. Focus your nursing assessment on family patterns vs. characteristics of individual members. Concentrate on patterns and processes that are consistent with reaching and maintaining family and individual health. For example, in the case of family caregiving, assess who are the family caregivers for a patient, their different roles, and how they interact to meet the patient's needs. Plan care to meet not only the patient's needs but also the changing needs of the family. Dealing with very complex family problems often requires an interdisciplinary approach. Always be aware of the limits of nursing practice and make referrals when appropriate.

Family As System

It is important to understand that, although you are able to make theoretical and practical distinctions between the family as context and the family as patient, they are not necessarily mutually exclusive. When you care for a family as a system, you are caring for each family member (family as context) and the family unit (family as patient), using all available environmental, social, psychological, and community resources.

The following clinical scenario illustrates three levels of approaches to family care.

> You are assisting with end-of-life care for David Daniels, who is 35 years old and at one time was a computer analyst. David and his wife, Lisa, have three school-age children. David expressed a wish to die at home and not in a hospital or an extended care facility. Lisa is on family leave from her job to help David through this period. Both Lisa and David are only children. David's parents are no longer living, but Lisa's mother is committed to staying with the family to help Lisa and David.

When you view this family as context, you focus first on the patient (David) as an individual. You assess and meet David's needs at end-of life, such as comfort, hygiene, and nutrition, as well as his social and emotional needs. You determine how David is coping with knowing his life is coming to an end and how he perceives it will affect his family. When viewing the family as patient, you assess and meet the needs of David's wife and children. Determine to what extent the family's basic needs for normal activity, comfort, and nutrition are being met and whether they have resources for emotional and social support. You determine the family's need for rest (especially the wife) and their stage of coping (the older child shows much anger and fear). It is important to determine the demands placed on David and the family, such as economic survival and well-being of the children. In addition, you need to continually assess the family's available resources such as time, coping skills, and energy level to support David through the end of life.

When viewing a family as system, you use elements from both of the previous perspectives, but you also assess the resources available to the family. Using the knowledge of the family as context, patient, and system, individualize care decisions based on the family assessment and your clinical judgment. For example, on the basis of your assessment, you determine that the family is not eating adequately. You also determine that Lisa is experiencing more stress, not sleeping well, and trying to "do it all" regarding her children's school and after-school activities. In addition, Lisa does not want to leave David's bedside when members of their church come to help. You recognize that this family is under enormous stress and that their basic needs such as meals, rest, and school activities are not adequately met. As a result, you determine that (1) the family needs help with meals, (2) Lisa needs time to rest, and (3) the family's church is eager to help with David's day-to-day care. On the basis of these decisions, you work with Lisa, David, and the family to set up a schedule among Lisa, her mother, and two close church members to provide Lisa with some time away from David's bedside. However, David and Lisa determine when this time will be. Because of the church involvement, members of the church begin to take responsibility for groceries and all meal preparation for the family. In addition, other members of the church help with the children's school and after-school activities.

NURSING PROCESS FOR THE FAMILY

Nurses interact with families in a variety of community-based and clinical settings. The nursing process is the same whether the focus is context, patient, or system. It is also the same as that used with individuals and incorporates the needs of the family and the patient. You use the nursing process to care for an individual within a family (e.g., the family as context) or the entire family (e.g., the family as patient).

BOX 10-3 Five Realms of Family Life: Family Health System—Family Assessment Plan

Interactive Processes
- Family relationships—Is the family a nuclear or blended family? Is it a single-parent family?
- Family communication—How do family members share ideas, concerns, problems?
- Family nurturing—How are family values set and communicated? How are house rules established?
- Intimacy expression—Does the family hug, touch, laugh, or cry together?
- Social support—Who in the community, school, or workplace is close to the family?
- Conflict resolution—How does conflict resolution occur? Who initiates it? What is the common conflict?
- Roles (instrumental and expressive)—What are the formal roles such as wage earner, disciplinarian, problem solver? What are the informal roles (e.g., peacekeeper)?
- Family leisure life—Vacations: what does the family do to relax? Do the parents have "date night?"

Developmental Processes
- Current family transitions—Recent death, divorces, children leaving/returning home, new births
- Family stage task completion or progression—Childbearing years, empty nesters, grandparenting
- Individual developmental issues that affect family development—Individuals in the family with social issues such as difficulty in school or legal issues who cannot participate in family development
- Development of health issue and family impact—Acute or chronic illnesses, high-risk pregnancies, delayed physical development

Coping Processes
- Problem solving—How did the family solve previous problems? Is there a single problem solver or a family resolution?
- Use of resources—Does the family use family or individual therapists, Alcoholics Anonymous, conflict-resolution resources, anger-management resources?
- Family life stressors and daily hassles—What are the family's financial concerns? Are the children overscheduled with activities? Who is the caregiver for older adults?
- Family coping strategies and effectiveness—How do the family and individual members cope (e.g., exercise, avoidance, overeating, arguing)?
- Past experiences with handling crises—How have past crises been managed (e.g., dealing with financial stress, illness, and legal problems).
- Family resistance resources—Does the family take measures to avoid stress (e.g., adhering to a budget, obtaining tutoring resources for their children)?

Integrity Processes
- Family values—What do the family consider as their important values (e.g., health, togetherness)?
- Family beliefs—What are the family beliefs about health/illness, end-of-life care, and advance directives?
- Family meaning—Ask the patient or a significant family member to describe what the family means to him or her.
- Family rituals—How does the family celebrate holidays, birthdays, weddings; how does the family cope with death (e.g., wakes, funerals)?
- Family spirituality—Ask what spirituality means. How does the family define their spirituality?
- Family culture and practices—Identify cultural customs and practices that impact health care.

Health Processes
- Family health beliefs and beliefs about health concerns or problems—Does the family practice health and illness prevention or wait until a problem occurs?
- Health behaviors of the family—How does the ill family member react? How does the family react to illness? Do the family members react the same way to an ill family member, or do they react differently when a homemaker vs. the wage earner is ill?
- Health patterns and health management activities—How do the family members manage their health? How do they manage care of a sick family member?
- Family caretaking responsibilities—When someone is ill, who is the caregiver? Is it always the same person?
- Disease conditions, treatments, and consequences for the family—Obtain current disease and treatment history for the family.
- Family illness stressors—What are these stressors (e.g., worsening of a chronic illness or when "Mom" is sick and cannot run the household)?
- Relationship with health care providers and health system access—Which type of health care provider does the family have (e.g., primary care, pediatrician)? How often does the family see the providers? Any hospitalizations?

Modified from Anderson KH, Friedemann ML: Strategies to teach family assessment and intervention through an online international curriculum, J Fam Nurs 16(2):213, 2010; and Anderson KH: The family health system approach to family systems nursing, *J Fam Nurs* 6(2):103, 2000.

When initiating the care of families, use these approaches to organize a family approach to the nursing process:

1. Assess all individuals within their family context.
2. Assess the family as patient.
3. Assess the family as a system.

Assessing the Needs of a Family

Family assessment is a priority to provide adequate family care and support. You have an essential role in helping families adjust to acute, chronic, and terminal illness; but first you need to understand the family unit and what a patient's illness means to the family members and family functioning (Anderson and Friedemann, 2010). You also need to understand how the illness affects the family structure and the support the family requires (Kaakinen et al., 2014). Although the family as a whole differs from individual members, the measure of family health is more than a summary of the health of all members. The form, structure, function, and health of the family are areas unique to family assessment. Box 10-3 lists the five areas of family life to include in an assessment.

During an assessment, incorporate knowledge of the patient's illness and assess the patient and the family. When focusing on the family, begin the family assessment by determining the patient's definition of and attitude toward the family. The concept of family is highly individualized. The patient's definition will influence how much you are able to incorporate the family into nursing care. To determine family form and membership, ask who the patient considers family or with whom the patient shares strong emotional feelings. If the patient is unable to express a concept of family, ask with whom he or she lives, spends time, and shares confidences and then ask whether he or she considers them to be family or like family. To further assess the family structure, ask questions that determine the power structure and patterning of roles and tasks (e.g., "Who decides where to go on vacation?"

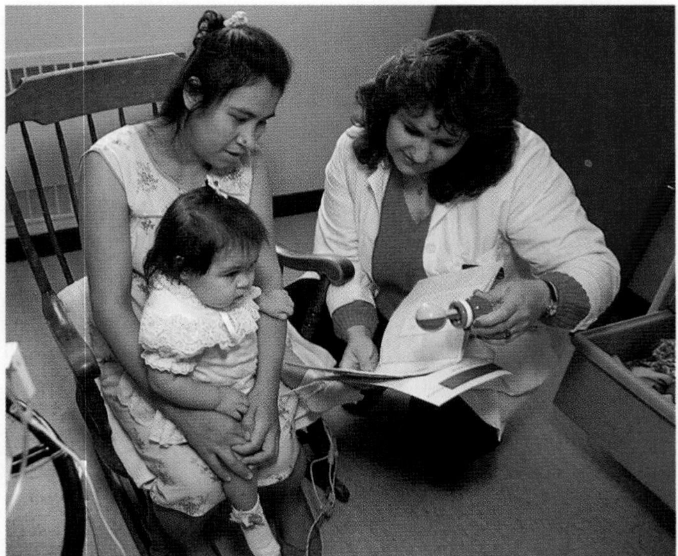

FIGURE 10-3 Nurse providing family education. (From Hockenberry MJ, Wilson D: *Wong's nursing care of infants and children,* ed 10, St Louis, 2015, Mosby.)

"How are tasks divided in your family?" "Who mows the lawn?" "Who usually prepares the meals?").

Assess family functions such as the ability to provide emotional support for members, the ability to cope with current health problems or situations, and the appropriateness of its goal setting and progress toward achievement of developmental tasks (Figure 10-3). Also determine whether the family is able to provide and distribute sufficient economic resources and whether its social network is extensive enough to provide support.

Cultural Aspects. Always recognize and respect a family's cultural background during your assessment (see Chapter 9). Culture is an important variable when assessing a family because race and ethnicity affect structure, function, health beliefs, values, and the way a family perceives events (Box 10-4). A comprehensive, culturally sensitive family assessment is critical to forming an understanding of family life, current changes in family life, overall goals and expectations, and planning family-centered care.

Forming conclusions about families' needs based on cultural backgrounds requires critical thinking. It is imperative to remember that categorical generalizations are often misleading. Overgeneralizations in terms of racial and ethnic group characteristics do not lead to greater understanding of a culturally diverse family. Culturally different families vary in meaningful and significant ways; however, neglecting to examine similarities leads to inaccurate assumptions and stereotyping (Giger, 2013).

Knowing about a family's culture and the meaning of that culture to a family's structure and functioning, health practices, and family celebrations helps to design family-centered care (see Chapter 9). To determine the influence of culture on a family, you ask the patient about his or her cultural background. Then ask questions concerning cultural practices. For example, "What type of foods do you eat?" "Who cares for sick family members?" "Have you or anyone in your family been hospitalized?" "Did family members remain at the hospital?" "Do you use any health practices of your culture such as acupuncture or meditation?" "What role do grandparents play in raising your children?"

BOX 10-4 CULTURAL ASPECTS OF CARE

Family Nursing

Families have unique perspectives and characteristics; and they have differences in values, beliefs, and philosophies. The cultural heritage of a family or member of the family affects religious, childrearing, and health care practices; recreational activities; and nutritional preferences. Be culturally sensitive and respectful when caring for multicultural patients. Incorporate individualized cultural preferences into your plan of care so it is culturally congruent. Design your care to integrate the personal values, life patterns, and beliefs of the patient and family into prescribed therapies.

Implications for Patient-Centered Care

- Focus on the needs of the family and understand the family's beliefs, values, customs, and roles when designing care (Brazil et al., 2012). Perception of certain events varies across cultural groups and has particular impact on families. For example, the care of the grandmother has a great significance to the extended family.
- Family caregiving values, practices, and roles vary across cultures (Plank et al., 2012).
- The family structure sometimes includes multiple generations living together. Intergenerational support and patterns of living arrangements are related to cultural background. For example, first-generation families are more likely to live in extended family households (Giger, 2013).
- In some cultures it is a sign of elder disrespect to place older adults in nursing homes, even when an older adult family member has severe dementia (Giger, 2013).
- Modesty is a strong value among many cultures. Some women bring female family members to health care visits, and a female health care provider must examine the woman.
- In the presence of a critical or terminal illness, some cultures come in groups to pray together with the family at the patient's bedside (Giger, 2013).
- Health beliefs differ among various cultures, which affect the decision of a family and its members about when and where to seek help.

A comprehensive, culturally sensitive family assessment is critical for you to understand family life, the current changes within it, and a family's overall goals and expectations (Campinha-Bacote, 2011). These data provide the foundation for family-centered nursing care (Anderson and Friedemann, 2010).

Discharge Planning. If a patient has been hospitalized or is in a rehabilitation setting, discharge planning begins with the initiation of care and includes the family. You are responsible for an accurate assessment of what will be needed for care in the home at the time of discharge, along with any shortcomings in the home setting. For example, if a postoperative patient is discharged to home and the older-adult husband does not feel comfortable with the dressing changes required, you need to find out if anyone else in the family or neighborhood is willing and able to do this. If not, you will need to arrange for a home care service referral. If the patient also needs exercise and strength training, you consult with the primary health care provider to recommend referral for physical therapy.

Family-Focused Care. Use a family-focused approach when assessing a patient and family to enhance your nursing care. When you establish a relationship with a patient and his or her family, it is important to identify potential and external resources. A complete assessment provides this information.

Collaboration with family members is essential, whether the family is the patient or the context of care. Collaborate closely with all appropriate family members when determining what they hope to achieve with regard to the family's health. You base a positive collaborative relationship on mutual respect and trust. The family needs to feel "in control" as much as possible.

Nursing Diagnosis

After assessing a patient's and family's needs and situation, you identify actual and at-risk nursing diagnoses. A number of diagnoses within the domain of role relationships are identified by the North American Nursing Diagnosis Association International (Herdman and Kamitsuru, 2014): caregiving roles and family relationships. Role relationships are defined by NANDA (Herdman and Kamitsuru, 2014, p. 277) as the "positive and negative connection or associations between people or groups of people and the means by which those connections are demonstrated." Examples of nursing diagnoses applicable to family care are:

- *Caregiver Role Strain*
- *Impaired Parenting*
- *Risk for Caregiver Role Strain*
- *Interrupted Family Processes*

Be sure to cluster appropriate risk factors or defining characteristics when making a nursing diagnosis. Diagnoses need to be relevant so that your plan of care is suitable to patient and family needs.

Planning Care

Once you identify pertinent nursing diagnoses, work together with patients and their families to develop plans of care that all members clearly understand and mutually agree to follow. The goals and outcomes you establish need to be concrete and realistic, compatible with a family's developmental stage, and acceptable to family members and their lifestyle.

By offering alternatives for care activities and asking family members for their own ideas and suggestions, you help to reduce their feelings of powerlessness. For example, offering options for how to prepare a low-fat diet or how to rearrange the furnishings of a room to accommodate a family member's disability gives a family an opportunity to express their preferences, make choices, and ultimately feel as though they have contributed. Collaborating with other disciplines increases the likelihood of a comprehensive approach to a family's health care needs, and it ensures better continuity of care. Using other disciplines is particularly important when discharge planning from a health care facility to home or an extended care facility is necessary (O'Shea et al., 2014; Tyrrell et al., 2012).

When you view a family as the patient, you need to support communication among all family members. This ensures that the family remains informed about the goals and interventions for health care. Often you participate in conflict resolution between family members so each member is able to confront and resolve problems in a healthy way. Help the family identify and use external and internal resources as necessary (Arestedt et al., 2013). For example, who in the family can run errands to get groceries while the patient is unable to drive? Are there members from the church who can come and provide respite care? Ultimately your aim is to help the family reach a point of optimal function, given the family's resources, capacities, and desire to become healthier.

Cultural sensitivity (see Chapter 9) in family nursing requires recognizing not only the diverse ethnic, cultural, and religious backgrounds of patients but also the differences and similarities within the same family. When planning family-centered care, recognize and integrate cultural practices, religious ceremonies, and rituals. Using effective and respectful communication techniques enables you to collaborate with the family to determine how best to integrate their beliefs and practices within the prescribed health care plan. For example, families holding traditions from Asian and Mexican American cultures frequently want to remain at the bedside around the clock and provide personal care for their loved ones. Integrating a family's values and needs into the care plan involves teaching family members how to provide simple, direct care measures, thus providing culturally sensitive and competent care. Together the nurse and the family blend the cultural and health care needs of the patient.

IMPLEMENTING FAMILY-CENTERED CARE

Whether caring for a patient with the family as context, directing care to the family as patient, or providing care to the family as system, nursing interventions aim to increase family members' abilities in certain areas, remove barriers to health care, and do things that the family is not able to do for itself. Assist the family in problem solving, provide practical services, and express a sense of acceptance and caring by listening carefully to family members' concerns and suggestions.

One of the roles you need to adopt is that of educator. Health education is a process by which a nurse and patient share information in a two-way fashion (see Chapter 25). Sometimes you recognize family/patient needs for information through direct questioning, but the methods for recognizing these needs are generally far more subtle (Plank et al., 2012). For example, you recognize that a new father is fearful of cleaning his newborn's umbilical cord or that an older-adult woman is not using her cane or walker safely. Respectful communication is necessary. Often you find the subtle needs for information by saying, "I notice you are trying to not touch the umbilical cord. I see that a lot." Or "You use the cane the way I did before I was shown a way to keep from falling or tripping over it; do you mind if I show you?" When you are confident and skillful instead of coming across as an authority on the subject, your patient's defenses are down, making him or her more willing to listen without feeling embarrassed. You will also recognize patient and family learning needs on the basis of a patient's health condition and physical and mental limitations. Your focus as an educator may be on the family caregiver, to prepare that person to manage the skills and processes needed to manage a patient's needs within the home.

Family Caregiving

Family support is a key driver in remaining in one's home and in the community, but it comes at substantial costs to the caregivers themselves, their families, and society. If family caregivers were no longer available, the economic cost to the U.S. health care and long-term service and support (LTSS) systems would increase astronomically (AARP, 2011). The economic value of family caregiving was estimated at $450 billion, which is more than total Medicaid spending ($361 billion) and approached the total expenditures in Medicare ($509 billion). These costs exceed the total sales of large companies (e.g., Wal-Mart [$408 billion]) (AARP, 2011).

There are approximately 42.1 million caregivers age 19 or older who are providing an average of 20 hours of care per week (AARP, 2011). Often they take on this responsibility without acknowledging the effect that it has on their lives and without realizing that relief is available (McDaniel and Allen, 2012).

The role of the family caregiver is multifaceted (Box 10-5). Family caregivers need preparation to meet these demands, including the physical care and psychological, social, and spiritual support (Grant and Ferrell, 2012). Family caregivers suffer emotionally. As a result, they may be at risk for a variety of physical conditions, ranging from

BOX 10-5 EVIDENCE-BASED PRACTICE

Caregiving Education for the Family Caregiver

PICO Question: Does a caregiving education program designed for family caregivers reduce caregiver stress and burnout?

Evidence Summary

When a family member has an illness or trauma that changes his or her physical or cognitive function, it is often a major life-changing event for the family and family caregiver. As a patient moves through hospitalization and rehabilitation and returns home, the family faces major changes in family dynamics, social interactions, financial commitments, and emotional support systems (Tyrrell et al., 2012; Tamayo et al., 2010). When the patient returns home, existing disabilities affect the primary caregiver and other members of the family. The family's and caregiver's social roles and activities, health-related activities and practices, and family dynamics all change (Bell, 2014). As a result, family members report stress and burnout related to the continual demands of the caregiving role (McDaniel and Allen, 2012). Caregiver preparation education programs help family caregivers identify methods to cope with the demands of caregiving and expand caregiving resources. Identifying interventions and resources helps the caregiver maintain a sense of hope, maintain his or her own health status, engage in more social activities, and have some respite from the day-to-day caregiving tasks (McDaniel and Allen, 2012).

Application to Nursing Practice

- Teach family caregivers how to identify potential stressors such as social isolation, physically demanding caregiving activities, behaviors of patient, and availability of resources (Sansoni et al., 2013).
- Identify the family's strengths (e.g., if some family members are good at helping their loved one exercise, involve them in physical rehabilitation activities) and use these strengths to reduce the potential for caregiver burnout (Sansoni et al., 2013; Tyrrell et al., 2012).
- Assess family caregiver's experience (e.g., has the caregiver observed any technical nursing care? Does the caregiver have a health care background? Has he or she provided care to another person?).
- Design an individualized caregiver education plan to reinforce experience and meet any knowledge gaps.
- Encourage family caregiver to set a routine family meeting to share joys and concerns with the family and identify caregiver needs for assistance (Bell, 2014).
- Encourage the caregiver to set a routine time for respite. The caregiver then knows when he or she can have some relaxation time or spouses can have a "date night."
- Teach family members how to be part of the support system. Show them how to participate in the care of a family member (Bell, 2014; Tamayo et al., 2010).

depression, cardiac illness, and eating disorders. In addition, the caregiver often puts his or her health needs on the back burner and misses routine primary care visits, routine screenings, and routine dental care (Dobrina et al., 2014; Kim et al., 2011).

Multiple national outreach programs such as the National Family Caregivers Association (www.thefamilycaregiver.org) and the National Alliance for Caregiving (www.caregiving.org) connect family caregivers to information and services that can help improve their lives and the level of care they can offer their loved ones.

Family caregiving is a family process that occurs in response to an illness and encompasses multiple cognitive, behavioral, and interpersonal processes. It typically involves the routine provision of services and personal care activities for a family member by spouses, siblings, friends, or parents. Caregiving activities include finding resources,

BOX 10-6 PATIENT TEACHING

Family Caregiving: Caregiver Role Strain

Objective

- Patient/family will adopt two interventions to reduce caregiver role strain.

Teaching Strategies

- Explain to all members of the family involved in caregiving that role strain may be present when the following occur:
  - There is a change in caregiver's appetite/weight, sleeping, or leisure activities. In addition, social withdrawal, irritability, anger, or changes in the caregiver's overall level of health can occur.
  - The caregiver is fearful when learning new therapies or administering new medications to the disabled/ill family member.
  - The caregiver loses interest in his or her personal appearance.
  - Signs of caregiver role strain may intensify if the loved one's health status changes or when institutional care is considered.
- Interventions for caregiver role strain
  - Help family members set up alternating schedules to give the primary caregiver some rest.
  - Design a schedule or other methods to provide groceries, meals, and housekeeping for the caregiver and patient.
  - Identify community resources for transportation, respite care, and support groups.
- Offer an opportunity to ask questions and, when possible, provide a phone number for questions and assistance.
- Provide family members with the contact information of the patient's health care provider and instruct them to call if the caregiver has health problems, the caregiver seems overly exhausted, or they observe changes in the caregiver's interactions and attention to normal activities.

Evaluation

- Ask the family to identify two or three indicators for caregiver role strain.
- Review with the family their plan to provide groceries, meals, and occasional respite care for the caregiver and patient.
- Ask the family where they keep the contact information of the patient's health care provider and when they would call the health care provider.

providing personal care (bathing, feeding, or grooming), monitoring for complications or side effects of an illness or treatment, providing instrumental activities of daily living (shopping or housekeeping), and the ongoing emotional support and decision making that is necessary. Family caregiving can create caregiver burden and strain. The physical and emotional demands are high, and the patient's disease itself creates changes in the family structure and roles (McDaniel and Allen, 2012). Family caregivers often feel ill prepared to take on the demands of care for their loved ones. Although the caregiver wants to care for the loved one, he or she often feels extreme pressure to do everything and do it correctly, including managing complex symptoms and medications and making accurate judgments about when to contact health professionals (Grant and Ferrell, 2012). Providing education to the family caregiver helps relieve some of the stress of caregiving (Box 10-6).

When an individual becomes dependent on another family member for care and assistance, significant stress affects both the caregiver and the care recipient. In addition, the caregiver needs to continue to meet the demands of his or her usual lifestyle (e.g., raising children, working full time, or dealing with personal problems or illness). In many instances adult children, the sandwich generation, are trying to take care of their parents while meeting the needs of their own family (see Box 10-6). Without adequate preparation and support from health care providers, caregiving puts the family at risk for serious problems, including a decline in the health of the caregiver and that of the care receiver and dysfunctional and even abusive relationships (McDaniel and Allen, 2012; Tamayo et al., 2010).

Providing care and support for family caregivers enhances patient safety and involves using available family and community resources. Establishing a caregiving schedule that enables all family members to participate, helping patients to identify extended family members who can share any financial burdens posed by caregiving, and having distant relatives send cards and letters communicating their support are very helpful. However, it is imperative to understand the relationship between potential caregivers and care recipients. If the relationship is not a supportive one, community services are often a better resource for the patient and family.

Use of community resources includes locating a service required by the family or providing respite care so the family caregiver has time away from the care recipient. Examples of services that are beneficial to families include caregiver support groups, housing and transportation services, food and nutrition services, housecleaning, legal and financial services, home care, hospice, and mental health resources. Before referring a family to a community resource, it is critical that the nurse understands the family's dynamics and knows whether the family wants support. Often a family caregiver resists help, feeling obligated to be the sole source of support to the care recipient. Be sensitive to family relationships and help caregivers understand the normalcy of caregiving demands. Given the appropriate resources, family caregivers are able to acquire the skills and knowledge necessary to effectively care for their loved ones within the context of the home while maintaining rich and rewarding personal relationships.

Despite its demands, family caregiving can be positive and rewarding. It is more than simply a series of tasks. Caregiving is an interactional process, whether it is a wife caring for a husband or a daughter caring for a mother. The interpersonal dynamics among family members influence the ultimate quality of caregiving. Thus you have a key role in helping them develop better communication and problem-solving skills to build the relationships needed for caregiving to be successful (Tamayo et al., 2010). Caregiving occurs in all aspects of care. As health care costs continue to increase, families are important caregivers. You can help them in their role as caregiver by showing them how to perform specific aspects of physical care (e.g., dressing changes) and helping them find home care equipment (e.g., oxygen therapy) and identify community resources. Preparing members of the family for care activities and responsibilities helps caregiving become a meaningful experience for both the caregiver and the patient.

Health Promotion

Although the family is the basic social context in which members learn health behaviors, the primary focus on health promotion has traditionally been on individuals. When implementing family nursing, health promotion interventions are designed to improve or maintain the physical, social, emotional, and spiritual well-being of the family unit and its members (Duhamel, 2010). Health promotion behaviors need to be tied to the developmental stage of a family (e.g., adequate prenatal care for the childbearing family or adherence to immunization schedules for the childrearing family). Your interventions need to enable individual members and the total family to reach their optimal levels of wellness.

One approach for meeting goals and promoting health is the use of family strengths. Families do often not look at their own system as one that has inherent, positive components. Family strengths include clear communication, adaptability, healthy childrearing practices, support and nurturing among family members, the use of crisis for growth, a commitment to one another and the family unit, a sense of well-being and cohesiveness, and spirituality (Kim et al., 2011). Help the family focus on their strengths instead of on problems and weaknesses. For example, point out that a couple's 30-year marriage has endured many crises and transitions. Therefore they are likely to be able to adapt to this latest challenge. Refer families to health promotion programs aimed at enhancing these attributes as needed. For example, some communities have low-cost fitness activities for school-age children that are designed to reduce the risk for obesity.

Acute Care

The family must be a central focus of nursing care, and it is crucial to emphasize family needs within the context of today's acute health care delivery system. For example, be aware of the implication of early discharge from a hospital for patients and their families. In many families all members of a household often are employed outside the home, and young adults who live at home are also involved with school and part-time jobs. In addition, some households may be multigenerational. These factors are both resources and challenges in preparing family members to help with health care or locate appropriate community resources. Do not assume because there are multiple people in the family that family caregiving is easier to attain. Often when family members assume the role of caregiver, they lose support from significant others and are at risk for caregiver role strain (Laitinen, et al., 2011). Always be sure that families are willing to assume care responsibilities once a patient returns home. Knowledge about a patient's and family's needs is essential to drive nursing interventions and maximize nursing outcomes.

QSEN QSEN: BUILDING COMPETENCY IN TEAMWORK AND COLLABORATION You are caring for the Carlson family. The father, Gary, is 47 years old with amyotrophic lateral sclerosis (Lou Gehrig's disease). He is a chemical engineer and recently took disability from his job. His disease has progressed to the point at which he needs a wheelchair because he tires easily. He is able to help with some of his physical care such as dressing but needs help with hygiene and toileting. His ability to swallow is diminished, and he needs help to eat to avoid the risk of aspiration. His wife, Kathy, is 48 years old and is an information technology specialist at a local company. They have two children. Karen is a college junior at a local university and lives in the residence hall. Kristen is a high school senior. The family is committed to helping Gary remain at home as long as possible. Kathy is working from home and will take a leave of absence if needed. Both girls have changed their schedules so one is home with their mother each evening. Using the family as patient, which assessment questions do you use to identify their strengths and their perceived challenges?

Answers to QSEN Activities can be found on the Evolve website.

In an acute care setting clear communication is essential. Help the family identify methods to maintain open lines of communication with you and the health care team to anticipate your patient's and family members' needs. For example, when a family member is ill, how will you use caring practices to help family members inform the nuclear and extended family about any progress or setbacks? Identify who makes decisions for the family and consistently go to the decision maker. In some situations the decision maker also needs assistance in developing a method to clearly communicate any decisions. In this electronic age, some families are using blogs on the Internet as a way of providing consistent information. Help the family determine if this is the best approach for their family needs and structure.

Likewise it is important that the health care team use communication techniques that are supportive and clear to understand and advocate for a family's expectations (Laitinen et al., 2011). In addition, clear communication from the health care team helps to untangle medical terminology and enables the family to understand the health care issues, types of decisions, and health care outcomes.

Restorative and Continuing Care

In restorative and continuing care settings, the challenge in family nursing is to try to maintain patients' functional abilities within the context of the family. This includes having home care nurses help patients remain in their homes following acute injuries or illnesses, surgery, or exacerbation of a chronic illness. It also requires finding ways to better the lives of chronically ill and disabled individuals and their families.

KEY POINTS

- Family structure and functions influence the lives of its individual members.
- Family members influence one another's health beliefs, practices, and status.
- The concept of family is highly individual; care focuses on a patient's attitude toward the family rather than on an inflexible definition of family.
- The family's structure, functioning, and relative position in society significantly influence its health and ability to respond to health problems.
- A nurse can view the family in three ways: as context, as patient, or as system.
- Measures of family health involve more than a summary of individual members' health.
- Family members as caregivers are often spouses who are either older adults themselves or adult children trying to work full-time and care for aging parents.
- Cultural sensitivity is vital to family nursing. Some members have differing beliefs, traditions, and restrictions, even within the same generation.
- Family caregiving is an interactive process that occurs within the context of the relationships among its members.

CLINICAL APPLICATION QUESTIONS

Preparing for Clinical Practice

A home health nurse is working with the Kline family. This is a family of four: Carol, a 45-year-old single mother; her two adolescent sons, Matt and Kent; and Sara, her 76-year-old mother, who is in the last stages of Alzheimer's disease. The mother has lived with Carol and her children for 10 years. Sara was a great support to Carol when her husband died 11 years ago. She helped Carol raise Matt and Kent. The family has decided to care for Sara in the home until she dies. Carol is the principal caregiver for Sara in the home.

1. Which type of assessments are important to determine family functioning and structure?
2. What should Carol assess to determine how the family can achieve their goal of caring for Sara?
3. How does Carol help the family determine their strengths, weaknesses, and resources?

ⓔ *Answers to Clinical Application Questions can be found on the Evolve website.*

REVIEW QUESTIONS

Are You Ready to Test Your Nursing Knowledge?

1. The Collins family includes a mother; stepfather, two teenage biological daughters of the mother; and a 25-year-old biological daughter of the father. The father's daughter just moved home following the loss of her job in another city. The family is converting a study into Stacey's bedroom and is in the process of distributing household chores. When you talk to members of the family, they all think that their family can adjust to lifestyle changes. This is an example of family:
   1. Diversity.
   2. Durability.
   3. Resiliency.
   4. Configuration.
2. What is the most common reason for calling on grandparents to raise their grandchildren?
   1. Single parenthood
   2. Legal interventions
   3. Dual-income families
   4. Increased divorce rate
3. Which of the following most greatly affects a family's access to adequate health care, opportunity for education, and sound nutrition?
   1. Development
   2. Family function
   3. Family structure
   4. Economic stability
4. You are caring for a family that consists of a father and 3-year-old boy who has well-managed asthma but misses care infrequently. They live in state-supported housing. The father is in school studying to be an information technology professional. His income and time are limited, and he admits to going to fast-food restaurants frequently for dinner. However, he and his son spend a lot of time together. The family receives state-supported health care for his son, but he does not have health insurance or a personal physician. He has his son enrolled in a government-assisted day care program. Which of the following are risks to this family's level of health? (Select all that apply.)
   1. Economic status
   2. Chronic illness
   3. Underinsured
   4. Government-assisted day care
   5. Frequency of fast-food dinners
   6. State-supported housing
5. Which of the following family assessments are most important for successful family caregiving? (Select all that apply.)
   1. Educational level of family members
   2. Cultural food preferences
   3. Collaboration between family members
   4. Social support
   5. Conflict resolution practices
6. Which of the following are possible outcomes with clear family communication? (Select all that apply.)
   1. Family goals
   2. Increased socialization
   3. Decision making
   4. Methods of discipline
   5. Improved education
   6. Impaired coping
7. A family has decided to care for a grandparent with terminal cancer in the daughter's home. Family caregiving is new to the

family. When helping this family as they begin to plan for their caregiving roles, what are the two top priority assessments to best learn about family functioning? (Select all that apply.)
   1. Communication
   2. Decision making
   3. Development
   4. Economic status
   5. Family structure
8. A family is facing job loss of the father, who is the major wage earner, and relocation to a new city where there is a new job. The children will have to switch schools, and his wife will have to resign from the job she likes. Which of the following contribute to this family's hardiness? (Select all that apply.)
   1. Family meetings
   2. Established family roles
   3. New neighborhood
   4. Willingness to change in time of stress
   5. Passive orientation to life
9. A family is undergoing a major change. Just as twins graduate from college and leave home to begin their careers, the husband loses his executive well-paying job. Because the family had two children in college at the same time, they did not save for retirement. They planned to save aggressively after the children left college. In this situation, which of the following demonstrate family resiliency? (Select all that apply.)
   1. Resuming full-time work when spouse loses job
   2. Increasing problems among siblings
   3. Developing hobbies when children leave home
   4. Placing blame on family members
   5. Expecting children to help financially
   6. Consulting a financial planner
10. In viewing the family as context, what is the primary focus?
    1. Family members within a system
    2. Family process and relationships
    3. Family relational and transactional concepts
    4. Health needs of an individual member
11. A hospice nurse is caring for a family that is providing end-of-life care for their grandmother, who has terminal breast cancer. When the nurse visits, the focus is on symptom management for the grandmother and helping the family with coping skills. This approach is an example of which of the following?
    1. Family as context
    2. Family as patient
    3. Family as system
    4. Family as structure
12. A new immigrant family consisting of a grandparent, two adults, and three school-age children has decided to receive their health promotion care at the Community Wellness Center. This is their first visit, and a family assessment, a health history, and a physical of each family member are needed. Which of the following are included in a family function assessment? (Select all that apply.)
    1. Cultural practices
    2. Decision making
    3. Neighborhood services
    4. Rituals and celebrations
    5. Neighborhood crime data
    6. Availability of parks
13. Two single mothers are active professionals and have teenage daughters. They also have busy social lives and date occasionally. Three years ago they decided to share a house and housing costs, living expenses, and child care responsibilities. The children consider one another as their family. What type of family form does this represent?
    1. Diverse family relationship
    2. Blended family relationships
    3. Extended family relationship
    4. Alternative family relationship
14. During a visit to a family clinic, a nurse teaches a mother about immunizations, car-seat use, and home safety for an infant and toddler. Which type of nursing interventions are these?
    1. Health promotion activities
    2. Acute care activities
    3. Restorative care activities
    4. Growth and development care activities
15. A family has decided to care for their father who is in the last stages of a debilitating neurological illness. Although he is alert, he cannot speak clearly or carry out self-care activities; he indicates that he wants to remain involved in family life as long as possible and loves spending time with his wife and two teenage children. Which best defines family caregiving? (Select all that apply.)
    1. Designing a nurturing family to raise children
    2. Providing physical and emotional care for a family member
    3. Establishing a safe physical environment for a family
    4. Monitoring for side effects of illness and treatments
    5. Reducing the use of community resources

Answers: 1. 3; **2.** 2; **3.** 4; **4.** 1, 3, 5; **5.** 3, 4, 5; **6.** 1, 3, 4; **7.** 1, 2; **8.** 1, 2, 4; **9.** 1, 3, 6; **10.** 4; **11.** 2; **12.** 1, 2, 4; **13.** 4; **14.** 1; **15.** 2, 3, 4.

ⓔ ***Rationales for Review Questions can be found on the Evolve website.***

REFERENCES

AARP Public Policy Institute: *Valuing the invaluable: 2011 Update: The growing contributions and costs of family caregiving*, 2011, http://assets.aarp.org/rgcenter/ppi/ltc/i51-caregiving.pdf. Accessed April 2015.

Anderson KH, Friedemann ML: Strategies to teach family assessment and intervention through an online international curriculum, *J Fam Nurs* 16(2):213, 2010.

Bell JM: Knowledge translation in family nursing: gazing into the promised land, *J Fam Nurs* 20(1):3, 2014.

Bell JM: Family nursing is more than family-centered care, *J Fam Nurs* 19(4):411, 2013.

Campinha-Bacote J: Delivering patient-centered care in the midst of a cultural conflict: the role of cultural competence, *Online J Issues Nurs* 16(2):5, 2011.

Children's Defense Fund (CDF): *The state of America's children 2014 report*, Washington DC, 2014, Children's Defense Fund. http://www.childrensdefense.org/library/state-of-americas-children/2014-soac.pdf. Accessed April 2015.

Copen CE, et al: First marriages in the United States: *Data from the 2006-2010 National Survey of Family Growth. National health statistics reports, No 49*, Hyattsville, MD, 2012, National Center for Health Statistics.

Duhamel F: Implementing family nursing: how do we translate knowledge into clinical practice? Part 2, *J Fam Nurs* 16(1):8, 2010.

Epley P, et al: Characteristics and trends in family-centered conceptualizations, *J Fam Social Work* 13:269, 2010.

Futures Without Violence: *National health resource center on domestic violence, futures without violence*, 2014, http://www.futureswithoutviolence.org/resources-events/get-the-facts. Accessed April 2015.

Giger J: *Transcultural nursing assessment and intervention*, ed 6, St Louis, 2013, Mosby.

Grant M, Ferrell B: Nursing role implications for family caregiving, *Semin Oncol Nurs* 28(4):279, 2012.

Herdman TH, Kamitsuru S, editors: *NANDA International nursing diagnoses: definitions & classification 2015-2017*, Oxford, 2014, Wiley Blackwell.

Kaakinen JR, et al: *Family health care nursing: theory, practice, and research*, ed 5, Philadelphia, 2014, FA Davis.

Kirk M: Introduction to genetics and genomics: a revised framework for nursing, *Nurs Stand* 28(8):37, 2013.

Laitinen H, et al: When time matters: the reality of patient care in acute care settings, *Int J Nurs Pract* 17:388, 2011.

Martin P, et al: Family health nursing: a response to the global health challenges, *J Fam Nurs* 19(1):99, 2013.

National Coalition for the Homeless: *Faces of homeless—the eCourse*, Washington, DC, 2014, The Coalition. http://homelessfaces.org/. Accessed April 2015.

Tobiano G, et al: Family member's perceptions of the nursing bedside handover, *J Clin Nurs* 22:192, 2012.

Touhy TA, Jett KF: *Ebersole and Hess: Gerontological nursing healthy aging*, ed 4, St Louis, 2014, Mosby.

US Bureau of the Census: *Population profile of the United States, 2009*, Washington, DC, 2011, The Bureau. http://www.census.gov/prod/2011pubs/acs-13.pdf. Accessed April 2015.

US Department of Health and Human Services (USDHHS): *Read the law*, 2014, http://www.hhs.gov/healthcare/rights/law/index.html. Accessed April 2015.

RESEARCH REFERENCES

Anderson KH: The family health system approach to family systems nursing, *J Fam Nurs* 6(2):103, 2000.

Arestedt L, et al: Living as a family in the midst of chronic illness, *Scand J Caring Sci* 28:29, 2013.

Biello KB, et al: Effect of teenage parenthood on mental health trajectories: does sex matter?, *Am J Epidemiol* 162(3):279, 2010.

Brazil K, et al: Family caregiver views on patient-centered care at the end of life, *Scand J Caring Sci* 26:513, 2012.

Calzone KA, et al: Survey of nursing integration of genomics into nursing practice, *J Nurs Scholarsh* 44(4):428, 2012.

Calzone KA, et al: A blueprint for genomic nursing science, *J Nurs Scholarsh* 45(1):96, 2013.

Dobrina R, et al: An overview of hospice and palliative care nursing models and theories, *Int J Palliat Nurs* 20(2):64, 2014.

Harper CC, et al: Abstinence and teenagers: prevention counseling practices of health care providers serving high-risk patients in the United States, *Perspect Sex Reprod Health* 42(2):125, 2010.

Kim SS, et al: Spirituality and psychological well-being: testing a theory of family interdependence among family caregivers and their elders, *Res Nurs Health* 34:103, 2011.

McCubbin MA, et al: Family hardiness index (FHI). In McCubbin HI, et al, editors: *Family assessment: resiliency, coping, and adaptation, inventories for research and practice*, Madison, 1996, University of Wisconsin Press.

McDaniel KR, Allen DG: Working and caregiving: the impact on caregiver stress, family-work conflict, and burnout, *J Life Care Planning* 10(4):21, 2012.

O'Shea F, et al: Family care experiences in nursing home facilities, *Nurs Older People* 26(2):26, 2014.

Plank A, et al: Becoming a caregiver: new family carers' experience during the transition from hospital to home, *J Clin Nurs* 21:2072, 2012.

Popejoy LL: Complexity of family caregiving and discharge planning, *J Fam Nurs* 17:61, 2011.

Reczek C, Umberson D: Gender, health behavior, and intimate relationships: lesbian, gay, and straight contexts, *Soc Sci Med* 74(1783):2012.

Sansoni J, et al: Caregiver of Alzheimer's patients and factors influencing institutionalization of loved ones: some considerations on existing literature, *Ann Ig* 25(3):235, 2013.

Tamayo GJ, et al: Caring for the caregiver, *Oncol Nurs Forum* 37(1):E50, 2010.

Tyrrell EF, et al: Nursing contributions to the rehabilitation of older patients: patient and family perspectives, *J Adv Nurs* 68(11):2466, 2012.

11

Developmental Theories

OBJECTIVES

- Discuss factors influencing growth and development.
- Describe biophysical developmental theories.
- Describe and compare the psychoanalytical/psychosocial theories proposed by Freud and Erikson.
- Describe Piaget's theory of cognitive development.
- Apply developmental theories when planning interventions in the care of patients throughout the life span.
- Discuss nursing implications for the application of developmental principles to patient care.

KEY TERMS

Biophysical development, p. 132
Conventional reasoning, p. 137
Erikson's theory of psychosocial development, p. 134
Freud's psychoanalytical model of personality development, p. 133
Kohlberg's theory of moral development, p. 137
Piaget's theory of cognitive development, p. 136
Postconventional reasoning, p. 137
Temperament, p. 135

MEDIA RESOURCES

http://evolve.elsevier.com/Potter/fundamentals/

- Review Questions
- Case Study with Questions
- Audio Glossary
- Content Updates

Understanding normal growth and development helps nurses predict, prevent, and detect deviations from patients' expected patterns. Growth encompasses the physical changes that occur from the prenatal period through older adulthood and also demonstrates both advancement and deterioration. Development refers to the biological, cognitive, and socioemotional changes that begin at conception and continue throughout a lifetime. Development is dynamic and includes progression. However, in some disease processes development is delayed or regresses.

Individuals have unique patterns of growth and development. The ability to progress through each developmental phase influences the overall health of the individual. The success or failure experienced within a phase affects the ability to complete subsequent phases. If individuals have repeated developmental failures, inadequacies sometimes result. However, when an individual experiences repeated successes, health is promoted. For example, a child who does not walk by 20 months demonstrates delayed gross motor ability that slows exploration and manipulation of the environment. In contrast, a child who walks by 10 months is able to explore and find stimulation in the environment.

When caring for patients, adopt a life span perspective of human development that takes into account all developmental stages. Traditionally development focused on childhood, but a comprehensive view of development also includes the changes that occur during the adult years. An understanding of growth and development throughout the life span helps in planning questions for health screening and health history, health promotion and maintenance, and health education for patients of all ages.

DEVELOPMENTAL THEORIES

Developmental theories provide a framework for examining, describing, and appreciating human development. For example, knowledge of Erikson's psychosocial theory of development helps caregivers understand the importance of supporting the development of basic trust in the infancy stage. Trust establishes the foundation for all future relationships. Developmental theories are also important in helping nurses assess and treat a person's response to an illness. Understanding the specific task or need of each developmental stage guides caregivers in planning appropriate individualized care for patients. Specific developmental theories that describe the aging process for adults are discussed in Chapters 13 and 14.

Human development is a dynamic and complex process that cannot be explained by only one theory. This chapter presents biophysical, psychoanalytical/psychosocial, cognitive, and moral developmental theories. Chapters 25 and 36 cover the areas of learning theory for patient teaching and spiritual development.

Biophysical Developmental Theories

Biophysical development is how our physical bodies grow and change. Health care providers are able to quantify and compare the changes that occur as a newborn infant grows against established norms. How does the physical body age? What are the triggers that move the body from the physical characteristics of childhood, through adolescence, to the physical changes of adulthood?

Gesell's Theory of Development. Fundamental to Gesell's theory of development is that each child's pattern of growth is unique

TABLE 11-1 **Comparison of Major Developmental Theories**

Developmental Stage/Age	Freud (Psychosexual Development)	Erikson (Psychosocial Development)	Piaget (Cognitive/ Moral Development)	Kohlberg (Development of Moral Reasoning)
Infancy (birth to 18 months)	Oral stage	Trust vs. mistrust Ability to trust others	Sensorimotor period Progress from reflex activity to simple repetitive actions	
Early childhood/toddler (18 months to 3 years)	Anal stage	Autonomy vs. shame and doubt Self-control and independence	Preoperational period—thinking using symbols Egocentric	Preconventional level Punishment-obedience orientation
Preschool (3-5 years)	Phallic stage	Initiative vs. guilt Highly imaginative	Use of symbols Egocentric	Preconventional level Premoral Instrumental orientation
Middle childhood (6-12 years)	Latent stage	Industry vs. inferiority Engaged in tasks and activities	Concrete operations period Logical thinking	Conventional level Good boy–nice girl orientation
Adolescence (12-19 years)	Genital stage	Identity vs. role confusion Sexual maturity, "Who am I?"	Formal operations period Abstract thinking	Postconventional level Social contract orientation
Young Adult		Intimacy vs. isolation Affiliation vs. love		
Adult		Generativity vs. self-absorption and stagnation		
Old Age		Integrity vs. despair		

and this pattern is directed by gene activity (Gesell, 1948). Gesell found that the pattern of maturation follows a fixed developmental sequence in humans. Sequential development is evident in fetuses, in which there is a specified order of organ system development. Today we know that growth in humans is both cephalocaudal and proximodistal. The cephalocaudal pattern describes the sequence in which growth is fastest at the top (e.g., head/brain develop faster than arm and leg coordination). The proximodistal growth pattern starts at the center of the body and moves toward the extremities (e.g., organ systems in the trunk of the body develop before arms and legs). Genes direct the sequence of development; but environmental factors also influence development, resulting in developmental changes. For example, genes direct the growth rate in height for an individual, but that growth is only maximized if environmental conditions are adequate. Poor nutrition or chronic disease often affects the growth rate and results in smaller stature, regardless of the genetic blueprint. However, adequate nutrition and the absence of disease cannot result in height beyond that determined by heredity.

Psychoanalytical/Psychosocial Theory

Theories of psychoanalytical/psychosocial development describe human development from the perspectives of personality, thinking, and behavior (Table 11-1). Psychoanalytical theory explains development as primarily unconscious and influenced by emotion. Psychoanalytical theorists maintain that these unconscious conflicts influence development through universal stages experienced by all individuals (Berger, 2011).

Sigmund Freud. Freud's psychoanalytical model of personality development development states that individuals go through five stages of psychosexual development and that each stage is characterized by sexual pleasure in parts of the body: the mouth, the anus, and the genitals. Freud believed that adult personality is the result of how an individual resolves conflicts between these sources of pleasure and the mandates of reality (Santrock, 2012b).

Stage 1: Oral (Birth to 12 to 18 Months). Initially sucking and oral satisfaction are not only vital to life but also extremely pleasurable in their own rights. Late in this stage the infant begins to realize that the mother/parent is something separate from self. Disruption in the physical or emotional availability of the parent (e.g., inadequate bonding or chronic illness) could affect an infant's development.

Stage 2: Anal (12 to 18 Months to 3 Years). The focus of pleasure changes to the anal zone. Children become increasingly aware of the pleasurable sensations of this body region with interest in the products of their effort. Through the toilet-training process the child delays gratification to meet parental and societal expectations.

Stage 3: Phallic or Oedipal (3 to 6 Years). The genital organs are the focus of pleasure during this stage. The boy becomes interested in the penis; the girl becomes aware of the absence of the penis, known as *penis envy*. This is a time of exploration and imagination as a child fantasizes about the parent of the opposite sex as his or her first love interest, known as the *Oedipus* or *Electra complex*. By the end of this stage the child attempts to reduce this conflict by identifying with the parent of the same sex as a way to win recognition and acceptance.

Stage 4: Latency (6 to 12 Years). In this stage Freud believed that children repress and channel sexual urges from the earlier Oedipal stage are repressed and channeled into productive activities that are socially acceptable. Within the educational and social worlds of the child, there is much to learn and accomplish.

Stage 5: Genital (Puberty Through Adulthood). In this final stage sexual urges reawaken and are directed to an individual outside the family circle. Unresolved prior conflicts surface during adolescence. Once the individual resolves conflicts, he or she is then capable of having a mature adult sexual relationship.

Freud believed that the components of the human personality develop in stages and regulate behavior. These components are the id, the ego, and the superego. The id (i.e., basic instinctual impulses driven to achieve pleasure) is the most primitive part of the personality and originates in the infant. The infant cannot tolerate delay and must have needs met immediately. The ego represents the reality component, mediating conflicts between the environment and the forces of the id. It helps people judge reality accurately, regulate impulses, and make good decisions. Ego is often referred to as one's sense of self. The third component, the superego, performs regulating, restraining, and prohibiting actions. Often referred to as the conscience, the superego is influenced by the standards of outside social forces (e.g., parent or teacher).

Some of Freud's critics contend that he based his analysis of personality development on biological determinants and ignored the influence of culture and experience. Others think that Freud's basic assumptions such as the Oedipus complex are not applicable across different cultures. Psychoanalysts today believe that the role of conscious thought is much greater than Freud imagined (Santrock, 2012a).

Erik Erikson. Freud had a strong influence on his psychoanalytical followers, including Erik Erikson (1902-1994), who constructed a theory of development that differed from Freud's in one main aspect: Erikson's stages emphasize a person's relationship to family and culture rather than sexual urges (Berger, 2011).

According to **Erikson's theory of psychosocial development**, individuals need to accomplish a particular task before successfully mastering the stage and progressing to the next one. Each task is framed with opposing conflicts, and tasks once mastered are challenged and tested again during new situations or at times of conflict (Hockenberry and Wilson, 2015). Erikson's eight stages of life are described here.

Trust vs. Mistrust (Birth to 1 Year). Establishing a basic sense of trust is essential for the development of a healthy personality. An infant's successful resolution of this stage requires a consistent caregiver who is available to meet his needs. From this basic trust in parents, an infant is able to trust in himself, in others, and in the world (Hockenberry and Wilson, 2015). The formation of trust results in faith and optimism. A nurse's use of anticipatory guidance helps parents cope with the hospitalization of an infant and the infant's behaviors when discharged to home.

Autonomy vs. Sense of Shame and Doubt (1 to 3 Years). By this stage a growing child is more accomplished in some basic self-care activities, including walking, feeding, and toileting. This newfound independence is the result of maturation and imitation. A toddler develops his or her autonomy by making choices. Choices typical for the toddler age-group include activities related to relationships, desires, and playthings. There is also opportunity to learn that parents and society have expectations about these choices. Limiting choices and/or enacting harsh punishment leads to feelings of shame and doubt. A toddler who successfully masters this stage achieves self-control and willpower. The nurse models empathetic guidance that offers support for and understanding of the challenges of this stage. Available choices for the child must be simple in nature and safe.

Initiative vs. Guilt (3 to 6 Years). Children like to pretend and try out new roles. Fantasy and imagination allow them to further explore their environment. Also at this time they are developing their superego, or conscience. Conflicts often occur between a child's desire to explore and the limits placed on his or her behavior. These conflicts sometimes lead to feelings of frustration and guilt. Guilt also occurs if a caregiver's responses are too harsh. Preschoolers learn to maintain a sense of initiative without imposing on the freedoms of others. Successful resolution of this stage results in direction and purpose. Teaching a child impulse control and cooperative behaviors helps a family avoid the risks of altered growth and development. Preschoolers frequently engage in animism, a developmental characteristic that makes them treat dolls or stuffed animals as if they have thoughts and feelings. Play therapy is also instrumental in helping a child successfully deal with the inherent threats related to hospitalization or chronic illness.

Industry vs. Inferiority (6 to 11 Years). School-age children are eager to apply themselves to learning socially productive skills and tools. They learn to work and play with their peers. They thrive on their accomplishments and praise. Without proper support for learning new skills or if skills are too difficult, they develop a sense of inadequacy and inferiority. Children at this age need to be able to experience real achievement to develop a sense of competency. Erikson believed that an adult's attitudes toward work are traced to successful achievement of this task (Erikson, 1963). During hospitalization it is important for a school-age child to understand the routines and participate as actively as possible in his or her treatment. For example, some children enjoy keeping a record of their intake and output.

Identity vs. Role Confusion (Puberty). Dramatic physiological changes associated with sexual maturation mark this stage. There is a marked preoccupation with appearance and body image. This stage, in which identity development begins with the goal of achieving some perspective or direction, answers the question, "Who am I?" Acquiring a sense of identity is essential for making adult decisions such as choice of a vocation or marriage partner. Each adolescent moves in his or her unique way into society as an interdependent member. There are also new social demands, opportunities, and conflicts that relate to the emergent identity and separation from family. Erikson held that successful mastery of this stage resulted in devotion and fidelity to others and to their own ideals (Hockenberry and Wilson, 2015). Elkind (1967) identified a notion of perceived invulnerability in adolescents that contributes to risk-taking behaviors. Nurses provide education and anticipatory guidance for parents about the changes and challenges to adolescents. Nurses also help hospitalized adolescents deal with their illness by giving them enough information to allow them to make decisions about their treatment plan.

Intimacy vs. Isolation (Young Adult). Young adults, having developed a sense of identity, deepen their capacity to love others and care for them. They search for meaningful friendships and an intimate relationship with another person. Erikson portrayed intimacy as finding the self and then losing it in another (Santrock, 2012a). If the young adult is not able to establish companionship and intimacy, isolation results because he or she fears rejection and disappointment (Berger, 2011). Nurses must understand that during hospitalization a young adults' need for intimacy remains present; thus young adults benefit from the support of their partner or significant other during this time.

Generativity vs. Self-Absorption and Stagnation (Middle Age). Following the development of an intimate relationship, an adult focuses on supporting future generations. The ability to expand one's personal and social involvement is critical to this stage of development. Middle-age adults achieve success in this stage by contributing to future generations through parenthood, teaching, mentoring, and community involvement. Achieving generativity results in caring for others as a basic strength. Inability to play a role in the development of the next generation results in stagnation (Santrock, 2012a). Nurses help physically ill adults choose creative ways to foster social development. Middle-age people often find a sense of fulfillment by volunteering in a local school, hospital, or church.

Integrity vs. Despair (Old Age). Many older adults review their lives with a sense of satisfaction, even with their inevitable mistakes. Others see themselves as failures, with their lives marked by despair and regret. Older adults often engage in a retrospective appraisal of their lives. They interpret their lives as a meaningful whole or experience regret because of goals not achieved (Berger, 2011). Because the aging process creates physical and social losses, some adults also suffer loss of status

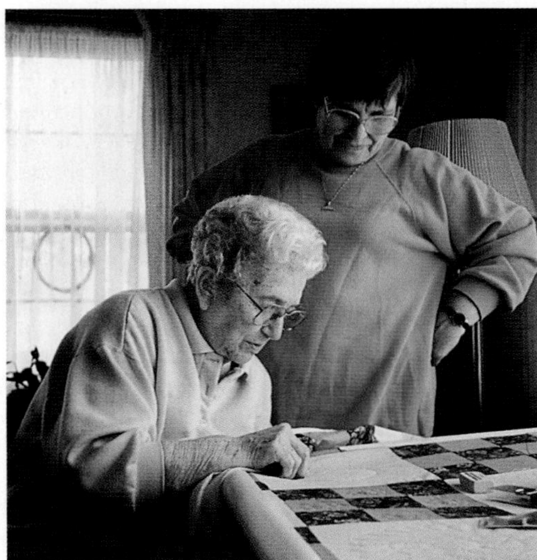

FIGURE 11-1 Quilting keeps this older adult active.

and function (e.g., through retirement or illness). These external struggles are met with internal struggles such as the search for meaning in life. Meeting these challenges creates the potential for growth and the basic strength of wisdom (Figure 11-1).

Nurses are in positions of influence within their communities to help people feel valued, appreciated, and needed. Erikson stated, "Healthy children will not fear life, if their parents have integrity enough not to fear death" (Erikson, 1963). Although Erikson believed that problems in adult life resulted from unsuccessful resolution of earlier stages, his emphasis on family relationships and culture offered a broad, life span view of development. As a nurse you will use this knowledge of development as you deliver care in any health care setting.

Theories Related to Temperament. Temperament is a behavioral style that affects an individual's emotional interactions with others (Santrock, 2012a). Personality and temperament are often closely linked, and research shows that individuals possess some enduring characteristics into adulthood. The individual differences that children display in responding to their environment significantly influence the way others respond to them and their needs. Knowledge of temperament helps parents better understand their child (Hockenberry and Wilson, 2015).

Psychiatrists Stella Chess (1914-2007) and Alexander Thomas (1914-2003) conducted a 20-year longitudinal study that identified three basic classes of temperament:

- *The easy child*—Easygoing and even-tempered. This child is regular and predictable in his or her habits. An easy child is open and adaptable to change and displays a mild to moderately intense mood that is typically positive.
- *The difficult child*—Highly active, irritable, and irregular in habits. Negative withdrawal toward others is typical, and the child requires a more structured environment. A difficult child adapts slowly to new routines, people, or situations. Mood expressions are usually intense and primarily negative.
- *The slow-to-warm up child*—Typically reacts negatively and with mild intensity to new stimuli. The child adapts slowly with repeated contact unless pressured and responds with mild but passive resistance to novelty or changes in routine.

Research on temperament and its stability has continued, with an emphasis on the individual's ability to make thoughtful decisions about behavior in demanding situations. Knowledge of temperament and how it impacts the parent-child relationship is critical when providing anticipatory guidance for parents. With the birth of a second child, most parents find that the strategies that worked well with the first child no longer work at all. The nurse individualizes counseling to greatly improve the quality of interactions between parents and children (Hockenberry and Wilson, 2015).

Perspectives on Adult Development

Early study of development focused only on childhood because scholars throughout history regarded the aging process as one of inevitable and irreversible decline. However, we now know that, although the changes come more slowly, people continue to develop new abilities and adapt to shifting environments. The life span perspective suggests that understanding adult development requires multiple viewpoints. Two of the ways researchers studied adult development were through the stage-crisis view and the life span approach. The most well-known stage theory is the one developed by Erik Erikson, which was discussed earlier. Another stage theory that contributed to understanding development throughout the life span was provided through the work of Robert Havinghurst.

Stage-Crisis Theory. Physicist, educator, and aging expert Robert Havinghurst (1900-1991) conducted extensive research and developed a theory of human development based on developmental tasks. Havinghurst's theory incorporates three primary sources for developmental tasks: tasks that surface because of physical maturation, tasks that evolve from personal values, and tasks that are a result of pressures from society. As with Erikson, Havinghurst believed that successful resolution of the developmental task was essential to successful progression throughout life. He identified six stages and six-to-ten developmental tasks for each stage: infancy and early childhood (birth to age 6), middle childhood (6 to 12 years), adolescence (13 to 18 years), early adulthood (19 to 30 years), middle adulthood (30 to 60 years), and late adulthood (60 and over). Havinghurst believed that the number of tasks differs in each age level for individuals because of the interrelationship among biology, society, and personal values. In later years he turned his focus to the study of aging. In response to the view that older adults should gradually withdraw from society, Havinghurst proposed an *activity theory,* which states that continuing an active, involved lifestyle results in greater satisfaction and well-being in aging (see Chapter 14).

Life Span Approach. The contemporary life-events approach takes into consideration the variations that occur for each individual. This view considers an individual's personal circumstances (health and family support), how a person views and adjusts to changes, and the current social and historical context in which an individual is living. The increase in life expectancy has made popular the life span approach to development (Santrock, 2012b). Paul Baltes (1939-2006), a life span development expert, viewed life span development as lifelong, multidimensional, multidirectional, plastic, multidisciplinary, and contextual. In Baltes' view development is constructed through an interaction of biological, sociocultural, and individual factors (Baltes et al., 2005). Current research on successful aging is much more consistent with a life span approach that emphasizes age-related goals that are relationship and socially oriented to support continued well-being (Reichstadt et al., 2010).

Cognitive Developmental Theory

Psychoanalytical/psychosocial theories focus on an individual's unconscious thought and emotions; cognitive theories stress how people

BOX 11-1 EVIDENCE-BASED PRACTICE

Applying Developmental Theory to Care of Infants

PICO Question: In infant patients does parental emotional involvement at bedtime result in improved quality and length of infant sleep?

Evidence Summary

Twenty to thirty percent of infants have difficulty falling asleep and staying asleep (Ball, 2014; Shapiro-Mendoza et al., 2015). Mother's emotional availability at bedtime has been linked to improved quality of sleep in infants, thought to be associated with infant feelings of safety and security. On the other hand, excessive parental involvement and physical soothing at bedtime is linked to frequent interruptions in sleep throughout the night. Mothers who have doubts of their parenting ability or who feel angry or helpless at their infant's demands may tend to be overintrusive at bedtime and report poor infant sleep quality (Cook et al., 2012). When mothers did not breastfeed at bedtime, Tikotzky et al. (2015) noted that increased participation by fathers during the bedtime ritual improved infant sleeping. It is important that nurses apply developmental theory and recognize the importance of parental engagement in the quality of infant sleep.

Application to Nursing Practice

- Educate parents how to realign their expectation regarding infant sleeping patterns (Ball, 2014).
- Be aware of the value of involving parents in infant care and feeding, particularly around bedtimes (Ball, 2014).
- Help breastfeeding parents set up a bedtime ritual that involves the father (Tikotzky et al., 2015).
- Understand an infant's need for parental involvement in developing a sense of safety and security to enhance quality of sleep.

learn to think and make sense of their world. As with personality development, cognitive theorists have explored both childhood and adulthood. Some of the theories highlight qualitative changes in thinking; others expand to include social, cultural, and behavioral dimensions.

Jean Piaget. Jean Piaget (1896-1980) was most interested in the development of children's intellectual organization: how they think, reason, and perceive the world. Piaget's theory of cognitive development includes four periods that are related to age and demonstrate specific categories of knowing and understanding (see also Chapter 12). He built his theory on years of observing children as they explored, manipulated, and tried to make sense out of the world in which they lived. Piaget believed that individuals move from one stage to the other seeking cognitive equilibrium or a state of mental balance and that they build mental structures to help adapt to the world (Santrock, 2012a). Within each of these primary periods of cognitive development are specific stages (see Table 11-1).

Period I: Sensorimotor (Birth to 2 Years). Infants develop a schema or action pattern for dealing with the environment (Box 11-1). These schemas include hitting, looking, grasping, or kicking. Schemas become self-initiated activities (e.g., the infant learning that sucking achieves a pleasing result generalizes the action to suck fingers, blanket, or clothing). Successful achievement leads to greater exploration. During this stage a child learns about himself and his environment through motor and reflex actions. He or she learns that he or she is separate from the environment and that aspects of the environment (e.g., parents or favorite toy) continue to exist even though they cannot always be seen. Piaget termed this understanding that objects continue to exist even when they cannot be seen, heard, or touched *object permanence* and considered it one of the child's most important accomplishments.

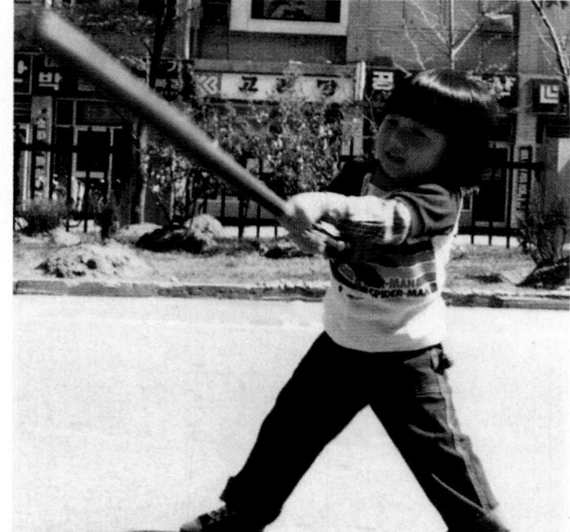

FIGURE 11-2 Play is important to a child's development.

Period II: Preoperational (2 to 7 Years). During this time children learn to think with the use of symbols and mental images. They exhibit "egocentrism" in that they see objects and people from only one point of view, their own. They believe that everyone experiences the world exactly as they do. Early in this stage children demonstrate "animism" in which they personify objects. They believe that inanimate objects have lifelike thought, wishes, and feelings. Their thinking is influenced greatly by fantasy and magical thinking. Children at this stage have difficulty conceptualizing time. Play becomes a primary means by which they foster their cognitive development and learn about the world (Figure 11-2). Nursing interventions during this period recognize the use of play as the way the child understands the events taking place. Play therapy is a nursing intervention that helps the child work through invasive and intrusive procedures that may occur during hospitalization. In addition, play therapy helps the ill child progress developmentally.

Period III: Concrete Operations (7 to 11 Years). Children now are able to perform mental operations. For example, the child thinks about an action that before was performed physically. Children are now able to describe a process without actually doing it. At this time they are able to coordinate two concrete perspectives in social and scientific thinking so they are able to appreciate the difference between their perspective and that of a friend. Reversibility is one of the primary characteristics of concrete operational thought. Children can now mentally picture a series of steps and reverse the steps to get back to the starting point. The ability to mentally classify objects according to their quantitative dimensions, known as *seriation,* is achieved. They are able to correctly order or sort objects by length, weight, or other characteristics. Another major accomplishment of this stage is conservation, or the ability to see objects or quantities as remaining the same despite a change in their physical appearance (Santrock, 2012b).

Period IV: Formal Operations (11 Years to Adulthood). The transition from concrete to formal operational thinking occurs in stages during which there is a prevalence of egocentric thought. This egocentricity leads adolescents to demonstrate feelings and behaviors characterized by self-consciousness: a belief that their actions and appearance are constantly being scrutinized (an "imaginary audience"), that their thoughts and feelings are unique (the "personal fable"), and that they are invulnerable (Santrock, 2012b). These feelings of invulnerability frequently lead to risk-taking behaviors, especially in early adolescence.

As adolescents share experiences with peers, they learn that many of their thoughts and feelings are shared by almost everyone, helping them to know that they are not so different. As they mature, their thinking moves to abstract and theoretical subjects. They have the capacity to reason with respect to possibilities. For Piaget this stage marked the end of cognitive development.

Piaget's work has been challenged over the years as researchers have continued to study cognitive development. For example, some aspects of objective performance emerge earlier than Piaget believed, and other cognitive abilities can surface later than he predicted. We now know that many adults may not become formal operational thinkers and remain at the concrete stage and others have cognitive development that goes beyond the stages that Piaget proposed (Santrock, 2012b). Assessment of cognitive ability becomes critical as you provide health care teaching to patients and families.

Research in Adult Cognitive Development. Research into cognitive development in adulthood began in the 1970s and continues today. It supports that adults do not always arrive at one answer to a problem but frequently accept several possible solutions. Adults also incorporate emotions, logic, practicality, and flexibility when making decisions. On the basis of these observations, developmentalists proposed a fifth stage of cognitive development termed *postformal thought.* Within this stage adults demonstrate the ability to recognize that answers vary from situation to situation and that solutions need to be sensible.

One of the earliest to develop a theory of adult cognition was William Perry (1913-1998), who studied college students and found that continued cognitive development involved increasing cognitive flexibility. As adolescents were able to move from a position of accepting only one answer to realizing that alternative explanations could be right, depending on one's perspective, there was a significant cognitive change. Adults change how they use knowledge, and the emphasis shifts from attaining knowledge or skills to using knowledge for goal achievement.

Moral Developmental Theory

Moral development refers to the changes in a person's thoughts, emotions, and behaviors that influence beliefs about what is right or wrong. It encompasses both *interpersonal* and *intrapersonal* dimensions as it governs how we interact with others (Santrock, 2012b). Although various psychosocial and cognitive theorists address moral development within their respective theories, the theories of Piaget and Kohlberg are more widely known (see Table 11-1).

Lawrence Kohlberg's Theory of Moral Development. Kohlberg's theory of moral development expands on Piaget's cognitive theory. Kohlberg interviewed children, adolescents, and eventually adults and found that moral reasoning develops in stages. From an examination of responses to a series of moral dilemmas, he identified six stages of moral development under three levels (Kohlberg, 1981).

Level I: Preconventional Reasoning. This is the premoral level, in which there is limited cognitive thinking and an individual's thinking is primarily egocentric. At this stage thinking is mostly based on likes and pleasures. This stage progresses toward having punishment guide behavior. A person's moral reason for acting, the "why," eventually relates to the consequences that the person believes will occur. These consequences come in the form of punishment or reward. It is at this level that children view illness as a punishment for fighting with their siblings or disobeying their parents. Nurses need to be aware of this egocentric thinking and reinforce that the child does not become ill because of wrongdoing.

Stage 1: Punishment and Obedience Orientation. In this first stage a child's response to a moral dilemma is in terms of absolute obedience to authority and rules. A child in this stage reasons, "I must follow the rules; otherwise I will be punished." Avoiding punishment or the unquestioning deference to authority is characteristic motivation to behave. Physical consequences guide right and wrong choices. If the child is caught, it must be wrong; if he or she escapes, it must be right.

Stage 2: Instrumental Relativist Orientation. In this stage the child recognizes that there is more than one right view; a teacher has one view that is different from that of the child's parent. The decision to do something morally right is based on satisfying one's own needs and occasionally the needs of others. The child perceives punishment not as proof of being wrong (as in stage 1) but as something that one wants to avoid. Children at this stage follow their parent's rule about being home in time for supper because they do not want to be confined to their room for the rest of the evening if they are late.

Level II: Conventional Reasoning. At level II, conventional reasoning, the person sees moral reasoning based on his or her own personal internalization of societal and others' expectations. A person wants to fulfill the expectations of the family, group, or nation and also develop a loyalty to and actively maintain, support, and justify the order. Moral decision making at this level moves from, "What's in it for me?" to "How will it affect my relationships with others?" Emphasis now is on social rules and a community-centered approach (Berger, 2011). Nurses observe this when family members make end-of-life decisions for their loved ones. Individual members often struggle with this type of moral dilemma. Grief support involves an understanding of the level of moral decision making of each family member (see Chapter 37).

Stage 3: Good Boy–Nice Girl Orientation. The individual wants to win approval and maintain the expectations of one's immediate group. "Being good" is important and defined as having positive motives, showing concern for others, and keeping mutual relationships through trust, loyalty, respect, and gratitude. One earns approval by "being nice." For example, a person in this stage stays after school and does odd jobs to win the teacher's approval.

Stage 4: Society-Maintaining Orientation. Individuals expand their focus from a relationship with others to societal concerns during stage 4. Moral decisions take into account societal perspectives. Right behavior is doing one's duty, showing respect for authority, and maintaining the social order. Adolescents choose not to attend a party where they know beer will be served, not because they are afraid of getting caught, but because they know that it is not right.

Level III: Postconventional Reasoning. The person finds a balance between basic human rights and obligations and societal rules and regulations in the level of postconventional reasoning. Individuals move away from moral decisions based on authority or conformity to groups to define their own moral values and principles. Individuals at this stage start to look at what an ideal society would be like. Moral principles and ideals come into prominence at this level (Berger, 2011).

Stage 5: Social Contract Orientation. Having reached stage 5, an individual follows the societal law but recognizes the possibility of changing the law to improve society. The individual also recognizes that different social groups have different values but believes that all rational people would agree on basic rights such as liberty and life. Individuals at this stage make more of an independent effort to determine what society *should* value rather than what the society as a group *would* value, as would occur in stage 4. The United States Constitution is based on this morality.

Stage 6: Universal Ethical Principle Orientation. Stage 6 defines "right" by the decision of conscience in accord with self-chosen ethical principles. These principles are abstract, like the Golden Rule, and appeal to logical comprehensiveness, universality, and consistency

(Kohlberg, 1981). For example, the principle of justice requires the individual to treat everyone in an impartial manner, respecting the basic dignity of all people, and guides the individual to base decisions on an equal respect for all. Civil disobedience is one way to distinguish stage 5 from stage 6. Stage 5 emphasizes the basic rights, the democratic process, and following laws without question; whereas stage 6 defines the principles by which agreements will be most just. For example, a person in stage 5 follows a law, even if it is not fair to a certain racial group. An individual in stage 6 may not follow a law if it does not seem just to the racial group. For example, Martin Luther King believed that, although we need laws and democratic processes, people who are committed to justice have an obligation to disobey unjust laws and accept the penalties for disobeying these laws (Crain, 1985).

Kohlberg's Critics. Kohlberg constructed a systemized way of looking at moral development and is recognized as a leader in moral developmental theory. However, critics of his work raise questions about his choice of research subjects. For example, most of Kohlberg's subjects were males raised in Western philosophical traditions. Research attempting to support Kohlberg's theory with individuals raised in the Eastern philosophies found that individuals raised in Eastern philosophies never rose above stages 3 or 4 of Kohlberg's model. To some, these findings suggest that people from Eastern philosophies have not reached higher levels of moral development, which is untrue. Others believe that Kohlberg's research design did not allow a way to measure those raised within a different culture.

Kohlberg has also been criticized for age and gender bias. Carol Gilligan criticizes Kohlberg for his gender biases. She believes that he developed his theory on the basis of a justice perspective that focused on the rights of individuals. In contrast, Gilligan's research looked at moral development from a care perspective that viewed people in their interpersonal communications, relationships, and concern for others (Gilligan, 1982; Santrock, 2012b). Other researchers have examined Gilligan's theory in studies with children and have not found evidence to support gender differences (Santrock, 2012b).

Moral Reasoning and Nursing Practice. Nurses need to know their own moral reasoning level. Recognizing your own moral developmental level is essential in separating your beliefs from others when helping patients with their moral decision-making process. It is also important to recognize the level of moral and ethical reasoning used by other members of the health care team and its influence on a patient's care plan. Ideally all members of the health care team are on the same level, creating a unified outcome. This is exemplified in the following scenario: The nurse is caring for a homeless person and believes that all patients deserve the same level of care. The case manager, who is responsible for resource allocation, complains about the patient's length of stay and the amount of resources being expended on this one patient. The nurse and the case manager are in conflict because of their different levels of moral decision making within their practices. They decide to hold a health care team conference to discuss their differences and the ethical dilemma of ensuring that the patient receives an appropriate level of care. Such ethical decisions should be examined through the ethical principles of autonomy; beneficence, nonmaleficence, and justice (see Chapter 22).

Developmental theories help nurses use critical thinking skills when asking how and why people respond as they do. From the diverse set of theories included in this chapter, the complexity of human development is evident. No one theory successfully describes all the intricacies of human growth and development. Today's nurse needs be knowledgeable about several theoretical perspectives when working with patients.

Your assessment of a patient requires a thorough analysis and interpretation of data to form accurate conclusions about his or her developmental needs. Accurate identification of nursing diagnoses relies on your ability to consider developmental theory in data analysis. You compare normal developmental behaviors with those projected by developmental theory. Examples of nursing diagnoses applicable to patients with developmental problems include *risk for delayed development, delayed growth and development,* and *risk for disproportionate growth.*

QSEN QSEN: BUILDING COMPETENCY IN SAFETY Sam is an 84-year-old patient hospitalized for acute abdominal pain. He does not have any local family and lives in an assisted–housing community. He is confused and disoriented. How would your knowledge of developmental theories guide your nursing care for Sam in ensuring his safety?

Answers to QSEN Activities can be found on the Evolve website.

Growth and development, as supported by a life span perspective, is multidimensional. The theories included are the basis for a meaningful observation of an individual's pattern of growth and development. They are important guidelines for understanding important human processes that allow nurses to begin to predict human responses and recognize deviations from the norm.

KEY POINTS

- Nurses administer care for individuals at various developmental stages. Developmental theory provides a basis for nurses to assess and understand the responses seen in their patients.
- Development is not limited to childhood and adolescence; people grow and develop throughout their life span.
- Developmental theories are a way to explain and try to predict human behavior.
- Growth refers to the quantitative changes that nurses measure and compare to norms.
- Development implies a progressive and continuous process of change, leading to a state of organized and specialized functional capacity. These changes are quantitatively measurable but are more distinctly measured in qualitative changes.
- Biophysical development theory explores theories of why individuals age from a biological standpoint, why development follows a predictable sequence, and how environmental factors can influence development.
- Cognitive development focuses on the rational thinking processes that include the changes in how children, adolescents, and adults perform intellectual operations.
- Developmental tasks are age-related achievements, the success of which leads to happiness; whereas failure often leads to unhappiness, disapproval, and difficulty in achieving later tasks.
- Developmental crisis occurs when a person is having great difficulty meeting tasks of the current developmental period.
- Psychosocial theories describe human development from the perspectives of personality, thinking, and behavior, with varying degrees of influence from internal biological forces and external societal/cultural forces.
- Temperament is a behavioral pattern that affects the individual's interactions with others.
- Moral development theory attempts to define how moral reasoning matures for an individual.

CLINICAL APPLICATION QUESTIONS

Preparing for Clinical Practice

1. Mrs. Banks is an 84-year-old woman who was recently diagnosed with breast cancer. She also has severe cardiovascular disease that limits her choices of treatment. She completed a series of radiation treatments that have left her exhausted and unable to participate in her usual activities. Her oncologist now recommends a cycle of chemotherapy treatments that her cardiologist believes would be fatal. Her family is urging her to do all that is recommended. The patient, who is in good spirits despite her diagnosis, decides against further medical treatment.
   a. How does Mrs. Banks' cognitive developmental stage impact her decision making related to her health care?
   b. Which of the psychosocial developmental theories helps explain her decision?
   c. Using your knowledge of her developmental stage, how can you help the family adjust to her choice?
2. Amanda Peters, 9 years old, was admitted to the unit yesterday with a new diagnosis of type I diabetes. Her mother spent the night with her and is arranging the food on Amanda's breakfast tray when you enter the room to check her blood sugar and administer her insulin. Although the diabetes educator will be meeting with Amanda and her family, as part of her care today you want to begin her discharge teaching.
   a. According to Piaget's theory, how will Amanda's cognitive development direct your teaching?
   b. Using Erikson's theory as a basis, which psychosocial factors will you consider when discussing home care with Amanda and her family?
   c. Based on her developmental stage, how can Amanda's family support her active participation in care?
3. You have been assigned to care for Daniel Jackson, a 17-year-old male who was in an automobile accident several days ago and sustained a fractured pelvis. He had a surgical repair and remains on bed rest. School is starting next month, and he was scheduled to begin football practice next week. During bedside report he refuses to make eye contact with the nursing staff or respond to any questions to help direct his care.
   a. How will you incorporate your knowledge of adolescent development as you establish priorities for his care?
   b. Thinking about Erikson's theory, which psychosocial concerns do you anticipate that Daniel might experience during his hospitalization and recovery period?
   c. How will Daniel's cognitive development contribute to his future planning?

ⓔ *Answers to Clinical Application Questions can be found on the Evolve website.*

REVIEW QUESTIONS

Are You Ready to Test Your Nursing Knowledge?

1. The nurse is aware that preschoolers often display a developmental characteristic that makes them treat dolls or stuffed animals as if they have thoughts and feelings. This is an example of:
   1. Logical reasoning.
   2. Egocentrism.
   3. Concrete thinking.
   4. Animism.
2. An 18-month-old child is noted by the parents to be "angry" about any change in routine. This child's temperament is most likely to be described as:
   1. Slow to warm up.
   2. Difficult.
   3. Hyperactive.
   4. Easy.
3. Nine-year-old Brian has a difficult time making friends at school and being chosen to play on the team. He also has trouble completing his homework and, as a result, receives little positive feedback from his parents or teacher. According to Erikson's theory, failure at this stage of development results in:
   1. A sense of guilt.
   2. A poor sense of self.
   3. Feelings of inferiority.
   4. Mistrust.
4. The nurse teaches parents how to have their children learn impulse control and cooperative behaviors. This would be during which of Erikson's stages of development?
   1. Trust versus mistrust
   2. Initiative versus guilt
   3. Industry versus inferiority
   4. Autonomy versus sense of shame and doubt
5. When Ryan was 3 months old, he had a toy train; when his view of the train was blocked, he did not search for it. Now that he is 9 months old, he looks for it, reflecting the presence of:
   1. Object permanence.
   2. Sensorimotor play.
   3. Schemata.
   4. Magical thinking.
6. When preparing a 4-year-old child for a procedure, which method is developmentally most appropriate for the nurse to use?
   1. Allowing the child to watch another child undergoing the same procedure
   2. Showing the child pictures of what he or she will experience
   3. Talking to the child in simple terms about what will happen
   4. Preparing the child through play with a doll and toy medical equipment
7. Which of the following are examples of the conventional reasoning form of cognitive development? (Select all that apply.)
   1. A 35-year-old woman is speaking with you about her recent diagnosis of a chronic illness. She is concerned about her treatment options in relation to her ability to continue to care for her family. As she considers the options and alternatives, she incorporates information, her values, and emotions to decide which plan will be the best fit for her.
   2. A young father is considering whether or not to return to school for a graduate degree. He considers the impact the time commitment may have on the needs of his wife and infant son.
   3. A teenage girl is encouraged by her peers to engage in shoplifting. She decides not to join her peers in this activity because she is afraid of getting caught in the act.
   4. A single mother of two children is unhappy with her employer. She has been unable to secure alternate employment but decides to quit her current job.
8. You are caring for a recently retired man who appears withdrawn and says he is "bored with life." Applying the work of Havinghurst, you would help this individual find meaning in life by:
   1. Encouraging him to explore new roles.
   2. Encouraging relocation to a new city.
   3. Explaining the need to simplify life.
   4. Encouraging him to adopt a new pet.

9. Place the following stages of Freud's psychosexual development in the proper order by age progression.
   1. Phallic
   2. Latent
   3. Oral
   4. Genital
   5. Anal
10. According to Piaget's cognitive theory, a 12-year-old child is most likely to engage in which of the following activities?
    1. Using building blocks to determine how houses are constructed
    2. Writing a story about a clown who wants to leave the circus
    3. Drawing pictures of a family using stick figures
    4. Writing an essay about patriotism
11. Allison, age 15 years, calls her best friend Laura and is crying. She has a date with John, someone she has been hoping to date for months, but now she has a pimple on her forehead. Laura firmly believes that John and everyone else will notice the blemish right away. This is an example of the:
    1. Imaginary audience.
    2. False-belief syndrome.
    3. Personal fable.
    4. Personal absorption syndrome.
12. Elizabeth, who is having unprotected sex with her boyfriend, comments to her friends, "Did you hear about Kathy? You know, she fools around so much; I heard she was pregnant. That would never happen to me!" This is an example of adolescent:
    1. Imaginary audience.
    2. False-belief syndrome.
    3. Personal fable.
    4. Sense of invulnerability.
13. Which of the following activities are examples of the use of activity theory in older adults? (Select all that apply.)
    1. Teaching an older adult how to use e-mail to communicate with a grandchild who lives in another state
    2. Introducing golf as a new hobby
    3. Leading a group walk of older adults each morning
    4. Engaging an older adult in a community project with a short-term goal
    5. Directing a community play at the local theater
14. Dave reports being happy and satisfied with his life. What do we know about him?
    1. He is in one of the later developmental periods, concerned with reviewing his life.
    2. He is atypical, since most people in any of the developmental stages report significant dissatisfaction with their lives.
    3. He is in one of the earlier developmental periods, concerned with establishing a career and satisfying long-term relationships.
    4. It is difficult to determine Dave's developmental stage since most people report overall satisfaction with their lives in all stages.
15. You are working in a clinic that provides services for homeless people. The current local regulations prohibit providing a service that you believe is needed by your patients. You adhere to the regulations but at the same time are involved in influencing authorities to change the regulation. This action represents __________ stage of moral development.

Answers: 1. 4; **2.** 2; **3.** 3; **4.** 2; **5.** 1; **6.** 4; **7.** 1, 2; **8.** 1; **9.** 3, 5, 1, 2, 4; **10.** 2; **11.** 1; **12.** 4; **13.** 1, 2, 4; **14.** 4; **15.** Social contract orientation.

ⓔ ***Rationales for Review Questions can be found on the Evolve website.***

REFERENCES

Baltes PB, et al: The psychological science of human aging. In Johnson ML, editor: *The Cambridge handbook of age and aging*, New York, 2005, Cambridge University Press, p 47.

Berger KS: *The developing person: through the life span*, ed 8, New York, 2011, Worth.

Crain WC: *Theories of development*, Upper Saddle River, NJ, 1985, Prentice Hall.

Elkind D: Egocentrism in adolescence, *Child Dev* 38:1025, 1967.

Erikson E: *Childhood and society*, New York, 1963, Norton.

Gesell A: *Studies in child development*, New York, 1948, Harper.

Gilligan C: *In a different voice: psychological theory and women's development*, Cambridge, 1982, Harvard University Press.

Hockenberry MJ, Wilson D: *Wong's nursing care of infants and children*, ed 10, St Louis, 2015, Mosby.

Kohlberg L: *The philosophy of moral development: moral stages and the idea of justice*, San Francisco, 1981, Harper & Row.

Reichstadt J, et al: Older adults' perspectives on successful aging: qualitative interviews, *Am J Geriatr Psychiatry* 18(7):567, 2010.

Santrock JW: *Life span development*, ed 13, New York, 2012a, McGraw-Hill.

Santrock JW: *A topical approach to life span development*, ed 6, New York, 2012b, McGraw-Hill.

RESEARCH REFERENCES

Ball HL: Reframing what we tell parents about normal infant sleep and how we support them, *Breastfeed Rev* 22(3):11, 2014.

Cook F, et al: Baby business: a randomized controlled trial of a universal parenting program that aims to prevent early infant sleep and cry problems and associated parental depression, *BMC Pediatr* 12:13, 2012.

Shapiro-Mendoza CK, et al: Trends in infant bedding use: National Infant Sleep Position study, 1993-2010, *Pediatrics* 135(1):10, 2015.

Tikotzky L, et al: Infant sleep development from 3 to 6 months postpartum: links with maternal sleep and paternal involvement, *Monogr Soc Res Child Dev* 80(1):107, 2015.

12

Conception Through Adolescence

OBJECTIVES

- Discuss common physiological and psychosocial health concerns during the transition of the child from intrauterine to extrauterine life.
- Describe characteristics of physical growth of the unborn child and from birth to adolescence.
- Describe cognitive and psychosocial development from birth to adolescence.
- Explain the role of play in the development of a child.
- Discuss ways in which a nurse is able to help parents meet their children's developmental needs.

KEY TERMS

Adolescence, p. 153
Apgar score, p. 142
Attachment, p. 142
Embryonic stage, p. 141
Fetal stage, p. 141
Fetus, p. 141
Inborn errors of metabolism (IEMs), p. 144
Infancy, p. 145
Molding, p. 143
Neonatal period, p. 142
Preembryonic stage, p. 141
Preschool period, p. 149
Puberty, p. 153
School-age, p. 151
Sexually transmitted infections (STIs), p. 152
Toddlerhood, p. 147

MEDIA RESOURCES

http://evolve.elsevier.com/Potter/fundamentals/

- Review Questions
- Case Study with Questions
- Audio Glossary
- Content Updates

STAGES OF GROWTH AND DEVELOPMENT

Human growth and development are continuous and complex processes that are typically divided into stages organized by age-groups such as from conception to adolescence. Although this chronological division is arbitrary, it is based on the timing and sequence of developmental tasks that the child must accomplish to progress to another stage. This chapter focuses on the various physical, psychosocial, and cognitive changes and health risks and health promotion concerns during the different stages of growth and development.

SELECTING A DEVELOPMENTAL FRAMEWORK FOR NURSING

Providing developmentally appropriate nursing care is easier when you base planning on a theoretical framework (see Chapter 11). An organized, systematic approach ensures that you assess the child appropriately and plan care that meets the child's and family's needs. If you deliver nursing care only as a series of isolated actions, you will overlook some of the child's developmental needs. A developmental approach encourages organized care directed at the child's current level of functioning to motivate self-direction and health promotion. For example, nurses encourage toddlers to feed themselves to advance their developing independence and thus promote their sense of autonomy. Another example involves a nurse understanding an adolescent's need to be independent and thus establishing a contract about the care plan and its implementation.

INTRAUTERINE LIFE

From the moment of conception until birth, human development proceeds at a predictive and rapid rate. During gestation or the prenatal period, the embryo grows from a single cell to a complex, physiological being. All major organ systems develop in utero, with some functioning before birth. Development proceeds in a cephalocaudal (head-to-toe) and proximal-distal (central-to-peripheral) pattern (Murray and McKinney, 2010).

Pregnancy that reaches full term is calculated to last an average of 38 to 40 weeks and is divided into three stages or trimesters. Beginning on the day of fertilization, the first 14 days are referred to as the **preembryonic stage**, followed by the **embryonic stage** that lasts from day 15 until the eighth week. These two stages are then followed by the **fetal stage** that lasts from the end of the eighth week until birth (Perry et al., 2014). Gestation is commonly divided into equal phases of 3 months called *trimesters*.

The placenta begins development at the third week of the embryonic stage and produces essential hormones that help maintain the pregnancy. The placenta functions as the fetal lungs, kidneys, gastrointestinal tract, and an endocrine organ. Because the placenta is extremely porous, noxious materials such as viruses, chemicals, and drugs also pass from mother to child. These agents are called *teratogens* and can cause abnormal development of structures in the embryo. The effect of teratogens on the **fetus** or unborn child depends on the developmental stage in which exposure takes place, individual genetic susceptibility, and the quantity of the exposure. The embryonic stage is the most vulnerable since all body organs are formed by the eighth week.

Some maternal infections can cross the placental barrier and negatively influence the health of the mother, fetus, or both. It is important to educate women about avoidable sources of teratogens and help them make healthy lifestyle choices before and during pregnancy.

Health Promotion During Pregnancy

The diet of a woman both before and during pregnancy has a significant effect on fetal development. Women who do not consume adequate nutrients and calories during pregnancy may not be able to meet the fetus' nutritional requirements. An increase in weight does not always indicate an increase in nutrients. In addition, the pattern of weight gain is important for tissue growth in a mother and fetus. For women who are at normal weight for height, the recommended weight gain is 25 to 35 lbs (11 to 15 kg) over three trimesters (Murray and McKinney, 2010). As a nurse you are in a key position to provide women with the education they need about nutrition before conception and throughout an expectant mother's pregnancy.

Pregnancy presents a developmental challenge that includes physiological, cognitive, and emotional states that are accompanied by stress and anxiety. The expectant woman will soon adopt a parenting role; and relationships within the family will change, whether or not there is a partner involved. Pregnancy can be a period of conflict or support; family dynamics impact fetal development. Parental reactions to pregnancy change throughout the gestational period, with most couples looking forward to the birth and addition of a new family member (Perry et al., 2014). Listen carefully to concerns expressed by a mother and her partner and offer support through each trimester.

The age of the pregnant woman sometimes plays a role in the health of the fetus and the overall pregnancy. Fetuses of older mothers are at risk for chromosomal defects, and older women may have more difficulty becoming pregnant. Studies indicate that pregnant adolescents often seek out less prenatal care than women in their 20s and 30s and are at higher risk for complications of pregnancy and labor. Infants of teen mothers are at increased risk for prematurity; low birth weight; and exposure to alcohol, drugs, and tobacco in utero and early childhood (USDHHS, 2014b). Adolescents who have been able to participate in prenatal classes may have improved nutrition and healthier babies.

Fetal growth and hormonal changes during pregnancy often result in discomfort for the expectant mother. Common concerns expressed include problems such as nausea and vomiting, breast tenderness, urinary frequency, heartburn, constipation, ankle edema, and backache. Always anticipate these discomforts and provide self-care education throughout the pregnancy. Discussing the physiological causes of these discomforts and offering suggestions for safe treatment can be very helpful for expectant mothers and contribute to overall health during pregnancy (Perry et al., 2014; USDHHS, 2014b).

Some complementary and alternative therapies such as herbal supplements can be harmful during pregnancy. Your assessment should include questions about use of these substances when providing education (Murray and McKinney, 2010). You can promote maternal and fetal health by providing accurate and complete information about health behaviors that support positive outcomes for pregnancy and childbirth.

TRANSITION FROM INTRAUTERINE TO EXTRAUTERINE LIFE

The transition from intrauterine to extrauterine life requires profound physiological changes in the newborn and occurs during the first 24 hours of life. Assessment of the newborn during this period is essential to ensure that the transition is proceeding as expected. Gestational age and development, exposure to depressant drugs before or during labor, and the newborn's own behavioral style also influence the adjustment to the external environment.

Physical Changes

An immediate assessment of the newborn's condition to determine the physiological functioning of the major organ systems occurs at birth. The most widely used assessment tool is the **Apgar score**. Heart rate, respiratory effort, muscle tone, reflex irritability, and color are rated to determine overall status of the newborn. The Apgar assessment generally is conducted at 1 and 5 minutes after birth and is sometimes repeated until the newborn's condition stabilizes. The most extreme physiological change occurs when the newborn leaves the utero circulation and develops independent circulatory and respiratory functioning.

Nursing interventions at birth include maintaining an open airway, stabilizing and maintaining body temperature, and protecting the newborn from infection. The removal of nasopharyngeal and oropharyngeal secretions with suction or a bulb syringe ensures airway patency. Newborns are susceptible to heat loss and cold stress. Because hypothermia increases oxygen needs, it is essential to stabilize and maintain a newborn's body temperature. A healthy newborn may be placed directly on the mother's abdomen and covered in warm blankets or provided warmth via a radiant warmer. Preventing infection is a major concern in the care of a newborn, whose immune system is immature. Good handwashing technique is the most important factor in protecting a newborn from infection. You can help prevent infection by instructing parents and visitors to wash their hands before touching the infant.

Psychosocial Changes

After immediate physical evaluation and application of identification bracelets, the nurse promotes the parents' and newborn's need for close physical contact. Early parent-child interaction encourages parent-child **attachment**. Merely placing the family together does not promote closeness. Most healthy newborns are awake and alert for the first half-hour after birth. This is a good time for parent-child interaction to begin. Close body contact, often including breastfeeding, is a satisfying way for most families to start bonding. If immediate contact is not possible, incorporate it into the care plan as early as possible, which means bringing the newborn to an ill parent or bringing the parents to an ill or premature child. Attachment is a process that evolves over the infant's first 24 months of life, and many psychologists believe that a secure attachment is an important foundation for psychological development in later life (Perry et al., 2014).

NEWBORN

The **neonatal period** is the first 28 days of life. During this stage the newborn's physical functioning is mostly reflexive, and stabilization of major organ systems is the primary task of the body. Behavior greatly influences interaction among the newborn, the environment, and caregivers. For example, the average 2-week-old smiles spontaneously and is able to look at the mother's face. The impact of these reflexive behaviors is generally a surge of maternal feelings of love that prompt the mother to cuddle the baby. You apply knowledge of this stage of growth and development to promote newborn and parental health. For example, the newborn's cry is generally a reflexive response to an unmet need (e.g., hunger, fatigue, or discomfort). Thus you help parents identify ways to meet these needs by counseling them to feed their baby on demand rather than on a rigid schedule.

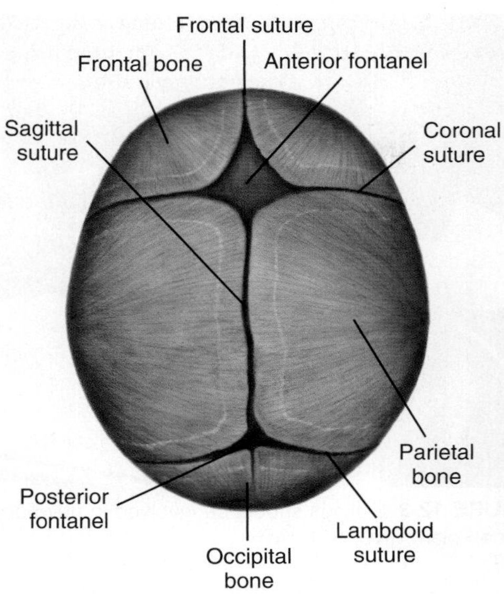

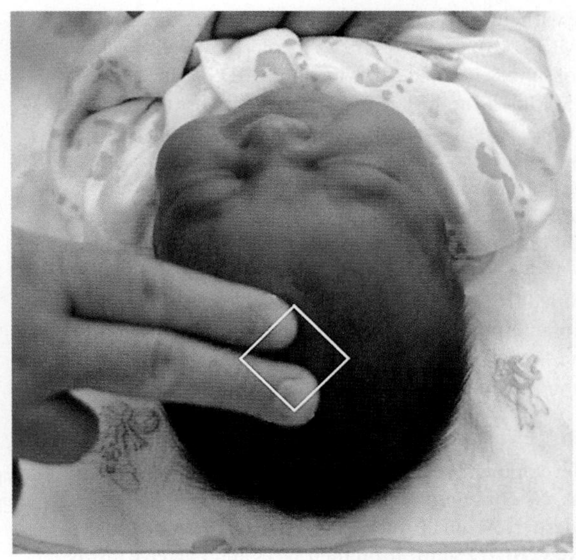

FIGURE 12-1 Fontanels and suture lines. (From Hockenberry MJ, Wilson D: *Wong's nursing care of infants and children,* ed 10, St Louis, 2015, Mosby.)

Physical Changes

The nurse performs a comprehensive nursing assessment as soon as the newborn's physiological functioning is stable, generally within a few hours after birth. At this time he or she measures height, weight, head and chest circumference, temperature, pulse, and respirations and observes general appearance, body functions, sensory capabilities, reflexes, and responsiveness. Following a comprehensive physical assessment, assess gestational age and interactions between infant and parent that indicate successful attachment (Hockenberry and Wilson, 2015).

The average newborn is 6 to 9 lbs (2700 to 4000 g), 19 to 21 inches (48 to 53 cm) in length, and has a head circumference of 13 to 14 inches (33 to 35 cm). Neonates lose up to 10% of birth weight in the first few days of life, primarily through fluid losses by respiration, urination, defecation, and low fluid intake. They usually regain birth weight by the second week of life; and a gradual pattern of increase in weight, height, and head circumference is evident. Accurate measurement as soon as possible after birth provides a baseline for future comparison (Hockenberry and Wilson, 2015).

Normal physical characteristics include the continued presence of lanugo on the skin of the back; cyanosis of the hands and feet for the first 24 hours; and a soft, protuberant abdomen. Skin color varies according to racial and genetic heritage and gradually changes during infancy. **Molding**, or overlapping of the soft skull bones, allows the fetal head to adjust to various diameters of the maternal pelvis and is a common occurrence with vaginal births. The bones readjust within a few days, producing a rounded appearance to the head. The sutures and fontanels are usually palpable at birth. Figure 12-1 shows the diamond shape of the anterior fontanel and the triangular shape of the posterior fontanel between the unfused bones of the skull. The anterior fontanel usually closes at 12 to 18 months, whereas the posterior fontanel closes by the end of the second or third month.

Assess neurological function by observing the newborn's level of activity, alertness, irritability, and responsiveness to stimuli and the presence and strength of reflexes. Normal reflexes include blinking in response to bright lights, startling in response to sudden loud noises or movement, sucking, rooting, grasping, yawning, coughing, sneezing, palmar grasp, swallowing, plantar grasp, Babinski, and hiccoughing.

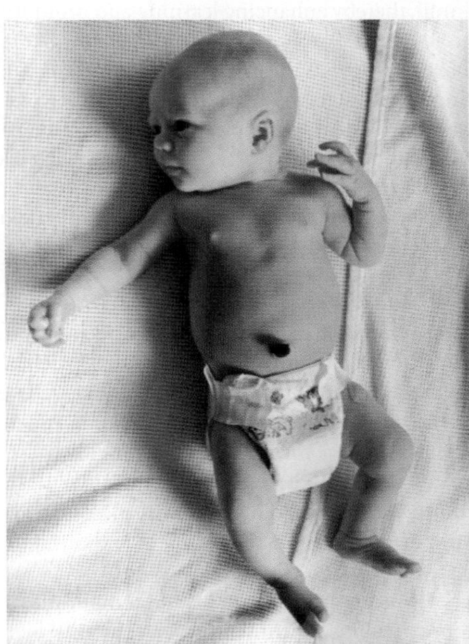

FIGURE 12-2 Tonic neck reflex. Newborns assume this position while supine. (From Hockenberry MJ, Wilson D: *Wong's nursing care of infants and children,* ed 10, St Louis, 2015, Mosby.)

Assessment of these reflexes is vital because the newborn depends largely on reflexes for survival and in response to its environment. Figure 12-2 shows the tonic neck reflex in the newborn.

Normal behavioral characteristics of the newborn include periods of sucking, crying, sleeping, and activity. Movements are generally sporadic, but they are symmetrical and involve all four extremities. The relatively flexed fetal position of intrauterine life continues as the newborn attempts to maintain an enclosed, secure feeling. Newborns normally watch the caregiver's face; have a nonpurposeful reflexive smile; and respond to sensory stimuli, particularly the primary caregiver's face, voice, and touch.

In accordance with the recommendations of the American Academy of Pediatrics (AAP, 2014b), position infants for sleep on their backs to decrease the risk of sudden infant death syndrome (SIDS) (Hockenberry and Wilson, 2015; Murray and McKinney, 2010). Newborns establish their individual sleep-activity cycle, and parents develop sensitivity to their baby's cues. Nurses play an important role in demonstrating to parents the correct positioning on the back to reduce the incidence of SIDS (Perry et al., 2014). Co-sleeping or bed sharing has also been reported to possibly be associated with an increased risk for SIDS (Hockenberry and Wilson, 2015). Safeguards include proper positioning; removing stuffed animals, soft bedding, and pillows; and avoiding overheating the infant. Individuals should avoid smoking during pregnancy and around the infant because it places the infant at greater risk for SIDS (Hockenberry and Wilson, 2015).

Cognitive Changes

Early cognitive development begins with innate behavior, reflexes, and sensory functions. Newborns initiate reflex activities, learn behaviors, and learn their desires. At birth infants are able to focus on objects about 8 to 10 inches (20 to 25 cm) from their faces and perceive forms. A preference for the human face is apparent. Teach parents about the importance of providing sensory stimulation such as talking to their babies and holding them to see their faces. This allows infants to seek or take in stimuli, thereby enhancing learning and promoting cognitive development.

For newborns crying is a means of communication to provide cues to parents. Some babies cry because their diapers are wet or they are hungry or want to be held. Others cry just to make noise or because they need a change in position or activity. The crying frustrates the parents if they cannot see an apparent cause. With the nurse's help parents learn to recognize infants' cry patterns and take appropriate action when necessary.

Psychosocial Changes

During the first month of life most parents and newborns normally develop a strong bond that grows into a deep attachment. Interactions during routine care enhance or detract from the attachment process. Feeding, hygiene, and comfort measures consume much of infants' waking time. These interactive experiences provide a foundation for the formation of deep attachments. Early on older siblings need to have opportunity to be involved in the newborn's care. Family involvement helps support growth and development and promotes nurturing (Figure 12-3).

If parents or children experience health complications after birth, this *may* compromise the attachment process. Infants' behavioral cues are sometimes weak or absent, and caregiving is possibly less mutually satisfying. Some tired or ill parents have difficulty interpreting and responding to their infants. Preterm infants and those born with congenital anomalies are often too weak to be responsive to parental cues and require special supportive nursing care. For example, infants born with heart defects tire easily during feedings. Nurses can support parental attachment by pointing out positive qualities and responses of the newborn and acknowledging how difficult the separation can be for parents and infant.

Health Promotion

Screening. Newborn screening tests are administered before babies leave the hospital to identify serious or life-threatening conditions before symptoms begin. Results of the screening tests are sent directly to an infant's pediatrician. If a screening test suggests a problem, the baby's physician usually follows up with further testing and may refer the infant to a specialist for treatment if needed. Blood tests help determine **inborn errors of metabolism (IEMs)**. These are genetic disorders caused by the absence or deficiency of a substance, usually an enzyme, essential to cellular metabolism that results in abnormal protein, carbohydrate, or fat metabolism. Although IEMs are rare, they account for a significant proportion of health problems in children. Neonatal screening is done to detect phenylketonuria (PKU), hypothyroidism, galactosemia, and other diseases to allow appropriate treatment that prevents permanent mental retardation and other health problems.

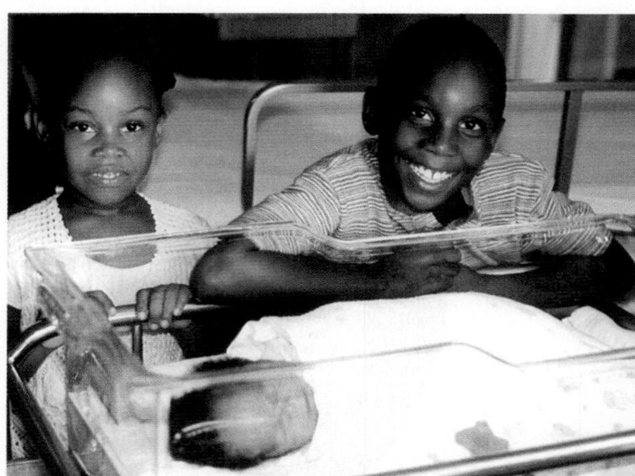

FIGURE 12-3 Siblings should be involved in newborn care. (Courtesy Elaine Polan, RNC, BSN, MS.)

The AAP recommends universal screening of newborn hearing before discharge since studies have indicated that the incidence of hearing loss is as high as 1 to 3 per 1000 normal newborns (Perry et al., 2014). If health care providers detect the loss before 3 months of age and intervention is initiated by 6 months, children are able to achieve normal language development that matches their cognitive development through the age of 5 (Hockenberry and Wilson, 2015).

Car Seats. An essential component of discharge teaching is the use of a federally approved car seat for transporting the infant from the hospital or birthing center to home. Automobile injuries are a leading cause of death in children in the United States. Many of these deaths occur when the child is not properly restrained (Hockenberry and Wilson, 2015). Parents need to learn how to fit the restraint to the infant properly and properly install the car seat. All infants and toddlers should ride in a rear-facing car safety seat until they are 2 years of age or until they reach the highest weight or height allowed by the manufacturer or their car safety seat (AAP, 2015a). Placing an infant in a rear-facing restraint in the front seat of a vehicle is extremely dangerous in any vehicle with a passenger-side air bag. Nurses are responsible for providing education on the use of a car seat before discharge from the hospital.

Cribs and Sleep. Federal safety standards were changed in 2011 to prohibit the manufacture or sale of drop-side rail cribs (AAP, 2014b). New cribs sold in the United States must meet these governmental standards for safety. Unsafe cribs that do not meet the safety standards should be disassembled and thrown away (AAP, 2014b). Parents also need to inspect an older crib to make sure the slats are no more than 6 cm (2.4 inches) apart. The crib mattress should fit snugly, and crib toys or mobiles should be attached firmly with no hanging strings or straps. Instruct parents to remove mobiles as soon as the infant is able to reach them (Hockenberry and Wilson, 2015). Also consider using a portable play yard, as long as it is not a model that has been recalled.

TABLE 12-1 Gross- and Fine-Motor Development in Infancy

Age	Gross-Motor Skill	Fine-Motor Skill
Birth to 1 month	Complete head lag persists No ability to sit upright Inborn reflexes predominant	Reflexive grasp
2 to 4 months	When prone, lifts head and chest and bears weight on forearms With support able to sit erect with good head control Can turn from side to back	Holds rattle for short periods Looks at and plays with fingers Able to bring objects from hand to mouth
4 to 6 months	Turns from abdomen to back at 5 months and then back to abdomen at 6 months Can support much of own weight when pulled to stand No head lag when pulled to sit	Grasps objects at will and can drop them to pick up another object Pulls feet to mouth to explore Can hold a baby bottle
6 to 8 months	Sits alone without support Bears full weight on feet and can hold on to furniture Can move from a sitting to kneeling position	Bangs objects together Pulls a string to obtain an object Transfers objects from hand to hand
8 to 10 months	Crawls or pulls entire body along floor using arms Pulls self to standing or sitting Creeps on hands and knees	Picks up small objects Uses pincer grasp well Shows hand preference
10 to 12 months	Stands alone Walks holding onto furniture Sits down from a standing position	Can place objects into containers Able to hold a crayon or pencil and make a mark on paper

Adapted from Hockenberry M, Wilson D: *Wong's nursing care of infants and children*, ed 10, St Louis, 2015, Mosby; Perry S et al: *Maternal child nursing care*, ed 5, St Louis, 2014, Mosby.

INFANT

During infancy, the period from 1 month to 1 year of age, rapid physical growth and change occur. This is the only period distinguished by such dramatic physical changes and marked development. Psychosocial developmental advances are aided by the progression from reflexive to more purposeful behavior. Interaction between infants and the environment is greater and more meaningful for the infant. During this first year of life the nurse easily observes the adaptive potential of infants because changes in growth and development occur so rapidly.

Physical Changes

Steady and proportional growth of an infant is more important than absolute growth values. Charts of normal age- and gender-related growth measurements enable a nurse to compare growth with norms for a child's age. Measurements recorded over time are the best way to monitor growth and identify problems. Size increases rapidly during the first year of life; birth weight doubles in approximately 5 months and triples by 12 months. Height increases an average of 2.5 cm (1 inch) during each of the first 6 months and about 1.2 cm (½ inch) each month until 12 months (Hockenberry and Wilson, 2015).

Throughout the first year an infant's vision and hearing continue to develop. Some infants as young as 3½ months are able to link visual and auditory stimuli (Hockenberry and Wilson, 2015). Patterns of body function also stabilize, as evidenced by predictable sleep, elimination, and feeding routines. Some reflexes that are present in the newborn such as blinking, yawning, and coughing remain throughout life; whereas others such as grasping, rooting, sucking, and the Moro or startle reflex disappear after several months.

Gross-motor skills involve large muscle activities and are usually closely monitored by parents who easily report recently achieved milestones. Newborns can only momentarily hold their heads up, but by 4 months most infants have no head lag. The same rapid development is evident as infants learn to sit, stand, and then walk. Fine-motor skills involve small body movements and are more difficult to achieve than gross-motor skills. Maturation of eye-and-hand coordination occurs over the first 2 years of life as infants move from being able to grasp a rattle briefly at 2 months to drawing an arc with a pencil by 24 months. Development proceeds at a variable pace for each individual but usually follows the same pattern and occurs within the same time frame (Table 12-1).

Cognitive Changes

The complex brain development during the first year is demonstrated by an infant's changing behaviors. As he or she receives stimulation through the developing senses of vision, hearing, and touch, the developing brain interprets the stimuli. Thus an infant learns by experiencing and manipulating the environment. Developing motor skills and increasing mobility expand an infant's environment and, with developing visual and auditory skills, enhance cognitive development. For these reasons Piaget (1952) named his first stage of cognitive development, which extends until around the third birthday, the sensorimotor period (see Chapter 11). In this stage of cognitive development, infants explore their world through senses. They learn by experimentation and trial and error. They shake and throw things and put things in their mouths. By the age of 7 to 9 months, they begin to realize that things still exist that that can no longer be seen. This is known as object permanence and is an important developmental milestone because it demonstrates that their memory is beginning to develop.

Infants need opportunities to develop and use their senses. Nurses need to evaluate the appropriateness and adequacy of these opportunities. For example, ill or hospitalized infants sometimes lack the energy to interact with their environment, thereby slowing their cognitive development. Infants need to be stimulated according to their temperament, energy, and age. The nurse uses stimulation strategies that maximize the development of infants while conserving their energy and orientation. An example of this is a nurse talking to and encouraging an infant to suck on a pacifier while administering the infant's tube feeding.

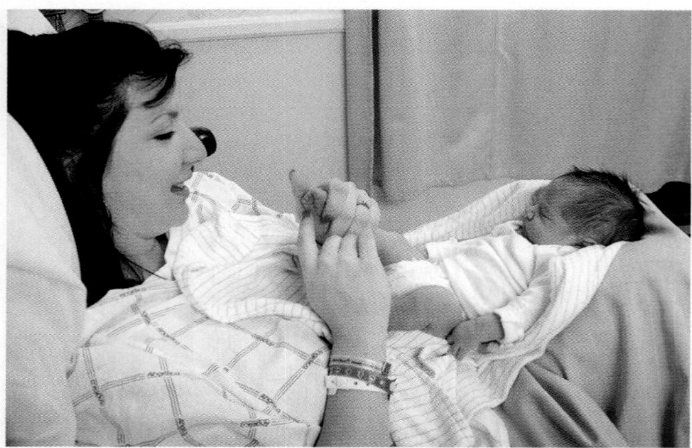

FIGURE 12-4 Smiling at and talking to an infant encourage bonding. (From Murray SS, McKinney ES: *Foundations of maternal-newborn and women's health nursing,* ed 6, St Louis, 2014, Saunders.)

Language. Speech is an important aspect of cognition that develops during the first year. Infants proceed from crying, cooing, and laughing to imitating sounds, comprehending the meaning of simple commands, and repeating words with knowledge of their meaning. According to Piaget this demonstrates that an infant is demonstrating some symbolic abilities. By 1 year infants not only recognize their own names but are able to say three to five words and understand almost 100 words (Hockenberry and Wilson, 2015). As a nurse, you promote language development by encouraging parents to name objects on which their infant's attention is focused. You also assess the infant's language development to identify developmental delays or potential abnormalities.

Psychosocial Changes

Separation and Individuation. During their first year infants begin to differentiate themselves from others as separate beings capable of acting on their own. Initially infants are unaware of the boundaries of self; but, through repeated experiences with the environment, they learn where the self ends and the external world begins. As they determine their physical boundaries, they begin to respond to others (Figure 12-4).

Two- and 3-month-old infants begin to smile responsively rather than reflexively. Similarly they recognize differences in people when their sensory and cognitive capabilities improve. By 8 months most infants are able to differentiate a stranger from a familiar person and respond differently to the two. Close attachment to their primary caregivers, most often parents, usually occurs by this age. Infants seek out these people for support and comfort during times of stress. The ability to distinguish self from others allows infants to interact and socialize more within their environments. For example, by 9 months infants play simple social games such as patty-cake and peek-a-boo. More complex interactive games such as hide-and-seek involving objects are possible by age 1.

Erikson (1963) describes the psychosocial developmental crisis for an infant as trust vs. mistrust. He explains that the quality of parent-infant interactions determines development of trust or mistrust. The infant learns to trust self, others, and the world through the relationship between the parent and child and the care the child receives (Hockenberry and Wilson, 2015). During infancy a child's temperament or behavioral style becomes apparent and influences the interactions between parent and child. You can help parents understand their child's temperament and determine appropriate childrearing practices (see Chapter 11).

BOX 12-1 Warning Signs of Abuse

- Physical evidence of abuse or neglect, including previous injuries
- Conflicting stories about the accident/trauma
- Injury blamed on sibling or another party
- Injury inconsistent with the history such as a concussion and a broken arm from falling off the bed
- History inconsistent with the child's developmental age (e.g., a 6-month-old burned by turning on the hot water)
- An initial complaint not associated with the signs and symptoms present (e.g., bringing the child to the clinic for a cold when there is evidence of physical trauma)
- Inappropriate response of the child, especially an older child (e.g., not wanting to be touched, looking at caregiver before answering any questions)
- Previous reports of abuse in the family
- Frequent emergency department or clinic visits

Adapted from Hockenberry MJ, Wilson D: *Wong's nursing care of infants and children,* ed 10, St Louis, 2015, Mosby.

Assess the availability and appropriateness of experiences contributing to psychosocial development. Hospitalized infants often have difficulty establishing physical boundaries because of repeated bodily intrusions and painful sensations. Limiting these negative experiences and providing pleasurable sensations are interventions that support early psychosocial development. Extended separations from parents complicate the attachment process and increase the number of caregivers with whom the infant must interact. Ideally the parents provide the majority of care during hospitalization. When parents are not present, either at home or in the hospital, make an attempt to limit the number of different caregivers who have contact with the infant and to follow the parents' directions for care. These interventions foster the infant's continuing development of trust.

Play. Play provides opportunities for development of cognitive, social, and motor skills. Much of infant play is exploratory as infants use their senses to observe and examine their own bodies and objects of interest in their surroundings. Adults facilitate infant learning by planning activities that promote the development of milestones and providing toys that are safe for infants to explore with their mouth and manipulate with their hands such as rattles, wooden blocks, plastic stacking rings, squeezable stuffed animals, and busy boxes.

Health Risks

Injury Prevention. Injury from motor vehicle accidents, aspiration, suffocation, falls, or poisoning is a major cause of death in children 6 to 12 months old. An understanding of the major developmental accomplishments during this time period allows for injury-prevention planning. As the child achieves gains in motor development and becomes increasingly curious about the environment, constant watchfulness and supervision are critical for injury prevention.

Child Maltreatment. Child maltreatment includes intentional physical abuse or neglect, emotional abuse or neglect, and sexual abuse (Hockenberry and Wilson, 2015). More children suffer from neglect than any other type of maltreatment. Children of any age can suffer from maltreatment, but the youngest are the most vulnerable. In addition, many children suffer from more than one type of maltreatment. No one profile fits a victim of maltreatment, and the signs and symptoms vary (Box 12-1).

A combination of signs and symptoms or a pattern of injury should arouse suspicion. It is important for the health care provider to be aware of certain disease processes and cultural practices. Lack of awareness of normal variants such as Mongolian spots causes the health care provider to assume that there is abuse. Children who are hospitalized for maltreatment have the same developmental needs as other children their age, and the nurse needs to support the child's relationship with the parents (Hockenberry and Wilson, 2015).

Health Promotion

Nutrition. The quality and quantity of nutrition profoundly influence an infant's growth and development. Many women have already selected a feeding method well before an infant's birth; others will have questions for the nurse later in the pregnancy. Nurses are in a unique position to help parents select and provide a nutritionally adequate diet for their infant. Understand that factors such as support, culture, role demands, and previous experiences influence feeding methods (Hockenberry and Wilson, 2015).

Breastfeeding is recommended for infant nutrition because breast milk contains the essential nutrients of protein, fats, carbohydrates, and immunoglobulins that bolster the ability to resist infection. Both the AAP and the U.S. Department of Health and Human Services (USDHHS) recommend human milk for the first year of life (Hockenberry and Wilson, 2015). However, if breastfeeding is not possible or if the parent does not desire it, an acceptable alternative is iron-fortified commercially prepared formula. Recent advances in the preparation of infant formula include the addition of nucleotides and long-chain fatty acids, which augment immune function and increase brain development. The use of whole cow's milk, 2% cow's milk, or alternate milk products before the age of 12 months is not recommended. The composition of whole cow's milk can cause intestinal bleeding, anemia, and increased incidence of allergies (Hockenberry and Wilson, 2015).

The average 1-month-old infant takes approximately 18 to 21 ounces of breast milk or formula per day. This amount increases slightly during the first 6 months and decreases after introducing solid foods. The amount of formula per feeding and the number of feedings vary among infants. The addition of solid foods is not recommended before the age of 6 months because the gastrointestinal tract is not sufficiently mature to handle these complex nutrients and infants are exposed to food antigens that produce food protein allergies. Developmentally infants are not ready for solid food before 6 months. The extrusion (protrusion) reflex causes food to be pushed out of the mouth. The introduction of cereals, fruits, vegetables, and meats during the second 6 months of life provides iron and additional sources of vitamins. This becomes especially important when children change from breast milk or formula to whole cow's milk after the first birthday. Solid foods should be offered one new food at a time. This allows for identification if a food causes an allergic reaction. The use of fruit juices and nonnutritive drinks such as fruit-flavored drinks or soda should be avoided since these do not provide sufficient and appropriate calories during this period (Hockenberry and Wilson, 2015). Infants also tolerate well-cooked table foods by 1 year. The amount and frequency of feedings vary among infants; thus be sure to discuss differing feeding patterns with parents.

Supplementation. The need for dietary vitamin and mineral supplements depends on an infant's diet. Full-term infants are born with some iron stores. The breastfed infant absorbs adequate iron from breast milk during the first 4 to 6 months of life. After 6 months iron-fortified cereal is generally an adequate supplemental source. Because iron in formula is less readily absorbed than that in breast milk, formula-fed infants need to receive iron-fortified formula throughout the first year.

Adequate concentrations of fluoride to protect against dental caries are not available in human milk; therefore fluoridated water or supplemental fluoride is generally recommended. A recent concern is the use of complementary and alternative medical therapies in children that may or may not be safe. Inquire about the use of such products to help the parent determine whether or not the product is truly safe for the child (Hockenberry and Wilson, 2015).

Immunizations. The widespread use of immunizations has resulted in the dramatic decline of infectious diseases over the past 50 years and therefore is a most important factor in health promotion during childhood. Although most immunizations can be given to people of any age, it is recommended that the administration of the primary series begin soon after birth and be completed during early childhood. Vaccines are among the safest and most reliable drugs used. Minor side effects sometimes occur; however, serious reactions are rare. Parents need instructions regarding the importance of immunizations and common side effects such as low-grade fever and local tenderness. The recommended schedule for immunizations changes as new vaccines are developed and advances are made in the field of immunology. Stay informed of the current policies and direct parents to the primary caregiver for their child's schedule. The AAP maintains the most current schedule on their Internet website, http://www.aap.org. Research over the past three decades has clearly indicated that infants experience pain with invasive procedures (e.g., injections) and that nurses need to be aware of measures to reduce or eliminate pain with any health care procedure (see Chapter 32).

Sleep. Sleep patterns vary among infants, with many having their days and nights reversed until 3 to 4 months of age. Thus it is common for infants to sleep during the day. By 6 months most infants are nocturnal and sleep between 9 and 11 hours at night. Total daily sleep averages 15 hours. Most infants take one or two naps a day by the end of the first year. Many parents have concerns regarding their infant's sleep patterns, especially if there is difficulty such as sleep refusal or frequent waking during the night. Carefully assess the individual problem before suggesting interventions to address their concern.

QSEN QSEN: BUILDING COMPETENCY IN INFORMATICS A pediatric unit is transitioning to an electronic health record. Describe the information that needs to be in an infant's chart for assessment and recording of development to support safe and effective care.

Answers to QSEN Activities can be found on the Evolve website.

TODDLER

Toddlerhood ranges from the time children begin to walk independently until they walk and run with ease, which is from 12 to 36 months. The toddler has increasing independence bolstered by greater physical mobility and cognitive abilities. Toddlers are increasingly aware of their abilities to control and are pleased with successful efforts with this new skill. This success leads them to repeated attempts to control their environments. Unsuccessful attempts at control result in negative behavior and temper tantrums. These behaviors are most common when parents stop the initial independent action. Parents cite these as the most problematic behaviors during the toddler years and at times express frustration with trying to set consistent and firm limits while simultaneously encouraging independence. Nurses and parents can deal with the negativism by limiting the opportunities for a "no" answer. For example, do not ask the toddler, "Do you want to take your medicine now?" Instead, tell the child that it is time to take medicine and offer a choice of water or juice to drink with it.

Physical Changes

The average toddler grows 7.5 cm (3 inches) in height and gains approximately 4 to 6 lbs (1.8 to 2.7 kg) each year (Hockenberry and Wilson, 2015). The rapid development of motor skills allows the child to participate in self-care activities such as feeding, dressing, and toileting. In the beginning the toddler walks in an upright position with a broad stance and gait, protuberant abdomen, and arms out to the sides for balance. Soon the child begins to navigate stairs, using a rail or the wall to maintain balance while progressing upward, placing both feet on the same step before continuing. Success provides courage to attempt the upright mode for descending the stairs in the same manner. Locomotion skills soon include running, jumping, standing on one foot for several seconds, and kicking a ball. Most toddlers ride tricycles, climb ladders, and run well by their third birthday.

Fine-motor capabilities move from scribbling spontaneously to drawing circles and crosses accurately. By 3 years the child draws simple stick people and is usually able to stack a tower of small blocks. Children now hold crayons with their fingers rather than with their fists and can imitate vertical and horizontal strokes. They are able to manage feeding themselves with a spoon without rotating it and can drink well from a cup without spilling. Toddlers can turn pages of a book one at a time and can easily turn doorknobs (Hockenberry and Wilson, 2015).

Cognitive Changes

Toddlers increase their ability to remember events and begin to put thoughts into words at about 2 years of age. They recognize that they are separate beings from their mothers, but they are unable to assume the view of another. A toddler's reasoning is based on their own experience of an event. They use symbols to represent objects, places, and people. Children demonstrate this function as they imitate the behavior of another that they viewed earlier (e.g., pretend to shave like daddy), pretend that one object is another (e.g., use a finger as a gun), and use language to stand for absent objects (e.g., request bottle).

Language. The 18-month-old child uses approximately 10 words. The 24-month-old child has a vocabulary of up to 300 words and is generally able to speak in two-word sentences, although the ability to understand speech is much greater than the number of words acquired (Hockenberry and Wilson, 2015). According to Piaget, the preoperational stage of development begins in toddlerhood. Children begin thinking about things more symbolically as their vocabulary develops (Piaget, 1952). "Who's that?" and "What's that?" are typical questions children ask during this period. Verbal expressions such as "me do it" and "that's mine" demonstrate the 2-year-old child's use of pronouns and desire for independence and control. By 36 months the child can use simple sentences, follow some grammatical rules, and learn to use five or six new words each day. Parents can facilitate language development best by talking to their children. Reading to children helps expand their vocabulary, knowledge, and imagination. Television should not be used to replace parent-child interaction, as it has been shown to delay language development (Hockenberry and Wilson, 2015).

Psychosocial Changes

According to Erikson (1963) a sense of autonomy emerges during toddlerhood. Children strive for independence by using their developing muscles to do everything for themselves and become the master of their bodily functions. Their strong wills are frequently exhibited in negative behavior when caregivers attempt to direct their actions. Temper tantrums result when parental restrictions frustrate toddlers. Parents need to provide toddlers with graded independence, allowing them to do things that do not result in harm to themselves or others. For example, young toddlers who want to learn to hold their own cups often benefit from two-handled cups with spouts and plastic bibs with pockets to collect the milk that spills during the learning process.

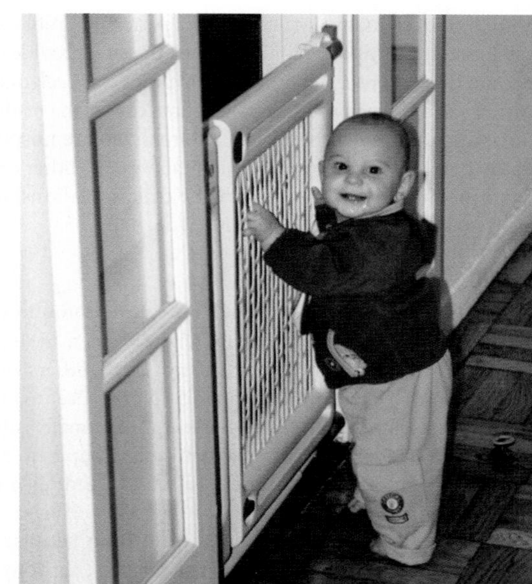

FIGURE 12-5 Safety precautions should be provided for toddlers. (Courtesy Elaine Polan, RNC, BSN, MS.)

Play. During the preoperational stage of development the child's imagination develops, and children begin to discern the difference between past and future, although they still do not grasp more complex concepts such as cause and effect (Piaget, 1952). Socially toddlers remain strongly attached to their parents and fear separation from them. In their presence they feel safe, and their curiosity is evident in their exploration of the environment. The child continues to engage in solitary play during toddlerhood but also begins to participate in parallel play, which is playing *beside* rather than *with* another child. Play expands the child's cognitive and psychosocial development. It is always important to consider if toys support development of the child, along with the safety of the toy.

Health Risks

The newly developed locomotion abilities and insatiable curiosity of toddlers make them at risk for injury. Toddlers need close supervision at all times and particularly when in environments that are not childproofed (Figure 12-5).

Poisonings occur frequently because children near 2 years of age are interested in placing any object or substance in their mouths to learn about it. The prudent parent removes or locks up all possible poisons, including plants, cleaning materials, and medications. These parental actions create a safer environment for exploratory behavior. Lead poisoning continues to be a serious health hazard in the United States, and children under the age of 6 years are most vulnerable (Hockenberry and Wilson, 2015).

Toddlers' lack of awareness regarding the danger of water and their newly developed walking skills make drowning a major cause of accidental death in this age-group. Limit setting is extremely important for toddlers' safety. Motor vehicle accidents account for half of all accidental deaths in children between the ages of 1 and 4 years. Some of these deaths are the result of unrestrained children, and some are attributed to injuries within the car resulting from not using car seat safety guidelines (Hockenberry and Wilson, 2015). Injury prevention is best accomplished by associating various injuries with the attainment of developmental milestones.

Toddlers who become ill and require hospitalization are most stressed by the separation from their parents. Nurses encourage parents to stay with their child as much as possible and actively participate in providing care. Creating an environment that supports parents helps greatly in gaining the cooperation of the toddler. Establishing a trusting relationship with the parents often results in toddler acceptance of treatment.

Health Promotion

Nutrition. Childhood obesity and the associated chronic diseases that result are sources of concern for all health care providers. Children establish lifetime eating habits in early childhood, and there is increased emphasis on food choices. They increasingly meet nutritional needs by eating solid foods. The healthy toddler requires a balanced daily intake of bread and grains, vegetables, fruit, dairy products, and proteins. Because the consumption of more than a quart of milk per day usually decreases a child's appetite for these essential solid foods and results in inadequate iron intake, advise parents to limit milk intake to 2 to 3 cups per day (Hockenberry and Wilson, 2015). Children should not be offered low-fat or skim milk until age 2 because they need the fat for satisfactory physical and intellectual growth.

Mealtime has psychosocial and physical significance. If the parents struggle to control toddlers' dietary intake, problem behavior and conflicts can result. Toddlers often develop "food jags," or the desire to eat one food repeatedly. Rather than becoming disturbed by this behavior, encourage parents to offer a variety of nutritious foods at meals and to provide only nutritious snacks between meals. Serving finger foods to toddlers allows them to eat by themselves and to satisfy their need for independence and control. Small, reasonable servings allow toddlers to eat all of their meals.

Toilet Training. Increased locomotion skills, the ability to undress, and development of sphincter control allow toilet training if a toddler has developed the necessary language and cognitive abilities. Parents often consult nurses for an assessment of readiness for toilet training. Recognizing the urge to urinate and or defecate is crucial in determining a child's mental readiness. The toddler must also be motivated to hold on to please the parent rather than letting go to please the self to successfully accomplish toilet training (Hockenberry and Wilson, 2015). As a nurse, remind parents that patience, consistency, and a nonjudgmental attitude, in addition to the child's readiness, are essential to successful toilet training.

PRESCHOOLERS

The preschool period refers to the years between ages 3 and 5. Children refine the mastery of their bodies and eagerly await the beginning of formal education. Many people consider these the most intriguing years of parenting because children are less negative, more accurately share their thoughts, and more effectively interact and communicate. Physical development occurs at a slower pace than cognitive and psychosocial development.

Physical Changes

Several aspects of physical development continue to stabilize in the preschool years. Children gain about 5 lbs (2.3 kg) per year; the average weight at 3 years is 32 lbs (14.5 kg); at 4 years, 37 lbs (16.8 kg); and at 5 years about 41 lbs (18.6 kg). Preschoolers grow 6.2 to 7.5 cm (2½ to 3 inches) per year, double their birth length around 4 years, and stand an average of 107 cm (43 inches) tall by their fifth birthday. The elongation of the legs results in more slender-appearing children. Little difference exists between the sexes, although boys are slightly larger with more muscle and less fatty tissue. Most children are completely toilet trained by the preschool years (Hockenberry and Wilson, 2015).

Large- and fine-muscle coordination improves. Preschoolers run well, walk up and down steps with ease, and learn to hop. By 5 years they usually skip on alternate feet, jump rope, and begin to skate and swim. Improving fine-motor skills allows intricate manipulations. They learn to copy crosses and squares. Triangles and diamonds are usually mastered between ages 5 and 6. Scribbling and drawing help to develop fine-muscle skills and the eye-hand coordination needed for the printing of letters and numbers.

Children need opportunities to learn and practice new physical skills. Nursing care of healthy and ill children includes an assessment of the availability of these opportunities. Although children with acute illnesses benefit from rest and exclusion from usual daily activities, children who have chronic conditions or who have been hospitalized for long periods need ongoing exposure to developmental opportunities. The parents and nurse weave these opportunities into the children's daily experiences, depending on their abilities, needs, and energy level.

Cognitive Changes

Maturation of the brain continues, with the most rapid growth occurring in the frontal lobe areas, where planning and organizing new activities and maintaining attention to tasks are paramount. Complete myelinization of the brain neurons does not occur until age 6 or 7 (Leifer, 2013).

Preschoolers demonstrate their ability to think more complexly by classifying objects according to size or color and by questioning. Children have increased social interaction, as is illustrated by the 5-year-old child who offers a bandage to a child with a cut finger. Children become aware of cause-and-effect relationships, as illustrated by the statement, "The sun sets because people want to go to bed." Early causal thinking is also evident in preschoolers. For example, if two events are related in time or space, children link them in a causal fashion. For example, the hospitalized child reasons, "I cried last night, and that's why the nurse gave me the shot." As children near age 5, they begin to use or learn to use rules to understand causation. They then begin to reason from the general to the particular. This forms the basis for more formal logical thought. The child now reasons, "I get a shot twice a day, and that's why I got one last night." Children in this stage also believe that inanimate objects have lifelike qualities and are capable of action, as seen through comments such as, "Trees cry when their branches get broken."

Preschoolers' knowledge of the world remains closely linked to concrete (perceived by the senses) experiences. Even their rich fantasy life is grounded in their perception of reality. The mixing of the two aspects often leads to many childhood fears, and adults sometimes misinterpret it as lying when children are actually presenting reality from their perspective. Preschoolers believe that, if a rule is broken, punishment results immediately. During these years they believe that a punishment is automatically connected to an act and do not yet realize that it is socially mediated (Perry et al., 2014).

The greatest fear of this age-group appears to be that of bodily harm; this is evident in children's fear of the dark, animals, thunderstorms, and medical personnel. This fear often interferes with their willingness to allow nursing interventions such as measurement of vital signs. Preschoolers cooperate if they are allowed to help the nurse measure the blood pressure of a parent or to manipulate the nurse's equipment.

Language. Preschoolers' vocabularies continue to increase rapidly; by the age of 6 children have 8000 to 14,000 words that they use to define familiar objects, identify colors, and express their desires and frustrations (Perry et al., 2014). Language is more social, and questions expand to "Why?" and "How come?" in the quest for information. Phonetically similar words such as *die* and *dye* or *wood* and *would* cause confusion in preschool children. Avoid such words when preparing them for procedures and assess comprehension of explanations.

Psychosocial Changes

The world of preschoolers expands beyond the family into the neighborhood where children meet other children and adults. Their curiosity and developing initiative lead to actively exploring the environment, developing new skills, and making new friends. Preschoolers have a surplus of energy that permits them to plan and attempt many activities that are beyond their capabilities such as pouring milk from a gallon container into their cereal bowls. Guilt arises within children when they overstep the limits of their abilities and think that they have not behaved correctly. Children who in anger wished that their sibling were dead experience guilt if that sibling becomes ill. Children need to learn that "wishing" for something to happen does not make it occur. Erikson (1963) recommends that parents help their children strike a healthy balance between initiative and guilt by allowing them to do things on their own while setting firm limits and providing guidance.

Sources of stress for preschoolers can include changes in caregiving arrangements, starting school, the birth of a sibling, parental marital distress, relocation to a new home, or an illness. During these times of stress preschoolers sometimes revert to bed-wetting or thumb sucking and want the parents to feed, dress, and hold them. These dependent behaviors are often confusing and embarrassing to parents. They benefit from the nurse's reassurance that they are the child's normal coping behaviors. Provide experiences that these children are able to master. Such successes help them return to their prior level of independent functioning. As language skills develop, encourage children to talk about their feelings. Play is also an excellent way for preschoolers to vent frustration or anger and is a socially acceptable way to deal with stress.

Play. The play of preschool children becomes more social after the third birthday as it shifts from parallel to associative play. Children playing together engage in similar if not identical activity; however, there is no division of labor or rigid organization or rules. Most 3-year-old children are able to play with one other child in a cooperative manner in which they make something or play designated roles such as mother and baby. By age 4 children play in groups of two or three, and by 5 years the group has a temporary leader for each activity.

During the preoperational stage of growth and development the child begins to engage in "make-believe" play (Piaget, 1952). Pretend play allows children to learn to understand others' points of view, develop skills in solving social problems, and become more creative. Some children have imaginary playmates. These playmates serve many purposes. They are friends when the child is lonely, they accomplish what the child is still attempting, and they experience what the child wants to forget or remember. Imaginary playmates are a sign of health and allow the child to distinguish between reality and fantasy.

Television (TV), videos, electronic games, and computer programs also help support development and the learning of basic skills. However, these should be only one part of the child's total play activities. The AAP (2014a) advises no more than 1 to 2 hours per day of educational, nonviolent TV programs, which should be supervised by parents or other responsible adults in the home. Limiting TV viewing will provide more time for children to read, engage in physical activity, and socialize with others (Hockenberry and Wilson, 2015).

Health Risks

As fine- and gross-motor skills develop and a child becomes more coordinated with better balance, falls become much less of a problem. Guidelines for injury prevention in the toddler also apply to the preschooler. Children need to learn about safety in the home, and parents need to continue close supervision of activities. Children at this age are great imitators; thus parental example is important. For instance, parental use of a helmet while bicycling sets an appropriate example for the preschooler.

Health Promotion

Little research has explored preschoolers' perceptions of their own health. Parental beliefs about health, children's bodily sensations, and their ability to perform usual daily activities help children develop attitudes about their health. Preschoolers are usually quite independent in washing, dressing, and feeding. Alterations in this independence influence their feelings about their own health.

Nutrition. Nutrition requirements for the preschooler vary little from those of the toddler. The average daily intake is 1800 calories. Parents often worry about the amount of food their child is consuming, and this is a relevant concern because of the problem of childhood obesity. However, the quality of the food is more important than quantity in most situations. Preschoolers consume about half of average adult portion sizes. Finicky eating habits are characteristic of the 4-year-old; however, the 5-year-old is more interested in trying new foods (CDC, 2014).

Sleep. Preschoolers average 12 hours of sleep a night and take infrequent naps. Sleep disturbances are common during these years. Disturbances range from trouble getting to sleep to nightmares to prolonging bedtime with extensive rituals. Frequently children have had an overabundance of activity and stimulation. Helping them slow down before bedtime usually results in better sleeping habits.

Vision. Vision screening usually begins in the preschool years and needs to occur at regular intervals. One of the most important tests is to determine the presence of nonbinocular vision or strabismus. Early detection and treatment of strabismus are essential by ages 4 to 6 to prevent amblyopia, the resulting blindness from disuse (Hockenberry and Wilson, 2015).

SCHOOL-AGE CHILDREN AND ADOLESCENTS

The developmental changes between ages 6 and 18 are diverse and span all areas of growth and development. Children develop, expand, refine, and synchronize physical, psychosocial, cognitive, and moral skills so the individual is able to become an accepted and productive member of society. The environment in which the individual develops skills also expands and diversifies. Instead of the boundaries of family and close friends, the environment now includes the school, community, and church. With age-specific assessment, you need to review the appropriate developmental expectations for each age-group. You can promote health by helping children and adolescents achieve a necessary developmental balance.

SCHOOL-AGE CHILDREN

During these "middle years" of childhood, the foundation for adult roles in work, recreation, and social interaction is laid. In industrialized countries this school-age period begins when the child starts elementary school around the age of 6 years. Puberty, around 12 years of age, signals the end of middle childhood. Children make great developmental strides during these years as they develop competencies in physical, cognitive, and psychosocial skills.

The school or educational experience expands the child's world and is a transition from a life of relatively free play to one of structured play, learning, and work. The school and home influence growth and development, requiring adjustment by the parents and child. The child learns to cope with rules and expectations presented by the school and peers. Parents have to learn to allow their child to make decisions, accept responsibility, and learn from the experiences of life.

Physical Changes

The rate of growth during these early school years is slow and consistent, a relative calm before the growth spurt of adolescence. The school-age child appears slimmer than the preschooler as a result of changes in fat distribution and thickness. The average increase in height is 5 cm (2 inches) per year, and weight increases by 4 to 7 lbs (1.8 to 3.2 kg) per year. Many children double their weight during these middle childhood years, and most girls exceed boys in both height and weight by the end of the school years (Hockenberry and Wilson, 2015).

School-age children become more graceful during the school years because their large-muscle coordination improves and their strength doubles. Most children practice the basic gross-motor skills of running, jumping, balancing, throwing, and catching during play, resulting in refinement of neuromuscular function and skills. Individual differences in the rate of mastering skills and ultimate skill achievement become apparent during their participation in many activities and games. Fine-motor skills improve; and, as children gain control over fingers and wrists, they become proficient in a wide range of activities.

Most 6-year-old children are able to hold a pencil adeptly and print letters and words; by age 12 a child is able to make detailed drawings and write sentences in script. Painting, drawing, playing computer games, and modeling allow children to practice and improve newly refined skills. The improved fine-motor capabilities of youngsters in middle childhood allow them to become very independent in bathing, dressing, and taking care of other personal needs. They develop strong personal preferences in the way these needs are met. Illness and hospitalization threaten children's control in these areas. Therefore it is important to allow them to participate in care and maintain as much independence as possible. Children whose care demands restriction of fluids cannot be allowed to decide the amount of fluids they will drink in 24 hours. However, they can help decide the type of fluids and help keep a record of their intake.

Assessment of neurological development is often based on fine-motor coordination. Fine-motor coordination is critical to success in the typical American school, where children have to hold pencils and crayons and use scissors and rulers. The opportunity to practice these skills through schoolwork and play is essential to learning coordinated, complex behaviors.

As skeletal growth progresses, a child's body appearance and posture change. Earlier the child's posture was stoop shouldered, with slight lordosis and a prominent abdomen. The posture of a school-age child is more erect. It is essential to evaluate children, especially girls after the age of 12 years, for scoliosis, the lateral curvature of the spine.

Eye shape alters because of skeletal growth. This improves visual acuity, and normal adult 20/20 vision is achievable. Screening for vision and hearing problems is easier, and results are more reliable because school-age children more fully understand and cooperate with the test directions. The school nurse typically assesses the growth, visual, and auditory status of school-age children and refers those with possible deviations to a health care provider such as their family practitioner or pediatrician.

Cognitive Changes

According to Piaget, children begin transitioning into the concrete-operational stage of growth and development around the age of 7 when they begin to demonstrate logical, more concrete thinking. They become less egocentric and begin to understand that their thoughts and feelings may not be shared by others (Piaget, 1952). Cognitive changes provide the school-age child with the ability to think in a logical manner about the here and now and to understand the relationship between things and ideas. They are now able to use their developed thinking abilities to experience events without having to act them out (Hockenberry and Wilson, 2015). Their thoughts are no longer dominated by their perceptions; thus their ability to understand the world greatly expands.

School-age children have the ability to concentrate on more than one aspect of a situation. They begin to understand that others do not always see things as they do and even begin to understand another viewpoint. They now have the ability to recognize that the amount or quantity of a substance remains the same even when its shape or appearance changes. For instance, two balls of clay of equal size remain the same amount of clay even when one is flattened and the other remains in the shape of a ball.

The young child is able to separate objects into groups according to shape or color, whereas the school-age child understands that the same element can exist in two classes at the same time. By 7 or 8 years these children develop the ability to place objects in order according to their increasing or decreasing size (Hockenberry and Wilson, 2015). School-age children frequently have collections such as baseball cards or stuffed animals that demonstrate this new cognitive skill.

Language Development. Language growth is so rapid during middle childhood that it is no longer possible to match age with language achievements. Children improve their use of language and expand their structural knowledge. They become more aware of the rules of syntax, the rules for linking words into phrases and sentences. They also identify generalizations and exceptions to rules. They accept language as a means for representing the world in a subjective manner and realize that words have arbitrary rather than absolute meanings. Children begin to think about language, which enables them to appreciate jokes and riddles. They are not as likely to use a literal interpretation of a word; rather they reason about its meaning within a context (Hockenberry and Wilson, 2015).

Psychosocial Changes

Erikson (1963) identifies the developmental task for school-age children as industry vs. inferiority. During this time children strive to acquire competence and skills necessary for them to function as adults. School-age children who are positively recognized for success feel a sense of worth. Those faced with failure often feel a sense of mediocrity

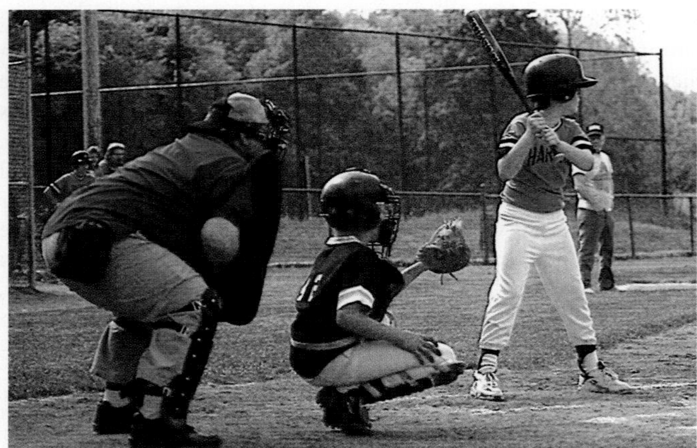

FIGURE 12-6 School-age children gain a sense of achievement working and playing with peers. (From Hockenberry MJ, Wilson D: *Wong's nursing care of infants and children,* ed 10, St Louis, 2015, Mosby.)

or unworthiness, which sometimes results in withdrawal from school and peers.

School-age children begin to define themselves on the basis of internal more than external characteristics. They begin to define their self-concept and develop self-esteem, an overall self-evaluation. Interaction with peers allows them to define their own accomplishments in relation to others as they work to develop a positive self-image (Perry et al., 2014).

According to Piaget, school-age children around the age of 11 may begin to enter the fourth and final stage of intellectual development, formal operations. In this stage they begin to ponder abstract relationships. They can formulate hypotheses and consider different possibilities. Piaget believed that this was the final stage of cognitive development and that the continued intellectual development in teenagers and adults depended on the accumulation of knowledge (Piaget, 1952).

Peer Relationships. Group and personal achievements become important to the school-age child. Success is important in physical and cognitive activities. Play involves peers and the pursuit of group goals. Although solitary activities are not eliminated, group play overshadows them. Learning to contribute, collaborate, and work cooperatively toward a common goal becomes a measure of success (Figure 12-6).

The school-age child prefers same-sex to opposite-sex peers. In general, girls and boys view the opposite sex negatively. Peer influence becomes quite diverse during this stage of development. Clubs and peer groups become prominent. School-age children often develop "best friends" with whom they share secrets and with whom they look forward to interacting on a daily basis. Group identity increases as the school-age child approaches adolescence.

Sexual Identity. Freud described middle childhood as the latency period because he believed that children of this period had little interest in their sexuality. Today many researchers believe that school-age children have a great deal of curiosity about their sexuality. Some experiment, but this play is usually transitory. Children's curiosity about adult magazines or meanings of sexually explicit words is also an example of their sexual interest. This is the time for them to have exposure to sex education, including sexual maturation, reproduction, and relationships (Hockenberry and Wilson, 2015).

Stress. Today's children experience more stress than children in earlier generations. Stress comes from parental expectations; peer expectations; the school environment; and violence in the family, school, or community. Some school-age children care for themselves before or after school without adult supervision. Latchkey children sometimes feel increased stress and are at greater risk for injury and unsafe behaviors (Hockenberry and Wilson, 2015). A nurse helps the child cope with stress by helping the parents and child identify potential stressors and designing interventions to minimize stress and the child's stress response. Deep-breathing techniques, positive imagery, and progressive relaxation of muscle groups are interventions that most children can learn (see Chapter 38). Include the parent, child, and teacher in the intervention for maximal success.

Health Risks

Accidents and injuries are a major health problem affecting school-age children. They now have more exposure to various environments and less supervision, but their developed cognitive and motor skills make them less likely to suffer from unintentional injury. Some school-age children are risk takers and attempt activities that are beyond their abilities. Motor vehicle injuries as a passenger or pedestrian and bicycle injuries are among the most common in this age-group.

Infections account for the majority of all childhood illnesses; respiratory infections are the most prevalent. The common cold remains the chief illness of childhood. Certain groups of children are more prone to disease and disability, often as a result of barriers to health care. Poverty and the prevalence of illness are highly correlated. Access to care is often very limited, and health promotion and preventive health measures are minimal.

Health Promotion

Perceptions. During the school-age years identity and self-concept become stronger and more individualized. Perception of wellness is based on readily observable facts such as presence or absence of illness and adequacy of eating or sleeping. Functional ability is the standard by which personal health and the health of others are judged. Six-year-olds are aware of their body and modest and sensitive about being exposed. Nurses need to provide for privacy and offer explanations of common procedures.

Health Education. The school-age period is crucial for the acquisition of behaviors and health practices for a healthy adult life. Because cognition is advancing during the period, effective health education must be developmentally appropriate. Promotion of good health practices is a nursing responsibility. Programs directed at health education are frequently organized and conducted in the school. Effective health education teaches children about their bodies and how the choices they make impact their health (Hockenberry and Wilson, 2015). During these programs focus on the development of behaviors that positively affect children's health status.

Health Maintenance. Parents need to recognize the importance of annual health maintenance visits for immunizations, screenings, and dental care. When their school-age child reaches 10 years of age, parents need to begin discussions in preparation for upcoming pubertal changes. Topics include introductory information regarding menstruation, sexual intercourse, reproduction, and **sexually transmitted infections (STIs)**. Human papilloma virus (HPV) is a widespread virus that will infect over 50% of males and females in their lifetime (AAP, 2015b). For many individuals HPV clears spontaneously, but for others it can cause significant consequences. Females can develop cervical, vaginal, and vulvar cancers and genital warts; and males can develop genital warts. Since it is not possible to determine who will or will not develop disease from the virus, the Centers for Disease Control and

Prevention (CDC, 2013b), along with the AAP, recommends routine HPV vaccination for girls ages 11 to 12 and for young women ages 13 through 26 who have not already been vaccinated. It is further recommended that HPV vaccine be given to boys and young men ages 9 to 26 years.

Safety. Because accidents such as fires and car and bicycle crashes are the leading cause of death and injury in the school-age period, safety is a priority health teaching consideration. Educate children about safety measures to prevent accidents. At this age encourage children to take responsibility for their own safety, such as wearing helmets during bike riding.

Nutrition. Growth often slows during the school-age period as compared to infancy and adolescence. School-age children are developing eating patterns that are independent of parental supervision. The availability of snacks and fast-food restaurants makes it increasingly difficult for children to make healthy choices. The prevalence of obesity among children 6 to 11 years of age increased from 6.5% in 1980 to 18% in 2012. In addition, the incidence of adolescents ages 12 to 19 years who were obese increased from 5% to almost 21% during the same period of time (CDC, 2014). Childhood obesity has become a prominent health problem, resulting in increased risk for hypertension, diabetes, coronary heart disease, fatty liver disease, pulmonary complications such as sleep apnea, musculoskeletal problems, dyslipidemia, and potential for psychological problems. Studies have found that overweight children are teased more often, less likely to be chosen as a friend, and more likely to be thought of as lazy and sloppy by their peers (Hockenberry and Wilson, 2015). Nurses contribute to meeting national policy goals by promoting healthy lifestyle habits, including nutrition. School-age children need to participate in educational programs that enable them to plan, select, and prepare healthy meals and snacks. Children need adequate caloric intake for growth throughout childhood accompanied by activity for continued gross-motor development.

ADOLESCENTS

Adolescence is the period during which the individual makes the transition from childhood to adulthood, usually between ages 13 and 20 years. The term *adolescent* usually refers to psychological maturation of the individual, whereas **puberty** refers to the point at which reproduction becomes possible. The hormonal changes of puberty result in changes in the appearance of the young person, and cognitive development results in the ability to hypothesize and deal with abstractions. Adjustments and adaptations are necessary to cope with these simultaneous changes and the attempt to establish a mature sense of identity. In the past many referred to adolescence as a stormy and stressful period filled with inner turmoil, but today it is recognized that most teenagers successfully meet the challenges of this period.

Your understanding of development provides a unique perspective for helping teenagers and parents anticipate and cope with the stresses of adolescence. Nursing activities, particularly education, promote healthy development. These activities occur in a variety of settings; and you can direct them at the adolescent, parents, or both. For example, a nurse conducts seminars in a high school to provide practical suggestions for solving problems of concern to a large group of students such as treating acne or making responsible decisions about drugs or alcohol use. Similarly a group education program for parents about how to cope with teenagers would promote parental understanding of adolescent development.

Physical Changes

Physical changes occur rapidly in adolescence. Sexual maturation occurs with the development of primary and secondary sexual characteristics. The four main physical changes are:

1. Increased growth rate of skeleton, muscle, and viscera.
2. Sex-specific changes such as changes in shoulder and hip width.
3. Alteration in distribution of muscle and fat.
4. Development of the reproductive system and secondary sex characteristics.

Wide variation exists in the timing of physical changes associated with puberty between sexes and within the same sex.

Girls generally have prepubescent changes 1 to 2 years before boys do. There is also evidence that African-American girls develop at a younger age than Caucasian girls. Although not clear, this phenomenon is believed to be influenced by being overweight and environmental factors (Perry et al., 2014). The rates of height and weight gain are usually proportional, and the sequence of pubertal growth changes is the same in most individuals.

Hormonal changes within the body create change when the hypothalamus begins to produce gonadotropin-releasing hormones that stimulate ovarian cells to produce estrogen and testicular cells to produce testosterone. These hormones contribute to the development of secondary sex characteristics such as hair growth and voice changes and play an essential role in reproduction. The changing concentrations of these hormones are also linked to acne and body odor. Understanding these hormonal changes enables you to reassure adolescents and educate them about body care needs.

Being like peers is extremely important for adolescents (Figure 12-7). Any deviation in the timing of their physical changes is extremely difficult for them to accept. Therefore provide emotional support for those undergoing early or delayed puberty. Even adolescents whose physical changes are occurring at the normal times seek confirmation of and reassurance about their normalcy.

Height and weight increases usually occur during the prepubertal growth spurt, which peaks in girls at about 12 years and boys at about 14 years. Girls' height increases 5 to 20 cm (2 to 8 inches), and weight increases by 15 to 55 lbs (6.8 to 25 kg). Boys' height increases approximately 10 to 30 cm (4 to 12 inches), and weight increases by 15 to 65 lbs (6.8 to 29.5 kg). Individuals gain the final 20% to 25% of their height and 50% of their weight during this time period (Hockenberry and Wilson, 2015).

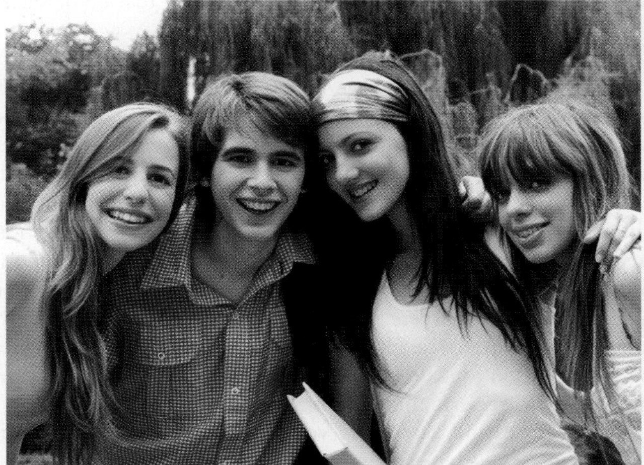

FIGURE 12-7 Peer interactions help increase self-esteem during puberty. (©Petrenko Andriy.)

Girls attain 90% to 95% of their adult height by menarche (the onset of menstruation) and reach their full height by 16 to 17 years of age, whereas boys continue to grow taller until 18 to 20 years of age. Fat is redistributed into adult proportions as height and weight increase, and gradually the adolescent torso takes on an adult appearance. Although individual and sex differences exist, growth follows a similar pattern for both sexes. Personal growth curves help the nurse assess physical development. However, the individual's sustained progression along the curve is more important than a comparison to the norm.

Cognitive Changes

The adolescent develops the ability to determine and rank possibilities, solve problems, and make decisions through logical operations. The teenager thinks abstractly and deals effectively with hypothetical problems. When confronted with a problem, the adolescent considers an infinite variety of causes and solutions. For the first time the young person moves beyond the physical or concrete properties of a situation and uses reasoning powers to understand the abstract. School-age individuals think about what is, whereas adolescents are able to imagine what might be.

Adolescents are now able to think in terms of the future rather than just current events. These newly developed abilities allow an individual to have more insight and skill in playing video, computer, and board games that require abstract thinking and deductive reasoning about many possible strategies. A teenager even solves problems requiring simultaneous manipulation of several abstract concepts. Development of this ability is important in the pursuit of an identity. For example, newly acquired cognitive skills allow the teenager to define appropriate, effective, and comfortable sex-role behaviors and to consider their impact on peers, family, and society. A higher level of cognitive functioning makes the adolescent receptive to more detailed and diverse information about sexuality and sexual behaviors. For example, sex education includes an explanation of physiological sexual changes and birth control measures.

Adolescents also develop the ability to understand how an individual's ideas or actions influence others. This complex development of thought leads them to question society and its values. Although adolescents have the capability to think as well as an adult, they do not have experiences on which to build. It is common for teenagers to consider their parents too narrow minded or materialistic. At this time adolescents believe that they are unique and the exception, giving rise to their risk-taking behaviors. In other words, they think that they are invincible. For example, an adolescent might state that he or she "is able to drive fast and not have an accident."

Language Skills. Language development is fairly complete by adolescence, although vocabulary continues to expand. The primary focus becomes communication skills that an adolescent uses effectively in various situations. Adolescents need to communicate thoughts, feelings, and facts to peers, parents, teachers, and other people of authority. The skills used in these diverse communication situations vary. Adolescents need to select the people with whom to communicate, decide on the exact message, and choose the way to transmit it. For example, how teenagers tell parents about failing grades is not the same as how they tell friends. Good communication skills are critical for adolescents in overcoming peer pressure and unhealthy behaviors. The following are some hints for communicating with adolescents:

- Do not avoid discussing sensitive issues. Asking questions about sex, drugs, and school opens the channels for further discussion.
- Ask open-ended questions (see Chapter 24).
- Look for the meaning behind their words or actions.
- Be alert to clues to their emotional state.
- Involve other individuals and resources when necessary.

Psychosocial Changes

The search for personal identity is the major task of adolescent psychosocial development. Teenagers establish close peer relationships or remain socially isolated. Erikson (1963) sees identity (or role) confusion as the prime danger of this stage and suggests that the cliquish behavior and intolerance of differences seen in adolescent behavior are defenses against identity confusion (Erikson, 1968). Adolescents work at becoming emotionally independent from their parents while retaining family ties. They are often described as being ambivalent. They love and hate their parents. In addition, they need to develop their own ethical systems based on personal values. They need to make choices about vocation, future education, and lifestyle. The various components of total identity evolve from these tasks and compose adult personal identity that is unique to the individual.

Sexual Identity. Physical changes of puberty enhance achievement of sexual identity. The physical evidence of maturity encourages the development of masculine and feminine behaviors. If these physical changes involve deviations, the person has more difficulty developing a comfortable sexual identity. Adolescents depend on these physical clues because they want assurance of maleness or femaleness and they do not wish to be different from peers. Without these physical characteristics, achieving sexual identity is difficult.

Group Identity. Adolescents seek a group identity because they need esteem and acceptance. Similarity in dress or speech is common in teenage groups. Peer groups provide the adolescent with a sense of belonging, approval, and the opportunity to learn acceptable behavior. Popularity with opposite-sex and same-sex peers is important. The strong need for group identity seems to conflict at times with the search for personal identity. It is as though adolescents require close bonds with peers so they later achieve a sense of individuality.

Family Identity. The movement toward stronger peer relationships is contrasted with adolescents' movements away from parents. Although financial independence for adolescents is not the norm in American society, many work part-time, using their income to bolster independence. When they cannot have a part-time job because of studies, school-related activities, and other factors, parents can provide allowances for clothing and incidentals, which encourage them to develop decision-making and budgeting skills.

Some adolescents and families have more difficulty during these years than others. Adolescents need to make choices, act independently, and experience the consequences of their actions. Nurses help families consider appropriate ways for them to foster the independence of their adolescent while maintaining family structure.

Health Identity. Another component of personal identity is perception of health. This component is of specific interest to health care providers. Healthy adolescents evaluate their own health according to feelings of well-being, ability to function normally, and absence of symptoms (Hockenberry and Wilson, 2015). They also often include health maintenance and health promotion behaviors as important concerns.

Therefore interventions to improve health perception concentrate on the adolescent period. The rapid changes during this period make health promotion programs especially crucial. Adolescents try new roles, begin to stabilize their identity, and acquire values and behaviors from which their adult lifestyle will evolve. They are able to identify behaviors such as smoking and substance abuse as threatening to health in general terms but frequently tend to underestimate the effect of the potentially negative consequences of their own actions (Hockenberry and Wilson, 2015).

Health Risks

Accidents. Accidents remain the leading cause of death in adolescence. Motor vehicle accidents, which are the most common cause of death, resulted in 74% of all unintentional deaths among teens 10 to 19 years (Hockenberry and Wilson, 2015). Such accidents are often associated with alcohol intoxication or drug abuse. Bicycling fatalities were 4 to 7 times more likely to occur in males than females. Other frequent causes of accidental death in teenagers are drowning and the use of firearms. Adolescents think that they are indestructible, which leads to risk-taking behaviors. The use of alcohol precedes many injuries, and adolescents continue to be both the victims and perpetrators of violence. An objective for Healthy People 2020 is to reduce the percentage of middle and public high schools that have violent incidents (USDHHS, 2014a).

Violence and Homicide. Homicide is the second leading cause of death in the 15- to 24-year-old age-group, and for African-American teenagers it is the most likely cause of death (National Institutes of Health, 2012). Results from the Youth Risk Behavior Surveillance System show that in 2013 17.9% of high school students had carried a weapon (e.g., gun, club, or knife) at some point during the preceding 30 days (CDC, 2013a). Individuals 12 years of age and older are most likely to be killed by an acquaintance or gang member and most often with a firearm. Because having a gun in the home raises the risk of homicide and suicide for adolescents, include assessment of gun presence in the home when counseling families (Hockenberry and Wilson, 2015).

Violence among adolescents has become a national concern (Box 12-2). Statistics show that in 2012 52 out of every 1000 high-school students were the victims of violence at school (USDEIES, 2012). This violence is not just limited to physical assaults and fighting, threats and intimidation, sexual harassment, or bullying. It can also include theft. Nurses working with adolescents need to be aware of the potential for school violence and include screening questions when providing health care, regardless of the setting.

Suicide. Suicide is a major leading cause of death in adolescents 15 to 24 years of age (CDC, 2011). In recent statistics reported by the CDC, 16% of high-school students indicated that they had seriously contemplated suicide in the previous 12 months (CDC, 2012). Depression and social isolation commonly precede a suicide attempt, but suicide probably results from a combination of several factors. Nurses must be able to identify the factors associated with adolescent suicide risk and precipitating events. The following warning signs often occur for at least a month before suicide is attempted:

- Decrease in school performance
- Withdrawal
- Loss of initiative
- Loneliness, sadness, and crying
- Appetite and sleep disturbances
- Verbalization of suicidal thought

Make immediate referrals to mental health professionals when assessment suggests that adolescents are considering suicide. Guidance helps them focus on the positive aspects of life and strengthen coping abilities.

BOX 12-2 EVIDENCE-BASED PRACTICE

Prevention Programs for School-Based Violence

PICO Question: For middle- and high-school students, are classroom-based curricular programs that promote prosocial behaviors and attitudes compared with efforts to improve the social and interpersonal climate of a school more effective in reducing school violence?

Evidence Summary

School violence is a complex issue and continues to be a problem in the United States. School safety research now includes a broader range of behaviors, including aggression, violence, and bullying (Astor et al., 2010). According to data from the Centers for Disease Control and Prevention (CDC, 2013a), the prevalence of being bullied on school property was as high as 27.9%. Bullying is considered to be one of the greatest public health concerns to youth in the United States. It not only poses one of the greatest health risks, but its effects are both immediate and long term and can developmentally affect the functioning of individuals across the life span (American Educational Research Association, 2013). Students who have been bullied experience higher rates of physical and mental health problems, including depression and anxiety. They also have issues with social adjustment, which can persist into adulthood (Ttofi et al., 2011). Bullying can encompass many forms such as physical or verbal aggression, including social exclusion or humiliation. It can be mild, moderate, or severe (Espelage et al., 2013). It can take place in face-to-face confrontations or through digital media (cyber-bullying). For instance, recent research has revealed that students who engage in school violence are also more likely to have insufficient sleep (Hildebrand et al., 2013).

One approach that schools take is to strengthen school safety through target hardening and zero-tolerance policies. Target hardening makes schools more difficult targets through architectural design, security cameras, and other safety measures (Astor et al., 2010). The other approach uses educational programs, including social skills training, conflict resolution and peer mediation, sleep interventions, programs to enhance school climate, and youth development programs that help students engage in community activities. Classroom-based curricular programs are more effective when offered to students in a positive school environment that fosters relationships between students and school personnel (Johnson et al., 2011).

Application to Nursing Practice

- Ongoing school violence assessment is critical to providing a healthy school environment (Johnson et al., 2011).
- Educate parents and children about the signs of cyber-bullying such as mean or hateful emails and inappropriate social media (Espelage et al., 2013).
- Teach parents how to place safety controls on home computers and smartphones and tablets (Espelage et al., 2013).
- Focus on the importance of a good night's sleep (Hildebrand et al., 2013)
- Work with educators and students to provide an environment that promotes adolescent health. (American Educational Research Association, 2013).

Substance Abuse. Substance abuse is a concern for all who work with adolescents. Adolescents often believe that mood-altering substances create a sense of well-being or improve level of performance. All adolescents are at risk for experimental or recreational substance use, but those who have dysfunctional families are more at risk for chronic use and physical dependency. Some adolescents believe that substance use makes them more mature. They further believe that they will look and feel better with drug use (Hockenberry and Wilson, 2015). Tobacco use continues to be a problem among adolescents; and, although its use is declining, 3 out of 10 adolescents are active smokers at the time of high-school graduation.

Eating Disorders. Adolescent overweight and obesity are current concerns in the United States, and most teens try dieting at some time to control weight. Unfortunately the number of eating disorders is on the rise in adolescent girls; thus the benefits of a healthy diet should be discussed with all adolescents. Routine nutritional screening should be a part of the health care provided to all adolescents. Areas to include in the assessment are past and present diet history, food records, eating habits, attitudes, health beliefs, and socioeconomic and psychosocial factors (Hockenberry and Wilson, 2015).

Anorexia nervosa and bulimia are two eating disorders that appear in adolescence. Anorexia nervosa is a clinical syndrome with both physical and psychosocial components that involves the pursuit of thinness through starvation. People with anorexia nervosa have an intense fear of gaining weight and refuse to maintain body weight at the minimal normal weight for their age and height. Bulimia nervosa is most identified with binge eating and behaviors to prevent weight gain. Behaviors include self-induced vomiting, misuse of laxatives and other medications, and excessive exercise. Unlike anorexia, bulimia occurs within a normal weight range; thus it is much more difficult to detect. Because adolescents rarely volunteer information about behaviors to prevent weight gain, it is important to take a thorough dietary history. If left undetected and untreated, these disorders lead to significant morbidity and mortality (Grodner et al., 2012; Hockenberry and Wilson, 2015).

Sexually Transmitted Infections. Sexually transmitted infections (STIs) annually affect 3 million sexually active adolescents. This high degree of incidence makes it imperative that sexually active adolescents be screened for STIs, even when they have no symptoms. The annual physical examination of a sexually active adolescent includes a thorough sexual history and a careful examination of the genitalia so STIs are not missed. Be proactive by using the interview process to identify risk factors in the adolescent and provide education to prevent STIs, including human immunodeficiency virus (HIV), HPV, and unwanted pregnancies (Hockenberry and Wilson, 2015). As discussed earlier for school-age children, immunization for HPV infection should be considered at this time if not already administered.

Pregnancy. Adolescent pregnancy continues to be a major social challenge for our nation. The United States has the highest rate of teenage pregnancy and childbearing annually compared to other industrialized nations (Hockenberry and Wilson, 2015). Adolescent pregnancy occurs across socioeconomic classes, in public and private schools, among all ethnic and religious backgrounds, and in all parts of the country. Teenage pregnancy with early prenatal supervision is less harmful to both mother and child than earlier believed. Pregnant teens need special attention to nutrition, health supervision, and psychological support. Adolescent mothers also need help in planning for the future and obtaining competent day care for their infants.

Health Promotion

Health Education. Community and school-based health programs for adolescents focus on health promotion and illness prevention. Nurses need to be sensitive to the emotional cues from adolescents before initiating health teaching to know when the teen is ready to discuss concerns. In addition, discussions with adolescents need to be private and confidential. Adolescents define health in much the same way as adults and look for opportunities to reach their physical, mental, and emotional potential. Large numbers of school-based clinics have been developed and implemented to respond to adolescents' needs. Adolescents are much more likely to use these health care services if they encounter providers who are caring and respectful (Hockenberry and Wilson, 2015).

Nurses play an important role in preventing injuries and accidental deaths. For example, urging adolescents to discuss alternatives to driving when under the influence of drugs or alcohol prepares them to consider alternatives when such an occasion arises. As a nurse, identify adolescents at risk for abuse, provide education to prevent accidents related to substance abuse, and provide counseling to those in rehabilitation.

Minority Adolescents. By the next century estimates predict that minorities as a group will become the majority. African-American, Hispanic, Latino, Asian, Native American, and Alaska Native American adolescents are the fastest-growing segment in the U.S. population. Minority adolescents experience a greater percentage of health problems and barriers to health care (Hockenberry and Wilson, 2015). Issues of concern for these adolescents living in a high-risk environment include learning or emotional difficulties, death related to violence, unintentional injuries, increased rate for adolescent pregnancy, STIs, HIV infection, and acquired immunodeficiency syndrome (AIDS). Poverty is a major factor negatively affecting the lives of minority adolescents. Limited access to health services is common. Nurses are able to make a significant contribution to improving access to appropriate health care for adolescents. With knowledge about various cultures and the means to care for minority adolescents, nurses act as advocates to ensure accessibility of appropriate services.

Gay, Lesbian, and Bisexual Adolescents. Researchers have studied development of a gay or lesbian identity in adults, but there are limited studies related to adolescents. It is widely known that, although some adolescents participate in same-gender sexual activity, they do not necessarily become homosexual as adults (Hockenberry and Wilson, 2015). Adolescents who believe that they have a homosexual or bisexual orientation often try to keep it hidden to avoid any associated stigma. This increases their vulnerability to depression and suicide. The teens who choose to disclose a homosexual or bisexual orientation become at risk for violence, harassment, and family abuse. If a teen chooses to disclose sexual orientation to you, help the adolescent construct a safety plan before telling his or her family or friends in case the response is not supportive (Hockenberry and Wilson, 2015). One of the Healthy People 2020 objectives is to increase the percentage of middle and high schools that prohibit harassment based on a student's sexual orientation or gender identity (USDHHS, 2014a).

KEY POINTS

- A developmental perspective helps a nurse understand commonalities and variations in each stage and the impact they have on a patient's health.
- During critical periods of development, a multitude of factors foster or hinder optimal physical, cognitive, and psychosocial development.
- In children, physiological, cognitive, and psychosocial development continues from conception through adolescence; thus be familiar with normal parameters to determine potential problems and identify ways to promote normal development.
- The most rapid period of growth and development occurs during infancy.

- The toddler's development of fine- and gross-motor skills supports the move toward independence.
- Preschoolers interpret language literally and are unable to see another's point of view.
- Physical growth during the school years is slow and steady until the skeletal growth spurt just before puberty.
- The major psychosocial developmental task of the school-age child is the development of a sense of industry or competency.
- Adolescence begins with puberty, when primary sexual characteristics begin to develop and secondary sexual characteristics complete development.
- Adolescents are able to solve complex mental problems, which includes use of deductive reasoning.
- Accidents are the major cause of death in all age-groups.
- Sexually transmitted diseases are the most common communicable diseases among adolescents.

CLINICAL APPLICATION QUESTIONS

Preparing for Clinical Practice

You are caring for 12-year-old Elizabeth who has been hospitalized for an appendectomy. Her mother tells you that she is concerned about her lack of physical development compared to her peers. As a nurse you know that adolescents are preoccupied with their bodies and develop individual images of what they think they should look like. You are also aware that adolescents define health in terms of not just absence of illness but also being able to live up to one's physical, mental, and social potential and they are influenced by their peers.

1. What would you want to discuss concerning the onset of puberty with Elizabeth?
2. How would you discuss smoking with Elizabeth?
3. How will Elizabeth's cognitive and psychosocial development direct your teaching?

ⓔ *Answers to Clinical Application Questions can be found on the Evolve website.*

REVIEW QUESTIONS

Are You Ready to Test Your Nursing Knowledge?

1. In an interview with a pregnant patient, the nurse discussed the three risk factors that have been cited as having a possible effect on prenatal development. They are:
   1. Nutrition, stress, and mother's age.
   2. Prematurity, stress, and mother's age.
   3. Nutrition, mother's age, and fetal infections.
   4. Fetal infections, prematurity, and placenta previa.
2. A parent has brought her 6-month-old infant in for a well-child check. Which of her statements indicates a need for further teaching?
   1. "I can start giving her whole milk at about 12 months."
   2. "I can continue to breastfeed for another 6 months."
   3. "I've started giving her plenty of fruit juice as a way to increase her vitamin intake."
   4. "I can start giving her solid food now."
3. The type of injury to which a child is most vulnerable at a specific age is most closely related to which of the following?
   1. Provision of adult supervision
   2. Educational level of the parent
   3. Physical health of the child
   4. Developmental level of the child
4. Which approach would be best for a nurse to use with a hospitalized toddler?
   1. Always give several choices.
   2. Set few limits to allow for open expression.
   3. Use noninvasive methods when possible.
   4. Establish a supportive relationship with the mother.
5. A nurse is providing information on prevention of sudden infant death syndrome (SIDS) to the mother of a young infant. Which of the following statements indicates that the mother has a good understanding? (Select all that apply.)
   1. "I won't use a pacifier to help my baby sleep."
   2. "I'll be sure that my baby doesn't spend any time sleeping on her abdomen."
   3. "I'll place my baby on her back for sleep."
   4. "I'll be sure to keep my baby's room cool."
   5. "I'll keep a crib bumper in the bed to prevent drafts."
6. Sequence the skills in the expected order of gross-motor development in an infant beginning with the earliest skill:
   1. Move from prone to sitting unassisted
   2. Sit down from standing position
   3. Sit upright without support
   4. Roll from abdomen to back
   5. Can turn from side to back
7. Parents are concerned about their toddler's negativism. To avoid a negative response, which of the following is the best way for a nurse to demonstrate asking the toddler to eat his or her lunch?
   1. Would you like to eat your lunch now?
   2. When would you like to eat your lunch?
   3. Would you like apple slices or applesauce with your sandwich?
   4. Would you like to sit at the big table to eat?
8. When nurses are communicating with adolescents, they should:
   1. Be alert to clues to their emotional state.
   2. Ask closed-ended questions to get straight answers.
   3. Avoid looking for meaning behind adolescents' words or actions.
   4. Avoid discussing sensitive issues such as sex and drugs.
9. Which of the following statements is most descriptive of the psychosocial development of school-age children?
   1. Boys and girls play equally with each other.
   2. Peer influence is not yet an important factor to the child.
   3. They like to play games with rigid rules.
   4. Children frequently have "best friends."
10. You are caring for a 4-year-old child who is hospitalized for an infection. He tells you that he is sick because he was "bad." Which is the most correct interpretation of his comment?
    1. Indicative of extreme stress
    2. Representative of his cognitive development
    3. Suggestive of excessive discipline at home
    4. Indicative of his developing sense of inferiority
11. At a well-child examination, the mother comments that her toddler eats little at mealtime, will only sit briefly at the table, and wants snacks all the time. Which of the following should the nurse recommend?
    1. Provide nutritious snacks.
    2. Offer rewards for eating at mealtimes.
    3. Avoid snacks so she is hungry at mealtime.
    4. Explain to her firmly why eating at mealtime is important.
12. An 8-year-old child is being admitted to the hospital from the emergency department with an injury from falling off her bicycle. Which of the following will most help her adjust to the hospital?

1. Explain hospital routines such as mealtimes to her.
2. Use terms such as "honey" and "dear" to show a caring attitude.
3. Explain when her parents can visit and why siblings cannot come to see her.
4. Since she is young, orient her parents to her room and hospital facility.

13. A school nurse is counseling an obese 10-year-old child. Which factors would be important to consider when planning an intervention to support the child's health? (Select all that apply.)

1. Consider both the child and the family when addressing the issue.
2. Consider the use of medications to suppress the appetite.
3. First plan for weight loss through dieting and then add activity as tolerated.
4. Plan food intake to allow for growth.
5. Consider consulting a bariatric surgeon if other measures fail.

14. You are working in an adolescent health center when a 15-year-old patient shares with you that she thinks she is pregnant and is worried that she may now have a sexually transmitted infection (STI). Her pregnancy test is negative. What is your next priority of care?

1. Contact her parents to alert them of her need for birth control.
2. Refer her to a primary health care provider to obtain a prescription for birth control.
3. Counsel her on safe sex practices.
4. Ask her to have her partner come to the clinic for sexually transmitted infection testing.

15. A 4-month-old infant has not been feeling well for 2 days. His mother has brought him to the clinic to be seen by his health care provider. Which number identifies the area of the infant's head where the nurse can assess for dehydration?

1. 1
2. 2
3. 3
4. 4
5. 5

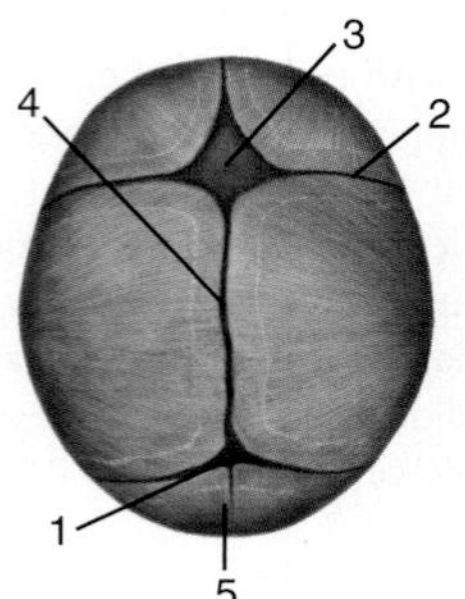

Answers: 1. 1; **2.** 3; **3.** 4; **4.** 4; **5.** 2, 3, 4; **6.** 5, 4, 3, 1, 2; **7.** 3; **8.** 1; **9.** 4; **10.** 2; **11.** 1; **12.** 1; **13.** 1, 4; **14.** 3; **15.** 3.

Rationales to Review Questions can be found on the Evolve website.

REFERENCES

American Academy of Pediatrics (AAP): *Healthy children: family life: where we stand: TV viewing time,* 2014a. http://www.healthychildren.org/English/family-life/Media/Pages/Where-We-Stand-TV-Viewing-Time.aspx. Accessed March 2015.

American Academy of Pediatrics (AAP): *Healthy children: safety and prevention: new crib standards: what parents need to know,* 2014b. http://www.healthychildren.org/English/ages-stages/baby/sleep/Pages/New-Crib-Standards-What-Parents-Need-to-Know.aspx. Accessed March 2015.

American Academy of Pediatrics (AAP): *Healthy children: safety and prevention: car seats: information for families for 2015,* 2015a. http://www.healthychildren.org/English/safety-prevention/on-the-go/pages/Car-Safety-Seats-Information-for-Families.aspx?nfstatus=401&nftoken=00000000-0000-0000-0000-000000000000&nfstatusdescription=ERROR%3a+No+local+token. Accessed March 2015.

American Academy of Pediatrics (AAP): *Healthy children: safety and prevention: HPV (Gardasil): what you need to know,* 2015b. http://www.healthychildren.org/english/safety-prevention/immunizations/pages/Human-Papillomavirus-HPV-Vaccine-What-You-Need-to-Know.aspx. Accessed March 2015.

Centers for Disease Control and Prevention (CDC): *Ten leading causes of death by age group, United States—2011,* 2011. http://www.cdc.gov/injury/wisqars/pdf/leading_causes_of_death_by_age_group_2011-a.pdf. Accessed March 2015.

Centers for Disease Control and Prevention (CDC): *Suicide facts at a glance 2012,* 2012. http://www.cdc.gov/violenceprevention/pdf/Suicide-DataSheet-a.pdf. Accessed March 2015.

Centers for Disease Control and Prevention (CDC): *MMWR surveillance summaries: youth risk behavior surveillance—United States, 2013,* 2013a. http://www.cdc.gov/mmwr/preview/mmwrhtml/ss6304a1.htm?s_cid=ss6304a1_w. Accessed March 2015.

Centers for Disease Control and Prevention (CDC): *HPV (human papillomavirus) Gardasil® vaccine information statement,* 2013b. http://www.cdc.gov/vaccines/hcp/vis/vis-statements/hpv-gardasil.html. Accessed March 2015.

Centers for Disease Control and Prevention (CDC): *Childhood obesity facts,* 2014. http://www.cdc.gov/healthyyouth/obesity/facts.htm. Accessed March 2015.

Erikson EH: *Childhood and society,* ed 2, New York, 1963, Norton.

Erikson EH: *Identity: youth and crises,* New York, 1968, Norton.

Grodner LR, et al: *Nutritional foundations and clinical applications: a nursing approach,* ed 5, St Louis, 2012, Mosby, VitalBook file. Pageburst Online.

Hockenberry M, Wilson D: *Wong's nursing care of infants and children,* ed 10, St Louis, 2015, Mosby.

Leifer G: *Growth and development across the lifespan,* ed 2, Philadelphia, 2013, Saunders, VitalBook file, Pageburst Online.

Murray SS, McKinney ES: *Foundations of maternal-newborn and women's health nursing,* ed 5, Philadelphia, 2010, Saunders, VitalBook file, Pageburst Online.

National Institutes of Health: US National Library of Medicine: *Death among children and adolescents,* 2012. http://www.nlm.nih.gov/medlineplus/ency/article/001915.htm. Accessed March 2015.

Perry S, et al: *Maternal child nursing care,* ed 5, St Louis, 2014, Mosby, VitalBook file, Pageburst Online.

Piaget J: *The origins of intelligence in children,* New York, 1952, International Universities Press.

US Department of Education Institute of Education Sciences (USDEIES) National Center for Education Statistics: *Number of non-fatal victimization against students 12-18 and rate of victimizations per 1000 students, by type of victimization, location and selected student characteristics: 2012,* 2012. http://nces.ed.gov/programs/digest/d13/tables/dt13_228.25.asp. Accessed August 2014.

US Department of Health and Human Services (USDHHS), Health Resources and Services Administration: *Adolesc Health,* 2014a. http://healthypeople.gov/2020/topicsobjectives2020/objectiveslist.aspx?topicId=2#16 Accessed March 2015.

US Department of Health and Human Services (USDHHS), Health Resources and Services Administration: *Child health USA 2013,* 2014b. http://mchb.hrsa.gov/chusa13. Accessed March, 2015.

RESEARCH REFERENCES

American Educational Research Association: *Prevention of bullying in schools, colleges, and universities: research report and recommendations,* Washington, DC, 2013, American Educational Research Association.

Astor RA, et al: How can we improve school safety research? *Educ Res* 39(1):69, 2010.

Espelage DL, et al: *Prevention of bullying in schools, colleges, and universities* (research report and recommendations), Washington, DC, 2013, American Educational Research Association.

Hildebrand AK, et al: Increased risk for school violence-related behaviors among adolescents with insufficient sleep, *J School Health* 83(6):408, 2013.

Johnson SL, et al: Prioritizing the school environment in school violence prevention efforts, *J Sch Health* 81(6):331, 2011.

Ttofi MM, et al: Do the victims of school bullies tend to become depressed later in life? A systematic review and meta-analysis of longitudinal studies, *J Aggress Confl Peace Res* 3:63, 2011.

13

Young and Middle Adults

OBJECTIVES

- Discuss developmental theories of young and middle adults.
- List and discuss major life events of young and middle adults and the childbearing family.
- Describe developmental tasks of the young adult, the childbearing family, and the middle adult.
- Discuss the significance of family in the life of the adult.
- Describe normal physical changes in young and middle adulthood and pregnancy.
- Discuss cognitive and psychosocial changes occurring during the adult years.
- Describe health concerns of the young adult, the childbearing family, and the middle adult.

KEY TERMS

Braxton Hicks contractions, p. 165
Climacteric, p. 166
Doula, p. 161
Emerging adulthood, p. 159
Infertility, p. 164
Lactation, p. 165
Menopause, p. 166
Prenatal care, p. 165
Puerperium, p. 161
Sandwich generation, p. 166

MEDIA RESOURCES

http://evolve.elsevier.com/Potter/fundamentals/
- Review Questions
- Case Study with Questions
- Audio Glossary
- Content Updates

Young and middle adulthood includes periods of challenges, rewards, and crises. Challenges often include the demands of working and raising families, although there are many rewards with these as well. Adults also face crises such as caring for their aging parents, the possibility of job loss in a changing economic environment, and dealing with their own developmental needs and those of their family members.

Classic works by developmental theorists such as Levinson et al. (1978), Diekelmann (1976), Erikson (1963, 1982), and Havighurst (1972) attempted to describe the phases of young and middle adulthood and related developmental tasks (see Chapter 11 for an in-depth discussion of developmental theories). More recent work has identified an additional phase of development in the young adult: emerging adulthood (Arnett, 2000; Grusec and Hastings, 2007; Jensen, 2011).

Faced with a societal structure that differs greatly from the norms of 20 or 30 years ago, both men and women are assuming different roles in today's society. Men were traditionally the primary supporter of the family. Today many women pursue careers and contribute significantly to their families' incomes. In 2012 59% of women 16 years and older participated in the U.S. labor force and constituted 46% of all U.S. workers in the U.S. labor force. Forty percent of employed women worked in management or professional occupations, and almost 30% of businesses in the United States were owned by women. In addition, 29% of women 25 years or older had completed four or more years of college, and 84.5% of women 18 years and older were living above the poverty level (Institute for Women's Policy Research [IWPR], 2014a). However, women in the United States are paid 77 cents for every dollar earned by men, a gender wage gap of 23% (IWPR, 2014b).

Developmental theories provide a basis for understanding the life events and developmental tasks of the young and middle adult. Patients present challenges to nurses who themselves are often young or middle adults coping with the demands of their respective developmental period. Nurses need to recognize the needs of their patients even if they are not experiencing the same challenges and events.

YOUNG ADULTS

Young adulthood is identified by some authors as the period between the late teens and the mid to late 30s (Edelman et al., 2014). In the past several decades, the period of life called **emerging adulthood** has been identified as lasting from about ages 18 to 25 (Grusec and Hastings, 2007; Jensen, 2011). This newly identified stage of development has been described as neither extended adolescence, since it is much freer from parental control and much more a period of independent exploration, nor young adulthood since most young people in their twenties have not made the transitions historically associated with adult status, especially marriage and parenthood. It is estimated that in 2013 young adults 20 to 34 years of age made up approximately 24% of the population (U.S. Census Bureau, 2014). According to the Pew Research Center (2011, 2013), today's young adults are history's first "always-connected" generation, with digital technology and social media major aspects of their lives. They adapt well to new experiences, are more ethnically and racially diverse than previous generations, and are the least overtly religious American generation in modern times. Young adults increasingly move away from their families of origin, establish career goals, and decide whether to marry or remain single and whether to begin families; however, often these goals may be delayed because increased numbers of young adults pursue higher education and economic conditions.

Physical Changes

The young adult usually completes physical growth by the age of 20. An exception to this is the pregnant or lactating woman. The physical, cognitive, and psychosocial changes and the health concerns of the pregnant woman and the childbearing family are extensive.

Young adults are usually quite active, experience severe illnesses less frequently than older age-groups, tend to ignore physical symptoms, and often postpone seeking health care. Physical strength typically peaks in early adulthood, and physical characteristics of young adults begin to change as middle age approaches. Physical changes are minimal during this developmental phase; however, weight and muscle mass may change as a result of diet, exercise, and lifestyle. Assessment findings are generally within normal limits unless an illness is present.

Cognitive Changes

Critical thinking habits increase steadily through the young- and middle-adult years. Formal and informal educational experiences, general life experiences, and occupational opportunities dramatically increase the individual's conceptual, problem-solving, and motor skills.

Identifying an occupational direction is a major task of young adults. When people know their skills, talents, and personality characteristics, educational preparation and occupational choices are easier and more satisfying. An associate's degree, bachelor's degree, or graduate degree is the most significant source of postsecondary education for many of the fastest-growing occupations (U.S. Department of Labor, 2014).

An understanding of how adults learn helps the nurse develop patient education plans (see Chapter 25). Adults enter the teaching-learning situation with a background of unique life experiences, including illness. Therefore always view them as individuals. Their adherence to regimens such as medications, treatments, or lifestyle changes such as smoking cessation involves decision-making processes. When determining the amount of information that an individual needs to make decisions about the prescribed course of therapy, consider factors that possibly affect his or her adherence to the regimen, including educational level, socioeconomic factors, and motivation and desire to learn.

Because young adults are continually evolving and adjusting to changes in the home, workplace, and personal lives, their decision-making processes need to be flexible. The more secure young adults are in their roles, the more flexible and open they are to change. Insecure people tend to be more rigid in making decisions.

Psychosocial Changes

The emotional health of a young adult is related to an individual's ability to address and resolve personal and social tasks. The young adult is often caught between wanting to prolong the irresponsibility of adolescence and assume adult commitments. However, certain patterns or trends are relatively predictable. Between the ages of 23 and 28, the person refines self-perception and ability for intimacy. From 29 to 34 the person directs enormous energy toward achievement and mastery of the surrounding world. The years from 35 to 43 are a time of vigorous examination of life goals and relationships. People make changes in personal, social, and occupational areas. Often the stresses of this reexamination results in a "midlife crisis" in which marital partner, lifestyle, and occupation change.

Ethnic and gender factors have a sociological and psychological influence in an adult's life, and these factors pose a distinct challenge for nursing care. Each person holds culture-bound definitions of health and illness. Nurses and other health professionals bring with them distinct practices for the prevention and treatment of illness. Knowing too little about a patient's self-perception or beliefs regarding health and illness creates conflict between a nurse and patient. Changes in the traditional role expectations of both men and women in young and middle adulthood also lead to greater challenges for nursing care. For example, women often continue to work during the childrearing years, and many women struggle with the enormity of balancing three careers: wife, mother, and employee. This is a potential source of stress for the adult working woman. Men are more aware of parental and household responsibilities and find themselves having more responsibilities at home while achieving their own career goals (Fortinash and Holoday Worret, 2012). An understanding of ethnicity, race, and gender differences enables a nurse to provide individualized care (see Chapter 9).

Support from a nurse, access to information, and appropriate referrals provide opportunities for achievement of a patient's potential. Health is not merely the absence of disease but involves wellness in all human dimensions. The nurse acknowledges the importance of a young adult's psychosocial needs and needs in all other dimensions. The young adult needs to make decisions concerning career, marriage, and parenthood. Although each person makes these decisions based on individual factors, a nurse needs to understand the general principles involved in these aspects of psychosocial development while assessing the young adult's psychosocial status.

Lifestyle. Family history of cardiovascular, renal, endocrine, or neoplastic disease increases a young adult's risk of illness. Your role in health promotion is to identify modifiable factors that increase the young adult's risk for health problems and provide patient education and support to reduce unhealthy lifestyle behaviors (Lin et al., 2014).

A personal lifestyle assessment (see Chapter 6) helps nurses and patients identify habits that increase the risk for cardiac, malignant, pulmonary, renal, or other chronic diseases. The assessment includes general life satisfaction, hobbies, and interests; habits such as diet, sleeping, exercise, sexual habits, and use of caffeine, tobacco, alcohol, and illicit drugs; home conditions and pets; economics, including type of health insurance; occupational environment, including type of work and exposure to hazardous substances; and physical or mental stress. Military records, including dates and geographical area of assignments, may also be useful in assessing the young adult for risk factors. Prolonged stress from lifestyle choices increases wear and tear on the adaptive capacities of the body. Stress-related diseases such as ulcers, emotional disorders, and infections sometimes occur (see Chapter 38).

Career. A successful vocational adjustment is important in the lives of most men and women. Successful employment not only ensures economic security; it also leads to fulfillment, friendships, social activities, support, and respect from co-workers.

Some young adults choose a two-career family, which has benefits and liabilities. In addition to increasing the family's financial base, the person who works outside the home is able to expand friendships, activities, and interests. However, stress exists in a two-career family as well. These stressors result from a transfer to a new city; increased expenditures of physical, mental, or emotional energy; child care demands; or household needs. To avoid stress in a two-career family, partners should share all responsibilities. For example, some families may decide to limit recreational expenses and instead hire someone to do routine housework. Others set up an equal division of household, shopping, and cooking duties.

Sexuality. The development of secondary sex characteristics occurs during the adolescent years (see Chapter 12). Physical development is accompanied by sexual maturation. The young adult usually has emotional maturity to complement the physical ability and therefore is able to develop mature sexual relationships and establish intimacy. Young adults who have failed to achieve the developmental task of personal integration sometimes develop relationships that are superficial and stereotyped (Fortinash and Holoday Worret, 2012).

The classic work of Masters and Johnson (1970) contributed important information about the physiological characteristics of the adult sexual response (see Chapter 35). The psychodynamic aspect of sexual activity is as important as the type or frequency of sexual intercourse to young adults. To maintain total wellness, encourage adults to explore various aspects of their sexuality and be aware that their sexual needs and concerns change. As the rate of early initiation of sexual intercourse continues to increase, young adults are at risk for sexually transmitted infections (STIs). Consequently there is an increased need for education regarding the mode of transmission, prevention, and symptom recognition and management for STIs.

Childbearing Cycle. Conception, pregnancy, birth, and the **puerperium** are major phases of the childbearing cycle. The changes during these phases are complex. Childbirth education classes can prepare pregnant women, their partners, and other support people to participate in the birthing process (Figure 13-1). Some health care agencies provide either professional labor support or a lay **doula**, a support person to be present during labor to assist women who have no other source of support. The stress that many women experience after childbirth may have a significant impact on postpartum women's health (Box 13-1).

Types of Families. During young adulthood most individuals experience singlehood and the opportunity to be on their own. Those who eventually marry or establish long-term partnerships encounter several changes as they take on new responsibilities. For example, many couples choose to become parents (Figure 13-2). Some young adults choose alternative lifestyles. Chapter 10 reviews forms of families.

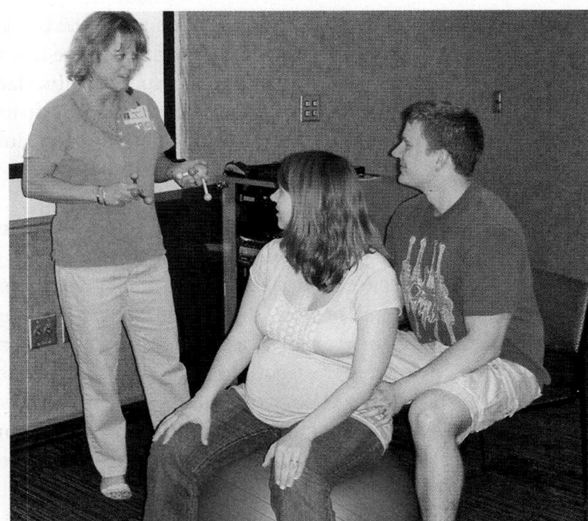

FIGURE 13-1 Nurse providing Lamaze class for expectant young adults.

Singlehood. Social pressure to get married is not as great as it once was, and many young adults do not marry until their late 20s or early 30s or not at all. For young adults who remain single, parents and siblings become the nucleus for a family. Some view close friends and associates as "family." One cause for the increased single population is the expanding career opportunities for women. Women enter the job market with greater career potential and have greater opportunities for financial independence. More single individuals are choosing to live together outside of marriage and become parents either biologically or

BOX 13-1 EVIDENCE-BASED PRACTICE

Assessing for Postpartum Depression

PICO Question: Do psychosocial factors have an influence on the prevalence of postpartum depression (PPD) in young adult women?

Evidence Summary

A woman often experiences dramatic physical and psychosocial changes during the postpartum period that impact health, with up to 85% of women experiencing some type of mood disturbance. For most women these transient symptoms are referred to as *postpartum blues* (Dennis C et al., 2012; Venkatesh et al., 2014). Common symptoms of postpartum blues, including rapidly fluctuating mood, tearfulness, irritability, and anxiety, are generally mild (Guille et al., 2013). Approximately 9% to 16% of women experience a more persistent form of postpartum depression (PPD) after the birth of a baby, and 0.1% to 0.2% of postpartum women experience postpartum psychosis (Drake et al., 2014; Glover et al., 2014). The onset of postpartum psychosis carries a high risk of suicide and infanticide (murder of an infant). The onset is abrupt and severe, with clinical manifestations of delusions, hallucinations, thoughts of harming or killing the baby, unwillingness to eat or sleep, frantic energy, risk of suicide, and severe depressive symptoms.

Research findings indicate several risk factors for the development of postpartum mood disorder, including stress, fatigue, quality of relationship with the father of the baby, social support, birth of a preterm or low-birth-weight infant, young maternal age, and race and ethnicity (Camp, 2013; Liu and Tronick, 2013). Studies also show that PPD may have a negative impact on the maternal-infant relationship, infant development, and long-term child behavior (Horowitz et al., 2013; Jarosinski and Pollard, 2014). Postpartum psychosis is an extremely serious and rare postpartum mood disorder, and it is considered a psychiatric emergency.

Successful treatment of PPD depends on early identification and intervention. Clinical assessment of pregnant and postpartum women that is guided by the major predictors of PPD can help nurses identify women most at risk. Subsequently intervention can be initiated before the occurrence of depressive symptoms.

Application to Nursing Practice

- Assess for potential postpartum stressors such as fatigue, first-time mother, previous postpartum stress, or feeling of social isolation (Camp, 2013; Liu and Tronick, 2013).
- Identify sources of social support for new mothers after they are discharged from the hospital with their babies such as new-mother visits, young-mother groups, and mom's–day out activities (Horowitz et al., 2013; Jarosinski and Pollard, 2014).
- Create culturally appropriate primary prevention strategies for stressors that new mothers encounter (Horowitz et al., 2013; Jarosinski and Pollard, 2014).
- Educate new mothers and their families on the risks for and signs and symptoms of postpartum stress and PPD (Camp, 2013).
- Provide new mothers with information on health care and community resources for use during the postpartum period.

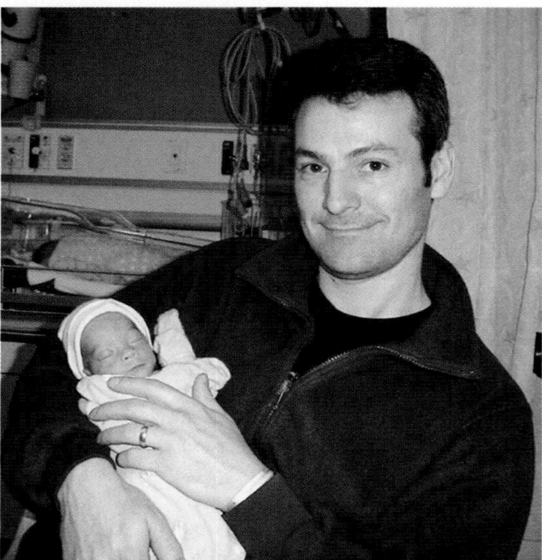

FIGURE 13-2 Parent-child nurturing is important in adapting to a newborn. (From Hockenberry MJ, Wilson D: *Wong's nursing care of infants and children,* ed 10, St Louis, 2015, Mosby.)

through adoption. Similarly many married couples choose to separate or divorce if they find their marital situation unsatisfactory.

Parenthood. The availability of contraception makes it easier for today's couples to decide when and if to start a family. Social pressures may encourage a couple to have a child or influence them to limit the number of children they have. Economic considerations frequently enter into the decision-making process because of the expense of childrearing. General health status and age are also considerations in decisions about parenthood because couples are getting married later and postponing pregnancies, which often results in smaller families.

Alternative Family Structures and Parenting. Changing norms and values about family life in the United States reveal basic shifts in attitudes about family structure. The trend toward greater acceptance of cohabitation without marriage is a factor in the greater numbers of infants being born to single women. In addition, approximately 6 million American children and adults have a lesbian, gay, bisexual, or transgender (LGBT) parent. More than 111,000 same-sex households include children under the age of 18 (Gates, 2013). The American Academy of Pediatrics (AAP), in recognizing the needs of gay and lesbian parents and their children, published a policy statement supporting adoption of children and the parenting role by same-sex parents (AAP, 2013). However, many times parents from alternative family structures still feel a lack of support and even bias from the health care system (Nicol et al., 2013).

Hallmarks of Emotional Health. Most young adults have the physical and emotional resources and support systems to meet the many challenges, tasks, and responsibilities they face. During psychosocial assessment of young adults, assess for 10 hallmarks of emotional health (Box 13-2) that indicate successful maturation in this developmental stage.

Health Risks

Health risk factors for a young adult originate in the community, lifestyle patterns, and family history. The lifestyle habits that activate the stress response (see Chapter 38) increase the risk of illness. Smoking is a well-documented risk factor for pulmonary, cardiac, and vascular diseases in smokers and the individuals who receive secondhand smoke. Inhaled cigarette pollutants increase the risk of lung cancer, emphysema, and chronic bronchitis. The nicotine in tobacco is a vasoconstrictor that acts on the coronary arteries, increasing the risk of angina, myocardial infarction, and coronary artery disease. Nicotine also causes peripheral vasoconstriction and leads to vascular problems.

BOX 13-2 Ten Hallmarks of Emotional Health

1. A sense of meaning and direction in life
2. Successful negotiation through transitions
3. Absence of feelings of being cheated or disappointed by life
4. Attainment of several long-term goals
5. Satisfaction with personal growth and development
6. When married, feelings of mutual love for partner; when single, satisfaction with social interactions
7. Satisfaction with friendships
8. Generally cheerful attitude
9. No sensitivity to criticism
10. No unrealistic fears

Family History. A family history of a disease puts a young adult at risk for developing it in the middle- or older-adult years. For example, a young man whose father and paternal grandfather had myocardial infarctions (heart attacks) in their 50s has a risk for a future myocardial infarction. The presence of certain chronic illnesses such as diabetes mellitus in the family increases the family member's risk of developing a disease. Regular physical examinations and screening are necessary at this stage of development. Since certain condition such as high blood pressure, high blood sugar, and high cholesterol levels may not have any symptoms in the early stages, having physical examinations and simple blood tests to screen for these conditions is important to assess the risk of current and future medical problems. Genomic science and resultant technologies have also facilitated new ways to identify people at risk for chronic disease through the use of genetic screening. Understanding the role genomics plays in the health of individuals and families enables clinicians to better advise young adults related to current and future health care.

Personal Hygiene Habits. As in all age-groups, personal hygiene habits in the young adult are risk factors. Sharing eating utensils with a person who has a contagious illness increases the risk of illness. Poor dental hygiene increases the risk of periodontal disease. Individuals avoid gingivitis (inflammation of the gums) and periodontitis (loss of tooth support) through oral hygiene (see Chapter 40).

Violent Death and Injury. Violence is a common cause of mortality and morbidity in the young-adult population. Factors that predispose individuals to violence, injury, or death include poverty, family breakdown, child abuse and neglect, drug involvement (dealing or illegal use), repeated exposure to violence, and ready access to guns. It is important for the nurse to perform a thorough psychosocial assessment, including such factors as behavior patterns, history of physical and substance abuse, education, work history, and social support systems to detect personal and environmental risk factors for violence. Death and injury primarily occur from physical assaults, motor vehicle or other accidents, and suicide attempts in young adults.

Intimate partner violence (IPV), formerly referred to as domestic violence, is a global public health problem. It exists along a continuum from a single episode of violence to ongoing battering (Dudgeon and Evanson, 2014). IPV often begins with emotional or mental abuse and may progress to physical or sexual assault. Each year women in the United States experience approximately 4.8 million intimate partner–related physical assaults and rapes, and men are the victims of approximately 2.9 intimate partner–related physical assaults. Physical injuries from IPV range from minor cuts and bruises to broken bones, internal bleeding, and head trauma. IPV is linked to such harmful health behaviors as smoking, alcohol abuse, drug use, and risky sexual activity. Risk factors for the perpetration of IPV include using drugs or alcohol, especially heavy drinking; unemployment; low self-esteem; antisocial or borderline personality traits; desire for power and control in relationships; and being a victim of physical or psychological abuse (Bonomi et al., 2014; DeWall and Way, 2014; Dudgeon and Evanson, 2014). The greatest risk of violence occurs during the reproductive years. A pregnant woman has a 35.6% greater risk of being a victim of IPV than a nonpregnant woman. Women experiencing IPV may be more likely to delay prenatal care and are at increased risk for multiple poor maternal and infant health outcomes such as low maternal weight gain, infections, high blood pressure, vaginal bleeding, and delivery of a preterm or low-birth-weight infant.

> **QSEN QSEN: BUILDING COMPETENCY IN PATIENT-CENTERED CARE** You are caring for Joan, a 25-year-old patient who has come to the clinic complaining of insomnia. Throughout the assessment interview Joan is slightly withdrawn, speaks quietly, and does not make eye contact. She does not work outside the home; and she acknowledges that her relationship with her husband, an engineer who lost his job as a result of downsizing 6 months ago, is "not going well." Physical examination reveals scratches and bruises on Joan's breasts, abdomen, and back. Which assessment questions, approaches, and tools do you use to determine whether Joan is a victim of IPV and, if so, how to help her?
>
> *Answers to QSEN Activities can be found on the Evolve website.*

Substance Abuse. Substance abuse directly or indirectly contributes to mortality and morbidity in young adults. Intoxicated young adults are often severely injured in motor vehicle accidents, resulting in death or permanent disability to other young adults.

Dependence on stimulant or depressant drugs sometimes results in death. Overdose of a stimulant drug ("upper") stresses the cardiovascular and nervous systems to the extent that death occurs. The use of depressants ("downers") leads to an accidental or intentional overdose and death.

Caffeine is a naturally occurring legal stimulant that is readily available in carbonated beverages; chocolate-containing foods; coffee and tea; and over-the-counter medications such as cold tablets, allergy and analgesic preparations, and appetite suppressants. It is the most widely ingested stimulant in North America. Caffeine stimulates catecholamine release, which in turn stimulates the central nervous system; it also increases gastric acid secretion, heart rate, and basal metabolic rate. This alters blood pressure, increases diuresis, and relaxes smooth muscle. Consumption of large amounts of caffeine results in restlessness, anxiety, irritability, agitation, muscle tremor, sensory disturbances, heart palpitations, nausea or vomiting, and diarrhea in some individuals.

Substance abuse is not always diagnosable, particularly in its early stages. Nonjudgmental questions about use of legal drugs (prescribed drugs, tobacco, and alcohol), soft drugs (marijuana), and more problematic drugs (cocaine or heroin) are a routine part of any health assessment. Obtain important information by making specific inquiries about past medical problems, changes in food intake or sleep patterns, or problems of emotional lability. Reports of arrests because of driving while intoxicated, wife or child abuse, or disorderly conduct are reasons to investigate the possibility of drug abuse more carefully.

Human Trafficking. Runaway and homeless youth and young adults have gained recognition as a significant and growing social problem (Benoit-Bryan, 2013). In particular, this population sometimes turns to illegal and dangerous activities to survive and may be at high risk for human trafficking (Derluyn, 2010; Pergamit and Ernst, 2010). The United Nations Office on Drugs and Crime (n.d.) defines human trafficking as the recruitment, transport, transfer, harboring, or receipt of a person by threat or use of force for the purpose of exploitation. Although human trafficking is often a hidden crime and accurate statistics are difficult to obtain, estimates indicate that over 80% of trafficking victims are female and 50% are children. Approximately 75% to 80% of human trafficking is for sex.

Unplanned Pregnancies. Unplanned pregnancies are a continued source of stress that may result in adverse health outcomes for the mother, infant, and family. Often young adults have educational and career goals that take precedence over family development. Interference with these goals affects future relationships and parent-child relationships.

Determination of situational factors that affect the progress and outcome of an unplanned pregnancy is important. Exploration of problems such as financial, career, and living accommodations; family support systems; potential parenting disorders; depression; and coping mechanisms is important in assessing the woman with an unplanned pregnancy.

Sexually Transmitted Infections. STIs are a major health problem in young adults. Examples of STIs include syphilis, chlamydia, gonorrhea, genital herpes, human papillomavirus (HPV), and acquired immunodeficiency syndrome (AIDS). STIs have immediate physical effects such as genital discharge, discomfort, and infection. They also lead to chronic disorders, terminal illnesses, infertility, or even death. They remain a major public health problem for sexually active people, with almost half of all new infections occurring in men and women younger than 24 years of age (USDHHS, CDC, 2014). In 2011 and 2012, 20- to 24-year-old men had the highest rate of chlamydia among men (1350.4 per 100,000 population); chlamydia rates in men of this age-group increased slightly from the previous year. Safe and effective vaccines have been developed for some STIs. For example HPV, which can cause several types of cancer, can be prevented through vaccination with Gardasil or Cervarix, both Food and Drug Administration (FDA)–approved vaccines for the prevention of HPV.

Environmental or Occupational Factors. A common environmental or occupational risk factor is exposure to work-related hazards or agents that cause diseases and cancer (Table 13-1). Examples include lung diseases such as silicosis from inhalation of talcum and silicon dust and emphysema from inhalation of smoke. Cancers resulting from occupational exposures may involve the lung, liver, brain, blood, or skin. Questions regarding occupational exposure to hazardous materials should be a routine part of your assessment.

Health Concerns

Health Promotion. Lifestyles (e.g., use of tobacco or alcohol) of young adults may put them at risk for illnesses or disabilities during their middle- or older-adult years. Young adults are also genetically susceptible to certain chronic diseases such as diabetes mellitus and familial hypercholesterolemia (Huether and McCance, 2013). Some

TABLE 13-1 Occupational Hazards/Exposures Associated with Diseases and Cancers

Job Category	Occupational Hazard/ Exposure	Work-Related Condition/Cancer
Agricultural workers	Pesticides, infectious agents, gases, sunlight	Pesticide poisoning, "farmer's lung," skin cancer
Anesthetists	Anesthetic gases	Reproductive effects, cancer
Automobile workers	Asbestos, plastics, lead, solvents	Asbestosis, dermatitis
Carpenters	Wood dust, wood preservatives, adhesives	Nasopharyngeal cancer, dermatitis
Cement workers	Cement dust, metals	Dermatitis, bronchitis
Dry cleaners	Solvents	Liver disease, dermatitis
Dye workers	Dyestuffs, metals, solvents	Bladder cancer, dermatitis
Glass workers	Heat, solvents, metal powders	Cataracts
Hospital workers	Infectious agents, cleansers, latex gloves, radiation	Infections, latex allergies, unintentional injuries
Insulators	Asbestos, fibrous glass	Asbestosis, lung cancer, mesothelioma
Jackhammer operators	Vibration	Raynaud's phenomenon
Lathe operators	Metal dusts, cutting oils	Lung disease, cancer
Office computer workers	Repetitive wrist motion on computers, eyestrain	Tendonitis, carpal tunnel syndrome, tenosynovitis

From Stanhope M, Lancaster J: *Foundations of nursing in the community,* ed 3, St Louis, 2010, Mosby.

diseases that may appear in later years are avoidable if identified early. Encourage adults to perform monthly skin, breast, or male genital self-examination (see Chapter 31). Breast cancer is the most common major cancer among women in the United States, with a steadily increasing incidence. A nurse's role is extremely important in educating female patients about breast self-examinations (BSEs) and the current breast screening recommendations. Encourage routine assessment of the skin for recent changes in color or presence of lesions and changes in their appearance. Prolonged exposure to ultraviolet rays of the sun by adolescents and young adults increase the risk for development of skin cancer later in life. Crohn's disease, a chronic inflammatory disease of the small intestine, most commonly occurs between 15 and 35 years of age. Many young adults have misconceptions regarding transmission and treatment of STIs. Encourage partners to know one another's sexual history and practices. Be alert for STIs when patients come to clinics with complaints of urological or gynecological problems (see Chapter 35). Assess young adults for knowledge and use of safe sex practices and genital self-examinations. Provide information on safe sex practice (e.g., use of condoms and having only one sex partner).

Psychosocial Health. The psychosocial health concerns of the young adult are often related to job and family stressors. As noted in Chapter 38, stress is valuable because it motivates a patient to change. However, if the stress is prolonged and the patient is unable to adapt to the stressor, health problems develop. Ninety percent of cases of eating disorders such as anorexia nervosa and bulimia nervosa begin during adolescence and young adulthood (Skinner et al., 2012). Some

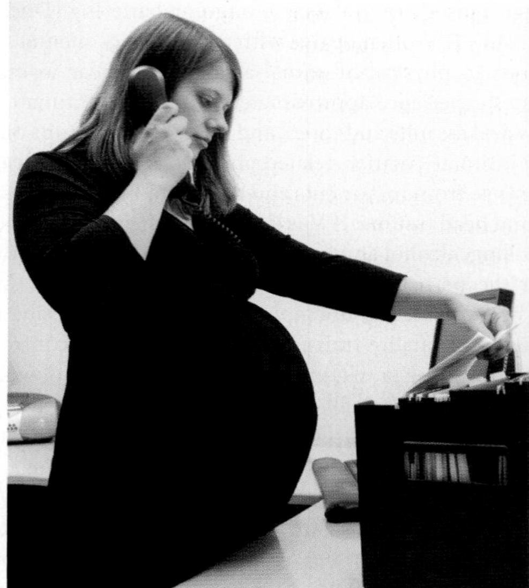

FIGURE 13-3 The ability to handle day-to-day challenges at work minimizes stress.

mental health disorders such as high levels of depression also begin in this age-group. These conditions may manifest during young adulthood, but symptoms and treatment may continue into middle adulthood and beyond (Smink et al., 2012).

Job Stress. Job stress can occur every day or from time to time. Most young adults are able to handle day-to-day crises (Figure 13-3). Situational job stress occurs when a new boss enters the workplace, a deadline is approaching, or the worker has new or greater numbers of responsibilities. A recent trend in today's business world and a risk factor for job stress is corporate downsizing, leading to increased responsibilities for employees with fewer positions within the corporate structure. Job stress also occurs when a person becomes dissatisfied with a job or the associated responsibilities. Because individuals perceive jobs differently, the types of job stressors vary from patient to patient. Your assessment of a young adult includes a description of the usual work performed. Job assessment also includes conditions and hours, duration of employment, changes in sleep or eating habits, and evidence of increased irritability or nervousness.

Family Stress. Because of the multiplicity of changing relationships and structures in the emerging young-adult family, stress is frequently high (see Chapter 10). Situational stressors occur during events such as births, deaths, illnesses, marriages, and job losses. Stress is often related to a number of variables, including the career paths of both husband and wife, and leads to dysfunction in the young-adult family. This is reflected in the fact that the highest divorce rate occurs during the first 3 to 5 years of marriage for young adults under the age of 30. When a patient seeks health care and presents stress-related symptoms, the nurse needs to assess for the occurrence of a life-change event.

Each family member has certain predictable roles or jobs. These roles enable a family to function and be an effective part of society. When they change as a result of illness, a situational crisis often occurs. Assess environmental and familial factors, including support systems and coping mechanisms commonly used by family members.

Infertility. According to the American Society for Reproductive Medicine (n.d.), an **infertility** evaluation is not undertaken until a couple has unprotected intercourse for about 12 months with the failure to conceive. An estimated 10% to 15% of reproductive couples are infertile, and many are young adults. However, approximately half of the couples evaluated and treated in infertility clinics become pregnant. In about 15% of infertile couples the cause is unknown. Female factors such as ovulatory dysfunction or a pelvic factor are responsible for infertility in 50% of couples, and infertility in 35% of couples is caused by a male factor such as sperm and semen abnormalities. For some infertile couples a nurse is the first resource they identify. Nursing assessment of the infertile couple includes comprehensive histories of both the male and female partners to determine factors that have affected fertility and pertinent physical findings (Murray and McKinney, 2014).

Obesity. Obesity is a major health problem in young adults and is recognized as a risk factor for other health problems later in life. It is influenced by poor diet and inactivity and has been linked to the development of conditions such as type 2 diabetes, hypertension, high cholesterol, asthma, joint problems, psoriatic arthritis, and poor health status (Berge et al., 2014; Vranian et al., 2013). Nursing assessment of diet and physical activity of young adults is an important part of data collection. All young adults should be counseled about the benefits of a healthful diet and physical activity.

Exercise. People of all ages, both male and female, benefit from regular physical activity; however, young adults are spending increasingly more time with technology and less time engaged in physical activity. Exercise in young adults is important to prevent or decrease the development of chronic health conditions such as high blood pressure, obesity, and diabetes that develop later in life. Exercise improves cardiopulmonary function by decreasing blood pressure and heart rate; increases the strength and size of muscles; and decreases fatigability, insomnia, tension, and irritability. Conduct a thorough musculoskeletal assessment and exercise history to develop a realistic exercise plan. Encourage regular exercise within the patient's daily schedule.

Pregnant Woman and the Childbearing Family. A developmental task for many young adult couples is the decision to begin a family. Although the physiological changes of pregnancy and childbirth occur only in the woman, cognitive and psychosocial changes and health concerns affect the entire childbearing family, including the baby's father, siblings, and grandparents. Single-parent families and young single mothers tend to be particularly vulnerable, both economically and socially.

Health Practices. Women who are anticipating pregnancy benefit from good health practices before conception; these include a balanced diet, folic acid, exercise, dental checkups, avoidance of alcohol, and cessation of smoking.

Prenatal Care. Prenatal care is the routine examination of the pregnant woman by an obstetrician or advanced practice nurse such as a nurse practitioner or certified nurse midwife. Prenatal care includes a thorough physical assessment of the pregnant woman during regularly scheduled intervals; provision of information regarding STIs, other vaginal infections, and urinary infections that adversely affect the fetus; and counseling about exercise patterns, diet, and child care. Regular prenatal care addresses health concerns that may arise during the pregnancy.

Physiological Changes. The physiological changes and needs of the pregnant woman vary with each trimester. Be familiar with them, their causes, and implications for nursing. All women experience some physiological changes in the first trimester. For example, they commonly have morning sickness, breast enlargement and tenderness, and fatigue. During the second trimester growth of the uterus and fetus results in some of the physical signs of pregnancy. During the third trimester increases in Braxton Hicks contractions (irregular, short contractions), fatigue, and urinary frequency occur.

Postpartum. Postpartum is a period of approximately 6 weeks after delivery. During this time the woman's body reverts to its prepregnant physical status. Determine the woman's knowledge of and ability to care for both herself and her newborn baby. Assessment of parenting skills and maternal-infant interactions is particularly important. The process of lactation or breastfeeding offers many advantages to both the new mother and baby. For the inexperienced mother breastfeeding can be a source of anxiety and frustration. Be alert for signs that the mother needs information and assistance.

Needs for Education. The entire childbearing family needs education about pregnancy, labor, delivery, breastfeeding, and integration of the newborn into the family structure.

Psychosocial Changes. Like the physiological changes of pregnancy, psychosocial changes occur at various times during the 9 months of pregnancy and in the puerperium. Table 13-2 summarizes the major categories of psychosocial changes and implications for nursing intervention.

TABLE 13-2 Major Psychosocial Changes During Pregnancy

Category	Implications for Nursing
Body image	Morning sickness and fatigue contribute to poor body image. Woman feels big, awkward, and unattractive during third trimester when fetus is growing more rapidly. Increase in breast size sometimes makes the woman feel more feminine and sexually appealing. Woman takes extra time with hygiene and grooming, trying new hairstyles and makeup. Woman begins to "show" during the second trimester and starts to plan maternity wardrobe. Woman has general feeling of well-being when she feels the baby move and hears the heartbeat.
Role changes	Both partners think about and have feelings of uncertainty about impending role changes. Both partners have feelings of ambivalence about becoming parents and concern about ability to be parents.
Sexuality	Woman needs reassurance that sexual activity will not harm fetus. Woman's desire for sexual activity is influenced by body image. Woman desires cuddling and holding rather than sexual intercourse.
Coping mechanisms	Woman needs reassurance that childbirth and childrearing are natural and positive experiences but are also stressful. Woman is often unable to cope with particular stressors such as finding new housing, preparing the nursery, or participating in childbirth classes.
Stresses during puerperium	Woman returns home from hospital fatigued and unfamiliar with infant care. Woman experiences physical discomfort or feelings of anxiety or depression. Woman must return to work soon after delivery with subsequent feelings of guilt, anxiety, or possibly a sense of freedom or relief.

Health Concerns. The pregnant woman and her partner have many health questions. For example, they wonder whether the pregnancy and baby will be normal. Proper prenatal care has the potential to identify risks and pregnancy problems and meet the majority of the expectant mother's emotional and physical health needs.

Acute Care. Young adults typically require acute care for accidents, substance abuse, exposure to environmental and occupational hazards, stress-related illnesses, respiratory infections, gastroenteritis, influenza, urinary tract infections, and minor surgery. An acute minor illness causes a disruption in life activities of young adults and increases stress in an already hectic lifestyle. Dependency and limitations posed by treatment regimens also increase frustration. To give them a sense of maintaining control of their health care choices, it is important to keep them informed about their health status and involve them in health care decisions.

Restorative and Continuing Care. Chronic conditions are not common in young adulthood, but they sometimes occur. Chronic illnesses such as hypertension, coronary artery disease, and diabetes have their onset in young adulthood but may not be recognized until later in life. Causes of chronic illness and disability in the young adult include accidents, multiple sclerosis, rheumatoid arthritis, AIDS, and cancer. Chronic illness or disability threatens a young adult's independence and results in the need to change personal, family, and career goals. Nursing interventions for the young adult faced with chronic illness or disability need to focus on problems related to sense of identity, establishing independence, reorganizing intimate relationships and family structure, and launching a chosen career.

MIDDLE ADULTS

The U.S. Census Bureau (2014) predicted that in 2013 39.6% of the population would be middle-age adults between the ages of 35 and 64. In middle adulthood an individual makes lasting contributions through involvement with others. Generally the middle-adult years begin around the early to mid-30s and last through the late 60s, corresponding to Levinson's developmental phases of "settling down" and the "payoff years." During this period personal and career achievements have often already been experienced. Many middle adults find particular joy in helping their children and other young people become productive and responsible adults (see Chapter 11 for Erikson's Theory of Psychosocial Development) (Figure 13-4). They also begin to help aging parents while being responsible for their own children, placing them in the sandwich generation. Using leisure time in satisfying and creative ways is a challenge that, if met satisfactorily, enables middle adults to prepare for retirement.

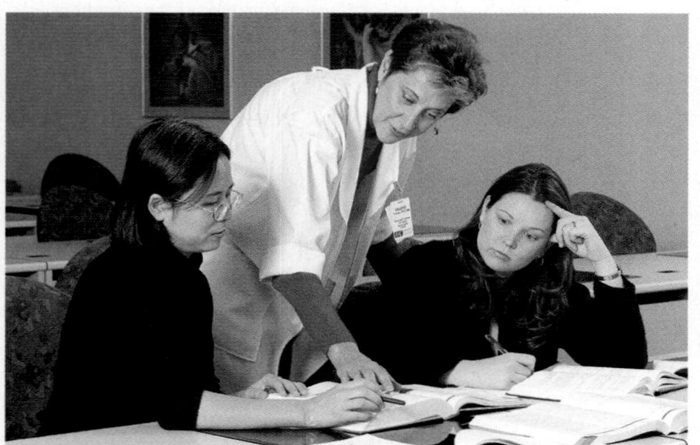

FIGURE 13-4 Middle adults enjoy helping young people become productive and responsible adults.

Although most middle adults have achieved socioeconomic stability, recent trends in corporate downsizing have left many either jobless or forced to accept lower-paying jobs. According to the U.S. Census Bureau (2013), the real median household income in the United States was not statistically different from 2011 to 2012; however, in 2012 the real median household income was 8.3% lower than in 2007, the year before the most recent recession, and the poverty rate was 2.5% higher.

Men and women need to adjust to inevitable biological changes. As in adolescence, middle adults use considerable energy to adapt self-concept and body image to physiological realities and changes in physical appearance. High self-esteem, a favorable body image, and a positive attitude toward physiological changes occur when adults engage in physical exercise, balanced diets, adequate sleep, and good hygiene practices that promote vigorous, healthy bodies.

Physical Changes

Major physiological changes occur between 40 and 65 years of age. Because of this it is important to assess the middle adult's general health status. A comprehensive assessment offers direction for health promotion recommendations and planning and implementing any acutely needed interventions. The most visible changes during middle adulthood are graying of the hair, wrinkling of the skin, and thickening of the waist. Decreases in hearing and visual acuity are often evident during this period. Often these physiological changes during middle adulthood have an impact on self-concept and body image. Table 13-3 summarizes abnormal findings to consider when conducting a physical examination (see Chapter 31). The most significant physiological changes during middle age are menopause in women and the climacteric in men.

Perimenopause and Menopause. Menstruation and ovulation occur in a cyclical rhythm in women from adolescence into middle adulthood. Perimenopause is the period during which ovarian function declines, resulting in a diminishing number of ova and irregular menstrual cycles; it generally lasts 1 to 3 years. Menopause is the disruption of this cycle, primarily because of the inability of the neurohormonal system to maintain its periodic stimulation of the endocrine system. The ovaries no longer produce estrogen and progesterone, and the blood levels of these hormones drop markedly. Menopause typically occurs between 45 and 60 years of age (see Chapter 35). Approximately 10% of women have no symptoms of menopause other than cessation of menstruation, 70% to 80% are aware of other changes but have no problems, and approximately 10% experience changes severe enough to interfere with activities of daily living.

Climacteric. The climacteric occurs in men in their late 40s or early 50s (see Chapter 35). Decreased levels of androgens cause climacteric. Throughout this period and thereafter a man is still capable of producing fertile sperm and fathering a child. However, penile erection is less firm, ejaculation is less frequent, and the refractory period is longer.

Cognitive Changes

Changes in the cognitive function of middle adults are rare except with illness or trauma. Some middle adults enter educational or vocational programs to prepare themselves with new skills and information for entering the job market or changing jobs.

TABLE 13-3 Abnormal Physical Assessment Findings in the Middle Adult

Body System	Assessment Findings
Integument	Very thin skin Rough, flaky, dry skin Lesions
Scalp and hair	Excessive generalized hair loss or patchy hair loss Excessive scaliness
Head and neck	Large, thick skull and facial bones Asymmetry in movement of head and/or neck Drooping of one side of the face
Eyes	Reduced peripheral vision Asymmetrical position of the light reflex Drooping of the upper lid (ptosis) Redness or crusting around the eyelids
Ears	Discharge of any kind Reddened, swollen ear canals
Nose, sinuses, and throat	Nasal tenderness Occlusion of nostril Swollen and pale pink or bluish-gray nasal mucosa Sinuses tender to palpation or on percussion Asymmetrical movement or loss of movement of uvula Tonsils red or enlarged
Thorax and lungs	Unequal chest expansion Unequal fremitus, hyperresonance, diminished or absent breath sounds Adventitious lung sounds such as crackles and wheezes
Heart and vascular system	Pulse inequality, weak pulses, bounding pulses, or variations in strength of pulse from beat to beat Bradycardia or tachycardia Hypertension Hypotension
Breasts—female	Recent increase in size of one breast Pigskin like or orange-peel appearance Redness or painful breasts
Breasts—male	Soft, fatty enlargement of breast tissue
Abdomen	Bruises, areas of local discoloration; purple discoloration; pale, taut skin Generalized abdominal distention Hypoactive, hyperactive, decreased, or absent bowel sounds
Female genitalia	Asymmetrical labia Swelling, pain, or discharge from Bartholin's glands Decreased tone of vaginal musculature Cervical enlargement or projection into the vagina Reddened areas or lesions in the vagina
Male genitalia	Rashes, lesions, or lumps on skin of shaft of penis Discharge from penis Enlarged scrotal sac Bulges that appear at the external inguinal ring or femoral canal when the patient bears down
Musculoskeletal system	Uneven weight bearing Decreased range of joint motion; swollen, red, or enlarged joint; painful joints Decreased strength against resistance
Neurological system	Lethargy Inadequate motor responses Abnormal sensory system responses: inability to smell certain aromas, loss of visual fields, inability to feel and correctly identify facial stimuli, absent gag reflex

Psychosocial Changes

The psychosocial changes in the middle adult involve expected events such as children moving away from home and unexpected events such as a marital separation or the death of a close friend.

You need to assess for major life changes and the impact that the changes have on the middle adult's state of health. Include individual psychosocial factors such as coping mechanisms and sources of social support in your assessment.

In the middle-adult years, as children depart from the household, the family enters the post-parental family stage. Time and financial demands on the parents decrease, and the couple faces the task of redefining their own relationship. It is during this period that many middle adults take on healthier lifestyles. Assessment of health promotion needs for the middle adult includes adequate rest, leisure activities, regular exercise, good nutrition, reduction or cessation in the use of tobacco or alcohol, and regular screening examinations. Assessment of the middle adult's social environment is also important, including relationship concerns; communication and relationships with children, grandchildren, and aging parents; and caregiver concerns with their own aging or disabled parents.

Career Transition. Career changes occur by choice or as a result of changes in the workplace or society. In recent decades middle adults change occupations more often for a variety of reasons, including limited upward mobility, decreasing availability of jobs, and seeking an occupation that is more challenging. In some cases downsizing, technological advances, or other changes force middle adults to seek new jobs. Such changes, particularly when unanticipated, result in stress that affects health, family relationships, self-concept, and other dimensions.

Sexuality. After the departure of their last child from the home, many couples recultivate their relationships and find increased marital and sexual satisfaction during middle age. The onset of menopause and the climacteric affect the sexual health of the middle adult. Some women may desire increased sexual activity because pregnancy is no longer possible. Menopausal women also experience vaginal dryness and dyspareunia or pain during sexual intercourse (see Chapter 35).

During middle age a man may notice changes in the strength of his erection and a decrease in his ability to experience repeated orgasm. Other factors influencing sexuality during this period include work stress, diminished health of one or both partners, and the use of prescription medications. For example, antihypertensive agents have side effects that influence sexual desire or functioning. Antihypertensive drugs represent one of the most implicated classes of drugs that cause erectile dysfunction (ED) in men. Patients who take beta blockers or diuretics exhibit significantly worse ED than patients receiving newer drugs such as angiotensin receptor blockers, angiotensin converting enzyme (ACE) inhibitors, and calcium antagonists for hypertension (Manolis and Doumas, 2012). Sometimes both partners experience sexual dysfunction caused by stresses related to sexual changes or a conflict between their sexual needs and self-perceptions and social attitudes or expectations (see Chapter 35).

Family Psychosocial Factors. Psychosocial factors involving the family include the stresses of singlehood, marital changes, transition of the family as children leave home, and the care of aging parents.

Singlehood. Many adults over 35 years of age in the United States have never been married. Many of these are college-educated people who have embraced the philosophy of choice and freedom, delayed marriage, and delayed parenthood. Some middle adults choose to remain single but also opt to become parents either biologically or through adoption. Many single middle adults have no relatives but share a family type of relationship with close friends or work associates. Consequently some single middle adults feel isolated during traditional "family" holidays such as Thanksgiving or Christmas. In times of illness middle adults who choose to remain single and childless have to rely on other relatives or friends, increasing caregiving demands of family members who also have other responsibilities. Nursing assessment of single middle adults needs to include a thorough assessment of psychosocial factors, including an individual's definition of family and available support systems.

Marital Changes. Marital changes occurring during middle age include death of a spouse, separation, divorce, and the choice of remarrying or remaining single. A widowed, separated, or divorced patient goes through a period of grief and loss in which it is necessary to adapt to the change in marital status. Normal grieving progresses through a series of phases, and resolution of grief often takes a year or more. You need to assess the level of coping of the middle adult to the grief and loss associated with certain life changes (see Chapter 37).

Family Transitions. The departure of the last child from the home is also a stressor. Many parents welcome freedom from childrearing responsibilities, whereas others feel lonely or without direction. *Empty nest syndrome* is the term used to describe the sadness and loneliness that accompany children leaving home. Eventually parents need to reassess their marriage and try to resolve conflicts and plan for the future. Occasionally this readjustment phase leads to marital conflicts, separation, and divorce (see Chapter 10).

Care of Aging Parents. Increasing life spans in the United States and Canada have led to increased numbers of older adults in the population. Therefore greater numbers of middle adults need to address the personal and social issues confronting their aging parents. Many middle adults find themselves caught between the responsibilities of caring for dependent children and those of caring for aging and ailing parents. Thus they find themselves in the sandwich generation, in which the challenges of caregiving can be stressful. The needs of family caregivers are being given more emphasis in the health care system.

Housing, employment, health, and economic realities have changed the traditional social expectations between generations in families. The middle-adult and older-adult parents often have conflicting relationship priorities when the older adult strives to remain independent. Negotiations and compromises help to define and resolve problems. Nurses deal with middle and older adults in the community, long-term care facilities, and hospitals. They help identify the health needs of both groups and assist the multigenerational family in determining the health and community resources available to them as they make decisions and plans. They evaluate family relationships to determine family members' perceptions of responsibility and loyalty in relation to caring for older-adult members. Assessment of environmental resources (e.g., number of rooms in the house or stairwells) in relation to the complexity of health care demands for the older adult is also important.

Health Concerns

Health Promotion and Stress Reduction. Because middle adults experience physiological changes and face certain health realities, their perceptions of health and health behaviors are often important factors in maintaining health. Today's complex world makes individuals more prone to stress-related illnesses such as heart attacks, hypertension, migraine headaches, ulcers, colitis, autoimmune disease, backache, arthritis, and cancer. When adults seek health care, nurses focus on the goal of wellness and guide patients to evaluate health behaviors, lifestyle, and environment.

Throughout life people have many stressors (see Chapter 38). After identifying these stressors, work with your patient to intervene and modify the stress response. Specific interventions for stress reduction fall into three categories. First minimize the frequency of stress-producing situations. Together with the patient identify approaches to preventing stressful situations such as habituation, change avoidance, time blocking, time management, and environmental modification. Second, increase stress resistance (e.g., increase self-esteem, improve assertiveness, redirect goal alternatives, and reorient cognitive appraisal). Finally avoid the physiological response to stress. Use relaxation techniques, imagery, and biofeedback to recondition the patient's response to stress.

Obesity. Obesity is a growing, expensive health concern for middle adults. It can reduce quality of life and increase risk for many serious chronic diseases and premature death. A new Healthy People 2020 (USDHHS, 2011) goal relates to improvement of health-related quality of life and well-being, including physical well-being. Health consequences of obesity include high blood pressure, high blood cholesterol, type 2 diabetes, coronary heart disease, osteoarthritis, and obstructive sleep apnea. Continued focus on the goal of health-related quality of life helps patients evaluate health behaviors and lifestyle that contribute to obesity during the middle-adult years. Counseling related to physical activity and nutrition is an important component of the plan of care for patients who are overweight and obese.

Forming Positive Health Habits. A habit is a person's usual practice or manner of behavior. Frequent repetition reinforces this behavior pattern until it becomes an individual's customary way of behaving. Some habits support health (e.g., exercise and brushing and flossing the teeth each day). Other habits involve risk factors to health (e.g., smoking or eating foods with little or no nutritional value. Evidence indicates that vitamin D and calcium play key roles in bone health and the prevention of osteopenia and osteoporosis in middle-age women (Institute of Medicine, 2011).

During assessment a nurse frequently obtains data indicating positive and negative health behaviors by a patient. Examples of positive health behaviors include regular exercise, adherence to good dietary habits, avoidance of excess consumption of alcohol, participation in routine screening and diagnostic tests for disease prevention and health promotion (e.g., laboratory screening for serum cholesterol or mammography), and lifestyle changes to reduce stress. You help patients maintain habits that protect health and offers healthier alternatives to poor habits.

Health teaching and counseling often focus on improving health habits. The more you understand the dynamics of behavior and habits, the more likely it is that your interventions will help patients achieve or reinforce health-promoting behaviors.

BOX 13-3 Barriers to Change

External Barriers
- Lack of facilities
- Lack of materials
- Lack of social supports
- Lack of motivation

Internal Barriers
- Lack of knowledge
- Insufficient skills to change health habits
- Undefined short- and long-term goals

To help patients form positive health habits, you act as a teacher and facilitator. By providing information about how the body functions and how patients form and change habits, patients' levels of knowledge regarding the potential impact of behavior on health are raised. You cannot change your patients' habits. They have control of and are responsible for their own behaviors. Explain psychological principles of changing habits and offer information about health risks. Offer positive reinforcement (such as praise and rewards) for health-directed behaviors and decisions. Such reinforcement increases the likelihood that the behavior will be repeated. However, ultimately a patient decides which behaviors will become habits of daily living.

Help middle adults consider factors such as avoidance of STIs, prevention of substance abuse, and accident prevention in relation to decreasing health risks. For example, provide patients with factual information on STI causes, symptoms, and transmission. Discuss methods of protection during sexual activity with a patient in an open and nonjudgmental manner and reinforce the importance of practicing safe sex (see Chapter 35). Provide counseling and support for patients seeking treatment for substance abuse. Help them recognize and alter unsafe and potential health hazards. In addition, encourage them to express their feelings so they become proficient in solving problems and recognizing risk factors themselves. Barriers to change exist (Box 13-3). Unless you minimize or eliminate these barriers, it is futile to encourage a patient to take action.

Health Literacy. Health literacy is defined as the cognitive and social skills that determine the motivation and ability of individuals to gain access to, understand, and use information in ways that promote and maintain good health (see Chapter 25). Health education materials such as medical instructions, consent forms, and questionnaires are often given to patients without consideration of their level of health literacy. It is estimated that nearly half of the American adult population functions at or below a basic health literacy level (Sorensen et al., 2012; Willens et al., 2013). A person with an adequate level of health literacy has the ability to take responsibility for his or her own health. Lower health literacy may impact the ability to understand basic written health information or read a prescription bottle correctly. People with low health literacy may not be able to self-manage their health with lifestyle risk-factor modification to prevent the development of chronic diseases (Dennis S et al., 2012).

Psychosocial Health

Anxiety. Anxiety is a critical maturational phenomenon related to change, conflict, and perceived control of the environment. Adults often experience anxiety in response to the physiological and psychosocial changes of middle age. Such anxiety motivates the adult to rethink life goals and stimulates productivity. However, for some adults this anxiety precipitates psychosomatic illness and preoccupation with death. In this case a middle adult views life as being half or more over and thinks in terms of the time left to live.

Clearly a life-threatening illness, marital transition, or job stressor increases the anxiety of a patient and family. Use crisis intervention or stress-management techniques to help a patient adapt to the changes of the middle-adult years (see Chapter 38).

Depression. Depression is a mood disorder that manifests itself in many ways. Although the most frequent age of onset is between ages 25 and 44, it is common among adults in the middle years and has many causes. The risk factors for depression include being female; disappointments or losses at work, at school, or in family relationships; departure of the last child from the home; and family history. In fact, the incidence of depression in women is twice that of men. People experiencing mild depression describe themselves as feeling sad, blue, downcast, down in the dumps, and tearful. Other symptoms include alterations in sleep patterns such as difficult sleeping (insomnia) or sleeping too much (hypersomnia), irritability, feelings of social disinterest, and decreased alertness. Physical changes such as weight gain or loss, headaches, or feelings of fatigue regardless of the amount of rest are also depressive symptoms. Individuals with depression that occurs during the middle years commonly experience moderate-to-high anxiety and have physical complaints. Mood changes and depression are common occurrences during menopause. The abuse of alcohol or other substances makes depression worse. Nursing assessment of a middle adult diagnosed with depression includes focused data collection regarding individual and family history of depression, mood changes, cognitive changes, behavioral and social changes, and physical changes. Collect assessment data from both the patient and the patient's family because family data are often particularly important, depending on the level of depression the middle adult is experiencing.

Community Health Programs. Community health programs offer services to prevent illness, promote health, and detect disease in the early stages. Nurses make valuable contributions to the health of the community by taking an active part in planning screening and teaching programs and support groups for middle adults (see Chapter 3).

Family planning, birthing, and parenting skills are program topics in which adults are usually interested. Health screening for diabetes, hypertension, eye disease, and cancer is a good opportunity for a nurse to perform assessment and provide health teaching and health counseling.

Health education programs promote changes in behavior and lifestyle. As a health teacher, offer information that enables patients to make decisions about health practices within the context of health promotion for young-to-middle adults. Make sure that educational programs are culturally appropriate. Changes to more positive health practices during young and middle adulthood lead to fewer or less complicated health problems as an older adult. During health counseling, collaborate with your patient to design a plan of action that addresses his or her health and well-being. Through objective problem solving you can help your patient grow and change.

Acute Care. Acute illnesses and conditions experienced in middle adulthood are similar to those of young adulthood. However, injuries and acute illnesses in middle adulthood require a longer recovery period because of the slowing of healing processes. In addition, they are more likely to become chronic conditions. For middle adults in the sandwich generation, stress levels also increase as they balance responsibilities related to employment, family life, care of children, and care of aging parents while recovering from an injury or acute illness.

Restorative and Continuing Care. Chronic illnesses such as diabetes mellitus, hypertension, rheumatoid arthritis, or multiple sclerosis affect the roles and responsibilities of a middle adult. Some results of chronic illness are strained family relationships, modifications in family activities, increased health care tasks, increased financial stress, the need for housing adaptation, social isolation, medical concerns, and grieving. The degree of disability and a patient's perception of both the illness and the disability determine the extent to which lifestyle changes occur. A few examples of the problems experienced by patients who develop debilitating chronic illness during adulthood include role reversal, changes in sexual behavior, and alterations in self-image. Along with the current health status of a middle adult living with a chronic illness, you need to assess the knowledge base of both the patient and family. This assessment includes the medical course of the illness and the prognosis for the patient. You need to determine the coping mechanisms of the patient and family. In addition, you need to assess adherence to treatment and rehabilitation regimens, evaluate the need for community and social services, and make appropriate referrals.

KEY POINTS

- Adult development involves orderly and sequential changes in characteristics and attitudes that adults experience over time.
- Many changes experienced by young adults are related to the natural process of maturation and socialization.
- Young adults are in a stable period of physical development, except for changes related to pregnancy.
- Cognitive development continues throughout the young- and middle-adult years.
- Emotional health of young adults is correlated with the ability to address and resolve personal and social problems.
- Pregnant women need to understand physiological changes occurring in each trimester.
- Psychosocial changes and health concerns during pregnancy and postpartum affect the parents, the siblings, and often the extended family.
- Midlife transition begins when a person becomes aware that physiological and psychosocial changes signify passage to another stage in life.
- Cognitive changes are rare in middle age except in cases of illness or physical trauma.
- Psychosocial changes for middle adults are often related to career transition, sexuality, marital changes, family transition, and care of aging parents.
- Health concerns of middle adults commonly involve stress-related illnesses, health assessment, adoption of positive health habits, and issues with health literacy.

CLINICAL APPLICATION QUESTIONS

Preparing for Clinical Practice

A 24-year-old patient who smokes two packs of cigarettes per day comes to a clinic to talk with you about quitting smoking. She began smoking when she was 14 years old. She states, "I just can't seem to kick the habit, no matter how hard I try. I'm smoking more now because of increased stress from my job."

1. What information do you need to know to help this patient quit smoking?
2. Which factors will have the greatest impact on health promotion related to smoking cessation in this patient?
3. Which steps should you take to help this patient decrease stress?

ⓔ *Answers to Clinical Application Questions can be found on the Evolve website.*

REVIEW QUESTIONS

Are You Ready to Test Your Nursing Knowledge?

1. With the exception of pregnant or lactating women, the young adult has usually completed physical growth by the age of:
   1. 18.
   2. 20.
   3. 25.
   4. 30.
2. A nurse is completing an assessment on a male patient, age 24. Following the assessment, the nurse notes that his physical and laboratory findings are within normal limits. Because of these findings, nursing interventions are directed toward activities related to:
   1. Instructing him to return in 2 years.
   2. Instructing him in secondary prevention.
   3. Instructing him in health promotion activities.
   4. Implementing primary prevention with vaccines.
3. When determining the amount of information that a patient needs to make decisions about the prescribed course of therapy, many factors affect his or her compliance with the regimen, including educational level and socioeconomic factors. Which additional factor affects compliance?
   1. Gender
   2. Lifestyle
   3. Motivation
   4. Family history
4. A patient is laboring with her first baby, who is about to be delivered 2 weeks early. Her husband is in the military and might not get back in time, and both families are unable to be with her during labor. The doctor decides to call in which of the following people employed by the birthing area as a support person to be present during labor?
   1. Nurse
   2. Midwife
   3. Geneticist
   4. Lay doula
5. A single young adult interacts with a group of close friends from college and work. They celebrate birthdays and holidays together. In addition, they help one another through many stressors. These individuals are viewed as:
   1. Family.
   2. Siblings.
   3. Substitute parents.
   4. Alternative family structure.
6. Sharing eating utensils with a person who has a contagious illness increases the risk of illness. This type of health risk arises from:
   1. Lifestyle.
   2. Community.
   3. Family history.
   4. Personal hygiene habits.
7. A 50-year-old woman has elevated serum cholesterol levels that increase her risk for cardiovascular disease. One method to control this risk factor is to identify current diet trends and

describe dietary changes to reduce the risk. This nursing activity is a form of:
1. Referral.
2. Counseling.
3. Health education.
4. Stress-management techniques.

8. A 34-year-old female executive has a job with frequent deadlines. She notes that, when the deadlines appear, she has a tendency to eat high-fat, high-carbohydrate foods. She also explains that she gets frequent headaches and stomach pain during these deadlines. The nurse provides a number of options for the executive, and she chooses yoga. In this scenario yoga is used as a (n):
   1. Outpatient referral.
   2. Counseling technique.
   3. Health promotion activity.
   4. Stress-management technique.
9. A 50-year-old male patient is seen in the clinic. He tells a nurse that he has recently lost his job and his wife of 26 years has asked for a divorce. He has a flat affect. Family history reveals that his father committed suicide at the age of 53. The nurse assesses for the following:
   1. Cardiovascular disease
   2. Depression
   3. Sexually transmitted infection
   4. Iron deficiency anemia
10. Middle-age adults frequently find themselves trying to balance responsibilities related to employment, family life, care of children, and care of aging parents. People finding themselves in this situation are frequently referred to as being a part of:
    1. The sandwich generation.
    2. The millennial generation.
    3. Generation X.
    4. Generation Y.
11. Intimate partner violence (IPV) is linked to which of the following factors? (Select all that apply.)
    1. Alcohol abuse
    2. Marriage
    3. Pregnancy
    4. Unemployment
    5. Drug use
12. Sexually transmitted infections (STIs) continue to be a major health problem in young adults. Men ages 20 to 24 years have the highest rate of which STI?
    1. Chlamydia
    2. Syphilis
    3. Gonorrhea
    4. Herpes zoster
13. Formation of positive health habits may prevent the development of chronic illness later in life. Which of the following are examples of positive health habits? (Select all that apply.)
    1. Routine screening and diagnostic tests
    2. Unprotected sexual activity
    3. Regular exercise
    4. Excess alcohol consumption
    5. Consistent seat belt use
14. Chronic illness (e.g., diabetes mellitus, hypertension, rheumatoid arthritis) may affect a person's roles and responsibilities during middle adulthood. When assessing the health-related knowledge base of both the middle-age patient with a chronic illness and his family, your assessment includes which of the following? (Select all that apply.)
    1. The medical course of the illness
    2. The prognosis for the patient
    3. Socioeconomic status
    4. Coping mechanisms of the patient and family
    5. The need for community and social services
15. A 45-year-old woman who is obese tells a nurse that she wants to lose weight. After conducting a thorough assessment, the nurse concludes that which of the following may be contributing factors to the woman's obesity? (Select all that apply.)
    1. The woman works in an executive position that is very demanding.
    2. The woman works out at the corporate gym at 5 AM two mornings per week.
    3. The woman says that she has little time to prepare meals at home and eats out at least four nights a week.
    4. The woman says that she tries to eat "low-cholesterol" foods to help lose weight.
    5. The woman says that she vacations annually to reduce stress.

Answers: 1. 2; **2.** 3; **3.** 3; **4.** 4; **5.** 1; **6.** 4; **7.** 3; **8.** 4; **9.** 2; **10.** 1; **11.** 1, 3, 4, 5; **12.** 1; **13.** 1, 3, 5; **14.** 1, 2, 4, 5; **15.** 1, 3, 4.

Rationales for Review Questions can be found on the Evolve website.

REFERENCES

American Academy of Pediatrics (AAP): *Policy statement: promoting the well-being of children whose parents are gay or lesbian*, 2013, www.pediatrics.aappublications.org/content/131/4/827. Accessed August 1, 2014.

American Society for Reproductive Medicine: *ReproductiveFacts.org*, n.d., http://www.reproductivefacts.org/Templates/SearchResults.aspx?q=Definition%20of%infertiliy&p=2. Accessed February 8, 2015.

Arnett J: Emerging adulthood: a theory of development from late teens through the twenties, *Am Psychol* 55(5):469, 2000.

Benoit-Bryan J: *National runaway safeline's 2013 reporter's source book on runaway and homeless youth*, Chicago, 2013, University of Illinois.

Bonomi A, et al: Intimate partner violence and neighborhood income: a longitudinal analysis, *Violence Against Women* 20(1):42, 2014.

Derluyn I, et al: Minors travelling alone: a risk group for human trafficking?, *Int Migration* 48(4):164, 2010.

DeWall C, Way B: A new piece to understanding the intimate partner violence puzzle: what role do genetics play?, *Violence Against Women* 20(4):414, 2014.

Diekelmann J: The young adult: the choice is health or illness, *Am J Nurs* 76:1276, 1976.

Dudgeon A, Evanson T: Intimate partner violence in rural U.S. areas: what every nurse should know, *Am J Nurs* 114(5):26, 2014.

Edelman C, et al: *Health promotion throughout the life span*, ed 8, St Louis, 2014, Elsevier.

Erikson E: *Childhood society*, ed 2, New York, 1963, WW Norton.

Erikson E: *The lifecycle completed: a review*, New York, 1982, WW Norton.

Fortinash K, Holoday Worret P: *Psychiatric mental health nursing*, ed 5, St Louis, 2012, Elsevier.

Gates G: *LGBT parenting in the United States, The Williams Institute*, 2013, www.williamsinstitute.law.ucla.edu/wp-content/uploads/LGBT-Parenting.pdf. Accessed August 15, 2014.

Grusec J, Hastings P: Socialization in emerging adulthood, *Handbook of socialization: theory and research*, New York, 2007, The Guilford Press.

Havighurst R: Successful aging. In Williams RH, et al, editors: *Process of aging*, vol 1, New York, 1972, Atherton.

Huether S, McCance K: *Understanding pathophysiology*, ed 5, St Louis, 2013, Mosby.

Institute for Women's Policy Research (IWPR): *State-by-state rankings and data on indicators of women's social and economic status, 2012*, June 2014a, www.iwpr.org/initiatives/states/state-by-state-rankings-and-data-on-indicators-of-womens-social-and-economic-status-201/view.

Institute for Women's Policy Research (IWPR): *Pay equity & discrimination*, 2014b, www.iwpr.org/initiatives/pay-equity-and-discrimination.

Institute of Medicine (IOM): *Dietary reference intakes: calcium, vitamin D*, Washington, DC, 2011, The National Academies Press.

Jensen L: *Bridging cultural and developmental approaches to psychology: new syntheses in theory, research, and policy*, New York, 2011, Oxford University Press.

Levinson D, et al: *The seasons of a man's life*, New York, 1978, Knopf.

Lin J, et al: Behavioral counseling to promote a healthy lifestyle in persons with cardiovascular risk factors: a systematic review for the U.S. Preventive Services Task Force, *Ann Intern Med* 161(8):568, 2014.

Masters W, Johnson V: *Human sexual response*, Boston, 1970, Little, Brown.

Murray S, McKinney E: *Foundations of maternal-newborn and women's health nursing*, ed 6, St Louis, 2014, Saunders.

Pergamit M, Ernst M: *Runaway youth's knowledge and access of services*, Chicago, 2010, The Urban Institute.

Pew Research Center: *Social networking sites and our lives*, 2011, www.pewinternet.org/files/old-media//Files/Reports/2011/PIP%20-%20Social%20networking%20sites%20and%20our%20lives.pdf/. Accessed August 23, 2014.

Pew Research Center: *Social networking fact sheet*, 2013, www.pewinternet.org/fact-sheets/social-networking-fact-sheet/. Accessed August 23, 2014.

United Nations Office on Drugs and Crime: *Human trafficking FAQs*, n.d., www.unodc.org/unodc/en/human-trafficking/faqs.html. Accessed February 7, 2015.

US Census Bureau: *Income, poverty and health insurance coverage in the United States: 2012*, 2013, http://www.census.gov/prod/2013pubs/p60-245.pdf. Accessed August 15, 2014.

US Census Bureau: *Annual estimates of the resident population for selected age-groups by sex for the United States, States, Counties, and Puerto Rico Commonwealth and Municipios: April 1, 2010 to July 1, 2013*, June 24, 2014, factfinder2.census.gov/faces/tableservices/jsf/pages/productview.xhtml?src=bkmk. Accessed August 23, 2014.

US Department of Health and Human Services (HHS): *Healthy People 2020*, 2011, www.healthypeople.gov/2020. Accessed August 12, 2014.

US Department of Health and Human Services (HHS), Centers for Disease Control and Prevention (CDC): *Sexually transmitted disease surveillance, 2012*, 2014.

US Department of Labor, Bureau of Labor Statistics: *The 2014-15 occupational outlook handbook*, January 9, 2014, www.bls.gov/ooh. Accessed August 23, 2014.

RESEARCH REFERENCES

Berge J, et al: Associations between relationship status and day-to-day health behaviors and weight among diverse young adults, *Fam Syst Health* 32(1):67, 2014.

Camp J: Postpartum depression 101: teaching and supporting the family, *Int J Childbirth Educ* 28(4):45, 2013.

Dennis C, et al: Epidemiology of postpartum depressive symptoms among Canadian women: regional and national results from a cross-sectional survey, *Can J Psychiatry* 57(9):537, 2012.

Dennis S, et al: Which providers can bridge the health literacy gap in lifestyle risk factor modification education: a systematic review and narrative synthesis, *BMC Pub Health* 13:44, 2012. http://www.biomedcentral.com/1471-22965/13/44. Accessed February 8, 2015.

Drake E, et al: Online screening and referral for postpartum depression: an exploratory study, *Community Ment Health J* 50:305, 2014.

Glover L, et al: Puerperal psychosis: a qualitative study of women's experiences, *J Reprod Infant Psychol* 32(3):254, 2014.

Guille C, et al: Management of postpartum depression, *J Midwifery Women's Health* 58(6):643, 2013.

Horowitz J, et al: Nurse home visits improve maternal/infant interaction and decrease severity of postpartum depression, *J Obstet Gynecol Neonatal Nurs* 42(3):287, 2013.

Jarosinski J, Pollard D: Postpartum depression: perceptions of a diverse sample of low-income women, *Issues Ment Health Nurs* 35:189, 2014.

Liu C, Tronick E: Rates and predictors of postpartum depression by race and ethnicity: results from the 2004 to 2007 New York City PRAMS survey (Pregnancy Risk Assessment Monitoring System), *Matern Child Health J* 17:1599, 2013.

Manolis A, Doumas M: Antihypertensive treatment and sexual dysfunction, *Curr Hypertens Rep* May:12, 2012.

Nicol P, et al: Tertiary paediatric hospital health professionals' attitudes to lesbian, gay, bisexual and transgender parents seeking health care for their children, *J Clin Nurs* 22(23–24):3396, 2013.

Skinner H, et al: A prospective study of overeating, binge eating, and depressive symptoms among adolescent and young adult women, *J Adolesc Health* 50:478, 2012.

Smink F, et al: Epidemiology of eating disorders: incidence, prevalence and mortality rates, *Curr Psychiatry Rep* 14:406, 2012.

Sorensen K, et al: Health literacy and public health: a systematic review and integration of definitions and models, *BMC Public Health* 12:80, 2012. http://www.biomedcentral.com/1471-2458/12/80. Accessed February 8, 2015.

Venkatesh K, et al: The relationship between parental stress and postpartum depression among adolescent mothers enrolled in a randomized controlled prevention trial, *Matern Child Health J* 18(6):1532, 2014.

Vranian M, et al: Impact of fitness versus obesity on routinely measured cardiometabolic risk in young, healthy adults, *Am J Cardiol* 111:991, 2013.

Willens D, et al: Association of brief health literacy screening and blood pressure in primary care, *J Health Com: Int Persp* 18(suppl):129, 2013.

14

Older Adults

OBJECTIVES

- Identify common myths and stereotypes about older adults.
- Discuss common developmental tasks of older adults.
- Describe common physiological changes of aging.
- Differentiate among delirium, dementia, and depression.
- Discuss issues related to psychosocial changes of aging.
- Describe the multifaceted aspects of elder mistreatment.
- Describe selected health concerns of older adults.
- Identify nursing interventions related to the physiological, cognitive, and psychosocial changes of aging.

KEY TERMS

Ageism, p. 174
Delirium, p. 179
Dementia, p. 179
Depression, p. 179
Elder mistreatment, p. 188
Gerontological nursing, p. 175
Gerontology, p. 174
Reality orientation, p. 189
Reminiscence, p. 189
Validation therapy, p. 189

MEDIA RESOURCES

http://evolve.elsevier.com/Potter/fundamentals/

- Review Questions
- Case Study with Questions
- Audio Glossary
- Content Updates

People who are 65 years old are in the lower boundary for "old age" in demographics and social policy within the United States. However, many older adults consider themselves to be "middle-age" well into their seventh decade. Chronological age often has little relation to the reality of aging for an older adult. Each person ages in his or her own way. Every older adult is unique, and as a nurse you need to approach each one as an individual.

The number of older adults in the United States is growing quickly. In 2013 there were 43.1 million adults over age 65 in the United States, representing 13.7% of the population or one in seven Americans (AOA, 2013). This represents an increase of 7.6 million or 21% since 2002. Part of this increase is caused by the increase of the average life span. The aging of the baby-boom generation and the growth of the population segment over age 85 contribute to the projected increase in the number of older adults. The baby boomers were born between 1946 and 1964. The first baby boomers reached age 65 in 2011. As the large number of baby boomers age, the social and health care programs necessary to meet their needs must dramatically reform their services. The diversity of the population over age 65 is also increasing. In 2012 minorities (African-Americans, Hispanics, Asians, American Indians/Eskimos/Aleuts, and other Pacific Islanders) made up 21% of the population over age 65 (AOA, 2013). As a nurse, you need to take cultural diversity into account as you care for older adults. The challenge is to gain new knowledge and skills to provide culturally sensitive and linguistically appropriate care (see Chapter 9).

VARIABILITY AMONG OLDER ADULTS

The nursing care of older adults poses special challenges because of great variation in their physiological, cognitive, and psychosocial health. Older adults also vary widely in their levels of functional ability. Most older adults are active and involved members of their communities. A smaller number have lost the ability to care for themselves, are confused or withdrawn, and/or are unable to make decisions concerning their needs. Most older adults live in noninstitutional settings. In 2012 57% of older adults in noninstitutional settings lived with a spouse (45% of older women, 71% of older men) (AOA, 2013), 28% lived alone (35% of older women, 19% of older men); and only 3.5% of all older adults resided in institutions such as nursing homes or centers.

Aging does not automatically lead to disability and dependence. Most older people remain functionally independent despite the increasing prevalence of chronic disease. Nursing assessment provides valuable clues to the effects of a disease or illness on a patient's functional status. Chronic conditions add to the complexity of assessment and care of the older adult. Most older people have at least one chronic condition, and many have multiple conditions. The physical and psychosocial aspects of aging are closely related. A reduced ability to respond to stress, the experience of multiple losses, and the physical changes associated with normal aging combine to place people at high risk for illness and functional deterioration. Although the interaction of these physical and psychosocial factors is often serious, do not assume that all older adults have signs, symptoms, or behaviors representing disease and decline or that these are the only factors you need to assess. You also need to identify an older adult's strengths and abilities during the assessment and encourage independence as an integral part of your plan of care (Kresevic, 2012).

MYTHS AND STEREOTYPES

Despite ongoing research in the field of gerontology, myths and stereotypes about older adults persist. These include false ideas about their physical and psychosocial characteristics and lifestyles. When health care providers hold negative stereotypes about aging, their action often negatively affect the quality of patient care. Although nurses are susceptible to these myths and stereotypes, they have the responsibility to replace them with accurate information.

Some people stereotype older adults as ill, disabled, and physically unattractive. Others believe that older adults are forgetful, confused, rigid, bored, and unfriendly and that they are unable to understand and learn new information. Yet specialists in the field of gerontology view centenarians, the oldest of the old, as having an optimistic outlook on life, good memories, broad social contacts and interests, and tolerance for others. Although changes in vision or hearing and reduced energy and endurance sometimes affect the process of learning, older adults are lifelong learners.

Stereotypes about lifestyles often include mistaken ideas about living arrangements and finances. Misconceptions about financial status range from beliefs that many are affluent to beliefs that many are poor. According to the U.S. Census Bureau, only 9.5% of people over age 65 had incomes below the poverty level. Older women report a significantly lower income than men. Poverty rates for older women are 11.6% compared with older men at 6.8% (U.S. Census Bureau, 2014).

In a society that values attractiveness, energy, and youth, these myths and stereotypes lead to the undervaluing of older adults. Some people equate worth with productivity; therefore they think that older adults become worthless after they leave the workforce. Others consider their knowledge and experience too outdated to have any current value. These ideas demonstrate ageism, which is discrimination against people because of increasing age, just as people who are racists and sexists discriminate because of skin color and gender. According to experts in the field of gerontology, ageism typically undermines the self-confidence of older adults, limits their access to care, and distorts caregivers' understanding of the uniqueness of each older adult. Always promote a positive perception regarding the aging process when you establish therapeutic relationships and show respect to older adults.

Current laws ban discrimination on the basis of age. The economic and political power of older adults challenges ageist views. Older adults are a significant proportion of the consumer economy. As voters and activists in various issues, they have a major influence in the formation of public policy. Their participation adds a unique perspective on social, economic, and technological issues because they have experienced almost a century of developments. In the past 100 years our nation has progressed from riding in horse-drawn carriages to tracking the adventures of the international space station. Gaslights and steam power have been replaced by electricity and nuclear power. Computers and copy machines replaced typewriters and carbon paper. Many older adults lived through or were born during the Great Depression of 1929. They also experienced two world wars and wars in Korea, Vietnam, and the Persian Gulf and are now experiencing the war on terrorism. They have seen changes in health care as the era of the family physician gave way to the age of specialization. After witnessing the government initiatives establishing the Social Security system, Medicare, and Medicaid, older adults are currently living with the changes imposed by health care reform and the uncertainty of the future of Social Security and Medicare. Living through all of these events and changes, they have stories and examples of coping with change to share.

NURSES' ATTITUDES TOWARD OLDER ADULTS

It is important for you to assess your own attitudes toward older adults; your own aging; and the aging of your family, friends, and patients. Nurses' attitudes come from personal experiences with older adults, education, employment experiences, and attitudes of co-workers and employing institutions. Given the increasing number of older adults in health care settings, forming positive attitudes toward them and gaining specialized knowledge about aging and the health care needs of older adults are priorities for all nurses. Positive attitudes are based in part on a realistic portrayal of the characteristics and health care needs of older adults. It is critical for you to respect older adults and actively involve them in care decisions and activities. In the past institutional settings such as hospitals and nursing centers often treated older adults as objects rather than independent, dignified people. The time has come for nurses to recognize and address ageism by questioning prevailing negative attitudes and stereotypes and reinforcing the realities of aging as they care for older adults in all care settings.

DEVELOPMENTAL TASKS FOR OLDER ADULTS

Theories of aging are closely linked to the concept of developmental tasks appropriate for distinct stages of life (see Chapter 11). Although no two individuals age in the same way, either biologically or psychosocially, researchers have developed frameworks outlining developmental tasks for older adults (Box 14-1). These developmental tasks are common to many older adults and are associated with varying degrees of change and loss. The more common losses are of health, significant others, a sense of being useful, socialization, income, and independent living. How older adults adjust to the changes of aging is highly individualized. For some adaptation and adjustment are relatively easy. For others coping with aging changes requires the assistance of family, friends, and health care professionals. Be sensitive to the effect of losses on older adults and their families and be prepared to offer support.

Older adults need to adjust to the physical changes that accompany aging. The extent and timing of these changes vary by individual but, as body systems age, changes in appearance and functioning occur. These changes are not associated with a disease; they are normal. The presence of disease sometimes alters the timing of the changes or their impact on daily life. The section on physiological changes describes structural and functional changes of aging.

Some older adults, both men and women, find it difficult to accept aging. This is apparent when they understate their ages when asked,

BOX 14-1 Developmental Tasks for Older Adults

- Adjusting to decreasing health and physical strength
- Adjusting to retirement and reduced or fixed income
- Adjusting to death of a spouse, children, siblings, friends
- Accepting self as aging person
- Maintaining satisfactory living arrangements
- Redefining relationships with adult children and siblings
- Finding ways to maintain quality of life

adopt younger styles of clothing, or attempt to hide physical evidence of aging with cosmetics. Others deny their aging in ways that are potentially problematic. For example, some older adults deny functional declines and refuse to ask for help with tasks, placing their safety at great risk. Others avoid activities designed for their benefit such as senior citizens' centers and senior health promotion activities and thus do not receive the benefits these programs offer. Acceptance of personal aging does not mean retreat into inactivity, but it does require a realistic review of strengths and limitations.

Older adults retired from employment outside the home need to cope with the loss of a work role. Older adults who worked at home and the spouses of those who worked outside the home also face role changes. Some welcome retirement as a time to pursue new interests and hobbies, volunteer in their community, continue their education, or start a new career. Retirement plans for others include changing residence by moving to a different city or state or to a different type of housing within the same area. Reasons other than retirement also lead to changes of residence. For example, physical impairments sometimes require relocation to a smaller, single-level home or nursing center. A change in living arrangements for the older adult usually requires an extended period of adjustment, during which assistance and support from health care professionals, friends, and family members are necessary.

The majority of older adults cope with the death of a spouse. In 2013 36% of all older women were widows, and 12% of older men were widowers (AOA, 2013). Some older adults must cope with the death of adult children and grandchildren. All experience the deaths of friends. These deaths represent both losses and reminders of personal mortality. Coming to terms with them is often difficult. By helping older adults through the grieving process (Chapter 37), you help them resolve issues posed by the deaths of those close to them.

The redefining of relationships with children that occurred as the children grew up and left home continues as older adults experience the challenges of aging. A variety of issues sometimes occur, including control of decision making, dependence, conflict, guilt, and loss. How these issues surface in situations and how they are resolved depend in part on the past relationship between the older adult and their adult children. All the involved parties have past experiences and powerful emotions. When adult children become their parents' caregivers, they have to find ways to balance the demands of their own children and careers with the many challenges of family caregiving. As adult children and aging parents negotiate the aspects of changing roles, nurses are in the position to act as counselors for the entire family. Helping older adults maintain their quality of life is often a priority. What defines quality of life is unique for each person.

COMMUNITY-BASED AND INSTITUTIONAL HEALTH CARE SERVICES

As a nurse you will encounter older-adult patients in a wide variety of community and institutional health care settings. Outside of an acute care hospital, nurses care for older adults in private homes and apartments, retirement communities, adult day care centers, assisted-living facilities, and nursing centers (extended care, intermediate care, and skilled nursing facilities). Chapter 2 describes these settings and the services provided in detail.

Nurses help older adults and their families by providing information and answering questions as they make choices among care options. Your assistance is especially valuable when patients and families need to make decisions about moving to a nursing center. Some family caregivers consider nursing center placement when in-home care becomes increasingly difficult or when convalescence (recovery) from hospitalization requires more assistance than the family is able to provide. Although the decision to enter a nursing center is never final and a nursing center resident is sometimes discharged to home or another less-acute facility, many older adults view the nursing center as their final residence. Results of state and federal inspections of nursing centers are available to the public at the nursing center, on-line, and at the inspectors' offices. The best way to evaluate the quality of a nursing center in a community is for the patient and family to visit that facility and inspect it personally. The Centers for Medicare and Medicaid (CMS website (http://www.Medicare.gov/NHcompare) is an excellent resource for you to learn about the quality rating of a nursing center on the basis of the health inspections, staffing, and quality measures of the facility. It also offers a nursing center checklist. Box 14-2 summarizes some features to look for in a nursing center.

BOX 14-2 FOCUS ON OLDER ADULTS

Selection of a Nursing Center or Home

An important step in the process of selecting a nursing center is to visit it. A quality nursing home has the following features:

- Does not feel like a hospital. It is a home, a place where people live. Residents are encouraged to personalize their rooms. Privacy is respected.
- Is Medicare and Medicaid certified.
- Has adequate, qualified staff members who have passed criminal background checks.
- Provides quality care, in addition to assistance with basic activities of daily living such as bathing, dressing, eating, oral hygiene, and toileting. Staff regularly help residents with social and recreational activities.
- Offers quality food and mealtime choices.
- Welcomes families when they visit the facility. Whether families wish to provide information, ask questions, participate in care planning, or help with social activities or physical care, staff always encourage family involvement.
- Is clean. There are no pervasive odors in the facility. The environment feels "homelike."
- Provides active communication from staff to patient and family.
- Attends quickly to resident requests. Staff are actively involved with assisting the residents. They focus on the person, not on the task.

Modified from the Centers for Medicare & Medicaid Services (CMS): *Your guide to choosing a nursing home or other long-term care,* Baltimore, MD, 2013, CMS, http://www.medicare.gov/Pubs/pdf/02174.pdf. Accessed March 25, 2015.

ASSESSING THE NEEDS OF OLDER ADULTS

Gerontological nursing requires creative approaches for maximizing the potential of older adults. With comprehensive assessment information regarding strengths, limitations, and resources, you and older adults identify needs and problems together. You select interventions with older adults to maintain their physical abilities and create environments for psychosocial and spiritual well-being (Chapter 36). To complete a thorough assessment, actively engage older adults and provide adequate time, allowing them to share important information about their health.

Nursing assessment takes into account three key points to ensure an age-specific approach: (1) the interrelation between physical and psychosocial aspects of aging, (2) the effects of disease and disability on functional status and, (3) tailoring the nursing assessment to an older person (Meiner, 2015). A comprehensive assessment of an older adult takes more time than the assessment of a younger adult because of the longer life and medical history and the potential complexity of the history. During the physical examination allow rest periods as needed or conduct the assessment in several sessions if a patient has reduced energy or limited endurance. Remember to review both prescribed and over-the-counter medications carefully with each patient.

A patient's sensory changes also affect data gathering. Your choice of communication techniques depends on an older adult's visual or hearing impairments. If an older adult is unable to understand your visual or auditory cues, your assessment data will likely be inaccurate or misleading, leading you to incorrectly conclude that the older adult is confused. When a person has a hearing impairment, speak directly to the patient in clear, low-pitched tones and move to a quiet area to reduce background noise. When caring for people with visual impairments, sit or stand at eye level and face them. Always encourage the use of assistive devices such as glasses and hearing aids. Chapter 49 explains in detail techniques to use when communicating with older adults who have sensory deficits.

Memory deficits, if present, affect the accuracy and completeness of your assessment. Information contributed by a family member or other caregiver is sometimes necessary to supplement an older adult's recollection of past medical events and information about current self-care habits, medication adherence, and history of allergies and immunizations. Use tact when involving another person in the assessment interview. The additional person supplements information with the consent of the older adult, but the older adult remains the primary source of the interview.

During all aspects of an assessment, you are responsible for providing culturally competent care. Your ability to recognize and process your own biases related to ageism, social norms, and racism affects your ability to provide culturally competent care. See Chapter 9 for a detailed description of the components of a cultural assessment. During an assessment, use caution when interpreting the signs and symptoms of diseases and laboratory values. Historically researchers used younger populations to establish these signs and norms. However, the classic signs and symptoms of diseases are sometimes absent, blunted, or atypical in older adults (Smith and Cotter, 2012). This is especially true in the cases of bacterial infection, pain, acute myocardial infarction, and heart failure. The masquerading of disease is possibly caused by age-related changes in organ systems and homeostatic mechanisms, progressive loss of physiological and functional reserves, or coexisting acute or chronic conditions. As a result an older adult with a urinary tract infection (UTI) sometimes presents with confusion, incontinence, and only a slight elevation of body temperature (within normal limits) instead of having fever, dysuria, frequency, or urgency. Some older adults with pneumonia have tachycardia, tachypnea, and confusion with decreased appetite and functioning, without the more common symptoms of fever and productive cough. Instead of crushing, substernal chest pain and diaphoresis, some older adults experience a sudden onset of dyspnea often accompanied by anxiety and confusion when having a myocardial infarction. Variations from the usual norms for laboratory values are sometimes caused by age-related changes in cardiac, pulmonary, renal, and metabolic function.

It is important to recognize early indicators of acute illness in older adults. Note changes in mental status, occurrence and reason for falls, dehydration, decrease in appetite, loss of function, dizziness, and incontinence because these symptoms are not frequently present in younger adults. A key principle of providing age-appropriate nursing care is timely detection of these cardinal signs of illness so early treatment can begin (Box 14-3). Mental status changes commonly occur as a result of disease and psychological issues. Some mental changes are often drug related, caused by drug toxicity or adverse drug events. Falls are complex and often cause injury. They are sometimes costly and can be a common event for an older adult. You need to investigate every fall carefully to find out if it was the result of environmental causes or the symptom of a new-onset illness. Problems with the cardiac, respiratory, musculoskeletal, neurological, urological, and sensory body systems sometimes present with a fall as a chief symptom of a new-onset condition. Dehydration is common in older adults because of decreased oral intake related to a reduced thirst response and less free water as a consequence of a decrease in muscle mass. When vomiting and diarrhea accompany the onset of an acute illness, an older adult is at risk for further dehydration. Decrease in appetite is a common symptom with the onset of pneumonia, heart failure, and UTI. Loss of functional ability occurs in a subtle fashion over a period of time; or it occurs suddenly, depending on the underlying cause. Thyroid

BOX 14-3 Examples of Altered Presentation of Illnesses in Older Adults Occurring in Various Health Care Settings

Hospital

- Confusion is not inevitable. Look for an acute illness, neurological events, new medication, or the presence of risk factors for delirium.
- Many hospitalized older adults suffer from chronic dehydration exacerbated by acute illness.
- Not all older adults have fevers with infection. Symptoms instead include increased respiratory rate, falls, incontinence, or confusion.

Nursing Home

- Health care providers often undertreat pain in older adults, especially those with dementia. Look for nonverbal cues or pain presence such as grimacing or resistance to care.
- Decline in functional ability (even a minor one such as the inability to sit upright in a chair) is a signal of new illness.
- Residents with less muscle mass—both the frail and the obese—are at a much higher risk for toxicity from protein-binding drugs such as phenytoin (Dilantin and others) and warfarin (Coumadin and others).
- New urinary and/or fecal incontinence is often a sign of the onset of a new illness.

Ambulatory Care

- Complaints of fatigue or decreased ability to do usual activities are often signs of anemia, thyroid problems, depression, or neurological or cardiac problems.
- Severe gastrointestinal problems in older adults do not always present with the same acute symptoms seen in younger patients. Ask about constipation, cramping sensations, and changes in bowel habits.
- Older adults reporting increased dyspnea and confusion, especially those with a cardiac history, need to go to the emergency department because these are the most common manifestations of myocardial infarction in this population.
- Depression is common among older adults with chronic illnesses. Watch for lack of interest in former activities, significant personal losses, or changes in role or home life.

Home Care

- Investigate all falls, focusing on balance, lower extremity strength, gait, and neurological issues (e.g., loss of sensation).
- Monitor older adults with late-stage heart disease for loss of appetite as an early symptom of impending heart failure.
- Drug-drug and drug-food interactions in older patients who are seeing more than one provider and taking multiple medications are common. Watch for signs of interactions.

disease, infection, cardiac or pulmonary conditions, metabolic disturbances, and anemia are common causes of functional decline. You play an essential role in early identification, referral, and treatment of health problems.

Physiological Changes

Perception of well-being defines quality of life. Understanding an older adult's perceptions about health status is essential for accurate assessment and development of clinically relevant interventions. Their concepts of health generally depend on personal perceptions of functional ability. Therefore older adults engaged in activities of daily living (ADLs) usually consider themselves healthy; whereas those who have physical, emotional, or social impairments that limit their activities perceive themselves as ill.

Some frequently observed physiological changes in older adults are normal (Table 14-1). The changes are not always pathological processes in themselves, but they make older adults more vulnerable to some common clinical conditions and diseases. Some older adults experience all of these changes, and others experience only a few. The body changes continuously with age; and specific effects on particular older adults depend on health, lifestyle, stressors, and environmental conditions. You need to understand these normal, more common changes to provide appropriate care for older adults and help with adaptation to associated changes.

General Survey. Your general survey begins during the initial nurse-patient encounter and includes a quick but careful head-to-toe scan of the older adult that you document in a brief description (see Chapter 31). An initial inspection reveals if eye contact and facial expression are appropriate to the situation and if universal aging changes (e.g., facial wrinkles, gray hair, loss of body mass in the extremities, an increase of body mass in the trunk) are present.

TABLE 14-1 Common Physiological Changes with Aging at a Glance

System	Common Changes
Integumentary	Loss of skin elasticity with fat loss in extremities; pigmentation changes; glandular atrophy (oil, moisture, sweat glands); thinning hair, with hair turning gray-white (facial hair: decreased in men, increased in women); slower nail growth; atrophy of epidermal arterioles
Respiratory	Decreased cough reflex; decreased cilia; increased anterior-posterior chest diameter; increased chest wall rigidity; fewer alveoli, increased airway resistance; increased risk of respiratory infections
Cardiovascular	Thickening of blood vessel walls, narrowing of vessel lumen, loss of vessel elasticity, lower cardiac output, decreased number of heart muscle fibers, decreased elasticity and calcification of heart valves, decreased baroreceptor sensitivity, decreased efficiency of venous valves, increased pulmonary vascular tension, increased systolic blood pressure, decreased peripheral circulation
Gastrointestinal	Periodontal disease; decrease in saliva, gastric secretions, and pancreatic enzymes; smooth-muscle changes with decreased peristalsis and small intestinal motility; gastric atrophy; decreased production of intrinsic factor; increased stomach pH; loss of smooth muscle in the stomach; hemorrhoids; rectal prolapse; and impaired rectal sensation.
Musculoskeletal	Decreased muscle mass and strength, decalcification of bones, degenerative joint changes, dehydration of intervertebral disks, fat tissue increases
Neurological	Degeneration of nerve cells, decrease in neurotransmitters, decrease in rate of conduction of impulses
Sensory	
Eyes	Decreased accommodation to near/far vision (presbyopia), difficulty adjusting to changes from light to dark, yellowing of the lens, altered color perception, increased sensitivity to glare, smaller pupils
Ears	Loss of acuity for high-frequency tones (presbycusis), thickening of tympanic membrane, sclerosis of inner ear, buildup of earwax (cerumen)
Taste	Often diminished; often fewer taste buds
Smell	Often diminished
Touch	Decreased skin receptors
Proprioception	Decreased awareness of body positioning in space
Genitourinary	Fewer nephrons, 50% decrease in renal blood flow by age 80, decreased bladder capacity Male—enlargement of prostate Female—reduced sphincter tone
Reproductive	Male—sperm count diminished, smaller testes, erections less firm and slow to develop Female—decreased estrogen production, degeneration of ovaries, atrophy of vagina, uterus, breasts
Endocrine	General—alterations in hormone production with decreased ability to respond to stress Thyroid—diminished secretions Cortisol, glucocorticoids—increased antiinflammatory hormone Pancreas—increased fibrosis, decreased secretion of enzymes and hormones, decreased sensitivity to insulin
Immune System	Thymus decreases in size and volume T-cell function decreases Core temperature elevation is lowered

Modified from Jett K: Physiological changes. In Touhy T, Jett K: *Ebersole and Hess' gerontological nursing and healthy aging,* ed 4, St Louis, 2014, Mosby.

Integumentary System. With aging the skin loses resilience and moisture. The epithelial layer thins, and elastic collagen fibers shrink and become rigid. Wrinkles of the face and neck reflect lifelong patterns of muscle activity and facial expressions, the pull of gravity on tissue, and diminished elasticity. Spots and lesions are often present on the skin. Smooth, brown, irregularly shaped spots (age spots or senile lentigo) initially appear on the backs of the hands and on forearms. Small, round, red or brown cherry angiomas occur on the trunk. Seborrheic lesions or keratoses appear as irregular, round or oval, brown, watery lesions. Years of sun exposure contribute to the aging of the skin and lead to premalignant and malignant lesions. You need to rule out these three malignancies related to sun exposure when examining skin lesions: melanoma, basal cell carcinoma, and squamous cell carcinoma (see Chapter 31).

Head and Neck. The facial features of an older adult sometimes become more pronounced from loss of subcutaneous fat and skin elasticity. Facial features appear asymmetrical because of missing teeth or improperly fitting dentures. In addition, common vocal changes include a rise in pitch and a loss of power and range.

Visual acuity declines with age. This is often the result of retinal damage, reduced pupil size, development of opacities in the lens, or loss of lens elasticity. Presbyopia, a progressive decline in the ability of the eyes to accommodate from near to far vision, is common. Ability to see in darkness and adapt to abrupt changes from dark to light areas (and the reverse) is reduced. More ambient light is necessary for tasks such as reading and other ADLs. Older adults have increased sensitivity to the effects of glare. Pupils are smaller and react slower. Objects do not appear bright, but older adults have difficulty when coming from bright to dark environments. Changes in color vision and discoloration of the lens make it difficult to distinguish between blues and greens and among pastel shades. Dark colors such as blue and black appear the same. Diseases of the older eye include cataract, macular degeneration, diabetic retinopathy, and retinal detachment. Cataracts, a loss of the transparency of the lens, are a prevalent disorder among older adults. They normally result in blurred vision, sensitivity to glare, and gradual loss of vision. Chapter 49 outlines nursing interventions for helping patients adapt to their visual changes.

Auditory changes are often subtle. Most of the time older adults ignore the early signs of hearing loss until friends and family members comment on compensatory attempts such as turning up the volume on televisions or avoiding social conversations. A common age-related change in auditory acuity is presbycusis. Presbycusis affects the ability to hear high-pitched sounds and conversational speech and is typically bilateral, affecting more men than women. Before the nurse assumes presbycusis, it is necessary to inspect the external auditory canal for the presence of cerumen. Impacted cerumen, a common cause of diminished hearing acuity, is easy to treat.

Salivary secretion is reduced, and taste buds atrophy and lose sensitivity. An older adult is less able to differentiate among salty, sweet, sour, and bitter tastes. The sense of smell also decreases, further reducing taste. Health conditions, treatments, and/or medications often alter taste. It is often a challenge to promote optimal nutrition in an older patient because of the loss of smell and changes in taste.

Thorax and Lungs. Because of changes in the musculoskeletal system, the configuration of the thorax sometimes changes. Respiratory muscle strength begins to decrease, and the anteroposterior diameter of the thorax increases. Vertebral changes caused by osteoporosis lead to dorsal kyphosis, the curvature of the thoracic spine. Calcification of the costal cartilage causes decreased mobility of the ribs. The chest wall gradually becomes stiffer. Lung expansion decreases, and the person is less able to cough deeply. If kyphosis or chronic obstructive lung disease is present, breath sounds become distant. With these changes an older adult is more susceptible to pneumonia and other bacterial or viral infections.

Heart and Vascular System. Decreased contractile strength of the myocardium results in decreased cardiac output. The decrease is significant when an older adult experiences anxiety, excitement, illness, or strenuous activity. The body tries to compensate for decreased cardiac output by increasing the heart rate during exercise. However, after exercise it takes longer for an older adult's rate to return to baseline. Systolic and/or diastolic blood pressures are sometimes abnormally high. Although a common chronic condition, hypertension is not a normal aging change and predisposes older adults to heart failure, stroke, renal failure, coronary heart disease, and peripheral vascular disease.

Peripheral pulses frequently are still palpable but weaker in lower extremities. Older adults sometimes complain that their lower extremities are cold, particularly at night. Changes in the peripheral pulses in the upper extremities are less common.

Breasts. As estrogen production diminishes, the milk ducts of the breasts are replaced by fat, making breast tissue less firm. Decreased muscle mass, tone, and elasticity result in smaller breasts in older women. In addition, the breasts sag. Atrophy of glandular tissue coupled with more fat deposits results in a slightly smaller, less dense, and less nodular breast. Gynecomastia, enlarged breasts in men, is often the result of medication side effects, hormonal changes, or obesity. Both older men and women are at risk of breast cancer.

Gastrointestinal System and Abdomen. Aging leads to an increase in the amount of fatty tissue in the trunk. As a result, the abdomen increases in size. Because muscle tone and elasticity decrease, it also becomes more protuberant. Gastrointestinal function changes include a slowing of peristalsis and alterations in secretions. An older adult experiences these changes by becoming less tolerant of certain foods and having discomfort from delayed gastric emptying. Alterations in the lower gastrointestinal tract lead to constipation, flatulence, or diarrhea.

Reproductive System. Changes in the structure and function of the reproductive system occur as the result of hormonal alterations. Women experience a reduced responsiveness of the ovaries to pituitary hormones and a resultant decrease in estrogen and progesterone levels. This can cause dryness of the vaginal mucosa, causing irritation and pain with intercourse, and may also cause a decreased libido. Aging men typically experience an erection that is less firm and shorter acting and have a less forceful ejaculation (Yeager, 2015).

Testosterone lessens with age and sometimes leads to a loss of libido. Spermatogenesis begins to decline during the fourth decade and continues into the ninth. However, for both men and women sexual desires, thoughts, and actions continue throughout all decades of life. Less frequent sexual activity often results from illness, death of a sexual partner, or decreased socialization.

Urinary System. Hypertrophy of the prostate gland is frequently seen in older men. This hypertrophy enlarges the gland and places pressure on the neck of the bladder. As a result, urinary retention, frequency, incontinence, and UTIs occur. In addition, prostatic hypertrophy results in difficulty initiating voiding and maintaining a urinary stream. Benign prostatic hypertrophy is different from cancer of the prostate. Cancer of the prostate is the second leading cause of cancer death in American men, behind only lung cancer. In 2014 the American Cancer Society estimated that one in seven men will be diagnosed with prostate cancer and 1 in 38 will die (ACS, 2015).

Urinary incontinence is an abnormal and typically embarrassing condition. Some men are afraid to discuss incontinence with their health care providers because they think that it is a "woman's disease." Older women, particularly those who have had children, experience stress incontinence, an involuntary release of urine that occurs when they cough, laugh, sneeze, or lift an object. This is a result of a weakening of the perineal and bladder muscles. Other types of urinary incontinence are urgency, overflow, functional, and mixed incontinence. The risk factors for urinary incontinence include age, menopause, diabetes, hysterectomy, stroke, and obesity.

Musculoskeletal System. With aging, muscle fibers become smaller. Muscle strength diminishes in proportion to the decline in muscle mass. Beginning in the 30s, bone density and bone mass decline in men and women. Older adults who exercise regularly do not lose as much bone and muscle mass or muscle tone as those who are inactive. Osteoporosis is a major public health threat. Fifty-four million Americans have osteoporosis or low bone mass, and approximately one in two women and one in four men over the age of 50 will break a bone because of osteoporosis (National Osteoporosis Foundation, n.d.). Postmenopausal women experience a greater rate of bone demineralization than older men. Women who maintain calcium intake throughout life and into menopause have less bone demineralization than women with low calcium intake. Older men with poor nutrition and decreased mobility are also at risk for bone demineralization.

Neurological System. A decrease in the number and size of neurons in the nervous system begins in the middle of the second decade. Neurotransmitters, chemical substances that enhance or inhibit nerve impulse transmission, change with aging as a result of the decrease in neurons. All voluntary reflexes are slower, and individuals often have less of an ability to respond to multiple stimuli. In addition, older adults frequently report alterations in the quality and the quantity of sleep (see Chapter 43), including difficulty falling asleep, difficulty staying asleep, difficulty falling asleep again after waking during the night, waking too early in the morning, and excessive daytime napping. These problems are believed to be caused by age-related changes in the sleep-wake cycle.

Functional Changes

Physical function is a dynamic process. It changes as individuals interact with their environments. Functional status in older adults includes the day-to-day ADLs involving activities within physical, psychological, cognitive, and social domains. A decline in function is often linked to illness or disease and its degree of chronicity. However, ultimately it is the complex relationship among all of these areas that influences an older adult's functional abilities and overall well-being.

Keep in mind that it may be difficult for older adults to accept the changes that occur in all areas of their lives, which in turn have a profound effect on functional status. Some deny the changes and continue to expect the same personal performance, regardless of age. Conversely some overemphasize them and prematurely limit their activities and involvement in life. The fear of becoming dependent is overwhelming for an older adult who is experiencing functional decline as a result of aging. Educate older adults to promote understanding of age-related changes, appropriate lifestyle adjustments, and effective coping. Factors that promote the highest level of function include a healthy, well-balanced diet; paced and appropriate activity; regularly scheduled visits with a health care provider; regular participation in meaningful activities; use of stress-management techniques; and avoidance of alcohol, tobacco, or illicit drugs.

Functional status in older adults refers to the capacity and safe performance of ADLs and instrumental ADLs (IADLs). It is a sensitive indicator of health or illness in the older adult. ADLs (such as bathing, dressing, and toileting) and IADLs (such as the ability to write a check, shop, prepare meals, or make phone calls) are essential to independent living; therefore carefully assess whether or not an older adult has changed the way he or she completes these tasks. Occupational and physical therapists are your best resources for a comprehensive assessment. A sudden change in function, as evidenced by a decline or change in an older adult's ability to perform any one or combination of ADLs, is often a sign of the onset of an acute illness (e.g., pneumonia, UTI, or electrolyte imbalance) or worsening of a chronic problem (e.g., diabetes or cardiovascular disease) (Kresevic, 2012).

Consult with other health care providers who work in a range of different settings and are experts in functional assessment. Several standardized functional assessment tools are widely available. An online collection of the tools used most commonly with older adults is available at the geriatric nursing website of the Hartford Institute for Geriatric Nursing, www.ConsultGeriRN.org.

When you identify a decline in a patient's function, focus your nursing interventions on maintaining, restoring, and maximizing an older adult's functional status to maintain independence while preserving dignity.

Cognitive Changes

A common misconception about aging is that cognitive impairments are widespread among older adults. Because of this misconception, older adults often fear that they are, or soon will be, cognitively impaired. Younger adults often assume that older adults will become confused and no longer able to handle their affairs. Forgetfulness as an expected consequence of aging is a myth. Some structural and physiological changes within the brain are associated with cognitive impairment. Reduction in the number of brain cells, deposition of lipofuscin and amyloid in cells, and changes in neurotransmitter levels occur in older adults both with and without cognitive impairment. Symptoms of cognitive impairment such as disorientation, loss of language skills, loss of the ability to calculate, and poor judgment *are not* normal aging changes and require you to further assess patients for underlying causes. There are standard assessment forms for determining a patient's mental status, including the Mini-Mental State Exam-2 (MMSE-2), the Mini-Cog, and the Clock Drawing Test (Jett, 2014).

The three common conditions affecting cognition are **delirium**, **dementia**, and **depression** (Table 14-2). Distinguishing among these three conditions is challenging. Complete a careful and thorough assessment of older adults with cognitive changes to distinguish among them. Select appropriate nursing interventions that are specific to the cause of the cognitive impairment.

Delirium. Delirium, or acute confusional state, is a potentially reversible cognitive impairment that often has a physiological cause. Physiological causes include electrolyte imbalances, untreated pain, infection, cerebral anoxia, hypoglycemia, medication effects, tumors, subdural hematomas, and cerebrovascular infarction or hemorrhage. Delirium in older adults sometimes accompanies systemic infections and is often the presenting symptom for pneumonia or UTI. Sometimes it is also caused by environmental factors such as sensory deprivation or overstimulation, unfamiliar surroundings, or sleep deprivation or psychosocial factors such as emotional distress. Although it occurs in any setting, an older adult in the acute care setting is especially at risk because of predisposing factors (physiological, psychosocial, and

TABLE 14-2 Comparison of Clinical Features of Delirium, Dementia, and Depression

Clinical Feature	Delirium	Dementia	Depression
Onset	Sudden/abrupt; depends on cause	Insidious/slow and often unrecognized	Happens with major life changes; often abrupt but can be gradual
Course	Short, daily fluctuations in symptoms; worse at night, in darkness, and on awakening	Long, no diurnal effects; symptoms progressive yet relatively stable over time; some deficits with increased stress	Diurnal effects, typically worse in the morning; situational fluctuations but less than with delirium
Progression	Abrupt	Slow over months and years	Variable; rapid or slow but even
Duration	Hours to less than 1 month; longer if unrecognized and untreated	Months to years	At least 6 weeks; sometimes several months to years
Consciousness	Reduced/disturbed	Awake	Awake
Alertness	Fluctuates; lethargic or hypervigilant	Generally normal	Normal
Attention	Impaired; fluctuates; inattention; distractible	Generally normal	Minimal impairment but is easily distracted
Orientation	Generally impaired; severity varies	Generally normal to person but not to place or time	Selective disorientation
Memory	Recently and immediately impaired; forgetful; unable to recall or follow directions	Recent memory worsens first in disease process, and remote memory becomes progressively impaired	Selective or "patchy" impairment; "islands" of intact memory; evaluation often difficult because of low motivation
Thinking	Disorganized, distorted, fragmented, illogical; incoherent speech, either slow or accelerated	Difficulty with abstraction; thoughts diminished; judgment impaired; words difficult to find	Intact but with themes of hopelessness, helplessness, or self-deprecation
Perception	Distorted perceptions often accompanied by delusions and hallucinations; difficulty distinguishing between reality and misperceptions	Misperceptions usually absent	Intact; delusions and hallucinations absent except in severe cases
Psychomotor behavior	Variable; hypoactive, hyperactive, or mixed	Normal; some have apraxia	Variable; psychomotor retardation or agitation
Sleep/wake cycle	Disturbed; cycle reversed	Fragmented	Disturbed; usually early morning awakening
Associated features	Variable affective changes; symptoms of autonomic hyperarousal; exaggeration of personality type; associated with acute physical illness	Affect tends to be superficial, inappropriate, and labile (changing); attempts to hide deficits in intellect; personality changes, aphasia, agnosia sometimes present; lacks insight and has poor judgment	Affect depressed; dysphoric mood; exaggerated and detailed complaints; preoccupied with personal thoughts; insight present; verbal elaboration; somatic complaints; poor hygiene; neglect of self
Assessment	Distracted from task; makes numerous errors	Failings highlighted by family, frequent "near-miss" answers; struggles with test; great effort to find an appropriate reply; frequent requests for feedback on performance	Failings highlighted by individual, frequent "don't knows"; poor motivation, frequently gives up; indifferent toward test; does not care or attempt to find answer

Modified from Milisen K et al: Assessing cognitive function. In Boltz M et al: *Evidence-based geriatric nursing protocols for best practice,* ed 4, New York, 2012, Springer.

environmental) in combination with underlying medical conditions. Dementia is an additional risk factor that greatly increases the risk for delirium; it is possible for delirium and dementia to occur in a patient at the same time. The presence of delirium is a medical emergency and requires prompt assessment and intervention. Nurses are at the bedside 24/7 and in a position to recognize delirium development and report it. The cognitive impairment usually reverses once health care providers identify and treat the cause of delirium.

Dementia. Dementia is a generalized impairment of intellectual functioning that interferes with social and occupational functioning. It is an umbrella term that includes Alzheimer's disease, Lewy body disease, frontal-temporal dementia, and vascular dementia. Cognitive function deterioration leads to a decline in the ability to perform basic ADLs and IADLs. Unlike delirium, a gradual, progressive, irreversible cerebral dysfunction characterizes dementia. Because of the similarity between delirium and dementia, you need to assess carefully to rule out the presence of delirium whenever you suspect dementia.

Nursing management of older adults with any form of dementia always considers the safety and physical and psychosocial needs of the older adult and the family. These needs change as the progressive nature of dementia leads to increased cognitive deterioration. To meet the needs of older adults, individualize nursing care to enhance quality of life and maximize functional performance by improving cognition, mood, and behavior. Box 14-4 lists general nursing principles for care of older adults with cognitive changes. Support and education about Alzheimer's disease for patients, families, and professionals can be found at the Alzheimer's Association website (www.alz.org).

BOX 14-4 Principles for Nursing Care of Adults Who Are Cognitively Impaired

- Provide a comprehensive assessment to differentiate between a progressive or reversible etiology.
- Institute medical measures to correct underlying physiological alterations (e.g., infection, electrolyte imbalances, pain).
- Maximize safe function. Keep a routine, encourage activity and mobility, limit choices (e.g., clothes for dressing, what to eat), allow for rest.
- Provide unconditional positive regard. Be respectful and provide positive nonverbal communication.
- Use behaviors to gauge activity and stimulation. Watch for nonverbal signs of anxiety.
- Teach caregivers to listen to the behaviors that show stress (e.g., verbalizations such as repetition).
- Make sure that the environment is safe for mobility and promote wayfinding with pictures or cues. Try to identify patients who wander and remove the cause (e.g., pain, thirst, unfamiliar surroundings, new noises).
- Promote social interaction on the basis of abilities.
- Compensate for sensory deficits (e.g., hearing aids, glasses, dentures).
- Encourage fluid intake (make sure that fluids are accessible) and avoid long periods of giving nothing orally.
- Be vigilant for drug reactions or interactions; consider onset of new symptoms as an adverse reaction.
- Activate bed and chair alarms.
- Provide ongoing assistance to family caregivers; educate them in nursing care techniques and inform them about community resources.

Modified from Fletcher K: Dementia. In Capezuti et al: *Evidence-based geriatric nursing protocols for best practice,* ed 4, New York, 2012, Springer.

Depression. Older adults sometimes experience late-life depression, but it is not a normal part of aging. Depression is the most common, yet most undetected and untreated, impairment in older adulthood. It sometimes exists and is exacerbated in patients with other health problems such as stroke, diabetes, dementia, Parkinson's disease, heart disease, cancer, and pain-provoking diseases such as arthritis. Loss of a significant loved one or admission to a nursing center sometimes causes depression. Clinical depression is treatable. Treatment includes medication, psychotherapy, or a combination of both. Electroconvulsant therapy (ECT) is sometimes used for treatment of resistant depression when medications and psychotherapy do not help. Of special note, suicide attempts in older adults are often successful. In fact, white men age 85 and older have the highest suicide rate in the United States (National Institute of Mental Health, n.d.).

Psychosocial Changes

The psychosocial changes occurring during aging involve life transitions and loss. The longer people live, the more transitions and losses they experience. Life transitions, of which loss is a major component, include retirement and the associated financial changes, changes in roles and relationships, alterations in health and functional ability, changes in one's social network, and relocation. But the universal loss for older adults usually revolves around the loss of relationships through death.

It is important to assess both the nature of the psychosocial changes that occur in older adults as a result of life transitions and the loss and the adaptations to the changes. During your assessment ask how an older adult feels about self, self in relation to others, and self as one who is aging and which coping methods and skills have been beneficial. Areas to address during the assessment include family, intimate relationships, past and present role changes, finances, housing, social networks, activities, health and wellness, and spirituality. Specific topics related to these areas include retirement, social isolation, sexuality, housing and environment, and death.

Retirement. Many often mistakenly associate retirement with passivity and seclusion. In actuality it is a stage of life characterized by transitions and role changes and may occupy 30 or more years of one's life. This transition requires letting go of certain habits and structure and developing new ones (Touhy, 2012). The psychosocial stresses of retirement are usually related to role changes with a spouse or within the family and to loss of the work role. Sometimes problems related to social isolation and finances are present. The age of retirement varies; but, whether it occurs at age 55, 65, or 75, it is one of the major turning points in life.

Preretirement planning is an important advisable task. People who plan in advance for retirement generally have a smoother transition. Preretirement planning is more than financial planning. Planning begins with consideration of the "style" of retirement desired and includes an inventory of interests, current skills, and general health. Meaningful retirement planning is critical as the population continues to age.

Retirement affects more than just the retired. It affects the spouse, adult children, and even grandchildren. When the spouse is still working, the retired person faces time alone. There may be new expectations of the retired person. For example, a working spouse has new ideas about the amount of housework expected of the retired person. Problems develop when the plans of the retired person conflict with the work responsibilities of the working spouse. The roles of the retiree and the working spouse need clarification. Some adult children expect the retired person to always care for the grandchildren, forgetting that this is a time for the retired person to pursue other personal interests.

Loss of the work role has a major effect on some retired people. When so much of life has revolved around work and the personal relationships at work, the loss of the work role is sometimes devastating. Personal identity is often rooted in the work role, and with retirement individuals need to construct a new identity. They also lose the structure imposed on daily life when they no longer have a work schedule. The social exchanges and interpersonal support that occur in the workplace are lost. In the adjustment to retirement an older adult has to develop a personally meaningful schedule and a supportive social network.

Factors that influence a retired person's satisfaction with life are health status and sufficient income. Positive preretirement expectations also contribute to satisfaction in retirement. You can help the older adult and family prepare for retirement by discussing with them several key areas, including relations with spouse and children; meaningful activities and interests; building social networks; issues related to income; health promotion and maintenance; and long-range planning, including wills and advance directives.

Social Isolation. Many older adults experience social isolation. Isolation is sometimes a choice, the result of a desire not to interact with others. It is also a response to conditions that inhibit the ability or the opportunity to interact such as the lack of access to transportation. Although some older adults choose isolation or a lifelong pattern of reduced interaction with others, older adults who experience social isolation become vulnerable to its consequences. An older adult's vulnerability increases in the absence of the support of other adults, as occurs with loss of the work role or relocation to unfamiliar surroundings. Impaired sensory function, reduced mobility, and cognitive changes all contribute to reduced interaction with others and often place an older adult at risk for isolation.

You assess patients' potential for social isolation by identifying their social network, access to transportation, and willingness and desire to interact with others. Use your findings to help a lonely older adult rebuild social networks and reverse patterns of isolation. Many communities have outreach programs designed to make contact with isolated older adults such as Meals on Wheels, which provides nutritional meals. Outreach programs such as daily telephone calls by volunteers or needs for activities such as social outings also meet socialization needs. Social service agencies in most communities welcome older adults as volunteers and provide the opportunity for them to serve while meeting their socialization or other needs. Churches, colleges, community centers, and libraries offer a variety of programs for older adults that increase the opportunity to meet people with similar activities, interests, and needs.

Sexuality. All older adults, whether healthy or frail, need to express their sexual feelings. Sexuality involves love, warmth, sharing, and touching, not just the act of intercourse. It plays an important role in helping the older adult maintain self-esteem. To help an older adult achieve or maintain sexual health, you need to understand the physical changes in a person's sexual response (see Chapter 35). You need to provide privacy for any discussion of sexuality and maintain a nonjudgmental attitude. Open-ended questions inviting an older adult to explain sexual activities or concerns elicit more information than a list of closed-ended questions about specific activities or symptoms. Include information about the prevention of sexually transmitted infections when appropriate. Sexuality and the need to express sexual feelings remain throughout the human life span.

When considering an older adult's need for sexual expression, do not ignore the important need to touch and be touched. Touch is an overt expression with many meanings and is an important part of intimacy (Yeager, 2015). Touch complements traditional sexual methods or serves as an alternative sexual expression when physical intercourse is not desired or possible. Knowing an older adult's sexual needs allows you to incorporate this information into the nursing care plan. The sexual preferences of older adults are as diverse as those of the younger population. Clearly not all older adults are heterosexual; and research is emerging on older adult, lesbian, gay, bisexual, and transgender individuals and their health care needs. Nurses often find that they are called on to help other health care professionals understand the sexual needs of older adults and advise them. Not all nurses feel comfortable counseling older adults about sexual health and intimacy-related needs. Be prepared to refer older adults to an appropriate professional counselor.

Housing and Environment. The extent of older adults' ability to live independently influences housing choices. Changes in social roles, family responsibilities, and health status influence their living arrangements. Some choose to live with family members. Others prefer their own homes or other housing options near their families. Leisure or retirement communities provide older people with living and social opportunities in a one-generation setting. Federally subsidized housing, where available, offers apartments with communal, social, and in some cases food-service arrangements.

The goal of your assessment of a patient's environment is to consider resources that promote independence and functional ability. When helping older adults with housing needs, assess their activity level, financial status, access to public transportation and community activities, environmental hazards, and support systems. When helping patients consider housing choices, anticipate their future needs as much as possible. For example, a housing unit with only one floor and without exterior steps is a prudent choice for an older adult with severe arthritis who has already had lower-extremity joint replacement surgery and anticipates the need for future operations. Assessment of safety, a major component of an older adult's environment, includes risks within the environment and the older adult's ability to recognize and respond to the risks (see Chapter 27). Safety risks in the home include factors leading to injury such as water heaters set at excessively hot temperatures or environmental barriers such as throw rugs or slippery floor surfaces that contribute to falls. Assess if a person has a pet that could easily move around the person's feet to cause a fall. Assess lighting in the home. Is the light bright enough to see walkways and stairs, and is there a lit path to the bathroom at night? Assess the safety of the home and environment with a family caregiver present if possible (Touhy, 2014).

Housing and environment affect the health of older adults. The environment supports or hinders physical and social functioning, enhances or drains energy, and complements or taxes existing physical changes such as vision and hearing. For example, furnishings with red, orange, and yellow colors are easiest for older adults to see. Shiny waxed floors may appear to be wet or have a hole in them. Ensure that door frames and baseboards are an appropriate color that contrasts with the color of the wall to improve perception of the boundaries of halls and rooms, keeping in mind that older adults often have difficulty distinguishing among pastel shades and between green and blue. Walkways leading to the house need to be flat and even, and stairs need to have a color contrast at the edge of the step so an older person knows where the stair ends. Glare from highly polished floors, metallic fixtures, and a window is difficult for an older adult to tolerate.

Furniture needs to be comfortable and safe. Older adults need to examine furniture carefully for size, comfort, and function before purchasing it. They need to be able to easily get into and out of the furniture, and it needs to provide adequate back support. Test dining room chairs for comfort during meals and for height in relation to the table. Many older adults find that chairs with armrests make it easier while getting into and out of the chair. Older adults often prefer transferring out of a wheelchair to another chair for meals because some styles of wheelchairs do not allow a person to sit close enough to the table to eat comfortably. Raising the table to clear the wheelchair arms brings the table closer to the older adult but makes it too high to eat comfortably. To make getting out of bed easier and safer, ensure that the height of the bed allows an older adult's feet to be flat on the floor when he or she is sitting on the side of the bed.

QSEN QSEN: BUILDING COMPETENCY IN SAFETY Mr. Sousa is an energetic 76-year-old man who is ready for discharge from the hospital. He does not "look" 76 as he appears very fit and states that he is active in social activities and volunteering. He was admitted to the hospital 3 days ago for a right total knee replacement and is doing well after surgery; he now walks with the assistance of one person and is using a walker. He is able to walk to the bathroom and has walked 125 feet in the hallway 3 times today. He will get home health care and home physical therapy rather than going to the hospital rehabilitation unit. He insists on going home because of his dog, Benji, a black Labrador retriever. Mr. Sousa's daughter is going to pick up Benji from the boarding kennel and take him home. Mr. Sousa's wife of 50 years died recently, leaving him alone at home, but he has been getting along well. His daughter lives within 25 miles of his home and will visit him daily. When considering safety for this patient in the home setting, which assessment questions and teaching approaches and resources can you use to enhance his safety in the home environment?

Answers to QSEN Activities can be found on the Evolve website.

Death. Part of one's life history is the experience of loss through the death of relatives and friends (see Chapter 37). This includes the loss of the older generations of families and sometimes, sadly, the loss of a child. However, death of a spouse or significant other is the loss that most affects the lives of older people. The death of a spouse affects older women more than men, a trend that will probably continue in the future. In spite of these experiences, do not assume that an older adult is comfortable with death. You play a key role in helping older adults understand the meaning of and cope with loss.

Current evidence supports that older people have a wide variety of attitudes and beliefs about death but fear of their own death is uncommon. Rather they are concerned with fear of being a burden, experiencing suffering, being alone, and the use of life-prolonging measures (Morgan and Upadhyaya, 2015). The stereotype that the death of an older adult is a blessing does not apply to every older adult. Even as death approaches, many older adults still have unfinished business and are not prepared for it. Families and friends are not always ready to let go of their older significant others. Older adults and family members or friends will often turn to you for assistance. Thus you need knowledge of the grieving process (see Chapter 37); excellent communication skills (see Chapter 24); understanding of legal issues and advance care planning (see Chapter 23); familiarity with community resources; and awareness of one's own feelings, limitations, and strengths as they relate to care of those confronting death.

Learning Needs

The complexities associated with managing chronic disease and the cognitive and sensory changes that may be associated with aging add to the challenges of teaching older adults. As you assess the various physical, cognitive, functional and psychosocial problems of older adults, it is important to also assess their associated learning needs. For example, during a cognitive and psychosocial assessment, you will learn information that indicates a patient's ability to follow a recommended treatment plan. When assessing a patient's medication history, have the patient describe when he or she takes the medication at home and what is the dosage. If a patient has slow responses or reaction time when performing physical activities, it will be necessary to consider these limitations when teaching new psychomotor skills. Older adults learn new information at a slower rate than younger adults due to a decline in fluid intelligence, which is defined as the reasoning and processing components of learning (Speros, 2009). In addition, an older adult has difficulty processing multiple bits of information at one moment. During your assessment, carefully consider a patient's learning needs and capability to learn.

ADDRESSING THE HEALTH CONCERNS OF OLDER ADULTS

As the population ages and life expectancy increases, emphasis on health promotion and disease prevention increases (see Chapter 6). The number of older adults becoming enthusiastic and motivated about these aspects of health is increasing. A number of national programs and projects address preventive practices in the older-adult population. The national initiative *Healthy People 2020* (Office of Disease Prevention and Health Promotion, 2015) has a number of major goals affecting the older adult population, including the following:

- Increase the number of older adults with one or more chronic conditions who report confidence in maintaining their conditions.
- Reduce the proportion of older adults who have moderate-to-severe functional limitations.
- Increase the proportion of older adults with reduced physical or cognitive function who engage in light, moderate, or vigorous leisure-term physical activities.
- Increase the proportion of older adults who receive diabetes self-management benefits.
- Increase the proportion of the health care workforce with geriatric certification.

The challenges of health promotion and disease prevention for older adults are complex and affect health care providers as well. Previous health care experiences, personal motivation, health beliefs, culture, health literacy, and non–health-related factors such as transportation and finances often create barriers for older adults. Barriers for health care providers include beliefs and attitudes about which services and programs to provide, their effectiveness and the lack of consistent guidelines, and absence of a coordinated approach. Your role is to focus interventions on maintaining and promoting patients' function and quality of life. You can empower older adults to make their own health care decisions and realize their optimum level of health, function, and quality of life (Meiner and Benzel-Lindley, 2015). Always be open to recognizing an older adult's concerns so you can adjust a plan of care accordingly. Although various interventions cross all three levels of care (i.e., health promotion, acute care, and restorative care), some approaches are unique to each level.

Educating Older Adults

Inadequate health literacy disproportionately affects older adults in the United States, causing misunderstanding of health information and subsequent nonadherence (Speros, 2009). The World Health Organization (2015) defines health literacy as the cognitive and social skills that determine the motivation and ability of individuals to gain access to, understand, and use information in ways that promote and maintain good health. To enhance comprehension and bring about positive health behavior changes, a nurse must use *more than words* when teaching older adults (Speros, 2009). Instead a nurse must know how to adapt routine patient education strategies to effectively meet the specific learning needs of elderly patients. Consider the need for learning new medications. Retrieving prescriptions and referrals, selecting providers from a list of names and addresses, calculating when to take multiple medications, interpreting medical terminology, comparing different insurance plans, and sifting through the myriad of health-related information available in magazines, on the Internet, and on television are just a few of the complex thought processes involved in selecting, understanding, and using health-related information about medications (Speros, 2009).

Box 14-5 summarizes teaching strategies to use for promoting an older adult's learning.

Health Promotion and Maintenance: Physiological Concerns

The desire of older adults to participate in health promotion activities varies. Therefore use an individualized approach, taking into account a person's beliefs about the importance of staying healthy and remaining independent. The Federal Interagency Forum on Aging-Related Statistics (2012) reported that 36% of older people 65 years and older reported a functional limitation (i.e., difficulty in hearing, vision, cognition, ambulation, self-care, or independent living), with older women reporting higher levels of functional limitations than men. Some of these disabilities are relatively minor, but others cause people to require assistance to meet important personal needs. The incidence of disability increases with age. Limitations in ADLs limit the ability to live independently. The ADL limitations most often reported include

BOX 14-5 PATIENT TEACHING

Adapting Instruction for Older Adults with Health Literacy Limitations

Objectives

- Patient will verbalize understanding of instructional content using Teach Back.
- Patient will demonstrate psychomotor skills.

Teaching Strategies

- Schedule teaching sessions in midmorning, when energy levels are high. Several brief teaching sessions on different days are more appropriate than one lengthy session that might fatigue the patient.
- Minimize use of medical terminology and replace with lay terms when possible.
- Allow additional time for the older adult to process new information by pausing after presenting each new concept or bit of information.
- Link new knowledge or skills to clearly identifiable past experiences. Reminiscing and storytelling help the older adult reconnect with lived experiences and serve as a valuable strategy to facilitate learning (e.g., explaining the use of an assist device and reviewing what occurred when a spouse had to a learn similar skill).
- Keep the content practical and relevant to the older adult's daily activities, social structure, and physical function. Emphasize safety and maintaining independence.
- Help the older adult focus during each interaction by minimizing distractions, limiting the message to a few (five or fewer) essential key points, and avoiding extraneous information.
- Speak slowly, but not so slowly that the patient becomes distracted or bored. Face the patient when speaking, and sit at the same level as the patient.
- Encourage the older adult to invite a family member or trusted friend to attend and actively participate in each teaching session.

Evaluation

- Validate understanding by using the Teach Back technique before moving on.
- Be sure the patient is able to demonstrate and do psychomotor skills independently.

Modified from Speros CI: More than words: promoting health literacy in older adults. *Online J Issue Nurs* 14(3):Manuscript 5, Sept 30, 2009; and Touhy T: Social, psychological, spiritual, and cognitive aspects of aging. In Touhy T, Jett K: *Ebersole and Hess' gerontological nursing and healthy aging*, ed 4, St Louis, 2014, Mosby.

walking, showering and bathing, getting in and out of bed and chair, dressing, toileting, and eating. There is a strong relationship between disability status and reported health status. The effect of chronic conditions on the lives of older adults varies widely, but in general chronic conditions further diminish well-being and a sense of independence. Direct nursing interventions at managing these conditions and educating family caregivers in ways to give appropriate support. You also need to focus interventions on prevention. General preventive measures to recommend to older adults include:

- Participation in screening activities (e.g., blood pressure, mammography, Papanicolaou [Pap] smears, depression, vision and hearing, colonoscopy)
- Regular exercise
- Weight reduction if overweight
- Eating a low-fat, well-balanced diet
- Moderate alcohol use

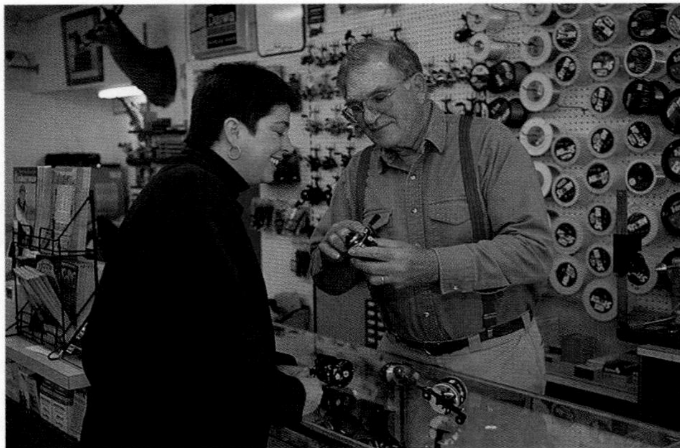

FIGURE 14-1 This older adult works part time at a sporting goods store.

- Regular dental visits
- Smoking cessation
- Stress management
- Socialization
- Good handwashing
- Regular check-ups with health care providers
- Immunization for seasonal influenza, tetanus, diphtheria and pertussis, shingles, and pneumococcal disease

Those who die from influenza are predominately older adults. Providers strongly recommend annual immunization of all older adults for influenza, with special emphasis on residents of nursing homes or residential or long-term care facilities. Not all older adults are current with their booster injections, and some never received the primary series of injections. Ask them about the current status of all immunizations, provide information about the immunizations, and make arrangements for them to receive immunizations as needed.

Most older adults are interested in their health and are capable of taking charge of their lives. They want to remain independent and prevent disability (Figure 14-1). Initial screenings establish baseline data that you use to determine wellness, identify health needs, and design health maintenance programs. Following initial screening sessions, share with older adults information on nutrition, exercise, medications, and safety precautions. You can also provide information on specific conditions such as hypertension, arthritis, or self-care procedures such as foot and skin care. By providing information about health promotion and self-care, you significantly improve the health and well-being of older adults.

Heart Disease. Heart disease is the leading cause of death in older adults, followed by cancer, chronic lung disease, and stroke (Murphy et al., 2013). Common cardiovascular disorders are hypertension and coronary artery disease. Hypertension is a silent killer because older adults are often unaware that their pressure is elevated (see Chapter 30). The fact that hypertension is common does not make it normal or harmless. Although one in three of Americans have elevated blood pressure, only one half of those have the condition under control. Treatment is linked to reduced incidence of myocardial infarction, chronic kidney disease, stroke, and heart failure. In coronary artery disease, partial or complete blockage of one or more coronary arteries leads to myocardial ischemia and myocardial infarction. The risk factors for both hypertension and coronary artery disease include smoking, obesity, lack of exercise, and stress. Additional risk factors for coronary artery disease include hypertension, hyperlipidemia, and diabetes mellitus. Nursing interventions for hypertension and coronary artery disease address weight reduction, exercise, dietary changes, limiting salt and fat intake, stress management, and smoking cessation. Patient teaching also includes information about medication management, blood-pressure monitoring, and the symptoms indicating the need for emergency care.

Cancer. Malignant neoplasms are the second most common cause of death among older adults. Nurses educate older adults about early detection, treatment, and cancer risk factors. Examples include smoking cessation, teaching breast self-examination (see Chapter 31), and encouraging all older adults to have annual screening for fecal occult blood with a rectal examination. It is also important to educate older adults about the signs of cancer and encourage prompt reporting of nonhealing skin lesions, unexpected bleeding, change in bowel habits, nagging cough, lump in breast or another part of body, change in a mole, difficulty swallowing, and unexplained weight loss. Cancer is difficult to detect because providers often mistake symptoms as part of the normal aging process or signs of a person's chronic disease. You need to carefully distinguish between signs of normal aging and signs of pathological conditions.

Chronic Lung Disease. Chronic lung disease, specifically chronic obstructive pulmonary disease (COPD) is the third leading cause of death in those 65 and older. More women than men die from COPD (American Lung Association, 2014). Lung injury from tobacco smoke leads to the development of COPD, causing airflow blockage and breathing-related difficulty. Tobacco smoke is a key factor in the development and progression of COPD. It is important to provide patients with information about quit smoking programs. In addition, depending on the severity of a patient's disease, you will teach a patient about proper exercise, how to use inhalers, and techniques for the removal of mucus from the airways (see Chapter 41). Exercise training is a major component of pulmonary rehabilitation programs today and is an established safe and effective intervention for improving patients' physical capacity and quality of life (American College of Sports Medicine, n.d.).

Stroke (Cerebrovascular Accident). Cerebrovascular accidents (CVAs) are the fourth leading cause of death in the United States and occur as brain ischemia (inadequate blood supply to areas of brain caused by arterial blockage) or brain hemorrhage (subarachnoid or intercerebral bleeds). Risk factors include hypertension, hyperlipidemia, diabetes mellitus, history of transient ischemic attacks, and family history of cardiovascular disease. CVAs often impair a person's functional abilities and lead to loss of independence and nursing home admission. The scope of nursing interventions ranges from teaching older adults about risk-reduction strategies to teaching family caregivers the early warning signs of a stroke and ways to support a patient during recovery and rehabilitation.

Smoking. Cigarette smoking is a risk factor for the four most common causes of death: heart disease, cancer, lung disease, and stroke. Smoking is the most preventable cause of disease and death in the United States. Smoking cessation is a health promotion strategy for older adults just as it is for younger adults. Older smokers still benefit from smoking cessation. In addition to reducing risk, it sometimes stabilizes existing conditions such as COPD and coronary artery disease. Smoking cessation after age 50 reduces the risk of dying prematurely by 50% compared with those who continue to smoke (NCI, 2014). Smoking cessation programs include individual, group, and telephone counseling and the use of nicotine (gum and patch) or non-nicotine medications. If a patient rejects smoking cessation, suggest at least a reduction in smoking. Finally set a quit or reduction date and a follow-up visit with the older adult to discuss the quit attempt. At follow-up visits, offer encouragement and assistance in modifying the plan as necessary.

Alcohol Abuse. Alcoholism is sometimes found in older adults. Studies of alcohol abuse in older adults report two patterns: a lifelong pattern of continuous heavy drinking and a pattern of heavy drinking that begins late in life. Frequently cited causes of excessive alcohol use include depression, loneliness, and lack of social support.

Alcohol abuse is often under-identified in older adults. The clues to creating suspicion of alcohol abuse are subtle; coexisting dementia or depression sometimes complicates your assessment. Your suspicion of alcohol abuse increases when there is a history of repeated falls and accidents, social isolation, recurring episodes of memory loss and confusion, failure to meet home and work obligations, a history of skipping meals or medications, and difficulty managing household tasks and finances. When you suspect that an older adult is abusing alcohol, realize that a variety of treatment needs are available. Treatment includes age-specific approaches that acknowledge the stresses experienced by an older adult and encourage involvement in activities that match his or her interests and increase feelings of self-worth. Identifying and treating coexisting depression is also important. The continuum of interventions ranges from simple education about risks to formalized treatment programs that include pharmacotherapy, psychotherapy, and rehabilitation.

Nutrition. Lifelong eating habits and situational factors influence how older adults meet their needs for good nutrition. Lifelong eating habits based in tradition, cultural habits and preferences, and religion influence food choices and how people prepare their food. Situational factors affecting nutrition include access to grocery stores, finances, physical and cognitive capability for food preparation, and a place to store food and prepare meals. Older adults' levels of activity and clinical conditions affect their nutritional needs. Level of activity has implications for the total amount of required calories. Older adults who are sedentary usually need fewer calories than those who are more active. However, activity alone does not determine caloric requirements. Patients often need additional calories in clinical situations such as recovery from surgery, whereas fewer calories are necessary when an older adult has diabetes or is overweight. Always consult with a clinical dietitian when planning nutritional interventions for your patients.

Healthy nutrition for older adults includes appropriate caloric intake and limited intake of fat, salt, refined sugars, and alcohol. Protein intake is sometimes lower than recommended if older adults have reduced financial resources or limited access to grocery stores. Difficulty chewing meat because of poor dentition or poor-fitting dentures also limits protein intake. Fat and sodium intake is sometimes higher than usual because of quick and convenient frozen meals or the substitution of fast-food restaurant meals for meals prepared at home. Home-prepared meals that are fried or made with canned goods also are high in fat and sodium. Some use extra salt and sugar while cooking or at the table to compensate for a diminished sense of taste. Older adults with dementia have special nutritional needs. As their memory and functional skills decline with the progression of dementia, they lose the ability to remember when to eat, how to prepare food, and how to feed themselves. Caloric needs sometimes increase because of the energy expended in pacing and wandering activities. When caring for older adults with dementia, routinely monitor weight and food intake, serve food that is easy to eat such as finger foods (e.g., chicken strips, sandwiches, cut-up vegetables, and fruit), provide assistance with eating, and offer food supplements that the patient likes and are easy to swallow. Home-delivered meals are an excellent source of nutrition for older adults.

Dental Problems. Dental problems with natural teeth and dentures are common in older adults. Dental caries, gingivitis, broken or missing teeth, and ill-fitting or missing dentures affect nutritional adequacy, cause pain, and lead to infection. Dentures are a frequent problem because the cost is not covered by Medicare and dentures tend to be quite expensive. Help prevent dental and gum disease through education about routine dental care (see Chapter 40).

Exercise. Encourage older adults to maintain physical exercise and activity. The primary benefits of exercise include maintaining and strengthening functional ability and promoting a sense of enhanced well-being. Regular daily exercise such as walking builds endurance, increases muscle tone, improves joint flexibility, strengthens bones, reduces stress, and contributes to weight loss. Other benefits include improvement of cardiovascular function, improved plasma lipoprotein profiles, increased metabolic rate, increased gastrointestinal transit time, prevention of depressive illness, and improved sleep quality. Older adults who participate in group exercise programs, individually tailored balance and strength programs, or planned walking programs often experience improved mobility, gait, and balance, resulting in fewer falls (CDC, 2015a).

Consult with physical therapists and a patient's health care provider to plan an exercise program that meets physical needs and is one the patient enjoys. Consider a patient's physical limitations and encourage him or her to stick with the exercise program. Many factors influence an individual's willingness to participate in an exercise program. These include general beliefs about benefits of exercise, past experiences with exercise, personal goals, personality, and any unpleasant sensations associated with exercise.

Walking is the preferred exercise of many older adults (Figure 14-2). Walking and other low-impact exercises such as riding a stationary exercise bicycle or water exercises in a swimming pool protect the musculoskeletal system and joints. Include other exercises in the older adult's ADLs. For example, have an older adult perform arm and leg circles while watching television. Before beginning an exercise program, all older adults need to have a physical examination. Exercise programs for sedentary older adults who have not been exercising regularly need to begin conservatively and progress slowly. Safety considerations include wearing good support shoes and appropriate clothing, drinking water before and after exercising, avoiding outdoor exercise when the weather is very warm or very cold, and exercising with a partner. Instruct older adults to stop exercising and seek help if they experience chest pain or tightness, shortness of breath, dizziness or lightheadedness, joint pain, or palpitations during exercise.

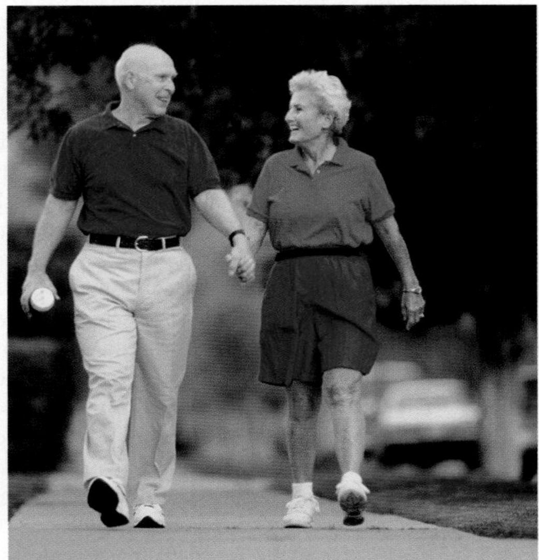

FIGURE 14-2 This couple enjoys walking together.

Falls. Falls are a safety concern of many older adults. A large research study of over 12,000 people over the age of 65 living in the community found that approximately 23% fell, yet less than half discussed it with their health care provider (Stevens et al., 2012). Fall-related injuries are often associated with a patient's preexisting medical conditions such as osteoporosis and bleeding tendencies. Hospitalization and placement in a nursing center for rehabilitation or long-term placement is sometimes necessary after a fall. In 2013 2.5 million nonfatal falls among older adults were treated in emergency departments, and more than 734,000 of these patients were hospitalized. The direct medical costs of those falls adjusted for inflation was $34 billion (CDC, 2015b). The most common injuries in older adults include fractures of the spine, hip, forearm, leg, ankle, pelvis, upper arm, and hand. Older adults who have fallen will often develop a fear of falling, which in turn often causes them to walk less naturally or to limit their activities, leading to reduced mobility and loss of physical fitness. See Chapter 39 for a complete description of fall-prevention interventions. Box 14-6 summarizes both intrinsic and extrinsic risk factors leading to falls.

Sensory Impairments. Because of common sensory impairments experienced by older adults, you need to promote existing sensory function and be sure that patients live in safe environments. Whenever you provide care activities, make sure that patients wear assist devices such as a hearing aid or glasses so they can fully

BOX 14-6 Risk Factors for Falls in Older Adults

Intrinsic Factors

- History of a previous fall
- Impaired vision
- Postural hypotension or syncope
- Conditions affecting mobility such as arthritis, lower extremity muscle weakness, peripheral neuropathy, foot problems
- Conditions affecting balance and gait
- Alterations in bladder function such as frequency or urge incontinence and nocturia
- Cognitive impairment, agitation, and confusion
- Adverse medication reactions (sedatives, hypnotics, anticonvulsants, opioids)
- Slowed reaction times
- Deconditioning

Extrinsic Factors

- Environmental hazards outside and within the home such as poor lighting, slippery or wet flooring, items on floor that are easy to trip over, furniture placement and other obstacles to ambulation, and sidewalks and stairs in poor repair
- Inappropriate footwear
- Unfamiliar environment of a hospital room that contains barriers to movement (e.g., clutter, equipment, poor lighting at night)
- Improper use of assistive devices (e.g., canes, walkers, crutches)

participate in care. Chapter 49 describes in detail the nursing interventions used to maintain and improve sensory function.

Pain. Pain is not a normal part of healthy aging. It is a symptom and a sensation of distress, alerting a person that something is wrong. It is prevalent in the older-adult population and may be acute or chronic. The consequences of persistent pain include depression, loss of appetite, sleep difficulties, changes in gait and mobility, and decreased socialization. Many factors influence the management of pain, including cultural influences on the meaning and expression of pain for older adults, fears related to the use of analgesic medications, and the problem of pain assessment with older adults who are cognitively impaired. Nurses caring for older adults have to advocate for appropriate and effective pain management (see Chapter 44). Again, the goal of nursing management of pain in older adults is to maximize function and improve quality of life.

Medication Use. One of the greatest challenges for older adults is safe medication use. Medication categories such as analgesics, anticoagulants, antidepressants, antihistamines, antihypertensives, sedative-hypnotics, and muscle relaxants create a high likelihood of adverse effects in older adults. They are at risk for adverse medication effects because of age-related changes in the absorption, distribution, metabolism, and excretion of drugs, collectively referred to as the process of pharmacokinetics (see Chapter 32). Medications sometimes interact with one another, adding or negating the effect of another drug. Examples of adverse effects include confusion, impaired balance, dizziness, nausea, and vomiting. Because of these effects, some older adults are unwilling to take medications; others do not adhere to the prescribed dosing schedule, or they try to medicate themselves with herbal and over-the-counter medications.

Polypharmacy, the concurrent use of many medications, increases the risk for adverse drug effects (Box 14-7). Although polypharmacy often reflects inappropriate prescribing, the concurrent use of multiple medications is often necessary when an older adult has multiple acute and chronic conditions. For example, it is common for a patient to take more than one medication to control hypertension. Your role as a nurse is to ensure the greatest therapeutic benefit with the least amount of harm by educating patients about safe medication use. You need to question the efficacy and safety of combinations of prescribed medications by conferring with pharmacists or health care providers. Advocate for the older adult to prevent adverse reactions. Older adults often use over-the-counter or herbal medications. The mix of over-the-counter and herbal medications with prescription medications can create adverse reactions.

For some older adults safely managing medications is complex and often becomes overwhelming. This problem is even more complicated when limited health literacy is an issue. Some take their medications incorrectly because they do not understand the administration instructions, thereby complicating your assessment of medication effects and side effects. Medications that need to be taken more than once or twice a day are a concern because a patient may not remember to take them as scheduled. As a nurse you are in a position to help older-adult patients as they carry out this important self-care activity (see Chapter 32).

The cost of prescriptions is often prohibitive. The Medicare Prescription Drug Benefit, Medicare Part D, was created in 2003 as part of the Medicare Modernization Act of 2003. This is not one plan but a designation of many plans that are approved by the Center for Medicare and Medicaid Services (CMS, 2015). Although accompanied by a deductible dependent on the number and expense of the medications prescribed, this benefit is of great help to aging adults. In

BOX 14-7 EVIDENCE-BASED PRACTICE

Polypharmacy in Older Adults

PICO Question: Do older community-living adults experience fewer adverse outcomes when they are on a limited medication therapy compared with older adults who are exposed to polypharmacy?

Evidence Summary

Polypharmacy is an important factor for numerous health problems in older adults, including the risk for adverse drug events (ADEs), the inappropriate use of medications, functional decline, and falls. In a study sample of 1503 community-dwelling older adults that recorded 1650 falls, 42% were judged to be at risk for falls because of polypharmacy (Boffin et al., 2014). Another study of older adults found a correlation between functional decline and older adults with dementia taking five or more medications (Lau et al., 2011). Polypharmacy causes a higher incidence of drug-to-drug interactions, especially in older adults, because of changes in pharmacokinetics, including changes with drug distribution and absorption, metabolism, and liver and renal clearance of drugs. A study of Canadian emergency department visits found that 21.5% of older adults presenting to the emergency department with an ADE were admitted to the hospital. In addition, the study identified that the drug classes most often associated with causing harm and occurring out of proportion to the frequency prescribed were anticoagulants, opioids, antibiotics, cardiovascular drugs, and nonsteroidal antiinflammatory drugs (Bayoumi et al., 2014). Over-the-counter supplemental herbals, vitamins, and drugs may also precipitate an ADE. Many supplements contain active ingredients that can have strong effects in the body. Although many prescriptions may be needed for some individuals, more prudent care is needed to lessen the risks. Two tools are especially helpful to providers to guide appropriate prescribing for older adults. *Beers Criteria for Potentially Inappropriate Medication Use in Older Adults,* a guideline developed originally in 1991 by the American Geriatrics Society and updated in 2012, (American Geriatrics Society, 2012) helps health care providers recognize drugs that have high association with ADEs. A Screening Tool of Older Person's Prescriptions and a Screening Tool to Alert Doctors to Right Treatment (STOPP-START) also screen for drug interactions and potentially inappropriate prescribing in older adults (Lam and Cheung, 2012). Using both sets of criteria, a study of 624 patients age 65 and older at time of hospital discharge showed that 22.9% had a potentially inappropriate prescription (PIP) using the Beer's criteria and 38.4% had a PIP using the STOPP-START criteria. PIP frequency also increased with the number of drugs prescribed (Hudhra et al., 2014).

Application to Nursing Practice

- Have patients and family caregivers ensure that one provider knows all medications that a patient is prescribed. This is especially important if a patient sees several physicians.
- Consider a possible ADE when a patient develops a new behavior or clinical change; consult the physician and a clinical pharmacist.
- Reconcile medications at the time of hospital admission and discharge to identify potentially inappropriate prescriptions.
- Review herbal supplements, vitamins, and over-the-counter medications in combination with prescription drugs for potential ADEs.
- Review older adults' medications in long-term settings routinely (e.g., monthly).
- Use nonpharmacological treatments known to be effective when possible.

addition, you advocate for patients who need certain medications by working with pharmacies or drug companies to provide the needed medication at less cost. Often a generic medication that will provide the desired effect is available at a reduced cost.

Work collaboratively with older adults to ensure safe and appropriate use of all medications, both prescribed and over-the-counter. Teach an older adult the names of all medications that he or she is taking, when and how to take them, and desirable and undesirable effects. Pill organizers and medication calendars help older adults track their doses. Explain how to avoid adverse effects and/or interactions of medications and how to establish and follow an appropriate self-administration pattern. Strategies for reducing the risk for adverse medication effects include reviewing the medications with older adults at each visit, examining for potential interactions with food or other medications, simplifying and individualizing medication regimens, taking every opportunity to inform older adults and their family caregivers about all aspects of medication use, and encouraging older adults to question their health care providers about all prescribed and over-the-counter medications.

When health care providers use medications to manage confusion, special care is necessary. Sedatives and tranquilizers sometimes prescribed for older adults who are acutely confused often cause or exacerbate confusion and increase risks for falls or other injuries. Carefully monitor patients who receive these medications, taking into account age-related changes in body systems that affect pharmacokinetic activity. When confusion has a physiological cause (such as an infection), health care providers need to treat the cause rather than the confused behavior. When confusion varies by time of day or is related to environmental factors, use creative, nonpharmacological measures such as making the environment more meaningful, providing adequate light, encouraging use of assistive devices, or even calling friends or family members to let older adults hear reassuring voices.

Health Promotion and Maintenance: Psychosocial Health Concerns

Interventions supporting the psychosocial health of older adults resemble those for other age-groups. However, some interventions are more crucial for older adults experiencing social isolation; cognitive impairment; or stresses related to retirement, relocation, or approaching death.

Elder Mistreatment. Elder mistreatment is complex and multifaceted and encompasses a broad range of abuses. It is found across all areas of nursing practice and socioeconomic settings. Consequently there is a strong likelihood that you will encounter elder mistreatment. Your ability to screen and assess for it is essential to the safety, health, and well-being of the older adult.

Elder mistreatment is defined as "intentional actions that cause harm or create serious risk of harm (whether harm is intended) to a vulnerable elder by a caregiver or other person who is in a trust relationship to the elder" (NRC, 2003). Types of elder mistreatment include physical abuse, emotional abuse, financial exploitation, sexual abuse, neglect (intentional and unintentional), and abandonment (Table 14-3). Although cases remain under-reported, data suggest that 10% of older adults in the United States experience some form of elder mistreatment (IOM and NRC, 2014). It is also common for vulnerable older adults to experience a combination of the various types of abuse.

Most perpetrators are relative caregivers, making abuse cases more complex to identify because of denial, fear of reporting, and the refusal of community services. Higher rates of elder mistreatment occur when there is a greater reliance on the caregiver because of functional and cognitive impairment. Low social support affects reports of mistreatment. One study found that reports of mistreatment tripled when there were poor social supports in place such as low income,

TABLE 14-3 Elder Mistreatment—Types, Descriptions, and Examples

Type	Description	Examples
Physical abuse	Inflicting or threatening to inflict physical pain or injury on a vulnerable older adult or depriving him or her of a basic need	Hitting, beating, pushing, slapping, kicking, physical restraint, inappropriate use of drugs, fractures, lacerations, rope burns, untreated injuries
Psychosocial/ emotional abuse	Verbal and nonverbal acts that inflict mental pain, anguish, and distress	Insults, threats, humiliation, intimidation, harassment, social isolation
Financial exploitation	Illegal taking, misuse, or concealment of funds, property, or assets of a vulnerable elder	Cashing check without authorization or permission, forging a signature, stealing money or possessions, coercing a signature on a financial document, forcing or improper use of guardianship or power of attorney, unpaid bills
Sexual abuse	Nonconsensual sexual contact or activity of any kind; coercing an elder to witness sexual behaviors	Unwanted touching, rape, sodomy, forced watching of pornography, coerced nudity, sexually explicit photography
Caregiver neglect	Refusal or failure by those responsible to fulfill caregiving activities, duties, protection, or obligations; may be intentional or unintentional because of lack of resources or education	Refusal or failure to provide basic necessities such as food, water, clothing, shelter, personal hygiene, or medication; unsafe and unclean living conditions, soiled bedding, animal or insect infestation
Abandonment	Desertion of a vulnerable elder by anyone who has assumed the responsibility for care or custody of that person	Desertion at a hospital, nursing facility, or public location such as a shopping center
Self-neglect	Behavior of an older adult that threatens his or her own well-being or safety; disregard of one's personal health or environment, causing unmet needs	Refusal or failure to provide oneself with basic necessities such as food, water, clothing, shelter, personal hygiene, medication, safety

Modified from the National Center on Elder Abuse, Administration on Aging: *Frequently asked questions,* n.d. http://www.ncea.aoa.gov/faq/index.aspx. Accessed March 30, 2015; and Fulmer T, Greenbery S: *Elder mistreatment & abuse,* 2015, http://consultgerirn.org/resources. Accessed March 30, 2015.

unemployment in the family, traumatic events, and little or no involvement of social services (Acierno et al., 2010). Vulnerable older adults may not reach out for help for fear of further retribution, fear of nursing home placement, or because they have become completely isolated from others. They may feel foolish or blame themselves for allowing someone to mistreat them or not want to get caregivers in legal or financial trouble (Bond and Butler, 2013).

Elder mistreatment has become the focus of national and international organizations, public and social policy, and research. Established by the U.S. Administration on Aging, the National Center for Elder Abuse (NCEA) is a resource center dedicated to the prevention of elder mistreatment. The Elder Justice Act of 2009 is widely regarded as the most comprehensive bill ever passed to address and battle elder mistreatment, providing federal funding to state Adult Protective Services (APS). In most states APS caseworkers are the first responders to reports of abuse, neglect, and exploitation of vulnerable adults. Services include receiving reports of adult abuse, exploitation or neglect, investigating these reports, case management, monitoring, and evaluation. In addition to casework services, APS arranges medical, social, economic, legal, housing, and law enforcement or other protective emergency or supportive services (National Center on Elder Abuse, n.d.).

As a nurse you are in a unique position to screen for elder mistreatment and assess for physical and emotional signs of abuse. A necessary part of your assessment is completing the interview and assessment privately away from the caregiver. It is definitely a "red flag" if the caregiver refuses to leave the room or area so you can ask questions confidentially. State laws differ on reporting and investigation of elder mistreatment. However, if you suspect that an older adult is being mistreated, it is your responsibility to know the reporting provisions of your jurisdiction (Falk et al., 2012).

Therapeutic Communication. Therapeutic communication skills enable you to perceive and respect the older adult's uniqueness and health care expectations. Attentive nurses provide care in a timely fashion, meeting a patient's expressed or unexpressed needs. A caring nurse expresses attitudes of concern, kindness, and compassion. Knowledgeable nurses not only demonstrate procedural competence but recognize needs and relay information skillfully. Patients accept and respect nurses who meet these expectations and communicate effectively about concern for the older adult's welfare. However, you cannot simply enter an older adult's environment and immediately establish a therapeutic relationship. First you have to be knowledgeable and skilled in communication techniques (see Chapter 24). Sitting down and engaging an older adult eye to eye goes a long way in establishing a therapeutic relationship.

Touch. Touch is a therapeutic tool that you use to help comfort older adults. It provides sensory stimulation, induces relaxation, provides physical and emotional comfort, conveys warmth, and communicates interest. It is a powerful physical expression of a relationship. In addition, gentle touch is a technique to use when administering any type of procedure that requires physical contact or repositioning and moving a patient.

Older adults are often deprived of touch when separated from family or friends. An older adult who is isolated, dependent, or ill; who fears death; or who lacks self-esteem has a greater need for touch. You recognize touch deprivation by behaviors as simple as an older adult reaching for the nurse's hand or standing close to the nurse. Unfortunately older men are sometimes wrongly accused of sexual advances when they reach out to touch others. When you use touch, be aware of cultural variations and individual preferences (see Chapters 7 and 9). Use touch to convey respect and sensitivity. Do not use it in a condescending way such as patting an older adult on the head. When you reach out to an older adult, do not be surprised if he or she reciprocates.

Reality Orientation. **Reality orientation** is a communication technique that makes an older adult more aware of time, place, and person. The purposes of reality orientation include restoring a sense of reality; improving the level of awareness, promoting socialization; elevating independent functioning; and minimizing confusion, disorientation, and physical regression. Although you use reality orientation techniques in any health care setting, they are especially useful in the acute care setting. The older adult experiencing a change in environment, surgery, illness, or emotional stress is at risk for becoming disoriented. Environmental changes such as bright lights, unfamiliar noises, and lack of windows in specialized units of a hospital often lead to disorientation and confusion. Absence of familiar caregivers is also disorienting. The use of anesthesia, sedatives, tranquilizers, analgesics, and physical restraints in older patients increases disorientation. Anticipate and monitor for disorientation and confusion as possible consequences of hospitalization, relocation, surgery, loss, or illness and incorporate interventions on the basis of reality orientation into the plan of care.

The principles of reality orientation offer useful guidelines for communicating with individuals who are acutely confused. The key elements of reality orientation include frequent reminders of person, place, and time; the use of familiar environmental aids such as clocks, calendars, and personal belongings; and stability of the environment, routine, and staff. However, do not continue to reorient older adults with chronic cognitive impairment. Communication is always respectful, patient, and calm. Answer questions from the older adult simply and honestly with sensitivity and a caring attitude.

Validation Therapy. **Validation therapy** is an alternative approach to communication with an older adult who is confused. Whereas reality orientation insists that the confused older adult agree with statements of time, place, and person, validation therapy accepts the description of time and place as stated by the older adult. Older adults with dementia are less likely to benefit and more likely to become agitated by a caregiver's insistence on the "correct" time, place, and person. In validation therapy you do not challenge or argue with statements and behaviors of the older adult. They represent an inner need or feeling. For example, a patient insists that the day is actually a different day because of high anxiety. The appropriate nursing intervention is to recognize and address that inner need or feeling. Validation does not involve reinforcing the older adult's misperceptions; it reflects sensitivity to hidden meanings in statements and behaviors. By listening with sensitivity and validating what the patient is expressing, you convey respect, reassurance, and understanding. Validating or respecting older adults' feelings in the time and place that is real to them is more important than insisting on the literally correct time and place.

Reminiscence. **Reminiscence** is recalling the past. Many older adults enjoy sharing past experiences. As a therapy, reminiscence uses the recollection of the past to bring meaning and understanding to the present and resolve current conflicts. Looking back to positive resolutions of problems reminds an older adult of coping strategies used successfully in the past. Reminiscing is also a way to express personal identity. Reflection on past achievements supports self-esteem. For some older adults the process of looking back on past events uncovers new meanings for those events.

During the assessment process use reminiscence to assess self-esteem, cognitive function, emotional stability, unresolved conflicts, coping ability, and expectations for the future. For example, have a patient talk about a previous loss to assess coping. You can also reminisce during direct care activities. Taking time to ask questions about past experiences and listening attentively conveys to an older adult your attitudes of respect and concern.

Although many use reminiscence in a one-on-one situation, it is also used as a group therapy for older adults who are cognitively impaired or depressed. You begin by organizing the group and selecting strategies to start a conversation. For example, you ask the group to discuss family activities or childhood memories, adapting questions to the group's size, structure, process, goals, and activities to meet its members' needs.

Body-Image Interventions. The way that older adults present themselves influences body image and feelings of isolation (see Chapter 34). Some physical characteristics of older adulthood such as distinguished-looking gray hair are socially desirable. Other features such as a lined face that displays character or wrinkled hands that show a lifetime of hard work are also impressive. However, too often society sees older people as incapacitated, deaf, obese, or shrunken in stature. Consequences of illness and aging that threaten an older adult's body image include invasive diagnostic procedures, pain, surgery, loss of sensation in a body part, skin changes, and incontinence. The use of devices such as dentures, hearing aids, artificial limbs, indwelling catheters, ostomy devices, and enteral feeding tubes also affects body image.

You need to consider the importance to an older adult of presenting a socially acceptable image. When older adults have acute or chronic illnesses, the related physical dependence makes it difficult for them to maintain body image. You influence an older adult's appearance by helping with grooming and hygiene. It takes little effort to help an older adult comb hair, clean dentures, shave, or change clothing. He or she does not choose to have an objectionable appearance. Be sensitive to odors in the environment. Odors created by urine and some illnesses are often present. By controlling odors you may prevent visitors from shortening their stay or not coming at all.

OLDER ADULTS AND THE ACUTE CARE SETTING

Older adults in the acute care setting need special attention to help them adjust to the acute care environment and meet their basic needs. The acute care setting poses increased risk for adverse events such as delirium, dehydration, malnutrition, health care–associated infections (HAIs), urinary incontinence, and falls. The risk for delirium increases when hospitalized older adults experience immobilization, sleep deprivation, infection, dehydration, pain, sensory impairment, drug interactions, anesthesia, and hypoxia. Nonmedical causes of delirium include placement in unfamiliar surroundings, unfamiliar staff, bed rest, separation from supportive family members, and stress. Impaired vision or hearing contributes to confusion and interferes with attempts to reorient an older adult. When the prevention of delirium fails, nursing management begins with identifying and treating the cause. Supportive interventions include encouraging family visits, providing memory cues (clocks, calendars, and name tags), and compensating for sensory deficits. Reality orientation techniques are often useful.

Older adults are at greater risk for dehydration and malnutrition during hospitalization because of standard procedures such as limiting food and fluids in preparation for diagnostic tests and medications that decrease appetite. The risk for dehydration and malnutrition increases when older adults are unable to reach beverages or feed themselves while in bed or connected to medical equipment. Interventions include getting the patient out of bed, providing beverages and snacks frequently, and including favorite foods and beverages in the diet plan.

The increased risk for HAIs in older adults is associated with the decreased immune system response related to advancing age in addition to other chronic conditions that make older adults more susceptible. UTIs are the most common type of HAI. Approximately 75% of UTIs acquired in hospitals result from the use of urinary catheters (CDC, 2015c). Other HAIs include central-line bloodstream infection, surgical site infection, *Clostridium difficile,* and hospital-acquired pneumonia. The leading preventive measure is hand hygiene combined with proper isolation policy and procedures to prevent and control the transmission of infection (see Chapter 29).

Older hospitalized adults are at risk for becoming incontinent of urine (transient incontinence). Causes of incontinence include delirium, untreated UTI, medications, restricted mobility, or need for assistance to get to the bathroom. Interventions to decrease incontinence include individualized care planning to provide voiding opportunities and modification of the environment to improve access to the toilet. Avoid indwelling urinary catheterization and promote measures to prevent skin breakdown (see Chapter 46).

The increased risk for skin breakdown and the development of pressure ulcers is related to changes in aging skin and to situations that occur in the acute care setting such as immobility, incontinence, and malnutrition. The key points in the prevention of skin breakdown are avoiding pressure with proper positioning and use of a support surface on the basis of risk status, reducing shear forces and friction, providing meticulous skin care and moisture management, and providing nutritional support (see Chapter 48).

Older adults in the acute care setting are also at greater risk for falling and sustaining injuries. The cause of a fall is typically multifactorial and composed of intrinsic or extrinsic factors (see Box 14-6). Sedative and hypnotic medications increase unsteadiness. Lower extremity weakness and general fatigue and deconditioning can make it difficult for a patient to get out of bed. Once the patient does get out of bed, often he or she is very unsteady and prone to falling. Medications causing orthostatic hypotension also increase the risk for falls because the blood pressure drops when an older adult gets out of a bed or chair. The increase in urine output from diuretics increases the risk for falling by increasing the number of attempts to get out of bed to void. Attempts to get out of bed when physically restrained sometimes lead to injury when an older adult becomes entangled in the restraint. Equipment such as wires from monitors, intravenous tubing, urinary catheters, and other medical devices become obstacles to safe ambulation. Impaired vision prevents an older adult from seeing tripping hazards such as trash cans. Many hospitals have significantly decreased restraint use and the incidence of falls by implementing frequent hourly rounds focusing on toileting needs, pain management, and personal needs of the patients. Other interventions to reduce the risk for falling in a health care setting are discussed in Chapter 39.

OLDER ADULTS AND RESTORATIVE CARE

Restorative care refers to two types of ongoing care: the continuation of the recovery from acute illness or surgery that began in the acute care setting and support of chronic conditions that affect day-to-day functioning. Both types of restorative care take place in private homes and long-term care settings.

Interventions during convalescence from acute illness or surgery aim at regaining or improving patients' prior level of independence in ADLs. Continue interventions that began in the acute care setting and later modify them as convalescence progresses. To achieve this continuation, ensure that discharge information provided by the acute care setting includes information on required ongoing interventions (e.g., exercise routines, wound care routines, medication schedules, and blood glucose monitoring). Interventions also need to address the restoration of interpersonal relationships and activities at either their previous level or the level desired by the older adult. When restorative care addresses chronic conditions, the goals of care include stabilizing the chronic condition, promoting health, and promoting independence in ADLs.

Interventions to promote independence in ADLs address a person's physical and cognitive ability and safety. The physical ability to perform ADLs requires strength, flexibility, and balance. You need to make accommodations for impairments of vision, hearing, and touch. The cognitive ability to perform ADLs requires the ability to recognize, judge, and remember. Cognitive impairments such as dementia interfere with safe performance of ADLs, although an older adult is still physically capable of the activities. Adapt interventions to promote independence in ADLs to meet the needs and lifestyle of the older adult. Although safety is paramount, an older adult needs to be able to perform ADLs with a level of risk that is acceptable to him or her. Collaborate with an occupational therapist, who is trained in selecting the correct type of assist devices for patients.

Beyond basic ADLs, you need to support an older adult's ability to perform IADLs such as using a telephone, doing laundry, cleaning the home or apartment, handling money, paying bills, and driving an automobile. To live independently at home or in an apartment, older adults need to be able to perform IADLs, purchase services by outside workers, or have a supportive network of family and friends who help with these tasks. Occupational therapists are an important resource for helping people adapt when IADLs are difficult to perform. Also, it might be appropriate to have a family caregiver assume more responsibility by completing IADLs for patients.

Restorative care measures focus on activities that allow older adults to remain functional within their living environments. Collaborate with an older adult to establish priorities of care and patient goals, determine expected outcomes, and select appropriate interventions. Patient collaboration promotes a patient's understanding about care and minimizes conflicts. Consideration of an older adult's lifetime experiences, values, and sociocultural patterns serves as the basis for planning individual care. When an older adult's cognitive status prevents participation in health care decisions, you need to include the family caregivers. Family and friends are rich sources of data because they knew the older adult before the impairment. Frequently they provide explanations for the older adult's behaviors and suggest methods of management. Thoughtful assessment and planning lead to goals of care that consider the influence of normal aging changes, facilitate an optimal level of comfort and coping, and promote independence in self-care activities.

KEY POINTS

- Nursing care of older adults poses special challenges because of great variation in their physiological, cognitive, and psychosocial health.
- When health care providers hold negative stereotypes about aging, these stereotypes can negatively affect the quality of patient care.
- The best way to evaluate the quality of a nursing center in a community is for a patient and family to visit that facility and inspect it personally.
- A comprehensive assessment of an older adult may take more time than the assessment of a younger adult because of the longer life and medical history, the potential complexity of the history, and the time it takes for an older adult to respond to questions.
- Classic signs and symptoms of diseases are sometimes absent, blunted, or atypical in older adults.
- Normal physiological changes of aging are not pathological processes, but they make older adults more vulnerable to some common clinical conditions and diseases.
- A sudden change in function, as evidenced by a decline or change in an older adult's ability to perform any one or combination of ADLs or IADLs, is often a sign of the onset of an acute illness.
- Symptoms of cognitive impairment such as disorientation, loss of language skills, and poor judgment are not normal aging changes and require you to further assess patients for underlying causes.
- Assess a patient's potential for social isolation by identifying social networks, access to transportation, and willingness and desire to interact with others.
- General preventive health measures for older adults include routine health screening; regular exercise; weight reduction if overweight; eating a low-fat, well-balanced diet; moderate alcohol use; regular dental visits; smoking cessation; and immunization.
- Polypharmacy, the concurrent use of many medications, increases the risk for adverse drug effects, inappropriate use of medications, and falls in older adults.
- Elder mistreatment is found across all areas of nursing practice and socioeconomic settings and includes physical, emotional, and sexual abuse; financial exploitation; caregiver neglect; self neglect; and abandonment.
- Reminiscence uses the recollection of the past to bring meaning and understanding to the present and resolve current conflicts.
- Acute care settings place older adults at risk for delirium, dehydration, malnutrition, HAIs, and falls.
- Restorative nursing interventions stabilize chronic conditions, promote health, and promote independence in basic and instrumental ADLs.

CLINICAL APPLICATION QUESTIONS

Preparing for Clinical Practice

Mrs. Kaven is an alert 81-year-old woman who is admitted to the hospital following emergency surgery for a hip pinning of a hip fracture secondary to a fall at her home. Her other medical problems are hypertension, hypothyroidism, and anxiety disorder for which she takes a diuretic and thyroid replacement medication. She has had bilateral knee replacements in the past. She is a retired bookkeeper, a widow living independently at her home, and usually very active. She drives, plays cards weekly with her friends, and participates in church activities twice a week. She hires help for household cleaning and yard work. She wears glasses, has uncorrected cataracts, and uses a cane.

You are assigned to care for her on her first postoperative day after the hip pinning. You learn in report that Mrs. Kaven has been receiving opioids for postoperative pain, with her last pain rating a 5 on a scale of 0 to 10. She has intravenous fluids for hydration for the first 24 hours. She has an indwelling urinary catheter. The night nurse reports that Mrs. Kaven was restless all night and slept very little and that she had even tried to get out of bed. Her ordered pain medication did not help her to sleep. You enter Mrs. Kaven's room and find her picking at the air and talking to herself as she tries to eat her breakfast. She is not wearing her glasses. She is oriented to self only. As you do your shift assessment, you recognize signs of delirium.

1. During your assessment, which conditions prompt you to suspect that the patient has delirium?
2. Mrs. Kaven's good friend comes to visit. She is concerned that Mrs. Kaven is confused. She asks you if there is anything she can do to help Mrs. Kaven be less confused. How do you respond to the friend?
3. Explain the approach that Mrs. Kaven's health care providers will use to reverse her delirium. Give some examples of these approaches.

ⓔ ***Answers to Clinical Application Questions can be found on the Evolve website.***

REVIEW QUESTIONS

Are You Ready to Test Your Nursing Knowledge?

1. A nursing student is caring for a 78-year-old patient with multiple sclerosis. The patient has had an indwelling Foley catheter in for 3 days. Eight hours ago the patient's temperature was 37.1° C (98.8° F). The student reports her recent assessment to the registered nurse (RN): the patient's temperature is 37.2° C (99° F); the Foley catheter is still in place, draining dark urine; and the patient is uncertain what time of day it is. From what the RN knows about presentation of symptoms in older adults, what should he recommend first?
   1. Tell the student that temporary confusion is normal and simply requires reorientation
   2. Tell the student to increase the patient's fluid intake since the urine is concentrated
   3. Tell the student that her assessment findings are normal for an older adult
   4. Tell the student that he will notify the patient's health care provider of the findings and recommend a urine culture
2. A patient's family member is considering having her mother placed in a nursing center. The nurse has talked with the family before and knows that this is a difficult decision. Which of the following criteria does the nurse recommend in choosing a nursing center? (Select all that apply.)
   1. The center needs to be clean, and rooms should look like a hospital room.
   2. Adequate staffing is available on all shifts.
   3. Social activities are available for all residents.
   4. The center provides three meals daily with a set menu and serving schedule.
   5. Staff encourage family involvement in care planning and assisting with physical care.
3. A nurse conducted an assessment of a new patient who came to the medical clinic. The patient is 82 years old and has had osteoarthritis for 10 years and diabetes mellitus for 20 years. He is alert but becomes easily distracted during the assessment. He recently moved to a new apartment, and his pet beagle died just 2 months ago. He is most likely experiencing:
   1. Dementia.
   2. Depression.
   3. Delirium.
   4. Hypoglycemic reaction.
4. The nurse is completing a health history with the daughter of a newly admitted patient who is confused and agitated. The daughter reports that her mother was diagnosed with Alzheimer's disease 1 year ago but became extremely confused last evening and was hallucinating. She was unable to calm her, and her mother thought she was a stranger. On the basis of this history, the nurse suspects that the patient is experiencing:
   1. Delirium.
   2. Depression.
   3. New-onset dementia.
   4. Worsening dementia.
5. Sexuality is maintained throughout our lives. Which of the following answers best explains sexuality in an older adult?
   1. When the sexual partner passes away, the survivor no longer feels sexual.
   2. A decrease in an older adult's libido occurs.
   3. Any outward expression of sexuality suggests that the older adult is having a developmental problem.
   4. All older adults, whether healthy or frail, need to express sexual feelings.
6. Older adults frequently experience a change in sexual activity. Which best explains this change?
   1. The need to touch and be touched is decreased.
   2. The sexual preferences of older adults are not as diverse.
   3. Physical changes usually do not affect sexual functioning.
   4. Frequency and opportunities for sexual activity may decline.
7. The nurse sees a 76-year-old woman in the outpatient clinic. She states that she recently started noticing a glare in the lights at home. Her vision is blurred; and she is unable to play cards with her friends, read, or do her needlework. The nurse suspects that the woman may have:
   1. Presbyopia.
   2. Presbycusis
   3. Cataract(s).
   4. Depression.
8. A nurse is caring for a patient preparing for discharge from the hospital the next day. The patient does not read. His family caregiver will be visiting before discharge. What can the nurse do to facilitate the patient's understanding of his discharge instructions? (Select all that apply.)
   1. Yell so the patient can hear you.
   2. Sit facing the patient so he is able to watch your lip movements and facial expressions.
   3. Present one idea or concept at a time.
   4. Send a written copy of the instructions home with him and tell him to have the family review them.
   5. Include the family caregiver in the teaching session.
9. A 63-year-old patient is retiring from his job at an accounting firm where he was in a management role for the past 20 years. He has been with the same company for 42 years and was a dedicated employee. His wife is a homemaker. She raised their five children, babysits for her grandchildren as needed, and belongs to numerous church committees. What are the major concerns for this patient? (Select all that apply.)
   1. The loss of his work role
   2. The risk of social isolation
   3. A determination if the wife will need to start working
   4. How the wife expects household tasks to be divided in the home in retirement
   5. The age the patient chose to retire
10. A nurse is assessing an older adult brought to the emergency department following a fall and wrist fracture. She notes that the patient is very thin and unkempt, has a stage 3 pressure ulcer to her coccyx, and has old bruising to the extremities in addition to her new bruises from the fall. She defers all of the questions to her caregiver son who accompanied her to the hospital. The nurse's next step is to:
    1. Call social services to begin nursing home placement.
    2. Ask the son to step out of the room so she can complete her assessment.

3. Call adult protective services because you suspect elder mistreatment.
4. Assess patient's cognitive status.

11. A nurse is participating in a health and wellness event at the local community center. A woman approaches and relates that she is worried that her widowed father is becoming more functionally impaired and may need to move in with her. The nurse inquires about his ability to complete activities of daily living (ADLs). ADLs include independence with: (Select all that apply.)
    1. Driving.
    2. Toileting.
    3. Bathing.
    4. Daily exercise.
    5. Eating.
12. During a home health visit a nurse talks with a patient and his family caregiver about the patient's medications. The patient has hypertension and renal disease. Which of the following findings place him at risk for an adverse drug event? (Select all that apply.)
    1. Taking two medications for hypertension
    2. Taking a total of eight different medications during the day
    3. Having one physician who reviews all medications
    4. Patient's health history of renal disease
    5. Involvement of the caregiver in helping with medication administration
13. The nurse is completing an admission assessment with an 80-year-old man who experienced a hip fracture following a fall. He is alert, lives alone, and has very poor hygiene. He reports a 20-pound weight loss in the last 6 months following his wife's death, as well as estrangement from his only child. He admits to falls before this most recent fall. What should the nurse suspect?
    1. Dementia.
    2. Elder abuse.
    3. Delirium.
    4. Alcohol abuse.
14. The nurse is working with an older adult after an acute hospitalization. The goal is to help this person be more in touch with time, place, and person. Which intervention will likely be most effective?
    1. Reminiscence
    2. Validation therapy
    3. Reality orientation
    4. Body image interventions
15. A 71-year-old patient enters the emergency department after falling down stairs in the home. The nurse is conducting a fall history with the patient and his wife. They live in a one-level ranch home. He has had diabetes for over 15 years and experiences some numbness in his feet. He wears bifocal glasses. His blood pressure is stable at 130/70. The patient does not exercise regularly and states that he experiences weakness in his legs when climbing stairs. He is alert, oriented, and able to answer questions clearly. What are the fall risk factors for this patient? (Select all that apply.)
    1. Impaired vision
    2. Residence design
    3. Blood pressure
    4. Leg weakness
    5. Exercise history

Answers: 1. 4; **2.** 2, 3, 5; **3.** 2; **4.** 1; **5.** 4; **6.** 4; **7.** 3; **8.** 2, 3, 5; **9.** 1, 4; **10.** 2; **11.** 2, 3, 5; **12.** 2, 4; **13.** 4; **14.** 3; **15.** 1, 4, 5.

Rationales for Review Questions can be found on the Evolve website.

REFERENCES

Administration on Aging (AOA): *A profile of older Americans,* 2013. http://www.aoa.acl.gov/Aging_Statistics/Profile/2013/docs/2013_Profile.pdf. Accessed June 13, 2015.

American Cancer Society (ACS): *Prostate cancer,* 2015. http://www.cancer.org/cancer/prostatecancer/. Accessed June 13, 2015.

American College of Sports Medicine: *Exercise for persons with chronic obstructive pulmonary disease,* n.d. http://www.acsm.org/docs/current-comments/exerciseforpersonswithcopd.pdf. Accessed July 11, 2015.

American Geriatrics Society 2012 Beers Criteria Update Expert Panel: American Geriatrics Society updated Beers Criteria for Potentially Inappropriate Medication Use in Older Adults, *J Am Geriatr Soc* 60(4):616, 2012.

American Lung Association: *Chronic obstructive pulmonary disease (COPD) fact sheet,* 2014. http://www.lung.org/lung-disease/copd/resources/facts-figures/COPD-Fact-Sheet.html. Accessed June 13, 2015.

Bond M, Butler K: Elder abuse and neglect: definitions, epidemiology, and approaches to emergency department screening, *Clin Geriatr Med* 29(1):257, 2013.

Centers for Disease Control and Prevention (CDC): *Preventing falls: a guide to implementing effective community-based fall prevention programs,* ed 2, 2015a. http://www.cdc.gov/homeandrecreationalsafety/pdf/falls/fallpreventionguide-2015-a.pdf. Accessed July 11, 2015.

Centers for Disease Control and Prevention (CDC): *Falls among older adults-an overview,* 2015b. http://www.cdc.gov/homeandrecreationalsafety/Falls/adultfalls.html. Accessed June 13, 2015.

Centers for Disease Control and Prevention (CDC): *Catheter-associated UTIs—CAUTI,* 2015c. http://www.cdc.gov/HAI/ca_uti/uti.html. Accessed June 13, 2015.

Centers for Medicare and Medicaid Services (CMS): *Drug coverage—Part D,* 2015. http://www.medicare.gov/part-d/index.html. Accessed June 13, 2015.

Falk N, et al: Elder mistreatment and Elder Justice Act, *Online J Nurs* 17(3):7, 2012.

Federal Interagency Forum on Aging-Related Statistics: *Older Americans 2012: key indicators of well-being,* 2012. http://www.agingstats.gov/Agingstatsdotnet/Main_Site/Data/2012_Documents/Docs/EntireChartbook.pdf. Accessed June 13, 2015.

Institute of Medicine (IOM) and National Research Council (NRC): *Elder abuse and its prevention: workshop summary,* Washington, DC, 2014, National Academies Press.

Jett K: Assessment and documentation for optimal care. In Touhy T, Jett K, editors: *Ebersole and Hess' gerontological nursing and healthy aging,* ed 4, St Louis, 2014, Mosby.

Kresevic D: Assessment of physical function. In Boltz M, et al, editors: *Evidence-based geriatric nursing protocols for best practice,* ed 4, New York, 2012, Springer.

Meiner S: Gerontologic assessment. In Meiner S, editor: *Gerontologic nursing,* ed 5, 2015, Mosby.

Meiner S, Benzel-Lindley J: Health promotion and illness/disability prevention. In Meiner S, editor: *Gerontologic nursing,* ed 5, 2015, Mosby.

Morgan C, Upadhyaya R: Loss and end-of-life issues. In Meiner S, editor: *Gerontologic nursing,* ed 5, 2015, Mosby.

Murphy S, et al: Deaths: final data for 2010, *Natl Vital Stat Rep* 61(4):May 8, 2013. http://www.cdc.gov/nchs/data/nvsr/nvsr61/nvsr61_04.pdf. Accessed June 13, 2015.

National Cancer Institute (NCI): *US National Cancer Institute fact sheet: harms of smoking and health benefits of quitting,* 2014. http://www.cancer.gov/cancertopics/factsheet/Tobacco/cessation. Accessed June 13, 2015.

National Center on Elder Abuse, Administration on Aging: *Adult protective services,* n.d. http://www.ncea.aoa.gov/Stop_Abuse/Partners/APS/index.aspx. Accessed June 13, 2015.

National Institute of Mental Health: *Older adults and depression,* n.d. http://www.nimh.nih.gov/health/publications/older-adults-and-depression/index.shtml. Accessed June 13, 2015.

National Osteoporosis Foundation: *Learn about osteoporosis,* n.d. http://www.nof.org/learn/basics. Accessed June 13, 2015.

National Research Council (NRC): *Elder mistreatment: abuse, neglect, and exploitation in an aging America, panel to review risk and prevalence of elder abuse and neglect,* Washington, DC, 2003, National Academics Press.

Office of Disease Prevention and Health Promotion: *Healthy People 2020, older adults,* 2015. http://www.healthypeople.gov/2020/topics-objectives/topic/older-adults. Accessed July 11, 2015.

Smith M, Cotter V: Age-related changes in health. In Boltz M, et al, editors: *Evidence-based geriatric nursing protocols for best practice*, ed 4, New York, 2012, Springer.

Speros CI: More than words: promoting health literacy in older adults, *Online J Issue Nurs* 14(3), Manuscript 5, Sept 30, 2009.

Touhy T: Relationships, roles, and transitions. In Touhy T, Jett K, editors: *Ebersole and Hess' toward healthy aging: human needs and nursing response*, ed 8, St Louis, 2012, Mosby.

Touhy T: Promoting safety. In Touhy T, Jett K, editors: *Ebersole and Hess' gerontological nursing and healthy aging*, ed 4, St Louis, 2014, Mosby.

U.S. Census Bureau: *Income and poverty in the United States: 2013, Current Population Reports,* 2014. https://www.census.gov/content/dam/Census/library/publications/2014/demo/p60-249.pdf. Accessed July 10, 2015.

World Health Organization: *Health Promotion: Health literacy and health behavior*, 2015. http://www.who.int/healthpromotion/conferences/7gchp/track2/en/. Accessed July 11, 2015.

Yeager J: Sexuality and aging. In Meiner S, editor: *Gerontologic nursing*, ed 5, 2015, Mosby.

RESEARCH REFERENCES

Acierno R, et al: Prevalence and correlates of emotional, physical, sexual, and financial abuse and potential neglect in the United States: the national elder mistreatment study, *Am J Public Health* 100(2):292, 2010.

Bayoumi I, et al: Medication-related emergency department visits and hospitalizations among older adults, *Can Fam Physician* 60(4):e217, 2014.

Boffin N, et al: Falls among older general practice patients: a 2-year nationwide surveillance study, *Fam Pract* 31(3):281, 2014.

Hudhra K, et al: Frequency of potentially inappropriate prescriptions in older people at discharge according to Beers and STOPP criteria, *Int J Clin Pharm* 36(3):596, 2014.

Lam MP, Cheung BM: The use of STOPP/START criteria as a screening tool for assessing the appropriateness of medications in the elderly population, *Expert Rev Clin Pharmacol* 5(2):187, 2012.

Lau DT, et al: Functional decline associated with polypharmacy and potentially inappropriate medications in community-dwelling older adults with dementia, *Am J Alzheimers Dis Other Demen* 26(8):606, 2011.

Stevens J, et al: Gender differences in seeking care for falls in the aged Medicare population, *Am J Prev Med* 12(43):59, 2012.

15

Critical Thinking in Nursing Practice

OBJECTIVES

- Discuss a nurse's responsibility in making clinical decisions.
- Discuss how reflection improves a nurse's capacity for making future clinical decisions.
- Describe the components of a critical thinking model for clinical decision making.
- Discuss critical thinking skills used in nursing practice.
- Explain the relationship between clinical experience and critical thinking.
- Discuss the critical thinking attitudes used in clinical decision making.
- Explain how professional standards influence a nurse's clinical decisions.
- Discuss the importance of managing stress when making clinical decisions.
- Discuss the relationship of the nursing process to critical thinking.

KEY TERMS

Clinical decision making, p. 200
Concept map, p. 205
Critical thinking, p. 196
Decision making, p. 199
Diagnostic reasoning, p. 199
Evidence-based knowledge, p. 196
Inference, p. 199
Knowing the patient, p. 200
Nursing process, p. 201
Problem solving, p. 199
Reflection, p. 196
Scientific method, p. 198

MEDIA RESOURCES

http://evolve.elsevier.com/Potter/fundamentals/

- Review Questions
- Case Study with Questions
- Audio Glossary
- Content Updates

As a nursing student you are just beginning to learn how to make clinical judgments or decisions about the patients and their families in your care. Clinical judgment is an essential skill that involves the interpretation of a patient's needs, concerns, or health problems and the decision to take action or not, to use or modify standard approaches, or to improvise new approaches on the basis of a patient's response (Tanner, 2006). Harjai and Tiwari (2009) explain it this way, "Contemporary nursing practice needs effective thinkers and decision makers who are capable of analyzing clinical data, medical and nursing knowledge, and environmental data, translating the analyses into life-saving interventions" (p. 305). Sound clinical judgment is associated with your ability to think critically. You apply it each day in your practice as a nurse.

Consider this example of critical thinking. The computer you are using flashes an error warning on the screen. You think about the steps you made before the error; consider the possible problem; and correct a key stroke, change a function, or maybe reboot the computer on the basis of your logic and reasoning skills. You consider what you know about computing, your past experiences in using computers, your experience with the same error in the past, and how you feel at the moment (stressed or hurried, calm and insightful) as you decide how to correct the error. You use a very similar critical thinking approach when you care for patients. However, you apply knowledge, clinical experiences, and professional standards when thinking critically and making decisions about patient care.

As you develop professionally, it is important to acquire critical thinking skills that allow you to face each new patient care experience or problem with open-mindedness, creativity, confidence, and continual inquiry. When a patient develops a new set of symptoms, asks you to offer comfort, or requires a procedure, it is important to think critically and make sensible judgments so the patient receives the best nursing care possible. Critical thinking is not a simple step-by-step, linear process that you learn overnight. It is a process gained only through experience, commitment, and an active curiosity toward learning. Thus this chapter leads you to think about and understand the thinking processes used in clinical judgment to help you improve your decision making and the ability to identify patient problems (Croskerry and Nimmo, 2011).

CLINICAL JUDGMENT IN NURSING PRACTICE

Registered nurses (RNs) are responsible for making accurate and appropriate clinical decisions or judgments. Clinical decision making separates RNs from technicians. For example, an RN observes for changes in patients, recognizes potential problems, identifies new problems as they arise, and takes immediate action when a patient's clinical condition worsens. Technical personnel are directed by nurses to perform certain aspects of care and report back any important observations to keep RNs informed. The RN is responsible for making decisions on the basis of clinical information. An RN relies on knowledge and experience when deciding if a patient is having complications that call for notification of a health care provider or if a teaching plan for a patient is ineffective and needs revision. Tanner (2006) describes clinical judgment or decision making as complex, requiring flexibility and the ability to know and recognize subtle changes or aspects of an undefined clinical situation. When a clinical situation develops (such as a patient experiencing pain, an adverse effect of a medication, or a serious drop in blood pressure), the RN must learn to recognize it, interpret the meaning, and respond appropriately.

Most patients have health care problems for which there are no clear textbook solutions. Each patient's health problems are unique, a product of the patient's physical health, lifestyle, culture, relationship with family and friends, living environment, and experiences. Thus as a nurse you do not always have a clear picture of a patient's needs and the appropriate actions to take when first meeting a patient. Instead you must learn to question, wonder, and explore different perspectives and interpretations to find a solution that benefits the patient. With experience you learn to creatively seek new knowledge, act quickly when events change, and make quality decisions for patients' well-being. You will find nursing to be rewarding and fulfilling through the clinical judgments you make.

CRITICAL THINKING DEFINED

Mr. Lawson is a 68-year-old patient who had abdominal surgery for a colon resection and removal of a tumor yesterday. His nurse, Tonya, finds the patient lying supine in bed with arms held tightly over his abdomen. His facial expression is tense. When Tonya checks the patient's surgical wound, she notes that he winces when she gently places her hands to palpate around the surgical incision. She asks Mr. Lawson when he last turned onto his side, and he responds, "Not since last night." Tonya asks Mr. Lawson if he is having pain around his incision, and he nods yes, saying, "It hurts too much to move." Tonya assesses Mr. Lawson with a pain-rating scale and finds that his pain is at a 7 on a scale of 0 to 10. Tonya considers the information she observed and learned from the patient to determine that he is in pain and has reduced mobility because of it. She decides to take action by administering an analgesic to relieve his pain so she can turn him more frequently and begin to get him out of bed for his recovery.

In the case example Tonya observes the patient's clinical situation; asks questions; considers knowledge gained from caring for previous patients with colon resection, postoperative pain, and risks from immobility; and takes action. Tonya makes a clinical decision by applying **critical thinking**, the ability to think in a systematic and logical manner with openness to question and reflect on the reasoning process. Critical thinking involves open-mindedness, continual inquiry, and perseverance, combined with a willingness to look at each unique patient situation and determine which identified assumptions are true and relevant. A nurse learns to recognize that a patient problem exists, analyzes information about the problem (e.g., clinical data, observation of patient behavior), evaluates the information (reviewing assumptions and evidence), and makes conclusions so he or she can act appropriately. A critical thinker considers what is important in each clinical situation, imagines and explores alternatives, considers ethical principles, and makes informed decisions about the care of patients.

Critical thinking is a way of thinking about a situation that always asks "Why?", "What am I missing?", "What do I really know about this patient's situation?", and "What are my options?" *Tonya knew that pain was likely going to be a problem because Mr. Lawson had extensive surgery. Her review of her observations and the patient's report of pain confirmed her knowledge that pain was a problem. Her options include giving Mr. Lawson an analgesic and waiting until it takes effect so she is able to reposition and make him more comfortable. Once he has less acute pain, Tonya offers to teach Mr. Lawson some relaxation exercises to maintain his comfort.*

You begin to learn how to think critically early in your practice. For example, as you learn about administering baths and other hygiene measures, take time to read your textbook, on-line resources, and the scientific literature about the concept of comfort. What are the criteria for comfort? How does a patient's culture affect perceptions of comfort? What are the many factors that promote comfort? The use of **evidence-based knowledge**, or knowledge based on research or clinical expertise, makes you an informed critical thinker. Thinking critically and learning about the concept of comfort prepares you to better anticipate your patients' needs, identify comfort problems quickly, and offer appropriate care. Critical thinking requires cognitive skills and the habit of asking questions, staying well informed, being honest in facing personal biases, and always being willing to reconsider and think clearly about issues (Facione, 1990). When core critical thinking skills are applied to nursing, they show the complex nature of clinical decision making (Table 15-1). Being able to apply all of these skills takes practice. You also need to have a sound knowledge base and thoughtfully consider what you learn when caring for patients.

Nurses who apply critical thinking in their work are able to see the big picture from all possible perspectives. They focus clearly on options for solving problems and making decisions rather than quickly and carelessly forming quick solutions (Kataoka-Yahiro and Saylor, 1994). Nurses who work in crisis situations such as the emergency department often act quickly when patient problems develop. However, even these nurses exercise discipline in decision making to avoid premature and inappropriate decisions. Learning to think critically helps you care for patients as their advocate, or supporter, and make better-informed choices about their care. Facione and Facione (1996) identified concepts for thinking critically (Table 15-2). Critical thinking is more than just problem solving. It is a continuous attempt to improve how to apply yourself when faced with problems in patient care.

Reflection

The ability to act on the basis of critical thinking comes with experience. When you care for patients, begin by thinking about previous situations and considering relevant issues: What did I notice before? How did I act? What could I have done differently? What should I do next time in the same situation? This is **reflection**, turning over a subject in the mind and thinking about it seriously. It involves purposeful thinking back or recalling a situation to discover its purpose or meaning. *For example, before Tonya makes a conclusion about Mr. Lawson's problems she thinks about previous surgical patients for whom she cared and how they responded to incisional pain. She recalls a patient who had a serious pulmonary embolus (clot in the lung) after surgery and how that pain differed from incisional pain. Reflecting on previous clinical situations prepares Tonya to act knowledgeably and quickly in caring for Mr. Lawson.* Research has shown that, when nurses reflect on past experiences, they perceive that their knowledge increases and their critical thinking moves to a higher level (Kaddoura, 2013).

Reflection is like instant replay. It is not intuitive. It involves playing back a situation in your mind and taking time to honestly review everything you remember about it. Reflective reasoning improves the accuracy of making diagnostic conclusions (Mamede et al., 2012). This means that, when you gather information about a patient, reflection on the meaning of your findings and exploration about what the

TABLE 15-1 Critical Thinking and Clinical Judgment Skills

Skill	Nursing Practice Applications
Interpretation	Be orderly in collecting data about patients. Apply reasoning while looking for patterns to emerge. Categorize the data (e.g., nursing diagnoses [see Chapter 17]). Gather additional data or clarify any data about which you are uncertain.
Analysis	Be open-minded as you look at information about a patient. Do not make careless assumptions. Does the data reveal a problem or trend that you believe is true, or are there other options?
Inference	Look at the meaning and significance of findings. Are there relationships among findings? Does the data about the patient help you see that a problem exists?
Evaluation	Look at all situations objectively. Use criteria (e.g., expected outcomes, pain characteristics, learning objectives) to determine results of nursing actions. Reflect on your own behavior.
Explanation	Support your findings and conclusions. Use knowledge and experience to choose strategies to use in the care of patients.
Self-regulation	Reflect on your experiences. Be responsible for connecting your actions with outcomes. Identify the ways you can improve your own performance. What will make you believe that you have been successful?

Modified from Facione P: *Critical thinking: a statement of expert consensus for purposes of educational assessment and instruction. The Delphi report: research findings and recommendations prepared for the American Philosophical Association,* ERIC Doc No. ED 315, Washington, DC, 1990, ERIC.; and Tanner CA: Thinking like a nurse: a research-based model of clinical judgment in nursing, *J Nurs Educ* 45(6):204, 2006.

TABLE 15-2 Concepts for a Critical Thinker

Concept	Critical Thinking Behavior
Truth seeking	Seek the true meaning of a situation. Be courageous, honest, and objective about asking questions.
Open-mindedness	Be tolerant of different views; be sensitive to the possibility of your own prejudices; respect the right of others to have different opinions.
Analyticity	Analyze potentially problematic situations; anticipate possible results or consequences; value reason; use evidence-based knowledge.
Systematicity	Be organized, focused; work hard in any inquiry.
Self-confidence	Trust in your own reasoning processes.
Inquisitiveness	Be eager to acquire knowledge and learn explanations even when applications of the knowledge are not immediately clear. Value learning for learning's sake.
Maturity	Multiple solutions are acceptable. Reflect on your own judgments; have cognitive maturity.

Modified from Facione N, Facione P: Externalizing the critical thinking in knowledge development and clinical judgment, *Nurs Outlook* 44(3):129, 1996.

BOX 15-1 Tips on Using Reflection

- Stop and think about what is going on with your patient. What do your assessment findings mean on the basis of what you have observed before with other patients? How do the findings compare with normal or baseline findings for the patient?
- Reflect carefully on any critical incidents (e.g., safety episodes, cardiac arrests, medication error, complex-care patient). What occurred? Which actions did you take? How did the patient respond? Did you think of taking any other options?
- Think about your feelings and the painful experiences you sometimes have. Realize that these emotions are real. How do they affect your care for others?
- At the end of each day after caring for a patient, take time to reflect. Ask yourself whether you achieved your original plan of care. If you did, why were you successful? If you did not, what were the barriers or problems? What would you do differently or the same?
- Keep all written care plans or clinical notes and papers. Use them frequently as a resource for care of future patients.
- Keep a personal journal and describe your feelings and experiences.

findings might mean improve your ability to problem solve. Reflection lessens the likelihood that reasoning is based on assumptions or guesswork. By reviewing your previous actions you see successes and opportunities for improvement. Always be cautious in using reflection. Reliance on it can block thinking and not allow you to look at newer evidence or subtle aspects of situations that you have not encountered. Box 15-1 summarizes tips on how to use reflection.

LEVELS OF CRITICAL THINKING IN NURSING

Your ability to think critically grows as you gain new knowledge and experience in nursing practice. Kataoka-Yahiro and Saylor (1994) developed a critical thinking model (Figure 15-1) that includes three levels: basic, complex, and commitment.

Basic Critical Thinking

As a beginning student you make a conscious effort to apply critical thinking because initially you are more task oriented and trying to learn how to organize nursing care activities. At the basic level of critical thinking a learner trusts that experts have the right answers for every problem. Thinking is concrete and based on a set of rules or principles. For example, as a nursing student you use a hospital procedure manual to confirm how to change an intravenous (IV) dressing. You likely follow the procedure step by step without adjusting it to meet a patient's unique needs (e.g., positioning to minimize the patient's pain or mobility restrictions). You do not have enough experience to anticipate how to individualize the procedure when problems arise. At this level answers to complex problems seem to be either right or wrong (e.g., when the IV is not infusing correctly, it must not be positioned in the vein). Although there are other explanations, basic critical thinkers tend to think that one right answer usually exists for each problem. Basic critical thinking is an early step in developing reasoning (Kataoka-Yahiro and Saylor, 1994). A basic critical thinker learns to accept the diverse opinions and values of experts (e.g., instructors and staff nurse preceptors). However, inexperience, weak competencies, and inflexible attitudes restrict a person's ability to move to the next level of critical thinking.

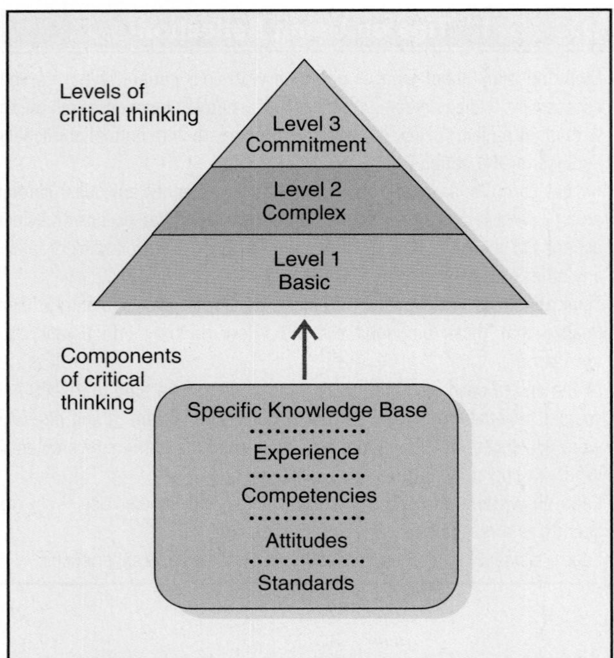

FIGURE 15-1 Critical thinking model for nursing judgment. (Redrawn from Kataoka-Yahiro M, Saylor C: A critical thinking model for nursing judgment, *J Nurs Educ* 33(8):351, 1994. Modified from Glaser E: *An experiment in the development of critical thinking,* New York, 1941, Bureau of Publications, Teachers College, Columbia University; Miller M, Malcolm N: Critical thinking in the nursing curriculum, *Nurs Health Care* 11:67, 1990; Paul RW: The art of redesigning instruction. In Willsen J, Blinker AJA, editors: *Critical thinking: how to prepare students for a rapidly changing world,* Santa Rosa, Calif, 1993, Foundation for Critical Thinking; and Perry W: *Forms of intellectual and ethical development in the college years: a scheme,* New York, 1979, Holt, Rinehart, & Winston.)

Complex Critical Thinking

Complex critical thinkers begin to separate themselves from experts. For example, while inserting a feeding tube, you recognize that your patient cannot swallow easily. Thus you adapt how you insert it. You analyze the clinical situation and examine choices more independently. A person's thinking abilities and initiative to look beyond expert opinion begin to change. As a nurse you learn that alternative and perhaps conflicting solutions exist.

Consider Mr. Lawson's case. His pain was partially relieved after receiving an analgesic (rating of 4 on scale of 0 to 10), and Tonya has helped him out of bed and into a chair. However, the patient becomes restless, cannot get comfortable, and begins to feel short of breath. Tonya wonders if something other than the incision is causing Mr. Lawson's discomfort. She sits down next to him and asks, "Is the pain you're feeling now different from before I gave you your medication?" The patient tells her that the pain feels sharper, in his chest. Tonya quickly takes a set of vital signs. His heart rate, which was 88 and regular 1 hour ago, is now 102 and irregular. Tonya calls the physician and notifies her of the changes in Mr. Lawson's condition. Tonya thought outside of the box. Rather than assume that Mr. Lawson's continued pain was from his incision, she gathered more data and recognized that the patient possibly was experiencing a life-threatening condition, a pulmonary embolus.

In complex critical thinking each solution has benefits and risks that you weigh before making a final decision. There are options. Thinking becomes more creative and innovative. The complex critical thinker is willing to consider different options from routine procedures when complex situations develop. You learn to gather additional information and take a variety of different approaches for the same therapy.

Commitment

The third level of critical thinking is commitment (Kataoka-Yahiro and Saylor, 1994). At this level you anticipate when to make choices without assistance from others and accept accountability for decisions made. As a nurse you do more than just consider the complex alternatives that a problem poses. At the commitment level you choose an action or belief that is based on the available alternatives and support it. Sometimes an action is to not act or to delay an action until a later time. You choose to delay as a result of your experience and knowledge. Because you take accountability for the decision, you consider the results of the decision and determine whether it was appropriate.

CRITICAL THINKING COMPETENCIES

Critical thinking competencies are the cognitive processes a nurse uses to make judgments about the clinical care of patients (Kataoka-Yahiro and Saylor, 1994). These include general critical thinking, specific critical thinking in clinical situations, and specific critical thinking in nursing. General critical thinking processes are not unique to nursing. They include the scientific method, problem solving, and decision making. Specific critical thinking competencies include diagnostic reasoning, clinical inference, and clinical decision making. The specific critical thinking competency in nursing is the nursing process, which involves each of the other three specific critical thinking competencies.

General Critical Thinking

Scientific Method. The scientific method is a methodical way to solve problems using reasoning. It is a systematic, ordered approach to gathering data and solving problems used by a variety of health care professionals. This approach looks for the truth or verifies that a set of facts agrees with reality. Nurse researchers use the **scientific method** when testing research questions (see Chapter 5). The scientific method has five steps:

1. Identify the problem.
2. Collect data.
3. Formulate a question or hypothesis.
4. Test the question or hypothesis.
5. Evaluate results of the test or study.

Box 15-2 offers an example of a nursing practice issue solved by applying the scientific method in a research study.

Problem Solving. Patients routinely present problems in nursing practice. For example, a home care nurse learns that a patient has difficulty taking her medications regularly. The patient is unable to describe which medications she has taken for the last 3 days. The medication bottles are labeled and filled. The nurse has to solve the problem of why the patient is not adhering to or following her medication schedule. The nurse knows that, when the patient was discharged from the hospital, she had five medications ordered. The patient tells the nurse that she also takes two over-the-counter medications regularly. When the nurse asks her to show the medications that she takes in the morning, the nurse notices that the patient has difficulty seeing the medication labels. The patient is able to describe the medications that she is to take but is uncertain about the times of administration.

BOX 15-2 Using the Scientific Method to Solve Nursing Practice Questions

Clinical Problem: Heart failure commonly results in 30-day hospital readmissions among hospitalized older adults. The Affordable Care Act, which includes two separate pieces of legislation—the Patient Protection and Affordable Care Act (P.L. 111-148) and the Health Care and Education Reconciliation Act of 2010 (P.L. 111-152), contains provisions that increase hospitals' financial accountability for preventable readmissions. If patients are inappropriately readmitted, hospitals receive less financial reimbursement. Are preventable readmissions in some way related to the level of care patients receive?

Identify the Problem: Are nurse staffing levels and nurse education associated with 30-day readmissions among Medicare patients with heart failure?

Collect Data: The researcher reviews the literature about heart failure readmissions and previous studies examining the effects that baccalaureate-prepared nurses have on discharge planning.

The researcher also reviews information about how a nursing work environment affects care delivery.

Form a Research Question to Study the Problem: What is the relationship between hospital nursing factors (defined as nurse work environment, nurse staffing levels, and nurse education) and 30-day readmissions among Medicare patients with heart failure?

Answer the Question: Analysis of data from three states in the United States included hospital nursing (i.e., work environment, patient-to-nurse ratios, and proportion of nurses holding a BSN degree), patient discharge data, and the American Hospital Association Annual Survey data.

Evaluate the Results of the Study. Is the Research Question Answered? Statistical methods estimated the relationship between nursing factors and 30-day readmission. Nearly 1 quarter of patients admitted to the hospital with heart failure (23.3% [n=39,954]) were readmitted within 30 days. Each additional patient assigned per nurse in the average nurse's workload was associated with 7% higher risk for readmission for heart failure. Care in a hospital with a good-versus-poor work environment was associated with odds of readmission that were 7% lower for heart failure (McHugh and Ma, 2013).

The nurse recommends having the patient's pharmacy relabel the medications in larger lettering. In addition, the nurse shows the patient examples of pill organizers that will help her sort her medications by time of day for a period of 7 days.

Effective problem solving involves evaluating a situation over time, identifying possible solutions, and trying a solution over time to make sure that it is effective. It becomes necessary to try different options if a problem recurs. From the previous example, during a follow-up visit the nurse finds that the patient has organized her medications correctly and is able to read the labels without difficulty. The nurse obtained information that correctly clarified the cause of the patient's problem and tested a solution that proved successful. Having solved a problem in one situation adds to a nurse's experience in practice, which allows the nurse to apply that knowledge in future patient situations.

Decision Making. When you face a problem or situation and need to choose a course of action from several options, you are making a decision. Decision making is a product of critical thinking that focuses on problem resolution. Following a set of criteria helps you make a thorough and thoughtful decision. The criteria may be personal; based on an organizational policy; or, in the case of nursing, a professional standard. For example, decision making occurs when a person decides on the choice of a health care provider. To make a decision, an individual has to recognize and define the problem or situation (need for a certain type of health care provider to provide medical care) and assess all options (consider recommended health care providers or choose one whose office is close to home). The person has to weigh each option against a set of personal criteria (experience, friendliness, and reputation), test possible options (talk directly with the different health care providers), consider the consequences of the decision (examine pros and cons of selecting one health care provider over another), and make a final decision. Although the set of criteria follows a sequence of steps, decision making involves moving back and forth when considering all criteria. It leads to informed conclusions that are supported by evidence and reason. Examples of decision making in the clinical area include determining which patient care priority requires the first response, choosing a type of dressing for a patient with a surgical wound, or selecting the best teaching approach for a family caregiver who will assist a patient who is returning home after a stroke.

Specific Critical Thinking

Diagnostic Reasoning and Inference. Once you gather information about a patient, as Tonya did in collecting information about Mr. Lawson's discomfort, diagnostic reasoning begins. It is the analytical process for determining a patient's health problems (Harjai and Tiwari, 2009). Accurate recognition of a patient's problems is necessary before you decide on solutions and implement action. It requires you to assign meaning to the behaviors and physical signs and symptoms presented by a patient. For example, what does Mr. Lawson's restlessness, shortness of breath, and developing chest pain indicate? Diagnostic reasoning begins when you interact with a patient or make physical or behavioral observations. An expert nurse sees the context of a patient situation (e.g., Mr. Lawson just had major surgery; has been inactive; and is at risk for blood pooling in the lower extremities, which can cause clots to form in the circulation), observes patterns and themes (e.g., symptoms that include shortness of breath, sharp chest pain, and irregular heart rate), and makes decisions quickly (e.g., a clot may have dislodged and traveled to the patient's lung, requiring a quick medical response). The information that a nurse collects and analyzes leads to a diagnosis of a patient's condition. Nurses do not make medical diagnoses, but they do assess and monitor each patient closely and compare a patient's signs and symptoms with those that are common to a medical diagnosis (e.g., in the case of Mr. Lawson, a pulmonary embolus). Diagnostic reasoning helps health care providers pinpoint the nature of a problem more quickly and select proper therapies.

Part of diagnostic reasoning is clinical inference, the process of drawing conclusions from related pieces of evidence and previous experience with the evidence. When making an inference, you form patterns of information from data before making a diagnosis. *In the initial scenario Tonya noted that Mr. Lawson was lying in a position to splint movement of his incision, had a tense facial expression, and experienced tenderness when his wound was palpated. Tonya infers that Mr. Lawson has a level of discomfort.* She demonstrates diagnostic reasoning by identifying the nursing diagnosis *Acute Pain* (see Chapter 17).

In diagnostic reasoning Tonya used patient data that she gathered and analyzed logically to recognize a problem. As a student, confirm any judgments such as when you make nursing diagnoses or believe that a medical problem is developing with experienced nurses. At times you may be wrong, but consulting with nurse experts gives you feedback to build on future clinical situations.

Often you cannot make a precise diagnosis during your first meeting with a patient. Sometimes you sense that a problem exists but do not have enough data to make a specific diagnosis. Some patients' physical conditions limit their ability to tell you about symptoms. Some choose to not share sensitive and important information during your initial assessment. Some patients' behaviors and physical responses become observable only under conditions not present during your initial assessment. When uncertain of a diagnosis, continue data collection. You have to critically analyze changing clinical situations until you are able to determine a patient's unique situation. Any diagnostic conclusions that you make will help health care providers identify the nature of a problem more quickly and select appropriate medical therapies.

Clinical Decision Making. As in the case of general decision making, clinical decision making is a problem-solving activity. It goes beyond diagnostic reasoning when you focus on defining a problem or diagnosis and selecting appropriate nursing interventions. When you approach a clinical problem such as a patient who is less mobile and develops an area of redness over the hip, you make a decision that identifies the problem (impaired skin integrity in the form of a pressure ulcer) and choose the best nursing interventions (skin care, special bed surface, and a turning schedule). Nurses make clinical decisions all the time to improve a patient's health or maintain wellness. This means reducing the severity of the problem or resolving the problem completely. **Clinical decision making** requires careful reasoning (i.e., choosing the options for the best patient outcomes on the basis of a patient's condition and the priority of the problem).

Skilled clinical decision making occurs through **knowing the patient** (Zolnierek, 2014). Knowing the patient is an in-depth knowledge of a patient's patterns of responses within a clinical situation and knowing the patient as a person (Tanner et al., 1993). It has two components: a nurse's understanding of a specific patient and his or her subsequent selection of interventions. Knowing the patient relates to a nurse's experience with caring for patients, time spent in a specific clinical area, and having a sense of closeness with patients (Radwin, 1996). For example, an expert nurse who has worked on a general surgery unit for many years has been caring for a patient the last 2 days. The nurse is familiar with how the patient is progressing physically and mentally. When the patient begins to experience a change (e.g., a slight fall in blood pressure, becoming less responsive), the nurse knows that something is wrong, suspects the patient may be bleeding internally, and takes action. Because of her clinical experience and knowing the patient, the expert nurse can make a clinical decision and act more quickly than a new nurse can be expected to act.

Knowing the patient is central to individualizing nursing care so a patient feels cared for and cared about (Zolnierek, 2014). Knowing offers a nurse "the big picture" and "knowing the whole person" so he or she can make suitable decisions to protect patients from harm. Henneman et al. (2010) found that knowing the patient enabled nurses to identify problems and potential errors and thus rescue their patients from potential adverse events. A critical aspect to knowing patients and thus being able to make timely and appropriate decisions is spending time establishing relationships with them (Zolnierek, 2014). A study found that work relationships with patients, families, and colleagues are most strongly associated with nurses' expertise (Roche et al., 2009).

Build your ability to make clinical decisions by fostering knowing your patients. Follow these tips:

- Spend more time during initial patient assessments to observe patient behavior and measure physical findings as a way to improve knowledge of your patients. Determine what is important to them and make an emotional connection. Patients perceive meaningful time as that involving personal rather than task-oriented conversation.
- When talking with patients, listen to their accounts of their experiences with illness, watch them, and come to understand how they typically respond (Tanner, 2006).
- Consistently check on patients to assess and monitor problems to help you identify how clinical changes develop over time.
- Ask to have the same patient assigned to you over consecutive days. Researchers have noted that a nurse-patient relationship develops from getting to know a patient and building a foundation for connecting on the first day of care, to deepening understanding of the patient and sustaining a connection by the second day, to being comfortable with the patient by the third day (Lotzkar and Bottorff, 2010).
- Social conversation and continuity are important for developing knowing and nurse-patient relationships (Zolnierek, 2014).

Always keep a patient as your center of focus as you try to solve clinical problems. Making accurate clinical decisions allows you to set priorities for the interventions to implement first (see Chapter 18). Do not assume that certain health situations produce automatic priorities. For example, a patient who has surgery is anticipated to experience a certain level of postoperative pain, which often becomes a priority for care. However, if a patient is experiencing severe anxiety that increases pain perception, you need to focus on ways to relieve the anxiety before pain-relief measures will be effective.

Critical thinking and clinical decision making are complicated because nurses care for multiple patients in fast-paced and unpredictable environments. When you work in a busy setting, use criteria that includes the clinical condition of the patient, Maslow's hierarchy of needs (see Chapter 6), the risks involved in treatment delays, environmental factors (staff resources available), and patients' expectations of care to determine which patients have the greatest priorities for care. For example, a patient who is having a sudden drop in blood pressure along with a change in consciousness requires your attention immediately as opposed to a patient who needs you to collect a urine specimen or one who needs your help to walk down the hallway. Critical thinking in decision making allows you to attend to a patient whose condition is changing quickly and delegate the specimen collection and ambulation to nursing assistive personnel. For you to manage the wide variety of problems associated with groups of patients, skillful, prioritized clinical decision making is critical (Box 15-3).

BOX 15-3 Clinical Decision Making for Groups of Patients

- Identify the nursing diagnoses and collaborative problems of each patient (see Chapter 17).
- Analyze the diagnoses/problems and decide which are most urgent on the basis of basic needs, the patients' changing or unstable status, and problem complexity (see Chapter 18).
- Consider the time it will take to care for patients whose problems are of high priority (e.g., do you have the time to restart a critical intravenous [IV] line when medication is due for a different patient?).
- Consider resources you have to manage each problem, nursing assistive personnel assigned with you, other health care providers, and patients' family members.
- Involve patients and/or their family as decision makers and participants in care.
- Decide how to combine activities to resolve more than one patient problem at a time.
- Decide which, if any, nursing care procedures to delegate to assistive personnel so you are able to spend your time on activities requiring professional nursing knowledge.
- Discuss complex cases with other members of the health care team to ensure a smooth transition in care requirements.

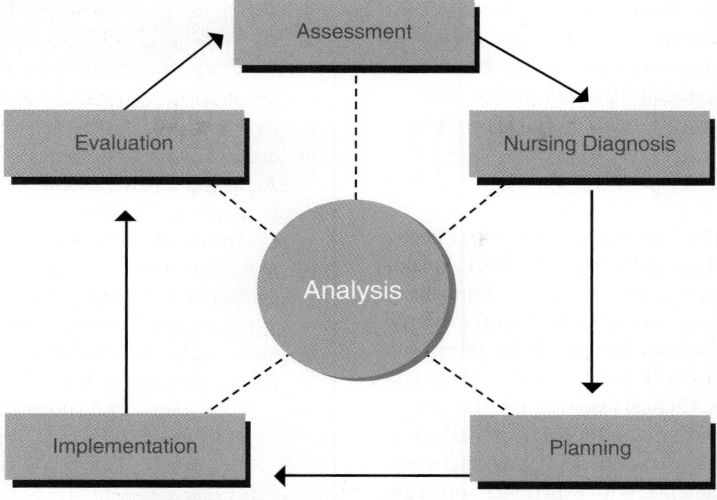

FIGURE 15-2 Five-step nursing process model.

> **QSEN: BUILDING COMPETENCY IN QUALITY IMPROVEMENT** A competency needed to improve the quality and safety of health care is quality improvement. A nursing unit has had an increase in the number of patient falls over the last 3 months. Explain how the nurses on the unit practice committee use critical thinking and clinical decision making to improve the quality of care in reducing patient falls on the nursing unit.
>
> *Answers to QSEN Activities can be found on the Evolve website.*

Nursing Process as a Competency

Nurses apply the **nursing process** as a competency when delivering patient care (Kataoka-Yahiro and Saylor, 1994). The American Nurses Association (ANA) (2010) developed standards that set forth the framework necessary for critical thinking in the application of the five-step nursing process: assessment, diagnosis, planning, implementation, and evaluation. The purpose of the nursing process is to diagnose and treat human responses (e.g., patient symptoms, need for knowledge) to actual or potential health problems (ANA, 2010). Use of the process allows nurses to help patients meet agreed-on outcomes for better health (Figure 15-2). The nursing process requires a nurse to use the general and specific critical thinking competencies described earlier to focus on a particular patient's unique needs. The format for the nursing process is unique to the discipline of nursing and provides a common language and process for nurses to "think through" patients' clinical problems (Kataoka-Yahiro and Saylor, 1994). Unit III describes the nursing process.

A CRITICAL THINKING MODEL FOR CLINICAL DECISION MAKING

Thinking critically is at the core of professional nursing competence. The ability to think critically, improve clinical practice, and decrease errors in clinical judgments is an aim of nursing practice. This text offers a model to help you develop critical thinking. Models help to explain concepts. Because critical thinking in nursing is complex, a model explains what is involved as you make clinical decisions and judgments about your patients. Kataoka-Yahiro and Saylor (1994) developed a model of critical thinking for nursing judgment based in part on previous work by a number of nurse scholars and researchers (Miller and Malcolm, 1990; Paul, 1993) (see Figure 15-1). The model defines the outcome of critical thinking: nursing judgment that is relevant to nursing problems in a variety of settings. According to this model, there are five components of critical thinking: knowledge base, experience, critical thinking competencies (with emphasis on the nursing process), attitudes, and standards. The elements of the model combine to explain how nurses make clinical judgments that are necessary for safe, effective nursing care (see Box 15-3). Throughout this text the model shows you how to apply critical thinking as part of the nursing process. Graphic illustration of the critical thinking model in our clinical chapters shows you how to apply elements of critical thinking in assessing patients, planning the interventions you provide, and evaluating the results. Consistently applying each element of this model in the way you think about patients will help you become a more confident and effective professional.

Specific Knowledge Base

The first component of the critical thinking model is a nurse's specific knowledge base. Knowledge prepares you to better anticipate and identify patients' problems by understanding their origin and nature. Nurses' knowledge varies according to educational experience and includes basic nursing education, continuing education courses, and additional college degrees. In addition, it includes the initiative you show in reading the nursing literature to remain current in nursing science. A nurse's knowledge base is continually changing as science progresses (Swinny, 2010). As a nurse your knowledge base includes information and theory from the basic sciences, humanities, behavioral sciences, and nursing. Nurses use their knowledge base in a different way than other health care disciplines because they think holistically about patient problems. For example, a nurse's broad knowledge base offers a physical, psychological, social, moral, ethical, and cultural view of patients and their health care needs. The depth and extent of knowledge influence your ability to think critically about nursing problems.

Tonya previously earned a bachelor's degree in education and taught high school for 1 year. She is now in her second year as a nurse. She is taking prerequisites to further her education, including courses in health ethics and population health. Her experience as a staff nurse has allowed her to develop knowledge about a variety of surgical procedures, the effects of different medications, and responses patients typically show to their treatment. Although she is still new to nursing, her experiences as a teacher and her preparation and knowledge base in nursing help her know how to interact and form relationships with patients that help her make clinical decisions about patients' health promotion practices.

Experience

Nursing is a practice discipline. Clinical learning experiences are necessary to acquire clinical decision-making skills. Swinny (2010) explains that knowledge itself is not necessarily related to the development of critical thinking. Instead knowledge combined with clinical expertise from experience defines critical thinking. In clinical situations you learn from observing, sensing, talking with patients and families, and reflecting actively on all experiences. Clinical experience is the laboratory for developing and testing approaches that you safely adapt or revise to fit the setting, a patient's unique qualities, and the experiences you have from caring for previous patients. With experience you begin to understand clinical situations, anticipate and recognize cues of patients' health patterns, and interpret the cues as relevant or irrelevant. Perhaps the best lesson a new nursing student can learn is to value all patient experiences, which become stepping-stones for building new knowledge and inspiring innovative thinking.

When Tonya was finishing her last year in nursing school, she worked as a nurse assistant in a nursing home. This experience provided valuable time for interacting with older-adult patients and giving basic nursing care. Each patient provided her with valuable learning experiences that she applies with other patients. Specifically she developed good interviewing skills, understands the importance of the family in an individual's health, and learned to become a patient advocate. She also learned that older adults need more time to perform activities such as eating, bathing, and grooming; therefore she has adapted these skill techniques. Finally Tonya's previous experience as a teacher helps her apply educational principles in her nursing role.

Your practice improves from what you learn personally. The opportunities you have to experience different emotions, crises, and successes in your lives and relationships with others build your experience as a nurse.

The Nursing Process Competency

The nursing process competency is the third component of the critical thinking model. In your practice you will apply critical thinking components during each step of the nursing process. Chapters 16 through 20 describe each step of the nursing process.

Attitudes for Critical Thinking

The fourth component of the critical thinking model is attitudes. Eleven attitudes define the central features of a critical thinker and how a successful critical thinker approaches a problem (Paul, 1993) (Box 15-4). For example, when a patient complains of anxiety before a diagnostic procedure, a curious nurse seeks an explanation and information by asking several questions to learn what the patient does not know and the nature of the patient's concerns (Kaddoura, 2013). The nurse shows discipline in forming questions and collecting a thorough assessment to find the source of the patient's anxiety. Attitudes of inquiry involve an ability to recognize that problems exist and that there is a need for evidence to support the truth in what you think is true. Critical thinking attitudes are guidelines for how to approach a problem or decision-making situation. Important parts of critical thinking are interpreting, evaluating, and making judgments about the adequacy of various arguments and available data. Knowing when you need more information, knowing when information is misleading, and recognizing your own knowledge limits are examples of how critical thinking attitudes guide decision making. Table 15-3 summarizes the use of critical thinking attitudes in nursing practice.

BOX 15-4 Components of Critical Thinking in Nursing

I. Specific knowledge base in nursing
II. Experience
III. Critical thinking competencies
  A. General critical thinking
  B. Specific critical thinking
  C. Specific critical thinking in nursing: nursing process
IV. Attitudes for critical thinking
  Confidence, independence, fairness, responsibility, risk taking, discipline, perseverance, creativity, curiosity, integrity, humility
V. Standards for critical thinking
  A. Intellectual standards
    Clear—Plain and understandable (e.g., clarity in how one communicates).
    Precise—Exact and specific (e.g., focusing on one problem and possible solution).
    Specific—To mention, describe, or define in detail
    Accurate—True and free from error; getting to the facts (objective and subjective)
    Relevant—Essential and crucial to a situation (e.g., a patient's changing clinical status)
    Plausible—Reasonable or probable
    Consistent—Expressing consistent beliefs or values
    Logical—Engaging in correct reasoning from what one believes in a given instance to the conclusions that follow
    Deep—Containing complexities and multiple relationships
    Broad—Covering multiple viewpoints (e.g., patient and family)
    Complete—Thoroughly thinking and evaluating
    Significant—Focusing on what is important and not trivial
    Adequate (for purpose)—Satisfactory in quality or amount
    Fair—Being open-minded and impartial
  B. Professional standards
    1. Ethical criteria for nursing judgment
    2. Criteria for evaluation
    3. Professional responsibility

Modified from Kataoka-Yahiro M, Saylor C: A critical thinking model for nursing judgment, *J Nurs Educ* 33(8):351, 1994. Data from Paul RW: The art of redesigning instruction. In Willsen J, Blinker AJA, editors: *Critical thinking: how to prepare students for a rapidly changing world,* Santa Rosa, Calif, 1993, Foundation for Critical Thinking.

Confidence. Confidence is the belief in oneself, one's judgment and psychomotor skills, and one's possession of the knowledge and the ability to think critically and draw appropriate conclusions (Etheridge, 2007). When you are confident, you feel certain about accomplishing a task or goal such as performing a procedure or making a diagnosis. Confidence grows with experience in recognizing your strengths and limitations. You shift your focus from your own needs (e.g., remembering what assessment data means or how to perform a procedure) to a patient's needs. When you are not confident in knowing if a patient is clinically changing or in performing a nursing skill, you become

TABLE 15-3 Critical Thinking Attitudes and Applications in Nursing Practice

Critical Thinking Attitude	Application in Practice
Confidence	Learn how to introduce yourself to a patient; speak with conviction when you begin a treatment or procedure. Do not lead a patient to think that you are unable to perform care safely. Always be well prepared before performing a nursing activity. Encourage a patient to ask questions.
Thinking independently	Read the nursing literature, especially when there are different views on the same subject. Talk with other nurses and share ideas about nursing interventions.
Fairness	Listen to both sides in any discussion. If a patient or family member complains about a co-worker, listen to the story and speak with the co-worker as well. If a staff member labels a patient uncooperative, assume the care of that patient with openness and a desire to meet the patient's needs.
Responsibility and authority	Ask for help if you are uncertain about how to perform a nursing skill. Refer to a policy and procedure manual to review steps of a skill. Report any problems immediately. Follow standards of practice in your care.
Risk taking	If your knowledge causes you to question a health care provider's order, do so. Be willing to recommend alternative approaches to nursing care when colleagues are having little success with patients.
Discipline	Be thorough in whatever you do. Use known scientific and practice-based criteria for activities such as assessment and evaluation. Take time to be thorough and manage your time effectively.
Perseverance	Be cautious of an easy answer. If co-workers give you information about a patient and some fact seems to be missing, clarify the information or talk to the patient directly. If problems of the same type continue to occur on a nursing division, bring co-workers together, look for a pattern, and find a solution.
Creativity	Look for different approaches if interventions are not working for a patient. For example, a patient in pain may need a different positioning or distraction technique. When appropriate, involve the patient's family in adapting your approaches to care methods used at home.
Curiosity	Always ask why. A clinical sign or symptom often indicates a variety of problems. Explore and learn more about a patient so as to make appropriate clinical judgments.
Integrity	Recognize when your opinions conflict with those of a patient; review your position and decide how best to proceed to reach outcomes that will satisfy everyone. Do not compromise nursing standards or honesty in delivering nursing care.
Humility	Recognize when you need more information to make a decision. When you are new to a clinical division, ask for an orientation to the area. Ask registered nurses (RNs) regularly assigned to the area for assistance with approaches to care.

anxious about not knowing what to do. This prevents you from giving attention to the patient. Always be aware of what you know and what you don't know. If you question the meaning of a clinical situation and you don't know if the information you have is important, discuss it with your nursing instructor first. Never perform a procedure unless you have the knowledge base and feel confident. Patient safety is of the upmost importance. When you show confidence, your patients recognize it by how you communicate and the way you perform nursing care. Confidence builds trust between you and your patients.

Thinking Independently. As you gain new knowledge, you learn to consider a wide range of ideas and concepts before forming an opinion or making a judgment. This does not mean that you ignore other people's ideas. Instead you learn to consider all sides of a situation. A critical thinker does not accept another person's ideas without question. When thinking independently, you challenge the ways that others think and look for rational and logical answers to problems. You begin to raise important questions about your practice. For example, why is one type of surgical dressing ordered over another, why do patients on your nursing unit fall, and what can you do to help patients with literacy problems learn about their medications? When nurses ask questions and look for the evidence behind clinical problems, they are thinking independently; this is an important step in evidence-based practice (see Chapter 5). Independent thinking and reasoning are essential to the improvement and expansion of nursing practice.

Fairness. A critical thinker deals with situations justly. This means that bias or prejudice does not enter into a decision. For example, regardless of how you feel about obesity, you do not allow personal attitudes to influence the way you care for a patient who is overweight. Look at a situation objectively and consider all viewpoints to understand the situation completely before making a decision. Having a sense of imagination helps you develop an attitude of fairness. Imagining what it is like to be in your patient's situation helps you see it with new eyes and appreciate its complexity.

Responsibility and Accountability. Responsibility is the knowledge that you are accountable for your decisions, actions, and critical thinking (Etheridge, 2007). When caring for patients, you are responsible for correctly performing nursing care activities on the basis of standards of practice. Standards of practice are the minimum level of performance accepted to ensure high-quality care. For example, you do not take shortcuts (e.g., failing to identify a patient, preparing medication doses for multiple patients at the same time) when administering medications. A professional nurse is responsible for competently performing nursing therapies and making clinical decisions about patients. As a nurse you are answerable or accountable for your decisions and the outcomes of your actions. This means that you are accountable for recognizing when nursing care is ineffective and you know the limits and scope of your practice.

Risk Taking. People often associate taking risks with danger. Driving 30 miles an hour over the speed limit is a risk that sometimes results in injury to the driver and an unlucky pedestrian. But risk taking does not always have negative outcomes. Risk taking is desirable, particularly when the result is a positive outcome. A critical thinker is willing to take risks when trying different ways to solve problems. The willingness to take risks comes from experience with similar problems. Risk taking often leads to advances in patient care. In the past nurses have taken risks when trying different approaches to skin and wound care and pain management, to name a few. When taking a risk, consider all options; follow safety guidelines; analyze any potential dangers to a patient; and act in a well-reasoned, logical, and thoughtful manner.

Discipline. A disciplined thinker misses few details and is orderly or systematic when collecting information, making decisions, or taking action. For example, you have a patient who is in pain. Instead of only asking the patient, "How severe is your pain on a scale of 0 to 10?", you also ask more specific questions about the character of pain. For example, "What makes the pain worse? Where does it hurt? How long have you noticed it?" Being disciplined helps you identify problems more accurately and select the most appropriate interventions.

Perseverance. A critical thinker is determined to find effective solutions to patient care problems. This is especially important when problems remain unresolved or recur. Learn as much as possible about a problem and try various approaches to care. Persevering means to keep looking for more resources until you find a successful approach. For example, a patient who is unable to speak following throat surgery poses challenges for the nurse to be able to communicate effectively. Perseverance leads the nurse to try different communication approaches (e.g., message boards or alarm bells) until he or she finds a method that the patient is able to use. A critical thinker who perseveres is not satisfied with minimal effort but works to achieve the highest level of quality care.

Creativity. Creativity involves original thinking. This means that you find solutions outside of the standard routines of care while still following standards of practice. Creativity motivates you to think of options and unique approaches. A patient's clinical problems, social support systems, and living environment are just a few examples of factors that make the simplest nursing procedure more complicated. For example, a home care nurse has to find a way to help an older patient with arthritis have greater mobility in the home. The patient has difficulty lowering and raising herself in a chair because of pain and limited range of motion in her knees. The nurse uses wooden blocks to elevate the chair legs so the patient is able to sit and stand with little discomfort while making sure that the chair is safe to use.

Curiosity. A critical thinker's favorite question is "Why?" In any clinical situation you learn a great deal of information about a patient. As you analyze patient information, data patterns appear that are not always clear. Having a sense of curiosity (asking yourself, "What if?") motivates you to inquire further (e.g., question family or physician, review the scientific literature) and investigate a clinical situation so you get all the information you need to make a decision.

Integrity. Critical thinkers question and test their own knowledge and beliefs. Your personal integrity as a nurse builds trust from your co-workers. Nurses face many dilemmas or problems in everyday clinical practice, and everyone makes mistakes at times. A person of integrity is honest and willing to admit to mistakes or inconsistencies in his or her own behavior, ideas, and beliefs. A professional nurse always tries to follow the highest standards of practice.

Humility. It is important for you to admit to any limitations in your knowledge and skill. Critical thinkers admit what they do not know and try to find the knowledge needed to make proper decisions. It is common for a nurse to be an expert in one area of clinical practice but a novice in another because the knowledge in all areas of nursing is unlimited. A patient's safety and welfare are at risk if you do not admit your inability to deal with a practice problem. You have to rethink a situation; learn more; and use the new information to form opinions, draw conclusions, and take action.

Mr. Lawson continues to have chest pain and shortness of breath. As Tonya waits for the medical team to arrive, she knows that she is responsible for his welfare until treatment can be initiated. Tonya acts independently by keeping Mr. Lawson comfortable in the chair, not moving him (to avoid worsening of his condition), and gathering additional assessment data. She displays discipline in further assessing Mr. Lawson's condition: rechecking vital signs, observing his abdominal wound and incision, and talking with him to notice if there is a change in consciousness. Tonya knows that she cannot diagnose medically. When the physician arrives, she objectively reports what happened with Mr. Lawson once he sat up in the chair, the symptoms he displayed, and how those symptoms have changed.

Standards for Critical Thinking

The fifth component of the critical thinking model includes intellectual and professional standards (Kataoka-Yahiro and Saylor, 1994).

Intellectual Standards. Paul (1993) identified 14 intellectual standards (see Box 15-4) universal for critical thinking. An intellectual standard is a principle for rational thought. You apply these standards during all steps of the nursing process. For example, when you consider a patient problem, apply the intellectual standards of preciseness, accuracy, and consistency to make sure that you have all the data you need to make sound clinical decisions. During planning, apply standards such as being logical and significant so that the plan of care is meaningful and relevant to a patient's needs. A thorough use of intellectual standards in clinical practice prevents you from performing critical thinking haphazardly.

The physician orders a lung scan, chest x-ray and places Mr. Lawson on bed rest. Blood tests are also ordered in anticipation of placing the patient on anticoagulation (to prevent further clot formation). Tonya asks the physician if there are risks to be considered regarding Mr. Lawson's wound should the patient receive an anticoagulant (relevant question). She also asks if she can give additional pain medication at this time to manage the patient's surgical incision pain during the x-ray procedures (logical decision). By applying intellectual standards, Tonya is a competent partner in managing the patient's care, showing her ability to anticipate possible clinical problems.

Professional Standards. Professional standards for critical thinking refer to ethical criteria for nursing judgments, evidence-based criteria used for evaluation, and criteria for professional responsibility (Paul, 1993). Application of professional standards requires you to use critical thinking for the good of individuals or groups (Kataoka-Yahiro and Saylor, 1994). Professional standards promote the highest level of quality nursing care.

Excellent nursing practice is a reflection of ethical standards (see Chapter 22). Patient care requires more than just the application of scientific knowledge. Being able to focus on a patient's values and beliefs helps you make clinical decisions that are just, faithful to a patient's choices, and beneficial to a patient's well-being. Critical thinkers maintain a sense of self-awareness through conscious awareness of their beliefs, values, and feelings and the multiple perspectives that patients, family members, and peers present in clinical situations. Critical thinking also requires the use of evidence-based criteria for making clinical judgments. These criteria are sometimes scientifically based on research findings (see Chapter 5) or practice based on standards developed by clinical experts and performance improvement initiatives of an institution. Examples are the clinical practice guidelines developed by individual clinical agencies and national organizations such as the Agency for Healthcare Research and Quality (AHRQ). A clinical practice guideline includes standards for the treatment of select clinical conditions such as stroke, deep vein thrombosis, and pressure ulcers. Another example is clinical criteria used to categorize clinical conditions such as the criteria for staging pressure ulcers (see Chapter 48) and rating phlebitis (see Chapter 42). Evidence-based evaluation criteria set the minimum requirements necessary to ensure appropriate and high-quality care.

Nurses routinely use evidence-based criteria to assess patients' conditions and determine the efficacy of nursing interventions. For example, accurate assessment of symptoms such as pain includes use of assessment criteria, including the duration, severity, location, aggravating or relieving factors, and effects on daily lifestyle (see Chapter 44). In this case assessment criteria allow you to accurately determine the nature of a patient's symptoms, select appropriate therapies, and evaluate if the therapies are effective. The standards of professional responsibility that a nurse tries to achieve are the standards cited in Nurse Practice Acts, institutional practice guidelines, and professional organizations' standards of practice (e.g., The ANA Standards of Professional Performance (see Chapter 1). These standards "raise the bar" for the responsibilities and accountabilities that a nurse assumes in guaranteeing quality health care to the public.

CRITICAL THINKING SYNTHESIS

Critical thinking is a reasoning process by which you reflect on and analyze your thoughts, action, and knowledge. As a beginning nurse it is important to learn the steps of the nursing process and incorporate the elements of critical thinking (Figure 15-3). The two processes go hand in hand in making quality decisions about patient care. This text provides a model to show you how important critical thinking is in the practice of the nursing process.

DEVELOPING CRITICAL THINKING SKILLS

To develop critical thinking skills you learn how to connect knowledge and theory with day-to-day practices. The ability to make sense of what you learn in the classroom, from reading, or from having dialogue with other students and then to apply it during patient care is challenging.

Reflective Journaling

Reflective journal writing is a tool for developing critical thought and reflection by clarifying concepts. These concepts are embedded in the day-to-day clinical situations and problems you face. Reflective writing gives you the chance to define and express clinical experiences in your own words. Always begin by recording notes after a clinical experience. The use of a journal improves your observation and descriptive skills and ultimately your clinical decision making. Use these tips for reflecting on a clinical experience to explore its meaning:

1. Which experience, situation, or information in your clinical experience is confusing, difficult, or interesting?
2. What is the meaning of the experience? What feelings did you have? What feelings did your patient or family have? What influenced the experience?
3. Do the feelings, guesses, or questions remind you of any experiences from the past or something that you think is a desirable future experience? How does it relate?
4. What are the connections between what is being described and what you have learned about nursing science and theory?

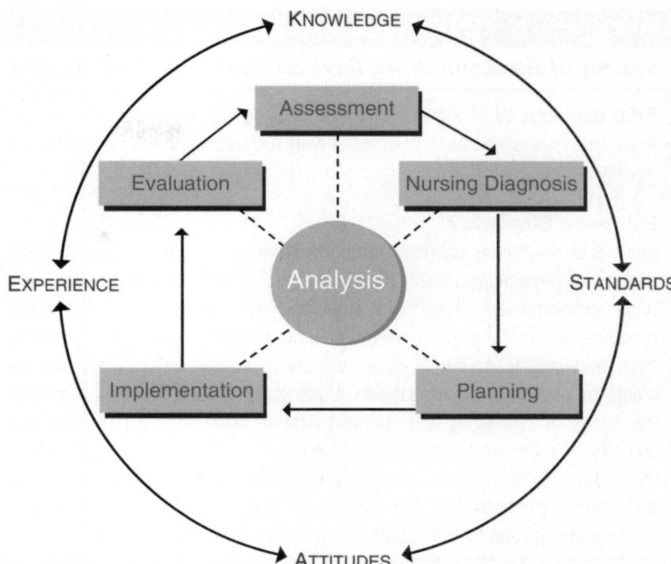

FIGURE 15-3 Synthesis of critical thinking with the nursing process competency.

Meeting with Colleagues

Nurses depend on others to help them think like nurses (Etheridge, 2007). A way to develop critical thinking skills is regularly meeting with colleagues such as faculty members or preceptors to discuss and examine work experiences and validate decisions. Connecting with others will help you learn that you do not need to know everything because support is available from other colleagues. When nurses have a formal means to discuss their experiences such as a staff meeting or unit practice council, the dialogue allows for questions, differing viewpoints, and sharing experiences. When they are able to discuss their practices, the process validates good practice and also offers challenges and constructive criticism. Much can be learned by drawing from others' experiences and perspectives to promote reflective critical thinking.

Concept Mapping

As a nurse you will care for patients who have multiple nursing diagnoses or collaborative problems. A **concept map** is a visual representation of patient problems and interventions that shows their relationships to one another. It is a nonlinear picture of a patient to be used for comprehensive care planning. The primary purpose of concept mapping is to better synthesize relevant data about a patient, including assessment data, nursing diagnoses, health needs, nursing

BOX 15-5 EVIDENCE-BASED PRACTICE

Impact of Stressful Work Environments on Thinking and Decision Making

PICO Question: What are the effects on thinking and decision making among acute care nurses who work in stressful work environments versus nonstressful environments?

Evidence Summary

Regions of the cortex, amygdala, and brainstem of the brain interact between mental and physiological states (Critchley et al., 2013). Thus cognitive and emotional processes are affected by autonomic mechanisms during the stress response. Stress is a common condition in the health care workplace, resulting from workload, leadership/management style, professional conflict, and the emotional cost of caring for patients. Understanding the relationship between the stress of caregiving and cognitive and decision-making processes and empathy is important for nursing practice (Critchley et al., 2013). Stress alters the ability to problem solve accurately, speak fluently and clearly, remember, and manage emotions. Negative mood and stress often affects what and how nurses communicate to one another (Pfaff, 2012). During stress there is greater likelihood for cynicism and frustration and inaccurate information being conveyed.

Application to Nursing Practice

- Learn to recognize when you are feeling stressed: your muscles will tense, you become reactive when others communicate with you, you have trouble concentrating, and you feel very tired.
- Take a time out. Try to find a way to relax by doing a quick relaxation exercise or finding a place where colleagues are not bombarding you with questions.
- Discuss the difficult and stressful patient care experiences that you are having with your colleagues with someone you trust. Realizing that your concerns are shared by others relieves stress.
- Participate in opportunities to make decisions about practice activities.
- Attend a stress-management class at work.

interventions, and evaluation measures. Through drawing a concept map, you learn to organize or connect information in a unique way so the diverse information that you have about a patient begins to form meaningful patterns and concepts. You begin to see a more holistic view of a patient. When you see the relationship between the various patient diagnoses and the data that support them, you better understand a patient's clinical situation. Concept maps can be found in the clinical chapters of this text (see Units V and VI).

MANAGING STRESS

The connection between stress in a health care setting and its effects on a nurse's mental and physiological state is receiving more attention. Autonomic control of decision making, error detection, speech, memory, and emotions during stressful situations are disrupted because of continued sympathetic nervous system stimulation. Research has shown that the stress of working 12-hour shifts, for example, impairs medical judgment, in part because of the way stress affects attention (McClelland et al., 2013). The work of professional nursing is difficult as you see patients endure suffering from disease and painful therapies and as you try to manage care responsibilities in busy, fast-paced work settings. Stress over a prolonged period or when extreme can lead to poor work productivity, impaired decision making and communication, and reduced ability to cope with clinical situations (Donovan et al., 2013). Box 15-5 offers perspectives on ways to better manage stress so you can make clear, thoughtful decisions and communicate effectively with health care colleagues (see Chapter 38).

KEY POINTS

- Clinical decision making involves judgment that includes critical and reflective thinking and action and application of scientific and practical logic.
- Nurses who apply critical thinking in their work focus on options for solving problems and making decisions rather than rapidly and carelessly forming quick, single solutions.
- Reflection involves purposeful thinking back or recalling a situation to discover its purpose or meaning.
- Following a procedure step by step without adjusting to a patient's unique needs is an example of basic critical thinking.
- In complex critical thinking a nurse learns that alternative and perhaps conflicting solutions exist.
- In diagnostic reasoning you collect patient data and analyze them to determine the patient's problems.
- The critical thinking model combines a nurse's knowledge base, experience, competence in the nursing process, attitudes, and standards to explain how nurses make clinical judgments that are necessary for safe, effective nursing care.
- Clinical learning experiences are necessary for you to acquire clinical decision-making skills.
- Critical thinking attitudes help you know when more information is necessary and when it is misleading and to recognize your own knowledge limits.
- The use of intellectual standards during assessment ensures that you obtain a complete database of information.
- Professional standards for critical thinking refer to ethical criteria for nursing judgments, evidence-based criteria for evaluation, and criteria for professional responsibility.
- Meeting regularly with colleagues allows you to discuss anticipated and unanticipated outcomes in any clinical situation to continually learn and develop your expertise.
- Stress over a prolonged period or when extreme can cause distress, leading to poor work productivity and impaired decision making and communication.

CLINICAL APPLICATION QUESTIONS

Preparing for Clinical Practice

Medical treatment stabilized Mr. Lawson's condition. He had a pulmonary embolus, but he is now on anticoagulants, medications that will reduce likelihood of more clot formation. Knowing that Mr. Lawson is on anticoagulants and has had recent surgery and the processes of normal wound healing (see Chapter 48), Tonya believes that the patient is at risk for bleeding from his surgical wound. She acts by increasing assessments of the wound and teaching Mr. Lawson how to avoid placing stress on the wound

1. Describe the critical thinking skill that Tonya is demonstrating.

   After Tonya assesses the wound, she enters a note in the medical record. She describes the appearance of the incision in detail, reports on the length of the incision, and notes that one suture is loose but there is no drainage.

2. Identify the three intellectual standards that Tonya uses in making a note in the record.
3. Mr. Lawson complains of more discomfort after lying on his right side for 30 minutes. Tonya asks him to describe the pain; it is focused more on his right shoulder and ribs. Tonya sees that the drainage tubing exiting the surgical wound is caught underneath the patient. She moves it, questions the patient further to find out that he has a history of arthritis in the shoulder, and then repositions and aligns him. This is an example of which critical thinking competencies?

ⓔ ***Answers to Clinical Application Questions can be found on the Evolve website.***

REVIEW QUESTIONS

Are You Ready to Test Your Nursing Knowledge?

1. Two patient deaths have occurred on a medical unit in the last month. The staff notices that everyone feels pressured and team members are getting into more arguments. As a nurse on the unit, what will best help you manage this stress?
   1. Keep a journal
   2. Participate in a unit meeting to discuss feelings about the patient deaths
   3. Ask the nurse manager to assign you to less difficult patients
   4. Review the policy and procedure manual on proper care of patients after death
2. A nurse has seen many cancer patients struggle with pain management because they are afraid of becoming addicted to the medicine. Pain control is a priority for cancer care. By helping patients focus on their values and beliefs about pain control, a nurse can best make clinical decisions. This is an example of:
   1. Creativity.
   2. Fairness.
   3. Clinical reasoning.
   4. Applying ethical criteria.
3. A nurse prepares to insert a Foley catheter. The procedure manual calls for the patient to lie in the dorsal recumbent position. The patient complains of having back pain when lying on her back. Despite this, the nurse positions the patient supine with knees flexed as the manual recommends and begins to insert the catheter. This is an example of:
   1. Accuracy.
   2. Reflection.
   3. Risk taking.
   4. Basic critical thinking.
4. A nurse is preparing medications for a patient. The nurse checks the name of the medication on the label with the name of the medication on the doctor's order. At the bedside the nurse checks the patient's name against the medication order as well. The nurse is following which critical thinking attitude:
   1. Responsible
   2. Complete
   3. Accurate
   4. Broad
5. A nurse on a busy medicine unit is assigned to four patients. It is 10 AM. Two patients have medications due and one of those has a specimen of urine to be collected. One patient is having complications from surgery and is being prepared to return to the operating room. The fourth patient requires instructions about activity restrictions before going home this afternoon. Which of the following should the nurse use in making clinical decisions appropriate for the patient group? (Select all that apply.)
   1. Consider availability of assistive personnel to obtain the specimen
   2. Combine activities to resolve more than one patient problem
   3. Analyze the diagnoses/problems and decide which are most urgent based on patients' needs
   4. Plan a family conference for tomorrow to make decisions about resources the patient will need to go home
   5. Identify the nursing diagnoses for the patient going home
6. By using known criteria in conducting an assessment such as reviewing with a patient the typical characteristics of pain, a nurse is demonstrating which critical thinking attitude?
   1. Curiosity
   2. Adequacy
   3. Discipline
   4. Thinking independently
7. A nurse just started working at a well-baby clinic. One of her recent experiences was to help a mother learn the steps of breastfeeding. During the first clinic visit the mother had difficulty positioning the baby during feeding. After the visit the nurse considers what affected the inability of the mother to breastfeed, including the mother's obesity and inexperience. The nurse's review of the situation is called:
   1. Reflection.
   2. Perseverance.
   3. Intuition.
   4. Problem solving.
8. Place the steps of the scientific method in their correct order with number 1 being the first step of the process.
   1. Formulate a question or hypothesis.
   2. Evaluate results of the study.
   3. Collect data.
   4. Identify the problem.
   5. Test the question or hypothesis.
9. A nurse changed a patient's surgical wound dressing the day before and now prepares for another dressing change. The nurse had difficulty removing the gauze from the wound bed yesterday, causing the patient discomfort. Today he gives the patient an analgesic 30 minutes before the dressing change. Then he adds some sterile saline to loosen the gauze for a few minutes before removing it. The patient reports that the procedure was much more comfortable. Which of the following describes the nurse's approach to the dressing change? (Select all that apply.)
   1. Clinical inference
   2. Basic critical thinking
   3. Complex critical thinking
   4. Experience
   5. Reflection
10. Which of the following describes a nurse's application of a specific knowledge base during critical thinking? (Select all that apply.)
    1. Initiative in reading current evidence from the literature
    2. Application of nursing theory
    3. Reviewing policy and procedure manual
    4. Considering holistic view of patient needs
    5. Previous time caring for a specific group of patients
11. **Fill in the Blank.** When a nurse tries to understand a patient's and family caregiver's perspective of why a patient is falling at home, the nurse applies the intellectual standard of ________________________ to understand all viewpoints.

12. An aspect of clinical decision making is knowing the patient. Which of the following is the most critical aspect of developing the ability to know the patient?
   1. Working in multiple health care settings
   2. Learning good communication skills
   3. Spending time establishing relationships with patients
   4. Relying on evidence in practice

13. In which of the following examples is a nurse applying critical thinking skills in practice? (Select all that apply.)
   1. The nurse thinks back about a personal experience before administering a medication subcutaneously.
   2. The nurse uses a pain-rating scale to measure a patient's pain.
   3. The nurse explains a procedure step by step for giving an enema to a patient care technician.
   4. The nurse gathers data on a patient with a mobility limitation to identify a nursing diagnosis.
   5. A nurse offers support to a colleague who has witnessed a stressful event.

14. A nurse enters a 72-year-old patient's home and begins to observe her behaviors and examine her physical condition. The nurse learns that the patient lives alone and notices bruising on the patient's leg. When watching the patient walk, the nurse notes that she has an unsteady gait and leans to one side. The patient admits to having fallen in the past. The nurse identifies the patient as having the nursing diagnosis of Risk for Falls. This scenario is an example of:
   1. Inference.
   2. Basic critical thinking.
   3. Evaluation.
   4. Diagnostic reasoning.

15. Match the concepts for a critical thinker on the right with the application of the term on the left.

Term Application	Concepts for Critical Thinkers
a. Anticipate how a patient might respond to a treatment.	___ 1. Truth seeking
b. Organize assessment on the basis of patient priorities.	___ 2. Open-mindedness
c. Be objective in asking questions of a patient.	___ 3. Analyticity
d. Be tolerant of the patient's views and beliefs.	___ 4. Systematicity

Answers: 1. 2; **2.** 4; **3.** 4; **4.** 1; **5.** 1, 2, 3; **6.** 3; **7.** 1; **8.** 4, 3, 1, 5, 2; **9.** 3, 4; **10.** 1, 2, 4; **11.** Broad; **12.** 3; **13.** 1, 2, 4; **14.** 4; **15.** 1c, 2d, 3a, 4b.

ⓔ *Rationales for Review Questions can be found on the Evolve website.*

REFERENCES

American Nurses Association (ANA): *Nursing's social policy statement: the essence of the profession*, Washington, DC, 2010, The Association.

Croskerry P, Nimmo GR: Better clinical decision making and reducing diagnostic error, *J R Coll Physicians Edinb* 41(2):155, 2011.

Facione N, Facione P: Externalizing the critical thinking in knowledge development and clinical judgment, *Nurs Outlook* 44:129, 1996.

Harjai PK, Tiwari R: Model of critical diagnostic reasoning: achieving expert clinician performance, *Nurs Educ Perspect* 30(5):305, 2009.

Kataoka-Yahiro M, Saylor C: A critical thinking model for nursing judgment, *J Nurs Educ* 33(8):351, 1994.

Miller M, Malcolm N: Critical thinking in the nursing curriculum, *Nurs Health Care* 11:67, 1990.

Paul RW: The art of redesigning instruction. In Willsen J, Blinker AJA, editors: *Critical thinking: how to prepare students for a rapidly changing world*, Santa Rosa, Calif, 1993, Foundation for Critical Thinking.

Swinny B: Assessing and developing critical thinking skills in the intensive care unit, *Crit Care Nurs Q* 33(1):2, 2010.

RESEARCH REFERENCES

Critchley HD et al: Interaction between cognition, emotion, and the autonomic nervous system, *Handb Clin Neurol* 117:597, 2013.

Donovan RO et al.: The effect of stress on health and its implications for nursing, *Br J Nurs* 22(16):969, 2013.

Etheridge SA: Learning to think like a nurse: stories from new nurse graduates, *J Contin Educ Nurs* 38(1):24, 2007.

Facione P: *Critical thinking: a statement of expert consensus for purposes of educational assessment and instruction. The Delphi report: research findings and recommendations prepared for the American Philosophical Association, ERIC Doc No. ED 315-423*, Washington, DC, 1990, ERIC.

Henneman EA et al: Strategies used by critical care nurse to identify, interrupt, and correct medical errors, *Am J Crit Care* 19:500, 2010.

Kaddoura M: New graduate nurses' perceived definition of critical thinking during their first nursing experience, *Educ Res Q* 36(3):3, 2013.

Lotzkar M, Bottorff JL: An observational study of the development of a nurse-patient relationship, *Clin Nurs Res* 10:275, 2010.

Mamede S et al: Exploring the role of salient distracting clinical features in the emergence of diagnostic errors and the mechanisms through which reflection counteracts mistakes, *BMJ Qual Saf* 21(4):295, 2012.

McClelland LE et al: Changes in nurses' decision making during a 12-h day shift, *Occup Med* 63(1):60, 2013.

McHugh MD, Ma C: Hospital nursing and 30-day readmissions among Medicare patients with heart failure, acute myocardial infarction, and pneumonia, *Med Care* 51(1):52, 2013.

Pfaff M: Negative affect reduces team awareness: the effects of mood and stress on computer-mediated team communication, *Human Factors* 54(4):5601, 2012.

Radwin LE: Knowing the patient: a review of research on an emerging concept, *J Adv Nurs* 23:1142, 1996.

Roche J et al: Testing a work empowerment–work relationship model to explain expertise in experienced acute care nurses, *J Nurs Admin* 39:115, 2009.

Tanner CA: Thinking like a nurse: a research-based model of clinical judgment in nursing, *J Nurs Educ* 45(6):204, 2006.

Tanner CA et al: The phenomenology of knowing the patient, *J Nurs Scholarsh* 25:273, 1993.

Zolnierek CD: An integrative review of knowing the patient, *J Nurs Scholarsh* 46(1):3, 2014.

16

Nursing Assessment

OBJECTIVES

- Discuss the relationship between critical thinking and nursing assessment.
- Describe how developing relationships with patients fosters the assessment process.
- Describe how courtesy, comfort, connection, and confirmation establish a foundation for patient assessment.
- Differentiate between subjective and objective data.
- Explain ways to make an assessment patient centered.
- Describe the methods of data collection.
- Discuss how to conduct a patient-centered interview.
- Describe the components of a nursing history.
- Explain the relationship between data interpretation and validation.
- Conduct a nursing assessment.

KEY TERMS

Assessment, p. 210
Back channeling, p. 217
Closed-ended questions, p. 217
Concomitant symptoms, p. 219
Cue, p. 212
Functional health patterns, p. 212
Inference, p. 212
Nursing health history, p. 217
Nursing process, p. 209
Objective data, p. 214
Open-ended questions, p. 217
Review of systems (ROS), p. 220
Subjective data, p. 213
Validation, p. 220

MEDIA RESOURCES

http://evolve.elsevier.com/Potter/fundamentals/

- Review Questions
- Concept Map Creator
- Case Study with Questions
- Audio Glossary
- Content Updates

The **nursing process** is a critical thinking five-step process (Figure 16-1) that professional nurses use to apply the best available evidence to caregiving and promoting human functions and responses to health and illness (ANA, 2010). It is the fundamental blueprint for how to care for patients. A patient-centered care approach is holistic and essential when applying the nursing process. Such an approach enhances patient assessment and education, family centeredness, patient adherence to interventions, and patient outcomes (Bertakis and Azari, 2011). The Quality and Safety Education for Nurses (QSEN) institute (2014) defines patient-centered care as "recognizing a patient or designee as the source of control and full partner in providing compassionate and coordinated care based on respect for a patient's preferences, values, and needs." Thus assessment is an important first step for learning as much as you can about each patient's health condition and health problems by partnering together in a therapeutic relationship. Consider the following scenario that was also described in Chapter 15.

Mr. Lawson is a 62-year-old patient who had abdominal surgery for a colon resection and removal of a tumor 2 days ago. His nurse, Tonya, implemented pain-control strategies in an effort to help him become more mobile so recovery could proceed. Up until now he was getting out of bed and rating his pain at a level of 4 on a scale of 0 to 10. The patient still tends to guard his incision by placing his hand over the wound when moving.

Mr. Lawson weighs 109 kg (240 lbs) and is 5 ft 11 inches tall. He has tried to cough more during his postoperative deep-breathing exercises. Tonya is caring for him for the third day in a row and begins the morning shift by inspecting his surgical wound. The wound is approximately 15 cm (6 inches) in length and closed with steel sutures. Tonya notices separation of the wound between two sutures at the bottom of the incision. There is a small amount of serous drainage. The area is inflamed, and she asks the patient if the incision is tender when she gently palpates around the area. Mr. Lawson states, "Ow, that feels sore there. I think I pulled it when I coughed last night." He also rates pain at this time as being at a level of 5. Tonya checks Mr. Lawson's vital signs and notes that his temperature is 37.5° C (99.6° F), slightly above his average temperature of 37.2° C (99.0° F). Tonya also inspects the intravenous (IV) access device in the patient's left forearm. It is intact, and there are no signs of phlebitis at the IV site.

Each time you meet a patient, you apply the nursing process, as Tonya does while caring for Mr. Lawson. The first step of the nursing process, assessment, involves the gathering and analysis of information about a patient's health status. *In the case example Tonya gathers information*

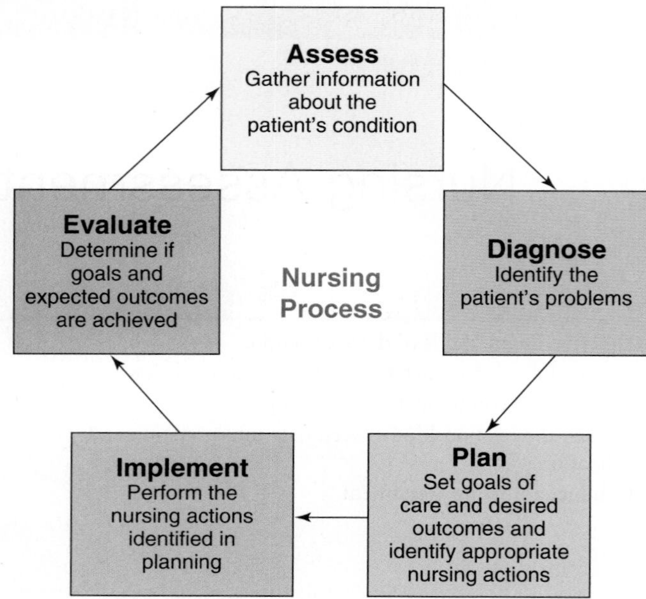

FIGURE 16-1 Five-step nursing process.

by looking at the patient's wound (inspection) to note its character (length, presence of sutures) and condition (slight separation with drainage and inflammation at site). She also checks the patient's vital signs and compares data with temperature measurements previously obtained. Inspection of the IV site involves further assessment.

As a nurse you learn to make clinical judgments from assessment data to identify a patient's level of wellness and desire for health promotion or to identify existing health problems. An individual's undesirable responses to a health condition or his or her desire to increase well-being is identified in the form of either nursing diagnoses or collaborative problems (see Chapter 17) (Herdman and Kamitsuru, 2014). Assessment must be complete, relevant to a patient's condition, and accurate for you to correctly identify a person's desire to improve his or her health or identify any health problem. A comprehensive assessment leads to making accurate nursing diagnoses, allowing you to then create an appropriate plan of care for a patient. The next step, implementation, involves performing the planned interventions or collaboration. After implementation you evaluate the patient's responses and whether the interventions were effective. The nursing process is central to your ability to provide timely and appropriate care to your patients.

The nursing process is a form of scientific reasoning. Initially you will learn how to apply the process step by step. However, as you gain more clinical experience and care for more patients, you learn to move back and forth through the steps of the process, critically making judgments about your patients' clinical situations and individualizing your approaches to care (O'Neill et al., 2011). Practicing the five steps of the nursing process allows you to organize and conduct your practice in a systematic way. You learn to make inferences about the meaning of a patient's responses to a health problem or generalize about his or her functional state of health. The data collected during assessment forms patterns that help lead to diagnostic conclusions. *For example, the condition of Mr. Lawson's incision leads Tonya to infer that wound healing is possibly impaired. Tonya gathers more information (e.g., checking temperature, noting Mr. Lawson's reaction to wound palpation) until she makes an accurate classification of the patient's problem.*

Clearly defining your patient's problems on the basis of assessment ensures that you can plan care, implement appropriate nursing interventions, and evaluate the outcomes of care.

A CRITICAL THINKING APPROACH TO ASSESSMENT

Assessment is the deliberate and systematic collection of information about a patient to determine the patient's current and past health and functional status and his or her present and past coping patterns (Carpenito-Moyet, 2013). Nursing assessment includes two steps:

1. Collection of information from a primary source (a patient) and secondary sources (e.g., family or friends, health professionals, and the medical record)
2. The interpretation and validation of data to ensure a complete database

In the case study Tonya collected information from the patient through observation and asking questions. She saw the inflammation in the incisional area and validated its presence by asking the patient if it was tender. She interpreted her data: an open area of an incision, draining fluid, and the resultant tenderness around the site indicating a pattern of altered wound healing. She also measured the body temperature to see if an early sign of a more serious systemic infection was present.

When a plumber comes to your home to repair a problem that you describe as a "leaking faucet," the plumber checks the faucet, its attachments to the water line, and the water pressure in the system to determine the real problem. When a patient presents an initial health problem, you conduct an assessment that will allow you to identify the problem correctly. However, patients are different from leaky faucets in that their clinical situation changes over time, sometimes quickly. *For example, Mr. Lawson presents with signs of altered wound healing. Tonya reports these findings to the patient's surgeon, who orders antibiotics intravenously for 24 hours but also plans for the patient's discharge tomorrow. Mr. Lawson's clinical condition has changed from immediate recovery from surgery to planning for discharge home. Tonya wants to continue to try to control the patient's pain but now has to conduct further assessment of the patient's knowledge, observe his behaviors, ask questions about his ability to care for his wound when he goes home, observe the nonverbal cues he provides, and determine if there are problems that will affect discharge planning.*

Once a plumber knows the source of the leaking faucet, he is able to repair it. Once you know the nature and source of a patient's specific health needs or problems (such as Mr. Lawson's *Risk for Infection* and his need to be prepared for discharge), you are able to provide interventions that will restore, maintain, or improve the patient's health.

Critical thinking is a vital part of assessment (see Chapter 15). While gathering data about a patient, you synthesize relevant knowledge, recall prior clinical experiences, apply critical thinking standards and attitudes, and use professional standards of practice to direct your assessment in a meaningful and purposeful way (Figure 16-2). Your knowledge from the physical, biological, and social sciences allows you to ask relevant questions and collect relevant history and physical assessment data related to a patient's presenting health care needs. *For example, Tonya knows that Mr. Lawson had part of his colon removed to remove a cancerous tumor. She reviewed her medical-surgical textbook and learned how a colectomy alters gastrointestinal function and poses risks for blood clots in the legs after surgery. This knowledge leads her to assess Mr. Lawson's bowel sounds, ask him if he is passing flatus, and assess the status of circulation in his legs. Tonya has learned from previous experience caring for patients with abdominal surgery that they will be given activity restrictions after surgery to reduce strain on the incision. Mr. Lawson's incision has a small separation; thus Tonya knows that she needs to assess what he has learned so far about the activity restrictions. Using good communication skills through interviewing and applying critical thinking intellectual standards (such as relevance [which activities the patient performs at home]), and broad (including patient's wife in*

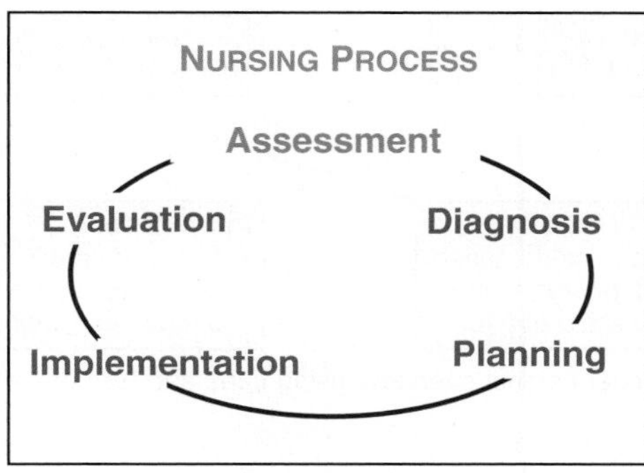

FIGURE 16-2 Critical thinking and the assessment process.

assessing home environment) will enable Tonya to collect complete, accurate, and relevant data.

Developing the Nurse-Patient Relationship for Data Collection

An assessment is necessary for you to gather information to make accurate judgments about a patient's current condition. Your information comes from:

- The patient through interview, observations, and physical examination.
- Family members or significant others' reports and response to interviews.
- Other members of the health care team.
- Medical record information (e.g., patient history, laboratory work, x-ray film results, multidisciplinary consultations).
- Scientific and medical literature (evidence about disease conditions, assessment techniques, and standards).

Typically there is a lot of information to consider about a patient. Where should you begin? Start by taking quality time to be with a patient, even if it is for a few minutes. Establishing a nurse-patient therapeutic relationship allows you to know a patient as a person. This occurs during admission of a patient to your unit, during rounds when you begin a shift of care, or in any encounter with a patient. Chapter 24 explains details of how you develop a therapeutic relationship. In this chapter patient assessment is explained as part of the working phase of a nurse-patient relationship. Patricia Benner (1984) described in her early research the importance of a healing relationship established between nurse and patient. This relational process mobilizes hope for a patient and nurse; allows for an acceptable interpretation and understanding of a patient's illness, pain, fear, and anxiety; and helps a patient use support from health care providers (Benner, 1984).

Connecting with a patient by showing interest in his or her problems and concerns helps you collect a relevant database. Research shows that hearing accounts of patients' health and illness experiences, watching them, and coming to understand how they typically respond develops a type of knowing that fosters good clinical judgments (Tanner, 2006). Visiting a hospitalized patient at set intervals (called *rounding*) allows you to address essential care needs and patient experiences and helps organize your workload on your work unit (Ministry of Health, 2013). Rounding is a vital opportunity to build trust with patients, increasing the likelihood that you will gain more information that will help you identify and communicate their health care problems more accurately and effectively.

Types of Assessments

Remember that assessment is all about accurate and thorough data collection. You will learn to conduct different types of assessments: the patient-centered interview during a nursing health history, a physical examination, and the periodic assessments you make during rounding or administering care. For example, when you bathe a patient or change a dressing, you are always using your skills of observation and physical examination (see Chapter 31) to gather data about him or her.

When you begin assessment, think critically about what to assess for that specific patient in that specific situation. As you are forming your relationship and connecting with a patient, the patient will begin to share information. Determine which questions or measurements are appropriate on the basis of what you initially learn from a patient about his or her health concerns and history, your clinical knowledge,

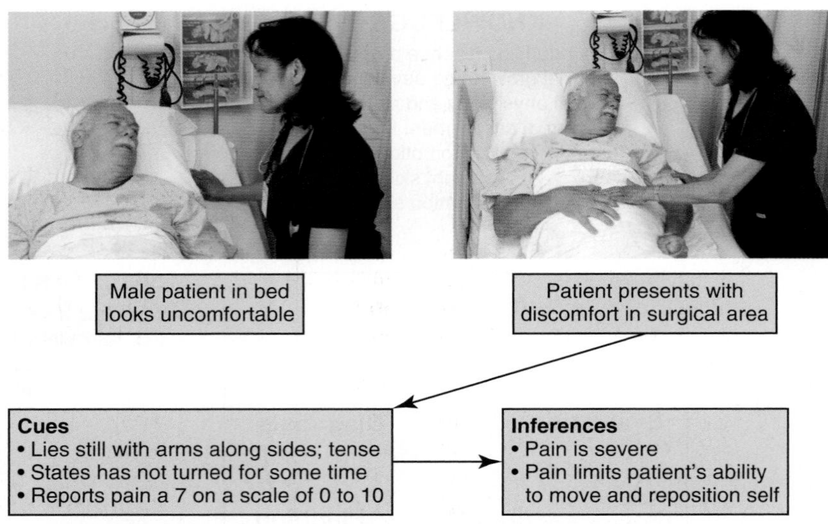

FIGURE 16-3 Observational overview using cues and forming inferences.

and your experience with other patients. In most cases a patient will reveal information that directs you to conduct a quick screening. This is common when you make rounds on a patient. For example, an emergency department nurse uses the ABC (airway-breathing-circulation) approach when a patient develops respiratory distress; and a medical-surgical nurse focuses on a patient's symptoms after returning from surgery, the expected healing response, and signs of potential complications. *For Mr. Lawson, Tonya focuses on the condition of the patient's surgical wound, looking for signs of healing. She later expands her assessment to determine how Mr. Lawson is adjusting emotionally to his surgery and whether he is prepared for discharge.*

You learn to differentiate important data from the total data you collect. A **cue** is information that you obtain through use of the senses. An **inference** is your judgment or interpretation of these cues (Figure 16-3). For example, a patient crying is a cue that possibly implies fear, pain, or sadness. You ask the patient about any concerns and make known any nonverbal expressions that you notice in an effort to direct the patient to share his or her feelings. It is possible to miss important cues during an initial overview. However, always try to interpret cues from the patient to know how in depth to make your assessment. Remember, thinking is human and imperfect. You will acquire appropriate thinking processes the more you conduct assessments, but sometimes you will make mistakes and miss important cues. Assessment is dynamic and allows you to freely explore relevant patient problems as you discover them.

When you conduct a more comprehensive patient history (i.e., a detailed assessment of a patient's physical, psychological, social, cultural, and spiritual needs), there are two approaches to this assessment. One involves use of a structured database format on the basis of an accepted theoretical framework or practice standard. Watson and Foster's model of "The Attending Caring Nurse" (2003), Nola Pender's "Health Promotion Model" (2011), and Gordon's model of 11 **functional health patterns** (1994) are examples. A theory or practice standard provides categories of information for you to assess. Pender's model is outlined in Chapter 6. Watson's model supports a comprehensive assessment of caring needs and concerns from a patient's frame of reference. It uses caring theory as a guide for identifying caring needs and assessing the meaning of both subjective and objective concerns (Watson and Foster, 2003). Gordon's functional health patterns model offers a holistic framework for assessment of any health problem (Box 16-1). *For example, Tonya plans to direct further assessment of Mr. Lawson to the cognitive-perceptual pattern to learn more about what the patient knows about recovering from surgery, any restrictions recommended by the surgeon, and how Mr. Lawson prefers to learn and make decisions about his care.* A theoretical or standard-based assessment

BOX 16-1 Typology of 11 Functional Health Patterns

- **Health perception–health management pattern:** Describes patient's self-report of health and well-being, how patient manages health (e.g., frequency of health care provider visits, adherence to therapies at home), knowledge of preventive health practices
- **Nutritional-metabolic pattern:** Describes patient's daily/weekly pattern of food and fluid intake (e.g., food preferences or restrictions, special diet, appetite), actual weight, weight loss or gain
- **Elimination pattern:** Describes patterns of excretory function (bowel, bladder, and skin)
- **Activity-exercise pattern:** Describes patterns of exercise, activity, leisure, and recreation; ability to perform activities of daily living
- **Sleep-rest pattern:** Describes patterns of sleep, rest, and relaxation
- **Cognitive-perceptual pattern:** Describes sensory-perceptual patterns: language adequacy, memory, decision-making ability
- **Self-perception–self-concept pattern:** Describes patient's self-concept pattern and perceptions of self (e.g., self-concept/worth, emotional patterns, body image)
- **Role-relationship pattern:** Describes patient's patterns of role engagements and relationships
- **Sexuality-reproductive pattern:** Describes patient's patterns of satisfaction and dissatisfaction with sexuality pattern, patient's reproductive patterns, premenopausal and postmenopausal problems
- **Coping–stress tolerance pattern:** Describes patient's ability to manage stress, previous coping responses, sources of support, effectiveness of coping patterns in terms of stress tolerance
- **Value-belief pattern:** Describes patterns of values, beliefs (including spiritual practices), and goals that guide patient's choices or decisions

Data from Gordon M: *Nursing diagnosis: process and application,* ed 3, St Louis, 1994, Mosby; and Carpenito-Moyet LJ: *Nursing diagnosis: application to clinical practice,* ed 13, Philadelphia, 2009, Lippincott Williams & Wilkins.

provides for a comprehensive review of a patient's health care problems.

A comprehensive assessment moves from the general to the specific. For example, start by assessing a patient using all of Gordon's 11 functional health patterns and then determine if patterns or problems appear in your data. Typically certain aspects of a situation stand out as most important. You then ask more focused questions on the basis of a patient's responses and physical signs. The data lead you to clarify which problems exist. You begin to see patterns of behavior and physiological responses that relate to a functional health category. You cannot understand one health pattern without knowledge of the other patterns (Gordon, 1994). Ultimately your assessment identifies functional (patient strengths) and dysfunctional (nursing diagnoses) patterns that help you develop the nursing care plan (see Chapter 18).

The second approach for conducting a comprehensive assessment is problem oriented. You focus on a patient's presenting situation and begin with problematic areas such as incisional pain or limited understanding of postoperative recovery. You ask the patient follow-up questions to clarify and expand your assessment so you can understand the full nature of the problem. Later your physical examination focuses on the same problem areas to further confirm your observations. Table 16-1 offers an example of a problem-focused assessment.

Whatever approach you use to collect data, you cluster cues, make inferences, and identify emerging patterns and potential problem areas. To do this well you critically anticipate, which means that you continuously think about what the data tell you and decide if more data are needed. Remember to always have supporting cues before you make an inference. Your inferences direct you to further questions. Once you ask a patient a question or make an observation, patterns form, and the information branches to an additional series of questions or observations (Figure 16-4). Knowing how to probe and frame questions is a skill that grows with experience. You learn to decide which questions are relevant to a situation and attend to accurate data interpretation on the basis of inferences and experience.

Types of Data

There are two primary sources of data: subjective and objective. **Subjective data** are your patients' verbal descriptions of their health problems. For example, Mr. Lawson's self-report of pain at the area where his incision slightly separated is an example of subjective data. Subjective data include patients' feelings, perceptions, and self-report of symptoms. Only patients provide subjective data relevant to their health condition. The data often reflect physiological changes, which you further explore through objective review of body systems.

TABLE 16-1 Example of Problem-Focused Patient Assessment: Pain

Problem and Associated Factors	Questions	Physical Assessment
Nature of pain	Describe your pain. Place your hand over the area that hurts or is uncomfortable.	Observe nonverbal cues. Observe where patient points to pain; note if it radiates or is localized.
Precipitating factors	Do you notice if pain worsens during any activities or specific time of day? Is pain associated with movement?	Observe if patient demonstrates nonverbal signs of pain during movement, positioning, swallowing.
Severity	Rate your pain on a scale of 0 to 10.	Inspect area of discomfort; palpate for tenderness.

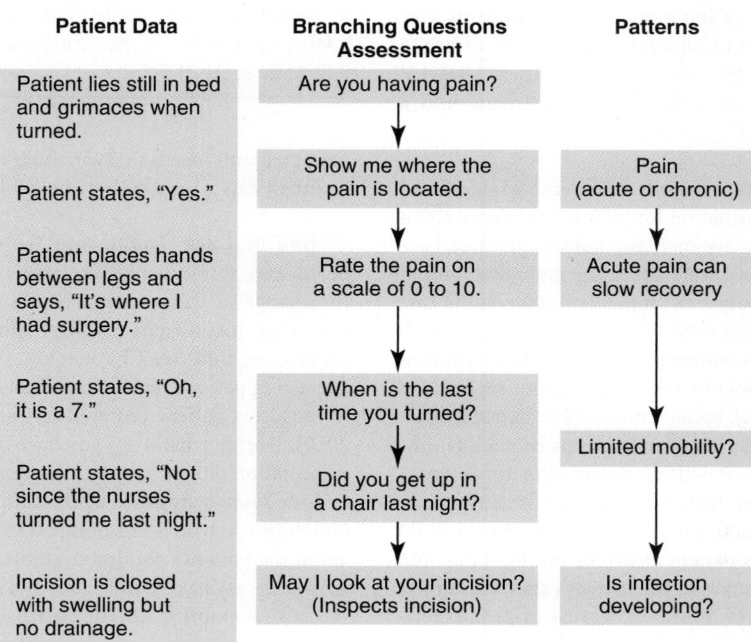

FIGURE 16-4 Example of branching logic for selecting assessment questions.

Objective data are observations or measurements of a patient's health status. Inspecting the condition of a surgical incision or wound, describing an observed behavior, and measuring blood pressure are examples of objective data. Objective data is measured on the basis of an accepted standard such as the Fahrenheit or Celsius measure on a thermometer, inches or centimeters on a measuring tape, or a rating scale (e.g., pain). When you collect objective data, apply critical thinking intellectual standards (e.g., clear, precise, and consistent) so you can correctly interpret your findings.

Sources of Data

A variety of sources provide information about a patient's current level of wellness and functional status, anticipated prognosis, risk factors for any health problems, health practices and goals, cultural background, responses to previous treatment, and patterns of health and illness.

Patient. A patient is usually your best source of information. Patients who are conscious, alert, and able to answer questions without cognitive impairment provide the most accurate information. You learn through the eyes of patients their health care needs, cultural and lifestyle patterns, present and past illnesses, perception of symptoms, responses to treatment, and changes in activities of daily living. Always consider the setting for your assessment and your patient's condition. A patient having acute symptoms in an emergency department will not offer as much information as one who comes to an outpatient clinic for a routine checkup. Also know your patient's health literacy level. A patient with limited literacy has difficulty obtaining, processing, and understanding basic health information (AHRQ, 2014). This means that patients do not always understand some of the questions you use to assess their conditions, especially if you use more clinically focused words or terms or do not speak their language. You will not gather accurate information if a patient does not understand your assessment questions (Box 16-2).

An older adult may require more time for assessment than someone younger if hearing or cognitive deficits exist. Use short (but not leading) questions, keep your language uncomplicated, and listen to a patient's perspective carefully (Ball et al., 2015) (Box 16-3). Always be attentive, engaged, and show a caring presence with patients (see Chapter 7). Patients are less likely to fully reveal the nature of health care problems when you show little interest or are easily distracted by activities around them such as entering an assessment into a computer.

BOX 16-2 EVIDENCE-BASED PRACTICE

Health Literacy Assessment

PICO Question: In adults does the use of literacy screening tools versus an assessment of patients' educational or occupational level assess level of health literacy?

Evidence Summary

Several assessment tools are available for assessing health literacy in adults, including the Rapid Estimate of Adult Literacy in Medicine—Short form (REALM-S); the Shortened Test of Functional Health Literacy in Adults (S-TOFHLA); and the Newest Vital Sign (NVS), a tool that consists of a nutrition label and only six questions (Mottus et al., 2014; Weiss et al., 2005). A thorough assessment of a patient's health literacy is not measured consistently by health care providers because of the time it takes to complete existing literacy assessment tools. The NVS has been tested among adults and geriatric patients (Johnson and Weiss, 2008; Patel et al., 2011). It takes on average 3 minutes for adults to complete the NVS but a longer period of time (11 minutes) for African-American older adults (Johnson and Weiss, 2008; Patel et al., 2011). A study by Mottus et al. (2014) tested the associations between health literacy (using the REALM, S-TOFLHA, and NVS tools) and three objective health outcomes in older people (physical fitness, body mass index (BMI), and count of natural teeth). The study found that cognitive ability in old age and childhood and educational and occupational levels accounted for the majority of the outcome associations (as much as health literacy scores).

Application to Nursing Practice

Knowing the level of patient's health literacy may help physicians and nurses deliver health information in a way that patients can understand (Patel et al., 2011).

When literacy assessment tools are not available, you need to include a review of general cognitive ability and educational and/or occupational levels in your nursing assessment.

Lower health literacy is associated with poorer health outcomes. Measure literacy levels to help patients obtain information, apply the information in real-life situations, and understand the information and services needed to make health decisions.

Asking the single question "How confident are you in filling out medical forms by yourself?" is often successful in detecting limited health literacy (Wallace et al., 2006).

Family and Significant Others. Family members and significant others are primary sources of information for infants or children, critically ill adults, and patients who are mentally handicapped or have cognitive impairment. In cases of severe illness or emergency situations, families are often the only sources of information for health care providers. The family and significant others are also important secondary sources of information. They confirm findings or identify patterns that a patient provides (e.g., whether he takes medications regularly at home or how well he sleeps or eats). Include the family when appropriate. Patients do not always want you to question or involve their family; thus some facilities require oral or written permission to do so. A spouse or close friend who sits in during an assessment can provide his or her view of the patient's health problems or needs. Not only do they supply information about a patient's current health status, but they are also able to tell when changes in the patient's status occurred. Family members are often very well informed because of their experiences living with a patient and observing how health problems affect daily living activities. Family and friends make important observations about patients' needs that can affect the way care is delivered (e.g., how a patient eats a meal or how he or she makes choices).

Health Care Team. You frequently communicate with other health care team members to assess patients. In the acute care setting the change-of-shift report, bedside rounds, and patient hand-off are ways that nurses from one shift communicate information to nurses on the next shift (see Chapter 26). A hand-off is an interactive process of passing patient-specific information from one caregiver to another for ensuring patient-centered care and patient safety (Chaboyer et al., 2010). During a hand-off you have the chance to collect the first set of information about patients assigned to your care. Ideally during bedside rounds the nurse who is completing care for a shift, the patient, and the nurse who is assuming care for the next shift share information about the patient's condition, status of problems, and treatment plan. In many settings rounds are multidisciplinary. Nurses, physicians, physical therapists, social workers, or other staff collaborate and consult on a patient's condition and share information about how he or she is reacting to treatments, the result of diagnostic procedures or

BOX 16-3 FOCUS ON OLDER ADULTS

Approaches for Gathering an Older-Adult Assessment

- Listen patiently; older adults are a rich source of wisdom and perspective.
- Allow for pauses and time for patients to tell their story.
- Recognize normal changes associated with aging (see Chapter 31). Older-adult symptoms are often less dramatic, vague, or nonspecific compared with those of younger adults (Ball et al., 2015).
- If patient has a proxy (person who legally represents him or her), gather history information from that individual.
- If patient has limited hearing or visual deficits, use nonverbal communication when conducting a patient-centered interview.
    - **Patient-directed eye gaze:** This allows a nurse or patient who is speaking to check whether information is understood. It is a signal for readiness to initiate interaction with a patient. Eye contact shows interest in what the other person is saying.
    - **Affirmative head nodding:** This has an important social function. It regulates an interaction (especially when alternate people speak), supports spoken language, and allows for comment on the interaction.
    - **Smiling:** Smiling is positive and considered as a sign of good humor, warmth, and immediacy. It helps when first establishing the nurse-patient relationship.
    - **Forward leaning:** This shows awareness, attention, and immediacy. During an interaction it also clearly suggests interest in that person.

therapies, and the future plan of care. Every member of the team is a source of information for identifying and verifying essential information about a patient.

Medical Records. The medical record is a source for a patient's medical history, laboratory and diagnostic test results, current physical findings, and the primary health care provider's treatment plan. The record is a valuable tool for checking the consistency and similarities of data with your personal observations. Data in the records offer a baseline and ongoing information about a patient's response to illness and progress to date. The Health Insurance Portability and Accountability Act (HIPAA) of 1996, made effective in 2003, has the privacy rule to set standards for the protection of health information (USDHHS, 2014). Information in a patient's record is confidential. Each health care agency has policies governing how a patient's health information can be shared among health care providers (see Chapter 26). Only individuals involved in a patient's care can access medical records (see agency policies).

Other Records and the Scientific Literature. Educational, military, and employment records often contain significant health care information (e.g., immunizations). If a patient received services at a community clinic or a different hospital, you need written permission from the patient or guardian to access the record. The HIPAA regulations protect access to patients' health information. The privacy rule allows health care providers to share protected information as long as they use reasonable safeguards. Consult agency policies and participate in annual HIPAA training as required.

Reviewing recent nursing, medical, and pharmacological literature about a patient's illness completes a patient's assessment database. This review increases your knowledge about a patient's diagnosed problems, expected symptoms, treatment, prognosis, and established standards of therapeutic practice. The scientific literature offers evidence (see Chapter 5) to direct you on how and why to conduct assessments for particular patient conditions. A knowledgeable nurse obtains relevant, accurate, and complete information for a patient's assessment.

Nurse's Experience. Your experiences in caring for patients are a source of data. Through clinical experience you observe other patients' behaviors and physical signs and symptoms; track trends and recognize clinical changes; and learn the types of questions to ask, choosing the questions that will give the most useful information. This experience builds your ability to know patients (i.e., knowing the patient's pattern of responses and knowing the patient as a person) (Tanner, 2006). A nurse's expertise develops after testing and refining questions with patients who have similar conditions or problems. *While caring for Mr. Lawson, Tonya has learned what a colectomy incision looks like and how a patient responds to the associated discomfort. She also is gaining knowledge about what an incision looks like when separation begins. During future care of patients Tonya will more quickly recognize behaviors of patients in acute pain and the signs of impaired wound healing.*

Practical experience and the opportunity to make clinical decisions strengthen your critical thinking.

THE PATIENT-CENTERED INTERVIEW

When a patient is admitted to a health care agency or when it is necessary to gather detailed information about a patient, you will collect an assessment using interview and observational skills. A patient-centered interview is relationship based and is an organized conversation focused on learning about the well and the sick as they seek care (Ball et al., 2015). A primary objective during an initial history taking is to discover details about a patient's concerns, explore expectations for the encounter you are having, and display genuine interest and partnership. A patient-centered interview becomes the basis for forming trust and effective long-term therapeutic relationships with patients (see Chapter 24).

One type of patient-centered interview is motivational interviewing. It is a technique used often in counseling that allows you to become a helper in the change process (see Chapter 38). Motivational interviewing is a process that addresses a patient's ambivalence to medically indicated behavior change and supports patients in making health care decisions in cases in which there is more than one reasonable option (Elwyn et al., 2014).

Effective communication with patients during an assessment interview requires the following communication skills (Ball et al., 2015):

- *Courtesy:* Greet patients by the name by which they prefer to be addressed. Ask, "Would you prefer I call you by Mrs. Silver or your first name?" Introduce yourself and explain your role (if it is the first time you have met) such as gathering an admission history or exploring a recent symptom or problem. Meet and acknowledge any visitors in a patient's room and learn their names. Remember to ask the patient's permission to conduct the interview in visitors' presence. Assure the patient that the information will be kept confidential among his or her health care providers (Ball et al., 2015). HIPAA regulations require patients to sign an authorization before you collect personal health data (USDHHS, 2014) (see agency policy).
- *Comfort:* If a patient is having symptoms such as pain, nausea or fatigue, it is difficult for you to gather a thorough and accurate history. In a hospital setting perform any necessary comfort measures before beginning the interview. Maintain privacy by closing room curtains or doors. Be sure the room temperature is comfortable and ensure good lighting. In the home choose a location that is quiet and free of interruptions. Timing is

important in avoiding interruptions. If possible, set aside a 10- to 15-minute period when no other activities are planned but realize that this is difficult to plan when you have multiple patients. Avoid overtiring a patient; you can always return for another visit to gather more information (Ball et al., 2015).

- *Connection:* It is so important to make a good first impression. If you begin collecting a history by staring at a computer screen to fill in required data fields or talking on a cell phone, patients will perceive you as uncaring or uninterested in hearing their stories. Patients know if you care. Establish eye contact and sit at eye level if possible during an interview. Do not dominate a discussion or assume that you know the nature of a patient's problems. Start with open-ended questions: "How have you been feeling?" or "What questions would you like to discuss?" Listen and be attentive. Use your observational skills—what is the patient's tone of voice, posture, level of energy when talking? Respect silence and be flexible; let the patient's needs, concerns, or questions guide your follow-up questions. Health problems can have multiple causes; do not leap to one cause too quickly (Ball et al., 2015).
- *Confirmation:* At the end of an interview, ask the patient to summarize the discussion so there are no uncertainties. Be open to further clarification or discussion; ask the patient "Is there anything else you would like to share"? If there are questions you cannot answer, say so and promise that you will return with a follow-up if possible (Ball et al., 2015).

Interview Preparation

Before you begin an interview, be prepared. Review a patient's medical record when information is available. If your interview is performed at patient admission, there may be little information in the medical record except for an admitting diagnosis. In other cases review the previous medical or nurse's note entry. Were problems identified that perhaps need clarification or follow-up? Does a patient's admitting diagnosis or other diagnoses suggest lines of questions for you to ask? The information you share with another nurse during hand-off at the beginning of a shift helps frame a clinical problem about which you want to learn more.

Phases of an Interview

An interview is an approach for gathering subjective and objective data from a patient through an organized conversation. An initial interview involves collecting a nursing health history and gathering information about a patient's condition (Ball et al., 2015). Later interviews have a different focus; you assess more about a patient's presenting situation and discuss specific problem areas. All patient-centered interviews follow three phases.

Orientation and Setting an Agenda. Begin an interview by introducing yourself and your position and explaining the purpose of the interview. Explain why you are collecting data and assure patients that all of the information will be confidential. Your aim is to set an agenda for how you will gather information about a patient's current chief concerns or problems. Remember, the best clinical interview focuses on a patient's goals, preferences, and concerns and not on your agenda. Explain your purpose (such as collecting a brief assessment or a nursing history) and ask a patient for his or her list of concerns or problems. This is the time that allows a patient to feel comfortable speaking with you and become an active partner in decisions about care. The professionalism and competence that you show when interviewing patients strengthens the nurse-patient relationship.

Tonya is doing a follow-up interview to learn more about Mr. Lawson's home situation. She explains, "Mr. Lawson, it looks like your doctor wants to send you home tomorrow. It's important for us to know more about how you care for yourself at home. Will your wife be able to help you when necessary? Are you comfortable and can I take a few minutes to talk about your discharge?" Mr. Lawson replies, "I feel a bit better, and yes, I've been thinking about some questions I want to ask." Tonya replies, "Good, we'll start there."

Working Phase—Collecting Assessment or Nursing Health History. Start an assessment or a nursing health history with open-ended questions that allow patients to describe more clearly their concerns and problems. For example, begin by having a patient explain symptoms or physical concerns and describe what he or she knows about the health problem or ask him or her to describe health care expectations. Use attentive listening and other therapeutic communication techniques (see Chapter 24) that encourage a patient to tell his or her story. The verbal cues that a patient expresses will help you stay focused so you can direct the assessment appropriately. Do not rush a patient. An initial interview (e.g., the one you collect to complete a nursing history) is more extensive. You gather information about a patient's concerns and then complete all relevant sections of the nursing history. Ongoing interviews, which occur each time you interact with your patient, do not need to be as extensive. An ongoing interview allows you to update a patient's status and concerns, focus on changes previously identified, and review new problems. In the case study Tonya gathers information to plan postoperative teaching and discharge planning for Mr. Lawson.

Tonya: "Mr. Lawson, you said you had some questions. Can you tell me what they are?"

Mr. Lawson: "Well, the doctor told me that I would not be able to lift anything heavy for a while, and I'm not sure if I understand. The way my incision looks, will I need to do something to it?

Tonya: Let's start with your question about lifting. First of all, what types of things do you lift regularly at home (for example, children, a pet, groceries)?

Mr. Lawson: "Well, when our grandchildren visit, they do like to be picked up. We have a pet schnauzer, but he just jumps up on the chair with me. My wife does the grocery shopping, but I come out to unload the car."

Tonya: "Ok, and about your incision, yes you will need to care for it. Do you know the signs of infection?

Mr. Lawson: "Not sure I do, but I guess it would hurt more. Is infection common?"

Tonya: "No, but you need to know the signs so, if something happens once you return home, you can call your doctor quickly. Has your doctor talked about ways to care for your incision?"

Mr. Lawson: "No, he hasn't mentioned anything about that yet."

Tonya: "Ok, I'll explain everything you need to know. Do you learn best by reading information or listening to explanations?"

Mr. Lawson: "I think I do okay with both."

Tonya's assessment focuses on the patient's questions and how they pertain to the information he will need to learn to go home and assume self-care.

Terminating an Interview. Termination of an interview requires skill. You summarize your discussion with a patient and check for accuracy of the information collected. Give your patient a clue that the interview is coming to an end. For example, say, "I have just two more questions. We'll be finished in a few more minutes." This helps a patient maintain direct attention without being distracted by wondering when the interview will end. This approach also gives him or her an opportunity to ask additional questions. End the interview in a friendly manner, telling the patient when you will return to provide care.

Tonya: "You've given me a good idea of which topics we need to cover to prepare you for going home. And we'll include your wife in these discussions. I'll return after checking on two other patients,"
Mr. Lawson: "You've been helpful already."

A skillful interviewer adapts interview strategies on the basis of a patient's responses. You successfully gather relevant health data when you are prepared for an interview and able to carry out each interview phase with minimal interruption.

Interview Techniques

How you conduct an interview is just as important as the questions you ask. During an interview you are responsible for directing the flow of the discussion so patients have the opportunity to freely contribute stories about their health problems to enable you to get as much detailed information as possible. Remember, some interviews are focused; others are comprehensive. Listen and consider the information shared because this helps you direct a patient to provide more detail or discuss a topic that might reveal a possible problem. Because a patient's report includes subjective information, validate data from the interview later with objective data. For example, if a patient reports difficulty breathing, this will lead you to further assess respiratory rate and lung sounds during the physical examination.

Observation. Observation is powerful. Observe a patient's nonverbal communication such as use of eye contact, body language, or tone of voice. While observing nonverbal behavior, appearance, and interaction with the environment, you determine whether the data you obtained are consistent with what the patient states verbally. Your observations lead you to pursue further objective information to form accurate conclusions. Patients also obtain information during interviews. If you establish a trusting nurse-patient relationship, the patient feels comfortable asking you questions about the health care environment, planned treatments, diagnostic testing, and available resources. A patient needs this information to partner in making decisions and planning the goals of care.

Open-Ended Questions. In a patient-centered interview you try to find out, in the patient's own words, his or her health goals and any concerns or problems that exist and their probable cause. Patients are the best resources for talking about their symptoms or relating their health history. Begin by asking a patient an *open-ended question* to elicit his or her story. An open-ended question gives a patient discretion about the extent of his or her answer (Ball et al., 2015). For example, "So, tell me more about ....." or "What are your concerns about this?" or "Tell me how you're feeling." An open-ended question does not presuppose a specific answer. The use of **open-ended questions** prompts patients to describe a situation in more than one or two words. This technique leads to a discussion in which patients actively describe their health status and strengthens your relationship with them. Open-ended questions show that you want to hear a patient's thoughts and feelings. Remember to encourage and let your patient tell the entire story.

Leading Question. These questions are the most risky because of possibly limiting the information provided to what a patient thinks you want to know (Ball et al., 2015). Examples include, "It seems to me this is bothering you quite a bit. Is that true?" or "Now, that wasn't very hard to do, was it?"

Back Channeling. Reinforce your interest in what a patient has to say through the use of good eye contact and listening skills. Also use **back channeling**, which includes active listening prompts such as "all right," "go on," or "uh-huh." These indicate that you have heard what a patient says, are interested in hearing the full story, and are encouraging the patient to give more details.

Probing. As a patient tells his or her story, encourage a full description without trying to control the direction the story takes. This requires you to probe with further open-ended statements such as "Is there anything else you can tell me?" or "What else is bothering you?" Each time a patient offers more detail, probe again until the patient has nothing else to say and has told the full story. Always stay observant. If a patient becomes fatigued or uncomfortable, know that it is time to postpone an interview.

Direct Closed-Ended Questions. As you learn information from a patient, you will ask direct questions to seek specific information. This problem-seeking technique gives details to identify a patient's problems accurately. This approach takes the information provided in a patient's story and more fully describes and identifies specific problem areas. For example, a patient reports experiencing indigestion over the course of several days and acknowledges having some diarrhea and loss of appetite. The patient's explanation for the cause relates to a recent series of trips that changed his eating habits. The nurse focuses on the symptoms the patient identifies and the general indigestion problem by asking **closed-ended questions** that limit answers to one or two words such as "yes" or "no" or a number or frequency of a symptom. For example, ask, "How often does the diarrhea occur?" or "Do you have pain or cramping?" Closed-ended questions require short answers and clarify previous information or provide additional information. The questions do not encourage the patient to volunteer more information than you request. The technique allows you to acquire specific information about health problems such as symptoms, precipitating factors, or relief measures.

A good interviewer leaves with a complete story that contains enough details for understanding a patient's perceptions of his or her health status and the information needed to help identify nursing diagnoses and/or collaborative health problems (see Chapter 17). Always clarify or validate any information about which you are unclear. Make no assumptions.

NURSING HEALTH HISTORY

You gather a **nursing health history** during an initial or early contact with a patient. The history is a key component of a comprehensive assessment. Most health history forms (manual and electronic) are structured. However, on the basis of information you gain as you conduct the patient-centered interview, you learn which components of the history to explore fully and which require less detail. A good assessor learns to refine and broaden questions as needed to correctly assess a patient's unique needs. Time and patient priorities determine how complete a history will be. A comprehensive history covers all health dimensions (Figure 16-5), allowing you to develop a complete plan of care.

Cultural Considerations

Obtaining a nursing health history requires cultural competence. This involves self-awareness, reflective practice, and knowledge of a patient's

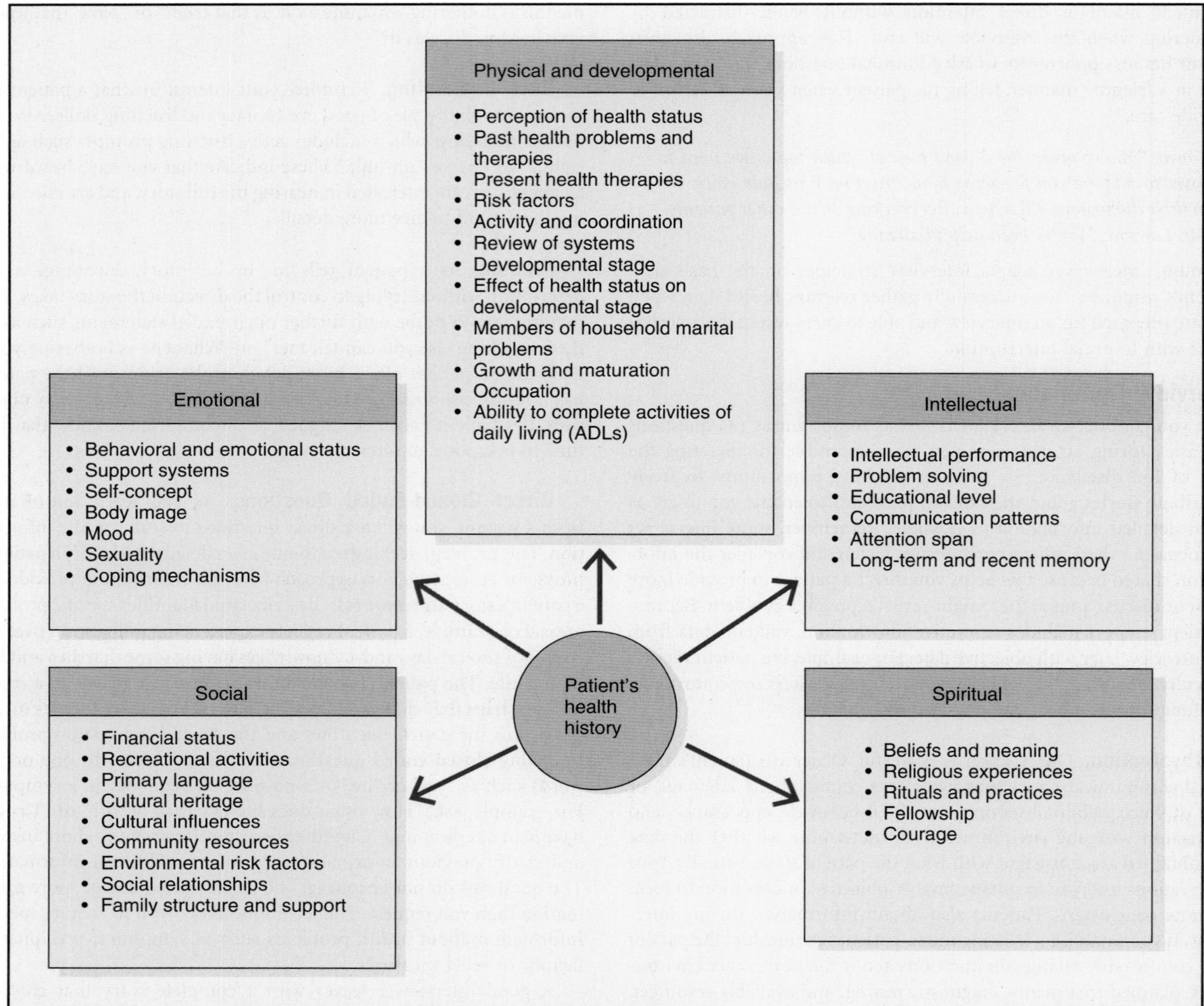

FIGURE 16-5 Dimensions for gathering data for a health history.

core cultural issues (Ball et al., 2015). Adapt each assessment to the unique needs of patients of backgrounds and cultures different from your own. Be respectful; understand these differences; and do not impose your own attitudes, biases, and beliefs (e.g., attitudes towards aging, obesity, or lifestyle). Having a genuine curiosity about a patient's beliefs and values lays a foundation for a trusting patient-nurse relationship (Ball et al., 2015). To conduct an accurate and complete assessment, consider a patient's cultural background. For clarity, explain the intent of any questions you have. Avoid making stereotypes; the assumptions tied to stereotypes (e.g., obese patients do not exercise regularly) can lead you to collect inaccurate information. Draw on knowledge from your assessment and ask questions in a constructive and probing way to allow you to truly know who a patient is (Box 16-4). Be sure to grasp exactly what a patient means and gain feedback to know if what a patient thinks you mean is accurate. If you are unsure about what a patient is saying, clarify to prevent making the wrong diagnostic conclusion. Do not form stereotypes and do not assume that you know a patient's cultural beliefs and behaviors without validation from the patient.

Components of the Nursing Health History

Most health histories contain the same components. Do not let a history form shape your assessment entirely. Decide what information you need on the basis of your patient's needs, responses to your questions, and changing status during the interview.

Biographical Information. Biographical information is factual demographic data that include a patient's age, address, occupation, and working status; marital status; source of health care; and types of insurance. The staff in an admitting office usually collects this information.

Chief Concern or Reason for Seeking Health Care. This is the information you gather when you initially set an agenda during a patient-centered interview. You learn a patient's chief concerns or problems. Compare what you learn from the patient with the "chief complaint," which is often typed on the patient's admission sheet. Often you learn much more. Ask a patient why he or she is seeking

BOX 16-4 CULTURAL ASPECTS OF CARE

Developing a Patient-Centered Approach

To successfully explore a patient's illness or health care problems, use a patient-centered approach. Elicit patient values, preferences, and expressed needs as part of your clinical interview (QSEN Institute, 2014). Ensure the interview is inclusive. Remove barriers to having families present on the basis of patient preferences.

Implications for Patient-Centered Care

- When talking about a patient's illness, try to understand it "through the patient's eyes."
  - What do you think is wrong with you?
  - What worries you most about your illness?
- When talking about treatments, value a patient's expertise with own health and symptoms.
  - What should we do to eliminate your problem?
  - Which types of treatment do you use?
  - What benefit do you expect from the treatment?
- If there is a cross-cultural difference between you and your patient, ask yourself these questions (Suhonen et al., 2011).
  - What is unique to your patient's culture and its impact on the treatment plan?
  - What potential is there to have a cultural misunderstanding? If one exists, try to correct it.
  - Which types of treatments or health practices do you use?

health care (e.g., "Tell me, Mr. Lynn, what brought you to the clinic today"). You record the patient's response in quotations to indicate the subjective response. As you explore a patient's reason for seeking health care, you will learn the chronological and sequential history of his or her health problems (Ball et al., 2015). A patient's statement is not diagnostic; instead it is his or her perception of reasons for seeking health care. Clarification of a patient's perception identifies potential needs for symptom management, education, counseling, or referral to community resources.

Patient Expectations. It is important to assess a patient's expectations of health care providers (e.g., being diagnosed correctly, receiving comfort measures, or being treated successfully for a disease). Patient satisfaction, a standard measure of quality for all hospitals throughout the country, can be perceived by patients as poor if their expectations are unmet (see Chapter 2). Patients typically have expectations of receiving information about their treatments and prognosis and a plan of care for returning home. In addition, they expect relief of pain and other symptoms and caring expressed by health care providers. During the initial interview a patient expresses expectations when entering the health care setting. Later, as a patient interacts with health care providers, assess whether these expectations have changed or been met.

Present Illness or Health Concerns. If a patient presents with an illness, collect essential and relevant data about the symptoms and their effects on the patient's health. Apply critical thinking intellectual standards (see Box 15-4) and use the acronym (PQRST) to guide an assessment:

- **P—Provokes** (e.g., precipitating and relieving factors): What causes symptom? What makes it better or worse? Are there activities (e.g., exercise) that affect it?
- **Q—Quality:** What does the symptom feel like? If patient cannot describe, offer probes such as "Is it sharp? Dull? Burning?"
- **R—Radiate:** Where is the symptom located? Is it in one place? Does it go anywhere else? Have patient be as precise as possible.
- **S—Severity:** Ask a patient to rate the severity of a symptom on a scale of 0 to 10. This gives you a baseline with which to compare in follow-up assessments.
- **T—Time:** Assesses onset and duration of symptom. When did it start? Does it come and go? If so, how often and for how long? What time of day or day of the week?

Also assess if the patient has **concomitant symptoms**. Does he or she experience other symptoms along with the primary symptom? For example, does nausea accompany pain?

Health History. A health history provides a holistic view of a patient's health care experiences and current health habits (see Figure 16-5). Assess whether a patient has ever been hospitalized or injured or has had surgery. Include a complete medication history (including herbal and over-the-counter [OTC] drugs). Also essential are descriptions of allergies, including allergic reactions to food, latex, drugs, or contact agents (e.g., soap). Asking patients if they have had problems with medications or food helps to clarify the type and amount of agent, the specific reaction, and whether a patient has required treatment. If the patient has an allergy, note the specific reaction and treatment on the assessment form and special armband provided.

The history also includes a description of a patient's habits and lifestyle patterns. Assessing for the use of alcohol, tobacco, caffeine, or recreational drugs (e.g., methamphetamine or cocaine) determines a patient's risk for diseases involving the liver, lungs, heart, or nervous system. It is essential to gather information about the type of habit and the frequency and duration of use. Assessing patterns of sleep (see Chapter 43), exercise (see Chapter 39), and nutrition (see Chapter 45) are also important when planning nursing care. Ultimately your aim is to match a patient's lifestyle patterns with approaches in the plan of care as much as possible.

Family History. The family history includes data about immediate and blood relatives. Your objective is to determine whether a patient is at risk for illnesses of a genetic or familial nature and to identify areas of health promotion and illness prevention (see Chapter 6). The family history also reveals information about family structure, interaction, support, and function that often is useful in planning care (see Chapter 10). *For example, Tonya assesses the level of support that Mrs. Lawson is willing to provide. Mrs. Lawson tells Tonya that the two have been married 32 years and states, "I feel I can do whatever is needed for him." Tonya's assessment shows a pattern that Mrs. Lawson is supportive and able to help her husband adjust to any initial limitations in activity when he returns home. Her assessment ultimately allows her to incorporate Mrs. Lawson into the patient teaching portion of the patient's plan of care* (see Chapter 18). If a patient's family is not supportive, it is better not to involve the family in care. Stressful family relationships are sometimes a significant barrier when you try to help patients with problems involving loss, self-concept, spiritual health, and personal relationships.

QSEN: BUILDING COMPETENCY IN PATIENT-CENTERED CARE Describe how to approach an interview with Mrs. Lawson using a patient-centered approach. Describe how you would interview Mrs. Lawson about her husband's pending wound care treatment at home.

Answers to QSEN Activities can be found on the Evolve website.

Psychosocial History. A psychosocial history provides information about a patient's support system, which often includes a spouse or partner, children, other family members, and close friends. The history also includes information about ways that a patient and family typically cope with stress (see Chapter 38). Behaviors that patients use at home to cope with stress such as walking, reading, or talking with a friend can also be used as nursing interventions if the patient experiences stress while receiving health care. In addition, you need to learn if the patient has experienced any recent losses that create a sense of grief (see Chapter 37).

Spiritual Health. Life experiences and events shape a person's spirituality. The spiritual dimension represents the totality of one's being and is difficult to assess quickly (see Chapter 36). Review with patients their beliefs about life, their source for guidance in acting on beliefs, and the relationship they have with family in exercising their faith. Also assess rituals and religious practices that patients use to express their spirituality. Patients may request availability of these practices while in a health care setting.

Review of Systems. The review of systems (ROS) is a systematic approach for collecting subjective information from patients about the presence or absence of health-related issues in each body system (Ball et al., 2015). For example, the review of the skin, hair, and nails includes assessment of whether a patient has noticed any rash or skin lesions or has itching or abnormal nail or hair growth. When using an admission form, you probably will not cover all of the questions for each body system every time you collect a history. You include questions about each system to explore any unexpected signs or symptoms that a patient mentions. In this case explore the system more in depth. The systems you assess thoroughly depend on a patient's condition and the urgency in starting care. During the ROS ask the patient about the normal functioning of each body system and any noted changes. Such changes are subjective data because they are described as perceived by the patient.

Along with the ROS, a nurse conducts a physical examination (see Chapter 31) to further explore and confirm patient information. The examination involves use of the techniques of inspection, palpation, percussion, auscultation, and smell.

Observation of Patient Behavior

Throughout a patient-centered interview and physical examination it is important to closely observe a patient's verbal and nonverbal behaviors. The information adds depth to your objective database. You learn to determine if data obtained by observation matches what a patient communicates verbally. For example, a patient expresses no concern about an upcoming diagnostic test but shows poor eye contact, shakiness, and restlessness, all suggesting anxiety and verbal and nonverbal data conflict. Observations direct you to gather additional objective information to form accurate conclusions about the patient's condition.

An important aspect of observation includes a patient's level of function: the physical, developmental, psychological, and social aspects of everyday living. Observation of level of function differs from observations you make during an interview. You assess level of function by watching what a patient does when eating or making a decision about preparing a medication rather than what the patient tells you that he or she can do. Observation of function often occurs in the home or in a health care setting during a return demonstration.

Diagnostic and Laboratory Data

The results of diagnostic and laboratory tests provide further explanation of alterations or problems identified during the health history and physical examination. For example, during the history a patient reports having a bad cold for 6 days and at present has a productive cough with brown sputum and mild shortness of breath. On physical examination you notice an elevated temperature, increased respirations, and decreased breath sounds in the right lower lobe. You review the results of a complete blood count and note that the white blood cell count is elevated (indicating an infection). You report your results to the patient's health care provider, who orders a chest x-ray film. When the results of the x-ray film show the presence of a right lower lobe infiltrate, the health care provider makes the medical diagnosis of pneumonia. Your assessment leads to the associated nursing diagnosis of *Impaired Gas Exchange.*

Some patients collect and monitor laboratory data in the home. For example, patients with diabetes mellitus often measure blood glucose daily. Ask patients about their routine results to determine their response to illness and information about the effects of treatment measures. Compare laboratory data with the established norms for a particular test, age-group, and gender.

Interpreting and Validating Assessment Data

Assessment involves the continuous interpretation of information. This is a critical thinking aspect of assessment. The successful ongoing interpretation and validation of assessment data ensures that you have collected a complete database. Ultimately this leads you to the second step of the nursing process, in which you make clinical decisions in your patient's care. These decisions are either in the form of nursing diagnoses or collaborative problems that require treatment from all collaborative disciplines (Carpenito-Moyet, 2013) (see Chapter 17).

Interpretation. When critically interpreting assessment information, you determine the presence of abnormal findings, recognize that further observations are needed to clarify information, and begin to identify a patient's health problems. This is clinical reasoning. You begin to see patterns of data that direct you to collect more information and clarify what you have. The patterns of data reveal meaningful and usable clusters. A data cluster is a set of signs or symptoms that you group together in a logical way (Box 16-5). The clusters begin to clearly identify a patient's health problems.

Data Validation. Before you complete data interpretation, validate the information you have collected to avoid making incorrect inferences. Validation of assessment data is the comparison of data with another source to determine data accuracy. For example, you observe a patient crying and logically infer that it is related to hospitalization or a medical diagnosis. Making such an initial inference is not wrong, but problems result if you do not validate the inference with the patient. Instead ask, "I notice that you have been crying. Can you tell me about it?" By validating you discover the real reason for the patient's crying behavior. Ask patients to validate unclear information obtained during an interview and history. Validate findings from the physical examination and observation of patient behavior by comparing data in the medical record and consulting with other nurses or health care team members. Often family or friends validate your assessment information.

Validation opens the door for gathering more assessment data because it involves clarifying vague or unclear data. Occasionally you need to reassess previously covered areas of the nursing history or gather further physical examination data. Continually analyze to make concise, accurate, and meaningful interpretations. Critical thinking applied to assessment enables you to fully understand a patient's problems, judge the extent of the problems carefully, and discover possible relationships between the problems.

BOX 16-5 Recognizing Data Clusters

Interpret how data form patterns or trends.

- Patient uncomfortable: remains still in bed
  - Limits turning
  - Grimaces when moving
- Mobility limited: limits turning
  - Only out of bed once after surgery
- Knowledge about postoperative care: asks questions about restrictions and expresses concerns about incision
  - Unsure about dressing care
  - Asks about risk of infection
- Appears anxious or uneasy: poor eye contact at times
  - Restless
  - Asks numerous questions

Tonya has gathered assessment data to better understand Mr. Lawson's health care needs. The focus of her assessment switched from pain to that of physical characteristics of the surgical incision because the patient's condition changed. Her findings suggest a problem that the patient is at risk for infection. She also assessed the patient's knowledge and learning needs so she can adequately formulate a plan of care to prepare him for discharge. She applied critical thinking in her assessment as she considered the need to include Mr. Lawson's wife in the assessment. In addition, she reflected on her knowledge base concerning surgical colectomies and anticipated what she needed to assess to eventually plan Mr. Lawson's instruction. When Tonya saw the need for more information, she directed her assessment to learn more about Mr. Lawson's concerns about the success of his surgery and what to expect during recovery.

Data Documentation

Record the results of the nursing health history and physical examination in a clear, concise manner using appropriate terminology. This information becomes the baseline to identify patient health problems, plan and implement care, and evaluate a patient's response to interventions. Standardized forms, especially electronic forms, make it easy to enter assessment data as a patient responds to questions. A timely, clear, concise record is necessary for use by other health care professionals (see Chapter 26). If you do not record an assessment finding or problem interpretation, it is lost and unavailable to anyone else caring for the patient. If information is not specific, the reader is left with only general impressions. Observing and recording patient status are legal and professional responsibilities. The Nurse Practice Acts in all states and the American Nurses Association Nursing's Social Policy Statement (ANA, 2010) require accurate data collection and recording as independent functions essential to the role of the professional nurse.

Being factual is easy after it becomes a habit. The basic rule is to record all observations succinctly. When recording data, pay attention to facts and be as descriptive as possible. You need to report anything you hear, see, feel, or smell precisely. Record objective information in accurate terminology (e.g., weighs 77.2 kg (170 lbs), abdomen is soft and nontender to palpation). Record any subjective information by using quotation marks. Do not generalize or form judgments through written communication when entering data. Conclusions about such data become nursing diagnoses and thus must be factual and accurate. As you gain experience and become familiar with clusters and patterns of signs and symptoms, you will correctly conclude the existence of a health problem. Review Chapter 26 for details on documentation.

Concept Mapping

Most patients for whom you care will present with more than one health problem. A concept map is a visual representation that allows you to graphically show the connections among a patient's many health problems. The concept map is a strategy that develops critical thinking skills by helping a learner understand the relationships that exist among patient problems (Bittencourt et al., 2013). Concept maps foster reflection and help students evaluate critical thinking patterns and see the reasons for nursing care. Your first step in concept mapping is to organize the assessment data you collect. Placing all of the cues together into the clusters that form patterns leads you to the next step of the nursing process, nursing diagnosis (see Chapter 17). Through concept mapping you obtain a holistic perspective of your patient's health care needs, which ultimately leads you to making better clinical decisions. Figure 16-6 shows the first step in a concept map that Tonya develops for Mr. Lawson as a result of her nursing assessment. *Tonya begins to identify patterns reflecting Mr. Lawson's problems. As a result of the assessment she has continuing discomfort over the incision, the risk for infection developing, and need for instruction about surgical postoperative care.* The next step (see Chapter 17) is to identify specific nursing diagnoses so you can plan appropriate nursing interventions.

KEY POINTS

- The nursing process is a variation of scientific reasoning that involves five steps: assessment, nursing diagnosis, planning, implementation, and evaluation.
- Assessment is an important first step of the nursing process for learning as much as you can about each patient by partnering together in a therapeutic relationship.
- Assessment involves collecting information from a patient and secondary sources (e.g., health care providers, family members) along with interpreting and validating the information to form a complete database.
- Establishing a nurse-patient therapeutic relationship allows you to know a patient as a person.
- There are two approaches to gathering a comprehensive assessment: use of a structured database format and use of a problem-focused approach.
- Effectively communicating with patients during an assessment interview requires communication skills built on courtesy, comfort, connection, and confirmation.
- Once a patient provides subjective data, explore the findings further by collecting objective data.
- During assessment critically anticipate and use an appropriate branching set of questions or observations to collect data and cluster cues of assessment information to identify emerging patterns and problems.
- In a patient-centered interview an organized conversation with a patient allows the patient to set the initial focus and initiate discussion about his or her health problems.
- An initial patient-centered interview involves: (1) setting the stage, (2) gathering information about the patient's problems and setting an agenda, (3) collecting the assessment or a nursing health history, and (4) terminating the interview.
- When literacy assessment tools are not available, a review of general cognitive ability and educational and/or occupational levels needs to be part of nursing assessment.

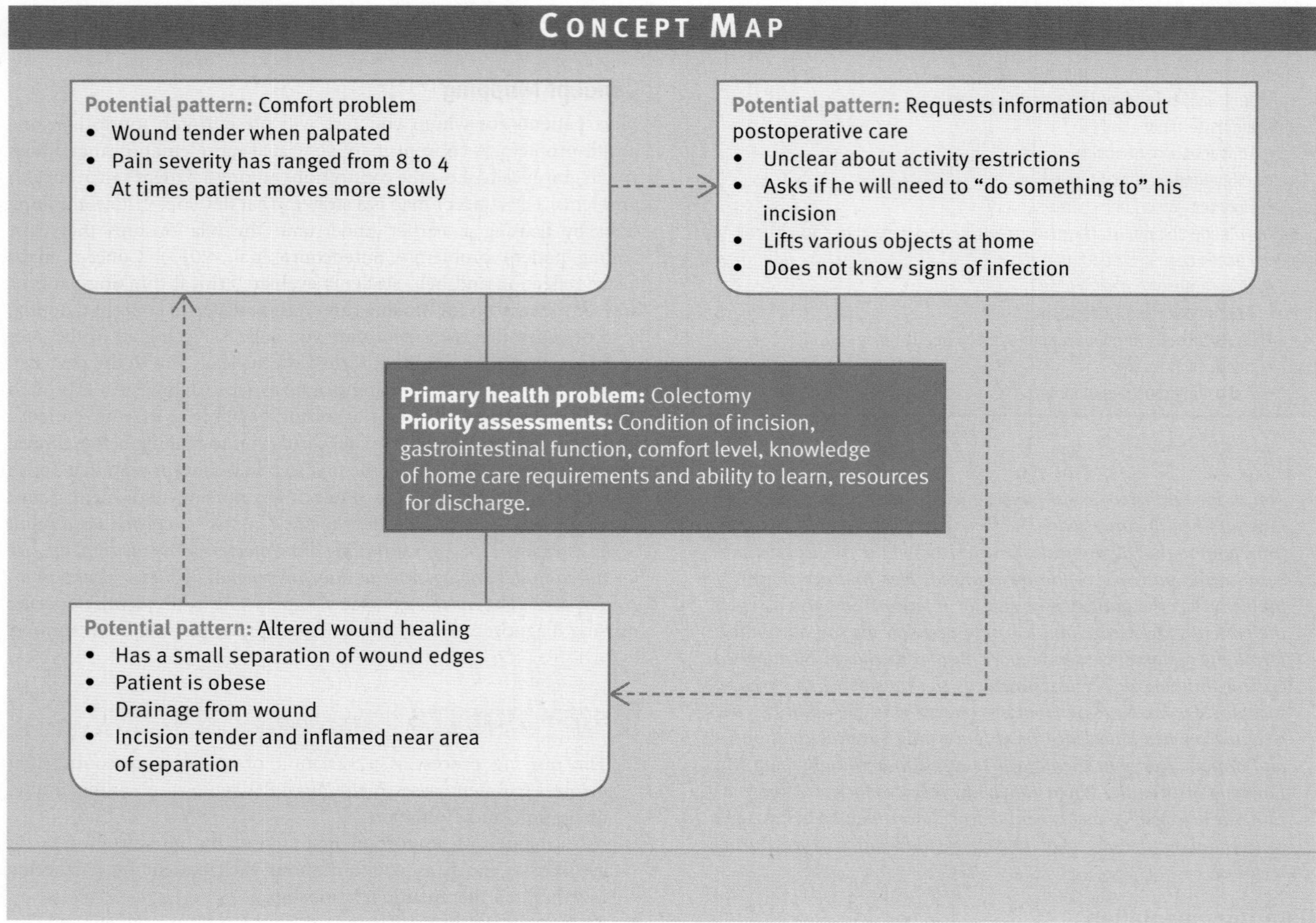

FIGURE 16-6 Concept map for Mr. Lawson: Assessment.

- An assessment needs to adapt to the unique needs of patients of backgrounds and cultures different from your own.
- When collecting a complete nursing history, let the patient's story guide you in fully exploring the components related to his or her problems.
- Successful interpretation and validation of assessment data ensure that you have collected a complete database.

CLINICAL APPLICATION QUESTIONS

Preparing for Clinical Practice

Tonya is planning to return to Mr. Lawson's room and spend more time discussing his concerns about going home and what to expect. She knows that Mrs. Lawson usually comes to visit around 11 AM, just before lunchtime. Tonya believes that Mrs. Lawson will be an important source of support in providing Mr. Lawson's ongoing home care. The surgeon has ordered directions for wound care and standard activity restrictions.

1. Tonya goes to Mr. Lawson's room and asks the patient, "What concerns do you and your wife have about cleaning the wound?" Which type of assessment question is this and why has Tonya asked it?
2. Tonya and Mr. Lawson have the following interaction:
   Tonya: Mr. Lawson, What do you understand about the reason for the activity restrictions your doctor ordered?
   Mr. Lawson: I think it will prevent me from not hurting myself.
   Tonya: Uh huh … go on.
   Mr. Lawson: I think the doctor said I could pull my stitches.
   Tonya's phrase "uh huh … go on" is an example of which interviewing technique? Explain why it is useful.
3. Tonya returns to Mr. Lawson's room to discuss his discharge instructions, but she notes as she enters the room that the patient is grimacing. She asks him, "Tell me where the pain is." Mr. Lawson is asked to rate the pain on a scale of 0 to 10 and rates it a 6. Tonya looks at the patient's surgical wound and notes that the area of separation is still inflamed. Match the assessment technique on the left with the type of measurement on the right.

1. Patient rates pain 6 on a 0 to 10 scale.	___ **A.** Determining location of a symptom
2. Tell me where the pain is.	___ **B.** Observation
3. Patient is seen grimacing.	___ **C.** Inspection
4. Nurse looks at condition of wound.	___ **D.** Determining severity of a symptom

ⓔ ***Answers to Clinical Application Questions can be found on the Evolve website.***

REVIEW QUESTIONS

Are You Ready to Test Your Nursing Knowledge?

1. Which of the following examples are steps of nursing assessment? (Select all that apply.)
   1. Collection of information from patient's family members
   2. Recognition that further observations are needed to clarify information
   3. Comparison of data with another source to determine data accuracy
   4. Complete documentation of observational information
   5. Determining which medications to administer based on a patient's assessment data
2. A nurse assesses a patient who comes to the pulmonary clinic. "I see that it's been over 6 months since you've been here, but your appointment was for every 2 months. Tell me about that. Also I see from your last visit that the doctor recommended routine exercise. Can you tell me how successful you've been in following his plan?" The nurse's assessment covers which of Gordon's functional health patterns?
   1. Value-belief pattern
   2. Cognitive-perceptual pattern
   3. Coping–stress-tolerance pattern
   4. Health perception–health management pattern
3. When a nurse conducts an assessment, data about a patient often comes from which of the following sources? (Select all that apply.)
   1. An observation of how a patient turns and moves in bed
   2. The unit policy and procedure manual
   3. The care recommendations of a physical therapist
   4. The results of a diagnostic x-ray film
   5. Your experiences in caring for other patients with similar problems
4. The nurse observes a patient walking down the hall with a shuffling gait. When the patient returns to bed, the nurse checks the strength in both of the patient's legs. The nurse applies the information gained to suspect that the patient has a mobility problem. This conclusion is an example of:
   1. Cue.
   2. Reflection.
   3. Clinical inference.
   4. Probing.
5. A 72-year-old male patient comes to the health clinic for an annual follow-up. The nurse enters the patient's room and notices him to be diaphoretic, holding his chest and breathing with difficulty. The nurse immediately checks the patient's heart rate and blood pressure and asks him, "Tell me where your pain is." Which of the following assessment approaches does this scenario describe?
   1. Review of systems approach
   2. Use of a structured database format
   3. Back channeling
   4. A problem-oriented approach
6. The nurse asks a patient, "Describe for me a typical night's sleep. What do you do to fall asleep? Do you have difficulty falling or staying asleep? This series of questions would likely occur during which phase of a patient-centered interview?
   1. Orientation
   2. Working phase
   3. Data validation
   4. Termination
7. A nurse is assigned to a 42-year-old mother of 4 who weighs 136.2 kg (300 lbs), has diabetes, and works part time in the kitchen of a restaurant. The patient is facing surgery for gallbladder disease. Which of the following approaches demonstrates the nurse's cultural competence in assessing the patient's health care problems?
   1. "I can tell that your eating habits have led to your diabetes. Is that right?"
   2. "It's been difficult for people to find jobs. Is that why you work part time?"
   3. "You have four children; do you have any concerns about going home and caring for them?"
   4. "I wish patients understood how overeating affects their health."
8. Which type of interview question does the nurse first use when assessing the reason for a patient seeking health care?
   1. Probing
   2. Open-ended
   3. Problem-oriented
   4. Confirmation
9. A nurse gathers the following assessment data. Which of the following cues together form(s) a pattern suggesting a problem? (Select all that apply.)
   1. The skin around the wound is tender to touch.
   2. Fluid intake for 8 hours is 800 mL.
   3. Patient has a heart rate of 78 beats/min and regular.
   4. Patient has drainage from surgical wound.
   5. Body temperature is 38.3° C (101° F).
   6. Patient states, "I'm worried that I won't be able to return to work when I planned."
10. A nurse is checking a patient's intravenous line and, while doing so, notices how the patient bathes himself and then sits on the side of the bed independently to put on a new gown. This observation is an example of assessing:
    1. Patient's level of function.
    2. Patient's willingness to perform self-care.
    3. Patient's level of consciousness.
    4. Patient's health management values.
11. A nurse makes the following statement during a change-of-shift report to another nurse. "I assessed Mr. Diaz, my 61-year-old patient from Chile. He fell at home and hurt his back 3 days ago. He has some difficulty turning in bed, and he says that he has pain that radiates down his leg. He rates his pain at a 6, and he moves slowly as he transfers to a chair." What can the nurse who is beginning a shift do to validate the previous nurse's assessment findings when she conducts rounds on the patient? (Select all that apply.)
    1. The nurse asks the patient to rate his pain on a scale of 0 to 10.
    2. The nurse asks the patient what caused his fall.
    3. The nurse asks the patient if he has had pain in his back in the past.
    4. The nurse assesses the patient's lower-limb strength.
    5. The nurse asks the patient what pain medication is most effective in managing his pain.
12. A patient who visits the surgery clinic 4 weeks after a traumatic amputation of his right leg tells the nurse practitioner that he is worried about his ability to continue to support his family. He tells the nurse he feels that he has let his family down after having an auto accident that led to the loss of his left leg. The nurse listens and then asks the patient, "How do you see yourself now?" On the basis of Gordon's functional health patterns, which pattern does the nurse assess?
    1. Health perception–health management pattern
    2. Value-belief pattern
    3. Cognitive-perceptual pattern
    4. Self-perception–self-concept pattern

13. A nurse is conducting a patient-centered interview. Place the statements from the interview in the correct order, beginning with the first statement a nurse would ask.
    1. "You say you've lost weight. Tell me how much weight you've lost in the last month."
    2. "My name is Todd. I'll be the nurse taking care of you today. I'm going to ask you a series of questions to gather your health history."
    3. "I have no further questions. Thank you for your patience."
    4. "Tell me what brought you to the hospital."
    5. "So, to summarize, you've lost about 6 lbs in the last month, and your appetite has been poor—correct?"
14. During a visit to the clinic, a patient tells the nurse that he has been having headaches on and off for a week. The headaches sometimes make him feel nauseated. Which of the following responses by the nurse is an example of probing?
    1. So you've had headaches periodically in the last week and sometimes they cause you to feel nauseated—correct?
    2. Have you taken anything for your headaches?
    3. Tell me what makes your headaches begin.
    4. Uh huh, tell me more.
15. The nurse enters the room of an 82-year-old patient for whom she has not cared previously. The nurse notices that the patient wears a hearing aid. The patient looks up as the nurse approaches the bedside. Which of the following approaches are likely to be effective with an older adult? (Select all that apply.)
    1. Listen attentively to the patient's story.
    2. Use gestures that reinforce your questions or comments.
    3. Stand back away from the bedside.
    4. Maintain direct eye contact.
    5. Ask questions quickly to reduce the patient's fatigue.

Answers: 1. 1, 2, 3; **2.** 4; **3.** 1, 3, 4; **4.** 3; **5.** 4; **6.** 2; **7.** 3; **8.** 2; **9.** 1, 4, 5; **10.** 1; **11.** 1, 4; **12.** 4; **13.** 2, 4, 1, 5, 3; **14.** 3; **15.** 1, 2, 4.

Rationales for Review Questions can be found on the Evolve website.

REFERENCES

Agency for Healthcare Research and Quality (AHRQ): *Health literacy measurement tools* (revised), 2014, http://www.ahrq.gov/professionals/quality-patient-safety/quality-resources/tools/literacy/. Accessed September 3, 2015.

American Nurses Association (ANA): *Nursing's social policy statement: the essence of the profession*, ed 3, Washington, DC, 2010, The Association.

Ball JW, et al: *Seidel's guide to physical examination*, ed 8, St Louis, 2015, Mosby.

Benner P: *From novice to expert: excellence and power in clinical nursing practice*, Menlo Park, 1984, Addison-Wesley Publishing.

Bertakis KD, Azari R: Determinants and outcomes of patient-centered care, *Patient Educ Couns* 85(10):46, 2011.

Carpenito-Moyet LJ: *Nursing diagnosis: application to clinical practice*, ed 14, Philadelphia, 2013, Lippincott, Williams & Wilkins.

Elwyn G, et al: Shared decision making and motivational interviewing: achieving patient-centered care across the spectrum of health care problems, *Ann Fam Med* 12(3):270, 2014.

Gordon M: *Nursing diagnosis: process and application*, ed 3, St Louis, 1994, Mosby.

Ministry of Health: *National Guideline on Ward Rounds*, 2013, http://www.health.gov.mv/standards/21_1381125641_National_Guideline_on_Ward_Rounds.pdf. Accessed September 3, 2015.

O'Neill S, et al: Nursing works: the application of lean thinking to nursing process, *J Nurs Adm* 41(12):546, 2011.

Pender NJ, et al: *Health promotion in nursing practice*, ed 6, Upper Saddle River, NJ, 2011, Prentice Hall.

QSEN Institute: *Pre-licensure KSAS*, http://qsen.org/competencies/pre-licensure-ksas/. Accessed September 3, 2015.

US Department of Health and Human Services (USDHHS): *Health information privacy, the privacy rule*, 2014, http://www.hhs.gov/ocr/privacy/hipaa/administrative/privacyrule/. Accessed September 3, 2015.

Watson J, Foster R: The Attending Nurse Caring Model: integrating theory, evidence and advanced caring–healing therapeutics for transforming professional practice, *J Clin Nurs* 12:360, 2003.

RESEARCH REFERENCES

Bittencourt GK, et al: Concept maps of the graduate programme in nursing: experience report, *Rev Gaucha Enferm* 34(2):172, 2013.

Chaboyer W, et al: Bedside nursing handover: a case study, *Int J Nurs Pract* 16(1):27, 2010.

Herdman TH, Kamitsuru S, editors: *NANDA International nursing diagnoses: definitions & classification 2015-2017*, Oxford, 2014, Wiley Blackwell.

Johnson K, Weiss BD: How long does it take to assess literacy skills in clinical practice? *J Am Board Fam Med* 21(3):211, 2008.

Mottus R, et al: Towards understanding the links between health literacy and physical health, *Health Psychol* 33(2):164, 2014.

Patel PJ, et al: Testing the utility of the newest vital sign (NVS) health literacy assessment tool in older African-American patients, *Patient Educ Couns* 85(3):505, 2011.

Suhonen R, et al: Nurses' perceptions of indivualised care: an international comparison, *J Adv Nurs* 67(9):1895, 2011.

Tanner CA: Thinking like a nurse: a research-based model of clinical judgment in nursing, *J Nurs Educ* 45(6):204, 2006.

Wallace L, et al: Brief report: screening items to identify patients with limited health literacy skills, *J Gen Intern Med* 21(8):874, 2006.

Weiss BD, et al: Quick assessment of literacy in primary care: the newest vital sign, *Ann Fam Med* 3(6):514, 2005.

17

Nursing Diagnosis

OBJECTIVES

- Discuss how a nursing diagnosis guides nursing practice.
- Differentiate among a nursing diagnosis, medical diagnosis, and collaborative problem.
- Discuss the relationship of critical thinking to the nursing diagnostic process.
- Describe the steps of the nursing diagnostic process.
- Explain how defining characteristics and the etiological factor individualize a nursing diagnosis.
- Describe the differences among health promotion, problem-focused, and risk nursing diagnoses.
- Describe sources of diagnostic errors.
- Identify nursing diagnoses from a nursing assessment.

KEY TERMS

Collaborative problem, p. 225
Data cluster, p. 230
Defining characteristics, p. 227
Diagnostic label, p. 231
Health promotion nursing diagnosis, p. 227
Medical diagnosis, p. 225
North American Nursing Diagnosis Association International (NANDA-I), p. 226
Nursing diagnosis, p. 225
Problem-focused nursing diagnosis, p. 227
Related factor, p. 227
Risk nursing diagnosis, p. 227

MEDIA RESOURCES

http://evolve.elsevier.com/Potter/fundamentals/

- Review Questions
- Concept Map Creator
- Case Study with Questions
- Audio Glossary
- Content Updates

During the nursing assessment process (see Chapter 16) you gather information about a patient from a variety of sources. As you collect and analyze the data you begin to recognize cues that form patterns of data that indicate either a patient's level of wellness and desire for health promotion or his or her existing health problems. When you identify patterns accurately, they form diagnostic conclusions. A diagnosis is a clinical judgment made on the basis of information. Diagnostic conclusions include problems treated primarily by nurses (nursing diagnoses) and those treated by several disciplines (collaborative problems). Together nursing diagnoses and collaborative problems represent the range of patient conditions that require nursing care (Carpenito-Moyet, 2013).

When physicians and certified advanced practice nurses identify common medical diagnoses such as diabetes mellitus or osteoarthritis, they all know the meaning of the diagnoses and the standard approaches for treatment. A **medical diagnosis** is the identification of a disease condition based on a specific evaluation of physical signs and symptoms, a patient's medical history, and the results of diagnostic tests and procedures. A medical diagnosis stays constant as a condition remains. Physicians are licensed to treat diseases and conditions described in medical diagnostic statements. An advanced practice nurse can also treat medical diagnoses but does not perform surgery.

Nursing has a similar diagnostic language. Nursing diagnosis, the second step of the nursing process (Figure 17-1), classifies health problems within the domain of nursing (i.e., the problems that nurses can treat and manage). A **nursing diagnosis** is a clinical judgment concerning a human response to health conditions/life processes, or vulnerability for that response by an individual, family, or community that a nurse is licensed and competent to treat (Herdman and Kamitsuru, 2014). For example, acute pain is a response to an injury such as a surgical procedure or chemical burn. Nurses are licensed to treat acute pain. A nursing diagnosis can be problem focused or a state of health promotion or potential risk (Herdman and Kamitsuru, 2014). What makes the nursing diagnostic process unique is having patients actively involved, when possible, in the process. Nursing diagnoses are ever changing on the basis of a patient's needs.

A **collaborative problem** is an actual or potential physiological complication that nurses monitor to detect the onset of changes in a patient's health status (Carpenito-Moyet, 2013). When collaborative problems develop, nurses intervene in collaboration with personnel from other health care disciplines. The Canadian Interprofessional Health Collaborative (2010) defines interprofessional collaboration as a partnership between a team of health care providers (such as nurses, therapists, dietitians, and physicians) and a patient in a participatory collaborative and coordinated approach for shared decision making around health issues. Nurses manage collaborative problems such as hemorrhage, infection, and paralysis using medical, nursing, and allied health (e.g., physical therapy) interventions. For example, a patient with a surgical wound is at risk for developing an infection; thus a physician or advanced practice nurse prescribes antibiotics. The nurse monitors the patient for fever and other signs of infection and implements appropriate wound care measures. A dietitian recommends a therapeutic diet high in protein and nutrients to promote wound healing. The patient collaborates in learning hand

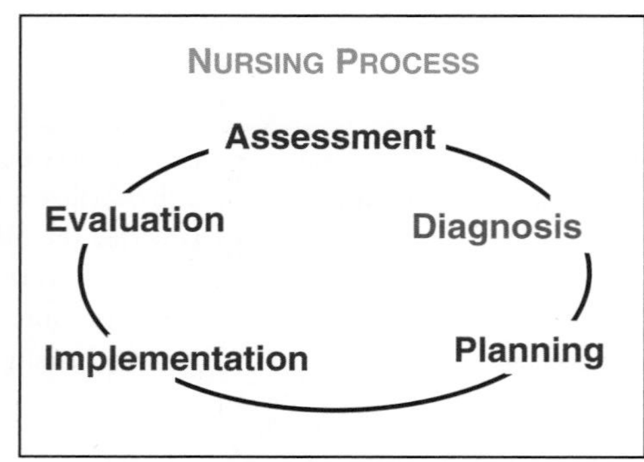

FIGURE 17-1 Critical thinking and the nursing diagnostic process.

hygiene, the signs of infection, and wound care to perform wound care at home.

Selecting the correct nursing diagnosis on the basis of an assessment involves diagnostic expertise (i.e., being able to make quick and accurate conclusions from patient data) (Cho et al., 2010). This is essential because accurate diagnosis of actual or potential patient responses to health conditions or life processes ensures that you select more effective and efficient nursing interventions. Diagnostic expertise improves with clinical experience. Consider the case study involving Mr. Lawson and his nurse, Tonya.

During her assessment Tonya gathered information suggesting that Mr. Lawson possibly has a number of health problems. The data about Mr. Lawson are cues that form patterns in three areas: comfort, requesting information about postoperative care for impending discharge, and the potential for infection at his wound site. Selecting specific diagnostic labels for these problem areas will allow Tonya to develop a relevant and appropriate plan of care. For example, with respect to Mr. Lawson's request for information, there are two accepted nursing diagnostic labels for problems related to knowledge: ***Deficient Knowledge*** *and* ***Readiness for Enhanced Knowledge.*** *Knowing the difference between these two diagnoses and identifying which one applies to Mr. Lawson is essential to allow Tonya to select the right type of interventions for his problem. Knowing the difference between diagnoses is critical for health care providers who need to rule out diagnoses such as rheumatoid arthritis versus osteoarthritis to be sure that patients receive the right form of medical treatment. Tonya needs to use a critical thinking approach to identify the correct diagnosis that applies to Mr. Lawson's condition.*

HISTORY OF NURSING DIAGNOSIS

Nursing diagnosis was first introduced in the nursing literature in 1950 (McFarland and McFarlane, 1989). Fry (1953) proposed the formulation of nursing diagnoses and an individualized nursing care plan to better define nursing practice and science. This emphasized a nurse's independent practice (e.g., patient education and symptom relief) compared with the dependent practice driven by physicians' orders (e.g., medication administration and intravenous fluids). Initially professional nursing did not support nursing diagnoses. The *Model Nurse Practice Act* of the American Nurses Association (ANA) (1955) excluded diagnosis. As a result, few nurses used nursing diagnoses in their practice.

When Yura and Walsh (1967) developed the theory of the nursing process, it included four parts: assessment, planning, implementation, and evaluation. However, nurse educators soon recognized that assessment data needed to be analyzed and clustered into patterns and interpreted before nurses could complete the remaining steps of the process (NANDA-I, 2012). Soon diagnosis became part of the five-step nursing process. You cannot plan and intervene correctly for patients if you do not know the problems with which you are dealing. The same holds true when a physician or advanced practice nurse does not know a patient's medical diagnosis. In 1973 the first national conference on nursing diagnosis was held. Nurse leaders identified and defined 80 nursing diagnoses at that conference (Gebbie, 1998). Today the list contains several hundred diagnoses and continues to grow on the basis of nursing research and the work of members of the North American Nursing Diagnosis Association International (NANDA-I) (Herdman and Kamitsuru, 2014).

Nurses make diagnostic conclusions using nursing diagnosis to form clinical decisions necessary for safe and effective nursing practice.

BOX 17-1 EVIDENCE-BASED PRACTICE

Nursing Diagnosis—Validation and Reliability

PICO Question: Is the use of nursing diagnosis being researched to determine if the diagnoses apply to adult patients with different medical conditions?

Evidence Summary

For nursing diagnosis to be useful in nursing practice it must be diagnostically efficient and relevant, meaning that the defining characteristics are clinical indicators that apply to problems experienced by diverse patient groups. Various researchers are testing components of specific nursing diagnoses to determine if they apply to patients with specific medical conditions. Guedes et al. (2013) studied patients with hypertension and found that some clinical indicators (defining characteristics) have been identified for the nursing diagnosis *Sedentary Lifestyle,* whereas others have been added on the basis of their work. Escalada et al. (2013) reviewed studies involving nursing work in mental health and found that the most prevalent diagnosis was *Impaired Social Interaction.* Both studies encourage more research in application of nursing diagnosis.

Application to Nursing Practice

- Use of nursing diagnosis offers an approach to ensure more comprehensive nursing assessment and identification of patient health problems.
- Use of nursing diagnosis can improve selection of nursing interventions by nurses in all practice settings.
- Contributions from research will build on the evidence for use of defining characteristics and nursing diagnoses in identification of patients' health care problems.

The ANA's paper *Scope of Nursing Practice* (1987) defined nursing as the diagnosis and treatment of human responses to health and illness, strengthening the definition of nursing diagnosis. In 1980 and 1995 the ANA included diagnosis as a separate activity in its publication *Nursing: A Social Policy Statement* (ANA, 2003). It continues today in the ANA's most recent policy statement (ANA, 2010). Today most state Nurse Practice Acts includes nursing diagnosis as part of the domain of nursing practice.

There is one exception in reference to use of the term *nursing diagnosis* as part of the nursing process. The National Council of State Boards of Nursing (NCSBN, 2013), which administers the NCLEX examination, defines the nursing process as a scientific, clinical reasoning approach to patient care that includes assessment, *analysis,* planning, implementation, and evaluation. The use of the term *analysis* instead of diagnosis places emphasis on the analytical work needed to form correct nursing diagnoses.

Research in the field of nursing diagnosis continues to grow (Box 17-1). As a result, NANDA-I continually develops and adds new diagnostic labels to the list (Box 17-2). The use of standard formal nursing diagnostic statements serves several purposes in nursing practice:

- Provides a precise definition of a patient's responses to health problems that gives nurses and other members of the health care team a common language for understanding a patient's needs
- Allows nurses to communicate (e.g., written and electronic) what they do among themselves with other health care professionals and the public
- Distinguishes the nurse's role from that of other health care providers
- Helps nurses focus on the scope of nursing practice
- Fosters the development of nursing knowledge
- Promotes creation of practice guidelines that reflect the essence and science of nursing

TYPES OF NURSING DIAGNOSES

NANDA-I nursing diagnoses include three types: problem-focused, risk, and health promotion (Herdman and Kamitsuru, 2014). A **problem-focused nursing diagnosis** describes a clinical judgment concerning an undesirable human response to a health condition/life process that exists in an individual, family, or community. There are **defining characteristics** (observable assessment cues such as patient behavior, physical signs) that support each problem-focused diagnostic judgment (Herdman and Kamitsuru, 2014). The selection of a problem-focused nursing diagnosis indicates that there are sufficient assessment data from the defining characteristics to establish the nursing diagnosis. In addition, a problem-focused nursing diagnosis includes a related factor. A **related factor** is an etiological or causative factor for the diagnosis (i.e., the data that appear to show some type of patterned relationship with a nursing diagnosis) (Herdman and Kamitsuru, 2014). A related factor allows you to individualize a problem-focused nursing diagnosis for a specific patient need. *Tonya assessed Mr. Lawson initially in Chapter 15 as having discomfort from the colectomy incision. He rated pain at 7 on a 10-point rating scale and was grimacing. He guarded the incisional area that was tender. Mr. Lawson was also hesitant to move actively in bed. Tonya selected* ***Acute Pain*** *as a problem-focused nursing diagnosis on the basis of the patient's self-report of pain intensity, guarding behavior, and the expression of grimacing.* ***Acute Pain*** *related to trauma of surgical incision adds the related factor of trauma of surgical incision, allowing nurses who care for Mr. Lawson to focus interventions at measures to relieve incisional pain.* Examples of other problem-focused diagnoses include *Impaired Bed Mobility, Nausea, Sexual Dysfunction,* and *Impaired Skin Integrity.*

A **risk nursing diagnosis** is a clinical judgment concerning the vulnerability of an individual, family, group, or community for developing an undesirable human response to health conditions/life processes (Herdman and Kamitsuru, 2014). These diagnoses do not have defining characteristics or related factors because they have not yet occurred. Instead a risk diagnosis has risk factors. Risk factors are the environmental, physiological, psychological, genetic, or chemical elements that place a person at risk for a health problem. *For example, in Mr. Lawson's case the presence of his incision, the separation of an area between the stitches, and being hospitalized and exposed to sources of infection pose risks for a hospital-acquired wound infection.* The key assessment for a risk diagnosis is the presence of risk factors (e.g., an incision and the hospital environment) that support a patient's vulnerability. The risk factors are the diagnostic-related factors that help in planning preventive health care measures. In Mr. Lawson' case *Risk for Infection* is appropriate for his condition. Other examples of risk nursing diagnoses include *Risk for Loneliness* and *Risk for Ineffective Peripheral Tissue Perfusion.*

A **health promotion nursing diagnosis** is a clinical judgment concerning a patient's motivation and desire to increase well-being and actualize human health potential (Herdman and Kamitsuru, 2014). You make this type of diagnosis when patients in any health state express a readiness to enhance specific health behaviors. Health promotion diagnoses may apply to an individual, family, group, or community. The diagnoses have only defining characteristics, although you may use a related factor to improve understanding of the diagnosis (Herdman and Kamitsuru, 2014). *Tonya analyzes her information about Mr. Lawson and identifies that he has limited knowledge about infection or experience with postoperative wound care and freely asks questions*

BOX 17-2 NANDA International Nursing Diagnoses

Activity intolerance
Risk for **Activity** intolerance
Ineffective **Activity** Planning
Risk for Ineffective **Activity** Planning
Decreased Intracranial **Adaptive Capacity**
Ineffective **Airway** Clearance
Risk for **Allergy** Response
Anxiety
Risk for **Aspiration**
Risk for Impaired **Attachment**
Autonomic Dysreflexia
Risk for **Autonomic** Dysreflexia
Disorganized Infant **Behavior**
Risk for Enhanced Organized Infant **Behavior**
Risk for Disorganized Infant **Behavior**
Risk for **Bleeding**
Risk for Unstable **Blood** Glucose Level
Disturbed **Body** Image
Risk for Imbalanced **Body** Temperature
Readiness for Enhanced **Breastfeeding**
Ineffective **Breastfeeding**
Interrupted **Breastfeeding**
Insufficient **Breast** Milk
Ineffective **Breathing** Pattern
Decreased **Cardiac** Output
Risk for Decreased **Cardiac** Output
Risk for Impaired **Cardiovascular** Function
Caregiver Role Strain
Risk for **Caregiver** Role Strain
Ineffective **Childbearing** Process
Readiness for Enhanced **Childbearing** Process
Risk for Ineffective **Childbearing** Process
Impaired **Comfort**
Readiness for Enhanced **Comfort**
Readiness for Enhanced **Communication**
Acute **Confusion**
Chronic **Confusion**
Risk for Acute **Confusion**
Constipation
Perceived **Constipation**
Risk for **Constipation**
Chronic Functional **Constipation**
Risk for Chronic Functional **Constipation**
Contamination
Risk for **Contamination**
Compromised Family **Coping**
Defensive **Coping**
Disabled Family **Coping**
Ineffective **Coping**
Ineffective Community **Coping**
Readiness for Enhanced **Coping**
Readiness for Enhanced Community **Coping**
Readiness for Enhanced Family **Coping**
Death Anxiety
Readiness for Enhanced **Decision Making**
Decisional Conflict
Ineffective **Denial**
Impaired **Dentition**
Risk for Delayed **Development**
Diarrhea
Risk for **Disuse** Syndrome
Deficient **Diversional** Activity
Risk for **Dry** Eye
Risk for **Electrolyte** Imbalance
Impaired **Emancipated** Decision Making
Readiness for Enhanced **Emancipated** Decision Making
Risk for Impaired **Emancipated** Decision Making
Labile **Emotional** Control
Risk for **Falls**
Dysfunctional **Family** Processes
Interrupted **Family** Processes
Readiness for Enhanced **Family** Processes
Fatigue
Fear
Ineffective Infant **Feeding** Pattern
Readiness for Enhanced **Fluid** Balance
Deficient **Fluid** Volume
Excess **Fluid** Volume
Risk for Deficient **Fluid** Volume
Risk for Imbalanced **Fluid** Volume
Frail Elderly Syndrome
Risk for **Frail** Elderly Syndrome
Impaired **Gas** Exchange
Dysfunctional **Gastrointestinal** Motility
Risk for Dysfunctional **Gastrointestinal** Motility
Risk for Ineffective **Gastrointestinal** Perfusion
Grieving
Complicated **Grieving**
Risk for Complicated **Grieving**
Risk for Disproportionate **Growth**
Deficient Community **Health**
Risk-Prone **Health** Behavior
Ineffective **Health** Maintenance
Ineffective **Health** Management
Readiness for Enhanced **Health** Management
Ineffective Family **Health** Management
Impaired **Home** Maintenance
Readiness for Enhanced **Hope**
Hopelessness
Risk for Compromised **Human** Dignity
Hyperthermia
Hypothermia
Risk for **Hypothermia**
Risk for Perioperative **Hypothermia**
Ineffective **Impulse** Control
Functional Urinary **Incontinence**
Overflow Urinary **Incontinence**
Reflex Urinary **Incontinence**
Stress Urinary **Incontinence**
Urge Urinary **Incontinence**
Risk for Urge Urinary **Incontinence**
Bowel **Incontinence**
Risk for Sudden **Infant** Death Syndrome
Risk for **Infection**
Risk for **Injury**
Risk for Corneal **Injury**
Risk for Perioperative-Positioning **Injury**
Risk for Thermal **Injury**
Risk for Urinary Tract **Injury**
Insomnia

BOX 17-2 NANDA International Nursing Diagnoses—cont'd

Neonatal **Jaundice**
Risk for Neonatal **Jaundice**
Deficient **Knowledge**
Readiness for Enhanced **Knowledge**
Latex Allergy Response
Risk for **Latex** Allergy Response
Sedentary **Lifestyle**
Risk for Impaired **Liver** Function
Risk for **Loneliness**
Risk for Disturbed **Maternal/Fetal Dyad**
Impaired **Memory**
Impaired Bed **Mobility**
Impaired Physical **Mobility**
Impaired Wheelchair **Mobility**
Impaired **Mood** Regulation
Moral Distress
Nausea
Unilateral **Neglect**
Noncompliance
Imbalanced **Nutrition:** Less than Body Requirements
Readiness for Enhanced **Nutrition**
Obesity
Impaired **Oral** Mucous Membrane
Risk for Impaired **Oral** Mucous Membrane
Overweight
Risk for **Overweight**
Acute **Pain**
Chronic **Pain**
Labor **Pain**
Chronic **Pain** Syndrome
Impaired **Parenting**
Readiness for Enhanced **Parenting**
Risk for Impaired **Parenting**
Risk for **Peripheral** Neurovascular Dysfunction
Disturbed **Personal** Identity
Risk for Disturbed **Personal** Identity
Risk for **Poisoning**
Post-Trauma Syndrome
Risk for **Post-Trauma** Syndrome
Readiness for Enhanced **Power**
Powerlessness
Risk for **Powerlessness**
Risk for **Pressure** Ulcer
Ineffective **Protection**
Rape-Trauma Syndrome
Risk for **Reaction** to Iodinated Contrast Media
Ineffective **Relationship**
Risk for Ineffective **Relationship**
Readiness for Enhanced **Relationship**
Impaired **Religiosity**
Readiness for Enhanced **Religiosity**
Risk for Impaired **Religiosity**
Relocation Stress Syndrome
Risk for **Relocation** Stress Syndrome
Risk for Ineffective **Renal** Perfusion
Impaired **Resilience**
Readiness for Enhanced **Resilience**
Risk for Impaired **Resilience**
Parental **Role** Conflict
Ineffective **Role** Performance
Readiness for Enhanced **Self-Care**
Bathing **Self-Care** Deficit
Dressing **Self-Care** Deficit
Feeding **Self-Care** Deficit
Toileting **Self-Care** Deficit
Readiness for Enhanced **Self-Concept**
Chronic Low **Self-Esteem**
Risk for Chronic Low **Self-Esteem**
Situational Low **Self-Esteem**
Risk for Situational Low **Self-Esteem**
Self-Mutilation
Risk for **Self-Mutilation**
Self-Neglect
Sexual Dysfunction
Ineffective **Sexuality** Pattern
Risk for **Shock**
Impaired **Sitting**
Impaired **Skin** Integrity
Risk for Impaired **Skin** Integrity
Sleep Deprivation
Readiness for Enhanced **Sleep**
Disturbed **Sleep** Pattern
Impaired **Social** Interaction
Social Isolation
Chronic **Sorrow**
Spiritual Distress
Risk for **Spiritual** Distress
Readiness for Enhanced **Spiritual** Well-Being
Impaired **Standing**
Stress Overload
Risk for **Suffocation**
Risk for **Suicide**
Delayed **Surgical** Recovery
Risk for Delayed **Surgical** Recovery
Impaired **Swallowing**
Ineffective **Thermoregulation**
Impaired **Tissue** Integrity
Risk for Impaired **Tissue** Integrity
Ineffective Peripheral **Tissue** Perfusion
Risk for Ineffective Peripheral **Tissue** Perfusion
Risk for Decreased Cardiac **Tissue** Perfusion
Risk for Ineffective Cerebral **Tissue** Perfusion
Impaired **Transfer** Ability
Risk for **Trauma**
Risk for Vascular **Trauma**
Impaired **Urinary** Elimination
Readiness for Enhanced **Urinary** Elimination
Urinary Retention
Risk for Self-Directed **Violence**
Risk for Other-Directed **Violence**
Dysfunctional **Ventilatory** Weaning Response
Impaired Spontaneous **Ventilation**
Impaired **Verbal** Communication
Impaired **Walking**
Wandering

From Herdman TH, Kamitsuru S (Editors): *NANDA International nursing diagnoses: definitions & classification 2015-2017,* Oxford, 2014, Wiley Blackwell.

*with the desire to enhance his learning. His desire to ask questions is a critical defining characteristic that leads Tonya to select **Readiness for Enhanced Knowledge,** a health promotion diagnosis.* Examples of other health promotion nursing diagnoses include:

- *Readiness for Enhanced Family Coping*
- *Readiness for Enhanced Nutrition*

CRITICAL THINKING AND THE NURSING DIAGNOSTIC PROCESS

The diagnostic process requires you to use critical thinking (see Chapter 15). You will learn to apply your knowledge, experience, critical thinking attitudes and intellectual standards when you collect and analyze assessment data to identify nursing diagnoses. Routinely applying critical thinking will make you more competent in making nursing diagnoses (Lunney, 2010).

In the practice of nursing it is important for you to know the nursing diagnostic labels, their definitions, the defining characteristics or risk factors for making diagnoses, related factors pertinent to the diagnoses, and the interventions suited for treating the diagnoses (Herdman and Kamitsuru, 2014). This means that you need to know how to access this information easily within the agency in which you work because the information is too extensive for you to memorize. Sources of information about nursing diagnoses include faculty, advanced practice nurses, documentation systems, and practice guidelines. Experience is essential in being competent at forming nursing diagnoses. Learn from your patients because this helps you think more carefully about your assessment information and what it means. Critical thinking helps you to be thorough, comprehensive, and accurate when identifying nursing diagnoses that apply to your patients.

The diagnostic reasoning process involves using the assessment data you gather about a patient to logically explain a clinical judgment, in this case a nursing diagnosis. The diagnostic process flows from the assessment process and includes decision-making steps (Figure 17-2). These steps include data clustering, identifying patient health problems, and formulating the diagnosis.

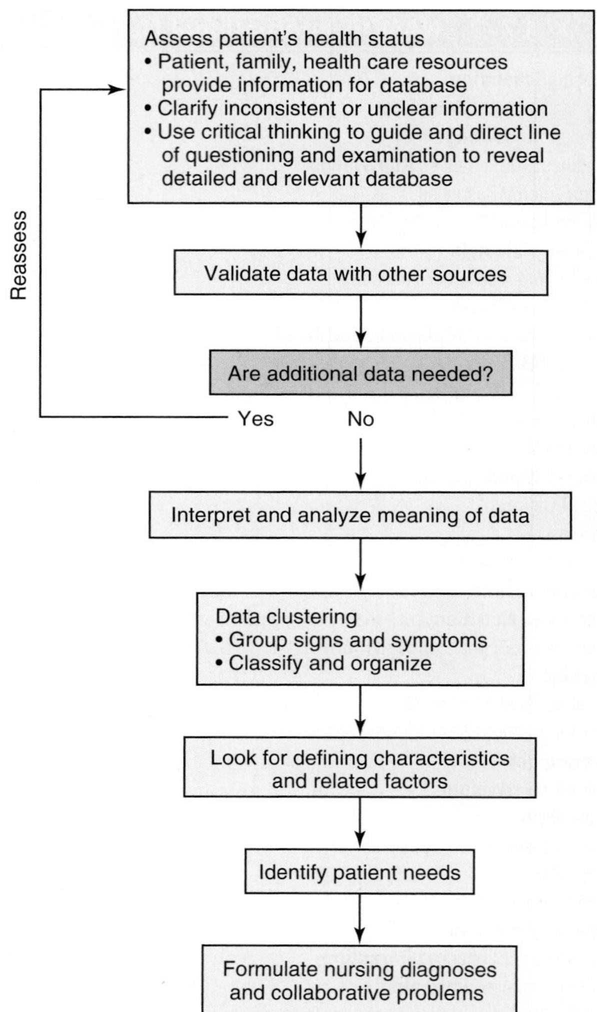

FIGURE 17-2 Nursing diagnostic process.

Data Clustering

Analysis and interpretation of assessment data begin by organizing all of a patient's data into meaningful and usable **data clusters**. A data cluster is a set of cues, the signs or symptoms gathered during assessment. Each cue is an objective or subjective sign, symptom, or risk factor that, when analyzed with other cues, begins to lead to diagnostic conclusions. A nurse collects cues intentionally or unintentionally (Herdman and Kamitsuru, 2014). Intentional assessment is the deliberate collection of data through physical examination or interviewing. Unintentional assessment is noticing cues that are important without planning to do so (Herdman and Kamitsuru, 2014). For example, an unintentional cue is noticing a patient grimace as you help him out of bed or hearing a patient's tone of voice while speaking with a visitor. You recognize the existence of cues and then cluster or group them together in a logical way to reveal how a patient is responding to a health condition or life process. During clustering of cues, your analysis makes you alert to thinking less about individual data points and instead to begin to see a pattern form. *For example, as Mr. Lawson begins to recover from surgery, he has questions. His knowledge of activity restrictions and signs of infection is unclear. Tonya clusters the cues she has learned from the patient, analyzes the cues, and recognizes the pattern of a knowledge problem.*

Data analysis and interpretation involve recognizing patterns in the clustered data, comparing them with standards, and coming to a reasoned conclusion about a patient's response to a health problem. The NANDA-I classification of nursing diagnoses provides the standards for the patterns of data for each nursing diagnosis (Herdman and Kamitsuru, 2014). These standards are the defining characteristics or risk factors described earlier. Defining characteristics are the observable assessment cues that cluster as manifestations of a problem-focused or health promotion nursing diagnosis. The cues have been found through research to support a specific NANDA-I approved nursing diagnosis. Each NANDA-I–approved health promotion or problem-focused nursing diagnosis has an identified set of defining characteristics that support identification of the nursing diagnosis (Herdman and Kamitsuru, 2014). Your recognition of a cue or defining characteristic as a cue with special meaning depends on your knowledge and experience. You learn to recognize patterns of defining characteristics, comparing current data with expected data for a nursing diagnosis, and then select the correct diagnosis.

Working with similar patients over a period of time helps you recognize clusters of defining characteristics; but remember that each patient is unique and requires an individualized diagnostic approach. Box 17-3 shows two examples of nursing diagnoses and their associated defining characteristics. The first diagnosis, *Deficient Knowledge,* is a problem-focused diagnosis. The second, *Readiness for Enhanced Knowledge,* is a health promotion diagnosis. The defining

BOX 17-3 Examples of NANDA International–Approved Nursing Diagnoses with Defining Characteristics

Diagnosis: Deficient Knowledge	Diagnosis: Readiness for Enhanced Knowledge
Defining Characteristics	***Defining Characteristics***
• Inaccurate follow-through of instruction	• Expresses a desire to increase or enhance learning
• Inaccurate performance on a test	
• Inappropriate behavior (e.g., hysterical, hostile, agitated, apathetic)	
• Insufficient knowledge	

From Herdman TH, Kamitsuru S (Editors): *NANDA International nursing diagnoses: definitions & classification 2015-2017,* Oxford, 2014, Wiley Blackwell.

characteristics in both have similarities such as patient behaviors and self-reported information. However, *Deficient Knowledge* results from the absence or deficiency of information about a topic. The second diagnosis of *Readiness for Enhanced Knowledge* applies when a patient wants to learn more about a topic. As you gather cues and see clusters of data forming patterns, confirm your data with your source of information on NANDA-I diagnoses.

When assessment cues reveal risk factors (i.e., the factors that increase an individual's vulnerability to an unhealthy event), you will recognize patterns, compare the patterns with expected data for a risk diagnosis, and then select the correct risk nursing diagnosis.

Data Interpretation

While analyzing clusters of defining characteristics or risk factors, you consider a patient's responses to health conditions. Your interpretation of the information allows you to select among various diagnoses that may apply to your patient. Often there are numerous possible diagnoses or explanations to consider (Herdman and Kamitsuru, 2014). You compare defining characteristics or risk factors in your database with the different diagnoses in NANDA-I. To be more accurate, review all characteristics or risk factors, eliminate irrelevant ones, and confirm the relevant ones.

It is critical to select the correct diagnostic label for a patient's need. Usually from assessment to diagnosis you move from general information to specific. The patterns of assessment cues point you toward identifying a general health care problem, and the formulation of the nursing diagnosis becomes the specific health problem. *For example, after analyzing Mr. Lawson's problem with knowledge, Tonya began to identify data needed for a specific nursing diagnosis,* ***Readiness for Enhanced Knowledge.***

Often a patient has defining characteristics or risk factors that apply to more than one diagnosis. There is no rule for the number necessary to form a diagnosis. It will depend on the diagnosis. *In Chapter 16 Mr. Lawson reported the following, "Well, the doctor did tell me that I wouldn't be able to lift anything heavy for a while; not sure if I understand. But with my incision looking the way it is, will I need to do something to it?"* This information might be interpreted as the patient reporting a problem, but the patient also expresses an interest in learning by asking a question. Just on the basis of this information, Tonya might choose *Deficient Knowledge* or *Readiness for Enhanced Knowledge* as nursing diagnoses, but she reviews her other findings. *Tonya assessed Mr. Lawson's knowledge of his problem, "Do you know what the signs of infection are? And the patient's response was, "Not sure I do, but I guess it would hurt more. Is infection common?" The assessment revealed Mr. Lawson's ability to explain knowledge of the topic of wound infection.* When interpreting data to form a diagnosis, remember that the absence of certain defining characteristics suggests that you reject a diagnosis under consideration. *In the same example Tonya's assessment fails to reveal inappropriate behavior on the part of Mr. Lawson, and there are no exaggerated behaviors; thus it is more likely that Mr. Lawson has* ***Readiness for Enhanced Knowledge,*** *the correct diagnosis.*

While focusing on patterns of defining characteristics, compare a patient's pattern of data with information that is consistent with normal, healthy patterns. Use accepted norms as the basis for comparison and judgment such as laboratory and diagnostic test values, professional standards, and normal anatomical or physiological limits already established. When comparing patterns, judge whether the grouped signs and symptoms are expected for a patient (e.g., consider current condition, history) and whether they are within the range of healthy responses. Isolate any defining characteristics not within healthy norms to allow you to identify a specific problem.

Nursing diagnoses provide the basis for selection of nursing interventions to achieve outcomes for which you, as a nurse, are accountable (Herdman and Kamitsuru, 2014). A nursing diagnosis focuses on a patient's actual or potential response to a health condition rather than on the physiological event, complication, or disease. A nurse cannot independently treat a medical diagnosis such as a tumor of the prostate. *However, Tonya manages Mr. Lawson's postoperative care, monitoring his postoperative progress and wound care, intravenous fluid administration, and medication therapy to prevent collaborative problems from developing.* Collaborative problems occur or probably will occur in association with a specific disease process, trauma, or treatment (Carpenito-Moyet, 2013). *For example, Tonya monitors Mr. Lawson in an effort to prevent him from developing infection.* You need nursing knowledge to assess a patient's specific risk for these problems, identify the problems early, and take preventive action (Figure 17-3). Critical thinking is necessary in identifying nursing diagnoses and collaborative problems so you appropriately individualize care for your patients.

Formulating a Nursing Diagnostic Statement

After clustering assessment data and interpreting the meaning, your aim is to select the correct nursing diagnostic statement. If you make an incorrect nursing diagnosis, a patient is likely to receive inappropriate or unnecessary care. For example, your approach to *Acute Pain* related to a surgical incision will be very different from *Acute Pain* related to a traumatic injury. An accurate nursing diagnostic statement requires you to identify the correct diagnostic label with associated defining characteristics or risk factors and a related factor (when applicable).

The **diagnostic label** is the name of the nursing diagnosis as approved by NANDA-I (see Box 17-2). It describes the essence of a patient's response to health conditions in as few words as possible. All NANDA-I approved diagnoses have a definition. The definition describes the characteristics of the human response identified and helps to select the correct diagnosis. *For example, Mr. Lawson just had surgery, is scheduled for discharge, and has ongoing self-care needs (wound care, activity restrictions) once he returns home. He shows interest in learning, and his wife is willing and able to help him at home.* The definition for *Readiness for Enhanced Knowledge* is "A pattern of cognitive information related to a specific topic, or its acquisition, which can be strengthened" (Herdman and Kamitsuru, 2014, p. 258). The definition helps to provide a context for understanding the assessment information gathered about Mr. Lawson's knowledge, and it is used in making a final diagnosis. Placing a diagnosis into the context of a

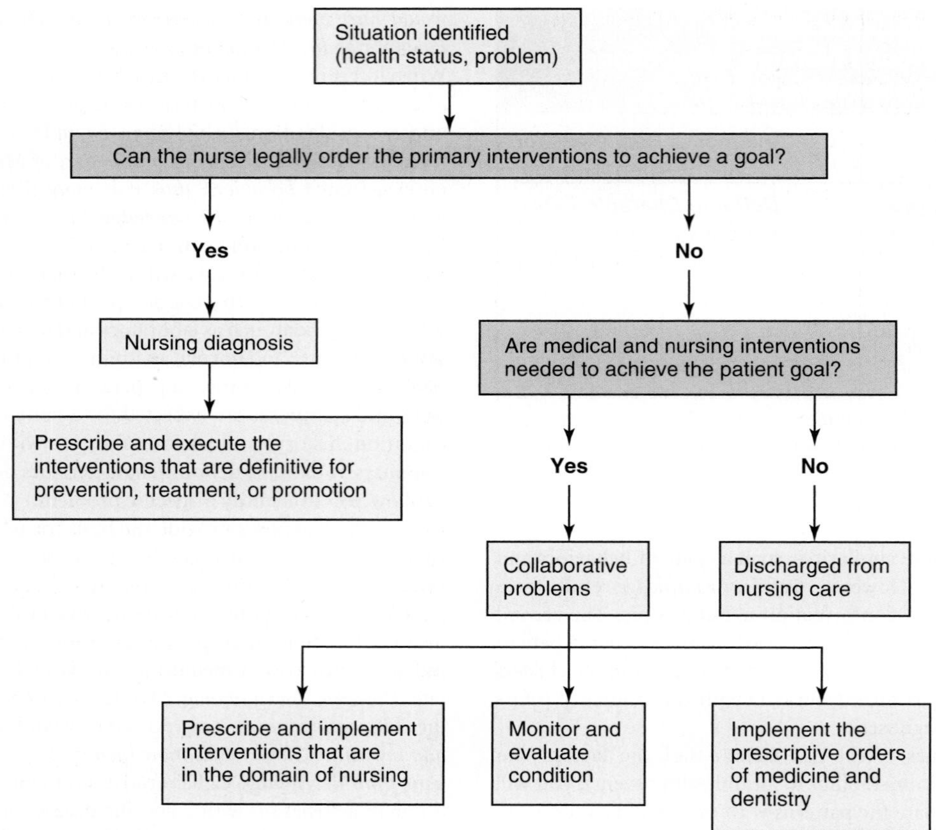

FIGURE 17-3 Differentiating nursing diagnoses from collaborative problems. (©1990, 1988, 1985 Lynda Juall Carpenito. Redrawn from Carpenito LJ: *Nursing diagnosis: application to clinical practice,* ed 6, Philadelphia, 1995, Lippincott.)

TABLE 17-1 Comparison of Interventions for Nursing Diagnoses with Different Related Factors

Nursing Diagnoses	Related Factor	Interventions
Patient A		
Anxiety	Uncertainty over surgery	Provide detailed instructions about the surgical procedure, recovery process, and postoperative care activities. Plan formal time for patient to ask questions.
Impaired Physical Mobility	Acute pain	Administer analgesics 30 minutes before planned exercise. Instruct patient how to splint painful site during activity.
Patient B		
Anxiety	Loss of job	Consult with social worker to arrange for job counseling. Encourage patient to continue health promotion activities (e.g., exercise, routine social activities).
Impaired Physical Mobility	Musculoskeletal injury	Have patient perform active range-of-motion exercises to affected extremity every 2 hours. Instruct patient on use of three-point crutch gait.

patient's situation clarifies the nature of a patient's health problem. *Tonya considers the nature of Mr. Lawson's situation and identifies his diagnosis as **Readiness for Enhanced Knowledge.***

A complete diagnostic statement will also include a related factor (appropriate for problem-based and some health promotion diagnoses). You identify the related factor from the patient's assessment data. The related factor is associated with a patient's actual or potential response to a health problem and can change by using specific nursing interventions (Table 17-1). Related factors for NANDA-I diagnoses include four categories: pathophysiological (biological or psychological), treatment-related, situational (environmental or personal), and maturational (Carpenito-Moyet, 2013). The "related to" phrase is not a cause-and-effect statement. It indicates that the etiology contributes to or is associated with the patient's diagnosis (Figure 17-4). *Tonya selects the related factor impending discharge with self-care needs because it explains Mr. Lawson's response to a knowledge problem.* In this case, adding the related factor to the health promotion diagnosis provides an etiology that can be targeted through instruction. *When Tonya is ready to form her plan of care and select nursing interventions, the concise nursing diagnosis with related factor allows her to select therapies for actively involving the patient and his wife in postoperative instruction.*

When communicating a nursing diagnosis, through either discussions with health care colleagues or documentation of your care, use the language adopted within an agency. Most settings use a two-part format in labeling health promotion and problem-focused nursing diagnoses: the NANDA-I diagnostic label followed by a statement of a related factor (Table 17-2). The two-part format provides a diagnosis meaning and relevance for a particular patient (Table 17-3).

However, some agencies prefer a three-part nursing diagnostic label. In this case the diagnostic label consists of the NANDA-I label, the related factor, and the defining characteristics (Ackley and Ladwig, 2011). NANDA-I believes that a problem-focused nursing diagnosis, including a diagnosis label and the related factor as exhibited by defining characteristics, to be best practice (Herdman and Kamitsuru, 2014). This structure makes a diagnosis even more patient specific. Throughout this text you will more commonly find the two-part diagnostic statement to include the diagnosis label and related factor.

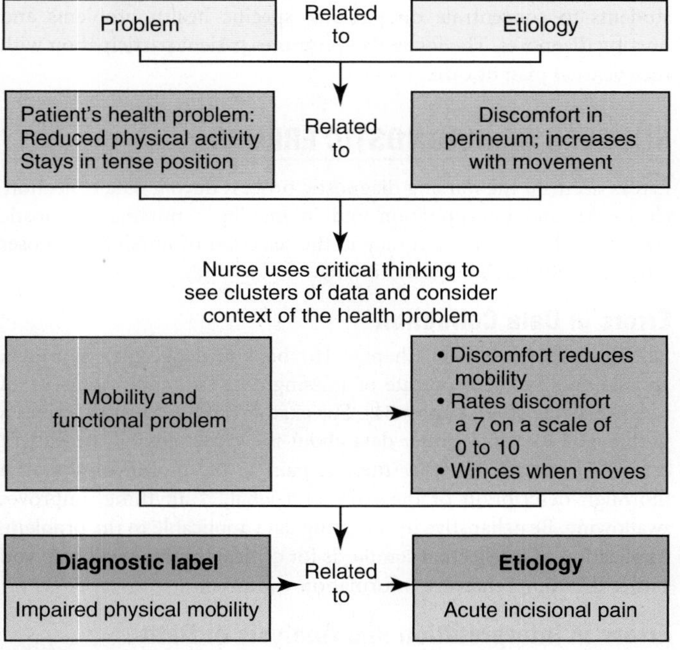

FIGURE 17-4 Relationship between a diagnostic label and related factor (etiology).

To write a three-part nursing diagnosis, the acronym PES, which stands for *p*roblem, *e*tiology, and *s*ymptoms, is helpful.

- **P** (problem)—NANDA-I label—Example: *Impaired Physical Mobility*
- **E** (etiology or related factor)—Example: incisional pain
- **S** (symptoms or defining characteristics)—Briefly lists defining characteristic(s) that show evidence of the health problem. Example: evidenced by restricted turning and positioning

Full three-part diagnostic statement: *Impaired Physical Mobility* related to incisional pain as evidenced by restricted turning and positioning.

Cultural Relevance of Nursing Diagnoses

When you select nursing diagnoses, consider your patients' cultural diversity, including values, beliefs, health practices, ethnicity, and gender (see Chapter 9). This also includes knowing the cultural differences that affect how patients define health and illness and their requests or choices for treatment. For example, Lai et al. (2013) explored how NANDA-I nursing diagnoses affect the quality of professional nursing from the perspective of Taiwanese nurses. Their work found that certain diagnoses were difficult for nurses to apply considering the cultural beliefs of a traditional Chinese health care setting, which emphasizes holistic harmony and balance. Nursing diagnoses are internationally accepted as a part of systematic and individualized nursing care (Herdman and Kamitsuru, 2014; ANA, 2010). However,

TABLE 17-2 NANDA International Two-Part Nursing Diagnosis Format

Diagnostic Label	Examples of Related Factors
Acute Pain	Biological (e.g., limited blood flow to an organ), chemical (skin burn), physical (traumatic injury, trauma of surgical incision), or psychological injury (primary traumatic stress) agents. Example: *Acute Pain* related to trauma of surgical incision.
Impaired Physical Mobility	Activity intolerance, decrease in muscle strength, joint stiffness, cultural belief regarding appropriate activity, malnutrition, pain. Example: *Impaired Physical Mobility* related to incisional pain.
Impaired Memory	Alteration in fluid volume, anemia, decrease in cardiac output, neurological impairment. Example: *Impaired Memory* related to dehydration

TABLE 17-3 Developing a Two-Part Nursing Diagnosis Label

Assessment Activities	Defining Characteristics (Clustering Cues)	Etiologies ("Related To")	Nursing Diagnosis
Ask patient to rate severity of pain on a scale from 0 to 10.	Verbal report of pain at a level of 7	Physical; swelling from incisional trauma	**Acute Pain** related to trauma of incision
Observe patient's positioning in bed.	Lies flat, avoids turning		
Ask patient to describe what he knows about surgery.	Has no knowledge about postoperative wound care	Inexperience; first time to have surgery	**Readiness for Enhanced Knowledge**
Observe his interactions.	Asks questions about activity restrictions; shows interest in learning what to expect		
Question wife's role in postoperative care and her level of knowledge.	Wife to provide support within the home; no knowledge of how to manage wound		

it is important to consider your patient's culture and your own cultural competence to accurately identify a patient's health care problems.

Consider the example of the nursing diagnosis *Sedentary Lifestyle*. The definition for the diagnosis is a patient reporting a habit of life that is characterized by a low physical activity level (Herdman and Kamitsuru, 2014). It would be easy to apply cultural bias in selecting this diagnosis for a patient, depending on your own exercise habits and the values that you hold regarding healthy behavior. However, the definition for the diagnosis stresses "patient report." The inappropriate selection of this diagnosis on the basis of your values or beliefs potentially results in the implementation of interventions that a patient likely will not accept. Consider asking these questions to make culturally competent nursing diagnoses:

- How has this health problem affected you and your family?
- What do you believe will help or fix the problem?
- What worries you the most about this problem?
- What do you expect from us, your nurses, to help maintain some of your values or practices for staying healthy?
- Which cultural practices do you observe to keep yourself and your family well?

When you ask questions such as these, you use a patient-centered approach that allows you to see a patient's health situation through his or her eyes. This is necessary to identify relevant cues pertaining to a patient's health problem. When making a nursing diagnosis, consider how culture influences the related factor for the diagnostic statement. For example, *Noncompliance* related to patient value system reflects a diagnostic conclusion that considers a patient's unique cultural needs.

CONCEPT MAPPING NURSING DIAGNOSES

In Chapter 16 you learned how concept mapping offers a graphic look at the connections among patient's multiple health problems. Once you enter practice as a graduate nurse, you will care for multiple patients. Then it becomes especially challenging to prioritize and focus on all patients' diagnoses. A concept map helps you critically think about a patient's diagnoses and how they relate to one another (Chabeli, 2010; Pilcher, 2011). Concept mapping helps you organize and link data about a patient's multiple diagnoses in a logical way. It graphically represents the connections among concepts (e.g., nursing diagnoses and the interventions later selected) that relate to a central subject (e.g., the patient's primary health problem).

In Figure 17-5, the concept map for Mr. Lawson, Tonya uses data gathered from her assessment of Mr. Lawson and now replaces patterns of problems with nursing diagnoses. *Tonya's assessment included Mr. Lawson's perspective of his health problems and the objective and subjective data she collected through observation and examination. She validated findings and added to the database as she learned new information. As Tonya begins to see patterns of defining characteristics, she places labels to identify three nursing diagnoses that apply to Mr. Lawson. She is also able to see the relation among the diagnoses and connects them on the concept map. If Mr. Lawson does not receive pain relief, Tonya knows from her experience in caring for patients with* ***Acute Pain*** *that he will not be attentive or receptive in her efforts to educate him about home care. Tonya wants to provide instruction about postoperative care, an intervention that will be planned later for* ***Readiness for Enhanced Knowledge.*** *The patient's* ***Risk for Infection*** *requires Tonya to address infection prevention strategies along with wound care and activity restrictions when she instructs Mr. and Mrs. Lawson.*

Concept mapping organizes and links information to allow you to see a dynamic holism and complexity of individualized patient care. The advantage of a concept map is its central focus on a patient rather than on a disease or health alteration. This encourages nursing students to concentrate on patients' specific health problems and nursing diagnoses. The focus also promotes patient participation with the eventual plan of care.

BOX 17-4 Sources of Diagnostic Error

Collecting
- Lack of knowledge or skill
- Inaccurate data
- Missing data
- Disorganization
- Failure to validate

Interpreting
- Inaccurate interpretation of cues
- Failure to consider conflicting cues
- Using an insufficient number of cues
- Using unreliable or invalid cues
- Failure to consider cultural influences or developmental stage

Clustering
- Insufficient cluster of cues
- Premature or early closure
- Incorrect clustering

Labeling
- Wrong diagnostic label selected
- Evidence that another diagnosis is more likely
- Condition is a collaborative problem
- Failure to validate nursing diagnosis with patient
- Failure to seek guidance

SOURCES OF DIAGNOSTIC ERRORS

Errors occur in the nursing diagnostic process during data collection, clustering, and interpretation and in making a nursing diagnostic statement (Box 17-4). Accuracy in the selection of nursing diagnoses requires methodical critical thinking.

Errors in Data Collection

During assessment (see Chapter 16) be knowledgeable, thorough, and skillful. Avoid inaccurate or missing data and collect data in an organized way (see Chapter 31). For example, if a patient describes a problem swallowing, gather data about the types of food the patient can or cannot eat; whether there is pain in the mouth or throat; a thorough description of the pain; and what, if anything, improves swallowing. Be exhaustive in collecting data applicable to the problem. Application of intellectual standards for critical thinking will help you gather the comprehensive information you need.

Errors in Interpretation and Analysis of Data

Following data collection, review your database to decide if it is accurate and complete. Validate that measurable, objective physical findings support subjective data. For example, when a patient reports "difficulty breathing," you also listen to lung sounds, assess respiratory rate, and measure the patient's chest excursion (see Chapter 31). When you are unable to validate data, it signals an inaccurate match between clinical cues and the nursing diagnosis. Begin interpretation by identifying and organizing relevant assessment patterns to support the presence of patient problems. Be careful to consider conflicting cues or decide if there are insufficient cues to form a diagnosis. It is important to consider a patient's cultural background or developmental stage when interpreting the meaning of cues. For example, a male patient may express pain differently than a female patient. Thus misinterpreting how a male patient expresses pain could easily lead to an inaccurate diagnosis.

Errors in Data Clustering

Errors occur when you cluster data prematurely, incorrectly, or not at all. Premature clustering occurs when you make a nursing diagnosis

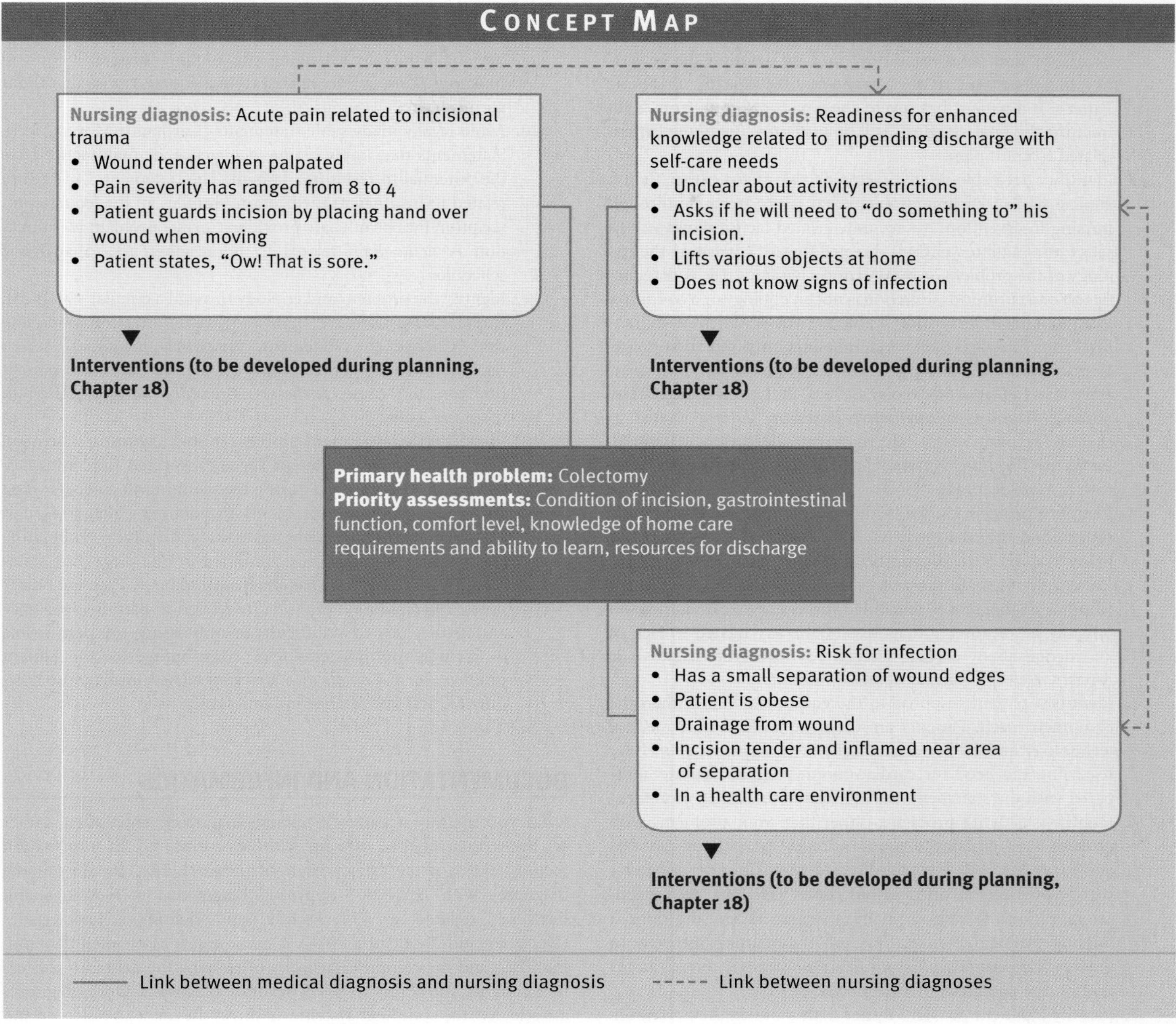

FIGURE 17-5 Concept map for Mr. Lawson: Nursing Diagnoses.

before grouping all data. For example, a patient has urinary incontinence and states that he has dysuria. You cluster the available data and identify *Impaired Urinary Elimination* as a probable nursing diagnosis. Incorrect clustering occurs when you try to make a diagnosis fit the signs and symptoms that you obtain. In this example further assessment reveals that the patient also has bladder distention and dribbling; thus the correct diagnosis is *Urinary Retention*. Always identify a nursing diagnosis from the data, not the reverse. An incorrect nursing diagnosis affects quality of patient care.

Errors in the Diagnostic Statement

Clinical reasoning leads to a higher-quality level of nursing diagnosis, which eventually leads to etiology-specific interventions and enhanced patient outcomes (Muller-Staub et al., 2008). The correct selection of a diagnostic statement is more likely to result in the appropriate selection of interventions and outcomes (Herdman and Kamitsuru, 2014) during planning and implementation (see Chapters 18 and 19). Reduce errors by selecting appropriate, concise, and precise language using NANDA-I terminology. Be sure that the etiology portion of the diagnostic statement is within the scope of nursing to diagnose and treat. Additional guidelines to reduce errors in the diagnostic statement follow.

1. Identify a patient's response, not the medical diagnosis (Carpenito-Moyet, 2013). Because a medical diagnosis requires medical interventions, it is legally inadvisable to include it in the nursing diagnosis. Change the diagnosis *Acute Pain* related to colectomy to *Acute Pain* related to trauma of a surgical incision.
2. Identify a NANDA-I diagnostic statement rather than the symptom. Identify nursing diagnoses from a cluster of defining characteristics and not just a single symptom. One defining characteristic is insufficient for problem identification. For

example, dyspnea alone does not definitively lead you to a diagnosis. However, the pattern of dyspnea, reduced chest excursion, and rapid respiratory rate are defining characteristics that lead you to the diagnosis of *Ineffective Breathing Pattern*. If a patient has severe chest pain resulting from a rib fracture, the final diagnosis will be *Ineffective Breathing Pattern* related to chest pain.

3. Identify a treatable related factor or risk factor rather than a clinical sign or chronic problem that is not treatable through nursing intervention. An accurate related factor allows you to select nursing interventions directed toward correcting the etiology of the problem or minimizing a patient's risk. A diagnostic test or a chronic dysfunction is not an etiology or a condition that a nursing intervention is able to treat. A patient with fractured ribs likely has pain when inhaling; impaired chest excursion; and slower, shallow respirations. An x-ray film may show atelectasis (collapse of alveolar air sacs) in the area affected. The nursing diagnosis of *Ineffective Breathing Pattern* related to shallow respirations is an incorrect diagnostic statement. *Ineffective Breathing Pattern* related to chest pain from rib fracture is more accurate.
4. Identify a problem caused by the treatment or diagnostic study rather than the treatment or study itself. Patients experience many responses to diagnostic tests and medical treatments. These responses are the area of nursing concern. The patient who has angina and is scheduled for a cardiac catheterization possibly has a nursing diagnosis of *Anxiety* related to lack of knowledge about cardiac testing. An incorrect diagnosis is *Anxiety* related to cardiac catheterization.
5. Identify a patient response to the equipment rather than the equipment itself. Patients are often unfamiliar with medical technology and its use. The diagnosis of *Deficient Knowledge* regarding the need for cardiac monitoring is accurate compared with the statement *Anxiety* related to cardiac monitor.
6. Identify a patient's problems rather than your problems with nursing care. Nursing diagnoses are always patient centered and form the basis for goal-directed care. Consider a patient with a peripheral intravenous line. *Potential Intravenous Complications* related to poor vascular access indicates a nursing problem in initiating and maintaining intravenous therapy. The diagnosis *Risk for Infection* properly centers attention on the patient's potential needs.
7. Identify a patient problem rather than a nursing intervention. You plan nursing interventions after identifying a nursing diagnosis. The intervention, "offer bedpan frequently because of altered elimination patterns," is not a diagnostic statement. Instead, with the proper assessment data the correct diagnostic statement would be *Diarrhea* related to food intolerance. This corrects the misstatement and allows proper implementation of the nursing process. More appropriate interventions are selected rather than a single intervention that alone will not solve the problem.
8. Identify a patient problem rather than the goal of care. You establish goals during the planning step of the nursing process (see Chapter 18). Goals based on accurate identification of a patient's problems serve as a basis to determine problem resolution. Change the goal-phrased statement, "Patient needs high-protein diet related to potential alteration in nutrition," to *Imbalanced Nutrition: Less Than Body Requirements* related to inadequate protein intake.
9. Make professional rather than prejudicial judgments. Base nursing diagnoses on subjective and objective patient data and do not include your personal beliefs and values. Remove your judgment from *Impaired Skin Integrity* related to poor hygiene habits by changing the nursing diagnosis to read *Impaired Skin Integrity* related to inadequate knowledge about perineal care.
10. Avoid legally inadvisable statements (Carpenito-Moyet, 2013). Statements that imply blame, negligence, or malpractice have the potential to result in a lawsuit. The statement, "*Acute Pain* related to insufficient medication," implies an inadequate prescription by a health care provider. Correct problem identification is *Acute Pain* related to poor adherence to analgesic schedule.
11. Identify the problem and etiology to avoid a circular statement. Circular statements are vague and give no direction to nursing care. Change the statement, "*Impaired Breathing Pattern* related to shallow breathing," to identify the real patient problem and cause, *Ineffective Breathing Pattern* related to incisional pain.
12. Identify only one patient problem in the diagnostic statement. Every problem has different specific expected outcomes (see Chapter 18). Confusion during the planning step occurs when you include multiple problems in a nursing diagnosis. For example, *Pain and Anxiety* related to difficulty in ambulating are two nursing diagnoses combined in one diagnostic statement. A more accurate statement would be two separate diagnoses: *Impaired Physical Mobility* related to pain in right knee and *Anxiety* related to difficulty in ambulating. It is permissible to include multiple etiologies contributing to one patient problem, as in *Complicated Grieving* related to diagnosed terminal illness and change in family role.

DOCUMENTATION AND INFORMATICS

Once you identify a patient's nursing diagnoses, enter them either on the written plan of care or in the electronic health information record (EHR) of the agency. State-of-the-art EHRs contain nursing diagnoses with NANDA-I approved diagnoses, interventions and outcomes, related or risk factors, and defining characteristics (Herdman and Kamitsuru, 2014). A nurse enters assessment data into the EHR, and the computer helps by organizing the data into clusters that enhance the ability to select accurate diagnoses. Once diagnoses are selected, the computer system will direct the nurse to outcome and intervention options to select for a patient. This makes building a care plan more theoretically based.

There are agencies with EHRs that do not use NANDA-I terminology. This makes entry of NANDA-I diagnoses more tedious. However it is important to know why to use NANDA-I terminology in a medical record entry (Herdman and Kamitsuru, 2014):

- NANDA-I diagnoses have a broad literature base, with many diagnoses being evidence based. Patient safety requires accurate documentation of health problems.
- NANDA-I classifications are the most comprehensive.
- NANDA-I diagnoses are under continual refinement and development by professional nurses.

In an agency, list nursing diagnoses chronologically as you identify them. When initiating an original care plan, place the highest-priority nursing diagnosis first. This will depend on a patient's condition and the nature of the nursing diagnosis. Thereafter add nursing diagnoses to the list. Date a nursing diagnosis at the time of initiation. When caring for a patient, review the list and identify nursing diagnoses with the greatest priority, regardless of chronological order.

QSEN QSEN: BUILDING COMPETENCY IN INFORMATICS
Refer to Mr. Lawson's concept map and consider that you are using a computer to enter assessment data relating to his knowledge problem. The data form a cluster leading to the nursing diagnosis of *Readiness for Enhanced Knowledge.*

How do you apply critical thinking in the use of an electronic health record to be sure that you have individualized your diagnostic approach?

Answers to QSEN Activities can be found on the Evolve website.

NURSING DIAGNOSES: APPLICATION TO CARE PLANNING

Nursing diagnosis is a universal means for communication among professional nurses and across other health care disciplines. Diagnoses direct the planning process and the selection of nursing interventions to achieve desired outcomes for patients. Just as a medical diagnosis of diabetes leads a health care provider to prescribe a low-carbohydrate diet and medication for blood glucose control, the nursing diagnosis of *Impaired Skin Integrity* directs a nurse to apply a support surface to a patient's bed and initiate a turning schedule. In Chapter 18 you will learn how unifying the languages of NANDA-I with the Nursing Interventions Classification (NIC) and Nursing Outcomes Classification (NOC) facilitates the process of matching nursing diagnoses with accurate and appropriate interventions and outcomes. The care plan (see Chapter 18) is a map for nursing care and demonstrates your accountability for patient care. By making accurate nursing diagnoses, your subsequent care plan communicates a patient's health care problems to other professionals and ensures that you select relevant and appropriate nursing interventions.

KEY POINTS

- The diagnostic process is a clinical judgment that involves reviewing assessment information, recognizing cues, clustering cues into patterns of data, and identifying a patient's specific health care problems.
- Diagnostic conclusions include problems treated primarily by nurses (nursing diagnoses) and those requiring treatment by several disciplines (collaborative problems).
- Nurses manage collaborative problems by using medical, nursing, and allied health interventions.
- The use of standard formal nursing diagnostic statements provides a precise definition of a patient's problem that gives nurses and other members of the health care team a common language for understanding a patient's needs.
- Data analysis and interpretation involve recognizing patterns in clustered data, comparing them with standards such as the NANDA-I classification of nursing diagnoses and defining characteristics, and coming to a reasoned conclusion about a patient's response to a health problem.
- Accurate diagnosis of patient problems ensures the selection of more effective and efficient nursing interventions.
- Defining characteristics are the subjective and objective clinical cues that a nurse gathers intentionally and unintentionally, clusters, and uses to form a diagnostic conclusion.
- When an assessment reveals defining characteristics that apply to more than one nursing diagnosis, gather more information to clarify your interpretation.
- Absence of defining characteristics suggests that you reject a proposed diagnosis.
- A problem-focused nursing diagnosis is usually written in a two-part format, including a diagnostic label and an etiological or related factor.
- A three-part diagnostic statement includes defining characteristics that apply to a patient's condition.
- Assessing the cultural differences that affect how patients define health and illness and want or choose to be treated will assist in making correct diagnostic conclusions.
- The "related to" factor of a diagnostic statement helps you to individualize problem-focused and health promotion nursing diagnoses and provides direction for your selection of appropriate interventions.
- Risk factors serve as cues to indicate that a risk nursing diagnosis applies to a patient's condition.
- A concept map is a visual representation of a patient's nursing diagnoses and their relationship with one another.
- Nursing diagnostic errors occur by errors in data collection, interpretation and analysis of data, clustering of data, or the diagnostic statement.

CLINICAL APPLICATION QUESTIONS

Preparing for Clinical Practice

Tonya begins to discuss Mr. and Mrs. Lawson's questions about caring for a wound at home. The patient lives in his own home. Mrs. Lawson has no restrictions to her activity and believes that she can help the patient with any physical limits. As they talk, Mr. Lawson shares with Tonya, "I'm worried about being able to return to work on time." When instructing the patient an hour ago, Tonya noticed that he was having trouble concentrating on what she had to say. He seemed more concerned about how his incision felt. Mrs. Lawson tells Tonya, "His office has been laying off workers; that's why he's concerned."

1. Consider Mr. Lawson's behaviors and statements in this case study and identify three pieces of assessment data that cluster together to form defining characteristics.
2. Tonya clusters the defining characteristics to select the diagnostic label of *Anxiety*. What would you identify as the related factor for this diagnosis?
3. If Tonya identified the patient's diagnosis as *Anxiety* related to need to perform wound care, would this be an accurate nursing diagnosis? Explain.

Answers to Clinical Application Questions can be found on the Evolve website.

REVIEW QUESTIONS

Are You Ready to Test Your Nursing Knowledge?

1. A nurse identified that a patient has difficulty turning in bed, moves slowly when assisted into a chair, and expresses having breathlessness after walking to the bathroom and back. The patient has been in the hospital for over 4 days. Write a three-part nursing diagnostic statement using the PES format.
2. Review the following problem-focused nursing diagnoses and identify the diagnoses that are stated correctly. (Select all that apply.)
   1. *Impaired Skin Integrity* related to physical immobility
   2. *Fatigue* related to heart disease
   3. *Nausea* related to gastric distention
   4. Need for improved *Oral Mucosa Integrity* related to inflamed mucosa
   5. *Risk for Infection* related to surgery

3. A nurse reviews data gathered regarding a patient's ability to cope with loss. The nurse compares the defining characteristics for *Ineffective Coping* with those for *Readiness for Enhanced Coping* and selects *Ineffective Coping* as the correct diagnosis. This is an example of the nurse avoiding an error in: (Select all that apply.)
   1. Data collection.
   2. Data clustering.
   3. Data interpretation.
   4. Making a diagnostic statement.
   5. Goal setting.
4. The nursing diagnosis *Impaired Parenting* related to mother's developmental delay is an example of a(n):
   1. Risk nursing diagnosis.
   2. Problem-focused nursing diagnosis.
   3. Health promotion nursing diagnosis.
   4. Wellness nursing diagnosis.
5. A nurse interviewed and conducted a physical examination of a patient. Among the assessment data the nurse gathered were an increased respiratory rate, the patient reporting difficulty breathing while lying flat, and pursed-lip breathing. This data set is an example of:
   1. Collaborative data set.
   2. Diagnostic label.
   3. Related factors.
   4. Data cluster.
6. In which of the following examples are nurses making diagnostic errors? (Select all that apply.)
   1. The nurse who observes a patient wincing and holding his left side and gathers no additional assessment data
   2. The nurse who measures joint range of motion after the patient reports pain in the left elbow
   3. The nurse who considers conflicting cues in deciding which diagnostic label to choose
   4. The nurse who identifies a diagnosis on the basis of a patient reporting difficulty sleeping
   5. The nurse who makes a diagnosis of *Ineffective Airway Clearance* related to pneumonia.
7. A nurse is reviewing a patient's list of nursing diagnoses in the medical record. The most recent nursing diagnosis is *Diarrhea* related to intestinal colitis. For which of the following reasons is this an incorrectly stated diagnostic statement?
   1. Identifying the clinical sign instead of an etiology
   2. Identifying a diagnosis on the basis of prejudicial judgment
   3. Identifying the diagnostic study rather than a problem caused by the diagnostic study
   4. Identifying the medical diagnosis instead of the patient's response to the diagnosis.
8. A nurse is assigned to a new patient admitted to the nursing unit following admission through the emergency department. The nurse collects a nursing history and interviews the patient. Place the following steps for making a nursing diagnosis in the correct order, beginning with the first step.
   1. Considers context of patient's health problem and selects a related factor
   2. Reviews assessment data, noting objective and subjective clinical information
   3. Clusters clinical cues that form a pattern
   4. Chooses diagnostic label
9. A nursing student reports to a lead charge nurse that his assigned patient seems to be less alert and his blood pressure is lower, dropping from 140/80 to 110/60. The nursing student states, "I believe this is a nursing diagnosis of *Deficient Fluid Volume*." The lead charge nurse immediately goes to the patient's room with the student to assess the patient's orientation, heart rate, skin turgor, and urine output for last 8 hours. The lead charge nurse suspects that the student has made which type of diagnostic error?
   1. Insufficient cluster of cues
   2. Disorganization
   3. Insufficient number of cues
   4. Evidence that another diagnosis is more likely
10. A nurse in a mother-baby clinic learns that a 16-year-old has given birth to her first child and has not been to a well-baby class yet. The nurse's assessment reveals that the infant cries when breastfeeding and has difficulty latching on to the nipple. The infant has not gained weight over the last 2 weeks. The nurse identifies the patient's nursing diagnosis as *Ineffective Breastfeeding*. Which of the following is the best "related to" factor?
    1. Infant crying at breast
    2. Infant unable to latch on to breast correctly
    3. Mother's deficient knowledge
    4. Lack of infant weight gain
11. A nurse is getting ready to assess a patient in a neighborhood community clinic. He was newly diagnosed with diabetes just a month ago. He has other health problems and a history of not being able to manage his health. Which of the following questions reflects the nurse's cultural competence in making an accurate diagnosis? (Select all that apply.)
    1. How is your diabetic diet affecting you and your family?
    2. You seem to not want to follow health guidelines. Can you explain why?
    3. What worries you the most about having diabetes?
    4. What do you expect from us when you do not take your insulin as instructed?
    5. What do you believe will help you control your blood sugar?
12. A nurse assesses a young woman who works part time but also cares for her mother at home. The nurse reviews clusters of data that include the patient's report of frequent awakenings at night, reduced ability to think clearly at work, and a sense of not feeling well rested. Which of the following diagnoses is in the correct PES format?
    1. *Disturbed Sleep Pattern* evidenced by frequent awakening
    2. *Disturbed Sleep Pattern* related to family caregiving responsibilities
    3. *Disturbed Sleep Pattern* related to need to improve sleep habits
    4. *Disturbed Sleep Pattern* related to caregiving responsibilities as evidenced by frequent awakening and not feeling rested
13. A nursing student is working with a faculty member to identify a nursing diagnosis for an assigned patient. The student has assessed that the patient is undergoing radiation treatment and has had liquid stool and the skin is clean and intact; therefore she selects the nursing diagnosis *Impaired Skin Integrity*. The faculty member explains that the student has made a diagnostic error for which of the following reasons?
    1. Incorrect clustering
    2. Wrong diagnostic label
    3. Condition is a collaborative problem.
    4. Premature closure of clusters
14. The use of standard formal nursing diagnostic statements serves several purposes in nursing practice, including which of the following? (Select all that apply.)
    1. Defines a patient's problem, giving members of the health care team a common language for understanding the patient's needs
    2. Allows physicians and allied health staff to communicate with nurses how they provide care among themselves

3. Helps nurses focus on the scope of nursing practice
4. Creates practice guidelines for collaborative health care activities
5. Builds and expands nursing knowledge

15. Which of the following nursing diagnoses is stated correctly? (Select all that apply.)
    1. *Fluid Volume Excess* related to heart failure
    2. *Sleep Deprivation* related to sustained noisy environment
    3. *Impaired Bed Mobility* related to postcardiac catheterization
    4. *Ineffective Protection* related to inadequate nutrition
    5. *Diarrhea* related to frequent, small, watery stools.

Answers: 1. See Evolve; **2.** 1, 3; **3.** 1, 3; **4.** 2; **5.** 4; **6.** 1, 4, 5; **7.** 4; **8.** 2, 3, 4, 1; **9.** 3; **10.** 3; **11.** 1, 3, 5; **12.** 4; **13.** 2; **14.** 1, 3, 5; **15.** 2, 4.

Rationales for Review Questions can be found on the Evolve website.

REFERENCES

Ackley BJ, Ladwig GB: *Nursing diagnosis handbook*, ed 9, St Louis, 2011, Mosby.

American Nurses Association (ANA): *Scope of nursing practice*, Washington, DC, 1987, The Association.

American Nurses Association (ANA): *Model nurse practice act*, Washington, DC, 1955, The Association.

American Nurses Association (ANA): *Nursing's social policy statement*, ed 2, Washington, DC, 2003, The Association.

American Nurses Association (ANA): *Nursing's social policy statement*, ed 3, Washington, DC, 2010, The Association.

Canadian Interprofessional Health Collaborative: *A national interprofessional competency framework*, February 2010. http://www.cihc.ca/files/CIHC_IPCompetencies_Feb1210.pdf. Accessed August 15, 2015.

Carpenito-Moyet LJ: *Nursing diagnoses: application to clinical practice*, ed 14, Philadelphia, 2013, Lippincott, Williams & Wilkins.

Chabeli MM: Concept-mapping as a teaching method to facilitate critical thinking in nursing education: a review of the literature, *Health SA Gesondheid* 15(1):Art rew, 2010.

Fry VS: The creative approach to nursing, *Am J Nurs* 53:301, 1953.

Gebbie K: Utilization of a classification of nursing diagnosis, *Nurs Diagn* 9(2 Suppl):17, 1998.

Herdman TH, Kamitsuru S, editors: *NANDA International nursing diagnoses: definitions & classification 2015-2017*, Oxford, 2014, Wiley Blackwell.

McFarland GK, McFarlane EA: *Nursing diagnosis and intervention: planning for patient care*, St Louis, 1989, Mosby.

NANDA International (NANDA-I): *Nursing diagnoses: definitions and classification, 2012-2014*, Oxford, 2012, Wiley-Blackwell.

National Council of State Boards of Nursing: *NCLEX RN detailed test plan*, April 2013. https://www.ncsbn.org/2013_NCLEX_RN_Detailed_Test_Plan_Educator.pdf. Accessed November 18, 2014.

Pilcher J: Teaching and learning with concept maps, *Neonatal Netw* 30(5):336, 2011.

Yura H, Walsh M: *The nursing process*, Norwalk, CT, 1967, Appleton-Century-Crofts.

RESEARCH REFERENCES

Cho I, et al: Nurses' responses to differing amounts and information content in a diagnostic computer-based decision support application, *Comput Inform Nurs* 28(2):95, 2010.

Escalada H, et al: Nursing care for psychiatric patients defined by NANDA-NIC-NOC terminology; a literature review, *Rev Enferm* 36(3):14, 19–25, 2013.

Guedes NG, et al: Review of nursing diagnosis sedentary lifestyle in individuals with hypertension: conceptual analysis, *Rev Esc Enferm USP* 47(3):742, 2013.

Lai W, et al: Does one size fit all? Exploring the cultural applicability of NANDA-I nursing diagnoses to Chinese nursing practice, *J Transcult Nurs* 24(1):43, 2013.

Lunney M: Use of critical thinking in the diagnostic process, *Int J Nurs Terminol Classif* 21(2):82, 2010.

Muller-Staub M, et al: Implementing nursing diagnostics effectively: cluster randomized trial, *J Adv Nurs* 63(3):291, 2008.

18

Planning Nursing Care

OBJECTIVES

- Explain the relationship of planning to assessment and nursing diagnosis.
- Describe how use of a PICOT question can influence a patient's plan of care.
- Discuss criteria used in priority setting.
- Explain the benefits of using the nursing outcomes classification.
- Discuss the difference between a goal and an expected outcome.
- Explain the SMART approach to writing goal and outcome statements.
- Correctly write an outcome for a goal of care.
- Develop a plan of care from a nursing assessment.
- Discuss the differences among independent, dependent, and collaborative nursing interventions.
- Discuss the process of selecting nursing interventions during planning.
- Describe the role that communication plays in planning patient-centered care.
- Describe the consultation process.

KEY TERMS

Collaborative interventions, p. 246
Consultation, p. 253
Dependent nursing interventions, p. 246
Expected outcome, p. 242
Goal, p. 242
Independent nursing interventions, p. 246
Interdisciplinary care plans, p. 248
Long-term goal, p. 245
Nursing care plan, p. 248
Nursing Outcomes Classification, p. 244
Nursing Interventions Classification, p. 246
Nursing-sensitive patient outcome, p. 244
Patient-centered goal, p. 244
Planning, p. 240
Priority setting, p. 241
Scientific rationale, p. 249
Short-term goal, p. 245

MEDIA RESOURCES

http://evolve.elsevier.com/Potter/fundamentals/

- Review Questions
- Concept Map Creator
- Case Study with Questions
- Audio Glossary
- Content Updates

Tonya conducted a thorough assessment of Mr. Lawson's health status and identified three nursing diagnoses: Acute Pain related to trauma of surgical incision, Readiness for Enhanced Knowledge related to impending discharge, and Risk for Infection. Tonya is responsible for the initial planning of Mr. Lawson's nursing care after identifying relevant nursing diagnoses. The care that she plans will continue throughout the course of Mr. Lawson's hospital stay by the other nurses involved in Mr. Lawson's' care. If Tonya plans well, the individualized interventions that she selects will prepare the patient for a smooth transition home. Collaboration with the patient and his wife will be critical for a plan of care to be successful. Using input from Mr. Lawson, Tonya identifies the goals and expected outcomes for each of his nursing diagnoses. The goals and outcomes direct Tonya in selecting appropriate therapeutic nursing interventions. Tonya knows that Mrs. Lawson must be involved in her husband's care because of the ongoing support that she provides and because she will be a key care provider once Mr. Lawson returns home. Consultation with other health care providers such as home health ensures that the right resources will be used in planning care. In addition, Tonya poses a PICOT question about Mr. Lawson: Does the use of visual aids compared with standard discharge literature affect adult patients' ability to learn infection control principles? Tonya will use results of her literature search to build interventions for Mr. Lawson's care. Careful planning involves seeing the relationships among a patient's problems, recognizing that certain problems take precedence over others, identifying the most appropriate interventions, and proceeding with planning a safe and efficient approach to care.

After making a medical diagnosis, a health care provider will choose interventions and communicate the plan to the health care team. For example, after making a diagnosis of diabetes mellitus, a health care provider will prescribe a treatment plan that includes an insulin regimen, specific caloric diet, blood glucose monitoring, and an exercise plan. The health care provider establishes the plan with the goal of achieving blood glucose control. Outcomes for determining if the goal is met include blood glucose levels and hemoglobin A1c test measures.

After identifying a patient's nursing diagnoses and collaborative problems, the nurse prioritizes the diagnoses, sets patient-centered goals and expected outcomes, and chooses nursing interventions appropriate for each diagnosis. This is the third step of the nursing process, **planning**. The nurse collaborates with a patient and family (as appropriate) and the rest of the health care team to determine the urgency of the identified problems and prioritizes patient needs (Ackley and Ladwig, 2014). Planning requires critical thinking applied through deliberate decision making and problem solving. Perhaps the most important principle to learn about planning is the need to individualize a plan of care for a patient's unique needs. This requires communicating closely with patients, their families, and the health care team and ongoing consultation with team members. The nursing diagnoses that you identify direct your selection of individualized nursing interventions and the goals and outcomes you hope to achieve (Suhonen et al., 2011). Know that a plan of care is dynamic and changes as a patient's needs change.

ESTABLISHING PRIORITIES

A single patient often has multiple nursing diagnoses and collaborative problems. When you enter nursing practice, you will care for multiple patients. You must be able to set priorities for these patients carefully and wisely to ensure safe, timely, and effective care. **Priority setting** is the ordering of nursing diagnoses or patient problems using notions of urgency and importance to establish a preferential order for nursing interventions. Priority setting is not the ordering of a list of care tasks, but an organization of a vision of desired outcomes for a patient.

Symptom pattern recognition from your assessment database and certain knowledge triggers help you understand which diagnoses require intervention and the associated time frame to intervene effectively (Ackley and Ladwig, 2014). An example is a patient who suddenly spikes a fever. Coupling this symptom with other symptoms of purulent drainage from a surgical wound and an inflamed incision tells the nurse that an infection has developed, and the nurse recognizes the symptoms as an immediate cause for action.

As you care for a patient or multiple patients, you must deal with certain aspects of care before others. By ranking a patient's nursing diagnoses in order of importance and always monitoring changing signs and symptoms (defining characteristics) of patient problems, you attend to each patient's most important needs and better organize ongoing care activities. Priorities help you to anticipate and sequence nursing interventions when a patient has multiple nursing diagnoses and collaborative problems. You also set priorities by selecting mutually agreed-on priorities with a patient on the basis of the urgency of the problems, the patient's safety and desires, the nature of the treatment indicated, and the relationship among the diagnoses. Priority setting is not a matter of numbering the nursing diagnoses on the basis of severity or physiological importance. Such a numbering system does not always reflect actual clinical changes in patients. You must establish priorities in relation to their ongoing clinical importance.

Classify patients' priorities as high, intermediate, or low importance. Nursing diagnoses that, if untreated, result in harm to a patient or others (e.g., those related to airway status, circulation, safety, and pain) have the highest priorities. One way to consider nursing diagnoses of high priority is to consider Maslow's hierarchy of needs (see Chapter 6). For example, *Risk for Other-Directed Violence, Impaired Gas Exchange,* and *Decreased Cardiac Output* are examples of high-priority nursing diagnoses that drive the priorities of safety, adequate oxygenation, and adequate circulation. However, it is always important to consider each patient's unique situation. Avoid classifying only physiological nursing diagnoses as high priority. *Consider Mr. Lawson's case. Among his nursing diagnoses,* ***Acute Pain*** *was an initial priority because Tonya knew that she needed to relieve Mr. Lawson's acute pain for him to be responsive to discharge education. Now that his pain has been controlled reasonably well,* ***Readiness for Enhanced Knowledge*** *has become a priority because of the patient's expressed desire to learn and the urgency of preparing him adequately for pending discharge.*

Intermediate-priority nursing diagnoses involve nonemergent, nonlife-threatening needs of patients. In Mr. Lawson's case, *Risk for Infection* is an intermediate diagnosis. The nursing staff will continue to monitor his wound healing, and it is important for Mr. and Mrs. Lawson to learn the signs of infection and understand what to observe once the patient returns home. In this case focused and individualized instruction from all members of the health care team about infection prevention is necessary throughout the patient's hospitalization.

Low-priority nursing diagnoses are not always directly related to a specific illness or prognosis but affect a patient's future well-being. Many low-priority diagnoses focus on a patient's long-term health care needs. You learned in Chapter 17 that Mr. Lawson shares a concern with Tonya, "I'm worried about being able to return to work on time." When instructing the patient, Tonya noticed that he was having trouble attending to what she had to say. Tonya has not yet identified a nursing diagnosis related to Mr. Lawson's concern about returning to work. She will need to assess more fully, but a nursing diagnosis such as *Anxiety* may be of low priority compared to others. However, if the patient's anxiety is left unaddressed, it could become a higher priority if it interferes with his ability to learn discharge information.

The order of priorities changes as a patient's condition and needs change, sometimes within a matter of minutes. Each time you begin a sequence of care such as at the beginning of a hospital shift or during a clinic visit, it is important to reorder priorities. For example, when Tonya first met Mr. Lawson, his *Acute Pain* was rated at a 7, and it was apparent that administering an analgesic and repositioning the patient were greater priorities than trying to prepare him for instruction. Later, after receiving the analgesic, Mr. Lawson's pain lessened to a level of 4; and Tonya was able to gather more assessment information and begin to focus on his problem of *Readiness for Enhanced Knowledge.* Ongoing patient assessment is critical to determine the status of your patient's nursing diagnoses. The appropriate ordering of priorities ensures that you meet a patient's needs in a safe, timely, and effective way.

Priority setting begins when you identify and prioritize a patient's main diagnoses or problems. The next step is to prioritize the specific nursing interventions that you plan to use to help a patient achieve desired goals and outcomes. For example, as Tonya considers the high-priority diagnosis of *Acute Pain* for Mr. Lawson, she includes in her plan of care these options: administering an analgesic, repositioning, and teaching relaxation exercises. With each clinical encounter, Tonya applies critical thinking to prioritize which intervention to use. Tonya knows that a certain degree of pain relief is necessary before a patient can participate in relaxation exercises. When she is in the patient's room, she might decide to turn and reposition Mr. Lawson first and then prepare the analgesic. However, if Mr. Lawson expresses that pain is a high level and he is too uncomfortable to turn, Tonya chooses obtaining and administering the analgesic as her first priority. Later, with Mr. Lawson's pain more under control, she considers whether relaxation is appropriate.

Involve patients in priority setting whenever possible. Patient-centered care requires you to know a patient's preferences, values, and expressed needs. In some situations a patient assigns priorities differently from those you select. Resolve any conflicting values concerning health care needs and treatments with open communication, informing the patient of all options and consequences. Consulting with and knowing a patient's concerns do not relieve you of the responsibility to act in a patient's best interests. Always assign priorities on the basis of good nursing judgment. Ethical care is a part of priority setting (see Chapter 22). Nurses decide about priorities on the basis of their fundamental disposition of what is good and right (Benner et al., 1996). Often these values remain unspoken and perhaps unrecognized, but nevertheless they profoundly influence what nurses attend to in a

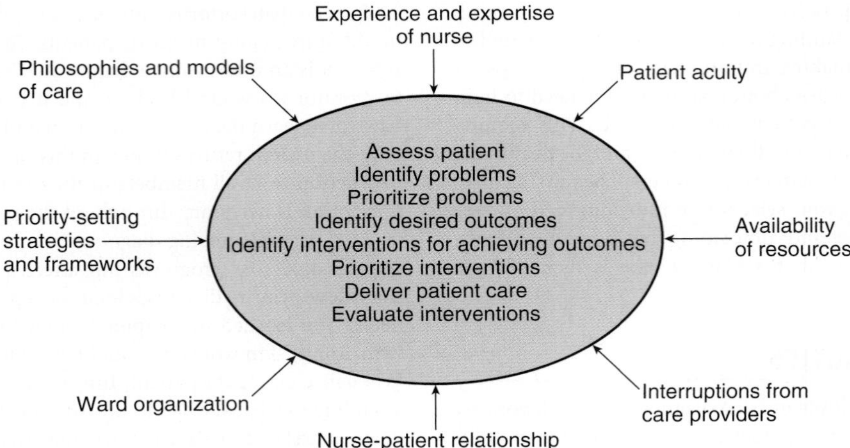

FIGURE 18-1 A model for priority setting. (Modified from Hendry C, Walker A: Priority setting in clinical nursing practice, *J Adv Nurs* 47(4):427, 2004.)

particular clinical situation and the options they consider in making decisions and taking action (Tanner, 2006). When ethical issues make priorities less clear, it is important to have an open discussion with a patient, the family, and other health care providers. For example, when caring for patients with cancer and other disabling illnesses, discuss the situation with them and understand their expectations, understand your professional responsibility in protecting the patients from harm, know their health care provider's therapeutic or palliative goals, and then form appropriate plans of care.

Priorities in Practice

Many factors within the health care environment affect your ability to set priorities (Figure 18-1). For example, in a hospital setting the model for delivering care (see Chapter 21), the workflow routine of the nursing unit, staffing levels, and interruptions from other care providers affect the minute-by-minute determination of patient care priorities. In the home health setting the number of visits scheduled for a day and the availability of family caregivers and resources within a patient's home affect them. Available resources (e.g., nurse specialists and dietitians), policies and procedures, and supply access also affect priorities. Patients' conditions are always changing; thus priority setting is always changing.

Successful priority setting also involves working well with the health care team. When you work with nursing assistive personnel (NAP), discuss the purpose of each patient's hospitalization, the picture of how the patient should look at the end of the shift, the plan for achieving desired outcomes, and the part you and the NAP will play. You agree on priorities at the beginning of a shift, but they are usually reshuffled several times before the next shift. Patients' needs change, some patients are discharged, and new patients are admitted (Nelson et al., 2006).

The same factors that influence your minute-by-minute ability to prioritize nursing actions affect the ability to prioritize nursing diagnoses and plan care for groups of patients. The nature of nursing work challenges your ability to cognitively attend to a given patient's priorities when you care for more than one patient. The nursing care process is nonlinear (Potter et al., 2005). Often you complete an assessment and identify nursing diagnoses for one patient, leave the room to perform an intervention for a second patient, and move on to consult on a third patient. Nurses exercise "cognitive shifts" (i.e., shifts in attention from one patient to another during the conduct of the nursing process). This shifting of attention occurs in response to changing patient needs, new procedures being ordered, or environmental processes interacting (Potter et al., 2005). Because of these cognitive shifts, it becomes important to stay organized and know your patients' priorities. Work from your plan of care and use patients' priorities to organize the order for delivering interventions and organizing documentation of care.

CRITICAL THINKING IN SETTING GOALS AND EXPECTED OUTCOMES

When you start nursing school, your goal is to graduate. Success in meeting that goal is measured by grades and the outcomes of your class work. A baseball team strives to achieve the goal of winning the World Series. The team achieves that goal through the outcome of winning more games than other teams. The use of goals and outcomes in patient care is designed to help focus the efforts of all health care team members to a common purpose: helping a patient achieve or maintain a desired level of health. In the case of Mr. Lawson, Tonya sets the goal of the patient being "infection free." The expected outcomes for achieving that goal include the patient remaining afebrile, without wound drainage, and with wound edges healing. Expected outcomes are time limited, measurable ways of determining if a goal is met (Table 18-1).

After identifying a patients' nursing diagnoses and collaborative problems, ask yourself, "What do I plan to achieve?" and "How will I know when I have achieved what I want?" During planning you select goals and expected outcomes for each nursing diagnosis or problem to provide clear direction for the type of interventions needed to care for your patient and to then evaluate the effectiveness of these interventions. A **goal** is a broad statement that describes a desired change in a patient's condition, perceptions, or behavior. Mr. Lawson has the diagnosis of *Readiness for Enhanced Knowledge.* A goal of care for this diagnosis includes, "Patient will understand postoperative risks." The goal requires making Mr. Lawson aware of the risks associated with his type of surgery. It gives Tonya a clear focus on the topics to include in her instruction. For Tonya to know if Mr. Lawson does understand postoperative risks, the patient must meet expected outcomes. An **expected outcome** is the measurable change (patient behavior, physical state, or perception) that must be achieved to reach a goal. In Mr. Lawson's case, after Tonya provides an educational intervention, the expected outcome would be, "Patient identifies signs and symptoms of wound infection before discharge." Tonya might measure along a continuum of no correct answers versus three correct to determine if Mr. Lawson identifies signs and symptoms correctly. Sometimes several

TABLE 18-1 Examples of Goal Setting with Expected Outcomes for Mr. Lawson

Nursing Diagnoses	Goals	Expected Outcomes
Acute Pain related to trauma of surgical incision	Mr. Lawson will achieve pain relief by day of discharge.	Mr. Lawson reports pain at a level of 3 or below by discharge. Mr. Lawson transfers from bed to chair with no increase in pain in 48 hours. Mr. Lawson's incisional area shows signs of wound healing by discharge.
Readiness for Enhanced Knowledge related to impending discharge with self-care needs	Mr. Lawson will express understanding of postoperative risks in 24 hours.	Mr. Lawson describes activity restrictions to follow by discharge. Mr. Lawson demonstrates how to cleanse surgical wound by discharge. Mr. Lawson describes three risks for infection in 24 hours.
Risk for Infection	Mr. Lawson will remain infection free by discharge.	Mr. Lawson remains afebrile by discharge. Mr. Lawson's wound shows no purulent drainage by discharge. Mr. Lawson's wound closes at site of incision separation by discharge

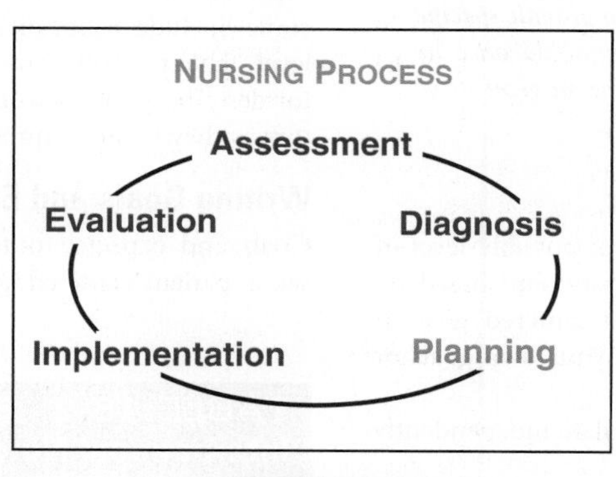

FIGURE 18-2 Critical thinking and the process of planning care.

expected outcomes must be met for a single goal. In all cases the goal and expected outcomes align with the patient's nursing diagnoses.

In health care today the terms *goals* and *outcomes* are sometimes interchanged, and this can be confusing. Significant importance is placed on outcome measurement within health care institutions; however, even the way electronic health records (EHRs) label the categories that nurses use to complete plans of care can be unclear. But again, think of a goal as an ultimate outcome and expected outcomes as the measurable changes that must be achieved to reach a goal.

Planning nursing care requires you to critically evaluate the identified nursing diagnoses, the urgency or priority of the problems, and the resources of the patient and the health care delivery system (Figure 18-2). Apply knowledge from the medical, sociobehavioral, and nursing sciences to plan patient care. When Tonya selected her PICOT question about approaches for teaching infection control, she applied the knowledge she gained in selecting a specific teaching approach. The selection of goals, expected outcomes, and interventions requires consideration of your previous experience with similar patient problems and any established standards for clinical problem management. The goals and outcomes need to meet established intellectual standards by being relevant to patient needs, specific, singular, observable, measurable, and time limited. You also use critical thinking attitudes in selecting interventions with the greatest likelihood of success.

Role of the Patient in Goal/Outcome Setting

Always partner with patients when setting their individualized goals. Mutual goal setting includes a patient and family (when appropriate) in prioritizing the goals of care and developing a plan of action. For patients to participate in goal setting, they need to be alert and have some degree of independence in completing activities of daily living, problem solving, and decision making. They also need to understand the priority problems and have a willingness/motivation to resolve those problems. Unless goals are mutually set and there is a clear plan of action, patients may not fully participate in the plan of care, leading to suboptimal outcomes. Patients need to understand and see the value of nursing therapies, even though they are often totally dependent on you as the nurse. When setting goals, act as an advocate or support for the patient to select nursing interventions that promote his or her return to health or prevent further deterioration when possible.

*Tonya has a discussion with Mr. Lawson and his wife together about setting the plan for the diagnosis of **Readiness for Enhanced Knowledge.** Tonya explains the topics that they need to discuss so the couple understands Mr. Lawson's postoperative risks. In addition, she talks about the use of a DVD program on infection control that the couple can watch in their room. Tonya applied knowledge learned from her PICOT question literature search and chose the visual aid strategy. They plan for the couple to view the DVD when Mrs. Lawson visits. Mr. Lawson asks Tonya to also provide specific instruction about the activities he can and cannot do once he returns home. Tonya agrees and consults with the surgeon to be sure that her information is accurate and realistic.*

Selecting Goals and Expected Outcomes

A **patient-centered goal** reflects a patient's highest possible level of wellness and independence in function. It is realistic and based on patient needs, abilities, and resources. A patient-centered goal or outcome reflects a patient's specific behavior, not your own goals or interventions.

- A correct goal statement: "Patient will ambulate independently in 3 days."
- A correct outcome statement: "Patient ambulates in the hall 3 times a day by 4/22."
- A common error is to write an intervention: "Ambulate patient in the hall 3 times a day."

A patient-centered goal represents a predicted resolution of a diagnosis or problem, progress toward improved health status, or continued maintenance of good health or function (Carpenito-Moyet, 2013). Nurses monitor and manage patient conditions and diagnose problems that are amenable to nursing intervention. The clinical reasoning and decision making of nurses is a key part of quality health care (Moorhead et al., 2013). Thus it becomes important to select and measure patient outcomes that are influenced by nursing care. A **nursing-sensitive patient outcome** is a measurable patient, family, or community state, behavior, or perception largely influenced by and sensitive to nursing interventions (Moorhead et al., 2013). Examples of nursing-sensitive outcomes include reduction in pain frequency and severity, incidence of pressure ulcers, and incidence of falls. In comparison, medical outcomes are largely influenced by medical interventions. Examples include patient mortality, surgical wound infection, and hospital readmissions. For the nursing profession to become a full participant in clinical evaluation research, policy development, and interdisciplinary work, nurses need to identify and measure patient outcomes influenced by nursing interventions.

The Iowa Intervention Project has shown the link between nursing diagnoses and outcomes. It publishes the **Nursing Outcomes Classification** (NOC), which link outcomes to NANDA International (NANDA-I) nursing diagnoses (Moorhead et al., 2013). This resource is an option that you can use in selecting goals and outcomes for your patients. For each NANDA-I nursing diagnosis there are multiple NOC suggested outcomes. The outcomes have labels for describing the focus of nursing care and include indicators (expected outcomes) to use in evaluating the success with nursing interventions. The indicators for each NOC outcome allow measurement of the outcomes at any point on a five-point Likert scale from most negative to most positive (Moorhead et al., 2013). Such a rating system adds objectivity to judging a patient's progress. Many health care institutions use NOC as part of the infrastructure of their documentation system. Using standardized nursing terminologies such as NOC makes it more possible to measure aspects of nursing care on a national and international level (Park, 2013). For example, when researchers compare databases that have used the standard terminologies from NOC, they can determine which common nursing interventions favorably impact outcomes.

What NOC describes as an outcome such as anxiety level, appetite, or physical comfort is a very abstract term, which in real clinical practice comes closer to a goal statement. For example, in NOC terminology the outcome for the nursing diagnosis of *Acute Pain* is described as "pain control" or pain relief, the goal set for Mr. Lawson. The NOC outcome indicators are the same for what most clinicians set as expected outcomes. In the example of pain control, the expected outcomes include symptom severity measured on a pain scale or mobility level. Table 18-2 offers more examples of how to use NOC terminology for describing the focus or goals of nursing care and outcome indicators as they relate to nursing diagnoses.

Writing Goals and Expected Outcomes

Goals and expected outcomes direct your nursing care. Once you set a patient-centered goal for a nursing diagnosis, the expected

TABLE 18-2 Examples of NANDA International Nursing Diagnoses and Suggested NOC Linkages

Nursing Diagnosis	Examples of NOC Outcomes (Consider as Goal Statements)	Outcome Indicators (Examples)
Impaired Oral Mucous Membrane	Oral Health	Knowledge of infection management Self-care oral hygiene
	Tissue Integrity	Hydration Infection severity
Activity Intolerance	Activity Tolerance	Oxygen saturation with activity Pulse rate with activity Respiratory rate with activity
	Self-Care Status	Bathes self Dresses self Prepares food and fluid for eating

NOC, Nursing Outcomes Classification.

outcomes provide the desired physiological, psychological, social, developmental, or spiritual responses that indicate resolution of the patient's health problems. Usually you develop several expected outcomes for each nursing diagnosis and goal. For a patient to resolve a goal, several measurable outcomes are needed to ensure that the goal is met. In the case of Mr. Lawson's diagnosis of *Risk for Infection,* Tonya knows that more than one outcome is needed to ensure that the patient is infection free.

The SMART acronym (*S*pecific, *M*easurable, *A*ttainable, *R*ealistic, *T*imed) is a useful approach for writing goals and outcome statements more effectively (Ackley and Ladwig, 2013).

Specific or Singular Goal or Outcome. You need to be precise when you evaluate a patient's response to a nursing intervention during the evaluation phase of the nursing process (see Chapter 20). Each goal and outcome addresses only one behavior, perception, or physiological response. The example, "Patient will administer a self-injection and demonstrate infection control measures," is incorrect because the statement includes two different behaviors, administer and demonstrate. Instead word each goal separately as follows, "Patient will administer a self-injection by discharge," and "Patient will demonstrate infection control measures at home."

Expected outcomes must also be singular. For example, consider the expected outcome, "Patient's lungs are clear to auscultation, and respiratory rate is 20 breaths/min by 8/22." It will be difficult to measure if the patient has achieved the goal of "Improved respiratory status" by using a combined outcome statement. When you evaluate that the lungs are clear but the respiratory rate is 28 breaths/min, the patient did not achieve the expected outcome because only one of the desired physical changes was achieved. By splitting the statement into two parts, "Lungs will be clear to auscultation by 8/22," and "Respiratory rate will be 20 breaths/min by 8/22," you are able to determine if and when the patient achieves each outcome. Specificity allows you to decide if there is a need to modify the plan of care.

Measurable. Goals and expected outcomes are the standards against which to measure or observe a patient's response to nursing care. You need to be able to measure or observe if change takes place in a patient's status. Changes occur in physiological findings and in a patient's knowledge, perceptions, and behavior. Examples such as, "Body temperature will remain 98.6° F (37° C)," and "Apical pulse will remain between 60 and 100 beats/min" allow you to objectively measure physical changes in a patient's status. The outcome statement, "Patient's pain is less than 4 on a scale of 0 to 10 in 48 hours" allows you to objectively measure patient perception using a pain-rating scale. Do not use vague qualifiers such as "normal," "acceptable," or "stable" in an expected outcome statement. Vague terms result in guesswork in determining a patient's response to care. Terms describing quality, quantity, frequency, length, or weight allow you to evaluate outcomes precisely.

Attainable. For a patient's health to improve, he or she must be able to attain the outcomes of care that are set. A goal and an outcome likely are attainable when mutually set with the patient. This ensures that a patient and nurse agree on the direction and time limits of care. Mutually set attainable goals and outcomes (e.g., distance to walk, topics to learn about medications) increase a patient's motivation and cooperation. As a patient advocate, apply standards of practice, evidence-based knowledge, safety principles, and basic human needs when helping patients set goals. Your knowledge background helps to select goals and outcomes that your patients should meet on the basis of typical responses to clinical interventions. Always consider patients' desires to recover and their physical and psychological condition to set goals and outcomes to which they can agree.

Realistic. Set goals and expected outcomes that a patient is able to realistically reach. Your assessment of a patient will reveal a patient's condition and willingness and ability to be a care participant. For example, a patient who just experienced a stroke and has left-sided weakness in the arm has the goal of "assuming self-care with bathing." The patient will be limited by what he or she can do independently during the first several days and weeks ahead. You set realistic time-specific goals and outcomes within the patient's limitations and abilities. For example, an initial goal is, "Patient will wash hands and face in 72 hours." Your assessment and collaboration with occupational therapy will determine if the goal is realistic for the level of the patient's weakness.

Setting realistic goals and outcomes often requires you to communicate these goals and outcomes to caregivers in other settings who will assume responsibility for patient care (e.g., home health, rehabilitation). Realistic goals give patients a sense of hope. To establish realistic goals, assess the resources of a patient, health care facility, and family. Be aware of the patient's physiological, emotional, cognitive, and sociocultural potential and the economic cost and resources available to reach expected outcomes in a timely manner.

Timed. Each goal and outcome is time limited so the health care team has a common time frame for problem resolution. For example, the goal of "patient will achieve pain relief" for Mr. Lawson is complete by adding the time frame "by day of discharge." With this goal in place, all members of the nursing team will aim to manage and reduce the patient's pain while he is hospitalized. At the time of discharge, evaluation of expected outcomes (e.g., pain-rating score, signs of grimacing, level of movement) show if the goal was met. The time frame depends on the nature of the problem, etiology, overall condition of the patient, and treatment setting. A **short-term goal** is an objective behavior or response that you expect a patient to achieve in a short time, usually less than a week. In an acute care setting you often set goals for over a course of just a few hours. A **long-term goal** is an objective behavior or response that you expect a patient to achieve over a longer period, usually over several days, weeks, or months (e.g., "Patient will be tobacco free within 60 days"). Always collaborate with patients to set realistic and reasonable time frames. Time frames help you and a patient determine if the patient is making progress at a reasonable rate. If not, you must revise the plan of care. Time frames also promote accountability in delivering and managing nursing care.

CRITICAL THINKING IN PLANNING NURSING CARE

Part of the planning process is selecting nursing interventions for meeting a patient's goals and outcomes. Once you identify nursing diagnoses and select goals and outcomes, you choose interventions individualized for a patient's situation. Nursing interventions are any treatments or actions based on clinical judgment and knowledge that nurses perform to enhance patient outcomes (Bulechek et al., 2013). During planning you select interventions designed to help a patient move from the present level of health to the level described in the goal and measured by the expected outcomes. The actual implementation of these interventions occurs during the implementation phase of the nursing process (see Chapter 19). Choosing suitable nursing interventions involves applying the best evidence for a patient's health problems and using good clinical judgment.

Tonya identified a PICOT question to help her select instructional interventions for enhancing Mr. and Mrs. Lawson's knowledge about infection control. She also chooses interventions on the basis of what she has learned about the etiologies behind his learning needs. Mr. Lawson has not experienced postoperative care, he is facing restrictions with which he is unfamiliar, and the condition of his incision requires wound care at home. Tonya will plan instructional topics to address postoperative risks in a way that will be relevant to Mr. Lawson and his usual routines at home. The instruction will include Mrs. Lawson since she is a reliable resource for Mr. Lawson.

Types of Interventions

There are three categories of nursing interventions: nurse-initiated, health care provider-initiated, and collaborative interventions. Some patients require all three categories, whereas others need only nurse- and health care provider-initiated interventions.

Nurse-initiated interventions are the **independent nursing interventions** or actions that a nurse initiates without supervision or direction from others. Examples include positioning patients to prevent pressure ulcer formation, instructing patients in side effects of medications, or providing skin care to an ostomy site. Independent nursing interventions do not require an order from another health care provider. Nurse-initiated interventions are autonomous actions based on scientific rationale. Such interventions benefit a patient in a predicted way related to nursing diagnoses and patient goals (Bulechek et al., 2013). Each state within the United States has Nurse Practice Acts that define the legal scope of nursing practice (see Chapter 23). According to the Nurse Practice Acts in a majority of states, independent nursing interventions pertain to activities of daily living, health education and promotion, and counseling. *For Mr. Lawson Tonya selects the following nursing interventions to resolve his acute pain: positioning, relaxation therapy, and exercise promotion.*

Health care provider–initiated interventions are **dependent nursing interventions**, or actions that require an order from a health care provider. The interventions are based on the health care provider's response to treating or managing a medical diagnosis. Advanced practice nurses who work under collaborative agreements with physicians or who are licensed independently by state practice acts are also able to write dependent interventions. As a nurse you intervene by carrying out the health care provider's written and/or verbal orders. Administering a medication, implementing an invasive procedure (e.g., inserting a Foley catheter, starting an intravenous [IV] infusion) and preparing a patient for diagnostic tests are examples of health care provider-initiated interventions.

Each health care provider-initiated intervention requires specific nursing responsibilities and technical nursing knowledge. You are often the one performing the intervention, and you must know the types of observations and precautions to take for the intervention to be delivered safely and correctly. For example, when administering a medication you are responsible for not only giving the medicine correctly, but also knowing the classification of the drug; its physiological action, normal dosage, and side effects; and nursing interventions related to its action or side effects (see Chapter 32). You are responsible for knowing when an invasive procedure is necessary, the clinical skills necessary to complete it, and its expected outcome and possible side effects. You are also responsible for adequate preparation of a patient and proper communication of the results. You perform dependent nursing interventions, like all nursing actions, with appropriate knowledge, clinical reasoning, and good clinical judgment.

Collaborative interventions, or interdependent interventions, are therapies that require the combined knowledge, skill, and expertise of multiple health care providers. Typically when you plan care for a patient, you review the necessary interventions and determine if the collaboration of other health care disciplines is necessary. A patient care conference with an interdisciplinary health care team results in selection of interdependent interventions.

In the case study involving Mr. Lawson, Tonya plans independent interventions to help relieve Mr. Lawson's pain and begin teaching him about postoperative care activities. Among the dependent interventions Tonya plans to implement are the administration of an analgesic and ordered wound care. Tonya's collaborative intervention involves consulting with the unit discharge coordinator, who will help Mr. and Mrs. Lawson plan for their return home, and the home health department to ensure that the Lawsons have home health visits.

When preparing for health care provider-initiated or collaborative interventions, do not automatically implement the therapies but determine whether they are appropriate for each patient. Every nurse faces an inappropriate or incorrect order at some time. The nurse with a strong knowledge base and clinical experience recognizes an error and seeks to correct it. The ability to recognize incorrect therapies is particularly important when administering medications or procedures. Errors occur in writing orders or transcribing them to a documentation form or computer screen. Clarifying an order is competent nursing practice, and it protects a patient and members of the health care team. When you carry out an incorrect or inappropriate intervention, it is as much your error as the person who wrote or transcribed the original order. You are legally responsible for any complications resulting from an error (see Chapter 23).

Selection of Interventions

During planning do not select interventions randomly. For example, patients with the diagnosis of *Anxiety* do not always need care in the same way with the same interventions. You treat *Anxiety related to the uncertainty of surgical recovery* very differently than *Anxiety related to a threat to loss of job*. When choosing interventions, consider six important factors: (1) desired patient outcomes, (2) characteristics of the nursing diagnosis, (3) research base knowledge for the intervention, (4) feasibility for doing the intervention, (5) acceptability to the patient, and (6) your own competency (Bulechek et al., 2013) (Box 18-1).

When developing a plan of care, review resources such as the scientific literature, standard protocols or guidelines, the Nursing Outcomes Classification (NOC) and **Nursing Interventions Classification (NIC)**, policy or procedure manuals, or textbooks. Collaboration with other health professionals is also useful. As you select interventions, review your patient's needs, priorities, and previous experiences to select the interventions that have the best potential for achieving the expected outcomes.

Nursing Interventions Classification. Just as with the standardized NOC, the Iowa Intervention Project has developed a set of nursing interventions that provides a level of standardization to enhance communication of nursing care across all health care settings and compare outcomes (Bulechek et al., 2013). The NIC model includes three levels: domains, classes, and interventions for ease of use. The seven domains are the highest level (level 1) of the model, using broad terms (e.g., safety and basic physiological) to organize the more specific classes and interventions (Table 18-3). The second level of the model includes 30 classes, which offer useful clinical categories to reference when selecting interventions. The third level of the model includes the 554 interventions, defined as any treatment based on

BOX 18-1 Choosing Nursing Interventions

Desired Patient Outcomes
- Outcome serves as the criteria against which to judge efficacy of intervention.
- Nursing Outcomes Classification (NOC) outcomes are linked to Nursing Interventions Classification (NIC) interventions. NIC is designed to show the link to NOC (Moorhead et al., 2013). Use these resources to develop care plans.

Characteristics of the Nursing Diagnosis
- Choose interventions to alter the etiological (related to) factor or causes of the diagnosis. **Example:** Acute Pain related to trauma of surgical incision—choose interventions for Mr. Lawson that relieve swelling and strain on incision site (positioning and turning measures) and lower pain reception (analgesic).
- When an etiological factor cannot change, direct the interventions toward treating the signs and symptoms (e.g., defining characteristics for a diagnosis). **Example:** Readiness for Enhanced Knowledge related to impending discharge with self-care needs—choose interventions that provide information that answers Mr. and Mrs. Lawson's questions about recovery procedures, wound care, and what to observe.
- For risk diagnoses, direct interventions at altering or eliminating the risk factors for the diagnosis. **Example:** Risk for Infection requires interventions for keeping Mr. Lawson's incisional area clean, free from further trauma, and for maintaining good nutrition.

Research Base
- Be familiar with the research evidence for an intervention and use it for the appropriate patient group and/or setting (see Chapter 5).
- Research evidence in support of a nursing intervention will indicate the effectiveness of using the intervention with certain types of patients.
- When research is not available, use scientific principles (e.g., infection control, learning) or consult a clinical expert about your patient.

Feasibility
- A specific intervention has the potential to interact with other interventions provided by the nurse and other health professionals.
- Know and be involved in a patient's total plan of care.
- Consider cost of an intervention and the amount of time required for implementation. **Example:** If you plan to get a patient up into a chair 3 times a day, will there be staff to assist with the transfer?

Acceptability to the Patient
- When possible, offer a patient a choice of interventions to assist in reaching outcomes.
- Promote informed choice; give patients information about each intervention and how they are expected to participate.
- Consider a patient's values, beliefs, and culture for a patient-centered approach to selecting interventions.

Capability of the Nurse
- Have knowledge of the scientific rationale for the intervention.
- Have the necessary psychosocial and psychomotor skills to complete the intervention.
- Be able to function within the specific setting to effectively use health care resources.

Modified from Bulechek GM, et al: *Nursing interventions classification (NIC)*, ed 6, St Louis, 2013, Mosby.

BOX 18-2 Example of Interventions for Physical Comfort Promotion

Class: Physical Comfort Promotion (Level 2)
Interventions to promote comfort using physical techniques

Interventions (Examples)
Aromatherapy
Cutaneous Stimulation
Environmental Management
Heat/Cold Application
Nausea Management
Pain Management
Progressive Muscle Relaxation

Examples of Linked Nursing Diagnoses
Acute Pain
Chronic Pain

From Bulechek GM, et al: *Nursing interventions classification (NIC)*, ed 6, St Louis, 2013, Mosby.

BOX 18-3 Example of an Intervention and Associated Nursing Activities

Intervention—Environmental Management: Comfort
Examples of Activities
- Create a calm and supportive environment.
- Provide a single room if it is the patient's preference to offer quiet and rest.
- Adjust room temperature to that most comfortable for the individual.
- Provide a safe and clean environment.
- Determine sources of discomfort: damp dressing, positioning on tubing, wrinkled linen.
- Provide hygiene measures for comfort (e.g., skin creams, oral care).
- Provide prompt attention to call lights, which should always be within reach.

From Bulechek GM, et al: *Nursing interventions classification (NIC)*, ed 6, St Louis, 2013, Mosby.

clinical judgment and knowledge that a nurse performs to enhance patient outcomes (Bulechek et al., 2013) (Box 18-2). Each intervention then includes a variety of nursing activities from which to choose (Box 18-3) and which a nurse commonly uses in a plan of care. NIC interventions are also linked with NANDA-I nursing diagnoses for ease of use (NANDA-I, 2012). For example, if a patient has a nursing diagnosis of *Acute Pain,* there are 20 recommended interventions, including pain management, cutaneous stimulation, and anxiety reduction. Each of the recommended interventions has a variety of activities for nursing care. For example, cutaneous stimulation activities include selection of massage, cold or heat. NIC is a valuable resource for selecting appropriate interventions and activities for your patient. It is evolving and practice oriented. The classification is comprehensive, including independent and collaborative interventions. It remains your decision to determine which interventions and activities best suit your patient's individualized needs and situation.

TABLE 18-3 Nursing Interventions Classification (NIC) Taxonomy

Domain 1	Domain 2	Domain 3
Level 1 Domains		
1. Physiological: Basic Care that supports physical functioning	**2. Physiological: Complex** Care that supports homeostatic regulation	**3. Behavioral** Care that supports psychosocial functioning and facilitates lifestyle changes
Level 2 Classes		
A *Activity and Exercise Management:* Interventions to organize or assist with physical activity and energy conservation and expenditure B *Elimination Management:* Interventions to establish and maintain regular bowel and urinary elimination patterns and manage complications caused by altered patterns C *Immobility Management:* Interventions to manage restricted body movement and the sequelae D *Nutrition Support:* Interventions to modify or maintain nutritional status E *Physical Comfort Promotion:* Interventions to promote comfort using physical techniques F *Self-Care Facilitation:* Interventions to provide or assist with routine activities of daily living	G *Electrolyte and Acid-Base Management:* Interventions to regulate electrolyte/acid-base balance and prevent complications H *Drug Management:* Interventions to facilitate desired effects of pharmacological agents I *Neurological Management:* Interventions to optimize neurological functions J *Perioperative Care:* Interventions to provide care before, during, and immediately after surgery K *Respiratory Management:* Interventions to promote airway patency and gas exchange L *Skin/Wound Management:* Interventions to maintain or restore tissue integrity M *Thermoregulation:* Interventions to maintain body temperature within a normal range N *Tissue Perfusion Management:* Interventions to optimize circulation of blood and fluids to the tissue	O *Behavior Therapy:* Interventions to reinforce or promote desirable behaviors or alter undesirable behaviors P *Cognitive Therapy:* Interventions to reinforce or promote desirable cognitive functioning or alter undesirable cognitive functioning Q *Communication Enhancement:* Interventions to facilitate delivering and receiving verbal and nonverbal messages R *Coping Assistance:* Interventions to assist another to build on own strengths, adapt to a change in function, or achieve a higher level of function S *Patient Education:* Interventions to facilitate learning T *Psychological Comfort Promotion:* Interventions to promote comfort using psychological techniques

From Bulechek GM, et al: *Nursing interventions classification (NIC)*, ed 5, St Louis, 2013, Mosby.

SYSTEMS FOR PLANNING NURSING CARE

In any health care setting a nurse is responsible for providing a nursing plan of care for all patients. The plan of care can take several forms (e.g., nursing Kardex, computerized plans, and standardized care plans). With the growth of EHRs within health care institutions, documentation systems typically include software programs for nursing care plans. Many of these software programs use the NANDA, NOC, and NIC taxonomies, enabling nurses to clearly identify a plan of care using appropriate nursing diagnoses, outcomes, and interventions. There is value in using standardized nursing terminologies in EHRs (Lundberg et al., 2008). Patients benefit from continuity of care being facilitated through the use of standardized terminologies that offer improved and clear communication between clinicians. Health care organizations benefit by measuring nursing care and its effects on patient care through queries of patient records instead of costly manual chart audits. The use of standardized nursing terminologies allows health care institutions to determine the impact of nursing and thus validate the contribution of nursing to health care and patient safety (Lundberg et al., 2008).

A **nursing care plan** includes nursing diagnoses, goals and/or expected outcomes, specific nursing interventions, and a section for evaluation findings so any nurse is able to quickly identify a patient's clinical needs and situation. Nurses revise a plan when a patient's status changes. Preprinted standardized care plans and EHR care plans follow a standardized format, but you can individualize each plan to a patient's unique needs (see Chapter 26). The plan gives all nurses a central document that outlines a patient's diagnoses/problems, the plan of care for each diagnosis/problem, and the outcomes for monitoring and evaluating patient progress.

In hospitals and community-based settings, patients receive care from more than one nurse, health care provider, or allied health professional. Thus more institutions are developing **interdisciplinary care plans**, which include contributions from all disciplines involved in patient care. The interdisciplinary plan focuses on patient priorities and improves the coordination of all patient therapies and communication among all disciplines.

A well-planned, comprehensive nursing care plan reduces the risk for incomplete, incorrect, or inaccurate care. As a patient's problems and status change, so does the plan. A nursing care plan is a guideline for coordinating nursing care, promoting continuity of care, and listing outcome criteria to be used later in evaluation (see Chapter 20). The plan of care communicates nursing care priorities to nurses and other health care providers. It also identifies and coordinates resources for delivering nursing care. For example, in a care plan you list specific supplies necessary to use in a dressing change or names of clinical nurse specialists who are consulting for a patient.

The nursing care plan enhances the continuity of nursing care by listing specific nursing interventions needed to achieve the goals of care. All nurses who care for a given patient carry out these nursing interventions (e.g., throughout each day during a patient's length of stay [in a hospital] or during weekly visits to the home [home health nursing]). A correctly formulated nursing care plan makes it easy to continue care from one nurse to another. The Nursing Care Plan is an example of a care plan for Mr. Lawson, using the format found throughout this text.

A care plan includes a patient's short- and long-term goals and outcomes, making it an important part of discharge planning. Thus you need to involve the family in planning care if the patient is agreeable. The family is often a resource to help a patient meet health care goals.

Domain 4	Domain 5	Domain 6	Domain 7
4. Safety	**5. Family**	**6. Health System**	**7. Community**
Care that supports protection against harm	Care that supports the family	Care that supports effective use of the health care delivery system	Care that supports the health of the community
U *Crisis Management:* Interventions to provide immediate short-term help in both psychological and physiological crises V *Risk Management:* Interventions to initiate risk-reduction activities and continue monitoring risks over time	W *Childbearing Care:* Interventions to assist in understanding and coping with the psychological and physiological changes during the childbearing period Z *Childrearing Care:* Interventions to assist in rearing children X *Life Span Care:* Interventions to facilitate family unit functioning and promote the health and welfare of family members throughout the life span	Y *Health System Mediation:* Interventions to facilitate the interface between patient/family and the health care system a *Health System Management:* Interventions to provide and enhance support services for the delivery of care b *Information Management:* Interventions to facilitate communication among health care providers	c *Community Health Promotion:* Interventions that promote the health of the whole community d *Community Risk Management:* Interventions that assist in detecting or preventing health risks to the whole community

In addition, meeting some of the family's needs can improve a patient's level of wellness. Discharge planning is especially important for a patient with a disability or injury that was not present before hospitalization. As a result, the patient must undergo long-term rehabilitation in the community and often will require home health care. Same-day surgeries and earlier discharges from hospitals require you to begin planning discharge from the moment the patient enters the health care agency. The complete care plan is the blueprint for nursing action.

Hand-off Reporting

Part of planning is transferring essential information (along with responsibility and authority) from one nurse to the next during transitions in care (e.g., end of shift, during a patient transfer to a new care unit, discharge to another setting). Hand-off reporting offers the opportunity to ask questions, clarify, and confirm important details about a patient's progress and continuing care needs. A hand-off report is the standard practice used by a nurse to communicate information about a patient's plan of care to oncoming patient care personnel. During a hand-off report always provide accurate, up-to-date, and pertinent information to the next nurse assuming patient care. The hand-off is a critical time for ensuring continuity of care for a patient and preventing errors or delays in providing nursing interventions. Recent research identifies approaches to use for effective hand-offs and barriers to their effectiveness (Riesenberg, 2012; Riesenberg et al., 2010) (Box 18-4). Written care plans organize information exchanged by nurses in hand-off reports (see Chapter 26). You learn to focus your reports on the nursing care and treatments completed, patient responses, and expected outcomes documented in the care plans.

Student Care Plans

Student care plans help you learn problem-solving techniques, the nursing process, skills of written communication, and organizational skills for nursing care. Most important, a student care plan helps you apply scientific knowledge gained from the scientific literature and the classroom to a practice situation. Students typically write a care plan for each nursing diagnosis. The student care plan is more elaborate than a care plan used in a hospital or community agency because its purpose is to teach the process of planning care. Each school uses a different format for student care plans. Often the format used is similar to the one used by the health care agency that provides students from that school their clinical experiences.

One example of a form of care plan developed by students is the five-column format. Starting from left to right, the five columns include: (1) assessment data relevant to corresponding diagnosis, (2) goals/outcomes identified for the patient, (3) implementation (selected interventions) for the plan of care, (4) a **scientific rationale** (the reason that you chose a specific nursing action, based on supporting evidence), and (5) a section to evaluate your care. The following questions help you design a plan:

- *What* is the intervention, and is it evidence based?
- *When* should each intervention be implemented?
- *How* should the intervention be performed for this specific patient?
- *Who* should be involved in each aspect of intervention?

Each scientific rationale that you use to support a nursing intervention needs to include a reference, whenever possible, to document the source from the scientific literature. This reinforces the importance of evidence-based nursing practice. It is also important that each intervention be specific and unique to a patient's situation. Nonspecific nursing interventions result in incomplete or inaccurate nursing care, lack of continuity among caregivers, and poor use of resources. Common omissions that nurses make in writing nursing interventions include action, frequency, quantity, method, or person to perform them. These errors occur when nurses are unfamiliar with the

NURSING CARE PLAN

Anxiety

ASSESSMENT

Mr. Lawson is a 62-year-old patient who had abdominal surgery for a colon resection and removal of a tumor 3 days ago. The patient has a 7.5 to 8.75 cm (3- to 3½-inch) surgical incision in the left abdominal quadrant. Previous assessment revealed a separation in the wound edges between two sutures at the bottom of the incision. Mr. Lawson knows that he will have activity restrictions. His wife will be a resource to him once he returns home. His discharge has been planned tentatively. His family still depends on his income. Now he begins to share concerns with Tonya about being able to return to work after surgery. Tonya senses that a new diagnosis might be applicable to Mr. Lawson and knows that she needs to gather additional information.

*Assessment Activities**	*Findings/Defining Characteristics*
Ask patient to clarify concerns he has about surgery.	Patient **reports concern** about his wound not healing and keeping him from being able to return to work on time. He is to return to work in 6 weeks.
Assess patient's cognitive function.	Patient **does not attend** to Tonya's explanation of risk factors for infection and shows **poor eye contact** when discussing condition.
Observe patient's emotions.	Patient is **irritable** with technicians who enter room for a blood sample.

***Defining characteristics** are shown in bold type.

NURSING DIAGNOSIS: Anxiety related to uncertainty over ability to return to work

PLANNING

Goals	*Expected Outcomes (NOC)*[†]
	Anxiety Level
Mr. Lawson will explain types of activity restrictions in context of resuming self-care at home by day of discharge.	Patient maintains attention during instruction about activity restrictions within 24 hours. Patient shows eye contact during scheduled instructional sessions within 24 hours. Patient shows less facial tension during discussions in 24 hours.
	Information Processing
Mr. Lawson will demonstrate proper wound care approach (see plan for knowledge enhancement) by day of discharge.	Patient describes reason for activity restriction by day of discharge. Patient describes steps of wound care 24 hours before discharge.
	Coping
Mr. Lawson will verbalize acceptance of need to gain full recovery before returning to work by day of discharge.	Patient shares concerns about work with wife by day of discharge.

[†]Outcomes classification labels from Moorhead S, et al: *Nursing outcomes classification (NOC),* ed 5, St Louis, 2013, Mosby.

INTERVENTIONS (NIC)[‡]	**RATIONALE**
Anxiety Reduction	
Use a calm, reassuring approach during discussions and instruction.	For patient to be able to express concerns and ask questions, he must see nurse as being nonthreatening, reliable, and understanding (Vacarolis and Halter, 2014).
Encourage Mrs. Lawson to stay with her husband as much as possible; include her in discussions.	A support system benefits a patient experiencing stress. Strong families tend to have good problem-solving skills and a commitment to one another (Schumacher et al., 2006).
Collaborate with health care provider to provide factual information concerning activity restrictions, progress of wound healing, and expectations for ability to return to work.	Facts provide patient with a more objective view of feasibility of returning to work as anticipated.
Confirm with patient that following postoperative care guidelines will improve likelihood of recovery and ability to return to work.	When comparing people with similar degrees of functional impairment, people with optimistic expectations recover more quickly by using coping strategies and have a higher quality of life (Conversano et al., 2010).

[‡]Intervention classification labels from Bulechek GM, et al: *Nursing interventions classification (NIC),* ed 6, St Louis, 2013, Mosby.

EVALUATION

Nursing Actions	*Patient Response/Finding*	*Achievement of Outcome*
Ask Mr. Lawson to explain the types of activity restrictions he will have when going home.	Mr. Lawson reports that his surgeon has told him that he must limit lifting objects greater than 30 lbs for 6 weeks to reduce stress on the suture line.	Outcome achieved.
Have Mr. Lawson explain his thoughts about needing to recover fully before returning to work. Observe his behavior during discussion.	Mr. Lawson is able to attend to discussion about his recovery and shows good eye contact. He has some worries about whether he will be able to perform normally at his job.	Patient's level of anxiety is declining. Continue discussion about what he will be able to do at 6 weeks.

BOX 18-4 EVIDENCE-BASED PRACTICE

Nursing Hand-off Reports

PICO Question: Does the use of bedside hand-off communication compared with traditional end-of shift report between nurses in acute care settings reduce errors?

Evidence Summary

A nursing hand-off during change of shift involves a nurse-to-nurse verbal exchange of information about patients. The Agency for Healthcare Research and Quality (AHRQ, 2011) surveyed 1032 hospitals, with over 50% of staff respondents agreeing that important patient care information is often lost during shift changes. Athwal et al. (2009) found that a combination of a written update along with a bedside hand-off report reduced the total time expended for shift report, reduced nurse overtime hours, and led to fewer times patients used call lights. A systematic review of scientific articles discussing nursing hand-offs identified strategies for and barriers to effective hand-offs (Riesenberg et al., 2010). Research suggests that there is no evidence pointing to the best nursing hand-off practices and whether errors are reduced. However, hand-offs have multiple purposes, including information transfer, shared decision making, review of treatment options, and shared planning (Riesenberg, 2012). Carefully consider the following strategies and decide if they are useful and if they fit your own institutional setting and resources.

Application to Nursing Practice

Strategies for Effective Nursing Hand-offs

- Do prework; manage your time so you are prepared to give report and be concise.
- Keep report patient centered; ask questions and clarify.
- Standardize the process using tools, forms, and checklists and be sure that essential information is consistently included.
- During walking rounds include patient and family in discussion of goals.
- Limit interruptions and distraction.
- Acknowledge information received and transfer of responsibility (Riesenberg, 2012)

Barriers to Effective Nursing Hand-offs

- Communication barriers, including omissions (missing or incomplete information), errors (incorrect, extraneous, duplicate), disorganized report or one that is routine and not individualized
- Social problems, including a culture of blame on unit that inhibits questioning
- Complexity of cases and high patient care load—increased volume of patient information and inadequate time to report

TABLE 18-4 Frequent Errors in Writing Nursing Interventions

Type of Error	Incorrectly Stated Nursing Intervention	Correctly Stated Nursing Intervention
Failure to precisely or completely indicate nursing actions	Perform exercises on left lower extremity.	Perform ROM for flexion and extension of right knee; plantar flexion and dorsiflexion of right ankle 3 times a day.
Failure to indicate frequency	Perform blood glucose measurements.	Measure blood glucose before each meal: 0700—1100—1700.
Failure to indicate quantity	Irrigate wound once a shift: 0600—1400—2000.	Irrigate wound with 100 mL normal saline until clear: 0600—1400—2000.
Failure to indicate method	Change patient's dressing daily.	Apply a transparent dressing to skin tear site daily.

ROM, Range of motion.

planning process. Table 18-4 illustrates these types of errors by showing incorrect and correct statements of nursing interventions. The fifth column of the care plan includes a section for you to evaluate the plan of care: was each goal/outcome fully or only partially met? Use the evaluation column to document whether the plan requires revision or when outcomes are met, thus indicating when a particular nursing diagnosis is no longer relevant to a patient's plan of care (see Chapter 20).

Care Plans for Community-Based Settings. Planning care for patients in community-based settings (e.g., clinics, community centers, or patients' homes) applies the same principles of nursing practice. However, in these settings you need to complete a more comprehensive community, home, and family assessment. Ultimately a patient/family unit must be able to provide the majority of health care independently. You design a plan to (1) educate the patient/family about the necessary care techniques and precautions, (2) teach a patient/family how to integrate care within family activities, and (3) guide the patient/family on how to assume a greater percentage of care over time. Finally the plan includes nurses' and the patient's/family's evaluation of expected outcomes.

Concept Maps

Chapter 16 first described concept maps and their use in the nursing process. Because you care for patients who have multiple health problems and related nursing diagnoses, it is often not realistic to have a written columnar plan developed for each nursing diagnosis. In addition, the columnar plans do not contain a means to show the association between different nursing diagnoses and different nursing interventions. A concept map is a visual representation of all of a patient's nursing diagnoses and allows you to diagram interventions for each. Research shows that use of concept maps help nursing students make better clinical decisions and develop better clinical judgment skills (Gerdeman et al., 2013). A map shows you the relationship within the nursing process (i.e., how nursing interventions often apply to more than one nursing diagnosis). Concept maps group and categorize nursing concepts to give you a holistic view of your patient's health care needs.

In Chapter 17 you learned how to add nursing diagnostic labels to a concept map. When planning care for each nursing diagnosis, analyze the relationships among the diagnoses. Draw dotted lines between nursing diagnoses to indicate their relationship to one another (Figure 18-3). It is important for you to make meaningful associations between

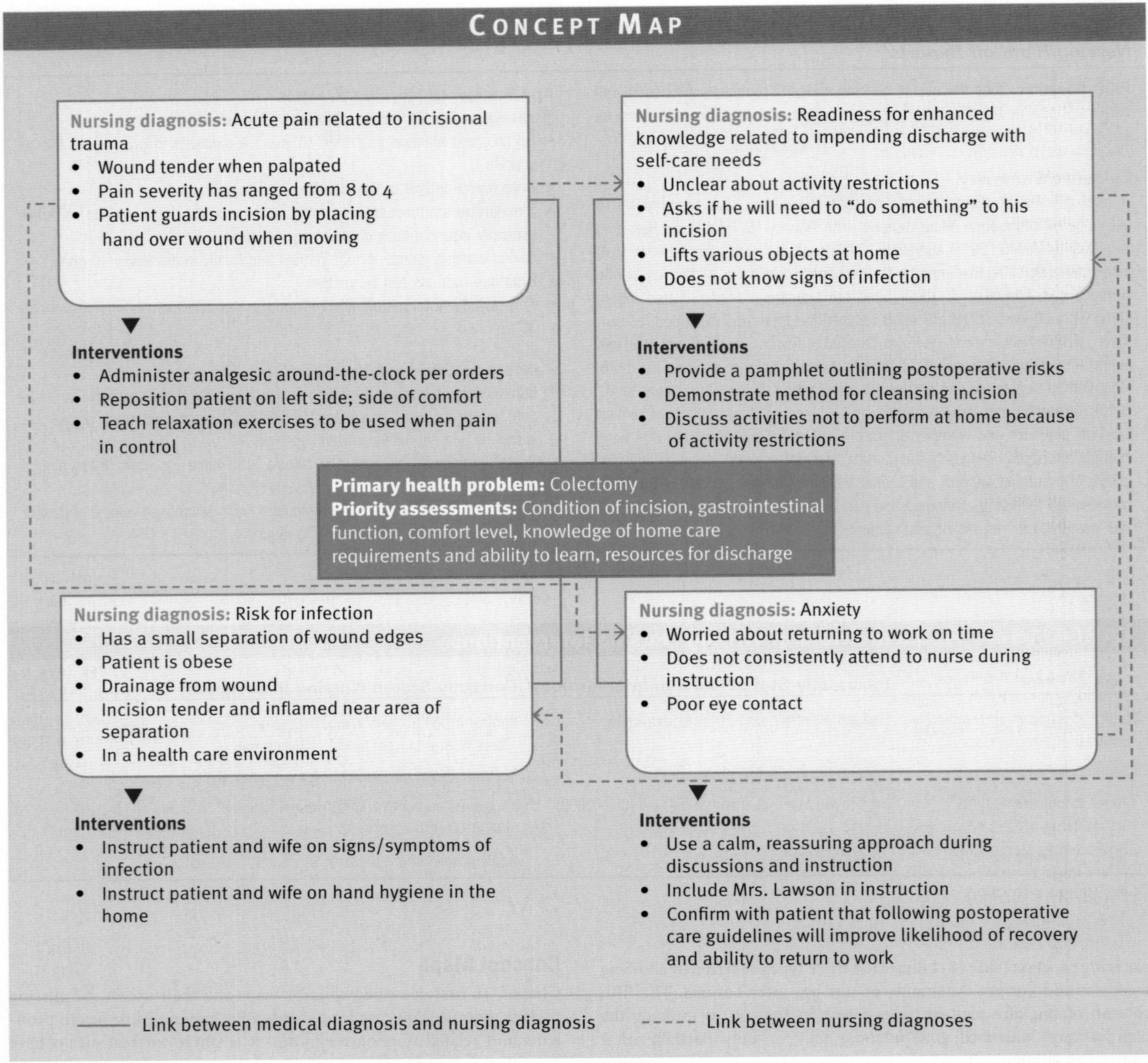

FIGURE 18-3 Concept map for Mr. Lawson: Planning.

one concept and another. The links need to be accurate, meaningful, and complete so you can explain why nursing diagnoses are related. Mr. Lawson's concept map has a new, fourth nursing diagnosis, *Anxiety*. Mr. Lawson's *Anxiety* and *Acute Pain* are interrelated; in addition, *Acute Pain* has an influence on his *Readiness for Enhanced Learning*.

Finally, on a separate sheet of paper or on the map itself, list nursing interventions to attain the measurable outcomes for each nursing diagnosis. This step corresponds to the planning phase of the nursing process. While caring for a patient, use the map to write his or her responses to each nursing activity. Also write your clinical impressions and inferences regarding the patient's progress toward expected outcomes and the effectiveness of interventions. Keep the concept map with you throughout the clinical day. As you revise the plan, take notes and add or delete nursing interventions. Use the information recorded on the map to document patient care. Critical thinkers learn by organizing and relating cognitive concepts. Concept maps help you learn the interrelationships among nursing diagnoses to create a unique meaning and organization of information collected.

CONSULTING WITH OTHER HEALTH CARE PROFESSIONALS

Planning involves consultation with members of the health care team when you face problems in providing nursing or collaborative care. Consultation occurs at any step in the nursing process, but you consult most often during planning and implementation. During these times you are more likely to identify a problem requiring additional knowledge, skills, or resources. One way to consult is using the SBAR approach, a mechanism for framing conversations, especially critical ones, requiring a clinician's immediate attention and action (see Chapter 26). SBAR is an acronym for *S*ituation, *B*ackground, *A*ssessment, and *R*ecommendation.

Consultation requires you to be aware of your strengths and limitations as a team member. During a **consultation** you seek the expertise of a specialist such as your nursing instructor, a health care provider, or a clinical nurse educator to identify ways to handle problems in patient management or the planning and implementation of therapies. The consultation process is important so all health care providers are focused on common patient goals and outcomes. Be prepared before you make a consultation. Consultation is based on the problem-solving approach, and the consultant is the stimulus for change.

An experienced nurse is a valuable consultant when you face an unfamiliar patient care situation such as a new procedure or a patient presenting a set of symptoms that you cannot identify. In clinical nursing consultation helps to solve problems in the delivery of nursing care. For example, a nursing student consults a clinical specialist for wound care techniques or an educator for useful teaching resources. Nurses are consulted for their clinical expertise, patient education skills, or staff education skills. Nurses also consult with other members of the health care team such as physical therapists, nutritionists, and social workers.

QSEN QSEN: BUILDING COMPETENCY IN TEAMWORK AND COLLABORATION Mr. Lawson's concept map includes the nursing diagnosis of *Anxiety related to uncertainty over ability to return to work.* How would you apply principles of teamwork and collaboration in planning interventions for this diagnosis?

Answers to QSEN Activities can be found on the Evolve website.

When to Consult

Consultation occurs when you identify a problem that you are unable to solve using personal knowledge, skills, and resources. The process requires good interprofessional collaboration. Consultation with other care providers increases your knowledge about a patient's problems and helps you learn skills and obtain resources. A good time to consult with another health care provider is when the exact problem remains unclear. An objective consultant enters a clinical situation and more clearly assesses and identifies the nature of a problem, whether it is patient, personnel, or equipment oriented. Most often you consult with health care providers who are working in your clinical area. However, sometimes you consult over the telephone (Box 18-5).

How to Consult

Begin with your own understanding of a patient's clinical problems. The first step in making a consultation is to assess the situation and identify the general problem area. Second, direct the consultation to the right professional such as another nurse or social worker. Third, provide a consultant with relevant information about the problem area and seek a solution. Include a brief summary of the problem, methods used to resolve the problem so far, and outcomes of these methods. Also share information from the patient's medical record, conversations with other nurses, and the patient's family. Fourth, do not prejudice or influence consultants. Consultants are in the clinical setting to help identify and resolve a nursing problem, and biasing or prejudicing them blocks problem resolution. Avoid bias by not overloading consultants with subjective and emotional conclusions about the patient and the problem.

BOX 18-5 Tips for Making Phone Consultations

- Have the information you need available BEFORE you make a call. At a minimum have the medical record, medication sheets (if the consultation is about a medicine), and any notes on recent care activities.
- Assess the patient yourself before making the call. For example, when you consult with health care providers, they rely heavily on your assessment so they can give appropriate advice.
- Address both the clinical history and patient's perspective, including social and cultural context.
- Give a diagnosis or interpretation of the patient's problem with an explanation or a summary. Use of the SBAR (*S*ituation-*B*ackground-*A*ssessment-*R*ecommendation) approach in reporting is helpful (see Chapter 26).
- Understand why you are calling for consultation and think through some possible solutions. Your experience in caring for the patient allows you to make useful suggestions.

Data from Maison D: Effective communications are more important than ever: a health care provider's perspective, *J Home Care Hospice Professional* 24(3):178, 2006; Males T: In the dark: risks of telephone consultations, *Sessional GP* 4(2):2012, http://www.medicalprotection.org/docs/default-source/pdfs/uk-sessional-gp/oct-2012.pdf. Accessed July 21, 2014.

Fifth, be available to discuss a consultant's findings and recommendations. Provide a private, comfortable atmosphere for the consultant and patient to meet. However, this does not mean that you leave the environment. A common mistake is turning the whole problem over to the consultant. The consultant is not there to take over the problem but to help you resolve it. When possible, request the consultation for a time when both you and the consultant are able to discuss the patient's situation with minimal interruptions or distractions. Finally, incorporate the consultant's recommendations into the care plan. The success of the advice depends on the implementation of the problem-solving techniques. Always give the consultant feedback regarding the outcome of the recommendations.

KEY POINTS

- After identifying a patient's nursing diagnoses and collaborative problems, establish a plan of care that prioritizes the diagnoses and establishes nursing interventions, patient-centered goals, and expected outcomes.
- Planning involves individualizing a plan of care for a patient's unique needs.
- Priority setting is the ordering of nursing diagnoses or patient problems using notions of urgency and importance to establish a preferential order for nursing actions.
- Priorities help you anticipate and sequence nursing interventions when a patient has multiple nursing diagnoses and collaborative problems.
- A patient-centered goal or outcome reflects a patient's specific behavior, not your own goals or interventions.
- The use of goals and outcomes in patient care is designed to focus the efforts of all health care team members on a common purpose.
- Outcomes provide the desired physiological, psychological, social, developmental, or spiritual responses that indicate resolution of a patient's health problems.
- When writing goals and outcomes, use the SMART acronym: *S*pecific, *M*easurable, *A*ttainable, *R*ealistic, and *T*imed.

- During planning select interventions designed to help a patient move from the present level of health to the level described in the goal and measured by the expected outcomes.
- Independent nursing interventions are actions that a nurse initiates without supervision or direction from others, are autonomous based on scientific rationale, and do not require an order from another health care provider.
- Health care provider-initiated interventions require specific nursing responsibilities and technical nursing knowledge.
- Care plans increase communication among nurses and facilitate the continuity of care from one nurse to another and from one health care setting to another.
- A nurse hand-off transfers essential information (along with responsibility and authority) from one nurse to the next during transitions in care and allows you to ask questions, clarify, and confirm important details.
- A concept map is a visual representation of a patient's nursing diagnoses with links to nursing interventions, helping you learn to make better clinical decisions.
- The NIC taxonomy provides a standardization to help nurses select suitable interventions for patients' problems.
- Correctly written nursing interventions include actions, frequency, quantity, method, and the person to perform them.

CLINICAL APPLICATION QUESTIONS

Preparing for Clinical Practice

Tonya formally plans Mr. Lawson's care. For the nursing diagnosis of *Acute Pain related to trauma of surgical incision,* Tonya identifies the goal of "Patient will use relaxation technique after ambulation"; and the outcome she lists is, "Patient reports pain below level of 4 and does not splint incision when moving within 48 hours." The interventions she selects for her plan include administering the ordered analgesic, progressive relaxation, and splinting the incision when the patient gets out of bed.

1. Critique the goal and outcomes that Tonya set and explain if they were written correctly. If they are incorrect, how could you reword them so they are correctly stated?
2. Among the interventions that Tonya selected, which ones are independent, dependent, and collaborative?
3. If Tonya were to write on the patient's care plan, "use progressive relaxation," would that be an accurate way of writing an intervention? If not, which error(s) has been made?

Ⓔ *Answers to Clinical Application Questions can be found on the Evolve website.*

REVIEW QUESTIONS

Are You Ready to Test Your Nursing Knowledge?

1. A nurse enters the room of a 32-year-old patient newly diagnosed with cancer at the beginning of the 0700 evening/night shift. The nurse noted in the patient's nursing history that this is her first hospitalization. She is scheduled for surgery in the morning to remove a tumor and has questions about what to expect after surgery. She is observed talking with her mother and is crying. The patient says, "This is so unfair." An order has been written for an enema to be given this evening in preparation for the surgery. The nurse establishes priorities for which of the following situations first?
   1. Giving the enema on time
   2. Talking with the patient about her past experiences with illness
   3. Talking with the patient about her concerns and acknowledging her sense of unfairness
   4. Beginning instruction on postoperative procedures
2. A 62-year-old patient had a portion of the large colon removed and a colostomy created for drainage of stool. The nurse has had repeated problems with the patient's colostomy bag not adhering to the skin and thus leaking. The nurse wants to consult with the wound care nurse specialist. Which of the following should the nurse do? (Select all that apply.)
   1. Assess condition of skin before making the call
   2. Rely on the nurse specialist to know the type of surgery the patient likely had
   3. Explain the patient's response emotionally to the repeated leaking of stool
   4. Describe the type of bag being used and how long it lasts before leaking
   5. Order extra colostomy bags currently being used
3. It is time for a nurse hand-off between the night nurse and nurse starting the day shift. The night nurse checks the most recent laboratory results for the patient and then begins to discuss the patient's plan of care to the day nurse using the standard checklist for reporting essential information. The patient has been seriously ill, and his wife is at the bedside. The nurse asks the wife to leave the room for just a few minutes. The night nurse completes the summary of care before the day nurse is able to ask a question. Which of the following activities are strategies for an effective hand-off? (Select all that apply.)
   1. Using a standardized checklist for essential information
   2. Asking the wife to briefly leave the room
   3. Completing the hand-off without inviting questions
   4. Doing prework such as checking laboratory results before giving a report
   5. Including the wife in the hand-off discussion
4. A nurse assesses a 78-year-old patient who weighs 108.9 kg (240 lbs) and is partially immobilized because of a stroke. The nurse turns the patient and finds that the skin over the sacrum is very red and the patient does not feel sensation in the area. The patient has had fecal incontinence on and off for the last 2 days. The nurse identifies the nursing diagnosis of *Risk for Impaired Skin Integrity*. Which of the following outcomes is appropriate for the patient?
   1. Patient will be turned every 2 hours within 24 hours.
   2. Patient will have normal bowel function within 72 hours.
   3. Patient's skin integrity will remain intact through discharge.
   4. Erythema of skin will be mild to none within 48 hours.
5. Which of the following factors does a nurse consider in setting priorities for a patient's nursing diagnoses? (Select all that apply.)
   1. Numbered order of diagnosis on the basis of severity
   2. Notion of urgency for nursing action
   3. Symptom pattern recognition suggesting a problem
   4. Mutually agreed on priorities set with patient
   5. Time when a specific diagnosis was identified
6. A home health nurse visits a 42-year-old woman with diabetes who has a recurrent foot ulcer. The ulcer has prevented the woman from working for over 2 weeks. The patient has had diabetes for 10 years. The ulcer has not been healing; it has drainage with a foul-smelling odor. As the nurse examines the patient, she learns that the patient is not following the ordered diabetic diet. Which of the following is considered a low-priority goal for this patient?
   1. Achieving wound healing of the foot ulcer
   2. Enhancing patient knowledge about the effects of diabetes

3. Providing a dietitian consultation for diet retraining
4. Improving patient adherence to diabetic diet

7. The nurse writes an expected outcome statement in measurable terms. An example is:
   1. Patient will have normal stool evacuation.
   2. Patient will have fewer bowel movements.
   3. Patient will take stool softener every 4 hours.
   4. Patient will report stool soft and formed with each defecation.
8. A patient has the nursing diagnosis of *Nausea*. The nurse develops a care plan with the following interventions. Which are examples of collaborative interventions? (Select all that apply.)
   1. Providing mouth care every 4 hours
   2. Maintaining intravenous (IV) infusion at 100 mL/hr
   3. Administering prochlorperazine (Compazine) via rectal suppository
   4. Consulting with dietitian on initial foods to offer patient
   5. Controlling aversive odors or unpleasant visual stimulation that triggers nausea
9. An 82-year-old patient who resides in a nursing home has the following three nursing diagnoses: *Risk for Fall, Impaired Physical Mobility related to pain,* and *Imbalanced Nutrition: Less Than Body Requirements related to reduced ability to feed self.* The nursing staff identified several goals of care. Match the goals on the left with the appropriate outcome statements on the right.

Goals	**Outcomes**
1. _____ Patient will ambulate independently in 3 days.	a. Patient expresses fewer nonverbal signs of discomfort within 24 hrs.
2. _____ Patient will be injury free for 1 month.	b. Patient increases calorie intake to 2500 daily.
3. _____ Patient will achieve 5-lb weight gain in 1 month.	c. Patient walks 20 feet using a walker in 24 hrs.
4. _____ Patient will achieve pain relief by discharge.	d. Patient identifies barriers to remove in the home within 1 week.

10. Which of the following factors does a nurse consider for a patient with the nursing diagnosis of *Disturbed Sleep Pattern related to noisy home environment* in choosing an intervention for enhancing the patient's sleep? (Select all that apply.)
    1. The intervention should be directed at reducing noise.
    2. The intervention should be one shown to be effective in promoting sleep on the basis of research.
    3. The intervention should be one commonly used by the patient's sleep partner.
    4. The intervention should be one acceptable to the patient.
    5. The intervention should be one you used with other patients in the past.
11. A nurse begins the night shift being assigned to five patients. She learns that the floor will be a registered nurse (RN) short as a result of a call in. A patient care technician from another area is coming to the nursing unit to assist. The nurse is required to do hourly rounds on all patients, so she begins rounds on the patient who has recently asked for a pain medication. As the nurse begins to approach the patient's room, a nurse stops her in the hallway to ask about another patient. Which factors in this nurse's unit environment will affect her ability to set priorities? (Select all that apply.)
    1. Policy for conducting hourly rounds
    2. Staffing level
    3. Interruption by staff nurse colleague
    4. RN's years of experience
    5. Competency of patient care technician
12. A nursing student is reporting during hand-off to the registered nurse (RN) assuming her patient's care. The student states, "Mr. Roarke had a good day, his intravenous (IV) fluid is infusing at 124 mL/hr with D_5½NS infusing in right forearm. The IV site is intact, and no complaints of tenderness. I ambulated him twice during the shift; he tolerated well walking to end of hall and back with no shortness of breath. He still uses his cane without difficulty. Mr. Roarke said he slept better last night after I closed his door and gave him a chance to be uninterrupted. If the nurse's goal for Mr. Roarke was to improve activity tolerance, which expected outcomes were shared in the hand-off? (Select all that apply.)
    1. IV site not tender
    2. Uses cane to walk
    3. Walked to end of hall
    4. No shortness of breath
    5. Slept better during night
13. A nursing student is reporting during hand-off to the RN assuming her patient's care. She explains, "I ambulated him twice during the shift; he tolerated well walking to end of hall and back with no shortness of breath. Mr. Roarke said he slept better last night after I closed his door and gave him a chance to be uninterrupted. I changed the dressing over his intravenous (IV) site and started a new bag of D_5½NS. Which intervention is a dependent intervention?
    1. Reporting hand-off at change of shift
    2. Ambulating patient down hallway
    3. Sleep hygiene
    4. IV fluid administration
14. A nursing student knows that all patients should be ambulated regularly. The patient to which she is assigned has had reduced activity tolerance. She followed orders to ambulate the patient twice during the shift of care. In what way can the nursing student make the goal of improving the patient's activity tolerance a patient-centered effort?
    1. Engage the patient in setting mutual outcomes for distance he is able to walk
    2. Confirm with the patient's health care provider about ambulation goals
    3. Have physical therapy assist with ambulation
    4. Refer to medical record regarding nature of patient's physical problem
15. A patient signals the nurse by turning on the call light. The nurse enters the room and finds the patient's drainage tube disconnected, 100 mL of fluid remaining in the intravenous (IV) line, and the patient asking questions about whether his doctor is coming. Which of the following does the nurse perform first?
    1. Reconnect the drainage tubing
    2. Inspect the condition of the IV dressing
    3. Obtain the next IV fluid bag from the medication room
    4. Explain when the health care provider is likely to visit

Answers: 1. 3; **2.** 1, 3, 4; **3.** 1, 4, 5; **4.** 4; **5.** 2, 3, 4; **6.** 2; **7.** 4; **8.** 2, 4; **9.** 1c, 2d, 3b, 4a; **10.** 1, 2, 4; **11.** 1, 2, 3; **12.** 3, 4; **13.** 4; **14.** 1; **15.** 1.

Rationales for Review Questions can be found on the Evolve website.

REFERENCES

Ackley BJ, Ladwig GB: *Nursing diagnosis handbook*, ed 10, St Louis, 2014, Mosby.

Agency for Healthcare Research and Quality (AHRQ): *Hospital survey on patient safety culture: 2011 user comparative database report*, 2011, http://www.ahrq.gov/professionals/quality-patient-safety/patientsafetyculture/hospital/2011/index.html. Accessed July 21, 2014.

Bulechek GM, et al: *Nursing interventions classification (NIC)*, ed 6, St Louis, 2013, Mosby.

Carpenito-Moyet LJ: *Nursing diagnoses: application to clinical practice*, ed 14, Philadelphia, 2013, Lippincott, Williams & Wilkins.

Conversano C, et al: Optimism and its impact on mental and physical well-being, *Clin Pract Epidemiol Ment Health* 6:25, 2010.

Lundberg C, et al: Selecting a standardized terminology for the electronic health record that reveals the impact of nursing on patient care, *Online J Nurs Inform* 12(2):2008. Available at: http://www.ojni.org/12_2/lundberg.pdf. Accessed February 15, 2015.

Moorhead S, et al: *Nursing outcomes classification*, ed 5, St Louis, 2013, Mosby.

NANDA International (NANDA-I): *Nursing diagnoses: definitions and classification 2012–2014*, United Kingdom, 2012, Wiley-Blackwell.

Nelson JL, et al: Teaching prioritization skills, *J Nurses Staff Dev* 22(4):172, 2006.

Schumacher K, et al: Family caregivers, *Am J Nurs* 106(8):40, 2006.

Vacarolis EM, Halter MJ: *Essentials of psychiatric mental health nursing: a communication approach to evidence-based care*, ed 7, St Louis, 2014, Saunders.

RESEARCH REFERENCES

Athwal P, et al: Standardization of change-of-shift report, *J Nurs Care Qual* 24(2):143, 2009.

Benner P, et al: *Expertise in nursing practice: caring, clinical judgment and ethics*, New York, 1996, Springer.

Gerdeman JL, et al: Using concept mapping to build clinical judgment skills, *Nurse Educ Pract* 13(1):11, 2013.

Park H: Nursing-sensitive outcome change scores for hospitalized older adults with heart failure: a preliminary descriptive study, *Res Gerontol Nurs* 6(4):234, 2013.

Potter P, et al: Understanding the cognitive work of nursing in the acute care environment, *J Nurs Adm* 35(7/8):327, 2005.

Riesenberg LA: Shift-to-shift handoff research: Where do we go from here? *J Grad Med Educ* 4(1):4, 2012.

Riesenberg LA, et al: Nursing handoffs: a systematic review of the literature, *Am J Nurs* 110(4):24, 2010.

Suhonen R, et al: Nurses' perceptions of individualised care: an international comparison, *J Adv Nurs* 67(9):1895, 2011.

Tanner CA: Thinking like a nurse: a research-based model of clinical judgment in nursing, *J Nurs Educ* 45(6):2004, 2006.

19

Implementing Nursing Care

OBJECTIVES

- Explain the relationship of implementation to the nursing diagnostic process.
- Describe the association between critical thinking and selecting nursing interventions.
- Discuss the differences between protocols and standing orders.
- Discuss the influence of organizational culture on interdisciplinary collaboration.
- Discuss the value of the Nursing Interventions Classification system in documenting nursing care.
- Discuss the steps for revising a plan of care before performing implementation.
- Define the three implementation skills.
- Describe and compare direct and indirect nursing interventions.
- Select appropriate interventions for a patient.

KEY TERMS

Activities of daily living (ADLs), p. 264
Adverse reaction, p. 265
Clinical practice guideline, p. 258
Counseling, p. 265
Direct care, p. 257
Implementation, p. 257
Indirect care, p. 257
Instrumental activities of daily living (IADLs), p. 264
Interdisciplinary care plans, p. 266
Lifesaving measure, p. 264
Nursing intervention, p. 257
Patient adherence, p. 267
Preventive nursing actions, p. 266
Standing order, p. 258

MEDIA RESOURCES

http://evolve.elsevier.com/Potter/fundamentals/

- Review Questions
- Concept Map Creator
- Case Study with Questions
- Audio Glossary
- Content Updates

You first met Tonya and Mr. Lawson in Chapter 15. Mr. Lawson is a 68-year-old patient who had abdominal surgery for a colon resection and is preparing to be discharged soon from the hospital. His nurse Tonya developed a plan of care to address four different nursing diagnoses: ***Acute Pain, Anxiety, Readiness for Enhanced Knowledge,*** *and* ***Risk for Infection.*** *Mr. Lawson is interested in learning about his postoperative activity restrictions and being able to care for his incision, which had a small separation. He also shared with Tonya that he is worried about being able to return to work after surgery. Tonya and the other nursing staff have consistently applied the nursing process. Tonya identified the diagnosis of* ***Anxiety*** *while planning for Mr. and Mrs. Lawson's education. During implementation Tonya will provide planned interventions, along with her health care colleagues, to achieve the goals and expected outcomes identified in Mr. Lawson's plan of care. Critical thinking, which includes good clinical decision making, is important for the successful implementation of nursing interventions.*

Implementation, the fourth step of the nursing process, formally begins after you develop a plan of care. With a care plan based on clear and relevant nursing diagnoses, you initiate interventions designed to help a patient achieve the goals and expected outcomes needed to support or improve the patient's health status. A **nursing intervention** is any treatment based on clinical judgment and knowledge that a nurse performs to enhance patient outcomes (Bulechek et al., 2013). Ideally nursing interventions are evidence based (see Chapter 5), providing the most current, up-to-date, and effective approaches for delivering patient-centered care. Nursing interventions include direct and indirect care measures aimed at individuals, families, and/or the community.

Direct care interventions are treatments performed through interactions with patients (Bulechek et al., 2013). For example, a patient receives direct intervention in the form of medication administration, insertion of a urinary catheter, discharge instruction, or counseling during a time of grief. **Indirect care** interventions are treatments performed away from a patient but on behalf of the patient or group of patients (e.g., managing a patient's environment [e.g., safety and infection control]), documentation, and interdisciplinary collaboration (Bulechek et al., 2013). Both direct and indirect care measures fall under the intervention categories described in Chapter 18: nurse-initiated, health care provider–initiated, and collaborative. For example, the direct intervention of patient education is a nurse-initiated intervention. The indirect intervention of consultation is a collaborative intervention.

Dr. Patricia Benner (1984) defined the domains of nursing practice, which explain the nature and intent of the many ways nurses intervene for patients (Box 19-1). These domains are current today. However, the extent of organizational and work role competencies in health care has become more complex, making it a challenge to fulfill each domain of practice. Nurses are required to have effective organizational skills and maintain competencies in advanced nursing care.

BOX 19-1 Domains of Nursing Practice

- The Helping Role
- The Teaching-Coaching Function
- The Diagnostic and Patient-Monitoring Function
- Effective Management of Rapidly Changing Situations
- Administering and Monitoring Therapeutic Interventions and Regimens
- Monitoring and Ensuring the Quality of Health Care Practices
- Organizational and Work-Role Competencies

From Benner P: *From novice to expert,* Menlo Park, CA, 1984, Addison Wesley.

In addition, nurses must be able to manage conflict and effectively advocate for patients in challenging interdisciplinary relationships. Thus it is important for implementation to be patient-centered. Nursing is an art and a science. It is not simply a task-based profession. You must learn to intervene for a patient within the context of his or her unique situation. Consider these factors during implementation: Who is the patient? How do a patient's attitudes, values, and cultural background affect how you provide care? What does an illness mean to a patient and his or her family? Which clinical situation requires you to intervene? How does a patient perceive the interventions that you will deliver? In what way do you best support or show caring as you intervene? The answers to these questions enable you to deliver care compassionately and effectively with the best outcomes for your patients.

STANDARD NURSING INTERVENTIONS

Health care settings offer various ways for nurses to create and individualize patients' care plans. It is critical for each patient to have his or her unique set of interventions. However, many health care systems have mechanisms for standardizing the more common types of interventions. Many patients have common health problems; thus standardized interventions make it quicker and easier for nurses to intervene. More important, if the standards are evidence-based, you are likely to deliver the most clinically effective care that will result in the best patient outcomes (see Chapter 5). As a nurse, you are accountable for individualizing standardized interventions as necessary.

Standardized interventions most often set a level of clinical excellence for practice. Nurse- and health care provider–initiated standardized interventions are available in the form of clinical guidelines or protocols, preprinted (standing) orders, and Nursing Interventions Classification (NIC) interventions. At a professional level the American Nurses Association (ANA) defines standards of professional nursing practice, which include standards for the implementation step of the nursing process. The Quality and Safety Education for Nurses (QSEN) defines skills competencies. These standards are authoritative statements of the duties that all registered nurses (RNs) are expected to perform competently, regardless of role, patient population they serve, or specialty (ANA, 2010) (see Chapter 1).

Clinical Practice Guidelines and Protocols

A clinical practice guideline or protocol is a systematically developed set of statements that helps nurses, physicians, and other health care providers make decisions about appropriate health care for specific clinical situations (Manchikanti et al., 2010). Evidence-based research provides the basis for sound clinical practice guidelines and associated recommendations that often improves quality of care (AHRQ, 2014a). A guideline establishes interventions for specific health care problems or conditions. A nurse individualizes how to apply interventions for each unique patient. The National Guidelines Clearinghouse (NGC) is a public resource for evidence-based clinical practice guidelines (AHRQ, 2014b). The NGC guidelines are linked to a particular term derived from the U.S. National Library of Medicine (NLM) Medical Subject Headings (MeSH), a controlled vocabulary for disease/condition, treatment/intervention, and health services administration. You can access guidelines for patients with a wide variety of conditions and problems such as arthritis, wounds and injuries, and pain management. These guidelines are readily available to any clinician or health care institution.

Clinicians within a health care agency sometimes review the scientific literature and their own standard of practice to develop guidelines and protocols in an effort to improve the standard of care at their facility. For example, a hospital develops a rapid-assessment protocol to improve the identification and early treatment of patients suspected of having a stroke or sepsis. Many times clinicians will develop guidelines that incorporate standards unique to their organizational processes and guidelines from national health groups such as the National Institutes of Health (NIH) and the NGC. Another valuable source for nursing practice guidelines is the University of Iowa (n.d.) Hartford Center, which develops evidence-based practice (EBP) guidelines for geriatric nursing. The center has numerous clinical guidelines, including ones for acute confusion and delirium, acute pain management, and fall prevention for older adults.

Advanced practice nurses (APNs) who provide primary care for patients in a variety of settings frequently follow diagnostic and treatment protocols for their interventions. A collaborative agreement with a physician identifies protocols for the medical conditions that APNs are permitted to treat such as controlled hypertension and the types of treatment that they are permitted to administer such as antihypertensive medications. These state-derived protocols vary from state to state. APNs are also able to act independently, developing and applying clinical protocols that outline independent nursing interventions. For example, in the long-term setting scientifically based protocols for incontinence, pressure ulcers, depression, and aggressive behavior are common. Databases such as Up-to-Date and the Cochrane library provide valuable treatment guidelines supported by rigorous systematic reviews to provide evidence-based treatment guidelines.

Standing Orders

A standing order is a preprinted document containing orders for routine therapies, monitoring guidelines, and/or diagnostic procedures for specific patients with identified clinical problems. A standing order directs patient care in a specific clinical setting. Licensed prescribing health care providers in charge of care at the time of implementation approve and sign standing orders. These orders are common in critical care settings and other specialized acute care settings where patients' needs change rapidly and require immediate attention. An example of such a standing order is one specifying certain medications such as diltiazem (Cardizem) and amiodarone (Cordarone) for an irregular heart rhythm. A critical care nurse compares assessment data to the protocol criteria and implements the protocol without first notifying the physician. The physician's initial standing order covers the nurse's action. After completing a standing order, the nurse notifies the physician in case further treatment is needed. Standing orders are also common in community health settings, where nurses face situations that do not permit immediate contact with a health care provider. Standing orders give nurses legal protection to intervene appropriately in the best interests of patients with rapidly changing needs.

BOX 19-2 Purposes of Nursing Interventions Classification (NIC)

1. Standardizing the nomenclature (e.g., labeling, describing) of nursing interventions; standardizes the language nurses use to describe sets of actions in delivering patient care
2. Expanding nursing knowledge about connections among nursing diagnoses, treatments, and outcomes; connections determined through the study of actual patient care using a database that the classification generates
3. Developing NIC language into software of health care information systems
4. Teaching decision making to nursing students; defining and classifying nursing interventions to teach beginning nurses how to determine a patient's need for care and respond appropriately
5. Determining the cost of services provided by nurses
6. Standardizing a clear and consistent language to communicate the unique functions of nursing
7. Linking with the classification systems of other health care providers

From Bulechek GM, et al: *Nursing interventions classification (NIC)*, ed 6, St Louis, 2013, Mosby.

Nursing Interventions Classification Interventions

The NIC system developed by the University of Iowa differentiates nursing practice from that of other health care disciplines (Box 19-2) by offering a language that nurses can use to describe sets of actions in delivering nursing care. The NIC interventions offer a level of standardization to enhance communication of nursing care across settings and to compare outcomes. Many health care information systems have incorporated the NIC system. By using NIC you will learn the common interventions recommended for the various NANDA-International (NANDA-I) nursing diagnoses. Chapter 18 describes the NIC system in more detail.

Standards of Practice

Nurses use the ANA Standards of Professional Nursing Practice (ANA, 2010) as evidence of the standard of care provided to patients (see Chapter 1). The standards are formally reviewed on a regular basis. The newest standards include competencies for establishing professional and caring relationships, using evidence-based interventions and technologies, providing ethical holistic care across the life span to diverse groups, and using community resources and systems. In addition, the standards emphasize implementing a timely plan following patient safety goals (ANA, 2010).

Quality and Safety Education for Nurses (QSEN)

The QSEN Institute established standard competencies in knowledge, skills, and attitudes (KSAs) for the preparation of future nurses (QSEN, 2014). The goal of QSEN is to prepare nurses so they can continuously improve the quality and safety of the health care systems within which they work. Examples of QSEN skills include providing patient-centered care with sensitivity and respect for the diversity of the human experience, initiating effective treatments to relieve pain and suffering, and participating in building consensus or resolving conflict in the context of patient care (QSEN, 2014).

CRITICAL THINKING IN IMPLEMENTATION

Clinical judgment includes making appropriate interpretations or conclusions about the interventions used to address a patient's human response to health conditions or life processes. It requires a nurse to use or modify standard approaches and to sometimes improvise new ones (ideally based on evidence) to respond appropriately (Tanner,

BOX 19-3 EVIDENCE-BASED PRACTICE

Interdisciplinary Practices

PICO Question: In health care settings how does interdisciplinary teamwork compared with multidisciplinary models of care affect patient care delivery?

Evidence Summary

Teamwork is a standard of care in all health care settings. However, interdisciplinary involvement in patient care does not guarantee multidimensionality in health care interventions (Klarare et al, 2013). Just because there is input from various disciplines, a patient's final plan of care may not reflect interventions from all disciplines. Organizational culture affects how well teams collaborate. Organizational culture includes leadership, communication processes, shared beliefs about the quality of clinical guidelines, and conflict resolution (Dodek et al., 2010). A culture that bolsters collaboration among nurses, physicians, and other health care providers is needed to merge the unique strengths of all disciplines into opportunities to improve patient outcomes (Nair et al., 2012). As a beginning nurse you will not be considered a leader of the health care team, but your input as an interdisciplinary team member is critical.

Application to Nursing Practice

- Remain competent in your ability to provide clinical care; this will develop trust among other health care providers (McDonald et al., 2012).
- Good communication between other health care providers builds trust and is related to the acceptance of your role in the health care team (McDonald et al., 2012).
- Understand the roles of each health care provider and what each can contribute to a patient's care.

2006). The critical thinking model discussed in Chapter 15 provides a framework for how to make decisions when implementing nursing care. You learn how to implement nursing care by applying appropriate knowledge, experience, attitudes, and standards of care (Figure 19-1). The delivery of nursing interventions is complex. It is based on the knowledge you have about a patient and the social context of the unit where you work. Interdisciplinary relationships, particularly those between nurses and health care providers, contribute to nursing judgments in the degree to which you pursue understanding a patient's problem and intervene effectively (Box 19-3). The context in which you deliver care to each patient and the many interventions required result in decision-making approaches for each clinical situation. Critical thinking allows you to consider the complexity of interventions, changing priorities, alternative approaches, and the amount of time available to act.

Tonya identified four relevant nursing diagnoses for Mr. Lawson: ***Acute Pain related to trauma of surgical incision, Readiness for Enhanced Knowledge related to impending discharge with self-care needs, Risk for Infection,*** *and* ***Anxiety related to uncertainty over ability to return to work.*** *The diagnoses are interrelated, and sometimes a planned intervention (e.g., promoting relaxation exercises) treats or modifies more than one of the patient's health problems (anxiety and acute pain). Tonya applies critical thinking and uses her time with Mr. Lawson wisely by anticipating his priorities, applying the knowledge she has about his problems and the interventions planned, and implementing care strategies skillfully.*

As you implement interventions, use critical thinking to confirm whether the interventions are correct and still appropriate. Be sure that

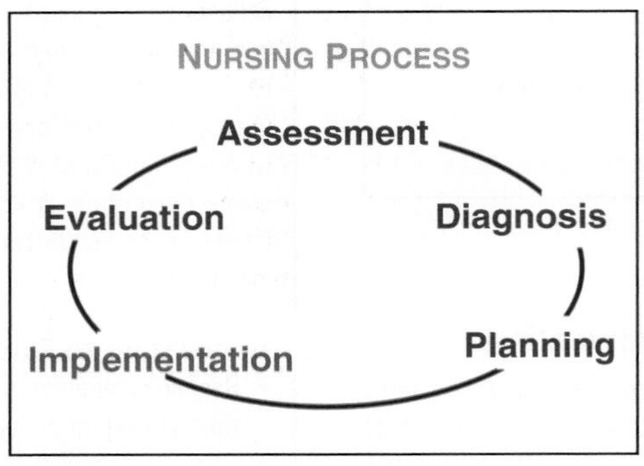

FIGURE 19-1 Critical thinking and the process of implementing care. *AHRQ,* Agency for Healthcare Research Quality; *ANA,* American Nurses Association; *APS,* American Pain Society.

you understand a patient's clinical situation. Always be aware of a patient's changing condition and what you would expect after caring for patients with similar conditions. You will "reflect-in-action" (i.e., what Tanner [2006] describes as being able to read a patient and how he or she is responding to your interventions) and then adjust the interventions on the basis of ongoing assessment.

Critical thinking requires you to make correct judgments as you care for multiple patients with different needs and whose priorities can change quickly. You need to maintain critical thinking, organization, and time management skills to provide safe and effective care to patients (see Chapter 21).

Even though you plan a set of interventions for a patient, you have to exercise critical judgment and decision making while delivering each intervention. Always think before you act. Consider the resources you have and the scheduling of activities on a nursing unit, which often dictate when and how to complete an intervention. Many factors influence your decision on how and when to intervene. You are responsible for having the necessary knowledge and clinical competency to perform interventions for your patients safely and effectively. Follow these tips for making decisions during implementation:

- Review the set of all possible nursing interventions for a patient's problem (e.g., for Mr. Lawson's pain Tonya considered analgesic administration, positioning and splinting, progressive relaxation, and other nonpharmacological approaches).
- Review all possible consequences associated with each possible nursing action (e.g., Tonya considers that the analgesic will relieve pain; have little or insufficient effect; or cause an adverse reaction, including sedating the patient and increasing the risk of falling).
- Determine the probability of all possible consequences (e.g., if Mr. Lawson's pain continues to decrease with analgesia and positioning and there have been no side effects, it is unlikely that adverse reactions will occur, and the intervention will be successful; however, if the patient continues to remain highly anxious, his pain may not stay relieved, and Tonya needs to consider an alternative).
- Judge the value of the consequence to the patient (e.g., if the administration of an analgesic is effective, Mr. Lawson will likely become less anxious and more responsive to postoperative instruction and counseling about his anxiety).

Selecting nursing interventions for a patient is part of clinical decision making. It is important to know the purpose of an intervention, the steps in performing the intervention correctly, the current medical condition of the patient, and his or her expected response. Always prepare well before providing any intervention. With experience you become more proficient in anticipating what to expect in a given clinical situation and how to modify your approach. As you gain clinical experience, you are able to consider patterns of responses from similar patients and the interventions that did or did not work previously and why. It also helps to know the clinical standards of practice for your agency.

QSEN QSEN: BUILDING COMPETENCY IN EVIDENCE-BASED PRACTICE Explain how Tonya would use current evidence in selecting interventions for Mr. Lawson's nursing diagnoses. Is a prn medication the best approach to treat his pain? Are there evidence-based relaxation exercises that Tonya might use?

Answers to QSEN Activities can be found on the Evolve website.

As you perform a nursing intervention, apply intellectual standards, which are the guidelines for rational thought and responsible action (see Chapter 15). *For example, before Tonya begins to teach Mr. Lawson, she considers how to make her instructions relevant, clear, logical, and complete to promote patient learning.* A critical thinker applies critical thinking attitudes when intervening. For example, show confidence in performing an intervention. When you are unsure of how to perform a procedure, be responsible. Seek assistance from others. Confidence in performing interventions builds trust with patients. Creativity and self-discipline are attitudes that guide you in reviewing, modifying, and implementing interventions. As a beginning nursing student, seek out supervision from instructors or experienced nurses or review agency policy and procedures to guide you in the decision-making process for implementation.

IMPLEMENTATION PROCESS

Preparation for implementation ensures efficient, safe, and effective nursing care. Five preparatory activities are reassessing the patient, reviewing and revising the existing nursing care plan, organizing resources and care delivery, anticipating and preventing complications, and implementing nursing interventions.

Tonya returns to Mr. Lawson's room to begin instruction. His wife is present, and Mr. Lawson reports that his incisional pain is currently a level of 3. Tonya helps the patient sit up in a chair. She gets the teaching DVD program identified in her review of evidence and the booklets she wants to use to prepare the patient and his wife for infection control, wound care, and activity restrictions in the home. She knows that Mr. Lawson still has concerns about returning to work and thus wants to incorporate discussion about wound care with expected postoperative recovery. Tonya sees the opportunity of using Mr. Lawson's desire to return to work to increase the likelihood of his adherence to postoperative restrictions. If Mrs. Lawson understands how she can help Mr. Lawson in recovery, positive outcomes should be achieved.

Reassessing a Patient

Assessment is a continuous process that occurs each time you interact with a patient. When you collect new data about a patient, you sometimes identify a new nursing diagnosis or determine the need to modify the care plan. Creating a concept map helps you better understand the relationship between different nursing diagnoses and interventions appropriate to a patient's care (Figure 19-2). During the initial phase of implementation reassess the patient to be sure that you have selected appropriate interventions. The reassessment often focuses on one primary nursing diagnosis, or one dimension of a patient such as level of comfort, or one system such as the cardiovascular system. The reassessment helps you decide if the proposed nursing actions are still appropriate for a patient's level of wellness. Reassessment is not the evaluation of care or determination of a patient's response to an intervention (see Chapter 20), but it is the gathering of additional information to ensure that the plan of care is still appropriate. *For example, Tonya begins to talk with Mr. and Mrs. Lawson about wound care and the patient's activity restrictions. Mrs. Lawson shares that Mr. Lawson's employer called to ask how he was doing. Tonya notices that Mr. Lawson begins to show more anxiety; as Tonya explains lifting restrictions, the patient is not able to teach back what he can and cannot do. Tonya decides to redirect the discussion. She says to Mr. Lawson, "Let's talk about going back to work. Tell me more about when they expect you to return and what your work actually involves." Tonya realizes that to be effective with instruction she needs an attentive learner. Gaining more detail about the patient's work will help him express his concerns while at the same time allow Tonya to explain how activity restrictions fit into daily routines.*

Reviewing and Revising the Existing Nursing Care Plan

Reassessment allows you to validate a patient's nursing diagnoses, review the care plan, and determine whether the nursing interventions remain the most appropriate for a patient's needs. If a patient's status has changed and the nursing diagnosis and related nursing interventions are no longer appropriate, modify the nursing care plan. An out-of-date or incorrect care plan compromises the quality of nursing care. Review and modification enable you to provide timely nursing interventions to best meet a patient's needs. Modification of an existing written care plan includes four steps:

1. Revise data in the assessment column to reflect the patient's current status. Date any new data to inform other members of the health care team of the time that the change occurred.
2. Revise the nursing diagnoses. Delete nursing diagnoses that are no longer relevant and add and date any new diagnoses. Revise related factors and the patient's goals, outcomes, and priorities. Date any revisions.
3. Revise specific interventions that correspond to the new nursing diagnoses and goals. Be sure that revisions reflect the patient's present status.
4. Choose the method of evaluation for determining whether the patient achieved his or her outcomes.

As Tonya continues to prepare Mr. Lawson for discharge, she reassesses his pain status. His pain has been controlled well on around-the-clock analgesics. In consultation with the physician and in preparation for discharge, the physician decides to order an analgesic prn. Tonya also decides to include Mrs. Lawson as a coach to facilitate relaxation exercises for Mr. Lawson.

Preparing for Implementation

A nurse organizes time and resources in preparation for implementing nursing care. Always be sure that a patient is physically and psychologically ready for any interventions or procedures.

Time Management. Nurses practice within work environments that are part of the social-cultural context of health care organizations. As a result, they must assume dual roles: that of a patient care provider and an organizational employee (Jones, 2010). Your focus on providing individualized patient care can compete with the focus of standardization, efficiency, and cost control of the organization. Inadequate nursing time contributes to poor quality of patient care, and excess nursing time contributes to high costs of care (Aiken, 2008; Storfjell et al., 2008). Time devoted to nursing care has three components: physical (the physical amount of time consumed in the completion of nursing activities), psychological (what nursing care patients experience and how they experience it), and sociological (the sequential ordering of events within the daily routines of a practice setting) (Jones, 2010). All components of time occur within the context of an organization and the resources available. As a new nurse, understand that the decisions you make about how your time is allocated, prioritized, and sequenced are always interpreted by the patients you serve (Jones, 2010). Delayed and hurried responses convey disinterest,

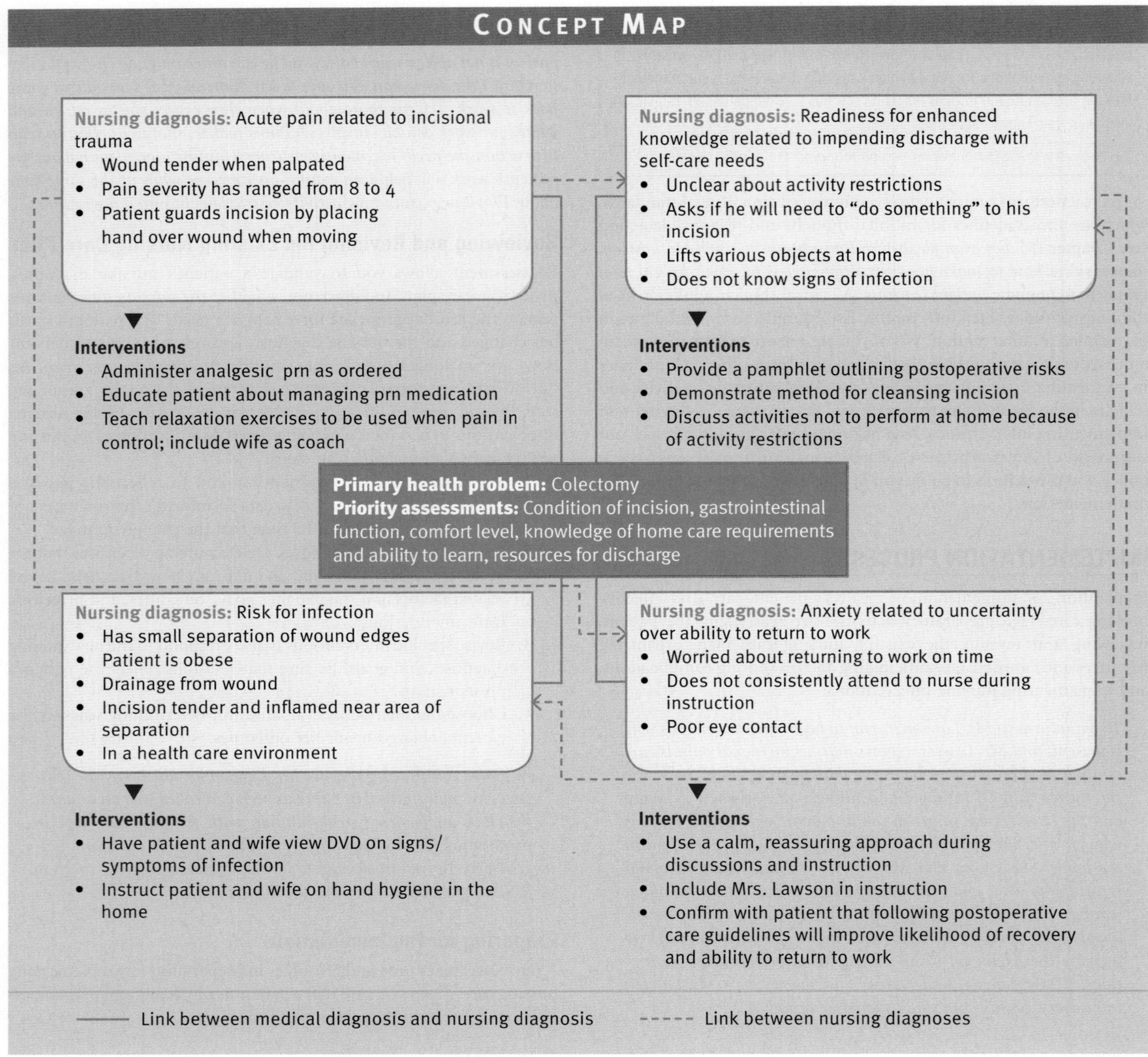

FIGURE 19-2 Concept map for Mr. Lawson: Implementation.

whereas timely interaction conveys care and concern. Be aware of factors affecting time with patients and apply time-management principles (see Chapter 21).

Equipment. Most nursing procedures require some equipment or supplies. Before performing an intervention, decide which supplies you need and determine their availability. Is the equipment in working order to ensure safe use, and do you know how to use it? Place supplies in a convenient location to provide easy access during a procedure. Keep extra supplies available in case of errors or mishaps, but do not open them unless you need them. This controls health care costs, allowing you to be a fiscally responsible member of the health care team. After a procedure return any unopened supplies to storage areas.

Personnel. Nursing care delivery models determine how nursing personnel deliver patient care (see Chapter 21). A nurse's role in a team nursing model differs from that in a primary nursing model. As a nurse you are responsible for deciding whether to perform an intervention, delegate it to an unlicensed member of the nursing team, or have an RN colleague assist you. Your ongoing assessments of your patients, the priorities of each, and not an intervention alone, direct your decision about delegation. You have a legal duty to follow delegation guidelines and only delegate interventions within the delegate's training and ability according to the state Nurse Practice Act.

Patient care staff work together as patients' needs demand it. If a patient makes a request such as use of a bedpan or assistance in feeding, help the patient if you have time rather than trying to find a nursing assistive personnel (NAP) who is in a different room. Nursing staff respect colleagues who show initiative; collaborate together; and communicate with one another on an ongoing, reciprocal basis as patients' needs change (Potter et al., 2010). When interventions are complex or physically difficult, you will need assistance from colleagues. For example, you and the NAP more effectively change a dressing in a large gaping wound when you apply the dressing and the NAP assists with patient positioning and handing off of supplies.

Environment. A patient's care environment needs to be safe and conducive to implementing therapies. Patient safety is your first concern. If a patient has sensory deficits, physical disabilities, or an alteration in level of consciousness, arrange the environment to prevent injury. For example, provide a patient's assist devices (e.g., walker or eyeglasses), rearrange furniture and equipment when ambulating a patient, or make sure that the water temperature is not too warm before a bath. Patients benefit most from nursing interventions when surroundings are compatible with care activities. When you need to expose a patient's body parts, do so privately by closing room doors or curtains because the patient will then be more relaxed. Ask visitors to leave as you complete care. Reduce distractions during teaching to enhance a patient's learning opportunities. Make sure that lighting is adequate to perform procedures correctly.

Patient. Before you implement interventions, make sure that your patients are physically and psychologically comfortable. Control noise, temperature, and lighting for maximal comfort. Physical symptoms such as nausea, dizziness, fatigue, or pain often interfere with a patient's full concentration and ability to cooperate. Offer comfort measures before initiating interventions to help patients participate more fully. If you need a patient to be alert, administer a dose of pain medication strong enough to relieve discomfort but not to impair mental faculties (e.g., ability to follow instruction and communication). If a patient is fatigued, delay ambulation or transfer to a chair until after he or she has had a chance to rest. Also consider a patient's level of endurance and plan only the amount of activity that he or she is able to tolerate comfortably.

Awareness of a patient's psychosocial needs helps you create a favorable emotional climate. *Do not rush your care.* Some patients feel reassured by having a significant other present to lend encouragement and moral support. Other strategies include planning sufficient time or multiple opportunities for a patient to work through and ventilate feelings and anxieties. Adequate preparation allows a patient to obtain maximal benefit from each intervention.

Anticipating and Preventing Complications

As a nurse, always stay alert for the risks posed by a patient's illness and treatments. If a patient's condition changes, adapt your choice of interventions to the situation, evaluate the relative benefit of the treatment versus the risk, and take risk-prevention measures. Many conditions place patients at risk for complications. For example, a patient with preexisting left-sided paralysis following a stroke 2 years earlier is at risk for developing a pressure ulcer following orthopedic surgery that requires traction and bed rest. A patient with obesity and diabetes mellitus who has major abdominal surgery is at risk for poor wound healing. Nurses are often the first ones to detect and document changes in patients' conditions. Expert nurses learn to anticipate breakdown and deterioration of patients even before confirming diagnostic signs develop.

Your knowledge of pathophysiology and experience with previous patients help in identifying the risk of complications that can occur. A thorough assessment reveals the level of a patient's current risk. The evidence or scientific rationales for how interventions (e.g., pressure-relief devices, repositioning, or wound care) prevent or minimize complications help you select the most appropriate preventive measures. For example, if a patient who is obese has uncontrolled postoperative pain, the risk for pressure ulcer development increases because the patient is unwilling or unable to change position frequently. The nurse anticipates when a patient's pain will increase, administers ordered analgesics, and then positions the patient to remove pressure on the skin and underlying tissues. If a patient continues to have difficulty turning or repositioning, the nurse selects a pressure-relief device to place on the patient's bed.

Some nursing procedures pose risks. Be aware of potential complications and take precautions. For example, a patient who has a feeding tube is at risk for aspiration. Position the patient in high-Fowler's position, check for residual, and check tube position before administering a feeding.

Identifying Areas of Assistance. Certain patient care situations require you to obtain assistance by seeking additional personnel, knowledge, and/or nursing skills. Before beginning care, review the plan to determine the need for assistance and the type required. Sometimes you need assistance in performing a procedure, providing comfort measures, or preparing a patient for a diagnostic test. Do not take shortcuts if assistance is not immediately available since this increases risk of injury to you and the patient. For example, when you care for a patient who is overweight and immobilized, you require additional personnel and transfer equipment to turn and position the patient safely. Be sure to determine the number of additional personnel and if you need them in advance. Discuss your need for assistance with other nurses or the NAP.

You require additional knowledge and skills in situations in which you are less experienced. Because of the continual growth in health care technology, you may lack the skills to perform a procedure. When you are asked to administer a new medication, operate a new piece of equipment, or administer a procedure with which you are unfamiliar, follow these steps.

1. Seek the information you need to be informed about a procedure. Check the scientific literature for evidence-based information, review resource manuals and the procedure book of the agency, or consult with experts (e.g., pharmacists, clinical nurse specialists).
2. Collect all equipment necessary for the procedure.
3. Have another nurse (e.g., staff nurse, faculty, clinical nurse specialist) who has completed the procedure correctly and safely provide assistance and guidance. Requesting assistance occurs frequently in all types of nursing practice. It is a learning process that continues throughout educational experiences and into professional development. One tip is to verbalize with an instructor or staff nurse the steps you will take before actually performing the procedure to improve your confidence and ensure accuracy.

Implementation Skills

Nursing practice requires cognitive, interpersonal, and psychomotor (technical) skills to implement direct and indirect nursing interventions. You are responsible for knowing when one type of implementation skill is preferred over another and for having the necessary knowledge and skill to perform each.

Cognitive Skills. Cognitive skills include the critical thinking and decision-making skills described earlier. Always use good judgment and sound clinical decision making when performing any intervention. This ensures that no nursing action is automatic. Grasp each clinical situation at hand, interpret the information you observe, and anticipate a patient's response so you individualize patient care appropriately. Know the rationale for therapeutic interventions and understand normal and abnormal physiological and psychological responses. Also know the evidence in nursing science to ensure that you deliver current and relevant nursing interventions.

Tonya knows the pathophysiology of colon cancer, the anatomy of the abdomen and surrounding structures, and the normal mechanisms for pain. She considers each of these as she observes Mr. Lawson, noting how the patient's movement and position either aggravate or lessen his incisional pain. Tonya focused initially on relieving Mr. Lawson's acute pain with an analgesic; but, now that pain has become well managed, she considers additional nonpharmacological approaches to keep him comfortable and also help lessen any anxiety.

Interpersonal Skills. Interpersonal communication is essential for effective nursing action. Develop a trusting relationship, express a level of caring, and communicate clearly with patients and their families (see Chapter 24). Good interpersonal communication keeps patients informed and engaged in decision making, provides individualized instruction, and supports patients who have challenging emotional needs. Proper use of interpersonal skills enables you to be perceptive of a patient's verbal and nonverbal communication. As a member of the health care team, communicate patient problems and needs clearly, intelligently, and in a timely way.

Psychomotor Skills. Psychomotor skills require the integration of cognitive and motor activities. For example, when giving an injection you need to understand anatomy and pharmacology (cognitive) and use good coordination and precision to administer the injection correctly (motor). With time and practice you learn to perform skills correctly, smoothly, and confidently. This is critical in establishing patient trust. You are responsible for acquiring necessary psychomotor skills through your experience in the nursing laboratory, the use of interactive instructional technology, or actual hands-on care of patients. When performing a new skill, assess your level of competency and obtain the necessary resources to ensure that your patient receive safe treatment.

DIRECT CARE

Nurses provide a wide variety of direct care measures through patient interactions. How a nurse interacts affects the success of any direct care activity. Remain sensitive to a patient's clinical condition, previous experiences, expectations, and cultural views. All direct care measures require competent safe practice. Show a caring approach each time you provide direct care.

Activities of Daily Living

Activities of daily living (ADLs) are usually performed in the course of a normal day; they include ambulation, eating, dressing, bathing, and grooming. A patient's need for assistance with ADLs is temporary, permanent, or rehabilitative. For example, a patient with impaired physical mobility because of bilateral arm casts temporarily needs assistance. After the casts are removed, the patient gradually regains the strength and range of motion needed to perform ADLs. In contrast, a patient with an irreversible cervical spinal cord injury is paralyzed and has a permanent need for assistance. It is unrealistic to plan rehabilitation with a goal of becoming independent with ADLs for this patient. Instead the patient learns new ways to perform ADLs independently through rehabilitation. Occupational and physical therapists play a key role in rehabilitation to restore ADLs function.

When a patient is experiencing fatigue, a limitation in mobility, confusion, and/or pain, assistance with ADLs is likely. For example, a patient who experiences shortness of breath avoids eating because of associated fatigue. Help the patient by setting up meals and offering to cut up food and plan for more frequent, small meals to maintain his or her nutrition. Assistance with ADLs ranges from partial assistance to complete care. Remember to always respect a patient's wishes and determine his or her preferences. Patients from some cultures prefer receiving assistance with ADLs from family members. As long as a patient is stable and alert, it is appropriate to allow family to help with care. Most patients want to remain independent in meeting their basic needs. Allow a patient to participate to the level that he or she is able. Involving patients in planning the timing and types of interventions boosts their self-esteem and willingness to become more independent.

Instrumental Activities of Daily Living

Illness or disability sometimes alters a patient's ability to be independent in society. Instrumental activities of daily living (IADLs) include skills such as shopping, preparing meals, housecleaning, writing checks, and taking medications. Nurses within home care and community health settings frequently help patients adapt ways to perform IADLs. Occupational therapists are specially educated to adapt approaches for patients to use when performing IADLs. Often family and friends are excellent resources for helping patients. In acute care it is important to anticipate how patients' illnesses will affect their ability to perform IADLs so you can make appropriate referrals to be sure that they have resources they need at home.

Physical Care Techniques

You routinely perform a variety of physical care techniques when caring for patients. Physical care techniques involve the safe and competent administration of nursing procedures (e.g., turning and positioning, inserting a feeding tube, administering medications, and providing comfort measures). The specific knowledge and skills needed to perform these procedures are in subsequent clinical chapters of this text. All physical care techniques require you to protect yourself and patients from injury, use safe patient-handling techniques, use proper infection control practices, stay organized, and follow applicable practice guidelines.

To carry out a procedure you need to be knowledgeable about the procedure itself, the standard frequency, the associated risks, and the necessary assessments before, during, and after performing the skill. Always remain thoughtful of a patient's condition and how the patient has responded to the procedure in the past. Know how the procedure is going to affect the patient and which expected outcomes you desire. In a hospital you perform many procedures each day, often for the first time. Before performing a new procedure, assess the situation and your personal competencies to determine if you need assistance, new knowledge, or new skills. Performing any procedure correctly requires critical thinking and thoughtful decision making.

Lifesaving Measures

A lifesaving measure is a physical care technique that you use when a patient's physiological or psychological state is threatened (see Chapters 38 and 41). The purpose of lifesaving measures is to restore physiological or psychological homeostasis. Such measures include administering emergency medications, instituting cardiopulmonary resuscitation, intervening to protect a confused or violent patient, and obtaining immediate counseling from a crisis center for a severely anxious patient. If an inexperienced nurse faces a situation requiring emergency measures, the proper nursing actions are to stay with the patient, maintain support, and have another staff member obtain an experienced professional.

Counseling

Counseling is a direct care method that helps patients use problem-solving processes to recognize and manage stress and facilitate interpersonal relationships. As a nurse you counsel patients to accept actual or impending changes resulting from stress (see Chapter 38). Examples include patients who are facing terminal illness or chronic disease. Counseling involves emotional, intellectual, spiritual, and psychological support. A patient and family who need nurse counseling have normal adjustment difficulties and are upset or frustrated, but they are not necessarily psychologically disabled. An example is the stress that a young woman faces when caring for her aging mother. Family caregivers need assistance in adjusting to the physical and emotional demands of caregiving. Sometimes they need respite (i.e., a break from providing care). The recipient of care also needs assistance in adjusting to his or her disability. Patients with psychiatric diagnoses require therapy from nurses specializing in psychiatric nursing or social workers, psychiatrists, or psychologists.

Many counseling techniques foster cognitive, behavioral, developmental, experiential, and emotional growth in patients. Counseling encourages individuals to examine available alternatives and decide which choices are useful and appropriate. When patients are able to examine alternatives, they develop a sense of control and are able to better manage stress.

Teaching

Patient education is key to patient-centered care (see Chapter 25). A teaching plan is essential, especially when patients are inexperienced and being asked to manage health problems they are facing for the first time. Counseling and teaching closely align. Both involve using good interpersonal skills to create a change in a patient's knowledge and behavior. Counseling results in changes in the development of new attitudes, behaviors, and feelings; whereas teaching focuses on intellectual growth or the acquisition of psychomotor skills.

When you educate patients, respect their expertise with their own health and symptoms, their daily routines, the diversity of their human experiences, their values and preferences as to how they learn, and the importance of shared decision making. As an educator you present health care principles, procedures, and techniques to inform patients about their health status in such a way that patients can adapt what they learn to their daily routines at home to achieve self-care. Emphasis has been placed on patient education in acute care recently because of the Hospital Consumer Assessment of Healthcare Providers and Systems (HCAHPS), a standardized survey used across the country by hospitals to measure patients' perspectives on hospital care (HCAHPS, 2014). The survey results currently are a standard for measuring and comparing quality of hospitals. Hospitals stress the importance of nurses addressing the topics covered by the survey, including patient education. Examples of questions on the HCAHPS include:

- How often did nurses explain things in a way you could understand?
- During this hospital stay did you get information in writing about which symptoms or health problems to look for after you left the hospital?
- Before giving you new medicine, how often did staff describe possible side effects in a way you could understand?

The HCAHPS initiative stresses the importance of patient education. But remember, teaching is an ongoing process of keeping patients

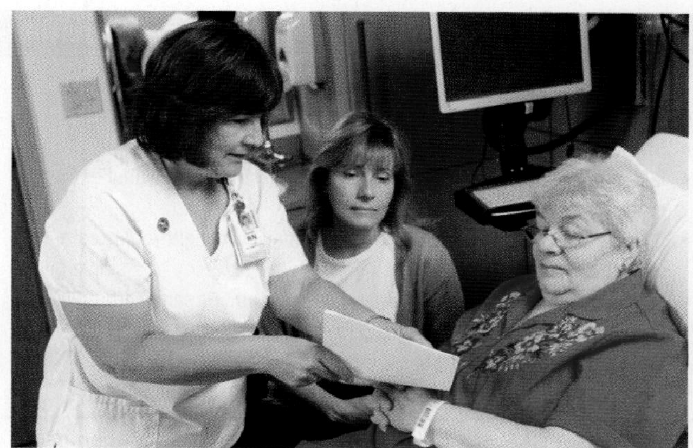

FIGURE 19-3 Nurse providing discharge instructions to patient and family.

informed. Patients want to know why you do what you do. When performing a procedure, engage your patient and explain the procedure, why it is being done and the expected outcomes, and any problems to look for afterwards. Encourage patients to ask questions. Here is an example of incorporating teaching in your daily work. When starting an intravenous (IV) infusion, explain what the IV fluid bag contains, how long the bag should last, sensations the patient will feel if the IV site becomes inflamed, the fact that a small flexible catheter is in the arm, and any potential side effects of medications in the bag.

Teaching takes place in all health care settings (Figure 19-3). As a nurse you are accountable for the quality of education you deliver. Know your patient; be aware of the cultural and social factors that influence a patient's willingness and ability to learn. It is also important to know your patient's health literacy level (see Chapter 25). Can he or she read directions or make calculations that often are necessary with self-care skills? Do not assume that patients understand their illness or disease. If they seem uneasy or refuse a treatment, simply ask what concerns them. This gives you the chance to provide further teaching and correct knowledge deficiencies.

Controlling for Adverse Reactions

An **adverse reaction** is a harmful or unintended effect of a medication, diagnostic test, or therapeutic intervention. Adverse reactions can result from any nursing intervention; thus learn to anticipate and know which adverse reactions to expect. Nursing actions that control for adverse reactions reduce or counteract a reaction. For example, when applying a moist heat compress, you know that burning the patient's skin is a possible adverse reaction unless you protect the skin. First assess the condition of the area where you plan to place the compress. Following application of the compress, inspect the area every 5 minutes for any adverse reaction such as excessive reddening of the skin from the heat or skin maceration from the moisture (see Chapter 48). Taking the right precautions can prevent adverse reactions.

When completing a health care provider–directed intervention such as medication administration, always know the potential side effects of the drug. After you administer a medication, evaluate the patient for adverse effects. Also be aware of drugs that counteract the side effects. For example, a patient has an unknown hypersensitivity to penicillin and develops hives after three doses. You record the reaction, stop further administration of the drug, and consult with the physician. You then administer an ordered dose of diphenhydramine (Benadryl), an antihistamine and antipruritic medication, to reduce the allergic response and relieve the itching.

BOX 19-4 Examples of Indirect Care Activities

- Documentation (electronic or written)
- Delegation of care activities to nursing assistive personnel (NAP)
- Medical order transcription
- Infection control (e.g., proper handling and storage of supplies, use of protective isolation)
- Environmental safety management (e.g., making patient rooms safe, strategically assigning patients in a geographical proximity to a single nurse)
- Telephone consultations with physicians and other health care providers
- Hand-off reports to other health care team members
- Collecting, labeling, and transporting specimens
- Transporting patients to procedural areas and other nursing units

From Bulechek GM, et al: *Nursing interventions classification (NIC)*, ed 6, St Louis, 2013, Mosby.

When caring for patients who undergo diagnostic tests, you need to understand the test and any potential adverse effects. For example, a patient has not had a bowel movement in 24 hours after a barium enema. Because bowel impaction is a potential side effect of a barium enema, you increase fluid intake and instruct the patient to let a nurse know when a bowel movement occurs. Although adverse effects are not common, they do occur. It is important that you recognize the signs and symptoms of an adverse reaction and intervene in a timely manner.

Preventive Measures

Preventive nursing actions promote health and prevent illness to avoid the need for acute or rehabilitative health care (see Chapter 2). Changes in the health care system are leading to greater emphasis on health promotion and illness prevention. Primary prevention aimed at health promotion includes health education programs, immunizations, and physical and nutritional fitness activities. Secondary prevention focuses on people who are experiencing health problems or illnesses and who are at risk for developing complications or worsening conditions. It includes screening techniques and treating early stages of disease. Tertiary prevention involves minimizing the effects of long-term illness or disability, including rehabilitation measures.

INDIRECT CARE

Indirect care measures are nursing actions that manage the patient care environment and interdisciplinary collaborative actions that support the effectiveness of direct care interventions (Bulechek et al., 2013). Many of the measures are managerial in nature such as emergency cart maintenance and environmental and supply management (Box 19-4). Nurses spend much time in indirect and unit management activities. Communication of information about patients (e.g., hand-off report, hourly rounding, and consultation) is critical, ensuring that direct care activities are planned, coordinated, and performed with the proper resources. Delegation of care to NAP is another indirect care activity (see Chapter 21). When performed correctly, delegation ensures that the right care provider performs the right tasks so the nurse and NAP work together most efficiently for a patient's benefit.

Communicating Nursing Interventions

Any intervention that you provide for a patient is communicated in an electronic, written, or oral format (see Chapter 26). Electronic health records (EHRs) or written charts have sections for individualized interventions that are part of the nursing care plan (see Chapter 18) and a patient's permanent medical record. The record entry usually includes a brief description of pertinent assessment findings, the specific intervention(s), and the patient's response. An EHR or written record validates that you performed a procedure and provides valuable information to subsequent caregivers about the approaches needed to provide successful care. Some institutions have **interdisciplinary care plans** (i.e., plans representing the contributions of all disciplines caring for a patient). You enter nursing interventions into the plan, documenting the treatment and patient's response (see Chapter 26).

Effective communication and good teamwork are ways to reduce medical errors and prevent adverse patient outcomes (ECRI, 2015). Miscommunication is often the root cause for most reported adverse or sentinel events that occur in health care organizations. Communication with other health care professionals needs to be timely, accurate, and relevant to a patient's clinical situation. Ineffective or incomplete communications result in caregivers being uninformed, interventions possibly duplicated needlessly, procedures possibly delayed, or tasks possibly left undone. Chapter 26 explains the approach for effective hand-off communication between two care providers. Always be clear, concise, and to the point when you communicate nursing interventions.

Delegating, Supervising, and Evaluating the Work of Other Staff Members

A nurse who develops a patient's care plan frequently does not perform all of the nursing interventions. Some activities you coordinate and delegate to other members of the health care team (see Chapter 21). Delegation requires clinical judgment and accountability for patient care (Weydt, 2010). The frequency and manner in which nursing care activities are delegated often depends on a nursing unit delivery of care model. Koloroutis et al. (2007) describe three approaches for delegation based on the way RN and NAP assignments are made.

- Unit-based scenario—NAP serves the unit. The NAP works off a task list usually found in the job description and has minimal direction from or interaction with RNs. Limited 1 : 1 delegation occurs. Lack of communication can cause conflicts.
- Pairing—One RN works with a licensed practical nurse (LPN) and/or a NAP for a shift. The RN and LPN and/or NAP are not intentionally scheduled to work the same shift each day. For a given shift they work together, or are paired, and care for the same group of patients. Delegation usually increases with pairing.
- Partnering—Involves one RN and one LPN and/or NAP who are consistently scheduled to work together. The partners commit to healthy interpersonal relationships, trust in one another, and advance each other's knowledge. It is recognized that the RN has the authority to make the delegation decisions.

Delegation allows you to use your time more wisely and to have NAP assist by performing noninvasive and frequently repetitive interventions such as skin care, ambulation, vital signs on stable patients, and hygiene measures. When you delegate tasks to NAP, you are responsible for ensuring that you assign each task appropriately and that the NAP completes each task according to the standard of care. You must be sure that any delegated action was completed correctly, documented, and evaluated. You only delegate direct care interventions to personnel who are competent.

ACHIEVING PATIENT GOALS

You implement interventions to achieve patient goals and expected outcomes. In most clinical situations multiple interventions are needed to achieve select outcomes. In addition, patients' conditions often change minute by minute. Therefore it is important to apply principles of care coordination such as good time management, organizational skills, and appropriate use of resources to ensure that you deliver interventions effectively and meet desired outcomes (see Chapter 21). Priority setting is critical in successful implementation. Priorities help you to anticipate and sequence nursing interventions when a patient has multiple nursing diagnoses and collaborative problems (see Chapter 18).

Another way to help patients achieve their goals is to help them adhere to their treatment plan. Patient adherence means that patients and families invest time in carrying out required treatments. To ensure that patients have a smooth transition across different health care settings (e.g., hospital to home and clinic to home to assisted living), it is important to introduce interventions that patients are willing and able to follow. Adequate and timely discharge planning and education of a patient and family are the first steps in promoting a smooth transition from one health care setting to another or to the home. Effective discharge planning and education involve individualizing your care and taking into consideration the various factors that influence a patient's health beliefs (see Chapter 6). *For example, for Tonya to effectively help Mr. Lawson follow the activity limitations required after surgery, she needs to know if Mr. Lawson understands the risks to wound healing if limitations are not followed. His anxiety about being able to return to work on time will likely improve his motivation to adhere.* You are responsible for delivering interventions in a way that reflects your understanding of a patient's health beliefs, culture, lifestyle pattern, and patterns of wellness. In addition, reinforcing successes with the treatment plan encourages a patient to follow his or her care plan.

KEY POINTS

- Implementation, the fourth step of the nursing process, formally begins after a nurse develops a plan of care. The nurse then initiates interventions that are designed to achieve patient goals and expected outcomes.
- A direct care intervention is a treatment performed through interactions with a patient that include nurse-initiated, health care provider–initiated and collaborative approaches.
- Always think first and determine if an intervention is correct and appropriate and if you have the resources needed to implement it.
- Clinical guidelines or protocols are evidence-based documents that guide decisions and interventions for specific health care problems.
- Remaining competent and using good communication skills build your ability to participate in interdisciplinary practices.
- A clinical practice guideline establishes evidence-based interventions for specific health care problems or conditions.
- The implementation of nursing care often requires additional knowledge, nursing skills, and personnel resources.
- Before performing an intervention, make sure that a patient is as physically and psychologically comfortable as possible.
- Use good judgment during implementation to ensure that no nursing action is automatic.
- Know the purpose of each intervention, the associated preassessment and postassessment risks, steps in performing the intervention correctly, the current medical condition of a patient, and his or her expected response so you can anticipate what to expect in a given clinical situation and how to modify your approach.
- To anticipate and prevent complications, identify risks to a patient, adapt interventions to the situation, evaluate the relative benefit of a treatment versus the risk, and initiate risk-prevention measures.
- When you administer physical care techniques, protect yourself and the patient from injury, use proper infection control practices, stay organized, and follow applicable practice guidelines.
- When you delegate aspects of a patient's care, you are responsible for ensuring that each task is assigned appropriately and completed according to the standard of care.

CLINICAL APPLICATION QUESTIONS

Preparing for Clinical Practice

Tonya responds to Mr. Lawson's call light and finds that he has questions about his medications before his discharge. She conducts further assessment and asks Mr. Lawson which questions he has regarding his home medication therapy. Tonya determines Mr. Lawson's knowledge of the medications and assesses his routines for eating meals and going to bed at home. Tonya positions the patient comfortably and checks his abdominal incision; she notices that the drainage has not increased. She explains the purpose, doses, and times for administration of the medicines. She asks Mr. Lawson to explain to her when he should take the medicines once he is at home. Tonya also reviews the signs and symptoms of wound infection.

1. Why does Tonya inspect the patient's incision when Mr. Lawson asked about his medications?
2. Why does Tonya assess Mr. Lawson's routines for eating meals and going to bed?
3. Tonya's explanation of the signs and symptoms of wound infection was an example of which aspect of organizing resources and care delivery?

ⓔ ***Answers to Clinical Application Questions can be found on the Evolve website.***

REVIEW QUESTIONS

Are You Ready to Test Your Nursing Knowledge?

1. A nurse working on a surgery floor is assigned five patients and has a patient care technician assisting her. Which of the following shows the nurse's understanding and ability to safely delegate to the patient care tech? (Select all that apply.)
   1. The nurse considers the time available to gather routine vital signs on one patient before checking on a second patient arriving from a diagnostic test.
   2. Determining what is the patient care technician's current workload.
   3. The nurse chooses to delegate the measurement of a stable patient's vital signs and not the assessment of the patient arriving from a diagnostic test.
   4. The nurse reviews with the NAP, newly hired to the floor, her experience in measuring a blood pressure.
   5. The nurse confers with another registered nurse about organizing priorities.
2. The nurse administers a tube feeding via a patient's nasogastric tube. This is an example of which of the following?
   1. Physical care technique
   2. Activity of daily living
   3. Indirect care measure
   4. Lifesaving measure
3. A nurse is caring for a complicated patient 3 days in a row. The nurse attends an interdisciplinary conference to discuss the

patient's plan of care. In which ways can the nurse develop trust with members of the conference team? (Select all that apply.)
1. Is willing to challenge other members' ideas because the nurse disagrees with their rationale
2. Shows competence in how to monitor patients' clinical status and inform the physician of critical changes
3. Asks a more experienced nurse to attend the conference
4. Listens to opinions of members of interdisciplinary team and expresses recommendations for care clearly
5. During the meeting focus on similar problems the nurse has had in delivering care to other patients.

4. Which principle is most important for a nurse to follow when using a clinical practice guideline for an assigned patient?
1. Knowing the source of the guideline
2. Reviewing the evidence used to develop the guideline
3. Individualizing how to apply the clinical guideline for a patient
4. Explaining to a patient the purpose of the guideline

5. A nurse is visiting a patient in the home and is assessing the patient's adherence to medications. While talking with the family caregiver, the nurse learns that the patient has been missing doses. The nurse wants to perform interventions to improve the patient's adherence. Which of the following will affect how this nurse will make clinical decisions about how to implement care for this patient? (Select all that apply.)
1. Reviewing the family caregiver's availability during medication administration times
2. Making a judgment of the value of improved adherence for the patient
3. Reviewing the number of medications and time each is to be taken
4. Determining all consequences associated with the patient missing specific medicines
5. Reviewing the therapeutic actions of the medications

6. The nurse enters a patient's room and finds that the patient was incontinent of liquid stool. Because the patient has recurrent redness in the perineal area, the nurse worries about the risk of the patient developing a pressure ulcer. The nurse cleanses the patient, inspects the skin, and applies a skin barrier ointment to the perineal area. The nurse consults the ostomy and wound care nurse specialist for recommended skin care measures. Which of the following correctly describe the nurse's actions? (Select all that apply.)
1. The application of the skin barrier is a dependent care measure.
2. The call to the ostomy and wound care specialist is an indirect care measure.
3. The cleansing of the skin is a direct care measure.
4. The application of the skin barrier is an instrumental activity of daily living.
5. Inspecting the skin is a direct care activity.

7. During the implementation step of the nursing process, a nurse reviews and revises a patient's plan of care. Place the following steps of review and revision in the correct order.
1. Modify care plan as needed.
2. Decide if the nursing interventions remain appropriate.
3. Reassess the patient.
4. Compare assessment findings to validate existing nursing diagnoses.

8. Before consulting with a physician about a female patient's need for urinary catheterization, the nurse considers the fact that the patient has urinary retention and has been unable to void on her own. The nurse knows that evidence for alternative measures to promote voiding exists, but none has been effective, and that before surgery the patient was voiding normally. This scenario is an example of which implementation skill?
1. Cognitive
2. Interpersonal
3. Psychomotor
4. Consultative

9. Match the category of direct care on the left with the specific direct care activity on the right.

1. Counseling ___	a. Assisting patient with oral care
2. Lifesaving measure ____	b. Discussing a patient's options in choosing palliative care
3. Physical care technique ___	c. Protecting a violent patient from injury
4. Activity of daily living ____	d. Using safe patient handling during positioning of a patient

10. What is the importance of the Hospital Consumer Assessment of Healthcare Providers and Systems (HCAHPS) survey?
1. Measures a nurse's competency in interdisciplinary care
2. Measures the number of adverse events in a hospital
3. Measures quality of care within hospitals
4. Measures referrals to a health care agency

11. **Fill in the Blank.** A nurse administered an antibiotic 30 minutes ago and returns to the patient's room to determine if the patient is having any unexpected symptoms. This is an example of assessing for a(n) ________________.

12. Which measures does a nurse follow when being asked to perform an unfamiliar procedure? (Select all that apply.)
1. Checks scientific literature or policy and procedure
2. Reassesses the patient's condition
3. Collects all necessary equipment
4. Delegates the procedure to a more experienced nurse
5. Considers all possible consequences of the procedure

13. A nurse is conferring with another nurse about the care of a patient with a stage II pressure ulcer. The two decide to review the clinical practice guideline of the hospital for pressure ulcer management. The use of a standardized guideline achieves which of the following? (Select all that apply.)
1. Makes it quicker and easier for nurses to intervene
2. Sets a level of clinical excellence for practice
3. Eliminates need to create an individualized care plan for the patient
4. Delivers evidence-based interventions for stage II pressure ulcer
5. Summarizes the various approaches used for the practice concern or problem

14. A nurse reviews all possible consequences before helping a patient ambulate such as how the patient ambulated last time; how mobile the patient was before admission to the health care facility; or any current clinical factors affecting the patient's ability to stand, remain balanced, or walk. Which of the following is an example of a nurse's review of this situation?
1. Critical thinking
2. Managing an adverse event
3. Exercising self-discipline
4. Time management

15. A nurse collects equipment needed to administer an enema to a patient. Previously the nurse reviewed the procedure in the policy manual. The nurse raises the patient's bed and adjusts the room lighting to illuminate the work area. A patient care technician comes into the room to assist. Which aspect of organizing resources and care delivery did the nurse omit?

1. Environment
2. Personnel
3. Equipment
4. Patient

Answers: 1. 1, 3, 4; **2.** 1; **3.** 2, 4; **4.** 3; **5.** 2, 4; **6.** 2, 3; **7.** 3, 4, 2, 1; **8.** 1; **9.** 1b, 2c, 3d, 4a; **10.** 3; **11.** Adverse reaction; **12.** 1, 2, 3, 5; **13.** 1, 2, 4; **14.** 1; **15.** 4.

Rationales for Review Questions can be found on the Evolve website.

REFERENCES

Agency for Healthcare Research and Quality (AHRQ): *Clinical guidelines and recommendations*, 2014a, http://www.ahrq.gov/professionals/clinicians-providers/guidelines-recommendations/index.html. Accessed September 27, 2015.

Agency for Healthcare Research and Quality (AHRQ): *National Guidelines Clearinghouse*, 2014b, http://www.guideline.gov/browse/by-topic.aspx. Accessed September 27, 2015.

Aiken LH: Economics of nursing, *Policy Polit Nurs Pract* 9(2):73, 2008.

American Nurses Association (ANA): *Scope and standards of practice: nursing*, ed 2, Silver Spring, MD, 2010, American Nurses Association.

Bulechek GM, et al: *Nursing interventions classification (NIC)*, ed 6, St Louis, 2013, Mosby.

ECRI Institute: *Top 10 patient safety concerns for 2015*, 2015, https://www.ecri.org/Pages/PStop10_ThankYou.aspx. Accessed September 27, 2015.

Hospital Consumer Assessment of Healthcare Providers and Systems (HCAHPS): *HCAHPS*, 2014, http://www.hcahpsonline.org/home.aspx. Accessed September 27, 2014.

Jones TL: A holistic framework for nursing time: implications for theory, practice and research, *Nurs Forum* 45(3):185, 2010.

Koloroutis M, et al: *Field guide: relationship-based care visions, strategies, tools and exemplars for transforming practice*, Minneapolis, MN, 2007, Creative Health Care Management.

Manchikanti L, et al: A critical review of the American Pain Society clinical practice guidelines for interventional techniques. Part 1, Diagnostic interventions, *Pain Physician* 13(3):E141, 2010.

QSEN Institute: *Pre-Licensure KSAS*, 2014, http://qsen.org/competencies/pre-licensure-ksas/. Accessed September 27, 2014.

Storfjell JL, et al: The balancing act: patient care time versus cost, *J Nurs Adm* 38(5):244, 2008.

Weydt A: Developing delegation skills, *Online J Issues Nurs* 15(2):1, 2010.

RESEARCH REFERENCES

Benner P: *From novice to expert*, Menlo Park, CA, 1984, Addison-Wesley.

Dodek P, et al: The relationship between organizational culture and implementation of clinical practice guidelines: a narrative review, *JPEN J Parenter Enteral Nutr* 34(6):669, 2010.

Klarare A, et al: Team interactions in specialized palliative care teams: a qualitative study, *J Palliat Care* 16(9):1062, 2013.

McDonald J, et al: The influence of power dynamics and trust on multidisciplinary collaboration: a qualitative case study of type 2 diabetes mellitus, *BMC Health Serv Res* 12:63, 2012.

Nair DM, et al: Frequency of nurse-physician collaborative behaviors in an acute care hospital, *J Interprof Care* 26(2):115, 2012.

Potter P, et al: Delegation practices between registered nurses and nursing assistive personnel, *J Nurs Manag* 18(2):157, 2010.

Tanner C: Thinking like a nurse: a research-based model of clinical judgment in nursing, *J Nurs Educ* 45(6):204, 2006.

University of Iowa: *Evidence-based practice guidelines*, n.d., University of Iowa, http://www.nursing.uiowa.edu/excellence/evidence-based-practice-guidelines. Accessed September 27, 2014.

20

Evaluation

OBJECTIVES

- Discuss the relationship between critical thinking and evaluation.
- Describe the indicators of a nurse's ability to evaluate nursing care.
- Explain the relationship among goals of care, expected outcomes, and evaluative measures when evaluating nursing care.
- Explain the importance of using accurate evaluation measures.
- Explain the process of evaluating the outcomes of care for a patient.
- Describe how evaluation leads to discontinuation, revision, or modification of a plan of care.

KEY TERMS

Evaluation, p. 270
Evaluative measures, p. 271
Nurse-sensitive patient outcomes, p. 272
Standard of care, p. 275

MEDIA RESOURCES

http://evolve.elsevier.com/Potter/fundamentals/

- Review Questions
- Case Study with Questions
- Audio Glossary
- Content Updates

Critical thinking in nursing practice influences a nurse's workplace performance and reflects his or her ability to resolve patients' health-related problems (Shu-Yuan et al., 2013). When you apply the nursing process to identify patient problems and select and deliver relevant interventions, the evaluation step determines if patient problems are resolved. The outcomes of nursing practice are the measurable conditions of patient, family, or community status; behavior; or perception. These outcomes are the criteria used to judge success in delivering nursing care.

When a repairman comes to a home to fix a leaking faucet, he turns the faucet on to determine the problem, changes or adjusts parts, and rechecks the faucet to determine if the leak is fixed. After a patient diagnosed with pneumonia completes a course of antibiotics, the health care provider often has him or her return to the office to have a chest x-ray film examination to determine if the pneumonia has resolved. When a nurse provides wound care, including application of a warm compress, several steps are involved. He or she assesses the appearance of the wound, determines its severity, applies the appropriate form of compress, and returns later to inspect the wound to determine if the condition has improved. These three scenarios depict what ultimately occurs during the process of evaluation. The repairman rechecks the faucet, the health care provider orders a chest x-ray film, and the nurse reinspects the patient's wound. Through the process of evaluation you determine if a patient has improved, resulting in a desired outcome.

The previous chapters on the nursing process describe how you apply critical thinking to gather patient data, form nursing diagnoses, develop a plan of care, and implement interventions. **Evaluation**, the final step of the nursing process, is crucial to determine whether, after application of the first four steps of the nursing process, a patient's condition or well-being improves. *You conduct evaluative measures to determine if your patients met expected outcomes, not if nursing interventions were completed.* The expected outcomes established during planning are the standards against which you judge whether goals have been met and if care is successful.

In the continuing case study Mr. Lawson is going home in a couple of hours. Tonya organizes her care so she can take the time needed to evaluate the outcomes of her plan of care. Mr. Lawson took two doses of the prn analgesic ordered for his pain over the last 8 hours. Thirty minutes after the last dose he rated his pain a 3 on a scale of 0 to 10. He states, "I only really notice now when I move too quickly." Mrs. Lawson is in the room, so Tonya takes time to inspect and evaluate Mr. Lawson's wound, describes what she sees, and asks the Lawsons to explain the signs of infection and how to care for the wound at home. Tonya gives the Lawsons the discharge instruction sheet that is part of the standard of care of her nursing unit. She asks Mr. Lawson to explain the types of activity he needs to avoid for the first 2 weeks that he is home.

CRITICAL THINKING IN EVALUATION

Critical thinking is key to evaluation (Figure 20-1). In Chapter 15 you learned that clinical decision making is complex, requiring flexibility and the ability to know and recognize subtle changes or aspects of a patient's condition. In an extensive literature review of studies examining critical thinking indicators, Shu-Yuan et al. (2013) identified four indicators reflecting a nurse's ability to perform evaluation:

- Examine the results according to clinical data collected.
- Compare achieved effect with goals and expected outcomes.
- Recognize errors.
- Understand a patient situation, participate in self-reflection, and correct errors.

KNOWLEDGE
Characteristics of improved physiological, psychological, spiritual, and sociocultural status
Expected outcomes of pharmacological, medical, nutritional, and other therapies
Unexpected outcomes of pharmacological, medical, nutritional, and other therapies
Characteristics of improved family and group dynamics
Community resources

EXPERIENCE
Previous patient care experience

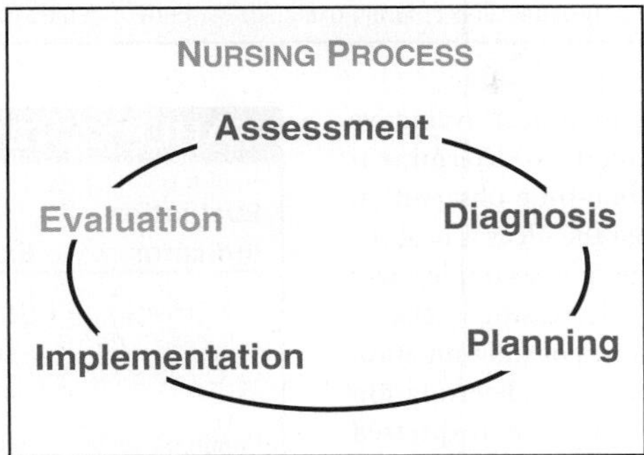

STANDARDS
Expected outcomes of care
Specialty standards of practice (e.g., American Pain Society; University of Iowa Evidence-Based Protocols, Intravenous Nursing Society)
Intellectual standards

ATTITUDES
Creativity
Responsibility
Perseverance
Humility

FIGURE 20-1 Critical thinking and evaluation.

These indicators show that the evaluation process is comprehensive. It requires more than making a quick check of a patient to be sure that he or she is stable or without further problems. It is a methodical approach for determining if nursing implementation effectively influenced a patient's progress or condition favorably.

Examine Results

Evaluation is an ongoing process that occurs whenever you have contact with a patient. Once you deliver an intervention, you continuously examine results by gathering subjective and objective data from a patient, family, and health care team members. Tanner (2006) calls this *reflection-in-action* (i.e., a nurse is able to "read" a patient by reviewing assessment data and determine how the patient is responding). At the same time you review knowledge regarding a patient's current condition, the treatment, and the resources available for recovery. By reflecting on previous experiences caring for similar patients, you are in a better position to know how to evaluate your patient. You can anticipate what to evaluate.

The effective examination of results requires you to have an open mind, keen observation skills, and the ability to exhibit a neutral perspective (Shu-Yuan et al., 2013). Do not form a judgment about a patient's progress or response without gathering data pertinent to the health care problem. *For example, because Mr. Lawson is being discharged and there have been no delays, Tonya might assume that his pain is under control. However, until Tonya reassesses the patient's pain character and severity, evaluation is not complete.* Be thorough in gathering all clinical information needed to adequately evaluate a patient's condition.

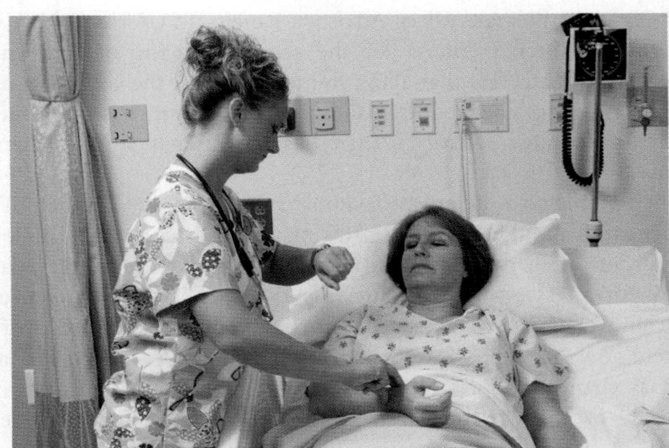

FIGURE 20-2 Evaluative measures. Nurse evaluates patient's vital signs.

Evaluative Measures. You examine the results of care by using **evaluative measures**, which are assessment skills and techniques (e.g., observations, physiological measurements, use of measurement scales, patient interview) (Figure 20-2). In fact, evaluative measures are the same as assessment measures, but you perform them at the point of care when you make decisions about a patient's status and progress (Table 20-1). The intent of assessment is to identify which, if any, problems exist. The intent of evaluation is to determine if the known problems have remained the same, improved, worsened, or otherwise changed.

TABLE 20-1 Evaluative Measures to Determine the Success of Goals and Expected Outcomes

Goals	Evaluative Measures	Expected Outcomes
Patient's pressure ulcer will heal within 7 days.	Inspect color, condition, and location of pressure ulcer. Measure diameter of ulcer daily. Note odor and color of drainage from ulcer.	Erythema is reduced in 2 days. Diameter of ulcer decreases in 5 days. Ulcer has no drainage in 2 days. Skin overlying ulcer is closed in 7 days.
Patient will tolerate ambulation to end of hall by 11/20.	Palpate patient's radial pulse before exercise. Palpate patient's radial pulse 10 minutes after exercise. Assess respiratory rate during exercise. Observe patient for dyspnea or breathlessness during exercise.	Pulse remains below 110 beats/min during exercise. Pulse rate returns to resting baseline within 10 minutes after exercise. Respiratory rate remains within two breaths of patient's baseline rate. Patient denies feeling of breathlessness.

In many clinical situations it is important to collect evaluative measures over a period of time. You look for trends to determine if a pattern of improvement or change exists. A one-time observation of a pressure ulcer is insufficient to determine that the ulcer is healing. It is important to note a consistency in change. For example, over a period of 3 days is the pressure ulcer gradually decreasing in size, is the amount of drainage declining, and is the redness of inflammation resolving? Recognizing a pattern of improvement or deterioration allows you to reason and decide whether a patient's problems (expressed in nursing diagnoses) are resolved. This is very important in the home care or nursing home setting. It may take weeks or even months to determine if interventions led to a pattern of improvement. For example, when evaluating a patient's risk for falls over time, has the patient, family, or health care team successfully reduced fall risks in the home such as eliminating barriers in the home, removing factors impairing the person's vision, or providing direction for proper use of assistive devices?

It is important to use the right evaluative measure. For example, pain scales have been shown to be valid and reliable for assessing pain severity (see Chapter 44) and change over time. The European and National Pressure Ulcer Advisory Panels (EPUAP and NPUAP, 2009) have specific criteria for the accurate staging of a pressure ulcer (see Chapter 48) that allow you to identify if the condition of a treated ulcer has changed. By using the right measure you are more likely to accurately identify if there has been a change in a patient's condition.

Being able to evaluate behavioral change is more difficult. The information about behavior (e.g., taking medications correctly, following a diet) often relies on a patient's self-report. An example is any survey or interview that evaluates a patient's ability to perform self-care and achieve self-management. Self-report is a measure of a patient's own perceptions or beliefs and may not truly reflect if behavior has changed. Your willingness to use self-report as an outcome measure of behavior reflects trust in the patient. When using self-report, it is very important that the patient understands questions posed and why his or her response is important to gauge behavior change.

Much emphasis in health care today is on patients and their family caregivers to achieve self-management to improve the quality of their lives. The aim of self-management is to minimize the impact of chronic disease or sudden acute illness on physical health status and functioning and to enable people to cope with the psychological effects of an illness. *In Mr. Lawson's case, Tonya has planned and implemented educational interventions designed to improve his ability to adopt the behaviors needed for self-care, specifically to follow activity restrictions and perform correct wound care. Tonya evaluates the patient's ability by measuring what he is able to either explain or demonstrate.* There are relevant, objective, and appropriate evaluative indicators of self-management, including self-efficacy, health behavior or attitude, health status, health service use, quality of life, and psychological indicators (Du and Yuan, 2010) (Table 20-2).

TABLE 20-2 Self-Management Evaluation

Evaluation Indicator	Examples of Measures
Self-Efficacy	General self-efficacy (GSE) scale, disease-specific self-efficacy scales (e.g., arthritis, cardiac); medication-adherence self-efficacy scale
Health Behavior	Adherence to medication schedule (e.g., pill count), demonstrated psychomotor skill (e.g., dressing change, self-injection), adherence to medical follow-up visits
Health Status	Clinical indicators (e.g., exercise tolerance, blood pressure control, blood glucose control (HgA1C)
Health Service Utilization	Readmission to hospital in 30 days Admission to Emergency Department
Quality of Life	Quality-of-life scales (e.g., for chronic illness, cancer, chronic pain)
Psychological Indicators	Perceived-stress scale, self-control (e.g., Impulsivity Teen Conflict survey),

During planning a valuable resource for selecting outcomes is the Nursing Outcomes Classification (NOC) (see Chapter 18). The classification offers a language for the evaluation step of the nursing process. The purposes of NOC are (1) to identify, label, validate, and classify **nurse-sensitive patient outcomes**; (2) to field test and validate the classification; and (3) to define and test measurement procedures for the outcomes and indicators using clinical data (Moorhead et al., 2013). Within the NOC taxonomy you can select outcomes specific for nursing interventions that relate to nursing diagnoses. The NOC classification offers nurse-sensitive outcomes for NANDA-International (NANDA-I) nursing diagnoses (Table 20-3). For each outcome there are specific recommended evaluative measures, called *evaluation indicators* (i.e., the patient's physical condition, behaviors, or perceptions that are measures of outcome achievement).

QSEN QSEN: BUILDING COMPETENCY IN INFORMATICS

Explain how the use of the NOC classification in an electronic health record could improve patient safety. How would such a system help you monitor patient outcomes?

Answers to QSEN Activities can be found on the Evolve website.

Compare Achieved Effect with Goals and Outcomes. In Chapter 18 you learned that an expected outcome is a state, behavior, or perception that is measured along a continuum in response to a nursing intervention (Moorhead et al., 2013). During evaluation you perform evaluative measures that allow you to compare clinical data, patient behavior measures, and patient self-report measures collected before implementation with the evaluation findings gathered after administering nursing care. Next you evaluate whether the results of care match the expected outcomes and goals set for a patient. If outcomes are met, the overall goals for the patient also are met. Critical thinking directs you to analyze the findings from evaluation (Figure 20-3). Has the patient's condition improved? Is the patient able to improve, or are there physical factors preventing recovery? To what degree does this patient's motivation or willingness to pursue healthier behaviors influence responses to therapies?

TABLE 20-3 Linkages Between Nursing Outcomes Classification and Nursing Diagnoses

Nursing Diagnosis	Suggested Outcomes	Indicators (Examples)
Anxiety	Anxiety level	Ability to attend or concentrate Ability to learn Level of verbalized anxiety
Deficient Knowledge	Knowledge: treatment procedures Adherence behavior	Description of treatment procedures Description of prescribed activity Use of strategies to optimize health Performance of activities of daily living consistent with energy and tolerance

Adapted from Moorhead S, et al: *Nursing outcomes classification (NOC)*, ed 5, St Louis, 2013, Mosby.

Outcomes are statements of progressive, step-by-step physical, emotional, or behavioral responses that a patient needs to accomplish to achieve the goals of care. When your patients achieve outcomes, the related factors for a nursing diagnosis usually no longer exist. *In Mr. Lawson's case the nursing diagnosis of **Anxiety related to uncertainty over ability to return to work** has the goal of "Mr. Lawson will be able to assume activity restrictions at home." Tonya has planned and implemented nursing care to prepare Mr. Lawson for a smooth postoperative recovery. She implements interventions to minimize his anxiety and provides instruction about his activity restrictions so he will adhere to his treatment plan. The aim is to achieve adherence so return to work is a reasonable goal. Two of the expected outcomes for Mr. Lawson's goal include that the patient will maintain attention during instructional sessions and that patient will explain how activity restrictions aid recovery. Tonya uses evaluative measures, including observation of the patient's behavior during instruction and then patient self-report of what he understands about his activity restrictions. If Tonya's plan of care is successful, the related factor of "uncertainty over ability to return to work" was managed. Tonya will know that, because Mr. Lawson was able to attend during instruction and explain how adherence to activity restrictions will hasten his recovery, one source of anxiety has lessened.*

Interpreting and Summarizing Findings. A patient's clinical condition often changes during an acute illness. In contrast, chronic illness results in slow, subtle changes, although acute exacerbations can occur. When you evaluate the effect of interventions, you interpret or learn to recognize relevant evidence about a patient's condition, even evidence that sometimes does not match clinical expectations. By applying your clinical knowledge and experience, you recognize complications or adverse responses to illness and treatment in addition to expected outcomes.

Careful monitoring and early detection of problems are a nurse's first line of defense. Always make clinical judgments on the basis of your observations of what is occurring with a specific patient and not merely on what happens to patients in general. It is important to be detailed with your evaluation measures because change frequently

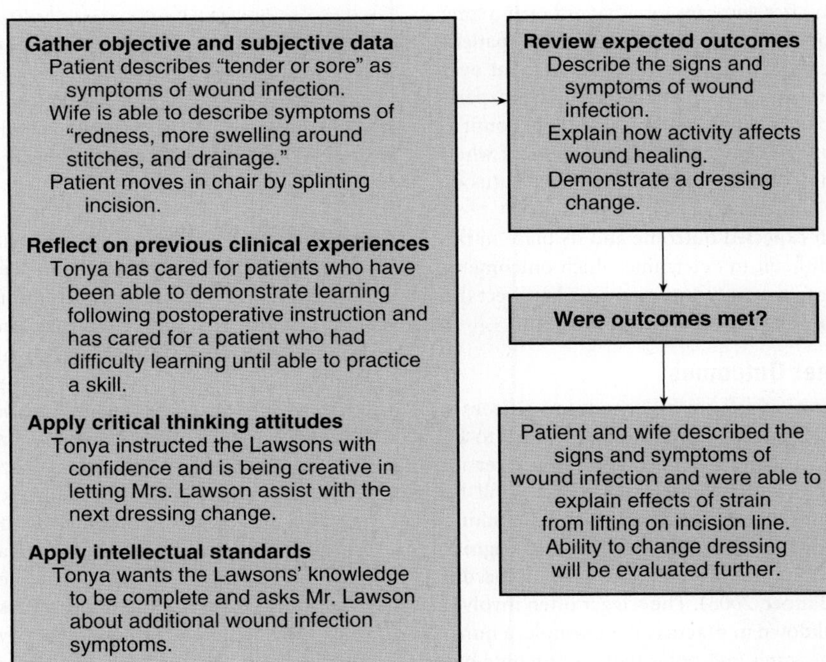

FIGURE 20-3 Critical thinking and the evaluation process.

TABLE 20-4 Examples of Objective Evaluation of Goal Achievement

Goals	Outcome Criteria	Patient Response	Evaluation Findings
Patient will change surgical dressing correctly by 12/18.	Patient demonstrates correct hand hygiene by 12/16. Patient describes material to use in dressing change by 12/17. Patient demonstrates dressing change by 12/18.	Patient used antiseptic hand rub correctly to wash hands. Patient applied clean gauze correctly and taped securely in place over incision.	Patient shows progression toward outcomes and achieved desired behavior.
Patient's lungs will be free of secretions by 11/30.	Coughing is nonproductive by 11/29. Lungs are clear to auscultation by 11/30. Respirations are 20/min by 11/30.	Patient coughed frequently and productively on 11/29 following nebulization. Lungs were clear to auscultation on 11/30. Respirations were 18/min on 11/29.	Patient will require continued nebulizer therapy. Condition is improving.

is not obvious. Evaluations are patient specific, made on the basis of a close familiarity with each patient's behavior, physical status, and reaction to caregivers. Perceptive clinical judgment involves matching the results of evaluative measures with expected outcomes to determine whether or not a patient's status is improving. When interpreting findings, you compare a patient's behavioral responses, perceptions, and the physiological signs and symptoms you expect to see with those actually seen from your evaluation. Comparing expected and actual findings allows you to interpret and judge a patient's condition and whether predicted changes occurred (Table 20-4). Perform the following steps to objectively evaluate the degree of success in achieving outcomes of care:

1. Examine the outcome criteria to identify the exact desired patient behavior or response.
2. Evaluate a patient's actual behavior or response.
3. Compare the established outcome criteria with the actual behavior or response.
4. Judge the degree of agreement between outcome criteria and the actual behavior or response.
5. If there is no agreement (or only partial agreement) between the outcome criteria and the actual behavior or response, what is/are the barrier(s)? Why did they not agree?

Evaluation is easier to perform after you care for a patient over a long period. You are then able to make subtle comparisons of patient responses and behaviors. When you have not cared for a patient over an extended time, evaluation improves by referring to previous experiences or asking colleagues who are familiar with the patient to confirm evaluation findings. The accuracy of any evaluation improves when you are familiar with a patient's behavior and physiological status or have cared for more than one patient with a similar problem.

Remember to evaluate each expected outcome and its place in the sequence of care. If not, it is difficult to determine which outcome in the sequence was not met; therefore you cannot revise and redirect the plan of care at the most appropriate time.

Recognize Errors or Unmet Outcomes

During evaluation the recognition of errors or unmet outcomes requires you to have an open mind, to actively pursue truth, to be patient and confident, and to engage in self-reflection (Shu-Yuan et al., 2013). You cannot assume that your treatment approaches will be successful. You must apply your observational skills, critical thinking intellectual standards (see Chapter 15), and knowledge to recognize the actual results of your care. Reflection-in-action typically occurs when there is a trigger event (Tanner, 2006). The trigger often involves a breakdown or perceived breakdown in practice. For example, a nurse reviews results of evaluative measures and notes that an outcome has not been met. Or a nurse observes how a patient reacts to a treatment (e.g., exercise, positioning, or teaching) and realizes that the approach is ineffective. A final example is a nurse reviewing a patient's progress and identifying that planned interventions were not completed, often described in the literature as "missed care" (Box 20-1). Reflection-in-action involves a nurse's ability to recognize how a patient is responding and then adjust interventions as a result (Tanner, 2006). A nurse will change the frequency of an intervention, change how the intervention is delivered, or select a new intervention.

The nursing process is a systematic, problem-solving approach to individualized patient care, but many factors affect each patient with health care problems. Often you will discover patients who have unmet needs. Patients with the same health care problem are not treated the same way. As a result you sometimes make errors in judgment. The systematic use of evaluation provides a way for you to catch these errors. By consistently incorporating evaluation into practice, you minimize errors and ensure that a patient's plan of care is appropriate and relevant and changes according to met and unmet needs.

BOX 20-1 EVIDENCE-BASED PRACTICE

Missed Care

PICO Question: In acute care settings which factors contribute to missed care involving adult patients?

Evidence Summary

Missed nursing care is any aspect of required patient care that is omitted or delayed (Kalisch et al., 2009). When nurses face the need to rethink priorities, manage the complexity of the nursing process for multiple patients, and deal with internal perceptions and values, the result is often delay in care, abbreviated care, or missed care. In a study by Kalisch and Lee (2010), teamwork alone accounted for about 11% of missed nursing care. In a study involving focus groups with staff nurses, nine themes of regularly missed nursing care included ambulation, turning, feedings, patient teaching, discharge planning, emotional support, hygiene, intake and output, documentation, and surveillance (evaluation) (Kalisch, 2006). These areas of omitted nursing care can influence patient outcomes negatively.

Application to Nursing Practice

- Work with team members and assign patients by acuity and geographical proximity rather than just by number.
- Learn to delegate effectively (see Chapter 21) and manage conflict when disagreements develop between colleagues.
- Teamwork requires accountability; responsibility; and a commitment to ongoing, clear communication.
- Review your plan of care routinely to minimize delays or omissions.

Self-Reflection and Correction of Errors

Reflection-in-action and subsequent clinical learning are also important parts of evaluation. What a nurse gains from caring for patients and carefully evaluating the outcomes of care later contributes to ongoing clinical knowledge development and capacity for making clinical judgments in the future (Tanner, 2006). Reflective reasoning improves the accuracy of making diagnostic conclusions (Mamede et al., 2012). This means that, when you gather evaluative measures about a patient, reflection on the findings and exploration about what the findings mean improve your ability to problem solve. Reflection lessens the likelihood that reasoning is based on assumptions or guesswork and increases the likelihood that it is based on objective critical thinking.

Care Plan Revision

As you evaluate patient care, your reflection-in-action helps you determine if the plan of care continues or if revisions are necessary. If your patient meets a goal successfully, discontinue that part of the care plan. Unmet and partially met goals require you to continue intervention. It also may be appropriate to modify or add nursing diagnoses for a new plan of care with appropriate goals, expected outcomes, and interventions. You must sometimes redefine priorities according to changes in patient condition, evaluation findings, or changes in the medical plan of care. An important step in critical thinking is knowing how a patient is progressing and how problems resolve, change, or worsen.

Tonya evaluates Mr. Lawson's understanding of how activity restrictions aid recovery. The patient explained the following, "My doctor doesn't want me to do any heavy lifting." As Tonya listens to Mr. and Mrs. Lawson discuss going home, Mrs. Lawson comments, "It will be great for my husband to see the grandkids soon. He's really close to them. He loves playing with the 3-year-old." Tonya uses the evaluative measure of patient self-report to determine what Mr. Lawson understands about his activity restrictions. She recognizes that playing with grandkids could involve picking up the children. *Tonya decides to modify her plan of care by reassessing the types of activities Mr. Lawson does at home (e.g., type of lifting, exercise, manual work) and adapting her instructions to be more comprehensive.*

Discontinuing a Care Plan. After you determine that your patient met expected outcomes and goals, confirm your evaluation with the patient when possible. If you and the patient agree, you discontinue that part of the care plan. Documentation of a discontinued plan ensures that other nurses will not unnecessarily continue interventions. Continuity of care assumes that care provided to patients is relevant and timely. You waste much time and energy when you do not communicate achieved goals with other nurses.

Modifying a Care Plan. When patients do not meet goals and outcomes, you identify the factors that interfere with their achievement. Usually a change in a patient's condition, needs, or abilities makes alteration of the care plan necessary. For example, when teaching self-administration of insulin, a nurse discovers that a patient has developed a new problem, a tremor associated with a side effect of a medication. The patient is unable to draw medication from a syringe or inject the needle safely. As a result, the original outcomes, "Patient correctly prepares insulin in a syringe," and "Patient administers insulin injection independently," are no longer appropriate because they cannot be met. The nurse introduces new interventions (instructing a family member in insulin preparation and administration) and revises outcomes, "Family caregiver correctly prepares insulin in syringe," and "Family caregiver administers insulin injection correctly," to meet the goal of care.

At times a lack of goal achievement results from an error in nursing judgment or failure to follow each step of the nursing process. Patients often have multiple and complex problems. Always remember the possibility of overlooking or misjudging something. When a goal is not met, no matter what the reason, repeat the nursing process sequence for that nursing diagnosis. Reassess the patient; determine accuracy of the nursing diagnosis; and establish a plan with new goals, expected outcomes, and appropriate priority interventions.

Reassessment. If a nursing diagnosis is unresolved or if you determine that perhaps a new problem has developed, reassessment is necessary. A complete reassessment of patient factors relating to an existing nursing diagnosis and etiology is necessary when modifying a plan. Apply critical thinking while comparing new data about a patient's condition with previously assessed information. Knowledge from previous experiences helps you direct the reassessment process. Caring for patients and families who have had similar health problems gives you a strong background of knowledge to use for anticipating patient needs and knowing what to assess. Reassessment ensures that the database is accurate and current. It also reveals a missing link (i.e., a critical piece of new information that was overlooked and thus interfered with goal achievement). You sort, validate, and cluster all new data to analyze and interpret differences from the original database (see Chapter 16). You also document reassessment data to alert other nursing staff and collaborative health care providers to the patient's status.

Redefining Diagnoses. After reassessment determine which nursing diagnoses are accurate for the situation. Ask yourself whether you selected the correct diagnosis and if the etiological factor is accurate and current. Then revise the problem list to reflect the patient's changed status. Sometimes you form a new diagnosis, or the prioritizing of diagnoses change. You base your nursing care on an accurate list of nursing diagnoses. Accuracy is more important than the number of diagnoses selected. As a patient's condition changes, the diagnoses also change.

Goals and Expected Outcomes. When revising a care plan, review the goals and expected outcomes for necessary changes. For example, does the time frame for outcomes need to be revised? Have certain outcomes been met and others only partially met? Does your reassessment reveal a goal that is unrealistic? Examine the appropriateness of goals for any unchanged nursing diagnoses and remember that a change in one health care problem sometimes affects the goals for others. *In Mr. Lawson's case, if his anxiety were to worsen again, Tonya likely would not only have to revise the plan for managing the anxiety but also consider if her selection of teaching strategies also needs to be changed.* Determining that each goal and expected outcome is realistic for the problem, etiology, and time frame is particularly important. Unrealistic expected outcomes and time frames make goal achievement difficult.

Clearly document goals and expected outcomes for new or revised nursing diagnoses so all team members are aware of the revised care plan. When the goal is still appropriate but has not yet been met, try changing the evaluation criteria to allow more time. You may also decide at this time to change interventions that are more individualized to a patient need or status.

Interventions. The evaluation of interventions examines two factors: the appropriateness of the intervention selected and the correct application of the intervention. Appropriateness is based on the standard of care for a patient's health problem. A **standard of care** is the minimum level of care accepted to ensure high quality of patient care. Standards of care define the types of therapies typically administered to patients with defined problems or needs. For example, if a patient who is receiving chemotherapy for leukemia has the nursing diagnosis

Acute pain related to oral mucosa inflammation from mucositis, the standard of care established by the nursing department for this problem includes pain-control measures, mouth care guidelines, and diet therapy. Professional organizations such as the Oncology Nursing Society often have clinical guidelines as standards of care for select health problems. The nurse reviews the standard of care and decides which interventions have been chosen and whether additional ones are required to achieve expected outcomes.

Increasing or decreasing the frequency of interventions is another approach to ensure appropriate application of an intervention. You adjust interventions on the basis of a patient's actual response to therapy and your previous experience with similar patients. For example, if a patient continues to have congested lung sounds, you increase the frequency of coughing and deep-breathing exercises to remove secretions and add positioning to ensure airway clearance.

During evaluation you find that some planned interventions are designed for an inappropriate level of nursing care. If you need to change the level of care, substitute a different action verb such as *assist* in place of *provide* or *demonstrate* in place of *instruct.* For example, assisting a patient to walk requires a nurse to be at the patient's side during ambulation, whereas providing an assistive device (e.g., a cane or walker) suggests that the patient is more independent. In addition, demonstration requires you to show a patient how a skill is performed rather than simply telling the patient how to perform it. Sometimes the level of care is appropriate, but the interventions are unsuitable because of a change in the expected outcome. In this example discontinue the interventions and plan new ones.

Make any changes in the plan of care on the basis of the nature of a patient's unfavorable response. Consulting with other health care team members often yields suggestions for improving the care delivery approach. Experienced nurses are often excellent resources and can provide valuable insight. Simply changing a care plan is not enough. Implement the new plan and reevaluate the patient's response to the nursing actions. *Evaluation is continuous, occurring through each step of the nursing process.*

STANDARDS FOR EVALUATION

Nursing care helps patients resolve actual health problems, prevent the occurrence of potential problems, and maintain a healthy state. Evaluation is an integral step to that end. The American Nurses Association (ANA) defines standards of professional nursing practice (see Chapter 1), which include standards for the evaluation step of the nursing process. The standards are authoritative statements of the duties that all registered nurses, regardless of role, patient population they serve, or specialty, are expected to perform competently (ANA, 2010). The competencies for evaluation include being systematic and using criterion-based evaluation, collaborating with patients and health care professionals, using ongoing assessment data to revise a plan, and communicating results to patients and families. Always deliver interventions responsibly and appropriately to minimize unwarranted or unwanted treatment (ANA, 2010).

Collaborate and Evaluate Effectiveness of Interventions

An important aspect of evaluation is collaboration. Patient-centered care is only achieved when a patient and family are actively involved in the evaluation process. This requires you to consider what is important to your patients, including their values, preferences, and expressed needs. When you develop patient care goals and expected outcomes with patients, they are an important resource for being able to tell you if outcomes are being met. They are able to share their perspective of whether an intervention is successful. For example, a patient knows best if pain has lessened or if breathing is easier. The same holds true for the family, who often can recognize changes in patient behavior sooner than you can because of their familiarity with the patient.

It is essential for nurses to collaborate closely with all members of the health care team during evaluation. Successful collaboration involves interactions in which professionals work together cooperatively with shared responsibility and interdependence toward achieving patient outcomes. Members of the health care team who contribute to the patient's care also gather evaluative findings. Communicating openly and on a regular basis with the health care team improves the likelihood of staying informed about a patient's responses to care.

Proper evaluation determines the effectiveness of nursing interventions. It is also important to evaluate whether each patient reaches a level of wellness or recovery that the health care team and patient established in the goals of the care plan. In addition, have you met the patient's expectations of care? Ask patients about their perceptions of care such as, "Did you receive the type of pain relief you expected?" "Did you receive enough information to change your dressing when you return home?" This level of evaluation determines the patient's satisfaction with care and strengthens partnering between you and the patient.

Document Results

Documentation and reporting are important parts of evaluation because it is crucial to share information about a patient's progress and current status. Accurate information needs to be present in a patient's medical record and shared during hand-off communication so nurses and other health care team members know if a patient is progressing and to make ongoing clinical decisions. In settings in which the same nurse will not be providing care throughout a patient's stay, it becomes very important to have consistent, thorough documentation of a patient's progress toward expected outcomes. The use of nursing diagnostic language and the Nursing Interventions Classification (NIC) and NOC is becoming more common in electronic medical records, improving the quality, consistency, and accuracy of what is documented. In addition, electronic systems provide linkages to make it easier to interpret cues regarding whether interventions led to expected patient outcomes. When documenting a patient's response to your interventions, describe the interventions, the evaluative measures used, the outcomes achieved, and the continued plan of care. *Here is an example of Tonya's documentation of evaluation of care:*

> *1430: Instructed patient on importance of handwashing and need to observe surgical wound daily for signs of redness or drainage from incision. Discussed ways to reduce strain on suture line by avoiding lifting any object over 20 lbs. Asked patient to describe when it is necessary to call doctor about wound. Patient and wife were able to identify signs of infection and occurrence of pain as reasons to notify doctor. Wife was able to demonstrate proper handwashing technique. Patient was able to verbalize several examples of objects not to lift (grandchild, groceries, trash). Provided patient additional instruction in form of pamphlet with outline of wound care steps. Will recommend to home health need to observe patient and wife perform wound care at home.*

Your aim in documenting is to present a clear argument from the evaluative data as to whether a patient is progressing or not.

One of the ANA standards for evaluation is to share results of care with patients and their families according to federal and state regulations (ANA, 2010). Keep patients and families informed about the patients' progress. Be aware of guidelines of your agency for the type of clinical information (e.g., diagnostic findings, results of treatment) that you can communicate.

KEY POINTS

- Evaluation is a step of the nursing process that includes two components: an examination of a condition or situation and a judgment as to whether change has occurred.
- During evaluation apply critical thinking to make clinical decisions and redirect nursing care to best meet patient needs.
- Positive evaluations occur when your patient meets desired outcomes and goals.
- Criterion-based standards for evaluation are the physiological, emotional, and behavioral responses that are a patient's goals and expected outcomes.
- Evaluative measures are assessment skills or techniques that you use to collect data for determining if outcomes were met.
- It sometimes becomes necessary to collect evaluative measures over time to determine if a pattern of change exists.
- When interpreting findings, you compare a patient's behavioral responses and the physiological signs and symptoms that you expect to see with those actually seen from your evaluation and judge the degree of agreement.
- Documentation of evaluative findings allows all members of the health care team to know whether or not a patient is progressing.
- A patient's nursing diagnoses, priorities, and interventions sometimes change as a result of evaluation.
- Evaluation examines two factors: the appropriateness of the interventions selected and the correct application of the intervention.

CLINICAL APPLICATION QUESTIONS

Preparing for Clinical Practice

Tonya organizes herself so she can take the time needed to evaluate the outcomes of her plan of care. Mr. Lawson has the nursing diagnosis of *Acute Pain related to incisional trauma.* The patient has taken two doses of the prn analgesic ordered for his pain over the last 8 hours. Thirty minutes after the last dose Mr. Lawson rated his pain a 3 on a scale of 0 to 10; he states, "I only really notice now when I move too quickly." An outcome for the patient's goal of achieving pain relief is for pain scores to be at 4 or less. Mrs. Lawson is in the room, so Tonya takes time to give the Lawsons the discharge instruction sheet that is part of standard of care of her nursing unit. She asks Mr. Lawson to explain the types of activity he must avoid for the first 2 weeks he is at home.

1. Describe the type of evaluation measure Tonya uses when asking Mr. Lawson to explain the types of activities he should avoid. What limitations are there in using this type of evaluation measure?
2. Explain how Tonya can determine if the patient's nursing diagnosis of *Acute Pain* has been resolved. Describe how this affects her other priorities.
3. Explain how Tonya's evaluation of the patient's ability to learn about activity restrictions can be patient centered.

ⓔ *Answers to Clinical Application Questions can be found on the Evolve website.*

REVIEW QUESTIONS

Are You Ready to Test Your Nursing Knowledge?

1. For the nursing diagnosis of *Deficient Knowledge* a nurse selects an outcome from the Nursing Outcome Classification (NOC) of patient knowledge of arthritis treatment. Which of the following are examples of an outcome indicator for this outcome? (Select all that apply.)
   1. Nurse provides four teaching sessions before discharge.
   2. Patient denies joint pain following heat application.
   3. Patient describes correct schedule for taking antiarthritic medications.
   4. Patient explains situations for using heat application on inflamed joints.
   5. Patient explains role family caregiver plays in applying heat to inflamed joint.
2. A nurse in a community health clinic has been caring for a young teenager with asthma for several months. The nurse's goal of care for this patient is to achieve self-management of asthma medications. Identify appropriate evaluative indicators for self-management for this patient. (Select all that apply.)
   1. Quality of life
   2. Patient satisfaction
   3. Use of clinic services
   4. Adherence to use of inhaler
   5. Description of side effects of medications
3. A nurse caring for a patient with heart failure instructs the patient on foods to eat for a low-sodium diet. The nurse will perform which of the following evaluation measures to determine success of her instruction?
   1. Patient weight
   2. Asking patient to identify three low-sodium foods to eat for lunch
   3. A calorie count of food
   4. Patient description of how food selections are made
4. From the following list of indicators, determine which indicators are goals **(G)** and which indicators are outcomes **(O)**.
   1. _____ Will achieve pain relief
   2. _____ Ambulates 10 feet down hallway
   3. _____ Will remain free of infection
   4. _____ Will be afebrile
   5. _____ Reports pain severity reduced from 6 to a 4 on scale of 0 to 10
   6. _____ Will gain improved mobility
5. A nurse has been caring for a patient over 2 consecutive days. During that time the patient has had an intravenous (IV) catheter in the right forearm. At the end of shift on the second day the nurse inspects the catheter site, observes for redness, and asks if the patient feels tenderness when the site is palpated. This is an example of which indicator reflecting the nurse's ability to perform evaluation:
   1. Examining results of clinical data
   2. Comparing achieved effects with outcomes
   3. Recognizing error
   4. Self-reflection
6. A patient has been febrile and coughing thick secretions; adventitious lung sounds indicate rales in the left lower lobe of the lungs. The nurse decides to perform nasotracheal suction because the patient is not coughing. The nurse inspects the mucus that is suctioned, which is minimal. The nurse again auscultates for lung sounds. Auscultation and mucus inspection are examples of:
   1. Evaluative measures.
   2. Expected outcomes.
   3. Reassessments.
   4. Reflection.
7. After caring for a young man newly diagnosed with diabetes, a nurse is reviewing what was completed in his plan of care following discharge. She considers how she related to the patient and whether she selected interventions best suited to his educational level. It was the nurse's first time caring for a new patient with

diabetes. The nurse's behavior is an example of which of the following?
1. Reflection-in-action
2. Reassessment
3. Reprioritizing
4. Reflection-on-action

8. A nurse has been caring for a patient over the last 10 hours. The patient's plan of care includes the nursing diagnosis of *Nausea related to effects of postoperative anesthesia.* The nurse has been asking the patient to rate his nausea over the last several hours after administering antiemetics and using comfort measures such as oral hygiene. The nurse reviews the patient's responses over the past 10 hours and notes how the patient's self-report of nausea has changed. This review an example of:
   1. Comparing outcome criteria with actual response.
   2. Gathering outcome criteria.
   3. Evaluating the patient's actual response.
   4. Reprioritizing interventions.
9. A faculty member is reviewing a nursing student's plan of care, including the interventions the student provided for a patient with dementia. The student reviewed clinical guidelines on a professional website to identify interventions successful in reducing wandering in patients with dementia. The faculty member should evaluate which of the following? (Select all that apply.)
   1. Number of interventions
   2. Appropriateness of the intervention for the patient
   3. The prior use of interventions by other nursing staff
   4. Correct application of the intervention for the patient care setting
   5. The time it takes to provide interventions
10. A nurse enters a patient's room and begins a conversation. During this time the nurse evaluates how a patient is tolerating a new diet plan. The nurse decides to also evaluate the patient's expectations of care. Which statement is appropriate for evaluating a patient's expectations of care?
   1. On a scale of 0 to 10 rate your level of nausea.
   2. The nurse weighs the patient.
   3. The nurse asks, "Did you believe that you received the information you needed to follow your diet?"
   4. The nurse states, "Tell me four different foods included in your diet."
11. A nurse checks an intravenous (IV) solution container for clarity of the solution, noting that it is infusing into the patient's left arm. The IV solution of 9% NS is infusing freely at 100 mL/hr as ordered. The nurse reviews the nurses' notes from the previous shift to determine if the dressing over the site was changed as scheduled per standard of care. While in the room the nurse inspects the condition of the dressing and notes the date on the dressing label. In which ways did the nurse evaluate the condition of the IV site? (Select all that apply.)
   1. Checked the IV infusion rate
   2. Checked the type of IV solution
   3. Confirmed from nurses' notes the time of dressing change
   4. Inspected the condition of the IV dressing at the site
   5. Checked clarity of IV solution
12. A patient is being discharged after treatment for colitis (inflammation of the colon). The patient has had no episodes of diarrhea or abdominal pain for 24 hours. Following instruction, the patient identified correctly the need to follow a low-residue diet and the types of food to include if a bout of diarrhea develops at home. These behaviors are examples of:
   1. Evaluative measures.
   2. Expected outcomes.
   3. Reassessments.
   4. Standards of care.
13. Which of the following does a nurse perform when discontinuing a plan of care for a patient?
   1. Confirms with the patient that expected outcomes and goals have been met
   2. Talks with the patient about reprioritizing interventions in the plan of care
   3. Changes the frequency of interventions provided
   4. Reassesses how goals were met
14. Purposes of the Nursing Outcomes Classification (NOC) include which of the following? (Select all that apply.)
   1. To identify and label nurse-sensitive patient outcomes
   2. To test the classification in clinical settings
   3. To establish health care reimbursement guidelines
   4. To identify nursing interventions for linked nursing diagnoses
   5. To define measurement procedures for outcomes
15. Which of the following statements correctly describes the evaluation process? (Select all that apply.)
   1. Evaluation is an ongoing process.
   2. Evaluation usually reveals obvious changes in patients.
   3. Evaluation involves making clinical decisions.
   4. Evaluation requires the use of assessment skills.
   5. Evaluation is only done when a patient's condition changes.

Answers: 1. 3, 4; **2.** 1, 3, 4; **3.** 2; **4.** 1-goal, 2-outcome, 3-goal, 4-goal, 5-outcome, 6-goal; **5.** 1; **6.** 1; **7.** 4; **8.** 1; **9.** 2, 4; **10.** 3; **11.** 1, 4; **12.** 2; **13.** 1; **14.** 1, 2, 5; **15.** 1, 3, 4.

Rationales for Review Questions can be found on the Evolve website.

REFERENCES

American Nurses Association (ANA): *Scope and standards of practice: nursing*, ed 2, Silver Spring, MD, 2010, American Nurses Association.

European Pressure Ulcer Advisory Panel (EPUAP) and National Pressure Ulcer Advisory Panel (NPUAP): *Prevention of pressure ulcers: quick reference guide*, Washington DC, 2009, National Ulcer Advisory Panel, http://www.epuap.org/guidelines/Final_Quick_Prevention.pdf. Accessed September 14, 2014.

Moorhead S, et al: *Nursing outcomes classification (NOC)*, ed 5, St Louis, 2013, Mosby.

RESEARCH REFERENCES

Du S, Yuan C: Evaluation of patient self-management outcomes in health care: a systematic review, *Int Nurs Rev* 57(2):159, 2010.

Kalisch BJ: Missed nursing care: a qualitative study, *J Nurs Care Qual* 21(4):306, 2006.

Kalisch BJ, Lee KH: The impact of teamwork on missed nursing care, *Nurs Outlook* 58(5):233, 2010.

Kalisch BJ, et al: Missed nursing care: a concept analysis, *J Adv Nurs* 65(7):1509, 2009.

Mamede S, et al: Exploring the role of salient distracting clinical features in the emergence of diagnostic errors and the mechanisms through which reflection counteracts mistakes, *BMJ Qual Saf* 21(4):295, 2012.

Shu-Yuan C, et al: Identifying critical thinking indicators and critical thinker attributes in nursing practice, *J Nurs Res* 21(3):204, 2013.

Tanner CA: Thinking like a nurse: a research-based model of clinical judgment in nursing, *J Nurs Educ* 45(6):204, 2006.

21

Managing Patient Care

OBJECTIVES

- Differentiate among the types of nursing care delivery models.
- Describe the elements of shared decision making.
- Describe the characteristics and traits of a transformational leader.
- Discuss the ways in which a nurse manager supports staff involvement in a decentralized decision-making model.
- Discuss ways to apply clinical care coordination skills in nursing practice.
- Discuss principles to follow in the appropriate delegation of patient care activities.

KEY TERMS

Accountability, p. 282
Authority, p. 282
Autonomy, p. 282
Case management, p. 281
Delegation, p. 286
Empowered, p. 279
Interprofessional, p. 283
Patient- and family-centered care, p. 281
Responsibility, p. 282
Shared governance, p. 283
Total patient care, p. 281
Transformational leadership, p. 279

MEDIA RESOURCES

http://evolve.elsevier.com/Potter/fundamentals/

- Review Questions
- Case Study with Questions
- Audio Glossary
- Content Updates

As a nursing student it is important for you to acquire the necessary knowledge and competencies that ultimately allow you to practice as an entry-level staff nurse. The National Council of State Boards of Nursing (NCSBN) identified competencies that registered nurses (RNs) and licensed practical nurses (LPNs)/licensed vocational nurses (LVNs) need on entry to practice (Kearney, 2009) (Box 21-1). Regardless of the type of setting in which you eventually choose to work as a staff nurse, you will be responsible for using organizational resources, participating in organizational routines while providing direct patient care, using time productively and setting priorities, collaborating with all members of the health care team, and using certain leadership skills to manage others on the nursing team. The delivery of nursing care within a health care system is a challenge because of the changes that influence health professionals, patients, and health care organizations (see Chapter 2). However, change offers opportunities. As you develop the knowledge and skills to become a staff nurse, you learn what it takes to effectively manage the patients for whom you care and to take the initiative in becoming a leader among your professional colleagues.

BUILDING A NURSING TEAM

Nurses want to work within an institutional and unit culture that promotes autonomy and quality (Kramer et al., 2011). Nurses are self-directed and, with proper leadership and motivation, are able to solve most complex problems. A nurse's education and commitment to practicing within established standards and guidelines ensures a rewarding professional career. As a nurse it is also important to work in an empowering environment as a member of a solid and strong nursing team. A strong nursing team works together to achieve the best outcomes for patients. Effective team development requires team building and training, trust, communication, and a workplace that facilitates collaboration (Huber, 2014). Patient care units where teamwork is stronger had fewer reports and incidents of missed nursing care, leading to improved quality and safety of nursing care for patients (Kalisch and Lee, 2010). Stronger levels of teamwork among staff members have been found to contribute to higher levels of job satisfaction among nurses (Kalisch et al., 2010).

Building an **empowered** nursing team begins with the nurse executive, who is often a vice president or director of nursing. The executive's position within an organization is critical in uniting the strategic direction of an organization with the philosophical values and goals of nursing. The nurse executive is a clinical and business leader who is concerned with maximizing quality of care and cost-effectiveness while maintaining relationships and professional satisfaction of the staff. Perhaps the most important responsibility of the nurse executive is to establish a philosophy for nursing that enables managers and staff to provide quality nursing care. Box 21-2 identifies the characteristics of an effective nurse leader.

The nurse manager is critical to developing a successful unit that works together as a healthy team (LeBlanc, 2014). The nurse manager who uses **transformational leadership** is focused on change and innovation through team development, motivates and empowers staff to function at a high level of performance, and serves as a role model for the nurses on the unit (Smith, 2011). The TEEAMS approach is an approach that the nurse manager may use. In this approach the nurse manager spends *time* on the unit with the staff sharing ideas, *empowers* the staff, is *enthusiastic* about seeking opportunities to enhance the

BOX 21-1 Entry-Level Nurse Competencies

- Possess a systems focus to see the big picture.
- Understand the environment of care.
- Manage the care of patients.
- Prioritize basic patient care needs.
- Be able to critically think as demonstrated by assessment of problem, identification of solution, implementation of solution, evaluation of care, and follow-up of care.
- Communicate effectively with physicians and health care team members.
- Demonstrate nursing knowledge and display confidence in knowledge base.
- Work as a team member collaborating with health care team members.
- Have a patient orientation and focus with actions focused on patient and patient needs.
- Respect the rights, beliefs, wishes, and values of patients.
- Be a patient advocate.
- Recognize own limitations and see support of validation of decisions as needed.
- Demonstrate knowledge of roles, responsibilities, and functions of a nurse.

Modified from Kearney MH: Report of the findings from the post-entry competence study, Chicago, 2009, National Council of State Boards of Nursing; National Council of State Boards of Nursing: 2009 Tuning analysis: a comparison of US and international nursing educational competencies, Chicago, 2010, National Councils State Boards of Nursing.

BOX 21-2 Characteristics of an Effective Leader

- Is an effective communicator
- Is consistent in managing conflict
- Is knowledgeable and competent in all aspects of delivery of care
- Is a role model for staff
- Uses participatory approach in decision making
- Shows appreciation for a job well done
- Delegates work appropriately
- Sets objectives and guides staff
- Displays caring, understanding, and empathy for others
- Motivates and empowers others
- Is proactive and flexible
- Focuses on team development

Modified from Dunham-Taylor J: Quantum leadership: love one another. In Dunham-Taylor J, Pinczak JZ: *Financial management for nurse managers*, ed 2, Boston, 2010, Jones & Bartlett Publishers; Huber DL: *Leadership & nursing care management*, ed 5, St Louis, 2014, Elsevier.

team, shows *appreciation* and recognizes team members for a job well done, *manages* the team and holds team members accountable, and provides *support* in the stressful health care environment (LeBlanc, 2014). Together a manager and the nursing staff have to share a philosophy of care for their work unit. A philosophy of care includes the professional nursing staff's values and concerns for the way they view and care for patients. For example, a philosophy addresses the purpose of the nursing unit, how staff works with patients and families, and the standards of care for the work unit. Selection of a nursing care delivery model and a management structure that supports professional nursing practice are essential to the philosophy of care.

The nurse manager's leadership style impacts the work environment and patient outcomes. Nursing units where nurse managers use transformational leadership styles have a shared vision that leads the unit to work toward the unit goals together, and staff members have job clarity that improves productivity and staff motivation (Holly and Igwee, 2011). Research supports that, on nursing units where the nurse manager uses transformational leadership, there is an increased level of patient satisfaction, a lower patient mortality rate, and a lower rate of medication errors (Wong et al., 2013). Transformational leadership practices of the nurse manager also lead to increased staff satisfaction, decreased stress and burnout in staff nurses, increased overall staff feeling of well-being, and staff retention (Weberg, 2010). Nurse managers who use these relational leadership styles create a positive work environment by providing support, encouragement, and constructive feedback to staff through open communication (Wong et al., 2013). A positive work environment engages nurses in their practice, promotes good working relationships among colleagues and a high morale level, and prompts nurses to take responsibility for their career development morale level (Fasoli, 2010) (Box 21-3).

BOX 21-3 EVIDENCE-BASED PRACTICE

Nurses Work Engagement

PICO Question: In hospitals are nurses who are highly engaged in their work more likely to remain in nursing than nurses who have lower levels of work engagement?

Evidence Summary

Work engagement is "a positive, fulfilling state of mind about work that is characterized by vigor, dedication and absorption" (Bargagliotti, 2012, p. 1414). Nurses who trust in an organization, the nurse leader or manager, and colleagues and have a high degree of nursing autonomy contribute to the nurses' work engagement (Bargagliotti, 2012; Cowden et al., 2011). Nurses who are engaged in their work were less likely to consider leaving their current position (Carter and Tourangeau, 2012; Cowden et al., 2011). Nurse leaders who use meaningful recognition as a way to recognize the extraordinary contributions of their nursing staff help develop a healthy work culture where nurses are more engaged (Lefton, 2012). Work engagement of nurses has a positive impact on a nursing unit and health care organization. Research has shown that, when there is a highly engaged nursing workforce, nurses had higher levels of personal initiative, making work engagement contagious. This contagiousness and spread of work engagement often leads to a decrease in patient mortality and complications and an increase in financial profitability of the health care organization (Bargagliotti, 2012). Work engagement is an important factor in the delivery of safe patient care.

Application to Nursing Practice

- Build positive relationships with colleagues on the nursing unit (Fasoli, 2010).
- Work with nurse leaders on the unit to develop a meaningful recognition program for nurses' extraordinary work (Lefton, 2012).
- Nurse managers need to focus on meeting needs of nursing staff (Cowden et al., 2011).
- Participate in shared governance and decision making at the unit level (Cowden et al., 2011)
- Participate in professional development activities that stimulate personal growth (Carter and Tourangeau, 2012).

Magnet Recognition

One way of creating an empowering work environment is through the Magnet Recognition Program (see Chapter 2). The Magnet Recognition Program is based on five model components—transformational leadership; structural empowerment; exemplary professional practice, new knowledge, innovation, and improvements; and empirical quality results. A hospital that is Magnet certified has a transformed culture with a practice environment that is dynamic, autonomous, collaborative, and positive for nurses. The culture focuses on concern for patients. Typically a Magnet hospital has clinical promotion systems and research and evidence-based practice programs. The nurses have professional autonomy over their practice and control over the practice environment (Kramer et al., 2010). A Magnet hospital empowers a nursing team to make changes and be innovative. Professional nurse councils at the organizational and unit level are one way to create an empowerment model. This culture and empowerment combine to produce a strong collaborative relationship among team members and improve patient quality outcomes (ANCC, 2014).

Nursing Care Delivery Models

Ideally the philosophy that nurses greatly contribute to the quality care of patients guides the selection of a care delivery model. However, too often a lack of nursing resources and the goals of the business plan of the hospital influence the final choice of a model. A care delivery model needs to help nurses achieve desirable outcomes for their patients in the way that work is organized, the roles that each care provider assumes, or the way a nurse's responsibilities are defined. Nursing care delivery models contain the common components of nurse-patient relationship, clinical decision making, patient assignments and work allocation, interprofessional communication, and management of the environment of care (Huber, 2014).

Two traditional models that sometimes are used today in some health care institutions are team nursing and primary nursing. Team nursing developed in response to the severe nursing shortage following World War II. By 2000 the interprofessional team was a more common model (Yoder-Wise, 2014). In team nursing the RN is the leader who leads a team of other RNs, practical nurses, and nursing assistive personnel (NAP) who provide direct patient care. The primary nursing model of care delivery was developed to place RNs at the bedside and improve the accountability of nursing for patient outcomes and the professional relationships among staff members (Yoder-Wise, 2014). The model became more popular in the 1970s and early 1980s as hospitals began to employ more RNs. Primary nursing supports a philosophy regarding nurse and patient relationships. It is typically not practiced today because of the high cost of an all RN staffing model.

More common models used today are patient-centered care, total patient care, and case management. **Patient- and family-centered care** is a model of nursing care in which mutual partnerships among the patient, family, and health care team are formed to plan, implement, and evaluate the nursing and health care delivered (IPFCC, 2010; Mastro et al., 2014). At the center of patient-centered care is the patient or family member as the source of control and full partner in providing care (QSEN Institute, 2014). The Institute for Patient-and Family-Centered Care identified four core concepts for patient-centered care (IPFCC, 2010; Mastro et al., 2014): (1) *respect and dignity,* ensuring that the care provided is given on the basis of a patient's and family's knowledge, values, beliefs, and cultural backgrounds; (2) *information sharing,* meaning that health care providers communicate and share information so patients and families receive timely, complete, and accurate information to effectively participate in care and decision making; (3) *participation,* whereby patients and families are encouraged and supported in participating in care and decision-making; and (4) *collaboration,* demonstrated by the health care leaders collaborating with patients and families in policy and program development, implementation, and evaluation and patients who are fully engaged in their health care. Nurses support and promote patient engagement and empowerment through the use of patient- and family-centered communication, bedside shift report, and patient- and family-centered interprofessional rounds (Mastro et al., 2014).

Total patient care delivery was the original care delivery model developed during Florence Nightingale's time. In this model the RN is responsible for all aspects of care for one or more patients during a shift of care, working directly with patients, families, and health team members. There is a high degree of collaboration among health care team members. The model disappeared in the 1930s and became popular again during the 1970s and 1980s when the number of RNs increased; it is primarily found in critical care areas (Yoder-Wise, 2014).

Case management is a care-management approach designed to coordinate and link health care services across all levels of care for patients and their families while streamlining costs and maintaining quality (Yoder-Wise, 2014) (see Chapter 2). The case-management system is focused on achieving patient outcomes within effective time frames and with available resources (Huber, 2014). The Case Management Society of America (2012) defines case management as "a collaborative process of assessment, planning, facilitation, and advocacy for options and services to meet an individual's health needs through communication and available resources to promote quality cost-effective outcomes." Effective case management delivery is important; and there have been many initiatives to support case management because of hospitals' need to improve patient outcomes such as reduction of 30-day readmissions. Case management is unique because clinicians, either as individuals or as part of a collaborative group, oversee the management of patients with specific, complex health problems or are held accountable for some standard of cost management and quality.

For example, a case manager coordinates a patient's acute care in the hospital and follows up with the patient after discharge, either to home, rehabilitation, or a long-term care setting. Case managers do not provide direct care but instead work with and collaborate with direct-care providers about the care delivered by other staff and health care team members and actively coordinate patient discharge planning. Ongoing communication with team members facilitates a patient's transition to home. In this situation the case manager helps the patient identify health needs, determine the services and resources that are available, and make cost-efficient choices (Yoder-Wise, 2014). The case manager frequently oversees a caseload of patients with complex nursing and medical problems. Often he or she is an advanced practice nurse who, through specific interventions, helps to improve patient outcomes, optimize patient safety by facilitating care transitions, decrease length of stay, and lower health care costs.

Decision Making

With a philosophy for nursing established, it is the manager who directs and supports staff in the realization of that philosophy. The nurse executive supports managers by establishing a structure that helps to achieve organizational goals and provide appropriate support to care delivery staff. It takes a committed nurse executive, an excellent manager, and an empowered nursing staff to create an enriching work environment in which nursing practice thrives. Decision-making is a critical component of an effective leader and manager (Huber, 2014).

Decentralization is a component of the hierarchical level of decision making found in health care institutions (Huber, 2014). Higher degrees of decentralization take the decision making down to the lower levels of the health care institution and have less supervision of the decision-making process (Huber, 2014). More and more health care institutions have moved the decision making down to the level of staff. This type of decision-making structure has the advantage of creating an environment in which managers and staff become more actively

BOX 21-4 Responsibilities of a Nurse Manager

- Help staff establish annual goals for the unit and systems needed to accomplish goals.
- Monitor professional nursing standards of practice on the unit.
- Develop an ongoing staff development plan, including one for new employees.
- Recruit new employees (interview and hire).
- Conduct routine staff evaluations.
- Establish self as a role model for positive customer service (customers include patients, families, and other health care team members).
- Submit staffing schedules for the unit.
- Conduct regular patient rounds and problem solve patient or family complaints.
- Establish, monitor, and implement a unit performance/quality improvement plan.
- Review and recommend new equipment for the unit.
- Conduct regular staff meetings.
- Make rounds with health care providers.
- Establish and support staff and interprofessional committees.

involved in shaping the identity and determining the success of a health care organization. Working in a decentralized structure has the potential for greater collaborative effort, increased competency of staff, increased staff motivation, and ultimately a greater sense of professional accomplishment and satisfaction.

Progressive organizations achieve more when employees at all levels are empowered and actively involved. As a result, the role of a nurse manager is critical in the management of effective nursing units or groups. Box 21-4 highlights the diverse responsibilities of nursing managers. To make shared decision making work, managers need to know how to move it down to the lowest level possible. On a nursing unit it is important for all nursing staff members (RNs, LPNs, and LVNs), nursing assistants, and unit secretaries to become engaged. They need to be kept well informed. They also need to be given the opportunity by managers to participate in problem-solving activities related to direct patient care and unit activities. This high level of employee engagement in shared governance is a key factor in promoting teamwork and collaboration on the nursing unit (LeBlanc, 2014; Smith, 2011). Important elements of the decision-making process are responsibility, autonomy, authority, and accountability (Yoder-Wise, 2014).

Responsibility refers to the duties and activities that an individual is employed to perform. A position description outlines a professional nurse's responsibilities. Nurses meet these responsibilities through participation as members of a nursing unit.

Responsibility reflects ownership. An individual who manages employees distributes responsibility, and the employees have to accept the manager's direction. Managers need to ensure that staff clearly understand their responsibilities, particularly in the face of change. For example, when hospitals participate in work redesign, patient care delivery models change significantly. A manager is responsible for clearly defining an RN's role within a new care delivery model. If decentralized decision making is in place, the professional nursing staff has a voice in identifying the new RN role. Each RN on the team is responsible for knowing his or her role and how to perform that role on the busy nursing unit. For example, nurses are responsible for completing a nursing assessment of all assigned patients and developing a plan of care that addresses each of the patient's nursing diagnoses (see Chapters 15 to 20). As the staff implements the plan of care, the nurse evaluates whether the plan is successful. This responsibility becomes a work ethic for the nurse in delivering excellent patient care.

Autonomy is freedom of choice and responsibility for the choices (Yoder-Wise, 2014). Autonomy consistent with the scope of professional nursing practice maximizes a nurse's effectiveness (Yoder-Wise, 2014). With clinical autonomy a professional nurse makes independent decisions about patient care (i.e., planning nursing care for a patient within the scope of professional nursing practice). The nurse implements independent nursing interventions (see Chapter 19). Another type of autonomy for nurses is work autonomy. In work autonomy a nurse makes independent decisions about the work of the unit such as scheduling or unit governance. Autonomy is not an absolute; it occurs in degrees. For example, a nurse has the autonomy to develop and implement a discharge teaching plan on the basis of specific patient needs for any hospitalized patient. He or she also provides nursing care that complements the prescribed medical therapy. Clear communication and organization of work to allow a nurse to act on nursing decisions using clinical judgment help to promote autonomy (Weston, 2010).

Authority refers to formal legitimate power to give commands and make final decisions specific to a given position (Huber, 2014). For example, a nurse managing the care of a patient discovers that one of the members of the health care team, the registered dietitian, did not follow through on a discharge teaching plan for an assigned patient. A nurse has the authority to consult a dietitian to learn why the recommendations on the plan of care were not implemented and to review the established plan with him or her to ensure that the recommended patient teaching is completed. The nurse is able to choose and recommend appropriate teaching strategies for the patient and for the other health care team members. The nurse has the final authority in selecting the best course of action for the patient's care.

Accountability refers to individuals being answerable for their actions. It means that as a nurse you take responsibility to provide excellent patient care by following standards of practice and institutional policies and procedures. You assume responsibility for the outcomes of the actions, judgments, and omissions in providing that care (Krautscheid, 2014). A nurse demonstrates accountability by doing his or her best each day. You are not accountable for the overall outcomes of patient care, but you are accountable for what you do (i.e., performing the nursing process, communicating effectively with health care team colleagues, and staying current on nursing practice issues).

A successful nursing unit supports the four elements of decision making: responsibility, autonomy, authority, and accountability. An effective nurse manager sets the same expectations for the staff in how decisions are made. The strong nurse manager is key in producing the environment that supports autonomy (Weston, 2010). Staff routinely meet to discuss and negotiate how to maintain an equality and balance in the elements. Staff members need to feel comfortable in expressing differences of opinion and challenging ways in which the team functions while recognizing their own responsibility, autonomy, authority, and accountability. Ultimately decentralized decision making helps create the philosophy of professional nursing care for the unit.

Staff Involvement. When transformational leadership and decentralized decision making exist on a nursing unit, all staff members actively participate in unit activities (Figure 21-1). Because the work environment promotes participation, all staff members benefit from the knowledge and skills of the entire work group. If the staff learns to value the pursuit of knowledge and the contributions of co-workers, better patient care is an outcome. Recognition of nurses' exceptional work with patients helps to reinforce these behaviors and create and maintain a healthy work environment (Lefton, 2012). Healthy work

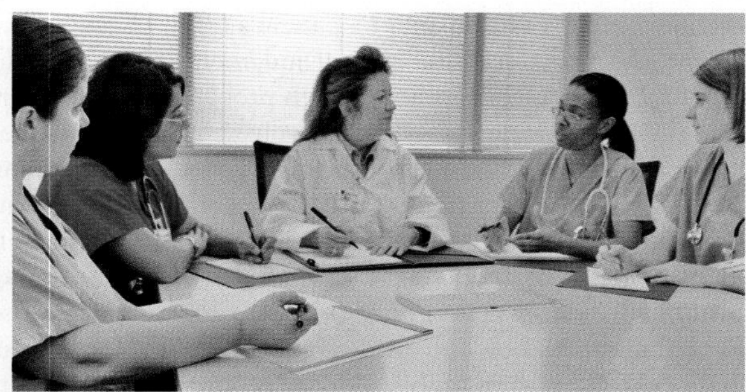

FIGURE 21-1 Staff collaborating on practice issues. (From Yoder-Wise P: *Leading and managing in nursing*, ed 6, St Louis, 2015, Mosby.)

environments have nurses who are skilled in communication, true collaboration among health care team members in decision making, appropriate levels of staffing to meet patient needs, meaningful recognition of nurses, and a nurse leader engaged in authentic leadership (AACN, 2005). The use of transformational leadership practices positively impacts the work environment, resulting in greater nurse empowerment, improved culture and climate, increased nurses' research utilization, better teamwork between nurses and physicians, greater role clarity, and reduced conflict and ambiguity (Cummings et al., 2010). The nursing manager supports staff involvement through a variety of approaches:

1. **Establishing nursing practice through problem-solving committees or professional shared governance councils.** Chaired by senior clinical staff nurses, these groups establish and maintain care standards for nursing practice on their work unit. Shared governance is a dynamic process that promotes decision making, accountability, and empowerment in staff nurses and enables them to control their nursing practice (Huber, 2014; Kramer et al., 2010). Participation in shared governance empowers a nurse to make decisions and increases nurses' confidence in decision making and their autonomy (Huber, 2014; Newman, 2011). The committees review ongoing clinical care issues, identify problems, apply evidence-based practice in establishing standards of care, develop policy and procedures, resolve patient satisfaction issues, or develop new documentation tools. It is important for the committees to focus on patient outcomes rather than only work issues to ensure quality care on the unit. Quality of care is further improved when nurses control their own practice. The committee establishes methods to ensure that all staff have input or participation on practice issues. Managers do not always sit on a committee, but they receive regular reports of committee progress. The nature of work on the nursing unit determines committee membership. At times members of other disciplines (e.g., pharmacy, respiratory therapy, or clinical nutrition) participate in practice committees or shared governance councils.
2. **Interprofessional collaboration among nurses and health care providers.** Interprofessional collaboration among nurses and health care providers (e.g., medical doctors [MDs], physical therapists [PTs], respiratory therapists [RTs]) is critical to the delivery of quality, safe patient care and the creation of a positive work culture for practitioners (Andreatta, 2010; IECEP, 2011). Interprofessional collaboration involves bringing representatives of various disciplines together to work with patients and families to deliver quality care (see Figure 21-1) (IECEP, 2011). It involves more than having members of other disciplines present. Interprofessional collaboration involves all professions bringing different points of view to the table to identify, clarify, and solve complex patient problems together, providing integrated and cohesive patient care (Legare et al., 2011). The nurse plays a unique role within the team and is often viewed as the team leader because it is the nurse who takes on the responsibilities of coordination of communication and patient care (Burzotta and Noble, 2011; Halabisky et al., 2010). Open communication, cooperation, trust, mutual respect, and understanding of team member roles and responsibilities are critical for successful interprofessional collaboration (Andreatta, 2010; Burzotta and Noble, 2011). A change in education and team training of health care practitioners is needed to build effective teams to improve interprofessional collaboration (Andreatta, 2010; Halabisky et al., 2010). The IECEP (2011) identified four competencies that health care practitioners need to bring to professional practice to be effective team members in interprofessional collaboration. The development of these competencies comes through interprofessional education. Competencies needed for effective interpersonal collaboration include:
   - Work with individuals of other professions to maintain a climate of mutual respect and shared values.
   - Use the knowledge of one's own role and those of other professions to appropriately assess and address the health care needs of patients and populations served.
   - Communicate with patients, families, communities, and other health care professionals in a responsive and responsible manner that supports patient-centered care and a team approach to the maintenance of health and treatment of disease.

   New graduate nurses often lack self-confidence and knowledge and experience fear when communicating with physicians and other members of the health care team (Plaff et al., 2014). Education, training, and role modeling are effective strategies that frequently help new graduates improve interprofessional collaboration (Robichaud et al., 2012). Apply relationship-building values and the principles of team dynamics to perform effectively in different team roles to plan and deliver patient- and population-centered care that is safe, timely, efficient, effective, and equitable.
3. **Interprofessional rounding.** Many institutions that are focused on patient- and family-centered care conduct interprofessional rounding to involve a patient and family in planning care and improving patient care coordination and communication among the health care team (Mastro et al., 2014). During rounding members of the team meet and share patient information, answer questions asked by other team members, discuss the patient's clinical progress and plans for discharge, and focus all team members on the same patient goals (Sharp, 2013). Interprofessional rounding helps decrease medical errors, decrease patient readmission rates, impact patient satisfaction, and improve quality of care (Begue et al, 2012; Townsend-Gervais et al., 2014). For interprofessional rounding to be successful, health care team members need to be flexible and open to ideas, questions, and suggestions offered by others.
4. **Staff communication.** A manager's greatest challenge, especially if a work group is large, is communication with staff. It is difficult to make sure that all staff members receive the same message (i.e., the correct message). In the present health care environment, staff quickly become uneasy and distrusting if they fail to hear about planned changes on their work unit. However, a manager cannot assume total responsibility for all communication. An effective manager uses a variety of

approaches to communicate quickly and accurately to all staff. For example, many managers distribute biweekly or monthly newsletters of ongoing unit or agency activities. Minutes of committee meetings are usually in an accessible location for all staff to read or are sent to individuals via email. When the team needs to discuss important issues regarding the operations of the unit, the manager conducts staff meetings. When the unit has practice- or quality-improvement committees, each committee member has the responsibility to communicate directly to a select number of staff members. Thus all staff members are contacted and given the opportunity for input.

5. **Staff education.** A professional nursing staff needs to always grow in knowledge. It is impossible to remain knowledgeable about current medical and nursing practice trends without ongoing education. A nurse manager is responsible for making learning opportunities available so staff members remain competent in their practice and empowered in their decision making (LeBlanc, 2014). This involves planning in-service programs, sending staff to continuing education classes and professional conferences, and having staff present case studies or evidence-based practice issues during staff meetings. Staff members are responsible for pursuing educational opportunities for relicensure/recertification and changing information regarding their patient population.

LEADERSHIP SKILLS FOR NURSING STUDENTS

It is important that as a nursing student you prepare yourself for leadership roles. This does not mean that you have to quickly learn how to lead a team of nursing staff. Instead first learn to become a dependable and competent provider of patient care. As a nursing student you are responsible and accountable for the care you give to your patients. Learn to become a leader by consulting with instructors and nursing staff to obtain feedback in making good clinical decisions, learning from mistakes and seeking guidance, working closely with professional nurses, and trying to improve your performance during each patient interaction. These skills require you to think critically and solve problems in the clinical setting. Thinking critically allows nurses to provide higher-quality care, meet the needs of patients while considering their preferences, consider alternatives to problems, understand the rationale for performing nursing interventions, and evaluate the effectiveness of interventions. Clinical experiences develop these critical thinking skills (Benner et al., 2010). Important leadership skills to learn include clinical care coordination, team communication, delegation, and knowledge building.

Clinical Care Coordination

You acquire necessary skills so you can deliver patient care in a timely and effective manner. In the beginning this often involves only one patient, but eventually it will involve groups of patients. Clinical care coordination includes clinical decision making, priority setting, use of organizational skills and resources, time management, and evaluation. The activities of clinical care coordination require use of critical reflection, critical reasoning, and clinical judgment (Benner et al., 2010). They are important first steps in developing a caring relationship with a patient. Use a critical thinking approach, applying previous knowledge and experience to the decision-making process (see Chapter 15).

Clinical Decisions. Your ability to make clinical decisions depends on application of the nursing process (see Chapters 16 to 20). When you begin a patient assignment, the first activity involves a focused but complete assessment of a patient's condition so you know the patient and make accurate clinical judgments about his or her nursing diagnoses and collaborative health problems (see Chapter 16) (Tanner, 2006). Knowing the patient involves more than gathering formal assessment data. It requires learning a patient's typical patterns of responses and his or her current situation and knowing the patient as an individual (Tanner, 2006). The initial contact with a patient is an important first step in developing a caring relationship. Encouraging patients to share their narrative of their health problems is very useful, such as "Tell me about how you are dealing with ...", or "Can you share what has been your biggest problem since becoming ill?" After obtaining a thorough assessment and identifying a patient's diagnoses and problems, you develop a plan of care, implement nursing interventions, and evaluate patient outcomes. The process requires clinical decision making using a critical thinking approach (see Chapter 15).

If you do not make accurate clinical decisions about a patient, undesirable outcomes will probably occur. A patient's condition worsens or remains the same when you lose the potential for improvement. An important lesson in organizational skills is to be thorough. Learn to attend and listen to the patient, look for any cues (obvious or subtle) that point to a pattern of findings, and direct the assessment to explore the pattern further. Accurate clinical decision making keeps you focused on the proper course of action. Never hesitate to ask for assistance when a patient's condition changes.

Priority Setting. After forming a picture of a patient's total needs, you set priorities by deciding which patient needs or problems need attention first (see Chapter 18). Priority setting is not the ordering of a list of care tasks but an organization of a vision of desired outcomes for a patient. Symptom pattern recognition from your assessment database and certain knowledge triggers help you understand which diagnoses require intervention and the associated time frame to intervene effectively (Ackley and Ladwig, 2014). It is important to prioritize in all caregiving situations because it allows you to see relationships among patient problems and avoid delays in taking action that can lead to serious complications for a patient. If a patient is experiencing serious physiological or psychological problems, the priority becomes clear. You need to act immediately to stabilize his or her condition. Classify patient problems in three priority levels:

- High priority—An immediate threat to a patient's survival or safety such as a physiological episode of obstructed airway, loss of consciousness, or a psychological episode of an anxiety attack.
- Intermediate priority—Nonemergency, nonlife-threatening actual or potential needs that a patient and family members are experiencing. Anticipating teaching needs of patients related to a new drug and taking measures to decrease postoperative complications are examples of intermediate priorities.
- Low priority—Actual or potential problems that are not directly related to a patient's illness or disease. These problems are often related to developmental needs or long-term health care needs. An example of a low-priority problem is a patient at admission who will eventually be discharged and needs teaching for self-care in the home.

Many patients have all three types of priorities, requiring you to make careful judgments in choosing a course of action. Obviously high-priority needs demand immediate attention. When a patient has diverse priority needs, it helps to focus on his or her basic needs. For example, a patient who has just completed ambulation down the hall is short of breath. The dietary assistant arrives in the room to deliver a meal tray. Instead of immediately helping the patient with the meal, you position him comfortably in bed, offer basic hygiene measures, and then evaluate his breathlessness. The patient likely becomes more interested in eating after he is more comfortable. He also is more receptive to any instruction you need to provide.

Eventually you will be required to meet the priority needs of a group of patients. This means that you need to know the priorities of each patient within the group, assessing each patient's needs as soon as possible while addressing high priorities first. To identify which patients require assessment first, rely on information from the change-of-shift report, your own most recent assessment of the patient, and information from the medical record. Over time you learn to spontaneously rank patients' needs by priority or urgency. Priorities do not remain stable but change as a patient's condition changes. It is important to think about the resources available, be flexible in recognizing that priority needs often change, and consider how to use time wisely.

You also make priorities on the basis of patient expectations. Sometimes you have established an excellent plan of care; however, if a patient is resistant to certain therapies or disagrees with the approach, you have very little success. Working closely with a patient and showing a caring attitude are important. Share the priorities you have defined with the patient to establish a level of agreement and cooperation.

Organizational Skills. Implementing a plan of care requires you to be effective and efficient. Effective use of time means doing the right things, whereas efficient use of time means doing things right. Learn to become efficient by combining various nursing activities (i.e., doing more than one thing at a time). For example, during medication administration or while obtaining a specimen, combine therapeutic communication, teaching interventions, and assessment and evaluation. Always establish and strengthen relationships with patients and use any patient contact as an opportunity to convey important information. Patient interaction gives you the chance to show caring and interest. Always attend to a patient's behaviors and responses to therapies to assess if new problems are developing and evaluate responses to interventions.

A well-organized nurse approaches any planned procedure by having all of the necessary equipment available and making sure that the patient is prepared. If the patient is comfortable and well informed, the likelihood that the procedure will go smoothly increases. Sometimes you require the assistance of colleagues to perform or complete a procedure. Keep the work area organized and complete preliminary steps before asking co-workers for assistance.

As you deliver care on the basis of established priorities, events sometimes occur within the health care setting that interfere with plans. For example, just as you begin to provide morning hygiene for a hospitalized patient, an x-ray film technician enters to take a chest x-ray film. Once the technician completes the x-ray film examination, a phlebotomist arrives to draw a blood sample. In this case your priorities conflict with the priorities of other health care personnel. It is important to always keep a patient's needs at the center of attention. If the patient experienced symptoms earlier that required a chest x-ray film and laboratory work, it is important to be sure that the diagnostic tests are completed. In another example a patient is waiting to visit family, and a chest x-ray film is a routine order from 2 days earlier. The patient's condition has stabilized, and the x-ray technician is willing to return later to shoot the film. In this case attending to the patient's hygiene and comfort so family members can visit is more of a priority.

Use of Resources. Appropriate use of resources is an important aspect of clinical care coordination. Resources in this case include members of the health care team. In any setting the administration of patient care occurs more smoothly when staff members work together. Never hesitate to have staff help you, especially when there is an opportunity to make a procedure or activity more comfortable and safer for patients. For example, assistance in turning, positioning, and ambulating patients is frequently necessary when patients are unable to move. Having a staff member such as NAP assist with handling equipment and supplies during complicated procedures such as catheter insertion or dressing changes makes procedures more efficient. In addition, you need to recognize personal limitations and use professional resources for assistance. For example, you assess a patient and find relevant clinical signs and symptoms but are unfamiliar with the physical condition. Consulting with an experienced RN confirms findings and ensures that you take the proper course of action for the patient. A leader knows his or her limitations and seeks professional colleagues for guidance and support.

Time Management. Shorter hospital stays, early discharges, same-day surgeries, and increasing complexity of patients are examples that create stress for nurses as they work to meet patient needs. One way to manage this stress is through the use of time-management skills. These skills involve learning how, where, and when to use your time. Because you have a limited amount of time with patients, it is essential to remain goal oriented and use it wisely. You quickly learn the importance of using patient goals as a way to identify priorities. However, also learn how to establish personal goals and time frames. For example, you are caring for two patients on a busy surgical nursing unit. One had surgery the day before, and the other will be discharged the next day. Clearly the first patient's goals center on restoring physiological function impaired as a result of the stress of surgery. The second patient's goals center on adequate preparation to assume self-care at home. In reviewing the therapies required for both patients, you learn how to organize your time so the activities of care and patient goals are achieved. You need to anticipate when care will be interrupted for medication administration and diagnostic testing and when is the best time for planned therapies such as dressing changes, patient education, and patient ambulation. Delegation of tasks is another way to help improve time management.

One useful time-management skill involves making a priority to-do list (Thomack, 2012). When you begin working with a patient or patients, it helps to make a list that sequences the nursing activities you need to perform. The change-of-shift report helps to sequence activities on the basis of what you learn about a patient's condition and the care provided before you arrived on the unit. It is helpful to consider activities that have specific time limits in terms of addressing patient needs such as administering a pain medication before a scheduled procedure or instructing patients before their discharge home. You also analyze the items on the list that are scheduled by agency policies or routines (e.g., medications or intravenous [IV] tubing changes). Note which activities need to be done on time and which activities you can do at your discretion. You have to administer medication within a specific schedule, but you are also able to perform other activities while in the patient's room. Finally, estimate the amount of time needed to complete the various activities. Activities requiring the assistance of other staff members usually take longer because you have to plan around their schedules.

Good time management also involves setting goals to help you complete one task before starting another (Thomack, 2012). If possible, complete the activities started with one patient before moving on to the next. Care is less fragmented, and you are better able to focus on what you are doing for each patient. As a result, it is less likely that you will make errors. Time management requires you to anticipate the

BOX 21-5 Principles of Time Management

Goal setting: Review a patient's goals of care for the day and any goals you have for activities such as completing documentation, attending a patient care conference, giving a hand-off report, or preparing medications for administration.

Time analysis: Reflect on how you use your time. While working on a clinical area, keep track of how you use your time in different activities. This provides valuable information to reveal how well organized you really are.

Priority setting: Set the priorities that you have established for patients within set time frames. For example, determine when is the best time to have teaching sessions, plan ambulation, and provide rest periods on the basis of what you know about the patient's condition. For example, if a patient is nauseated or in pain, it is not a good time for a teaching session.

Interruption control: Everyone needs time to socialize or discuss issues with colleagues. However, do not let this interrupt important patient care activities such as medication administration (see Chapter 32), ordered treatments, or teaching sessions. Use time during report, mealtime, or team meetings to your advantage. In addition, plan time to help fellow colleagues so it complements your patient care schedule.

Evaluation: At the end of each day take time to think and reflect about how effectively you used your time. If you are having difficulties, discuss them with an instructor or a more experienced staff member.

activities of the day and combine activities when possible. When you practice good time management, you focus on organization and setting priorities. Other strategies include keeping your work area clean and clutter free and trying to decrease interruptions as you are completing tasks (Thomack, 2012). Box 21-5 summarizes principles of time management.

Evaluation. Evaluation is one of the most important aspects of clinical care coordination (see Chapter 20). It is a mistake to think that evaluation occurs at the end of an activity. It is ongoing, just like other steps of the nursing process. Once you assess a patient's needs and begin therapies directed at a specific problem area, immediately evaluate whether therapies are effective and the patient's response. The process of evaluation compares actual patient outcomes with expected outcomes. For example, a clinic nurse assesses a foot ulcer of a patient who has diabetes to determine if healing has progressed since the last clinic visit. When expected outcomes are not met, evaluation reveals the need to continue current therapies for a longer period, revise approaches to care, or introduce new therapies. As you care for a patient throughout the day, anticipate when to return to the bedside to evaluate care (e.g., 30 minutes after a medication was administered, 15 minutes after an IV line has begun infusing, or 60 minutes after discussing discharge instructions with the patient and family).

Keeping a focus on evaluation of a patient's progress lessens the chance of becoming distracted by the tasks of care. It is common to assume that staying focused on planned activities ensures that you will perform care appropriately. However, task orientation does not ensure positive patient outcomes. Learn that at the heart of good organizational skills is the constant inquiry into a patient's condition and progress toward an improved level of health.

Team Communication

Effective communication is critical to all teams (Haynes and Strickler, 2014). As a part of a nursing team, you are responsible for using open, professional communication. Regardless of the setting, an enriching professional environment is one in which staff members respect one another's ideas, share information, and keep one another informed. On a busy nursing unit this means keeping colleagues informed about patients with emerging problems, physicians or other health care providers who have been called for consultation, and unique approaches that solved a complex nursing problem. Strategies to improve your communication with health care providers include addressing the colleague by name, having the patient and chart available when discussing patient issues, focusing on the patient problem, and being professional and assertive but not aggressive or confrontational. In a clinic setting it may mean sharing unusual diagnostic findings or conveying important information regarding a patient's source of family support. One way of fostering good team communication is by setting expectations of one another. A professional nurse treats colleagues with respect, listens to the ideas of other staff members without interruption, explores the way other staff members think, and is honest and direct while communicating. Part of good communication is clarifying what others are saying and building on the merits of co-workers' ideas (Yoder-Wise, 2014). An efficient team knows that it is able to count on all members when needs arise. Sharing expectations of what, when, and how to communicate is a step toward establishing a strong work team. Examples of communication tools that improve communication include briefings or short discussions among team members; group rounds on patients; callouts to share critical information such as vital signs with all team members at the same time; check backs to restate what a person has said to verify understanding of information; the two-challenge rule that allows concerns to be voiced twice, which allows all team members to voice concerns about safety; "CUS" words, which means "I'm ***C***oncerned, I'm ***U***ncomfortable, I don't feel this is ***S***afe; and the use of Situation-Background-Assessment-Recommendation (SBAR) when sharing information (see Chapter 26) (Haynes and Strickler, 2014). When using electronic communication, it is important to communicate the appropriate information to the correct person, always maintaining patient privacy and confidentiality (NCSBN, 2011).

QSEN QSEN: BUILDING COMPETENCY IN TEAMWORK AND COLLABORATION The unit on which you are working just received the results of the Employee Opinion Survey that all staff members completed. The staff rated communication among team members as important, but satisfaction with communication was rated low. The unit nursing council has been charged with developing a plan to improve team communication. Which strategies does the council include in the plan?

Answers to QSEN Activities can be found on the Evolve website.

Delegation

The art of effective delegation is a skill that you need to observe and practice to improve your own management skills. The American Nurses Association (ANA, 2012) defines **delegation** as transferring responsibility for the performance of an activity or task while retaining accountability for the outcome. The Nurse Practice Act of your state, along with principles of authority, accountability, and responsibility, is the basis for effective delegation (Plawecki and Amrhein, 2010; Weydt, 2010). Effective delegation results in achievement of quality, safe patient care; improved efficiency; increased productivity; empowered staff; and skill development of others (Mueller and Vogelsmeier, 2013). Asking a staff member to obtain an ordered specimen while you attend to a patient's pain medication request effectively prevents a delay in the patient gaining pain relief and accomplishes two tasks related to the patient. Delegation also provides job enrichment. You show trust in colleagues by delegating tasks to them and showing staff members that they are important players in the delivery of care.

Successful delegation is important to the quality of the RN-NAP relationship and their willingness to work together (Potter et al., 2010). Never delegate a task that you dislike doing or would not do yourself because this creates negative feelings and poor working relationships. For example, if you are in the room when a patient asks to be placed on a bedpan and there are no urgent care issues, you assist the patient rather than leave the room to find the nurse assistant. Remember that, even though the delegation of a task transfers the responsibility and authority to another person, you are accountable for the delegated task.

As a nurse you are responsible and accountable for providing care to patients and delegating care activities to the NAP. However, you do not delegate the steps of the nursing process of assessment, diagnosis, planning, and evaluation because these steps require nursing judgment (Duffy and McCoy, 2014). Patient teaching is also the responsibility of an RN and should not be delegated. Recognize that, when you delegate to the NAP, you delegate tasks, not patients. Do not give the NAP sole responsibility for the care of patients. Instead it is you as the professional nurse in charge of patient care who decides which activities the NAP performs independently and which the RN and NAP perform in partnership. One way to accomplish this is to have the RN and NAP conduct rounds together. You assess each patient as the NAP attends to basic patient needs. Care is delegated on the basis of assessment findings and priority setting. As an RN, you are always responsible for the assessment of a patient's ongoing status; but, if a patient is stable, you delegate vital sign monitoring to the NAP.

In most settings the RN is the one who decides when delegation is appropriate. The NCSBN (1995) provides some guidelines for delegation of tasks in accordance with an RN's legal scope of practice (Box 21-6). As the leader of the health care team, the RN gives clear instructions, effectively prioritizes patient needs and therapies, and gives staff timely and meaningful feedback. NAPs respond positively when you include them as part of the nursing team.

BOX 21-6 The Five Rights of Delegation

Right Task

The right tasks to delegate are ones that are repetitive, require little supervision, are relatively noninvasive, have results that are predictable, and have potential minimal risk (e.g., simple specimen collection, ambulating a stable patient, preparing a room for patient admission).

Right Circumstances

Consider the appropriate patient setting, available resources, and other relevant factors. In an acute care setting patients' conditions often change quickly. Use good clinical decision making to determine what to delegate.

Right Person

The right person is delegating the right tasks to the right person to be performed on the right person. A registered nurse (RN) knows which tasks to delegate to nursing assistive personnel (NAP) for each specific patient.

Right Direction/Communication

Give a clear, concise description of a task, including its objective, limits, and expectations. Communication needs to be ongoing between the RN and NAP during a shift of care.

Right Supervision/Evaluation

Provide appropriate monitoring, evaluation, intervention as needed, and feedback. NAP need to feel comfortable asking questions and seeking assistance.

Modified from The Council and American Nurses Association (ANA) and National Council of State Boards of Nursing (NCSBN): Joint statement on delegation, 2006, https://www.ncsbn.org/Delegation_joint_statement_NCSBN-ANA.pdf. Accessed March 28, 2015.

Appropriate delegation begins with knowing which skills you are able to delegate. This requires you to be familiar with the Nurse Practice Act of your state, institutional policies and procedures, and the job description for NAPs provided by the institution (Duffy and McCoy, 2014). These standards help to define the necessary level of competency of the NAP and contain specific guidelines regarding which tasks or activities a nurse is able to delegate. The job description identifies any required education and the types of tasks the NAP can perform, either independently or with RN direct supervision. Institutional policy defines the amount of training required for the NAP. Procedures detail who is qualified to perform a given nursing procedure, whether supervision is necessary, and the type of reporting required. You need to have a means to easily access policies or have supervisory staff who inform you about the NAP's job duties.

As a professional nurse you cannot simply assign the NAP tasks without considering the implications. Assess the patient and determine a plan of care before identifying which tasks someone else is able to perform. When directing the NAP, determine how much supervision is necessary. Is it the first time the NAP performed the task? Does the patient present a complicating factor that makes the RN's assistance necessary? Does the NAP have prior experience with a particular type of patient in addition to having received training on the skill? The final responsibility is to evaluate whether the NAP performed the task properly and whether the desired outcomes were met.

Efficient delegation requires constant communication (i.e., sending clear messages and listening so all participants understand expectations regarding patient care) (Mueller and Vogelsmeier, 2013). Provide clear instructions and desired outcomes when delegating tasks. These instructions initially focus on the procedure itself, what will be accomplished, when it should be completed, and the unique needs of the patient. The RN also communicates when and which information to report such as expected observations and specific patient concerns (NCSBN, 2005). Communication is a two-way process in delegation; thus the NAP needs to have the chance to ask questions and have your expectations made clear (ANA and NCSBN, 2005; NCSBN, 2005). Conflict, which often impacts quality and patient safety, occurs between RNs and NAPs when there is little or poor communication (Kalisch, 2011; Potter et al., 2010). Hand-off disconnects from team member to team member, lack of knowledge about the workload of team members, and difficulties dealing with conflict are examples of communication failures that often result in delegation ineffectiveness and omissions of nursing care (Gravlin and Bittner, 2010). As you become more familiar with a staff member's competency, trust builds, and the staff member needs fewer instructions; but clarification of patients' specific needs is always necessary.

Important steps in delegation are evaluation of a staff member's performance, achievement of the patient's outcomes, the communication process used, and any problems or concerns that occurred (NCSBN, 2005). When a NAP performs a task correctly and does a good job, it is important to provide praise and recognition. If a staff member's performance is not satisfactory, give constructive and appropriate feedback. As a nurse, always give specific feedback regarding any mistakes that staff members make, explaining how to avoid the mistake or a better way to handle the situation. Giving feedback in private is the professional way and preserves the staff member's dignity. When giving feedback, make sure to focus on things that can be changed, choose only one issue at a time, and give specific details. Frequently when a NAP's performance does not meet expectations, it is the result of inadequate training or assignment of too many tasks. You may discover the need to review a procedure with staff and offer demonstration or even recommend that additional training be scheduled with the education department. If too many tasks are being delegated, this might be a nursing practice issue. All staff need to discuss the appropriateness of delegation on their unit. Sometimes NAP need help to learn how to prioritize. In some cases you discover that you are overdelegating. It is your responsibility to complete documentation of the delegated task. Here are a few tips on appropriate delegation (Mueller and Vogelsmeier, 2013):

- *Assess the knowledge and skills of the delegatee:* Assess the knowledge and skills of the NAP by asking open-ended questions that elicit conversation and details about what he or she knows (e.g., "How do you usually apply the cuff when you measure a blood pressure?" or "Tell me how you prepare the tubing before you give an enema.")
- *Match tasks to the delegatee's skills:* Know which tasks and skills are in the scope of practice and job description for the team members to whom you delegate in your agency. Determine if personnel have learned critical thinking skills such as knowing when a patient is in harm or the difference between normal clinical findings and changes to report.
- *Communicate clearly:* Always provide clear directions by describing a task, the desired outcome, and the time period within which the NAP needs to complete the task. Never give instructions through another staff member. Make the person feel as though he or she is part of the team. Begin requests for help with please and end with thank you. For example, "I'd like you to please help me by getting Mr. Floyd up to ambulate before lunch. Be sure to check his blood pressure before he stands and write your finding on the graphic sheet. OK? Thanks."
- *Listen attentively:* Listen to the NAP's response after you provide directions. Does he or she feel comfortable in asking questions or requesting clarification? If you encourage a response, listen to what the person has to say. Be especially attentive if the staff member has a deadline to meet for another nurse. Help sort out priorities.
- *Provide feedback:* Always give the NAP feedback regarding performance, regardless of outcome. Let them know of a job well done. A "thank you" increases the likelihood of the NAP helping in the future. If an outcome is undesirable, find a private place to discuss what occurred, any miscommunication, and how to achieve a better outcome in the future.

Knowledge Building

As a professional nurse, recognize the importance of pursuing knowledge to remain competent. As an accountable nurse, you are responsible for lifelong learning and maintaining competency (Krautscheid, 2014). You need to maintain and continually improve your knowledge and skills. Lifelong learning allows you to continuously provide safe, effective, quality care. A leader recognizes that there is always something new to learn. Opportunities for learning occur with each patient interaction, each encounter with a professional colleague, and each meeting or class session in which health care professionals meet to discuss clinical care issues. People always have different experiences and knowledge to share. Ongoing development of skills in delegation, communication, and teamwork helps maintain and build competency (Gravlin and Bittner, 2010). In-service programs, workshops, professional conferences, professional reading, and collegiate courses offer innovative and current information on the rapidly changing world of health care. To be a safe and competent nurse you need to actively pursue learning opportunities, both formal and informal, and to share knowledge with the professional colleagues you encounter.

KEY POINTS

- A manager sets a philosophy for a work unit, ensures appropriate staffing, mobilizes staff and institutional resources to achieve objectives, motivates staff members to carry out their work, sets standards of performance, and empowers staff to achieve objectives.
- Patient- and family-centered care is composed of the core concepts of respect and dignity, information sharing, participation of family members and collaboration.
- A transformational leader develops effective teams on the nursing unit, empowers staff members, communicates effectively with the nursing team, and guides and supports the nursing team in their shared decision making.
- An empowered nursing staff has decision-making authority to change how they practice.
- Nursing care delivery models vary according to the responsibility and autonomy of the RN in coordinating care delivery and the roles other staff members play in assisting with care.
- Critical to the success of decision making is making staff members aware that they have the responsibility, authority, autonomy, and accountability for the care they give and the decisions they make.
- A nurse manager encourages shared decision making by establishing nursing practice committees, supporting interprofessional collaboration, setting and implementing quality improvement plans, and maintaining timely staff communication.
- Clinical care coordination involves accurate clinical decision making, establishing priorities, efficient organizational skills, appropriate use of resources and time-management skills, and an ongoing evaluation of care activities.
- In an enriched professional environment, each member of a nursing team is responsible for open, professional communication.
- Effective delegation requires the use of good communication skills.
- When done correctly, delegation improves job efficiency, productivity, and job enrichment.
- An important responsibility for the nurse who delegates nursing care is evaluation of the staff member's performance and patient outcomes.

CLINICAL APPLICATION QUESTIONS

Preparing for Clinical Practice

You are a staff nurse on a 32-bed cardiac step-down unit. You are assigned as the preceptor for Tony, RN, a new graduate nurse, who just started his nursing career on your floor.

1. You and Tony just received morning shift report on your patients. You are assigned the following patients. Which patient do you and Tony need to see first? Explain your answer.
    1. Mr. Dodson, a 52-year-old patient who was admitted yesterday with a diagnosis of angina pectoris. He is scheduled for a cardiac stress test at 0900.
    2. Mrs. Wallace, a 60-year-old patient who was transferred out of intensive care at 0630 today. She had uncomplicated coronary artery bypass surgery yesterday.
    3. Mr. Workman, a 45-year-old patient who experienced a myocardial infarction 2 days ago. He is complaining of chest pain rated as 6 on a scale of 0 to 10.
    4. Mrs. Harris, a 76-year-old patient who had a permanent pacemaker inserted yesterday. She is complaining of incision pain rated as a 5 on a scale of 0 to 10.
2. As you work with Tony on your unit, you notice that he has trouble with time-management skills when providing patient care. Which

strategies will you suggest to Tony to help him improve organization of his delivery of patient care?

3. Sonya, a nursing assistive personnel (NAP), is paired to work with you and Tony. You overhear Tony giving Sonya directions for what she needs to do. Tony says, "Sonya, assist Mrs. Harris in room 418 with her afternoon walk. Take her pulse before and after she walks and record it in her chart. I'll check with you when you're finished to see how she did." On the basis of what you know about delegation, did Tony give appropriate or inappropriate directions to Sonya? Provide rationale for your answer.

Answers to Clinical Application Questions can be found on the Evolve website.

REVIEW QUESTIONS

Are You Ready to Test Your Nursing Knowledge?

1. At 1200 the registered nurse (RN) says to the nursing assistive personnel (NAP), "You did a good job walking Mrs. Taylor by 0930. I saw that you recorded her pulse before and after the walk. I saw that Mrs. Taylor walked in the hallway barefoot. For safety, the next time you walk a patient, you need to make sure that the patient wears slippers or shoes. Please walk Mrs. Taylor again by 1500." Which characteristics of positive feedback did the RN use when talking to the nursing assistant? (Select all that apply.)
   1. Feedback is given immediately.
   2. Feedback focuses on one issue.
   3. Feedback offers concrete details.
   4. Feedback identifies ways to improve.
   5. Feedback focuses on changeable things.
   6. Feedback is specific about what is done incorrectly only.
2. As a nurse, you are assigned to four patients. Which patient do you need to see first?
   1. The patient who had abdominal surgery 2 days ago who is requesting pain medication
   2. A patient admitted yesterday with atrial fibrillation with decreased level of consciousness
   3. A patient with a wound drain who needs teaching before discharge in the early afternoon
   4. A patient going to surgery for a mastectomy in 3 hours who has a question about the surgery
3. A nurse asks a nursing assistive personnel (NAP) to help the patient in room 418 walk to the bathroom right now. The nurse tells the NAP that the patient needs the assistance of one person and the use of a walker. The nurse also tells the NAP that the patient's oxygen can be removed while he goes to the bathroom but to make sure that it is put back on at 2 L. The nurse also instructs the NAP to make sure the side rails are up and the bed alarm is reset after the patient gets back in bed. Which of the following components of the "Five Rights of Delegation" were used by the nurse? (Select all that apply.)
   1. Right task
   2. Right circumstances
   3. Right person
   4. Right direction/communication
   5. Right supervision/evaluation
4. A patient asks a nurse what the patient-centered care model for the hospital means. What is the nurse's best answer?
   1. "This model ensures that all patients have private rooms when they are admitted to the hospital."
   2. "In this model you and the health care team are full partners in decisions related to your health care."
   3. "This model focuses on making the patient experience a good one by providing amenities such as restaurant-style food service."
   4. "Patients and families sign a document providing them full access to their medical charts."
5. While administering medications, a nurse realizes that a prescribed dose of a medication was not given. The nurse acts by completing an incident report and notifying the patient's health care provider. The nurse is exercising:
   1. Authority.
   2. Responsibility.
   3. Accountability.
   4. Decision making.
6. The staff on the nursing unit are discussing implementing interprofessional rounding. Which of the following statements correctly describe interprofessional rounding? (Select all that apply.)
   1. Allows team members to share information about patients to improve care
   2. Provides an opportunity for early patient discharge planning
   3. Improves communication among health care team members
   4. Allows each of the health care team members to identify separate patient goals
   5. Allows each health care provider an opportunity to delegate a task.
7. After a nurse receives a change-of-shift report on his assigned patients, he prioritizes the tasks that need to be completed. This is an example of a nurse displaying which practice?
   1. Organizational skills
   2. Use of resources
   3. Time management
   4. Evaluation
8. A nurse is teaching a patient about wound care that will need to be done daily at home after the patient is discharged. This is which priority nursing need for this patient?
   1. Low priority
   2. High priority
   3. Intermediate priority
   4. Nonemergency priority
9. A registered nurse (RN) is providing care to a patient who had abdominal surgery 2 days ago. Which task is appropriate to delegate to the nursing assistant?
   1. Helping the patient ambulate in the hall
   2. Changing surgical wound dressing
   3. Irrigating the nasogastric tube
   4. Providing brochures to the patient on health diet
10. Which task is appropriate for a registered nurse (RN) to delegate to a nursing assistant?
    1. Explaining to the patient the preoperative preparation before the surgery in the morning
    2. Administering the ordered antibiotic to the patient before surgery
    3. Obtaining the patient's signature on the surgical informed consent
    4. Helping the patient to the bathroom before leaving for the operating room
11. Which of the following are components of interprofessional collaboration? (Select all that apply.)
    1. Interprofessional education does not impact the collaboration among interprofessional team members.
    2. Nurses are often viewed as the team leader because of their coordination of patient care.

3. Effective interprofessional collaboration requires mutual respect and trust from all team members.
4. Open communication improves the collaboration among the interprofessional team members.
5. The goal of interprofessional collaboration is to improve the quality of patient care.

12. A registered nurse performs the following four steps in delegating a task to a nursing assistant. Place the steps in the order of appropriate delegation.
    1. Do you have any questions about walking Mr. Malone?
    2. Before you take him for his walk to the end of the hallway and back, please take and record his pulse rate.
    3. In the next 30 minutes please assist Mr. Malone in room 418 with her afternoon walk.
    4. I will make sure that I check with you in about 40 minutes to see how the patient did.
13. Which example demonstrates a nurse performing the skill of evaluation?
    1. The nurse explains the side effects of the new blood pressure medication ordered for the patient.
    2. The nurse asks a patient to rate pain on a scale of 0 to 10 before administering the pain medication.
    3. After completing the teaching, the nurse observes a patient draw up and administer an insulin injection.
    4. The nurse changes a patient's leg ulcer dressing using aseptic technique.
14. The nurse manager from the surgical unit was awarded the nursing leadership award for practice of transformational leadership. Which of the following are characteristics or traits of transformational leadership displayed by award winner? (Select all that apply.)
    1. The nurse manager regularly rounds on staff to gather input on unit decisions.
    2. The nurse manager sends thank-you notes to staff in recognition of a job well done.
    3. The nurse manager sends memos to staff about decisions that the manager has made regarding unit policies.
    4. The nurse manager has an "innovation idea box" to which staff are encouraged to submit ideas for unit improvements.
    5. The nurse develops a philosophy of care for the staff.
15. A nurse assesses patients and uses assessment findings to identify patient problems and develop an individualized plan of care. The nurse is displaying:
    1. Organizational skills.
    2. Use of resources.
    3. Priority setting.
    4. Clinical decision making.

Answers: 1. 2, 3, 4, 5; **2.** 2; **3.** 1, 2, 3, 4; **4.** 2; **5.** 3; **6.** 1, 2, 3; **7.** 3; **8.** 3; **9.** 1; **10.** 4; **11.** 2, 3, 4, 5; **12.** 3, 2, 4, 1; **13.** 3; **14.** 1, 2, 4; **15.** 4.

Rationales to Review Questions can be found on the Evolve website.

REFERENCES

Ackley BJ, Ladwig G: *Nursing diagnosis handbook*, ed 10, St Louis, 2014, Mosby.

American Association of Colleges of Nursing (AACN): *AACN standards for establishing and sustaining healthy work environments: a journey to excellence, executive summary*, 2005, http://www.aacn.org/wd/hwe/docs/execsum.pdf. Accessed September 3, 2015.

American Nurses Association (ANA): *Principles for delegation by registered nurses to unlicensed assistive personnel (UAP)*, Silver Springs, MD, 2012, ANA.

American Nurses Association (ANA); National Council of State Boards of Nursing (NCSBN): *Joint statement on delegation*, 2005, https://www.ncsbn.org/Delegation_joint_statement_NCSBN-ANA.pdf. Accessed September 3, 2015.

American Nurses Credentialing Center (ANCC). *Magnet Recognition Program*, 2014, http://www.nursecredentialing.org/Magnet.aspx. Accessed September 3, 2015.

Andreatta PB: A typology for health care teams, *Health Care Manage Rev* 35(4):345, 2010.

Benner P, et al: *Educating nurses: a call for radical transformation*, San Francisco, CA, 2010, Josey-Bass.

Burzotta L, Noble H: The dimensions of interprofessional practice, *Br J Nurs* 20(3):310, 2011.

Case Management Society of America: *What is a case manager?* 2012, http://www.cmsa.org/Home/CMSA/whatisacasemanager/tabid/224/Default.aspx. Accessed September 3, 2015.

Duffy M, McCoy SF: *Delegation and YOU: when to delegate and to whom*, Silver Springs, MD, 2014, American Nurses Association.

Fasoli DR: The culture of nursing engagement: a historical perspective, *Nurs Admin Q* 34(1):18, 2010.

Halabisky B, et al: eLearning, knowledge brokering and nursing strengthening collaborative practice in long-term care, *CIN: Comput Informat Nurs* 28(5):24, 2010.

Haynes J, Strickler J: Team STEPPS makes strides for better communication, *Nursing* 44(1):62, 2014.

Huber DL: *Leadership and nursing care management*, ed 5, St Louis, 2014, Saunders.

Institute for Patient and Family Centered Care (IPFCC): *Frequently asked questions*, 2010, http://www.ipfcc.org/faq.html. Accessed September 3, 2015.

Interprofessional Education Collaborative Expert Panel (IECEP): *Core competencies for interprofessional collaborative practice: report of an expert panel*, Washington, DC, 2011, Interprofessional Education Collaborative.

LeBlanc P: Leadership by design: creating successful "TEEAMS", *Nurs Manage* 45(3):49, 2014.

Mueller C, Vogelsmeier A: Effective delegation: understanding responsibility, authority and accountability, *J Nurs Regulation* 4(3):20, 2013.

National Council of State Boards of Nursing (NCSBN): *Delegation: concepts and decision-making process*, Chicago, 1995, The Council.

National Council of State Boards of Nursing (NCSBN): *Working with others: a position paper*, Chicago, 2005, The Council.

National Council of State Boards of Nursing (NCSBN): *White paper: a nurse's guide to the use of social media*, Chicago, 2011, National Council of State Boards of Nursing, https://www.ncsbn.org/11_NCSBN_Nurses_Guide_Social_Media.pdf. Accessed September 3, 2015.

Newman K: Transforming organizational culture through nursing shared governance, *Nurs Clin North Am* 46(45):2011.

Plawecki LH, Amrhein DW: A question of delegation: unlicensed assistive personnel and the professional nurse, *J Gerontol Nurs* 36(8):18, 2010.

QSEN Institute: *Prelicensure KSASs*, 2014, http://qsen.org/competencies/pre-licensure-ksas/. Accessed September 3, 2015.

Sharp H: Multidisciplinary team rounding: engaging patients and improving communication at the bedside, *New Hampshire Nurs News* January, February, March(14):2013.

Smith MA: Are you a transformational leader?, *Nurs Manage* 42(9):44, 2011.

Thomack B: Time management for today's workforce demands, *Workplace Health Safety* 60(5):201, 2012.

Weston MJ: Strategies for enhancing autonomy and control over nursing, *Online J Issues Nurs* 15(1):10, 2010.

Weydt A: Developing delegation skills, *Online J Issues Nurs* 15(2):1, 2010.

Yoder-Wise PS: *Leading and managing in nursing*, ed 5, St Louis, 2014, Mosby.

RESEARCH REFERENCES

Bargagliotti LA: Work engagement: a concept analysis, *J Adv Nurs* 68(6):1414, 2012.

Begue A, et al: Retrospective study of multidisciplinary rounding on a thoracic surgical oncology unit, *Clin J Oncol Nurs* 16(6):E198, 2012.

Carter MR, Tourangeau AE: Staying in nursing: what factors determine whether nurses intend to remain employed, *J Adv Nurs* 68(7):1589, 2012.

Cowden T, et al: Leadership practices and staff nurses' intent to stay: a systematic review, *J Nurse Manage* 19:461, 2011.

Cummings GG, et al: Leadership styles and outcome patterns for the nursing workforce and work environment: a systematic review, *Int J Nurs Stud* 47:363, 2010.

Gravlin G, Bittner NP: Nurses' and nursing assistants' reports of missed care and delegation, *J Nurs Admin* 40(7/8):329, 2010.

Holly C, Igwee G: A systematic review of the influence of transformational leadership style on nursing staff in acute care hospitals, *International J Evid-based Healthc* 9(3):301, 2011.

Kalisch BJ: The impact of RN-UAP relationships on quality and safety, *Nurs Manage* 42(9):16, 2011.

Kalisch BJ, Lee KH: The impact of teamwork on missed nursing care, *Nurs Outlook* 58(5):233, 2010.

Kalisch BJ, et al: Nursing staff teamwork and job satisfaction, *J Nurs Manage* 18:938, 2010.

Kearney MH: *Report of the findings from the post-entry competence study, National Council of State Boards of Nursing*, Chicago, 2009.

Kramer M, et al: Nine structures and leadership practices essential for a magnetic (healthy) work environment, *Nurs Admin Q* 34(1):4, 2010.

Kramer M, et al: Clinical nurses in Magnet hospitals confirm productive, healthy unit work environments, *J Nurse Manage* 19:5, 2011.

Krautscheid LC: Defining professional nursing accountability: a literature review, *J Prof Nurs* 30(1):43, 2014.

Lefton C: Strengthening the workforce through meaningful recognition, *Nurs Econ* 30(6):331, 2012.

Legare F, et al: Interprofessionalism and shared decision-making in primary care: a stepwise approach towards a new model, *J Interprof Care* 25:18, 2011.

Mastro KA, et al: Patient- and family-centered care: a call to action for new knowledge and innovation, *J Nurs Admin* 44(9):446, 2014.

Plaff K, et al: An integrative review of the factors influencing new graduate nurse engagement in interprofessional collaboration, *J Adv Nurs* 70(1):4, 2014.

Potter PA, et al: Delegation practices between registered nurses and nursing assistive personnel, *J Nurs Manage* 18:157, 2010.

Robichaud P, et al: The value of quality improvement project in promoting interprofessional collaboration, *J Interprof Care* 26:158, 2012.

Tanner CA: Thinking like a nurse: a research-based model of clinical judgment in nursing, *J Nurs Educ* 45(6):204, 2006.

Townsend-Gervais M, et al: Interprofessional rounds and structured communication reduce re-admissions and improve some patient outcomes, *West J Nurs Res* 36(7):917, 2014.

Weberg D: Transformational leadership and staff retention: an evidence review with implications for healthcare systems, *Nurs Admin Q* 34(3):246, 2010.

Wong CA, et al: The relationship between nursing leadership and patient outcomes: a systematic review update, *J Nurse Manage* 21:709, 2013.

22

Ethics and Values

OBJECTIVES

- Discuss the role of ethics in professional nursing.
- Discuss the role of values in the study of ethics.
- Examine and clarify personal values.
- Understand basic philosophies of health care ethics.
- Explain a nursing perspective in ethics.
- Apply critical thinking to ethical dilemmas.
- Discuss contemporary ethical issues.

KEY TERMS

Accountability, p. 293
Advocacy, p. 293
Autonomy, p. 292
Beneficence, p. 293
Casuistry, p. 295
Code of ethics, p. 293
Confidentiality, p. 293
Consequentialism, p. 295
Deontology, p. 295
Ethics, p. 292
Ethics of care, p. 295
Feminist ethics, p. 295
Fidelity, p. 293
Justice, p. 293
Nonmaleficence, p. 293
Responsibility, p. 293
Teleology, p. 295
Utilitarianism, p. 295
Value, p. 294

MEDIA RESOURCES

http://evolve.elsevier.com/Potter/fundamentals/

- Review Questions
- Case Study with Questions
- Audio Glossary
- Content Updates

Ethics is the study of conduct and character. It is concerned with determining what is good or valuable for individuals, groups, and society at large. Acts that are ethical reflect a commitment to standards that individuals, professions, and societies strive to meet. When decisions must be made about health care, understandable disagreement can occur among health care providers, families, patients, friends, and people in the community. The right thing to do can be hard to determine when ethics, values, and perceptions about health care collide. This chapter describes concepts that will help you embrace the role of ethics in your professional life and promote resolution when an ethical dilemma develops.

BASIC TERMS IN HEALTH ETHICS

Your understanding of the terms common in ethical discourse will help you participate thoughtfully in discussions with others and may even help you shape your own thoughts about ethical issues.

Autonomy

Autonomy refers to freedom from external control. In health care the concept applies to provider respect for the autonomy of patients. It can also apply to institutional respect for the autonomy of providers. A commitment to respect the autonomy of others is a fundamental principle of ethical practice.

Respect for patient autonomy refers to the commitment to include patients in decisions about all aspects of care. It is a key feature of patient-centered care. In respecting patient autonomy, you acknowledge and protect a patient's independence. Respect for autonomy is a relatively new concept and reflects a movement away from paternalistic patient care in which the physician made all decisions. The movement was in part a reaction to the Tuskegee Syphilis Study in which many African-American men were infected with the bacteria without their knowledge. When the story surfaced in the news media in 1972, the outcry resulted in reinforcement of informed consent, especially for research (Reverby, 2013).

Involving patients in decisions about their care is now standard practice. Providers are obligated to inform patients about risks and benefits of treatment plans and then to ensure that they understand and agree with their plan. In many cases (e.g., surgery and diagnostic procedures), the consent of a patient must be documented by the patient's signature. Out of respect for patient autonomy, you will support patients who raise questions about procedures by ensuring that they get the answers they request. As a nurse you will respect patient autonomy in all of your patient care by taking time to explain nursing procedures such as obtaining a blood pressure or administering medications.

Respect for provider autonomy refers to provider relationships to institutions. What happens when a provider is asked to perform duties that conflict with a religious or personal belief? Institutions have developed policies that accommodate respect for providers by finding a way to reassign duties when this conflict occurs. However, the reassignment is conducted so the patient is protected from abandonment and only when patient care is not compromised. What happens when an individual provider takes issue with policies or practices of an institution and is concerned that a practice is unsafe? Institutional whistle blower protections prohibit reprisal against an employee who makes a legitimate report about clinical safety issues. These protections represent expressions of respect for provider autonomy.

Beneficence

Beneficence refers to taking positive actions to help others. The principle of beneficence is fundamental to the practice of nursing and medicine. The agreement to act with beneficence implies that the best interests of the patient remain more important than self-interest. It implies that nurses practice primarily as a service to others, even in the details of daily work.

Nonmaleficence

Maleficence refers to harm or hurt. Nonmaleficence refers to the avoidance of harm or hurt. In health care ethical practice involves not only the will to do good but the equal commitment to do no harm. A health care professional tries to balance the risks and benefits of care while striving at the same time to do the least harm possible. A bone marrow transplant procedure may offer a chance at cure; but the process involves periods of suffering, and it may not be possible to guarantee a positive outcome. Decisions about the best course of action can be difficult and uncertain precisely because nurses agree to avoid harm at the same time as they commit to promoting benefit.

Justice

Justice refers to fairness. The term is most often used in discussions about access to health care resources, including the just distribution of scarce resources. Discussions about health insurance, hospital locations and services, and even organ transplants generally refer to issues of justice. The term itself is open to interpretation about how best to ensure justice. Does the principle of just distribution mean that health care resources should be available to as many people as possible? Or is it more important to remain concerned about equality by ensuring that all people receive resources equally? Especially as health care costs continue to rise, the issue of justice remains a critical part of the discussion about health care reform and access to care.

The term *just culture* refers to the promotion of open discussion without fear of recrimination whenever mistakes, especially those involving adverse events, occur or nearly occur. Blame is withheld at least at first so system issues and other elements can be investigated for their contributions to the error. By fostering open discussion about errors, members of the health care team become more richly informed participants, able to design new systems that prevent harm.

Fidelity

Fidelity refers to the agreement to keep promises. As a nurse you keep promises by following through on your actions and interventions. If you assess a patient for pain and offer a plan to manage the pain, the standard of fidelity encourages you to monitor the patient's response to the plan. Professional practice includes a willingness to revise the plan as necessary to try to keep the promise to reduce pain. Fidelity also refers to the unwillingness to abandon patients regardless of the circumstances, even when personal beliefs differ as they may when dealing with drug dealers, members of the gay community, women who received an abortion, or prisoners.

PROFESSIONAL NURSING CODE OF ETHICS

A code of ethics is a set of guiding principles that all members of a profession accept. It is a collective statement about the group's expectations and standards of behavior. The American Nurses Association (ANA) established the first code of nursing ethics decades ago. The ANA reviews and revises the code periodically; but principles of responsibility, accountability, advocacy, and confidentiality remain constant (ANA, 2015).

Advocacy

Advocacy refers to the support of a particular cause. As a nurse you advocate for the health, safety, and rights of patients, including their right to privacy and their right to refuse treatment. Your special relationship with patients provides you with knowledge that is specific to your role as a registered nurse and as such with the opportunity to make a unique contribution to understanding a patient's point of view.

Responsibility

The word responsibility refers to a willingness to respect one's professional obligations and to follow through. An example is following an agency's policies and procedures. As a nurse you are responsible for your actions and the actions of those to whom you delegate tasks. You agree to take responsibility to remain competent to practice so you can follow through on your responsibilities reliably.

Accountability

Accountability refers to the ability to answer for one's actions. You ensure that your professional actions are explainable to your patients and your employer. Health care institutions also exercise accountability by monitoring individual and institutional compliance with national standards established by agencies such as The Joint Commission (TJC). TJC establishes national patient safety guidelines to ensure patient and workplace safety through consistent, effective nursing practices (TJC, 2015). The ANA promotes ethical decision making by setting standards for collaborative practice through multidisciplinary discourse (ANA, 2015).

Confidentiality

Federal legislation known as the Health Insurance Portability and Accountability Act of 1996 (HIPAA) mandates confidentiality about and protection of patients' personal health information. The legislation defines the rights and privileges of patients for protection of privacy. It establishes fines for violations (USDHHS, 2013). In practice you cannot share information about a patient's medical condition or personal information to anyone not involved in the care of the patient. See Chapter 26 for details on HIPAA regulations governing communication of patient information contained in medical records, both hardcopy and electronic.

Social Networking

The online presence of social networks presents ethical challenges for nurses. On one hand social networks can be a supportive source of information about patient care or professional nursing activities. Social media can provide you emotional support when you encounter hardships at work with colleagues or patients. On the other hand, the risk to patient privacy is great. Even if you post an image of a patient without any obvious identifiers, the nature of shared media reposting can result in the image surfacing in a place where just the context of the image provides clues for friends or family to identify the patient.

Becoming friends in online chat rooms, on Facebook, or on other public sites interferes with your ability to maintain a therapeutic relationship. Friendship with a patient always comes with the risk of clouding your ability to remain objective in your clinical perceptions. The public nature of online relationships poses the additional risk that other patients may see and learn more than they should know about you and other patients. They may not trust you to remain impartial (i.e., available equally to each patient in your assignment).

Workplace policies will help to answer questions you have about when and where it is appropriate to engage in social media regarding workplace stories or issues. The ANA and the National Council of State Boards of Nursing (NCSBN) have crafted a joint White Paper on Social Media for guidance. As the joint statement puts it, "Effective nurse-patient relationships are built on trust. Patients need to be confident that their most personal information and their basic dignity will be protected by the nurse" (ANA/NCSBN, 2011).

VALUES

Nursing is a work of intimacy. Nursing practice requires you to be in contact with patients physically, emotionally, psychologically, and spiritually. In most other intimate relationships you choose to enter the relationship precisely because you anticipate that your values will be shared with the other person. But as a nurse you agree to provide care to your patients solely on the basis of their need for your services. The ethical principles of beneficence and fidelity shape the practice of health care and distinguish it from other common human relationships such as friendship, marriage, and employer-employee. But by its very nature relationships in health care sometimes can occur in the presence of conflicting values.

A **value** is a personal belief about the worth of a given idea, attitude, custom, or object that sets standards that influence behavior. Inevitably you will work with patients and colleagues whose values differ from yours. To negotiate differences of value, it is important to be clear about your own values: what you value, why, and how you respect your own values even as you try to respect those of others whose values differ from yours (see Chapter 9). The values that an individual holds reflect cultural and social influences, and these values vary among people and develop over time. For example, in some cultures decisions about health care flow from group or family-based discussion rather than independent decisions by one person. Such a practice may challenge your commitment to respect patient autonomy. Your effort to resolve differing opinions and maintain your cultural competence becomes the hallmark of your commitment to ethical practice.

Values Clarification

Ethical dilemmas almost always occur in the presence of conflicting values. To resolve ethical dilemmas one needs to distinguish among value, fact, and opinion. Sometimes people have such strong values that they consider them to be facts, not just opinion. Sometimes people are so passionate about their values that they become judgmental in a way that intensifies conflict. Clarifying values—your own, your patients', your co-workers'—is an important and effective part of ethical discourse. In the process of values clarification, you learn to tolerate differences in a way that often (although not always) becomes the key to the resolution of ethical dilemmas.

Examine the cultural values exercise in Box 22-1. The values in the exercise are in neutral terms so you can appreciate how differing values need not indicate "right" or "wrong." For example, for some people it is important to remain silent and stoic in the presence of great pain, and for others it is important to talk about it to understand and control it. Identifying values as something separate from facts can help you find tolerance for others, even when differences among you seem worlds apart.

BOX 22-1 Cultural Values Exercise

The column on the right contains statements describing an opinion; the column on the left contains statements describing the opposite opinion. Neither statement is right, nor is it wrong. These statements reflect opinion, not necessarily fact. If people from a variety of cultures were given this questionnaire, some would strongly agree with the beliefs on the right, and others with the opinions on the left. Read each statement and reflect on your own values and opinions. Circle 1 if you strongly agree with the statement on the left and 2 if you moderately agree. Circle 4 if you strongly agree with the statement on the right and 3 if you moderately agree.

Statement	Rank	Statement
Preparing for the future is an important activity and reflects maturity.	1 2 3 4	Life has a predestined course. The individual should follow that course.
Vague answers are dishonest and confusing.	1 2 3 4	Vague answers are sometimes preferred because they avoid embarrassment and confrontation.
Punctuality and efficiency are characteristics of a person who is both intelligent and concerned.	1 2 3 4	Punctuality is not as important as maintaining a relaxed atmosphere, enjoying the moment, and being with family and friends.
When in severe pain, it is important to remain strong and not to complain too much.	1 2 3 4	When in severe pain, it is better to talk about the discomfort and express frustration.
It is self-centered and unwise to accept a gift from someone you do not know well.	1 2 3 4	It is an insult to refuse a gift when it is offered.
Addressing someone by his or her first name shows friendliness.	1 2 3 4	Addressing someone by his or her first name is disrespectful.
Direct questions are usually the best way to gain information.	1 2 3 4	Direct questioning is rude and could cause embarrassment.
Direct eye contact shows interest.	1 2 3 4	Direct eye contact is intrusive.
Ultimately the independence of the individual must come before the needs of the family.	1 2 3 4	The needs of the individual are always less important than the needs of the family.

Modified from Renwick GW, Rhinesmith SH: *An exercise in cultural analysis for managers,* Chicago, 1995, Intercultural Press.

ETHICS AND PHILOSOPHY

Historically health care ethics constituted a search for fixed standards that would determine correct actions. Over time ethics has grown into a field of study that is more flexible and is filled with differences of opinion and deeply meaningful efforts to understand human interaction. The following review introduces you to a variety of philosophical approaches to ethics that you may encounter during ethical discussions in health care settings.

Deontology

Deontology proposes a system of ethics that is perhaps most familiar to health care practitioners. Its foundations come from the work of an eighteenth-century philosopher, Immanuel Kant (1724-1804). **Deontology** defines actions as right or wrong on the basis of their "right-making characteristics" such as fidelity to promises, truthfulness, and justice (Beauchamp and Childress, 2012). It specifically does not look at consequences of actions to determine right or wrong. Instead, deontology examines a situation for the existence of essential right or wrong. For example, if you try to make a decision about the ethics of a controversial medical procedure, deontology guides you to focus on how the procedure ensures fidelity to the patient, truthfulness, justice, and beneficence. You focus less on the consequences (ethically speaking). If the medical procedure in the example is just, respects autonomy, and provides good, it will be right, and it will be ethical according to this philosophy. If it provides good, but only to a limited number of people, it could be deemed unjust and therefore unethical.

Deontology depends on a mutual understanding of justice, autonomy, and goodness. But it still leaves room for confusion to surface. The principle of respect for autonomy can be complicated when dealing with children. For example, pediatricians recommend vaccinations against measles. But parents may refuse the recommendation, thinking that they are protecting the child from perceived harm. Whose autonomy should receive the respect—the parents'? What about the child's need to be protected from measles? What about the community's need to be protected from an epidemic? When is it acceptable to step in for a parent when seeking to speak for the child's best interest? A commitment to respect the "rightness" of autonomy is a guiding principle in deontology, but adherence to the principle alone does not always provide clear answers for complicated situations.

Utilitarianism

A utilitarian system of ethics proposes that the value of something is determined by its usefulness. This philosophy is also known as **consequentialism** because its main emphasis is on the outcome or consequence of action. A third term associated with this philosophy is **teleology**, from the Greek word telos, meaning "end," or the study of ends or final causes. John Stuart Mill (1806-1873), a British philosopher, first proposed its philosophical foundations. The greatest good for the greatest number of people is the guiding principle for determining right action in this system. As with deontology, **utilitarianism** relies on the application of a certain principle (i.e., measures of "good" and "greatest") (Beauchamp and Childress, 2012). The difference between utilitarianism and deontology is the focus on outcomes. Utilitarianism measures the effect that an act will have; deontology looks to the presence of principles regardless of outcome.

People have conflicting definitions of "greatest good." For example, research suggests that education about safe sex practices reduces the spread of human immunodeficiency virus (HIV). Reducing the incidence of HIV is good for a great number of people. For some, education about sex is best provided within a family setting rather than in school because it promotes family values. For others, using the same "greatest good" logic, sex education in public schools would be the best solution because it would educate the greatest number of people in an efficient and standard way. As with deontology, utilitarianism provides guidance, but it does not guarantee agreement.

Feminist Ethics

On the basis of their concerns about the unanswered questions that come with application of deontology and utilitarianism, scholars who focused on differences between genders, especially women's points of view, developed a critique of conventional ethical philosophies. Called **feminist ethics**, it looks to the nature of relationships to guide participants in making difficult decisions, especially relationships in which power is unequal or in which a point of view has become ignored or invisible (Beauchamp and Childress, 2012). Writers with a feminist perspective tend to concentrate more on practical solutions than on theory. For example, when deciding whether to perform a possibly futile procedure on a dying patient, feminist ethics might guide us to look at the patient's relationships with family and friends as a way to determine the ethically right thing to do. How would the patient's ability to engage in relationships be affected? If the patient is a parent, how would the patient's relationship to the children be affected by the intervention? These questions might surface less often if the discussion is framed solely by conventional ethical principles.

Critics of feminist ethics worry about the lack of appeal to traditional ethical principles. Without guidance from principles such as autonomy and beneficence, they argue, solutions to ethical questions will depend too much on subjective judgment.

Ethics of Care

The ethics of care and feminist ethics are closely related. Both promote a philosophy that focuses on understanding relationships, especially personal narratives.

An early proponent of the ethics of care, Nel Noddings, used the term *the one-caring* to identify the individual who provides care and *the cared-for* to refer to the patient. In adopting this language Noddings hoped to emphasize the role of feelings. **Ethics of care** also strives to address issues beyond individual relationships by raising ethical concerns about the structures within which individual caring occurs—structures such as hospitals or universities (Noddings, 2013).

Casuistry

Casuistry, or case-based reasoning, turns away from conventional principles of ethics as a way to determine best actions and focuses instead on an "intimate understanding of particular situations" (Beauchamp and Childress, 2012). This approach to ethical discourse depends on finding consensus more than an appeal to philosophical principle. Building consensus is an act of discovery in which collective wisdom guides a group to the best possible decision. As a strategy for solving dilemmas, consensus building promotes respect and agreement rather than a particular philosophy or moral system itself.

NURSING POINT OF VIEW

All patients in health care systems interact with nurses at some point, and they interact in ways that are unique to nursing. Nurses generally engage with patients over longer periods of time than other disciplines. They are involved in intimate physical acts such as bathing, feeding, and special procedures. As a result, patients and families may feel more comfortable in revealing information not always shared with physicians or other health care providers. Details about family life, information about coping styles, personal preferences, and details about fears and insecurities are likely to come out during the course of nursing interventions. Your ability to shape your care on the basis of this special knowledge provides an indispensable contribution to the overall care of your patient.

The care of any patient involves the collaboration of many disciplines. Managers and administrators from many different professional backgrounds contribute to ethical discourse with their knowledge of systems, distribution of resources, financial possibilities and limitations (Figure 22-1).

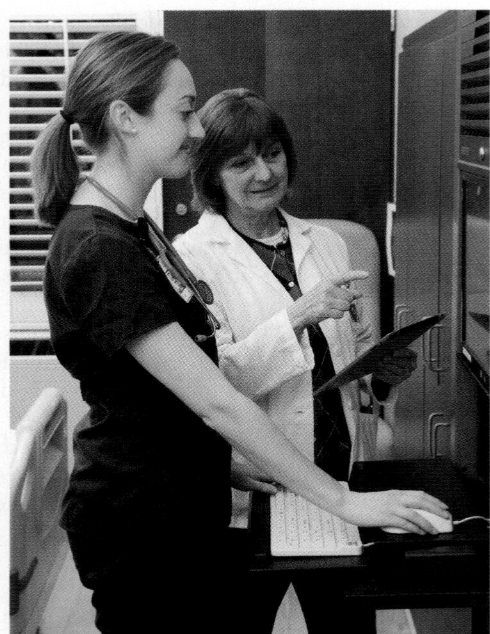

FIGURE 22-1 Nurses collaborate with other professionals in making ethical decisions.

Processing an Ethical Dilemma

Ethical dilemmas cause distress and controversy for both patients and professional caregivers. To minimize distress, participants strive to process ethical issues carefully and deliberately. The process should promote the free expression of feelings and opinions. However, you do not resolve an ethical dilemma by considering only what people want and feel (Zoloth, 2010).

Resolving an ethical dilemma is similar to the nursing process in its methodical approach to a clinical issue. But it differs from the nursing process in that it requires negotiation of differences of opinion and clarity about situations that are confusing and not easily solved by appealing to the usual ethical principles. Finding clarity and consensus can occur when the following elements remain essential to the process: the presumption of good will on the part of all participants, strict adherence to confidentiality, patient-centered decision making, and the welcome participation of families and primary caregivers (Zoloth, 2010).

The process begins with determining if an ethical dilemma exists. If the question is perplexing and the answer has relevance for several areas of human concern, an ethical dilemma exists. You then gather all pertinent information about the case, including review of the medical record for recent clinical evaluations. Examining your personal values at this point can help to differentiate between fact and opinion, an important part of the process. Once information is gathered, getting consensus on a statement about the dilemma will facilitate discussion. Next, listing all possible courses of action will guide the discussion toward a possible solution and help to identify areas of dissent and consensus. As a group you consider and evaluate alternatives with respect for all differences of opinion. Most of the time people in an ethical conflict come to a resolution and implement a plan. Evaluation of the plan follows (Box 22-2).

If the process involves a family conference or changes in the treatment plan, you document all relevant information in the medical record. Some institutions use a special ethics consultation form to structure documentation. However, if the ethical concern does not directly affect patient care, you may document the discussion in meeting minutes or in a memorandum to those involved in the discussion.

BOX 22-2 Key Steps in the Resolution of an Ethical Dilemma

Step 1: Ask the question, Is this an ethical dilemma?

Step 2: Gather information relevant to the case. Patient, family, institutional, and social perspectives are important sources of relevant information.

Step 3: Clarify values. Distinguish among fact, opinion, and values.

Step 4: Verbalize the problem. A clear, simple statement of the dilemma is not always easy, but it helps to ensure effectiveness in the final plan and facilitates discussion.

Step 5: Identify possible courses of action.

Step 6: Negotiate a plan. Negotiation requires a confidence in one's own point of view and a deep respect for the opinions of others.

Step 7: Evaluate the plan over time.

You have been taking care of a patient with a terminal illness for the last 3 weeks. The patient has just revealed to you that she is ready to explore Do Not Resuscitate (DNR) status. However, she has not been willing or able to express these sentiments to the attending physician. The physician has been taking care of the patient for the last 6 weeks. You ask the physician if he would conduct a patient care conference to talk about DNR, but he declines. You are challenged with how to proceed.

Step 1. Ask the question, Is this an ethical dilemma?

The question is perplexing. Your situation meets the criteria for an ethical dilemma. The disagreement does not revolve around whether the patient is in a terminally ill state; thus further clinical information will not change the basic question. Should the patient have an opportunity to discuss DNR orders at this time? You and the physician disagree on an assessment of the patient's readiness to confront difficult issues related to dying. If she is not ready, raising the issues could cause anguish and fear in the patient and her family. But she has expressed interest in discussing the topic. If she is ready and the team avoids discussion, she could suffer unnecessarily physically and emotionally. If she is very close to death, the lack of a DNR order necessitates the application of cardiopulmonary resuscitation (CPR) in a futile situation.

Step 2. Gather as much information as possible that is relevant to the case. Resolution of dilemmas can come from unlikely sources. Helpful information may include test results, the clinical state of the patient, and current literature about the diagnosis or condition of the patient. The patient's religious, cultural, and family situations are also essential to the assessment.

Since the dilemma exists because two professionals, you and the physician, disagree about the patient's state of mind, it is helpful to reassess the patient. An independent assessment could help resolve differences of opinion. Family members or significant others in the patient's life often hold important clues to a patient's state of mind.

Step 3. Examine and determine your values about the issues. Part of the goal is to accurately identify your own opinion, and an equally critical goal is to form respect for others' opinions.

Reflect on your values. You think that this patient wants a DNR order in place. But does this opinion accurately represent the patient's wishes or possibly your own idea about what is best for her? In addition, you understand that the attending physician has not had time to know this patient well. You continue to believe that the patient is capable of a discussion, in spite of her statements to the physician. In fact, you believe that she will benefit from a discussion, regardless of the final decision. Perhaps the combination of an unfamiliar caretaker and declining physical health has silenced her, even though her fears and concerns persist.

Step 4. Verbalize the problem. By agreeing to a statement of the problem, the group is able to conduct a focused discussion.

Is a DNR order a right or wrong thing for this patient? And is she ready to discuss the options?

Step 5. Consider possible courses of action. Which options are possible in this situation?

You could turn to your supervisor for advice. You could initiate a discussion with the physician, independent of the patient. You might consult with the ethics council in your workplace. Your goal is to find the best place to resolve the dilemma, and discourse is the most common avenue to resolution. Questions you might bring up to discuss with others: Is it in the patient's best interest to facilitate a DNR order? How can one determine what the patient really does want? What happens when, in good faith, professionals disagree about the patient's assessment? The answers to these questions can be elusive because they depend on an understanding of patient feelings and values that are not necessarily obvious.

Step 6. Negotiate the outcome. Negotiations can happen in a variety of settings: at the bedside, in an office, in a conference room. Sometimes a formal ethics meeting provides a useful resource. Wherever negotiations occur, the nurse has an obligation to articulate a personal point of view and at the same time to show respect for the points of views of others at the table.

If an ethics committee meeting occurs, the discussion usually involves participants from other disciplines and should include the patient and patient family. A facilitator or chairperson ensures that the group examines all points of view and identifies all relevant issues. In the best circumstances participants discover a course of action that meets criteria for consensus or acceptance by all. However, occasionally they leave the discussion disappointed or even opposed to the decision. But in a successful discussion all members will have agreed on an action.

The principles involved during an ethics committee discussion include beneficence and nonmaleficence: Which plan provides the most good for this patient, a DNR order or no order? A separate question addresses the patient's point of view and a respect for her autonomy: Would a discussion with the patient promote well-being or anguish? The commitment to respect a patient's autonomy reveals that a troublesome question remains: Does the patient want something different from what she is expressing?

With several members of the health care team present, the discussion proceeds. You present your point of view. You continue to sense that the patient is ready to discuss DNR orders. But you also respect the attending physician and his perception that the patient is reluctant to talk freely about it. In the end the team proposes the following: a formal meeting with the patient in which you, the attending physician, and a respected family member are present. You support this proposal because you believe that it maximizes comfort from the patient's network of friends and family. In addition, you recognize that in a trusting environment the patient is most likely to express herself freely. You suggest that, rather than asking if the patient wants a DNR order, perhaps the team could wait for her to initiate the discussion. In this way the team would be sure of her consent and willingness to address the difficult questions about dying.

Step 7. Evaluate the action.

At the meeting the patient brings up the DNR order. She expresses relief at the chance to explore her options and feelings. The physician clarifies pain-management issues that she poses. She wants to discuss a DNR order but requests a visit from her priest before making a final decision. At the end of the meeting you ask the patient if her expectations were met, and she says, "Yes, I am so glad you gave me the chance to talk about this. I feel I am ready to die."

Institutional Resources

An ethics committee devoted to the teaching and processing of ethical issues and dilemmas is required in most hospitals. A committee involves individuals from different disciplines and backgrounds who support health care institutions with three major functions: providing clinical ethics consultation, developing and/or revising policies pertaining to clinical ethics and hospital policy (e.g., advance directives, withholding and withdrawing life-sustaining treatments, informed consent, organ procurement), and facilitating education about topical issues in clinical ethics (University of Washington, 2013). Any person involved in seeking ethical advice, including nurses, physicians, health care providers, patients, and family members, can request access to an ethics committee.

You may also process ethical issues in settings other than a committee. Nurses provide insight about ethical problems at family conferences, staff meetings, or even in one-on-one meetings.

When ethical problems are not processed well, moral distress can result. Moral distress occurs when people feel misled or are not aware of their options and do not know when or how to speak up about their concerns. As a member of a health care community, regardless of your work setting, you can reduce the risk for moral distress by promoting discourse even when disagreements or confusion are profound. Ethics committees offer a valuable resource for nurturing discourse and strengthening relationships (Box 22-3).

QSEN QSEN: BUILDING COMPETENCY IN PATIENT-CENTERED CARE You have been assigned to care for a 27-year-old patient. He is obese and is newly diagnosed with hypertension and diabetes. You learn that he does not have health insurance. He works full time with a steady income, but he thought he was "too young and too healthy to need health insurance." He is about to be discharged to home. Without insurance, he will not be able to afford clinic visits or the new medications that have been prescribed. How will a focus on patient-centered care help you better meet your ethical and professional obligations?

Answers to QSEN Activities can be found on the Evolve website.

ISSUES IN HEALTH CARE ETHICS

Ethical issues change as society and technologies change, but common denominators remain: the basic process used to address the issues and your responsibility to deal with them. The following section describes examples of current issues in which ethical concerns arise.

BOX 22-3 EVIDENCE-BASED PRACTICE

Moral Distress

PICO Question: Which ethical actions diminish distress and promote compassionate care for nurses experiencing moral distress when caring for dying patients?

Evidence Summary

Moral distress describes the anguish experienced when a person feels unable to act according to closely held core values. Evidence indicates that underlying problems of poor communication, inadequate collaboration, and perceived powerlessness contribute to recurrent moral distress (Ulrich et al., 2010). Reliable tools to measure moral distress, tested for reliability and validity, continue to evolve as researchers focus on the experience of moral distress, especially in critical care units (Hamric et al., 2012). In guided interviews with intensive care unit (ICU) providers, researchers demonstrated how "feeling powerless, difficult family dynamics, and recognition of suffering predicted the development of moral distress" (McAndrew and Leske, 2015).

Application to Nursing Practice

Since moral distress is a shared experience, collaborative efforts to alleviate it are most successful. Research suggests that the following interventions can reduce risk for moral distress:

- Interdisciplinary ethics education, in which nurses and physicians learn together about ethical discourse (Ulrich et al., 2010; McAndrew and Leske, 2015)
- Development of workplace support groups for nurses and physicians
- Increasing opportunities for collegial practice such as routine multidisciplinary rounds
- Engaging in constructive and multidisciplinary conversation, which is key (McAndrew and Leske, 2015)

Quality of Life

Quality of life represents something deeply personal. Health care researchers use quality-of-life measures to define scientifically the value and benefits of medical interventions. Increasingly scientists incorporate not just observed measurement but patient self-reports about quality of life and other outcomes, referred to as Patient Reported Outcomes (Basch, 2014). Quality-of-life measures may take into account the age of a patient, the patient's ability to live independently, his or her ability to contribute to society in a gainful way, and other nuanced measures of quality. Still a definition remains deeply individual and difficult to predict. Nussbaum (2011) proposes that quality of life is not just a measurable entity but a shared responsibility that we owe to one another as members of a community. As Nussbaum (2011) describes it, the good life "begins with a commitment to the equal dignity of all people, whatever their class, religion, caste, race, or gender. It is committed to the attainment, for all, of lives that are worthy of that equal dignity." The question of quality of life is central to discussions about quality of care, outcome measures, care at the end of life, futile care, cancer therapy, and health care provider–assisted suicide.

Disabilities

Approximately 56.7 million people (18.7% in the civilian noninstitutionalized population) had a disability in 2010 (Brault, 2012). This includes people who have a disability in the communicative (e.g., blind, deaf), physical (e.g., use of assist device, chronic disease or acute injury affecting mobility), or mental (e.g., learning disability, dementia) domains. The population of disabled people in the United States and elsewhere has reshaped the discussion about quality of life. The national movement to respect the abilities of all, regardless of their functional status, has inspired a reconsideration of the definition of quality of life. Many school districts no longer separate physically or mentally challenged children but rather integrate them into mainstream classrooms. Public places such as restaurants and buses are accessible to people who use wheelchairs. Antidiscrimination laws enhance the economic security of people with physical, mental, or emotional challenges. These changes result in the greater integration of disabled people into general society.

Philosophically the conversation has shifted from one about a focus on what is wrong when a person has a disability to a conversation about how best to nurture capabilities of all humans regardless their circumstances. Sometimes referred to as a *capabilities approach,* it "begins with a commitment to the equal dignity of all people, whatever their class, religion, caste, race, or gender, and it is committed to the attainment, for all, of lives that are worthy of that equal dignity" (Nussbaum, 2011).

Care at the End of Life

Predictions about health outcomes are not always accurate. Even when they are, opinions about the value or worth of the outcome differ. For example, patients at risk for breast cancer occasionally request a mastectomy before any symptoms of breast disease have appeared, fearful of a family history and thinking that it will prevent future suffering. Physicians may be understandably reluctant to provide this intervention on the basis of knowledge of risk factors and their commitment to "do no harm." On the other hand, a physician might recommend that a patient undergo a liver transplantation for end-stage liver disease, even though the likelihood of a cure is uncertain. The patient may hold the opinion that the transplant is pointless (i.e., unlikely to produce benefit that justifies the suffering that he or she anticipates). Agreement on what is best is often elusive.

Difficult emotional and spiritual challenges resulting in moral distress can characterize the management of care at the end of life. The term *futile* refers to something that is hopeless or serves no useful purpose. In health care discussions the term refers to interventions unlikely to produce benefit for a patient. The concept is slippery when applied to clinical situations.

If a patient is dying of a condition with little or no hope of recovery, almost any intervention beyond symptom management and comfort measures is seen as futile. In this situation an agreement to label an intervention as futile can help providers, families, and patients turn to palliative care measures as a more constructive approach to the situation (see Chapter 37).

Health Care Reform

The Affordable Care Act (ACA), implemented January 2012, facilitated access to care for millions of formerly uninsured in the United States. Access to care is essentially an ethical issue of justice. A Rand corporation survey estimates that at least 9.3 million more adults in the United States now have health coverage as compared to coverage before ACA implementation (Carman and Eibner, 2014). The legislation also incorporates a promotion of wellness by proposing changes in payment for services and by rewarding practices that reduce harm and promote quality outcomes.

Adjustment to the ACA remains ongoing. Some states did not implement it in full (i.e., declined to accept expansion of Medicaid coverage for low-income residents). Many residents who did enroll are first-time users of health insurance and are still learning how to access it. In a poll conducted 6 months after ACA implementation, a quarter

BOX 22-4 CULTURAL ASPECTS OF CARE

Access to Affordable Health Care

Since the implementation of the Affordable Care Act, more residents in the United States have access to care than ever before. But according to the National Healthcare Disparities Report (NHDR), people of color, ethnic minorities, and low-income residents are "disproportionately represented among those with access problems." Reports from the National Healthcare Quality Report and NHDR reveal that lack of health insurance is the most significant contributing factor to poor quality of care. According to the authors of the report, "Uninsured people were less likely to get recommended care for disease prevention such as cancer screening, dental care, counseling about diet and exercise, and flu vaccination. They also were less likely to get recommended care for disease management such as diabetes care management" (AHRQ, 2013).

Implications for Patient-Centered Care

- Issues of justice and the just distribution of resources help to inform the discussion about access to care and its effect on health care outcomes.
- Health outcomes often correlate directly to health care access.
- Know and respect patient's cultural practices regarding health promotion and health care needs (Chapter 9).
- Identify culturally appropriate resources for patients and families in their community

of respondents incorrectly believed that they had enrolled in a single government plan (Hamel, 2014).

How people access health care in the United States will continue to evolve. Staying knowledgeable about affordable care in your community as a way to ensure healthy outcomes is an important part of your role as advocate for your patients and will reflect your ethical commitment to justice (Box 22-4).

• • •

The courage and intelligence to act as both an advocate for patients and a professional member of the health care community come from a committed effort to learn and understand ethical principles. As a professional nurse you provide a unique point of view regarding patients, the systems that support patients, and the institutions that make up the health care system. You have a duty and a privilege to articulate that point of view. Learning the language of ethical discourse is a part of the skill necessary to exercise this privilege. Review and consideration of various ethical principles help you form personal points of view, a necessary skill in the negotiation of difficult ethical situations.

KEY POINTS

- Ethics is the study of conduct and character. It is concerned with determining what is good or valuable for individuals and society at large.
- The ANA code of ethics provides a foundation for professional nursing.
- Professional nursing promotes accountability, responsibility, advocacy, and confidentiality.
- Principles of ethics in health care include autonomy, beneficence, nonmaleficence, justice, and fidelity.
- The process of values clarification helps you explore values and feelings and decide how to act on personal beliefs and respect values of others, even if they differ from yours.
- Ethical problems arise in the presence of differences in values, changing professional roles, technological advances, and social issues that influence quality of life.
- A process for resolving ethical dilemmas that respects differences of opinions and all participants equally helps health care providers resolve conflict about right actions.
- A nurse's point of view offers a unique voice in the resolution of ethical dilemmas.

CLINICAL APPLICATION QUESTIONS

Preparing for Clinical Practice

You are caring for a 17-year-old female patient with sickle cell disease who has been admitted for treatment of sickle cell crisis. Sickle cell disease is a genetic abnormality that affects hemoglobin in the red blood cells. In a sickle cell crisis weakened red blood cells clump together and impede blood flow, causing extreme pain. To prevent stroke and manage the pain of the crisis, your patient needs aggressive fluid and comfort management. At the change-of-shift report, you learn that, even though she is receiving pain medication around the clock, she continues to report acute pain at a level of 10 on a scale of 0 to 10. She complains about almost everything: her roommate, the food, even the intravenous line that delivers the fluids and pain medications. Her home is far from the hospital, and her family and friends are not able to visit.

During shift report the nurse from the past shift describes the patient as manipulative. On the basis of her concern about a risk for addiction, she has declined to increase the dose of pain medication.

1. Describe this case in terms of the ethical principles that it raises. Refer to the nursing code of ethics to compose your response.
2. How could a values clarification exercise promote an ethical response to this case?
3. In trying to better understand sickle cell disease, you join a chat room online where people with sickle cell disease discuss their problems. Hoping to protect patient privacy, you use only your first name and the patient's first name. You mention the name of the hospital where you work. On the basis of your reading of the ANA White Paper on Social Media, describe benefits and risks of participating in social media in this situation.

ⓔ ***Answers to Clinical Application Questions can be found on the Evolve website.***

REVIEW QUESTIONS

Are You Ready to Test Your Nursing Knowledge?

1. The patient for whom you are caring needs a liver transplant to survive. This patient has been out of work for several months and doesn't have health insurance or enough cash. Even though several ethical principles are at work in this case, list the principles from highest to lowest priority.
    1. Accountability: You as the nurse are accountable for the well-being of this patient.
    2. Respect for autonomy: This patient's autonomy will be violated if he does not receive the liver transplant.
    3. Ethics of care: The caring thing that a nurse could provide this patient is resources for a liver transplant.
    4. Justice: The greatest question in this situation is how to determine the just distribution of resources.
2. **Fill in the Blank.** The point of the ethical practice is an agreement to reassure the public that in all ways the health care team not only

works to heal patients but agrees to do this in the least painful and harmful way possible. This principle is commonly called the principle of ________?

3. A child's immunization may cause discomfort during administration, but the benefits of protection from disease, both for the individual and society, outweigh the temporary discomforts. Which principle is involved in this situation?
   1. Fidelity
   2. Beneficence
   3. Nonmaleficence
   4. Respect for autonomy
4. When designing a plan for pain management for a postoperative patient, the nurse assesses that the patient's priority is to be as free of pain as possible. The nurse and patient work together to identify a plan to manage the pain. The nurse continually reviews the plan with the patient to ensure that the patient's priority is met. Which principle is used to encourage the nurse to monitor the patient's response to the pain?
   1. Fidelity
   2. Beneficence
   3. Nonmaleficence
   4. Respect for autonomy
5. A patient is admitted to a medical unit. The patient is fearful of hospitals. The nurse carefully assesses the patient to determine the exact fears and then establishes interventions designed to reduce these fears. In this setting how is the nurse practicing patient advocacy?
   1. Seeking out the nursing supervisor to talk with the patient
   2. Documenting patient fears in the medical record in a timely manner
   3. Working to change the hospital environment
   4. Assessing the patient's point of view and preparing to articulate it
6. The application of utilitarianism does not always resolve an ethical dilemma. Which of the following statements best explains why?
   1. Utilitarianism refers to usefulness and therefore eliminates the need to talk about spiritual values.
   2. In a diverse community it can be difficult to find agreement on a definition of usefulness, the focus of utilitarianism.
   3. Even when agreement about a definition of usefulness exists in a community, laws prohibit an application of utilitarianism.
   4. Difficult ethical decisions cannot be resolved by talking about the usefulness of a procedure.
7. The *ethics of care* suggests that ethical dilemmas can best be solved by attention to relationships. How does this differ from other ethical practices? (Select all that apply.)
   1. Ethics of care pays attention to the environment in which caring occurs.
   2. Ethics of care pays attention to the stories of the people involved in the ethical issue.
   3. Ethics of care is used only in nursing practice.
   4. Ethics of care focuses only on the code of ethics for nurses
   5. Ethics of care focuses only on understanding relationships.
8. In most ethical dilemmas in health care, the solution to the dilemma requires negotiation among members of the health care team. Why is the nurse's point of view valuable?
   1. Nurses understand the principle of autonomy to guide respect for a patient's self-worth.
   2. Nurses have a scope of practice that encourages their presence during ethical discussions.
   3. Nurses develop a relationship with the patient that is unique among all professional health care providers.
   4. The nurse's code of ethics recommends that a nurse be present at any ethical discussion about patient care.
9. Ethical dilemmas often arise over a conflict of opinion. Reliance on a predictable series of steps can help people in conflict find common ground. All of the following actions can help resolve conflict. What is the best order of these actions in order to promote the resolution of an ethical dilemma?
   1. List the actions that could be taken to resolve the dilemma.
   2. Agree on a statement of the problem or dilemma that you are trying to resolve.
   3. Agree on a plan to evaluate the action over time.
   4. Gather all relevant information regarding the clinical, social, and spiritual aspects of the dilemma.
   5. Take time to clarify values and distinguish between facts and opinions—your own and those of others involved.
   6. Negotiate a plan.
10. The ANA code of nursing ethics articulates that the nurse "promotes, advocates for, and strives to protect the health, safety, and rights of the patient." This includes the protection of patient privacy. On the basis of this principle, if you participate in a public online social network such as Facebook, could you post images of a patient's x-ray film if you obscured or deleted all patient identifiers?
    1. Yes, because patient privacy would not be violated since patient identifiers were removed
    2. Yes, because respect for autonomy implies that you have the autonomy to decide what constitutes privacy
    3. No, because, even though patient identifiers are removed, someone could identify the patient on the basis of other comments that you make online about his or her condition and your place of work
    4. No, because the principle of justice requires you to allocate resources fairly
11. What are the correct steps to resolve an ethical dilemma on a clinical unit? Place the steps in correct order.
    1. Clarify values.
    2. Ask the question, Is this an ethical dilemma?
    3. Verbalize the problem.
    4. Gather information.
    5. Identify course of action.
    6. Evaluate the plan.
    7. Negotiate a plan
12. Resolution of an ethical dilemma involves discussion with the patient, the patient's family, and participants from all health care disciplines. Which of the following best describes the role of the nurse in the resolution of ethical dilemmas?
    1. To articulate the nurse's unique point of view, including knowledge based on clinical and psychosocial observations.
    2. To study the literature on current research about the possible clinical interventions available for the patient in question.
    3. To hold a point of view but realize that respect for the authority of administrators and physicians takes precedence over personal opinion.
    4. To allow the patient and the physician to resolve the dilemma on the basis of ethical principles without regard to personally held values or opinions.
13. It can be difficult to agree on a common definition of the word *quality* when it comes to quality of life. Why? (Select all that apply.)
    1. Average income varies in different regions of the country.
    2. Community values influence definitions of quality, and they are subject to change over time.

3. Individual experiences influence perceptions of quality in different ways, making consensus difficult.
4. The value of elements such as cognitive skills, ability to perform meaningful work, and relationship to family is difficult to quantify using objective measures.
5. Statistical analysis is difficult to apply when the outcome cannot be quantified.
6. Whether or not a person has a job is an objective measure, but it does not play a role in understanding quality of life.

14. Which of the following properly applies an ethical principle to justify access to health care? (Select all that apply.)
1. Access to health care reflects the commitment of society to principles of beneficence and justice.
2. If low income compromises access to care, respect for autonomy is compromised.
3. Access to health care is a privilege in the United States, not a right.
4. Poor access to affordable health care causes harm that is ethically troubling because nonmaleficence is a basic principle of health care ethics.
5. Providers are exempt from fidelity to people with drug addiction because addiction reflects a lack of personal accountability.
6. If a new drug is discovered that cures a disease but at great cost per patient, the principle of justice suggests that the drug should be made available to those who can afford it.

15. Match the examples with the professional nursing code of ethics:

1. You see an open medical record on the computer and close it so no one else can read the record without proper access.	**a.** Advocacy
2. You administer a once-a-day cardiac medication at the wrong time, but nobody sees it. However, you contact the primary care provider and your head nurse and follow agency procedure.	**b.** Responsibility
3. A patient at the end of life wants to go home to die, but the family wants every care possible. The nurse contacts the primary care provider about the patient's request.	**c.** Accountability
4. You tell your patient that you will return in 30 minutes to give him his next pain medication.	**d.** Confidentiality

Answers: 1. 4, 2, 3, 1; **2.** Nonmaleficence; **3.** 2; **4.** 1; **5.** 4; **6.** 2; **7.** 1, 2, 5; **8.** 3; **9.** 4, 5, 2, 1, 6, 3; **10.** 3; **11.** 2, 4, 1, 3, 5, 7, 6; **12.** 1; **13.** 2, 3, 4, 5; **14.** 1, 2, 4; **15.** 1d, 2c, 3a, 4b.

Rationales for Review Questions can be found on the Evolve website.

REFERENCES

Agency for Healthcare Research and Quality (AHRQ): *National Healthcare Disparities Report*, 2013, http://www.ahrq.gov/research/findings/nhqrdr/nhdr13/chap10.html, revised May 2014. Accessed February 2015.

American Nurses Association (ANA): *Code of ethics*, revised 2015, http://www.nursingworld.org/MainMenuCategories/EthicsStandards/CodeofEthicsforNurses/Code-of-Ethics-For-Nurses.html. Accessed February 2015.

American Nurses Association (ANA) and National Council of State Boards of Nursing (NCSBN): *White paper: a nurse's guide to the use of social media*, revised 2011, https://www.ncsbn.org/Social_Media.pdf. Accessed February 2015.

Basch E: New frontiers in patient-reported outcomes: adverse event reporting, comparative effectiveness, and quality assessment, *Annu Rev Med* 65:307, updated 2014. http://www.annualreviews.org/doi/abs/10.1146/annurev-med-010713-141500. Accessed July 28, 2015.

Beauchamp T, Childress J: *Principles of biomedical ethics*, ed 7, New York, 2012, Oxford University Press.

Brault MW: Americans with disabilities: 2010: Current population reports; Household economics, *US Census Bureau, Washington DC*, Available at http://www.census.gov/prod/2012pubs/p70-131.pdf. Accessed August 1, 2015.

Carman GC, Eibner C: *Survey estimates net gain of 9.3 million adults with health insurance*, revised July 2014, Rand Corporation, 2014, http://www.rand.org/blog/2014/04/survey-estimates-net-gain-of-9-3-million-american-adults.html. Accessed February 2015.

Hamel L, et al: *Kaiser health tracking poll*, July 2014, http://kff.org/health-reform/poll-finding/kaiser-health-tracking-poll-july-2014/, revised August 1, 2014. Accessed July 28, 2015.

Noddings N: *Caring: a relational approach to ethics and moral education*, Berkeley, 2013, University of California Press.

Nussbaum M: What makes a good life, *The Nation*, May 2, 2011.

Reverby SM: *Tuskegee Syphilis Study*, updated April 2013, http://www.encyclopediaofalabama.org/face/Article.jsp?id=h-1116. Accessed February 2015.

The Joint Commission (TJC): *Joint Commission hospital national patient safety goals*, 2015, http://www.jointcommission.org/hap_2015_npsgs/. Accessed February 2015.

University of Washington: Ethics committees, programs and consultations, *Ethics in Medicine 2013*. Available at https://depts.washington.edu/bioethx/topics/ethics.html. Accessed July 31, 2015.

US Department of Health and Human Services (USDHHS): *Understanding health information privacy*, last revised January 2013, http://www.hhs.gov/ocr/privacy/hipaa/understanding/index.html. Accessed February 2015.

Zoloth L: Learning a practice of uncertainty: clinical ethics and the nurse. In Cowen PS, Moorhead S, editors: *Current issues in nursing*, ed 7, St Louis, 2010, Mosby.

RESEARCH REFERENCES

Hamric AB, et al: Development and testing of an instrument to measure moral distress in healthcare professionals, *AJOB Prim Res* 3(2):1, 2012.

McAndrew NS, Leske JS: A balancing act: experiences of nurses and physicians when making end-of-life decisions in intensive care units, *Clin Nurs Res* 24(4):357, 2015.

Ulrich CM, et al: Moral distress: a growing problem in the health professions?, *Hastings Cent Rep* 40(1):20, 2010.

23

Legal Implications in Nursing Practice

OBJECTIVES

- Describe the legal obligations and role of the nurse regarding federal and state laws that affect health care.
- Explain the legal concepts of standard of care and informed consent.
- List sources of standards of care for nurses.
- Describe the nurse's role regarding a "do not resuscitate" (DNR) order.
- Analyze legal aspects of nurse-patient, nurse–health care provider, nurse-nurse, and nurse-employer relationships.
- List the elements needed to establish negligence.
- Analyze nursing actions most often associated in a breach of nursing practice.

KEY TERMS

Administrative law, p. 302
Assault, p. 308
Battery, p. 308
Civil laws, p. 303
Common law, p. 303
Confidentiality, p. 306
Criminal laws, p. 303
Defamation of character, p. 308
Durable power of attorney for health care (DPAHC), p. 305
False imprisonment, p. 308
Felony, p. 303
Good Samaritan laws, p. 307
Informed consent, p. 309
Intentional torts, p. 308
Invasion of privacy, p. 308
Libel, p. 309
Living wills, p. 305
Malpractice, p. 309
Misdemeanor, p. 303
Negligence, p. 309
Never events, p. 312
Nurse Practice Acts, p. 302
Occurrence report, p. 312
Privacy, p. 306
Quasi-intentional torts, p. 308
Regulatory law, p. 302
Risk management, p. 312
Slander, p. 308
Standards of care, p. 303
Statutory law, p. 302
Torts, p. 308
Unintentional torts, p. 308

MEDIA RESOURCES

http://evolve.elsevier.com/Potter/fundamentals/
- Review Questions
- Case Study with Questions
- Audio Glossary
- Content Updates

Safe and competent nursing practice requires clinical reasoning and an understanding of the legal framework of health care, the specific state's Nurse Practice Act, and the scope and standards of nursing care. Frequently nurses practice under several sources and jurisdictions of health care law simultaneously. Understanding the legal implications of nursing practice demands clinical judgment skills to protect patient's rights and the nurse from liability. Society expects safe health care delivery, especially from nurses who typically are perceived as being part of the most ethical and trusted profession. As patient care practice innovations and new health care technologies emerge, the principles of negligence and malpractice liability are being applied to challenging new situations. Thus you need to practice nursing armed with the skills that are the outcomes of informed critical thinking.

LEGAL LIMITS OF NURSING

As a professional nurse you need to understand the legal limits of nursing and the professional standards of care that affect nursing practice. Knowledge of these responsibilities allows you to be a patient advocate and protect patients from harm. If you have specific questions, consult your own attorney or the attorney for your agency.

Sources of Law

The legal guidelines that nurses follow originally were derived from constitutional law, statutory law, regulatory law, and common law. Elected legislative bodies such as state legislatures and the U.S. Congress create **statutory law**. An example of state statutes are the Nurse Practice Acts found in all 50 states (see Chapter 1). **Nurse Practice Acts** describe and define the legal boundaries of nursing practice within each state. The Nurse Practice Act of each state defines the scope of nursing practice and expanded nursing roles, sets education requirements for nurses, and distinguishes between nursing and medical practice. **Regulatory law**, or **administrative law**, reflects decisions made by administrative bodies such as State Boards of Nursing when rules and regulations are passed. An example of a regulatory law is the requirement to report incompetent or unethical nursing conduct to the State

Board of Nursing. Common law results from judicial decisions made by courts when individual legal cases are decided. An example of a common law includes informed consent, a patient's right to refuse treatment, negligence, and malpractice.

Statutory law is either civil or criminal. Civil laws protect the rights of individuals and provide for fair and equitable treatment when civil wrongs or violations occur (Guido, 2014). The consequences of civil law violations are fines or specific performance of good works such as public service. Nursing negligence or malpractice is an example of a civil law violation. Criminal laws protect society as a whole and provide punishment for crimes, which are defined by municipal, state, and federal legislation (Garner, 2014). Criminal laws are separated into misdemeanors or felonies. A misdemeanor is a crime that causes injury but does not inflict serious harm (Shilling, 2011). For example, parking in a no-parking zone is a misdemeanor violation of traffic laws. A misdemeanor usually has a penalty of a monetary fine, forfeiture, or brief imprisonment. A felony is a serious offense that results in significant harm to another person or society in general. Felony crimes carry penalties of monetary restitution, imprisonment for greater than 1 year, or death (Guido, 2014). Examples of Nurse Practice Act violations that often carry criminal penalties include misuse of a controlled substance or practicing without a license.

Standards of Care

Standards of care are the legal requirements for nursing practice that describe minimum acceptable nursing care. Standards reflect the knowledge and skill ordinarily possessed and used by nurses actively practicing in the profession (Guido, 2014) (see Chapter 1). The American Nurses Association (ANA) (2010) develops standards for nursing practice, policy statements, and similar resolutions. These standards outline the scope, function, and role of the nurse in practice. Nursing standards of care are described in the Nurse Practice Act of every state, in the federal and state laws regulating hospitals and other health care agencies, by professional and specialty nursing organizations, and by the policies and procedures established by the health care agency where nurses work (Guido, 2014). In a malpractice lawsuit a nurse's actual conduct is compared to nursing standards of care to determine whether the nurse acted as any reasonably prudent nurse would act under the same or similar circumstances (Philo et al., 2015). For example, if a patient receives a burn from a warm compress application, negligence is determined by reviewing if the nurse followed the correct procedure for applying the compress. A breach of the nursing standard of care is one element that must be established in a claim of nursing negligence or malpractice (Westrick, 2014).

Nurse Practice Acts define the scope of nursing practice, distinguishing between nursing and medical practice and establishing education and licensure requirements for nurses. The rules and regulations enacted by a State Board of Nursing or a Nursing Commission define the practice of nursing more specifically. For example, State Boards of Nursing develop rules regarding intravenous therapy. Another example involves the use of nursing assistive personnel (NAP) (e.g., nurse assistants). Some State Boards of Nursing or Commissions define responsibilities of the registered nurse (RN) specifically and develop position statements and guidelines to help licensed nurses delegate safely to NAP (NCSBN, 2005). All nurses are responsible for knowing the provisions of the Nurse Practice Act of the state in which they work and the rules and regulations enacted by the State Board of Nursing and other regulatory administrative bodies.

The Joint Commission (TJC) (2014) requires accredited hospitals to have written nursing policies and procedures. These internal standards of care are specific to the agency and need to be accessible on all nursing units. For example, a policy/procedure outlining the steps to follow when changing a dressing or administering medication provides specific information about how nurses are to perform these tasks. Some hospitals currently are using commercially published procedural textbooks and online references to represent the general policies and procedures of the agency. You need to know the policies, procedures, and protocols of your employing agency so you use the same standard of care as the other nurses in your agency. Agency policies and procedures need to conform to state and federal laws and community standards and cannot conflict with legal guidelines that define acceptable standards of care (Guido, 2014).

In a lawsuit for malpractice or negligence, a nursing expert may testify to the jury about the standards of nursing care as applied to the facts of the case (Box 23-1). The nurse may be asked to give evidence in a deposition; statements made by the nurse will be analyzed by the nursing expert *before* a trial (Guido, 2014; Westrick, 2014). Nurse experts base their opinions on existing standards of practice established by Nurse Practice Acts, federal and state hospital licensing laws, TJC standards, professional organizations, institutional policies and procedures, job descriptions, and current nursing evidence-based literature (Guido, 2014). Usually nurses are responsible for meeting the same standards as other nurses practicing in similar settings. Specialized nurses such as certified nurse anesthetists, operating room (OR) nurses, intensive care nurses, nurse practitioners, or certified nurse-midwives have specially defined standards of care and skills. Ignorance of the law or of standards of care is not a defense against malpractice (Guido, 2014). Nurses are required to know valid, reliable, and credible evidence that is applicable to their practice and the settings in which they work, including current standards of care and the policies and procedures of their employing agency (ANA, 2014; Melnyk and Fineout-Overholt, 2014). The jury uses the standards of care to determine whether the nurse acted appropriately.

One of the first and most important cases to discuss a nurse's liability was Darling v Charleston Community Memorial Hospital (1965). It involved an 18-year-old man with a fractured leg. The emergency department physician applied a cast with insufficient padding. The man's toes became swollen and discolored, and he developed decreased sensation. He complained to the nursing staff many times. Although the nurses recognized the symptoms as signs of impaired circulation, they failed to tell their supervisor that the physician did not respond to their calls or the patient's needs. Gangrene developed, and the man's leg was amputated. Although the physician was held liable for incorrectly applying the cast, the nursing staff was also held liable for failing to adhere to the standards of care for monitoring and reporting the patient's symptoms. Even though the nurses attempted to contact the physician, the jury and subsequent judges held that, when the physician fails to respond, the nurse must continue to use the agency chain of command (e.g., charge nurse, nursing supervisor, department director or chief medical officer) to make sure that the patient receives appropriate care. Almost every state uses this 1965 Illinois Supreme Court case as legal precedence.

FEDERAL STATUTORY ISSUES IN NURSING PRACTICE

Patient Protection and Affordable Care Act

The Patient Protection and Affordable Care Act (PPACA or ACA, 2010), is characterized by four themes embedded in nursing practice: (1) consumer rights and protections; (2) affordable health care coverage; (3) increased access to care; and (4) stronger Medicare to improve care for those most vulnerable in our society.

PPACA created a new Patient's Bill of Rights that prohibited patients from being denied health care coverage because of prior existing

BOX 23-1 Anatomy of a Lawsuit

Pleadings Phase

Petition: Elements of the claim. The plaintiff outlines what the defendant nurse did wrong and, as a result of that alleged negligence, how the plaintiff was injured.

Answer: The nurse admits or denies each allegation in the petition. The plaintiff must prove anything that the nurse does not admit.

Discovery: The process of discovering all the facts of the case involves using interrogatories, full access to the medical records in question, and the depositions. The patient and the health care staff are asked questions by counsel for the defense. They answer under oath, and their testimony is recorded and kept for reference.

Interrogatories: Written questions requiring answers under oath. Typically opposing counsel requests a list of possible witnesses, insurance experts, and which health care providers the plaintiff saw before and after the event.

Requests for productions: Opposing parties request relevant documents, pictures, or related materials such as medical records for treatment before and after the event.

Depositions: Questions are posed to opposing parties, witnesses, and experts under oath to obtain all relevant, nonprivileged information about the case. Experts establish the elements of the case and the applicable standard of care.

Medical records: The defendant obtains all of the plaintiff's relevant medical records for treatment before and after the event. Everything written by the nurses and the health care provider in the medical record is open to examination by both the plaintiff and the defendants.

Witnesses' deposition: Questions are posed to the witnesses under oath to obtain all relevant, nonprivileged information about the case.

Parties' depositions: The plaintiff and defendants (health care provider, nurse, and hospital personnel) are almost always deposed.

Other witnesses: Factual witnesses, both neutral and biased, are deposed to obtain information about their version of the case. They may include family members on the plaintiff's side and other medical personnel (e.g., nurses) on the defendant's side.

Experts: The plaintiff selects experts to establish the essential legal elements of the case against the defendant. The defendant selects experts to establish the appropriateness of the nursing case. Nursing experts are asked to testify to the reasonableness or inappropriate actions of the health care staff once the patient's condition began to change. The expert is asked to compare the actions of the nursing staff to the standard of care.

Trial: The trial usually occurs at least 1 to 3 years after the filing of the petition.

Proof of Negligence

- The nurse owed a duty of care to the patient.
- The nurse did not carry out the duty or breached it (failed to use that degree of skill and learning ordinarily used under the same or similar circumstances by members of the profession).
- The patient was physically injured.
- The patient's injury resulted in compensable damages that can be qualified as medical bills, lost wages, and pain and suffering.
- The patient's injury was caused by the nurse's failure to carry out that duty.

conditions, limits on the amount of care for those conditions, and/or an accidental mistake in paperwork when a patient got sick (PPACA, 2010). Starting in 2014 more than 17.6 million children with preexisting conditions became eligible for health care; and more than 105 million Americans no longer have lifetime limits to receive care when they are ill.

PPACA is also intended to reduce overall care costs to the consumer by (1) providing tax credits; (2) increasing insurance company accountability for premiums and rate increases; and (3) increasing the number of choices patients have to select an insurer that best meets their needs. In addition, PPACA increased access to health care. Patients now receive recommended preventive services such as screenings for cancer, blood pressure, and diabetes without having to pay copays or deductibles. As of 2014 at least 54 million Americans with private health insurance have received care under this provision of the law. Many have benefited from PPACA; anyone under 26 years of age may now continue to receive coverage under his or her parents' insurance plan. More than 3.1 million adults are now receiving health care under this clause. In addition, because of increased access to health care exchanges and insurers, as of 2014 many adults who had preexisting conditions are now also eligible for care (USDHHS, 2015).

PPACA improves Medicare coverage for vulnerable populations by improving access to care and prescriptions, decreasing costs of medications, extending the life of the Medicare Trust Fund until 2024, and addressing fraud and abuse in billing practices.

Americans with Disabilities Act

The Americans With Disabilities Act (ADA) of 1990 and as amended in 2008 is a civil rights statute that protects the rights of people with physical or mental disabilities (Dupler et al., 2012). The ADA prohibits discrimination and ensures equal opportunities for people with disabilities in employment, state and local government services, public accommodations, commercial facilities, and transportation. As defined by the statute and the U.S. Supreme Court, a disability is a mental or physical condition that substantially limits a major life activity, including seeing, hearing, speaking, walking, breathing, performing manual tasks, learning, caring for oneself, and/or working. Under the ADA employers are required to construe the definition of a person's disability to the maximum intent allowed under the ADA. For example, as expanded under the ADA, an employer must consider the needs of a person with diabetes mellitus as a potential disability and reasonably accommodate that person's needs. A person with a disability makes the choice whether to tell others of his or her disability. By exception, several cases have held that a health care provider must disclose if he or she has human immunodeficiency virus (HIV). Despite these rulings and as enforced by the Office of Equal Employment Opportunity, the ADA protects health care workers in the workplace with disabilities such as HIV infection. Likewise, health care workers cannot discriminate against HIV-positive patients (Guido, 2014).

Emergency Medical Treatment and Active Labor Act

As a result of patients being transferred from private to public hospitals without appropriate screening and stabilization (referred to as patient dumping), Congress enacted the Emergency Medical Treatment and Active Labor Act (EMTALA) in 1986. This act provides that, when a patient comes to the emergency department or the hospital, an appropriate medical screening occurs within the capacity of the hospital. If an emergency condition exists, staff must evaluate the patient and may not discharge or transfer him or her until the patient's condition stabilizes. Exceptions to this provision include if a patient requests transfer or discharge in writing after receiving information about the benefits and risks or if a health care provider certifies that the benefits of transfer outweigh the risks.

Mental Health Parity Act as Enacted Under PPACA

The Mental Health Parity Act of 1996 (MHPA) required insurance companies to offer the same level of coverage for mental health care that they provide for medical and surgical care. The MHPA was replaced by the Paul Wellstone and Pete Domenici Mental Health Parity and Addiction Equity Act of 2008 (MHPAEA). The MHPAEA requires health insurance companies to provide equal coverage for mental health and substance abuse treatment. PPACA extended these requirements to small group and individual health insurance plans. It also requires Americans to obtain health insurance that includes these mental health benefits (Federal Register, 2013). PPACA requires parity (the state or condition of being equal) in provision of 10 specific services, including mental health, behavioral health, and substance use services. Insurers may not discriminate or deny coverage to patients with mental illness because of preexisting conditions; and patients may remain on their parent's health insurance until they are 26 years old. Insurers who are not required to comply with all provisions or who may be "grandfathered" into the law may exclude some treatments, especially expensive mental health treatments, from plans that provide lower-level coverage. And because PPACA does not clearly define mental illness other than to require that a "minimum level of mental health services must be covered by all insurance plans," some believe that many patients with mental illness will not be able to afford or will not be provided needed treatment.

Currently admission of a patient to a mental health unit occurs involuntarily or on a voluntary basis. Involuntary admission usually occurs when a patient is determined to be a danger either to himself or herself or others by a mental health professional (MHP). Subsequently the MHP, a court-appointed guardian ad litem, or a family member or other interested party files a petition with the court within 96 hours of the patient's admission to the hospital. A judge may determine that the patient remains a danger to himself or herself or others, in which case the judge grants the involuntary detention, and the patient can be hospitalized for 21 more days for psychiatric treatment. From a legal perspective this may be viewed as depriving the patient of his or her constitutional rights; thus nurses must clearly document the patient's behaviors to support the court's actions and decisions (Guido, 2014; Westrick, 2014).

Potentially suicidal patients are admitted to mental health units. If the patient's history and medical records indicate suicidal tendencies, the patient must be kept under supervision. Lawsuits result from patients' attempts at suicide within a hospital. The allegations in the lawsuits are that the health care provider failed to provide adequate supervision and appropriately implement agency policies and procedures to safeguard a patient while residing in this setting. Documentation of suicide precautions is essential (e.g., safety sitter).

Advance Directives

Advance directives include living wills, health care proxies, and durable powers of attorney for health care (Blais and Hayes, 2011). They are based on values of informed consent, patient autonomy over end-of-life decisions, truth telling, and control over the dying process. The Patient Self-Determination Act (PSDA) enacted in 1991 requires health care institutions to provide written information to patients concerning their rights under state law to make decisions, including the right to refuse treatment and formulate advance directives. Under PSDA a patient's record needs to document whether or not the patient has signed an advance directive. For living wills or durable powers of attorney for health care to be enforced, a patient must be declared legally incompetent or lack the capacity to make decisions regarding his or her own health care treatment. When legal competency needs clarification, a judge makes that determination. The health care provider and family usually make the determination of decisional capacity. Decisional capacity is the ability to make choices for oneself as they relate to medical care. Be familiar with the policies of your institution that comply with the PSDA. Likewise check the state laws to see if a state honors an advance directive that originates in another state (Guido, 2014; Westrick, 2014).

Living Wills. Living wills represent written documents that direct treatment in accordance with a patient's wishes in the event of a terminal illness or condition. With this document a patient is able to declare which medical procedures he or she wants or does not want when terminally ill or in a persistent vegetative state. Living wills are often difficult to interpret and not clinically specific in unforeseen circumstances. Thus you are required to know how your state interprets living wills and under which circumstances a nurse implements them (Guido, 2014).

Health Care Proxies or Durable Power of Attorney for Health Care. A health care proxy or durable power of attorney for health care (DPAHC) is a legal document that designates a person or people of one's choosing to make health care decisions when a patient is no longer able to make decisions on his or her own behalf. This agent makes health care treatment decisions on the basis of the patient's wishes (Blais and Hayes, 2011; Westrick, 2014).

In addition to federal statutes, the ethical doctrine of autonomy ensures the patient the right to refuse medical treatment. Courts upheld the right to refuse medical treatment in the Bouvia v Superior Court case (1986). They have also upheld the right of a legally competent patient to refuse medical treatment for religious reasons. Some groups may refuse or accept medical treatment on the basis of religious beliefs. The U.S. Supreme Court stated in the Cruzan v Director of Missouri Department of Health case (1990) that "we assume that the U.S. Constitution would grant a constitutionally protected competent person the right to refuse lifesaving hydration and nutrition." In cases involving a patient's right to refuse or withdraw medical treatment, the courts balance the patient's interest with the interest of the state in protecting life, preserving medical ethics, preventing suicide, and protecting innocent third parties. Children are generally innocent third parties. Although the courts will not force adults to undergo treatment refused for religious reasons, they will grant an order allowing hospitals and health care providers to treat children of abusive or negligent parents or groups who have denied consent for treatment of their minor children for religious reasons. This is based on the legal doctrine of *parens patriae* in which the state or government makes decisions on behalf of those who are unable to make decisions for themselves.

In addition to patient refusals of treatment, a nurse frequently encounters a "do not resuscitate" (DNR) or "no code" DNR order. In 1986, New York state was the first to develop legislation based on the recommendations of the New York State Task Force on Life and the Law. These recommendations went into effect in 1988, which allowed an adult with capacity, in conjunction with his or her physician, to authorize a DNR order (Golden, 1988). Documentation that the health care provider has consulted with the patient and/or family is required before attaching a DNR order to the patient's medical record (Guido, 2014). The health care provider needs to review DNR orders routinely in case the patient's condition demands a change. If a patient does not have a DNR order, health care providers need to make every effort to revive him or her. Some states offer DNR Comfort Care and DNR Comfort Care Arrest protocols. Protocols in these instances list specific actions that health care providers will take when providing cardiopulmonary resuscitation (CPR).

CPR is an emergency treatment provided without patient consent. Health care providers perform CPR when needed unless there is a DNR order in the patient's chart. The statutes assume that all patients will be resuscitated unless there is a written DNR order in the medical record. Legally competent adult patients consent to a DNR order verbally or in writing after receiving the appropriate information by the health care provider. Be familiar with the DNR protocols of your state.

Uniform Anatomical Gift Act

An individual who is at least 18 years of age has the right to make an organ donation (defined as a "donation of all or part of a human body to take effect upon or after death"). Donors need to make the gift in writing with their signature. In many states adults sign the back of their driver's license, indicating consent to organ donation.

In most states Required Request laws mandate that, at the time of admission to a hospital, a qualified health care provider has to ask each patient over age 18 whether he or she is an organ or tissue donor. If the answer is affirmative, the health care provider obtains a copy of the document. If the answer is negative, the health care provider discusses the option to make or refuse an organ donation and places such documentation in the patient's medical record. In most states there is a law requiring that at the time of death a qualified health care provider ask a patient's family members to consider organ or tissue donation (National Organ Transplant Act, 1984). Individuals are approached in the following order: (1) spouse, (2) adult son or daughter, (3) parent, (4) adult brother or sister, (5) grandparent, and (6) guardian. The person in the highest class makes the donation unless they are aware of conflicting indications by the decedent (Uniform Anatomical Gift Act, 1987). The health care provider who certifies death is not involved in the removal or transplantation of organs (see Chapter 37).

The National Organ Transplant Act (1984) prohibits the purchase or sale of organs. The act provides civil and criminal immunity to the hospital and health care provider who perform in accordance with the act. The act also protects the donor's estate from liability for injury or damage that results from the use of the gift. Organ transplantation is extremely expensive. Patients in end-stage renal disease are eligible for Medicare coverage for a kidney transplant. Sometimes private insurance pays for other transplants. The United Network for Organ Sharing (UNOS) has a contract with the federal government and sets policies and guidelines for the procurement of organs. Patients who require organ transplantation are on a waiting list for an organ in their geographical area that gives priority to patients who demonstrate the greatest need. Be familiar with the policies and procedures of your agency regarding organ donation.

Health Insurance Portability and Accountability Act

The Health Insurance Portability and Accountability Act (HIPAA, 1996) provides rights to patients and protects employees. It protects individual employees from losing their health insurance when changing jobs by providing portability. It allows individual employees to change jobs without losing coverage as a result of preexisting coverage exclusion as long as they have had 12 months of continuous group health insurance coverage (Mortensen et al., 2014).

In the privacy section of the HIPAA there are standards regarding accountability in the health care setting. These rules create patient right to consent to the use and disclosure of their protected health information, to inspect and copy one's medical record, and to amend mistaken or incomplete information. It limits who is able to access a patient's record. It establishes the basis for privacy and confidentiality concerns, viewed as two basic rights within the U.S. health care setting. **Privacy** is the right of patients to keep personal information from being disclosed. **Confidentiality** protects private patient information once it is disclosed in health care settings. Patient confidentiality is a sacred trust. Nurses help organizations protect patients' rights to confidentiality. Although HIPAA does not require extreme measures such as soundproof rooms in hospitals, it does mean that nurses and all health care providers need to avoid discussing patients in public hallways and provide reasonable levels of privacy when communicating with and about patients in any manner. Message boards used in patients' hospital rooms to post daily nursing care information can no longer contain information revealing a patient's medical condition.

Health care information privacy is also protected by standards set by the Health Care Financing Administration (HCFA) for hospitals and health care providers who participate in Medicare and Medicaid (Guido, 2014). These standards require that hospitals and health care providers give notice to patients of their rights to decisions about their care, grievances regarding their care management, personal freedom and safety, confidentiality, access to their own medical records, and freedom from restraints that are not clinically necessary. In addition, many state laws allow patients to access their medical records. Exceptions apply to psychotherapy notes or when a health care provider has determined that access would result in harm to the patient or another party (Privacy Rights Clearinghouse, 2014).

Health Information Technology Act

The Health Information Technology for Economic and Clinical Health Act (HITECH Act, 2009) was passed in conjunction with HIPPA in response to new technology and social media. In particular, HITECH expands the principles extended under the HIPAA, especially when a security breach of personal health information (PHI) occurs. Under the HITECH Act nurses must ensure that patient PHI is not inadvertently conveyed on social media and in particular that protected data are not disclosed other than as permitted by the patient (Box 23-2). Civil and criminal sanctions may be brought against both the nurse and the organization should either or both violate either the HIPPA or the HITECH Act.

Restraints

A physical restraint is any manual method, physical or mechanical device, or material or equipment that immobilizes or reduces the ability of a patient to move freely (CMS, 2008). The Omnibus Reconciliation Act (1987) includes chemical restraint as a form of

BOX 23-2 EVIDENCE-BASED PRACTICE

Social Media and Legal Liability

PICO Question: Can social media be used by nurses without creating legal liability?

Evidence Summary

Social media is used today to reach millions of patients, colleagues, and peers. It is a useful tool for promoting collaboration, disseminating and sharing information, and providing education. It is essential that nurses be responsible and accountable for understanding the use, implications, and guidelines associated with the use of social media (Scruth et al., 2015). The NCSBN (2011) and the International Nurse Regulators Collaborative (INRC) identified nurses' behaviors for appropriate use of social media.

Application to Nursing Practice

- Understand the risks and benefits of using social media
- Maintain professional boundaries
- Present a professional image in all social media interactions
- Maintain privacy and confidentiality
- Understand the implications of identifying yourself as a nurse
- Know state laws governing use of social media

restraint. The use of restraints has been associated with serious complications and even death. You need to know when and how to use and safely apply restraints. The Centers for Medicare and Medicaid Services (CMS) (2008), ANA (2001), and TJC (2014) set standards to reduce the use of all types of restraints in health care settings (i.e., that all patients have the right to be free from seclusion and physical or chemical restraints, except to ensure the patient's safety in emergency situations). They also describe the procedures to follow to restrain a patient, including who orders the restraints, when to write the order, and how often to renew the written order. Restraints can be used (1) only to ensure the physical safety of the patient or other patients, (2) when less restrictive interventions are not successful, and (3) only on the written order of a health care provider (TJC, 2014). The regulations also describe documentation of restraint use and follow-up assessments. Litigation from improper restraint use is a common nursing legal issue (Guido, 2014). Knowing when and how to use restraints correctly is key (Chapter 27). Liability for improper or unlawful restraint lies with the nurse and the health care agency.

STATE STATUTORY ISSUES IN NURSING PRACTICE

Licensure

A State Board of Nursing or Nursing Commission licenses all RNs in the state in which they practice. The requirements for licensure vary among states. All states use the National Council Licensure Examinations (NCLEX®) for RNs and licensed practical nurse examinations. Licensure permits people to offer special skills to the public, and it also provides legal guidelines for protection of the public.

The State Board of Nursing suspends or revokes a license if a nurse's conduct violates the Nurse Practice Act, which is a state law. For example, nurses who perform illegal acts such as selling or taking controlled substances often lose their license. Because a license is a property right, the State Board of Nursing must provide notice and follow due process before revoking or suspending a license. Due process means that the state is required to notify nurses of the charges brought against them. Nurses need to have an opportunity to defend themselves in a hearing. Hearings for suspension or revocation of a license do not occur in court. Usually a panel of professionals conducts the hearing. Nurses can choose to be represented by an attorney. They are allowed opportunities to provide evidence in support of their opinion regarding the charges, and they may call witnesses to testify on their behalf. Most states provide administrative and judicial review of these cases after nurses have exhausted all other forms of appeal. Actions and decisions by State Boards of Nursing are published and accessible by health care agencies and the general public.

Good Samaritan Laws

All states have **Good Samaritan laws** to encourage health care professionals to assist in emergencies (Westrick, 2014). These laws limit liability and offer legal immunity if a nurse helps at the scene of an accident. For example, if you stop at the scene of an automobile accident and give appropriate emergency care such as applying pressure to stop hemorrhage, you are acting within accepted standards, even though proper equipment is not available. If the patient subsequently develops complications as a result of your actions, you are immune from liability as long as you acted without gross negligence (Good Samaritan Act, 1997). Although Good Samaritan laws provide immunity to a nurse who does what is reasonable to save a person's life, if you perform a procedure exceeding your scope of practice and for which you have no training, you are liable for injury that may result from that act. You should only provide care that is consistent with your level of expertise. In addition, once you have committed to providing emergency care to a patient, you must stay with that patient until you can safely transfer his or her care to someone who can provide needed care such as emergency medical technicians (EMTs) or emergency department staff. If you leave the patient without properly transferring or handing him or her off to a capable person, you may be liable for patient abandonment and responsible for any injury suffered after you leave him or her (Westrick, 2014).

Public Health Laws

Nurses, especially those employed in community health settings; need to understand public health laws. State legislatures enact statutes under health codes, which describe the requirements for reporting communicable diseases, school immunizations, and other conditions intended to promote health and reduce health risks in communities. The Centers for Disease Control and Prevention (CDC) (http://www.CDC.gov) and the Occupational Health and Safety Act (OHSA) (http://www.osha.gov) provide guidelines on a national level for safe and healthy communities and work environments. Public health laws protect populations, advocate for the rights of people, regulate health care and health care financing, and ensure professional accountability for care provided. Community and public health nurses have the legal responsibility to enforce laws enacted to protect public health (see Chapter 3). These laws include reporting suspected abuse and neglect such as child abuse, elder abuse, or domestic violence; reporting communicable diseases; ensuring that patients in the community have received required immunizations; and reporting other health-related issues to protect public health. In most states nurses are mandatory reporters of suspected abuse or neglect of patients. Any health care professional who does not report suspected child abuse or neglect may be liable for civil or criminal legal action. Some State Boards of Nursing are now requiring mandatory continuing education on child abuse and neglect for license renewal or before obtaining a new nursing license.

The Uniform Determination of Death Act

Many legal issues surround the event of death, including a basic definition of the actual point at which a person is legally dead. There are two standards for the determination of death. The cardiopulmonary standard requires irreversible cessation of circulatory and respiratory functions. The whole-brain standard requires irreversible cessation of all functions of the entire brain, including the brainstem. The reason for the development of different definitions is to facilitate recovery of organs for transplantation. Even though the patient is legally "brain dead," the patient's organs are sometimes healthy for donation to other patients. Most states have statutes similar to the Uniform Determination of Death Act (1980). It states that health care providers can use either the cardiopulmonary or the whole-brain definition to determine death. Be aware of legal definitions of death in your state because you need to document all events that occur when the patient is in your care. Nurses have a specific legal obligation to treat the deceased person's remains with dignity (see Chapter 37). Wrongful handling of a deceased person's remains causes emotional harm to the surviving family.

Autopsy

An autopsy or postmortem examination is sometimes requested by the patient or patient's family (Autopsy Consent, 1998). In addition, an autopsy is requested as a part of agency policy; or it is sometimes required under the laws of your state. Some statutes specify that, when there are reasonable grounds to believe that a patient died as a result of violence, homicide, suicide, accident, or death in an unusual or suspicious manner, you need to notify the medical examiner (Autopsy Consent, 1998). When a patient's death is not subject to a medical examiner review, consent must be obtained. The priority for giving consent is (1) the patient, in writing before death; (2) durable power of attorney; (3) surviving spouse; and (4) surviving child, parent, or sibling in the order named. You also notify the medical examiner if a patient's death is unforeseen and sudden and a heath care provider has not seen the patient in over 36 hours.

Death with Dignity or Physician-Assisted Suicide

Providing end-of-life care in today's world is challenging for health care professionals because people are living longer (see Chapter 37). The Oregon Death With Dignity Act (1994) was the first statute that legislatively defined "death with dignity," more commonly called *physician-assisted suicide*. The statute stated that a competent individual with a terminal disease could make an oral and written request for medication to end his or her life in a humane and dignified manner. A terminal disease is defined as an "incurable and irreversible disease that has been medically confirmed and will, within reasonable medical judgment, produce death within 6 months."

The ANA (2013) believes that nurses' participation in assisted suicide violates the code of ethics for nurses. The American Association of Colleges of Nursing (AACN) supports the International Council of Nurses' mandate to ensure an individual's peaceful end of life (Guido, 2014). The positions of these two national organizations are not considered contradictory and require nurses to approach a patient's end of life with openness to listening to the patient's expressions of fear and to attempt to control the patient's pain during his or her last months of life. You need to know your state's laws and ensure your practice falls within the laws' requirements.

CIVIL AND COMMON LAW ISSUES IN NURSING PRACTICE

Torts

Nursing practice is also regulated by common law or judicial case law of torts. **Torts** are civil wrongful acts or omissions made against a person or property. They are classified as intentional, quasi-intentional, or unintentional. **Intentional torts** are deliberate acts that violate another's rights such as assault, battery, and false imprisonment. **Quasi-intentional torts** are acts in which intent is lacking but volitional action and direct causation occur such as in invasion of privacy and defamation of character. The third classification of tort is the **unintentional tort**, which includes negligence or malpractice.

Intentional Torts

Assault. **Assault** is an intentional threat toward another person that places the person in reasonable fear of harmful, imminent, or unwelcome contact (Shilling, 2011). No actual contact is required for an assault to occur. For example, it is an assault for a nurse to threaten to give a patient an injection or to threaten to restrain a patient for an x-ray film procedure when the patient has refused consent. Likewise, it is an assault for a patient to threaten a nurse (Guido, 2014).

Battery. **Battery** is any intentional offensive touching without consent or lawful justification (Shilling, 2011). The contact can be harmful to the patient and cause an injury, or it merely can be offensive to the patient's personal dignity. In the example of a nurse threatening to give a patient an injection without the patient's consent, if the nurse actually gives the injection, it is battery. Battery also results if the health care provider performs a procedure that goes beyond the scope of a patient's consent. For example, if a patient gives consent for an appendectomy and the surgeon performs a tonsillectomy, battery has occurred. The key component is the patient's consent.

In some situations consent is implied. For example, if a patient gets into a wheelchair or transfers to a stretcher after receiving advice that it is time to be taken for an x-ray film procedure, the patient has given implied consent to the procedure. If a patient learns that he or she will have an x-ray film of the head instead of the foot and the patient refuses to have the x-ray film taken, the consent has been revoked or withdrawn.

False Imprisonment. The tort of **false imprisonment** occurs with unjustified restraint of a person without a legal reason. This occurs when nurses restrain a patient in a confined area to keep the person from freedom. False imprisonment requires that the patient be aware of the confinement. An unconscious patient has not been falsely imprisoned (Guido, 2014).

Quasi-Intentional Torts

Invasion of Privacy. The tort of **invasion of privacy** protects a patient's right to be free from unwanted intrusion into his or her private affairs. HIPAA and HITECH Act privacy standards have raised awareness of the need for health care professionals to provide confidentiality and privacy. Typically invasion of privacy is the release of a patient's medical information to an unauthorized person such as a member of the press, the patient's employer, or the patient's family or online. The information that is in a patient's medical record is a confidential communication that may be shared with health care providers for the purpose of medical treatment only.

Do not disclose a patient's confidential medical information without his or her consent. A patient must authorize the release of information and designate to whom the health care information may be released. For example, respect the wish not to inform a patient's family of an illness. Similarly, do not assume that a patient's spouse or family members know all of the patient's history, particularly with respect to private issues such as mental illness, medications, pregnancy, termination of pregnancy, birth control, or sexually transmitted infections.

An individual's right to privacy sometimes conflicts with the public's right to know. In one case a television crew filmed a married couple who were participating in a hospital program. The couple had previously told no one but their immediate family that they were involved in the in vitro fertilization program and had received assurance that there would be no publicity or public exposure. After the newscast they received phone calls and embarrassing questions. The couple filed a lawsuit. The court held that the husband and wife stated a claim for invasion of privacy and that, even though the in vitro fertilization program was of public interest, the identity of the plaintiffs was a private matter (YG v Jewish Hospital, 1990).

Many states, through their respective public health departments, require that hospitals report certain infectious or communicable diseases. Sometimes the patient is a public figure whose physical condition is newsworthy (Guido, 2014). There are also cases in which information about a scientific discovery or a major medical breakthrough is newsworthy, as with the first heart transplant case or the first artificial heart recipient. If an event falls into any of these categories, never speak to the media; guide information through the public relations department of the institution to ensure that invasion of privacy does not occur. It is not the nurse's responsibility to decide independently the legality of disclosing information.

Defamation of Character. **Defamation of character** is the publication of false statements that result in damage to a person's reputation. **Slander** occurs when one speaks falsely about another. For example, if a nurse tells people erroneously that a patient has gonorrhea and the disclosure affects the patient's business, the nurse is liable for slander. Libel is the written defamation of character (e.g., charting false entries in a medical record) (Philo et al., 2015).

Unintentional Torts

Negligence. Negligence is conduct that falls below the generally accepted standard of care of a reasonably prudent person (Karno, 2011). The law establishes the standard of care to protect others against an unreasonably great risk of harm (Westrick, 2014). Negligent acts such as hanging the wrong intravenous solution for a patient often result in disciplinary action by the State Board of Nursing and a lawsuit for negligence against both the nurse and his or her employer.

Malpractice. Malpractice is one type of negligence and often referred to as professional negligence. When nursing care falls below a standard of care, nursing malpractice results. Certain criteria are necessary to establish nursing malpractice: (1) the nurse (defendant) owed a duty of care to the patient (plaintiff), (2) the nurse did not carry out or breached that duty, (3) the patient was injured, and (4) the nurse's failure to carry out the duty caused the injury. Even though nurses do not intend to injure patients, some patients file claims of malpractice if nurses give care that does not meet the appropriate standards. Malpractice sometimes involves failing to check a patient's identification correctly before administering blood and then giving the blood to the wrong patient. It also involves administering a medication to a patient even though the medical record contains documentation that the patient has an allergy to that medication. In general, courts define nursing malpractice as the failure to use that degree of skill or learning ordinarily used under the same or similar circumstances by members of the nursing profession (Box 23-3) (Keenan et al., 2013).

The best way for nurses to avoid malpractice is to follow standards of care, give competent care, and communicate with other health care providers. You also avoid malpractice by developing a caring rapport with the patient and documenting assessments, interventions, and evaluations fully. Nurses need to know the current nursing literature in their areas of practice. Know and follow the policies and procedures of the agency where you work. Be sensitive to common sources of patient injury such as falls and medication errors. Finally, communicate with the patient, explain all tests and treatments, document that you provided specific explanations to him or her, and listen to his or her concerns about treatments. You are accountable for timely reporting of any significant changes in the patient's condition to the health care provider and documenting these changes in the medical record (see Chapter 26). Timely and truthful documentation is important to provide the communication necessary among health care team members. Be certain that documentation is legible and signed (Westrick, 2014).

A number of courts have stated that, when a health care provider negligently alters or loses medical records relevant to a malpractice claim, the health care provider needs to demonstrate why these events occurred. An agency has a duty to maintain nursing records. Statutes and accreditation regulations establish these duties. Nursing notes contain substantial evidence needed to understand the care received by a patient. If records are lost or incomplete, there is a presumption that the care was negligent and therefore the cause of the patient's injuries. In addition, incomplete or illegible records make a health care provider less credible or believable. Especially when using electronic medical records, it is important to determine changes in patient conditions documented by prior nursing staff and document timely responses to those changes. In addition, it is essential to provide and document patient decision making—the patient is the primary decision maker, regardless of setting, when care is provided.

BOX 23-3 Common Sources of Negligence

Be aware of the common negligent acts that have resulted in lawsuits against hospitals and nurses.

- Failure to assess and/or monitor, including making a nursing diagnosis
  - Failure to observe, assess, correctly diagnose or treat in a timely manner
  - Failure to use, calibrate, or replace equipment required to safely care for the patient
  - Failure to document care and evaluation of care provided to the patient in a timely manner
- Failure to notify the health care provider of significant changes in a patient's status
- Failure to respond to or correctly implement new and existing orders
- Failure to follow the six rights of medication administration
- Failure to convey discharge instructions to the patient, his or her family, or providers who are assuming responsibility for the patient
- Failure to ensure patient safety, especially patients who have a history of falling, are sedated or confused, are frail, are mentally impaired, get up in the night, or are uncooperative
- Failure to follow policies and procedures
- Failure to properly delegate and supervise

Consent

A patient's signed consent form is necessary for admission to a health care agency, invasive procedures such as intravenous central line insertion, surgery, some treatment programs such as chemotherapy, and participation in research studies (Guido, 2014). A patient signs a general consent form for treatment when admitted to a health care agency or other health care facility. A patient or the patient's representative needs to sign separate special consent or treatment forms before the performance of a specialized procedure. State laws designate individuals who are legally able to give consent to medical treatment (Medical Patient Rights Act, 1994). Nurses need to know the law in their states and be familiar with the policies and procedures of their employing agency regarding consent (Box 23-4). Special consideration is used when a patient is deaf or illiterate or speaks a foreign language. An official interpreter must be present to explain the terms of consent. A family member or acquaintance who speaks a patient's language should not interpret health information. Make every effort to help the patient make an informed choice.

When a competent patient refuses care or treatment, it is important to recognize that this act is legally his or her right. You inform the health care provider of the patient's refusal to receive care and document this in the medical record.

Informed Consent. Informed consent is a patient's agreement to have a medical procedure after receiving full disclosure of risks, benefits, alternatives, and consequences of refusal (Westrick, 2014). Informed consent requires a health care provider to disclose information in terms a patient is able to understand to make an informed choice (Guido, 2014). Failure to obtain consent in situations other than emergencies can result in a claim of battery.

Informed consent is part of the health care provider–patient relationship. It must be obtained and witnessed when the patient is not under the influence of medication such as opioids. Because nurses do not perform surgery or direct medical procedures, in most situations obtaining patients' informed consent does not fall within the nurse's responsibility. The person responsible for performing the procedure is responsible for obtaining the informed consent.

BOX 23-4 Statutory Guidelines for Legal Consent for Medical Treatment

Those who may consent to medical treatment are governed by state law but generally include the following:

I. Adults
   A. Any competent individual 18 years of age or older for himself or herself
   B. Any parent for his or her unemancipated minor
   C. Any guardian for his or her ward
   D. Any adult for the treatment of his or her minor brother or sister (if an emergency and parents are not present)
   E. Any grandparent for a minor grandchild (in an emergency and if parents are not present)

II. Minors
   A. Ordinarily minors may not consent to medical treatment without a parent. However, emancipated minors may consent to medical treatment without a parent. Emancipated minors include:
      1. Minors who are designated emancipated by a court order
      2. Minors who are married, divorced, or widowed
      3. Minors who are in active military service
   B. Unemancipated minors may consent to medical treatment if they have specific medical conditions
      1. Pregnancy and pregnancy-related conditions (Various states differ in characterizing a pregnant minor as either emancipated or unemancipated. Know your state rules in this matter.)
      2. A minor parent for his or her custodial child
      3. Sexually transmitted infection (STI) information and treatment
      4. Substance abuse treatment
      5. Outpatient and/or temporary sheltered mental health treatment
   C. The issue of emancipated or unemancipated minors does not relieve the health care provider's duty to attempt to obtain meaningful informed consent (Guido, 2014).

Key elements of informed consent include the following: (1) the patient receives an explanation of the procedure or treatment; (2) the patient receives the names and qualifications of people performing and assisting in the procedure; (3) the patient receives a description of the serious harm, including death, that may occur as a result of the procedure and anticipated pain and/or discomfort; (4) the patient receives an explanation of alternative therapies to the proposed procedure/treatment and the risks of doing nothing; (5) the patient knows that he or she has the right to refuse the procedure/treatment without discontinuing other supportive care; (6) the patient knows that he or she may refuse the procedure/treatment even after the procedure has begun (Westrick, 2014).

The nurse's signature as a witness to the consent means that the patient voluntarily gave consent, the patient's signature is authentic, and the patient appears to be competent to give consent (Guido, 2014). When nurses provide consent forms for patients to sign, they must ask the patients if they understand the procedure for which they are giving consent. If patients deny understanding or you suspect that they do not understand, notify the health care provider or nursing supervisor. Health care providers must inform a patient refusing surgery or other medical treatment about any harmful consequences of refusal. If the patient continues to refuse the treatment, the nurse should again ensure that documentation of the rejection is written, signed, and witnessed. It is important to note that nursing students cannot and should not be responsible for or asked to witness consent forms because of the legal nature of the document.

Parents are usually the legal guardians of pediatric patients; therefore they typically are the people who sign consent forms for treatment. Occasionally a parent or guardian refuses treatment for a child. In these cases the court sometimes intervenes on the child's behalf. Courts generally consider the child's ultimate safety and well-being as the most important factors.

In some instances obtaining informed consent is difficult. For example, if a patient is unconscious, you must obtain consent from a person legally authorized to give it on the patient's behalf. Sometimes a patient has legally designated surrogate decision makers through special power of attorney documents or court guardianship procedures. In emergencies, if it is impossible to obtain consent from the patient or an authorized person, a health care provider may perform a procedure required to benefit the patient or save a life without liability for failure to obtain consent. In such cases the law assumes that the patient would wish to be treated.

Patients with mental illnesses must also give consent. They retain the right to refuse treatment until a court has determined legally that they are incompetent to decide for themselves.

Termination of Pregnancy or Abortion Issues

In 1973 in the case of Roe v Wade, the U.S. Supreme Court ruled that there is a fundamental right to privacy, which includes a woman's decision to terminate a pregnancy. The court ruled that during the first trimester a woman could end her pregnancy without state regulation because the risk of natural mortality from abortion is less than with normal childbirth. During the second trimester the state has an interest in protecting maternal health, and it enforces regulations regarding the person terminating the pregnancy and the facility where it is done. By the third trimester, when the fetus becomes viable, the interest of the state is to protect the fetus; therefore it prohibits termination except when necessary to save the mother.

In Webster v Reproductive Health Services (1989) the court substantially narrowed Roe v Wade. Some states require viability tests before conducting abortions if the fetus is over 28 weeks' gestational age; others consider 26 weeks' gestational age or less when terminating a pregnancy. Some states also require a minor's parental consent or a judicial decision that the minor is mature and can self-consent. Others do not require parental consent; thus again it is critical to know the law in your state related to termination of pregnancy before working in this area of practice.

Nursing Students

Nursing students are liable if their actions exceed their scope of practice and cause harm to patients. If a student harms a patient as a direct result of his or her actions or lack of action, the student, instructor, hospital, or health care agency and the university or educational institution generally share the liability for the incorrect action. Nursing students should never be assigned to perform tasks for which they are unprepared, and instructors should supervise them carefully as they learn new skills. Although nursing students are not employees of the hospital, the agency has a responsibility to monitor their acts. They are expected to perform as professional nurses would in providing safe patient care. Faculty members are usually responsible for instructing and observing students, but in some situations staff nurses serving as preceptors share these responsibilities. Every nursing school should provide clear definitions of preceptor and faculty responsibility. It is equally important that nursing preceptors be aware of state laws applicable to nursing students, faculty, and the educational institution when supervising students.

When students work as nursing assistants or nurse's aides when not attending classes, they should not perform tasks that do not appear in a job description for a nurse's aide or assistant. For example, even if a student has learned to administer intramuscular medications in class, the student now working as a nurse's aide may not perform this task. If a staff nurse overseeing the nursing assistant or aide knowingly assigns work without regard for the person's ability to safely conduct the task defined in the job description, the staff nurse is also liable. If someone requests that a student employed in the agency as a nurse's aide performs tasks that he or she is not prepared to complete safely, the student employee needs to bring this information to the supervisor's attention so the task can be assigned to an appropriate health care professional.

Malpractice Insurance

Malpractice or professional liability insurance is a contract between a nurse and an insurance company. This insurance provides both malpractice and professional defense coverage for individual nurses. Malpractice insurance provides for a defense when a nurse is in a lawsuit. The insurance company pays for costs, attorney's fees and settlement, and other related fees generated in the representation of the nurse. Nurses employed by health care agencies generally are covered by insurance provided by the agency; however, it is important to remember that the lawyer is representing your employer and not you. The insurance provided by the employing agency only covers nurses while they are working within the scope of their employment.

Nurses are also investigated by the State Board of Nursing or Nursing Commission to determine whether the alleged breach in care violated the Nurse Practice Act. This investigation typically is separate from the malpractice action and not covered under the employer's insurance coverage. Without individual insurance coverage, the nurse will be required to personally pay all costs and attorney fees incurred by him or her in the defense against these claims. Typically these costs exceed more than $10,000; therefore nurses should ensure that they have the means or personal liability to defend any action against their license to ensure their ongoing employment as a nurse.

Abandonment and Assignment Issues

Abandonment of a patient occurs when a nurse refuses to provide care for a patient after having established a patient-nurse relationship. Before having established that relationship, a nurse may refuse an assignment when (1) the nurse lacks the knowledge or skill to provide competent care; (2) care exceeding the Nurse Practice Act is expected; (3) health of the nurse or her unborn child is directly threatened by the type of assignment; (4) orientation to the unit has not been completed and safety is at risk; (5) the nurse clearly states and documents a conscientious objection on the basis of moral, ethical, or religious grounds; or (6) the nurse's clinical judgment is impaired as a result of fatigue, resulting in a safety risk for the patient (Westrick, 2014).

When refusing an assignment, it is important to give your immediate supervisor specific reasons for the refusal and determine if other alternatives such as reassignment are available. Be sure that you document in your personal notes specifics of the incident, to whom you reported it, and actions you took to ensure that patients were safe and that you did not abandon your patients (Westrick, 2014).

Short Staffing. During nursing shortages or staff downsizing periods, the issue of inadequate staffing occurs. The Community Health Accreditation Program (CHAP) and other state and federal standards require agencies to have guidelines for determining the number (staffing ratios) of nurses required to give care to a specific number of patients. Legal issues occur when there are not enough nurses available to provide competent care or when nurses work excessive overtime. One such example is in a class-action suit, Spires v Hospital Corporation of America, filed on April 10, 2006. The wife claimed there was poor patient care related to insufficient RN staffing and that the poor nurse-staffing levels led to the resultant death of her husband. This suit emphasized the potential seriousness of short staffing and the importance of nurses' asserting employee rights.

In an attempt to address the short-staffing problem, many states now require that nursing committees in acute care settings determine safe staffing on the basis of the needs of patients admitted to their facilities. In California fixed nurse-patient ratios are required in acute care settings. The safe staffing ratio debate is occurring throughout the country and demands close attention by all nurses (ANA, 2014).

The ANA in conjunction with professional nursing organizations has supported federal legislation titled the Registered Nurse Safe Staffing Act (ANA, 2014). This act supports recent evidence linking ratios of RN staffing to improved patient mortality and better patient outcomes. Under this act Medicare-certified facilities nationally would be required to establish staffing committees comprised of 55% direct-care nurses who would determine adequacy of staffing on the basis of patients admitted to specific units that provide predetermined types of care. Under this act, nurses become an integral part of ensuring that patients receive care from nurses qualified to meet their needs and that care is provided in a safe environment.

Floating. Nurses are sometimes required to "float" from the area in which they normally practice to other nursing units on the basis of census load and patient acuities. Nurses who float must inform the supervisor of any lack of experience in caring for the type of patients on the nursing unit. They should request and receive an orientation to the unit. Supervisors are liable if they give a staff nurse an assignment that he or she cannot handle safely. Before accepting employment, learn the policies of the agency regarding floating and understand what is expected (Guido, 2014).

Health Care Providers' Orders. The health care provider (physician or advanced practice nurse) is responsible for directing medical treatment. Nurses follow health care providers' orders unless they believe that the orders are in error, violate agency policy, or are harmful to the patient. Therefore you need to assess all orders; if you find one to be erroneous or harmful, further clarification from the health care provider is necessary. If the health care provider confirms an order and you still believe that it is inappropriate, use the agency chain of command to inform your direct supervisor. The supervising nurse should help resolve the questionable order. A medical consultant sometimes helps clarify its appropriateness or inappropriateness. A nurse carrying out an inaccurate or inappropriate order is legally responsible for any harm the patient suffers.

In a malpractice lawsuit against a health care provider and a hospital, one of the most frequently litigated issues is whether the nurse kept the health care provider informed of the patient's condition. To inform a health care provider properly, you perform a competent nursing assessment of the patient to determine the signs and symptoms that are significant related to the attending health care provider's tasks of diagnosis and treatment. Be certain to document that you notified the health care provider and his or her response, your follow-up, and the patient's response.

Make sure that all the health care provider orders are in writing, dated and timed appropriately, and transcribed correctly. Verbal or telephone orders are not recommended because they leave the possibilities for error. If a verbal or telephone order is necessary during an emergency, it is signed by the health care provider as soon as possible, usually within 24 hours (TJC, 2016).

RISK MANAGEMENT AND QUALITY ASSURANCE

The rationale for risk-management and quality improvement programs is the development of an organizational system of ensuring appropriate, quality health care by identifying potential hazards and eliminating them before harm occurs (Guido, 2014). Risk management involves several components, including identifying possible risks, analyzing them, acting to reduce the risks, and evaluating the steps taken to reduce them (Miller, 2011). TJC (2016) requires the use of quality improvement and risk-management procedures.

Both quality improvement and risk management require thorough documentation. One tool used in risk management is the occurrence report or incident report. Occurrence reporting provides a database for further investigation in an attempt to determine deviations from standards of care, to identify corrective measures needed to prevent recurrence, and to alert risk management to a potential claim situation. Examples of an occurrence include patient or visitor falls or injury; failure to follow health care provider orders; a significant complaint by patient, family, health care provider, or other hospital department; an error in technique or procedure; and a malfunctioning device or product. Agencies generally have specific guidelines to direct health care providers in how to complete the occurrence report. The report is confidential and separate from the medical record; however, it is often discoverable during a legal proceeding. As a nurse you are responsible for providing information in the medical record about the occurrence. Never document in the patient's medical record that you completed an occurrence report.

Risk management also requires complete documentation. A nurse's documentation is often the evidence of care received by a patient and establishes support that the nurse acted reasonably and safely. When a lawsuit is filed, very often the nurses' notes are the first thing an attorney reviews. The nurse's assessments and the reporting of significant changes in the assessments are very important factors in defending a lawsuit. Therefore it is critical for you to document the health care provider contacted, the information communicated to the health care provider, and the health care provider's response.

QSEN QSEN: BUILDING COMPETENCY IN QUALITY IMPROVEMENT You are a member of your unit's task force focusing on quality improvement and reduction in sentinel events. The chairperson explains to the task force that quality improvement relates to data collection, evaluation, and improvement in outcomes. One of the nurses asks, "How can we reduce the number of occurrence reports being filed on the unit related to patient falls?" How would you respond?

Answers to QSEN Activities can be found on the Evolve website.

One area of potential risk is associated with the use of electronic monitoring devices. No monitor is reliable at all times; therefore do not depend on them completely. Continual assessment of a patient is necessary to help document the accuracy of electronic monitoring. There are also electrical hazards to the nurse and the patient. Biomedical engineers check equipment to ensure that it is in proper working order and that a patient will not receive an electrical shock. Document when calibration of equipment occurs.

Nurses on the units are risk managers. For example, surgeons rely on OR nurses to compare the consent form with the indicated and prepped surgical site for accuracy. Because of errors with patients undergoing the wrong surgery or having surgery performed on the wrong site, TJC's Universal Protocol includes guidelines for preventing such mishaps (TJC, 2016) and now require mandatory time-outs before beginning the surgery. Implement this protocol whenever an invasive surgical procedure is to be performed, regardless of the location (hospital, ambulatory surgical center [ASC], or health care provider office). The three principles of the protocol are: (1) preoperative verification that relevant documents and studies are available before the start of the procedure and that these documents are consistent with the patient's expectations; (2) marking the operative site with indelible ink to mark left and right distinction, multiple structures (e.g., fingers), and levels of the spine; and (3) a *time-out* just before starting the procedure for final verification of the correct patient, procedure, site, and any implants.

Patient safety and improved care are the goals of quality improvement and risk management. TJC (2016) and groups such as the Institute of Medicine have a focus on patient safety as major goals. Never events are preventable errors, which may include falls, urinary tract infections from improper use of catheters, and pressure ulcers (AHRQ, 2015). The federal government and health care insurance companies have developed policies to withhold reimbursement for preventable medical errors (AHRQ, 2015). Know your agency policies and procedures to help develop a system and culture of patient safety.

Professional Involvement

Become involved in professional organizations and committees that define the standards of care for nursing practice. If current laws, rules and regulations, or policies under which nurses practice are not evidence based, advocate to ensure that the scope of nursing practice is defined accurately. Be willing to represent nursing and the patient's perspective in the community as well. The voice of nursing is powerful and effective when the organizing focus is the protection and welfare of the public entrusted to nurses' care (Blais and Hayes, 2011).

KEY POINTS

- RNs and licensed practical nurses are licensed by the state in which they practice; licensing is based on educational requirements, the passing of an examination, and other criteria.
- The civil law system is concerned with the protection of a person's private rights, and the criminal law system deals with the rights of individuals and society as defined by legislative statutes.
- A nurse is liable for malpractice if the nurse (defendant) owed a duty to the patient (plaintiff), the nurse did not carry out that duty, the patient was injured, and the nurse's failure to carry out the duty caused the patient's injury.
- All patients are entitled to confidential health care and freedom from unauthorized release of information.
- Under the law, practicing nurses must follow standards of care, the guidelines of professional organizations, and the written policies and procedures of the employing agency.
- Nurses who witness consents are responsible for confirming that patients have given informed consent for any surgery or other medical procedure voluntarily before the procedure is performed.
- Nurses are responsible for performing all procedures correctly and exercising professional judgment as they carry out health care providers' orders.
- Nurses follow health care providers' orders unless they believe the order to be in error, that it violates agency policy, or that it can harm patients.
- Staffing standards determine the ratio of nurses to patients; if the nurse has to care for more patients than is reasonable, he or she needs to make a formal protest to the nursing administration.
- Legal issues involving death include documenting all events surrounding the death and treating a deceased person with dignity.

- All nurses need to know the laws that apply to their area of practice.
- Depending on state laws, nurses are required to report possible criminal activities such as child abuse and certain communicable diseases.
- Nurses are patient advocates and ensure quality of care through risk management and lobbying for safe nursing practice standards.
- Nurses file incident/occurrence reports for all errors even when someone is not injured.

CLINICAL APPLICATION QUESTIONS

Preparing for Clinical Practice

You are working the first shift on the hematology-oncology unit and receive report on your assigned team of three patients. You have a nursing assistive personnel (NAP) assigned to help you with routine care. You make quick rounds on your patients to ensure that there are no immediate needs before you begin checking medications. Patient No. 1 is scheduled for surgery later in the morning for a biopsy and needs the surgical consent signed. Patient No. 2 is receiving blood products for a human immunodeficiency virus (HIV) complication and needs frequent vital sign monitoring. You find patient No. 3, an 83-year-old confused man, lying on the floor. He states that he needed to go to the restroom and no one was there to help.

1. The nurse prepares the surgical consent form for patient No. 1. Which key points does he or she need to ensure that the patient received before witnessing informed consent?
2. The son of patient No. 2 calls to talk to the nurse caring for his father. The son asks questions about the reason for the blood administration. Which guidelines does the nurse follow in responding to the son's questions about the father's condition? Which federal statutes are involved in this scenario?
3. One week after discharge from the hospital, the hospital received a written complaint from the family of patient No. 3 about the incident related to the fall and the intent to take legal action.
   a. What must patient No. 3 establish to prove negligence against the nurse?
   b. Describe situations in which restraints may be applied legally to prevent falls.

ⓔ *Answers to Clinical Application Questions can be found on the Evolve website.*

REVIEW QUESTIONS

Are You Ready to Test Your Nursing Knowledge?

1. A nurse is caring for a patient who recently had coronary bypass surgery and now is on the postoperative unit. Which are legal sources of standards of care that the nurse uses to deliver safe health care? (Select all that apply.)
   1. Information provided by the head nurse
   2. Policies and procedures of the employing hospital
   3. State Nurse Practice Act
   4. Regulations identified in The Joint Commission manual
   5. The American Nurses Association standards of nursing practice
2. A nurse is sued for negligence due to failure to monitor a patient appropriately after a procedure. Which of the following statements are correct about this lawsuit? (Select all that apply.)
   1. The nurse does not need any representation.
   2. The patient must prove injury, damage, or loss occurred.
   3. The person filing the lawsuit has to show a compensable damage, such as lost wages, occurred.
   4. The patient must prove that a breach in the prevailing standard of care caused an injury.
   5. The burden of proof is always the responsibility of the nurse.
3. A nurse stops to help in an emergency at the scene of an accident. The injured party files a suit, and the nurse's employing institution insurance does not cover the nurse. What would probably cover the nurse in this situation?
   1. The nurse's automobile insurance
   2. The nurse's homeowner's insurance
   3. The Good Samaritan law, which grants immunity from suit if there is no gross negligence
   4. The Patient Care Partnership, which may grant immunity from suit if the injured party consents
4. A nurse is planning care for a patient going to surgery. Who is responsible for informing the patient about the surgery along with possible risks, complications, and benefits?
   1. Family member
   2. Surgeon
   3. Nurse
   4. Nurse manager
5. A woman has severe life-threatening injuries and is hemorrhaging following a car accident. The health care provider ordered 2 units of packed red blood cells to treat the woman's anemia. The woman's husband refuses to allow the nurse to give his wife the blood for religious reasons. What is the nurse's responsibility?
   1. Obtain a court order to give the blood
   2. Coerce the husband into giving the blood
   3. Call security and have the husband removed from the hospital
   4. More information is needed about the wife's preference and if the husband has her medical power of attorney
6. A nurse notes that an advance directive is on a patient's medical record. Which statement represents the best description of an advance directive guideline that the nurse will follow?
   1. A living will allows an appointed person to make health care decisions when the patient is in an incapacitated state.
   2. A living will is invoked only when the patient has a terminal condition or is in a persistent vegetative state.
   3. The patient cannot make changes in the advance directive once admitted to the hospital.
   4. A durable power of attorney for health care is invoked only when the patient has a terminal condition or is in a persistent vegetative state.
7. A nurse notes that the health care unit keeps a listing of the patient names at the front desk in easy view for health care providers to more efficiently locate the patient. The nurse talks with the nurse manager because this action is a violation of which act?
   1. Patient Protection and Affordable Care Act (PPACA)
   2. Patient Self-Determination Act (PSDA)
   3. Health Insurance Portability and Accountability Act (HIPAA)
   4. Emergency Medical Treatment and Active Labor Act
8. Which of the following actions, if performed by a registered nurse, would result in both criminal and administrative law sanctions against the nurse? (Select all that apply.)
   1. Taking or selling controlled substances
   2. Refusing to provide health care information to a patient's child
   3. Reporting suspected abuse and neglect of children
   4. Applying physical restraints without a written physician's order
   5. Completing an occurrence report on the unit
9. The nurse received a hand-off report at the change of shift in the conference room from the night shift nurse. The nursing student assigned to the nurse asks to review the medical records of the

patients assigned to them. The nurse begins assessing the assigned patients and lists the nursing care information for each patient on each individual patient's message board in the patient rooms. The nurse also lists the patients' medical diagnoses on the message board. Later in the day the nurse discusses the plan of care for a patient who is dying with the patient's family. Which of these actions describes a violation of the Health Insurance Portability and Accountability Act (HIPAA)?
   1. Discussing patient conditions in the nursing report room at the change of shift
   2. Allowing nursing students to review patient charts before caring for patients to whom they are assigned
   3. Posting medical information about the patient on a message board in the patient's room
   4. Releasing patient information regarding terminal illness to family when the patient has given permission for information to be shared

10. A patient has a fractured femur that is placed in skeletal traction with a fresh plaster cast applied. The patient experiences decreased sensation and a cold feeling in the toes of the affected leg. The nurse observes that the patient's toes have become pale and cold but forgets to document this because one of the nurse's other patients experienced cardiac arrest at the same time. Two days later the patient in skeletal traction has an elevated temperature, and he is prepared for surgery to amputate the leg below the knee. Which of the following statements regarding a breach of duty apply to this situation? (Select all that apply.)
    1. Failure to document a change in assessment data
    2. Failure to provide discharge instructions
    3. Failure to follow the six rights of medication administration
    4. Failure to use proper medical equipment ordered for patient monitoring
    5. Failure to notify a health care provider about a change in the patient's condition
11. A homeless man enters the emergency department seeking health care. The health care provider indicates that the patient needs to be transferred to the City Hospital for care. This action is most likely a violation of which of the following laws?
    1. Health Insurance Portability and Accountability Act (HIPAA)
    2. Americans with Disabilities Act (ADA)
    3. Patient Self-Determination Act (PSDA)
    4. Emergency Medical Treatment and Active Labor Act (EMTALA) without triage completed
12. You are the night shift nurse caring for a newly admitted patient who appears to be confused. The family asks to see the patient's medical record. What is the priority nursing action?
    1. Give the family the record
    2. Discuss the issues that concern the family with them
    3. Call the nursing supervisor
    4. Determine from the medical record if the family has been granted permission by the patient to access his or her medical information
13. A home health nurse notices significant bruising on a 2-year-old patient's head, arms, abdomen, and legs. The patient's mother describes the patient's frequent falls. What is the best nursing action for the home health nurse to take?
    1. Document her findings and treat the patient
    2. Instruct the mother on safe handling of a 2-year-old child
    3. Contact a child abuse hotline
    4. Discuss this story with a colleague
14. Which of the following statements indicate that the new nursing graduate understands ways to remain involved professionally? (Select all that apply.)
    1. "I am thinking about joining the health committee at my church."
    2. "I need to read newspapers, watch news broadcasts, and search the Internet for information related to health."
    3. "I will join nursing committees at the hospital after I have completed orientation and better understand the issues affecting nursing."
    4. "Nurses do not have very much voice in legislation in Washington, DC, because of the nursing shortage."
    5. "I will go back to school as soon as I finish orientation."
15. You are floated to work on a nursing unit where you are given an assignment that is beyond your capability. Which is the best nursing action to take first?
    1. Call the nursing supervisor to discuss the situation
    2. Discuss the problem with a colleague
    3. Leave the nursing unit and go home
    4. Say nothing and begin your work

Answers: 1. 2, 3, 4, 5; **2.** 2, 3, 4; **3.** 3; **4.** 2; **5.** 4; **6.** 2; **7.** 3; **8.** 1, 4; **9.** 3; **10.** 1, 5; **11.** 4; **12.** 4; **13.** 3; **14.** 1, 2, 3; **15.** 1.

ⓔ ***Rationales for Review Questions can be found on the Evolve website.***

REFERENCES

Agency for Healthcare Research and Quality (AHRQ): *Never events*, 2015, US Department of Health and Human Services. http://psnet.ahrq.gov/primer.aspx?primerID=3. Accessed August 2015.

American Nurses Association: *Position statement: reduction of patient restraint and seclusion in health care settings*, Silver Spring, MD, 2001, Author.

American Nurses Association (ANA): *Nursing: scope and standards of practice*, ed 2, Silver Spring, MD, 2010, The Association.

American Nurses Association (ANA): *Position statement: euthanasia, assisted suicide, and aid in dying*, 2013, http://www.nursingworld.org/euthanasiaanddying. Accessed August 2015.

American Nurses Association (ANA): *Safe staffing: the Registered Nurse Safe Staffing Act*, https://www.congress.gov/bill/113th-congress/house-bill/1821, 2014. Accessed August 2015.

Blais K, Hayes JS: *Professional nursing practice: concepts and perspectives*, ed 6, Upper Saddle River, NJ, 2011, Pearson Prentice Hall.

Centers for Medicare and Medicaid Services (CMS): *Revisions to Medicare conditions of participation, 482.13*, Bethesda, Md, 2008, US Department of Health and Human Services.

Dupler A, et al: Leveling the playing field for nursing students with disabilities: implications of the amendments to the American With Disabilities act, *J Nurs Educ* 51:144, 2012.

Garner B: *Black's law dictionary, pocket*, ed 11, St Paul, 2014, Thomson West Publishing.

Golden S: Do not resuscitate orders: a matter of life and death in New York, *Contemp. Health L. & Poly* 449:4, 1988.

Guido G: *Legal and ethical issues in nursing*, ed 6, Upper Saddle River, NJ, 2014, Prentice Hall.

Karno S: Nursing malpractice/negligence and liability. In Grant P, Ballard D, editors: *Law for nurse leaders: a comprehensive reference*, New York, 2011, Springer.

Keenan G, et al: Challenges to nurses' efforts of retrieving, documenting, and communicating patient care information, *JAMIA* 20(2):245, 2013.

Melnyk BM, Fineout-Overholt E: *Evidence-based practice in nursing and healthcare: a guide to best practice*, ed 3, Philadelphia, 2014, Lippincott Williams & Wilkins.

Miller P: Risk management. In Grant P, Ballard D, editors: *Law for nurse leaders: a comprehensive reference*, New York, 2011, Springer.

Mortensen K, Serwing A: *Health care privacy and security*, Eagan, MN, 2014, Thomson West Publishing.

National Council of State Boards of Nursing (NCSBN): *Working with others: a position paper*, 2005,

http://www.ncsbn.org/pdfs/Working_with_Others.pdf. Accessed August 2015.
National Council of State Boards of Nursing (NCSBN): *White paper: a nurse's guide to the use of social media*, 2011, https://www.ncsbn.org/Social_Media.pdf. Accessed August 2015.
Philo H, et al: *Lawyers desk reference*, ed 9, Eagan, MN, 2015, Thomson West Publishing.
Privacy Rights Clearinghouse: *Understanding health and medical privacy*, 2014. https://www.privacyrights.org/content/understanding-health-and-medical-privacy. Accessed August 2015.
Shilling D: *Lawyer's desk book*, Austin, TX, 2011, Wolters Kluwer.
The Joint Commission (TJC): *Comprehensive accreditation manual for hospitals: the official handbook*, Oak Brook Terrace, IL, 2014, The Joint Commission.
The Joint Commission (TJC): *2016 National Patient Safety Goals*, Oak Brook Terrace, IL, 2016, The Commission. Available at http://www.jointcommission.org/standards_information/npsgs.aspx. Accessed November 2015.
The Registered Nurse Safe Staffing Act, 2014, https://www.congress.gov/bill/113th-congress/senate-bill/2353. Accessed August 2015.
US Department of Health and Human Services (USDHHS): *Key features of the affordable care act by year*, 2015, HHS.gov/HealthCare. http://www.hhs.gov/healthcare/facts/timeline/timeline-text.html. Accessed August 2015.
US Department of the Treasury, US Department of Labor, US Department of Health and Human Services (USDHHS): *Final rules under the Paul Wellstone and Pete Domenici Mental Health Parity and Addiction Equity Act of 2008; technical amendment to external review for multi-state plan program; final rule*. Available at http://www.gpo.gov/fdsys/pkg/FR-2013-11-13/pdf/2013-27086.pdf. Accessed September 28, 2015.
Westrick SJ: *Essentials of nursing law*, ed 2, Boston, MA, 2014, Jones & Bartlett.

RESEARCH REFERENCE

Scruth E, et al: Electronic and social media: the legal and ethical issues for healthcare, *Clin Nurse Spec* 29(1):10, 2015.

STATUTES

Americans with Disabilities Act (ADA), 42 USC §§121.010-12213 (1990)
Autopsy Consent, Mo Rev Stat, {194.115 (1998)
Emergency Medical Treatment and Active Labor Act (EMTALA), 42 USC §1395 (dd) (1986)
Good Samaritan Act, IL Compiled Statutes, 745 ILCS 49/ (1997)
Health Insurance Portability and Accountability Act of 1996 (HIPAA), Public Law No. 104 (1996)
Health Information Technology for Economic and Clinical Health Act (HITECH Act) 45 C.F.R. § 164.304.n8 Health Information Technology for Economic and Clinical Health Act (HITECH Act), Pub. L. No. 111-5, 123 Stat. 115 (Feb. 17, 2009), § 13401(a) (codified at 42 U.S.C. § 17931(a); 45 C.F.R. § 160.103).
Medical Patient Rights Act, IL Compiled Statutes, 410 ILCS 50 (1994)
Mental Health Parity Act of 1996, 29 USC §1885 (1996)
National Organ Transplant Act, Public Law 98-507 (1984)
Omnibus Budget Reconciliation Act of 1987 (Federal Nursing Home Reform Act). Retrieved from https://www.govtrack.us/congress/bills/99/hr5300.
Oregon Death With Dignity Act, Ore Rev Stat §§127.800-127.897 (1994)
Patient Protection and Affordable Care Act, 42 USC 18001 (2010)
Patient Self-Determination Act, 42 CFR 417 (1991)
Uniform Anatomical Gift Act (1987)
Uniform Determination of Death Act (1980)

CASES

Bouvia v Superior Court, 225 Cal Rptr 297 (1986)
Cruzan v Director of Missouri Department of Health, 497 U.S. 261 (1990)
Darling v Charleston Community Memorial Hospital, 33 Ill 2d 326 (Ill 1965)
Roe v Wade, 410 U.S. 113 (1973)
Spires v Hospital Corporation of America, 28 U.S.C. §1391(b) Kansas (2006), http://www.kansas.com/multimedia/kansas/archive/pdfs/041106spireshca.pdf
Webster v Reproductive Health Services, 492 U.S. 490 (1989)
YG v Jewish Hospital, 795 SW2d 488 (Mo App 1990)

24

Communication

OBJECTIVES

- Identify ways to apply critical thinking to the communication process.
- Use the five levels of communication with patients.
- Describe features of the circular transactional communication process.
- Incorporate features of a helping relationship when interacting with patients.
- Identify a nurse's communication approaches within the four phases of a nurse-patient helping relationship.
- Identify desired outcomes of nurse–health care team member relationships.
- Demonstrate qualities, behaviors, and communication techniques of professional communication while interacting with patients.
- Identify opportunities to improve communication with patients while giving care.
- Engage in effective communication techniques for older patients.
- Offer alternative communication devices when appropriate to promote communication with patients who have impaired communication.
- Implement nursing care measures for patients with special communication needs.

KEY TERMS

Active listening, p. 327
Assertiveness, p. 325
Autonomy, p. 324
Channels, p. 319
Circular transactional communication process, p. 319
Circular transactional model, p. 319
Communication, p. 316
Complementary, p. 319
Electronic communication, p. 319
Emotional intelligence, p. 317
Empathy, p. 328
Environment, p. 320
Feedback, p. 319
Interpersonal communication, p. 318
Interpersonal variables, p. 320
Intrapersonal communication, p. 318
Lateral violence, p. 324
Message, p. 319
Metacommunication, p. 321
Motivational interviewing, p. 323
Nonverbal communication, p. 320
Perceptual biases, p. 317
Public communication, p. 318
Receiver, p. 319
Referent, p. 319
Sender, p. 319
Small-group communication, p. 318
Stereotypes, p. 317
Symmetrical, p. 319
Therapeutic communication, p. 327
Verbal communication, p. 320

MEDIA RESOURCES

http://evolve.elsevier.com/Potter/fundamentals/

- Review Questions
- Case Study with Questions
- Audio Glossary
- Content Updates

COMMUNICATION AND NURSING PRACTICE

Communication is a lifelong learning process. Nurses make the intimate journey with patients and their families from the miracle of birth to the mystery of death. As a nurse you communicate with patients and families to develop meaningful relationships. Within those relationships you collect relevant assessment data, provide education, and interact during nursing interventions. The use of therapeutic communication promotes personal growth and attainment of patients' health-related goals. Despite the complexity of technology and the multiple demands on nurses' time, it is the intimate moment of connection that makes all the difference in the quality of care and meaning for a patient and a nurse. Communication is the key to nurse-patient relationships and the ability to deliver patient-centered care.

Patient safety also requires effective communication among members of the health care team as patients move from one caregiver to another or from one care setting to another. Good communication skills help to reduce the risk of errors. These skills promote improved patient outcomes and increased patient satisfaction (Lang, 2012). Effective team communication and collaboration skills are essential to ensure patient safety and optimum patient care (Lazure et al., 2014). Competency in communication maintains effective relationships within the entire sphere of professional practice and meets legal, ethical, and clinical standards of care.

The qualities, behaviors, and therapeutic communication techniques described in this chapter characterize professionalism in caring relationships. Although the term *patient* is often used, the same principles apply when communicating with any person in any nursing situation.

Communication and Interpersonal Relationships

Caring relationships formed among a nurse and those affected by the nurse's practice are at the core of nursing (see Chapter 7). Communication establishes these caring healing relationships. All behavior communicates, and all communication influences behavior. For these reasons communication is essential to the nurse-patient relationship. Nurses with expertise in communication express caring by (Ryan, 2005; Watson, 1985):

- Becoming sensitive to self and others.
- Promoting and accepting the expression of positive and negative feelings.
- Developing caring relationships.
- Instilling faith and hope.
- Promoting interpersonal teaching and learning.
- Providing a supportive environment.
- Assisting with gratification of human needs.
- Allowing for spiritual expression.

A nurse's ability to relate to others is important for interpersonal communication. This includes the ability to take initiative in establishing and maintaining communication, to be authentic (one's self), and to respond appropriately to the other person. Effective interpersonal communication also requires a sense of mutuality (i.e., a belief that the nurse-patient relationship is a partnership and that both are equal participants). Nurses honor the fact that people are very complex and ambiguous. Often more is communicated than first meets the eye, and patient responses are not always what you expect. Each patient is a unique individual, with specific communication needs. Most nurses embrace the view that the profession has of the wholistic nature of people and their need for effective, supportive communication and human interaction. When patients and nurses work together, much can be accomplished. The Joint Commission (TJC) recognized the need to promote effective communication for patient- and family-centered care, cultural competence, and improved patient safety. TJC initiated a set of standards for hospitals that promote these improvements in communication, and they became part of the TJC requirements (TJC, 2011).

Therapeutic communication occurs within a healing relationship between a nurse and patient (Arnold and Boggs, 2011). Like any powerful therapeutic agent, a nurse's communication can result in both harm and good. Every nuance of posture, every small expression and gesture, every word chosen, every attitude held—all have the potential to hurt or heal, affecting others through the transmission of human energy. Knowing that intention and behavior directly influence health gives nurses the ethical responsibility to do no harm to those entrusted to their care. Respect the potential power of communication and do not misuse communication carelessly to hurt, manipulate, or coerce others. Skilled communication empowers others to express what they believe and make their own choices; these are essential aspects of the individualized healing process. Nurses have wonderful opportunities to bring about good things for themselves, their patients, and their colleagues through therapeutic communication.

Developing Communication Skills

Gaining expertise in communication requires both an understanding of the communication process and reflection about one's communication experiences as a nurse. Nurses who develop critical thinking skills make the best communicators. They form therapeutic relationships to gather relevant and comprehensive information about their patients. Then they draw on theoretical knowledge about communication and integrate this knowledge with knowledge previously learned through personal clinical experience. They interpret messages received from others to obtain new information, correct misinformation, promote patient understanding, and assist with planning patient-centered care (Arnold and Boggs, 2011).

Critical thinking attitudes and ethical standards of care promote effective communication. When you consider a patient's problems, it is important to apply critical thinking and critical reasoning skills to improve communication in assessment and care of the patient (Arnold and Boggs, 2011). For example, curiosity motivates a nurse to communicate and know more about a person. Patients are more likely to communicate with nurses who express an interest in them. Perseverance and creativity are also attitudes conducive to communication because they motivate a nurse to communicate and identify innovative solutions. A self-confident attitude is important because a nurse who conveys confidence and comfort while communicating more readily establishes an interpersonal caring relationship. In addition, an independent attitude encourages a nurse to communicate with colleagues and share ideas about nursing interventions. Integrity allows nurses to recognize when their opinions conflict with those of their patients, review positions, and decide how to communicate to reach mutually beneficial decisions. It is also very important for a nurse to communicate responsibly and ask for help if uncertain or uncomfortable about an aspect of patient care. An attitude of humility is necessary to recognize when you need to better communicate and intervene with patients, especially related to their cultural needs (Issacson, 2014).

It is challenging to understand human communication within interpersonal relationships. Each individual bases his or her perceptions about information received through the five senses of sight, hearing, taste, touch, and smell (Arnold and Boggs, 2011). An individual's culture and education also influence perception. Critical thinking helps nurses overcome **perceptual biases** or **stereotypes** that interfere with accurately perceiving and interpreting messages from others. People often incorrectly assume that they understand an individual's culture. They tend to distort or ignore information that goes against their expectations, preconceptions, or stereotypes (Issacson, 2014). By thinking critically about personal communication habits, you learn to control these tendencies and become more effective in interpersonal relationships.

You become more competent in the nursing process as your communication skills develop. You learn to integrate communication skills throughout the nursing process as you collaborate with patients and health care team members to achieve goals (Box 24-1). Use communication skills to gather, analyze, and transmit information and accomplish the work of each step of the process. Assessment, diagnosis, planning, implementation, and evaluation all depend on effective communication among nurse, patient, family, and others on the health care team. Although the nursing process is a reliable framework for patient care, it does not work well unless you master the art of effective interpersonal communication.

Patients often experience high levels of anxiety when they are ill or receiving treatment. **Emotional intelligence** (EI) is an assessment and communication technique that allows nurses to better understand and perceive the emotions of themselves and others. EI enables a nurse to use self-awareness, motivation, empathy, and social skills to build therapeutic relationships with patients (Marquis and Huston, 2015). Patients' emotions can negatively impact their self-care behaviors. If a nurse understands a patient's perceptions and motivations, he or she can help the patient make healthy behavior changes. Patients feel more comfortable addressing their poor health habits when this approach is used. This can lead to enhanced self-care behaviors and improved patient outcomes (Fox, 2013; Shanta and Connolly, 2013).

The nature of the communication process requires you to constantly decide what, when, where, why, and how to convey a message.

BOX 24-1 Communication Throughout the Nursing Process

Assessment
- Verbal interviewing and history taking
- Visual and intuitive observation of nonverbal behavior
- Visual, tactile, and auditory data gathering during physical examination
- Written medical records, diagnostic tests, and literature review

Nursing Diagnosis
- Intrapersonal analysis of assessment findings
- Validation of health care needs and priorities via verbal discussion with patient
- Documentation of nursing diagnosis

Planning
- Interpersonal or small-group health care team planning sessions
- Interpersonal collaboration with patient and family to determine implementation methods
- Written documentation of expected outcomes
- Written or verbal referral to health care team members

Implementation
- Delegation and verbal discussion with health care team
- Verbal, visual, auditory, and tactile health teaching activities
- Provision of support via therapeutic communication techniques
- Contact with other health resources
- Written documentation of patient's progress in medical record

Evaluation
- Acquisition of verbal and nonverbal feedback
- Comparison of actual and expected outcomes
- Identification of factors affecting outcomes
- Modification and update of care plan
- Verbal and/or written explanation of care plan revisions to patient

A nurse's decision making is always contextual (i.e., the unique features of any situation influence the nature of the decisions made). For example, the explanation of the importance of following a prescribed diet to a patient with a newly diagnosed medical condition differs from the explanation to a patient who has repeatedly chosen not to follow diet restrictions. Effective communication techniques are easy to learn, but their application is difficult. Deciding which techniques best fit each unique nursing situation is challenging. Communication with patients and families about illness such as cancer or advance care planning can be stressful. Nurses may experience grief and fatigue related to emotional exhaustion when discussing these topics, especially when they have developed a bond with patients or families. However, discussion of these important and sensitive topics is linked to an increased quality of life for the patients and or family members (Moore and Reynolds, 2013).

Throughout this chapter brief clinical examples will guide you in the use of effective communication techniques. Situations that challenge a nurse's decision-making skills and call for careful use of therapeutic techniques often involve a variety of human behaviors described in Box 24-2. Because the best way to acquire skill is through practice, it is useful for you to discuss and role-play these scenarios before experiencing them in the clinical setting.

Levels of Communication

Nurses use different levels of communication in their professional role. A competent nurse uses a variety of techniques in each level.

BOX 24-2 Challenging Communication Situations

- People who are silent, withdrawn, and have difficulty expressing feelings or needs
- People who are sad and depressed
- People who require assistance with visual or speech disabilities (special needs)
- People who are angry or confrontational and cannot listen to explanations
- People who are uncooperative and resent being asked to help others
- People who are talkative or lonely and want someone to be with them all the time
- People who are demanding and expect others to meet their requests
- People who are frightened, anxious, and having difficulty coping
- People who are confused and disoriented
- People who speak and/or understand little English
- People who are flirtatious or sexually inappropriate

Intrapersonal communication is a powerful form of communication that you use as a professional nurse. This level of communication is also called *self-talk.* People's thoughts and inner communications strongly influence perceptions, feelings, behavior, and self-esteem. Always be aware of the nature and content of your own thinking. Positive self-talk provides a mental rehearsal for difficult tasks or situations so individuals deal with them more effectively and with increased confidence (Arnold and Boggs, 2011). Nurses use intrapersonal communication to develop self-awareness and a positive self-esteem that enhances appropriate self-expression. Positive self-talk can help you diminish cognitive distortions that lead to a decrease in self-esteem and impact your ability to work with patients. Transforming statements from "I'm scared to work with this type of patient" into "This is my opportunity to learn about this patient and I can ask for help when it's needed" is an example of positive self-talk.

Interpersonal communication is one-on-one interaction between a nurse and another person that often occurs face to face. It is the level most frequently used in nursing situations and lies at the heart of nursing practice. It takes place within a social context and includes all the symbols and cues used to give and receive meaning. Because meaning resides in people and not in words, messages received are sometimes different from intended messages. Nurses work with people who have different opinions, experiences, values, and belief systems; thus it is important to validate meaning or mutually negotiate it between participants. For example, use interaction to assess understanding and clarify misinterpretations when teaching a patient about a health concern. Meaningful interpersonal communication results in an exchange of ideas, problem solving, expression of feelings, decision making, goal accomplishment, team building, and personal growth.

Small-group communication is the interaction that occurs when a small number of people meet. This type of communication is usually goal directed and requires an understanding of group dynamics. When nurses work on committees with nurses or other disciplines and participate in patient care conferences, they use a small-group communication process. Communication in these situations should be organized, concise, and complete. All participating disciplines are encouraged to contribute and provide feedback. Good communication skills help each participant better meet a patient's needs and promote a safer care environment.

Public communication is interaction with an audience. Nurses often speak with groups of consumers about health-related topics, present scholarly work to colleagues at conferences, or lead classroom discussions with peers or students. Public communication requires special adaptations in eye contact, gestures, voice inflection, and use of media materials to communicate messages effectively. Effective public communication increases audience knowledge about health-related topics, health issues, and other issues important to the nursing profession.

Electronic communication is the use of technology to create ongoing relationships with patients and their health care team. Secure messaging provides an opportunity for frequent and timely communication with a patient's physician or nurse via a patient portal. An electronic portal enables patients to stay engaged and informed and build a therapeutic relationship with the health care team (Facchiano and Snyder, 2011; Rodriguez, 2010).

ELEMENTS OF THE COMMUNICATION PROCESS

Communication is an ongoing and continuously changing process. You are changing, the people with whom you are communicating are changing, and your environment is also continually changing. Figure 24-1 shows an example of a **circular transactional communication process** model. The model shows the situational contextual inputs, channels of communication, interpersonal contextual concepts, and factors affecting the sender and receiver. Nursing situations have many unique aspects that influence the nature of communication and interpersonal relationships. As a professional you will use critical thinking to focus on each aspect of communication so your interactions are purposeful and effective.

Circular Transactional Model

The **circular transactional model** includes several elements: the referent, sender and receiver, message, channels, context or environment in which the communication process occurs, feedback, and interpersonal variables (see Figure 24-1). In this model each person in the communication interaction is both a speaker and a listener and can be simultaneously sending and receiving messages. Both parties view the perceptions, attitudes, and potential reactions to a sent message. Communication becomes a continuous and interactive activity. Feedback from the receiver or environment enables the communicators to correct or validate the communication. This model also describes the role relationship of the communicators as **complementary** and **symmetrical**. Complementary role relationships function with one person holding an elevated position over the other person. Symmetrical relationships are more equal. For example, a nurse provides education to a patient about a new medication. This would be a complementary role. A group of patients discussing their plans after discharge would be a symmetrical role relationship (Arnold and Boggs, 2011).

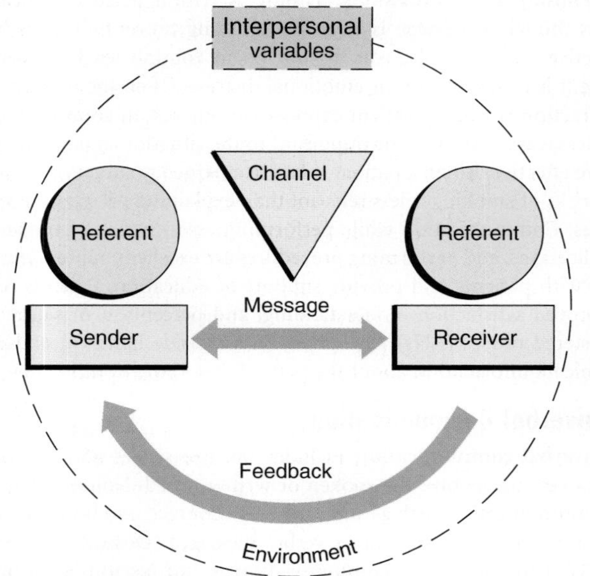

FIGURE 24-1 Circular transactional model of communication.

Referent. The **referent** motivates one person to communicate with another. In a health care setting sights, sounds, sensations, perceptions, and ideas are examples of cues that initiate the communication process. Knowing a stimulus or referent that initiates communication allows you to develop and organize messages more efficiently. For example, a patient request for help prompted by his difficulty breathing causes a different response than a patient request resulting from hunger.

Sender and Receiver. The **sender** is the person who encodes and delivers a message, and the **receiver** is the person who receives and decodes the message. The sender puts the message into verbal and nonverbal symbols that the receiver can understand (Arnold and Boggs, 2011). The sender's message acts as a referent for the receiver. Transactional communication involves the role of sender and receiver switching back and forth between nurse and patient. A decoding process includes the receiver interpreting the meaning of the word symbols. Active listening is important to accurately decode and understand a message. The more the sender and receiver have in common and the closer the relationship, the more likely they will accurately perceive one another's meaning and respond accordingly (Arnold and Boggs, 2011). Establishing a rapport with a patient ensures more effective communication.

Message. The **message** is the content of the communication. It contains verbal and nonverbal expressions of thoughts and feelings. Effective messages are clear, direct, and in understandable language. Individuals with communication barriers may need assistance via clarification devices such as hearing aids, interpreters, or pictures to ensure that messages sent and received are understandable. Personal perceptions may also distort the receiver's interpretation of a message. As a nurse you send effective messages by expressing clearly, directly, and in a manner familiar to a patient. You determine the need for clarification by watching the patient listen for nonverbal cues that suggest confusion or misunderstanding. Communication is difficult when participants have different levels of education and experience. For example, statements such as "Your incision is well approximated without purulent drainage" means the same as "Your wound edges are close together, and there are no signs of infection"; but the latter is easier to understand. You can also send messages in writing, but make sure that patients are able to read.

Channels. Communication **channels** are means of sending and receiving messages through visual, auditory, and tactile senses. Facial expressions send visual messages; spoken words travel through auditory channels. Touch uses tactile channels. Individuals usually understand a message more clearly when the sender uses more channels to send it.

Feedback. **Feedback** is the message a sender receives from the receiver. It indicates whether the receiver understood the meaning of the sender's message. Feedback occurs continuously between a sender and receiver. A sender seeks verbal and nonverbal feedback to evaluate the receiver's response and effectiveness of a communicated message. The type of feedback a sender or receiver gives depends on factors such as their background, prior experiences, attitudes, cultural beliefs, and self-esteem. A sender and receiver need to be sensitive and open to one another's messages, to clarify the messages, and to modify behavior accordingly for successful communication.

Interpersonal Variables. Interpersonal variables are factors within both the sender and receiver that influence communication. Perception provides a uniquely personal view of reality formed by an individual's culture, expectations, and experiences. Each person senses, interprets, and understands events differently. A nurse says, "You haven't been talking very much since your family left. Is there something on your mind?" One patient may perceive the nurse's question as caring and concerned; another perceives the nurse as invading privacy and is less willing to talk. Cultural sensitivity enables you to explore the interpersonal variables such as educational and developmental level, sociocultural background, values and beliefs, emotions, gender, physical health status, and roles and relationships that affect how a patient communicates. Interpersonal variables associated with illness such as pain, anxiety, and medication effects also affect nurse-patient communication.

Environment. The environment is the setting for sender-receiver interaction. An effective communication setting provides participants with physical and emotional comfort and safety. Noise, temperature extremes, distractions, and lack of privacy or space create confusion, tension, and discomfort. Environmental distractions are common in health care settings and interfere with messages sent between people. You control the environment as much as possible to create favorable conditions for effective communication.

FORMS OF COMMUNICATION

Messages are conveyed verbally and nonverbally, concretely and symbolically. As people communicate, they express themselves through words, movements, voice inflection, facial expressions, and use of space. These elements work in harmony to enhance a message or conflict with one another to contradict and confuse it.

Verbal Communication

Verbal communication uses spoken or written words. Verbal language is a code that conveys specific meaning through a combination of words. The most important aspects of verbal communication are presented in the following paragraphs.

Vocabulary. Communication is unsuccessful if senders and receivers cannot translate one another's words and phrases. When you care for a patient who speaks another language, a professional interpreter is necessary. Even those who speak the same language use subcultural variations of certain words (e.g., *dinner* means a noon meal to one person and the last meal of the day to another). Medical jargon (technical terminology used by health care providers) sounds like a foreign language to patients unfamiliar with the health care setting. Limiting use of medical jargon to conversations with other health care team members improves communication. Children have a more limited vocabulary than adults and often use special words to describe bodily functions or a favorite blanket or toy. Teenagers often use words in unique ways that are unfamiliar to adults.

Denotative and Connotative Meaning. Some words have several meanings. Individuals who use a common language share the denotative meaning: *baseball* has the same meaning for everyone who speaks English, but *code* denotes cardiac arrest primarily to health care providers. The connotative meaning is the shade or interpretation of the meaning of a word influenced by the thoughts, feelings, or ideas that people have about the word. For example, health care providers tell a family that a loved one is in serious condition and they believe that death is near; but to nurses *serious* simply describes the nature of the illness. You need to select words carefully, avoiding easily misinterpreted words, especially when explaining a patient's medical condition or therapy. Even a much-used phrase such as "I'm going to take your vital signs" may be unfamiliar to an adult or frightening to a child. "I'm going to check your blood pressure, heart rate, and temperature" may be more appropriate.

Pacing. Conversation is more successful at an appropriate speed or pace. Speak slowly and enunciate clearly. Talking rapidly, using awkward pauses, or speaking slowly and deliberately conveys an unintended message. Long pauses and rapid shifts to another subject give the impression that you are hiding the truth. Think before speaking and develop an awareness of the rhythm of your speech to improve pacing.

Intonation. Tone of voice dramatically affects the meaning of a message. Depending on intonation, even a simple question or statement expresses enthusiasm, anger, concern, or indifference. Be aware of voice tone to avoid sending unintended messages. If a patient interprets a nurse's patronizing tone of voice as condescending, this will inhibit further communication. A patient's tone of voice provides information about his or her emotional state or energy level.

Clarity and Brevity. Effective communication is simple, brief, and direct. For certain populations such as the elderly, fewer words result in less confusion. Speak slowly, enunciate clearly, and use examples to make explanations easier to understand. Repeating important parts of a message also clarifies communication. Phrases such as "you know" or "OK?" at the end of every sentence detract from clarity. Use sentences and words that express an idea simply and directly. "Where is your pain?" is much better than "I would like you to describe for me the location of your discomfort."

Timing and Relevance. Timing is critical in communication. Even though a message is clear, poor timing prevents it from being effective. For example, you do not begin routine teaching when a patient is in severe pain or emotional distress. Often the best time for interaction is when a patient expresses an interest in communicating. If messages are relevant or important to the situation at hand, they are more effective. When a patient is facing emergency surgery, discussing the risks of smoking is less relevant than explaining presurgical procedures. Communication while performing assessments, administering medications, and performing procedures are excellent opportunities to talk with patients and provide support or education. Patients report improved satisfaction, understanding, and perception of safety with registered nurses (RNs) who provided a bedside hand-off and communicate information about the plan of care (Ford et al., 2014).

Nonverbal Communication

Nonverbal communication includes the five senses and everything that does not involve the spoken or written word. Nonverbal aspects of communication such as voice tone, eye contact, and body positioning are often as important as verbal messages (Dossey and Keegan, 2013). Thus nonverbal communication is unconsciously motivated and more accurately indicates a person's intended meaning than spoken words (Stuart, 2013). When there is incongruity between verbal and nonverbal communication, the receiver usually "hears" the nonverbal message as the true message.

All kinds of nonverbal communication are important, but interpreting them is often problematic. Sociocultural background is a major influence on the meaning of nonverbal behavior. In the United States, with its diverse cultural communities, nonverbal messages between people of different cultures are easily misinterpreted. Because the meaning attached to nonverbal behavior is so subjective, it is imperative that you verify it (Dossey and Keegan, 2013; Stuart, 2013). Assessing nonverbal messages is an important nursing skill.

Personal Appearance. Personal appearance includes physical characteristics, facial expression, and manner of dress and grooming. These factors communicate physical well-being, personality, social status, occupation, religion, culture, and self-concept. In the health care setting research has shown that patients prefer nurses to have their hair back and off their shoulders and to not have long fingernails (Johnson et al., 2008). Many health care agencies have restrictions in the form of a dress code that requires a certain color and type of uniform, limitations on jewelry to wear, and whether tattoos need to be covered. Remember, first impressions are largely based on appearance. Nurses learn to develop a general impression of patient health and emotional status through appearance, and patients develop a general impression of the nurse's professionalism and caring in the same way.

Posture and Gait. Posture and gait (manner or pattern of walking) are forms of self-expression. The way people sit, stand, and move reflects attitudes, emotions, self-concept, and health status. For example, an erect posture and a quick, purposeful gait communicate a sense of well-being and confidence. Leaning forward conveys attention. A slumped posture and slow shuffling gait indicates depression, illness, or fatigue.

Facial Expression. The face is the most expressive part of the body. Facial expressions convey emotions such as surprise, fear, anger, happiness, and sadness. Some people have an expressionless face, or flat affect, which reveals little about what they are thinking or feeling. An inappropriate affect is a facial expression that does not match the content of a verbal message (e.g., smiling when describing a sad situation). People are sometimes unaware of the messages their expressions convey. For example, a nurse frowns in concentration while doing a procedure, and the patient interprets this as anger or disapproval. Patients closely observe nurses. Consider the impact a nurse's facial expression has on a person who asks, "Am I going to die?" The slightest change in the eyes, lips, or facial muscles reveals the nurse's feelings. Although it is hard to control all facial expressions, try to avoid showing shock, disgust, dismay, or other distressing reactions in a patient's presence.

Eye Contact. People signal readiness to communicate through eye contact. Maintaining eye contact during conversation shows respect and willingness to listen. Eye contact also allows people to closely observe one another. Lack of eye contact may indicate anxiety, defensiveness, discomfort, or lack of confidence in communicating. However, people from some cultures consider eye contact intrusive, threatening, or harmful and minimize or avoid its use (see Chapter 9). Always consider a person's culture when interpreting the meaning of eye contact. Eye movements communicate feelings and emotions. Looking down on a person establishes authority, whereas interacting at the same eye level indicates equality in the relationship. Rising to the same eye level as an angry person helps establish autonomy.

Gestures. Gestures emphasize, punctuate, and clarify the spoken word. Gestures alone carry specific meanings, or they create messages with other communication cues. A finger pointed toward a person communicates several meanings; but, when accompanied by a frown and stern voice, the gesture becomes an accusation or threat. Pointing to an area of pain is sometimes more accurate than describing its location.

Sounds. Sounds such as sighs, moans, groans, or sobs also communicate feelings and thoughts. Combined with other nonverbal communication, sounds help to send clear messages. They have several interpretations: moaning conveys pleasure or suffering; and crying communicates happiness, sadness, or anger. Validate nonverbal messages with patients to interpret them accurately.

Territoriality and Personal Space. Territoriality is the need to gain, maintain, and defend one's right to space. Territory is important because it provides people with a sense of privacy, identity, security, and control. It is sometimes separated and made visible to others such as a fence around a yard or a curtain around a bed in a hospital room. Personal space is invisible, individual, and travels with a person. During interpersonal interaction people maintain varying distances between one another, depending on their culture, the nature of their relationship, and the situation. When personal space becomes threatened, people respond defensively and communicate less effectively. Situations dictate whether the interpersonal distance between nurse and patient is appropriate. Box 24-3 provides examples of nursing actions within communication zones (Stuart, 2013). Nurses frequently move into patients' territory and personal space because of the nature of caregiving. You need to convey confidence, gentleness, and respect for privacy, especially when your actions require intimate contact or involve a patient's vulnerable zone.

Metacommunication

Metacommunication is a broad term that refers to all factors that influence communication. Awareness of influencing factors helps people better understand what is communicated (Arnold and Boggs, 2011). For example, a nurse observes a young patient holding his body rigidly, and his voice is sharp as he says, "Going to surgery is no big deal." The nurse replies, "You say having surgery doesn't bother you, but you look and sound tense. I'd like to hear more about how you're feeling." Awareness of the tone of the verbal response and the nonverbal behavior results in further exploration of the patient's feelings and concerns.

PROFESSIONAL NURSING RELATIONSHIPS

A nurse's application of knowledge, understanding of human behavior and communication, and commitment to ethical behavior create professional relationships. Having a philosophy based on caring and respect for others helps you be more successful in establishing relationships of this nature.

Nurse-Patient Caring Relationships

Caring relationships are the foundation of clinical nursing practice. In such relationships you assume the role of a professional who cares about each patient and his or her unique health needs, human responses, and patterns of living. Therapeutic relationships promote a psychological climate that facilitates positive change and growth. Therapeutic communication between you and your patients allows the attainment of health-related goals (Arnold and Boggs, 2011). The goals of a therapeutic relationship focus on a patient achieving optimal

BOX 24-3 Zones of Personal Space

Zones of Personal Space

Intimate Zone (0-8 inches)

- Holding a crying infant
- Performing physical assessment
- Bathing, grooming, dressing, feeding, and toileting a patient
- Changing a patient's surgical dressing

Personal Zone (18 inches-4 feet)

- Sitting at a patient's bedside
- Taking a patient's nursing history
- Teaching an individual patient

Socio-Consultative Zone (9-12 feet)

- Giving directions to visitors in the hallway
- Asking if families need assistance from the patient doorway
- Giving verbal report to a group of nurses

Public Zone (12 feet and more)

- Speaking at a community forum
- Lecturing to a class of students
- Testifying at a legislative hearing

Special Zones of Touch

Social Zone (Permission Not Needed)

Hands, arms, shoulders, back

Consent Zone (Permission Needed)

Mouth, wrists, feet

Vulnerable Zone (Special Care Needed)

Face, neck, front of body

Intimate Zone (Permission and Great Sensitivity Needed)

Genitalia, rectum

personal growth related to personal identity, ability to form relationships, and ability to satisfy needs and achieve personal goals (Stuart, 2013). There is an explicit time frame, a goal-directed approach, and a high expectation that what you discuss together is kept confidential among only members of the health care team involved in the patient's care. A nurse establishes, directs, and takes responsibility for the interaction; and a patient's needs take priority over a nurse's needs. Your nonjudgmental acceptance of a patient is an important characteristic of the relationship. Acceptance conveys a willingness to hear a message or acknowledge feelings. It does not mean that you always agree with the other person or approve of the patient's decisions or actions. A caring relationship between you and a patient does not just happen: you create it with skill and trust.

There is a natural progression of four goal-directed phases that characterize the nurse-patient relationship (Box 24-4). The relationship often begins before you meet a patient and continues until the caregiving relationship ends. Even a brief interaction uses an abbreviated version of preinteraction, orientation, working, and termination (Stuart, 2013). For example, a nursing student gathers patient information to prepare in advance for caregiving, meets the patient and establishes trust, accomplishes health-related goals through use of the nursing process, and says goodbye at the end of the day.

Socializing is an important initial component of interpersonal communication. It helps people get to know one another and relax. It is easy, superficial, and not deeply personal; whereas therapeutic interactions are often more intense, difficult, and uncomfortable. A nurse often uses social conversation to lay a foundation for a closer relationship: "Hi, Mr. Simpson, I hear it's your birthday today. How old are you?" A friendly, informal, and warm communication style establishes trust, but you have to move beyond social conversation to talk about issues or concerns affecting the patient's health. During social conversation some patients ask personal questions such as those about your family or place of residence. Students often wonder whether it is appropriate to reveal such information. The skillful nurse uses judgment about what to share and provides minimal information or

BOX 24-4 Phases of the Helping Relationship

Preinteraction Phase

Before meeting a patient:

- Review available data, including the medical and nursing history.
- Talk to other caregivers who have information about the patient.
- Anticipate health concerns or issues that arise.
- Identify a location and setting that fosters comfortable, private interaction.
- Plan enough time for the initial interaction.

Orientation Phase

When the nurse and patient meet and get to know one another:

- Set the tone for the relationship by adopting a warm, empathetic, caring manner.
- Recognize that the initial relationship is often superficial, uncertain, and tentative.
- Expect the patient to test your competence and commitment.
- Closely observe the patient and expect to be closely observed by the patient.
- Begin to make inferences and form judgments about patient messages and behaviors.
- Assess the patient's health status.
- Prioritize the patient's problems and identify his or her goals.
- Clarify the patient's and your roles.
- Form contracts with the patient that specify who will do what.
- Let the patient know when to expect the relationship to be terminated.

Working Phase

When the nurse and patient work together to solve problems and accomplish goals:

- Encourage and help the patient express feelings about his or her health.
- Encourage and help the patient with self-exploration.
- Provide information needed to understand and change behavior.
- Encourage and help the patient set goals.
- Take action to meet the goals set with the patient.
- Use therapeutic communication skills to facilitate successful interactions.
- Use appropriate self-disclosure and confrontation.

Termination Phase

During the ending of the relationship:

- Remind the patient that termination is near.
- Evaluate goal achievement with the patient.
- Reminisce about the relationship with the patient.
- Separate from the patient by relinquishing responsibility for his or her care.
- Achieve a smooth transition for the patient to other caregivers as needed.

deflects such questions with gentle humor and refocuses conversation back to the patient.

In a therapeutic relationship it may be helpful to encourage patients to share personal stories. Sharing stories is called *narrative interaction*. Through listening to stories you begin to understand the context of others' lives and learn what is meaningful for them from their perspective. For example, a nurse listens to a patient's perception of what it means to refuse medication treatment for breast cancer and is then better able to articulate the patient's wishes (Gidman, 2013). Listen to patients' stories to better understand their concerns, experiences, and challenges. This information is not usually revealed with a standard history form that elicits short answers.

As a nurse you can also tell stories to enhance patient education. Telling good stories frames important messages you wish to send and makes messages memorable for your patients. Purposeful storytelling brings across factual information along with a human interest perspective that draws on an individual's emotions such as a patient's desire to get well or feel a sense of hope. Emotions play a significant role in helping adults learn the ability to grasp new ideas.

Motivational Interviewing

Motivational interviewing (MI) is a technique that holds promise for encouraging patients to share their thoughts, beliefs, fears, and concerns with the aim of changing their behavior. MI provides a way of working with patients who may not seem ready to make behavior changes that are considered necessary by their health practitioners. It can potentially be used to evoke change talk, which links to improved patient outcomes (Copeland et al., 2015). For example, an interviewer uses information about a patient's personal goals and values to promote the patient's adherence to a new medication or exercise plan. The interviewing is delivered in a nonjudgmental, guided communication approach. When using MI, a nurse tries to understand a patient's motivations and values using an empathic and active listening approach. The nurse identifies differences between the patient's current health goals and behaviors and his or her current health status. The patient is supported even though a phase of resistance and ambivalence often occurs. Communication then focuses on recognizing the patient's strengths and supporting those strengths in an effort to make positive changes. This can result in dramatic improvements in health outcomes and patient satisfaction (Stawnychy et al., 2014; Stuart, 2013).

Nurse-Family Relationships

Many nursing situations, especially those in community and home care settings, require you to form caring relationships with entire families. The same principles that guide one-on-one helping relationships also apply when the patient is a family unit, although communication within families requires additional understanding of the complexities of family dynamics, needs, and relationships (see Chapter 10).

Nurse–Health Care Team Relationships

Communication with other members of the health care team affects patient safety and the work environment. Breakdown in communication, lack of patient education, and poor health care provider accountability is a frequent cause of serious injuries in health care settings (TJC Resources, 2012). When patients move from one nursing unit to another or from one provider to another, there is a risk for miscommunication. To address this risk health care providers provide detailed hand-off reports at end of shifts or when patients transfer off care units to ensure that patients have a safe and smooth transition in care. TJC Resources recommends that the entire health care team collaborate and coordinate during patient transition. Standardized discharge or transfer procedures and forms reduce the risk of errors during patient transitions. Timely follow-up after discharge or transfer is also encouraged (TJC Resources, 2012).

Use of a common language such as the SBAR technique for communicating critical information improves perception of communication and information about patients between health care providers (De Meester et al., 2013). The SBAR technique is a popular communication tool that standardizes communication. SBAR is the acronym for *S*ituation, *B*ackground, *A*ssessment, and *R*ecommendation (see Chapter 26). The use of this easy-to-remember, orderly technique is to relay relevant information in a structured and timely manner (Marquis and Huston, 2015). Evidence identifies nursing actions that increase effectiveness of nurse-to-nurse interaction and interprofessional communication (Box 24-5).

Some organizations have added an introduction step (ISBAR) into the SBAR process. The introduction step is used when health care providers do not actively know one another. They start with an introduction, a description of their location, and their role in caring for the patient (Marquis and Huston, 2015).

Lateral Violence. Professional nursing care requires nurses to interact with members of the nursing team and interprofessional

BOX 24-5 EVIDENCE-BASED PRACTICE

Safe and Effective Interprofessional Communication

PICO Question: Does the SBAR communication technique compared with standard end-of-shift narrative report among hospital health care team members improve patient outcomes?

Evidence Summary

Nurses are taught to be detailed and descriptive in their conversations but not to "medically" diagnose a problem or situation. Physicians express themselves in brief statements, providing only the specific facts (Haig et al., 2006). Disconnect in communication styles leads to dysfunctional physician-nurse communication and a significant increase in errors in patient care. Mutual respect and trust enable clarification and clear communication. Practitioners need an understanding and appreciation of interprofessional collaboration to promote effective team functioning necessary for optimum patient care (Lazure et al., 2014). Use of communication techniques such as SBAR (*S*ituation, *B*ackground, *A*ssessment, and *R*ecommendation) provides a framework for structure and accurate communication among health care providers that fosters patient safety. In a study involving 16 hospital units, nurses were trained to use SBAR to communicate with physicians in cases of deteriorating patient status. As a result, nurses had an increased perception of effective communication and collaboration between nurses and physicians (De Meester et al., 2013). Most important, the study found a decrease in unexpected deaths. Effective communication practices using SBAR and the Communication During Patient Handover (CDPH) approach minimize risk and improve hand-off communication between health care providers (Adams and Osborne-McKenzie, 2012).

Application to Nursing Practice

- Work in interprofessional teams to develop understanding and respect for other disciplines.
- Use a standardized approach (e.g., SBAR, CDPH, or a D-BANQ format) for report when patients are transferred to other units or facilities (Adams and Osborne-McKenzie, 2012).
- SBAR is not a document but rather a verbal technique that requires education for nurses and physicians (Compton et al., 2012).
- Provide the opportunity for questions and confirmation of understanding of communication.

QSEN QSEN BUILDING COMPETENCY IN TEAMWORK AND COLLABORATION You are facilitating the transfer of Mrs. Jones from the orthopedic unit to the rehabilitation (Rehab) unit. Mrs. Jones is 5 days' postoperative from total hip replacement surgery. She experienced an allergic reaction to hydrocodone/acetaminophen (Vicodin) yesterday. You found out that you will be giving report to a nurse who is known to be critical and demeaning with new nurses. You rush through a verbal report and forget to tell the Rehab nurse about the allergic reaction. Hydrocodone/acetaminophen is given to the patient after transfer. Mrs. Jones suffers a severe allergic reaction and is transferred to the intensive care unit (ICU). What could have been done to prevent this event?

Answers to QSEN Activities can be found on the Evolve website.

health care providers. Communication focuses on team building, facilitating group processes, collaborating, consulting, delegating, supervising, leading, and managing (see Chapter 21). Social, informational, and therapeutic interactions help team members build morale, accomplish goals, and strengthen working relationships. Lateral violence or workplace bullying between colleagues sometimes occurs and includes behaviors such as withholding information, backbiting, making snide remarks or put downs, and nonverbal expressions of disapproval such as raising eyebrows or making faces. Lateral violence adversely effects the work environment, leading to job dissatisfaction, a decreased sense of value, poor teamwork, poor retention of qualified nurses, and nurses leaving the profession. New nurses are especially prone to bullying behavior (Frederick, 2014). Lateral violence can be a symptom of compassion fatigue, wherein health care workers perceive a threat during interactions with colleagues and react emotionally rather than communicating intentionally in a professional manner.

Lateral violence interferes with effective health care team communication and jeopardizes patient safety (Marquis and Huston, 2015). Intimidation decreases the likelihood that a nurse will report a near-miss, question an order, or take action to improve the quality of patient care. There must be zero tolerance of lateral violence. Develop skills in conflict management and assertive communication to stop the spread of lateral violence in the workplace. Requesting a mentor can help the new nurse learn skills to address the perpetrators of bullying. The mentor can also be a personal support for the nurse and serve as a role model for the department (Frederick, 2014). The nurse experiencing lateral violence can also use additional techniques such as the following:

- Address the behavior when it occurs in a calm manner.
- Describe how the behavior affects your functioning.
- Ask for the abuse to stop.
- Notify the manager to get support for the situation.
- Make a plan for taking action in the future.
- Document the incidences in detail.

Nurse-Community Relationships

Many nurses form relationships with community groups by participating in local organizations, volunteering for community service, or becoming politically active. As a nurse, learn to establish relationships with your community to be an effective change agent. Providing clear and accurate information to members of the public is the best way to prevent errors, reduce resistance, and promote change. Communication within the community occurs through channels such as neighborhood newsletters, health fairs, public bulletin boards, newspapers, radio, television, and electronic information sites. Use these forms of communication to share information and discuss issues important to community health (see Chapter 3).

ELEMENTS OF PROFESSIONAL COMMUNICATION

Professional appearance, demeanor, and behavior are important in establishing trustworthiness and competence. A professional is expected to be clean, neat, well groomed, conservatively dressed, and odor free. Visible tattoos and piercings may not be considered acceptable in some professional settings. Professional behavior reflects warmth, friendliness, confidence, and competence. Professionals speak in a clear, well-modulated voice; use good grammar; listen to others; help and support colleagues; and communicate effectively. Being on time, organized, well prepared, and equipped for the responsibilities of the nursing role also communicate professionalism.

Courtesy

Common courtesy is part of professional communication. To practice courtesy, say hello and goodbye to patients and knock on doors before entering. State your purpose, address people by name, and say "please" and "thank you" to team members. Introduce yourself and state your title. When a nurse is discourteous, others perceive him or her as rude or insensitive. It sets up barriers to forming helping relationships between nurse and patient and causes friction among team members.

Use of Names

Always introduce yourself. Failure to give your name and status (e.g., nursing student, RN, or licensed practical nurse) or acknowledge a patient creates uncertainty about an interaction and conveys an impersonal lack of commitment or caring. Making eye contact and smiling recognize others. Addressing people by name conveys respect for human dignity and uniqueness. Because using last names is respectful in most cultures, nurses usually use a patient's last name in an initial interaction and then use the first name if the patient requests it. Ask how your patients and co-workers prefer to be addressed and honor their personal preferences. Using first names is appropriate for infants, young children, patients who are confused or unconscious, and close team members. Avoid terms of endearment such as "honey," "dear," "grandma," or "sweetheart." Even the closest nurse-patient relationships rarely progress to identities outside of first names. Avoid referring to patients by diagnosis, room number, or other attribute, which is demeaning and sends the message that you do not care enough to know the person as an individual.

Trustworthiness

Trust is relying on someone without doubt or question. Being trustworthy means helping others without hesitation. To foster trust, communicate warmth and demonstrate consistency, reliability, honesty, competence, and respect. Sometimes it isn't easy for a patient to ask for help. Trusting another person involves risk and vulnerability; but it also fosters open, therapeutic communication and enhances the expression of feelings, thoughts, and needs. Without trust a nurse-patient relationship rarely progresses beyond social interaction and superficial care. Avoid dishonesty at all costs. Withholding key information, lying, or distorting the truth violates both legal and ethical standards of practice. Sharing personal information or gossiping about others sends the message that you cannot be trusted and damages interpersonal relationships.

Autonomy and Responsibility

Autonomy is being self-directed and independent in accomplishing goals and advocating for others. Professional nurses make choices and accept responsibility for the outcomes of their actions (Townsend, 2012). They take initiative in problem solving and communicate in a way that reflects the importance and purpose of a therapeutic conversation (Arnold and Boggs, 2011). Professional nurses also recognize their patients' autonomy.

Assertiveness

Assertiveness allows you to express feelings and ideas without judging or hurting others. Assertive behavior includes intermittent eye contact; nonverbal communication that reflects interest, honesty, and active listening; spontaneous verbal responses with a confident voice; and culturally sensitive use of touch and space. An assertive nurse communicates self-assurance; communicates feelings; takes responsibility for choices; and is respectful of others' feelings, ideas, and choices (Stuart, 2013; Townsend, 2012). Assertive behavior increases self-esteem and self-confidence, increases the ability to develop satisfying interpersonal relationships, and increases goal attainment. Assertive individuals make decisions and control their lives more effectively than nonassertive individuals. They deal with criticism and manipulation by others and learn to say no, set limits, and resist intentionally imposed guilt. Assertive responses contain "I" messages such as "I want," "I need," "I think," or "I feel" (Townsend, 2012). Nurses may experience ethical issues that make it difficult to use their assertiveness skills for fear of retaliation (e.g., identifying an error made by another health care provider). In such a situation the individual would need to take steps to resolve this ethical dilemma (see Chapter 22).

AIDET® is a technique developed by the Studer Group to enable health care workers to provide accurate and timely communication to patients and families while focusing on excellent patient service. It is a technique commonly used in hospitals today. The acronym stands for *A*cknowledge, *I*ntroduce, *D*uration, *E*xplain, and *T*hank you. When using AIDET, a health care worker first acknowledges the person standing in front of him or her with a positive attitude and makes the person feel comfortable. The worker introduces himself or herself and lets the person know what his or her role is in the department and the person's care. It is important to always wear a name badge when working in a health care setting. When possible, the worker gives the patient or family an idea of how long a procedure may take. This keeps the patient informed of any delays that may occur. It is also helpful to let a patient know how long it will take to get results if they are related to testing. When explaining procedures, describe what the patient will experience with the treatment, procedure, or test. Inform him or her of any safety precautions. The worker using AIDET thanks the patient for coming to this organization for care and lets the patient know how much he or she enjoyed working with him or her (Rubin, 2014).

NURSING PROCESS

The nursing process provides a clinical decision-making approach for you to develop and implement an individualized plan of care. It guides care for patients who need special assistance with communication. Use therapeutic communication techniques as an intervention in an interpersonal nursing situation.

Assessment

During the assessment process thoroughly assess each patient and critically analyze findings to ensure that you make patient-centered clinical decisions required for safe nursing care.

Through the Patient's Eyes. Patient-centered care requires careful assessment of a patient's values; preferences; and cultural, ethnic, and social backgrounds (Harvey and Ahmann, 2014). During assessment a nurse also explores any personal biases and experiences that might affect his or her ability to form a therapeutic relationship. If the nurse cannot resolve his or her bias related to a patient, care should be transferred to another individual. Internal and external factors also affect a patient's ability to communicate (Box 24-6). Assessing these factors keeps a focus on the patient and helps you make patient-centered decisions during the communication process.

BOX 24-6 Assessment: Factors Influencing Communication

Psychophysiological Context (Internal Factors Affecting Communication)
- Physiological status (e.g., pain, hunger, nausea, weakness, dyspnea)
- Emotional status (e.g., anxiety, anger, hopelessness, euphoria)
- Growth and development status (e.g., age, developmental tasks)
- Unmet needs (e.g., safety/security, love/belonging)
- Attitudes, values, and beliefs (e.g., meaning of illness experience)
- Perceptions and personality (e.g., optimist/pessimist, introvert/extrovert)
- Self-concept and self-esteem (e.g., positive or negative)

Relational Context (Nature of the Relationship Among Participants)
- Social, helping, or working relationship
- Level of trust among participants
- Level of caring expressed
- Level of self-disclosure among participants
- Shared history of participants
- Balance of power and control

Situational Context (Reason for Communication)
- Information exchange
- Goal achievement
- Problem resolution
- Expression of feelings

Environmental Context (Physical Surroundings in Which Communication Occurs)
- Privacy level
- Noise level
- Comfort and safety level
- Distraction level

Cultural Context (Sociocultural Elements That Affect an Interaction)
- Educational level of participants
- Language and self-expression patterns
- Customs and expectations

Physical and Emotional Factors. It is especially important to assess the psychophysiological factors that influence communication. Many altered health states and human responses limit communication. People with hearing or visual impairments often have difficulty receiving messages (see Chapter 49). Facial trauma, laryngeal cancer, or endotracheal intubation often prevents movement of air past vocal cords or mobility of the tongue, resulting in inability to articulate words. An extremely breathless person needs to use oxygen to breathe rather than speak. People with aphasia after a stroke or in late-stage Alzheimer's disease cannot understand or form words. Some mental illnesses such as psychoses or depression cause patients to jump from one topic to another, constantly verbalizing the same words or phrases or exhibiting a slowed speech pattern. People with high anxiety are sometimes unable to perceive environmental stimuli or hear explanations. Finally patients who are unresponsive or heavily sedated cannot send or respond to verbal messages.

Review of a patient's medical record provides relevant information about his or her ability to communicate. The medical history and physical examination document physical barriers to speech, neurological deficits, and pathophysiology affecting hearing or vision. Reviewing a patient's medication record is also important. For example, opiates, antidepressants, neuroleptics, hypnotics, or sedatives may cause a patient to slur words or use incomplete sentences. The nursing progress notes in the electronic health record (EHR) sometimes reveal other factors that contribute to communication difficulties such as the absence of family members to provide more information about a confused patient.

Assessment includes communicating directly with patients to determine their ability to attend to, interpret, and respond to stimuli. If patients have difficulty communicating, it is important to assess the effect of the problem. Patients who are unable to speak are at risk for injury unless nurses identify an alternate communication method. If barriers exist that make it difficult to communicate directly with patients, family or friends become important sources concerning the patients' communication patterns and abilities.

Developmental Factors. Aspects of a patient's growth and development also influence nurse-patient interaction. For example, an infant's self-expression is limited to crying, body movement, and facial expression; whereas older children express their needs more directly. Adapt communication techniques to the special needs of infants and children and their parents. Depending on a child's age, include the parents, child, or both as sources of information about the child's health. Giving a young child toys or other distractions allows parents to give you their full attention. Children are especially responsive to nonverbal messages; sudden movements, loud noises, or threatening gestures are frightening. They prefer to make the first move in interpersonal contacts and do not like adults to stare or look down at them. A child who has received little environmental stimulation possibly is behind in language development, thus making communication more challenging.

Age alone does not determine an adult's capacity for communication. Hearing loss and visual impairments are changes that may occur during aging that contribute to communication barriers (NIH, 2014). Communicate with older adults on an adult level and avoid patronizing or speaking in a condescending manner. Simple measures facilitate communication with older individuals who have hearing loss (Box 24-7).

Sociocultural Factors. Culture influences thinking, feeling, behaving, and communicating. Be aware of the typical patterns of interaction that characterize various ethnic groups, but do not allow this information to bias your response. Know each patient individually (e.g., does he or she feel comfortable with eye contact or in sharing information with others). You will approach a patient very differently if he or she is open and willing to discuss private family matters versus others who are reluctant to reveal personal or family information to strangers.

Foreign-born people do not always speak or understand English. Those who speak English as a second language often experience difficulty with self-expression or language comprehension. To practice cultural sensitivity in communication, understand that people of different ethnic origins use different degrees of eye contact, personal space, gestures, loud voice, pace of speech, touch, silence, and meaning of language. Make a conscious effort not to interpret messages through your cultural perspective, but consider the communication within the context of the other individual's background. Avoid stereotyping, patronizing, or making fun of other cultures. Language and cultural barriers are not only frustrating but also dangerous, causing delay in care (Box 24-8).

Gender. Gender influences how we think, act, feel, and communicate. Men tend to use less verbal communication but are more likely to initiate communication and address issues more directly. They are also more likely to talk about issues. Women tend to disclose more personal information and use more active listening, answering with responses that encourage the other person to continue the conversation. It is important for you to recognize a patient's gender communication pattern. Being insensitive blocks therapeutic nurse-patient relationships. Assess communication patterns of each individual and

BOX 24-7 FOCUS ON OLDER ADULTS

Tips for Improved Communication with Older Adults Who Have Hearing Loss (Arnold and Boggs, 2011)

- Make sure the patient knows that you are talking.
- Face the patient, be sure that your face/mouth is visible to him or her, and do not chew gum or talk while chewing.
- Speak clearly but do not exaggerate lip movement or shout.
- Speak a little more slowly but not excessively slow.
- Check if patient uses hearing aids, glasses, or other adaptive equipment.
- Choose a quiet, well-lit environment with minimal distractions.
- Allow time for the patient to respond. Do not assume that patient is being uncooperative if he or she does not reply or takes a long time to reply.
- Give the patient a chance to ask questions.
- Keep communication short and to the point. Ask one question at a time.

BOX 24-8 CULTURAL ASPECTS OF CARE

Communication with Non–English-Speaking Patients

Patients who speak little or no English present challenges for nurse-patient communication. Federal and state laws require that hospitals that receive federal funding, including Medicare, Medicaid, and SCHIP, are required to provide language access services for their patients. For hospitals unable to provide onsite interpreters, telephone interpretation services must be available (Marcus, 2014). Use of family members, friends, or bilingual staff members to interpret for patients is strongly discouraged. Sometimes communication with patients is needed in sudden crucial interactions. Use family members or friends cautiously when there is a delay in acquiring interpretive services. Use of family members, children, or auxiliary personnel poses legal liabilities. Language is not the only barrier. Cultural differences also lead to misunderstanding. Developing cultural competence increases understanding (Dossey and Keegan, 2013; Weldon et al., 2014).

Implications for Patient-Centered Care

- Understand your own cultural values and biases.
- Assess the patient's primary language and level of fluency in English.
- Provide a professional interpreter for the patient and health care providers to communicate with one another. Do not use a family member as an interpreter.
- Speak directly to the patient even if an interpreter is present.
- Nodding or statements such as "OK" do not necessarily mean that the patient understands.
- Provide written information in English and primary language.
- Learn about other cultures, especially those commonly encountered in your work area.
- Incorporate the patient's communication methods or need into plan of care.

do not make assumptions simply on the basis of gender, race, sexuality, or cultural differences.

◆ Nursing Diagnosis

Most individuals experience difficulty with some aspect of communication. Patients sometimes lack skills in attending, listening, responding, and self-expression as a result of illness, treatment effects, or cultural or language barriers. The primary nursing diagnostic label used to describe a patient with limited or no ability to communicate verbally is *Impaired Verbal Communication.* This is the state in which an individual experiences a decreased, delayed, or absent ability to receive, process, transmit, and use symbols for a variety of reasons. The defining characteristics for this diagnosis include the inability to articulate words, inappropriate verbalization, difficulty forming words, and difficulty comprehending, which you cluster together to form the diagnosis (Sparks and Taylor, 2014). This diagnosis is useful for a wide variety of patients with special problems and needs related to communication such as impaired perception, reception, and articulation. Although a patient's primary problem is *Impaired Verbal Communication,* the associated difficulty in self-expression or altered communication patterns may also contribute to other nursing diagnoses such as:

- *Anxiety*
- *Social Isolation*
- *Ineffective Coping*
- *Compromised Family Coping*
- *Powerlessness*
- *Impaired Social Interaction*

The related factors for *Impaired Verbal Communication* focus on the causes of a communication disorder. In the case of *Impaired Verbal Communication,* these are physiological, mechanical, anatomical, psychological, cultural, or developmental in nature. Accuracy in identifying related factors is necessary so you select interventions that effectively resolve the diagnostic problem. For example, you manage the diagnosis of *Impaired Verbal Communication related to cultural difference (Hispanic heritage)* very differently than the diagnosis of *Impaired Verbal Communication related to hearing loss.*

◆ Planning

Once you have identified the nature of a patient's communication issues, consider several factors when designing the care plan. Motivation is a factor in improving communication, and patients often require encouragement to try different approaches that involve significant change. It is especially important to involve the patient and family in decisions about the plan of care to determine whether suggested methods are acceptable. Consider ways to meet basic comfort and safety needs before introducing new communication methods and techniques. Allow adequate time for practice. Participants need to be patient with themselves and one another to achieve effective communication. When the focus is on practicing communication, arrange for a quiet, private place that is free of distractions such as television or visitors.

Goals and Outcomes. Once a diagnosis has been identified, select a goal that is relevant and achievable for the patient such as being able to express needs or achieving understanding of physical condition. Next select expected outcomes that are very specific and measurable. Outcomes identify ways to determine if a broader goal is met. For example, outcomes for the patient possibly include the following:

- Patient initiates conversation about diagnosis or health care problem.
- Patient is able to attend to appropriate stimuli.
- Patient conveys clear and understandable messages with health care team.
- Patient expresses increased satisfaction with the communication process.

At times you care for patients whose difficulty in sending, receiving, and interpreting messages interferes with healthy interpersonal relationships. In this case impaired communication is a contributing factor to other nursing diagnoses such as *Impaired Social Interaction* or *Ineffective Coping.* Plan interventions to help these patients improve their communication skills. Expected outcomes for a patient in this situation possibly include demonstrating the ability to appropriately express needs, feelings, and concerns; communicating thoughts and feelings more clearly; engaging in appropriate social conversation with peers and staff; and increasing feelings of autonomy and assertiveness.

Setting Priorities. It is essential to always maintain an open line of communication so a patient is able to express emergent needs or problems. This sometimes involves an intervention as simple as keeping a call light in reach for a patient restricted to bed or providing communication augmentative devices (e.g., message board or Braille computer). When you plan to have lengthy interactions with a patient, it is important to address physical care priorities first so the discussion is not interrupted. Make the patient comfortable by ensuring that any symptoms are under control and elimination needs have been met.

Teamwork and Collaboration. To ensure an effective plan of care, you sometimes need to collaborate with other health care team members who have expertise in communication strategies. Speech language pathologists help patients with aphasia, professional interpreters are necessary for patients who speak a foreign language, and mental health nurse specialists help angry or highly anxious patients to communicate more effectively.

◆ Implementation

In carrying out any plan of care, use communication techniques that are appropriate for a patient's individual needs. Before learning how to adapt communication methods to help patients with serious communication impairments, it is necessary to learn the communication techniques that serve as the foundation for professional communication. It is also important to understand communication techniques that create barriers to effective interaction.

Therapeutic Communication Techniques. Therapeutic communication techniques are specific responses that encourage the expression of feelings and ideas and convey acceptance and respect. These techniques apply in a variety of different situations. Although some of the techniques seem artificial at first, skill and comfort increase with practice. Tremendous satisfaction results from developing therapeutic relationships that achieve desired patient outcomes.

Active Listening. Active listening means being attentive to what a patient is saying both verbally and nonverbally. It facilitates patient communication. Inexperienced nurses sometimes feel the need to talk to prove that they know what they are doing or to decrease anxiety (Stuart, 2013). It is often difficult at first to be quiet and really listen. Active listening enhances trust because you communicate acceptance and respect for a patient. Several nonverbal skills facilitate attentive listening, using the acronym SOLER (Townsend, 2012):

S—Sit facing the patient. This posture conveys the message that you are there to listen and are interested in what the patient is saying.

O—Open position (i.e., keep arms and legs uncrossed). This position suggests that you are "open" to what the patient says. A "closed" position such as crossing arms conveys a defensive attitude, possibly provoking a similar response in the patient.

L—*Lean* toward the patient. This position conveys that you are involved and interested in the interaction.

E—*Eye* contact—Establish and maintain intermittent eye contact to convey your involvement in and willingness to listen to what the patient is saying. Absence of eye contact or shifting the eyes gives the message that you are not interested in what the patient is saying.

R—*Relax*. It is important to communicate a sense of being relaxed and comfortable with the patient. Restlessness communicates a lack of interest and a feeling of discomfort to the patient.

Sharing Observations. Nurses make observations by commenting on how the other person looks, sounds, or acts. Stating observations often helps a patient communicate without the need for extensive questioning, focusing, or clarification. This technique helps start a conversation with quiet or withdrawn persons. Do not state observations that will embarrass or anger a patient such as telling someone, "You look a mess!" Even if you make such an observation with humor, the patient can become resentful.

Sharing observations differs from making assumptions, which means drawing unnecessary conclusions about the other person without validating them. Making assumptions puts a patient in the position of having to contradict you. Examples include interpreting a patient's fatigue as depression or assuming that untouched food indicates lack of interest in meeting nutritional goals. Making observations is a gentler and safer technique: "You look tired …," "You seem different today …," or "I see you haven't eaten anything."

Sharing Empathy. Empathy is the ability to understand and accept another person's reality, accurately perceive feelings, and communicate this understanding to the other. This is a therapeutic communication technique that enables you to understand a patient's situation, feelings, and concerns (Dinkins, 2011). To express empathy you reflect that you understand and feel the importance of the other person's communication. Empathetic understanding requires you to be sensitive and imaginative, especially if you have not had similar experiences. Strive to be empathetic in every situation because it is a key to unlocking concern and communicating support for others. Statements reflecting empathy are highly effective because they tell a person that you heard both the emotional and the factual content of the communication. Empathetic statements are neutral and nonjudgmental and help establish trust in difficult situations. For example, a nurse says to an angry patient who has low mobility after a stroke, "It must be very frustrating to not be able to do what you want."

Sharing Hope. Nurses recognize that hope is essential for healing and learn to communicate a "sense of possibility" to others. Appropriate encouragement and positive feedback are important in fostering hope and self-confidence and for helping people achieve their potential and reach their goals. You give hope by commenting on the positive aspects of the other person's behavior, performance, or response. Sharing a vision of the future and reminding others of their resources and strengths also strengthen hope. Reassure patients that there are many kinds of hope and that meaning and personal growth can come from illness experiences. For example, a nurse says to a patient discouraged about a poor prognosis, "I believe that you'll find a way to face your situation because I've seen your courage and creativity."

Sharing Humor. Humor is an important but often underused resource in nursing interactions. It is a coping strategy that can reduce anxiety and promote positive feelings (Rose et al., 2013). It is a perception and attitude in which a person can experience joy even when facing difficult times. It provides emotional support to patients and professional colleagues and humanizes the illness experience. It enhances teamwork, relieves tension, and helps nurses develop a bond between people who laugh together. Patients use humor to release tension, cope with fear related to pain and suffering, communicate a fear or need, or cope with an uncomfortable or embarrassing situation (Dossey and Keegan, 2013). The goals of using humor as a health care provider are to bring hope and joy to a situation and enhance a patient's well-being and the therapeutic relationship. It makes you seem more warm and approachable (Feagai, 2011). Use humor during the orientation phase to establish a therapeutic relationship and during the working phase as you help a patient cope with a situation.

Today it is common to care for patients from different cultural backgrounds. When you interact with patients be sensitive and realize that they may misunderstand or misinterpret jokes and statements meant to be humorous. It is never appropriate, with any patient, to joke about sexual orientation, race, economic status, disability, or any cultural attribute.

Health care professionals sometimes use a kind of dark, negative humor after difficult or traumatic situations as a way to deal with unbearable tension and stress. This coping humor has a high potential for misinterpretation as uncaring by people not involved in the situation. For example, nursing students are sometimes offended and wonder how staff are able to laugh and joke after unsuccessful resuscitation efforts. When nurses use coping humor within earshot of patients or their loved ones, great emotional distress results.

Sharing Feelings. Emotions are subjective feelings that result from one's thoughts and perceptions. Feelings are not right, wrong, good, or bad, although they are pleasant or unpleasant. If individuals do not express feelings, stress and illness may worsen. Help patients express emotions by making observations, acknowledging feelings, encouraging communication, giving permission to express "negative" feelings, and modeling healthy emotional self-expression. At times patients will direct their anger or frustration prompted by their illness toward you. Do not take such expressions personally. Acknowledging patients' feelings communicates that you listened to and understood the emotional aspects of their illness situation.

When you care for patients, be aware of your own emotions because feelings are difficult to hide. Students sometimes wonder whether it is helpful to share feelings with patients. Sharing emotion makes nurses seem more human and brings people closer. It is appropriate to share feelings of caring or even cry with others, as long as you are in control of the expression of these feelings and express them in a way that does not burden the patient or break confidentiality. Patients are perceptive and sense your emotions. It is usually inappropriate to discuss negative personal emotions such as anger or sadness with patients. A social support system of colleagues is helpful; and employee assistance programs, peer group meetings, and the use of interprofessional teams such as social work and pastoral care provide other means for nurses to safely express feelings away from patients.

Using Touch. Because of modern fast-paced technical environments in health care, nurses face major challenges in bringing the sense of caring and human connection to their patients (see Chapter 7). Touch is one of the most potent and personal forms of communication. It expresses concern or caring to establish a feeling of connection and promote healing (Stuart, 2013). Touch conveys many messages such as affection, emotional support, encouragement, tenderness, and personal attention. Comfort touch such as holding a hand is especially important for vulnerable patients who are experiencing severe illness with its accompanying physical and emotional losses (Figure 24-2).

Students initially may find giving intimate care to be stressful, especially when caring for patients of the opposite gender. They learn to cope with intimate contact by changing their perception of the

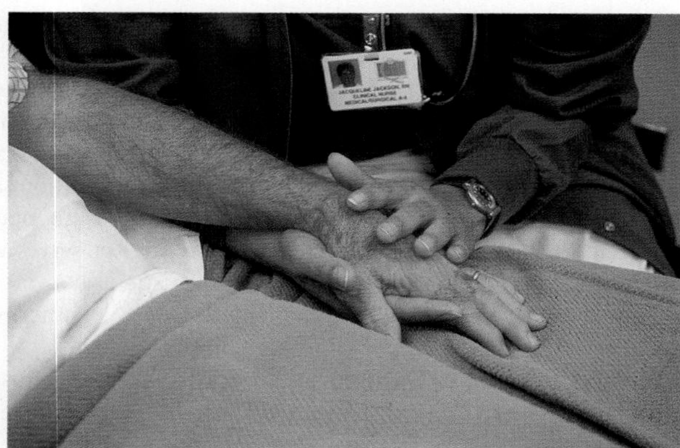

FIGURE 24-2 The nurse uses touch to communicate.

situation. Since much of what nurses do involves touching, you need to learn to be sensitive to others' reactions to touch and use it wisely. It should be as gentle or as firm as needed and delivered in a comforting, nonthreatening manner. Sometimes you withhold touch for highly suspicious or angry persons who respond negatively or even violently to you.

Nurses need to be aware of patients' nonverbal cues and ask permission before touching them to ensure that touch is an acceptable way to provide comfort. Some individuals may be sensitive to physical closeness and uncomfortable with touch. When this is the case, share the information with other nurses who will care for the patient. Nurses should be aware of a patient's concern and act accordingly. A nod, gesture, body position, or eye contact can also convey interest and acceptance of touch, which promotes a bonding moment with a patient (Stuart, 2013).

Using Silence. It takes time and experience to become comfortable with silence. Most people have a natural tendency to fill empty spaces with words, but sometimes these spaces really allow time for a nurse and patient to observe one another, sort out feelings, think about how to say things, and consider what has been communicated. Silence prompts some people to talk. It allows a patient to think and gain insight (Stuart, 2013). In general, allow a patient to break the silence, particularly when he or she has initiated it.

Silence is particularly useful when people are confronted with decisions that require much thought. For example, it helps a patient gain the necessary confidence to share the decision to refuse medical treatment. It also allows the nurse to pay particular attention to nonverbal messages such as worried expressions or loss of eye contact. Remaining silent demonstrates patience and a willingness to wait for a response when the other person is unable to reply quickly. Silence is especially therapeutic during times of profound sadness or grief.

Providing Information. Providing relevant information tells other people what they need or want to know so they are able to make decisions, experience less anxiety, and feel safe and secure. It is also an integral aspect of health teaching (see Chapter 25). It usually is not helpful to hide information from patients, particularly when they seek it. If a health care provider withholds information, the nurse clarifies the reason with him or her. Patients have a right to know about their health status and what is happening in their environment. Information of a distressing nature needs to be communicated with sensitivity, at a pace appropriate to a patient's ability to absorb it, and in general terms at first: "John, your heart sounds have changed from earlier today, and so has your blood pressure. I'll let your doctor know." A nurse provides information that enables others to understand what is happening and what to expect: "Mrs. Evans, John is getting an echocardiogram right now. This test uses painless sound waves to create a moving picture of his heart structures and valves and should tell us what's causing his murmur."

Clarifying. To check whether you understand a message accurately, restate an unclear or ambiguous message to clarify the sender's meaning. In addition, ask the other person to rephrase it, explain further, or give an example of what the person means. Without clarification you may make invalid assumptions and miss valuable information. Despite efforts at paraphrasing, sometimes you do not understand a patient's message. Let the patient know if this is the case: "I'm not sure I understand what you mean by 'sicker than usual.' What is different now?"

Focusing. Focusing involves centering a conversation on key elements or concepts of a message. If conversation is vague or rambling or patients begin to repeat themselves, focusing is a useful technique. Do not use focusing if it interrupts patients while they are discussing important issues. Rather use it to guide the direction of conversation to important areas: "We've talked a lot about your medications; now let's look more closely at the trouble you're having in taking them on time."

Paraphrasing. Paraphrasing is restating another's message more briefly using one's own words. Through paraphrasing you send feedback that lets a patient know that he or she is actively involved in the search for understanding. Accurate paraphrasing requires practice. If the meaning of a message is changed or distorted through paraphrasing, communication becomes ineffective. For example, a patient says, "I've been overweight all my life and never had any problems. I can't understand why I need to be on a diet." Paraphrasing this statement by saying, "You don't care if you're overweight," is incorrect. It is more accurate to say, "You're not convinced that you need a diet because you've stayed healthy."

Validation. This is a technique that nurses use to recognize and acknowledge a patient's thoughts, feelings, and needs. Patients and families know they are being heard and taken seriously when the caregiver addresses their issues (Harvey and Ahmann, 2014). For example, a nurse validates the patient's stated comments by asking, "Tell me if I understand your concerns regarding your surgery. You're worried that you will not be able to return to your usual way of life." This type of statement enables a nurse to convey empathy and interest in the patient's thoughts, feelings, and perceptions.

Asking Relevant Questions. Nurses ask relevant questions to seek information needed for decision making. Ask only one question at a time and fully explore one topic before moving to another area. During patient assessment questions follow a logical sequence and usually proceed from general to more specific. Open-ended questions allow patients to take the conversational lead and introduce pertinent information about a topic. For example, "What's your biggest problem at the moment?" Use focused questions when more specific information is needed in an area: "How has your pain affected your life at home?" Allow patients to respond fully to open-ended questions before asking more-focused questions. Closed-ended questions elicit a yes, no, or one-word response: "How many times a day are you taking pain medication?" Although they are helpful during assessment, they are generally less useful during therapeutic exchanges.

Asking too many questions is sometimes dehumanizing. Seeking factual information does not allow a nurse or patient to establish a meaningful relationship or deal with important emotional issues. It is a way for a nurse to ignore uncomfortable areas in favor of more comfortable, neutral topics. A useful exercise is to try conversing without asking the other person a single question. By using techniques such as giving general leads ("tell me about it …"), making observations, paraphrasing, focusing, and providing information, you discover important information that would have remained hidden if you limited the communication process to questions alone.

Summarizing. Summarizing is a concise review of key aspects of an interaction. It brings a sense of satisfaction and closure to an individual conversation and is especially helpful during the termination phase of a nurse-patient relationship. By reviewing a conversation, participants focus on key issues and add relevant information as needed. Beginning a new interaction by summarizing a previous one helps a patient recall topics discussed and shows him or her that you analyzed their communication. Summarizing also clarifies expectations, as in this example of a nurse manager who has been working with an unsatisfied employee, "You've told me a lot of things about why you don't like this job and how unhappy you've been. We've also come up with some possible ways to make things better, and you've agreed to try some of them and let me know if any help."

Self-Disclosure. Self-disclosures are subjectively true personal experiences about the self that are intentionally revealed to another person. This is not therapy for a nurse; rather it shows a patient that the nurse understands his experiences and that they are not unique. You choose to share experiences or feelings that are similar to those of the patient and emphasize both the similarities and differences. This kind of self-disclosure is indicative of the closeness of the nurse-patient relationship and involves a particular kind of respect for the patient. You offer it as an expression of sincerity and honesty, and it is an aspect of empathy (Stuart, 2013). Self-disclosures need to be relevant and appropriate and made to benefit the patient rather than yourself. Use them sparingly so the patient is the focus of the interaction.

Confrontation. When you confront someone in a therapeutic way, you help the other person become more aware of inconsistencies in his or her feelings, attitudes, beliefs, and behaviors (Stuart, 2013). This technique improves patient self-awareness and helps him or her recognize growth and deal with important issues. Use confrontation only after you have established trust, and do it gently with sensitivity: "You say you've already decided what to do; yet you're still talking a lot about your options."

Nontherapeutic Communication Techniques. Certain communication techniques hinder or damage professional relationships. These specific techniques are referred to as *nontherapeutic* or *blocking* and often cause recipients to activate defenses to avoid being hurt or negatively affected. Nontherapeutic techniques discourage further expression of feelings and ideas and engender negative responses or behaviors in others.

Asking Personal Questions. "Why don't you and John get married?" Asking personal questions that are not relevant to a situation simply to satisfy your curiosity is not appropriate professional communication. Such questions are nosy, invasive, and unnecessary. If patients wish to share private information, they will. To learn more about a patient's interpersonal roles and relationships, ask questions such as: "How would you describe your relationship with John?"

Giving Personal Opinions. "If I were you, I'd put your mother in a nursing home." When a nurse gives a personal opinion, it takes decision making away from the other person. It inhibits spontaneity, stalls problem solving, and creates doubt. Personal opinions differ from professional advice. At times people need suggestions and help to make choices. Suggestions that you present are options; the other person makes the final decision. Remember that the problem and its solution belong to the other person and not to you. A much better response is, "Let's talk about which options are available for your mother's care." The nurse also should not make promises to a patient about situations that require collaboration. For example, "I can't recommend that you stop taking the medications because of your side effects, but I would be happy to inform your primary care provider and ask if a change in medication is appropriate."

Changing the Subject. "Let's not talk about your problems with the insurance company. It's time for your walk." Changing the subject when another person is trying to communicate his or her story is rude and shows a lack of empathy. It blocks further communication, and the sender then withholds important messages or fails to openly express feelings. In some instances changing the subject serves as a face-saving maneuver. If this happens, reassure the patient that you will return to his or her concerns, "After your walk let's talk some more about what's going on with your insurance company."

Automatic Responses. "Older adults are always confused." "Administration doesn't care about the staff." Stereotypes are generalized beliefs held about people. Making stereotyped remarks about others reflects poor nursing judgment and threatens nurse-patient or team relationships. A cliché is a stereotyped comment such as "You can't win them all" that tends to belittle the other person's feelings and minimize the importance of his or her message. These automatic phrases communicate that you are not taking concerns seriously or responding thoughtfully. Another kind of automatic response is parroting (i.e., repeating what the other person has said word for word). Parroting is easily overused and is not as effective as paraphrasing. A simple "oh?" gives you time to think if the other person says something that takes you by surprise.

A nurse who is task oriented automatically makes the task or procedure the entire focus of interaction with patients, missing opportunities to communicate with them as individuals and meet their needs. Task-oriented nurses are often perceived as cold, uncaring, and unapproachable. When students first perform technical skills, it is difficult to integrate therapeutic communication because of the need to focus on the procedure. In time you learn to integrate communication with high-visibility tasks and accomplish several goals simultaneously.

False Reassurance. "Don't worry, everything will be all right." When a patient is seriously ill or distressed, you may be tempted to offer hope to him or her with statements such as "You'll be fine" or "There's nothing to worry about." When a patient is reaching for understanding, false reassurance discourages open communication. Offering reassurance not supported by facts or based in reality does more harm than good. Although you are trying to be kind, it has the secondary effect of helping you avoid the other person's distress, and it tends to block conversation and discourage further expression of feelings. A more facilitative response is, "It must be difficult not to know what the surgeon will find. What can I do to help?"

Sympathy. "I'm so sorry about your mastectomy; you probably feel devastated." Sympathy is concern, sorrow, or pity felt for another person. A nurse often takes on a patient's problems as if they were his or her own. Sympathy is a subjective look at another person's world that prevents a clear perspective of the issues confronting that person. If a nurse over-identifies with a patient, objectivity is lost, and the nurse is not able to help the patient work through the situation (Townsend, 2012). Although sympathy is a compassionate response to another's situation, it is not as therapeutic as empathy. A nurse's own emotional issues sometimes prevent effective problem solving and impair good judgment. A more empathetic approach is: "The loss of a breast is a major change. Do you feel comfortable talking about how it will affect your life?"

Asking for Explanations. "Why are you so anxious?" Some nurses are tempted to ask patients why they believe, feel, or act in a certain way. Patients frequently interpret "why" questions as accusations or think nurses know the reasons and are simply testing them. Regardless of a patient's perception of your motivation, asking "why" questions causes resentment, insecurity, and mistrust. If you need additional information, it is best to phrase a question to avoid using the word "why." For example, "You seem upset. What's on your mind?" is more likely to help an anxious patient communicate.

Approval or Disapproval. "You shouldn't even think about assisted suicide; it's not right." Do not impose your own attitudes, values, beliefs, and moral standards on others while in the professional helping role. Other people have the right to be themselves and make their own decisions. Judgmental responses often contain terms such as *should, ought, good, bad, right,* or *wrong.* Agreeing or disagreeing sends the subtle message that you have the right to make value judgments about patient decisions. Approving implies that the behavior being praised is the only acceptable one. Often a patient shares a decision with you, not in an effort to seek approval but to provide a means to discuss feelings. Disapproval implies that the patient needs to meet your expectations or standards. Instead help patients explore their own beliefs and decisions. The response, "I'm surprised you're considering assisted suicide. Tell me more about it," gives the patient a chance to express ideas or feelings without fear of being judged.

Defensive Responses. "No one here would intentionally lie to you." Becoming defensive in the face of criticism implies that the other person has no right to an opinion. The sender's concerns are ignored when the nurse focuses on the need for self-defense, defense of the health care team, or defense of others. When patients express criticism, listen to what they have to say. Listening does not imply agreement. Listen nonjudgmentally to discover reasons for a patient's anger or dissatisfaction. By avoiding a defensive attitude you are able to defuse anger and uncover deeper concerns, "You believe that people are dishonest with you. It must be hard to trust anyone."

Passive or Aggressive Responses. "Things are bad, and there's nothing I can do about it." "Things are bad, and it's all your fault." Passive responses serve to avoid conflict or sidestep issues. They reflect feelings of sadness, depression, anxiety, powerlessness, and hopelessness. Aggressive responses provoke confrontation at the other person's expense. They reflect feelings of anger, frustration, resentment, and stress. Nurses who lack assertive skills also use triangulation (i.e., complaining to a third party rather than confronting the problem or expressing concerns directly to the source). This lowers team morale and draws others into the conflict situation. Assertive communication is a far more professional approach for a nurse to take.

Arguing. "How can you say you didn't sleep a wink when I heard you snoring all night long?" Challenging or arguing against perceptions denies that they are real and valid. A skillful nurse gives information or presents reality in a way that avoids argument, "You feel like you didn't get any rest at all last night, even though I thought you slept well since I heard you snoring."

Adapting Communication Techniques for the Patient with Special Needs. With our aging population more patients have difficulty communicating. Hearing loss increases with age. Approximately one in three people between the ages 65 and 74 has hearing loss. Vision loss affects communication and presents a challenge for many individuals, particularly over the age of 65. This trend continues to increase. Rates of vision loss are predicted to double by the year 2030 as the population ages (Special Report on Aging, 2013).

Interacting with people who have conditions that impair communication requires special thought and sensitivity. For example, patients who have had a stroke or laryngectomy may require communication aids such as a writing or picture board or a special call system. Such patients benefit greatly when you adapt communication techniques to their unique circumstances, developmental level, or cognitive and sensory deficits. For example, a nurse caring for a patient with *Impaired Verbal Communication related to cognitive impairment* can use several techniques to enable the patient to understand the caregiver. The nurse can use pictures, drawings, or demonstration such as eating behavior to help the patient understand the verbal direction (NIH, 2014).

A nurse directs actions toward meeting the goals and expected outcomes identified in the plan of care, addressing both the communication impairment and its contributing factors. Box 24-9 lists methods available to encourage, enhance, restore, or substitute for verbal communication. Be sure that a patient is physically able to use the chosen method and that it does not cause frustration by being too complicated or difficult. Non-English speaking patients and families need assistance with communication. Interpretation services can be used to better facilitate communication, which improves patient safety and patient outcomes (Weldon et al., 2014).

Because nursing care of the older adult ideally is delivered through an interprofessional model, the primary goal is to establish a reliable communication system that all health care team members can understand easily. Effective communication involves adapting special needs resulting from sensory, motor, or cognitive impairments. Encouraging older adults to share life stories and reminisce about the past has a therapeutic effect and increases their sense of well-being. Avoid sudden shifts from subject to subject. It is helpful to include a patient's family and friends and become familiar with a patient's favorite topics for conversation.

◆ Evaluation

Evaluate the effectiveness of your own communication by videotaping practice sessions with peers or by making process recordings—written records of your verbal and nonverbal interactions with patients. Process recording analysis reveals how to improve personal communication techniques to make them more effective. Box 24-10 contains a sample communication analysis of such a record. Analysis of a process recording enables you to evaluate the following:

- Determine whether you encouraged openness and allowed the patient to "tell his story," expressing both thoughts and feelings.
- Identify any missed verbal or nonverbal cues or conversational themes.
- Examine whether nursing responses facilitated or blocked the patient's efforts to communicate.
- Determine whether nursing responses were positive and supportive or superficial and judgmental.
- Examine the type and number of questions asked.
- Determine the type and number of therapeutic communication techniques used.
- Discover any missed opportunities to use humor, silence, or touch.

Through the Patient's Eyes. You and your patient determine the success of the plan of care by evaluating patient communication outcomes together. You determine which strategies or interventions were effective and which patient changes (behaviors or perceptions) resulted because of the interventions. Ask the patient if you and other members of the interprofessional health care team met his or her expectations. For example, does the patient believe that nurses responded in a timely way when the call light was turned on? Does the patient feel able to express his needs clearly? Is the patient satisfied with the information that has been provided about his condition or hospitalization? Successful nursing care related to patients' communication needs results in clear and effective communication between patients and all members of the health care team and can favorably impact patient satisfaction and the delivery of safe care.

BOX 24-9 Communicating with Patients Who Have Special Needs

Patients Who Cannot Speak Clearly (Aphasia, Dysarthria, Muteness)

- Listen attentively, be patient, and do not interrupt.
- Ask simple questions that require "yes" or "no" answers.
- Allow time for understanding and response.
- Use visual cues (e.g., words, pictures, and objects) when possible.
- Allow only one person to speak at a time.
- Encourage patient to converse.
- Let patient know if you have not understood him or her.
- Collaborate with speech therapist as needed.
- Use communication aids: letter boards, flash cards, computer-generated speech program),

Patients Who Are Cognitively Impaired

- Use simple sentences and avoid long explanations.
- Ask one question at a time.
- Allow time for patient to respond.
- Be an attentive listener.
- Include family and friends in conversations, especially in subjects known to patient.
- Use picture or gestures that mimic the action desired.

Patients Who Are Hearing Impaired

- Check for hearing aids and glasses.
- Reduce environmental noise.
- Get patient's attention before speaking.
- Face patient with mouth visible.
- Do not chew gum.
- Speak at normal volume—do not shout.
- Rephrase rather than repeat if misunderstood.
- Provide a sign-language interpreter if indicated.

Patients Who Are Visually Impaired

- Check for use of glasses or contact lenses.
- Identify yourself when you enter room and notify patient when you leave room.
- Speak in a normal tone of voice.
- Do not rely on gestures or nonverbal communication.
- Use indirect lighting, avoiding glare.
- Use at least 14-point print.

Patients Who Are Unresponsive

- Call patient by name during interactions.
- Communicate both verbally and by touch.
- Speak to patient as though he or she can hear.
- Explain all procedures and sensations.
- Provide orientation to person, place, and time.
- Avoid talking about patient to others in his or her presence.

Patients Who Do Not Speak English

- Speak to patient in normal tone of voice.
- Establish method for patient to ask for assistance (call light or bell).
- Provide a professional interpreter as needed.
- Avoid using family members, especially children, as interpreters.
- Use communication board, pictures, or cards.
- Translate words from native language into English list for patient to make basic requests.
- Have dictionary (e.g., English/Spanish) available if patient can read.

BOX 24-10 Sample Communication Analysis

Nurse: Good morning, Mr. Simpson."
(Smiles, approaches bed holding clipboard)
Acknowledged by name, social greeting to begin conversation
Patient: "What's good about it?"
(Arms crossed over chest, frowning, direct stare)
Nonverbal signs of anger
Nurse: "You sound unhappy."
(Pulls up chair and sits at bedside)
Sharing observation, nonverbal communication of availability
Patient: "You'd be unhappy, too, if nobody would answer your questions. That girl wouldn't tell me my blood sugar."
(Angry voice tone, challenging expression)
Further expression of feelings facilitated by nurse making accurate observation
Nurse: "This hospital has a fine staff, Mr. Simpson. I'm sure no one would intentionally keep information from you."
Feeling threatened and being defensive, a nontherapeutic technique
Nurse: "I'm going to test your glucose in a minute, and I'll tell you the results."
(Does test) "Your blood sugar was 350."
Providing information, demonstrating trustworthiness
Patient: "I'm so afraid complications will set in since my blood sugar is high."
(Stares out window)
Feels free to express deeper concerns, but they are hard to face
Nurse: "What kinds of things are you worried about?"
Open-ended question to seek information
Patient: "I could lose a leg, like my mother did, or go blind or have to live hooked up to a kidney machine for the rest of my life.
Nurse: "You've been thinking about all kinds of things that could go wrong, and it adds to your worry not to be told what your blood sugar is."
Summarizing to let patient "hear" what he has communicated
Patient: "I always think the worst."
(Shakes head in exasperation)
Expressing insight into his "inner dialogue"
Nurse: "I'll pass along to the technician that it's OK to tell you your glucose levels. And later this afternoon I'd like us to talk more about some things you can do to help avoid these complications and set some goals for controlling your glucose."
Providing information, encouraging collaboration and goal setting

Patient Outcomes. If expected outcomes for the patient's plan of care are not met or if progress is not satisfactory, you determine which factors influenced the outcomes and modify the plan of care. If your evaluation data indicate that a patient perceives difficulty in communicating, you explore contributing factors so they can be addressed. For example, if using a pen and paper is frustrating for a nonverbal patient whose handwriting is shaky, you revise the care plan to include use of a picture board instead. Possible questions you ask when a patient does not meet expected outcomes include:

- You seem to be having difficulty communicating right now. What do you think is contributing to this?
- You're telling me that you don't feel anxious right now, but your face appears tense. Help me better understand how you're feeling right now.
- You seem frustrated with the use of pencil and paper to communicate. Would you like to try a letter board or a picture board and see if either of these is easier for you to use?

Evaluation of the communication process helps nurses gain confidence and competence in interpersonal skills. Becoming an effective communicator greatly increases your professional satisfaction and success. There is no skill more basic, no tool more powerful.

KEY POINTS

- Communication is a powerful therapeutic tool and an essential nursing skill that influences others and achieves positive health outcomes.
- Effective interprofessional communication is essential to provide safe transitions in care.
- Effective team communication and collaboration skills are necessary to ensure safe patient care.
- Critical thinking and critical reasoning skills promote more effective communication and patient assessment.
- Communication is most effective when the receiver and sender accurately perceive the meaning of one another's messages via feedback loops and validation.
- The sender and receiver's physical and developmental status, perceptions, values, emotions, knowledge, sociocultural background, roles, and environment all influence message transmission.
- Effective verbal communication requires appropriate intonation, clear and concise phrasing, proper pacing of statements, and proper timing and relevance of a message.
- Effective nonverbal communication complements and strengthens the message conveyed by verbal communication.
- Nurses use intrapersonal, interpersonal, small-group, electronic communication and public interaction to achieve positive change and health goals.
- Nurses strengthen caring relationships by establishing trust, empathy, autonomy, confidentiality, and professional competence.
- Effective communication techniques are facilitative and tend to encourage the other person to openly express ideas, feelings, or concerns.
- Ineffective communication techniques are inhibiting and tend to block the other person's willingness to openly express ideas, feelings, or concerns.
- Blend social and informational interactions with therapeutic communication techniques to help your patients explore feelings and manage health issues.
- Older adults with sensory, motor, or cognitive impairments require the adaptation of communication techniques to compensate for their loss of function and special needs.
- Lateral violence can be a symptom of compassion fatigue, leading to nurse dissatisfaction and decreased sense of value. This interferes with team communication and jeopardizes patient safety.
- Assessment and communication techniques such as MI and EI assessment enable a nurse to better understand and motivate patients toward more positive health practices.

CLINICAL APPLICATION QUESTIONS

Preparing for Clinical Practice

Mr. Simpson is a 78-year-old patient whose wife died last year. He has been living alone. He has limited cooking skills; thus he eats out a lot. Since his wife died, his blood sugar has been poorly controlled. To help Mr. Simpson gain better blood sugar control, the dietitian came to see him. After she left, Mr. Simpson was angry and stated his desire to leave the hospital right now. He stated, "That diet person came to see me, and she doesn't know anything."

1. How would you approach Mr. Simpson? Which communication techniques would you use and which would you avoid?
2. You talk with the dietitian and learn that she gave the patient information about his diet and recipes that he could try. As you talk further with Mr. Simpson, you learn that the physician told him he might not be able to live alone anymore. You realize that he doesn't know how to cook. Knowing this, how would you respond to him?
3. After talking with Mr. Simpson, you determine that he is able to care for himself at home but will need some assistance. He is willing to consider various options for meal preparation. You call the physician to discuss this. Your hospital has established SBAR (Situation-Background-Assessment-Recommendation) as a standard communication tool. How do you effectively communicate your concerns and the patient's need to the physician using SBAR?

ⓔ ***Answers to Clinical Application Questions can be found on the Evolve website.***

REVIEW QUESTIONS

Are You Ready to Test Your Nursing Knowledge?

1. When working with an older adult who is hearing-impaired, the use of which techniques would improve communication? (Select all that apply.)
   1. Check for needed adaptive equipment.
   2. Exaggerate lip movements to help the patient lip read.
   3. Give the patient time to respond to questions.
   4. Keep communication short and to the point.
   5. Communicate only through written information.
2. Nurses must communicate effectively with the health care team for which of the following reasons? (Select all that apply.)
   1. Improve the nurse's status with the health team members
   2. Reduce the risk of errors to the patient
   3. Provide optimum level of patient care
   4. Improve patient outcomes
   5. Prevent issues that need to be reported to outside agencies
3. A new nurse complains to her preceptor that she has no time for therapeutic communication with her patients. Which of the following is the best strategy to help the nurse find more time for this communication?
   1. Include communication while performing tasks such as changing dressings and checking vital signs.
   2. Ask the patient if you can talk during the last few minutes of visiting hours.
   3. Ask Pastoral care to come back a little later in the day.
   4. Remind the nurse to complete all her tasks and then set up remaining time for communication.
4. Motivational interviewing (MI) is a technique that applies understanding a patient's values and goals in helping the patient make behavior changes. What are other benefits of using MI techniques? (Select all that apply.)
   1. Gaining an understanding of patient's motivations
   2. Focusing on opportunities to avoid poor health choices
   3. Recognizing patient's strengths and supporting their efforts
   4. Providing assessment data that can be shared with families to promote change
   5. Identifying differences in patient's health goals and current behaviors
5. A nurse is talking with a young-adult patient about the purpose of a new medication. The nurse says, "I want to be clear. Can you tell me in your words the purpose of this medicine?" This exchange

is an example of which element of the transactional communication process?
1. Message
2. Obtaining feedback
3. Channel
4. Referent

6. A patient who is Spanish-speaking does not appear to understand the nurse's information on wound care. Which action should the nurse take?
1. Arrange for a Spanish-speaking social worker to explain the procedure
2. Ask a fellow Spanish-speaking patient to help explain the procedure
3. Use a professional interpreter to provide wound care education in Spanish
4. Ask the patient to write down questions that he or she has for the nurse

7. A nurse prepares to contact a patient's physician about a change in the patient's condition. Put the following statements in the correct order using SBAR (Situation, Background, Assessment, and Recommendation) communication.
1. "She is a 53-year-old female who was admitted 2 days ago with pneumonia and was started on Levaquin at 5 PM yesterday. She complains of a poor appetite."
2. "The patient reported feeling very nauseated after her dose of Levaquin an hour ago."
3. "Would you like to make a change in antibiotics, or could we give her a nutritional supplement before her medication?"
4. "The patient started complaining of nausea yesterday evening and has vomited several times during the night."

8. A nurse is assigned to care for a patient for the first time and states, "I don't know a lot about your culture and want to learn how to better meet your health care needs." Which therapeutic communication technique did the nurse use in this situation?
1. Validation
2. Empathy
3. Sarcasm
4. Humility

9. A new nurse is experiencing lateral violence at work. Which steps could the nurse take to address this problem?
1. Challenge the nurses in a public forum to embarrass them and change their behavior
2. Talk with the department secretary and ask if this has been a problem for other nurses
3. Talk with the preceptor or manager and ask for assistance in handling this issue
4. Say nothing and hope things get better

10. A nurse has been gathering physical assessment data on a patient and is now listening to the patient's concerns. The nurse sets a goal of care that incorporates the patient's desire to make treatment decisions. This is an example of the nurse engaged in which phase of the nurse-patient relationship?
1. Working phase
2. Preinteraction phase
3. Termination phase
4. Orientation phase

11. A patient is evaluated in the emergency department after causing an automobile accident while being under the influence of alcohol. While assessing the patient, which statement would be the most therapeutic?
1. "Why did you drive after you had been drinking?"
2. "We have multiple patients to see tonight as a result of this accident."
3. "Tell me what happened before, during, and after the automobile accident tonight."
4. "It will be okay. No one was seriously hurt in the accident."

12. A nursing student is reviewing a process recording with the instructor. The student engaged the patient in a discussion about availability of family members to provide support at home once the patient is discharged. The student reviews with the instructor whether the comments used encouraged openness and allowed the patient to "tell his story." This is an example of which step of the nursing process?
1. Planning
2. Assessment
3. Intervention
4. Evaluation

13. Which strategies should a nurse use to facilitate a safe transition of care during a patient's transfer from the hospital to a skilled nursing facility? (Select all that apply.)
1. Collaboration between staff members from sending and receiving departments
2. Requiring that the patient visit the facility before a transfer is arranged
3. Using a standardized transfer policy and transfer tool
4. Arranging all patient transfers during the same time each day
5. Relying on family members to share information with the new facility

14. A nurse is explaining to a patient how to follow infection control practices at home. During the discussion the nurse touches the patient on the shoulder. Explain which zone of touch the nurse should be practicing and what problems the action might cause.

15. The nurse uses silence as a therapeutic communication technique. What is the purpose of the nurse's silence? (Select all that apply.)
1. Prevent the nurse from saying the wrong thing
2. Prompt the patient to talk when he or she is ready
3. Allow the patient time to think and gain insight
4. Allow time for the patient to drift off to sleep
5. Determine if the patient would prefer to talk with another staff member

Answers: 1. 1, 3, 4; **2.** 2, 3, 4; **3.** 1; **4.** 1, 3, 5; **5.** 2; **6.** 3; **7.** 4S, 1B, 2A, 3R; **8.** 4; **9.** 3; **10.** 1; **11.** 3; **12.** 4; **13.** 1, 3; **14.** See Evolve; **15.** 2, 3.

Rationales to Review Questions can be found on the Evolve website.

REFERENCES

Arnold E, Boggs KU: *Interpersonal relationships: professional communication skills for nurses*, ed 6, St Louis, 2011, Saunders.

Dinkins CS: Ethics: Beyond patient care: practicing empathy in the workplace, *Online J Issues Nurs* 16(2):11, 2011.

Dossey BM, Keegan L: *Wholistic nursing: a handbook for practice*, ed 6, Burlington, 2013, Jones & Bartlett Learning.

Facchiano L, Snyder C: Challenges surrounding provider/client electronic-mail communication, *J Nurse Pract* 7(4):309, 2011.

Feagai HE: Let humor lead your nursing practice, *Nurse Leader* 9(4):44, 2011.

Fox M: Putting emotional intelligence to work, *J Acad Nutr Diet* 113(9):1138, 2013.

Frederick D: Bullying, mentoring and patient care, *AORN J* 99(5):587, 2014.

Harvey P, Ahmann E: Validation: a family-centered communication skill, *Pediatr Nurs* 40(3):143, 2014.

Issacson M: Clarifying concepts: cultural humility or competency, *J Prof Nurs* 30(3):251, 2014.

Lang EV: *A better patient experience through better communication: association or radiologic and imaging nursing*, 2012, http://dx.dol.org f/10.1016/j.jradnu.2012.08.001. Accessed August 16, 2014.

Marcus V: *Are hospitals required to provide language access services?* NWI Global, August 2014, http://www.nwiglobal.com/blog/hospitals-required-provide-language-access-services/. Accessed January 31, 2015.

Marquis BL, Huston CJ: *Leadership roles and management functions in nursing: theory and application*, ed 8, Philadelphia, 2015, LWW.

Moore CD, Reynolds AM: Clinical update: communication issues and advance care planning, *Semin Oncol Nurs* 29(4):e1, 2013.

National Institutes of Health (NIH): *Hearing loss and older adults*, NIH Publication No. 13(4913), 2013, updated 2014.

Rodriguez ES: Using a patient portal for electronic communication with patients with cancer: implications for nurses, *Oncol Nurs Forum* 37(6):667, 2010.

Rubin R: *AIDET® in the medical practice: more important than ever*, 2014, https://www.studergroup.com/resources/news-media/healthcare-publications-resources/insights/november-2014/aidet-in-the-medical-practice-more-important-than. Accessed August 30, 2015.

Ryan LA: *The journey to integrate Watson's caring theory with clinical practice*, 2005, http://watsoncaringscience.org/files/PDF/JourneytoIntegrate.pdf. Accessed January 31, 2015.

Shanta LL, Connolly M: Using King's interacting systems theory to link emotional intelligence with nursing practice, *J Prof Nurs* 29(3):174, 2013.

Sparks RS, Taylor CM: *Nursing diagnosis reference manual*, ed 9, Philadelphia, 2014, Wolters Kluwer Health/Lippincott-Williams & Wilkins.

Special report on aging and vision loss—American Foundation for the Blind, January 2013, http://www.afb.org/info/blindness-statistics/special-report-on-aging-and-vision-loss/25. Accessed January 29, 2015.

Stawnychy M, et al: Using brief motivational interviewing to address the complex needs of a challenging patient with heart failure, *J Cardiovasc Nurs* 29(5):E1, Wolters Kluwer Health/Lippincott Williams & Williams, 2014.

Stuart GW: *Principles and practice of psychiatric nursing*, ed 10, St Louis, 2013, Mosby.

The Joint Commission (TJC): *R3 Report Issue 1: Patient-centered communication*, Issue 1, February 2011, http://www.jointcommission.org/topics/default.aspx?k=898&b=. Accessed December 23, 2014.

The Joint Commission (TJC) Resources: *transitions of care: the need for more effective approach to continuing patient care*, June 2012, http://www.jointcommission.org/hot_topics_toc/. Accessed January 31, 2015.

Townsend MC: *Psychiatric mental health nursing: concepts of care*, ed 7, Philadelphia, 2012, FA Davis.

Watson J: *Nursing: human science and health care*, Norwalk, Conn, 1985, Appleton-Century-Crofts.

Weldon JM, et al: Special needs populations: overcoming language barriers for pediatric surgical patients and their family members, *AORN J* 99(5):616, 2014.

RESEARCH REFERENCES

Adams J, Osborne-McKenzie T: Advancing the evidence base for standardized provider handover structure: using staff nurse descriptions of information needed to deliver competent care, *J Contin Educ Nurs* 43(6):261, 2012.

Compton J, et al: Implementing SBAR across a large multihospital health system, *Jt Comm J Qual Patient Saf* 38(6):261, 2012.

Copeland L, et al: Mechanisms of change within motivational interviewing in relation to health behavior outcomes: a systematic review, *Patient Educ Couns* 98(4):401, 2015.

De Meester K, et al: SBAR improves nurse-physician communication and reduces unexpected death: a pre and post intervention study, *Resuscitation* 84(9):1192, 2013.

Ford Y, et al: Patients' perceptions of bedside handoff: the need for a culture of always, *J Nurs Care Qual* 29(4):1, 2014.

Gidman J: Listening to stories: valuing knowledge from patient experience, *Nurse Educ Pract* 13(3):192, 2013.

Haig KM, et al: SBAR: a shared mental model for improving communication between clinicians, *Jt Comm J Qual Patient Saf* 32(3):167, 2006.

Johnson K, et al: An evidence-based approach to creating a new nursing dress code, *Am Nurse Today* 3(1):2008. http://www.americannursetoday.com/an-evidence-based-approach-to-creating-a-new-nursing-dress-code/. Accessed January 31, 2015.

Lazure P, et al: Communication-the foundation for collaborative relationships amongst providers and between providers and patients: a case in breast and colorectal cancer, *J Commun Healthc* 7(1):41, 2014.

Rose SL, et al: The use of humor in patients with recurrent ovarian cancer: a phenomenological study, *Int J Gynecol Cancer* 23(4):775, 2013.

25

Patient Education

OBJECTIVES

- Identify the appropriate topics that address a patient's health education needs.
- Describe the similarities and differences between teaching and learning.
- Identify the role of the nurse in patient education.
- Identify the purposes of patient education.
- Describe appropriate communication principles when providing patient education.
- Describe the domains of learning.
- Identify basic learning principles.
- Discuss how to integrate education into patient-centered care.
- Differentiate factors that determine readiness to learn from those that determine ability to learn.
- Compare and contrast the nursing and teaching process.
- Write learning objectives for a teaching plan.
- Establish an environment that promotes learning.
- Include patient teaching while performing routine nursing care.
- Use appropriate methods to evaluate learning.

KEY TERMS

Affective learning, p. 339
Analogies, p. 349
Cognitive learning, p. 339
Functional illiteracy, p. 345
Health literacy, p. 344
Learning, p. 337
Learning objective, p. 338
Motivation, p. 340
Psychomotor learning, p. 339
Reinforcement, p. 348
Return demonstration, p. 349
Self-efficacy, p. 340
Teach Back, p. 351
Teaching, p. 337

MEDIA RESOURCES

http://evolve.elsevier.com/Potter/fundamentals/

- Review Questions
- Case Study with Questions
- Audio Glossary
- Content Updates

Patient education is one of the most important nursing interventions in any health care setting. Shorter hospital stays, increased demands on nurses' time, increase in the number of chronically ill patients, and the need to give acutely ill patients meaningful information quickly emphasize the importance of quality patient education. As nurses try to find the best way to educate patients, the general public has become more assertive in seeking knowledge, understanding health, and finding resources available within the health care system. Nurses provide patients with information needed for self-management of acute and chronic conditions to ensure continuity of care from the hospital to the home (Lorig et al., 2013; Falvo, 2011). Part of the patient education process is designing patient-centered action plans, which are an essential component of chronic disease self-management and are associated with improved health outcomes (Lorig et al., 2014a; 2014b).

Patients have the right to know and be informed about their diagnoses, prognoses, and available treatments to help them make intelligent, informed decisions about their health and lifestyle. Part of patient-centered care is to integrate educational approaches that acknowledge patients' understanding of their own health. The goals of a well-designed, comprehensive teaching plan include providing a good fit with each patient's unique learning needs, reducing health care costs, improving quality of care, and ultimately changing behaviors to improve patient outcomes. In due course this helps patients make informed decisions about their care and become healthier and more independent (Edelman et al., 2014; Friedman et al., 2011).

STANDARDS FOR PATIENT EDUCATION

Patient education has long been a standard for professional nursing practice. All state Nurse Practice Acts recognize that patient teaching falls within the scope of nursing practice (Bastable, 2014). In addition, various accrediting agencies set guidelines for providing patient education in health care institutions. For example, The Joint Commission (TJC, 2015a) sets standards for patient and family education. These standards require nurses and all health care providers to assess patients' learning needs and provide education on a variety of topics, including medications, nutrition, use of medical equipment, pain management, and the patient's plan of care. Successful fulfillment of the standards requires collaboration among health care professionals and enhances patient safety. Ensure that your educational efforts are patient centered by taking into consideration your patients' own education and experience; their desire to actively participate in the educational process; and their psychosocial, spiritual, and cultural values. It is important to document patient education interventions and a patient's response to teaching in the medical record. Standards such as these help to direct patient education and ensure best possible outcomes.

PURPOSES OF PATIENT EDUCATION

The goal of educating others about their health is to help individuals, families, or communities achieve optimal levels of health (Edelman et al., 2014). Patient education is an essential component of providing safe, patient-centered care (QSEN, 2014). In addition, providing education about preventive health care helps reduce health care costs and hardships on individuals and those surrounding them. Patients now know more about health and want to be actively involved in their health maintenance. Comprehensive patient education includes three important purposes, each involving a separate phase of health care: health promotion and illness prevention, health restoration, and coping.

Maintenance and Promotion of Health and Illness Prevention

As a nurse you are a visible, competent resource for patients who want to improve their physical and psychological well-being. In the school, home, clinic, or workplace you provide information and skills to help patients adopt healthier behaviors. For example, in childbearing classes you teach expectant parents about physical and psychological changes in a woman. After learning about normal childbearing, the mother who applies new knowledge is more likely to eat healthy foods, engage in physical exercise, and avoid substances that can harm the fetus. Promoting healthy behavior through education allows patients to assume more responsibility for their own health (Thom et al., 2013). Greater knowledge results in better health maintenance habits. In addition, when patients become more health conscious, they are more likely to seek early diagnosis of health problems (Hawkins et al., 2011).

Restoration of Health

Injured or ill patients need information and skills to help them regain or maintain their levels of health. Patients recovering from and adapting to changes resulting from illness or injury often seek information about their conditions. However, some patients find it difficult to adapt to illness and become passive and disinterested in learning. As the nurse you learn to identify patients' willingness to learn and motivate interest in learning (Bastable, 2014). The family often is a vital part of a patient's return to health. Family caregivers usually require as much education as the patient, including information on how to perform skills within the home. If you exclude a family from a teaching plan, conflicts can occur. However, do not assume that a family should be involved; assess the patient-family relationship before providing education for family caregivers.

Coping with Impaired Functions

Not all patients fully recover from illness or injury. In addition, patients with preexisting mental illness are also challenged during recovery (Lorig et al., 2014b). Many have to learn to cope with permanent health alterations. New knowledge and skills are often necessary for patients to continue activities of daily living. For example, a patient loses the ability to speak after larynx surgery and has to learn new ways of communicating. Changes in function are physical or psychosocial. In the case of serious disability such as following a stroke or a spinal cord injury, the patient's family needs to understand and accept many changes in his or her physical capabilities. The family's ability to provide support results in part from education, which begins as soon as you identify the patient's needs and the family displays a willingness to help. Teach family members to help the patient with health care management (e.g., giving medications through gastric tubes and doing passive range-of-motion exercises). Families of patients with alterations such as alcoholism, mental retardation, or drug dependence learn to adapt to the emotional effects of these chronic conditions and provide psychosocial support to facilitate the patient's health. Comparing the desired level of health with the actual state of health enables you to plan effective teaching programs.

TEACHING AND LEARNING

It is impossible to separate teaching from learning. **Teaching** is the concept of imparting knowledge through a series of directed activities. It consists of a conscious, deliberate set of actions that help individuals gain new knowledge, change attitudes, adopt new behaviors, or perform new skills (Billings and Halstead, 2012). An educator needs to be knowledgeable about the subject matter and patient teaching principles in order to provide individuals with guidance, appropriately set the learning pace, and creatively introduce concepts to successfully achieve the desired learning objectives.

Learning is the purposeful acquisition of new knowledge, attitudes, behaviors, and skills through an experience or external stimulus (Bastable, 2014). It is a process of both understanding and applying newly acquired concepts. A new mother exhibits learning when she demonstrates how to bathe her newborn. The mother shows transfer of learning when she uses the principles she learned about bathing a newborn when she bathes her older child. Teaching and learning generally begin when a person identifies a need for knowing or acquiring an ability to do something. Teaching is most effective when it responds to the learner's needs. An educator assesses these needs by asking questions and determining a learner's interests. Interpersonal communication is essential for successful teaching to occur (see Chapter 24).

Role of the Nurse in Teaching and Learning

Nurses have an ethical responsibility to teach their patients (Heiskell, 2010). In The Patient Care Partnership, the American Hospital Association (2003) indicates that patients have the right to make informed decisions about their care. The information required to make informed decisions must be accurate, complete, and relevant to patients' needs, language, and literacy.

The Joint Commission's Speak Up Initiatives helps patients understand their rights when receiving medical care (TJC, 2015b). The assumption is that patients who ask questions and are aware of their rights have a greater chance of getting the care they need when they need it. The program offers the following Speak Up tips to help patients become more involved in their treatment:

- *S*peak up if you have questions or concerns. If you still do not understand, ask again. It is your body, and you have a right to know.
- *P*ay attention to the care you get. Always make sure that you are getting the right treatments and medicines by the right health care professionals. Do not assume anything.
- *E*ducate yourself about your illness. Learn about the medical tests that are prescribed and your treatment plan.
- *A*sk a trusted family member or friend to be your advocate (advisor or supporter).
- *K*now which medicines you take and why you take them. Medication errors are the most common health care mistakes.
- *U*se a hospital, clinic, surgery center, or other type of health care organization that has been checked out carefully. For example, TJC visits hospitals to see if they are meeting TJC quality standards.
- *P*articipate in all decisions about your treatment. You are the center of the health care team.

In addition, patients are advised that they have a right to be informed about the care they will receive, obtain information about care in their preferred language, know the names of their caregivers, receive treatment for pain, receive an up-to-date list of current medications, and expect that they will be heard and treated with respect.

Teach information that patients and their families need. You frequently clarify information provided by health care providers and are the primary source of information that patients need to adjust to health problems (Bastable, 2014). However, it is also important to understand patients' preferences for what they wish to learn. For example, a patient requests information about a new medication, or family members question the reason for their mother's pain. Identifying the need for teaching is easy when patients request information. However, a patient's need for teaching is often less obvious. To be an effective educator, the nurse has to do more than just pass on facts. Carefully determine what patients need to know and find the time to educate them when they are ready to learn. When you value and provide education, patients are better prepared to assume health care responsibilities. Nursing research about patient education supports the positive impact of patient education on patient outcomes (Box 25-1).

Teaching as Communication

The teaching process closely parallels the communication process (see Chapter 24). Effective teaching depends in part on effective interpersonal communication. An educator applies each element of the communication process while providing information to learners. Thus the educator and learner become involved together in a teaching process that increases the learner's knowledge and skills.

The steps of the teaching process are similar to those of the communication process. You use patient requests for information or perceive a need for information because of a patient's health restrictions or the recent diagnosis of an illness. Then you identify specific **learning objectives** to describe the behaviors the learner will exhibit as a result of successful instruction (Bastable, 2014).

The nurse is the sender who conveys a message to the patient. Many intrapersonal variables influence your style and approach. Attitudes, values, emotions, cultural perspective, and knowledge influence the way information is delivered. Past experiences with teaching are also helpful for choosing the best way to present necessary content.

The receiver in the teaching-learning process is the learner. A number of intrapersonal variables affect motivation and ability to learn. Patients are ready to learn when they express a desire to do so and are more likely to receive your message when they understand the content. Attitudes, anxiety, and values influence the ability to understand a message. The ability to learn depends on factors such as emotional and physical health, education, cultural perspective, patients' values about their health, the stage of development, and previous knowledge.

Effective communication involves feedback. An effective educator provides a mechanism for evaluating the success of a teaching plan and then provides positive reinforcement (Bastable, 2014). This type of response reinforces health behavior and promotes continued self-management. You need to provide feedback both during and at the completion of each instructional encounter. Feedback needs to demonstrate the success of the learner in achieving objectives (i.e., the learner verbalizes information or provides a return demonstration of skills learned). Feedback you receive from the learner is equally important because it indicates the effectiveness of instruction and whether or not you need to modify your approach.

DOMAINS OF LEARNING

Learning occurs in three domains: cognitive (understanding), affective (attitudes), and psychomotor (motor skills) (Bastable, 2014). Health topics involve one or all domains or any combination of the three. You often work with patients who need to learn in each domain. For example, patients diagnosed with diabetes need to learn how diabetes affects the body and how to control blood glucose levels for healthier lifestyles (cognitive domain). In addition, patients begin to accept the chronic nature of diabetes by learning positive coping mechanisms (affective domain). Finally many patients living with diabetes learn to test their blood glucose levels at home. This requires learning how to use a glucose meter (psychomotor domain). The characteristics of learning within each domain influence your teaching and evaluation methods. Understanding each learning domain prepares you to select proper teaching techniques and apply the basic principles of learning (Box 25-2).

BOX 25-1 EVIDENCE-BASED PRACTICE

The Effectiveness of Individualized Patient Education in Self-Management of Diabetes

PICO Question: In patients with poorly controlled diabetes, does individualized patient education result in better glucose control compared with patients who participate in group education and those who receive no assigned education?

Evidence Summary

As of 2012, 29.1 million people in the world have diabetes (CDC, 2014). The majority of these people do not receive any formal diabetes education. Diabetes self-management education (DSME) is an essential element of care for people with diabetes to gain the knowledge necessary to manage the disease and prevent many of its potential complications (Haas et al., 2013). Although there are many approaches to diabetes education, little literature is available that supports one model over another, and systematic reviews on DSME have rated its quality as moderate to poor. Research that compared individual education (IE) to group education (GE) and usual care (no assigned education) found that participants who received IE resulted in better glucose control outcomes and more improved psychosocial and behavioral outcomes than did those assigned to group education or usual care (Sperl-Hillen et al., 2011). Quality DSME curricula contain the following seven components: physical activity, healthy eating, taking medications, monitoring blood glucose, problem solving, risk reduction, and healthy coping. However, to be successful it is necessary that content be tailored to match the specific needs of an individual and modified on the basis of the patient's medical history, age, cultural background, literacy level, support system, and financial status. Nurses who account for these variables when creating a new educational program will deliver content that is more relevant and engaging and can lead to improved patient outcomes (Haas et al., 2013; Sperl-Hillen et al., 2011).

Application to Nursing Practice

- Individuals with poorly controlled diabetes who receive IE often experience better patient outcomes, including improved overall blood glucose control, improved physical activity and nutrition scores, and greater patient satisfaction.
- The process of DSME needs to be patient centered and address the entire range of each participant's personal profile and medical history.
- Work with your patients to create a personalized agenda and select discussion topics that align with individual goals and values.
- You need to ensure that all information and educational materials are delivered at an appropriate literacy level and make use of interpreters when necessary.

BOX 25-2 Appropriate Teaching Methods Based on Domains of Learning

Cognitive
- Discussion (one-on-one or group)
  - Involves nurse and one patient or a nurse with several patients
  - Promotes active participation and focuses on topics of interest to patient
  - Allows peer support
  - Enhances application and analysis of new information
- Lecture
  - Is more formal method of instruction because it is educator controlled
  - Helps learner acquire new knowledge and gain comprehension
- Question-and-answer session
  - Addresses patient's specific concerns
  - Helps patient apply knowledge
- Role play, discovery
  - Allows patient to actively apply knowledge in controlled situation
  - Promotes synthesis of information and problem solving
- Independent project (computer-assisted instruction), field experience
  - Allows patient to assume responsibility for completing learning activities at own pace
  - Promotes analysis, synthesis, and evaluation of new information and skills

Affective
- Role play
  - Allows expression of values, feelings, and attitudes
- Discussion (group)
  - Allows patient to receive support from others in group
  - Helps patient learn from others' experiences
  - Promotes responding, valuing, and organization
- Discussion (one-on-one)
  - Allows discussion of personal, sensitive topics of interest or concern

Psychomotor
- Demonstration
  - Provides presentation of procedures or skills by nurse
  - Permits patient to incorporate modeling of nurse's behavior
  - Allows nurse to control questioning during demonstration
- Practice
  - Gives patient opportunity to perform skills using equipment in a controlled setting
  - Provides repetition
- Return demonstration
  - Permits patient to perform skill as nurse observes
  - Provides excellent source of feedback and reinforcement
  - Assists in determining patient's ability to correctly perform a skill or technique
- Independent projects, games
  - Requires teaching method that promotes adaptation and origination of psychomotor learning
  - Permits learner to use new skills

Cognitive Learning

Cognitive learning requires thinking and encompasses the acquisition of knowledge and intellectual skills (Billings and Halstead, 2012; Krau, 2011). The revised taxonomy of six cognitive behaviors is hierarchical and increases in complexity as in the following list:

- Remembering: Learning new facts or information and being able to recall them
- Understanding: Ability to understand the meaning of learned material
- Applying: Using abstract, newly learned ideas in an actual situation
- Analyzing: Breaking down information into organized parts
- Evaluating: Ability to judge the value of something for a given purpose
- Creating: Ability to apply knowledge and skills to create something new

Affective Learning

Affective learning deals with expression of feelings and development of values, attitudes, and beliefs (Billings and Halstead, 2012; Krau, 2011). Values clarification (see Chapter 22) is an example of affective learning. The simplest behavior in the hierarchy is receiving, and the most complex is characterizing. Affective learning includes the following:

- Receiving: Learner is passive and needs only to pay attention and receive information
- Responding: Requires active participation through listening and reacting verbally and nonverbally
- Valuing: Attaching worth and value to the acquired knowledge as demonstrated by the learner's behavior
- Organizing: Developing a value system by identifying and organizing values according to their worth
- Characterizing: Acting and responding with a consistent value system; requires introspection and self-examination of one's own values in relation to an ethical issue or particular experience

Psychomotor Learning

Psychomotor learning involves acquiring motor skills that require coordination and the integration of mental and physical movements such as the ability to walk or use an eating utensil (McDonald, 2014). The simplest behavior in the hierarchy is perception, whereas the most complex is origination. Psychomotor learning includes the following:

- Perception: Being aware of objects or qualities through the use of sensory stimulation
- Set: Readiness to take a particular action; there are three sets: mental, physical, and emotional
- Guided response: Early stages of learning a particular skill under the guidance of an instructor that involves imitation and practice of a demonstrated act
- Mechanism: Higher level of behavior in which a person gains confidence and proficiency in performing a skill that is more complex or involves several more steps than a guided response
- Complex overt response: Smoothly and accurately performing a motor skill that requires complex movement patterns
- Adaptation: Motor skills are well developed and movements can be modified when unexpected problems occur
- Origination: Using existing psychomotor skills to create new movement patterns and perform them as needed in response to a particular situation or problem

BASIC LEARNING PRINCIPLES

To teach effectively and efficiently, you must first be aware of the factors that influence how a person learns (Bastable, 2014). Achievement of the desired learning outcomes depends on a number of factors, including an individual's motivation and ability to learn and the context and environment where learning will take place. Motivation underlies a person's desire or willingness to learn. Previous knowledge, experience, attitudes, and sociocultural factors all influence a person's motivation. The ability to learn depends on physical and cognitive attributes, developmental level, physical wellness, and intellectual thought processes. Both a patient's willingness and ability to become involved in learning influence your teaching approach.

A person's learning style affects his or her preferences for learning. People process information in a number of ways: through seeing and hearing, reflecting and acting, reasoning logically and intuitively, and analyzing and visualizing. Effective teaching plans incorporate a combination of activities that target a variety of learning styles (Billings and Halstead, 2012). When you tailor your teaching approach to meet your patient's needs and learning style, you will optimize the learning experience at the individual level.

Motivation to Learn

Attentional Set. An attentional set is the mental state that allows the learner to focus on and comprehend a learning activity. Before learning anything, patients must give attention to, or concentrate on, the information to be learned. Physical discomfort, anxiety, and environmental distractions influence the ability to focus. Therefore determine a patient's level of comfort before beginning a teaching plan and ensure that the patient is able to focus on the information.

As anxiety increases, a patient's ability to pay attention often decreases. Anxiety is uneasiness or worry resulting from anticipating a threat or danger. When faced with change or the need to act differently, a person often feels anxious. A mild level of anxiety motivates learning. However, a high level of anxiety prevents learning from occurring. It incapacitates a person, creating an inability to focus on anything other than relieving the anxiety. Assess for and moderate the patient's anxiety (see Chapter 38) before educating to improve his or her comprehension and understanding of the information given (Bastable, 2014).

Motivation. Motivation is a force that acts on or within a person (e.g., an idea, emotion, or a physical need) to cause the person to behave in a particular way (Miller and Stoeckel, 2015). If a person does not want to learn, it is unlikely that learning will occur. You assess a patient's motivation to learn and what the patient needs to know to promote adherence to his or her prescribed therapy. Unfortunately not all people are interested in maintaining health. Many do not adopt new health behaviors or change unhealthy behaviors unless they perceive a disease as a threat, overcome barriers to changing health practices, and see the benefits of adopting a healthy behavior. For example, some patients with lung disease continue to smoke. No therapy has an effect unless a person believes that health is important and that the therapy will improve health.

Use of Theory to Enhance Motivation and Learning. Health education often involves changing attitudes and values that are not easy to change simply through transfer of information. Therefore it is important for you to use various theory-based interventions when developing patient education plans. Learning theories focus on how individuals learn and can facilitate the teaching-learning process by creating the desired climate and guiding the selection of instructional strategies. Because of the complexity of patient education, different theories and models are available to guide patient education. Using a theory that matches a patient's needs and personal learning preferences allows the patient to become an active participant, leading to effective instruction. Social learning theory provides one of the most useful approaches to patient education because it considers the personal characteristics of the learner, behavior patterns, and the environment and guides the educator in developing effective teaching interventions that result in improved motivation and enhanced learning (Bastable, 2014; Sanderson et al., 2012).

According to social learning theory, a person's state of mind and intrinsic motivational factors (i.e., sense of accomplishment, pride, or confidence) reinforce behaviors and influence learning (Burkhart et al., 2012). This type of internal reward system allows a person to attain desired outcomes and avoid undesired outcomes, resulting in improved motivation. Self-efficacy, a concept included in social learning theory, refers to a person's perceived ability to successfully complete a task. When people believe that they are able to execute a particular behavior, they are more likely to perform the behavior consistently and correctly.

Self-efficacy beliefs come from four sources: enactive mastery experiences, vicarious experiences, verbal persuasion, and physiological and affective states (Bandura, 1997). Understanding the four sources of self-efficacy allows you to develop interventions to help patients adopt healthy behaviors. For example, a nurse who is wishing to teach a child recently diagnosed with asthma how to correctly use an inhaler expresses personal belief in the child's ability to use the inhaler (verbal persuasion). Then the nurse demonstrates how to use the inhaler (vicarious experience). Once the demonstration is complete, the child uses the inhaler (enactive mastery experience). As the child's wheezing and anxiety decrease after the correct use of the inhaler, he or she experiences positive feedback, further enhancing his or her confidence to use it (physiological and affective states). Interventions such as these enhance perceived self-efficacy, which in turn improves the achievement of desired outcomes.

Self-efficacy is a concept included in many health promotion theories because it often is a strong predictor of healthy behaviors and because many interventions improve self-efficacy, resulting in improved lifestyle choices (Bandura, 1997). Because of its use in theories and research studies, many evidence-based teaching interventions include a focus on self-efficacy. When nurses implement interventions to enhance self-efficacy, their patients frequently experience positive outcomes. For example, researchers associated interventions that included self-efficacy with effective management of diabetes and glycemic control (Tan et al., 2011), self-management of asthma in school-age children (Burkhart et al., 2012), and improved functioning along with a reduction in symptoms related to anxiety and depression (Brown et al., 2014).

Psychosocial Adaptation to Illness. A temporary or permanent loss of health is often difficult for patients to accept. They need to grieve, and the process of grieving gives them time to adapt psychologically to the emotional and physical implications of their illnesses. The stages of grieving (see Chapter 37) include a series of responses that patients experience during a loss such as illness. They experience these stages at different rates and sequences, depending on their self-concept before illness, the severity of the illness, and the changes in lifestyle that the illness creates. Effective, supportive care guides the patient through the grieving process.

Readiness to learn is related to the stage of grieving (Table 25-1). Patients cannot learn when they are unwilling or unable to accept the reality of illness. However, properly timed teaching facilitates adjustment to illness or disability. Identify a patient's stage of grieving on the basis of his or her behaviors. When a patient enters the stage of acceptance, the stage compatible with learning, introduce a teaching plan. Continuous assessment of a patient's behaviors determines the stages of grieving. Teaching continues as long as the patient remains in a stage conducive to learning.

Active Participation. Learning occurs when a patient is actively involved in an educational session (Edelman et al., 2014). A patient's

TABLE 25-1 Relationship Between Psychosocial Adaptation to Illness, Grief, and Learning

Stage	Patient's Behavior	Learning Implications for Nurse and Family Caregiver	Rationale
Denial or disbelief	Patient avoids discussion of illness ("I'm fine; there's nothing wrong with me"), withdraws from others, and disregards physical restrictions. Patient suppresses and distorts information that has not been presented clearly.	Provide support, empathy, and careful explanations of all procedures while they are being done. Let patient know that you are available for discussion. Explain situation to family or significant other if appropriate. Teach in present tense (e.g., explain current therapy).	Patient is not prepared to deal with problem. Any attempt to convince or tell patient about illness results in further anger or withdrawal. Provide only information patient pursues or absolutely requires.
Anger	Patient blames and complains and often directs anger toward nurse or others.	Do not argue with patient but listen to concerns. Teach in present tense. Reassure family and significant others that patient's anger is normal.	Patient needs opportunity to express feelings and anger; he or she is still not prepared to face future.
Bargaining	Patient offers to live better life in exchange for promise of better health. ("If God lets me live, I promise to quit smoking.")	Continue to introduce only reality. Teach only in present tense.	Patient is still unwilling to accept limitations.
Resolution	Patient begins to express emotions openly, realizes that illness has created changes, and begins to ask questions.	Encourage expression of feelings. Begin to share information needed for future and set aside formal times for discussion.	Patient begins to perceive need for assistance and is ready to accept responsibility for learning.
Acceptance	Patient recognizes reality of condition, actively pursues information, and strives for independence.	Focus teaching on future skills and knowledge required. Continue to teach about present occurrences. Involve family/significant other in teaching information for discharge.	Patient is more easily motivated to learn. Acceptance of illness reflects willingness to deal with its implications.

involvement in learning implies an eagerness to acquire knowledge or skills. It also improves the opportunity for the patient to make decisions during teaching sessions. For example, when teaching car-seat safety during a parenting class, hold a teaching session in the parking lot where the participants park their cars. Encourage active participation by providing the learners with several different car seats for them to place in their cars. At the completion of this session, the parents are able to determine which type of car seat fits best in their cars and which is the easiest to use. This provides participants with the information needed to purchase the appropriate car seat.

Ability to Learn

Developmental Capability. Cognitive development influences a patient's ability to learn. You can be a competent educator, but if you do not consider a patient's intellectual abilities, teaching is unsuccessful. Learning, like developmental growth, is an evolving process. You need to know a patient's level of knowledge and intellectual skills before beginning a teaching plan. Learning occurs more readily when new information complements existing knowledge. For example, measuring liquid or solid food portions requires the ability to perform mathematical calculations. Reading a medication label or discharge instructions requires reading and comprehension skills. Learning to regulate insulin dosages requires problem-solving skills.

Learning in Children. The capability for learning and the type of behaviors that children are able to learn depend on the child's maturation. Without proper physiological, motor, language, and social development, many types of learning cannot take place. However, learning occurs in children of all ages. Intellectual growth moves from the concrete to the abstract as the child matures. Therefore information presented to children needs to be understandable, and the expected outcomes must be realistic based on the child's developmental stage (Box 25-3). Use teaching aids that are developmentally appropriate (Figure 25-1). Learning occurs when behavior changes as a result of experience or growth (Hockenberry and Wilson, 2015).

Adult Learning. Teaching adults differs from teaching children. Adults are able to reflect on their current situation critically but sometimes need help to see their problems and change their perspectives. Because adults become independent and self-directed as they mature, they are often able to identify their own learning needs (Billings and Halstead, 2012). Learning needs come from problems or tasks that result from real-life situations. Although adults tend to be self-directed learners, they often become dependent in new learning situations. The amount of information you provide and the amount of time you spend with an adult patient varies, depending on the patient's personal situation and readiness to learn. An adult's readiness to learn is often associated with his or her developmental stage and other events that are occurring in his or her life. Resolve any needs or issues that a patient perceives as extremely important so learning can occur.

Adults have a wide variety of personal and life experiences. Therefore patient learning will be enhanced if they perceive the information to be relevant and are asked to use past experiences to solve real-life problems (Billings and Halstead, 2012). Furthermore, you make education patient centered by developing educational topics and goals in collaboration with the adult patient. Adult patients ultimately are responsible for changing their own behavior. Assessing what an adult patient currently knows, teaching what the patient wants to know, and setting mutual goals improve the outcomes of patient education (Bastable, 2014).

Physical Capability. The ability to learn often depends on a patient's level of physical development and overall physical health. To learn psychomotor skills a patient needs to possess a certain level of strength, coordination, and sensory acuity. For example, it is useless to teach a patient to transfer from a bed to a wheelchair if he or she has

BOX 25-3 Teaching Methods Based on Patient's Developmental Capacity

Infant
- Keep routines (e.g., feeding, bathing) consistent.
- Hold infant firmly while smiling and speaking softly to convey sense of trust.
- Have infant touch different textures (e.g., soft fabric, hard plastic).

Toddler
- Use play to teach procedure or activity (e.g., handling examination equipment, applying bandage to doll).
- Offer picture books that describe story of children in hospital or clinic.
- Use simple words such as cut instead of laceration to promote understanding.

Preschooler
- Use role play, imitation, and play to make learning fun.
- Encourage questions and offer explanations. Use simple explanations and demonstrations.
- Encourage children to learn together through pictures and short stories about how to perform hygiene.

School-Age Child
- Teach psychomotor skills needed to maintain health. (Complicated skills such as learning to use a syringe take considerable practice.)
- Offer opportunities to discuss health problems and answer questions.

Adolescent
- Help adolescent learn about feelings and need for self-expression.
- Use teaching as collaborative activity.
- Allow adolescents to make decisions about health and health promotion (safety, sex education, substance abuse).
- Use problem solving to help adolescents make choices.

Young or Middle Adult
- Encourage participation in teaching plan by setting mutual goals.
- Encourage independent learning.
- Offer information so adult understands effects of health problem.

Older Adult
- Teach when patient is alert and rested.
- Involve adult in discussion or activity.
- Focus on wellness and person's strength.
- Use approaches that enhance patient's reception of stimuli when they have a sensory impairment (see Chapter 49).
- Keep teaching sessions short.

insufficient upper body strength. An older patient with poor eyesight or the inability to grasp objects tightly cannot learn to apply an elastic bandage. Therefore do not overestimate the patient's physical development or status. The following physical characteristics are necessary to learn psychomotor skills:

- Size (patient's height and weight should match the task to be performed or the equipment being used)
- Strength (ability of the patient to follow a strenuous exercise program)
- Coordination (dexterity needed for complicated motor skills such as using utensils or changing a bandage)
- Sensory acuity (visual, auditory, tactile, gustatory, and olfactory; sensory resources needed to receive and respond to messages taught)

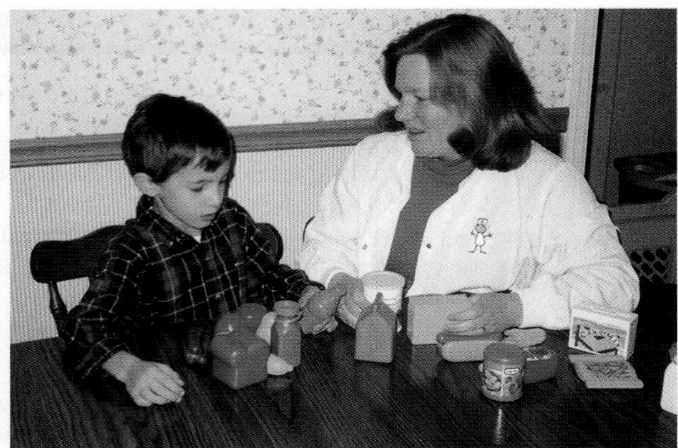

FIGURE 25-1 The nurse uses developmentally appropriate food models to teach healthy eating behaviors to the school-age child.

Any condition (e.g., pain or fatigue) that depletes a person's energy also impairs the ability to learn. For example, a patient who spends a morning having rigorous diagnostic studies is unlikely to be able to learn later in the day because of fatigue. Postpone teaching when an illness becomes aggravated by complications such as a high fever or respiratory difficulty. As you work with a patient, assess energy level by noting the patient's willingness to communicate, the amount of activity initiated, and responses to questions. Temporarily stop teaching if the patient needs rest. You achieve greater teaching success when patients are physically able to actively participate in learning.

Learning Environment

Factors in the physical environment where teaching takes place make learning either a pleasant or a difficult experience (Bastable, 2014). The ideal setting helps a patient focus on the learning task. The number of people included in the teaching session; the need for privacy; the room temperature; and the lighting, noise, ventilation, and furniture in the room are important factors when choosing the setting. The ideal environment for learning is well lit and has good ventilation, appropriate furniture, and a comfortable temperature. A darkened room interferes with a patient's ability to watch your actions, especially when demonstrating a skill or using visual aids such as posters or pamphlets. A room that is cold, hot, or stuffy makes a patient too uncomfortable to focus on the information being presented.

It is also important to choose a quiet setting. A quiet setting offers privacy; infrequent interruptions are best. Provide privacy even in a busy hospital by closing cubicle curtains or taking the patient to a quiet spot. Family caregivers often need to share in discussions in the home. However, patients who are reluctant to discuss the nature of the illness when others are in the room benefit from receiving education in a room separate from household activities such as a bedroom.

Teaching a group of patients requires a room that allows everyone to be seated comfortably and within hearing distance of the educator. Make sure that the size of the room does not overwhelm the group. Arranging the group to allow participants to observe one another further enhances learning. More effective communication occurs as learners observe others' verbal and nonverbal interactions.

❖ NURSING PROCESS

Apply the nursing process and use a critical thinking approach in your care of patients. The nursing process provides a clinical decision-making approach for you to develop and implement an individualized plan of care. There are distinct similarities between the nursing process

TABLE 25-2 Comparison of the Nursing and Teaching Processes

Basic Steps	Nursing Process	Teaching Process
Assessment	Collect data about patient's physical, psychological, social, cultural, developmental, and spiritual needs from patient, family, diagnostic tests, medical record, nursing history, and literature.	Gather data about patient's learning needs, motivation, ability to learn, health literacy, and teaching resources from patient, family, learning environment, medical record, nursing history, and literature.
Nursing diagnosis	Identify appropriate nursing diagnoses on basis of assessment findings.	Identify patient's learning needs on basis of three domains of learning. Identify conditions that may interfere with learning.
Planning	Develop an individualized care plan. Set diagnosis priorities on basis of patient's immediate needs, expected outcomes, and patient-centered goals. Collaborate with patient on care plan.	Establish learning objectives stated in behavioral terms. Identify priorities regarding learning needs. Collaborate with patient about teaching plan. Identify type of teaching method to use.
Implementation	Perform nursing care therapies. Include patient as active participant in care. Involve family/significant other in care as appropriate.	Implement teaching methods. Actively involve patient in learning activities. Include family caregiver as appropriate.
Evaluation	Identify success in meeting desired outcomes and goals of nursing care. Alter interventions as indicated when goals are not met.	Determine outcomes of teaching-learning process. Measure patient's achievement of learning objectives. Reinforce information as needed.

and the teaching process. During the assessment phase of the nursing process, determine a patient's health care needs (see Unit 3). During this phase a patient's need for health care information sometimes emerges. When education becomes a part of the care plan, the teaching process begins. Like the nursing process, the teaching process requires assessment—in this case analyzing a patient's learning needs, motivation, and ability to learn. A diagnostic statement specifies the information or skills that a patient requires or identifies factors interfering with learning. Develop specific learning objectives, implement appropriate patient-centered teaching strategies, and use learning principles to ensure that your patient acquires the necessary knowledge and skills. Finally the teaching process requires an evaluation of learning based on learning objectives.

The nursing and teaching processes differ when the nursing process requires assessment of all sources of data to determine a patient's total health care needs. The teaching process focuses on a patient's learning needs and willingness and capability to learn. Table 25-2 compares the teaching and nursing processes.

◆ Assessment

Through the Patient's Eyes. When providing patient education, it is important to partner with the patient to ensure safe, compassionate, and coordinated care (QSEN, 2014). During the assessment process thoroughly assess a patient and critically analyze your findings to ensure that you make patient-centered clinical decisions required for safe nursing care. To be successful in teaching a patient, you need to assess all factors that will influence the choice of relevant teaching topics and your approach. This includes the patient's learning needs, motivation to learn, and ability to learn; the teaching environment; the resources available; and any health literacy and learning disabilities. By seeing health care situations "through the patient's eyes," you gain a better appreciation of your patient's knowledge, expectations, and preferences for learning.

Learning Needs. Learning needs, identified by both you and the patient, determine the choice of teaching content. An effective assessment provides the basis for individualized patient teaching (Olsen, 2010). Box 25-4 summarizes examples of specific assessment questions to use in determining a patient's unique learning needs.

Sometimes nurses use formal educational assessment tools to determine their patients' perceived learning needs. Other times they simply identify their patients' expectations during routine assessments. Patients often identify their own learning needs on the basis of the implications of living with their illness. To meet these learning needs, assess what patients view as important information to know. When a patient has a need to know something, he or she is likely to be receptive to information presented. For example, many parents need to know how to care for their new baby. Therefore they are often very receptive to information about infant care (e.g., how to feed the infant and make sure that he or she gets enough sleep).

BOX 25-4 Nursing Assessment Questions

Previous Learning and Identification of Learning Needs and Preferences

- What do you want to know about ______________?
- What do you know about your illness and your treatment plan?
- Which experiences have you had in the past that are similar to those you are experiencing now?
- Together we can choose the best way for you to learn about your disease. How can I best help you?
- When you learn new information, do you prefer to have it given to you in pictures or written down in words?
- When you give someone directions to your house, do you tell the person how to get there, write out the instructions, or draw a map?

Self-Management

- How does (or will) your illness affect your current lifestyle?
- Which barriers currently exist that prevent you from managing your illness the way you would like to manage it?
- What role do you believe your health care providers should take in helping you manage your illness or maintain health?
- How involved do you want a family member to be in the management of your illness? Who is that family member?

Cultural and Spiritual Influences

- Which cultural or spiritual beliefs do you have regarding your illness and the prescribed treatment?

For Family Caregivers

- When are you available to help, and how do you plan to help your loved one?
- Your spouse needs some help. How do you feel about learning how to assist him or her?
- Tell me how you feel about performing the care activities that your family member requires.

Determine information that is critical for patients to learn. Learning needs change, depending on a patient's current health status. Because health status is dynamic, assessment is an ongoing activity. Assess the following:

- Information or skills needed by a patient to perform self-care and to understand the implications of a health problem: Health care team members anticipate learning needs related to specific health problems. For example, you teach a young man who has just entered high school how to prevent sexually transmitted infections (STIs).
- Patient experiences (e.g., new or recurring problem, past hospitalization) that influence the need to learn.
- Information that family caregivers require to support the patient's needs: The amount of information needed depends on the extent of a family member's role in helping the patient.

Motivation to Learn. Ask questions to identify and define the patient's motivation. These questions help to determine if a patient is prepared and willing to learn. Assess the following motivational factors:

- Behavior (e.g., attention span, tendency to ask questions, memory, and ability to concentrate during the teaching session)
- Health beliefs and sociocultural background: Norms, values, experiences, and traditions all influence a patient's beliefs and values about health and various therapies, communication patterns, and perceptions of time (see Chapter 9).
- Perception of the severity and susceptibility of a health problem and the benefits and barriers to treatment
- Perceived ability to perform needed health behaviors
- Desire to learn
- Attitudes about health care providers (e.g., role of patient and nurse in making decisions)
- Learning style preference: As the nurse, any educational effort will be more effective if the chosen method of instruction aligns with your patient's preferred learning style (Billings and Halstead, 2012). Patients who are visual-spatial learners enjoy learning through pictures, visual charts, or any exercise that allows them to visualize concepts. The verbal/linguistic learner demonstrates strength in the language arts and therefore prefers learning by listening or reading information. Kinesthetic learners process knowledge by moving and participating in hands-on activities. Role-play and return demonstrations are popular activities for the kinesthetic learner. Patients who learn through logical-mathematical reasoning think in terms of cause and effect and respond best when required to predict logical outcomes. Specific teaching strategies could include open-ended questioning or problem-solving exercises. Assess and inquire about your patient's learning preferences when planning your instruction.

Ability to Learn. Determine a patient's physical and cognitive ability to learn. Health care providers often underestimate patients' cognitive deficits. Many factors impair the ability to learn, including preexisting physical or mental illness, fatigue, body temperature, electrolyte imbalance, oxygenation status, and blood glucose level. In any health care setting several of these factors often influence a patient at the same time. Assess the following factors related to the ability to learn:

- Physical strength, endurance, movement, dexterity, and coordination: Determine the extent to which a patient can perform skills by having him or her practice with equipment that will be used in self-care at home.
- Sensory deficits (see Chapter 49) that affect a patient's ability to understand or follow instruction
- Patient's reading level: This is often difficult to assess because patients who are functionally illiterate are often able to conceal it by using excuses such as not having the time or not being able to see. One way to assess a patient's reading level and level of understanding is to ask the patient to read instructions from an educational handout and then explain their meaning (see the discussion of health literacy below).
- Patient's developmental level: This influences the selection of teaching approaches (see Box 25-3).
- Patient's cognitive function, including memory, knowledge, association, and judgment
- Pain, fatigue, depression, anxiety, or other physical or psychological symptoms that interfere with the ability to maintain attention and participate: In acute care settings a patient's physical condition can easily prevent a patient from learning.

Teaching Environment. The environment for a teaching session needs to be conducive to learning. Assess the following environmental factors:

- Distractions or persistent noise: A quiet area is essential for focusing on the topic and effective learning.
- Comfort of the room, including ventilation, temperature, lighting, furniture, and size
- Room facilities and available equipment

Resources for Learning. A patient frequently requires the support of family members or significant others. If this support is necessary, assess the readiness and ability of family caregivers to learn the information necessary for the care of the patient. Also review resources within the home environment. Assess the following:

- Patient's willingness to have family caregivers involved in the teaching plan and provide health care: Information about a patient's health care is confidential unless the patient chooses to share it. Sometimes it is difficult for a patient to accept the help of family caregivers, especially when bodily functions are involved.
- Family caregiver's perceptions and understanding of a patient's illness and its implications: Family caregivers' perceptions should match those of the patient; otherwise conflicts occur in the teaching plan.
- Family caregiver's willingness and ability to participate in care: If a patient chooses to share information about his or her health status with family members, they need to be responsible, willing, and physically and cognitively able to assist in care activities such as bathing or administering medications. Not all family members meet these requirements.
- Resources: These include financial or material resources such as having the ability to obtain health care equipment.
- Teaching tools, including brochures, audiovisual materials, or posters: Printed material needs to present current information that is written clearly and logically and matches the patient's reading level.

Health Literacy and Learning Disabilities. Research shows that health literacy is a strong predictor of a person's health status (Osborn et al., 2011). The World Health Organization (WHO, 2015) defines **health literacy** as the cognitive and social skills that determine the motivation and ability of individuals to gain access to, understand, and use information in ways that promote and maintain good health. Health literacy pertains not only to a patient's ability to read and comprehend health-related information, but to having the skills to problem solve, articulate, and make appropriate health care decisions as well (Ingram, 2011). People most likely to be at risk for low health literacy include the elderly (age 65 years and older), minority populations, immigrant populations, people of low income, and people with chronic mental and/or physical health conditions. For example, approximately half of Medicare/Medicaid recipients read below the fifth-grade level (National Network of Libraries of Medicine, 2014).

Functional illiteracy, the inability to read above a fifth-grade level, is a major problem in America today. The National Assessment of Adult Literacy Survey (NAALS), conducted in 2003 by the National Center for Education Statistics, assessed the extent of literacy skills in Americans over the age of 16 (Kutner et al., 2006). Results from a 2015 survey by the U.S. Department of Education, National Institute of Literacy (U.S. Department of Education, 2015) found that 32 million American adults had below-basic levels of health literacy. Older adults, men, people who did not speak English before entering school, people living below poverty level, and people without a high school education tended to have lower health literacy scores.

To compound the problem, the readability of printed health education material is often above the patient's reading level, which can lead to misinterpretation and prevent patients from asking for help (Gargoum and O'Keeffe, 2014; Protheroe et al., 2015). This discrepancy results in unsafe care. Health literacy is one of the most important predictors of health outcomes. Studies have shown that patients with low literacy levels are 1.5 to 3 times more likely to experience adverse health outcomes and an increased risk for hospitalization than those with higher literacy levels (Kasabwala et al., 2012). To ensure patient safety, all health care providers need to ensure that information is presented clearly and in a culturally sensitive manner (TJC, 2015a). Both the American Medical Association (AMA) and National Institutes of Health (NIH) recommend that patient education materials be written at the sixth-grade level or lower (Kasabwala et al., 2012).

Because health literacy influences how you deliver teaching strategies, it is critical for you to assess a patient's health literacy before providing instruction. Assessing health literacy is challenging, especially in busy clinical settings where often there is little time to conduct a thorough health literacy assessment. However, all health care providers need to identify problems and provide appropriate education to people who have special health literacy needs (TJC, 2015a). Research shows that many Americans read and understand information that is 3 to 5 years below their last year of formal education.

To assess health literacy, ask patients to perform simple literacy skills. For example, can a patient read a medication label back to you correctly? After you give a simple 1-minute explanation of a diet or exercise program, can the patient explain it back to you? Can a patient correctly describe in his or her own words the information in a written handout? Most people with low health literacy say they are good readers even if they cannot read (Lee et al., 2010). A variety of screening tools are available to test literacy. The Wide Range Achievement Test (WRAT 3) is a word-recognition screening test that evaluates reading, spelling, and arithmetic skills for patients from 5 to 74 years of age. The Rapid Estimate of Adult Literacy in Medicine (REALM) uses pronunciation of health care terms to determine a patient's ability to read medical vocabulary. The Cloze test, used to assess comprehension of health education materials, asks patients to fill in the blanks that are in a written paragraph.

In addition to illiteracy, assess patients for learning disabilities. For example, many self-care behaviors require an understanding of mathematics, including computation and fractions. If a learning disability impairs a patient's ability to effectively use mathematics skills, teaching is challenging, especially when trying to teach him or her about complex medication dosages and frequencies. Although not considered a learning disability, attention-deficit hyperactivity disorder (ADHD) also affects a patient's ability to learn. Patients with ADHD frequently experience inattention, hyperactivity, and impulsivity, which makes it difficult for them to stay focused during educational sessions, making learning challenging (Learning Disabilities Association of America, 2015).

Patients who have low health literacy or learning disabilities may be ashamed of not being able to understand you and often try to mask their inability to comprehend information. Therefore make sure that you are sensitive and maintain a therapeutic relationship with your patients while assessing their ability to learn. Appreciating the unique qualities of your patients helps to ensure safe and effective patient care (QSEN, 2014).

BOX 25-5 Nursing Diagnostic Process

Deficient Knowledge (Psychomotor) Regarding Use of Crutches Related to Lack of Experience

Assessment Activities	Defining Characteristics
Have patient describe how to walk with crutches.	Patient states that he or she has not received information about use of crutches. Patient asks questions about how to use crutches.
Have patient demonstrate three-point crutch walking on level surfaces and up stairs.	Patient uses crutches inappropriately. Patient cannot go up or down stairs on crutches.

◆ Nursing Diagnosis

After assessing information related to the patient's ability and need to learn, interpret data and cluster-defining characteristics to form diagnoses that reflect his or her specific learning needs or factors affecting the ability to learn (Box 25-5). This ensures that teaching will be goal directed and individualized. If a patient has several learning needs, the nursing diagnoses guide priority setting. When the nursing diagnosis is *Deficient Knowledge,* the diagnostic statement describes the specific type of learning need and its cause (e.g., *Deficient Knowledge* regarding a surgical procedure related to lack of recall and exposure to information). Patients often require education to support resolution of their various health problems. Examples of nursing diagnoses that indicate a need for education include the following:

- *Decisional Conflict*
- *Deficient Knowledge (Affective, Cognitive, Psychomotor)*
- *Ineffective Health Maintenance*
- *Noncompliance*
- *Readiness for Enhanced Health Management*
- *Self-Neglect*

When you can manage or eliminate health care problems through education, the related factor of a diagnostic statement is *Deficient Knowledge.* For example, an older adult is having difficulty managing a medication regimen that involves a number of newly prescribed medications that she has to take at different times of the day. The nursing diagnosis is *Ineffective Health Maintenance related to deficient knowledge regarding scheduling of medications.* In this case educating the patient about her medications and the correct dosage schedules improves her ability to schedule and take them as directed. When you identify conditions that cause barriers to effective learning (e.g., nursing diagnosis of *Acute Pain* or *Activity Intolerance*), teaching is inappropriate. In these cases delay teaching until the nursing diagnosis is resolved or the health problem controlled.

◆ Planning

After determining the nursing diagnoses that identify a patient's learning needs, develop a teaching plan, determine goals and expected outcomes, and involve the patient in selecting learning experiences (see the Nursing Care Plan). Expected outcomes of an education plan are learning objectives. They guide the choice of teaching strategies and approaches with a patient. Patient participation ensures a more relevant, meaningful plan.

Goals and Outcomes. Goals of patient education identify what a patient needs to achieve to gain a better understanding of the information provided and better manage his or her illness (e.g., "achieves ostomy self-care"). Outcomes describe behaviors that identify a patient's ability to do something on completion of teaching such as empties colostomy bag or administers an injection. When developing outcomes, conditions or time frames need to be realistic and meet the patient's needs (e.g., "will identify the side effects of aspirin by discharge"). Consider conditions under which the patient or family will typically perform the behavior (e.g., "will walk from bedroom to bathroom using crutches"). If possible, include the patient when establishing learning goals and outcomes and serve as a resource in setting the minimum criteria for success.

In some health care settings nurses develop written teaching plans. The teaching plan includes topics for instruction, resources (e.g., equipment, teaching booklets, and referrals to special educational programs), recommendations for involving family, and objectives of the teaching plan. Some plans are very detailed, whereas others are in outline form. Detailed chronic disease self-management plans (CDSMP), such as those used with patients who have type 2 diabetes, have been shown to result in significant improvements in health indicators and behaviors (Lorig et al., 2013). Use the plan to provide continuity of instruction. The more specific the plan, the easier it is to follow.

The setting influences the complexity of any teaching plan. In an acute care setting plans are concise and focused on the primary learning needs of the patient because there is limited time for teaching. Home care and outpatient clinic teaching plans are usually more comprehensive in scope because you often have more time to instruct patients and patients are often less anxious in outpatient settings.

Setting Priorities. Include the patient when determining priorities for patient education. Base priorities on a patient's immediate needs, nursing diagnoses, and the goals and outcomes established for him or her. Priorities also depend on what a patient perceives to be most important, his or her anxiety level, and the amount of time available to teach. A patient's learning needs are set in order of priority. For example, a patient recently diagnosed with coronary artery disease has *Deficient Knowledge related to the illness and its implications*. The patient benefits most by first learning about the correct way to take nitroglycerin and how long to wait before calling for help when chest pain occurs. Once you assist in meeting patient needs related to basic survival, you can discuss other topics such as exercise and nutritional changes.

Timing. When is the right time to teach? Before a patient enters a hospital? When a patient first enters a clinic? At discharge? At home? Each is appropriate because patients continue to have learning needs as long as they stay in the health care system. Plan teaching activities for a time when a patient is most attentive, receptive, and alert and organize the patient's activities to provide time for rest and teaching-learning interactions.

Timing is sometimes difficult because the emphasis is often on a patient's discharge from a hospital. For example, it takes several days after surgery for a patient to be alert and comfortable enough to learn. By the time a patient feels ready to learn, discharge is already scheduled. Therefore, to improve patient outcomes, anticipate patients' educational needs before they occur and involve family if possible.

Although prolonged sessions cause concentration and attentiveness to decrease, make sure that teaching sessions are not too brief. A patient needs time to comprehend the information and give feedback. It is easier for patients to tolerate and retain interest in the material during frequent sessions lasting 10 to 15 minutes. However, factors such as shorter hospital stays and lack of insurance reimbursement for outpatient education sessions often necessitate longer teaching sessions.

The frequency of sessions depends on a learner's abilities and the complexity of the material. For example, a child newly diagnosed with diabetes requires more visits to an outpatient center than the older adult who has had diabetes for 15 years and lives at home. Make sure that intervals between teaching sessions are not so long that the patient forgets information. Home care nurses frequently reinforce learning during home visits when patients are discharged from the hospital.

Organizing Teaching Material. An effective educator carefully considers the order of information to present. When a nurse has an ongoing relationship with a patient, as in the case of home health or case management, an outline of content helps organize information into a logical sequence. Material needs to progress from simple to complex because a person must learn the simple facts and concepts before learning how to make associations or complex interpretations of ideas. Staff nurses in an acute care setting often focus on the simpler, more essential concepts, whereas home health nurses can better address complex issues. For example, to teach a woman how to feed her husband who has a gastric tube, the nurse first teaches the wife how to measure the tube feeding and manipulate the equipment. Once the wife has accomplished this, the process of administering the feeding occurs.

Begin instruction with essential content because patients are more likely to remember information that you teach early in the teaching session. For example, immediately after surgical removal of a malignant breast tumor, a patient has many learning needs. To ensure that all essential material is covered, start with content considered to be high priority such as how to monitor the incision site for signs of infection; deal with the emotional aspects of a cancer diagnosis and complete the teaching session with informative but less critical content. Repetition reinforces learning. A concise summary of key content helps the learner remember the most important information (Bastable, 2014).

Teamwork and Collaboration. During planning choose appropriate teaching methods, encourage the patient to offer suggestions, and make referrals to other health care professionals (e.g., dietitians and physical, speech, or occupational therapists) when appropriate. As a nurse you are the member of the health care team primarily responsible for ensuring that all patient educational needs are met. However; sometimes patient needs are highly complex. In these cases identify appropriate health education resources within the health care system or the community during planning. Examples of resources for patient education include diabetes education clinics, cardiac rehabilitation programs, prenatal classes, and support groups. When patients receive education and support from these types of resources, the nurse obtains a referral order if necessary, encourages patients to attend educational sessions, and reinforces information taught. Resources that specialize in a particular health need (e.g., wound care or ostomy specialists) are integral to successful patient education.

NURSING CARE PLAN

Deficient Knowledge: Surgical Procedure

ASSESSMENT

Connie, a nurse in a surgeon's office, is preparing Mr. Holland for a colon resection, which is scheduled in 1 week. Mr. Holland is 75 years old and was recently diagnosed with colorectal cancer. Connie's assessment focuses on Mr. Holland's readiness to learn and factors that affect his ability to understand the procedure and related postoperative care.

*Assessment Activities**	*Findings/Defining Characteristics*
Assess Mr. Holland's readiness to learn and ask what his primary doctor has already told him about the surgery.	Mr. Holland responds, "**I can't remember what the doctor told me when I saw him last week,** but I need to know how to take care of myself. My surgery is scheduled for next week."
Ask Mr. Holland to explain what he knows about postoperative care, including performing a return demonstration of deep breathing and coughing.	**Mr. Holland is unable to describe postoperative care or provide a return demonstration of deep breathing and coughing.**
Observe Mr. Holland's behavior during the office visit.	Mr. Holland states he is anxious but asks appropriate questions. He maintains good contact with the nurse.
Ask patient how he prefers to learn.	Mr. Holland says, "I am a visual learner."

***Defining characteristics** are shown in bold type.

NURSING DIAGNOSIS: Deficient Knowledge: surgical procedure related to lack of recall and exposure to information

PLANNING

Goals	*Expected Outcomes (NOC)*[†] *Knowledge: Treatment Procedure*
Mr. Holland will describe preoperative and postoperative care activities before surgery.	Mr. Holland verbalizes understanding of the surgical procedure, postoperative monitoring, and activity planned on the day of surgery.
Mr. Holland will participate in postoperative care during hospitalization.	Mr. Holland demonstrates deep breathing and coughing.
	Mr. Holland advances his level of physical activity after his surgery.

[†]Outcome classification labels from Moorhead S et al: *Nursing outcomes classification (NOC),* ed 5, St Louis, 2013, Mosby.

INTERVENTIONS (NIC)[‡]	**RATIONALE**
Learning Readiness Enhancement	
Provide a nonthreatening environment in the consultation area. Sit with the patient and encourage any questions during instruction.	The adult patient's learning is enhanced when the patient is ready to learn and when he or she perceives the information to be important (Bastable, 2014).
Learning Facilitation	
Offer Mr. Holland teaching modalities that match his learning preference (e.g., brochures and DVDs describing preoperative and postoperative care) while explaining preoperative and postoperative care.	Providing patients with educational methods that use multiple senses is effective in educating older adults. Older adults prefer written handouts in large fonts (Meiner, 2014).
Explain postoperative care activities, including frequent monitoring; demonstrate deep breathing and coughing; and have Mr. Holland perform return demonstration.	Improving self-efficacy by using role modeling and having the patient perform behaviors enhance the successful adoption of healthy behaviors (Bandura, 1997).

[‡]Intervention classification labels from Bulechek GM, Butcher HK, and Dochterman JM: *Nursing interventions classification (NIC),* ed 6, St Louis, 2013, Mosby.

EVALUATION

Nursing Actions	*Patient Response/Finding*	*Achievement of Outcome*
Ask Mr. Holland to describe what will happen before and after surgery.	Mr. Holland is able to state understanding of preoperative and postoperative care activities.	Mr. Holland's anxiety level has decreased, and he reports that he is ready for surgery.
Observe patient as he demonstrates deep breathing and coughing and advances his activity after surgery.	Mr. Holland is able to deep breathe and cough after surgery, but he is hesitant to advance his activity level.	Patient has not totally achieved outcome of advancing activity after surgery. Manage barriers inhibiting attainment of this outcome (e.g., pain) and continue to encourage and educate patient.

◆ Implementation

The implementation of patient education depends on your ability to critically analyze assessment data to form diagnoses that identify patient learning needs. On the basis of the diagnoses, you develop a teaching plan (see Care Plan). Carefully evaluate the learning objectives and determine which teaching and learning principles most effectively and efficiently help the patient meet expected goals and outcomes. Implementation involves believing that each interaction with a patient is an opportunity to teach. Use evidence-based interventions to create an effective learning environment.

Maintaining Learning Attention and Participation. Active participation is key to learning. People learn better when more than one of the senses is stimulated. Audiovisual aids and role play are good teaching strategies. By actively experiencing a learning event, a person is more likely to retain knowledge. An educator's actions also increase learner attention and interest. When conducting a discussion with a learner, an educator stays active by changing the tone and intensity of his or her voice, making eye contact, and using gestures that accentuate key points of discussion. An effective educator engages learners and talks and moves among a group rather than remaining stationary behind a lectern or table. A learner remains interested in an educator who is actively enthusiastic about the subject under discussion.

Building on Existing Knowledge. A patient learns best on the basis of preexisting cognitive abilities and knowledge. Thus an educator is more effective when he or she presents information that builds on a learner's existing knowledge. A patient quickly loses interest if a nurse begins with familiar information. For example, a patient who has lived with multiple sclerosis for several years is beginning a new medication that is given subcutaneously. Before teaching the patient how to prepare the medication and give the injection, the nurse asks him or her about previous experience with injections. On assessment the nurse learns that the patient's father had diabetes and the patient administered the insulin injections. The nurse individualizes the teaching plan by building on the patient's previous knowledge and experience with insulin injections.

Teaching Approaches. A nurse's approach in teaching is different from teaching methods. Some situations require an educator to be directive. Others require a nondirective approach. An effective educator concentrates on the task and uses teaching approaches according to the learner's needs. A learner's needs and motives frequently change over time. Thus the effective educator is always aware of the need to modify teaching approaches.

Telling. Use the telling approach when teaching limited information (e.g., preparing a patient for an emergent diagnostic procedure). If a patient is highly anxious but it is vital for information to be given, telling is effective. When using telling, the nurse outlines the task that a patient will perform and gives explicit instructions. There is no opportunity for feedback with this method.

Participating. In the participating approach a nurse and patient set objectives and become involved in the learning process together. The patient helps decide content, and the nurse guides and counsels the patient with pertinent information. In this method there is opportunity for discussion, feedback, mutual goal setting, and revision of the teaching plan. For example, a parent caring for a child with leukemia learns how to care for the child at home and recognize problems that need to be reported immediately. The parent and nurse collaborate on developing an appropriate teaching plan. After each teaching session is completed, the parent and nurse review the objectives together, determine if the objectives were met, and plan what will be covered in the next session.

Entrusting. The entrusting approach provides a patient the opportunity to manage self-care. The patient accepts responsibilities and performs tasks correctly and consistently. The nurse observes the patient's progress and remains available to assist without introducing more new information. For example, a patient has been managing type 2 diabetes well for 10 years with oral medications, diet, and exercise. However, 1 year ago his diabetes changed, and it was difficult to control his glucose level. As a result, the oral medications were discontinued and insulin was added to his self-management plan.

Because of arthritis in his hips, the patient now needs to walk instead of jog during exercise. The patient understands how to adjust insulin when exercising to prevent hypoglycemia. The nurse instructs the patient about the newly prescribed exercise therapy and allows him or her to adjust insulin dosages independently.

Reinforcing. **Reinforcement** requires the use of a stimulus to increase the probability of a desired response. A learner who receives reinforcement before or after a desired learning behavior is more likely to repeat that behavior. Reinforcers can be positive or negative. Positive reinforcement such as a smile or verbal praise promotes desired behaviors. Although negative reinforcement such as frowning or criticizing can decrease an undesired response, it may also discourage participation and cause the learner to withdraw (Bastable, 2014). The effects of negative reinforcement are less predictable and often undesirable.

Reinforcers come in the form of social acknowledgments (e.g., nods, smiles, words of encouragement), pleasurable activities (e.g., walks or play time), and tangible rewards (e.g., toys or food). Choosing an appropriate reinforcer to alter behavior requires careful observation of an individual's response to specific stimuli. When a nurse works with a patient, most reinforcers are social; however, material reinforcers may work well with young children. In adults reinforcement is more effective when the nurse has established a therapeutic relationship with the patient. Whatever the form, it is important that reinforcement closely follow the desired behavior. Timing is essential so that a clear correlation between the desired behavior and reward is established (Bastable, 2014).

Incorporating Teaching with Nursing Care. Many nurses find that they are able to teach more effectively while delivering nursing care. This becomes easier as you gain confidence in your clinical skills. For example, while hanging blood you explain to the patient why the blood is necessary and the symptoms of a transfusion reaction that need to be reported immediately. Another example is explaining the side effects of a medication while administering it. An informal, unstructured style relies on the positive therapeutic relationship between nurse and patient, which fosters spontaneity in the teaching-learning process. Teaching during routine care is efficient and cost-effective (Figure 25-2).

Instructional Methods. Choose instructional methods that match a patient's learning needs, the time available for teaching, the setting, the resources available, and your comfort level with teaching. Skilled educators are flexible in altering teaching methods according to a learner's responses. An experienced educator uses a variety of techniques and teaching aids. Do not expect to be an expert educator

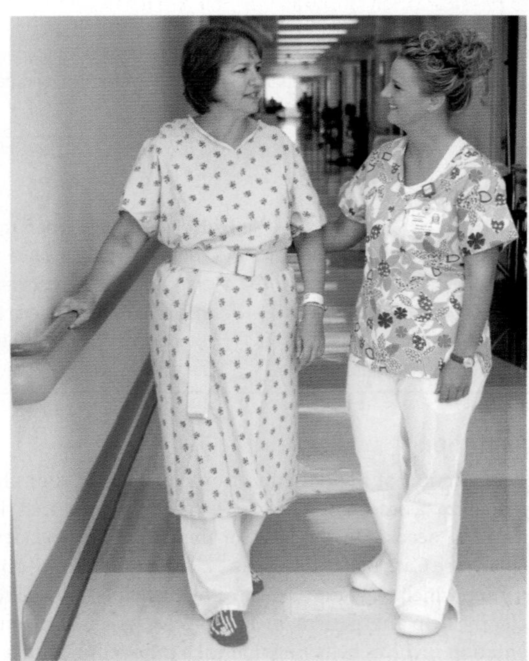

FIGURE 25-2 Teaching postoperative care while walking with the patient uses time efficiently.

when first entering nursing practice. Learning to become an effective educator takes time and practice.

When first starting to teach patients, it helps to remember that patients perceive you as an expert. However, this does not mean that they expect you to have all of the answers. It simply means that they expect that you will keep them appropriately informed. Effective nurses keep the teaching plan simple and focused on patients' needs.

One-on-One Discussion. Perhaps the most common method of instruction is one-on-one discussion. When teaching a patient at the bedside, in a health care provider's office, or in the home, the nurse shares information directly. You usually give information in an informal manner, allowing the patient to ask questions or share concerns. Use various teaching aids such as models or diagrams during the discussion, depending on the patient's learning needs. Use unstructured and informal discussions when helping patients understand the implications of illness and ways to cope with health stressors.

Group Instruction. You may choose to teach patients in groups because of the advantages associated with group teaching. Groups are an economical way to teach a number of patients at one time, and patients are able to interact with one another and learn from the experiences of others. Learning in a group of six or less is most effective and avoids distracting behaviors. Group-based instruction also results in improvement in patient satisfaction and self-management skills (Steinsbekk et al., 2012). Group instruction often involves both lecture and discussion. Lectures are highly structured and efficient in helping groups of patients learn standard content about a subject. A lecture does not ensure that learners are actively thinking about the material presented; thus discussion and practice sessions are essential. After a lecture, learners need the opportunity to share ideas and seek clarification. Group discussions allow patients and families to learn from one another as they review common experiences. A productive group discussion helps participants solve problems and arrive at solutions toward improving each member's health. To be an effective group leader, you guide participation. Acknowledging a look of interest, asking questions, and summarizing key points foster group involvement. However, not all patients benefit from group discussions; sometimes the physical or emotional level of wellness makes participation difficult or impossible.

Preparatory Instruction. Patients frequently face unfamiliar tests or procedures that create significant anxiety about the procedure and outcome. Providing information about procedures often decreases anxiety because this gives patients a better idea of what to expect during their procedures, which provides them a sense of control. The known is less threatening than the unknown. Use the following guidelines for giving preparatory explanations:

- Describe physical sensations during a procedure. For example, when drawing a blood specimen, explain that the patient will feel a sticking sensation as the needle punctures the skin.
- Describe the cause of the sensation, preventing misinterpretation of the experience. For example, explain that a needlestick burns because the alcohol used to clean the skin enters the puncture site.
- Prepare patients only for aspects of the experience that others have commonly noticed. For example, explain that it is normal for a tight tourniquet to cause a person's hand to tingle and feel numb.
- Be sure the patients know when the results will be available and who will give them the results of their tests and/or procedures.

Demonstrations. Use demonstrations when teaching psychomotor skills such as preparing a syringe, bathing an infant, crutch walking, or taking a pulse. Demonstrations are most effective when learners first observe the educator and during a **return demonstration** have the chance to practice the skill. Combine a demonstration with discussion to clarify concepts and feelings. An effective demonstration requires advanced planning:

1. Be sure that the learner can see each step of the demonstration easily. Position the learner to provide a clear view of the skill being performed.
2. Assemble and organize the equipment. Make sure that all equipment works.
3. Perform each step slowly and accurately in sequence while analyzing the knowledge and skills involved and allow the patient to handle the equipment.
4. Review the rationale and steps of the procedure.
5. Encourage the patient to ask questions so he or she understands each step.
6. Judge proper speed and timing of the demonstration on the basis of the patient's cognitive abilities and anxiety level.
7. To demonstrate mastery of the skill, have the patient perform a return demonstration under the same conditions that will be experienced at home or in the place where the skill is to be performed. For example, when a patient needs to learn to walk with crutches, stimulate the home environment. If the patient's home has stairs, the patient practices going up and down a staircase in the hospital.

Analogies. Learning occurs when an educator translates complex language or ideas into words or concepts that a patient understands. **Analogies** supplement verbal instruction with familiar images that make complex information more real and understandable. For example, when explaining arterial blood pressure, use an analogy of the flow of water through a hose. Follow these general principles when using analogies:

- Be familiar with the concept.
- Know the patient's background, experience, and culture.
- Keep the analogy simple and clear.

Role Play. During role play people are asked to play themselves or someone else. Patients learn required skills and feel more confident in being able to perform them independently. The technique involves rehearsing a desired behavior. For example, a nurse who is teaching a parent how to respond to a child's behavior pretends to be a child who is having a temper tantrum. The parent responds to the nurse who is pretending to be the child. Afterward the nurse evaluates the parent's response and determines whether an alternative approach would have been more appropriate.

Simulation. Simulation is a useful technique for teaching problem solving, application, and independent thinking. During individual or group discussion you pose a pertinent problem or situation for patients to solve. For example, patients with heart disease plan a meal that is low in cholesterol and fat. The patients in the group decide which foods are appropriate. You ask the group members to present their diet, providing an opportunity to identify mistakes and reinforce correct information.

Illiteracy and Other Disabilities. Implications of low health literacy, illiteracy, and learning disabilities include an impaired ability to analyze instructions or synthesize information. In addition, many of these patients have not acquired or are unable to acquire the problem-solving skills of drawing conclusions and inferences from experience, and they do not ask questions to obtain or clarify information that has been presented. Using strategies to promote health literacy creates a more patient-centered approach to health education and can have a significant impact on patient outcomes (Edelman et al., 2014). You can promote health literacy by creating a safe, shame-free environment, using clear and purposeful communication techniques, using visual

BOX 25-6 PATIENT TEACHING

Teaching a Patient with Literacy or Learning Disability Problems

Objective

- Patient will perform desired behaviors accurately.

Teaching Strategies

- Establish trust with patient before beginning the teaching-learning session.
- Speak slowly and encourage questions.
- Use simple terminology and avoid medical jargon. If necessary, explain medical terms using basic one- or two-syllable words.
- Keep teaching sessions short and to the point and minimize distractions. Include the most important information at the beginning of the session.
- Teach in increments and organize information into sections.
- Provide teaching materials that reflect reading level of patient, with attention given to short words and sentences, large type, and simple format (generally information written on a fifth-grade reading level is recommended for adult learners).
- Relate practical information to personal experiences or real-life situations.
- Use visual aids when appropriate and simple analogies or stories to personalize messages.
- Model appropriate behavior and use role-play to help patient learn how to ask questions and ask for help effectively.
- Frequently ask patient for feedback to determine if he or she comprehends information.
- Ask for return demonstrations, use the Teach Back method, and clarify instructions when needed.
- Keep motivation high and recognize progress with positive reinforcement.
- Reinforce the most important information at the end of the session.
- Schedule teaching sessions at frequent intervals.

Evaluation

- Observe and evaluate patient's ability to perform desired behaviors.
- Use **Teach Back:** To determine patient's and family's understanding about a topic or ability to demonstrate a procedure. Teach Back determines patient's and family caregiver's level of understanding of instructional topic. Always revise your instruction or develop a plan for revised patient teaching if patient is not able to teach back correctly.

Data from Bastable S: *Nurse as educator: principles of teaching and learning for nursing practice,* ed 4, Burlington, 2014, Jones & Bartlett.

aids to reinforce spoken material, and taking special care to evaluate patient understanding of the content. Face a patient when speaking and sit at his or her level to maintain eye contact. Because medical jargon can be confusing, it is important to use words that a patient is able to understand. Printed information, including hospital forms, legal documents, and patient education materials, must be written using plain language in a clear and concise manner. Encourage questions and verify understanding of content following any teaching intervention. Box 25-6 summarizes interventions to use when caring for patients who have literacy or learning disability problems.

Sometimes patients have sensory deficits that affect how you present information (see Chapter 49). For example, patients who are deaf may require a sign language interpreter. Not all people who are deaf read lips. Therefore it is very important to provide clear written materials that match the patients' reading level. Visual impairments also affect the teaching strategy you use. Many people who are blind have acute listening skills. Avoid shouting and announce your presence to patients with visual impairments before approaching them. If the patient has partial vision, use colors and a print font size (14-point font or greater) that the patient is able to see. Be sure to use proper lighting. Other helpful interventions include audio recording teaching sessions and providing structured, well-organized instructions (Bastable, 2014).

BOX 25-7 CULTURAL ASPECTS OF CARE

Patient Education

Patient education needs to be patient centered and culturally sensitive for learning to occur. Sociocultural norms, values, and traditions often determine the importance of different health education topics and the preference of one learning approach over another. Educational efforts are especially challenging when patients and educators do not speak the same language or when written materials are not culturally sensitive and are written above patients' reading abilities.

Implications for Patient-Centered Care

- Develop a cultural awareness to establish and maintain respectful relationships with culturally diverse patients to encourage trust and communication (Ingram, 2011) (see Chapter 9).
- Sociocultural factors influence a patient's perception of health and illness and how patients seek health care information (Campinha-Bacote, 2011).
- Carefully assess a patient's cultural needs and preferences for instructional methods to enhance learning and compliance.
- Nurses need to have access to a variety of culturally diverse health care resources and select teaching strategies that are relevant to the individual patient.
- When you and the patient do not speak the same language, professional translators are necessary.

QSEN QSEN: BUILDING COMPETENCY IN PATIENT-CENTERED CARE. You are doing a home visit with Bob, a 47-year-old patient with hyperlipidemia and hypothyroidism. Bob was recently diagnosed with type 2 diabetes and is having difficulty following a complicated medication schedule at home. He needs to take three different medications to control his hyperlipidemia and hypothyroidism. Now he has been prescribed two new oral medications to control his blood glucose. During your assessment you find that he has difficulty understanding printed teaching sheets. He admits, "I had to drop out of school when I was in eighth grade, and my vision is not as good as it used to be." When you ask Bob where he keeps his medications, he shows you the prescription bottles in a kitchen cabinet. Which additional assessment questions and teaching strategies, approaches, and tools do you use to enhance Bob's learning and ability to take his medications as ordered?

Answers to QSEN Activities can be found on the Evolve website.

Cultural Diversity. You should appreciate the patient's cultural background and belief system and gauge his or her ability to understand instructions in a language that may be different from his or her native language (see Chapter 9 and Box 25-7). Assess and determine a patient's personal beliefs, values, and customs as they relate to health (Campinha-Bacote, 2011; Ingram, 2011). However, be careful not to generalize or stereotype patients solely on the basis of their culture. Collaborate with other nurses and educators to develop appropriate teaching approaches and ask people from their cultural group to help by sharing their values and beliefs. Ethnic nurses are excellent resources who are able to provide input through their experiences to improve the care provided to members of their own community (Bastable, 2014). When patients cannot understand English, use trained and certified health care interpreters to provide health care information.

In addition, be aware of intergenerational conflict of values. This occurs when immigrant parents uphold their traditional values and their children, who are exposed to American values in social encounters, develop beliefs similar to those of their American peers. Consider this conflict in values when providing information to families or groups who have members from different generations. To enhance patient education in culturally diverse populations, know when and how to provide education while respecting cultural values. Modify teaching to accommodate for cultural differences. Effective educational strategies require you to use culturally tailored, interactive instructional methods that involve the family and community in the learning process (Chin et al., 2012).

Using Teaching Tools. Many teaching tools are available for patient education. Selection of the right tool depends on the instructional method, a patient's learning needs, and the ability to learn (Table 25-3). For example, a printed pamphlet is not the best tool to use for a patient with poor reading comprehension, but an audio recording is a good choice for a patient with visual impairment. Health care facilities often provide clinicians with access to a variety of teaching resources. Be knowledgeable about what is available in your facility to better serve your patients.

Special Needs of Children and Older Adults. Children, adults, and older adults learn differently. You adapt teaching strategies to each learner. Children pass through several developmental stages (see Unit 2). In each developmental stage children acquire new cognitive and psychomotor abilities that respond to different types of teaching methods (Figure 25-3). Incorporate parental input in planning health education for children.

Older adults experience numerous physical and psychological changes as they age (see Chapter 14). These changes not only increase their educational needs but also create barriers to learning unless adjustments are made in nursing interventions. Sensory changes such as visual and hearing changes require adaptation of teaching methods to enhance functioning. Older adults learn and remember effectively if you pace the learning properly and if the material is relevant to the learner's needs and abilities. Although many older adults have slower cognitive function and reduced short-term memory, you facilitate learning in several ways to support behaviors that maximize the individual's capacity for self-care (Box 25-8).

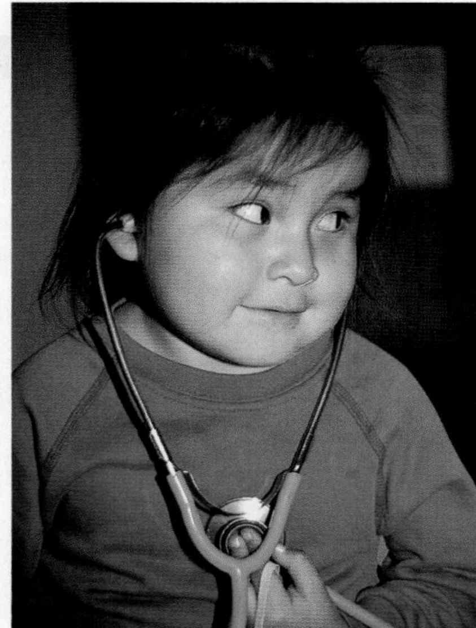

FIGURE 25-3 The preschool child learns not to be afraid of medical equipment by being allowed to handle the stethoscope and imitating its use.

Establish short-term goals when teaching older patients. Include family members who assume care for the patient. However, be sensitive to a patient's desire for assistance because offering unwanted support often results in negative outcomes and perceptions of nagging and interference. Furthermore, not all relationships between older adults and other family members are therapeutic. Because of the high incidence of abuse and neglect of older adults, assess family dynamics before including family members in educational sessions.

◆ Evaluation

Through the Patient's Eyes. Patient education is not complete until you evaluate outcomes of the teaching-learning process (see Care Plan). Engage patients in the evaluation process to determine if they have learned essential material. It is also important to determine if patients believe that they have the information necessary to continue self-care activities within the home. This is why it is important to evaluate through the patient's eyes, respecting the type of situations to which patients return after receiving care. Evaluation reinforces correct behavior, helps learners realize how to change incorrect behavior, and helps the educator determine adequacy of teaching.

Patient Outcomes. The nurse is legally responsible for providing accurate, timely patient information that promotes continuity of care; therefore it is essential to document the outcomes of teaching. Documentation of patient teaching also supports quality improvement efforts, meets TJC standards, and promotes third-party reimbursement. Teaching flow sheets and written plans of care (e.g., CareMaps) are excellent records that document the plan, implementation, and evaluation of learning.

You evaluate success by observing a patient's performance of each expected behavior. Success depends on a patient's ability to meet the established goals and outcomes. Questions should be phrased carefully to ensure that the learner understands them and that objectives are truly measured. Examples of questions to ask when evaluating patient education include the following:

- Were the patient's goals or outcomes realistic and observable?
- Is the patient able to perform the behavior or skill in the natural setting (e.g., home)?
- How well is the patient able to answer questions about the topic?
- Does the patient continue to have problems understanding the information or performing a skill? If so, how can you change the interventions to enhance knowledge or skill performance?

Teach Back. The ability of the patient to recall and comprehend information that has been taught is a predictor of patient adherence to health and disease management (Xu, 2012). One way to evaluate patient understanding is with the Teach Back method. **Teach Back** is a closed-loop communication technique that assesses patient retention of the information imparted during a teaching session. To perform Teach Back, ask the patient to explain material that was discussed, such as the role of diet and exercise in managing blood glucose levels, or to demonstrate a skill, such as self-monitoring blood glucose. The response allows you to determine the degree to which the patient remembers and understands what was taught or demonstrated. If the patient has difficulty recalling the material or demonstrating a skill,

TABLE 25-3 Teaching Tools for Instruction

Description	Learning Implications
Written Materials	
Printed Material and Online Materials	
Written teaching tools available in print or online as pamphlets, booklets, brochures	Material needs to be easy to read. Information needs to be accurate and current. Method is ideal for understanding complex concepts and relationships.
Programmed Instruction	
Written sequential presentation of learning steps requiring that learners answer questions and educators tell them whether they are right or wrong	Instruction is primarily verbal, but the educator sometimes uses pictures or diagrams. Method requires active learning, giving immediate feedback, correcting wrong answers, and reinforcing right answers. Learner works at own pace.
Computer Instruction	
Use of programmed instruction format in which computers store response patterns for learners and select further lessons on basis of these patterns (programs can be individualized)	Method requires reading comprehension, psychomotor skills, and familiarity with computer.
Nonprint Materials	
Diagrams	
Illustrations that show interrelationships by means of lines and symbols	Method demonstrates key ideas, summarizes, and clarifies key concept.
Graphs (Bar, Circle, or Line)	
Visual presentations of numerical data	Graphs help learner grasp information quickly about single concept.
Charts	
Highly condensed visual summary of ideas and facts that highlights series of ideas, steps, or events	Charts demonstrate relationship of several ideas or concepts. Method helps learners know what to do.
Pictures	
Photographs or drawings used to teach concepts in which the third dimension of shape and space is not important	Photographs are more desirable than diagrams because they more accurately portray the details of the real item.
Physical Objects	
Use of actual equipment, objects, or models to teach concepts or skills	Models are useful when real objects are too small, large, or complicated or are unavailable. Allows learners to manipulate objects that they will use later in skill.
Other Audiovisual Materials	
Slides, audiotapes, television, and videotapes used with printed material or discussion	Materials are useful for patients with reading comprehension problems and visual deficits.

BOX 25-8 FOCUS ON OLDER ADULTS

Providing Patient Education

Facilitate learning by using the following teaching strategies when providing patient education to older adults:

- Promote concentration and learner readiness by scheduling teaching sessions when the patient is comfortable and well rested. Provide medication for pain relief when necessary.
- Create a casual and relaxed learning environment.
- Establish personalized, realistic short-term learning goals.
- Provide sufficient lighting with low glare.
- If using visual aids or written materials to supplement instruction, assess the patient's reading ability and make sure that information is printed in a large font size and color that contrasts the background (e.g., black 14-point print on matte white paper). Avoid blues and greens because these colors can become more difficult to distinguish with age.
- To accommodate for hearing loss, present information slowly, in a clear, low tone of voice. Eliminate any extraneous noises and directly face the learner when speaking.
- Encourage the use of prosthesis (i.e., glasses, hearing aid) and ensure proper fit and working condition.
- Allow sufficient time to process and comprehend new information.
- Build on existing knowledge and present content in a way that relates to relevant past life experiences.
- Make information meaningful by using concrete examples that apply to current situations.
- Only present the most significant information to avoid overwhelming the learner. Use repetition to reinforce content.
- When giving instructions or teaching a new skill, give concise, step-by-step directions. Assess understanding of each step before moving ahead.
- Provide regular positive reinforcement.
- Keep teaching sessions short and allow for frequent breaks. Schedule follow-up sessions as needed to ensure learning.
- Conclude with a brief summary and allow sufficient time for questions and feedback.

Data from Touhy TA, Jett KF: *Ebersole and Hess' toward healthy aging,* ed 8, St Louis, 2012, Mosby; Edelman CL, et al: *Health promotion throughout the lifespan,* ed 8, St Louis, 2014, Mosby.

modify and repeat the content and reassess his or her retention. Patient understanding is confirmed when the patient can accurately restate the information in his or her own words (Tamura-Lis, 2013).

KEY POINTS

- The nurse ensures that patients, families, and communities receive information needed to promote, restore, and maintain optimal health.
- Teaching is most effective when it is responsive to a learner's needs.
- Teaching is a form of interpersonal communication, with the educator and learner actively involved in a process that increases the learner's knowledge and skills.
- The ability to learn depends on a person's physical and cognitive attributes.
- The ability to attend to the learning process depends on physical comfort, anxiety levels, and the presence of environmental distraction.
- A person's health beliefs influence the willingness to gain knowledge and skills necessary to maintain health.
- Use of a theory (e.g., social learning theory) or theoretical concepts (e.g., self-efficacy) enhances learning.
- Time teaching so it occurs when a patient is ready to learn.
- Patients of different age-groups require different teaching strategies because of developmental capabilities.
- Involve patients actively in all aspects of teaching plans.
- Use learning objectives to set learning priorities.
- A combination of teaching methods improves the learner's attentiveness and involvement.
- An educator is more effective when presenting information that builds on a learner's existing knowledge.
- Effective educators use positive reinforcement.
- Older adults learn most effectively when information is slower paced and presented in small amounts.
- Evaluate a patient's learning by observing performance of expected learning behaviors under desired conditions.
- Effective documentation describes the entire process of patient education, promotes continuity of care, and demonstrates that educational standards have been met.

CLINICAL APPLICATION QUESTIONS

Preparing for Clinical Practice

While Connie is providing preoperative teaching, she provides Mr. Holland with several teaching brochures that explain what colorectal cancer is and what to expect before, during, and after the surgery. Mr. Holland reads through the brochures and nods his head as if he understands the material.

1. To evaluate Mr. Holland's learning, Connie states, "I want to be sure you understand the brochure. Can you tell me in your own words what you read in the brochure?" He has trouble describing it. Connie asks him questions about information in the brochures and discovers that he misunderstood much of the information. What do the assessment data suggest about Mr. Holland's health literacy? Which special considerations does Connie need to implement at this time?
2. The surgeon comes to see Mr. Holland after surgery. A new nurse, John, is in the hospital room at this time. The surgeon tells Mr. Holland that his cancer is aggressive and that he will probably need to have chemotherapy once the incision is healed. The surgeon leaves the room. John sits in a chair to talk with Mr. Holland. Mr. Holland states, "I'm sure the doctor is wrong. After all, he's a surgeon, not an oncologist." How is Mr. Holland accepting this diagnosis? What approach should John take in planning education for him?
3. Mr. Holland is discharged. In planning discharge teaching, John reviews the medications that Mr. Holland will be taking at home. He notices that his physician prescribed three new medications. When John asks Mr. Holland what he understands about them, Mr. Holland states, "I've never heard of these medications." When John asks him to explain when he should take the medications, Mr. Holland is unable to do so correctly. What is the nursing diagnosis for this situation?

ⓔ ***Answers to Clinical Application Questions can be found on the Evolve website.***

REVIEW QUESTIONS

Are You Ready to Test Your Nursing Knowledge?

1. A patient needs to learn to use a walker. Which domain is required for learning this skill?
   1. Affective domain
   2. Cognitive domain
   3. Attentional domain
   4. Psychomotor domain
2. The nurse is planning to teach a patient about the importance of exercise. When is the best time for teaching to occur? (Select all that apply.)
   1. When there are visitors in the room
   2. When the patient states that he or she is pain free
   3. Just before lunch, when the patient is most awake and alert
   4. When the patient is talking about current stressors in his or her life
   5. When the patient is being transported for a procedure
3. A patient newly diagnosed with cervical cancer is going home. The patient is avoiding discussion of her illness and postoperative orders. What is the nurse's best plan in teaching this patient?
   1. Teach the patient's spouse
   2. Focus on knowledge the patient will need in a few weeks
   3. Provide only the information that the patient needs to go home
   4. Convince the patient that learning about her health is necessary
4. The ______________ is a closed-loop communication technique used to evaluate patient understanding and retention of material.
5. When planning for instruction on cardiac diets to a patient with heart failure, which of the following instructional methods would be the most appropriate for someone identified as a visual/spatial learner?
   1. Printed pamphlets on cardiovascular disease and dietary recommendations from the American Heart Association
   2. A role-play activity requiring the patient to select proper foods from a wide selection
   3. Colored visual diagrams that categorize foods according to fat and sodium content
   4. A lecture-style discussion on heart healthy diet options
6. A patient with chest pain is having an emergency cardiac catheterization. Which teaching approach does the nurse use in this situation?
   1. Telling approach
   2. Selling approach

3. Entrusting approach
4. Participating approach

7. The nurse is organizing a disease prevention program for a specific cultural group. To effectively meet the needs of this group the nurse will: (Select all that apply.)
   1. Assess the needs of the community in general.
   2. Involve those affected by the problem in the planning process.
   3. Develop generalized goals and objectives for the program.
   4. Use educational materials that are simplistic and have many pictures.
   5. Assess commonly held health beliefs among the cultural group.
   6. Educate the specific cultural group about Western concepts of health and illness.
   7. Include cultural practices that are relevant to the specific community.
8. An older adult is being started on a new antihypertensive medication. In teaching the patient about the medication, the nurse:
   1. Speaks loudly.
   2. Presents the information once.
   3. Expects the patient to understand the information quickly.
   4. Allows the patient time to express himself or herself and ask questions.
9. A patient needs to learn how to administer a subcutaneous injection. Which of the following reflects that the patient is ready to learn?
   1. Describing difficulties a family member has had in taking insulin
   2. Expressing the importance of learning the skill correctly
   3. Being able to see and understand the markings on the syringe
   4. Having the dexterity needed to prepare and inject the medication
10. A patient who is hospitalized has just been diagnosed with diabetes. He is going to need to learn how to give himself injections. Which teaching method does the nurse use?
    1. Simulation
    2. Demonstration
    3. Group instruction
    4. One-on-one discussion
11. When a nurse is teaching a patient about how to administer an epinephrine injection in case of a severe allergic reaction, the nurse tells the patient to hold the injection like a dart. Which of the following instructional methods did the nurse use?
    1. Telling
    2. Analogy
    3. Demonstration
    4. Simulation
12. A nurse needs to teach a young woman newly diagnosed with asthma how to manage her disease. Which of the following topics does the nurse teach first?
    1. How to use an inhaler during an asthma attack
    2. The need to avoid people who smoke to prevent asthma attacks
    3. Where to purchase a medical alert bracelet that says she has asthma
    4. The importance of maintaining a healthy diet and exercising regularly
13. A nurse is teaching a group of young college-age women the importance of using sunscreen when going out in the sun. Which type of content is the nurse providing?
    1. Simulation
    2. Restoring health
    3. Coping with impaired function
    4. Health promotion and illness prevention
14. A nurse is planning a teaching session about healthy nutrition with a group of children who are in first grade. The nurse determines that after the teaching session the children will be able to name three examples of foods that are fruits. This is an example of:
    1. A teaching plan.
    2. A learning objective.
    3. Reinforcement of content.
    4. Enhancing the children's self-efficacy.
15. A nurse is teaching a 27-year-old gentleman how to adjust his insulin dosages on the basis of his blood sugar results. This type of activity addresses learning in the cognitive domain at the level of ___________.

Answers: 1. 4; **2.** 2, 3; **3.** 3; **4.** Teach Back method; **5.** 3; **6.** 1; **7.** 2, 5, 7; **8.** 4; **9.** 2; **10.** 2; **11.** 2; **12.** 1; **13.** 4; **14.** 2; **15.** Application.

ⓔ *Rationales for Review Questions can be found on the Evolve website.*

REFERENCES

American Hospital Association: *The patient care partnership: understanding expectations, rights, and responsibilities*, 2003. http://www.aha.org/aha/issues/Communicating-With-Patients/pt-care-partnership.html. Accessed August 16, 2014.

Bandura A: *Self-efficacy: the exercise of control*, New York, 1997, WH Freeman.

Bastable SB: *Nurse as educator: principles of teaching and learning for nursing practice*, ed 4, Burlington, 2014, Jones & Bartlett.

Billings DM, Halstead JA: *Teaching in nursing: a guide for faculty*, ed 4, St Louis, 2012, Saunders.

Campinha-Bacote J: Delivering patient-centered care in the midst of cultural conflict: the role of cultural competence, *Online J Issues Nurs* 16(2):5, 2011.

Centers for Disease Control and Prevention (CDC): *National Diabetes Statistics Report*, 2014. http://www.cdc.gov/diabetes. Accessed November 11, 2015.

Edelman C, et al: *Health promotion throughout the life span*, ed 8, St Louis, 2014, Mosby.

Falvo DR: *Effective patient education: a guide to increased compliance*, ed 4, Sudbury, MA, 2011, Jones & Bartlett.

Heiskell H: Ethical decision-making for the utilization of technology-based patient/family education, *Online J Nurs Inform* 14(1):1, 2010.

Hockenberry M, Wilson D: *Wong's nursing care of infants and children*, ed 10, St Louis, 2015, Mosby.

Krau SD: Creating educational objectives for patient education using the new Bloom's taxonomy, *Nurs Clin North Am* 46(3):299, 2011.

Learning Disabilities Association of America: *ADHD*, 2015. http://ldaamerica.org/types-of-learning-disabilities/adhd/. Accessed June 8, 2015.

McDonald ME: *The nurse educator's guide to assessing learning outcomes*, ed 3, Burlington, 2014, Jones & Bartlett.

Meiner SA: *Gerontologic nursing*, ed 5, St Louis, 2014, Mosby.

Miller M, Stoeckel P: *Client education: theory and practice*, ed 2, Sudbury, MA, 2015, Jones & Bartlett.

National Network of Libraries of Medicine: *Health literacy*, 2014. http://nnlm.gov/outreach/consumer/hlthlit.html. Accessed June 8, 2015.

Olsen L: Patient assessment: building a foundation for optimal patient discharge outcomes, *Care Manage* 16(3):11, 2010.

Quality and Safety Education for Nurses (QSEN): *Competency KSAs (pre-licensure)*, 2014. http://qsen.org/competencies/pre-licensure-ksas/#patient-centered_care. Accessed June 8, 2015.

Sanderson BK, et al: Writing for publication: faculty development initiative using social learning theory, *Nurse Educ* 37(5):206, 2012.

Tamura-Lis W: Teach-back for quality education and patient safety, *Urol Nurs* 33(6):267, 2013.

The Joint Commission (TJC): *Comprehensive accreditation manual for hospitals: the official handbook* (E-dition), 2015a, The Joint Commission.

The Joint Commission (TJC): *Speak up initiatives*, 2015b. http://www.jointcommission.org/speakup.aspx. Accessed June 8, 2015.

US Department of Education: *Adult education and literacy*, 2015. http://www2.ed.gov/about/offices/list/ovae/pi/AdultEd/index.html. Accessed June 25, 2015.

World Health Organization (WHO): *Health promotion. Track 2: Health literacy and health behavior*, 2015. http://www.who.int/healthpromotion/conferences/7gchp/track2/en/. Accessed June 7, 2015.

Xu P: Using teach back for patient education and self-management, *Am Nurs Today* 7(3), 2012.

RESEARCH REFERENCES

Brown LA, et al: Changes in self-efficacy (SE) and outcome expectancy (OE) as predictors of anxiety outcomes from the calm study, *Depress Anxiety* 31(8):678, 2014.

Burkhart PV, et al: Asthma self-management for school-age children, *Curr Pediatr Rev* 8(1):45, 2012.

Chin MH, et al: A roadmap and best practices for organizations to reduce racial and ethnic disparities in health care, *J Gen Intern Med* 27(8):992, 2012.

Friedman AJ, et al: Effective teaching strategies and methods of delivery for patient education: a systematic review and practice guideline recommendations, *J Cancer Educ* 26(1):12, 2011.

Gargoum FS, O'Keeffe ST: Readability and content of patient information leaflets for endoscopic procedures, *Ir J Med Sci* 183(3):429, 2014.

Haas L, et al: National standards for diabetes self-management education and support, *Diabetes Care* 36(4):S100, 2013.

Hawkins N, et al: Why the PAP test? Awareness and use of the PAP test among women in the United States, *J Womens Health* 20(4):511, 2011.

Ingram RR: Using Campinha-Bacote's process of cultural competence model to examine the relationship between health literacy and cultural competence, *J Adv Nurs* 68(3):695, 2011.

Kasabwala K, et al: Readability assessment of patient education materials from the American academy of otolaryngology-head and neck surgery foundation, *Otolaryngol Head Neck Surg* 147(3):466, 2012.

Kutner M, et al: *The health literacy of America's adults: results from the 2003 National Assessment of Adult Literacy (NCES 2006-2483)*, Washington, DC, 2006, US Department of Education, National Center for Education Statistics. http://nces.ed.gov/pubs2006/2006483.pdf.

Lee SY, et al: Short assessment of health literacy—Spanish and English: a comparable test of health literacy for Spanish and English speakers, *Health Serv Res* 45(4): 1105, 2010.

Lorig K, et al: Effectiveness of a generic chronic disease self-management program for people with type 2 diabetes: A translation study, *Diabetes Educ* 39(5):655, 2013.

Lorig K, et al: The components of action planning and their associations with behavior and health outcomes, *Chronic Illn* 12(1):59, 2014a.

Lorig K, et al: Effectiveness of the chronic disease self-management program for persons with a serious mental illness: A translation study, *Community Ment Health J* 50:96, 2014b.

Osborn CY, et al: The mechanisms linking health literacy to behavior and health status, *Am J Health Behav* 35(1):118, 2011.

Protheroe J, et al: Patient information materials in general practices and promotion of health literacy: an observational study of their effectiveness, *Br J Gen Pract* 65(632):e192, 2015.

Sperl-Hillen J, et al: Comparing effectiveness of patient education methods for type 2 diabetes, *Arch Intern Med* 171(22):2001, 2011.

Steinsbekk A, et al: Group based diabetes self-management education compared to routine treatment for people with type 2 diabetes mellitus: a systematic review with meta-analysis, *BMC Health Serv Res* 12:213, 2012.

Tan MY, et al: A brief structured education programme enhances self-care practices and improves glycaemic control in Malaysians with poorly controlled diabetes, *Health Educ Res* 26(5):896, 2011.

Thom DH, et al: Impact of peer health coaching on glycemic control in low-income patients with diabetes: a randomized controlled trial, *Ann Fam Med* 11(2):137, 2013.

26

Documentation and Informatics

OBJECTIVES

- Identify purposes of a health care record.
- Discuss legal guidelines for documentation.
- Identify ways to maintain confidentiality of electronic and written records.
- Describe five quality guidelines for documentation.
- Discuss the relationship between documentation and financial reimbursement for health care.
- Describe the different methods used in record keeping.
- Discuss the advantages of standardized documentation forms.
- Identify elements to include when documenting a patient's discharge plan.
- Identify important aspects of home care and long-term care documentation.
- Discuss the relationship between informatics and quality health care.
- Describe the advantages of a nursing information system.
- Identify ways to reduce data entry errors.

KEY TERMS

Accreditation, p. 361
Acuity ratings, p. 366
Case management, p. 364
Charting by exception (CBE), p. 364
Clinical decision support system (CDSS), p. 368
Clinical information system (CIS), p. 368
Clinical practice guidelines (CPG), p. 365
Computerized provider order entry (CPOE), p. 367
Critical pathways, p. 364
DAR, p. 364
Diagnosis-related group (DRG), p. 357
Documentation, p. 356
Electronic health record (EHR), p. 359
Electronic medical record (EMR), p. 359
Firewall, p. 360
Flow sheets, p. 365
Focus charting, p. 364
Health informatics, p. 367
Incident (occurrence) report, p. 367
Information technology (IT), p. 367
Nursing clinical information system (NCIS), p. 368
Nursing informatics, p. 368
PIE, p. 364
Problem-oriented medical record (POMR), p. 364
SOAP, p. 364
SOAPIE, p. 364
Standardized care plans, p. 365
Variances, p. 364

MEDIA RESOURCES

http://evolve.elsevier.com/Potter/fundamentals/

- Review Questions
- Case Study with Questions
- Audio Glossary
- Content Updates

Documentation is a nursing action that produces a written account of pertinent patient data, nursing clinical decisions and interventions, and patient responses in a health record (O'Toole, 2013). Documentation in a patient's medical record is a vital aspect of nursing practice. Nursing documentation needs to be accurate and comprehensive. Nursing documentation systems need to be flexible enough to retrieve clinical data, facilitate continuity of care, track patient outcomes, and reflect current standards of nursing practice. Information in a patient's record provides a detailed account of the level of quality of care delivered. Effective documentation helps ensure continuity of care, saves time, and minimizes the risk of errors. The quality of care, the standards of regulatory agencies and nursing practice, the reimbursement structure in the health care system, and legal guidelines make documentation and reporting an extremely important nursing responsibility.

PURPOSES OF THE MEDICAL RECORD

A patient's medical record is a valuable source of data for all members of the health care team. Data entered into the medical record facilitate interdisciplinary communication; provide a legal record of care provided; justify financial billing/reimbursement; and allow for auditing, monitoring, and evaluation of care provided. Medical records also serve as sources of research data and as learning resources for nursing and health care education.

Communication

A patient's medical record is one way that members of the health care team communicate about patients' needs and responses to care, clinical decision making, individual therapies, content of consultations, patient education, and discharge planning. The record is the most current and accurate continuous source of information about a patient's health care status; the plan of care needs to be clear to anyone who accesses the record (see Unit 3). Information communicated in a patient's record allows health care providers to know a patient thoroughly, facilitating safe, effective, timely, and patient-centered clinical decision making. To enhance communication and promote safe patient care, document assessment findings and patient information as soon as possible after you provide care (e.g., immediately after providing a nursing intervention or completing a patient assessment).

Legal Documentation

Accurate documentation is one of the best defenses for legal claims associated with nursing care (see Chapter 23). You need to document in a timely manner. Documentation needs to indicate clearly that a patient received individualized, goal-directed nursing care on the basis of your nursing assessment. When documenting, describe exactly what happened to a patient and follow agency standards. Documenting the nursing process is a critical nursing responsibility that limits nursing liability by providing evidence that you maintained nursing practice standards while providing patient care (Lewis et al., 2014).

Mistakes in documentation that commonly result in malpractice include (1) failing to record pertinent health or drug information, (2) failing to record nursing actions, (3) failing to record medication administration, (4) failing to record drug reactions or changes in patients' conditions, (5) incomplete or illegible records, and (6) failing to document discontinued medications. Table 26-1 provides guidelines for legally sound documentation.

Reimbursement

Documentation by all members of the health care team is used to determine the severity of illness, the intensity of services received, and the quality of care provided during an episode of care. Insurance companies use this information to determine payment or reimbursement for health care services (ANA, 2010). **Diagnosis-related groups (DRGs)** are classifications based on a patient's primary and secondary medical diagnoses that are used as the basis for establishing Medicare reimbursement for patient care (O'Toole, 2013). Hospitals are reimbursed a predetermined dollar amount by Medicare for each DRG. Detailed recording establishes diagnoses for determining a DRG. A medical record audit reviews financial charges accrued throughout an episode of patient care. Private insurance carriers and auditors from federal agencies review records to determine the reimbursement that a patient or a health care agency receives. Accurate nursing documentation of services provided and supplies and equipment used in a patient's care clarifies the type of treatment a patient received and supports accurate and timely reimbursement to a health care agency and/or patient.

Auditing and Monitoring

Hospitals establish quality improvement programs for conducting objective, ongoing reviews of patient care and to keep nurses informed of standards of nursing practice to maintain excellence in nursing care. Accrediting agencies such as The Joint Commission (TJC, 2015) require quality improvement programs and set standards for the information needed in patient records, including evidence of an individualized plan of care developed with a patient's input, discharge planning, and patient education. Nurses periodically audit records to determine the degree to which standards of care are met and identify areas needing improvement and staff development. Health care agencies use these reports to make institutional changes to positively affect patient care. TJC requires self-regulation and quality improvement actions; one example is that nurses are required to review nursing outcomes (see Chapter 5). Nurses share deficiencies and successes identified during monitoring with all members of the nursing staff to make changes in policy or practice.

Research

After securing appropriate agency and institutional review board (IRB) approval, researchers use patient records to gather statistical data on the incidence and prevalence of health problems, complications, use and effectiveness of specific medical and nursing interventions, outcomes in recovery from illness, and deaths. Data analysis contributes to evidence-based nursing practice and quality health care (see Chapter 5). For example, a nurse researcher wants to compare use of a new method of pain control with use of a standard pain control protocol in two separate groups of patients. The investigator plans to collect data from patient health records that describe the types and doses of analgesic medications administered, objective assessment data, and patients' subjective reports of pain relief. The researcher compares findings from both groups to determine if the new method of pain control is more effective than the standard pain-control protocol.

Education

One way to learn the nature of an illness and an individual's response to it is to read a patient care record. A patient's record contains a variety of information, including diagnoses, signs and symptoms of disease, successful and unsuccessful therapies, diagnostic findings, and patient behaviors. No two patients have identical records, but in the course of clinical training nursing and other health care students review records of patients who have similar health problems to identify patterns of information and anticipate the type of care required for a patient.

The Shift to Electronic Documentation

Traditionally health care professionals documented on paper medical records. Paper records are episode oriented, with a separate record for each patient visit to a health care agency. Key information such as patient allergies, current medications, and complications from treatment are sometimes lost from one episode of care (e.g., hospitalization or clinic visit) to the next, jeopardizing a patient's safety (Hebda and Czar, 2013).

To enhance communication among health care providers and thus patient safety, the American Recovery and Reinvestment Act (ARRA) of 2009 set a goal that all medical records will be kept electronically as of 2014. Since 2011 the Health Information Technology for Economic and Clinical Health Act (HITECH), enacted under Title XIII of ARRA, has been a major driver in the adoption and use of the electronic health record across the United States. HITECH established provisions to promote the meaningful use of health information technology (HIT) to improve the quality and value of health care. These included the appropriation of a total of $2 billion in discretionary funding and incentive payments under the Medicare and Medicaid programs that reward providers for the adoption and meaningful use of certified EHR technology (Dacey and Bholat, 2012).

The CMS Medicare and Medicaid EHR incentive programs evolved into three stages of the implementation of meaningful use. Stage 1 began in 2011 and set the basic functionalities of EHRs; requirements focused on the capture of patient data and the ability of providers to share that data with patients and other health care professionals. Stage 2 began in 2014; requirements focused on the exchange of health information among providers and the promotion of patient engagement through secure online access to personal health information. Stage 3, which includes recommendations for the expansion of the meaningful use objective to improve health care outcomes, is scheduled to begin in 2016 (HITECH Answers, 2015).

TABLE 26-1 **Legal Guidelines for Documentation**

Guidelines for Electronic and Written Documentation	Rationale	Correct Action
Do not document retaliatory or critical comments about a patient or care provided by another health care professional. Do not enter personal opinions.	Statements can be used as evidence for nonprofessional behavior or poor quality of care.	Enter only objective and factual observations of a patient's behavior or the actions of another health care professional. Quote all patient statements.
Correct all errors promptly.	Errors in recording can lead to errors in treatment or may imply an attempt to mislead or hide evidence.	Avoid rushing to complete documentation; be sure that information is accurate and complete.
Record all facts.	Record must be accurate, factual, and objective.	Be certain that each entry is factual and thorough. A person reading your documentation needs to be able to determine that a patient received adequate care.
Document discussions with providers that you initiate to seek clarification regarding an order that is questioned.	If you carry out an order that is written incorrectly, you are just as liable for prosecution as the health care provider.	Do not record "physician made error." Instead document that "Dr. Smith was called to clarify order for analgesic." Include the date and time of the phone call, with whom you spoke, and the outcome.
Document only for yourself.	You are accountable for information that you enter into a patient's record.	Never enter documentation for someone else (exception: if caregiver has left unit for the day and calls with information that needs to be documented; include date and time of entry and reference specific date and time to which you are referring and name of source of information in entry; include that information was provided via telephone).
Avoid using generalized, empty phrases such as "status unchanged" or "had good day."	This type of documentation is subjective and does not reflect patient assessment.	Use complete, concise descriptions of assessments and care provided so documentation is objective and factual.
Begin each entry with date and time and end with your signature and credentials.	Ensures that the correct sequence of events is recorded; signature documents who is accountable for care delivered.	Do not wait until the end of shift to record important changes that occurred several hours earlier; sign each entry according to agency policy (e.g., M. Marcus, RN).
Protect the security of your password for computer documentation.	Maintains security and confidentiality of patient medical records.	Once logged into a computer, do not leave computer screen unattended. Log out when you leave the computer. Make sure that a computer screen is not accessible for public viewing.
Guidelines Specific to Written Documentation	**Rationale**	**Correct Action**
Do not erase, apply correction fluid, or scratch out errors made while recording.	Charting becomes illegible: it appears as if you were attempting to hide information or deface a written record.	Draw single line through error, write word error above it, and sign your name or initials and date it. Then record note correctly.
Do not leave blank spaces or lines in a written nurses' progress note.	Allows another person to add incorrect information in open space.	Chart consecutively, line by line; if space is left, draw a line horizontally through it and place your signature and credentials at the end.
Record all written entries legibly and in black ink. Do not use felt-tip pens or erasable ink.	Illegible entries are easily misinterpreted, causing errors and lawsuits; ink from felt-tip pen can smudge or run when wet and may destroy documentation; erasures are not permitted in clinical documentation; black ink is more legible when records are photocopied or scanned.	Never use pencil to document in a written clinical record. Never erase entries, use correction fluid, or use pencil. To indicate an error in written documentation, place a single line through the inaccurate information and write your signature with credentials at the end of the text that has been crossed out.

Although ARRA's goal to keep all medical records electronically by 2014 was not realized, EHR adoption has accelerated rapidly since the passage of HITECH. As of May 2013 more than 293,000 eligible medical providers and over 3900 eligible hospitals received incentive payments from the Medicare and Medicaid EHR incentive programs, and more than 220,000 of the nation's eligible professionals and over 3000 of the nation's eligible hospitals achieved the requirements for stage I meaningful use of electronic patient data. These numbers represent nearly 80% of eligible hospitals and over half of physicians and other eligible professionals (Mostashari, 2013).

As of now evidence that the EHR will be an effective, if not essential, element to improving health care quality is not conclusive (Fontenot, 2013; Kelley et al., 2011). Englebright et al. (2014) reported a first step in using computerized nursing documentation to capture meaningful data at a 170-bed community hospital in the central United States. These authors describe the development of a definition of basic nursing care that includes ten activities classified under "assess and monitor," "perform or provide," "teach," and "manage" that are provided to all hospitalized adult patients. The list of activities was coded using the Clinical Care Classification (CCC) taxonomy system and built into the nursing information system of the hospital. Many other professional organizations and accrediting body initiatives also support initiation of the **electronic health record (EHR)**. Ultimately experts believe that implementing EHRs across the health care delivery system will decrease costs and improve the quality of patient care.

Although the terms *EHR* and **electronic medical record (EMR)** frequently are used interchangeably in practice, there are differences between them. An EHR is a digital version of patient data that is found in traditional paper records. The term *EHR* is used increasingly to refer to a longitudinal (lifetime) record of all health care encounters for an individual patient (Hebda and Czar, 2013). An EMR is the legal record that describes a single encounter or visit created in hospitals and outpatient health care settings that is the source of data for the EHR (Hebda and Czar, 2013).

To meet agreed-on standards, EHRs are expected to have the following attributes or components (Hebda and Czar, 2013):

- Provide a longitudinal or lifetime patient record by linking all patient data from previous health care encounters
- Include a problem list indicating current clinical problems for each health care encounter, the number of occurrences associated with all past and current problems, and the current status of each problem
- Require the use of accepted, standardized measures to evaluate and record health status and functional levels
- Provide a method for documenting the clinical reasoning or rationale for diagnoses and conclusions that allows clinical decision making to be tracked by all providers who access the record
- Support confidentiality, privacy, and audit trails
- Provide continuous access to authorized users at any time
- Allow multiple health care providers access to customized views of patient data at the same time
- Support links to local or remote information resources such as databases using the Internet or intranet resources based within an organization
- Support the use of decision analysis tools
- Support direct entry of patient data by physicians
- Include mechanisms for measuring the cost and quality of care
- Support existing and evolving clinical needs by being flexible and expandable

The promise of the EHR is twofold: (1) making a positive impact on the quality of patient care through interprofessional collaboration with improved data availability and information synthesis, and (2) improving patient safety through the use of clinical decision support (Saleem et al., 2013). The EHR provides access to a patient's health record information at the time and place that clinicians need it. A unique feature of an EHR is its ability to integrate all patient information into one record, regardless of the number of times a patient enters a health care system. An EHR also includes results of diagnostic studies that may include diagnostic images (e.g., x-ray film or ultrasound images) and decision support software programs. Because an unlimited number of patient records potentially can be stored within an EHR system, health care providers can access clinical data to identify quality issues, link interventions with positive outcomes, and make evidence-based decisions. Here is an example of how an EHR works: A patient with a complex medical history sees multiple specialists to manage his or her health such as an endocrinologist to address diabetes, a pulmonologist to manage emphysema, and a cardiologist to manage heart failure and atrial fibrillation. Each of these providers is able to access patient data from the EMR at the same time.

The development of an EHR for all patients has the potential to benefit every member of the health care team. As of 2013 approximately 80% of all eligible hospitals and critical-access hospitals and more than half of physicians and other eligible professionals in the United States received an incentive payment for adopting, implementing, upgrading, or meaningfully using an EHR (USDHHS, 2013).

Accurate documentation within an EHR facilitates interprofessional communication; helps to meet professional, regulatory, and legal requirements; and aids in quality improvement efforts and health care research (Blair and Smith, 2012). Members of the health care team use EHRs to improve continuity of health care from one episode of illness to another. A clinician accesses relevant and timely information about a patient and focuses on the priority problems to make timely, well-informed clinical decisions. An EHR includes tools to guide and critique medication administration (see Chapter 32) and basic decision-support tools such as physician order sets and interdisciplinary treatment plans. The key advantages of an EHR for nursing include a means for nurses to compare current clinical data about a patient with data from previous health care encounters and to maintain an ongoing record of health education provided to a patient and the patient's response to that information.

INTERPROFESSIONAL COMMUNICATION WITHIN THE MEDICAL RECORD

The quality of patient care depends on your ability to communicate with other members of the health care team. Regardless of whether documentation is entered electronically or on paper, each member of the health care team needs to document patient information in an accurate, timely, concise, and effective manner to develop and maintain an effective, organized, and comprehensive plan of care. When a plan is not communicated to all members of the health care team, care becomes fragmented, tasks are repeated, and delays or omissions in care often occur.

The health care environment creates many challenges for accurately documenting and reporting the care delivered to patients. Whether the transfer of patient information occurs through verbal reports, electronic records, or written documents, you need to follow some basic principles.

CONFIDENTIALITY

Nurses are legally and ethically obligated to keep information about patients confidential. Only members of the health care team who are directly involved in a patient's care have legitimate access to the medical record. Thus you only discuss a patient's diagnosis, treatment, assessment, and/or any personal conversations with members of the health care team who are involved in a patient's care. Do not share information with other patients or health care team members who are not caring for a patient. Patients have the right to request copies of their medical records and read the information. Each institution has policies that describe how medical records are shared with patients or other people who request them. In most situations patients are required to give written permission for release of medical information.

The Health Insurance Portability and Accountability Act (HIPAA) of 1996 was the first federal legislation providing protection for patient records; it governs all areas of patient information and management of that information. To eliminate barriers that possibly delay access to care, HIPAA requires providers to notify patients of privacy policies and obtain written acknowledgment from patients indicating that they received this information. Under HIPAA the Privacy Rule requires that disclosure or requests regarding health information be limited to the specific information required for a particular purpose (Hebda and Czar, 2013). For example, if you need a patient's home telephone number to reschedule an appointment, access to the medical records is limited solely to telephone information. Of equal importance under HIPAA is the Security Rule, which specifies administrative, physical, and technical safeguards for 18 defined elements of protected health information (PHI) in electronic form (Administrative Committee of the Federal Registrar, 2014).

Sometimes nurses use health care records for data gathering, research, or continuing education. As long as a nurse uses a record as specified and permission is granted, this is permitted. When you are a student in a clinical setting, confidentiality and compliance with HIPAA are part of professional practice. You can review your patients' medical records only for information needed to provide safe and effective patient care. For example, when you are assigned to care for a patient, you need to review the patient's medical record and plan of care. You do not share this information with classmates (except for clinical conferences) and do not access the medical records of other patients on the unit. Access to EHRs is traceable through user log-in information. Not only is it unethical to view medical records of other patients, but breaches of confidentiality lead to disciplinary action by employers and dismissal from work or nursing school. To protect patient confidentiality, ensure that written or electronic materials used in your student clinical practice do not include patient identifiers (e.g., room number, date of birth, demographic information) and never print material from an EHR for personal use.

Privacy, Confidentiality, and Security Mechanisms

Electronic documentation has legal risks. It is possible for anyone to access a computer station within a health care agency and gain information about almost any patient. Therefore protection of information and computer systems is a top priority. Under HIPAA ensuring appropriate access to and confidentiality of PHI is the responsibility of all people working in health care. PHI includes individually identifiable health information such as demographic data; facts that relate to an individual's past, present, or future physical or mental health condition; provision of care; and payment for the provision of care that identifies the individual (Hebda and Czar, 2013).

Most security mechanisms for computerized information systems use a combination of logical and physical restrictions to protect information. For example, an automatic sign-off is a safety mechanism that logs a user off a computer system after a specified period of inactivity (Hebda and Czar, 2013). Other security measures include firewalls and the installation of antivirus and spyware-detection software. A **firewall** is a combination of hardware and software that protects private network resources (e.g., the information system of the hospital) from outside hackers, network damage, and theft or misuse of information.

Physical security measures include placing computers or file servers in restricted areas or using privacy filters for computer screens visible to visitors or others without access. This form of security has limited benefit, especially if an organization uses mobile wireless devices such as notebooks, tablets, personal computers (PCs), and personal digital assistants (PDAs). These devices are easily misplaced or lost, falling into the wrong hands. Some organizations use motion detectors or alarms with these devices to help prevent theft.

Access or log-in codes along with passwords are frequently used for authenticating authorized access to electronic records. A password is a collection of alphanumeric characters that a user types into a computer before accessing a program after the entry and acceptance of an access code or user name. Strong passwords use combinations of letters, numbers, and symbols that are difficult to guess. When using a health care agency computer system, it is essential that you do not share your computer password with anyone under any circumstances. A good system requires frequent, random changes in personal passwords to prevent unauthorized people from tampering with records. A password does not appear on the computer screen when it is typed, nor should it be known to anyone but the user and information system administrators (Hebda and Czar, 2013). In addition, most health care personnel are only given access to patients in their work area. Some staff (e.g., administrators or risk managers) have authority to access all patient records. To protect patient privacy, health care agencies track who accesses patient records and when they access them. Disciplinary action, including loss of employment, occurs when nurses or other health care personnel inappropriately access patient information.

Handling and Disposing of Information

Maintaining the confidentiality of medical records is an essential responsibility of all members of the health care team. It is equally important to safeguard any information that is printed from the record or extracted for report purposes. For example, you print a copy of a nursing-activities work list to use as a day planner while providing patient care. You refer to information on the list and write notes to enter later into the computer. Information on the list is PHI; you do not leave it out for view by unauthorized people. Destroy (e.g., shred) anything that is printed when the information is no longer needed. Nursing students must write down patient data needed for clinical paperwork directly from a patient's medical record on the computer screen or the physical chart. You need to de-identify all patient data when you write it onto forms or include it in papers written for nursing courses. Do not remove patient information that is printed out from a clinical agency. If you need to remove printed information from a clinical setting, de-identify all PHI, keep the documents secure, and destroy documents by shredding or disposing of them in a locked receptacle as soon as possible.

Historically the primary sources for inadvertent, unauthorized disclosure of PHI occurred when information was printed from a patient record and/or faxed to other health care providers. Thus you destroy all papers containing PHI (e.g., Social Security number, date of birth or age, patient's name or address) immediately after you use or fax them. Most agencies have shredders or locked receptacles for shredding and incineration. Some nurses work in settings where they are responsible for erasing files from a computer hard drive that contain calendars, surgery or diagnostic procedure schedules, or other daily records that contain PHI (Hebda and Czar, 2013). Know and follow the disposal policies for records in the institution where you work.

Health care facilities and departments have policies for the use of fax machines, which specify the types of information that can be faxed, allowable recipients of the information, where information is sent, and the process used to verify that information was sent to and received by the appropriate person(s). Only fax the amount of information that is requested or required for immediate clinical needs. The following are some steps to take to enhance fax security (Hebda and Czar, 2013):

- Confirm that fax numbers are correct before sending to be sure that you direct information properly.
- Use a cover sheet to eliminate the need for the recipient to read the information to determine who gets it. This is especially important if a fax machine serves a number of different users.
- Authenticate at both ends before data transmission to verify that source and destination are correct. Use the cover sheet to list intended recipient(s), the sender, and the phone and fax

numbers. Verify the fax number on the transmittal confirmation sheet.
- Use programmed speed-dial keys to eliminate the chance of a dialing error and misdirected information.
- Use the encryption feature on the fax machine. Encoding transmissions makes it impossible to read confidential information without the encryption key.
- Place fax machines in a secure area and limit machine access to designated individuals.
- Log fax transmissions. This feature is often available electronically on the machine.

QSEN QSEN: BUILDING COMPETENCY IN INFORMATICS. Nurses and nursing students are responsible for maintaining the confidentiality of patient records. A group of nurses working at a physician's office where an EHR is being implemented are having a discussion about how electronic records are kept confidential.
- If you were part of this group, which suggestions would you add to the discussion?
- Which specific measures need to be taken to safeguard patient data from being viewed electronically?
- Which additional measures are needed when you print data from an EHR?

Answers to QSEN Activities can be found on the Evolve website.

STANDARDS

Each health care organization has standards that govern the type of information you document and for which you are accountable. Institutional standards or policies often dictate the frequency of documentation such as how often you record a nursing assessment or a patient's level of pain. Know the standards of your health care organization to ensure complete and accurate documentation. Nurses are expected to meet the standard of care for every nursing task they perform. A court of law uses patient records to demonstrate whether nursing standards of practice were or were not met (ANA, 2010).

In addition, your documentation needs to conform to the standards of the National Committee for Quality Assurance (NCQA) and accrediting bodies such as TJC to maintain institutional **accreditation** and minimize liability. Usually an organization incorporates accreditation standards into its policies and revises documentation forms to suit these standards. Current documentation standards require that all patients admitted to a health care facility have an assessment of physical, psychosocial, environmental, self-care, knowledge level, and discharge planning needs. According to current standards your documentation needs to demonstrate application of the nursing process and include evidence of patient and family teaching and discharge planning (TJC, 2015). Other standards such as HIPAA include those that are directed by state and federal regulatory agencies and are enforced through the Department of Justice and the Centers for Medicare and Medicaid Services (ANA, 2010).

Patient care requires effective communication among members of the health care team. The medical record is an important means of communication because it is a confidential, permanent, legal documentation of information relevant to a patient's health care. The record is a continuing account of a patient's health care status and is available to all members of the health care team. All medical records contain the following information:

- Patient identification and demographic data
- Existence of "Living Will" or "Durable Power of Attorney for Healthcare" documents
- Informed consent for treatment and procedures
- Admission data
- Nursing diagnoses or problems and the nursing or interdisciplinary care plan
- Record of nursing care treatment and evaluation
- Medical history
- Medical diagnoses
- Therapeutic orders, including code status (i.e., provider order for "Do Not Resuscitate")
- Medical and interdisciplinary progress notes
- Physical assessment findings
- Diagnostic study results
- Patient education
- Summary of operative procedures
- Discharge summary and plan

GUIDELINES FOR QUALITY DOCUMENTATION

High-quality documentation is necessary to enhance efficient, individualized patient care. Quality documentation has five important characteristics: it is factual, accurate, complete, current, and organized. It is easier to maintain these characteristics if you continually seek to express ideas clearly and succinctly by (Beach and Oates, 2014):

- Sticking to the facts.
- Writing in short sentences.
- Using simple, short words.
- Avoiding the use of jargon or abbreviations.

Factual

A factual record contains descriptive, objective information about what a nurse observes, hears, palpates, and smells. Avoid vague terms such as appears, seems, or apparently. These words suggest that you are stating an opinion; they do not communicate facts accurately and do not inform another caregiver of the details regarding the behaviors exhibited by a patient. Objective data are obtained through direct observation and measurement (e.g., "B/P 80/50, patient diaphoretic, heart rate 102 and regular"). Objective documentation includes the description of a patient's behaviors. The only subjective data that you include in the record is what a patient says. When recording subjective data, you document the patient's exact words within quotation marks whenever possible. Include objective data to support subjective data so your charting is as descriptive as possible. For example, instead of documenting "the patient seems anxious," provide objective signs of anxiety and document the patient's statement about the feeling(s) experienced (e.g., "the patient's pulse rate is 110 beats/min, respiratory rate is slightly labored at 22 breaths/min, and the patient states 'I feel very nervous'").

Accurate

The use of exact measurements establishes accuracy and helps you determine if a patient's condition has changed in a positive or negative way. For example, a description such as "intake, 360 mL of water" is more accurate than "Patient drank an adequate amount of fluid." Charting that an abdominal incision is "approximated, 5 cm in length without redness, drainage, or edema" is more descriptive than "large abdominal incision healing well." Documentation of concise data is clear and easy to understand. It is essential to avoid the use of unnecessary words and irrelevant detail. For example, the fact that the patient is watching television is only necessary when this activity is significant to the patient's status and plan of care.

To ensure patient safety use abbreviations carefully to avoid misinterpretation. TJC's "do not use" list of abbreviations (see Chapter 32)

TABLE 26-2 Examples of Criteria for Documentation and Reporting

Topic	Criteria to Report or Record
Subjective assessment data	Patient's description of episode in quotation marks (e.g., *"I feel like an elephant is sitting on my chest, and I can't catch my breath."*) Describe in patient's own words the onset, location, description of condition (severity, duration, frequency, precipitating, aggravating, and relieving factors) (e.g., *"The pain in my left knee started last week after I knelt on the ground. Every time I bend my knee, I have a shooting pain on the inside of the knee."*).
Objective assessment data (e.g., rash, tenderness, breath sounds, or descriptions of patient behavior [e.g., anxiety, confusion, hostility])	Onset, location, description of condition (e.g., 11:00: 2-cm raised pale, red area noted on back of left hand). Onset, precipitating factors, behaviors exhibited (e.g., pacing in room, avoiding eye contact with nurse), patient statements (e.g., repeatedly stating, *"I have to go home now."*)
Nursing interventions, treatments, and evaluation (e.g., enema, bath, dressing change)	Time administered, equipment used, patient's response (subjective and objective response) compared to previous treatment (e.g., denied incisional pain during abdominal dressing change, ambulated 300 feet in hallway without assistance)
Medication administration	At time of administration when using a computerized bar-code medication administration program (or immediately after administration), document: time medication given, medication name, dose, route, preliminary assessment (e.g., pain level, vital signs), patient response, or effect of medication (e.g., 1500: Reports *"throbbing headache all over my head."* Rates pain at 6 (scale 0 to 10). Tylenol 650 mg given PO. 1530: Patient reports pain level 2 (scale 0 to 10) and states, *"the throbbing has stopped."*
Patient and/or family teaching	Information presented; method of instruction (e.g., discussion, demonstration, videotape, booklet); and patient response, including questions and evidence of understanding such as Teach Back, return demonstration, or change in behavior
Discharge planning	Measurable patient goals or expected outcomes, progress toward goals, need for referrals.

is used by all health care providers to promote patient safety. In addition, TJC (2015) requires that health care institutions develop a list of standard abbreviations, symbols, and acronyms to be used by all members of the health care team when documenting or communicating patient care and treatment. To minimize errors, spell out abbreviations in their entirety when they become confusing.

Correct spelling demonstrates a level of competency and attention to detail. Many terms are easily misinterpreted (e.g., dysphagia or dysphasia and dram or gram). Some spelling errors result in serious treatment errors (e.g., the names of certain look alike–sound alike medications such as Lamictal and Lamisil or hydromorphone and hydrocodone are similar). Transcribe medication names carefully to ensure that patients receive the correct medications.

You need to date and time all entries in medical records, and there needs to be a method to identify the authors of all entries (TJC, 2015). Each entry in a patient's record ends with the caregiver's full name or initials and credentials/title/role such as "Jane Woods, RN." If initials are used in a signature, the full name and credentials/title/role of the individual need to be documented at least once in the medical record to allow others to readily identify the individual. As a nursing student enter your full name and nursing student (NS) abbreviation such as "David Jones, NS. The abbreviation for nursing student varies between NS for nursing student or SN for student nurse. Include your educational institution when required by agency policy.

Complete

You need to ensure that the information within a recorded entry or a report is complete, containing appropriate and essential information. Follow established criteria and standards for thorough communication within the medical record or when reporting certain health problems or nursing activities (Table 26-2). Your written entries in a patient's medical record describe the nursing care you administer and a patient's response. An example of a thorough nurse's note follows:

19:15 Verbalizes sharp, throbbing pain localized along lateral side of right ankle, which began approximately 15 minutes ago after twisting his foot on the stairs. Rates pain as 8 on a scale of 0 to 10. Pain increases with movement, is slightly relieved with elevation and rest. Pedal pulses equal bilaterally. Right ankle circumference 1 cm larger than left. Bilateral lower extremities warm, pale pink, skin intact, responds to tactile stimulation, capillary refill less than 3 seconds. Ice applied to right ankle. Percocet 2 tabs (PO) given for pain. Dr. M. Smith notified. Lee Turno, RN

19:45 States pain was somewhat relieved with ice and now rates pain as a 3 on a scale of 0 to 10. States, "The pain medication really helped." Lee Turno, RN

You frequently use flow sheets or graphic records to document routine activities such as daily hygiene care, vital signs, and pain assessments. Describe these data in greater detail when they are relevant such as when a change in functional ability or status occurs. For example, if your patient's blood pressure, pulse, and respirations are elevated above expected values following a walk down the hall, document additional description about the patient's status and response to the walk in the appropriate place in the medical record (e.g., nurse's notes).

Current

Timely entries are essential in a patient's ongoing care. Delays in documentation lead to unsafe patient care. To increase accuracy and decrease unnecessary duplication, many health care agencies keep records or computers near a patient's bedside to facilitate immediate documentation of information as it is collected. Document the following activities or findings at the time of occurrence:

- Vital signs
- Pain assessment
- Administration of medications and treatments

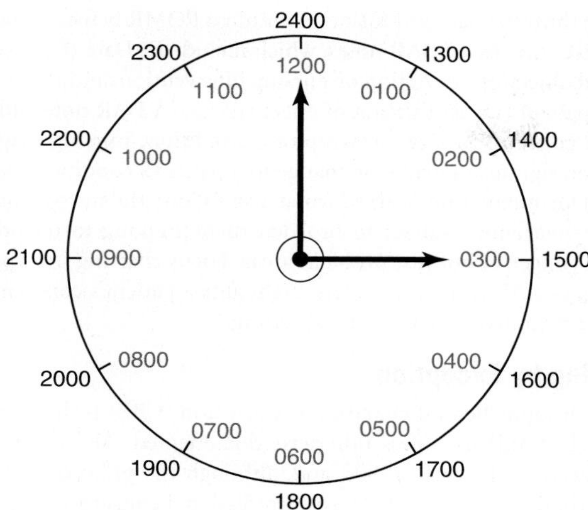

FIGURE 26-1 Comparison of 24 hours of military time with the hourly positions for civilian time on the clock face.

- Preparation for diagnostic tests or surgery, including preoperative checklist
- Change in patient status and who was notified (e.g., physician, manager, patient's family)
- Admission, transfer, discharge, or death of a patient
- Treatment for sudden change in patient status
- Patient's response to treatment or intervention

Most health care agencies use military time, a 24-hour system that avoids misinterpretation of AM and PM times (Figure 26-1). Instead of two 12-hour cycles in standard time, the military clock is one 24-hour time cycle. The military clock ends with midnight at 2400 and begins at one minute after midnight as 0001. For example, 10:22 AM is 10:22 military time; 3:00 PM is 15:00 military time.

Organized

Information entered into a medical record facilitates communication when it is documented in a logical order. Documentation is also more effective when notes are concise, clear, and to the point. To document notes about complex situations in an organized fashion, think about the situation and make a list of what you need to include before beginning to enter data in the medical record. Applying your critical thinking skills and the nursing process gives logic and order to nursing documentation. For example, an organized entry describes a patient's pain, your assessment and interventions, and the patient's response.

BOX 26-1 Examples of a Nursing Progress Note Written in Different Formats

Narrative Note

Patient stated, "I'm worried about the surgery. Last time I had a lot of pain when I got out of bed." Discussed importance of postoperative ambulation and demonstrated turning, coughing, deep-breathing (TCDB) exercises. Patient set postoperative pain-rating goal at 4 on scale of 0 to 10. Discussed analgesic plan of care and reassured that analgesics will be offered around the clock as ordered. Encouraged to tell nursing staff as soon as possible if pain is not relieved. Provided with teaching booklet on postoperative care. Stated, "I feel less anxious about my pain now." Verbalized understanding of the importance of postoperative ambulation and confidence in the plan of care.

SOAP (Subjective—Objective—Assessment—Plan) Note

S: "I'm worried about the surgery. Last time I had a lot of pain when I got out of bed."
O: Asking multiple questions about how postoperative pain will be addressed.
A: *Anxiety related to perceived threat of postoperative pain* as evidenced by statement of prior experience with uncontrolled postoperative pain.
P: Explain routine postoperative analgesic plan of care. Encourage to inform nursing staff as soon as possible if pain is not relieved. Explain rationale for early postoperative ambulation and demonstrate TCDB exercises. Provide teaching booklet on postoperative nursing care.

PIE (Problem—Intervention—Evaluation) Note

P: *Anxiety related to perceived threat of postoperative pain* as evidenced by statement of prior experience with uncontrolled postoperative pain.
I: Explained importance of postoperative ambulation and demonstrated TCDB exercises. Described analgesic plan of care. Encouraged to inform nursing staff as soon as possible if pain is not relieved. Provided teaching booklet on postoperative nursing care.
E: Stated, "I feel less anxious about postoperative pain now" and performed return demonstration of TCDB exercises correctly. Needs review of postoperative nursing care.

Focus Charting (Data—Action—Response) Note

D: Patient stated, "I'm worried about the surgery. Last time I had a lot of pain when I got out of bed." Asking frequent questions about postoperative pain management.
A: Discussed importance of postoperative ambulation and demonstrated TCDB exercises. Described postoperative analgesic plan of care that is in place. Provided teaching booklet on postoperative nursing care.
R: Demonstrated TCDB exercises correctly. Needs review of postoperative nursing care. States, "I feel better knowing how my pain will be treated."

METHODS OF DOCUMENTATION

There are several documentation methods for recording patient assessment data and progress notes (Box 26-1). Regardless of whether documentation is entered electronically or on paper, each health care agency selects a documentation system that reflects its philosophy of nursing. The same system is used throughout a specific agency and is sometimes used throughout a health care system as well.

Narrative Documentation

Narrative documentation is the method traditionally used to record patient assessment and nursing care provided. It is simply the use of a storylike format to document information. In an electronic nursing information system, this is accomplished through use of free text entry or menu selections (Hebda and Czar, 2013). Narrative documentation tends to be time consuming and repetitious. It requires the reader to sort through a lot of information to locate desired data. However, some nurses believe that in certain situations use of this method provides better detail of individual patient assessment findings and/or complex patient situations (Kerr, 2013). Physicians and other health care providers review nursing documentation for details about changes in a patient's condition (Penoyer et al., 2014). One of the limitations of electronic documentation is the limited use of narrative documentation. Some areas of the EMR are designed to use multiple checkboxes or drop-down lists, which some believe may not adequately convey the details of significant events that result in a change in patient condition (Kerr, 2013; Penoyer et al., 2014). EMRs that incorporate options for narrative descriptions in a format that is easily retrieved and reviewed may enhance clinician communication and interdisciplinary understanding for patient care.

Problem-Oriented Medical Record

The problem-oriented medical record (POMR) is a system of organizing documentation to place the primary focus on patients' individual problems. Data are organized by problem or diagnosis. Ideally each member of the health care team contributes to a single list of identified patient problems, which coordinates a common plan of care. The POMR has the following major sections: database, problem list, care plan, and progress notes.

Database. The database section contains all available assessment information pertaining to a patient (e.g., history and physical examination, nursing admission history and ongoing assessment, physical therapy assessment, laboratory reports, and radiological test results). The database provides the foundation for identifying patient problems and planning care. As new data become available, the database is revised. It accompanies patients through successive hospitalizations or clinic visits.

Problem List. After analyzing data, health care team members identify problems and make a single problem list. The problem list includes a patient's physiological, psychological, social, cultural, spiritual, developmental, and environmental needs. Team members list the problems in chronological order and file the list in the patient's record to serve as an organizing guide for patient care. Team members add and date new problems as they arise. When a problem is resolved, the text of that problem is highlighted, or lined out, and the date is recorded.

Care Plan. Disciplines involved in a patient's care develop a care plan or plan of care for each problem (see Chapter 18). Nurses document the plan of care in a variety of formats; generally all of these formats include nursing diagnoses, expected outcomes, and interventions.

Progress Notes. Health care team members monitor and record the progress made toward resolving a patient's problems in progress notes. Health care providers write progress notes in one of several formats or structured notes within a POMR (see Box 26-1).

One method is the SOAP note. The acronym SOAP stands for: *S:* Subjective data (verbalizations of the patient), *O:* Objective data (that which is measured and observed), *A:* Assessment (diagnosis based on the data), and *P:* Plan (what the caregiver plans to do). An "I" and an "E" are added (i.e., SOAPIE) in some institutions. The *I* stands for intervention, and the *E* represents evaluation. The logic of the SOAPIE note format is similar to that of the nursing process. You collect data about a patient's problems, draw conclusions, develop a plan of care, and then evaluate the outcome(s). Each SOAP note is numbered and titled according to the problem on the list that it addresses.

A second progress note used in the POMR is the PIE format. It is similar to SOAP charting in its problem-oriented nature. However, a PIE note differs from a SOAP note in that it has a nursing origin. *P:* Identifies a nursing diagnosis, *I:* Describes the interventions that will be used to address the problem, and *E:* Is the evaluation. The format simplifies documentation by unifying the care plan and progress notes. PIE notes also differ from SOAP notes because the narrative does not include assessment information. A nurse's daily assessment data appear on flow sheets, preventing duplication of data. PIE notes are also numbered or labeled according to the patient's problems. Problems that are resolved are dropped from daily documentation after a nurse's review. Nurses document about continuing problems daily with a PIE note for each problem.

The third format used for notes within a POMR is focus charting. It involves the use of DAR notes, which include *D:* Data (both subjective and objective), *A:* Action or nursing intervention, and *R:* Response of the patient (i.e., evaluation of effectiveness). A DAR note addresses patient concerns: a sign or symptom, condition, nursing diagnosis, behavior, significant event, or change in a patient's condition (see Box 26-1). Documentation in this format also follows the nursing process. This format allows nurses to broaden their thinking to include any patient concerns, not just problem areas. Focus charting incorporates all aspects of the nursing process, highlights a patient's concerns, and can be integrated into any clinical setting.

Charting by Exception

The philosophy behind charting by exception (CBE) is that a patient meets all standards unless otherwise documented. The method was introduced in the early 1980s; and, although the philosophy behind the method has consistently raised professional concern (Kerr, 2013), many computerized nursing documentation systems use a CBE design. Exception-based documentation systems incorporate standards of care, evidence-based interventions, and clearly defined criteria for nursing assessment and documentation of "normal" findings. The predefined statements used to document nursing assessment of body systems are called *within defined limits (WDL)* or *within normal limits (WNL)* definitions. They consist of written criteria for a "normal" assessment for each body system. Automated documentation within a computerized documentation system allows nurses to select a WDL statement or to choose other statements from a drop-down menu that allow description of any assessment findings that deviate from the WDL definition or that are unexpected (Hebda and Czar, 2013). You only write a progress note when a patient's assessment does not meet the standardized criteria for "normal" in one or more body systems. When changes in a patient's condition develop, you need to include a thorough and precise description of the effects of the change(s) on the patient and the actions taken to address the change(s) in the progress note.

Case Management and Use of Critical Pathways

The case management model of delivering care (see Chapter 2) incorporates an interprofessional approach to documenting patient care. Critical pathways (also known as clinical pathways, practice guidelines, critical pathways, or CareMap® tools) are interprofessional care plans that identify patient problems, key interventions, and expected outcomes within an established time frame (American Health Consultants, 2015). The document facilitates the integration of care because all health care team members use the same critical pathway to monitor a patient's progress during each shift or, in the case of home care, every visit (Chan and Webster, 2013). Many organizations summarize the standardized plan of care into critical pathways for a specific disease or condition. For example, in cancer care some pathways focus on malignancies that have a higher incidence such as breast, colon, prostate, and lung cancers and certain types of blood cancers (DeMartino and Larsen, 2012). Evidence-based critical pathways improve patient outcomes. For example, one critical pathway to manage pain caused by vascular-occlusive crisis in patients with sickle cell disease significantly improved the time interval between patient triage and administration of first analgesic dose and the likelihood of ketorolac administration in a pediatric emergency department (Ender et al., 2014).

A critical pathway eliminates nurses' notes, flow sheets, and nursing care plans because the document integrates all relevant information. Unexpected outcomes, unmet goals, and interventions not specified within the critical pathway are called variances. A variance occurs

BOX 26-2 Example of Variance Documentation

You are using a critical pathway for "Routine Postoperative Care" for a 56-year-old man who had abdominal surgery yesterday. One of the expected outcomes for postoperative day 1 on the critical pathway document is "Afebrile with lungs clear bilaterally." This patient has an elevated temperature, his breath sounds are decreased bilaterally in the bases of both lobes of the lungs, and he is slightly confused.

The following is an example of how you document this variance on the pathway:

"Breath sounds diminished bilaterally at the bases. T-100.4; P-92; R-28/min; pulse oximetry 84% on room air. Daughter states he is "confused" and did not recognize her when she arrived a few minutes ago. Oxygen 2 L nasal cannula started per standing orders. Oxygen saturation improved to 92% after 5 minutes. Dr. Lopez notified of change in status. Daughter remains at bedside."

when the activities on the critical pathway are not completed as predicted or a patient does not meet the expected outcomes. A positive variance occurs when a patient progresses more rapidly than expected (e.g., use of a Foley catheter is discontinued a day early). An example of a negative variance is when a patient develops pulmonary complications after surgery, requiring oxygen therapy and monitoring with pulse oximetry. You document all variances on the critical pathway (Box 26-2). Analysis of variances identifies trends and provides data to develop an effective action plan to respond to identified patient problems. Variances sometimes result from changes in a patient's health or because of other health complications not associated with the primary reason for which a patient requires care. Once you identify a variance, you modify the patient's care to meet the needs associated with the variance. Over time health care teams revise critical pathways when similar variances recur.

COMMON RECORD-KEEPING FORMS

Nurses use a variety of electronic or paper forms for the type of information routinely documented. The categories or data fields within a form are usually derived from institutional standards of practice or guidelines established by accrediting agencies.

Admission Nursing History Form

A nurse completes a nursing history form when a patient is admitted to a nursing unit. The fields in the form guide you through a comprehensive assessment to identify relevant nursing diagnoses or problems (see Chapters 16 and 17). Completion of this form provides baseline data that you use for comparison when a patient's condition changes.

Flow Sheets and Graphic Records

Acute and critical care nurses commonly use **flow sheets** and graphic records to document physiological data and routine care. Within a computerized documentation system these forms allow you to quickly and easily enter assessment data about a patient such as vital signs, admission and or daily weights, and percentage of meals eaten. They also facilitate the documentation of the provision of routine, repetitive care such as hygiene measures, ambulation, and safety and restraint checks. These documents provide current patient information accessible to all members of the health care team and help team members quickly see patient trends over time. You explain any occurrence on a flow sheet that is unusual or represents a significant change in a patient's condition in detail in a progress note. For example, if a patient's blood pressure becomes dangerously high, you first complete and record a focused assessment and then document the action taken in a progress note.

Patient Care Summary

Many computerized documentation systems have the ability to generate a patient care summary document that you review and sometimes print for each patient at the beginning and/or end of each shift. The document automatically updates and provides the most current information that has been entered into the EHR and usually includes the following information:

- Basic demographic data (e.g., age, religion)
- Health care provider's name
- Primary medical diagnosis
- Medical and surgical history
- Current orders from health care provider (e.g., dressing changes, ambulation, glucose monitoring)
- Nursing care plan
- Nursing orders (e.g., education needed, symptom relief measures, counseling)
- Scheduled tests and procedures
- Safety precautions used in the patient's care
- Factors that affect patient independence with activities of daily living
- Nearest relative/guardian or person to contact in an emergency
- Emergency code status (e.g., indication of "do not resuscitate" order)
- Allergies

Standardized Care Plans

Many computerized documentation systems include **standardized care plans** or **clinical practice guidelines (CPGs)** to facilitate the creation and documentation of a nursing and or interprofessional plan of care. Each CPG facilitates safe and consistent care for an identified problem by describing or listing institutional standards and evidence-based guidelines that are easily accessed and included in a patient's EHR. After completing a nursing assessment, the nurse identifies the CPGs that are appropriate for the patient and selects each one to be included in an individualized plan of care within the EHR. Most computer documentation systems allow CPGs to be modified, allowing you to individualize interventions, goals, and/or outcomes for each patient.

Standardized care plans or CPGs are useful when conducting quality improvement audits. They also improve continuity of care among professional nurses. When they are used, the nurse remains responsible for providing individualized care to each patient. Standardized care plans or CPGs cannot replace a nurse's professional judgment and decision making. Update care plans or CPGs on a regular basis to ensure that the documents are appropriate and evidence based.

Discharge Summary Forms

Nurses help ensure cost-effective care and appropriate reimbursement by preparing patients for an effective, timely discharge from a health care institution. The development of a comprehensive plan for safe discharge relies on interprofessional discharge planning. This process includes identification of key clinical outcomes and appropriate timelines for reaching them, the appropriate level of care for discharge, and all necessary resources.

Ideally discharge planning begins at admission. By identifying discharge needs early, nursing and other health care professionals begin planning for discharge to the appropriate level of care, which sometimes includes support services such as home care and equipment

BOX 26-3 Guidelines for Information to Include on a Discharge Summary

- Use clear, concise descriptions in the patient's own language.
- Provide step-by-step instructions for how to perform any procedure that the patient or family will be doing independently (e.g., emptying a urinary catheter drainage bag or self-administration of an injectable medication).
- Identify precautions to follow when performing self-care or administering medications.
- List signs and symptoms of complications that a patient needs to report to a health care provider.
- List names and phone numbers of health care providers and community resources that the patient can contact.
- Identify any unresolved problems, including plans for follow-up and continuous treatment.
- List actual time of discharge, mode of transportation, and who accompanied the patient.

needs. Involve the patient and family in the discharge planning process so they have the necessary information and resources to return home. Discharge documentation includes medications, diet, community resources, follow-up care, and who to contact in case of an emergency or for questions. All of this information is included in a discharge summary that is printed out and given to the patient on discharge but remains in the EHR as a record of the discharge teaching that was provided (Box 26-3).

ACUITY RATING SYSTEMS

Nurses use acuity ratings to determine the hours of care and number of staff required for a given group of patients every shift or every 24 hours. A patient's acuity level, usually determined by assessment data entered into a computer program by a registered nurse, is based on the type and number of nursing interventions (e.g., intravenous [IV] therapy, wound care, or ambulation assistance) required by a patient over a 24-hour period. Although acuity ratings are not part of a patient's medical record, nursing documentation within the medical record provides evidence to support the assessment of an acuity rating for an individual patient.

The acuity level is a classification used to compare one or more patients to another group of patients. For example, an acuity system classifies bathing patients from 1 (independent in all but one or two aspects of care; almost ready for discharge) to 5 (totally dependent in all aspects of care; requiring intensive care). Using this system, a patient returning from surgery requiring frequent monitoring and extensive care has an acuity level of 3 compared with another patient awaiting discharge after a successful recovery from surgery who has an acuity level of 1. Accurate acuity ratings justify the number and qualifications of staff needed to safely care for patients. The patient-to-staff ratios established for a unit depend on a composite gathering of 24-hour acuity data for all patients receiving care.

DOCUMENTATION IN THE HOME HEALTH CARE SETTING

Documentation in the home care setting is different from other areas of nursing. Medicare has specific guidelines to establish eligibility for home care reimbursement. Information used for reimbursement is gathered from documentation of care provided in the home care setting. Documentation is both the quality control and the justification for reimbursement from Medicare, Medicaid, or private insurance companies. Information in the home care medical record includes patient assessment, referral and intake forms, interprofessional plan of care, a list of medications, and reports to third-party payers. Nurses must document all of their services for payment (e.g., direct skilled care, patient teaching, skilled observation, and evaluation visits) (TJC, 2015).

The use of laptop and tablet computers makes it possible for home health care records to be available in multiple locations (the patient's home and the home care agency), improving accessibility to information and facilitating interprofessional collaboration.

Nurses use two different data sets to document the clinical assessments and care provided in the home care setting: the Outcome and Assessment Information Set (OASIS) and the Omaha System (Monsen et al., 2012). The Centers for Medicare and Medicaid Services (CMS) mandates the use of OASIS for collecting and reporting patient assessments and outcomes in the home care setting. OASIS includes a comprehensive admission assessment and calculates clinical, functional, and service scores to provide justification for reimbursement of services (Allender et al., 2014). The Omaha System consists of three components: Problem Classification Scheme, Intervention Scheme, and Problem Rating Scale for Outcomes (Monsen et al., 2012). It provides a useful model for the comprehensive evaluation of nursing care and evaluates the quality of nursing care provided in the home care setting (Allender et al., 2014).

DOCUMENTATION IN THE LONG-TERM HEALTH CARE SETTING

The long-term health care setting includes skilled nursing facilities (SNFs) in which patients receive 24-hour-a-day care, which includes housing, meals, specialized (skilled) nursing care, and treatment services, and long-term care facilities in which patients with chronic conditions receive 24–hour-a-day care, which includes housing, meals, personal care, and basic nursing care. Individual state regulations, TJC, and The CMS govern documentation requirements in these facilities. The Resident Assessment Instrument (RAI), which includes the Minimum Data Set (MDS) and the Care Area Assessment (CAA), is the data set that is federally mandated for use in long-term care facilities by CMS. MDS assessment forms are completed on admission and then periodically, within specific guidelines and time frames for all residents in certified nursing homes (American Health Information Management Association, 2010).

The MDS also determines the reimbursement level under the prospective payment system for Medicare Part A residents in an SNF. On the basis of the MDS scoring, a resource utilization group (RUG) is assigned, which determines the per-diem payment (American Health Information Management Association, 2010). Communication among nurses; social workers; dietitians; and recreational, speech, physical, and occupational therapists is essential. Documentation in the long-term care setting supports an interprofessional approach to the assessment and planning process for all patients. Compliance with state and federal requirements and reimbursement for care provided in a long-term care facility depend on accurate completion of the required documentation to justify the care provided (Hebda and Czar, 2013).

DOCUMENTATNG COMMUNICATION WITH PROVIDERS AND UNIQUE EVENTS

Telephone Calls Made to a Provider

Document every phone call you make to a health care provider. Your documentation includes when the call was made, who made it (if you

BOX 26-4 Guidelines for Telephone and Verbal Orders

- Clearly determine the patient's name, room number, and diagnosis.
- Use clarification questions to avoid misunderstandings.
- Write TO (telephone order) or VO (verbal order), including date and time, name of patient, the complete order; sign the name of the physician or health care provider and nurse.
- Read back any prescribed orders to the physician or health care provider.
- Follow agency policies; some institutions require telephone (and verbal) orders to be reviewed and signed by two nurses.

did not make the call), who was called, to whom information was given, what information was given, and what information was received. An example follows: *"10/16/2015 (20:30): Called Dr. Morgan's office. Spoke with S. Thomas, RN, who will inform Dr. Morgan that Mr. Wade's potassium level drawn at 21:00 was 5.9 mEq/dL. Informed that Dr. Morgan will call back after he is finished seeing his current patient. D. Markle, RN."*

Telephone and Verbal Orders

Telephone orders (TOs) occur when a health care provider gives therapeutic orders over the phone to a registered nurse. Verbal orders (VOs) occur when a health care provider gives therapeutic orders to a registered nurse while they are standing in proximity to one another. TOs and VOs usually occur at night or during emergencies; they should be used only when absolutely necessary and not for the sake of convenience. In some situations it is prudent to have a second person listen to TOs. Check agency policy. Box 26-4 provides guidelines that promote accuracy when receiving TOs or VOs.

The nurse receiving a TO or VO enters the complete order into the computer using the **computerized provider order entry (CPOE)** software or writes it out on a physician's order sheet for entry in the computer as soon as possible. After you have taken the order, read it back using the "read-back" process and document that you did this to provide evidence that the information received (such as call-back instructions and/or therapeutic orders) was verified with the provider. An example follows: *"10/16/2015 (08:15), Change IV fluid to Lactated Ringers with potassium 20 mEq per liter to run at 125 mL / hour. TO: Dr. Knight/J. Woods, RN, read back."* The health care provider later verifies the TO or VO legally by signing it within a set time (e.g., 24 hours) as set by hospital policy.

Incident or Occurrence Reports

An incident or occurrence is any event that is not consistent with the routine, expected care of a patient or the standard procedures in place on a health care unit. Examples include patient falls, needlestick injuries, a visitor losing consciousness, medication administration errors, accidental omission of ordered therapies, and any circumstances that lead to injury or pose a risk for patient injury. You complete **incident (or occurrence) reports** whenever an incident occurs. They are an important part of the quality improvement program of a unit (see Chapter 2). A "near miss" is an incident in which no property was damaged and no patient or personnel were injured; but, given a slight shift in time or position, damage or injury could have occurred easily (OSHA, n.d.). When an incident occurs, document an objective description of what happened; what you observed; and the follow-up actions taken, including notification of the patient's health care provider in the patient's medical record. Remember to evaluate and document the patient's response to the incident.

Incident reports contain confidential information; distribution of the report is limited to those responsible for reviewing the forms. Follow agency policy when making an incident report and file the report with the risk-management department of your agency. Analysis of incident reports helps identify trends in an organization that provide justification for changes in policies and procedures or for in-service programs. Do not include any reference to an incident in the medical record. A notation about an incident report in a patient's medical record makes it easier for a lawyer to argue that the reference makes the incident report part of the medical record and therefore subject to attorney review.

INFORMATICS AND INFORMATION MANAGEMENT IN HEALTH CARE

Information technology (IT) refers to the management and processing of information, generally with the assistance of computers. **Health informatics** is the "application of computer and information science in all basic and biomedical sciences to facilitate the acquisition, processing, interpretation, optimal use, and communication of health-related data. The focus is the patient and the process of care, and the goal is to enhance the quality and efficiency of care provided" (Hebda and Czar, 2013, p. 6). A health care information system (HIS) is a group of systems used within a health care organization to support and enhance health care. A HIS consists of two major types of information systems: clinical information systems and administrative information systems. Together the two systems operate to make the entry and communication of data and information more efficient. You will find that any single health care agency uses one or several of these systems.

Nursing competence in health care informatics is becoming a priority as health care providers and facilities across the United States implement electronic documentation. You need informatics competencies to deliver safer and more efficient care, to add to the nursing professional knowledge base, and to facilitate the growth of evidence-based practice. Professional organizations such as the Institute of Medicine, The Robert Wood Johnson Foundation, and the National League for Nursing recommend that all nurses acquire a minimal level of awareness and competence in informatics and use of IT. The American Association of Colleges of Nursing established a framework that outlines curricular goals and outcomes in informatics for baccalaureate, masters, and doctoral programs of nursing (Hebda and Czar, 2013).

The Technology Informatics Guiding Education Reform (TIGER) Initiative began as a grassroots program in 2006 and was supported by over 70 contributing organizations, two grants from the Robert Wood Johnson Foundation, and one personal endowment. TIGER is focused on better preparing the clinical workforce to use technology and informatics to improve the delivery of patient care. On September 22, 2014, TIGER transitioned to the Healthcare Information and Management Systems Society (HIMSS). Under the direction of HIMSS, the momentum of the grass roots initiative will benefit from the robust volunteer structure that HIMSS can provide so strategies for the recruitment, retention, and training of current and future workforces for informatics education, practice, and research can be advanced (Healthcare Information and Management Systems Society, 2015).

Competence in informatics is not the same as computer competency. To become competent in informatics you need to be able to use evolving methods of discovering, retrieving, and using information in practice (Hebda and Czar, 2013). This means that you learn to recognize when information is needed and have the skills to find, evaluate, and use that information effectively. As a nurse you also need to know how to use clinical databases within your institution and apply the information so you can deliver high-quality, appropriate patient care.

Nursing Informatics

Nursing informatics is broadly defined as the "use of information and computer technology to support all aspects of nursing practice, including direct delivery of care, administration, education, and research," (Hebda and Czar, 2013, p. 6). All nurses deal with data, information, and knowledge. It is important that you know how to record, interpret, and report data and critically think and apply that knowledge when providing patient care. Data include numbers, characters, or facts that you collect according to a perceived need for analysis and possible action. You gain knowledge from gathering and using information from several sources. An example is a nurse's review of several, consecutive assessments of a wound documented within the EHR. Reviewing changes in the descriptions of the edges of the wound, color of drainage, and measurements over several days allows the nurse to evaluate and identify a pattern that indicates that the wound is not healing (information). On the basis of evidence available in the scientific literature, the nurse applies knowledge of wound care principles and intervenes to manage the patient's wound to promote healing.

Nursing informatics is also recognized as a specialty area of nursing practice. Informatics nurses have advanced preparation in information management and demonstrate proficiency with informatics to support all areas of nursing practice, including quality improvement, research, project management, and system design (Hebda and Czar, 2013). Through the application of nursing informatics, technology is put to practical use to enhance bedside care and education. The application of nursing informatics results in an efficient and effective nursing information system that facilitates the integration of data, information, and knowledge to support patients, nurses, and other providers in decision making in all roles and settings.

Clinical Information Systems

All members of the interprofessional health care team, including nurses, physicians, pharmacists, social workers, and therapists, use programs available on a clinical information system (CIS). These programs include monitoring systems; order entry systems; and laboratory, radiology, and pharmacy systems. A monitoring system includes devices that automatically monitor and record biometric measurements (e.g., vital signs, oxygen saturation, cardiac index, and stroke volume) in acute care, critical care, and specialty areas. The devices electronically send measurements directly to the nursing documentation system.

Order-entry systems allow nurses to order supplies and services from another department. An example is a computer program that provides the ability to order sterile supplies from the central supply department. This eliminates the use of written order forms and expedites the delivery of needed supplies to a nursing unit. Computerized provider order entry (CPOE) systems allow health care providers to directly enter orders for patient care into hospital information system. In advanced systems CPOE has built-in reminders and alerts that help a health care provider select the most appropriate medication or diagnostic test. The direct entry of orders eliminates issues related to illegible handwriting and transcription errors. In addition, a CPOE system potentially speeds the implementation of ordered diagnostic tests and treatments, which improves staff productivity and saves money because the unit secretary no longer transcribes a written order onto a nursing order form (Hebda and Czar, 2013). Orders made through CPOE are integrated within the record and sent to the appropriate departments (e.g., pharmacy or radiology).

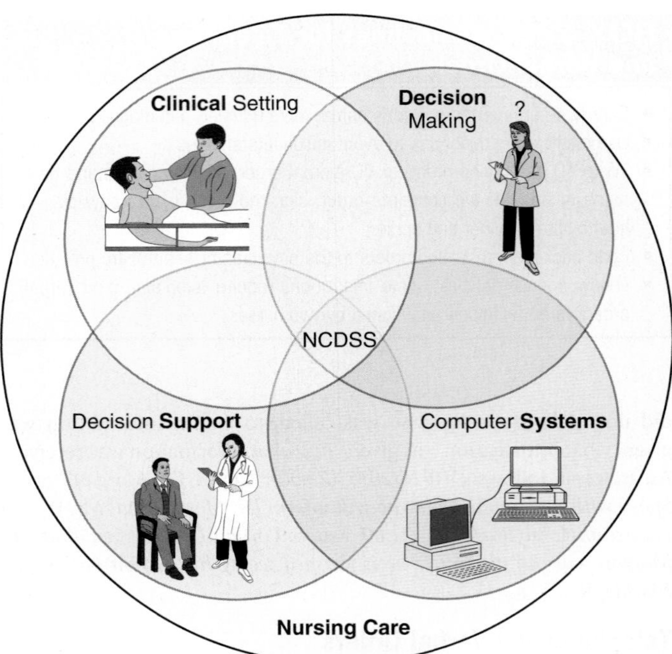

FIGURE 26-2 Model of a nursing clinical decision support system (CDSS).

Clinical decision support systems (CDSSs) are computerized programs used within the health care setting to aid and support clinical decision making. When used to support nursing decisions it is called a nursing CDSS (Figure 26-2). The knowledge base within a CDSS contains rules and logic statements that link information required for clinical decisions to generate tailored recommendations for individual patients, which are presented to nurses as alerts, warnings, or other information for consideration (Lee, 2013). For example, an effective CDSS notifies health care providers of patient allergies before ordering a medication, which enhances patient safety during the medication ordering process. CDSSs also improve nursing care. When patient assessment data are combined with patient care guidelines, nurses are better able to implement evidence-based nursing care, resulting in improved patient outcomes (Box 26-5).

Nursing Clinical Information Systems

A well-designed nursing clinical information system (NCIS) incorporates the principles of nursing informatics to support the work that nurses do by facilitating documentation of nursing process activities and offering resources for managing nursing care delivery. As a nurse you need to access a computer program easily, review a patient's medical history and health care provider orders, and then go to the patient's bedside to conduct a comprehensive assessment. Once you complete an assessment, enter data into the computer terminal at the patient's bedside and develop a plan of care from the information gathered. This allows you to quickly share the plan of care with your patient. Periodically return to the computer to check on laboratory test results and document the care you deliver. The computer screens and optional pop-up windows make it easy to locate information, enter and compare data, and make changes.

NCISs have two designs. The nursing process design is the most traditional. It organizes documentation within well-established formats such as admission and postoperative assessment problem lists,

BOX 26-5 EVIDENCE-BASED PRACTICE

Effect of Clinical Decision Support Systems on Patient Outcomes

PICO Question: Do nurses who work at health care agencies that use clinical decision support systems (CDSSs) provide safer and more effective patient care when compared with nurses who work at agencies that do not use CDSSs?

Evidence Summary

Nurses who provide evidence-based care at the bedside provide safe and effective care. However, one barrier to implementing evidence-based practice is getting information to nurses at the bedside when they need it. Several studies investigated the effect of the CDSS on patient outcomes. Harrison et al. (2013) examined the impact of a nursing CDSS integrated with the electronic heart record developed to facilitate adherence to guidelines for the management of hypoglycemia. Data were collected and reviewed 6 months before implementation, 6 months following implementation, and 7 to 12 months after implementation of the CDSS. The findings of this study demonstrated a statistically significant improvement in adherence to use of the clinical guideline. The study also showed that the protocol was almost 3 times as likely to be followed 7 to 12 months after implementation of the CDSS. Current evidence also shows that use of CDSS improves adherence to implementation of evidence-based sepsis care in intensive care units (Giuliano et al., 2011) and completion of screening for osteoporosis in primary care settings (DeJesus et al., 2012). These studies show that CDSSs that provide automatic decision support at the time and place nurses need it enhance the quality and safety of patient care. CDSSs also help nurses initiate evidence-based care faster and with more accuracy, improving patient outcomes.

Application to Nursing Practice

- CDSSs enhance the implementation of evidence-based practice into nursing care because they remind nurses which interventions need to be implemented for specific patients at the time the care is needed.
- Nurses need to be involved in the design and selection of CDSSs to ensure that they provide clinical decision support effectively and efficiently.
- Nurses need to evaluate patient outcomes when CDSSs are used. They also need to be involved in developing solutions to improve the effectiveness of CDSSs when opportunities for improvement are identified.

care plans, intervention lists or notes, and discharge planning instructions. The nursing process design facilitates the following:

- Generation of a nursing work list that outlines routine scheduled activities related to the care of each patient
- Documentation of routine aspects of patient care such as hygiene, positioning, fluid intake and output, wound care measures, and blood glucose measurements
- Progress note entries using narrative notes, charting by exception, and/or flow-sheets
- Documentation of medication administration (see Chapter 32)

More advanced systems incorporate standardized nursing languages such as the North American Nursing Diagnosis Association–International (NANDA-I) nursing diagnoses, the Nursing Interventions Classification (NIC), and the Nursing Outcomes Classification (NOC) into the software.

The other model for an NCIS is the protocol or critical pathway design (Hebda and Czar, 2013). This design facilitates interdisciplinary management of information because all health care providers use evidenced-based protocols or critical pathways to document the care they provide. The information system allows a user to select one or more appropriate protocols for a patient. An advanced system merges multiple protocols, using a master protocol or path to direct patient care activities. Standard health care provider order sets are included in the protocols and automatically processed. The system integrates appropriate information into the medication delivery process to enhance patient safety. In addition, the system identifies variances of the anticipated outcomes on the protocols as documentation is entered. This provides all caregivers the ability to analyze variances and offer an accurate clinical picture of a patient's progress.

Advantages of a Nursing Clinical Information System. Anecdotal reports and descriptive studies suggest that NCISs offer important advantages to nurses in practice. According to Hebda and Czar (2013), some specific advantages include:

- Better access to information.
- Enhanced quality of documentation through prompts.
- Reduced errors of omission.
- Reduced hospital costs.
- Increased nurse job satisfaction.
- Compliance with requirements of accrediting agencies (e.g., TJC).
- Development of a common clinical database.
- Enhanced ability to track records.

Many NCIS's include content-importing technologies that allow the use of templates, macros, automated data points, and the ability to copy forward either parts of or entire nursing shift assessments that enable nurses to quickly document their assessment or the care they provided. These features have benefits and risks associated with their use. When allergy and current medication lists are automatically imported into nursing admission documentation from a previous hospital encounter, you need to meticulously review this information for accuracy and update it as needed to avoid documentation errors and patient safety concerns. When nursing shift assessment data is copied forward from a previous shift or day, it must be updated so it accurately reflects a patient's current clinical status (Weis and Levy, 2014).

QSEN QSEN: BUILDING COMPETENCY IN INFORMATICS. You are using the bar-code medication administration (BCMA) system at the hospital where you work to document administration of a dose of warfarin (Coumadin) 7.5 mg PO to one of your patients. When you scan the dose of medication, an alert pops up on the computer screen in the patient's room, which requires you to enter the patient's current international normalized ratio (INR) result before you can give the patient the medication and complete the documentation of the administration of the medication.

At your hospital the normal range for INR is 0.8 to 1.1, and the therapeutic range for INR for patient's taking Warfarin (Coumadin) is 2.5 to 3.0. Your patient's INR result for today is 4.2 (much higher than the therapeutic range desired). What will you do in response to the alert that popped up on the computer screen?

Answers to QSEN Activities can be found on the Evolve website.

KEY POINTS

- The electronic (or paper-based) medical record is a legal document that contains information describing the care delivered to a patient.
- The medical record is also a financial record that serves as the basis for reimbursement.
- All information contained in the medical record is confidential; access to patient records is limited to individuals involved in the care of the patient.

- Interdisciplinary communication among members of the health care team is essential, and the medical record is one tool that supports and facilitates that communication.
- Accurate record keeping requires an objective interpretation of data with precise measurements, correct spelling, and proper use of abbreviations.
- To keep medical records accurate, any change in a patient's condition warrants immediate documentation about the event and the action that was taken to address the change.
- A nurse's electronic or handwritten signature on an entry in a record designates accountability for the contents of that entry.
- Protection of the confidentiality of patients' health information and the security of computer systems are top priorities that include log-in processes, audit trails, firewalls, data-recovery processes, and policies about handling and disposing of data to protect patient information.
- POMRs are organized by the patient's health care problems.
- SOAP, SOAPIE, PIE, or DAR charting formats organize entries in the progress notes according to the nursing process.
- Medicare guidelines establish the requirements for documentation by nurses working in the home care setting that supports and justifies reimbursement for care delivered.
- Long-term care documentation is interdisciplinary and closely linked with fiscal requirements of outside agencies.
- Always verify patient care information communicated to providers through telephone orders by using and documenting use of the "read-back" process.
- A hospital information system consists of two major types of information systems: CIS and administrative information systems.
- Computerized information systems provide information about patients in an organized and easily accessible fashion.
- Nursing informatics facilitates the integration of data, information, and knowledge to support clinical decision making of nurses and other providers in all roles and settings.

CLINICAL APPLICATION QUESTIONS

Preparing for Clinical Practice

David Page, an 80-year-old man, is admitted to the hospital with a diagnosis of possible pneumonia. He states that he is not feeling well and has a frequent cough, which produces thick, light tan sputum. Vital signs are: blood pressure, 150/90 mm Hg; pulse rate, 92 beats/min; respirations, 22 breaths/min. During your initial assessment he coughs violently for 40 to 45 seconds. His lungs have wheezes and rhonchi in both bases but are otherwise clear. He states, "My chest hurts when I cough, and the pain radiates into my shoulders."

1. Which data do you document as objective?
2. Which data are subjective?
3. This assessment information was documented electronically in narrative format. Discuss the benefits and negatives associated with this format of documentation.

ⓔ *Answers to Clinical Application Questions can be found on the Evolve website.*

REVIEW QUESTIONS

Are You Ready to Test Your Nursing Knowledge?

1. A manager is reviewing the nursing documentation entered by a staff nurse in a patient's electronic medical record and finds the following entry, "Patient is difficult to care for, refuses suggestion for improving appetite." Which of the following statements is most appropriate for the manager to make to the staff nurse who entered this information?
   1. "Avoid rushing when documenting an entry in the medical record."
   2. "Use correction fluid to remove the entry."
   3. "Draw a single line through the statement and initial it."
   4. Enter only objective and factual information about a patient in the medical record.
2. A preceptor observes a new graduate nurse discussing changes in a patient's condition with a physician over the phone. The new graduate nurse accepts telephone orders for a new medication and for some laboratory tests from the physician at the end of the conversation. During the conversation the new graduate writes the orders down on a piece of paper to enter them into the electronic medical record when a computer terminal is available. At this hospital new medication orders entered into the electronic medical record can be viewed immediately by hospital pharmacists, and hospital policy states that all new medications must be reviewed by a pharmacist before being administered to patients. Which of the following actions requires the preceptor to intervene? The new nurse:
   1. Reads the orders back to the health care provider to verify accuracy of transcribing the orders after receiving them over the phone.
   2. Documents the date and time of the phone conversation, the name of the physician, and the topics discussed in the electronic record.
   3. Gives a newly ordered medication before entering the order in the patient's medical record.
   4. Asks the preceptor to listen in on the phone conversation.
3. As the nurse enters a patient's room, the nurse notices that the patient is anxious. The patient quickly states, "I don't know what's going on; I can't get an explanation from my doctor about my test results. I want something done about this." Which of the following is the most appropriate way for the nurse to document this observation of the patient?
   1. "The patient has a defiant attitude and is demanding test results."
   2. "The patient appears to be upset with the nurse because he wants his test results immediately."
   3. "The patient is demanding and is complaining about the doctor."
   4. "The patient stated feelings of frustration from the lack of information received regarding test results."
4. The nurse is reviewing the Health Insurance Portability and Accountability Act (HIPAA) regulations with the patient during the admission process. The patient states, "I'm not familiar with these HIPAA regulations. How will they affect my care?" Which of the following is the best response?
   1. HIPAA allows all hospital staff access to your medical record.
   2. HIPAA limits the information that is documented in your medical record.
   3. HIPAA provides you with greater protection of your personal health information.
   4. HIPAA enables health care institutions to release all of your personal information to improve continuity of care.
5. A patient states, "I would like to see what is written in my medical record." What is the nurse's best response?
   1. "Only your family can read your medical record."
   2. "You have the right to read your record."
   3. "Patients are not allowed to read their records."
   4. "Only health care workers have access to patient records."

6. Which of the following documentation entries is most accurate?
   1. "Patient walked up and down hallway with assistance, tolerated well."
   2. "Patient up, out of bed, walked down hallway and back to room, tolerated well."
   3. "Patient up, walked 50 feet and back down hallway with assistance from nurse. Spouse also accompanied patient during the walk."
   4. "Patient walked 50 feet and back down hallway with assistance from nurse; HR 88 and regular before exercise, HR 94 and regular following exercise."
7. Label each line of documentation with the appropriate SOAP category (Subjective [S], Objective [O], Assessment [A], Plan [P]).
   1. ______ Repositioned patient on right side. Encouraged patient to use patient-controlled analgesia (PCA) device.
   2. ______ "The pain increases every time I try to turn on my left side."
   3. ______ *Acute pain related to tissue injury from surgical incision.*
   4. ______ Left lower abdominal surgical incision, 3 inches in length, closed, sutures intact, no drainage. Pain noted on mild palpation.
8. **Fill in the Blank.** While working on a unit within a hospital, the nurse was able to access a patient's medical record and review the education that other nurses provided during an initial hospitalization and three subsequent clinic visits that occurred in different provider's offices over the past 6 months. This type of feature is most common in a(n) ________________________.
9. The nurse is transferring a patient to a long-term, skilled care facility and has just given a telephone report to a registered nurse (RN) who works at that facility and who will be receiving the patient. In documenting this call, the nurse begins by writing the date and time the report was given and the name of the RN taking the report. Which of the following pieces of information does the nurse include in the documentation of this telephone call? (Select all that apply.)
   1. The patient's name, age, and admitting diagnoses
   2. The discussion of any allergies to food and medications that the patient has
   3. That the nurse receiving the report was advised that the patient is "needy" and "on the call light all the time"
   4. That the patient's pain rating went from 8 to 2 on a scale of 1 to 10 after receiving 650 mg of Tylenol
   5. Description of any unresolved problems and current interventions in place
10. The nurse is supervising a beginning nursing student and allowing the student to complete documentation of care under direct observation. Which of the following actions are not appropriate and would require intervention? The nursing student: (Select all that apply.)
    1. Documents a medication given by another nursing student.
    2. Includes the date and time of the entry into the medical record.
    3. Enters assessment data into the electronic medical record using the computer mounted on the wall in the patient's room.
    4. Leaves a slip of paper with her user name and password in the patient's room.
    5. Starts to enter "Docusate sodium 100 mg ordered at 08:00 held. Patient declined to take dose stating, "I had several loose stools yesterday, and I'm afraid if I take this dose the problem will get worse," as a narrative comment.
11. A group of nurses is discussing the advantages of using computerized provider order entry (CPOE). Which of the following statements indicates that the nurses understand the major advantage of using CPOE?
    1. "CPOE reduces transcription errors."
    2. "CPOE reduces the time needed for health care providers to write orders."
    3. "CPOE eliminates verbal and telephone orders from health care providers."
    4. "CPOE reduces the time nurses use to communicate with health care providers."
12. The nurse is working the evening shift at a hospital that uses military time for documentation. The nurse administered morphine 2 mg intravenously (IV) for pain at 3:45 PM, changed the dressing over the patient's abdominal incision at 5:34 PM, and administered Ancef 1 g IV at 8:00 PM. Using correct military time, label the documentation for each task with the time that it was completed.
    1. ______ Morphine 2 mg IV given for pain rating of 8/10
    2. ______ Dressing changed over midline abdominal incision using aseptic technique
    3. ______ Ancef 1 g given IVPB over 30 minutes.
13. The nurse is caring for a patient with a nasogastric feeding tube who is receiving a continuous tube feeding at a rate of 45 mL per hour. The nurse enters the patient assessment data and information that the head of the patient's bed is elevated to 20 degrees. An alert appears on the computer screen warning that this patient is at a high risk for aspiration because the head of the bed is not elevated enough. This warning is known as which type of system?
    1. Electronic health record
    2. Clinical documentation
    3. Clinical decision support system
    4. Computerized physician order entry
14. While reviewing the pulmonary assessment entered by a nurse in a patient's electronic medical record (EMR), a physician notices that the only information documented in that section is "WDL" (within defined limits). The physician also is not able to find a narrative description of the patient's respiratory status in the nurse's progress notes. What is the most likely reason for this?
    1. The nurse caring for the patient forgot to document on the pulmonary system.
    2. The EMR uses a charting-by-exception format.
    3. The computer shut down unexpectedly when the nurse was documenting the assessment.
    4. Because of HIPAA regulations, physicians are not authorized to view the nursing assessment.
15. What is the appropriate way for a nurse to dispose of information printed out from a patient's electronic health record?
    1. Rip the papers up into small pieces and place the pieces into a standard trash can
    2. Place all papers in the flip-top binder designated for that patient that is located in the nurse's station on the patient care unit
    3. Place papers with patient information in a secure canister marked for shredding
    4. Burn documents with patient information in the steel sink located within the dirty supply room on the patient care unit

Answers: 1. 4; **2.** 3; **3.** 4; **4.** 3; **5.** 2; **6.** 4; **7.** 1=P, 2=S, 3=A, 4=O; **8.** Electronic health record; **9.** 1, 2, 4, 5; **10.** 1, 4; **11.** 1; **12.** 1=15:45, 2=17:34, 3=20:00; **13.** 3; **14.** 2; **15.** 3.

Rationales for Review Questions can be found on the Evolve website.

REFERENCES

Administrative Committee of the Federal Registrar: *Electronic Code of Federal Regulations (eCFR)*, 2014, National Archives and Records Administrations Office of the Federal Register & Government Printing Office, http://www.ecfr.gov/cgi-bin/text-idx?c=ecfr&tpl=/ecfrbrowse/Title45/45cfr164_main_02.tpl. Accessed April 29, 2015.

Allender JA, et al: *Community & public health nursing: promoting the public's health*, ed 8, Philadelphia, 2014, Wolters Kluwer: Lippincott Williams & Wilkins.

American Health Consultants: They're back! Clinical pathways are in favor again, *Hosp Case Manag* 23(2):13, 2015.

American Health Information Management Association: *Documentation in the long-term care record*, October 2010, http://ahimaltcguidelines.pbworks.com/w/page/46508844/Documentation%20in%20the%20Long%20Term%20Care%20Record. Accessed April 29, 2015.

American Nurses Association (ANA): *ANA's Principles for nursing documentation: guidance for nurses*, Silver Spring, MD, 2010, American Nurses Association.

Beach J, Oates J: Maintaining best practice in record-keeping and documentation, *Nurs Stand* 28(36):45, 2014.

Blair W, Smith B: Nursing documentation: frameworks and barriers, *Contemp Nurse* 41(2):160, 2012.

Dacey B, Bholat MA: Health information technology: medical record documentation issues in the electronic era, *Prim Care* 39(4):633, 2012.

DeMartino JK, Larsen JK: Equity in cancer care: pathways, protocols, and guidelines, *J Natl Comp Cancer Netw* 10(Suppl 1):S1, 2012.

Fontenot SF: The affordable care act and electronic health care records, *Physician Executive J* November–December:72, 2013.

Healthcare Information and Management Systems Society: *The TIGER initiative: technology informatics guiding education reform*, 2015, http://www.thetigerinitiative.org/. Accessed April 29, 2015.

Hebda T, Czar P: *Handbook of informatics for nurses & healthcare professionals*, ed 5, Upper Saddle River, NJ, 2013, Pearson Education.

HITECH Answers: *Meaningful use*, 2015, http://www.hitechanswers.net/ehr-adoption-2/meaningful-use/. Accessed April 29, 2015.

Lee S: Features of computerized clinical decision support systems supportive of nursing practice, *Comput Inform Nurs* 31(10):477, 2013.

Lewis SL, et al: *Medical-surgical nursing: assessment and management of clinical problems*, ed 9, St Louis, 2014, Elsevier.

Mostashari F: *Statement by Farzad Mostashari, MD, ScM, National Coordinator, Office of the National Coordinator for Health Information Technology, U.S. Department of Health and Human Services (HHS) on Health IT before Committee on Finance, U.S. Senate*, Wednesday, July 17, 2013, http://www.hhs.gov/asl/testify/2013/07/t20130717b.html. Accessed April 29, 2015.

Occupational Safety and Health Administration (OSHA): *Accident/incident investigation*, n.d., https://www.osha.gov/SLTC/etools/safetyhealth/mod4_factsheets_accinvest.html. Accessed April 29, 2015.

O'Toole M, editor: *Mosby's dictionary of medicine, nursing & health professions*, ed 9, St Louis, 2013, Elsevier.

Saleem JJ, et al: The next-generation electronic health record: perspectives of key leaders from the US Department of Veterans Affairs, *J Am Med Inform Assoc* 20(e1):e175, 2013.

The Joint Commission (TJC): *Comprehensive accreditation manual for hospitals: the official handbook*, Oak Brook, IL, 2015, The Joint Commission.

US Department of Health and Human Services (USDHHS): *2013 News: doctors and hospitals' use of health IT more than doubles since 2012*, May 22, 2013, http://www.hhs.gov/news/press/2013pres/05/20130522a.html. Accessed May 3, 2015.

Weis JM, Levy PC: Copy, paste, and cloned notes in electronic health records, *Chest* 145(3):632, 2014.

RESEARCH REFERENCES

Chan RJ, Webster J: End-of-life care pathways for improving outcomes in caring for the dying, *Cochrane Database Syst Rev* (11):CD008006.pub3, 2013. DOI: 10.1002/14651858.

DeJesus RS, et al: Use of clinical decision support system to increase osteoporosis screening, *J Eval Clin Pract* 18:89, 2012.

Ender KL, et al: Use of a clinical pathway to improve the acute management of vaso-occlusive crisis pain in pediatric sickle cell disease, *Pediatr Blood Cancer* 61:693, 2014.

Englebright J, et al: Defining and incorporating basic nursing care actions into the electronic health record, *J Nurs Sch* 46(1):50, 2014.

Giuliano KK, et al: Impact of protocol watch on compliance with the surviving sepsis campaign, *Am J Crit Care* 20(4):313, 2011.

Harrison RL, et al: Use of a clinical decision support system to improve hypoglycemia management, *MEDSURG Nurs J Adult Health* 22(4):250, 263, 2013.

Kelley TF, et al: Electronic nursing documentation as a strategy to improve quality of patient care, *J Nurs Scholars* 43(2):154, 2011.

Kerr N: Creating a protective picture: a grounded theory of RN decision-making when using a charting-by-exception documentation system, *MEDSURG Nurs: J Adult Health* 22(2):110, 2013.

Monsen KA, et al: Exploring the value of clinical data standards to predict hospitalization of home care patients, *Appl Clin Inform* 3:419, 2012.

Penoyer DA, et al: Use of electronic health record documentation by healthcare workers in an acute care hospital system, *J Healthc manage* 59(2):130, 2014.

27

Patient Safety and Quality

OBJECTIVES

- Discuss the importance of consensus standards for public reporting of patient safety events.
- Describe environmental hazards that pose risks to a person's safety.
- Discuss methods to reduce physical hazards and the transmission of pathogens.
- Discuss the specific risks to safety related to developmental age.
- Identify the factors to assess when a patient is in restraints.
- Describe the four categories of safety risks in a health care agency.
- Describe assessment activities designed to identify a patient's physical, psychosocial, and cognitive status as it pertains to his or her safety.
- Identify relevant nursing diagnoses associated with risks to safety.
- Develop a nursing care plan for patients whose safety is threatened.
- Describe nursing interventions specific to a patients' age for reducing risk of falls, fires, poisonings, and electrical hazards.
- Define the knowledge, skills, and attitudes necessary to promote safety in a health care setting.

KEY TERMS

Aura, p. 393
Food and Drug Administration (FDA), p. 374
Immunization, p. 375
Pathogen, p. 375
Poison, p. 375
Pollutant, p. 376
Restraint, p. 391
Seizure, p. 393
Seizure precautions, p. 393
Status epilepticus, p. 393

MEDIA RESOURCES

http://evolve.elsevier.com/Potter/fundamentals/

- Review Questions
- Video Clips
- Concept Map Creator
- Case Study with Questions
- Skills Performance Checklists
- Audio Glossary
- Content Updates

Safety, often defined as freedom from psychological and physical injury, is a basic human need. Health care provided in a safe manner and a safe community environment is essential for a patient's survival and well-being. A safe environment reduces the risk for illness and injury and helps to contain the cost of health care by preventing extended lengths of treatment and/or hospitalization, improving or maintaining a patient's functional status, and increasing a patient's sense of well-being. The Institute of Medicine's report *To Err Is Human: Building a Safer Health System* (IOM, 2000) was a pivotal publication that brought patient safety to the forefront of health care in the United States. This report indicated that 44,000 to 98,000 people die each year as a result of preventable medical errors. In an effort to improve patient safety, many organizations became devoted to developing and monitoring key health care safety initiatives and providing information to health care organizations and the public. Health care organizations foster a patient-centered safety culture by continually focusing on performance-improvement endeavors, risk-management findings, and safety reports; providing current reliable technology; integrating evidence-based practice into procedures; designing a safe work environment and atmosphere; and providing continuing education and access to appropriate resources for staff (Box 27-1).

As part of the health care team, nurses are professionally responsible for engaging in activities that support a patient-centered safety culture. The IOM defined patient-centered care as health care that establishes a partnership among practitioners, patients, and their families (when appropriate) to ensure that decisions respect patients' wants, needs, and preferences and that patients have the education and support they need to make decisions and participate in their own care (IOM, 2001). Considerable emphasis is placed on improving the education of nursing students so they become competent in promoting safe health care practices.

The Quality and Safety Education for Nurses (QSEN) project was developed to meet the challenge of preparing future nurses who will have the knowledge, skills, and attitudes necessary to continuously improve the quality and safety of the health care systems within which they work (QSEN, 2014). The QSEN safety competency for a nurse is defined as "Minimizes risk of harm to patients and providers through both system effectiveness and individual performance." As a nurse you are responsible for incorporating critical thinking skills when using the nursing process, assessing each patient and his or her environment for hazards that threaten safety, and planning and intervening appropriately to maintain a safe environment. By doing this you become a

BOX 27-1 Resources Related to Safety and Safety Initiatives

- The Joint Commission http://www.jointcommission.org/
- The Agency for Healthcare Research and Quality http://www.ahrq. gov/
- The Institute for Healthcare Improvement http://www.ihi.org/
- The U.S. Department of Veterans Affairs http://www.patientsafety.va.gov
- Centers for Medicare and Medicaid Services http://www.cms.gov
- ECRI Institute http://www.ecri.org
- U.S. Department of Health and Human Services http://www.hospitalcompare.hhs.gov

provider of safe acute, restorative, and continuing care and an active participant in health promotion.

SCIENTIFIC KNOWLEDGE BASE

Environmental Safety

A patient's environment includes physical and psychosocial factors that influence or affect the life and survival of that patient. This broad definition of environment crosses the continuum of care for settings in which the nurse and patient interact such as the hospital, long-term care facility, clinic, community center, school, and home. A safe environment protects the staff as well, allowing them to function optimally. Vulnerable groups who often require help in achieving a safe environment include infants, children, older adults, the ill, the physically and mentally disabled, the illiterate, and the poor. A safe environment includes meeting basic needs, reducing physical hazards and the transmission of pathogens, and controlling pollution.

Basic Needs. Physiological needs, including the need for sufficient oxygen, nutrition, and optimum temperature, influence a person's safety. According to Maslow's hierarchy of needs, these basic needs must be met before physical and psychological safety and security can be addressed (see Chapter 6).

Oxygen. Supplemental oxygen is sometimes required to meet a person's oxygenation needs. Oxygen is not flammable, but it is combustible. This means that fire needs oxygen to start and to keep burning. When more oxygen is in the air, a fire burns hotter and faster. Strict codes regulate the use and storage of medical oxygen in health care facilities. This is not necessarily true in the home environment. Hospital emergency departments see approximately 1190 thermal burns per year caused by ignitions associated with home medical oxygen (NFPA, 2008). Smoking is the leading cause of burns, reported fires, deaths, and injuries involving home medical oxygen.

Be aware of factors in a patient's environment that decrease the amount of available oxygen. A common environmental hazard in the home is an improperly functioning heating system. A furnace, stove, or fireplace that is not properly vented introduces carbon monoxide into the environment (NFPA, 2014a). Carbon monoxide affects a person's oxygenation by binding with hemoglobin, preventing the formation of oxyhemoglobin and thus reducing the supply of oxygen delivered to tissues (see Chapter 41). Low concentrations cause nausea, dizziness, headache, and fatigue. Very high concentrations cause death after 1 to 3 minutes of exposure (Mayo Clinic, 2014).

Nutrition. Meeting nutritional needs adequately and safely requires environmental controls and knowledge (see Chapter 45). Health care facilities and restaurants are required to meet State Board of Health regulations. To protect consumers, commercially processed and packaged foods are subject to Food and Drug Administration (FDA) regulations. The FDA is a federal agency responsible for the enforcement of federal regulations regarding the manufacture, processing, and distribution of foods, drugs, and cosmetics to protect consumers against the sale of impure or dangerous substances. Although food supply in the United States is one of the safest in the world, about 48 million illnesses occur annually, more than 128,000 people are hospitalized, and 3000 die from foodborne illness (CDC, 2014a). Groups at the highest risk are children, pregnant women, older adults, and people with compromised immune systems. Foods that are inadequately prepared or stored or subject to unsanitary conditions increase a patient's risk for infections and food poisoning.

Temperature. A person's comfort zone is usually between 18.3° and 23.9° C (65° and 75° F). Temperature extremes that frequently occur during the winter and summer affect comfort, productivity, and safety. Exposure to severe cold for prolonged periods causes frostbite and accidental hypothermia. Older adults, the young, patients with cardiovascular conditions, patients who have ingested drugs or alcohol in excess, and people who are homeless are at high risk for hypothermia. Exposure to extreme heat changes the electrolyte balance of the body and raises the core body temperature, resulting in heatstroke or heat exhaustion. Chronically ill patients, older adults, and infants are at greatest risk for injury from extreme heat. These patients need to avoid extremely hot, humid environments (see Chapter 30).

Physical Hazards. On average 33.5 million injuries take place each year (CDC, 2010). Physical hazards in the environment threaten a person's safety and often result in physical or psychological injury or death. Unintentional injuries are the fifth leading cause of death for Americans of all ages (National Center for Injury Prevention and Control, 2010a, 2010b). Motor vehicle accidents are the leading cause, followed by poisonings and falls. Additional hazards consist of fire and disasters. Nurses play a role in educating patients about common safety hazards and how to prevent injury while placing emphasis on hazards to which patients are more vulnerable.

Motor Vehicle Accidents. Vehicle design and equipment such as seat belts, air bags, and laminated windshields (remain in one piece when impacted) have improved safety for vehicle occupants. State-specific laws relating to young driver licensing, safety belt use, child restraint use, and motorcycle helmets exist for protection. Child safety seats and booster seats appropriate for a child's age and weight and the type of car need to be used. The American Academy of Pediatrics (AAP, 2011a) recommends that all infants and toddlers ride in the back seat with a rear-facing-only seat and rear-facing convertible seat until they are 2 years of age or they reach the highest weight or height allowed by the manufacturer of the car safety seat. Toddlers and preschoolers or any child who has outgrown the rear-facing weight or height limit for his convertible car seat should use a forward-facing car seat. The website of the AAP, Healthy Children, http://www.healthychildren.org/English/safety-prevention/on-the-go/Pages/Car-Safety-Seats-Information-for-Families.aspx, has information for children of all ages and the type of safety seat to use. The back seat of a car is the safest part of the vehicle in the event of a crash and prevents injury from deployment of passenger and side air bags.

According to the CDC (2014b), the risk of motor vehicle accidents is higher among 16- to 19-year-old drivers than any other age-group. Teens are more likely to underestimate dangerous situations or not be able to recognize hazardous situations, speed and allow shorter headways, ride with intoxicated drivers, and drive after using alcohol and drugs. Teens also have the lowest rate of seat belt use. Older drivers are keeping their licenses longer and driving more miles than in the past. Per mile traveled, fatal crash rates increase starting at age 75 and increase markedly after age 80 (Insurance Institute for Highway Safety, 2015). An older adult is not always able to quickly observe situations in which an accident is likely to occur. Decreased hearing acuity alters the ability to hear emergency vehicle sirens or vehicle horns. A decreased nervous system response prevents older adults from being able to react as quickly as they once could to avoid an accident. A decline in these skills accounts for the most common types of accidents, including right-of-way and turning accidents.

Poison. A **poison** is any substance that impairs health or destroys life when ingested, inhaled, or absorbed by the body. Almost any substance is poisonous if too much is taken. Sources in a person's home include drugs, medicines, other solid and liquid substances, and gases and vapors. Poisons often impair the function of every major organ system. Health care providers are at risk from chemicals such as toxic cleaning agents. In the home accidental poisoning is a greater risk for toddlers, preschoolers, and young school-age children, who often ingest household cleaning solutions, medications, or personal hygiene products. Emergency treatment is necessary when a person ingests a poisonous substance or comes in contact with a chemical that is absorbed through the skin. In 2014 more than 2000 people a day were seen in emergency departments after a poison incident (CDC, 2014c). A poison control center is the best resource for patients and parents needing information about the treatment of an accidental poisoning.

Although lead has not been used in house paint or plumbing materials since the U.S. Consumer Product Safety Commission banned it in 1978, older homes in poorer communities continue to contain high lead levels. Soil and water systems are sometimes contaminated. Poisoning occurs from swallowing or inhaling lead. Fetuses, infants, and children are more vulnerable to lead poisoning than adults because their bodies absorb lead more easily and small children are more sensitive to the damaging effects of lead. Exposure to excessive levels of lead affects a child's growth or causes learning and behavioral problems and brain and kidney damage (Agency for Toxic Substances and Disease Registry, 2014).

Falls. Falls are a major public health problem. Among adults 65 years and older, falls are the leading cause of both fatal and nonfatal injuries (CDC, 2015a). Numerous factors increase the risk of falls, including a history of falling, being age 65 or over, reduced vision, orthostatic hypotension, lower-extremity weakness, gait and balance problems, urinary incontinence, improper use of walking aids, and the effects of various medications (e.g., anticonvulsants, diuretics, hypnotics, sedatives, certain analgesics) (Deandrea et al., 2010). Common physical hazards that lead to falls in the home include inadequate lighting, barriers along normal walking paths and stairways, loose rugs and carpeting, and a lack of safety devices in the home. Falls are also a common problem in health care settings (Spoelstra et al., 2011). Hospitals throughout the country carefully monitor the incidence of falls and fall-related injuries as part of their ongoing performance improvement work. Falls are often a combination of individual and transient risk factors, the physical environment (e.g., poor lighting, high bed position, improper equipment), and the riskiness of a person's behavior (unwilling to call for assistance when getting up) (Spoelstra et al., 2011). Falls often lead to serious injuries such as fractures or internal bleeding. Patients most at risk for injury are those with bleeding tendencies resulting from disease or medical treatments and osteoporosis.

Fire. A total of 487,500 structure fires were reported in the United States in 2013, resulting in 2855 deaths and 14,075 injuries (NFPA, 2014b). The leading cause of fire-related death is careless smoking, especially when people smoke in bed at home. However, the U.S. Consumer Product Safety Commission estimates that more than 25,000 residential fires every year are associated with the use of space heaters, resulting in more than 300 deaths (Energy.gov, 2014). The improper use of cooking equipment and appliances, particularly stoves, is a main source for in-home fires and fire injuries. Smoke detectors and carbon monoxide detectors need to be placed strategically throughout a home. Multipurpose fire extinguishers need to be near the kitchen and any workshop areas. Advise families to only purchase newer-model space heaters that have all of the current safety features.

Disasters. Natural disasters such as floods, tsunamis, hurricanes, tornadoes, and wildfires are a major cause of death and injury. These types of disasters result in death and leave many people homeless. Every year millions of Americans face disaster and its terrifying consequences. Bioterrorism is another cause of disaster. Threats of this type come in the form of biological, chemical, and radiological attacks. Bioterrorism, or the use of biological agents such as anthrax, smallpox, and botulism to create fear or threat, is the most likely form of a terrorist attack to occur (CDC, 2014d).

Transmission of Pathogens. Pathogens and parasites pose a threat to patient safety (see Chapter 29). A **pathogen** is any microorganism capable of producing an illness. The most common means of transmission of pathogens is by the hands. For example, if an individual infected with hepatitis A does not wash his or her hands thoroughly after having a bowel movement, the risk for transmitting the disease during food preparation is great. One of the most effective methods for limiting the transmission of pathogens is the medically aseptic practice of hand hygiene (see Chapter 29). It is important to educate your patients and their family caregivers about the importance of hand hygiene. Hand hygiene is used in all aspects of life, not just in food preparation practices or when caring for a sick family member. Teach all family members to wash their hands after activities such as play, coming home from work, working in the garden, and car maintenance. Hand hygiene is a simple and effective measure to reduce the transmission of pathogens and the risk of subsequent illness.

The human immunodeficiency virus (HIV), the pathogen that causes acquired immunodeficiency syndrome (AIDS), and the hepatitis B virus are transmitted through blood and other select body fluids. High-risk behaviors such as sexual contact and drug use are common risk factors for HIV. People who abuse drugs often share syringes and needles, which increases the risk of acquiring these viruses. Some states and many nonprofit organizations fund syringe-exchange programs as a means to slow down the spread of infectious diseases obtained through needle sharing (Coalition for Safe Community Needle Disposal, 2015).

Immunization reduces, and in some cases prevents, the transmission of disease from person to person. Great progress has been made in the United States over the last 50 years in the use of vaccines to prevent serious and infectious diseases. However, frequently issues about vaccine safety and the increasing complexity of immunization schedules have fostered doubts among parents about the necessity of vaccinations (Kennedy et al., 2011). You are responsible as a nurse to educate parents about the benefits of immunization. A survey conducted in 2010 found that over half of the parents expressed concerns that their child would have a serious reaction from the vaccine or that the vaccine might not be safe. The researchers found that these concerns were predictive of the parents delaying future immunizations for their children (Opel et al., 2013). However, a 2011 survey of over 300 parents found that the majority surveyed reported that they had either already vaccinated (83%) or planned to vaccinate (11%) their children with all recommended vaccines (Kennedy et al., 2011). Lack of immunization puts children and adults at risk.

Pollution. A healthy environment is free of pollution. A pollutant is a harmful chemical or waste material discharged into the water, soil, or air. People commonly think of pollution only in terms of air, land, or water pollution; but excessive noise is also a form of pollution that presents health risks. Air pollution is the contamination of the atmosphere with a harmful chemical. Prolonged exposure to industrial waste and vehicle exhaust increases the risk of pulmonary disease. In the home, school, or workplace, cigarette smoke is the primary cause of air pollution. Improper disposal of radioactive and bioactive waste products (e.g., dioxin) can cause land pollution. Water pollution is the contamination of lakes, rivers, and streams, usually by industrial pollutants. If water becomes contaminated, the public needs to use bottled or boiled water for drinking and cooking. Flooding damages water-treatment stations and also requires the use of bottled or boiled water.

NURSING KNOWLEDGE BASE

Factors Influencing Patient Safety

In addition to being knowledgeable about the home and health care environment and the inherent safety risks, nurses need to know a patient's developmental level; mobility, sensory, and cognitive status; lifestyle choices; and knowledge of common safety precautions. They also need to be aware of the special risks to safety that are found in health care settings.

Risks at Developmental Stages. A patient's developmental stage creates threats to safety as a result of lifestyle, cognitive and mobility status, sensory impairments, and safety awareness. With this information you tailor safety prevention programs to the needs, preferences, and life circumstances of particular age-groups. Unfortunately all age-groups are subject to abuse. Child abuse, domestic violence, and elder abuse are serious threats to safety (see Chapters 11 to 14).

Infant, Toddler, and Preschooler. Injuries are the leading cause of death in children over age 1 and cause more death and disabilities than do all diseases combined (Hockenberry and Wilson, 2015). The nature of the injury sustained is closely related to normal growth and development. For example, the incidence of lead poisoning is highest in late infancy and toddlerhood. Children at this stage explore the environment and, because of their increased level of oral activity, put objects in their mouths. This increases risk for poisoning and choking. Fire often results from their curiosity in playing with matches. In addition, limited physical coordination contributes to falls from bicycles and playground equipment. Additional injuries at this age are related to riding unrestrained in a motor vehicle, drowning, and head trauma from objects. Accidents involving children are largely preventable, but parents need to be aware of specific dangers at each stage of growth and development. Thus accident prevention requires health education for parents and the removal of dangers whenever possible.

School-Age Child. When a child enters school, the environment expands to include the school, transportation to and from school, school friends, and after-school activities. School-age children are learning how to perform more complicated motor activities and often are uncoordinated. Parents, teachers, and nurses need to instruct children in safe practices to follow at school or play, including what to do if approached by strangers. Teach school-age children involved in team and contact sports the rules for playing safely and how to use protective safety equipment such as helmets and other protective gear. Head injuries are a major cause of death, with bicycle accidents being one of the major causes of such injuries (Hockenberry and Wilson, 2015). Bikes need to be the proper size for the child, and helmets must be worn (Figure 27-1). Parents need to be reminded of the importance of a helmet for tricycles, scooters, and motorized toys. Additional injuries in this age-group are decreased by using seat belts and booster seats in motor vehicles properly and providing pedestrian safety education.

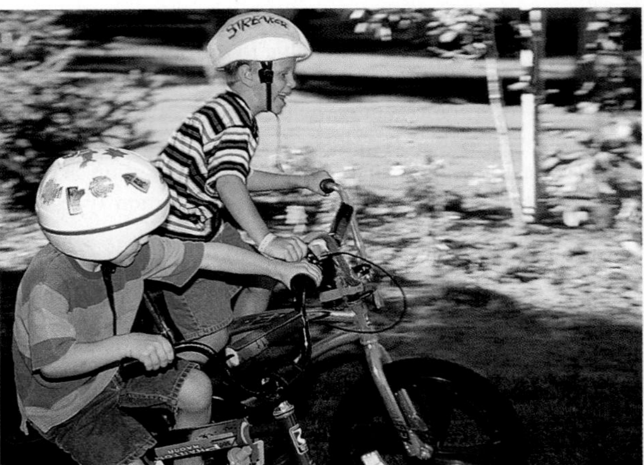

FIGURE 27-1 Proper bicycle safety equipment for school-age child.

Adolescent. Adolescents develop greater independence and begin to develop a sense of identity and their own values. The adolescent begins to separate emotionally from his or her family, and peers generally have a stronger influence. Wide variations that swing from child-like to mature behavior are characteristic of adolescent behavior (Hockenberry and Wilson, 2015). In an attempt to relieve the tensions associated with physical and psychosocial changes and peer pressures, some adolescents engage in risk-taking behaviors such as smoking, drinking alcohol, and using drugs. This increases the incidence of accidents such as drowning and motor vehicle accidents. When adolescents learn to drive, their environment expands, and so does their potential for injury. Teen motor vehicle crashes are preventable by avoiding distractions such as using cell phones, texting, eating, and drinking while driving.

To assess for possible substance abuse, have parents look for environmental and psychosocial clues from their children. Environmental clues include the presence of drug-oriented magazines, beer and liquor bottles, drug paraphernalia and blood spots on clothing, and the continual wearing of long-sleeved shirts in hot weather and dark glasses indoors. Psychosocial clues include failing grades, change in dress, increased absenteeism from school, isolation, increased aggressiveness, and changes in interpersonal relationships. Because adolescence is a time when mature sexual physical characteristics develop, some adolescents begin to have physical relationships with others that present the risk of sexually transmitted infections.

Adult. The threats to an adult's safety are frequently related to lifestyle habits. For example, a person who uses alcohol excessively is at greater risk for motor vehicle accidents. People who smoke long-term have a greater risk of cardiovascular or pulmonary disease as a result of the inhalation of smoke and the effect of nicotine on the circulatory system. Likewise, the adult experiencing a high level of stress is more likely to have an accident or illness such as headaches, gastrointestinal (GI) disorders, and infections.

Older Adult. The physiological changes associated with aging, effects of multiple medications, psychological and cognitive factors, and the effects of acute or chronic disease increase an older adult's risk for falls and other types of accidents. The risk of being seriously injured in a fall increases with age. Patients who wander have special safety challenges. Wandering is the meandering, aimless, or repetitive locomotion that exposes a person to harm and is often in conflict with boundaries (such as doors), limits, or obstacles (Herdman and

Kamitsuru, 2014). Individuals can walk away from home or off care units or enter restricted or closed areas without the knowledge of caregivers. This is a common problem in patients who are confused or disoriented. Interrupting a wandering patient can increase his or her distress.

Older patients are more likely to fall in the bedroom, bathroom, and kitchen in their homes. Environmental factors such as broken stairs, icy sidewalks, inadequate lighting, throw rugs, and exposed electrical cords cause many of the accidents. Inside falls most often occur while transferring from beds, chairs, and toilets; getting into or out of bathtubs; tripping over items such as cords covered by rugs or carpets, carpet edges, or doorway thresholds; slipping on wet surfaces; and descending stairs. Fear of falling is a concern of community-dwelling older adults, and many avoid activities because of their fear. Main risk factors for developing fear of falling are at least one fall, being female, and being older (Scheffer et al., 2008).

Multiple trials and systemic review provide clear evidence that falls in the community can be reduced through regular exercise (Sherrington et al., 2011). Falls can be decreased by group exercise, tai chi, and having cataract surgery. Decreasing hazards in the home that increase falls is also effective (Gillespie et al., 2012). Clinicians in hospital settings continue to struggle to find consistent and reliable approaches for fall reduction. Interventions shown to reduce hospital fall rates include developing a culture of safety, conducting fall risk assessments, and multifactorial interventions (e.g., equipment upgrades, removing hazards, identifying high-risk patients, low beds) (Spoelstra et al., 2011).

Individual Risk Factors. Other risk factors posing threats to safety include lifestyle, impaired mobility, sensory or communication impairment, and the lack of safety awareness. Know your patients' risks when you plan their nursing care.

Lifestyle. Some lifestyle choices increase safety risks. People who drive or operate machinery while under the influence of chemical substances (drugs or alcohol), work at inherently dangerous jobs, or are risk takers are at greater risk of injury. In addition, people experiencing stress, anxiety, fatigue, or alcohol or drug withdrawal or those taking prescribed medications are sometimes more accident prone. Because of these factors, some people are too preoccupied to notice the source of potential accidents such as cluttered stairs or a stop sign.

Impaired Mobility. A patient with impaired mobility has many kinds of safety risks. Muscle weakness, paralysis, and poor coordination or balance are major factors in falls. Immobilization predisposes patients to additional physiological and emotional hazards, which in turn further restrict mobility and independence. People who are physically challenged are at greater risk for injury when entering motor vehicles and buildings that are not handicap accessible.

Sensory or Communication Impairment. Cognitive impairments associated with delirium, dementia, and depression contribute to altered concentration and attention span, impaired memory, and orientation changes. Patients with these alterations become easily confused about their surroundings and are more likely to have falls and burns. Patients with visual, hearing, tactile, or communication impairment such as aphasia or a language barrier are not always able to perceive a potential danger or express their need for assistance (see Chapter 49).

Lack of Safety Awareness. Some patients are unaware of safety precautions such as keeping medicine or poisons away from children or reading the expiration date on food products. A nursing assessment that includes a home inspection helps you identify a patient's level of knowledge about home safety so you can correct deficiencies with an individualized nursing care plan.

BOX 27-2 The Joint Commission 2015 National Patient Safety Goals for Critical Access Hospitals

- Identify patients correctly.
- Improve staff communication.
- Use medicines safely.
- Use alarms safely.
- Prevent infection.
- Prevent mistakes in surgery.

Risks in the Health Care Agency. Patient safety continues to be one of the most pressing health care challenges in the nation. Medical errors happen when something that was planned as part of medical care doesn't work out or when the wrong plan was used. They occur in all health care settings. You must be aware of regulatory and organizational safety initiatives and individual patient risk factors. The Agency for Healthcare Research and Quality lists 20 tips to help prevent medical errors (AHRQ, 2014). You can view these tips at the AHRQ website, http://www.ahrq.gov/patients-consumers/care-planning/errors/20tips/.

The Joint Commission (TJC) and the Centers for Medicare and Medicaid Services (CMS) emphasize error prevention and patient safety. Their "Speak Up" campaign encourages patients to take a role in preventing health care errors by becoming active, involved, and informed participants on the health care team. For example, patients are encouraged to ask health care workers if they have washed their hands before providing care. The National Patient Safety Goals of TJC (2016) are specifically directed to reduce the risk of medical errors (Box 27-2). The goals highlight specific improvements in patient safety and ongoing problematic areas in health care. These evidence-based recommendations require health care facilities to focus their attention on a series of specific actions.

The mission of the National Quality Forum (NQF) (2011a) is improving the quality of health care in America by:

- Building consensus on national priorities and goals for performance improvement and working in partnership to achieve them;
- Endorsing national consensus standards for measuring and publicly reporting on performance; and
- Promoting the attainment of national goals through education and outreach programs.

Recently the NQF released its *National Voluntary Consensus Standards for Public Reporting of Patient Safety Events* (NQF, 2011b). The report provides a framework for publicly reporting patient safety information, including events, indicators, and measures, about health care organizations to consumers. It is important for nurses to understand the NQF standards and their intent since ultimately they influence the types of priorities that patient care organizations (e.g., hospitals, community health centers) set to improve the quality of care delivered to patients. Many of the NQF measures of patient safety (e.g., patient falls with injury, incidence of pressure ulcers, and central line bloodstream infection) are standards for judging the quality of care of health care organizations. The measures are also used by other organizations such as TJC and the CMS. Among the safety measures, the NQF endorsed a select list of serious reportable events (SREs), which was updated in 2006. The 28 events (Box 27-3) are a major focus of health care providers for patient safety initiatives. The CMS names select SREs as *Never Events* (i.e., adverse events that should never occur in a health care

BOX 27-3 The National Quality Forum List of Serious Reportable Events

Surgical Events

A. Surgery performed on the wrong body part
B. Surgery performed on the wrong patient
C. Wrong surgical procedure performed on a patient
D. Unintended retention of foreign object in a patient after surgery or procedure
E. Intraoperative or immediately postoperative death

Patient-Protection Events

A. Infant discharged to wrong person
B. Patient death or serious disability associated with patient elopement
C. Patient suicide or attempted suicide resulting in serious disability during care in a health care facility

Care-Management Events

A. Patient death or serious disability associated with medication error
B. Patient death or serious disability associated with hemolytic reaction as a result of administration of ABO/HLA–incompatible blood or blood products
C. Maternal death or serious disability associated with labor or delivery in a low-risk pregnancy during care in a health care facility
D. Patient death or serious disability associated with hypoglycemia, the onset of which occurs during care in a health care facility
E. Death or serious disability associated with failure to identify and treat hyperbilirubinemia in neonates
F. Stage III or IV pressure ulcers acquired after admission to a health care facility
G. Patient death or serious disability caused by spinal manipulative therapy
H. Artificial insemination with wrong donor sperm or wrong egg

Product or Device Events

A. Patient death or serious disability associated with use of contaminated drugs, devices, or biologicals provided by the health care facility
B. Patient death or serious disability associated with use or function of a device in patient care when the device is used for functions other than as intended
C. Patient death or serious disability associated with intravascular air embolism that occurs during care in a health care facility

Environmental Events

A. Patient death or serious disability associated with an electric shock during care in a health care facility
B. Any incident in which a line designated for oxygen or other gas to be delivered to a patient contains the wrong gas or is contaminated by toxic substances
C. Patient death or serious disability associated with burn incurred from any source during care in a health care facility
D. Patient death or serious disability associated with fall during care in a health care facility
E. Patient death or serious disability associated with use of restraints or bedrails during care in a health care facility

Criminal Events

A. Care provided by someone impersonating a health care provider
B. Abduction of patient of any age
C. Sexual assault on patient within or on the grounds of a health care facility
D. Death or significant injury resulting from a physical assault that occurs within or on the grounds of the facility

BOX 27-4 The 2014 Centers for Medicare and Medicaid Services Hospital-Acquired Conditions (Present-on-Admission Indicator)

- Foreign object retained after surgery
- Air embolism
- Blood incompatibility
- Pressure ulcer stages III and IV
- Falls and trauma (fracture, dislocation, intracranial injury, crushing injury, burn, electric shock)
- Catheter-associated urinary tract infections
- Vascular catheter-associated infections
- Manifestations of poor glycemic control (diabetic ketoacidosis, nonketotic hyperosmolar coma, hypoglycemic coma, secondary diabetes with ketoacidosis, secondary diabetes with hyperosmolarity)
- Surgical site infections following:
  - Mediastinitis following coronary artery bypass graft
  - Certain orthopedic procedures (spine, neck, shoulder, elbow)
  - Bariatric surgery for obesity (laparoscopic gastric bypass, gastroenterostomy, laparoscopic gastric restrictive surgery)
  - Cardiac implantable medical device
  - Deep-vein thrombosis (DVT)/pulmonary embolism (PE) following certain orthopedic procedures (total knee replacement, hip replacement)
  - Iatrogenic pneumothorax with venous catheterization

From Centers for Medicare and Medicaid Services (CMS): *Hospital-acquired conditions,* 2015, http://www.cms.gov/HospitalAcqCond/06_Hospital-Acquired_Conditions.asp. Accessed September 2015.

setting) (DHHS, 2008). The CMS (2015) denies hospitals higher payment for any hospital-acquired condition resulting from or complicated by the occurrence of certain Never Events (Box 27-4). Many of the hospital-acquired conditions (e.g., fall or stage III pressure ulcer) are nurse-sensitive indicators, meaning that a nurse directly affects their development. The NQF (2011c) also released 34 safe practices for better health care. Evidence supports the effectiveness of these practices in reducing the occurrence of adverse health care events.

Being aware of and engaged in activities focused on the prevention of these conditions not only enhances patient safety but also contributes to the overall success of the health care facility. The CMS believes that the Never Events will strengthen incentives by hospitals to develop safety practices and reduce health care costs in the long term. Health care facilities often conduct a failure mode and effect analysis (FMEA) to identify problems with processes and products before they occur.

When an actual or potential adverse event occurs, the nurse or health care provider involved completes an incident or occurrence report. An incident report is a confidential document that completely describes any patient accident occurring on the premises of a health care agency (see Chapter 23). Reporting allows an organization to identify trends/patterns throughout the facility and areas to improve. Focusing on the root cause of an event instead of the individual involved promotes a "culture of safety" that helps in specifically identifying what contributed to an error. The probability of an accident occurring declines when health care providers adhere to evidence-based principles of safety (Taylor-Adams et al., 2009).

Nurses face specific environmental risks in health care facilities. An example is exposure to various forms of chemicals. Chemicals found in some medications (e.g., chemotherapy), anesthetic gases, cleaning solutions, and disinfectants are potentially toxic if ingested, absorbed into the skin, or inhaled. Material safety data sheets (MSDSs) are required resources available in any health care agency (OSHA, 2014). The MSDS provides detailed information about the chemical, health hazards imposed, first aid guidelines, and precautions for safe handling and use. MSDSs give information on the steps to take in case the material is released or spilled. Be aware of the location of the MSDSs and be knowledgeable about hazardous chemicals in your environment. Spread of pathogens also presents a risk to both nurses and other patients. Therefore always follow standard and transmission-based isolation precautions and use proper hand hygiene (see Chapter 29).

Specific risks to a patient's safety within the health care environment include falls, patient-inherent accidents, procedure-related accidents, and equipment-related accidents. The nurse assesses for these four potential problem areas and, considering the developmental level of the patient, takes steps to prevent or minimize accidents.

Falls. Falls result in minor-to-severe injuries such as bruises, hip fractures, or head trauma that result in reduced mobility and independence and increase the risk for premature death. Patients who have underlying disease states are more susceptible to fall-related injuries (Grundstrom et al., 2012). For example, a patient with a bleeding disorder is more likely to have an intracranial bleed; a patient with osteoporosis has a greater chance for fracture. The unfamiliar environment, effects of acute illness or surgery, impaired mobility, effects of medications and treatments, and placement of various tubes and catheters place patients of any age at risk of falling. Nurses can implement multifactorial interventions, including assessment and communication about patient risks, staff assignments in close proximity, signage, improved patient hand-offs, nurse toilet and comfort safety rounds, and involving the patient and family (Spoelstra et al., 2011). Injuries from falls often extend a patient's length of stay in the health care environment, placing them at an even greater risk for other complications.

Patient-Inherent Accidents. Patient-inherent accidents are accidents (other than falls) in which a patient is the primary reason for the accident. Examples include self-inflicted cuts, injuries, and burns; ingestion or injection of foreign substances; self-mutilation or fire setting; and pinching fingers in drawers or doors. One of the more common precipitating factors for a patient-inherent accident is a seizure.

Procedure-Related Accidents. Procedure-related accidents are caused by health care providers and include medication and fluid administration errors, improper application of external devices, and accidents related to improper performance of procedures such as dressing changes or urinary catheter insertion. Nurses are able to prevent many procedure-related accidents by adhering to organizational policy and procedures and standards of nursing practice. For example, proper preparation and administration of medications, use of patient and medication bar coding, and "smart" intravenous (IV) pumps reduce medication errors (see Chapters 32 and 42). All staff need to be aware that distractions and interruptions contribute to procedure-related accidents and need to be limited, especially during high-risk procedures such as medication administration. The potential for infection is reduced when surgical asepsis is used for sterile dressing changes or any invasive procedure such as insertion of a urinary catheter. Finally, correct use of safe patient handling techniques and equipment reduces the risk of injuries when moving and lifting patients (see Chapter 39).

Equipment-Related Accidents. Accidents that are equipment related result from the malfunction, disrepair, or misuse of equipment or from an electrical hazard. To avoid rapid infusion of IV fluids, all general-use and patient-controlled analgesic pumps need to have free-flow protection devices. To avoid accidents, do not operate monitoring or therapy equipment without adequate instruction. If you find a piece of faulty equipment, place a tag on it to prevent it from being used on another patient and promptly report any malfunctions. Assess potential electrical hazards to reduce the risk of electrical fires, electrocution, or injury from faulty equipment. In health care settings the clinical engineering staff make regular safety checks of equipment. Facilities must report all suspected medical device–related deaths to both the FDA and the manufacturer of the product if known (USFDA, 2015). This is usually done in conjunction with the risk-management department after tagging and removing the piece of equipment.

QSEN QSEN: BUILDING COMPETENCY IN SAFETY. A nurse is caring for a patient who is receiving chemotherapy. The patient becomes confused, pulls out her IV line, and the chemotherapy drug leaks into the bed linens and all over the floor. What risks are posed for this patient? What risks are posed for the nurse? How should the nurse handle the situation?

Answers to QSEN Activities can be found on the Evolve website.

CRITICAL THINKING

Successful critical thinking requires a synthesis of knowledge, experience, critical thinking attitudes, and intellectual and professional standards. Clinical judgments require nurses to anticipate necessary information, analyze the data, and make decisions regarding patient care. Critical thinking is an ongoing process. During assessment (Figure 27-2) consider all critical thinking elements and information about a specific patient to make appropriate nursing diagnoses.

In the case of safety, a nurse integrates knowledge from nursing and other scientific disciplines, previous experiences in caring for patients who were at risk for or had an injury, critical thinking attitudes such as responsibility and discipline, and any standards of practice that are applicable. For example, the American Nurses Association (ANA) standards for nursing practice address the nurse's responsibility in maintaining patient safety. TJC (2016) also provides standards for safety. Apply this information and your experience as you conduct a detailed assessment of a specific patient. For example, while assessing a patient's home environment, you consider typical locations within the home where dangers commonly exist. If a patient has a visual impairment, you apply previous experiences in caring for patients with visual changes to anticipate how to thoroughly assess his or her needs. Critical thinking directs you to anticipate what you need to assess and how to make conclusions about available data.

NURSING PROCESS

Apply the nursing process and use a critical thinking approach in your care of patients. The nursing process provides a clinical decision-making approach for you to develop and implement an individualized plan of safe patient care.

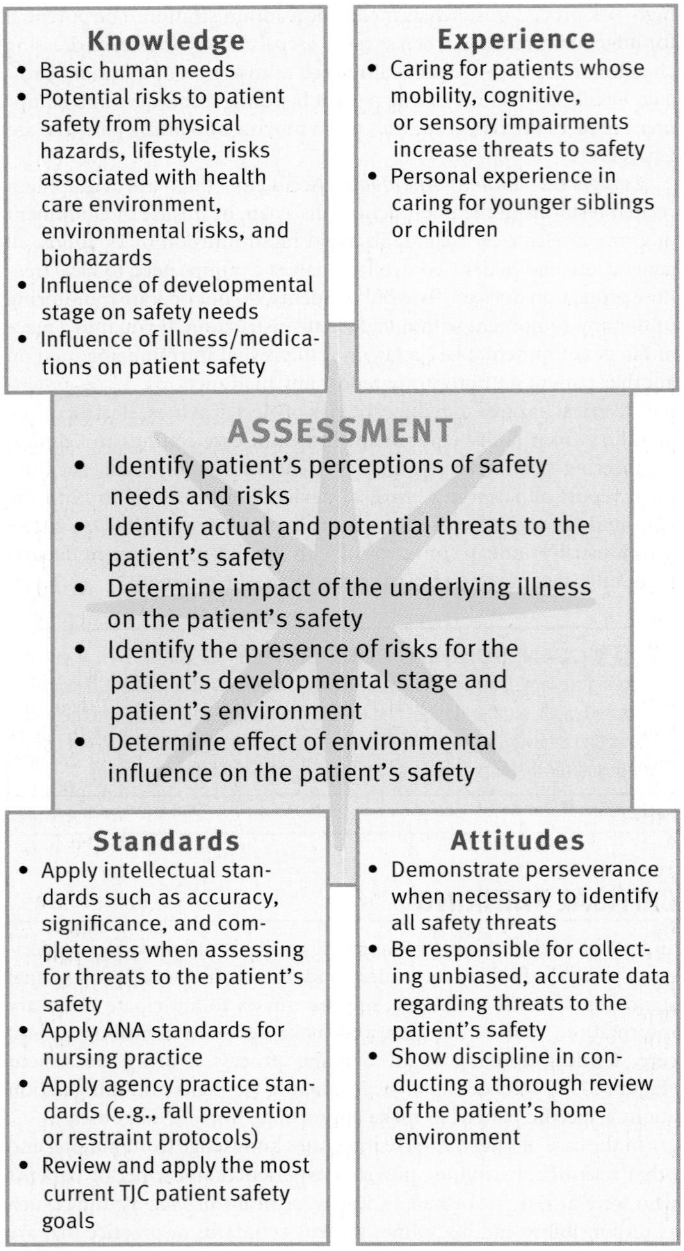

Knowledge
- Basic human needs
- Potential risks to patient safety from physical hazards, lifestyle, risks associated with health care environment, environmental risks, and biohazards
- Influence of developmental stage on safety needs
- Influence of illness/medications on patient safety

Experience
- Caring for patients whose mobility, cognitive, or sensory impairments increase threats to safety
- Personal experience in caring for younger siblings or children

ASSESSMENT
- Identify patient's perceptions of safety needs and risks
- Identify actual and potential threats to the patient's safety
- Determine impact of the underlying illness on the patient's safety
- Identify the presence of risks for the patient's developmental stage and patient's environment
- Determine effect of environmental influence on the patient's safety

Standards
- Apply intellectual standards such as accuracy, significance, and completeness when assessing for threats to the patient's safety
- Apply ANA standards for nursing practice
- Apply agency practice standards (e.g., fall prevention or restraint protocols)
- Review and apply the most current TJC patient safety goals

Attitudes
- Demonstrate perseverance when necessary to identify all safety threats
- Be responsible for collecting unbiased, accurate data regarding threats to the patient's safety
- Show discipline in conducting a thorough review of the patient's home environment

FIGURE 27-2 Critical thinking model for safety assessment. *ANA,* American Nurses Association; *TJC,* The Joint Commission.

◆ Assessment

During the assessment process thoroughly assess each patient and critically analyze findings to ensure that you make patient-centered clinical decisions required for safe patient care.

Through the Patient's Eyes. Patients generally expect to be safe in health care settings and in their homes. However, sometimes a patient's view of what is safe does not agree with that of the nurse and the standards he or she hopes to enforce. For this reason your assessment needs to be patient centered and include the patient's own perceptions of his or her risk factors, concerns about being in a health care setting, knowledge of how to adapt to any safety risks, and previous experience with any accidents (Box 27-5). This is important if you need to make changes in the patient's environment. Patients usually do not purposefully put themselves in jeopardy. When they are uninformed or inexperienced, threats to their safety occur. You always need to consult patients or family members about ways to reduce hazards in their environment. To conduct a thorough patient assessment, consider possible threats to the patient's safety, including the immediate environment and any individual risk factors.

BOX 27-5 Nursing Assessment Questions

Activity and Exercise
- Do you use any assistive devices such as a wheelchair, walker, or cane to help you move or get around? Did someone show you how to use them safely?
- Do you have any difficulty bathing? Dressing? Eating?
- Do you need assistance in using the bathroom? Getting out of bed or a chair?
- What type of exercise or physical activity do you get? How often?
- How do you handle meal preparation (e.g., use stove and appliances safely)?
- Do you do your own laundry? How do you do this, and where are these appliances located?
- Do you drive a car or motorcycle? When do you normally drive? How far?
- How often do you wear a safety belt when in the car or a helmet when on your bike?

Medication History
- Which medications (prescription, over-the-counter, herbal) do you take?
- Has your doctor or pharmacist reviewed your medicines with you?
- Do any medications make you dizzy or light-headed?

History of Falls
- Have you ever fallen or tripped over anything in your home? Have you had any near misses? (If so, describe)
- Have you ever suffered an injury from a fall? What was it and how did it happen?
- Did you have any symptoms right before you fell? What were they?
- Which activity were you performing before the fall?

Home Maintenance and Safety
- Who does your simple home maintenance or minor home repairs?
- Who shovels your snow? Mows your lawn?
- Do you feel safe in your home? Which things in your environment make you feel unsafe?
- Do you have someone to call in case of an emergency?
- How do you feel about modifying your home to make it safer? Do you need help finding resources to help you do this?

Nursing History. A nursing history (see Chapter 31) includes data about a patient's level of wellness to determine if any underlying conditions exist that pose threats to safety. For example, give special attention to assessing a patient's gait, lower-body muscle strength and coordination, and balance by having the patient walk in his or her room. Consider a review of the patient's developmental status as you analyze assessment information. Also review if the patient is taking any medications or undergoing any procedures that pose risks. For example, use of diuretics increases the frequency of voiding and results in the patient having to use toilet facilities more often. Falls often occur with patients who have to get out of bed quickly because of urinary urgency.

Health Care Environment. When caring for patients within a health care facility, determine if any hazards exist in the immediate care environment. Does the placement of equipment (e.g., drainage bags,

IV pumps) or furniture pose barriers when the patient tries to ambulate? Does positioning of the patient's bed allow him or her to reach items on a bedside table or stand easily? Does the patient need help with ambulation? Are there multiple tubes or IV lines? Is the call bell within reach? Contact the clinical engineering staff if there are questions as to whether equipment is functioning properly and in good condition.

Risk for Falls. Assessment of a patient's risk factors for falling is essential to determine specific needs and develop targeted interventions to prevent falls. Many different fall risk–assessment instruments are available; use the tool chosen by your health care agency. Most tools include categories on age, fall history, elimination habits, high-risk medications, mobility, and cognition. At a minimum the assessment needs to be completed on admission, following a change in a patient's condition, after a fall, and when transferred. If it is determined that a patient is at risk for falling, regular assessment always continues. In many cases family members are important resources in assessing a patient's fall risk. Families often are able to report on the patient's level of confusion and ability to ambulate. On the basis of the results of a fall risk assessment, you implement multiple evidence-based interventions. It is very important to inform a patient and family members about a patient's risks. Often younger patients are not aware of how medications and treatments cause dizziness, orthostatic hypotension, or changes in balance. When patients are unaware of their risks, they are less likely to ask for assistance. If family members are informed, they will often call for help (when they are visiting patients) to be sure that patients have appropriate assistance.

Risk for Medical Errors. Be alert to factors within your own work environment that create conditions in which medical errors are more likely to occur. Studies show that overwork and fatigue, particularly when working consecutive 12 hour-shifts, cause a significant decrease in alertness and concentration, leading to errors (Geiger-Brown et al., 2012). It is important for you to be aware of these factors and include checks and balances when working under stress. For example, to reduce chances for a medical error, it is essential that you check the patient's identification by using two identifiers (e.g., name and birthday or name and medical record number) according to agency policy before beginning any procedure or administering a medication (see Chapter 32).

Disasters. Hospitals must be prepared to respond to and care for a sudden influx of patients at the time of a community disaster. Although the occurrence of a bioterrorist attack has been limited to the anthrax deaths following September 11, 2001, the threat is very real. Be prepared to make accurate and timely assessments in any type of setting. A bioterrorist attack will likely resemble a natural outbreak initially. Acutely ill patients representing the earliest cases after a covert attack seek care in emergency departments. Patients less ill at the onset of an illness possibly seek care in primary care settings. Rapid detection of a bioterrorism attack occurs through syndrome surveillance and specific clinical reporting of suspected cases. The early signs of a bioterrorism-related illness often include nonspecific symptoms (e.g., nausea, vomiting, diarrhea, skin rash, fever, confusion) that may persist for several days before the onset of more severe disease. Patients with prodromal illnesses seek outpatient care and are assigned nonspecific diagnoses such as "viral syndrome." Data on patients fitting various syndromic criteria are then transferred to a health department and tested. Be alert for these types of cases in your practice.

Patient's Home Environment. When caring for a patient in the home, a home hazard assessment is necessary. A thorough hazard assessment covers topics such as adequacy of lighting (inside and outdoors), presence of safety devices, placement of furniture or other items that can create barriers, condition of flooring, and safety in the kitchen and bathrooms. Know where medications and cleaning supplies are located. Walk through the home with the patient and discuss how he or she normally conducts daily activities and whether the environment poses problems. Assess for the presence of locks on doors and windows that make the home less susceptible to intruders. When assessing the adequacy of lighting, inspect the areas where the patient moves and works such as outside walkways, steps, interior halls, and doorways. Getting a sense of a patient's routines helps you recognize less obvious hazards.

Assessment for risk of food infection or poisoning includes assessing a patient's knowledge of food preparation and storage practices. For example, does a patient know to check expiration dates of prepared food and milk products? Does he or she keep foods in the refrigerator that are fresh and not spoiled? Does the patient clean fresh fruits and vegetables correctly before eating them? Assess for clinical signs of infection by conducting an examination of GI and central nervous system function, observing for a fever, and analyzing the results of cultures of feces and emesis. In the home inspect suspected food and water sources and assess the patient's handwashing practices. It is useful to ask patients when they routinely wash their hands. This then prompts a helpful discussion about the purpose and importance of handwashing.

Assessment of the environmental comfort of a patient's home includes a review of when the patient normally has heating and cooling systems serviced. Does the patient have a functional furnace or space heater? Does the home have air conditioning or fans? Inform patients who use space heaters of the risk for fires. Are smoke detectors and carbon monoxide detectors up-to-date and functional, and are fire extinguishers present and placed strategically throughout the home and checked routinely?

When patients live in older homes, encourage them to have inspections for the presence of lead in paint, dust, or soil. Because lead also comes from the solder or plumbing fixtures in a home, patients need to have water from each faucet tested. Local health offices will help homeowners locate a trained lead inspector who takes samples from various locations and has them analyzed at a laboratory for lead content.

It is important that your assessment help individuals focus on avoiding losses and reducing their risk for injury associated with disasters. The Federal Emergency Management Agency (http://www.fema.gov/) and the American Red Cross (http://www.redcross.org/) provide nationwide education to help community members prepare for disasters of all types.

◆ Nursing Diagnosis

Gather data from your nursing assessment and analyze clusters of defining characteristics or risk factors to identify relevant nursing diagnoses. Include specific related or contributing factors to individualize your nursing care (Box 27-6). For example, the nursing diagnosis *Risk for Falls* is associated with altered mobility or sensory alteration (e.g., visual) risk factors. Altered mobility leads you to select such nursing interventions as range-of-motion (ROM) exercises; more frequent supervised ambulation; or teaching the proper use of safety devices such as side rails, canes, or crutches. Also consult with a physician about a physical therapy referral. If visual impairment is the risk factor, select different interventions such as keeping the area well lit; orienting the patient to the surroundings; or keeping eye glasses clean, handy, and well protected. When you do not identify the correct risk factors for the diagnosis *Risk for Falls*, the use of inappropriate interventions may increase a patient's risk for falling. For example, not evaluating the home environment for hazards can result in sending a hospitalized

BOX 27-6 Nursing Diagnostic Process

Risk for Falls

Assessment Activities	Defining Characteristics
Observe patient's posture, range of motion, strength, balance, and body alignment.	Decrease in lower-extremity strength, difficulty with gait, impaired balance
Assess patient's visual acuity, ability to read, identify distant objects.	Reports difficulty seeing at night Vision blurred, unable to identify near objects
Complete a home hazard appraisal.	Poorly lighted home Rooms filled with small items Excessive amount of furniture for size of room Rugs not secure

patient home only to return with an additional injury. Examples of additional nursing diagnoses for patients with safety risk include the following:

- *Risk for Injury*
- *Impaired Home Maintenance*
- *Deficient Knowledge*
- *Risk for Poisoning*
- *Risk for Suffocation*
- *Risk for Trauma*

◆ Planning

Patients with actual or potential risks to safety require a nursing care plan with interventions that prevent and minimize threats to their safety. Design your interventions to help a patient feel safe to move about and interact freely within the environment. The total plan of care addresses all aspects of patient needs and uses resources of the health care team and the community when appropriate. Critically synthesize information from multiple sources (Figure 27-3). Critical thinking ensures that a patient's plan of care integrates all that you learned about the patient and the key critical thinking elements. For example, you reflect on knowledge regarding the services that other health professions (e.g., occupational therapy, case management) provide to help patients return to their home environments safely. Also reflect on previous experiences when patients benefited from safety interventions. Such experience helps you adapt approaches with each new patient. Applying critical thinking attitudes such as creativity helps you to collaborate with a patient in planning interventions that are relevant and most useful, particularly when making changes in the home environment.

Goals and Outcomes. You collaborate with a patient, family, and other members of the health care team when setting goals and expected outcomes during the planning process (see the Nursing Care Plan). The patient who actively participates in reducing threats to safety becomes more alert to potential hazards and is more likely to adhere to the plan. Make sure that goals and outcomes for each nursing diagnosis are measurable and realistic, with consideration of the resources available to the patient. For example, in the case of the nursing diagnosis of *Impaired Physical Mobility related to left-sided paralysis,* the goal is the patient "will remain free of injury throughout hospitalization." Examples of expected outcomes include:

- Patient uses tripod cane correctly within 24 hours.
- Patient describes approach to rise up from bed correctly with assistance by end of the teaching session today.

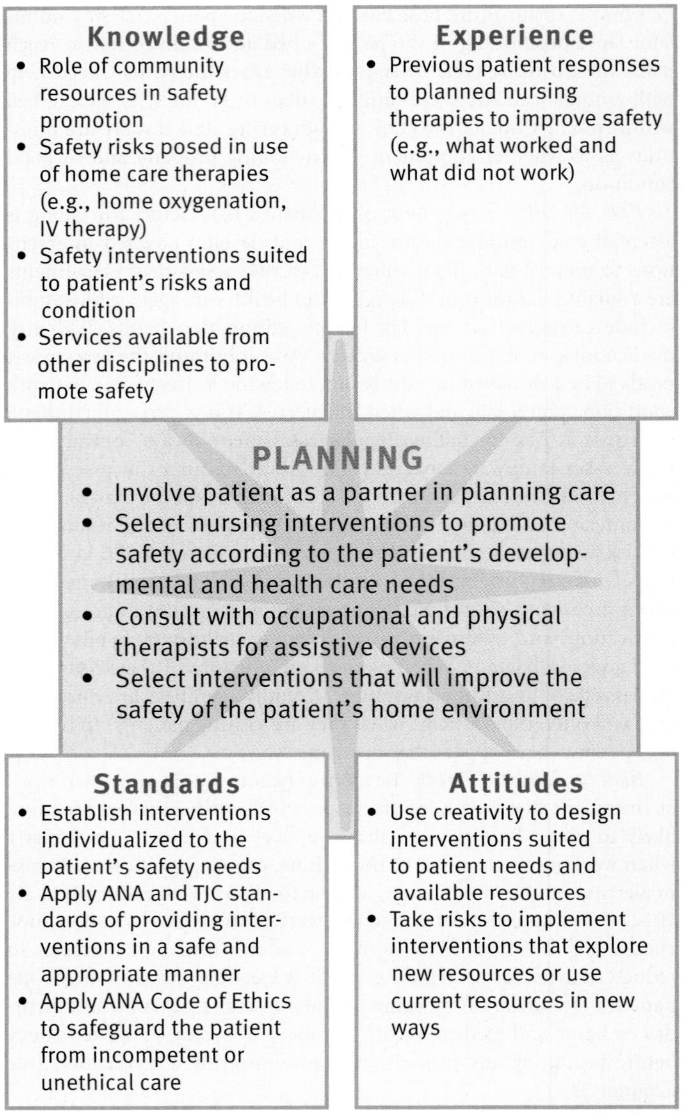

Knowledge
- Role of community resources in safety promotion
- Safety risks posed in use of home care therapies (e.g., home oxygenation, IV therapy)
- Safety interventions suited to patient's risks and condition
- Services available from other disciplines to promote safety

Experience
- Previous patient responses to planned nursing therapies to improve safety (e.g., what worked and what did not work)

PLANNING
- Involve patient as a partner in planning care
- Select nursing interventions to promote safety according to the patient's developmental and health care needs
- Consult with occupational and physical therapists for assistive devices
- Select interventions that will improve the safety of the patient's home environment

Standards
- Establish interventions individualized to the patient's safety needs
- Apply ANA and TJC standards of providing interventions in a safe and appropriate manner
- Apply ANA Code of Ethics to safeguard the patient from incompetent or unethical care

Attitudes
- Use creativity to design interventions suited to patient needs and available resources
- Take risks to implement interventions that explore new resources or use current resources in new ways

FIGURE 27-3 Critical thinking model for safety planning. *ANA,* American Nurses Association; *IV,* intravenous; *TJC,* The Joint Commission.

Setting Priorities. Prioritize a patient's nursing diagnoses and interventions to provide safe and efficient care. For example, the concept map (Figure 27-4) has several nursing diagnoses that apply to Ms. Cohen in the care plan. The patient's mobility problem is an obvious priority because of its influence on risk for falls and skin integrity. Plan individualized interventions on the basis of the severity of risk factors and the patient's developmental stage, level of health, lifestyle, and cultural needs (Box 27-7). Planning involves an understanding of the patient's need to maintain independence within physical and cognitive capabilities. Collaborate to establish ways of maintaining the patient's active involvement within the home and health care environment. Education of the patient and family is also an important intervention to plan for reducing safety risks over the long term.

Teamwork and Collaboration. Collaboration with the patient, family, and other health professions such as social work and occupational and physical therapy becomes an important part of a patient's plan of care. For example, a hospitalized patient may need to go to a rehabilitation facility to gain strength and endurance before being discharged home. Communication is essential. You communicate risk

NURSING CARE PLAN

Risk for Falls

ASSESSMENT

Mr. Key, a home health nurse, is seeing Ms. Cohen, an 85-year-old woman, at her home. The patient is recovering from a mild stroke affecting her left side. Ms. Cohen lives alone but receives regular assistance from her daughter Peggy and son Michael, who both live within 10 miles. Mr. Key's assessment included a discussion of Ms. Cohen's health problem and how the stroke has affected her, a pertinent physical examination, and home hazard assessment.

Assessment Activities*	***Findings/Defining Characteristics***
Ask how the stroke has affected her mobility.	She responds, "**I bump into things,** and **I'm afraid I'm going to fall.**"
Conduct a home hazard assessment.	Cabinets in kitchen are **cluttered** and full of breakable items that could fall out. **Throw rugs are on floors;** bathroom **lighting is poor** (40-watt bulbs); bathtub **lacks safety strips** or grab bars; **home is cluttered** with furniture and small objects.
Observe gait and posture.	She has **kyphosis** and a **hesitant, uncoordinated gait;** frequently holds walls for support.
Assess muscle strength.	**Left arm and leg are weaker** than right.
Assess visual acuity with corrective lenses.	She has **trouble reading and seeing familiar objects at a distance** while wearing current glasses.

*__Defining characteristics__ are shown in bold type.

NURSING DIAGNOSIS: Risk for falls

PLANNING

Goals	***Expected Outcomes (NOC)***[†]
	Risk Control
Ms. Cohen's family will modify the home to eliminate hazards within 1 month.	Family members will reduce modifiable hazards in kitchen and hallway within 1 week. Family members will modify bathroom in 1 month.
	Knowledge: Personal Safety
Ms. Cohen and family will be knowledgeable of potential hazards for Ms. Cohen's age-group within 1 week.	Ms. Cohen and daughter will identify risks for falls and prevention methods to avoid falls in home at conclusion of teaching session next week.
	Fall Prevention Behavior
Ms. Cohen will express greater sense of feeling safe from falling in 1 month.	Ms. Cohen will report improved vision with the aid of new eyeglasses in 2 weeks.
Ms. Cohen will be free of injury within 1 week.	Ms. Cohen will safely ambulate throughout the home within 1 week.

[†]Outcome classification labels from Moorhead S et al: *Nursing outcomes classification (NOC)*, ed 5, St Louis, 2013, Mosby.

INTERVENTIONS (NIC)[‡] ***Fall Prevention***	**RATIONALE**
Review findings from home hazard assessment with Ms. Cohen and her children and collaborate on proposed changes.	Home hazard assessment highlights extrinsic factors that lead to falls and that can be changed.
Establish a list of priorities to modify and have Ms. Cohen's son help to install bathroom safety devices.	Implementing home modifications based on home assessment decreases falls (Chase et al., 2012).
Discuss with Ms. Cohen and daughter the normal changes of aging, effects of recent stroke, associated risks for injury, and how to reduce risks.	Education regarding hazards reduces fear of falling (Olsen and Bergland, 2014).
Encourage daughter to schedule vision testing for new prescription within 2 to 4 weeks.	Improved visual acuity reduces incidence of falls (Chase et al., 2012).
Refer to physical therapist to assess need for strengthening and endurance training and use of assistive devices for kyphosis, left-sided weakness, and gait.	Exercise is effective in reducing falls and needs to include a comprehensive program combining muscle strengthening, balance, and/or endurance training for a minimum of 12 weeks (Sherrington et al., 2011).

[‡]Intervention classification labels from Bulechek GM et al: *Nursing interventions classification (NIC)*, ed 6, St Louis, 2013, Mosby.

EVALUATION

Nursing Actions	***Patient Response/Finding***	***Achievement of Outcome***
Ask Ms. Cohen and family to identify fall risks.	Ms. Cohen and family are able to identify risks during a walk through the home and express a greater sense of safety as a result of changes made.	Ms. Cohen and family are more knowledgeable of potential hazards.
Observe environment for elimination of hazards.	Throw rugs were removed. Lighting was increased to 75 watts except in bathroom and bedroom.	Environmental hazards are partially reduced.
Reassess Ms. Cohen's visual acuity.	Ms. Cohen has new glasses and says she is able to read better and see distant objects more clearly.	Ms. Cohen's vision has improved, enabling her to ambulate more safely.
Observe Ms. Cohen's gait and posture.	Ms. Cohen's gait remains hesitant and uncoordinated; she reports that her daughter has limited time to take her to the physical therapist.	Outcome of safe ambulation is not totally achieved; help daughter develop a schedule that allows her time to take her mother to physical therapy appointments.

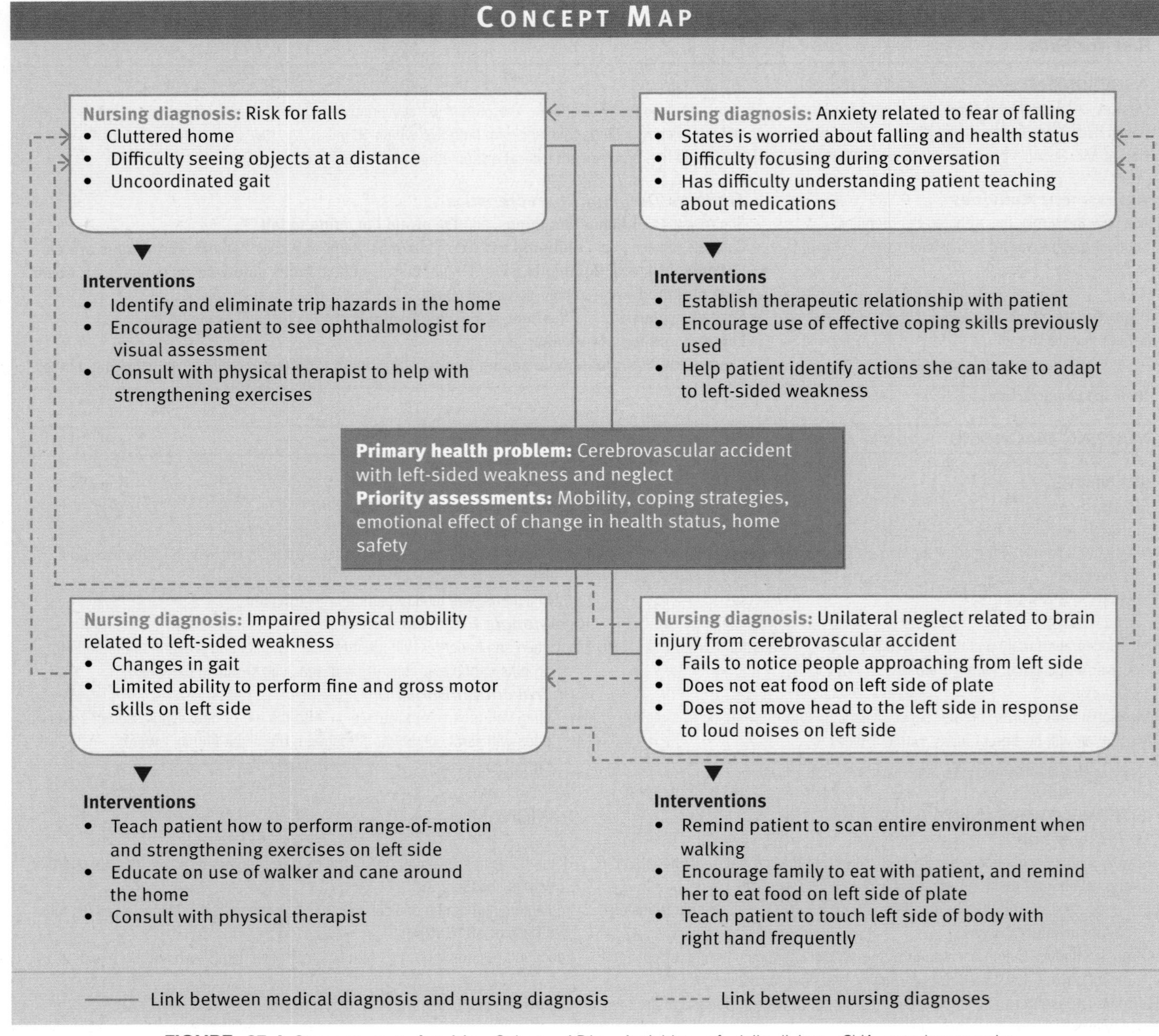

FIGURE 27-4 Concept map for Ms. Cohen. *ADLs,* Activities of daily living; *CVA,* cerebrovascular accident.

factors and the plan of care with the patient, family, and other health care providers, including other disciplines and nurses on other shifts. Permanent dry-erase boards in the patient's room with patient information such as activity and level of assistance communicate information to all health care providers. A standard approach to communication such as SBAR (*S*ituation, *B*ackground, *A*ssessment, *R*ecommendation) helps you obtain and organize information (see Chapter 26).

> **QSEN QSEN: BUILDING COMPETENCY IN PATIENT-CENTERED CARE.** Mr. Key, the nurse for Ms. Cohen, needs to provide a hand-off report to the nurse who will be assuming primary responsibility for the oversight of Ms. Cohen's care. Using the SBAR format, write out a comprehensive report that will allow the new nurse to care for Ms. Cohen safely with a thorough understanding of her needs related to her care plan and concept map around her risk for falls.
>
> *Answers to QSEN Activities can be found on the Evolve website.*

Patients need to be able to identify, select, and know how to use resources within their community (e.g., neighborhood block homes, local police departments, and neighbors willing to check on their well-being) that enhance safety. Make sure that the patient and family understand the need for these resources and are willing to make changes that promote their safety.

◆ Implementation

The QSEN project (2014) outlines recommended skills to ensure nurse competency in patient safety. Among these skills are those involving safe nursing practice during direct care:

- Demonstrate effective use of technology and standardized practices that support safety and quality.

BOX 27-7 CULTURAL ASPECTS OF CARE

A Patient-Centered Care Approach

Hospitalization places patients at risk for injury in an unfamiliar and confusing environment. The experience is usually at least minimally frightening. Normal life cues such as a bed without side rails and the direction one usually takes to the bathroom are absent. Thought processes and coping mechanisms are affected by illness and its accompanying emotions. Thus patients are more vulnerable to injury. This vulnerability is often intensified for patients of diverse backgrounds. It is a nurse's responsibility to diligently protect all patients, regardless of their socioeconomic status and cultural background. Most untoward events are related to failures of communication. It has been estimated that more than 300 languages are spoken in the United States and more than 90 million Americans have low health literacy, creating challenges during your assessment and efforts at implementing safe care measures (TJC, 2016). Screen all patients for health literacy. Ensure that you use an approach that recognizes a patient's cultural background so you ask appropriate questions to reveal health behaviors and risks. Also be aware of cultural beliefs about restraints when caring for patients who need restraints. Safety is enhanced when you consider patients in light of the whole person and value seeing each care situation through "the patient's eyes" and not just through your own perspective. Some specific patient-centered safety guidelines about the use of restraints follow.

Implications for Patient-Centered Care

- When restraints are needed, assess their meaning to the patient and the family. Some cultures may find restraints to be disrespectful. Similarly some survivors of war or persecution or those suffering from post-traumatic stress disorder may view restraints as imprisonment or punishment.
- Collaborate with family members in accommodating a patient's cultural perspectives about restraints. Removing the restraints when family members are present shows respect and caring for the patient.
- Define the protocol of the nursing unit on the use of restraints. Identify potential areas for negotiation with the patient's/family's preferences for using restraints, including having family members stay with the patient.

- Demonstrate effective use of strategies to reduce risk of harm to self or others.
- Use appropriate strategies to reduce reliance on memory (e.g., forcing functions, checklists).

Direct your nursing interventions toward maintaining a patient's safety in all types of settings. You implement health promotion and illness prevention measures in the community setting, whereas prevention is a priority in the acute care setting.

Health Promotion. To promote an individual's health, it is necessary for the individual to be in a safe environment and practice a lifestyle that minimizes risk of injury. Edelman and Mandle (2013) describe passive and active strategies aimed at health promotion. Passive strategies include public health and government legislative interventions (e.g., sanitation and clean water laws) (see Chapter 3). Active strategies are those in which an individual is actively involved through changes in lifestyle (e.g., engaging in better nutritional health or exercise programs, wearing seat belts) and participation in wellness programs.

Nurses promote individual and community health by supporting legislation, acting as positive role models, and working in community-based settings. Because environmental and community values have the greatest influence on health promotion, community and home health nurses are able to assess and recommend safety measures in the home, school, neighborhood, and workplace.

Developmental Interventions

Infant, Toddler, and Preschooler. Growing, curious children need adults to protect them from injury. Children are trusting of their environment and do not perceive themselves to be in danger. Educate parents or guardians about reducing risks of injuries to children and ways to promote safety in the home (Table 27-1). Nurses working in prenatal and postpartum settings easily incorporate safety into the care plans of childbearing families. Community health nurses assess the home and show parents how to promote safety. Educate parents about the importance of immunizations and how they protect a child from life-threatening disease.

TABLE 27-1 Interventions to Promote Safety for Children and Adolescents

Intervention	Rationale
Infants and Toddlers	
Have infants sleep on their back or side. Teach parents the mnemonic "back to sleep."	Placing infants on their back confers the lowest risk of sudden infant death syndrome (SIDS) and is the preferred position (AAP, 2011b).
Infants should be immunized.	Evidence suggests that immunization reduces the risk of SIDS by 50% (AAP, 2011b).
Do not fill cribs with pillows, bumper pads, large stuffed toys, or comforters. Use snug-fitting sheets.	Possibility exists for these items to cause potential risk of suffocation, strangulation, or entrapment.
Do not attach pacifiers to string or ribbon and place around a child's neck.	String or ribbon around the neck increases risk for choking.
Follow all instructions for preparing and storing formula.	Proper formula preparation and storage prevent contamination. Following product directions ensures proper concentration of formula. Undiluted formula causes fluid and electrolyte disturbances; much diluted formula does not provide sufficient nutrients.
Use large, soft toys without small parts such as buttons.	Small parts become dislodged, and choking and aspiration can occur.
Do not leave the mesh sides of playpens lowered; spaces between crib slats need to be less than 2⅜ inches (6 cm) apart.	Possibility exists for a child's head to become wedged in the lowered mesh side or between crib slats, and asphyxiation may occur.
Never leave crib sides down or babies unattended on changing tables or in infant seats, swings, strollers, or high chairs.	Infants and toddlers roll or move and fall from changing tables or out of accessories such as infant seats or swings.

Continued

TABLE 27-1 Interventions to Promote Safety for Children and Adolescents—cont'd

Intervention	Rationale
Discontinue using accessories such as infant seats and swings when the child becomes too active or physically too big and/or according to the manufacturer's directions.	When physically active or too big, the child can fall out of or tip over these accessories and suffer an injury.
Never leave a child alone in the bathroom, tub, or near any water source (e.g., pool).	Supervision reduces risk for accidental drowning.
Baby-proof the home; remove small or sharp objects and toxic or poisonous substances, including plants; install safety locks on floor-level cabinets.	Babies explore their world with their hands and mouth. Choking and poisoning can occur.
Remove plastic bags from the cleaners or grocery store from the home.	Removal reduces risk for suffocation from plastic bags.
Cover electrical outlets.	Covers reduce opportunity for crawling babies to insert objects into outlets and experience an electrical shock.
Place window guards on all windows.	Guards prevent children from falling out of windows.
Install keyless locks (e.g., deadbolts) on doors above a child's reach, even when they are standing on a chair.	Deadbolts prevent a toddler from leaving the house and wandering off. Keyless locks allow for rapid exit in case of fire.
Put children weighing less than 80 lbs or under 8 years of age in an age/weight–appropriate car seat that has been installed according to manufacturer's instructions. This includes car seats and booster seats. In cars with a passenger air bag, children under 12 need to be in the back seat. All passengers need to wear seat belts.	In case of a sudden stop or crash, an unrestrained child suffers severe head injuries and death.
Caregivers need to learn cardiopulmonary resuscitation (CPR) and the Heimlich maneuver.	Caregivers need to be prepared to intervene in acute emergencies such as choking.
Preschoolers	
Teach children to swim at an early age but always provide supervision near water.	Learning to swim is a useful skill that can someday save a child's life. However, all children need constant supervision.
Teach children how to cross streets and walk in parking lots. Instruct them to never run out after a ball or toy.	Pedestrian accidents involving young children are common.
Teach children not to talk to, go with, or accept any item from a stranger.	Avoiding strangers reduces the risk of injury and stranger abduction.
Teach children basic physical safety rules such as proper use of safety scissors, never running with an object in their mouth or hand, and never attempting to use the stove or oven unassisted.	Risk of injury is lower if children know basic safety procedures.
Teach children not to eat items found in the street or grass.	Avoiding these items reduces risk for possible poisoning.
Remove doors from unused refrigerators and freezers. Instruct children not to play or hide in a car trunk or unused appliances.	If a child cannot freely exit from appliances and car trunks, asphyxiation can occur.
School-Age Children	
Teach children the safe use of equipment for play and work.	The child needs to learn the safe, appropriate use of implements to avoid injury.
Teach children proper bicycle safety, including use of helmet and rules of the road.	Reduces injuries from falling off a bike or being hit by a car.
Teach children proper techniques for specific sports and the need to wear proper safety gear (e.g., helmets, eyewear, mouth guards).	Using proper techniques, correct equipment, and protective gear prevents injuries.
Teach children not to operate electrical equipment while unsupervised.	If an electrical mishap were to occur, no one would be available to help.
Do not allow children access to firearms or other weapons. Keep all firearms in locked cabinets.	Children are often fascinated by firearms and often try to play with them.
Adolescents	
Encourage enrollment in driver education classes.	Many injuries in this age-group are related to motor vehicle accidents.
Provide information about the effects of using alcohol and drugs.	Adolescents are prone to risk-taking behaviors and are subject to peer pressures.
Refer adolescents to community and school-sponsored activities.	The adolescent needs to socialize with peers, yet needs some supervision.
Encourage mentoring relationships between adults and adolescents.	Adolescents are in need of role models after whom they can pattern their behavior.
Teach them safe use of the Internet.	Avoids overuse and possible exposure to inappropriate websites.

Modified from Hockenberry M, Wilson D: *Wong's nursing care of infants and children,* ed 10th, St Louis, 2015, Mosby.

School-Age Child. School-age children increasingly explore their environment (see Chapter 12). They have friends outside their immediate neighborhood; and they become more active in school, church, and community activities. The school-age child needs specific teaching regarding safety in school and at play. See Table 27-1 for nursing interventions to help guide parents in providing for the safety of school-age children.

Adolescent. Risks to the safety of adolescents involve many factors outside the home because much of their time is spent away from home and with their peer group (see Chapter 12). Adults serve as role models for adolescents and, by providing examples, setting expectations, and providing education, help them minimize risks to their safety. This age-group has a high incidence of suicide because of feelings of decreased self-worth and hopelessness. Be aware of the risks posed at this time and be prepared to teach adolescents and their parents measures to prevent accidents and injury.

Adult. Risks to young and middle-age adults frequently result from lifestyle factors such as childrearing, high stress levels, inadequate nutrition, use of firearms, excessive alcohol intake, and substance abuse (see Chapter 13). In this fast-paced society there also appears to be more expression of anger, which can quickly precipitate accidents related to "road rage." Help adults understand their safety risks and guide them in making lifestyle modifications by referring them to resources such as classes to help quit smoking and for stress management, including employee-assistance programs. Also encourage adults to exercise regularly, maintain a healthy diet, practice relaxation techniques, and get adequate sleep.

Older Adult. Nursing interventions for older adults reduce patients' risks of falls and other accidents and compensate for the physiological changes of aging (Box 27-8). The American Geriatric Society (2015) developed an algorithm for fall prevention (Figure 27-5). Provide information about neighborhood resources to help an older adult maintain an independent lifestyle. Older adults frequently relocate to new neighborhoods and need to become acquainted with new resources such as modes of transportation, church schedules, and food resources (e.g., Meals on Wheels).

Educate older adults about safe driving tips (e.g., driving shorter distances or only in daylight, using side and rearview mirrors carefully, and looking behind them toward their "blind spot" before changing lanes). If hearing is a problem, encourage the patient to keep a window rolled down while driving or reduce the volume of the radio. Counseling is often necessary to help older patients make the decision of when to stop driving. At that time help locate resources in the community that provide transportation.

Burns and scalds are also more apt to occur with older people because they sometimes forget and leave hot water running or become confused when turning the dials on a stove or other heating appliance. Nursing measures for preventing burns minimize the risk from impaired vision. Hot-water faucets and dials are color coded to make it easier for an adult to know which is hot and which is cold. Reducing the temperature of the hot water heater is also very beneficial.

Many older adults love to walk. Reduce pedestrian accidents for older adults and all other age-groups by persuading people to wear reflectors on garments when walking at night; stand on the sidewalk and not in the street when waiting to cross a street; always cross at corners and not in the middle of the block (particularly if the street is a major one); cross with the traffic light and not against it; and look left, right, and left again before entering the street or crosswalk. Also encourage people to assess their walking route for hazards such as unequal or damaged walk ways, unrestrained dogs, and excessive toys; all of these increase the risk for falls.

BOX 27-8 FOCUS ON OLDER ADULTS

Physiological Changes of Aging and Their Effect on Patient Safety

As people age physiological changes occur. They experience visual and hearing alterations; slowed reaction time; and decreased range of motion, flexibility, and strength. In addition, reflexes are slowed, and the ability to respond to multiple stimuli is reduced. Memory can become impaired, and nocturia and incontinence are more frequent in older adults. The family plays a significant role in the care of older adults. Over 66 million unpaid caregivers for adults are mostly family members (i.e., nearly 40% of the U.S. adult population) (National Alliance for Caregiving, 2015). Encourage the family to allow the older adult to remain as independent as possible and provide help only for those things that are especially stressful or depleted.

The high prevalence of chronic conditions in older adults results in the use of a high number of prescription and over-the-counter medications. Coupled with age-related changes in pharmacokinetics, there is a greater risk of serious adverse effects. Medications typically prescribed for older adults include anticholinergics, diuretics, anxiolytic and hypnotic agents, antidepressants, antihypertensives, vasodilators, analgesics, and laxatives, all of which pose risks or interact to increase the risk for falls.

Implications for Practice

- Encourage annual vision and hearing examinations and frequent cleaning of glasses and hearing aids as a means of preventing falls and burns.
- Teach patients safety tips for avoiding automobile accidents. Sometimes driving needs to be restricted to daylight hours or temporarily or permanently suspended.
- Encourage supervised exercise classes for older adults and teach them to seek assistance with household tasks as needed. Safety features such as grab bars in the bathroom are often necessary.
- Be sure that adults know how to use assist devices (e.g., walkers and canes) correctly. Consult with a physical therapy staff member.
- Institute a regular toileting schedule for the patient. A recommended frequency is every 3 hours. Give diuretics in the morning. Provide assistance, along with adequate lighting, to patients who need to go to the bathroom at night.
- Encourage patients to use medication organizers, which can be purchased at any drugstore at a very reasonable cost. Fill these dispensers once a week with the proper medications to be taken at a specific time during the day.
- Review the patient's drug profile to ensure that these drugs are used cautiously and assess the patient regularly for any adverse effects that increase fall risk.

Environmental Interventions. Nursing interventions directed at eliminating environmental threats include those associated with a person's basic needs and general preventive measures.

Basic Needs. Nurses contribute to a safer environment by helping patients meet basic needs related to oxygen, nutrition, and temperature. When oxygen is in use, take appropriate precautions to prevent fire. Contact with heat or a spark is required to trigger combustion; therefore certain precautions are necessary, regardless of the setting where oxygen is in use. Post "No Smoking" and "Oxygen in Use" signs in patient rooms. Do not use oxygen around electrical equipment or flammable products. Store oxygen tanks upright in carts or stands to prevent tipping or falling or place the tanks flat on the floor when not in use. Check tubing for kinks that affect the oxygen flow. Maintain oxygen at the prescribed liter flow and do not change without a health care provider's order. Additional precautions are indicated for liquid or pressurized oxygen and when traveling with home oxygen. Refer to

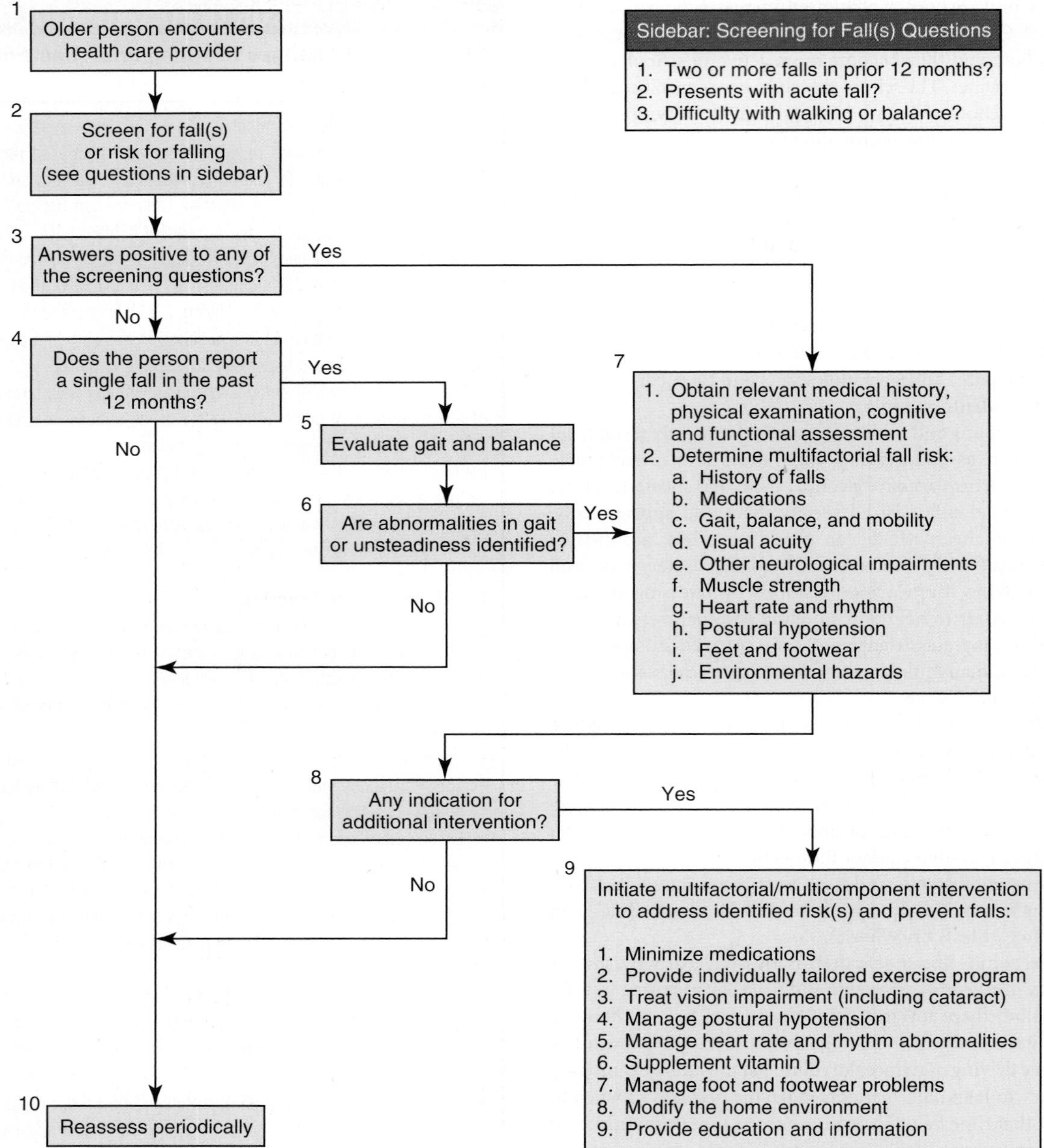

FIGURE 27-5 American Geriatrics Society Clinical Practice Guideline Fall Prevention Algorithm 2010. (From American Geriatrics Society/British Geriatrics Society: *Clinical practice guideline for prevention of falls in older persons,* 2010, http://www.medcats.com/FALLS/frameset.htm. Accessed August 14, 2015.)

the oxygen supplier. Recommend that the patient have annual inspections of heating systems, chimneys, and fuel-burning appliances in the home. Carbon monoxide detectors are available at a reasonable cost but are not a replacement for proper use and maintenance of fuel-burning appliances.

Teach basic techniques for food handling and preparation:

- Properly refrigerate, store, and prepare food to decrease the risk of foodborne illness. Store perishable foods in refrigerators to maintain freshness.
- Wash hands before and after preparing foods.
- Rinse fruits and vegetables thoroughly.
- Pay attention to prevent cross-contamination of one food with another during food preparation, especially with poultry. Use separate cutting boards.
- Use a separate cutting board for vegetables, meats, and poultry.
- Adequately cook foods to kill any residual organisms. Refrigerate leftovers promptly. Bacteria grow quickly at room temperature.
- Have family caregivers label the date when leftovers are saved.

General Preventive Measures. Adequate lighting and security measures in and around the home, including the use of night-lights, exterior lighting, and locks on windows and doors, enable patients to reduce the risk of injury from crime. The local police department and community organizations often have safety classes available for residents to learn how to take precautions to minimize the chance of becoming involved in a crime. For example, some useful tips include always parking the car near a bright light or busy public area, carrying a whistle attached to the car keys, keeping car doors locked while

BOX 27-9 PATIENT TEACHING

Prevention of Electrical Hazards

Objective

- Patient will recognize and eliminate electrical hazards in the home.

Teaching Strategies

- Discuss importance of checking for grounding of electrical appliances and other equipment.
- Provide examples of common hazards: frayed cords, damaged equipment, and overloaded outlets.
- Discuss guidelines to prevent electrical shocks:
  - Use extension cords only when necessary and use electrical tape to secure the cord to the floor, preferably against baseboards.
  - Do not run wires under carpeting.
  - Grasp the plug, not the cord, when unplugging items.
  - Keep electrical items away from water.
  - Do not operate unfamiliar equipment.
  - Disconnect items before cleaning.

Evaluation

- Have patient list electrical hazards existing in the home.
- Review steps the patient will take to eliminate these hazards.
- Observe the home environment after the patient has had an opportunity to eliminate hazards.

BOX 27-10 PATIENT TEACHING

Correct Use of a Fire Extinguisher in the Home

Objective

- Patient will use a fire extinguisher in the home correctly.

Teaching Strategies

- Discuss how to choose a correct location for an extinguisher. It is recommended that one be placed on each level of the home, near an exit, in clear view, away from stoves and heating appliances, and above the reach of small children. Keep a fire extinguisher in the kitchen, near the furnace, and in the garage.
- Make sure that patients read instructions after purchasing the extinguisher and how often to review the instructions.
- Describe the steps to take before using the extinguisher. Attempt to fight the fire only when all occupants have left the home, the fire department has been called, the fire is confined to a small area, there is an exit route readily available, the extinguisher is the right type for the fire (see discussion in text for a description of the types of extinguishers), and the patient knows how to use it.
- Instruct the patient to memorize the mnemonic PASS: *P*ull the pin to unlock handle, *A*im low at the base of the fire, *S*queeze the handles, and *S*weep the unit from side to side (see Figure 27-9).

Evaluation

- Patient is able to describe when it is appropriate to use a home fire extinguisher.
- Patient correctly lists the steps to take before attempting to use an extinguisher.
- Patient demonstrates correct use of the extinguisher while reciting the instructions with the mnemonic PASS.

driving, and always paying attention while driving to notice if anyone starts to follow the car.

Modifications in the environment easily reduce the risk of falls. To reduce the risk of injury in the home, remove all obstacles from halls and other heavily traveled areas. Necessary objects such as clocks, glasses, or tissues remain on bedside tables within reach of the patient but out of the reach of children. Take care to ensure that end tables are secure and have stable, straight legs. Place nonessential items in drawers to eliminate clutter. Patients who have problems stumbling or tripping should never have small area rugs in the home. If small area rugs are used, secure them with a nonslip pad or skid-resistant adhesive strips. Make sure that carpeting on the stairs is secured with carpet tacks. If patients have a history of falling and live alone, recommend that they wear an electronic safety alert device. When activated by the wearer, this device alerts a monitoring site to call emergency services for assistance.

Accidental home fires typically result from smoking in bed, placing cigarettes in trash cans, grease fires, improper use of candles or space heaters, or electrical fires resulting from faulty wiring or appliances. Teach patients and families how to reduce the risk of electrical injury in the home (Box 27-9) and how to use a home fire extinguisher (Box 27-10). To reduce the risk of fires in the home, instruct patients to quit smoking or smoke outside the home. Have them inspect the condition of cooking equipment and appliances, particularly irons and stoves. Have patients with visual deficits install dials with large numbers or symbols on temperature controls. Make sure that smoke detectors are in strategic positions throughout the home so the alarm will alert the occupants in a home in case of fire. All patients, even young children, need to know the phrase "stop, drop, and roll," which describes what to do when a person's clothing or skin is burning.

Help parents reduce the risk of accidental poisoning by teaching them to keep hazardous substances such as medications, cleaning fluids, and batteries out of the reach of children. Drug and other substance poisonings in adolescents and adults are commonly related to suicide attempts or drug experimentation. Teach parents that calling a poison control center for information before attempting home remedies will save their child's life. Guidelines for accepted interventions for accidental poisonings are available to teach a parent or guardian (Box 27-11). Older adults are also at risk for poisoning because diminished eyesight may cause an accidental ingestion of a toxic substance. In addition, the impaired memory of some older adults results in an accidental overdose of prescription medications. In health care settings it is important for you to know how to respond when exposure to a poisonous substance occurs. In addition, adhere to guidelines for intervening in accidental poisoning.

Be sure that a patient's home medications are kept in their original containers and labeled in large print. Recommend the use of medication organizers that are filled once a week by the patient and/or family caregiver. Have patients keep poisonous substances out of the bathroom and discard old or unused medications appropriately.

To prevent the transmission of pathogens, nurses teach aseptic practices. Medical asepsis, which includes hand hygiene and environmental cleanliness, reduces the transfer of organisms (see Chapter 29). Patients and family members need to learn how to perform thorough hand hygiene (handwashing or use of a hand rub) and when to use it (i.e., before and after caring for a family member, before food preparation, before preparing a medication for a family member, after using the bathroom, and after contacting any body fluids). Patients also need to know how to dispose of infected material such as wound dressings and used needles in the home setting. Heavy plastic containers such as hard, colored plastic liquid detergent bottles are excellent for needle disposal. The Environmental Protection Agency (EPA) encourages disposal of used needles by way of community drop-off programs,

BOX 27-11 Intervening in Accidental Poisoning

1. If the person is conscious and alert, call the local poison control center or the national toll-free poison control center number (1-800-222-1222) before trying any intervention. Be sure that this number is posted and easy to access in the home. Poison control centers have information needed to treat poisoned patients or offer referral to treat. *The administration of ipecac syrup or induction of vomiting is no longer recommended for routine home treatment of poisoning.*
2. Assess for signs or symptoms of ingestion of harmful substance such as nausea, vomiting, foaming at the mouth, drooling, difficulty breathing, sweating, and lethargy.
3. Stop exposure to the poison. Have the person empty his or her mouth of pills, plant parts, or other material.
4. If poisoning is caused by skin or eye contact, irrigate the skin or eye with copious amounts of cool tap water for 15 to 20 minutes. In the case of an inhalation exposure, safely remove the victim from the potentially dangerous environment.
5. Identify the type and amount of substance ingested to help determine the correct type and amount of antidote needed.
6. If the victim has collapsed or stopped breathing, call 911. Initiate CPR if indicated until emergency personnel arrive. Ambulance personnel can provide emergency measures if needed. In addition, a parent or guardian is sometimes too upset to drive safely.
7. Position the victim with head turned to side to reduce risk for aspiration.
8. Never induce vomiting if the victim has ingested the following poisonous substances: lye, household cleaners, hair care products, grease or petroleum products, furniture polish, paint thinner, or kerosene.

Modified from Hockenberry MJ, Wilson D: *Wong's essentials of pediatric nursing,* ed 10, St Louis, 2015, Mosby; American Academy of Pediatrics, Committee on Injury, Violence and Poison Prevention: Gastrointestinal decontamination of the poisoned patient, *Pediatr Emerg Care* 24(3):176, 2008.
CPR, Cardiopulmonary resuscitation.

BOX 27-12 EVIDENCE-BASED PRACTICE

Effects of Nursing Rounds on Patient Safety and Patient Satisfaction

PICO Question: In the hospitalized adult patient, will hourly rounding compared with standard practice decrease patient falls and improve patient's perception of nurse responsiveness?

Evidence Summary

Patient falls are considered a nurse-sensitive indicator. Nurses have the opportunity to reduce this adverse outcome on the basis of evidence-based nursing actions. Hospitalized patients often require assistance with basic activities of daily living such as toileting and mobility. Not meeting patient needs in a timely fashion decreases patient satisfaction and places patients at greater risk for injury when they attempt to move unassisted (Mitchell et al., 2014). Current evidence supports a patient-centered approach to nursing care by implementing purposeful hourly rounding (Ford, 2010). A recent systematic review looked at 16 studies and found moderately strong evidence to support that hourly rounding programs reduce patient falls and call-light use and increase their perception of nursing responsiveness. Most of the programs used every hour or every 2-hour rounds and used the 5 Ps: *p*ain, *p*otty, *p*osition, *p*ossessions, and *p*lan of care as the focus (Mitchell et al., 2014).

Application to Nursing Practice

- Implementation of purposeful, hourly nursing rounds with nurses visiting patients improves outcomes by reducing patient falls (Mitchell et al., 2014).
- Purposeful rounding includes specific nursing actions such as addressing toileting, assessing pain level, turning, and ensuring that possessions are within reach.
- Nurses and nursing assistive personnel often share rounding responsibilities (e.g., alternating every other hour).
- Nurse responsiveness to call lights is an important factor in a patient's hospital experience and leads to improved patient satisfaction.

household hazardous waste facilities, sharps mail-back programs, or home needle destruction devices (CDC, 2011)

Acute and Restorative Care. Within hospital and long-term care settings nurses take various measures to maintain patient safety, including fall-prevention strategies, prevention of injuries from use of restraints and side rails, and precautions to prevent fires and exposure to poisoning and electrical hazards. Special precautions are also necessary to prevent injury in patients susceptible to having seizures. Radiation injuries are also a specific safety concern in hospitals.

Nurses use standard precautions for all patients to protect themselves from contact with blood and other potentially infectious body fluids (see Chapter 29). Additional specific safety measures are applicable to patients in the acute care environment. Nurses are responsible for making a patient's bedside safe. Explain and demonstrate to patients how to use the call light or intercom system and always place the call device close to the patient at the conclusion of every nurse-patient interaction. Respond quickly to call lights and bed/chair alarms. Keep the environment free from clutter around the bedside.

Fall Prevention. TJC recommends that hospitals have formal fall-reduction programs (TJC, 2015). A fall-reduction program includes a fall risk assessment of every patient conducted on admission and routinely (see hospital policy) until a patient's discharge. Many health care organizations are implementing hourly rounding to reduce falls (Box 27-12). In addition, most organizations apply yellow color-coded wristbands to patients' wrists to communicate to all health care providers that a patient is a fall risk. In 2008 the American Hospital Association issued an advisory recommending that hospitals standardize wristband colors: red for patient allergies, yellow for fall risk, and purple for do-not-resuscitate preferences (American Hospital Association, 2008). This recommendation came after a near-miss incident in which a nurse working in two different hospitals placed a wrong-colored band on a patient. Many state hospital associations and communities are now standardizing colors to reduce confusion both within and across the health care organizations.

Patient-centered care is important, with nurses making patients and families their partners in recognizing fall risks and taking preventive action. Most hospitals and long-term care facilities have fall-prevention protocols for those patients at risk for falling. A patient assessed as being at fall risk receives a fall risk identification bracelet (yellow in color), is given information about personal fall risks, and receives additional individualized nursing interventions (see Skill 27-1 on pp. 395-399). For example, if a patient has postural hypotension, a nurse chooses a low bed and the practice of dangling the patient for 5 minutes on the side of the bed before ambulating. Or a patient with a history of urinary urgency or incontinence benefits from a bedside commode instead of being expected to walk to the bathroom unassisted. Other interventions include established elimination schedules, placement of a fall pad on the floor along the bed, and use of bed safety alarms or motion detectors. A gait belt provides a secure way to steady or guide patients who need assistance with ambulation when

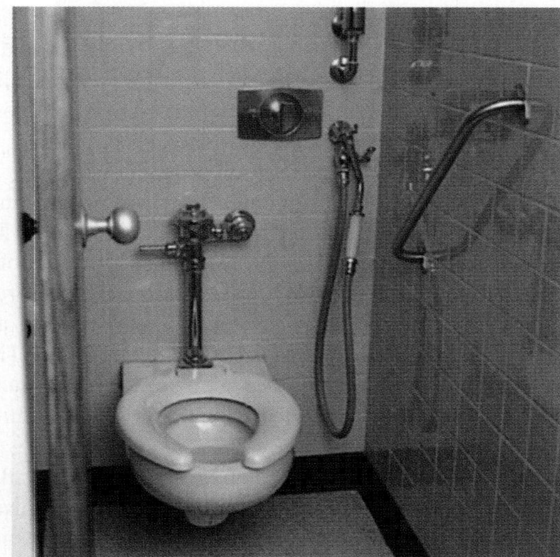

FIGURE 27-6 Safety bars around toilets and showers.

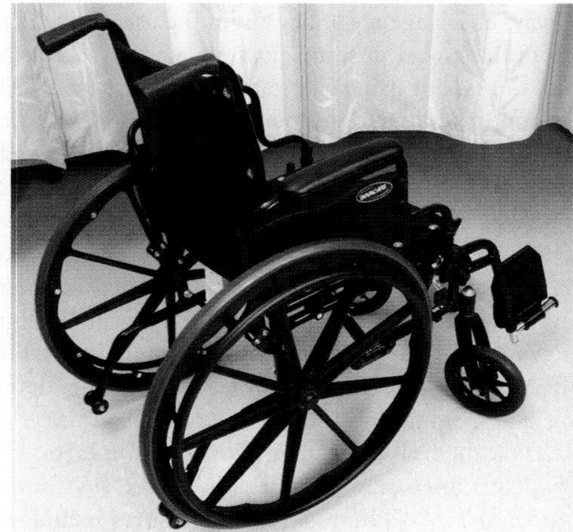

FIGURE 27-7 Wheelchair with safety locks and anti-tip bars.

transferring or walking. Use additional safety equipment as needed when moving patients (see Chapter 39).

When patients use assistive aids such as canes, crutches, or walkers, it is important to routinely check the condition of rubber tips and the integrity of the aid. Also be sure that patients use their devices correctly. Remove excess furniture and equipment and make sure that patients wear rubber-soled shoes or slippers for walking or transferring. Safety bars near toilets (Figure 27-6), locks on beds and wheelchairs (Figure 27-7), and call lights are additional safety features found in health care settings.

Another area of fall risk includes wheelchair-related falls involving older adults or patients with disabilities. Patients are at risk for falls during transfer tasks and reaching while seated in a wheelchair. An example of a wheelchair characteristic that increases risk for falls is having smaller and harder front wheels that cause a chair to tip when striking uneven terrain (such as uneven floor surface moving into an elevator). Tripping over the front foot or leg rest and leaning over the back of a wheelchair to engage or disengage the wheel lock are common causes of injury.

Restraints. Patients who are confused or disoriented and who wander or repeatedly fall or try to remove medical devices (e.g., oxygen equipment, IV lines, or dressings) often require the temporary use of restraints to keep them safe. *However, remember, the use of alternatives to restraints is preferred.* Current nursing home laws prohibit the unnecessary use of restraints; except in emergencies, nursing homes cannot use restraints without a resident's consent (CANHR, 2015).

Physical and chemical restraints restrict a patient's physical activity or normal access to the body and are not a usual part of treatment indicated by a patient's condition or symptoms. Thus restraints are not a solution to a patient problem but rather a temporary means to maintain patient safety. The CMS set the standard that restraints may be imposed only to ensure the immediate physical safety of a patient and must be discontinued at the earliest possible time (Department of Health and Human Services, Office of Inspector General, 2008).

A physical **restraint** is any manual method or physical or mechanical device (such as full set of side rails), material, or equipment that immobilizes or reduces the ability of a patient to move his or her arms, legs, body, or head freely (TJC, 2015). Chemical restraints are medications such as anxiolytics and sedatives used to manage a patient's behavior and are not a standard treatment or dosage for the patient's condition. A restraint does not include devices such as orthopedically prescribed devices, surgical dressings or bandages, protective helmets, or other methods that involve physically holding a patient to conduct routine physical examinations or tests, protecting the patient from falling out of bed, or permitting the patient to participate in activities without the risk of physical harm (TJC, 2015).

The use of restraints is associated with serious complications resulting from immobilization such as pressure ulcers, pneumonia, constipation, and incontinence. In some cases death has resulted because of restricted breathing and circulation. Patients have been strangled while trying to get out of bed while restrained in a jacket or vest restraint. As a result, many health care facilities have eliminated the use of the jacket (vest) restraint (Capezuti et al., 2008). Loss of self-esteem, humiliation, and agitation are also serious concerns. Legislation emphasizes reducing the use of restraints. Regulatory agencies such as TJC and the CMS enforce standards for the safe use of restraint devices. The optimal goal for all patients is a restraint-free environment.

Always consider and implement alternatives to restraints first. Individualize your approaches for each patient. Restraint alternatives include more frequent observations, social interaction such as involvement of family during visitation, frequent reorientation, regular exercise, and the introduction of familiar and meaningful stimuli (e.g., involve in hobbies such as knitting or crocheting or looking at family photos) within the environment. These interventions reduce behaviors such as wandering that often lead to restraint use. In nursing homes evidence shows that outcomes related to behavior issues, cognitive performance, falls, walking dependence, activities of daily living, pressure ulcers, and contractures are significantly worse when a restraint is used compared to no restraint (Castle, 2009). An interdisciplinary approach that includes individualized assessments and development of structured treatment plans reduces restraint use.

The use of restraints involves a psychological adjustment for the patient and family. If restraints are necessary, the nurse assists family members and patients by explaining their purpose, expected care while the patient is restrained, precautions taken to avoid injury, and that the restraint is temporary and protective. Informed consent from family members is required before using restraints in long-term care settings.

For legal purposes know agency-specific policy and procedures for appropriate use and monitoring of restraints. The use of a restraint must be clinically justified and a part of the patient's prescribed medical treatment and plan of care. A physician's order is required, based on a face-to-face assessment of the patient. The order must be current, state the type and location of restraint, and specify the duration and circumstances under which it will be used. Orders for restraint used to protect the physical safety of the nonviolent or non-self-destructive patient are written and renewed in accordance with hospital policy (TJC, 2017). In the case of management of violent or self-destructive behavior that jeopardizes the immediate physical safety of a patient, staff, or others, orders for restraints may be renewed within the following limits: 4 hours for adults 18 years of age or older and 2 hours for children and adolescents 9 to 17 years of age (TJC, 2017). These orders may be renewed, according to the time limits, for a maximum of 24 consecutive hours. Restraints are not to be ordered prn (as needed). Routine ongoing assessment is required of patients restrained. Documentation of behaviors that necessitated restraint application, the procedure used in restraining, the condition of the body part restrained (e.g., circulation to hand), and the evaluation of the patient response, is required. Restraints must be removed periodically, and the nurse assesses the patient to determine if they continue to be necessary. Skill 27-2 on pp. 399-403 includes guidelines for the proper use and application of restraints. Their use must meet one of the following objectives:

- Reduce the risk of patient injury from falls
- Prevent interruption of therapy such as traction, IV infusions, nasogastric (NG) tube feeding, or Foley catheterization
- Prevent patients who are confused or combative from removing life-support equipment
- Reduce the risk of injury to others by the patient

In keeping with current safety trends, electronic devices are alternatives to restraints. Weight and motion sensor mats placed on patients' beds or chairs emit silent or audible alarms when pressure is released off the mat. An alarm signals at the central nurses' station or sends a text message to a staff member's phone so staff is alerted quickly when a patient is moving and getting up and out of bed. Alarms on doors also alert staff or family members when a patient who is confused, disoriented, or prone to wandering opens a door.

A less-restrictive restraint is the Posey bed (Figure 27-8). It is a soft-sided, self-contained enclosed bed that is much less restrictive than chemical or physical restraints. It allows for freedom of movement and thus reduces the side effects such as pressure ulcers and loss of dignity caused by physical restraints. A vinyl top covers the padded upper frame of the bed, and the nylon-net canopy surrounds the mattress and completely encloses the patient in the bed. Zippers on the four sides of the enclosure provide access to the patient. The Posey bed enclosure works well for patients who are restless and unpredictable, cognitively impaired, and at risk for injury if they were to fall or get out of bed such as patients on anticoagulant therapy at risk for intracranial bleed. The bed is also a safer alternative to side rails.

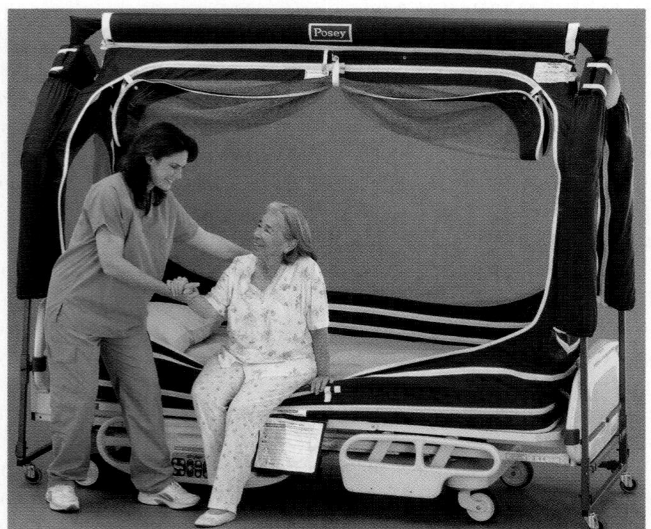

FIGURE 27-8 Posey Bed All-Care Model. (Courtesy JT Posey Co, Arcadia, CA.)

Side Rails. Side rails help to increase a patient's mobility and/or stability when repositioning or moving in bed or moving from bed to chair. They are the most commonly used physical restraint. However, many deaths and injuries related to entrapment and falls for both adult portable bedrail products and hospital bed rails have been reported to the U.S. Consumer Product Safety Commission (CPSC) and the U.S. Food and Drug Administration (FDA) (USFDA, 2014). The FDA recommends that all bedrails be used with caution, especially with older adults and people with altered cognition, physical limitations, and certain medical conditions.

There are a variety of beds with different side rail designs. Basically a patient needs to have a route to exit a bed safely and move freely within the bed; in this case side rails are not considered a restraint. For example, raising only the top two side rails of a four rail system gives a patient room to exit a bed safely. Side rails used to prevent a patient, such as one who is sedated, from falling out of bed are not considered a restraint. Always check agency policy about the use of side rails. Be sure that a bed is in the lowest position possible when side rails are raised. Always assess the risk of using side rails compared to not using them. Check their condition; bars between the bedrails need to be closely spaced to prevent entrapment, the space between bedrails and mattress and between headboard and mattress is filled to prevent patients from falling in between, and latches securing bedrails are stable.

The use of side rails alone for a patient who is disoriented usually causes more confusion and further injury. A patient who is determined to get out of bed attempts to climb over the side rail or climbs out at the foot of the bed. Either attempt usually results in a fall or injury. Nursing interventions to reduce a patient's confusion first focus on determining and eliminating the cause of the confusion such as a response to a new medication, dehydration, or pain. Frequently nurses mistake a patient's attempt to explore his or her environment or to self-toilet as confusion. Additional safety measures include the use of a low bed with a nonskid mat placed alongside the bed on the floor. A low bed reduces the distance between the bed and floor, facilitating a roll rather than a fall from the bed.

Fires. Although smoking is not allowed in most hospital and long-term care settings, smoking-related fires continue to pose a significant risk because of unauthorized smoking in the bed or bathroom. Institutional fires often result from an electrical fire. The best intervention is to prevent fires. Nursing measures include complying with the smoking policies and keeping combustible materials away from heat sources. Box 27-13 discusses additional fire-intervention

BOX 27-13 Fire Intervention Guidelines

- Keep the phone number for reporting fires visible on the telephone at all times.
- Know the fire drill and evacuation plan of the agency.
- Know the location of all fire alarms, exits, extinguishers, and oxygen shut-off in your work area.
- Use the mnemonic RACE to set priorities in case of fire:
  R—Rescue and remove all patients in immediate danger.
  A—Activate the alarm. Always do this before attempting to extinguish even a minor fire.
  C—Confine the fire by closing doors and windows and turning off oxygen and electrical equipment.
  E—Extinguish the fire with an appropriate extinguisher (see Figure 27-9).

guidelines in health care agencies. Regardless of where a fire occurs, it is important to have an evacuation plan in place. Know where fire extinguishers and gas shut-off valves are located and how to activate a fire alarm.

If a fire occurs in a health care agency, protect patients from immediate injury, report the exact location of the fire, contain it, and extinguish it if possible. Some agencies have fire doors that are held open by magnets and close automatically when a fire alarm sounds. It is important to keep equipment from blocking these doors. All personnel evacuate patients when appropriate. Patients who are close to a fire, regardless of its size, are at risk of injury and need to be moved to another area. If a patient is on life support, maintain his or her respiratory status manually with a bag-valve-mask device (e.g., Ambu-bag) (see Chapter 41) until he or she is moved away from the fire. Direct all ambulatory patients to walk by themselves to a safe area. In some cases they are able to help move patients in wheelchairs. Move bedridden patients from the scene of a fire by a stretcher, their bed, or a wheelchair. If none of these methods is appropriate, they need to be carried from the area. If you have to carry a patient, do so correctly (e.g., two-man carry). If you overextend your physical limits for lifting, injuring yourself results in further injury to the patient. If fire department personnel are on the scene, they help evacuate the patients.

After a fire is reported and patients are out of danger, health care personnel take measures to contain or extinguish it such as closing doors and windows, placing wet towels along the base of doors, turning off sources of oxygen and electrical equipment, and using a fire extinguisher. Fire extinguishers are categorized as type A, used for ordinary combustibles (e.g., wood, cloth, paper, and many plastic items); type B, used for flammable liquids (e.g., gasoline, grease, paint, and anesthetic gas); and type C, used for electrical equipment. Figure 27-9 demonstrates the process of using an extinguisher.

Electrical Hazards. Much of the equipment used in health care settings is electrical and must be well maintained. The clinical engineering departments of hospitals inspect biomedical equipment such as hospital beds, infusion pumps, or ventilators regularly. You know that a piece of equipment is safe to use when you see a safety inspection sticker with an expiration date. Decrease the risk for electrical injury and fire by using properly grounded and functional electrical equipment. The ground prong of an electrical outlet carries any stray electrical current back to the ground. Remove equipment that is not in proper working order or that sparks when plugged in for service and notify the appropriate hospital staff.

Seizures. Patients who have experienced some form of neurological injury or metabolic disturbance are at risk for a seizure. A **seizure** is hyperexcitation and disorderly discharge of neurons in the brain leading to a sudden, violent, involuntary series of muscle contractions that is paroxysmal and episodic, causing loss of consciousness, falling, tonicity (rigidity of muscles), and clonicity (jerking of muscles). A generalized tonic-clonic, or grand mal, seizure lasts approximately 2 minutes (no longer than 5) and is characterized by a cry and loss of consciousness with falling, tonicity, clonicity, and incontinence. During a fall or as a result of muscle jerking, musculoskeletal injuries can occur. Before a convulsive episode a few patients report an aura, which serves as a warning or sense that a seizure is about to occur. An **aura** is often a bright light, smell, or taste. During a seizure the patient often experiences shallow breathing, cyanosis, and loss of bladder and bowel control. A postictal phase follows the seizure, during which the patient has amnesia or confusion and falls into a deep sleep. A person in the community needs to be taken to a medical facility immediately if he or she has repeated seizures; if a single seizure lasts longer than 5 minutes without any sign of slowing down or is unusual in some way; if the person has trouble breathing afterwards or appears to be injured or in pain; or if recovery is different from usual (Epilepsy Foundation, 2014). Instruct family members in steps to take when a patient experiences a seizure. Assess a patient's home for environmental hazards in light of a seizure condition.

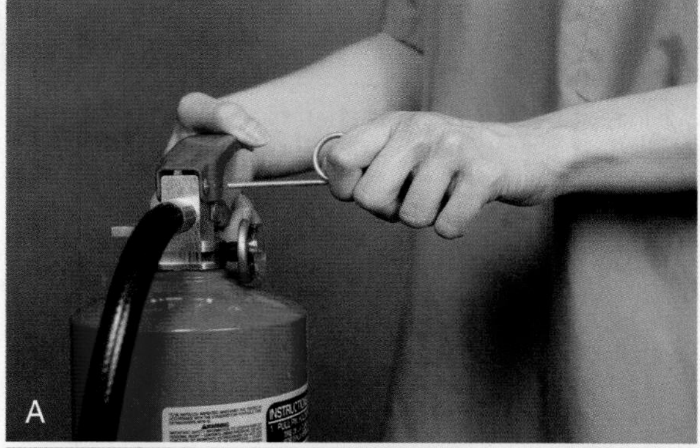

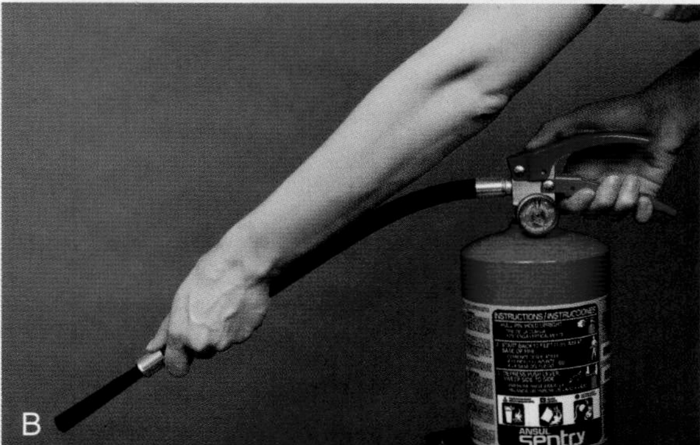

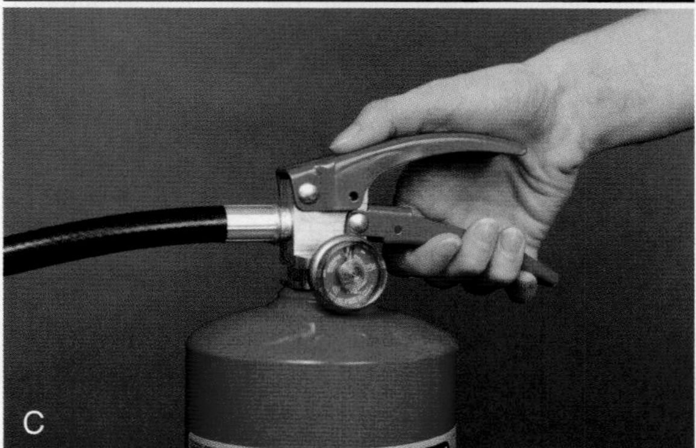

FIGURE 27-9 Correct use of a fire extinguisher. **A, *P***ull pin. **B, *A***im at base of fire. **C, *S***queeze handles and ***S***weep from side to side to coat area evenly.

Prolonged or repeated seizures indicate **status epilepticus**, a medical emergency that requires intensive monitoring and treatment. It is important that you observe the patient carefully before, during, and after the seizure so you are able to document the episode accurately. **Seizure precautions** encompass all nursing interventions to protect a patient from traumatic injury, position for adequate ventilation and drainage of oral secretions, and provide privacy and support following the seizure (Box 27-14).

Radiation. Radiation and radioactive materials used in the diagnosis and treatment of patients is a health hazard in health care settings. Hospitals have strict guidelines for the care of patients who receive

BOX 27-14 Tips for Protecting Patients During a Seizure

1. When seizure begins, note time, stay with patient, and call for help. Track duration of seizure. Notify health care provider immediately.
2. Position patient safely. If standing or sitting, guide patient to floor and protect head by cradling in your lap or placing a pad under head.
3. Do not lift patient from floor to bed while seizure is in progress. Clear surrounding area of furniture. If patient is in bed, remove pillows and raise side rails.
4. If possible, turn patient onto one side, head tilted slightly forward.
5. Do not restrain patient; hold limbs loosely if they are flailing. Loosen clothing.
6. Never force apart a patient's clenched teeth. Do not place any objects into patient's mouth such as fingers, medicine, tongue depressor, or airway when teeth are clenched. **Insert a bite-block or oral airway in advance only if you recognize the possibility of a tonic-clonic seizure.**
7. Stay with patient, observing sequence and timing of seizure activity.
8. As patient regains consciousness reorient and reassure. Assist patient to position of comfort in bed with side rails up (one rail down for easy exit) and bed in lowest position.
9. Conduct a head-to-toe evaluation, including an inspection of oral cavity for breaks in mucous membranes from bites or broken teeth; look for bruising of skin or injury to bones and joints.

radiation and are exposed to radioactive materials. Be familiar with established agency protocols. To reduce your exposure to radiation, limit the time spent near the source, make the distance from the source as great as possible, and use shielding devices such as lead aprons. Staff who work regularly near radiation wear devices that track the accumulative exposure to radiation.

Disasters. As a nurse you need to be prepared to respond and care for a sudden influx of patients during a disaster. TJC (2016) requires hospitals to have an emergency-management plan that addresses identifying possible emergency situations and their probable impact, maintaining adequate amount of supplies, and a formal response plan that includes actions to be taken by staff and steps to restore essential services and resume normal operations following the emergency.

Infection control practices are critical in the event of a biological attack. Therefore you manage all patients with suspected or confirmed bioterrorism-related illnesses using standard precautions (see Chapter 29). For certain diseases such as smallpox or pneumonic plague, additional precautions such as airborne or contact isolation precautions are necessary. Most infections associated with biological agents are not transmissible from patient to patient. Transport and move patients only when it is essential for treatment and care. An important aspect of care for patients who have a bioterrorism-related illness is postexposure management.

◆ Evaluation

Through the Patient's Eyes. Patient-centered care involves a thorough evaluation of a patient's perspective related to safety and whether his or her expectations have been met. Ask the patient questions such as "Are you satisfied with the changes made to your home? Do you feel safer as a result of the changes? Have you had any falls or injury? Are you still afraid of falling?" Involve the family in your evaluation, especially if they live with the patient and provide assistance in the home.

Patient Outcomes. Evaluation involves monitoring the actual care delivered by the health care team on the basis of the expected outcomes (Figure 27-10). For each nursing diagnosis measure whether the outcomes of care have been met. If your patient meets the goals, the diagnosis is resolved, and your nursing interventions were effective and appropriate. If not, determine whether new safety risks to the patient have developed or whether previous risks remain. For example, if the patient has a recurrent fall, reassess the conditions surrounding that fall and determine whether contributing factors can be removed or managed. The patient and family need to participate to find permanent ways to reduce risks to safety. When patient outcomes are not met, ask the following questions:

- What factors led to your fall/injury?
- Help me understand what makes you feel unsafe in your environment.
- What questions do you have about your safety?
- Do you need help locating community resources to help make your home safer?
- What changes have you recently experienced that you believe contribute to your risk for falling or lack of safety?

Continually reassess a patient's and family's need for additional support services such as home care, physical therapy, counseling, and further teaching. A safe environment is essential to promoting, maintaining, and restoring health. Overall your expected outcomes include a safe physical environment and a patient whose expectations have been met, who is knowledgeable about safety factors and precautions, and who is free of injury.

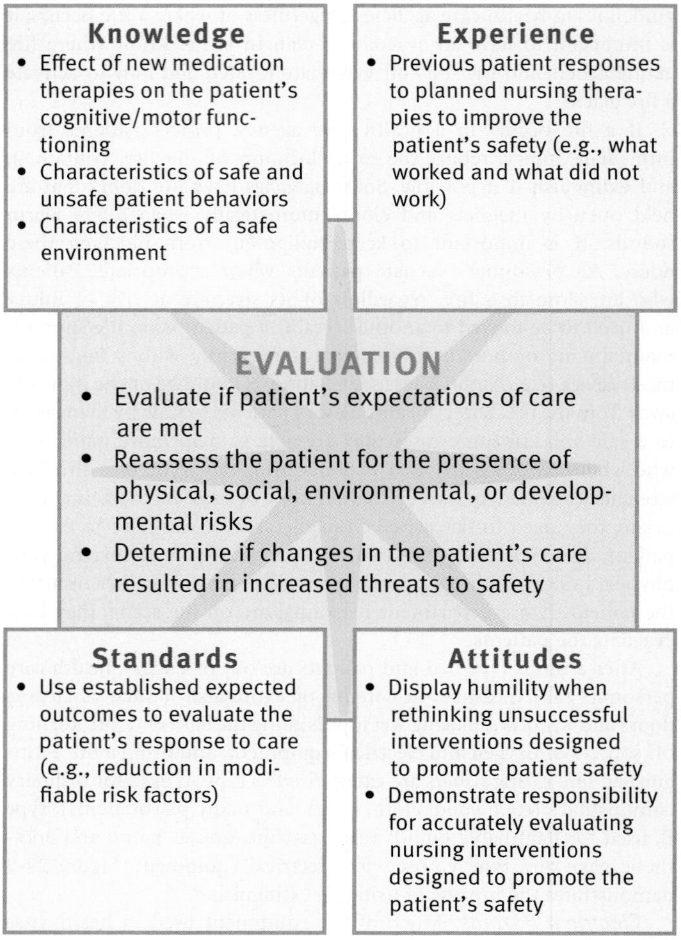

Knowledge
- Effect of new medication therapies on the patient's cognitive/motor functioning
- Characteristics of safe and unsafe patient behaviors
- Characteristics of a safe environment

Experience
- Previous patient responses to planned nursing therapies to improve the patient's safety (e.g., what worked and what did not work)

EVALUATION
- Evaluate if patient's expectations of care are met
- Reassess the patient for the presence of physical, social, environmental, or developmental risks
- Determine if changes in the patient's care resulted in increased threats to safety

Standards
- Use established expected outcomes to evaluate the patient's response to care (e.g., reduction in modifiable risk factors)

Attitudes
- Display humility when rethinking unsuccessful interventions designed to promote patient safety
- Demonstrate responsibility for accurately evaluating nursing interventions designed to promote the patient's safety

FIGURE 27-10 Critical thinking model for safety evaluation.

SAFETY GUIDELINES FOR NURSING SKILLS

Ensuring patient safety is an essential role of the professional nurse. To ensure patient safety, communicate clearly with members of the health care team, assess and incorporate the patient's priorities of care and preferences, and use the best evidence when making decisions about your patient's care. When performing the skills in this chapter, remember the following points to ensure safe, individualized patient care:

- On the basis of your assessment and knowledge of physiological and behavioral factors, anticipate a patient's fall risks when choosing fall prevention strategies.
- Involve patients and families in selection of fall prevention strategies.
- Always try restraint alternatives before using a restraint. Involve family in your approach.
- Protect patients from injury. Follow assessment guidelines while patients are restrained to avoid injury from inappropriate placement.
- Protect patients from falling by implementing fall prevention protocols and providing patient and family education about fall prevention.

SKILL 27-1 FALL PREVENTION IN HEALTH CARE SETTINGS

DELEGATION AND COLLABORATION

The skill of assessing and communicating a patient's risk for falling cannot be delegated to nursing assistive personnel (NAP). Skills used to prevent falls can be delegated. The nurse instructs NAP to:

- Use fall prevention measures that match a patient's mobility limitations.
- Use specific environmental safety precautions (e.g., bed locked in low position, call light within reach).
- Report to the nurse any patient behaviors (e.g., disorientation, wandering) that are precursors to falls.

EQUIPMENT

- Fall risk assessment tool
- Hospital bed with side rails; *option*—low bed
- Call light/intercom system
- Gait belt
- Wheelchair (as needed)
- Additional safety devices (e.g., bed alarm pad, wedge cushion)

STEP	RATIONALE
ASSESSMENT	
1. Identify patient using two identifiers (e.g., name and birthday or name and medical record number) according to agency policy.	Ensures correct patient. Complies with The Joint Commission standards and improves patient safety (TJC, 2016).
2. Assess patient's fall risks using an agency fall risk assessment tool. Assess patient's age (over 65), number of co-morbidities, impaired memory and cognition, incontinence or urinary frequency/urgency, decreased hearing, decreased vision, orthostatic hypotension, impaired gait, weak lower extremities, poor balance, fatigue, need for transfer assistance, decreased peripheral sensation (Spoelstra, 2011; Viera et al., 2011).	A variety of physiological factors predispose patients to fall.
3. Determine if patient has a history of recent falls or other injuries within the home. Assess previous falls, using the acronym SPLATT (Touhy and Jett, 2014). • *S*ymptoms at time of fall • *P*revious fall • *L*ocation of fall • *A*ctivity at time of fall • *T*ime of fall • *T*rauma after fall	*Key symptoms are helpful in identifying cause for falls. Onset, location, and activity* associated with a fall provide further details on causative factors and how to prevent future falls.
4. Review patient's medications (including over-the-counter [OTC] medications and herbal products) for use of antidepressants, anticonvulsants, antipsychotics, hypnotics (especially benzodiazepines), anxiolytics, diuretics, antihypertensives, antihistamines, anti-Parkinson drugs, hypoglycemics, muscle relaxants, analgesics, and laxatives. Also assess for polypharmacy (i.e., over six medications, duplicate medications, drugs inappropriate for condition) (Bushardt et al., 2008).	Effects of certain medications and use of multiple medications increase risk for falls and injury (Chang et al., 2011; Gribbin et al., 2010; Kojima et al., 2011).

CLINICAL DECISION: *If patient takes multiple medications, confer with health care provider on possibility of reducing or adjusting number of medications.*

STEP	RATIONALE
5. Assess patient for fear of falling: those higher at risk are over 75 years of age, female, lower income, or single and have poor perceived general health or history of falling in last 3 months (Boyd and Stevens, 2009).	Fear of falling is interrelated with incidence of falls.

SKILL 27-1 FALL PREVENTION IN HEALTH CARE SETTINGS—cont'd

STEP	RATIONALE
6. Perform the "Timed Get-up and Go" (TUG) if patient is able to ambulate. At a minimum observe patient walk in room (with or without assistance). Steps for TUG dual assessment: • Give patient verbal instructions to stand up from a chair, walk 10 feet (3 meters) as quickly and safely as possible (cross a line marked on the floor), turn around, walk back, and sit down. • Have patient rise from straight back chair without using arms for support. • Begin counting. • Look for unsteadiness in patient's gait. • Have patient return to chair and sit down without using arms for support. Check time elapsed. For accuracy, a patient should have one practice trial that is not included in the score. Patient must use the same assistive device each time he or she is tested to be able to compare scores.	The Timed Get-up and Go (TUG) is a revision to the original Get-up and Go test (Podsiadlo and Richardson, 1991). It quantifies a patient's functional mobility. Observing a patient walk allows you to determine if gait and posture are normal. The TUG is a measure of physical and cognitive performance. A patient's ability to follow simple instructions measures cognitive function. An older adult who takes 12 seconds or longer to complete the TUG is at high risk for falling (CDC, 2015b). Balance function is scored on a five-point scale: 1 = Normal; 2 = Very slightly abnormal; 3 = Mildly abnormal; 4 = Moderately abnormal; 5 = Severely abnormal (Mathias et al., 1986). A score of 3 or more on the balance scale indicates a patient is at risk for falling (Mathias et al., 1986). **Note:** The TUG has been found to have limited ability to predict falls in community-dwelling elderly and should not be used in isolation to identify individuals at high risk for falls in this setting (Barry et al., 2014).
7. Assess risk factors for falls in health care facility (e.g., being attached to equipment such as sequential compression hose, intravenous [IV] line, or oxygen tubing; improperly lighted room; clutter; obstructed walkway to bathroom; and frequently needed items that are difficult to reach.	Environmental barriers pose risk for falls.
8. Assess condition of equipment (i.e., legs on bedside commode, tips of walker).	Equipment in poor repair increases the risk for fall.
9. Assess patient's medical history for osteoporosis, being on anticoagulants, history of previous fracture, cancer, and recent chest or abdominal surgery.	Factors increase likelihood of injury from a fall.
10. Use a patient-centered approach. Determine what patient knows about risks for falling and steps that he or she can take to prevent falls.	Knowledge of fall risks influences one's ability to take needed precautions in reducing falling.
11. If patient is assessed to be a fall risk, apply color-coded wristband (see illustration). Some agencies institute fall risk signs on doors.	Color-coded yellow bands are easily recognizable.
PLANNING	
1. Gather equipment and perform hand hygiene.	Organizes care. Reduces transmission of microorganisms.
2. Explain what you plan to do. Specifically discuss reasons that patient is at risk for falling. Include family caregivers (as appropriate) in discussion. Provide privacy. Be sure that patient is comfortable.	Reduces patient anxiety and promotes cooperation. Results in fall prevention measures that are patient centered and not just routine. Younger patients are very independent and often believe that they are not likely to fall.
IMPLEMENTATION	
1. A adjust bed to low position with wheels locked (see illustration). *Option:* Place nonslip padded floor mats at exit side of bed.	Height of bed allows ambulatory patient to get in and out of bed easily and safely. Pads provide nonslippery surface on which to stand.
2. Encourage the use of properly fitted skid-proof footwear.	Prevents falls from slipping on floor.

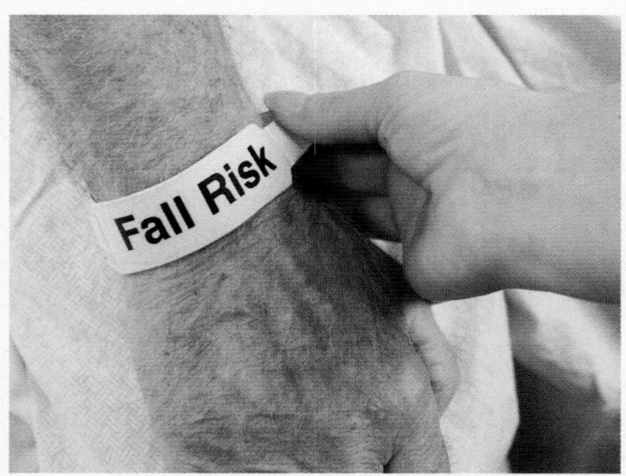

STEP 11 Arm band alerts nursing staff to patient's risk of falling.

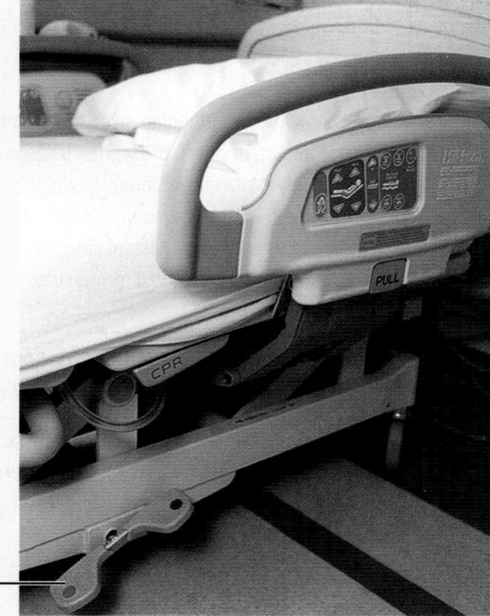

STEP 1 Hospital bed should be kept in lowest position with wheels locked and side rails up as appropriate.

STEP	RATIONALE
3. Orient patient to surroundings, call light, and routines to expect in plan of care.	Orientation to room and plan of care provides familiarity with environment and activities to anticipate.
a. Provide patient's hearing aid and glasses. Be sure that each is functioning/clean.	Enables patient to remain alert to conditions in environment.
b. Be sure that call light/bed control system is in an accessible location within patient's reach. Explain and demonstrate how to turn call light/intercom system on and off at bedside and in bathroom (see illustration). Have patient perform a return demonstration.	Knowledge of location and use of call light is essential for patient to be able to call for assistance quickly. Reaching for an object when in bed can lead to an accidental fall.
c. Explain to patient/family caregiver when and why to use call system (e.g., report pain, get out of bed, go to bathroom). Provide clear instructions to patient/family caregiver regarding mobility restrictions.	Increases likelihood that patient will call for help and of nurse being able to respond to patient's needs in a timely way.
4. Safe use of side rails	
a. Explain to patient and family members the reason for using side rails: moving and turning self in bed.	Promotes cooperation.
b. Check agency policy regarding side-rail use.	Side rails are restraint devices if they immobilize or reduce ability of a patient to move his or her arms, legs, body, or head freely.
• Dependent, less mobile patients: In a two-side rail bed, keep both rails up. (NOTE: Rails on newer hospital beds allow for room at foot of bed for patient to safely exit bed.) In a four-side rail bed, leave two upper rails up.	
• Patient able to get out of bed independently: In a four-side rail bed, leave two upper side rails up. In a two-side rail, keep only one rail up.	Allows for safe exit from bed.
5. Make the patient's environment safe.	
a. Remove excess equipment, supplies, and furniture from rooms and halls.	Reduces likelihood of falling or tripping over objects.
b. Keep floors clutter and obstacle free, particularly the path to the bathroom.	Reduces likelihood of falling or tripping over objects.
c. Coil and secure excess electrical, telephone, and any other cords or tubing.	Reduces the risk of entanglement.
d. Clean all spills promptly. Post a sign indicating a wet floor. Remove the sign when the floor is dry (usually done by housekeeping).	Reduces the risk of falling on slippery, wet surfaces.
e. Ensure adequate glare-free lighting; use a night-light at night.	Glare may be a problem for older adults because of vision changes.
f. Have assistive devices (e.g., cane, walker, bedside commode) on exit side of bed. Have chair back of commode placed against wall of room if possible.	Provides added support when transferring out of bed. Stabilizes commode.
g. Arrange personal items (e.g., water pitcher, telephone, reading materials, dentures) within patient's easy reach and in a logical way.	Facilitates independence and self-care; prevents falls related to reaching for hard-to-reach items.
h. Secure locks on beds, stretchers, and wheelchairs.	Prevents accidental movement of devices during patient transfer.
6. Additional interventions for patients at moderate-to-high risk for falling (based on fall risk assessment)	
a. Prioritize call-light responses to patients at high risk, using a team approach with all staff knowing responsibility to respond.	Ensures rapid response by a health care provider when patient calls for assistance.
b. Establish elimination schedule, using bedside commode when appropriate.	Proactive toileting keeps patients from being unattended with sudden urge to use toilet.

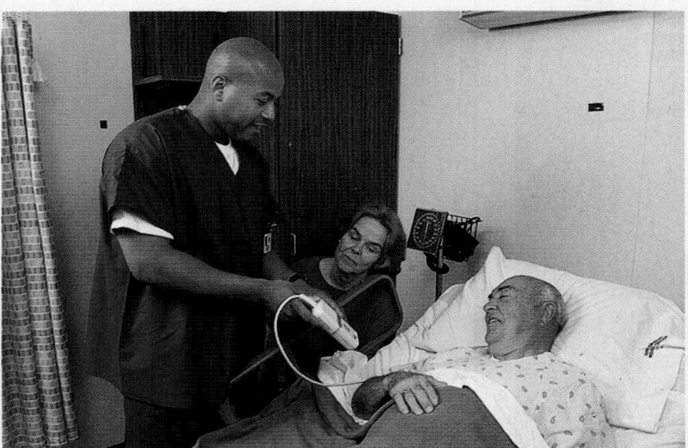

STEP 3b Nurse demonstrates use of call light to patient.

SKILL 27-1 FALL PREVENTION IN HEALTH CARE SETTINGS—cont'd

STEP	RATIONALE
CLINICAL DECISION: *Getting out of bed for toileting is a common event leading to a patient's fall (Tzeng, 2010), especially during evening or night hours when a room is darkened.*	
c. Stay with patient during toileting (standing outside bathroom door).	Patients often try to get up to stand and walk back to their bed from the bathroom without assistance.
d. Place patient in a geri chair or wheelchair with wedge cushion. Use wheelchair only for transport, not for sitting an extended time.	Maintains alignment and comfort and makes it difficult to exit chair.
e. Use a low bed that has low height above floor and apply floor mats.	Reduces fall-related injuries.
f. Activate a bed alarm for patient.	Alarm activates when patient rises off a sensor. Alarm sounds an alert to staff.
g. Confer with physical therapy on feasibility of gait training, weight-bearing activities, balance exercise, and strengthening exercises.	Exercise can reduce falls, fall-related fractures, and several risk factors for falls in individuals with low bone density and in older adults (deKam et al., 2009; Schubert, 2011).
h. Use sitters or restraints only when alternatives are exhausted.	A sitter is a nonprofessional staff member or volunteer who stays in a patient room to closely observe patients who are at risk for falling. Restraints should be used only as a final option (see Skill 27-2).
7. When ambulating a patient, have patient wear a gait belt and walk along patient's side (see Chapter 39).	Gait belt gives you a secure hold on patient during ambulation.
8. Safe Transport Using a Wheelchair.	
a. Determine level of assistance needed to transfer patient to wheelchair. Position wheelchair on same side of bed as patient's strong or unaffected side (see Chapter 39).	Patient's condition may require more than a one-person assist. Positioning of chair facilitates patient's ability to assist in transfer.
b. Place wedge cushion in chair (see illustration.)	Prevents patient from slipping out of chair.
c. Securely lock brakes on both wheels when transferring patient into or out of wheelchair.	Keeps chair steady and secure.
d. Raise footplates before transfer to chair; then lower footplates, placing patient's feet on them after he or she is seated.	Prevents tripping over footplate.
e. Have patient sit with buttocks well back in seat. *Option:* Apply a quick-release seat belt.	Prevents patient from sliding out of chair.
f. Back wheelchair into and out of elevator or door, leading with large rear wheels first (see illustration).	Prevents smaller front wheels from catching in crack between elevator and floor, causing chair to tip.
9. Remove unnecessary supplies. Perform hand hygiene.	Reduces transmission of microorganisms.
EVALUATION	
1. Conduct hourly rounds.	Hourly rounding programs reduce patient falls, and call light use increases patients' perception of nursing responsiveness.
2. Evaluate patient's ability to use assistive devices such as walker or bedside commode.	Adjustments in devices may become necessary.
3. Evaluate for changes in motor, sensory, and cognitive status and review if any falls or injuries have occurred.	May require different interventions to be added. Fall outcomes determine success of plan.

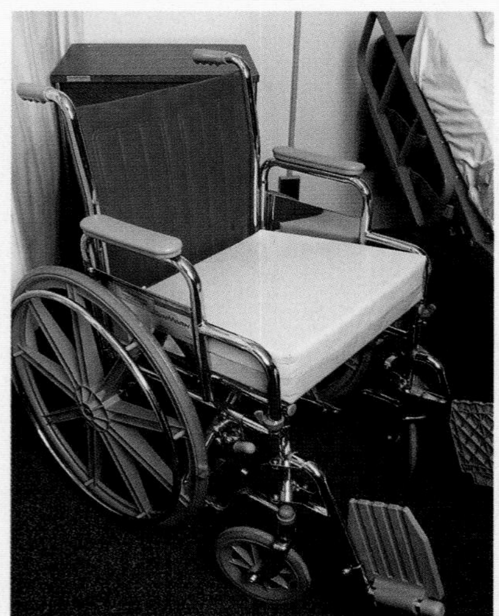

STEP 8b Wheelchair with footplates raised and a wedge cushion in place.

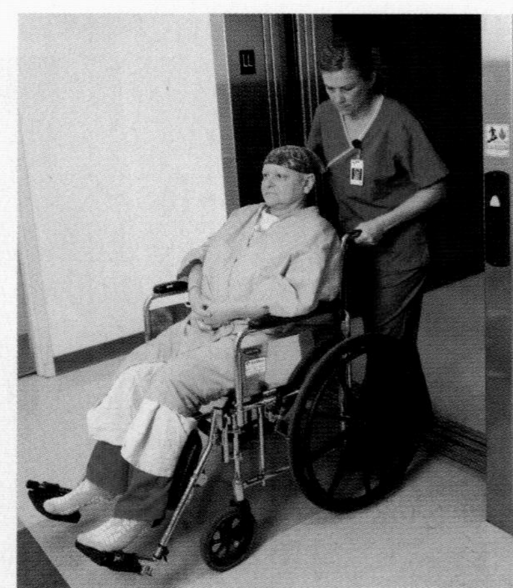

STEP 8f Nurse backing wheelchair into elevator.

STEP	RATIONALE
4. Use ***Teach Back:*** State to the patient and family caregiver, "I want to be sure I explained clearly to you why you are more likely to fall than other patients. Can you tell me some of those reasons?" Evaluate whether patient/caregiver is able to explain fall risks. Revise your instruction now or develop plan for revised patient teaching to be implemented at an appropriate time if patient/caregiver is not able to teach back correctly.	Evaluates what patient and family caregiver are able to explain or demonstrate.

UNEXPECTED OUTCOMES AND RELATED INTERVENTIONS

1. Patient starts to fall while ambulating with a nurse.
   - Put both arms around patient's waist or grasp gait belt.
   - Stand with feet apart to provide a broad base of support (see Figure 39-11, *A*).
   - Extend one leg and let patient slide against it to the floor (see Figure 39-11, *B*).
   - Bend knees and lower body as patient slides to floor (see Figure 39-11, *C*).
2. Patient falls.
   - Call for assistance. Assess patient for injury and stay with patient until assistance arrives to help lift him or her to bed or wheelchair.
   - Reinforce explanation of identified risks with patient and review safety measures needed to prevent a fall.
   - Monitor patient closely after the fall since injuries are not always immediately apparent.
3. Patient/family caregiver is unable to explain fall risks.
   - Offer re-explanation, using plain language, and consider use of printed materials if available.

RECORDING AND REPORTING

- Record in plan of care specific interventions to prevent falls and promote safety.
- Document your evaluation of patient learning.
- Report patient's fall risks and measures taken to reduce risks to all health care personnel.
- Report immediately to physician or health care provider if the patient sustains a fall or an injury.
- Complete an agency safety event or incident report noting objective details of fall (time, location, patient's condition, treatment, treatment response). Do not place report in patient medical record.
- Record events related to the fall and treatment in medical record.

HOME CARE CONSIDERATIONS

- Assess the patient's home environment for hazards and institute safety measures as appropriate, with patient and family partnering on decisions.
- Keep personal items in their familiar positions and within easy reach in rooms frequently used.
- If patient has a history of falls and lives alone, recommend that he or she wear an electronic Safe Patient Care device. The device is turned on by the wearer to alert a monitoring site to call emergency services for help.

SKILL 27-2 APPLYING PHYSICAL RESTRAINTS

DELEGATION AND COLLABORATION

The skill of assessing a patient's behavior, orientation to the environment, need for restraints, and appropriate use cannot be delegated. The application and routine checking of a restraint can be delegated to nursing assistive personnel (NAP). TJC (2009) requires training on first aid for anyone who monitors patients in restraints. The nurse instructs the NAP about:

- Appropriate restraint to use and correct placement of restraint.
- When and how to change patient's position and provide range-of-motion exercises, hydration, toileting, skin care, and time for socialization.
- When to report signs and symptoms of patient not tolerating restraint (e.g., agitation, change in skin integrity, circulation of extremities, or patient's breathing) and what to do.

EQUIPMENT

- Proper restraint
- Padding (if needed)

STEP	RATIONALE
ASSESSMENT	
1. Identify patient using two identifiers (e.g., name and birthday or name and medical record number) according to agency policy.	Ensures correct patient. Complies with The Joint Commission standards and improves patient safety (TJC, 2016).
2. Assess patient's behavior (e.g., confusion; disorientation; agitation; restlessness; combativeness; inability to follow directions or repeated removal of tubing, dressing, or other therapeutic devices). Does patient create a risk to other patients?	If patient's behavior continues despite treatment or restraint alternatives, use of restraint is indicated. You use the least restrictive type of restraint.

SKILL 27-2 APPLYING PHYSICAL RESTRAINTS—cont'd

STEP	RATIONALE
3. Determine failure of restraint alternatives. Review facility policies and state laws regarding restraints. Check for a current health care provider's order. The licensed health care provider assesses the patient in person within 1 hour of initiation of restraints (TJC, 2009). Order must include purpose, type, location, and time or duration of restraint. Determine if signed consent for use of restraint is necessary (long-term care). Orders for non-violent or non-self destructive-patients are written and renewed according to agency policy. Orders for self-destructive or violent patients are limited to select time limits and only renewed for a maximum of 24 consecutive hours (TJC, 2017).	A health care provider's order for the least restrictive type of restraint is required.

CLINICAL DECISION: *A licensed independent health care provider responsible for the care of the patient evaluates the patient in person within 1 hour of the initiation of restraint used for the management of violent or self-destructive behavior that jeopardizes the physical safety of the patient, staff, or others. A registered nurse or a physician assistant may conduct the in-person evaluation if trained in accordance with the requirements and consultations with the previously mentioned health care provider after the evaluation as determined by hospital policy (TJC, 2016).*

STEP	RATIONALE
4. Review manufacturer's instructions for restraint application before entering patient's room. Determine most appropriate size restraint.	You need to be familiar with all devices used for patient care and protection. Incorrect application of restraint device results in patient injury or death.
PLANNING	
1. Gather equipment and perform hand hygiene.	Promotes organization and reduces transmission of microorganisms.
2. Explain what you plan to do. Provide privacy. Be sure that patient is comfortable and in correct anatomical position.	Reduces patient anxiety and promotes cooperation; positioning prevents contractures and neurovascular impairment.
IMPLEMENTATION	
1. Adjust bed to proper height and lower side rail on side of patient contact. Be sure that patient is comfortable and in proper body alignment.	Allows you to use proper body mechanics and prevents injury during restraint application. Positioning prevents contractures and neurovascular injury while restraint is in place.
2. Inspect area where restraint is to be placed. Note if there is any nearby tubing or device. Assess condition of skin, sensation, adequacy of circulation, and range of joint motion.	Restraints sometimes compress and interfere with functioning of devices or tubes. Assessment provides baseline to monitor patient's response to restraint.
3. Pad skin and bony prominences (as necessary) that will be under restraint.	Reduces friction and pressure from restraint to skin and underlying tissue.
4. Apply proper-size restraint. NOTE: Refer to manufacturer's directions.	
a. *Belt restraint:* Have patient in sitting position in bed. Apply belt over clothes, gown, or pajamas. Be sure to place restraint at waist, not chest or abdomen. Remove wrinkles or creases in clothing. Bring ties through slots in belt. Help patient lie down in bed. Have patient roll to side and avoid applying belt too tightly (see illustrations). *Option: Apply a belt restraint net.*	Restrains center of gravity and prevents patient from rolling off stretcher or sitting up while on stretcher or from falling out of bed. Tight application interferes with ventilation if belt moves up over abdomen or chest.
b. *Extremity (ankle or wrist) restraint:* Restraint made of soft quilted material or sheepskin with foam padding. Wrap limb restraint around wrist or ankle with soft part toward skin and secure snugly (not tightly) in place by Velcro strap or quick-release buckle. Insert two fingers under secured restraint (see illustration).	Restraint designed to immobilize one or all extremities. Maintain immobilization of extremity to protect patient from fall or accidental removal of therapeutic device (e.g., intravenous [IV] tube, Foley catheter). Tight application interferes with circulation and potentially causes neurovascular injury.

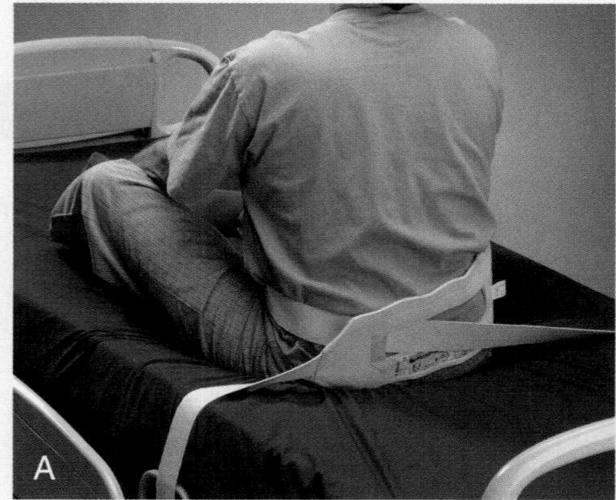

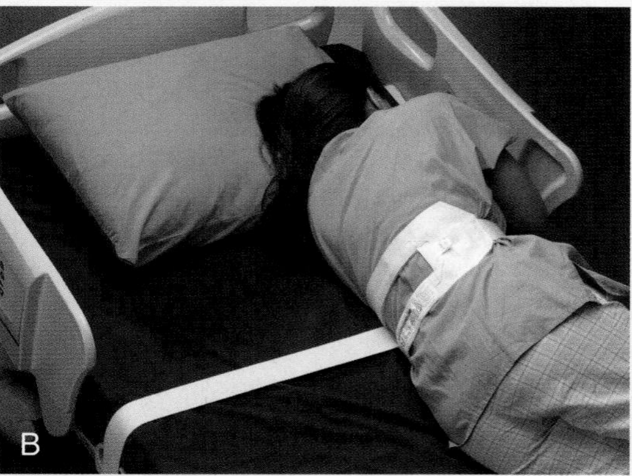

STEP 4a A, Apply belt restraint with patient sitting. **B,** A properly applied belt restraint allows patient to turn in bed. (Courtesy Posey Company, Arcadia, CA.)

STEP	RATIONALE

CLINICAL DECISION: *Patient with wrist and ankle restraints is at risk for aspiration if positioned supine. Place patient in lateral position or with head of bed elevated rather than supine.*

STEP	RATIONALE
c. *Mitten restraint:* Thumbless mitten device restrains patient's hands. Place hand in mitten, being sure that Velcro strap is around wrist and not forearm (see illustration).	Prevents patient from dislodging invasive equipment, removing dressings, or scratching but allows greater movement than a wrist restraint. It is considered a restraint alternative if untethered and patient is physically and cognitively able to remove it.
d. *Elbow restraint (freedom splint):* Restraint consists of rigidly padded fabric that wraps around the arm and is closed with Velcro. The upper end has a clamp that hooks to the sleeve of a patient's gown or shirt (see illustration). Insert arm so elbow joint rests against padded area, keeping joint extended.	Commonly used with infants and children to prevent elbow flexion (e.g., with IV line placed in antecubital fossa). Restraint keeps elbow extended.

CLINICAL DECISION: *This text does not address application of vest restraints. Many health care agencies ban the use of jacket (vest) restraints because of their association with fatal injuries.*

STEP	RATIONALE
5. Attach restraint straps to portion of bedframe that moves when raising or lowering head of bed (see illustrations). Be sure that straps are secure. *Do not attach to side rails.* Attach restraint to chair frame for patient in chair or wheelchair, being sure that tie is out of patient's reach.	Properly positioned strap does not tighten and restrict circulation when bed is raised or lowered.

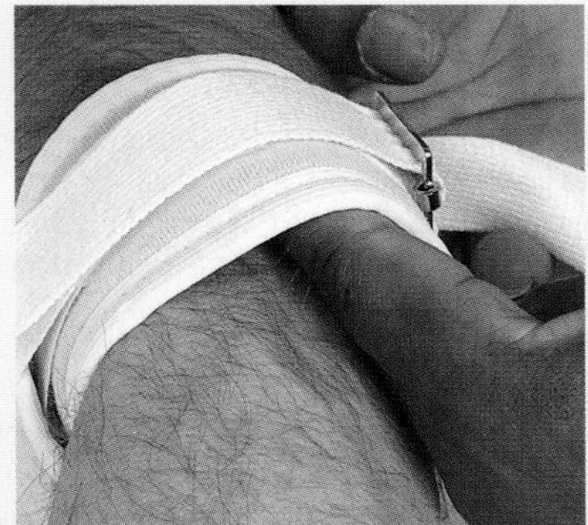

STEP 4b Insert two fingers under restraint to check for constriction.

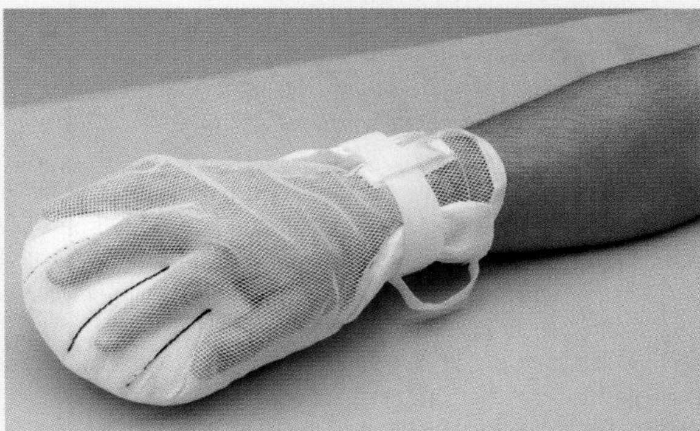

STEP 4c Mitten restraint. (Courtesy Posey Company, Arcadia, CA.)

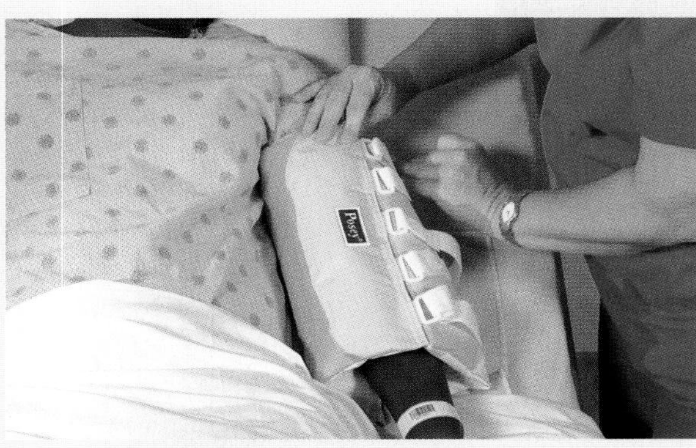

STEP 4d Freedom elbow restraint.

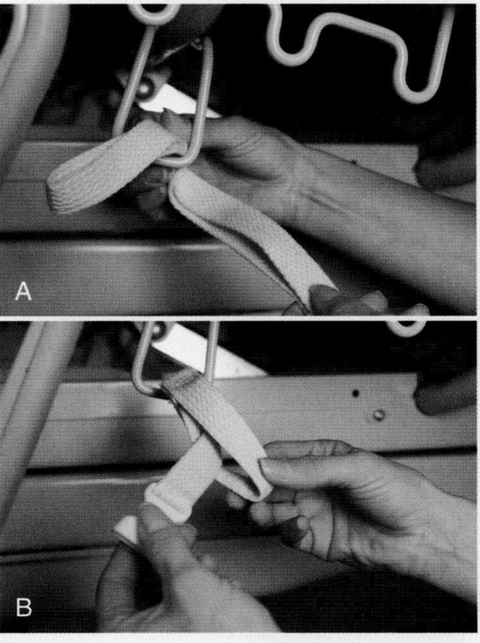

STEP 5 Attaching restraint buckle and strap to bedframe.

SKILL 27-2 APPLYING PHYSICAL RESTRAINTS—cont'd

STEP	RATIONALE
6. Secure restraints with quick-release buckle (see illustrations). *Do not tie strap in a knot.* Be sure that buckle is out of patient reach.	Allows for quick release in an emergency.
7. Double-check and insert two fingers under secured restraint. Assess proper placement of restraint, including skin integrity, pulses, skin temperature and color, and sensation of restrained body part.	Provides baseline assessment data if injury develops from restraint.
8. Remove restraint at least every 2 hours (TJC, 2016) or more frequently as determined by agency policy. Reposition patient, provide comfort and toileting measures, evaluate patient condition each time. If patient is violent or noncompliant, remove one restraint at a time and/or have staff assist while removing restraints.	Provides an opportunity to attend to patient's basic needs and determine need for continuation.
9. Secure call light or intercom system within reach.	Allows patient, family, or caregiver to obtain assistance quickly.
10. Leave bed or chair with wheels locked. Keep bed in lowest position.	Prevents bed or chair from moving if patient tries to get out. If patient falls with bed in lowest position, this reduces chance of injury.
11. Perform hand hygiene.	Reduces transmission of microorganisms.

EVALUATION

STEP	RATIONALE
1. After application, evaluate patient for signs of injury every 15 minutes (e.g., circulation, vital signs, range of motion, physical and psychological status, and readiness for discontinuation. Perform visual checks if patient is too agitated to approach (TJC, 2015).	Frequent evaluation prevents injury to patient and ensures removal of restraint at earliest possible time. Frequency of monitoring guides staff in determining appropriate intervals for evaluation on the basis of patient's needs and condition, type of restraint used, risk associated with use of chosen intervention, and other relevant factors.
2. Evaluate patient's need for toileting, nutrition and fluids, hygiene, and elimination and release restraint at least every 2 hours.	Prevents injury to patient and attends to basic needs.
3. Evaluate patient for any complications of immobility.	Early detection of skin irritation, restricted breathing, or reduction in mobility prevents serious adverse events.
4. The licensed health care provider or registered nurse trained according to CMS requirements needs to evaluate patient within either 1 or 4 hours after initiation of restraints, depending on Medicare status of hospital (see agency policy).	Determines patient's immediate situation, reaction to restraints, medical and behavioral condition, and need to continue or terminate restraints (CMS, 2007).
5. After 24 hours, before writing a new order, the health care provider who is responsible for patient's care must see and assess patient.	Ensures that restraint application continues to be medically appropriate.
6. Observe IV catheters, urinary catheters, and drainage tubes to determine that they are positioned correctly and that therapy remains uninterrupted.	Reinsertion is uncomfortable and increases risk for infection or interrupts therapy.
7. Observe patient's behavior and reaction to presence of restraint.	Restraints can increase restlessness and agitation, resulting in harm.

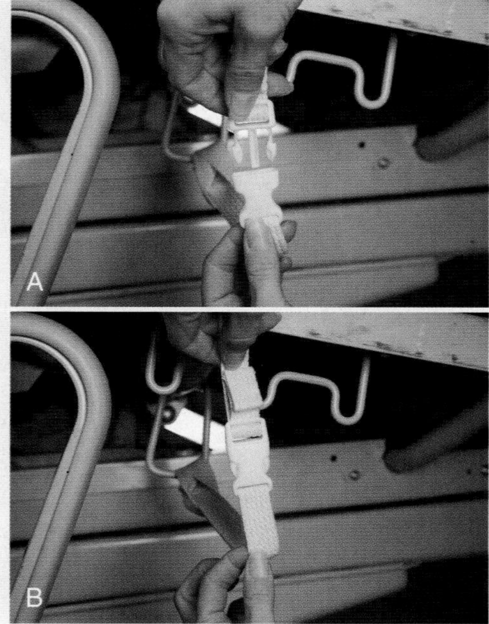

STEP 6 Connecting the quick-release buckle.

UNEXPECTED OUTCOMES AND RELATED INTERVENTIONS

1. Skin underlying restraint becomes reddened or damaged.
   - Provide appropriate skin/wound care (see Chapter 48).
   - Notify health care provider and reassess need for continued use of restraint or if you can use alternative measures.
   - Be sure that restraint is applied correctly and has adequate padding.
   - Remove restraints more frequently. Change wet or soiled restraints.
2. Patient has altered neurovascular status of an extremity such as cyanosis, pallor, and coldness of skin or complains of tingling, pain, or numbness.
   - Remove restraint immediately and notify health care provider. Stay with patient.
3. Patient becomes confused or agitated.
   - Identify reason for change in behavior and try to eliminate cause.
   - Use restraint alternatives.

RECORDING AND REPORTING

- Record nursing interventions, including restraint alternatives tried, in nurses' notes.
- Record patient's behavior before restraints were applied, level of orientation, and patient or family's understanding of application.
- Document your evaluation of patient/family learning.
- Record purpose for restraint, type and location of restraint used, time applied and discontinued, times restraint was released, and routine observations (e.g., skin color, pulses, sensation, vital signs, behavior) in nurses' notes and flow sheets.
- Record patient's level of orientation and behavior after restraint application. Record times patient was evaluated, attempts to use alternatives, and patient's response when restraint was removed.

HOME CARE CONSIDERATIONS

- A physical restraint is a device that requires a physician's order. Do not send a patient home with intent of restraining unless device is necessary to protect patient from injury. If patient's family wishes to use restraint at home, a physician's order is required, and you need to give clear instructions regarding proper application, care needed while in restraints, and complications for which to look. Carefully assess the family for competency and understanding of intent for using restraint.

KEY POINTS

- In the community a safe environment means that basic needs are achievable, physical hazards are reduced, transmission of pathogens and parasites is reduced, pollution is controlled, and sanitation is maintained.
- A safe health care environment is one that reduces the risk of injury, including minimizing falls, patient-inherent accidents, procedure-inherent accidents, and equipment-related accidents.
- Reduction of physical hazards in the environment includes providing adequate lighting, decreasing clutter, and securing the home.
- Reduce the transmission of pathogens through medical and surgical asepsis, immunization, adequate food sanitation, and appropriate disposal of human waste.
- Every developmental age involves specific safety risks.
- Children younger than 5 years of age are at greatest risk for home accidents that result in severe injury and death.
- Patient safety continues to be one of the most pressing health care challenges in the nation.
- Adolescents are at risk for injury from automobile accidents, suicide, and substance abuse.
- Threats to an adult's safety are frequently associated with lifestyle habits.
- Risks for injury for older patients are directly related to the physiological changes of the aging process.
- Nursing interventions for promoting safety are individualized for patients' developmental stage, lifestyle, and environment.
- Continually evaluate a patient's safety risk and update the nursing care plan appropriately.
- Fall risk prevention strategies are implemented on the basis of patients' risk factors, medical history, and condition of patient's environment.
- Use physical restraints only as a last resort, when patients' behavior places them or others at risk for injury.

CLINICAL APPLICATION QUESTIONS

Preparing for Clinical Practice

Ms. Cohen is hospitalized for repair of a fractured hip after a fall at home. She requires intravenous (IV) antibiotics after surgery. Shortly after the first dose she became restless and started picking at her IV line and frequently tried to get out of bed. Several restraint alternatives were attempted; but, because of her restlessness, she was successful at pulling out her IV line and getting out of bed. It becomes necessary to restrain Ms. Cohen.

1. You know that a health care provider's order is required for the restraint. What are essential components of the restraint order?
2. Which assessments do you need to perform on Ms. Cohen while she is restrained?
3. The physician orders a belt restraint. Your assessment of Ms. Cohen the next day reveals that during the day she is alert and pleasantly confused but not attempting to get out of bed. Do you continue use of the restraint? Explain.

ⓔ ***Answers to Clinical Application Questions can be found on the Evolve website.***

REVIEW QUESTIONS

Are You Ready to Test Your Nursing Knowledge?

1. A patient has been newly admitted to a medicine unit with a history of diabetes and advanced heart failure. The nurse is assessing the patient's fall risks. Place the following steps for measuring the "Timed Get-up and Go Test" (TUG) in the correct order:
   1. Have patient rise from straight-back chair without using arms for support.
   2. Begin timing.
   3. Tell patient to walk 10 feet as quickly and safely as possible to a line you marked on the floor, turn around, walk back, and sit down.
   4. Check time elapsed.
   5. Look for unsteadiness in patient's gait.
   6. Have patient return to chair and sit down without using arms for support.
2. A nurse knows that the people most at risk for accidental hypothermia are: (Select all that apply.)
   1. People who are homeless.
   2. People with respiratory conditions.
   3. People with cardiovascular conditions.
   4. The very old.
   5. People with kidney disorders.
3. A parent calls the pediatrician's office to ask about directions for using a car seat. Which of the following is the most correct set of instructions the nurse gives to this parent?
   1. Only infants and toddlers need to ride in the back seat.
   2. All toddlers can move to a forward facing car seat when they reach age 2.
   3. Toddlers must reach age 2 and the height/weight requirement before they ride forward facing.
   4. Toddlers must reach age 2 or the height or weight requirement before they ride forward facing.
4. The nursing assessment of a 78-year-old woman reveals orthostatic hypotension, weakness on the left side, and fear of falling. On the basis of the patient's data, which one of the following nursing diagnoses indicates an understanding of the assessment findings?
   1. *Activity Intolerance*
   2. *Impaired Bed Mobility*
   3. *Acute Pain*
   4. *Risk for Falls*
5. A couple who is caring for their aging parents are concerned about factors that put them at risk for falls. Which factors are most likely to contribute to an increase in falls in the elderly? (Select all that apply.)
   1. Inadequate lighting
   2. Throw rugs
   3. Multiple medications
   4. Doorway thresholds
   5. Cords covered by carpets
   6. Staircases with handrails
6. You are caring for a patient who frequently tries to remove his intravenous catheter and feeding tube. You have an order from the health care provider to apply a wrist restraint. Place the steps for applying a wrist restraint in the correct order.
   1. Be sure that patient is comfortable with arm in anatomic alignment.
   2. Wrap wrist with soft part of restraint toward skin and secure snugly.
   3. Identify patient using two identifiers.
   4. Introduce self and ask patient about his feelings of being restrained.
   5. Assess condition of skin where restraint will be placed.
7. The family of a patient who is confused and ambulatory insists that all four side rails be up when the patient is alone. What is the best action to take in this situation? (Select all that apply.)
   1. Contact the nursing supervisor.
   2. Restrict the family's visiting privileges.
   3. Ask the family to stay with the patient if possible.
   4. Inform the family of the risks associated with side-rail use.
   5. Thank the family for being conscientious and put the four rails up.
   6. Discuss alternatives that are appropriate for this patient with the family.
8. You are conducting an education class at a local senior center on safe-driving tips for seniors. Which of the following should you include? (Select all that apply.)
   1. Drive shorter distances
   2. Drive only during daylight hours
   3. Use the side and rearview mirrors carefully
   4. Keep a window rolled down while driving if has trouble hearing
   5. Look behind toward the blind spot
   6. Stop driving at age 75
9. The nursing assessment of an 80-year-old patient who demonstrates some confusion but no anxiety reveals that the patient is a fall risk because she continues to get out of bed without help despite frequent reminders. The initial nursing intervention to prevent falls for this patient is to:
   1. Place a bed alarm device on the bed.
   2. Place the patient in a belt restraint.
   3. Provide one-on-one observation of the patient.
   4. Apply wrist restraints.
10. A nurse is evaluating a patient who is in soft wrist restraints. Which of the following activities does the nurse perform? (Select all that apply.)
    1. Check the patient's peripheral pulse in the restrained extremity
    2. Evaluate the patient's need for toileting
    3. Offer the patient fluids if appropriate
    4. Release both limbs at the same time to perform range of motion (ROM)
    5. Inspect the skin under each restraint
11. You are admitting Mr. Jones, a 64-year-old patient who had a right hemisphere stroke and a recent fall. His wife stated that he has a history of high blood pressure, which is controlled by an antihypertensive and a diuretic. Currently he exhibits left-sided neglect and problems with spatial and perceptual abilities and is impulsive. He has moderate left-sided weakness that requires the assistance of two and the use of a gait belt to transfer to a chair. He currently has an intravenous (IV) line and a urinary catheter in place. Which factors increase his fall risk at this time? (Select all that apply.)
    1. Smokes a pack a day
    2. Used a cane to walk at home
    3. Takes antihypertensive and diuretics
    4. History of recent fall
    5. Neglect, spatial and perceptual abilities, impulsive
    6. Requires assistance with activity, unsteady gait
    7. IV line, urinary catheter
12. At 12 noon the emergency department nurse hears that an explosion has occurred in a local manufacturing plant. Which action does the nurse take first?

1. Prepare for an influx of patients
2. Contact the American Red Cross
3. Determine how to resume normal operations
4. Evacuate patients per the disaster plan

13. The nurse is caring for a patient who is having a seizure. Which of the following measures will protect the patient and the nurse from injury? (Select all that apply.)
1. If patient is standing, attempt to get him or her back in bed.
2. With patient on floor, clear surrounding area of furniture or equipment.
3. If possible, keep patient lying supine.
4. Do not restrain patient; hold limbs loosely if they are flailing.
5. Never force apart a patient's clenched teeth.

14. What is your role as a nurse during a fire? (Select all that apply.)
1. Help to evacuate patients
2. Shut off medical gases
3. Use a fire extinguisher
4. Single carry patients out
5. Direct ambulatory patients

15. A nurse is educating parents to look for clues in teenagers for possible substance abuse. Which environmental and psychosocial clues should the nurse include? (Select all that apply.)
1. Blood spots on clothing
2. Long-sleeved shirts in warm weather
3. Changes in relationships
4. Wearing dark glasses indoors
5. Increased computer use

Answers: 1. 3, 1, 2, 5, 6, 4; **2.** 1, 3, 4; **3.** 4; **4.** 4; **5.** 1, 2, 3, 4, 5; **6.** 3, 4, 1, 5, 2; **7.** 3, 4, 6; **8.** 1, 2, 3, 4, 5; **9.** 1; **10.** 1, 2, 3, 5; **11.** 3, 4, 5, 6, 7; **12.** 1; **13.** 2, 4, 5; **14.** 1, 2, 3, 5; **15.** 1, 2, 3, 4.

Rationales for Review Questions can be found on the Evolve website.

REFERENCES

Agency for Healthcare Research and Quality (AHRQ): *20 tips to help prevent medical errors: a patient fact sheet*, 2014, http://www.ahrq.gov/patients-consumers/care-planning/errors/20tips/index.html. Accessed September 2015.

Agency for Toxic Substances and Disease Registry: *Lead: toxFAQs*, 2014, http://www.atsdr.cdc.gov/toxfaqs/tf.asp?id=93&tid=22. Accessed September 2015.

American Academy of Pediatrics (AAP): *Car safety seats: information for families for 2011, healthy children*, 2011a, http://www.aap.org/en-us/about-the-aap/aap-press-room/Pages/AAP-Updates-Recommendation-on-Car-Seats.aspx. Accessed September 2015.

American Academy of Pediatrics (AAP): *AAP expands guidelines for infant sleep safety and SIDS risk reduction*, 2011b, http://www.aap.org/en-us/about-the-aap/aap-press-room/Pages/AAP-Expands-Guidelines-for-Infant-Sleep-Safety-and-SIDS-Risk-Reduction.aspx. Accessed September, 2015.

American Geriatric Society: *Clinical practice guideline fall prevention in older persons*, 2015, http://www.americangeriatrics.org/health_care_professionals/clinical_practice/clinical_guidelines_recommendations/prevention_of_falls_summary_of_recommendations. Accessed September 2015.

American Hospital Association: *Quality advisory: implementing standardized colors for patient alert wristbands*, 2008, http://www.aha.org/advocacy-issues/tools-resources/advisory/2008/080904-quality-adv.pdf. Accessed September 2015.

Barry E, et al: Is the Timed Up and Go test a useful predictor of risk of falls in community dwelling older adults: a systematic review and meta-analysis, *BMC Geriatr* 14:14, 2014.

California Advocates for Nursing Home Reform (CANHR): *Restraint-free care*, 2015, http://www.canhr.org/factsheets/nh_fs/html/fs_RestraintFreeCare.htm. Accessed September 2015.

Capezuti E, et al: Least restrictive or least understood? Waist restraints, provider practices, and risk of harm, *J Aging Soc Policy* 20(3):305, 2008.

Centers for Disease Control and Prevention (CDC): *Bloodborne infectious diseases: HIV/AIDS, hepatitis B, hepatitis C: safe community needle disposal*, 2011, http://www.cdc.gov/niosh/topics/bbp/disposal.html. Accessed September 2015.

Centers for Disease Control and Prevention (CDC): *Percentage distribution of injuries by place of occurrence, among males and females—national health interview survey, United States, 2004–2007*, (Morbidity and Mortality Weekly Report) Atlanta, Ga, 2010, Office of Surveillance, Epidemiology and Laboratory Services, CDC, US Department of Health and Human Services.

Centers for Disease Control and Prevention (CDC): *Food safety*, 2014a, http://www.cdc.gov/foodsafety/. Accessed September 2015.

Centers for Disease Control and Prevention (CDC): *Injury prevention and control: motor vehicle safety*, 2014b, http://www.cdc.gov/Motorvehiclesafety/teen_drivers/teendrivers_factsheet.html. Accessed September 2015.

Centers for Disease Control and Prevention (CDC): *Poisoning prevention*, 2014c, http://www.cdc.gov/HealthyHomes/ByTopic/Poisoning.html. Accessed September 2015.

Centers for Disease Control and Prevention (CDC): *Bioterrorism*, 2014d, http://www.bt.cdc.gov/bioterrorism/factsheets.asp. Accessed September 2015.

Centers for Disease Control and Prevention (CDC): *Important facts about falls*, 2015a, http://www.cdc.gov/HomeandRecreationalSafety/Falls/adultfalls.html. Accessed September 2015.

Centers for Disease Control and Prevention (CDC): *STEADI older adult fall prevention tests: The Timed Get Up and Go Test (TUG)*, 2015 Available at http://www.cdc.gov/homeandrecreationalsafety/pdf/steadi-2015.04/TUG_Test-a.pdf. Accessed October 25, 2015.

Centers for Medicare and Medicaid Services (CMS): *Revisions to Medicare conditions of participation, 482.13*, Bethesda, MD, 2007, US Department of Health and Human Services.

Centers for Medicare and Medicaid Services (CMS): *Hospital-acquired conditions*, 2015, http://www.cms.gov/HospitalAcqCond/06_Hospital-Acquired_Conditions.asp. Accessed September 2015.

Coalition for Safe Community Needle Disposal: *Safe needle disposal*, 2015, http://www.safeneedledisposal.org/. Accessed September 2015.

Department of Health and Human Services (DHHS), Office of Inspector General: *Adverse events in hospitals: overview of key issues*, OEI-06-07-00470, Washington DC, 2008, DHHS.

Department of Health and Human Services (DHHS): *Interpretive guidelines for hospitals*, 482.13(e) *Standard: restraint or seclusion*, 2008, http://cms.gov/Regulations-and-Guidance/Guidance/Transmittals/downloads/R37SOMA.pdf. Accessed September 2015.

Edelman CL, Mandle CL: *Health promotion throughout the life span*, ed 8, St Louis, 2013, Mosby.

Energy.gov: *Portable heaters*, 2014, http://energy.gov/energysaver/articles/portable-heaters. Accessed March 28, 2015.

Epilepsy Foundation: *Seizure first aid*, 2014, http://www.epilepsy.com/learn/treating-seizures-and-epilepsy/seizure-first-aid. Accessed September 2015.

Herdman TH, Kamitsuru S, editors: *NANDA International nursing diagnoses: definitions and classification, 2015–2017*, ed 10, Oxford, 2014, Wiley-Blackwell.

Hockenberry MJ, Wilson D: *Wong's essentials of pediatric nursing*, ed 8, St Louis, 2015, Mosby.

Institute of Medicine (IOM) Committee on Quality of Health Care in America: *To err is human: building a safer health system*, Washington, DC, 2000, National Academies Press.

Institute of Medicine (IOM): *Envisioning the National Health Care Quality Report*, Washington, D.C., 2001, National Academies Press.

Insurance Institute for Highway Safety: *Highway safety topics*, 2015, http://www.iihs.org/research/fatality_facts_2008/olderpeople.html. Accessed September 2015.

Kennedy A, et al: Confidence about vaccines in the United States: understanding parents' perceptions, *Health Aff* 30(6):1151, 2011.

Mathias S, et al: Balance in elderly patients: the "Get-up and Go" test, *Arch Phys Med Rehabil* 67(6):387, 1986.

Mayo Clinic: *Carbon monoxide poisoning*, 2014, http://www.mayoclinic.org/diseases-conditions/carbon-monoxide/basics/definition/con-20025444. Accessed September 2015.

National Alliance for Caregiving: *Research*, 2015, http://www.caregiving.org/research/. Accessed September 2015.

National Center for Injury Prevention and Control: *1999–2007, United States unintentional injuries ages 65–85+, all races, both sexes*, 2010b, http://webappa.cdc.gov/sasweb/ncipc/leadcaus10.html. Accessed September 2014.

National Center for Injury Prevention and Control: *10 leading causes of death, United States 1999–2007*, 2010a, http://webappa.cdc.gov/sasweb/ncipc/leadcaus10.html. Accessed September 2015.

National Fire Protection Association (NFPA): *Fires and burns involving home medical oxygen*, Quincy, MA, 2008, NFPA. http://www.nfpa.org/~/media/Files/Research/NFPA%20reports/Major%20Causes/osoxygen.pdf. Accessed September 2015.

National Fire Protection Association (NFPA): *Carbon monoxide safety tips*, 2014a, http://www.nfpa.org/safety-information/for-consumers/fire-and-safety-equipment/carbon-monoxide/carbon-monoxide-safety-tips. Accessed September 2015.

National Fire Protection Association (NFPA): *Structure fires*, 2014b, http://www.nfpa.org/research/reports-and-statistics/fires-in-the-us/overall-fire-problem/structure-fires. Accessed September 2015.

National Quality Forum (NQF): *Mission and vision*, Washington DC, 2011a, http://www.qualityforum.org/About_NQF/Mission_and_Vision.aspx. Accessed September 2015.

National Quality Forum (NQF): *National voluntary consensus standards for public reporting of patient safety events*, Washington DC, 2011b. http://www.qualityforum.org/Publications/2011/02/National_Voluntary_Consensus_Standards_for_Public_Reporting_of_Patient_Safety_Event_Information.aspx. Accessed September 2015.

National Quality Forum (NQF): *National Quality Forum safe practices for better healthcare—2010 update*, Washington DC, 2011c, https://www.qualityforum.org/Publications/2010/04/Safe_Practices_for_Better_Healthcare_%E2%80%93_2010_Update.aspx. Accessed September 2015.

Occupational Safety and Health Administration (OSHA): *Hazard communication*, 2014, https://www.osha.gov/dsg/hazcom/. Accessed September 2015.

Podsiadlo D, Richardson S: The timed "Up & Go": a test of basic functional mobility for frail elderly persons, *J Am Geriatr Soc* 39(2):142, 1991.

Quality and Safety Education for Nurses (QSEN): *University of North Carolina at Chapel Hill*, Chapel Hill, NC, 2014, http://www.qsen.org/. Accessed September 2015.

Taylor-Adams S, et al: Safety skills for clinicians: an essential component of patient safety, *J Patient Safety* 4(3):141, 2009.

The Joint Commission (TJC): *Provision of care, treatment and services: restraint /seclusion for hospitals that use The Joint Commission for deemed status purposes*, 2009, http://www.jointcommission.org/mobile/standards_information/jcfaqdetails.aspx?StandardsFAQId=260&StandardsFAQChapterId=78. Accessed September 2015.

The Joint Commission (TJC): *Comprehensive accreditation manual for hospitals*, Chicago, 2015, TJC.

The Joint Commission (TJC): *2016 National Patient Safety Goals*, Oakbrook Terrace, IL, 2016, The Commission. http://www.jointcommission.org/standards_information/npsgs.aspx. Accessed November 2015.

The Joint Commission (TJC): *Joint Commission Resources Quality & Safety Network (JCRQSN) resource guide; Be prepared: Maximizing behavioral healthcare-related tracer activities*, Oakbrook Terrace, IL, 2017, The Commission.

Touhy T, Jett K: *Ebersole and Hess' Gerontological nursing & health care*, ed 4, St Louis, 2014, Elsevier.

Tzeng HM: Understanding the prevalence of inpatient falls associated with toileting in adult acute care settings, *J Nurs Care Qual* 25(1):22, 2010.

University of Iowa: *Get-up and Go Test*, n.d., https://www.healthcare.uiowa.edu/igec/tools/mobility/getUpAndGo.pdf. Accessed October 14, 2015.

US Food and Drug Administration (FDA): *Bed rail safety*, 2014, http://www.fda.gov/MedicalDevices/ProductsandMedicalProcedures/HomeHealthandConsumer/ConsumerProducts/BedRailSafety/default.htm. Accessed September 2015.

US Food and Drug Administration (FDA): *Medical device reporting*, 2015, http://www.fda.gov/MedicalDevices/Safety/ReportaProblem/default.htm. Accessed September 2015.

RESEARCH REFERENCES

Boyd R, Stevens JA: Falls and fear of falling: burden, beliefs and behaviors, *Age Ageing* 38(4):423, 2009.

Bushardt RL, et al: Polypharmacy: misleading but manageable, *Clin Interv Aging* 3(2):383, 2008.

Castle NG: The health consequences of using physical restraints in nursing homes, *Med Care* 47(11):1164, 2009.

Chang CM, et al: Medical conditions and medications as risk factors of falls in inpatient older people: a case-controlled study, *Int J Geriatr Psychiatry* 26(6):602, 2011.

Chase CA, et al: Systematic review of the effect of home modification and fall prevention programs on falls and the performance of community-dwelling older adults, *Am J Occup Ther* 66(3):284, 2012.

Deandrea S, et al: Risk factors for falls in community dwelling older people: a systematic review and meta-analysis, *Epidemiology* 21(5):658, 2010.

de Kam D, et al: Exercise interventions to reduce fall-related fractures and their risk factors in individuals with low bone density: a systematic review of randomized controlled trials, *Osteoporos Int* 20(12):2111, 2009.

Ford BM: Hourly rounding: a strategy to improve patient satisfaction scores, *Medsurg Nurs* 19(3):188, 2010.

Geiger-Brown J, et al: Sleep, sleepiness, fatigue, and performance of 12-hour shift nurses, *Chronobiol Int* 29(2):211, 2012.

Gillespie LD, et al: Interventions for preventing falls in older people living in the community, *Cochrane Database Syst Rev* (9):CD007146, 2012.

Gribbin J, et al: Risk of falls associated with antihypertensive medication: population-based case-control study, *Age Ageing* 39(5):592, 2010.

Grundstrom AC, et al: Risk factors for falls and fall-related in adults 85 years of age and older, *Arch Gerontol Geriatr* 54(3):421, 2012.

Khazzani H, et al: The relationship between physical performance measures, bone mineral density, falls, and the risk of peripheral fracture: a cross sectional analysis, *BMC Public Health* 9:297, 2009.

Kojima T, et al: Association of polypharmacy with fall risk among geriatric outpatients, *Geriatr Gerontol Int* 11(4):438, 2011.

Mitchell MD, et al: Hourly rounding to improve nursing responsiveness: a systematic review, *J Nurs Adm* 44(9):462, 2014.

Olsen CF, Bergland A: The effect of exercise and education on fear of falling in elderly women with osteoporosis and a history of vertebral fracture: results of a randomized controlled trial, *Osteoporos Int* 25(8):2017, 2014.

Opel DJ, et al: The relationship between parent attitudes about childhood vaccines survey scores and future child immunization status: a validation study, *JAMA Pediatr* 167(11):1065, 2013.

Scheffer AC, et al: Fear of falling: measurement strategy, prevalence, risk factors and consequences among older persons, *Age Ageing* 37(1):19, 2008.

Schubert TE: Evidence-based exercise prescription for balance and falls prevention: a current review of the literature, *J Geriatr Phys Ther* 34(3):100, 2011.

Sherrington C, et al: Exercise to prevent falls in older adults: an updated meta-analysis and best practice recommendations, *N S W Public Health Bull* 22(3-4):78, 2011.

Spoelstra SL, et al: Fall prevention in hospitals: an integrative review, *Clin Nurs Res* published online 2011. http://cnr.sagepub.com/content/21/1/92. Accessed October 14, 2015.

Viera ER, et al: Risk factors for geriatric patients falls in rehabilitation hospital settings: a systematic review, *Clin Rehabil* 25(9):788, 2011.

28

Immobility

OBJECTIVES

- Discuss physiological and pathological influences on mobility.
- Identify changes in physiological and psychosocial function associated with immobility.
- Assess for correct and impaired body alignment and mobility.
- Formulate appropriate nursing diagnoses for patients with impaired mobility.
- Develop individualized nursing care plans for patients with impaired mobility.
- Compare and contrast active and passive range-of-motion exercises.
- Describe interventions for improving or maintaining patients' mobility.
- Evaluate patient outcomes as a result of a nursing plan for improving or maintaining mobility.

KEY TERMS

MEDIA RESOURCES

http://evolve.elsevier.com/Potter/fundamentals/

- Review Questions
- Video Clips
- Concept Map Creator
- Case Study with Questions
- Audio Glossary
- Content Updates

People are mobile for many purposes (e.g., expression of emotions with nonverbal gestures and meeting basic needs). Mobility is also essential for self-defense, activities of daily living (ADLs), and recreational activities. Many functions of the body depend on mobility. Intact musculoskeletal and nervous systems are necessary for optimal physical mobility and functioning. Clinical nursing practices related to mobility and immobility require the incorporation of scientific and nursing knowledge and skills to provide competent care.

SCIENTIFIC KNOWLEDGE BASE

Nature of Movement

Movement is a complex process that requires coordination between the musculoskeletal and nervous systems. As a nurse you will consider how a patient's physical and psychological condition affect body movement. **Body mechanics** is a term that describes the coordinated efforts of the musculoskeletal and nervous systems. Knowing how patients initiate movement and understanding your own movements requires a basic understanding of the physics surrounding body mechanics. The body mechanics applied in the lifting techniques historically used in nursing practice often cause debilitating injuries to nurses and other health care staff (Burnfield et al., 2013; Griffis, 2012). Today nurses use evidence-based information about body alignment, balance, gravity, and friction when implementing nursing interventions such as positioning patients, determining the risk of patient falls, and selecting the safest way to move or transfer patients (Healey and Darowski, 2012).

Alignment and Balance. The terms *body alignment* and **posture** are similar and refer to the positioning of the joints, tendons, ligaments, and muscles while standing, sitting, and lying. **Body alignment** means that an individual's center of gravity is stable. Correct body alignment reduces strain on musculoskeletal structures, aids in maintaining adequate muscle tone, promotes comfort, and contributes to balance and conservation of energy. Without balance control the center of gravity is displaced.

Individuals require balance for maintaining a static position (e.g., sitting) and moving (e.g., walking). Disease, injury, pain, physical development (e.g., age), and life changes (e.g., pregnancy) compromise the ability to remain balanced. Medications that cause dizziness and prolonged immobility affect balance. Impaired balance is a major threat to mobility and physical safety and contributes to a fear of falling and self-imposed activity restrictions (McMahon and Fleury, 2012) (see Chapter 39).

Gravity and Friction. Weight is the force exerted on a body by gravity. The force of weight is always directed downward, which is why an unbalanced object falls. Unsteady patients fall if their center of gravity becomes unbalanced because of the gravitational pull on their weight.

To lift safely the lifter has to overcome the weight of the object and know its center of gravity. In symmetrical inanimate objects the center of gravity is at the exact center of the object. However, people are not geometrically perfect; their centers of gravity are usually at 55% to 57% of standing height and are in the midline, which is why only using principles of body mechanics in lifting patients often leads to injury of a nurse or other health care professional (see Chapter 39).

Friction is a force that occurs in a direction to oppose movement. The greater the surface area of the object that is moved, the greater is the friction. A larger object produces greater resistance to movement. In addition, the force exerted against the skin while the skin remains stationary and the bony structures move is called **shear**. Unfortunately a common example is when the head of a hospital bed is elevated beyond 60 degrees and gravity pulls a patient so that the bony skeleton moves toward the foot of the bed while the skin remains against the sheets. The blood vessels in the underlying tissue are stretched and damaged, resulting in impeded blood flow to the deep tissues. Ultimately pressure ulcers often develop within the undermined tissue; the surface tissue appears less affected (see Chapter 48). To decrease surface area and reduce friction when patients are unable to assist with moving up in bed, nurses use an ergonomic assistive device such as a full-body sling. This sling mechanically lifts a patient off the surface of a bed, thereby preventing friction, tearing, or shearing his or her delicate skin, and protects the nurse and other staff from injury (Burnfield et al., 2013).

Skeletal System. The skeletal system provides attachments for muscles and ligaments and the **leverage** necessary for mobility. Thus the skeleton is the supporting framework of the body and is made up of four types of bones: long, short, flat, and irregular. Bones are important for mobilization because they are firm, rigid, and elastic. The aging process changes the components of bone, which impacts mobility.

Firmness results from inorganic salts such as calcium and phosphate that are in the bone matrix. It is related to the rigidity of the bone, which is necessary to keep long bones straight, and enables bones to withstand weight bearing. Elasticity and skeletal flexibility change with age. For example, a newborn has a large amount of cartilage and is highly flexible but is unable to support weight. A toddler's bones are more pliable than those of an older person and are better able to withstand falls. Older adults, especially women, are more susceptible to bone loss (resorption) and osteoporosis, which increase the risk of fractures.

The skeletal system has several functions. It protects vital organs (e.g., the skull around the brain and the ribs around the heart and lungs) and aids in calcium regulation. Bones store calcium and release it into the circulation as needed. Patients who have decreased calcium regulation and metabolism and who are immobile are at risk for developing osteoporosis and **pathological fractures** (fractures caused by weakened bone tissue) (see Chapter 39).

In addition, the internal structure of long bones contains bone marrow, participates in red blood cell (RBC) production, and acts as a reservoir for blood. Patients with altered bone marrow function or diminished RBC production tire easily because of reduced hemoglobin and oxygen-carrying ability. This fatigue decreases their mobility and increases the risk for falling.

Joints. Joints are the connections between bones. Each joint is classified according to its structure and degree of mobility. There are three classifications of joints: cartilaginous, fibrous, and synovial (McCance and Huether, 2014) (see Chapter 39).

Ligaments, Tendons, and Cartilage. Ligaments are white, shiny, flexible bands of fibrous tissue that bind joints together, connect bones and cartilages, and aid joint flexibility and support. Tendons are white, glistening, fibrous bands of tissue that connect muscle to bone and are strong, flexible, and inelastic. Cartilage is nonvascular (without blood vessels) supporting connective tissue located chiefly in the joints and thorax, trachea, larynx, nose, and ear. The characteristics of the cartilage change with the aging process (see Chapter 39).

Skeletal Muscle. Movement of bones and joints involves active processes that are carefully integrated to achieve coordination. Skeletal muscles, because of their ability to contract and relax, are the working elements of movement. Anatomical structure and attachment to the skeleton enhance contractile elements of the skeletal muscle (see Chapter 39).

Nervous System. The nervous system regulates movement and posture. The precentral gyrus, or motor strip, is the major voluntary motor area and is in the cerebral cortex. A majority of motor fibers descend from the motor strip and cross at the level of the medulla. Movement is impaired by disorders that alter neurotransmitter production, transfer of impulses from the nerve to the muscle, or activation of muscle activity (see Chapter 39).

Pathological Influences on Mobility

Many pathological conditions affect mobility. Although a complete description of each is beyond the scope of this chapter, an overview of four pathological influences is presented.

Postural Abnormalities. Congenital or acquired postural abnormalities affect the efficiency of the musculoskeletal system and body alignment, balance, and appearance. During assessment observe body alignment and ROM (see Chapter 39). Postural abnormalities can cause pain, impair alignment or mobility, or both. Knowledge about the characteristics, causes, and treatment of common postural abnormalities is necessary for lifting, transfer, and positioning (Table 28-1). Some postural abnormalities limit ROM. Nurses intervene to maintain maximum ROM in unaffected joints and then often collaborate with physical therapists to design interventions to strengthen affected muscles and joints, improve the patient's posture, and adequately use affected and unaffected muscle groups. Referral to and/or collaboration with a physical therapist enhances the nurse's interventions for a patient with a postural abnormality.

TABLE 28-1 Postural Abnormalities

Abnormality	Description	Cause	Possible Treatments* (McCance and Huether, 2014)
Torticollis	Inclining head to affected side, in which sternocleidomastoid muscle is contracted	Congenital or acquired condition	Surgery, heat, support, or immobilization, depending on cause and severity; gentle ROM
Lordosis	Exaggeration of anterior convex curve of lumbar spine	Congenital condition; temporary condition (e.g., pregnancy)	Spine-stretching exercises (based on cause)
Kyphosis	Increased convexity in curvature of thoracic spine	Congenital condition; rickets, osteoporosis; tuberculosis of spine	Spine-stretching exercises, sleeping without pillows, using bed board, bracing, surgical spinal fusion (based on cause and severity)
Scoliosis	Lateral S- or C-shaped spinal column with vertebral rotation, unequal heights of hips and shoulders	Sometimes a consequence of numerous congenital, connective tissue, and neuromuscular disorders	Approximately half of children with scoliosis require surgery Nonsurgical treatment is with braces and exercises
Congenital hip dysplasia	Hip instability with limited abduction of hips and occasionally adduction contractures (head of femur does not articulate with acetabulum because of abnormal shallowness of acetabulum)	Congenital condition (more common with breech deliveries)	Maintenance of continuous abduction of thigh so head of femur presses into center of acetabulum; abduction splints, casting, surgery
Knock-knee (genu valgum)	Legs curved inward so knees come together as person walks	Congenital condition; rickets	Knee braces; surgery if not corrected by growth
Bowlegs (genu varum)	One or both legs bent outward at knee, which is normal until 2 to 3 years of age	Congenital condition; rickets	Slowing rate of curving if not corrected by growth; with rickets, increase of vitamin D, calcium, and phosphorus intake to normal ranges
Clubfoot	*95%:* Medial deviation and plantar flexion of foot (equinovarus) *5%:* Lateral deviation and dorsiflexion (calcaneovalgus)	Congenital condition	Casts, splints such as Denis Browne splint, and surgery (based on degree and rigidity of deformity)
Footdrop	Inability to dorsiflex and invert foot because of peroneal nerve damage	Congenital condition; trauma; improper position of immobilized patient	None (cannot be corrected); prevention through physical therapy; bracing with ankle-foot orthotic (AFO)
Pigeon toes	Internal rotation of forefoot or entire foot; common in infants	Congenital condition; habit	Growth; wearing reversed shoes

ROM, Range of motion.
*Severity of condition and cause dictate treatment, which is individualized to the patient's needs.

Muscle Abnormalities. Injury and disease lead to numerous alterations in musculoskeletal function. For example, the muscular dystrophies are a group of familial disorders that cause degeneration of skeletal muscle fibers. They are the most prevalent of the muscle diseases in childhood. Patients with muscular dystrophy experience progressive, symmetrical weakness and wasting of skeletal muscle groups, with increasing disability and deformity (McCance and Huether, 2014).

Damage to the Central Nervous System. Damage to any component of the central nervous system that regulates voluntary movement results in impaired body alignment, balance, and mobility. Trauma from a head injury, ischemia from a stroke (cerebrovascular accident [CVA]), or bacterial infection such as meningitis can damage the cerebellum or the motor strip in the cerebral cortex. Damage to the cerebellum causes problems with balance, and motor impairment is directly related to the amount of destruction of the motor strip. For example, a person with a right-sided cerebral hemorrhage with necrosis has destruction of the right motor strip that results in left-sided hemiplegia. Trauma to the spinal cord also impairs mobility. For example, a complete transection of the spinal cord results in a bilateral loss of voluntary motor control below the level of the trauma because motor fibers are cut.

Direct Trauma to the Musculoskeletal System. Direct trauma to the musculoskeletal system results in bruises, contusions, sprains, and fractures. A fracture is a disruption of bone tissue continuity. Fractures most commonly result from direct external trauma, but they also occur as a consequence of some deformity of the bone (e.g., pathological fractures of osteoporosis, Paget's disease, or osteogenesis imperfecta). Young children are usually able to form new bone more easily than adults and, as a result, have few complications after a fracture. Treatment often includes positioning the fractured bone in proper alignment and immobilizing it to promote healing and restore function. Even this temporary immobilization results in some muscle atrophy, loss of muscle tone, and joint stiffness.

NURSING KNOWLEDGE BASE

Fully understanding movement and mobility requires more than an overview of movement and the physiology and regulation of movement by the musculoskeletal and nervous systems. You need to know how to apply these scientific principles in the clinical setting to determine the safest way to move patients and to understand the effect of immobility on the physiological, psychosocial, and developmental aspects of patient care.

Factors Influencing Mobility-Immobility

To determine how to move patients safely, you will assess their ability to move. **Mobility** refers to a person's ability to move about freely, and **immobility** refers to the inability to do so. Think of mobility as a continuum, with mobility on one end, immobility on the other, and varying degrees of partial immobility between the end points. Some patients move back and forth between mobility and immobility, but for others immobility is absolute and continues indefinitely. The terms *bed rest* and *impaired physical mobility* are used frequently when discussing patients on the mobility-immobility continuum.

Bed rest is an intervention that restricts patients to bed for therapeutic reasons. Although it is much less commonly used, health care providers most often prescribe this intervention. Bed rest has many different interpretations among health care professionals. The duration of bed rest depends on the illness or injury and a patient's prior state of health.

The effects of muscular deconditioning associated with lack of physical activity are often apparent in a matter of days. This cluster of symptoms is often referred to as the "hazards of immobility." The individual of average weight and height without a chronic illness on bed rest loses muscle strength from baseline levels at a rate of 3% a day. Immobility also is associated with cardiovascular, skeletal, and other organ changes. The term *disuse atrophy* describes the tendency of cells and tissue to reduce in size and function in response to prolonged inactivity resulting from bed rest, trauma, casting of a body part, or local nerve damage (McCance and Huether, 2014).

Periods of immobility due to disability or injury or prolonged bed rest during hospitalization cause major physiological, psychological, and social effects. These effects are gradual or immediate and vary from patient to patient. The greater the extent and the longer the duration of immobility, the more pronounced the consequences. The patient with complete mobility restrictions is continually at risk for the hazards of immobility. When possible, it is imperative that patients, especially older adults, have limited bed rest and that their activity is more than bed to chair. Loss of walking independence increases hospital stays, need for rehabilitation services, or nursing home placement. In addition, the deconditioning related to reduced walking increases the risk for patient falls (AAN, 2015; Pashikanti and Von Ah, 2012).

Systemic Effects.

All body systems work more efficiently with some form of movement. Exercise has positive outcomes for all major systems of the body. When there is an alteration in mobility, each body system is at risk for impairment. The severity of the impairment depends on a patient's overall health, degree and length of immobility, and age. For example, older adults with chronic illnesses develop pronounced effects of immobility more quickly than do younger patients with the same immobility problem.

Metabolic Changes. Changes in mobility alter endocrine metabolism, calcium resorption, and functioning of the gastrointestinal system. The endocrine system, composed of hormone-secreting glands, maintains and regulates vital functions such as (1) response to stress and injury; (2) growth and development; (3) reproduction; (4) maintenance of the internal environment; and (5) energy production, use, and storage.

When injury or stress occurs, the endocrine system triggers a series of responses aimed at maintaining blood pressure and preserving life. It is important in maintaining homeostasis. Tissues and cells live in an internal environment that the endocrine system helps regulate through maintenance of sodium, potassium, water, and acid-base balance. It also regulates energy metabolism. Thyroid hormone increases the basal metabolic rate (BMR), and energy becomes available to cells through the integrated action of gastrointestinal and pancreatic hormones (McCance and Huether, 2014).

Immobility disrupts normal metabolic functioning, decreasing the metabolic rate; altering the metabolism of carbohydrates, fats, and proteins; causing fluid, electrolyte, and calcium imbalances; and causing gastrointestinal disturbances such as decreased appetite and slowing of peristalsis. However, in the presence of an infectious process, immobilized patients often have an increased BMR as a result of fever or wound healing because these increase cellular oxygen requirements (McCance and Huether, 2014).

A deficiency in calories and protein is characteristic of patients with a decreased appetite secondary to immobility. The body is constantly synthesizing proteins and breaking them down into amino acids to form other proteins (see Chapter 45). When the patient is immobile, his or her body often excretes more nitrogen (the end product of amino acid breakdown) than it ingests in proteins, resulting in **negative nitrogen balance**. Weight loss, decreased muscle mass, and weakness result from tissue catabolism (tissue breakdown) (McCance and Huether, 2014).

Another metabolic change associated with immobility is calcium resorption (loss) from bones. Immobility causes the release of calcium into the circulation. Normally the kidneys excrete the excess calcium. However, if they are unable to respond appropriately, hypercalcemia results. Pathological fractures occur if calcium resorption continues as a patient remains on bed rest or continues to be immobile (McCance and Huether, 2014).

Impairments of gastrointestinal functioning caused by decreased mobility vary. Difficulty in passing stools (constipation) is a common symptom, although pseudodiarrhea often results from a fecal impaction (accumulation of hardened feces). Be aware that this finding is not normal diarrhea, but rather liquid stool passing around the area of impaction (see Chapter 47). Left untreated, fecal impaction results in a mechanical bowel obstruction that partially or completely occludes the intestinal lumen, blocking normal propulsion of liquid and gas. The resulting fluid in the intestine produces distention and increases intraluminal pressure. Over time intestinal function becomes depressed, dehydration occurs, absorption ceases, and fluid and electrolyte disturbances worsen.

Respiratory Changes. Regular aerobic exercise enhances respiratory functioning. In contrast, lack of movement and exercise places patients at risk for respiratory complications. Patients who are immobile are at high risk for developing pulmonary complications such as **atelectasis** (collapse of alveoli) and **hypostatic pneumonia** (inflammation of the lung from stasis or pooling of secretions). Both decreased oxygenation and prolonged recovery add to patients' discomfort (Lewis et al., 2013). In atelectasis secretions block a bronchiole or a bronchus; and the distal lung tissue (alveoli) collapses as the existing air is absorbed, producing hypoventilation. The site of the blockage affects the severity of atelectasis. Sometimes an entire lung lobe or a whole lung collapses. At some point in the development of these complications, there is a proportional decline in the patient's ability to cough productively. Ultimately the distribution of mucus in the bronchi increases, particularly when the patient is in the supine, prone, or lateral position. Mucus accumulates in the dependent regions of the airways (Figure 28-1). Hypostatic pneumonia frequently results because mucus is an excellent place for bacteria to grow.

Cardiovascular Changes. Immobilization also affects the cardiovascular system, frequently resulting in orthostatic hypotension,

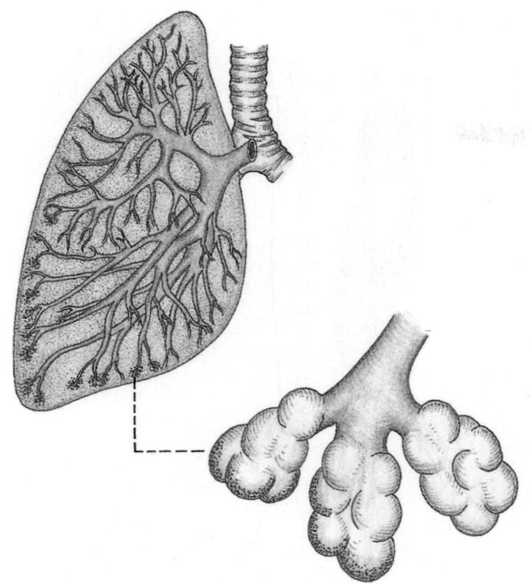

FIGURE 28-1 Pooling of secretions in dependent regions of lungs in supine position.

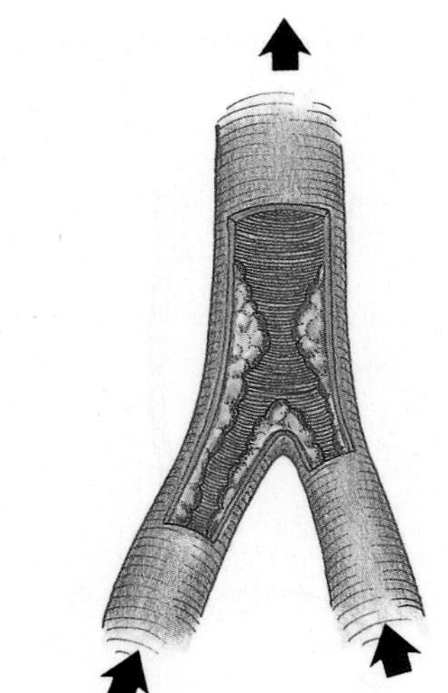

FIGURE 28-2 Thrombus formation in a vessel.

increased cardiac workload, and thrombus formation. **Orthostatic hypotension** is a drop of blood pressure greater than 20 mm Hg in systolic pressure or 10 mm Hg in diastolic pressure and symptoms of dizziness, light-headedness, nausea, tachycardia, pallor, or fainting when the patient changes from the supine to standing position (Ball et al., 2015). In the immobilized patient decreased circulating fluid volume, pooling of blood in the lower extremities, and decreased autonomic response occur. These are especially evident in the older adult.

As the workload of the heart increases, so does its oxygen consumption. Therefore the heart works harder and less efficiently during periods of prolonged rest. As immobilization increases, cardiac output falls, further decreasing cardiac efficiency and increasing workload.

Patients who are immobile are also at risk for thrombus formation. A **thrombus** is an accumulation of platelets, fibrin, clotting factors, and the cellular elements of the blood attached to the interior wall of a vein or artery, which sometimes occludes the lumen of the vessel (Figure 28-2). Three factors contribute to venous thrombus formation: (1) damage to the vessel wall (e.g., injury during surgical procedures), (2) alterations of blood flow (e.g., slow blood flow in calf veins associated with bed rest), and (3) alterations in blood constituents (e.g., a change in clotting factors or increased platelet activity). These three factors are often referred to as *Virchow's triad* (McCance and Huether, 2014). As a nurse you will practice in numerous situations when deep vein thrombosis (DVT) must be prevented, especially during perioperative care (see Chapter 50).

Musculoskeletal Changes. Immobility affects the musculoskeletal system by causing permanent or temporary impairment or permanent disability. Restricted mobility sometimes results in loss of endurance, strength, and muscle mass and decreased stability and balance. Other effects of restricted mobility affecting the skeletal system are impaired calcium metabolism and joint mobility.

Muscle Effects. Because of protein breakdown, a patient loses lean body mass during immobility. The reduced muscle mass makes it difficult for patients to sustain activity without increased fatigue. If immobility continues and the patient does not exercise, there is further loss of muscle mass. Prolonged immobility often leads to disuse atrophy. Loss of endurance, decreased muscle mass and strength, and joint instability (see Skeletal Effects) place patients at risk for falls (see Chapter 39).

Skeletal Effects. Immobilization causes two skeletal changes: impaired calcium metabolism and joint abnormalities. Because immobilization results in bone resorption, the bone tissue is less dense or atrophied, and **disuse osteoporosis** results. When disuse osteoporosis occurs, a patient is at risk for pathological fractures.

Osteoporosis is a major health concern in this country. It is predicted that by 2025 it will be responsible for approximately three million fractures and $25.3 billion in costs each year. Furthermore, the National Osteoporosis Foundation (2014) reports that about 54 million Americans have osteoporosis and low bone mass. Studies suggest that approximately one in two women and up to one in four men age 50 and older will break a bone as a result of osteoporosis. Although primary osteoporosis is different in origin from the osteoporosis that results from immobility, it is imperative that nurses recognize that immobilized patients are at high risk for accelerated bone loss if they have primary osteoporosis.

Immobility can lead to joint contractures. A **joint contracture** is an abnormal and possibly permanent condition characterized by fixation of a joint. It is important to note that flexor muscles for joints are stronger than extensor muscles and therefore contribute to the formation of contractures. Disuse, atrophy, and shortening of the muscle fibers cause joint contractures. When a contracture occurs, the joint cannot achieve full ROM. Contractures sometimes leave a joint or joints in a nonfunctional position, as seen in patients who are permanently curled in a fetal position. Early prevention of contractures is essential (Box 28-1) (Clavet et al., 2011).

One common and debilitating contracture is footdrop (Figure 28-3). When **footdrop** occurs, the foot is permanently fixed in plantar flexion. Ambulation is difficult with the foot in this position because the patient cannot dorsiflex the foot. A patient with footdrop is unable to lift the toes off the ground. Patients who have suffered CVAs with resulting right- or left-sided paralysis (hemiplegia) are at risk for footdrop.

Urinary Elimination Changes. Immobility alters a patient's urinary elimination. In the upright position urine flows out of the renal pelvis and into the ureters and bladder because of gravitational forces. When a patient is recumbent or flat, the kidneys and ureters move toward a more level plane. Urine formed by the kidney needs to enter the bladder unaided by gravity. Because the peristaltic contractions of the ureters are insufficient to overcome gravity, the renal pelvis fills before urine enters the ureters (Figure 28-4). This condition is called **urinary stasis** and increases the risk of urinary tract infection and renal calculi

BOX 28-1 EVIDENCE-BASED PRACTICE

Patient Contractures and Treatments to Reduce Future Contractures for At-Risk Patients

PICO Question: Can the use of early correct positioning, range-of-motion (ROM) exercises, and mechanical treatment modalities such as dynamic and static splints reduce joint contractures in the lower extremities in patients with at-risk conditions compared with patients who do not have any early intervention?

Evidence Summary

Joint contractures are common preventable disorders that can result in significant long-term morbidity and reduced patient independence. Contracture is the shortening of the connective tissue and is an abnormal and possibly permanent condition characterized by decreased range of joint motion and/or fixation of the joint. Contractures occur following prolonged joint positioning (immobility), neurological disorders, and surgical joint manipulation (Furia et al., 2013). Evidence shows that early prevention of contractures is essential (Furia et al., 2013; Clavet et al., 2011). A systematic review of contracture reduction by Furia et al (2013) reported on the success of early intervention with splinting procedures. They noted that prompt use of splinting with prescribed range-of-motion exercises reduced contractures and improved active range of joint motion in affected lower extremities.

Application to Nursing Practice

- In conjunction with an interprofessional health care team, develop an early intervention protocol using prescribed positioning, range-of-motion exercises, and/or splints to reduce the risk for contracture formation (Furia et al., 2013).
- Health care agencies need to provide equipment (e.g., splints) and appropriate education for staff to reduce the risk of contractures.
- A collaborative plan of care, including a discharge plan, with a contracture prevention and muscle strengthening protocol must be developed on patient admission (Clavet et al., 2011).
- Use positioning, ROM exercises, and ROM devices according to the individualized need of the patient and as ordered (Furia et al., 2013).

ROM, Range of motion.

(see Chapter 46). Renal calculi are calcium stones that lodge in the renal pelvis or pass through the ureters. Immobilized patients are at risk for calculi because they frequently have hypercalcemia.

As the period of immobility continues, fluid intake often diminishes. When combined with other problems such as fever, the risk for dehydration increases. As a result, urinary output declines on or about the fifth or sixth day after immobilization, and the urine becomes concentrated. This concentrated urine increases the risk for calculi formation and infection. Another cause of urinary tract infections in immobilized patients is the use of an indwelling urinary catheter.

Integumentary Changes. The changes in metabolism that accompany immobility add to the harmful effect of pressure on the skin in immobilized patients. This makes immobility a major risk factor for pressure ulcers. Any break in the integrity of the skin is difficult to heal. Preventing a pressure ulcer is much less expensive than treating one; therefore preventive nursing interventions are imperative (WOCN, 2010).

A pressure ulcer is an impairment of the skin as a result of prolonged ischemia (decreased blood supply) in tissues (see Chapter 48). An ulcer is characterized initially by inflammation and usually forms over a bony prominence. Ischemia develops when the pressure on the skin is greater than the pressure inside the small peripheral blood vessels supplying blood to the skin.

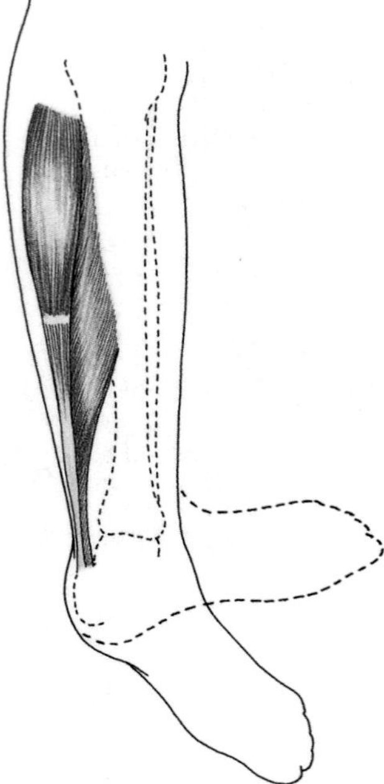

FIGURE 28-3 Footdrop. Ankle is fixed in plantar flexion. Normally ankle is able to flex *(dotted line)*, which eases walking.

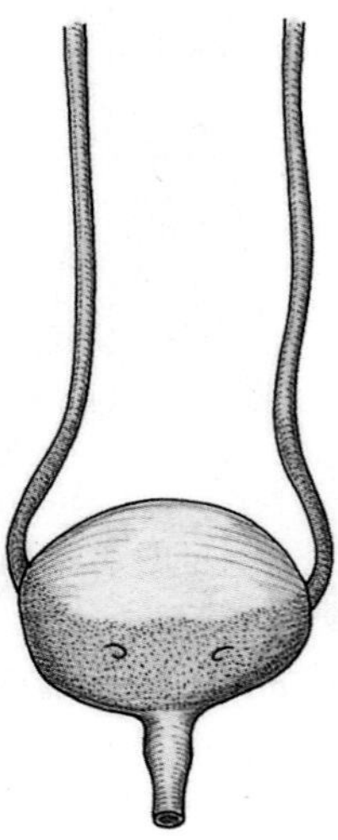

FIGURE 28-4 Stasis of urine with reflux to ureters.

Tissue metabolism depends on the supply of oxygen and nutrients to and the elimination of metabolic wastes from the blood. Pressure affects cellular metabolism by decreasing or totally eliminating tissue circulation. When a patient lies in bed or sits in a chair, the weight of the body is on bony prominences. The longer the pressure is applied, the longer is the period of ischemia and therefore the greater the risk of skin breakdown. The prevalence of pressure ulcers is highest in long-term care facilities, whereas hospital-acquired pressure ulcers are the highest in adult intensive care units (Peterson et al., 2013).

Psychosocial Effects. Immobilization often leads to emotional and behavioral responses, sensory alterations, and changes in coping. Illnesses that result in limited or impaired mobility can cause social isolation and loneliness (Parker, 2012). Every patient responds to immobility differently.

Patients with restricted mobility may have some depression. Depression is an affective disorder characterized by exaggerated feelings of sadness, melancholy, dejection, worthlessness, emptiness, and hopelessness out of proportion to reality. It results from worrying about present and future levels of health, finances, and family needs. Because immobilization removes a patient from a daily routine, he or she has more time to worry about disability. Worrying quickly increases a patient's depression, causing withdrawal. Withdrawn patients often do not want to participate in their own care.

Developmental Changes

Immobility often leads to developmental changes in the very young and in older adults. The immobilized young or middle-age adult who has been healthy experiences few, if any, developmental changes. However, there are exceptions. For example, a mother with complications following birth has to go on bed rest and as a result cannot interact with her newborn as expected.

Infants, Toddlers, and Preschoolers. The newborn infant's spine is flexed and lacks the anteroposterior curves of the adult (see Chapter 12). As the baby grows, musculoskeletal development permits support of weight for standing and walking. Posture is awkward because the head and upper trunk are carried forward. Because body weight is not distributed evenly along a line of gravity, posture is off balance, and falls occur often. When an infant, toddler, or preschooler becomes immobilized, it is usually because of trauma or the need to correct a congenital skeletal abnormality. Prolonged immobilization delays a child's gross motor skills, intellectual development, and musculoskeletal development.

Adolescents. The adolescent stage usually begins with a tremendous increase in growth (see Chapter 12). When the activity level is reduced because of trauma, illness, or surgery, the adolescent is often behind peers in gaining independence and accomplishing certain skills such as obtaining a driver's license. Social isolation is a concern for this age-group when immobilization occurs.

Adults. An adult who has correct posture and body alignment feels good, looks good, and generally appears self-confident. The healthy adult also has the necessary musculoskeletal development and coordination to carry out ADLs (see Chapter 13). When periods of prolonged immobility occur, all physiological systems are at risk. In addition, the role of the adult often changes with regard to the family or social structure. Some adults lose their jobs, which affects their self-concept (see Chapter 34).

Older Adults. A progressive loss of total bone mass occurs with older adults. Some of the possible causes of this loss include decreased physical activity, hormonal changes, and bone resorption. The effect of bone loss is weaker bones. Older adults often walk more slowly, take smaller steps, and appear less coordinated. Prescribed medications alter their sense of balance or affect their blood pressure when they change position too quickly, increasing their risk for falls and injuries (see Chapter 14). The outcomes of a fall include not only possible injury but also hospitalization, loss of independence, psychological effects, and quite possibly death (McMahon and Fleury, 2012).

Older adults often experience functional status changes secondary to hospitalization and altered mobility status (Box 28-2). Immobilization of older adults increases their physical dependence on others and accelerates functional losses (Padula et al., 2009). Immobilization of some older adults results from a degenerative disease, neurological trauma, or chronic illness. In some it occurs gradually and progressively; in others, especially those who have had a stroke, it is sudden. When providing nursing care for an older adult, encourage the patient to perform as many self-care activities as possible, thereby maintaining the highest level of mobility. Sometimes nurses inadvertently contribute to a patient's immobility by providing unnecessary help with activities such as bathing and transferring.

BOX 28-2 FOCUS ON OLDER ADULTS

Functional Decline in Hospitalized Immobile Older Adults

For many older adults, admission to a hospital often results in functional decline despite the treatment for which they were admitted. Some older adults have problems related to mobility and quickly regress to a dependent state. Usual aging is associated with decreased muscle strength and aerobic capacity, which become exacerbated if a patient's nutritional state is poor.

- A nutritional assessment needs to be included in the plan of care for the older adult experiencing immobility.
- Anorexia and insufficient assistance with eating lead to malnutrition, which contributes to the known problems associated with immobility.
- Improved nutrition increases patient's ability to perform physical reconditioning exercises (Padula et al., 2009).
- There is a direct relationship between the success of older adults' rehabilitation and their nutritional status.

NURSING PROCESS

Apply the nursing process and use a critical thinking approach in your care of patients. The nursing process provides a clinical decision-making approach for you to develop and implement an individualized plan of care. Patients with preexisting mobility impairments and those who are at risk for immobility will greatly benefit from a care plan that improves the patient's functional status, promotes self-care, maintains psychological well-being, and reduces the hazards of immobility.

Assessment

Your assessment of a patient must consider his or her normal mobility status, the effects of any diseases or conditions on mobility, and the patient's risks for mobility alterations as a result of treatments. Critically analyze findings to ensure that you make patient-centered clinical decisions required for safe nursing care.

Through the Patient's Eyes. Usually you will assess a patient's degree of mobility and immobility during the history interview and physical examination (Box 28-3). Keep in mind that the patient is a full partner in providing information and designing the plan of care. It is important to understand how any limitations in mobility are perceived by the patient. Has the patient had a disability for an extended period of time, and is he or she well adapted to the use of an assist device or even a wheelchair? Is the limitation in mobility sudden and unexpected, causing the patient to be fearful or full of questions? Always convey respect for the patient's preferences, values, and needs during assessment and when designing a plan of care (Ackley and Ladwig, 2014).

Mobility. Assessment of patient mobility focuses on ROM, gait, exercise and activity tolerance, and body alignment. When unsure of a patient's abilities, begin assessment of mobility with the patient in the most supportive position and move to higher levels according to his or her tolerance. Generally the assessment of movement starts while the patient is lying and proceeds to assessing sitting positions in

BOX 28-3 Nursing Assessment Questions

Mobility
- Describe any changes you've noticed in your ability to walk and take care of yourself on a daily basis.
- Have you experienced any stiffness, swelling of a joint, muscle or joint pain, or difficulty with moving? If so, describe how you are affected.
- Have you noticed any shortness of breath; if so, does it worsen when walking?

Immobility
- Describe your normal daily activity. Has this changed recently?
- How have your appetite and diet changed since you've had problems moving around?
- Describe what you eat in a normal day.
- Does your day seem very long?
- Are you sleeping well at night?
- Have you noticed any places on your skin that are reddened or have any open sores?
- Describe any changes you've noticed in urinating and/or having bowel movements.

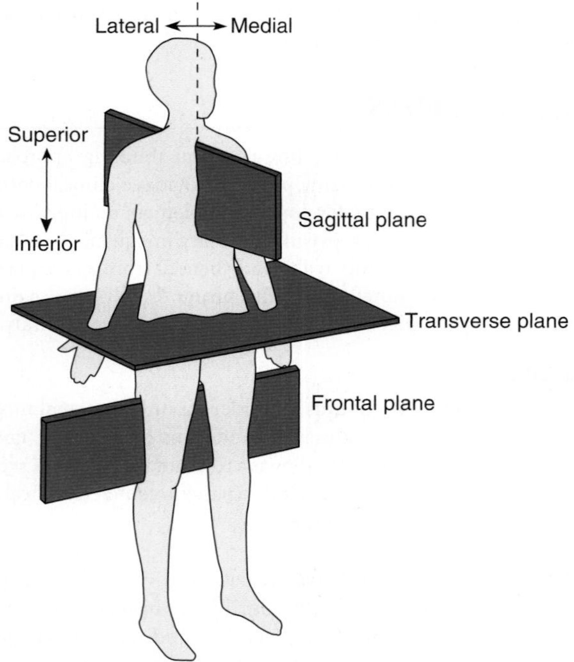

FIGURE 28-5 Planes of body.

bed, transfers to chair, and finally walking. This helps to protect the patient's safety.

Range of Motion. Range of motion (ROM) is the maximum amount of movement available at a joint in one of the three planes of the body: sagittal, transverse, or frontal (Figure 28-5). The sagittal plane is a line that passes through the body from front to back, dividing it into a left and right side. The frontal plane passes through the body from side to side and divides it into front and back. The transverse plane is a horizontal line that divides the body into upper and lower portions.

Ligaments, muscles, and the nature of the joint limit joint mobility in each of the planes. However, some joint movements are specific to each plane. In the sagittal plane, movements are flexion and extension (e.g., fingers and elbows), dorsiflexion, and plantar flexion (feet) and extension (e.g., hip). In the frontal plane movements are abduction and adduction (e.g., arms and legs) and eversion and inversion (feet). In the transverse plane movements are pronation and supination (hands) and internal and external rotation (hips).

Assessment of ROM is important as a baseline measure to determine a patient's mobility status and to later compare and evaluate whether a loss in joint mobility has occurred as a result of clinical changes or treatments. When assessing ROM, ask questions about and physically examine the patient for stiffness, swelling, pain, limited movement, and unequal movement. Chapter 31 describes specific techniques for measuring the degrees of motion in a joint. Patients whose mobility is restricted require ROM exercises to reduce the hazards of immobility. Limited ROM often indicates inflammation such as arthritis, fluid in the joint, altered nerve supply, or contractures. Increased mobility (beyond normal) of a joint sometimes indicates connective tissue disorders, ligament tears, or possible joint fractures.

Assess the type of ROM exercise that a patient is able to perform. First consider the medical plan of care and if active ROM exercises are appropriate; then assess the patient's ability to engage in active ROM exercises. ROM exercises are active (the patient moves all joints through his or her ROM unassisted), passive (the patient is unable to move independently, and the nurse moves each joint through its ROM), or somewhere in between (Table 28-2). For example, you might need to provide support for a weak patient while he or she performs most of the joint movement. Some patients are able to move some joints actively, whereas you will passively move others. Your assessment will help to determine the patient's need for assistance, teaching, or reinforcement. In general, exercises need to be as active as health and mobility allow. Contractures develop in joints that are not moved periodically through their full ROM. Assessment data from patients with limited joint movements vary on the basis of the area affected.

Neck. A flexion contracture of the neck is a serious disability because the patient's neck is permanently flexed with the chin close to or actually touching the chest. Assessment reveals altered body alignment, changes in the visual field, and decreased level of independent functioning.

Shoulder. One feature of the shoulder that sets it apart from other joints in the body is that the strongest muscle controlling it, the deltoid, is in complete elongation in the normal position. No other muscle exerts its full strength when in complete elongation. Patients with limited movement in the shoulder have difficulty moving their arms.

Elbow. The elbow functions optimally at an angle of approximately 90 degrees. An elbow fixed in full extension is disabling and limits a patient's independence.

Forearm. Most functions of the hand are best carried out with the forearm in moderate pronation. When the forearm is fixed in a position of full supination, the patient's use of the hand is limited.

Wrist. The primary function of the wrist is to place the hand in slight dorsiflexion, the position of functioning. When the wrist is fixed in even a slightly flexed position, the grasp is weakened.

Fingers and Thumb. The ROM in the fingers and thumb enables a patient to perform ADLs and activities requiring fine-motor skills such as carpentry, needlework, drawing, and painting. The functional position of the fingers and thumb is slight flexion of the thumb in opposition to the fingers.

Hip. Because the lower extremities are concerned chiefly with locomotion and weight bearing, stability of the hip joint is more important than its mobility. For example, if one hip has no mobility but is fixed in a neutral position and fully extended, it is possible to walk without a significant limp. However, contractures often fix the hip in positions

TABLE 28-2 Range-of-Motion Exercises

Body Part	Type of Joint	Type of Movement	Range (Degrees)	Primary Muscles
Neck, cervical spine	Pivotal	*Flexion:* Bring chin to rest on chest.	45	Sternocleidomastoid
		Extension: Return head to erect position.	45	Trapezius
		Hyperextension: Bend head back as far as possible.	10	Trapezius
		Lateral flexion: Tilt head as far as possible toward each shoulder.	40-45	Sternocleidomastoid
		Rotation: Turn head as far as possible in circular movement.	180	Sternocleidomastoid, trapezius
Shoulder	Ball and socket	*Flexion:* Raise arm from side position forward to position above head.	180 45-60	Coracobrachialis, biceps brachii, deltoid, pectoralis major
		Extension: Return arm to position at side of body.	180	Latissimus dorsi, teres major, triceps brachii
		Hyperextension: Move arm behind body, keeping elbow straight.	45-60	Latissimus dorsi, teres major, deltoid
		Abduction: Raise arm to side to position above head with palm away from head.	180	Deltoid, supraspinatus
		Adduction: Lower arm sideways and across body as far as possible.	320	Pectoralis major
		Internal rotation: With elbow flexed, rotate shoulder by moving arm until thumb is turned inward and toward back.	90	Pectoralis major, latissimus dorsi, teres major, subscapularis
		External rotation: With elbow flexed, move arm until thumb is upward and lateral to head.	90	Infraspinatus, teres major, deltoid
		Circumduction: Move arm in full circle (Circumduction is combination of all movements of ball-and-socket joint.)	360	Deltoid, coracobrachialis, latissimus dorsi, teres major
Elbow	Hinge	*Flexion:* Bend elbow so lower arm moves toward its shoulder joint and hand is level with shoulder.	150	Biceps brachii, brachialis, brachioradialis
		Extension: Straighten elbow by lowering hand.	150	Triceps brachii
Forearm	Pivotal	*Supination:* Turn lower arm and hand so palm is up.	70-90	Supinator, biceps brachii
		Pronation: Turn lower arm so palm is down.	70-90	Pronator teres, pronator quadratus
Wrist	Condyloid	*Flexion:* Move palm toward inner aspect of forearm.	80-90	Flexor carpi ulnaris, flexor carpi radialis
		Extension: Move fingers and hand posterior to midline.	80-90	Extensor carpi radialis brevis, extensor carpi radialis longus, extensor carpi ulnaris
		Hyperextension: Bring dorsal surface of hand back as far as possible.	80-90	Extensor carpi radialis brevis, extensor carpi radialis longus, extensor carpi ulnaris
		Abduction: Place hand with palm down and extend wrist laterally toward fifth finger.	Up to 30	Flexor carpi radialis, extensor carpi radialis brevis, extensor carpi radialis longus
		Adduction: Place hand with palm down and extend wrist medially toward thumb.	30-50	Flexor carpi ulnaris, extensor carpi ulnaris
Fingers	Condyloid hinge	*Flexion:* Make fist.	90	Lumbricales, interosseus volaris, interosseus dorsalis
		Extension: Straighten fingers.	90	Extensor digiti quinti proprius, extensor digitorum communis, extensor indicis proprius
		Hyperextension: Bend fingers back as far as possible.	30-60	Extensor digitorum
		Abduction: Spread fingers apart.	30	Interosseus dorsalis
		Adduction: Bring fingers together.	30	Interosseus volaris
Thumb	Saddle	*Flexion:* Move thumb across palmar surface of hand.	90	Flexor pollicis brevis
		Extension: Move thumb straight away from hand.	90	Extensor pollicis longus, extensor pollicis brevis
		Abduction: Extend thumb laterally (usually done when placing fingers in abduction and adduction).	30	Abductor pollicis brevis
		Adduction: Move thumb back toward hand.	30	Adductor pollicis obliquus, adductor pollicis transversus
		Opposition: Touch thumb to each finger of same hand.		Opponens pollicis, opponens digiti minimi

Continued

TABLE 28-2 Range-of-Motion Exercises—cont'd

Body Part	Type of Joint	Type of Movement	Range (Degrees)	Primary Muscles
Hip	Ball and socket	*Flexion:* Move leg forward and up.	90-120	Psoas major, iliacus, sartorius
		Extension: Move back beside other leg.	90-120	Gluteus maximus, semitendinosus, semimembranosus
		Hyperextension: Move leg behind body.	30-50	Gluteus maximus, semitendinosus, semimembranosus
		Abduction: Move leg laterally away from body.	30-50	Gluteus medius, gluteus minimus
		Adduction: Move leg back toward medial position and beyond if possible.	30-50	Adductor longus, adductor brevis, adductor magnus
		Internal rotation: Turn foot and leg toward other leg.	90	Gluteus medius, gluteus minimus, tensor fasciae latae
		External rotation: Turn foot and leg away from other leg.	90	Obturatorius internus, obturatorius externus
		Circumduction: Move leg in circle.		Psoas major, gluteus maximus, gluteus medius, adductor magnus
Knee	Hinge	*Flexion:* Bring heel back toward back of thigh.	120-130	Biceps femoris, semitendinosus, semimembranosus, sartorius
		Extension: Return leg to floor.	120-130	Rectus femoris, vastus lateralis, vastus medialis, vastus intermedius
Ankle	Hinge	*Dorsal flexion:* Move foot so toes are pointed upward.	20-30	Tibialis anterior
		Plantar flexion: Move foot so toes are pointed downward.	45-50	Gastrocnemius, soleus
Foot	Gliding	*Inversion:* Turn sole of foot medially.	10 or less	Tibialis anterior, tibialis posterior
		Eversion: Turn sole of foot laterally.	10 or less	Peroneus longus, peroneus brevis
Toes	Condyloid	*Flexion:* Curl toes downward.	30-60	Flexor digitorum, lumbricalis pedis, flexor hallucis brevis
		Extension: Straighten toes.	30-60	Extensor digitorum longus, extensor digitorum brevis, extensor hallucis longus
		Abduction: Spread toes apart.	15 or less	Abductor hallucis, interosseus dorsalis
		Adduction: Bring toes together.	15 or less	Adductor hallucis, interosseus plantaris

of deformity. Excessive abduction makes the affected leg appear too short, whereas excessive adduction makes it appear too long. In either case the patient has limited locomotion and walks with an obvious limp. Internal and external rotation contractures cause an abnormal and unbalanced gait.

Knee. A primary function of the knee is stability, which is achieved by ligaments and muscles supporting the joint. However, the knees cannot remain stable under weight-bearing conditions unless there is adequate quadriceps power to maintain them in full extension. An immobile knee joint results in serious disability. The degree of disability depends on the position in which the knee is stiffened. If it is fixed in full extension, the person needs to sit with the leg out in front. When the knee is flexed, the person limps while walking. The greater the flexion, the greater is the limp.

Ankle and Foot. Without full ROM of the ankle, gait deviations occur. If the joint is not stable, the person falls. When the person relaxes as in sleep or coma, the foot relaxes and assumes a position of plantar flexion. As a result, it becomes fixed in plantar flexion (footdrop), which impairs the ability to walk independently and increases the risk for falls.

Toes. Excessive flexion of the toes results in clawing. When this is a permanent deformity, the foot is unable to rest flat on the floor, and the patient is unable to walk properly. Flexion contractures are the most common foot deformity associated with reduced joint mobility.

Gait. The term **gait** describes a particular manner or style of walking. It is a coordinated action that requires the integration of sensory function, muscle strength, proprioception, balance, and a properly functioning CNS (vestibular system and cerebellum). A gait cycle begins with the heel strike of one leg and continues to the heel strike of the other leg. Assessing a patient's gait allows you to draw conclusions about balance, posture, and the ability to walk without assistance, all of which affect the risk for falling. Here are a few ways to assess a patient's gait:

1. Observe the patient entering the room, and note speed, stride, and balance.
2. Ask the patient to walk across the room, turn, and come back.
3. Ask the patient to walk heel-to-toe in a straight line. This may be difficult for older patients even in the absence of disease, so stay at the patient's side during the walk.

Exercise and Activity Tolerance. **Exercise** is physical activity for conditioning the body, improving health, and maintaining fitness. Nurses use it as therapy to correct a deformity or restore the overall body to a maximal state of health. When a person exercises, beneficial physiological changes occur in numerous body systems (see Chapter 39). You will assess a patient's exercise history by asking what exercise he or she normally engages in and the normal amount of exercise performed daily and weekly. For example, if a patient walks, what distance does he or she typically walk, and how often? If a patient does not exercise regularly, you will want to focus on his or her activity tolerance.

Activity tolerance is the type and amount of exercise or work that a person is able to perform without undue exertion or possible injury. Assessment of activity tolerance is necessary when planning activity such as walking, ROM exercises, or ADLs. Activity tolerance assessment includes data from physiological, emotional, and developmental domains (see Chapter 39).

When a patient begins to walk, monitor for symptoms such as dyspnea, fatigue, or chest pain. If such symptoms develop, assess for a change in vital signs (heart rate and blood pressure). A weak or debilitated patient is unable to sustain even slight changes in activity because of the increased demand for energy. Seemingly simple tasks such as eating and moving in bed often result in extreme fatigue. When the patient experiences decreased activity tolerance, carefully assess how much time he or she needs to recover. Decreasing recovery time indicates improving activity tolerance.

People who are depressed, worried, or anxious are frequently unable to tolerate exercise. Depressed patients tend to withdraw rather than participate. Patients who worry or are frequently anxious expend a tremendous amount of mental energy and often report feeling fatigued. Because of this, they also experience physical and emotional exhaustion.

Developmental changes also affect activity tolerance. As an infant enters the toddler stage, the activity level increases, and the need for sleep declines. The child entering preschool or primary grades expends mental energy in learning and often requires more rest after school or before strenuous play. The adolescent going through puberty requires more rest because much body energy is expended for growth and hormone changes (see Chapter 43).

Changes still occur through the adult years, but many of them are related to work and lifestyle choices. Pregnancy causes fluctuations in a woman's activity tolerance, especially during the first and third trimesters, when she experiences increased fatigue. Hormonal changes and fetal development use body energy, and the woman is sometimes unable or unmotivated to carry out physical activities. During the last trimester fetal development consumes a great deal of the mother's energy; and the size and location of the fetus limit the ability to take a deep breath, resulting in less oxygen being available for physical activities.

As a person grows older, activity tolerance changes. Muscle mass is reduced, and posture and bone composition change. Changes in the cardiorespiratory system such as decreased maximum heart rate and lung compliance, which affect the intensity of exercise, often occur. As age progresses, some older individuals still exercise but do so at a reduced intensity. The more inactive a patient is, the more pronounced are these activity changes.

Body Alignment. Perform assessment of body alignment with the patient standing, sitting, or lying down. This assessment has the following objectives:

- Determining normal physiological changes in body alignment resulting from growth and development for each patient
- Identifying deviations in body alignment caused by incorrect posture
- Providing opportunities for patients to observe their posture
- Identifying learning needs of patients for maintaining correct body alignment
- Identifying trauma, muscle damage, or nerve dysfunction
- Obtaining information concerning other factors that contribute to incorrect alignment such as fatigue, malnutrition, and psychological problems

The first step in assessing body alignment is to put patients at ease so they do not assume unnatural or rigid positions. When assessing the body alignment of an immobilized or unconscious patient, remove pillows and positioning supports from the bed and place the patient in the supine position.

Standing. Characteristics of correct body alignment for the standing patient include the following:

1. The head is erect and midline.
2. When observed posteriorly, the shoulders and hips are straight and parallel.
3. When observed posteriorly, the vertebral column is straight.
4. When observed laterally, the head is erect, and the spinal curves are aligned in a reversed S pattern. The cervical vertebrae are anteriorly convex, the thoracic vertebrae are posteriorly convex, and the lumbar vertebrae are anteriorly convex.
5. When observed laterally, the abdomen is comfortably tucked in, and the knees and ankles are slightly flexed. The person appears comfortable and does not seem conscious of the flexion of knees or ankles.
6. The arms hang comfortably at the sides.
7. The feet are slightly apart to achieve a base of support, and the toes are pointed forward.
8. When viewing the patient from behind, the center of gravity is in the midline, and the line of gravity is from the middle of the forehead to a midpoint between the feet. Laterally the line of gravity runs vertically from the middle of the skull to the posterior third of the foot (Figure 28-6).

Sitting. Characteristics of correct alignment of the sitting patient include the following:

1. The head is erect, and the neck and vertebral column are in straight alignment.
2. The body weight is distributed evenly on the buttocks and thighs.
3. The thighs are parallel and in a horizontal plane.
4. Both feet are supported on the floor (Figure 28-7), and the ankles are flexed comfortably. With patients of short stature, use a footstool to ensure that ankles are flexed comfortably.
5. A 2.5- to 5-cm (1- to 2-inch) space is maintained between the edge of the seat and the popliteal space on the posterior surface

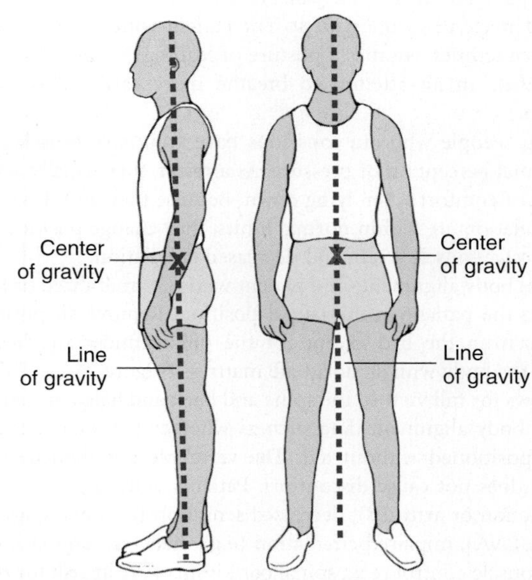

FIGURE 28-6 Correct body alignment when standing.

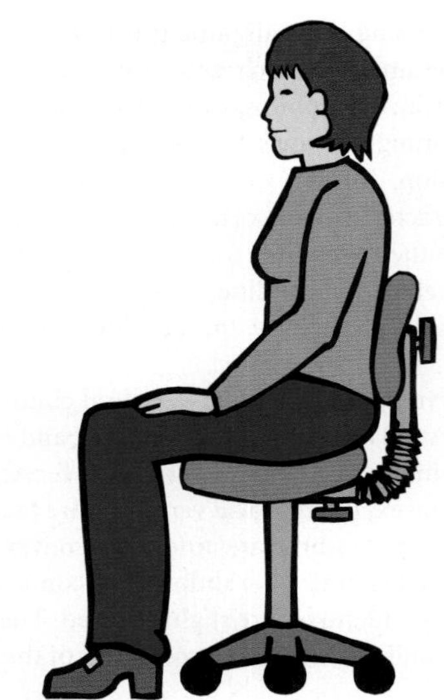

FIGURE 28-7 Correct body alignment when sitting.

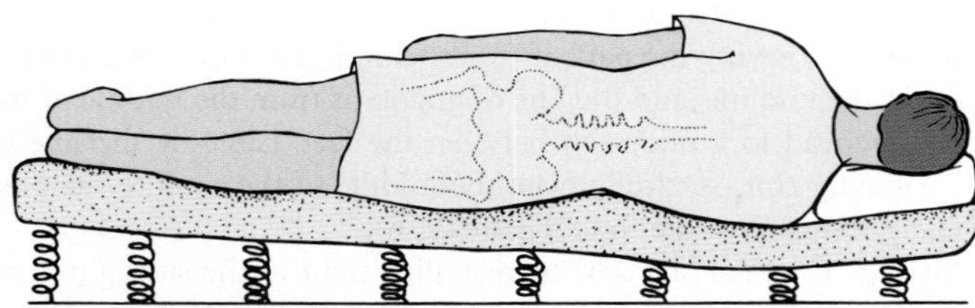

FIGURE 28-8 Correct body alignment when lying down.

of the knee. This space ensures that there is no pressure on the popliteal artery or nerve to decrease circulation or impair nerve function.

6. The patient's forearms are supported on the armrest, in the lap, or on a table in front of the chair.

It is particularly important to assess alignment when sitting if the patient has muscle weakness, muscle paralysis, or nerve damage. Patients who have these problems have diminished sensation in the affected area and are unable to perceive pressure or decreased circulation. Proper alignment while sitting reduces the risk of musculoskeletal system damage in such a patient. The patient with severe respiratory disease sometimes assumes a posture of leaning on the table in front of the chair in an attempt to breathe more easily. This is called *orthopnea.*

Lying. People who are conscious have voluntary muscle control and normal perception of pressure. As a result, they usually assume a position of comfort when lying down. Because their ROM, sensation, and circulation are within normal limits, they change positions when they perceive muscle strain and decreased circulation.

Assess body alignment for a patient who is immobilized or bedridden with the patient in the lateral position. Remove all positioning supports from the bed except for the pillow under the head and support the body with an adequate mattress (Figure 28-8). This position allows for full view of the spine and back and helps provide other baseline body alignment data such as whether the patient is able to remain positioned without aid. The vertebrae are aligned, and the position does not cause discomfort. Patients with impaired mobility (e.g., traction or arthritis), decreased sensation (e.g., hemiparesis following a CVA), impaired circulation (e.g., diabetes), and lack of voluntary muscle control (e.g., spinal cord injury) are at risk for damage when lying down.

TABLE 28-3 Assessment of the Physiological Hazards of Immobility

System	Assessment Techniques	Abnormal Findings
Metabolic	Inspection	Slowed wound healing, abnormal laboratory data
	Inspection	Muscle atrophy
	Anthropometric measurements (mid-upper arm circumference, triceps skinfold measurement)	Decreased amount of subcutaneous fat
	Palpation	Generalized edema
Respiratory	Inspection	Asymmetrical chest wall movement, dyspnea, increased respiratory rate
	Auscultation	Crackles, wheezes
Cardiovascular	Auscultation	Orthostatic hypotension
	Auscultation, palpation	Increased heart rate, third heart sound, weak peripheral pulses, peripheral edema
Musculoskeletal	Inspection, palpation	Decreased range of motion, erythema, increased diameter in calf or thigh
	Palpation	Joint contracture
	Inspection	Activity intolerance, muscle atrophy, joint contracture
Skin	Inspection, palpation	Break in skin integrity
Elimination	Inspection	Decreased urine output, cloudy or concentrated urine, decreased frequency of bowel movements
	Palpation	Distended bladder and abdomen
	Auscultation	Decreased bowel sounds

Immobility. Assess the patient for the physiologic hazards of immobility while performing a head-to-toe physical assessment (Table 28-3) (see Chapter 31). In addition, focus on the patient's psychosocial and developmental dimensions.

Metabolic System. When assessing metabolic functioning, use **anthropometric measurements** (measures of height, weight, and skinfold thickness) to evaluate muscle atrophy. In addition, analyze intake and output records for fluid balance. Does intake equal output? Intake and output measurements help to determine whether a fluid imbalance exists (see Chapter 42). Dehydration and edema increase the rate of skin breakdown in a patient who is immobilized. Monitoring laboratory data such as levels of electrolytes, serum protein (albumin and total protein), and blood urea nitrogen (BUN) help you to determine metabolic functioning.

Monitoring food intake and elimination patterns and assessing wound healing help to determine altered gastrointestinal functioning and potential metabolic problems. If the patient has a wound, the rate of healing is affected by nutritional intake and nutrient absorption. Normal progression of healing indicates that metabolic needs of injured tissues are being met. Anorexia commonly occurs in patients who are immobilized. Assess the patient's food intake before the meal tray is removed to determine the amount eaten. Assess his or her dietary patterns and food preferences at the onset of immobilization to help prevent nutritional imbalances (see Chapter 45).

Respiratory System. Perform a respiratory assessment at least every 2 hours for patients with restricted activity. Inspect chest wall movements during the full inspiratory-expiratory cycle. If a patient has an atelectatic area, chest movement is often asymmetrical. Auscultate the entire lung region to identify diminished breath sounds, crackles, or wheezes. Focus auscultation on the dependent lung fields because pulmonary secretions tend to collect in these lower regions. Assessment findings that indicate pneumonia include productive cough with greenish yellow sputum; fever; pain on breathing; and crackles, wheezes, and dyspnea.

Cardiovascular System. Cardiovascular nursing assessment of a patient who is immobilized includes blood pressure monitoring, evaluation of apical and peripheral pulses, and observation for signs of venous stasis (e.g., edema and delayed wound healing).

Although not all patients experience orthostatic hypotension, nurses monitor their vital signs during the first few attempts at sitting or standing (see Chapter 30), especially after periods of immobilization. Move a patient gradually during position changes and monitor him or her closely for dizziness while assessing the orthostatic blood pressures. The longer the period of immobility, the greater is the risk of hypotension when the patient stands (McCance and Huether, 2014).

Also assess apical and peripheral pulses (see Chapter 31). Recumbent positions increase cardiac workload and result in an increased pulse rate. In some patients, particularly older adults, the heart does not tolerate the increased workload, and a form of cardiac failure develops. A third heart sound, heard at the apex, is an early indication of congestive heart failure. Monitoring peripheral pulses allows you to evaluate the ability of the heart to pump blood. Immediately document and report the absence of a peripheral pulse in the lower extremities to the patient's health care provider, especially if the pulse was present previously.

Edema sometimes develops in patients who have had injury or whose heart is unable to handle the increased workload of bed rest. Because edema moves to dependent body regions, assessment of the patient experiencing immobility includes inspection of the sacrum, legs, and feet. If the heart is unable to tolerate the increased workload, peripheral body regions such as the hands, feet, nose, and earlobes are colder than central body regions. To assess for a deep vein thrombosis (DVT), remove the patient's elastic stockings and/or sequential compression devices (SCDs) every 8 hours (or according to agency policy) and observe the calves for redness, warmth, and tenderness. Homans' sign, or calf pain on dorsiflexion of the foot, is contraindicated in patients when a DVT is suspected and is no longer considered a reliable indicator in assessing for DVT.

Measure bilateral calf circumference and record it daily as an alternative assessment for DVT. To do this, mark a point on each calf 10 cm (3.9 inches) down from the midpatella. Measure the circumference each day using the mark for placement of the tape measure. Unilateral increases in calf circumference are an early indication of thrombosis. Because DVTs also occur in the thigh, take thigh measurements daily if the patient is prone to thrombosis. A dislodged venous thrombus, called an **embolus**, can travel through the circulatory system to the lungs and impair circulation and oxygenation, resulting in tachycardia and shortness of breath. Venous emboli that travel to the lungs are sometimes life threatening. More than 90% of all pulmonary emboli begin in the deep veins of the lower extremities (McCance and Huether, 2014).

Musculoskeletal System. Major musculoskeletal abnormalities to identify during nursing assessment include decreased muscle tone and strength, loss of muscle mass, reduced ROM, and contractures. The anthropometric measurements described previously indicate losses in muscle mass. During assessment of ROM (described earlier) you can detect muscle tone by asking the patient to relax and then passively moving each limb at several joints to get a feeling for any resistance or rigidity that may be present. You assess for muscle strength by having the patient assume a stable position and then performing maneuvers to demonstrate strength of the major muscle groups (see Chapter 31).

Physical assessment cannot identify disuse osteoporosis. However, patients on prolonged bed rest, postmenopausal women, patients taking steroids, and people with increased serum and urine calcium levels have a greater risk for bone demineralization. Consider the risk of disuse osteoporosis when planning nursing interventions. Although some falls result in injury, others occur because of pathological fractures secondary to osteoporosis.

Integumentary System. Continually assess the patient's skin for breakdown and color changes such as pallor or redness. Consistently use a standardized tool such as the Braden Scale. The screening tool identifies patients with a high risk for impaired skin integrity or early changes in the condition of patients' skin. Early identification allows for early intervention. Observe the skin often during routine care (e.g., when the patient is turned, during hygiene measures, and when providing for elimination needs). Frequent skin assessment, which can be as often as every hour and is based on patients' mobility, hydration, and physiological status, is essential to promptly identify changes in their skin and underlying tissues (see Chapter 48).

Elimination System. To determine the effects of immobility on elimination, assess the patient's total intake and output each shift and every 24 hours. Compare the amounts over time. Determine that the patient is receiving the correct amount and type of fluids orally or parenterally (see Chapter 42). Inadequate intake and output or fluid and electrolyte imbalances increase the risk for renal system impairment, ranging from recurrent infections to kidney failure. Dehydration also increases the risk for skin breakdown, thrombus formation, respiratory infections, and constipation.

Immobility impairs gastrointestinal peristalsis. Assessment of bowel elimination status includes the adequacy of a patient's dietary choices, bowel sounds, and the frequency and consistency of bowel movements (see Chapter 47). Accurate assessment enables you to intervene before constipation and fecal impaction occur.

Psychosocial Assessment. Many alterations in developmental functioning are related to immobility. Often these problems are interrelated, and it is imperative that nursing care focus on all dimensions. Often the focus of immobility is on the easily visible physical problems such as skin impairment, but do not overlook its psychosocial and developmental aspects.

Abrupt changes in personality often have a physiological cause such as surgery, a medication reaction, a pulmonary embolus, or an acute infection. For example, the primary symptom of compromised older patients with an acute urinary tract infection or fever is confusion. Identifying confusion is an important component of a nurse's assessment. Acute confusion in older adults is not normal; a thorough nursing assessment is the priority (Touhy and Jett, 2012).

Common reactions to immobilization include boredom and feelings of isolation, depression, and anger. Observe for changes in a patient's emotional status and listen carefully to family if they report emotional changes. Examples of change that indicate psychosocial concerns are a cooperative patient who becomes less cooperative or an independent patient who asks for more help than is necessary. Investigate reasons for such alterations. Identifying how the patient usually copes with loss is vital (see Chapters 36 and 37). A change in mobility status, whether permanent or not, causes a grief reaction. Families are a key resource for information about behavior changes.

Identify and correct unexplained changes in the sleep-wake cycle. Nurses prevent or minimize most stimuli that interrupt the sleep-wake cycle (e.g., nursing activities, a noisy environment, or discomfort). However, some medications such as analgesics, sleeping pills, or cardiovascular drugs also cause sleep disturbances (see Chapter 43).

Because psychosocial changes usually occur gradually, observe the patient's behavior on a daily basis. If behavioral changes occur, determine the cause(s) and evaluate the changes. Identifying the cause helps you to design appropriate nursing interventions.

Developmental Assessment. Include a developmental assessment of patients who are immobilized. When caring for a young child, determine whether he or she is able to meet developmental tasks and is progressing normally. The child's development sometimes regresses or slows because he or she is immobilized. Design nursing interventions that maintain normal development and provide physical and psychosocial stimuli after identifying a child's developmental needs and assure the parents that developmental delays are usually temporary (see Chapter 12).

Immobilization of a family member changes family functioning. The family's response to this change often leads to problems, stress, and anxieties. When children see parents who are immobile, they sometimes have difficulty understanding what is occurring and coping.

Immobility has a significant effect on the older adult's levels of health, independence, and functional status. Nursing assessment enables the nurse to determine the patient's ability to meet needs independently and adapt developmental changes such as declining physical functioning and altered family and peer relationships. A decline in developmental functioning needs prompt investigation to determine why the change occurred and interventions that can return the patient to an optimal level of functioning as soon as possible. Activities that reduce immobility and promote participation in ADLs are vital to preventing functional decline (Nagarkar et al., 2014).

QSEN QSEN: BUILDING COMPETENCY IN QUALITY IMPROVEMENT Ms. Cavallo's skilled care unit is implementing a quality improvement (QI) project focused on prevention of falls. The unit has been experiencing a notable increase in the number of falls over the past several months. A review of the literature notes that the consequences of falls are many, including the need for additional care, psychological effects, and even death. You recognize the need to develop a collaborative plan of care that includes all health care professionals that work on the unit, the patients, and their families. What is the best method(s) for you to communicate your findings and strategies for fall prevention to all health care providers and family participating in Ms. Cavallo's care? How do you identify gaps between the unit and best practice? Which measures could you use to evaluate if change has taken place?

Answers to QSEN Activities can be found on the Evolve website.

◆ Nursing Diagnosis

A patient who is experiencing an alteration in mobility often has one or more nursing diagnoses. The two diagnoses most directly related to mobility problems are *Impaired Physical Mobility* and *Risk for Disuse Syndrome.* The diagnosis of *Impaired Physical Mobility* applies to the patient who has some limitation but is not completely immobile. The diagnosis of *Risk for Disuse Syndrome* applies to the patient who is immobile and at risk for multisystem problems because of inactivity. Beyond these diagnoses, the list of potential diagnoses is extensive,

BOX 28-4 Nursing Diagnostic Process

Impaired Physical Mobility Related to Left Hip/Leg Pain

Assessment Activities	Defining Characteristics
Measure ROM during extension and flexion of the hip.	Patient has limited ROM in left hip/leg.
Observe patient attempt to move her left leg.	Patient has impaired movement attempting to move her left hip and leg.
Ask patient about perception of pain.	Patient complains of sharp pain (8 on scale of 0 to 10) in hip and leg when she tries to move it.
Ask patient about endurance and activity tolerance.	Patient reports no muscle strength in left leg. "I can't move it by myself."

ROM, Range of motion.

because immobility affects multiple body systems. Possible nursing diagnoses include the following:

- *Ineffective Airway Clearance*
- *Ineffective Coping*
- *Impaired Physical Mobility*
- *Impaired Urinary Elimination*
- *Risk for Impaired Skin Integrity*
- *Risk for Disuse Syndrome*
- *Social Isolation*

Assessment reveals clusters of data that indicate whether a patient is at risk or if a problem-focused diagnosis exists. The clusters of data reveal at-risk factors or defining characteristics that are observable assessment cues to support a problem-focused diagnostic label. In the case of a problem-focused diagnosis, the assessment data will reveal a related factor or causative factor for the diagnosis. Identifying the related factor allows you to identify the most appropriate interventions to manage or eliminate the related factor. Accurate identification of nursing diagnoses is important to planning patient-centered goals and subsequent nursing interventions that will best help the patient.

Impaired Physical Mobility related to reluctance to initiate movement requires slightly different interventions than *Impaired Physical Mobility* related to pain in the left shoulder. Thus it is critical that nursing assessment activities identify and cluster defining characteristics that ultimately support the nursing diagnosis selected (Box 28-4). The diagnosis related to reluctance to initiate movement requires interventions aimed at keeping the patient as mobile as possible and encouraging him or her to perform self-care and ROM. The diagnosis related to pain requires the nurse to assist the patient with comfort measures so he or she is then willing and more able to move. In both situations the nurse explains how activity enhances healthy body functioning.

Often the physiological dimension is the major focus of nursing care for patients with impaired mobility. Thus the psychosocial and developmental dimensions are neglected. Yet all dimensions are important to health. During immobilization some patients experience decreased social interaction and stimuli. These patients frequently use the nurse's call bell to request minor physical attention when their real need is greater socialization. Nursing diagnoses for health needs in developmental areas reflect changes from the patient's normal activities. Immobility leads to a developmental crisis if the patient is unable to resolve problems and continue to mature.

Immobility also leads to multiple complications (e.g., renal calculi, DVT, pulmonary emboli, or pneumonia). If these conditions develop, collaborate with the health care provider or nurse practitioner for prescribed therapy to intervene. Be alert for and prevent these potential complications when possible.

◆ Planning

During planning, a nurse synthesizes information from resources such as knowledge of the role of respiratory and physical therapy, standards such as skin care guidelines from the Agency for Healthcare Research and Quality (Chou et al., 2013) and the Wound, Ostomy and Continence Nurses Society (WOCN, 2010), protocols for patients at risk for falls (AACN, 2014), attitudes such as creativity and perseverance, and past experiences with immobilized patients. Critical thinking ensures that the patient's plan of care integrates all that you know about the individual and key critical thinking elements. Professional standards are especially important to consider when you develop a plan of care. These standards often establish scientifically proven guidelines for selecting effective nursing interventions. Finally, as stated earlier, the patient is a full partner in designing the plan of care, and this input must be reflected when establishing the goals and outcomes.

Goals and Outcomes. Develop an individualized plan of care for each nursing diagnosis (see the Nursing Care Plan). Set realistic expectations for care and include the patient and family when possible. Set goals that are individualized, realistic, and measurable. The goals focus on preventing problems or risks to impaired body alignment and mobility.

Develop goals and expected outcomes to help patients achieve their highest level of mobility and reduce the hazards of immobility. For example, a patient who has left-sided paralysis following a stroke has two long-term goals. The first, directed toward improved mobility, is "Patient will use walker to ambulate safely in the home." A parallel goal directed toward the hazards of immobility is "Patient's skin will remain intact." Both of these goals are essential to restoring the patient's maximal mobility.

Because the patient has impaired sensation, both the patient and caregivers need to be aware of the patient's need to have the skin free of pressure. Expected outcomes for the goal of the skin remaining intact include the following:

- Patient's skin color and temperature return to normal baseline within 20 minutes of position change.
- Patient changes position at least every 2 hours.

Setting Priorities. The effect that problems have on a patient's mental and physical health determines the immediacy of any problem. Set priorities when planning care to ensure that immediate needs are met first. This is particularly important when patients have multiple diagnoses. Plan therapies according to severity of risks to the patient; and individualize the plan according to the patient's developmental stage, level of health, and lifestyle.

It is especially important in priority setting to make sure that you do not overlook potential complications. Many times actual problems such as pressure ulcers and disuse syndrome are addressed only after they develop. Therefore monitor the patient often, reinforcing prevention techniques to both the patient and other caregivers and supervising nursing assistive personnel in carrying out activities aimed at preventing complications of impaired mobility.

Teamwork and Collaboration. Care of the patient experiencing alterations in mobility requires a team approach. Nurses often delegate select interventions that are appropriate for nursing assistive personnel to perform. For example, in the case of postoperative patients who are at risk for respiratory problems from temporary immobility, nursing assistive personnel (NAP) can encourage the patient to do leg exercises, use the incentive spirometer, and cough and deep breathe (see Chapter 41). When patients have limited mobility as a result of paralysis, NAP can turn and position patients and apply elastic stockings. They can also help the nurse measure leg circumferences and height and weight.

Collaborate with other health care team members such as physical or occupational therapists when it is essential to consider mobility needs. Understanding the need for and having open communications with other members of the interdisciplinary care team results in better patient outcomes and hopefully prevents the hazards of immobility. It is through these collaborative efforts and teamwork that patients benefit most. For example, physical therapists are a resource for planning ROM or strengthening exercises, and occupational therapists are a resource for planning ADLs that patients need to modify or relearn. Wound care specialists and respiratory therapists are often involved in patient care, especially with patients who are experiencing complications related to their immobility. Consult a registered dietitian when the patient is experiencing nutritional problems; and refer him or her to a mental health advanced practice nurse, licensed social worker, or psychologist to assist with coping or other psychosocial issues.

Discharge planning begins when a patient enters the health care system. In anticipation of the patient's discharge from an institution, make appropriate referrals or consult a case manager or a discharge planner to ensure that the patient's needs are met at home. Consider the patient's home environment when planning therapies to maintain or improve body alignment and mobility. Referrals to home care or outpatient therapy are often needed.

◆ Implementation

Health Promotion. Health promotion activities include a variety of interventions such as education, prevention, and early detection. Examples of health promotion activities that address mobility and immobility include prevention of work-related injury, fall prevention measures, exercise, and early detection of scoliosis.

Prevention of Work-Related Musculoskeletal Injuries. The rate of work-related injuries in health care settings has increased in recent years. In 2006 there were 4.4 cases per 100 full-time workers who experienced occupational injury and illness compared with 5 cases per 100 for private industry overall. The rate for nursing homes was 10.1 cases per 100 workers (USDL, 2014). Most of these injuries occurred as a result of overexertion, which resulted in back injuries and other musculoskeletal problems. Back injuries are often the direct result of improper lifting and bending. The most common back injury is strain on the lumbar muscle group, which includes the muscles around the lumbar vertebrae. Injury to these areas affects the ability to bend forward, backward, and from side to side and limits the ability to rotate the hips and lower back. Research has demonstrated that ergonomic programs in health care facilities reduce costs, injuries to employees, and missed work days (Hunter et al., 2010).

Nurses and other health care staff are especially at risk for injury to lumbar muscles when lifting, transferring, or positioning immobilized patients. Therefore be aware of agency policies and protocols that protect staff and patients from injury. When lifting, assess the weight you will lift and determine the assistance you will need. Current evidence supports that using mechanical or other ergonomic assistive devices is the safest way to reposition and lift patients who are unable to do these activities themselves. Many agencies have developed special patient lift teams and have instituted a no-lift policy (see Chapter 39).

Exercise. Although many diseases and physical problems cause or contribute to immobility, it is important to remember that exercise programs enhance feelings of well-being and improve endurance,

NURSING CARE PLAN

Impaired Physical Mobility

ASSESSMENT

Ms. Carmella Cavallo, a 97-year-old patient, is admitted to a skilled care unit for rehabilitation 10 days after the surgical procedure of fixation of a fractured left hip. She has a history of smoking but stopped 40 years ago. She has no cardiac problems and no hypertension. She experiences "aches" and "stiffness" in her knees but usually says that she "has no pain" when asked. The three small incisions are clean, dry, and intact. Staples were removed yesterday.

Assessment Activities	*Findings/Defining Characteristics*[*]
Ask Ms. Cavallo to rate her pain on a scale of 0 to 10.	She rates her pain as a 2 on a scale of 0 to 10 at rest, but it **increases to an 8** with any movement of her left leg.
Assess Ms. Cavallo's ability to transfer.	She is **not able to transfer, even** with help from chair to bed.
Ask Ms. Cavallo how her surgery has affected her mobility.	She responds that she wants to get out of bed but, when she moves her left leg, her nonverbal signs indicate that she is in severe pain. She says that it is a **"sharp, stabbing pain."**

[*]**Defining characteristics** are shown in bold type.

NURSING DIAGNOSIS: Impaired physical mobility related to musculoskeletal impairment from surgery and pain with movement

PLANNING

Goals	*Expected Outcomes*[†]
	Pain Control
Ms. Cavallo will have more pain relief during activity.	Ms. Cavallo's pain is less than 6 during activity.
	Body Positioning: Self-initiated
Ms. Cavallo will be able to transfer with assistive device by discharge.	Ms. Cavallo is able to move from her bed to her chair and back again using her walker and assist ×1 within 5 days.
	Ms. Cavallo is able to transfer from her chair to her bedside commode using her walker within 5 days.
	Ambulation
Ms. Cavallo will walk 100 feet using her walker by discharge.	Ms. Cavallo walks to her door and around her room with her walker within 10 days.
	Ms. Cavallo walks 100 feet at a slow pace using her walker 3 times a day in 14 days and increases the distance that she walks by 100 feet every day after that.

[†]Nursing outcomes classification from Moorhead S et al., editors: *Nursing outcomes classification (NOC)*, ed 5, St Louis, 2013, Mosby.

INTERVENTIONS[‡]	RATIONALE
Exercise Therapy: Ambulation	
Consult with physical therapist on selection of transfer technique.	Ensures safe transfer technique with less risk of patient injury.
Instruct Ms. Cavallo on safe transfer and ambulation techniques in an environment with few distractions. Provide written materials and the use of the Teach Back method to reinforce verbal instructions.	Providing instruction in a quiet environment and the use of the Teach Back method enhances learning (Winifred, 2013).
Establish realistic increments for transferring and increasing distance for ambulation.	Physiotherapy exercises, physical activity, and setting realistic goals for ambulation encourage activity in older adults (Schiller et al., 2015).
Pain Management	
Administer pain medication on the basis of your assessment of Ms. Cavallo's needs and on a schedule rather than prn if patient exhibits signs of being in pain but does not request pain medication and dose is not relieving her pain.	Obtain order to adjust (increase or decrease dose) on the basis of her report of pain severity or her ability to perform activities of daily living (ADLs) (Botti et al., 2014).
Observe for overt and covert signs of pain when she is moving or attempting to implement plan from physical therapy (PT) and have prn dose of pain medication ordered if additional pain medication is needed for PT activities.	It is important for you to have "as needed" dose of pain medication for patient in case requires a supplemental dose.

[‡]Intervention classification labels from Bulechek GM et al., editors: *Nursing interventions classification (NIC)*, ed 6, St Louis, 2013, Mosby.

EVALUATION

Nursing Actions	*Patient Response/Finding*	*Achievement of Outcome*
Ask Mrs. Cavallo to rate her level of pain.	Ms. Cavallo reports pain at 5 during activity.	Ms. Cavallo has achieved improved pain control.
Ask Ms. Cavallo if her mobility has improved after therapy. Observe her transfer from bed to chair.	Ms. Cavallo is able to transfer from bed to chair using her walker and stand-by assistance of nurse.	Ms. Cavallo has achieved goal of transferring with walker and assistance.
Assess Ms. Cavallo as she walks in the hall; measure how far she walks.	Ms. Cavallo is able to walk 200 feet in the hall with her walker.	Activity level is improving. Continue interventions and continue to encourage ambulation.

 BOX 28-5 CULTURAL ASPECTS OF CARE

Cultural Influences on Mobility

Many activities are specifically linked to an individual's culture such as time orientation, health care practices, nutritional habits, religious rituals, and family systems. Less attention has been given to the impact of culture on mobility. However, cultural influences have an important role in exercise and physical activity.

Culture influences an individual's preferences for activity and exercise. Certain cultures discourage involvement in organized recreational physical activities such as basketball, running, and aerobics. Ethnic dancing is an effective activity that is acceptable in many countries. Other cultures emphasize exercise in terms of activities of daily living such as walking, gardening, and prayer/meditation.

A sedentary lifestyle places an individual at risk for being overweight. Children from many cultures who live in the United States are becoming more sedentary. Therefore a national health approach is needed for communities to provide social and physical environments that promote healthy choices. From the earliest age preventive health practices should be included in the education process.

Implications for Patient-Centered Care

- Assess patterns of daily living and culturally prescribed activities before suggesting specific forms of exercise to patients.
- Help patients plan physical activities that are culturally acceptable.
- Exercise programs need to be flexible and accommodate family and community responsibilities of the culture.
- Encourage culturally specific and individually tailored interventions to facilitate commitment to exercise.
- Educate patients of all ages on the importance of exercise in preserving health and correct any misconceptions.

BOX 28-6 PATIENT TEACHING

Teaching Patients with Osteoporosis

Objective

- Patient will verbalize strategies to prevent or limit the severity of osteoporosis.

Teaching Strategies

- Instruct patient and/or family caregiver about common risk factors and how to modify lifestyle (e.g., smoking, caffeine, alcohol, hormone replacement as recommended by health care provider).
- Teach patient and/or caregiver the current recommended dietary allowances for calcium and review foods high in calcium (e.g., milk fortified with vitamin D, leafy green vegetables, yogurt, and cheese).
- Instruct patient and/or caregiver in appropriate types of weight-bearing exercises as recommended by health care provider or physical therapist to prevent injury or fractures.
- Teach patient and/or caregiver about safety, fall prevention, and strategies to create a safe home environment (e.g., remove scatter rugs; ensure that hallways, steps, and rooms are well lit) (McMahon and Fleury, 2012).
- Instruct patient and/or caregiver in self-administration of prescribed medication used to treat osteoporosis.
- Promote positive self-image in patient by providing realistic yet optimistic and positive feedback about changes in appearance and mobility.

Evaluation

- Patient and/or caregiver can verbalize *three lifestyle modifications* such as stopping smoking, reducing caffeine or alcohol intake, or increasing dietary calcium.
- Patient and/or caregiver can verbalize *at least four* foods high in calcium and vitamin D.
- Patient and/or caregiver can *demonstrate appropriate weight-bearing exercises* and plan times for exercise.
- Patient and/or caregiver verbalize *three safety strategies* that they can implement at home to prevent falls.
- Patient and/or caregiver verbalize *knowledge* about dosage schedule and side effects of osteoporosis medications.
- Patient and/or caregiver express positive but realistic feedback regarding effects of disease.

strength, and health. Exercise reduces the risk of many health problems such as cardiovascular disease, diabetes, and osteoporosis. It is important to give patients options for how to stay active and how to change their behavior if exercise has not been their routine. The Stanford Medicine (2015) chronic disease self-management program encourages appropriate exercise for maintaining and improving strength, flexibility, and endurance. As a nurse you can encourage all patients to find a type of exercise that meets their lifestyle and particular health-related needs. For example, a patient with severe arthritis of the knees might benefit from aquatic therapy (exercise in a pool) rather than walking. Encourage hospitalized patients to perform stretching, ROM exercises, and light walking within the limits of their condition (see Chapter 39). Collaboration with a physical therapist is recommended.

Nurses contribute to promoting health for many patients by encouraging or starting managed exercise programs. Exercise is a key prescription for health promotion of all patients, regardless of their age. In older adults routine exercise or activity helps maintain ROM and functional mobility and improves balance (Touhy and Jett, 2012; Edelman et al., 2013; Elliott, 2011). Take cultural preferences into consideration when helping patients design exercise plans (Box 28-5).

Bone Health in Patients with Osteoporosis. Patients at risk for or diagnosed with osteoporosis have special health promotion needs. Encourage patients at risk to be screened for osteoporosis and assess their diets for calcium and vitamin D intake. Patients who have lactose intolerance need dietary teaching about alternative sources of calcium.

For patients diagnosed with osteoporosis, early evaluation, consultation with, and referral to health care providers, dietitians, and physical therapists are important interventions, especially when they become immobilized. The goal of the patient with osteoporosis is to maintain independence with ADLs. Assistive ambulatory devices, adaptive clothing, and safety bars help the patient maintain independence. Patient teaching needs to focus on limiting the severity of the disease through diet and activity (Box 28-6).

Acute Care. Patients in acute care settings who experience altered physical mobility usually have some problems associated with the hazards of immobility such as impaired respiratory status, orthostatic hypotension, and impaired skin integrity. Therefore design nursing interventions to reduce the impact of immobility on body systems and prepare the patient for the restorative phase of care.

Metabolic System. Because the body needs protein to repair injured tissue and rebuild depleted protein stores, give the immobilized patient a high-protein, high-calorie diet. A high-calorie intake provides sufficient fuel to meet metabolic needs and replace subcutaneous tissue. Also ensure that the patient is taking vitamin B and C supplements when necessary. Supplementation with vitamin C is needed for skin integrity and wound healing; vitamin B complex assists in energy metabolism.

If the patient is unable to eat, nutrition must be provided parenterally or enterally. Total parenteral nutrition refers to delivery of nutritional supplements through a central or peripheral intravenous catheter. Enteral feedings include delivery through a nasogastric, gastrostomy, or jejunostomy tube of high-protein, high-calorie solutions with complete requirements of vitamins, minerals, and electrolytes (see Chapter 45).

Respiratory System. Patients who are immobilized and have reduced ventilation can benefit from a variety of nursing interventions that promote lung expansion and removal of pulmonary secretions. Patients need to frequently fully expand their lungs to maintain their elastic recoil property. In addition, secretions accumulate in the dependent areas of the lungs. Often patients with restricted mobility experience weakness, and as this progresses the cough reflex gradually becomes inefficient. All of these factors put the patient at risk of developing pneumonia. The stasis of secretions in the lungs is life threatening for an immobilized patient.

Deep-breathing exercises, incentive spirometry, controlled coughing, and chest physiotherapy are among the nursing interventions available to expand the lungs, dislodge and mobilize stagnant secretions, and clear the lungs (Chapters 41 and 50). All of these interventions help reduce the risk of pneumonia. It is essential to implement pulmonary interventions early in all patients with limited mobility, even those who do not have pneumonia.

Encourage an immobile patient to deep breathe and cough every 1 to 2 hours. Teach alert patients to deep breathe or yawn every hour or to use an incentive spirometer (when ordered). Controlled coughing, a common therapy for postoperative patients, involves taking in three deep breaths and then coughing with the third exhalation.

Chest physiotherapy (CPT) (percussion and postural drainage) is another effective method for preventing pneumonia and keeping the airways clear (see Chapter 41). It helps the patient drain secretions from specific segments of the bronchi and lungs into the trachea so he or she is able to cough and expel them. Respiratory assessment findings identify areas of the lungs requiring CPT.

Ensure that patients who are immobile have an adequate fluid intake. Unless there is a medical contraindication, an adult needs to drink at least 1100 to 1400 mL of noncaffeinated fluids daily. This helps keep mucociliary clearance normal. Expect pulmonary secretions to be removed easily with coughing and appear thin, watery, and clear. Without adequate hydration, pulmonary secretions become thick and tenacious and difficult to remove. Offering fluids that patients prefer on a regularly timed schedule also helps with bowel and urine elimination and aids in maintaining circulation and skin integrity.

Cardiovascular System. The effects of bed rest or immobilization on the cardiovascular system include orthostatic hypotension, increased cardiac workload, and thrombus formation. Design nursing therapies to minimize or prevent these alterations.

Reducing Orthostatic Hypotension. When patients who are on bed rest or have been immobile move to a sitting or standing position, they often experience orthostatic hypotension. They have an increased pulse rate, a decreased pulse pressure, and a drop in blood pressure. If symptoms become severe enough, the patient can faint (McCance and Huether, 2014). To prevent injury, nurses implement interventions that reduce or eliminate the effects of orthostatic hypotension. Mobilize the patient as soon as the physical condition allows, even if this only involves dangling at the bedside or moving to a chair. This activity maintains muscle tone and increases venous return. Isometric exercises (i.e., activities that involve muscle tension without muscle shortening) have no beneficial effect on preventing orthostatic hypotension, but they improve activity tolerance. When getting an immobile patient up for the first time, assess the situation using a safe patient-handling algorithm (VISN8, 2015). This is a precautionary step that protects the nurse and patient from injury and also allows the patient to do as much of the transfer as possible.

Reducing Cardiac Workload. A nursing intervention that reduces cardiac workload involves instructing patients to avoid using a Valsalva maneuver when moving up in bed, defecating, or lifting household objects. During a Valsalva maneuver a patient holds his or her breath and strains, which increases intrathoracic pressure and in turn decreases venous return and cardiac output. When the strain is released, venous return and cardiac output immediately increase, and systolic blood pressure and pulse pressure rise. These pressure changes produce a reflex bradycardia and possible decrease in blood pressure that can result in sudden cardiac death in patients with heart disease. Teach patients to breathe out while defecating, lifting, or moving side-to-side or up in bed and to not hold their breath and strain.

Preventing Thrombus Formation. The Centers for Medicare and Medicaid Services identified ten "Never Events" in 2008. A Never Event is a hospital-acquired event for which Medicare and other third-party payors will no longer pay hospitals at a higher rate for the increased costs of care. Deep vein thrombosis (DVT) is one of these Never Events. The most cost-effective way to address DVT is through an aggressive program of prophylaxis. Prevention of DVT is critical to reduce the risk of fatal and nonfatal pulmonary embolism. A prophylaxis program begins with identification of patients at risk and continues throughout their immobilization. This requires a collaborative role between nurses and health care providers. You will identify patient risk factors from the nursing assessment. There are nursing interventions you can employ to reduce the risk of thrombus formation in immobilized patients. Early ambulation; leg, foot, and ankle exercises; regularly provided fluids; frequent position changes; and patient teaching need to begin when a patient becomes immobile (see Chapter 50).

Prophylaxis also includes anticoagulation, mechanical prevention with graduated compression stockings, intermittent pneumatic compression devices, and foot pumps. Anticoagulation may include the use of aspirin, although this is somewhat controversial. Anticoagulants most often used include unfractionated heparin (UFH) (usually given as 5000 units two or three times daily), low-molecular-weight heparins (LMWH) (e.g., enoxaparin or dalteparin), vitamin K antagonists (e.g., warfarin, but also acenocoumarol, phenindione, and dicoumarol), and fondaparinux (a selective factor Xa inhibitor) (Cayley, 2007). Because bleeding is a potential side effect of anticoagulant medications, continually assess the patient for signs of bleeding such as hematuria, bruising, coffee ground–like vomitus or gastrointestinal aspirate, guaiac-positive stools, and bleeding gums.

SCDs and intermittent pneumatic compression (IPC) are used to prevent blood clots in the lower extremities. These consist of sleeves or stockings made of fabric or plastic that are wrapped around the leg and secured with Velcro (Box 28-7). Once they are applied, connect the sleeves to a pump that alternately inflates and deflates the stocking around the leg. A typical cycle is inflation for 10 to 15 seconds and deflation for 45 to 60 seconds. Inflation pressures average 40 mm Hg. Use of SCD/IPC on the legs decreases venous stasis by increasing venous return through the deep veins of the legs. For optimal results begin use of SCD/IPC as soon as possible and maintain it until the patient becomes fully ambulatory.

Elastic stockings (sometimes called *antiembolitic stockings*) also aid in maintaining external pressure on the muscles of the lower extremities and thus promote venous return (see Box 28-7). To obtain the correct size, measure the patient's calf, thigh, and leg length accurately. When considering applying graded compression stockings, first assess the patient's suitability for wearing them. Do not apply them if he or she has a local condition affecting the leg (e.g., any skin lesion, gangrenous condition, or recent vein ligation) because application

BOX 28-7 PROCEDURAL GUIDELINES

Applying Sequential Compression Devices and Elastic Stockings

Delegation Considerations

The skill of applying elastic stockings and sequential compression devices (SCDs) can be delegated to nursing assistive personnel (NAP). The nurse initially determines the size of elastic stockings and assesses the patient's lower extremities for signs and symptoms of DVT or impaired circulation. Instruct NAP to:

- Remove SCD sleeves before allowing patient to get out of bed.
- Notify nurse if patient complains of pain in leg or if discoloration develops in extremities.
- When applying elastic stockings, instruct patient to avoid activities that promote venous stasis (e.g., crossing legs, wearing garters).
- Elevate legs while sitting and before applying stockings to improve venous return.
- Take precautions and **Do Not** massage patient's legs.
- Avoid wrinkles in elastic stockings.

Equipment

Tape measure, powder or cornstarch (optional), Elastic or compression stockings, SCD insufflator with air hoses attached, adjustable Velcro compression stockings/SCD disposable sleeve(s), hygiene supplies

Steps

1. Identify patient using two identifiers (e.g., name and birthday or name and medical record number) according to agency policy.
2. Assess for risk factors in Virchow's triad:
   a. Hypercoagulability (e.g., clotting disorders [laboratory test results], fever, dehydration)
   b. Venous wall abnormalities found in patient medical history (i.e., history of orthopedic surgery, atherosclerosis)
   c. Blood stasis (e.g., immobility, obesity, pregnancy)

   CLINICAL DECISION: Clinical signs of thrombophlebitis vary according to the size and location of the thrombus. Signs and symptoms of superficial thrombosis include palpable veins and surrounding areas that are tender to the touch, reddened, and warm. Temperature elevation and edema may or may not be present. Signs and symptoms of deep vein thrombosis (DVT) include swollen extremity; pain; warm, cyanotic skin; and temperature elevation. Homans' sign (pain in the calf on dorsiflexion of the foot) is no longer considered a reliable indicator (Ball et al., 2015; Grinage and Werner, 2013).

3. Assess condition of patient's skin and circulation to the legs (e.g., presence of pedal pulses, edema, discoloration of skin, skin temperature, capillary refill, presence of lesions or cuts). Assess for contraindications for use of elastic stockings or SCDs:
   a. Dermatitis or open skin lesions
   b. Recent skin graft
   c. Decreased arterial circulation in lower extremities as evidenced by cyanotic, cool extremities.
4. Obtain health care provider order.
5. When applying elastic stockings, use tape measure to measure patient's legs to determine proper stocking size.
6. Perform hand hygiene. Also provide hygiene to patient's lower extremities as needed.
7. Assemble and prepare equipment.
8. Explain procedure and reason for applying SCDs or elastic stockings.
9. Position patient in supine position. Elevate head of bed to comfortable level.
10. *Option:* When applying elastic stockings, apply a small amount of powder or cornstarch to legs provided that patient does not have sensitivity to either. Powder eases application of stockings.
11. Apply SCD Sleeve(s):
    a. Remove SCD sleeves from plastic cover; unfold and flatten.
    b. Arrange sleeve under patient's leg according to leg position indicated on inner lining of sleeve.
    c. Place patient's leg on SCD sleeve. Back of ankle should line up with ankle marking on inner lining of sleeve.
    d. Position back of knee with popliteal opening on the sleeve (see Illustration).
    e. Wrap SCD sleeve securely around patient's leg. Check fit of SCD sleeve by placing two fingers between patient's leg and sleeve (see illustration).

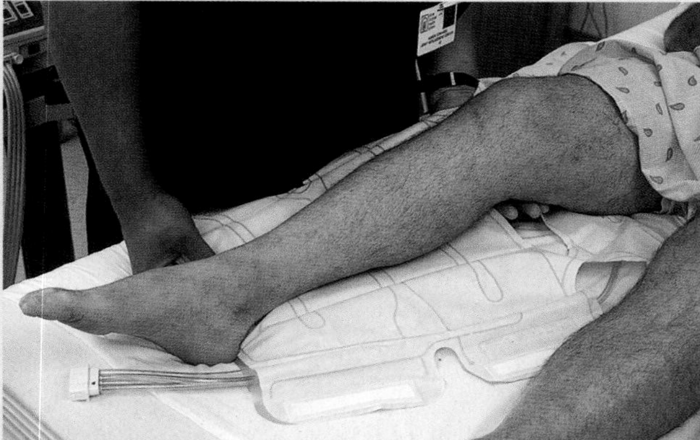

STEP 11d Position back of patient's knee with the popliteal opening.

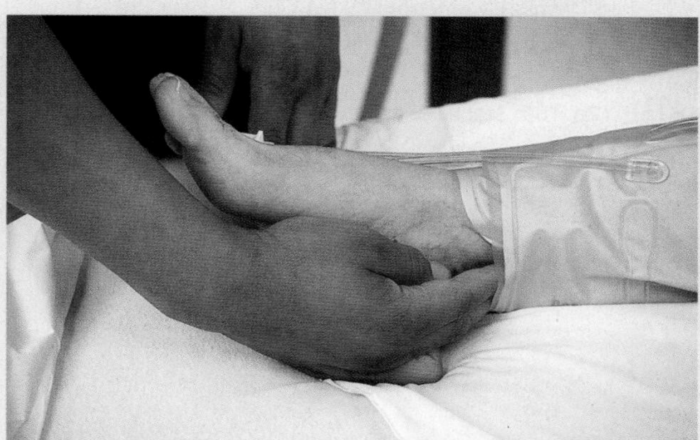

STEP 11e Check fit of SCD sleeve.

Continued

BOX 28-7 PROCEDURAL GUIDELINES

***Applying Sequential Compression Devices and Elastic Stockings*—cont'd**

f. Attach SCD sleeve connector to plug on mechanical unit. Arrows on connector line up with arrows on plug from unit (see illustration).
g. Turn mechanical unit on. Green light indicates that unit is functioning. Monitor functioning SCD through one full cycle of inflation and deflation. A typical cycle is inflation for 10 to 15 seconds and deflation for 45 to 60 seconds. Inflation pressures average 40 mm Hg.
h. Reposition patient for comfort and perform hand hygiene.
i. Remove compression stockings at least once per shift.
j. Monitor skin integrity and circulation to patient's lower extremities as ordered or as recommended by SCD manufacturer.

12. Apply Elastic Stocking:
    a. Turn elastic stocking inside out by placing one hand into the sock, holding toe of sock with hand. Using other hand, pull sock over hand until reaching the heel (see illustration).
    b. Place patient's toes into foot of elastic stocking, making sure that stocking is smooth (see illustration).
    c. Slide remaining portion of stocking over patient's foot, being sure that toes are covered. Make sure that foot fits into toe and heel position of stocking (see illustration).
    d. Slide stocking up over patient's calf until stocking is completely extended. Be sure that stocking is smooth and that no ridges or wrinkles are present, particularly behind knee (see illustration).
    e. Instruct patient not to roll stockings partially down because constricting ring around leg can occlude circulation.
    f. Instruct patient not to massage legs.
    g. Reposition patient for comfort and perform hand hygiene.
    h. Remove stockings at least once per shift.
    i. Inspect stockings for wrinkles or constriction.
    j. Inspect elastic stockings to determine that there are no wrinkles, rolls, or binding.

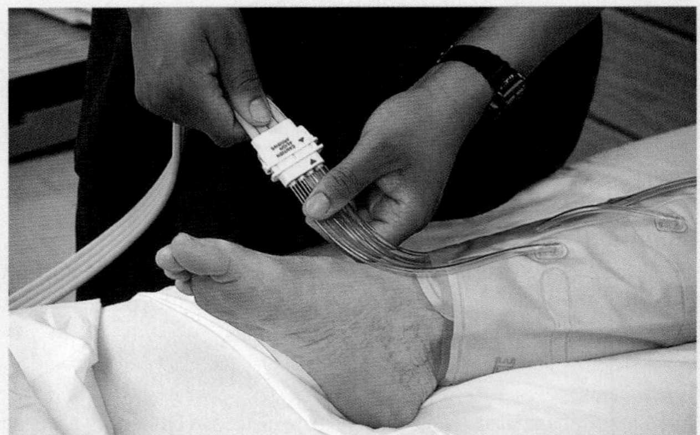

STEP 11f Align arrows when connecting SCD to mechanical unit.

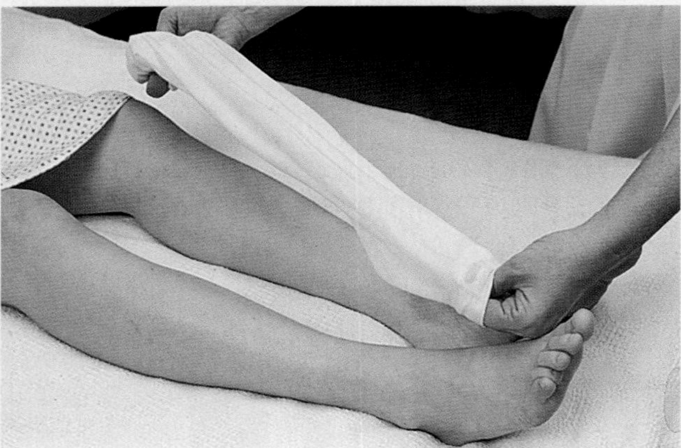

STEP 12a Turn stocking inside out: hold toe and pull through.

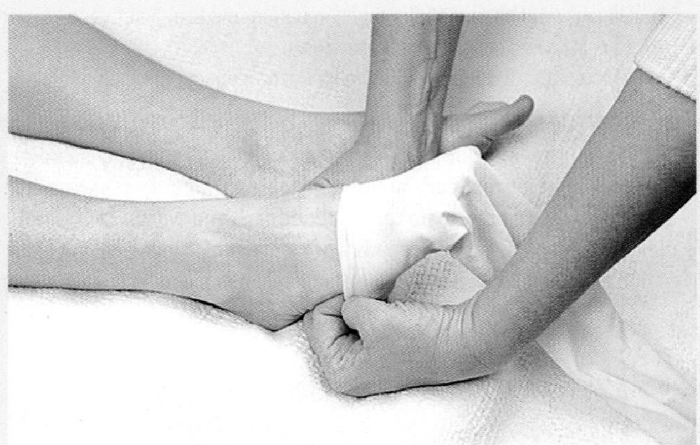

STEP 12b Place toes into foot of stocking.

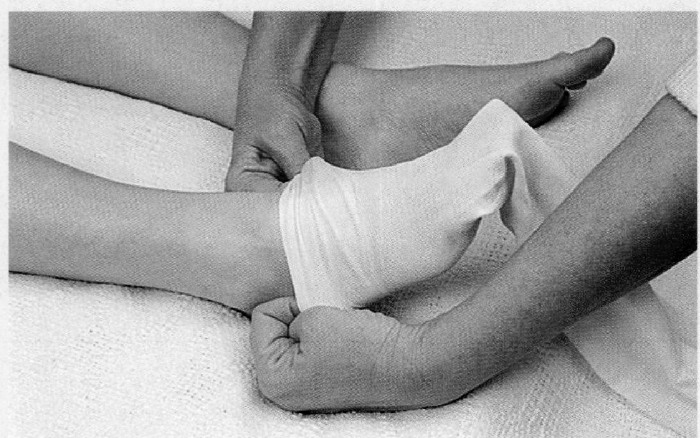

STEP 12c Slide remaining portion of stocking over foot.

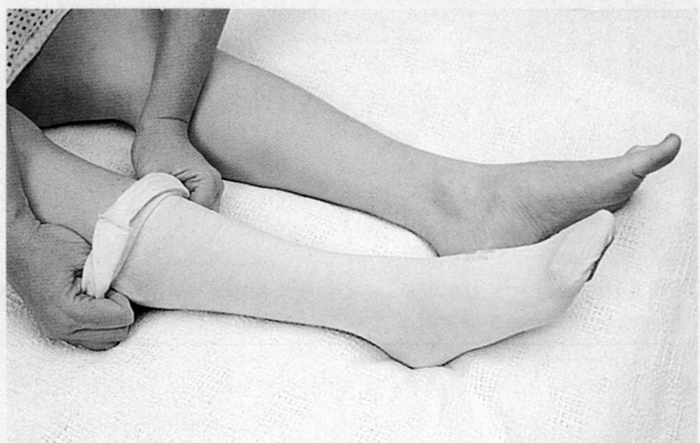

STEP 12d Slide stocking up leg until completely extended.

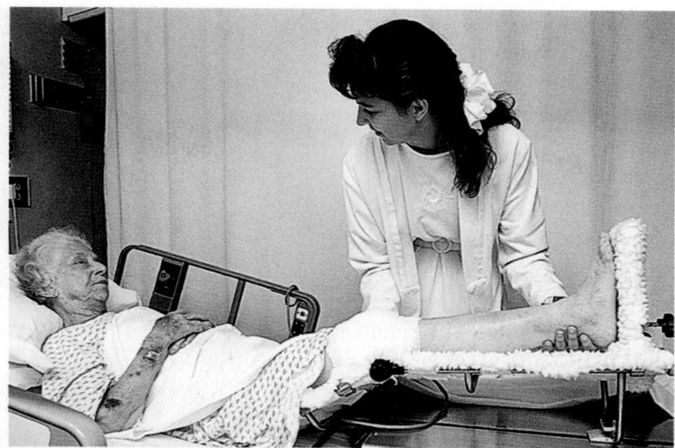

FIGURE 28-9 Continuous passive range-of-motion machine.

compromises circulation. Apply them properly and remove them at least once per shift. Be sure to assess circulation at the toes to ensure that the stockings are not too tight. Another device for preventing DVT is the venous plexus foot pump. It promotes circulation by mimicking the natural action of walking.

Proper positioning reduces a patient's risk of thrombus formation because compression of the leg veins is minimized. Therefore, when positioning patients, use caution to prevent pressure on the posterior knee and deep veins in the lower extremities. Teach patients to avoid the following: crossing the legs, sitting for prolonged periods of time, wearing clothing that constricts the legs or waist, and massaging the legs. Report suspected DVT immediately to the patient's health care provider. Elevate the leg but avoid pressure on the suspected thrombus area. Instruct the family, patient, and all health care personnel not to massage the area because of the danger of dislodging the thrombus.

ROM exercises reduce the risk of contractures and aid in preventing thrombi. Activity causes contraction of the skeletal muscles, which in turn exerts pressure on the veins to promote venous return, thereby reducing venous stasis. Specific exercises that help prevent thrombophlebitis are ankle pumps, foot circles, and knee flexion. Ankle pumps, sometimes called *calf pumps,* include alternating plantar flexion and dorsiflexion. Foot circles require the patient to rotate the ankle. Encourage patients to make the letters of the alphabet with their feet every 1 to 2 hours. Knee flexion involves alternately extending and flexing the knee. These exercises are sometimes referred to as *antiembolic exercises* and need to be done hourly while awake.

Musculoskeletal System. Exercises to prevent excessive muscle atrophy and joint contractures help maintain musculoskeletal function. If a patient is unable to move part or all of the body, perform passive ROM exercises for all immobilized joints while bathing the patient and at least 2 or 3 more times a day. If one extremity is paralyzed, teach the patient to put each joint independently through its ROM. Patients on bed rest need to have active ROM exercises incorporated into their daily schedules. Teach patients to also integrate exercises during ADLs.

Some orthopedic conditions require more frequent passive ROM exercises to restore the function of the injured joint after surgery. Patients with such conditions may use automatic equipment (continuous passive motion [CPM]) for passive ROM exercises) (Figure 28-9). The CPM machine moves an extremity to a prescribed angle for a prescribed period. Researchers continuously investigate uses for CPM. Patients who had a rotator cuff repair and received CPM therapy to their affected shoulder reported a decrease in pain in one study and improved muscle strength in another (DuPlessis et al., 2011). However, in a recent systematic review, CPM was shown to not have clinically important effects on active knee flexion, ROM, pain, function, or quality of life to justify its routine use for patients who undergo a total knee arthroplasty (Harvey, et al., 2014).

Integumentary System. The major risk to the skin from restricted mobility is the formation of pressure ulcers. Early identification of high-risk patients helps prevent pressure ulcers (see Chapter 48). Interventions aimed at prevention include turning and positioning and the use of therapeutic support surfaces to relieve pressure. Regular skin care (cleansing of soiled areas and use of moisturizers) aims to maintain the condition of the skin. Change the immobilized patient's position according to his or her activity level, perceptual ability, treatment protocols, and daily routines. For example, an obese patient or a very thin patient, both of whom have bowel incontinence, will require more frequent turning than standard practice. Although turning every 1 to 2 hours is standard practice for preventing ulcers, it is sometimes necessary to use support surface devices (e.g., air loss mattresses, heel boots, floatation mattresses) for relieving pressure.

Usually the time that a patient sits uninterrupted in a chair is limited to 1 hour. This interval is shortened in patients who are at very high risk for skin breakdown. Reposition patients frequently because uninterrupted pressure causes skin breakdown. Teach patients to shift their weight in a chair every 15 minutes. Chair-bound patients need to have a device for the chair that reduces pressure (Chou et al., 2013).

Elimination System. The nursing interventions for maintaining optimal urinary functioning are directed at keeping the patient well hydrated and preventing urinary stasis, calculi, and infections without causing bladder distention. Adequate hydration (e.g., at least 1100 to 1400 mL of noncaffeinated fluids daily) helps prevent renal calculi and urinary tract infections. The well-hydrated patient needs to void large amounts of dilute urine that is approximately equal to fluid intake. Also record the frequency and consistency of bowel movements. Provide a diet rich in fluids, fruits, vegetables, and fiber to facilitate normal peristalsis. If a patient is unable to maintain regular bowel patterns, stool softeners, cathartics, or enemas are sometimes necessary. If the patient is incontinent, modify the care plan to include toileting aids and a hygiene schedule so the increased urinary output does not cause skin breakdown.

Psychosocial Changes. Use assessment data to identify the psychosocial effects of prolonged immobilization. People who have a tendency toward depression or mood swings are at greater risk for developing psychosocial effects during bed rest or immobilization.

Anticipate changes in the patient's psychosocial status and provide routine and informal socialization. Observe the patient's ability to cope with restricted mobility. In institutional health care settings do not schedule nursing care activities between 10:00 PM and 7:00 AM to minimize sleep interruptions. For example, administer medications and assess vital signs when you enter the room to turn the patient or provide special skin care. If the nursing care plan is not improving coping patterns, consult a clinical nurse specialist, counselor, social worker, spiritual adviser, or other health care professional. Incorporate their recommendations into the care plan.

Nurses provide meaningful stimuli to maintain a patient's orientation. Plan nursing activities so a patient is able to talk and interact with staff. If possible, place him or her in a room with others who are mobile and interactive. If a private room is required, ask staff members to visit throughout the shift to provide meaningful interaction. A daily newspaper helps the patient keep track of events and time. Bedside conversations at appropriate moments familiarize him or her with nursing activities, meals, and visiting hours. Books help occupy the patient when he or she is alone. The patient can participate in craft activities. iPods, MP3 players, radio, television, and videotapes provide stimulation and help pass the time.

Involve patients in their care whenever possible. For example, encourage the patient to determine when the bed should be made. Some patients rest better during the night when fresh sheets are put on in the evening rather than in the morning. The patient needs to provide as much self-care as possible. Keep hygiene and grooming articles within easy reach. Encourage patients to wear their glasses or artificial teeth and shave or apply makeup. People use these activities to maintain their body image, thus improving their outlook.

Developmental Changes. Ideally immobilized patients continue normal development. Nursing interventions can help. Nursing care needs to provide mental and physical stimulation, particularly for a young child. Incorporate play activities into the care plan. For example, completing puzzles helps a child to develop fine-motor skills, and reading helps him or her develop cognitively. Encourage parents to stay with a child who is hospitalized. Place a child who is immobilized with children of the same age who are not immobilized unless a contagious disease is present. Allow the child to participate in nursing interventions such as dressing changes, cast care, and care of traction. The nurse needs to recognize significant changes from normal behavioral patterns and consult with a pediatric clinical nurse specialist, counselor, or other health care professional.

Restricted mobility of older patients presents unique nursing problems. Older patients who are frail or have chronic illnesses are often at increased risk for the psychosocial hazards of immobility. Maintaining a calendar and clock with a large dial, conversing about current events and family members, and encouraging visits from significant others reduce the risk of social isolation. Spending time in the room talking and listening to the patient also helps reduce the risk of social isolation.

Nurses need to encourage older immobilized patients to perform as many ADLs as independently as possible. Patients need to continue to perform personal grooming if they did so before their mobility was restricted. This type of activity preserves the patient's dignity and gives him or her a sense of accomplishment.

Positioning Techniques. Patients with impaired nervous, skeletal, or muscular system functioning and increased weakness and fatigue often require help from nurses for positioning and maintenance of proper body alignment while in bed or sitting (see Skill 28-1 on pp. 432-438). Several positioning devices are available for maintaining good body alignment for patients. Pillows are positioning aids and are sometimes readily available. Before using a pillow, determine whether it is the proper size. A thick pillow under a patient's head increases cervical flexion, which is not desirable. A thin pillow under bony prominences does not protect skin and tissue from damage caused by pressure. When additional pillows are unavailable or if they are an improper size, use folded sheets, blankets, or towels as positioning aids.

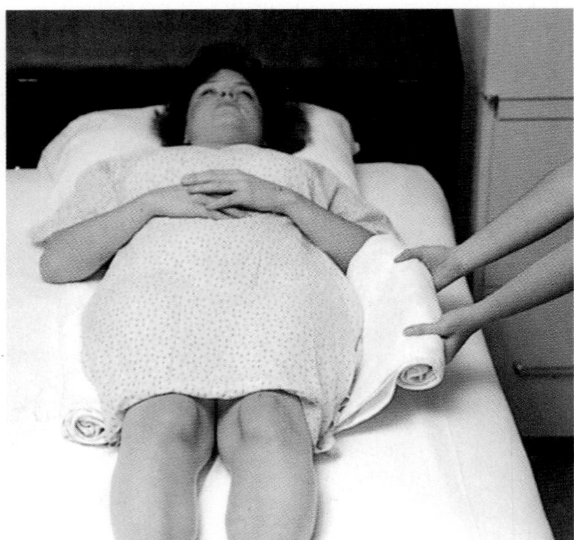

FIGURE 28-10 Trochanter roll.

Apply positioning boots to prevent footdrop by maintaining the feet in dorsiflexion. Ankle-foot orthotic (AFO) devices also help maintain dorsiflexion. Patients who wear positioning boots or AFOs need to have these removed periodically (e.g., 2 hours on, 2 hours off).

A **trochanter roll** prevents external rotation of the hips when a patient is in a supine position. To form a trochanter roll, fold a cotton bath blanket lengthwise to a width that extends from the greater trochanter of the femur to the lower border of the popliteal space (Figure 28-10). Place the blanket under the buttocks and roll it counterclockwise until the thigh is in neutral position or inward rotation. When the hip is aligned correctly, the patella faces directly upward. Use sandbags in place of or in addition to trochanter rolls. Sandbags are sand-filled plastic tubes or bags that are shaped to body contours. Hand rolls maintain the thumb in slight adduction and in opposition to the fingers, which maintain a functional position. Evaluate the hand roll to make sure that the hand is indeed in a functional position. Hand rolls are most often used with patients whose arms are paralyzed or who are unconscious. Do not use rolled washcloths as hand rolls because they do not keep the thumb well abducted, especially in patients who have a spastic paralysis. Hand-wrist splints are individually molded for a patient to maintain proper alignment of the thumb (slight adduction) and wrist (slight dorsiflexion). Use splints only on the patient for whom they were made and follow the splint schedule (e.g., wear for 2 hours, remove for 2 hours).

The **trapeze bar** is a triangular device that hangs down from a securely fastened overhead bar that is attached to the bedframe. It allows a patient to pull with the upper extremities to raise the trunk off the bed, assist in transfer from bed to wheelchair, or perform upper-arm exercises (Figure 28-11). It increases independence, maintains upper-body strength, and decreases the shearing action from sliding across or up and down in bed.

Although each procedure for positioning has specific guidelines, there are universal steps to follow for patients who require positioning assistance. Following the guidelines reduces the risk of injury to the musculoskeletal system when a patient is sitting or lying. When joints

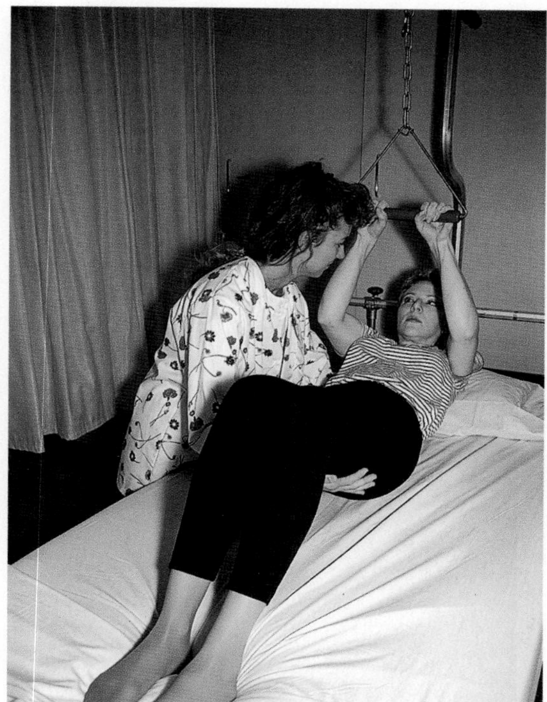

FIGURE 28-11 Patient using trapeze bar.

are unsupported, their alignment is impaired. Likewise, if joints are not positioned in a slightly flexed position, their mobility is decreased. During positioning also assess for pressure points. When actual or potential pressure areas exist, nursing interventions involve removal of the pressure, thus decreasing the risk for development of pressure ulcers and further trauma to the musculoskeletal system. In these patients use the 30-degree lateral position.

Supported Fowler's Position. In the supported Fowler's position the head of the bed is elevated 45 to 60 degrees, and the patient's knees are slightly elevated without pressure to restrict circulation in the lower legs. The patient's illness and overall condition influence the angle of head and knee elevation and the length of time that the patient needs to remain in the supported Fowler's position. Supports need to permit flexion of the hips and knees and proper alignment of the normal curves in the cervical, thoracic, and lumbar vertebrae. The following are common trouble areas for a patient in the supported Fowler's position:

- Increased cervical flexion because the pillow at the head is too thick and the head thrusts forward
- Extension of the knees, allowing the patient to slide to the foot of the bed
- Pressure on the posterior aspect of the knees, decreasing circulation to the feet
- External rotation of the hips
- Arms hanging unsupported at the patient's sides
- Unsupported feet or pressure on the heels
- Unprotected pressure points at the sacrum and heels
- Increased shearing force on the back and heels when the head of the bed is raised greater than 60 degrees

Supine Position. Patients in the supine position rest on their backs. In the supine position the relationship of body parts is essentially the same as in good standing alignment, except that the body is in the horizontal plane. Use pillows, trochanter rolls, and hand rolls or arm splints to increase comfort and reduce injury to the skin or musculoskeletal system. The mattress needs to be firm enough to support the cervical, thoracic, and lumbar vertebrae. Shoulders are supported, and the elbows are slightly flexed to control shoulder rotation. A foot support prevents footdrop and maintains proper alignment. The following are some common trouble areas for patients in the supine position:

- Pillow at the head that is too thick, increasing cervical flexion
- Head flat on the mattress
- Shoulders unsupported and internally rotated
- Elbows extended
- Thumb not in opposition to the fingers
- Hips externally rotated
- Unsupported feet
- Unprotected pressure points at the occipital region of the head, vertebrae, coccyx, elbows, and heels

Prone Position. The patient in the prone position lies face or chest down. Often his or her head is turned to the side; but, if a pillow is under the head, it needs to be thin enough to prevent cervical flexion or extension and maintain alignment of the lumbar spine. Placing a pillow under the lower leg permits dorsiflexion of the ankles and some knee flexion, which promote relaxation. If a pillow is unavailable, the ankles need to be in dorsiflexion over the end of the mattress. Although the prone position is seldom used in practice, consider this as an alternative, especially in patients who normally sleep in this position. The prone position also may have some benefits in patients with acute respiratory distress syndrome and acute lung injury (Barbas et al., 2012). Specialty beds that safely position acutely ill patients in the prone position are available. Assess for and correct any of the following potential trouble points with patients in the prone position:

- Neck hyperextension
- Hyperextension of the lumbar spine
- Plantar flexion of the ankles
- Unprotected pressure points at the chin, elbows, female breasts, hips, knees, and toes

Side-Lying Position. In the side-lying (or lateral) position the patient rests on the side with the major portion of body weight on the dependent hip and shoulder. A 30-degree lateral position is recommended for patients at risk for pressure ulcers (see Chapter 48) (Chou et al., 2013). Trunk alignment needs to be the same as in standing. The patient needs to maintain the structural curves of the spine, the head needs to be supported in line with the midline of the trunk, and rotation of the spine needs to be avoided. The following trouble points are common in the side-lying position:

- Lateral flexion of the neck
- Spinal curves out of normal alignment
- Shoulder and hip joints internally rotated, adducted, or unsupported
- Lack of foot support
- Lack of protection for pressure points at the ear, shoulder, anterior iliac spine, trochanter, and ankles
- Excessive lateral flexion of the spine if the patient has large hips and a pillow is not placed superior to the hips at the waist

Sims' Position. Sims' position differs from the side-lying position in the distribution of the patient's weight. In Sims' position the patient places the weight on the anterior ileum, humerus, and clavicle. Trouble points common in Sims' position include the following:

- Lateral flexion of the neck
- Internal rotation, adduction, or lack of support to the shoulders and hips
- Lack of foot support
- Lack of protection for pressure points at the ileum, humerus, clavicle, knees, and ankles

Moving Patients. When moving a patient during repositioning, a safe transfer is the first priority. Patients require various levels of assistance to move up in bed, move to the side-lying position, or sit up at the side of the bed. For example, a young, healthy woman may need support as she sits at the side of the bed for the first time after childbirth, whereas an older man may need help from two or more nurses to do the same task 1 to 2 days after surgery.

Always ask patients to help to their fullest extent possible. To determine what a patient is able to do alone and how many people are needed to help move him or her in bed, assess him or her to determine whether the illness contradicts exertion (e.g., cardiovascular disease). Next determine whether the patient comprehends what is expected. For example, a patient recently medicated for postoperative pain is too lethargic to understand instructions; thus to ensure safety two nurses are necessary to move him or her. Then determine his or her comfort level. It is important to evaluate your personal strength and knowledge of the procedure. Finally determine whether the patient is too heavy or immobile for you to move alone (VISN8, 2015) (see Chapter 39).

Restorative and Continuing Care. The goal of restorative care for the patient who is immobile is to maximize functional mobility and independence and reduce residual functional deficits such as impaired gait and decreased endurance. The focus in restorative care is not only on ADLs that relate to physical self-care but also on instrumental activities of daily living (IADLs). IADLs are activities that are necessary to be independent in society beyond eating, grooming, transferring, and toileting and include such skills as shopping, preparing meals, banking, and taking medications.

Nurses use many of the same interventions as described in the health promotion and acute care sections, but the emphasis is on working collaboratively with patients and their significant others and with other health care professionals to facilitate the patient's return to maximal functional ability in both ADLs and IADLs.

Intensive specialized therapy such as occupational or physical therapy is common. If the patient is in a rehabilitation institution, he or she likely goes to the therapy department 2 to 3 times a day. The nurse's role is to work collaboratively with these professionals and reinforce exercises and teaching. For example, after a stroke, a patient likely receives gait training from a physical therapist; speech rehabilitation from a speech therapist; and help from an occupational therapist for ADLs such as dressing, bathing and toileting, or household chores. The therapy is not always able to restore total functional health, but it often helps the patient adapt to the mobility limitations or complications. Equipment frequently used to help patients adapt to mobility limitations includes walkers, canes, wheelchairs, and assistive devices such as toilet seat extenders, reaching sticks, special silverware, and clothing with Velcro closures.

Range-of-Motion Exercises. To ensure adequate joint mobility, teach the patient about ROM exercises. Walking also increases joint mobility. Patients with restricted mobility are unable to perform some or all ROM exercises independently. Provide ROM exercises to maintain maximum joint mobility. To ensure that patients routinely receive ROM exercises, schedule them at specific times, perhaps with another nursing activity such as during the patient's bath. This enables the nurse to systematically reassess mobility while improving the patient's ROM. In addition, bathing usually requires that extremities and joints are put through complete ROM.

Passive ROM exercises begin as soon as a patient's ability to move an extremity or joint is lost. Carry out movements slowly and smoothly, just to the point of resistance; ROM should not cause pain. **Never force a joint beyond its capacity.** Each movement needs to be repeated 5 times during a session.

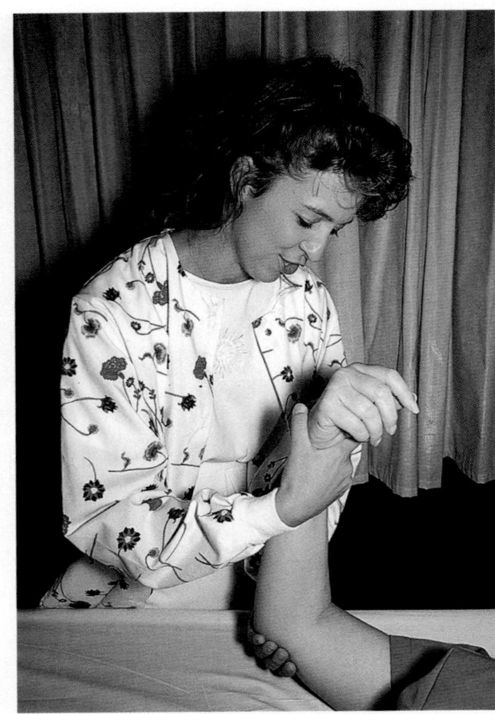

FIGURE 28-12 Supporting joint by holding distal and proximal areas adjacent to joint.

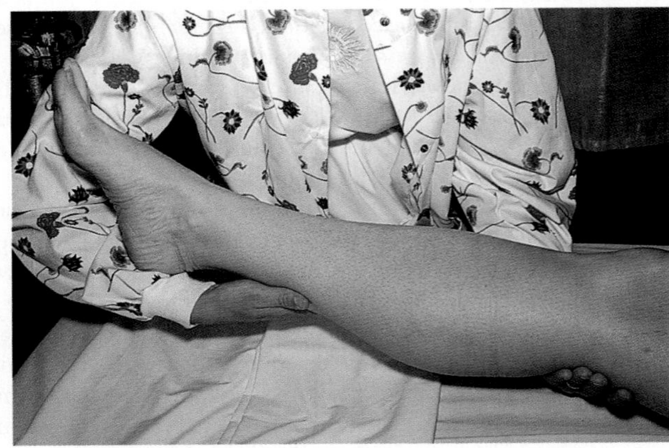

FIGURE 28-13 Cradling distal portion of extremity.

When performing passive ROM exercises, stand at the side of the bed closest to the joint being exercised. Use a head-to-toe sequence and move from larger to smaller joints. If an extremity is to be moved or lifted, place a cupped hand under the joint to support it, support the joint by holding the adjacent distal and proximal areas (Figure 28-12), or support the joint with one hand and cradle the distal portion of the extremity with the remaining arm (Figure 28-13). See Table 28-2 for detailed ROM for each joint. Appropriate ROM exercises are based on the patient and the affected joint.

Walking. When a patient has a limited ability to walk, assess his or her activity tolerance, tolerance to the upright position (orthostatic hypotension), strength, the presence of pain, coordination, and balance to determine the amount of assistance needed. Explain how far the

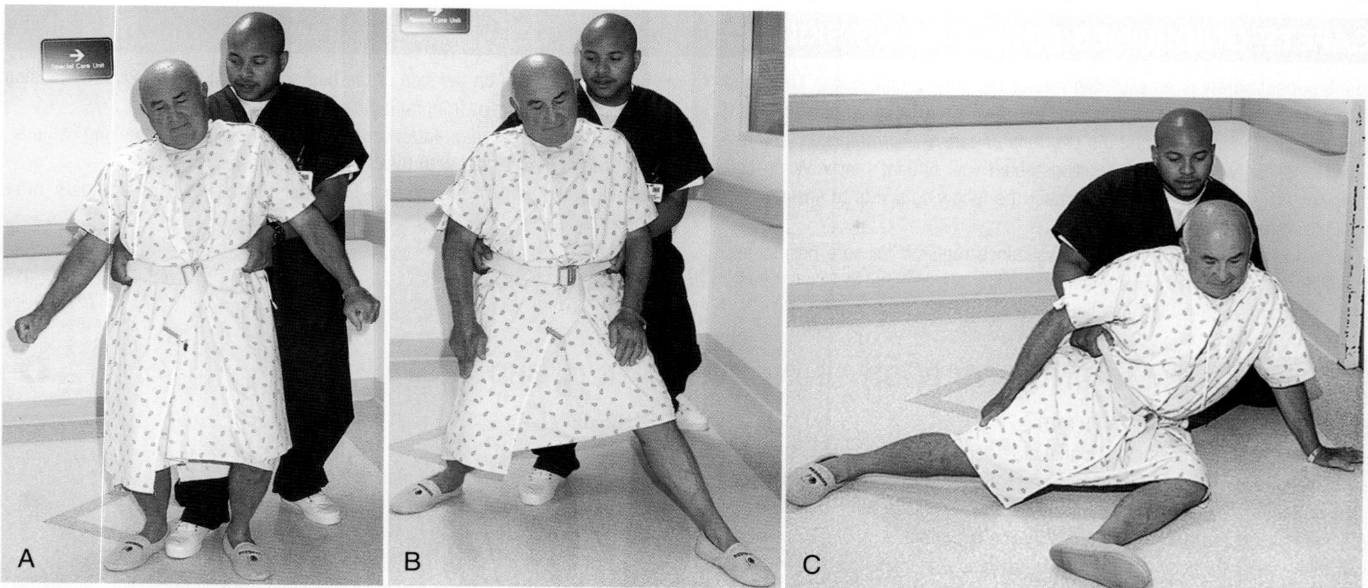

FIGURE 28-14 **A,** Stand with feet apart to provide broad base of support. **B,** Extend one leg and let patient slide against it to the floor. **C,** Bend knees to lower body as patient slides to floor.

patient should try to walk, who is going to help, when the walk will take place, and why walking is important. Some settings have distances marked along hallways to measure a patient's progress. Other facilities use accelerometers to measure distance walked. In addition, determine with the patient how much independence he or she can assume.

Check the environment to be sure that there are no obstacles in the patient's path. Clear chairs, over-bed tables, and wheelchairs out of the way so the patient has ample room to walk safely. Before starting, establish rest points in case activity tolerance is less than estimated or the patient becomes dizzy. For example, place a chair in the hall for the patient to rest if needed. A nurse who does not have a lot of strength and who is unable to ambulate a patient alone needs to request help and ensure that the patient has an assistive device such as a walker (see Chapter 39). A nurse stands on either side of the patient, and each holds one side of the gait belt.

Provide support at the waist by using a **gait belt** so the patient's center of gravity remains midline. While walking, the patient should not lean to one side because this alters the center of gravity, distorts balance, and increases the risk of falling. Return a patient who at any point appears unsteady or complains of dizziness to a nearby bed or chair. If the patient faints or begins to fall, assume a wide base of support with one foot in front of the other, thus supporting the body weight (Figure 28-14, *A, B, C*). Then gently lower the patient to the floor, protecting the head. Although lowering a patient to the floor is not difficult, the nursing student needs to practice this technique with a friend or classmate before attempting it in a clinical setting.

Patients with **hemiplegia** (one-sided paralysis) or **hemiparesis** (one-sided weakness) often need assistance with walking. When an assistive device is used, stand on the patient's affected side and support him or her with a gait belt. Providing support by holding the patient's arm is incorrect because the nurse cannot easily support the patient's weight to lower him or her to the floor if he or she faints or falls. In addition, if the patient falls with the nurse holding an arm, a shoulder joint may be dislocated.

◆ Evaluation

Through the Patient's Eyes. Just as it was important to include the patient during the assessment and planning phase of the care plan, it is essential to have the patient's evaluation of the plan of care. Were the goals met, or is more work required? You must now determine with the patient and others involved with care if the goals or outcomes established with and for the patient have indeed been met; what still needs to be achieved from the patient's perspective; and whether it is necessary to revise a new plan of care. In other words, how have the patient's expectations changed and in what ways?

Patient Outcomes. From your perspective as the nurse, you are to evaluate expected outcomes and a patient's response to nursing care and compare the patient's actual outcomes with the outcomes selected during planning such as his or her ability to maintain or improve body alignment, joint mobility, walking, moving, or transferring. Evaluate the effectiveness of specific interventions designed to promote body alignment, improve mobility, and protect the patient from the hazards of immobility. Evaluate the patient's and family's understanding of all teaching provided as well. The continuous nature of evaluation allows you to determine whether new or revised therapies are required and if new nursing diagnoses have developed.

When outcomes are not met, consider asking the following questions:

- Are there ways we can assist you to increase your activity?
- Which activities are you having trouble completing right now?
- How do you feel about not being able to dress yourself and make your own meals?
- Which exercises do you find most helpful?
- What goals for your activity would you like to set now?

Once these questions have been asked and you have addressed the limited mobility and its associated problems through the patient's eyes, you are prepared to adjust the plan of care to address the remaining clinical problems that your patient is experiencing related to immobility.

SAFETY GUIDELINES FOR NURSING SKILLS

Ensuring patient safety is an essential role of the professional nurse. To ensure patient safety, communicate clearly with the members of the health care team, assess and incorporate the patient's priorities of care and preferences, and use the best evidence when making decisions about your patient's care. When performing the skills in this chapter, remember the following points to ensure safe, individualized patient-centered care.

- Determine the amount and type of assistance required for safe positioning, including any transfer equipment and the number of personnel to safely transfer and prevent harm to patient and health care providers.
- Raise the side rail on the side of the bed opposite of where you are standing to prevent the patient from falling out of bed on that side.
- Arrange equipment (e.g., intravenous lines, feeding tube, indwelling catheter) so it does not interfere with the positioning process.
- Evaluate the patient for correct body alignment and pressure risks after repositioning.

SKILL 28-1 MOVING AND POSITIONING PATIENTS IN BED 

DELEGATION CONSIDERATIONS

The skill of moving and positioning patients in bed can be delegated to nursing assistive personnel (NAP). The nurse is responsible for assessing the patient's level of comfort and for any hazards of immobility. Instruct NAP about:

- Any moving and positioning imitations unique to patient.
- Individual needs for body alignment (e.g., patient with spinal cord injury).
- Scheduled times to reposition patient through the shift.
- When to request assistance (e.g., if the patient has a spinal cord injury, when the patient is unable to assist the nurse, has a lot of equipment, or is confused).

EQUIPMENT

- Pillows, drawsheet
- Therapeutic boots, splints if needed
- Trochanter roll
- Hand rolls
- Side rails
- Appropriate safe patient–handling assistive device (e.g., friction-reducing device)

STEP	RATIONALE
ASSESSMENT	
1. Identify patient using two identifiers (e.g., name and birthday or name and medical record number), according to agency policy.	Ensures correct patient. Complies with The Joint Commission standards and improves patient safety (TJC, 2016).
2. Assess patient's body alignment and comfort level while he or she is lying down.	Provides baseline data for later comparisons. Determines ways to improve position and alignment.
3. Assess for risk factors that contribute to complications of immobility:	Increased risk factors require more frequent repositioning.
a. Paralysis, hemiparesis resulting from a cerebrovascular accident (CVA); decreased sensation	Paralysis impairs movement; muscle tone changes; sensation is often affected. Because of difficulty in moving and poor awareness of involved body part, patient is unable to protect and position body part for self (Lewis et al., 2013).
b. Impaired mobility from traction, arthritis, or other contributing disease processes	Traction or arthritic changes of affected extremity result in decreased range of motion (ROM).
c. Impaired circulation	Decreased circulation to skin and underlying tissue predisposes patient to pressure ulcers.
d. *Age:* Very young, older adults	Premature and young infants require frequent turning because their skin is fragile. Normal physiological changes associated with aging predispose older adults to greater risks for developing complications of immobility (Drake et al., 2012).
e. *Sensation:* Decreased from CVA, paralysis, neuropathy.	Because of poor awareness of body part or reduced sensation, patient is unable to protect and position body part from pressure.
f. Level of consciousness and mental status	Determines need for special aids or devices. Patients with altered levels of consciousness may not understand instructions or be able to help during positioning.
4. Assess patient's physical ability to help with moving and positioning:	Enables nurse to use patient's mobility, coordination, and strength; determines need for additional help. Ensures patient's and nurse's safety (VISN8, 2015).
a. Age	Some older adults move more slowly with less strength.
b. Disease process	Cardiopulmonary disease requires patient to have head of bed elevated.
c. Strength, coordination	Determines amount of assistance provided by patient during position change.
d. ROM	Limited ROM contraindicates certain positions.
5. Assess patient's height, weight, and body shape.	Devices used for safe patient handling have different weight restrictions; bariatric patients require special beds, lifts, wheelchairs, and toileting and bathing equipment (Pierson and Fairchild, 2013).
6. Assess health care provider's orders before positioning. Clarify whether any positions are contraindicated because of patient's condition (e.g., spinal cord injury; respiratory difficulties; certain neurological conditions; presence of incisions, drains, and tubing).	Placing patient in an inappropriate position causes injury.
7. Assess for presence of tubes, incisions, and equipment (e.g., traction).	Alters positioning procedure and affects patient's ability to independently change positions.

STEP	RATIONALE
8. Assess condition of patient's skin (see Chapter 31).	Provides baseline to determine effects of positioning.
9. Assess ability and motivation of patient and family caregivers to participate in moving and positioning patient in bed in anticipation of discharge to home.	Determines ability of patient and caregivers to help with positioning.
PLANNING	
1. Collect appropriate equipment. Get extra help as needed. Close door to room or bedside curtains.	Having appropriate number of people to position patient prevents patient and nurse injury. Provides for patient privacy.
2. Perform hand hygiene.	Reduces transfer of microorganisms.
3. Raise level of bed to comfortable working height. Remove all pillows and devices used for positioning.	Raises work toward nurse's center of gravity. Reduces any interference during positioning.
4. Explain procedure to patient.	Helps to relieve anxiety and allows patient to participate more actively.
IMPLEMENTATION	
1. Assist Patient in Moving Up in Bed	
a. ***Can patient assist?***	Determines degree of risk in repositioning patient and technique required to safely assist patient.
(1) Fully able to assist, nurse assistance not needed; nurse stands by to assist.	
(2) Partially able to assist; patient can assist with nurse using positioning cues or aids (e.g., drawsheet or friction-reducing device).	
CLINICAL DECISION: *Before lowering head of bed to flatten bed, account for all tubing, drains, and equipment to prevent dislodgement or tipping if caught in mattress or bedframe as bed is lowered.*	
b. ***Assist patient moving up in bed, using a drawsheet (two or three nurses).***	This is not a one-person task. Helping a patient move up in bed without help from other co-workers or without the aid of an assistive device (i.e., friction-reducing pad) is not recommended or considered safe for the patient or nurse (ANA, 2010; CDC, 2009). If the patient is unable to fully assist, refer to Step 1c.
(1) Place patient supine with head of bed flat. A nurse stands on each side of bed.	Enables nurse to assess body alignment. Reduces pull of gravity on patient's upper body.
(2) Remove pillow from under head and shoulders and place it at head of bed.	Prevents striking patient's head against head of bed.
(3) Turn patient side to side to place drawsheet under patient, extending from shoulders to thighs.	Supports patient's body weight and reduces friction during movement.
(4) Return patient to supine position.	Even distribution of patient's weight makes lifting and positioning easier.
(5) Fanfold drawsheet on both sides, with each nurse grasping firmly near patient.	Provides strong handles to grip drawsheet without slipping.
CLINICAL DECISION: *Protect patient's heels from shearing force by having a third nurse lift heels while moving patient up in bed.*	
(6) Nurses place their feet apart with forward-backward stance. Flex knees and hips. On the count of three, shift weight from front to back leg and move patient and drawsheet to desired position in bed (see illustration).	Facing direction of movement ensures proper balance. Shifting weight reduces force needed to move load. Flexing knees lowers center of gravity and uses thigh muscles instead of back muscles.

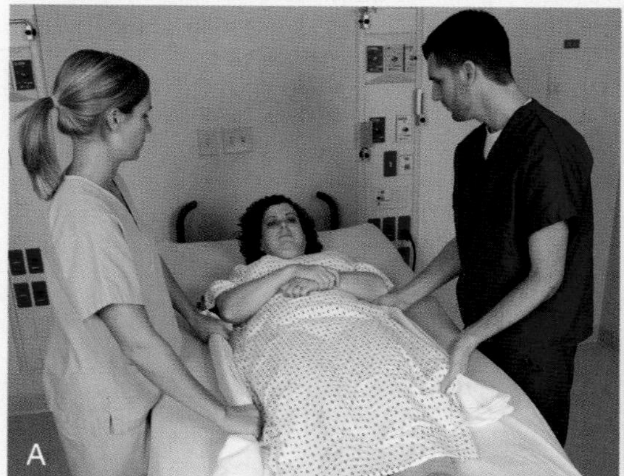
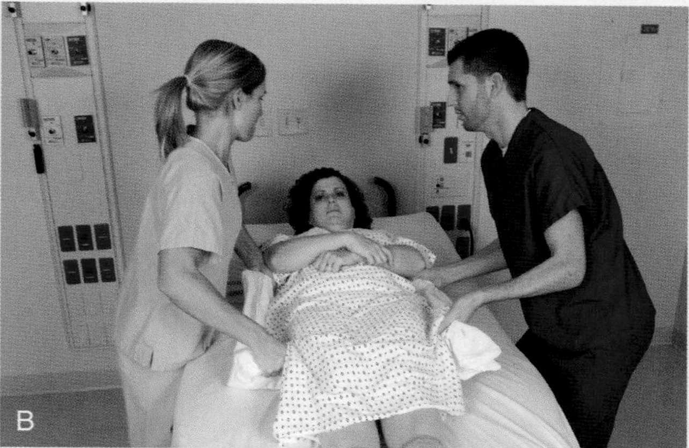

STEP 1b(6) A and **B,** Moving immobile patient up in bed with drawsheet.

SKILL 28-1 MOVING AND POSITIONING PATIENTS IN BED—cont'd

STEP	RATIONALE
c. ***Assist moving up in bed using a friction-reducing device (three nurses assist).***	Patients weighing less than 200 pounds require at least three nurses; patients over 200 pounds require mechanical assist device.
(1) Position patient as in Steps 1b (1-3).	Prepares patient for placement of friction-reducing device.
(2) With patient already on side, place friction-reducing device under drawsheet and then have patient turn over to other side.	Prevents friction from contact of skin with board.
(3) Move patient up in bed by having two nurses grasp drawsheet and one hold on to friction-reducing device. Follow Steps 1b(5-6), moving patient up in bed.	The slide board remains stationary, provides a slippery surface to reduce friction, and allows the patient to move easily up in bed.
2. Position patient in one of the following positions using correct body alignment to protect pressure areas. Begin with patient lying supine and move up in bed following either Steps 1b or 1c.	Prevents injury to the patient's musculoskeletal system
a. ***Positioning patient in supported Fowler's position (see illustration):***	
(1) With patient supine, elevate head of bed 45 to 60 degrees if not contraindicated.	Increases comfort, improves ventilation, and increases patient's opportunity to socialize or relax.
(2) Rest head against mattress or on small pillow.	Prevents flexion contractures of cervical vertebrae.
(3) Use pillows to support arms and hands if patient does not have voluntary control or use of hands and arms.	Prevents shoulder dislocation from effect of downward pull of unsupported arms, promotes circulation by preventing venous pooling, and prevents flexion contractures of arms and wrists.
(4) Position small pillow at lower back.	Supports lumbar vertebrae and decreases flexion of vertebrae.
(5) Place small pillow under thigh. Support calves with pillows.	Prevents hyperextension of knee and occlusion of popliteal artery from pressure from body weight. Heels should not be in contact with bed to prevent prolonged pressure of mattress on heels. This is sometimes referred to as "floating" heels.
(6) *Option:* Use a heel pressure–relieving device (pillow or heel boot).	Pressure on the heels must be relieved by off-loading, which is done by regular repositioning or using a purpose-made pressure-relieving device. When pillows are used, they must be repositioned each time the patient moves (Bangova, 2013).

CLINICAL DECISION: *To keep feet in proper alignment and prevent footdrop, use foot support devices (check agency policy). In addition, a foot cradle is often used for patients with poor peripheral circulation as a means of reducing pressure on the tips of patient's toes.*

STEP	RATIONALE
b. ***Positioning hemiplegic patient in supported Fowler's position:***	
(1) Elevate head of bed 45 to 60 degrees. Adjust head of bed according to patient's condition. For example, those with increased risk of pressure ulcers remain at 30-degree angle (semi-Fowler's) (see Chapter 48).	Increases comfort, improves ventilation, and increases patient's opportunity to relax.
(2) Position patient in sitting position as straight as possible.	Counteracts tendency to slump toward affected side. Improves ventilation and cardiac output; decreases intracranial pressure. Improves patient's ability to swallow and helps to prevent aspiration of food, liquids, and gastric secretions.
(3) Position head on small pillow with chin slightly forward. If patient is totally unable to control head movement, avoid hyperextension of neck.	Prevents hyperextension of neck. Too many pillows under head cause or worsen neck flexion contracture.
(4) Provide support for involved arm and hand on overbed table in front of patient. Place arm away from patient's side and support elbow with pillow.	Paralyzed muscles do not automatically resist pull of gravity as they do normally. As a result, shoulder subluxation, pain, and edema may occur.

CLINICAL DECISION:

- *Position flaccid hand in normal resting position with wrist slightly extended, arches of hand maintained, and fingers partially flexed; use section of rubber ball cut in half; clasp patient's hands together.*
- *Position spastic hand with wrist in neutral position or slightly extended; extend fingers with palm down or leave them in relaxed position palm up. At times it is difficult to position spastic hands without the use of specially made splints for the patient.*

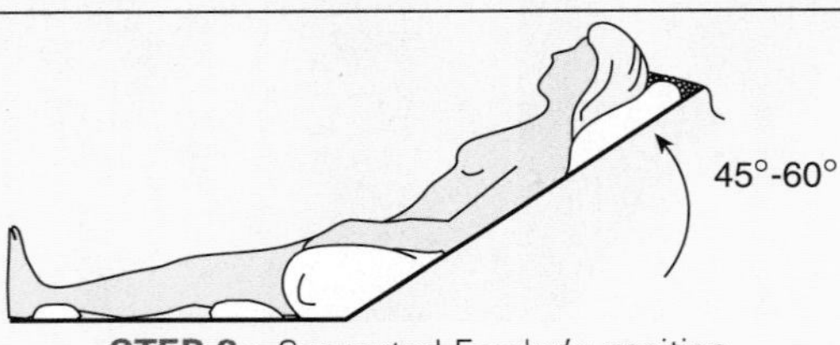

STEP 2a Supported Fowler's position.

STEP	RATIONALE
(5) Place trochanter rolls (rolled blanket) alongside of patient's legs.	Reduces external rotation of hip.
(6) If needed, support feet in dorsiflexion with therapeutic boots or splints (check agency policy) (see illustration).	Maintains foot in dorsiflexion and prevents footdrop. Pillows prevent stimulation to ball of foot by hard surface, which has a tendency to increase muscle tone in patient with extensor spasticity of lower extremity.
c. *Positioning patient in supported supine position:*	
(1) Be sure that patient is comfortable on back with head of bed flat.	Some patients' physical conditions do not tolerate supine position.
(2) Place small rolled towel under lumbar area of back.	Provides support for lumbar spine.
(3) Place pillow under upper shoulders, neck, or head.	Maintains correct alignment and prevents flexion contractures of cervical vertebrae.
(4) Place trochanter rolls or sandbags parallel to lateral surface of patient's thighs if patient is immobile.	Reduces external rotation of hip.
(5) Position patient's heels in heel boots or other heel pressure-relief device (check agency policy).	Heel pressure-relief devices are more effective than pillows for consistently reducing pressure from the mattress on the heels.
(6) If needed, support feet in dorsiflexion with foot support devices (check agency policy).	Maintains foot in dorsiflexion and prevents footdrop. Pillows prevent stimulation to ball of foot by hard surface, which has tendency to increase muscle tone in patient with extensor spasticity of lower extremity.
(7) Place pillows under pronated forearms, keeping upper arms parallel to patient's body (see illustration).	Reduces internal rotation of shoulder and prevents extension of elbows. Maintains correct body alignment.
(8) Place hand rolls in patient's hands. Consider physical therapy referral for use of hand splints.	Reduces extension of fingers and abduction of thumb. Maintains thumb slightly adducted and in opposition to fingers.
d. *Positioning hemiplegic patient in supine position:*	
(1) Be sure that patient is comfortable on back with head of bed flat.	Some patients' physical conditions do not tolerate supine position.
(2) Place folded towel or small pillow under shoulder of affected side.	Decreases possibility of pain, joint contracture, and subluxation. Maintains mobility in muscles around shoulder to permit normal movement patterns.
(3) Keep affected arm away from body with elbow extended and palm up. (Alternate position is to place arm out to side, with elbow bent and hand toward head of bed.)	Maintains mobility in arm, joints, and shoulder to permit normal movement patterns. (Alternate position counteracts limitation of ability of arm to rotate outward at shoulder [external rotation]. Need external rotation to raise arm overhead without pain.)

CLINICAL DECISION: *Position affected hand in one of the recommended positions for flaccid or spastic hand.*

STEP	RATIONALE
(4) Place folded towel under hip of involved side.	Diminishes effect of spasticity in entire leg by controlling hip position.
(5) Flex affected knee 30 degrees by supporting it on pillow or folded blanket.	Slight flexion breaks up abnormal extension pattern of leg. Extensor spasticity is most severe when patient is supine.
(6) If needed, support feet in dorsiflexion with foot support devices (check agency policy).	Maintains foot in dorsiflexion and prevents footdrop. Pillows prevent stimulation to ball of foot by hard surface, which has tendency to increase muscle tone in patient with extensor spasticity of lower extremity.
e. *Positioning patient in prone position, using two to three nurses:*	In certain patients with pulmonary conditions such as acute respiratory distress syndrome, the use of the prone position can help improve oxygenation.
(1) With head of bed flat and one nurse standing on each side of bed, roll patient to one side while placing arm on side to be turned along side of body.	Prepares patient for positioning.

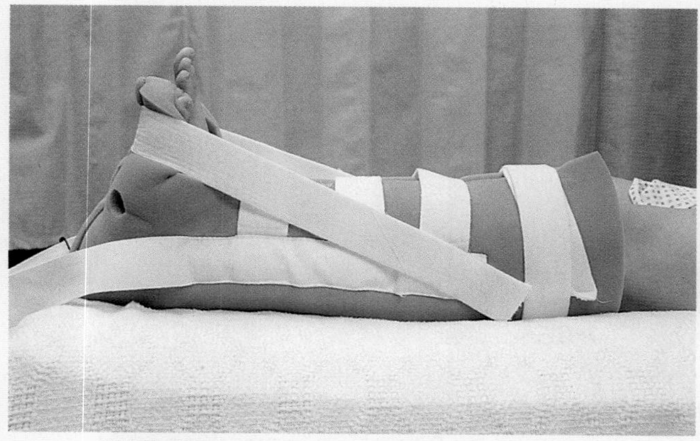

STEP 2b(6) Foot boot with lower leg extension.

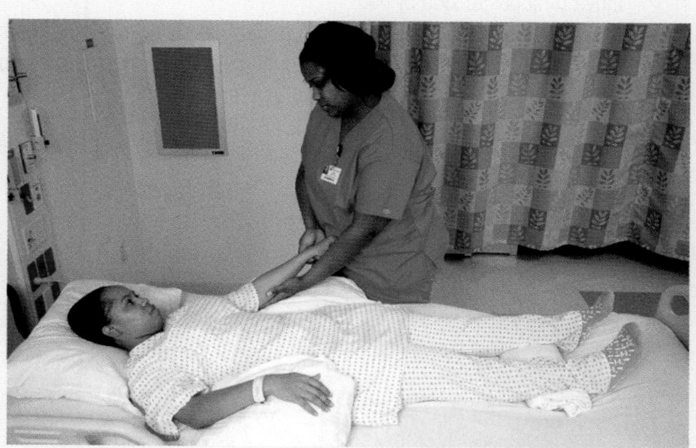

STEP 2c(7) Supported supine position with pillows in place.

SKILL 28-1 MOVING AND POSITIONING PATIENTS IN BED—cont'd

STEP	RATIONALE
(2) Roll patient over arm positioned close to body, with elbow straight and hand under hip. Position on abdomen in center of bed.	Positions patient correctly so alignment can be maintained.
(3) Turn patient's head to one side and support it with small pillow (see illustration).	Reduces flexion or hyperextension of cervical vertebrae.
(4) Place small pillow under patient's abdomen below level of diaphragm.	Reduces pressure on breasts of some female patients and decreases hyperextension of lumbar vertebrae and strain on lower back. Improves breathing by reducing mattress pressure on diaphragm.
(5) Support arms in flexed position level at shoulders.	Maintains proper body alignment. Support reduces risk of joint dislocation.
(6) Support lower legs with pillows to elevate toes.	Prevents footdrop. Reduces external rotation of hips. Eliminates mattress pressure on toes.
f. ***Positioning patient in 30-degree lateral (side-lying) position (one nurse):***	
(1) Lower head of bed completely or as low as patient can tolerate.	Provides position of comfort for patient and removes pressure from bony prominences on back.
(2) Position patient in supine position on side of bed opposite direction toward which patient is to be turned. Move upper trunk, supporting shoulders first, followed by moving lower trunk, supporting hips. Raise side rails and move to opposite side of bed.	Provides room for patient to turn to side. Use of safe patient-handling equipment reduces workload of caregivers and enhances safety (Burnfield et al., 2013; Griffis, 2012).
(3) Prepare to turn patient onto side. Flex patient's knee that will not be next to mattress. Place one hand on patient's knee and one hand on patient's shoulder.	Use of leverage makes turning to side easy.
(4) Roll patient onto side toward you.	Rolling decreases trauma to tissues. In addition, patient is positioned so leverage on hip makes turning easy.
(5) Place pillow under patient's head and neck.	Maintains alignment. Reduces lateral neck flexion. Decreases strain on sternocleidomastoid muscle.
(6) Bring dependent shoulder blade forward.	Prevents patient's weight from resting directly on shoulder joint.
(7) Position both arms in slightly flexed position. Support upper arm by pillow level with shoulder; support the other arm with mattress.	Decreases internal rotation and adduction of shoulder. Supporting both arms in slightly flexed position protects joint and improves ventilation because chest is able to expand more easily.
(8) Place your hands under patient's hips and bring dependent hip slightly forward so angle from hip to mattress is approximately 30 degrees.	The 30-degree lateral position reduces pressure on trochanter.
(9) Place small tuck-back pillow behind patient's back. (Make by folding pillow lengthwise. Smooth area is slightly tucked under patient's back.)	Provides support to maintain patient on side.
(10) Place pillow under semiflexed upper leg level at hip from groin to foot (see illustration).	Flexion prevents hyperextension of leg. Maintains leg in correct alignment. Prevents pressure on bony prominences.
(11) Support feet in dorsiflexion with foot support devices (check agency policy).	Maintains foot in dorsiflexion and prevents footdrop. Pillows prevent stimulation to ball of foot by hard surface, which has tendency to increase muscle tone in patient with extensor spasticity of lower extremity.
g. ***Positioning patient in Sims' (semi-prone) position (one nurse):***	
(1) Position patient in supine position on side of bed opposite direction toward which patient is to be turned. Move upper trunk, supporting shoulders first; move lower trunk, supporting hips. Raise side rails and move to opposite side of bed.	Prepares patient for positioning.
(2) Move to other side of bed and turn patient on side. Position in lateral position, lying partially on abdomen, with dependent shoulder lifted out and arm placed at patient's side.	Patient is rolled only partially on abdomen.

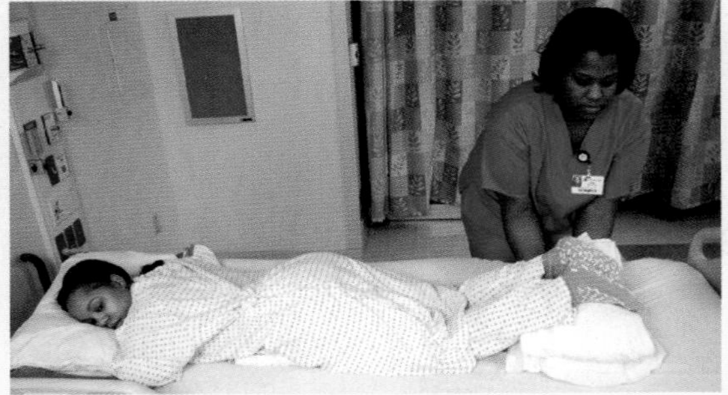

STEP 2e(3) Prone position with pillows supporting lower legs.

STEP	RATIONALE
(3) Place small pillow under patient's head.	Patient is rolled only partially on abdomen.
(4) Place pillow under flexed upper arm, supporting arm level with shoulder.	Maintains proper alignment and prevents lateral neck flexion. Prevents internal rotation of shoulder.
(5) Place pillow under flexed upper leg, supporting leg level with hip.	Prevents internal rotation of hip and adduction of leg. Flexion prevents hyperextension of leg. Reduces mattress pressure on knees and ankles.
(6) Support feet in dorsiflexion with foot support devices (check agency policy).	Maintains foot in dorsiflexion and prevents footdrop. Pillows prevent stimulation to ball of foot by hard surface, which has tendency to increase muscle tone in patient with extensor spasticity of lower extremity.

h. ***Logrolling patient (three nurses):***

CLINICAL DECISION: *Supervise and assist NAP when there is a health care provider's order to logroll a patient. Patients who have suffered from spinal cord injury or are recovering from neck, back, or spinal surgery often need to keep the spinal column in straight alignment to prevent further injury.*

STEP	RATIONALE
(1) Place patient in supine position on side of bed opposite direction to be turned.	Prepares patient for turning onto side.
(2) Place small pillow between patient's knees.	Prevents tension on spinal column and adduction of hip.
(3) Cross patient's arms on chest.	Prevents injury to arms.
(4) Position two nurses or other staff members on side of bed to which patient will be turned. Position third nurse or staff member on other side of bed (see illustration). If needed, four nurses are used; fourth nurse stands on same side as third nurse.	Distributes weight equally among nurses.
(5) Fanfold or roll drawsheet alongside of patient.	Provides strong handles to grip the drawsheet or pull sheet without slipping.
(6) With one nurse grasping drawsheet at lower hips and thighs and the other nurse grasping drawsheet at patient's shoulders and lower back, roll patient as one unit in a smooth, continuous motion on the count of three (see illustration).	This maintains proper alignment by moving all body parts at the same time, preventing tension or twisting of the spinal column.

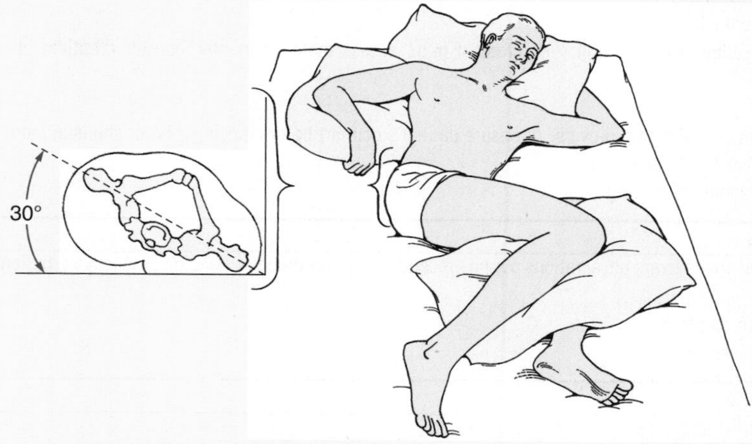

STEP 2f(10) Thirty-degree lateral position with pillows in place.

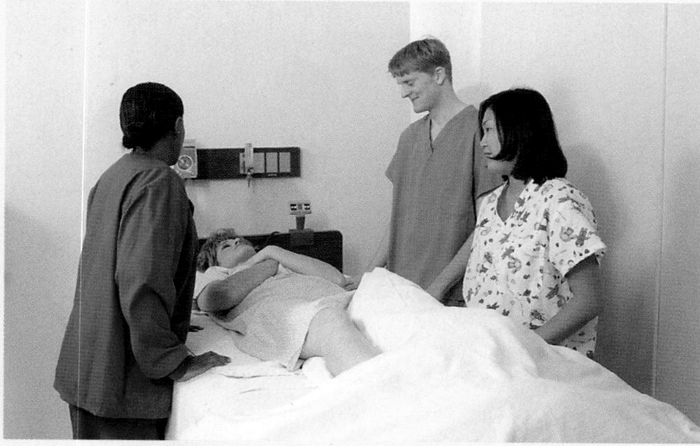
STEP 2h(4) Preparing patient for logroll.

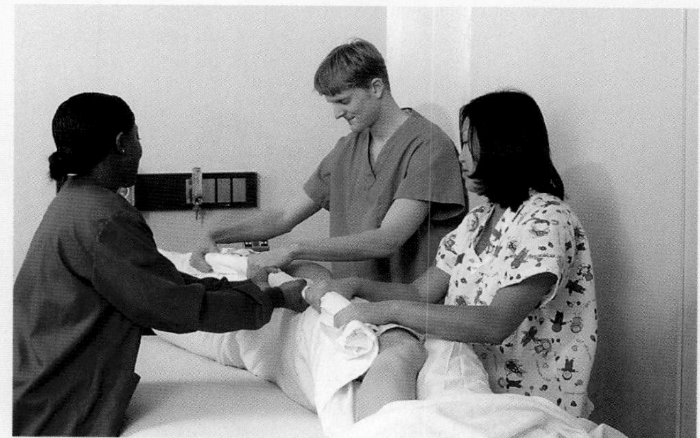
STEP 2h(6) Move patient as a unit, logrolling onto side.

SKILL 28-1 MOVING AND POSITIONING PATIENTS IN BED—cont'd

STEP	RATIONALE
(7) Nurse on opposite side of bed places pillows along length of patient (see illustration).	Pillows keep patient aligned.
(8) Gently lean patient as a unit back toward pillows for support (see illustration).	Ensures continued straight alignment of spinal column, preventing injury.
3. Perform hand hygiene.	Reduces transmission of microorganisms.

EVALUATION

1. Evaluate patient's body alignment, position, and level of comfort (using pain scale). Patient's body should be supported by adequate mattress, and vertebral column is properly aligned.	Determines effectiveness of positioning. Patients who have adequate pain control and are comfortable maintain proper positioning.
2. Measure ROM.	Determines if joint contracture is developing.
3. Observe skin for areas of erythema or breakdown, especially under bony prominences.	Indicates complications of immobility or improper positioning of body part. Determines if need exists for increasing frequency of repositioning patient.
4. Use ***Teach Back*** to determine patient and family understanding of moving and positioning. State, "I want to be sure I explained how proper moving and positioning prevents risk for injury while providing you safe care. Can you explain to me why it is important we move and position you often?" Revise your instruction now or develop plan for revised patient teaching if patient is not able to teach back correctly.	Evaluates what the patient is able to explain or demonstrate.

UNEXPECTED OUTCOMES AND RELATED INTERVENTIONS

1. Joint contractures develop or worsen.
   - Consult physical and/or occupational therapy.
   - Ensure that activity and ROM orders are implemented consistently.
2. Skin shows areas of erythema and breakdown.
   - Increase frequency of turning and repositioning
   - Place turning schedule above patient's bed.
   - Implement other activities per agency skin care policy or protocol (e.g., assess more frequently, consult dietitian, place patient on pressure-relieving mattress).
3. Patient avoids moving.
   - Administer analgesia as ordered by a health care provider to ensure patient's comfort before moving if he or she is in pain.
   - Allow pain medication to take effect before proceeding.
   - Provide patient education about benefits of moving.

RECORDING AND REPORTING

- Document repositioning or turning and any relevant observations during procedure (e.g., condition of skin, joint movement, patient's ability to assist with positioning) in nurses' notes.
- Report observations at change of shift hand-off.
- Document your evaluation of patient learning.

HOME CARE CONSIDERATIONS

- Teach family how to use safe patient-handling equipment if necessary.
- Teach patient and family about the signs of skin breakdown and the importance of safety during positioning for patients with decreased sensation.

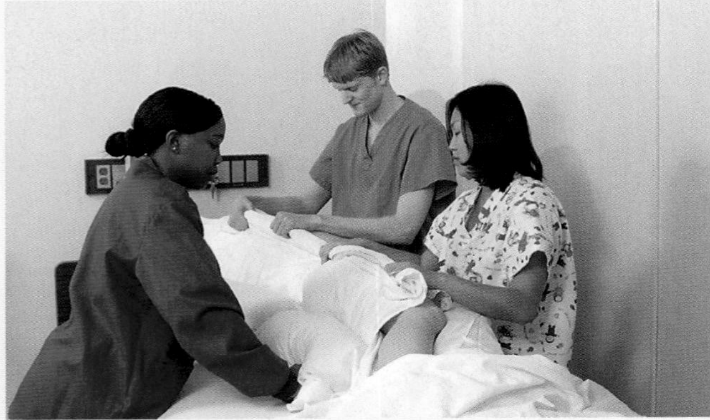

STEP 2h(7) Place pillows along patient's back for support.

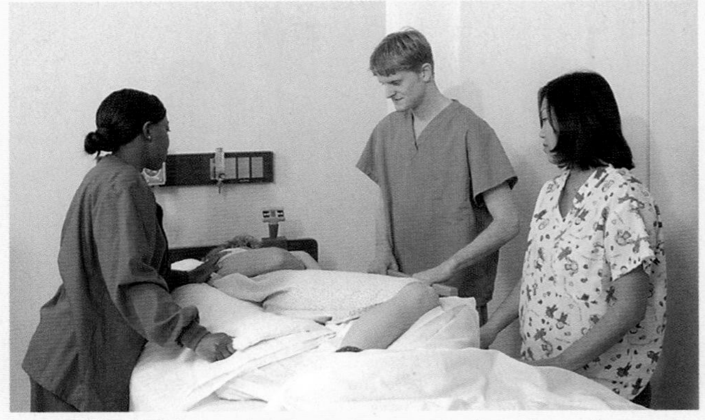

STEP 2h(8) Gently lean patient as a unit against pillows.

KEY POINTS

- Use findings from evidence-based nursing research about safe patient handling to prevent injuries to nurses and patients when moving and transferring.
- Coordination and regulation of muscle groups depend on muscle tone; activity of antagonistic, synergistic, and antigravity muscles; and neural input to muscles.
- Body alignment is the condition of joints, tendons, ligaments, and muscles in various body positions.
- Balance occurs when there is a wide base of support, the center of gravity falls within the base of support, and a vertical line falls from the center of gravity through the base of support.
- Developmental stages influence body alignment and mobility; the greatest impact of physiological changes on the musculoskeletal system is observed in children and older adults.
- The risk of disabilities related to immobilization depends on the extent and duration of immobilization and the patient's overall level of health.
- Immobility presents hazards in the physiological, psychological, and developmental dimensions.
- The nursing process and critical thinking assist you in providing care for patients who are experiencing or are at risk for the adverse effects of impaired body alignment and immobility.
- Patients with impaired body alignment require nursing care to maintain correct positioning such as the supported Fowler's, supine, prone, side-lying, and Sims' positions.
- Patient movement algorithms serve as assessment tools and guide safe patient handling and movement.
- Appropriate friction-reducing assistive devices and mechanical lifts need to be used for patient transfers when applicable.
- No-lift policies benefit all members of the health care system: patients, nurses, and administration.

CLINICAL APPLICATION QUESTIONS

Preparing for Clinical Practice

Ms. Cavallo, 97 years of age, has been a resident at the rehabilitation unit for 6 weeks. She has been receiving rehabilitation therapy following the repair of her fractured left hip. The nursing assistive personnel (NAP) tells you that Ms. Cavallo has not been finishing her meals over the past 2 days because of poor appetite. As you enter her room with a food tray today, she states, "Go away and take that tray of food with you. I'm tired of all of this, and I just want to stay in bed today." You explore why she feels this way. You discover that she does not like the foods that are being prepared for her and she does not feel strong enough to use her walker. She states, "I'm afraid that I'm going to fall because I don't feel strong enough to get out of bed and use my walker."

1. On the basis of these data, you develop a nursing diagnosis of *Deficient Knowledge (Imbalanced Nutrition: Less Than Body Requirements) related to lack of information*. Identify one goal, two expected outcomes, and three related nursing interventions with rationales that will help her meet the identified goal and outcomes.
2. You finish teaching Ms. Cavallo about the importance of a balanced diet and how it will help her regain strength to ambulate. As you are doing her morning assessment, you notice that she has a reddened area on her coccyx.
   a. Which risk factors contribute to this finding?
   b. In addition to a balanced diet, which other nursing interventions would be good to include in her plan of care?
3. You convince Ms. Cavallo to eat a balanced diet of three meals and two snacks high in protein. Describe the decision-making process you use to ensure that Ms. Cavallo continues to recognize the importance of a balanced diet. Include essential assessment data that you need to ensure that she continues to have an intake of proper foods.

ⓔ ***Answers to Clinical Application Questions can be found on the Evolve website.***

REVIEW QUESTIONS

Are You Ready to Test Your Nursing Knowledge?

1. An older adult has limited mobility as a result of a total knee replacement. During assessment you note that the patient has difficulty breathing while lying flat. Which of the following assessment data support a possible pulmonary problem related to impaired mobility? (Select all that apply.)
   1. B/P = 128/84
   2. Respirations 26/min on room air
   3. HR 114
   4. Crackles over lower lobes heard on auscultation
   5. Pain reported as 3 on scale of 0 to 10 after medication
2. A patient has been on bed rest for over 4 days. On assessment, the nurse identifies the following as a sign associated with immobility:
   1. Decreased peristalsis
   2. Decreased heart rate
   3. Increased blood pressure
   4. Increased urinary output
3. The nurse puts elastic stockings on a patient following major abdominal surgery. The nurse teaches the patient that the stockings are used after a surgical procedure to ______________________.
4. A nurse is teaching a community group about ways to minimize the risk of developing osteoporosis. Which of the following statements reflect understanding of what was taught? (Select all that apply.)
   1. "I usually go swimming with my family at the YMCA 3 times a week."
   2. "I need to ask my doctor if I should have a bone mineral density check this year."
   3. "If I don't drink milk at dinner, I'll eat broccoli or cabbage to get the calcium that I need in my diet."
   4. "I'll check the label of my multivitamin. If it has calcium, I can save money by not taking another pill."
   5. "My lactose intolerance should not be a concern when considering my calcium intake."
5. A nurse is caring for an older adult who has had a fractured hip repaired. In the first few postoperative days, which of the following nursing measures will best facilitate the resumption of activities of daily living for this patient?
   1. Encouraging use of an overhead trapeze for positioning and transfer
   2. Frequent family visits
   3. Assisting the patient to a wheelchair once per day
   4. Ensuring that there is an order for physical therapy
6. An older-adult patient has been bedridden for 2 weeks. Which of the following complaints by the patient indicates to the nurse that he or she is developing a complication of immobility?
   1. Loss of appetite
   2. Gum soreness

3. Difficulty swallowing
4. Left ankle joint stiffness

7. A patient is receiving 5000 units of heparin subcutaneously every 12 hours while on prolonged bed rest to prevent thrombophlebitis. Because bleeding is a potential side effect of this medication, the nurse should continually assess the patient for the following signs of bleeding: (Select all that apply.)
   1. Bruising
   2. Pale yellow urine
   3. Bleeding gums
   4. Coffee ground–like vomitus
   5. Light brown stool
8. The nurse is caring for a patient whose calcium intake must increase because of high risk factors for osteoporosis. Which of the following menus should the nurse recommend?
   1. Cream of broccoli soup with whole wheat crackers, cheese, and tapioca for dessert
   2. Hot dog on whole wheat bun with a side salad and an apple for dessert
   3. Low-fat turkey chili with sour cream with a side salad and fresh pears for dessert
   4. Turkey salad on toast with tomato and lettuce and honey bun for dessert
9. The nurse evaluates that the NAP has applied a patient's sequential compression device (SCD) appropriately when which of the following is observed? (Select all that apply.)
   1. Initial patient measurement is made around the calves
   2. Inflation pressure averages 40 mm Hg
   3. Patient's leg placed in SCD sleeve with back of knee aligned with popliteal opening on the sleeve.
   4. Stockings are removed every 2 hours during application.
   5. Yellow light indicates SCD device is functioning.
10. A patient on prolonged bed rest is at an increased risk to develop this common complication of immobility if preventive measures are not taken:
    1. Myoclonus
    2. Pathological fractures
    3. Pressure ulcers
    4. Pruritus
11. The effects of immobility on the cardiac system include which of the following? (Select all that apply.)
    1. Thrombus formation
    2. Increased cardiac workload
    3. Weak peripheral pulses
    4. Irregular heartbeat
    5. Orthostatic hypotension
12. To prevent complications of immobility, what would be the most effective activity on the first postoperative day for a patient who has had abdominal surgery?
    1. Turn, cough, and deep breathe every 30 minutes while awake
    2. Ambulate patient to chair in the hall
    3. Passive range of motion 4 times a day
    4. Immobility is not a concern the first postoperative day
13. Which of the following nursing interventions should be implemented to maintain a patent airway in a patient on bed rest?
    1. Isometric exercises
    2. Administration of low-dose heparin
    3. Suctioning every 4 hours
    4. Use of incentive spirometer every 2 hours while awake
14. Place the following options in the order in which elastic stockings should be applied.
    1. Identify patient using two identifiers.
    2. Smooth any creases or wrinkles.
    3. Slide the remainder of the stocking over the patient's heel and up the leg
    4. Turn the stocking inside out until heel is reached.
    5. Assess the condition of the patient's skin and circulation of the legs.
    6. Place toes into foot of the stocking.
    7. Use tape measure to measure patient's legs to determine proper stocking size.
15. Which of the following are physiological outcomes of immobility?
    1. Increased metabolism
    2. Reduced cardiac workload
    3. Decreased lung expansion
    4. Decreased oxygen demand

Answers: 1. 2, 3, 4; **2.** 1; **3.** Promote venous return to the heart; **4.** 1, 2, 3; **5.** 1; **6.** 4; **7.** 1, 3, 4; **8.** 1; **9.** 2, 3; **10.** 3; **11.** 1, 2, 5; **12.** 2; **13.** 4; **14.** 1, 5, 7, 4, 6, 3, 2; **15.** 3.

Rationales for Review Questions can be found on the Evolve website.

REFERENCES

Ackley BJ, Ladwig GB: *Nursing diagnosis handbook: an evidence-based guide to planning care*, ed 10, St Louis, 2014, Mosby.

American Association of Critical-Care Nurses (AACN): Prevention of falls: applying AACN's healthy work environment standards to a fall campaign, *Crit Care Nurse* 34(5):75, 2014.

American Nurses Association (ANA): *Statement of the American Nurses Association for the committee on Health, Education, Labor, and Pensions of the United States Senate subcommittee on Employment and Workplace Safety*, 2010. http://www.nursingworld.org/DocumentVault/GOVA/Federal/Testimonies/SPH-Testimony.pdf. Accessed September 2015.

Ball JE, et al: *Seidel's guide to physical examination*, ed 8, St Louis, 2015, Mosby.

Bangova A: Prevention of pressure ulcers in nursing home residents, *Nurs Stand* 27(24):54, 2013.

Barbas C, et al: Goal-oriented respiratory management for critically ill patients with acute respiratory distress syndrome, *Crit Care Res Pract* 2012:952168, 2012.

Cayley WE Jr: Preventing deep vein thrombosis in hospital inpatients, *BMJ* 335(7611):147–151, 2007.

Centers for Disease Control and Prevention (CDC): *Safe patient handling training for schools of nursing: curricular materials*, 2009. http://www.cdc.gov/niosh/docs/2009-127/pdfs/2009-127.pdf. Accessed September 2015.

Edelman CL, et al: *Health promotion throughout the life span*, ed 8, St Louis, 2013, Mosby.

Elliott M: Taking control of osteoporosis to cut down on risk of fracture, *Nurs Older People* 23(3):30, 2011.

Griffis H: Adverse risk: a dynamic interaction model of patient moving and handling, *J Nurs Manag* 20(6):713, 2012.

Harvey LA, et al: Continuous passive motion following total knee arthroplasty in people with arthritis, *Cochrane Database Syst Rev* (2):CD004260, 2014.

Healey F, Darowski A: Older patients and falls in hospitals, *Clin Risk* 18(5):170, 2012.

Hunter B, et al: Saving costs, saving health care providers' backs, and creating a safe patient environment, *Nurs Econ* 23(2):130, 2010.

Lewis SL, et al: *Medical-surgical nursing assessment and management of clinical problems*, ed 9, St Louis, 2013, Mosby.

McCance KL, Huether SE: *Pathophysiology: the biologic basis for disease in adults and children*, ed 7, St Louis, 2014, Mosby.

National Osteoporosis Foundation: *Get the facts*, Washington, DC, 2014, 2015. http://nof.org/learn/basics. Accessed September 11, 2015.

Parker K: Psychosocial effects of living with a leg ulcer, *Nurs Stand* 26(45):52, 2012.

Pierson F, Fairchild S: *Principles & techniques of patient care*, ed 5, St Louis, 2013, Saunders.

The Joint Commission (TJC): *2016 National Patient Safety Goals*. Oakbrook Terrace, IL, 2016, The Commission.

Available at http://www.jointcommission.org/standards_information/npsgs.aspx. Accessed November 2015.
Touhy TA, Jett K: *Toward healthy aging: human needs and nursing response*, ed 8, St Louis, 2012, Mosby.
US Department of Labor (USDL): *Bureau of Labor Statistics*, 2014. http://www.bls.gov/news.release/osh.nr0.htm. Accessed March 2015.
VISN8 Patient Safety Center (VISN8): *Algorithms for safe patient handling and movement*, 2015. http://www.visn8.va.gov/patientsafetycenter/safepthandling/. Accessed March 2015.
Winifred T-L: Teach-back for quality education and patient safety, *Urol Nurs* 33(6):267, 2013.
Wound, Ostomy and Continence Nurses Society (WOCN): *Guidelines for prevention and management of pressure ulcers*, 2010. http://www.guideline.gov/popups/printView.aspx?id=23868. Accessed September 2015.

RESEARCH REFERENCES

American Academy Of Nursing (AAN): Choosing wisely campaign, five things nurses and patients should question, *Nurs Outlook* 63:96, 2015.
Botti M, et al: Development of a management algorithm for post-operative pain (MAPP) after total knee and total hip replacement: study rationale and design, *Implement Sci* 9(1):1, 2014.
Burnfield J, et al: Comparative kinematic and electromagnetic assessment of clinician- and device-assisted sit-to-stand transfers in patients with stroke, *Phys Ther* 93(10):1331, 2013.
Chou R, et al: *Pressure ulcer risk assessment and prevention: comparative effectiveness*, 2013, Agency for Healthcare Research and Quality (AHRQ). http://www.ncbi.nlm.nih.gov/books/NBK143579/?term=Pressure%20ulcer%20risk%20assessment%20and%20prevention%3A%20comparative%20effectiveness. Accessed September 2015.
Clavet H, et al: Joint contractures in the intensive care unit: association with resource utilization and ambulatory status at discharge, *Disabil Rehabil* 33(2):105, 2011.
Drake J, et al: Pediatric skin care: what do nurses really know? *J Spec Pediatr Nurs* 17:329, 2012.
DuPlessis M, et al: The effectiveness of continuous passive motion on range of motion, pain, and muscle strength following rotator cuff repair: a systematic review, *Clin Rehabil* 26:291, 2011.
Furia JP, et al: Systematic review of contracture reduction in the lower extremity with dynamic splinting, *Adv Ther* 30:763, 2013.
Grinage JA, Werner CM: *The human's sign for DVT: use caution with interpretation*, Advanced Healthcare Network for NPs and Pas, August 28, 2013. http://nurse-practitioners-and-physician-assistants.advanceweb.com/Features/Articles/The-Homans-Sign-for-DVT.aspx. Accessed September 2015.
McMahon S, Fleury J: External validity of physical activity interventions for community-dwelling older adults with fall risk: a quantitative systematic literature review, *J Adv Nurs* 68(10):2140, 2012.
Nagarkar AK, et al: Chronic diseases and functional decline: a cross-sectional study among older adults in India, *Indian J Gerontol* 28(1):37, 2014.
Padula CA, et al: Impact of a nurse-driven mobility protocol on functional decline in hospitalized older adults, *J Nurs Care Qual* 24(4):325, 2009.
Pashikanti L, Von Ah D: Impact of early mobilization protocol on medical-surgical inpatient population, *Clin Nurse Spec* 26(2):97, 2012.
Peterson M, et al: Patient repositioning and pressure ulcer risk—monitoring interface pressures of at-risk patients, *J Rehabil Res Dev* 50(4):477, 2013.
Schiller C, et al: Words of wisdom—patient perspectives to guide recovery for older adults after hip fracture: a qualitative study, *Patient Prefer Adherence* 9:57, 2015.
Stanford Medicine: *Patient education: chronic disease self-management program*, 2015. Available at http://patienteducation.stanford.edu/programs/cdsmp.html. Accessed September 14, 2015.

29

Infection Prevention and Control

OBJECTIVES

- Explain the relationship between the infection chain and transmission of infection.
- Give an example of preventing infection for each element of the infection chain.
- Identify the normal defenses of the body against infection.
- Discuss the events in the inflammatory response.
- Identify patients most at risk for infection.
- Describe the signs/symptoms of a localized infection and those of a systemic infection.
- Explain conditions that promote the transmission of health care–associated infection.
- Explain the difference between medical and surgical asepsis.
- Explain the rationale for standard precautions.
- Perform proper procedures for hand hygiene.
- Explain how infection control measures differ in the home versus the hospital.
- Properly apply a surgical mask, sterile gown, and sterile gloves.
- Explain procedures for each isolation category.
- Understand the definition of occupational exposure.
- Explain the postexposure process.

KEY TERMS

Aerobic, p. 443
Anaerobic, p. 444
Asepsis, p. 455
Asymptomatic, p. 443
Bactericidal, p. 444
Bacteriostasis, p. 444
Broad-spectrum antibiotics, p. 446
Colonization, p. 443
Communicable disease, p. 443
Cough etiquette, p. 456
Disinfection, p. 455
Edema, p. 446
Endogenous infection, p. 448
Epidemiology, p. 466
Exogenous infection, p. 448
Exudates, p. 446
Granulation tissue, p. 446
Hand hygiene, p. 458
Handwashing, p. 458
Health care–associated infections (HAIs), p. 447
Iatrogenic infections, p. 448
Immunocompromised, p. 443
Infection, p. 443
Infectious, p. 443
Invasive, p. 442
Localized, p. 445
Medical asepsis, p. 455
Multidrug-resistant organism, p. 447
Necrotic, p. 446
Normal floras, p. 446
Pathogens, p. 443
Purulent, p. 446
Reservoir, p. 443
Sanguineous, p. 446
Serous, p. 446
Standard precautions, p. 458
Sterile field, p. 469
Sterilization, p. 455
Suppurative, p. 451
Suprainfection, p. 446
Surgical asepsis, p. 467
Susceptibility, p. 445
Symptomatic, p. 443
Systemic, p. 445
Vector, p. 445
Virulence, p. 443

MEDIA RESOURCES

http://evolve.elsevier.com/Potter/fundamentals/

- Review Questions
- Video Clips
- Concept Map Creator
- Concept Care Map
- Case Study with Questions
- Skills Performance Checklists
- Audio Glossary
- Content Updates

The incidence of patients developing infections as the direct result of contact during health care is increasing. Based on a large sample of U.S. acute care hospitals, a Center for Disease Control and Prevention (CDC) survey found that, on any given day, about 1 in 25 hospital patients has at least one health care–associated infection (CDC, 2015a). Current trends, public awareness, and rising costs of health care have increased the importance of infection prevention and control. The Joint Commission (TJC) (2016) views this as a patient safety issue. Infection prevention and control are essential for creating a safe health care environment for patients, families, and health care staff. Nurses are essential in infection prevention and control. Patients in all health care settings are at risk for acquiring infections because of lower resistance to pathogens; increased exposure to pathogens, some of which may be resistant to most antibiotics; and invasive procedures. Health care workers are at risk for exposure to pathogens as a result of contact with patient blood, body fluids, and contaminated equipment and surfaces. By practicing basic infection prevention and control techniques, you avoid spreading pathogens to patients and sustaining an exposure when providing direct care.

Patients and their families need to be able to recognize sources of infection and understand measures used to protect themselves. Patient teaching must include basic information about infection, the various modes of transmission, and appropriate methods of prevention such as hand hygiene and covering a cough.

Health care workers protect themselves from contact with infectious material, sharps injury, and/or exposure to a communicable disease by applying knowledge of the infectious process and using appropriate personal protective equipment (PPE). Increases in multidrug-resistant organisms (MDROs), health care–acquired infections (HAIs), and concern about diseases such as hepatitis B virus (HBV) and hepatitis C virus (HCV), human immunodeficiency virus (HIV) infection, and tuberculosis (TB) require a greater emphasis on infection prevention and control techniques (CDC, 2006, 2007, 2013a).

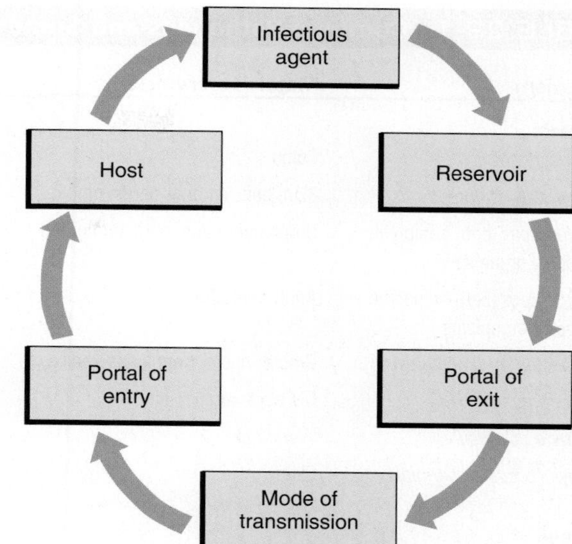

FIGURE 29-1 Chain of infection.

SCIENTIFIC KNOWLEDGE BASE

Nature of Infection

An **infection** is the invasion of a susceptible host (e.g., human being) by **pathogens** or microorganisms, resulting in disease. It is important to know the difference between an infection and colonization. **Colonization** is the presence and growth of microorganisms within a host but without tissue invasion or damage (Tweeten, 2014). Disease or infection results only if the pathogens multiply and alter normal tissue function. Some **infectious** diseases such as viral meningitis and pneumonia have a low or no risk for transmission. Although these illnesses can be serious for patients, they do not pose a risk to others, including caregivers.

If an infectious disease can be transmitted directly from one person to another, it is termed a **communicable disease** (Tweeten, 2014). If the pathogens multiply and cause clinical signs and symptoms, the infection is **symptomatic**. If clinical signs and symptoms are not present, the illness is termed **asymptomatic**. HCV is an example of a communicable disease that can be asymptomatic. It is most efficiently transmitted through the direct passage of blood into the skin from a percutaneous exposure, even if the source patient is asymptomatic (CDC, 2010a).

Chain of Infection

The presence of a pathogen does not mean that an infection will occur. Infection occurs in a cycle that depends on the presence of all of the following elements:

- An infectious agent or pathogen
- A reservoir or source for pathogen growth
- A port of exit from the reservoir
- A mode of transmission
- A port of entry to a host
- A susceptible host

Infection can develop if this chain remains uninterrupted (Figure 29-1). Preventing infections involves breaking the chain of infection.

Infectious Agent. Microorganisms include bacteria, viruses, fungi, and protozoa (Table 29-1). Microorganisms on the skin are either resident or transient flora. Resident organisms (normal flora) are permanent residents of the skin and within the body, where they survive and multiply without causing illness (CDC, 2008a; WHO, 2009). The potential for microorganisms or parasites to cause disease depends on the number of microorganisms present; their **virulence**, or ability to produce disease; their ability to enter and survive in a host; and the susceptibility of the host. Resident skin microorganisms are not virulent. However, these skin microorganisms can cause serious infection when surgery or other invasive procedures allow them to enter deep tissues or when a patient is severely **immunocompromised** (has an impaired immune system).

Transient microorganisms attach to the skin when a person has contact with another person or object during normal activities. For example, when you touch a contaminated gauze dressing or cleanse a patient following diarrheal episode, transient bacteria adhere to your skin. These organisms may be readily transmitted unless removed using hand hygiene (Ellingson et al., 2014). If hands are visibly soiled with proteinaceous material or care is being provided to a patient with *Clostridium difficile (C. difficile),* washing with soap and water is the preferred practice (Oughton et al., 2009). If hands are not visibly soiled, use of an alcohol-based hand product or handwashing with soap and water is acceptable for disinfecting hands of health care workers. Hand hygiene is the most effective way to break the chain of infection (CDC, 2008a; WHO, 2009).

Reservoir. A **reservoir** is a place where microorganisms survive, multiply, and await transfer to a susceptible host. Common reservoirs are humans and animals (hosts), insects, food, water, and organic matter on inanimate surfaces (fomites). Frequent reservoirs for HAIs include health care workers, especially their hands; patients; equipment; and the environment. Human reservoirs are divided into two types: those with acute or symptomatic disease and those who show no signs of disease but are carriers of it. Humans can transmit microorganisms in either case. Animals, food, water, insects, and inanimate objects can also be reservoirs for infectious organisms. To thrive organisms require a proper environment, including appropriate food, oxygen, water, temperature, pH, and light.

Food. Microorganisms require nourishment. Some such as *Clostridium perfringens,* the microbe that causes gas gangrene, thrive on organic matter. Others such as *Escherichia coli* consume undigested foodstuff in the bowel. Carbon dioxide and inorganic material such as soil provide nourishment for other organisms.

Oxygen. **Aerobic** bacteria require oxygen for survival and for multiplication sufficient to cause disease. Aerobic organisms cause more infections in humans than anaerobic organisms. An example of an

TABLE 29-1 Common Pathogens and Some Infections or Diseases They Produce

Organism	Major Reservoir(s)	Major Infections/Diseases
Bacteria		
Escherichia coli	Colon	Gastroenteritis, urinary tract infection
Staphylococcus aureus	Skin, hair, anterior nares, mouth	Wound infection, pneumonia, food poisoning, cellulitis
Streptococcus (beta-hemolytic group A) organisms	Oropharynx, skin, perianal area	"Strep throat," rheumatic fever, scarlet fever, impetigo, wound infection
Streptococcus (beta-hemolytic group B) organisms	Adult genitalia	Urinary tract infection, wound infection, postpartum sepsis, neonatal sepsis
Mycobacterium tuberculosis	Droplet nuclei from lungs, larynx	Tuberculosis
Neisseria gonorrhoeae	GU tract, rectum, mouth	Gonorrhea, pelvic inflammatory disease, infectious arthritis, conjunctivitis
Rickettsia rickettsii	Wood tick	Rocky Mountain spotted fever
Staphylococcus epidermidis	Skin	Wound infection, bacteremia
Viruses		
Hepatitis A virus	Feces	Hepatitis A
Hepatitis B virus	Blood and certain body fluids, sexual contact	Hepatitis B
Hepatitis C virus	Blood, certain body fluids, sexual contact	Hepatitis C
Herpes simplex virus (type 1)	Lesions of mouth or skin, saliva, genitalia	Cold sores, aseptic meningitis, sexually transmitted disease, herpetic whitlow
Human immunodeficiency virus (HIV)	Blood, semen, vaginal secretions via sexual contact	Acquired immunodeficiency syndrome (AIDS)
Fungi		
Aspergillus organisms	Soil, dust, mouth, skin, colon, genital tract	Aspergillosis, pneumonia, sepsis
Candida albicans	Mouth, skin, colon, genital tract	Candidiasis, pneumonia, sepsis
Protozoa		
Plasmodium falciparum	Blood	Malaria

Modified from Brown M: Microbiology basics. In Grota P, editor: *APIC text of infection control and epidemiology,* Washington, DC, 2014, Association for Professionals in Infection Control and Epidemiology.

aerobic organism is *Staphylococcus aureus*. **Anaerobic** bacteria thrive where little or no free oxygen is available. Anaerobes typically cause infections deep within the pleural cavity, in a joint, or in a deep sinus tract. An example of an anaerobic organism is *Bacteroides fragilis,* an organism that is part of the normal flora of the human colon but can cause infection if displaced into the bloodstream or surrounding tissue following surgery or injury.

Water. Most organisms require water or moisture for survival. For example, a frequent place for microorganisms is the moist drainage from a surgical wound. Some bacteria assume a form, called a *spore,* which is resistant to drying, and can live on inanimate surfaces for long periods of time. A common spore-forming bacterium is *C. difficile,* an organism that causes antibiotic-induced diarrhea.

Temperature. Microorganisms can live only in certain temperature ranges. Each species of bacteria has a specific temperature at which it grows best. The ideal temperature for most human pathogens is 20° to 43°C (68° to 109°F). For example, *Legionella pneumophila* grows best in water at 25° to 42°C (77° to 108°F). Cold temperatures tend to prevent growth and reproduction of bacteria (**bacteriostasis**). A temperature or chemical that destroys bacteria is **bactericidal**.

pH. The acidity of an environment determines the viability of microorganisms. Most microorganisms prefer an environment within a pH range of 5.0 to 7.0. Bacteria in particular thrive in urine with an alkaline pH.

Light. Microorganisms thrive in dark environments such as those under dressings and within body cavities.

Portal of Exit. After microorganisms find a site to grow and multiply, they need to find a portal of exit if they are to enter another host and cause disease. Portals of exit include sites such as blood, skin and mucous membranes, respiratory tract, genitourinary (GU) tract, gastrointestinal (GI) tract, and transplacental (mother to fetus). Some viruses such as Ebola virus are transmitted through direct contact with the blood or body fluids of a person who is sick with Ebola. However, droplets (e.g., splashes or sprays) of respiratory or other secretions from a person who is sick with Ebola could also be infectious. Therefore certain precautions (called standard, contact, and droplet precautions) are recommended for use in health care settings to prevent the transmission of the virus from patients who are sick with Ebola to health care personnel and other patients or family members (CDC, 2015b).

Skin and Mucous Membranes. The skin is considered a portal of exit because any break in the integrity of the skin and mucous membranes allows pathogens to exit the body. This may be exhibited by the presence of purulent drainage.

Respiratory Tract. Pathogens that infect the respiratory tract such as the influenza virus are released from the body when an infected person sneezes or coughs.

Urinary Tract. Normally urine is sterile. However, when a patient has a urinary tract infection (UTI), microorganisms exit during urination.

Gastrointestinal Tract. The mouth is one of the most bacterially contaminated sites of the human body, but most of the organisms are normal floras. Organisms that are normal floras in one person can be pathogens in another. For example, organisms exit when a person expectorates saliva. In addition, gastrointestinal portals of exit include emesis, bowel elimination, drainage of bile via surgical wounds, or drainage tubes.

Reproductive Tract. Organisms such as *Neisseria gonorrhea* and HIV exit through a man's urethral meatus or a woman's vaginal canal during sexual contact.

Blood. The blood is normally a sterile body fluid; however, in the case of communicable diseases such as HBV, HCV, or HIV, it becomes a reservoir for pathogens. Organisms exit from wounds, venipuncture sites, hematemesis, and bloody stool.

Modes of Transmission. Each disease has a specific mode of transmission. Many times you are able to do little about the infectious agent or the susceptible host; but, by practicing infection prevention and control techniques such as hand hygiene, you interrupt the mode of transmission (Box 29-1). The same microorganism is sometimes transmitted by more than one route. For example, varicella zoster (chickenpox) is spread by the airborne route in droplet nuclei or by direct contact.

The major route of transmission for pathogens identified in the health care setting is the unwashed hands of the health care worker (CDC, 2008a; Ellingson et al., 2014; WHO, 2009). Equipment used within the environment (e.g., a stethoscope, blood pressure cuff, or bedside commode) often becomes a source for the transmission of pathogens.

Portal of Entry. Organisms enter the body through the same routes they use for exiting. For example, during venipuncture when a needle pierces a patient's skin, organisms enter the body if proper skin preparation is not performed first. Factors such as a depressed immune system that reduce body defenses enhance the chances of pathogens entering the body.

Susceptible Host. Susceptibility to an infectious agent depends on an individual's degree of resistance to pathogens. Although everyone is constantly in contact with large numbers of microorganisms, an infection does not develop until an individual becomes susceptible to the strength and numbers of the microorganisms. A person's natural defenses against infection and certain risk factors (e.g., age, nutritional status, presence of chronic disease, trauma, and smoking) affect susceptibility (resistance) (Roach, 2014). Organisms such as *S. aureus* with resistance to key antibiotics are becoming more common in all health care settings, but especially acute care. The increased resistance is associated with the frequent and sometimes inappropriate use of antibiotics over the years in all settings (i.e., acute care, ambulatory care, clinics, and long-term care) (Arnold, 2014).

THE INFECTIOUS PROCESS

By understanding the chain of infection, you have knowledge that is vital in preventing infections. When the patient acquires an infection, observe for signs and symptoms of infection and take appropriate actions to prevent its spread. Infections follow a progressive course (Box 29-2).

BOX 29-1 Modes of Transmission

Contact

Direct

- Person-to-person (fecal, oral) physical contact between source and susceptible host (e.g., touching patient feces and then touching your inner mouth or consuming contaminated food)

Indirect

- Personal contact of susceptible host with contaminated inanimate object (e.g., needles or sharp objects, dressings, environment)

Droplet

- Large particles that travel up to 3 feet during coughing, sneezing, or talking and come in contact with susceptible host

Airborne

- Droplet nuclei or residue or evaporated droplets suspended in air during coughing or sneezing or carried on dust particles

Vehicles

- Contaminated items
- Water
- Drugs, solutions
- Blood
- Food (improperly handled, stored, or cooked; fresh or thawed meats)

Vector

- External mechanical transfer (flies)
- Internal transmission such as parasitic conditions between **vector** and host such as:
  - Mosquito
  - Louse
  - Flea
- Tick

Modified from Tweeten S: General principles of epidemiology. In Grota P, editor: *APIC text of infection control and epidemiology,* Washington, DC, 2014, Association for Professionals in Infection Control and Epidemiology.

If an infection is localized (e.g., a wound infection), a patient usually experiences localized symptoms such as pain, tenderness, warmth, and redness at the wound site. Use standard precautions, appropriate PPE, and hand hygiene when assessing the wound. The use of these precautions and hand hygiene blocks the spread of infection to other sites or other patients. An infection that affects the entire body instead of just a single organ or part is systemic and can become fatal if undetected and untreated.

The course of an infection influences the level of nursing care provided. The nurse is responsible for properly administering antibiotics, monitoring the response to drug therapy (see Chapter 32), using proper hand hygiene, and standard precautions. Supportive therapy includes providing adequate nutrition and rest to bolster defenses of the body against the infectious process. The course of care for the patient often has additional effects on body systems affected by the infection.

Defenses Against Infection

The body has natural defenses that protect against infection. Normal floras, body system defenses, and inflammation are all nonspecific defenses that protect against microorganisms regardless of prior

BOX 29-2 Course of Infection by Stage

Incubation Period

Interval between entrance of pathogen into body and appearance of first symptoms (e.g., chickenpox, 14 to 16 days after exposure; common cold, 1 to 2 days; influenza, 1 to 4 days; measles, 10 to 12 days; mumps, 16 to 18 days; Ebola 2 to 21 days (CDC, 2015b).

Prodromal Stage

Interval from onset of nonspecific signs and symptoms (malaise, low-grade fever, fatigue) to more specific symptoms. (During this time microorganisms grow and multiply, and patient may be capable of spreading disease to others.) For example, herpes simplex begins with itching and tingling at the site before the lesion appears.

Illness Stage

Interval when patient manifests signs and symptoms specific to type of infection. For example, strep throat is manifested by sore throat, pain, and swelling; mumps is manifested by high fever, parotid and salivary gland swelling.

Convalescence

Interval when acute symptoms of infection disappear. (Length of recovery depends on severity of infection and patient's host resistance; recovery may take several days to months.)

exposure. If any of these body defenses fail, an infection usually occurs and leads to a serious health problem.

Normal Floras. The body normally contains microorganisms that reside on the surface and deep layers of skin, in the saliva and oral mucosa, and in the GI and GU tracts. A person normally excretes trillions of microbes daily through the intestines. **Normal floras** do not usually cause disease when residing in their usual area of the body but instead participate in maintaining health.

Normal floras of the large intestine exist in large numbers without causing illness. They also secrete antibacterial substances within the walls of the intestine. The normal floras of the skin exert a protective, bactericidal action that kills organisms landing on the skin. The mouth and pharynx are also protected by floras that impair growth of invading microbes. Normal floras maintain a sensitive balance with other microorganisms to prevent infection. Any factor that disrupts this balance places a person at increased risk for acquiring a disease. For example, the use of **broad-spectrum antibiotics** for the treatment of infection can lead to **suprainfection**. A suprainfection develops when broad-spectrum antibiotics eliminate a wide range of normal flora organisms, not just those causing infection. When normal bacterial floras are eliminated, body defenses are reduced, which allows disease-producing microorganisms to multiply, causing illness (Arnold, 2014).

Body System Defenses. A number of body organ systems have unique defenses against infection (Table 29-2). The skin, respiratory tract, and GI tract are easily accessible to microorganisms. Pathogenic organisms can adhere to the surface skin, be inhaled into the lungs, or be ingested with food. Each organ system has defense mechanisms physiologically suited to its specific structure and function. For example, the lungs cannot completely control the entrance of microorganisms. However, the airways are lined with moist mucous membranes and hairlike projections, or cilia, that rhythmically beat to move mucus or cellular debris up to the pharynx to be expelled through swallowing.

Inflammation. The cellular response of the body to injury, infection, or irritation is termed *inflammation*. Inflammation is a protective vascular reaction that delivers fluid, blood products, and nutrients to an area of injury. The process neutralizes and eliminates pathogens or dead (**necrotic**) tissues and establishes a means of repairing body cells and tissues. Signs of localized inflammation include swelling, redness, heat, pain or tenderness, and loss of function in the affected body part. When inflammation becomes systemic, other signs and symptoms develop, including fever, increased white blood cells (WBCs), malaise, anorexia, nausea, vomiting, lymph node enlargement, or organ failure.

Physical agents, chemical agents, or microorganisms trigger the inflammatory response. Mechanical trauma, temperature extremes, and radiation are examples of physical agents. Chemical agents include external and internal irritants such as harsh poisons or gastric acid. Sometimes microorganisms also trigger this response.

After tissues are injured, a series of well-coordinated events occurs. The inflammatory response includes vascular and cellular responses, formation of inflammatory **exudates** (fluid and cells that are discharged from cells or blood vessels [e.g., pus or serum]), and tissue repair.

Vascular and Cellular Responses. Acute inflammation is an immediate response to cellular injury. Rapid vasodilation occurs, allowing more blood near the location of the injury. The increase in local blood flow causes the redness and localized warmth at the site of inflammation.

Injury causes tissue damage and possibly necrosis. As a result the body releases chemical mediators that increase the permeability of small blood vessels; and fluid, protein, and cells enter interstitial spaces. The accumulation of fluid appears as localized swelling (**edema**). Another sign of inflammation is pain, which is caused by the swelling of inflamed tissues that increases pressure on nerve endings. As a result of the physiological inflammatory response, the involved body part may have a temporary loss of function. For example, a localized infection of the hand causes the fingers to become swollen, painful, and discolored. Joints become stiff as a result of swelling, but function of the fingers returns when inflammation subsides.

The cellular response of inflammation involves WBCs arriving at the site. WBCs pass through blood vessels and into the tissues. Phagocytosis is a process that involves the destruction and absorption of bacteria. Through the process of phagocytosis, specialized WBCs, called neutrophils and monocytes, ingest and destroy microorganisms or other small particles. If inflammation becomes systemic, other signs and symptoms develop. Leukocytosis, or an increase in the number of circulating WBCs, is the response of the body to WBCs leaving blood vessels. In the adult a serum WBC count is normally 5,000 to 10,000/mm^3 but typically rises to 15,000 to 20,000/mm^3 and higher during inflammation. Fever is caused by phagocytic release of pyrogens from bacterial cells, which causes a rise in the hypothalamic set point (see Chapter 30).

Inflammatory Exudate. Accumulation of fluid, dead tissue cells, and WBCs forms an exudate at the site of inflammation. Exudate may be **serous** (clear, like plasma), **sanguineous** (containing red blood cells), or **purulent** (containing WBCs and bacteria). Usually the exudate is cleared away through lymphatic drainage. Platelets and plasma proteins such as fibrinogen form a meshlike matrix at the site of inflammation to prevent its spread.

Tissue Repair. When there is injury to tissue cells, healing involves the defensive, reconstructive, and maturative stages (see Chapter 48). Damaged cells eventually are replaced with healthy new cells. The new cells undergo a gradual maturation until they take on the same structural characteristics and appearance as the previous cells. If inflammation is chronic, tissue defects sometimes fill with fragile **granulation**

TABLE 29-2 Natural Defense Mechanisms Against Infection

Defense Mechanisms	Action	Factors That May Alter Defense Mechanisms
Skin		
Intact multilayered surface (first line of defense against infection)	Provides barrier to microorganisms and antibacterial activity	Cuts, abrasions, puncture wounds, areas of maceration
Shedding of outer layer of skin cells	Removes organisms that adhere to outer layers of skin	Failure to bathe regularly, improper handwashing technique
Sebum	Contains fatty acid that kills some bacteria	Excessive bathing
Mouth		
Intact multilayered mucosa	Provides mechanical barrier to microorganisms	Lacerations, trauma, extracted teeth
Saliva	Washes away particles containing microorganisms Contains microbial inhibitors (e.g., lysozyme)	Poor oral hygiene, dehydration
Eye		
Tearing and blinking	Provides mechanisms to reduce entry (blinking) or help wash away (tearing) particles containing pathogens, thus reducing dose of organisms	Injury, exposure—splash/splatter of blood or other potentially infectious material into eye
Respiratory Tract		
Cilia lining upper airway, coated by mucus	Traps inhaled microbes and sweeps them outward in mucus to be expectorated or swallowed	Smoking, high concentration of oxygen and carbon dioxide, decreased humidity, cold air
Macrophages	Engulf and destroy microorganisms that reach alveoli of lung	Smoking
Urinary Tract		
Flushing action of urine flow	Washes away microorganisms on lining of bladder and urethra	Obstruction to normal flow by urinary catheter placement, obstruction from growth or tumor, delayed micturition
Intact multilayered epithelium	Provides barrier to microorganisms	Introduction of urinary catheter, continual movement of catheter in urethra can facilitate migration of organisms to bladder
Gastrointestinal Tract		
Acidity of gastric secretions	Prevents retention of bacterial contents	Administration of antacids
Rapid peristalsis in small intestine		Delayed motility resulting from impaction of fecal contents in large bowel or mechanical obstruction by masses
Vagina		
At puberty normal flora causing vaginal secretions to achieve low pH	Inhibit growth of many microorganisms	Antibiotics and oral contraceptives disrupting normal flora

tissue that eventually takes the form of a scar at the completion of the healing process. The scar and surrounding tissues are not as strong as normal tissue and may be more susceptible to injury from pressure, shear, or friction, which increase the risk for pressure ulcer development (see Chapter 48).

Health Care–Associated Infections

Patients in health care settings, especially hospitals and long-term care facilities, have an increased risk of acquiring infections. **Health care–associated infections (HAIs)** result from the delivery of health services in a health care facility. They occur as the result of invasive procedures, antibiotic administration, the presence of **multidrug-resistant organisms** (MDROs), and breaks in infection prevention and control activities. The number of health care employees having direct contact with a patient, the type and number of invasive procedures, the therapy received, and the length of hospitalization influence the risk of infection. Major sites for HAIs include surgical or traumatic wounds, urinary and respiratory tracts, and the bloodstream (Box 29-3).

HAIs significantly increase costs of health care. Older adults have increased susceptibility to these infections because of their affinity to chronic disease and the aging process itself (Box 29-4). Extended stays in health care institutions, increased disability, increased costs of antibiotics, and prolonged recovery times add to the expenses both of the patient and the health care institution and funding bodies (e.g., Medicare). Costs for HAIs are often not reimbursed; as a result, prevention has a beneficial financial impact and is an important part of managed care. TJC lists several national safety goals focusing on the care of older adults (e.g., ensuring that older adults receive influenza and pneumonia vaccines, preventing infection after surgery) (TJC, 2016).

BOX 29-3 Examples of Sites for and Causes of Health Care–Associated Infections

Improperly performing hand hygiene increases patient risk for all types of health care–associated infections.

Urinary Tract

- Unsterile insertion of urinary catheter
- Improper positioning of the drainage tubing
- Open drainage system
- Catheter and tube becoming disconnected
- Drainage bag port touching contaminated surface
- Improper specimen collection technique
- Obstructing or interfering with urinary drainage
- Urine in catheter or drainage tube being allowed to reenter bladder (reflux)
- Repeated catheter irrigations
- Improper perineal hygiene

Surgical or Traumatic Wounds

- Improper skin preparation before surgery (e.g., shaving versus clipping hair; not performing a preoperative bath or shower)
- Failure to clean skin surface properly
- Failure to use aseptic technique during operative procedures and dressing changes
- Use of contaminated antiseptic solutions

Respiratory Tract

- Contaminated respiratory therapy equipment
- Failure to use aseptic technique while suctioning airway
- Improper disposal of secretions

Bloodstream

- Contamination of intravenous (IV) fluids by tubing
- Insertion of drug additives to IV fluid
- Addition of connecting tube or stopcocks to IV system
- Improper care of needle insertion site
- Contaminated needles or catheters
- Failure to change IV access at first sign of infection or at recommended intervals
- Improper technique during administration of multiple blood products
- Improper care of peritoneal or hemodialysis shunts
- Improperly accessing an IV port

BOX 29-4 FOCUS ON OLDER ADULTS

Risks for Infection

- An age-related functional deterioration in immune system function, termed *immune senescence,* increases the susceptibility of the body to infection and slows overall immune response (Larbi et al., 2013).
- Older adults are less capable of producing lymphocytes to combat challenges to the immune system. When antibodies are produced, the duration of their response is shorter, and fewer cells are produced (Roach, 2014).
- Risks associated with the development of infections or HAIs in older patients include poor nutrition, unintentional weight loss, lack of exercise, poor social support, and low serum albumin levels (Meiner, 2014).
- Flu and pneumonia vaccinations are recommended for the older-adult population to reduce their risk for infectious diseases.
- Teach older adults and their families how to reduce the risk for infections by using proper hand hygiene practices.

Patients who develop HAIs often have multiple illnesses, are older adults, or are poorly nourished and may have a compromised immune system; thus they are more susceptible to infections. In addition, many patients have a lowered resistance to infection because of underlying medical conditions (e.g., diabetes mellitus or cancer) that impair or damage the immune response of the body. Invasive treatment devices such as intravenous (IV) catheters or indwelling urinary catheters impair or bypass the natural defenses of the body against microorganisms. Critical illness increases patients' susceptibility to infections, especially multidrug-resistant bacteria. Meticulous hand hygiene practices, the use of chlorhexidine washes for bathing and personal hygiene care, and advances in intensive care unit (ICU) infection prevention help to prevent these infections (Doyle et al., 2011; Kassakian et al., 2011).

HAI infections are either exogenous or endogenous. An **exogenous infection** comes from microorganisms found outside the individual, such as *Salmonella, Clostridium tetani,* and *Aspergillus.* These microorganisms do not exist as normal floras. An **endogenous infection** occurs when part of the patient's flora becomes altered and an overgrowth results (e.g., staphylococci, enterococci, yeasts, and streptococci). This often happens when a patient receives broad-spectrum antibiotics that alter the normal floras. When sufficient numbers of microorganisms normally found in one body site move to another site, an endogenous infection develops. The number of microorganisms needed to cause an HAI depends on the virulence of the organism, the susceptibility of the host, and the body site affected.

Iatrogenic infections are a type of HAI caused by an invasive diagnostic or therapeutic procedure. For example, procedures such as a bronchoscopy and treatment with broad-spectrum antibiotics increase the risk for certain infections (Arnold, 2014; Day, 2014). Use critical thinking when practicing aseptic techniques during the performance of procedures. Follow basic infection prevention and control policies and procedures to reduce the risk of HAIs. Always consider the patient's risks for infection and anticipate how the approach to care increases or decreases the risk.

NURSING KNOWLEDGE BASE

Body substances such as feces, urine, and wound drainage contain potentially infectious microorganisms. Health care workers are at risk for exposure to microorganisms in the hospital and/or home setting (Fiutem, 2014). The meticulous use of specific infection prevention practices reduces the risk of cross-contamination and transmission of infection to other patients when caring for a patient with a known or suspected infection (CDC, 2007).

Serious infections are ongoing challenges to clinicians, and they create feelings of anxiety, frustration, loneliness, and anger in patients and/or their families (Nesher et al., 2014). These feelings worsen when patients are isolated to prevent transmission of a microorganism to other patients or health care staff. Isolation disrupts normal social relationships with visitors and caregivers. Patient safety is usually an additional risk for the patient on isolation precautions (Monsees, 2014). For example, an older patient with a chronic illness is more at risk for a HAI. When family members fear the possibility of developing the infection, they may avoid contact with the patient. Some patients perceive the simple procedures of proper hand hygiene and gown and glove use as evidence of rejection. Help patients and families reduce some of these feelings by discussing the disease process; explaining isolation procedures; and maintaining a friendly, understanding manner.

When establishing a plan of care, it is important to know how a patient reacts to an infection or infectious disease. The challenge is to identify and support behaviors that maintain human health or prevent infection.

Factors Influencing Infection Prevention and Control

Multiple factors influence a patient's susceptibility to infection. It is important to understand how each of these factors alone or in combination increases this risk. When more than one factor is present, a patient's susceptibility often increases, which affects length of stay, recovery time, and/or overall level of health following an illness. Understanding these factors helps to assess and care for a patient who has an infection or is at risk for one.

Age. Throughout life a person's susceptibility to infection changes. For example, an infant has immature defenses against infection. Born with only the antibodies provided by the mother, the infant's immune system is incapable of producing the necessary immunoglobulins and WBCs to adequately fight some infections. However, breastfed infants often have greater immunity than bottle-fed infants because they receive their mother's antibodies through the breast milk. As the child grows the immune system matures; but the child is still susceptible to organisms that cause the common cold; intestinal infections; and infectious diseases such as mumps, measles, and chickenpox (if not vaccinated).

The young or middle-age adult has refined defenses against infection. Viruses are the most common cause of communicable illness in young or middle-age adults. Since 2000 there has been a major effort to vaccinate all children against all infectious diseases for which vaccines are available. Vaccine-preventable disease levels are at or near record lows (CDC, 2011a).

Defenses against infection change with aging (Larbi et al., 2013). The immune response, particularly cell-mediated immunity, declines. Older adults also undergo alterations in the structure and function of the skin, urinary tract, and lungs. For example, the skin loses its turgor, and the epithelium thins. As a result it is easier to tear or abrade the skin, which increases the potential for invasion by pathogens. In addition, older adults who are hospitalized or reside in an assisted-living or residential care facility are at risk for airborne infections. Ensuring that health care workers are vaccinated against influenza reduces the transmission of this illness in older adults (Thomas et al., 2013).

Nutritional Status. A patient's nutritional health directly influences susceptibility to infection. A reduction in the intake of protein and other nutrients such as carbohydrates and fats reduces body defenses against infection and impairs wound healing (see Chapter 48). Patients with illnesses or problems that increase protein requirements, such as extensive burns and febrile conditions, are at further risk. For example, patients who have undergone surgery require increased protein. A thorough diet history is necessary. Determine a patient's normal daily nutrient intake and whether preexisting problems such as nausea, impaired swallowing, or oral pain alter food intake. Confer with a dietitian to assist in calculating the calorie count of foods ingested.

Stress. The body responds to emotional or physical stress by the general adaptation syndrome (see Chapter 38). During the alarm stage the basal metabolic rate increases as the body uses energy stores. Adrenocorticotropic hormone increases serum glucose levels and decreases unnecessary antiinflammatory responses through the release of cortisone. If stress continues or becomes intense, elevated cortisone levels result in decreased resistance to infection. Continued stress leads to exhaustion, which causes depletion in energy stores, and the body has no resistance to invading organisms. The same conditions that increase nutritional requirements such as surgery or trauma also increase physiological stress.

Disease Process. Patients with diseases of the immune system are at particular risk for infection. Leukemia, acquired immunodeficiency syndrome (AIDS), lymphoma, and aplastic anemia are conditions that compromise a host by weakening defenses against infectious organisms. For example, patients with leukemia are unable to produce enough WBCs to ward off infection. Patients with HIV are often unable to ward off simple infections and are prone to opportunistic infections.

Patients with chronic diseases such as diabetes mellitus and multiple sclerosis are also more susceptible to infection because of general debilitation and nutritional impairment. Diseases that impair body system defenses such as emphysema and bronchitis (which impair ciliary action and thicken mucus), cancer (which alters the immune response), and peripheral vascular disease (which reduces blood flow to injured tissues) increase susceptibility to infection. Patients with burns have a high susceptibility to infection because of the damage to skin surfaces. The greater the depth and extent of the burns, the higher is the risk for infection.

❖ NURSING PROCESS

Apply the nursing process and use a critical thinking approach in your care of patients. The nursing process provides a clinical decision-making approach for you to develop and implement an individualized plan of care.

◆ Assessment

During the assessment process thoroughly assess each patient and critically analyze findings to ensure that you make patient-centered clinical decisions required for safe nursing care. Determine how the patient feels about the illness or risk for infection. Assess his or her defense mechanisms, susceptibility, and knowledge of how infections are transmitted (Table 29-3). Conduct a review of systems and travel history with the patient and family to reveal any risks for exposure to a communicable disease. Immunization and vaccination history is also very useful. It is important to be thorough in assessing a patient's clinical condition. A medication history is necessary to identify medications that increase a patient's susceptibility to infection. An analysis of laboratory findings provides information about a patient's defense against infection. The early recognition of infection or risk factors helps you make the correct nursing diagnosis and establish a treatment plan.

Through the Patient's Eyes. Some patients with infection have a variety of problems. It is important to ask specific questions to determine the patient's and family's needs related to the risk for infection or disease status (Box 29-5). These needs vary from patient to patient and include physical, psychological, social, or economic needs. Patients with chronic or serious infection, especially communicable infections such as TB or AIDS, experience psychological and social problems from self-imposed isolation or rejection by friends and family. Ask the patient how the infection affects the ability to maintain relationships and perform activities of daily living. Determine whether chronic infection has drained the patient's financial resources. Ask about his or her expectations of care and determine how much he or she wants to be involved in planning care. Some patients and their families wish to know more about the disease process, whereas others only want to know the interventions necessary to treat the infection. In addition,

TABLE 29-3 Assessing the Risk of Infection in Adults

Risk Factor	Causes	Outcome
Chronic disease	COPD, heart failure, diabetes	Pneumonia, skin breakdown, venous stasis ulcers
Lifestyle—high-risk behaviors	Exposure to communicable/infectious diseases, use of IV drugs and other drugs/substances	STIs, HIV, HBV, HCV, opportunistic infections, viral infections, yeast infections, liver failure
Occupation	Health care worker; miner, unemployed, homeless	Exposure to blood and body fluids increase risk of infection; black lung disease, pneumonia, TB, poor nutritional intake; lack of access to medical care; stress
Diagnostic procedures	Invasive radiology, transplant	Multiple IV lines, immunosuppressive drugs
Heredity	Sickle cell disease, diabetes	Anemia, delayed healing
Travel history	West Nile virus, SARS, avian flu, *Hantavirus*	Meningitis, acute respiratory distress
Trauma	Fractures, internal bleeding	Sepsis, secondary infection
Nutrition	Obesity, anorexia	Impaired immune response

Modified from Tweeten SM: General principles of epidemiology. In Grota P, editor: *APIC text of infection control and epidemiology,* Washington, DC, 2014, Association for Professionals in Infection Control and Epidemiology. *COPD,* Chronic obstructive pulmonary disease; *HBV,* hepatitis B virus; *HCV,* hepatitis C virus; *HIV,* human immunodeficiency virus; *IV,* intravenous; *SARS,* severe acute respiratory syndrome; *STIs,* sexually transmitted infections; *TB,* tuberculosis.

BOX 29-5 Nursing Assessment Questions

Risk Factors
- Do you have any recent cuts or lacerations? Show me the location.
- Describe for me any illnesses or diseases that you have and those for which you receive treatment.
- Tell me about any recent diagnostic testing you have undergone, such as colonoscopy or cystoscopy?

Possible Existing Infections
- Do you have or feel like you have a fever?
- Do you have any cuts or wounds with drainage?
- Do you have any pain/burning during urination?
- Do you have a cough? Is there any sputum?

Recent Travel History
- Have you traveled outside the United States in the past 6 months?
- Are you a resident of or have you travelled within the last 21 days to a country where an Ebola outbreak is occurring (CDC, 2015c)?
- Were any of the people you visited or traveled with ill?

Medication History
- List for me the medications you are currently taking.
- Describe any over-the-counter medications or herbals that you are currently taking.

Stressors
- Tell me about any major lifestyle change occurring such as the loss of employment or place of residence, divorce, or disability.

there are emerging infections throughout the globe, and it is important to also obtain travel history from your patients. Encourage patients to verbalize their expectations so you are able to establish interventions to meet patients' priorities.

Status of Defense Mechanisms. Review physical assessment findings (see Chapter 31) and the patient's medical condition to determine the status of normal defense mechanisms against infection. For example, any break in the skin such as an ulcer on the foot of a patient who has diabetes is a potential site for infection. Any reduction in the primary or secondary defenses of the body against infection such as a weakened ability to cough places a patient at increased risk.

Patient Susceptibility. As noted previously, assess the patient's age, nutritional status, presence of chronic illnesses, stress, and disease process to identify factors that influence susceptibility to infection. Gather information about each factor through your interview and the patient's and family's medical history.

Medical Therapy. Some drugs and medical therapies compromise immunity to infection. Assess your patient's medication history to determine whether he or she takes any medications that increase infection susceptibility. These include any over-the-counter medications and herbal supplements. A review of therapies received within the health care setting further reveals risks. For example, adrenal corticosteroids, prescribed for several conditions, are antiinflammatory drugs that cause protein breakdown and impair the inflammatory response against bacteria and other pathogens. Cytotoxic and antineoplastic drugs attack cancer cells but also cause the side effects of bone marrow depression and normal cell toxicity, which affects the response of body against pathogens.

Clinical Appearance. The signs and symptoms of infection may be local or systemic. Localized infections are most common in areas of skin or mucous membrane breakdown such as surgical and traumatic wounds, pressure ulcers, oral lesions, and abscesses.

To assess an area for localized infection, first inspect it for redness, warmth, and swelling caused by inflammation. Because there may be drainage from open lesions or wounds, wear clean gloves. Infected drainage may be yellow, green, or brown, depending on the pathogen. For example, green nasal secretions often indicate a sinus infection. Ask the patient about pain or tenderness around the site. Some patients complain of tightness and pain caused by edema. If the infected area is large enough, movement is restricted. Gentle palpation of an infected area usually results in some degree of tenderness. Wear protective eyewear and a surgical mask when there is a risk for splash or spray with blood or body fluids.

Systemic infections cause more generalized symptoms than local infection. These symptoms often include fever, fatigue, nausea/

vomiting, and malaise. Lymph nodes that drain the area of infection often become enlarged, swollen, and tender during palpation. For example, an abscess in the peritoneal cavity causes enlargement of lymph nodes in the groin. An infection of the upper respiratory tract causes cervical lymph node enlargement. If an infection is serious and widespread, all major lymph nodes may enlarge.

Systemic infections sometimes develop after treatment for localized infection has failed. Be alert for changes in a patient's level of activity and responsiveness. As systemic infections develop, an elevation in body temperature can lead to episodes of increased heart and respiratory rates and low blood pressure. Involvement of major body systems produces specific symptoms. For example, a pulmonary infection results in a productive cough with purulent sputum. A UTI results in cloudy, foul-smelling urine.

An infection does not always present with typical signs and symptoms in all patients. For example, some older adults have an advanced infection before it is identified. Because of the aging process, there is a reduced inflammatory and immune response. Older adults have increased fatigue and diminished pain sensitivity. A reduced or absent fever response often occurs from chronic use of aspirin or nonsteroidal antiinflammatory drugs. Atypical symptoms such as confusion, incontinence, or agitation may be the only symptoms of an infectious illness (Roach, 2014). For example, as many as 20% of older adults with pneumonia do not have the typical signs and symptoms of fever, shaking, chills, and colored productive sputum. Often the only symptoms are an unexplained increase in heart rate, confusion, or generalized fatigue. A pneumonia vaccine is available and recommended for all people with chronic respiratory problems and those over 65 years of age.

Laboratory Data. Review laboratory data as soon as the results are available. Laboratory values such as increased WBCs and/or a positive blood culture often indicate infection (Table 29-4). However, laboratory values are not enough to detect infection. It is possible that a contaminated specimen was collected because of poor technique (e.g., a blood sample is mixed with IV fluid because it is improperly collected from an indwelling line; a urine specimen is contaminated because of poor perineal cleansing). You need to assess other clinical signs of infection. A culture result may show growth of an organism in the absence of infection. For example, in the older adult bacterial growth in urine without clinical symptoms does not always indicate the presence of a UTI (Roach, 2014). Also know that laboratory values often vary from laboratory to laboratory. Be sure to know the standard range of laboratory values for the laboratory in your facility.

◆ Nursing Diagnosis

During assessment gather objective data such as inspection of an open incision or a reduced caloric intake record and subjective data such as a patient's complaint of tenderness over a surgical wound site. Review the data carefully, looking for clusters of defining characteristics or risk factors that create a pattern. This pattern suggests a specific nursing diagnosis (Box 29-6). The following are examples of nursing diagnoses that often apply to patients with infection:

- *Risk for Infection*
- *Imbalanced Nutrition: Less Than Body Requirements*
- *Impaired Oral Mucous Membrane*
- *Risk for Impaired Skin Integrity*
- *Social Isolation*
- *Impaired Tissue Integrity*

It is necessary to validate data such as inspecting the integrity of a wound more carefully and to review laboratory findings to confirm a diagnosis. Success in planning appropriate nursing interventions depends on the accuracy of the diagnostic statement and the ability to meet the patient's needs. A patient will have defining characteristics for a problem focused diagnosis, and it is individualized with the addition of an accurate *related* factor in the diagnostic statement. For example, minimizing the risk for infection in a patient with a diagnosis of *Impaired Oral Mucous Membrane related to mouth breathing* requires frequent and proper oral hygiene measures. Minimizing the risk for infection in a patient with a nursing diagnosis of *Imbalanced Nutrition: Less Than Body Requirements related to inability to absorb nutrients* requires good nutritional support and fluid balance. At-risk diagnoses

TABLE 29-4 Laboratory Tests to Screen for Infection

Laboratory Value	Normal (Adult) Values	Indication of Infection
White blood cell (WBC) count	5000-10,000/mm³	Increased in acute infection, decreased in certain viral or overwhelming infections
Erythrocyte sedimentation rate	Up to 15 mm/hr for men and 20 mm/hr for women	Elevated in presence of inflammatory process
Iron level	80-180 mcg/mL for men 60-160 mcg/ml for women	Decreased in chronic infection
Cultures of urine and blood	Normally sterile, without microorganism growth	Presence of infectious microorganism growth
Cultures and Gram stain of wound, sputum, and throat	No WBCs on Gram stain, possible normal flora	Presence of infectious microorganism growth and WBCs on Gram stain
Differential Count (Percentage of Each Type of White Blood Cell)		
Neutrophils	55%-70%	Increased in acute **suppurative** (pus-forming) infection, decreased in overwhelming bacterial infection (older adult)
Lymphocytes	20%-40%	Increased in chronic bacterial and viral infection, decreased in sepsis
Monocytes	2%-8%	Increased in protozoan, rickettsial, and tuberculosis infections
Eosinophils	1%-4%	Increased in parasitic infection
Basophils	0.5%-1.5%	Normal during infection

Adapted from Pagana KD, Pagana TJ: *Mosby's diagnostic and laboratory test reference,* ed 12, St Louis, 2015, Elsevier.

BOX 29-6 Nursing Diagnostic Process

Risk for Infection

Assessment Activities	Defining Characteristics
Check results of laboratory tests.	WBC count 5000/mm^3
Review current medications.	Patient receiving antibiotics and oral antidiabetic medications
Identify potential sites of infection.	IV catheter in right forearm, in place for 3 days Foley catheter draining cloudy amber-colored urine

IV, Intravenous; *WBC*, white blood cell.

such as *Risk for Infection* require careful identification of relevant risk factors.

◆ Planning

Goals and Outcomes. The patient's care plan is based on each nursing diagnosis and related factor (see the Nursing Care Plan). Develop a plan that sets realistic outcomes so interventions are purposeful, direct, and measurable. For example, when you care for a patient with broken skin and obesity, the nursing diagnosis of *Risk for Infection* would require you to implement skin and wound care measures to promote healing. The expected outcome of "absence of drainage" sets a target for measuring the patient's improvement. Common goals of care applicable to patients with infection often include the following:

- Preventing further exposure to infectious organisms
- Controlling or reducing the extent of infection
- Maintaining resistance to infection
- Verbalizing understanding of infection prevention and control techniques (e.g., hand hygiene)

Patients often have multiple nursing diagnoses that are interrelated, and one diagnosis affects other diagnoses. A concept map for Mrs. Andrews helps to show the relationships among multiple nursing diagnoses (Figure 29-2).

Setting Priorities. Establish priorities for each diagnosis and related goals of care. For example, you are caring for a patient with cancer who develops an open wound and is unable to tolerate solid foods. The priority of administering therapies to promote wound healing such as improved nutritional intake overrides the goal of educating the patient to assume self-care therapies at home. When the patient's condition improves, the priorities change, and patient education will then become an essential intervention. Patient priorities can change quickly in the acute care environment.

Teamwork and Collaboration. The development of a care plan includes prevention and infection control practices provided by multiple disciplines. Select interventions in collaboration with the patient, the family caregiver, and health care providers such as the dietitian or respiratory therapist. Know the patient's sociocultural preferences to help you identify the most appropriate types of interventions (Box 29-7). In addition, consult with an expert in infection control in planning the patient's care. Before discharge consult with case management to complete a home assessment and identify home health needs. Case managers work with the patient, family, and home care services to ensure that a safe discharge plan is in place.

BOX 29-7 CULTURAL ASPECTS OF CARE

Implications for Infection Control and Isolation Procedures

Various cultural practices and beliefs present challenges to health care providers when infection control and isolation procedures are needed. Patients' health care practices and beliefs influence their decisions to seek treatment for an infection or to use methods to prevent infections. In the United States cities and rural areas have immigrant populations that hold on to the health care practices of their country of origin. Some of the immigrant population may come from war-torn countries where health care was limited and infections were rampant. In addition, some of these patients may fear isolation equipment, which for some may indicate that they have a deadly disease or that harm will come to them or their family. It is important to meet the cultural needs of the patients but also to integrate best practices related to infection control and, when needed, isolation procedures. Although gender-congruent caregivers are important for many cultures, the cultural aspects of care for infection control must expand beyond that premise.

Implications for Patient-Centered Care

- Identify the best method for communication and patient teaching for the patient and family. This may include a community elder, an interpreter, or a family member.
- Determine initially if the patient has any signs of fear, anxiety, or confusion about his condition and treatment plan.
- Reinforce that infection control and isolation procedures are designed for patient safety. Use simple language to explain.
- Explain each item used for infection control and isolation procedures and obtain feedback from the patient to determine his or her level of understanding.
- Be aware that in some cultures touch from a person who is not a family member is not appropriate. Thus prepare the patient by explaining why you need to touch and, when possible, ask permission. For example, "I need to check your arm that has an IV line. May I do that now?"
- If the patient seems fearful of the isolation equipment, continually reinforce why you are wearing the equipment.
- Culturally sensitive care is necessary to identify unique approaches to help patients who are on isolation precautions to understand why the precautions are necessary, answer any questions, and allay patient's and/or family's fear.

IV, Intravenous.

When care continues into the patient's home, the home care nurse plans to ensure that the home environment supports good infection prevention and control practices. For example, if a patient does not have running water yet requires wound care, even simple hand hygiene with soap and water is difficult to achieve. Home health nurses instruct patients to perform hand hygiene with either bottled water and soap or alcohol-based hand products.

◆ Implementation

By identifying and assessing a patient's risk factors and implementing appropriate measures, you can effectively reduce the risk of infection.

Health Promotion. Use your critical thinking skills to prevent an infection from developing or spreading. In the home and community settings, review with and teach patients and their family caregivers about ways to strengthen a potential host's defenses against infection. Nutrition support, rest, personal hygiene, maintenance of

NURSING CARE PLAN

Risk for Infection

ASSESSMENT

Mrs. Andrews has diabetes mellitus, urinary incontinence, and degenerative disk disease. She had surgery on her lower spine late last night. She is currently experiencing pain along her incision and is having difficulty walking. Cody is the nursing student assigned to care for Mrs. Andrews. During hand-off report, Cody finds out that Mrs. Andrews needs to wear a brace when she is out of bed, is having difficulty turning herself when she is in bed, and needs incisional dressing change because of contamination from urine following an episode of incontinence. The surgeon comes in before Cody's assessment and removes the dressing, leaving the incision open to air. The physical therapist plans to help Mrs. Andrews transfer into a chair after breakfast.

Assessment Activities	*Findings/Defining Characteristics**
Review Mrs. Andrews' chart for laboratory data that reflects infection (e.g., white blood cell [WBC] count).	The **WBC count is 9500.**
Inspect incision area.	**Incision** edges are slightly pink; edges approximated but edematous; no drainage noted.
Review risk factors for infection.	Has had **diabetes mellitus** for past 16 years; states blood sugars have been "poorly controlled" for the past year. Dietary assessment reflects malnutrition before surgery. Is **taking a glucocorticosteroid,** which reduces inflammation and suppresses the immune system.

***Defining characteristics** are shown in bold type.

NURSING DIAGNOSIS: Risk for infection

PLANNING

Goals	*Expected Outcomes (NOC)*†
	Immune Status
Mrs. Andrews will remain free from symptoms of infection.	Mrs. Andrews remains afebrile.
	Mrs. Andrews has no signs or symptoms of infection (e.g., incision intact; edges approximated; no redness, swelling, or drainage).
	Knowledge: Infection Management
Mrs. Andrews will describe ways to prevent infection before discharge.	Mrs. Andrews identifies signs and symptoms of infection by the end of today.
	Mrs. Andrews demonstrates appropriate hand hygiene before discharge.
	Mrs. Andrews identifies who will help assess incisional site when she goes home.

†Outcome classification labels from Moorhead S et al.: *Nursing outcomes classification (NOC),* ed 5, St Louis, 2013, Mosby.

INTERVENTIONS (NIC)‡	RATIONALE
Infection Protection	
Teach Mrs. Andrews how to perform hand hygiene correctly.	Meticulous hand hygiene reduces bacterial counts on the hands (Hass, 2014). Patient can easily come in contact with organisms in the health care environment that can cause infection.
Monitor Mrs. Andrews frequently to prevent urine contamination of the incision site.	Offer bedpan/restroom frequently to decrease risk for incontinence.
Provide Mrs. Andrews with incontinence panties that she wears at home.	Absorbent padding will wick away urine from Mrs. Andrew's incision.
Help Mrs. Andrews identify a family member to check the incision until it is healed and teach Mrs. Andrews and the family member signs and symptoms of infection.	Mrs. Andrews will be unable to visualize incision since it is on her back; she will need a family member to help monitor healing of the surgical site.

‡Intervention classification labels from Bulecheck GM et al.: *Nursing interventions classification (NIC),* ed 6, St Louis, 2013, Mosby.

EVALUATION

Nursing Actions	*Patient Response/Finding*	*Achievement of Outcome*
Compare Mrs. Andrews' body temperature with baseline.	Mrs. Andrews has an oral temperature of 38° C (100.4° F).	Mrs. Andrews is suspected to have infection at this time.
Ask Mrs. Andrews to describe signs and symptoms to report to health care provider.	Mrs. Andrews is unable to identify temperature range to report; unable to identify signs of wound infection.	Mrs. Andrews has minimal understanding of signs and symptoms to report. Will require additional instruction and include an information sheet on signs and symptoms of infection.
Observe for signs of infection at incisional site (e.g., redness, warmth, and wound discharge).	Incision shows has signs of infection: redness, warmth, and a small amount of tan drainage.	Incision is showing signs of infection at this time.

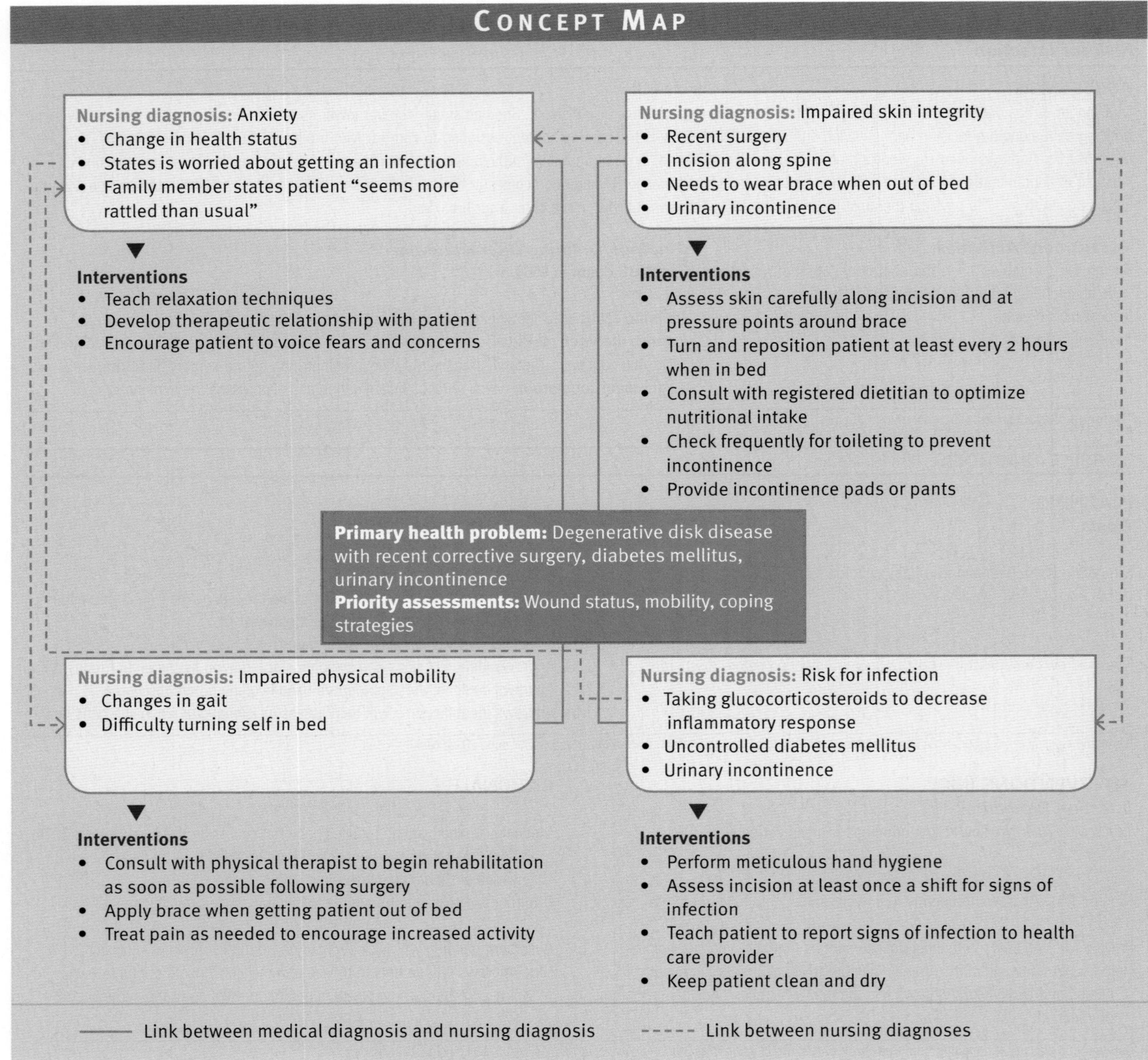

FIGURE 29-2 Concept map for Mrs. Andrews.

physiological protective mechanisms, and recommended immunizations protect patients. Explain infection prevention and control principles such as hand hygiene and methods for proper disposal of medical waste. Based on your assessment of a patient's cultural practices, integrate infection prevention and control measures into the patient's daily lifestyle practices.

Nutrition. Nutritional requirements for your patients will vary depending on their age and condition. A proper diet helps the immune system function and consists of a variety of foods from all food groups (see Chapter 45). Collaborate with registered dietitians, the patient, and the family to select the correct foods. Recommend ways to prepare foods that the patient will enjoy. Teach patients the importance of a proper diet in maintaining immunity and preventing infection.

Hygiene. Personal hygiene measures (see Chapter 40) reduce microorganisms on the skin and maintain the integrity of mucous membranes such as the mouth and vagina. Patients and family caregivers need to understand techniques for cleansing the skin and how to avoid spread of microorganisms in body secretions or excretions. For example, teach female patients how to wash their perineum from clean to dirty, from the urethra down toward the rectum, using a clean washcloth with each wipe.

Immunization. Immunization programs for infants and children have decreased the occurrence of childhood diphtheria, whooping cough, and measles. For example, according to the CDC (2015d), DTaP vaccination for whooping cough is effective for up to 8 or 9 out of 10 children who receive it, but protection fades over time. About 7 out of

10 children are fully protected 5 years after getting their last dose of DTaP. Getting a vaccine is recommended because children who still get whooping cough are much more likely to have a mild illness compared with those who never received the vaccine (CDC, 2015d). More recently developed vaccines for hepatitis A and chickenpox (varicella) provide immunity to adults and children. Advise parents about the advantages of immunizations; but also make them aware of the contraindications for certain vaccines, especially in pregnant and lactating women. You can access the most current immunization schedule at http://www.cdc.gov/vaccines/schedules/hcp/index.html.

Adequate Rest and Regular Exercise. Adequate rest and regular exercise help prevent infection. Physical exercise increases lung capacity, circulation, energy, and endurance. It also decreases stress and improves appetite, sleeping, and elimination. Help patients with a schedule that balances regular exercise with the need for rest and sleep.

Acute Care. Treatment of an infectious process includes eliminating the infectious organisms and supporting a patient's defenses. To identify the causative organisms, you will collect specimens of body fluids such as sputum or drainage from infected body sites for cultures. When the disease process or causative organism is identified, the health care provider prescribes the most effective treatment (e.g., antimicrobials).

Systemic infections require measures to prevent complications of fever (see Chapter 30). Maintaining intake of fluids prevents dehydration resulting from diaphoresis. The patient's increased metabolic rate requires an adequate nutritional intake, which may be provided through intravenous parenteral nutrition. Rest preserves energy for the healing process.

Localized infections often require measures to assist removal of debris to promote healing. You apply principles of wound care to remove infected drainage from wound sites and support the integrity of healing wounds (see Chapter 48). When changing a dressing, wear a mask and goggles or a mask with a face shield if splashing or spraying with blood or body fluids is anticipated. Apply gloves to reduce the transmission of microorganisms into the wound. Apply special dressings to facilitate removal of drainage and promote healing of wound margins. Sometimes a surgeon will insert drainage tubes to remove infected drainage from body cavities (see Chapter 48). Use medical and surgical aseptic techniques to manage wounds and ensure correct handling of all drainage or body fluids.

During the course of infection, support the patient's body defense mechanisms. For example, if a patient has diarrhea, maintain skin integrity by frequent cleansing, application of a skin-barrier cream, and frequent repositioning to prevent breakdown and the entrance of additional microorganisms. Other routine hygiene measures such as cleaning the oral cavity and bathing protect the skin and mucous membranes from invasion and overgrowth of organisms.

Medical Asepsis. Asepsis is the absence of pathogenic (disease-producing) microorganisms. Aseptic technique refers to the practices/procedures that help reduce the risk for infection. The two types of aseptic technique are medical and surgical asepsis. Basic medical aseptic techniques break the chain of infection. Use these techniques for all patients, even when no infection is diagnosed. Aggressive preventive measures are highly effective in reducing HAIs. Hand hygiene, barrier techniques, and routine environmental cleaning are examples of medical asepsis. Principles of medical asepsis are also commonly followed in the home; examples are performing hand hygiene with soap and water before preparing food, after using the bathroom, or after touching what are interpreted as dirty objects. It is important to include cultural or social beliefs of the patient and family.

Control or Elimination of Infectious Agents. With the increased use of disposable equipment, nurses are often less aware of disinfection and sterilization procedures. The proper cleaning, disinfection, and sterilization of contaminated objects significantly reduce and/or eliminate microorganisms (CDC, 2008b; Rutala and Weber, 2014). In health care facilities a sterile processing department is responsible for the disinfection and sterilization of reusable supplies and equipment. However, nurses sometimes need to perform these functions in the home care setting. Many principles of cleaning and disinfection also apply to the home, so it becomes your role to educate patients and family caregivers on these techniques.

Cleaning. Cleaning is the removal of organic material (e.g., blood) or inorganic material (e.g., soil) from objects and surfaces (Rutala and Weber, 2014). In general, cleaning involves the use of water, a detergent/disinfectant, and proper mechanical scrubbing. Cleaning occurs before disinfection and sterilization procedures.

When an object comes in contact with an infectious or potentially infectious material, it is contaminated. If the object is disposable, it is discarded. Reusable objects need to be cleaned thoroughly before reuse and then either disinfected or sterilized according to manufacturer recommendations. Failure to follow manufacturer recommendations transfers liability from the manufacturer to the health care facility or agency if an infection results from improper processing.

Apply protective eyewear (or a face shield) and utility (dishwashing style) gloves when cleaning equipment that is soiled by organic material such as blood, fecal matter, mucus, or pus. Protective barriers provide protection from potentially infectious organisms. A brush and detergent or soap are necessary for cleaning. The following steps ensure that an object is clean:

1. Rinse the contaminated object or article with cold running water to remove organic material. Hot water causes the protein in organic material to coagulate and stick to objects, making removal difficult.
2. After rinsing, wash the object with soap and warm water. Soap or detergent reduces the surface tension of water and emulsifies dirt or remaining material. Rinse the object thoroughly.
3. Use a brush to remove dirt or material in grooves or seams. Friction dislodges contaminated material for easy removal. Open hinged items for cleaning.
4. Rinse the object in warm water.
5. Dry the object and prepare it for disinfection or sterilization if indicated by classification of the item (i.e., critical, semicritical, or noncritical).
6. The brush, gloves, and sink used to clean the equipment are considered contaminated and are cleaned and dried according to policy.

Disinfection and Sterilization. Disinfection and sterilization use both physical and chemical processes that disrupt the internal functioning of microorganisms by destroying cell proteins. Disinfection describes a process that eliminates many or all microorganisms, with the exception of bacterial spores, from inanimate objects (Rutala and Weber, 2014). There are two types of disinfection: (1) the disinfection of surfaces, and (2) high-level disinfection, which is required for some patient care items such as endoscopes and bronchoscopes. Sterilization eliminates or destroys all forms of microbial life, including spores (Rutala and Weber, 2014). Sterilization methods include processing items using steam, dry heat, hydrogen peroxide plasma, or ethylene oxide (ETO). The decision to clean, clean and disinfect, or sterilize depends on the intended use of a contaminated item (Box 29-8). Be familiar with the health care facility or agency policy and procedures for cleaning, handling, and delivering care items for eventual disinfection and sterilization. Workers in the central processing area who are

BOX 29-8 Categories for Sterilization, Disinfection, and Cleaning

Critical Items

Items that enter sterile tissue or the vascular system present a high risk of infection if they are contaminated with microorganisms, especially bacterial spores. *Critical items* must be *sterile.* These items include:

- Surgical instruments
- Cardiac or intravascular catheters
- Urinary catheters
- Implants

Semicritical Items

Items that come in contact with mucous membranes or nonintact skin also present a risk. These objects must be free of all microorganisms (except bacterial spores). *Semicritical items* must be *high-level disinfected (HLD)* or *sterilized.* These items include:

- Respiratory and anesthesia equipment
- Endoscopes
- Endotracheal tubes
- GI endoscopes
- Diaphragm fitting rings

After rinsing, dry items and store in a manner to protect from damage and contamination.

Noncritical Items

Items that come in contact with intact skin but not mucous membranes must be clean. *Noncritical items* must be *disinfected.* These items include:

- Bedpans
- Blood pressure cuffs
- Bedrails
- Linens
- Stethoscopes
- Bedside trays and patient furniture
- Food utensils

TABLE 29-5 Examples of Disinfection and Sterilization Processes

Characteristics	Examples of Use
Moist Heat	
Steam is moist heat under pressure. When exposed to high pressure, water vapor reaches a temperature above boiling point to kill pathogens and spores.	Autoclave sterilizes heat-tolerant surgical instruments and semi-critical patient care items.
Chemical Sterilants—High-Level Disinfection (HLD)	
A number of chemical disinfectants are used in health care. These include alcohols, chlorines, formaldehyde, glutaraldehyde, hydrogen peroxide, iodophors, phenolics, and quaternary ammonium compounds. Each product performs in a unique manner and is used for a specific purpose.	Chemicals disinfect heat-sensitive instruments and equipment such as endoscopes and respiratory therapy equipment.
Ethylene Oxide (ETO) Gas	
This gas destroys spores and microorganisms by altering the metabolic processes of cells. Fumes are released within an autoclave-like chamber. ETO gas is toxic to humans, and aeration time varies with products.	This gas sterilizes most medical materials.
Boiling Water	
Boiling is least expensive for use in the home. Bacterial spores and some viruses resist boiling. It is not used in health care facilities.	Boiling is commonly used in the home for items such as urinary catheters, suction tubes, and drainage collection devices.

specially trained in disinfection and sterilization perform most of the procedures. The following factors influence the efficacy of the disinfecting or sterilizing method:

- *Concentration of solution and duration of contact.* A weakened concentration or shortened exposure time lessens its effectiveness.
- *Type and number of pathogens.* The greater the number of pathogens on an object, the longer the required disinfecting time.
- *Surface areas to treat.* All dirty surfaces and areas need to be fully exposed to disinfecting and sterilizing agents. The type of surface is an important factor. Is the surface porous or nonporous?
- *Temperature of the environment.* Disinfectants tend to work best at room temperature.
- *Presence of soap.* Soap causes certain disinfectants to be ineffective. Thorough rinsing of an object is necessary before disinfecting.
- *Presence of organic materials.* Disinfectants become inactivated unless blood, saliva, pus, or body excretions are washed off.

Table 29-5 lists processes for disinfection and sterilization and their characteristics. Some delicate instruments requiring sterilization cannot tolerate steam and must be processed with gas or plasma.

Protection of the Susceptible Host. A patient's resistance to infection improves as you protect normal body defenses against infection. Intervene to maintain the normal reparative processes of the body (Box 29-9). Nurses also protect themselves and others through the use of isolation precautions.

Control or Elimination of Reservoirs of Infection. In order to control or eliminate the numbers and types of organisms in reservoir sites, eliminate sources of body fluids, drainage, or solutions that possibly harbor microorganisms. Eliminating reservoirs of infection (e.g., emptying urinary drainage bags), controlling portals of exit and entry (e.g., using antiseptic wipes on IV tubing ports), and avoiding actions that transmit microorganisms prevent bacteria from finding a new site in which to grow (Box 29-10). Be aware of the state regulations for the handling and disposal of medical (infectious) waste. Occupational Safety and Health Administration (OSHA) regulations address the handling and disposal of blood and body fluids that potentially pose a risk for the transmission of bloodborne pathogens. These regulations defer to state laws and regulations (OSHA, 2011b).

Control of Portals of Exit/Entry. To control organisms exiting via the respiratory tract, cover your mouth or nose when coughing or sneezing. Teach patients, health care staff, patient's families, and visitors about respiratory hygiene or **cough etiquette**. The use of posters and written material explaining cough etiquette to learners

BOX 29-9 Infection Prevention and Control: Protecting the Susceptible Host

Protecting Natural Defense Mechanisms

- Regular bathing removes transient microorganisms from the surface of the skin. Lubrication helps keep the skin hydrated and intact. In some situations a chlorhexidine (CHG) wash is required if there is a risk for *methicillin-resistant Staphylococus aureus* (MRSA) or other resistant bacteria (CDC, 2013b).
- Perform regular oral hygiene. Saliva contains enzymes that promote digestion and has a bactericidal action to maintain control of bacteria. Flossing removes tartar and plaque that cause germ infection.
- Maintenance of adequate fluid intake promotes normal urine formation and a resultant outflow of urine to flush the bladder and urethral lining of microorganisms.
- For patients who are physically dependent or immobilized, encourage routine coughing and deep breathing to keep lower airways clear of mucus.
- Encourage proper immunization of children or adult patients who are exposed to certain infectious microorganisms. Children are vaccinated for measles, mumps, rubella, chickenpox, diphtheria, and other vaccine-preventable diseases. Adults receive one booster of tetanus-diphtheria-acellular pertussis (Tdap), annual flu vaccine, and others as recommended by the Centers for Disease Control and Prevention (CDC) (2010a). Older adults should receive a pneumococcal vaccine and an annual influenza vaccine.

Maintaining Healing Processes

- Promote intake of adequate fluids and a well-balanced diet containing essential proteins, vitamins, carbohydrates, and fats. The nurse also uses measures to increase the patient's appetite.
- Promote a patient's comfort and sleep so energy stores are replaced daily.
- Help the patient learn techniques to reduce stress.

is beneficial. Cough etiquette has become more important because of concerns for transmission of respiratory infections such as *Mycobacterium tuberculosis,* severe acute respiratory syndrome (SARS), and H1N1 influenza (CDC, 2007, 2010b). The elements of a respiratory hygiene or cough etiquette is summarized in Table 29-6 (CDC, 2007).

Another way of controlling the exit of microorganisms is by using Standard Precautions (see Table 29-6) when handling body fluids such as urine, feces, and wound drainage. Wear clean gloves if there is a chance of contact with any blood or body fluids and perform hand hygiene after providing care. Be sure to bag contaminated items (e.g., linen) appropriately.

Many measures that control the exit of microorganisms also control their entrance. Maintaining the integrity of skin and mucous membranes reduces the chances of microorganisms reaching a host. Keep a patient's skin well lubricated by using lotion as appropriate. Patients who are immobilized and debilitated are particularly susceptible to skin breakdown. Do not position patients on tubes or objects that cause breaks in the skin. It is important to turn and position patients before their skin becomes reddened. Frequent oral hygiene prevents drying of mucous membranes. A water-soluble ointment keeps the patient's lips well lubricated.

After elimination instruct women to clean the rectum and perineum by wiping from the urinary meatus toward the rectum. Cleaning in a direction from the least to the most contaminated area helps reduce GU infections. Meticulous and frequent perineal care is especially important in older-adult women who wear disposable incontinence pads.

BOX 29-10 Infection Prevention and Control to Reduce Reservoirs of Infection

Bathing

- Use soap and water to remove drainage, dried secretions, or excess perspiration.

Dressing Changes

- Change dressings that become wet and/or soiled (see Chapter 48).

Contaminated Articles

- Place tissues, soiled dressings, or soiled linen in fluid-resistant bags for proper disposal.

Contaminated Sharps

- Place all needles, safety needles, and needleless systems into puncture-proof containers, which should be located at the site of use. Federal law requires the use of needle-safe technology. Blood tube holders are single use only (OSHA, 2012).

Bedside Unit

- Keep table surfaces clean and dry.

Bottled Solutions

- Do not leave bottled solutions open.
- Keep solutions tightly capped.
- Date bottles when opened and discard in 24 hours.

Surgical Wounds

- Keep drainage tubes and collection bags patent to prevent accumulation of serous fluid under the skin surface.

Drainage Bottles and Bags

- Wear gloves and protective eyewear if splashing or spraying with contaminated blood or body fluids is anticipated.
- Empty and dispose of drainage suction bottles according to agency policy.
- Empty all drainage systems on each shift unless otherwise ordered by a health care provider.
- Never raise a drainage system (e.g., urinary drainage bag) above the level of the site being drained unless it is clamped off.

Another cause for entrance of microorganisms into a host is improper handling and management of urinary catheters and drainage sets (see Chapter 46). Keep the point of connection between a catheter and drainage tube closed and intact. As long as such systems are closed, their contents are considered sterile. Outflow spigots on drainage bags should also remain closed to prevent entrance of bacteria. Minimize movement of the catheter at the urethra by stabilizing it with tape or a securing device to reduce chances of microorganisms ascending the urethra into the bladder. Do not share urine-measuring containers among patients. Sometimes you care for patients with closed drainage systems that collect wound drainage, bile, or other body fluids. Make sure that the site from which a drainage tube exits remains clear of excess moisture or accumulated drainage. Keep all tubing connected throughout use and only open drainage receptacles when it is necessary to discard or measure the volume of drainage (see Chapter 48).

Control of Transmission. Effective prevention and control of infection requires you to remain aware of the modes of transmission of microorganisms and ways to control them. In any health care setting a patient usually has a personal set of care items. Sharing bedpans, urinals, bath basins, and eating utensils among patients easily leads to cross-infection. When using a stethoscope, always wipe off the bell, diaphragm, and ear tips with a disinfectant such as an alcohol wipe before proceeding to the next patient. Ear tips are a common location for staphylococcal organisms (Whittington et al., 2009). In facilities where HAI diarrhea occurs, electronic thermometers are not recommended for rectal temperatures. You usually use oral or tympanic thermometers to assess temperature. Do not use electronic thermometers for patients on contact isolation.

Always be careful when handling exudate such as urine, feces, emesis, and blood. Contaminated fluids easily splash while being discarded in toilets or hoppers. Urinals and bedpans need to be emptied at water level to reduce the risk of splash or splatter, and gloves and protective eyewear are worn. Appropriately dispose of disposable soiled items in trash bags. Dispose of items contaminated with large amounts of blood in biohazard bags. Know the location of biohazard bags; it may differ among facilities. Handle laboratory specimens from all patients as if they were infectious and place them in designated biohazard containers or bags for transport or disposal. Because certain microorganisms travel easily through the air, do not shake linens or bedclothes. Dust with a treated or dampened cloth to prevent dust particles from entering the air.

To prevent transmission of microorganisms through individual contact, do not allow soiled items and equipment to touch your clothing. A common error is to carry dirty linen in the arms against your uniform. Use fluid-resistant linen bags or carry soiled linen with hands held out from the body. Cover laundry hampers and empty them before they become overloaded. **Never put clean or soiled linens on the floor.**

You will learn to follow **standard precautions** to prevent and control infection transmission. Standard precautions apply to contact with blood, body fluid, nonintact skin, and mucous membranes from all patients. These precautions protect patients and provide protection for health care workers.

Hand Hygiene. The most effective basic technique in preventing and controlling the transmission of infection is hand hygiene (see Skill 29-1 on pp. 471-473) (Mathur, 2011; WHO, 2009). **Hand hygiene** is a general term that applies to four techniques: handwashing, antiseptic hand wash, antiseptic hand rub, or surgical hand antisepsis. **Handwashing** is defined by the CDC (2008a) as the vigorous, brief rubbing together of all surfaces of lathered hands, followed by rinsing under a stream of warm water for 15 seconds. The fundamental principle behind handwashing is removing microorganisms mechanically from the hands and rinsing with water. Handwashing does not kill microorganisms. An antiseptic hand wash means washing hands with warm water and soap or other detergents containing an antiseptic agent, Some antiseptics kill bacteria and some viruses. An antiseptic hand rub means applying an antiseptic hand-rub product to all surfaces of the hands to reduce the number of microorganisms present. Ethanol-based hand antiseptics containing 60% to 90% alcohol appear to be the most effective against common pathogens found on the hands (CDC, 2008a). Alcohol-based products are more effective for standard handwashing or hand antisepsis (nonsoiled hands) by health care workers than regular soap or antimicrobial soaps (CDC, 2008a). Surgical hand antisepsis is an antiseptic hand-wash or hand-rub technique that surgical personnel perform before surgery to eliminate transient and reduce resident hand flora. Antiseptic detergent preparations have persistent antimicrobial activity (CDC, 2008a; WHO, 2009).

According to the World Health Organization (2009), hand cleansing practices are likely established in the first 10 years of a person's life. This imprinting affects an individual's attitudes about hand cleansing throughout life. This is called inherent hand hygiene (WHO, 2009). Attitudes toward handwashing in situations such as the delivery of health care are called elective handwashing practices (WHO, 2009). In many patient populations, inherent and elective handwashing are influenced by cultural factors. Thus hand hygiene is often performed for hygienic reasons, rituals, and symbolic reasons. It is important to learn the significance hand hygiene holds for an individual.

The use of alcohol-based hand rubs is recommended by the CDC (2008a) to improve hand hygiene practices, protect health care workers' hands, and reduce the transmission of pathogens to patients and personnel in health care settings. Alcohols have excellent germicidal activity and are as effective as soap and water. However, alcohol-based hand antiseptics are not effective on hands that are visibly dirty or are contaminated with organic materials (CDC, 2013). Boyce et al. (2002) and the WHO (2009) recommend the following hand hygiene guidelines:

1. When hands are visibly dirty, when hands are soiled with blood or other body fluids, before eating, and after using the toilet, wash hands with water and either a nonantimicrobial or antimicrobial soap.
2. Wash hands if exposed to spore-forming organisms such as *C. difficile, Bacillus anthracis, or Norovirus* (CDC, 2014).
3. If hands are not visibly soiled (WHO, 2009), use an alcohol-based, waterless antiseptic agent for routinely decontaminating hands in the following clinical situations:
   - Before, after, and between direct patient contact (e.g., taking a pulse, lifting a patient)
   - Before putting on sterile gloves and before inserting invasive devices such as a peripheral vascular catheter or urinary catheter
   - After contact with body fluids or excretions, mucous membranes, nonintact skin, and wound dressings (even if gloves are worn)
   - When moving from a contaminated to a clean body site during care
   - After contact with surfaces or objects in the patient's room (e.g., overbed table, IV pump)
   - After removing gloves (CDC, 2008a)

Remember, contaminated hands of health care workers are a primary source of infection transmission in health care settings. It is recommended that health care workers have well-manicured nails and refrain from wearing artificial nails to reduce microorganism transmission.

Infection can easily be transmitted by visitors of patients in health care settings. A study by Birnbach (2012) and colleagues showed that a coordinated effort is needed to increase visitor hand hygiene compliance, including an evaluation of access to an alcohol-based hand sanitizer, education of visitors on the importance of hand hygiene, and evaluation of corresponding changes in hand hygiene behavior. Instruct patients and visitors about proper hand hygiene technique, the reason for it, and the times for performing it. If health care is to continue at home, teach patients and family caregivers to wash their hands before eating or handling food; after handling contaminated equipment, linen, or organic material; and after elimination. In health care settings, encourage visitors to wash their hands before eating or handling food; after coming in contact with infected patients; and after handling contaminated equipment, patient furniture, or organic material (Gould et al., 2011).

You are responsible for providing the patient and family with a safe environment. Recently the CDC (2015e) launched its Clean Hands Save Lives Campaign. It highlights for consumers the five simple and effective steps (Wet, Lather, Scrub, Rinse, Dry) to take to reduce the spread of diarrheal and respiratory illnesses and thus to stay healthy. Many hospitals encourage patients to follow the recommendations of TJC's "Speak Up" campaign. TJC together with the Centers for Medicare and Medicaid Services urge patients to take a role in preventing health care errors by becoming active, involved, and informed participants on the health care team. The program features brochures, posters, and buttons on a variety of patient safety topics. One recommendation is to have patients speak up to be sure the health care provider has cleaned his or her hands or wears gloves when providing care.

The effectiveness of infection prevention practices such as hand hygiene depends on the conscientiousness and consistency in using proper technique by all health care providers. It is human nature to forget key procedural steps or, when hurried, to take shortcuts that break aseptic procedures. However, failure to comply with basic procedures places patients at risk for infections that can seriously impair recovery or lead to death.

Isolation and Isolation Precautions. In 2007 the Hospital Infection Control Practices Advisory Committee (HICPAC) of the CDC published revised guidelines for isolation precautions. HICPAC recommended that facilities modify the guidelines according to need and as dictated by federal, state, or local regulations. The guidelines contain recommendations for respiratory hygiene/cough etiquette as part of Standard Precautions. The CDC recommendations contain two tiers of precautions (Table 29-6). The first and most important tier is called *Standard Precautions,* which are designed to be used for the care of all patients, in all settings, regardless of risk or presumed infection

TABLE 29-6 Centers for Disease Control and Prevention Isolation Guidelines

Standard Precautions (Tier One) for Use with All Patients

- Standard precautions apply to blood, blood products, all body fluids, secretions, excretions (except sweat), nonintact skin, and mucous membranes.
- Perform hand hygiene before, after, and between direct contact with patients. (Examples of between-contact activities are cleaning hands after a patient care activity, moving to a non–patient care activity, and cleaning hands again before returning to perform patient contact.)
- Perform hand hygiene after contact with blood, body fluids, mucous membranes, nonintact skin, secretions, excretions, or wound dressings; after contact with inanimate surfaces or articles in a patient room; and immediately after gloves are removed.
- When hands are visibly soiled or contaminated with blood or body fluids, wash them with either a nonantimicrobial or an antimicrobial soap and water.
- When hands are not visibly soiled or contaminated with blood or body fluids, use an alcohol-based, waterless antiseptic agent to perform hand hygiene (WHO, 2009).
- Wash hands with nonantimicrobial soap and water if contact with spores (e.g., *Clostridium difficile*) is likely to have occurred.
- Do not wear artificial fingernails or extenders if duties include direct contact with patients at high risk for infection and associated adverse outcomes.
- Wear gloves when touching blood, body fluids, secretions, excretions, nonintact skin, mucous membranes, or contaminated items or surfaces is likely. Remove gloves and perform hand hygiene between patient care encounters and when going from a contaminated to a clean body site.
- Wear personal protective equipment (PPE) when the anticipated patient interaction indicates that contact with blood or body fluids may occur.
- A private room is unnecessary unless the patient's hygiene is unacceptable (e.g., uncontained secretions, excretions, or wound drainage).
- Discard all contaminated sharp instruments and needles in a puncture-resistant container. Health care facilities must make available needleless devices. Any needles should be disposed of uncapped, or a mechanical safety device is activated for recapping.
- *Respiratory hygiene/cough etiquette:* Have patients cover the nose/mouth when coughing or sneezing; use tissues to contain respiratory secretions and dispose in nearest waste container; perform hand hygiene after contacting respiratory secretions and contaminated objects/materials; contain respiratory secretions with procedure or surgical mask; spatial separation of at least 3 feet away from others if coughing.

Transmission-Based Precautions (Tier Two) for Use with Specific Types of Patients

Category	Infection/Condition	Barrier Protection
Airborne precautions (droplet nuclei smaller than 5 microns)	Measles, chickenpox (varicella), disseminated varicella zoster, pulmonary or laryngeal tuberculosis	Private room, negative-pressure airflow of at least 6 to 12 exchanges per hour via high-efficiency particulate air (HEPA) filtration; mask or respiratory protection device, N95 respirator (depending on condition)
Droplet precautions (droplets larger than 5 microns; being within 3 feet of the patient)	Diphtheria (pharyngeal), rubella, streptococcal pharyngitis, pneumonia or scarlet fever in infants and young children, pertussis, mumps, *Mycoplasma* pneumonia, meningococcal pneumonia or sepsis, pneumonic plague	Private room or cohort patients; mask or respirator required (depending on condition) (refer to agency policy)
Contact precautions (direct patient or environmental contact)	Colonization or infection with multidrug-resistant organisms such as VRE and MRSA, *Clostridium difficile,* shigella, and other enteric pathogens; major wound infections; herpes simplex; scabies; varicella zoster (disseminated); respiratory syncytial virus in infants, young children, or immunocompromised adults	Private room or cohort patients (see agency policy), gloves, gowns (Patients may leave their room for procedures or therapy if infectious material is contained or covered, placed in a clean gown, and if hands are cleaned.)
Protective environment	Allogeneic hematopoietic stem cell transplants	Private room; positive airflow with 12 or more air exchanges per hour; HEPA filtration for incoming air; mask to be worn by patient when out of room during times of construction in area

Adapted from Centers for Disease Control and Prevention, Hospital Infection Control Practice Advisory Committee: Guidelines for isolation precautions in hospitals, *MMWR Morb Mortal Wkly Rep* 57/RR-16:39, 2007.
MRSA, Methicillin-resistant *Staphylococcus aureus; VRE,* vancomycin-resistant enterococcus.

status. Standard Precautions are the primary strategies (including barrier precautions) for prevention of infection transmission and apply to contact with blood, body fluids, nonintact skin, mucous membranes, and equipment or surfaces contaminated with potentially infectious materials. Basically, in the acute care setting a nurse will follow standard precautions in all aspects of care. This includes barrier precautions and the appropriate use of PPE such as gowns, gloves, masks, eyewear, and other protective devices or clothing. The choice of barriers depends on the task being performed and the patient's disease. Standard precautions applies to all patients because every patient has the potential to transmit infection via blood and body fluids, and the risk for infection transmission is unknown. Respiratory hygiene/cough etiquette applies to any person with signs of respiratory infection, including cough, congestion, rhinorrhea, or increased production of respiratory secretions when entering a health care site. Educating health care staff, patients, and visitors to follow respiratory hygiene/cough etiquette protect both patients and health care workers.

The second tier of precautions (see Table 29-6) includes precautions designed for the care of patients who are known or suspected to be infected or colonized with microorganisms transmitted by droplet, airborne, or contact routes (CDC, 2007; Brisko, 2009). There are four types of transmission-based precautions, which are based on the mode of transmission of a disease: ***Airborne, Droplet, Contact,*** and ***Protective Environment Precautions.*** These precautions are for patients with highly transmissible pathogens. The protective environment category is designed for patients who have undergone transplants and gene therapy (CDC, 2007).

- *Contact precautions:* Used for direct and indirect contact with patients and their environment. Direct contact refers to the care and handling of contaminated body fluids. Contact precautions require a gown and gloves. An example includes blood or other body fluids from an infected patient that enter the health care worker's body through direct contact with compromised skin or mucous membranes. Indirect contact involves the transfer of an infectious agent through a contaminated intermediate object such as contaminated instruments or hands of health care workers. The health care worker may transmit microorganisms from one patient site to another if hand hygiene is not performed between patients (CDC, 2007).
- *Droplet precautions:* Focus on diseases that are transmitted by large droplets (greater than 5 microns) expelled into the air and by being within 3 feet of a patient. Droplet precautions require the wearing of a surgical mask when within 3 feet of the patient, proper hand hygiene, and some dedicated-care equipment. An example is a patient with influenza.
- *Airborne precautions:* Focus on diseases that are transmitted by smaller droplets, which remain in the air for longer periods of time. This requires a specially equipped room with a negative air flow referred to as an *airborne infection isolation room.* Air is not returned to the inside ventilation system but is filtered through a high-efficiency particulate air (HEPA) filter and exhausted directly to the outside. All health care personnel wear an N95 respirator every time they enter the room.
- *Protective environment:* Focuses on a very limited patient population. This form of isolation requires a specialized room with positive airflow. The airflow rate is set at greater than 12 air exchanges per hour, and all air is filtered through a HEPA filter. Patients must wear masks when out of their room during times of construction in area.

Health care facilities are required to have the capability of isolating patients. However, not all communicable diseases require placing a patient in a special private room. You can conduct many isolation practices in standard rooms using barrier precautions.

Because of the resurgence of TB, the CDC (2007) developed guidelines to prevent its transmission to health care workers and stresses the importance of isolation for the patient with known or suspected TB in a special negative pressure room. Close the doors to the patient's room to control direction of airflow. You must wear a special high-filtration particulate respirator on entering a respiratory isolation rooms. A respirator must be fitted to your facial size and characteristics. When worn correctly, particulate respirators and masks have a tighter face seal and filter at a higher level than routine surgical masks.

Multidrug-resistant organisms (MDROs) such as methicillin-resistant *Staphylococcus aureus* (MRSA), vancomycin-resistant enterococcus (VRE) and *Clostridium difficile* (*C. diff*) are more common as a cause of colonization and HAIs. MDROs have developed a resistance to one or more broad spectrum antibiotics, making the organisms hard to treat effectively. Major efforts have been in place for a number of years to reduce the incidence of HAIs caused by these dangerous organisms. For example, evidence shows that the percentage of central line bloodstream infections (see Chapter 42) caused by MRSA, VRE, and gram-negative bacteria have declined (CDC, 2011b). Unlike MRSA and VRE, *C. difficile* (which is transmitted by the fecal-oral route) is harder to eliminate from the environment. It is a spore-forming microorganism, meaning it can remain on surfaces (e.g., bedside table, stethoscope) in a dormant state for long periods of time. To reduce the risk of cross-contamination among patients, use Contact Precautions in addition to Standard Precautions when caring for patients with MDROs.

Regardless of the type of isolation or barrier protection you use, follow these basic principles when caring for patients:

- Understand how certain diseases are transmitted and which protective barriers to use.
- Use thorough hand hygiene before entering and leaving the room of a patient in isolation.
- Dispose of contaminated supplies and equipment in a manner that prevents spread of microorganisms to other people as indicated by the mode of transmission of the organism.
- Protect all people who might be exposed during transport of a patient outside the isolation room.

Psychological Implications of Isolation. The psychological effects of being in an isolation room must be considered in your care of patients. Many patients find positive aspects of being accommodated in a single room; however, the overall experience of isolation is commonly viewed negatively (Barratt, 2010). Isolation imposes barriers to the expression of a patient's identity and normal interpersonal relationships and affects the delivery of quality care. When a patient requires isolation in a private room, a sense of loneliness sometimes develops because normal social relationships become disrupted. This situation can be psychologically harmful, especially for children. A study noted that patients in isolation suffered more depression and anxiety and were less satisfied with their care (Abad et al., 2010). Patients' body images become altered as a result of the infectious process. Some feel unclean, rejected, lonely, or guilty. Infection prevention and control practices further intensify these beliefs of difference or undesirability. Isolation disrupts normal social relationships with visitors and caregivers. Take the opportunity to listen to a patient's concerns or interests. If you rush care or show a lack of interest in a patient's needs, he or she feels rejected and even more isolated.

Before you institute isolation measures, the patient and family need to understand the nature of the disease or condition, the purposes of isolation, and steps for following specific precautions. If they are able to participate in maintaining infection prevention and control practices, the chances of reducing the spread of infection increase. Teach the patient and family to perform hand hygiene and use barrier protection if appropriate. Demonstrate each procedure; be sure to give the patient and family an opportunity for practice. It is also important to explain how infectious organisms are transmitted so the patient and family understand the difference between contaminated and clean objects. Explaining and demonstrating these procedures, especially hand hygiene, help the family to consistently practice correct hand hygiene and prescribed isolation measures (Gould et al., 2011).

Take measures to improve a patient's sensory stimulation during isolation. Make sure that the room environment is clean and pleasant. Open drapes or shades and remove excess supplies and equipment. Listen to the patient's concerns or interests. Mealtime is a particularly good opportunity for conversation. Providing comfort measures such as repositioning, a back massage, or a warm sponge bath increase physical stimulation. Depending on the patient's condition, encourage him or her to walk around the room or sit up in a chair. Recreational activities such as board games, reading, or cards are options for keeping a patient mentally stimulated.

Explain to the family the patient's risk for depression or loneliness (Abad et al., 2010). Encourage visiting family members to avoid expressions or actions that convey revulsion or disgust related to infection prevention and control practices. Discuss ways to provide meaningful stimulation.

The Isolation Environment. Private rooms used for isolation sometimes provide negative-pressure airflow to prevent infectious particles from flowing out of a room to other rooms and the air handling system. Special rooms with positive-pressure airflow are also used for highly susceptible immunocompromised patients such as recipients of transplanted organs. On the door or wall outside the room a nurse posts a card listing precautions for the isolation category in use according to health care facility policy. The card is a handy reference for health care personnel and visitors and alerts anyone who might enter the room accidentally that special precautions must be followed.

An area immediately outside an isolation room or an adjoining anteroom needs to contain hand hygiene and PPE supplies. Soap and antiseptic (antimicrobial) solutions are also available. Personnel and visitors perform hand hygiene before entering a patient's room and again before leaving the room. If toilet facilities are unavailable, there are special procedures for handling portable commodes, bedpans, or urinals.

All patient care rooms, including those used for isolation, should contain an impervious bag for soiled or contaminated linen and a trash container with plastic liners. Impervious receptacles prevent transmission of microorganisms by preventing leaking and soiling of the outside surface. A disposable rigid container needs to be available in the room to discard used sharps such as safety needles and syringes.

Remain aware of infection prevention and control techniques while working with patients in protected environments. You need to feel comfortable performing all procedures and yet remain conscious of infection prevention and control principles. Depending on the microorganism and mode of transmission, evaluate which articles or equipment to take into an isolation room. For example, the CDC (2007) recommends the dedicated use of articles such as stethoscopes, sphygmomanometers, and thermometers in the isolation room of a patient infected or colonized with VRE. Do not use these devices on other patients unless they are first adequately cleaned and disinfected. Box 29-11 describes the procedures to perform when using shared equipment.

Personal Protective Equipment. The PPE, specialized clothing or equipment (e.g., gowns, masks or respirators, protective eyewear and gloves) that you wear for protection against exposure to infectious materials, should be readily available in a patient care area (CDC, 2007). You choose the equipment to use depending on the task to be performed.

Gowns. The primary reason for gowning is to prevent soiling clothes during contact with a patient. Gowns or cover-ups protect health care personnel and visitors from coming in contact with infected material and blood or body fluids. Gowns are often required, depending on the expected amount of exposure to infectious material. Gowns used for barrier protection are made of a fluid-resistant material. Change gowns immediately if damaged or heavily contaminated.

Isolation gowns usually open at the back and have ties or snaps at the neck and waist to keep the gown closed and secure. Gowns need to be long enough to cover all outer garments. Long sleeves with tight-fitting cuffs provide added protection. No special technique is required for applying clean gowns as long as they are fastened securely. However, carefully remove gowns to minimize contamination of the hands and uniform and discard them after removal.

BOX 29-11 PROCEDURAL GUIDELINES

Caring for a Patient on Isolation Precautions

Delegation Considerations

The skill of caring for a patient on isolation precautions can be delegated to nursing assistive personnel (NAP). However, it is the nurse who assesses the patient's status and isolation indications. Instruct NAP about:

- Reason patient is on isolation precautions.
- Precautions about bringing equipment into the patient's room.
- Special precautions regarding individual patient needs such as transportation to diagnostic tests.

Equipment

Personal protective equipment (PPE) determined by type of isolation—gloves, gowns, masks, protective eyewear, or face shield—that may be needed; supplies depend on procedures performed in room; sharps container; disposable blood pressure (BP) cuff.

Steps

1. Assess isolation indications (e.g., patient's medical history for exposure, laboratory tests, and wound drainage).
2. Review laboratory test results to identify type of microorganism for which the patient is isolated and if patient is immunocompromised.
3. Review agency policies and precautions necessary for the specific isolation system and consider care measures you will perform while in patient's room.
4. Review nurses' notes or speak with colleagues regarding patient's emotional state and adjustment to isolation.
5. Determine if patient has latex allergy to avoid sensitivity or allergic reaction.
6. Perform hand hygiene and prepare all equipment that you need to take into patient's room. In some cases equipment remains in the room (stethoscope

Continued

BOX 29-11 PROCEDURAL GUIDELINES

***Caring for a Patient on Isolation Precautions*—cont'd**

or BP cuff). Decide which isolation equipment is necessary before entering the patient's room. For example, decide if you need a gown and gloves for a patient in contact precautions or a special respirator mask for a patient on airborne precautions.

7. Prepare for entrance into isolation room:
   a. Apply cover gown, being sure that it covers all outer garments. Pull sleeves down to wrist. Tie securely at neck and waist (see illustration).

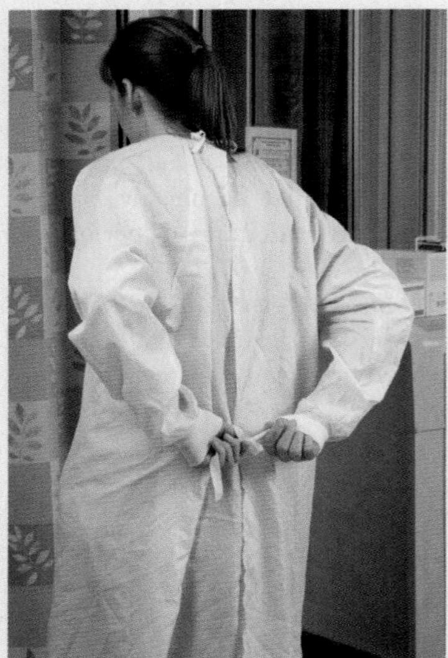

STEP 7a Tie gown at waist.

   b. Apply either surgical mask or fitted respirator around mouth and nose. (Type depends on type of precautions and agency policy.) The nurse must have a medical evaluation and be fit tested before using a respirator (OSHA, 2011a).
   c. If needed, apply eyewear or goggles snugly around face and eyes. If prescription glasses are worn, side shield may be used.
   d. Apply clean gloves. (NOTE: Wear unpowdered latex-free gloves if patient has a history of latex allergy.) Wear gloves within gown; bring glove cuffs over edge of gown sleeves (see illustration).

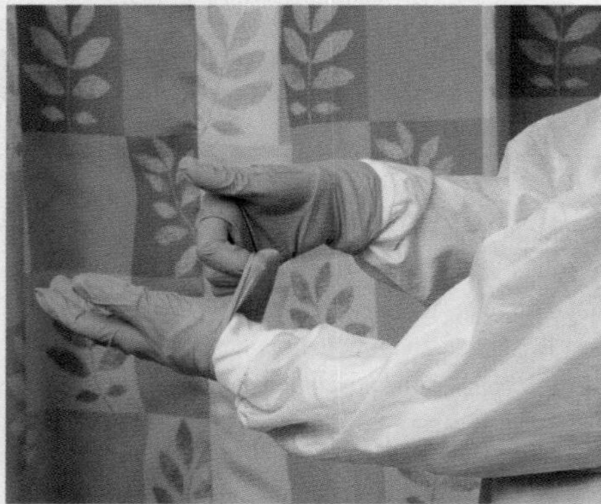

STEP 7d Apply gloves over gown sleeves.

8. Enter patient's room. Arrange supplies and equipment. (If equipment will be removed from room for reuse, place on clean paper towel.)
9. Explain purpose of isolation and necessary precautions to patient and family. Offer opportunity to ask questions. Discuss types of activities patient may wish to try to stay occupied. Assess for evidence of emotional problems that can occur from isolation.
10. Assess vital signs (see Chapter 30).
    a. If patient is infected or colonized with a resistant organism (e.g., VRE, MRSA, or C. diff), equipment remains in room. This includes stethoscope and BP cuff.
    b. If stethoscope is to be reused, clean diaphragm or bell with alcohol. Set aside on clean surface.
    c. Use individual electronic or disposable thermometer.

CLINICAL DECISION: If disposable thermometer indicates a fever, assess for other signs/symptoms. Confirm fever using an alternative thermometer. Do not use electronic thermometer if patient is suspected or confirmed to have *Clostridium difficile* (Cohen et al., 2010)

11. Administer medications (see Chapter 32).
    a. Give oral medication in wrapper or cup.
    b. Dispose of wrapper or cup in plastic-lined receptacle.
    c. Wear gloves when administering an injection.
    d. Discard safety needle and syringe or uncapped needle into sharps container.
    e. Place reusable syringe (e.g., Carpujet) on a clean towel for eventual removal and disinfection.
    f. If you are not wearing gloves and hands come into contact with contaminated article or body fluids, perform hand hygiene as soon as possible.
12. Administer hygiene, encouraging patient to discuss questions or concerns about isolation. Provide informal teaching at this time.
    a. Avoid allowing gown to become wet. Carry wash basin out away from gown; avoid leaning against any wet surface.
    b. Remove linen from bed; avoid contact with gown. Place in linen bag according to agency policy.
    c. Provide clean bed linen and a set of towels.
    d. Change gloves and perform hand hygiene if they become solid and further care is necessary.
13. Collect specimens.
    a. Place specimen containers on clean paper towel in patient's bathroom. Follow procedure for collecting specimen of body fluids.
    b. Transfer specimen to container without soiling outside of container. Place container in plastic bag and place label on outside of bag or per agency policy. Label specimen in front of patient (TJC, 2016).
    c. Perform hand hygiene and reglove if additional procedures are needed.
    d. Check label on specimen for accuracy (warning labels are often used, depending on agency policy). Send to laboratory. Label containers with a biohazard label (see illustration).

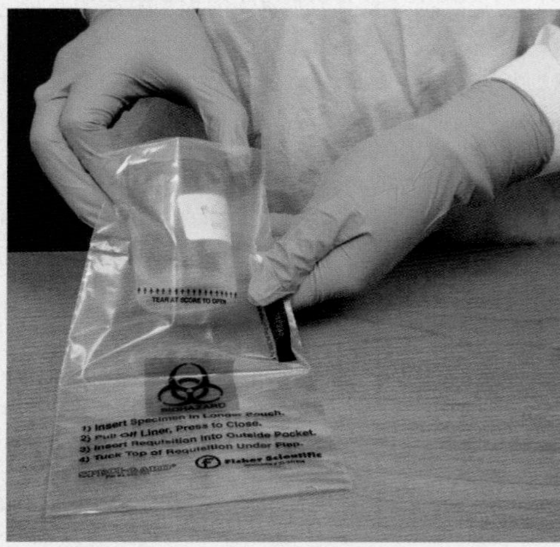

STEP 13d Specimen container placed in biohazard bag.

BOX 29-11 PROCEDURAL GUIDELINES

***Caring for a Patient on Isolation Precautions*—cont'd**

14. Dispose of linen and trash bags as they become full.
    a. Use sturdy, moisture-resistant single bags to contain soiled articles. Use double bag if outside of bag is contaminated.
    b. Tie bags securely at top in knot (see illustration).

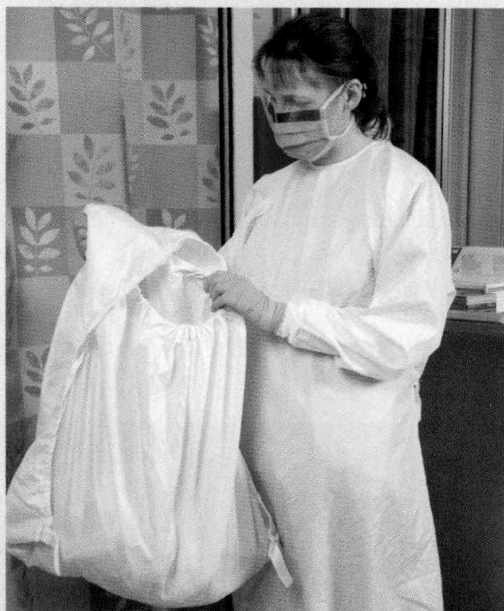

STEP 14b Tie trash bag securely.

15. Remove all reusable equipment. Clean any contaminated surfaces (see health care facility or agency policy).
16. Resupply room as needed. Have a staff member outside isolation room hand you new supplies.
17. Explain to patient when you plan to return to room. Ask whether patient requires any personal care items, books, or magazines.
18. Leave isolation room. The order for removing PPE depends on what was needed for the type of isolation. The sequence listed is based on full PPE being required.
    a. Remove gloves. Remove one glove by grasping cuff and pulling glove inside out over hand. With ungloved hand tuck finger inside cuff of remaining glove and pull it off, inside out (see illustration).

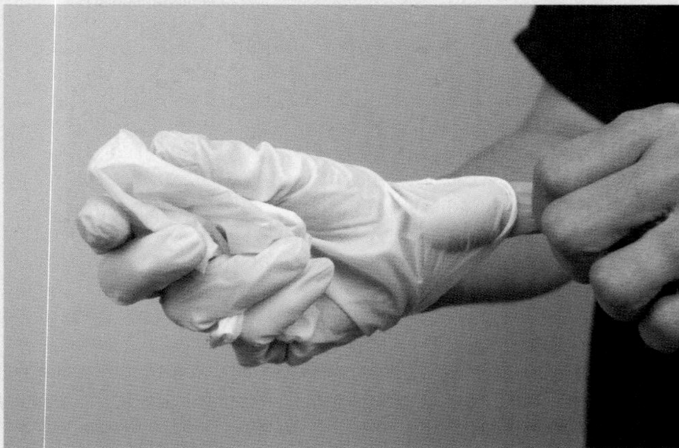

STEP 18a Remove glove.

    b. Remove eyewear/face shield or goggles.
    c. Untie waist and neck strings of gown. Allow gown to fall from shoulders. Remove hands from sleeves without touching outside of gown. Hold gown inside at shoulder seams and fold inside out. Discard in laundry bag if fabric or in trash can if gown is disposable.
    d. Remove mask: If mask loops over your ears, remove from ears and pull away from face. For a tie-on mask, untie *top* mask strings; hold strings; untie bottom strings, pull mask away from face, and drop it into trash receptacle. Do not touch outer surface of mask (see illustrations).

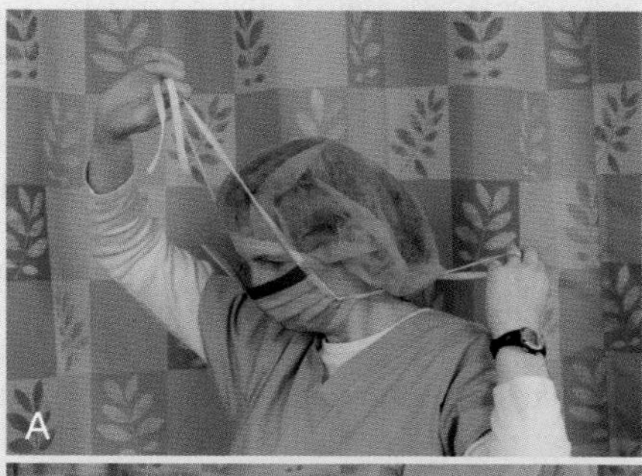

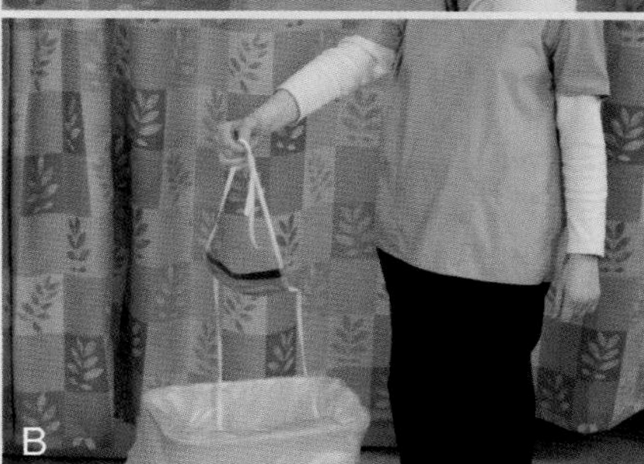

STEP 18d A, Untie top strings of mask. **B,** Drop mask into trash.

    e. Perform hand hygiene.
    f. Leave room and close door if necessary. (Make sure that door is closed if patient is on airborne precautions.)
    g. Dispose of all contaminated supplies and equipment in a manner that prevents spread of microorganisms to other people (see health care facility or agency policy).

Masks. Masks provide respiratory protection. Wear full-face protection (with eyes, nose, and mouth covered) when you anticipate splashing or spraying of blood or body fluid into the face. Also wear masks when working with a patient placed on airborne or droplet precautions. If a patient is on airborne precautions for TB, apply an OSHA-approved respirator-style mask. The mask protects you from inhaling microorganisms and small-particle droplet nuclei that remain suspended in the air from a patient's respiratory tract. The surgical mask protects a wearer from inhaling large-particle aerosols that travel short distances (3 feet). When caring for patients on droplet or airborne precautions, apply a mask (surgical or respirator) when entering the isolation room.

At times a patient who is susceptible to infection wears a mask to prevent inhalation of pathogens. Patients on droplet or airborne precautions who are transported outside of their rooms need to wear a surgical mask to protect other patients and personnel. Masks prevent transmission of infection by direct contact with mucous membranes (CDC, 2005a). A mask discourages the wearer from touching the eyes, nose, or mouth (Box 29-12).

A properly applied mask fits snugly over the mouth and nose so pathogens and body fluids cannot enter or escape through the sides. If a person wears glasses, the top edge of the mask fits below the glasses so they do not cloud over as the person exhales. Keep talking to a minimum while wearing a mask to reduce respiratory airflow. A mask that has become moist does not provide a barrier to microorganisms and is ineffective. You need to discard it. Never reuse a disposable mask. Warn patients and family members that a mask can cause a sensation of smothering. If family members become uncomfortable, they should leave the room and discard the mask.

Specially fitted respiratory protective devices (N95 respirator masks) are required when caring for patients on airborne precautions such as patients with known or suspected TB (Figure 29-3) (CDC, 2005a). The mask must have a higher filtration rating than regular surgical masks and be fitted snugly to prevent leakage around the sides. Be aware of health care facility policy regarding the type of respiratory protective device required. Special fit testing is required to establish the size and ability of the nurse to wear this type of mask (CDC, 2005a).

Eye Protection. Use either special glasses or goggles when performing procedures that generate splash or splatter. Examples of such procedures include irrigation of a large abdominal wound or insertion of an arterial catheter when the nurse assists a health care provider. A

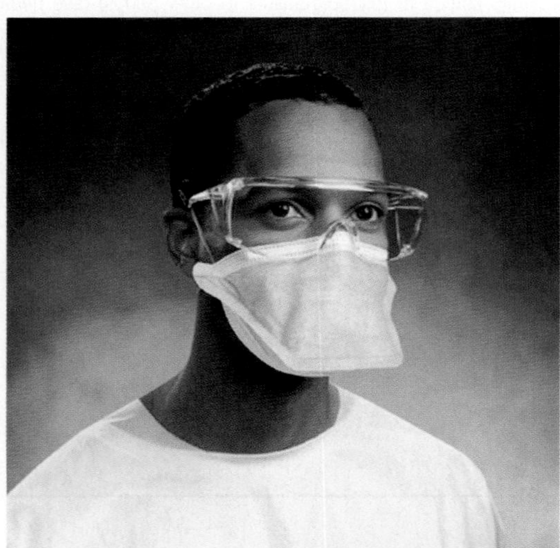

FIGURE 29-3 N95 respirator mask with protective eyewear. (Courtesy Kimberly-Clark Health Care, Roswell, Ga.)

BOX 29-12 PROCEDURAL GUIDELINES

Applying a Surgical Type of Mask

Delegation Considerations

The skill of applying a surgical mask can be delegated when NAP are trained in required sterile procedure. The nurse informs NAP to:

- Put on the mask following the appropriate steps.
- Change the mask if it becomes moist or contaminated.
- Remove the mask when leaving the patient's room.

Equipment

Disposable mask

Steps

1. Find top edge of mask (some have a thin metal strip along edge). Pliable metal fits snugly against bridge of nose. Others offer an occlusive fit that does not require an adjustment.
2. Hold mask by top two strings or loops. Secure two top ties at top of back of head (see illustration), with ties above ears. (*Alternative:* Slip loops over each ear.)

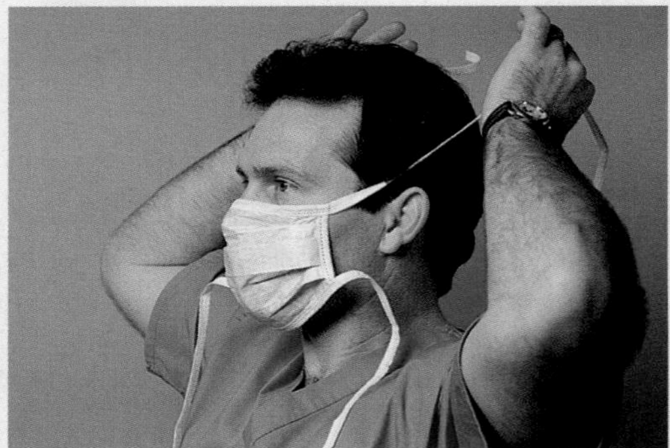

STEP 2 Securing top two ties of a tie-on mask.

3. Tie two lower ties snugly around neck with mask well under chin (see illustration).

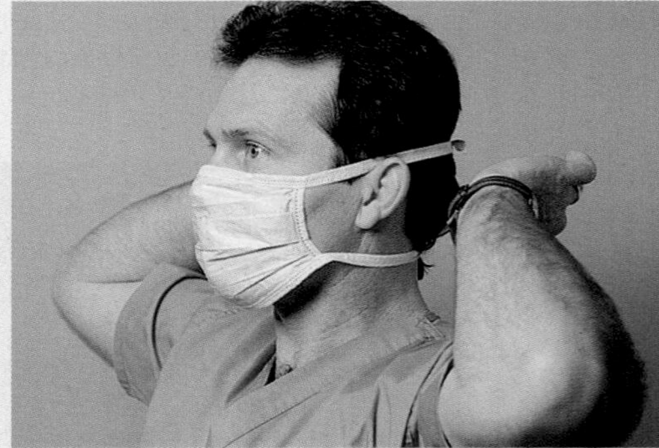

STEP 3 Securing lower ties of a tie-on mask.

4. Gently pinch upper metal band around bridge of nose.
   NOTE: Change mask if wet, moist, or contaminated.
5. Remove mask by untying *bottom* mask strings and then top strings; pull mask away from face and drop into trash receptacle. (Do not touch outer surface of mask.)

nurse who wears prescription glasses uses removable, reusable, or disposable side shields over them (OSHA, 2011b). Eyewear is available in the form of plastic glasses or goggles. The eyewear needs to fit snugly around the face so fluids cannot enter between the face and the glasses.

Gloves. Gloves help to prevent the transmission of pathogens by direct and indirect contact. The CDC (2007) notes that you need to wear clean gloves when touching blood, body fluid, secretions, excretions (except sweat), moist mucous membranes, nonintact skin, and contaminated items or surfaces. Change gloves and perform hand hygiene between tasks and procedures on the same patient after contact with material that contains a high concentration of microorganisms. Remove gloves promptly after use, before touching noncontaminated items and environmental surfaces, and before going to another patient. Perform hand hygiene immediately to avoid transfer of microorganisms to other patients or environments. Because of allergy or sensitivity to latex gloves, facilities provide nonlatex gloves to reduce the incidence of health care providers developing latex allergy or sensitivity. Most facilities are working to become latex free to protect health care providers and patients.

When full PPE is necessary, first perform hand hygiene, then apply a gown, apply mask and eyewear or goggles (as needed), and end with applying gloves. Clean gloves are easy to apply and fit either hand. Pull the cuffs of the glove up over the wrists or over the cuffs of the gown. If you notice a break or tear in a glove while providing care, change gloves. If you do not plan to have additional contact with the patient, reapplying gloves is unnecessary. Perform hand hygiene when gloves are removed.

Instruct family members visiting patients on isolation precautions how to apply gloves properly. Demonstrate application of gloves to family members and explain the reason for the use of gloves. Emphasize the importance of performing hand hygiene after removing gloves.

Specimen Collection. Many laboratory studies are often necessary when a patient is suspected of having an infectious or communicable disease (Box 29-13). You collect body fluids and secretions suspected of containing infectious organisms for culture and sensitivity tests. After a specimen is sent to a laboratory, the laboratory technologist identifies the microorganisms growing in the culture. Additional test results indicate antibiotics to which the organisms are resistant or sensitive. Sensitivity reports determine which antibiotics used in treatment are effective and need to be ordered for treatment.

Obtain all culture specimens using clean gloves and sterile equipment. Collecting fresh material such as wound drainage from the site of infection ensures that neighboring microbes do not contaminate a specimen. Seal all specimen containers tightly to prevent spillage and contamination of the outside of the container.

Bagging Trash or Linen. Bagging contaminated items prevents accidental exposure of personnel and contamination of the surrounding environment. Double bagging is not recommended. Studies demonstrate that this procedure is not necessary to prevent and control infection (CDC, 2007). The use of a single, intact, standard-size linen bag that is not overfilled and tied securely is adequate to prevent infection transmission. Check the color code of bag that your facility uses for bagging these items.

Transporting Patients. Before transferring patients to wheelchairs or stretchers, give them clean gowns to serve as robes. Patients infected with organisms transmitted by the airborne route normally leave their rooms only for essential purposes such as diagnostic procedures or surgery. When a patient has an airborne infection, he or she must wear a mask when leaving the room. Notify personnel in diagnostic or procedural areas or the operating room of the type of isolation precautions the patient requires. Some patients being transported drain body fluids onto a stretcher or wheelchair. Use an extra layer of sheets to cover the stretcher or seat of the wheelchair. Be sure to clean the equipment with an approved germicide after patient use and before another patient uses the shared equipment.

BOX 29-13 Specimen Collection Techniques*

Ensure that all specimen containers used have the biohazard symbol on the outside (Pagana and Pagana, 2014). Also follow agency policy in confirming proper labeling of all specimen containers (i.e., labelling in front of patient).

Wound Specimen

Perform hand hygiene and apply clean gloves. Clean site with sterile water or saline before wound specimen collection with a clean swab. Wipe from edges outward to remove old exudate (see Chapter 48). Remove gloves, perform hand hygiene, and apply gloves and use sterile cotton-tipped swab or syringe to collect as much drainage as possible. Have clean test tube or culture tube on clean paper towel. After swabbing center of wound site, grasp collection tube with a paper towel. Carefully insert swab without touching outside of tube. After securing top of tube, label specimen container with patient name and identifying information, then transfer tube into labeled biohazard bag for transport and perform hand hygiene.

Blood Specimen

(This procedure is often performed by a laboratory technician.)

Wearing gloves, clean venipuncture site with antiseptic swab; move the first swab back and forth on horizontal plane, another swab on the vertical plane, and the last swab in a circular motion from site outward for 5 cm (2 inches) lasting a total of 30 seconds. Allow area to dry. Clean tops of culture bottles for 15 seconds with agency-approved cleansing solution. Use a 20-mL needle-safe syringe and collect up to 10 to 15 mL of blood per culture bottle (check health care facility or agency policy). Perform venipuncture at two different sites to decrease likelihood of both specimens being contaminated with skin flora. Place blood culture bottles on a clean paper towel on bedside table or other surface; swab off bottle tops with alcohol. Inject an appropriate amount of blood into each bottle. If collecting aerobic and anaerobic specimens, inject blood into the aerobic bottle (first) and the anaerobic bottle (second). Transfer labeled specimen into clean, labeled biohazard bag for transport. Remove gloves and perform hand hygiene.

Stool Specimen

Wearing gloves, use clean cup with seal top (need not be sterile) and a tongue blade to collect a small amount, approximately 2 to 3 cm (1 inch) of stool. Place cup on clean paper towel in patient's bathroom. Using tongue blade, collect needed amount of feces from patient's bedpan. Transfer feces to cup without touching outside surface of cup. Dispose of tongue blade and place seal on cup. Transfer labeled specimen into clean labeled biohazard bag for transport. Remove gloves and perform hand hygiene.

Urine Specimen

Apply gloves, cleanse needleless port on urinary catheter and, using a needleless safety syringe, collect 1 to 5 mL of urine. Fill sterile specimen tube and place on clean towel in patient's bathroom. Instruct patient to follow procedure to obtain a clean voided specimen (see Chapter 46) if not catheterized. Secure top of transfer container, label container in front of patient, and place in a biohazard bag with label attached. Remove gloves and perform hand hygiene.

*Health care facility or agency policies may differ on type of containers and amount of specimen material required.

Role of the Infection Control Professional. An infection control professional is a valuable resource for helping nurses control HAIs. These professionals are specially trained in infection prevention

QSEN QSEN: BUILDING COMPETENCY IN EVIDENCE-BASED PRACTICE You notice that, although a number of patients on your unit are in isolation for *C. difficile,* many unit staff are not following agency protocol of gowning and gloving before entering an isolation room. When you bring this to your co-workers' attention, their response is that the precautions are not really necessary because they are not in contact with the patient's stool. You have heard that the organism is very hardy and can live on inanimate objects such as bedrails and door knobs but are unsure of how you know this or how the isolation protocol was developed within your organization. Where could you find evidence to help your colleagues understand why contact precautions are necessary at all times?

Answers to QSEN Activities can be found on the Evolve website.

and control. They are responsible for advising health care personnel regarding infection prevention and control practices and monitoring infections within the hospital. An infection control professional's responsibilities often include:

- Identifying and recommending adoption of evidence-based practices for prevention of HAIs
- Providing staff and patient education on infection prevention and control.
- Developing and reviewing infection prevention and control policies and procedures
- Recommending appropriate isolation procedures for specific patients.
- Screening patient records for community-acquired infections that are reportable to the public health department.
- Consulting with employee health departments concerning recommendations to prevent and control the spread of infection among personnel such as TB testing.
- Gathering statistics regarding the epidemiology (cause and effect) of HAIs.
- Notifying the public health department of incidences of communicable diseases within the facility.
- Consulting with all hospital departments to investigate unusual events or clusters of infection.
- Monitoring antibiotic-resistant organisms in the institution.

Infection Prevention and Control for Hospital Personnel. Health care workers are continually at risk for exposure to infectious microorganisms. Numerous efforts have been made by health care agencies to improve health care provider compliance with hand hygiene, including increased access to automatic alcohol-based hand sanitizers, posted reminders, and sensor monitoring of sanitizer use (Box 29-14). The World Health Organization recently released a new initiative for improving compliance of health care workers with hand hygiene. The WHO's Five Moments for Hand Hygiene has emerged from the WHO Guidelines on Hand Hygiene in Health Care to add value to any hand hygiene improvement strategy (WHO, 2015). The Five Moments defines the key moments for hand hygiene, overcoming misleading language and complicated descriptions.

Patient Education. Often patients need to learn to use infection prevention and control practices at home (Box 29-15). Preventive technique becomes almost second nature to the nurse who practices it daily. However, patients are less aware of factors that promote the spread of infection or ways to prevent its transmission. The home environment may not always lend itself to infection prevention and control. Often you help a patient adapt according to the resources available to maintain hygienic techniques. Generally patients in a home care setting have a decreased risk of infection because of decreased exposure to resistant organisms such as those found in a health care facility and fewer invasive procedures. However, it is important to educate patients and their family caregivers about infection prevention and control techniques.

BOX 29-14 EVIDENCE-BASED PRACTICE

Health Care Worker Compliance with Hand Hygiene

PICO Question: Does the use of bundled evidence-based interventions compared with standard practice improve health care worker compliance in performing hand hygiene?

Evidence Summary

There have been numerous studies examining the use of bundled interventions for improving hand hygiene (HH), including combinations of interventions such as staff education, reminders (e.g., posters, electronic voice prompts), performance feedback, administrative support, and access to alcohol-based hand rub (e.g., wall-mounted dispensers, pocket size bottles, or both) (Schweizer et al., 2014). Most studies have been conducted in Intensive Care units or acute care units, however other study locations have included long-term care facilities and outpatient clinics. Evidence for the use of bundled interventions to improve HH compliance is promising, but higher quality studies are needed to validate these results and examine questions such as which specific interventions should be included in a bundle (Schweizer et al., 2014). A systematic review of studies by Luangasanatip et al. (2015) suggests that the WHO-5 Moments for Hand Hygiene is effective and that compliance can be further improved by adding interventions including goal setting, reward incentives, and accountability. In a number of the studies analyzed, improvements in hand hygiene were associated with reductions in at least one measure of hospital acquired infection and/or resistance rates (Luangasanatip et al., 2015).

Application to Nursing Practice

- Follow the WHO-5 Moments:

  Before Patient Contact

  WHEN? Clean your hands before touching a patient when approaching him or her.

  WHY? To protect the patient against harmful germs carried on your hands.

  Before an Aseptic Task

  WHEN? Clean your hands immediately before any aseptic task.

  WHY? To protect the patient against harmful germs, including the patient's own germs, entering his or her body.

  After Body Fluid Exposure Risk

  WHEN? Clean your hands immediately after an exposure risk to body fluids (and after glove removal).

  WHY? To protect yourself and the health care environment from harmful patient germs.

  After Patient Contact

  WHEN? Clean your hands after touching a patient and his or her immediate surroundings when leaving.

  WHY? To protect yourself and the health care environment from harmful patient germs.

  After Contact with Patient Surroundings

  WHEN? Clean your hands when leaving after touching any object or furniture in the patient's immediate surroundings, even without touching the patient.

  WHY? To protect yourself and the health care environment from harmful patient germs.
- Adding supplemental interventions, including goal setting, reward incentives, and accountability to the WHO-5 Moments strategy leads to additional improvements in hand hygiene compliance.

BOX 29-15 PATIENT TEACHING

Infection Prevention and Control

Objective
- Patient and/or caregiver will use proper infection prevention and control practices when performing a clean dressing change.

Teaching Strategies
- Demonstrate proper hand hygiene, explaining that patient and/or caregiver needs to perform it before and after all treatments and when infected body fluids are contacted.
- Instruct patient and/or caregiver about the signs and symptoms of wound infection and when to notify the health care provider.
- Instruct patient and/or caregiver to place contaminated dressings and other disposable items containing infectious body fluids in impervious plastic or brown paper bags. Place needles in metal or hard plastic containers such as coffee cans or laundry detergent bottles and tape the openings shut. *Some states have specific requirements for sharps disposal. Check local regulations.*
- Instruct patient and/or caregiver to separate linen soiled with wound drainage from other laundry. Wash in warm water with detergent. There are no special recommendations for setting a dryer temperature (CDC, 2007).

Evaluation
- Ask patient or caregiver to describe techniques used to reduce transmission of infection.
- Have patient or caregiver demonstrate hand hygiene and dressing change techniques.
- Ask patient or caregiver to describe signs of a wound infection.
- Ask patient or caregiver when to notify the health care provider if signs and symptoms of infection are present.

Surgical Asepsis. Surgical asepsis or sterile technique prevents contamination of an open wound, serves to isolate an operative area from the unsterile environment, and maintains a sterile field for surgery. Surgical asepsis includes procedures used to eliminate all microorganisms, including pathogens and spores, from an object or area (Rutala and Weber, 2014). In surgical asepsis an area or object is considered contaminated if touched by any object that is not sterile. It demands the highest level of aseptic technique and requires that all areas be kept free of infectious microorganisms.

Use surgical asepsis in the following situations:
- During procedures that require intentional perforation of the patient's skin, such as insertion of peripheral IV catheters or a central intravenous line
- When the integrity of the skin is broken as a result of trauma, surgical incision, or burns
- During procedures that involve invasive procedures such as insertion of a urinary catheter or surgical instruments into sterile body cavities such as insertion of a wound drain

Although surgical asepsis is common in the operating room, labor and delivery area, and major diagnostic areas, you also use surgical aseptic techniques at the patient's bedside (e.g., when inserting IV or urinary catheters, suctioning the tracheobronchial airway, and sterile dressing changes). A nurse in an operating room follows a series of steps to maintain sterile technique, including applying a mask, protective eyewear, and a cap; performing a surgical hand scrub; and applying a sterile gown and gloves. In contrast, a nurse performing a dressing change at a patient's bedside only performs hand hygiene and applies gloves. For certain procedures (e.g., changing a central line dressing) the nurse also uses a mask and gown (see agency policy). Regardless of the procedures followed or the setting, the nurse always recognizes the importance of strict adherence to aseptic principles (Iwamoto and Post, 2014).

Patient Preparation for a Sterile Procedure. Because surgical asepsis requires exact techniques, you need to have the patient's full cooperation. Therefore assess a patient's understanding of the sterile procedure and explain the reasons for not moving or interfering with the procedure. Certain patients fear moving or touching objects during a sterile procedure, whereas others try to help. Explain how you will perform a procedure and what the patient can do to avoid contaminating sterile items, including the following:
- Avoid sudden movements of body parts covered by sterile drapes.
- Refrain from touching sterile supplies, drapes, or the nurse's gloves and gown.
- Avoid coughing, sneezing, or talking over a sterile area.

Certain sterile procedures last an extended time. Assess a patient's needs and anticipate factors that may disrupt a procedure. If a patient is in pain, administer ordered analgesics about a half an hour before a sterile procedure begins. Ask a patient if he or she needs to use the bathroom or a bedpan. Often patients have to assume relatively uncomfortable positions during sterile procedures. Help a patient assume the most comfortable position possible. Finally a patient's condition sometimes results in actions or events that contaminate a sterile field. For example, a patient with a respiratory infection transmits organisms by coughing or talking. Anticipate such a problem and place a surgical mask on him or her before the procedure begins.

Principles of Surgical Asepsis. Performing sterile aseptic procedures requires a work area in which objects can be handled with minimal risk of contamination. A sterile field provides a sterile surface for placement of sterile equipment. It is an area considered free of microorganisms and consists of a sterile kit or tray, a work surface draped with a sterile towel or wrapper, or a table covered with a large sterile drape (Murphy, 2014). When beginning a surgically aseptic procedure, nurses follow certain principles to ensure maintenance of asepsis. Failure to follow these principles places patients at risk for infection. The following principles are important:

1. *A sterile object remains sterile only when touched by another sterile object.* This principle guides a nurse in placement of sterile objects and how to handle them.
   a. Sterile touching sterile remains sterile (e.g., use sterile gloves or sterile forceps to handle objects on a sterile field).
   b. Sterile touching clean becomes contaminated (e.g., if the tip of a syringe or other sterile object touches the surface of a clean disposable glove, the object is contaminated).
   c. Sterile touching contaminated becomes contaminated (e.g., when a nurse touches a sterile object with an ungloved hand, the object is contaminated).
   d. Sterile state is questionable (e.g., when you find a tear or break in the covering of a sterile object). Discard it regardless of whether the object itself appears untouched.
2. *Only sterile objects may be placed on a sterile field.* All items are properly sterilized before use. Sterile objects are kept in clean, dry storage areas. The package or container holding a sterile object must be intact and dry. A package that is torn, punctured, wet, or open is considered unsterile.
3. *A sterile object or field out of the range of vision or an object held below a person's waist is contaminated.* Nurses never turn their back on a sterile field or tray or leave it unattended. Contamination can occur accidentally by a dangling piece of clothing or an unknowing patient touching a sterile object. Any object held below waist level is considered contaminated

because it cannot be viewed at all times. Keep sterile objects in front with the hands as close together as possible.

4. *A sterile object or field becomes contaminated by prolonged exposure to air.* Avoid activities that create air currents such as excessive movements or rearranging linen after a sterile object or field becomes exposed. When you open sterile packages, it is important to minimize the number of people walking into an area. Microorganisms also travel by droplet through the air. Do not talk, laugh, sneeze, or cough over a sterile field or when gathering and using sterile equipment. When opening sterile packages, hold the item or piece of equipment as close as possible to the sterile field without touching the sterile surface.
5. *When a sterile surface comes in contact with a wet, contaminated surface, the sterile object or field becomes contaminated by capillary action.* If moisture leaks through the protective covering of a sterile package, microorganisms travel to the sterile object. When stored sterile packages become wet, discard the objects immediately or send the equipment for resterilization. When working with a sterile field or tray, you may have to pour sterile solutions. Any spill is a source of contamination unless on a sterile surface that moisture cannot penetrate. Urinary catheterization trays contain sterile supplies that rest in a sterile, plastic container. In contrast, if you place a piece of sterile gauze in its wrapper on a patient's bedside table and the table surface is wet, the gauze is considered contaminated.
6. *Fluid flows in the direction of gravity.* A sterile object becomes contaminated if gravity causes a contaminated liquid to flow over the surface of the object. To avoid contamination during a surgical hand scrub, hold your hands above your elbows. This allows water to flow downward without contaminating your hands and fingers. The principle of water flow by gravity is also the reason for drying from fingers to elbows, with hands held up, after the scrub.
7. *The edges of a sterile field or container are considered to be contaminated.* Frequently you place sterile objects on a sterile towel, drape, or tray (Figure 29-4). Because the edge of the drape touches an unsterile surface such as a table or bed linen, a 2.5-cm (1-inch) border around the drape is considered contaminated. Objects placed on the sterile field need to be inside this border. The edges of sterile containers become exposed to air after they are open and thus are contaminated. After you remove a sterile needle from its protective cap or forceps from a container, the objects must not touch the edge of the container.

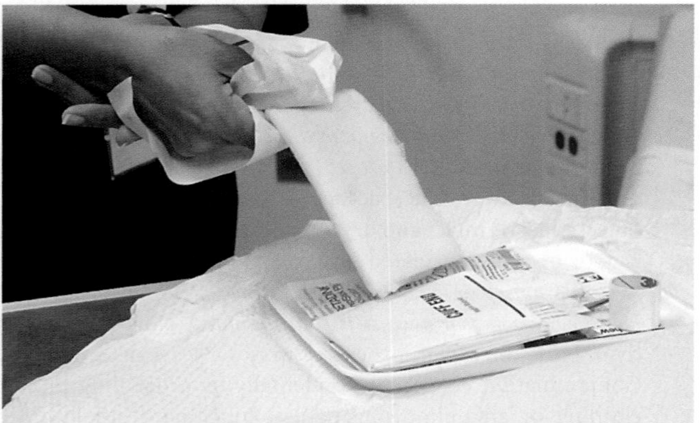

FIGURE 29-4 Placing sterile item on sterile field.

Performing Sterile Procedures. Assemble all of the equipment that will be needed before a procedure. Have a few extra supplies available in case objects accidentally become contaminated. Do not leave a sterile area. Before a sterile procedure, explain each step so the patient can cooperate fully. If an object becomes contaminated during the procedure, do not hesitate to discard it immediately.

Donning and Removing Caps, Masks, and Eyewear. Wear a surgical mask and eyewear without a cap for any sterile procedures on a general nursing unit. Eyewear is worn as a part of standard precautions if there is a risk of fluid or blood splashing into your eyes. For sterile surgical procedures, you first apply a clean cap that covers all of your hair and then the surgical mask and eyewear. A mask must fit snugly around the face and nose. After wearing a mask for several hours, the area over the mouth and nose often becomes moist. Because moisture promotes the growth of microorganisms, change the mask if it becomes moist.

Protective glasses or goggles fit snugly around the forehead and face to fully protect the eyes. Wear eyewear only for procedures that create the risk of body fluids splashing into the eyes. Remove PPE in the following order: gloves, face shield or goggles, gown, and mask or respirator (CDC, 2005b). After removing all PPE, perform hand hygiene.

Opening Sterile Packages. Sterile items such as syringes, gauze dressings, or catheters are packaged in paper or plastic containers and are impervious to microorganisms as long as they are dry and intact. Some institutions wrap reusable supplies (e.g., operating room instruments) in a double thickness of paper, linen, or muslin. These packages are permeable to steam and thus allow for steam autoclaving. Sterile items are kept in clean, enclosed storage cabinets and separated from dirty equipment.

Sterile supplies have chemical tapes indicating that a sterilization process has taken place. The tapes change color during the process. Failure of the tapes to change color means that the item is not sterile. Health care facilities follow the principles of event-related sterility, a concept that items are considered sterile if the packaging is uncompromised (Jefferson and Young, 2014). Never use a sterile item if the packaging is open or soiled or shows evidence that the package had been wet. Before opening a sterile item, perform hand hygiene. Inspect the supplies for package integrity and sterility and assemble the supplies in the work area such as the bedside table or treatment room before opening packages. A bedside table or countertop provides a large, clean working area for opening items. Keep the work area above waist level. Do not open sterile supplies in a confined space where contamination might occur.

Opening a Sterile Item on a Flat Surface. You must open sterile packages without contaminating the contents. Commercially packaged items are usually designed so you only have to tear away or separate the paper or plastic cover. Hold the item in one hand while pulling the wrapper away with the other (Figure 29-5). Take care to keep the inner contents sterile before use. You may use a sterile wrapper from a commercial kit or a sterile paper or linen wrapper from an institutional pack to create a sterile field on which to work. Use the inner surface of the package (except for the 2.5 cm [1-inch] border around the edges) as a sterile field to add sterile items. You can grasp the 2.5 cm (1-inch) border to maneuver the field on a table surface (see Skill 29-2 on pp. 473-476).

Opening a Sterile Item While Holding It. To open a small sterile item, hold the package in your nondominant hand while opening the top flap and pulling it away from you. Using the dominant hand, carefully open the sides and innermost flap away from the enclosed sterile item in the same order previously mentioned. You open the item in a hand so you can pass it to a person wearing sterile gloves or transfer it to a sterile field.

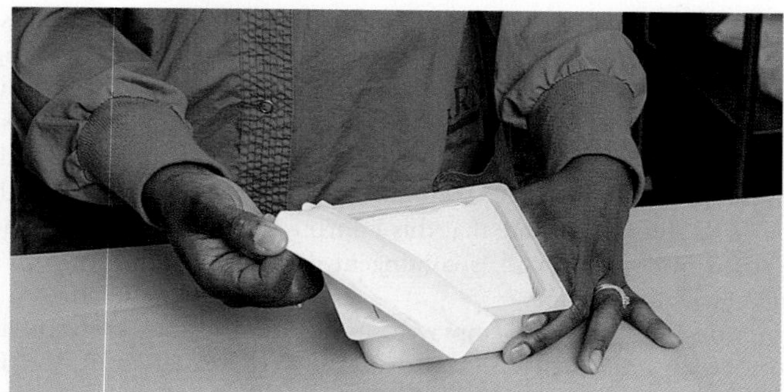

FIGURE 29-5 Nurse opens sterile package on work area above waist level.

Preparing a Sterile Field. When performing sterile procedures, you need a sterile work area that provides room for handling and placing sterile items. A **sterile field** is an area free of microorganisms and prepared to receive sterile items. You prepare the field by using the inner surface of a sterile wrapper as the work surface or by using a sterile drape or dressing tray. After creating the surface for the sterile field, add sterile items by placing them directly on the field or transferring them with a sterile forceps (see Skill 29-2). Discard an object that comes in contact with the 2.5 cm (1-inch) border.

Sometimes you will wear sterile gloves while preparing items on a sterile field. If you do this, you can touch the entire drape, but sterile items must be handed over by an assistant. The gloves cannot touch the wrappers of sterile items.

Pouring Sterile Solutions. Often you have to pour sterile solutions into sterile containers. A bottle containing a sterile solution is sterile on the inside and contaminated on the outside; the neck of the bottle is also contaminated, but the inside of the bottle cap is considered sterile. After you remove the cap or lid, you hold it in your hand or place its sterile side (inside) up on a clean surface. This means that you are able to see the inside of the lid as it rests on the table surface. Never rest a bottle cap or lid on a sterile surface, even though the inside of the cap is sterile. The outer edge of the cap is unsterile and contaminates the surface. Placing a sterile cap down on an unsterile surface increases the chances of the inside of the cap becoming contaminated.

Hold the bottle with its label in the palm of the hand to prevent the possibility of the solution wetting and fading the label. Before pouring the solution into the container, pour a small amount (1 to 2 mL) into a disposable cap or plastic-lined waste receptacle. The discarded solution cleans the lip of the bottle. Keep the edge of the bottle away from the edge or inside of the receiving container. Pour the solution slowly to avoid splashing the underlying drape or field. Never hold the bottle so high above the container that even slow pouring causes splashing. Hold the bottle outside the edge of the sterile field.

Surgical Scrub. Patients undergoing operative procedures are at an increased risk for infection. Nurses working in operating rooms perform surgical hand antisepsis (see Skill 29-3 on pp. 476-478) to decrease and suppress the growth of skin microorganisms under the gloved hand in case of glove tears. A surgical hand scrub must eliminate the transient flora and reduce the resident flora on the hands. For maximum elimination of bacteria, remove all jewelry and keep the nails clean and short. Do not wear chipped nail polish, artificial nails, or extenders because they often hold a greater number of bacteria (AORN, 2014; WHO, 2009). Nurses who have active skin infections, open lesions or cuts, or respiratory infections should be excluded from the surgical team.

During surgical hand antisepsis the nurse scrubs from fingertips to elbows with an antiseptic soap before each surgical procedure. Research studies vary on the optimum duration of a surgical hand scrub (WHO, 2009). Chlorhexidine gluconate has been found to be more effective than povidone iodine as a cleansing agent, although both can be found in health care agencies. Thus the type of product used for cleansing will influence the time required for hand antisepsis (CDC, 2008a; WHO 2009). The traditional scrub time in the United States for both the initial and the subsequent scrub is 5 minutes, but research has shown effectiveness can be gained when scrubs are performed for 2, 3 and 6 minutes (WHO, 2009). Follow manufacturer recommendation for scrub solutions. For many years preoperative handwashing protocols required nurses to scrub with a brush. However, this practice damages the skin. Scrubbing with a disposable sponge or combination sponge-brush reduces bacterial counts on the hands as effectively as scrubbing with a brush. However, several studies suggest that neither a brush nor a sponge is necessary to reduce bacterial counts on the hands, especially when using an alcohol-based product (CDC, 2008a).

Applying Sterile Gloves. Sterile gloves are an additional barrier to bacterial transfer. There are two gloving methods: open and closed. Nurses who work on general nursing units use open gloving before procedures such as dressing changes or urinary catheter insertions. The closed-gloving method, which you perform after applying a sterile gown, is practiced in operating rooms and special treatment areas (see Skills 29-4 and 29-5 on pp. 479-482). Make sure to select the proper glove size; the glove should not stretch so tightly that it can tear easily, yet it must be tight enough that you can pick up objects easily.

Donning a Sterile Gown. Nurses wear sterile gowns when assisting at the sterile field in the operating room, delivery room, and special treatment areas. It allows the nurse to handle sterile objects and also be comfortable with less risk of contamination. The sterile gown acts as a barrier to decrease shedding of microorganisms from skin surfaces into the air and thus prevents wound contamination. Nurses caring for patients with large open wounds or assisting health care providers during major invasive procedures (e.g., inserting an arterial catheter) also wear sterile gowns. The circulating nurse generally does not wear one.

The nurse does not apply a sterile gown until after applying a mask and surgical cap and completing surgical handwashing. He or she picks up the gown from a sterile pack, or an assistant hands the gown to the nurse. Only a certain portion of the gown (i.e., the area from the anterior waist to, but not including, the collar and the anterior surface of the sleeves) is considered sterile. The back of the gown, the area under the arms, the collar, the area below the waist, and the underside of the sleeves are not sterile because the nurse cannot keep these areas in constant view and ensure their sterility (see Skill 29-4 on pp. 479-480).

Exposure Issues. Patients and health care personnel, including housekeepers and maintenance personnel, are at risk for acquiring infections from accidental needlesticks. In the past, a stray needle lying in bed linen or carelessly thrown into a wastebasket served as a prime source for exposure to bloodborne pathogens. With the passage of the Needlestick Safety and Prevention Act in 2000 (OSHA, 2012) and the implementation of safety needle devices, the incidence rate of sharps injuries has decreased. All sharps must now be either needle safe or needleless. After administering an injection or inserting an IV catheter, place the used needle safety device in a puncture-resistant box (see Chapter 32). Sharps boxes must be at the site of use; this is an Occupational Safety and Health Administration (OSHA) requirement.

HBV and HCV are the infections most commonly transmitted by contaminated needles (Box 29-16). Report any contaminated

BOX 29-16 Hepatitis B Vaccination and Follow-Up After Hepatitis C and Human Immunodeficiency Virus Exposure

1. Health care employers shall make available the hepatitis B vaccine and vaccination series to all employees who may have occupational exposures. If an employee declines the vaccine, he or she must sign a declination form. Evaluation and follow-up care is available to all employees who have been exposed.
2. Hepatitis B vaccinations are made available to employees within 10 working days of assignment—this means before starting to provide patient care and after receiving education and training on the vaccine.
3. A blood test (titer) is offered in some facilities 1 to 2 months after completing the three-dose vaccine series (check the health care facility or agency policy).
4. Vaccine is offered at no cost to employees. At present the vaccine does not require any boosters.
5. After exposure no treatment is needed if there is a positive blood titer on file. If no positive titer is on file, follow CDC guidelines.

Exposure to Hepatitis C Virus

1. If the source patient is positive for hepatitis C virus (HCV), the employee receives a baseline test.
2. At 4 weeks after exposure the employee should be offered an HCV-RNA test to determine if he or she contracted HCV.
3. If positive, the employee starts treatment.
4. There is no prophylactic treatment for HCV after exposure.
5. Early treatment for infection can prevent chronic infection.

Exposure to Human Immunodeficiency Virus

1. If the patient is positive for human immunodeficiency virus (HIV) infection, a viral load study should be performed to determine the amount of virus present in the blood.
2. If the exposure meets the CDC criteria for HIV prophylactic treatment (PEP), it should be started as soon as possible, preferably within 24 hours after the exposure (CDC, 2005b).

All medical evaluations and procedures, including the vaccine and vaccination series and evaluation after exposure (prophylaxis), are made available at no cost to at-risk employees.

A confidential written medical evaluation will be available to employees with exposure incidents.

From Occupational Safety and Health Administration: Occupational Safety and Health Act of 2001, 2001, 2005, http://www.cdc.gov. *CDC,* Centers for Disease Control and Prevention; *RNA,* ribonucleic acid; *PEP,* postexposure prophylaxis.

needlestick immediately. Additional criteria for exposure reporting include blood or other potentially infectious materials (OPIMs) in direct contact with an open area of the skin, blood or OPIM that is splashed into a health care worker's eye or mouth or up the nose, and cuts with a sharp object that is covered with blood or OPIM.

Follow-up for risk of acquiring infection begins with source patient testing. Access to testing the source patient is stated in the testing law for each state. Some states have deemed consent, which means that the state has granted the patient's consent to be tested. Other states require that the patient consent to testing for the presence of bloodborne pathogens. Know the testing policies in the facility and state in which you practice. Health care facilities and agencies and workers' compensation require exposed employees to complete an injury report and seek appropriate treatment if needed. The need for treatment is linked to the results of a risk assessment and the testing of the patient. Test the patient for HIV, HBV, and HCV. If positive for HIV or HCV, testing for syphilis may be indicated because of the incidence of coinfection (CDC, 2005b, 2010a). It is required that an exposed employee be given the patient's testing results. This is *not* a violation of the Health Insurance Portability and Accountability Act (HIPAA) of 1996. Both the CDC and OSHA state that this information must be given to the exposed health care worker contingent on the health care worker's willingness to be tested.

Testing the exposed employee at the time of the exposure is not needed immediately unless required by the state testing law. If the patient tests positive for a bloodborne pathogen or if the source patient is unknown, prophylactic treatment is recommended for the employee.

Exposures also occur involving non-bloodborne pathogens. Airborne and droplet diseases pose a risk to the nonimmune nurse. The CDC (2010c) has published a list of recommended immunizations and vaccinations for health care workers, including hepatitis B vaccine; TB testing; annual influenza vaccine; measles, mumps, rubella (MMR); chickenpox vaccine; and tetanus, diphtheria, and pertussis. Employee health should review your health history and offer appropriate prevention. Declination forms are needed if these are declined (OSHA, 2011b).

◆ Evaluation

Measure the success of infection prevention and control techniques by determining whether you achieved the goals for reducing or preventing infection. Document the patient's response to therapies for infection prevention and control. A clear description of any signs and symptoms of systemic or local infection is necessary to give all nurses a baseline for comparative evaluation.

Through the Patient's Eyes. Patients generally expect to be safe and protected when receiving health care. A patient at risk for infection needs to understand the measures needed to reduce or prevent microorganism growth and spread. Providing patients and/or family caregivers the opportunity to discuss infection prevention and control measures or to demonstrate procedures such as hand hygiene reveals their ability to comply with therapy. Be sure that you understand the patient's perceptions of how infection spreads, his or her expectations for self-care, and how it can affect him or her as you evaluate the results of your instruction. Sometimes patients require new information, or previously instructed information needs reinforcement.

Patient Outcomes. A comparison of a patient's response before and after an infection control measure, such as the absence of fever or wound infection, is an example of an expected outcome for measuring the success of nursing interventions. Observe wounds during dressing changes to determine the degree of wound healing. Monitor patients, especially those at risk, for signs and symptoms of infection. For example, a patient who has undergone a surgical procedure is at risk for infection at the surgical site and other invasive sites such as the venipuncture site or central line sites. In addition, the patient is at risk for a respiratory tract infection as a result of decreased mobility and for a UTI if an indwelling catheter is present. Observe all invasive and surgical sites for swelling, erythema, or purulent drainage. Monitor breath sounds for changes and observe sputum character for change in color or consistency. Review laboratory test results for leukocytes. For example, leukocytosis in the urine often indicates a UTI. The absence of signs or symptoms of infection is the expected outcome of infection prevention and control.

SAFETY GUIDELINES FOR NURSING SKILLS

Ensuring patient safety is an essential role of the professional nurse. To ensure patient safety, communicate clearly with members of the health care team, assess and incorporate the patient's priorities of care and preferences, and use the best evidence when making decisions about your patient's care. When performing the skills in this chapter, remember the following points to ensure safe, individualized patient care.

- Use clean gloves when you anticipate contact with body fluids and nonintact skin or mucous membranes when there is a risk of drainage.
- Use gown, mask, and eye protection when there is a risk for splash.
- Keep bedside table surfaces clutter free, clean, and dry when performing aseptic procedures.
- Clean all equipment that is shared between patients.
- Ensure that patients cover mouth and nose when coughing or sneezing, use tissues to contain respiratory secretions, and dispose of tissues in waste receptacle.

SKILL 29-1 HAND HYGIENE

DELEGATION CONSIDERATIONS

The skill of hand hygiene is performed by all caregivers. Instruct all caregivers to use proper hand hygiene.

EQUIPMENT

- Antiseptic hand rub
  - Alcohol-based, waterless, antiseptic-containing emollient
- Handwashing
  - Easy-to-reach sink with warm running water
  - Antimicrobial or nonantimicrobial soap
  - Paper towels or air dryer
  - Disposable nail cleaner (optional)

STEP	RATIONALE
1. Inspect surface of your hands for breaks or cuts in skin or cuticles. Cover any skin lesions with a dressing before providing care. If lesions are too large to cover, you may be restricted from direct patient care (CDC, 2008a).	Open cuts or wounds can harbor high concentrations of microorganisms. Health care facility or agency policy often prevents nurses from caring for high-risk patients if open lesions are present on hands.
2. Inspect hands for visible soiling.	If hands are visibly soiled, you will use soap and water until soil is removed.
3. Inspect condition of nails. Natural tips need to be less than ¼ inch long and free of artificial nails, extenders, or polish (especially cracked polish). Check agency policy.	Subungual areas of hands harbor high concentrations of bacteria. Long nails and chipped or old polish increase the number of bacteria residing on hands. Artificial applications increase microbial load on hands (CDC, 2008a).
4. Push wristwatch and long uniform sleeves above wrists. Avoid wearing rings.	Provides complete access to fingers, hands, and wrists. Some studies show that skin underneath rings carries a higher bacterial load. Gram-negative bacilli, enterobacteria, and *Staphylococcus aureus* are more common under rings (Messano, 2013).
5. Antiseptic hand rub	
a. Following manufacturer directions apply an ample amount of product to palm of one hand (see illustration).	Enough product is needed to thoroughly cover the hands.
b. Rub hands together, covering all surfaces of hands and fingers with antiseptic (see illustration).	Covering all aspects of the hands kills transient bacteria; ensures complete antimicrobial action.
c. Rub hands together for several seconds until alcohol is completely dry. Allow hands to dry before applying gloves.	Provides enough time for antimicrobial solution to be effective.

CLINICAL DECISION: *If hands feel dry after rubbing hands together for 10 to 15 seconds, an insufficient volume of product likely was applied (Boyce et al., 2002).*

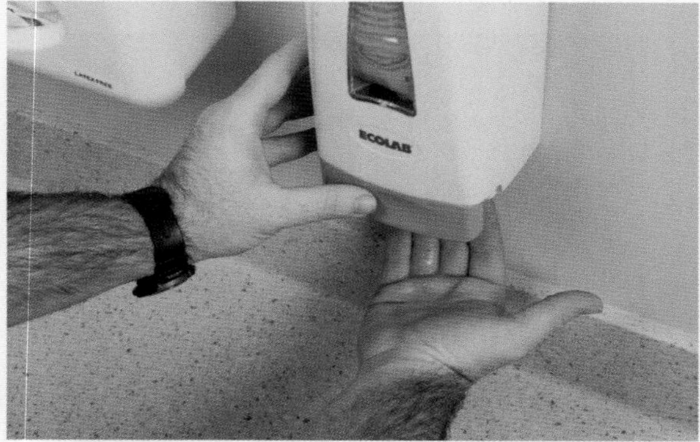

STEP 5a Apply waterless antiseptic to hands.

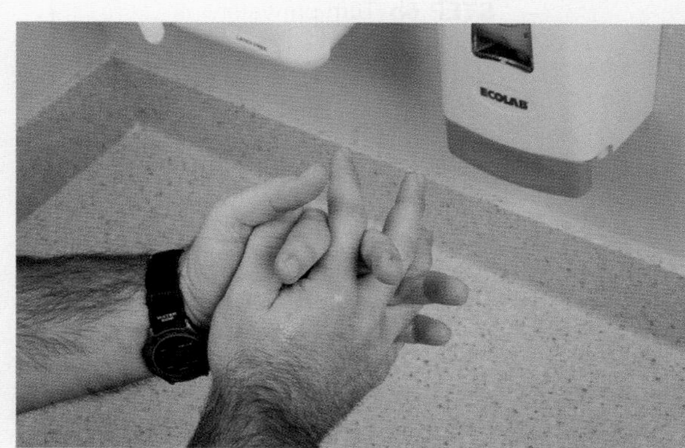

STEP 5b Rub hands thoroughly.

SKILL 29-1 HAND HYGIENE—cont'd

STEP	RATIONALE
6. Handwashing with antiseptic soap	
a. Stand in front of sink, keeping hands and uniform away from sink surface. (If hands touch sink during handwashing, repeat process.)	Inside of sink is a contaminated area. Reaching over sink increases risk of touching edge, which is contaminated.
b. Turn on water. Turn faucet on or push knee pedals laterally or press pedals with foot to regulate flow and temperature (see illustration).	Knee pedals within the operating room and treatment areas are preferred to prevent hand contact with faucet. Faucet handles are likely to be contaminated with organic debris and microorganisms (AORN, 2014).
c. Avoid splashing water against uniform.	Microorganisms travel and grow in moisture.
d. Regulate flow of water so temperature is warm.	Warm water removes less of the protective oils than hot water.
e. Wet hands and wrists thoroughly under running water. Keep hands and forearms lower than elbows during washing.	Hands are the most contaminated parts to be washed. Water flows from least to most contaminated area, rinsing microorganisms into the sink.
f. Apply 3 to 5 mL of antiseptic soap and rub hands together vigorously, lathering thoroughly (see illustration).	Ensures that all surface areas of the hands and fingers are cleaned.

CLINICAL DECISION: *The decision whether to use a nonantimicrobial soap, antimicrobial soap, or alcohol-based hand antiseptic depends on the procedure, the patient's immune status, and the type of infection the patient has (CDC, 2008a).*

STEP	RATIONALE
g. Wash hands using plenty of lather and friction for at least 15 seconds. Interlace fingers and rub palms and back of hands with circular motion at least 5 times each. Keep fingertips down to facilitate removal of microorganisms.	Soap cleans by emulsifying fat and oil and lowering surface tension. Friction and rubbing mechanically loosen and remove dirt and transient bacteria. Interlacing fingers and thumbs ensures that all surfaces are cleansed. Adequate time is needed to expose skin surfaces to antimicrobial agent.
h. Areas under fingernails are often soiled. Clean them with fingernails of other hand and additional soap with an orangewood stick (optional).	Areas under nails are often highly contaminated, which increases the risk of infection for the nurse or patient.
i. Rinse hands and wrists thoroughly, keeping hands down and elbows up (see illustration).	Rinsing mechanically washes away dirt and microorganisms.
j. Dry hands thoroughly from fingers to wrists and forearms with paper towel, single-use cloth, or warm air dryer.	Drying from cleanest (fingertips) to least clean (forearms) area avoids contamination. Drying hands prevents chapping and roughened skin.
k. If used, discard paper towel in proper receptacle.	Prevents transfer of microorganisms.
l. Turn off water with foot or knee pedals. To turn off hand faucet, use clean, dry paper towel; avoid touching handles with hands (see illustration).	Wet towel and hands allow transfer of pathogens from faucet to hands. Faucet handles are contaminated.

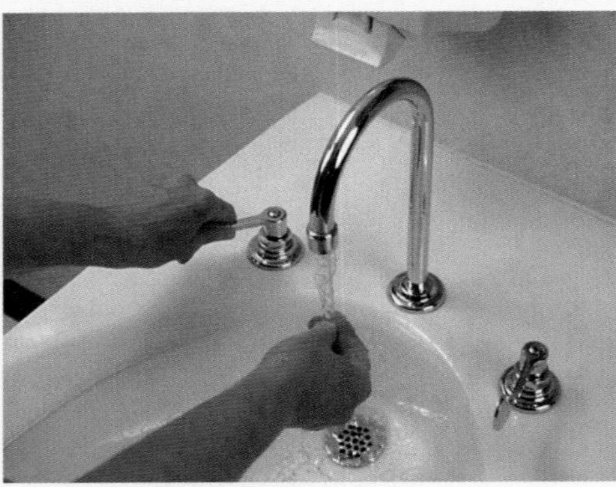

STEP 6b Turn on water.

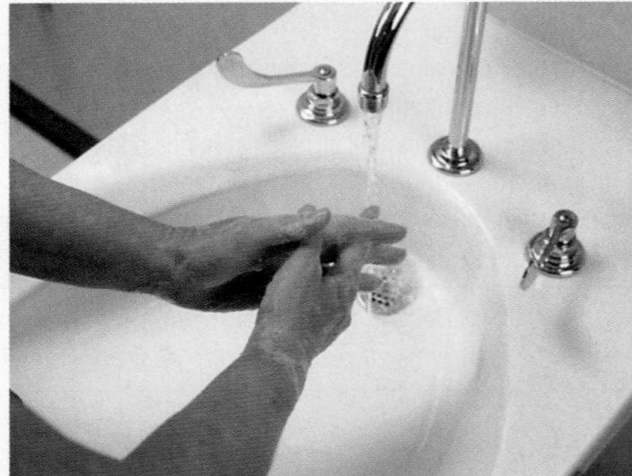

STEP 6f Lather hands thoroughly.

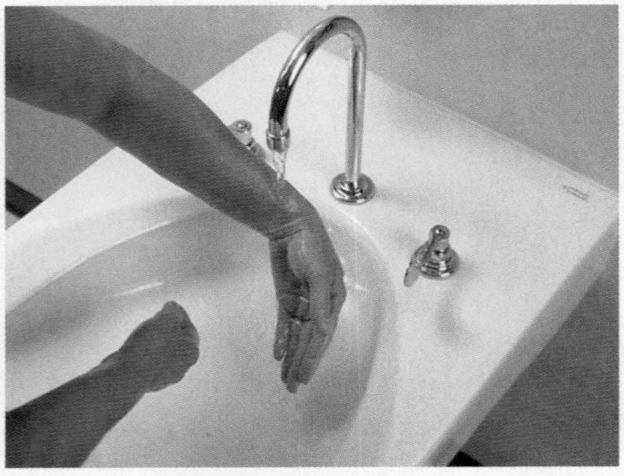

STEP 6i Rinse hands.

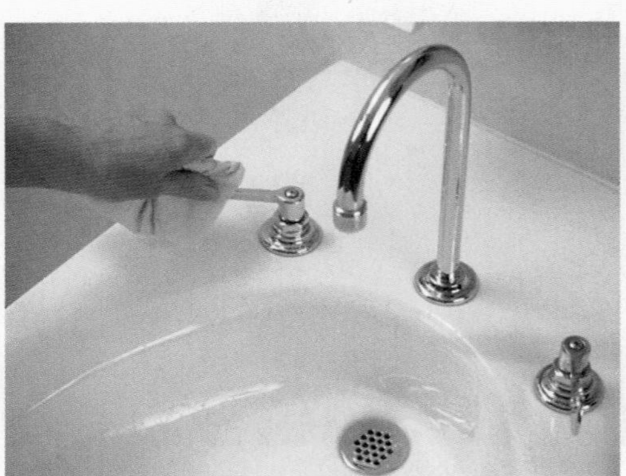

STEP 6l Turn off faucet.

HOME CARE CONSIDERATIONS

- Evaluate the handwashing facilities in a patient's home, including the availability of warm running water and soap, to determine the potential for contamination, how close the facilities are to the patient, and available supplies in the area.
- Anticipate the need for alternative handwashing products such as alcohol-based hand rubs and/or detergent-containing towels.
- Instruct the patient and primary caregiver in proper techniques and situations for handwashing.

SKILL 29-2 PREPARATION OF STERILE FIELD

DELEGATION CONSIDERATIONS

The skill of preparing a sterile field cannot be delegated to nursing assistive personnel (NAP). A surgical technician may prepare a sterile field as indicated by health care facility policy.

EQUIPMENT

- Sterile pack (commercial or institution wrapped)
- Sterile drape to be used as a sterile field
- Sterile gloves (optional, check agency policy)
- Sterile solution and equipment specific to the procedure
- Waist-high table or countertop surface
- Appropriate personal protective equipment (PPE) (see agency policy)

STEP	RATIONALE
1. Complete all priority care tasks before beginning procedure.	Sterile field should be prepared as close as possible to time of use (AORN, 2014).
2. Ask visitors to step out of room briefly during procedure.	Traffic and movement increase potential for spread of microorganisms through air currents.
3. Select a clean, dry work surface above waist level.	A sterile object held below the waist is contaminated.
4. Assemble necessary equipment and check expiration dates or labels and condition of supply packaging for sterility of equipment.	Preparation of equipment in advance prevents break in technique. Equipment that has evidence of previously being open, soiled, or wet is considered unsterile.
5. Apply PPE as needed (consult agency policy).	Controls the spread of microorganisms.
6. Perform hand hygiene.	Reduces transmission of microorganisms.
7. Prepare sterile field.	
a. Prepare sterile commercial kit or tray containing sterile items	
(1) Place sterile kit or pack containing sterile items on work surface above waist level.	Ensures sterility of packaged drape.
(2) Open outside cover and remove kit from dust cover. Place on work surface.	Inner kit remains sterile.
(3) Grasp outer edge of tip of outermost flap.	Outer surface of package is considered unsterile. There is a 2.5-cm (1-inch) border around any sterile drape or wrap that is considered unsterile.
(4) Open outermost flap away from body, keeping arm outstretched and away from the sterile field (see illustration).	Reaching over sterile field contaminates it.
(5) Grasp outer edge of first side of flap.	Outer border is considered unsterile.
(6) Open side flap, pulling to side and allowing it to lie flat on table surface (see illustration). Keep arm to the side and do not extend it over sterile surface.	Drape or flap should lie flat so it will not accidentally rise up and contaminate inner surface or sterile items placed on its surface.

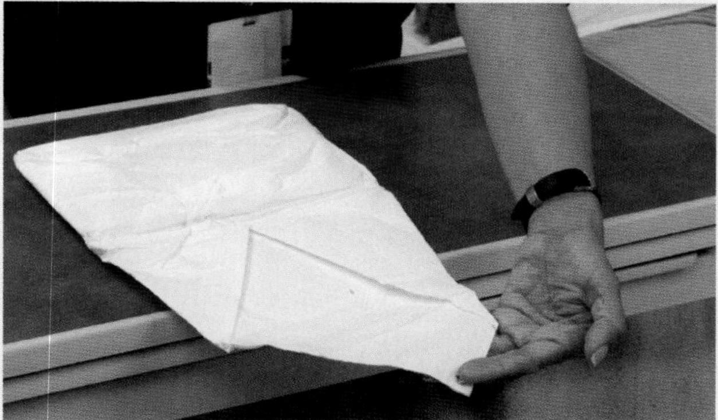

STEP 7a(4) Open outermost flap of sterile kit away from body.

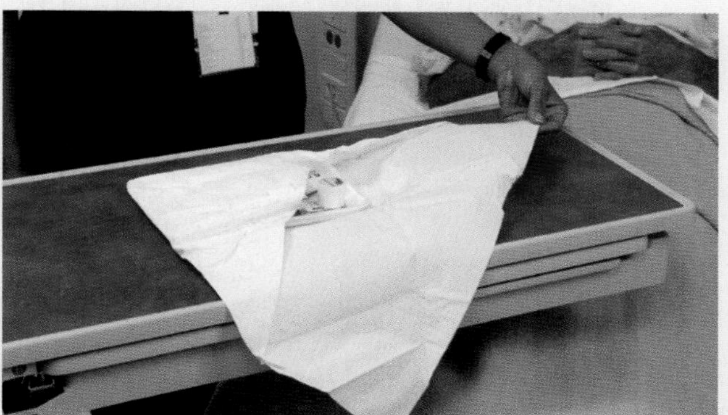

STEP 7a(6) Open first side flap, pulling to side.

SKILL 29-2 PREPARATION OF STERILE FIELD—cont'd

STEP	RATIONALE
(7) Grasp outer edge of second side flap. Repeat for opening second side of package, pulling out to side (see illustration).	
(8) Grasp outer edge of last and innermost flap.	
(9) Stand away from sterile package and pull flap back, allowing it to fall flat on work surface (see illustration).	Reaching over sterile field contaminates it.
b. Sterile linen-wrapped package	
(1) Place package on flat work surface.	
(2) Remove sterilization tape and seal and unwrap both layers, following Steps 7a(1-9) as with sterile kit (see illustrations).	Tape and seal confirms sterility.
(3) Use opened package wrapper as sterile field.	Inner surface of wrapper is considered sterile.
c. Sterile drape	
(1) Place pack containing sterile drape on work surface. Follow Steps 7a(1-9) to open.	Ensures sterility of packaged drape.

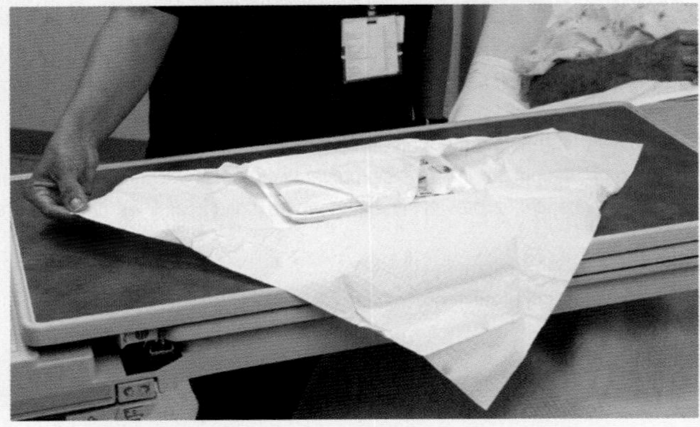

STEP 7a(7) Open second side flap, pulling to side.

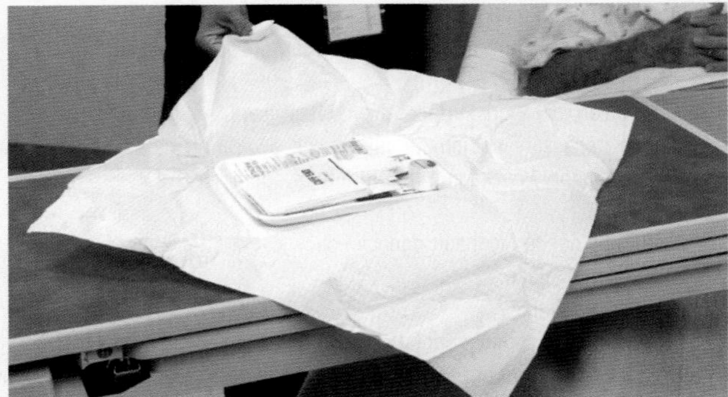

STEP 7a(9) Open last and innermost flap, standing away from sterile field.

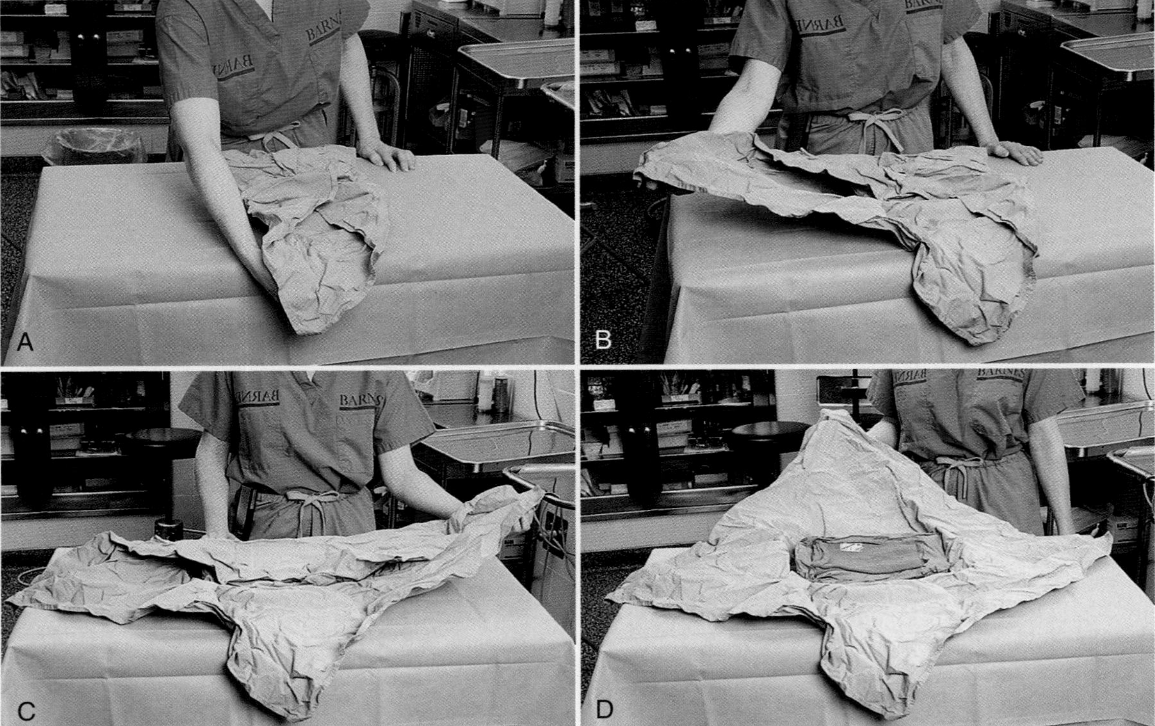

STEP 7b(2) A, Nurse opens top flap away from body. **B,** Nurse's arm is kept out away from sterile field while opening a side flap. **C,** Nurse opens second side flap, keeping arm away from sterile field. **D,** Nurse opens back flap.

STEP	RATIONALE
(2) Apply sterile glove. NOTE: This is an option, depending on health care facility policy. You may touch outer 2.5-cm (1-inch) border of drape without wearing gloves.	
(3) Grasp folded top edge of drape with fingertips of one hand. Gently lift drape up from its wrapper without touching any object.	If sterile object touches any nonsterile object, it becomes contaminated.
(4) Allow drape to unfold, keeping it above waist and work surface and away from body. (Carefully discard outer wrapper with other hand.)	Object held below person's waist or above chest is contaminated.
(5) With other hand grasp adjacent corner of drape. Hold drape straight over work surface (see illustration).	Drape can now be placed properly with two hands.
(6) Holding drape, first position bottom half over top half of intended work surface (see illustration).	Prevents nurse from reaching over sterile field.
(7) Allow top half of drape to be placed over bottom half of work surface (see illustration).	A flat sterile surface is now available for placement of sterile items.
8. Adding sterile items	
a. Open sterile item (following package directions) while holding outside wrapper in nondominant hand.	Frees dominant hand for unwrapping outer wrapper.
b. Carefully peel wrapper onto nondominant hand.	Item remains sterile. Inner surface of wrapper covers hand, making it sterile.
c. Being sure wrapper does not fall down on sterile field, place item onto field at angle. *Do not hold arm over sterile field* (see illustration).	Prevents reaching over field and contaminating its surface.
d. Dispose of outer wrapper.	Prevents accidental contamination of sterile field.

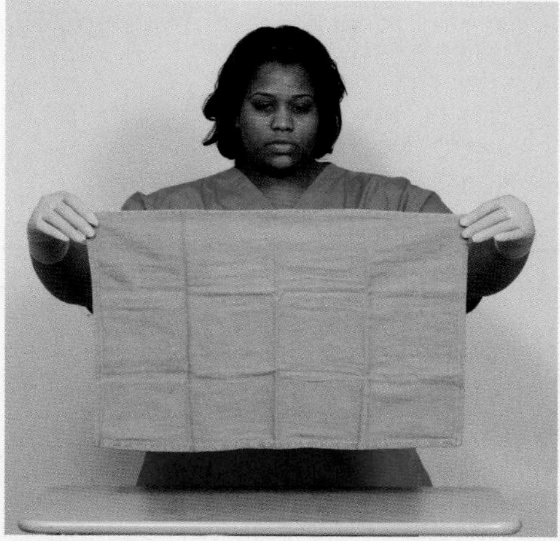

STEP 7c(5) Hold drape straight up and away from body.

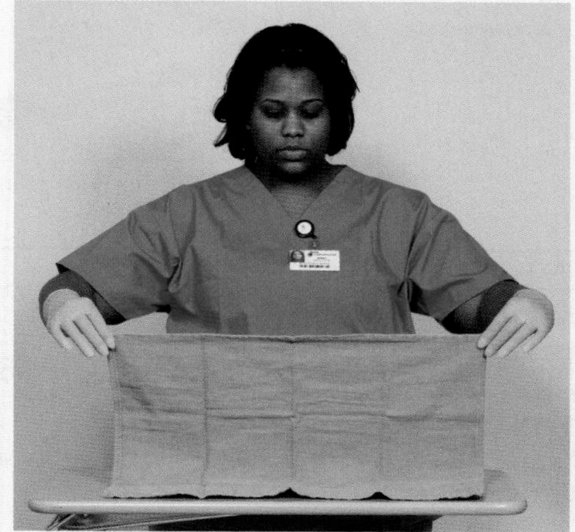

STEP 7c(6) Lay bottom half over work surface.

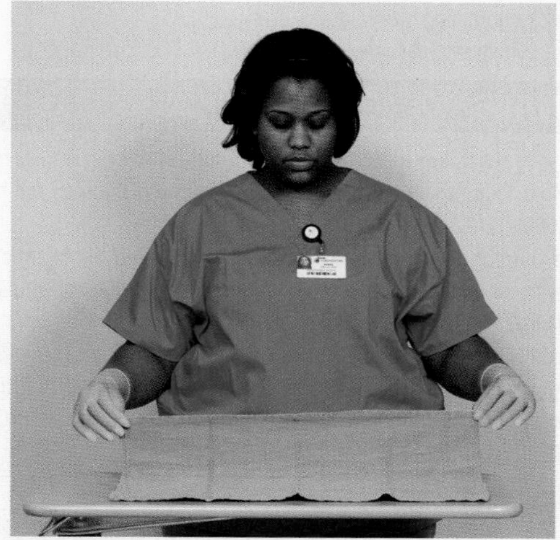

STEP 7c(7) Place top half of drape over work surface.

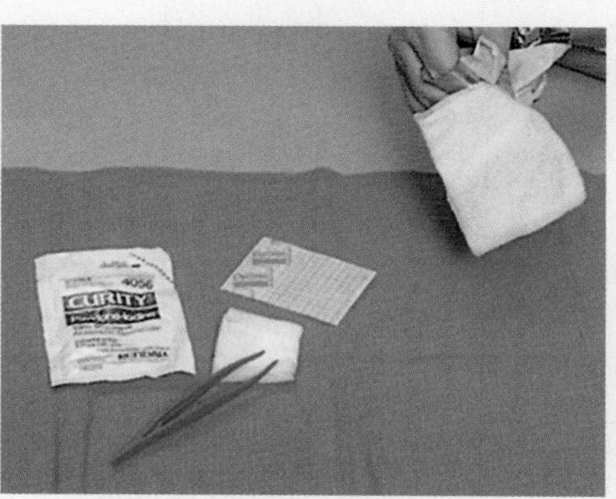

STEP 8c Add item to sterile field.

SKILL 29-2 PREPARATION OF STERILE FIELD—cont'd

STEP	RATIONALE
9. Pour sterile solution.	
a. Verify contents and expiration date of solution.	Ensures proper solution and sterility of contents.
b. Be sure that receptacle for solution is located near or on sterile work surface edge. Sterile kits have cups or plastic molded sections into which you can pour fluids.	Prevents reaching over sterile field.
c. Remove sterile seal and cap from bottle in an upward motion. With solution bottle held away from sterile field, with the label facing up and the bottle lip 1 to 2 inches above inside of receiving container, slowly pour contents into container (see illustration).	Prevents contamination of bottle lip and keeps inside of cap sterile. Edge and outside of bottle are considered contaminated. Slow pouring prevents splashing liquids, which causes fluid permeation of sterile barrier (called *strike through*) and results in contamination.
10. Perform procedure using sterile technique.	Prevents transmission of infection to patient.

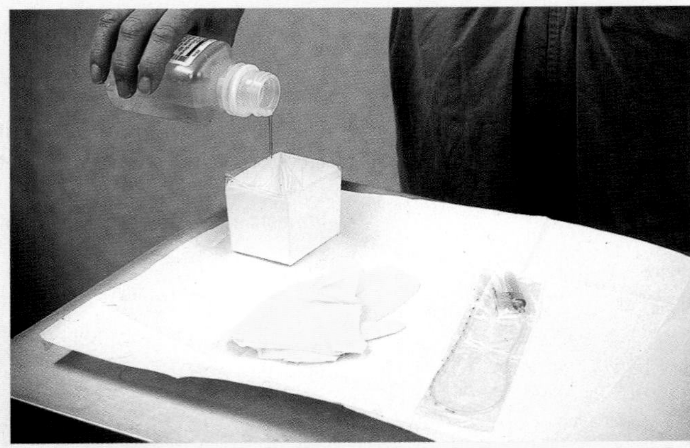

STEP 9c Pour solution into receiving container on sterile field.

RECORDING AND REPORTING

- It is not necessary to record or report this procedure.

SKILL 29-3 SURGICAL HAND ASEPSIS

DELEGATION CONSIDERATIONS

The skill of surgical hand asepsis can be delegated to properly trained surgical technicians (know the state Nurse Practice Act).

EQUIPMENT

- Deep sink with foot or knee controls for dispensing water and soap (faucets should be high enough for hands and forearms to fit comfortably)
- Antimicrobial agent approved by the health care facility
- Surgical scrub sponge with plastic nail pick (optional)
- Paper face mask, cap or hood, surgical shoe covers
- Sterile towel
- Sterile pack containing sterile gown
- Protective eyewear (glasses or goggles)

STEP	RATIONALE
1. Consult manufacturer policy regarding required length of time and antiseptic to use for hand antisepsis. Chlorhexidine has been found to be more effective than povidone iodine (WHO, 2009).	Guidelines vary regarding ideal time needed and antiseptic to use for surgical scrub. Most facilities in the United States follow 5 minutes for hand scrub (WHO, 2009).
2. Remove bracelets, rings, and watches.	Jewelry may harbor or protect microorganisms from removal. Allergic skin reactions may occur as a result of scrub agent or glove powder accumulating under jewelry (Messano, 2013).
3. Be sure that fingernails are short, clean, and healthy. Artificial nails should be removed. Natural nails should be less than ¼ inch long from fingertip.	Long nails and chipped or old polish increase number of bacteria residing on nails. Long fingernails can puncture gloves, causing contamination. Artificial nails are known to harbor gram-negative microorganisms and fungus (AORN, 2014; CDC, 2008a).

CLINICAL DECISION: *Remove nail polish if chipped or worn longer than 4 days because it likely will harbor microorganisms (AORN, 2014).*

STEP	RATIONALE
4. Inspect condition of cuticles, hands, and forearms for abrasions, cuts, or open lesions.	These conditions increase likelihood of more microorganisms residing on skin surfaces. Broken skin permits microorganisms to enter layers of the skin, providing deeper microbial breeding grounds (AORN, 2014).
5. Apply surgical shoe covers, cap or hood, face mask, and protective eyewear.	Mask prevents escape into air of microorganisms that can contaminate hands. Other protective wear prevents exposure to blood and body fluid splashes during the procedure.
6. Turn on water using knee or foot controls and adjust to comfortable temperature.	Knee or foot controls prevent contamination of hands after scrub.
7. Prescrub wash/rinse: Wet hands and arms under running lukewarm water and lather with detergent to 5 cm (2 inches) above elbows. (Hands need to be above elbows at all times.)	Water runs by gravity from fingertips to elbows. Hands become cleanest part of upper extremity. Keeping hands elevated allows water to flow from least to most contaminated areas. Washing a wide area reduces risk of contaminating overlying gown that the nurse later applies.
8. Rinse hands and arms thoroughly under running water. Remember to keep hands above elbows.	Rinsing removes transient bacteria from fingers, hands, and forearms.
9. Under running water clean under nails of both hands with nail pick. Discard after use (see illustration).	Removes dirt and organic material that harbor large numbers of microorganisms.
10. Surgical hand scrub (with sponge or sponge brush)	
a. Wet clean sponge and apply antimicrobial agent. Visualize each finger, hand, and arm as having four sides. Wash all four sides effectively. Scrub the nails of one hand with 15 strokes. Scrub the palm, each side of thumb and fingers, and posterior side of hand with 10 strokes each (see illustration).	Friction loosens resident bacteria that adhere to skin surfaces. Ensures coverage of all surfaces. Scrubbing is performed from cleanest area (hands) to marginal area (upper arms).
b. Divide the arm mentally into thirds: scrub each third 10 times (AORN, 2014) (see illustration). Some health care facility policies require scrub by total time (e.g., 5 minutes) rather than number of strokes. Rinse brush and repeat sequence for the other arm. A two-sponge method may be substituted (check health care facility policy).	Eliminates transient microorganisms and reduces resident hand flora.
c. Discard brush. Flex arms and rinse from fingertips to elbows in one continuous motion, allowing water to run off at elbow (see illustration).	Hands remain the cleanest part of upper extremities.

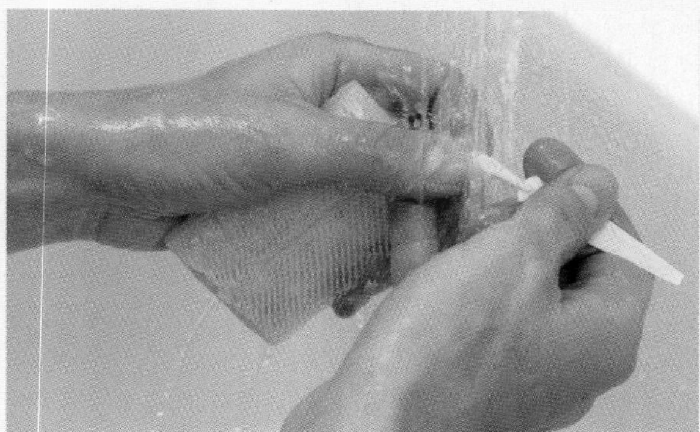

STEP 9 Clean under fingernails.

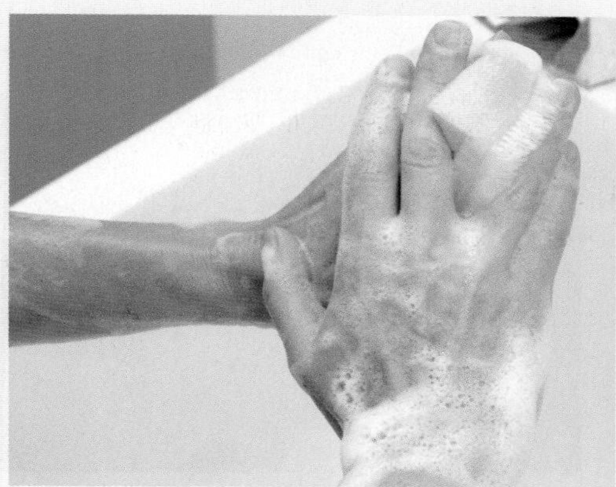

STEP 10a Scrub side of fingers.

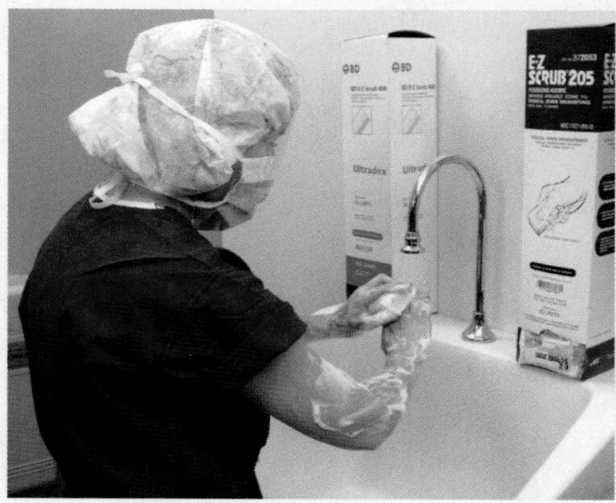

STEP 10b Scrub forearms.

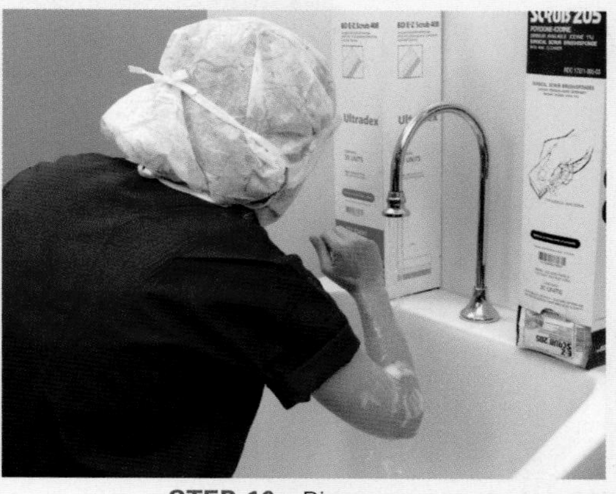

STEP 10c Rinse arms.

SKILL 29-3 SURGICAL HAND ASEPSIS—cont'd

STEP	RATIONALE
d. Turn off water with foot or knee control, with hands elevated in front of and away from body. Enter operating room suite by backing into room.	Keeps hands free of microorganisms.
e. Approach sterile setup; grasp sterile towel, taking care not to drip water onto sterile setup.	Water contaminates sterile setup.
f. Bending slightly at waist, keeping hands and arms above waist and outstretched, grasp one end of sterile towel and dry one hand, moving from fingers to elbow in a rotating motion (see illustrations).	Avoids sterile towel from contacting unsterile scrub attire and transferring contamination to hands. Dry skin from cleanest (hands) to least clean (elbows).
g. Repeat drying method for other hand by carefully reversing towel or using a new sterile towel.	Prevents accidental contamination.
h. Drop towel into linen hamper or circulating nurse's hand.	Prevents accidental contamination.
11. *Optional:* Brushless antiseptic hand rub	
a. After prescrub wash (see Step 7), dry hands and forearms thoroughly with paper towel.	Promotes reduction in microorganisms on all surfaces of hands and arms.
b. Dispense 2 mL of antimicrobial agent hand preparation into palm of one hand. Dip fingertips of opposite hand into hand preparation and work it under nails. Spread remaining hand preparation over hand and up to just above elbow, covering all surfaces (see illustrations).	
c. Using another 2 mL of hand preparation, repeat with other hand.	
d. Dispense another 2 mL of hand preparation into either hand and reapply to all aspects of both hands up to wrist. Allow to dry thoroughly before donning gloves.	Ensures complete antiseptic coverage of all hand surfaces.
12. Proceed with sterile gowning (see Skill 29-4).	

RECORDING AND REPORTING

- It is not necessary to record or report this procedure.
- Report any skin dermatitis to employee health or infection control per agency policy.

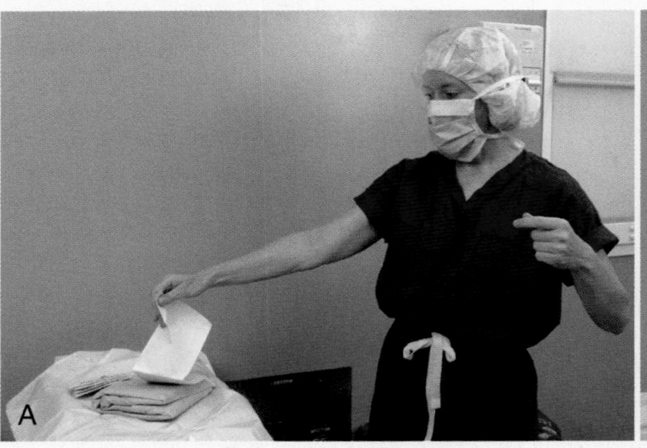

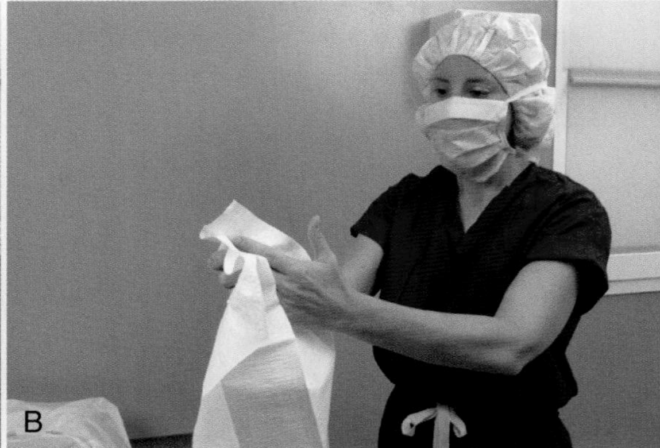

STEP 10f A, Grasp sterile towel. **B,** Drying sequence.

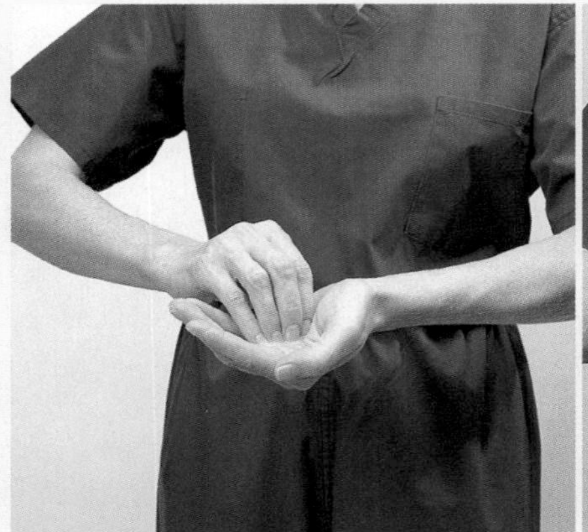

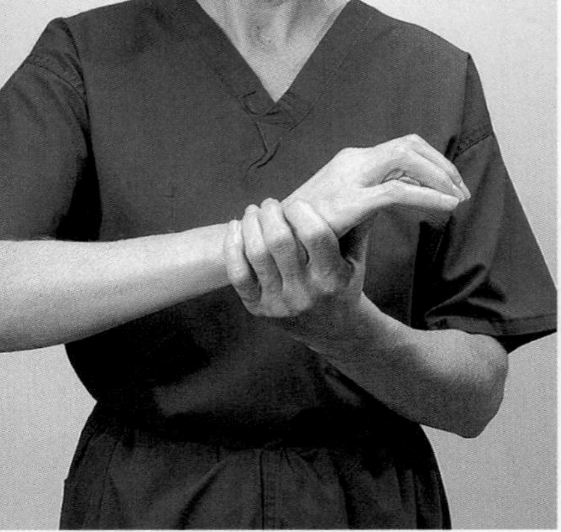

STEP 11b Application of antimicrobial agent for brushless hand scrub. Nurse using 3M Avagard. (Photos courtesy 3M Health Care.)

SKILL 29-4 APPLYING A STERILE GOWN AND PERFORMING CLOSED GLOVING

DELEGATION CONSIDERATIONS

Applying a sterile gown and closed gloving can be delegated to a properly trained surgical technician (know the state Nurse Practice Act).

EQUIPMENT

- Package of proper-size sterile gloves (latex free if nurse or patient has sensitivity or allergy)
- Sterile pack containing sterile gown
- Clean, flat, dry surface
- Paper face masks, cap or hood, surgical shoe covers
- Protective eyewear/face shield

STEP	RATIONALE
APPLYING STERILE GOWN	
1. Before entering operating room or treatment area, apply cap, face mask, eyewear, and foot covers (paper or cloth covers fit over work shoes).	Prevents hair and air droplet nuclei from contaminating sterile work areas. Eyewear protects mucous membranes of eye. Foot covers reduce contamination from shoes.
2. Perform thorough surgical hand wash (see Skill 29-3).	Removes transient and resident bacteria from fingers, hands, and forearms.
3. Circulating nurse assists by opening sterile pack containing sterile gown (folded inside out).	Outer surface of gown remains sterile.
4. Circulating nurse prepares glove package by peeling outer wrapper open while keeping inner contents sterile. Places inner glove package on sterile field created by sterile outer wrapper.	Keeps gloves sterile and allows nurse who has scrubbed to handle sterile items.
5. Reach down to sterile gown package; lift folded gown directly upward and step back away from table.	Provides wide margin of safety, avoiding contamination of gown.
6. Holding folded gown, locate neckband. With both hands grasp inside front of gown just below neckband.	Clean hands can touch inside of gown without contaminating outer surface.
7. Allow gown to unfold, keeping inside of gown toward body. Do not touch outside of gown with bare hands.	Outside of gown is sterile surface.
8. With hands at shoulder level, slip both arms into armholes simultaneously (see illustration). Ask circulating nurse to bring gown over your shoulders by reaching inside to arm seams and pulling gown on, leaving sleeves covering hands.	Careful application prevents contamination. Gown covers hands to prepare for closed gloving.
9. Have circulating nurse securely tie back of gown at neck and waist (see illustration). (If gown is wraparound style, do not touch sterile flap to cover it until you are gloved.)	Gown must completely enclose underlying garments.
PERFORMING CLOSED GLOVING	
10. Closed gloving	
a. With hands covered by gown sleeves, open inner sterile glove package (see illustration).	Hands remain clean. Sterile gown cuff touches sterile glove surface.

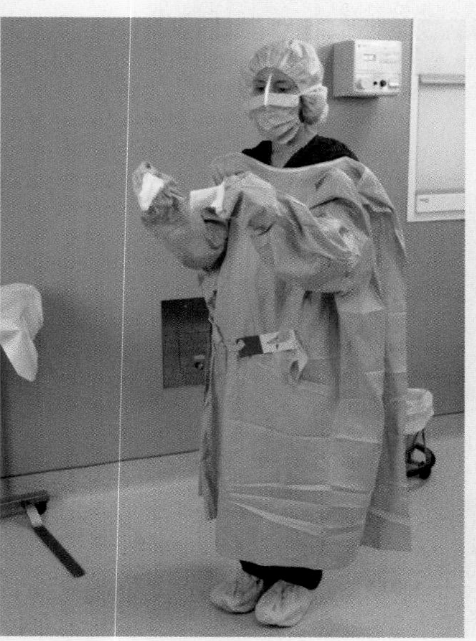

STEP 8 Place arms in sleeves.

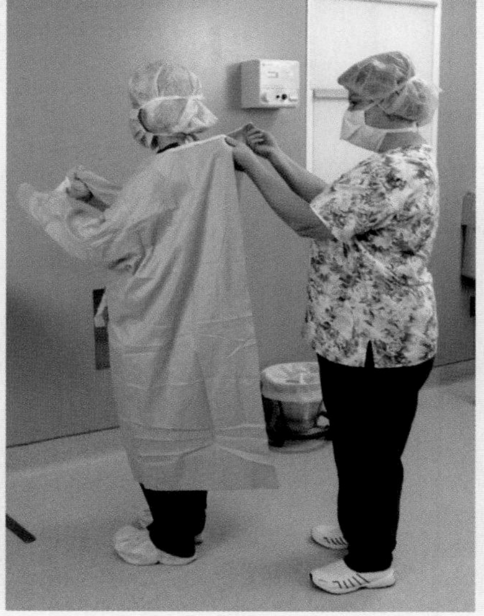

STEP 9 Circulating nurse ties scrub gown.

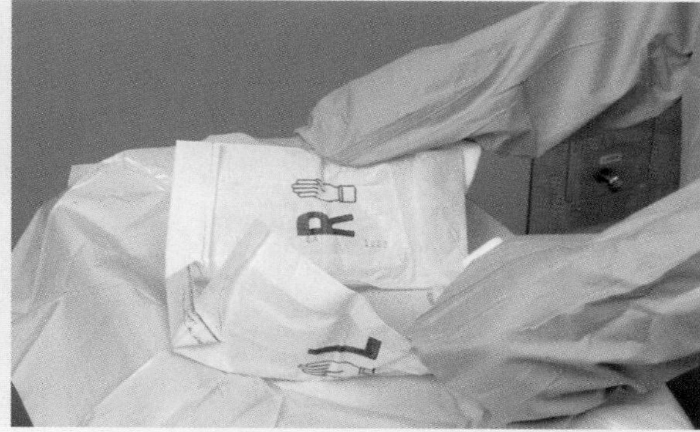

STEP 10a Scrub nurse opens glove package.

SKILL 29-4 APPLYING A STERILE GOWN AND PERFORMING CLOSED GLOVING—cont'd

STEP	RATIONALE
b. With dominant hand inside gown cuff, pick up glove for nondominant hand by grasping folded cuff.	Sterile gown touches sterile glove.
c. Extend nondominant forearm with palm up and place palm of glove against palm of nondominant hand. Glove fingers point toward elbow.	Positions glove for application over cuffed hand, keeping glove sterile.
d. Grasp back of glove cuff with covered dominant hand and turn glove cuff over end of nondominant hand and gown cuff (see illustration).	Seal created by glove cuff over gown prevents exit of microorganisms over operative sterile field.
e. Grasp top of glove and underlying gown sleeve with covered dominant hand. Carefully extend fingers into glove, being sure that glove cuff covers gown cuff.	
f. Glove dominant hand in same manner, reversing hands (see illustration). Use gloved nondominant hand to pull on glove. Keep hand inside sleeve (see illustration).	Sterile touches sterile.
g. Be sure that fingers are fully extended into both gloves.	Ensures that nurse has full dexterity while using gloved hand.
11. For wraparound sterile gowns: take gloved hand and release fastener or ties in front of gown.	Front of gown is sterile.
12. Hand paper tab connected to sterile tie to circulating nurse, who is nonsterile (see illustration). Circulating nurse stands still as you turn completely around to left, allowing for margin of safety as gown wraps around and covers your back. Take back sterile tie from circulating nurse and secure tie to gown.	Contact with team member could contaminate gown and gloves. Gown must enclose undergarments.

RECORDING AND REPORTING

- It is not necessary to record or report this procedure.

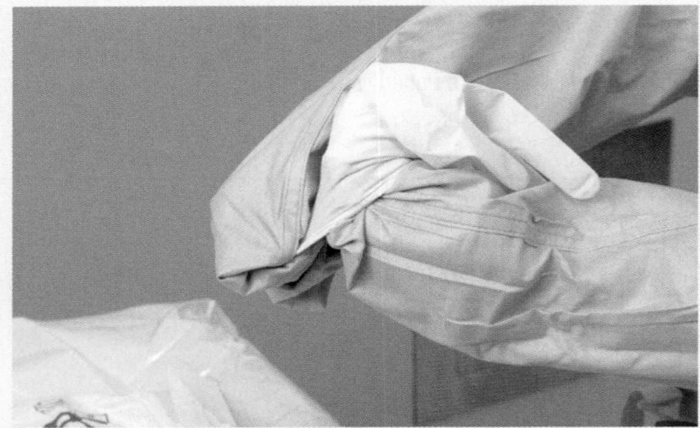

STEP 10d Glove is applied to left hand as right hand remains inside cuff.

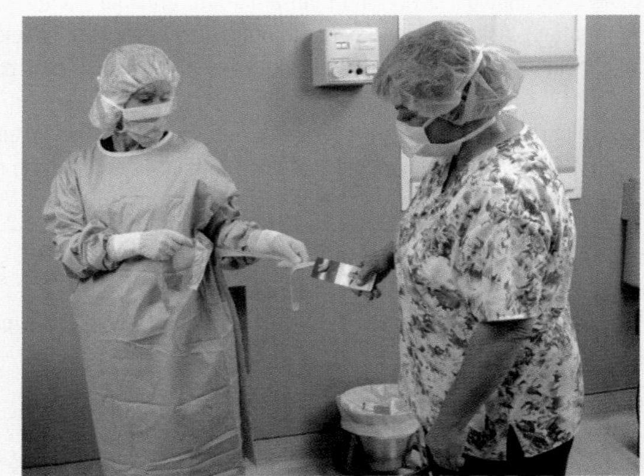

STEP 12 Hand tie to sterile team member.

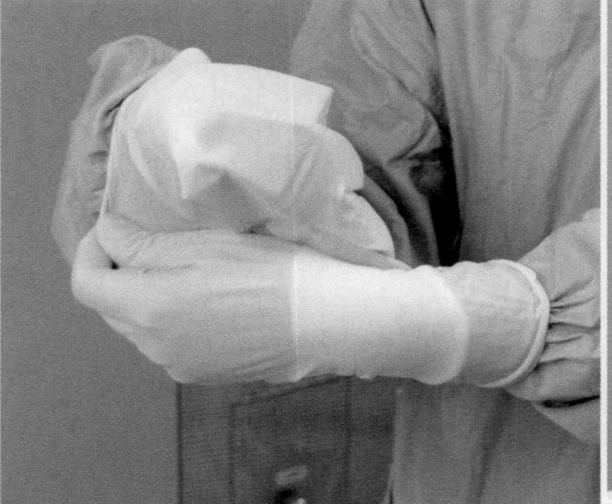

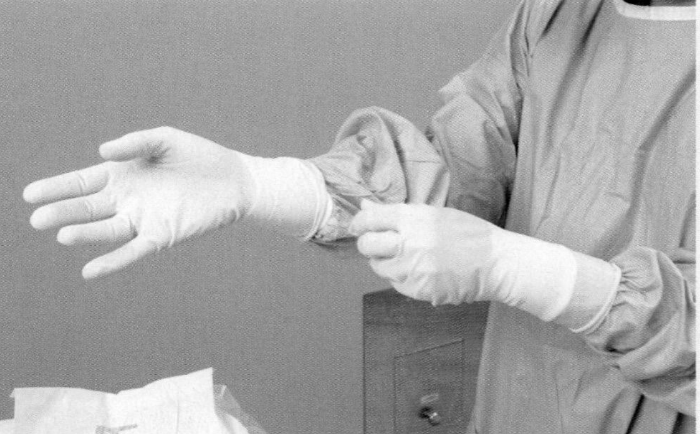

STEP 10f Second glove is applied.

SKILL 29-5 OPEN GLOVING

DELEGATION CONSIDERATIONS

The skill of open gloving can be delegated when personnel are trained to perform a sterile procedure.

EQUIPMENT

- Sterile gloves (proper size)

STEP	RATIONALE
1. Perform thorough hand hygiene.	Removes bacteria from skin surfaces and reduces transmission of infection.
2. Remove outer glove package wrapper by carefully separating and peeling apart sides.	Prevents inner glove package from accidentally opening and touching contaminated objects.
3. Grasp inner package and lay it on clean, flat surface just above waist level. Open package, keeping gloves on wrappers inside surface (see illustration).	Sterile object held below waist is contaminated. Inner surface of glove package is sterile.
4. Identify right and left glove. Each glove has cuff approximately 5 cm (2 inches) wide. Glove dominant hand first.	Proper identification of gloves prevents contamination by improper fit. Gloving of dominant hand first improves dexterity.
5. With thumb and first two fingers of nondominant hand, grasp edge of cuff of glove for dominant hand. Touch only inside surface of glove.	Inner edge of cuff lies against skin and thus is not sterile.
6. Carefully pull glove over dominant hand, leaving cuff and being sure that it does not roll up wrist. Be sure that thumb and fingers are in proper spaces (see illustration).	If outer surface of glove touches hand or wrist, it is contaminated.
7. With gloved dominant hand, slip fingers underneath cuff of second glove (see illustration).	Cuff protects gloved fingers. Sterile touching sterile prevents glove contamination.

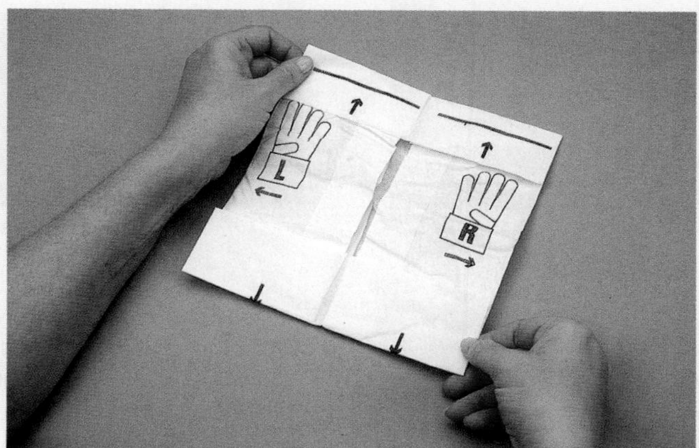

STEP 3 Open package.

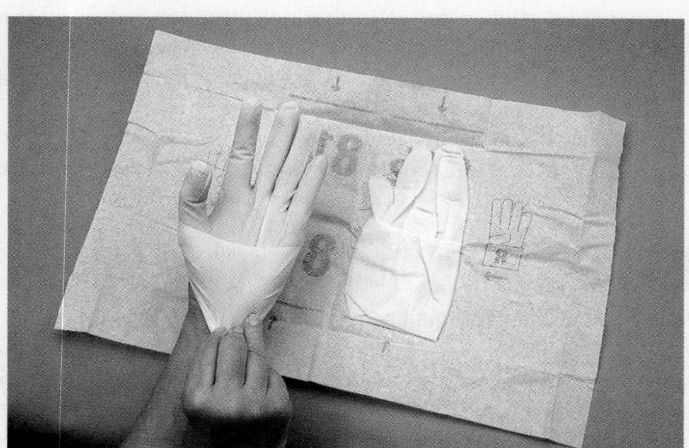
STEP 6 Pull glove over dominant hand.

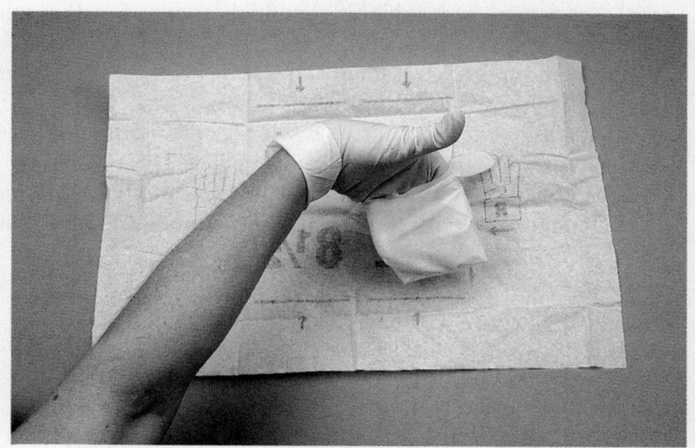
STEP 7 Slip fingers underneath cuff of second glove.

SKILL 29-5 OPEN GLOVING—cont'd

STEP	RATIONALE
8. Carefully pull second glove over nondominant hand. Do not allow fingers and thumb of gloved dominant hand to touch any part of exposed nondominant hand. Keep thumb of dominant hand abducted back (see illustration).	Contact of gloved hand with exposed hand results in contamination.
9. After second glove is on, interlock fingers of gloved hands and hold away from body above waist level until beginning procedure (see illustration).	Prevents accidental contamination from hand movement.
GLOVE DISPOSAL	
10. Grasp outside of one cuff with other gloved hand; avoid touching wrist. Pull halfway down palm of hand. Take thumb of half-ungloved hand and place under cuff of other glove.	Minimizes contamination of underlying skin.
11. Pull glove off, turning it inside out. Discard in receptacle.	Outside of glove does not touch skin surface.
12. Take fingers of bare hand and tuck inside remaining glove cuff. Peel glove off, inside out. Discard in receptacle.	

RECORDING AND REPORTING

- It is not necessary to record or report this procedure.

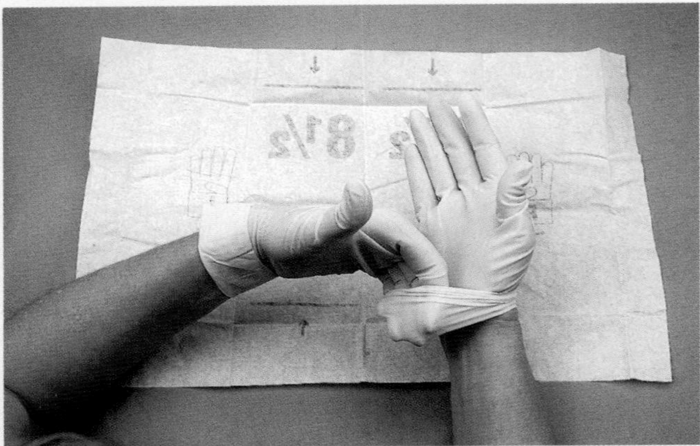

STEP 8 Pull second glove over nondominant hand.

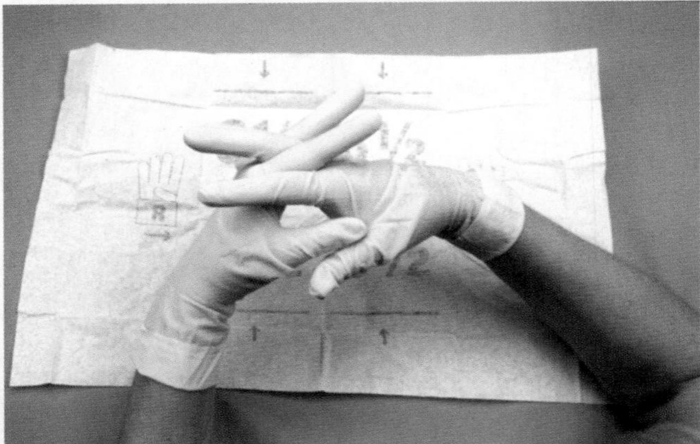

STEP 9 Hands are interlocked.

KEY POINTS

- Hand hygiene practices are the most important techniques to use in the prevention and control of infection.
- The potential for microorganisms to cause disease depends on the number of organisms, virulence, and ability to enter and survive in a host and susceptibility of the host.
- Normal body floras help to resist infection by releasing antibacterial substances and inhibiting multiplication of pathogenic microorganisms.
- An infection can develop as long as the six elements composing the infection chain are uninterrupted.
- Microorganisms are transmitted by direct and indirect contact, airborne spread, and vectors and contaminated articles.
- Increasing age, poor nutrition, stress, inherited conditions, chronic disease, and treatments or conditions that compromise the immune response increase susceptibility to infection.
- The major sites for HAIs include the urinary and respiratory tracts, bloodstream, and surgical or traumatic wounds.
- Invasive procedures, medical therapies, long hospitalization, and contact with health care personnel increase a hospitalized patient's risk for acquiring an HAI.
- Isolation practices may prevent personnel and patients from acquiring infections and transmitting microorganisms to other people.
- Standard precautions involve the use of generic barrier techniques when caring for all patients.
- Proper cleaning requires mechanical removal of all soil from an object or area.
- The overall experience of isolation is commonly viewed negatively due to barriers affecting the expression of a patient's identity and normal interpersonal relationships.
- An infection prevention and control professional monitors the incidence of infection within an institution, introduces evidence-based practices and provides educational and consulting services.
- Surgical asepsis requires more stringent techniques than medical asepsis and is directed at eliminating microorganisms.
- If the skin is broken or if an invasive procedure into a body cavity normally free of microorganisms is performed, follow surgical aseptic practices.

CLINICAL APPLICATION QUESTIONS

Preparing for Clinical Practice

Mrs. Andrews shares that she has had some wetness on her back and has been using tissues to wipe off and scratch her back. She also is having increased incision pain. She attributes her symptoms to the back brace because "it makes me sweat and itch." Her daughter noted that the incision was reddened with a small amount of drainage coming from the site. Mrs. Andrews was seen by the surgeon, and an incision and drainage of the back wound were performed.

1. What do you need to include when assessing the wound for infection?
2. If Mrs. Andrews were to develop a systemic infection as a result of the localized wound infection, which assessments would you expect to find? Explain your answers.
3. Which methods of infection control do you need to use when caring for Mrs. Andrews?

ⓔ ***Answers to Clinical Application Questions can be found on the Evolve website.***

REVIEW QUESTIONS

Are You Ready to Test Your Nursing Knowledge?

1. What is the most effective way to control transmission of infection?
   1. Isolation precautions
   2. Identifying the infectious agent
   3. Hand hygiene practices
   4. Vaccinations
2. A patient who has been isolated for *Clostridium difficile (C. difficile)* asks you to explain what he should know about this organism. What is the most appropriate information to include in patient teaching? (Select all that apply.)
   1. The organism is usually transmitted through the fecal-oral route.
   2. Hands should always be cleaned with soap and water versus alcohol-based hand sanitizer.
   3. Everyone coming into the room must be wearing a gown and gloves.
   4. While the patient is in contact precautions, he cannot leave the room.
   5. *C. difficile* dies quickly once outside the body.
3. Your assigned patient has a leg ulcer that has a dressing on it. During your assessment you find that the dressing is saturated with purulent drainage. Which action would be best on your part?
   1. Reinforce dressing with a clean, dry dressing and call the health care provider.
   2. Remove wet dressing and apply new dressing using sterile procedure.
   3. Put on gloves before removing the old dressing; then obtain a wound culture.
   4. Remove saturated dressing with gloves, remove gloves, then perform hand hygiene and apply new gloves before putting on a clean dressing.
4. A patient is diagnosed with methicillin-resistant *Staphylococcus aureus* (MRSA) pneumonia. Which type of isolation precaution is *most* appropriate for this patient?
   1. Reverse isolation
   2. Droplet precautions
   3. Standard precautions
   4. Contact precautions
5. A family member is providing care to a loved one who has an infected leg wound. What should the nurse instruct the family member to do after providing care and handling contaminated equipment or organic material?
   1. Wear gloves before eating or handling food.
   2. Place any soiled materials into a bag and double bag it.
   3. Have the family member check with the health care provider about need for immunization.
   4. Perform hand hygiene after care and/or handling contaminated equipment or material.
6. A patient is isolated for pulmonary tuberculosis. The nurse notes that the patient seems to be angry, but he knows that this is a normal response to isolation. Which is the best intervention?
   1. Provide a dark, quiet room to calm the patient.
   2. Reduce the level of precautions to keep the patient from becoming angry.
   3. Explain the reasons for isolation procedures and provide meaningful stimulation.
   4. Limit family and other caregiver visits to reduce the risk of spreading the infection.
7. When should a nurse wear a mask? (Select all that apply.)
   1. The patient's dental hygiene is poor.
   2. The nurse is assisting with an aerosolizing respiratory procedure such as suctioning.
   3. The patient has acquired immunodeficiency syndrome (AIDS) and a congested cough.
   4. The patient is in droplet precautions.
   5. The nurse is assisting a health care provider in the insertion of a central line catheter.
8. Which type of personal protective equipment are staff required to wear when caring for a pediatric patient who is placed into airborne precautions for confirmed chickenpox/herpes zoster? (Select all that apply.)
   1. Disposable gown
   2. N 95 respirator mask
   3. Face shield or goggles
   4. Surgical mask
   5. Gloves
9. The infection control nurse has asked the staff to work on reducing the number of iatrogenic infections on the unit. Which of the following actions on your part would contribute to reducing health care–acquired infections? (Select all that apply.)
   1. Teaching correct handwashing to assigned patients
   2. Using correct procedures in starting and caring for an intravenous infusion
   3. Providing perineal care to a patient with an indwelling urinary catheter
   4. Isolating a patient who has just been diagnosed as having tuberculosis
   5. Decreasing a patient's environmental stimuli to decrease nausea
10. Which of the following actions by the nurse comply with core principles of surgical asepsis? (Select all that apply.)
    1. Set up sterile field before patient and other staff come to the operating suite.
    2. Keep the sterile field in view at all times.
    3. Consider the outer 2.5 cm (1 inch) of the sterile field as contaminated.
    4. Only health care personnel within the sterile field must wear personal protective equipment.
    5. The sterile gown must be put on before the surgical scrub is performed.
11. A patient has an indwelling urinary catheter. Why does an indwelling urinary catheter present a risk for urinary tract infection? (Select all that apply.)
    1. It allows migration of organisms into the bladder.
    2. The insertion procedure is not done under sterile conditions.
    3. It obstructs the normal flushing action of urine flow.
    4. It keeps an incontinent patient's skin dry.
    5. The outer surface of the catheter is not considered sterile.

12. Put the following steps for removal of protective barriers after leaving an isolation room in order.
    1. Remove gloves.
    2. Perform hand hygiene.
    3. Remove eyewear or goggles.
    4. Untie top and then bottom mask strings and remove from face.
    5. Untie waist and neck strings of gown. Remove gown, rolling it onto itself without touching the contaminated side.
13. What does it mean when a patient is diagnosed with a multidrug-resistant organism in his or her surgical wound? (Select all that apply.)
    1. There is more than one organism in the wound that is causing the infection.
    2. The antibiotics the patient has received are not strong enough to kill the organism.
    3. The patient will need more than one type of antibiotic to kill the organism.
    4. The organism has developed a resistance to one or more broad-spectrum antibiotics, indicating that the organism will be hard to treat effectively.
    5. There are no longer any antibiotic options available to treat the patient's infection.
14. A patient's surgical wound has become swollen, red, and tender. The nurse notes that the patient has a new fever, purulent wound drainage, and leukocytosis. Which interventions would be appropriate and in what order?
    1. Notify the health care provider of the patient's status.
    2. Reassure the patient and recheck the wound later.
    3. Support the patient's fluid and nutritional needs.
    4. Use aseptic technique to change the dressing.
15. Which of these statements are true regarding disinfection and cleaning? (Select all that apply.)
    1. Proper cleaning requires mechanical removal of all soil from an object or area.
    2. General environmental cleaning is an example of medical asepsis.
    3. When cleaning a wound, wipe around the wound edge first and then clean inward toward the center of the wound.
    4. Cleaning in a direction from the least to the most contaminated area helps reduce infections.
    5. Disinfecting and sterilizing medical devices and equipment involve the same procedures.

Answers: 1. 3; **2.** 1, 2, 3; **3.** 4; **4.** 2; **5.** 4; **6.** 3; **7.** 2, 4, 5; **8.** 1, 2, 5; **9.** 1, 2, 3; **10.** 2, 3; **11.** 1, 3; **12.** 1, 3, 5, 4, 2; **13.** 2, 4; **14.** 4, 2, 1, 3; **15.** 1, 2, 4.

Rationales for Review Questions can be found on the Evolve website.

REFERENCES

Arnold F: *Antimicrobials and resistance.* In Grota P, editor: *APIC text of infection control and epidemiology*, Washington, DC, 2014, Association for Professionals in Infection Control and Epidemiology.

Boyce JM, et al: Guideline for hand hygiene in health-care settings: recommendations of the Healthcare Infection Control Practices Advisory Committee and the HICPAC/SHEA/APIC/IDSA Hand Hygiene Task Force, *MMWR Recomm Rep* 51(RR–16):1, 2002.

Brisko V: Isolation precautions. In Carrico R, et al., editors: *APIC text of infection control and epidemiology*, ed 3, Washington, DC, 2009, Association for Professionals in Infection Control and Epidemiology (APIC).

Centers for Disease Control and Prevention (CDC): *Guideline for preventing the transmission of* Mycobacterium tuberculosis *in health-care facilities*, Washington, DC, 2005a, CDC.

Centers for Disease Control and Prevention (CDC): *Updated US Public Health Service guidelines for the management of occupational exposures to HIV and recommendations for post exposure prophylaxis*, Washington, DC, 2005b, CDC.

Centers for Disease Control and Prevention (CDC): *Management of multidrug-resistant organisms in healthcare settings*, 2006, CDC.

Centers for Disease Control and Prevention (CDC): *Guideline for isolation precautions: preventing transmission of infectious agents in healthcare settings—recommendations to the Healthcare Infection Control Practices Advisory Committee (HICPAC)*, Washington, DC, 2007, CDC. http://www.cdc.gov/hicpac/2007IP/2007isolationPrecautions.html. Accessed April 12, 2015.

Centers for Disease Control and Prevention (CDC), Hospital Infection Control Practice Advisory Committee and the HICPAC/SHEA/APIC/IDSA: *Hand Hygiene Task Force Guidelines for hand hygiene in health care settings*, Atlanta, 2008a, Centers for Disease Control and Prevention.

Centers for Disease Control and Prevention (CDC) and the Hospital Infection Control Practice Advisory Committee, Rutal W, Weber D, and the Healthcare Infection Control Practices and Advisory Committee: *Guidelines for disinfection and sterilization in healthcare facilities*, 2008b. http://www.cdc.gov/ncidod/eid/vol7no2/rutala.html. Accessed October 5, 2015.

Centers for Disease Control and Prevention (CDC): Sexually transmitted diseases treatment guidelines (includes chapter on hepatitis C), *MMWR Morb Mortal Wkly Rep* 59(RR–12):1, 2010a.

Centers for Disease Control and Prevention (CDC): *Interim guidance for infection control for care of patients with confirmed or suspected swine influenza A (H1N1) virus infection in a healthcare setting*, 2010b. http://www.cdc.gov/h1n1flu/guideline_infectioncontrol.htm. Accessed August 15, 2014.

Centers for Disease Control and Prevention: *Immunization schedules, CDC*, 2010c. http://www.cdc.gov/vaccines/recs/schedules/default.htm. Accessed August 20, 2011.

Centers for Disease Control and Prevention (CDC): *Vaccines and preventable diseases, CDC*, 2011a. http://www.cdc.gov/vaccines/vpd-vac/default.htm. Accessed August 15, 2014.

Centers for Disease Control and Prevention (CDC): *CDC vital signs: Making healthcare safer*, 2011b. Available at: http://www.cdc.gov/vitalsigns/pdf/2011-03-vitalsigns.pdf. Accessed October 25, 2015.

Centers for Disease Control and Prevention (CDC): *Wash your hands*, 2013a. http://www.cdc.gov/features/handwashing. Accessed April 12, 2015.

Centers for Disease Control and Prevention (CDC): *Precautions to prevent the spread of MRSA in healthcare settings*, 2013b. http://www.cdc.gov/mrsa/index.html. Accessed April 2015.

Centers for Disease Control and Prevention (CDC): *Show me the science—when to use hand sanitizers*, 2014. http://www.cdc.gov/handwashing/show-me-the-science-hand-sanitizer.html. Accessed April 12, 2015.

Centers for Disease Control and Prevention (CDC): *Healthcare associated infections*, 2015a. http://www.cdc.gov/HAI/surveillance/. Accessed October 24, 2015.

Centers for Disease Control and Prevention (CDC): *Ebola virus disease*, August 2015b. http://www.cdc.gov/vhf/ebola/index.html. Accessed October 3, 2015.

Centers for Disease Control and Prevention (CDC): *Fact Sheet: Screening and monitoring travelers to prevent the spread of Ebola*, September 2015c. http://www.cdc.gov/vhf/ebola/travelers/ebola-screening-factsheet.html. Accessed October 3, 2015.

Centers for Disease Control and Prevention (CDC): *Long-term effectiveness of whooping cough vaccines*, June 2015d. http://www.cdc.gov/pertussis/pregnant/mom/vacc-effectiveness.html. Accessed October 3, 2015.

Centers for Disease Control and Prevention (CDC): *Handwashing: Clean hands saves lives*, 2015e. http://www.cdc.gov/handwashing/. Accessed October 23, 2015.

Cohen S, et al: Clinical Practice Guidelines for *Clostridium difficile* infection in adults: 2010 update from the Society for Healthcare Epidemiology of America and the Infectious Diseases Society of America, *Infect Control Hosp Epidemiol* 31(5):431, 2010.

Day M: Endoscopy. In Grota P, editor: *APIC text of infection control and epidemiology*, Washington, DC, 2014, Association for Professionals in Infection Control and Epidemiology.

Ellingson K, et al: Strategies to prevent healthcare-associated infections through hand hygiene, *Infect Control Hosp Epidemiol* 35(8):937, 2014.

Fiutem C: *Risk factors facilitating transmission of infectious agents.* In Grota P, editor: *APIC text of infection control and epidemiology*, Washington, DC, 2014, Association for Professionals in Infection Control and Epidemiology.

Hass J: Hand hygiene. In Grota P, editor: *APIC text of infection control and epidemiology*, Washington, DC,

2014, Association for Professionals in Infection Control and Epidemiology.
Iwamoto P, Post M: *Aseptic technique*. In Grota P, editor: *APIC text of infection control and epidemiology*, Washington, DC, 2014, Association for Professionals in Infection Control and Epidemiology.
Jefferson J, Young M: *Sterile Processing*. In Grota P, editor: *APIC text of infection control and epidemiology*, Washington, DC, 2014, Association for Professionals in Infection Control and Epidemiology.
Larbi A, et al: The immune system in the elderly: a fair fight against diseases? *Aging Health* 9(1):35, 2013.
Mathur P: Hand hygiene: back to the basics of infection control, *Indian J Med Res* 134(5):611–620, 2011.
Meiner S: *Gerontologic nursing*, ed 5, St Louis, 2014, Mosby.
Monsees E: Patient safety. In Grota P, editor: *APIC text of infection control and epidemiology*, Washington, DC, 2014, Association for Professionals in Infection Control and Epidemiology.
Murphy R: Surgical services. In Grota P, editor: *APIC text of infection control and epidemiology*, Washington, DC, 2014, Association for Professionals in Infection Control and Epidemiology.
Nesher L, et al: The current spectrum of infection in cancer patients with chemotherapy-related neutropenia, *Infection* 42:5, 2014.
Occupational Safety and Health Administration (OSHA): *Respiratory protective devices: final rules and notice, Fed Regist* 33606, 2011a.
Occupational Safety and Health Administration (OSHA): *Enforcement procedures for the occupational exposure to bloodborne injury final rule, Fed Regist* 33606, 2011b.
Occupational Safety and Health Administration (OSHA): *Needlestick Safety and Prevention Act, Fed Regist 19934*, 2012.
Pagana KD, Pagana TJ: *Manual of diagnostic and laboratory tests*, ed 5, St Louis, 2014, Mosby.
Roach R: Geriatrics. In Grota P, editor: *APIC text of infection control and epidemiology*, Washington, DC, 2014, Association for Professionals in Infection Control and Epidemiology.
Rutala W, Weber DJ: *Cleaning, disinfection and sterilization*. In Grota P, editor: *APIC text of infection control and epidemiology*, Washington, DC, 2014, Association for Professionals in Infection Control and Epidemiology.
The Joint Commission (TJC): *2016 National Patient Safety Goals*, Oakbrook Terrace, IL, 2016, The Commission. Available at http://www.jointcommission.org/standards_information/npsgs.aspx. Accessed November 2015.
Tweeten SM: *General principles of epidemiology*. In Grota P, editor: *APIC text of infection control and epidemiology*, Washington, DC, 2014, Association for Professionals in Infection Control and Epidemiology.
World Health Organization (WHO): *WHO guidelines on hand hygiene in healthcare*, Geneva, Switzerland, 2009, WHO Press.
World Health Organization (WHO): *Five Moments for Hand Hygiene*, 2015. http://www.who.int/gpsc/tools/Five_moments/en/. Accessed October 24, 2015.

RESEARCH REFERENCES

Abad C, et al: Adverse effects of isolation in hospitalised patients: a systematic review, *J Hosp Infect* 76(2):97, 2010.
Association of Operating Room Nurses (AORN): *Standards, recommended practices, and guidelines*, Denver, 2014, The Association.
Barratt R: Behind barriers: patient's perceptions of source isolation for methicillin resistant *Staphylococcus aureus* (MRSA), *Austral J Adv Nsng* 28(2):53, 2010.
Birnbach DJ, et al: Do hospital visitors wash their hands? Assessing the use of alcohol-based hand sanitizer in a hospital lobby, *Am J Infect Control* 40(4):340, 2012.
Doyle JS, et al: Epidemiology of infections acquired in intensive care units, *Semin Respir Crit Care Med* 32(2):115, 2011.
Gould D, et al: *Interventions to improve hand hygiene compliance in patient care, Cochrane Database Syst Rev* volume 8, *The Cochrane Library*, 2011, The Cochrane Collaboration.
Kassakian SZ, et al: Impact of chlorhexidine bathing on hospital-acquired infections among general medical patients, *Infec Control Hosp Epidemiol* 32(3):238, 2011.
Luangasanatip N, et al: Comparative efficacy of interventions to promote hand hygiene in hospital: systematic review and network meta-analysis, *BMJ* 351:h3728, 2015.
Messano GA: Bacterial and fungal contamination of dental hygienists' hands with and without finger rings, *Acta Stomatologica Naissi* 29:1260, 2013.
Oughton M, et al: Hand hygiene with soap and water is superior to alcohol rub and antiseptic wipes for removal of *Clostridium difficile*, *Infect Control Hosp Epidemiol* 30(10):939, 2009.
Schweizer ML, et al: Searching for an optimal hand hygiene bundle: a meta-analysis, *Clin Infect Dis* 58(2):248, 2014.
Thomas R, et al: *Influenza vaccination for healthcare workers who work care for people aged 60 or older living in long-term care settings*, The Cochrane Library, Issue 7, 2013, The Cochrane Collaboration. http://onlinelibrary.wiley.com/doi/10.1002/14651858.CD005187.pub4/pdf. Accessed October 3, 2015.
Whittington AM, et al: Bacterial contamination of stethoscopes on the intensive care unit, *Anaesthesia* 64(6):620, 2009.

30

Vital Signs

OBJECTIVES

- Explain the principles and mechanisms of thermoregulation.
- Describe nursing measures that promote heat loss and heat conservation.
- Discuss physiological changes associated with fever.
- Accurately assess body temperature, pulse, respirations, oxygen saturation, and blood pressure.
- Explain the physiology of normal regulation of blood pressure, pulse, oxygen saturation, and respirations.
- Describe factors that cause variations in body temperature, pulse, oxygen saturation, respirations, capnography, and blood pressure.
- Describe cultural and ethnic variations with blood pressure assessment.
- Identify ranges of acceptable vital sign values for an infant, a child, and an adult.
- Explain variations in technique used to assess an infant's, a child's, and an adult's vital signs.
- Describe the benefits and precautions involving self-measurement of blood pressure.
- Identify when to measure vital signs.
- Accurately record and report vital sign measurements.
- Appropriately delegate measurement of vital signs to nursing assistive personnel.

KEY TERMS

Afebrile, p. 491
Antipyretics, p. 496
Auscultatory gap, p. 508
Basal metabolic rate (BMR), p. 488
Blood pressure, p. 503
Bradycardia, p. 499
Capnography, p. 501
Cardiac output, p. 497
Conduction, p. 489
Convection, p. 489
Core temperature, p. 488
Diaphoresis, p. 489
Diastolic pressure, p. 503
Diffusion, p. 500
Dysrhythmia, p. 499
Eupnea, p. 500
Evaporation, p. 489
Febrile, p. 490
Fever, p. 490
Fever of unknown origin (FUO), p. 491
Frostbite, p. 491
Heat exhaustion, p. 491
Heatstroke, p. 491
Hematocrit, p. 503
Hypertension, p. 504
Hyperthermia, p. 491
Hypotension, p. 505
Hypothermia, p. 491
Hypoxemia, p. 500
Malignant hyperthermia, p. 491
Nonshivering thermogenesis, p. 488
Orthostatic hypotension, p. 505
Oxygen saturation, p. 502
Perfusion, p. 500
Postural hypotension, p. 505
Pulse deficit, p. 499
Pulse pressure, p. 503
Pyrexia, p. 490
Pyrogens, p. 490
Radiation, p. 489
Shivering, p. 488
Sphygmomanometer, p. 506
Systolic pressure, p. 503
Tachycardia, p. 499
Thermoregulation, p. 488
Ventilation, p. 500
Vital signs, p. 486

ⓔ MEDIA RESOURCES

http://evolve.elsevier.com/Potter/fundamentals/

- Review Questions
- Video Clips
- Case Study with Questions
- Skills Performance Checklists
- Audio Glossary
- Content Updates

The most frequent and routine measurements obtained by health care providers are those of temperature, pulse, blood pressure (BP), respiratory rate, and oxygen saturation. As indicators of health status, these measures indicate the effectiveness of circulatory, respiratory, neural, and endocrine body functions. Because of their importance, they are referred to as **vital signs.** Pain, a subjective symptom, is often called another vital sign and is frequently measured with the others (see Chapter 44).

Measurement of vital signs provides data to determine a patient's usual state of health (baseline data). Many factors such as the temperature of the environment, the patient's physical exertion, and the effects of illness cause vital signs to change, sometimes outside an acceptable range. Assessment of vital signs provides data to identify nursing diagnoses, implement planned interventions, and evaluate outcomes of care. An alteration in vital signs signals a change in physiological function and the need for medical or nursing intervention.

Vital signs are a quick and efficient way of monitoring a patient's condition or identifying problems and evaluating his or her response to intervention. When you learn the physiological variables influencing vital signs and recognize the relationship of their changes to one another and to other physical assessment findings, you can make precise determinations about a patient's health problems. Vital signs and other physiological measurements are the basis for clinical decision making and problem solving. Many facilities adopt Early Warning Scores determined by vital sign data entered into the electronic medical record to alert nurses to potential changes in their patients' conditions.

GUIDELINES FOR MEASURING VITAL SIGNS

Vital signs are a part of the assessment database. You include them in a complete physical assessment (see Chapter 31) or obtain them individually to assess a patient's condition. Establishing a database of vital signs during a routine physical examination serves as a baseline for future assessments. A patient's needs and condition determine when, where, how, and by whom vital signs are measured. You need to measure them correctly, and at times you appropriately delegate their measurement. You also need to know expected values (Box 30-1), interpret your patient's values, communicate findings appropriately, and begin interventions as needed. Use the following guidelines to incorporate measurements of vital signs into nursing practice:

- Measuring vital signs is your responsibility. You may delegate measurement of vital signs in selected situations (e.g., in stable patients). However, it is your responsibility to review vital sign data, interpret their significance, and critically think through decisions about interventions.
- Assess equipment to ensure that it is working correctly and provides accurate findings.
- Select equipment on the basis of the patient's condition and characteristics (e.g., do not use an adult-size BP cuff for a child).
- Know the patient's usual range of vital signs. These values can differ from the acceptable range for that age or physical state. The patient's usual values serve as a baseline for comparison with later findings. Thus you are able to detect a change in condition over time.
- Know your patient's medical history, therapies, and prescribed medications. Some illnesses or treatments cause predictable changes in vital signs. Some medications affect one or more vital signs.
- Control or minimize environmental factors that affect vital signs. For example, assessing a patient's temperature in a warm, humid room may yield a value that is not a true indicator of his or her condition.
- Use an organized, systematic approach when taking vital signs. Each procedure requires a step-by-step approach to ensure accuracy.
- On the basis of a patient's condition, collaborate with health care providers to decide the frequency of vital sign assessment. In the hospital health care providers order a minimum frequency of vital sign measurements for each patient. Following surgery or treatment intervention you measure vital signs more frequently to detect complications. In a clinic or outpatient setting you take vital signs before the health care provider examines the patient and after any invasive procedures. As a patient's physical condition worsens, it is often necessary to monitor vital signs as often as every 5 to 10 minutes. The nurse is responsible for judging whether more frequent assessments are necessary (Box 30-2).
- Use vital sign measurements to determine indications for medication administration. For example, give certain cardiac drugs only within a range of pulse or BP values. Administer antipyretics when temperature is elevated outside of the acceptable range for the patient. Know the acceptable ranges for your patients before administering medications.
- Analyze the results of vital sign measurement on the basis of patient's condition and past medical history.
- Verify and communicate significant changes in vital signs. Baseline measurements provide a starting point for identifying and accurately interpreting possible changes. When vital signs appear abnormal, have another nurse or health care provider repeat the measurement to verify readings. Inform the charge

BOX 30-1 Vital Signs

Acceptable Ranges for Adults

Temperature Range

Average temperature range: 36° to 38° C (96.8° to 100.4° F)

Average oral/tympanic: 37° C (98.6° F)

Average rectal: 37.5° C (99.5° F)

Axillary: 36.5° C (97.7° F)

Pulse

60 to 100 beats/min, strong and regular

Pulse Oximetry (SpO_2)

Normal: SpO_2 ≥95%

Respirations

Adult: 12 to 20 breaths/min, deep and regular

Blood Pressure

Systolic <120 mm Hg

Diastolic <80 mm Hg

Pulse pressure: 30 to 50 mm Hg

Capnography ($EtCO_2$)

Normal: 35-45 mm Hg

BOX 30-2 When to Measure Vital Signs

- On admission to a health care facility
- When assessing a patient during home care visits
- In a hospital on a routine schedule according to the health care provider's order or hospital standards of practice before, during, and after a surgical procedure or invasive diagnostic procedure
- Before, during, and after a transfusion of blood products
- Before, during, and after the administration of medication or therapies that affect cardiovascular, respiratory, or temperature-control functions
- When a patient's general physical condition changes (e.g., loss of consciousness or increased intensity of pain)
- Before, during, and after nursing interventions influencing a vital sign (e.g., before a patient previously on bed rest ambulates or before a patient performs range-of-motion exercises)
- When a patient reports nonspecific symptoms of physical distress (e.g., feeling "funny" or "different")

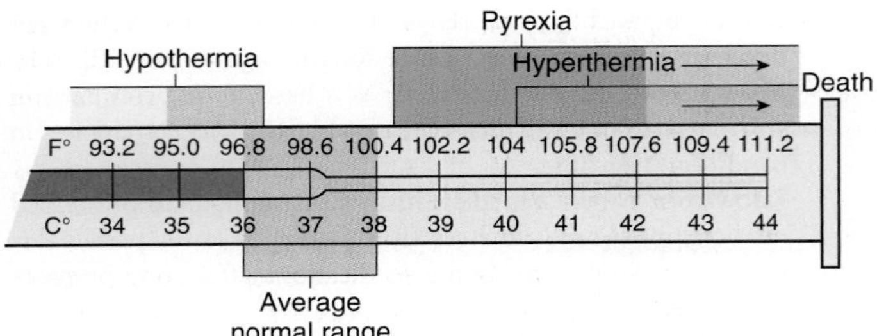

FIGURE 30-1 Ranges of normal temperature values and abnormal body temperature alterations.

nurse or health care provider immediately, document findings in your patient's record, and report vital sign changes to nurses during hand-off communication (TJC, 2016)

- Instruct the patient or family caregiver in vital sign assessment and the significance of findings.

BODY TEMPERATURE

Physiology

Body temperature is the difference between the amount of heat produced by body processes and the amount lost to the external environment.

Heat Produced − Heat Lost = Body Temperature

Despite extremes in environmental conditions and physical activity, temperature-control mechanisms of humans keep body core temperature (temperature of the deep tissues) relatively constant (Figure 30-1). However, surface temperature varies, depending on blood flow to the skin and the amount of heat lost to the external environment. Body tissues and cells function efficiently within a narrow range, from 36° to 38° C (96.8° to 100.4° F), but no single temperature is normal for all people.

The site of temperature measurement (oral, rectal, tympanic membrane, temporal artery, esophageal, pulmonary artery, axillary, or even urinary bladder) is one factor that determines a patient's temperature. For healthy young adults the average oral temperature is 37° C (98.6° F). In the elderly population the average core temperature ranges from 35° to 36.1° C (95° to 97° F) as a result of decreased immunity (Touhy and Jett, 2014). The time of day also affects body temperature, with the lowest temperature at 6:00 AM and the highest temperature at 4:00 PM in healthy people. Invasive measurements such as with a pulmonary artery catheter are considered core temperatures; whereas axillary temperatures are reflective of the surface temperature of the body. It is important to remember that a consistent body temperature measurement from a single site allows you to monitor patterns of your patient's body temperature. As you assess these temperature trends, you can collaborate with the health care team to determine if a body temperature measurement site is more appropriate.

Body Temperature Regulation. Physiological and behavioral mechanisms regulate the balance between heat lost and heat produced, or thermoregulation. For the body temperature to stay constant and within an acceptable range, various mechanisms maintain the relationship between heat production and heat loss. Apply knowledge of temperature-control mechanisms to promote temperature regulation.

Neural and Vascular Control. The hypothalamus, located between the cerebral hemispheres, controls body temperature the same way a thermostat works in the home. A comfortable temperature is the "set point" at which a heating system operates. In the home a drop in environmental temperature activates the furnace, whereas a rise in temperature shuts the system down.

The hypothalamus senses minor changes in body temperature. The anterior hypothalamus controls heat loss, and the posterior hypothalamus controls heat production. When nerve cells in the anterior hypothalamus become heated beyond the set point, impulses are sent out to reduce body temperature. Mechanisms of heat loss include sweating, vasodilation (widening) of blood vessels, and inhibition of heat production. The body redistributes blood to surface vessels to promote heat loss.

If the posterior hypothalamus senses that body temperature is lower than the set point, the body initiates heat-conservation mechanisms. Vasoconstriction (narrowing) of blood vessels reduces blood flow to the skin and extremities. Compensatory heat production is stimulated through voluntary muscle contraction and muscle shivering. When vasoconstriction is ineffective in preventing additional heat loss, shivering begins. Disease or trauma to the hypothalamus or the spinal cord, which carries hypothalamic messages, causes serious alterations in temperature control.

Heat Production. Temperature regulation depends on normal heat production processes. Heat produced by the body is a by-product of metabolism, which is the chemical reaction in all body cells. Food is the primary fuel source for metabolism. Activities requiring additional chemical reactions increase the metabolic rate. As metabolism increases, additional heat is produced. When metabolism decreases, less heat is produced. Heat production occurs during rest, voluntary movements, involuntary shivering, and nonshivering thermogenesis.

- Basal metabolism accounts for the heat produced by the body at absolute rest. The average basal metabolic rate (BMR) depends on the body surface area. Thyroid hormones also affect the BMR. By promoting the breakdown of body glucose and fat, thyroid hormones increase the rate of chemical reactions in almost all cells of the body. When large amounts of thyroid hormones are secreted, the BMR can increase 100% above normal. The absence of thyroid hormones reduces the BMR by half, causing a decrease in heat production. The male sex hormone testosterone increases BMR. Men have a higher BMR than women.
- Voluntary movements such as muscular activity during exercise require additional energy. The metabolic rate increases during activity, sometimes causing heat production to increase up to 50 times normal.
- Shivering is an involuntary body response to temperature differences in the body. The skeletal muscle movement during shivering requires significant energy. Shivering sometimes increases heat production 4 to 5 times greater than normal. The heat that is produced helps equalize the body temperature, and the shivering ceases. In vulnerable patients shivering seriously drains energy sources, resulting in further physiological deterioration.
- Nonshivering thermogenesis occurs primarily in neonates. Because neonates cannot shiver, a limited amount of vascular brown tissue, present at birth, is metabolized for heat production.

Heat Loss. Heat loss and heat production occur simultaneously. The structure of the skin and exposure to the environment result in constant, normal heat loss through radiation, conduction, convection, and evaporation.

Radiation is the transfer of heat from the surface of one object to the surface of another without direct contact between the two. As much as 85% of the surface area of the human body radiates heat to the environment. Peripheral vasodilation increases blood flow from the internal organs to the skin to increase radiant heat loss. Peripheral vasoconstriction minimizes radiant heat loss. Radiation increases as the temperature difference between the objects increases. Radiation heat loss can be considerable during surgery when the patient's skin is exposed to a cool environment. However, if the environment is warmer than the skin, the body absorbs heat through radiation.

The patient's position enhances radiation heat loss (e.g., standing exposes a greater radiating surface area, and lying in a fetal position minimizes heat radiation). Help promote heat loss through radiation by removing clothing or blankets. Covering the body with dark, closely woven clothing decreases the amount of heat lost from radiation.

Conduction is the transfer of heat from one object to another with direct contact. Solids, liquids, and gases conduct heat through contact. When the warm skin touches a cooler object, heat is lost. Conduction normally accounts for a small amount of heat loss. Applying an ice pack or bathing a patient with a cool cloth increases conductive heat loss. Applying several layers of clothing reduces conductive loss. The body gains heat by conduction when it makes contact with materials warmer than skin temperature (e.g., application of an aquathermia pad).

Convection is the transfer of heat away by air movement. A fan promotes heat loss through convection. The rate of heat loss increases when moistened skin comes into contact with slightly moving air.

Evaporation is the transfer of heat energy when a liquid is changed to a gas. The body continuously loses heat by evaporation. Approximately 600 to 900 mL a day evaporates from the skin and lungs, resulting in water and heat loss. By regulating perspiration or sweating, the body promotes additional evaporative heat loss. When body temperature rises, the anterior hypothalamus signals the sweat glands to release sweat through tiny ducts on the surface of the skin. Sweat evaporates, resulting in heat loss. During physical exercise over 80% of the heat produced is lost by evaporation.

Diaphoresis is visible perspiration primarily occurring on the forehead and upper thorax, although you can see it in other places on the body. For each hour of exercise in hot conditions ½ to 2 L of body fluid can be lost in sweat (Rowland, 2011). Excessive evaporation causes skin scaling and itching and drying of the nares and pharynx. A lowered body temperature inhibits sweat gland secretion. People who have a congenital absence of sweat glands or a serious skin disease that impairs sweating are unable to tolerate warm temperatures because they cannot cool themselves adequately.

Skin in Temperature Regulation. The skin regulates temperature through insulation of the body, vasoconstriction (which affects the amount of blood flow and heat loss to the skin), and temperature sensation. The skin, subcutaneous tissue, and fat keep heat inside the body. People with more body fat have more natural insulation than do slim and muscular people.

The way the skin controls body temperature is similar to the way an automobile radiator controls engine temperature. An automobile engine generates a great deal of heat. Water is pumped through the engine to collect the heat and carry it to the radiator, where a fan transfers the heat from the water to the outside air. In the human body the internal organs produce heat; during exercise or increased sympathetic stimulation (such as in the stress response) the amount of heat produced is greater than the usual core temperature. Blood flows from the internal organs, carrying heat to the body surface. The skin has many blood vessels, especially the areas of the hands, feet, and ears. Blood flow through these vascular areas of the skin varies from minimal flow to as much as 30% of the blood ejected from the heart. Heat transfers from the blood, through vessel walls, to the surface of the skin and is lost to the environment through the heat-loss mechanisms. The core temperature of the body remains within safe limits.

The degree of vasoconstriction determines the amount of blood flow and heat loss to the skin. If the core temperature is too high, the hypothalamus inhibits vasoconstriction. As a result, blood vessels dilate, and more blood reaches the surface of the skin. On a hot, humid day the blood vessels in the hands are dilated and easily visible. In contrast, if the core temperature becomes too low, the hypothalamus initiates vasoconstriction, and blood flow to the skin lessens to conserve heat.

Behavioral Control. Healthy individuals are able to maintain comfortable body temperature when exposed to temperature extremes. The ability of a person to control body temperature depends on (1) the degree of temperature extreme, (2) the person's ability to sense feeling comfortable or uncomfortable, (3) thought processes or emotions, and (4) the person's mobility or ability to remove or add clothes. Individuals are unable to control body temperature if any of these abilities is lost. For example, infants are able to sense uncomfortable warm conditions but need help to change their environment. Older adults sometimes need help to detect cold environments and minimize heat loss. Illnesses, a decreased level of consciousness, or impaired thought processes result in an inability to recognize the need to change behavior for temperature control. When temperatures become extremely hot or cold, health-promoting behaviors such as removing or adding clothing have a limited effect on controlling temperature.

Factors Affecting Body Temperature

Many factors affect body temperature. Changes in body temperature within an acceptable range occur when physiological or behavioral mechanisms alter the relationship between heat production and heat loss. Be aware of these factors when assessing temperature variations and evaluating deviations from normal.

Age. At birth the newborn leaves a warm, relatively constant environment and enters one in which temperatures fluctuate widely. Temperature-control mechanisms are immature. An infant's temperature responds drastically to changes in the environment. Take extra care to protect newborns from environmental temperatures. Provide adequate clothing and avoid exposing infants to temperature extremes. A newborn loses up to 30% of body heat through the head and therefore needs to wear a cap to prevent heat loss. When protected from environmental extremes, the newborn's body temperature is usually within 35.5° to 37.5° C (95.9° to 99.5° F).

Temperature regulation is unstable until children reach puberty. The usual temperature range gradually drops as individuals approach older adulthood. The older adult has a narrower range of body temperatures than the younger adult. Oral temperatures of 35° C (95° F) are sometimes found in older adults in cold weather. However, the average body temperature of older adults is approximately 35° to 36.1° C (95° to 97° F). Older adults are particularly sensitive to temperature extremes because of deterioration in control mechanisms, particularly poor vasomotor control (control of vasoconstriction and vasodilation), reduced amounts of subcutaneous tissue, reduced sweat gland activity, and reduced metabolism.

Exercise. Muscle activity requires an increased blood supply and carbohydrate and fat breakdown. Any form of exercise increases metabolism and heat production and thus body temperature. Prolonged strenuous exercise such as long-distance running temporarily raises body temperature.

Hormone Level. Women generally experience greater fluctuations in body temperature than men. Hormonal variations during the menstrual cycle cause body temperature fluctuations. Progesterone levels rise and fall cyclically during the menstrual cycle. When progesterone levels are low, the body temperature is a few tenths of a degree below the baseline level. The lower temperature persists until ovulation occurs. During ovulation greater amounts of progesterone enter the circulatory system and raise the body temperature to previous baseline levels or higher. These temperature variations help to predict a woman's most fertile time to achieve pregnancy.

Body temperature changes also occur in women during menopause (cessation of menstruation). Women who have stopped menstruating often experience periods of intense body heat and sweating lasting from 30 seconds to 5 minutes. During these periods often intermittent skin temperature increases up to 4° C (7.2° F), referred to as hot flashes. This is caused by the instability of the vasomotor controls for vasodilation and vasoconstriction.

Circadian Rhythm. Body temperature normally changes 0.5° to 1° C (0.9° to 1.8° F) during a 24-hour period. However, temperature is one of the most stable rhythms in humans. The temperature is usually lowest between 1:00 and 4:00 AM (Figure 30-2). During the day body temperature rises steadily to a maximum temperature value at about 4:00 PM and then declines to early-morning levels. Temperature patterns are not automatically reversed in people who work at night and sleep during the day. It takes 1 to 3 weeks for the cycle to reverse. In general the circadian temperature rhythm does not change with age.

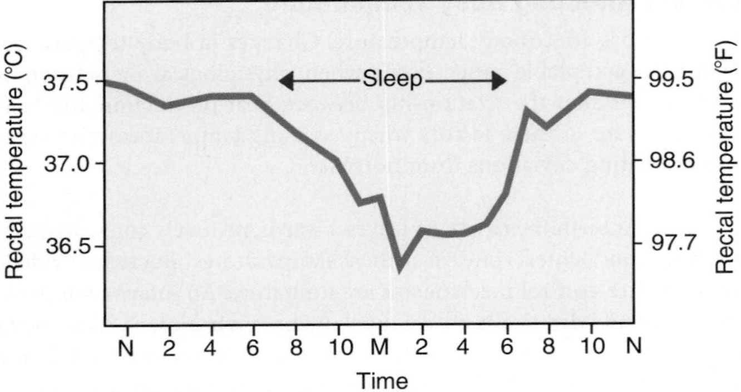

FIGURE 30-2 Temperature cycle for 24 hours.

Stress. Physical and emotional stress increase body temperature through hormonal and neural stimulation (see Chapter 38). These physiological changes increase metabolism, which increases heat production. A patient who is anxious about entering a hospital or a health care provider's office often has a higher normal temperature.

Environment. Environment influences body temperature. When placed in a warm room a patient may be unable to regulate body temperature by heat-loss mechanisms, and the body temperature may elevate. If the patient is outside in the cold without warm clothing, body temperature may be low as a result of extensive radiant and conductive heat loss. Environmental temperatures affect infants and older adults more often because their temperature-regulating mechanisms are less efficient.

Temperature Alterations. Changes in body temperature outside the usual range are related to excessive heat production, excessive heat loss, minimal heat production, minimal heat loss, or any combination of these alterations.

Fever. Fever, or pyrexia, occurs because heat-loss mechanisms are unable to keep pace with excessive heat production, resulting in an abnormal rise in body temperature. A fever is usually not harmful if it stays below 39° C (102.2° F) in adults or below 40° C (104° F) in children. A single temperature reading does not always indicate a fever. In addition to physical signs and symptoms of infection, fever determination is based on several temperature readings at different times of the day compared with the usual value for that person at that time.

A true fever results from an alteration in the hypothalamic set point. Pyrogens such as bacteria and viruses elevate body temperature. They act as antigens, triggering immune system responses. The hypothalamus reacts to raise the set point, and the body responds by producing and conserving heat. Several hours pass before the body temperature reaches the new set point. During this period a person experiences chills, shivers, and feels cold, even though the body temperature is rising (Figure 30-3). The chill phase resolves when the new set point, a higher temperature, is achieved. During the next phase, the plateau, the chills subside, and the person feels warm and dry. If the new set point is "overshot" or the pyrogens are removed (e.g., destruction of bacteria by antibiotics), the third phase of a febrile episode

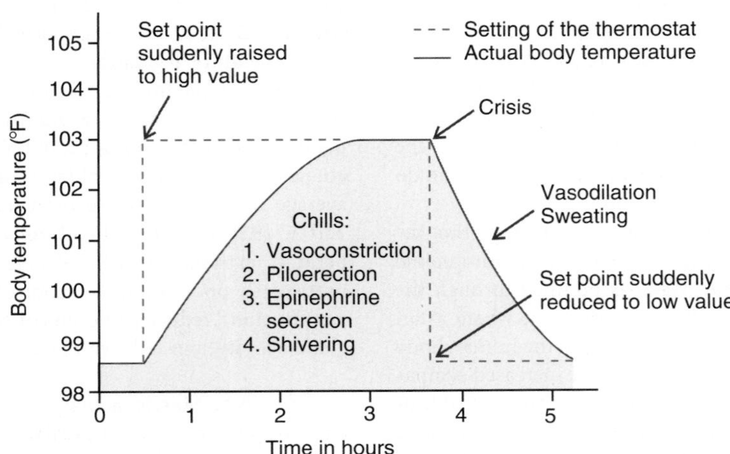

FIGURE 30-3 Effect of changing set point of hypothalamic temperature control during a fever. (Modified from Guyton AC, Hall JE: *Textbook of medical physiology,* ed 12, Philadelphia, 2011, Saunders.)

BOX 30-3 Patterns of Fever

Sustained: A constant body temperature continuously above 38° C (100.4° F) that has little fluctuation

Intermittent: Fever spikes interspersed with usual temperature levels (Temperature returns to acceptable value at least once in 24 hours.)

Remittent: Fever spikes and falls without a return to acceptable temperature levels.

Relapsing: Periods of febrile episodes and periods with acceptable temperature values (Febrile episodes and periods of normothermia are often longer than 24 hours.)

occurs. The hypothalamus set point drops, initiating heat-loss responses. The skin becomes warm and flushed because of vasodilation. Diaphoresis assists in evaporative heat loss. When the fever "breaks," the patient becomes afebrile.

Fever is an important defense mechanism. Mild temperature elevations as high as 39°C (102.2°F) enhance the immune system of the body. During a febrile episode white blood cell production is stimulated. Increased temperature reduces the concentration of iron in the blood plasma, suppressing the growth of bacteria. Fever also fights viral infections by stimulating interferon, the natural virus-fighting substance of the body.

Fevers and fever patterns serve a diagnostic purpose. Fever patterns differ, depending on the causative pyrogen (Box 30-3). The increase or decrease in pyrogen activity results in fever spikes and declines at different times of the day. The duration and degree of fever depend on the strength of the pyrogen and the ability of the individual to respond. The term fever of unknown origin (FUO) refers to a fever with an undetermined cause.

During a fever cellular metabolism increases, and oxygen consumption rises. Body metabolism increases 10% for every degree Celsius of temperature elevation. Heart and respiratory rates increase to meet the metabolic needs of the body for nutrients. The increased metabolism uses energy that produces additional heat. If a patient has a cardiac or respiratory problem, the stress of a fever is great. A prolonged fever weakens a patient by exhausting energy stores. Increased metabolism requires additional oxygen. If the body cannot meet the demand for additional oxygen, cellular hypoxia (inadequate oxygen) occurs. Myocardial hypoxia produces angina (chest pain). Cerebral hypoxia produces confusion. Interventions during a fever include oxygen therapy. When water loss through increased respiration and diaphoresis is excessive, the patient is at risk for fluid volume deficit. Dehydration is a serious problem for older adults and children with low body weight. Maintaining optimum fluid volume status is an important nursing action (see Chapter 42).

Hyperthermia. An elevated body temperature related to the inability of the body to promote heat loss or reduce heat production is hyperthermia. Whereas fever is an upward shift in the set point, hyperthermia results from an overload of the thermoregulatory mechanisms of the body. Any disease or trauma to the hypothalamus impairs heat-loss mechanisms. Malignant hyperthermia is a hereditary condition of uncontrolled heat production that occurs when susceptible people receive certain anesthetic drugs.

Heatstroke. Heat depresses hypothalamic function. Prolonged exposure to the sun or a high environmental temperature overwhelms the heat-loss mechanisms of the body. These conditions cause heatstroke, defined as a body temperature of 40°C (104°F) or more (Goforth and Kazman, 2015). Heatstroke is a dangerous heat emergency with a high mortality rate. Patients at risk include the very young or very old and those who have cardiovascular disease, hyperthyroidism, diabetes, or alcoholism. Also at risk are those who take medications that decrease the ability of the body to lose heat (e.g., phenothiazines, anticholinergics, diuretics, amphetamines, and beta-adrenergic receptor antagonists) and those who exercise or work strenuously (e.g., athletes, construction workers, and farmers).

TABLE 30-1 Classification of Hypothermia

	Celsius	Fahrenheit
Mild	34°-36°	93.2°-96.8°
Moderate	30°-34°	86.0°-93.2°
Severe	<30°	<86°

Signs and symptoms of heatstroke include giddiness, confusion, delirium, excess thirst, nausea, muscle cramps, visual disturbances, and even incontinence. Vital signs reveal a body temperature sometimes as high as 45°C (113°F), with an increase in heart rate (HR) and lowering of BP. The most important sign of heatstroke is hot, dry skin. Victims of heatstroke do not sweat because of severe electrolyte loss and hypothalamic malfunction. If the condition progresses, a patient with heatstroke becomes unconscious, with fixed, nonreactive pupils. Permanent neurological damage occurs unless cooling measures are rapidly started.

Heat Exhaustion. Heat exhaustion occurs when profuse diaphoresis results in excess water and electrolyte loss. Caused by environmental heat exposure, a patient exhibits signs and symptoms of deficient fluid volume (see Chapter 42). First aid includes transporting him or her to a cooler environment and restoring fluid and electrolyte balance.

Hypothermia. Heat loss during prolonged exposure to cold overwhelms the ability of the body to produce heat, causing hypothermia. Hypothermia is classified by core temperature measurements (Table 30-1). It is sometimes unintentional such as falling through the ice of a frozen lake. Occasionally hypothermia is intentionally induced during surgical or emergency procedures to reduce metabolic demand and the need of the body for oxygen.

Accidental hypothermia usually develops gradually and goes unnoticed for several hours. When skin temperature drops below 34°C (93.2°F), the patient suffers uncontrolled shivering, loss of memory, depression, and poor judgment. As the body temperature falls lower, HR, respiratory rate, and BP fall. The skin becomes cyanotic. Patients experience cardiac dysrhythmias, loss of consciousness, and unresponsiveness to painful stimuli if hypothermia progresses. In cases of severe hypothermia a person demonstrates clinical signs similar to those of death (e.g., lack of response to stimuli and extremely slow respirations and pulse). When you suspect hypothermia, assessment of core temperature is critical. A special low-reading thermometer is required because standard devices do not register below 35°C (95°F).

Frostbite occurs when the body is exposed to subnormal temperatures. Ice crystals form inside the cells, and permanent circulatory and tissue damage occurs. Areas particularly susceptible to frostbite are the earlobes, tip of the nose, and fingers and toes. The injured area becomes white, waxy, and firm to the touch. The patient loses sensation in the affected area. Interventions include gradual warming measures, analgesia, and protection of the injured tissue.

❖ NURSING PROCESS

Apply the nursing process and use a critical thinking approach in your care of patients. The nursing process provides a clinical decision-making approach for you to develop and implement an individualized plan of care.

Knowledge of the physiology of body temperature regulation is essential to assess and evaluate a patient's response to temperature alterations and intervene safely. Implement independent measures to increase or minimize heat loss, promote heat conservation, and increase comfort. These measures complement the effects of medically ordered therapies during illness. You also provide education to family members, parents of children, or other caregivers.

◆ Assessment

During the assessment process thoroughly assess each patient and critically analyze findings to ensure that you make patient-centered clinical decisions required for safe nursing care.

Through the Patient's Eyes. Identify your patient's values, beliefs, current treatments, and expectations regarding fever management. When possible, select the temperature site preferred by the patient. Include the patient's preferences when selecting nonpharmacological interventions for hyperthermia (e.g., cooling blankets, tepid baths, fans).

Sites. Core and surface body temperature can be measured at several sites. Intensive care units use the core temperatures of the pulmonary artery, esophagus, and urinary bladder. These measurements require the use of continuous invasive devices placed in body cavities or organs and continually display readings on an electronic monitor.

Use a thermometer to obtain intermittent temperature measurements from the mouth, rectum, tympanic membrane, or temporal artery. Axillary temperature measurements, obtained by placing a thermometer under the axillae, are not recommended in adults because they have been shown to be inaccurate and poorly reflect core temperature (Haugan et al., 2012; Reynolds et al., 2014). However, axillary measurements have been shown to be as reliable as rectal temperature measurement in stable infants (Charafeddine et al., 2014). You can apply noninvasive chemically prepared thermometer patches to the skin. Oral, rectal, and skin temperature sites rely on effective blood circulation at the measurement site. The heat of the blood is conducted to the thermometer probe. Tympanic temperature relies on the radiation of body heat to an infrared sensor. Because the tympanic membrane shares the same arterial blood supply as the hypothalamus, it is a core temperature. Temporal artery measurements detect the temperature of cutaneous blood flow.

To ensure accurate temperature readings, measure each site correctly (see Skill 30-1 on pp. 512-517). The temperature obtained varies, depending on the site used, but it is usually between 36° C (96.8° F) and 38° C (100.4° F). Rectal temperatures are usually 0.5° C (0.9° F) higher than oral temperatures. Each of the common temperature measurement sites has advantages and disadvantages (Box 30-4). Choose the safest and most accurate site for each patient. When possible, use the same site when repeated measurements are necessary.

Thermometers. Two types of thermometers are available for measuring body temperature: electronic and disposable. The mercury-in-glass thermometer, once the standard device, has been eliminated from health care facilities because of the environmental hazards of mercury. However, some patients still use mercury-in-glass thermometers at home. When you find a mercury-in-glass thermometer in the home, teach the patient about safer temperature devices and encourage the disposal of mercury products at appropriate neighborhood hazardous disposal locations. Disposable digital thermometers are readily available for use in the home setting. Home disposable thermometers are useful for temperature screening but are not as accurate as nondisposable electronic thermometers (Counts et al., 2014).

Each device measures temperature using the Celsius or Fahrenheit scale. Electronic thermometers convert the temperature scales by activating a switch. When it is necessary to convert temperature readings, use the following formulas:

1. To convert Fahrenheit to Celsius, subtract 32 from the Fahrenheit reading and multiply the result by 5/9.

$$C = (F - 32) \times 5/9$$
$$\text{Example: } 40°C = (104°F - 32) \times 5/9$$

2. To convert Celsius to Fahrenheit, multiply the Celsius reading by 9/5 and add 32 to the product.

$$F = (9/5 \times °C) + 32$$
$$\text{Example: } 104°F = (9/5 \times 40°C) + 32°$$

Electronic Thermometer. The electronic thermometer consists of a rechargeable battery-powered display unit, a thin wire cord, and a temperature-processing probe covered by a disposable probe cover (Figure 30-4). Separate unbreakable probes are available for oral and rectal use. Electronic thermometers provide two modes of operation: a 4-second predictive temperature and a 3-minute standard temperature. Nurses use the 4-second predictive mode, which improves measurement accuracy. A sound signals, and a reading appears on the display unit when the peak temperature reading has been measured.

Another form of electronic thermometer is used exclusively for tympanic temperature. An otoscope-like speculum with an infrared sensor tip detects heat radiated from the tympanic membrane. Within seconds of placement in the auditory canal, a sound signals, and a reading appears on the display unit when the peak temperature reading has been measured.

Another form of electronic thermometer measures the temperature of the superficial temporal artery. A handheld scanner with an infrared sensor tip detects the temperature of cutaneous blood flow by sweeping the sensor across the forehead and just behind the ear (Figure 30-5). After scanning is complete, a reading appears on the display unit. Temporal artery temperature is a reliable noninvasive measure of core temperature.

The greatest advantages of electronic thermometers are that their readings appear within seconds and they are easy to read. The plastic sheath is unbreakable and ideal for children. Their expense is a major disadvantage. Maintaining cleanliness of the probes is an important consideration. For example, if not properly cleaned between patients, gastrointestinal contamination of the rectal probe causes disease transmission. Wipe the thermometer daily with alcohol and the thermometer probe with an alcohol swab after each patient, paying particular attention to the ridges where the probe cover is secured to the probe.

Chemical Dot Thermometers. Single-use or reusable chemical dot thermometers (Figure 30-6) are thin strips of plastic with a temperature sensor at one end. The sensor consists of a matrix of chemically impregnated dots that change color at different temperatures. In the Celsius version there are 50 dots, each representing a temperature increment of 0.1° C, over a range of 35.5° C to 40.4° C. The Fahrenheit version has 45 dots with increments of 0.2° F and a range of 96° F to 104.8° F. Chemical dots on the thermometer change color to reflect temperature reading, usually within 60 seconds. Most are for single use. In one reusable brand for a single patient the chemical dots return to the original color within a few seconds. Chemical dot thermometers are usually for oral temperatures. You also use them for rectal temperatures when covered by a plastic sheath and placed for 3 minutes. Chemical dot thermometers are useful for screening temperatures, especially in infants, young children, and patients who are intubated.

BOX 30-4 Advantages and Disadvantages of Select Temperature Measurement Sites

Site Advantages	Site Limitations
Oral	
Easily accessible—requires no position change Comfortable for patient Provides accurate surface temperature reading Reflects rapid change in core temperature Reliable route to measure temperature in patients who are intubated	Causes delay in measurement if patient recently ingested hot/cold fluids or foods, smoked, or is receiving oxygen by mask/cannula Not for patients who had oral surgery, trauma, history of epilepsy, or shaking chills Not for infants, small children, or patients who are confused, unconscious, or uncooperative Risk of body fluid exposure
Tympanic Membrane	
Easily accessible site Minimal patient repositioning required Obtained without disturbing, waking, or repositioning patients Used for patients with tachypnea without affecting breathing Sensitive to core temperature changes Very rapid measurement (2 to 5 seconds) Unaffected by oral intake of food or fluids or smoking Used in newborns to reduce infant handling and heat loss (Ozdemir et al., 2011) Not influenced by environmental temperatures (Schey et al., 2010)	More variability of measurement than with other core temperature devices Requires removal of hearing aids before measurement Requires disposable sensor cover with only one size available Otitis media and cerumen impaction distorts readings Not used in patients who have had surgery of the ear or tympanic membrane Does not accurately measure core temperature changes during and after exercise Does not obtain continuous measurement Affected by ambient temperature devices such as incubators, radiant warmers, and facial fans When used in neonates, infants, and children under 3 years old, use care to position device correctly because anatomy of ear canal makes it difficult to position Inaccuracies reported caused by incorrect positioning of handheld unit
Rectal	
Argued to be more reliable when oral temperature is difficult or impossible to obtain	Lags behind core temperature during rapid temperature changes Not for patients with diarrhea, rectal disorders, or bleeding tendencies or those who had rectal surgery Requires positioning and is often source of patient embarrassment and anxiety Risk of body fluid exposure and injury to rectal lining Requires lubrication Not for routine vital signs in newborns Readings influenced by impacted stool
Skin	
Inexpensive Provides continuous reading Safe and noninvasive Used for neonates	Measurement lags behind other sites during temperature changes, especially during hyperthermia Adhesion impaired by diaphoresis or sweat Reading affected by environmental temperature Cannot be used for patients with allergy to adhesives
Temporal Artery	
Easy to access without position change Very rapid measurement Comfortable with no risk of injury to patient or nurse Eliminates need to disrobe or be unbundled Comfortable for patient Used in premature infants, newborns, and children (Reynolds et al., 2014) Reflects rapid change in core temperature Sensor cover not required	Inaccurate with head covering or hair on forehead Affected by skin moisture such as diaphoresis or sweating
Axillary	
Safe and inexpensive Reliable in stable term and preterm infants (Charafeddine et al., 2014)	Long measurement time Requires continuous positioning Measurement lags behind core temperature during rapid temperature changes Not recommended for detecting fever Requires exposure of thorax that can result in temperature loss, especially in newborns Affected by exposure to environment, including time to place the thermometer Underestimates core temperature

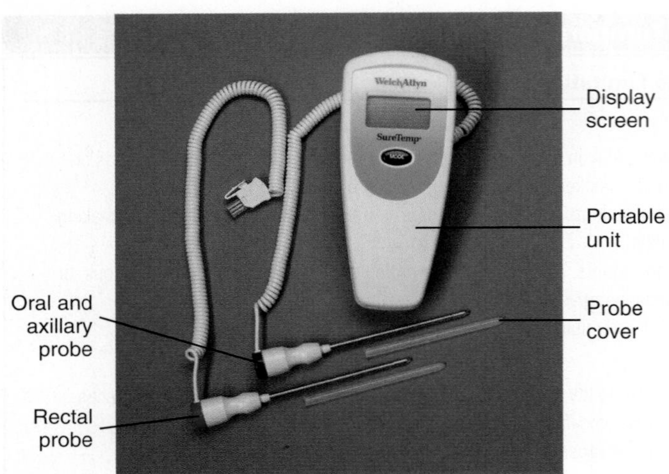

FIGURE 30-4 Electronic thermometer. Blue probe is for oral use. Red probe is for rectal use.

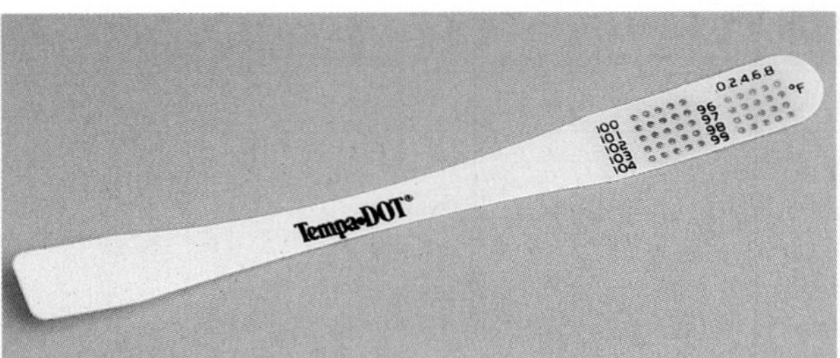

FIGURE 30-6 Disposable, single-use thermometer strip.

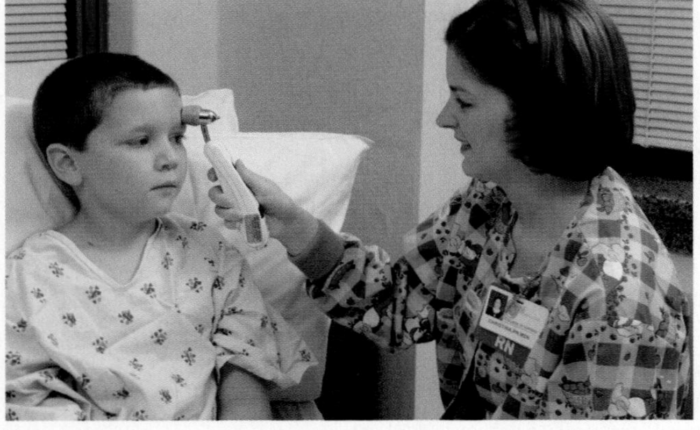

FIGURE 30-5 Temporal artery thermometer scanning child's forehead.

BOX 30-5 Nursing Diagnostic Process

Ineffective Thermoregulation Related to Aging and Inability to Adapt to Environmental Temperature

Assessment Activities	Defining Characteristics
Obtain vital signs, including temperature, pulse (see Skill 30-2), respirations (see Skill 30-3), SpO_2 (see Skill 30-4).	Increased body temperature above usual range Tachycardia Tachypnea Hypoxemia
Palpate skin.	Warm, dry skin
Observe patient's appearance and behavior while talking and resting.	Restlessness Confusion Flushed appearance
Review medical history.	Found in unventilated apartment during heat wave; 85 years old with history of dementia

Because they often underestimate oral temperature by 0.4°C (0.7°F) or more, use electronic thermometers to confirm measurements made with a chemical dot thermometer when treatment decisions are involved. Chemical dot thermometers are useful when caring for patients on protective isolation to avoid the need to take electronic instruments into patient rooms (see Chapter 29).

Another disposable thermometer useful for screening temperature is a temperature-sensitive patch or tape. Applied to the forehead or abdomen, chemical sensitive areas of the patch change color at different temperatures. This type of thermometer can also be affected by environmental temperatures.

◆ Nursing Diagnosis

After concluding your assessment, cluster defining characteristics to form a nursing diagnosis (Box 30-5). For example, an increase in body temperature, flushed skin, skin warm to touch, and tachycardia indicate the diagnosis of *hyperthermia.* State a nursing diagnosis as either an at-risk or problem-focused temperature alteration. Implement actions to minimize or eliminate the risk factors if the patient has an at-risk diagnosis. Examples of nursing diagnoses for patients with body temperature alterations include the following:

- *Risk for Imbalanced Body Temperature*
- *Hyperthermia*
- *Hypothermia*
- *Ineffective Thermoregulation*
- *Risk for Hypothermia*

Once you determine a diagnosis, accurately select the related factor for problem-focused diagnoses. The related factor allows you to develop/set appropriate patient goals and select appropriate nursing interventions. In the example of hyperthermia, a related factor of *vigorous activity* results in much different interventions than a related factor of *decreased ability to perspire.*

NURSING CARE PLAN

Hyperthermia

ASSESSMENT

Mr. Coburn is a 56-year-old school teacher who arrives at the outpatient clinic with malaise. His medical history includes a past urinary tract infection. Several of his students have been out of school lately with colds. He has been feeling poorly for the past 3 days.

Assessment Activities	*Findings/Defining Characteristics**
Palpate skin.	Mr. Coburn's skin is **warm and dry** to touch.
Observe patient's behavior while talking and resting.	Mr. Coburn's breathing is labored; he's using his neck accessory muscles. His face is **flushed.**
Obtain vital signs.	Blood pressure right arm 116/62 mm Hg, left arm 114/64 mm Hg; right radial pulse **128 beats/min,** regular and bounding; respiratory rate **26 breaths/min, breaths deep and regular;** SpO_2 98% on room air; oral temperature **39.2° C** (102.6° F).
Review medical history.	He admits to smoking one pack of cigarettes per day and recently began expectorating **yellow-green sputum.** He has been **tired** for the past 3 days and on rising in the morning has been dizzy.

***Defining characteristics** are shown in bold type.

NURSING DIAGNOSIS: Hyperthermia related to infectious process

PLANNING

Goals	*Expected Outcomes (NOC)*† *Thermoregulation*
Mr. Coburn will regain normal range of body temperature within next 24 hours.	Body temperature declines at least 1° C (1.8° F) within next 8 hours.
Mr. Coburn will state a sense of comfort and rest within next 48 hours.	Patient verbalizes increased satisfaction with rest and sleep pattern. Patient reports increase in energy level within next 3 days.
Mr. Coburn's fluid and electrolyte balance will be maintained during next 3 days.	Intake equals output within next 24 hours. No evidence of postural hypotension during ambulation.

†Outcome classification labels from Moorhead S et al: *Nursing outcomes classification (NOC),* ed 5, St Louis, 2013, Mosby.

INTERVENTIONS (NIC)‡ *Fever Treatment*	**RATIONALE**
Instruct Mr. Coburn to reduce external coverings and keep clothing and bed linen dry.	Promotes heat loss through conduction and convection.
Instruct Mr. Coburn to use ordered antipyretic medications safely when needed for comfort.	Antipyretics reduce set point (Lehne, 2013).
Instruct Mr. Coburn to limit physical activity and increase to two rest periods per day over next 2 days.	Activity and stress increase metabolic rate, contributing to heat production.
Instruct Mr. Coburn to increase oral fluids of choice to 8 to 10 8-oz glasses of fluid daily.	Increased metabolic rate and diaphoresis associated with fever cause loss of body fluids.

‡Intervention classification labels from Bulechek GM et al: *Nursing interventions classification (NIC),* ed 6, St Louis, 2013, Mosby.

EVALUATION

Nursing Actions	*Patient Response/Finding*	*Achievement of Outcome*
Obtain body temperature measurement.	Body temperature is 37.8° C (100.0° F).	Body temperature within normal limits
Obtain orthostatic blood pressure measurements.	Blood pressure measurements lying, sitting, and standing are within 5 mm Hg of each other.	No evidence of postural hypotension
Ask Mr. Coburn if his energy level has changed since the last visit.	He responds, "I'm sleeping much better and have returned to work with a lot more energy."	Improved rest and sleep pattern and increased energy level

◆ Planning

During planning integrate the knowledge gathered from assessment and the patient history to develop an individualized plan of care (see the Nursing Care Plan). Match the patient's needs with interventions that are supported and recommended in the clinical research literature.

Goals and Outcomes. The plan of care for a patient with alteration in temperature includes realistic and individualized goals along with relevant outcomes. This requires collaboration with the patient and family in setting goals and outcomes and selecting nursing interventions. Establish expected outcomes to gauge progress toward returning the body temperature to an acceptable range. In cases in which the temperature alteration requires helping patients modify their environment, goals may be long term (e.g., obtaining appropriate clothing to wear in cold weather). Short-term goals such as regaining normal range of body temperature improve patient health. In the example of a patient who has an elevated fever and excessive diaphoresis, the goal of care is attaining fluid and electrolyte balance. The outcome is that patient intake and output are balanced for the next 24 hours.

Setting Priorities. Set priorities of care with regard to the extent that the temperature alteration affects a patient. The severity of a temperature alteration and its effects, together with the patient's general health status, influence your priorities in his or her care. Safety is a top priority. Often other medical problems complicate the care plan. For instance, body temperature imbalance affects body requirements for fluids. Patients with heart problems often have difficulty tolerating required fluid replacement therapy.

Teamwork and Collaboration. Patients at risk for imbalanced body temperature require an individualized care plan directed at maintaining normothermia and reducing risk factors. For example, it is important to establish the outcome that the patient can explain appropriate actions to take and available community resources to use (e.g., cooling stations) during a heat wave. Teach the patient and caregiver the importance of thermoregulation and actions to take during excessive environmental heat. Education is particularly important for parents, who need to know how to take action at home and whom to call (e.g., health care provider's office, home care nurse) when an infant or child develops a temperature imbalance.

BOX 30-6 Nursing Interventions for Patients with a Fever

Interventions (Unless Contraindicated)

- Obtain blood cultures (before beginning antibiotics) if ordered. Obtain blood specimens to coincide with temperature spikes when the antigen-producing organism is most prevalent.
- Minimize heat production: reduce frequency of activities that increase oxygen demand such as excessive turning and ambulation; allow rest periods; limit physical activity.
- Maximize heat loss: reduce external covering on patient's body without causing shivering; keep patient, clothing, and bed linen dry.
- Satisfy requirements for increased metabolic rate: provide supplemental oxygen therapy as ordered to improve oxygen delivery to body cells; provide measures to stimulate appetite and offer well-balanced meals; provide fluids (at least 8-to-10 8-oz glasses for patients with normal cardiac and renal function) to replace fluids lost through insensible water loss and sweating.
- Promote patient comfort: encourage oral hygiene because oral mucous membranes dry easily from dehydration; control temperature of the environment without inducing shivering; apply damp cloth to patient's forehead.
- Identify onset and duration of febrile episode phases: examine previous temperature measurements for trends.
- Initiate health teaching as indicated.
- Control environmental temperature to 21° to 27° C (70° to 80° F).

◆ Implementation

Health Promotion. By maintaining balance between heat production and heat loss you promote the health of patients at risk for imbalanced body temperature. Consider patient activity, temperature of the environment, and clothing. Teach patients to avoid strenuous exercise in hot, humid weather; drink fluids such as water or clear fruity juices before, during, and after exercise; and wear light, loose-fitting, light-colored clothes. Also teach patients to avoid exercising in areas with poor ventilation, wear a protective covering over the head when outdoors, and expose themselves to hot climates gradually.

Prevention is key for patients at risk for hypothermia. It involves educating patients, family members, and friends. Patients at risk include the very young; the very old; and people debilitated by trauma, stroke, diabetes, drug or alcohol intoxication, and sepsis. Patients who are mentally ill or handicapped sometimes fall victim to hypothermia because they are unaware of the dangers of cold conditions. People without adequate home heating, shelter, diet, or clothing are also at risk. Fatigue, dark skin color, malnutrition, and hypoxemia also contribute to the risk of frostbite.

Acute Care

Fever. When an elevated body temperature develops, initiate interventions to treat fever. The objective of therapy is to increase heat loss, reduce heat production, and prevent complications. The choice of interventions depends on the cause; adverse effects; and the strength, intensity, and duration of the temperature elevation. Nurses are essential in assessing and implementing temperature-reducing strategies (Box 30-6). The health care provider attempts to determine the cause of the elevated temperature by isolating the causative pyrogen. Sometimes it is necessary to obtain culture specimens for laboratory analysis such as urine, blood, sputum, and wound sites (see Chapter 29). Some antibiotic medications are ordered to be given after the cultures have been obtained. Administering antibiotics destroys pyrogenic bacteria and eliminates body stimulus for the elevated temperature.

Most fevers in children are of a viral origin, last only briefly, and have limited effects. However, children still have immature temperature-control mechanisms, and temperatures can rise rapidly. Dehydration and febrile seizures occur during rising temperatures of children between 6 months and 3 years of age. Febrile seizures are unusual in children more than 5 years of age. The extent of the temperature, often exceeding 38.8° C (101.8° F), seems to be a more important factor than the rapidity of the temperature increase. Children are at particular risk for fluid volume deficit because they can quickly lose large amounts of fluids in proportion to their body weight. It is important to maintain accurate intake and output records, weigh the patient daily, encourage fluids, and provide regular mouth/oral care.

Sometimes a fever is a hypersensitivity response to a drug. Drug fevers are often accompanied by other allergy symptoms such as rash or pruritus (itching). Treatment involves withdrawing the medication, treating any skin integrity impairment, and educating the patient and family about the allergy.

Antipyretics are medications that reduce fever. Acetaminophen and nonsteroidal antiinflammatory drugs such as ibuprofen, salicylates, and indomethacin reduce fever by increasing heat loss. Although not used to treat fever, corticosteroids reduce heat production by interfering with the hypothalamic response. It is important to remember that steroids mask signs and symptoms of infection by suppressing the immune system. Therefore patients who are prescribed steroids need to be monitored closely, especially if they are at risk for infection.

Nonpharmacological therapy for fever uses methods that increase heat loss by evaporation, conduction, convection, or radiation. Make sure that nursing measures to enhance body cooling do not stimulate shivering. Shivering is counterproductive and increases energy expenditure up to 400%. Tepid sponge baths, bathing with alcohol-water solutions, applying ice packs to axillae and groin areas, and cooling fans were previously used to reduce fever; however, avoid these therapies because they lead to shivering. There is no advantage of these methods over antipyretic medications.

Blankets cooled by circulating water delivered by motorized units increase conductive heat loss. Follow manufacturer instructions for applying these hypothermia blankets because of the risk for skin breakdown and "freeze burns." Placing a bath blanket between the patient and the hypothermia blanket and wrapping distal extremities (fingers, toes, and genitalia) reduces the risk of injury to the skin and tissue from hypothermia therapy. Wrapping the patient's extremities reduces the incidence and intensity of shivering. Medications such as meperidine or butorphanol reduce shivering.

Heatstroke. Heatstroke is an emergency situation. First aid treatment includes moving the patient to a cooler environment; removing excess body clothing; placing cool, wet towels over the skin; and using oscillating fans to increase convective heat loss. Emergency medical treatment includes intravenous (IV) fluids, irrigating the stomach and lower bowel with cool solutions, and hypothermia blankets.

Hypothermia. The priority treatment for hypothermia is to prevent a further decrease in body temperature. Removing wet clothes, replacing them with dry ones, and wrapping patients in blankets are key nursing interventions. In emergencies away from a health care setting, have the patient lie under blankets next to a warm person. A conscious patient benefits from drinking hot liquids such as soup and avoiding alcohol and caffeinated fluids. It is also helpful to keep the head covered, place the patient near a fire or in a warm room, or place heating pads next to areas of the body (head and neck) that lose heat the quickest.

Restorative and Continuing Care. Educate the patient with a fever about the importance of taking and continuing any antibiotics as directed until the course of treatment is completed. Children and older adults are at risk for deficient fluid volume because they can quickly lose large amounts of fluids in proportion to their body weight. Identifying preferred fluids and encouraging oral fluid intake are important ongoing nursing interventions.

◆ Evaluation

Through the Patient's Eyes. Evaluate your patient's perspectives about the care provided. Is he or she satisfied with the outcomes of care or does the care plan need to be modified? Including the patient in the evaluation demonstrates that you value his or her perspective and contributes to patient safety.

Patient Outcomes. Evaluate all nursing interventions by comparing the patient's actual response to the expected outcomes of the care plan. Determine if goals of care were met and make revisions to the care plan when necessary. After an intervention, measure the patient's temperature to evaluate for change. In addition, use other evaluative measures such as palpating the skin and assessing pulse and respirations. If therapies are effective, body temperature returns to an acceptable range, other vital signs stabilize, and the patient reports a sense of comfort.

PULSE

The pulse is the palpable bounding of blood flow in a peripheral artery. Blood flows through the body in a continuous circuit. The pulse is an indirect indicator of circulatory status.

Physiology and Regulation

Electrical impulses originating from the sinoatrial (SA) node travel through heart muscle to stimulate cardiac contraction. Approximately 60 to 70 mL of blood enters the aorta with each ventricular contraction (stroke volume [SV]). With each SV ejection, the walls of the aorta distend, creating a pulse wave that travels rapidly toward the distal ends of the arteries. The pulse wave moves 15 times faster through the aorta and 100 times faster through the small arteries than the ejected volume of blood. When a pulse wave reaches a peripheral artery, you can feel it by palpating the artery lightly against underlying bone or muscle. The number of pulsing sensations occurring in 1 minute is the pulse rate.

The volume of blood pumped by the heart during 1 minute is the **cardiac output**, the product of HR and the SV of the ventricle. In an adult the heart normally pumps 5000 mL of blood per minute. A change in HR or SV does not always change the output of the heart or the amount of blood in the arteries. For example, if a person's HR is 70 beats/min and the SV is 70 mL, the cardiac output is 4900 mL/min (70 beats/min × 70 mL/beat). If the HR drops to 60 beats/min and the SV rises to 85 mL/beat, the cardiac output increases to 5100 mL or 5.1 L/min (60 beats/min × 85 mL/beat).

Mechanical, neural, and chemical factors regulate the strength of ventricular contraction and its SV. But when these factors are unable to alter SV, a change in HR causes a change in cardiac output, which affects BP. As HR increases, there is less time for the ventricular chambers of the heart to fill. As HR increases without a change in SV, BP decreases. As HR slows, filling time is increased, and BP increases. The inability of BP to respond to increases or decreases in HR indicates a possible health problem. Report this to the health care provider.

An abnormally slow, rapid, or irregular pulse alters cardiac output. Assess the ability of the heart to meet the demands of body tissue for nutrients by palpating a peripheral pulse or using a stethoscope to listen to heart sounds (apical rate).

Assessment of Pulse

You can assess any artery for pulse rate, but you typically use the radial artery because it is easy to palpate. When a patient's condition suddenly worsens, the carotid site is recommended for quickly finding and assessing the pulse. The heart continues delivering blood through the carotid artery to the brain as long as possible. When cardiac output declines significantly, peripheral pulses weaken and are difficult to palpate.

The radial and apical locations are the most common sites for pulse rate assessment. Use the radial pulse to teach patients how to monitor their own HRs (e.g., athletes, people taking heart medications, and patients starting a prescribed exercise regimen). If the radial pulse is abnormal or intermittent resulting from dysrhythmias or if it is inaccessible because of a dressing or cast, assess the apical pulse. When a patient takes medication that affects the HR, the apical pulse provides a more accurate assessment of heart function. The brachial or apical pulse is the best site for assessing an infant's or a young child's pulse because other peripheral pulses are deep and difficult to palpate accurately.

Assessment of other peripheral pulse sites such as the brachial or femoral artery is unnecessary when routinely obtaining vital signs. You assess other peripheral pulses when conducting a complete physical, when surgery or treatment has impaired blood flow to a body part, or when there are clinical indications of impaired peripheral blood flow (see Chapter 31). Table 30-2 summarizes pulse sites and criteria for measurement. Skill 30-2 on pp. 517-521 outlines pulse rate assessment.

TABLE 30-2 Pulse Sites

Site	Location	Assessment Criteria
Temporal	Over temporal bone of head, above and lateral to eye	Easily accessible site used to assess pulse in children
Carotid	Along medial edge of sternocleidomastoid muscle in neck	Easily accessible site used during physiological shock or cardiac arrest when other sites are not palpable
Apical	Fourth to fifth intercostal space at left midclavicular line	Site used to auscultate for apical pulse
Brachial	Groove between biceps and triceps muscles at antecubital fossa	Site used to assess status of circulation to lower arm and auscultate blood pressure
Radial	Radial or thumb side of forearm at wrist	Common site used to assess character of pulse peripherally and status of circulation to hand
Ulnar	Ulnar or little finger side of forearm at wrist	Site used to assess status of circulation to hand; also used to perform an Allen's test
Femoral	Below inguinal ligament, midway between symphysis pubis and anterior superior iliac spine	Site used to assess character of pulse during physiological shock or cardiac arrest when other pulses are not palpable; used to assess status of circulation to leg
Popliteal	Behind knee in popliteal fossa	Site used to assess status of circulation to lower leg
Posterior tibial	Inner side of ankle, below medial malleolus	Site used to assess status of circulation to foot
Dorsalis pedis	Along top of foot, between extension tendons of great and first toe	Site used to assess status of circulation to foot

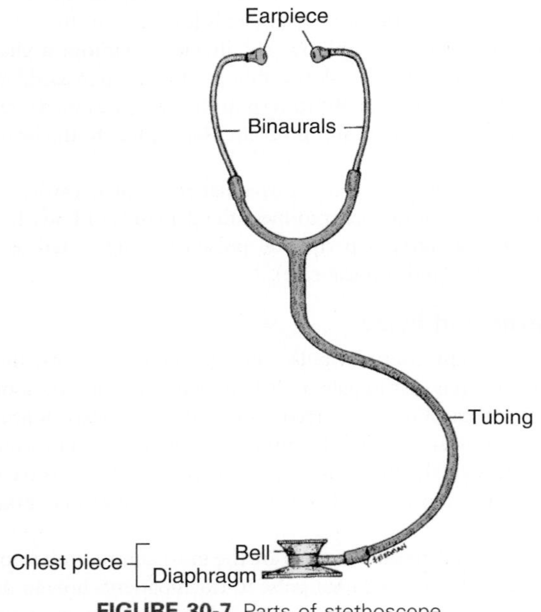

FIGURE 30-7 Parts of stethoscope.

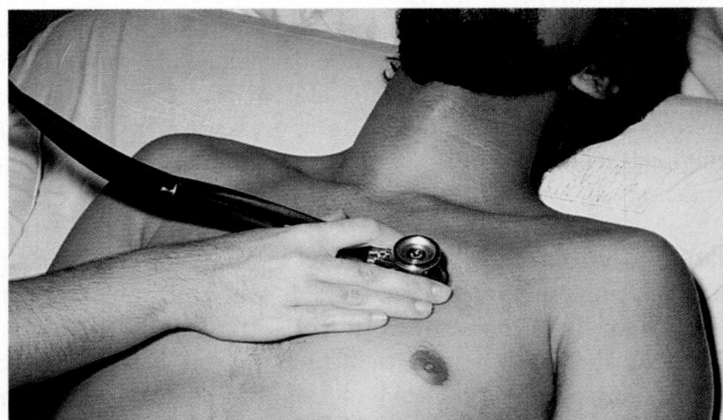
FIGURE 30-8 Positioning diaphragm of stethoscope firmly and securely when auscultating high-pitched heart sounds.

Use of a Stethoscope. Assessing the apical rate requires a stethoscope. The five major parts of the stethoscope are the earpieces, binaurals, tubing, bell chest piece, and diaphragm chest piece (Figure 30-7).

The plastic or rubber earpieces should fit snugly and comfortably in your ears. The binaurals should be angled and strong enough so the earpieces stay firmly in the ears without causing discomfort. To ensure the best reception of sound, the earpieces follow the contour of the ear canal pointing toward the face when the stethoscope is in place.

The polyvinyl tubing is flexible and 30 to 40 cm (12 to 18 inches) in length. Longer tubing decreases the transmission of sound waves. Thick-walled and moderately rigid tubing eliminates transmission of environmental noise and prevents the tubing from kinking, which distorts sound-wave transmission. Stethoscopes have single or dual tubes.

The chest piece consists of a bell and a diaphragm that you rotate into position. The diaphragm or bell needs to be in proper position during use to hear sounds through the stethoscope. With the earpieces in your ears, tap lightly on the diaphragm to determine which side of the chest piece is functioning. The diaphragm is the circular, flat portion of the chest piece covered with a thin plastic disk. It transmits high-pitched sounds created by the high-velocity movement of air and blood. Auscultate bowel, lung, and heart sounds with the diaphragm. Always place the stethoscope directly on the skin because clothing obscures the sound. Position the diaphragm to make a tight seal and press firmly against the patient's skin (Figure 30-8). Do not use your thumb to hold the diaphragm in place because you may hear the pulse being transmitted through it.

The bell is the bowl-shaped chest piece usually surrounded by a rubber ring. The ring avoids chilling patients with cold metal when placed on the skin. The bell transmits low-pitched sounds created by the low-velocity movement of blood. Auscultate heart and vascular sounds with the bell. Apply the bell lightly, resting the chest piece on the skin (Figure 30-9).

TABLE 30-3 Acceptable Ranges of Heart Rate

Age	Heart Rate (beats/min)
Infant	120-160
Toddler	90-140
Preschooler	80-110
School-age child	75-100
Adolescent	60-90
Adult	60-100

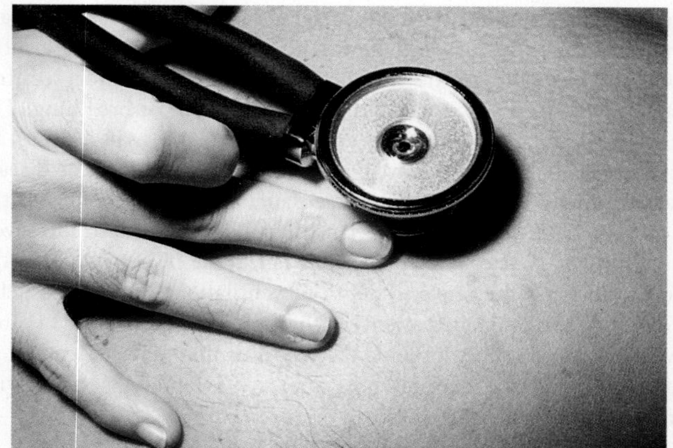

FIGURE 30-9 Positioning bell of stethoscope lightly on skin to hear low-pitched heart sounds.

Compressing the bell against the skin reduces low-pitched sound amplification and creates a "diaphragm of skin." Some stethoscopes have one chest piece that combines features of the bell and diaphragm. When you use light pressure, the chest piece is a bell; exerting more pressure converts the bell into a diaphragm.

The stethoscope is a delicate instrument and requires proper care for optimal function. Remove the earpieces regularly and clean them of cerumen (earwax). Clean the bell and diaphragm between patients with an antiseptic swab to remove microorganisms. Clean the tubing regularly with mild soap and water.

Character of the Pulse

Assessment of the radial pulse includes measuring the rate, rhythm, strength, and equality. When auscultating an apical pulse, assess rate and rhythm only.

Rate. Before measuring a pulse, review the patient's baseline rate for comparison (Table 30-3). Some practitioners prefer to make baseline measurements of the pulse rate as a patient assumes a sitting, standing, and lying position. Postural changes affect the pulse rate because of alterations in blood volume and sympathetic activity. The HR temporarily increases when a person changes from a lying to a sitting or standing position.

When assessing the pulse, consider the variety of factors influencing the pulse rate (Table 30-4). A single factor or a combination of these factors often causes significant changes. If you detect an abnormal rate while palpating a peripheral pulse, the next step is to assess the apical rate. The apical rate requires auscultation of heart sounds, which provides a more accurate assessment of cardiac contraction.

Assess the apical rate by listening to heart sounds (see Chapter 31). Identify the first and second heart sounds (S_1 and S_2). At normal slow rates S_1 is low pitched and dull, sounding like a "lub." S_2 is higher pitched and shorter, creating the sound "dub." Count each set of "lub-dub" as one heartbeat. Using the diaphragm or bell of the stethoscope, count the number of lub-dubs occurring in 1 minute.

TABLE 30-4 Factors Influencing Pulse Rate

Factor	Increases Pulse Rate	Decreases Pulse Rate
Exercise	Short-term exercise	Heart conditioned by long-term exercise, resulting in lower resting pulse and quicker return to resting level after exercise
Temperature	Fever and heat	Hypothermia
Emotions	Sympathetic stimulation increased by acute pain and anxiety, affecting heart rate; effect of chronic pain on heart rate varies	Parasympathetic stimulation increased by unrelieved severe pain affecting heart rate; relaxation
Medications	Positive chronotropic drugs such as epinephrine	Negative chronotropic drugs such as digitalis; beta-adrenergic and calcium channel blockers
Hemorrhage	Sympathetic stimulation increased by loss of blood	
Postural changes	Standing or sitting	Lying down
Pulmonary conditions	Diseases causing poor oxygenation such as asthma, chronic obstructive pulmonary disease (COPD)	

Peripheral and apical pulse rate assessment often reveals variations in HR. Two common abnormalities in pulse rate are tachycardia and bradycardia. **Tachycardia** is an abnormally elevated HR, above 100 beats/min in adults. **Bradycardia** is a slow rate, below 60 beats/min in adults.

An inefficient contraction of the heart that fails to transmit a pulse wave to the peripheral pulse site creates a **pulse deficit**. To assess a pulse deficit you and a colleague assess radial and apical rates simultaneously and then compare rates. The difference between the apical and radial pulse rates is the pulse deficit. For example, an apical rate of 92 with a radial rate of 78 leaves a pulse deficit of 14 beats. Pulse deficits are often associated with abnormal rhythms.

Rhythm. Normally a regular interval occurs between each pulse or heartbeat. An interval interrupted by an early or late beat or a missed beat indicates an abnormal rhythm or **dysrhythmia**. A dysrhythmia threatens the ability of the heart to provide adequate cardiac output, particularly if it occurs repetitively. You identify a dysrhythmia by palpating an interruption in successive pulse waves or auscultating an interruption between heart sounds. If a dysrhythmia is present, assess the regularity of its occurrence and auscultate the apical rate (see Chapter 31). Dysrhythmias are described as regularly irregular or irregularly irregular.

To document a dysrhythmia, the health care provider often orders an electrocardiogram (ECG), Holter monitor, or telemetry monitor. An ECG records the electrical activity of the heart for a 12-second interval. This test requires placement of electrodes across a patient's chest followed by recording of the heart rhythm. A patient wears the Holter monitor, which records and stores 24 hours of electrical activity. Access to the information recorded is not available until after the 24 hours have passed and the data are reviewed. Cardiac telemetry provides continuous monitoring of the electrical activity of the heart transmitted to a stationary monitor. Telemetry permits continuous observation of heart rhythm during all of a patient's daily activities and thus allows for immediate treatment if the rhythm becomes erratic or unstable.

Children often have a sinus dysrhythmia, which is an irregular heartbeat that speeds up with inspiration and slows with expiration. This is a normal finding that you can verify by having the child hold his or her breath; the HR usually becomes regular.

Strength. The strength or amplitude of a pulse reflects the volume of blood ejected against the arterial wall with each heart contraction and the condition of the arterial vascular system leading to the pulse site. Normally the pulse strength remains the same with each heartbeat. Document the pulse strength as bounding (4); full or strong (3); normal and expected (2); diminished or barely palpable (1); or absent (0). Include assessment of pulse strength in the assessment of the vascular system (see Chapter 31).

Equality. Assess radial pulses on both sides of the peripheral vascular system, comparing the characteristics of each. A pulse in one extremity is sometimes unequal in strength or absent in many disease states (e.g., thrombus [clot] formation, aberrant blood vessels, cervical rib syndrome, or aortic dissection). Assess all symmetrical pulses simultaneously except for the carotid pulse. Never measure the carotid pulses simultaneously because excessive pressure occludes blood supply to the brain.

Nursing Process and Pulse Determination

Pulse assessment determines the general state of cardiovascular health and the response of the body to other system imbalances. Tachycardia, bradycardia, and dysrhythmias are defining characteristics of many nursing diagnoses, including the following:

- *Activity Intolerance*
- *Anxiety*
- *Decreased Cardiac Output*
- *Deficient/Excess Fluid Volume*
- *Impaired Gas Exchange*
- *Acute Pain*
- *Ineffective Peripheral Tissue Perfusion*

The nursing care plan includes interventions based on the nursing diagnosis identified and the related factors. For example, the defining characteristics of an abnormal HR, exertional dyspnea, and a patient's verbal report of fatigue lead to a diagnosis of *Activity Intolerance.* When the related factor is *inactivity following a prolonged illness,* interventions focus on increasing the patient's daily exercise routine. Once the plan is implemented, evaluate patient outcomes, including assessment of his or her pulse.

RESPIRATION

Human survival depends on the ability of oxygen (O_2) to reach body cells and carbon dioxide (CO_2) to be removed from the cells. Respiration is the mechanism the body uses to exchange gases between the atmosphere and the blood and the blood and the cells. Respiration involves **ventilation** (the movement of gases in and out of the lungs), **diffusion** (the movement of oxygen and carbon dioxide between the alveoli and the red blood cells), and **perfusion** (the distribution of red blood cells to and from the pulmonary capillaries). Analyzing respiratory efficiency requires integrating assessment data from all three processes. Assess ventilation by determining respiratory rate, depth, rhythm and end-tidal carbon dioxide ($ETCO_2$) value. Assess diffusion and perfusion by determining oxygen saturation.

Physiological Control

Breathing generally is a passive process. Normally a person thinks little about it. The respiratory center in the brainstem regulates the involuntary control of respirations. Adults normally breathe in a smooth, uninterrupted pattern 12 to 20 times a minute.

The body regulates ventilation using levels of CO_2, O_2, and hydrogen ion concentration (pH) in the arterial blood. The most important factor in the control of ventilation is the level of CO_2 in the arterial blood. An elevation in the CO_2 level causes the respiratory control system in the brain to increase the rate and depth of breathing. The increased ventilatory effort removes excess CO_2 (hypercarbia) by increasing exhalation. However, patients with chronic lung disease have ongoing hypercarbia. For these patients chemoreceptors in the carotid artery and aorta become sensitive to **hypoxemia**, or low levels of arterial O_2. If arterial oxygen levels fall, these receptors signal the brain to increase the rate and depth of ventilation. Hypoxemia helps to control ventilation in patients with chronic lung disease. Because low levels of arterial O_2 provide the stimulus that allows a patient to breathe, administration of high oxygen levels is fatal for patients with chronic lung disease.

Mechanics of Breathing

Although breathing is normally passive, muscular work is involved in moving the lungs and chest wall. Inspiration is an active process. During inspiration the respiratory center sends impulses along the phrenic nerve, causing the diaphragm to contract. Abdominal organs move downward and forward, increasing the length of the chest cavity to move air into the lungs. The diaphragm moves approximately 1 cm ($\frac{4}{10}$ inch), and the ribs retract upward from the midline of the body approximately 1.2 to 2.5 cm ($\frac{1}{2}$ to 1 inch). During a normal, relaxed breath, a person inhales 500 mL of air. This amount is referred to as the tidal volume. During expiration the diaphragm relaxes, and the abdominal organs return to their original positions. The lung and chest wall return to a relaxed position (Figure 30-10). Expiration is a passive process. Sighing interrupts the normal rate and depth of ventilation, **eupnea**. The sigh, a prolonged deeper breath, is a protective

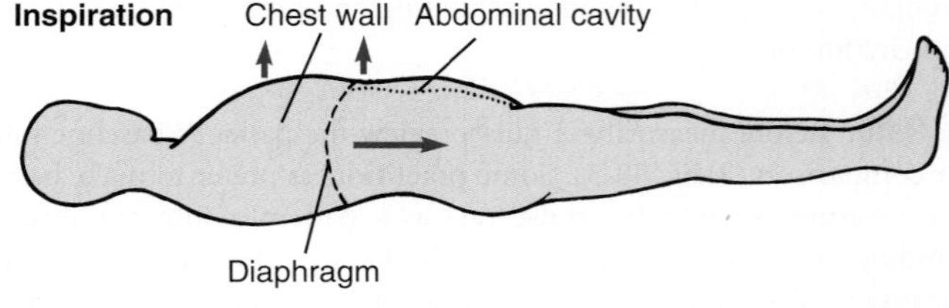

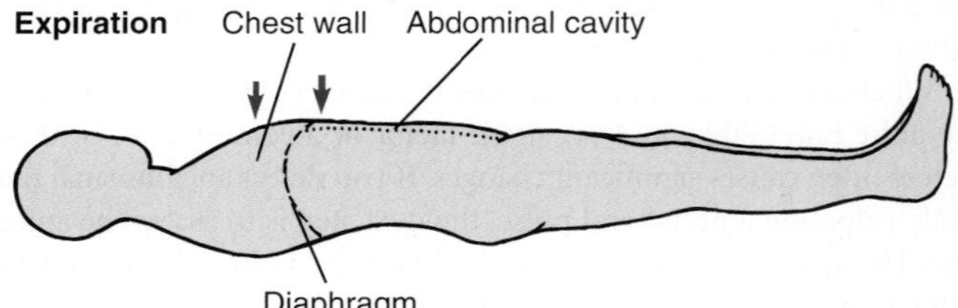

FIGURE 30-10 Illustration of diaphragmatic and chest wall movement during inspiration and expiration.

physiological mechanism for expanding small airways and alveoli not ventilated during a normal breath.

The accurate assessment of respirations depends on the recognition of normal thoracic and abdominal movements. During quiet breathing the chest wall gently rises and falls. Contraction of the intercostal muscles between the ribs or contraction of the muscles in the neck and shoulders (the accessory muscles of breathing) is not visible. During normal quiet breathing diaphragmatic movement causes the abdominal cavity to rise and fall slowly.

Assessment of Ventilation

Respirations are the easiest of all vital signs to assess, but they are often the most haphazardly measured. Do not estimate respirations. Accurate measurement requires observation and palpation of chest wall movement.

A sudden change in the character of respirations is important. Because respiration is tied to the function of numerous body systems, consider all variables when changes occur (Box 30-7). For example, a drop in respirations occurring in a patient after head trauma often signifies injury to the brainstem. Abdominal trauma injures the phrenic nerve, which is responsible for diaphragmatic contraction.

Do not let a patient know that you are assessing respirations. A patient aware of the assessment can alter the rate and depth of breathing. Assess respirations immediately after measuring pulse rate, with your hand still on the patient's wrist as it rests over the chest or abdomen. When assessing a patient's respirations, keep in mind the patient's usual ventilatory rate and pattern, the influence any disease or illness has on respiratory function, the relationship between respiratory and cardiovascular function, and the influence of therapies on respirations. The objective measurements of respiratory status include the rate and depth of breathing and the rhythm of ventilatory movements (see Skill 30-3 on pp. 521-523).

Capnography is the measurement of exhaled carbon dioxide throughout exhalation. At the end of exhalation, the $ETCO_2$ measurement approximates the $PaCo_2$ in a healthy patient, normally 35 to 45 mm Hg. In nonintubated patients $ETCO_2$ can be obtained from a special nasal cannula connected to a monitor that detects the percentage of carbon dioxide exhaled at the end of respiratory cycle. The $ETCO_2$ can be used to evaluate respiratory and cardiac status, whereas interpretation of a continuous recording, or capnogram, can detect changes in ventilation.

Respiratory Rate. Observe a full inspiration and expiration when counting ventilation or respiration rate. The usual respiratory rate varies with age (Table 30-5). The usual range of respiratory rate declines throughout life. A respiratory rate above 27 breaths/min is an important risk factor for cardiac arrest (Parkes, 2011)

The apnea monitor is a device that aids respiratory rate assessment. This device uses leads attached to a patient's chest wall; the leads sense movement. The absence of chest wall movement triggers the apnea alarm. Apnea monitoring is used often with infants in the hospital and at home to observe the risk for prolonged apneic events.

Ventilatory Depth. Assess the depth of respirations by observing the degree of excursion or movement in the chest wall. Describe ventilatory movements as deep or shallow, normal or labored. A deep respiration involves a full expansion of the lungs with full exhalation. Respirations are shallow when only a small quantity of air passes through the lungs and ventilatory movement is difficult to see. Use more objective techniques if you observe that chest excursion is unusually shallow (see Chapter 31). Table 30-6 summarizes types of breathing patterns.

Ventilatory Rhythm. Determine breathing pattern by observing the chest or the abdomen. Diaphragmatic breathing results from the contraction and relaxation of the diaphragm, and you observe it best

BOX 30-7 Factors Influencing Character of Respirations

Exercise

- Exercise increases rate and depth to meet the need of the body for additional oxygen and to rid the body of CO_2.

Acute Pain

- Pain alters rate and rhythm of respirations; breathing becomes shallow.
- Patient inhibits or splints chest wall movement when pain is in area of chest or abdomen.

Anxiety

- Anxiety increases respiration rate and depth as a result of sympathetic stimulation.

Smoking

- Chronic smoking changes pulmonary airways, resulting in increased rate of respirations at rest when not smoking.

Body Position

- A straight, erect posture promotes full chest expansion.
- A stooped or slumped position impairs ventilatory movement.
- Lying flat prevents full chest expansion.

Medications

- Opioid analgesics, general anesthetics, and sedative hypnotics depress rate and depth.
- Amphetamines and cocaine sometimes increase rate and depth.
- Bronchodilators slow rate by causing airway dilation.

Neurological Injury

- Injury to brainstem impairs respiratory center and inhibits respiratory rate and rhythm.

Hemoglobin Function

- Decreased hemoglobin levels (anemia) reduce oxygen-carrying capacity of the blood, which increases respiratory rate.
- Increased altitude lowers amount of saturated hemoglobin, which increases respiratory rate and depth.
- Abnormal blood cell function (e.g., sickle cell disease) reduces ability of hemoglobin to carry oxygen, which increases respiratory rate and depth.

TABLE 30-5 Acceptable Ranges of Respiratory Rate

Age	Rate (breaths/min)
Newborn	30-60
Infant (6 months)	30-50
Toddler (2 years)	25-32
Child	20-30
Adolescent	16-20
Adult	12-20

TABLE 30-6 Alterations in Breathing Pattern

Alteration	Description
Bradypnea	Rate of breathing is regular but abnormally slow (less than 12 breaths/min).
Tachypnea	Rate of breathing is regular but abnormally rapid (greater than 20 breaths/min).
Hyperpnea	Respirations are labored, increased in depth, and increased in rate (greater than 20 breaths/min) (occurs normally during exercise).
Apnea	Respirations cease for several seconds. Persistent cessation results in respiratory arrest.
Hyperventilation	Rate and depth of respirations increase. Hypocarbia sometimes occurs.
Hypoventilation	Respiratory rate is abnormally low, and depth of ventilation is depressed. Hypercarbia sometimes occurs.
Cheyne-Stokes respiration	Respiratory rate and depth are irregular, characterized by alternating periods of apnea and hyperventilation. Respiratory cycle begins with slow, shallow breaths that gradually increase to abnormal rate and depth. The pattern reverses; breathing slows and becomes shallow, concluding as apnea before respiration resumes.
Kussmaul's respiration	Respirations are abnormally deep, regular, and increased in rate.
Biot's respiration	Respirations are abnormally shallow for two to three breaths, followed by irregular period of apnea.

by watching abdominal movements. Healthy men and children usually demonstrate diaphragmatic breathing. Women tend to use thoracic muscles to breathe, assessed by observing movements in the upper chest. Labored respirations usually involve the accessory muscles of respiration visible in the neck. When something such as a foreign body interferes with the movement of air in and out of the lungs, the intercostal spaces retract during inspiration. A longer expiration phase is evident when the outward flow of air is obstructed (e.g., asthma, chronic obstructive lung disease (COPD).

With normal breathing a regular interval occurs after each respiratory cycle. Infants tend to breathe less regularly. The young child often breathes slowly for a few seconds and then suddenly breathes more rapidly. While assessing respirations, estimate the time interval after each respiratory cycle. Respiration is regular or irregular in rhythm.

Assessment of Diffusion and Perfusion

Evaluate the respiratory processes of diffusion and perfusion by measuring the oxygen saturation of the blood. Blood flow through the pulmonary capillaries delivers red blood cells for oxygen attachment. After oxygen diffuses from the alveoli into the pulmonary blood, most of the oxygen attaches to hemoglobin molecules in red blood cells. Red blood cells carry the oxygenated hemoglobin molecules through the left side of the heart and out to the peripheral capillaries, where the oxygen detaches, depending on the needs of the tissues.

The percent of hemoglobin that is bound with oxygen in the arteries is the percent of saturation of hemoglobin (or SaO_2). It is usually between 95% and 100%. It is affected by factors that interfere with ventilation, perfusion, or diffusion (see Chapter 41). The saturation of venous blood (SvO_2) is lower because the tissues have removed some of the oxygen from the hemoglobin molecules. Factors that interfere with or increase tissue oxygen demand affect the usual value for SvO_2, which is 70%.

Measurement of Arterial Oxygen Saturation. A pulse oximeter permits the indirect measurement of oxygen saturation (see Skill 30-4 on pp. 523-535). The pulse oximeter is a probe with a light-emitting diode (LED) connected by cable to an oximeter (Figure 30-11). The LED emits light wavelengths that the oxygenated and deoxygenated hemoglobin molecules absorb differently. A photodetector in the probe detects the amount of oxygen bound to hemoglobin molecules, and the oximeter calculates the pulse saturation (SpO_2).

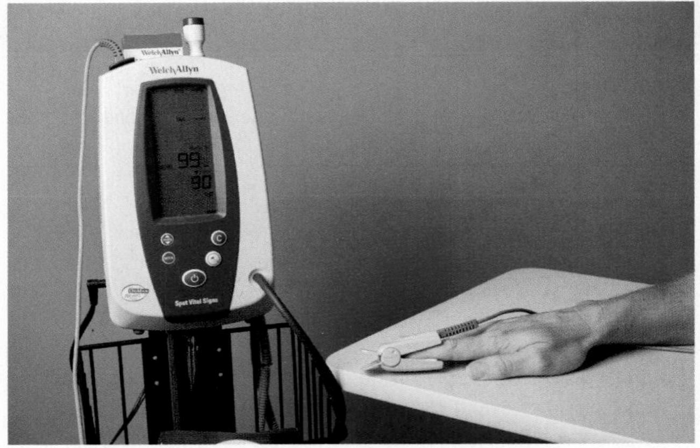

FIGURE 30-11 Portable pulse oximeter with digit probe.

SpO_2 is a reliable estimate of SaO_2 when the SaO_2 is over 70%. A saturation of less than 90% is a clinical emergency (WHO, 2011). Values obtained with pulse oximetry are less accurate at saturations less than 70%.

The photodetector is in the oximeter probe. Selecting the appropriate probe is important to reduce measurement error. Digit probes are spring loaded and conform to various sizes. Earlobe probes have greater accuracy at lower saturations and are least affected by peripheral vasoconstriction. You can apply disposable sensor pads to a variety of sites, including the forehead, the bridge of an adult's nose, or the sole of an infant's foot. Oxygen saturation measurement using a forehead probe is quicker than finger probes (Yont et al., 2011) and more accurate in conditions that decrease blood flow (Nesseler et al., 2012). Factors that affect light transmission or peripheral arterial pulsations affect the ability of the photodetector to measure SpO_2 correctly (Box 30-8). An awareness of these factors allows accurate interpretation of abnormal SpO_2 measurements.

Nursing Process and Respiratory Vital Signs

Measurement of respiratory rate, pattern, and depth, along with SpO_2, assesses ventilation, diffusion, and perfusion. You also conduct other assessments to measure respiratory status (see Chapter 31). Use assessment data to determine the nature of a patient's problem. Respiratory

BOX 30-8 Factors Affecting Determination of Pulse Oxygen Saturation (SpO_2)

Interference with Light Transmission

- Outside light sources interfere with ability of oximeter to process reflected light.
- Carbon monoxide (caused by smoke inhalation or poisoning) artificially elevates SpO_2 by absorbing light similar to oxygen.
- Patient motion interferes with ability of oximeter to process reflected light.
- Jaundice interferes with ability of oximeter to process reflected light.
- Intravascular dyes (methylene blue) absorb light similar to deoxyhemoglobin and artificially lower saturation.
- Black or brown nail polish or metal studs in nails and thickened nails can interfere with light absorption and the ability of the oximeter to process reflected light (Chan et al., 2013).
- Dark skin pigment sometimes results in signal loss or overestimation of saturation.

Interference with Arterial Pulsations

- Peripheral vascular disease (atherosclerosis) reduces pulse volume.
- Hypothermia at assessment site decreases peripheral blood flow.
- Pharmacological vasoconstrictors (e.g., epinephrine) decrease peripheral pulse volume.
- Low cardiac output and hypotension decrease blood flow to peripheral arteries.
- Peripheral edema obscures arterial pulsation.
- Tight probe records venous pulsations in finger that compete with arterial pulsations.

assessment data are defining characteristics of many nursing diagnoses, including the following:

- *Activity Intolerance*
- *Ineffective Airway Clearance*
- *Anxiety*
- *Ineffective Breathing Pattern*
- *Impaired Gas Exchange*
- *Acute Pain*
- *Ineffective Peripheral Tissue Perfusion*
- *Dysfunctional Ventilatory Weaning Response*

The nursing care plan includes interventions based on the nursing diagnosis identified and the related factors. For example, the defining characteristics of tachycardia, changes in depth of respirations, dyspnea, and a decline in CO_2 level lead to a diagnosis of *Impaired Gas Exchange*. Related factors could include *alveolar capillary membrane changes from infection or a ventilator-perfusion imbalance*. You select interventions on the basis of the related factor. After intervening, evaluate patient outcomes by assessing the respiratory rate, ventilatory depth, rhythm, and SpO_2.

BLOOD PRESSURE

Blood pressure is the force exerted on the walls of an artery by the pulsing blood under pressure from the heart. Blood flows throughout the circulatory system because of pressure changes. It moves from an area of high pressure to one of low pressure. Systemic or arterial BP, the BP in the system of arteries in the body, is a good indicator of cardiovascular health. The contraction of the heart forces the blood under high pressure into the aorta. The peak of maximum pressure when ejection occurs is the **systolic pressure**. When the ventricles relax, the blood remaining in the arteries exerts a minimum or **diastolic pressure**. Diastolic pressure is the minimal pressure exerted against the arterial walls at all times.

The standard unit for measuring BP is millimeters of mercury (mm Hg). The measurement indicates the height to which the BP raises a column of mercury. Record BP with the systolic reading before the diastolic reading (e.g., 120/80). The difference between systolic and diastolic pressure is the **pulse pressure**. For example, for a BP of 120/80, the pulse pressure is 40.

Physiology of Arterial Blood Pressure

Blood pressure reflects the interrelationships of cardiac output, peripheral vascular resistance, blood volume, blood viscosity, and artery elasticity. Your knowledge of these hemodynamic variables helps in the assessment of BP alterations.

Cardiac Output. The BP depends on the cardiac output. When volume increases in an enclosed space such as a blood vessel, the pressure in that space rises. Thus as cardiac output increases, more blood is pumped against arterial walls, causing the BP to rise. Cardiac output increases as a result of an increase in HR, greater heart muscle contractility, or an increase in blood volume. Changes in HR occur faster than changes in heart muscle contractility or blood volume. A rapid or significant increase in HR decreases the filling time of the heart. As a result BP decreases.

Peripheral Resistance. The BP depends on peripheral vascular resistance. Blood circulates through a network of arteries, arterioles, capillaries, venules, and veins. Arteries and arterioles are surrounded by smooth muscle that contracts or relaxes to change the size of the lumen. The size of arteries and arterioles changes to adjust blood flow to the needs of local tissues. For example, when a major organ needs more blood, the peripheral arteries constrict, decreasing their supply of blood. More blood becomes available to the major organ because of the resistance change in the periphery. Normally arteries and arterioles remain partially constricted to maintain a constant flow of blood. Peripheral vascular resistance is the resistance to blood flow determined by the tone of vascular musculature and diameter of blood vessels. The smaller the lumen of a vessel, the greater is the peripheral vascular resistance to blood flow. As resistance rises, arterial BP rises. As vessels dilate and resistance falls, BP drops.

Blood Volume. The volume of blood circulating within the vascular system affects BP. Most adults have a circulating blood volume of 5000 mL. Normally the blood volume remains constant. However, an increase in volume exerts more pressure against arterial walls. For example, the rapid, uncontrolled infusion of IV fluids elevates BP. When a person's circulating blood volume falls, as in the case of hemorrhage or dehydration, the BP falls.

Viscosity. The thickness or viscosity of blood affects the ease with which blood flows through small vessels. The **hematocrit**, or percentage of red blood cells in the blood, determines blood viscosity. When the hematocrit rises and blood flow slows, arterial BP increases. The heart contracts more forcefully to move the viscous blood through the circulatory system.

Elasticity. Normally the walls of an artery are elastic and easily distensible. As pressure within the arteries increases, the diameter of vessel walls increases to accommodate the pressure change. Arterial distensibility prevents wide fluctuations in BP. However, in certain diseases such as arteriosclerosis, the vessel walls lose their elasticity and are replaced by fibrous tissue that cannot stretch well. Reduced

TABLE 30-7 Average Optimal Blood Pressure for Age

Age	Blood Pressure (mm Hg)
Newborn (3000 g [6.6 lb])	40 (mean)
1 month	85/54
1 year	95/65
6 years*	105/65
10-13 years*	110/65
14-17 years*	119/75
18 years and older	<120/<80

From James PA et al: 2014 evidence-based guideline for the management of high blood pressure in adults: report by the panel appointed to the Eighth Joint National Committee (JNC 8), *JAMA* 31:507, 2014.

*In children and adolescents hypertension is defined as blood pressure that on repeated measurement is at the 95th percentile or greater adjusted for age, height, and gender (NHBPEP, 2003).

TABLE 30-8 Classification of Blood Pressure for Adults Ages 18 and Older

Category	Systolic (mm Hg)*		Diastolic (mm Hg)*
Normal	<120		<80
Prehypertension†	120-139	Or	80-89
Stage 1 hypertension	≥140	Or	≥90
Stage 2 hypertension	≥160	Or	≥90

Data from James PA, et al: 2014 evidence-based guideline for the management of high blood pressure in adults: report by the panel appointed to the Eighth Joint National Committee (JNC 8), *JAMA* 31:507, 2014.

*Treatment based on highest category.

†Based on the average of two or more readings taken at each of two or more visits after an initial screening. Patient should not be taking antihypertensive drugs or be acutely ill. When systolic and diastolic blood pressures fall into different categories, select the higher category to classify the individual's blood pressure status. For example, classify 160/92 mm Hg as stage 2 hypertension.

elasticity results in greater resistance to blood flow. As a result, when the left ventricle ejects its SV, the vessels no longer yield to pressure. Instead a given volume of blood is forced through the rigid arterial walls, and the systemic pressure rises. Systolic pressure is more significantly elevated than diastolic pressure as a result of reduced arterial elasticity.

Each hemodynamic factor significantly affects the others. For example, as arterial elasticity declines, peripheral vascular resistance increases. The complex control of the cardiovascular system normally prevents any single factor from permanently changing the BP. For example, if the blood volume falls, the body compensates with an increased vascular resistance.

Factors Influencing Blood Pressure

BP is not constant. Many factors continually influence it. One measurement cannot adequately reflect a patient's usual BP. Even under the best conditions, it changes from heartbeat to heartbeat. BP trends, not individual measurements, guide nursing interventions. Understanding these factors ensures a more accurate interpretation of BP readings.

Age. Normal BP levels vary throughout life (Table 30-7). BP increases during childhood. Evaluate the level of a child's or adolescent's BP with respect to body size and age. An infant's BP ranges from 65 to 115/42 to 80 mm Hg. The normal BP for a 7-year-old is 87 to 117/48 to 64 mm Hg. Larger children (heavier and/or taller) have higher BPs than smaller children of the same age. During adolescence BP continues to vary according to body size.

An adult's BP tends to rise with advancing age. The optimal BP for a healthy, middle-age adult is less than 120/80 mm Hg. Values of 120 to 139 systolic and 80 to 89 diastolic mm Hg are considered prehypertension (James et al., 2014) (Table 30-8). Older adults often have a rise in systolic pressure related to decreased vessel elasticity; however, BP greater than 140/90 mm Hg is defined as hypertension and increases the risk for hypertension-related illness.

Stress. Anxiety, fear, pain, and emotional stress result in sympathetic stimulation, which increases HR, cardiac output, and vascular resistance. The effect of sympathetic stimulation increases BP. Anxiety raises BP as much as 30 mm Hg.

Ethnicity. The incidence of hypertension (high BP) is higher in African-Americans than in European Americans. African-Americans tend to develop more severe hypertension at an earlier age and have twice the risk for complications such as stroke and heart attack. Genetic and environmental factors are often contributing factors. Hypertension-related deaths are also higher among African-Americans.

Gender. There is no clinically significant difference in BP levels between boys and girls. After puberty males tend to have higher BP readings. After menopause women tend to have higher BP levels than men of similar age.

Daily Variation. Blood pressure varies throughout the day, with lower BP during sleep between midnight and 3:00 AM. Between 3:00 AM and 6:00 AM there is a slow and steady rise in BP. When a patient awakens, there is an early-morning surge. It is highest during the day between 10:00 AM and 6 PM. No two people have the same pattern or degree of variation.

Medications. Some medications directly or indirectly affect BP. Before BP assessment ask whether the patient is receiving antihypertensive, diuretic, or other cardiac medications, which lower BP (Table 30-9). Another class of medications affecting BP is opioid analgesics, which can also lower it. Vasoconstrictors and an excess volume of IV fluids increase it.

Activity and Weight. A period of exercise can reduce BP for several hours afterwards. An increase in oxygen demand by the body during activity increases BP. Inadequate exercise frequently contributes to weight gain, and obesity is a factor in the development of hypertension.

Smoking. Smoking results in vasoconstriction, a narrowing of blood vessels. BP rises when a person smokes and returns to baseline about 15 minutes after stopping smoking.

Hypertension

The most common alteration in BP is **hypertension**. Hypertension is often asymptomatic. Prehypertension is diagnosed in adults when an

TABLE 30-9 Antihypertensive Medications

Medication Type	Example	Action
Diuretics	Furosemide (Lasix), spironolactone (Aldactone), metolazone, polythiazide, hydrochlorothiazide	Lowers blood pressure by reducing resorption of sodium and water by the kidneys, thus lowering circulating fluid volume
Beta-adrenergic blockers	Atenolol (Tenormin), nadolol (Corgard), timolol maleate (Blocadren), metoprolol (Lopressor)	Combines with beta-adrenergic receptors in the heart, arteries, and arterioles to block response to sympathetic nerve impulses; reduces heart rate and thus cardiac output
Vasodilators	Hydralazine hydrochloride (Apresoline), minoxidil (Loniten)	Acts on arteriolar smooth muscle to cause relaxation and reduce peripheral vascular resistance
Calcium channel blockers	Diltiazem (Cardizem, Dilacor XR), verapamil hydrochloride (Calan SR), nifedipine (Procardia), nicardipine (Cardene)	Reduces peripheral vascular resistance by systemic vasodilation
Angiotensin-converting enzyme (ACE) inhibitors	Captopril (Capoten), enalapril (Vasotec), lisinopril (Prinivil, Zestril), benazepril (Lotensin)	Lowers blood pressure by blocking the conversion of angiotensin I to angiotensin II, preventing vasoconstriction; reduces aldosterone production and fluid retention, lowering circulating fluid volume
Angiotensin-II receptor blockers (ARBs)	Losartan (Cozaar), olmesartan (Benicar)	Lowers blood pressure by blocking the binding of angiotensin II, which prevents vasoconstriction

TABLE 30-10 Recommendations for Blood Pressure Follow-Up

Initial Blood Pressure	Follow-up Recommended*
Normal	Recheck in 2 years.
Prehypertension	Recheck in 1 year.†
Stage 1 hypertension	Evaluate therapy within 1 month (James et al., 2014).†
Stage 2 hypertension	Evaluate therapy within 1 month (James et al., 2014). For those with higher pressure (e.g., >180/110 mm Hg), evaluate and treat immediately or within 1 week, depending on clinical situation and complications.

Data from James PA et al. 2014 evidence-based guideline for the management of high blood pressure in adults: report by the panel appointed to the Eighth Joint National Committee (JNC 8), *JAMA* 31:507, 2014.

*Modify the scheduling of follow-up according to reliable information about past blood pressure measurements, other cardiovascular risk factors, or target organ damage.

†Provide advice about lifestyle modifications.

average of two or more readings on at least two subsequent visits is between 120 and 139 mm Hg systolic and 80 and 89 mm Hg diastolic. Diastolic readings greater than 90 mm Hg and systolic readings greater than 140 mm Hg define hypertension (James et al., 2014). Categories of hypertension have been developed (Table 30-10) and determine medical intervention. One elevated BP measurement does not qualify as a diagnosis of hypertension. However, if a high reading during the first BP measurement (e.g., 150/90 mm Hg) is obtained, the patient is encouraged to return for another checkup within 2 months.

Hypertension is associated with thickening and loss of elasticity in the arterial walls. Peripheral vascular resistance increases within thick and inelastic vessels. The heart continually pumps against greater resistance. As a result blood flow to vital organs such as the heart, brain, and kidney decreases.

People with a family history of hypertension are at significant risk. Modifiable risk factors include obesity, cigarette smoking, heavy alcohol consumption, and high sodium (salt) intake. Sedentary lifestyle and continued exposure to stress are also linked to hypertension. The incidence of hypertension is greater in patients with diabetes, older adults, and African-Americans. It is a major factor underlying deaths from strokes and is a contributing factor to myocardial infarctions (heart attacks). When patients are diagnosed with hypertension, educate them about BP values, long-term follow-up care and therapy, the usual lack of symptoms (the fact that it may not be "felt"), the ability of therapy to control but not cure it, and a consistently followed treatment plan that ensures a relatively normal lifestyle (James et al., 2014).

Hypotension

Hypotension is present when the systolic BP falls to 90 mm Hg or below. Although some adults have a low BP normally, for most people low BP is an abnormal finding associated with illness.

Hypotension occurs because of the dilation of the arteries in the vascular bed, the loss of a substantial amount of blood volume (e.g., hemorrhage), or the failure of the heart muscle to pump adequately (e.g., myocardial infarction). Hypotension associated with pallor, skin mottling, clamminess, confusion, increased HR, or decreased urine output is life threatening and is reported to a health care provider immediately.

Orthostatic hypotension, also referred to as **postural hypotension**, occurs when a normotensive person develops symptoms and a drop in systolic pressure by at least 20 mm Hg or a drop in diastolic pressure by at least 10 mm Hg within 3 minutes of rising to an upright position (Shibao et al., 2013). When a healthy individual changes from a lying–to sitting–to standing position, the peripheral blood vessels in the legs constrict. When standing, the lower-extremity vessels constrict, preventing the pooling of blood in the legs caused by gravity. Thus an individual normally does not feel any symptoms when standing. In contrast, when patients have a decreased blood volume, their blood vessels are already constricted. When a patient with volume depletion stands, there is a significant drop in BP with an increase in HR to compensate for the drop in cardiac output. Patients who are dehydrated, anemic, or have

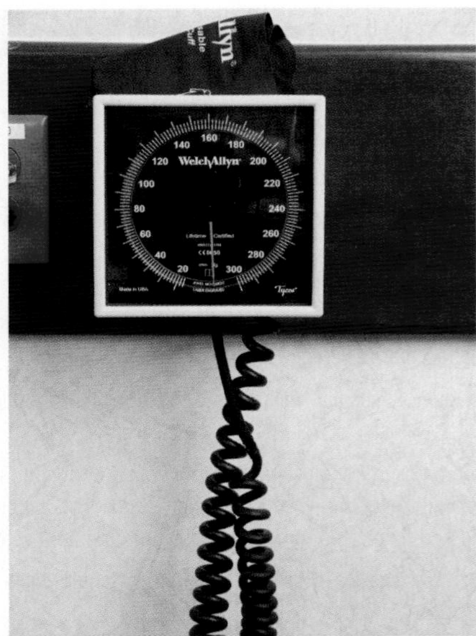

FIGURE 30-12 Wall-mounted aneroid sphygmomanometer.

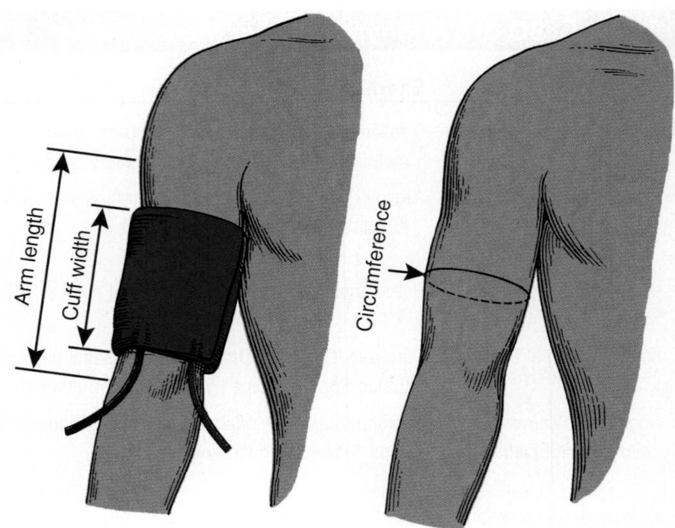

FIGURE 30-13 Guidelines for proper blood pressure cuff size. Cuff width 20% more than upper-arm diameter or 40% of circumference and two thirds of arm length.

experienced prolonged bed rest or recent blood loss are at risk for orthostatic hypotension, particularly in the morning (Shibao et al., 2013). Some medications cause orthostatic hypotension if misused, especially in older adults or young patients. Always measure BP before administering such medications.

Assess for orthostatic hypotension during measurements of vital signs by obtaining BP and pulse in sequence with the patient supine, sitting, and standing. Obtain BP readings within 3 minutes after the patient changes position. In most cases orthostatic hypotension is detected within a minute of standing. If it occurs, help the patient to a lying position and notify the health care provider or nurse in charge. While obtaining orthostatic measurements, observe for other symptoms of hypotension such as fainting, weakness, blurred vision, or light-headedness. Orthostatic hypotension is a risk factor for falls, especially among elderly patients with hypertension (Angelousi et al., 2014). When recording orthostatic BP measurements, record the patient's position in addition to the BP measurement (e.g., 140/80 mm Hg supine, 132/72 mm Hg sitting, 108/60 mm Hg standing). The skill of orthostatic measurements requires critical thinking and ongoing nursing judgment when determining a patient's response to repositioning. Do not delegate this procedure.

Measurement of Blood Pressure

Arterial BP measurements are obtained either directly (invasively) or indirectly (noninvasively). The direct method requires the insertion of a thin catheter into an artery. Tubing connects the catheter with electronic hemodynamic monitoring equipment. The monitor displays a constant arterial pressure waveform and reading. Because of the risk of sudden blood loss from an artery, invasive BP monitoring is used only in intensive care settings. The common indirect method requires a sphygmomanometer and stethoscope. Auscultation or palpation with auscultation is the most widely used technique (see Skill 30-5 on pp. 525-529).

Blood Pressure Equipment. Before assessing BP, make sure that you are comfortable using a sphygmomanometer and stethoscope. A **sphygmomanometer** includes a pressure manometer, an occlusive cuff that encloses an inflatable rubber bladder, and a pressure bulb with a release valve that inflates the bladder (Figure 30-12). The aneroid manometer has a glass-enclosed circular gauge containing a needle that registers millimeter calibrations. Before using the aneroid model, make sure that the needle points to zero and that the manometer is correctly calibrated. Aneroid sphygmomanometers require biomedical calibration every 6 months to verify their accuracy.

The occlusive cuff comes in different sizes. The size selected is proportional to the circumference of the limb being assessed (Figure 30-13). Ideally the width of the cuff is 40% of the circumference (or 20% wider than the diameter) of the midpoint of the limb on which the cuff is used to measure BP. The inflatable bladder, contained in the occlusive cuff, encircles at least 80% of the upper arm of an adult and the entire arm of a child (James et al., 2014). Place the lower edge of the cuff above the antecubital fossa, allowing room for positioning the stethoscope bell or diaphragm. Many adults require a large adult cuff. Using the forearm when a larger cuff is not readily available is not recommended and can result in an overestimate of systolic blood pressure up to 20 mm Hg (Schimanski et al, 2014). An improperly fitting cuff causes inaccurate BP measurements (Table 30-11).

The release valve of the sphygmomanometer needs to be clean and freely movable in either direction. A closed valve holds the pressure constant. A sticky valve makes pressure cuff deflation hard to regulate.

Auscultation. The best environment for BP measurement by auscultation is a quiet room at a comfortable temperature. Although the patient may lie or stand, sitting is the preferred position. In most cases BP readings obtained with the patient in the supine, sitting, and standing positions are similar.

The patient's position during routine BP determination needs to be the same during each measurement to permit a meaningful comparison of values. Before obtaining the patient's BP, attempt to control factors responsible for artificially high readings such as pain, anxiety, or exertion. The patient's perception that the physical or interpersonal environment is stressful affects the BP measurement. BP measurements taken at the patient's place of employment or in a health care provider's office are often higher than those taken at the patient's home.

During the initial assessment obtain and record the BP in both arms. Normally there is a difference of 5 to 10 mm Hg between the arms. In subsequent assessments measure the BP in the arm with the higher pressure. Pressure differences greater than 10 mm Hg indicate

TABLE 30-11 Common Errors in Blood Pressure Assessment

Error	Effect
Bladder or cuff too wide	False-low reading
Bladder or cuff too narrow or too short	False-high reading
Cuff wrapped too loosely or unevenly	False-high reading
Deflating cuff too slowly	False-high diastolic reading
Deflating cuff too quickly	False-low systolic and false-high diastolic reading
Arm below heart level	False-high reading
Arm above heart level	False-low reading
Arm not supported	False-high reading
Stethoscope that fits poorly or impairment of examiner's hearing, causing sounds to be muffled	False-low systolic and false-high diastolic reading
Stethoscope applied too firmly against antecubital fossa	False-low diastolic reading
Inflating too slowly	False-high diastolic reading
Repeating assessments too quickly	False-high systolic reading
Inadequate inflation level	False-low systolic reading
Multiple examiners using different sounds for diastolic readings	False-high systolic and false-low diastolic reading

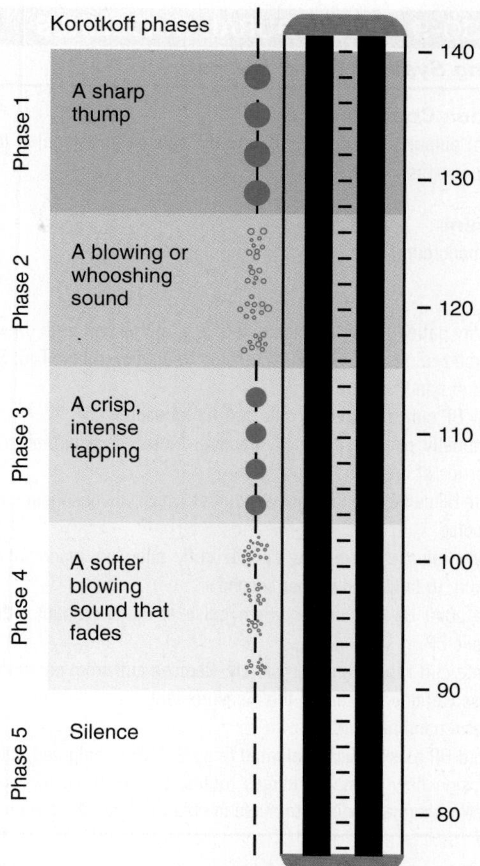

FIGURE 30-14 The sounds auscultated during blood pressure measurement can be differentiated into five phases. In this example blood pressure is 140/90 mm Hg.

vascular problems and are reported to the health care provider or nurse in charge.

Ask the patient to state his or her usual BP. If the patient does not know, inform him or her after measuring and recording it. This is a good opportunity to educate a patient about optimal values of BP, risk factors for developing hypertension, and dangers of hypertension.

Indirect measurement of arterial BP works on a basic principle of pressure. Blood flows freely through an artery until an inflated cuff applies pressure to tissues and causes the artery to collapse. After release of the cuff pressure, the point at which blood flow returns and sound appears through auscultation is the systolic pressure.

In 1905 Korotkoff, a Russian surgeon, first described the sounds heard over an artery distal to the BP cuff when the cuff was deflated. The first sound is a clear rhythmical tapping corresponding to the pulse rate that gradually increases in intensity. *Onset of the sound corresponds to the systolic pressure.* A blowing or swishing sound occurs as the cuff continues to deflate, resulting in the second sound. As the artery distends there is turbulence in blood flow. The third sound is a crisper and more intense tapping. The fourth sound becomes muffled and low pitched as the cuff is further deflated. At this point the cuff pressure has fallen below the pressure within the vessel walls; *this sound is the diastolic pressure in infants and children.* The fifth sound marks the disappearance of sound. *In adolescents and adults the fifth sound corresponds with the diastolic pressure* (Figure 30-14). In some patients the sounds are clear and distinct. In others only the beginning and ending sounds are clear.

The American Heart Association recommends recording two numbers for a BP measurement: the point on the manometer when you hear the first sound for systolic and the point on the manometer when you hear the fifth sound for diastolic. Some institutions recommend recording the point when you hear the fourth sound as well, especially for patients with hypertension. Divide the numbers by slashed lines (e.g., 120/70 or 120/100/70). Note the arm used to measure the BP (e.g., right arm [RA] 130/70) and the patient's position (e.g., sitting).

BP assessment results in many medical decisions and nursing interventions. Obtaining an accurate measurement is essential. There are several sources for error (see Table 30-11). When you are unsure of a reading, have a colleague reassess the BP.

Assessment in Children. All children 3 years of age through adolescence need to have BP checked at least annually. BP in children changes with growth and development. Help parents understand the importance of this routine screening to detect children who are at risk for hypertension. The measurement of BP in infants and children is difficult for several reasons:

- Different arm size requires careful and appropriate cuff size selection. Do not choose a cuff on the basis of the name of the cuff. An "infant" cuff is often too small for some infants.
- Readings are difficult to obtain in restless or anxious infants and children. Allow at least 15 minutes for children to recover from recent activities and become less apprehensive. The child's cooperation is increased when you or the parent have prepared him or her for the unusual sensation of the BP cuff. Most children understand the analogy of a "tight hug on your arm."
- Placing the stethoscope too firmly on the antecubital fossa causes errors in auscultation. Sounds are difficult to hear in children because of low frequency and amplitude. A pediatric stethoscope bell is often helpful.

BOX 30-9 PROCEDURAL GUIDELINES

Palpating Systolic Blood Pressure

Delegation Considerations

The skill of palpation of blood pressure (BP) cannot be delegated to nursing assistive personnel.

Equipment

Sphygmomanometer

Steps

1. Identify patient using two identifiers (e.g., name and birth date or name and medical record number) according to agency policy (TJC, 2016).
2. Perform hand hygiene.
3. Apply BP cuff to extremity selected for measurement.
4. Continually palpate pulse of brachial, radial, or popliteal artery with fingertips of one hand.
5. Inflate BP cuff 30 mm Hg above point at which you no longer can palpate the pulse.
6. Slowly release valve and deflate cuff, allowing manometer needle mercury to fall 2 mm Hg per second.
7. Note point on manometer when pulse is again palpable; this is the systolic BP.
8. Deflate cuff rapidly and completely. Remove cuff from patient extremity unless you need to repeat the measurement.
9. Perform hand hygiene.
10. Record BP as systolic/-, palpated (e.g., BP 108/-, palpated, location) on vital sign flow sheet, in nurses' notes, or electronic medical record. Report abnormal findings to nurse in charge or health care provider.

Ultrasonic Stethoscope. When you are unable to auscultate sounds because of a weakened arterial pulse, you can use an ultrasonic stethoscope (see Chapter 31). This stethoscope allows you to hear low-frequency systolic sounds. You frequently use this device when measuring the BP of infants and children and low BP in adults.

Palpation. Indirect measurement of BP by palpation is useful for patients whose arterial pulsations are too weak to create sounds. Severe blood loss and decreased heart contractility are examples of conditions that result in BPs too low to auscultate accurately. In these cases you can assess the systolic BP by palpation (Box 30-9). The diastolic BP is difficult to determine by palpation. When using the palpation technique, record the systolic value and how you measured it (e.g., RA 90/-, palpated, supine).

You can use the palpation technique along with auscultation. In some patients with hypertension the sounds usually heard over the brachial artery when the cuff pressure is high disappear as pressure is reduced and then reappear at a lower level. This temporary disappearance of sound is the **auscultatory gap**. It typically occurs between the first and second sounds. The gap in sound covers a range of 40 mm Hg and thus causes an underestimation of systolic pressure or overestimation of diastolic pressure. The examiner needs to be certain to inflate the cuff high enough to hear the true systolic pressure before the auscultatory gap. Palpation of the radial artery helps to determine how high to inflate the cuff. The examiner inflates the cuff 30 mm Hg above the pressure at which the radial pulse was palpated. Record the range of pressures in which the auscultatory gap occurs (e.g., BP RA 180/94 mm Hg with an auscultatory gap from 180 to 160 mm Hg, sitting).

Lower-Extremity Blood Pressure. Dressings, casts, IV catheters, or arteriovenous fistulas or shunts make the upper extremities inaccessible for BP measurement. You then need to obtain the BP in a lower extremity. Comparing upper-extremity BP with that in the legs is also necessary for patients with certain cardiac and BP abnormalities. The popliteal artery, palpable behind the knee in the popliteal space, is the site for auscultation. The cuff needs to be wide and long enough to allow for the larger girth of the thigh. Placing the patient in a prone position is best. If such a position is impossible, ask the patient to flex the knee slightly for easier access to the artery. Position the cuff 2.5 cm (1 inch) above the popliteal artery, with the bladder over the posterior aspect of the midthigh (Figure 30-15). The procedure is identical to brachial artery auscultation. Systolic pressure in the legs is usually higher by 10 to 40 mm Hg than in the brachial artery, but the diastolic pressure is the same (Frese et al., 2011).

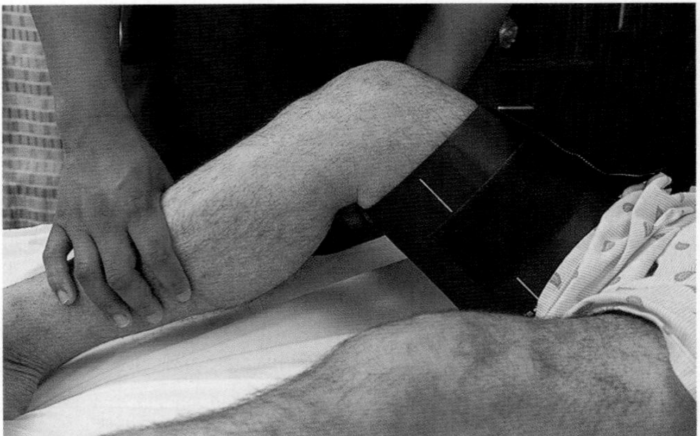

FIGURE 30-15 Lower-extremity blood pressure cuff positioned above popliteal artery at midthigh with knee flexed.

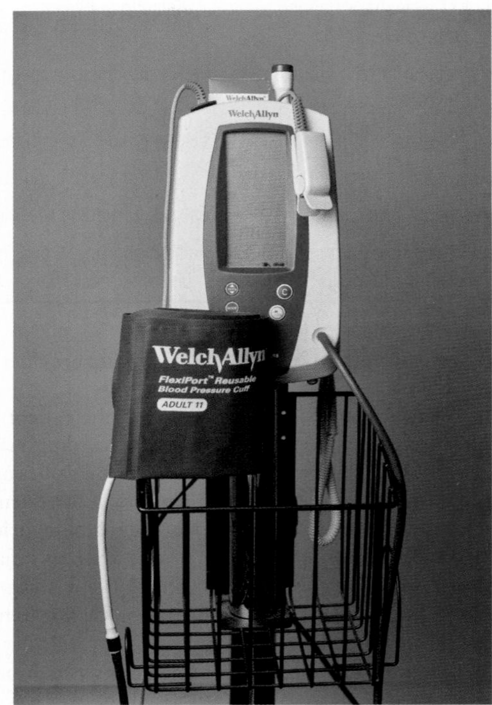

FIGURE 30-16 Automatic blood pressure monitor.

Electronic Blood Pressure Devices. Many different styles of electronic BP machines are available to determine BP automatically (Figure 30-16). Electronic BP machines rely on an electronic sensor to

BOX 30-10 PROCEDURAL GUIDELINES

Electronic Blood Pressure Measurement

Delegation Considerations

The skill of obtaining an electronic blood pressure (BP) measurement can be delegated to nursing assistive personnel (NAP). However, the nurse must first verify that the patient is stable and does not need to be monitored closely for evaluating response to medications or other therapies. Instruct the NAP to:

- Obtain BP at appropriate times as determined by agency policy, health care provider's order, or patient's condition such as frequent postoperative measurements.
- Consider patient-specific factors that affect patient's usual values.
- Obtain the BP on the appropriate limb using the correct size cuff considering the patient's history such as presence of intravenous (IV) sites.
- Immediately report significant BP changes as specified by the nurse.

Equipment

Electronic BP machine, BP cuff of appropriate size as recommended by manufacturer

Steps

1. Identify patient using two identifiers (e.g., name and birth date or name and medical record number) according to agency policy (TJC, 2016).
2. Determine appropriateness of using electronic BP measurement. Patients with irregular heart rate, peripheral vascular disease, seizures, tremors, and shivering are not candidates for this device (Suokhrie et al., 2013).
3. Determine best site for cuff placement (see Skill 30-5).
4. Perform hand hygiene. Help patient to comfortable position, either lying or sitting. Plug in device and place it near patient, ensuring that connector hose between cuff and machine will reach.
5. Locate on/off switch and turn machine on to enable device to self-test computer systems.
6. Select appropriate cuff size for patient extremity (see Table 30-11) and appropriate cuff for machine. Electronic BP cuff and machine are matched by the manufacturer and are not interchangeable.
7. Prepare BP cuff by manually squeezing all the air out of cuff and attaching cuff to connector hose.
8. Remove any constricting clothing to ensure proper cuff application. BP cuff may be placed over a light shirt sleeve (Pinar et al., 2010).
9. Wrap flattened cuff snugly around extremity, verifying that only one finger fits between cuff and patient's skin. Make sure that "artery" arrow marked on outside of cuff is placed correctly (see illustration for Skill 30-5, Step 4).
10. Verify that connector hose between cuff and machine is not kinked. Kinking prevents proper inflation and deflation of cuff.
11. Following manufacturer directions, set frequency control of automatic or manual and press start button. The first BP measurement pumps cuff to pressure of approximately 180 mm Hg. After this pressure is reached, the machine begins a deflation sequence that determines BP. The first reading determines peak pressure inflation for additional measurements.

CLINICAL DECISION: If unable to obtain BP with electronic device, verify machine connections (e.g., plugged into working electrical outlet, hose-cuff connections tight, machine on, correct cuff). Wait at least 1 minute but not more than 2 minutes to repeat electronic BP; if unable to obtain, use auscultatory technique (see Skill 30-5).

12. When deflation is complete, digital display provides most recent values and flashes time in minutes that have elapsed since measurement occurred.
13. Set frequency of BP measurements and upper and lower alarm limits for systolic, diastolic, and mean BP readings. Intervals between BP measurements are set from 1 to 90 minutes.
14. Determine measurement frequency and alarm limits on the basis of patient's acceptable range of BP, nursing judgment, and health care provider order.
15. Obtain additional readings at any time by pressing start button. (Sometimes you need additional readings for unstable patients.) Pressing cancel button immediately deflates cuff.
16. If frequent BP determinations are necessary, leave cuff in place. Remove cuff at least every 2 hours to assess underlying skin integrity and, if possible, alternate BP sites. Patients with abnormal bleeding tendencies are at risk for microvascular rupture from repeated inflations. When you are finished using the electronic BP machine, clean BP cuff according to agency policy to reduce transmission of microorganisms.
17. Compare electronic BP readings with auscultatory BP to verify accuracy of electronic BP measurement.
18. Record BP and site assessed on vital sign flow sheet, in nurses' notes, or electronic medical record (per agency policy). Record any signs of BP alterations in nurses' notes.
19. Report abnormal findings to nurse in charge or health care provider.

detect the vibrations caused by the rush of blood through an artery (Box 30-10). Use electronic devices when frequent BP assessment is necessary such as in patients who are critically ill or unstable, during or after invasive procedures, or when therapies require frequent monitoring (e.g., IV heart and BP medications). Box 30-11 lists conditions that are not appropriate for automatic BP devices.

The advantages of automatic devices are the ease of use and efficiency when repeated or frequent measurements are indicated. The ability to use a stethoscope is not necessary. However, automatic devices are not recommended for hypertensive patients, patients with irregular heart rates, or those who have experienced trauma (Skirton et al., 2011). Most electronic BP devices are unable to process sounds or vibrations of low BP. The range of device sophistication also makes BP measurement comparisons difficult.

Self-Measurement of Blood Pressure. Improved technology in electronic monitoring devices allows individuals to measure their own BPs in their home with the push of a button. The portable home

BOX 30-11 Patient Conditions Not Appropriate for Electronic Blood Pressure Measurement

- Irregular heart rate
- Peripheral vascular obstruction (e.g., clots, narrowed vessels)
- Shivering
- Seizures
- Excessive tremors
- Inability to cooperate
- Blood pressure less than 90 mm Hg systolic

devices include the aneroid sphygmomanometer and electronic digital readout devices that do not require use of a stethoscope. The electronic devices are easier to manipulate but require frequent recalibration, more than once a year. Because of their sensitivity, improper cuff placement or movement of the arm causes electronic devices to give incorrect readings.

Stationary automatic BP devices are often found in public places such as grocery stores, fitness clubs, airports, or work sites. Users simply rest their arms within the inflatable cuff of the machine, which contains a pressure sensor. A visual display tells users their BP within 60 to 90 seconds. The reliability of the stationary machines is limited. BP values vary by 5 to 10 mm Hg or more (for both systolic and diastolic values) compared with pressures taken with a manual sphygmomanometer.

Self-measurement of BP has several benefits. Sometimes elevated BP is detected in people previously unaware of a problem. People with prehypertension provide information about the pattern of BP values to their health care provider. Patients with hypertension benefit from participating actively in their treatment through self-monitoring, which helps adherence with treatment. The disadvantages of self-measurement include improper use of the device and risk of inaccurate readings. Some patients are needlessly alarmed with one elevated reading. Some patients with hypertension become overly conscious of their BP and inappropriately self-adjust medications.

Consumers can learn to use self-measurement devices if they have the information needed to perform the procedure correctly and if they know when to seek medical attention. Advise patients of possible inaccuracies in the BP devices, help them understand the meaning and implications of readings, and teach them proper measurement techniques. Encourage them to record the date of their BP readings to assess BP over time and share findings with their health care provider.

Nursing Process and Blood Pressure Determination

The assessment of BP along with pulse assessment evaluates the general state of cardiovascular health and responses to other system imbalances. Hypotension, hypertension, orthostatic hypotension, and narrow or wide pulse pressures are defining characteristics of certain nursing diagnoses, including the following:

- *Activity Intolerance*
- *Anxiety*
- *Decreased Cardiac Output*
- *Deficient/Excess Fluid Volume*
- *Risk for Injury*
- *Acute Pain*
- *Ineffective Peripheral Tissue Perfusion*

The nursing care plan includes interventions based on the nursing diagnosis identified and the related factors. For example, the defining characteristics of hypotension, dizziness, pulse deficit, and dysrhythmia lead to a diagnosis of *Decreased Cardiac Output.* Related factors might include *poor oral intake, excessive heat exposure,* and a *history of valvular heart disease.* The related factor guides the choice of nursing interventions. Evaluate patient outcomes by assessing the BP following each intervention.

HEALTH PROMOTION AND VITAL SIGNS

The emphasis on health promotion and maintenance and discharge from hospital settings has resulted in an increase in the need for patients and their families to monitor vital signs in the home. Teaching considerations affect all vital sign measurements. Incorporate them within the patient's plan of care (Box 30-12).

When considering how to teach patients and their families about vital sign measurements and their importance and significance, a patient's age is an important factor. With an increase in the older-adult population there is a greater need for family caregivers to be aware of changes that are unique to older adults. Box 30-13 identifies some of these variations.

BOX 30-12 PATIENT TEACHING

Health Promotion

Objective

- Patient identifies measures to promote health.

Teaching Strategies

- Instruct patient about the importance of diet, exercise, and remaining tobacco free.
- Instruct patient on risk factors for hypothermia, frostbite, and heat stroke.
- Demonstrate self-assessment of heart rate using the carotid pulse. Patients taking certain prescribed cardiac medications need to learn to assess their own pulse rate to detect side effects of medications. Patients undergoing cardiac rehabilitation need to learn to assess their own pulse rate to determine their response to exercise.
- Instruct patient about normal blood pressure values, risk factors for hypertension, and usual lack of hypertension symptoms.
- Demonstrate how to obtain blood pressure to the patient's family caregiver using an appropriate-size blood pressure cuff for home use at the same time each day, after patient has had a brief rest, and in the same position and arm each time pressure is taken.

Evaluation

- Ask patient to state three activities to promote health.
- Observe patient obtaining carotid pulse rate.
- Observe family caregiver's measurement of blood pressure.

RECORDING VITAL SIGNS

Special electronic and paper graphic flow sheets exist for recording vital signs (see Chapter 26). Identify institution procedure for documenting on a graphic. In addition to the actual vital sign values, record in the nurses' notes any accompanying or precipitating symptoms such as chest pain and dizziness with abnormal BP, shortness of breath with abnormal respirations, cyanosis with hypoxemia, or flushing and diaphoresis with elevated temperature. Document any interventions initiated as a result of vital sign measurement such as administration of oxygen therapy, hydration, or an antihypertensive medication.

Patients being managed on critical paths often have vital sign values listed as outcomes. If a vital sign value is above or below the anticipated outcomes, write a variance note to explain the nature of the variance and the nursing course of action. For example, a path for a patient who has undergone lung surgery often has an outcome during the postoperative period of "afebrile." If the patient has a fever, the nurse's variance note addresses possible sources of fever (e.g., retained pulmonary secretions) and nursing interventions (e.g., increased suctioning, postural drainage, or hydration).

BOX 30-13 FOCUS ON OLDER ADULTS

Factors Affecting Vital Signs of Older Adults

Temperature

- The temperature of older adults is at the lower end of the normal temperature range, 36° to 36.8° C (96.8° to 98.3° F) orally and 36.6° to 37.2° C (98° to 99° F) rectally. Therefore temperatures considered within normal range sometimes reflect a fever in an older adult. In an older adult fever is present when a single oral temperature is over 37.8° C (100° F); repeated oral temperatures are over 37.2° C (99° F); rectal temperatures are over 37.5° C (99.5° F); or temperature has increased more than 1° C (2° F) over baseline.
- Older adults are very sensitive to slight changes in environmental temperature because their thermoregulatory systems are not as efficient.
- A decrease in sweat gland reactivity in the older adult results in a higher threshold for sweating at high temperatures, which leads to hyperthermia and heatstroke.
- Be especially attentive to subtle temperature changes and other manifestations of fever in this population such as tachypnea, anorexia, falls, delirium, and overall functional decline.
- Older adults without teeth or with poor muscle control may be unable to close their mouths tightly to obtain accurate oral temperature readings.

Pulse Rate

- If it is difficult to palpate the pulse of an obese older adult, a Doppler device provides a more accurate reading.
- Pedal pulses are often difficult to palpate in older adults.
- The older adult has a decreased heart rate at rest.
- It takes longer for the heart rate to rise in the older adult to meet sudden increased demands that result from stress, illness, or excitement. Once elevated, the pulse rate takes longer to return to normal resting rate.
- Heart sounds are sometimes muffled or difficult to hear in older adults because of an increase in air space in the lungs.

Blood Pressure

- Older adults who have lost upper arm mass, especially the frail elderly, require special attention to selection of a smaller size blood pressure cuff.
- Older adults sometimes have an increase in systolic pressure related to decreased vessel elasticity, whereas the diastolic pressure remains the same, resulting in a wider pulse pressure.
- Instruct older adults to change position slowly and wait after each change to avoid postural hypotension and prevent injuries.
- Skin of older adults is more fragile and susceptible to cuff pressure during frequent measurements. More frequent assessment of skin under the cuff or rotating blood pressure sites is recommended.

Respirations

- Aging causes ossification of costal cartilage and downward slant of ribs, resulting in a more rigid rib cage, which reduces chest wall expansion. Kyphosis and scoliosis that occur in older adults also restrict chest expansion and decrease tidal volume.
- Older adults depend more on accessory abdominal muscles during respiration than on weaker thoracic muscles.
- The respiratory system matures by the time a person reaches 20 years of age and begins to decline in healthy people after the age of 25. Despite this decline older adults are able to breathe effortlessly as long as they are healthy. However, sudden events that require an increased demand for oxygen (e.g., exercise, stress, illness) create shortness of breath in the older adult.
- Identifying an acceptable pulse oximeter probe site is difficult with older adults because of the likelihood of peripheral vascular disease, decreased cardiac output, cold-induced vasoconstriction, and anemia.

QSEN QSEN: BUILDING COMPETENCY IN INFORMATICS. The team leader notifies you that your patient has achieved a critical Early Warning Score, a computer-generated value that reflects a patient's condition on the basis of the vital signs entered by the nursing assistive personnel within the past 15 minutes. After completing a focused assessment of the patient, you review the vital signs and compare the most recent with baseline readings. Which vital signs that are included in the Early Warning Score indicate a potential change in the patient's condition? Which actions should you take next?

Baseline Vital Signs	Vital Signs During the Past 15 Minutes
Heart rate 86 and regular	Heart rate 92 and regular
Blood pressure 120/84 in right arm via electronic blood pressure machine	Blood pressure 92/76 in right arm via electronic blood pressure machine
Oxygen saturation 95% on 2 L nasal cannula	Oxygen saturation 89% on 2 L nasal cannula
Respiratory rate 16, regular and deep	Respiratory rate 22, regular and deep
Temperature 37.2° C via temporal artery	Temperature 37.6° C via temporal artery

Answers to QSEN Activities can be found on the Evolve website.

SAFETY GUIDELINES FOR NURSING SKILLS

Ensuring patient safety is an essential role of the professional nurse. To ensure patient safety, communicate clearly with the members of the health care team, assess and incorporate the patient's priorities of care and preferences and use the best evidence when making decisions about your patient's care. When performing the skills in this chapter, remember the following points to ensure safe, individualized patient-centered care.

- Devices for measuring vital signs are often shared among patients. Cleaning each device carefully between patients decreases patients' risk of infection.
- Blood pressure cuffs and pulse oximetry sensors can apply excessive pressure on fragile skin. Rotating sites during repeated measurements decreases risk for skin breakdown.
- Analyze the trends for measuring vital signs and report abnormal findings to the health care provider.
- Determine frequency of measuring vital signs on the basis of the patient's condition.

SKILL 30-1 MEASURING BODY TEMPERATURE

DELEGATION CONSIDERATIONS

The skill of temperature measurement can be delegated to nursing assistive personnel (NAP). Instruct the NAP about:

- Using the appropriate route, device, and frequency for temperature measurement.
- Implementing appropriate precautions when positioning the patient for rectal temperature measurement.
- Considering specific patient-related factors that falsely raise or lower temperature.
- Obtaining temperature measurements at appropriate times as determined by agency policy, health care provider's orders, or patient condition such as when a patient is shivering or feels warm.
- Knowing the usual temperature values for patient.
- Immediately reporting abnormalities to the nurse for further assessment.

EQUIPMENT

- Appropriate thermometer (see Box 30-4)
- Soft tissue or wipe
- Alcohol wipe
- Lubricant (for rectal measurements only)
- Pen, vital sign flow sheet or record, or patient's electronic medical record
- Clean gloves, plastic thermometer sleeve, disposable probe or sensor cover
- Towel

STEP	RATIONALE
ASSESSMENT	
1. Assess for signs and symptoms of temperature alterations and factors that accompany body temperature alterations. *Hyperthermia:* Decreased skin turgor; tachycardia; hypotension; concentrated urine *Heatstroke:* Hot, dry skin; tachycardia; hypotension; excessive thirst; muscle cramps; visual disturbances; confusion or delirium *Hypothermia:* Pale skin; skin cool or cold to touch; bradycardia and dysrhythmias; uncontrolled shivering; reduced level of consciousness; shallow respirations	Physical signs and symptoms indicate abnormal temperature. Enables you to accurately assess the nature of variations.
2. Determine previous activity that interferes with accuracy of temperature measurement. When taking oral temperature, wait 20 to 30 minutes before measuring temperature if patient has smoked or ingested hot or cold liquids or foods.	Smoking, mouth breathing, and oral intake cause false oral temperature readings (Lu et al., 2010).
3. Assess pertinent laboratory values, including complete blood count (CBC).	A white blood cell count (WBC) greater than 12,000/mm^3 in a nonpregnant adult suggests the presence of infection, which can lead to hyperthermia; a WBC count less than 5000/mm^3 suggests that the ability to fight an infection is compromised, which can lead to ineffective thermoregulation.
4. Identify any medications or treatments that may influence body temperature.	Antiinflammatory medications, steroids, and warming or cooling blankets affect body temperature.
5. Determine appropriate temperature site and device for patient.	Site is chosen on the basis of advantages and disadvantages of each site (see Box 30-4). Use disposable single-use thermometer for patient on isolation precautions.
6. Obtain previous baseline temperature and measurement site from patient's medical record.	Allows for assessment of change in patient's condition with future measurements.
PLANNING	
1. Identify patient using two identifiers (e.g., name and birth date or name and medical record number) according to agency policy.	Ensures correct patient. Complies with The Joint Commission standards and improves patient safety (TJC, 2016).
2. Explain route by which temperature will be taken and importance of maintaining proper position until reading is complete.	Patients often are curious about such measurements and need to be cautioned against prematurely removing thermometer to read results.
IMPLEMENTATION	
1. Perform hand hygiene.	Reduces transmission of microorganisms.
2. Help patient assume comfortable position that provides easy access to temperature measurement site.	Ensures comfort and accuracy of temperature reading.
3. Obtain temperature reading.	
a. Oral temperature measurement with electronic thermometer	
(1) Apply clean gloves (optional) when there are respiratory secretions or facial or mouth wound drainage.	Use of oral probe cover, which you can remove without physical contact, minimizes need to wear gloves.
(2) Remove thermometer pack from charging unit. Attach oral thermometer probe stem (blue tip) to thermometer unit. Grasp top of probe stem, being careful not to apply pressure on ejection button.	Charging provides battery power. Ejection button releases plastic probe cover from probe stem.
(3) Slide disposable plastic probe cover over thermometer probe stem until cover locks in place (see illustrations).	Soft plastic cover will not break in patient's mouth and prevents transmission of microorganisms between patients.

STEP	RATIONALE
(4) Ask patient to open mouth; gently place thermometer probe under tongue in posterior sublingual pocket lateral to center of lower jaw (see illustration).	Heat from superficial blood vessels in sublingual pocket produces temperature reading. With electronic thermometer, temperatures in right and left posterior sublingual pocket are significantly higher than in area under front of tongue.
(5) Ask patient to hold thermometer probe with lips closed.	Closed lips maintain proper position of thermometer during recording.
(6) Leave thermometer probe in place until audible signal indicates completion and temperate reading appears on digital display; remove thermometer probe from under patient's tongue.	Probe needs to stay in place until signal occurs to ensure accurate reading.
(7) Push ejection button on thermometer probe stem to discard plastic probe cover into appropriate receptacle.	Reduces transmission of microorganisms.
(8) Return thermometer probe stem to storage position of recording unit.	Storage position protects probe stem. Returning probe stem automatically causes digital reading to disappear.
(9) If gloves are worn, remove and dispose in appropriate receptacle. Perform hand hygiene.	Hand hygiene reduces transmission of microorganisms.
(10) Return thermometer to charger.	Charger maintains battery charge.
b. Rectal temperature measurement with electronic thermometer	
(1) Draw curtain around bed and/or close room door. Help patient to Sims' position with upper leg flexed. Move aside bed linen to expose only anal area. Keep patient's upper body and lower extremities covered with sheet or blanket.	Maintains patient's privacy, minimizes embarrassment, and promotes comfort. Exposes anal area for correct thermometer placement.

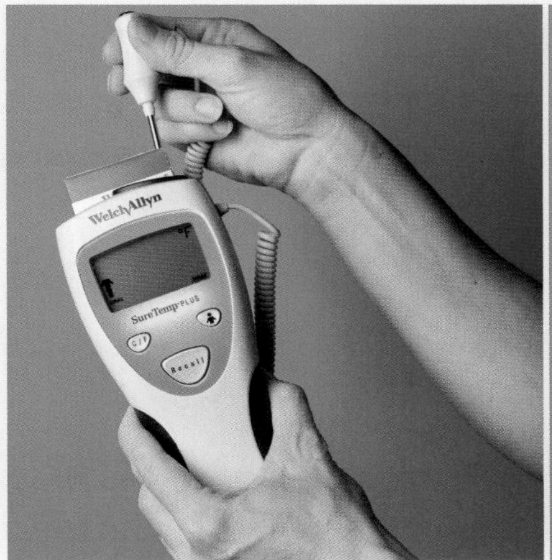

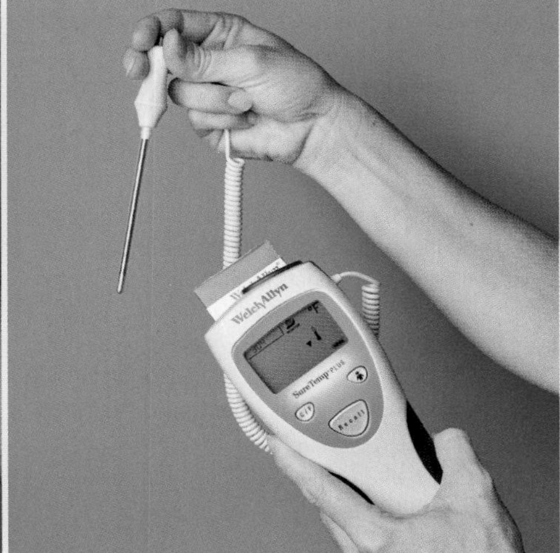

STEP 3a(3) Disposable plastic cover is placed over probe.

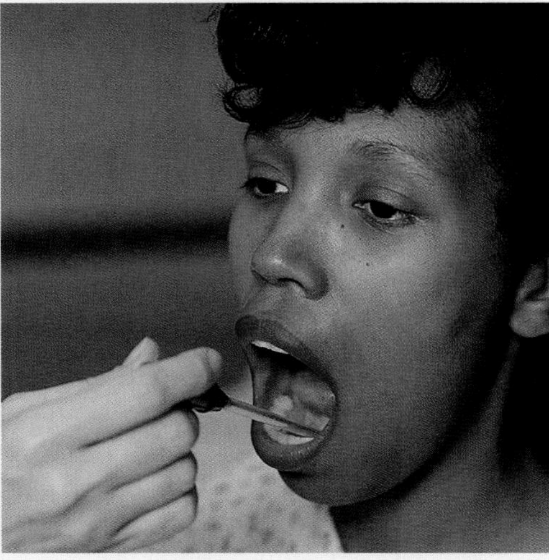

STEP 3a(4) Probe under tongue in posterior sublingual pocket.

SKILL 30-1 MEASURING BODY TEMPERATURE—cont'd

STEP	RATIONALE
(2) Apply clean gloves. Cleanse anal region when feces and/or secretions are present. Remove soiled gloves and reapply clean gloves.	Maintains standard precautions when exposed to items soiled with body fluids (e.g., feces).
(3) Remove thermometer pack from charging unit. Attach rectal probe stem (red tip) to thermometer unit. Grasp top of probe stem, being careful not to apply pressure ejection button.	Charging provides battery power. Ejection button releases plastic cover from probe stem.
(4) Slide disposable plastic probe cover over thermometer probe stem until cover locks in place.	Soft plastic probe cover prevents transmission of microorganisms between patients.
(5) Squeeze liberal portion of lubricant on tissue. Dip end of probe cover into lubricant, covering 2.5 to 3.5 cm (1 to 1½ inches) for adult.	Lubrication minimizes trauma to rectal mucosa during insertion. Tissue avoids contamination of remaining lubricant in container.
(6) With nondominant hand separate patient's buttocks to expose anus. Ask patient to breathe slowly and relax.	Fully exposes anus for thermometer insertion. Relaxes anal sphincter for easier thermometer insertion.
(7) Gently insert thermometer probe into anus in direction of umbilicus 2.5 to 3.5 cm (1 to 1½ inches) for adult. Do not force thermometer.	Ensures adequate exposure against blood vessels in rectal wall.

CLINICAL DECISION: *If you cannot adequately insert thermometer into rectum, remove it and consider alternative method for obtaining temperature.*

STEP	RATIONALE
(8) Once positioned, hold thermometer probe in place (see illustration) until audible signal indicates completion and patient's temperature appears on digital display; remove thermometer probe from anus.	Probe needs to stay in place until signal occurs to ensure accurate reading. Holding probe in place prevents movement.
(9) Push ejection button on thermometer stem to discard plastic probe cover into appropriate receptacle. Wipe probe stem with alcohol swab, paying particular attention to ridges where probe stem cover connects to probe.	Reduces transmission of microorganisms.
(10) Return thermometer probe stem to storage position of recording unit.	Protects probe stem from damage. Returning probe stem automatically causes digital reading to disappear.
(11) Wipe patient's anal area with soft tissue to remove lubricant or feces and discard tissue. Help patient assume a comfortable position.	Provides for comfort and hygiene.
(12) Remove and dispose of gloves in appropriate receptacle. Perform hand hygiene.	Reduces transmission of microorganisms.
(13) Return thermometer to charger. Verify that charger and probes are wiped with alcohol daily.	Maintains battery charge of thermometer unit. Reduces transmission of microorganisms.
c. Tympanic membrane temperature with electronic infrared thermometer	
(1) Help patient assume comfortable position with head turned toward side away from you. If patient has been lying on one side, use upper ear.	Ensures comfort and exposes auditory canal for accurate temperature measurement. Heat trapped in lower ear causes false-high temperature readings.
(2) Note if there is obvious earwax in patient's ear canal.	Earwax on lens cover blocks a clear optical pathway. It can lower tympanic temperature by 0.3° C (0.6° F). Switch to other ear or select alternative measurement site if needed.

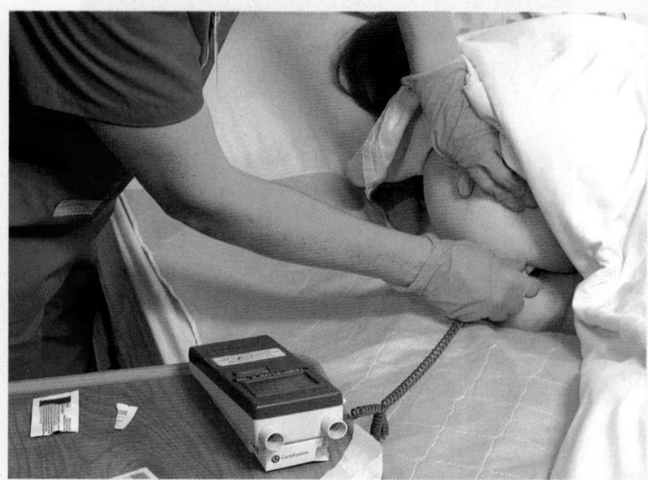

STEP 3b(8) Probe positioned in anus. (Copyright © Mosby's Clinical Skills: Essentials Collection.)

STEP	RATIONALE
(3) Remove thermometer handheld unit from charging base.	Base provides battery power. Removal of handheld unit from base prepares it to measure temperature.
(4) Slide clean disposable speculum cover over otoscope-like lens tip until it locks into place. Be careful not to apply pressure to ejection button and not to touch lens cover.	Soft plastic probe cover prevents transmission of microorganisms between patients. Ejection button releases plastic probe cover from thermometer tip. Lens cover needs to be free of dust, fingerprints, or earwax to ensure clear optical pathway.
(5) Insert infrared speculum into ear canal following manufacturer instructions for tympanic probe positioning:	Ear tug straightens external auditory canal, allowing maximum exposure of tympanic membrane to correctly position speculum (Hockenberry and Wilson, 2015).
(a) Pull ear pinna backward, up, and out for an adult. For children 3 years and younger, point covered probe toward midpoint between eyebrow and side burns. For children older than 3 years, pull pinna up and back (Hockenberry and Wilson, 2015).	Correctly positioning speculum tip with respect to ear canal ensures accurate readings.
(b) Move thermometer in a figure-eight pattern (see manufacturer directions).	Some manufacturers recommend movement of the speculum tip in a figure-eight pattern, which allows the sensor to detect maximum tympanic membrane heat radiation.
(c) Fit speculum tip snugly into canal and do not move (see illustration), pointing speculum tip toward nose.	Gentle pressure seals ear canal from ambient temperature, which alters readings as much as 2.8° C (5° F). Operator error leads to false-low temperatures.
(6) Once positioned, press scan button on handheld unit. Leave speculum in place until audible signal indicates completion and patient's temperature appears on digital display.	Pressing scan button causes detection of infrared energy. Speculum probe tip needs to stay in place until device has detected infrared energy noted by audible signal.
(7) Carefully remove speculum from auditory meatus.	Prevents rubbing of sensitive outer ear lining.
(8) Push ejection button on handheld unit to discard speculum cover into appropriate receptacle.	Reduces transmission of microorganisms. Automatically causes digital reading to disappear.
(9) If temperature is abnormal or a second reading is necessary, replace speculum cover and wait 2 to 3 minutes before repeating measurement in same ear. Repeat measurement in other ear or try an alternative temperature site or instrument.	Time allows ear canal to regain usual temperature.
(10) Return handheld unit to charging base.	Protects sensor tip from damage.
(11) Help patient get into a comfortable position.	Restores comfort and sense of well-being.
(12) Perform hand hygiene.	Reduces transmission of microorganisms.
d. **Temporal artery temperature measurement with electronic infrared thermometer**	
(1) Ensure that forehead is dry; wipe with towel if needed.	Moist skin interferes with thermometer sensor.
(2) Place sensor flush on patient's forehead above eyebrow (see illustration).	Contact avoids measurement of ambient temperature.
(3) Press red scan button with your thumb. Slowly slide thermometer straight across forehead while keeping sensor flush on skin.	Scanning for highest temperature continues until you release scan button.
(4) Keeping scan button pressed, lift sensor from forehead and touch sensor to skin on neck, just behind earlobe. Peak temperature occurs when clicking sound during scanning stops (see illustration). Release scan button and note reading.	Sensor confirms highest temperature behind earlobe.

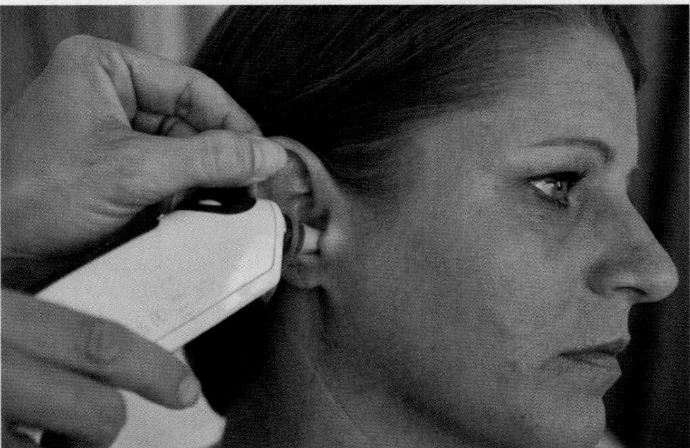

STEP 3c(5)(c) Tympanic thermometer with probe cover inserted into auditory canal.

SKILL 30-1 MEASURING BODY TEMPERATURE—cont'd

STEP	RATIONALE
(5) Clean sensor with alcohol swab.	Prevents transmission of microorganisms.
(6) Return thermometer to charger or thermometer base.	Maintains battery charge of thermometer unit.
e. Axillary temperature measurement with electronic thermometer	
(1) Draw curtain around bed or close room door. Help patient to supine or sitting position. Move clothing or gown away from shoulder and arm.	Maintains patient's privacy, minimizes embarrassment, and promotes comfort. Exposes axilla for correct thermometer probe placement.
(2) Remove thermometer pack from charging unit. Attach oral thermometer probe stem (blue tip) to thermometer unit. Grasp top of thermometer probe stem, being careful not to apply pressure on ejection button.	Ejection button releases plastic cover from probe.
(3) Slide disposable plastic probe cover over thermometer stem until cover locks in place.	Probe cover prevents transmission of microorganisms between patients.
(4) Raise patient's arm away from torso. Inspect for skin lesions and excessive perspiration. Insert thermometer probe into center of axilla (see illustration). Lower arm over probe and place arm across patient's chest.	Do not use axillar if skin lesions are present because local skin temperature may be altered or area may be painful to touch. Axillary temperature is not reliable in adults but can be used in infants.

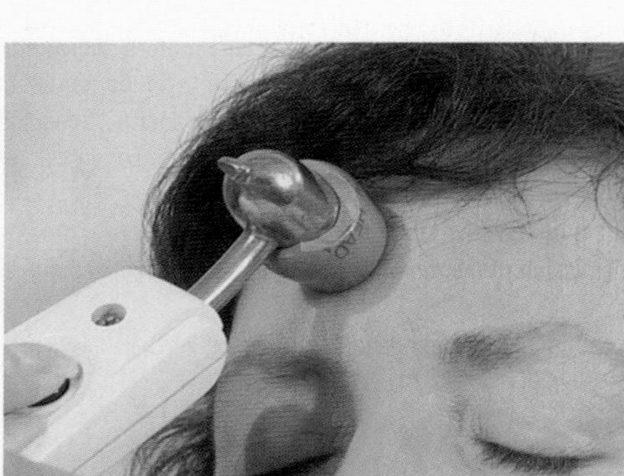

STEP 3d(2) Scanning the forehead. (Copyright © Mosby's Clinical Skills: Essentials Collection.)

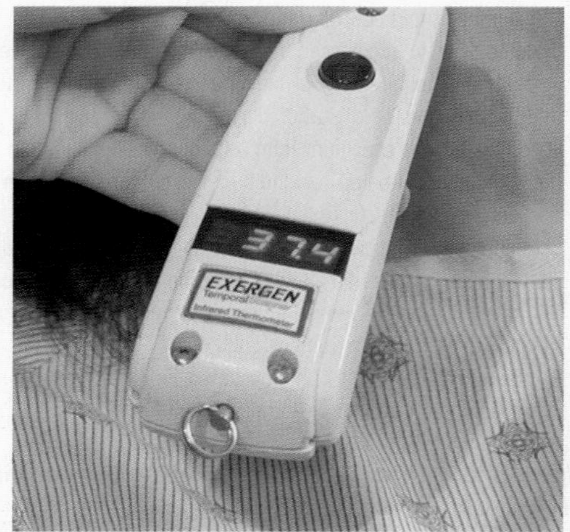

STEP 3d(4) Digital reading shown on display unit. (Copyright © Mosby's Clinical Skills: Essentials Collection.)

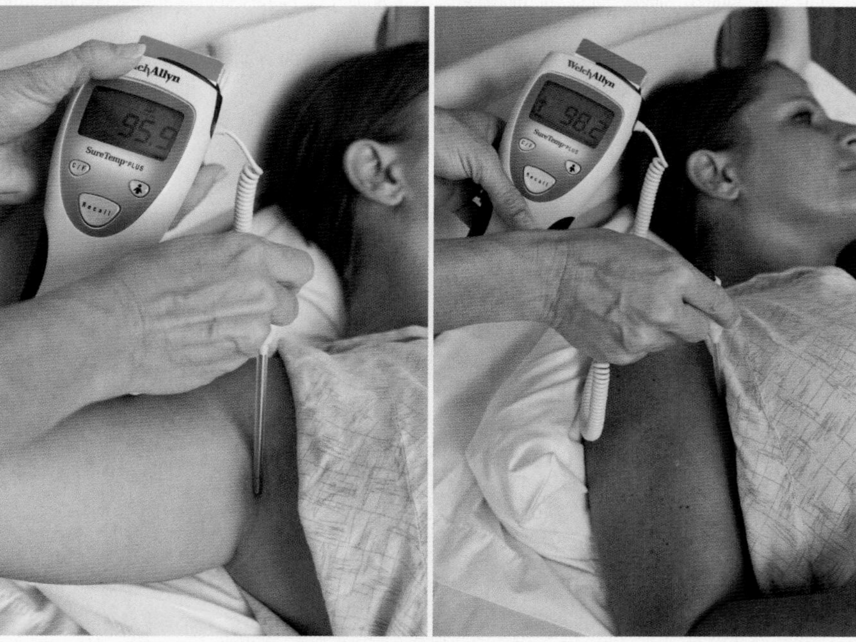

STEP 3e(4) Place thermometer in axilla.

STEP	RATIONALE
(5) Once positioned, hold thermometer probe in place until audible signal indicates completion and patient's temperature appears on digital display. Remove thermometer probe from axilla.	Thermometer probe needs to stay in place until signal sounds to ensure accurate reading.
(6) Push ejection button on thermometer stem to discard plastic probe cover into appropriate receptacle.	Reduces transmission of microorganisms.
(7) Return thermometer stem to storage position/charger of recording unit.	Returning thermometer stem to storage unit position automatically causes digital reading to disappear. Storage position protects stem.
4. Discuss findings with patient and explain significance.	Promotes participation in care and understanding of health status.
EVALUATION	
1. If temperature is assessed for first time, establish temperature as baseline if it is within normal range.	Used to compare future temperature measurements.
2. Compare temperature reading with patient's previous baseline and acceptable temperature range for his or her age-group.	Body temperature fluctuates within narrow range; comparison reveals presence of abnormality. Improper placement or movement of thermometer causes inaccuracies. Second measurement confirms initial findings of abnormal body temperature.

UNEXPECTED OUTCOMES AND RELATED INTERVENTIONS

1. Temperature 1° C (1.8° F) above usual range
   - Assess possible sites (e.g., central line catheter, wounds) for localized infection and related data suggesting a systemic infection.
   - Follow interventions listed in Box 30-7.
2. Fever persists or reaches unacceptable level as defined by health care provider.
   - Notify health care provider and administer antipyretics and antibiotics as ordered.
3. Temperature 1° C (1.8° F) below usual range
   - Remove any drafts, wet clothing, or linen.
   - Apply extra blankets and, unless contraindicated, offer warm liquids.
   - Monitor apical pulse rate and rhythm because hypothermia causes bradycardia and dysrhythmias.

RECORDING AND REPORTING

- Record temperature in nurses' notes or vital sign flow sheet or EHR. Document measurement of temperature after administration of specific therapies in narrative form in nurses' notes.
- Report abnormal findings to nurse in charge or health care provider.

HOME CARE CONSIDERATIONS

- Assess temperature and ventilation of patient's environment to determine existence of any environmental condition that influences patient's temperature.

SKILL 30-2 ASSESSING RADIAL AND APICAL PULSES

DELEGATION CONSIDERATIONS

The skill of pulse measurement can be delegated to nursing assistive personnel (NAP) if the patient is stable and not at high risk for acute or serious cardiac problems. The nurse instructs the NAP to:

- Consider factors related to patient's history, usual values, and risk for abnormally slow or irregular pulse.
- Obtain appropriate pulse measurement frequency at appropriate times as determined by agency policy, health care provider's order, or patient condition such as presence of chest pain or dizziness.
- Immediately report significant changes or abnormalities to nurse for further assessment.

EQUIPMENT

- Stethoscope (apical pulse only)
- Wristwatch with second hand or digital display
- Pen, vital sign flow sheet, or patient's electronic health record
- Alcohol swab

STEP	RATIONALE
ASSESSMENT	
1. Determine need to assess radial or apical pulse:	Nurse uses clinical judgment to determine need for assessment.
a. Assess for any risk factors for pulse alterations. • History of heart disease • Cardiac dysrhythmias • Onset of sudden chest pain or acute pain from any site • Invasive cardiovascular diagnostic tests • Surgery • Sudden infusion of large volume of intravenous (IV) fluid • Internal or external hemorrhage, dehydration • Administration of medications that alter cardiac function	These conditions place patients at risk for pulse alterations. A history of peripheral vascular disease often alters pulse rate and quality.

SKILL 30-2 ASSESSING RADIAL AND APICAL PULSES—cont'd

STEP	RATIONALE
b. Assess for signs and symptoms of altered stroke volume and cardiac output such as dyspnea, fatigue, chest pain, orthopnea, syncope, palpitations (person's unpleasant awareness of heartbeat), jugular venous distention, edema of dependent body parts, cyanosis, or pallor of skin (see Chapter 41).	Physical signs and symptoms indicate alteration in cardiac function.
c. Assess for signs and symptoms of peripheral vascular disease such as pale, cool extremities; thin, shiny skin with decreased hair growth; thickened nails.	Physical signs and symptoms indicate alteration in local arterial blood flow.
2. Assess for factors that influence pulse rate and rhythm: age, exercise, position changes, fluid balance, medications, temperature, and sympathetic stimulation.	Allows for accurate assessment of presence and significance of pulse alterations. Acceptable range of pulse rate changes with age (see Table 30-3).
3. Assess pertinent laboratory values, including serum potassium and complete blood count (CBC).	Elevated or decreased potassium levels can cause dysrhythmias. Low values for hemoglobin are associated with reduced oxygen transport, which can increase pulse rate.
4. Determine patient's previous baseline pulse rate if available in his or her medical record.	Allows for accurate assessment of change in condition and provides comparison with future apical pulse measurements.
5. Determine if patient has latex allergy.	If patient has latex allergy, verify that stethoscope is latex free.
PLANNING	
1. Identify patient using two identifiers (e.g., name and birth date or name and medical record number) according to agency policy.	Ensures correct patient. Complies with The Joint Commission standards and improves patient safety (TJC, 2016).
2. Explain that you will assess pulse or heart rate. Encourage patient to relax and not speak. If patient was active, wait 5 to 10 minutes before assessing pulse.	Activity and anxiety elevate heart rate. Patient's voice interferes with your ability to hear sound when assessing apical rate. Obtaining pulse rates at rest allows for objective comparison of values.
IMPLEMENTATION	
1. Perform hand hygiene.	Reduces transmission of microorganisms.
2. Draw curtain around bed and/or close door.	Maintains privacy.
3. Obtain pulse measurement.	
a. Radial pulse	
(1) Help patient get into supine or sitting position.	Provides easy access to pulse sites.
(2) If supine, place patient's forearm straight alongside body or across lower chest or upper abdomen with wrist extended straight (see illustration). If sitting, bend patient's elbow 90 degrees and support lower arm on chair or on your arm.	Relaxed position of lower arm and slight flexion of wrist promote exposure of artery to palpation without restriction.
(3) Place tips of first two or middle three fingers of hand over groove along radial or thumb side of patient's inner wrist. Slightly extend or flex wrist with palm down until you note strongest pulse (see illustration).	Fingertips are most sensitive parts of hand to palpate arterial pulsation. Your thumb has a pulsation that interferes with accuracy.
(4) Lightly compress pulse against radius, losing pulse initially, and then relax pressure so pulse becomes easily palpable.	Pulse is assessed more accurately with moderate pressure. Too much pressure occludes pulse and impairs blood flow.
(5) Determine strength of pulse. Note whether thrust of vessel against fingertips is bounding (4), full/strong (3), normal or expected (2), diminished or barely palpable (1), or absent (0).	Strength reflects volume of blood ejected against arterial wall with each heart contraction. Accurate description of strength improves communication among nurses and other health care providers.

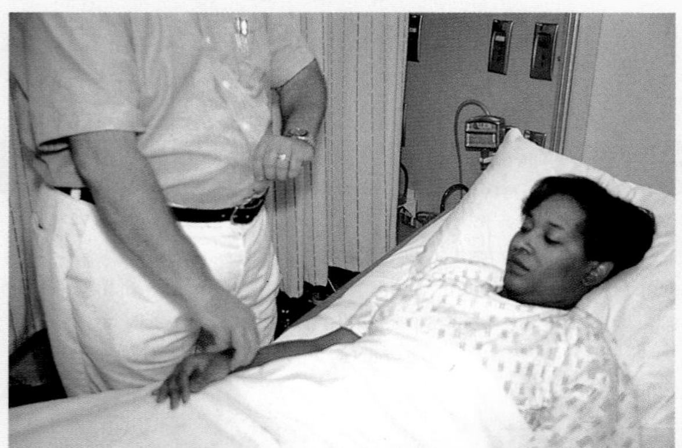

STEP 3a(2) Pulse check with patient's forearm at side with wrist flexed.

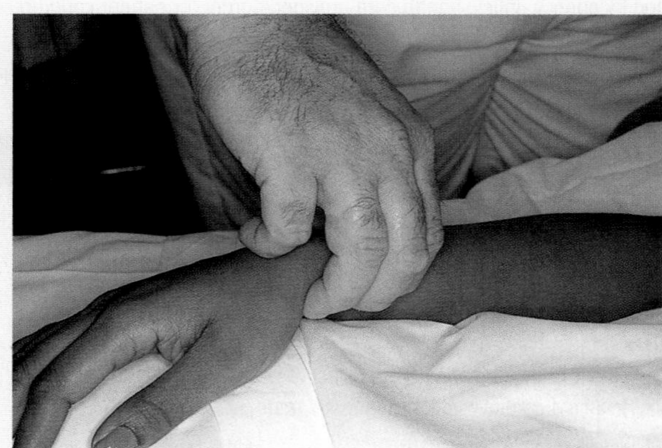

STEP 3a(3) Hand placement for pulse checks.

STEP	RATIONALE
(6) After feeling a regular pulse, look at second hand of a watch and begin to count rate: count the first beat after the second hand hits the number on the dial; count as one, then two, and so on.	Determine rate only after knowing that you can palpate pulse. Timing begins with zero. Count of one is first beat palpated after timing begins.
(7) If pulse is regular, count rate for 30 seconds and multiply total by 2.	A 30-second count is accurate for rapid, slow, or regular pulse rates.
(8) If pulse is irregular, count rate for 1 minute (60 seconds). Assess frequency and pattern of irregularity. Compare radial pulses bilaterally.	Inefficient contraction of heart fails to transmit pulse wave, interfering with cardiac output, resulting in irregular pulse. Longer time ensures accurate count.

CLINICAL DECISION: *If pulse is irregular, do an apical/radial pulse assessment to detect a pulse deficit. Count apical pulse (see Step 3b) while a colleague counts radial pulse. Begin apical pulse count out loud to simultaneously assess pulses. If pulse count differs by more than 2, a pulse deficit exists, which sometimes indicates alterations in cardiac output.*

STEP	RATIONALE
b. Apical pulse	
(1) Clean earpieces and diaphragm of stethoscope with alcohol swab. Perform hand hygiene.	Reduces transmission of microorganisms.
(2) Draw curtain around bed and/or close door.	Provides privacy and minimizes embarrassment.
(3) Help patient to supine or sitting position. Move aside bed linen and gown to expose sternum and left side of chest.	Exposes portion of chest wall for selection of auscultatory site. Stethoscope diaphragm must touch skin to best hear sounds.
(4) Locate anatomical landmarks to identify point of maximal impulse (PMI), also called *apical impulse* (see illustrations A-D). Heart is located behind and to left of sternum with base at top and apex at bottom. Find angle of Louis just below suprasternal notch between sternal body and manubrium; feels like bony prominence (illustration A). Slip fingers down each side of angle to find second intercostal space (ICS) (illustration B). Carefully move fingers down left side of sternum to fifth ICS (illustration C) and laterally to left midclavicular line (MCL) (illustration D). A light tap felt within an area 1 to 2 cm (½ to 1 inch) of PMI is reflected from apex of heart.	Use of anatomical landmarks allows correct placement of stethoscope over apex of heart, enhancing ability to hear heart sounds clearly. If unable to palpate PMI, reposition patient on left side. In presence of serious heart disease, PMI is located to left of MCL or at sixth ICS.

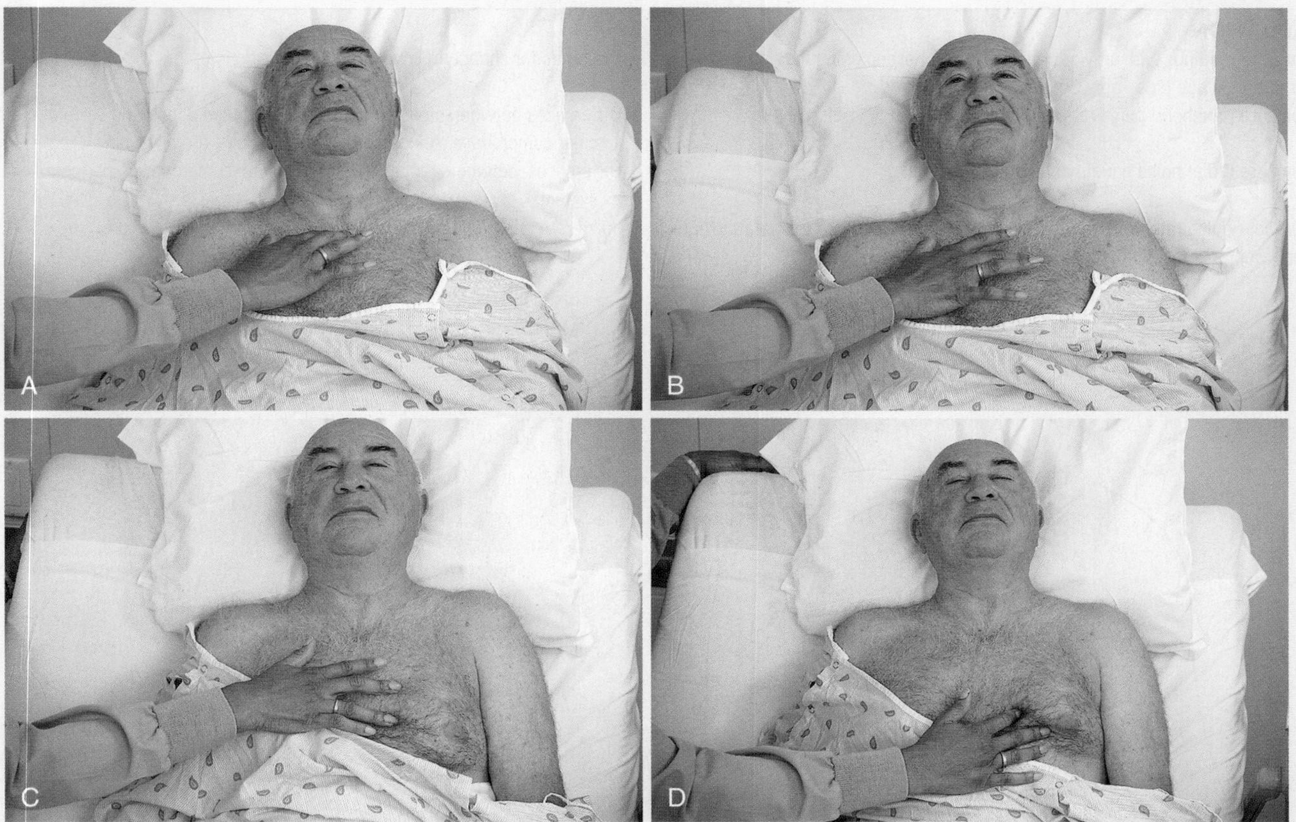

STEP 3b(4) A, Locating angle of Louis. **B,** Locating second intercostal space (ICS). **C,** Locating fifth ICS. **D,** Identifying midclavicular line (MCL).

SKILL 30-2 ASSESSING RADIAL AND APICAL PULSES—cont'd

STEP	RATIONALE
CLINICAL DECISION: *When assessing the apical rate of an older woman, lift the breast tissue gently, and place the stethoscope at the fifth intercostal space (ICS) or the lower edge of the breast.*	
(5) Place diaphragm of stethoscope in palm of hand for 5 to 10 seconds.	Warming of metal or plastic diaphragm prevents patient from being startled and promotes comfort.
(6) Place diaphragm of stethoscope over PMI at fifth ICS at left MCL and auscultate for normal S_1 and S_2 heart sounds (heard as "lub-dub") (see illustrations).	Allow stethoscope tubing to extend straight without kinks that would distort sound transmission. Normal sounds S_1 and S_2 are high pitched and best heard with the diaphragm.
(7) When you hear S_1 and S_2 with regularity, use second hand of watch and begin to count rate; when sweep hand hits number 12 on dial, start counting with zero, then one, two, and so on.	Determine apical rate accurately only after you are able to auscultate sounds clearly. Timing begins with zero. Count of one is first sound auscultated after timing begins.
(8) If apical rate is regular, count for 30 seconds and multiply by 2.	The first time the apical rate is measured, it should be counted for 60 seconds. If the rate is regular, subsequent measurements will be accurate for 30 seconds.
CLINICAL DECISION: *If heart rate is irregular or patient is receiving cardiovascular medication, count for 1 minute (60 seconds). Irregular rate is assessed more accurately when measured over a longer interval.*	
(9) Note if heart rate is irregular and describe pattern or irregularity (S_1 and S_2 occurring early or later after previous sequence of sounds [e.g., every third or every fourth beat is skipped]).	Irregular heart rate indicates dysrhythmia. Regular occurrence of dysrhythmia within 1 minute indicates inefficient contraction of heart and alteration in cardiac output.
(10) Replace patient's gown and bed linen; help patient return to comfortable position.	Restores comfort and promotes sense of well-being.
(11) Perform hand hygiene.	Reduces transmission of microorganisms.
(12) Clean earpieces and diaphragm of stethoscope with alcohol swab routinely after each use.	Prevents transmission of microorganisms.
4. Discuss findings with patient as needed.	Promotes participation in care and understanding of health status.
EVALUATION	
1. Compare readings with previous baseline and/or acceptable range of heart rate for patient's age (see Table 30-3).	Evaluates for change in condition and alterations.
2. Compare peripheral pulse rate with apical rate and note discrepancy.	Differences between measurements indicate pulse deficit and warn of cardiovascular compromise. Abnormalities often require therapy.
3. Compare radial pulse equality and note discrepancy.	Differences between radial arteries indicate compromised peripheral vascular system.
4. Correlate pulse rate with data obtained from blood pressure and related signs and symptoms (palpitations, dizziness).	Pulse rate and blood pressure are interrelated.

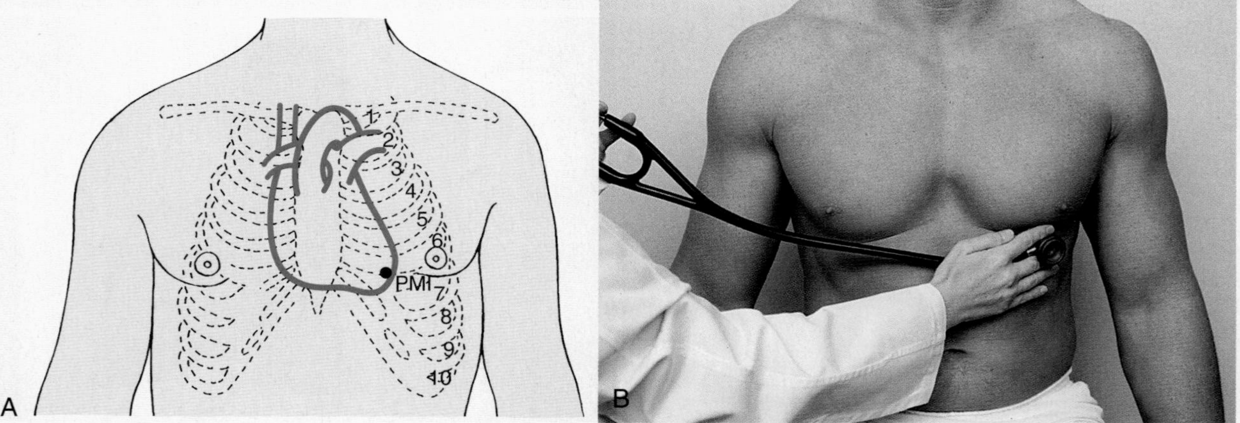

STEP 3b(6) A, Location of point of maximal impulse (PMI) in adult. **B,** Stethoscope diaphragm over PMI.

UNEXPECTED OUTCOMES AND RELATED INTERVENTIONS

1. Radial pulse is less than expected value, weak, thready, or difficult to palpate.
   - Assess both radial pulses and compare findings. Local obstruction to one extremity (e.g., clot, edema) decreases peripheral blood flow.
   - Assess for swelling in surrounding tissues or other reason causing decreased peripheral blood flow (e.g., dressing, cast).
   - Perform complete assessment of all peripheral pulses (see Chapter 31).
   - Observe for symptoms associated with decreased tissue perfusion, including pallor and cool skin temperature of tissue distal to the weak pulse.
   - Measure apical and radial pulse simultaneously to determine presence of pulse deficit.
   - Have a second nurse assess pulses.
2. Apical pulse is greater than expected normal value (e.g., rate greater than 100 beats/min [tachycardia] in an adult; see Table 30-3).
   - Identify related data, including fever, anxiety, pain, recent exercise, hypotension, decreased oxygenation, or dehydration.
   - Observe for signs and symptoms of inadequate cardiac output, including fatigue, chest pain, orthopnea, cyanosis, and dizziness.
3. Apical pulse is less than expected normal value (e.g., rate less than 60 beats/min [bradycardia] in an adult; see Table 30-3).
   - Assess for factors that alter heart rate such as beta-blockers and antidysrhythmic medications.
   - Observe for signs and symptoms of inadequate cardiac output, including fatigue, chest pain, orthopnea, cyanosis, dizziness.

RECORDING AND REPORTING

- Record pulse rate with assessment site in nurses' notes or vital signs flow sheet. Document pulse rate after administration of specific therapies in narrative form in nurses' notes.
- Report abnormal findings to nurse in charge or health care provider immediately.

HOME CARE CONSIDERATIONS

- Assess home environment to determine room that affords quiet environment for auscultating apical rate.

SKILL 30-3 ASSESSING RESPIRATIONS

DELEGATION CONSIDERATIONS

The skill of respiration measurement can be delegated to nursing assistive personnel (NAP) unless the patient is considered unstable. The nurse instructs the NAP to:

- Obtain the appropriate frequency of respirations as determined by patient history and risk for respiratory rate, rhythm, or depth alternations.
- Consider specific patient factors related to history or risk for increased or decreased respiratory rate or irregular respirations.
- Immediately report significant changes or abnormalities to the nurse immediately for further assessment.

EQUIPMENT

- Wristwatch with second hand or digital display
- Pen, vital sign flow sheet or record, or electronic health record

STEP	RATIONALE
ASSESSMENT	
1. Determine need to assess patient's respirations:	Nurse uses clinical judgment to determine need for assessment.
a. Identify risk factors for respiratory alterations, including: • Fever, pain, anxiety • Diseases of chest wall or muscles • Constrictive chest or abdominal dressings • Gastric distention • Pulmonary disease (emphysema, bronchitis, asthma, pneumonia, acute bronchitis) • Traumatic injury to chest wall with or without collapse of underlying lung tissue; thoracic or abdominal surgery • Presence of chest tube • Pulmonary edema and emboli • Head injury with damage to brainstem • Anemia	Conditions that place patient at risk for ventilatory and respiratory alterations are detected by changes in respiratory rate, depth, and rhythm.
b. Assess for signs and symptoms of respiratory alterations such as bluish or cyanotic appearance of nail beds, lips, mucous membranes, and skin; restlessness, irritability, confusion, reduced level of consciousness; pain during inspiration; labored or difficult breathing; adventitious breath sounds (see Chapter 31) or inability to breathe spontaneously; thick, frothy, blood-tinged, or copious sputum produced on coughing.	Physical signs and symptoms indicate alterations in respiratory status.

SKILL 30-3 ASSESSING RESPIRATIONS—cont'd

STEP	RATIONALE
2. Assess pertinent laboratory values:	
a. Arterial blood gases (ABGs): Normal ABGs (values vary slightly among institutions): • pH: 7.35-7.45 • $PaCO_2$: 35-45 mm Hg • PaO_2: 80-100 mm Hg • SaO_2: 95%-100%	ABGs measure arterial blood pH; partial pressure of O_2 and CO_2; and arterial O_2 saturation, which reflects patient's oxygenation status.
b. Pulse oximetry (SpO_2): Acceptable SpO_2 ranges from 95% to 100%; a value of less than 90% is considered hypoxemia; however, values below 90% may be acceptable for certain chronic disease conditions (see Skill 30-4).	SpO_2 less than 90% is often accompanied by changes in respiratory rate, depth, and rhythm.
c. Complete blood count (CBC): Normal CBC for adults (values vary among institutions): • *Hemoglobin:* 14 to 18 g/100 mL, males; 12 to 16 g/100 mL, females • *Hematocrit:* 42% to 52%, males; 37% to 47%, females • *Red blood cell count:* 4.7 to 6.1 million/mm^3, males; 4.2 to 5.4 million/mm^3, females (Pagana and Pagana, 2015)	Complete blood count measures red blood cell count; volume of red blood cells; and concentration of hemoglobin, which reflects patient's capacity to carry O_2.
3. Assess for factors that influence respirations (see Box 30-7).	Allows you to control for factors that can affect measurement.
4. Determine previous baseline respiratory rate (if available) from patient's record.	Allows you to assess for change in condition. Provides comparison with future respiratory measurements.
PLANNING	
1. Identify patient using two identifiers (e.g., name and birth date or name and medical record number) according to agency policy.	Ensures correct patient. Complies with The Joint Commission standards and improves patient safety (TJC, 2016).
2. Plan to assess respirations after measuring pulse in an adult.	Inconspicuous assessment of respirations immediately after pulse assessment prevents patient from consciously or unintentionally altering rate and depth of breathing.
IMPLEMENTATION	
1. Perform hand hygiene. Draw curtain around bed and/or close door.	Prevents transmission of microorganisms. Maintains privacy.
2. Be sure that patient is in comfortable position, preferably sitting or lying with head of bed elevated 45 to 60 degrees. Be sure that patient's chest is visible. If necessary, move bed linen or gown.	Sitting erect promotes full ventilatory movement. Ensures clear view of chest wall and abdominal movements.
3. Place patient's arm in relaxed position across abdomen or lower chest or place your hand directly over patient's upper abdomen.	A similar position used during pulse assessment allows respiratory rate assessment to be inconspicuous. Patient's hand or your hand rises and falls during respiratory cycle.
4. Observe complete respiratory cycle (one inspiration and one expiration).	Rate is accurately determined only after you have observed a respiratory cycle.
5. After observing a cycle, look at second hand of watch and begin to count rate; when sweep hand hits number on dial, begin time frame, counting one with first full respiratory cycle.	Timing begins with count of one. Respirations occur more slowly than pulse; thus timing does not begin with zero.
6. If rhythm is regular, count number of respirations in 30 seconds and multiply by 2. If rhythm is irregular, less than 12, or greater than 20, count for 1 full minute.	Respiratory rate is equivalent to number of respirations per minute. Suspected irregularities require assessment for at least 1 minute (see Table 30-6).
7. Note depth of respirations subjectively assessed by observing degree of chest wall movement while counting rate. You also objectively assess depth by palpating chest wall excursion or auscultating posterior thorax after rate has been counted (see Chapter 31). Describe depth as shallow, normal, or deep.	Character of ventilatory movement reveals specific disease states that restrict volume of air from moving into and out of the lungs.
8. Note rhythm of ventilatory cycle. Normal breathing is regular and uninterrupted. Do not confuse sighing with abnormal rhythm.	Character of ventilations reveals specific types of alterations. Periodically people unconsciously take single deep breaths or sighs to expand small airways prone to collapse.
9. Observe for any increased effort to inhale and exhale. Ask patient to describe subjective experience of breathing compared with usual breathing pattern.	Patients with chronic lung disease may experience difficulty breathing all the time and can best describe their own discomfort from shortness of breath.

CLINICAL DECISION: *An irregular respiratory pattern or occurrence of periods of apnea (cessation of respiration for several seconds) is a symptom of underlying disease in the adult and must be reported to the nurse in charge or health care provider. The patient requires further assessment (see Chapter 31) and needs immediate intervention. An irregular respiratory rate and short apneic spells are normal for newborns.*

STEP	RATIONALE
10. Replace bed linen and patient's gown.	Restores comfort and promotes sense of well-being.
11. Perform hand hygiene.	Reduces transmission of microorganisms.
12. Discuss findings with patient as needed.	Promotes participation in care and understanding of health status.

STEP	RATIONALE
EVALUATION	
1. If assessing respirations for first time, establish rate, rhythm, and depth as baseline if within normal range.	Used to compare future respiratory assessment.
2. Compare respirations with patient's previous baseline and normal rate, rhythm, and depth.	Allows nurse to assess for changes in patient's condition and presence of respiratory alterations.
3. Correlate respiratory rate, depth, and rhythm with data obtained from pulse oximetry and ABG measurements if available.	Ventilation, perfusion, and diffusion are interrelated.

UNEXPECTED OUTCOMES AND RELATED INTERVENTIONS

1. Patient has respiratory rate that is outside of expected normal values (e.g., less than 12 (bradypnea) or above 20 (tachypnea) breaths/min in an adult; see Table 30-5). Breathing pattern is irregular. Depth of respirations increases or decreases: patient complains of dyspnea.
- Observe for related factors such as obstructed airway; assess for abnormal breath sounds, productive cough, restlessness, irritability, anxiety, confusion (see Chapter 31).
- Help patient to supported sitting position (semi- or high-Fowler's) unless contraindicated, which improves ventilation.
- Provide oxygen as ordered (see Chapter 31).
- Assess for environmental factors that influence patient's respiratory rate such as secondhand smoke and poor room ventilation and make corrections.

RECORDING AND REPORTING

- Record respiratory rate and character in nurses' notes or vital sign flow sheet.
- Record abnormal depth and rhythm in narrative form in nurses' notes.
- Document measurement of respiratory rate after administration of specific therapies in narrative form in nurses' notes.
- Indicate type and amount of oxygen therapy if used by patient during assessment. Document respiratory assessment after administration of specific therapies in narrative form in nurses' notes.
- Report abnormal findings to nurse in charge or health care provider immediately.

HOME CARE CONSIDERATIONS

- Assess for environmental factors in the home that influence patient's respiratory rate such as secondhand smoke, poor ventilation, gas or fireplace fumes, dust, and pets.

SKILL 30-4 MEASURING OXYGEN SATURATION (PULSE OXIMETRY)

DELEGATION CONSIDERATIONS

The skill of oxygen saturation measurement can be delegated to nursing assistive personnel (NAP) unless patient is unstable. The nurse instructs the NAP about:
- The frequency, probe location, and patient position for oxygen saturation measurement based on patient condition such as onset of dyspnea, labored breathing, or cyanosis.
- The appropriate sensor site, probe, and patient position for measurement of oxygen saturation.
- Refraining from using pulse oximetry as an assessment of heart rate because oximeter will not detect an irregular pulse.
- Need to immediately report any significant changes or abnormalities and any SpO_2 reading lower than 90% to nurse immediately.

EQUIPMENT

- Oximeter
- Oximeter probe appropriate for patient and recommended by manufacturer
- Acetone or nail polish remover if needed
- Pen, vital sign flow sheet or record form, or patient's electronic medical record

STEP	RATIONALE
ASSESSMENT	
1. Determine need to measure patient's oxygen saturation:	Clinical judgment determines need for assessment.
a. Identify risk factors of decreased oxygen saturation, including acute or chronic compromised respiratory function, recovery from general anesthesia or conscious sedation, traumatic injury to chest wall with or without collapse of underlying lung tissue, ventilator dependence, changes in supplemental oxygen therapy.	Certain conditions place patients at risk for decreased oxygen saturation.
b. Assess for signs and symptoms of alterations in oxygen saturation such as altered respiratory rate, depth, or rhythm; adventitious breath sounds (see Chapter 31); cyanotic appearance of nail beds, lips, mucous membranes, and skin; restlessness, irritability, confusion; reduced level of consciousness; labored or difficult breathing.	Physical signs and symptoms often indicate abnormal oxygen saturation.
2. Assess for factors that normally influence measurement of SpO_2 (see Box 30-8) in addition to oxygen therapy, hemoglobin level, body temperature, and medications such as bronchodilators.	Allows you to accurately assess oxygen saturation variations.

SKILL 30-4 MEASURING OXYGEN SATURATION (PULSE OXIMETRY)—cont'd

STEP	RATIONALE
3. Determine previous baseline SpO_2 (if available) from patient's record.	Baseline information provides basis for comparison and helps in assessment of current status and evaluation of interventions.
4. Determine most appropriate patient-specific site (e.g., finger, earlobe, forehead) for sensor probe placement by measuring capillary refill (see Chapter 31). If capillary refill is greater than 2 seconds, select alternate site.	Sensor requires pulsating vascular bed to identify hemoglobin molecules that absorb emitted light. Changes in SpO_2 are reflected in circulation of finger capillary bed within 30 seconds and capillary bed of earlobe within 5-10 seconds. Forehead sensors are preferred for critically ill patients requiring vasopressors (Nesseler et al., 2012).
a. Site must have adequate local circulation and be free of moisture.	Moisture prevents sensor from detecting SpO_2 levels.
b. Place probe on finger free of polish or artificial nail.	Black or brown nail polish color alters readings (Chan et al., 2013).
c. If tremors are present, use earlobe as site.	Motion artifact is most common cause of inaccurate readings (Chan et al., 2013).
d. If patient is obese, clip-on probe may not fit properly; obtain single-use (tape-on) probe.	
5. Determine if patient has latex allergy.	Do not use adhesive sensors if patient has latex allergy.
PLANNING	
1. Identify patient using two identifiers (e.g., name and birth date or name and medical record number) according to agency policy.	Ensures correct patient. Complies with The Joint Commission standards and improves patient safety (TJC, 2016).
2. Explain purpose of procedure and how you measure oxygen saturation to patient. Instruct patient to breathe normally.	Promotes patient cooperation and increases compliance. Prevents large fluctuations in minute ventilation and possible error in SpO_2 readings.
IMPLEMENTATION	
1. Perform hand hygiene.	Reduces transmission of microorganisms.
2. Position patient comfortably. When using finger as monitoring site, support lower arm.	Ensures probe positioning and decreases motion artifact that interferes with SpO_2 determination.
3. Instruct patient to breathe normally.	Prevents large fluctuations in respiratory rate and depth and possible changes in SpO_2.
4. When using finger as monitoring site, remove fingernail polish on one finger with acetone or polish remover. Acrylic nails without polish do not interfere with SpO_2 determination.	Ensures accurate readings. Nail polish may falsely alter saturation (Chan et al., 2013).
5. Attach sensor probe to monitoring site. Instruct patient that clip-on probe feels like a clothespin on finger but will not hurt.	Pressure spring tension of sensor probe on peripheral digit or earlobe is unexpected.

CLINICAL DECISION: *Do not attach probe to finger, ear, forehead, or bridge of nose if area is edematous or skin integrity is compromised. Do not attach probe to fingers that are hypothermic. Select forehead, ear, or bridge of nose if adult patient has history of peripheral vascular disease. Do not use earlobe and bridge of nose sensors for infants and toddlers because of skin fragility. Do not use disposable adhesive probes if patient has latex allergy. Do not place sensor on same extremity as electronic blood pressure cuff because blood flow to finger is interrupted temporarily when cuff inflates and causes inaccurate readings that trigger alarms.*

STEP	RATIONALE
6. Once sensor is in place, turn on oximeter by activating power. Observe pulse waveform/intensity display and audible beep. Correlate oximeter pulse rate with patient's radial pulse. Differences require reevaluation of oximeter probe placement and may require reassessment of pulse rates.	Pulse waveform/intensity display enables detection of valid pulse or presence of interfering signal. Pitch of audible beep is proportional to SpO_2 value. Double-checking pulse rate ensures oximeter accuracy. Oximeter pulse rate, patient's radial pulse, and apical pulse rate should be the same. Any difference requires reevaluation of oximeter sensor probe placement and reassessment of pulse rates.
7. Leave probe in place until oximeter readout reaches constant value and pulse display reaches full strength during each cardiac cycle. Inform patient that oximeter will alarm if probe falls off or patient moves probe. Read SpO_2 on digital display.	Reading takes 10-30 seconds, depending on site selected.
8. If continuous SpO_2 monitoring is necessary, verify SpO_2 alarm limits and volume, which are preset by manufacturer at low of 85% and high of 100%. Determine limits for SpO_2 and pulse rate alarms on basis of each patient's condition. Verify that alarms are on. Assess skin integrity every 2 hours under sensor probe. Relocate sensor probe at least every 24 hours or more frequently if skin integrity is altered or tissue perfusion compromised.	Alarms are set at appropriate limits and volumes to avoid frightening patients and visitors. Sensor probe tension and sensitivity to disposable sensor probe adhesive cause skin irritation and lead to disruption of skin integrity.
9. Help patient return to comfortable position.	Restores comfort and promotes sense of well-being.
10. Perform hand hygiene.	Reduces transmission of microorganisms.
11. Discuss findings with patient as needed.	Promotes participation in care and understanding of health status.
12. If planning intermittent or spot-checking SpO_2 measurements, remove probe and turn oximeter power off. Store probe in appropriate location.	Batteries will run out if oximeter is left on. Sensor probes are expensive and vulnerable to damage.

STEP	RATIONALE
EVALUATION	
1. Compare SpO_2 readings with patient baseline and acceptable values. Note use of oxygen therapy, which can affect SpO_2.	Comparison reveals presence of abnormality.
2. Correlate SpO_2 with SaO_2 obtained from ABG measurements (see Chapter 42) if available.	Documents reliability of noninvasive assessment.
3. Correlate SpO_2 reading with data obtained from respiratory rate, depth, and rhythm assessment (see Skill 30-3).	Measurements assessing ventilation, perfusion, and diffusion are interrelated.
4. During continuous monitoring assess skin integrity underneath probe at least every 2 hours on basis of patient's peripheral circulation.	Prevents tissue ischemia.

UNEXPECTED OUTCOMES AND RELATED INTERVENTIONS

1. SpO_2 is less than 90%.
   - Verify that oximeter probe is intact and outside light transmission does not influence measurement.
   - Observe for signs and symptoms of decreased oxygenation: anxiety, restlessness, tachycardia, cyanosis.
   - Verify that supplemental oxygen delivery system is delivered as ordered and functioning properly.
   - Observe for and minimize factors that decrease SpO_2 such as lung secretions, increased activity, and hyperthermia.
   - Help patient to a position that maximizes ventilatory effort (e.g., place obese patient in high-Fowler's position).
   - Notify nurse in charge or health care provider immediately.
2. Pulse rate indicated on the oximeter is less than patient's radial or apical pulse.
   - Reposition sensor probe to an alternative site with increased blood flow.
   - Assess patient for signs of altered cardiac output (e.g., decreased blood pressure, cool skin, confusion).

RECORDING AND REPORTING

- Record SpO_2 value on nurses' notes or vital sign flow sheet.
- Indicate type and amount of oxygen therapy used by patient during assessment.
- Record signs and symptoms of oxygen desaturation in nurses' notes.
- Report abnormal findings to nurse in charge or health care provider immediately.
- Document oxygen saturation after administration of specific therapies in narrative form in nurses' notes.
- Record in nurses' notes patient's use of continuous or intermittent pulse oximetry (documents use of equipment for third-party payers).

HOME CARE CONSIDERATIONS

- Pulse oximetry is used in home care to noninvasively monitor oxygen therapy or changes in oxygen therapy.
- Instruct family caregivers to examine oximeter site before applying sensor.
- Instruct family caregivers on procedure to implement when oxygen saturation is not within acceptable values.

SKILL 30-5 MEASURING BLOOD PRESSURE

DELEGATION CONSIDERATIONS

The skill of blood pressure (BP) measurement can be delegated to nursing assistive personnel (NAP) unless the patient is considered unstable. The nurse instructs the NAP about:

- The appropriate times to obtain BP measurements as determined by agency policy, health care provider's order, or patient condition.
- The patient-specific factors related to the patient's history that may alter BP, such as previous surgery or risk for orthostatic hypotension.
- The appropriate limb to use for BP measurement.
- The appropriate size BP cuff to use for designated limb and equipment (electronic or manual).
- When to report any significant changes or abnormalities to the nurse for further assessment.

EQUIPMENT

- Aneroid sphygmomanometer
- Cloth or disposable vinyl pressure cuff of appropriate size for patient's extremity
- Stethoscope
- Alcohol swab
- Pen, vital sign flow sheet or record form, or electronic medical record

STEP	RATIONALE
ASSESSMENT	
1. Determine need to assess patient's BP:	Use clinical judgment to determine need for assessment.
a. Identify risk factors, including: • History of cardiovascular, cerebrovascular or renal disease, diabetes • Circulatory shock (hypovolemic, septic, cardiogenic, or neurogenic) • Acute or chronic pain • Rapid intravenous infusion of fluids or blood products • Increased intracranial pressure • Toxemia of pregnancy	Conditions place patients at risk for BP alteration.

SKILL 30-5 MEASURING BLOOD PRESSURE—cont'd

STEP	RATIONALE
b. Observe for signs and symptoms of BP alterations:	Physical signs and symptoms often indicate alterations in BP.
(1) High BP (hypertension): headache (usually occipital), flushing of face, nosebleed, and fatigue in older adults	High BP is often asymptomatic until pressure is very high.
(2) Low BP (hypotension): dizziness, mental confusion; restlessness; pale, dusky, or cyanotic skin and mucous membranes; cool, mottled skin over extremities	
2. Assess for factors that affect BP (see Table 30-11).	Allows you to ensure that BP measurement is accurate.
3. Determine best site for BP assessment. Avoid applying cuff to an extremity where intravenous fluids are infusing, a peripherally inserted central catheter (PICC) line has been inserted, an arteriovenous shunt or fistula is present, breast or axillary surgery has been performed on that side, or extremity has been traumatized or diseased or requires a cast or bulky bandage. Use lower extremities when brachial arteries are inaccessible.	Inappropriate site selection results in poor amplification of sounds, causing inaccurate readings. Application of pressure from inflated cuff temporarily restricts blood flow and further compromises circulation in extremity that already has impaired blood flow.
4. Determine previous baseline BP (if available) from patient's record.	Allows you to assess for change in condition. Provides comparison with future BP measurements.
5. Determine if patient has latex allergy.	Verify that stethoscope and BP cuff are latex free if patient has latex allergy.
PLANNING	
1. Identify patient using two identifiers (e.g., name and birth date or name and medical record number) according to agency policy.	Ensures correct patient. Complies with The Joint Commission standards and improves patient safety (TJC, 2016).
2. Explain to patient that you will assess BP. Have patient rest at least 5 minutes before measuring BP sitting or lying down; wait 1 minute if patient is standing. When possible, have patient sit in a chair with legs uncrossed (James et al., 2014; NHBPEP, 2003). Ask patient not to speak while measuring BP and breathe normally.	Allows patient to relax and helps to avoid falsely elevated readings. When assessed at rest, BP readings taken at different times are comparable. Talking increases BP readings (Zheng et al., 2012). Deep breath lowers blood pressure.
3. Be sure that patient has not ingested caffeine or smoked 20 to 30 minutes before BP measurement.	Caffeine or nicotine causes false BP elevations. Smoking immediately increases BP and lasts up to 15 minutes; caffeine increases BP up to 3 hours.
4. Help patient to sitting position with legs uncrossed at knees (Adiyaman, 2007) if appropriate. Be sure that room is warm, quiet, and relaxing.	Maintains patient comfort during measurement. Sitting is preferred to lying. Diastolic pressure measured with sitting is approximately 5 mm Hg higher than when measured supine. Patient perceptions of stressful environment affect BP measurement. Talking and background noise result in inaccurate measurements.
5. Select appropriate cuff size.	Improper cuff size results in inaccurate readings (see Table 30-11). If cuff is too small, it tends to come loose when being inflated or results in false-high readings. If cuff is too large, you may obtain false-low readings (Mourad et al., 2013).
IMPLEMENTATION	
1. Perform hand hygiene and clean stethoscope earpieces and diaphragm with alcohol swab.	Reduces transmission of microorganisms.
2. Position patient.	
a. Arm: Position patient sitting or lying; position his or her forearm at heart level (see illustration). Turn palm up. If sitting, instruct patient to keep feet flat on floor without crossing legs. **b.** Thigh: Position patient lying with thigh flat (provide support as needed). Have knee slightly flexed.	If arm is extended and not supported, patient performs isometric exercise that increases diastolic pressure. Placing arm above level of heart causes false-low reading 2 mm Hg for each inch above heart level. Leg crossing falsely increases systolic BP. Even in the supine position a diastolic pressure increases BP up to 3-4 mm Hg for each 5-cm (1.97-in) change in heart level.
3. Expose extremity (arm or leg) fully by removing constricting clothing. Cuff may be placed over shirt sleeve as long as stethoscope rests on skin of antecubital space (Box 30-14).	Ensures proper cuff application. Tight clothing causes congestion of blood and can falsely elevate BP readings.

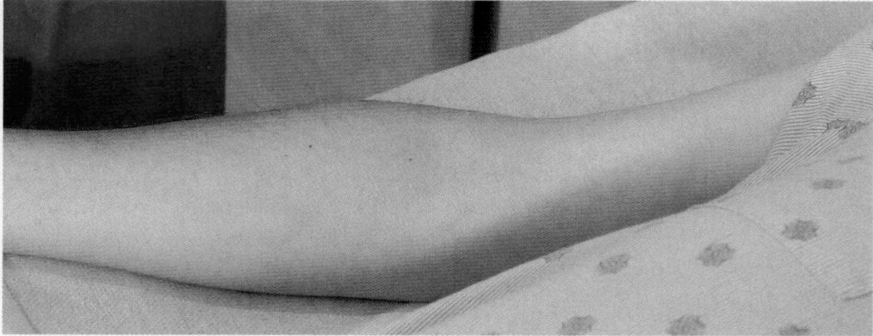

STEP 2a Patient's forearm supported in bed. (Copyright © Mosby's Clinical Skills: Essentials Collection.)

STEP	RATIONALE
4. Palpate brachial artery (arm) (see illustration) or popliteal artery (leg). With cuff fully deflated, apply bladder of cuff above artery by centering arrows marked on cuff over artery. If there are no center arrows on cuff, estimate center of bladder and place it over artery. Position cuff 2.5 cm (1 inch) above site of pulsation (antecubital or popliteal space). Wrap cuff evenly and snugly around extremity (see illustrations).	Inflating bladder directly over artery ensures that proper pressure is applied during inflation. Loose-fitting cuff causes false-high readings.
5. Position manometer gauge vertically at eye level and no farther than 1 m (approximately 1 yard) away.	Looking up or down at scale results in inaccurate readings.
6. Measure BP.	
a. Two-step method	
(1) Relocate brachial or popliteal pulse. Palpate artery distal to cuff with fingertips of nondominant hand while inflating cuff rapidly to pressure 30 mm Hg above point at which pulse disappears. Slowly deflate cuff and note point when pulse reappears. Deflate cuff fully and wait 30 seconds.	Estimating systolic pressure prevents false-low readings. Determine maximal inflation point for accurate reading by palpation. If unable to palpate artery because of weakened pulse, use an ultrasonic stethoscope (see Chapter 31). Completely deflating cuff prevents venous congestion and false-high readings.
(2) Place stethoscope earpieces in ears and be sure that sounds are clear, not muffled.	Each earpiece follows angle of ear canal to facilitate hearing.
(3) Relocate brachial or popliteal artery and place bell or diaphragm chest piece of stethoscope over it. Do not allow chest piece to touch cuff or clothing (see illustration).	Proper stethoscope placement ensures best sound reception. Stethoscope improperly positioned causes muffled sounds that often result in false-low systolic and false-high diastolic readings.
(4) Close valve of pressure bulb clockwise until tight.	Tightening valve prevents air leak during inflation.
(5) Quickly inflate cuff to 30 mm Hg above palpated systolic pressure (patient's estimated systolic pressure) (see illustration).	Rapid inflation ensures accurate measurement of systolic pressure.
(6) Slowly release pressure bulb valve and allow needle of manometer gauge to fall at rate of 2-3 mm Hg/sec. Make sure that there are no extraneous sounds.	Too-rapid or too-slow decline in pressure causes inaccurate readings (Zheng et al., 2011). Noise interferes with precise assessment of sounds.
(7) Note point on manometer when you hear first clear sound. Sound slowly increases in intensity.	First sound reflects systolic BP.

BOX 30-14 EVIDENCE-BASED PRACTICE

Effect of Clothes on Blood Pressure Measurements

PICO Question: Does placing the blood pressure cuff over clothes compared to a bare arm effect blood pressure measurement?

Evidence Summary

Obtaining blood pressure measurements has traditionally required exposing a bare upper arm either by rolling up the shirt sleeve or removing upper garments. Sleeve rolling has the potential to constrict the underlying vessels. Some patients may be uncomfortable disrobing, which lacks dignity and privacy and can infringe on religious beliefs. Most cotton shirts are less than 2 mm thick and provide little resistance to the pressure generated by an inflated blood pressure cuff. A study obtained two manual auscultatory blood pressure readings on a nonsleeved arm, sleeved arm, and again on a nonsleeved arm of 258 hypertensive patients (Pinar et al., 2010). There was no significant difference among the six measurements. A similar study (Ki et al., 2013) compared sleeved, rolled sleeve, and bare arm blood pressure measurements using an automatic oscillometric sphygmomanometer on 141 clinic patients. There was no difference among the groups in systolic or diastolic measurements.

Application to Nursing Practice

- Blood pressure cuffs applied over sleeves will save time during routine blood pressure screenings and disasters.
- Allowing the patient to remain robed can provide culturally congruent care in some settings.
- Consider patient privacy and cultural beliefs when repositioning clothing for blood pressure measurement.

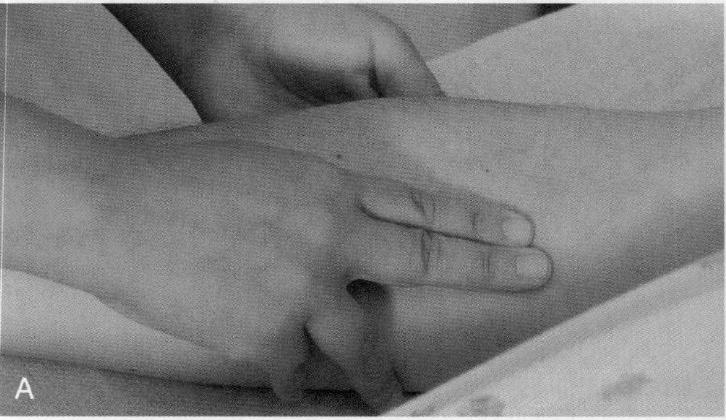

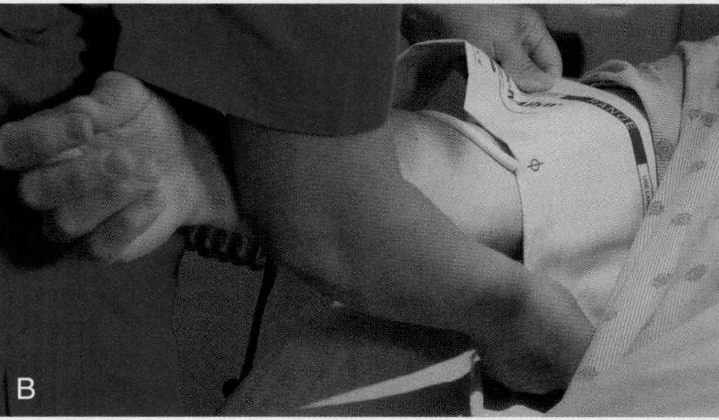

STEP 4 A, Palpate the brachial artery. **B,** Align blood pressure cuff arrow with the brachial artery. (Copyright © Mosby's Clinical Skills: Essentials Collection.)

SKILL 30-5 MEASURING BLOOD PRESSURE—cont'd

STEP	RATIONALE
(8) Continue to deflate cuff, noting point at which muffled or dampened sound appears.	Fourth sound involves distinct muffling of sounds and is an indicator of diastolic pressure in children (Kaplan et al., 2014).
(9) Continue to deflate cuff gradually, noting point at which sound disappears in adults. Listen for 10-20 mm Hg after last sound and allow remaining air to escape quickly.	Beginning of fifth sound is indicator of diastolic pressure in adults (Kaplan et al., 2014). Continuous cuff inflation causes arterial occlusion, resulting in numbness and tingling of patient's arm.
b. **One-step method**	
(1) Place stethoscope earpieces in ears and be sure that sounds are clear, not muffled.	Each earpiece follows angle of ear canal to facilitate hearing.
(2) Relocate brachial or popliteal artery and place bell or diaphragm chest piece of stethoscope over it. Do not allow chest piece to touch cuff or clothing.	Proper stethoscope placement ensures optimal sound reception. Stethoscope improperly positioned causes muffled sounds that result in false-low systolic and false-high diastolic readings.
(3) Close valve of pressure bulb clockwise until tight.	Tightening of valve prevents air leak during inflation.
(4) Quickly inflate cuff to 30 mm Hg above patient's usual systolic pressure.	Inflation above systolic level ensures accurate measurement of systolic BP.
(5) Slowly release pressure bulb valve and allow needle of manometer gauge to fall at rate of 2 to 3 mm Hg/sec.	Too-rapid or too-slow decline in pressure causes inaccurate readings (Zheng et al., 2011).
(6) Note point on manometer when you hear first clear sound. Sound slowly increases in intensity.	First sound reflects systolic pressure.
(7) Continue to deflate cuff, noting point at which muffled or dampened sound appears.	In children fourth sound involves distinct muffling of sounds and indicates diastolic pressure (Hockenberry and Wilson, 2015).
(8) While gradually deflating cuff, note point at which sound disappears in adults. Listen for 10 to 20 mm Hg after last sound and allow remaining air to escape quickly.	Beginning of last or fifth sound indicates diastolic pressure in adults. Continuous cuff inflation causes arterial occlusion, resulting in numbness and tingling of patient's arm.
7. American Heart Association recommends average of two sets of BP measurement, 2 minutes apart. Use second set of BP measurements as baseline. If readings are different by more than 5 mm Hg, additional readings are necessary.	Two sets of BP measurements help to prevent false-positives based on patient's sympathetic response (alert reaction). Averaging minimizes effect of anxiety, which often causes first reading to be higher than subsequent measurements (Kaplan et al., 2014).
8. Remove cuff from extremity unless you need to repeat measurement. If this is first assessment of patient, repeat BP assessment on other extremity.	Comparison of BP in both extremities detects circulation problems. (Normal difference of 5-10 mm Hg exists between extremities.) Use arm with higher pressure for repeated measurements (Frese et al., 2011).
9. Help patient return to comfortable position and cover upper arm if previously clothed.	Restores comfort and promotes sense of well-being.
10. Discuss findings with patient as needed.	Promotes participation in care and understanding of health status.
11. Perform hand hygiene. Wipe cuff with facility-approved cleaning agent if used between patients.	Reduces transmission of microorganisms.

EVALUATION

1. Compare reading with previous baseline and/or acceptable value of BP for patient's age.	Evaluates for change in condition and cardiovascular alterations.
2. Compare BP in both arms or both legs.	If using upper extremities, use arm with higher pressure for subsequent assessments unless contraindicated.
3. Correlate BP with data obtained from pulse assessment and related cardiovascular signs and symptoms.	BP and heart rate are interrelated.

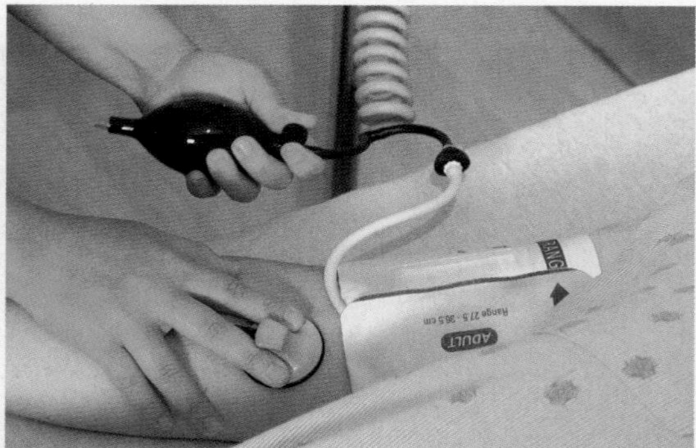

STEP 6a(3) Stethoscope over brachial artery to measure BP. (Copyright © Mosby's Clinical Skills: Essentials Collection.)

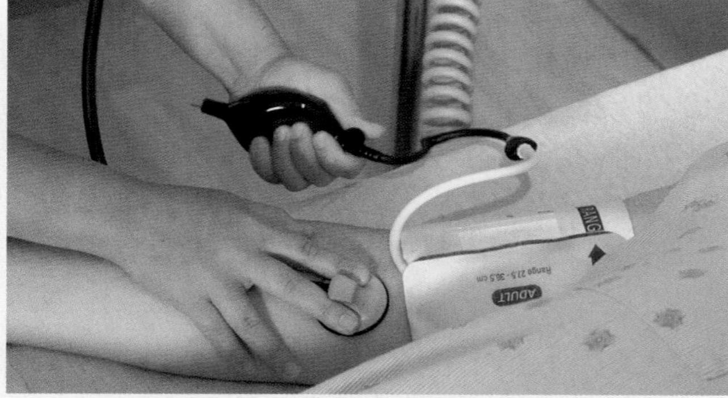

STEP 6a(5) Inflating BP cuff. (Copyright © Mosby's Clinical Skills: Essentials Collection.)

UNEXPECTED OUTCOMES AND RELATED INTERVENTIONS

1. Unable to obtain BP reading
   - Determine that no immediate crisis is present by obtaining pulse and respiratory rate.
   - Assess for signs of decreased cardiac output; if present, notify nurse in charge or health care provider immediately.
   - Use alternative sites or procedures to obtain BP: auscultate BP in lower extremity, use a Doppler ultrasonic instrument, implement palpation method to obtain systolic BP.
   - Repeat BP measurement with sphygmomanometer. Electronic BP devices are less accurate in low–blood flow conditions.
2. BP is not sufficient for adequate perfusion and oxygenation of tissues.
   - Compare BP value to baseline. A systolic reading of 90 mm Hg is an acceptable value for some patients.
   - Position patient in supine position to enhance circulation and restrict activity if it is decreasing BP.
   - Assess for signs and symptoms of hypotension such as tachycardia; weak, thready pulse; weakness, dizziness, confusion; cool, pale, dusky or cyanotic skin.
   - Notify nurse in charge or health care provider immediately.
   - Increase rate of intravenous infusion or administer vasoconstricting drugs if ordered.
3. BP is above acceptable range.
   - Repeat BP measurement in other arm and compare findings. Verify correct size and placement of cuff.
   - Ask nurse colleague to repeat measurement in 1 to 2 minutes.
   - Observe for related symptoms, although symptoms are sometimes not apparent until BP is extremely elevated.
   - Report elevated BP to nurse in charge or health care provider to initiate appropriate evaluation and treatment.
   - Administer antihypertensive medications as ordered.
4. Patient has a difference of more than 20 mm Hg systolic or diastolic when comparing BP measurements on upper extremities.
   - Report abnormal findings to nurse in charge or health care provider.

RECORDING AND REPORTING

- Record BP in nurses' notes or vital sign flow sheet. BP measurement after administration of specific therapies needs to be documented in narrative form in nurses' notes.
- Record any signs or symptoms of BP alterations in narrative form in nurses' notes.
- Document measurement of BP after administration of specific therapies in narrative form in nurses' notes.
- Report abnormal findings to nurse in charge or health care provider immediately.

HOME CARE CONSIDERATIONS

- Assess home noise level to determine room that provides most quiet environment for assessing BP.
- Consider electronic BP cuff for home if patient has hearing difficulties, sufficient financial resources, and adequate dexterity.

KEY POINTS

- Measurement of vital signs includes the physiological measurement of temperature, pulse, BP, respirations, and oxygen saturation.
- Nurses measure vital signs as part of a complete physical examination or in a review of a patient's condition.
- Nurses assess changes in vital signs with other physical assessment findings, using clinical judgment to determine measurement frequency.
- Knowledge of the factors influencing vital signs helps to determine and evaluate abnormal values.
- Vital signs provide a basis for evaluating response to nursing interventions.
- Measure vital signs when the patient is inactive and the environment is controlled for comfort.
- Nurses help patients maintain body temperature by initiating interventions that promote heat loss, production, or conservation.
- A fever is one of the normal defense mechanisms of the body.
- Measurement of temperature using the temporal artery is the least invasive, most accurate method of obtaining core temperature.
- Respiratory assessment includes determining the effectiveness of ventilation, perfusion, and diffusion.
- Assessment of respiration involves observing ventilatory movements through the respiratory cycle.
- Variables affecting ventilation, perfusion, and diffusion influence oxygen saturation.
- To assess cardiac function, it is easy to measure pulse rate and rhythm using the radial or apical pulses.
- Hypertension is diagnosed only after an average of readings made during two or more subsequent visits reveals an elevated BP.
- Improper selection and application of the BP measurement cuff result in errors in BP measurement.
- Changes in one vital sign often influence characteristics of the other vital signs.

CLINICAL APPLICATION QUESTIONS

Preparing for Clinical Practice

Mr. Coburn, the 56-year-old school teacher who was seen earlier in the week for hyperthermia, arrives at the walk-in health center complaining of feeling dizzy and nauseated. You immediately note that he appears to be having some difficulty catching his breath during coughing spells. A new graduate nurse takes Mr. Coburn's admitting vital signs as: pulse 122 and regular, RR 22 and easy, BP 88/50 RA, tympanic temperature 38° C (100.4° F), SpO_2 92%. As you enter Mr. Coburn's room, the electronic blood pressure (BP) machine alarm is sounding with cuff on right arm. You note that it is flashing "72 systolic" with no diastolic reading. Mr. Coburn is turned on his right side, and his eyes are closed. His respirations appear labored.

1. List in order of priority your first five interventions.
2. Which vital signs should you reassess and which methods should you use?
3. Which hourly vital signs should you delegate to a nursing assistive personnel (NAP)?

ⓔ ***Answers to Clinical Application Questions can be found on the Evolve website.***

REVIEW QUESTIONS

Are You Ready to Test Your Nursing Knowledge?

1. A 52-year-old woman is admitted with dyspnea and discomfort in her left chest with deep breaths. She has smoked for 35 years and recently lost over 10 lbs. Her vital signs on admission are: HR 112, BP 138/82, RR 22, tympanic temperature 36.8° C (98.2° F), and oxygen saturation 94%. She is receiving oxygen at 2 L via a nasal cannula. Which vital sign reflects a positive outcome of the oxygen therapy?
   1. Temperature: 37° C (98.6° F)
   2. Radial pulse: 112
   3. Respiratory rate: 24
   4. Oxygen saturation: 96%
   5. Blood pressure: 134/78
2. The licensed practical nurse (LPN) provides you with the change-of-shift vital signs on four of your patients. Which patient do you need to assess first?
   1. 84-year-old man recently admitted with pneumonia, RR 28, SpO_2 89%
   2. 54-year-old woman admitted after surgery for fractured arm, BP 160/86 mm Hg, HR 72
   3. 63-year-old man with venous ulcers from diabetes, temperature 37.3° C (99.1° F), HR 84
   4. 77-year-old woman with left mastectomy 2 days ago, RR 22, BP 148/62
3. A 55-year-old female patient was in a motor vehicle accident and is admitted to a surgical unit after repair of a fractured left arm and left leg. She also has a laceration on her forehead. An intravenous (IV) line is infusing in the right antecubital fossa, and pneumatic compression stockings are on the right lower leg. She is receiving oxygen via a simple face mask. Which sites do you instruct the nursing assistant to use for obtaining the patient's blood pressure and temperature?
   1. Right antecubital and tympanic membrane
   2. Right popliteal and rectal
   3. Left antecubital and oral
   4. Left popliteal and temporal artery
4. The nurse observes a nursing student taking a blood pressure (BP) on a patient. The nurse notes that the student very slowly deflates the cuff in an attempt to hear the sounds. The patient's BP range over the past 24 hours is 132/64 to 126/72 mm Hg. Which of the following BP readings made by the student is most likely caused by an incorrect technique?
   1. 96/40 mm Hg
   2. 110/66 mm Hg
   3. 130/90 mm Hg
   4. 156/82 mm Hg
5. As you are obtaining the oxygen saturation on a 19-year-old college student with severe asthma, you note that she has black nail polish on her nails. You remove the polish from one nail, and she asks you why her nail polish had to be removed. What is the best response?
   1. Nail polish attracts microorganisms and contaminates the finger sensor.
   2. Nail polish increases oxygen saturation.
   3. Nail polish interferes with sensor function.
   4. Nail polish creates excessive heat in sensor probe.
6. A patient has been hospitalized for the past 48 hours with a fever of unknown origin. His medical record indicates tympanic temperatures of 38.7° C (101.6° F) (0400), 36.6° C (97.9° F) (0800), 36.9° C (98.4° F) (1200), 37.6° C (99.6° F) (1600), and 38.3° C (100.9° F) (2000). How would you describe this pattern of temperature measurements?
   1. Usual range of circadian rhythm measurements
   2. Sustained fever pattern
   3. Intermittent fever pattern
   4. Resolving fever pattern
7. A patient presents in the clinic with dizziness and fatigue. The nursing assistant reports a slow but regular radial pulse of 44. What is your priority intervention?
   1. Request that the nursing assistant repeat the pulse check
   2. Call for a stat electrocardiogram (ECG)
   3. Assess the patient's apical pulse and evidence of a pulse deficit
   4. Prepare to administer cardiac-stimulating medications
8. Which patient is at highest risk for tachycardia?
   1. A healthy basketball player during warmup exercises
   2. A patient admitted with hypothermia
   3. A patient with a fever of 39.4° C (103° F)
   4. A 90-year-old male taking beta blockers
9. Which of the following patients are at most risk for tachypnea? (Select all that apply.)
   1. Patient just admitted with four rib fractures
   2. Woman who is 9 months' pregnant
   3. Adult who has consumed alcoholic beverages
   4. Adolescent waking from sleep
   5. Three-pack–per-day smoker with pneumonia
10. Which number marks the location where you would auscultate the point of maximal impulse (PMI)?
    1. 1
    2. 2
    3. 3
    4. 4
    5. 5
    6. 6

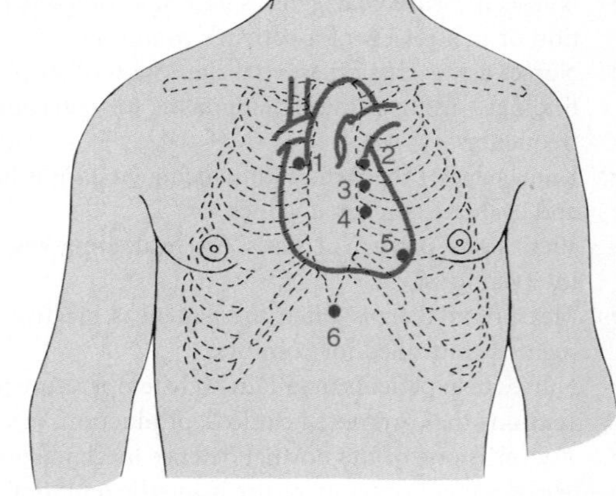

11. A patient has been admitted for a cerebrovascular accident (stroke). She cannot move her right arm, and she has a right-sided facial droop. She is able to eat with her dentures in place and

swallow safely. The nursing assistive personnel (NAP) reports to you that the patient will not keep the oral thermometer probe in her mouth. What direction do you provide to the NAP?
1. Direct the NAP to hold the thermometer in place with her gloved hand
2. Direct the NAP to switch the thermometer probe to the left sublingual pocket
3. Direct the NAP to obtain a right tympanic temperature
4. Direct the NAP to use a temporal artery thermometer from right to left

12. The nursing assistive personnel (NAP) reports to you that the blood pressure (BP) of the patient in Question 11 is 140/76 on the left arm and 128/72 on the right arm. What actions do you take on the basis of this information? (Select all that apply.)
    1. Notify the health care provider immediately
    2. Repeat the measurements on both arms using a stethoscope
    3. Ask the patient if she has taken her blood pressure medications recently
    4. Obtain blood pressure measurements on lower extremities
    5. Verify that the correct cuff size was used during the measurements
    6. Review the patient's record for her baseline vital signs
    7. Compare right and left radial pulses for strength
13. The nursing assistive personnel (NAP) informs you that the electronic blood pressure machine on the patient who has recently returned from surgery following removal of her gallbladder is flashing a blood pressure of 65/46 and alarming. Place your care activities in priority order.
    1. Press the start button of the electronic blood pressure machine to obtain a new reading.
    2. Obtain a manual blood pressure with a stethoscope.
    3. Check the patient's pulse distal to the blood pressure cuff.
    4. Assess the patient's mental status.
    5. Remind the patient not to bend her arm with the blood pressure cuff.
14. A healthy adult patient tells the nurse that he obtained his blood pressure in "one of those quick machines in the mall" and was alarmed that it was 152/72 when his normal value ranges from 114/72 to 118/78. The nurse obtains a blood pressure of 116/76. What would account for the blood pressure of 152/92? (Select all that apply.)
    1. Cuff too small
    2. Arm positioned above heart level
    3. Slow inflation of the cuff by the machine
    4. Patient did not remove his long-sleeved shirt
    5. Insufficient time between measurements
15. A patient is admitted for dehydration caused by pneumonia and shortness of breath. He has a history of heart disease and cardiac dysrhythmias. The nursing assistant reports his admitting vital signs to the nurse. Which measurements should the nurse reassess? (Select all that apply.)
    1. Right arm BP: 118/72
    2. Radial pulse rate: 72 and irregular
    3. Temporal temperature: 37.4°C (99.3°F)
    4. Respiratory rate: 28
    5. Oxygen saturation: 99%

Answers: 1. 4; **2.** 1; **3.** 1; **4.** 3; **5.** 3; **6.** 3; **7.** 3; **8.** 3; **9.** 1, 2, 5; **10.** 5; **11.** 4; **12.** 2, 6; **13.** 4, 1, 3, 2, 5; **14.** 1, 5; **15.** 2, 4, 5.

Rationales for Review Questions can be found on the Evolve website.

REFERENCES

Frese EM, et al: Blood pressure measurement guidelines for physical therapists, *Cardiopulmon Phys Ther J* 22(2):5, 2011.

Goforth CW, Kazman JB: Exertional heat stroke in Navy and Marine personnel: a hot topic, *Crit Care Nurse* 35(1):52, 2015.

Hockenberry MJ, Wilson D: *Wong's nursing care of infants and children*, ed 10, St Louis, 2015, Mosby.

James P, et al: 2014 Evidence-based guideline for the management of high blood pressure in adults: report from the panel members appointed to the Eighth Joint National Committee (JNC8), *JAMA* 311:507, 2014.

Kaplan N, et al: *Overview of hypertension in adults*, *UpToDate*, 2014. http://www.uptodate.com/contents/overview-of-hypertension-in-adults. Accessed June 10, 2015.

Lehne R: *Pharmacology for nursing care*, ed 8, Philadelphia, 2013, Elsevier.

National High Blood Pressure Education Program (NHBPEP): National Heart, Lung, and Blood Institute; National Institutes of Health (NIH): The seventh report of the Joint National Committee on Detection, Evaluation, and Treatment of High Blood Pressure, *JAMA* 289(19):2560, 2003.

Pagana KD, Pagana TJ: *Mosby's diagnostic and laboratory test reference*, ed 12, St Louis, 2015, Mosby.

Parkes R: Rate of respiration: the forgotten vital sign, *Emerg Nurse* 19:12, 2011.

Shibao C, et al: Evaluation and treatment of orthostatic hypotension, *J Am Soc Hypertens* 7:317, 2013.

The Joint Commission (TJC): *2016 National Patient Safety Goals*, Oakbrook Terrace, IL, 2016, The Commission. Available at http://www.jointcommission.org/standards_information/npsgs.aspx. Accessed November 2015.

Touhy TA, Jett KF: *Ebersole and Hess' Gerontological nursing & healthy aging*, ed 4, 2014, Mosby.

World Health Organization (WHO): *WHO pulse oximetry training manual*, ©2011. http://www.who.int/patientsafety/safesurgery/pulse_oximetry/who_ps_pulse_oxymetry_training_manual_en.pdf. Accessed June 10, 2015.

RESEARCH REFERENCES

Adiyaman A: The effect of crossing legs on blood pressure, *Blood Press Monit* 12(3):189, 2007.

Angelousi A, et al: Association between orthostatic hypotension and cardiovascular risk, cerebrovascular risk, cognitive decline and falls, as well as overall mortality: a systematic review and meta-analysis, *J Hypertens* 32:1562, 2014.

Chan E, et al: Pulse oximetry: understanding its basic principles facilitates appreciation of its limitations, *Respir Med* 107:789, 2013.

Charafeddine L, et al: Axillary and rectal thermometry in the newborn: Do they agree? *BMC Res Notes* 31(7):584, 2014.

Counts D, et al: Evaluation of temporal artery and disposable digital oral thermometers in acutely ill patients, *Medsurg Nurs* 23(4):239, 2014.

Haugan B, et al: Can we trust the new generation of infrared tympanic thermometers in clinical practice? *J Clin Nurs* 22:698, 2012.

Ki J, et al: Differences in blood pressure measurements obtained using an automatic oscillometric sphygmomanometer depending on clothes-wearing status, *Korean J Fam Med* 34:145, 2013.

Lu S, et al: A systematic review of body temperature variations in older people, *J Clin Nurs* 19:4, 2010.

Mourad J, et al: Impact of miscuffing during home blood pressure measurement on the prevalence of masked hypertension, *Am J Hypertens* 26:1205, 2013.

Nesseler N, et al: Pulse oximetry and high-dose vasopressors: a comparison between forehead reflectance and finger transmission sensors, *Intensive Care Med* 38:1718, 2012.

Ozdemir H, et al: A comparison of different methods of temperature measurements in sick newborns, *J Trop Pediatr* 57:418, 2011.

Pinar R, et al: The effect of clothes on sphygmomanometric blood pressure measurement in hypertensive patients, *J Clin Nurs* 19:1861, 2010.

Reynolds M, et al: Are temporal artery temperatures accurate enough to replace rectal temperature measurement in pediatric ED patients? *J Emerg Nurs* 40:46, 2014.

Rowland T: Fluid replacement requirements for child athletes, *Sports Med* 41:279, 2011.

Schey BM, et al: Skin temperature and core-peripheral temperature gradient as markers of hemodynamic status in crucially ill patients: a review, *Heart Lung* 39(1):27, 2010.

Schimanski K, et al: Comparison study of upper arm and forearm non-invasive blood pressures in adult emergency department patients, *Int J Nurs Studies* 51(12):1575, 2014.

Skirton H, et al: A systematic review of variability and reliability of manual and automated blood pressure readings, *J Clin Nurs* 20:614, 2011.

Suokhrie L, et al: Differences in automated and manual blood pressure measurement in hospitalized psychiatric patients, *J Psychosoc Nurs* 51(3):32, 2013.

Yont GH, et al: Comparison of oxygen saturation values and measurement times by pulse oximetry in various parts of the body, *Appl Nurs Res* 24(4):e39, 2011.

Zheng D, et al: How important is the recommended slow cuff pressure deflation rate for blood pressure measurement? *Ann Biomed Eng* 39:2584, 2011.

Zheng D, et al: Effect of respiration, talking and small body movements on blood pressure measurement, *J Human Hypertens* 26:458, 2012.

31

Health Assessment and Physical Examination

OBJECTIVES

- Discuss the purposes of physical assessment.
- Discuss how cultural diversity influences a nurse's approach to and findings from a health assessment.
- List techniques for preparing a patient physically and psychologically before and during an examination.
- Describe interview techniques used to enhance communication during history taking.
- Make environmental preparations before an examination.
- Identify data to collect from the nursing history before an examination.
- Demonstrate the techniques used with each physical assessment skill.
- Discuss normal physical findings in a young, middle-age, and older adult.
- Discuss ways to incorporate health promotion and health teaching into an examination.
- Identify ways to use physical assessment skills during routine nursing care.
- Describe physical measurements made in assessing each body system.
- Identify self-screening examinations commonly performed by patients.
- Identify preventive screenings and the appropriate age(s) for each screening to occur.

KEY TERMS

Adventitious sounds, p. 570
Alopecia, p. 549
Aphasia, p. 601
Apical impulse or point of maximal impulse (PMI), p. 572
Arcus senilis, p. 556
Atrophied, p. 598
Auscultation, p. 540
Borborygmi, p. 588
Bruit, p. 576
Cerumen, p. 558
Clubbing, p. 578
Conjunctivitis, p. 556
Cyanosis, p. 546
Distention, p. 587
Dysrhythmia, p. 574
Ectropion, p. 555
Edema, p. 547
Entropion, p. 555
Erythema, p. 547
Excoriation, p. 561
Goniometer, p. 596
Hypertonicity, p. 596
Hypotonicity, p. 598
Indurated, p. 547
Inspection, p. 539
Integumentary system, p. 544
Jaundice, p. 546
Kyphosis, p. 595
Lordosis, p. 595
Malignancy, p. 564
Murmurs, p. 574
Nystagmus, p. 555
Olfaction, p. 539
Orthopnea, p. 568
Osteoporosis, p. 595
Ototoxicity, p. 559
Palpation, p. 539
Percussion, p. 540
Peristalsis, p. 588
PERRLA, p. 556
Petechiae, p. 547
Pigmentation, p. 546
Polyps, p. 561
Ptosis, p. 555
Scoliosis, p. 595
Stenosis, p. 575
Striae, p. 587
Syncope, p. 575
Thrill, p. 574
Turgor, p. 547
Ventricular gallop, p. 574
Vocal or tactile fremitus, p. 569

MEDIA RESOURCES

http://evolve.elsevier.com/Potter/fundamentals/

- Review Questions
- Video Clips
- Case Study with Questions
- Audio Glossary
- Content Updates

The health assessment and physical examination are important steps toward providing safe and competent nursing care. As a nurse, you are in a unique position to determine each patient's current health status, distinguish variations from the norm, and recognize improvements or deterioration in his or her condition. As a nurse you must be able to recognize and interpret each patient's behavioral and physical presentation. By performing health assessments and physical examinations, you identify health patterns and evaluate each patient's response to treatments and therapies.

Nurses gather assessment data about patients' past and current health conditions in a variety of ways, using a comprehensive or focused approach, depending on the patient situation. Assessments are performed at health fairs, at screening clinics, in a health provider's office, in acute care agencies, or in patients' homes. Depending on the outcome of an assessment, a nurse considers evidence-based recommendations for care on the basis of a patient's values, the health provider's clinical expertise, or own personal experience.

A complete health assessment involves a nursing history (see Chapter 16) and behavioral and physical examination. Through the health history interview you gather subjective data about a patient's condition. You obtain objective data while observing a patient's behavior and overall presentation. You identify additional objective data through a head-to-toe body system review during the physical examination. Your clinical judgments are made on the basis of all of the gathered data to create a plan of care for each situation. With accurate data you create a patient-centered care plan, identifying the nursing diagnoses, desired patient outcomes, and nursing interventions. Continuity in health care improves when you evaluate a patient by making ongoing, objective, and comprehensive assessments.

PURPOSES OF THE PHYSICAL EXAMINATION

A physical examination is conducted as an initial evaluation in triage for emergency care; for routine screening to promote wellness behaviors and preventive health care measures; to determine eligibility for health insurance, military service, or a new job; or to admit a patient to a hospital or long-term care facility. After considering a patient's current condition, a nurse selects a focused physical examination on a specific system or area. For example, when a patient is having a severe asthma episode, the nurse first focuses on the pulmonary and cardiovascular systems so treatments can begin immediately. When the patient is no longer at risk for a bad outcome or injury, the nurse performs a more comprehensive examination of other body systems.

For patients who are hospitalized, a nurse integrates the collection of physical assessment data during routine patient care, validating findings with what is known about the patient's health history. For example, on entering a patient's room a nurse may notice behavioral patient cues that indicate comfort, anxiety, or sadness; assess the skin during the bed bath; or assess physical movements and swallowing abilities while administering medications. Use physical examination to do the following:

- Gather baseline data about the patient's health status.
- Supplement, confirm, or refute subjective data obtained in the nursing history.
- Identify and confirm nursing diagnoses.
- Make clinical decisions about a patient's changing health status and management.
- Evaluate the outcomes of care.

Cultural Sensitivity

Respect the cultural differences among patients from a variety of backgrounds when completing an examination. It is important to remember that cultural differences influence patient behaviors. Consider the patient's health beliefs, use of alternative therapies, nutrition habits, relationships with family, and comfort with physical closeness during the examination and history. These factors will affect both your approach and the type of findings you might expect.

Be culturally aware and avoid stereotyping on the basis of gender, race, education or other cultural factors. There is a difference between cultural and physical characteristics. Learn to recognize common characteristics and disorders among members of ethnic populations within the community. It is equally important to recognize variations in physical characteristics such as in the skin and musculoskeletal system, which are related to racial variables. Consider the patient's cultural beliefs as you assess how the person receives, processes, and understands health care information and how he or she makes health care decisions (Ingram, 2012). By recognizing cultural diversity, you show respect for each patient's uniqueness, leading to higher-quality care and improved clinical outcomes (see Chapter 9).

PREPARATION FOR EXAMINATION

Physical examination is a routine part of a nurse's patient assessment. In many care settings a head-to-toe physical assessment is required daily. You perform a reassessment when a patient's condition changes as it improves or worsens. In some health care settings such as during a home health visit a focused physical examination is preferred. Proper preparation of the environment, equipment, and patient ensures a smooth physical examination with few interruptions. A disorganized approach causes errors and incomplete findings. Safety for confused patients should be a priority; never leave a confused or combative patient alone during an examination.

Infection Control

Some patients present with open skin lesions, infected wounds, or other communicable diseases. Use standard precautions throughout an examination (see Chapter 29). When an open sore or microorganism is present, wear gloves to reduce contact with contaminants. If a patient has excessive drainage or there is a risk of splattering from a wound, additional personal protective equipment such as an isolation gown or eye shield should be used. Follow agency hand hygiene policies before initiating and after completing a physical assessment.

Although most health care agencies make nonlatex gloves available, it is your responsibility to identify latex allergies in patients and use equipment items that are latex free. By recognizing risk factors for latex allergies, patients remain free of a natural rubber latex (NRL) allergy response. Two types of allergic responses appear with NRL. The most immediate is an immunological reaction type 1 response, for which the body develops antibodies known as *immunoglobulin E* that can lead to an anaphylactic response. Atopy occurs when there is an increased tendency for the body to form antibodies as a result of the immune response. The second is the allergic contact dermatitis type 4 response, which causes a delayed reaction that appears 12 to 48 hours after exposure (Huether and McCance, 2012). Both require prior exposure to the substance to which the body reacts. The severity of the response varies among individuals. Table 31-1 provides a short list of products that contain latex and suggests available alternatives.

Environment

A respectful, considerate physical examination requires privacy. In the acute setting nurses perform assessments in a patient's room. Examination rooms are used in clinics or office settings. In the home the examination is performed in a space where privacy can be established such as the patient's bedroom.

Examination spaces need to be well equipped for any procedures. Adequate lighting is necessary to properly illuminate body parts. The hospital patient room can be secured for privacy so patients are comfortable discussing their condition. Eliminate extra noise and take precautions to prevent interruptions from others. The room must be warm enough to maintain comfort.

Depending on the body part being assessed, it may be difficult to perform a selected assessment skill when a patient is in bed or on a stretcher. Special examination tables make positioning easier and body areas more easily accessible. By helping patients on and off

TABLE 31-1 Products Containing Latex and Nonlatex Substitutes*

Products Containing Latex	Nonlatex Substitutes
Medical Equipment	
Disposable gloves	Vinyl, nitrile, or neoprene gloves
Blood pressure cuffs	Covered cuffs
Stethoscope tubing	Covered tubing
Intravenous injection ports	Needleless system, stopcocks, covered latex ports
Tourniquets	Latex-free or cloth-covered tourniquets
Syringes	Glass syringes
Adhesive tape	Nonlatex tapes
Oral and nasal airways	Nonlatex tubes
Endotracheal tubes	Hard plastic tubes
Catheters	Silicone catheters
Eye goggles	Silicone eye goggles
Anesthesia masks	Silicone masks
Respirators	Nonlatex respirators
Rubber aprons	Cloth-covered aprons
Wound drains	Silicone drains
Medication vial stoppers	Stoppers removed
Household Items	
Rubber bands	String; latex-free bands
Erasers	Silicone erasers
Motorcycle and bicycle handgrips	Handgrips removed or covered
Carpeting	Other types of flooring
Swimming goggles	Silicone construction
Shoe soles	Leather shoes
Expandable fabric (e.g., waistbands)	Fabric removed or covered
Dishwashing gloves	Vinyl gloves
Condoms	Nonlatex condoms
Diaphragms	Synthetic rubber diaphragms
Balloons	Mylar balloons
Pacifiers and baby bottle nipples	Silicone, plastic, or nonlatex pacifiers and nipples

Modified from American Latex Allergy Association: *Literature review on latex-food cross-reactivity, 1991-2006*, 2011, http://latexallergyresources.org/sites/default/files/attachments/Latex-food%20cross-reactivity%20review.pdf. Accessed November 13, 2014; and Seidel HM et al: *Mosby's guide to physical examination*, ed 8, St Louis, 2015, Mosby;

*This list is intended to provide examples of products and alternatives. It is not complete.

examination tables, injury can be avoided, and falls prevented. Examination tables can be uncomfortable; elevate the head of the table about 30 degrees. A small pillow helps with head and neck comfort. If the examination is completed in the patient room, raise the patient's bed to be able to reach him or her more easily.

BOX 31-1 Equipment and Supplies for Physical Assessment

- Cervical brush or broom devices (if needed)
- Cotton applicators
- Disposable pad/paper towels
- Drapes/cover
- Eye chart (e.g., Snellen chart)
- Flashlight and spotlight
- Forms (e.g., physical, laboratory)
- Nonlatex gloves (clean)
- Gown for patient
- Ophthalmoscope
- Otoscope
- Papanicolaou (Pap) liquid preparation (if needed)
- Percussion (reflex) hammer
- Pulse oximeter
- Ruler
- Scale with height measurement rod
- Specimen containers, slides, wooden or plastic spatula, and cytological fixative (if needed)
- Sphygmomanometer and cuff
- Sterile swabs
- Stethoscope
- Tape measure
- Thermometer
- Tissues
- Tongue depressors
- Tuning fork
- Vaginal speculum (if needed)
- Water-soluble lubricant
- Watch with second hand or digital display

Equipment

Perform hand hygiene thoroughly before handling equipment and starting an examination. Arrange any necessary equipment so it is readily available and easy to use. Prepare equipment as appropriate (e.g., warm the diaphragm of the stethoscope between the hands before applying it to the skin). Be sure that equipment functions properly before using it (e.g., ensure that the ophthalmoscope and otoscope have good batteries and light bulbs). Box 31-1 lists typical equipment used during a physical examination.

Physical Preparation of the Patient

To show respect for a patient, ensure that physical comfort needs are met. Before starting, ask if the patient needs to use the restroom. An empty bladder and bowel facilitate examination of the abdomen, genitalia, and rectum. You will collect urine or fecal specimens at this time if needed.

Physical preparation involves making certain that patient privacy is maintained with proper dress and draping. The patient in the hospital likely is wearing only a simple gown. In the clinic or health care provider's office the patient needs to undress and usually is provided a disposable paper cover or paper gown. If the examination is limited to certain body systems, it is not always necessary for the patient to undress completely. Provide the patient privacy and plenty of time to undress to avoid embarrassment. After changing into the recommended gown or cover, the patient sits or lies down on the examination table with a light drape over the lap or lower trunk. Make sure that he or she stays warm by eliminating drafts, controlling room temperature, and providing warm blankets. Routinely ask if he or she is comfortable.

Positioning. During the examination ask the patient to assume proper positions so body parts are accessible and he or she stays comfortable. Table 31-2 lists the preferred positions for each part of the examination and contains figures illustrating the positions. Patients' abilities to assume positions depend on their physical strength, mobility, ease of breathing, age, and degree of wellness. After explaining a position, help the patient to assume it correctly. Take care to maintain respect and show consideration by adjusting the drapes so only the area examined is accessible. During the examination a patient may need to assume more than one position. To decrease the number of

TABLE 31-2 Positions for Examination

Position	Areas Assessed	Rationale	Limitations
Sitting	Head and neck, back, posterior thorax and lungs, anterior thorax and lungs, breasts, axillae, heart, vital signs, and upper extremities	Sitting upright provides full expansion of lungs and better visualization of symmetry of upper body parts.	Physically weakened patient sometimes is unable to sit. Use supine position with head of bed elevated instead.
Supine	Head and neck, anterior thorax and lungs, breasts, axillae, heart, abdomen, extremities, pulses	This is most normally relaxed position. It provides easy access to pulse sites.	If patient becomes short of breath easily, raise head of bed.
Dorsal recumbent	Head and neck, anterior thorax and lungs, breasts, axillae, heart, abdomen	Position is for abdominal assessment because it promotes relaxation of abdominal muscles.	Patients with painful disorders are more comfortable with knees flexed.
Lithotomy*	Female genitalia and genital tract	Position provides maximal exposure of female genitalia and facilitates insertion of vaginal speculum.	Lithotomy position is embarrassing and uncomfortable; thus examiner minimizes time that patient spends in it. Keep patient well draped.
Sims'	Rectum and vagina	Flexion of hip and knee improves exposure of rectal area.	Joint deformities hinder patient's ability to bend hip and knee.
Prone	Musculoskeletal system	Position is only for assessing extension of hip joint, skin, and buttocks.	Patients with respiratory difficulties do not tolerate this position well.
Lateral recumbent	Heart	Position aids in detecting murmurs.	Patients with respiratory difficulties do not tolerate this position well.
Knee-chest*	Rectum	Position provides maximal exposure of rectal area.	This position is embarrassing and uncomfortable.

*Some patients with arthritis or other joint deformities are unable to assume this position.

position changes, organize the examination so all techniques requiring a sitting position are completed first, followed by those that require a supine position next, and so forth. Use extra care when positioning older adults with disabilities and limitations.

Psychological Preparation of a Patient

Many patients find an examination stressful or tiring, or they experience anxiety about possible findings. A thorough explanation of the purpose and steps of each assessment lets a patient know what to expect and how to cooperate. Adapt explanations to the patient's level of understanding and encourage him or her to ask questions and comment on any discomfort. Convey an open, professional approach while remaining relaxed. A quiet, formal demeanor inhibits a patient's ability to communicate, but a style that is too casual may cause him or her to doubt an examiner's competence (Ball et al., 2015).

Consider cultural or social norms when performing an examination on a person of the opposite gender. When this situation occurs, another person of the patient's gender or a culturally approved family member needs to be in the room. By taking this step you demonstrate cultural awareness for a patient's individual needs. As a side benefit, the second person acts as a witness to the conduct of the examiner and the patient should any question arise.

During the examination watch the patient's emotional responses by observing whether his or her facial expressions show fear or concern or if body movements indicate anxiety. When you remain calm, the patient is more likely to relax. Especially if the patient is weak or elderly, it is necessary to pace the examination, pausing at intervals to ask how he or she is tolerating the assessment. If the patient feels alright, the examination can proceed. However, do not force the patient to cooperate based on your schedule. Postponing the examination is advantageous because the findings may be more accurate when the patient can cooperate and relax.

Assessment of Age-Groups

It is necessary to use different interview styles and approaches to physical examination for patients of different age-groups. Your approach will vary with each group. When assessing children, show sensitivity and anticipate the child's perception of the examination as a strange and unfamiliar experience. Routine pediatric examinations focus on health promotion and illness prevention, particularly for well children who receive competent parenting and have no serious health problems (Hockenberry and Wilson, 2015). This examination focuses on growth and development, sensory screening, dental examination, and behavioral assessment. Children who are chronically ill or disabled and foster, foreign-born, or adopted children sometimes require additional examination visits. When examining children, the following tips help in data collection:

- Gather all or part of the history on infants and children from parents or guardians. Use open-ended questions to allow parents to share more information and describe more of the children's problems. This also allows observation of parent-child interactions. You can interview older children, who often provide details about their health history and severity of symptoms.
- Gain a child's trust before doing any type of an examination. Perform the examination in a nonthreatening area. Talk and play with the child first. Do the visual parts of the examination before actually touching the child. Start the examination from the periphery and then move to the center (e.g., start with the extremities before moving to the chest).
- Because parents sometimes think the examiner is testing them, offer support during the examination and do not pass judgment.
- Call children by their first name and address the parents as "Mr., Mrs., or Ms." rather than by their first name unless instructed differently.
- Treat adolescents as adults and individuals because they tend to respond best when treated as such. Remember that adolescents have the right to confidentiality. After talking with parents about historical information, speak alone with adolescents.

A comprehensive health assessment and examination of older adults includes physical data; developmental stage; family relationships; religious and occupational pursuits; and a review of the patient's cognitive, affective, and social level. An important aspect is to assess the patient's ability to perform basic activities of daily living (e.g., bathing, grooming) and complex instrumental activities of daily living (e.g., making phone call).

Throughout an examination recognize that with advancing age the body does not demonstrate obvious injury or disease as vigorously as younger patients and older adults do not always exhibit the expected signs and symptoms (Touhy and Jett, 2014). Characteristically older adults present with subtle or atypical signs and symptoms. Principles to follow during examination of an older adult include the following:

- Do not stereotype about aging patients' level of cognition. Most older adults are able to adapt to change and learn about their health. Similarly most are reliable historians.
- Recognize that some older adults have sensory or physical limitations that affect how quickly they can be interviewed and examinations can be conducted. It might be necessary to plan for more than one examination session. Sometimes it helps to give patients an initial health questionnaire before they come to a clinic or office.
- Perform the examination with adequate space; this is especially important for patients with mobility aids such as a cane or walker.
- During the examination use patience, allow for pauses, and observe for details. Recognize normal physiological and behavioral changes that are characteristic of later life.
- Certain types of health information are stressful for older patients to give. Some view illness as a threat to independence and a step toward institutionalization.
- Be aware of the location of the closest bathroom facility in case the patient has an urgent need to eliminate.
- Be alert to signs of increasing fatigue such as sighing, grimacing, irritability, leaning against objects for support, and drooping head and shoulders.

ORGANIZATION OF THE EXAMINATION

You conduct a physical examination by assessing each body system. Use judgment to ensure that an examination is relevant and includes the correct assessments. Patients with focused symptoms or needs require only parts of an examination; thus, when a patient comes to a clinic with symptoms of a severe chest cold, a neurological assessment should not be required. A patient entering the emergency department with acute abdominal symptoms requires assessment of the body systems most at risk for being abnormal. However, when a patient is admitted to the hospital, you perform a complete examination at the time of admission and at least once each day to maintain and monitor the patient's baseline. Agency guidelines may define the components of a complete examination (see agency policy). A patient in the community seeks screening for specific conditions, often dependent on his or her age or health risks listed in Table 31-3.

TABLE 31-3 **Recommended Preventive Screenings**

Disease/Condition	Age-Group	Screening Measures
Breast cancer* (Women at average risk)	Ages 40-44	Should have the choice to start annual breast cancer screening with mammograms if they wish to do so. The risks of screening as well as the potential benefits should be considered. Monthly BSE dependent on health care provider recommendations (not recommended by ACS)
	Ages 45-54	Monthly BSE dependent upon health care provider recommendations (not recommended by ACS) Should get mammogram every year
	Ages 55 and older	Should switch to mammograms every 2 years or have the choice to continue yearly screening.
	Women with a personal history of breast cancer, a family history of breast cancer, a genetic mutation known to increase the risk of breast cancer (such as *BRCA*), and women who have had radiation therapy to the chest before the age of 30 are at a higher risk for breast cancer, not average risk. These women require earlier and more extensive screening.	
Colon/rectal cancer**	Ages 50 and up	Men and women need to have one of the following: fecal occult blood test (FOBT) or fecal immunochemical test (FIT) annually or flexible sigmoidoscopy (FSIG) every 5 years; the combination of FOBT or FIT annually and an FSIG every 5 years is preferred over either of the previous options; or double-contrast barium enema every 5 years; or colonoscopy every 10 years. They also need a digital rectal examination at the same time. Earlier screening is necessary if risk factors exist.
Ear disorders	All ages	Periodic hearing checks as needed
	Over age 65	Regular hearing checks
Eye disorders	Age 40 and under	Complete eye examination every 3 to 5 years (more if positive history for eye disease [e.g., diabetes])
	Ages 40 to 64	Complete eye examination every 2 years to screen for conditions that may go unnoticed (e.g., glaucoma) Annual eye examinations if patient has diabetes
	Age 65 and up	Complete eye examination every year
Heart/vascular disorders	Men age 45 to 65 Women age 45 to 65	Regular measurement of total blood cholesterol levels, lipids, and triglycerides; blood pressure screenings (If patient has risk factors for coronary artery disease [CAD], blood pressure screening needs to begin at age 20-35 for men, 20-45 for women.)
Obesity	All ages	Periodic height and weight measurements
Oral cavity/pharyngeal disorders/cancer	All ages (children, adults, older adults)	Regular dental examinations every 6 months
Ovarian cancer**	Age 18 and up or on becoming sexually active	Annual pelvic examinations by health care provider (This screening occasionally detects ovarian cancer in its advanced stage. Those at high risk need to have a thorough pelvic examination, a transvaginal ultrasound, and a blood test [tumor marker CA 125].)
Prostate cancer**	Ages 50 and up	Men who have at least a 10-year life expectancy need to have a digital rectal examination (DRE) and prostate-specific antigen (PSA) blood test annually. Men at high risk require earlier screening.
Skin cancer**	Ages 20 to 40	See specialist every 3 years
	Over 40	Annual skin checkups with biopsy of suspicious lesions
Testicular cancer**	Age 15 and up	Monthly testicular self-examination (TSE)
Uterine cancer**	Screening begins 3 years after having vaginal intercourse but not later than age 21	Annual pelvic examination by health care provider plus annual Papanicolaou (Pap) test
Cervical cancer	An **annual** Pap test is no longer recommended by the United States Preventive Services Task Force (USPSTF) (2012) and the American Cancer Society (ACS).	
	Ages 21-29	Pelvic examination by health care provider plus Pap test with cytology every 3 years; human papillomavirus (HPV) needed only if Pap test is abnormal (USPSTF, 2012; ACS, 2012)
	Ages 30-65	Pap test with cytology every 3 years. Women who want to lengthen the screening interval: pelvic exam with a combination of cytology and HPV testing every 5 years (USPSTF, 2012; ACS, 2012)
	Over 65	No testing needed if previous regular testing was normal and not otherwise at high risk for cervical cancer (USPSTF, 2012; ACS, 2012). Women diagnosed with cervical precancer should continue to be screened
Endometrial cancer	Same as for cervical cancer	Endometrial biopsy at age 35 for high-risk patients (those with or at risk for hereditary nonpolyposis colon cancer [HNPCC]) (At menopause women at average and high risk need to be informed about signs and symptoms to report.)

*Data from American Cancer Society (ACS): American Cancer Society recommendations for early breast cancer detection in women without breast symptoms, http://www.cancer.org/cancer/breastcancer/moreinformation/breastcancerearlydetection/breast-cancer-early-detection-acs-recs. Accessed October 26, 2015.

**Data from American Cancer Society (ACS): *American Cancer Society guidelines for the early detection of cancer,* 2014, http://www.cancer.org/healthy/findcancerearly/cancerscreeningguidelines/american-cancer-society-guidelines-for-the-early-detection-of-cancer. Accessed November 12, 2014; Agency for Healthcare Research and Quality: *Guide to clinical preventive services,* AHRQ Publication No. 14-05158, Rockville, MD, 2014, http://www.ahrq.gov/professionals/clinicians-providers/guidelines-recommendations/guide/cpsguide.pdf. Accessed November 13, 2014.

Any physical examination should follow a systematic routine to avoid missing important findings. A head-to-toe approach includes all body systems, and the examiner recalls and performs each step in a predetermined order. For an adult the examination begins with an assessment of the head and neck and progresses methodically down the body to incorporate all body systems. The following tips help keep an examination well organized:

- Compare both sides of the body for symmetry. A degree of asymmetry is normal (e.g., the biceps muscles in the dominant arm are sometimes more developed than the same muscles in the nondominant arm).
- If the patient is seriously ill, first assess the systems of the body most at risk for being abnormal. For example, a patient with chest pain first undergoes a cardiovascular assessment.
- If the patient becomes fatigued, offer rest periods between assessments.
- Perform painful procedures near the end of an examination.
- Record assessments in specific terms in the electronic or paper record. A standard form allows for recording information in the same sequence that it is gathered.
- Use common and accepted medical terms and abbreviations to keep notes accurate, brief, and concise.
- Record quick notes during the examination to avoid delays. Complete any larger documentation notes at the end of the examination.

TECHNIQUES OF PHYSICAL ASSESSMENT

The four techniques used in a physical examination are inspection, palpation, percussion, and auscultation.

Inspection

To inspect, carefully look, listen, and smell to distinguish normal from abnormal findings. To do so, you must be aware of any personal visual, hearing, or olfactory deficits. It is important to deliberately practice this skill and learn to recognize all of the possible pieces of data that can be gathered through inspection alone. **Inspection** occurs when interacting with a patient, watching for nonverbal expressions of emotional and mental status. Physical movements and structural components can also be identified in such an informal way. Most important, be deliberate and pay attention to detail. Follow these guidelines to achieve the best results during inspection:

- Make sure that adequate lighting is available, either direct or tangential.
- Use a direct lighting source (e.g., a penlight or lamp) to inspect body cavities.
- Inspect each area for size, shape, color, symmetry, position, and abnormality.
- Position and expose body parts as needed so all surfaces can be viewed but privacy can be maintained.
- When possible, check for side-to-side symmetry by comparing each area with its match on the opposite side of the body.
- Validate findings with the patient.

While assessing a patient, recognize the nature and source of body odors (Table 31-4). An unusual odor often indicates an underlying pathology. **Olfaction** helps to detect abnormalities that cannot be recognized by any other means. For example, when a patient's breath has a sweet, fruity odor, assess for signs of diabetes. Continue to inspect various parts of the body during the physical examination. Palpation may be used concurrently with inspection, or it may follow in a more deliberate fashion.

TABLE 31-4 Assessment of Characteristic Odors

Odor	Site or Source	Potential Causes
Alcohol	Oral cavity	Ingestion of alcohol, diabetes
Ammonia	Urine	Urinary tract infection, renal failure
Body odor	Skin, particularly in areas where body parts rub together (e.g., underarms and under breasts)	Poor hygiene, excess perspiration (hyperhidrosis), foul-smelling perspiration (bromhidrosis)
	Wound site	Wound abscess
	Vomitus	Abdominal irritation, contaminated food
Feces	Vomitus/oral cavity (fecal odor)	Bowel obstruction
	Rectal area	Fecal incontinence
Foul-smelling stools in infant	Stool	Malabsorption syndrome
Halitosis	Oral cavity	Poor dental and oral hygiene, gum disease
Sweet, fruity ketones	Oral cavity	Diabetic acidosis
Stale urine	Skin	Uremic acidosis
Sweet, heavy, thick odor	Draining wound	*Pseudomonas* (bacterial) infection
Musty odor	Casted body part	Infection inside cast
Fetid, sweet odor	Tracheostomy or mucus secretions	Infection of bronchial tree (*Pseudomonas* bacteria)

Palpation

Palpation involves using the sense of touch to gather information. Through touch you make judgments about expected and unexpected findings of the skin or underlying tissue, muscle, and bones. For example, you palpate the skin for temperature, moisture, texture, turgor, tenderness, and thickness and the abdomen for tenderness, distention, or masses. Use different parts of the hand to detect different characteristics (Table 31-5). The palmar surface of the hand and finger pads is more sensitive than the fingertips and should be used to determine position, texture, size, consistency, masses, fluid, and crepitus (Figure 31-1, *A*). Assess body temperature by using the dorsal surface or back of the hand (Figure 31-1, *B*). The palmar surface of the hand and fingers (Figure 31-1, *C*) is more sensitive to vibration. Measure position, consistency, and turgor by lightly grasping the body part with the fingertips.

Touching a patient is a personal experience for both you and the patient. Display respect and concern throughout an examination. Before palpating consider the patient's condition and ability to tolerate the assessment techniques, paying close attention to areas that are painful or tender. In addition, always be conscious of the environment and any threats to the patient's safety.

Prepare for palpation by warming hands, keeping fingernails short, and using a gentle approach. Palpation proceeds slowly, gently, and deliberately. The patient needs to be guided to relax and feel comfortable since tense muscles make assessment more difficult. To promote

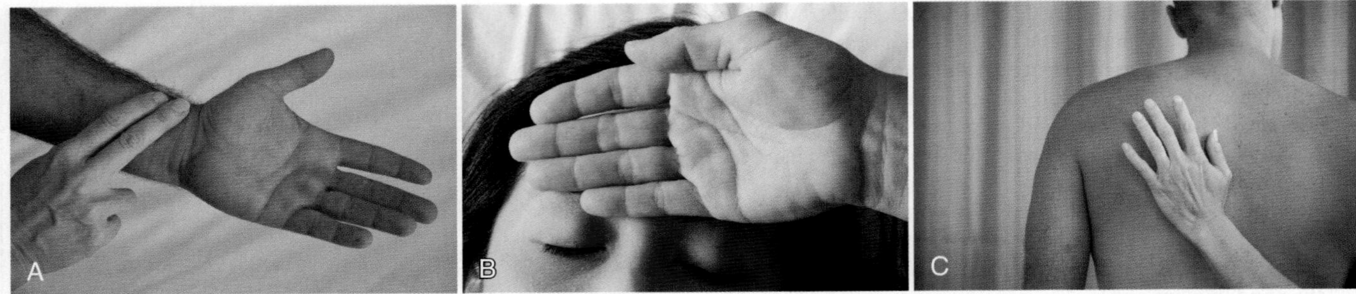

FIGURE 31-1 **A,** Radial pulse is detected with pads of fingertips, the most sensitive part of the hand. **B,** Dorsum of hand detects temperature variations in skin. **C,** Bony part of palm at base of fingers detects vibrations.

TABLE 31-5 Examples of Characteristics Measured by Palpation

Area Examined	Criteria Measured	Portion of Hand to Use
Skin	Temperature	Dorsum of hand/fingers
	Moisture	Palmar surface
	Texture	Palmar surface
	Turgor and elasticity	Grasping with fingertips
	Tenderness	Finger pads/palmar surface of fingers
	Thickness	Palmar surface
Organs (e.g., liver and intestine)	Size Shape Tenderness Absence of masses	Entire palmar surface of hand or palmar surface of fingers
Glands (e.g., thyroid and lymph)	Swelling Symmetry and mobility	Pads of fingertips
Blood vessels (e.g., carotid or femoral artery)	Pulse amplitude Elasticity Rate Rhythm	Palmar surface/pads of fingertips
Thorax	Excursion	Palmar surface
	Tenderness	Finger pads/palmar surface of fingers
	Fremitus	Palmar or ulnar surface of entire hand

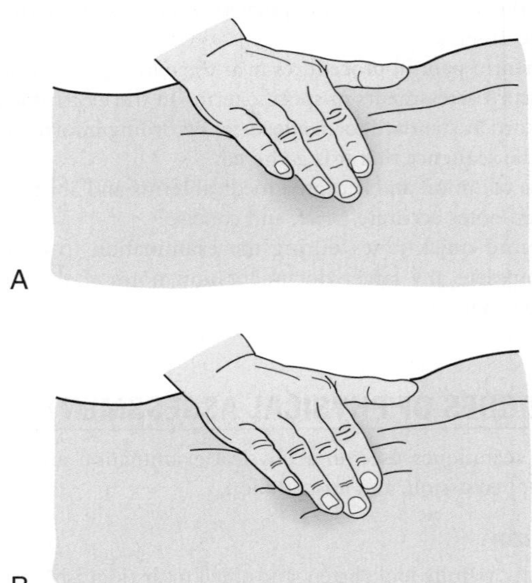

FIGURE 31-2 **A,** During light palpation gentle pressure against underlying skin and tissues can detect areas of irregularity and tenderness. **B,** During deep palpation depress tissue to assess condition of underlying organs.

relaxation, have him or her take slow, deep breaths and place both arms along the sides of the body. Ask the patient to point to more sensitive areas, watching for nonverbal signs of discomfort. *Palpate tender areas last.*

Two types of palpation are used for physical examination, light and deep. Perform light palpation by placing the hand on the body part being examined; it also involves pressing inward about 1 cm (½ inch). Light, superficial palpation of structures such as the abdomen gives the patient the chance to identify areas of tenderness (Figure 31-2, *A*). Inquire about areas of tenderness and assess them further for potentially serious pathologies. Use deep palpation to examine the condition of organs such as those in the abdomen (Figure 31-2, *B*). Depress the area under examination approximately 4 cm (2 inches) (Ball et al., 2015), using one or both hands (bimanually). When using bimanual palpation, relax one hand (sensing hand) and place it lightly over the patient's skin. The other hand (active hand) helps apply pressure to the sensing hand. The lower hand does not exert pressure directly and thus remains sensitive to detect organ characteristics. For safety deep palpation should be observed by your clinical instructor when you first attempt the procedure.

Percussion

Percussion involves tapping the skin with the fingertips to vibrate underlying tissues and organs. The vibration travels through body tissues, and the character of the resulting sound reflects the density of the underlying tissue. The denser the tissue, the quieter is the sound. By knowing how various densities influence sound, it is possible to locate organs or masses, map their edges, and determine their size. An abnormal sound suggests a mass or substance such as air or fluid within an organ or body cavity. The skill of percussion is used more often by advanced practice nurses than by nurses in daily practice at the bedside.

Auscultation

Auscultation involves listening to sounds the body makes to detect variations from normal. Some sounds such as speech and coughing can be heard without additional equipment, but a stethoscope is necessary to hear internal body sounds.

Internal body sounds are created by blood, air, or gastric contents as they move against the body structures. For example, normal heart sounds are created when the heart valves close, moving blood to the next part of the cardiovascular system. Normal sounds for each body system are discussed later in this chapter. Learn to recognize abnormal sounds after learning normal variations. Becoming more proficient in auscultation occurs by knowing the types of sounds each body structure makes and the location in which the sounds are heard best.

To auscultate internal sounds you need to hear well, have a good stethoscope, and know how to use it properly. Nurses with hearing disorders can obtain stethoscopes with extra sound amplification. Chapter 30 describes the parts of the stethoscope and its general use. The bell is best for hearing low-pitched sounds such as vascular and certain heart sounds, and the diaphragm is best for listening to high-pitched sounds such as bowel and lung sounds.

By practicing with the stethoscope, you become proficient at using it and realize when sounds are clear and when there are extraneous sounds. Extraneous sounds created by rubbing against the tubing or chest piece interfere with auscultation of body organ sounds. By deliberately producing these sounds, you learn to recognize and disregard them during the actual examination. Box 31-2 contains ways to practice using and techniques for caring for the stethoscope. Describe any sound you hear using the following characteristics:

- Frequency indicates the number of sound wave cycles generated per second by a vibrating object. The higher the frequency, the higher the pitch of a sound and vice versa.
- Loudness refers to the amplitude of a sound wave. Auscultated sounds range from soft to loud.
- Quality refers to sounds of similar frequency and loudness from different sources. Terms such as *blowing* or *gurgling* describe the quality of sound.
- Duration means the length of time that sound vibrations last. The duration of sound is short, medium, or long. Layers of soft tissue dampen the duration of sounds from deep internal organs.

Auscultation requires concentration and practice. While listening, know which sounds are expected in certain parts of the body and what causes the sounds. Expected sounds are discussed in each body system section of this chapter. After understanding the cause and character of normal auscultated sounds, it becomes easier to recognize abnormal sounds and their origins.

BOX 31-2 Use and Care of the Stethoscope

- Ensure that the earpiece follows the contour of the ear canals. Learn which fit is best for you by comparing amplification of sounds with the earpieces in both directions.
- Place the earpieces in your ears with the tips turned toward the face. *Lightly* blow into the diaphragm. Again place the earpieces in your ears, this time with the ends turned toward the back of the head. *Lightly* blow into the diaphragm. You will find that you hear clearer sounds with the earpiece turned toward the face. After you have learned the right fit for the loudest amplification, wear the stethoscope the same way each time.
- Put on the stethoscope and *lightly* blow into the diaphragm. If the sound is barely audible, *lightly* blow into the bell. Sound is carried through only one part of the chest piece at a time. If the sound is greatly amplified through the diaphragm, the diaphragm is in position for use. If the sound is barely audible through the diaphragm, the bell is in position for use. Rotation of the diaphragm and bell places the chest piece in the desired position. Leave the diaphragm in position for the next exercise.
- Place the diaphragm over the anterior part of your chest. Ask a friend to speak in a normal conversational tone. Environmental noise seriously detracts from hearing the noise created by body organs. When using a stethoscope, the patient and the examiner need to remain quiet.
- Put on the stethoscope and gently tap the tubing. It is often difficult to avoid stretching or moving the stethoscope tubing. The examiner is in a position so the tubing hangs free. Moving or touching the tubing creates extraneous sounds.
- *Care of the stethoscope:* Remove earpieces regularly and clean; remove cerumen (earwax). Keep the bell and diaphragm free of dust, lint, and body oils. Keep the tubing away from any body oils. Avoid draping the stethoscope around the neck next to the skin. Clean daily or after soiling by wiping the entire stethoscope (e.g., diaphragm, tubing) with alcohol. Be sure to dry all parts thoroughly. Follow manufacturer recommendations.
- *Infection control:* Harmful bacteria such as gram-positive bacilli, methicillin-resistant *Staphylococcus aureus* (MRSA), nonaureus *Staphylococcus, Enterobacter cloacae,* and methicillin-sensitive *S. aureus* can be transferred from patient to patient when using portable equipment such as stethoscopes. Clean the stethoscope (diaphragm/bell) *before* reuse on another patient. Using a disinfectant such as isopropyl alcohol (with or without chlorhexidine), benzalkonium, or sodium hypochlorite is effective in reducing the number of bacterial colonies. Hand foam serves this purpose well. Earpieces of stethoscopes are sources of transferable bacteria. When you inadvertently touch your ears and care for the patient, potential pathogens could contaminate the earpieces. Using hand hygiene before and after patient contact decreases the risk of transmitting microorganisms from your ear to your patient. Follow institution infection control guidelines, especially contact precautions, to decrease this risk.

GENERAL SURVEY

When a patient first enters an examination room, observe his or her walk and general appearance and be attentive to his or her behavior and dress. A general survey, or appraisal, of the patient's presentation and behavior provides information about characteristics of an illness, the patient's ability to function independently, body image, emotional state, recent changes in weight, and developmental status. If there are abnormalities or problems, assess the affected body system more closely during the full examination.

General Appearance and Behavior

Assess appearance and behavior while preparing the patient for the examination. For this review include:

- *Gender and race:* A person's gender affects the type of examination performed and the order of the assessments. Different physical features are related to gender and race. Certain illnesses are more likely to affect a specific gender or race (e.g., the incidence of skin cancer is more common in whites than in blacks, prostate cancer is higher in black men than in white men, and cancer of the bladder is higher in men than women) (ACS, 2015a).
- *Age:* Age influences normal physical characteristics and a person's ability to participate in some parts of the examination.
- *Signs of distress:* Sometimes obvious signs or symptoms indicate pain (grimacing, splinting painful area), difficulty breathing (shortness of breath, sternal retractions), or anxiety. Set priorities and examine the related physical areas first.
- *Body type:* Observe if the patient appears trim and muscular, obese, or excessively thin. Body type reflects the level of health, age, and lifestyle.
- *Posture:* Normal standing posture shows an upright stance with parallel alignment of the hips and shoulders. Normal sitting

posture involves some degree of rounding of the shoulders. Observe whether the patient has a slumped, erect, or bent posture, which reflects mood or pain. Changes in older adult physiology often result in a stooped, forward-bent posture, with the hips and knees somewhat flexed and the arms bent at the elbows.

- *Gait:* Observe as the patient walks into the room or stands at the bedside (if the patient is ambulatory). Note whether movements are coordinated or uncoordinated. A person normally walks smoothly, with the arms swinging freely at the sides and the head and face leading the body.
- *Body movements:* Observe whether movements are purposeful, noting any tremors involving the extremities. Determine if any body parts are immobile.
- *Hygiene and grooming:* Note the patient's level of cleanliness by observing the appearance of the hair, skin, and fingernails. Determine if his or her clothes are clean. Grooming depends on the patient's cognitive and emotional function, daily or social activities, and occupation. Observe for excessive use of cosmetics or colognes that could indicate a change in self-perception.
- *Dress:* Culture, lifestyle, socioeconomic level, and personal preference affect the selection and wearing of clothing. However, you should assess whether or not the clothing is appropriate for the temperature, weather conditions, or setting. Depressed or mentally ill people may not be able to select proper clothing, and an older adult might tend to wear extra clothing because of sensitivity to cold.
- *Body odor:* An unpleasant body odor can result from physical exercise, poor hygiene, or certain disease states. Validate any odors that might indicate a health problem.
- *Affect and mood:* Affect is how a person appears to others. Patients express mood or emotional state verbally and nonverbally. Determine whether or not verbal expressions match nonverbal behavior and if the mood is appropriate for the situation. By maintaining eye contact you can observe facial expressions while asking questions.
- *Speech:* Normal speech is understandable and moderately paced and shows an association with the person's thoughts. However, emotions or neurological impairment sometimes causes rapid or slowed speech. Observe whether the patient speaks in a normal tone with clear inflection of words.
- *Signs of patient abuse:* During the examination observe if the patient fears his or her spouse or partner, a caregiver, a parent, or an adult child. Abuse of children, women, and older adults is a growing health problem. Consider any obvious physical injury or neglect as signs of possible abuse (e.g., evidence of malnutrition or presence of bruising on the extremities or trunk) (WHO, 2015). Abuse occurs in many forms: physical, mental or emotional, sexual, social, and financial or economic. Observe the behavior of the individual for any signs of frustration, explanations that do not fit his or her physical presentation, or signs of injury. Most states mandate a report to a social service center when abuse or neglect is suspected (Box 31-3). It is difficult to detect abuse because victims often do not complain or report that they are in abusive situations. If abuse is suspected, find a way to interview the patient in private; patients are more likely to reveal any problems when the suspected abuser is absent from the room. It is imperative that you help the patient find safe housing or seek protection from the abuser since the risk for further abuse is high once the victim has reported it or tries to leave the abusive situation.
- *Substance abuse:* Unusual or inconsistent behavior may be an indicator of substance abuse, which can affect all socioeconomic groups. Although a single patient visit to a clinic does not always reveal the problem, unusual behaviors should be investigated further to reveal behaviors that should be confirmed with a well-focused history and physical examination. Always approach the patient in a caring and nonjudgmental way; substance abuse involves both emotional and lifestyle issues. Box 31-4 lists characteristics of patients who should be further assessed for potential substance abuse. If you suspect abuse or addiction in people 18 years of age or older, a tool such as the NIDA Quick Screen V1.0 helps to identify the level or risks associated with substance abuse (NIDA, 2012). If you suspect that alcohol abuse is a major problem, the CAGE questionnaire provides a useful set of questions to guide assessment. CAGE is an acronym for the following:
    - Have you ever felt the need to **Cut down** on your drinking or drug use?
    - Have people **Annoyed** you by criticizing your drinking or drug use?
    - Have you ever felt bad or **Guilty** about your drinking or drug use?
    - Have you ever used or had a drink first thing in the morning as an **Eye-opener** to steady your nerves or feel normal?

Among older adults risk factors for development of alcohol-related problems include chronic medical disorders, sleep disorders, social isolation, loneliness, bereavement, and acute or chronic pain. When assessing adolescents use the T-ACE modification to assess a patient's degree of tolerance (e.g., how many drinks does it take to make you feel high?) (Burns et al., 2010).

Vital Signs

After completing the general survey, measure the patient's vital signs (see Chapter 30). Measurement of vital signs is more accurate if completed before beginning positional changes or movements. If there is a chance that the vital signs are skewed when first measured, recheck them later during the rest of the examination. Pain, considered the fifth vital sign, should also be assessed.

Height and Weight

The relationship of height and weight reflects a person's general health status. Assess every patient to identify if he or she is at a healthy weight, overweight, or obese. Weight is routinely measured during health screenings, visits to physicians' offices or clinics, and on admission to the hospital. Infants and children are measured for both height and weight at each health care visit to assess for healthy growth and development. If older adults are underweight, difficulty with feeding and other functional activities is a possibility. Measuring height and weight of older adults, along with obtaining a dietary history (Box 31-5), shows risk factors for chronic diseases.

Assess trends in weight changes compared with height for signs of poor health. Assessments screen for abnormal weight changes. A patient's weight normally varies daily because of fluid loss or retention. However, a downward trend in a frail older adult indicates that there is a serious reduction in nutritional reserves. The nursing history helps to focus on possible causes for a change in weight (Table 31-6). Ask the patient to report current height and weight, along with a history of any substantial weight gain or loss. A weight gain of 5 lbs (2.3 kg) in 1 day indicates fluid-retention problems. A weight loss is considered significant if the patient has lost more than 5% of body weight in a month or 10% in 6 months.

BOX 31-3 Clinical Indicators of Abuse

Physical Findings	Behavioral Findings
Child Abuse	
Vaginal or penile discharge	Problem sleeping or eating, anxiety, depression
Blood on underclothing	Fear of certain people or places
Pain, itching, or unusual odor in genital area	Play activities recreate the abuse situation
Genital injuries	Regressed behavior
Difficulty sitting or walking	Sexual acting out
Pain while urinating; recurrent urinary tract infections	Knowledge of explicit sexual matters
Foreign bodies in rectum, urethra, or vagina	Preoccupation with others' or own genitals
Sexually transmitted infections	Profound and rapid personality changes
Pregnancy in young adolescent	Rapidly declining school performance
	Poor relationship with peers
Intimate Partner Violence	
Injuries and trauma inconsistent with reported cause	Overuse of health services
Multiple injuries involving head, face, neck, breasts, abdomen, and genitalia (black eyes, orbital fractures, broken nose, fractured skull, lip lacerations, broken teeth, vaginal tears)	Thoughts of or attempted suicide Eating or sleeping disorders Anxiety and panic attacks
X-ray films showing old and new fractures in different stages of healing	Pattern of substance abuse (follows physical abuse)
Abrasions, lacerations, bruises/welts	Low self-esteem
Burns from cigarettes or other	Depression, problems with eating or sleeping
Human bites	Sense of helplessness
Unexplained injuries (e.g., bruises, fractures, and welts)	Guilt
Strangulation marks on neck from rope burns or bruises; throat pain, voice changes, trouble swallowing; damage to hyoid bone	Smoking Stress-related complaints (headache, anxiety)
Stress-related disorders such as irritable bowel syndrome, exacerbation of asthma, or chronic pain	Financial dependence on abuser Isolation from others
	Unsafe sexual behaviors
Older-Adult Abuse	
Injuries and trauma inconsistent with reported cause (scratch, bruise, or bite)	Dependent on caregiver
Hematomas, bruises at various stages of resolution	Physically and/or cognitively impaired
Unexplained bruises or welts, pattern bruises	Combative, verbally aggressive
Burns	Wandering
Bruises, chafing, excoriation on wrist or legs (restraints)	Minimal social support
Fractures inconsistent with cause described	Prolonged interval between injury and medical treatment
Dried blood	Life circumstances do not match size of patient's estate
Overmedication or undermedication	Uncommunicative or isolated
Exposure to severe weather, cold or hot	
Torn, bloody underwear or vaginal and anal bruises	
Sunken eyes or loss of weight	
Extreme thirst	
Bed sores	

Data from Cooper C et al: The prevalence of elder abuse and neglect: a systematic review, *Age Aging* 37(2):151, 2008; Hockenberry MJ, Wilson P: *Wong's nursing care of infants and children*, ed 10, St Louis, 2015, Mosby; World Health Organization (WHO): Intimate partner violence, 2012, http://www.who.int/reproductivehealth/publications/violence/rhr12_36/en/index.html. Accessed October 26, 2015.

When a patient is hospitalized, daily weight is measured at the same time of day, on the same scale, with approximately the same clothes (Byrd et al., 2011). This allows an objective comparison of subsequent weights. Accuracy of weight measurement is important because health care providers base medical and nursing decisions (e.g., drug dosage, medications) on changes.

Several different scales are available for use. Patients capable of bearing their own weight use a standing scale. You calibrate a standard platform scale by moving the large and small weights to zero. By adjusting the calibrating knob, the balance beam is leveled and steadied. The patient stands on the scale platform and remains still as the nurse adjusts the largest solid weight to the 50-lb or 22.5-kg increment under the patient's weight. Next the smaller weight is moved to balance the scale at the nearest ¼ lb or 0.1 kg (Ball et al., 2015). Electronic scales are calibrated automatically each time they are used and automatically display the weight within seconds.

Bed and chair scales are available for patients who are unable to bear weight. Newer electronic hospital beds have built-in electronic scales for weighing patients who are not able to get out of bed.

You can use a basket or platform scale to weigh infants. After removing the infant's clothing, weigh him or her in dry disposable diapers. Adjust the measurement later for the weight of the diaper, ensuring an accurate reading. Keep the room warm to prevent chills. Place a light cloth or paper on the surface of the infant scale to prevent

BOX 31-4 Behaviors That are Suspicious for Substance Abuse

Among adolescents and adults: Agitation; inappropriate behavior; problems thinking clearly, remembering, and paying attention; poor coordination; seizure; respiratory depression; coma; asphyxiation; aspiration; pulmonary edema; cardiac arrhythmias; immune system impairment, self-inflicted trauma; and suicidal ideation

Red flags:

- The risk of suicide, seizures, and violent behavior is high among substance abusers.
- Intoxicated patients, particularly those with phencyclidine (PCP) or methamphetamine intoxication, are at significant risk for becoming agitated and violent, placing themselves and others at risk for injury.
- Observe for combinations or repetition of these behaviors:
- Frequently misses appointments
- Frequently requests written excuses for absence from school or work
- Drops out of school
- Chief complaints of insomnia, "bad nerves," or pain that does not fit a particular pattern
- Reports lost prescriptions (e.g., tranquilizers or pain medications) or asks for frequent refills
- Frequent emergency department visits
- History of changing health care providers or brings in medication bottles prescribed by several different providers
- History of gastrointestinal bleeds, peptic ulcers, pancreatitis, cellulitis, or frequent pulmonary infections
- Frequent sexually transmitted infections (STIs), complicated pregnancies, multiple abortions, or sexual dysfunction
- Complaints of chest pains or palpitations or has a history of admissions to rule out heart attacks
- History of activities that place the patient at risk for human immunodeficiency virus (HIV) infections (multiple partners, multiple rapes)
- Family history of addiction; history of childhood sexual, physical, or emotional abuse; or social and financial or marital problems
- Intimate partner violence

Data from American Psychiatric Association: *Diagnostic and statistical manual of mental disorders*, ed 4, text revision, Washington, DC, 2000, The Association; American Society of Addiction Medicine and Widlitz M, Marin D: Substance abuse in older adults: an overview, *Geriatrics* 57(12):29, 2002; and Walsh K et al: Examining the interface between substance misuse and intimate partner violence, *Substance Abuse Res Treatment* 3:25, 2009; and National Institute on Drug Abuse: *Drugs, brains and behavior: the science of addiction*, 2014, https://www.drugabuse.gov/publications/drugs-brains-behavior-science-addiction/introduction. Accessed October 26, 2015.

BOX 31-5 Dietary History for Older Adults

- Does the older adult need or have help shopping for or preparing meals?
- Is income adequate for food purchasing? Food stamps or public assistance required?
- Does the patient ever skip meals?
- Are the five primary food groups from MyPlate (fruits, grains, protein, vegetables, dairy) represented in the daily diet (see Chapter 45) (USDA, 2011)?
- Does the older adult take nutritional supplements such as multivitamins?
- Does the older adult take any medication affecting appetite or absorption of nutrients?
- Does the older adult have any religious or cultural beliefs and practices that influence diet?
- Does the older adult have a special diet, food intolerances, or allergies? Does the patient's diet contain an unusual amount of alcohol, sweets, or fried food?
- Does the older adult have problems with chewing, swallowing, or salivation?
- Does the older adult have gastrointestinal problems that interfere with food intake?

Data from Meiner SE: *Gerontologic nursing*, ed 4, St Louis, 2011, Mosby; and US Department of Agriculture and US Department of Health and Human Services: *Dietary guidelines for Americans, 2010*, ed 7, Washington, DC, 2010, US Government Printing Office.

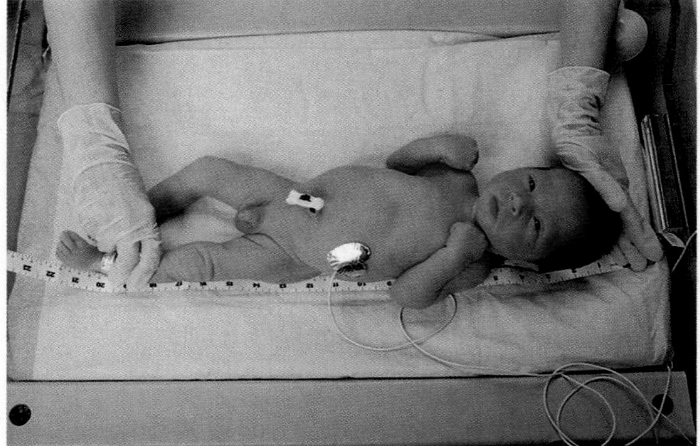

FIGURE 31-3 Measurement of infant length. (From Murray SS, McKinney ES: *Foundations of maternal-newborn and women's health nursing*, ed 5, St Louis, 2010, Saunders.)

cross-infection from urine or feces. When placing an infant in a basket or on a platform, hold a hand lightly above him or her to detect movements and prevent accidental falls. Measure an infant's weight in both ounces and grams.

In patients who are able to stand, measure height by having them remove their shoes. The standing surface should be clean. Use a measuring rod attached vertically to a weight scale, or use a tape ruler on the wall. As the patient stands erect, place a flat surface on his or her head that is even with the vertical measure. Then read the number on the scale or ruler that indicates his or her height in centimeters or inches.

Remove the shoes of a non–weight-bearing patient and position the patient (such as an infant) supine on a firm surface. When measuring an infant, hold his or her head and make sure that his or her legs are straight at the knees. After positioning the infant, use a tape measure to measure length from the head to the bottom of the feet (Figure 31-3). Record the infant's length to the nearest 0.5 cm or ¼ inch.

SKIN, HAIR, AND NAILS

The **integumentary system** refers to the skin, hair, scalp, and nails. To assess the integument, you first gather a health history to guide your examination and use the techniques of inspection and palpation.

Skin

Begin an assessment of the skin by focusing on the health history questions found in Table 31-7. The physical examination begins with an inspection of all visible skin surfaces; the less visible surfaces are assessed when you examine other body systems. Use the senses of

TABLE 31-6 Nursing History for Weight Assessment

Assessment	Rationale
Ask about total weight lost or gained; compare with usual weight; note time period for loss and whether it was planned (e.g., gradual, sudden, desired, or undesired).	Assessment determines severity of problem and reveals if weight change is related to disease process, change in eating pattern, or pregnancy.
If weight loss desired, ask about eating habits, diet plan followed, food preparation, calorie intake, appetite, exercise pattern, support group participation, weight goal.	Assessment helps to determine appropriateness of diet plan followed.
If weight loss undesired, ask about anorexia; vomiting; diarrhea; thirst; frequent urination; and change in lifestyle, activity, and stress levels.	Assessment focuses on problems that cause weight loss (e.g., gastrointestinal problems).
Assess if patient has noted changes in social aspects of eating: more meals in restaurants, rushing to eat meals, stress at work, or skipping meals.	Lifestyle changes sometimes contribute to weight changes.
Assess if patient takes chemotherapy, diuretics, insulin, fluoxetine, prescription and nonprescription appetite suppressants, laxatives, oral hypoglycemics, or herbal supplements (weight loss); steroids, oral contraceptives, antidepressants, insulin (weight gain).	Weight gain or loss is a side effect of these medications.
Assess for preoccupation with body weight or body shape such as fasting, never feeling thin enough, unusually strict caloric intake or restrictions, laxative abuse, induced vomiting, amenorrhea, excessive exercise, alcohol intake.	Excesses indicate an eating disorder.

TABLE 31-7 Nursing History for Skin Assessment

Assessment	Rationale
Ask patient about history of changes in skin: dryness, pruritus, sores, rashes, lumps, color, texture, odor, and lesion that does not heal.	Patient is best source to recognize change. Usually skin cancer is first noticed as a localized change in skin color.
Consider if patient has the following history: fair, freckled, ruddy complexion; light-colored hair or eyes; tendency to burn easily.	Characteristics are risk factors for skin cancer.
Determine whether patient works or spends excessive time outside. If so, ask whether patient wears sunscreen and the level of protection.	Exposed areas such as face and arms are more pigmented than rest of body. The American Cancer Society (2015a) recommends sun safety and use of sunscreen and lip balm with broad-spectrum protection and a sun protection factor (SPF) of 30 or higher.
Determine whether patient has noted lesions, rashes, or bruises.	Most skin changes do not develop suddenly. Change in character of lesion can indicate cancer. Bruising indicates trauma or bleeding disorder.
Question patient about frequency of bathing and type of soap used.	Excessive bathing and use of harsh soaps cause dry skin.
Ask if patient has had recent trauma to skin.	Some injuries cause bruising and changes in skin texture.
Determine whether patient has history of allergies.	Skin rashes commonly occur from allergies.
Ask if patient uses topical medications or home remedies on skin.	Incorrect use of topical agents causes inflammation or irritation.
Ask if patient goes to tanning parlors, uses sunlamps, or takes tanning pills.	Overexposure of skin to these irritants can cause skin cancer.
Ask if patient has family history of serious skin disorders such as skin cancer or psoriasis.	Family history can reveal information about patient's condition.
Determine if patient works with creosote, coal, tar, petroleum products, arsenic compounds, or radium.	Exposure to these agents creates risk for skin cancer.

sight, smell, and touch while performing inspection and palpation of the skin.

Assessment of the skin reveals the patient's health status related to oxygenation, circulation, nutrition, local tissue damage, and hydration. Check the condition of the patient's integument to determine the need for nursing care. For example, assessment findings can help determine the type of hygiene measures required to maintain integrity of the integument (see Chapter 40). For example, vigorous towel drying significantly impairs the barrier function of the skin in adults, whereas using no-rinse cleansers and cleaning cloths results in less damage to the skin (Cowdell, 2011). Adequate nutrition and hydration become goals of therapy if there is an alteration in the integumentary status (see Chapter 45).

Every patient has a risk for skin impairment during administration of care in a hospital setting. Risk increases if there is pressure against the skin when the patient is immobile, from reactions to various medications used in treatment, and from moisture if the patient is incontinent or has wound drainage. At high risk are patients who are neurologically impaired or chronically ill or have had orthopedic or vascular injuries. Also at higher risk are patients with diminished mental status, poor tissue oxygenation, low cardiac output, or inadequate nutrition. Patients who are homebound or in nursing homes or extended care facilities are often at risk for pressure ulcers, depending on their level of mobility and the presence of chronic illness. Routinely assess the skin of all at-risk patients to look for primary or initial lesions that develop. Without proper care primary lesions can deteriorate to become secondary lesions that require more extensive nursing care. For example, the development of a pressure ulcer lengthens a hospital stay unless it is prevented or discovered and treated early (see Chapter 48).

Adequate lighting is required when assessing the skin. Daylight is the best choice to identify variations in skin color, especially for detecting skin changes in dark-skinned patients. When sunlight is not available, fluorescent lighting is the next best choice. Room temperature also affects skin assessment. A room that is too warm causes superficial vasodilation, resulting in increased redness of the skin. A cool environment causes the sensitive patient to develop cyanosis around the lips and nail beds (Ball et al., 2015).

Although you inspect the skin over each part of the body during an examination, it is helpful to make a brief but careful overall visual sweep of the entire body. This approach provides a good idea of the distribution and extent of any lesions and the overall symmetry of skin color. Inspect all skin surfaces, making a point to do so when examining other body systems. Often overlooked, inspection of the feet is absolutely essential for patients with poor circulation or diabetes. If any abnormalities are found during an examination, palpate the involved areas. Use disposable gloves for palpation if open, moist, or draining lesions are present.

Throughout the examination remain alert for skin odors. White and black adolescents and adults ordinarily have body odor because they have a greater number of functioning apocrine glands. In contrast, Asians and Native Americans/American Indians often do not (Ball et al., 2015). Figure 31-4 illustrates a normal cross-section of the skin.

Color. Skin color varies from body part to body part and from person to person. Despite individual variations, it is usually uniform over the body. Table 31-8 lists common variations. Normal skin pigmentation ranges in tone from ivory or light pink to ruddy pink in light skin and from light to deep brown or olive in dark skin. In older adults **pigmentation** increases unevenly, causing discolored skin. While inspecting the skin be aware that cosmetics or tanning agents sometimes mask normal skin color.

The assessment of color first involves areas of the skin not exposed to the sun such as the palms of the hands. Note if the skin is unusually pale or dark. Areas exposed to the sun such as the face and arms are darker. It is more difficult to note changes such as pallor or cyanosis in patients with dark skin. Usually color hues are most evident in the palms, soles of the feet, lips, tongue, and nail beds. Areas of increased (hyperpigmentation) and decreased (hypopigmentation) color are common. Skin creases and folds are darker than the rest of the body in the dark-skinned patient.

Inspect sites where abnormalities are more easily identified. For example, pallor is more evident in the face, buccal (mouth) mucosa, conjunctiva, and nail beds. Observe for **cyanosis** (bluish discoloration) in the lips, nail beds, palpebral conjunctivae, and palms. In recognizing pallor in the dark-skinned patient, observe that normal brown skin appears to be yellow-brown and normal black skin appears to be ashen gray. Also assess the lips, nail beds, and mucous membranes for generalized pallor; if pallor is present, the mucous membranes are ashen gray. Assessment of cyanosis in the dark-skinned patient requires observing areas where pigmentation occurs the least (conjunctiva, sclera, buccal mucosa, tongue, lips, nail beds, and palms and soles). In addition, verify these findings with clinical manifestations (Ball et al., 2015).

The best site to inspect for **jaundice** (yellow-orange discoloration) is on the patient's sclera. You can see normal reactive hyperemia, or redness, most often in regions exposed to pressure such as the sacrum, heels, and greater trochanter. Inspect for any patches or areas

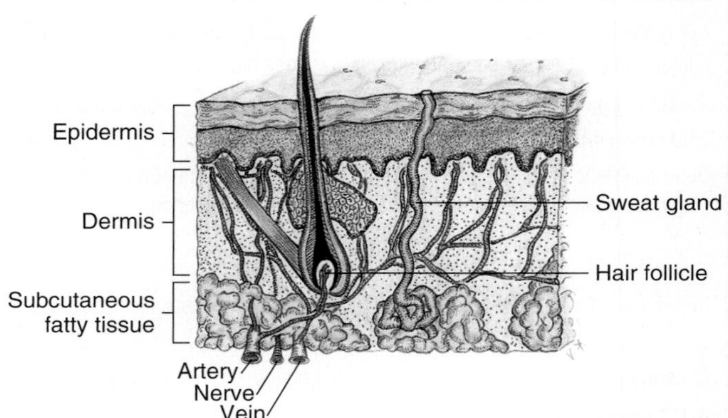

FIGURE 31-4 Cross-section of skin reveals three layers: epidermis, dermis, and subcutaneous fatty tissues.

TABLE 31-8 Skin Color Variations

Color	Condition	Causes	Assessment Locations
Bluish (cyanosis)	Increased amount of deoxygenated hemoglobin (associated with hypoxia)	Heart or lung disease, cold environment	Nail beds, lips, mouth, skin (severe cases)
Pallor (decrease in color)	Reduced amount of oxyhemoglobin Reduced visibility of oxyhemoglobin resulting from decreased blood flow	Anemia Shock	Face, conjunctivae, nail beds, palms of hands Skin, nail beds, conjunctivae, lips
Loss of pigmentation	Vitiligo	Congenital or autoimmune condition causing lack of pigment	Patchy areas on skin over face, hands, arms
Yellow-orange (jaundice)	Increased deposit of bilirubin in tissues	Liver disease, destruction of red blood cells	Sclera, mucous membranes, skin
Red (erythema)	Increased visibility of oxyhemoglobin caused by dilation or increased blood flow	Fever, direct trauma, blushing, alcohol intake	Face, area of trauma, sacrum, shoulders, other common sites for pressure ulcers
Tan-brown	Increased amount of melanin	Suntan, pregnancy	Areas exposed to sun: face, arms, areolas, nipples

TABLE 31-9 Physical Findings of the Skin Indicative of Substance Abuse

Skin Finding	Commonly Associated Drug
Diaphoresis	Sedative hypnotic (including alcohol)
Spider angiomas	Alcohol, stimulants
Burns (especially fingers)	Alcohol
Needle marks	Opioids
Contusion, abrasions, cuts, scars	Alcohol, other sedative hypnotics, intravenous (IV) opioids
"Homemade" tattoos	Cocaine, IV opioids (prevents detection of injection sites)
Vasculitis	Cocaine
Red, dry skin	Phencyclidine (PCP)

Modified from Lehne RA: *Pharmacology for nursing care*, ed 8, St Louis, 2013, Saunders; Ries R, Wilford B: *Principles of addiction medicine*, ed 4, Chevy Chase, MD, 2009, Lippincott Williams & Wilkins.

of skin color variation. Localized skin changes such as pallor or **erythema** (red discoloration) indicate circulatory changes. For example, an area of erythema is caused by localized vasodilation resulting from a sunburn, inflammation, or fever. It is difficult to observe erythema in the dark-skinned patient; thus palpate the area for heat and warmth to note the presence of skin inflammation. Compare the area with a different part of the skin to detect a difference in temperature. An area of an extremity that appears unusually pale results from arterial occlusion or edema. Be sure to ask if the patient has noticed any changes in skin coloring.

There is also a pattern of findings associated with patients who are chemically dependent or intravenous (IV) drug abusers (Table 31-9). It is sometimes difficult to recognize signs and symptoms through an isolated examination. A patient who takes repeated IV injections has edematous, reddened, and warm areas along the arms and legs. This pattern suggests recent injections. Evidence of old injection sites appears as hyperpigmented and shiny or scarred areas.

Moisture. The hydration of skin and mucous membranes helps to reveal body fluid imbalances, changes in the environment of the skin, and regulation of body temperature. Moisture refers to wetness and oiliness. The skin is normally smooth and dry. Skinfolds such as the axillae are normally moist. Minimal perspiration or oiliness is often present (Ball et al., 2015). Increased perspiration can be associated with activity, exposure to warm environments, obesity, anxiety, or excitement. Use ungloved fingertips to palpate skin surfaces. Observe for dullness, dryness, crusting, and flaking that resembles dandruff when the skin surface is lightly rubbed. Excessively dry skin is common in older adults and people who use excessive amounts of soap during bathing (Cowdell, 2011). Other factors causing dry skin include lack of humidity, exposure to sun, smoking, stress, excessive perspiration, and dehydration. Excessive dryness worsens existing skin conditions such as eczema and dermatitis. Patients with large abdominal skinfolds are at high risk for moisture within the skinfolds. This moisture promotes the growth of bacteria and fungi, which contribute to rashes and infection (Rush and Muir, 2012). Excessive moisture may cause maceration of the skin or softening of the tissues, resulting in an increased risk for breakdown (see Chapter 48).

Temperature. The temperature of the skin depends on the amount of blood circulating through the dermis. Increased or decreased skin temperature indicates an increase or decrease in blood flow. An increase in skin temperature often accompanies localized erythema or redness of the skin. A reduction in skin temperature often accompanies pallor and reflects a decrease in blood flow. It is important to remember that a cold or excessively warm examination room can cause changes in the patient's skin temperature and color.

Accurately assess temperature by palpating the skin with the dorsum or back of the hand. Compare symmetrical body parts. Normally the skin temperature is warm. Sometimes it is the same throughout the body, and other times it varies in one area. Always assess skin temperature for patients at risk of having impaired circulation such as after a cast application or vascular surgery. You can identify a stage I pressure ulcer early by noting warmth over an area of erythema on the skin (see Chapter 48).

Texture. Texture refers to the character of the surface of the skin and how the deeper layers feel. By palpating lightly with the fingertips, you determine whether the patient's skin is smooth or rough, thin or thick, tight or supple, and **indurated** (hardened) or soft. The texture of the skin is normally smooth, soft, even, and flexible in children and adults. However, the texture is usually not uniform throughout, with thicker texture over the palms of the hand and soles of the feet. In older adults the skin becomes wrinkled and leathery because of a decrease in collagen, subcutaneous fat, and sweat glands.

Localized skin changes result from trauma, surgical wounds, or lesions. When there are irregularities in texture such as scars or indurations, ask the patient about recent injury to the skin. Deeper palpation sometimes reveals irregularities such as tenderness or localized areas of induration, which can be caused by repeated injections.

Turgor. **Turgor** refers to the elasticity of the skin. Normally the skin loses its elasticity with age, but fluid balance can also affect skin turgor. Edema or dehydration diminishes turgor. To assess skin turgor, grasp a fold of skin on the back of the forearm or sternal area with the fingertips and release (Figure 31-5). Since the skin on the back of the hand is normally loose and thin, turgor is not assessed reliably at that site (Ball et al., 2015). Normally the skin lifts easily and falls immediately back to its resting position. When turgor is poor, it stays pinched and shows tenting. Evaluate the ease with which the skin moves and the speed at which it returns to its resting state. Failure of the skin to reassume its normal contour or shape indicates dehydration. The patient with poor skin turgor does not have resilience to the normal wear and tear on the skin, and a decrease in turgor predisposes him or her to skin breakdown.

Vascularity. The circulation of the skin affects color in localized areas and leads to the appearance of superficial blood vessels. Vascularity occurs in localized pressure areas when patients remain in one position. Vascularity appears reddened, pink, or pale (see Chapter 48). With aging capillaries become fragile and more easily injured. **Petechiae** are nonblanching, pinpoint-size, red or purple spots on the skin caused by small hemorrhages in the skin layers. Many petechiae have no known cause; but some may indicate serious blood-clotting disorders, drug reactions, or liver disease.

Edema. Areas of the skin become swollen or edematous from a buildup of fluid in the tissues. Direct trauma and impairment of venous return are two common causes of **edema**. Inspect edematous areas for location, color, and shape. The formation of edema separates the surface of the skin from the pigmented and vascular layers, masking skin color. Edematous skin also appears stretched and shiny. Palpate edematous areas to determine mobility, consistency, and tenderness. When pressure from the examiner's fingers leaves an indentation in the edematous area, it is called *pitting edema*. To assess the degree of pitting edema, press the edematous area firmly with the thumb for several seconds and release. The depth of pitting, recorded in millimeters, determines the degree of edema (Ball et al., 2015). For example, 1+ edema equals a 2-mm depth, 2+ edema equals a 4-mm depth, 3+ equals 6 mm, and 4+ equals 8 mm (Figure 31-6).

Lesions. The term *lesion* refers broadly to any unusual finding of the skin surface. Normally the skin is free of lesions, except for common freckles or age-related changes such as skin tags, senile keratosis (thickening of skin), cherry angiomas (ruby red papules), and atrophic warts. Lesions that are primary occur as an initial spontaneous sign of a pathological process such as with an insect bite. Secondary lesions result from later formation or trauma to a primary lesion such as occurs with a pressure ulcer. When you find a lesion, collect standard information about its color, location, texture, size, shape, type, grouping (clustered or linear), and distribution (localized or generalized). Next observe for any exudate, odor, amount, and consistency. Measure the size of the lesion in centimeters by using a small, clear, flexible ruler. Measure each lesion for height, width, and depth.

Palpation helps determine the mobility, contour (flat, raised, or depressed), and consistency (soft or indurated) of a lesion. Certain types of lesions present characteristic patterns. For example, a tumor is usually an elevated, solid lesion larger than 2 cm (1 inch). Primary lesions such as macules and nodules come from some stimulus to the skin (Box 31-6). Secondary lesions such as ulcers occur as alterations in primary lesions. After you identify a lesion, closely inspect it in good lighting. Palpate gently, covering the entire area of the lesion. If it is moist or draining fluid, wear gloves during palpation and pay attention to whether or not the patient identifies any areas of tenderness.

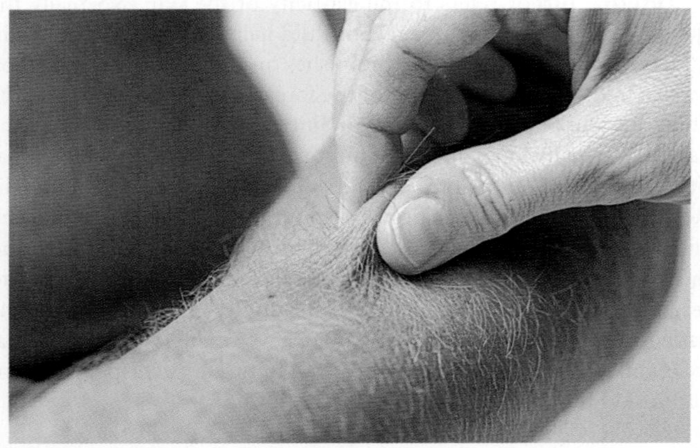

FIGURE 31-5 Assessment for skin turgor. (From Ball JW et al: *Seidel's guide to physical examination,* ed 8, St Louis, 2015, Mosby.)

Skin (cutaneous) malignancies are the most common neoplasms in patients. For this reason the examiner should incorporate a thorough skin assessment on all patients. Cancerous lesions have distinct features and over time undergo changes in color and size (Box 31-7). Basal cell carcinoma is most common in sun-exposed areas and frequently occurs with a history of sun-damaged skin; it almost never spreads to other parts of the body. Squamous cell carcinoma is more serious than basal cell and develops on the outer layers of sun-exposed skin; these cells may travel to lymph nodes and throughout the body. Malignant melanoma, a skin cancer that develops from melanocytes, begins as a mole or other area that has changed in appearance and is usually located on normal skin (**NOTE:** melanoma also can originate in noncutaneous primary sites including mucosal epithelium (GI tract), retinas, and leptomeninges). In African-Americans (more than in other races) it can also appear under fingernails or on the palms of the hands and soles of the feet. Use the *ABCD* mnemonic to assess the skin for any type of carcinoma (ACS, 2015a):

- *A*symmetry—Look for an uneven shape. One half of mole does not match other half.
- *B*order irregularity—Look for edges that are blurred, notched, or ragged.
- *C*olor—Look for pigmentation that is not uniform; variegated areas of blue, black, and brown and areas of pink, white, gray, blue, or red are abnormal.
- *D*iameter—Look for areas greater than 6 mm (about the size of a typical pencil eraser).

Report abnormal lesions to the health care provider for further examination. Since ultraviolet light of the sun or tanning beds increase the risk for development of skin cancers, teach patients about the risks that exist. They should be taught how to perform a skin self-examination, using the best-quality teaching materials.

Hair and Scalp

Two types of hair cover the body: soft, fine, vellus hair, which covers the body; and coarse, long, thick terminal hair, which is easily visible on the scalp, axillae, and pubic areas and in the facial beard on men. First obtain health history information listed in Table 31-10. Prepare to inspect the condition and distribution of hair and the integrity of the scalp by first obtaining a good light source. In addition, hair assessment occurs during all parts of the examination.

Inspection. During inspection explain that it is necessary to separate parts of the hair to detect abnormalities. Wear a pair of clean gloves if open lesions or lice are noted.

First inspect the color, distribution, quantity, thickness, texture, and lubrication of body hair. Scalp hair is coarse or fine and curly or straight; and it should be shiny, smooth, and pliant. While separating

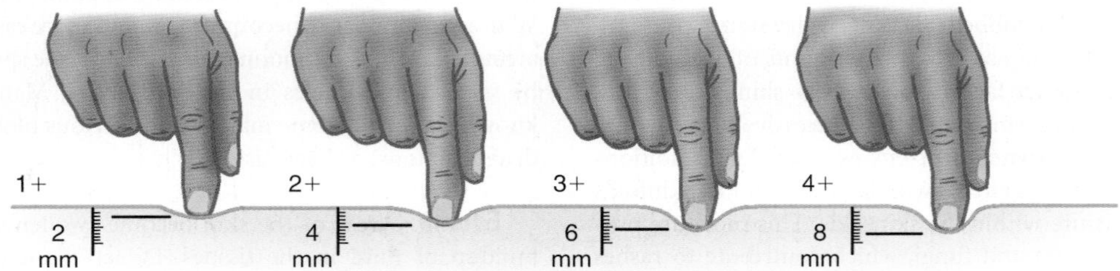

FIGURE 31-6 Assessing for pitting edema. (From Ball JW et al: *Seidel's guide to physical examination,* ed 8, St Louis, 2015, Mosby.)

BOX 31-6 Types of Primary Skin Lesions

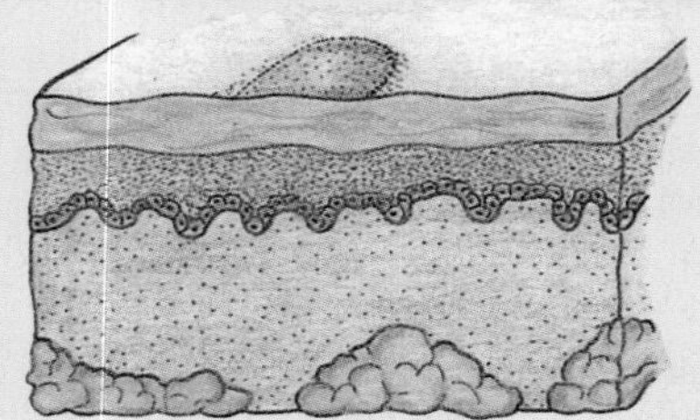

Macule: Flat, nonpalpable change in skin color; smaller than 1 cm (e.g., freckle, petechiae)

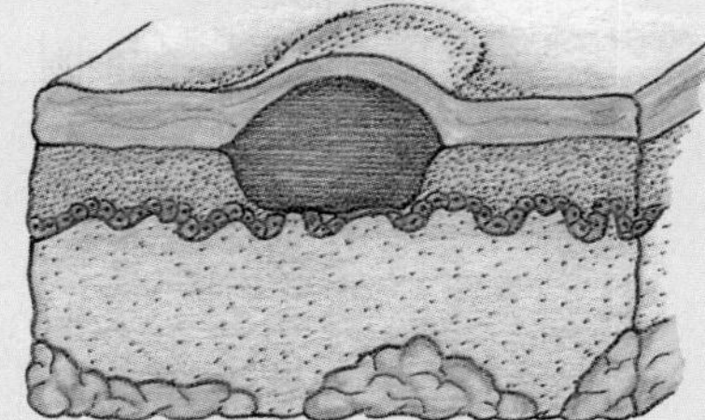

Papule: Palpable, circumscribed, solid elevation in skin; smaller than 1 cm (e.g., elevated nevus)

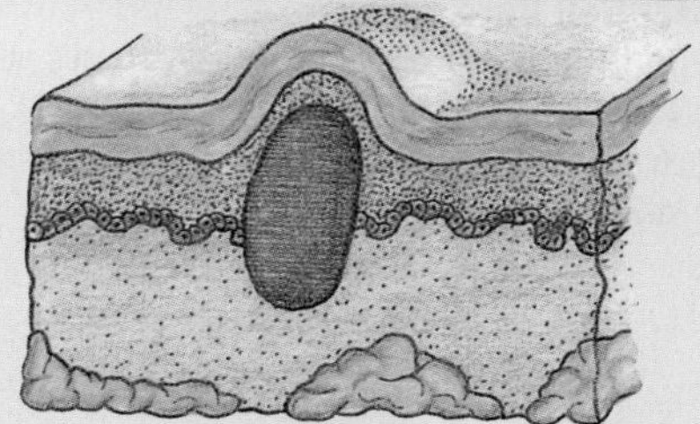

Nodule: Elevated solid mass, deeper and firmer than papule; 1-2 cm (e.g., wart)

Tumor: Solid mass that extends deep through subcutaneous tissue; larger than 1-2 cm (e.g., epithelioma)

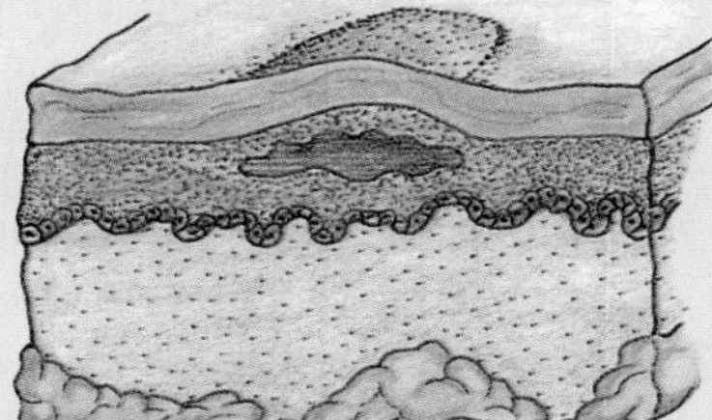

Wheal: Irregularly shaped, elevated area or superficial localized edema; varies in size (e.g., hive, mosquito bite)

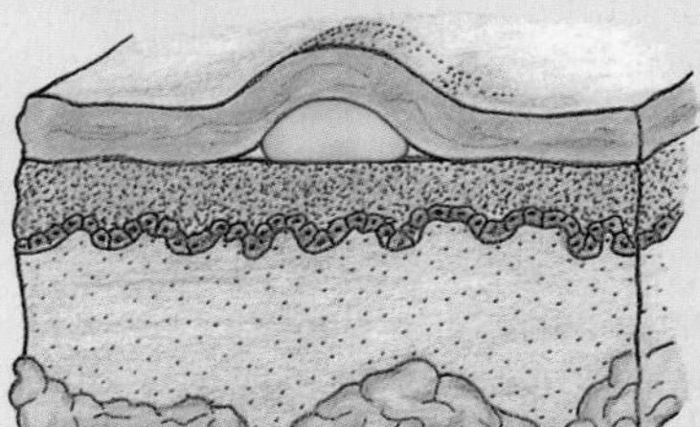

Vesicle: Circumscribed elevation of skin filled with serous fluid, smaller than 1 cm (e.g., herpes simplex, chickenpox)

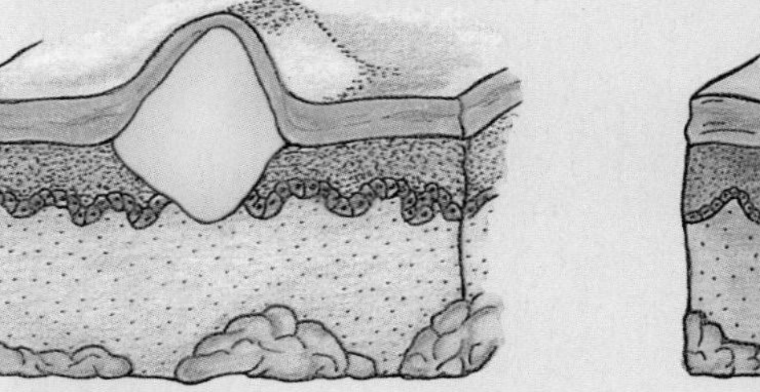

Pustule: Circumscribed elevation of skin similar to vesicle but filled with pus; varies in size (e.g., acne, staphylococcal infection)

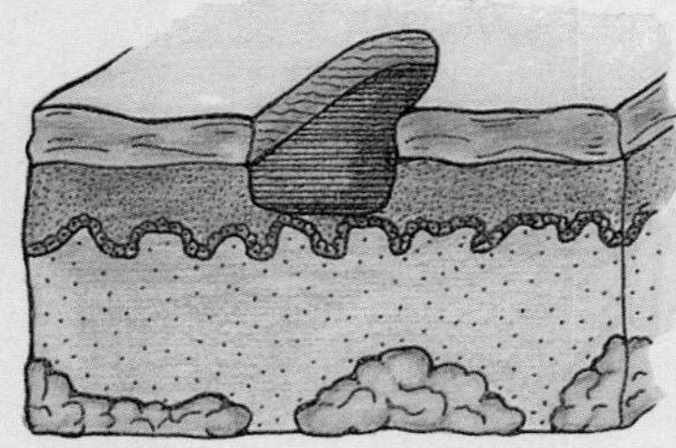

Ulcer: Deep loss of skin surface that extends to dermis and frequently bleeds and scars; varies in size (e.g., venous stasis ulcer)

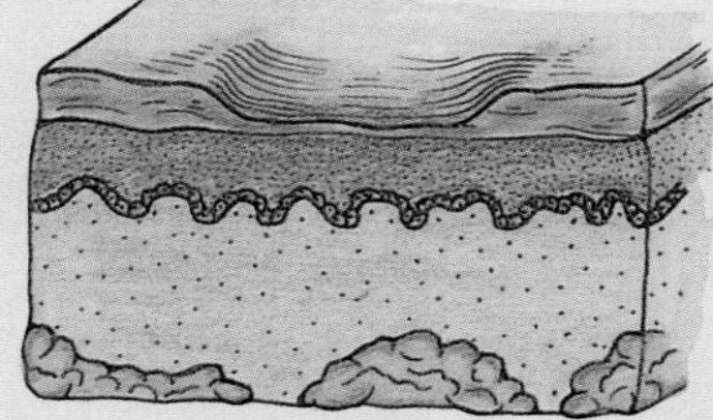

Atrophy: Thinning of skin with loss of normal skin furrow, with skin appearing shiny and translucent; varies in size (e.g., arterial insufficiency)

sections of scalp hair, observe characteristics of color and coarseness. Color varies from very light blond to black to gray and is sometimes altered by rinses or dyes. In older adults the hair becomes dull gray, white, or yellow.

Be aware of the normal distribution of hair growth in a man and a woman. At puberty an increase in the amount and distribution of hair occurs for both genders. During the aging process the hair may thin over the scalp, axillae, and pubic areas. Facial hair of older men decreases. A woman with hirsutism has hair growth on the upper lip, chin, and cheeks, with vellus hair becoming coarser over the body. This may be related to an endocrine disorder. For some a change in hair growth negatively affects body image and emotional well-being. The amount of hair covering the extremities is sometimes reduced as a result of aging, or it could result from arterial insufficiency that could reduce hair growth over the lower extremities. In the United States and some other cultures, women commonly shave their legs and axilla, although shaving remains a matter of personal preference among women from all cultures.

Assess for causes of changes in the thickness, texture, and lubrication of scalp hair. At times these are a result of febrile illnesses or scalp diseases that result in hair loss. Conditions such as thyroid disease alter the condition of the hair, making it fine and brittle. Hair loss (**alopecia**) or thinning of the hair is usually related to genetic tendencies or endocrine disorders such as diabetes, thyroiditis, and even menopause. Poor nutrition causes stringy, dull, dry, and thin hair. The oil of sebaceous glands lubricates the hair, but excessively oily hair is associated with androgen hormone stimulation. Dry, brittle hair occurs with aging and excessive use of chemical agents.

Normally the scalp is smooth and inelastic with even coloration. Carefully separate strands of hair and thoroughly inspect the scalp for lesions, which are not easy to notice in thick hair. Note the characteristics of any scalp lesion. For lumps or bruises, ask if the patient has experienced recent head trauma. Moles on the scalp are common, but they can bleed as a result of vigorous combing or brushing. Dandruff or psoriasis frequently causes scaliness or dryness of the scalp.

Careful inspection of hair follicles on the scalp and pubic areas can reveal lice or other parasites. The three types of lice are *Pediculus humanus capitis* (head lice), *Pediculus humanus corporis* (body lice), and *Pediculus pubis* (crab lice). The presence of lice does not mean that a person practices poor hygiene. Lice spread easily, especially among children who play closely together. Head and crab lice attach their eggs to hair. The tiny eggs look like oval particles of dandruff, although the

BOX 31-7 Skin Malignancies

Basal Cell Carcinoma

0.5- to 1-cm crusted lesion that is flat or raised and has a rolled, somewhat scaly border

Frequently appearance of underlying, widely dilated blood vessels within the lesion

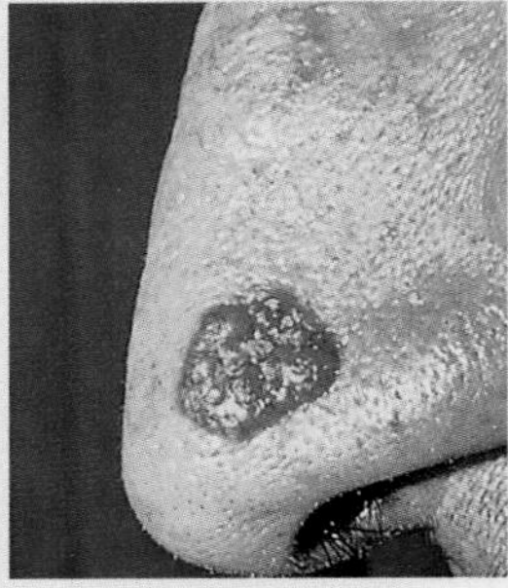

Squamous Cell Carcinoma

Occurs more often on mucosal surfaces and nonexposed areas of skin than basal cell

0.5- to 1.5-cm scaly lesion sometimes ulcerated or crusted; appears frequently and grows more rapidly than basal cell

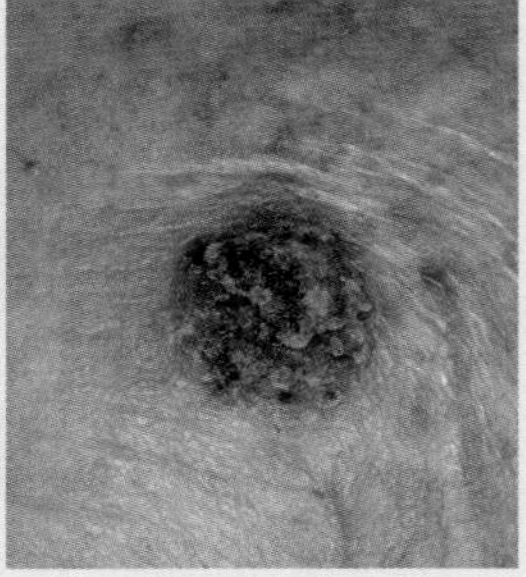

Melanoma

0.5- to 1-cm brown, flat lesion; appears on sun-exposed or nonexposed skin; variegated pigmentation, irregular borders, and indistinct margins

Ulceration, recent growth, or recent changes in long-standing mole are ominous signs

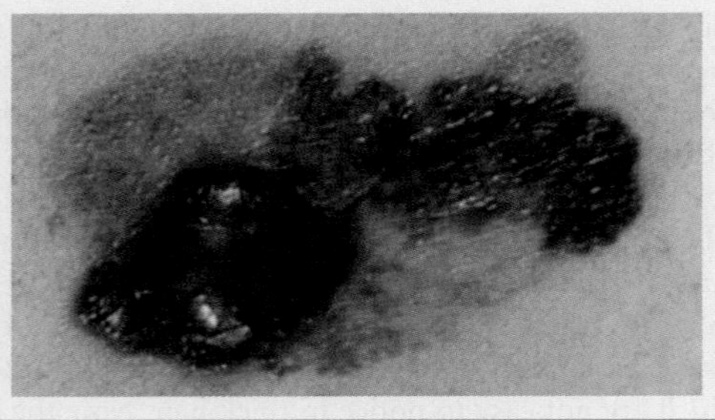

Illustrations from Belcher AE: *Cancer nursing,* St Louis, 1992, Mosby; Habif TP: *Clinical dermatology: a color guide to diagnosis and therapy,* ed 3, St Louis, 1996, Mosby; and Zitelli BJ, McIntyre SC, Nowalk AJ: *Zitelli and Davis' atlas of pediatric physical diagnosis,* ed 6, St Louis, 2012, Saunders.

lice themselves are difficult to see (Figure 31-7). Head and body lice are very small with grayish-white bodies, whereas crab lice have red legs. To better identify infestations, observe for small, red, pustular eruptions in the hair follicles and areas where skin surfaces meet, such as behind the ears and in the groin. A person often has intense itching of the scalp, especially on the back of the head or neck. Combing with a fine-tooth comb reveals the small oval-shaped lice; discovery of lice requires immediate treatment. Teach the patient to perform best hair and scalp hygiene practices (Box 31-8).

TABLE 31-10 Nursing History for Hair and Scalp Assessment

Assessment	Rationale
Ask patient if he or she is wearing a wig or hairpiece and ask him or her to remove it.	Wigs or hairpieces interfere with inspection of hair and scalp. (Patient sometimes requests to omit this part of examination.)
Determine if patient has noted change in growth, loss of hair, or change in texture or color.	Change often occurs slowly over time.
Identify type of hair-care products used for grooming.	Excessive use of chemical agents and burning of hair causes drying and brittleness.
Determine if patient has had chemotherapy (drugs that cause hair loss) recently or taken a vasodilator (minoxidil) for hair growth.	Chemotherapeutic agents kill cells that rapidly multiply such as tumor and normal hair cells. Minoxidil causes excessive hair growth.
Has patient noted changes in diet or appetite?	Nutrition influences condition of hair.

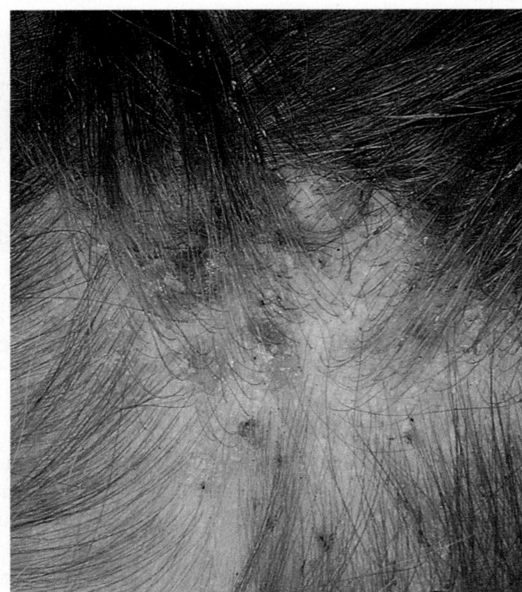

FIGURE 31-7 Head lice infestation. (From Habif TP: *Clinical dermatology: a color guide to diagnosis and therapy,* ed 4, Philadelphia, 2004, Mosby.)

Nails

The condition of the nails reflects a person's general health, state of nutrition, occupation, and habits of self-care. Before assessing the nails, gather a brief history (Table 31-11). The most visible part of the nail is the nail plate, the transparent layer of epithelial cells covering the nail bed (Figure 31-8). The vascularity of the nail bed creates the underlying color of the nail. The semilunar whitish area at the base of the nail bed is called the *lunula,* from which the nail plate grows.

BOX 31-8 PATIENT TEACHING

Hair and Scalp Assessment

Objective

- Patient will perform proper hygiene practices for care of hair and scalp.

Teaching Strategies

- Instruct patient about basic hygiene practices for hair and scalp care.
- Instruct patients who have head lice to shampoo thoroughly with pediculicide (shampoo available at drugstores) in cold water at a basin or sink. Do not use a tub or shower, where the medication can reach other body parts. Comb thoroughly with a fine-tooth comb (following product directions) and discard comb. *Caution: Do not use products containing Lindane, a toxic ingredient known to cause adverse reactions.* Repeat shampoo treatment 12 to 24 hours later.
- After shampooing, remove any detectable nits or nit cases with tweezers or a metal nit comb. A dilute solution of vinegar and water helps loosen nits.
- Instruct patients and parents about ways to reduce transmission of lice:
  - Do not share hair brushes, combs, hairpieces, hats, bedding, towels, or clothing with someone who has head lice.
  - Vacuum all rugs, car seats, pillows, furniture, and flooring thoroughly and discard vacuum bag.
  - Seal nonwashable items in plastic bags for 14 days if unable to dry-clean or vacuum.
  - Use thorough hand hygiene practices.
  - Launder all clothing, linen, and bedding in hot water and detergent; then dry in a hot dryer for at least 31 minutes. Dry-clean nonwashable items.
  - Do not use insecticide.
  - Instruct patient to notify his or her partner if lice were sexually transmitted.
  - Avoid physical contact with infested individuals and their belongings, especially clothing and bedding.
  - Soak any comb or brush used to remove lice for 15 minutes in very hot ammonia water (1 tsp ammonia to 2 cups hot water) or boiling water for 10 minutes.

Evaluation

- Have patient describe methods used to care for hair and scalp.
- Have patient explain the steps to take to reduce lice transmission in the home.

Inspection and Palpation. Inspect the nail bed for color, length, symmetry, cleanliness, and configuration. The shape and condition of the nails can give clues to pathophysiological problems. Assess the thickness and shape of the nail, its texture, the angle between the nail and the nail bed, and the condition of the lateral and proximal nail folds around the nail. When inspecting the nails you gather a sense of the patient's hygiene practices. The nails are normally transparent, smooth, well rounded, and convex, with a nail bed angle of about 160 degrees (Box 31-9). A larger angle and softening of the nail bed indicate chronic oxygenation problems. The surrounding cuticles are smooth, intact, and without inflammation. When you assess for basic care of the nails, you recognize that nail biting, stains, and jagged edges either represent poor nail care or are caused by habits or occupational exposure to grease or dirt. Jagged, bitten, or broken nail edges or cuticles predispose a patient to localized infection.

When palpating, expect to find a firm nail base and check for any abnormalities such as erythema or swelling. For patients with impaired circulation, especially observe for early signs of infection or open lesions. To palpate, gently grasp the patient's finger and observe the color of the nail bed. The nail bed and nails appear pink with white nail tips in white patients. In darker-skinned patients the nail beds are darkly pigmented with a blue or reddish hue. A brown or black pigmentation is normal with longitudinal streaks (Figure 31-9). Trauma, cirrhosis, diabetes mellitus, and hypertension cause splinter hemorrhages. Vitamin, protein, and electrolyte changes cause various lines or bands to form on the nail beds.

Nails normally grow at a constant rate, but direct injury or generalized disease changes growth patterns. With aging the nails of the fingers and toes become harder and thicker. Longitudinal striations develop, and the rate of nail growth slows. Nails become more brittle, dull, and

TABLE 31-11 Nursing History for Nail Assessment

Assessment	Rationale
Ask if patient has experienced recent trauma or changes in nails (splitting, breaking, discoloration, thickening).	Trauma changes shape and growth of nail. Systemic conditions cause changes in color, growth, and shape.
Has patient had other symptoms of pain, swelling, presence of systemic disease with fever, or psychological or physical stress?	Alterations sometimes occur slowly over time.
Question patient's nail care practices. Determine if patient has acrylic nails or silk wraps.	Change in nails can be caused by local or systemic problem. Acrylic nails and silk wraps are areas for fungal growth.
Determine if patient has risks for nail or foot problems (e.g., diabetes, peripheral vascular disease, older adulthood, obesity).	Chemical agents cause drying of nails. Improper care damages nails and cuticles. Vascular changes associated with diabetes and peripheral vascular disease reduce blood flow to peripheral tissues; foot lesions and thickened nails are common. Some older adults have trouble performing foot and nail care because of poor vision, lack of coordination, or inability to bend over. Obese patients have difficulty bending.

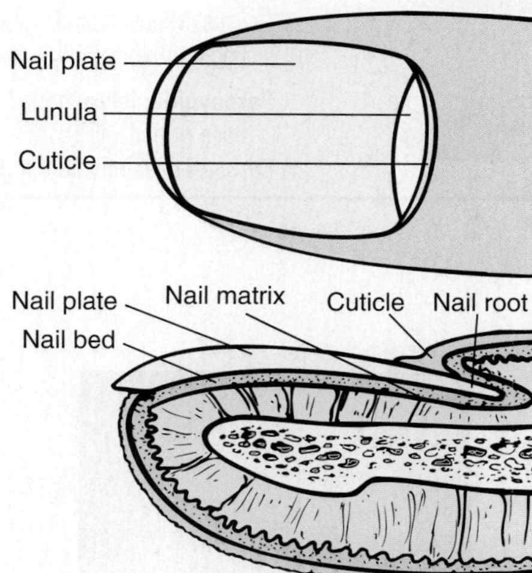

FIGURE 31-8 Components of nail unit. (From Lewis SL et al: *Medical-surgical nursing,* ed 9, St Louis, 2014, Mosby.)

BOX 31-9 Abnormalities of the Nail Bed

Normal nail: Approximately 160-degree angle between nail plate and nail

Clubbing: Change in angle between nail and nail base (eventually larger than 180 degrees); nail bed softening with nail flattening; often enlargement of fingertips
Causes: Chronic lack of oxygen: heart or pulmonary disease

Beau's lines: Transverse depressions in nails indicating temporary disturbance of nail growth (nail grows out over several months).
Causes: Systemic illness such as severe infection; nail injury

Koilonychia (spoon nail): Concave curves
Causes: Iron deficiency anemia, syphilis, use of strong detergents

Splinter hemorrhages: Red or brown linear streaks in nail bed
Causes: Minor trauma, subacute bacterial endocarditis, trichinosis

Paronychia: Inflammation of skin at base of nail
Causes: Local infection, trauma

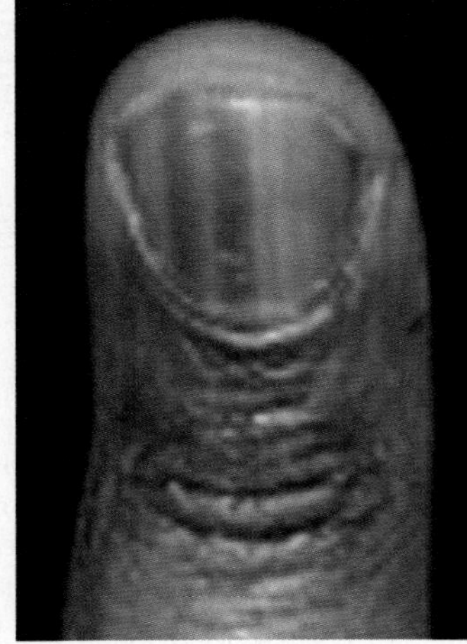

FIGURE 31-9 Pigmented bands in nail of patient with dark skin. (From Habif TP: *Clinical dermatology: a color guide to diagnosis and therapy,* ed 5, St Louis, 2010, Mosby.)

BOX 31-10 PATIENT TEACHING

Nail Assessment

Objective

- Patient will properly care for fingernails, feet, and toenails.

Teaching Strategies

- Instruct patient to cut nails only after soaking them about 10 minutes in warm water. (*Exception:* Patients with diabetes or peripheral vascular disease are warned against soaking nails because this can cause maceration of the skin, leading to infection. Long-term soaking also dries out the hands and feet; dry, cracked skin leads to infection.)
- Caution patient against over-the-counter preparations to treat corns, calluses, or ingrown toenails.
- Instruct patient to cut nails straight across and even with tops of fingers or toes. If patient has diabetes, tell him or her to file rather than cut nails (see Chapter 40).
- Instruct patient to shape nails with a file or emery board.
- If patient has diabetes:
  - Wash feet daily in warm water and carefully dry them, especially between toes. Inspect feet each day in good lighting, looking for dry places and cracks in skin. Soften dry feet by applying a cream or lotion such as Nivea, Eucerin, or Alpha Keri.
  - Do not put lotion between toes; moisture between toes allows microorganisms to grow, leading to infections.
  - Caution patient against using sharp objects to poke or dig under toenail or around the cuticle.
  - Have patient see a podiatrist for treatment of ingrown toenails and nails that are thick or tend to split.

Evaluation

- Inspect nails during the next home visit.
- Have patient explain steps to take to avoid injury.

opaque and turn yellow in older adults with insufficient calcium. In addition, the cuticle becomes less thick and wide.

Calluses and corns commonly are found on the toes or fingers. A callus is flat and painless, resulting from a thickening of the epidermis. Friction and pressure from shoes cause corns, usually over bony prominences. During the examination instruct the patient in proper nail care (Box 31-10).

HEAD AND NECK

An examination of the head and neck includes assessment of the head, eyes, ears, nose, mouth, pharynx, and neck (lymph nodes, carotid arteries, thyroid gland, and trachea). During assessment of peripheral arteries also assess the carotid arteries. Assessment of the head and neck uses inspection, palpation, and auscultation, with inspection and palpation often used simultaneously.

Head

Inspection and Palpation. The nursing history screens for intracranial injury and local or congenital deformities (Table 31-12). Inspect the patient's head, noting the position, size, shape, and contour. The head is normally held upright and midline to the trunk. Holding it tilted to one side acts as a behavioral indicator of a potential unilateral hearing or visual loss or is a physical indicator of muscle weakness in the neck. A horizontal jerking or bobbing indicates a tremor.

Note the patient's facial features, looking at the eyelids, eyebrows, nasolabial folds, and mouth for shape and symmetry. It is normal for slight asymmetry to exist. If there is facial asymmetry, note if all features on one side of the face are affected or if only a part of the face is involved. Various neurological disorders (e.g., facial nerve paralysis) affect different nerves that innervate muscles of the face.

Examine the size, shape, and contour of the skull. The skull is generally round with prominences in the frontal area anteriorly and the occipital area posteriorly. Trauma typically causes local skull deformities. In infants a large head results from congenital anomaly or the buildup of cerebrospinal fluid in the ventricles (hydrocephalus). Some adults have enlarged jaws and facial bones resulting from acromegaly, a disorder caused by excessive secretion of growth hormone. Palpate the skull for nodules or masses. Gently rotate the fingertips down the midline of the scalp and along the sides of the head to identify abnormalities. Palpate the temporomandibular joint (TMJ) space bilaterally. Place the fingertips just anterior to the tragus of each ear. The fingertips should slip into the joint space as the patient's mouth opens to gently palpate the joint spaces. Normally the movements should be smooth, although it is not unusual to hear or feel a clicking, grating or snapping in the TMJ, indicating degenerative joint disease (Ball et al., 2015).

TABLE 31-12 Nursing History for Head Assessment

Assessment	Rationale
Determine if patient experienced recent head trauma. If so, assess state of consciousness after injury (immediately on return and 5 minutes later), duration of unconsciousness, and predisposing factors (e.g., seizure, poor vision, blackout).	Trauma is major cause for lumps, bumps, cuts, bruises, or deformities of scalp or skull. Loss of consciousness following head injury indicates possible brain injury.
Ask if patient has history of headache; note onset, duration, character, pattern, and associated symptoms.	Character of headache helps to reveal causative factors such as sinus infection, migraine, or neurological disorders.
Determine length of time patient has experienced neurological symptoms.	Duration of signs or symptoms reveals severity of problem.
Review patient's occupational history for use of safety helmets.	Nature of some occupations creates a risk for head injury.
Ask if patient participates in contact sports, cycling, rollerblading, or skateboarding.	These activities require use of safety helmets.

Eyes

Examination of the eyes includes assessment of visual acuity, visual fields, extraocular movements, and external and internal eye structures. Figure 31-10 shows a cross-section of the eye. The eye assessment detects visual alterations and determines the general level of assistance that patients require when ambulating or performing self-care activities. Some patients with visual problems also need special aids for reading educational materials or instructions (e.g., medication labels). Table 31-13 reviews the nursing history for an eye examination. Box 31-11 describes common types of visual problems.

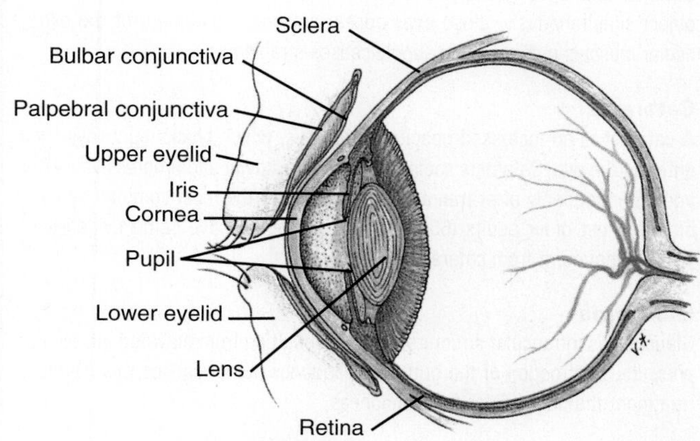

FIGURE 31-10 Cross-section of eye.

TABLE 31-13 Nursing History for Eye Assessment

Assessment	Rationale
Determine if patient has history of eye disease (e.g., glaucoma, retinopathy, cataracts), eye trauma, diabetes, hypertension, or eye surgery.	Some diseases or trauma cause risk for partial or complete visual loss. Patient may have had surgery for a visual disorder.
Determine problems that prompted patient to seek health care. Ask patient about eye pain, photophobia (sensitivity to light), burning or itching, excess tearing or crusting, diplopia (double vision) or blurred vision, awareness of a "film" or "curtain" over field of vision, floaters (small, black spots that seem to float across field of vision), flashing lights, or halos around lights.	Common symptoms of eye disease indicate need for health care provider.
Determine whether there is family history of eye disorders or diseases.	Certain eye problems such as glaucoma or retinitis pigmentosa are inherited.
Review patient's occupational history and recreational hobbies. Are safety glasses worn?	Performance of close, intricate work causes eye fatigue. Working with computers causes eye strain. Certain occupational tasks (e.g., working with chemicals) and recreational activities (e.g., fencing, motorcycle riding) place people at risk for eye injury unless they take precautions.
Ask patient if he or she wears glasses or contacts and, if so, how often.	Patients need to wear glasses or contacts during certain parts of examination for accurate assessment.
Determine when patient last visited ophthalmologist or optometrist.	Date of last eye examination reveals level of preventive care patient takes.
Assess medications patient is taking, including eyedrops or ointment.	Determines need to assess patient's knowledge of medications. Certain medications cause visual symptoms.

BOX 31-11 Common Eye and Vision Problems

Hyperopia
Hyperopia is farsightedness, a refractive error in which rays of light enter the eye and focus behind the retina. People are able to clearly see distant objects but not close objects.

Myopia
Myopia is nearsightedness, a refractive error in which rays of light enter the eye and focus in front of the retina. People are able to clearly see close objects but not distant objects.

Presbyopia
Presbyopia is impaired near vision in middle-age and older adults caused by loss of elasticity of the lens and associated with the aging process.

Retinopathy
Retinopathy is a noninflammatory eye disorder resulting from changes in retinal blood vessels. It is a leading cause of blindness.

Strabismus
Strabismus is a (congenital) condition in which both eyes do not focus on an object simultaneously; these eyes appear crossed. Impairment of the extraocular muscles or their nerve supply causes strabismus.

Cataracts
A cataract is an increased opacity of the lens, which blocks light rays from entering the eye. Cataracts sometimes develop slowly and progressively after age 35 or suddenly after trauma. They are one of the most common eye disorders. Most older adults (65 years old and older) have some evidence of visual impairment from cataracts.

Glaucoma
Glaucoma is intraocular structural damage resulting from elevated intraocular pressure. Obstruction of the outflow of aqueous humor causes this. Without treatment the disorder leads to blindness.

Macular Degeneration
Macular degeneration is associated with aging and results in damaging sharp and central vision. There are two types of macular degeneration: wet and dry. Wet AMD occurs when abnormal blood vessels behind the retina start to grow under the macula, ultimately leading to blood and fluid leakage. Dry AMD occurs when the macula thins over time as part of the aging process, gradually blurring central vision (CDC, 2013). Macular degeneration is one of the leading causes of blindness and low vision in the United States (CDC, 2013). There is no cure.

Visual Acuity. The assessment of visual acuity (i.e., the ability to see small details) tests central vision. The easiest way to assess near vision is to ask patients to read printed material under adequate lighting. If patients wear glasses, make sure that they wear them during the assessment. Determine the language the patient speaks and his or her reading ability. Asking patients to read aloud helps to determine literacy. If the patient has difficulty reading, move to the next step.

Assessment of distant vision requires using a Snellen chart (paper chart or projection screen). The chart should be well lit. Test vision without corrective lenses first. Have the patient sit or stand 6.1 m (20 feet) away from the chart and try to read all of the letters beginning at any line with both eyes open. Then have the patient read the line with each eye separately (patient covers the opposite eye with an index card or eye cover to avoid applying pressure to the eye). Note the smallest line for which the patient is able to read all of the letters correctly and record the visual acuity for that line. Repeat the test with the patient wearing corrective lenses. Complete the test rapidly enough so the patient does not memorize the chart (Ball et al., 2015). If a patient is unable to read, use an *E* chart or one with pictures of familiar objects. Instead of reading letters, patients tell which direction each *E* is pointing or the name of the object.

The Snellen chart has standardized numbers at the end of each line of the chart. The numerator is the number 20, or the distance the patient stands from the chart. The denominator is the distance from which the normal eye is able to read the chart. Normal visual acuity is 20/20. The larger the denominator, the poorer the patient's visual acuity. For example, a value of 20/40 means that the patient, standing 20 feet away, can read a line that a person with normal vision can read from 40 feet away. Record visual acuity for each eye and both eyes and record whether the test was performed with or without correction (including glasses or contact lenses).

If patients cannot read even the largest letters or figures of a Snellen chart, test their ability to count upraised fingers or distinguish light. Hold a hand 31 cm (1 foot) from the patient's face and have him or her count the upraised fingers. To check light perception shine a penlight into the eye and turn off the light. If the patient notes when the light is turned on or off, light perception is intact.

Assess near vision by asking the patient to read a handheld card containing a vision screening chart. The patient holds the card a comfortable distance (5 to 6 cm [about 12½ to 14 inches]) from the eyes and reads the smallest line possible. This part of the examination is a good time to discuss the need for routine eye examinations (Box 31-12).

BOX 31-12 PATIENT TEACHING

Eye Assessment

Objective
- Patient will follow recommendations for regular eye examinations and prevention of injury.

Teaching Strategies
- Explain recommended frequency for eye testing with a Snellen chart and examination (see Table 31-3).
- Describe the typical symptoms of eye disease.
- Instruct older adult to take the following precautions because of normal vision changes: avoid or use caution while driving at night, increase lighting in the home to reduce risk of falls, and paint the first and last steps of a staircase and the edge of each of the other steps a bright color to aid depth perception.
- Remind patient that wearing protective eyewear prevents injury from debris and splashes.

Evaluation
- Ask patient or family member to report on patient's most recent visit to an ophthalmologist.
- Have patient describe when to have an eye examination.
- Ask patient to describe common symptoms of eye disease.
- Observe the home environment of a patient with visual deficits.

Modified from Agency for Healthcare Research and Quality: *Guide to clinical preventive services,* AHRQ Publication No. 14-05158, 2014, Rockville, MD, http://www.ahrq.gov/professionals/clinicians-providers/guidelines-recommendations/guide/cpsguide.pdf. Accessed November 13, 2014.

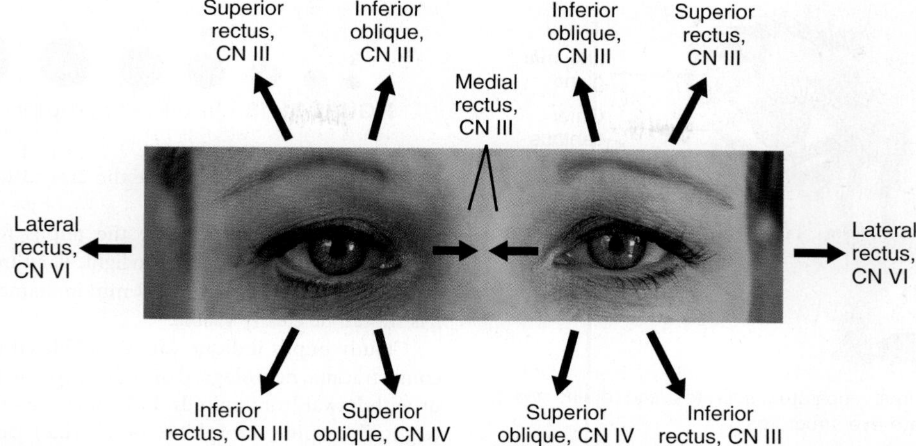

FIGURE 31-11 Six directions of gaze. Direct patient to follow finger movement through each gaze. *CN,* Cranial nerve.

Extraocular Movements. Six small muscles guide the movement of each eye. Both eyes move parallel to one another in each of the six directions of gaze (Figure 31-11). To assess extraocular movements, a patient sits or stands, and the nurse faces the patient from 60 cm (2 feet) away. The nurse holds a finger at a comfortable distance (15 to 31 cm [6 to 12 inches]) from the patient's eyes. While the patient maintains his or her head in a fixed position facing forward, the nurse directs him or her to follow with the eyes only as the nurse's finger moves to the right, left, and diagonally up and down to the left and right. The nurse moves the finger smoothly and slowly within the normal field of vision.

As the patient gazes in each direction, observe for parallel eye movement, the position of the upper eyelid in relation to the iris, and the presence of abnormal movements. As the eyes move through each direction of gaze, the upper eyelid covers the iris only slightly. Nystagmus, an involuntary, rhythmical oscillation of the eyes, occurs as a result of local injury to eye muscles and supporting structures or a disorder of the cranial nerves innervating the muscles. Initiate nystagmus in patients with normal eye movements by having them gaze to the far left or right.

Visual Fields. As a person looks straight ahead, he or she normally is able to see all objects in the periphery. To assess visual fields direct the patient to stand or sit 60 cm (2 feet) away at eye level. The patient gently closes or covers one eye (e.g., the left) and looks at your eye directly opposite. You close your opposite eye (in this case the right) so the field of vision is superimposed on that of the patient. Next move a finger equidistant between you and the patient outside the field of vision and slowly bring it back into the visual field. The patient reports when he or she is able to see the finger. If you see the finger before the patient does, a part of the patient's visual field is reduced. To test temporal field vision, hold an object or your finger slightly behind the patient. Repeat the procedure for each field of vision for the other eye. Patients with visual field problems are at risk for injury because they cannot see all of the objects in front of them. Older adults commonly have loss of peripheral vision caused by changes in the lens.

External Eye Structures. To inspect external eye structures, stand directly in front of the patient at eye level and ask him or her to look at your face.

Position and Alignment. Assess the position of the eyes in relation to one another. Normally they are parallel to one another. Bulging eyes (exophthalmos) usually indicate hyperthyroidism. Crossed eyes (strabismus) result from neuromuscular injury or inherited abnormalities. Tumors or inflammation of the orbit often cause abnormal eye protrusion.

For the remainder of the eye examination have the patient remove contact lenses.

Eyebrows. Inspect the eyebrows for size, extension, texture of hair, alignment, and movement. Normally the eyebrows are symmetrical. Coarseness of hair and failure to extend beyond the temporal canthus possibly reveals hypothyroidism. Thin brows may be a result of waxing or plucking. Aging causes loss of the lateral third of the eyebrows. To assess movement, ask the patient to raise and lower the eyebrows. The brows normally raise and lower symmetrically. An inability to move them indicates a facial nerve paralysis (cranial nerve VII).

Eyelids. Inspect the eyelids for position; color; condition of the surface; condition and direction of the eyelashes; and the patient's ability to open, close, and blink. When the eyes are open in a normal position, the lids cover the sclera above the iris but not the pupil. The lids are also close to the eyeball. An abnormal drooping of the lid over the pupil is called ptosis (pronounced "toe-sis"), caused by edema or impairment of the third cranial nerve. In the older adult ptosis results from a loss of elasticity that accompanies aging. You observe for defects in the position of the lid margins. An older adult frequently has lid margins that turn out (ectropion) or in (entropion). Entropion sometimes leads to the lashes of the lid irritating the conjunctiva and cornea, increasing the risk of infection. Normally the eyelashes are distributed evenly and curved outward away from the eye. An erythematous or yellow lump (hordeolum or sty) on the follicle of an eyelash indicates an acute suppurative inflammation.

To inspect the surface of the upper lids ask the patient to close his or her eyes while observing for lid tremors. Normally the lids are smooth and the same color as the surrounding skin. Redness indicates inflammation or infection. Lid edema is sometimes caused by allergies or heart or kidney failure. Edema of the eyelids prevents them from closing. Inspect any lesions for typical characteristics and discomfort or drainage. Wear clean gloves if drainage is present.

The lids normally close symmetrically. Their failure to close exposes the cornea to drying. This condition is common in unconscious patients or those with facial nerve paralysis. To inspect the lower lids, ask the patient to open the eyes again while you look for the same characteristics noted for the upper lids. Normally a patient blinks involuntarily and bilaterally up to 20 times a minute. The blink reflex

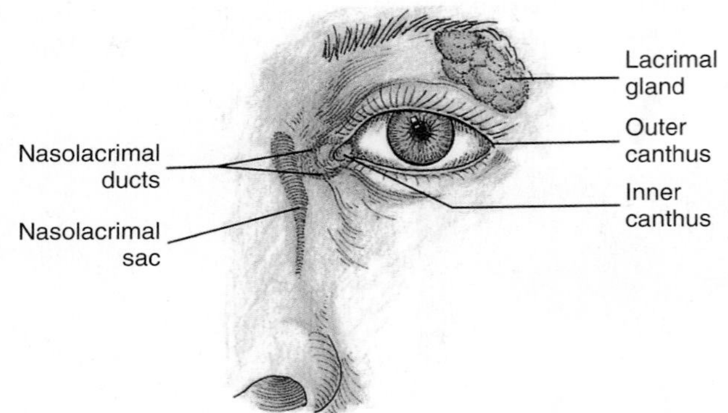

FIGURE 31-12 The lacrimal apparatus secretes and drains tears, which moisten and lubricate eye structures.

lubricates the cornea. Report absent, infrequent, rapid, or monocular (one-eyed) blinking.

Lacrimal Apparatus. The lacrimal gland (Figure 31-12), located in the upper outer wall of the anterior part of the orbit, is responsible for tear production. Tears flow from the gland across the surface of the eye to the lacrimal duct, which is in the nasal corner or inner canthus of the eye. The lacrimal gland is sometimes the site of tumors or infections and should be inspected for edema and redness. Palpate the gland gently to detect tenderness; normally tenderness cannot be felt.

The nasolacrimal duct sometimes becomes obstructed, blocking the flow of tears. Observe for evidence of edema in the inner canthus. Gentle palpation of the duct at the lower eyelid just inside the lower orbital rim causes a regurgitation of tears.

Conjunctivae and Sclerae. The bulbar conjunctiva covers the exposed surface of the eyeball up to the outer edge of the cornea. Observe the sclera under the bulbar conjunctiva; normally it has the color of white porcelain in light-skinned patients and is light yellow in dark-skinned patients. Sclerae become pigmented and appear either yellow or green if liver disease is present.

Take care when inspecting the conjunctivae. For adequate exposure of the bulbar conjunctiva, retract the eyelids without placing pressure directly on the eyeball. Gently retract both lids, with the thumb and index finger pressed against the lower and upper bony orbits. Ask the patient to look up, down, and from side to side. Many patients begin to blink, making the examination difficult. Inspect for color, texture, and the presence of edema or lesions. Normally the conjunctivae are free of erythema. The presence of redness indicates an allergic or infectious conjunctivitis. Bright red blood in a localized area surrounded by normal-appearing conjunctiva usually indicates subconjunctival hemorrhage. Conjunctivitis is a highly contagious infection. It is easy to spread the crusty drainage that collects on eyelid margins from one eye to the other. Wear clean gloves during the examination. Performing proper hand hygiene is necessary before and after the examination.

Corneas. The cornea is the transparent, colorless part of the eye covering the pupil and iris. From a side view it looks like the crystal of a wristwatch. While the patient looks straight ahead, inspect the cornea for clarity and texture while shining a penlight obliquely across its entire surface. The cornea is normally shiny, transparent, and smooth. In older adults it loses its luster. Any irregularity in the surface indicates an abrasion or tear that requires further examination by a health care provider. Both conditions are very painful. Note the color and details of the underlying iris. In an older adult the iris becomes faded. A thin white ring along the margin of the iris, called an arcus senilis, is common with aging but is abnormal in anyone under age 40. To test for the corneal blink reflex, see the cranial nerve test section of this chapter.

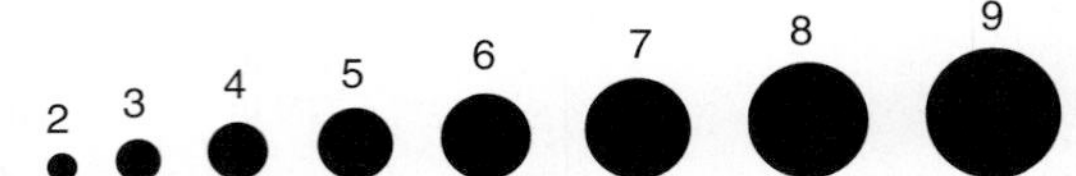

FIGURE 31-13 Chart depicting pupillary size in millimeters.

Pupils and Irises. Observe the pupils for size, shape, equality, accommodation, and reaction to light. They are normally black, round, regular, and equal in size (3 to 7 mm in diameter) (Figure 31-13). The iris should be clearly visible.

Cloudy pupils indicate cataracts. Dilated pupils result from glaucoma, trauma, neurological disorders, eye medications (e.g., atropine), or withdrawal from opioids. Inflammation of the iris or use of drugs (e.g., pilocarpine, morphine, or cocaine) causes constricted pupils. Pinpoint pupils are a common sign of opioid intoxication. Shining a beam of light through the pupil and onto the retina stimulates the third cranial nerve, causing the muscles of the iris to constrict. Any abnormality along the nerve pathways from the retina to the iris alters the ability of the pupils to react to light. Changes in intracranial pressure, lesions along the nerve pathways, locally applied ophthalmic medications, and direct trauma to the eye alter pupillary reaction.

Test pupillary reflexes (to light and accommodation) in a dimly lit room. Instruct the patient to avoid looking directly at the light. While the patient looks straight ahead, bring a penlight from the side of his or her face, directing the light onto the pupil (Figure 31-14). A directly illuminated pupil constricts, and the opposite pupil constricts consensually. Observe the quickness and equality of the reflex. Repeat the examination for the opposite eye.

To test for accommodation, ask the patient to gaze at a distant object (the far wall) and then at a test object (finger or pencil) held approximately 10 cm (4 inches) from the bridge of his or her nose. The pupils normally converge and accommodate by constricting when looking at close objects. The pupillary responses are equal. Testing for accommodation is only important if the patient has a defect in the pupillary response to light (Ball et al., 2015). If assessment of pupillary reaction is normal in all tests, record the abbreviation PERRLA (pupils equal, round, reactive to light, and accommodation).

Internal Eye Structures. The examination of the internal eye structures through the use of an ophthalmoscope is beyond the scope of new graduate nurses' practice. Advanced nurse practitioners use the ophthalmoscope to inspect the fundus (Figure 31-15), which includes the retina, choroid, optic nerve disc, macula, fovea centralis, and retinal vessels. Patients in greatest need of an examination are those with diabetes, hypertension, and intracranial disorders.

Ears

The ear assessment determines the integrity of ear structures and hearing acuity. The three parts of the ear are the external, middle, and inner ear (Figure 31-16). Inspect and palpate external ear structures, which consist of the auricle, outer ear canal, and tympanic membrane (eardrum). The ear canal is normally curved and approximately 2.5 cm (1 inch) long in an adult. It is lined with skin containing fine hairs, nerve endings, and glands secreting cerumen. The middle ear is inspected with an otoscope. It is an air-filled cavity containing the three bony ossicles (malleus, incus, and stapes). The eustachian tube connects the middle ear to the nasopharynx. Pressure between the outer atmosphere and the middle ear is stabilized through this tube. Finally the inner ear is tested by measuring a patient's hearing acuity. The inner ear contains the cochlea, vestibule, and semicircular canals.

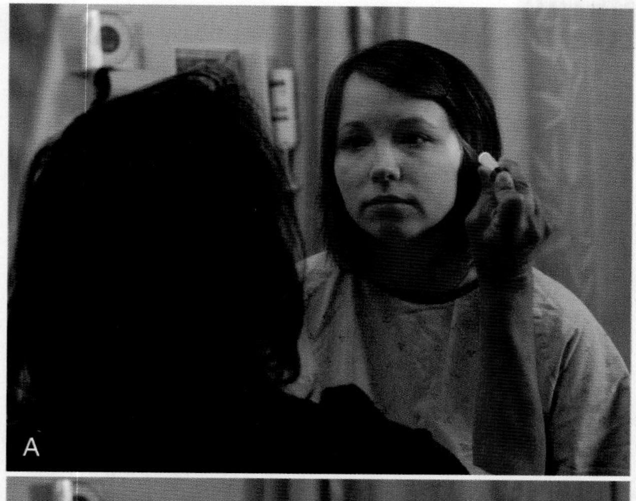

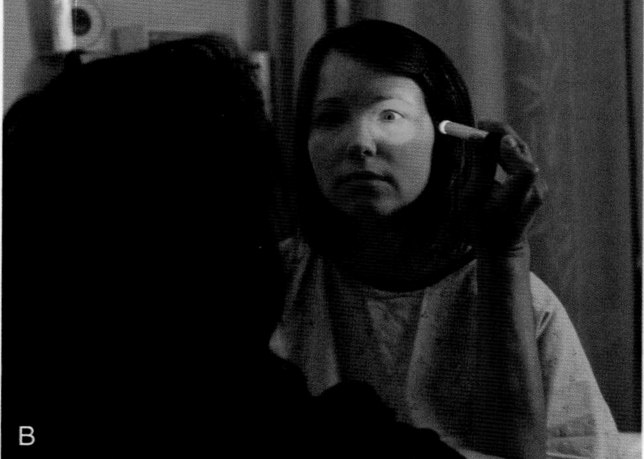

FIGURE 31-14 **A,** To check pupillary reflexes the nurse first holds penlight to side of patient's face. **B,** Illumination of pupil causes pupillary constriction.

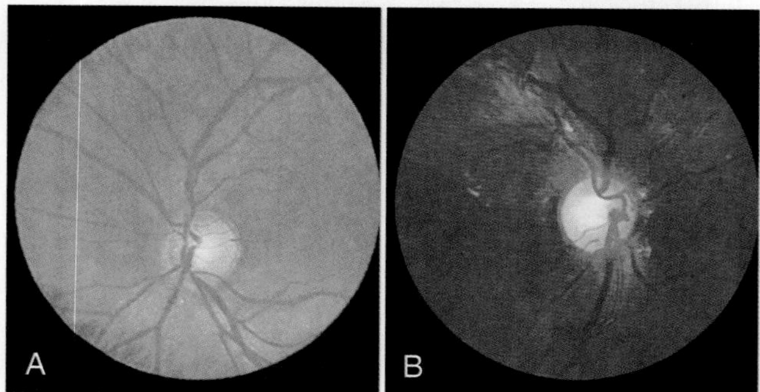

FIGURE 31-15 Fundus of white patient **(A)** and black patient **(B).** (Courtesy MEDCOM, Cypress, CA.)

Assessing the ears determines the integrity of ear structures and the condition of hearing. Use nursing history data to identify patients' risks for hearing disorders (Table 31-14).

Understanding the mechanisms for sound transmission helps identify the nature of hearing disorders. Sound travels through the ear by air and bone conduction. Nerve impulses from the cochlea travel to the auditory nerve (eighth cranial nerve) and the cerebral cortex. Disorders of the ear result from several types of problems, including mechanical dysfunction (blockage by cerumen or foreign body), trauma (foreign bodies or noise exposure), neurological disorders (auditory nerve damage), acute illnesses (viral infection), and toxic effects of medications.

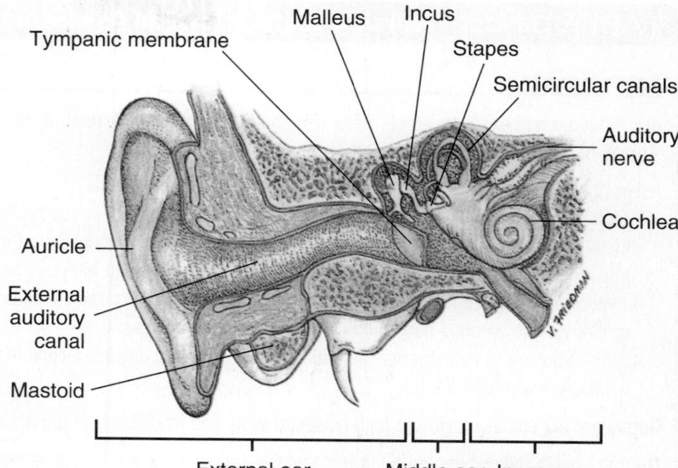

FIGURE 31-16 Structures of external, middle, and inner ear.

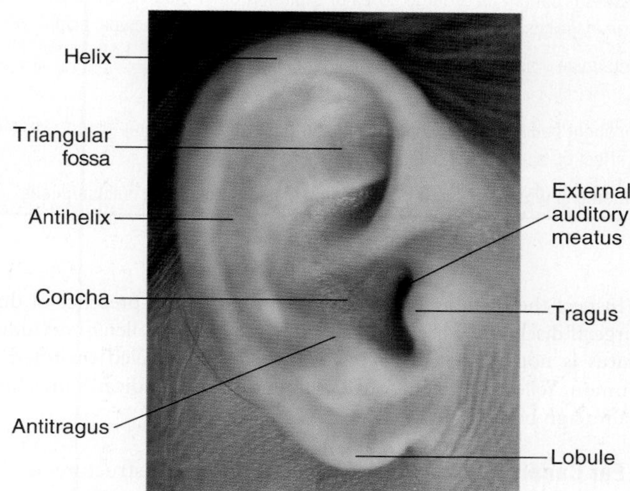

FIGURE 31-17 Anatomical structures of auricle.

Auricles. With the patient sitting comfortably, inspect the size, shape, symmetry, landmarks, position, and color of the auricle (Figure 31-17). The auricles are normally of equal size and level with one another. The upper point of attachment is in a straight line with the lateral canthus, or corner of the eye. The position of the auricle is almost vertical. Ears that are low set or at an unusual angle are a sign of chromosome abnormality such as Down syndrome. Ear color is usually the same as that of the face, without moles, cysts, deformities, or nodules. Redness is a sign of inflammation or fever. Extreme pallor indicates frostbite.

Palpate the auricles for texture, tenderness, and skin lesions. Auricles are normally smooth and without lesions. If a patient complains of pain, gently pull the auricle, press on the tragus, and palpate behind the ear over the mastoid process. If palpating the external ear increases the pain, an external ear infection is likely. If palpating the auricle and tragus does not influence the pain, the patient can have a middle ear infection. Tenderness in the mastoid area indicates mastoiditis.

TABLE 31-14 Nursing History for Ear Assessment

Assessment	Rationale
Ask if patient has experienced ear pain, itching, discharge, vertigo, tinnitus (ringing in ears), or change in hearing.	These signs and symptoms indicate infection or hearing loss.
Assess risks for hearing problem. *Infants/children:* Hypoxia at birth, meningitis, birth weight less than 1500 g, family history of hearing loss, congenital anomalies of skull or face, nonbacterial intrauterine infections (rubella, herpes), maternal drug use, excessively high bilirubin, head trauma *Adolescents:* Frequent exposure to loud music from concerts, car radios, and cell phone or iPods while wearing headphone, earbuds, or other devices *Adults:* Exposure to industrial or recreational noise, genetic disease (Ménière's disease), neurodegenerative disorder	Risk factors predispose patient to permanent hearing loss. It is difficult to assess infant's hearing status with examination only.
Determine patient's exposure to loud noises at work and availability of protective devices.	Prolonged noise exposure causes temporary or permanent hearing loss.
Note behaviors indicative of hearing loss such as failure to respond when spoken to, requests to repeat comments, leaning forward to hear, and child's inattentiveness or use of monotonous voice tone.	People with hearing loss cope with sensory deficit through a variety of behavioral cues.
Assess if patient takes large doses of aspirin or other ototoxic drugs (e.g., aminoglycosides, furosemide, streptomycin, cisplatin, ethacrynic acid).	Medications have side effects of hearing loss.
Determine whether patient uses hearing aid.	Determination allows you to assess patient's ability to care for device and adjust voice tone to communicate.
If patient had recent hearing problem, note onset, contributing factors, affected ear, and effect on activities of daily living.	Helps determine nature and severity of hearing problem.
Determine whether patient has repeated history of cerumen buildup in ear.	Cerumen impaction is common cause for conduction deafness.

Inspect the opening of the ear canal for size and presence of discharge. If discharge is present, wear clean gloves. A swollen or occluded meatus is not normal. A yellow, waxy substance called **cerumen** is common. Yellow or green, foul-smelling discharge indicates infection or a foreign body.

Ear Canals and Eardrums. Observe the deeper structures of the external and middle ear with the use of an otoscope. A special ear speculum attaches to the handle of the ophthalmoscope. For best visualization select the largest speculum that fits comfortably in the patient's ear. Before inserting the speculum, check for foreign bodies in the opening of the auditory canal.

Make sure that the patient avoids moving the head during the examination to avoid damage to the canal and tympanic membrane. Infants and young children might need to be held securely to prevent movement. Lay infants supine with head turned to one side and arms held securely at the sides. Have young children sit on their parents' laps with their legs held between the parents' knees.

Turn on the otoscope by rotating the dial at the top of the handle. To insert the speculum properly, ask the patient to tip the head slightly toward the opposite shoulder. Hold the handle of the otoscope in the space between the thumb and index finger, supported on the middle finger. This leaves the ulnar side of the hand to rest against the patient's head, stabilizing the otoscope as you insert it into the canal (Ball et al., 2015). There are two ways to grip the otoscope: (1) hold the handle along the patient's face with the fingers against the face or neck; and (2) lightly brace the inverted otoscope against the side of the patient's head or cheek. This latter grip, used with children, prevents accidental movement of the otoscope deeper into the ear canal. Insert the scope while pulling the auricle upward and backward in the adult and older child (Figure 31-18). This maneuver straightens the ear canal. For infants the auricle should be pulled down and back.

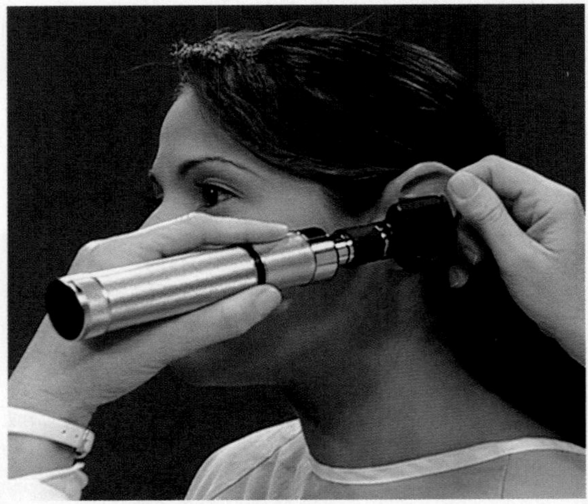

FIGURE 31-18 Otoscopic examination. (From Ball JW et al: *Seidel's guide to physical examination,* ed 8, St Louis, 2015, Mosby.)

Insert the speculum slightly down and forward 1 to 1.5 cm (½ inch) into the ear canal. Take care not to scrape the sensitive lining, which is painful. The ear canal normally has little cerumen and is uniformly pink with tiny hairs in the outer third of the canal. Observe for color, discharge, scaling, lesions, foreign bodies, and cerumen. Normally cerumen is dry (light brown to gray and flaky) or moist (dark yellow or brown) and sticky. Dry cerumen is common in Asians and Native Americans (Ball et al., 2015). A reddened canal with discharge is a sign of inflammation or infection. In other adults accumulated cerumen is a common problem; buildup creates a mild hearing loss. During the examination ask the patient about methods he or she uses to clean the ear canal (Box 31-13).

BOX 31-13 PATIENT TEACHING

Ear Assessment

Objective

- Patient will follow preventive guidelines for screening of hearing loss and proper cleaning technique for the ears.

Teaching Strategies

- Explain that noise-induced hearing loss can lead to communication difficulties, learning difficulties, pain or ringing in the ears (tinnitus), distorted or muffled hearing, and an inability to hear some environmental sounds and warning signals.
- Apply cultural sensitivity in encouraging patients to adopt behaviors to protect their hearing (CDC, 2015a):
  - Avoid or limit exposure to excessively loud sounds
  - Turn down the volume of music systems
  - Move away from the source of loud sounds when possible
  - Use hearing protection devices when it is not feasible to avoid exposure to loud sounds or to reduce them to a safe levels
- Instruct patient in the proper way to clean the outer ear (see Chapter 40), avoiding use of cotton-tipped applicators and sharp objects such as hairpins, which cause impaction of cerumen deep in the ear canal or trauma.
- Tell patient to avoid inserting pointed objects into the ear canal.
- Encourage patients over age 65 to have regular hearing checks. Explain that a reduction in hearing is a normal part of aging (see Chapter 49).
- Instruct family members of patients with hearing loss to avoid shouting; speak in slower, low tones; and be sure that patient is able to see the speaker's face.

Evaluation

- Have patient describe ways he or she can protect hearing at home.
- Ask patient to explain the proper technique for cleaning the ears.
- In a follow-up visit question patient about frequency of hearing checks.
- Observe patient with hearing loss interacting with family members.

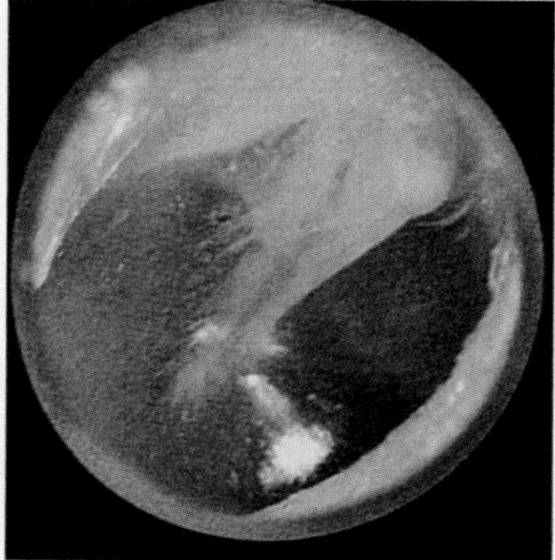

FIGURE 31-19 Normal right tympanic membrane. (Courtesy Dr. Richard A. Buckingham, Abraham Lincoln School of Medicine, University of Illinois, Chicago.)

The light from the otoscope allows visualization of the tympanic membrane. Know the common anatomical landmarks and their appearances (Figure 31-19). Gently move the otoscope so the entire tympanic membrane and its periphery are visible. Because the tympanic membrane is angled away from the ear canal, the light from the otoscope appears as a cone shape rather than a circle. A ring of fibrous cartilage surrounds the oval membrane. The umbo is near the center of the membrane, behind which is the attachment of the malleus. The underlying short process of the malleus creates a knoblike structure at the top of the drum. Check carefully to make sure that there are no tears or breaks in the membrane. The normal tympanic membrane is translucent, shiny, and pearly gray. It is free from tears or breaks. A pink or red bulging membrane indicates inflammation. A white color reveals pus behind it. The membrane is taut, except for the small triangular pars flaccida near the top. If cerumen is blocking the tympanic membrane, warm water irrigation safely removes the wax.

Hearing Acuity. A patient with a hearing loss often fails to respond to conversation. The three types of hearing loss are conduction, sensorineural, and mixed. A conduction loss interrupts sound waves as they travel from the outer ear to the cochlea of the inner ear because the sound waves are not transmitted through the outer and middle ear structures. For example, causes of a conduction loss include swelling of the auditory canal and tears in the tympanic membrane. A sensorineural loss involves the inner ear, auditory nerve, or hearing center of the brain. Sound is conducted through the outer and middle ear structures, but the continued transmission of sound becomes interrupted at some point beyond the bony ossicles. A mixed loss involves a combination of conduction and sensorineural loss. Patients working or living around loud noises and those who listen to loud music are at risk for hearing loss. According to the CDC (2015a) an estimated 12.5% of children and adolescents 6 to 19 years of age (approximately 5.2 million) and 17% of adults 20 to 69 years of age (approximately 26 million) have suffered permanent damage to their hearing from excessive exposure to noise.

Older adults experience an inability to hear high-frequency sounds and consonants (e.g., *S, Z, T,* and *G*). Deterioration of the cochlea and thickening of the tympanic membrane cause older adults to gradually lose hearing acuity. They are especially at risk for hearing loss caused by **ototoxicity** (injury to auditory nerve) resulting from high maintenance doses of antibiotics (e.g., aminoglycosides).

To conduct a hearing assessment, have the patient remove any hearing aid if worn. Note his or her response to questions. Normally he or she responds without excessive requests to have the questions repeated. If a hearing loss is suspected, check the patient's response to the whispered voice. Test one ear at a time while the patient occludes the other ear with a finger. Ask him or her to gently move the finger up and down during the test in response to the whispered sound. While standing 31 to 60 cm (1 to 2 feet) from the testing ear, speak while covering the mouth so the patient is unable to read lips. After exhaling fully, whisper softly toward the unoccluded ear, reciting random numbers with equally accented syllables such as *nine-four-ten.* If necessary, gradually increase voice intensity until the patient correctly repeats the numbers. Then test the other ear for comparison. Ball et al. (2015) report that patients normally hear numbers clearly when whispered, responding correctly at least 50% of the time.

If a hearing loss is present, test the hearing using a tuning fork. A tuning fork of 256 to 512 hertz (Hz) is most commonly used. The tuning fork allows for comparison of hearing by bone conduction with that of air conduction. Hold the base of the tuning fork with one hand without touching the tines. Tap the fork lightly against the palm of the other hand to set it in vibration (Table 31-15).

Nose and Sinuses

Use inspection and palpation to assess the integrity of the nose and sinuses. The patient sits during the examination. A penlight allows for gross examination of each naris. A more detailed examination requires use of a nasal speculum to inspect the deeper nasal turbinates. Do not use a speculum unless a qualified practitioner such as a nurse educator or an advanced practice nurse is present. Table 31-16 lists components of the nursing history.

TABLE 31-15 Tuning Fork Tests

Tests and Steps	Rationale
Weber's Test (Lateralization of Sound) Hold fork at its base and tap it lightly against heel of palm. Place base of vibrating fork on midline vertex of patient's head or middle of forehead (see illustration *A*). Ask patient if he or she hears the sound equally in both ears or better in one ear (lateralization).	Patient with normal hearing hears sound equally in both ears. In conduction deafness sound is heard best in impaired ear. In sensorineural hearing loss, sound is heard better in normal ear.
Rinne Test (Comparison of Air and Bone Conduction) Place stem of vibrating tuning fork against patient's mastoid process (see illustration *B*). Begin counting the interval with your watch. Ask patient to tell you when he or she no longer hears the sound; note number of seconds. Quickly place still-vibrating tines 1 to 2 cm (½ to 1 inch) from ear canal and ask patient to tell you when he or she no longer hears the sound (see illustration *C*). Continue counting time the sound is heard by air conduction. Compare number of seconds the sound is heard by bone conduction versus air conduction.	Patient should hear air-conducted sound twice as long as bone-conducted sound (2 : 1 ratio). For example, if patient hears bone-conducted sound for 10 seconds, he or she should hear air-conducted sound for an additional 10 seconds. In conduction deafness patient hears bone conduction longer than air conduction in affected ear. In sensorineural loss patient hears air conduction longer than bone conduction in affected ear, but at less than a 2 : 1 ratio (Ball et al., 2015).

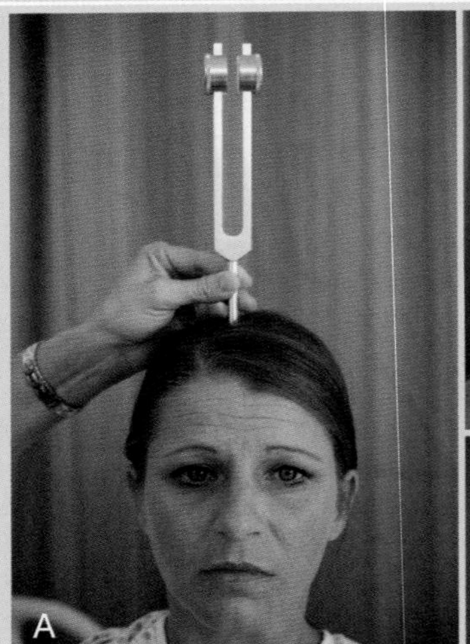

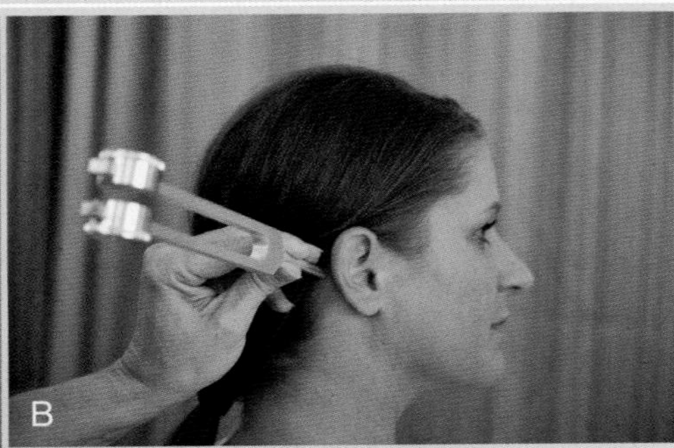

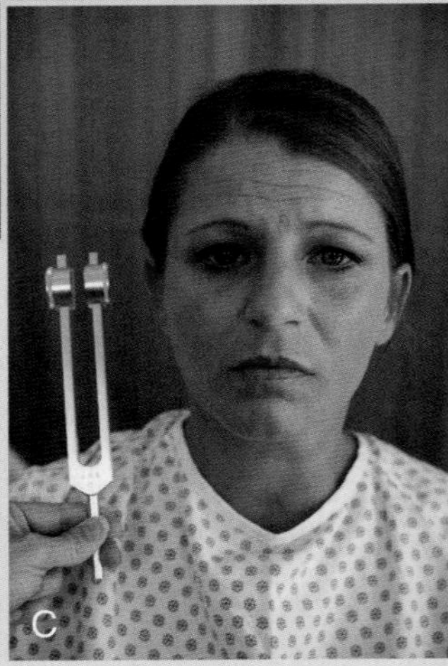

Nose. When inspecting the external nose, observe for shape, size, skin, color, and the presence of deformity or inflammation. The nose is normally smooth and symmetrical with the same skin color as the face. Recent trauma sometimes causes edema and discoloration. If swelling or deformities exist, gently palpate the ridge and soft tissue of the nose by placing one finger on each side of the nasal arch and gently moving the fingers from the nasal bridge to the tip. Note any tenderness, masses, or underlying deviations. Nasal structures are usually firm and stable.

Air normally passes freely through the nose when a person breathes. To assess patency of the nares, place a finger on the side of the patient's nose and occlude one naris. Ask the patient to breathe with the mouth closed. Repeat the procedure for the other naris.

While illuminating the anterior nares, inspect the mucosa for color, lesions, discharge, swelling, and evidence of bleeding. If discharge is present, apply gloves. Normal mucosa is pink and moist without lesions. Pale mucosa with clear discharge indicates allergy. A mucoid discharge indicates rhinitis. A sinus infection results in yellowish or

TABLE 31-16 Nursing History for Nose and Sinus Assessment

Assessment	Rationale
Ask if patient has had trauma to nose.	Trauma causes septal deviation and asymmetry of external nose.
Ask if patient has history of allergies, nasal discharge, epistaxis (nosebleeds), or postnasal drip.	History is useful in determining source or nature of nasal and sinus drainage.
If there is history of nasal discharge, assess color, amount, odor, duration, and associated symptoms (e.g., sneezing, nasal congestion, obstruction, or mouth breathing).	Aids in ruling out presence of infection, allergy, or drug use.
Assess for history of nosebleed, including site, frequency, amount of bleeding, treatment, and difficulty stopping bleeding.	Characteristics sometimes reveal trauma, medication use, or excessive dryness as causative factors.
Ask if patient uses nasal spray or drops, including amount, frequency, and duration of use.	Overuse of over-the-counter nasal preparations causes physical change in mucosa.
Ask if patient snores at night or has difficulty breathing.	Difficulty breathing or snoring indicates septal deviation or obstruction.

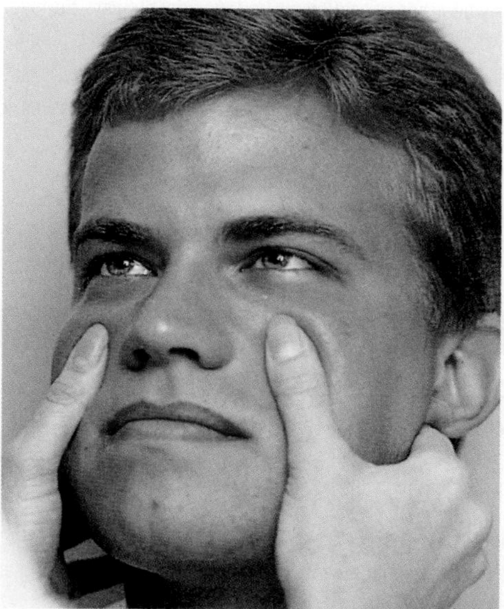

FIGURE 31-20 Palpation of maxillary sinuses.

greenish discharge. Habitual use of intranasal cocaine and opioids causes puffiness and increased vascularity of the nasal mucosa. For the patient with a nasogastric tube, routinely check for local skin breakdown (**excoriation**) of the naris, characterized by redness and skin sloughing.

To view the septum and turbinates, have the patient tip the head back slightly to provide a clear view. Illuminate the septum and observe for alignment, perforation, or bleeding. Normally the septum is close to the midline and thicker anteriorly than posteriorly. The turbinates are covered with mucous membranes that warm and moisten inspired air. Normal mucosa is pink and moist, without lesions. A deviated septum obstructs breathing and interferes with passage of a nasogastric tube. Perforation of the septum often occurs after repeated use of intranasal cocaine. Note any **polyps** (tumorlike growths) or purulent drainage.

Sinuses. Examination of the sinuses involves palpation. In cases of allergies or infection, the interior of the sinuses becomes inflamed and swollen. The most effective way to assess for tenderness is by externally palpating the frontal and maxillary facial areas (Figure 31-20). Palpate the frontal sinus by exerting pressure with the thumb up and under the patient's eyebrow. Gentle, upward pressure elicits tenderness easily if sinus irritation is present. Do not apply pressure to the eyes. If sinus tenderness is present, the sinuses may be transilluminated. However, this procedure requires advanced experience. Box 31-14 describes teaching guidelines during nose and sinus assessment.

BOX 31-14 PATIENT TEACHING

Nose and Sinus Assessment

Objective

- Patient will explain self-care measures to address and minimize loss of olfaction.

Teaching Strategies

- Caution patient against overuse of over-the-counter nasal sprays, which leads to "rebound" effect, causing excess nasal congestion.
- Instruct parents in care of a child with nosebleeds: have child sit up and lean forward to avoid aspiration of blood, apply pressure to the anterior nose with the thumb and forefinger as the child breathes through the mouth, and apply ice or a cold cloth to the bridge of the nose if pressure fails to stop bleeding.
- Instruct older adults with loss of olfaction to follow safety precautions:
  - Install smoke detectors on each floor of their home.
  - Ask others to advise them when food smells pungent.
- Instruct older adults to always check dated labels on food to ensure against spoilage.

Evaluation

- Have patient explain proper use of over-the-counter nasal sprays.
- Have parents demonstrate and describe technique for stopping a nosebleed.
- Inspect patient's home during visit and look for smoke detectors. Ask to check some food items in the refrigerator.

Mouth and Pharynx

Assess the mouth and pharynx to detect signs of overall health. Determine the patient's oral hygiene needs and therapies needed if he or she has dehydration, restricted intake, oral trauma, or oral airway obstruction. To assess the oral cavity use a penlight and tongue depressor or gauze square. Wear clean gloves during the examination. Have the patient sit or lie down. Assess the oral cavity also while

TABLE 31-17 Nursing History for Mouth and Pharyngeal Assessment

Assessment	Rationale
Determine if patient wears dentures or retainers and if they are comfortable.	Patient needs to remove dentures to visualize and palpate gums. Ill-fitting dentures chronically irritate mucosa and gums.
Determine if patient has had recent change in appetite or weight.	Symptoms result from painful mouth conditions or poor hygiene.
Determine if patient uses tobacco products: • Smoking cigarette, cigar, or pipe; smokeless tobacco; chewing tobacco and snuff • E-Cigarettes or vapor cigarettes	Tobacco use in any form (smoked and smokeless) increases the risk for oral-pharyngeal cancer (ACS, 2015a). Long-term snuff users have an increased risk for cancer of the gums and cheeks (ACS, 2015a). Exposure to addictive nicotine effects; unknown effects of inhalants on the oral cavity (Cancer Net, 2015)
Review history for alcohol consumption.	Oral and pharyngeal cancers are more common in alcohol users than nonalcohol users. Combine tobacco with heavy use of alcohol, and the risk is significantly increased because the two act synergistically (ACS, 2015a). Those who both smoke and drink have a 15 times greater risk of developing oral cancer than others (Oral Cancer Foundation, 2014). Effects of alcohol are also independent of tobacco use.
Assess dental hygiene practices, including use of fluoride toothpaste, frequency of brushing and flossing, and frequency of dental visits.	Assessment reveals patient's need for education and/or financial support. Periodontal disease has a higher prevalence in older adults who have history of high plaque buildup, use tobacco, and visit the dentist infrequently.
Ask if patient has pain from chewing or eating. If so, ask if mouth lesions are present, including duration and associated symptoms.	Pain is often associated with broken tooth, teeth grinding, or temporomandibular joint problems. Extra care is needed during oral hygiene administration.
Review the patient's medical history for a previous diagnosis of the human papilloma virus (HPV).	HPV, particularly HPV16, has been definitively implicated as a risk for oral cancers, particularly those that occur in the back of the mouth (oropharynx, base of tongue, tonsillar pillars and crypt, and the tonsils themselves) (Oral Cancer Foundation, 2014; ACS, 2015a).

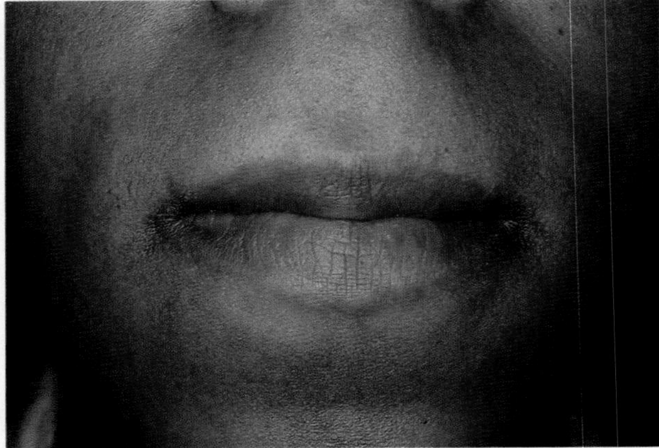

FIGURE 31-21 Lips are normally pink, symmetrical, smooth, and moist.

administering oral hygiene (see Chapter 40). Table 31-17 describes the nursing history for assessment of the mouth and pharynx.

Lips. Inspect the lips for color, texture, hydration, contour, and lesions. With the patient's mouth closed, view the lips from end to end. Normally they are pink, moist, symmetrical, and smooth (Figure 31-21). Lip color in the dark-skinned patient varies from pink to plum. Have female patients remove their lipstick before the examination. Anemia causes pallor of the lips, with cyanosis caused by respiratory or cardiovascular problems. Cherry-colored lips indicate carbon monoxide poisoning. When you inspect any lesion, consider the potential of it being an infection, irritation, or skin cancer.

Buccal Mucosa, Gums, and Teeth. Ask the patient to clench the teeth and smile to observe teeth occlusion. The upper molars normally rest directly on the lower molars, and the upper incisors slightly override the lower incisors. A symmetrical smile reveals normal facial nerve function.

Inspect the teeth to determine the quality of dental hygiene (Box 31-15). Note the position and alignment of the teeth. To examine the

BOX 31-15 PATIENT TEACHING

Mouth and Pharyngeal Assessment

Objective

- Patient will practice proper oral hygiene/dental care measures and identify symptoms of oral cancer.

Teaching Strategies

- Discuss proper techniques for oral hygiene, including brushing and flossing (see Chapter 40).
- Explain the early warning signs of oral cavity and pharynx cancer that should be checked by a health care professional, including a mouth sore that bleeds easily and does not heal, a lump or thickening in the cheek, a white or red patch on the mucosa that persists, a sore throat or a feeling that something is caught in the throat, numbness of the tongue or other area of the mouth, or a swelling of the jaw that causes dentures to not fit (Oral Cancer Foundation, 2014).
- Late symptoms of oral cancer are difficulty chewing, swallowing, or moving the tongue or jaw (ACS, 2015a).
- Encourage regular dental examination every 6 months for children, adults, and older adults.

Evaluation

- Ask patient to demonstrate brushing.
- Have patient identify when to have regular dental checkups.
- Have patient identify the warning signs of oral cavity and pharynx cancer that require further evaluation by a health care provider.

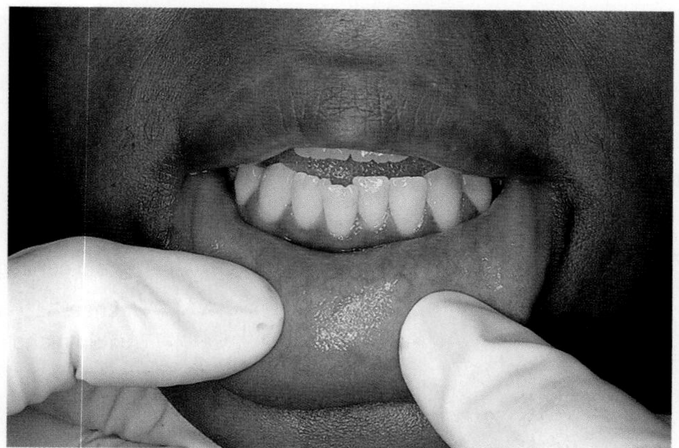

FIGURE 31-22 Inspection of inner oral mucosa of lower lip.

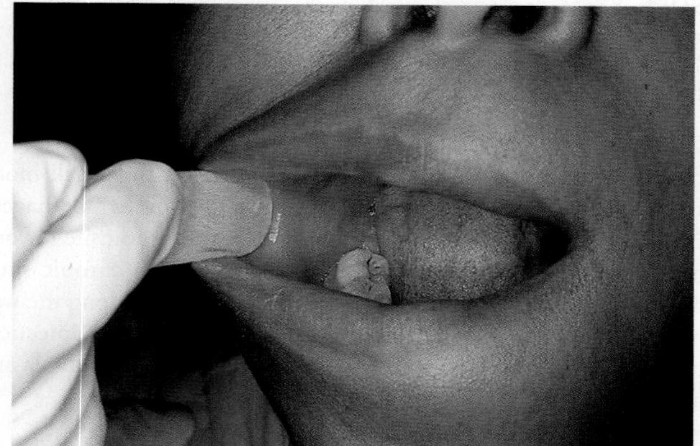

FIGURE 31-23 Retraction of buccal mucosa allows for clear visualization.

posterior surface of the teeth, have the patient open the mouth with the lips relaxed. Use a tongue depressor to retract the lips and cheeks, especially when viewing the molars. Note the color of teeth and presence of dental caries (cavities), tartar, and extraction sites. Normal, healthy teeth are smooth, white, and shiny. A chalky white discoloration of the enamel is an early indication of caries formation. Brown or black discolorations indicate the formation of caries. A stained yellow color is from tobacco use; coffee, tea, and colas cause a brown stain. In the older adult loose or missing teeth are common because bone resorption increases. An older adult's teeth often feel rough when tooth enamel calcifies. Yellow or darkened teeth are also common in the older adult because of the general wear and tear that exposes the darker underlying dentin.

To view the mucosa and gums, ask the patient to first remove any dental appliance. View the inner oral mucosa by having the patient open and relax the mouth slightly and then gently retract his or her lower lip away from the teeth (Figure 31-22). Repeat this process for the upper lip. Inspect the mucosa for color; hydration; texture; and lesions such as ulcers, abrasions, or cysts. Normally the mucosa is glistening, pink, smooth, and moist. Some common small, yellow-white raised lesions on the buccal mucosa and lips are Fordyce spots, or ectopic sebaceous glands (Ball et al., 2015). If lesions are present, palpate them gently with a gloved hand for tenderness, size, and consistency.

To inspect the buccal mucosa, ask the patient to open the mouth and then gently retract the cheeks with a tongue depressor (Figure 31-23). View the surface of the mucosa from right to left and top to bottom. A penlight illuminates the most posterior part of the mucosa. Normal mucosa is glistening, pink, soft, moist, and smooth. Varying shades of hyperpigmentation are normal in 10% of whites after age 50 and as many as 90% of blacks by the same age. For patients with normal pigmentation, the buccal mucosa is a good site to inspect for jaundice and pallor. In older adults the mucosa is normally dry because of reduced salivation. Thick white patches (leukoplakia) are often a precancerous lesion seen in heavy smokers and alcoholics. Palpate for any buccal lesions by placing the index finger within the buccal cavity and the thumb on the outer surface of the cheek. Patients who smoke cigarettes, cigars, or pipes and those who use smokeless tobacco have an increased risk of oral, pharyngeal, laryngeal, and esophageal cancer. These individuals may have leukoplakia or other lesions anywhere in their oral cavity (e.g., lips, gums, or tongue) at an early age.

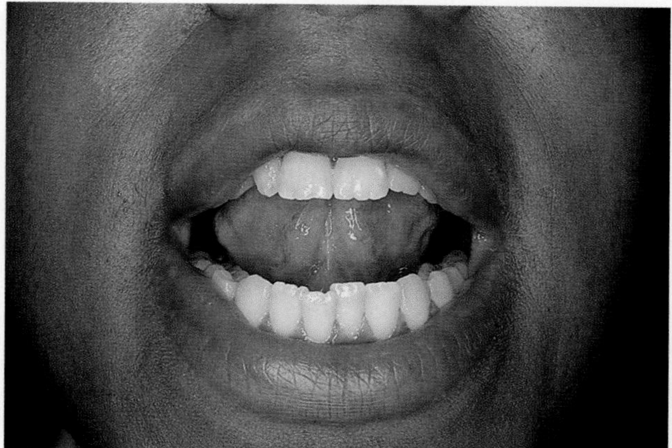

FIGURE 31-24 Undersurface of tongue is highly vascular.

Inspect the gums (gingivae) for color, edema, retraction, bleeding, and lesions while retracting the cheeks. Healthy gums are pink, smooth, and moist and fit tightly around each tooth. Dark-skinned patients often have patchy pigmentation. In older adults the gums are usually pale. Using clean gloves, palpate the gums to assess for lesions, thickening, or masses. Normally there is no tenderness. Spongy gums that bleed easily indicate periodontal disease and vitamin C deficiency. If a patient has loose or mobile teeth, swollen gums, or pockets containing debris at the tooth margins, a dental referral is necessary to check for periodontal disease or gingivitis.

Tongue and Floor of Mouth. Carefully inspect the tongue on all sides and the floor of the mouth. Have the patient relax the mouth and stick the tongue out halfway. Note any deviation, tremor, or limitation in movement. This tests hypoglossal nerve function. If a patient protrudes the tongue too far, it elicits the gag reflex. When the tongue protrudes, it lays midline. To test for tongue mobility, ask the patient to raise it up and move it from side to side. It should move freely.

Using a penlight for illumination, examine the tongue for color, size, position, texture, and coatings or lesions. A normal tongue is medium or dull red in color, moist, slightly rough on the top surface, and smooth along the lateral margins. The undersurface of the tongue and the floor of the mouth are highly vascular (Figure 31-24). Take extra care to inspect this area, a common site for oral cancer lesions. The patient lifts the tongue by placing its tip on the palate behind the upper incisors. Inspect for color, swelling, and lesions such as nodules or cysts. The ventral surface of the tongue is pink and smooth, with large veins between the frenulum folds. To palpate the tongue, explain the procedure and ask the patient to protrude it. Grasp the tip with a gauze square and gently pull it to one side. With a gloved hand palpate the full length of the tongue and the base for any areas of hardening

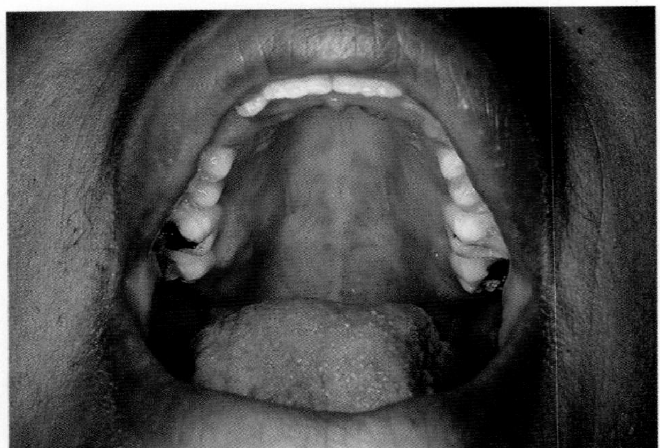

FIGURE 31-25 Hard palate is located anteriorly in roof of mouth.

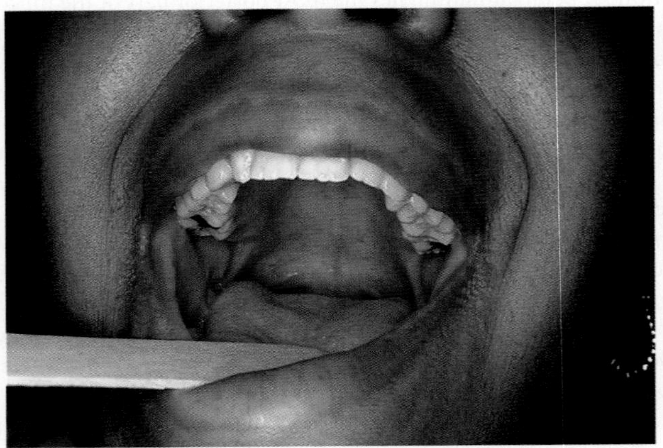

FIGURE 31-26 Penlight and tongue depressor allow visualization of uvula and posterior soft palate.

or ulceration. Varicosities (swollen, tortuous veins) are common in the older adult and rarely cause problems.

Palate. Have the patient extend the head backward, holding the mouth open to inspect the hard and soft palates. The hard palate, or roof of the mouth, is located anteriorly. The whitish hard palate is dome shaped. The soft palate extends posteriorly toward the pharynx. It is normally light pink and smooth. Observe the palates for color, shape, texture, and extra bony prominences or defects (Figure 31-25). A bony growth, or exostosis, between the two palates is common.

Pharynx. Perform an examination of pharyngeal structures to rule out infection, inflammation, or lesions. Have the patient tip the head back slightly, open the mouth wide, and say "ah" while you place the tip of a tongue depressor on the middle third of the tongue. Take care not to press the lower lip against the teeth. By placing the tongue depressor too far anteriorly, the posterior part of the tongue mounds up, obstructing the view. Placing the tongue depressor on the posterior tongue elicits the gag reflex.

With a penlight first inspect the uvula and soft palate (Figure 31-26). Both structures, which are innervated by the tenth cranial (vagus) nerve, should rise centrally as the patient says "ah." Examine the anterior and posterior pillars, soft palate, and uvula. View the tonsils in the cavities between the anterior and posterior pillars and note the presence or absence of tissue. The posterior pharynx is behind the pillars. Normally pharyngeal tissues are pink and smooth and well

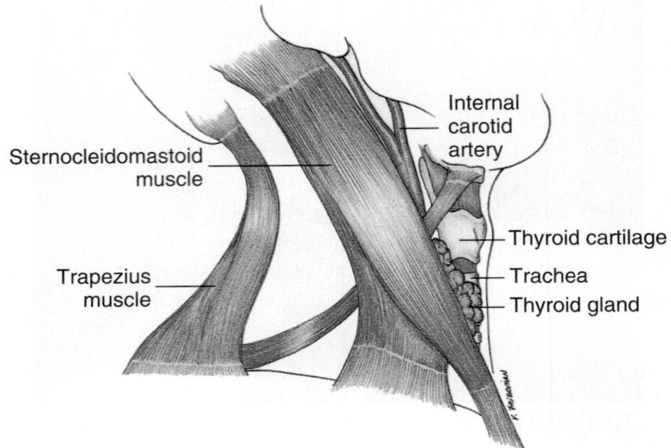

FIGURE 31-27 Anatomical position of major neck structures. Note triangles formed by sternocleidomastoid muscle, lower jaw, and anterior neck anteriorly and sternocleidomastoid muscle, trapezius muscle, and lower neck posteriorly.

hydrated. Small irregular spots of lymphatic tissue and small blood vessels are normal. Note edema, petechiae (small hemorrhages), lesions, or exudate. The back of the pharynx is a common site for oral cancer (Oral Cancer Foundation, 2014). Patients with chronic sinus problems frequently exhibit a clear exudate that drains along the wall of the posterior pharynx. Yellow or green exudate indicates infection. A patient with a typical sore throat has a red and edematous uvula and tonsillar pillars with possible presence of yellow exudate.

Neck

Assessment of the neck includes assessing the neck muscles, lymph nodes of the head and neck, carotid arteries, jugular veins, thyroid gland, and trachea (Figure 31-27). You may postpone the examination of the jugular veins and carotid arteries until the vascular system assessment. Inspect and palpate the neck to determine the integrity of its structures and examine the lymphatic system. An abnormality of superficial lymph nodes sometimes reveals the presence of an infection or malignancy. Examine the lymphatic system region by region during the assessment of other body systems (head and neck, breast, genitalia, and extremities). Examination of the thyroid gland and trachea also aids in ruling out malignancies. Perform this examination with the patient sitting. The sternocleidomastoid and trapezius muscles outline the areas of the neck, dividing each side of the neck into two triangles. The anterior triangle contains the trachea, thyroid gland, carotid artery, and anterior cervical lymph nodes. The posterior triangle contains the posterior lymph nodes. Table 31-18 reviews the nursing history for the head and neck examination.

Neck Muscles. First inspect the neck in the usual anatomical position, with slight hyperextension. Observe for symmetry of the neck muscles. Ask the patient to flex the neck with the chin to the chest, hyperextend the neck backward, and move the head laterally to each side and then sideways with the ear moving toward the shoulder. This tests the sternocleidomastoid and trapezius muscles. The neck normally moves without discomfort. Perform other tests for muscle strength and function during assessment of the musculoskeletal system.

Lymph Nodes. An extensive system of lymph nodes collects lymph from the head, ears, nose, cheeks, and lips (Figure 31-28). The

TABLE 31-18 Nursing History for Neck Assessment

Assessment	Rationale
Assess for history of recent cold, infection, or enlarged lymph nodes or exposure to radiation or toxic chemicals.	Colds or infections cause temporary or permanent lymph node enlargement. Lymph nodes are also enlarged in various diseases such as cancer.
If there is an enlarged lymph node, consider reviewing history of intravenous drug use, hemophilia, sexual contact with people infected with human immunodeficiency virus (HIV), history of blood transfusion, multiple and indiscriminate sexual contacts, or male with homosexual or bisexual activities.	These are risk factors for HIV infection.
Ask if patient has had history of neck pain with restriction in movement.	This indicates muscle strain, head injury, local nerve injury, or enlarged or swollen lymph node.
Ask if patient has had change in temperature preference (more or less clothing); swelling in neck; change in texture of hair, skin, or nails; or change in emotional stability.	Symptoms indicate thyroid disease.
Ask if patient has history of hypothyroidism or hyperthyroidism, takes thyroid medication, or has a family history of thyroid disease.	Disease or medications influence tissue growth of gland.
Review medical history of pneumothorax (collapsed lung) or bronchial tumor.	Conditions place patient at risk for tracheal displacement or lateral deviation.

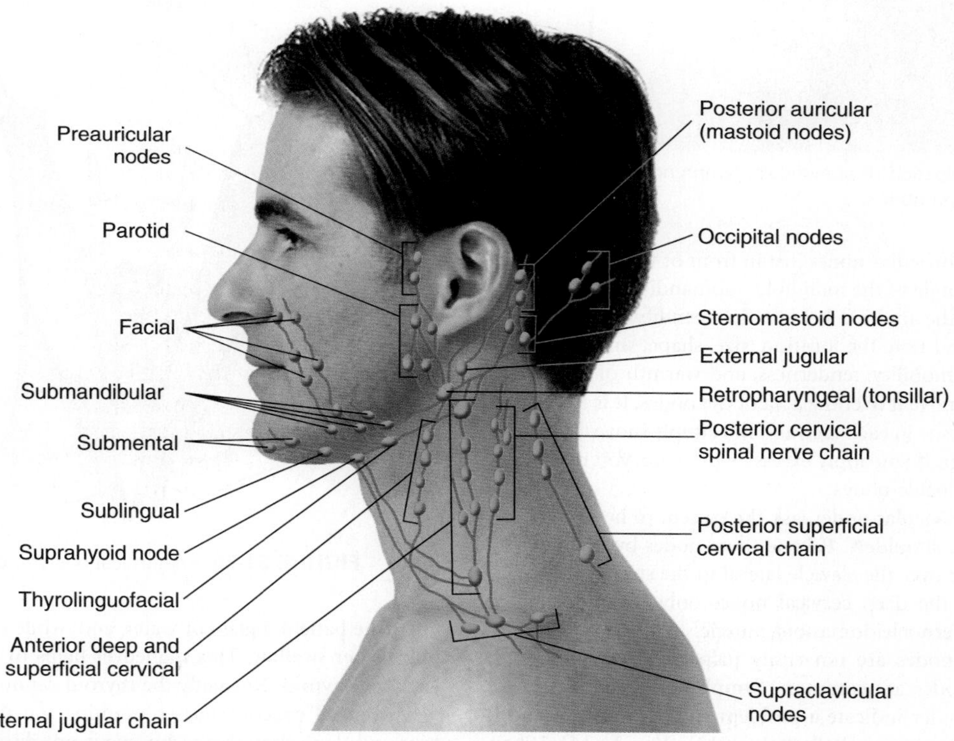

FIGURE 31-28 Palpable lymph nodes in head and neck. (From Ball JW et al: *Seidel's guide to physical examination,* ed 8, St Louis, 2015, Mosby.)

immune system protects the body from foreign antigens, removes damaged cells from the circulation, and provides a partial barrier to growth of malignant cells within the body. Assessing the lymph nodes requires competence when caring for patients with suspected immunoincompetence, which is often linked to allergies, human immunodeficiency virus (HIV) infection, autoimmune disease (e.g., lupus erythematosus), or serious infection.

With the patient's chin raised and head tilted slightly, first inspect the area where lymph nodes are distributed and compare both sides. This position stretches the skin slightly over any possible enlarged nodes. Inspect visible nodes for edema, erythema, or red streaks. Nodes normally are not visible.

Use a methodical approach to palpate the lymph nodes to avoid overlooking any single node or chain. The patient relaxes with the neck flexed slightly forward. Inspect and palpate both sides of the neck for comparison. During palpation either face or stand to the side of the patient for easy access to all nodes. Use the pads of the middle three fingers of each hand to gently palpate in a circular motion over the nodes (Figure 31-29). Check each node methodically in the following sequence: occipital nodes at the base of the skull, postauricular nodes

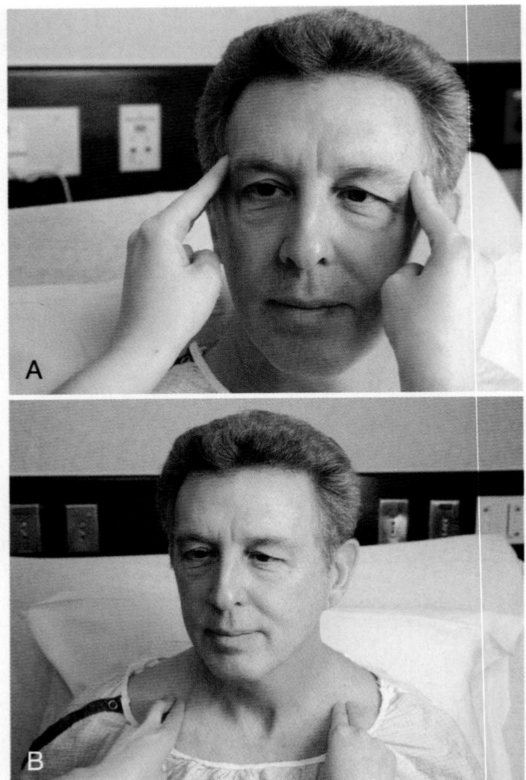

FIGURE 31-29 A, Palpation of preauricular lymph nodes. **B,** Palpation of supraclavicular lymph nodes.

over the mastoid, preauricular nodes just in front of the ear, retropharyngeal nodes at the angle of the mandible, submandibular nodes, and submental nodes in the midline behind the mandibular tip. Try to detect enlargement and note the location, size, shape, surface characteristics, consistency, mobility, tenderness, and warmth of the nodes. If the skin is mobile, move it over the area of the nodes. It is important to press underlying tissue in each area and not simply move the fingers over the skin. However, if you apply excessive pressure, you miss small nodes and destroy palpable nodes.

To palpate supraclavicular nodes, ask the patient to bend the head forward and relax the shoulders. Palpate these nodes by hooking the index and third finger over the clavicle lateral to the sternocleidomastoid muscle. Palpate the deep cervical nodes only with the fingers hooked around the sternocleidomastoid muscle.

Normally lymph nodes are not easily palpable. However, small, mobile, nontender nodes are common. Lymph nodes that are large, fixed, inflamed, or tender indicate a problem such as local infection, systemic disease, or neoplasm (Ball et al., 2015) (Box 31-16). When you find enlarged nodes, explore the adjacent areas and regions that they drain. Tenderness almost always indicates inflammation. A problem involving a lymph node of the head and neck means an abnormality in the mouth, throat, abdomen, breasts, thorax, or arms. These are the areas drained by the head and neck nodes.

Thyroid Gland. The thyroid gland lies in the anterior lower neck, in front of and to both sides of the trachea. The gland is fixed to the trachea, with the isthmus overlying the trachea and connecting the two irregular, cone-shaped lobes (Figure 31-30). Inspect the lower neck overlying the thyroid gland for obvious masses, symmetry, and any subtle fullness at the base of the neck. Ask the patient to hyperextend the neck, which helps tighten the skin for better visualization.

BOX 31-16 PATIENT TEACHING

Neck Assessment

Objective

- Patient will take proper preventive action if he or she notices a mass in the neck.

Teaching Strategies

- Stress importance of regular compliance with medication schedule to patients with thyroid disease.
- Instruct patient about the lymph nodes and how infection commonly causes node tenderness and mild enlargement.
- Instruct patient to call a health care provider when he or she notices a fixed, enlarged lump or mass in the neck.
- Teach patient risk factors for HIV infection and other sexually transmitted diseases.

Evaluation

- Have patient explain when to notify a physician about a neck mass.

HIV, Human immunodeficiency virus.

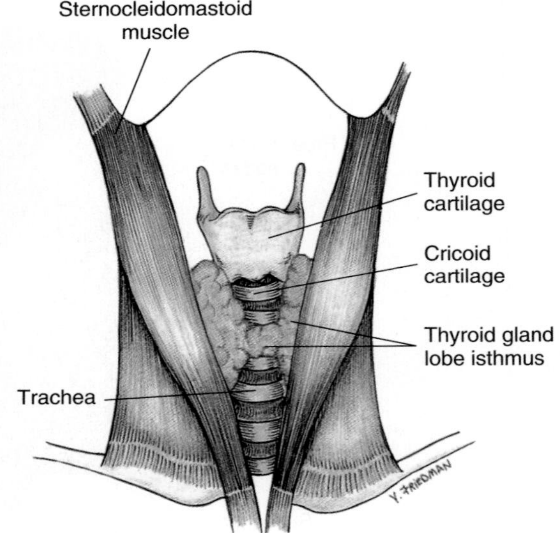

FIGURE 31-30 Anatomical position of thyroid gland.

Offer the patient a glass of water, and, while observing the neck, have him or her swallow. This maneuver helps to visualize an abnormally enlarged thyroid. Normally the thyroid cannot be visualized.

Advanced practice nurses examine the thyroid by palpating for more subtle masses; this technique is not discussed here.

Carotid Artery and Jugular Vein. This part of the examination is described under examination of the vascular system (see later section).

Trachea. The trachea is a part of the upper respiratory system that you directly palpate. It is normally located in the midline above the suprasternal notch. Masses in the neck or mediastinum and pulmonary abnormalities cause displacement laterally. Have the patient sit or lie down during palpation. Determine the position of the trachea by palpating at the suprasternal notch, slipping the thumb and index fingers to each side. Note if the finger and thumb shift laterally. Do not apply forceful pressure because this elicits coughing.

THORAX AND LUNGS

Accurate physical assessment of the thorax and lungs requires review of the ventilatory and respiratory functions of the lungs. If disease is affecting the lungs, it affects other body systems as well. For example, reduced oxygenation causes changes in mental alertness because of the sensitivity of the brain to lowered oxygen levels. Use data from all body systems to determine the nature of pulmonary alterations. You use inspection, palpation, and auscultation to examine the thorax and lungs. Diagnostic equipment such as x-ray films, magnetic resonance imaging (MRI), and computed tomography (CT) scans create little need for the use of percussion as an assessment measure. Risk factors for lung disease are reviewed at the time of respiratory assessment (Box 31-17).

Before assessing the thorax and lungs, be familiar with the landmarks of the chest (Figure 31-31, *A* to *C*). These landmarks help you identify findings and use assessment skills correctly. A patient's nipples, angle of Louis, suprasternal notch, costal angle, clavicles, and vertebrae are key landmarks that provide a series of imaginary lines for sign identification. Keep a mental image of the location of the lobes of the lung and the position of each rib (Figure 31-32, *A* to *C*). The proper orientation to anatomical structures ensures a thorough assessment of the anterior, lateral, and posterior thorax.

Locating the position of each rib is critical to visualizing the lobe of the lung being assessed. To begin, locate the angle of Louis at the manubriosternal junction. The angle is a visible and palpable angulation of the sternum and is the point at which the second rib articulates with the sternum. Count the ribs and intercostal spaces (between the ribs) from this point. The number of each intercostal space corresponds with that of the rib just above it. The spinous process of the third thoracic vertebra and the fourth, fifth, and sixth ribs helps to locate the lobes of the lung laterally. The lower lobes project laterally

BOX 31-17 PATIENT TEACHING

Lung Assessment

Objective

- Patients of all age-groups will practice preventive care measures for lung health.

Teaching Strategies

- Explain risk factors for chronic lung disease and lung cancer, including cigarette smoking, history of smoking for over 20 years; exposure to environmental pollution; and radiation exposure from occupational, medical, and environmental sources. Exposure to radon and asbestos also increases risk. Other risk factors include exposure to certain metals (e.g., arsenic, cadmium, chromium), some organic chemicals, and tuberculosis. Exposure to secondhand cigarette smoke increases risk for nonsmokers (ACS, 2015a).
- Share brochures on lung cancer, asthma, and COPD from American Cancer Society with patient and family.
- Instruct patient with asthma to identify and tell family members and friends which triggers cause asthma episodes.
- Discuss warning signs of lung cancer such as a persistent cough, sputum streaked with blood, chest pains, and recurrent attacks of pneumonia or bronchitis.
- Counsel older adult about benefits of receiving influenza and pneumonia vaccinations because of a greater susceptibility to respiratory infection.
- Instruct patient with COPD how to perform coughing and pursed-lip breathing exercises.
- Refer people at risk for tuberculosis to visit clinics or health care centers for skin testing.

Evaluation

- Have patient describe risk factors for lung disease and cancer.
- Ask patient to identify any known risks for cancer.
- Ask patient to name warning signs of lung cancer.
- In a follow-up visit review patient's immunization record.
- Observe patient performing breathing exercises and coughing.

COPD, chronic obstructive pulmonary disease.

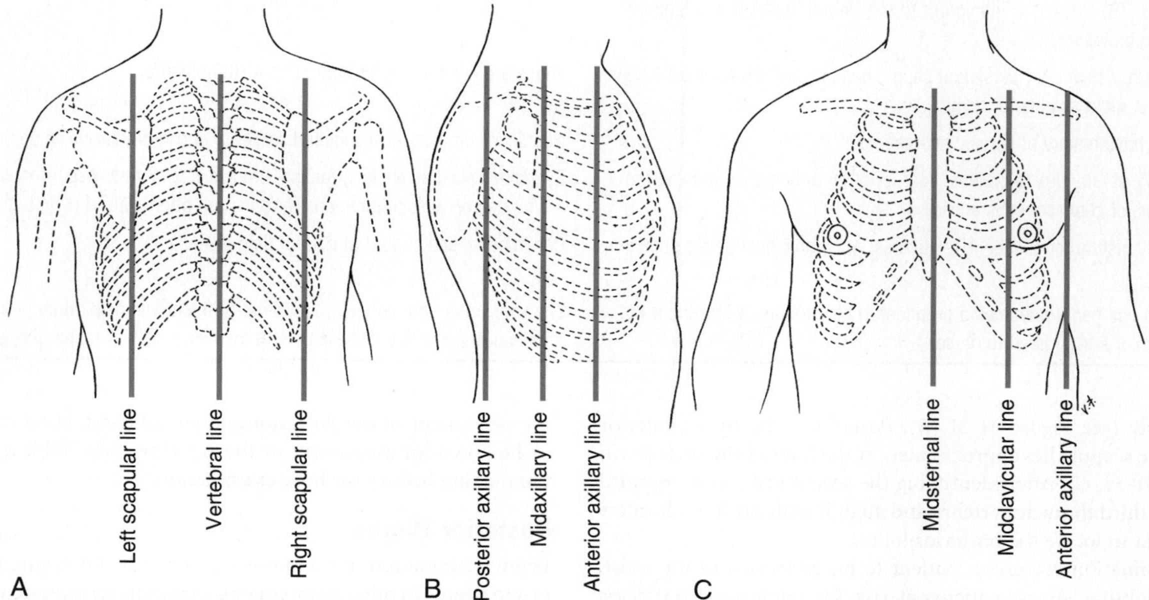

FIGURE 31-31 Anatomical chest wall landmarks. **A,** Posterior chest landmarks. **B,** Lateral chest landmarks. **C,** Anterior chest landmarks.

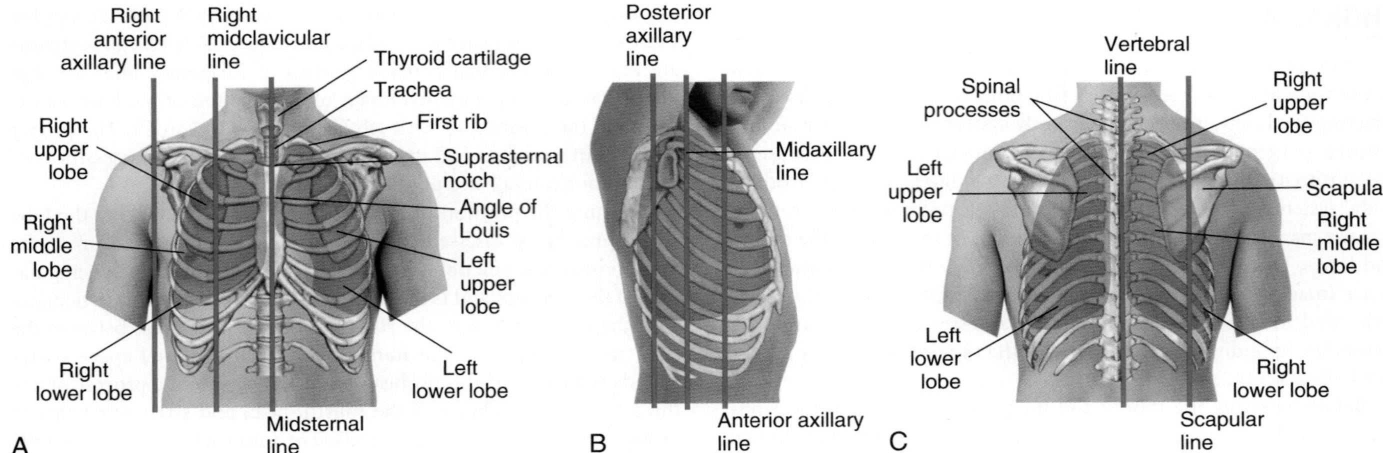

FIGURE 31-32 Position of lung lobes in relation to anatomical landmarks. **A,** Anterior position. **B,** Lateral position. **C,** Posterior position. (From Ball JW et al: *Seidel's guide to physical examination,* ed 8, St Louis, 2015, Mosby.)

TABLE 31-19 Nursing History for Lung Assessment

Assessment	Rationale
Assess history of tobacco or marijuana use, including type of tobacco, duration and amount (Pack-years = Number of years smoking × Number of packs per day), age started, efforts to quit, and length of time since smoking stopped.	Smoking is a risk factor for lung cancer, heart disease, cerebrovascular disease, emphysema, or chronic bronchitis. It accounts for a significant percentage of all cancer deaths. It increases the risk for 15 types of cancer (ACS, 2015a).
Ask if patient has had a *persistent cough* (productive or nonproductive), *sputum streaked with blood, voice change, chest pain,* shortness of breath, **orthopnea**, dyspnea during exertion or at rest, poor activity tolerance, or *recurrent attacks of pneumonia or bronchitis.*	Symptoms of cardiopulmonary alterations help localize objective physical findings. (Warning signals for lung cancer are in italic type.) The diaphragm of the lungs expands more easily when the individual is sitting upright, as for patients who must be in an upright position to breathe.
Determine if patient works in environment containing pollutants (e.g., asbestos, arsenic, coal dust) or requiring exposure to radiation. Does patient have exposure to secondhand smoke?	These risk factors increase chance for various lung diseases.
Review history for known or suspected human immunodeficiency virus (HIV) infection; substance abuse; low income; or being a resident or employee of nursing home or shelter, homeless, recent prison inmate, family member of tuberculosis (TB) patient, or immigrant to the United States from a country where TB is prevalent.	These are risk factors for TB.
Ask if patient has history of persistent cough, hemoptysis, unexplained weight loss, fatigue, night sweats, or fever.	These are risk factors for both TB and HIV infection.
Does patient have history of chronic hoarseness?	Hoarseness indicates laryngeal disorder or abuse of cocaine or opioids (sniffing).
Assess history of allergies to pollens, dust, or other airborne irritants and to foods, drugs, or chemical substances.	Symptoms such as choking feeling, bronchospasm with respiratory stridor, wheezes on auscultation, and dyspnea are often caused by allergic response.
Review family history for cancer, TB, allergies, or chronic obstructive pulmonary disease.	Conditions place patient at risk for lung disease.
Ask if patient has had a pneumonia or influenza vaccine and a TB test; if not, educate him or her on need to do so.	The very young, the very old, and those with chronic respiratory problems or immunosuppressive diseases are at increased risk for respiratory disease.

and anteriorly (see Figure 31-32, *B*). Posteriorly the tip or inferior margin of the scapula lies approximately at the level of the seventh rib (see Figure 31-32, *C*). After identifying the seventh rib, count upward to locate the third thoracic vertebra and align it with the inner borders of the scapula to locate the posterior lobes.

The examination requires a patient to be undressed to the waist, with good lighting. Assess patients at risk for pulmonary problems such as the patient confined to bed rest or with chest pain who cannot fully expand the lungs. The examination begins with the patient sitting for assessment of the posterior and lateral chest. Have him or her sit or lie down for assessment of the anterior chest. Table 31-19 reviews the nursing history for lung examination.

Posterior Thorax

Begin examination of the posterior thorax by observing for any signs or symptoms in other body systems that indicate pulmonary problems. Reduced mental alertness, nasal flaring, somnolence, and cyanosis are examples of assessed signs that indicate oxygenation problems. Inspect

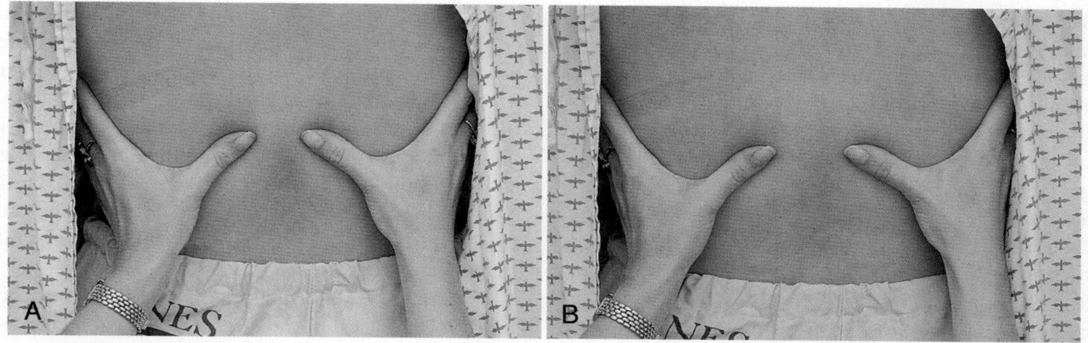

FIGURE 31-33 A, Hand position for palpation of posterior thorax excursion. **B,** As patient inhales, movement of chest excursion separates thumbs.

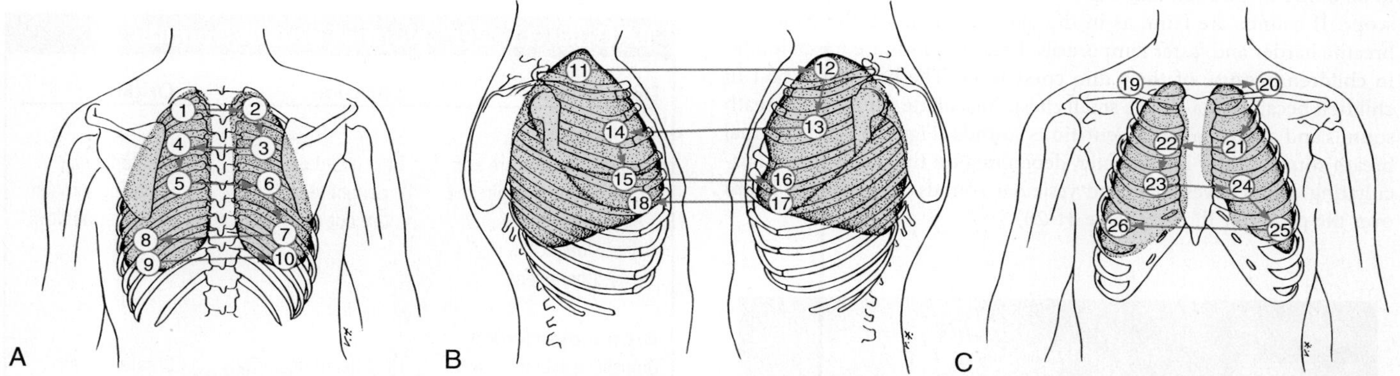

FIGURE 31-34 A to **C,** Systematic pattern (posterior-lateral-anterior) is followed when palpating and auscultating thorax.

the posterior thorax by observing the shape and symmetry of the chest from the patient's back and front. Note the anteroposterior diameter. Body shape or posture significantly impairs ventilatory movement. Normally the chest contour is symmetrical, with the anteroposterior diameter one third to one half of the transverse, or side-to-side, diameter. A barrel-shaped chest (anteroposterior diameter equals transverse diameter) characterizes aging and chronic lung disease. Infants have an almost round shape. Congenital and postural alterations cause abnormal contours. Some patients lean over a table or splint the side of the chest because of a breathing problem. Splinting or holding the chest wall because of pain causes a patient to bend toward the side affected. Such a posture impairs ventilatory movement.

Standing at a midline position behind the patient, look for deformities, position of the spine, slope of the ribs, retraction of the intercostal spaces during inspiration, and bulging of the intercostal spaces during expiration. The scapulae are normally symmetrical and closely attached to the thoracic wall. The normal spine is straight without lateral deviation. Posteriorly the ribs tend to slope across and down. The ribs and intercostal spaces are easier to see in a thin person. Normally no bulging or active movement occurs within the intercostal spaces during breathing. Bulging indicates that a patient is using great effort to breathe.

Also assess the rate and rhythm of breathing (see Chapter 30). Observe the thorax as a whole. It normally expands and relaxes regularly with equality of movement bilaterally. In healthy adults the normal respiratory rates vary from 12 to 20 respirations per minute.

Palpation of the posterior thorax provides further information about a patient's health status. Palpate the thoracic muscles and skeleton for lumps, masses, pulsations, and unusual movement. If the patient voices pain or tenderness, avoid deep palpation. Fractured rib fragments could be displaced against vital organs. Normally the chest wall is not tender. If there is a suspicious mass or swollen area, lightly palpate it for size, shape, and the typical qualities of a lesion.

To measure chest excursion or depth of breathing, stand behind the patient and place the thumbs along the spinal processes at the tenth rib, with the palms lightly contacting the posterolateral surfaces. Place thumbs 5 cm (2 inches) apart, pointing toward the spine with fingers pointing laterally (Figure 31-33, *A*). Press the hands toward the spine so a small skinfold appears between the thumbs. Do not slide the hands over the skin. Instruct the patient to exhale and then take a deep breath. Note movement of the thumbs during inhalation (see Figure 31-33, *B*). Chest excursion is symmetrical, separating the thumbs 3 to 5 cm (1¼ to 2 inches). Reduced chest excursion may be caused by pain, postural deformity, or fatigue. In older adults chest movement normally declines because of costal cartilage calcification and respiratory muscle atrophy.

During speech the sound created by the vocal cords is transmitted through the lungs to the chest wall. The sound waves create vibrations that you palpate externally. These vibrations are called **vocal or tactile fremitus**. The accumulation of mucus, the collapse of lung tissue, or the presence of one or more lung lesions blocks the vibrations from reaching the chest wall.

To palpate for tactile fremitus, place the palmar surfaces of the fingers or the ulnar part of the hand over symmetrical intercostal spaces, beginning at the lung apex (Figure 31-34, *A*) and using a firm, light touch. Ask the patient to say "ninety-nine" or "one-one-one." Palpate both sides simultaneously and symmetrically (from top to bottom) for comparison or use one hand, quickly alternating between the two sides (Ball et al., 2015). Normally a faint vibration is present as a patient speaks. If fremitus is faint, ask the patient to speak in a louder or lower tone of voice. Normally fremitus is symmetrical. Vibrations are strongest at the top, near the level of the tracheal bifurcation. Strong vibrations through the chest wall occur in crying infants.

Auscultation assesses the movement of air through the tracheobronchial tree and detects mucus or obstructed airways. Normally air flows through the airways in an unobstructed pattern. Recognizing the sounds created by normal airflow allows you to detect sounds caused by airway obstruction. Follow the same systematic approach when listening that was used for palpation (see Figure 31-34, *A*).

Place the diaphragm of the stethoscope firmly on the skin, over the posterior chest wall between the ribs (Figure 31-35). Have the patient fold the arms in front of the chest and keep the head bent forward while taking slow, deep breaths with the mouth slightly open. Listen to an entire inspiration and expiration at each position of the stethoscope. If sounds are faint, as in the obese patient, ask the patient to breathe harder and faster temporarily. Breath sounds are much louder in children because of their thin chest walls. The bell works best in children because of a child's small chest. Auscultate for normal breath sounds and abnormal or **adventitious sounds** (Figure 31-36). Normal breath sounds differ in character, depending on the area you are auscultating. Bronchovesicular and vesicular sounds are normally heard over the posterior thorax (Table 31-20).

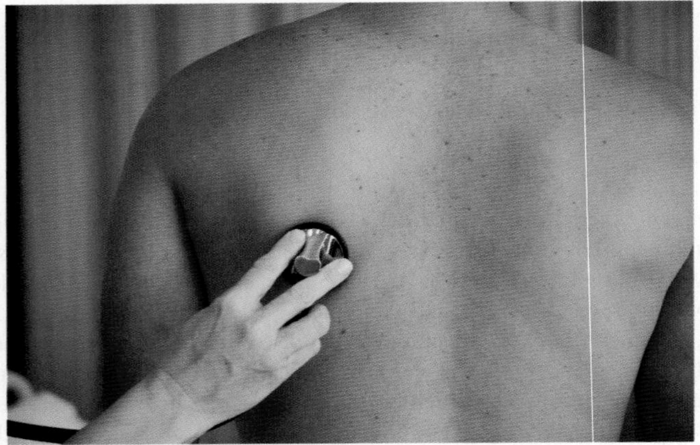

FIGURE 31-35 Use diaphragm of stethoscope to auscultate breath sounds.

Abnormal sounds result from air passing through moisture, mucus, or narrowed airways. They also result from alveoli suddenly reinflating or an inflammation between the pleural linings of the lung. Adventitious sounds often occur superimposed over normal sounds. The four types of adventitious sounds are crackles, rhonchi, wheezes, and pleural friction rub (see Figure 31-36). A specific entity causes each sound, and each has typical auditory features (Table 31-21). During auscultation note the location and characteristics of the sounds and listen for the absence of breath sounds (found in patients with collapsed or surgically removed lobes).

If there are abnormalities in tactile fremitus or auscultation, perform the vocal resonance tests (spoken and whispered voice sounds). Place the stethoscope over the same locations used to assess breath sounds and have the patient say "ninety-nine" in a normal voice tone. Normally the sound is muffled. If fluid is compressing the lung,

TABLE 31-20 Normal Breath Sounds

Description	Location	Origin
Vesicular		
Vesicular sounds are soft, breezy, and low pitched. Inspiratory phase is 3 times longer than expiratory phase.	Best heard over periphery of lung (except over scapula)	Created by air moving through smaller airways
Bronchovesicular		
Bronchovesicular sounds are blowing sounds that are medium pitched and of medium intensity. Inspiratory phase is equal to expiratory phase.	Best heard posteriorly between scapulae and anteriorly over bronchioles lateral to sternum at first and second intercostal spaces	Created by air moving through large airways
Bronchial		
Bronchial sounds are loud and high pitched with hollow quality. Expiration lasts longer than inspiration (3:2 ratio).	Heard only over trachea	Created by air moving through trachea close to chest wall

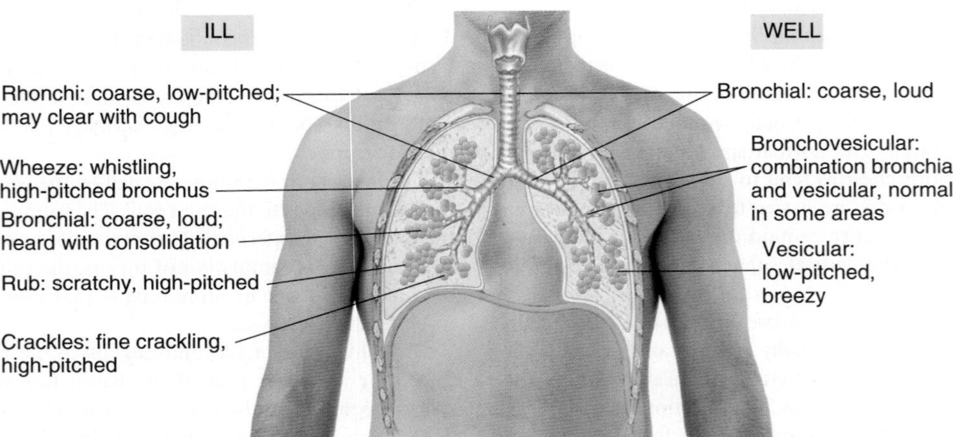

FIGURE 31-36 Schema of breath sounds in the ill and well patient. (From Ball JW et al: *Seidel's guide to physical examination,* ed 8, St Louis, 2015, Elsevier.)

TABLE 31-21 Adventitious Breath Sounds

Sound	Site Auscultated	Cause	Character
Crackles	Most common in dependent lobes: right and left lung bases	Random, sudden reinflation of groups of alveoli; disruptive passage of air through small airways	Fine crackles are high-pitched fine, short, interrupted crackling sounds heard during end of inspiration; usually not cleared with coughing. Medium crackles are lower, moister sounds heard during middle of inspiration; not cleared with coughing. Coarse crackles are loud, bubbly sounds heard during inspiration; not cleared with coughing.
Rhonchi (sonorous wheeze)	Primarily heard over trachea and bronchi; if loud enough, able to be heard over most lung fields	Muscular spasm, fluid, or mucus in larger airways; new growth or external pressure causing turbulence	Loud, low-pitched, rumbling, coarse sounds are heard either during inspiration or expiration; sometimes cleared by coughing.
Wheezes (sibilant wheeze)	Heard over all lung fields	High-velocity airflow through severely narrowed or obstructed airway	High-pitched, continuous musical sounds are like a squeak heard continuously during inspiration or expiration; usually louder on expiration.
Pleural friction rub	Heard over anterior lateral lung field (if patient is sitting upright)	Inflamed pleura; parietal pleura rubbing against visceral pleura	Dry, rubbing, or grating quality is heard during inspiration or expiration; does not clear with coughing; heard loudest over lower lateral anterior surface.

Data from Ball JW et al: *Seidel's guide to physical examination,* ed 8, St Louis, 2015, Mosby.

the vibrations from the patient's voice are transmitted to the chest wall, and the sound becomes clear (bronchophony). Then ask the patient to whisper "ninety-nine." The whispered voice is usually faint and indistinct. Certain lung abnormalities cause the whispered voice to become clear and distinct (whispered pectoriloquy).

Lateral Thorax

Extend the assessment of the posterior thorax to the lateral sides of the chest. The patient sits during examination of the lateral chest. Have the patient raise the arms to improve access to lateral thoracic structures. Use inspection, palpation, and auscultation skills to examine the lateral thorax (see Figure 31-34, *B*). Do not assess excursion laterally. Normally the breath sounds you hear are vesicular.

Anterior Thorax

Inspect the anterior thorax for the same features as the posterior thorax. The patient sits or lies down with the head elevated. Observe the accessory muscles of breathing: sternocleidomastoid, trapezius, and abdominal muscles. The accessory muscles move little with normal passive breathing. However, patients who use a great deal of effort to breathe as a result of strenuous exercise or pulmonary disease (e.g., chronic obstructive pulmonary disease) rely on the accessory and abdominal muscles to contract, thereby leading to inspiration and expiration. Some patients who require great effort produce a grunting sound.

Observe the width of the costal angle. It is usually larger than 90 degrees between the two costal margins. Observe the breathing pattern. Normal breathing is quiet and barely audible near the open mouth. You most often assess respiratory rate and rhythm anteriorly (see Chapter 30). The male patient's respirations are usually diaphragmatic, whereas a female's are more costal. Accurate assessment occurs as the patient breathes passively.

Palpate the anterior thoracic muscles and skeleton for lumps, masses, tenderness, or unusual movement. The sternum and xiphoid are relatively inflexible. Place the thumbs parallel approximately along the costal margin 6 cm (2½ inches) apart with the palms touching the anterolateral chest. Push the thumbs toward the midline to create a skinfold. As the patient inhales deeply, the thumbs normally separate approximately 3 to 5 cm (1¼ to 2 inches), with each side expanding equally.

Assess tactile fremitus over the anterior chest wall. Anterior findings differ from posterior findings because of the heart and female breast tissue. Fremitus is felt next to the sternum at the second intercostal space, at the level of the bronchial bifurcation. It decreases over the heart, lower thorax, and breast tissue.

Auscultation of the anterior thorax follows a systematic pattern (see Figure 31-34, *C*) comparing right and left sides. This is important so lung sounds in one region on one side of the body can be compared with sounds in the same region on the opposite side of the body.

If possible, have the patient sit to maximize chest expansion. Give special attention to the lower lobes, where mucus secretions commonly gather. Listen for bronchovesicular and vesicular sounds above and below the clavicles and along the lung periphery. In addition, auscultate for bronchial sounds, which are loud, high pitched, and hollow sounding, with expiration lasting longer than inspiration (3:2 ratio). This sound is normally heard over the trachea.

HEART

Compare the assessment of heart function with findings from the vascular assessment (see later section). Alterations in either system sometimes manifest as changes in the other. Some patients with signs or symptoms of heart (cardiac) problems have a life-threatening condition requiring immediate attention. In this case act quickly and conduct only the parts of the examination that are absolutely necessary. Conduct a more thorough assessment when the patient is more stable. The nursing history (Table 31-22) provides data to help interpret physical findings.

Assess cardiac function through the anterior thorax. Form a mental image of the exact location of the heart (Figure 31-37). In the adult it is located in the center of the chest (precordium), behind and to the left of the sternum, with a small section of the right atrium extending to the right of the sternum. The base of the heart is the upper part, and the apex is the bottom tip. The surface of the right ventricle

TABLE 31-22 Nursing History for Heart Assessment

Assessment	Rationale
Determine history of smoking, alcohol intake, caffeine intake, use of prescriptive and recreational drugs, exercise habits, and dietary patterns and intake (including fat and sodium intake).	Smoking; alcohol ingestion; cocaine use; lack of regular exercise; intake of foods high in carbohydrates, fats, and cholesterol are risk factors for cardiovascular disease. Caffeine can cause heart dysrhythmias.
Determine if patient is taking medications for cardiovascular function (e.g., antidysrhythmics, antihypertensives) and if he or she knows their purpose, dosage, and side effects.	Knowledge allows nurse to assess compliance with drug therapies. Medications sometimes affect vital sign values.
Assess for chest pain or discomfort, palpitations, excess fatigue, cough, dyspnea, leg pain or cramps, edema of feet, cyanosis, fainting, and orthopnea. Ask if symptoms occur at rest or during exercise.	These are key symptoms of heart disease. Cardiovascular function is sometimes adequate during rest but not during exercise. Positions affect how well lungs can expand.
If patient reports chest pain, determine if it is cardiac in nature. Anginal pain is usually a deep pressure or ache that is substernal and diffuse, radiating to one or both arms, neck, or jaw.	Assessment determines nature of pain and need to initiate care immediately.
Determine whether patient has stressful lifestyle. Which physical demands and/or emotional stress exist?	Repeated exposure to stress increases risk for heart disease.
Assess family history for heart disease, diabetes, high cholesterol levels, hypertension, stroke, or rheumatic heart disease.	Factors increase risk for heart disease.
Ask patient about history of heart trouble (e.g., heart failure, congenital heart disease, coronary artery disease, dysrhythmias, murmurs).	Knowledge reveals patient's level of understanding of condition. Preexisting condition influences examination techniques used and findings to expect.
Determine whether patient has preexisting diabetes, lung disease, obesity, or hypertension.	These disorders alter heart function.

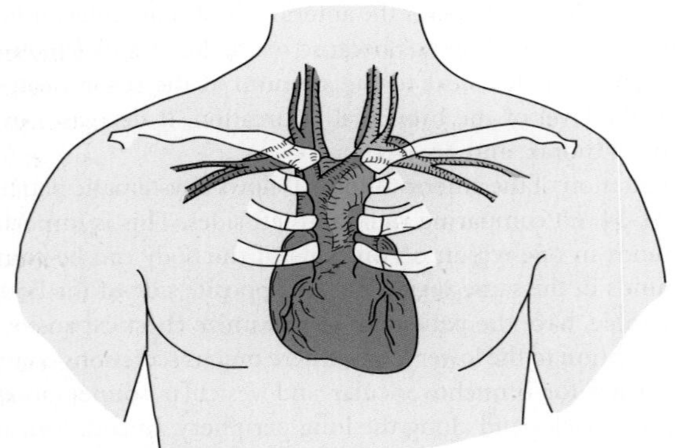

FIGURE 31-37 Anatomical position of heart.

composes most of the anterior surface of the heart. A section of the left ventricle shapes the left anterior side of the apex. The apex actually touches the anterior chest wall at approximately the fourth to fifth intercostal space just medial to the left midclavicular line. This is the **apical impulse or point of maximal impulse (PMI)**.

An infant's heart is positioned more horizontally. The apex of the heart is at the third or fourth intercostal space, just to the left of the midclavicular line. By the age of 7 a child's PMI is in the same location as the adult's. In tall, slender people the heart hangs more vertically and is positioned more centrally. In shorter or stockier individuals the heart tends to lie more to the left and horizontally (Ball et al., 2015).

To assess heart function, a clear understanding of the cardiac cycle and associated physiological events is of utmost importance (Figure 31-38). The heart normally pumps blood through its four chambers in a methodical, even sequence. Events on the left side occur just before those on the right. As blood flows through each chamber, the valves open and close, the pressures within chambers rise and fall, and the chambers contract. Each event creates a physiological sign. Both sides of the heart function in a coordinated fashion.

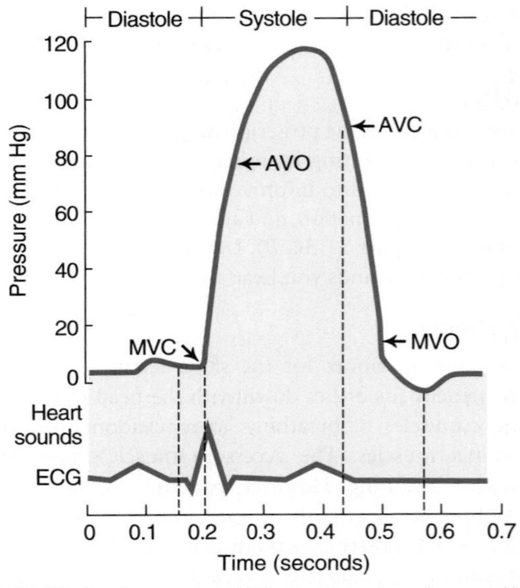

FIGURE 31-38 Cardiac cycle. *AVC,* Aortic valve closes; *AVO,* aortic valve opens; *ECG,* electrocardiogram; *MVC,* mitral valve closes; *MVO,* mitral valve opens.

There are two phases to the cardiac cycle: systole and diastole. During systole the ventricles contract and eject blood from the left ventricle into the aorta and from the right ventricle into the pulmonary artery. During diastole the ventricles relax, and the atria contract to move blood into the ventricles and fill the coronary arteries.

Heart sounds occur in relation to physiological events in the cardiac cycle. As systole begins, ventricular pressure rises and closes the mitral and tricuspid valves. Valve closure causes the first heart sound (S_1),

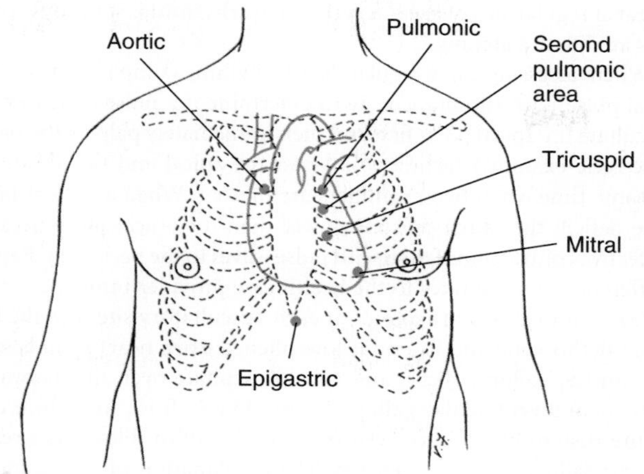

FIGURE 31-39 Anatomical sites for assessment of cardiac function.

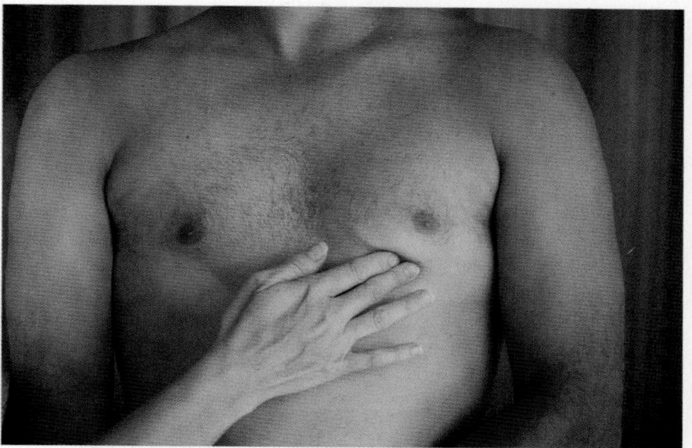

FIGURE 31-40 Palpation of apical pulse.

often described as "lub." The ventricles then contract, and blood flows through the aorta and pulmonary circulation. After the ventricles empty, ventricular pressure falls below that in the aorta and pulmonary artery. This allows the aortic and pulmonic valves to close, causing the second heart sound (S_2), described as "dub." As ventricular pressure continues to fall, it drops below that of the atria. The mitral and tricuspid valves reopen to allow ventricular filling. When the heart attempts to fill an already distended ventricle, a third heart sound (S_3) can be heard, as with heart failure. An S_3 is considered abnormal in adults over 31 years of age but can often be heard normally in children and young adults. It can also be present among women in the late stages of pregnancy. A fourth heart sound (S_4) occurs when the atria contract to enhance ventricular filling. An S_4 is often heard in healthy older adults, children, and athletes; but it is not normal in adults. Because S_4 also indicates an abnormal condition, report it to a health care provider.

Inspection and Palpation

Make the patient relaxed and comfortable before the examination. Explain the procedure to relieve his or her anxiety. An anxious or uncomfortable patient has mild tachycardia, which leads to inaccurate findings.

Use the skills of inspection and palpation simultaneously. Begin the examination with the patient in the supine position or the upper body elevated 45 degrees because patients with heart disease frequently suffer shortness of breath while lying flat. Stand at the patient's right side. Do not let the patient talk, especially when auscultating heart sounds. Good lighting in the room is essential.

Direct your attention to the anatomical sites best suited for assessment of cardiac function. During inspection and palpation look for visible pulsations and exaggerated lifts and palpate for the apical impulse and any source of vibrations (thrills). Follow an orderly sequence, beginning with assessment of the base of the heart and moving toward the apex. First inspect the angle of Louis, which lies between the sternal body and manubrium, and feel the ridge in the sternum approximately 5 cm (2 inches) below the sternal notch. Slip the fingers along the angle on each side of the sternum to feel adjacent ribs. The intercostal spaces are just below each rib. The second intercostal space allows identification of each of the six anatomical landmarks (Figure 31-39). The second intercostal space on the right is the *aortic area,* and the left second intercostal space is the *pulmonic area.* You need to use deeper palpation to feel the spaces in obese or heavily muscled patients. After locating the pulmonic area, move the fingers down the patient's left sternal border to the third intercostal space, called the *second pulmonic area.* The *tricuspid area* is located at the fourth or fifth intercostal space along the sternum. To find the *apical* or *mitral area,* locate the fifth intercostal space just to the left of the sternum and move the fingers laterally to the left midclavicular line. Locate the apical area with the palm of the hand or the fingertips. Normally you feel the apical impulse as a light tap in an area 1 to 2 cm (½ to 1 inch) in diameter at the apex (Figure 31-40). Another landmark is the epigastric area at the tip of the sternum. Palpate there if you suspect aortic abnormalities.

Locate the six anatomical landmarks of the heart and inspect and palpate each area. Look for the appearance of pulsations, viewing each area over the chest at an angle to the side. Normally pulsations are not seen, except perhaps at the PMI in thin patients or at the epigastric area as a result of abdominal aorta pulsation. Use the proximal halves of the four fingers together and alternate this with the ball of the hand to palpate for pulsations. Touch the areas gently to allow movements to lift the hand. Normally no pulsations or vibrations are felt in the second, third, or fourth intercostal spaces. Loud murmurs cause a vibration. Time palpated pulsations or vibrations and their occurrence in relation to systole or diastole by auscultating heart sounds simultaneously.

The apical impulse or PMI is felt easily. If you cannot locate it with the patient in a supine position, have him or her roll onto the left side, moving the heart closer to the chest wall. Estimate the size of the heart by noting the diameter of the PMI and its position relative to the midclavicular line. In cases of serious heart disease, the cardiac muscle enlarges, with the PMI found to the left of the midclavicular line. The PMI is sometimes difficult to find in the older adult because the chest deepens in its anteroposterior diameters. It is also difficult to find in muscular or overweight patients. An infant's PMI is located near the third or fourth intercostal space. It is easy to palpate because of the child's thin chest wall.

Auscultation

Auscultation of the heart detects normal heart sounds, extra heart sounds, and murmurs. Concentrate on detecting the normal low-intensity sounds created by valve closures. To begin auscultation eliminate all sources of room noise and explain the procedure to reduce the patient's anxiety. Follow a systematic pattern, beginning at the aortic area and inching the stethoscope across each of the anatomical sites. Listen for the complete cycle ("lub-dub") of heart sounds clearly at each location. Repeat the sequence with the bell of the stethoscope.

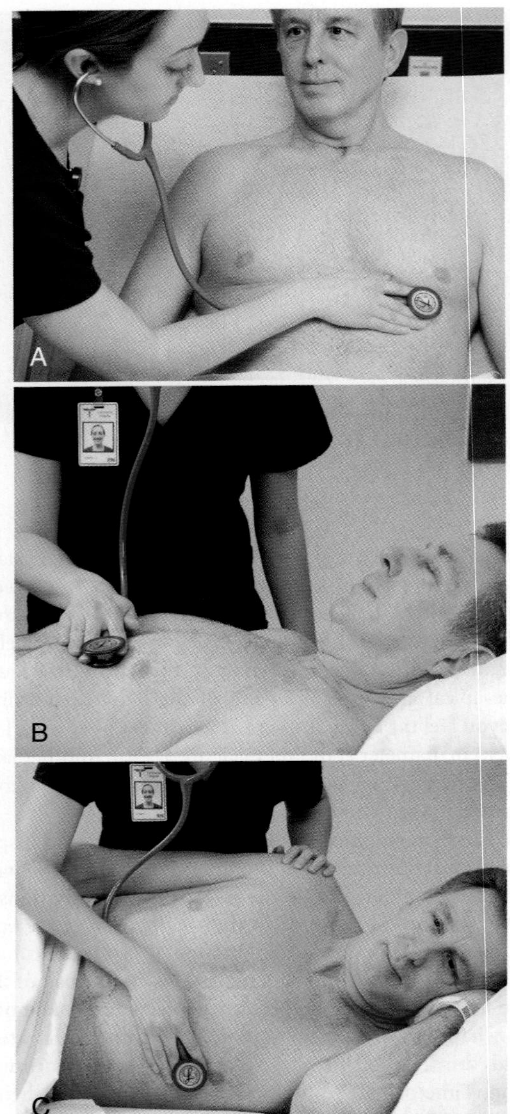

FIGURE 31-41 Sequence of patient positions for heart auscultation. **A,** Sitting. **B,** Supine. **C,** Left lateral recumbent.

Sometimes you will have a patient assume three different positions during the examination to hear sounds clearly (Figure 31-41, *A* to *C*): sitting up and leaning forward (good for all areas and to hear high-pitched murmurs), supine (good for all areas), and left lateral recumbent (good for all areas; best position to hear low-pitched sounds in diastole).

Learn to identify the first (S_1) and second (S_2) heart sounds. At normal rates S_1 occurs after the long diastolic pause and before the short systolic pause. S_1 is high pitched, dull in quality, and heard best at the apex. If it is difficult to hear S_1, time it in relation to the carotid pulsation. S_2 follows the short systolic pause and precedes the long diastolic pause; it is best heard at the aortic area.

Auscultate for rate and rhythm after hearing both sounds clearly. Each combination of S_1 and S_2 or "lub-dub" counts as one heartbeat. Count the rate for 1 minute and listen for the interval between S_1 and S_2 and then the time between S_2 and the next S_1. A regular rhythm involves regular intervals of time between each sequence of beats. There is a distinct silent pause between S_1 and S_2. Failure of the heart to beat at regular successive intervals is a **dysrhythmia**. Some dysrhythmias are life threatening.

When assessing an irregular heart rhythm, compare apical and radial pulse rates simultaneously to determine if a pulse deficit exists. Auscultate the apical pulse first and then immediately palpate the radial pulse (one-examiner technique). Assess the apical and radial rates at the same time when two examiners are present. When a patient has a pulse deficit, the radial pulse is slower than the apical pulse because ineffective contractions fail to send pulse waves to the periphery. Report a difference in pulse rates to the health care provider immediately.

Assess for extra heart sounds at each auscultatory site. Use the bell of the stethoscope and listen for low-pitched extra heart sounds such as S_3 and S_4 gallops, clicks, and rubs. Auscultate over all anatomical areas. S_3, or a **ventricular gallop**, occurs after S_2. It is caused by a premature rush of blood into a ventricle that is stiff or dilated as a result of heart failure and hypertension. The combination of S_1, S_2, and S_3 sounds like "Ken-TUCK-y".

S_4, or an atrial gallop, occurs just before S_1 or ventricular systole. The sound of an S_4 is similar to that of "TEN-nes-see" Physiologically it is caused by an atrial contraction pushing against a ventricle that is not accepting blood because of heart failure or other alterations. You can hear extra heart sounds more easily with the patient lying on the left side and the stethoscope at the apical site.

The final part of the examination includes assessment for heart murmurs. **Murmurs** are sustained swishing or blowing sounds heard at the beginning, middle, or end of the systolic or diastolic phase. They are caused by increased blood flow through a normal valve, forward flow through a stenotic valve or into a dilated vessel or heart chamber, or backward flow through a valve that fails to close. A murmur is asymptomatic or a sign of heart disease (Box 31-18). It is common in children. Keep the following factors in mind when auscultating to detect murmurs:

- When a murmur is detected, auscultate the mitral, tricuspid, aortic, and pulmonic valve areas for placement in the cardiac cycle (timing); the place it is heard best (location); radiation; loudness; pitch; and quality.
- If a murmur occurs between S_1 and S_2, it is a systolic murmur.
- If it occurs between S_2 and the next S_1, it is a diastolic murmur.
- The location of a murmur is not necessarily directly over the valves. Experience with hearing murmurs helps with better understanding of where each type of murmur is best heard. For example, mitral murmurs are best heard at the apex of the heart.
- To assess for radiation, listen over other areas in addition to where it is heard best. Murmurs can also be heard over the neck or back.
- Intensity or loudness is related to the rate of blood flow through the heart or the amount of blood regurgitated. Feel for a thrust or intermittent palpable sensation at the auscultation site in serious murmurs. A **thrill** is a continuous palpable sensation that resembles the purring of a cat. Intensity is recorded using the following grades (Ball et al., 2015):
  - *Grade 1:* Barely audible in a quiet room
  - *Grade 2:* Quiet but clearly audible
  - *Grade 3:* Moderately loud
  - *Grade 4:* Loud, with associated thrill
  - *Grade 5:* Very loud; thrill easily palpable
  - *Grade 6:* Very loud; audible with stethoscope not in contact with chest; thrill palpable and visible
- A murmur is low, medium, or high in pitch, depending on the velocity of blood flow through the valves. A low-pitched murmur is best heard with the bell of the stethoscope. If the murmur is best heard with the diaphragm, it is high pitched.

BOX 31-18 PATIENT TEACHING

Heart Assessment

Objective

- Patient will describe risk factors for heart disease and take appropriate steps to eliminate risks from lifestyle.

Teaching Strategies

- Explain risk factors for heart disease, including high dietary intake of saturated fat or cholesterol, lack of regular aerobic exercise, smoking, excess weight, stressful lifestyle, hypertension, and family history of heart disease.
- Refer patient (if appropriate) to resources available for controlling or reducing risks (e.g., nutritional counseling, exercise class, stress-reduction programs).
- Teach patient to reduce dietary intake of cholesterol and saturated fats. Explain that approximately 70% to 75% of saturated fatty acids come from meats, poultry, fish, and dairy products. The American Heart Association (AHA) (2014) recommends a diet that includes an intake that limits total fat to less than 35% of total calories, saturated fats to less than 10% of daily calories, trans fats to less than 1% of calories, and cholesterol to less than 310 mg/day.
- Encourage patient to have total blood cholesterol levels and triglycerides measured regularly. Desirable levels are less than 200 mg/dL. You need more than one cholesterol measurement to assess the blood cholesterol level accurately. Low-density lipoprotein (LDL) cholesterol is the major component of atherosclerotic plaques. Separate measurement of LDL cholesterol is wise in a patient with high total blood cholesterol levels. In an individual with no other risk factors, an LDL cholesterol level of 160 mg/100 dL or higher is high risk (AHA, 2014).
- Encourage patient to discuss with health care provider the need for periodic C-reactive protein (CRP) testing. CRP levels assess a patient's risk for cardiovascular disease.
- Advise patient to avoid cigarette smoke because nicotine causes vasoconstriction.
- Advise patient to quit smoking to lower the risk for coronary heart disease and coronary vascular disease.
- Patients who are at risk benefit from taking a daily low dose of aspirin. Consult health care provider before starting therapy.

Evaluation

- Ask patient to identify risk factors for heart disease.
- Have patient develop a meal plan low in saturated fat and cholesterol.
- Check patient's cholesterol level during follow-up appointments at the clinic or physician's office.
- Ask patient to describe ways he or she has chosen to reduce cardiac risk factors.

The quality of a murmur refers to its characteristic pattern and sound. A crescendo murmur starts softly and builds in loudness. A decrescendo murmur starts loudly and becomes less intense.

VASCULAR SYSTEM

Examination of the vascular system includes measuring the blood pressure (see Chapter 30) and assessing the integrity of the peripheral vascular system. Table 31-23 reviews the nursing history data collected before the examination. Use the skills of inspection, palpation, and auscultation. Perform parts of the vascular examination during other body system assessments. For example, check the carotid pulse after palpating the cervical lymph nodes. Note signs and symptoms of arterial and venous insufficiency when assessing the skin.

TABLE 31-23 Nursing History for Vascular Assessment

Assessment	Rationale
Determine if patient experiences leg cramps; numbness or tingling in extremities; sensation of cold hands or feet; pain in legs; or swelling or cyanosis of feet, ankles, or hand.	These signs and symptoms indicate vascular disease.
If patient experiences leg pain or cramping in lower extremities, ask if walking or standing for long periods or sleeping aggravates or relieves it.	Relationship of symptoms to exercise clarifies whether problem is vascular or musculoskeletal. Pain caused by vascular condition tends to increase with activity. Musculoskeletal pain usually is not relieved when exercise ends.
Ask patients if they wear tight-fitting garters, socks, or hosiery and sit or lie in bed with legs crossed.	Tight hosiery around lower extremities and crossing legs can impair venous return.
Reconsider previous heart risk factors (e.g., smoking, exercise, nutritional problems).	These predispose patient to vascular disease.
Assess medical history for heart disease, hypertension, phlebitis, diabetes, or varicose veins.	Circulatory and vascular disorders influence findings gathered during examination.

Blood Pressure

When auscultating blood pressure, know that readings between the arms vary by as much as 10 mm Hg and tend to be higher in the right arm (Ball et al., 2015). Always record the higher reading. Repeated systolic readings that differ by 15 mm Hg or more suggest atherosclerosis or disease of the aorta.

Carotid Arteries

When the left ventricle pumps blood into the aorta, the arterial system transmits pressure waves. The carotid arteries reflect heart function better than peripheral arteries because their pressure correlates with that of the aorta. The carotid artery supplies oxygenated blood to the head and neck (Figure 31-42). The overlying sternocleidomastoid muscle protects it.

To examine the carotid arteries, have the patient sit or lie supine with the head of the bed elevated 31 degrees. Examine one carotid artery at a time. If both arteries are occluded simultaneously during palpation, the patient loses consciousness as a result of inadequate circulation to the brain. *Do not palpate or massage the carotid arteries vigorously* because the carotid sinus is located at the bifurcation of the common carotid arteries in the upper third of the neck. This sinus sends impulses along the vagus nerve. Its stimulation causes a reflex drop in heart rate and blood pressure, which causes syncope or circulatory arrest. This is a particular problem for older adults.

Begin inspection of the neck for obvious pulsation of the artery. Have the patient turn the head slightly away from the artery being examined. Sometimes the wave of the pulse is visible. The carotid is the only site for assessing the quality of a pulse wave. An absent pulse wave indicates arterial occlusion (blockage) or stenosis (narrowing).

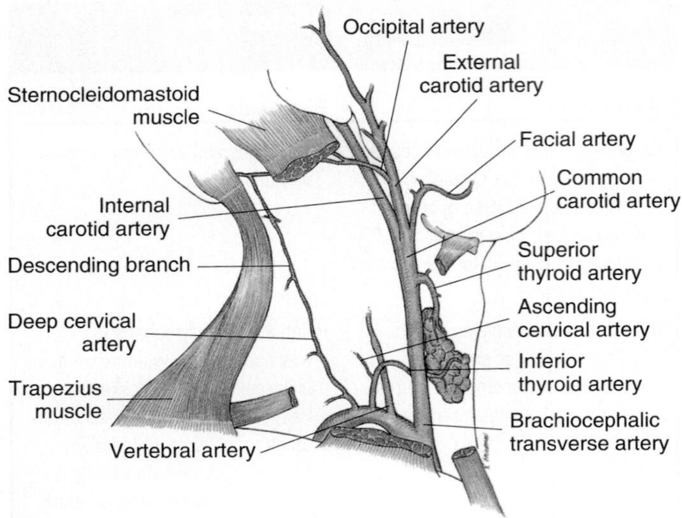

FIGURE 31-42 Anatomical position of carotid artery.

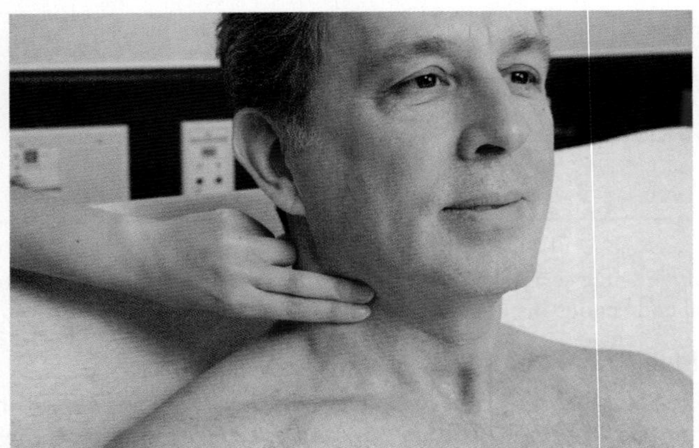

FIGURE 31-43 Palpation of internal carotid artery along margin of sternocleidomastoid muscle.

To palpate the pulse ask the patient to look straight ahead or turn the head slightly toward the side you are examining. Turning relaxes the sternocleidomastoid muscle. Slide the tips of the index and middle fingers around the medial edge of the sternocleidomastoid muscle. Gently palpate to avoid occlusion of circulation (Figure 31-43).

The normal carotid pulse is localized and strong rather than diffuse. It has a thrusting quality. As a patient breathes, no change occurs. Rotation of the neck or a shift from a sitting to a supine position does not change the quality of the carotid impulse. Both carotid arteries are normally equal in pulse rate, rhythm, and strength and are equally elastic. Diminished or unequal carotid pulsations indicate atherosclerosis or other forms of arterial disease.

The carotid is the most commonly auscultated pulse. Auscultation is especially important for middle-age or older adults or patients suspected of having cerebrovascular disease. When the lumen of a blood vessel is narrowed, it disturbs blood flow. As blood passes through the narrowed section, it creates turbulence, causing a blowing or swishing sound. The blowing sound is called a **bruit** (pronounced "brew-ee") (Figure 31-44).

Place the bell of the stethoscope over the carotid artery at the lateral end of the clavicle and the posterior margin of the sternocleidomastoid muscle. Have the patient turn his or her head slightly away from the side being examined (Figure 31-45). Ask him or her to hold the breath for a moment so breath sounds do not obscure a bruit. Normally you do not hear any sounds during carotid auscultation. Palpate the artery lightly for a thrill (palpable bruit) if you hear a bruit.

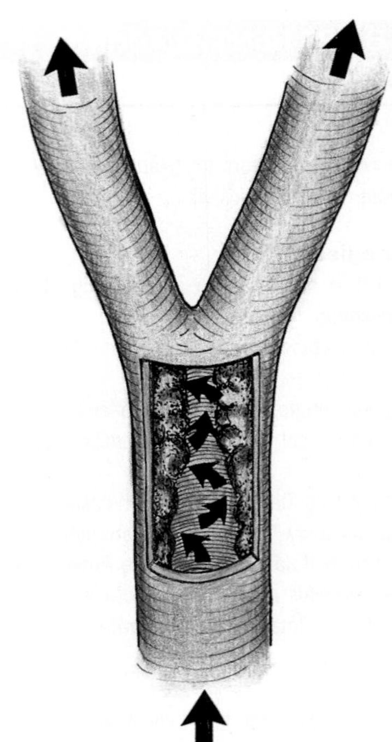

FIGURE 31-44 Occlusion or narrowing of the carotid artery disrupts normal blood flow. The resultant turbulence creates a sound (bruit) that is auscultated.

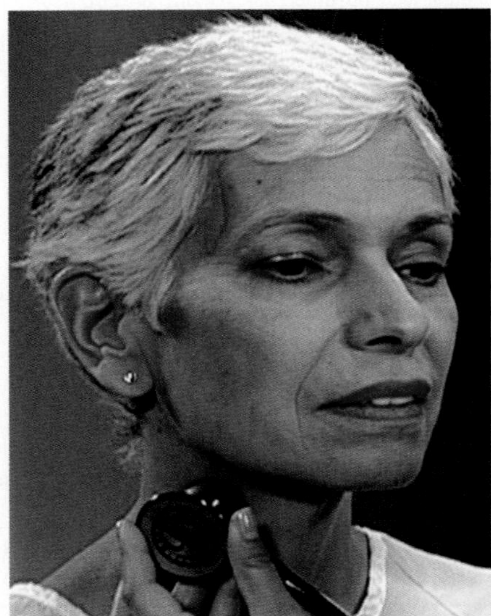

FIGURE 31-45 Auscultation for carotid artery bruit. (From Ball JW et al: *Seidel's guide to physical examination,* ed 8, St Louis, 2015, Mosby.)

Jugular Veins

The most accessible veins for examination are the internal and external jugular veins in the neck. Both veins drain bilaterally from the head and neck into the superior vena cava. The external jugular vein lies

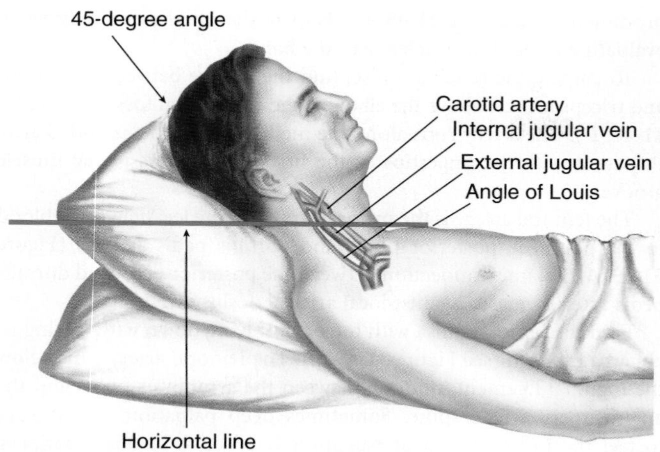

FIGURE 31-46 Position of patient to assess jugular vein distention. (From Thompson JM et al: *Mosby's manual of clinical nursing,* ed 5, St Louis, 2001, Mosby.)

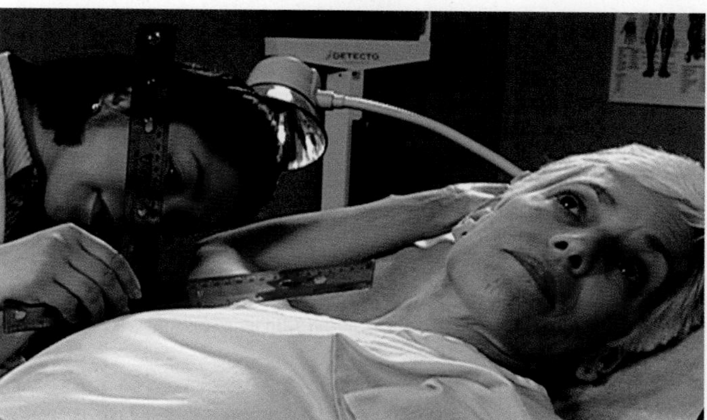

FIGURE 31-47 Measuring jugular venous pressure. (From Ball JW et al: *Seidel's guide to physical examination,* ed 8, St Louis, 2015, Mosby.)

superficially and is just above the clavicle. The internal jugular vein lies deeper, along the carotid artery.

It is best to examine the right internal jugular vein because it follows a more direct anatomical path to the right atrium of the heart. The column of blood inside the internal jugular vein serves as a manometer, reflecting pressure in the right atrium. The higher the column, the greater is the venous pressure. Raised venous pressure reflects right-sided heart failure.

Normally, when a patient lies in the supine position, the external jugular vein distends and becomes easily visible. In contrast, the jugular veins normally flatten when the patient changes to a sitting or standing position. However, for some patients with heart disease the jugular veins remain distended when sitting.

To measure venous pressure, first inspect the jugular veins. Venous pressure is influenced by blood volume (i.e., the capacity of the right atrium to receive blood and send it to the right ventricle and the ability of the right ventricle to contract and force blood into the pulmonary artery). Any factor resulting in greater blood volume within the venous system results in elevated venous pressure. Assess venous pressure by using the following steps:

1. Ask the patient to lie supine with the head elevated 31 to 45 degrees (semi-Fowler's position).
2. Expose the neck and upper thorax. Use a pillow to align the head. Avoid neck hyperextension or flexion to ensure that the vein is not stretched or kinked (Figure 31-46).
3. Usually pulsations are not evident with the patient sitting up. As he or she slowly leans back into a supine position, the level of venous pulsations begins to rise above the level of the manubrium as much as 1 or 2 cm ($\frac{1}{2}$ to 1 inch) as the patient reaches a 45-degree angle. Measure venous pressure by measuring the vertical distance between the angle of Louis and the highest level of the visible point of the internal jugular vein pulsation.
4. Use two rulers. Line up the bottom edge of a regular ruler with the top of the area of pulsation in the jugular vein. Then take a centimeter ruler and align it perpendicular to the first ruler at the level of the sternal angle. Measure in centimeters the distance between the second ruler and the sternal angle (Figure 31-47).
5. Repeat the same measurement on the other side. Bilateral pressures higher than 2.5 cm (1 inch) are considered elevated and are a sign of right-sided heart failure. One-sided pressure elevation is caused by obstruction.

TABLE 31-24 Indicators for Assessing Local Blood Flow

Indicator	Rationale
Systemic diseases (e.g., arteriosclerosis, atherosclerosis, diabetes)	Diseases result in changes in integrity of walls of arteries and smaller blood vessels.
Coagulation disorders (e.g., thrombosis, embolus)	Blood clot causes mechanical obstruction to blood flow.
Local trauma or surgery (e.g., contusion, fracture, vascular surgery)	Direct manipulation of vessels or localized edema impairs blood flow.
Application of constricting devices (e.g., casts, dressings, elastic bandages, restraints)	Constriction causes tourniquet effect, impairing blood flow to areas below site of constriction.

Peripheral Arteries and Veins

To examine the peripheral vascular system, first assess the adequacy of blood flow to the extremities by measuring arterial pulses and inspecting the condition of the skin and nails. Next assess the integrity of the venous system. Assess the arterial pulses in the extremities to determine sufficiency of the entire arterial circulation.

Factors such as coagulation disorders, local trauma or surgery, constricting casts or bandages, and systemic diseases impair circulation to the extremities (Table 31-24). Discuss risk factors and ways to monitor for circulatory problems with the patient (Box 31-19).

Peripheral Arteries. Examine each peripheral artery using the distal pads of your second and third fingers. The thumb helps anchor the brachial and femoral artery. Apply firm pressure but avoid occluding a pulse. When a pulse is difficult to find, it helps to vary pressure and feel all around the pulse site. Be sure not to palpate your own pulse.

Routine vital signs usually include assessment of the rate and rhythm of the radial artery because it is easily accessible. Count the pulse for either 31 seconds or a full minute, depending on the character of the pulse (see Chapter 30). Always count an irregular pulse for 60 seconds. With palpation normally feel the pulse wave at regular intervals. When an interval is interrupted by an early, a late, or a missed beat, the pulse rhythm is irregular. During cardiac emergencies health care providers usually assess the carotid artery because it is accessible

BOX 31-19 PATIENT TEACHING

Vascular Assessment

Objective

- Patient with vascular insufficiency will avoid activities that worsen circulatory status.

Teaching Strategies

- Instruct patient with risk or evidence of vascular insufficiency in the lower extremities to avoid tight clothing over the lower body or legs, avoid sitting or standing for long periods, avoid sitting with legs crossed, walk regularly, and elevate feet when sitting.
- Advise patient to avoid or stop smoking cigarettes, cigars, pipes or using nicotine products (e.g., chewing tobacco, nicotine patches or gum) because nicotine causes vasoconstriction. Offer a referral to a reliable stop-smoking program.
- Instruct patient with hypertension about the benefits of regular monitoring of blood pressure (daily, weekly, or monthly). Teach patient how to use home monitoring kits.

Evaluation

- Ask patient to identify if blood pressure reading is within normal limits for age.
- Have patient with vascular insufficiency describe precautions to take to avoid further circulatory deficiency.
- Have patient demonstrate self-monitoring of blood pressure.

and most useful in evaluating heart activity. To check local circulatory status of tissues (e.g., when a leg cast is in place or following vascular surgery), palpate the peripheral arteries long enough to note that a pulse is present.

Assess each peripheral artery for elasticity of the vessel wall, strength, and equality. The arterial wall normally is elastic, making it easily palpable. After depressing the artery, it springs back to shape when the pressure is released. An abnormal artery is hard, inelastic, or calcified.

The strength of a pulse is a measurement of the force at which blood is ejected against the arterial wall. Some examiners use a scale rating from 0 to 4 for the strength of a pulse (Ball et al., 2015):

0: Absent, not palpable
1: Pulse diminished, barely palpable
2: Expected
3: Full, increased
4: Bounding, aneurysmal

Measure all peripheral pulses for equality and symmetry. Compare the left radial pulse with that of the right and so on. Lack of symmetry indicates impaired circulation such as a localized obstruction or an abnormally positioned artery.

In the upper extremities the brachial artery channels blood to the radial and ulnar arteries of the forearm and hand. If circulation in this artery becomes blocked, the hands do not receive adequate blood flow. If circulation in the radial or ulnar arteries becomes impaired, the hand still receives adequate perfusion. An interconnection between the radial and ulnar arteries guards against arterial occlusion (Figure 31-48, *A*).

To locate pulses in the arm have the patient sit or lie down. Find the radial pulse along the radial side of the forearm at the wrist. Thin individuals have a groove lateral to the flexor tendon of the wrist. Feel the radial pulse with light palpation in the groove (see Figure 31-48, *B*). The ulnar pulse is on the opposite side of the wrist and feels less prominent (see Figure 31-48, *C*). Palpate the ulnar pulse only when evaluating arterial insufficiency to the hand.

To palpate the brachial pulse, find the groove between the biceps and triceps muscle above the elbow at the antecubital fossa (see Figure 31-48, *D*). The artery runs along the medial side of the extended arm. Palpate it with the fingertips of the first three fingers in the muscle groove.

The femoral artery is the primary artery in the leg, delivering blood to the popliteal, posterior tibial, and dorsalis pedis arteries (Figure 31-49, *A*). An interconnection between the posterior tibial and dorsalis pedis arteries guards against local arterial occlusion.

Find the femoral pulse with the patient lying down with the inguinal area exposed (see Figure 31-49, *B*). The femoral artery runs below the inguinal ligament, midway between the symphysis pubis and the anterosuperior iliac spine. Sometimes deep palpation is necessary to feel the pulse. Bimanual palpation is effective in obese patients. Place the fingertips of both hands on opposite sides of the pulse site. Feel a pulsatile sensation when the arterial pulsation pushes the fingertips apart.

The popliteal pulse runs behind the knee. Have the patient slightly flex the knee with the foot resting on the examination table or assume a prone position with the knee slightly flexed (see Figure 31-49, *C*). Instruct him or her to keep leg muscles relaxed. Palpate with the fingers of both hands deeply into the popliteal fossa, just lateral to the midline. The popliteal pulse is difficult to locate.

With the patient's foot relaxed, locate the dorsalis pedis pulse. The artery runs along the top of the foot in line with the groove between the extensor tendons of the great toe and first toe (see Figure 31-49, *D*). To find the pulse, place the fingertips between the first and second toes and slowly move up the dorsum of the foot. This pulse is sometimes congenitally absent.

Find the posterior tibial pulse on the inner side of each ankle (Figure 31-49, *E*). Place the fingers behind and below the medial malleolus (ankle bone). With the foot relaxed and slightly extended, palpate the artery.

Ultrasound Stethoscopes. If a pulse is difficult to palpate, an ultrasound (Doppler) stethoscope is a useful tool that amplifies the sounds of a pulse wave. Factors that weaken a pulse or make palpation difficult include obesity, reduction in the stroke volume of the heart, diminished blood volume, or arterial obstruction. Apply a thin layer of transmission gel to the patient's skin at the pulse site or directly onto the transducer tip of the probe. Turn on the volume control and place the tip of the transducer at a 45- to 90-degree angle on the skin (Figure 31-50). Move the transducer until you hear a pulsating "whooshing" sound that indicates that arterial blood flow is present.

Tissue Perfusion. The condition of the skin, mucosa, and nail beds offers useful data about the status of circulatory blood flow. Examine the face and upper extremities, looking at the color of the skin, mucosa, and nail beds. The presence of cyanosis requires special attention. Heart disease sometimes causes central cyanosis, which indicates poor arterial oxygenation. Some characteristics of this are a bluish discoloration of the lips, mouth, and conjunctivae. Blue lips, earlobes, and nail beds are signs of peripheral cyanosis, which indicates peripheral vasoconstriction. When cyanosis is present, consult with a health care provider to request laboratory testing of oxygen saturation to determine the severity of the problem. Examination of the nails involves inspection for **clubbing**, a bulging of the tissues at the nail base. Clubbing is caused by insufficient oxygenation at the periphery resulting from conditions such as chronic emphysema and congenital heart disease.

Inspect the lower extremities for changes in color, temperature, and condition of the skin, indicating either arterial or venous

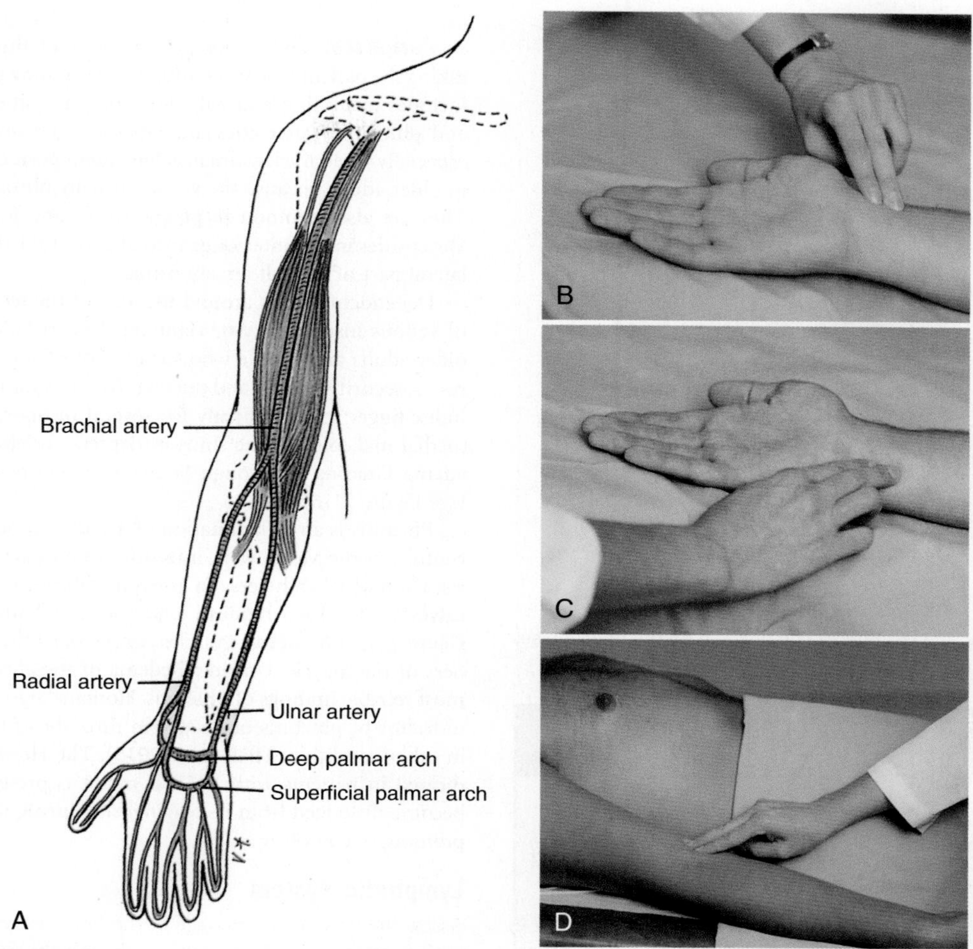

FIGURE 31-48 A, Anatomical positions of brachial, radial, and ulnar arteries. **B,** Palpation of radial pulse. **C,** Palpation of ulnar pulse. **D,** Palpation of brachial pulse.

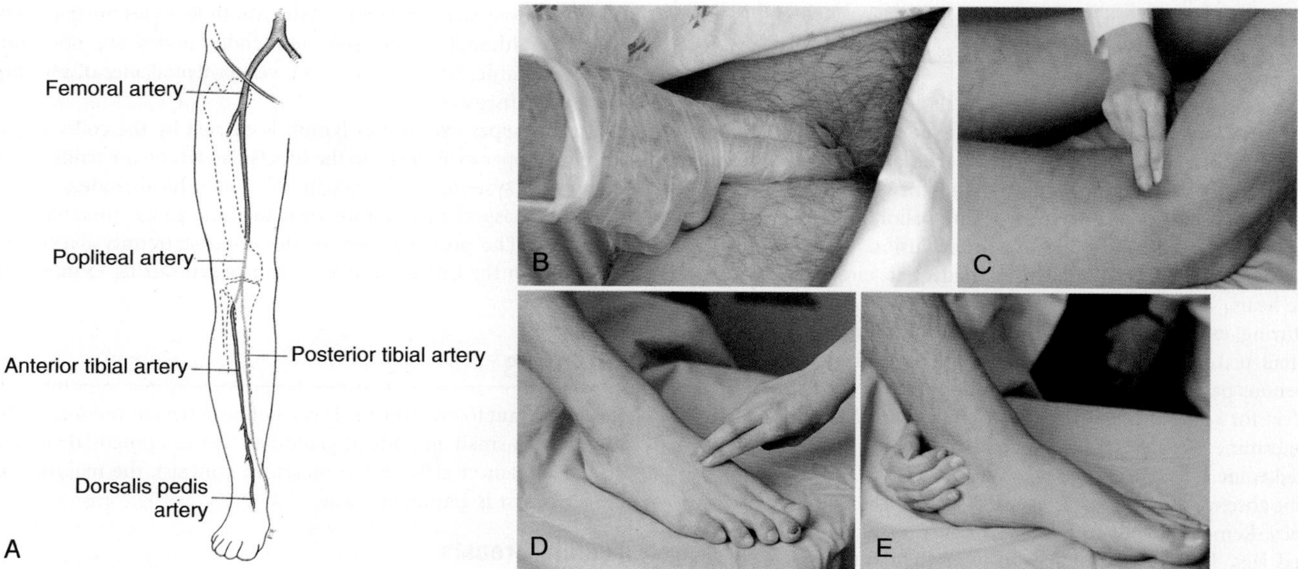

FIGURE 31-49 A, Anatomical position of femoral, popliteal, dorsalis pedis, and posterior tibial arteries. **B,** Palpation of femoral pulse. **C,** Palpation of popliteal pulse. **D,** Palpation of dorsalis pedis pulse. **E,** Palpation of posterior tibial pulse.

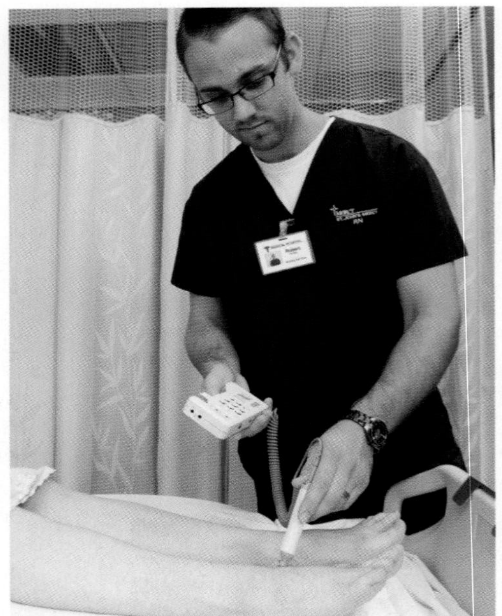

FIGURE 31-50 Ultrasound stethoscope in position on the pedal pulse.

TABLE 31-25 Signs of Venous and Arterial Insufficiency

Assessment Criterion	Venous	Arterial
Color	Normal or cyanotic	Pale; worsened by elevation of extremity; dusky red when extremity is lowered
Temperature	Normal	Cool (blood flow blocked to extremity)
Pulse	Normal	Decreased or absent
Edema	Often marked	Absent or mild
Skin changes	Brown pigmentation around ankles	Thin, shiny skin; decreased hair growth; thickened nails

alterations (Table 31-25). This is a good time to ask the patient about any history of pain in the legs. If an arterial occlusion is present, the patient has signs resulting from an absence of blood flow. Pain is distal to the occlusion. The five *Ps*—pain, pallor, pulselessness, paresthesias, and paralysis—characterize an occlusion. Venous congestion causes tissue changes that indicate an inadequate circulatory flow back to the heart.

During examination of the lower extremities, also inspect skin and nail texture; hair distribution on the lower legs, feet, and toes; the venous pattern; and scars, pigmentation, or ulcers. Palpate the legs and feet for color and temperature. Capillary refill, traditionally used to determine adequacy of peripheral blood flow to the digits, has limited value.

The absence of hair growth over the legs indicates circulatory insufficiency. Remember not to confuse absence of hair on the legs with shaved legs. In addition, men who wear tight-fitting dress socks or jeans may have less hair on their calves. Chronic recurring ulcers of the feet or lower legs are a serious sign of circulatory insufficiency and require a health care provider's intervention.

Peripheral Veins. Assess the status of the peripheral veins by asking the patient to assume sitting and standing positions. Assessment includes inspection and palpation for varicosities, peripheral edema, and phlebitis. Varicosities are superficial veins that become dilated, especially when the legs are in a dependent position. They are common in older adults because the veins normally fibrose, dilate, and stretch. They are also common in people who stand for prolonged periods. Varicosities in the anterior or medial part of the thigh and the posterolateral part of the calf are abnormal.

Dependent edema around the area of the feet and ankles is a sign of venous insufficiency or right-sided heart failure. It is common in older adults and people who spend a lot of time standing (e.g., waitresses, security guards, and nurses). To assess for pitting edema, use the index finger to press firmly for several seconds and release over the medial malleolus or the shins. A depression left in the skin indicates edema. Grading 1+ through 4+ characterizes the severity of the edema (see Figure 31-6).

Phlebitis is an inflammation of a vein that occurs commonly after trauma to the vessel wall, infection, immobilization, and prolonged insertion of IV catheters. To assess for phlebitis in the leg, inspect the calves for localized redness, tenderness, and swelling over vein sites. Gentle palpation of calf muscles reveals warmth, tenderness, and firmness of the muscle. Unilateral edema of the affected leg is one of the most reliable findings of phlebitis. Homans' sign is no longer a reliable indicator of phlebitis or deep vein thrombosis (DVT) and is present in other conditions (Ball et al., 2015). The Homans' sign is contraindicated in patients with DVT. If a clot is present in the leg, it may become dislodged from its original site during this test, resulting in a pulmonary embolism.

Lymphatic System

Assess the lymphatic drainage of the lower extremities during examination of the vascular system or during the female or male genital examination. Superficial and deep nodes drain the legs, but only two groups of superficial nodes are palpable. With the patient supine, palpate the area of the superficial inguinal nodes in the groin area (Figure 31-51, *A*). Then move the fingertips toward the inner thigh, feeling for any inferior nodes. Use a firm but gentle pressure when palpating over each lymphatic chain. Multiple nodes normally are not palpable, although a few soft, nontender nodes are not unusual. Enlarged, hardened, tender nodes reveal potential sites of infection or metastatic disease.

In the upper extremities lymph is carried by the collecting ducts from the upper extremities to the subclavian lymphatic trunk. To assess this lymph system, gently palpate the epitrochlear nodes, located on the medial aspect of the arms near the antecubital fossa (see Figure 31-51, *B*). The proximal part of the upper-extremity lymph system is located in the axilla and is usually assessed during examination of the breasts.

BREASTS

It is important to examine the breasts of both female and male patients. Men have a small amount of glandular tissue, a potential site for the growth of cancer cells, in the breast. In contrast, the majority of the female breast is glandular tissue.

Female Breasts

New cases of invasive breast cancer were predicted to affect an estimated 231,840 women in the United States during 2015; about 2,350 new cases were expected in men (ACS, 2015a). The disease is second

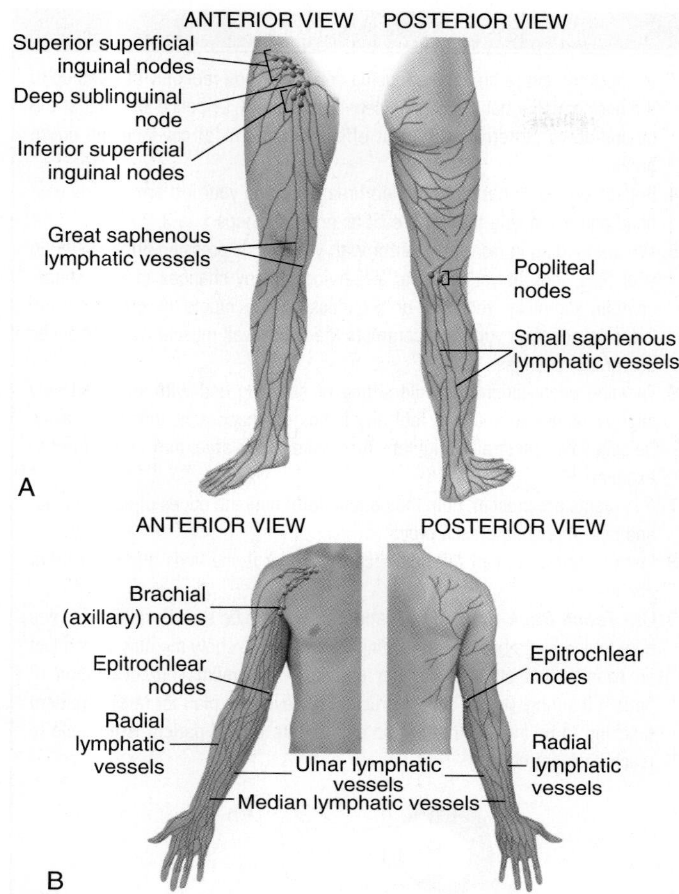

FIGURE 31-51 **A,** Lymphatic drainage for lower extremities. **B,** Lymphatic drainage for upper extremities. (From Ball JW et al: *Seidel's guide to physical examination,* ed 8, St Louis, 2015, Mosby.)

BOX 31-20 EVIDENCE-BASED PRACTICE

Detection of Breast Cancer

PICO Question: Does the use of a targeted intervention compared with standard teaching methods increase the rate of annual mammograms in African-American women?

Evidence Summary

The mortality rate from breast cancer is higher in African-American women than in other racial groups (Conway-Phillips and Janusek, 2014; Northington et al., 2011). This is often because of a low rate of breast cancer screening, leading to the diagnosis of breast cancer when it is in a more advanced stage (Brooks et al., 2013). A number of factors contribute to this low screening rate, including but not limited to lack of health insurance, preconceived beliefs or lack of knowledge about the importance of screening, attitudes toward screening, financial burden, low level of education or income, fear of radiation, and distrust of the health care system (Conway-Phillips and Janusek, 2014; Northington et al., 2011). Specific targeted interventions have been successful in increasing mammograms in this population. Khaliq et al. (2013) found that, in a group of high-risk breast cancer women from lower socioeconomic levels, inpatient hospital stays were an effective time to offer mammogram screening along with screening education. In this group a higher percentage of women agreed to have an inpatient screening mammogram while in the hospital if it was offered (Khaliq et al., 2013). Women who watched a narrative video from an African-American breast cancer survivor reported fewer barriers to mammography and increased confidence that mammograms were effective screening measures (Kreuter et al., 2010). Women with lower educational levels who watched the narrative video had higher mammogram rates than women who watched the standard information video (Kreuter et al., 2010). Research found that targeted postcard reminders were effective if barriers were removed. Likelihood of obtaining a mammogram was related to belief in preventive screening (Feldstein et al., 2011). Conway-Phillips and Janusek (2014) also found that spirituality was a strong predictor of likelihood of an African-American woman to obtain breast cancer screening.

Application to Nursing Practice

- Remember that it is important to identify barriers to breast cancer screening. Removal of the barriers is often necessary to be able to develop effective targeted strategies to increase screening (Conway-Phillips and Janusek, 2014; Northington et al., 2011).
- Discuss with the health care provider the opportunity to offer screening mammograms to hospitalized patients (Khaliq et al., 2013).
- Use inpatient hospitalizations as an opportunity to teach women about the importance of breast cancer screening (Khaliq et al., 2013).
- Collaborate with the faith community nurses in African-American churches to provide breast cancer screening education to church members (Conway-Phillips and Janusek, 2014).
- Develop and use narrative videos of African-American women who are breast cancer survivors as educational tools related to the importance of breast cancer screening (Kreuter et al., 2010).

to lung cancer as the leading cause of death in women with cancer. Early detection is the key to cure (Box 31-20). A major responsibility for nurses is to teach patients health behaviors such as breast self-examination (BSE) (Box 31-21).

Women need to be taught to know how their breasts usually look and feel and report changes to a health care professional. In addition, they need to know about the benefits and limitations of performing a systematic BSE. Once thought essential for early breast cancer detection, BSEs are now considered optional because there is limited evidence as to the benefits in locating cancerous tumors (ACS, 2015b). If a female patient already performs BSE, assess the method she uses and times she does the examination in relation to her menstrual cycle. The best time for a BSE is the fourth through seventh day of the menstrual cycle or right after the menstrual cycle ends, when the breast is no longer swollen or tender from hormone elevations. If the woman is postmenopausal, advise her to check her breasts on the same day each month. The pregnant woman should also check her breasts on a monthly basis.

Older women require special attention when reviewing the need for regular BSE. Fixed incomes limit many older women; thus they fail to pursue regular clinical breast examination and mammography. Unfortunately many older women ignore changes in their breasts, assuming that they are a part of aging. In addition, physiological factors affect the ease with which older women perform a BSE. Musculoskeletal limitations, diminished peripheral sensation, reduced eyesight, and changes in joint range of motion (ROM) limit palpation and inspection abilities. Find resources for older women, including free screening programs. Teach family members to perform the patient's examination.

Table 31-3 outlines the American Cancer Society (ACS, 2015b) guidelines for the early detection of breast cancer in women at average risk. Monthly BSE is no longer recommended by the ACS (2015b) for women at any age, but other health organizations encourage BSE as an important option for women (National Breast Cancer Foundation, 2015). Encourage women to ask their personal physician what he or she recommends in regards to screening.

BOX 31-21 Breast Self-Examination

There is recent controversy over the value of women performing breast self-examinations (BSE) to screen for cancer. In 2015, the American Cancer Society (ACS) reported that research does not show a clear benefit of physical breast exams done by either a health professional or by the individual woman (ACS, 2015b). Due to this lack of evidence, regular clinical breast exams and breast self-exams are not recommended by the ACS. However, many physicians argue that women should be familiar with how their breasts normally look and feel and report any changes to a health care provider right away. Thus many physicians still recommend regular BSE.

When instructing women about BSE, explain the benefits and limitations of breast self-examination (BSE) (National Breast Cancer Foundation, 2015). Emphasize the importance of prompt reporting of any new breast symptoms to a health care professional. Women who choose to do BSE should receive instruction and have their technique reviewed. BSE done once a month helps women become familiar with the usual appearance and feel of their breasts. Familiarity makes it easier to notice any changes in the breast from one month to another. Early discovery of a change from "normal" is the main idea behind BSE.

For women who menstruate, the best time to do BSE is the fourth through the seventh day of the menstrual cycle or right after the menstrual cycle ends, when the breasts are least likely to be tender or swollen. Women who no longer menstruate should pick a day such as the first day of the month to remind them to do BSE. Males should also examine their breast, areolas, nipples, and axillae for any swelling, nodules, or ulcerations.

When a woman has breast implants, it might be helpful for the surgeon to identify the edges of the implant. Women who are pregnant or breastfeeding should also do a BSE.

Procedure

1. Examine your right breast. Lie on your back and place your right arm behind your head (see illustration A). The examination is best completed lying down, not standing up, because when you lie down the breast tissue spreads evenly over the chest wall and is as thin as possible, making it much easier to feel all of it.
2. Use finger pads of the three middle fingers on your left hand to feel for lumps in the right breast (see illustration B). Use overlapping dime-size circular motions of the finger pads to feel the breast tissue. Use three different levels of pressure to feel all the breast tissue. Light pressure is needed to feel the tissue closest to the skin; medium pressure to feel a little deeper; and firm pressure to feel the tissue closest to the chest and ribs. It is normal to feel a firm ridge in the lower curve of each breast, but you should tell your health care provider if you feel anything else out of the ordinary. If you're not sure how hard to press, discuss this with your health care provider. Use each pressure level to feel the breast tissue before moving on to the next spot.
3. Move around the breast in an up-and-down pattern starting at an imaginary line drawn straight down your side from the under arm and moving across the breast to the middle of the chest bone (sternum or breastbone). Be sure to check the entire breast area, going down until you feel only ribs and up to the neck or collar bone (clavicle) (see illustration C). Evidence shows that the up-and-down pattern is the most effective pattern for covering the entire breast.
4. Repeat self-examination in the left breast, putting your left arm behind your head and examining the left breast as noted in Steps 1 to 3.
5. While standing in front of a mirror with your hands pressing firmly down on your hips, look at your breasts, observing for any changes in size, shape, contour, dimpling, redness, or scaliness of the nipple or breast tissue. Pressing down on your hips contracts the chest wall muscles and enhances any breast changes.
6. Examine each underarm while sitting or standing and with your arm only slightly raised so you can feel any lumps or changes in this area easily. Raising your arm straight tightens the tissue in this area, making it harder to examine.
7. If implants are present, help the patient determine the edges of each implant and how to evaluate each breast.
8. Instruct patient to call the health care provider if she finds a lump or other abnormality.
9. Use ***Teach Back.*** State to the patient, "I want to be sure I explained to you how to conduct a breast self-examination. Can you show me how to conduct an examination on both of your breasts?" Document your evaluation of patient learning. Revise your instruction or develop a plan for revised patient teaching to be implemented at an appropriate time if patient is not able to teach back correctly.

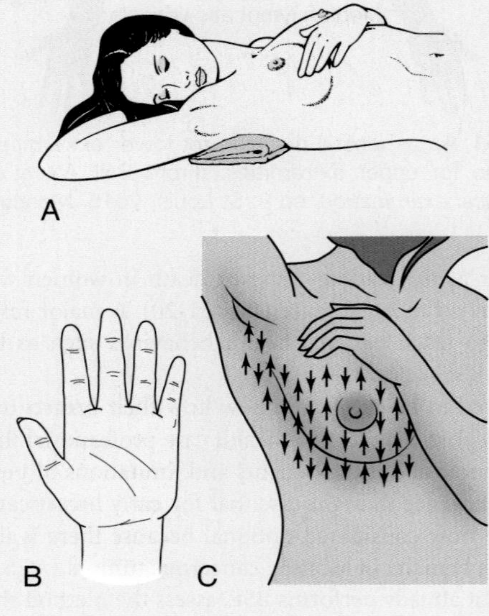

The ACS (2015b) recommends that women who are at high risk for breast cancer based on certain factors should get an MRI and a mammogram every year. This includes women who:

- Have a lifetime risk of breast cancer of about 20% to 25% or greater, according to risk assessment tools that are based mainly on family history
- Have a known *BRCA1* or *BRCA2* gene mutation
- Have a first-degree relative (parent, brother, sister, or child) with a *BRCA1* or *BRCA2* gene mutation and have not had genetic testing themselves
- Had radiation therapy to the chest when they were between the 10 and 30 years of age

The patient's history (Table 31-26) reveals normal developmental changes and signs of breast disease. Because of its glandular structure, the breast undergoes changes during a woman's life. Knowing these changes (Box 31-22) allows complete and accurate assessment. Encourage both men and women to observe their breasts for changes.

Inspection. Have the patient remove the top gown or drape to allow simultaneous visualization of both breasts. Have her stand or sit with her arms hanging loosely at her sides. If possible, place a mirror in front of her during inspection so she sees what to look for when performing a BSE. To recognize abnormalities the patient needs to

TABLE 31-26 Nursing History for Breast Assessment

Assessment	Rationale
Determine if woman is over age 40; has a personal or family history of breast cancer, especially with the BRCA1 or BRCA2 inherited gene mutations; early-onset menarche (before age 12) or late-age menopause (after age 55); has never had children or gave birth to first child after age 31; or has recently used oral contraceptives.	These are risk factors for breast cancer (ACS, 2015a).
Ask if patient (both sexes) has noticed lump, thickening, pain, or tenderness of breast; discharge, distortion, retraction, or scaling of the nipple; or change in size of breast.	Potential signs and symptoms of breast cancer allow nurse to focus on specific areas of breast during assessment.
Determine patient's use of medications (oral contraceptives, digitalis, diuretics, steroids, or estrogen). Determine his or her caffeine intake.	Some medications cause nipple discharge. Hormones and caffeine cause fibrocystic changes in breast.
Determine patient's level of activity, alcoholic intake, and weight.	Breast cancer incidence rates correlate with being overweight or obese (postmenopausal), physical inactivity, and consumption of one or more alcoholic beverages per day (ACS, 2015a).
Ask if patient performs monthly breast self-examination (BSE). If so, determine time of month she performs examination in relation to menstrual cycle. Have her describe or demonstrate method used.	Nurse's role is to educate patient about breast cancer and correct techniques for BSE.
If patient reports a breast mass, ask about length of time since she first noticed the lump. Does lump come and go, or is it always present? Have there been changes in the lump (e.g., size, relationship to menses), and are there associated symptoms?	Assessment helps to determine nature of mass (e.g., breast cancer versus fibrocystic disease).

BOX 31-22 Normal Changes in the Breast During a Woman's Life Span

Puberty (8 to 20 Years)
Breasts mature in five stages. One breast may grow more rapidly than the other. The ages at which changes occur and rate of developmental progression vary.

Stage 1 (Preadolescent)
This stage involves elevation of the nipple only.

Stage 2
The breast and nipple elevate as a small mound, and the areolar diameters enlarge.

Stage 3
There is further enlargement and elevation of the breast and areola, with no separation of contour.

Stage 4
The areola and nipple project into the secondary mound above the level of the breast (does not occur in all girls).

Stage 5 (Mature Breast)
Only the nipple projects, and the areola recedes (varies in some women).

Young Adulthood (20 to 31 Years)
Breasts reach full (nonpregnant) size. Shape is generally symmetrical. Breasts are sometimes unequal in size.

Pregnancy
Breast size gradually enlarges to 2 to 3 times the previous size. Nipples enlarge and become erect. Areolas darken, and diameters increase. Superficial veins become prominent. The nipples expel a yellowish fluid (colostrum).

Menopause
Breasts shrink. Tissue becomes softer, sometimes flabby.

Older Adulthood
Breasts become elongated, pendulous, and flaccid as a result of glandular tissue atrophy. The skin of the breasts tends to wrinkle, appearing loose and flabby.

Nipples become smaller and flatter and lose erectile ability. They sometimes invert because of shrinkage and fibrotic changes.

Data from Touhy TA, Jett KF: *Ebersole and Hess' gerontological nursing & healthy aging*, ed 4, St Louis, 2014, Elsevier; Hockenberry MJ, Wilson D: *Wong's nursing care of infants and children*, ed 10, St Louis, 2015, Mosby; and Ball JW et al: *Seidel's guide to physical examination*, ed 8, St Louis, 2015, Mosby.

be familiar with the normal appearance of her breasts. Describe observations or findings in relation to imaginary lines that divide the breast into four quadrants and a tail. The lines cross at the center of the nipple. Each tail extends outward from the upper outer quadrant (Figure 31-52).

Inspect the breasts for size and symmetry. Normally they extend from the third to the sixth ribs, with the nipple at the level of the fourth intercostal space. It is common for one breast to be smaller. However, inflammation or a mass causes a difference in size. As a woman ages, the ligaments supporting the breast tissue weaken, causing the breasts to sag and the nipples to lower.

Observe the contour or shape of the breasts and note masses, flattening, retraction, or dimpling. Breasts vary in shape from convex to pendulous or conical. Retraction or dimpling can result from invasion of underlying ligaments by tumors. The ligaments fibrose and pull the overlying skin inward toward the tumor. Edema also changes the contour of the breasts. To bring out retraction or changes in the shape of breasts, ask the patient to assume three positions: raise arms above the head, press hands against the hips, and extend arms straight ahead while sitting and leaning forward. Each maneuver causes a contraction of the pectoral muscles, which accentuates the presence of any retraction.

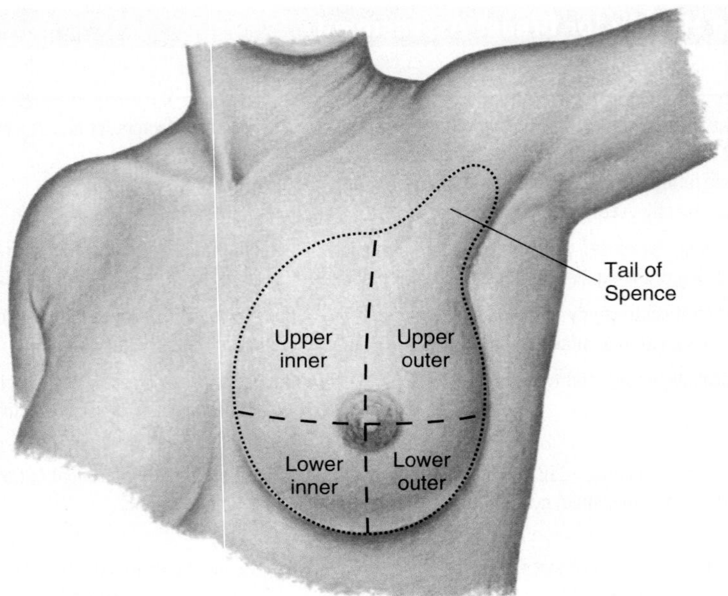

FIGURE 31-52 Quadrants of left breast and axillary tail of Spence. (From Ball JW et al: *Seidel's guide to physical examination,* ed 8, St Louis, 2015, Mosby.)

Carefully inspect the skin for color; venous pattern; and the presence of lesions, edema, or inflammation. Lift each breast when necessary to observe lower and lateral aspects for color and texture changes. The breasts are the color of neighboring skin, and venous patterns are the same bilaterally. Venous patterns are easily visible in thin or pregnant women. Women with large breasts often have redness and excoriation of the undersurfaces caused by rubbing of skin surfaces.

Inspect the nipple and areola for size, color, shape, discharge, and the direction in which the nipples point. The normal areolas are round or oval and nearly equal bilaterally. Color ranges from pink to brown. In light-skinned women the areola turns brown during pregnancy and remains dark. In dark-skinned women the areola is brown before pregnancy (Ball et al., 2015). Normally the nipples point in symmetrical directions, are everted, and have no drainage. If the nipples are inverted, ask if this has been a lifetime history. A recent inversion or inward turning of the nipple indicates an underlying growth. Rashes or ulcerations are not normal on the breast or nipples. Note any bleeding or discharge from the nipple. Clear yellow discharge 2 days after childbirth is common. While inspecting the breasts, explain the characteristics you see. Teach patients the significance of abnormal signs or symptoms.

Palpation. Palpation assesses the condition of underlying breast tissue and lymph nodes. Breast tissue consists of glandular tissue, fibrous supportive ligaments, and fat. Glandular tissue is organized into lobes that end in ducts that open onto the surface of the nipple. The largest part of glandular tissue is in the upper outer quadrant and tail of each breast. Suspensory ligaments connect to skin and fascia underlying the breast to support the breast and maintain its upright position. Fatty tissue is located superficially and to the sides of the breast.

A large part of lymph from the breasts drains into axillary lymph nodes. If cancerous lesions metastasize (spread), the nodes commonly become involved. Study the location of supraclavicular, infraclavicular, and axillary nodes (Figure 31-53). The axillary nodes drain lymph from the chest wall, breasts, arms, and hands. A tumor of one breast sometimes involves nodes on the same and opposite sides.

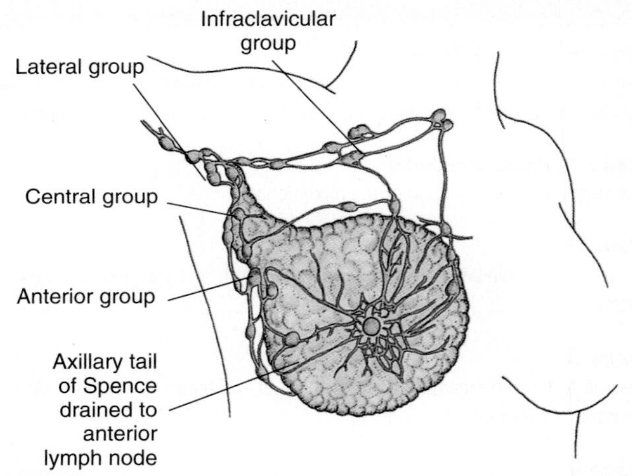

FIGURE 31-53 Anatomical position of axillary and clavicular lymph nodes.

To palpate the lymph nodes have the patient sit with her arms at her sides and muscles relaxed. While facing the patient and standing on the side you are examining, support her arm in a flexed position and abduct it from the chest wall. Place the free hand against the patient's chest wall and high in the axillary hollow. With the fingertips press gently down over the surface of the ribs and muscles. Palpate the axillary nodes with the fingertips, gently rolling soft tissue (Figure 31-54). Palpate four areas of the axilla: at the edge of the pectoralis major muscle along the anterior axillary line, the chest wall in the midaxillary area, the upper part of the humerus, and the anterior edge of the latissimus dorsi muscle along the posterior axillary line.

Normally lymph nodes are not palpable. Carefully assess each area and note their number, consistency, mobility, and size. One or two small, soft, nontender palpable nodes are normal. An abnormal palpable node feels like a small mass that is hard, tender, and immobile. Continue to palpate along the upper and lower clavicular ridges. Reverse the procedure for the patient's other side.

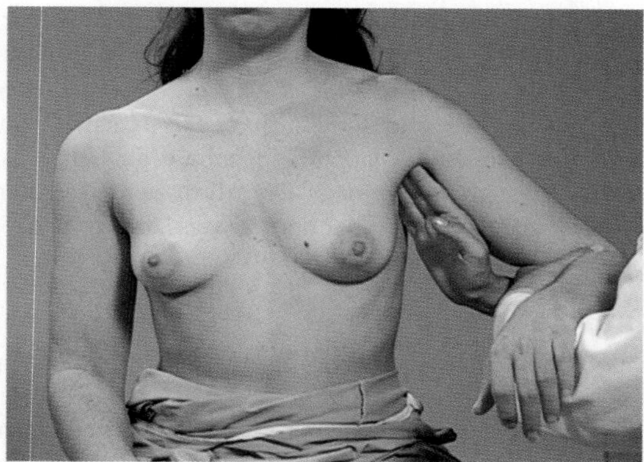

FIGURE 31-54 Support patient's arm and palpate axillary lymph nodes. (From Ball JW et al: *Seidel's guide to physical examination,* ed 8, St Louis, 2015, Mosby.)

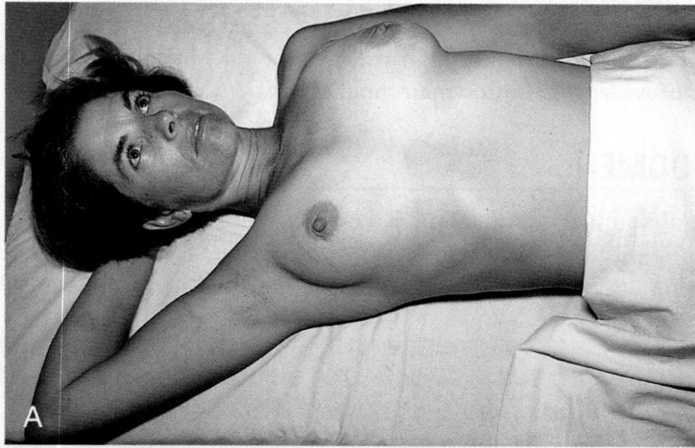

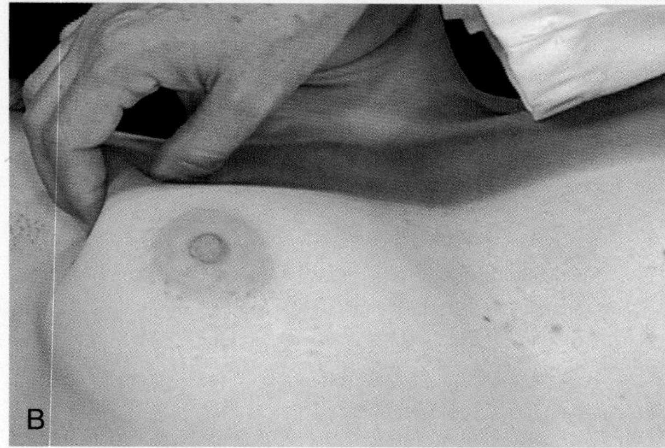

FIGURE 31-55 A, Patient lies flat with arm abducted and hand under head to help flatten breast tissue evenly over chest wall. **B,** Each breast is palpated in a systematic fashion. (From Ball JW et al: *Seidel's guide to physical examination,* ed 8, St Louis, 2015, Mosby.)

It is sometimes difficult for a patient to learn to palpate for lymph nodes. Lying down with the arm abducted makes the area more accessible. Instruct the patient to use her left hand for the right axillary and clavicular areas. Take the patient's fingertips and move them in the proper fashion. Then have the patient use her right hand to palpate for nodes on the left side.

With the patient lying supine and one arm under the head and neck (alternating with each breast), palpate her breast tissue. The supine position allows the breast tissue to flatten evenly against the chest wall. The position of the arm and hand further stretches and positions breast tissue evenly (Figure 31-55, *A*). Place a small pillow or towel under the patient's shoulder blade to further position breast tissue. Palpate the tail of Spence (see Figure 31-55, *B*).

BOX 31-23 PATIENT TEACHING

Female Breast Assessment

Objective

- Patient will follow prevention and detection practices to ensure breast health.

Teaching Strategies

- Have patient perform return demonstration of breast self-examination (BSE) and offer the opportunity to ask questions.
- Explain recommended frequency of mammography and assessment by the patient's health care provider.
- Discuss signs and symptoms of breast cancer.
- Discuss signs and symptoms of benign (fibrocystic) breast disease.
- Inform a woman who is obese or has a family history of breast cancer that she is at higher risk for the disease (ACS, 2015a). Encourage dietary changes, including limiting meat consumption to well-trimmed, lean beef, pork, or lamb; removing skin from cooked chicken before eating it; selecting tuna and salmon packed in water and not oil; and using low-fat dairy products.
- Encourage patient to reduce intake of caffeine and theophyllines. Although this approach is controversial, it can reduce symptoms of benign (fibrocystic) breast disease.

Evaluation

- Have patient demonstrate BSE.
- During follow-up visit determine whether patient has had mammography performed.
- Ask patient to explain frequency of mammography for her situation.
- Have patient describe signs and symptoms of breast cancer compared with benign (fibrocystic) breast disease.

The consistency of normal breast tissue varies widely. The breasts of a young patient are firm and elastic. In an older patient the tissue sometimes feels stringy and nodular. A patient's familiarity with the texture of her own breasts is very important. Patients gain familiarity through monthly BSE (Box 31-23).

If the patient complains of a mass, examine the opposite breast to ensure an objective comparison of normal and abnormal tissue. Use the pads of the first three fingers to compress breast tissue gently against the chest wall, noting tissue consistency. Perform palpation systematically in one of three ways: (1) using a vertical technique with the fingers moving up and down each quadrant; (2) clockwise or counterclockwise, forming small concentric circles with the fingers along each quadrant and the tail; or (3) palpating from the center of the breast in a radial fashion, returning to the areola to begin each spoke (Figure 31-56, *A* to *C*). Whichever approach you use, be sure to cover the entire breast and tail, directing attention to any areas of tenderness. Use a bimanual technique when palpating large, pendulous breasts. Support the inferior part of the breast in one hand while using the other hand to palpate breast tissue against the supporting hand.

During palpation note the consistency of breast tissue. It normally feels dense, firm, and elastic. With menopause breast tissue shrinks and becomes softer. The lobular feel of glandular tissue is normal. The lower edge of each breast sometimes feels firm and hard. This is the normal inframammary ridge and not a tumor. It helps to move the patient's hand so she can feel normal tissue variations. Palpate abnormal masses to determine location in relation to quadrants, diameter in centimeters, shape (e.g., round or discoid), consistency (soft, firm, or hard), tenderness, mobility, and discreteness (clear or unclear boundaries).

Cancerous lesions are hard, fixed, nontender, irregular in shape, and usually unilateral. A common benign condition of the breast is benign (fibrocystic) breast disease. Bilateral lumpy, painful breasts and sometimes nipple discharge characterize this condition. Symptoms are more apparent during the menstrual period. When palpated, the cysts (lumps) are soft, well differentiated, and movable. Deep cysts feel hard.

Give special attention to palpating the nipple and areola. Palpate the entire surface gently. Use the thumb and index finger to compress the nipple and note any discharge. During the examination of the nipple and areola, the nipple sometimes becomes erect with wrinkling of the areola. These changes are normal. Continue by positioning the patient and examining the other breast.

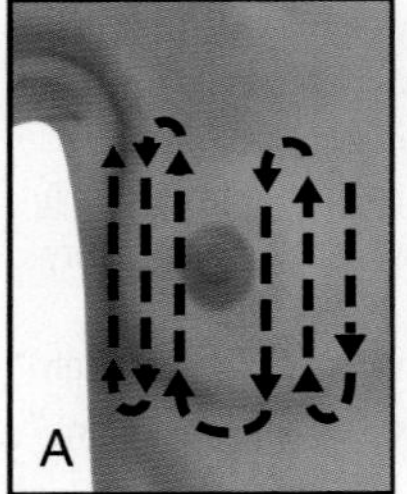

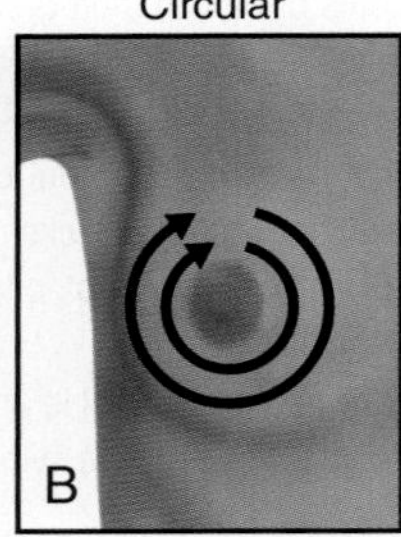

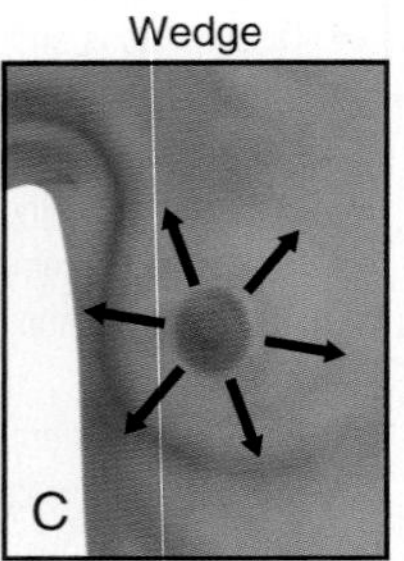

FIGURE 31-56 Various methods for palpation of breast. **A,** Palpate from top to bottom in vertical strips. **B,** Palpate in concentric circles. **C,** Palpate out from center in wedge sections. (From Ball JW et al: *Seidel's guide to physical examination,* ed 8, St Louis, 2015, Mosby.)

After completing the examination, have the patient demonstrate self-palpation. Observe the patient's technique and emphasize the importance of a systematic approach. Urge the patient to see her health care provider if she discovers an abnormal mass during BSE. She also needs to know all of the signs and symptoms of breast cancer.

Male Breasts

Examination of the male breast is relatively easy. Inspect the nipple and areola for nodules, edema, and ulceration. An enlarged male breast results from obesity or glandular enlargement. Breast enlargement in young males results from steroid use. Fatty tissue feels soft, whereas glandular tissue is firm. Use the same techniques to palpate for masses used in examination of the female breast. Because breast cancer in men is relatively rare, routine self-examinations are unnecessary. However, men who have a first-degree relative (e.g., mother or sister) with breast cancer are at risk for breast cancer and need to palpate their breasts at regular intervals. Men at high risk may be scheduled by their health care provider for routine mammograms.

ABDOMEN

The abdominal examination is complex because of the number of organs located within and near the abdominal cavity. A thorough nursing history (Table 31-27) helps interpret physical signs. The

TABLE 31-27 Nursing History for Abdominal Assessment

Assessment	Rationale
If patient has abdominal or low back pain, assess character of pain in detail (location, onset, frequency, precipitating factors, aggravating factors, type of pain, severity, course).	Pattern of characteristics of pain helps determine its source.
Carefully observe patient's movement and position, including lying still with knees drawn up, moving restlessly to find comfortable position, and lying on one side or sitting with knees drawn to chest.	Positions assumed by patient reveal nature and source of pain, including peritonitis, renal stone, and pancreatitis.
Assess normal bowel habits and stool character; ask if patient uses laxatives.	Data compared with physical findings help identify cause and nature of elimination problems.
Determine if patient has had abdominal surgery, trauma, or diagnostic tests of gastrointestinal (GI) tract.	Surgical or traumatic alterations of abdominal organs cause changes in expected findings (e.g., position of underlying organs). Diagnostic tests change character of stool.
Assess if patient has had recent weight changes or intolerance to diet (e.g., nausea, vomiting, cramping, especially in last 24 hours).	Data can indicate alterations in upper GI tract (stomach or gallbladder) or lower colon.
Assess for difficulty in swallowing, belching, flatulence (gas), bloody emesis (hematemesis), black or tarry stools (melena), heartburn, diarrhea, or constipation.	These characteristic signs and symptoms indicate GI alterations.
Ask if patient takes antiinflammatory medication (e.g., aspirin, ibuprofen, steroids) or antibiotics.	Pharmacological agents cause GI upset or bleeding.
Ask patient to locate tender areas before examination begins.	Assess painful areas last to minimize discomfort and anxiety.
Inquire about family history of cancer, kidney disease, alcoholism, hypertension, or heart disease.	Data can reveal risk for alterations identifiable during examination.
Determine if female patient is pregnant; note last menstrual period.	Pregnancy causes changes in abdominal shape and contour.
Assess patient's usual intake of alcohol.	Chronic alcohol ingestion causes GI and liver problems, including liver, colon and pancreatic cancer (ACS, 2015a).
Review patient's history for the following: health care occupation, hemodialysis, intravenous drug user, household or sexual contact with hepatitis B virus (HBV) carrier, heterosexual person with more than one sex partner in previous 6 months, sexually active homosexual or bisexual male, international traveler in area of high HBV infection rate.	Risk factors for HBV exposure.

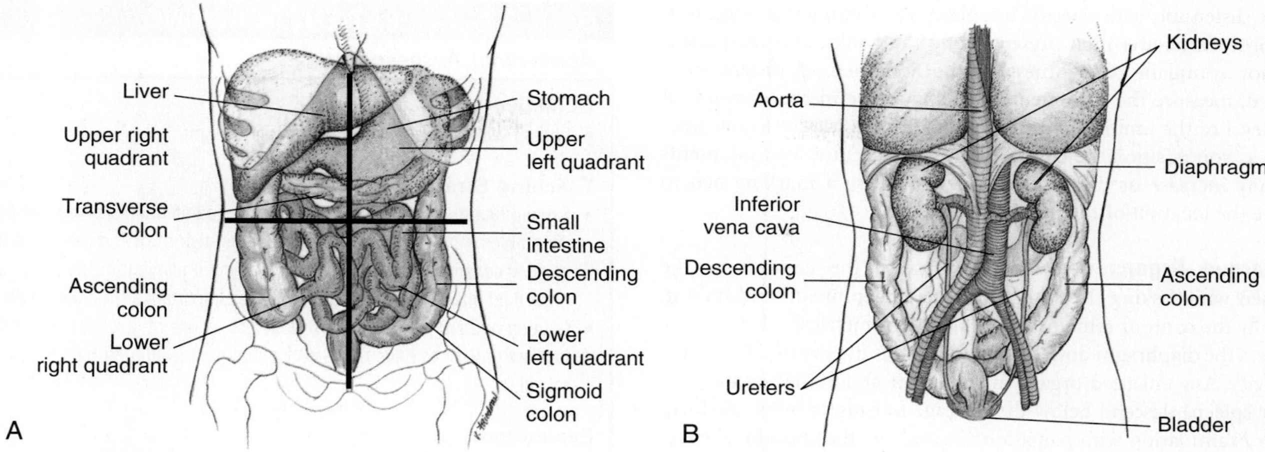

FIGURE 31-57 **A,** Anterior view of abdomen divided by quadrants. **B,** Posterior view of abdominal section.

examination includes an assessment of structures of the lower gastrointestinal (GI) tract in addition to the liver, stomach, uterus, ovaries, kidneys, and bladder. Abdominal pain is one of the most common symptoms that patients report when seeking medical care. An accurate assessment requires matching patient history data with a careful assessment of the location of physical symptoms.

Assess the organs anteriorly and posteriorly. A system of landmarks help map out the abdominal region. The xiphoid process (tip of the sternum) is the upper boundary of the anterior abdominal region. The symphysis pubis marks the lower boundary. Divide the abdomen into four imaginary quadrants (Figure 31-57, *A*); refer to assessment findings and record them in relation to each quadrant. Posteriorly the lower ribs and heavy back muscles protect the kidneys, which are located from the T12 to L3 vertebrae (see Figure 31-57, *B*). The costovertebral angle formed by the last rib and vertebral column is a landmark used during kidney palpation.

During the abdominal examination the patient needs to relax. A tightening of abdominal muscles hinders palpation. Ask the patient to void before beginning. Be sure that the room is warm and drape upper chest and legs. The patient lies supine or in a dorsal recumbent position with the arms at the sides and knees slightly bent. Place small pillows beneath the knees. If the patient places the arms under the head, the abdominal muscles tighten. Proceed calmly and slowly, being sure that there is adequate lighting. Expose the abdomen from just above the xiphoid process down to the symphysis pubis. Warm hands and stethoscope further promote relaxation. Ask the patient to report pain and point out tender areas. Assess tender areas last.

The order of an abdominal examination differs slightly from previous assessments. Begin with inspection and follow with auscultation. By using auscultation before palpation there is less chance of altering the frequency and character of bowel sounds. Be sure to have a tape measure and marking pen available during the examination.

Inspection

Make it a habit to observe the patient during routine care activities. Note his or her posture and look for evidence of abdominal splinting: lying with the knees drawn up or moving restlessly in bed. A patient free from abdominal pain does not guard or splint the abdomen. To inspect the abdomen for abnormal movement or shadows, stand on the patient's right side and inspect from above the abdomen. After sitting or stooping down to look across the abdomen, assess abdominal contour. Direct the examination light over the abdomen.

Skin. Inspect the skin over the abdomen for color, scars, venous patterns, lesions, and **striae** (stretch marks). The skin is subject to the same color variations as the rest of the body. Venous patterns are normally faint, except in thin patients. Striae result from stretching of tissue by obesity or pregnancy. Artificial openings indicate drainage sites resulting from surgery (see Chapter 50) or an ostomy (see Chapters 46 and 47). Scars reveal evidence of past trauma or surgery that has created permanent changes in underlying organ anatomy. Bruising indicates accidental injury, physical abuse, or a type of bleeding disorder. If needle marks or bruises are present, ask if the patient self-administers injections (e.g., low-molecular-weight heparin or insulin). Unexpected findings include generalized color changes such as jaundice or cyanosis. Shiny abdominal skin with a taut (tight) appearance can indicate ascites.

Umbilicus. Note the position; shape; color; and signs of inflammation, discharge, or protruding masses. A normal umbilicus is flat or concave, with the color the same as that of the surrounding skin. Underlying masses cause displacement of the umbilicus. An everted (pouched-out) umbilicus usually indicates distention. Hernias (protrusion of abdominal organs through the muscle wall) cause upward protrusion of the umbilicus. Normally the umbilical area does not emit discharge.

Contour and Symmetry. Inspect for contour, symmetry, and surface motion of the abdomen, noting any masses, bulging, or distention. A flat abdomen forms a horizontal plane from the xiphoid process to the symphysis pubis. A round abdomen protrudes in a convex sphere from the horizontal plane. A concave abdomen appears to sink into the muscular wall. Each of these findings is normal if the shape of the abdomen is symmetrical. In older adults there is often an overall increased distribution of adipose tissue. The presence of masses on only one side, or asymmetry, can indicate an underlying pathological condition.

Intestinal gas, a tumor, or fluid in the abdominal cavity causes **distention** (swelling). When distention is generalized, the entire abdomen protrudes. The skin often appears taut, as if it were stretched over the abdomen. When gas causes distention, the flanks (side muscles) do not bulge. However, if fluid is the source of the problem, the flanks bulge. Ask the patient to roll onto one side. A protuberance forms on the dependent side if fluid is the cause of the distention. Ask the patient if the abdomen feels unusually tight. Be careful not to confuse distention with obesity. In obesity the abdomen is large, rolls of adipose tissue are often present along the flanks, and the patient does not complain of tightness in the abdomen. If distention is expected, measure the abdomen by placing a tape measure around it at the level of the umbilicus (this may require the patient to roll side-to-side as you position the tape measure). Consecutive measurements show any increase or decrease in distention. Use a marking pen to indicate the location of the tape measure.

Enlarged Organs or Masses. Observe the contour of the abdomen while asking the patient to take a deep breath and hold it. Normally the contour remains smooth and symmetrical. This maneuver forces the diaphragm downward and reduces the size of the abdominal cavity. Any enlarged organs in the upper abdominal cavity (e.g., liver or spleen) descend below the rib cage to cause a bulge. Perform a closer examination with palpation. To evaluate the abdominal musculature have the patient raise the head. This position causes superficial abdominal wall masses, hernias, and muscle separations to become more apparent.

Movement or Pulsations. Inspect for movement. Normally men breathe abdominally, and women breathe more costally. A patient with severe pain has diminished respiratory movement and tightens the abdominal muscles to guard against the pain. Closely inspect for peristaltic movement and aortic pulsation by looking across the abdomen from the side. These movements are visible in thin patients; otherwise no movement is present.

Auscultation

Auscultate before palpation during the abdominal assessment because manipulation of the abdomen alters the frequency and intensity of bowel sounds. Ask patients not to talk. Patients with GI tubes connected to suction need them temporarily turned off before beginning an examination.

Bowel Motility. **Peristalsis**, or the movement of contents through the intestines, is a normal function of the small and large intestine. Bowel sounds are the audible passage of air and fluid that peristalsis creates. Place the warmed diaphragm of the stethoscope lightly over each of the four quadrants. Normally air and fluid move through the intestines, creating soft gurgling or clicking sounds that occur irregularly 5 to 35 times per minute (Ball et al., 2015). Sounds usually last ½ second to several seconds. It normally takes 5 to 20 seconds to hear a bowel sound. However, it takes 5 minutes of continuous listening before determining that bowel sounds are absent (Ball et al., 2015). Auscultate all four quadrants to be sure that you do not miss any sounds. The best time to auscultate is between meals. Sounds are generally described as normal, audible, absent, hyperactive, or hypoactive. Absent sounds indicate a lack of peristalsis, possibly the result of late-stage bowel obstruction; paralytic ileus; or peritonitis. Normally absent or hypoactive bowel sounds occur after surgery following general anesthesia. Hyperactive sounds are loud, "growling" sounds called **borborygmi**, which indicate increased GI motility. Inflammation of the bowel, anxiety, diarrhea, bleeding, excessive ingestion of laxatives, and reaction of the intestines to certain foods cause increased motility. Teach patients practices to promote normal elimination patterns (Box 31-24).

Vascular Sounds. Bruits indicate narrowing of the major blood vessels and disruption of blood flow. The presence of bruits in the abdominal area can reveal aneurysms or stenotic vessels. Use the bell of the stethoscope to auscultate in the epigastric region and each of the four quadrants. Normally there are no vascular sounds over the aorta (midline through the abdomen) or femoral arteries (lower quadrants). You can hear renal artery bruits by placing the stethoscope over each upper quadrant anteriorly or over the costovertebral angle posteriorly. Report a bruit immediately to a health care provider.

BOX 31-24 PATIENT TEACHING

Abdominal Assessment

Objective

- Patient will maintain normal bowel elimination.

Teaching Strategies

- Explain factors that promote normal bowel elimination such as diet (fruits, vegetables, fiber), regular exercise, limited use of over-the-counter drugs causing constipation, establishment of regular elimination schedule, and a good fluid intake (see Chapter 46). Stress importance for older adults.
- Caution patients about dangers of excessive use of laxatives or enemas.
- Instruct patient to have acute abdominal pain evaluated by a health care provider.

Evaluation

- Reassess patient's bowel elimination pattern and stool character after therapies begin.
- Observe patient using pain-relief measures and reassess character of pain.

Kidney Tenderness. With the patient sitting or standing erect, use direct or indirect percussion to assess for kidney inflammation. You might require an advanced practice nurse to help you with this skill. With the ulnar surface of the partially closed fist, percuss posteriorly the costovertebral angle at the scapular line. If the kidneys are inflamed, the patient feels tenderness during percussion.

Palpation

Palpation primarily detects areas of abdominal tenderness, distention, or masses. As your skill base increases, learn to palpate for specific organs by using light and deep palpation.

Use light palpation over each abdominal quadrant to detect areas of tenderness. Initially avoid areas previously identified as problem spots. Lay the palm of the hand with fingers extended and approximated lightly on the abdomen. Explain the maneuver to the patient and, with the palmar surface of the fingers, depress approximately 1.3 cm (½ inch) in a gentle dipping motion (Figure 31-58). Avoid quick jabs and use smooth, coordinated movements. If the patient is ticklish, first place his or her hand on the abdomen with your hand on the patient's; continue this until the patient tolerates palpation.

Use a systematic palpation approach for each quadrant and assess for muscular resistance, distention, tenderness, and superficial organs or masses. Observe the patient's face for signs of discomfort. The abdomen is normally smooth with consistent softness and nontender without masses. In contrast to firm muscles found among young adults, an older adult often lacks abdominal tone. Guarding or muscle tenseness sometimes occurs while palpating a sensitive area. If tightening remains after the patient relaxes, peritonitis, acute cholecystitis, or appendicitis is sometimes the cause. It is easy to detect a distended bladder with light palpation. Normally the bladder lies below the umbilicus and above the symphysis pubis. Routinely check for a distended bladder if the patient has been unable to void (e.g., because of anesthesia or sedation or has been incontinent or if an indwelling urinary catheter is not draining well.

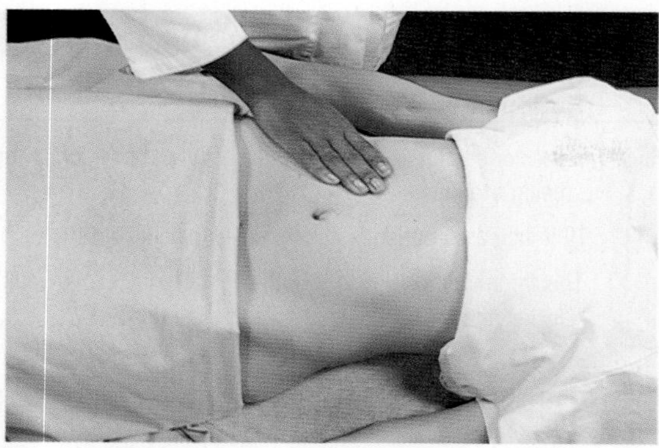

FIGURE 31-58 Light palpation of abdomen. (From Ball JW et al: *Seidel's guide to physical examination,* ed 8, St Louis, 2015, Mosby.)

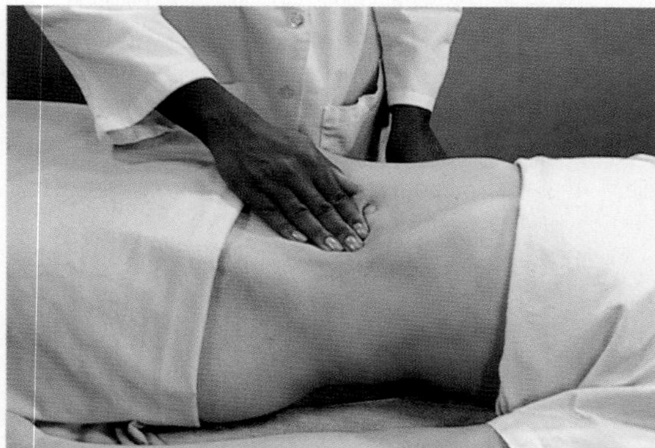

FIGURE 31-59 Deep palpation of abdomen. (From Ball JW et al: *Seidel's guide to physical examination,* ed 8, St Louis, 2015, Mosby.)

With practice and experience perform deep palpation to delineate abdominal organs and detect less obvious masses. You need short fingernails. It is important for the patient to be relaxed while the hands depress approximately 2.5 to 7.5 cm (1 to 3 inches) into the abdomen (Figure 31-59). Never use deep palpation over a surgical incision or over extremely tender organs. It is also unwise to use palpation on abnormal masses. Deep pressure causes tenderness in a healthy patient over the cecum, sigmoid colon, aorta, and the midline near the xiphoid process (Ball et al., 2015).

Survey each quadrant systematically. Palpate masses for size, location, shape, consistency, tenderness, pulsation, and mobility. Test for rebound tenderness by pressing a hand slowly and deeply into the involved area and letting go quickly. The test is positive if the patient feels pain with the release of the hand. Rebound tenderness occurs in patients with peritoneal irritation such as occurs in appendicitis; pancreatitis; or any peritoneal injury causing bile, blood, or enzymes to enter the peritoneal cavity.

Aortic Pulsation. Palpate with the thumb and forefinger of one hand deeply into the upper abdomen just left of the midline to assess aortic pulsation. Normally a pulsation is transmitted forward. If the aorta is enlarged because of an aneurysm (localized dilation of a vessel wall), the pulsation expands laterally. Do not palpate a pulsating abdominal mass. When enlargement from an aneurysm is present, palpate this area only lightly, referring the finding to the health care provider. In obese patients it is often necessary to palpate with both hands, one on each side of the aorta.

FEMALE GENITALIA AND REPRODUCTIVE TRACT

Examination of the female genitalia is embarrassing to a patient unless you use a calm, relaxed approach. The gynecological examination is one of the most difficult experiences for adolescents. A person's cultural background further adds to apprehension. For example, female Mexican-Americans have a strong social value that women do not expose their bodies to men or even to other women. Similarly, Chinese Americans believe that the examination of genitalia is offensive. Muslim women value respect for female modesty. Provide a thorough explanation of the reason for the procedures used in an examination. The lithotomy position assumed during the examination is an added source of embarrassment. A patient is more comfortable when you use correct positioning and draping. Be sure to explain each part of the examination in advance so patients anticipate necessary actions. Adolescents sometimes choose to have parents present in the examination room.

Sometimes a patient requires a complete examination of the female reproductive organs, including assessing the external genitalia and performing a vaginal examination. You can examine external genitalia while performing routine hygiene measures or when preparing to insert a urinary catheter. An internal examination is part of each woman's preventive health care because ovarian cancer causes more deaths than any other cancer of the female reproductive system (ACS, 2014b).

Adolescents and young adults are examined because of the growing incidence of sexually transmitted infections (STIs). The average age of menarche among young girls has declined, and the majority of male and female teenagers are sexually active by age 19 (Hockenberry and Wilson, 2015). It is important to assess a patient's level of anxiety when obtaining the nursing history (Table 31-28). Combine rectal and anal assessments with the pelvic examination since the patient is situated in a lithotomy or dorsal recumbent position.

Preparation of the Patient

As a new nurse, you are responsible for assisting a patient's health care provider with a pelvic examination. For a complete examination the following equipment is needed: examination table with stirrups, vaginal speculum of correct size, adjustable light source, sink, clean disposable gloves, sterile cotton swabs, glass slides, plastic or wooden spatula, cervical brush or broom device, cytological fixative, and culture plates or media (Ball et al., 2015).

Make sure that the equipment is ready before the examination begins. Ask the patient to empty her bladder so the uterus and ovaries are readily palpable. Often it is necessary to collect a urine specimen. Help the patient to the lithotomy position in bed or on an examination table for the external genitalia assessment. Assist her into stirrups for a speculum examination. Have a woman stabilize each foot in a stirrup and slide the buttocks down to the edge of the examining table. Place a hand at the edge of the table and instruct the patient to move until touching the hand. The patient's arms should be at her sides or folded across the chest to prevent tightening of abdominal muscles.

Some women suffering from pain or deformity of the joints are unable to assume a lithotomy position. In this situation it is necessary to have the patient abduct only one leg or have another assist in separating the patient's thighs. In addition, use the side-lying position with the patient on the left side with the right thigh and knee drawn up to her chest.

Give the patient a square drape or sheet. She holds one corner over her sternum, the adjacent corners fall over each knee, and the fourth corner covers the perineum. After the examination begins, lift the

TABLE 31-28 Nursing History for Female Genitalia and Reproductive Tract Assessment

Assessment	Rationale
Determine if patient has had previous illness or surgery involving reproductive organs, including STIs.	Illness or surgery influences appearance and position of organs being examined.
Determine if patient has received HPV vaccine.	HPV increases patient's risk for development of cervical cancer.
Review menstrual history, including age at menarche, frequency and duration of menstrual cycle, character of flow (e.g., amount, presence of clots), presence of dysmenorrhea (painful menstruation), pelvic pain, dates of last two menstrual periods, and premenstrual symptoms.	This information helps to reveal level of reproductive health, including normalcy of menstrual cycle.
Ask patient to describe obstetrical history, including each pregnancy and history of abortions or miscarriages.	Observed physical findings vary, depending on woman's history of pregnancy.
Determine whether patient uses safe sex practices; have patient describe current and past contraceptive practices and problems encountered. Discuss risk of STIs and HIV infection.	Use of certain types of contraceptives influences reproductive health (e.g., sensitivity reaction to spermicidal jelly). Sexual history reveals risk for and understanding of STIs.
Assess if patient has signs and symptoms of vaginal discharge, painful or swollen perianal tissues, or genital lesions.	These signs and symptoms may indicate STI or other pathological condition.
Determine if patient has symptoms or history of genitourinary problems, including burning during urination, frequency, urgency, nocturia, hematuria, incontinence, or stress incontinence (see Chapter 46).	Urinary problems are associated with gynecological disorders, including STIs.
Ask if patient has had signs of bleeding outside of normal menstrual period or after menopause or has had unusual vaginal discharge.	These are warning signs for cervical and endometrial cancer or vaginal infection.
Determine if patient has history of HPV (condyloma acuminatum, herpes simplex, or cervical dysplasia), has multiple sex partners, smokes cigarettes, has had multiple pregnancies, or was young at first intercourse.	These are risk factors for cervical cancer (ACS, 2015a).
A strong family history of breast or ovarian cancer, women who have had breast cancer or who have tested positive for inherited mutations in *BRCA1* or *BRCA2* genes are at increased risk. Other medical conditions associated with increased risk include pelvic inflammatory disease and Lynch syndrome. The use of estrogen alone as menopausal hormone therapy has been shown to increase risk. Tobacco smoking increases the risk of mucinous ovarian cancer. Heavier body weight may be associated with increased risk of ovarian cancer.	These are risk factors for ovarian cancer (ACS, 2015a).
Determine if patient is postmenopausal, is obese, has abdominal fat, or is infertile. Assess if patient received menopausal estrogen therapy, had late menopause, never had children, and had a history of polycystic ovary syndrome. Tamoxifen, a drug used to reduce breast cancer risk, increases the risk slightly because it has estrogen-like effects on the uterus. Medical conditions that increase the risk include Lynch syndrome and diabetes.	These are risk factors for endometrial cancer (ACS, 2015a).

HIV, Human immunodeficiency virus; *HPV,* human papillomavirus (HPV) vaccine; *STI,* sexually transmitted infection.

drape over the perineum. A male examiner always needs to have a female attendant present during the examination, whereas a female examiner may choose to work alone. An additional female should be present if the patient requests it.

External Genitalia

You can perform this examination independently of a health care provider. Make sure that the perineal area is well illuminated. Follow standard precautions and wear clean gloves to prevent contact with infectious organisms. The perineum is sensitive and tender; do not touch the area suddenly without warning a patient. It is best to touch the inner thigh first before touching the perineum.

While sitting at the end of the examination table or bed, inspect the quantity and distribution of hair growth. Preadolescents have no pubic hair. During adolescence hair grows along the labia, becoming darker, coarser, and curlier. In an adult hair grows in a triangle over the female perineum and along the medial surfaces of the thighs. The underlying skin is free of inflammation, irritation, or lesions.

Inspect surface characteristics of the labia majora. The skin of the perineum is smooth, clean, and slightly darker than other skin. The mucous membranes appear dark pink and moist. The labia majora can be gaping or closed, appear dry or moist, and are usually symmetrical. After childbirth the labia majora separate, causing the labia minora to become more prominent. When a woman reaches menopause, the labia majora become thinned; they become atrophied in older age. The labia majora are normally without inflammation, edema, lesions, or lacerations.

To inspect the remaining external structures, use your nondominant hand and gently place the thumb and index finger inside the labia minora and retract the tissues outwardly (Figure 31-60). Be sure to have a firm hold to avoid repeated retraction against the sensitive tissues. Use the other hand to palpate the labia minora between the thumb and second finger. On inspection the labia minora are normally thinner than the labia majora, and one side is sometimes larger. The tissue feels soft on palpation and without tenderness. The size of the clitoris varies, but it normally does not exceed 2 cm (1 inch) in length and 0.5 cm (¼ inch) in width. Look for atrophy, inflammation, or adhesions. If inflamed, the clitoris is a bright cherry red. In young women it is a common site for syphilitic lesions, or chancres, which appear as small open ulcers that drain serous material.

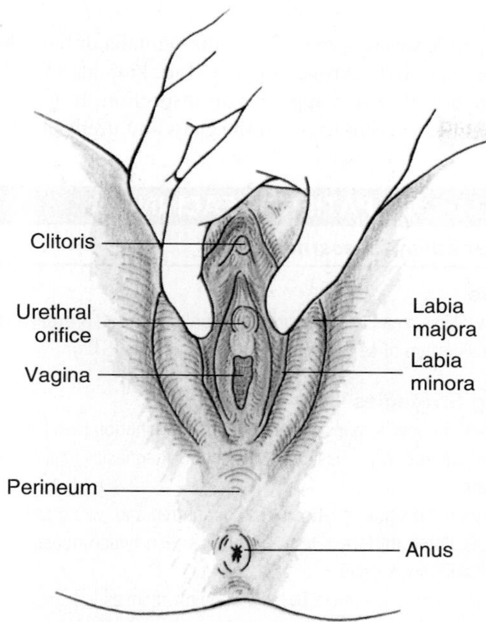

FIGURE 31-60 Female external genitalia.

Inspect the urethral orifice carefully for color and position. It is normally intact without inflammation. The urethral meatus is anterior to the vaginal orifice and is pink. It appears as a small slit or pinhole opening just above the vaginal canal. Note any discharge, polyps, or fistulas.

Inspect the vaginal orifice for inflammation, edema, discoloration, discharge, and lesions. Normally the opening is a thin, vertical slit; and the tissue is moist. While inspecting the vaginal orifice, note the condition of the hymen, which is just inside the opening. In the virgin female the hymen restricts the opening of the vagina, but the tissue retracts or disappears after sexual intercourse.

Inspect the anus, looking for lesions and hemorrhoids (see rectal examination). After completion of the external examination, dispose of examination gloves and offer the patient soft disposable cloths for perineal hygiene.

Patients who are at risk for contracting an STI need to learn to perform a genital self-examination (Box 31-25). The purpose of the examination is to detect any signs or symptoms of an STI. Many people do not know that they have an STI (e.g., chlamydia), and some STIs (e.g., syphilis) remain undetected for years.

Speculum Examination of Internal Genitalia

An examination of the internal genitalia requires much skill and practice. Advanced nurse practitioners and primary care providers perform this examination. As a nursing student you observe the procedure or assist the examiner by helping the patient with positioning, handing off specimen supplies, and providing emotional support for the patient.

The examination involves use of a plastic or metal speculum consisting of two blades and an adjustment device. The examiner inserts the speculum into the vagina to assess the internal genitalia for cancerous lesions and other abnormalities. During the examination the examiner collects a specimen for a Papanicolaou (Pap) test for cervical and vaginal cancer. The cervix is inspected for color, position, size, surface characteristics, and discharge (Ball et al., 2015).

BOX 31-25 PATIENT TEACHING

Female Genitalia and Reproductive Tract Assessment

Objective

- Patient will use measures to maintain sexual health and prevent acquisition and transmission of sexually transmitted infections (STIs).

Teaching Strategies

- Instruct patient about purpose and recommended frequency of Papanicolaou (Pap) smears and gynecological examinations. Explain that the Pap smear is relatively painless and needed annually with a pelvic examination for women who are sexually active or over the age of 21. Patients are screened more often if certain risk factors exist such as a weak immune system, multiple sex partners, smoking, and a history of infections (e.g., human papillomavirus [HPV]).
- Counsel patient with an STI about the implications of diagnosis and treatment.
- Counsel young males and females and their parents about genital HPV infection and the need to receive the HPV vaccine before becoming sexually active. The vaccine is recommended for preteen boys and girls at age 11 or 12 (CDC, 2015b). Adolescent boys and girls who did not start or finish the HPV vaccine series when they were younger should get it now. Young women can get an HPV vaccine through age 26, and young men can get vaccinated through age 21 (CDC, 2015b).
- Instruct in genital self-examination (GSE). Using a mirror, position self to examine the area covered by the pubic hair. Spread the hair apart, looking for bumps, sores, or blisters. Also look for any warts, which appear as small, bumpy spots and enlarge to fleshy, cauliflower-like lesions. Next spread the outer vaginal lips apart and look at the clitoris for bumps, blisters, sores, or warts. Look at both sides of the inner vaginal lips. Inspect the area around the urinary and vaginal opening for bumps, blisters, sores, or warts.
- Explain warning signs of STIs: pain or burning on urination, pain during sex, pain in pelvic area, bleeding between menstruation, itchy rash around vagina, and abnormal vaginal discharge.
- Teach measures to prevent STIs: male partner's use of condoms, restricting number of sexual partners, avoiding sex with people who have several other partners, and perineal hygiene measures.
- Tell patients with an STI to inform sexual partners of the need for an examination.
- Reinforce the importance of performing perineal hygiene (as appropriate).

Evaluation

- Determine if parents followed through in having their child immunized for HPV.
- Ask patient to explain when she should routinely have a gynecological examination and Pap test.
- Have patient describe ways to prevent transmission of STIs.
- For patient with an STI, determine during follow-up visit if she has followed safe sexual practices (use nonthreatening inquiry).

MALE GENITALIA

An examination of the male genitalia assesses the integrity of the external genitalia (Figure 31-61), inguinal ring, and canal. Because the incidence of STIs in adolescents and young adults is high, an assessment of the genitalia needs to be a routine part of any health maintenance examination for this age-group (Box 31-26). The examination begins by having the patient void. Make sure the examination room is warm. Have the patient lie supine with the chest, abdomen, and lower legs draped or stand during the examination. Apply clean gloves.

Use a calm, gentle approach to lessen the patient's anxiety. The position and exposure of the body during the examination is embarrassing for some men. To minimize his anxiety, it often helps to offer explanation of the steps of examination so he anticipates all actions. Manipulate the genitalia gently to avoid causing erection or discomfort. Obtain a thorough history (Table 31-29) before the examination, ensuring that the assessment is complete.

Sexual Maturity

First note the sexual maturity of the patient by observing the size and shape of the penis and testes; the size, color, and texture of the scrotal skin; and the character and distribution of pubic hair. The testes first increase in size in preadolescence. During this time there is no pubic hair. By the end of puberty, the testes and penis enlarge to adult size and shape, and scrotal skin darkens and becomes wrinkled. With puberty hair is coarse and abundant in the pubic area. The penis has no hair, and the scrotum has very little hair (Figure 31-62, *A* and *B*). Also inspect the skin covering the genitalia for lice, rashes, excoriations, or lesions. Normally it is clear, without lesions.

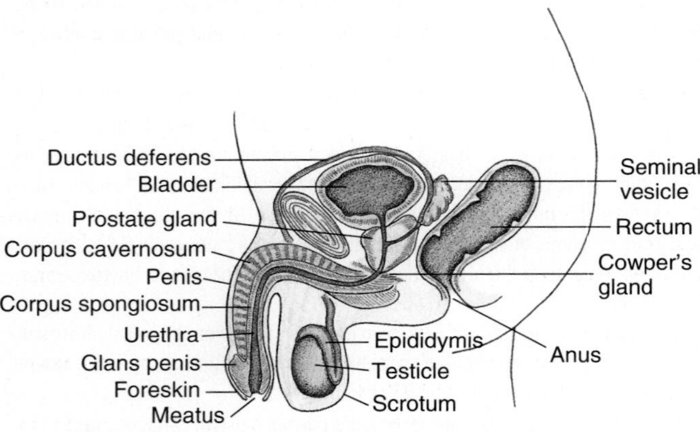

FIGURE 31-61 External and internal male sex organs.

Penis

To inspect penile surfaces, manipulate the genitalia or have the patient assist. Inspect the shaft, corona, prepuce (foreskin), glans, and urethral meatus. The dorsal vein is apparent on inspection. In uncircumcised males retract the foreskin to reveal the glans and urethral meatus. The

BOX 31-26 PATIENT TEACHING

Male Genitalia Assessment

Objective

- Patient will use measures to maintain sexual health and prevent acquisition and transmission of sexually transmitted infections (STIs).

Teaching Strategies

- Teach patient how to perform genital self-examination (see Box 31-27).
- Counsel patient who has an STI about diagnosis implications and treatment.
- Explain warning signs of STIs: pain on urination and during sex, abnormal penile discharge (different from usual), swollen lymph nodes, or rash or ulcer on skin or genitalia.
- Teach measures to prevent STIs: HPV immunization, use of condoms, avoiding sex with infected partner, restricting number of sexual partners, avoiding sex with people who have multiple partners, and using regular perineal hygiene.
- Recommend HPV vaccine for preteen boys age 11 or 12; young men can get vaccinated through age 21 (CDC, 2015b).
- Tell patients with an STI to inform their sexual partners of the need to have an examination.
- Instruct patient to seek treatment as soon as possible if partner becomes infected with an STI.

Evaluation

- Ask patient to describe methods for preventing and treating STIs.
- During a follow-up visit determine whether patient with an STI has used safe sex practices.
- Ask parents or patient if HPV vaccination was achieved.

TABLE 31-29 Nursing History for Male Genitalia Assessment

Assessment	Rationale
Review normal urinary elimination pattern, including frequency of voiding; history of nocturia; character and volume of urine; daily fluid intake; symptoms of burning, urgency, and frequency; difficulty starting stream; and hematuria (see Chapter 46).	Urinary problems are directly associated with genitourinary problems because of anatomical structure of men's reproductive and urinary systems.
Assess patient's sexual history and use of safe sex habits (multiple partners, infection in partners, failure to use condom).	Sexual history reveals risk for and understanding of sexually transmitted diseases (STIs) and human immunodeficiency virus (HIV).
Determine if patient has received the human papillomavirus (HPV) vaccine.	HPV is associated with genital warts in males and can lead to cervical cancer in females (CDC, 2014).
Determine if patient has had previous surgery or illness involving urinary or reproductive organs, including STI.	Alterations resulting from disease or surgery are sometimes responsible for symptoms or changes in organ structure or function.
Ask if patient has noted penile pain or swelling, genital lesions, or urethral discharge.	These signs and symptoms may indicate STI.
Determine if patient has noticed heaviness or painless enlargement of testis or irregular lumps.	These signs and symptoms are early warning signs for testicular cancer.
If patient reports an enlargement in inguinal area, assess if it is intermittent or constant, associated with straining or lifting, and painful; and whether pain is affected by coughing, lifting, or straining at stool.	Signs and symptoms reflect potential inguinal hernia.
Ask if patient has difficulty achieving erection or ejaculation; also review whether patient is taking diuretics, sedatives, antihypertensives, or tranquilizers.	These medications influence sexual performance.

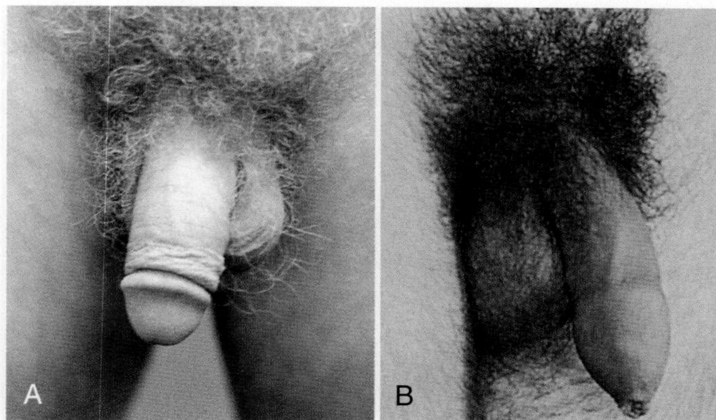

FIGURE 31-62 Appearance of male genitalia. **A,** Circumcised. **B,** Uncircumcised. (From Ball JW et al: *Seidel's guide to physical examination,* ed 8, St Louis, 2015, Mosby.)

foreskin usually retracts easily. A small amount of white, thick smegma sometimes collects under this foreskin. Obtain a culture if abnormal discharge is present. The urethral meatus is slitlike in appearance and positioned on the ventral surface just millimeters from the tip of the glans. In some congenital conditions the meatus is displaced along the penile shaft. The area between the foreskin and glans is a common site for venereal lesions. Gently compress the glans between the thumb and index finger; this opens the urethral meatus for inspection of lesions, edema, and inflammation. Normally the opening is glistening and pink without discharge. Palpate any lesion gently to note tenderness, size, consistency, and shape. When inspection and palpation of the glans is complete, pull the foreskin down to its original position.

Continue by inspecting the entire shaft of the penis, including the undersurface, looking for lesions, scars, or edema. Palpate the shaft between the thumb and first two fingers to detect localized areas of hardness or tenderness. A patient who has lain in bed for a prolonged time sometimes develops dependent edema in the penis shaft.

It is important for any male patient to learn to perform a genital self-examination to detect signs or symptoms of STIs, especially men who have had more than one sexual partner or whose partner has had other partners. Men may have an STI but not be aware of it; self-examination is a routine part of self-care (Box 31-27).

Scrotum

Be particularly cautious while inspecting and palpating the scrotum because the structures lying within the scrotal sac are very sensitive. The scrotum is divided internally into two halves. Each half contains a testicle, epididymis, and the vas deferens, which travels upward into the inguinal ring. Normally the left testicle is lower than the right. Inspect the size, shape, and symmetry of the scrotum while observing for lesions or edema. Gently lift the scrotum to view the posterior surface. The scrotal skin is usually loose, and the surface is coarse. The scrotal skin is more deeply pigmented than body skin. Tightening of the skin or loss of wrinkling reveals edema. The size of the scrotum normally changes with temperature variations because the dartos muscle contracts in cold and relaxes in warm temperatures. Lumps in the scrotal skin are commonly sebaceous cysts.

Testicular cancer is a solid tumor common in young men ages 18 to 34 years. Early detection is critical. Explain testicular self-examination (see Box 31-27) while examining the patient. The testes are normally sensitive but not tender. The underlying testicles are normally ovoid and approximately 2 to 4 cm (1 to 1½ inch) in size. Gently palpate the testicles and epididymis between the thumb and first two fingers. The testes feel smooth, rubbery, and free of nodules. The epididymis is resilient. Note the size, shape, and consistency of the organs. The most common symptoms of testicular cancer are a painless enlargement of one testis and the appearance of a palpable, small, hard lump, about the size of a pea, on the front or side of the testicle. In the older adult the testicles decrease in size and are less firm during palpation. Continue to palpate the vas deferens separately as it forms the spermatic cord toward the inguinal ring, noting nodules or swelling. It normally feels smooth and discrete.

Inguinal Ring and Canal

The external inguinal ring provides the opening for the spermatic cord to pass into the inguinal canal. The canal forms a passage through the abdominal wall, a potential site for hernia formation. A hernia is a protrusion of a part of intestine through the inguinal wall or canal. Sometimes an intestinal loop enters the scrotum. Have the patient stand during this part of the examination.

During inspection ask the patient to strain or bear down. The maneuver helps to make a hernia more visible. Look for obvious bulging in the inguinal area.

Complete the examination by palpating for inguinal lymph nodes. Normally small, nontender, mobile horizontal nodes are palpable. Any abnormality indicates local or systemic infection or malignant disease.

RECTUM AND ANUS

A good time to perform the rectal examination is after the genital examination. Usually this examination is not performed for young children or adolescents. It detects colorectal cancer in its early stages. The rectal examination also detects prostatic tumors in men. Collect a health history (Table 31-30) to detect the patient's risk for bowel or rectal disease (men and women) or prostate disease (men). Teach the patient about the purpose of the examination (Box 31-28).

The rectal examination is uncomfortable; thus explaining all steps helps a patient relax. Use a calm, slow-paced, gentle approach during the examination. Female patients remain in the dorsal recumbent position following genitalia examination or they assume a side-lying (Sims') position. The best way to examine men is to have the patient stand and bend over forward with hips flexed and upper body resting across an examination table. Examine a nonambulatory patient in the Sims' position. Use nonlatex clean gloves.

Inspection

Using the nondominant hand, gently retract the buttocks to view the perianal and sacrococcygeal areas. Perianal skin is smooth, more pigmented, and coarser than skin over the buttocks. Inspect anal tissue for skin characteristics, lesions, external hemorrhoids (dilated veins that appear as reddened protrusions), ulcers, fissures and fistulas, inflammation, rashes, or excoriation. Anal tissues are moist and hairless, and the voluntary external muscle sphincter holds the anus closed. Next ask a patient to bear down as though having a bowel movement. Any internal hemorrhoids or fissures appear at this time. Use clock reference (e.g., 3 o'clock or 8 o'clock) to describe location of findings. Normally there is no protrusion of tissue.

Digital Palpation

Examine the anal canal and sphincters with digital palpation, and in male patients palpate the prostate gland to rule out enlargement. Usually advanced practitioners perform this part of the examination. This technique is not discussed here.

BOX 31-27 Male Genital Self-Examination

All men 15 years and older need to perform this examination monthly using the following steps.

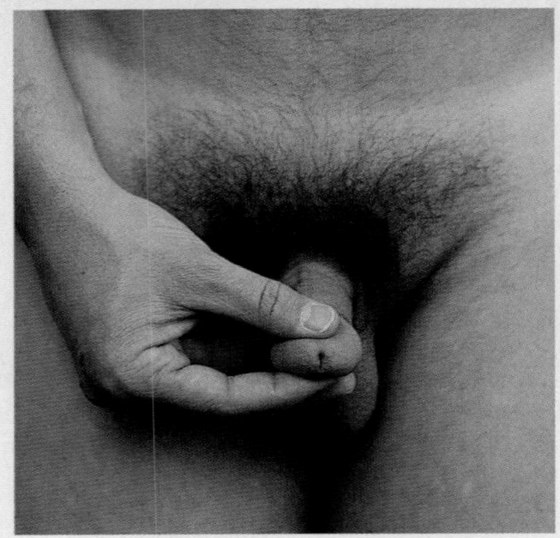

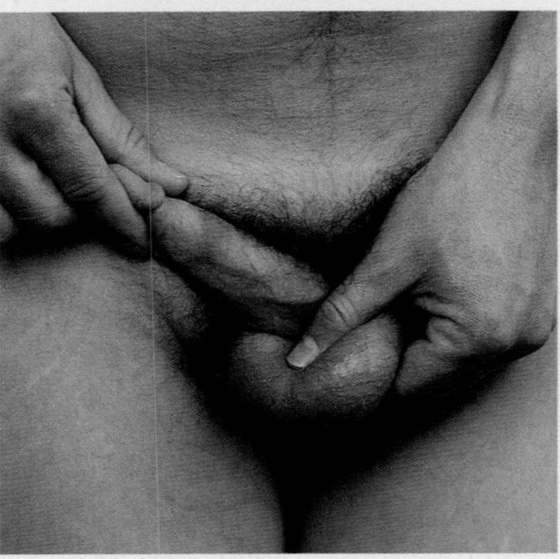

Genital Examination

- Perform the examination after a warm bath or shower when the scrotal skin is less thick.
- Stand naked in front of a mirror, hold the penis in your hand, and examine the head. Pull back the foreskin if uncircumcised to expose the glans.
- Inspect and palpate the entire head of the penis in a clockwise motion, looking carefully for any bumps, sores, or blisters (bumps and blisters may be light colored or red, resemble pimples).
- Look also for any genital warts (see illustration).
- Look at the opening (urethral meatus) at the end of the penis for discharge.
- Look along the entire shaft of the penis for the same signs.
- Be sure to separate pubic hair at the base of the penis and carefully examine the skin underneath.

Testicular Self-Examination

- Look for swelling or lumps in the skin of the scrotum while looking in the mirror.
- Use both hands, placing the index and middle fingers under the testicles and the thumb on top (see illustration).
- Gently roll the testicle, feeling for lumps, swelling, soreness, or a harder consistency.
- Find the epididymis (a cordlike structure on the top and back of the testicle; it is not a lump).
- Feel for small, pea-size lumps on the front and side of the testicle. Abnormal lumps are usually painless.
- Call your health care provider for abnormal findings.

Illustrations from Ball JW et al: *Seidel's guide to physical examination,* ed 8, St Louis, 2015, Mosby.

TABLE 31-30 Nursing History for Rectal and Anal Assessment

Assessment	Rationale
Determine whether patient has experienced bleeding from rectum, black or tarry stools (melena), rectal pain, or change in bowel habits (constipation or diarrhea).	These are warning signs of colorectal cancer* or other gastrointestinal alterations.
Determine whether patient has personal or strong family history of colorectal cancer, polyps, or chronic inflammatory bowel disease. Ask if patient is over age 40.	These are risk factors for colorectal cancer (ACS, 2014a).*
Assess dietary habits, including high fat intake, diet high in processed or red meats, or deficient fiber content (inadequate fruits and vegetables).	Bowel cancer is often linked to dietary intake of fat or insufficient fiber intake.*
Determine if patient is obese, is physically inactive, smokes, or consumes alcohol.	These are risk factors for colorectal cancer (ACS, 2014a).
Determine whether patient has undergone screening for colorectal cancer (digital examination, fecal occult blood test, flexible sigmoidoscopy, and colonoscopy).	Undergoing this screening reflects understanding and compliance with preventive health care measures.
Assess medication history for use of laxatives or cathartic medications.	Repeated use causes diarrhea and eventual loss of intestinal muscle tone.
Assess for use of codeine or iron preparations.	Codeine causes constipation. Iron turns the color of feces black and tarry.
Ask male patient if he has experienced weak or interrupted urine flow, inability to urinate, difficulty starting or stopping urine flow, polyuria, nocturia, hematuria, or dysuria. Does patient have continuing pain in lower back, pelvis, or upper thighs?	These are warning signs of prostate cancer.* Symptoms also suggest infection or prostate enlargement.

*Data from American Cancer Society: *Cancer facts and figures 2015,* Atlanta, 2015, The Society.

BOX 31-28 PATIENT TEACHING

Rectal and Anal Assessment

Objective

- Patient will be able to identify symptoms of colorectal and prostatic cancer.

Teaching Strategies

- Discuss the guidelines of the American Cancer Society (ACS, 2014a) for early detection of colorectal cancer. **Beginning at age 50,** both men and women of average risk should use one of these screening tests (ACS, 2015a):
  - Fecal occult blood test (FOBT) or fecal immunochemical test (FIT) annually
  - Stool DNA test performed every 3 years
  - Flexible sigmoidoscopy (FSIG): Visual inspection of the rectum and lower colon with a hollow, lighted tube performed by a health care provider every 5 years OR
  - Double-contrast barium enema every 5 years if recommended by health care provider
  - Colonoscopy every 10 years if recommended
  - Computed tomography (CT) colonoscopy every 5 years if recommended
- Individuals at increased risk should discuss options with their health care provider
- Discuss warning signs of colorectal cancer (see Table 31-30)
- Discuss with male patient the ACS guidelines (2015a) for early detection of prostate cancer:
- For men ages 50+, Digital rectal examination (DRE) and prostate-specific antigen test (PSA). The ACS recommends that men who have at least a 10-year life expectancy should have an opportunity to make an informed decision with their health care provider about whether to be screened for prostate cancer after receiving information about the potential benefits, risks, and uncertainties of testing.
- Discuss warning signs of prostate cancer.

Evaluation

- During follow-up visit determine whether patient has had appropriate screening tests performed.
- Have patient explain warning signs of colorectal and prostate cancer.

MUSCULOSKELETAL SYSTEM

The musculoskeletal assessment can be performed as a separate examination or integrated with other parts of the total physical examination. In addition, you can assess the patient's movements while performing other nursing care measures such as bathing or positioning. The assessment of musculoskeletal function focuses on determining range of joint motion, muscle strength and tone, and joint and muscle condition. Assessing musculoskeletal integrity is especially important when a patient reports pain or loss of function in a joint or muscle. Because muscular disorders are often the result of neurological disease, you may choose to perform a simultaneous neurological assessment.

While examining a patient's musculoskeletal function, visualize the anatomy of bone and muscle placement and joint structure (see Chapter 28). Joints vary in degree of mobility, depending on the type of joint.

For a complete examination expose the muscles and joints so they are free to move. Have the patient assume a sitting, supine, prone, or standing position while assessing specific muscle groups. Table 31-31 lists the information gathered in the nursing history.

General Inspection

Observe the patient's gait when he or she enters the examination room. When the patient is unaware of the nature of your observation, gait is more natural. Later a more formal test has the patient walk in a straight line away from and returning to the point of origin. Note how the patient walks, sits, and rises from a sitting position. Normally patients walk with the arms swinging freely at the sides and the head leading the body. Older adults often walk with smaller steps and a wider base of support. Note foot dragging, limping, shuffling, and the position of the trunk in relation to the legs.

Observe the patient from the side and while facing him or her in a standing position. The normal standing posture is upright with parallel alignment of the hips and shoulders (Figure 31-63, *A* to *C*). There is an even contour of the shoulders, level scapulae and iliac crests, alignment of the head over the gluteal folds, and symmetry of extremities. While observing from the side of the patient, note the normal cervical, thoracic, and lumbar curves. Holding the head erect is normal. As the patient sits, some degree of rounding of the shoulders is normal. Older adults tend to assume a stooped, forward-bent posture with the hips and knees somewhat flexed and arms bent at the elbows, raising the level of the arms.

Common postural abnormalities include kyphosis, lordosis, and scoliosis (Figure 31-64, *A* to *C*). **Kyphosis**, or hunchback, is an exaggeration of the posterior curvature of the thoracic spine. This postural abnormality is common in older adults. **Lordosis**, or swayback, is an increased lumbar curvature. A lateral spinal curvature is called **scoliosis**. Loss of height is frequently the first clinical sign of osteoporosis, in which height loss occurs in the trunk as a result of vertebral fracture and collapse. **Osteoporosis** is a systemic skeletal condition that is noted to have both decreased bone mass and deterioration of bone tissue, making bones fragile and at risk for fracture (Nelson et al., 2010). Osteopenia, characterized by low bone mass of the hip, puts people at risk for osteoporosis, fractures, and potential complications later in life. Approximately 80% of people with osteoporosis are women; approximately 20% of the time the disease affects men. It affects any age-group, including children. Patients should be taught ways to reduce the chance of developing this disease (Box 31-29).

During general inspection look at the extremities for overall size, gross deformity, bony enlargement, alignment, and symmetry. Normally there is bilateral symmetry in length, circumference, alignment, and position and in the number of skinfolds (Ball et al., 2015). A general review pinpoints areas requiring specialized assessment.

Palpation

Apply gentle palpation to all bones, joints, and surrounding muscles during a complete examination. For a focused assessment only examine the involved area. Note any heat, tenderness, edema, or resistance to pressure. The patient should not feel any discomfort when you palpate. Muscles should be firm.

Range of Joint Motion

The examination includes comparison of both active and passive ROM. Ask the patient to put each major joint through active and passive full ROM (see Chapter 28). Learn the correct terminology for the movements that the joints are capable of making (Table 31-32) and teach the patient how to move through each ROM. Demonstrate ROM to the patient when possible. To assess ROM passively, ask the patient to relax and then passively move the extremities through their ROM. Compare the same body parts for equality in movement. Figure 31-65, *A* to *F*, shows an example of ROM positions for the hand and wrist. Do not force a joint into a painful position. Know the normal range of each joint and the extent to which you can move the patient's joints.

TABLE 31-31 Nursing History for Musculoskeletal Assessment

Assessment	Rationale
Determine if patient is involved in competitive sports (particularly involving collision and contact), fails to warm up adequately, is in poor physical condition, or has had a rapid growth spurt (adolescents).	These are risk factors for sports injury.
Assess for risk factors of osteoporosis. Uncontrollable risk factors: • Over age 50 • Female • Nulliparous • Menopause before age 45 • Family history of osteoporosis • Low body weight/being small and thin/constant dieting • Broken bones or height loss Controllable risk factors: • Not getting enough calcium (less than 500 mg) and vitamin D • Not eating enough fruits and vegetables • Getting too much protein, sodium and caffeine • Having an inactive lifestyle • Smoking • Drinking too much alcohol • Losing weight Long-term use of certain medications: aluminum-containing antacids; antiseizure medicines such as Dilantin or Phenobarbital; aromatase inhibitors such as Arimidex, Aromasin, and Femara; cancer chemotherapeutic drugs, and heparin.	These are risk factors for osteoporosis (Walker, 2010: NOF, n.d.).
Ask patient to describe history of problems in bone, muscle, or joint function (e.g., recent fall, trauma, lifting of heavy objects, history of bone or joint disease with sudden or gradual onset, location of alteration).	History helps to assess nature of musculoskeletal problem.
Assess nature and extent of pain, including location, duration, severity, predisposing and aggravating factors, relieving factors, and type.	Pain frequently accompanies alterations in bone, joints, or muscle. This has implications not only for comfort, but also for ability to perform activities of daily living.
Assess patient's normal activity pattern, including type of exercise routinely performed.	Provides baseline in assessment. Sedentary lifestyle and lack of appropriate exercise increase bone loss and risk of fractures.
Determine how alteration influences ability to perform activities of daily living (e.g., bathing, feeding, dressing, toileting, ambulating) and social functions (e.g., household chores, work, recreation, sexual activities).	The extent to which patient is able to perform self-care determines the level of nursing care. Type and degree of restriction in continuing social activities influence topics for patient education and ability of nurse to identify alternative ways to maintain function.
Assess height loss of woman over age 50 by subtracting current height from recall of maximum adult height. Refer to physician for bone density exam (women 65 years and older).	Measurement is useful screening tool to predict osteoporosis. Bone density recommended by USPSTF (2011).

ROM is equal between contralateral joints. Ideally assess the patient's normal range to determine a baseline for assessing later change.

A **goniometer**, frequently used by physical and occupational therapists, measures the precise degree of motion in a particular joint and is mainly for patients who have a suspected reduction in joint movement. The instrument has two flexible arms with a 180-degree protractor in the center. Position the center of the protractor at the center of the joint you are measuring (Figure 31-66). The arms extend along the body parts on each side of the protractor. Measure the joint angle before moving the joint. After taking the joint through a full ROM, measure the angle again to determine the degree of movement. Compare the reading with the normal degree of joint movement.

Joints are typically free from stiffness, instability, swelling, or inflammation. There should be no discomfort when applying pressure to bones and joints. In older adults joints often become swollen and stiff with reduced ROM resulting from cartilage erosion and fibrosis of synovial membranes (see Chapter 28). If a joint appears swollen and inflamed, palpate it for warmth.

Muscle Tone and Strength

Assess muscle strength and tone during ROM measurement. Integrate these findings with those from the neurological assessment. Note muscle tone, the slight muscular resistance felt as you move the relaxed extremity passively through its ROM.

Ask the patient to allow an extremity to relax or hang limp. This is often difficult, particularly if the patient feels pain in it. Support the extremity and grasp each limb, moving it through the normal ROM (Figure 31-67). Normal tone causes a mild, even resistance to movement through the entire range.

If a muscle has increased tone, or **hypertonicity**, there is considerable resistance with any sudden passive movement of a joint. Continued movement eventually causes the muscle to relax. A muscle that has

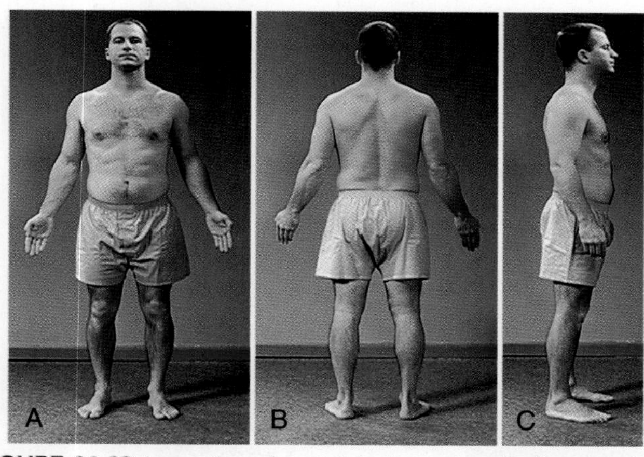

FIGURE 31-63 Inspection of overall body posture. **A,** Anterior view. **B,** Posterior view. **C,** Lateral view. (From Ball JW et al: *Seidel's guide to physical examination*, ed 8, St Louis, 2015, Mosby.)

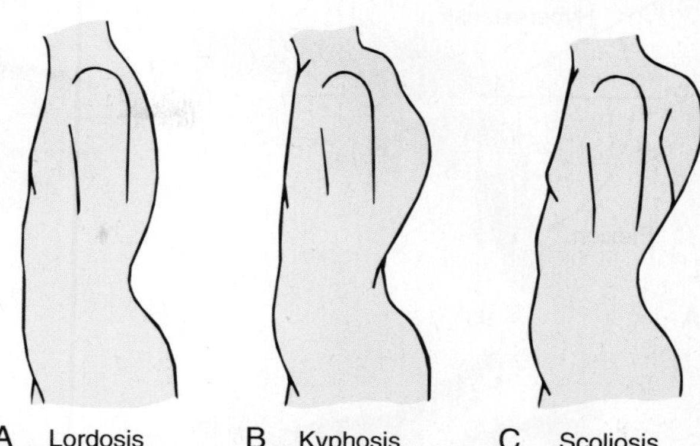

FIGURE 31-64 Common postural abnormalities. **A,** Lordosis. **B,** Kyphosis. **C,** Scoliosis.

BOX 31-29 PATIENT TEACHING

Health Promotion to Prevent Osteoporosis in Women

Objective
- Patient will follow measures to prevent or minimize osteoporosis.

Teaching Strategies
- Recommend women age 65 and older for routine screening for osteoporosis (USPSTF, 2011). Recommend men for screening as well; they are at risk for development of osteoporosis equally as they age.
- To reduce bone demineralization, instruct older adults in a proper exercise program (e.g., weight-bearing, muscle-strengthening, and balance-training exercises) to be followed 3 or more times a week.
- Encourage intake of calcium to meet the recommended daily allowance. Increased vitamin D aids calcium absorption.
- Recommendation for calcium supplements for adults over age 25 is 1000 to 1500 mg/day. Instruct patient to take no more than 500 mg of calcium at one time.
- Instruct older adults and those with osteoporosis in proper body mechanics and range-of-motion and moderate weight-bearing exercises (e.g., swimming and walking) to minimize trauma and subsequent fracture of bones.
- Instruct older patients to pace activities to compensate for loss in muscle strength.

Evaluation
- Observe patient's posture.
- Ask patient to describe therapies for preventing osteoporosis.
- Observe patient perform range-of-motion exercises.
- Have patient keep log of regular weight-training exercises.

TABLE 31-32 Terminology for Normal Range-of-Motion Positions

Term	Range of Motion	Examples of Joints
Flexion	Movement decreasing angle between two adjoining bones; bending of limb	Elbow, fingers, knee
Extension	Movement increasing angle between two adjoining bones	Elbow, knee, fingers
Hyperextension	Movement of body part beyond its normal resting extended position	Head
Pronation	Movement of body part so front or ventral surface faces downward	Hand, forearm
Supination	Movement of body part so front or ventral surface faces upward	Hand, forearm
Abduction	Movement of extremity away from midline of body	Leg, arm, fingers
Adduction	Movement of extremity toward midline of body	Leg, arm, fingers
Internal rotation	Rotation of joint inward	Knee, hip
External rotation	Rotation of joint outward	Knee, hip
Eversion	Turning of body part away from midline	Foot
Inversion	Turning of body part toward midline	Foot
Dorsiflexion	Flexion of toes and foot upward	Foot
Plantar flexion	Bending of toes and foot downward	Foot

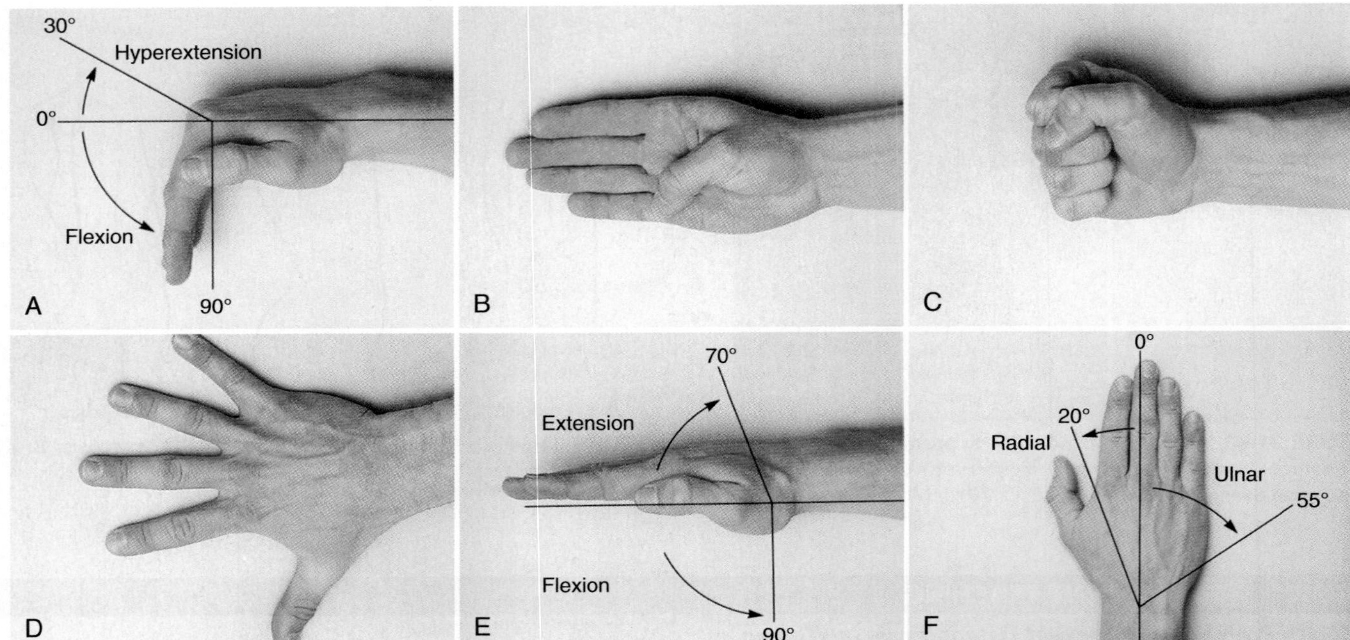

FIGURE 31-65 Range of motion of hand and wrist. **A,** Metacarpophalangeal flexion and hyperextension. **B,** Finger flexion: thumb to each fingertip and to base of little finger. **C,** Finger flexion, fist formation. **D,** Finger abduction. **E,** Wrist flexion and hyperextension. **F,** Wrist radial and ulnar movement. (From Ball JW et al: *Seidel's guide to physical examination,* ed 8, St Louis, 2015, Mosby.)

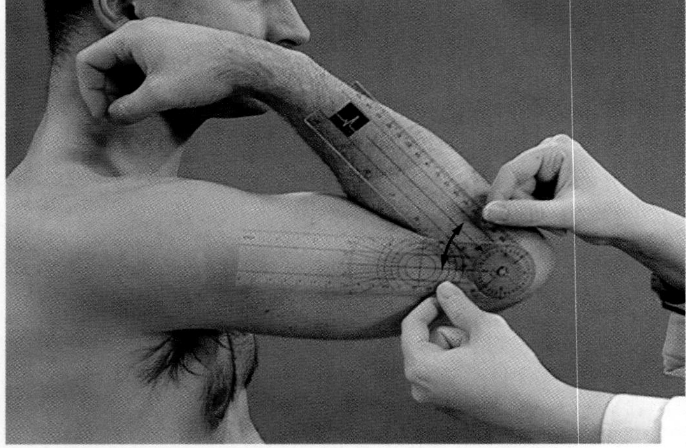

FIGURE 31-66 The patient flexes the arm; the goniometer measures joint range of motion. (From Ball JW et al: *Seidel's guide to physical examination,* ed 8, St Louis, 2015, Mosby.)

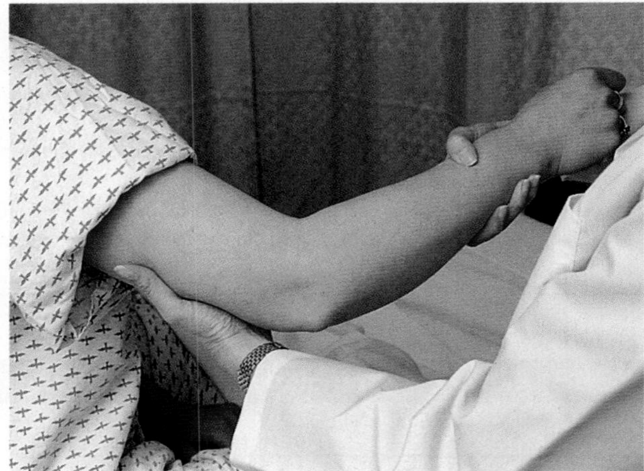

FIGURE 31-67 Assessing muscle tone.

little tone (hypotonicity) feels flabby. The involved extremity hangs loosely in a position determined by gravity.

For assessment of muscle strength, have the patient assume a stable position. He or she performs maneuvers demonstrating strength of major muscle groups (Table 31-33). Use a grading scale of "0 to 5" to compare symmetrical muscle pairs for strength (Table 31-34). The arm on the dominant side normally is stronger than the arm on the nondominant side. In older adults a loss of muscle mass causes bilateral weakness, but muscle strength remains greater in the dominant arm or leg.

Examine each muscle group. Ask the patient to first flex the muscle you are examining and then to resist when you apply an opposing force against that flexion. It is important to not allow the patient to move the joint. Gradually increase pressure to a muscle group (e.g., elbow extension). Have the patient resist the pressure you apply by attempting to move against resistance (e.g., elbow flexion) until instructed to stop. Vary the amount of pressure applied and observe the joint move. If you identify a weakness, compare the size of the muscle with its opposite counterpart by measuring the circumference of the muscle body with a tape measure. A muscle that has atrophied (reduced in size) feels soft and boggy when palpated.

NEUROLOGICAL SYSTEM

The neurological system is responsible for many functions, including initiation and coordination of movement, reception and perception of sensory stimuli, organization of thought processes, control of speech, and storage of memory. A close integration exists between the neurological system and all other body systems. For example, urine production relies in part on the adequacy of blood flow to the kidneys and on neural control, which affects the size of arterioles supplying the kidneys.

A full assessment of neurological function requires much time and attention to detail. For efficiency, integrate neurological measurements with other parts of the physical examination. For example, test cranial nerve function while assessing the head and neck. Observe mental and emotional status during the initial interview.

Consider many variables when deciding the extent of the neurological examination. A patient's level of consciousness influences his or her ability to follow directions. General physical status influences tolerance to assessment. A patient's chief complaint also helps determine the need for a thorough neurological assessment. If a patient complains of headache or a recent loss of function in an extremity, he or she needs a complete neurological review. Table 31-35 lists the data

TABLE 31-33 Maneuvers to Assess Muscle Strength

Muscle Group	Maneuver
Neck (sternocleidomastoid)	Place hand firmly against patient's upper jaw. Ask patient to turn head laterally against resistance.
Shoulder (trapezius)	Place hand over midline of patient's shoulder, exerting firm pressure. Have patient raise shoulders against resistance.
Elbow	
Biceps	Pull down on forearm as patient attempts to flex arm.
Triceps	As you flex patient's arm, apply pressure against forearm. Ask patient to straighten arm.
Hip	
Quadriceps	When patient is sitting, apply downward pressure to thigh. Ask patient to raise leg up from table.
Gastrocnemius	Patient sits while examiner holds shin of flexed leg. Ask patient to straighten leg against resistance.

TABLE 31-34 Muscle Strength

	SCALES		
Muscle Function Level	Grade	% Normal	Lovett Scale
No evidence of contractility	0	0	0 (zero)
Slight contractility, no movement	1	10	T (trace)
Full range of motion, gravity eliminated*	2	25	P (poor)
Full range of motion with gravity	3	50	F (fair)
Full range of motion against gravity, some resistance	4	75	G (good)
Full range of motion against gravity, full resistance	5	100	N (normal)

Modified from Ball JW et al: *Seidel's guide to physical examination*, ed 8, St Louis, 2015, Mosby; and Walker J: The role of the nurse in the management of osteoporosis, *Br J Nurs* 19(19):1243, 2010.
*Passive movement.

TABLE 31-35 Nursing History for Neurological Assessment

Assessment	Rationale
Determine if patient uses analgesics, alcohol, sedatives, hypnotics, antipsychotics, antidepressants, nervous system stimulants, or recreational drugs.	These medications alter level of consciousness or cause behavioral changes. Abuse sometimes causes tremors, ataxia, and changes in peripheral nerve function.
Determine if patient has recent history of seizures/convulsions: clarify sequence of events (aura, fall to ground, motor activity, loss of consciousness); character of any symptoms; and relationship of seizure to time of day, fatigue, or emotional stress.	Seizure activity often originates from central nervous system alteration. Characteristics of seizure help determine its origin.
Screen patient for symptoms of headache, tremors, dizziness, vertigo, numbness or tingling of body part, visual changes, weakness, pain, or changes in speech. Presence of any symptom requires more detailed review (onset, severity, precipitating factors or sequence of events).	These symptoms frequently originate from alterations in central or peripheral nervous system function. Identification of specific patterns aids in diagnosis of pathological condition.
Discuss with patient's family any recent changes in patient's behavior (e.g., increased irritability, mood swings, memory loss, change in energy level).	Behavioral changes sometimes result from intracranial pathological states.
Assess patient for history of change in vision, hearing, smell, taste, or touch.	Major sensory nerves originate from brainstem. These symptoms help to localize nature of problem.
If an older patient displays sudden acute confusion (delirium), review history for drug toxicity (anticholinergics, diuretics, digoxin, cimetidine, sedatives, antihypertensives, antiarrhythmics), serious infections, metabolic disturbances, heart failure, and severe anemia.	Delirium is one of the most common mental disorders in older people. Condition is always potentially reversible (see Box 31-31).
Review past history for head or spinal cord injury, meningitis, congenital anomalies, neurological disease, or psychiatric counseling.	Factors cause neurological symptoms or behavioral changes to develop, focusing assessment on possible cause.

collected in the nursing history. You will need the following items for a complete examination:

- Reading material
- Vials containing aromatic substances (e.g., vanilla extract and coffee)
- Opposite tip of cotton swab or tongue blade broken in half
- Snellen eye chart
- Penlight
- Vials containing sugar, salt, lemon with applicators
- Tongue blade
- Two test tubes, one filled with hot water and the other with cold water
- Cotton balls or cotton-tipped applicators
- Tuning fork
- Reflex hammer

Mental and Emotional Status

You learn a great deal about mental capacities and emotional state simply by interacting with a patient. Ask questions during an examination to gather data and observe the appropriateness of emotions and thoughts. Special assessment tools are designed to assess a patient's mental status. The Mini-Mental State Examination (MMSE) is an instrument developed by Folstein et al. (1975) that measures orientation and cognitive function. The questions in Box 31-30 offer examples of questions found on the MMSE. The maximum score on the MMSE is 31. Patients with scores of 21 or less generally reveal cognitive impairment requiring further evaluation.

To ensure an objective assessment, consider a patient's cultural and educational background, values, beliefs, and previous experiences. Such factors influence response to questions. An alteration in mental or emotional status reflects a disturbance in cerebral functioning. The cerebral cortex controls and integrates intellectual and emotional functioning. Primary brain disorders, medication, and metabolic changes are examples of factors that change cerebral function.

Delirium is an acute mental disorder that occurs among hospitalized patients. Obtain a thorough history of a patient's behavior before delirium develops to recognize the condition early. Family members are usually a good resource. Among older adults delirium most often presents within the first 48 to 72 hours of hospital admission (Rigney, 2010). It is an acute mental disorder characterized by confusion, disorientation, and restlessness. It is often a sign of an impending or underlying physical illness in older adults. The acute condition differs from dementia, a more progressive, organic mental disorder such as Alzheimer's disease. You need to recognize the difference so you can try to learn the underlying cause of delirium. Fortunately the condition often reverses when it is correctly assessed and the underlying cause is treated (i.e., central nervous system [CNS], metabolic, and cardiopulmonary disorders; systemic illnesses; and sensory deprivation or overload). To avoid misdiagnosis you need to adequately assess mental status. Frequently patients who develop delirium are labeled with "sundown syndrome" because the delirium frequently worsens at night. Many practitioners mistake this as being common with old age. Be aware that children are vulnerable to delirium from causes such as infection, drugs, serious trauma, autoimmune disorders, and general anesthesia and after transplant (Hatherill and Fisher, 2010). Box 31-31 summarizes clinical criteria for delirium.

Level of Consciousness. A person's level of consciousness exists along a continuum from full awakening, alertness, and cooperation to unresponsiveness to any form of external stimuli. Talk with the patient, asking questions about events involving his or her concerns about any health problems. A fully conscious patient responds to questions quickly and expresses ideas logically. With a lowering of a patient's consciousness, use the Glasgow Coma Scale (GCS) for an objective measurement of consciousness on a numerical scale (Table 31-36). The patient needs to be as alert as possible before testing. Take care when using the scale if the patient has sensory losses (e.g., vision or hearing). The GCS allows evaluation of a patient's neurological status over time.

BOX 31-30 Mini-Mental State Examination Sample Questions

- Orientation to time
  "What is the date?"
- Registration
  "Listen carefully. I am going to say three words. Say them back after I stop. Ready? Here they are . . .
  HOUSE (pause), CAR (pause), LAKE (pause). Now repeat these words back to me."
  (Repeat up to 5 times but score only the first trial.)
- Naming
  "What is this?" (Point to a pencil or pen.)
- Reading
  "Please read this and do what it says." (Show examinee the words on the stimulus form.)
  CLOSE YOUR EYES

BOX 31-31 Clinical Criteria for Delirium

Definition: An acute disturbance of consciousness that is accompanied by a change in cognition. It is not caused by a preexisting or evolving dementia. Delirium develops over a short period of time, usually hours to days, and tends to fluctuate during the course of the day. It is usually a direct physiological consequence of a general medical condition. It is most common in older adults but occasionally occurs in younger patients.

- There is reduced clarity of awareness of the environment.
- Ability to focus, sustain, or shift attention is impaired (questions must be repeated).
- Irrelevant stimuli easily distract the person.
- There is an accompanying change in cognition (memory impairment, disorientation, or language disturbance).
- Recent memory commonly is affected.
- Disorientation usually occurs, with patient disoriented to time, place, or person.
- Language disturbance involves impaired ability to name objects or ability to write; speech is sometimes rambling.
- Perceptual disturbances include misinterpretations, delusions, or visual and auditory hallucinations. Neurological signs include tremor, unsteady gait, asterixis, or myoclonus.

TABLE 31-36 Glasgow Coma Scale

(The total score is the sum of the scores in the three categories.)

Action	Response	Score
Eyes open	Spontaneously	4
	To speech	3
	To pain	2
	None	1
Best verbal response	Oriented	5
	Confused	4
	Inappropriate words	3
	Incomprehensible sounds	2
	None	1
Best motor response	Obeys commands	6
	Localized pain	5
	Flexion withdrawal	4
	Abnormal flexion	3
	Abnormal extension	2
	Flaccid	1
	TOTAL SCORE	**3 to 15**

The higher the score, the better the patient's neurological function. Ask short, simple questions such as "What is your name?" "Where are you?" and "What day is this?" Also ask the patient to follow simple commands such as "Move your toes."

If the patient is not conscious enough to follow commands, try to elicit the pain response. Apply firm pressure with the thumb over the root of the patient's fingernail. The normal response to the painful stimuli is withdrawal of the body part from the stimulus. A patient with serious neurological impairment exhibits abnormal posturing in response to pain. A flaccid response indicates the absence of muscle tone in the extremities and severe injury to brain tissue.

Behavior and Appearance. Behavior, moods, hygiene, grooming, and choice of dress reveal pertinent information about mental status. Remain perceptive of a patient's mannerisms and actions during the entire physical assessment. Note nonverbal and verbal behaviors. Does the patient respond appropriately to directions? Does his or her mood vary with no apparent cause? Does he or she show concern about appearance? Is his or her hair clean and neatly groomed, and are the nails trim and clean? The patient should behave in a manner expressing concern and interest in the examination. He or she should make eye contact with you and express appropriate feelings that correspond to the situation. Normally the patient shows some degree of personal hygiene.

Choice and fit of clothing reflect socioeconomic background or personal taste rather than deficiency in self-concept or self-care. Avoid being judgmental and focus assessment on the appropriateness of clothing for the weather. Older adults sometimes neglect their appearance because of a lack of energy, finances, or reduced vision.

Language. Normal cerebral function allows a person to understand spoken or written words and express the self through written words or gestures. Assess the patient's voice inflection, tone, and manner of speech. Normally a patient's voice has inflections, is clear and strong, and increases in volume appropriately. Speech is fluent. When communication is clearly ineffective (e.g., omission or addition of letters and words, misuse of words, or hesitations), assess for **aphasia**. Injury to the cerebral cortex results in aphasia.

The two types of aphasia are sensory (or receptive) and motor (or expressive). With receptive aphasia a person cannot understand written or verbal speech. With expressive aphasia a person understands written and verbal speech but cannot write or speak appropriately when attempting to communicate. A patient sometimes suffers a combination of receptive and expressive aphasia. Assess language capabilities when it is clear that a patient is communicating ineffectively. Some simple assessment techniques include the following:

- Point to a familiar object and ask the patient to name it.
- Ask the patient to respond to simple verbal and written commands such as "Stand up" or "Sit down."
- Ask the patient to read simple sentences out loud.

Normally a patient names objects correctly, follows commands, and reads sentences correctly.

Intellectual Function

Intellectual function includes memory (recent, immediate, and past), knowledge, abstract thinking, association, and judgment. Testing each aspect of function involves a specific technique. However, because cultural and educational background influences the ability to respond to test questions, do not ask questions related to concepts or ideas with which a patient is unfamiliar.

Memory. Assess immediate recall and recent and remote memory. Patients demonstrate immediate recall by repeating a series of numbers (e.g., *7, 4, 1*) in the order they are presented or in reverse order. Patients normally recall a series of five-to-eight digits forward and four-to-six digits backward.

First ask to test the patient's memory. Then state clearly and slowly the name of three unrelated objects. After mentioning all three, ask the patient to repeat each. Continue until he or she is successful. Later in the assessment ask the patient to repeat the three words again. He or she should be able to identify them. Another test for recent memory involves asking the patient to recall events occurring during the same day (e.g., what was eaten for breakfast). Validate information with a family member.

To assess past memory, ask the patient to recall his or her mother's maiden name, a birthday, or a special date in history. It is best to ask open-ended rather than simple yes-or-no questions. A patient usually has immediate recall of such information. With older adults do not interpret hearing loss as confusion. Good communication techniques are essential throughout the examination to ensure that a patient clearly understands all directions and testing.

Knowledge. Assess knowledge by asking how much the patient knows about his or her illness or the reason for seeking health care. A knowledge assessment allows you to determine a patient's ability to learn or understand. If there is an opportunity to teach, test a patient's mental status by asking for feedback during a follow-up visit.

Abstract Thinking. Interpreting abstract ideas or concepts reflects the capacity for abstract thinking. For an individual to explain common phrases such as "A stitch in time saves nine" or "Don't count your chickens before they're hatched" requires a higher level of intellectual function. Note whether a patient's explanations are relevant and concrete. A patient with altered mental status probably interprets the phrase literally or merely rephrases the words.

Association. Another higher level of intellectual functioning involves finding similarities or associations between concepts: a dog is to a beagle as a cat is to a Siamese. Name related concepts and ask the

TABLE 31-37 Cranial Nerve Function and Assessment

Number	Name	Type	Function	Method
I	Olfactory	Sensory	Sense of smell	Ask patient to identify different nonirritating aromas such as coffee and vanilla.
II	Optic	Sensory	Visual acuity	Use Snellen chart or ask patient to read printed material while wearing glasses.
III	Oculomotor	Motor	Extraocular eye movements: inward, up and inward, up and outward, down and outward	Assess six directions of gaze.
			Pupil constriction and dilation Opening the eye	Measure pupillary reaction to light reflex and accommodation.
IV	Trochlear	Motor	Downward, inward eye movements	Assess six directions of gaze.
V	Trigeminal	Sensory and motor	Sensory nerve to skin of face	Lightly touch cornea with wisp of cotton. Assess corneal reflex. Measure sensation of light pain and touch across skin of face.
			Motor nerve to muscles of jaw	Palpate temples as patient clenches teeth.
VI	Abducens	Motor	Lateral movement of eyeballs	Assess six directions of gaze.
VII	Facial	Sensory and motor	Facial expression	As patient smiles, frowns, puffs out cheeks, and raises and lowers eyebrows, look for asymmetry.
			Taste	Have patient identify salty or sweet taste on front of tongue.
VIII	Auditory	Sensory	Hearing	Assess ability to hear spoken word.
IX	Glossopharyngeal	Sensory and motor	Taste Ability to swallow	Ask patient to identify sour or sweet taste on back of tongue. Use tongue blade to elicit gag reflex.
X	Vagus	Sensory and motor	Sensation of pharynx Movement of vocal cords Parasympathetic innervation to glands of mucous membranes of the pharynx, larynx, organs in the neck, thorax (heart and lungs), and abdomen	Ask patient to say "ah." Observe movement of palate and pharynx. Assess speech for hoarseness. Assess heart rate, presence of peristalsis.
XI	Spinal accessory	Motor	Movement of head and shoulders	Ask patient to shrug shoulders and turn head against passive resistance.
XII	Hypoglossal	Motor	Position of tongue	Ask patient to stick out tongue to midline and move it from side to side.

patient to identify their associations. Ask questions that are appropriate to the patient's level of intelligence, using simple concepts.

Judgment. Judgment requires a comparison and evaluation of facts and ideas to understand their relationships and form appropriate conclusions. Attempt to measure the patient's ability to make logical decisions with questions such as "Why did you seek health care?" or "What would you do if you became ill at home?" Normally a patient makes logical decisions.

Cranial Nerve Function

To assess cranial nerve function, you may test all 12 cranial nerves, a single nerve, or a related group of nerves. A dysfunction in one nerve reflects an alteration at some point along the distribution of the cranial nerve. Measurements used to assess the integrity of organs within the head and neck also assess cranial nerve function. A complete assessment involves testing the 12 cranial nerves in their numerical order. To remember the order of the nerves, use this simple phrase, "On old Olympus' towering tops, a Finn and German viewed some hops." The first letter of each word in the phrase is the same as the first letter of the names of the cranial nerves listed in order (Table 31-37).

Sensory Function

The sensory pathways of the CNS conduct sensations of pain, temperature, position, vibration, and crude and finely localized touch. Different nerve pathways relay the sensations. Most patients require only a quick screening of sensory function unless there are symptoms of reduced sensation, motor impairment, or paralysis. The risk of skin breakdown is greater in a patient with impaired sensation. When assessing decreased sensation, complete a skin assessment of the area affected by the sensory loss. In addition, teach the patient to avoid pressure, thermal, and/or chemical trauma to the area.

Normally a patient has sensory responses to all stimuli that are tested. He or she feels sensations equally on both sides of the body in all areas. Assess the major sensory nerves by knowing the sensory dermatome zones (Figure 31-68, *A* and *B*). Some areas of the skin are innervated by specific dorsal root cutaneous nerves. For example, if assessment reveals reduced sensation when checking for light touch along an area of the skin (e.g., the lower neck), this determines in general where a neurological lesion exists (e.g., fourth cervical spinal cord segment).

Perform all sensory testing with the patient's eyes closed so he or she is unable to see when or where a stimulus touches the skin

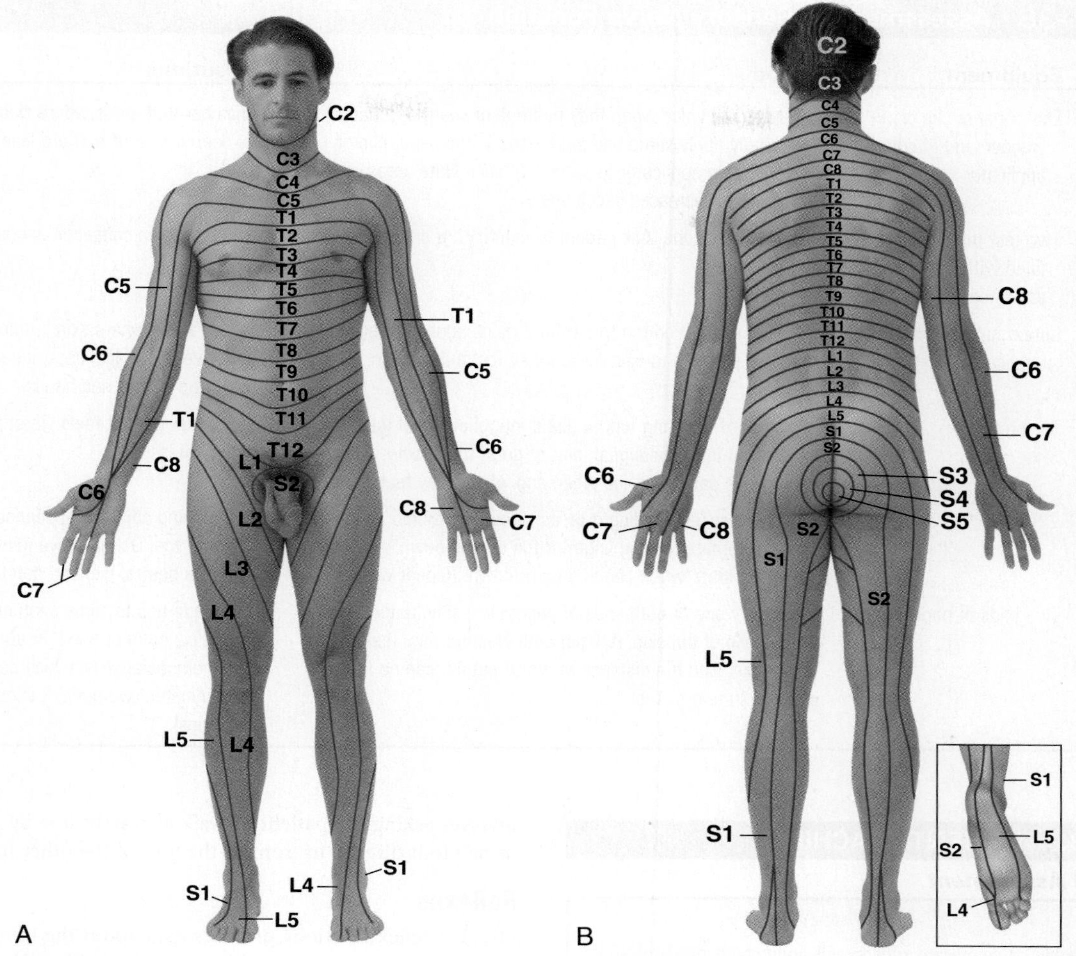

FIGURE 31-68 Dermatomes of body (body surface areas innervated by particular spinal nerves); C1 usually has no cutaneous distribution. **A,** Anterior view. **B,** Posterior view. It appears that there is a distinct separation of surface area controlled by each dermatome, but there is almost always overlap between spinal nerves. (From Ball JW et al: *Seidel's guide to physical examination,* ed 8, St Louis, 2015, Mosby.)

(Table 31-38). Then touch the patient's skin in a random, unpredictable order to maintain his or her attention and prevent detection of a predictable pattern. Ask the patient to describe when, what, and where he or she feels each stimulus. Compare symmetrical areas of the body while applying stimuli to the patient's arms, trunk, and legs.

Motor Function

An examination of motor function includes assessments made during the musculoskeletal examination. In addition, you assess the patient's cerebellar function. The cerebellum coordinates muscular activity, maintains balance and equilibrium, and controls posture.

Coordination. To avoid confusion, demonstrate each maneuver and have the patient repeat it, observing for smoothness and balance in his or her movements (Box 31-32). In older adults normally slow reaction time causes movements to be less rhythmical.

To assess fine-motor function, have the patient extend the arms out to the sides and touch each forefinger alternately to the nose (first with eyes open, then with eyes closed). Normally a patient alternately touches the nose smoothly. Performing rapid, rhythmical, alternating movements demonstrates coordination in the upper extremities. While sitting, the patient begins by patting the knees with both hands. Then he or she alternately turns up the palm and back of the hands while continuously patting the knees. Normally patients perform the maneuver smoothly and regularly with increasing speed.

An additional maneuver for upper-extremity coordination involves touching each finger with the thumb of the same hand in rapid sequence. A patient moves from the index finger to the little finger and back, with one hand tested at a time. The dominant hand is slightly less awkward when performing this movement. Movement is smooth and in succession.

Test lower-extremity coordination with the patient lying supine, legs extended. Place a hand at the ball of the patient's foot. The patient taps the hand with the foot as quickly as possible. Test each foot for speed and smoothness. The feet do not move as rapidly or evenly as the hands.

Balance. Use one or two of the following tests to assess balance and gross-motor function. When examining the older adult for balance and equilibrium, be aware of the risk for falls. Some older adults need help with this part of the examination.

Have the patient perform a Romberg's test by standing with feet together, arms at the sides, both with eyes open and eyes closed. Protect the patient's safety by standing at the side, observe for swaying. Expect

TABLE 31-38 Assessment of Sensory Nerve Function

Function	Equipment	Method	Precautions
Pain	End of paper clip or wooden end of cotton applicator	Ask patients to voice when they feel dull or sharp sensation. Alternately apply sharp and blunt ends of the paper clip or broken cotton applicator to surface of skin. Note areas of numbness or increased sensitivity.	Remember that areas where skin is thick such as heel or sole of foot are less sensitive to pain.
Temperature	Two test tubes, one filled with hot water and another with cold	Touch skin with tube. Ask patient to identify hot or cold sensation.	Omit test if pain sensation is normal.
Light touch	Cotton ball or cotton-tip applicator	Apply light wisp of cotton to different points along surface of skin. Ask patients to voice when they feel a sensation.	Apply at areas where skin is thin or more sensitive (e.g., face, neck, inner aspect of arms, top of feet and hands).
Vibration	Tuning fork	Apply stem of vibrating fork to distal interphalangeal joint of fingers and interphalangeal joint of great toe, elbow, and wrist. Have patients voice when and where they feel vibration.	Be sure that patient feels vibration and not merely pressure.
Position		Grasp finger or toe, holding it by its sides with thumb and index finger. Alternate moving finger or toe up and down. Ask patient to state when finger is up or down. Repeat with toes.	Avoid rubbing adjacent appendages as you move finger or toe. Do not move joint laterally; return to neutral position before moving again.
Two-point discrimination	Two ends of paper clips	Lightly apply one or both ends of paper clips simultaneously to the surface of the skin. Ask patients whether they feel one or two pricks. Find the distance at which patient can no longer distinguish two points.	Apply blade tips to same anatomical site (e.g., fingertips, palm of hand, or upper arms). Minimum distance at which patient discriminates two points varies (2 to 8 mm on fingertips).

BOX 31-32 PATIENT TEACHING

Neurological Assessment

Objective

- Patient and family or significant others will understand relationship of patient's behavioral and mental changes to physical status.

Teaching Strategies

- Explain to family caregiver the implications of any behavioral or mental impairment shown by patient.
- If patient has sensory or motor impairments, explain measures to ensure safety (e.g., wearing glasses or hearing aids, use of ambulation aids or safety bars in bathrooms or stairways) (see Chapter 49).
- Teach older adult to plan enough time to complete tasks because reaction time is slow.
- Teach older adult to observe skin surfaces for areas of trauma since pain perception is reduced.

Evaluation

- Ask family member to discuss patient behaviors that result from neurological impairments.
- Have patient explain safety measures used to avoid injury from sensory and motor limitations.
- Have older patient explain reason for inspecting skin surface routinely.

slight swaying of the body in the Romberg's test. A loss of balance (positive Romberg) causes a patient to fall to the side. Normally he or she does not break the stance.

Have the patient close the eyes, with arms held straight at the sides, and stand on one foot and then the other. Normally patients are able to maintain balance for 5 seconds with slight swaying. Another test involves asking the patient to walk a straight line by placing the heel of one foot directly in front of the toes of the other foot.

Reflexes

Eliciting reflex reactions provides data about the integrity of sensory and motor pathways of the reflex arc and specific spinal cord segments. Assessment of reflexes does not determine higher neural center functioning but helps to assess peripheral-spinal nerve function. Figure 31-69 traces the pathway of the reflex arc. Each muscle contains a small sensory unit called a *muscle spindle,* which controls muscle tone and detects changes in the length of muscle fibers. Tapping a tendon with a reflex hammer stretches the muscle and tendon, lengthening the spindle. The spindle sends nerve impulses along afferent nerve pathways to the dorsal horn of the spinal cord segment. Within milliseconds the impulses reach the spinal cord and synapse to travel to the efferent motor neuron in the spinal cord. A motor nerve sends the impulses back to the muscle, causing the reflex response.

The two categories of normal reflexes are deep tendon reflexes, elicited by mildly stretching a muscle and tapping a tendon, and cutaneous reflexes, elicited by stimulating the skin superficially. Grade reflexes as follows (Ball et al., 2015):

0: No response
1+: Sluggish or diminished
2+: Active or expected response
3+: More brisk than expected, slightly hyperactive
4+: Brisk and hyperactive with intermittent or transient clonus

When assessing reflexes, have the patient relax as much as possible to avoid voluntary movement or tensing of muscles. Position the limbs to slightly stretch the muscle being tested. Hold the reflex hammer loosely between the thumb and fingers so it is able to swing freely and tap the tendon briskly (Figure 31-70). Compare the responses on corresponding sides. Normally the older adult presents with diminished reflexes. Reflexes are hyperactive in patients with alcohol, cocaine, or

TABLE 31-39 Assessment of Common Reflexes

Type	Procedure	Normal Reflex
Deep Tendon Reflexes		
Biceps	Flex patient's arm up to 45 degrees at elbow with palms down. Place your thumb in antecubital fossa at base of biceps tendon and your fingers over biceps muscle. Strike biceps tendon with reflex hammer.	Flexion of arm at elbow
Triceps	Flex patient's arm at elbow, holding arm across chest, or hold upper arm horizontally and allow lower arm to go limp. Strike triceps tendon just above elbow.	Extension at elbow
Patellar	Have patient sit with legs hanging freely over side of table or chair or have him or her lie supine and support knee in a flexed 90-degree position. Briskly tap patellar tendon just below patella.	Extension of lower leg
Achilles	Have patient assume same position as for patellar reflex. Slightly dorsiflex patient's ankle by grasping toes in palm of your hand. Strike Achilles tendon just above heel at ankle malleolus.	Plantar flexion of foot
Cutaneous Reflexes		
Plantar	Have patient lie supine with legs straight and feet relaxed. Take handle end of reflex hammer and stroke lateral aspect of sole from heel to ball of foot, curving across ball of foot toward big toe.	Plantar flexion of all toes
Abdominal	Have patient stand or lie supine. Stroke abdominal skin with base of cotton applicator over lateral borders of rectus abdominis muscle toward midline. Repeat test in each abdominal quadrant.	Contraction of rectus abdominis muscle with pulling of umbilicus toward stimulated side

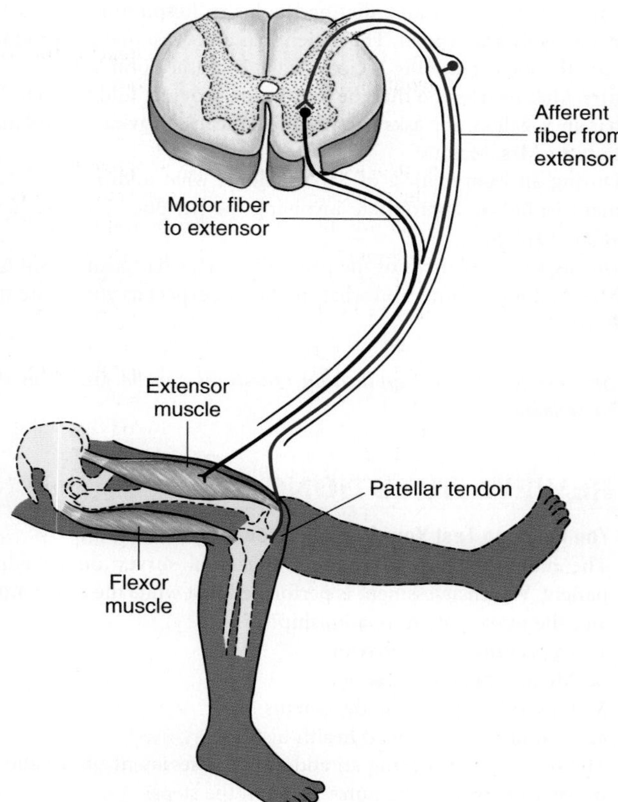

FIGURE 31-69 Pathway of reflex arc.

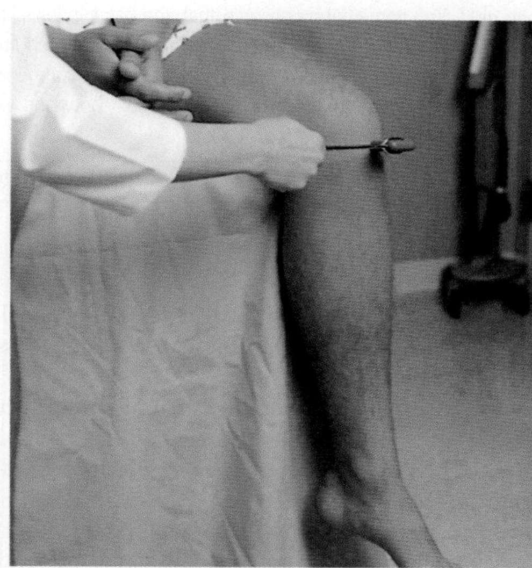

FIGURE 31-70 Position for eliciting patellar tendon reflex. Lower leg normally extends.

opioid intoxication. Table 31-39 summarizes common deep tendon and cutaneous reflexes.

AFTER THE EXAMINATION

Record findings from the physical assessment either during the examination or when it is completed. Special forms are available to record data both electronically and on printed forms. Review all findings before helping patients dress in case it is necessary to recheck any information or gather additional data. Integrate physical assessment findings into the plan of care.

After completing an assessment, give the patient time to dress. The hospitalized patient sometimes needs help with hygiene and returning to bed. When the patient is comfortable, it helps to share a summary of the assessment findings. If the findings have revealed serious abnormalities such as a mass or highly irregular heart rate, consult the patient's health care provider before revealing them. It is the health care provider's responsibility to make definitive medical diagnoses. Explain the type of abnormality found and the need for the health care provider to conduct an additional examination.

Delegate cleaning the examination area to support staff if needed. Use infection control practice to remove materials or instruments soiled with potentially infectious wastes. If the patient's bedside was the examination site, clear away soiled items from the bedside table and make sure that the bed linen is dry and clean. A patient appreciates a clean gown and the opportunity to wash the face and hands. Afterward be sure to perform hand hygiene.

Be sure to record a complete assessment. If you delayed entering any items into the assessment form, record them at this time to avoid forgetting any important information. If you made entries periodically during the examination, review them for accuracy and thoroughness. Communicate significant findings to appropriate medical and nursing personnel, either verbally or in the patient's written care plan.

QSEN QSEN: BUILDING COMPETENCY IN SAFETY You are preparing to examine a 75-year-old female who arrives at the clinic in a wheelchair. She explains, "I can't walk very well because my legs just won't carry me far anymore! I use this wheelchair so I don't wear out or lose my breath. I refuse to let these problems get in the way of doing what I want—getting out of the house and going places. I'm just not as spry as I was when I was young girl." You immediately observe that she has kyphosis. To climb onto the examination table, a patient needs to climb on a 6-inch step; turn around; and sit on an elevated, padded table surface. Which component findings from the general survey guide your decision about how and where to continue with the physical examination?

Answers to QSEN Activities can be found on the Evolve website.

KEY POINTS

- Baseline assessment findings reflect a patient's functional abilities and serve as the basis for comparison with subsequent assessment findings.
- Physical assessment of a child or infant requires the application of the principles of growth and development.
- Recognize that the normal process of aging affects physical findings collected from an older adult.
- Integrate patient teaching throughout an examination to help patients learn about health promotion, disease prevention, and skills to help with any current health issues.
- Inspection requires a careful, systematic approach that compares a body part with its counterpart on the opposite side of the body.
- Use auscultation to assess the character of sounds created in various body organs.
- Perform a physical examination only after proper preparation of the environment and equipment and after preparing a patient physically and psychologically.
- Throughout an examination keep the patient warm, comfortable, and informed of each step of the process.
- A competent examiner is systematic while combining assessment of different body systems simultaneously.
- Information from the history helps to focus on body systems likely to be affected.
- When assessing a seriously ill patient, first concentrate on the body systems most affected.
- Creating a mental image of internal organs in relation to external anatomical landmarks enhances accuracy in assessing the thorax, heart, and abdomen.
- When assessing heart sounds, imagine events occurring during the cardiac cycle.
- Never palpate both of the carotid arteries simultaneously.
- When examining a woman's breasts, explain the techniques for BSE.
- The order of the abdominal assessment is inspection, auscultation, percussion (if used), and palpation.
- During assessment of the genitalia explain the technique for genital self-examination.
- Conduct an assessment of musculoskeletal function when observing a patient ambulate or participate in other active movements.
- Assess mental and emotional status by interacting with a patient throughout the examination.
- At the end of the examination provide for the patient's comfort and then document a detailed summary of physical assessment findings.

CLINICAL APPLICATION QUESTIONS

Preparing for Clinical Practice

You receive morning report for Mrs. Malone, age 71, admitted to the hospital yesterday with fatigue, a cough, and dyspnea; she is diagnosed with chronic heart failure. She states that she had increasing difficulty with shortness of breath and swelling in her legs. Pedal pulses are +1 bilaterally. On auscultation you hear bilateral crackles in the lung bases and an S_3 gallop when auscultating the heart. Respiratory rate is 18; heart rate is 84 and regular. The patient has an occasional nonproductive cough. She is receiving 2 L of oxygen by nasal cannula.

1. Mrs. Malone tells you that the health care provider told her that she has an S_3 gallop. She asks you what this means. Provide an explanation for Mrs. Malone.
2. During an examination of Mrs. Malone, what additional assessment would be appropriate involving the peripheral arteries and veins? Explain.
3. During the assessment of the patient's heart, what position should Mrs. Malone assume, and what might you expect as you locate the PMI?

Answers to Clinical Application Questions can be found on the Evolve website.

REVIEW QUESTIONS

Are You Ready to Test Your Nursing Knowledge?

1. The nurse prepares to conduct a general survey on an adult patient. Which assessment is performed first while the nurse initiates the nurse-patient relationship?
   1. Appearance and behavior
   2. Measurement of vital signs
   3. Observing specific body systems
   4. Conducting a detailed health history
2. The nurse is performing an abdominal assessment on a patient. In what order does the nurse perform the steps?
   1. Percussion
   2. Inspection
   3. Auscultation
   4. Palpation
3. While auscultating the adult patient's lungs, the nurse hears loud, bubbly sounds during inspiration that did not disappear after the

patient coughed. Which finding should the nurse document from the lung assessment?

1. Rhonchi
2. Coarse crackles
3. Sibilant wheeze
4. Pleural friction rub

4. During assessment of the skin, the nurse assesses a lesion on the arm of the patient. The lesion is irregularly shaped, elevated with edema, and about 3 cm. What type of lesion does the patient have?
   1. Nodule
   2. Macule
   3. Wheal
   4. Pustule
5. Which number corresponds to the area of the chest where you would auscultate for the tricuspid valve?
   1. 1
   2. 2
   3. 3
   4. 4
   5. 5
   6. 6

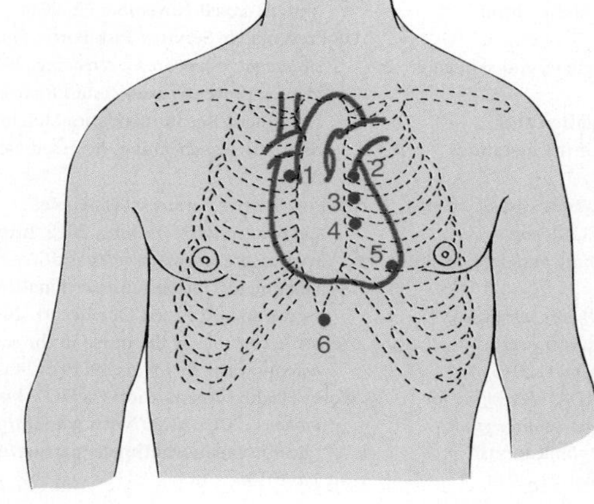

6. The nurse is assessing a patient who returned 1 hour ago from surgery for an abdominal hysterectomy. Which assessment finding would require immediate follow-up?
   1. Auscultation of an apical heart rate of 76
   2. Absence of bowel sounds on abdominal assessment
   3. Respiratory rate of 8 breaths/min
   4. Palpation of dorsalis pedis pulses with strength of +2
7. Which statement made by the patient indicates an understanding about teaching related to early detection of colorectal cancer?
   1. "I'll make sure to schedule my colonoscopy annually after the age of 60."
   2. "I'll make sure to have a computed tomography (CT) colonoscopy every 5 years."
   3. "I'll make sure to have a flexible sigmoidoscopy every year once I turn 55."
   4. "I'll make sure to have a fecal occult blood test annually once I turn 50."
8. The nurse is teaching a patient to prevent heart disease. Which information should the nurse include? (Select all that apply.)
   1. Limit intake of cholesterol to less than 400 mg/day.
   2. Talk with your health care provider about taking a daily low dose of aspirin.
   3. Work with your health care provider to develop a regular exercise program.
   4. Limit daily intake of fats to less than 25% to 35% of total calories.
   5. Review strategies to encourage the patient to quit smoking.
9. How should the patient be positioned to best palpate for lumps or tumors during an examination of the right breast?
   1. Supine with both arms overhead with palms upward
   2. Sitting with hands clasped just above the umbilicus
   3. Supine with the right arm abducted and hand under the head and neck
   4. Lying on the right side, adducting the right arm on the side of the body
10. The nurse is assessing the cranial nerves. Match the cranial nerve with its related function.

Cranial Nerves	**Cranial Nerve Function**
1. XII Hypoglossal	a. Motor innervation to the muscles of the jaw
2. V Trigeminal	b. Lateral movement of the eyeballs
3. VI Adducens	c. Sensation of the pharynx
4. IV Trochlear	d. Downward, inward eye movements
5. X Vagus	e. Position of the tongue

11. The nurse is teaching a patient how to perform a testicular self-examination. Which statement made by the patient indicates a need for further teaching?
    1. "I'll recognize abnormal lumps because they are very painful."
    2. "I'll start performing testicular self-examination monthly after I turn 15."
    3. "I'll perform the self-examination in front of a mirror."
    4. "I'll gently roll the testicle between my fingers."
12. The nurse is observing the student nurse perform a respiratory assessment on a patient. Which action by the student nurse requires the nurse to intervene?
    1. The student stands at a midline position behind the patient observing for position of the spine and scapula.
    2. The student palpates the thoracic muscles for masses, pulsations, or abnormal movements.
    3. The student places the bell of the stethoscope on the anterior chest wall to auscultate breath sounds.
    4. The student places the palm of the hand over the intercostal spaces and asks the patient to say "ninety-nine."
13. The nurse plans to assess the patient's memory. Which task should the nurse ask the patient to perform?
    1. "Tell me where you are."
    2. "What can you tell me about your illness?"
    3. "Repeat these numbers back to me: 7…5…8."
    4. "What does this mean: 'A stitch in time saves nine?'"
14. A patient has undergone surgery for a femoral artery bypass. The surgeon's orders include assessment of dorsalis pedis pulses. The nurse will use which of the following techniques to assess the pulses? (Select all that apply.)
    1. Place the fingers behind and below the medial malleolus.
    2. Have the patient slightly flex the knee with the foot resting on the bed.
    3. Have the patient relax the foot while lying supine.
    4. Palpate the groove lateral to the flexor tendon of the wrist.
    5. Palpate along the top of the foot in a line with the groove between extensor tendons of great and first toes.
15. The faith community nurse is teaching the community center women's group about breast cancer risk factors. Which factors does the nurse include? (Select all that apply.)
    1. First child at the age of 26 years
    2. Menopause onset at the age of 49 years
    3. Family history with BRCA1 inherited gene mutation
    4. Age over 40 years
    5. Onset of menses before the age of 12
    6. Recent use of oral contraceptives

Answers: 1. 1; **2.** 2, 3, 1, 4; **3.** 2; **4.** 3; **5.** 4; **6.** 3; **7.** 4; **8.** 2, 3, 4, 5; **9.** 3; **10.** 1e, 2a, 3b, 4d, 5c; **11.** 1; **12.** 3; **13.** 3; **14.** 3, 5; **15.** 3, 4, 5, 6.

Rationales for Review Questions can be found on the Evolve website.

REFERENCES

American Cancer Society (ACS): *Screening guidelines for the prevention and early detection of cervical cancer. CA: A Cancer Journal for Clinicians*, Atlanta, 2012, Author.

American Cancer Society (ACS): *Colorectal cancer: what are the risk factors for colorectal cancer?* 2014a. http://www.cancer.org/cancer/colonandrectumcancer/detailedguide/colorectal-cancer-risk-factors. Accessed November 12, 2014.

American Cancer Society (ACS): *Ovarian cancer,* 2014b. http://www.cancer.org/cancer/ovariancancer/detailedguide/ovarian-cancer-key-statistics. Accessed November 12, 2014.

American Cancer Society (ACS): *Cancer facts and figures,* 2015a. http://www.cancer.org/acs/groups/content/@editorial/documents/document/acspc-044552.pdf. Accessed October 30, 2015.

American Cancer Society (ACS): *American Cancer Society recommendations for early breast cancer detection in women without breast symptoms,* 2015b. http://www.cancer.org/cancer/breastcancer/moreinformation/breastcancerearlydetection/breast-cancer-early-detection-acs-recs. Accessed October 26, 2015.

American Heart Association (AHA): *Know Your Fats,* 2014. http://www.heart.org/HEARTORG/Conditions/Cholesterol/PreventionTreatmentofHighCholesterol/Know-Your-Fats_UCM_315628_Article.jsp. Accessed November 12, 2014.

Ball JW, et al: *Seidel's guide to physical examination*, ed 8, St Louis, 2015, Mosby.

Cancer Net: *Health risks of E-cigarettes, smokeless tobacco, and waterpipes, American Society of Clinical Oncology,* Alexandria, VA, 2015, The Association. http://www.cancer.net/navigating-cancer-care/prevention-and-healthy-living/tobacco-use/health-risks-e-cigarettes-smokeless-tobacco-and-waterpipes. Accessed April 19, 2015.

Centers for Disease Control and Prevention (CDC): *Vision health initiative: common eye disorders*, 2013. http://www.cdc.gov/visionhealth/basic_information/eye_disorders.htm. Accessed October 27, 2015.

Centers for Disease Control and Prevention (CDC): *Vaccines and immunizations: HPV vaccine questions and answers,* 2014. http://www.cdc.gov/vaccines/vpd-vac/hpv/vac-faqs.htm. Accessed November 12, 2014.

Centers for Disease Control and Prevention (CDC): *Healthy schools: noise induced hearing loss,* 2015a. http://www.cdc.gov/healthyschools/noise/index.htm. Accessed October 30, 2015.

Centers for Disease Control and Prevention (CDC): *HPV vaccines: vaccinating your preteen or teen,* 2015b. http://www.cdc.gov/hpv/parents/vaccine.html. Accessed October 31, 2015.

Cowdell F: Older people, personal hygiene, and skin care, *Medsurg Nurs* 20(5):235, 2011.

Hatherill S, Fisher AJ: Delirium in children and adolescents: a systematic review of the literature, *J Psychosoma Res* 68:337, 2010.

Hockenberry MJ, Wilson P: *Wong's nursing care of infants and children*, ed 10, St Louis, 2015, Mosby.

Huether SE, McCance KL: *Understanding pathophysiology*, ed 5, St Louis, 2012, Elsevier.

National Breast Cancer Foundation: *Breast self-exam,* 2015. http://www.nationalbreastcancer.org/breast-self-exam. Accessed October 31, 2015.

National Institute on Drug Abuse (NIDA): *Screening for drug use in general medical settings, resource guide,* 2012. http://www.drugabuse.gov/publications/resource-guide. Accessed November 21, 2014.

National Osteoporosis Foundation: *Are you at risk?* n.d. http://nof.org/articles/2. Accessed October 31, 2014.

Nelson HD, et al: Screening for osteoporosis: an update for the US Preventive Services Task Force, *Ann Intern Med* 153(2):1, 2010. http://www.annals.org.

Oral Cancer Foundation: *Oral cancer facts,* 2014. http://oralcancerfoundation.org/facts/index.htm. Accessed November 12, 2014.

Rush A, Muir M: Maintaining skin integrity in bariatric patients, *Br J Community Nurs* 17(4):154, 2012.

Touhy T, Jett K: *Ebersole and Hess' gerontological nursing & healthy aging*, ed 4, St Louis, 2014, Mosby.

US Department of Agriculture (USDA): *Let's eat for the health of it, Pub No: Home & Garden Bulletin No. 232-CP*, 2011. http://www.choosemyplate.gov/food-groups/downloads/MyPlate/DG2010Brochure.pdf. Accessed November 22, 2014.

US Preventative Services Task Force: *Final recommendation statement: osteoporosis: screening,* 2011. http://www.uspreventiveservicestaskforce.org/Page/Document/RecommendationStatementFinal/osteoporosis-screening. Accessed October 31, 2015.

US Preventative Services Task Force: *Cervical cancer: screening,* 2012. http://www.uspreventiveservicestaskforce.org/Page/Document/UpdateSummaryFinal/cervical-cancer-screening. Accessed October 31, 2012.

Walker J: The role of the nurse in the management of osteoporosis, *Br J Nurs* 19(19):1243, 2010.

World Health Organization (WHO): *Intimate partner violence*, 2015. http://www.who.int/gho/women_and_health/violence/intimate_partner/en/. Accessed April 20, 2015.

RESEARCH REFERENCES

Brooks SE, et al: Mobile mammography in underserved populations: analysis of outcomes of 3,923 women, *J Community Health* 38:900, 2013.

Burns E, et al: Brief screening questionnaires to identify problem drinking during pregnancy: a systematic review, *Addiction* 105:601, 2010.

Byrd J, et al: Research corner. Scale consistency study: how accurate are inpatient hospital scales? *Nursing* 41(11):21, 2011.

Conway-Phillips R, Janusek L: Influence of sense of coherence, spirituality, social support and health perception on breast cancer screening motivation and behaviors in African American women, *ABNF J* 25(3):72, 2014.

Feldstein AC, et al: Patient barriers to mammography identified during a reminder program, *J Womens Health* 20(3):421, 2011.

Folstein MF, et al: Mini-mental state: a practical method for grading the cognitive state of patients for the clinician, *J Psychiatr Res* 12:82, 1975.

Ingram RR: Using Campinha-Bacote's process of cultural competence model to examine the relationship between health literacy and cultural competence, *J Adv Nurs* 68(3):695, 2012.

Khaliq W, et al: Breast cancer screening preferences among hospitalized women, *J Womens Health* 22(7):637, 2013.

Kreuter MW, et al: Comparing narrative and informational videos to increase mammography in low-income African American women, *Patient Educ Couns* 81S:S6, 2010.

Northington L, et al: Integrated community education model: breast health awareness to impact late-stage breast cancer, *Clin J Oncol Nurs* 15(4):387, 2011.

Rigney T: Allostatic load and delirium in the hospitalized older adult, *Nurs Res* 59(5):322, 2010.

32

Medication Administration

OBJECTIVES

- Discuss nursing roles and responsibilities in medication administration.
- Describe the physiological mechanisms of medication action.
- Differentiate among different types of medication actions.
- Discuss developmental factors that influence pharmacokinetics.
- Discuss factors that influence medication actions.
- Discuss methods used to educate patients about prescribed medications.
- Compare and contrast the roles of the health care provider, pharmacist, and nurse in medication administration.
- Implement nursing actions to prevent medication errors.
- Describe factors to consider when choosing routes of medication administration.
- Calculate prescribed medication doses correctly.
- Discuss factors to include in assessing a patient's needs for and response to medication therapy.
- Identify the six rights of medication administration and apply them in clinical settings.
- Correctly and safely prepare and administer medications.

KEY TERMS

Absorption, p. 611
Adverse effects, p. 613
Anaphylactic reactions, p. 613
Biological half-life, p. 614
Biotransformation, p. 612
Buccal, p. 615
Detoxify, p. 612
Idiosyncratic reaction, p. 613
Infusions, p. 614
Injection, p. 611
Instillation, p. 617
Intraarticular, p. 616
Intracardiac, p. 616
Intradermal (ID), p. 615
Intramuscular (IM), p. 615
Intraocular, p. 617
Intravenous (IV), p. 615
Irrigations, p. 618
Medication allergy, p. 613
Medication error, p. 624
Medication interaction, p. 613
Medication reconciliation, p. 625
Metric system, p. 617
Nurse Practice Acts (NPAs), p. 610
Ophthalmic, p. 638
Parenteral administration, p. 615
Peak, p. 614
Pharmacokinetics, p. 611
Polypharmacy, p. 633
Prescriptions, p. 623
Pressurized metered-dose inhalers (pMDIs), p. 638
Side effects, p. 613
Solution, p. 618
Subcutaneous, p. 615
Sublingual, p. 615
Synergistic effect, p. 613
Therapeutic effect, p. 613
Toxic effects, p. 613
Transdermal disk, p. 616
Trough, p. 614
Verbal order, p. 621
Z-track method, p. 650

(e) MEDIA RESOURCES

http://evolve.elsevier.com/Potter/fundamentals/

- Review Questions
- Video Clips
- Concept Map Creator
- Case Study with Questions
- Skills Performance Checklists
- Audio Glossary
- Calculations Tutorial
- Content Updates

Patients with health problems use a variety of strategies to restore or maintain their health. One strategy they often use is medication, a substance used in the diagnosis, treatment, cure, relief, or prevention of health problems. No matter where patients receive health care (i.e., hospitals, clinics, or home), nurses play an essential role in preparing, administering, and evaluating the effects of medications. Family members, friends, or home care personnel often administer medications when patients cannot administer them themselves at home. In all settings nurses are responsible for evaluating the effects of medications on the patient's ongoing health status, teaching him or her about medications and side effects, encouraging adherence to the medication regimen, and evaluating the patient's and family caregiver's ability to administer medications.

SCIENTIFIC KNOWLEDGE BASE

Because medication administration and evaluation are a critical part of nursing practice, nurses need to understand the actions and effects of all medications taken by their patients. Administering medications safely requires an understanding of legal aspects of health care, pharmacology, pharmacokinetics, the life sciences, pathophysiology, human anatomy, and mathematics.

Medication Legislation and Standards

Federal Regulations. The U.S. government protects the health of the people by ensuring that medications are safe and effective. The first American law to regulate medications was the Pure Food and Drug Act. This law simply requires all medications to be free of impure products. Subsequent legislation created standards related to safety, potency, and efficacy. Currently the Food and Drug Administration (FDA) enforces medication laws that ensure that all medications on the market undergo vigorous testing before they are sold to the public. Federal medication laws also control medication sales and distribution; testing, naming, and labeling; and the use of controlled substances. Official publications such as the *United States Pharmacopeia* (USP) and the *National Formulary* set standards for medication strength, quality, purity, packaging, safety, labeling, and dose form. In 1993 the FDA instituted the MedWatch program. This voluntary program encourages nurses and other health care professionals to report when a medication, product, or medical event causes serious harm to a patient by completing the MedWatch form. The form is available on the MedWatch website (USFDA, 2015).

BOX 32-1 Guidelines for Safe Narcotic Administration and Control

- Store all narcotics in a locked, secure cabinet or container (e.g., computerized, locked cabinets are preferred).
- Maintain a running count of narcotics by counting them whenever dispensing them. If you find a discrepancy, correct and report it immediately.
- Use a special inventory record each time a narcotic is dispensed. Records are often kept electronically and provide an accurate ongoing count of narcotics used, wasted, and remaining.
- Use the record to document the patient's name, date, time of medication administration, name of medication, and dosage. If the agency keeps a paper record, the nurse dispensing the medication signs the record. If the agency uses a computerized system, the computer records the nurse's name.
- A second nurse witnesses disposal of the unused part if a nurse gives only part of a dose of a controlled substance. Computerized systems record the nurses' names electronically. If paper records are kept, both nurses sign their names on the form. Follow agency policy for appropriate waste of narcotics. Do not place wasted parts of medications in sharps containers.

State and Local Regulation of Medication. State and local medication laws must conform to federal legislation. States often have additional controls, including control of substances not regulated by the federal government. Local governmental bodies regulate the use of alcohol and tobacco.

Health Care Institutions and Medication Laws. Health care agencies establish individual policies to meet federal, state, and local regulations. The size of the agency, the services it provides, and the professional personnel it employs influence these policies. Agency policies are often more restrictive than governmental controls. For example, a common agency policy is the automatic discontinuation of narcotics after a set number of days. Although a health care provider can reorder the narcotic, this policy helps to control unnecessarily prolonged medication therapy because it requires the health care provider to regularly review the need for the medication.

Medication Regulations and Nursing Practice. State Nurse Practice Acts (NPAs) define the scope of nurses' professional functions and responsibilities. Most NPAs are purposefully broad so nurses' professional responsibilities are not limited. Health care agencies can interpret specific actions allowed under NPAs; but they cannot modify, expand, or restrict the intent of the act. The primary intent of NPAs is to protect the public from unskilled, undereducated, and unlicensed personnel.

A nurse is responsible for following legal provisions when administering controlled substances such as opioids, which are carefully controlled through federal and state guidelines. Violations of the Controlled Substances Act are punishable by fines, imprisonment, and loss of nurse licensure. Hospitals and other health care agencies have policies for the proper storage and distribution of narcotics (Box 32-1).

Pharmacological Concepts

Medication Names. Some medications have as many as three different names. The chemical name of a medication provides an exact description of its composition and molecular structure. Nurses rarely use chemical names in clinical practice. An example of a chemical name is *N*-acetyl-para-aminophenol, which is commonly known as Tylenol. The manufacturer who first develops the medication gives the generic or nonproprietary name, with United States Adopted Names (USAN) Council approval (AMA, 2015). Acetaminophen is an example of the generic name for Tylenol. The generic name becomes the official name listed in official publications such as the United States Pharmacopeia (USP). The trade name, brand name, or proprietary name is the name under which a manufacturer markets a medication. The trade name has the symbol (™) at the upper right of the name, indicating that the manufacturer has trademarked the name of the medication (e.g., Panadol™, and Tempra™).

Manufacturers choose trade names that are easy to pronounce, spell, and remember. Many companies produce the same medication, and similarities in trade names are often confusing. Therefore be careful to obtain the exact name and spelling for each medication you administer to your patients. Because similarities in drug names are a common cause of medical errors, the Institute for Safe Medication Practices (ISMP) (2015a) (http://www.ismp.org/Tools/confuseddrugnames.pdf) publishes a list of medications that are frequently confused with one another. The ISMP recommends the use of Food and Drug Administration (FDA)-approved tall-man or mixed-case letters when possible (e.g., aMILoride versus amLODIPine) to help health care providers easily recognize the difference between these commonly confused medications.

Classification. Medication classification indicates the effect of a medication on a body system, the symptoms a medication relieves, or its desired effect. Usually each class contains more than one medication that is used for the same type of health problem. For example, patients who have asthma often take a variety of medications to control their illness such as beta$_2$-adrenergic agonists. The *beta$_2$-adrenergic* classification contains more than 15 different medications (Lehne, 2013). Some medications are in more than one class. For example, aspirin is an analgesic, an antipyretic, and an antiinflammatory medication.

Medication Forms. Medications are available in a variety of forms, or preparations. The form of the medication determines its route of administration. The composition of a medication enhances its absorption and metabolism. Many medications come in several forms such as tablets, capsules, elixirs, and suppositories. When

TABLE 32-1 Forms of Medication

Form	Description
Medication Forms Commonly Prepared for Administration by Oral Route	
Solid Forms	
Caplet	Solid dosage form for oral use; shaped like capsule and coated for ease of swallowing
Capsule	Medication encased in gelatin shell
Tablet	Powdered medication compressed into hard disk or cylinder; in addition to primary medication, contains binders (adhesive to allow powder to stick together), disintegrators (to promote tablet dissolution), lubricants (for ease of manufacturing), and fillers (for convenient tablet size)
Enteric-coated tablet	Coated tablet that does not dissolve in stomach; coatings dissolve in intestine, where medication is absorbed
Liquid Forms	
Elixir	Clear fluid containing water and/or alcohol; often sweetened
Extract	Concentrated medication form made by removing the active part of medication from its other components
Aqueous solution	Substance dissolved in water and syrups
Aqueous suspension	Finely dissolved drug particles dispersed in liquid medium; when suspension is left standing, particles settle to bottom of container
Syrup	Medication dissolved in a concentrated sugar solution
Other Oral Forms and Terms Associated with Oral Preparations	
Troche (lozenge)	Flat, round tablets that dissolve in mouth to release medication; not meant for ingestion
Aerosol	Aqueous medication sprayed and absorbed in mouth and upper airway; not meant for ingestion
Sustained release	Tablet or capsule that contains small particles of a medication coated with material that requires a varying amount of time to dissolve
Medication Forms Commonly Prepared for Administration by Topical Route	
Ointment (salve or cream)	Semisolid, externally applied preparation, usually containing one or more medications
Liniment	Usually contains alcohol, oil, or soapy emollient applied to skin
Lotion	Semiliquid suspension that usually protects, cools, or cleanses skin
Paste	Thick ointment; absorbed through skin more slowly than ointment; often used for skin protection
Transdermal disk or patch	Medicated disk or patch absorbed through skin slowly over long period of time (e.g., 24 hours)
Medication Forms Commonly Prepared for Administration by Parenteral Route	
Solution	Sterile preparation that contains water with one or more dissolved compounds
Powder	Sterile particles of medication that are dissolved in a sterile liquid (e.g., water, normal saline) before administration
Medication Forms Commonly Prepared for Instillation Into Body Cavities	
Intraocular disk	Small, flexible oval (similar to contact lens) consisting of two soft, outer layers and a middle layer containing medication; slowly releases medication when moistened by ocular fluid
Suppository	Solid dosage form mixed with gelatin and shaped in form of pellet for insertion into body cavity (rectum or vagina); melts when it reaches body temperature, releasing medication for absorption

administering a medication, be certain to use the proper form (Table 32-1).

Pharmacokinetics As the Basis of Medication Actions

For a medication to be useful therapeutically, it must be taken into a patient's body; be absorbed and distributed to cells, tissues, or a specific organ; and alter physiological functions. **Pharmacokinetics** is the study of how medications enter the body, reach their site of action, metabolize, and exit the body. You use knowledge of pharmacokinetics when timing medication administration, selecting the route of administration, and evaluating a patient's response.

Absorption. **Absorption** occurs when medication molecules pass into the blood from the site of medication administration. Factors that influence absorption are the route of administration, ability of the medication to dissolve, blood flow to the site of administration, body surface area (BSA), and lipid solubility of medication.

Route of Administration. Each route of medication administration has a different rate of absorption. When applying medications on the skin, absorption is slow because of the physical makeup of the skin. Because orally administered medications pass through the gastrointestinal (GI) tract, the overall rate of absorption is usually slow. Medications placed on the mucous membranes and respiratory airways are absorbed quickly because these tissues contain many blood vessels. Intravenous (IV) **injection** produces the most rapid absorption because medications are available immediately when they enter the systemic circulation.

Ability of a Medication to Dissolve. The ability of an oral medication to dissolve depends largely on its form or preparation. The body absorbs solutions and suspensions already in a liquid state more readily than tablets or capsules. Acidic medications pass through the gastric mucosa rapidly. Medications that are basic are not absorbed before reaching the small intestine.

Blood Flow to the Site of Administration. The blood supply to the site of administration will determine how quickly the body can absorb a drug. Medications are absorbed as blood comes in contact with the site of administration. The richer the blood supply to the site of administration, the faster a medication is absorbed.

Body Surface Area. When a medication comes in contact with a large surface area, it is absorbed at a faster rate. This helps explain why the majority of medications are absorbed in the small intestine rather than the stomach (Lehne, 2013).

Lipid Solubility. Because the cell membrane has a lipid layer, highly lipid-soluble medications cross cell membranes easily and are absorbed quickly. Another factor that often affects medication absorption is whether or not food is in the stomach. Some oral medications are absorbed more easily when administered between meals because food changes the structure of a medication and sometimes impairs its absorption. When some medications are administered together, they interfere with one another, impairing the absorption of both medications.

Safe medication administration requires knowledge of factors that alter or impair absorption of prescribed medications. You need to understand medication pharmacokinetics, a patient's health history, physical examination data, and knowledge gained through daily patient interactions. Use your knowledge to plan medication administration times that will promote optimal absorption. For example, plan medication administration times around meals (e.g., before or after meals) when medications interact with food. When they interact with one another, make sure that you do not give them at the same time. Consult and collaborate with your patient's health care provider or a pharmacist when setting medication times to ensure that the patient achieves the therapeutic effect of all medications. Before administering any medication, check pharmacology books, drug references, or package inserts or consult with pharmacists to identify medication-medication or medication-food interactions.

Distribution. After a medication is absorbed, it is distributed within the body to tissues and organs and ultimately to its specific site of action. The rate and extent of distribution depend on the physical and chemical properties of the medication and the physiology of the person taking it.

Circulation. Once a medication enters the bloodstream, it is carried throughout the tissues and organs. How fast it reaches a site depends on the vascularity of the various tissues and organs. Conditions that limit blood flow or blood perfusion inhibit the distribution of a medication. For example, patients with heart failure have impaired circulation, which slows medication delivery to the intended site of action. Therefore the effectiveness of medications in these patients is often delayed or altered.

Membrane Permeability. Membrane permeability refers to the ability of a medication to pass through tissues and membranes to enter target cells. To be distributed to an organ, a medication has to pass through all of the tissues and biological membranes of the organ. Some membranes serve as barriers to the passage of medications. For example, the blood-brain barrier allows only fat-soluble medications to pass into the brain and cerebral spinal fluid. Therefore central nervous system infections often require treatment with antibiotics injected directly into the subarachnoid space in the spinal cord. Some older adults experience adverse effects (e.g., confusion) as a result of the change in the permeability of the blood-brain barrier, with easier passage of fat-soluble medications.

Protein Binding. The degree to which medications bind to serum proteins such as albumin affects their distribution. Most medications partially bind to albumin, reducing the ability of a drug to exert pharmacological activity. The unbound or "free" medication is its active form. Older adults and patients with liver disease or malnutrition have decreased albumin in the bloodstream. Because more medication is unbound in these patients, they are at risk for an increase in medication activity, toxicity, or both.

Metabolism. After a medication reaches its site of action, it becomes metabolized into a less active or an inactive form that is easier to excrete. Biotransformation occurs under the influence of enzymes that detoxify, break down, and remove biologically active chemicals. Most biotransformation occurs within the liver, although the lungs, kidneys, blood, and intestines also metabolize medications. The liver is especially important because its specialized structure oxidizes and transforms many toxic substances. The liver degrades many harmful chemicals before they become distributed to the tissues. If a decrease in liver function occurs such as with aging or liver disease, a medication is usually eliminated more slowly, resulting in its accumulation. Patients are at risk for medication toxicity if organs that metabolize medications are not functioning correctly. For example, a small sedative dose of a barbiturate sometimes causes a patient with liver disease to lapse into a coma.

Excretion. After medications are metabolized, they exit the body through the kidneys, liver, bowel, lungs, and exocrine glands. The chemical makeup of a medication determines the organ of excretion. Gaseous and volatile compounds such as nitrous oxide and alcohol exit through the lungs. Deep breathing and coughing (see Chapter 41) help patients eliminate anesthetic gases more rapidly after surgery. The exocrine glands excrete lipid-soluble medications. When medications exit through sweat glands, the skin often becomes irritated, requiring you to teach patients good hygiene practices (see Chapter 40). If a medication is excreted through the mammary glands, there is a risk that a nursing infant will ingest the chemicals. Check the safety of any medication used in breastfeeding women.

The GI tract is another route for medication excretion. Medications that enter the hepatic circulation are broken down by the liver and excreted into the bile. After chemicals enter the intestines through the biliary tract, the intestines resorb them. Factors that increase peristalsis (e.g., laxatives and enemas) accelerate medication excretion through the feces, whereas factors that slow peristalsis (e.g., inactivity and improper diet) often prolong the effects of a medication.

The kidneys are the main organs for medication excretion. Some medications escape extensive metabolism and exit unchanged in the urine. Others undergo biotransformation in the liver before the kidneys excrete them. Maintenance of an adequate fluid intake (50 mL/kg/hr) promotes proper elimination of medications for the average adult. If a patient's renal function declines, the kidneys cannot excrete medications adequately. Thus the risk for medication toxicity increases. Health care providers usually reduce medication doses when this happens.

Types of Medication Action

Medications vary considerably in the way they act and their types of action. Patients do not always respond in the same way to each successive dose of a medication. Sometimes the same medication causes very different responses in different patients. Therefore you need to understand all the effects that medications you administer have on patients.

Therapeutic Effects. The therapeutic effect is the expected or predicted physiological response caused by a medication. For example, nitroglycerin reduces cardiac workload and increases myocardial oxygen supply. Some medications have more than one therapeutic effect. For example, prednisone, a steroid, decreases swelling, inhibits inflammation, reduces allergic responses, and prevents rejection of transplanted organs. Knowing the desired therapeutic effect for each medication allows you to provide patient education and accurately evaluate the desired effect of a medication.

Adverse Effects. Every medication has the ability to harm a patient. Undesired, unintended, and often unpredictable responses to medication are referred to as adverse effects. Adverse drug effects range from mild to severe. Some happen immediately, whereas others develop over time. Be alert and assess for unusual individual responses to drugs, especially with newly prescribed medications. Patients most at risk for adverse medication reactions include the very young and older adults, women, patients taking multiple medications, patients extremely underweight or overweight, and patients with renal or liver disease. If adverse effects are mild and tolerable, patients often remain on the medications. However, if they are not tolerated and are potentially harmful, stop giving the medication immediately. When adverse responses to medications occur, the health care provider discontinues the medication immediately. Health care providers report adverse effects to the FDA using the MedWatch program (USFDA, 2015).

Side Effects. A side effect is a predictable and often unavoidable adverse effect produced at a usual therapeutic dose. For example, some antihypertensive medications cause impotence in men. Side effects range from being harmless to causing serious symptoms or injury. If the side effects are serious enough to negate the beneficial effects of the therapeutic action of the medication, the health care provider discontinues the medication. Patients often stop taking medications because of side effects, the most common of which are anorexia, nausea, vomiting, constipation, drowsiness, and diarrhea.

Toxic Effects. Toxic effects often develop after prolonged intake of a medication or when a medication accumulates in the blood because of impaired metabolism or excretion. Excess amounts of a medication within the body sometimes have lethal effects, depending on its action. For example, toxic levels of morphine, an opioid, cause severe respiratory depression and death. Antidotes are available to treat specific types of medication toxicity. For example, naloxone (Narcan), an opioid antagonist, reverses the effects of opioid toxicity.

Idiosyncratic Reactions. Medications sometimes cause unpredictable effects such as an idiosyncratic reaction, in which a patient overreacts or underreacts to a medication or has a reaction different from normal. For example, a child who receives diphenhydramine (Benadryl), an antihistamine, becomes extremely agitated or excited instead of drowsy. It is not always possible to predict if a patient will have an idiosyncratic response to a medication.

Allergic Reactions. Allergic reactions also are unpredictable responses to a medication. Some patients become immunologically sensitized to the initial dose of a medication. With repeated administration the patient develops an allergic response to it, its chemical preservatives, or a metabolite. The medication or chemical acts as an antigen, triggering the release of the antibodies in the body. A patient's medication allergy symptoms vary, depending on the individual and the medication (Table 32-2). Among the different classes of medications, antibiotics cause a high incidence of allergic reactions. Severe or anaphylactic reactions, which are life threatening, are characterized by sudden constriction of bronchiolar muscles, edema of the pharynx and larynx, and severe wheezing and shortness of breath. Immediate medical attention is required to treat anaphylactic reactions. A patient with a known history of an allergy to a medication needs to avoid taking that medication in the future and wear an identification bracelet or medal (Figure 32-1), which alerts nurses and other health care providers to the allergy if a patient is unable to communicate when receiving medical care.

TABLE 32-2 Mild Allergic Reactions

Symptom	Description
Urticaria (hives)	Raised, irregularly shaped skin eruptions with varying sizes and shapes; eruptions have reddened margins and pale centers
Rash	Small, raised vesicles that are usually reddened; often distributed over entire body
Pruritus	Itching of skin; accompanies most rashes
Rhinitis	Inflammation of mucous membranes lining nose; causes swelling and clear, watery discharge

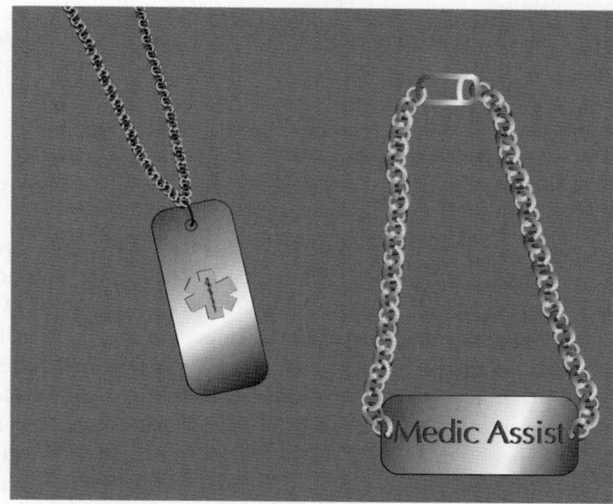

FIGURE 32-1 Allergy identification bracelet and medal.

Medication Interactions. When one medication modifies the action of another, a medication interaction occurs. Medication interactions are common when individuals take several medications. Some medications increase or diminish the action of others or alter the way another medication is absorbed, metabolized, or eliminated from the body. When two medications have a synergistic effect, their combined effect is greater than the effect of the medications when given separately. For example, alcohol is a central nervous system depressant that has a synergistic effect on antihistamines, antidepressants, barbiturates, and narcotic analgesics. Sometimes a medication interaction is desired. Health care providers often combine medications to create an interaction that has a beneficial effect. For example, a patient with high blood pressure takes several medications such as diuretics and vasodilators that act together to control blood pressure when one medication is not effective on its own.

Timing of Medication Dose Responses

Medications administered intravenously enter the bloodstream and act immediately, whereas those given in other routes take time to enter the bloodstream and have an effect. The quantity and distribution of a medication in different body compartments change constantly.

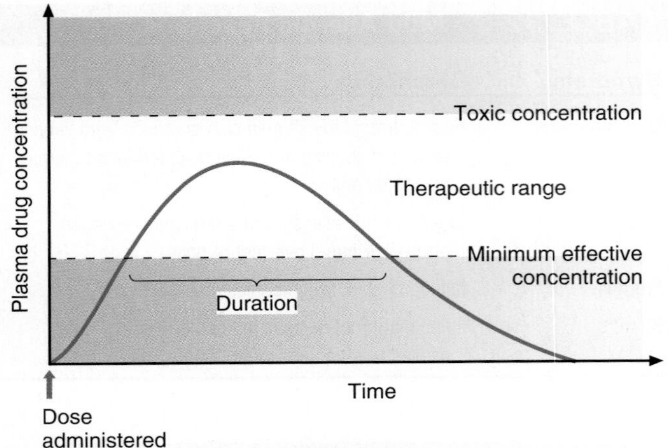

FIGURE 32-2 The therapeutic range of a medication occurs between the minimum effective concentration and the toxic concentration. (From Lehne RA: *Pharmacology for nursing care*, ed 8, St Louis, 2013, Saunders.)

Medications are ordered at various times, depending on when their response begins, becomes most intense, and ceases.

The minimum effective concentration (MEC) is the plasma level of a medication below which the effect of the medication does not occur. The toxic concentration is the level at which toxic effects occur. When a medication is prescribed, the goal is to achieve a constant blood level within a safe therapeutic range, which falls between the MEC and the toxic concentration (Figure 32-2). When a medication is administered repeatedly, its serum level fluctuates between doses. The highest level is called the **peak** concentration, and the lowest level is called the **trough** concentration. After reaching its peak, the serum concentration of the medication falls progressively. With IV **infusions** the peak concentration occurs quickly, but the serum level also begins to fall immediately. Some medication doses (e.g., vancomycin) are based on peak and trough serum levels. The trough level is generally drawn 30 minutes before administering the drug, and the peak level is drawn whenever the drug is expected to reach its peak concentration. The time it takes for a drug to reach its peak concentration varies, depending on the pharmacokinetics of the medication.

All medications have a **biological half-life**, which is the time it takes for excretion processes to lower the amount of unchanged medication by half. A medication with a short half-life needs to be given more frequently than a medication with a longer half-life. The half-life does not change, no matter how much medication is given. For example, if the nurse gives 1 g of a medication that has a half-life of 8 hours, the patient excretes 500 mg of the medication in 8 hours. In the next 8 hours the patient excretes 250 mg. This process continues until the medication is totally eliminated from the body.

To maintain a therapeutic plateau the patient must receive regular fixed doses. For example, pain medications for certain cancer patients are most effective when they are given around the clock (ATC) rather than when the patient intermittently complains of pain because ATC allows the body to maintain an almost constant level of pain medication. After an initial medication dose, a patient receives each successive dose when the previous dose reaches its half-life (Burchum and Rosenthal, 2016).

Safe drug administration involves adherence to prescribed doses and dosage schedules (Table 32-3). Some agencies set schedules for medication administration. However, nurses are able to alter this schedule on the basis of knowledge about a medication. For example, at some agencies medications that are to be taken once a day are given at 9:00 AM. However, if a medication works best when given before bedtime, the nurse administers it before the patient goes to sleep. In addition, acute care agencies use guidelines from the ISMP (CMS, 2011; ISMP, 2011) to determine safe, effective, and timely administration of scheduled medications. According to ISMP guidelines, hospitals need to determine which medications are time critical and which are non–time critical. Time-critical medications are medications in which early or delayed administration of maintenance doses (more than 30 minutes before or after the scheduled dose) will most likely result in harm or subtherapeutic responses in a patient. Non–time-critical medications include medications in which the timing of administration will most likely not affect the desired effect of the medication if given 1 to 2 hours before or after its scheduled time. You need to administer time-critical medications at a precise time or within 30 minutes before or after the scheduled time. You administer non–time-critical medications within 1 to 2 hours of their scheduled time. Follow the medication administration policies of your agency about the timing of medications to ensure that you administer medications at the right time (CMS, 2011; ISMP, 2011).

When you teach patients about medication schedules, use familiar language. For example, instruct a patient who needs to take a medication twice a day to take it in the morning and again in the evening. Use knowledge about time intervals and terms used to describe medication actions to anticipate the effect of a medication and educate the patient about when to expect a response (Table 32-4).

TABLE 32-3 Common Dosage Administration Schedules

Dosage Schedule (Meaning)	Abbreviation
Before meals	AC, ac
As desired	ad lib
Twice each day	BID, bid
After meals	PC, pc
Whenever there is a need	prn
Every morning, every AM	qam
Every hour	qh
Every day	Daily
Every 4 hours	Q4h
4 times per day	QID, qid
Give immediately	STAT, stat
3 times per day	TID, tid

QSEN QSEN: BUILDING COMPETENCY IN EVIDENCE-BASED PRACTICE. You are a member of the shared governance practice council in your hospital. The practice council is investigating evidence-based practices to reduce medication errors. The chairperson explains to the committee that evidence-based practice changes are based on the current best evidence, resources, nursing expertise, and patient preferences. One of the nurses asks, "How can we ensure that patient preferences are respected when we are administering medications?" How would you respond?

Answers to QSEN Activities can be found on the Evolve website.

TABLE 32-4 Terms Associated with Medication Actions

Term	Meaning
Onset	Time it takes after a medication is administered for it to produce a response
Peak	Time it takes for a medication to reach its highest effective concentration
Trough	Minimum blood serum concentration of medication reached just before the next scheduled dose
Duration	Time during which medication is present in concentration great enough to produce a response
Plateau	Blood serum concentration of medication reached and maintained after repeated fixed doses

Routes of Administration

The route prescribed for administering a medication depends on the properties and desired effect of the medication and the patient's physical and mental condition (Table 32-5). Work with the health care provider to determine the best route for a patient's medication.

Oral Routes. The oral route is the easiest and the most commonly used route of medication administration. Medications are given by mouth and swallowed with fluid. Oral medications have a slower onset of action and a more prolonged effect than parenteral medications. Patients generally prefer the oral route.

Sublingual Administration. Some medications (e.g., nitroglycerin) are readily absorbed after being placed under the tongue to dissolve (Figure 32-3). Instruct patients not to swallow a medication given by the sublingual route or drink anything until the medication is completely dissolved to ensure that the medication will have the desired effect.

Buccal Administration. Administration of a medication by the buccal route involves placing the solid medication in the mouth against the mucous membranes of the cheek until it dissolves (Figure 32-4). Teach patients to alternate cheeks with each subsequent dose to avoid mucosal irritation. Warn patients not to chew or swallow the medication or to take any liquids with it. A buccal medication acts locally on the mucosa or systemically as it is swallowed in a person's saliva.

Parenteral Routes. Parenteral administration involves injecting a medication into body tissues. The following are the four major sites of injection:

1. Intradermal (ID): Injection into the dermis just under the epidermis
2. Subcutaneous: Injection into tissues just below the dermis of the skin
3. Intramuscular (IM): Injection into a muscle
4. Intravenous (IV): Injection into a vein

Some medications are administered into body cavities through other routes, including epidural, intrathecal, intraosseous, intraperitoneal, intrapleural, and intraarterial. Nurses usually are not responsible for the administration of medications through these advanced techniques. Whether or not you actually administer a medication, you remain responsible for monitoring the integrity of the medication delivery system, understanding the therapeutic value of the medication, and evaluating a patient's response to the therapy.

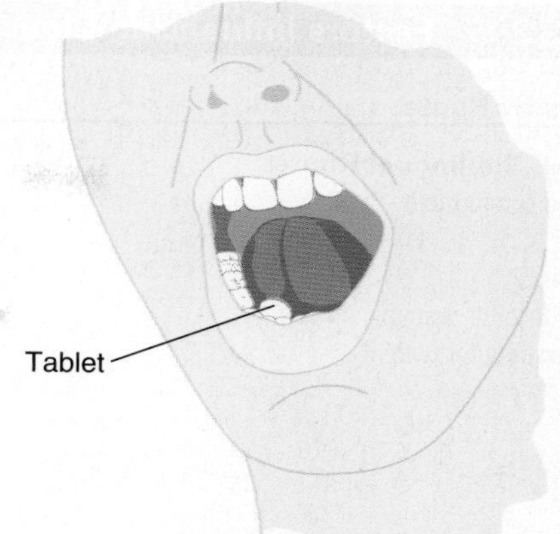

FIGURE 32-3 Sublingual administration of a tablet.

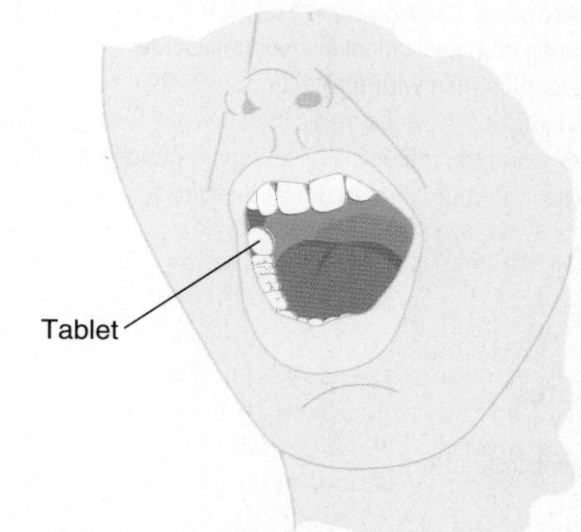

FIGURE 32-4 Buccal administration of a tablet.

Epidural. Epidural medications are administered in the epidural space via a catheter, which is placed by a nurse anesthetist or an anesthesiologist. This route is used for the administration of regional analgesia for surgical procedures (see Chapters 44 and 50). Nurses who have advanced education in the epidural route can administer medications by continuous infusion or a bolus dose.

Intrathecal. Physicians and specially educated nurses administer intrathecal medications through a catheter surgically placed in the subarachnoid space or one of the ventricles of the brain. Intrathecal medication administration often is a long-term treatment.

Intraosseous. This method of medication administration involves the infusion of medication directly into the bone marrow. It is used most commonly in infants and toddlers who have poor access to their intravascular space or when an emergency arises and IV access is impossible.

Intraperitoneal. Medications administered into the peritoneal cavity are absorbed into the circulation. Chemotherapeutic agents, insulin, and antibiotics are administered in this fashion.

Intrapleural. A syringe and needle or a chest tube is used to administer intrapleural medications directly into the pleural space. Chemotherapeutic agents are the most common medications administered via this method. Physicians also instill medications that help resolve persistent pleural effusion to promote adhesion between the visceral and parietal pleura. This is called *pleurodesis*.

Intraarterial. Intraarterial medications are administered directly into the arteries. Intraarterial infusions are common in patients who have arterial clots and receive clot-dissolving agents. A nurse manages

TABLE 32-5 Factors Influencing Choice of Administration Routes

Advantages by Route	Disadvantages/Contraindications
Oral, Buccal, Sublingual Routes	
Convenient and comfortable Economical Easy to administer Often produce local or systemic effects Rarely cause anxiety for patient	Oral route is avoided when patient has alterations in gastrointestinal (GI) function (e.g., nausea, vomiting), reduced GI motility (after general anesthesia or bowel inflammation), and surgical resection of the GI tract. Oral administration is contraindicated in patients unable to swallow (e.g., patients with neuromuscular disorders, esophageal strictures, mouth lesions). Oral administration is contraindicated in patients who are unconscious, confused, or unable or unwilling to swallow or hold medication under tongue. Oral medications cannot be administered when patients have gastric suction; are contraindicated before some tests or surgery. Oral medications sometimes irritate lining of GI tract, discolor teeth, or have unpleasant taste. Gastric secretions destroy some medications.
Parenteral Routes (Subcutaneous, Intramuscular, Intravenous, Intradermal)	
Can be used when oral medications are contraindicated More rapid absorption than with topical or oral routes Intravenous (IV) infusion provides medication delivery when patient is critically ill or long-term therapy is necessary; if peripheral perfusion is poor, IV route preferred over injections	There is risk of introducing infection. Some medications are expensive. Some patients experience pain from repeated needlesticks. Subcutaneous, intramuscular (IM), and intradermal (ID) routes are avoided in patients with bleeding tendencies. There is risk of tissue damage. IM and IV routes have higher absorption rates, thus placing patient at higher risk for reactions. They often cause considerable anxiety in many patients, especially children.
Topical Routes	
Skin	
Primarily provides local effect Painless Limited side effects	Patients with skin abrasions are at risk for rapid medication absorption and systemic effects. Medications are absorbed through skin slowly.
Transdermal	
Prolonged systemic effects with limited side effects	Medication leaves oily or pasty substance on skin and sometimes soils clothing.
Mucous Membranes*	
Therapeutic effects provided by local application to involved sites Aqueous solutions readily absorbed and capable of causing systemic effects Potential route of administration when oral medications are contraindicated	Mucous membranes are highly sensitive to some medication concentrations. Patients with ruptured eardrum cannot receive ear irrigations. Insertion of rectal and vaginal medication often causes embarrassment. Rectal suppositories contraindicated if patient has had rectal surgery or if active rectal bleeding is present.
Other Routes	
Inhalation	
Provides rapid relief for local respiratory problems Used for introduction of general anesthetic gases	Some local agents cause serious systemic effects.
Intraocular Disk	
Route advantageous because it does not require frequent administration as eyedrops do	Local reactions possible; expensive Patients must be taught to insert and remove disk Contraindicated in eye infections

*Includes eyes, ears, nose, vagina, rectum, and ostomy.

a continuous infusion of the clot-dissolving agent and carefully monitors the integrity of the infusion to prevent inadvertent disconnection of the system and subsequent bleeding.

Other methods of medication administration that are usually limited to physician administration are **intracardiac**, an injection of a medication directly into cardiac tissue, and **intraarticular**, an injection of a medication into a joint.

Topical Administration. Medications applied to the skin and mucous membranes generally have local effects. You apply topical medications to the skin by painting or spreading the medication over an area, applying moist dressings, soaking body parts in a solution, or giving medicated baths. Systemic effects often occur if a patient's skin is thin or broken down, the medication concentration is high, or contact with the skin is prolonged. A **transdermal disk** or patch (e.g., nitroglycerin, scopolamine, and estrogens) has systemic effects. The disk secures the medicated ointment to the skin. These topical applications are left in place for as little as 12 hours or as long as 7 days.

You apply topical medications to mucous membranes in the following ways:

1. Direct application of a liquid or ointment (e.g., eyedrops, gargling, or swabbing the throat)
2. Insertion of a medication into a body cavity (e.g., placing a suppository in rectum or vagina or inserting medicated packing into vagina)
3. Instillation of fluid into a body cavity (e.g., eardrops, nose drops, or bladder and rectal instillation [fluid is retained])
4. Irrigation of a body cavity (e.g., flushing eye, ear, vagina, bladder, or rectum with medicated fluid [fluid is not retained])
5. Spraying a medication into a body cavity (e.g., instillation into nose and throat)

Inhalation Route. The deeper passages of the respiratory tract provide a large surface area for medication absorption. Nurses administer inhaled medications through the nasal and oral passages or endotracheal or tracheostomy tubes. Endotracheal tubes enter the patient's mouth and end in the trachea, whereas tracheostomy tubes enter the trachea directly through an incision made in the neck. Inhaled medications are readily absorbed and work rapidly because of the rich vascular alveolar capillary network present in the pulmonary tissue. Many inhaled medications have local or systemic effects.

Intraocular Route. Intraocular medication delivery involves inserting a medication similar to a contact lens into a patient's eye. The eye medication disk has two soft outer layers that have medication enclosed in them. The nurse inserts the disk into the patient's eye, much like a contact lens. The medication remains in the eye for up to 1 week.

Systems of Medication Measurement

The proper administration of a medication depends on your ability to compute medication doses accurately and measure medications correctly. Fatal errors often occur when nurses make mistakes in calculating or measuring medications. As a nurse you are responsible for checking calculations carefully before giving a medication. Many agencies have policies related to the administration of high-risk medications (e.g., heparin and insulin) that may need a second nurse check before administration.

Medication therapy uses the metric, apothecary, and household systems of measurement. The apothecary system is used infrequently today. Although the U.S. Congress has not officially adopted the metric system, most health professionals in the United States use it.

Metric System. As a decimal system, the metric system is the most logically organized. You convert and compute metric units using simple multiplication and division. Each basic unit of measurement is organized into units of 10. Multiplying or dividing by 10 forms secondary units. In multiplication the decimal point moves to the right; in division the decimal moves to the left. For example:

$$10 \text{ mg} \times 10 = 100 \text{ mg}$$
$$10 \text{ mg} \div 10 = 1 \text{ mg}$$

The basic units of measurement in the metric system are the meter (length), the liter (volume), and the gram (weight). For medication calculations only use the volume and weight units. The metric system uses lowercase or capital letters or a combination of lowercase and capital letters to designate basic units:

Gram = g or Gm
Liter = l or L
Milligram = mg
Milliliter = mL

A system of Latin prefixes designates subdivision of the basic units: *deci-* (1/10 or 0.1), *centi-* (1/100 or 0.01), and *milli-* (1/1000 or 0.001). Greek prefixes designate multiples of the basic units: *deka-* (10), *hecto-* (100), and *kilo-* (1000). When writing medication doses in metric units, health care providers and nurses use fractions or multiples of a unit. Convert fractions to decimals.

500 mg or 0.5 g, *not* ½ g
10 mL or 0.01 L, *not* $\frac{1}{100}$ L

Many actual and potential medication errors happen with the use of fractions and decimal points. Follow practice standards when medications are ordered in fractions to prevent these errors. For example, to make the decimal point more visible, a leading zero is *always* placed in front of a decimal (e.g., use 0.25 *not* .25). *Never* use a trailing zero (i.e., a zero after a decimal point) because, if a health care worker does not see the decimal point, the patient may receive 10 times more medication than that prescribed (e.g., use 5 *not* 5.0) (ISMP, 2013a).

Household Measurements. Household units of measure are familiar to most people. Household measures include drops, teaspoons, tablespoons, and cups for volume and pints and quarts for weight. The advantage of household measurements is their convenience and familiarity. Their disadvantage is their inaccuracy if a patient uses household utensils such as teaspoons and cups. Encourage patients to never use household measuring devices to give liquid medicines. The devices are inaccurate and may deliver more or less than prescribed (Consumer Med Safety, 2015). Today's over-the-counter (OTC) liquid medicines almost always have their own measuring devices (Consumer Med Safety, 2015). Scales to measure pints or quarts are not well calibrated. To calculate medications accurately, you need to know common equivalents of metric and household units (Table 32-6).

TABLE 32-6 Equivalents of Measurement

Metric	Apothecary	Household
1 mL	15-16 minims*	15 drops (gtt)
5 mL	1 dram*	1 teaspoon (tsp)
15 mL	4 drams*	1 tablespoon (tbsp)
30 mL	1 fluid ounce	2 tablespoons (tbsp)
240 mL	8 fluid ounces	1 cup (c)
480 mL (approximately 500 mL)	1 pint (pt)	1 pint (pt)
960 mL (approximately 1 L)	1 quart (qt)	1 quart (qt)
3840 mL (approximately 4 L)	1 gallon (gal)	1 gallon (gal)

*Minims and drams are no longer acceptable units of measure for medication administration, although some medication cups and syringes still have them listed. Use mL for safe medication preparation (Morris, 2014).

Solutions. Nurses use solutions of various concentrations for injections, irrigations, and infusions. A solution is a given mass of solid substance dissolved in a known volume of fluid or a given volume of liquid dissolved in a known volume of another fluid. When a solid is dissolved in a fluid, the concentration is in units of mass per units of volume (e.g., g/L, mg/mL). You can also express a concentration of a solution as a percentage. For example, a 10% solution is 10 g of solid dissolved in 100 mL of solution. A proportion also expresses concentrations. A $\frac{1}{1000}$ solution represents a solution containing 1 g of solid in 1000 mL of liquid or 1 mL of liquid mixed with 1000 mL of another liquid.

NURSING KNOWLEDGE BASE

The Institute of Medicine (IOM) published the book *To Err Is Human: Building a Safer Health System* (IOM, 1999). This book created a new national awareness of problems within the health care system. It estimated that up to 98,000 people die in any given year from medical errors that occur in hospitals. This means that more people die from medical errors than from motor vehicle accidents, breast cancer, acquired immunodeficiency syndrome (AIDS), and workplace injuries. Health care experts estimate that medication-related errors for hospitalized patients cost more than $3.5 billion annually (CDC, 2012).

Nurses play an important role in patient safety, especially in the area of medication administration. The safe administration of medications is also an important topic for current nursing researchers (Box 32-2). As a nurse you need to know how to calculate medication doses accurately and understand the different roles that members of the health care team play in prescribing and administering medications. Apply your knowledge and think critically to ensure safe medication administration.

Clinical Calculations

To administer medications safely, you need to have an understanding of basic mathematics skills to calculate medication doses, mix solutions, and perform a variety of other activities. This is important because medications are not always dispensed in the unit of measure in which they are ordered. Medication companies package and bottle medications in standard dosages. For example, a patient's health care provider orders 20 mg of a medication that is available only in 40-mg vials. Nurses frequently convert available units of volume and weight to desired doses. Therefore it is important to be aware of equivalents in all major measurement systems. You use equivalents when performing other nursing actions such as when calculating patients' intake and output and IV flow rates.

Conversions Within One System. Converting measurements within one system is relatively easy; simply divide or multiply in the metric system. To change milligrams to grams, divide by 1000, moving the decimal 3 points to the left.

$$1000 \text{ mg} = 1 \text{ g}$$
$$350 \text{ mg} = 0.35 \text{ g}$$

To convert liters to milliliters, multiply by 1000 or move the decimal 3 points to the right.

$$1 \text{ L} = 1000 \text{ mL}$$
$$0.25 \text{ L} = 250 \text{ mL}$$

To convert units of measurement within the household system, consult an equivalent table. For example, when converting fluid ounces to quarts, you first need to know that 32 ounces is the equivalent of 1 quart. To convert 8 ounces to a quart measurement, divide 8 by 32 to get the equivalent, $\frac{1}{4}$ or 0.25 quart.

BOX 32-2 EVIDENCE-BASED PRACTICE

Reducing Errors During Medication Administration

PICO Question: In hospitals does the use of computerized prescription order entry (CPOE), automated medication dispensers (AMDs), and bar-code medication administration (BCMA) during medication administration decrease the incidence of medication errors made by nurses when compared with nurses who do not use these health technologies?

Evidence Summary

Medication administration is a highly complex process. Errors often result from problems within one or more parts of the process. Many errors occur either when a medication is ordered or when it is administered (Grou Volpe et al., 2014). Research shows that the implementation of medication administration technologies such as CPOE, AMD, and BCMA helps to decrease medication errors in various patient care settings (Ching et al., 2013; Cochran and Haynatzki, 2013; Cousein et al., 2014). However, health care agencies cannot rely on technology alone. Considering human factors such as staffing levels of nurses and pharmacists (Cochran and Haynatzki, 2013) and integrating technology into nursing work flow (Ching et al., 2013) are also essential in promoting medication safety.

Application to Nursing Practice

- The process of implementing medication administration technology is complex and needs to be well planned and involve health care staff, including nurses, to ensure successful implementation (Ching et al., 2013).
- Even though using CPOE, AMD, and BCMA reduces many medication errors, it does not eliminate all of them (Ching et al., 2013; Cousein et al., 2014). Therefore nurses need to remain vigilant and consistently follow medication administration policies and protocols to ensure safe medication administration.
- Because medication errors are often associated with high nursing workloads, increased complexity and acuity of patient care, and reduced pharmacy support, health care administrators, including nurse leaders, need to ensure appropriate nurse and pharmacist staffing levels that are based on patient acuity and workload (Cochran and Haynatzki, 2013; Grou Volpe et al., 2014).

Conversion Between Systems. Nurses frequently determine the proper dose of a medication by converting weights or volumes from one system of measurement to another. Thus sometimes you convert metric units to equivalent household measures for use at home. To calculate medications it is necessary to work with units in the same measurement system. Tables of equivalent measurements are available in all health care agencies. A pharmacist is also a good resource.

Before converting, compare the measurement system available with the system used when the medication was ordered. For example, a patient is ordered guaifenesin (Robitussin) 30 mL, but the patient only has tablespoons at home. To properly instruct him or her on how to prepare the dose, you convert mL to tablespoons, which requires you to know the equivalent or refer to a table such as Table 32-6.

Dose Calculations. Methods used to calculate medication doses include the ratio and proportion method, the formula method, and dimensional analysis. Before completing any calculation, make a mental estimate of the approximate and reasonable dosage. If the estimate does not match the calculated solution, recheck the calculation before preparing and administering the medication. Many nursing students are anxious when calculating medication doses. To enhance accuracy and reduce anxiety, think critically about the processes used during the calculation and practice doing calculations until you feel confident about your mathematics skills (Hunter Revell and McCurry, 2013). In addition, choose the method of calculation with which you are most comfortable and use it consistently (Morris, 2014). Most health care agencies require a nurse to double-check calculations with another nurse before giving medications, especially when the risk for giving the wrong medication is high (e.g., heparin, insulin). *Always* have another nurse double-check your work if you are unsure about the answer or if the answer to a medication calculation seems unreasonable or inappropriate.

The Ratio and Proportion Method. A ratio indicates the relationship between two numbers separated by a colon (:). The colon in the ratio indicates the need to use division. Think of a ratio as a fraction; the number to the left is the numerator, and the number to the right is the denominator. For example, the ratio 1:2 is the same as ½. A proportion is an equation that has two ratios of equal value. Write a proportion in one of three ways:

Example 1: $1:2 = 4:8$
Example 2: $1:2::4:8$
Example 3: $1/2 = 4/8$

In a proportion the first and last numbers are called the *extremes,* and the second and third numbers are called the *means.* When multiplying the extremes, the answer is the same when multiplying the means. For example, in the previous proportions, multiplying the extremes ($1 \times 8 = 8$) is the same result as multiplying the means ($2 \times 4 = 8$). Because of this relationship, if you know three of the numbers in the proportion, calculating the unknown fourth number is easy. The numbers need to all be in the same unit and system of measurement. To solve a calculation using the ratio and proportion method, first estimate the answer in your mind. Then set up the proportion, labeling all the terms. Put the terms of the ratio in the same sequence (e.g., mg : mL = mg : mL). Cross-multiply the means and the extremes and divide both sides by the number before the *x* to obtain the dosage. *Always* label the answer; if the answer is not close to the estimate, recheck the calculation.

Example: The health care provider orders 500 mg of amoxicillin to be administered in a gastric tube every 8 hours. The bottle of amoxicillin is labeled 400 mg/5 mL. Use the following steps to calculate how much amoxicillin to give:

1. **Estimate the answer:** The amount to be given is a little more than the labeled dose per 5 mL (unit dose) that is provided in the solution; therefore the answer is a little more than 5 mL.
2. **Set up the proportion:**

$$\frac{400 \text{ mg}}{5 \text{ mL}} = \frac{500 \text{ mg}}{x \text{ mL}}$$

3. **Cross-multiply the means and the extremes:**

$$400x = 500 \times 5$$
$$400x = 2500$$

4. **Divide both sides by the number before x:**

$$\frac{400x}{400} = \frac{2500}{400}$$
$$x = \frac{2500}{400}$$
$$x = 6.25 \text{ mL}$$

5. **Compare the estimate in Step 1 with the answer in Step 4:** The answer (6.25 mL) is close to the estimated amount (a little more than 5 mL). Therefore the answer is correct; prepare and administer 6.25 mL in the patient's gastric tube.

The Formula Method. Using this method requires you to first memorize the formula. Estimate the answer and then place all the information from the medication order into the formula. Label all the parts of the formula and ensure that all measures in the formula are in the same units and system of measurement before calculating the dosage. If the measures are not in the same measurement system, convert the numbers to the same system before calculating the dose. Calculate and label the answer and compare the answer with the estimated answer. If the estimate is not similar to the answer, recheck the calculation. Use the following basic formula when using the formula method:

$$\frac{\text{Dose ordered}}{\text{Dose on hand}} \times \text{Amount on hand} = \text{Amount to administer}$$

The dose ordered is the amount of medication prescribed. The dose on hand is the dose (e.g., mg, units) of medication supplied by the pharmacy. The amount on hand is the basic unit or quantity of the medication that contains the dose on hand. For solid medications the amount on hand is often one capsule; the amount of liquid on hand is sometimes 1 mL or 1 L, depending on the container. For example, a liquid medication comes in the strength of 125 mg per 5 mL. In this case 125 mg is the dose on hand, and 5 mL is the amount on hand. The amount to administer is the actual amount of medication the nurse administers. Always express the amount to administer in the same unit as the amount on hand.

Example: The health care provider orders morphine sulfate 2 mg IV. The medication is available in a vial containing 10 mg/mL. The formula is applied as follows:

1. **Estimate the answer:** The medication is a liquid; thus the answer will be in milliliters (mL). The amount to be given is less than ½ of the dose; thus the answer will be less than ½ mL.
2. **Set up the formula:**

$$\frac{\text{Dose ordered}}{\text{Dose on hand}} \times \text{Amount on hand} = \text{Amount to administer}$$
$$\frac{2 \text{ mg}}{10 \text{ mg}} \times 1 \text{ mL} = \text{Amount to administer}$$

3. **Calculate the answer:**

$$\frac{2 \text{ mg}}{10 \text{ mg}} \times 1 \text{ mL} = 0.2 \text{ mL}$$

4. **Compare the estimate in Step 1 with the answer in Step 3:** The answer is less than ½ mL; thus it is close to the estimated answer. Prepare 0.2 mL of the medication in a syringe and administer it to the patient.

Dimensional Analysis. Dimensional analysis is the factor-label or the unit-factor method. There is no need to memorize a formula since only one equation is needed and the same steps are used in solving every medication calculation. Nursing students who use dimensional analysis to calculate medication dosages often find it easier to calculate medications than when they use the formula method (Cookson, 2013). Use the following steps to calculate medication doses by dimensional analysis:

1. Identify the unit of measure that you need to administer. For example, if you are giving a pill, you usually give a tablet or a capsule; for parenteral or liquid oral medications, the unit is milliliters.
2. Estimate the answer.
3. Place the name or appropriate abbreviation for *x* on the left side of the equation (e.g., *x* tab, *x* mL).
4. Place available information from the problem in a fraction format on the right side of the equation. Place the abbreviation or unit that matches what you are going to administer (determined in Step 1) in the numerator.
5. Look at the medication order and add other factors into the problem. Set up the numerator so it matches the unit in the previous denominator.
6. Cancel out like units of measurement on the right side of the equation. You should end up with only one unit left in the equation, and it should match the unit on the left side of the equation.
7. Reduce to the lowest terms if possible and solve the problem or solve for *x*. Label your answer.
8. Compare your estimate from Step 1 with your answer in Step 2.

Example: The health care provider orders 0.45 g penicillin V potassium through a gastric tube. The vial label reads: penicillin V potassium 125 mg/5 mL.

1. **Identify the unit of measure that you need to administer.** This medication is given in a gastric tube, which is a liquid medication; therefore the answer will be in milliliters (mL).
2. **Estimate the answer.** The medication order is more than 3 times but less than 4 times the unit dose in the vial; thus the answer is more than 15 mL but less than 20 mL.
3. **Place the name or appropriate abbreviation for *x* on the left side of the equation.**

$$x \text{ mL} =$$

4. **Place available information from the problem in a fraction format on the right side of the equation.** Since the medication will be administered in milliliters, place mL in the numerator.

$$x \text{ mL} = \frac{5 \text{ mL}}{125 \text{ mg}}$$

5. **Look at the medication order and add other factors into the problem.** Set up the numerator so it matches the unit in the previous denominator. The order is for 0.45 g, and the medication is available in 125-mg bottles. Knowing that 1 g = 1000 mg, add this conversion to the calculation.

$$x \text{ mL} = \frac{5 \text{ mL}}{125 \text{ mg}} \times \frac{1000 \text{ mg}}{1 \text{ g}} \times \frac{0.45 \text{ g}}{1}$$

6. **Cancel out like units of measurement on the right side of the equation.**

$$x \text{ mL} = \frac{5 \text{ mL}}{125 \not{\text{mg}}} \times \frac{1000 \not{\text{mg}}}{1 \not{\text{g}}} \times \frac{0.45 \not{\text{g}}}{1}$$

7. **Reduce to the lowest terms if possible and solve the problem or solve for *x*.** Label your answer.

$$x \text{ mL} = \frac{5 \times 1000 \times 0.45}{125}$$

$$x = \frac{2250}{125}$$

$$x = 18 \text{ mL}$$

8. **Compare the estimate from Step 2 with the answer in Step 7.** The calculated answer is 18 mL, which is between 15 mL and 20 mL. This matches the estimate made in Step 2. Prepare and administer 18 mL of medication as ordered.

Pediatric Doses. Current evidence shows that children are at a much higher risk for experiencing a medication error than adults, and medication errors in children have a much greater chance of causing serious and even fatal consequences (Kaufmann et al., 2012; Rinke et al., 2014). Medication errors involving children frequently happen for the following reasons (Morris, 2014):

- Confusion between formulations for adults and children
- Availability of multiple pediatric concentrations of oral liquid medications
- Inaccurate preparation of medications that need to be diluted
- Similar packaging of medications and names of medications that look alike and sound alike
- Parents who do not understand how to prepare and administer medications correctly
- Errors in calculation and use of inaccurate measuring devices (e.g., household teaspoons and tablespoons) as opposed to devices made to measure small-volume doses

Calculating children's medication doses requires caution (Hockenberry and Wilson, 2015). Even small errors or discrepancies in medication amounts can affect a child's health negatively (Morris, 2014). A child's age, weight, and maturity of body systems affect the ability to metabolize and excrete medications. Nurses sometimes have difficulty evaluating a child's response to a medication, especially when he or she cannot communicate verbally. For example, a side effect of vancomycin is ototoxicity. If a child cannot talk yet, it is challenging to assess for ototoxicity. Use the following guidelines when calculating pediatric doses:

1. Most pediatric medications are ordered in milligrams per kilogram (mg/kg). Therefore weigh the patient in kilograms before administering medications. Avoid converting the patient's weight from pound to kilograms to prevent errors.
2. Pediatric doses are usually a lot smaller than adult doses for the same medication. You frequently use micrograms and small syringes (e.g., tuberculin or 1 mL).
3. IM doses are very small and usually do not exceed 1 mL in small children or 0.5 mL in infants.
4. Subcutaneous dosages are also very small and do not usually exceed 0.5 mL.
5. Most medications are not rounded off to the nearest tenth. Instead they are rounded to the nearest thousandth.
6. Measure dosages that are less than 1 mL in syringes that are marked in tenths of a milliliter if the dosage calculation comes out even and does not need to be rounded. Use a tuberculin syringe for medication preparation when the medication needs to be rounded to the nearest thousandth.
7. Estimate the patient's dose before beginning the calculation; label and compare the answer with the estimate before preparing the medication.
8. To determine if a dose is safe before giving the medication, compare and evaluate the amount of medication ordered over 24 hours with the recommended dosage.

Different formulas and methods are used to calculate drug dosages in children. The two most common methods of calculating pediatric dosages are based on a child's weight or BSA. BSA is used in rare situations (e.g., determining chemotherapy doses). Refer to a pediatric or pharmacology resource and consult with the patient's health care provider or the pharmacist if you have to calculate a medication based on BSA.

Most of the time you calculate medications based on a child's weight. You can use the ratio and proportion method, the formula method, or dimensional analysis to calculate a pediatric dose using body weight. Refer to the previous sections on ratio and proportion, formula method, and dimensional analysis to select a method easier for you to use.

Health Care Provider's Role

A physician, nurse practitioner, or physician's assistant prescribes medications by writing an order on a form in a patient's medical record, in an order book, or on a legal prescription pad. Some health care providers use a desktop, laptop, or handheld electronic device to enter medication orders. Many hospitals implement computerized physician order entry (CPOE) to handle medication orders to decrease medication errors (Ghaemmaghami, 2014). In these systems the health care provider completes all computerized fields before the order for the medication is filled, thus avoiding incomplete or illegible orders.

Sometimes a health care provider orders a medication by telephone or talking to a nurse in person. An order for a medication or medical treatment made over the telephone is called a *telephone order*. If the order is given verbally to the nurse, it is called a **verbal order**. When a verbal or telephone order is received, the nurse who took the order writes the complete order or enters it into a computer, reads it back, and receives confirmation from the health care provider to confirm accuracy. The nurse indicates the time and name of the health care provider who gave the order, signs it, and follows agency policy to indicate that it was read back. The health care provider countersigns the order at a later time, usually within 24 hours after giving it. Follow guidelines for taking telephone or verbal orders for medications safely (Box 32-3). Agency policies vary regarding personnel who can take telephone or verbal orders. Nursing students cannot take medication orders of any kind. They only give newly ordered medications after a registered nurse has written and verified the order.

Common abbreviations are often used when writing orders. Abbreviations indicate dosage frequencies or times, routes of administration, and special information for giving the medication (see Table 32-3). Medication errors frequently involve the use of abbreviations. Table 32-7 lists abbreviations that are associated with a high incidence of medication errors. Do *not* use these abbreviations when documenting medication orders or other information about medications (ISMP, 2013a; TJC, 2014a). Sometimes abbreviations used in different agencies vary. Check agency policy to determine which abbreviations are acceptable to use and their meaning.

BOX 32-3 Guidelines for Telephone and Verbal Orders

- Only authorized staff receive and record telephone or verbal orders. Agency identifies in writing the staff who are authorized.
- Clearly identify patient's name, room number, and diagnosis.
- Read back all orders to health care provider (TJC, 2016).
- Use clarification questions to avoid misunderstandings.
- Write "TO" (telephone order) or "VO" (verbal order), including date and time, name of patient, and complete order; sign the name of the health care provider and nurse.
- Follow agency policies; some agencies require documentation of the "read-back" or require two nurses to review and sign telephone or verbal orders.
- Health care provider co-signs the order within the time frame required by the agency (usually 24 hours; verify agency policy).

QSEN QSEN: BUILDING COMPETENCY IN SAFETY. Your patient's health care provider has written the following orders. Which orders do you need to clarify before administering the medication? Provide rationale for your answers and rewrite the order so it follows the ISMP current medication order safety guidelines.

Timolol .5% solution 1 drop OD BID
Losartan 12.50 mg QD
Insulin Lispro 6 u SC twice a day
Captopril 25 mg. PO three times a day, hold for systolic blood pressure <100

Answers to QSEN Activities can be found on the Evolve website.

Types of Orders in Acute Care Agencies

A medication cannot be given to a patient without a health care provider order. The frequency and urgency of medication administration forms the basis for medication orders. Some conditions change the status of a patient's medication orders. For example, in some agencies a patient's preoperative medications are discontinued automatically, and the health care provider writes new medication orders after surgery (see Chapter 50). Agency policies that surround medication orders vary. Nurses need to be aware of and follow these policies.

Standing Orders or Routine Medication Orders. A standing order is carried out until the health care provider cancels it by another order or a prescribed number of days elapse. Some standing orders indicate a final date or number of treatments or doses. Know your agency policies surrounding the discontinuation of standing orders. The following are examples of standing orders:

Tetracycline 500 mg PO q6h
Decadron 10 mg daily × 5 days

prn Orders. Sometimes the health care provider orders a medication to be given only when a patient requires it. This is a prn order. Use objective and subjective assessment (e.g., severity of pain, body temperature) and discretion in determining whether or not the patient needs the medication. An example of a prn order is:

Morphine sulfate 2 mg IV q2h prn for incisional pain

This order indicates that the patient needs to wait at least 2 hours between doses and can take the medication if experiencing pain at the incision. When administering prn medications, document assessment findings to show why the patient needs the medication and the time of administration. Frequently evaluate the effectiveness of the medication and record evaluation data appropriately. Unclear orders for prn medications that include a range (e.g., morphine sulfate IM 5-10 mg every 4-6 hours) are a source of medication errors. If a range order is written, ensure that the order follows agency policy for these types of orders. An example of a safer range order is to increase morphine dosage 50% to 100% if pain is moderate to severe based on use of the agency pain scale.

When multiple prn medications with the same action are ordered, the orders need to identify when to use each medication and how to use the medications in relationship to each other. The order below provides an example of a safe prn order for two medications used for treatment of constipation:

Docusate 100 mg PO TID prn constipation. Bisacodyl 10 mg suppository rectally daily prn constipation in addition to docusate if no bowel movement every 2 days

TABLE 32-7 Prohibited and Error-Prone Abbreviations*

The abbreviations, symbols, and dose designations found in this table have been reported to ISMP through the USP-ISMP Medication Error Reporting Program as being frequently misinterpreted and involved in harmful medication errors. They should NEVER be used when communicating medical information. This includes internal communications, telephone/verbal prescriptions, computer-generated labels, labels for drug storage bins, medication administration records, and pharmacy and prescriber computer order entry screens. The Joint Commission (TJC) has established a National Patient Safety Goal that specifies that certain abbreviations must appear on the do-not-use list of the accredited organization; they are highlighted with a double asterisk (**). However, we hope that you will consider others beyond the minimum TJC requirements. By using and promoting safe practices and educating one another about hazards, we can better protect our patients.

Abbreviations	Intended Meaning	Misinterpretation	Correction
µg	Microgram	Mistaken as "mg"	Use "mcg"
AD, AS, AU	Right ear, left ear, each ear	Mistaken as OD, OS, OU (right eye, left eye, each eye)	Use "right ear," "left ear," or "each ear"
OD, OS, OU	Right eye, left eye, each eye	Mistaken as AD, AS, AU (right ear, left ear, each ear)	Use "right eye," "left eye," or "each eye"
BT	Bedtime	Mistaken as "BID" (twice daily)	Use "bedtime"
HS	Half-strength	Mistaken as bedtime	Use "half-strength" or "bedtime"
hs	At bedtime, hours of sleep	Mistaken as half-strength	Use "bedtime" or "half-strength"
IU**	International unit	Mistaken as IV (intravenous) or 10 (ten)	Use "units"
o.d. or OD	Once daily	Mistaken as "right eye" (OD—oculus dexter), leading to oral liquid medications administered in the eye	Use "daily"
Per os	By mouth, orally	The "os" can be mistaken as "left eye" (OS—oculus sinister)	Use "PO," "by mouth," or "orally"
q.d. or QD**	Every day	Mistaken as q.i.d., especially if the period after the "q" or the tail of the "q" is misunderstood as an "I"	Use "daily"
qhs	Nightly at bedtime	Mistaken as "qhr" or every hour	Use "nightly"
SC, SQ, sub q	Subcutaneous	SC mistaken as SL (sublingual); SQ mistaken as "5 every"; the "q" in "sub q" has been mistaken as "every" (e.g., a heparin dose ordered "sub q 2 hours before surgery" misunderstood as every 2 hours before surgery)	Use "subcut" or "subcutaneously"
TIW or tiw	3 times a week	Mistaken as "3 times a day" or "twice in a week"	Use "3 times weekly"
U or u**	Unit	Mistaken as the number 0 or 4, causing a 10-fold overdose or greater (e.g., 4 U seen as "40" or 4 u seen as "44"); mistaken as "cc" so dose given in volume instead of units (e.g., 4 u seen as 4 cc)	Use "unit"
Dose Designations and Other Information	**Intended Meaning**	**Misinterpretation**	**Correction**
Trailing zero after decimal point (e.g., 1.0 mg)†	1 mg	Mistaken as 10 mg if the decimal point is not seen	Do not use trailing zeros for doses expressed in whole numbers
"Naked" decimal point (e.g., .5 mg)**	0.5 mg	Mistaken as 5 mg if the decimal point is not seen	Use zero before a decimal point when the dose is less than a whole unit
Abbreviations such as mg. or mL. with a period following the abbreviation	mg mL	The period is unnecessary and could be mistaken as the number 1 if written poorly	Use mg, mL, etc. without a terminal period
Drug Name Abbreviations	**Intended Meaning**	**Misinterpretation**	**Correction**
HCl	hydrochloric acid or hydrochloride	Mistaken as potassium chloride (The "H" is misinterpreted as "K")	Use complete drug name unless expressed as a salt of a drug
HCT	hydrocortisone	Mistaken as hydrochlorothiazide	Use complete drug name
HCTZ	hydrochlorothiazide	Mistaken as hydrocortisone (seen as HCT250 mg)	Use complete drug name

*Applies to all orders and medication-related documentation that is handwritten (including free-text computer entry or on preprinted forms).

**These abbreviations are included on The Joint Commission "minimum list" of dangerous abbreviations, acronyms, and symbols that must be included on the "Do Not Use" list of an organization, effective January 1, 2004.

†Exception: A "trailing zero" may be used only where required to show precision of a reported value (e.g., laboratory test results), in studies that report the size of lesions, or for catheter and tube sizes. A "trailing zero" cannot be used in medication orders or medication-related documentation (ISMP, 2013a).

TABLE 32-7 Prohibited and Error-Prone Abbreviations—cont'd

MgSO4**	magnesium sulfate	Mistaken as morphine sulphate	Use complete drug name
MS, MSO4**	morphine sulfate	Mistaken as magnesium sulphate	Use complete drug name
PCA	procainamide	Mistaken as patient-controlled analgesia	Use complete drug name
Stemmed Drug Names	**Intended Meaning**	**Misinterpretation**	**Correction**
"Nitro" drip	nitroglycerin infusion	Mistaken as sodium nitroprusside infusion	Use complete drug name
Symbols	**Intended Meaning**	**Misinterpretation**	**Correction**
ʒ	Dram	Symbol for dram mistaken as "3"	Use metric system
×3d	For three days	Mistaken as "3 doses"	Use "for three days"
> and <	Greater than and less than	Mistaken as opposite of intended; mistakenly use incorrect symbol; "<10" mistaken as "40"	Use "greater than" or "less than"
@	At	Mistaken as "2"	Use "at"
&	And	Mistaken as "2"	Use "and"
+	Plus or and	Mistaken as "4"	Use "and"
°	Hour	Mistaken as a zero (e.g., q2° seen as q20)	Use "hr," "h," or "hour"

From The Joint Commission (TJC): *Facts about the Official "Do Not Use" List of Abbreviations,* 2014, http://www.jointcommission.org/assets/1/18/Do_Not_Use_List.pdf. Accessed June 6, 2015. Reprinted with permission.

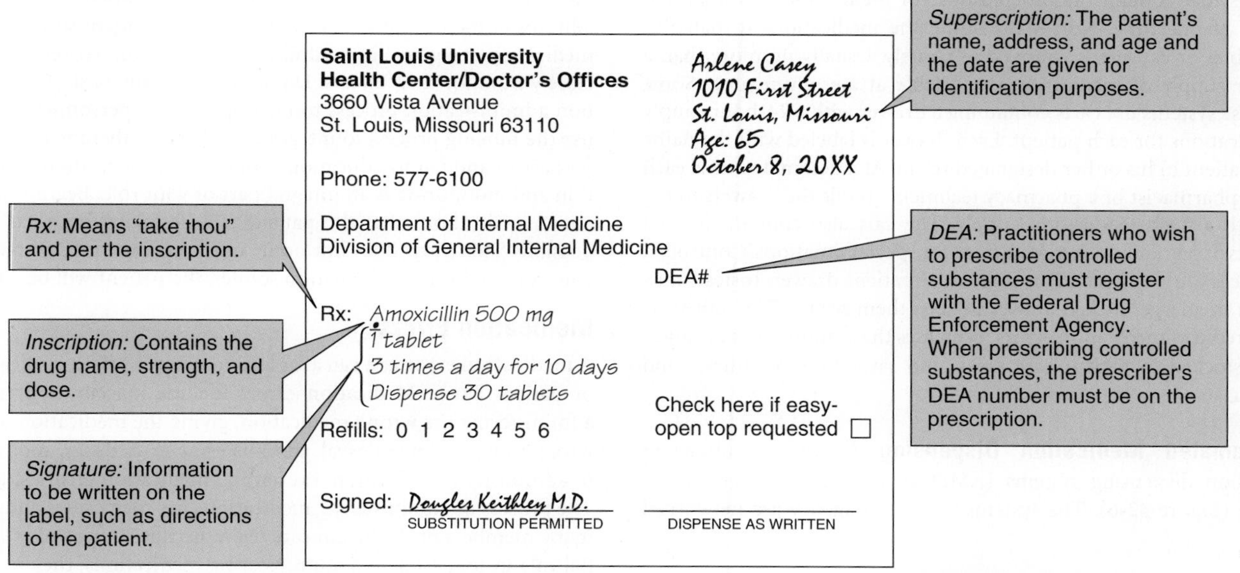

FIGURE 32-5 Example of a medication prescription. (Courtesy Saint Louis University Medical Center, St Louis, MO.)

Single (One-Time) Orders. Sometimes a health care provider orders a medication to be given once at a specified time. This is common for preoperative medications or medications given before diagnostic examinations. The following is an example of a single order:

Ativan 1 mg IV on call to MRI

STAT Orders. A STAT order signifies that a single dose of a medication is to be given immediately and only once. STAT orders are often written for emergencies when a patient's condition changes suddenly. For example:

Apresoline 10 mg IV STAT

Now Orders. A now order is more specific than a 1-time order and is used when a patient needs a medication quickly but not right away, as in a STAT order. When receiving a now order, the nurse has up to 90 minutes to administer the medication. Only administer now medications 1 time. For example:

Vancomycin 1 g IV piggyback now

Prescriptions. The health care provider writes **prescriptions** for patients who are to take medications outside of the hospital. The prescription includes more detailed information than a medication order because the patient needs to understand how to take the medication and when to refill the prescription if necessary. Some agencies require health care providers to write prescriptions for controlled substances on a special prescription pad that is different (e.g., a different color) than the prescription pad used for other medications. Figure 32-5 illustrates the parts of a prescription.

Pharmacist's Role

The pharmacist prepares and distributes prescribed medications. Pharmacists work with nurses, physicians, and other health care providers to evaluate the effectiveness of patients' medications. They are responsible for filling prescriptions accurately and being sure that prescriptions are valid. Pharmacists in health care agencies rarely mix compounds or solutions, except in the case of IV solutions. Most medication companies deliver medications in a form ready for use. Dispensing the correct medication, in the proper dosage and amount, with an accurate label is the pharmacist's main task. Pharmacists also provide information about medication side effects, toxicity, interactions, and incompatibilities.

Distribution Systems

Systems for storing and distributing medications vary. Health care agencies have a special area for stocking and dispensing medications. Examples of storage areas include special medication rooms, portable locked carts, computerized medication cabinets, and individual storage units next to patients' rooms. Medication storage areas need to be locked when unattended.

Unit Dose. A unit-dose system is a storage system that varies by health care agency. Pharmacists provide the medications in single-unit packages that contain the ordered dose of medication that a patient receives at one time. Nurses distribute the medications to patients. Each tablet or capsule is wrapped separately. Usually no more than a 24-hour supply of medication is available at any given time. Some unit-dose systems use carts containing a drawer with a 24-hour supply of medications for each patient. Each drawer is labeled with the name of the patient in his or her designated room. At a designated time each day the pharmacist or a pharmacy technician refills the drawers in the cart with a fresh medication supply. The cart also contains limited amounts of prn and stock medications for special situations. Controlled substances are not kept in an individual patient drawer. Instead they are kept in a larger locked drawer to keep them secure. The unit-dose system reduces medication errors, decreases the amount of medication that is stocked in patient care areas, and saves time for nurses and pharmacists.

Automated Medication Dispensing Systems. Automated medication dispensing systems (AMDSs) are used throughout the country (Figure 32-6). The systems within an agency are networked with one another and with other agency computer systems (e.g., computerized medical record). AMDSs control the dispensing of all medications, including narcotics. Each nurse accesses the system by entering a security code. Some systems require bio-identification as well. In these systems you place your finger on a screen to access the computer. You select the patient's name and his or her drug profile before the AMDS dispenses a medication. In these systems you are allowed to select the desired medication, dosage, and route from a list displayed on the computer screen. The system causes the drawer containing medication to open, records it, and charges it to the patient. Systems that are connected to the patient's computerized medical record then record information about the medication (e.g., medication name, dose, time) and the nurse's name in the patient's medical record. The bar-code medication administration (BCMA) system is often used with AMDSs. BCMA requires nurses to scan bar codes to identify the patient, the medication, and an identification tag of the nurse administering the medication before recording this information in the patient's computerized medical record. Agencies that implement AMDS with BCMA often reduce the incidence of medication errors (see Box 32-2).

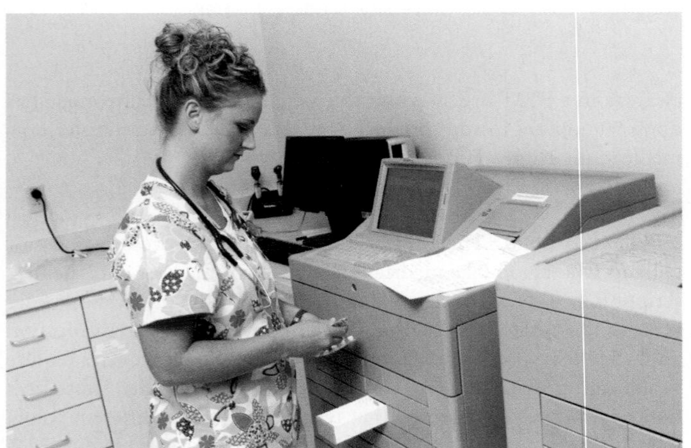

FIGURE 32-6 Automated medication dispensing system.

Nurse's Role

Administering medications requires unique nursing knowledge and skills. You first determine that the medication ordered is the correct medication. As a nurse you need to assess the patient's ability to self-administer medications, determine whether a patient should receive a medication at a given time, administer medications correctly, and then closely monitor their effects. Do not delegate any part of the medication administration process to nursing assistive personnel (NAP) and use the nursing process to integrate medication therapy into care.

Patient and family education about proper medication administration and monitoring is an integral part of your role. Begin instruction about medications that the patient will be taking home as soon as possible. This often does not occur until the day of discharge; but, if you can obtain this information sooner, the patient will benefit.

Medication Errors

A **medication error** can cause or lead to inappropriate medication use or patient harm. Medication errors include inaccurate prescribing, administering the wrong medication, giving the medication using the wrong route or time interval, administering extra doses, and/or failing to administer a medication. Preventing medication errors is essential. The process of administering medications has many steps and involves many members of the health care team. Because nurses play an essential role in preparing and administering medications, they need to be vigilant in preventing errors (Box 32-4). Advances in health care informatics have helped to decrease the occurrence of medication errors (Box 32-5).

Medication errors can be caused by many factors such as technology workarounds, the design of medication labels, and medication distribution systems. When an error occurs, the patient's safety and well-being are the top priorities. You first assess and examine the patient's condition and notify the health care provider of the incident as soon as possible. Once the patient is stable, report the incident to the appropriate person in the agency (e.g., manager or supervisor). You are responsible for preparing and filing an occurrence or incident report as soon as possible after the error occurs. The report includes patient identification information; the location and time of the incident; an accurate, factual description of what occurred and actions taken; and your signature. The occurrence report is not a permanent part of the medical record and is not referred to anywhere in a patient's medical record to legally protect the nurse and health care agency (see

BOX 32-4 Steps to Take to Prevent Medication Errors

- Prepare medications for only one patient at a time.
- Follow the six rights of medication administration.
- Be sure to read labels at least 3 times (comparing medication administration record [MAR] with label) before administering the medication.
- Use at least two patient identifiers and review the patient's allergies whenever administering a medication.
- Do not allow any other activity to interrupt administration of medication to a patient (e.g., phone call, pager, discussion with other staff) (Hopkinson and Jennings, 2013).
- Double-check all calculations and other high-risk medication administration processes (e.g., patient-controlled analgesia) and verify with another nurse.
- Do not interpret illegible handwriting; clarify with health care provider.
- Question unusually large or small doses.
- Document all medications as soon as they are given.
- When you have made an error, reflect on what went wrong and ask how you could have prevented the error. Complete an occurrence report per agency policy.
- Evaluate the context or situation in which a medication error occurred. This helps to determine if nurses have the necessary resources for safe medication administration.
- Attend in-service programs that focus on the medications commonly administered.
- Ensure that you are well rested when caring for patients. Nurses make more errors when they are tired (Murphy and While, 2012).
- Involve and educate patients when administering medications. Address patients' concerns about medications before administering them (e.g., concerns about their appearance or side effects).
- Follow established agency policies and procedures when using technology to administer medications (e.g., automated medication dispensers [AMDs] and bar-code scanning). Medication errors occur when nurses "work around" the technology (e.g., override alerts without thinking about them) (Voshall et al., 2013).

Chapters 23 and 26). Occurrence reports track incident patterns and indicate the need to implement quality improvement actions.

Report all medication errors that reach the patient, including those that do not cause harm. You also need to report near misses. For example, you are caring for a patient who has a urinary tract infection and is allergic to sulfa drugs. The patient's health care provider orders trimethoprim/sulfamethoxazole (TMP/SMZ). You know TMP/SMZ contains sulfa. You contact the health care provider before you administer the medication to obtain an order for a different medication. This type of medication error is a near miss because it did not actually reach the patient. All health care workers, including nurses, need to feel comfortable in reporting an error and not fear repercussions from managers or administrators. Even when a patient suffers no harm from a medication error, the agency can still learn why the mistake occurred and what can be done to avoid similar errors in the future.

Some medication errors happen when patients experience a transition in care such as when a patient is admitted or discharged from a hospital, is transferred from an intensive care unit to a general patient care unit, or sees a new health care provider. During these times the risk of unintended changes in medication orders increases. Thus reconciling medication information is a key Hospital National Patient Safety Goal (TJC, 2016). During **medication reconciliation** nurses, pharmacists, and other health care providers compare the medication that a patient is taking currently with what the patient should be taking and any newly ordered medications (Box 32-6). Throughout this

BOX 32-5 Informatics and Medication Safety

Many medication errors occur when a nurse incorrectly administers medications at the patient's bedside. The following innovations and advances in technology have helped reduce the number of medication errors in nursing practice.

- Networked computers allow all the patient's health care providers to see a current list of ordered and discontinued medications.
- Internet and intranet access allows nurses and other health care providers to access current information about medications (e.g., indications, desired effects, adverse effects) and specific agency policies that address medication administration (e.g., how fast to administer an intravenous [IV] push medication, how to administer medications through a nasogastric tube).
- In some agencies health care providers use computerized prescription order entry [CPOE], allowing them to enter medication orders directly into a networked computer system or a personal handheld computer.
- Automated medication dispensers [AMDs] and electronic medication administration records (eMARs) help with medication reconciliation, administration, and documentation.
- Bar-coding technology requires nurses to scan the medication, the patient's identification bracelet, and the nurse's identification badge before administering the medication, which helps ensure the six rights of medication administration.

Application to Nursing Practice

- Actively participate in selecting and evaluating advanced technologies and creating nursing policies and protocols used for medication administration.
- Always follow agency policies when administering medications.
- Implement agency policies when the technology cannot be used (e.g., during down time or power outages).
- Follow manufacturer guidelines for care of electronic equipment and report problems with technology immediately.

BOX 32-6 Process for Medication Reconciliation

1. **Obtain, Verify, Document:** Obtain a comprehensive and current list of a patient's medications whenever he or she experiences a change in health care setting (e.g., during admission, transfer, discharge). Include all current prescriptions and over-the-counter (OTC) medications.
2. **Consider and Compare:** Review what the patient was taking at home or preadmission and make sure that the list of medications, dosages, and frequencies is accurate. Compare this list to the current ordered medications and treatment plan to ensure accuracy. Include family caregiver in this discussion when appropriate.
3. **Reconcile:** Compare new medication orders with the current list; investigate any discrepancies with the patient's health care provider and document changes.
4. **Communicate:** Ensure that all the patient's health care providers have the most updated list of medications. Communicate and verify changes in medications as with the patient.

Data from Gleason KM et al; Agency for Healthcare Research and Quality: *Medications at transitions and clinical handoffs (MATCH) toolkit for medication reconciliation,* http://www.ahrq.gov/professionals/quality-patient-safety/patient-safety-resources/resources/match/match.pdf. Accessed June 6, 2015.

process you identify and resolve orders that are duplicated and omitted. You also evaluate the risk for unintended medication interactions. Creating and maintaining an accurate list of all patient medications helps to ensure safe and effective patient care (Gleason et al., 2012). For example, when you admit a patient who is having a hip replacement to an orthopedic unit, you compare the medications that the patient took at home with those ordered in the hospital. When the patient is discharged to a rehabilitation unit, you communicate the patient's current medications with the nurse who is accepting the patient. The nurse on the rehabilitation unit reconciles the patient's medications when the patient is discharged with the home health nurse. Many agencies have computerized or written forms to facilitate the process of medication reconciliation. The process is challenging and takes a lot of time and concentration. Eliminate distractions and go slowly when reconciling patients' medications. Always clarify information when needed and question for accuracy. Accurate medication reconciliation requires consulting with the patient, family caregivers, other clinicians, pharmacists, and other members of the health care team.

CRITICAL THINKING

Knowledge

You use knowledge from many disciplines when administering medications. Your knowledge helps you understand why a medication is prescribed for a patient and how it will alter the patient's physiology to have a therapeutic effect. For example, in physiology you learn that potassium is a major intracellular ion. When patients do not have enough potassium in their body (hypokalemia), they experience signs and symptoms such as muscle fatigue or weakness. In some cases severe hypokalemia is fatal as a result of associated cardiac dysrhythmias. Prescribed medications help to restore the patient's potassium level to normal, which relieves the signs and symptoms of hypokalemia. In another example knowledge about child development indicates that children often associate medication administration with a negative experience. Use principles from child development to ensure that the child cooperates with the medication experience.

Patients take a variety of medications, and new medications are constantly approved. As a result you will not always understand all the medications ordered for a patient. Critical thinkers admit what they do not know and acquire the knowledge needed to safely administer unfamiliar medications. This means that, when you do not know all the medications you need to administer, you will consult a reliable source (e.g., a more expert nurse, pharmacist, the health care provider, or a reference book) *before* administering the medication.

Experience

Nursing students have limited experience with medication administration as it applies to professional practice. Clinical experiences give you opportunities to use the nursing process as it applies to medication administration. As you gain experience, your psychomotor skills ("the how-to") become more refined. However, psychomotor skills represent a small part of medication administration. Patient attitudes, knowledge, physical and mental status, and responses make medication administration a complex responsibility.

Attitudes

Use your critical thinking skills to administer medications safely. Be disciplined and take adequate time to prepare and administer medications. Take the time to read your patient's medical record before administering medications and carefully review the patient's history, physical examination, and orders. Look up medications that you do not know in a medication reference and determine why each patient is taking each of the prescribed medications. Every step of safe medication administration requires a disciplined attitude and a comprehensive, systematic approach. Following the same procedure each time medications are administered ensures safe administration.

Responsibility and accountability are other critical thinking attitudes essential to safe medication administration. Accept full accountability and responsibility for all actions surrounding the administration of medications. Do not assume that a medication that is ordered for a patient is the correct medication or the correct dose. Be responsible for knowing that the medications and doses ordered are correct and appropriate. You are accountable if you give an ordered medication that is not appropriate for a patient. Therefore be familiar with each medication, including its therapeutic effect, usual dosage, anticipated changes in laboratory data, and side effects. You are also responsible for ensuring that patients or caregivers who administer medications have been properly informed about all aspects of self-administration (TJC, 2016). If you determine that a patient cannot self-administer medications safely, design interventions such as involving family caregivers to ensure safe administration.

Standards

Standards are actions that ensure safe nursing practice. Standards for medication administration are set by health care agencies and the nursing profession. Agency policy sets limits on a nurse's ability to administer medications in certain units of the acute care setting. Sometimes nurses are limited by certain medication routes or dosages. Most agencies have nursing procedure manuals that contain policies that define the types of medications nurses can and cannot administer. The types and dosages of some medications that nurses deliver vary from unit to unit within the same agency. For example, phenytoin (Dilantin), a medication for treating seizures, may be administered by mouth or IV push. In large dosages phenytoin affects heart rhythm. Therefore some agencies place limits on how much nurses can administer to a patient on a nursing unit that does not have the ability to monitor a patient's heart rate and rhythm. Not all health care providers are aware of the limitations and sometimes prescribe medications that nurses cannot give in a particular health care setting. Recognize these limitations and inform the health care provider accordingly. Take appropriate actions to ensure that patients receive medications as prescribed and within the time prescribed in the appropriate environment.

Professional standards such as *Nursing: Scope and Standards of Practice* (ANA, 2010) (see Chapters 1 and 23) apply to the activity of medication administration. To prevent medication errors, follow the six rights of medication administration consistently every time you administer medications. Many medication errors can be linked in some way to an inconsistency in adhering to these six rights:

1. The right medication
2. The right dose
3. The right patient
4. The right route
5. The right time
6. The right documentation

Right Medication. A medication order is required for every medication that you administer to a patient. Sometimes health care providers write orders by hand in the patient's medical record. Alternatively some agencies use CPOE. CPOE allows a health care provider to order medications electronically, eliminating the need for written orders and enhancing medication safety (Radley et al., 2013).

Regardless of how a nurse receives a medication order, he or she compares the health care provider's written orders with the medication administration record (MAR) or electronic MAR (eMAR) when it is ordered initially. Nurses verify medication information whenever new MARs are created or distributed or when patients transfer from one nursing unit or health care setting to another.

Once you determine that information on a patient's MAR is accurate, use it to prepare and administer medications. When preparing medications from bottles or containers, compare the label of the medication container with the MAR 3 times: (1) before removing the container from the drawer or shelf; (2) as the amount of medication ordered is removed from the container; and (3) at the patient's bedside before administering the medication to the patient. Never prepare medications from unmarked containers or containers with illegible labels (TJC, 2016). With unit-dose prepackaged medications, check the label with the MAR when taking medications out of the medication dispensing system. Finally verify all medications at the patient's bedside with the patient's MAR and use at least two identifiers before giving the patient any medications (TJC, 2016).

Patients who self-administer medications need to keep them in their original labeled containers, separate from other medications, to avoid confusion. Many hospitals require that nurses administer all medications rather than letting patients self-administer to enhance accuracy and patient safety. Because the nurse who administers the medication is responsible for any errors related to it, nurses administer only the medications they prepare. You cannot delegate preparation of medication to another person and then administer the medication to the patient. If a patient questions the medication, do not ignore these concerns. A patient or a family caregiver familiar with a patient's medications often knows whether a medication is different from those received before. In most cases a patient's medication order has changed; however, sometimes patient questions reveal an error. When this occurs, withhold the medication and recheck it against the health care provider's orders. If a patient refuses a medication, discard it rather than returning it to the original container. Unit-dose medications can be saved if they are not opened. If a patient refuses narcotics, follow proper agency procedure by having someone else witness the "wasted" medication.

Right Dose. The unit-dose system is designed to minimize errors. When preparing a medication from a larger volume or strength than needed or when the health care provider orders a system of measurement different from that which the pharmacy supplies, the chance of error increases. You need to have another qualified nurse check the calculated doses when performing medication calculations or conversions. Prepare medications using standard measurement devices such as graduated cups, syringes, and scaled droppers to measure medications accurately. At home educate patients to use similar measurement devices such as measuring spoons rather than household teaspoons and tablespoons, which are inaccurate.

Medication errors often occur when pills need to be split. To promote patient safety in inpatient settings, pharmacists split the medications, label and package them, and then send them to the nurse for administration. Because pill splitting is particularly problematic in the home care setting, the U.S. FDA (USFDA) (2013) developed suggestions to help with this process. They include ensuring that the tablet is designed to be split, using a tablet splitter and not splitting the entire prescription at one time, and determining if the patient has the motor dexterity or visual acuity to split tablets. If at all possible, health care providers need to avoid ordering medications that require splitting.

Tablets are sometimes crushed and mixed with food. Be sure to completely clean a crushing device before crushing the tablet. Remnants of previously crushed medications increase the concentration of a medication or result in the patient receiving part of a medication that was not prescribed. Mix crushed medications with very small amounts of food or liquid (e.g., a single tablespoon). Do not use a patient's favorite foods or liquids because medications alter their taste and decrease the patient's desire for them. This is especially a concern for pediatric patients.

Not all medications are suitable for crushing. Some medications (e.g., extended-release capsules) have special coatings to prevent them from being absorbed too quickly. These medications should not be crushed. Refer to the "Do Not Crush List" (ISMP, 2014a), http://www.ismp.org/tools/donotcrush.pdf) to ensure that a medication is safe to crush.

Right Patient. Medication errors often occur because a patient gets a drug intended for another patient. Therefore an important step in safe medication administration is being sure that you give the right medication to the right patient. It is difficult to remember every patient's name and face. Before administering a medication, use at least two patient identifiers (TJC, 2016). Acceptable patient identifiers include the patient's name, his or her medical record number assigned by a health care agency, or a telephone number. Do not use the patient's room number as an identifier. To identify a patient correctly, you usually compare the patient identifiers on the MAR with the patient's identification bracelet while at the patient's bedside. If an identification bracelet becomes smudged or illegible or is missing, obtain a new one. All agencies in all health care settings need to use a system that verifies the patient's identification with at least two identifiers before administering medications and other treatments.

Patients do not need to state their names and other identifiers when you administer medications. Collect patient identifiers reliably when he or she is admitted to a health care setting. Once the identifiers are assigned to the patient (e.g., putting identifiers on an armband and placing the armband on the patient), you use the identifiers to match the patient with the MAR, which lists the correct medications. Asking patients to state their full names and identification information provides a third way to verify that the nurse is giving medications to the right patient.

In addition to using two identifiers, some agencies use BCMA to help identify the right patient (Figure 32-7). This system requires

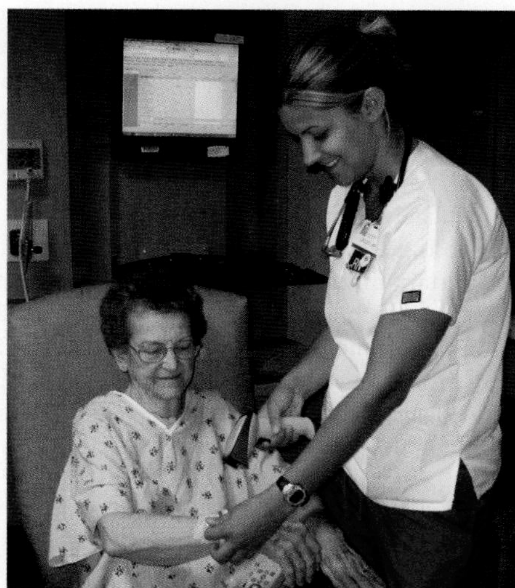

FIGURE 32-7 Nurse using bar-code scanner to identify patient during medication administration.

nurses to scan a personal bar code that is commonly placed on their name tag first. Then the nurse scans a bar code on the single-dose medication package. Finally the nurse scans the patient's armband. All this information is then stored in a computer for documentation purposes. This system helps eliminate medication errors because it provides another step to ensure that the right patient receives the right medication (Ching et al., 2013).

Right Route. Always consult the health care provider if an order does not include a route of administration. Likewise alert the health care provider immediately if the specified route is not the recommended route. Recent evidence shows that medication errors involving the wrong route are common. For example, when nurses need to prepare an oral medication in a syringe, the risk to administer the medication via the wrong route (e.g., intravenously) is very high and often results in fatal consequences. Thus the ISMP (2015b) recommends that pharmacists, *not nurses,* prepare all oral medications that are not prepared commercially as a unit product to enhance patient safety. The IV injection of a liquid designed for oral use produces local complications such as sterile abscess or fatal systemic effects. If you are in a setting that requires you to prepare oral medications, only use enteral syringes when preparing the medication. The enteral syringes are often a different color than the parenteral syringes and are clearly labeled for oral or enteral use. The syringe tips of enteral syringes will not connect with parenteral medication administration systems. Needles do not attach to the syringes, and the syringes cannot be inserted into any type of IV line. Label the syringe after preparing the medication and be sure to remove any caps from the tip of an oral syringe before administering the medication. Failure to remove the cap can result in the patient aspirating it, thus blocking the trachea.

Right Time. To administer medications safely, you need to know why a medication is ordered for certain times of the day and whether you are able to alter the time schedule. For example, two medications are ordered, one q8h (every 8 hours) and the other 3 times a day. Both medications are scheduled for 3 times within a 24-hour period. You need to give the q8h medication every 8 hours ATC to maintain therapeutic blood levels of the medication. In contrast, you need to give the 3-times-a-day medication at 3 different times while the patient is awake. Each agency has a recommended time schedule for medications ordered at frequent intervals. You can alter these recommended times if necessary or appropriate.

The health care provider often gives specific instructions about when to administer a medication. A preoperative medication to be given "on call" means that you give the medication when the operating room staff members notify you that they are coming to get a patient for surgery. Give a medication ordered PC (after meals) within half an hour after a meal, when a patient has a full stomach. Give a STAT medication immediately.

Give priority to time-critical medications that must act and therefore be given at certain times. Hospitals designate which medications are time critical and which are non–time critical (CMS, 2011; ISMP, 2011). You administer time-critical medications within 30 minutes before or after their scheduled time. For example, give insulin (a time-critical medication) at a precise interval before a meal. Give antibiotics 30 minutes before or after they are scheduled ATC to maintain therapeutic blood levels. Give all routinely ordered non–time-critical medications within 1 to 2 hours before or after the scheduled time or per agency policy (CMS, 2011; ISMP, 2011).

Some medications require a nurse's clinical judgment in deciding the proper time for administration. Administer a prn sleeping medication when a patient is prepared for bed. In addition, use judgment when administering prn analgesics. For example, you may need to obtain a STAT order from the health care provider if a patient requires a medication before the prn interval has elapsed. Always document when you call a patient's health care provider to obtain a change in a medication order.

Before discharge from the hospital setting, evaluate a patient's need for home care, especially if he or she was admitted to the hospital because of a problem with medication self-administration. Patients often leave the hospital with a basic knowledge of their medications but are unable to remember or implement this knowledge once back home. Before patients are discharged from the hospital, evaluate whether the medications are adequate or prescribed at therapeutic levels for them.

At home some patients take several medications throughout the day. Help to plan schedules on the basis of preferred medication intervals, the pharmacokinetics of the medications, and the patient's daily schedule. For patients who have difficulty remembering when to take medications, make a chart that lists the times to take each one or prepare a special container to hold each timed dose.

Right Documentation. Nurses and other health care providers use accurate documentation to communicate with one another. Many medication errors result from inaccurate documentation. Therefore always document medications accurately at the time of administration and verify any inaccurate documentation before giving medications.

Before administering a medication, ensure that the MAR clearly reflects a patient's full name; the full name of the ordered medication (no medication name abbreviations); the time the medication is to be administered; and the dosage, route, and frequency. Common problems with medication orders include incomplete information; inaccurate dosage form or strength; illegible order or signature; incorrect placement of decimals, leading to the wrong dosage; and nonstandard terminology. If there is any question about a medication order because it is incomplete, illegible, vague, or not understood, contact the health care provider before administering the medication. The health care provider is responsible to provide accurate, complete, and understandable medication orders. If he or she is unable to do this, nurses implement agency policy (usually a "chain of command" policy) to determine who to contact until they resolve issues related to patients' medications. You are responsible to begin this chain of command to ensure that patients receive the correct medication for documenting any preassessment data required of certain medications such as a blood pressure measurement for antihypertensive medications or laboratory values, as in the case of warfarin, before giving the drug.

After administering a medication, immediately document which medication was given on a patient's MAR per agency policy to verify that it was given as ordered. Inaccurate documentation such as failing to document giving a medication or documenting an incorrect dose leads to errors in subsequent decisions about patient care. For example, errors in documentation about insulin often result in negative patient outcomes. Consider the following situation: a patient receives insulin before breakfast, but the nurse who gave the insulin forgot to document it. The nurse caring for the patient goes home, and you are the patient's new nurse for the day. You notice that the insulin is not documented, you assume that the previous nurse did not give the insulin, and you give the patient another dose of insulin. Approximately 2 hours later, the patient experiences a low blood glucose level, which results in seizure activity. Accurate documentation and following up with the nurse from the previous shift to verify that the insulin was given as ordered would have prevented this situation from happening.

Never document that you have given a medication until you have actually given it. Document the name of the medication, the dose, the time of administration, and the route on the MAR. Also document the site of any injections and the patient's responses to medications, either positive or negative. Notify a patient's health care provider of any negative responses to medications and document the time, date, and name of the health care provider who was notified in the patient's medical record. The efforts you make to ensure proper documentation help provide safe care.

Maintaining Patients' Rights. In accordance with *The Patient Care Partnership* (American Hospital Association, 2003) and because of the potential risks related to medication administration, a patient has the following rights:

- To be informed of the name, purpose, action, and potential undesired effects of a medication
- To refuse a medication regardless of the consequences
- To have qualified nurses or physicians assess a medication history, including allergies and use of herbals
- To be properly advised of the experimental nature of medication therapy and give written consent for its use
- To receive labeled medications safely without discomfort in accordance with the six rights of medication administration
- To receive appropriate supportive therapy in relation to medication therapy
- To not receive unnecessary medications
- To be informed if medications are a part of a research study

Know these rights and handle all patient and family questions courteously and professionally. Do not become defensive if a patient refuses medication therapy, recognizing that every person of consenting age has a right to refusal.

NURSING PROCESS

Apply the nursing process and use a critical thinking approach in your care of patients. The nursing process provides a clinical decision-making approach for you to develop and implement an individualized plan of care.

Assessment

During the assessment process thoroughly assess each patient and critically analyze findings to ensure that you make patient-centered clinical decisions required for safe nursing care.

Through the Patient's Eyes. Use professional knowledge, skills, and attitudes to provide compassionate and coordinated care. Consider patients' preferences, values, and needs while determining their need for and possible responses to medication therapy. Assess their experiences and encourage them to express their beliefs, feelings, and concerns about their medications. For example, ask them how their religious or family backgrounds influence their beliefs about taking medications. Putting patients in the center of their care helps you to see the situation through their eyes and contributes to safe medication administration. Begin your assessment by asking a variety of questions to help you better understand your patients' current medication management routine, their ability to afford medications, and their beliefs and expectations about medications.

History. Before you administer medications, review a patient's medical history to help you understand the indications or contraindications for medication therapy. Some illnesses place patients at risk for adverse medication effects. For example, if a patient has a gastric ulcer, medications containing aspirin increase the likelihood of bleeding. Long-term health problems (e.g., diabetes or arthritis) require specific medications. This knowledge helps you anticipate the type of medications that a patient requires. A patient's surgical history also sometimes indicates the need for medications. For example, after a thyroidectomy a patient requires thyroid hormone replacement.

BOX 32-7 Nursing Assessment Questions

- Which prescription and nonprescription medications and herbal and nutritional supplements do you take? When do you take them? How do you take them? Do you have a list of medications from your pharmacy or health care provider's office?
- Why do you take these medications?
- Which side effects do you experience? Which of the side effects bother you or affect you negatively?
- What have you been told to do if a side effect develops?
- Have you ever stopped taking your medications? If so, why?
- What do you do to help remember to take your medications?
- Do you have any allergies to medications or foods? If so, which ones? Describe what happens when you take the medication or eat the food.
- Describe your normal eating patterns. Which foods and at what times do you normally eat?
- How do you pay for your medications? Do you sometimes have to stretch your budget to afford them or space them out to save money?
- What questions do you have about your medications?

Allergies. Inform the other members of the health care team if a patient has a history of allergies to medications and foods. Many medications have ingredients also found in food sources. For example, propofol (Diprivan), which is used for anesthesia and sedation, includes egg lecithin and soybean oil as inactive ingredients. Therefore patients who have an egg or soy allergy should not receive propofol (Skidmore-Roth, 2015). In most health care settings patients wear identification bands listing medication and food allergies. Ensure that all your patient's allergies and their allergic reactions are documented appropriately in the patient's medical record (e.g., history and physical, MAR) to facilitate communication of this essential information to members of the health care team.

Medications. Ask your patients questions to find out about each medication they take (Box 32-7). Possible questions include: How long have you been taking these medications? What is the current dosage of each medication? Do you experience side effects or adverse effects from your medications? In addition, review the action, purpose, normal dosage, routes, side effects, and nursing implications for administering and monitoring each medication. You often need to consult several resources such as pharmacology textbooks; medication manuals available on a computer, electronic tablet, or AMDS; nursing journals; the *Physician's Desk Reference* (PDR); medication package inserts; and pharmacists to gather necessary information. As a nurse you are responsible for knowing as much as possible about each medication your patients take.

Diet History. A diet history reveals a patient's normal eating patterns and food preferences. Use your patient's diet history to plan an effective and individualized medication dosage schedule. Teach your patient to avoid foods that interact with medications. In addition, provide education when your patients take medications that need to be taken before, with, or after meals.

Patient's Perceptual or Coordination Problems. Patients with perceptual, fine-motor, or coordination limitations often have difficulty self-administering medications. For example, a patient who takes insulin to manage blood glucose and has arthritis has difficulty manipulating a syringe. Assess the patient's ability to prepare doses and take medications correctly. If a patient is unable to self-administer medications, assess if family or friends are available to help or make a home care referral.

Patient's Current Condition. The ongoing physical or mental status of a patient affects whether a medication is given and how it is administered. *Assess a patient carefully before giving any medication.* For example, check a patient's blood pressure before giving an antihypertensive. A patient who is vomiting is unable to take medications by mouth. Notify the patient's health care provider when this happens. Assessment findings serve as a baseline in evaluating the effects of medication therapy.

Patient's Attitude About Medication Use. A patient's attitudes about medications (e.g., benefit, risk, likelihood to cure) sometimes reveals a level of medication dependence or drug avoidance. Some patients do not express their feelings about taking a particular medication, particularly if dependence is a problem. Listen carefully when a patient describes how he or she uses medications to identify evidence of dependence or avoidance. Also be aware that cultural beliefs about Western medicine sometimes interfere with medication adherence (Box 32-8; see Chapter 9).

Factors Affecting Adherence to Medication Therapy. Many complex factors affect a patient's ability to adhere to prescribed medication therapy. For example, a patient's knowledge and understanding of medication therapy influence the willingness or ability to follow a medication regimen. If a patient has a history of poor adherence (e.g., frequently missed doses or failure to fill prescriptions), investigate if he or she can afford prescribed medications and review resources available for purchase of medications if indicated. Also determine if the patient understands the purpose of the medication, the importance of regular dosage schedules, proper administration methods, and the possible side effects. Without adequate funding, knowledge, and motivation, adherence to medication schedules is unlikely (Viswanathan et al., 2012).

Patient's Learning Needs. Health-related information is difficult to understand because of the use of technical terminology. Serious errors can occur when patients do not understand information about their medications. Assess patients' health literacy regarding medication administration to determine their need for instruction (Weekes, 2012; Zullig et al., 2014) (see Chapter 25). Have the patient explain the medication schedule of a typical day. Have him or her read a medication label and explain what it includes. Health literacy also includes numeracy. Have a patient show how to give a medication dose if it is necessary to split a pill or give more than one in a container. Consider patient responses to your medication assessment questions such as those listed in Box 32-7. When a patient is unable to answer questions about medications appropriately, assess his or her health literacy.

◆ Nursing Diagnosis

Assessment provides data about the patient's condition, ability to self-administer medications, and medication adherence. Use these data to determine a patient's actual or potential problems with medication therapy. Certain data are defining characteristics that, when clustered together, reveal actual nursing diagnoses. For example, *Ineffective Health Management related to complexity of treatment regimen* is indicated when patients have a complex medication schedule and admit to having difficulty integrating their medications into their daily routine.

BOX 32-8 CULTURAL ASPECTS OF CARE

Influences in Medication Administration

Health beliefs vary by culture and often influence how patients manage and respond to drug therapy. Significant differences in values, beliefs, and attitudes affect a patient's adherence to drug therapy (Alhalaiqa et al., 2013). Some cultures attach different symbolic meanings to medications and drug therapy. Herbal remedies and alternative therapies are common in various cultures and ethnic groups and sometimes interfere with prescribed medications (Li et al., 2012). Some people stop taking medications when their symptoms are resolved, even if the medications are still needed for management of a chronic illness. In addition, health beliefs often differ markedly between health providers and patients, further affecting a patient's adherence to medical therapy (Polinski et al., 2014). In addition to the psychosocial aspect of medication therapy, pharmacological research has shown that differences in drug response, metabolism, and side effects may be affected by patients' ethnicity, genetics, gender, and age (Blazquez et al., 2012).

Implications for Patient-Centered Care

- Assess cultural beliefs, attitudes, and values when administering medications and teaching patients about self-administration.
- Establish trust with patients and resolve conflicts between medications and cultural beliefs to achieve optimal patient outcomes (Polinski et al., 2014).
- Investigate if the patient practices any alternative therapies or is taking any herbal preparations (Li et al., 2012).
- Consider cultural influences on drug response, metabolism, and side effects if a patient is not responding to drug therapy as expected. Confer with health care provider because a change in the patient's medication is sometimes necessary.
- Assess food preferences that may interfere with patients' medication therapy (Giger, 2013).

This list of nursing diagnoses may apply during medication administration in a variety of settings:

- *Anxiety*
- *Ineffective Health Maintenance*
- *Deficient Knowledge (Medication Self-Administration)*
- *Noncompliance (Medications)*
- *Impaired Swallowing*
- *Impaired Memory*
- *Caregiver Role Strain (Caregiving Activities)*

After selecting the diagnosis, identify the related factor (if applicable) that drives the selection of nursing interventions. In the example of *Noncompliance,* the related factors of *financial barriers* versus *insufficient knowledge about the regimen* require different interventions. If a patient's nursing diagnosis is related to inadequate finances, you collaborate with family members, social workers, case managers, or community agencies to connect the patient with necessary financial resources and develop a medication regimen the patient can afford. If the related factor is *insufficient knowledge,* you implement a teaching plan with appropriate follow-up.

◆ Planning

Always organize your care activities to ensure the safe administration of medications. Rushing to give patients medications leads to errors. It is important to minimize distractions or interruptions when preparing and administering medications (Ching et al., 2013; Donaldson et al., 2014). No-interruption zones (NIZs) have been recommended to reduce distractions and interruptions during medication administration (Yoder et al., 2015). NIZs are created by placing signs, red tape, or some type of borders on the floor around medication carts or areas. Nurses standing in these areas are not to be interrupted.

Goals and Outcomes. Setting goals and related outcomes contributes to patient safety and allows for effective use of time during medication administration. For example, a nurse establishes the following goal and related outcomes for a patient with newly diagnosed type 2 diabetes who has the diagnosis of *Deficient Knowledge related to insufficient information*:

Goal: The patient will safely self-administer all ordered medications before discharge.

Outcomes:

- The patient verbalizes understanding of desired and adverse effects of medications.
- The patient states signs, symptoms, and treatment of hypoglycemia.
- The patient is able to monitor blood glucose levels to determine if it is safe to take medication or if an alteration in dose is needed.
- The patient prepares a dose of ordered medication.
- The patient describes a daily routine that will integrate timing of medication with daily activities.

Setting Priorities. Prioritize care when administering medications. Use patient assessment data to determine which medications to give first, whether it is time to evaluate a patient's response to a medication, or if it is appropriate to administer prn medications. For example, if a patient is in pain, it is important to provide pain medication as soon as possible. If the patient's blood pressure is elevated, administer the blood pressure medication before other medications. Nurses also prioritize when providing patient education about medications. Provide the most important information about the medications first. For example, hypoglycemia is a serious side effect of insulin. A patient taking insulin needs to be able to identify and treat hypoglycemia immediately; thus first teach how to recognize and treat hypoglycemia before teaching about how to administer an injection.

Teamwork and Collaboration. Collaboration during medication administration is essential. You need to collaborate with a patient's family caregivers whenever possible. Family caregivers and significant others often reinforce the importance of medication schedules when a patient is at home. Nurses often collaborate with patients' health care providers, pharmacists, and case managers to ensure that patients are able to afford their medications. On discharge ensure that patients know where and how to obtain medications. Be sure that patients are able to read medication labels and medication teaching information. Some patients also need to understand how to calculate dosages and prepare complex medication regimens. Collaborate with community resources (e.g., agency on aging, public health department, medical interpreters) when patients have significant literacy issues or difficulty understanding medication instructions (see Chapter 25).

◆ Implementation

Health Promotion. In promoting or maintaining a patient's health, nurses identify factors that improve or diminish well-being. Health beliefs, personal motivation, socioeconomic factors, and habits influence a patient's adherence with medications. Several nursing interventions promote adherence to the medication regimen and foster independence. Teach a patient and family about the benefit of a medication and the knowledge needed to take it correctly. Integrate a patient's health beliefs and cultural practices into the treatment plan. Help a patient and family establish a medication routine that fits into the patient's normal schedule. Make referrals to community resources if a patient is unable to afford or cannot arrange transportation to obtain necessary medications.

Patient and Family Teaching. Some patients take medications incorrectly or not at all because they do not understand their medications. When this happens, you need to provide patient education using language your patient understands (see Chapter 25). Include information about the purpose, actions, timing, dosages, and side effects of medications. Many health care agencies offer easy-to-read teaching sheets written at the sixth grade level about specific types of medications. Patients need to know how to take medications properly and the risks associated when they fail to do so. For example, after receiving a prescription for an antibiotic, a patient needs to understand the importance of taking the full prescription. Failure to do this can lead to a worsening of the condition and the development of bacteria resistant to the medication. Current recommendations suggest the use of Teach Back as a method to confirm patient learning and improve health care provider education (Nouri and Rudd, 2015). Have the patient explain for you the topic about which you instructed him or her so you can confirm understanding.

Nurses teach patients how to administer their medications correctly. For example, teach a patient how to measure a liquid medication accurately. Provide special education to patients who depend on daily injections (Box 32-9). The patient learns to prepare and administer an injection correctly using aseptic technique. Teach family caregivers how to give injections in case the patient becomes ill or physically unable to handle a syringe. Provide specially designed equipment such as syringes with enlarged calibrated scales or medications with labels in braille when patients have visual alterations.

BOX 32-9 PATIENT TEACHING

Safe Insulin Administration

Objective

- Patient will correctly self-administer subcutaneous insulin.

Teaching Strategies

- Teach patient how to determine if insulin is expired.
- Instruct patient to keep medication in its original labeled container and refrigerated if needed.
- Demonstrate how to prepare insulin in a syringe, assessing visual acuity to ensure that patient is able to draw up the correct amount of insulin.
- Coach patient through the steps of administering subcutaneous insulin injection.
- Demonstrate how to rotate insulin injection sites.
- Help patient determine the amount of insulin required on the basis of the results of home capillary glucose monitoring as ordered by the health care provider.
- Show patient how to keep a daily log for insulin injections, including results of home capillary glucose monitoring, type and amount of insulin given, expiration date on insulin vial, time of insulin injection, and injection site used.

Evaluation

- Use Teach Back and ask patient to describe procedure used at home for determining the correct dose of insulin needed and injection site.
- Watch patient prepare insulin dose on the basis of results of capillary glucose monitoring, select injection site, and self-administer injection.
- Review information recorded in patient log for completeness.
- If patient is unable to prepare the correct amount of insulin or self-administer safely, instruct a family caregiver and notify the health care provider.

Patients need to know the symptoms of medication side effects or toxicity. For example, patients taking anticoagulants learn to notify their health care providers immediately when signs of bleeding or bruising develop. Inform family members or friends of medication side effects such as changes in behavior because they are often the first to recognize these effects. Patients cope better with problems caused by medications if they understand how and when to act. All patients need to learn the basic guidelines for medication safety, which ensure the proper use and storage of medications in the home.

Acute Care. Patients are often hospitalized to receive expert nursing observation and documentation of responses to medications. When a nurse receives a medication order, several nursing interventions are essential for safe and effective medication administration.

Receiving, Transcribing, and Communicating Medication Orders. An order is required to administer any medication. In the absence of CPOE, health care providers hand write orders onto order sheets in a patient's chart. If orders are handwritten, be sure that medication names, dosages, and symbols are legible. Clarify and then rewrite any unclear or illegible transcribed orders.

The process of verifying medical orders varies among health care agencies. Nurses follow agency policy and current national patient safety standards when receiving, transcribing, and communicating medication orders. *Nursing students are prohibited from transcribing or receiving verbal and telephone orders.*

Medication orders need to contain all of the elements in Box 32-10. If a medication order is incomplete, inform the health care provider and ensure completeness before carrying it out. Nurses read back verbal or telephone orders to health care providers to ensure that the correct order is obtained. The registered nurse follows agency policy regarding receiving, recording, and transcribing verbal and telephone orders. Generally the health care provider must sign them within 24 hours.

Nurses and pharmacists check all medication orders for accuracy and thoroughness several times during the transcription process. They also take patients' current problems, treatments, laboratory values, and other prescribed medications into consideration. Once the nurse and pharmacist determine that a medication order is safe and appropriate, it is placed on the appropriate medication form, usually called the *MAR*. The MAR is either printed on paper or available electronically. An electronic version of the MAR is called an *eMAR*. Whether it is handwritten, printed from a computer, or in an electronic version, it includes the patient's name, room, and bed number; medical record number; medical and food allergies; other patient identifiers (e.g., birthday); and medication name, dose, frequency, and route and time of administration. Each time a medication dose is prepared, the nurse refers to the MAR.

It is essential to verify the accuracy of every medication you give to your patients with the patients' orders. If the medication order is incomplete, incorrect, or inappropriate or if there is a discrepancy between the original order and the information on the MAR, consult with the health care provider. Do not give a medication until you are certain that you can follow the six rights of medication administration. When you give the wrong medication or an incorrect dose, *you* are legally responsible for the error.

Accurate Dose Calculation and Measurement. When measuring liquid medications, use standard measuring containers. Use a systematic procedure for medication measurement to lessen the chance of error. Calculate each dose when preparing a medication, pay close attention to the process of calculation, and avoid interruptions from other people or nursing activities. Ask another nurse to double-check your calculations against the original medication order if you are *ever* in doubt about the accuracy of your calculation or if you are calculating a dose for the first time or for a high-risk medication.

Correct Administration. For safe administration follow the six rights of medication administration. Verify the patient's identity by using at least two patient identifiers (TJC, 2016). In the acute care setting identifiers are usually on a patient's armband. Carefully compare patient identifiers with the MAR to ensure that you are giving the medication to the right patient. Use aseptic technique and proper procedures when handling and giving medications and perform necessary assessments (e.g., heart rate for antidysrhythmic medications) before administering a medication to a patient. Carefully monitor a patient's response to a medication, especially when the first dose of a new medication is administered.

Recording Medication Administration. Follow all agency policies when documenting medication administration. After administering a medication, appropriately document the name of the medication, dose, route, and exact time of administration immediately. Include the site of any injections per agency policy.

If a patient refuses a medication or is undergoing tests or procedures that result in a missed dose, explain the reason that a medication was not given in the nurses' notes. Some agencies require the nurse to circle the prescribed administration time on the medication record or to notify the health care provider when a patient misses a dose. Be aware of the effects that missing doses have on a patient (e.g., with hypertension or diabetes). Coordinating care with health care providers and other services when testing or diagnostic procedures are being completed helps ensure patient safety and therapeutic control of the disease.

Restorative Care. Because of the numerous types of restorative care settings, medication administration activities vary. Patients with functional limitations often require a nurse to fully administer all medications. In the home care setting patients usually administer their own medications or receive assistance from family caregivers. Regardless of the type of medication activity, the nurse is responsible

BOX 32-10 Components of Medication Orders

A medication order needs to have all of the following parts:

Patient's full name: A patient's full name distinguishes the patient from other people with the same last name. In the acute care setting patients are sometimes assigned special identification numbers (e.g., medical record number) to help distinguish patients with the same names. This number is often included on the order form.

Date and time that the order is written: The day, month, year, and time need to be included. Designating the time that an order is written clarifies when certain orders are to start and stop. If an incident occurs involving a medication error, it is easier to document what happened when this information is available.

Medication name: A health care provider orders a medication by its generic or trade name. Correct spelling is essential to prevent confusion with medications with similar spelling.

Dosage: The amount or strength of the medication is included.

Route of administration: A health care provider only uses accepted abbreviations for medication routes. Accuracy is important to ensure that patients receive medications by the intended route.

Time and frequency of administration: A nurse needs to know what time and how frequently to administer medications. Orders for multiple doses establish a routine schedule for medication administration.

Signature of health care provider: The signature makes an order a legal request.

for instructing patients and families in medication action, administration, and side effects. He or she is also responsible for monitoring adherence with medication and determining the effectiveness of medications that have been prescribed.

Special Considerations for Administering Medications to Specific Age-Groups. A patient's developmental level is a factor to consider when administering medications. Knowledge of developmental needs helps you anticipate responses to medication therapy.

Infants and Children. In many pediatric settings the standard of practice is to have another nurse verify all pediatric dose calculations before administration. All children require special psychological preparation before receiving medications. A child's parents are often valuable resources for determining the best way to give a child medication. Sometimes it is less traumatic for a child if a parent gives the medication and the nurse supervises. Supportive care is necessary if a child is expected to cooperate. Explain the procedure to a child, using words appropriate to his or her level of comprehension. Long explanations increase a child's anxiety, especially for painful procedures such as an injection. Providing a child with choices when possible can result in greater success. For example, saying, "It's time to take your pill now. Do you want it with water or juice?" allows a child to make a choice. Do not give the child the option of not taking a medication. After taking a medication, praise the child and offer a simple reward such as a star or token. Tips for administering medication to children are in Box 32-11.

Older Adults. Older adults also require special considerations during medication administration (Box 32-12). In addition to physiological changes of aging (Figure 32-8), behavioral and economic factors influence an older person's use of medications.

BOX 32-11 Tips for Administering Medications to Children

Oral Medications

- Liquids are safer to swallow than pills to avoid aspiration.
- Use droppers for administering liquids to infants; straws often help older children swallow pills.
- Offer juice, a soft drink, or frozen juice bar, if allowed, after the child swallows a drug.
- When mixing medications in other foods or liquids, use only a small amount. The child may refuse to take all of a larger mixture.
- Avoid mixing a medication in a child's favorite foods or liquids because the child may later refuse them.
- A plastic, disposable oral syringe is the most accurate device for preparing liquid doses, especially those less than 10 mL (cups, teaspoons, and droppers are inaccurate).

Injections

- Use caution when selecting intramuscular (IM) injection sites. Infants and small children have underdeveloped muscles. Follow agency policy.
- Children are sometimes unpredictable and uncooperative. Make sure that someone (preferably another nurse) is available to restrain a child if needed. Have the parent act as a comforter, not restrainer, if restraint is necessary.
- Always awaken a sleeping child before giving an injection.
- Distracting a child with conversation, bubbles, or a toy reduces pain perception.
- If time allows, apply a lidocaine ointment to an injection site before the injection to reduce pain perception during the injection.

Polypharmacy. Polypharmacy happens when a patient takes multiple medications or potentially inappropriate or unnecessary medications or when a medication does not match a diagnosis (Touhy and Jett, 2014). For example, polypharmacy exists when a patient takes two medications from the same chemical class to treat the same illness. Suspect polypharmacy if your patient uses two or more medications with the same or similar actions to treat several illnesses simultaneously and mixes nutritional supplements or herbal products with medications. Older adults also often experience polypharmacy when they seek relief from a variety of symptoms (e.g., pain, constipation, insomnia, and indigestion) by using OTC preparations. Sometimes polypharmacy is unavoidable. For example, some patients need to take more than one medication to control their high blood pressure. When a patient experiences polypharmacy, the risk of adverse reactions and medication interactions with other medications and food is increased.

Because many older adults suffer chronic health problems, polypharmacy is common. However, it is also becoming more common in children and patients with mental illnesses. Taking OTC medications frequently, lack of knowledge about medications, incorrect beliefs about medications, and visiting several health care providers to treat different illnesses increase the risk for polypharmacy. To minimize risks associated with polypharmacy, frequent communication among health care providers is essential to make sure that the patients' medication regimen is as simple as possible (Pasina et al, 2014).

◆ Evaluation

Evaluation of medication administration is an essential role of professional nursing that requires assessment skills; critical thinking; analysis; and knowledge of medications, physiology, and pathophysiology. You need to thoroughly and accurately gather data to complete a holistic evaluation. The goal of safe and effective medication administration is met when a patient responds appropriately to medication therapy and assumes responsibility for self-care. When patients do not experience expected outcomes of medication therapy, investigate possible reasons and determine appropriate revisions to the plan of care.

BOX 32-12 FOCUS ON OLDER ADULTS

Safety in Medication Administration

- Frequently review a patient's medication history, including use of over-the-counter medications, and consult with health care provider to simplify the drug therapy plan whenever possible (Pasina et al., 2014).
- Keep instructions clear and simple, provide memory aids (e.g., calendar, medication schedule), and ensure that written information about medications is in print large enough for a patient to see (Touhy and Jett, 2014).
- Assess functional status to determine if patient will require assistance in taking medications (Touhy and Jett, 2014).
- Some older adults have a greater sensitivity to drugs, especially those that act on the central nervous system. Therefore carefully monitor patients' responses to medications and anticipate dosage adjustments as needed (Touhy and Jett, 2014).
- If patient has difficulty swallowing a capsule or tablet, ask the health care provider to substitute a liquid medication or instruct patient to place medication on the front of the tongue and then swallow fluid to help wash it to the back of the throat. If the patient continues to have problems, have him or her try taking medication with a very small amount of semisolid food (e.g., applesauce) (Touhy and Jett, 2014).
- Teach alternatives to medications such as proper diet instead of vitamins and exercise instead of laxatives (Touhy and Jett, 2014).

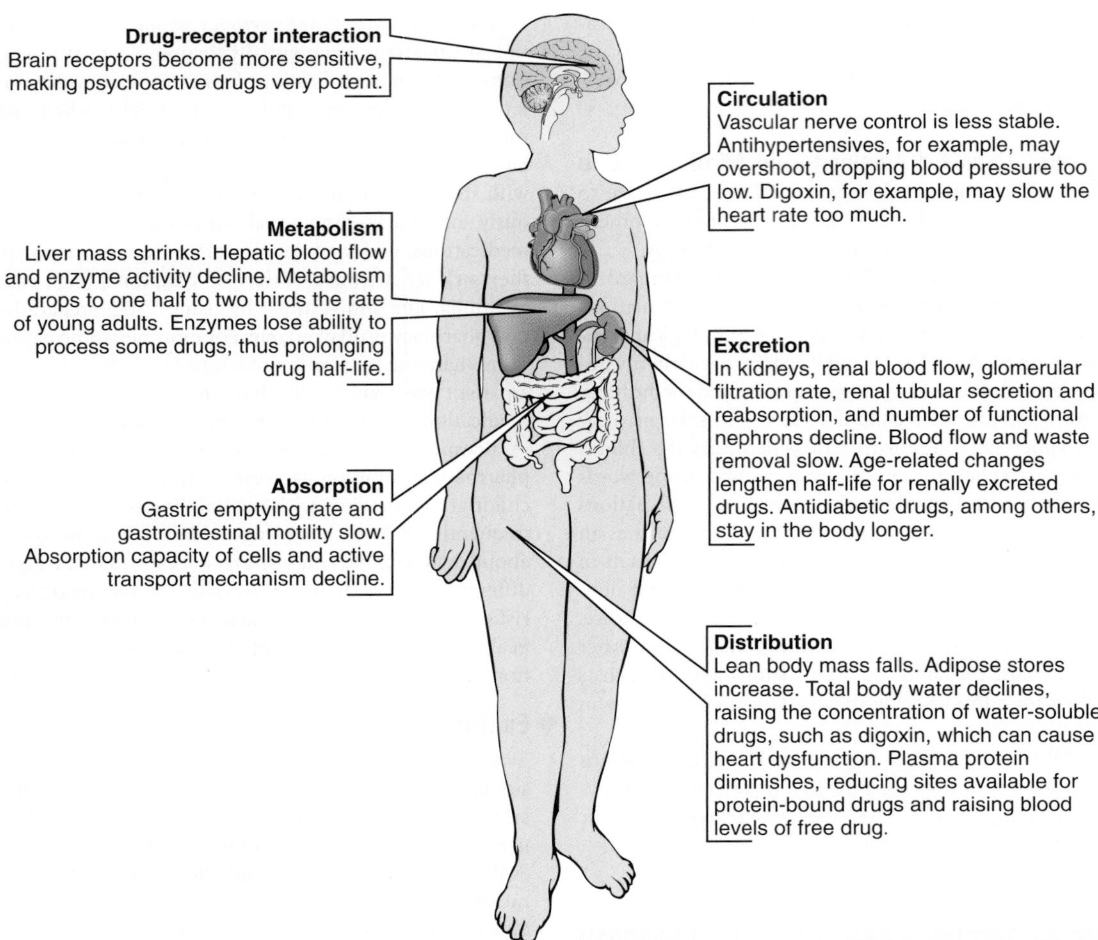

FIGURE 32-8 Effects of aging on medication metabolism. (From Lewis SM et al: *Medical-surgical nursing,* ed 9, St Louis, 2014, Mosby.)

Through the Patient's Eyes. Evaluation is more effective when you value your patients' participation. Therefore partner with your patients and include them in the evaluation process. Ensure that they understand and are able to safely administer their medications. For example, if you are caring for a child who needs an inhaler, be sure to watch the patient use the inhaler. To determine if patients understand their medication schedules, ask them to explain when they take their medications and if they are able to take them as prescribed. When patients struggle with their medication schedule, determine barriers to medication adherence (e.g., cost, lack of knowledge) and remove these barriers if possible. Also remember that patients have different values and define health differently. These values and beliefs influence their perception of the effectiveness of their medications. Therefore ask patients to describe this effectiveness. Ask if they are satisfied with their medications and how they make them feel. Use patients' statements and responses to questions (e.g., "I feel less anxious now") when determining the effectiveness of medications. Including patients in the evaluation process empowers them and helps them become more actively involved in their care.

Patient Outcomes. A patient's clinical condition can change minute by minute. Use knowledge of the desired effect and common side effects of each medication to compare expected outcomes with actual findings. A change in a patient's condition is often physiologically related to changes in health status or results from medications or both. Be alert for reactions in a patient taking several medications. Nurses use a variety of measures to evaluate patient responses to medications such as direct observation of physiological measures (e.g., blood pressure or laboratory values), behavioral responses (e.g., agitation), and rating scales (e.g., rating on a pain or nausea scale). The type of measurement used varies with the medication action being evaluated, the reading skill and knowledge level of the patient, and the patient's cognitive and psychomotor ability. The most common type of measurement is a physiological measure. Examples of physiological measures are blood pressure, heart rate, and visual acuity. Nurses also use patient statements as evaluative measures. Table 32-8 contains examples of goals, expected outcomes, and corresponding evaluative measures.

MEDICATION ADMINISTRATION

A sound knowledge base is required for medications to be administered safely. Nurses need to be prepared to administer medications using a variety of routes.

Oral Administration

The easiest and most desirable route for administering medications is by mouth (see Skill 32-1 on pp. 655-659). Patients usually are able to self-administer oral medications. Food sometimes affects their absorption so give them on an empty stomach if absorption is

TABLE 32-8 Example Evaluation for Patient Goals

Goal	Expected Outcomes	Evaluative Measure with Example
Patient and family will understand medication therapy.	Patient and family describe information about medication, dosage, schedule, purpose, and adverse effects.	Written measurement: Have patient write out medication schedule for a 24-hour period. Oral questioning: Use Teach Back and ask patient to describe purpose, dosage, and adverse effects of each prescribed medication.
	Patient and family identify situations that require medical intervention.	Oral questioning: Use Teach Back and have family describe what to do when a patient has adverse effects from a medication.
	Patient and family demonstrate appropriate administration technique.	Direct observation: Have patient complete return demonstration by filling insulin syringe and administering injection.
Patient will safely self-administer medications.	Patient follows prescribed treatment regimen.	Anecdotal notes: Have family keep log of patient's adherence to therapy for 1 week.
	Patient performs administration techniques correctly.	Direct observation: Observe patient instill eyedrops.
	Patient identifies available resources for obtaining necessary medication.	Oral questioning: Use Teach Back and ask family to identify how to contact local pharmacy or community clinic for necessary medications.

BOX 32-13 Protecting a Patient from Aspiration

- Allow patients to self-administer medications if possible.
- Know signs of dysphagia (difficulty swallowing): cough, change in voice tone or quality after swallowing, delayed swallowing, incomplete oral clearance or pocketing of food, regurgitation.
- Assess patient's ability to swallow and cough by checking for presence of gag reflex and then offering 50 mL of water in 5-mL allotments. Stop if patient begins to cough.
- Prepare oral medications in the form that is easiest to swallow.
- Position patient in an upright, seated position with feet on the floor, hips and knees at 90 degrees, head midline, and back erect if possible.
- If patient has unilateral weakness, place the medication in the stronger side of the mouth. Turning the head toward the weaker side helps the medication move down the stronger side of the esophagus.
- Administer pills one at a time, ensuring that each medication is swallowed properly before the next one is introduced.
- Thicken regular liquids or offer fruit nectars if patient cannot tolerate thin liquids.
- Some medications can be crushed and mixed with pureed foods if necessary. Refer to a medication reference to verify which medications are safe to crush.
- Avoid straws because they decrease the control patient has over volume intake, which increases the risk of aspiration.
- Have patient hold and drink from a cup if possible.
- Time medications to coincide with mealtimes or when patient is well rested and awake if possible.
- Administer medications using another route if risk of aspiration is severe.

decreased. Likewise give medications with meals if absorption is enhanced by food (Burchum and Rosenthal, 2016). Most tablets and capsules need to be swallowed and administered with approximately 60 to 240 mL of fluid (as allowed).

Oral medication administration is contraindicated in some situations (see Table 32-5). Many medications interact with nutritional and herbal supplements. You need to be knowledgeable about these interactions to determine the best time to give oral medications.

An important precaution to take when administering any oral preparation is to protect patients from aspiration. Aspiration occurs when food, fluid, or medication intended for GI administration inadvertently enters the respiratory tract. Protect a patient from aspiration by assessing his or her ability to swallow. Box 32-13 provides techniques that protect patients from aspiration. Proper positioning is essential. Position a patient in a seated position at a 90-degree angle when administering oral medications if not contraindicated by his or her condition. Usually having the patient slightly flex the head in a chin-down position reduces aspiration. Use a multidisciplinary approach (e.g., speech therapist, dietitian, and occupational therapist) to determine the best techniques for patients who have difficulty swallowing.

Special consideration is needed when administering medications to patients with enteral or small-bore feeding tubes (Box 32-14). Failing to follow current evidence-based recommendations from the American Society for Parenteral and Enteral Nutrition (ASPEN) can result in tube obstruction, reduced medication effectiveness, and increased risk of medication toxicity (Malone, 2014; Phillips and Endacott, 2011). Tubing misconnections continue to cause patient injury because tubes with different functions can be connected with Luer connectors (TJC, 2014b). In response to this issue the International Organization for Standardization (ISO) (ISMP, 2014b) has developed tubing connector standards in which the enteral connector will no longer be Luer compatible. A new enteral-only connector (ENFit) is available, and health care facilities have changed enteral nutrition practices, policies, procedures, and processes per the new guidelines (TJC, 2014b) (Box 32-15). Before giving a medication by this route, verify that the location of the tube (e.g., stomach or jejunum) is compatible with medication absorption. For example, iron dissolves in the stomach and is mostly absorbed in the duodenum. If it is administered through a jejunal tube, it has poor bioavailability.

Use liquid medications when possible. When liquid medications are not available, crush simple tablets or open capsules and dilute them in water. Pierce a gel cap with a sterile needle and empty contents into 30 mL of warm water or other solution as designated by the manufacturer of the medication. You can dissolve gel caps in warm water, but this often takes 15 to 20 minutes. Only use oral syringes when preparing medications for this route to prevent accidental parenteral administration. Flush tubes with at least 30 mL of water before and after giving medications. When administering more than one medication at a time, give each separately and flush between medications with 15 to 30 mL of water. Determine if medications need to be given on an empty stomach or if they are compatible with the patient's enteral feeding. If a medication needs to be given on an empty stomach or is not compatible with the feeding (e.g., phenytoin, carbamazepine [Tegretol], warfarin [Coumadin], fluoroquinolones, proton pump inhibitors), hold the feeding for at least 30 minutes before or 30 minutes after medication administration. Some of these medications may need up to 120 minutes to absorb (Guenter and Boullata, 2013). Verify the time with a drug reference or consult with a pharmacist.

BOX 32-14 PROCEDURAL GUIDELINES

Administering Medications Through an Enteral Tube (Nasogastric Tube, G-Tube, J-Tube, or Small-Bore Feeding Tube)

Delegation Considerations

The skill of giving medications through an enteral tube cannot be delegated to nursing assistive personnel (NAP). Instruct the NAP to:

- Keep the head of the bed elevated for a minimum of 30 degrees (preferably 45 degrees) for 1 hour after medication administration; follow agency policy.
- Immediately report coughing, choking, gagging, or drooling of liquid to the nurse.
- Report occurrence of side effects of medications to the nurse.

Equipment

60-mL oral syringe with appropriate tip (catheter tip for large-bore tube, Luer-Lok tip for small-bore tube) or enteral-only connector (ENFit) (see illustration), if available; gastric pH test strip (scale of 1.0 to 11.0); graduated container; medication to be administered; pill crusher if medication in tablet form; water or sterile water for immunocompromised patient; tongue blade or straw to stir dissolved medication; medication administration record (MAR) (electronic or printed); clean gloves; stethoscope (for evaluation)

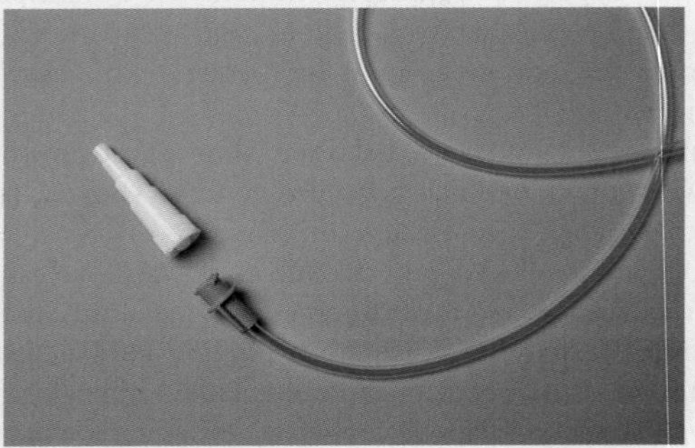

Steps

1. Check accuracy and completeness of each MAR with health care provider's medication order. Check patient's name and medication name, dosage, and route and time of administration. Recopy or reprint any part of printed MAR that is difficult to read.
2. Assess patient's knowledge about medication. Also assess medical history and for history or allergies to medications and foods. Make sure that patient's food and drug allergies are listed on the MAR and are prominently displayed on the patient's medical record per agency policy.
3. Avoid complicated medication schedules that frequently interrupt enteral feedings. Investigate options with health care provider and use alternative routes of medication administration if possible (e.g., intravenous [IV], transdermal, rectal).
   a. Evaluate where medication is absorbed and ensure that point of absorption is not bypassed by feeding tube. For example, some medications (e.g., antacids) are absorbed in the stomach. If the patient's tube is placed in the intestines, these medications are not absorbed because the tube bypasses the stomach (McIntyre and Monk, 2014; Prohaska and King, 2012).
   b. Determine if medication interacts with enteral feeding. If there is a risk for an interaction, stop the feeding for at least 30 minutes before giving the medication (see agency policy or consult with pharmacist or drug reference) (Phillips and Endacott, 2011).
4. Perform hand hygiene and prepare medication (see Skill 32-1, Steps 1a-g, 1l). Prepare medications in a liquid form when possible to prevent tube obstruction (Bankhead et al., 2009; Lohmann et al., 2015). Check label of medication with MAR 2 times for accuracy. *This is the first and second accuracy check.*
5. *Never* add medications directly to a container or bag of tube feeding (Bankhead et al., 2009). Sometimes the tube feeding needs to be held. Verify this and the amount of time that you hold a feeding with agency policy, a pharmacist, or a medication reference before administering the medication to maximize the therapeutic effect of the medication (Bankhead et al., 2009; Guenter and Boullata, 2013).
6. Take medications to patient at correct time (see agency policy). Give STAT, first-time or loading, and 1-time doses at the time ordered. Give time-critical scheduled medications no later than 30 minutes before or after scheduled dose. Give non–time-critical scheduled medications within 1-2 hours of scheduled dose (ISMP, 2011). Perform hand hygiene.
7. Identify patient using two identifiers (e.g., name and birthday or name and medical record number) according to agency policy. Compare identifiers with information on patient's MAR or medical record.
8. Compare label of medications against MAR one more time at patient's bedside. *This is the third accuracy check.*
9. Explain procedure and medications to patient.
10. Remember: Do not give whole or undissolved medications through the feeding tube.
11. Elevate head of bed to a minimum of 30 degrees (preferably 45 degrees) (unless contraindicated) or sit patient up in a chair (Bankhead et al., 2009).
12. Apply clean gloves. NOTE: If patient has a latex allergy, use latex-free gloves.
13. If an enteral tube feeding is infusing, adjust infusion pump to hold tube feeding. Verify placement of any feeding tube that enters the mouth or nose by observing gastric contents and checking pH of aspirated contents. A properly obtained pH value of less than 5.0 is a good indication of gastric placement (Clifford et al., 2015) (see Chapter 45).
14. Assess gastric residual volume (GRV). Draw up 30 mL air into 60-mL syringe, connect to feeding tube, and flush tube with air. Then pull back slowly to aspirate gastric contents (see Chapter 45). Determine GRV using either the scale on the syringe or graduated container. If GRV is 250 mL or less, return aspirated contents to stomach (see agency policy). If GRV is greater than 250 mL, hold medication and aspirated fluid and contact health care provider for orders (see agency policy) (Malone, 2014; Metheny et al., 2010).
15. Pinch or clamp enteral tube and remove syringe used to obtain GRV. Draw up 30 mL of water into syringe. Reinsert syringe tip into tube, release clamp, and flush tubing. Clamp tube again and remove syringe.
16. Administer medication
    a. **Syringe method:** Draw up liquid medication into syringe (do not mix medications); connect tip of syringe to end of enteral tubing. Push medication through tube. If resistance is felt when pushing medication through tube, stop administration and contact patient's health care provider.
    b. **Gravity method:** Remove bulb or plunger from syringe and reinsert syringe into tip of feeding tube. Do not insert into pigtail vent on nasogastric tube. Pour liquid medication or dissolved mixture of crushed medicine into feeding tube and allow it to flow into stomach or intestine freely using gravity. *Do not* mix medications together; administer each separately (Bankhead et al., 2009; Zhu and Zhou, 2013). If medication does not flow freely, raise the height of the syringe or have patient change position slightly. If medication still does not flow, attach bulb or plunger to syringe and follow Step 16a.
17. Flush tube with 15-30 mL of water between each medication (Klang et al., 2013).
18. After giving all the medications, flush tube again with 30-60 mL of water (Klang et al., 2013).

BOX 32-14 PROCEDURAL GUIDELINES

Administering Medications Through an Enteral Tube (Nasogastric Tube, G-Tube, J-Tube, or Small-Bore Feeding Tube)—cont'd

19. Restart tube feeding if appropriate. Clamp proximal end of tube if feeding is not being administered or needs to be held for 30 minutes or longer to avoid alterations in medication bioavailability (Bankhead et al., 2009).
20. Help patient to comfortable position and keep head of bed elevated for at least 1 hour (per agency policy). Clean area and put supplies away. Remove gloves and perform hand hygiene.
21. Document administration of medications, dose, route, and time on MAR.
22. Monitor patient for signs of aspiration such as choking, gurgling speech, or congested breath sounds during and after medication administration.
23. Evaluate patient's response to medication at times that correspond with onset, peak, and duration of medication. If desired effect is not achieved, a different medication or route of administration is probably indicated because of problems with drug bioavailability when given the enteral route.
24. Use ***Teach Back*** to determine patient's and family's understanding about enteral medications. State to patient, "I want to be sure I explained the medicines we're giving you through the feeding tube. Can you tell me why you're taking these medicines and what side effects you may develop?" If patient self-administers medications, state, "Show me how you're going to take these medications at home." Revise your instruction now or develop plan for revised teaching if patient or family is not able to teach back correctly.

BOX 32-15 The Joint Commission (TJC) Recommendations for New Enteral Tube Connectors

- Trace tubing or catheter from the patient to the point of origin:
  - Before connecting or reconnecting any device or infusion.
  - At any transition such as to a new setting or service.
  - As part of the hand-off process.
- Route tubes and catheters with different purposes in standard directions (e.g., toward the head, toward the feet) and label the tubes at both the proximal and distal ends.
- Use tubing and related equipment only for their intended use.
  - Never use standard Luer syringes for oral medications or enteral feedings.
  - Do not use intravenous (IV) tubing or IV pumps for enteral feedings.
  - Use distinctly different pumps for IV applications.
  - Eliminate the use of temporary adapters as soon as possible.
  - Do not force connections and avoid workarounds.
- Use safe practices for high-alert medications.
  - Label the tubing or catheter.
  - Do not use tubing or catheter with injection ports.
  - Use an independent double-check procedure.
- Educate staff.
  - Provide adequate staff education for anyone using this new equipment.
  - Provide a reference manual.
- Create a culture of safety and reporting of adverse events.

Adapted from The Joint Commission (TJC): *Sentinel alert event: managing risk during transition to new ISO connector standards,* 2014b, http://www.jointcommission.org/assets/1/6/SEA_53_Connectors_8_19_14_final.pdf. Accessed June 8, 2015.

Monitor the patient closely for adverse reactions. The risk for drug-drug interactions is high when two or more medications are given in this route because they can interact together as soon as they are administered.

Topical Medication Applications

Topical medications are medications that are applied locally, most often to intact skin. They come in many forms (see Table 32-1). They are also applied to mucous membranes.

Skin Applications. Because many locally applied medications such as lotions, pastes, and ointments create systemic and local effects, apply these medications with gloves and applicators. Use sterile technique if a patient has an open wound. Skin encrustation and dead tissues harbor microorganisms and block contact of medications with the tissues to be treated. Before applying medications, clean the skin thoroughly by washing the area gently with soap and water, soaking an involved site, or locally debriding tissue.

Apply each type of medication according to directions to ensure proper penetration and absorption. When applying ointments or pastes, spread the medication evenly over the involved surface and cover the area well without applying an overly thick layer. Health care providers sometimes order a gauze dressing to be applied over the medication to prevent soiling clothes and wiping away the medication. Lightly spread lotions and creams onto the surface of the skin; rubbing often causes irritation. Apply a liniment by rubbing it gently but firmly into the skin. Dust a powder lightly to cover the affected area with a thin layer.

Some topical medications are applied in the form of a transdermal patch that remains in place for an extended amount of time (e.g., 12 hours or 7 days). Before applying a new patch, don disposable gloves and remove the old one. Medication remains on the patch even after its recommended duration of use. Nurses and patients have inadvertently left old transdermal patches in place, resulting in the patient receiving an overdose of the medication. For example, patients who use fentanyl transdermal patches for pain management can experience respiratory depression, coma, and death when the patches are not removed. In addition, some people, especially children, have experienced life-threatening harm from accidental exposure to fentanyl patches that were not disposed of properly (USFDA, 2012). Many patches are clear, which makes them difficult to see. Therefore carefully assess the patient's skin and be sure to remove the existing patch before applying a new one. Follow these guidelines to ensure safe administration of transdermal or topical medications:

- When taking a medication history or reconciling medications, specifically ask patients if they take any medications in the forms of patches, topical creams, or any route other than the oral route.
- When applying a transdermal patch, ask the patient if he or she has an existing patch.
- Wear disposable gloves when removing and applying transdermal patches.
- If the dressing or patch is difficult to see (e.g., clear), apply a noticeable label to the patch.
- Document the location on the patient's body where the medication was placed on the MAR.
- Document removal of the patch or medication on the MAR. Fold sticky sides of the patch together and dispose of the patch in a child-proof container.

Nasal Instillation. Patients with nasal sinus alterations sometimes receive medications by spray, drops, or tampons (Box 32-16). The most commonly administered form of nasal instillation is decongestant spray or drops, used to relieve symptoms of sinus congestion and colds. Caution patients to avoid abuse of medications because overuse leads to a rebound effect in which the nasal congestion worsens. When excess decongestant solution is swallowed, serious systemic effects also develop, especially in children. Saline drops are safer than nasal preparations that contain sympathomimetics (e.g., Afrin or Neo-Synephrine) as a decongestant for children.

It is easier to have patients self-administer sprays because they are able to control the spray and inhale as the medication enters the nasal passages. For patients who use nasal sprays repeatedly, check the nares for irritation. When used to treat a sinus infection, position patients to permit the nasal medication to reach the affected sinus. Severe nosebleeds are usually treated with packing or nasal tampons, which are treated with epinephrine, to reduce blood flow. Usually a physician or advanced practice clinician places nasal tampons.

Eye Instillation. Some patients use OTC eyedrops and ointments such as artificial tears and vasoconstrictors (e.g., Visine and Murine). Other patients, especially older adults, receive prescribed **ophthalmic** medications for eye conditions such as glaucoma or after cataract extraction. Age-related problems, including poor vision, hand tremors, and difficulty grasping or manipulating containers, affect an older adult's ability to self-administer eye medications. Instruct patients and family members about the proper techniques for administering them (see Skill 32-2 on pp. 660-663). Determine a patient's and family caregiver's ability to self-administer through a return demonstration of the procedure. Show patients each step for instilling eyedrops to help them understand the procedure. Follow these principles when administering eye medications:

- Avoid instilling any form of eye medications directly onto the cornea. The cornea of the eye has many pain fibers and thus is very sensitive to anything applied to it.
- Avoid touching the eyelids or other eye structures with eyedroppers or ointment tubes. The risk of transmitting infection from one eye to the other is high.
- Use eye medication only for the patient's affected eye.
- Never allow a patient to use another patient's eye medications.

Intraocular Administration. One less common way to administer eye medications is by the intraocular route (see Skill 32-2). These medications resemble a contact lens. You place the medication into the conjunctival sac where it remains for up to 1 week. You need to teach patients how to insert and remove the disk and to monitor for adverse medication reactions.

Ear Instillation. Because internal ear structures are very sensitive to temperature extremes, you need to instill eardrops at room temperature to prevent vertigo, dizziness, or nausea. Although the structures of the outer ear are not sterile, sterile solutions are used in case the eardrum is ruptured. The entrance of nonsterile solutions into middle ear structures often results in infection. If a patient has ear drainage, be sure that the eardrum has not ruptured. Never occlude or block the ear canal with the dropper or irrigating syringe. Forcing medication into an occluded ear canal creates pressure that injures the eardrum. Box 32-17 provides guidelines for administering eardrops.

Vaginal Instillation. Vaginal medications are available as suppositories, foam, jellies, or creams. Solid, oval-shaped suppositories are packaged individually in foil wrappers and are sometimes stored in the refrigerator to prevent them from melting. After a suppository is inserted into the vaginal cavity, body temperature causes it to melt and be distributed and absorbed. Foam, jellies, and creams are administered with an applicator inserter (Box 32-18). Give a suppository with a gloved hand in accordance with standard precautions (see Chapter 29). Patients often prefer administering their own vaginal medications and need privacy. Because vaginal medications are often given to treat infection, discharge is usually foul smelling. Follow aseptic technique and offer the patient frequent opportunities to maintain perineal hygiene (see Chapter 40).

Rectal Instillation. Rectal suppositories are thinner and more bullet shaped than vaginal suppositories. The rounded end prevents anal trauma during insertion. Rectal suppositories contain medications that exert local effects such as promoting defecation or systemic effects such as reducing nausea. They are stored in a refrigerator until administered. Sometimes it is necessary to clear the rectum with a small cleansing enema before inserting a suppository (Box 32-19).

Administering Medications by Inhalation

Medications administered with handheld inhalers are dispersed through an aerosol spray, mist, or powder that penetrates lung airways. The alveolar-capillary network absorbs medications rapidly.

Pressurized metered-dose inhalers (pMDIs), breath-actuated metered-dose inhalers (BAIs), and dry powder inhalers (DPIs) deliver medications that produce local effects such as bronchodilation. Some medications create serious systemic side effects. pMDIs use a chemical propellant to push the medication out of the inhaler and require the patient to apply approximately 5 to 10 lbs of pressure to the top of the canister to administer the medication. Children or older adults with chronic respiratory diseases often use pMDIs. These two populations have diminished hand strength; therefore it is essential to assess if they

BOX 32-16 PROCEDURAL GUIDELINES

Administering Nasal Medications

Delegation Considerations

The skill of administering nasal medications cannot be delegated to nursing assistive personnel (NAP). Instruct the NAP to:

- Watch for potential side effects of medications and report their occurrence.

Equipment

Prepared medication with clean dropper or spray container, facial tissue, small pillow (optional), washcloth (optional), clean gloves (if patient has extensive nasal drainage), medication administration record (MAR) (electronic or printed), penlight

Steps

1. Check accuracy and completeness of each MAR with health care provider's medication order. Check patient's name and medication name, dosage, and route and time of administration. Recopy or reprint any part of printed MAR that is difficult to read.
2. Refer to the medical record to determine which sinus is affected if giving nasal drops.
3. Assess patient's medical history (e.g., history of hypertension, heart disease, diabetes mellitus, hyperthyroidism) and for history or allergies to medications and foods. Make sure that patient's food and drug allergies

BOX 32-16 PROCEDURAL GUIDELINES

Administering Nasal Medications—cont'd

are listed on the MAR and prominently displayed on his or her medical record per agency policy.

4. Perform hand hygiene. Using a penlight, inspect condition of nose and sinuses. Palpate sinuses for tenderness (see Chapter 31).
5. Assess patient's knowledge regarding use of and technique for nasal instillation and willingness to learn self-administration.
6. Review pertinent information related to medication: action, purpose, normal dose and route, side effects, time of onset and peak action, and nursing implications.
7. Perform hand hygiene and prepare medication (see Skill 32-1, Steps 1a-g, 1l). Compare medication label against MAR at least 2 times while preparing medication. *This is the first and second accuracy check.*
8. Take medication to patient at correct time (see agency policy). Give STAT, first-time or loading, and 1-time doses at the time ordered. Give time-critical scheduled medications no later than 30 minutes before or after scheduled dose. Give non–time-critical scheduled medications within 1-2 hours of scheduled dose (ISMP, 2011). Perform hand hygiene.
9. Identify patient using two identifiers (e.g., name and birthday or name and medical record number) according to agency policy. Compare identifiers with information on patient's MAR or medical record.
10. Compare names of medication on label with MAR one more time at patient's bedside. *This is the third accuracy check.*
11. Explain procedure to patient regarding positioning and sensations to expect such as burning or stinging of mucosa or choking sensation as medication trickles into throat.
12. Arrange supplies and medications at bedside. Apply clean gloves if patient has nasal drainage. NOTE: If patient has a latex allergy, use latex-free gloves.
13. Gently roll or shake container.
14. Instruct patient to clear or blow nose gently unless contraindicated (e.g., risk of increased intracranial pressure or nosebleeds). Teach patient about medication purpose, dose, time to instill, and possible side effects.
15. *Administer nasal drops:*
    a. Help patient to supine position and position head properly.
        (1) For access to posterior pharynx, tilt patient's head backward.
        (2) For access to ethmoid or sphenoid sinus, tilt head back over edge of bed or place small pillow under patient's shoulder and tilt head back (see illustration).

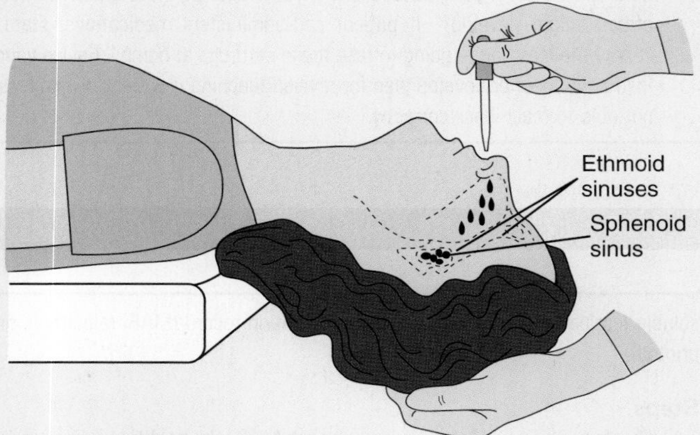

STEP 15a(2) Position for instilling nose drops into ethmoid or sphenoid sinus.

        (3) For access to frontal and maxillary sinus, tilt head back over edge of bed or pillow with head turned toward side to be treated (see illustration).

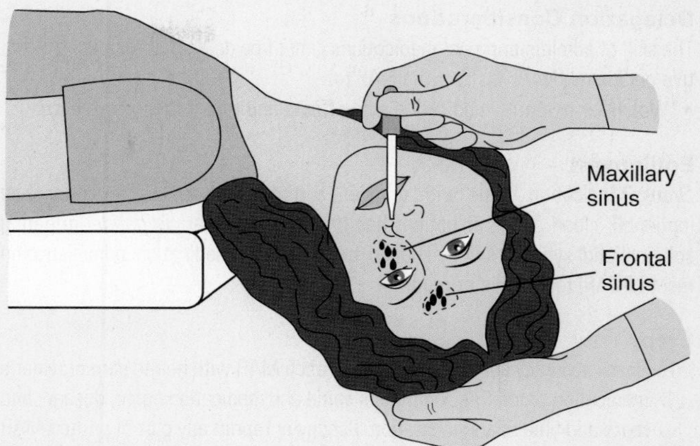

STEP 15a(3) Position for instilling nose drops into frontal and maxillary sinus.

    b. Support patient's head with nondominant hand.
    c. Instruct patient to breathe through mouth.
    d. Hold dropper 1 cm (½ inch) above nares and instill prescribed number of drops toward midline of ethmoid bone.
    e. Have patient remain in supine position 5 minutes.
    f. Offer facial tissue to blot runny nose but caution patient against blowing nose for several minutes.
16. *Administer nasal spray:*
    a. Prime nasal spray if indicated by manufacturer. Help patient to supine position and position head slightly tilted forward.
    b. Help patient place spray nozzle into appropriate nares, pointing nozzle to side and away from center of nose. Gently close opposite nostril with a finger.
    c. Have patient spray medication into nose while inhaling.
    d. Help patient take nozzle out of nose and instruct him or her to hold breath for a few seconds and then breathe out through the mouth.
    e. Offer facial tissue but caution patient against blowing nose for several minutes.
17. Help patient to a comfortable position after medication is absorbed.
18. Wipe tip of bottle with clean, dry tissue and replace the cap; dispose of soiled supplies in proper container; remove and dispose of gloves and perform hand hygiene.
19. Document name of medication, dose, route, and time of administration on MAR.
20. Observe patient for onset of side effects 15 to 30 minutes after administration. Ask if he or she is able to breathe through nose after decongestant administration. It may be necessary to have patient occlude one nostril at a time and breathe deeply.
21. Evaluate patient's response to medications at times that correlate with the onset, peak, and duration of the medication. Evaluate patient for both desired effect and adverse effects. Reinspect condition of nasal passages between instillations.
22. Use ***Teach Back*** to determine patient's and family's understanding about nasal medications. State to patient, "I want to be sure I explained your nasal spray correctly. Can you tell me the best time for you to use this spray? What side effects may you get from using the spray?" If patient self-administers medications at home, state, "Show me how you're going to take this medication at home." Revise your instruction now or develop plan for revised teaching if patient or family is not able to teach back correctly.

BOX 32-17 PROCEDURAL GUIDELINES

Administering Ear Medications

Delegation Considerations

The skill of administering ear medications cannot be delegated to nursing assistive personnel (NAP). Instruct the NAP to:

- Watch for potential medication side effects and report their occurrence.

Equipment

Drops: Medication bottle with dropper, cotton-tipped applicator, cotton ball (optional), clean gloves if patient has drainage from ear; *Irrigation:* irrigating solution and syringe, kidney-shaped basin, towel; medication administration record (MAR) (electronic or printed)

Steps

1. Check accuracy and completeness of each MAR with health care provider's medication order. Check patient's name and medication name, dosage, and route and time of administration. Recopy or reprint any part of printed MAR that is difficult to read.
2. Assess patient's medical history (e.g., history of dizziness, hearing loss); medication history; and history of allergies to medications, food, and latex.
3. Review pertinent information related to medication: action, purpose, normal dose and route (correct ear), side effects, time of onset and peak action, and nursing implications.
4. Assess patient's knowledge of medication.
5. Perform hand hygiene. Prepare medication (see Skill 32-1, Steps 1a-g, 1l). Check label of medication with MAR 2 times for accuracy. *This is the first and second accuracy check.*
6. Take medication to patient at correct time (see agency policy). Give STAT, first-time or loading, and 1-time doses at the time ordered. Give time-critical scheduled medications no later than 30 minutes before or after scheduled dose. Give non–time-critical scheduled medications within 1-2 hours of scheduled dose (ISMP, 2011). Perform hand hygiene.
7. Identify patient using two identifiers (e.g., name and birthday or name and medical record number) according to agency policy. Compare identifiers with information on the patient's MAR or medical record.
8. Compare names of medications on label with the MAR one more time at the patient's bedside. *This is the third accuracy check.* Hold medication container in hands for a few minutes to bring medication to body temperature.
9. Explain procedure to patient regarding positioning and sensations to expect such as hearing bubbling or feeling water in ear as medication trickles into ear.
10. Teach patient about action of medication, dose, time of instillation, and possible side effects.
11. Administer eardrops:
    a. Apply clean gloves and gently clean outer ear with washcloth if drainage is present. NOTE: If patient has a latex allergy, use latex-free gloves.
    b. Place patient in side-lying position (if not contraindicated by his or her condition) with ear to be treated facing up or have him or her sit in chair or at the bedside. If eardrops are a cloudy suspension, shake them for about 10 seconds.
    c. Straighten ear canal by pulling auricle down and back (children younger than 3 years) or upward and backward (children 3 years of age and older and adults).
    d. Instill prescribed drops holding dropper 1 cm (½ inch) above ear canal (see illustration).

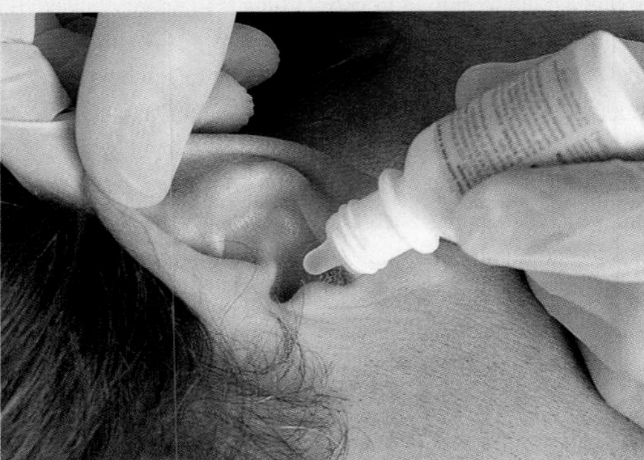

STEP 11d Instill prescribed drops above ear canal.

    e. Ask patient to remain in side-lying position 2 to 3 minutes. Apply gentle massage or pressure to tragus of ear with finger unless contraindicated because of pain.
    f. If cotton ball is needed, place it into outermost part of canal. Do not press cotton deep into canal. Remove it after 15 minutes.
12. Clean the area and put supplies away.
13. Remove gloves and perform hand hygiene.
14. Document medication administration on MAR.
15. Use ***Teach Back*** to determine patient's and family's understanding about ear medications. State to patient, "I want to be sure I explained your eardrops correctly. Can you tell me why you are taking these and what side effects might develop?" If patient self-administers medications, state, "Show me how you're going to take these eardrops at home." Revise your instruction now or develop plan for revised teaching if patient or family is not able to teach back correctly.

BOX 32-18 PROCEDURAL GUIDELINES

Administering Vaginal Medications

Delegation Considerations

The skill of administering vaginal medications cannot be delegated to nursing assistive personnel (NAP). Instruct the NAP to:

- Report new or increased vaginal discharge or bleeding and occurrence of side effects of medications.
- Offer to provide perineal care following medication administration.

Equipment

Vaginal cream, foam, jelly, or suppository with applicator (if required); clean gloves; towels and/or washcloth; perineal pad; drape or sheet; water-soluble lubricating jelly; medication administration record (MAR) (electronic or printed)

Steps

1. Check accuracy and completeness of each MAR with health care provider's medication order. Check patient's name and medication name, form (cream or suppository), dosage, and route and time of administration. Recopy or reprint any part of printed MAR that is difficult to read.
2. Assess patient's medical history (e.g., history of vaginal drainage); medication history; and history of allergies to medications, food, and latex.

BOX 32-18 PROCEDURAL GUIDELINES

Administering Vaginal Medications—cont'd

3. Review pertinent information related to medication: action, purpose, normal dose and route, side effects, time of onset and peak action, and nursing implications.
4. Assess patient's knowledge of medication.
5. Perform hand hygiene. Prepare medication (see Skill 32-1, Steps 1a-g, 1l). Check name of medication on label with MAR 2 times for accuracy. *This is the first and second accuracy check.*
6. Take medication to patient at the correct time (see agency policy). Give STAT, first-time or loading, and 1-time doses at the time ordered. Give time-critical scheduled medications no later than 30 minutes before or after scheduled dose. Give non–time-critical scheduled medications within 1-2 hours of scheduled dose (ISMP, 2011). Perform hand hygiene.
7. Identify patient using two identifiers (e.g., name and birthday or name and medical record number) according to agency policy. Compare identifiers with information on patient's MAR or medical record.
8. Compare names of medication on label with the MAR one more time at patient's bedside. *This is the third accuracy check.*
9. Teach patient about the action of medication, dose, time for instillation, and possible side effects. Explain procedure regarding positioning and sensations to expect such as feelings of moisture or wetness in the vaginal area. Be sure that patient understands the procedure if she plans to self-administer the medication.
10. Close room door or pull curtain to provide privacy. Determine patient's ability to manipulate applicator or suppository and ability to position self to insert medication.
11. Apply clean gloves. NOTE: If patient has a latex allergy, use latex-free gloves.
12. Help patient into dorsal recumbent position and keep abdomen and lower extremities draped.
13. Be sure that lighting is adequate to visualize vaginal opening. Inspect condition of external genitalia and vaginal canal (see Chapter 31), noting appearance of any discharge. Clean area with washcloth or towel if necessary (see Chapter 40).
14. Administer vaginal suppository:
    a. Remove suppository from foil wrapper and apply liberal amount of sterile, water-based lubricating jelly to smooth or rounded end. Lubricate gloved index finger of dominant hand.
    b. With nondominant gloved hand expose vaginal orifice by gently retracting labial folds.
    c. With dominant gloved hand gently insert rounded end of suppository along posterior wall of vaginal canal entire length of finger (7.5 to 10 cm [3 to 4 inches]) to ensure equal distribution of medication along walls of vaginal cavity (see illustration).

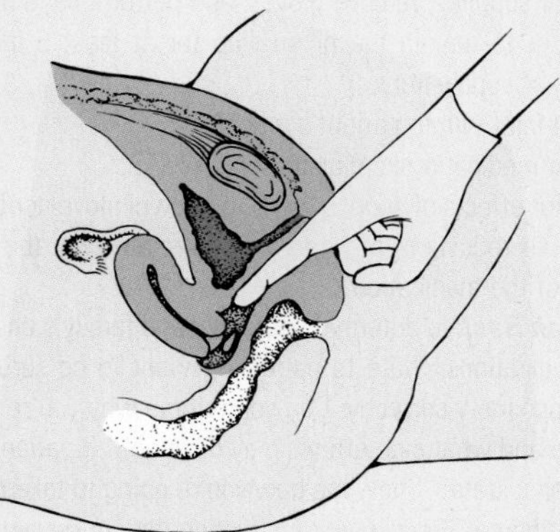

STEP 14c Insertion of suppository into vaginal canal.

    d. Withdraw finger and wipe away remaining lubricant from around orifice and labia.
15. Administer cream or foam:
    a. Fill cream or foam applicator following package directions.
    b. With nondominant gloved hand, expose vaginal orifice by gently retracting labial folds.
    c. With dominant gloved hand, insert applicator approximately 5 to 7.5 cm (2 to 3 inches). Push applicator plunger to deposit medication into vagina to allow equal distribution of medication (see illustration).

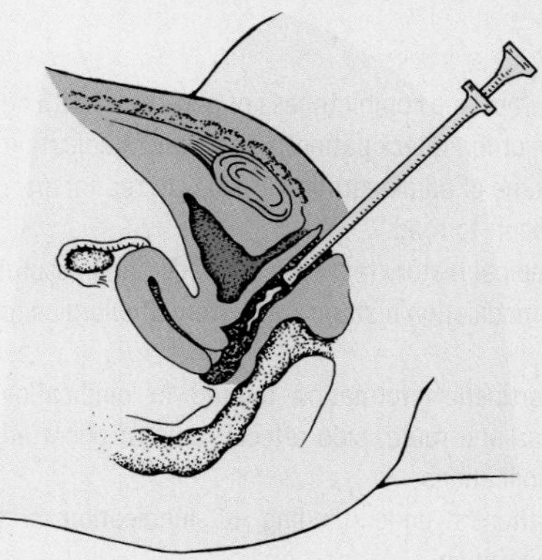

STEP 15c Instillation of medication in vaginal canal.

    d. Withdraw applicator and place on paper towel. Wipe off residual cream from labia or vaginal orifice.
16. Dispose of supplies, remove and dispose of gloves, and perform hand hygiene.
17. Instruct patient to remain on back for at least 10 minutes to allow medication to be distributed and absorbed evenly throughout vaginal cavity and not lost through orifice.
18. Document medication administration on MAR.
19. If using an applicator, wear gloves while washing with soap and warm water, rinse, and store for future use.
20. Offer patient perineal pad when she resumes ambulation.
21. Use ***Teach Back*** to determine patient and family's understanding about vaginal medications. State to patient, "I want to be sure I explained your vaginal medication correctly. Can you tell me why you're taking these suppositories and what type of side effects may develop?" If patient self-administers medications, state, "Show me how you're going to take your vaginal medications at home." Revise your instruction now or develop plan for revised teaching if patient or family is not able to teach back correctly.

BOX 32-19 PROCEDURAL GUIDELINES

Administering Rectal Suppositories

Delegation Considerations

The skill of administering rectal suppositories cannot be delegated to nursing assistive personnel (NAP). Instruct NAP to:

- Watch for and report fecal discharge or bowel movement.
- Report occurrence of medication side effects.
- Offer to provide perineal care following medication administration.

Equipment

Rectal suppository, water-soluble lubricating jelly, clean gloves, drape or sheet, tissue, medication administration record (MAR) (electronic or printed)

Steps

1. Check accuracy and completeness of each MAR with health care provider's medication order. Check patient's name and medication name, dosage, and route and time of administration. Recopy or reprint any part of printed MAR that is difficult to read.
2. Review medical history (e.g., hemorrhoids, anal fissures, rectal surgery, or bleeding); medication history; and history of allergies to medications, food, and latex.
3. Review pertinent information related to medication: action, purpose, normal dose and route, side effects, time of onset and peak action, and nursing implications.
4. Assess patient's understanding of medication and experience with self-administration.
5. Perform hand hygiene and prepare medication (see Skill 32-1, Steps 1a-g, 1l). Compare names of medication on label with the MAR 2 times for accuracy. *This is the first and second accuracy check.*
6. Take medication to patient at the correct time. Give STAT, first-time or loading, and 1-time doses at the time ordered. Give time-critical scheduled medications no later than 30 minutes before or after scheduled dose. Give non–time-critical scheduled medications within 1-2 hours of scheduled dose (ISMP, 2011). Perform hand hygiene.
7. Identify patient using two identifiers (e.g., name and birthday or name and medical record number) according to agency policy. Compare identifiers with information on patient's MAR or medical record.
8. Compare names of medication on label with the MAR one more time at patient's bedside. *This is the third accuracy check.*
9. Teach patient about the medication. Explain procedure regarding positioning and sensations to expect such as feelings of needing to defecate. Be sure that patient understands the procedure if he or she is going to self-administer the medication.
10. Close room door or pull curtain to ensure privacy.
11. Apply clean gloves. NOTE: If patient has a latex allergy, use latex-free gloves.
12. Help patient to Sims' position. Keep him or her draped with only anal area exposed.
13. Be sure that lighting is adequate to visualize anus. Examine condition of anus externally and palpate rectal walls as needed (see Chapter 31). Dispose of gloves in proper receptacle if soiled.
14. Apply new pair of clean gloves (if previous gloves were soiled). NOTE: If patient has a latex allergy, use latex-free gloves.
15. Remove suppository from wrapper and lubricate rounded end (see illustration) with sterile water-soluble lubricating jelly. Lubricate index finger of dominant hand with water-soluble lubricant.

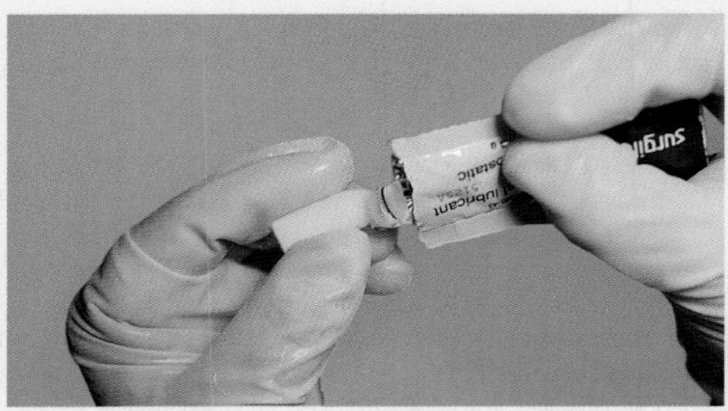

STEP 15 Remove suppository from wrapper.

16. Ask patient to take slow, deep breaths through mouth and relax anal sphincter.
17. Retract buttocks with nondominant hand. Insert suppository gently through anus, past internal sphincter and against rectal wall, 10 cm (4 inches) in adults, 5 cm (2 inches) in children and infants (see illustration). Apply gentle pressure to hold buttocks together momentarily if needed to keep medication in place.

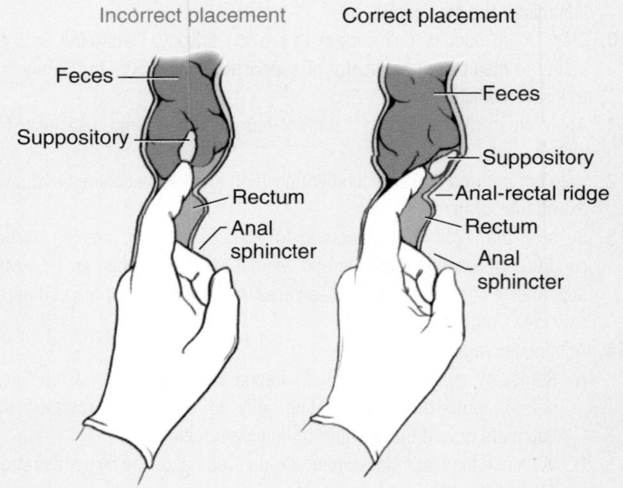

STEP 17 Inserting rectal suppository. (From deWit S: *Fundamental concepts and skills for nursing,* ed 4, Philadelphia, 2014, Saunders.)

18. Withdraw finger and wipe anal area with tissue.
19. Dispose of supplies, remove gloves, and perform hand hygiene.
20. Ask patient to remain flat or on side for at least 5 minutes to prevent expulsion of suppository.
21. Place call light within patient's reach.
22. Document medication administration on MAR.
23. Observe for effects of suppository (e.g., bowel movement, relief of nausea, temperature reduction) at times that correlate with the onset, peak, and duration of the medication.
24. Use ***Teach Back*** to determine patient's and family's understanding about rectal medications. State to patient, "I want to be sure I explained your rectal suppository correctly. Can you tell me why you're taking these suppositories and what side effects may develop?" If patient self-administers medications, state, "Show me how you're going to take these rectal medications at home." Revise your instruction now or develop plan for revised teaching if patient or family is not able to teach back correctly.

have enough strength to use the pMDI. BAIs release medication when a patient raises a lever and inhales. Release of the medication depends on the strength of the patient's breath on inspiration, and a BAI is a good choice for patients who have difficulty using pMDIs because it eliminates the need for hand-breath coordination (Ari and Restrepo, 2012).

DPIs hold dry powder medication and create an aerosol when the patient inhales through a reservoir that contains a dose of the medication. Some DPIs are unit dosed. These inhalers require patients to load a single dose of medication into the inhaler with each use. Other DPIs hold enough medication for 1 month. DPIs require less manual dexterity. Because the device is activated with the patient's breath, there is no need to coordinate puffs with inhalation. However, the medication inside the DPI can clump if the patient is in a humid climate, and some patients cannot inspire fast enough to administer the entire dose of the medication.

Patients who receive medications by inhalation frequently suffer chronic respiratory disease such as chronic asthma, emphysema, or bronchitis. Different respiratory problems require different inhaled medication. For example, patients with asthma usually receive antiinflammatory medications because asthma is primarily an inflammatory disease, whereas patients with chronic obstructive pulmonary disease (COPD) receive bronchodilators because they usually have problems with bronchoconstriction. Inhaled medications are also often described as "rescue" or "maintenance" medications. Rescue medications are short acting and taken for immediate relief of acute respiratory distress. Maintenance medications are used on a daily schedule to prevent acute respiratory distress. The effects of maintenance medications start within hours of administration and last for a longer period of time than rescue medications. Some inhalers contain combinations of rescue and maintenance medications. Because patients depend on inhaled medications for disease control and current evidence shows that many patients do not use their inhalers correctly, nurses need to teach and reteach their patients about their safe and effective use (Ari and Restrepo, 2012) (see Skill 32-3 on pp. 663-666).

Some patients use a spacer with the pMDI. The spacer is a 10- to 20-cm (4- to 8-inch) long tube that attaches to the pMDI and allows the particles of medication to slow down and break into smaller pieces, which improves drug absorption in a patient's airway. Spacers have a face mask for infants and children less than 4 years of age. They are especially helpful when a patient has difficulty coordinating the steps involved in self-administering inhaled medications. When patients do not use their inhalers and spacers correctly, they do not receive the full effect of the medication. Therefore patient education is essential. BAIs and DPIs do not require the use of spacers.

One important aspect of patient teaching is to help the patient determine when the MDI, BAI, or DPI is empty and needs to be replaced. Floating an MDI in water to determine how much medication is left is not recommended because extra propellant causes the container to float even if no medication remains in the inhaler. Devices that count down the number of remaining doses are available for MDIs. Some DPIs have mechanisms that indicate how many doses are left. However, these mechanisms are not always accurate. Therefore, to calculate how long medication in an inhaler will last, divide the number of doses in the container by the number of doses the patient takes per day. For example, a patient is to take albuterol 2 puffs 4 times a day. The canister has a total of 200 puffs. Complete the following calculation to determine how long the MDI will last:

$$2 \text{ puffs} \times 4 \text{ times a day} = 8 \text{ puffs per day}$$
$$200 \text{ puffs} \div 8 \text{ puffs per day} = 25 \text{ days}$$

The canister in this example will last 25 days. To ensure that the patient does not run out of medication, teach him or her to refill it at least 7 to 10 days before it runs out.

BOX 32-20 Preventing Infection During an Injection

- To prevent contaminating the solution, draw up medication quickly. Do not allow ampules to stand open.
- To prevent needle contamination, avoid letting a needle touch contaminated surfaces (e.g., outer edges of ampule or vial, outer surface of needle cap, nurse's hands, countertop, table surface).
- To prevent syringe contamination, avoid touching length of plunger or inner part of barrel. Keep tip of syringe covered with cap or needle.
- To prepare skin, wash with soap and water if soiled with dirt, drainage, or feces and dry. Use friction and a circular motion while cleaning with an antiseptic swab. Swab from center of site and move outward in a 5-cm (2-inch) radius.

Administering Medications by Irrigations

Some medications irrigate or wash out a body cavity and are delivered through a stream of solution. Irrigations most commonly use sterile water, saline, or antiseptic solutions on the eye, ear, throat, vagina, and urinary tract. Use aseptic technique if there is a break in the skin or mucosa. Use clean technique when the cavity to be irrigated is not sterile, as in the case of the ear canal or vagina. Irrigations cleanse an area, instill a medication, or apply hot or cold to injured tissue (see Chapter 48).

Parenteral Administration of Medications

Parenteral administration of medications is the administration of medications by injection into body tissues. This is an invasive procedure that is performed using aseptic techniques (Box 32-20). A risk of infection occurs after a needle pierces the skin. Each type of injection requires certain skills to ensure that the medication reaches the proper location. The effects of a parenteral medication develop rapidly, depending on the rate of medication absorption. You must closely observe a patient's response to parental medications.

Equipment. A variety of syringes and needles are available, each designed to deliver a certain volume of a medication to a specific type of tissue. Use nursing judgment when determining the syringe size or needle length and gauge that will be most effective.

Syringes. Syringes consist of a cylindrical barrel with a tip designed to fit the hub of a hypodermic needle and a close-fitting plunger. In general syringes are classified as being Luer-Lok or non–Luer-Lok. This terminology is based on the design of the tip of the syringe. Luer-Lok syringes have needles that are twisted onto the tip and lock themselves in place (Figure 32-9, *A* and *B*). This design prevents the inadvertent removal of the needle. Non–Luer-Lok syringes (Figure 32-9, C and *D*) have needles that slip onto the tip. Syringes have safety devices to prevent needlestick injury.

Syringes come in a number of sizes, from 0.5 to 60 mL. It is unusual to use a syringe larger than 5 mL for an injection. A 1- to 3-mL syringe is usually adequate for a subcutaneous or IM injection. A larger volume creates discomfort. Use larger syringes to administer certain IV medications and irrigate wounds or drainage tubes. Syringes often come prepackaged with a needle attached. However, you sometimes change a needle on the basis of the route of administration and size of a patient.

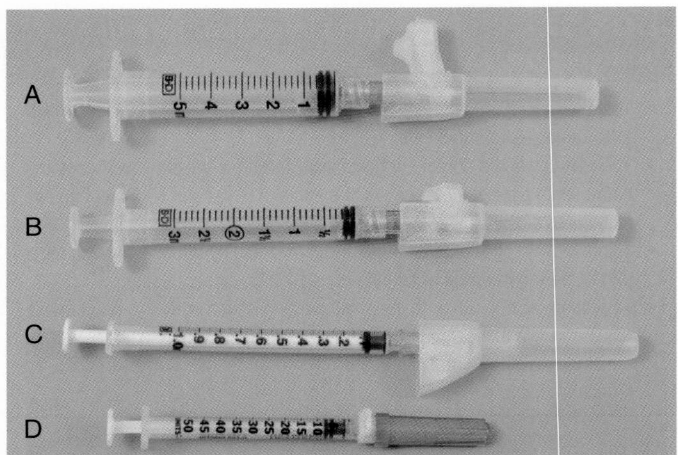

FIGURE 32-9 Types of syringes. **A,** 5-mL syringe. **B,** 3-mL syringe. **C,** Tuberculin syringe marked in 0.01 (hundredths) for doses less than 1 mL. **D,** Insulin syringe marked in units (50).

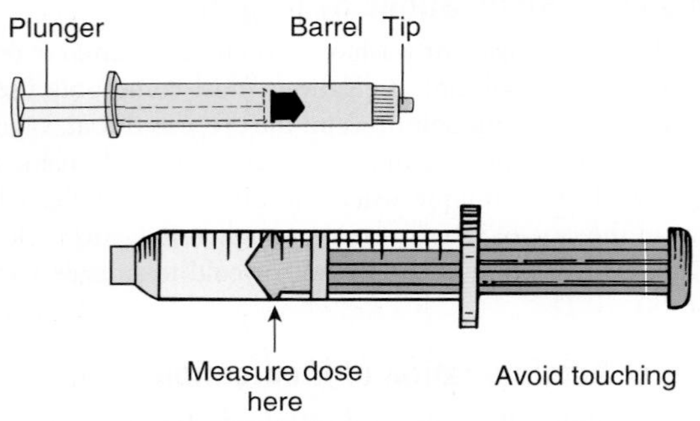

FIGURE 32-10 Parts of a syringe.

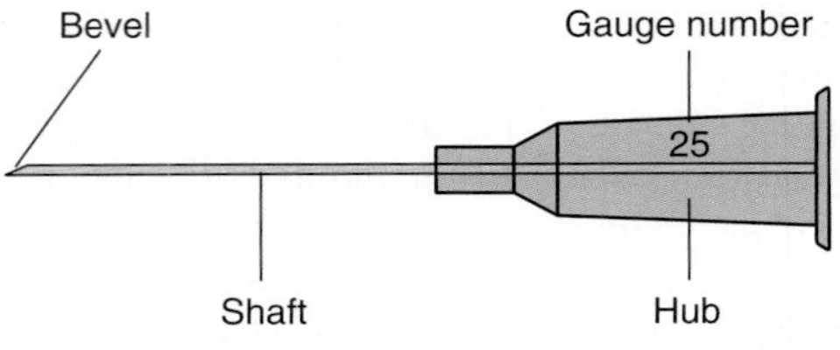

FIGURE 32-11 Parts of the needle.

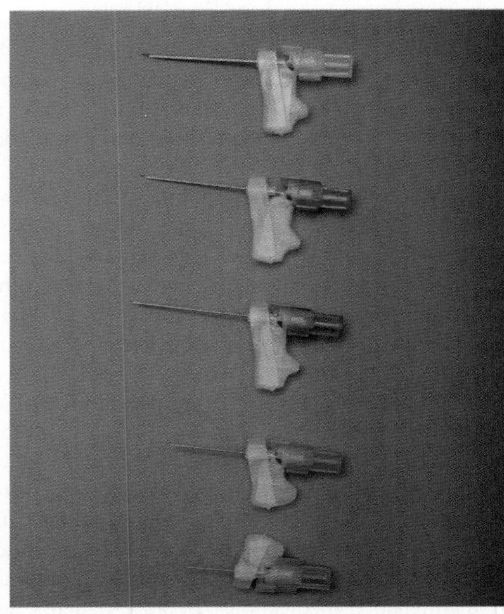

FIGURE 32-12 Hypodermic needles *(top to bottom)*: 18 gauge, 1½-inch length; 21 gauge, 1½-inch length; 22 gauge, 1½-inch length; 23 gauge, 1-inch length; and 25 gauge, ⅝-inch length.

The tuberculin syringe (see Figure 32-9, *C*) is calibrated in sixteenths of a minim and hundredths of a milliliter and has a capacity of 1 mL. Use a tuberculin syringe to prepare small amounts of medications (e.g., ID or subcutaneous injections). A tuberculin syringe is also useful when preparing small, precise doses for infants or young children.

Insulin syringes (see Figure 32-9, *D*) are available in sizes that hold 0.3 to 1 mL and are calibrated in units. Most insulin syringes are U-100s, designed to be used with U-100 strength insulin. Each milliliter of U-100 insulin contains 100 units of insulin.

Fill a syringe by pulling the plunger outward while the needle tip remains immersed in the prepared solution. Only touch the outside of the syringe barrel and the handle of the plunger to maintain sterility. Avoid letting any unsterile object touch the tip or inside of the barrel, the hub, the shaft of the plunger, or the needle (Figure 32-10).

Needles. Some needles come packaged in individual sheaths to allow flexibility in choosing the right needle for a patient, whereas others are preattached to standard-size syringes. Most needles are made of stainless steel, and all are disposable. A needle has three parts: the hub, which fits onto the tip of a syringe; the shaft, which connects to the hub; and the bevel, or slanted tip (Figure 32-11). The tip of a needle, or the bevel, is always slanted. The bevel creates a narrow slit when injected into tissue that quickly closes when the needle is removed to prevent leakage of medication, blood, or serum. Long, beveled tips are sharper and narrower, minimizing discomfort when entering tissue used for subcutaneous or IM injections.

Most needles vary in length from ¼ to 3 inches (Figure 32-12). Choose the needle length according to a patient's size and weight and the type of tissue into which the medication is to be injected. Current evidence suggests that needle length should be based on the patient's weight (Davidson and Rourke, 2013). There should be a 5-mm depth of muscle penetration to achieve an IM injection (Hibbard et al., 2015). A child or slender adult generally requires a shorter needle. Use longer needles (1 to 1½ inches) for IM injections and a shorter needle (⅜ to ⅝ inch) for subcutaneous injections. As the needle gauge becomes smaller, the diameter becomes larger. The selection of a gauge depends on the viscosity of fluid to be injected or infused.

Disposable Injection Units. Disposable, single-dose, prefilled syringes are available for some medications. Be careful to check the medication and concentration because prefilled syringes appear very similar. With these syringes you do not have to prepare medication doses, except perhaps to expel parts of unneeded medications.

The Tubex and Carpuject injection systems include reusable plastic mechanisms that hold prefilled, disposable, sterile cartridge-needle units (Figure 32-13). To assemble a prefilled system, place the cartridge barrel first into the plastic syringe holder. Following manufacturer directions, turn the plunger rod to the left (counterclockwise) and the lock to the right (clockwise) until it "clicks." Finally remove the needle guard and advance the plunger to expel air and excess medication as in a regular syringe. The glass cartridge can be used with needleless systems or safety needles. After giving the medication, safely dispose of the glass cartridge in a puncture-proof, leak-proof receptacle.

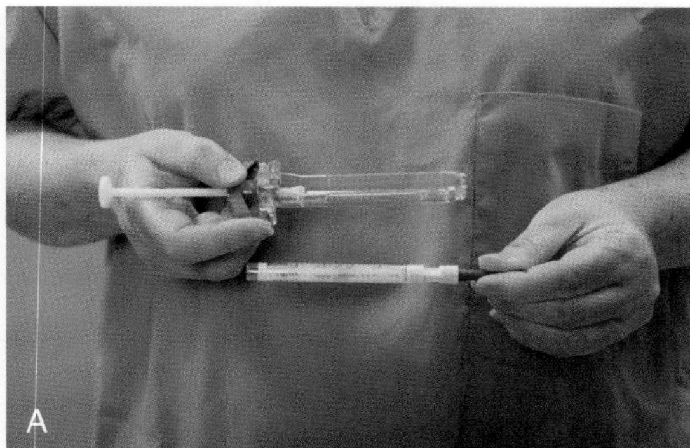

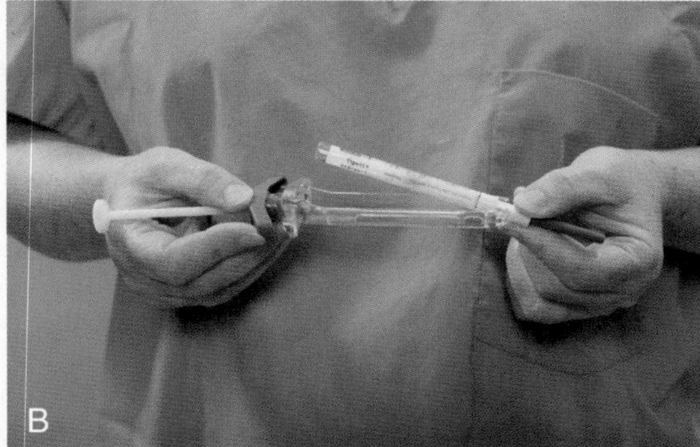

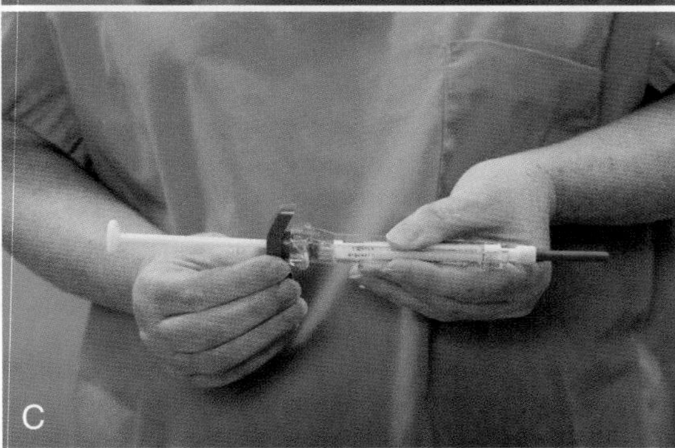

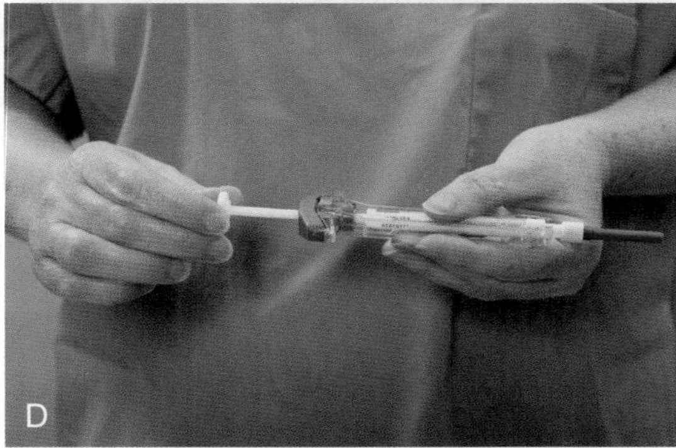

FIGURE 32-13 A, Carpuject syringe and prefilled sterile cartridge with needle. **B,** Assembling the Carpuject. **C,** Cartridge slides into syringe barrel. Turn and lock syringe into cartridge. **D,** Screw plunger into end of cartridge. Expel excess medication to obtain accurate dose *(not pictured).*

Preparing an Injection from an Ampule. Ampules contain single doses of medication in a liquid. They are available in several sizes, from 1 mL to 10 mL or more (Figure 32-14, *A*). An ampule is made of glass with a constricted neck that must be snapped off to allow access to the medication. A colored ring around the neck indicates where the ampule is prescored so you can break it easily. Carefully aspirate the medication into a syringe (see Skill 32-4 on pp. 666-670) with a filter needle. The use of a filter needle prevents particulate matter such as small glass fragments from entering the syringe (Alexander et al., 2014). Replace the filter needle with an appropriate-size needle or a needleless access device before administering the injection.

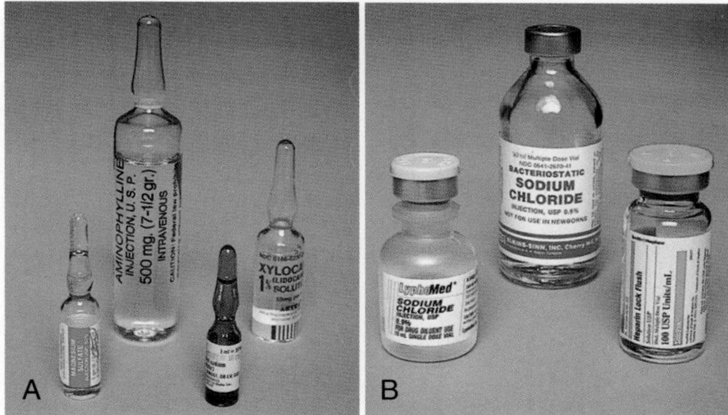

FIGURE 32-14 A, Medication in ampules. **B,** Medication in vials.

Preparing an Injection from a Vial. A vial is a single-dose or multidose container with a rubber seal at the top (see Figure 32-14, *B*). A metal cap protects the seal until it is ready for use. Vials contain liquid or dry forms of medications. Medications that are unstable in solution are packaged dry. The vial label specifies the solvent or diluent used to dissolve the medication and the amount of diluent needed to prepare a desired medication concentration. Normal saline and sterile distilled water are commonly used to dissolve medications.

Unlike the ampule, the vial is a closed system, and air needs to be injected into it to permit easy withdrawal of the solution. Failure to inject air when withdrawing creates a vacuum within the vial that makes withdrawal difficult. If concerned about drawing up parts of the rubber stopper or other particles into the syringe, use a filter needle when preparing medications from vials (Alexander et al., 2014). Some vials contain powder, which is mixed with a diluent during preparation and before injection (see Skill 32-4). After mixing multidose vials, make a label that includes the date and time of mixing and the concentration of medication per milliliter. Some multidose vials require refrigeration after the contents are reconstituted.

Mixing Medications. If two medications are compatible, it is possible to mix them in one injection if the total dose is within accepted limits. This prevents a patient from having to receive more than one injection at a time. Most nursing units have charts that list common compatible medications. If there is any uncertainty about medication compatibilities, consult a pharmacist or a medication reference.

Mixing Medications from a Vial and an Ampule. When mixing medication from both a vial and ampule, prepare medication from the vial first. Using the same syringe and filter needle, next withdraw medication from the ampule. Nurses prepare the combination in this order because it is not necessary to add air to withdraw medication from an ampule.

Mixing Medications from Two Vials. Apply these principles when mixing medications from two vials:

1. Do not contaminate one medication with another.
2. Ensure that the final dose is accurate.
3. Maintain aseptic technique.

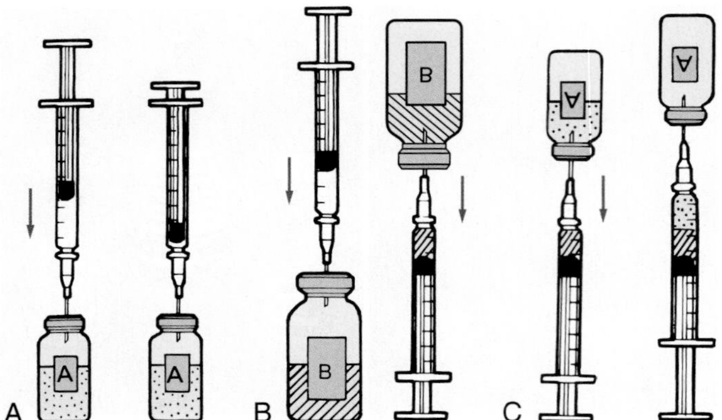

FIGURE 32-15 **A,** Injecting air into vial A. **B,** Injecting air into vial B and withdrawing dose. **C,** Withdrawing medication from vial A; medications are now mixed.

Use only one syringe with a needle or needleless access device attached to mix medications from two vials (Figure 32-15). Aspirate the volume of air equivalent to the dose of the first medication (vial A) (see Figure 32-15, *A*). Inject the air into vial A, making sure that the needle does not touch the solution. Withdraw the needle and aspirate air equivalent to the dose of the second medication (vial B). Inject the volume of air into vial B (see Figure 32-15, *B*). Immediately withdraw the medication from vial B into the syringe and insert the needle back into vial A, being careful not to push the plunger and expel the medication within the syringe into the vial. Withdraw the desired amount of medication from vial A into the syringe (see Figure 32-15, *C*). After withdrawing the necessary amount, withdraw the needle and apply a new safety needle or needleless access device suitable for injection.

Insulin Preparation. Insulin is the hormone used to treat diabetes mellitus. It is administered by injection because the GI tract breaks down and destroys an oral form of insulin. Most patients with diabetes mellitus who take insulin injections learn to administer their own injections. In the United States and Canada, health care providers usually prescribe insulin in concentrations of 100 units per milliliter of solution. This is called *U-100 insulin*. Insulin is also commercially available in concentrations of 500 units per milliliter of solution; it is called *U-500 insulin*. U-500 insulin is 5 times as strong as U-100 insulin and is used only in rare cases when patients are very resistant to insulin.

Use the correct syringe when preparing insulin. Use a 100-unit insulin syringe or an insulin pen to prepare U-100 insulin. Because there is no syringe currently designed to prepare U-500 insulin, many medication errors result with this kind of insulin. To prevent errors, ensure that the order for U-500 specifies units and volume (e.g., 150 units, 0.3 mL of U-500 insulin) and use tuberculin syringes to draw up the doses (ISMP, 2013b). Verify every injection you prepare with another nurse before administering it. Additional safety measures common with U-500 insulin include listing the insulin as being concentrated in computerized medication dispensing systems, making health care providers and pharmacists verify that a patient is to receive U-500 insulin when it is ordered, and only stocking U-500 insulin on patient care units when it is ordered for a specific patient (ISMP, 2013b).

Insulin is classified by rate of action, including rapid-acting, short-acting, intermediate-acting, and long-acting. To provide safe and effective care, you need to know the onset, peak, and duration for each of your patients' ordered insulin doses. Refer to a medication reference or consult with a pharmacist if you are unsure of this information.

BOX 32-21 Example of Correction Insulin Order

Give regular U-100 insulin subcutaneously:
2 units for glucose 150 to 200 mg/dL
4 units for glucose 201 to 275 mg/dL
Call for glucose greater than 275 mg/dL

Clinical scenario: Before lunch patient's blood glucose level is 201. After referring to patient's correction insulin order, the nurse administers 4 units of insulin to patient.

Regular insulin is the only type of insulin that can be given intravenously.

A patient with diabetes mellitus sometimes requires more than one type of insulin. For example, by receiving a short-acting (regular) and intermediate-acting (NPH) insulin, a patient receives more sustained control of blood glucose levels over 24 hours. The timing of insulin injections attempts to imitate the normal pattern of insulin release from the pancreas. Some insulins come in a stable premixed solution (e.g., 70/30 insulin is 70% NPH [intermediate] and 30% regular), eliminating the need to mix the insulins in a syringe. Other patients use an insulin pen. The insulin pen provides multiple doses and allows a patient to dial in the dose, avoiding the need to use a syringe for insulin preparation. Research shows that different types of a patient's blood cells can enter into the insulin pen after an injection. Several U.S. health care organizations recently reported that the same insulin pen was inadvertently used on multiple patients, exposing the patients to bloodborne illnesses (e.g., human immunodeficiency virus [HIV], hepatitis B, and hepatitis C). Thus the ISMP recommends that insulin pens only be used at home and that inpatient settings such as hospitals stop using them whenever possible (ISMP, 2013c).

Insulin is ordered by a specific dose at select times. Correction insulin, also known as sliding-scale insulin, provides a dose of insulin based on the patient's blood glucose level (Box 32-21). The term *correction insulin* is preferred because it indicates that small doses of rapid- or short-acting insulin are needed to correct a patient's elevated blood sugar. Reliance on correction insulin is unlikely to achieve long-term glucose control; therefore it should only be ordered on a temporary basis (ADA, 2015).

Before drawing up insulin doses, gently roll all cloudy insulin preparations between the palms of the hands to resuspend the insulin (Diggle, 2014). Do not shake insulin vials; shaking causes bubbles to form. Bubbles take up space in the syringe and alter the dose.

If more than one type of insulin is required to manage the patient's diabetes, you mix two different types of insulin into one syringe *if* they are compatible (Box 32-22). If regular and intermediate-acting insulins are ordered, prepare the regular insulin first to prevent it from becoming contaminated with the intermediate-acting insulin (Diggle, 2014). Use the following principles when mixing insulins (Diggle, 2014; McCulloch, 2015; Novo Nordisk, 2014):

- Patients whose blood glucose levels are well controlled on a mixed-insulin dose need to maintain their individual routine when preparing and administering their insulin.
- Do not mix insulin with any other medications or diluents unless approved by the health care provider.
- Never mix insulin glargine (Lantus) or insulin detemir (Levemir) with other types of insulin.
- Inject rapid-acting insulins mixed with NPH insulin within 15 minutes before a meal.
- Verify insulin doses with another nurse while you are preparing the injection.

BOX 32-22 PROCEDURAL GUIDELINES

Mixing Two Types of Insulin in One Syringe

Delegation Considerations

The skill of mixing two types of insulin in one syringe cannot be delegated to nursing assistive personnel (NAP).

Equipment

Insulin vials, insulin syringe, alcohol swabs, medication administration (MAR) (electronic or printed)

Steps

1. Check accuracy and completeness of each MAR with health care provider's medication order. Check patient's name and medication name, dosage, and route and time of administration. Recopy or reprint any part of printed MAR that is difficult to read.
2. Review medical history (e.g., type of diabetes, reason for elevated blood sugars) and allergies to medications, food, and latex.
3. Carefully verify insulin labels; compare labels against the MAR before preparing the dose to ensure that the correct type of insulin is prepared. *This is the first accuracy check.*
4. Perform hand hygiene.
5. If patient takes insulin that is cloudy, roll the bottle of insulin between the hands to resuspend the preparation.
6. Wipe off tops of both insulin vials with alcohol swabs.
7. Verify insulin dosages against MAR a second time. *This is the second accuracy check.*
8. If mixing rapid- or short-acting insulin with intermediate-acting insulin, take insulin syringe and aspirate volume of air equivalent to the dose of insulin to be withdrawn from intermediate-acting insulin first. If two intermediate-acting insulins are mixed, it makes no difference which vial you prepare first.
9. Insert needle and inject air into vial of intermediate-acting insulin. Do not let the tip of the needle touch the insulin.
10. Remove the syringe from the vial of intermediate-acting insulin without aspirating the insulin.
11. With the same syringe, inject air equal to the dose of insulin to be withdrawn into the vial of rapid- or short-acting insulin. Then withdraw the correct dose into the syringe.
12. Remove the syringe from the rapid- or short-acting insulin vial after carefully removing air bubbles in the syringe to ensure correct dose.
13. After verifying insulin dosages with MAR a third time, show insulin prepared in syringe to another nurse to verify that correct dosage was prepared. *This is the third accuracy check.* Determine which point on the syringe scale combined the units of insulin measured by adding the number of units of both insulins together (e.g., 3 units regular + 10 units NPH = 13 units total).
14. Place the needle of the syringe back into the vial of intermediate-acting insulin. Be careful not to push the plunger and inject insulin in syringe into the vial.
15. Invert vial and carefully withdraw the desired amount of insulin into the syringe.
16. Withdraw needle and check the fluid level in syringe. Keep needle of prepared syringe sheathed or capped until ready to administer medication. Show another nurse the syringe to verify that the correct dose was prepared.
17. Dispose of soiled supplies in proper receptacle. Place used vials in puncture-proof, leak-proof container and perform hand hygiene.
18. Because rapid- or short-acting insulin binds with intermediate-acting insulin, which reduces the action of the faster-acting insulin, administer mixture within 5 minutes of preparing it.

Modified from American Diabetes Association (ADA): *Insulin & other injectables*, 2013, http://www.diabetes.org/living-with-diabetes/treatment-and-care/medication/insulin. Accessed June 8, 2015; Dunning T: *Care of people with diabetes: a manual of nursing practice*, ed 4, Hoboken, NJ, 2013, Wiley-Blackwell.

Administering Injections

Each injection route differs based on the type of tissues the medication enters. The characteristics of the tissues influence the rate of medication absorption, affecting the onset of medication action. Before injecting a medication, know the volume of the medication to administer, the characteristics and viscosity of the medication, and the location of anatomical structures underlying injection sites (see Skill 32-5 on pp. 670-675).

If you do not administer injections correctly, negative patient outcomes result. Failure to select an injection site in relation to anatomical landmarks results in nerve or bone damage during needle insertion. Inability to maintain stability of the needle and syringe unit can result in pain and tissue damage. If you fail to aspirate the syringe before injecting an IM medication, the medication may be injected accidentally directly into an artery or vein. Injecting too large a volume of medication for the site selected causes extreme pain and results in local tissue damage.

Many patients, particularly children, fear injections. Patients with serious or chronic illness often are given several injections daily. Minimize discomfort in the following ways:

- Use a sharp-beveled needle in the smallest suitable length and gauge.
- Position a patient as comfortably as possible to reduce muscular tension.
- Select the proper injection site, using anatomical landmarks.
- Apply a vapocoolant spray (e.g., Fluori-Methane spray or ethyl chloride) or topical anesthetic (e.g., EMLA cream) to the injection site before giving the medication when possible.
- Divert the patient's attention from the injection through conversation using open-ended questioning.
- Insert the needle quickly and smoothly to minimize tissue pulling.
- Hold the syringe steady while the needle remains in tissues.
- Inject the medication slowly and steadily.

Subcutaneous Injections. Subcutaneous injections involve placing medications into the loose connective tissue under the dermis (see Skill 32-5). Because subcutaneous tissue is not as richly supplied with blood as the muscles, medication absorption is somewhat slower than with IM injections. However, medications are absorbed completely if the patient's circulatory status is normal. Because subcutaneous tissue contains pain receptors, a patient often experiences slight discomfort.

The best subcutaneous injection sites include the outer posterior aspect of the upper arms, the abdomen from below the costal margins to the iliac crests, and the anterior aspects of the thighs (Figure 32-16). The site most frequently recommended for heparin injections is the abdomen (Figure 32-17). Alternative subcutaneous sites for other medications include the scapular areas of the upper back and the upper ventral or dorsal gluteal areas. The injection site you choose needs to

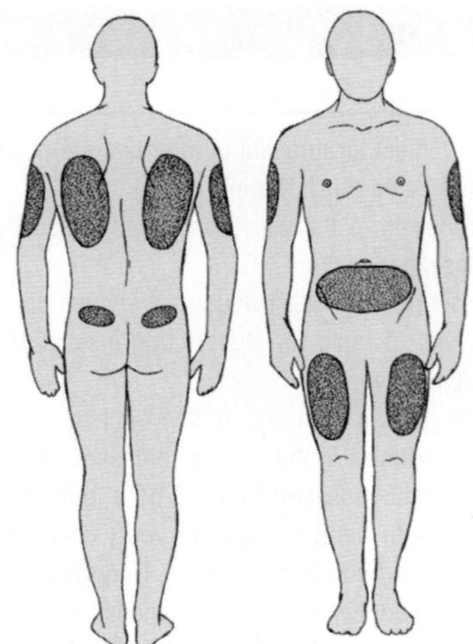

FIGURE 32-16 Sites recommended for subcutaneous injections.

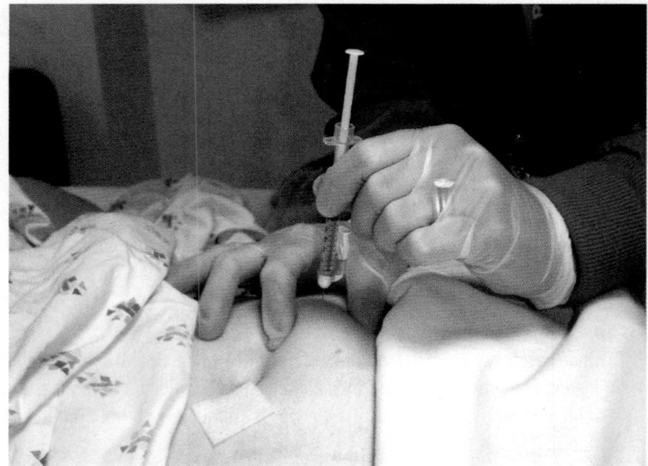

FIGURE 32-17 Giving subcutaneous heparin in abdomen.

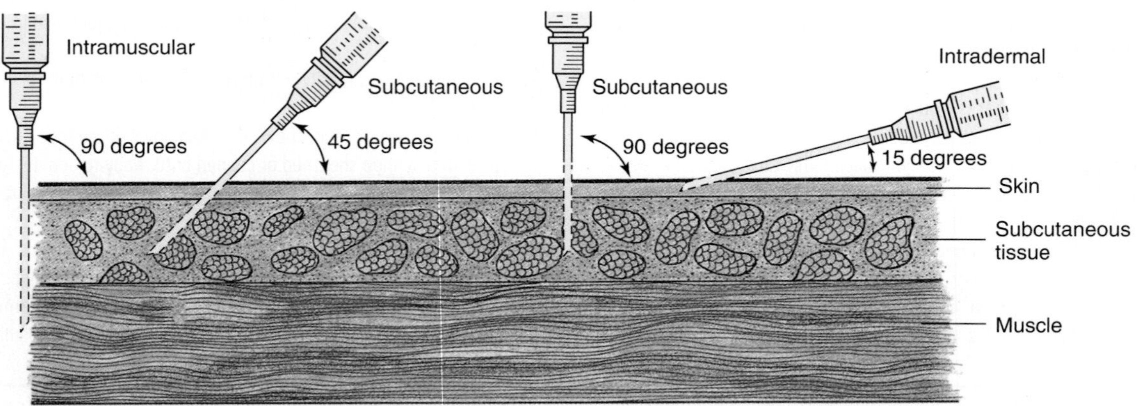

FIGURE 32-18 Comparison of angles of insertion for intramuscular (90 degrees), subcutaneous (45 to 90 degrees), and intradermal (15 degrees) injections.

be free of skin lesions, bony prominences, and large underlying muscles or nerves.

The administration of low-molecular-weight heparin (LMWH) (e.g., enoxaparin) requires special considerations. When injecting the medication, use the right or left side of the abdomen at least 2 inches from the umbilicus (the patient's "love handles") and pinch the injection site as you insert the needle. Administer LMWH in its prefilled syringe with the attached needle and do not expel the air bubble in the syringe before giving the medication. There is some new evidence to support a slower injection rate of 30 seconds to reduce bruising and pain (Akbari Sari et al, 2014; Sanofi-Aventis, 2014).

Use U-100 insulin syringes with preattached 32- to 25-gauge needles when giving U-100 insulin and 1-mL tuberculin syringes when giving U-500 insulin (ISMP, 2013b). Recommended sites for insulin injections include the upper arm and the anterior and lateral parts of the thigh, buttocks, and abdomen. Rotating injections within the same body part (intrasite rotation) provides more consistency in the absorption of the insulin. For example, if a patient receives morning insulin in the right arm, give the next injection in a different place in the same arm. The injections are to be given at least 2.5 cm (1 inch) away from the previous site. Injection sites should not be used again for at least 1 month. The rate of insulin absorption varies based on the site; the abdomen has the quickest absorption, followed by the arms, thighs, and buttocks (McCulloch, 2015).

Subcutaneous tissue is sensitive to irritating solutions and large volumes of medications. Thus you only administer small volumes (0.5 to 1.5 mL) of water-soluble medications subcutaneously to adults. You give smaller volumes up to 0.5 mL to children (Hockenberry and Wilson, 2015). Hardened, painful lumps called *sterile abscesses* occur under the skin if medication collects within the tissues.

A patient's body weight indicates the depth of the subcutaneous layer. Therefore choose the needle length and angle of insertion on the basis of a patient's weight and an estimation of the amount of subcutaneous tissue (Juip and Fitzner, 2012). Nurses typically use a 25-gauge, ⅝-inch (16-mm) needle inserted at a 45-degree angle (Figure 32-18) or a ½-inch (12-mm) needle inserted at a 90-degree angle to administer subcutaneous medications to a normal-size adult patient. Some children require only a ½-inch needle. If the patient is obese, pinch the tissue and use a needle long enough to insert through fatty tissue at the base of the skinfold. Thin patients often do not have sufficient tissue for subcutaneous injections; the upper abdomen is usually the best site in this case. To ensure that a subcutaneous medication reaches the subcutaneous tissue, follow this rule: If you can grasp 2 inches (5 cm) of tissue, insert the needle at a 90-degree angle; if you can grasp 2.5 cm (1 inch) of tissue, insert the needle at a 45-degree angle.

Newer research in insulin administration shows that insulin needles that are $\frac{5}{16}$ (8 mm) or longer often enter the muscles of men and people with a body mass index (BMI) of 25 or less. Shorter ($\frac{3}{16}$-inch

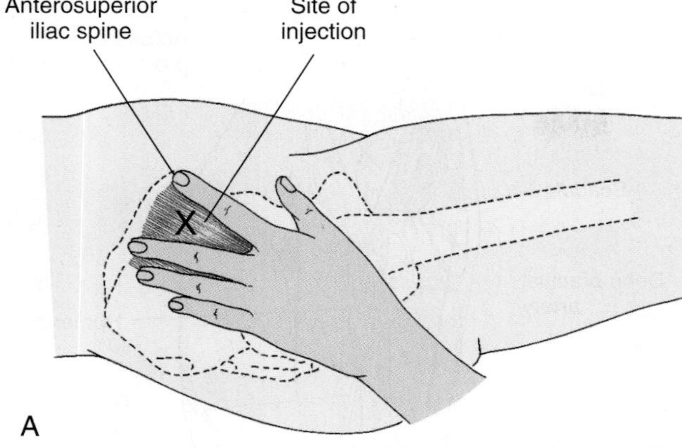

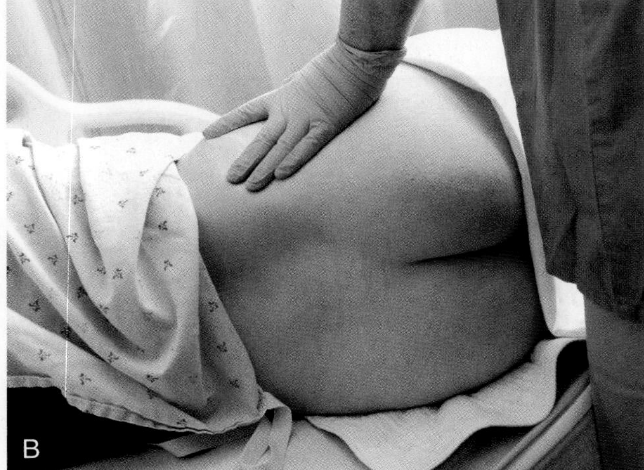

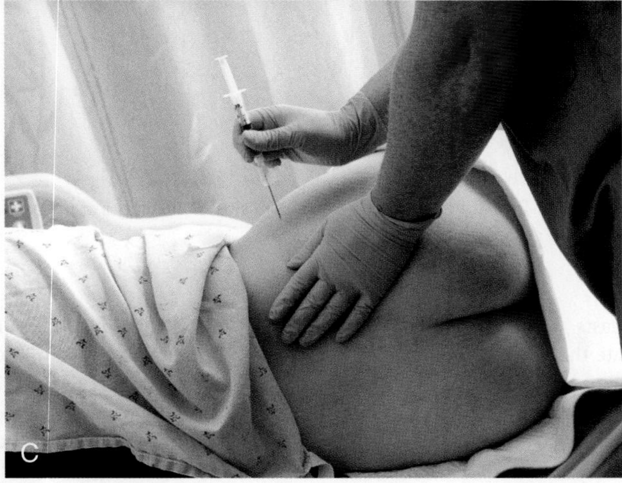

FIGURE 32-19 A, Landmarks for ventrogluteal site. **B,** Locating ventrogluteal site in patient. **C,** Giving intramuscular injection in ventrogluteal muscle using Z-track method.

or 4- to 5-mm) needles were associated with less pain, adequate control of blood sugars, and minimal leakage of medication (Diggle, 2014; Gibney et al., 2010; Hirsch et al., 2012; Hoffman et al., 2010). Thus, when administering insulin, needles of $\frac{3}{16}$ inch (4 to 5 mm) administered at a 90-degree angle should be used to reduce pain and achieve adequate control of blood sugars with minimal adverse effects for people of all BMIs, including children (AADE, 2013).

Intramuscular Injections. The IM route provides faster medication absorption than the subcutaneous route because of the greater vascularity of muscles. However, IM injections are associated with many risks. Therefore, whenever administering a medication by the IM route, first verify that the injection is justified (Nicoll and Hesby, 2002; WHO, 2015). Some medications such as hepatitis B and tetanus, diphtheria, and pertussis (Tdap) immunizations are only given intramuscularly.

Use a longer and heavier-gauge needle to pass through subcutaneous tissue and penetrate deep muscle tissue (see Skill 32-5). A patient's BMI and the amount of adipose tissue influence needle size selection. Many needles available in health care settings are not long enough to reach the muscle, especially in patients who are obese and females (Bhalla et al., 2013; Dayananda et al., 2014; Palma and Strohfus, 2013). Because most agencies have needles that range in length from only $\frac{5}{8}$ to $1\frac{1}{2}$ inches, investigate different medication routes, especially when IM injections are ordered for obese female patients.

The angle of insertion for an IM injection is 90 degrees (see Figure 32-18). Muscle is less sensitive to irritating and viscous medications. A normal, well-developed adult patient tolerates 2 to 5 mL of medication into a larger muscle without severe muscle discomfort (Hopkins and Arias, 2013: Nicoll and Hesby, 2002). However, larger volumes of medication (4 to 5 mL) are unlikely to be absorbed properly. Children, older adults, and thin patients tolerate only 2 mL of an IM injection. Do not give more than 1 mL to small children and older infants, and do not give more than 0.5 mL to smaller infants (Hockenberry and Wilson, 2015).

Assess a muscle before giving an injection. Properly identify the site for the IM injection by palpating bony landmarks and be aware of the potential complications associated with each site. The site needs to be free of tenderness because repeated injections in the same muscle cause severe discomfort. With the patient relaxed, palpate the muscle to rule out any hardened lesions. Minimize discomfort during an injection by helping a patient assume a position that helps to reduce muscle strain. Other interventions such as distraction and applying pressure to an IM site decrease pain during an injection.

Sites. When selecting an IM site, consider the following: Is the area free of infection or necrosis? Are there local areas of bruising or abrasions? What is the location of underlying bones, nerves, and major blood vessels? What volume of medication is to be administered? Each site has different advantages and disadvantages.

Ventrogluteal. The ventrogluteal muscle involves the gluteus medius; it is situated deep and away from major nerves and blood vessels. This site is the preferred and safest site for all adults, children, and infants, especially for medications that have larger volumes and are more viscous and irritating (Hockenberry and Wilson, 2015; Hopkins and Arias, 2013; Nicoll and Hesby, 2002). The ventrogluteal site is recommended for volumes greater than 2 mL (Hopkins and Arias, 2013; Nicoll and Hesby, 2002). Research shows that injuries such as fibrosis, nerve damage, abscess, tissue necrosis, muscle contraction, gangrene, and pain are associated with all the common IM sites *except* the ventrogluteal site (Hopkins and Arias, 2013).

Locate the ventrogluteal muscle by positioning the patient in a supine or lateral position. Flexing the knee and hip helps to relax this muscle. Place the palm of your hand over the greater trochanter of the patient's hip with the wrist perpendicular to the femur. Use the right hand for the left hip and the left hand for the right hip. Point the thumb toward the patient's groin and the index finger toward the anterior superior iliac spine; extend the middle finger back along the iliac crest toward the buttock. The index finger, the middle finger, and the iliac crest form a V-shaped triangle; the injection site is the center of the triangle (Figure 32-19, *A* to *C*).

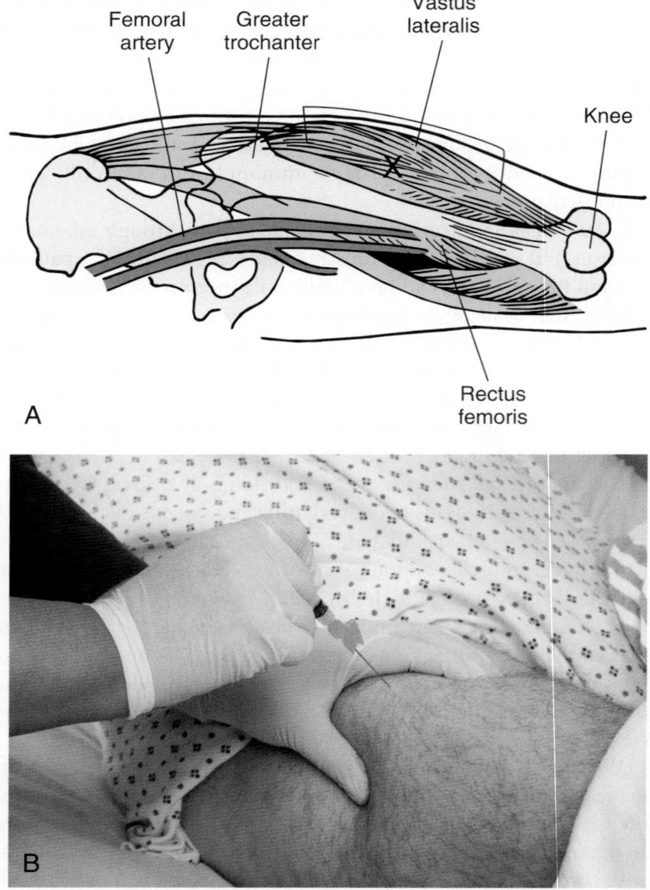

FIGURE 32-20 **A,** Landmarks for vastus lateralis site. **B,** Giving intramuscular injection in vastus lateralis muscle.

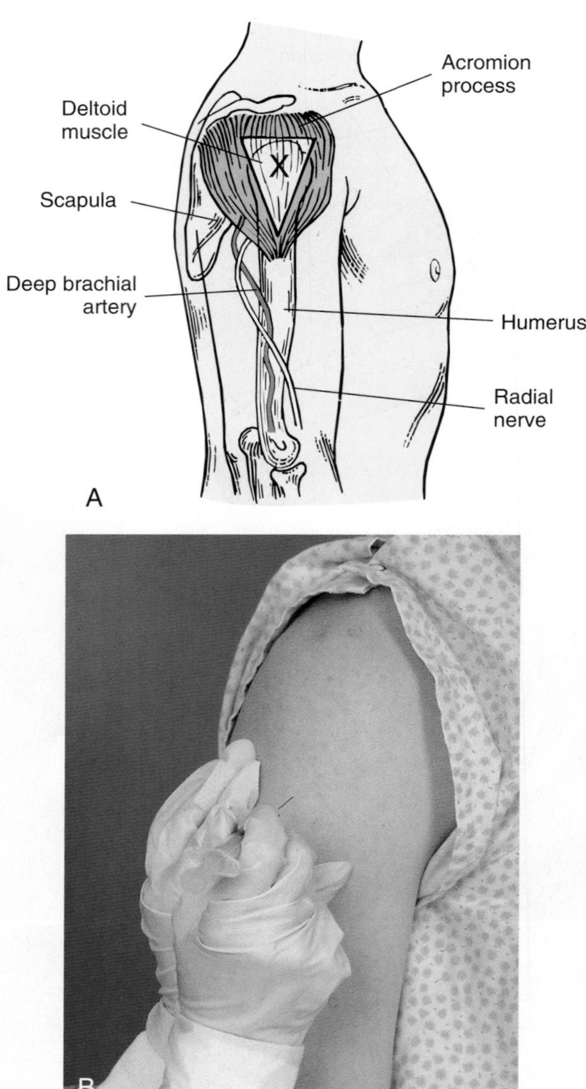

FIGURE 32-21 **A,** Landmarks for deltoid site. **B,** Giving intramuscular injection in deltoid muscle.

Vastus Lateralis. The vastus lateralis muscle is another injection site for adults and children. The muscle is thick and well developed, is located on the anterior lateral aspect of the thigh, and extends in an adult from a hand breadth above the knee to a hand breadth below the greater trochanter of the femur (Figure 32-20, *A* and *B*). Use the middle third of the muscle for injection. The width of the muscle usually extends from the midline of the thigh to the midline of the outer side of the thigh. With young children or cachectic patients, it helps to grasp the body of the muscle during injection to be sure that the medication is deposited in muscle tissue. To help relax the muscle, ask a patient to lie flat with the knee slightly flexed or in a sitting position. The vastus lateralis site is often used for infants, toddlers, and children receiving biologicals (e.g., immunoglobulins, vaccines, or toxoids) (Nicoll and Hesby, 2002).

Deltoid. Although the deltoid site is easily accessible, this muscle is not well developed in many adults. There is a potential for injury because the axillary, radial, brachial, and ulnar nerves and the brachial artery lie within the upper arm under the triceps and along the humerus. Use this site for small medication volumes (2 mL or less) (Hopkins and Arias, 2013; Nicoll and Hesby, 2002). Carefully assess the condition of the deltoid muscle, consult medication references for suitability of the medication, and carefully locate the injection site using anatomical landmarks (Figure 32-21, *A*). Use this site only for small medication volumes, when giving immunizations (e.g., hepatitis B, flu shots), or when other sites are inaccessible because of dressings or casts (Davidson and Rourke, 2013; Nicoll and Hesby, 2002). To locate the muscle, fully expose the patient's upper arm and shoulder. Do not roll up a tight-fitting sleeve. Have the patient relax the arm at the side and flex the elbow. The patient may sit, stand, or lie down (see Figure 32-21, *B*). Palpate the lower edge of the acromion process, which forms the base of a triangle in line with the midpoint of the lateral aspect of the upper arm. The injection site is in the center of the triangle, about 3 to 5 cm (1 to 2 inches) below the acromion process. You can also locate the site by placing four fingers across the deltoid muscle, with the top finger along the acromion process. The injection site is then three finger widths below the acromion process.

Use of the Z-Track Method in Intramuscular Injections. It is recommended that, when administering IM injections, the **Z-track method** be used to minimize local skin irritation by sealing the medication in muscle tissue (Hopkins and Arias, 2013; Nicoll and Hesby, 2002). To use the Z-track method, put a new needle on the syringe after preparing the medication so no solution remains on the outside needle shaft. Then select an IM site, preferably in a large, deep

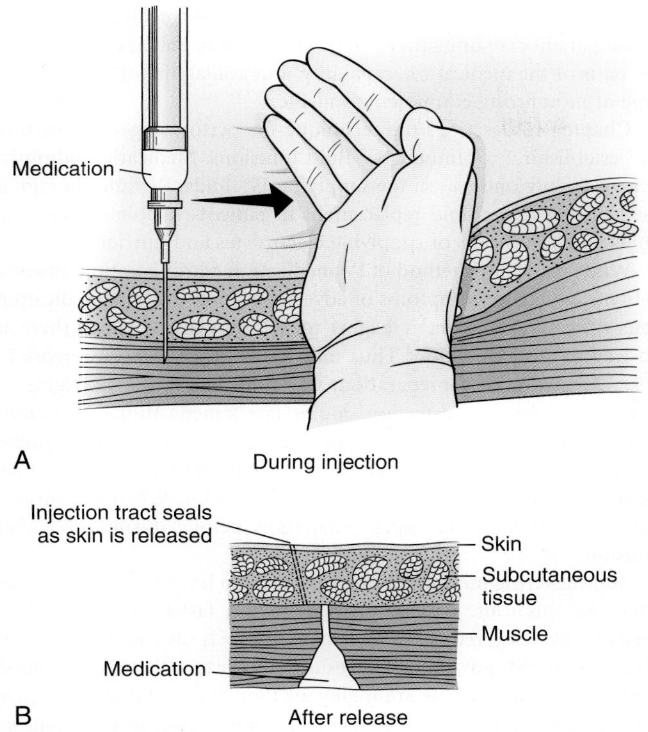

FIGURE 32-22 **A,** Pulling on overlying skin during intramuscular injection moves tissue to prevent later tracking. **B,** Z-track method of injection prevents deposit of medication into sensitive tissue.

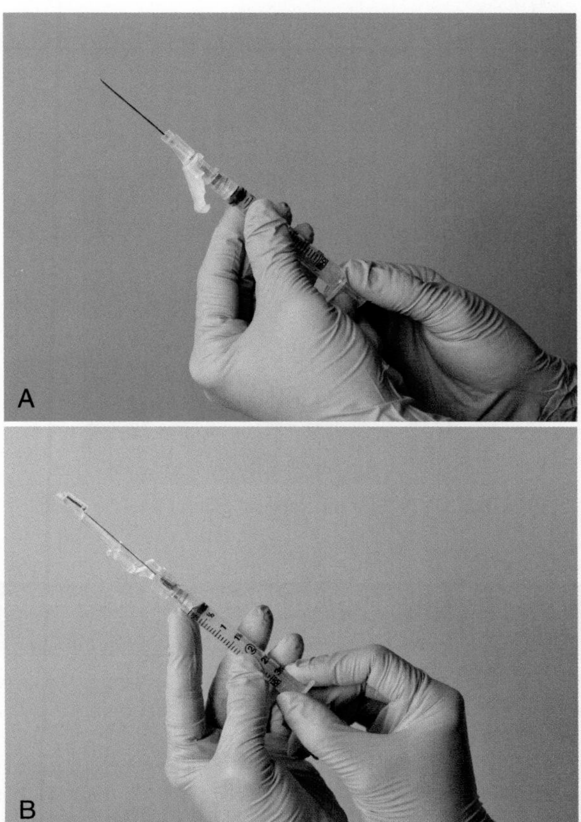

FIGURE 32-23 Needle with plastic guard to prevent needlesticks. **A,** Position of guard before injection. **B,** After injection guard locks in place, covering needle.

muscle such as the ventrogluteal muscle. Place the ulnar side of the nondominant hand just below the site and pull the overlying skin and subcutaneous tissues approximately 2 to 3 cm (1 to 1.2 inches) laterally or downward (Hopkins and Arias, 2013; Nicoll and Hesby, 2002). Hold the skin in this position until you administer the injection. After preparing the site with an antiseptic swab, inject the needle deep into the muscle. Grasp the barrel of the syringe with the thumb and index finger of the nondominant hand and slowly inject the medication if there is no blood return on aspiration. The Centers for Disease Control and Prevention (CDC) no longer recommends aspiration when administering immunizations to reduce discomfort (CDC, 2015; Hopkins and Arias, 2013). The needle remains inserted for 10 seconds to allow the medication to disperse evenly rather than channeling back up the track of the needle. Release the skin after withdrawing the needle. This leaves a zigzag path that seals the needle track where tissue planes slide across one another (Figure 32-22, *A* and *B*). The medication cannot escape from the muscle tissue.

Intradermal Injections. ID injections typically are used for skin testing (e.g., tuberculin screening and allergy tests). Because these medications are potent, they are injected into the dermis, where blood supply is reduced and medication absorption occurs slowly. Some patients have a severe anaphylactic reaction if medications enter the circulation too rapidly. You need to choose skin-testing sites that allow you to easily assess for changes in color and tissue integrity. Thus ID sites need to be lightly pigmented, free of lesions, and relatively hairless. The inner forearm and upper back are ideal locations.

Use a tuberculin or small hypodermic syringe for skin testing. The angle of insertion for an ID injection is 5 to 15 degrees (see Figure 32-18), and the bevel of the needle is pointed up. As you inject the medication, a small bleb resembling a mosquito bite appears on the surface of the skin. If a bleb does not appear or if the site bleeds after needle withdrawal, there is a good chance that the medication entered subcutaneous tissues. In this case test results will not be valid.

Safety in Administering Medications by Injection

Needleless Devices. Approximately 5.6 million health care workers in the United States are at risk of occupational exposure to bloodborne pathogens such as HIV and the hepatitis B virus (OSHA, n.d.). Occupational exposure often occurs through accidental needlesticks and sharps injuries. Needlestick injuries commonly occur when health care workers recap needles, mishandle IV lines and needles, or leave needles at a patient's bedside. Exposure to bloodborne pathogens is one of the deadliest hazards to which nurses are exposed on a daily basis. Most needlestick injuries are preventable with the implementation of safe needle devices. The Needlestick Safety and Prevention Act mandates the use of special needle safety devices to reduce the frequency of needlestick injuries.

Safety syringes have a sheath or guard that covers a needle immediately after it is withdrawn from the skin (Figure 32-23, *A* and *B*). This eliminates the chance for a needlestick injury. The syringe and sheath are disposed of together in a receptacle. Use needleless devices whenever possible to reduce the risk of needlestick and sharps injuries (OSHA, n.d.). Always dispose of needles and other instruments considered sharps into clearly marked, appropriate containers

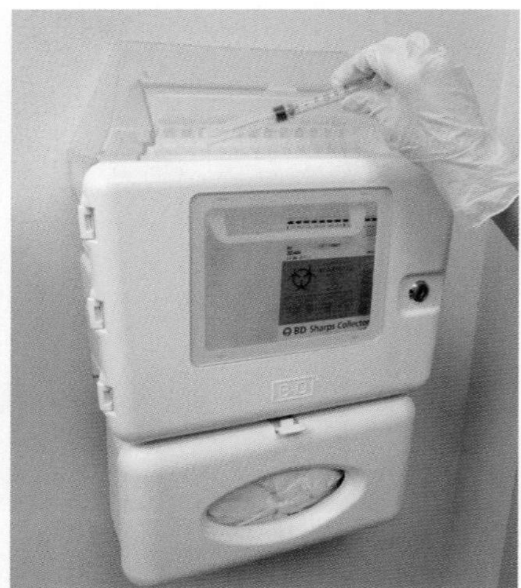

FIGURE 32-24 Sharps disposal using only one hand.

BOX 32-23 Recommendations for Prevention of Needlestick Injuries

- Avoid using needles when effective needleless systems or sharps with engineered sharps injury protection (SESIP) safety devices are available.
- Do not recap any needle after medication administration.
- Plan safe handling and disposal of needles before beginning a procedure.
- Immediately dispose of needles, needleless systems, and SESIP into puncture-proof, leak-proof sharps disposal containers.
- Maintain a sharps injury log that includes the following: type and brand of device involved in the incident, location of the incident (e.g., department or work area), description of the incident, and privacy of the employees who have had sharps injuries.
- Attend education offerings on bloodborne pathogens and follow recommendations for infection prevention, including receiving the hepatitis B vaccine.
- Participate in the selection and evaluation of SESIP devices with safety features within your agency whenever possible.

Data from Occupational Safety and Health Administration (OSHA): *Bloodborne pathogens and needlestick injuries, 77 FR 19934,* 2012, https://www.osha.gov/FedReg_osha_pdf/FED20120403.pdf. Accessed on January 15, 2015.

(Figure 32-24). Containers need to be puncture proof and leak proof. Never force a needle into a full needle disposal receptacle. Never place used needles and syringes in a wastebasket, in your pocket, on a patient's meal tray, or at the patient's bedside. Box 32-23 summarizes the recommendations for the prevention of needlestick injuries.

Intravenous Administration. Nurses administer medications intravenously by the following methods:

1. As mixtures within large volumes of IV fluids
2. By injection of a bolus or small volume of medication through an existing IV infusion line or intermittent venous access (heparin or saline lock)
3. By "piggyback" infusion of a solution containing the prescribed medication and a small volume of IV fluid through an existing IV line

In all three methods a patient has either an existing IV infusion running continuously or an IV access site for intermittent infusions. Most policies and procedures list who is able to give IV medications and in which patient care units they can be given. These policies are made on the basis of the medication, capability, and availability of staff and the type of monitoring equipment available.

Chapter 42 describes the technique for performing venipuncture and establishing continuous IV fluid infusions. Medication administration is only one reason for supplying IV fluids. IV fluid therapy is used primarily for fluid replacement in patients unable to take oral fluids and as a means of supplying electrolytes and nutrients.

When using any method of IV medication administration, observe patients closely for symptoms of adverse reactions. After a medication enters the bloodstream, it begins to act immediately, and there is no way to stop its action. Thus take special care to avoid errors in dose calculation and preparation. Carefully follow the six rights of safe medication administration, double-check medication calculations with another nurse, and know the desired action and side effects of every medication you give. If the medication has an antidote, make sure that it is available during administration. When administering potent medications, assess vital signs before, during, and after infusion.

Administering medications by the IV route has advantages. Nurses often use this route in emergencies when a fast-acting medication needs to be delivered quickly. The IV route is also best when it is necessary to give medications to establish constant therapeutic blood levels. Some medications are highly alkaline and irritating to muscle and subcutaneous tissue. These medications cause less discomfort when given intravenously. Because IV medications are immediately available to the bloodstream once they are administered, verify the rate of administration with a medication reference or a pharmacist before giving them to ensure that you give them safely over the appropriate amount of time. Patients experience severe adverse reactions if IV medications are administered too quickly.

Large-Volume Infusions. Of the three methods of administering IV medications, mixing them in large volumes of fluids is the safest and easiest. Because the medication is not in a concentrated form, the risk of side effects or fatal reactions is minimal when infused over the prescribed time frame. Medications are diluted in large volumes (500 or 1000 mL) of compatible IV fluids such as normal saline or lactated Ringer's solution. Vitamins and potassium chloride are two types of medications commonly added to IV fluids. There is a danger with continuous infusion: if the IV fluid is infused too rapidly, the patient is at risk for medication overdose and circulatory fluid overload.

In the past nurses mixed medications into IV fluids. However, current safety standards and evidence-based practice no longer support this practice on a routine basis (Alexander et al., 2014; ASHP, 2014; INS, 2011; TJC 2016). Many patient safety risks such as incorrect calculation, nonaseptic preparation, and incorrect labeling occur when nurses have to prepare medications in IV containers on patient care units. Current best practices include use of IV medications that come in standardized concentrations and dosages; standardized procedures for ordering, preparing, and administering IV medications; and ready-to-administer doses when possible (ASHP, 2014).

Nurses only mix medications into IV fluids in emergency situations. The nurse *never* prepares high-alert medications (e.g., heparin, dopamine, dobutamine, nitroglycerin, potassium, antibiotics, or magnesium) on a patient care unit. Check with a pharmacist before mixing a medication in an IV container. If a pharmacist confirms that you need to prepare the medication, ask another nurse to verify your medication calculations and have that nurse watch you during the entire procedure to ensure that you prepare the medication safely. First ensure that the IV fluid and medication are compatible. Then prepare the medication in a syringe (see Skill 32-4) using strict aseptic technique. Clean the injection port of the IV bag with an alcohol swab, remove the cap from the needle, and insert the needle through the IV port. Push the syringe plunger to instill medication into the IV fluid and mix the solution by turning the IV bag gently end to end. Finally attach a medication label following ISMP (2015b) safe-label guidelines. Administer the medication to the patient at the prescribed rate (see Chapter 42). *Do not* add medications to IV bags that are already hanging because there is no way to tell the exact concentration of the medication. Add medications *only* to new IV bags.

When administering medications in large IV infusions, regulate the IV rate according to the health care provider's order. Monitor patients closely for adverse reactions to the medication and fluid volume overload. Also check the site frequently for infiltration and phlebitis (see Chapter 42).

Intravenous Bolus. An IV bolus involves introducing a concentrated dose of a medication directly into the systemic circulation (see Skill 32-6 on pp. 675-679). Because a bolus requires only a small amount of fluid to deliver the medication, it is an advantage when the amount of fluid that the patient can take is restricted. The IV bolus, or "push," is the most dangerous method for administering medications because there is no time to correct errors. In addition, a bolus may cause direct irritation to the lining of blood vessels. Before administering a bolus confirm placement of the IV line. Never give a medication intravenously if the insertion site appears swollen or edematous or the IV fluid cannot flow at the proper rate. Accidental injection of a medication into the tissues around a vein causes pain, sloughing of tissues, and abscesses, depending on the composition of the medication. Medications that carry a risk of adverse effects if administered too quickly should be diluted and administered as a piggyback or via an infusion pump.

Determine the rate of administration of an IV bolus medication by the amount of medication that can be given each minute. For example, if a patient is to receive 4 mL of a medication over 2 minutes, give 2 mL of the IV bolus medication every minute. Look up each medication to determine the recommended concentration and rate of administration. The ISMP (2003) has recommended avoiding using terms such as "IV push," "IVP," or "bolus" in orders with drugs that require administration over 1 minute or longer. Use more descriptive terms such as "IV over 5 minutes." Remember, consider the purpose for which an IV medication is prescribed and any potential adverse effects related to the rate or route of administration.

Volume-Controlled Infusions. Another way of administering IV medications is through small amounts (50 to 100 mL) of compatible IV fluids. The fluid is within a secondary fluid container separate from the primary fluid bag. The container connects directly to the primary IV line or to separate tubing that inserts into the primary line (see Skill 32-7 on pp. 679-683). Three types of containers are volume-control administration sets (e.g., Volutrol or Pediatrol), piggyback sets, and syringe pumps. Using volume-controlled infusions has several advantages:

- It reduces risk of rapid-dose infusion by IV push. Medications are diluted and infused over longer time intervals (e.g., 30 to 60 minutes).
- It allows for administration of medications (e.g., antibiotics) that are stable for a limited time in solution.
- It allows for control of IV fluid intake.

Piggyback. A piggyback is a small (25 to 250 mL) IV bag or bottle connected to a short tubing line that connects to the *upper* Y-port of a primary infusion line or to an intermittent venous access (Figure 32-25). The label on the medication follows the ISMP IV piggyback medication label format (ISMP, 2015b) (Figure 32-26). The piggyback tubing is a microdrip or macrodrip system (see Chapter 42). The set is called a *piggyback* because the small bag or bottle is higher than the primary infusion bag or bottle. In the piggyback setup the main line does not infuse when the piggybacked medication is infusing. The port of the primary IV line contains a back-check valve that automatically stops flow of the primary infusion once the piggyback infusion flows. After the piggyback solution infuses and the solution within the tubing falls below the level of the primary infusion drip chamber, the back-check valve opens, and the primary infusion again flows.

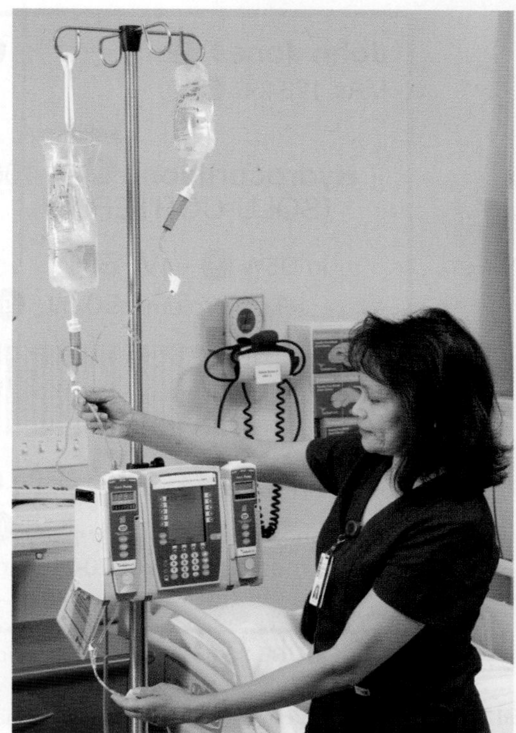
FIGURE 32-25 Piggyback setup.

Volume-Control Administration. Volume-control administration (e.g., Buretrol) sets are small (150-mL) containers that attach just below the primary infusion bag or bottle. The set is attached and filled in a manner similar to that used with a regular IV infusion. Follow package directions for priming sets (see Chapter 42).

Syringe Pump. The syringe pump is battery operated and allows medications to be given in very small amounts of fluid (5 to 60 mL) within controlled infusion times using standard syringes.

Intermittent Venous Access. An intermittent venous access (commonly called a *saline lock*) is an IV catheter capped off on the end with a small chamber covered by a rubber diaphragm or a specially designed cap. Special rubber-seal injection caps usually accept needle safety devices (see Chapter 42). Advantages to intermittent venous access include the following:

- Cost savings resulting from the omission of continuous IV therapy
- Effectiveness of nurse's time enhanced by eliminating constant monitoring of flow rates
- Increased mobility, safety, and comfort for the patient

Before administering an IV bolus or piggyback medication, assess the patency and placement of the IV site. After the medication has been administered through an intermittent venous access, the access must

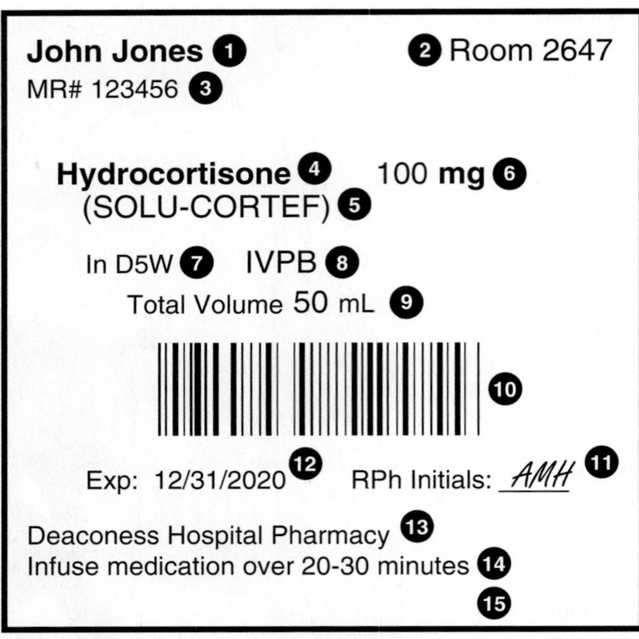

FIGURE 32-26 IV piggyback medication with label following ISMP safe-labeling guidelines.

be flushed with a solution to keep it patent. Generally normal saline is an effective flush solution for peripheral catheters. Some agencies require the use of heparin. Nurses need to verify and follow agency policies regarding the care and maintenance of the IV site.

Administration of Intravenous Therapy in the Home. Sometimes patients need IV therapy at home. Common infusions that patients receive include antibiotics, chemotherapy, total parenteral nutrition, analgesics, and blood transfusions. Most patients typically receive their home IV therapy through a long-term central venous catheter (CVC) (see Chapter 42). Home health nurses assess patients' responses to the medication, monitor the CVC site, and teach patients and their family caregivers how to administer infusions and maintain the CVC.

Carefully assess patients and their families to determine their ability to manage IV therapy at home. Begin instruction on IV care management as soon as you know that a patient will have IV therapy at home. Your instruction often begins while a patient is hospitalized. Patients and families need to learn how to recognize problems such as signs of infections and other complications related to IV therapy and what to do when these problems occur. Patients also need to know when to notify the home care nurse or health care provider. Plan to teach patients and their families how to maintain IV administration equipment, including the infusion pump.

SAFETY GUIDELINES FOR NURSING SKILLS

Ensuring patient safety is an essential role of a professional nurse. To ensure patient safety, communicate clearly with members of the health care team, assess and incorporate the patient's priorities of care and preferences, and use the best evidence when making decisions about your patient's care. When performing the skills in this chapter, remember the following points to ensure safe, individualized patient care.

- Be vigilant during the entire process of medication administration. Ensure that your patients receive the appropriate medications. Know why every medication is ordered for your patient, even if you are not administering the medication. Understand what you need to do before, during, and after medication administration. Evaluate the effectiveness and assess for adverse effects after your patients take their medications.
- Take care of yourself. You think as clearly and critically as possible when you are healthy. Healthy behaviors such as getting adequate sleep, making healthy food choices, and getting regular exercise or activity are positive ways to help you better process information and make safe decisions during medication administration.
- Set up and prepare medications in distraction-free, no-interruption zone (NIZ) areas.
- Verify expiration date of every medication during preparation. Do not administer expired medications. Return expired medication to pharmacy.
- Identify each patient using at least two identifiers before administering medications and check against the medication administration record (MAR).
- Clarify all unclear orders and ask for help whenever you are uncertain about a medication order or calculation. Consult with your peers, pharmacists, and other health care providers. Resolve all your concerns related to medication administration before preparing and giving medications.
- Use technology (e.g., bar-code scanning, electronic MARs) that is available to you when preparing and administering medications. Follow all policies related to the safe use of technology and do not use "work-arounds." Nurses who use "work-arounds" fail to follow agency protocols, policies, or procedures during medication administration in an attempt to administer medications to patients in a timelier manner. Failure to follow the standard of care greatly increases the risk for making a medication error, impairs patient safety, and places you at risk for malpractice and disciplinary action (see Chapter 23).
- Educate patients about their medications during medication administration. Patients are often able to identify inappropriate medications. Answer all patient questions and resolve their concerns before giving medications. Include family caregivers in medication education when appropriate.
- In most circumstances you cannot delegate medication administration. Ensure that you follow standards set by your state Nurse Practice Act and guidelines established by the health care agency. Nursing instructors or registered nurses

need to verify all medications and closely supervise nursing students throughout the entire medication preparation and administration process. Licensed practical nurses (LPNs) or licensed vocational nurses (LVNs) can usually administer medications given PO, subcutaneously, intramuscularly, and intradermally. In some cases they can give medications intravenously if they have had special training and if the medications are not high alert. Some states also allow certified medical assistants (CMAs) to administer some types of medications (e.g., PO medications) in some health care settings (e.g., long-term care facilities). The skills in this chapter assume that you are not in a setting where you can delegate medication administration to nursing assistive personnel (NAP). If you are practicing in a state and a health care setting that allow you to delegate medication administration, follow the guidelines for safe delegation (see Chapter 21), agency policies, and the standards outlined in the Nurse Practice Act in your state.

SKILL 32-1 ADMINISTERING ORAL MEDICATIONS

DELEGATION CONSIDERATIONS

The skill of administering oral medications cannot be delegated to nursing assistive personnel (NAP). Instruct the NAP about:

- Potential side effects of medications and the need to report their occurrence.
- Informing nurse if patient condition worsens (e.g., increased pain, change in behavior).

EQUIPMENT

- Automated, computer-controlled drug-dispensing system or medication cart
- Disposable medication cups
- Glass of water, juice, or preferred liquid and drinking straw
- Device for crushing or splitting tablets (optional)
- Clean gloves (if handling a medication)
- Medication administration record (MAR) (electronic or printed)
- Paper towels

STEP	RATIONALE
ASSESSMENT	
1. Check accuracy and completeness of each MAR with health care provider's medication order. Check patient's name, medication name and dosage, and route and time of administration. Recopy or reprint any part of printed MAR that is difficult to read.	The order sheet is the most reliable source and only legal record of medications that patient is to receive. Ensures that patient receives correct medications (Mandrack et al., 2012; Sulosaari et al., 2011). Illegible MARs are a source of medication errors (Alassaad et al., 2013).
2. Review pertinent information related to medication: action, purpose, normal dose and route, side effects, time of onset and peak action, and nursing implications.	Allows you to anticipate effects of drug and observe patient's response.
3. Assess for any contraindications to patient receiving oral medication, including being NPO (nothing by mouth), inability to swallow, nausea or vomiting, bowel inflammation or reduced peristalsis, recent gastrointestinal (GI) surgery, gastric suction, and decreased level of consciousness. Check patient's swallow, cough, and gag reflexes.	Alterations in GI function interfere with medication distribution, absorption, and excretion. Patients with GI suction do not receive benefit from oral medications because they are suctioned from the GI tract before they can be absorbed. Risk factors for aspiration include impaired swallowing, decreased level of consciousness (LOC), immobility, and poor functional status (Park et al., 2013).

CLINICAL DECISION: *If there are any contraindications to the patient receiving oral medications or if in doubt about the patient's ability to swallow oral medications, temporarily withhold medication and inform health care provider.*

STEP	RATIONALE
4. Assess patient's medical, medication, and diet history and history of allergies. List patient's food and drug allergies on each page of the MAR and prominently display it on the patient's medical record per agency policy. When patient has allergy, provide allergy bracelet.	Information reflects patient's need for and potential responses to medications. Information also indicates potential food and drug interactions. Communication of allergies is essential for safe, effective care.
5. Assess risk for aspiration using a dysphagia screening tool if available (see Skill 45-1).	Patients with dysphagia are at risk for aspirating oral medications. Early detection of dysphagia can improve patient outcomes (Speyer, 2013).
6. Gather physical examination and laboratory data that influence medication administration (e.g., vital signs, renal and liver function, laboratory values).	Data sometimes reveal need to hold medication or that medication is contraindicated. Poor liver and kidney function affects metabolism and excretion of medications (Burchum and Rosenthal, 2016).
7. Assess patient's knowledge regarding health and medication use.	Determines patient's need for medication education and guidance needed to achieve drug adherence. Assessment often reveals problems such as medication tolerance, nonadherence, abuse, addiction, or dependence.
8. Assess patient's preferences for fluids. Maintain fluid restrictions when applicable. Determine if medication can be given with preferred fluid.	Fluids ease swallowing and facilitate absorption from the GI tract. Some fluids interfere with absorption of medications.
PLANNING	
1. Collect appropriate equipment and MAR.	Enhances time management and efficiency.
2. Plan preparation to avoid interruptions. Do not take phone calls or talk with others. Follow agency policy.	Interruption contributes to medication errors. Use no-interruption zone (NIZ) when possible (Prakash et al., 2014; Yoder et al., 2015).

SKILL 32-1 ADMINISTERING ORAL MEDICATIONS—cont'd

STEP	RATIONALE
IMPLEMENTATION	
1. Prepare medications:	
a. Perform hand hygiene.	Reduces transfer of microorganisms.
b. If using a medication cart, move it outside patient's room. Option: Arrange medication cups in medication preparation area.	Organization of equipment saves time and reduces error.
c. Log into automated dispensing system (ADS) or unit-dose cart or unlock medicine drawer or cart.	Medications are safeguarded when locked in cabinet, cart, or computerized medication dispensing system.
d. Prepare medication for one patient at a time. Follow the six rights of medication administration. Keep all pages of MARs for one patient together or look at only one patient's medication administration computer screen at a time.	Preventing distractions limits preparation errors (Kim and Bates, 2013).
e. Select correct medication from stock supply, unit-dose drawer, or ADS. Compare name of medication on label with MAR (see illustration). Exit ADS after removing drug(s).	Reading labels and comparing them with transcribed order reduces error. *This is the first accuracy check.* Logging out of ADS ensures that no one else can use your identity to remove medications.
f. Check expiration date on each medication, one at a time. Return outdated drug to pharmacy.	Medications used past their expiration date may lose strength, be inactive, or harm patient.
g. Check or calculate medication dose as necessary. Double-check calculation. If needed, have another nurse verify calculations.	Double-checking reduces risk of error. Some agencies require nurses to double-check calculations of certain medications (e.g., insulin, heparin) with another nurse (Kim and Bates, 2013).
h. If preparing a controlled substance, check record for previous medication count and compare current count with supply available.	Controlled substance laws require nurses to carefully monitor and count dispensed narcotics.
i. Prepare solid forms of oral medications:	
(1) To prepare tablets or capsules from a floor stock bottle, pour required number into bottle cap and transfer medication to medication cup. Do not touch medication with fingers. Return extra tablets or capsules to bottle.	Avoids contamination and waste of medications.
(2) To prepare unit-dose tablets or capsules, place packaged tablet or capsule directly into medicine cup. Do not remove wrapper (see illustration).	Wrapper maintains cleanliness of medications and allows you to identify medication name and dose at patient's bedside.
(3) When using a blister pack, "pop" medications through foil or paper backing into a medication cup.	Packs provide 1-month supply, with each "blister" usually containing a single dose.
(4) If it is necessary to give half a tablet or pill, pharmacy should split, label package, and send medication to unit.	The ISMP (2006) recommends for inpatient settings that, if a pill must be split, a pharmacist splits the pill, repackages and labels it, and sends to nurse for administration. Nurses should not split pills.

CLINICAL DECISION: *Splitting tablets in half, even if they are prescored with a line down the middle, leads to medication errors (Niemann et al., 2015). Medications need to be provided in the correct dose whenever possible. If a pill must be split within inpatient settings, the pharmacist splits the pill with a splitting device, repackages and labels it, and sends it to the nurse for administration. Nurses should not split pills (USFDA, 2013).*

STEP	RATIONALE
(5) Place all tablets or capsules for patient in one medicine cup, except for those requiring preadministration assessments (e.g., pulse rate or blood pressure); keep medications in their wrappers.	Keeping medications that require preadministration assessments separate from others makes it easier to withhold medications as necessary.

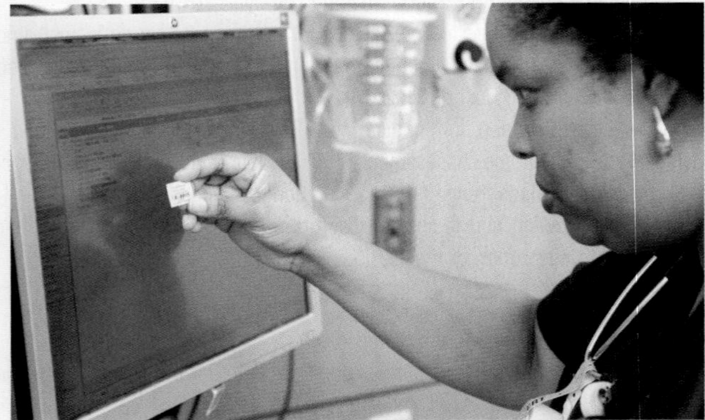

STEP 1e The nurse verifies each medication with medication administration record.

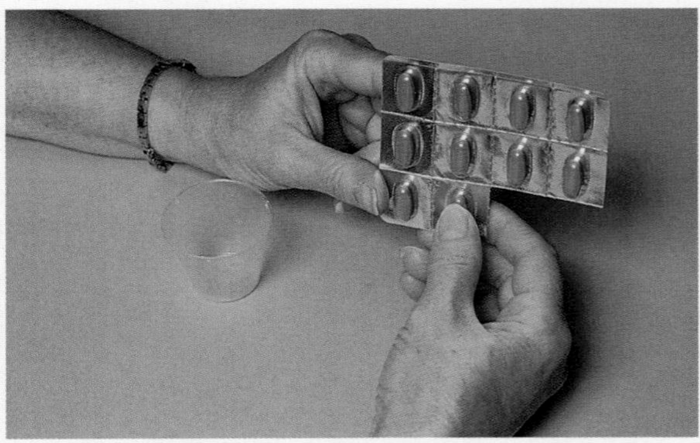

STEP 1i(2) Place tablet into medicine cup without removing wrapper.

STEP	RATIONALE
(6) If patient has difficulty swallowing and liquid medications are not an option, use pill-crushing device (see illustration). Clean crushing device before using it. If a pill-crushing device is not available, place tablet between two medication cups and grind with blunt instrument. Mix ground tablet in small amount (e.g., teaspoon) of soft food (custard or applesauce).	Large tablets are often difficult to swallow. Ground tablet mixed with palatable soft food is usually easier to swallow. Cleaning pill-crushing device ensures that contamination of medications does not occur.

CLINICAL DECISION: *Not all medications can be crushed (e.g., capsules, enteric-coated drugs). Consult with pharmacist and/or the "Do Not Crush List" when in doubt (ISMP, 2014a).*

STEP	RATIONALE
j. Prepare liquids:	
(1) Unit-dose container with correct amount of medication: Gently shake container. Administer liquid medication packaged in single-dose cup directly from the single-dose cup. Do not pour into medicine cup.	Using unit-dose container with correct dose of medication provides most accurate dose (ISMP, 2015c). Shaking container ensures that medication is mixed before administration.

CLINICAL DECISION: *On the basis of current best practice (ISMP, 2015c), liquid medications that are not available or are not in correct dose in a unit-dose container should be dispensed by the pharmacy in special oral syringes marked "Oral Use Only." These syringes do not connect to any type of parenteral (e.g., intravenous) tubing. In addition, current evidence shows that liquid measuring devices on patient care units result in inaccurate dosing. Having oral medications prepared in the pharmacy ensures that you give the most accurate dose of a medication possible and prevents parenteral administration of oral medications. Steps (2)-(4) that follow are included ONLY if you need to prepare your own liquid medications.*

STEP	RATIONALE
(2) Liquid medication in bottle or unit-dose container not available in dose ordered: If medication is in multidose bottle, remove bottle cap from container and place cap upside down. Hold multidose bottle with label against palm of hand while pouring.	Verify with pharmacy that you need to prepare your own dose before proceeding (ISMP, 2015c). Keeping cap upside down maintains cleanliness of cap. Spilled liquid does not soil or fade label.
(3) Place medication cup at eye level on hard surface (e.g., countertop). Fill to desired level on scale (see illustration A). Make sure that scale is even with fluid level at its surface or base of meniscus, not edges. Draw up volumes of less than 10 mL in syringe designed for oral medication use without needle (see illustration B). Do not use parenteral syringe to draw up oral medications. Place label on the medication.	Ensures accuracy of measurement. Use of special oral syringe for oral medications prevents accidental parenteral administration of oral medication and is more accurate for small doses of medication (ISMP, 2015c). Labeling ensures that you remember which medication is in the medicine cup or oral medication syringe.
(4) Discard any excess liquid into sink or place specially designated for wasting of medications. Wipe lip and neck of bottle with paper towel.	Prevents contamination of contents of bottle and prevents bottle cap from sticking.
k. Return stock containers or unused unit-dose medications to shelf or ADS drawer and read label again.	Reading label of medications in multiple-dose containers reduces administration errors.
l. Do not leave medications unattended.	Nurse is responsible for safekeeping of drugs.
m. Before going to patient's room, compare patient's name and name of medication on label of prepared drugs with MAR.	Reading labels second time reduces error. *This is the second accuracy check.*
2. Administer medications:	

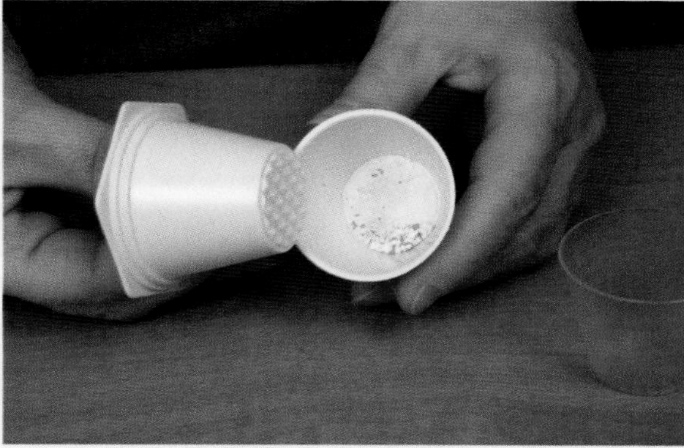

STEP 1i(6) Pill-crushing device used to crush pills when necessary.

SKILL 32-1 ADMINISTERING ORAL MEDICATIONS—cont'd

STEP	RATIONALE
a. Take medications to patient at correct time (see agency policy). Medications that require exact timing include STAT, first-time or loading, and 1-time doses. Give time-critical scheduled medications (e.g., antibiotics, anticoagulants, insulin, anticonvulsants, immunosuppressive agents) at exact time ordered (within 30 minutes before or after scheduled dose). Give non–time critical scheduled medications within a range of either 1 or 2 hours of scheduled does (ISMP, 2011). Apply the six rights of medication administration throughout medication administration. Perform hand hygiene.	Ensures intended therapeutic effect and complies with professional standards. Hospitals need to adopt a medication administration policy and procedure for timing of medication administration that considers patient needs, prescribed medication, and specific clinical indications (CMS, 2011; ISMP, 2011). Time-critical scheduled medications are medications in which early or delayed administration of maintenance doses of more than 30 minutes before or after the scheduled dose may cause harm or result in suboptimal therapy or pharmacological effect. Non–time-critical medications are medications in which early or delayed administration of 1-2 hours should not cause harm or result in suboptimal therapy or pharmacological effects (CMS, 2011; ISMP, 2011). Hand hygiene decreases transfer of microorganisms.
b. Identify patient using at least two identifiers (e.g., name and birthday or name and medical record number) according to agency policy. Compare identifiers with information on patient's MAR or medical record.	Ensures correct patient. Complies with The Joint Commission standards and improves patient safety (TJC, 2016).
CLINICAL DECISION: *Replace patient identification bracelets that are missing, illegible, or faded.*	
c. Compare names of medications on labels with MAR at patient's bedside.	Final check of medication labels against MAR at patient's bedside reduces medication administration errors. *This is the third check for accuracy.*
d. Explain purpose of each medication, its action, and possible adverse effects to patient. Explore concerns expressed by patient and verify orders if concerns about accuracy of medication orders arise.	Patient has right to be informed; questions often indicate need for teaching or possible nonadherence to therapy. Allows patient to express concerns regarding medications and possibly identifies potential errors in medication orders.
e. Perform necessary preadministration assessments (e.g., blood pressure, pulse). Verify allergies with patient.	Determines whether specific medications should be withheld at that time.
f. Help patient to sitting or Fowler's position. Use side-lying position if sitting is contraindicated. Have patient stay in this position for 30 minutes after administration.	Sitting position prevents aspiration during swallowing (Echevarria and Schwoebel, 2012).
g. Administer medications	
(1) For tablets: Some patients want to hold solid medications in hand or cup before placing in mouth. Offer water or juice to help patient swallow and give full glass if not contraindicated.	Patient becomes familiar with medications by seeing each drug. Choice of fluid can improve fluid intake.
(2) For orally disintegrating formulations (tablets or strips): Remove medication from blister packet just before use. Do not push the tablet through the foil. Place medication on top of patient's tongue and caution against chewing the medication.	These medications begin to dissolve when placed on the tongue. Water is not needed. Because they are thin and fragile, remove them carefully from packaging.
(3) For sublingual medications: Have patient place medication under tongue and allow it to dissolve completely (see Figure 32-3). Caution patient against swallowing tablet.	Medication is absorbed through blood vessels of undersurface of tongue. If swallowed, gastric juices destroy medication, or liver detoxifies it so rapidly that therapeutic blood levels are not attained.
(4) For buccal medications: Have patient place medication in mouth against mucous membranes of cheek until it dissolves (see Figure 32-4). Avoid administering liquids until buccal medication has dissolved.	Buccal medications act locally on mucosa or systemically as they are swallowed in saliva.

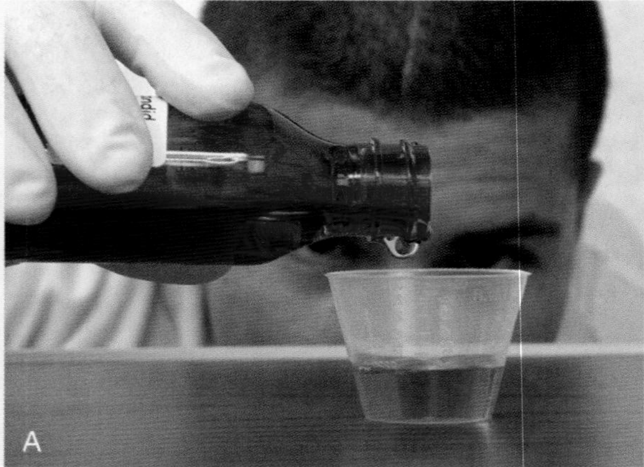

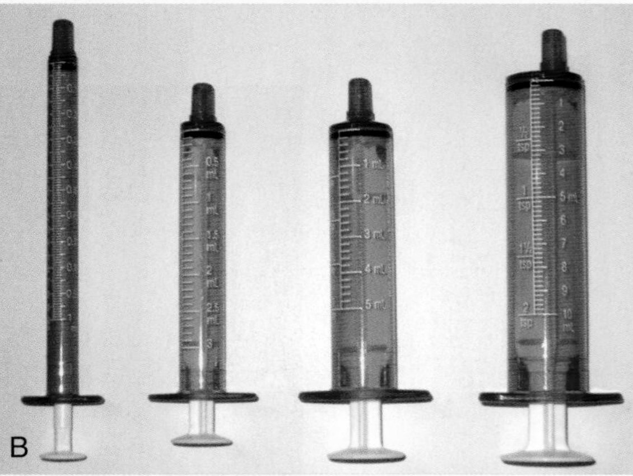

STEP 1j(3) A, Pour desired volume of liquid so base of meniscus is level with line on scale. **B,** Use special oral medication syringes to prepare small amounts of liquid medications.

STEP	RATIONALE
(5) **For powdered medications:** Mix with liquids at bedside and give to patient to drink.	When prepared in advance, powdered medications often thicken and even harden, making swallowing difficult.
(6) **For crushed medications mixed in food:** Give each medication separately in teaspoon of food.	Ensures that patient swallows all of medicine.
(7) **For lozenges:** Caution patient against chewing or swallowing lozenges.	Medication acts through slow absorption through oral mucosa, not gastric mucosa.
(8) **For effervescent medication:** Add tablet or powder to glass of liquid. Give immediately after dissolving.	Effervescence improves unpleasant taste and often relieves GI problems.
h. If patient is unable to hold medications, place medication cup to lips and gently introduce each drug into mouth, one at a time. Consider using spoon to place pills in mouth. Do not rush or force medications.	Administering single tablet or capsule eases swallowing and decreases risk of aspiration.

CLINICAL DECISION: *If tablet or capsule falls to the floor, discard it and repeat preparation. Medication is contaminated.*

STEP	RATIONALE
i. Stay until patient completely takes all medications by their prescribed route. Ask patient to open mouth if uncertain whether medication was swallowed.	You are responsible for ensuring that patient receives ordered dosage. If left unattended, some patients do not take dose or save medications, causing risk to health.
j. For highly acidic medications (e.g., aspirin), offer patient nonfat snack (e.g., crackers) if not contraindicated by his or her condition.	Reduces gastric irritation. The fat content of foods can delay medication absorption.
k. Help patient return to comfortable position.	Maintains patient's comfort.
l. Dispose of soiled supplies and perform hand hygiene.	Hand hygiene reduces transmission of microorganisms.
m. Replenish stock such as cups and straws, return cart to medication room if used, and clean work area.	Maintaining clean and organized workspace enhances efficiency of all staff.

EVALUATION

STEP	RATIONALE
1. Evaluate patient's response to medications at times that correlate with onset, peak, and duration of the medication.	Evaluates therapeutic benefit of medication and detects onset of side effects or allergic reactions.
2. Ask patient or family member to identify medication name and explain purpose, action, dosage schedule, and potential side effects of drug.	Determines level of knowledge gained by patient and family.
3. Use ***Teach Back*** to determine patient's and family's understanding about oral medications. State, "I want to be sure I explained how to take your (e.g., sublingual, tablet) medicines. Can you explain how to take these medicines?" Revise your instruction now or develop plan for revised teaching if patient or family is not able to teach back correctly.	Evaluates what the patient and family are able to explain or demonstrate.

UNEXPECTED OUTCOMES AND RELATED INTERVENTIONS

1. Patient exhibits adverse effects (side effect, toxic effect, allergic reaction) such as urticaria, rash, wheezing.
   - *Always* notify health care provider and pharmacy when patient exhibits adverse effects.
   - Withhold further doses and add allergy information to patient's medical record.
2. Patient refuses medication.
   - Explore reasons why patient does not want medication.
   - Educate if misunderstandings of medication therapy are apparent.
   - Do not force patient to take medication; patients have the right to refuse treatment. If patient continues to refuse medication despite educational attempts, record why the drug was withheld on his or her chart and notify health care provider.

RECORDING AND REPORTING

- Chart medication dose, route, and time and date given on MAR immediately after administering.
- Record the reason that any drug is withheld and follow agency policy for proper recording.
- Record and report evaluation of medication effect to health care provider if required (e.g., report urine output following administration of diuretic if ordered by health care provider).
- Document your evaluation of patient and family learning.

HOME CARE CONSIDERATIONS

- Instruct patients and family caregivers about all aspects of medication administration, including dosage, desired effect, when to take medications, proper storage of medications, anticipated side effects, and whether to take medication with or without food, to ensure safe medication administration at home.
- Evaluate patient's ability to safely self-administer medications. If unable to safely self-administer, attempt nursing interventions such as a chart or pillbox to assist in self-administration. If interventions fail and patient still is unable to administer medications safely, notify the health care provider.

SKILL 32-2 ADMINISTERING OPHTHALMIC MEDICATIONS 

DELEGATION CONSIDERATIONS

The skill of administering ophthalmic medications cannot be delegated to nursing assistive personnel (NAP). Instruct NAP about:

- Potential side effects of medications and to report their occurrence, including the potential for visual changes.

EQUIPMENT

- Medication bottle with sterile eyedropper, ointment tube, or medicated intraocular disk
- Cotton ball or tissue
- Wash basin filled with warm water and washcloth (if eyes have crust or drainage)
- Eye patch and tape (optional)
- Clean gloves
- Medication administration record (MAR) (electronic or printed)

STEP	RATIONALE
ASSESSMENT	
1. Check accuracy and completeness of each MAR with health care provider's medication order. Check patient's name, medication name and dosage (e.g., number of drops [if a liquid] and eye [right, left, or both eyes]), and route and time of administration. Recopy or reprint any part of MAR that is difficult to read.	The order sheet is the most reliable source and only legal record of medications that patient is to receive. Ensures that patient receives correct medications (Mandrack et al., 2012; Sulosaari et al., 2011). Illegible MARs are a source of medication errors (Alassaad et al, 2013).
2. Review pertinent information related to medication: action, purpose, normal dose and route, side effects, time of onset and peak action, and nursing implications.	Allows you to anticipate effects of drug and observe patient's response.
3. Assess condition of external eye structures (see Chapter 31). (You may also do this just before medication administration.)	Provides baseline to later determine if local response to medication occurs. Also indicates need to clean eye before medication application.
4. Assess patient's medical history, history of allergies (including latex), and medication history. If patient has latex allergy, use nonlatex gloves.	Factors in history influence how certain drugs act. Protects patient from risk of allergic medication response.
5. Determine whether patient has any symptoms of visual alterations.	Certain eye medications act to either lessen or increase these symptoms. Provides baseline assessment for recognizing change in patient's condition.
6. Assess patient's level of consciousness and ability to follow directions.	If patient becomes restless or combative during procedure, a greater risk of accidental eye injury exists.
7. Assess patient's knowledge regarding medication therapy and desire to self-administer medication.	Patient's level of understanding determines need for health teaching. Motivation influences teaching approach.
8. Assess patient's ability to manipulate and hold equipment necessary for eye medication (e.g., dropper, ointment tube).	Reflects patient's ability to learn to self-administer medication.
PLANNING	
1. Collect appropriate equipment and MAR.	Enhances time management and efficiency.
2. Plan preparation to avoid interruptions. Do not take phone calls. Follow agency policy.	Interruption contributes to medication errors. Use no-interruption zone (NIZ) when possible (Prakash et al., 2014; Yoder et al., 2015).
IMPLEMENTATION	
1. Perform hand hygiene and prepare medication (see Skill 32-1, Steps 1a-g). Preparation usually involves taking eyedrops out of refrigerator and rewarming to room temperature before administering to patient. Check expiration date on container. Be sure to check the label 2 times while preparing medication.	Hand hygiene reduces transmission of microorganisms. Warming eyedrops reduces eye irritation. Ensures that patient receives correct medication. Following medication policies and preparing medications in the same way every time helps to prevent medication errors (Murphy and While, 2012). *This is the first and second accuracy check.*
2. Take medications to patient at correct time (see agency policy). Medications that require exact timing include STAT, first-time, loading, and 1-time doses. Give time-critical scheduled medications (e.g., antibiotics, anticoagulants, insulin, anticonvulsants, immunosuppressive agents) at exact time ordered (within 30 minutes before or after scheduled dose). Give non–time-critical scheduled medications within a range of either 1 or 2 hours of scheduled does (ISMP, 2011). Apply the six rights of medication administration throughout medication administration. Perform hand hygiene.	Ensures intended therapeutic effect and complies with professional standards. Hospitals need to adopt a medication administration policy and procedure for timing of medication administration that considers patient needs, prescribed medication, and specific clinical indications (CMS, 2011; ISMP, 2011). Time-critical scheduled medications are medications in which early or delayed administration of maintenance doses of more than 30 minutes before or after the scheduled dose may cause harm or result in suboptimal therapy or pharmacological effect. Non–time-critical medications are medications in which early or delayed administration of 1-2 hours should not cause harm or result in suboptimal therapy or pharmacological effects (CMS, 2011; ISMP, 2011). Hand hygiene decreases transfer of microorganisms.
3. Identify patient using at least two identifiers (e.g., name and birthday or name and medical record number) according to agency policy. Compare identifiers with information on patient's MAR or medical record.	Ensures correct patient. Complies with The Joint Commission standards and improves patient safety (TJC, 2016).
4. Compare names of medications on labels with MAR at patient's bedside.	*Third check for accuracy* ensures that right medication is administered.

STEP	RATIONALE
5. Explain procedure to patient; describe positioning and sensations to expect such as burning or eye irritation. Discuss purpose, action, and possible adverse effects of each medication. Ask if patient has any questions.	Patient has right to be informed. Questions may reveal potentially incorrect medication orders. Relieves anxiety about medication being instilled into eye.
6. Arrange supplies at bedside; apply clean gloves.	Ensures organized procedure and reduces transmission of microorganisms.
7. Gently roll eyedrop container between your hands.	Ensures that medication is mixed before administration. Shaking bottle causes bubbles, which makes medication administration difficult.
8. Ask patient to lie supine or sit back in chair with head slightly hyperextended.	Position provides easy access to eye for medication instillation and minimizes drainage of medication through tear duct.

CLINICAL DECISION: *Do not hyperextend the neck of a patient with cervical spine injury.*

STEP	RATIONALE
9. If crusting or drainage is present along eyelid margins or inner canthus, gently wash away. Soak any crusts that are dried and difficult to remove by applying damp washcloth or cotton ball over eye for a few minutes. Always wipe clean from inner to outer canthus.	Crusts or drainage harbors microorganisms. Soaking allows easy removal and prevents pressure from being applied directly over eye. Cleaning from inner to outer canthus avoids entrance of microorganism into lacrimal duct.
10. Hold cotton ball or clean tissue in nondominant hand on patient's cheekbone just below lower eyelid.	Cotton or tissue absorbs medication that escapes eye.
11. With tissue or cotton resting below lower lid, gently press downward with thumb or forefinger against bony orbit.	Technique exposes lower conjunctival sac. Retraction against bony orbit prevents pressure and trauma to eyeball and fingers from touching eye.
12. Ask patient to look at ceiling.	Action retracts sensitive cornea up and away from conjunctival sac and reduces stimulation of blink reflex.
13. Instill ophthalmic drops:	
a. With dominant hand resting on patient's forehead, hold filled medication eyedropper or ophthalmic solution approximately 1 to 2 cm (½ to ¾ inches) above conjunctival sac (see illustration).	Helps prevent accidental contact of eyedropper with eye structures, thus reducing risk of injury to eye and transfer of infection to dropper. Ophthalmic medications are sterile.
b. Drop prescribed number of medication drops into conjunctival sac.	Conjunctival sac normally holds 1 or 2 drops. Provides even distribution of medication across eye.
c. If patient blinks or closes eye or if drops land on outer lid margins, repeat instillation.	Patient obtains therapeutic effect of drug only when drops enter conjunctival sac.
d. After instilling drops, ask patient to close eye gently.	Helps to distribute medication. Squinting or squeezing of eyelids forces medication from conjunctival sac (ASHP, 2013).
e. When administering medications that cause systemic effects, apply gentle pressure with your finger and clean tissue on patient's nasolacrimal duct for 30 to 60 seconds.	Prevents overflow of medication into nasal and pharyngeal passages. Prevents absorption into systemic circulation (ASHP, 2013).
f. If patient receives more than one eye medication to the same eye at the same time, wait at least 5 minutes before administering next medication and use a different cotton ball or tissue with each medication.	Avoids interaction between medications (ASHP, 2013).
14. Instill ophthalmic ointment:	
a. Holding ointment applicator above lower lid margin, apply thin stream of ointment evenly along inner edge of lower eyelid on conjunctiva (see illustration) from inner canthus to outer canthus.	Distributes medication evenly across eye and lid margin.
b. Have patient close eye and rub lid lightly in circular motion with cotton ball if rubbing is not contraindicated.	Distributes medication evenly across eye and lid margin.

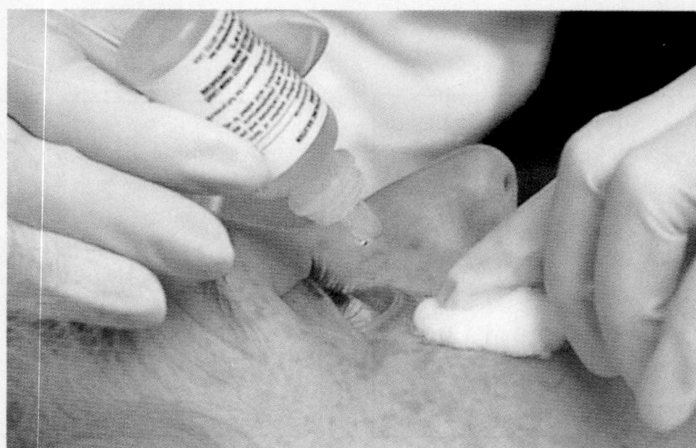

STEP 13a Hold eyedropper above conjunctival sac.

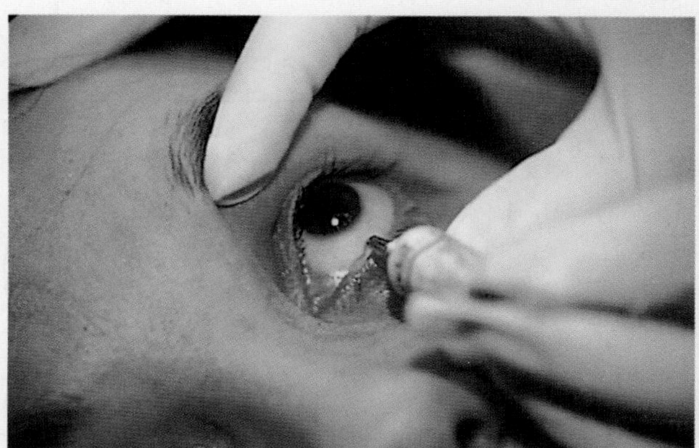

STEP 14a Apply ointment along lower eyelid.

SKILL 32-2 ADMINISTERING OPHTHALMIC MEDICATIONS—cont'd

STEP	RATIONALE
15. Administer intraocular disk:	
a. Open package containing disk. Gently press fingertip against disk so it adheres to finger. Position convex side of disk on fingertip (see illustration).	Allows you to inspect disk for damage or deformity.
b. With other hand gently pull patient's lower eyelid away from eye. Ask patient to look up.	Prepares conjunctival sac for receiving medicated disk.
c. Place disk in conjunctival sac so it floats on sclera between iris and lower eyelid (see illustration).	Ensures delivery of medication (Guzman-Aranguez et al., 2013).
d. Pull patient's lower eyelid out and over disk (see illustration). You should not be able to see disk at this time. Repeat Step 15 if you can see disk.	Ensures accurate medication delivery.
16. Removal of intraocular disk:	
a. Perform hand hygiene and apply clean gloves.	Prevents transfer of microorganisms.
b. Explain procedure to patient.	Relieves anxiety about manipulation of disk in eye.
c. Gently pull on patient's lower eyelid with nondominant hand.	Exposes intraocular disk.
d. Using forefinger and thumb of opposite hand, pinch disk, and lift it out of patient's eye (see illustration).	
17. If excess medication is on eyelid, gently wipe it from inner to outer canthus.	Promotes comfort and prevents trauma to eye (ASHP, 2013).
18. If patient had eye patch, apply clean one by placing it over affected eye so entire eye is covered. Tape securely without applying pressure to eye.	Clean eye patch reduces chance of infection.
19. Remove gloves, dispose of soiled supplies in proper receptacle, and perform hand hygiene.	Maintains neat environment at bedside and reduces transmission of microorganisms.

EVALUATION

1. Note patient's immediate response to instillation; ask if patient felt any discomfort.	Determines if procedure performed correctly and safely.
2. Observe response to medication by assessing visual changes and noting any side effects.	Evaluates effects of medication.
3. Use ***Teach Back*** to determine patient's and family's understanding about eye medications. State, "I want to be sure you understand what I explained about your eyedrops. Can you tell me the name of your eyedrops, why you are taking them, how much to take, and which side effects you might have?" Revise your instruction now or develop plan for revised teaching if patient or family is not able to teach back correctly.	Evaluates what patient and family are able to explain or demonstrate.

UNEXPECTED OUTCOMES AND RELATED INTERVENTIONS

1. Patient cannot instill eyedrops without supervision.
   - Reinforce teaching and allow patient to self-administer drops as much as possible to enhance confidence.
   - If patient cannot self-administer drops, teach family caregivers to instill them into patient's eye.
2. Patient displays signs of allergic reaction (e.g., tearing, reddened sclera) or systemic response (e.g., bradycardia) to medication.
   - Hold medication and speak with health care provider.
   - Follow agency policy or guidelines for reporting adverse or allergic reaction to medications.
   - Add information about allergy to medical record per agency policy.

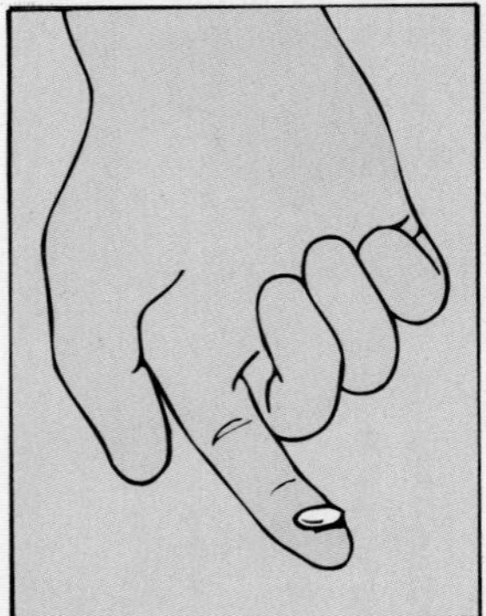

STEP 15a Gently position convex side of disk against fingertips.

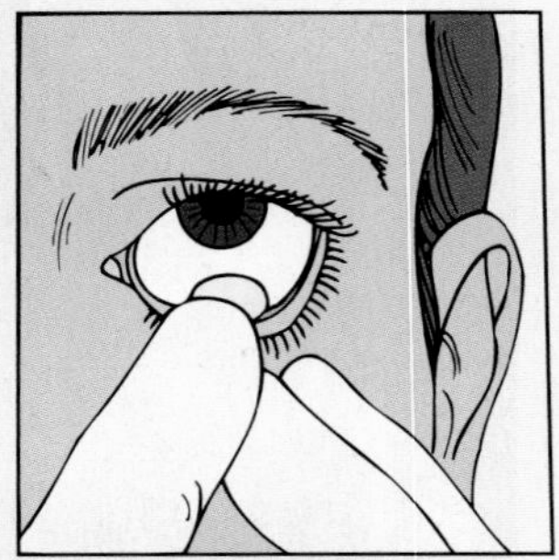

STEP 15c Place disk in conjunctival sac between iris and lower eyelid.

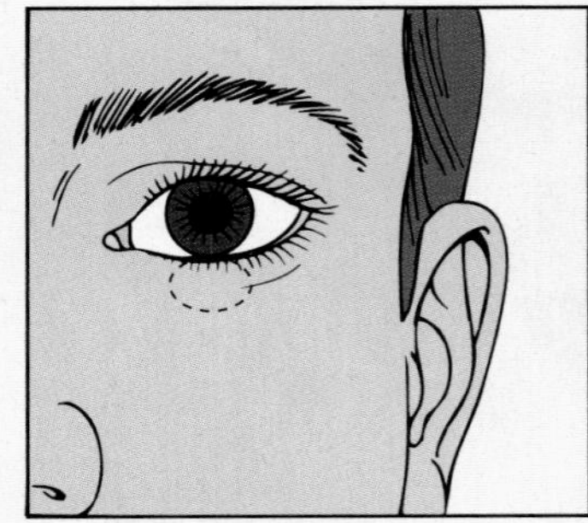

STEP 15d Gently pull lower eyelid over disk.

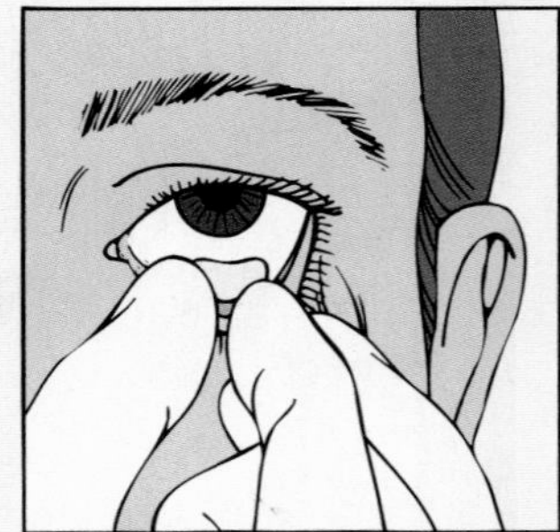

STEP 16d Carefully pinch disk to remove it from patient's eye.

RECORDING AND REPORTING

- Record medication, concentration, number of drops, time and date of administration, and eye (left, right, or both) that received medication on MAR.
- Record appearance of eye in nurses' notes.
- Document your evaluation of patient and family learning.

HOME CARE CONSIDERATIONS

- Have patients with chronic health care problems consult with their health care provider before using over-the-counter eye medication.
- When using eyedrops at home, patients should not share medications with other family members because risk of infection transmission is high.

SKILL 32-3 USING METERED-DOSE OR DRY POWDER INHALERS

DELEGATION CONSIDERATIONS

The skill of administering inhaled medications and supervision of patients who self-administer them cannot be delegated to nursing assistive personnel (NAP). Instruct NAP about:

- Potential side effects of medications, changes in patient's respiratory status (e.g., increased coughing, breathing difficulties), and need to report their occurrence.

EQUIPMENT

- Inhaler device with medication canister (metered-dose inhaler [MDI] or dry powder inhaler [DPI])
- Spacer device such as AeroChamber or InspirEase (optional with MDI)
- Facial tissues (optional)
- Wash basin or sink with warm water
- Paper towel
- Medication administration record (MAR) (electronic or printed)
- Stethoscope

STEP	RATIONALE
ASSESSMENT	
1. Check accuracy and completeness of each MAR with health care provider's medication order. Check patient's name, medication name and dosage (e.g., number of puffs), and route and time for administration. Recopy or reprint any part of MAR that is difficult to read.	The order sheet is the most reliable source and only legal record of medications that patient is to receive. Ensures that patient receives correct medications (Mandrack et al., 2012; Sulosaari et al., 2011). Illegible MARs are a source of medication errors (Alassaad et al, 2013).
2. Review pertinent information related to medication: action, purpose, normal dose and route, side effects, time of onset and peak action, and nursing implications.	Allows you to anticipate effects of drug and observe patient's response.
3. Assess patient's medical history, history of allergies, and medication history.	Factors influence how drugs act. Reveals patient's risk for allergic response.
4. Assess patient's respiratory pattern and auscultate breath sounds (Chapter 31).	Establishes baseline of airway status for comparison during and after treatment.
5. If previously instructed in self-administration, assess patient's ability to use inhaler (e.g., hold, manipulate, and depress canister; strength of inhalation).	Instruction sometimes requires reinforcement of previous learning. Inability to grasp container, breathe, or coordinate hand movement interferes with patient's ability to use MDI or DPI correctly.
6. Assess patient's readiness and ability to learn: patient asks questions about medication, disease, or complications; requests education in use of inhaler; is mentally alert, not fatigued or in pain, or in respiratory distress; and participates in own care.	Readiness affects patient's ability to understand explanations and actively participate in instruction. Mental or physical limitations affect patient's ability to learn and methods nurse uses for instruction (Bastable, 2014).
7. Assess patient's knowledge and understanding of disease and purpose and action of prescribed medications.	Knowledge of disease is essential for patient to realistically understand use of inhaler.
8. Determine medication schedule and number of inhalations prescribed for each dose.	Influences explanations you provide for inhaler use.
PLANNING	
1. Collect appropriate equipment and MAR. Plan preparation to avoid interruptions. Do not take phone calls. Follow agency policy.	Interruption contributes to medication errors. Use no-interruption zone (NIZ) when possible (Prakash et al., 2014; Yoder et al., 2015).
2. Provide adequate time for teaching session.	Prevents interruptions and enhances learning (Bastable, 2014).
IMPLEMENTATION	
1. Perform hand hygiene and prepare medication (see Skill 32-1, Steps 1a-g). Be sure to compare label of medication with MAR 2 times while preparing the medication.	Following the same routine when preparing medications, eliminating distractions, and checking the label of the medication with transcribed order reduce error (Murphy and While, 2012). *This is the first and second accuracy check.*

SKILL 32-3 USING METERED-DOSE OR DRY POWDER INHALERS—cont'd

STEP	RATIONALE
2. Take medications to patient at correct time (see agency policy). Medications that require exact timing include STAT, first-time, loading, and 1-time doses. Give time-critical scheduled medications (e.g., antibiotics, anticoagulants, insulin, anticonvulsants, immunosuppressive agents) at exact time ordered (within 30 minutes before or after scheduled dose). Give non–time-critical scheduled medications within a range of either 1 or 2 hours of scheduled doses (ISMP, 2011). Apply the six rights of medication administration throughout medication administration. Perform hand hygiene.	Ensures intended therapeutic effect and complies with professional standards. Hospitals need to adopt a medication administration policy and procedure for the timing of medication administration that considers patient needs, prescribed medication, and specific clinical indications (CMS, 2011; ISMP, 2011). Time-critical scheduled medications are medications in which early or delayed administration of maintenance doses of more than 30 minutes before or after the scheduled dose may cause harm or result in suboptimal therapy or pharmacological effect. Non–time-critical medications are medications in which early or delayed administration of 1-2 hours should not cause harm or result in suboptimal therapy or pharmacological effects (CMS, 2011; ISMP, 2011). Hand hygiene decreases transfer of microorganisms.
3. Identify patient using at least two identifiers (e.g., name and birthday or name and medical record number) according to agency policy. Compare identifiers with information on patient's MAR or medical record.	Ensures correct patient. Complies with The Joint Commission standards and improves patient safety (TJC, 2016).
4. Compare names of medications on labels with MAR at patient's bedside.	*This is the third accuracy check.*
5. Instruct patient in comfortable environment by sitting in chair in hospital room or at kitchen table in home.	Patient is more likely to remain receptive of your explanations if in a comfortable environment (Bastable, 2014).
6. Allow patient opportunity to manipulate inhaler, canister, and spacer device. Explain and demonstrate how canister fits into inhaler.	Patient needs to be familiar with how to use equipment.

CLINICAL DECISION: *If patient is using an MDI with or without a spacer and the inhaler is new or has not been used for several days, push a "test spray" into the air. You do not need to do this for a DPI.*

STEP	RATIONALE
7. Explain what metered dose is and warn patient about overuse of inhaler, including medication side effects.	Excessive inhalations increase risk of serious side effects. When patient takes medication in recommended doses, side effects are rare.
8. Explain steps for administering squeeze-and-breathe MDI without spacer (demonstrate steps when possible): **a.** Insert MDI canister into the holder. **b.** Remove mouthpiece cover from inhaler.	Use of simple, step-by-step explanations allows patient to ask questions at any point during procedure (Bastable, 2014).

CLINICAL DECISION: *Clean dirt or foreign objects from mouthpiece before using inhaler to avoid inhalation of unwanted material.*

STEP	RATIONALE
c. Shake inhaler vigorously 5 or 6 times. Hold inhaler upright in dominant hand.	Ensures that fine particles are aerosolized.
d. Have patient sit up or stand and take a deep breath and exhale.	Empties lungs and prepares patient's airway to receive medication.
e. Instruct patient to position inhaler in one of two ways.	Proper positioning of inhaler is essential to administering medication correctly.
(1) Close mouth around mouthpiece with opening toward back of throat (see illustration) and lips held tight around it.	Position directs aerosol toward airways.
(2) Alternative technique for using MDI: Position mouthpiece 2 to 4 cm (1 to 2 inches) in front of mouth (see illustration).	
f. With inhaler properly positioned, have patient readjust hold and have thumb at mouthpiece and index and middle fingers at top. This is called a three-point or lateral hand position.	Holding MDI with a three-point or lateral hand position helps patient activate canister effectively.

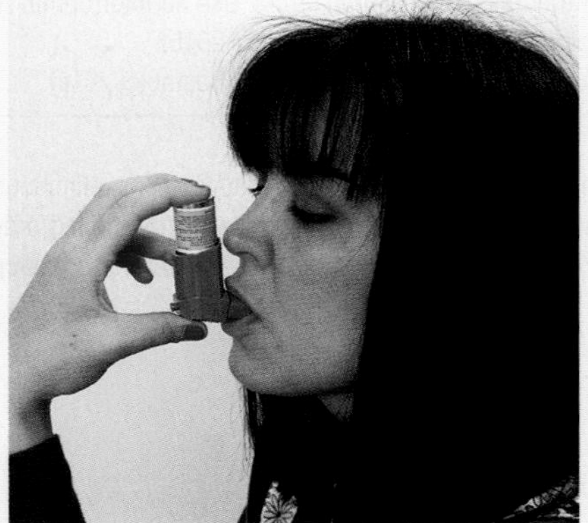

STEP 8e(1) Patient opens lips and places inhaler in mouth with opening toward back of throat.

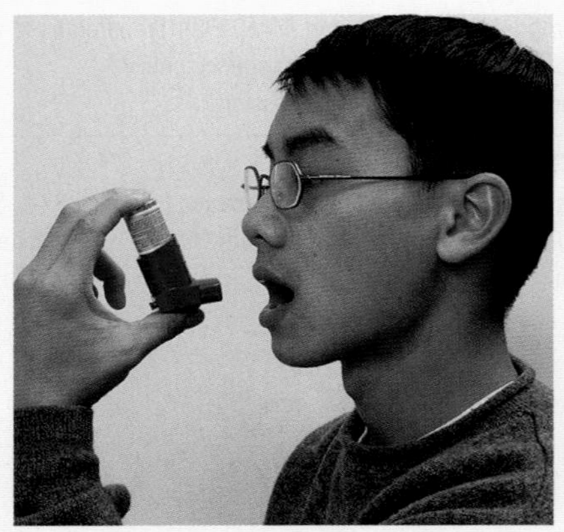

STEP 8e(2) Patient positions mouthpiece 1 to 2 inches away from mouth.

STEP	RATIONALE
g. Instruct patient to tilt head back slightly and inhale slowly and deeply through mouth for 3 to 5 seconds while depressing canister fully.	Distributes medication to airways during inhalation. Inhalation through mouth rather than nose draws medication more effectively into airways.
h. Have patient hold breath for about 10 seconds.	Allows tiny drops of aerosol spray to reach deeper branches of airways (MayoClinic.com, 2015b).
i. Remove MDI from mouth and exhale through pursed lips.	Keeps small airways open during exhalation.
9. Explain steps to administer MDI using a spacer such as an Aerochamber (demonstrate when possible):	Use of simple, step-by-step explanations allows patient to ask questions at any point during instruction (Bastable, 2014).
a. Insert canister into holder. Remove mouthpiece cover from MDI and mouthpiece of spacer. Inspect spacer for foreign objects and ensure that valve is intact if spacer has one.	Inhaler fits into end of spacer.
b. Shake MDI inhaler vigorously 5 or 6 times.	Ensures that fine particles are aerosolized.
c. Insert MDI into end of spacer.	Spacer traps medication released from MDI; patient then inhales drug from device. These devices break up and slow down medication particles, increasing amount of medication that goes into patient's lungs (MayoClinic.com, 2015a).
d. Instruct patient to place spacer mouthpiece into mouth and close lips. Do not insert beyond raised lip on mouthpiece. Avoid covering small exhalation slots with lips (see illustration).	Medication should not escape through mouth.
e. Have patient breathe in and exhale completely and then breathe normally through spacer mouthpiece.	Empties lungs and prepares for medication.
f. Have patient depress medication canister, spraying one puff into spacer.	Emits spray that allows finer particles to be inhaled. Large droplets are retained in spacer.
g. Instruct patient to inhale deeply and slowly through mouth for 3 to 5 seconds.	Maximizes amount of medication that enters lung.
h. Have patient hold breath for 10 seconds.	Ensures full medication distribution.
i. Remove MDI and spacer before exhaling.	Allows patient to exhale normally.
10. Explain steps to administer DPI or breath-activated MDI (demonstrate when possible):	
a. Remove cover from mouthpiece. Do not shake inhaler.	
b. Prepare medication as directed by manufacturer (e.g., hold inhaler upright and turn wheel to right and then to left until click is heard; load medication pellet).	Primes inhaler, ensuring that medication is delivered to patient (MayoClinic.com, 2015c).
c. Exhale away from inhaler before inhalation.	Prevents loss of powder.
d. Position mouthpiece between lips (see illustration).	Prevents medication from escaping through mouth.
e. Inhale deeply and forcefully through mouth.	Creates aerosol.
f. Hold breath for 5 to 10 seconds.	Ensures full medication distribution.
11. Instruct patient to wait at least 20 to 30 seconds between inhalations of the same medication and 2 to 5 minutes between inhalations of different medications or as ordered by health care provider.	Medications must be inhaled sequentially. Always give bronchodilators before steroids. First inhalation opens airways. Second or third inhalation reduces inflammation and/or penetrates deeper airways.

CLINICAL DECISION: *If patient uses a corticosteroid, have him or her rinse mouth out with water or salt water or brush teeth after inhalation to reduce risk of fungal infection. Also teach patient to inspect oral cavity daily for redness, sores, or white patches. Report abnormal assessment findings to the patient's health care provider (MayoClinic.com, 2015d).*

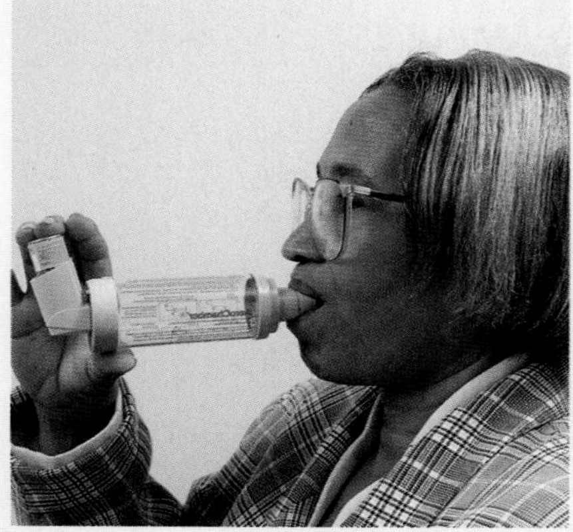

STEP 9d Have patient place mouthpiece in mouth and close lips, being careful to keep exhalation slots exposed.

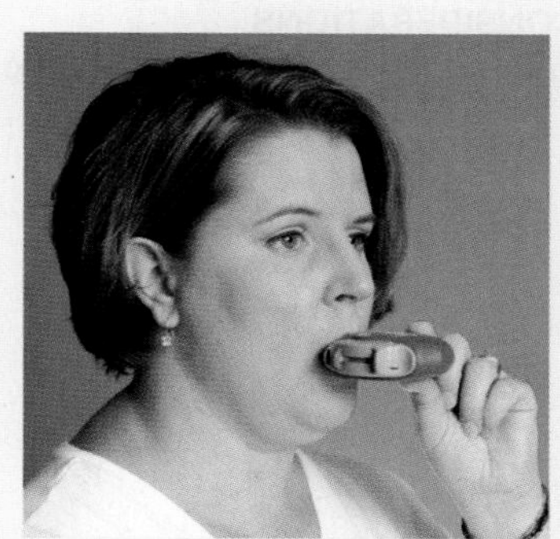

STEP 10d Have patient place mouthpiece of dry powdered inhaler between lips.

SKILL 32-3 USING METERED-DOSE OR DRY POWDER INHALERS—cont'd

STEP	RATIONALE
12. Instruct patient against repeating inhalations before next scheduled dose.	Medications are prescribed at intervals during day to provide constant drug levels and minimize side effects.
13. Explain that patient may feel gagging sensation in throat caused by droplets of medication on pharynx or tongue. Approximately 2 minutes after dose have patient rinse mouth out with warm water.	Results when inhalant is sprayed and inhaled incorrectly.
14. Instruct patient how to clean inhaler:	
a. Once a day remove canister from inhaler. Inhaler and cap need to be rinsed in warm running water. Inhaler needs to be completely dry before using.	Accumulation of spray around mouthpiece interferes with proper distribution during use.
b. Twice a week wash the L-shaped plastic mouthpiece with mild dishwashing soap and warm water. Rinse and dry well before putting canister back inside mouthpiece.	Removes residual medication. Do not place inhalers holding cromolyn, nedocromil, or hydrofluoroalkanes (HFAs) in water.
EVALUATION	
1. Observe patient demonstrate a self-inhalation. Ask if patient has any questions.	Clarifies misconceptions or misunderstanding.
2. Use ***Teach Back*** to determine patient's and family's understanding about inhaled medications. State, "I want to be sure you understand what I explained about how to use your inhaler. Please describe and show me how to use your inhaler." Revise your instruction now or develop plan for revised teaching if patient or family is not able to teach back correctly.	Evaluates what the patient and family are able to explain or demonstrate.
3. Ask patient or family caregiver to calculate how many days inhaler will last.	Helps patient determine when to reorder prescription.
4. Assess patient's respiratory status: ease of respirations, auscultation of lungs, and use of pulse oximetry (see Chapter 31).	Determines status of breathing pattern and adequacy of ventilation.

UNEXPECTED OUTCOMES AND RELATED INTERVENTIONS

1. Patient develops breathing difficulty and needs a bronchodilator more than every 4 hours.
   - Indicates respiratory problems; reassessment of type of medication and delivery methods is needed.
   - Notify health care provider if respiratory status does not improve.
2. Patient experiences cardiac dysrhythmias, light-headedness, and/or syncope, especially if receiving beta-adrenergics.
   - Withhold all further doses of medication.
   - Consult with health care provider.
3. Patient is not able to self-administer medication properly.
   - Explore alternative delivery routes or methods of medication administration.

RECORDING AND REPORTING

- Document skills taught and patient's ability to perform them.
- Document your evaluation of patient and family learning.
- Record medication, time and date of administration, route, and number of puffs on the MAR.
- Document patient's response to medication in nurses' notes.
- Report any undesirable effects from medication.

HOME CARE CONSIDERATIONS

- Remind patients to carry their prescribed inhalers to use emergently in case of an acute asthma attack.

SKILL 32-4 PREPARING INJECTIONS FROM VIALS AND AMPULES

DELEGATION CONSIDERATIONS

The skill of preparing injections cannot be delegated to nursing assistive personnel (NAP).

EQUIPMENT

Medication in an ampule

- Safety syringe, needle, and filter needle
- Small, sterile gauze pad or alcohol swab

Medication in a vial

- Safety syringe
- Needles:
  - Needleless blunt tip vial access cannula
  - Filter needle (if indicated)
  - Needle for drawing up medication (if needed)
- Small, sterile gauze pad or alcohol swab
- Diluent (e.g., normal saline or sterile water) (if indicated)

Both

- Medication administration record (MAR) (electronic or printed)
- Medication in vial or ampule
- Puncture-proof container for disposal of syringes, needles, and glass

STEP	RATIONALE
ASSESSMENT	
1. Check accuracy and completeness of each MAR with health care provider's medication order. Check patient's name, medication name and dosage (e.g., number of drops [if a liquid] and eye [right, left, or both eyes]), and route and time of administration. Recopy or reprint any part of MAR that is difficult to read.	The order sheet is the most reliable source and only legal record of medications that patient is to receive. Ensures that patient receives correct medications (Mandrack et al., 2012; Sulosaari et al., 2011). Illegible MARs are a source of medication errors (Alassaad et al, 2013).
2. Review pertinent information related to medication, including action, purpose, dose and route, side effects, and nursing implications.	Medication information is needed to administer medication properly and monitor patient's response.
3. Assess patient's medical history, history of allergies, and medication history.	Knowledge of medical history influences how some medications act. Protects patient from risk for allergic drug response.
4. Assess patient's body build, muscle size, and weight if giving subcutaneous or intramuscular injection.	Determines type and size of syringe and needles for injection.
PLANNING	
1. Collect appropriate equipment and MAR.	Enhances time management and efficiency.
2. Plan preparation to avoid interruptions. Do not take phone calls or talk with others. Follow agency policy.	Interruption contributes to medication errors. Use no-interruption zone (NIZ) when possible (Prakash et al., 2014; Yoder et al., 2015).
IMPLEMENTATION	
1. Perform hand hygiene.	Reduces transmission of microorganisms.
2. Prepare medication (see Skill 32-1, Steps 1a-h). Be sure to check label 2 times while preparing medication. Check expiration date on label to be sure not outdated.	Following the same routine when preparing medications, eliminating distractions, and checking label of medication with transcribed order reduce error (Murphy and While, 2012). *This is the first and second accuracy check.*
a. Ampule preparation	
(1) Tap top of ampule lightly and quickly with finger until fluid moves from neck of ampule (see illustration).	Dislodges any fluid that collects above neck of ampule. All solution moves into lower chamber.
(2) Place small gauze pad or unopened alcohol swab just above neck of ampule (see illustration).	Placing pad around neck of ampule protects your fingers from trauma as glass tip is broken off.
(3) Snap neck of ampule quickly and firmly away from hands (see illustration).	Protects your fingers and face from shattering glass.
(4) Draw up medication quickly, using filter needle long enough to reach bottom of ampule.	System is open to airborne contaminants. Needle needs to be long enough to access medication for preparation. Filter needles filter out any fragments of glass (Alexander et al., 2014).
(5) Hold ampule upside down or set it on flat surface with filter needle in center of ampule opening. Do not allow needle tip or shaft to touch rim of ampule.	Broken rim of ampule is considered contaminated. When ampule is inverted, solution comes out if needle tip or shaft touches rim of ampule.
(6) Aspirate medication into syringe by gently pulling back on plunger (see illustrations).	Withdrawal of plunger creates negative pressure within syringe barrel, which pulls fluid into syringe.

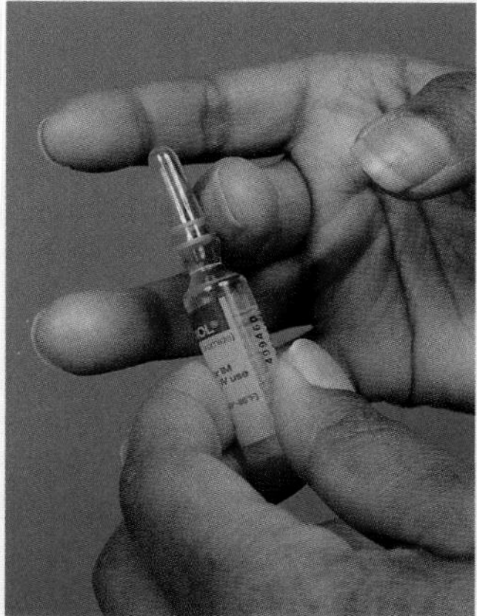
STEP 2a(1) Tapping ampule moves fluid down neck.

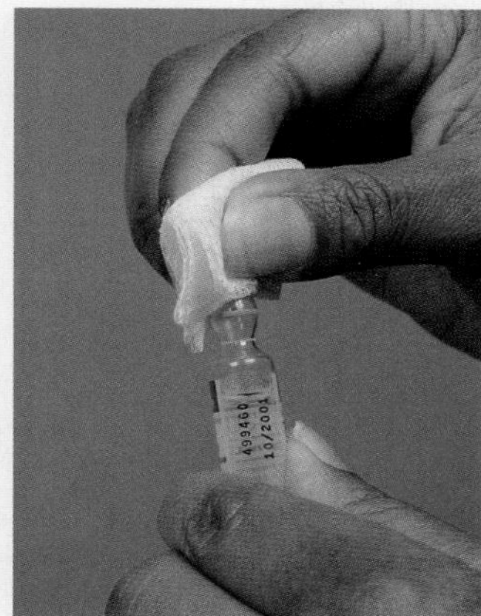
STEP 2a(2) Gauze pad placed just above neck of ampule.

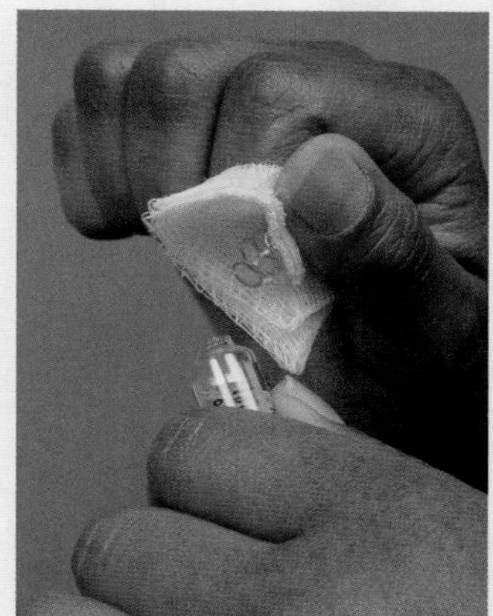
STEP 2a(3) Snapping neck away from hands.

SKILL 32-4 PREPARING INJECTIONS FROM VIALS AND AMPULES—cont'd

STEP	RATIONALE
(7) Keep needle tip under surface of liquid. Tip ampule to bring all fluid within reach of needle.	Prevents aspiration of air bubbles.
(8) If air bubbles are aspirated, do not expel air into ampule.	Air pressure forces liquid out of ampule, and medication is lost.
(9) To expel excess air bubbles, remove needle from ampule. Hold syringe with needle pointing up. Tap side of syringe to cause bubbles to rise toward needle. Draw back slightly on plunger and push plunger upward to eject air. Do not eject fluid.	Withdrawing plunger too far removes it from barrel. Holding syringe vertically allows fluid to settle in bottom of barrel. Pulling back on plunger allows fluid within needle to enter barrel so it is not expelled. Air at top of barrel and within needle is then expelled.
(10) If syringe contains excess fluid, use sink or other specially designated area for medication disposal. Hold syringe vertically with needle tip up and slanted slightly toward sink. Slowly eject excess fluid into sink. Recheck fluid level in syringe by holding it vertically.	Medication dose prepared accurately. Position of needle allows medication to be expelled without flowing down needle shaft. Rechecking fluid level ensures proper dose.
(11) Cover needle with its safety sheath or scoop needle to recap. Replace filter needle with safety needle or needleless access device for injection.	Prevents contamination of needle. Filter needles cannot be used for injection. Scooping technique prevents needlestick injury.
b. Vial containing a solution	
(1) Remove cap covering top of unused vial to expose sterile rubber seal, keeping rubber seal sterile. If a multi-dose vial has been used before, cap is already removed. Firmly and briskly wipe surface of rubber seal with alcohol swab and allow it to dry.	Vial comes packaged with seal that cannot be replaced after cap removal. Not all drug manufacturers guarantee that caps of unused vials are sterile. Therefore swab seals with alcohol before preparing medication. Allowing alcohol to dry prevents needle from being coated with alcohol and mixing with medication.
(2) Pick up syringe and remove needle cap or cap covering needleless vial access device (see illustration). Pull back on plunger to draw amount of air into syringe equal to volume of medication to be aspirated from vial.	Inject air first into vial to prevent buildup of negative pressure in vial when aspirating medication.

CLINICAL DECISION: *Some medications and agencies require use of a filter needle when preparing medications from a vial. See agency policy (Alexander et al., 2014). If you use a filter needle to aspirate the medication, you need to change it to a regular needle of suitable size to administer the medication.*

STEP	RATIONALE
(3) With vial on flat surface, insert tip of needle with beveled tip entering first or needleless access device through center of rubber seal (see illustration). Apply pressure to tip of needle during insertion.	Center of seal is thinner and easier to penetrate. Injecting beveled tip first and using firm pressure prevent coring of rubber seal, which could enter vial or needle.
(4) Inject air into air space of vial, holding on to plunger. Hold plunger with firm pressure; air pressure within vial sometimes forces plunger backward.	Injecting air before aspirating fluid creates vacuum needed to get medication to flow into syringe. Injecting into air space of vial prevents formation of bubbles and inaccuracy in dose.
(5) Invert vial while keeping firm hold on syringe and plunger. Hold vial between thumb and middle fingers of nondominant hand. Grasp end of syringe barrel and plunger with thumb and forefinger of dominant hand to counteract pressure in vial.	Inverting vial allows fluid to settle in lower half of container. Position of hands prevents forceful movement of plunger and permits easy manipulation of syringe.
(6) Keep tip of needle below fluid level.	Prevents aspiration of air.

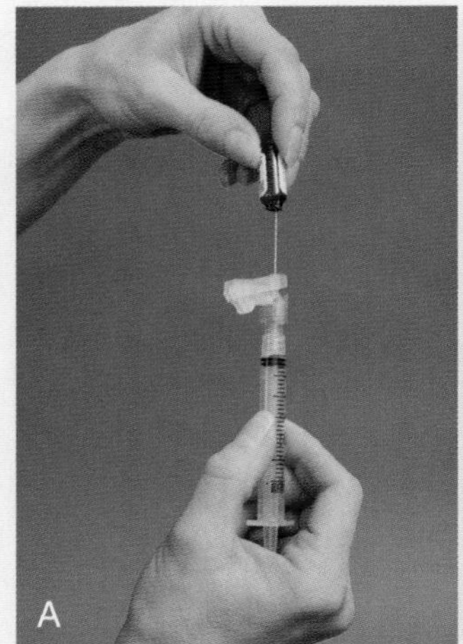

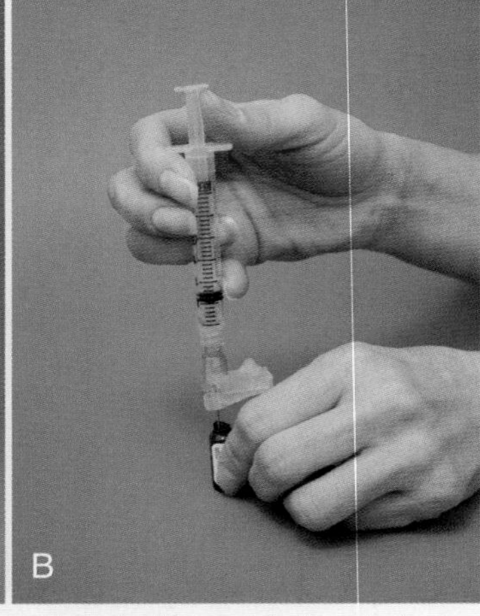

STEP 2a(6) A, Medication aspirated with ampule inverted. **B,** Medication aspirated with ampule on flat surface.

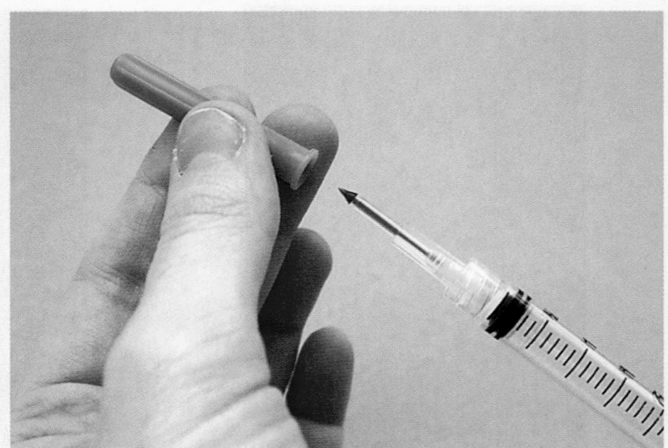

STEP 2b(2) Syringe with needleless adapter.

STEP	RATIONALE
(7) Allow air pressure from vial to fill syringe gradually with medication. If necessary, pull back slightly on plunger to obtain correct amount of solution (see illustration).	Positive pressure within vial forces fluid into syringe.
(8) When desired volume is obtained, position needle into air space of vial; tap side of syringe barrel carefully to dislodge any air bubbles. Eject any air remaining at top of syringe into vial.	Forcefully striking barrel while needle is inserted in vial bends needle. Accumulation of air displaces medication and causes dose errors.
(9) Remove needle or needleless vial access device from vial by pulling back on barrel of syringe.	Accidentally pulling plunger rather than barrel causes plunger to separate from barrel, resulting in loss of medication.
(10) Hold syringe at eye level at 90-degree angle to ensure correct volume and absence of air bubbles. Remove any remaining air by tapping barrel to dislodge air bubbles (see illustration). Draw back slightly on plunger; push plunger upward to eject air. Do not eject fluid. Recheck volume of medication.	Holding syringe vertically allows fluid to settle in bottom of barrel. Pulling back on plunger allows fluid within needle to enter barrel so it is not expelled. Air at top of barrel and within needle is then expelled.
(11) If medication will be injected into patient's tissue, change needle to appropriate gauge and length according to route of medication.	Inserting needle through rubber stopper dulls beveled tip. New needle is sharper. Because no fluid is along shaft, needle does not track medication through tissues.
(12) For multi-dose vial make label that includes date of mixing, concentration of medication per milliliter, and your initials.	Ensures that future doses will be prepared correctly. Some medications need to be discarded a certain number of days after mixing of vial.
c. Vial containing a powder (reconstituting medications)	
(1) Remove cap covering vial of powdered medication and cap covering vial of proper diluent. Firmly swab both seals with alcohol swab and allow to dry.	Not all drug manufacturers guarantee that caps of unused vials are sterile. Therefore seals must be swabbed with alcohol before preparing medication. Allowing alcohol to dry prevents needle from being coated with alcohol and mixing with medication.
(2) Draw up diluent into syringe following Steps 2b(2)-(10).	Prepares diluent for injection into vial containing powdered medication.
(3) Insert tip of safety needle or needleless access device through center of rubber seal of vial of powdered medication. Inject diluent into vial. Remove needle.	Diluent begins to dissolve and reconstitute medication.
(4) Mix medication thoroughly. Roll in palms. Do not shake.	Ensures proper dispersal of medication throughout solution. Shaking produces bubbles.
(5) Reconstituted medication in vial is ready to be drawn into new syringe. Read label carefully to determine dose after reconstitution.	Once diluent is added, concentration of medication (mg/mL) determines dose to be given. Read medication label carefully to avoid medication errors.
(6) Draw up reconstituted medication in syringe following Steps 2b(2)-(12).	

CLINICAL DECISION: *Some agencies require prepared parenteral medications to be verified for accuracy by another nurse. Check policies before administering medication.*

STEP	RATIONALE
3. Compare label of medication with MAR for final time at patient's bedside before administering medication.	*This is the third accuracy check.*
4. Return unused multi-dose medication vial to shelf, drawer, or refrigerator.	
5. Dispose of soiled supplies. Place broken ampule and/or used vials and used needle in puncture-proof, leak-proof container. Clean work area and perform hand hygiene.	Proper disposal of glass and needle prevents accidental injury to staff. Controls transmission of infection.

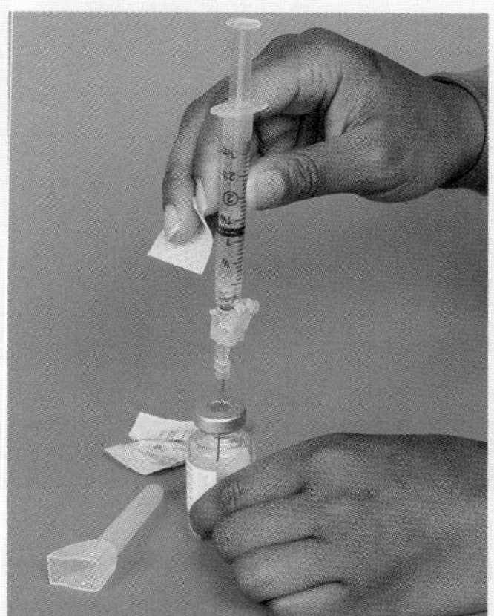

STEP 2b(3) Insert safety needle through center of vial diaphragm (with vial flat on table).

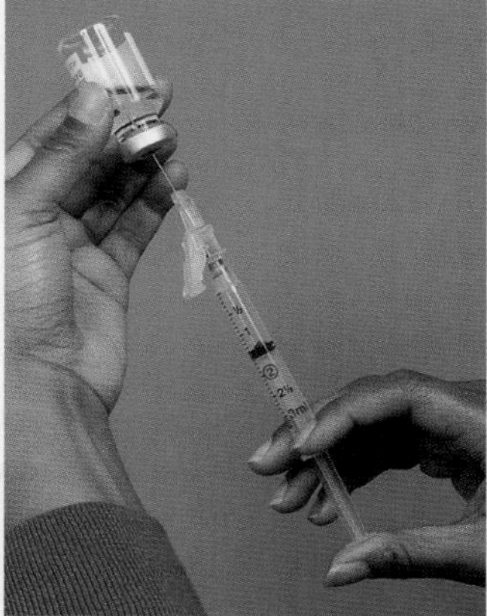

STEP 2b(7) Fluid withdrawn from vial.

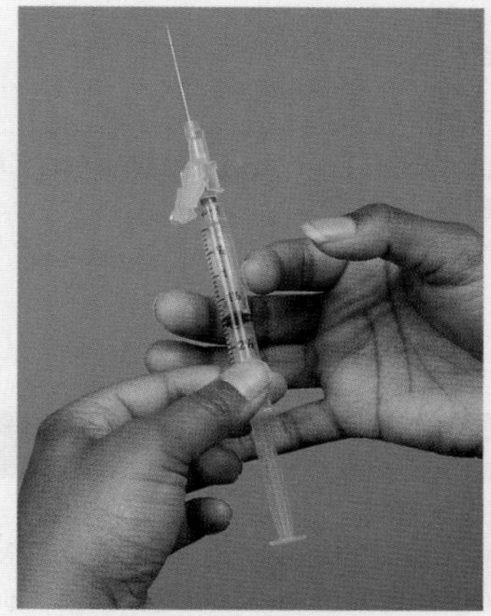

STEP 2b(10) Hold syringe upright; tap barrel to dislodge air bubbles.

SKILL 32-4 PREPARING INJECTIONS FROM VIALS AND AMPULES—cont'd

STEP	RATIONALE
EVALUATION	
1. Compare dose in syringe with desired dose.	Determines that dose is accurate.

UNEXPECTED OUTCOMES AND RELATED INTERVENTIONS

1. Air bubbles remain in syringe.
   - Expel air from syringe and add medication to syringe until correct dose is prepared.
2. Incorrect dose is prepared.
   - Discard prepared dose and prepare corrected new dose.

SKILL 32-5 ADMINISTERING INJECTIONS

DELEGATION CONSIDERATIONS

The skill of administering injections cannot be delegated to nursing assistive personnel (NAP). Instruct the NAP about:

- Potential medication side effects and the need to report their occurrence along with any changes in patient's vital signs or level of consciousness (e.g., sedation).

EQUIPMENT

- Proper-size safety syringe and sharps with engineered sharps injury protection (SESIP) needle:
  - *Subcutaneous:* Syringe (1 to 3 mL) and needle (25- to 27-gauge, 3/8- to 5/8-inch)
  - *Immunizations:* 5/8-inch, 23- to 25-gauge needle (CDC, 2015)
  - *Subcutaneous U-100 insulin:* Insulin syringe (1 mL) with preattached needle (28- to 31-gauge, 5/16- to 1/2-inch)
  - *Subcutaneous U-500 insulin:* 1-mL tuberculin syringe with needle (25- to 27-gauge, 1/2- to 5/8-inch)
  - *Intramuscular (IM):* Syringe 2 to 3 mL for adult, 0.5 to 1 mL for infants and small children
  - Needle length corresponds to site of injection, age, and size of patient. Refer to guidelines below; length needed may vary outside of these guidelines for patients who are smaller or larger than average.
  - Needle length for immunizations (see below)—based on CDC (2015) guidelines
  - Needle gauge often depends on length of needle. Administer most biologicals and medications in aqueous solutions with 20- to 25-gauge needle. Use 18- to 21-gauge needles for medications in oil-based solutions.
  - *Intradermal (ID):* 1-mL tuberculin syringe with needle (25- to 27-gauge, 1/2- to 5/8-inch)
- Small gauze pad
- Antiseptic swab
- Vial or ampule of medication or skin test solution
- Clean gloves
- Medication administration record (MAR) (electronic or printed)
- Puncture-proof container

NEEDLE LENGTH FOR SITE AND AGES

SITE	CHILD	ADULT
Ventrogluteal	1/2- to 1-inch	1 1/2-inch
Vastus lateralis	5/8- to 1-inch	5/8- to 1-inch
Deltoid	1/2- to 1-inch	1- to 1 1/2-inch

NEEDLE LENGTH FOR IMMUNIZATIONS

GENDER—MALE	GENDER—FEMALE	NEEDLE LENGTH
Less than 130 lbs	Less than 130 lbs	5/8-1-inch
130-152 lbs	130-152 lbs	1-inch
153-260 lbs	153-200 lbs	1-1.5-inches
260+ lbs	200+ lbs	1.5-inches

STEP	RATIONALE
ASSESSMENT	
1. Check accuracy and completeness of each MAR with health care provider's medication order. Check patient's name, medication name and dosage, and route and time of administration. Recopy or reprint any part of printed MAR that is difficult to read.	The order sheet is the most reliable source and only legal record of medications that patient is to receive. Ensures that patient receives correct medications (Mandrack et al., 2012; Sulosaari et al., 2011). Illegible MARs are a source of medication errors (Alassaad et al., 2013).

STEP	RATIONALE
2. Review pertinent information related to medication: action, purpose, normal dose and route, side effects, time of onset and peak action, nursing implications.	Allows you to anticipate effects of drug and observe patient's response.
3. Assess patient's medical and medication history and history of allergies. Know his or her normal response to an allergy. Assess patient symptoms or condition for which medication has been prescribed.	Reveals need for medication. Allows for early identification of patient risk for allergic response. May require different medication prescription. Do not administer medication to which patient is allergic. Provides baseline for determining patient's drug response.
4. Observe verbal and nonverbal responses toward receiving injection.	Injections are often painful. Some patients have anxiety, which increases pain.
5. Assess for contraindications.	
a. For subcutaneous injections	
(1) Assess for factors such as circulatory shock or reduced local tissue perfusion. Assess adequacy of patient's adipose tissue.	Reduced tissue perfusion interferes with medication absorption and distribution. Physiological changes of aging or patient illness often influence amount of subcutaneous tissue that patient possesses.
b. For IM injections	
(1) Assess for factors such as muscle atrophy, reduced blood flow, or circulatory shock.	Atrophied muscle absorbs medication poorly. Factors interfering with blood flow to muscles impair medication absorption.
6. Assess patient symptoms or condition for which medication has been prescribed.	Provides baseline to determine response to therapy.

CLINICAL DECISION: *Because of documented adverse effects of intramuscular (IM) injections, other routes of medication administration are safer. Verify that IM injection is necessary and explore alternative medication routes if possible (Nicoll and Hesby, 2002; World Health Organization [WHO], 2015).*

STEP	RATIONALE
7. Assess patient's knowledge about medication.	Determines if there is a need for patient education.
PLANNING	
1. Collect appropriate equipment and MAR.	Enhances time management and efficiency.
2. Plan preparation to avoid interruptions. Do not take phone calls or talk with others. Follow agency policy.	Interruption contributes to medication errors. Use no-interruption zone (NIZ) when possible (Prakash et al., 2014; Yoder et al., 2015).
IMPLEMENTATION	
1. Perform hand hygiene. Aseptically prepare correct medication dose from ampule or vial (see Skill 32-4). Check label of medication with MAR 2 times while preparing medication.	Ensures that medication is sterile. Following the same routine when preparing medications, eliminating distractions, and checking label of medication with transcribed order reduce error (Murphy and While, 2012). *This is the first and second accuracy check.*
2. Take medications to patient at correct time (see agency policy). Medications that require exact timing include STAT, first-time, loading, and 1-time doses. Give time-critical scheduled medications (e.g., antibiotics, anticoagulants, insulin, anticonvulsants, immunosuppressive agents) at exact time ordered (within 30 minutes before or after scheduled dose). Give non–time critical scheduled medications within a range of either 1 or 2 hours of scheduled doses (ISMP, 2011). Apply the six rights of medication administration throughout medication administration. Perform hand hygiene.	Ensures intended therapeutic effect and complies with professional standards. Hospitals need to adopt a medication administration policy and procedure for the timing of medication administration that considers patient needs, prescribed medication, and specific clinical indications (CMS, 2011; ISMP, 2011). Time-critical scheduled medications are medications in which early or delayed administration of maintenance doses of more than 30 minutes before or after the scheduled dose may cause harm or result in suboptimal therapy or pharmacological effect. Non–time-critical medications are medications in which early or delayed administration of 1-2 hours should not cause harm or result in suboptimal therapy or pharmacological effects (CMS, 2011; ISMP, 2011). Hand hygiene decreases transfer of microorganisms.
3. Close room curtain or door.	Provides privacy.
4. Identify patient using at least two identifiers (e.g., name and birthday or name and medical record number) according to agency policy. Compare identifiers with information on patient's MAR or medical record.	Ensures correct patient. Complies with The Joint Commission standards and improves patient safety (TJC, 2016).
5. Compare name of medication on label with MAR one more time at patient's bedside.	*This is the third accuracy check.*
6. Explain steps of procedure and tell patient that injection will cause slight burning or sting.	Helps minimize patient's anxiety.
7. Apply clean gloves. Note: If patient has latex allergy, use latex-free gloves.	Reduces transfer of microorganisms.
8. Keep sheet or gown draped over body parts not requiring exposure.	Respects dignity of patient while area to be injected is exposed.
9. Select appropriate injection site. Inspect skin surface over sites for bruises, inflammation, or edema.	Injection sites need to be free of abnormalities that interfere with medication absorption. Sites used repeatedly become hardened from lipohypertrophy (increased growth in fatty tissue). Do not use an area that is bruised or has signs associated with infection.

SKILL 32-5 ADMINISTERING INJECTIONS—cont'd

STEP	RATIONALE
a. Subcutaneous: Palpate sites for masses or tenderness. Avoid these areas. For daily insulin, rotate site within anatomical area. Be sure that needle is correct size by grasping skinfold at site with thumb and forefinger. Measure fold from top to bottom. Needle should be one-half length.	Subcutaneous injections are sometimes mistakenly given in muscle, especially in abdomen and thigh sites. Appropriate size of needle and angle of injection ensures that medication is injected in subcutaneous tissue (Hirsch et al., 2012; Hoffman et al., 2010).
b. IM: Note integrity and size of muscle and palpate for tenderness or hardness. Avoid these areas. If injections are given frequently, rotate sites. Use ventrogluteal site if possible.	Ventrogluteal site is preferred site for adults. This site is also preferred for children who are receiving viscous or irritating solutions (Hockenberry and Wilson, 2015; Nicoll and Hesby, 2002; Ogston-Tuck, 2014).
c. Intradermal (ID): Note lesions or discolorations of skin. If possible, select site three to four finger widths below antecubital space and a hand width above wrist. If you cannot use forearm, inspect upper back. If necessary, use sites for subcutaneous injections.	An ID site needs to be clear so you can see results of skin test and interpret them correctly (CDC, 2014a).
10. Help patient to comfortable position:	
a. Subcutaneous: Have patient relax arm, leg, or abdomen, depending on site chosen for injection.	Relaxation of site minimizes discomfort.
b. IM: Position patient depending on site chosen (e.g., sit or lie flat, on side, or prone).	Reduces strain on muscle and minimizes discomfort of injections.
c. ID: Have patient extend elbow and support it and forearm on flat surface.	Stabilizes injection site for easiest accessibility.
d. Have patient talk about subject of interest. Ask open-ended questions.	Distraction reduces anxiety.
CLINICAL DECISION: *Ensure that patient's position is not contraindicated by medical condition.*	
11. Relocate site using anatomical landmarks.	Injection into correct anatomical site prevents injury to nerves, bones, and blood vessels.
12. Clean site with an antiseptic swab. Apply swab at center of site and rotate outward in circular direction for approximately 5 cm (2 inches) (see illustration).	Mechanical action of swab removes secretions containing microorganisms.
13. Hold swab or gauze between third and fourth fingers of nondominant hand.	Gauze or swab remains readily accessible when needle is withdrawn.
14. Remove needle cap or sheath from needle by pulling it straight off.	Preventing needle from touching sides of cap prevents contamination.
15. Hold syringe between thumb and forefinger of dominant hand.	
a. Subcutaneous: Hold as dart, palm up (see illustration).	Quick, smooth injection requires proper manipulation of syringe parts.
b. IM: Hold as dart, palm down.	
c. ID: Hold bevel of needle pointing up.	With bevel up, medication is less likely to be deposited into tissues below dermis.
16. Administer injection:	
a. Subcutaneous	
(1) For average-size patient, pinch skin with nondominant hand.	Pinching skin elevates subcutaneous tissue and desensitizes area.
(2) Inject needle quickly and firmly at 45- to 90-degree angle. Release skin. Option: Continue to pinch skin and release after injecting medications.	Quick, firm insertion minimizes discomfort. (Injecting medication into compressed tissue irritates nerve fibers.) Correct angle prevents accidental injection into muscle.
(3) For obese patient pinch skin at site and inject needle at 90-degree angle below tissue fold.	Obese patients have fatty layer of tissue above subcutaneous layer.

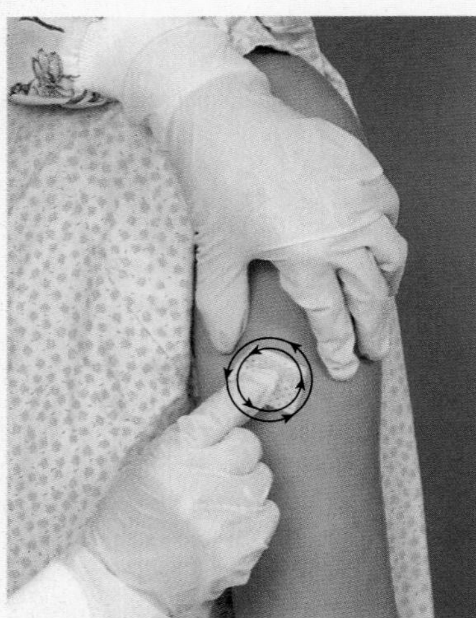

STEP 12 Clean site with circular motion.

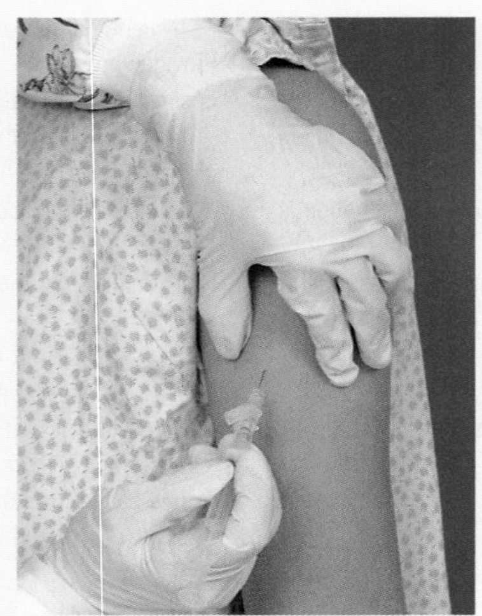

STEP 15a Hold syringe as if grasping a dart.

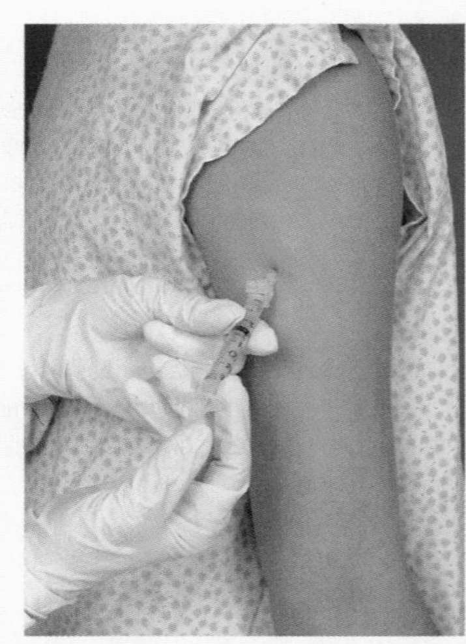

STEP 16a(4) Inject medication slowly.

STEP	RATIONALE

CLINICAL DECISION: *Piercing a blood vessel during a subcutaneous injection is very rare. Therefore aspiration is not necessary when administering subcutaneous injections (Lilley et al., 2011).*

STEP	RATIONALE
(4) Inject medication slowly (see illustration).	Minimizes discomfort.
b. Intramuscular	
(1) Position ulnar aspect of your nondominant hand just below site and pull skin approximately 2.5 to 3.5 cm (1 to 1.5 inches) down or laterally to administer in a Z-track. Hold position until medication is injected (see Figure 32-22). With dominant hand inject needle quickly at 90-degree angle into muscle.	Z-track creates zigzag path through tissues that seals needle track to avoid tracking of medication. Use Z-track for all IM injections (Hopkins and Arias, 2013; Nicoll and Hesby, 2002; Ogston-Tuck, 2014). A quick, dartlike injection reduces discomfort.
(2) Option: If patient's muscle mass is small, grasp body of muscle between thumb and fingers.	Ensures that medication reaches muscle mass (Hockenberry and Wilson, 2015).

CLINICAL DECISION: *When giving immunizations to adults: to avoid injection into subcutaneous tissue, spread the skin of the selected vaccine administration site taut between the thumb and forefinger, isolating the muscle (CDC, 2015).*

STEP	RATIONALE
(3) Insert needle into muscle with smooth, steady motion. After needle pierces skin, grasp lower end of syringe barrel with nondominant hand to stabilize syringe. Continue to hold skin tightly with nondominant hand. Move dominant hand to end of plunger. Do not move syringe.	Smooth, steady motion reduces pain at moment of injection. Smooth manipulation of syringe reduces discomfort from needle movement. Skin needs to remain pulled until after injecting medication to ensure Z-track administration.
(4) Pull back on plunger 5 to 10 seconds. If no blood appears, inject medicine slowly, at rate of 1 mL/10 seconds. **Note:** Do not aspirate if administering immunizations (CDC, 2015).	This time is necessary to ensure that needle is not in low-flow blood vessel (Nicoll and Hesby, 2002). Aspiration of blood into syringe indicates intravenous (IV) placement of needle. Slow injection rate reduces pain and tissue trauma and the chance of leakage of medication back through needle track (Hockenberry and Wilson, 2015; Nicoll and Hesby, 2002). The CDC (2015) no longer recommends aspiration when administering an immunization.

CLINICAL DECISION: *If blood appears in syringe, remove needle and dispose of medication and syringe properly. Prepare another dose of medication for injection.*

STEP	RATIONALE
(5) Wait 10 seconds. Then smoothly and steadily withdraw needle and release skin.	Allows for medication to absorb into muscle before removing syringe rather than leaking back out through track that needle created (Hopkins and Arias, 2013; Nicoll and Hesby, 2002).
c. Intradermal	
(1) With nondominant hand stretch skin over site with forefinger or thumb.	Needle pierces tight skin more easily.
(2) With needle almost against patient's skin, insert it slowly with bevel up at 5- to 15-degree angle until resistance is felt. Advance it through epidermis to approximately 3 mm (⅛ inch) below skin surface. You will see needle tip through skin.	Ensures that needle tip is in dermis. You obtain inaccurate results if you do not inject needle at correct angle and depth (CDC, 2014b).
(3) Inject medication slowly. Normally you feel resistance. If not, needle is too deep; remove and begin again. Nondominant hand can stabilize needle during the injection.	Slow injection minimizes discomfort at site. Dermal layer is tight and does not expand easily when solution is injected. Stabilizing needle prevents unnecessary movements and decreases patient discomfort.
(4) While injecting medication, notice that small bleb approximately 6 mm (¼ inch) in diameter (resembling mosquito bite) appears on surface of skin (see illustration). Instruct patient that this is normal finding.	Bleb indicates that medication is deposited in dermis.

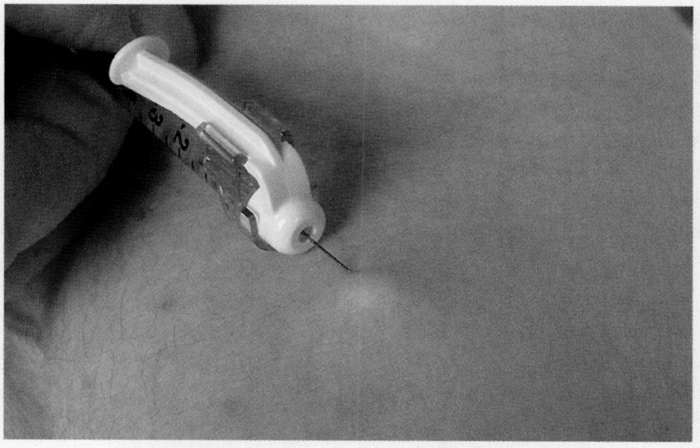

STEP 16c(4) Injection creates small bleb.

SKILL 32-5 ADMINISTERING INJECTIONS—cont'd

STEP	RATIONALE
17. Withdraw needle while applying alcohol swab or gauze gently over site.	Support of tissue around injection site minimizes discomfort during needle withdrawal. Dry gauze minimizes patient discomfort associated with alcohol on nonintact skin.
18. Apply gentle pressure. Do not massage site. Apply bandage if needed.	Massage causes underlying tissue damage. Massaging ID site disperses medication into underlying tissue layers and alters test results.
19. Help patient to comfortable position.	Gives patient sense of well-being.
20. Discard uncapped needle or needle enclosed in safety shield and attached syringe into puncture-proof, leak-proof receptacle.	Prevents injury to patient and health care personnel. Recapping needles increases risk of needlestick injury (OSHA, n.d.).
21. Remove gloves and perform hand hygiene.	Reduces transmission of microorganisms.
22. Stay with patient and observe for any allergic reactions.	Dyspnea, wheezing, and circulatory collapse are signs of severe anaphylactic reaction, which is life-threatening emergency.

EVALUATION

STEP	RATIONALE
1. Return to room and ask if patient feels any acute pain, burning, numbness, or tingling at injection site.	Continued discomfort often indicates injury to underlying bones or nerves.
2. Inspect site, noting any bruising or induration. Document bruising or induration if present. Notify health care provider and provide warm compress to site.	Bruising or induration indicates complication associated with injection.
3. Observe patient's response to medication at times that correlate with onset, peak, and duration of medication.	IM medications are absorbed rapidly. Adverse effects of parenteral medications develop rapidly. Nurse's observations determine efficacy of medication action.
4. Use ***Teach Back*** to determine patient's and family's understanding about injections. State, "I want to be sure you understand what I explained about your injection. Can you explain why you need this injection and the side effects to watch for and report to me if they occur?" Revise your instruction now or develop plan for revised teaching if patient is not able to teach back correctly.	Evaluates what patient and family are able to explain or demonstrate.
5. For ID injections: Use skin pencil and draw circle around perimeter of injection site. Read site within appropriate amount of time, designated by type of medication or skin test administered.	Pencil mark makes site easy to find. Results of skin testing are read at various times on the basis of type of medication used or type of skin testing completed. Refer to manufacturer directions to determine when to read results of test.

CLINICAL DECISION: *Read tuberculin test at 48 to 72 hours. Induration (hard, dense, raised area) of skin around injection site indicates positive reaction, as follows:*

- *15 mm or more in patients with no known risk factors for tuberculosis (TB)*
- *10 mm or more in patients who are recent immigrants; injection drug users; residents and employees of high-risk settings; mycobacteriology laboratory personnel; patients with clinical conditions placing them at high risk; children less than 4 years of age; and infants, children, and adolescents exposed to high-risk adults*
- *5 mm or more in patients who are human immunodeficiency virus (HIV) positive, have fibrotic changes on chest x-ray film consistent with previous TB infection, have had organ transplants, or are immunosuppressed (CDC, 2014b)*

UNEXPECTED OUTCOMES AND RELATED INTERVENTIONS

1. Raised, reddened, or hard zone (induration) forms around an ID test site.
   - Notify patient's health care provider.
   - Document sensitivity to injected allergen or positive test if tuberculin skin testing was completed.
2. Hypertrophy of skin develops from repeated subcutaneous injections.
   - Do not use this site for future injections.
   - Instruct patient not to use site for 6 months.
3. Patient develops signs and symptoms of allergy or side effects.
   - Follow agency policy or guidelines for appropriate response to adverse drug reactions.
   - Notify patient's health care provider immediately.
   - Add allergy information to patient's medical record.
4. Patient complains of localized pain, numbness, tingling, or burning at injection site, indicating possible injury to nerve or tissues.
   - Assess injection site.
   - Document findings.
   - Notify patient's health care provider.

RECORDING AND REPORTING

- Chart medication dose, route, site, and time and date given on MAR immediately after giving medication per agency policy.
- Document if scheduled medication is withheld and record the reason per agency policy.
- Report any undesirable effects from medication to health care provider.
- Record patient's response to medications in nurses' notes and report to health care provider if required.
- Document immunizations in patient's permanent record, including date of administration, vaccine manufacturer and lot number, expiration date, name and title of the person who administered the vaccine and the address of the agency where the permanent record will reside, vaccine information statement (VIS) and date printed on the VIS, and date VIS given to patient or parent/guardian (CDC, 2015).
- Document your evaluation of patient and family learning.

HOME CARE CONSIDERATIONS

- Assess patient's readiness to learn before instructing in self-injections. Some patients are hesitant to self-administer injections; thus relieve anxiety before teaching this skill.
- Some patients prefer to reuse their syringes to save costs. This practice is safe and practical if the needle is not contaminated during the preparation and administration of the injection. Teach patients to recap needles immediately after use.
- Patients can often purchase or obtain sharps boxes for home use. If this is not possible, they can use a hard plastic bottle that they cannot see through (e.g., a fabric softener bottle or detergent bottle) to safely store syringes after use. Disposal of needles used in the home varies among communities. Check with local authorities to verify how to dispose of needles.

SKILL 32-6 ADMINISTERING MEDICATIONS BY INTRAVENOUS BOLUS

DELEGATION CONSIDERATIONS

The skill of administering medications by intravenous (IV) bolus cannot be delegated to nursing assistive personnel (NAP). Inform NAP about:

- Potential side effects of medications and need to report their occurrence.
- The need to report discomfort at infusion site as soon as possible.
- When to obtain required vital signs and report these findings to the nurse.

EQUIPMENT

- Watch with second hand
- Clean gloves
- Antiseptic swab
- Medication in vial or ampule
- Proper-size syringes for medication and saline flush with needleless device or sharps with engineered sharps injury protection (SESIP) needle (21- to 25-gauge)
- Intravenous lock: Vial of normal saline flush solution (recommended [Alexander et al., 2014]); if agency continues to use heparin flush, most common concentration is 10 units/mL; see agency policy)
- Medication administration record (MAR) (electronic or printed)
- Puncture-proof container

STEP	RATIONALE
ASSESSMENT	
1. Check accuracy and completeness of each MAR with health care provider's medication order. Check patient's name, medication name and dosage, and route and time of administration. Recopy or reprint any part of printed MAR that is difficult to read.	The order sheet is the most reliable source and only legal record of medications that patient is to receive. Ensures that patient receives correct medications (Mandrack et al., 2012; Sulosaari et al., 2011). Illegible MARs are a source of medication errors (Alassaad et al., 2013).

CLINICAL DECISION: *Some IV medications can only be pushed safely when a patient is being monitored continuously for dysrhythmias, blood pressure changes, or other adverse effects. Therefore some medications can only be pushed in specific areas within a health care agency. See agency policy for special monitoring requirements before giving medication (Burchum and Rosenthal, 2016).*

STEP	RATIONALE
2. Review pertinent information related to medication: action, purpose, normal dose and route, side effects, time of onset and peak action, how slowly to give medication, compatibility with IV fluids, and nursing implications.	Allows you to give medication safely and monitor patient's response to therapy (Burchum and Rosenthal, 2016). Prevents incompatible drug reaction.
3. If pushing medication into an existing IV line, determine compatibility of medication with IV fluids and any additives within IV solution.	IV medications are not always compatible with IV solution and/or additives.
4. Perform hand hygiene. Assess IV or saline lock insertion site for signs of infiltration or phlebitis (see Chapter 42).	Confirming placement of IV catheter and integrity of surrounding tissue ensures that medication is administered safely. Do not administer medication if site is inflamed or edematous.
5. Check patient's medical history, medication history, and history of drug or latex allergies. Assess patient symptoms or condition for which medication has been prescribed.	Knowledge of medical history influences how some medications act. IV bolus delivers medication rapidly. Allergic reactions can be fatal. Provides baseline for determining patient's drug response.
6. Assess patient's understanding of purpose of medication therapy.	Reveals need for patient education.

SKILL 32-6 ADMINISTERING MEDICATIONS BY INTRAVENOUS BOLUS—cont'd

STEP	RATIONALE
PLANNING	
1. Collect appropriate equipment and MAR.	Enhances time management and efficiency.

CLINICAL DECISION: *Some IV medications require dilution before administration. Verify with agency policy. If a small amount of medication is given (e.g., less than 1 mL), dilute medication in 5 to 10 mL of normal saline or sterile water so medication does not collect in "dead spaces" (e.g., Y-site injection port, IV cap) of the IV delivery system. Verify that medication can be diluted by consulting medication reference or checking with pharmacist first.*

STEP	RATIONALE
2. Plan preparation to avoid interruptions. Do not take phone calls or talk with others. Follow agency policy.	Interruption contributes to medication errors. Use no-interruption zone (NIZ) when possible (Prakash et al., 2014; Yoder et al., 2015).
IMPLEMENTATION	
1. Perform hand hygiene. Prepare ordered medication from vial or ampule using aseptic technique (see Skill 32-4). Check label of medication carefully with MAR 2 times.	Ensures that medication is sterile. Following the same routine when preparing medications, eliminating distractions, and checking label of medication with transcribed order reduce error (Murphy and While, 2012). *This is the first and second accuracy check.*
2. Take medications to patient at correct time (see agency policy). Medications that require exact timing include STAT, first-time, loading, and 1-time doses. Give time-critical scheduled medications (e.g., antibiotics, anticoagulants, insulin, anticonvulsants, immunosuppressive agents) at exact time ordered (within 30 minutes before or after scheduled dose). Give non–time-critical scheduled medications within a range of either 1 or 2 hours of scheduled dose (ISMP, 2011). Apply the six rights of medication administration throughout medication administration. Perform hand hygiene.	Ensures intended therapeutic effect and complies with professional standards. Hospitals need to adopt a medication administration policy and procedure for the timing of medication administration that considers patient needs, prescribed medication, and specific clinical indications (CMS, 2011; ISMP, 2011). Time-critical scheduled medications are medications in which early or delayed administration of maintenance doses of more than 30 minutes before or after the scheduled dose may cause harm or result in suboptimal therapy or pharmacological effect. Non–time-critical medications are medications in which early or delayed administration of 1-2 hours should not cause harm or result in suboptimal therapy or pharmacological effects (CMS, 2011; ISMP, 2011). Hand hygiene decreases transfer of microorganisms.
3. Identify patient using at least two identifiers (e.g., name and birthday or name and medical record number) according to agency policy. Compare identifiers with information on patient's MAR or medical record.	Ensures correct patient. Complies with The Joint Commission standards and improves patient safety (TJC, 2016).
4. Compare names of medications on labels with MAR one more time at patient's bedside.	*Third check for accuracy* ensures that right medication is administered.
5. Explain procedure to patient. Encourage patient to report symptoms of discomfort at IV site. Provide instruction on purpose and action of medication and possible side effects.	Keeps patient informed and ensures patient-centered care. Helps identify possible infiltration early.
6. Apply clean gloves. NOTE: If patient has latex allergy, use latex-free gloves.	Reduces transmission of microorganisms. During IV bolus administration there is risk of blood exposure.
7. IV push (existing line):	
a. Select injection port of IV tubing closest to patient. Whenever possible, injection port should accept a needleless syringe. Use IV filter if required by medication reference or agency policy.	Follows provisions of Needle Safety and Prevention Act of 2001 (OSHA, n.d.).

CLINICAL DECISION: *Never administer IV medications through tubing that is infusing blood, blood products, or parenteral nutrition solutions.*

STEP	RATIONALE
b. Clean injection port with antiseptic swab. Allow to dry.	Prevents introduction of microorganisms during needle insertion. Drying enhances effects of antiseptic.
c. Connect syringe to port of IV line. Insert needleless tip or small-gauge needle of syringe containing prepared drug through center of injection port (see illustration).	Prevents damage to diaphragm of port and subsequent leakage.
d. Occlude IV line by pinching tubing just above injection port (see illustration). Pull back gently on syringe plunger to aspirate blood return.	Final check that medication is being delivered into bloodstream.

CLINICAL DECISION: *In some cases, especially with a smaller-gauge IV needle, blood return is not aspirated, even if IV is patent. If IV site shows no signs of infiltration and IV fluid is infusing without difficulty, proceed with IV push slowly.*

STEP	RATIONALE
e. Release tubing and inject medication within amount of time recommended by agency policy, pharmacist, or medication reference manual. Use watch to time administration (see illustration). You can pinch IV line while pushing medication and release when not pushing it. Allow IV fluids to infuse when not pushing medication.	Ensures safe medication infusion. Rapid injection of IV medication can be fatal (Burchum and Rosenthal, 2016). Allowing IV fluids to infuse while pushing IV drug enables medications to be delivered to patient at prescribed rate.

STEP	RATIONALE

CLINICAL DECISION: *When IV medication is incompatible with IV fluids, stop the IV fluids, clamp the IV line above the injection site, flush with 10 mL of normal saline or sterile water, give the IV bolus over the appropriate amount of time, flush with another 10 mL of normal saline or sterile water at the same rate as the medication was administered, and restart the IV fluids at the prescribed rate. If IV line that is currently hanging contains a medication (e.g., ranitidine), disconnect it and administer IV push as outlined in Step 8 to avoid giving a sudden bolus of the medication in existing IV line. Some IV medications and fluids cannot be stopped. Verify agency policy regarding temporarily stopping IV fluids or continuous IV medications. If unable to stop IV infusion, start a new IV site (see Chapter 42) and administer medication using the IV lock method.*

STEP	RATIONALE
f. After injecting medication, release tubing, withdraw syringe, and recheck fluid infusion rate.	Injection of bolus alters rate of fluid infusion. Rapid fluid infusion causes circulatory overload.
8. IV push (IV lock):	
a. Prepare two syringes with 2 to 3 mL of normal saline (0.9%) in syringe.	

CLINICAL DECISION: *Current evidence reflects that saline flushes are effective in maintaining patency of IV lines and do not carry risk of thrombocytopenia associated with heparin flushes.*

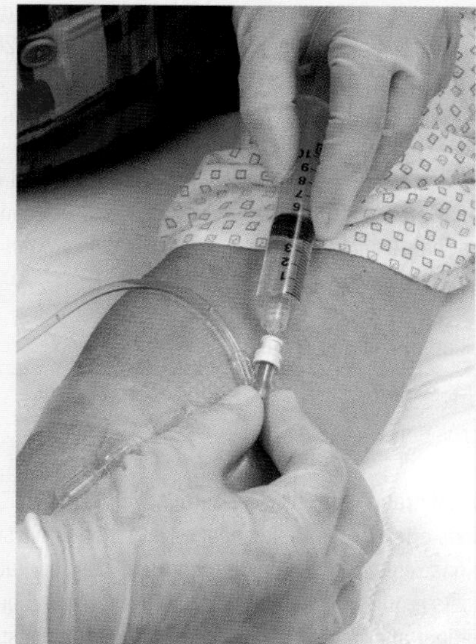
STEP 7c Connecting syringe to IV line with blunt needleless cannula tip.

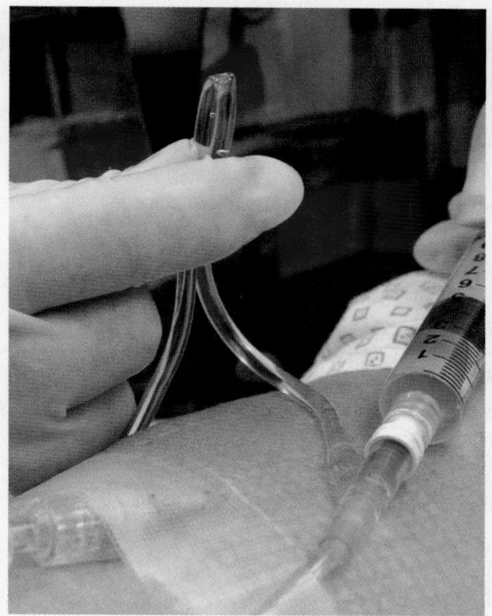
STEP 7d Occluding IV tubing above injection port.

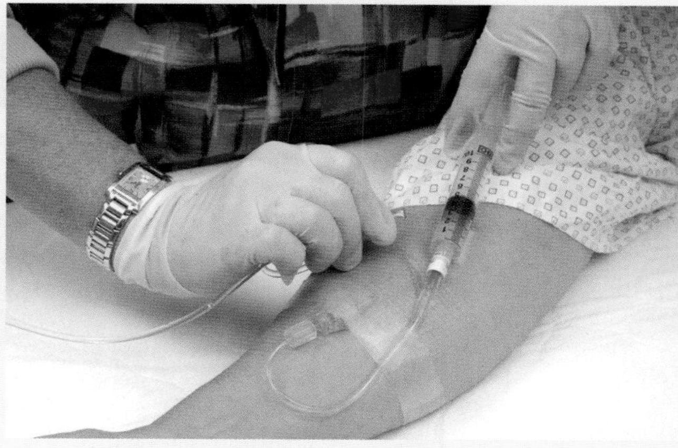
STEP 7e Using watch to time IV push medication.

SKILL 32-6 ADMINISTERING MEDICATIONS BY INTRAVENOUS BOLUS—cont'd

STEP	RATIONALE
b. Administer medication:	
(1) Clean injection port of lock with antiseptic swab. Allow to dry.	Prevents introduction of microorganisms during needle insertion. Drying enhances effects of antiseptic.
(2) Insert syringe containing normal saline (0.9%) into injection port of IV lock (see illustration).	
(3) Pull back gently on syringe plunger and look for blood return.	Determines whether IV needle or catheter is positioned in vein.

CLINICAL DECISION: *At times a blood return is not aspirated even though lock is patent. If IV site does not show signs of infiltration and flushes without difficulty, proceed with IV push.*

STEP	RATIONALE
(4) Flush IV lock with normal saline by pushing slowly on plunger.	Clears IV lock of blood.

CLINICAL DECISION: *Observe area of skin above IV catheter closely. Note any puffiness or swelling as IV lock is flushed, which indicates infiltration into vein, requiring removal of catheter.*

STEP	RATIONALE
(5) Remove saline flush syringe.	
(6) Clean injection port of lock with antiseptic swab.	Prevents transmission of infection.
(7) Insert syringe containing prepared medication into injection port of IV lock.	
(8) Inject medication within amount of time recommended by agency policy, pharmacist, or medication reference manual. Use watch to time administration.	Rapid injection of IV medication can result in death. Following guidelines for IV push rates promotes patient safety (Burchum and Rosenthal, 2016).
(9) After administering bolus, withdraw syringe.	
(10) Clean injection port of lock with antiseptic swab.	Prevents transmission of microorganisms.
(11) Flush injection port by attaching syringe with normal saline. Inject normal saline flush at same rate medication was delivered.	Irrigation with saline prevents occlusion of IV access device and ensures that all medication is delivered. Flushing IV site at same rate as medication ensures that any medication remaining within IV needle is delivered at correct rate.
9. Dispose of uncapped needles and syringes in puncture-proof, leak-proof container.	Reduces accidental needlesticks (OSHA, n.d.).
10. Remove and dispose of gloves. Perform hand hygiene.	Reduces transmission of microorganisms.

EVALUATION

STEP	RATIONALE
1. Observe patient closely for adverse reaction as drug is administered and for several minutes thereafter.	IV medications act rapidly.
2. Observe IV site during injection for sudden swelling.	Swelling indicates infiltration into tissues surrounding vein.
3. Assess patient's status after giving medication to evaluate its effectiveness.	IV bolus medications often cause rapid changes in patient's physiological status. Some medications require careful monitoring and possibly laboratory testing (e.g., vasopressors require monitoring of blood pressure and heart rate).
4. Use ***Teach Back*** to determine patient's and family's understanding about intravenous medications. State, "I want to be sure you understand what I explained about your intravenous medicine. Can you explain why you need to take this medicine and side effects that you need to watch for and let me know if they occur?" Revise your instruction now or develop plan for revised teaching if patient or family is not able to teach back correctly.	Evaluates what patient and family are able to explain or demonstrate.

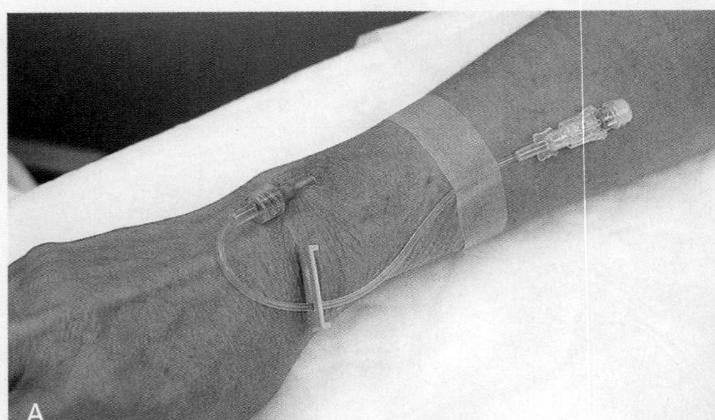

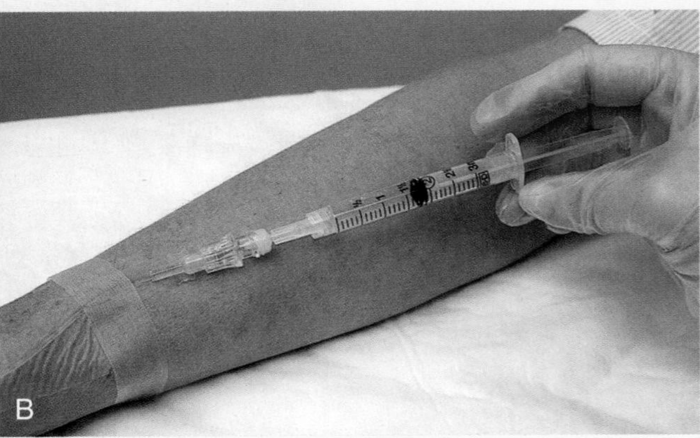

STEP 8b(2) A, IV catheter with saline lock adapter. **B,** Syringe inserted into injection port.

UNEXPECTED OUTCOMES AND RELATED INTERVENTIONS

1. Patient develops adverse reaction to medication.
   - Stop delivering medication immediately, be sure that IV continues to infuse, and follow agency policy or guidelines for appropriate response and reporting of adverse drug reactions.
   - Add allergy information to patient's medical record.
2. IV site shows symptoms of infiltration or phlebitis (see Chapter 42).
   - Stop infusing medication.
   - Treat IV site as indicated by agency policy.
   - Insert new IV site if continuing IV therapy.
3. Patient is unable to explain medication information.
   - Patient requires reinstruction or is unable to learn at this time.

RECORDING AND REPORTING

- Record medication, dose, time and date, and route of administration.
- Report any adverse reactions immediately to health care provider. Patient's response may indicate need for additional medical therapy.
- Record patient's response to medication in nurses' notes.
- Document your evaluation of patient and family learning.

SKILL 32-7 ADMINISTERING INTRAVENOUS MEDICATIONS BY PIGGYBACK, INTERMITTENT INTRAVENOUS INFUSION SETS, AND SYRINGE PUMPS

DELEGATION CONSIDERATIONS

The skill of administering intravenous (IV) medications by piggyback, intermittent IV infusion sets, and syringe pumps cannot be delegated to nursing assistive personnel (NAP). Instruct NAP about:

- Potential side effects of medications and need to report their occurrence to the nurse immediately.
- Reporting patient's verbalization of discomfort at infusion site.
- Reporting changes in patient's condition or vital signs.

EQUIPMENT

- Adhesive tape (optional)
- Antiseptic swab
- IV pole
- Medication administration record (MAR) (electronic or printed)
- Clean gloves
- Piggyback or mini-infusion pump
  - Medication prepared in 5- to 250-mL labeled infusion bag or syringe
  - Prefilled syringe containing normal saline flush solution (for saline lock)
  - Short microdrip, macrodrip, or mini-infusion IV tubing set, with blunt-end needleless cannula attachment
  - Needleless access device
  - Mini-infusion pump if needed
- Volume-control administration set
  - Buretrol
  - Infusion tubing with blunt-end needleless cannula attachment
  - Syringe (1- to 20-mL)
  - Vial or ampule of ordered medication

STEP	RATIONALE
ASSESSMENT	
1. Check accuracy and completeness of each MAR with health care provider's medication order. Check patient's name, medication name and dosage, and route and time of administration. Recopy or reprint any part of printed MAR that is difficult to read.	The order sheet is the most reliable source and only legal record of medications that patient is to receive. Ensures that patient receives correct medications (Mandrack et al., 2012; Sulosaari et al., 2011). Illegible MARs are a source of medication errors (Alassaad et al., 2013).
2. Review patient's medical history, medication history, and history of allergies. Assess patient symptoms or condition for which medication has been prescribed.	Helps you anticipate therapeutic effect of medication. IV bolus delivers medication rapidly. Allergic reactions can be fatal. Provides baseline to determine patient's response to medication.
3. Review pertinent information related to medication: action, purpose, normal dose and route, side effects, time of onset and peak action, compatibility with existing IV fluids, and nursing implications.	Allows you to give medication safely and monitor patient's response to therapy.
4. Assess patency of patient's existing IV infusion line by noting infusion rate of main IV line (see Chapter 42).	IV line must be patent, and fluids need to infuse easily for medication to reach venous circulation effectively.

SKILL 32-7 ADMINISTERING INTRAVENOUS MEDICATIONS BY PIGGYBACK, INTERMITTENT INTRAVENOUS INFUSION SETS, AND SYRINGE PUMPS—cont'd

STEP	RATIONALE
CLINICAL DECISION: *If the patient's IV site is saline locked, clean the port with alcohol and assess the patency of the IV line by flushing it with 2 to 3 mL of sterile normal saline. Attach appropriate IV tubing to the saline lock and administer the medication via piggyback, tandem, mini-infusion, or volume-control administration set. When the infusion is completed, disconnect the tubing, clean the port with alcohol, and flush the IV line with 2 to 3 mL of sterile normal saline. Maintain sterility of IV tubing between intermittent infusions.*	
5. Perform hand hygiene. Assess IV insertion site for signs of infiltration or phlebitis: redness, pallor, swelling, and tenderness on palpation.	Confirmation of placement of IV needle or catheter and integrity of surrounding tissues ensures safe medication administration.
6. Assess patient's understanding of purpose of medication therapy.	Reveals need for education.
PLANNING	
1. Collect appropriate equipment and MAR.	Enhances time management and efficiency.
2. Plan preparation to avoid interruptions. Do not take phone calls or speak with others. Follow agency policy.	Interruption contributes to medication errors. Use no-interruption zone (NIZ) when possible (Prakash et al., 2014; Yoder et al., 2015).
IMPLEMENTATION	
1. Perform hand hygiene. Prepare medication from ampule or vial (see Skill 32-4). Be sure to compare label of medication with MAR 2 times while preparing the medication.	Ensures that medication is sterile. Following the same routine when preparing medications, eliminating distractions, and checking label of medication with transcribed order reduce error (Murphy and While, 2012). *This is the first and second accuracy check.*
2. Take medications to patient at correct time (see agency policy). Medications that require exact timing include STAT, first-time, loading, and 1-time doses. Give time-critical scheduled medications (e.g., antibiotics, anticoagulants, insulin, anticonvulsants, immunosuppressive agents) at exact time ordered (within 30 minutes before or after scheduled dose). Give non–time-critical scheduled medications within a range of either 1 or 2 hours of scheduled doses (ISMP, 2011). Apply the six rights of medication administration throughout medication administration. Perform hand hygiene.	Ensures intended therapeutic effect and complies with professional standards. Hospitals need to adopt a medication administration policy and procedure for the timing of medication administration that considers patient needs, prescribed medication, and specific clinical indications (CMS, 2011; ISMP, 2011). Time-critical scheduled medications are medications in which early or delayed administration of maintenance doses of more than 30 minutes before or after the scheduled dose may cause harm or result in suboptimal therapy or pharmacological effect. Non–time-critical medications are medications in which early or delayed administration of 1-2 hours should not cause harm or result in suboptimal therapy or pharmacological effects (CMS, 2011; ISMP, 2011). Hand hygiene decreases transfer of microorganisms.
3. Identify patient using at least two identifiers (e.g., name and birthday or name and medical record number) according to agency policy. Compare identifiers with information on patient's MAR or medical record.	Ensures correct patient. Complies with The Joint Commission standards and improves patient safety (TJC, 2016).
4. Explain purpose of medication and side effects to patient. Explain that you will give medication through existing IV line. Encourage patient to report symptoms of discomfort at site immediately.	Keeps patient informed of planned therapies, minimizing anxiety. Patients who verbalize pain at IV site help detect infiltrations early.
5. Compare names of medications on labels with MAR one more time at patient's bedside.	*This is the third accuracy check.*
6. Apply clean gloves. NOTE: If patient has latex allergy, use latex-free gloves.	Reduces transmission of microorganisms. During IV administration there is a risk of blood exposure.
7. Administer medications. **a.** Piggyback infusion	
CLINICAL DECISION: *Never administer IV medications through tubing that is infusing blood, blood products, or parenteral nutrition solutions.*	
(1) Connect infusion tubing to medication bag (see Chapter 42). Allow solution to fill tubing by opening regulator flow clamp. Once tubing is full, close clamp and cap end of tubing.	Infusion tubing needs to be filled with solution and free of air bubbles to prevent air embolus. Capping keeps line sterile.
(2) Hang piggyback medication bag above level of primary fluid bag (use hook to lower main bag) (see Figure 32-25).	Height of fluid bag affects rate of flow to patient.
(3) Wipe off needleless port of main IV line with antiseptic swab and allow to air dry. Connect tubing of piggyback infusion to appropriate connector on upper Y-port of primary infusion line: **(a)** Needleless system: Remove cap and insert cannula tip of piggyback infusion tubing to appropriate connector on primary infusion line (see illustration).	Use needleless connections to prevent accidental needlestick injuries (OSHA, n.d.). Establishes route for IV medication to enter main IV line.

STEP	RATIONALE
(b) Saline (IV) lock: Follow Steps 8a(1)-8b(5) in Skill 32-6 to flush and prepare lock. Then wipe off port of lock with antiseptic swab and allow to dry. Remove cap and insert tip of infusion tubing via needless access to port of saline lock. Ensure that end of IV tubing system is sterile. Change tubing if it is not sterile.	Flushing lock ensures patency; IV fluids and medications must be administered aseptically.
(4) Regulate flow rate of medication solution by adjusting regulator clamp or IV pump infusion rate (see Chapter 42). Infusion times vary. Refer to medication reference or agency policy for safe flow rate.	Provides slow, intermittent infusion of medication and maintains therapeutic blood levels.
(5) After medication has infused:	
(a) Continuous infusion: Check flow rate of primary infusion. Primary infusion automatically begins to flow after piggyback solution is empty.	Back-check valve on piggyback stops flow of primary infusion until second medication infuses. Checking flow rate ensures proper administration of IV fluids.
(b) Saline lock: Disconnect tubing and apply cap. Cleanse port with antiseptic swab, let dry and flush IV line with 2-3 mL of sterile 0.9% sodium chloride. Maintain sterility of IV tubing between intermittent infusions.	Helps to ensure that lock remains patent.
(6) Regulate main infusion line to desired rate if necessary.	Infusion of piggyback sometimes interferes with main-line infusion rate.
(7) Leave IV piggyback bag and tubing in place for future medication administration or discard in appropriate containers.	Establishment of secondary line produces route for microorganisms to enter main line. Repeated changes in tubing increase risk of infection transmission (see agency policy).
b. Mini-infusion administration	
(1) Connect prefilled syringe to mini-infusion tubing.	Special tubing designed to fit syringe delivers medication to main IV line.
(2) Carefully apply pressure to syringe plunger, allowing tubing to fill with medication.	Ensures that tubing is free of air bubbles to prevent air embolus.
(3) Place syringe into mini-infusion pump (follow product directions). Be sure that syringe is secured (see illustration).	
(4) Wipe off needleless port of IV tubing with antiseptic swab and allow to dry. Connect mini-infusion tubing to main IV following Step 7a(3)(a or b).	
(5) Hang infusion pump with syringe on IV pole alongside main IV bag. Set pump to deliver medication within time recommended by agency policy, pharmacist, or medication reference manual. Use alarm if medication is delivered into heparin/saline lock. Press button on pump to begin infusion.	Pump automatically delivers medication at safe, constant rate on basis of volume in syringe.

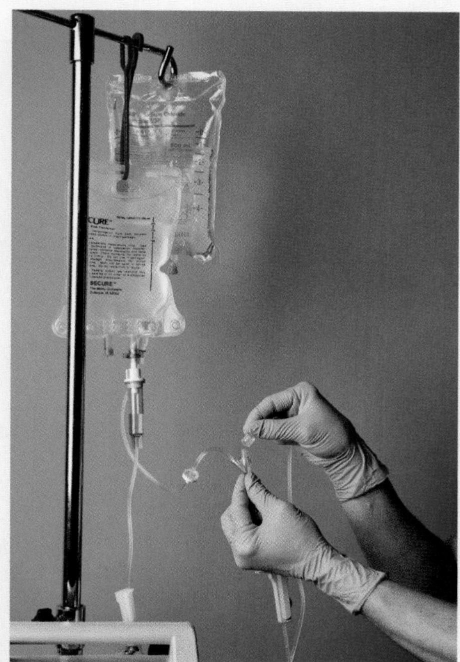

STEP 7a(3)(a) For needleless system insert tip of piggyback infusion tubing into port.

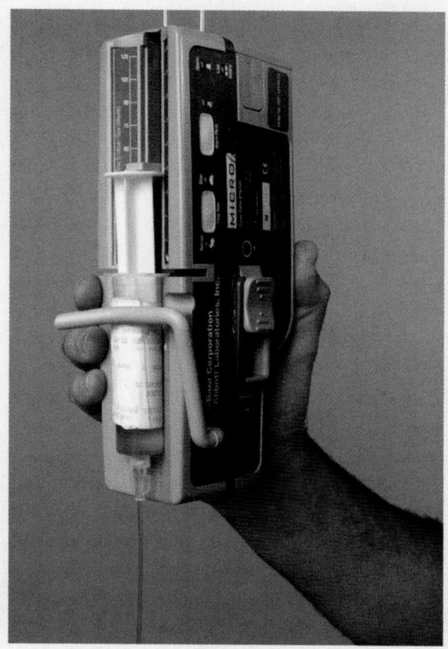

STEP 7b(3) Ensure that syringe is secure after placing it into syringe pump.

SKILL 32-7 ADMINISTERING INTRAVENOUS MEDICATIONS BY PIGGYBACK, INTERMITTENT INTRAVENOUS INFUSION SETS, AND SYRINGE PUMPS—cont'd

STEP	RATIONALE
(6) After medication has infused, check flow rate on primary infusion or re-establish saline lock following Steps 7a(5)(a or b).	Maintains patency of primary IV line.
c. Volume-control administration set (e.g., Buretrol)	
(1) Fill Buretrol with desired amount of fluid (50 to 100 mL) by opening clamp between Buretrol and main IV bag (see illustrations).	Small volume of fluid dilutes IV medication and reduces risk of too-rapid infusion.
(2) Close clamp and check to be sure that clamp on air vent of Buretrol chamber is open.	Prevents additional leakage of fluid into Buretrol. Air vent allows fluid in Buretrol to exit at regulated rate.
(3) Clean injection port on top of Buretrol with antiseptic swab and allow to dry.	Prevents introduction of microorganisms during needle insertion.
(4) Remove needle cap or sheath, insert syringe needle through port, and inject medication (see illustrations). Gently rotate Buretrol between hands.	Rotating mixes medication with solution in Buretrol to ensure equal distribution.
(5) If Buretrol tubing is not already connected to patient's IV site, connect it to patient's saline lock following Step 7a(3)(b).	
(6) Regulate IV infusion rate to allow medication to infuse in time recommended by agency policy, pharmacist, or medication reference manual.	For optimal therapeutic effect, medication needs to infuse in prescribed time interval.
(7) Label Buretrol with name of medication, dosage, and total volume, including diluent and time of administration following ISMP (2015b) safe medication label format (see Figure 32-26).	Alerts nurses to medication being infused. Prevents other medications from being added to Buretrol.
(8) After medication has infused, check flow rate on primary infusion or re-establish saline lock following Steps 7a(5)(a or b).	Ensures appropriate fluid balance and maintains IV site.
(9) Dispose of uncapped needle or needle enclosed in safety shield and syringe in proper container.	Prevents accidental needlesticks (OSHA, n.d.).
(10) Discard supplies in appropriate container and perform hand hygiene.	Reduces transmission of microorganisms.

EVALUATION

STEP	RATIONALE
1. Assess patient's status after administering medication.	Evaluates effect of medication.
2. Observe patient for signs of adverse reactions.	IV medications act rapidly.
3. During infusion periodically check infusion rate and condition of IV site.	IV line needs to remain patent for proper medication administration. Development of infiltration necessitates discontinuing infusion.

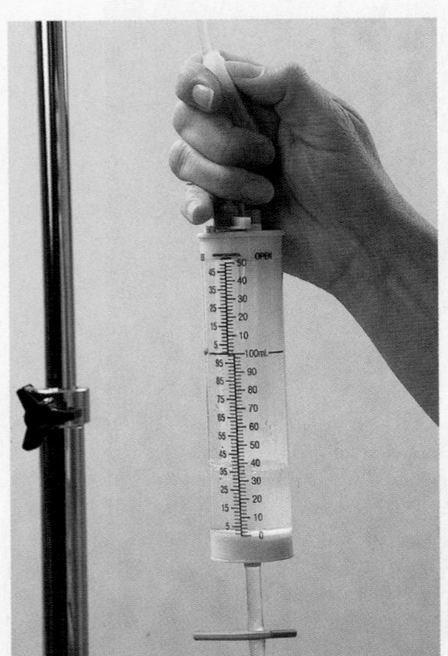

STEP 7c(1) Filling volume-control administration device.

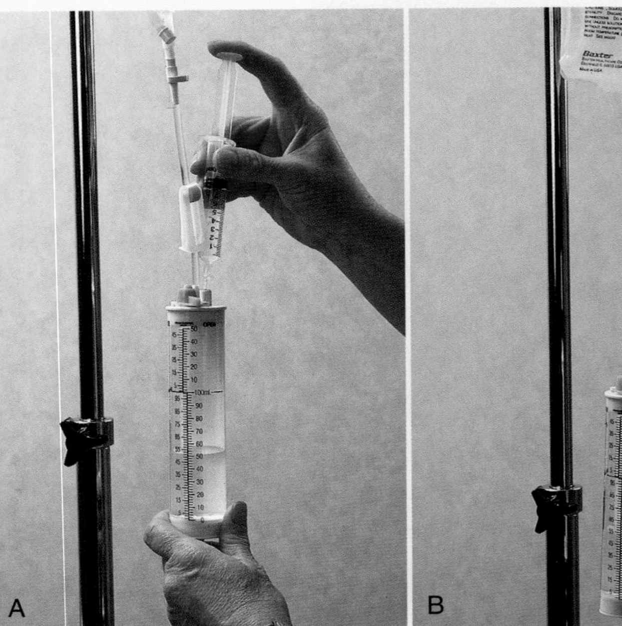

STEP 7c(4) A, Medication injected into device. **B,** Prepared device.

STEP	RATIONALE
4. Use ***Teach Back*** to determine patient's and family's understanding about intravenous piggyback medications. State, "I want to be sure you understand what I explained about your IV piggyback medicine. Can you explain why you need to take this IV medicine and any side effects you need to watch for and let me know if they occur?" Revise your instruction now or develop plan for revised teaching if patient or family is not able to teach back correctly.	Evaluates what the patient and family are able to explain or demonstrate.

UNEXPECTED OUTCOMES AND RELATED INTERVENTIONS

1. Patient develops adverse drug reaction.
   - Stop medication infusion immediately. Be sure that main IV line is infusing.
   - Follow agency policy or guidelines for appropriate response and reporting of adverse drug reactions.
   - Document allergy in patient's medical record.
2. Medication does not infuse over desired period.
   - Determine reason (e.g., improper calculation of flow rate, malpositioning of IV needle at insertion site, or infiltration).
   - Take corrective action as indicated (see Chapter 42).
3. IV site shows signs of phlebitis or infiltration (see Chapter 42).
   - See related interventions in Skill 32-6.

RECORDING AND REPORTING

- Record medication, dose, route, and time and date administered on MAR.
- Record volume of fluid in medication bag or Buretrol on intake and output form.
- Report adverse reactions to patient's health care provider.
- Document your evaluation of patient and family learning.

HOME CARE CONSIDERATIONS

- Teach patient and family caregiver how to dispose of needles and contaminated equipment in puncture-proof containers (e.g., coffee can).
- Instruct family caregiver about community resources to obtain supplies.

KEY POINTS

- Learning medication classifications improves understanding of nursing implications for administering medications with similar characteristics.
- All controlled substances are handled according to strict procedures that account for each medication.
- A nurse applies understanding of the physiology of medication action when timing administration, selecting routes, initiating actions to promote medication efficacy, and observing responses to medications.
- The older adult's body undergoes structural and functional changes that alter medication actions and influence the manner in which nurses provide medication therapy.
- Verify medication calculations with another nurse to ensure accuracy.
- Medications given parenterally are absorbed more quickly than those administered by other routes.
- Each medication order needs to include the patient's name, order date, medication name, dosage, route, time of administration, drug indication, and health care provider's signature.
- A medication history reveals allergies, medications a patient is taking, and the patient's adherence to therapy.
- The six rights of medication administration contribute to accurate preparation and administration of medication doses.
- The six rights of medication administration are the right medication, right dose, right patient, right route, right time, and right documentation.
- Nurses need to avoid distractions, use NIZs, and follow the same routine when preparing medications to reduce medication errors.
- Nurses administer only medications they prepare, and prepared medications are never left unattended.
- Document medications immediately after administration.
- A nurse uses clinical judgment regarding a patient's clinical status in determining the best time to administer prn medications.
- A nurse reports a medication error immediately.
- When preparing medications, a nurse checks the medication container label against the MAR 3 times.
- The Z-track method for IM injections protects subcutaneous tissues from irritating parenteral fluids.
- Failure to select injection sites by anatomical landmarks leads to tissue, bone, or nerve damage.

CLINICAL APPLICATION QUESTIONS

Preparing for Clinical Practice

Kyle, a nursing student, is caring for Maria, a 48-year-old who is being treated for multiple fractures after a motorcycle accident. Maria's health care provider writes a new medication order for morphine sulfate liquid suspension 20 mg orally STAT and then q4h as needed for pain. Maria is having difficulty swallowing pills as a result of her trauma; thus her medications are ordered in liquid suspension.

1. What does Kyle need to know about morphine sulfate before administering it?
2. Four unit-dose containers of liquid morphine sulfate arrive on the patient care unit. The labels on the medication say: "10 mg morphine sulfate/5 mL." Using dimensional analysis, how much medication should Kyle administer?
3. Kyle collects the appropriate equipment to administer the medication, performs hand hygiene, prepares the medication, takes it to

Maria at the correct time, and uses two patient identifiers to ensure that she is the right patient. Which step does Kyle need to take next in administering the medication?

ⓔ *Answers to Clinical Application Questions can be found on the Evolve website.*

REVIEW QUESTIONS

Are You Ready to Test Your Nursing Knowledge?

1. You are a new graduate nurse completing your orientation on a very busy intensive care unit. You cannot read a health care provider's order for one of your patient's medications. You have heard from more experienced nurses that this health care provider does not like to be called, and you know that another of the health care provider's patients is very unstable. What is the most appropriate next step for you to take?
   1. Call the health care provider to clarify the order
   2. Talk with your preceptor to help you interpret the order
   3. Refer to a medication manual before giving the medication
   4. Use your best judgment and critical thinking and administer the dose you think the health care provider ordered
2. A toddler is to receive 2.5 mL of an antipyretic by mouth. Which equipment is the most appropriate for medication administration for this child?
   1. A medication cup
   2. A teaspoon
   3. A 5-mL syringe
   4. An oral-dosing syringe
3. What statement made by a 4-year-old patient's mother indicates that she understands how to administer her son's eardrops?
   1. "To straighten his ear canal, I need to pull the outside part of his ear down and back."
   2. "I need to straighten his ear canal before administering the medication by pulling his ear upward and outward."
   3. "I need to put my son in a chair and make sure that he's sitting up with his head tilted back before I give him the eardrops."
   4. "After I'm done giving him his eardrops, I need to make sure that my son remains sitting straight up for at least 10 minutes."
4. A health care provider ordered enalapril (Vasotec) 2 mg IV push for a patient with hypertension. The pharmacy sent vials marked 1.25 mg enalapril/mL. How many mL does the nurse administer? ___ mL
5. A nurse admits a 72-year-old patient with a medical history of hypertension, heart failure, renal failure, and depression to a general medical patient care unit. The nurse reviews the patient's medication orders and notes that the patient has three health care providers who have ordered a total of 13 medications. What is the most appropriate action for the nurse to take next?
   1. Give the medications after identifying the patient using two patient identifiers
   2. Provide medication education to the patient to help with adherence to the medical plan
   3. Review the list of medications with the health care providers to ensure that the patient needs all 13 medications
   4. Set up a medication schedule for the patient that is least disruptive to the expected treatment schedule in the hospital
6. The nurse is administering an intravenous (IV) push medication to a patient who has a compatible IV fluid running through intravenous tubing. Place the following steps in the appropriate order.
   1. Release tubing and inject medication within amount of time recommended by agency policy, pharmacist, or medication reference manual. Use watch to time administration.
   2. Select injection port of intravenous (IV) tubing closest to patient. Whenever possible, injection port should accept a needleless syringe. Use IV filter if required by medication reference or agency policy.
   3. After injecting medication, release tubing, withdraw syringe, and recheck fluid infusion rate.
   4. Connect syringe to port of intravenous (IV) line. Insert needleless tip or small-gauge needle of syringe containing prepared drug through center of injection port.
   5. Clean injection port with antiseptic swab. Allow to dry.
   6. Occlude intravenous (IV) line by pinching tubing just above injection port. Pull back gently on syringe plunger to aspirate blood return.
7. A nursing student is administering ampicillin PO. The expiration date on the medication wrapper was yesterday. What is the appropriate action for the nursing student to take next?
   1. Ask the nursing professor for advice
   2. Return the medication to pharmacy and get another tablet
   3. Call the health care provider after discussing this situation with the charge nurse
   4. Administer the medication since medications are good for 30 days after their expiration date
8. A nursing student is administering medications to a patient through a gastric tube (G-tube). Which of the following actions taken by the nursing student requires the nursing instructor to intervene?
   1. The nursing student places all the patient's medications in different medicine cups.
   2. The nursing student evaluates each medication and holds the tube feeding before administering a medication that needs to be administered on an empty stomach.
   3. The nursing student flushes the tube with 30 mL of water between each medication.
   4. The nursing student crushes a nifedipine extended-release tablet and mixes it with water before administering it.
9. A pediatric nurse takes a medication to a 12-year-old female patient. The patient tells the nurse to take it away because she is not going to take it. What is the nurse's next action?
   1. Ask the patient's reason for refusal
   2. Consult with the patient's parents for advice
   3. Take the medication away and chart the patient's refusal
   4. Tell the patient that her health care provider knows what is best for her
10. A nurse caring for a patient on a general surgical unit notes the following medication order in the patient's medical record:
    3 March 2016 1415 Administer 25 mg hydrochlorothiazide PO BID D. Anderson, MD
    What should the nurse do next?
11. After receiving an intramuscular (IM) injection in the deltoid, a patient states, "My arm really hurts. It's burning and tingling where I got my injection. What should the nurse do next? (Select all that apply.)
    1. Assess the injection site
    2. Administer an oral medication for pain
    3. Notify the patient's health care provider of assessment findings
    4. Document assessment findings and related interventions in the patient's medical record
    5. This is a normal finding so nothing needs to be done
    6. Apply ice to the site for relief of burning pain

12. You are working in a health clinic on a college campus. You need to administer medroxyprogesterone acetate intramuscularly (IM) to a female patient for birth control. You look up this medication in a reference manual and determine that it is viscous and injections can be painful. On the basis of this information, you plan which of the following when administering this medication? (Select all that apply.)
    1. Inject the medication over 3 minutes to reduce pain associated with the injection
    2. Administer the medication in the ventral gluteal site
    3. Use the Z-track method when administering the medication
    4. Use the deltoid site for medication administration
    5. Ask the patient questions about her major and which classes she is taking during the injection to provide distraction
13. After seeing a patient, the health care provider starts to give a nursing student a verbal order for a new medication. The nursing student first needs to:
    1. Follow ISMP guidelines for safe medication abbreviations.
    2. Explain to the health care provider that the order needs to be given to a registered nurse.
    3. Write down the order on the patient's order sheet and read it back to the health care provider.
    4. Ensure that the six rights of medication administration are followed when giving the medication.
14. A nurse accidently gives a patient the medications that were ordered for the patient's roommate. What is the nurse's first priority?
    1. Complete an occurrence report.
    2. Notify the health care provider.
    3. Inform the charge nurse of the error.
    4. Assess the patient for adverse effects.
15. A child is taking albuterol through a pressurized metered-dose inhaler (pMDI) that contains a total of 64 puffs. The dose is 2 puffs every 6 hours. How many days will the pMDI last? ___________ days.

Answers: 1. 1; **2.** 4; **3.** 2; **4.** 1.6 mL; **5.** 3; **6.** 2, 5, 4, 6, 1, 3; **7.** 2; **8.** 4; **9.** 1; **10.** See Evolve; **11.** 1, 3, 4; **12.** 2, 3, 5; **13.** 2; **14.** 4; **15.** 8.

Rationales for Review Questions can be found on the Evolve website.

REFERENCES

Alexander M, et al: *Core curriculum for infusion nursing*, ed 4, Philadelphia, 2014, Williams & Wilkins.

American Association of Diabetes Educators (AADE): *Teaching injection technique to people with diabetes*, 2013, http://www.diabeteseducator.org/export/sites/aade/_resources/pdf/research/InjectionEducationPracticeGuide.pdf. Accessed January 11, 2015.

American Diabetes Association (ADA): Diabetes care in the hospital, nursing home, and skilled nursing facility, *Diabetes Care* 38(S1):S80, 2015. http://care.diabetesjournals.org/content/38/Supplement_1/S80.full. Accessed January 11, 2015.

American Hospital Association: *The patient care partnership*, 2003, http://www.aha.org/advocacy-issues/communicatingpts/pt-care-partnership.shtml. Accessed November 28, 2014.

American Medical Association (AMA): *Generic naming*, 2015, http://www.ama-assn.org/ama/pub/physician-resources/medical-science/united-states-adopted-names-council/generic-drug-naming-explained.page. Accessed June 18, 2015.

American Nurses Association (ANA): *Nursing: scope and standards of practice*, ed 2, Silver Spring, Md, 2010, The Association.

American Society of Health-System Pharmacists (ASHP): *How to use eyedrops properly*, 2013, http://www.safemedication.com/safemed/MedicationTipsTools/HowtoAdminister/HowtoUseEyeDropsProperly. Accessed June 8, 2015.

American Society of Health-System Pharmacists [ASHP]: *ASHP guidelines: compounding sterile preparations*, 2014, http://www.ashp.org/DocLibrary/BestPractices/PrepGdlCSP.aspx. Accessed June 8, 2015.

Bankhead R, et al: Enteral nutrition practice recommendations, *JPEN J Parenter Enteral Nutr* 33:1, 2009.

Bastable S: *Nurse as educator: principles of teaching and learning for nursing practice*, ed 4, Sudbury, Mass, 2014, Jones & Bartlett.

Burchum J, Rosenthal L: *Lehne's pharmacology for nursing care*, ed 9, St Louis, 2016, Saunders.

Centers for Disease Control and Prevention (CDC): *Medication safety basics*, 2012, http://www.cdc.gov/medicationsafety/basics.html. Accessed June 6, 2015.

Centers for Disease Control and Prevention (CDC): *Vaccine administration: recommendations and guidelines*, 2014a, http://www.cdc.gov/vaccines/recs/vac-admin/default.htm?s_cid=. Accessed June 7, 2015.

Centers for Disease Control and Prevention (CDC): *Tuberculosis (TB)*, 2014b, http://www.cdc.gov/tb/. Accessed June 7, 2015.

Centers for Disease Control and Prevention (CDC): *Vaccine administration: epidemiology and prevention of vaccine-preventable diseases*, 2015, http://www.cdc.gov/vaccines/pubs/pinkbook/vac-admin.html. Accessed June 15, 2015.

Centers for Medicare and Medicaid Services (CMS): 2011, http://www.ismp.org/download/files/Updated_IGs_Medication_Adminis_Nov-18-11.pdf. Accessed June 6, 2015.

Consumer Med Safety: Tips for measuring liquid medicines safely, *Institute for Safe Medicine Practices*, 2015, http://www.consumermedsafety.org/tools-and-resources/medication-safety-tools-and-resources/taking-your-medicine-safely/measure-liquid-medications. Accessed June 11, 2015.

Cookson KL: Dimensional analysis: calculate dosages the easy way, *Nursing* 43(6):57, 2013.

Davidson K, Rourke L: Teaching best evidence: deltoid intramuscular injection technique, *J Nurs Educ Pract* 3(7):122, 2013.

Diggle D: Are you FIT for purpose? The importance of getting injection technique right, *J Diabetes Nurs* 18:50, 2014.

Echevarria IM, Schwoebel A: Development of an intervention model for the prevention of aspiration pneumonia in high-risk patients on a medical-surgical unit, *Medsurg Nurs* 21(5):303, 2012.

Ghaemmaghami V: Computerized provider order entry: advancing technology today, saving lives tomorrow, *AORN J* 100(6):683, 2014.

Giger JL: *Transcultural nursing: assessment and intervention*, ed 6, St Louis, 2013, Mosby.

Gleason KM, et al; Agency for Healthcare Research and Quality: *Medications at transitions and clinical handoffs (MATCH) toolkit for medication reconciliation*, 2012, http://www.ahrq.gov/professionals/quality-patient-safety/patient-safety-resources/resources/match/match.pdf. Accessed June 6, 2015.

Guenter P, Boullata J: Drug administration by enteral feeding tube, *Nursing* 43(12):26, 2013.

Guzman-Aranguez A, et al: Contact lenses: promising devices for ocular drug delivery, *J Ocular Pharmacol Ther* 29(2):189, 2013.

Hockenberry MJ, Wilson D: *Wong's nursing care of infants and children*, ed 10, St Louis, 2015, Mosby.

Hopkins U, Arias C: *Large-volume IM injections: a review of best practices*, 2013, http://www.oncologynurseadvisor.com/chemotherapy/large-volume-im-injections-a-review-of-best-practices/article/281208/. Accessed June 7, 2015.

Infusion Nurses Society: INS): Infusion nursing standards of practice, *J Infus Nurs* 34(1 Suppl):S1, 2011.

Institute for Safe Medication Practices (ISMP): *How fast is too fast for IV push medications: acute care ISMP medication safety alert*, May 15, 2003, http://www.ismp.org/newsletters/acutecare/articles/20030515.asp. Accessed June 13, 2015.

Institute for Safe Medication Practices (ISMP): *Tablet splitting: do it only if you "half" to and then do it safely: acute Care ISMP medication safety alert*, May 18, 2006, https://www.ismp.org/newsletters/acutecare/articles/20060518.asp. Accessed June 13, 2015.

Institute for Safe Medication Practices (ISMP): *ISMP acute care guidelines for timely administration of scheduled medications*, 2011, http://www.ismp.org/Tools/guidelines/acutecare/tasm.pdf. Accessed June 6, 2015.

Institute for Safe Medication Practices (ISMP): *ISMP's list of error-prone abbreviations, symbols, and dose designations*, 2013a, http://www.ismp.org/Tools/errorproneabbreviations.pdf. Accessed June 6, 2015.

Institute for Safe Medication Practices (ISMP): *As U-500 insulin safety concerns mount, it's time to rethink safe use of strengths above U-100*, 2013b, https://www.ismp.org/newsletters/acutecare/showarticle.aspx?id=62. Accessed June 8, 2015.

Institute for Safe Medication Practices (ISMP): *Ongoing concern about insulin pen reuse shows hospitals need to consider transitioning away from them*, 2013c, http://www.ismp.org/newsletters/acutecare/showarticle.aspx?id=41. Accessed January 11, 2015.

Institute for Safe Medication Practices (ISMP): *Oral dosage forms that should not be crushed*, 2014a, http://www.ismp.org/tools/donotcrush.pdf. Accessed November 28, 2014.

Institute for Safe Medication Practices (ISMP): Medication safety alert: *Acute Care* 19(16):2, 2014b.

Institute for Safe Medication Practices (ISMP): *ISMP's list of confused drug names*, 2015a, http://www.ismp.org/Tools/confuseddrugnames.pdf. Accessed June 8, 2015.

Institute for Safe Medication Practices (ISMP): *Principles of designing a medication label for intravenous piggyback medication for patient specific, inpatient use*, 2015b, http://www.ismp.org/tools/guidelines/labelFormats/IVPB.asp. Accessed January 17, 2015.

Institute for Safe Medication Practices (ISMP): *2014-2015 targeted medication safety best practices for hospitals*, 2015c, http://www.ismp.org/Tools/BestPractices/default.aspX Accessed June 8, 2015.

Institute of Medicine (IOM): *Report brief, to err is human: building a safer health system*, 1999, http://iom.edu/Reports/1999/To-Err-is-Human-Building-A-Safer-Health-System.aspx. Accessed June 8, 2015.

Juip M, Fitzner K: A problem-solving approach to effective insulin injection for patients at either end of the body mass index, *Popul Health Manag* 15(3):168, 2012.

Lehne RA: *Pharmacology for nursing care*, ed 8, St Louis, 2013, Saunders.

Lilley LL, et al: *Pharmacology and the nursing process*, ed 6, St Louis, 2011, Mosby.

Mandrack M, et al: Nursing best practices using automated dispensing cabinets: nurses' key role in improving medication safety, *Medsurg Nurs* 21(3):134, 2012.

MayoClinic.com: *Asthma inhalers: which one's right for you?* 2015a, http://www.mayoclinic.com/health/asthma-inhalers/HQ01081. Accessed June 8, 2015.

MayoClinic.com: *Using a metered-dose asthma inhaler and spacer*, 2015b, http://www.mayoclinic.com/health/asthma/MM00608. Accessed June 8, 2015.

MayoClinic.com: *How to use a dry powder disk inhaler*, 2015c, http://www.mayoclinic.org/diseases-conditions/asthma/multimedia/asthma/vid-20084733. Accessed June 8, 2015.

MayoClinic.com: *Prednisone and other corticosteroids*, 2015d, http://www.mayoclinic.org/steroids/art-20045692?pg=1. Accessed June 8, 2015.

McCulloch D: General principles of insulin therapy in diabetes mellitus, *UpToDate*, 2015, http://www.uptodate.com/contents/general-principles-of-insulin-therapy-in-diabetes-mellitus. Accessed June 7, 2015.

Morris DG: *Calculate with confidence*, ed 6, St Louis, 2014, Mosby.

Nouri S, Rudd R: Health literacy in the "oral exchange": an important element of patient provider communication, *Patient Educ Couns* 98(5):565, 2015.

Novo Nordisk: *Levemir*, 2014, http://www.levemir.com/. Accessed January 11, 2015.

Occupational Safety and Health Administration (OSHA): *Bloodborne pathogens and needlestick prevention*, n.d., https://www.osha.gov/SLTC/bloodbornepathogens/index.html. Accessed June 8, 2015.

Ogston-Tuck S: Intramuscular injection technique: an evidence based approach, *Nurs Stand* 29(4):55, 2014.

Sanofi-Aventis: *Lovenox® subcutaneous injection*, 2014, http://www.lovenox.com/hcp_default.aspx. Accessed January 11, 2015.

Skidmore-Roth L: *Mosby's 2015 nursing drug reference*, ed 28, St Louis, 2015, Mosby.

Speyer R: Oropharyngeal dysphagia: screening and assessment, *Otolaryngol Clin North Am* 46(6):989, 2013.

The Joint Commission (TJC): *Facts about the official "Do Not Use" list of abbreviations*, 2014a, http://www.jointcommission.org/assets/1/18/Do_Not_Use_List.pdf. Accessed June 6, 2015.

The Joint Commission (TJC): *Sentinel alert event: managing risk during transition to new ISO connector standards*, 2014b, http://www.jointcommission.org/assets/1/6/SEA_53_Connectors_8_19_14_final.pdf. Accessed June 8, 2015.

The Joint Commission (TJC): *2016 National Patient Safety Goals*, Oakbrook Terrace, IL, 2016, The Commission. Available at http://www.jointcommission.org/standards_information/npsgs.aspx. Accessed November 2015.

Touhy TA, Jett KF: *Ebersole and Hess' gerontological nursing & healthy aging*, ed 4, St Louis, 2014, Elsevier.

US Food and Drug Administration (USFDA): *FDA reminds the public about the potential for life-threatening harm from accidental exposure to fentanyl transdermal systems ("patches")*, 2012, http://www.fda.gov/Drugs/DrugSafety/ucm300747.htm. Accessed June 8, 2015.

US Food and Drug Administration (USFDA): *Best practices for tablet splitting*, 2013, http://www.fda.gov/Drugs/ResourcesForYou/Consumers/BuyingUsingMedicineSafely/EnsuringSafeUseofMedicine/ucm184666.htm. Accessed June 7, 2015.

US Food and Drug Administration (USFDA): *MedWatch: the FDA safety information and adverse event reporting program*, 2015, http://www.fda.gov/safety/medwatch/default.htm. Accessed June 6, 2015.

World Health Organization (WHO): *Injection safety*, 2015, http://www.who.int/injection_safety/en/. Accessed January 12, 2015.

Yoder M, et al: The effect of a safe zone on nurse interruptions, distractions, and medication administration errors, *J Infus Nurs* 38(2):140, 2015.

RESEARCH REFERENCES

Akbari Sari A, et al: Slow versus fast subcutaneous heparin injections for preventing bruising and site-pain intensity, *Cochrane Database Syst Rev* (7):CD008077, 2014.

Alhalaiqa F, et al: Hypertensive patients' experience with adherence therapy for enhancing medication compliance: a qualitative exploration, *J Clin Nurs* 22(13/14):2039, 2013.

Alassaad A, et al: Prescription and transcription errors in multidose-dispensed medication on discharge from hospital: an observational and interventional study, *J Eval Clin Pract* 19(1):185, 2013.

Ari A, Restrepo RD: Aerosol delivery device selection for spontaneously breathing patients, *Respir Care* 57(4):613, 2012.

Bhalla MC, et al: Predictors of epinephrine autoinjector needle length inadequacy, *Am J Emerg Med* 31(12):1671, 2013.

Blazquez A, et al: Fluoxetine pharmacogenetics in child and adult populations, *Eur Child Adolesc Psychiatry* 21(11):599, 2012.

Ching JM, et al: Using lean "automation with a human touch" to improve medication safety: a step closer to the "perfect dose," *Jt Comm J Qual Patient Saf* 40(8):341, 2013.

Clifford P, et al: Following the evidence: enteral tube placement and verification in neonates and young children, *J Perinat Neonatal Nurs* 29(2):149, 2015.

Cochran GL, Haynatzki G: Comparison of medication safety effectiveness among nine critical access hospitals, *Am J Health Syst Pharm* 70(24):2218, 2013.

Cousein E, et al: Effect of automated drug distribution systems on medication error rates in a short-stay geriatric unit, *J Eval Clin Pract* 20(5):678, 2014.

Dayananda L, et al: Intended intramuscular gluteal injections: are they truly intramuscular? *J Postgrad Med* 60(2):175, 2014.

Donaldson N, et al: Predictors of unit-level medication administration accuracy, *J Nurs Adm* 44(6):353, 2014.

Gibney MA, et al: Skin and subcutaneous adipose layer thickness in adults with diabetes at sites used for insulin injections: implications for needle length recommendations, *Curr Med Res Opin* 26(6):1519, 2010.

Grou Volpe CR, et al: Medication errors in a public hospital in Brazil, *Br J Nurs* 23(11):552, 2014.

Hibbard P, et al: Approach to immunizations in healthy adults, *UpToDate*, 2015, http://www.uptodate.com/contents/approach-to-immunizations-in-healthy-adults. Accessed June 7, 2015.

Hirsch LJ, et al: Glycemic control, reported pain and leakage with a 4 mm × 32 G pen needle in obese and non-obese adults with diabetes: a post hoc analysis, *Curr Med Res Opin* 28(8):1305, 2012.

Hoffman PL, et al: Defining the ideal injection techniques when using 5-mm needles in children and adults, *Diabetes Care* 33(9):1940, 2010.

Hopkinson SG, Jennings BM: Interruptions during nurses' work: a state-of-the-science review, *Res Nurs Health* 36(1):38, 2013.

Hunter Revell SM, McCurry MK: Effective pedagogies for teaching math to nursing students: a literature review, *Nurse Educ Today* 33(11):1352, 2013.

Kaufmann J, et al: Medication errors in pediatric emergencies: a systematic analysis, *Dtsch Arztebl Int* 109(38):609, 2012.

Kim J, Bates DW: Medication administration errors by nurses: adherence to guidelines, *J Clin Nurs* 22(3/4):590, 2013.

Klang M, et al: Osmolality, pH, and compatibility of selected oral liquid medications with an enteral nutrition product, *JPEN J Parenter Enteral Nutr* 37(5):689, 2013.

Li W, et al: Factors related to medication non-adherence for patients with hypertension in Taiwan, *J Clin Nurs* 21(13/14):1816, 2012.

Lohmann K, et al: More than just crushing: a prospective pre-post intervention study to reduce drug preparation errors in patients with feeding tubes, *J Clin Pharm Ther* 40(2):220, 2015.

Malone A: Clinical guidelines from the American Society for Parenteral and Enteral Nutrition: best practice recommendations for patient care, *J Infus Nurs* 37(3):179, 2014.

McIntyre CM, Monk HM: Medication absorption considerations in patients with postpyloric enteral feeding tubes, *Am J Health Syst Pharm* 71(7):549, 2014.

Metheny NA, et al: Effectiveness of an aspiration risk-reduction protocol, *Nurs Res* 59(1):18, 2010.

Murphy M, While A: Medication administration practices among children's nurses: a survey, *Br J Nurs* 21(15):928, 2012.

Nicoll LH, Hesby A: Intramuscular injection: an integrative research review and guideline for evidence-based practice, *Appl Nurs Res* 16(2):149, 2002.

Niemann D, et al: A prospective three-step intervention study to prevent medication errors in drug handling in paediatric care, *J Clin Nurs* 24(1–2):101–114, 2015.

Palma S, Strohfus P: Are IM injections IM in obese and overweight females? A study in injection technique, *Appl Nurs Res* 26(4):e1, 2013.

Park YH, et al: Prevalence and associated factors of dysphagia in nursing home residents, *Geriatr Nurs* 34(3):212, 2013.

Pasina L, et al: Medication non-adherence among elderly patients newly discharged and receiving polypharmacy, *Drugs Aging* 31(4):283, 2014.

Phillips NM, Endacott R: Medication administration via enteral tubes: a survey of nurses' practices, *J Adv Nurs* 67(12):2586, 2011.

Polinski JM, et al: A matter of trust: patient barriers to primary medication adherence, *Health Educ Res* 29(5):755, 2014.

Prakash V, et al: Mitigating errors caused by interruptions during medication verification and administration: interventions in a simulated ambulatory chemotherapy setting, *BMJ Qual Saf* 23(11):884, 2014.

Prohaska ES, King AR: Administration of antiretroviral medication via enteral tubes, *Am J Health Syst Pharm* 69(24):2140, 2012.

Radley DC, et al: Reduction in medication errors in hospitals due to adoption of computerized provider order entry systems, *BMJ* 20(3):470, 2013.

Rinke ML, et al: Interventions to reduce pediatric medication errors: a systematic review, *Pediatrics* 134(2):338, 2014.

Sulosaari V, et al: An integrative review of the literature on registered nurses' medication competence, *J Clin Nurs* 20(3):464, 2011.

Viswanathan M, et al: Interventions to improve adherence to self-administered medications for chronic diseases in the United States: a systematic review, *Ann Intern Med* 157(11):785, 2012.

Voshall B, et al: Barcode medication administration work-arounds, *J Nurs Adm* 43(10):530, 2013.

Weekes CV: African Americans and health literacy: a systematic review, *ABNF J* 23(4):76, 2012.

Zhu LL, Zhou Q: Therapeutic concerns when oral medications are administered nasogastrically, *J Clin Pharm Ther* 38(4):272, 2013.

Zullig L, et al: A health literacy pilot intervention to improve medication adherence using medication technology, *Patient Educ Couns* 95(2):288, 2014.

33

Complementary and Alternative Therapies

OBJECTIVES

- Differentiate between complementary and alternative therapies.
- Describe the clinical applications of relaxation therapies.
- Discuss the relaxation response and its effect on somatic ailments.
- Identify the principles and effectiveness of imagery, meditation, and breathwork.
- Describe the purpose and principles of biofeedback.
- Describe the methods of and the psychophysiological responses to therapeutic touch.
- Describe safe and unsafe herbal therapies.

KEY TERMS

Acupoints, p. 694
Acupuncture, p. 694
Allopathic or biomedicine, p. 688
Alternative therapies, p. 689
Biofeedback, p. 693
Chiropractic therapy, p. 689
Complementary therapies, p. 688
Creative visualization, p. 693
Cupping, p. 695
Imagery, p. 693
Integrative health care, p. 689
Integrative nursing, p. 689
Meditation, p. 692
Moxibustion, p. 695
Passive relaxation, p. 692
Progressive relaxation, p. 692
***Qi gong*, p. 695**
Relaxation response, p. 691
Stress response, p. 691
Tai chi, p. 695
Therapeutic touch (TT), p. 694
Traditional Chinese medicine (TCM), p. 689
Vital energy (*qi*), p. 694
Whole medical systems, p. 689
Yin and yang, p. 694

MEDIA RESOURCES

http://evolve.elsevier.com/Potter/fundamentals/

- Review Questions
- Case Study with Questions
- Audio Glossary
- Content Updates

The general health of North American people has steadily improved over the course of the last century as evidenced by lower mortality rates and increased life expectancies (CDC, 2014). Changes in science and health care have provided the knowledge and technology to successfully alter the course of many illnesses. Despite the success of **allopathic or biomedicine** (conventional western medicine), many conditions such as chronic back and neck pain, arthritis, gastrointestinal problems, allergies, headache, and anxiety continue to be difficult to treat. As a result, more patients are exploring alternative methods to relieve their symptoms. Researchers estimate that up to 75% of patients seek care from their primary care providers for stress, pain, and health conditions for which there are no known causes or cures (Rakel, 2012). Although biomedicine is quite effective in treating numerous physical ailments (e.g., bacterial infections, chronic diseases, structural abnormalities, and acute illnesses/emergencies), it is generally less effective in decreasing stress-induced illnesses, managing symptoms of chronic disease, caring for the emotional and spiritual needs of individuals, and improving quality of life and general well-being.

The number of patients seeking unconventional treatments has risen considerably over the past decade. In part this increase is caused by (1) a desire for less invasive, less toxic, "more natural" treatments; (2) lack of satisfaction with biomedical treatments; (3) an increasing desire by patients to take a more active role in their treatment process; (4) beliefs that a combination of treatments (biomedical and complementary) results in better overall results; (5) the increased number of research articles in journals such as *Journal of Alternative and Complementary Medicine* and the *Journal of Holistic Nursing;* and (6) beliefs and values that are consistent with an approach to health that incorporates the mind, body, and spirit or a holistic approach (Koithan, 2009).

COMPLEMENTARY, ALTERNATIVE, AND INTEGRATIVE APPROACHES TO HEALTH

The National Institutes of Health/National Center for Complementary and Integrative Health (NIH/NCCIH, 2015a) defines complementary and alternative medicine (CAM) as "an array of health care approaches with a history of use or origins outside of mainstream medicine." **Complementary therapies** are therapies used in addition to or together with conventional treatment recommended by a person's health care provider. As the name implies, complementary therapies complement conventional treatments. Many of them such as therapeutic touch contain diagnostic and therapeutic methods that require special training. Others such as guided imagery and breathwork are easily learned and applied. Complementary therapies also include relaxation; exercise; massage; reflexology; prayer; biofeedback; hypnotherapy; creative therapies, including art, music, or dance therapy; meditation; **chiropractic therapy**; and herbs/supplements (Lindquist et al., 2014). Another term that is used to describe interventions used in this fashion, particularly by licensed health care providers, is *integrative therapies.*

Alternative therapies sometimes include the same interventions as complementary therapies; but they become the primary treatment (Table 33-1). For example, a person with chronic pain uses yoga to encourage flexibility and relaxation at the same time that nonsteroidal antiinflammatory or opioid medications are prescribed. Both sets of interventions are based on conventional pathophysiology and anatomy while acknowledging the mind-body connection that contributes to the physiological pain response. In this case yoga is used as a complementary intervention. In contrast, another patient decides that a meditative practice that includes yoga and other lifestyle changes is more helpful than an allopathic approach to chronic pain. This patient studies these practices more deeply, adhering to one of the many schools or traditions, and decides to use them as the primary approach to manage chronic pain. In this case yoga is an alternative treatment. Several therapies are always considered alternative because they are based on completely different philosophies and life systems than those used by allopathic medicine. These are identified by the NIH/NCCIH as **whole medical systems** and include practices such as **traditional Chinese medicine (TCM)**, Ayurveda, and naturopathy (see Table 33-1).

Because of the increased interest in complementary therapies, many health care programs, including medical and nursing schools, have integrated conventional "biomedical" education with programs that incorporate complementary and alternative therapy content. Integrative health care practitioners recommend that patients receive a full spectrum of possible treatments, both biomedical and complementary. **Integrative health care** emphasizes the importance of the relationship between practitioner and patient; focuses on the whole person; is informed by evidence; and makes use of appropriate therapeutic approaches, health care professionals, and disciplines to achieve optimal health (Rakel, 2012). In an integrative health care system consumers are treated by a team of providers consisting of both biomedical and complementary practitioners.

Historically nurses have practiced in an integrative fashion; a review of nursing theory (see Chapter 4) reveals the values of holism, relational care, and informed practice. Until recently nursing identified its practice as holistic rather than integrated. Holistic nursing treats the mind-body-spirit of patients, using interventions such as relaxation therapy, music therapy, touch therapies, and guided imagery (Dossey and Keegan, 2012). The American Holistic Nurses Association (AHNA) maintains Standards of Holistic Nursing Practice, which defines and establishes the scope of holistic practice and describes the level of care expected from a holistic nurse (AHNA/ANA, 2013).

In 2014 Kreitzer and Koithan challenged the nursing profession to embrace its long-standing roots of integrative care, standing alongside our physician colleagues to transform the current health care system and offer whole-person care that is patient centered, relationship based, and supported by evidence, incorporating the best of all possible interventions. Grounded in six principles, **integrative nursing** is defined as "a way of being-knowing-doing that advances the health and well-being of people, families, and communities through caring-healing relationships. Integrative nurses use evidence to inform traditional and emerging interventions that support "whole person/whole systems healing" (Kreitzer and Koithan, 2014, p. 4).

Increasing interest in integrative health care is evident in the increased number of publications in respected health care journals and continued support of research and discovery. The mission of the NIH/NCCIH supports the investigation of the benefits and safety of integrative health solutions. Although the body of evidence about CAM is growing, limited data make it difficult to establish the specific benefits of complementary therapies. Reasons vary but reflect the growing and developing nature of the science. Therefore you need to weigh the risk and benefits of each intervention and consider the following when recommending complementary therapies: (1) the history of each

TABLE 33-1 Complementary and Integrative Therapies

Types	Definitions
Biologically Based Therapies *(Natural Products)*	
Dietary supplements	Defined by the Dietary Supplement Health and Education Act of 1994 and used to supplement dietary/nutritional intake by mouth; contain one or more dietary ingredients, including vitamins, minerals, herbs, or other botanical products
Herbal medicines	Plant-based therapies used in whole systems of medicine or as individual preparations by allopathic providers and consumers for specific symptoms or issues
Mycotherapies	Fungi-based (mushroom) products
Probiotics	Live microorganisms (in most cases, bacteria) that are similar to beneficial microorganisms found in the human gastrointestinal system; also called *good bacteria*
Energy Therapies *(Use or Manipulation of Energy Fields)*	
Healing touch	Biofield therapy; uses gentle touch directly on or close to body to influence and support the human energy system and bring balance to the whole body (physical, spiritual, emotional, and mental); a formal educational and certification system provides credentials for practitioners
Reiki therapy	Biofield therapy derived from ancient Buddhist rituals; practitioner places hands on or above a body area and transfers "universal life energy," providing strength, harmony, and balance to treat a patient's health disturbances
Therapeutic touch	Biofield therapy involving direction of a practitioner's balanced energies in an intentional manner toward those of a patient; practitioner's hands lay on or close to a patient's body

Continued

TABLE 33-1 Complementary and Integrative Therapies—cont'd

Types	Definitions
Manipulative and Body-Based Methods ***(Involve Movement of Body with Focus on Body Structures and Systems)***	
Acupressure	Applying digital pressure in a specified way on designated points on the body to relieve pain, produce analgesia, or regulate a body function
Chiropractic medicine	Manipulating the spinal column; includes physiotherapy and diet therapy
Craniosacral therapy	Assessing the craniosacral motion for rate, amplitude, symmetry, and quality and attuning/aligning the spinal column, cerebrospinal fluid, and rhythmic processes, releasing restrictions or abnormal barriers to motion
Massage therapy	Manipulating soft tissue through stroking, rubbing, or kneading to increase circulation, improve muscle tone, and provide relaxation
Mind-Body Interventions ***(Honor Connections Between Thoughts and Physiological Functioning Using Emotion to Influence Health and Well-Being)***	
Biofeedback	Process providing a person with visual or auditory information about autonomic physiological functions of the body such as muscle tension, skin temperature, and brain wave activity through the use of instruments
Breathwork	Using a variety of breathing patterns to relax, invigorate, or open emotional channels
Guided imagery	Concentrating on an image or series of images to treat pathological conditions
Meditation	Self-directed practice for relaxing the body and calming the mind with focused rhythmic breathing
Music therapy	Using music to address physical, psychological, cognitive, and social needs of individuals with disabilities and illnesses; improves physical movement and/or communication, develops emotional expression, evokes memories, and distracts people who are in pain.
Tai chi	Incorporating breath, movement, and meditation to cleanse, strengthen, and circulate vital life energy and blood; stimulate the immune system; and maintain external and internal balance
Yoga	Focuses on body musculature, posture, breathing mechanisms, and consciousness; goal is attainment of physical and mental well-being through mastery of body achieved through exercise, holding of postures, proper breathing, and meditation
Movement Therapies ***(Eastern or Western Approaches to Promote Well-Being)***	
Dance therapy	Intimate and powerful medium because it is a direct expression of the mind and body; treats people with social, emotional, cognitive, or physical problems
Pilates	Method of body movement used to strengthen, lengthen, and improve the voluntary control of muscles and muscle groups, especially those used for posture and core strengthening
Whole Medical Systems ***(Complete Systems of Theory and Practice That Have Evolved Independently from or Parallel to Allopathic [Conventional] Medicine)***	
Ayurvedic medicine	One of the oldest systems of medicine practiced in India since the first century AD. Treatments balance the doshas with a combination of dietary and lifestyle changes, herbal remedies and purgatives, massage, meditation, and exercise.
Homeopathic medicine	Developed in Germany and practiced in the United States since the mid-1800s. It is a system of medical treatments based on the theory that certain diseases can be cured by giving small, highly diluted doses of substances made from naturally occurring plant, animal, or mineral substances that stimulate the vital force of the body so it can heal itself.
Latin American traditional healing	*Curanderismo* is a Latin American traditional healing system that includes a humoral model for classifying food, activity, drugs, and illnesses and a series of folk illnesses. The goal is to create a balance between the patient and his or her environment, thereby sustaining health.
Native American traditional healing	Tribal traditions are individualistic, but similarities across traditions include the use of sweating and purging, herbal remedies, and ceremonies in which a shaman (a spiritual healer) makes contact with spirits to ask their direction in bringing healing to people to promote wholeness and healing.
Naturopathic medicine	A system of therapeutics focused on treating the whole person and promoting health and well-being rather than an individual disease. Therapeutics include herbal medicine, nutritional supplementation, physical medicine, homeopathy, lifestyle counseling, and mind-body therapies with an orientation toward assisting the person's internal capacity for self-healing (vitalism).
Traditional Chinese medicine (TCM)	An ancient healing tradition identified in the first century AD focused on balancing yin/yang energies. It is a set of systematic techniques and methods, including acupuncture, herbal medicines, massage, acupressure, moxibustion (use of heat from burning herbs), Qi gong (balancing energy flow through body movement), cupping, and massage. Fundamental concepts are from Taoism, Confucianism, and Buddhism.

BOX 33-1 EVIDENCE-BASED PRACTICE

Pain in Hospitalized Children

PICO Question: Do complementary therapies safely and effectively reduce pain and discomfort in hospitalized children?

Evidence Summary

Pain is a complex phenomenon for children, involving psychological, biological, and sociological factors. Hospitalization and pain are often linked in the minds of children. Despite advances in pediatric pain management, recent studies demonstrate that many children continue to have uncontrolled moderate-to-severe pain when they are in the hospital. Several systematic analyses focusing on the use of alternative therapies to control pain show that many complementary and nonpharmacological therapies such as relaxation, distraction, focused breathing, imagery, art therapy, and humor are effective in reducing discomfort in children who are hospitalized (Birnie et al., 2014; Thrane, 2013; Uman et al., 2013). Barriers to the use of complementary therapies included nurses' heavy workloads and the need for further education about how to use these techniques.

Application to Nursing Practice

- Children who are hospitalized often respond positively to complementary therapies, experience reduced pain, and need fewer medications to control their pain.
- Instructing parents on specific complimentary therapies used for their child's pain control (e.g., breathing techniques, art therapy) allows the parents to use these techniques.
- Nurses need to learn about and use complementary therapies such as breathing techniques and distraction to alleviate the pain associated with painful and stressful procedures, especially among children.

therapy (many have been used by cultures for thousands of years to support health and reduce suffering); (2) history and experience of nursing with a particular therapy; (3) outcomes and safety data, including case study and qualitative research (Box 33-1); and (4) the cultural influences and context for certain patient populations.

Open communication is essential to ensure safe and effective use of complementary and alternative therapies. People choose these therapies based on many reasons, including personal preference, experience of a family or friend, desire for a more holistic approach to their care, and/or a feeling that traditional medicine alone is not effective. It is important to first assess why the person chose the therapy and his or her understanding of it. For example, if it is an herbal therapy, it is important to determine if the person is taking it correctly and that the side effects or potential interaction with other medicine is known.

This chapter discusses several types of complementary and alternative therapies, including a description, the clinical applications, and the limitations of each therapy. The therapies are organized into two categories. The first are nursing-accessible therapies that you can learn and implement in patient care. The second category includes training-specific therapies such as therapeutic touch or acupressure that a nurse cannot perform without additional training and/or certification.

NURSING-ACCESSIBLE THERAPIES

Some complementary therapies and techniques are general in nature and use natural processes (e.g., breathing, thinking and concentration, presence, movement) to help people feel better and cope with both acute and chronic conditions. Ongoing assessment and evaluation of your patients' responses to these interventions will determine both the appropriateness and usefulness of these complementary therapies. Sometimes changes to physician-prescribed therapies such as medication doses are needed when complementary therapies alter physiological responses and lead to improved therapeutic responses (Kreitzer and Koithan, 2014).

Complementary therapies teach behavioral modifications that often alter physical responses to stress and improve symptoms such as muscle tension, gastrointestinal discomfort, pain, or sleep disturbances. Active involvement is a primary principle for these therapies; individuals achieve better responses if they practice the techniques or exercises daily. Therefore to achieve effective outcomes, therapeutic strategies need to be matched with an individual's lifestyle, beliefs and values, and treatment preferences.

It is important to remember that all therapies have the potential to interact with medication or other therapies currently in use. Patients need to understand what the therapy is, how it is used, and what benefits and side effects can occur. Informed consent is needed for many therapies, and the nurse needs to ensure that institutional policy is followed. Although a therapy may not be invasive, such as an injection of medication, all therapies have potential side effects.

Relaxation Therapy

People face situations in everyday life that evoke the **stress response** (see Chapter 38). The mind varies the biochemical functions of the major organ systems in response to feedback. Thoughts and feelings influence the production of chemicals (i.e., neurotransmitters, neurohormones, and peptides) that circulate throughout the body and convey messages via cells to various systems within the body. The stress response is a good example of the way in which systems cooperate to protect an individual from harm. Physiologically the cascade of changes associated with the stress response causes increased heart and respiratory rates; tightened muscles; increased metabolic rate; and a general sense of foreboding, fear, nervousness, irritability, and negative mood. Other physiological responses include elevated blood pressure; dilated pupils; stronger cardiac contractions; and increased levels of blood glucose, serum cholesterol, circulating free fatty acids, and triglycerides. Although these responses prepare a person for short-term stress, the effects on the body of long-term stress sometimes include structural damage and chronic illness such as angina, tension headaches, cardiac arrhythmias, pain, ulcers, and atrophy of the immune system organs (Kreitzer and Koithan, 2014).

The **relaxation response** is the state of generalized decreased cognitive, physiological, and/or behavioral arousal. Relaxation also involves arousal reduction. The process of relaxation elongates the muscle fibers, reduces the neural impulses sent to the brain, and thus decreases the activity of the brain and other body systems. Decreased heart and respiratory rates, blood pressure, and oxygen consumption and increased alpha brain activity and peripheral skin temperature characterize the relaxation response. It occurs through a variety of techniques that incorporate a repetitive mental focus and the adoption of a calm, peaceful attitude (Lindquist et al., 2014).

Relaxation helps individuals develop cognitive skills to reduce the negative ways in which they respond to situations within their environment. Cognitive skills include the following:

- Focusing (the ability to identify, differentiate, maintain attention on, and return attention to simple stimuli for an extended period)
- Passivity (the ability to stop unnecessary goal-directed and analytic activity)
- Receptivity (the ability to tolerate and accept experiences that are uncertain, unfamiliar, or paradoxical).

The long-term goal of relaxation therapy is for people to continually monitor themselves for indicators of tension and consciously let go and release the tension contained in various body parts.

Progressive relaxation training teaches an individual how to effectively rest and reduce tension in the body. The person learns to detect subtle localized muscle tension sequentially, one muscle group at a time (e.g., the upper arm muscles, the forearm muscles). In doing so, an individual learns to differentiate between high-intensity tension, subtle tension, and relaxation, by practicing with different muscle groups (Dossey and Keegan, 2012). One active progressive relaxation technique involves the use of slow, deep abdominal breathing while tightening and relaxing an ordered succession of muscle groups, focusing on the associated bodily sensations while letting go of extraneous thoughts. Choose a logical order when guiding a patient through progressive relaxation. For example, begin with the muscles in the face, followed by those in the arms, hands, abdomen, legs, and feet; or begin with the feet and work up the body.

The goal of **passive relaxation** is to still the mind and body intentionally without the need to tighten and relax any particular body part. One effective passive relaxation technique incorporates slow, abdominal breathing exercises while imagining warmth and relaxation flowing through specific body parts such as the lungs or hands.

Clinical Applications of Relaxation Therapy. Research shows that relaxation techniques effectively lower blood pressure and heart rate, decrease muscle tension, improve well-being, and reduce symptom distress in people experiencing a variety of situations (e.g., complications from medical treatments, chronic illness, or loss of a significant other) (Bloch et al., 2010; Jones et al., 2013). Research also indicates that relaxation, alone or in combination with imagery, yoga (Figure 33-1), and music, reduces pain and anxiety while improving well-being (Nightingale et al., 2013; Weeks and Nilsson, 2011). Other benefits of relaxation include the reduction of hypertension (Nagele et al., 2014); depression (Jorm et al., 2008); and menopausal symptoms, including vasomotor responses, insomnia, mood, and musculoskeletal pain (Innes et al., 2010).

Relaxation enables individuals to exert control over their lives. Some experience a decreased feeling of helplessness and a more positive psychological state overall. Relaxation also reduces workplace stress on nursing units, often leading to improved staff satisfaction, staff relationships and communication, and workload perceptions (Clarke et al., 2009).

Limitations of Relaxation Therapy. During relaxation training individuals learn to differentiate between low and high levels of muscle tension. During the first months of training sessions, when the person is learning how to focus on body sensations and tensions, there are reports of increased sensitivity in detecting muscle tension. Usually these feelings are minor and resolve as the person continues with the training. However, be aware that on occasion some relaxation techniques result in continued intensification of symptoms or the development of altogether new symptoms (Dossey and Keegan, 2012).

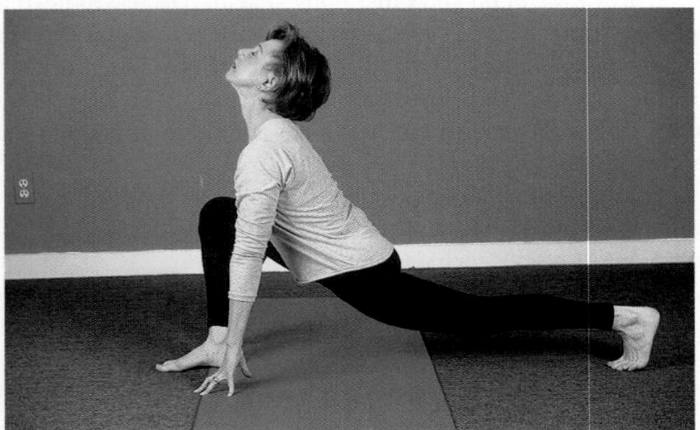

FIGURE 33-1 Yoga is a discipline that focuses on muscles, posture, breathing, and consciousness.

An important consideration when choosing a relaxation technique is the physiological and psychological status of the individual. Some patients with chronic illness such as cancer seek relaxation training to reduce their stress response. However, techniques such as active progressive relaxation require a moderate expenditure of energy, which often increases fatigue and limits an individual's ability to complete relaxation sessions and practice. Therefore active progressive relaxation is not appropriate for patients with advanced disease or decreased energy reserves. Passive relaxation or guided imagery is more appropriate for these individuals.

Meditation and Breathing

Meditation is any activity that limits stimulus input by directing attention to a single unchanging or repetitive stimulus so the person is able to become more aware of self (Lindquist et al., 2014). It is a general term for a wide range of practices that involve relaxing the body and stilling the mind. The root word, *meditari,* means to consider or pay attention to something. Although meditation has its roots in eastern religious practices (Hindu, Buddhism, and Taoism), conventional health care practitioners began to recognize its healing potential in the early 1970s (Lindquist et al., 2014). The four components of meditation were identified by Benson (1975) as (1) a quiet space, (2) a comfortable position, (3) a receptive attitude, and (4) a focus of attention. Meditation is a process that anyone can use to calm down; cope with stress; and, for those with spiritual inclinations, feel one with God or the universe.

Meditation is different from relaxation; its purpose is to become "mindful," increasing our ability to live freely and escape destructive patterns of negativity. It is self-directed; it does not necessarily require a teacher and can be learned from books or audiotapes (Kabat-Zinn, 2011). Most meditation techniques involve slow, relaxed, deep, abdominal breathing that evokes a restful state, lowers oxygen consumption, reduces respiratory and heart rates, and reduces anxiety (Chiesa and Serretti, 2010).

Clinical Applications of Meditation. Several studies support the clinical benefits of meditation. For example, meditation reduces overall systolic and diastolic blood pressures and significantly reduces hypertensive risk (Nidich et al., 2009). It has also been shown to reduce relapses in alcohol treatment programs (Bowen et al., 2009). Patients with cancer who use mindfulness-based cognitive therapies often experience less depression, anxiety, and distress and report an improved quality of life (Musial et al., 2011). Patients suffering from posttraumatic stress disorders and chronic pain also benefit from mindfulness meditation (Kim et al., 2013). In addition, meditation increases productivity, improves mood, increases sense of identity, and lowers irritability (Dossey and Keegan, 2012).

Considerations for the appropriateness of meditation include a person's degree of self-discipline; it requires ongoing practice to achieve lasting results. Most meditation activities are easy to learn and do not require memorization or particular procedures. Patients typically find mindfulness and meditation self-reinforcing. The peaceful, positive mental state is usually pleasurable and provides an incentive for individuals to continue meditating.

Limitations of Meditation. Although meditation contributes to improvement in a variety of physiological and psychological ailments, it is contraindicated for some people. For example, a person who has a strong fear of losing control can perceive it as a form of mind control and thus will be resistant to learning the technique. Some individuals also become hypertensive during meditation and require a much shorter session than the average 15- to 20-minute session.

Meditation sometimes increases the effects of certain drugs. Therefore monitor individuals learning meditation closely for physiological changes with respect to their medications. Prolonged practice of meditation techniques sometimes reduces the need for antihypertensive, thyroid-regulating, and psychotropic medications (e.g., antidepressants and antianxiety agents). In these cases adjustment of the medication is necessary.

Imagery

Imagery or visualization is a mind-body therapy that uses the conscious mind to create mental images to stimulate physical changes in the body, improve perceived well-being, and/or enhance self-awareness. Frequently imagery, combined with some form of relaxation training, facilitates the effect of the relaxation technique. Imagery can be self-directed, in which individuals create their mental images, or guided, during which a practitioner leads an individual through a particular scenario (Lindquist et al., 2014). When guiding an imagery exercise, direct a patient to begin slow abdominal breathing while focusing on the rhythm of breathing. Then direct the patient to visualize a specific image such as ocean waves coming to shore, walking along a country road with birds chirping, or sitting by a running stream with each inspiration and receding with each exhalation. Next instruct the patient to take notice of the smells, sounds, and temperatures that he or she is experiencing. As the imagery session progresses, instruct the patient to visualize warmth entering the body during inspiration and tension leaving the body during exhalation.

Imagery often evokes powerful psychophysiological responses such as alterations in gastric secretions, body chemistry, blood flow, wound healing, and heart rate (Pincus and Sheikh, 2009). Most imagery techniques involve visual images; some also include auditory, proprioceptive, gustatory, and olfactory senses. An example of this involves visualizing a lemon being sliced in half and squeezing the lemon juice on the tongue. This visualization produces increased salivation as effectively as the actual event. Creative visualization is self-directed imagery based on the principle of mind-body connectivity (i.e., every mental image leads to physical or emotional changes) (Gawain, 2002). Box 33-2 lists teaching strategies for helping patients adopt creative visualization. People typically respond to their environment according to the way they perceive it and by their own visualizations and expectancies. Therefore you need to individualize imagery for each patient (Lindquist et al., 2014).

Clinical Applications of Imagery. You can use imagery in a number of pediatric and adult patient populations. For example, it helps control or relieve pain, decrease nightmares, and improve sleep (Pincus and Sheikh, 2009). It also aids in the treatment of chronic conditions such as asthma, cancer, sickle cell anemia, migraines, autoimmune disorders, atrial fibrillation, functional urinary disorders, menstrual and premenstrual syndromes, gastrointestinal disorders such as irritable bowel syndrome and ulcerative colitis, and rheumatoid arthritis (Lindquist et al., 2014).

Limitations of Imagery. Imagery is a behavioral intervention that has relatively few side effects (Roffe et al., 2005). Yet increased anxiety and fear sometimes occur when it is used to treat post-

BOX 33-2 PATIENT TEACHING

Creative Visualization

Objective

- The patient will demonstrate skills in creative visualization.

Teaching Strategies

- Set goals the patient can meet. Success achieves confidence and increased self-esteem.
- Create a clear image. Although it is sometimes difficult to develop a visual image, if the patient views the goals of the imagery with clear thoughts and in the present tense, he or she will be more successful in creating an effective image.
- Have the patient frequently visualize the image during relaxing states and throughout the day but particularly before bedtime or on wakening, when his or her mind usually is more relaxed.
- Have the patient repeat encouraging statements while focusing on the image. This alleviates any doubts about his or her ability to achieve established goals.

Evaluation

- Observe patient behaviors for presence of anxiety or increased discomfort.
- Ask patient to describe the helpfulness of the visualization experience.
- Ask how the patient is coping with daily stressors.

traumatic stress and social anxiety disorders (Cook et al., 2010). Some patients with chronic obstructive pulmonary disease (COPD) and asthma experience increased airway constriction when using guided imagery (Reed, 2007). Thus you need to monitor patients closely when beginning this therapy.

TRAINING-SPECIFIC THERAPIES

Training-specific therapies are CAM treatments that nurses administer only after completing a specific course of study and training. These therapies require postgraduate certificates or degrees indicating completion of additional education and training, national certification, or additional licensure beyond the registered nurse (RN) to practice and administer them. Several training-specific therapies (e.g., biofeedback and acupuncture) are very effective and often recommended by western health care practitioners (NIH/NCCIH, 2015b; Giggins et al., 2013). Although many of these complementary therapies elicit positive effects, all therapies carry some risk, particularly when used in conjunction with conventional medical therapies. Therefore you need advanced knowledge to talk about them effectively with patients and provide education about their safe use.

Biofeedback

Biofeedback is a mind-body technique that uses instruments to teach self-regulation and voluntary self-control over specific physiological responses. Electronic or electromechanical instruments measure, process, and provide information to patients about their muscle tension, cardiac activity, respiratory rates, brain-wave patterns, and autonomic nervous system activity. This feedback is given in physical, physiological, auditory, and/or visual feedback signals that increase a person's awareness of internal processes that are linked to illness and distress. Biofeedback therapies can change thinking, emotions, and behaviors, which in turn support beneficial physiological changes, resulting in improved health and well-being. For example, patients connected to a biofeedback device sometimes hear a sound if their

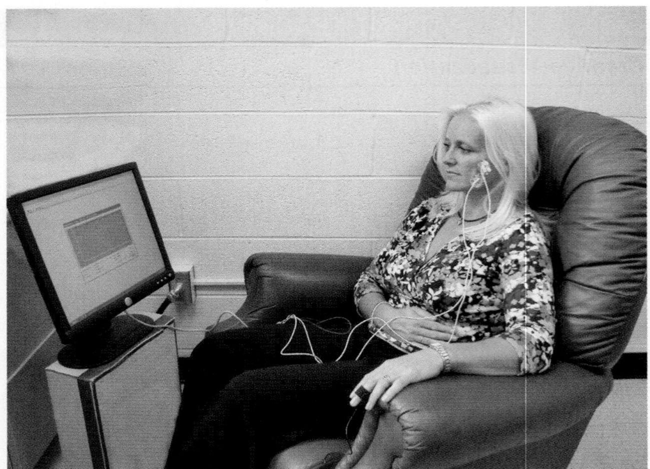

FIGURE 33-2 A patient using biofeedback can visually see how relaxation affects physiologic functions. (From Okeson JP: *Management of temporomandibular disorders and occlusion,* ed 7, St Louis, 2013, Elsevier.)

pulse rate or blood pressure increases out of their therapeutic zone. Practitioners then help patients interpret these sounds and use a variety of breathing, relaxation, and imaging exercises to gain voluntary control over their racing heart or their increasing systolic blood pressure (Lindquist et al., 2014).

Biofeedback is an effective addition to more traditional relaxation programs because it immediately demonstrates to patients their ability to control some physiological responses and the relationship among thoughts, feelings, and physiological responses. It helps individuals focus on and monitor specific body parts by providing immediate feedback about which stress-relaxation behaviors work most effectively. Eventually patients notice positive physiological changes without the need for instrument feedback. One of the most critical components of any behavioral program is adherence to a treatment regimen. Patients who are compliant have more positive results.

Biofeedback is used in numerous situations (Figure 33-2). Studies suggest that it may be helpful in stroke recovery, smoking cessation, attention deficit hyperactivity disorder (ADHD), epilepsy, headache disorders, and a variety of gastrointestinal and urinary tract disorders (Arns et al., 2009; Schoenberg and David, 2014). Although biofeedback produces effective outcomes in many patients, there are several precautions, particularly in those with psychological or neurological conditions. During biofeedback sessions repressed emotions or feelings sometimes surface. For this reason practitioners who offer biofeedback need to be trained in more traditional psychological methods or have qualified professionals available for referral. In addition, long-term use of biofeedback sometimes lowers blood pressure, heart rates, and other physiological parameters. As with other biobehavioral interventions, monitor patients closely to determine the need for medication adjustments.

Acupuncture

As a key component of TCM, **acupuncture** is one of the oldest practices in the world. When used outside of TCM, it is viewed as a mind-body therapy and is called *medical acupuncture.* In the United States medical acupuncture is often provided by specially trained health care providers.

Acupuncture regulates or realigns the **vital energy *(qi)***, which flows like a river through the body in channels that form a system of 20 pathways called meridians. An obstruction in these channels blocks energy flow in other parts of the body. Acupuncturists insert needles into the skin in specific areas along the channels called **acupoints**, through which the *qi* can be influenced and flow reestablished.

Current evidence shows that acupuncture modifies the response of the body to pain and how pain is processed by central neural pathways and cerebral function (NIH/NCCIH, 2015b). It is effective for a variety of health problems such as low back pain, myofascial pain (e.g., temporomandibular joint disorder and trigeminal neuralgia), hot flashes, simple and migraine headaches, osteoarthritis, plantar heel pain, and chronic shoulder pain (Frisk et al., 2014; Ang and Kaptchuk, 2011).

Acupuncture is a safe therapy when the practitioner has the appropriate training and uses sterilized needles. Although needle complications occur (e.g., infection, fainting), they are rare if the practitioner takes appropriate precautions. In addition, caution patients about the use of acupuncture in cases of pregnancy, history of seizures, and immunosuppression. Treatment is contraindicated in people who have bleeding disorders and skin infections.

Therapeutic Touch

Therapeutic touch (TT), developed in the 1970s, is one of the "touch therapies" identified by NCCIH. It affects the energy fields that surround and penetrate the human body with the conscious intent to help or heal (Dossey and Keegan, 2012). Blending ancient eastern traditions with modern nursing theory, TT uses the energy of the provider to positively influence the patient's energy field.

TT consists of placing a practitioner's open palms either on or close to the body of a person (Figure 33-3). It occurs in five phases: centering, assessing, unruffling, treating, and evaluating. To begin, the practitioner centers physically and psychologically, becoming fully present in the moment and quieting outside distractions. Then he or she scans the body of the patient with the palms (roughly 5 to 15 cm [2 to 6 inches] from the body) from head to toe. While assessing the patient's energetic biofield, the practitioner focuses on the quality of the *qi* and areas of energy obstructions, redirecting the energy to harmonize and move. Using long, downward strokes over the energy fields of the body, the practitioner touches the body or maintains the hands in a position a few inches away from the body. The final phase consists of evaluating the patient, ensuring that energy is flowing freely, and determining additional outcomes and responses to the treatment.

The evidence supporting the effectiveness of TT is inconclusive, although it may be effective in treating pain in adults and children, dementia, trauma, and anxiety during acute and chronic illnesses (O'Mathúna and Ashford, 2012). Box 33-3 summarizes the importance of touch in older adults. Although the use of TT causes very few complications or side effects, it is contraindicated in situations when patients are sensitive to human interaction and touch (e.g., those who have been physically abused or have psychiatric disorders).

Traditional Chinese Medicine

TCM is a whole system of medicine that began approximately 3600 years ago. Chinese medicine views health as "life in balance," which manifests as lustrous hair, a radiant complexion, engaged interactions, a body that functions without limitations, and emotional balance. Health promotion encourages healthy diet, moderate regular exercise, regular meditation/introspection, healthy family and social relationships, and avoidance of environmental toxins such as cigarette smoke.

Several concepts and principles guide the TCM system of assessment, diagnosis, and intervention. The most important of these is the concept of **yin and yang**, which represent opposing yet complementary phenomena that exist in a state of dynamic equilibrium. Examples are night/day, hot/cold, and shady/sunny. Yin represents shade, cold, and inhibition; whereas yang represents fire, light, and excitement. Yin

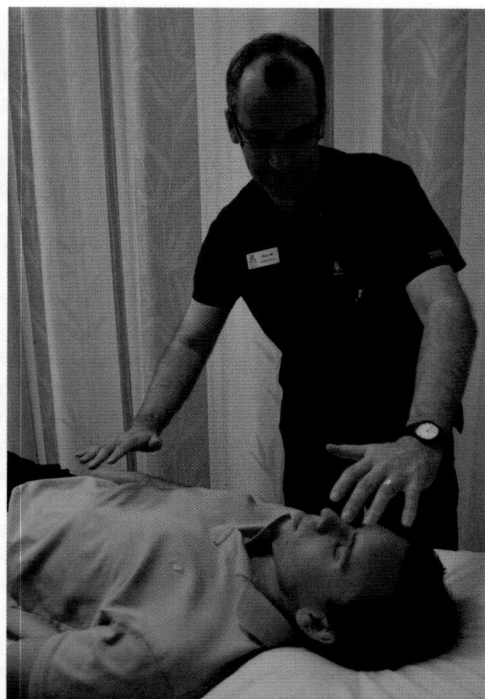

FIGURE 33-3 During a therapeutic touch session, the practitioner intentionally directs energy to facilitate the patient's healing process.

BOX 33-3 FOCUS ON OLDER ADULTS

The Importance of Touch

- Touch is a primal need, as necessary as food, growth, or shelter. It is like a nutrient transmitted through the skin, and "skin hunger" is like a form of malnutrition that has reached epidemic proportions in the United States, especially among older adults (Fontaine, 2014).
- Older adults need touch as much as or more than any other age-group. However, the elderly often experience "skin hunger." Older adults often have fewer family members or friends to touch them, especially when other senses are reduced (Dossey and Keegan, 2012).
- Simple touch helps older adults feel more connected to and accepted by those around them and more in tune with their environment. Touch enhances self-esteem and sense of worth.
- Nurses who react adversely to skin changes caused by aging often find it difficult to touch older adults. This reluctance communicates a negative message to the older adult (Dossey and Keegan, 2012). Therefore be aware of your own reactions to touch when caring for older adults to ensure a therapeutic approach to patient-centered care.

also represents the inner part of the body, specifically the viscera, liver, heart, spleen, lung, and kidney; whereas yang represents the outer part, specifically the bowels, stomach, and bladder. Harmony and balance in every aspect of life are the keys to health, including yin/yang balance. Practitioners believe that disease occurs when there is an imbalance in these two paired opposites. Imbalance occurs as excess or deficiencies in three areas: external, internal, or neither internal nor external (Table 33-2). It ultimately leads to disruption of vital energy, *qi,* which then compromises the body-mind-spirit of the person, causing *"disease."* Disruptions in *qi* along the meridians can be evaluated systematically and treated by TCM practitioners.

TCM practitioners use four methods to evaluate a patient's condition: observing, hearing/smelling, asking/interviewing, and touching/

TABLE 33-2 Three Causes of Disease According to Traditional Chinese Medicine

Cause of Disease	Influences
Internal causes	Internal causes originate in emotions and affect different organs: anger (liver), joy (heart), fear (kidney), grief/sadness (lung), pensiveness/worry (spleen), and shock (heart/kidney).
External causes	Six "evils" primarily linked to weather and climate (wind, cold, fire, damp, summer heat, and dryness) are manifested as linked patterns such as wind-cold, wind-heat, fire-toxin.
Nonexternal, noninternal causes	Additional causes of disharmony include congenital weak constitutions (birth defects), trauma, overexertion, excessive sexual activity, poor-quality diet, and parasites and poisons.

palpating. In Chinese medicine outward manifestations reflect the internal environment. For example, the color, shape, and coating of the tongue reflect the general condition of the internal organs. The pulses provide information about the condition and balance of *qi,* blood, yin and yang, and internal organs. Therapeutic modalities include acupuncture, Chinese herbs, tui na massage, **moxibustion** (burning moxa, a cone or stick of dried herbs that has healing properties on or near the skin) **cupping** (placing a heated cup on the skin to create a slight suction), **tai chi** (originally a martial art that is now viewed as a moving meditation in which patients move their bodies slowly, gently, and with awareness while breathing deeply), ***qi gong*** (originally a martial art, now viewed as a series of carefully choreographed movements or gestures that are designed to promote and manipulate the flow of *qi* within the body), lifestyle modifications, and dietary changes.

In spite of widespread use of TCM in Asia, evidence about its effectiveness is limited. Most research in this field focuses on the study of individual treatment components of TCM such as acupuncture and herbal therapies. However, some evidence shows that TCM is helpful in treating fibromyalgia (Cao et al., 2010) and addressing symptoms associated with menopause (Taylor-Swanson et al., 2014).

There is some concern about the safety of Chinese herbal treatments that are used in teas, remedies, and supplements. The U.S. Food and Drug Administration (FDA) does not regulate, inspect, or ensure that the ingredients of these herbs are safe and without toxins. Recent reports about these products suggest that many Chinese herbs are contaminated with drugs, toxins, or heavy metals or that many ingredients may not be clearly listed or labeled. Further, these herbs can be very powerful, interacting with drugs and causing serious complications. When assessing a person using TCM, you need to ask him or her about the therapies he or she receives, including the types of herbs that he or she is using. Some patients consider these as teas or dietary additives, powders, or supplements and not as over-the-counter medications.

Natural Products and Herbal Therapies

Researchers estimate that approximately 25,000 plant species are used medicinally throughout the world. It is the oldest form of medicine known to man, and archeological evidence suggests that herbal remedies have been used for over 60,000 years. Herbal medicines are a prominent part of health care worldwide.

A natural product is a chemical compound or substance produced by a living organism and includes herbal medicines (also known as botanicals), dietary supplements, vitamins, minerals, mycotherapies (fungi-based products), essential oils (aromatherapy), and probiotics. Many are sold over the counter as dietary supplements. The most frequently used products are garlic, echinacea, saw palmetto, ginkgo biloba, cranberry, soy, ginseng, black cohosh, St. John's wort, glucosamine, peppermint, fish oil/omega 3, soy, and milk thistle.

Herbal medicines are not approved for use as drugs and are not regulated by the FDA. For this reason many are sold as food or food supplements. The Dietary Supplement Health and Education Act of 1994 allows companies to sell herbs as dietary supplements as long as their labels do not contain health claims. Natural products in the United States are prepared primarily from plant materials. They are provided as tinctures or extracts, elixirs, syrups, capsules, pills, tablets, lozenges, powders, ointments or creams, drops, and suppositories.

A number of herbs are safe and effective for a variety of conditions (Table 33-3). Nurses have used cranberry juice to treat urinary tract infections for decades. Research now supports the use of cranberry supplements to prevent urinary tract infections because cranberry molecules bind with the iron that bacteria need to grow and reproduce and substances in cranberry block adherence of bacteria to the walls of the bladder (Wang et al., 2012). Chamomile is a plant substance that has been widely used in teas to promote sleep and relaxation and treat mild gastrointestinal disturbances and premenstrual symptoms. Clinical trials have recently found that chamomile may have modest benefits for people with mild-to-moderate generalized anxiety disorder (Ross, 2013).

Simply because a product is "natural" does not make it "safe." Although herbal medicines provide beneficial effects for a variety of conditions, a number of problems exist. Because they are not regulated, concentrations of the active ingredients vary considerably. Contamination with other herbs or chemicals, including pesticides and heavy metals, is also problematic. Not all companies follow strict quality control and manufacturing guidelines that set standards for acceptable levels of pesticides, residual solvents, bacterial levels, and heavy metals. For this reason, teach patients to purchase herbal medicines only from reputable manufacturers. Labels on herbal products need to contain the scientific name of the botanical, the name and address of the actual manufacturer, a batch or lot number, the date of manufacture, and the expiration date. Using natural products that have been verified by the U.S. Pharmacopeia (USP) is another way to ensure product safety, quality, and purity. Look for the USP Verified Dietary Supplement mark on product labels when buying or recommending natural products.

Some herbs also contain toxic products that have been linked to cancer. Table 33-4 lists several unsafe herbs. Some herbal substances contain powerful chemicals. As with any other medication, examine herbs for interaction and compatibility with other prescribed or over-the-counter substances that are being used simultaneously.

THE INTEGRATIVE NURSING ROLE

Interest in complementary/integrative therapies continues to increase. Most people using and seeking information about these therapies are well educated and have a strong desire to actively participate in decision making about their health care. This increased interest comes not only from health care consumers but also from mainstream physicians who have increasing concerns that current conventional medicine is not meeting the needs of their patients. Although many physicians do not refer their patients for complementary therapies because they are not familiar with them, others are beginning to recognize their benefits. Yet providers continue to have reservations about them because many have not been tested or researched adequately.

In North America and Europe professional groups are increasingly supporting the use of complementary and alternative therapies and monitoring research in this area. Priorities include assessing the public use of complementary therapies, teaching the principles of integrative health care across all professional educational programs, teaching the public to inform health care providers when using various therapeutics as self-care and health promotion strategies, improving public education about complementary therapies, and supporting studies that examine the safety and effectiveness of these therapies in a way that ensures improved quality of care. For example, if health care providers want to recommend the best treatment option for each health condition or symptom cluster, providers need to be aware of the evidence supporting complementary therapies and how to safely refer patients to complementary therapy providers. On the other hand, complementary therapy providers need to participate in the research process, working with scientists to demonstrate the effectiveness of these therapies on patient outcomes within the more rigorous framework of western science. All providers, including nurses, need to encourage open, honest dialogue about the use of complementary therapies by patients and better understand the benefits of therapies that encourage active participation by their patients in preventing or managing illness rather than relying solely on surgery or drugs.

Integrative health care, a strategy that is gaining popularity, involves interprofessional group practices in which patients receive care simultaneously from more than one type of practitioner. Patients have the option to choose the type of practitioner that they believe is beneficial for their particular health problem. Patients with the most to gain are those who have chronic health problems (e.g., fibromyalgia, chronic fatigue syndrome, or chronic pain) that have historically been difficult to treat with traditional biomedical approaches. An interprofessional group practice represents a truly integrated system in which all practitioners work side by side to improve the well-being of their patients.

This integrative approach is patient-centered and is focused on the whole person well-being and health. Nurses should be essential participants in this type of health care delivery system because many already practice the use of touch, relaxation techniques, imagery, and breathwork using the principles of integrative nursing (Kreitzer and Koithan, 2014). Familiarize yourself with the evidence in each modality that you incorporate into your practice. Know which patient is most likely to benefit from each therapy, when to use the various therapies, which complications might occur, and which precautions are needed when using these therapies.

QSEN QSEN: BUILDING COMPETENCY IN PATIENT-CENTERED CARE You are caring for a 48-year-old woman, Carmen, with stage 3 breast cancer who has returned to the hospital after being discharged after a mastectomy. She developed an infection in her suture line and around her drain site. Just before changing her dressings, you notice that she is more withdrawn and unwilling to speak more than one or two words and only to answer direct questions. When you question her further, she states that she can't stop thinking about her future and fears that "this will be how it's going to be…one hospital visit after another." She also says that she's concerned about the amount of pain medication that she's taking and that she's "tired of feeling drowsy and out-of-it" when her family comes to visit but doesn't know how else to manage her fear and pain. Which techniques could you offer Carmen to alleviate her suffering? Are there strategies that would help address her fears of the future and begin to view it in a more positive light?

Answers to QSEN Activities can be found on the Evolve website.

TABLE 33-3 Select Herbs and Corresponding Effects

Common Name and Uses	Effects	Potential Drug Interactions
Aloe		
Skin disorders, including inflammation and acute injuries (used topically)	Acceleration of wound healing	Furosemide (Lasix) and loop diuretics
GI ulcerations, including Crohn's disease and ulcerative colitis (taken orally)	Unknown mechanism, although there is a known laxative effect	May enhance effects of laxatives when taken orally
Chamomile		
Inflammatory diseases of GI and upper respiratory tracts	Antiinflammatory	Drugs that cause drowsiness (alcohol, barbiturates, benzodiazepines, narcotics, antidepressants)
Generalized anxiety disorder	Calming agent	
Echinacea		
Upper respiratory tract infections	Stimulant of immune system	Antirejection and other drugs that weaken immune system; may interact with antiretrovirals and other drugs used in treatment of HIV/AIDS
Feverfew		
Wound healing	Antiinflammatory	Warfarin (Coumadin) and blood thinners
Arthritis	Inhibition of serotonin and prostaglandins	Aspirin and ibuprofen
Garlic		
Elevated cholesterol levels	Inhibition of platelet aggregation	Warfarin and blood thinners
Hypertension		Saquinavir (Fortovase) and other anti-HIV drugs
Ginger		
Nausea and vomiting	Antiemetic	Warfarin and blood thinners Aspirin and NSAIDs
Gingko Biloba		
Alzheimer's disease and dementia	Memory improvement, although these effects are in question given results in two clinical trials (Solomon et al., 2002; Snitz et al., 2009)	Warfarin and anticoagulants; aspirin and NSAIDs
Ginseng		
Age-related diseases	Increased physical endurance, improved immune function	Warfarin and anticoagulants; aspirin and NSAIDs; MAO inhibitors
Licorice		
GI disorders, including gastric ulcers and hepatitis C	Unknown	Corticosteroids and other immunosuppressive drugs; digoxin; antihypertensive drugs
Saw Palmetto		
Benign prostatic hyperplasia	Prevention of conversion of testosterone to dihydrotestosterone (needed for prostate cell multiplication)	Finasteride (Propecia) and antiandrogen drugs
Chronic pelvic pain	Unknown mechanism	None known
Valerian		
Sleep disorders, mild anxiety, and restlessness	Central nervous system depression	Barbiturates and other sleep medications; alcohol; antihistamines

Data from National Institutes of Health/National Center for Complementary and Alternative Medicine: *Herbs at a glance*, 2014, http://nccam.nih.gov/health/herbsataglance.htm. Accessed August 19, 2014.
AIDS, Acquired immunodeficiency disease; *GI*, gastrointestinal; *HIV*, human immunodeficiency virus; *MAO*, monoamine oxidase; *NSAID*, nonsteroidal antiinflammatory drug.

TABLE 33-4 Unsafe Herbs

Common Name	Effects	Comments
Calamus (Indian type most toxic)	Fever Digestive aid	Contains varying amounts of carcinogenic *cis*-isoasarone Documented cases of kidney damage and seizures with oral preparations
Chaparral	Anticancer Used for bronchitis in traditional healing systems (Native American and Hispanic folk medicine) Found in "natural" weight-loss products	No proven efficacy Induces severe liver toxicity in some cases and severe uterine contractions
Coltsfoot	Antitussive	Contains carcinogenic pyrrolizidine alkaloids Hepatotoxic
Comfrey	Wound healing and acute injuries Used for antiinflammatory effects in osteoarthritis and rheumatoid arthritis	Contains carcinogenic pyrrolizidine alkaloids May induce venoocclusive disease Hepatotoxic
Ephedra (ma huang)	Central nervous system stimulant Bronchodilator Cardiac stimulation Weight loss	Unsafe for people with hypertension, diabetes, or thyroid disease Avoid consumption with caffeine
Life root	Menstrual flow stimulant	Hepatotoxic
Pokeweed	Antirheumatic Anticancer	Do not use with children, but many websites state that it is safe with observation, monitoring, and proper dosing; often used with folk remedies and in Native American healing

Data from National Institutes of Health/National Center for Complementary and Alternative Medicine: *Herbs at a glance,* 2014, http://nccam.nih.gov/health/herbsataglance.htm. Accessed August 19, 2014; Natural Standard, 2014, https://naturalmedicines.therapeuticresearch.com/databases/food,-herbs-supplements.aspx. Accessed August 31, 2014; US Pharmacopeia, 2014, http://www.usp.org/. Accessed July 28, 2014.

In addition, you need enough knowledge to discuss the full range of possible therapeutic options, both biomedical and complementary, so you can help patients make informed health care decisions. Always ask patients directly about their use of complementary therapies, including self-care activities such as yoga, meditation, or dietary supplements. Be knowledgeable about the evidence for different complementary therapies so you can make appropriate therapy recommendations for patients. Know about the different credentialing processes and how to refer patients to competent providers. Understand thoroughly the potential benefits and risks so you clearly and fully disclose information. Be knowledgeable so you can give advice to patients about when to seek conventional care and when it is safe to consider complementary care services. For example, if a patient complains of right lower abdominal pain, nausea, and vomiting, be suspicious of appendicitis and recommend a physician consultation. However, if the patient has a chronic gastrointestinal disorder and has a diagnosis of irritable bowel syndrome, he or she may benefit from relaxation and herbal therapy. Be aware of the safety precautions for each complementary therapy and incorporate these in your teaching plans. Finally understand your state Nurse Practice Act with regard to complementary therapies and practice only within the scope of these laws.

Nurses work very closely with their patients and are in the unique position of becoming familiar with the patient's spiritual and cultural viewpoints. They are often able to determine which complementary therapies are more appropriately aligned with these beliefs and offer recommendations accordingly. Being knowledgeable about CAM therapies will help you provide accurate information to patients and other health care professionals.

KEY POINTS

- Integrative health care programs use the full complement of treatment approaches (biomedical and complementary) when providing patient-centered care to patients.
- The stress response is an adaptive response that allows individuals to respond to stressful situations.
- Complementary therapies require commitment and regular involvement by a patient to be most effective and have prolonged beneficial outcomes.
- Choose complementary therapies appropriately according to a patient's overall health status, presenting symptom severity and distress, beliefs and cultural values, access to health care options, and insurance coverage/ability to pay.
- Continuously evaluate a patient's response to complementary therapies because medication doses may need to change on the basis of physiological responses.
- Complementary therapies accessible to nursing include relaxation, meditation and mindfulness techniques, and imagery.
- Many complementary therapies require additional education and certification, including biofeedback, touch therapies, and acupuncture.
- Although there is increasing evidence to support the use of complementary therapies, additional research of sufficient quality and rigor is needed.

CLINICAL APPLICATION QUESTIONS

Preparing for Clinical Practice

1. Margaret Thompson is a 76-year-old Catholic woman who was diagnosed with a slow-growing renal tumor. She is scheduled for surgery. You are responsible for the admission assessment and initial care for this patient. Which assessment questions about complementary and alternative therapies will you include during this preoperative period?
2. During the initial assessment Ms. Thompson asks many questions. "Is it cancer? Will the surgery result in a disability? What can I expect? Will I have to be in the intensive care unit (ICU)?" You conclude that she is afraid of both the surgical procedure and the

outcome. Which types of specific nursing-accessible complementary therapies will you offer her during the preoperative period to reduce her anxiety and help her prepare for surgery?

3. In the days following surgery you are assigned to care for Ms. Thompson. Although physically she is recovering quite well from the procedure, you note that she is becoming more despondent and depressed. Preparing for discharge, which complementary and alternative medicine (CAM) therapies do you recommend to help her deal with her depression and cancer diagnosis?

ⓔ *Answers to Clinical Application Questions can be found on the Evolve website.*

REVIEW QUESTIONS

Are You Ready to Test Your Nursing Knowledge?

1. When planning patient education, it is important to remember that patients with which of the following illnesses often find relief in complementary therapies?
   1. Lupus and diabetes
   2. Ulcers and hepatitis
   3. Heart disease and pancreatitis
   4. Chronic back pain and arthritis
2. Which complementary therapies are most easily learned and applied by a nurse? (Select all that apply.)
   1. Massage therapy
   2. Traditional Chinese medicine
   3. Progressive relaxation
   4. Breathwork and guided imagery
   5. Therapeutic touch
3. Which statement best describes the evidence associated with complementary therapies as a whole?
   1. Many clinical trials in complementary therapies support their effectiveness in a wide range of clinical problems.
   2. It is difficult to find funding for studies about complementary therapies. Therefore we should not expect to find evidence supporting its use.
   3. The science supporting the effectiveness of complementary therapies is early in its development.
   4. Most of the research examining complementary and alternative therapies has found little evidence, suggesting that, although people like them, they are not effective.
4. While planning care for a patient, a nurse understands that providing integrative care includes treating which of the following?
   1. Disease, spirit, and family interactions
   2. Desires and emotions of the patient
   3. Mind-body-spirit of patients and their families
   4. Muscles, nerves, and spine disorders
5. In addition to an adequate patient assessment, when a nurse uses one of the nursing-accessible complementary therapies, he or she must ensure that which of the following has occurred?
   1. The family has provided permission.
   2. The patient has provided permission and consent.
   3. The health care provider has given approval or provided orders for the therapy.
   4. He or she has documented that the patient has a complete understanding of complementary and alternative medicine.
6. What role do patients have in complementary and alternative therapies?
   1. Submissive to the practitioner
   2. Actively involved in the treatment
   3. Allow practitioner to experiment
   4. Total believer in what is being taught
7. A nurse is caring for a patient experiencing a stress response. The nurse plans care with the knowledge that systems respond to stress in what manner? (Select all that apply.)
   1. Always fail and cause illness and disease
   2. Cause negative responses over time
   3. React the same way for all individuals
   4. Protect an individual from harm in the short term
8. Meditation may compound the effects of which of these medications?
   1. Prednisone and antibiotics
   2. Insulin and vitamins
   3. Cough syrups and aspirin
   4. Antihypertensive and thyroid-regulating medications
9. A patient who has been using relaxation wants a better response. The nurse recommends the addition of biofeedback. What is the expected outcome related to using this additional modality?
   1. To eat less food
   2. To control diabetes
   3. To live longer with acquired immunodeficiency syndrome (AIDS)
   4. To learn how to control some autonomic nervous system responses
10. Which of the following statements best explains the actions of therapeutic touch (TT)?
    1. Intentionally mobilizes energy to balance, harmonize, and repattern the recipient's biofield
    2. Intentionally heals specific diseases or corrects certain symptoms
    3. Is overwhelmingly effective in many conditions
    4. Is completely safe and does not warrant any special precautions
11. Traditional Chinese medicine (TCM) is used by many patients. Which statement most accurately describes intervention(s) offered by TCM providers?
    1. Uses acupuncture as its primary intervention modality
    2. Uses many modalities based on the individual's needs
    3. Uses primarily herbal remedies and exercise
    4. Is the equivalent of medical acupuncture
12. A nurse is planning care for a group of patients who have requested the use of complementary health modalities. Which patient is not a good candidate for guided imagery?
    1. Pregnant patient
    2. Hypertensive patient
    3. Patient with post-traumatic stress disorder (PTSD)
    4. A pediatric patient
13. Several nurses on a busy unit are using relaxation strategies while at work. What is the desired workplace outcome from this intervention? (Select all that apply.)
    1. Improved health among the staff
    2. Increased patient safety
    3. Improved staff satisfaction
    4. Improved staff relationships
    5. Fewer overtime assignments
14. A nursing professor is teaching a nursing student about caring patients who use herbal preparations in addition to prescribed medications. Which of the following statements made by the student indicates that the student understands herbal preparations?
    1. "Herbal preparations are regulated by the Food and Drug Administration (FDA); therefore I need to tell patients that they are completely safe."
    2. "They are natural products and therefore are safe as long as you use them for the conditions that are indicated."
    3. "These preparations are covered by insurance, including Medicare, Medicaid, and private payers."

4. "We need to treat herbal preparations as though they are "drugs" because many have active ingredients that can interact with other medications and change physiological responses."

15. The nurse manager of a community clinic arranges for staff in-services about various complementary therapies available in the community. What is the purpose of this training? (Select all that apply.)
    1. Nurses have a long history of providing some of these therapies and need to be knowledgeable about their positive outcomes.
    2. Nurses are often asked for recommendations and strategies that promote well-being and quality of life.
    3. Nurses play an essential role in patient education to provide information about the safe use of these healing strategies.
    4. Nurses appreciate the cultural aspects of care and recognize that many of these complementary strategies are part of a patient's life.
    5. Nurses play an essential role in the safe use of complementary therapies.
    6. Nurses learn how to provide all of the complementary modalities during their basic education.

Answers: 1. 4; **2.** 3, 4; **3.** 3; **4.** 3; **5.** 2; **6.** 2; **7.** 2, 4; **8.** 4; **9.** 4; **10.** 1; **11.** 2; **12.** 3; **13.** 3, 4; **14.** 4; **15.** 1, 2, 3, 4, 5.

Rationales for Review Questions can be found on the Evolve website.

REFERENCES

American Holistic Nursing Association/American Nurses Association (AHNA/ANA): *Holistic nursing: scope and standards of practice*, ed 2, Silver Spring, MD, 2013, American Nurses Publishing.

Benson H: *The relaxation response*, New York, 1975, Avon.

Dossey B, Keegan L: *Holistic nursing: a handbook for practice*, ed 6, Boston, MA, 2012, Jones & Bartlett.

Fontaine K: *Complementary and alternative therapies for nursing practice, healing practices: alternative therapies for nursing*, ed 4, Upper Saddle River, NJ, 2014, Prentice Hall.

Gawain S: *Creative visualization: use the power of your imagination to create what you want in your life*, Novato, CA, 2002, New World Library.

Kabat-Zinn J: *Mindfulness for beginners*, Boulder, CO, 2011, Sounds True Publishing.

Koithan M: Let's talk about complementary and alternative therapies, *J Nurse Pract* 5(3):214, 2009.

Kreitzer MJ, Koithan M: *Integrative Nursing*, New York, 2014, Oxford Press.

Lindquist R, et al: *Complementary and alternative therapies in nursing*, ed 7, New York, 2014, Springer.

National Institutes of Health/National Center for Complementary and Integrative Health (NIH/NCCIH): *Complementary, alternative, or integrative health: what's in a name?*, 2015a, https://nccih.nih.gov/health/integrative-health/. Accessed June 29, 2015.

National Institutes of Health/National Center for Complementary and Integrative Health (NIH/NCCIH): *Acupuncture: what you need to know*, 2015b, https://nccih.nih.gov/health/acupuncture/introduction. Accessed June 29, 2015.

Pincus D, Sheikh AA: *Imagery for pain relief: a scientifically grounded guidebook for clinicians*, New York, 2009, Routledge, Taylor & Francis Group.

Rakel D: *Integrative medicine*, ed 3, Philadelphia, PA, 2012, Elsevier.

RESEARCH REFERENCES

Ang L, Kaptchuk TJ: The case of acupuncture for chronic low back pain: when efficacy and comparative effectiveness conflict, *Spine* 36(3):181, 2011.

Arns M, et al: Efficacy of neurofeedback treatment in ADHD: the effects on inattention, impulsivity and hyperactivity: a meta-analysis, *Clin EEG Neurosci* 40(3):180, 2009.

Birnie KA, et al: Systematic review and meta-analysis of distraction and hypnosis for needle-related pain and distress in children and adolescents, *J Pediatr Psychol* 39(8):783, 2014.

Bloch B, et al: The effects of music relaxation on sleep quality and emotional measures in people living with schizophrenia, *J Music Ther* 47(1):27, 2010.

Bowen S, et al: Mindfulness-based relapse prevention for substance use disorders: a pilot efficacy trial, *Subst Abuse* 30(4):295, 2009.

Cao H, et al: Traditional Chinese medicine for treatment of fibromyalgia: a systematic review of randomized controlled trials, *J Altern Complement Med* 16(4):397, 2010.

Centers for Disease Control and Prevention (CDC): *NCHS data brief: mortality in the United States, 2012*, 2014, http://www.cdc.gov/nchs/data/databriefs/db168.htm. Accessed August 6, 2015.

Chiesa A, Serretti A: A systematic review of neurobiological and clinical features of mindfulness meditations, *Psychol Med* 40(8):1239, 2010.

Clarke PN, et al: From theory to practice: caring science according to Watson and Brewer, *Nurs Sci Q* 22(4):339, 2009.

Cook JM, et al: Imagery rehearsal for posttraumatic nightmares: a randomized controlled trial, *Trauma Stress* 23(5):553, 2010.

Frisk JW, et al: How long do the effects of acupuncture on hot flashes persist in cancer patients?, *Support Care Cancer* 22(5):1409, 2014.

Giggins OM, et al: Biofeedback in rehabilitation, *J Neuroeng Rehabil* 10(60):2013.

Innes KE, et al: Mind-body therapies for menopausal symptoms: a systematic review, *Maturitas* 66(2):135, 2010.

Jones M, et al: Breathing exercises for dysfunctional breathing/hyperventilation syndrome in adults, *Cochrane Database Syst Rev* (5):CD009041, 2013.

Jorm AF, et al: Relaxation for depression, *Cochrane Database Syst Rev* (4):CD007142, 2008.

Kim SH, et al: Mind-body practices for posttraumatic stress disorder, *J Investig Med* 61(5):827, 2013.

Musial F, et al: Mindfulness-based stress reduction for integrative cancer care: a summary of evidence, *Forsch Komplementmed* 18(4):192, 2011.

Nagele E, et al: Clinical effectiveness of stress-reduction techniques in patients with hypertension: systematic review and meta-analysis, *J Hypertens* 32(10):1936, 2014.

Nidich SI, et al: A randomized controlled trial on effects of the transcendental meditation program on blood pressure, psychological distress, and coping in young adults, *Am J Hypertens* 22(12):1326, 2009.

Nightingale CL, et al: The impact of music interventions on anxiety for adult cancer patients: a meta-analysis and systematic review, *Integr Cancer Ther* 12(5):393, 2013.

O'Mathúna DP, Ashford RL: Therapeutic touch for healing acute wounds, *Cochrane Database Syst Rev* 13(6):CD002766, 2012.

Reed T: Imagery in the clinical setting: a tool for healing, *Nurs Clin North Am* 42(2):261, 2007.

Roffe L, et al: A systematic review of guided imagery as an adjuvant cancer therapy, *Psycho-Oncol* 14(8):607, 2005.

Ross S: Efficacy of standardized matricaria recutita (German chamomile) extract in the treatment of generalized anxiety disorder, *Holist Nurs Pract* 27(6):366, 2013.

Schoenberg PL, David AS: Biofeedback for psychiatric disorders: a systematic review, *Appl Psychophysiol Biofeedback* 39(2):109, 2014.

Snitz BE, et al: Ginkgo biloba for preventing cognitive decline in older adults: a randomized trial, *JAMA* 302(24):2663, 2009.

Solomon PR, et al: Ginkgo for memory enhancement: a randomized controlled trial, *JAMA* 288(7):835, 2002.

Taylor-Swanson L, et al: Effects of traditional Chinese medicine on symptom clusters during the menopausal transition, *Climacteric* 18(2):1, 2014.

Thrane S: Effectiveness of integrative modalities for pain and anxiety in children and adolescents with cancer: a systematic review, *J Pediatr Oncol Nurs* 30(6):320, 2013.

Uman LS, et al: Psychological interventions for needle-related procedural pain and distress in children and adolescents, *Cochrane Database Syst Rev* (10):CD005179, 2013.

Wang CH, et al: Cranberry-containing products for prevention of urinary tract infections in susceptible populations: a systematic review and meta-analysis of randomized controlled trials, *Arch Intern Med* 172(13):988, 2012.

Weeks BP, Nilsson U: Music interventions in patients during coronary angiographic procedures: a randomized controlled study of the effect on patients' anxiety and well-being, *Eur J Cardiovasc Nurs* 10(2):88, 2011.

34

Self-Concept

OBJECTIVES

- Discuss factors that influence the components of self-concept.
- Identify stressors that affect self-concept and self-esteem.
- Describe the components of self-concept as related to psychosocial and cognitive developmental stages.
- Explore ways in which a nurse's self-concept and nursing actions affect a patient's self-concept and self-esteem.
- Discuss evidence-based practices applicable for identity confusion, disturbed body image, low self-esteem, and role conflict.
- Examine cultural considerations that affect self-concept.
- Apply the nursing process to promote a patient's self-concept.

KEY TERMS

Body image, p. 703
Identity, p. 703
Identity confusion, p. 705
Role ambiguity, p. 705
Role conflict, p. 705
Role overload, p. 706
Role performance, p. 704
Role strain, p. 706
Self-concept, p. 701
Self-esteem, p. 704
Sick role, p. 705

MEDIA RESOURCES

http://evolve.elsevier.com/Potter/fundamentals/

- Review Questions
- Concept Map Creator
- Case Study with Questions
- Audio Glossary
- Content Updates

Self-concept is an individual's view of self. It is subjective and involves a complex mixture of unconscious and conscious thoughts, attitudes, and perceptions. Self-concept, or how a person *thinks* about oneself, directly affects self-esteem, or how one *feels* about oneself. Although these two terms often are used interchangeably, nurses need to differentiate the two so they correctly and completely assess a patient and develop an individualized plan of care on the basis of the patient's needs.

Patients face a variety of health problems that threaten their self-concept and self-esteem. The loss of bodily function, decline in activity tolerance, and difficulty managing a chronic illness are examples of situations that change a patient's self-concept. You will help patients adjust to alterations in self-concept and strengthen components of self-concept to promote successful coping and positive health outcomes.

SCIENTIFIC KNOWLEDGE BASE

The development and maintenance of self-concept and self-esteem begin at a young age and continue across the life span. Parents and other primary caregivers influence the development of a child's self-concept and self-esteem. In addition, individuals learn and internalize cultural influences on self-concept and self-esteem in childhood and adolescence. There is a significant emphasis on fostering a school-age child's self-concept. In general young children tend to rate themselves higher than they rate other children, suggesting that their view of themselves is positively inflated. Adolescence is a particularly critical developmental period when many variables, including school, family, and friends, affect self-concept and self-esteem (Mantilla et al., 2014). The adolescent experience can adversely affect self-esteem, often more strongly for girls than for boys. For example, some adolescent girls are more sensitive about their appearance and how others view them. Thus it is important to assess changes in identity formation and self-esteem among early, middle, and late adolescence because changes in self-concept occur over time (Figure 34-1).

Job satisfaction and overall performance in adulthood are also linked to self-esteem. Self-expanding opportunities such as exploring new ideas, solving problems in creative ways, and learning new skills predict job satisfaction and commitment and promote self-concept clarity and self-esteem (McIntyre et al., 2014). Sometimes when individuals lose a job, their sense of self diminishes, they lose motivation to be socially active, and they even become depressed. They lose their job identity, and this alters their self-perceptions and self-care practices. Establishing a stable sense of self that transcends relationships and situations is a developmental goal of adulthood.

Cultural variations in self-concept and self-esteem across the life span can impact health behaviors. In adolescent girls cultural pride and self-esteem serve as protective factors against risk behaviors, including intentions to have sexual intercourse (Pai and Lee, 2012). Cultural identity of older adults is one of the major elements of self-concept and a key aspect of self-esteem (Touhy and Jett, 2014). Be aware of the cultural perspectives of aging when providing patient care. Sensitivity to factors that affect self-concept and self-esteem in diverse cultures is essential to ensure an individualized approach to health care.

How individuals view themselves and their perception of their health are closely related. Lower self-esteem is a risk factor that leaves

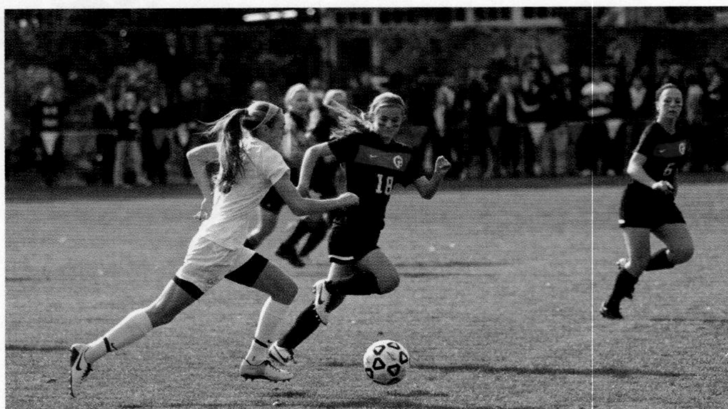

FIGURE 34-1 Adolescents' participation in group activities can foster self-esteem. (iStock.com/Bastiaan Slabbers.)

one vulnerable to health problems, whereas higher self-esteem and strong social relationships support good health. A patient's belief in personal health often enhances his or her self-concept. Statements such as, "I can get through anything" or "I've never been sick a day in my life" indicate that a person's thoughts about personal health are positive. Illness, hospitalization, and surgery affect self-concept. Chronic illness often affects the ability to provide financial support and maintain relationships, which then affects an individual's self-esteem and perceived roles within the family. Negative perceptions regarding health status are reflected in such statements as, "It's not worth it anymore" or "I'm a burden to my family." Furthermore, chronic illness affects identity and body image as reflected by verbalizations such as, "I'll never get any better" or "I can't stand to look at myself anymore."

What individuals think and how they feel about themselves affect the way in which they approach self-care physically and emotionally and how they care for others. Furthermore, a person's behaviors are generally consistent with both self-concept and self-esteem. Individuals who have a poor self-concept often do not feel in control of situations and worthy of care, which influences decisions regarding health care. Patients often have difficulty making even simple decisions such as what to eat. Knowledge of variables that affect self-concept and self-esteem is critical to provide effective treatment.

BOX 34-1 Self-Concept: Developmental Tasks

Trust versus Mistrust (Birth to 1 Year)
- Develops trust following consistency in caregiving and nurturing interactions
- Distinguishes self from environment

Autonomy versus Shame and Doubt (1 to 3 Years)
- Begins to communicate likes and dislikes
- Increasingly independent in thoughts and actions
- Appreciates body appearance and function (e.g., dressing, feeding, talking, and walking)

Initiative versus Guilt (3 to 6 Years)
- Identifies with a gender
- Enhances self-awareness
- Increases language skills, including identification of feelings

Industry versus Inferiority (6 to 12 Years)
- Incorporates feedback from peers and teachers
- Increases self-esteem with new skill mastery (e.g., reading, mathematics, sports, music)
- Aware of strengths and limitations

Identity versus Role Confusion (12 to 20 Years)
- Accepts body changes/maturation
- Examines attitudes, values, and beliefs; establishes goals for the future
- Feels positive about expanded sense of self

Intimacy versus Isolation (Mid-20s to Mid-40s)
- Has stable, positive feelings about self
- Experiences successful role transitions and increased responsibilities

Generativity versus Self-Absorption (Mid-40s to Mid-60s)
- Able to accept changes in appearance and physical endurance
- Reassesses life goals
- Shows contentment with aging

Ego Integrity versus Despair (Late 60s to Death)
- Feels positive about life and its meaning
- Interested in providing a legacy for the next generation

NURSING KNOWLEDGE BASE

In providing evidence-based practices to patients, incorporate professional nursing knowledge developed from the humanities, sciences, nursing research, and clinical practice. A broad knowledge base allows nurses to have a holistic view of patients, thus promoting quality patient care that best meets the self-concept needs of each patient and family. Understanding a patient's self-concept is a necessary part of all nursing care (Stuart, 2013).

Factors Influencing the Development of Self-Concept

The development of self-concept is a complex lifelong process that involves many factors. Erikson's psychosocial theory of development (1963) remains beneficial in understanding key tasks that individuals face at various stages of development. Each stage builds on the tasks of the previous stage. Successful mastery of each stage leads to a solid sense of self (Box 34-1).

Learn to recognize an individual's failure to achieve an age-appropriate developmental stage or his or her regression to an earlier stage in a period of crisis. This understanding allows you to individualize care and determine appropriate nursing interventions. Self-concept is always changing and is based on the following:

- Sense of competency
- Perceived reactions of others to one's body
- Ongoing perceptions and interpretations of the thoughts and feelings of others
- Personal and professional relationships
- Academic and employment-related identity
- Personality characteristics that affect self-expectations
- Perceptions of events that have an impact on self
- Mastery of prior and new experiences
- Cultural identity

Self-esteem is often highest in childhood, fluctuates during adolescence, gradually rises throughout adulthood, and either diminishes or increases again in old age, depending on self-concept clarity (Diehl and Hay, 2011; Stuart, 2013). Although this pattern varies, in general it holds true across gender, socioeconomic status, and culture. Children often report high self-esteem because their sense of self is inflated by a variety of extremely positive sources, and periodic declines may be associated with shifts to more realistic information about the self. Adolescence is a time of marked maturational changes and shifting levels of self-esteem that set the stage for rises in self-concept in young adulthood (Maldonado et al., 2013).

Erikson's emphasis on the generativity stage (1963) (see Chapter 11) explains the rise in self-esteem and self-concept in adulthood. The individual focuses on being increasingly productive and creative at work while at the same time promoting and guiding the next generation. On the basis of Erikson's stages of development, a decline in self-concept in later adulthood reflects a diminished need for self-promotion and a shift in self-concept to a more modest and balanced view of self. Many report a decline in self-esteem in later adulthood caused in part by physical and emotional changes associated with aging, but older adults with self-concept clarity demonstrate psychological well-being (Diehl and Hay, 2011; Touhy and Jett, 2014). When aging is associated with deterioration of health, nursing interventions must focus on health behavior changes to promote self-care and self-concept (Wurm et al., 2013). Identifying specific nursing interventions to address the unique needs of patients at various life stages is essential.

Components and Interrelated Terms of Self-Concept

A positive self-concept gives a sense of meaning, wholeness, and consistency to a person. A healthy self-concept has a high degree of stability, which generates positive feelings toward self. The components of self-concept are identity, body image, and role performance. Because how one thinks about oneself (self-concept) affects how one feels about oneself (self-esteem), both concepts need to be evaluated.

Identity. Identity involves the internal sense of individuality, wholeness, and consistency of a person over time and in different situations. It implies being distinct and separate from others. Being "oneself" or living an authentic life is the basis of true identity. Children learn culturally accepted values, behaviors, and roles through identification and modeling. They often gain an identity from self-observations and from what individuals tell them. An individual first identifies with parenting figures and later with other role models such as teachers or peers. Relationships with parents, teachers, and peers have unique and combined effects on young children's general, academic, and social self-concept (Verschueren et al., 2012). To form an identity, a child must be able to bring together learned behaviors and expectations into a coherent, consistent, and unique whole (Erikson, 1963).

The achievement of identity is necessary for intimate relationships because individuals express identity in relationships with others (Stuart, 2013). Sexuality is a part of identity, and its focus differs across the life span. For example, as an adult ages the focus shifts from procreation to companionship, physical and emotional intimacy, and pleasure seeking (Touhy and Jett, 2014). Gender identity is a person's private view of maleness or femaleness; gender role is the masculine or feminine behavior exhibited. This image and its meaning depend on culturally determined values (see Chapters 9 and 22).

Cultural differences in identity exist (Box 34-2). Cultural identity develops from identification and socialization within an established group and through the experience of integrating the response of individuals outside the group into one's self-concept. Differences in cultural identity (e.g., Mexican American or Cuban American, homosexual or heterosexual) exist through identification with traditions, customs, and rituals within one's cultural group (e.g., Hispanic, Latino, gender identity). When cultural identity is central to self-concept and is positive, cultural pride and self-esteem tend to be strong (Rhea and Thatcher, 2013). An individual who experiences discrimination, prejudice, or environmental stressors such as low-income or high-crime neighborhoods often conceptualizes himself or herself differently than an individual who experiences better living conditions.

BOX 34-2 CULTURAL ASPECTS OF CARE

Promoting Self-Concept and Self-Esteem in Culturally Diverse Patients

Cultural identity is an important component of a person's self-concept and self-esteem. Early in growth and development an individual develops this identity within the context of family. As an individual matures, the cultural aspects of his or her self-concept are reinforced through social, family, or cultural experiences. In addition, a person's self-concept is strengthened or questioned through political, social, or cultural influences experienced in the home, school, and workplace environments. Positive or negative cultural role modeling, identity, and past experiences influence self-care, self-concept, and self-esteem (Rhea and Thatcher, 2013).

Implications for Patient-Centered Care

- Develop an open, nonrestrictive attitude for assessing and encouraging cultural practices to improve patients' self-concept.
- Understand that the relationship among self-esteem, stress, and social support can facilitate the development of nursing strategies to promote effective coping in culturally diverse adolescents (Rhea and Thatcher, 2013).
- Ask patients what they think is important to help them feel better or gain a stronger sense of self.
- Encourage cultural identity and pride by individualizing self-care practices and offering treatment choices to meet patients' self-concept needs.
- Facilitate culturally sensitive health promotion activities that address at-risk behaviors identified through evidence-based practice (e.g., smoking, drinking, eating disorder risks, premature sexual experiences, excessive and violent video gaming (Dudovitz et al., 2013).

Body Image. Body image involves attitudes related to the body, including physical appearance, structure, or function. Feelings about body image include those related to sexuality, femininity and masculinity, youthfulness, health, and strength. These mental images are not always consistent with a person's actual physical structure or appearance. Some body image distortions have deep psychological origins such as the eating disorder anorexia nervosa. Other alterations occur as a result of situational events such as the loss or change in a body part. Be aware that most men and women experience some degree of dissatisfaction with their bodies, which affects body image and overall self-concept. Individuals often exaggerate disturbances in body image when a change in health status occurs. The way others view a person's body and the feedback offered are also influential. For example, a controlling, violent husband tells his wife that she is ugly and that no one else would want her. Over the years of marriage she incorporates this devaluation into her self-concept.

Cognitive growth and physical development also affect body image. Normal developmental changes such as puberty and aging have a more apparent effect on body image than on other aspects of self-concept. Hormonal changes during adolescence influence body image. The development of secondary sex characteristics and the changes in body fat distribution have a tremendous impact on an adolescent's self-concept. For both male and female adolescents, negative body image is a risk factor for many psychological conditions that impact health behaviors. For example, an adolescent girl may have a distorted body image and view herself as fat, which signals an eating disorder. Your assessment may reveal that an adolescent engages in self-harmful

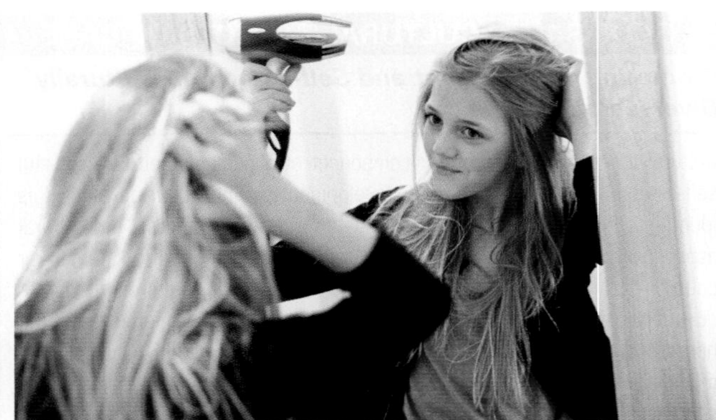

FIGURE 34-2 An individual's appearance influences self-concept. (iStock.com/stocknroll.)

behaviors such as cutting; self-mutilation can indicate self-concept and self-esteem issues that warrant nursing intervention (Rissanen et al., 2011). A threat to body image and overall self-concept can affect adherence to recommended health regimens, including diet, exercise, health screening practices, and taking medications as prescribed. Changes associated with aging (e.g., menopause; wrinkles; graying hair; and decrease in visual acuity, hearing, and mobility) also affect body image in an older adult.

Cultural and societal attitudes and values influence body image. Culture and society dictate the accepted norms of body image and influence one's attitudes (Figure 34-2). Cultural background plays an integral role in body satisfaction in adolescent girls and is reflected in differences in body satisfaction among groups. For example, identification with and pride in their cultural background can act as a partial buffer against advertisements, magazines, television, and movies depicting the thin-ideal white image and help Latina teenage girls feel more comfortable with themselves and their appearance (Schooler and Daniels, 2014). Furthermore, body image is more favorable in cultures in which girls describe more reasonable views about physical appearance, report less social pressure for thinness, and have less tendency to base self-esteem on body image. Low self-concept clarity increases a women's vulnerability to body image issues as a result of the internalization of the thin-ideal and appearance-related social comparisons (Vartanian and Dey, 2013). Values such as ideal body weight and shape and attitudes toward piercing and tattoos are culturally based. American society emphasizes youth, beauty, and wholeness. Western cultures have been socialized to dread the normal aging process, whereas eastern cultures view aging very positively and respect older adults. Body image issues are often associated with impaired self-concept and self-esteem.

Role Performance. Role performance is the way in which individuals perceive their ability to carry out significant roles (e.g., parent, supervisor, partner, or close friend). Normal changes associated with maturation result in changes in role performance. For example, when a man has a child, he becomes a father. The new role of father requires many changes in behavior if the man is going to be successful. Roles that individuals follow in given situations involve socialization, expectations, or standards of behavior. The patterns are stable and change only minimally during adulthood.

Ideal societal role behaviors are often hard to achieve in real life. Individuals have multiple roles and personal needs that sometimes conflict. Successful adults learn to distinguish between ideal role expectations and realistic possibilities. To function effectively in multiple roles, a person must know the expected behavior and values, desire to conform to them, and be able to meet the role requirements. Fulfillment of role expectations leads to an enhanced sense of self. Difficulty or failure to meet role expectations leads to deficits and often contributes to decreased self-esteem or altered self-concept.

Self-Esteem. Self-esteem is an individual's overall feeling of self-worth or the emotional appraisal of self-concept. It is the most fundamental self-evaluation because it represents the overall judgment of personal worth or value. Self-esteem is positive when one feels capable, worthwhile, and competent. A person's self-esteem is related to his or her evaluation of his or her effectiveness at school, within the family, and in social settings. The evaluation of others also is likely to have a profound influence on a person's self-esteem.

Considering the relationship between a person's actual self-concept and his or her ideal self enhances understanding of that person's self-esteem. The ideal self consists of the aspirations, goals, values, and standards of behavior that a person considers ideal and strives to attain. In general, a person whose self-concept comes close to matching the ideal self has high self-esteem, whereas a person whose self-concept varies widely from the ideal self suffers from low self-esteem (Stuart, 2013). Once established, basic feelings about the self tend to be constant, even though a situational crisis can temporarily affect self-esteem.

Factors Influencing Self-Concept

A self-concept stressor is any real or perceived change that threatens identity, body image, or role performance (Figure 34-3). An individual's perception of the stressor is the most important factor in determining his or her response. The ability to reestablish balance following a stressor is related to numerous factors, including the number of stressors, duration of the stressor, and health status (see Chapter 38). Stressors challenge a person's adaptive capacities. Changes that occur in physical, spiritual, emotional, sexual, familial, and sociocultural health affect self-concept. Being able to successfully adapt to stressors is likely to lead to a positive sense of self, whereas failure to adapt often leads to a negative self-concept.

Any change in health is a stressor that potentially affects self-concept. A physical change in the body sometimes leads to an altered body image, affecting identity and self-esteem. Chronic illnesses often alter role performance, which change an individual's identity and self-esteem. An essential process in the adjustment to loss is the development of a new self-concept. A loss of a partner can lead to a loss of identity and a lower self-esteem. Unlike the loss in self-esteem shown in vulnerable older adults, the resiliency demonstrated in some older adults may reflect more sophisticated cognitive strategies to manage losses.

The stressors created as a result of a crisis also affect a person's health. If the resulting identity confusion, disturbed body image, low self-esteem, or role conflict is not relieved, illness can result. For example, the diagnosis of cancer places additional demands on a person's established living pattern. It changes his or her appraisal of and satisfaction with the current level of physical, emotional, and social functioning. Assess self-esteem, effectiveness of coping strategies, and social support in all patients. During self-concept crises, supportive and educative resources are valuable in helping a person learn new ways of coping with and responding to the stressful event or situation to maintain or enhance self-concept.

Identity Stressors. Stressors affect an individual's identity throughout life, but individuals are particularly vulnerable during adolescence. Adolescents are trying to adjust to the physical, emotional, and mental changes of increasing maturity, which results in insecurity

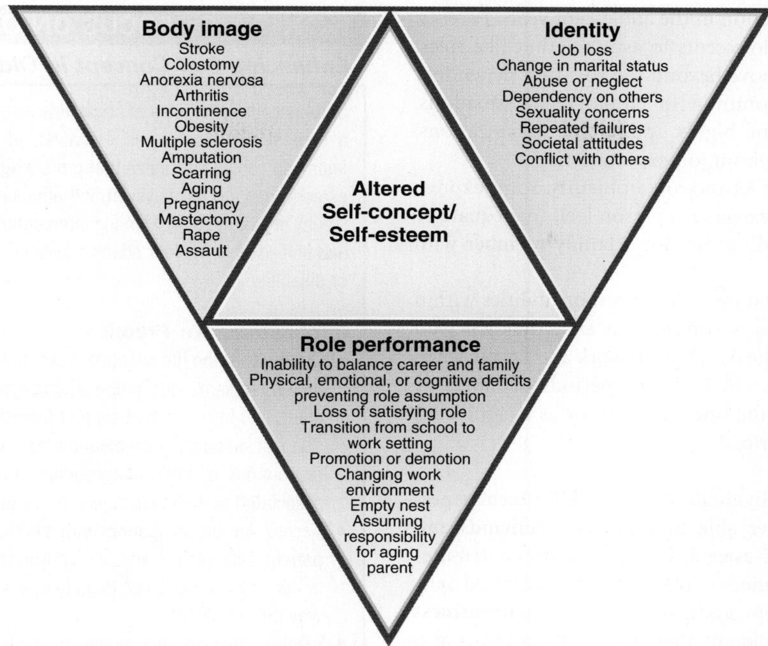

FIGURE 34-3 Common stressors that influence self-concept.

and anxiety. It is also a time when the adolescent is developing academic and psychosocial competence (Preckel et al., 2013).

Compared to an adolescent, an adult generally has a more stable identity and thus a more firmly developed self-concept. Cultural and social stressors rather than personal stressors have more impact on an adult's identity. For example, an adult has to balance career and family or make choices regarding honoring religious traditions from one's family of origin. **Identity confusion** results when people do not maintain a clear, consistent, and continuous consciousness of personal identity. Inability to adapt to identity stressors can result in identity confusion regardless of stage of life.

Body Image Stressors. A change in the appearance, structure, or function of a body part requires an adjustment in body image. An individual's perception of the change and the relative importance placed on body image affects the significance of a loss of function or change in appearance. For example, if a woman's body image incorporates reproductive organs as the ideal, a hysterectomy needed because of a diagnosis of uterine cancer is a significant alteration and can result in a perceived loss of femininity or wholeness. Changes in the appearance of the body such as an amputation, facial disfigurement, or scars from burns are obvious stressors affecting body image. Mastectomy and colostomy are surgical procedures that alter the appearance and function of the body, yet the changes typically are not apparent to others when the individual is dressed. Although potentially undetected by others, these changes significantly impact the individual. Even some elective changes such as breast augmentation or reduction affect body image. Chronic illnesses such as heart and renal disease affect body image because the body no longer functions at an optimal level. The patient has to adjust to a decrease in activity tolerance that impacts his or her ability to perform normal activities of daily living. In addition, pregnancy, significant weight gain or loss, pharmacological management of illness, or radiation therapy changes body image. Negative body image often leads to adverse health outcomes.

The response of society to physical changes in an individual often depends on the conditions surrounding the alteration. Some social changes have allowed the public to respond more favorably to illness and altered body image. For example, the media frequently presents positive stories about people adjusting in a healthy manner following serious injuries (e.g., surfer Bethany Hamilton's loss of a limb) or adapting to a debilitating illness (e.g., actor Michael J. Fox's Parkinson's disease). These stories change public awareness and the perception of what constitutes a disability and provide positive role models for individuals undergoing self-concept stressors and their families, friends, and society as a whole. In view of the growing epidemic of obesity in western cultures, parents and health care providers need to address weight-management issues without causing further injury to body image. Providing a social environment that focuses on health and fitness rather than a drive for thinness for girls or muscularity for boys can potentially increase adolescent satisfaction with their bodies.

Role Performance Stressors. Throughout life a person undergoes numerous role changes. Situational transitions occur when parents, spouses, children, or close friends die or people move, marry, divorce, or change jobs. It is important to recognize that a shift along the continuum from illness to wellness is as stressful as a shift from wellness to illness. Any of these transitions may lead to role conflict, role ambiguity, role strain, or role overload.

Role conflict results when a person has to simultaneously assume two or more roles that are inconsistent, contradictory, or mutually exclusive. For example, when a middle-age woman with teenage children assumes responsibility for the care of her older parents, conflicts occur in relation to being both a parent to her children and the child of her parents. Negotiating a balance of time and energy between her children and parents creates role conflicts. The perceived importance of each conflicting role influences the degree of conflict experienced. The **sick role** involves the expectations of others and society regarding how an individual behaves when sick. Role conflict occurs when general societal expectations (take care of yourself, and you will get better) and the expectations of co-workers (need to get the job done regardless of illness) collide. The conflict of taking care of oneself while getting everything done is often a major challenge.

Role ambiguity involves unclear role expectations, which makes people unsure about what to do or how to do it, creating stress and confusion. Role ambiguity is common in the adolescent years. Parents, peers, and the media pressure adolescents to assume adult-like roles; yet many lack the resources to move beyond the role of a dependent child. Role ambiguity is also common in employment situations. In complex, rapidly changing, or highly specialized organizations, employees often become unsure about job expectations.

Role strain combines role conflict and role ambiguity. Some express role strain as a feeling of frustration when a person feels inadequate or unsuited to a role such as providing care for a family member with Alzheimer's disease.

Role overload involves having more roles or responsibilities within a role than are manageable. This is common in an individual who unsuccessfully attempts to meet the demands of work and family while carving out some personal time. Often during periods of illness or change, those involved either as the one who is ill or as a significant other find themselves in role overload.

Self-Esteem Stressors. Individuals with high self-esteem generally are more resilient and better able to cope with demands and stressors than those with low self-esteem. Low self-worth contributes to feeling unfulfilled and disconnected from others. Decreased self-worth potentially can result in depression and unremitting uneasiness or anxiety. Illness, surgery, or accidents that change life patterns also influence feelings of self-worth. Chronic illnesses such as diabetes, arthritis, and cardiac disease require changes in accepted and long-assumed behavioral patterns. Female children and adolescents with chronic illness such as chronic fatigue syndrome and chronic headaches are particularly vulnerable to low self-esteem (Pinquart, 2012). The more the chronic illness interferes with the person's ability to engage in activities contributing to feelings of worth or success, the more it affects self-esteem.

Self-esteem stressors vary with developmental stages. Perceived inability to meet parental expectations, harsh criticism, inconsistent discipline, and unresolved sibling rivalry reduce the level of self-worth of children. A developmental milestone such as pregnancy introduces unique self-concept stressors and has significant health care implications. For some economically disadvantaged youth, safe sex behaviors are not always valued, and pregnancy is an affirmation of cultural identity. Low self-esteem during adolescence also has significant real-world consequences in adulthood, including poor health, criminal behavior, and limited economic prospects compared to adolescents with high self-esteem. Self-esteem and health behaviors are intertwined. Self-concept guides health behaviors and organizes health-related actions (Thomas and Moring, 2014). Stressors affecting the self-esteem of an adult include failure in work and unsuccessful relationships. Self-concept stressors in older adults include health problems, declining socioeconomic status, spousal loss or bereavement, loss of social support, and decline in achievement experiences following retirement (Box 34-3).

BOX 34-3 FOCUS ON OLDER ADULTS

Enhancing Self-Concept in Older Adults

Self-concept sometimes is negatively affected in older adulthood because of a number of life changes. However, in some individuals aging promotes improved coping strategies that protect against the declining feelings of self-esteem, despite the physical and emotional changes associated with aging (Touhy and Jett, 2014). Nursing interventions aimed at enhancing self-concept and self-esteem in older adults is essential, particularly during illness, injury, or disability.

Implications for Practice

- Clarify what the life changes mean and the effect on self-concept. Discuss health problems, declining socioeconomic status, spousal loss or bereavement, and loss of social support following retirement.
- Conduct supportive conversations to understand challenges to the patient's perceptions of body image adjustments as part of aging and changes associated with illness, injury, or disability.
- Assess for preoccupation with physical complaints. Thoroughly assess patient's complaints and, if no physical explanation exists, encourage him or her to verbalize needs (e.g., fear, insecurity, loneliness) in a nonphysical way (Stuart, 2013).
- Identify positive and negative coping mechanisms. Support effective strategies.
- Provide resources to help patient learn new positive coping mechanisms.
- Encourage the use of storytelling and review of old photographs.
- Modify nursing interventions with patients experiencing dementia to support self-concept; recognize that self-concept in early dementia is largely intact (Clare et al., 2012).
- Communicate that the older adult is worthwhile by actively listening to and accepting the person's feelings, being respectful, and praising healthy behaviors.
- Allow additional time to complete tasks. Reinforce the older adult's efforts at independence (Touhy and Jett, 2014).

Family Effect on Self-Concept Development

The family plays a key role in creating and maintaining the self-concepts of its members. Children develop a basic sense of who they are from their family caregivers. A child also gains accepted norms for thinking, feeling, and behaving from family members. Sometimes well-meaning parents cultivate negative self-concepts in children. Some literature suggests that parents are the most important influences on a child's development, yet variations in parenting approach depend on the culture. Specifically a child's positive self-esteem and school achievement are fostered by parents who respond in a firm, consistent, and warm manner. High parental support and parental monitoring are related to greater self-esteem and lower risk behaviors. Parents who are harsh, inconsistent, or have low self-esteem themselves often behave in ways that foster negative self-concepts in their children. Positive communication and social support foster self-esteem and well-being in adolescence. To reverse a patient's negative self-concept, first assess the family's style of relating (see Chapter 10). Family and cultural factors sometimes influence negative health practices such as excessive drinking (Box 34-4). Self-concept change demands an evidence-based practice approach supported by the entire health care team.

Nurse's Effect on Patient's Self-Concept

Your acceptance of a patient with an altered self-concept can promote positive change. Often this simply involves sitting with a patient and forming a therapeutic relationship. When a patient's physical appearance has changed, it is likely that both the patient and the family look to nurses and observe their verbal and nonverbal responses and reactions to the changed appearance. You need to remain aware of your own feelings, ideas, values, expectations, and judgments. Self-awareness is critical in understanding and accepting others. Nurses derive their self-concepts and professional identity from their public image; work environment; education; and their professional, social, and cultural values (Ten Hoeve et al., 2014). They need to assess and clarify the following self-concept issues about themselves:

- Thoughts and feelings about lifestyle, health, and illness
- Awareness of how their own nonverbal communication affects patients and families
- Personal values and expectations and how these affect patients

BOX 34-4 EVIDENCE-BASED PRACTICE

Self-Concept and the Impact on Adolescent Drinking Behaviors

PICO Question: How does self-concept influence drinking behaviors in at-risk adolescents?

Evidence Summary

Low self-concept may precede or perhaps even motivate adolescent drinking (Dudovitz et al., 2013). Because many teens engage in behaviors that increase the potential for morbidity and mortality, helping youth develop a healthy self-concept may prevent health risk behaviors, including teen drinking (CDC, 2014). In 2013 two thirds of high school students reported drinking; 34.9% reported current alcohol use, and 20.8% endorsed binge drinking (CDC, 2014). Overall the prevalence of current drinking in both males and females was higher among white students, followed by Hispanic, and then black students. Identifying risk and protective factors is important when creating drinking-prevention programs. Enhancing opportunities to learn communication skills and engage in alternative behaviors may make drinking less of an adolescent risk behavior.

Application to Nursing Practice

- Drinking-prevention efforts should include stress management and improving self-esteem.
- A priority nursing action is the assessment of child and adolescent coping strategies. Appropriate techniques include effective communication, conflict resolution, and stress management (Dudovitz et al., 2013).
- Families, peers, teachers, and health care providers should instill students' cultural pride, which promotes self-concept and the use of protective factors against risk behaviors such as drinking.
- Family, social, and behavioral factors are important issues to address during preadolescence and adolescence.
- Identifying risk factors for early drug and alcohol use, including genetic predisposition, family environment, and cultural identity, needs to be a priority for health care providers (CDC, 2014).

- Ability to convey a nonjudgmental attitude toward patients and families
- Preconceived attitudes toward cultural differences in self-concept and self-esteem

Some patients with a change in body appearance or function are extremely sensitive to the verbal and nonverbal responses of the health care team. A positive, matter-of-fact approach to care provides a model for the patient and family to follow. For example, when you observe a positive change in a patient's behavior, note it and allow the patient to establish its meaning. Nurses have a significant effect on patients by conveying genuine interest and acceptance. Including self-concept issues in the planning and delivery of care can influence patient outcomes positively. Building a trusting nurse-patient relationship that incorporates both the patient and family in the decision-making process enhances self-concept and self-esteem. You can individualize your approach by highlighting a patient's unique needs and incorporating alternative health care practices or methods of spiritual expression into the plan of care. It is important that health care providers understand the degree to which self-esteem and sexuality affect patient outcomes.

Your nursing care significantly affects a patient's body image. For example, the body image of a woman following a mastectomy is positively influenced by showing acceptance of the mastectomy scar. On the other hand, a nurse who has a shocked or disgusted facial expression contributes to the woman developing a negative body image. Patients closely watch the reactions of others to their wounds and scars, and it is very important to be aware of your responses toward the patient. Statements such as, "This wound is healing nicely" or "This tissue looks healthy" are affirmations for the body image of the patient. Nonverbal behaviors convey the level of caring that exists for a patient and affect self-esteem. Anticipate personal reactions, acknowledge them, and focus on the patient instead of the unpleasant task or situation. Nurses who put themselves in the patient's situation incorporate measures to ease embarrassment, frustration, anger, and denial.

Preventive measures, early identification, and appropriate treatment minimize the intensity of self-esteem stressors and the potential effects for a patient and his or her family. Learn to design specific self-concept interventions to fit a patient's profile of risk factors. It is essential to assess a patient's perception of a problem and work collaboratively to resolve self-concept issues. Interventions designed to promote active living and healthy eating may be beneficial for preventing childhood obesity, improving self-esteem, preventing chronic diseases, and improving health outcomes in adulthood.

QSEN QSEN: BUILDING COMPETENCY IN PATIENT-CENTERED CARE. You are a third-year nursing student who feels insecure in the clinical setting. You are caring for Mrs. Johnson who had a bilateral mastectomy. This is your first time caring for this type of patient, and you hope that your clinical instructor won't ask you questions about your patient because you "forget" everything when your assigned faculty approaches; you feel embarrassed that you sometimes "hide" or "look busy" to avoid interacting with your instructor. You wonder, "How can I attend to my patient's physical care and self-concept and self-esteem issues when I can't even deal with my own?" Which actions must you take to improve your self-esteem and self-concept as a student nurse?

Answers to QSEN Activities can be found on the Evolve website.

CRITICAL THINKING

Successful critical thinking requires a synthesis of knowledge, experience, information gathered from patients and families, critical thinking attitudes, and intellectual and professional standards. Clinical judgments require you to anticipate information, analyze the data, and make decisions regarding your patient's care. During assessment consider all elements that build toward making an appropriate nursing diagnosis.

In the case of self-concept, it is essential to integrate knowledge from nursing and other disciplines, including self-concept theory, communication principles, and a consideration of cultural and developmental factors. Previous experience in caring for patients with self-concept alterations helps to individualize care. Self-concept profoundly influences a person's response to illness. A critical thinking approach to care is essential.

NURSING PROCESS

Apply the nursing process and use a critical thinking approach in your care of patients. The nursing process provides a clinical decision-making approach for you to develop and implement an individualized plan of care. Use of the nursing process is continuous until the patient's self-concept is improved, restored, or maintained.

Assessment

During the assessment process thoroughly assess each patient and critically analyze findings to ensure that you make patient-centered

BOX 34-5 Behaviors Suggestive of Altered Self-Concept

- Avoidance of eye contact
- Slumped posture
- Unkempt appearance
- Overly apologetic
- Hesitant speech
- Overly critical or angry
- Frequent or inappropriate crying
- Negative self-evaluation
- Excessively dependent
- Hesitant to express views or opinions
- Lack of interest in what is happening
- Passive attitude
- Difficulty in making decisions
- Self-harm behaviors

BOX 34-6 Nursing Assessment Questions

Nature of the Problem
- How would you describe yourself?
- Which aspects of your appearance do you like?
- Tell me about the things you do that make you feel good about yourself.
- Tell me about your primary roles. How effective are you at carrying out each of these roles?

Onset and Duration
- When did you start to think or feel differently about yourself?
- How long have you struggled with _____ (specify identity, body image, role performance, or self-esteem)?
- Can you remember a time when you felt good about yourself?

Effect on Patient
- Tell me how your self-concept affects your ability to take care of yourself.
- What impact does your self-esteem have on relationships?
- How does your self-esteem affect other areas of your life?
- Have you considered hurting yourself (specify self-mutilation, suicidal gestures)?

clinical decisions required for safe nursing care. In assessing self-concept and self-esteem, first focus on each component of self-concept (identity, body image, and role performance). Assessment needs to include looking for the range of behaviors suggestive of an altered self-concept or self-esteem (Box 34-5), actual and potential self-concept stressors (see Figure 34-3), and coping patterns. Gathering comprehensive assessment data requires the critical synthesis of information from multiple sources (Figure 34-4). In addition to direct questioning (Box 34-6), gather much of the data regarding self-concept through observation of the patient's nonverbal behavior and by paying attention to the content of the patient's conversations. Take note of the manner in which patients talk about the people in their lives because this provides clues to both stressful and supportive relationships and key roles the patient assumes. Use knowledge of developmental stages to determine which areas are likely to be important to the patient and inquire about these aspects of the person's life. For example, ask a 70-year-old patient about his life and what has been important to him. The individual's conversation likely provides data relating to role performance, identity, self-esteem, stressors, and coping patterns.

Through the Patient's Eyes. An important factor in assessing self-concept is the person's viewpoint of his or her health condition and its influence on self-concept. Give patients the opportunity to tell their stories of how they perceive their illness or condition affecting their identity, their image of themselves, and their ability to lead a normal lifestyle. Assess their expectations of health care by asking them how interventions will make a difference. This is also an opportunity to discuss the patient's goals. For example, a nurse working with a patient who is experiencing anxiety related to an upcoming diagnostic study asks the patient about his expectations of the relaxation exercise that they have been practicing together. The patient's response gives the nurse valuable information about his beliefs and attitudes regarding the efficacy of the interventions and the potential need to modify the nursing approach.

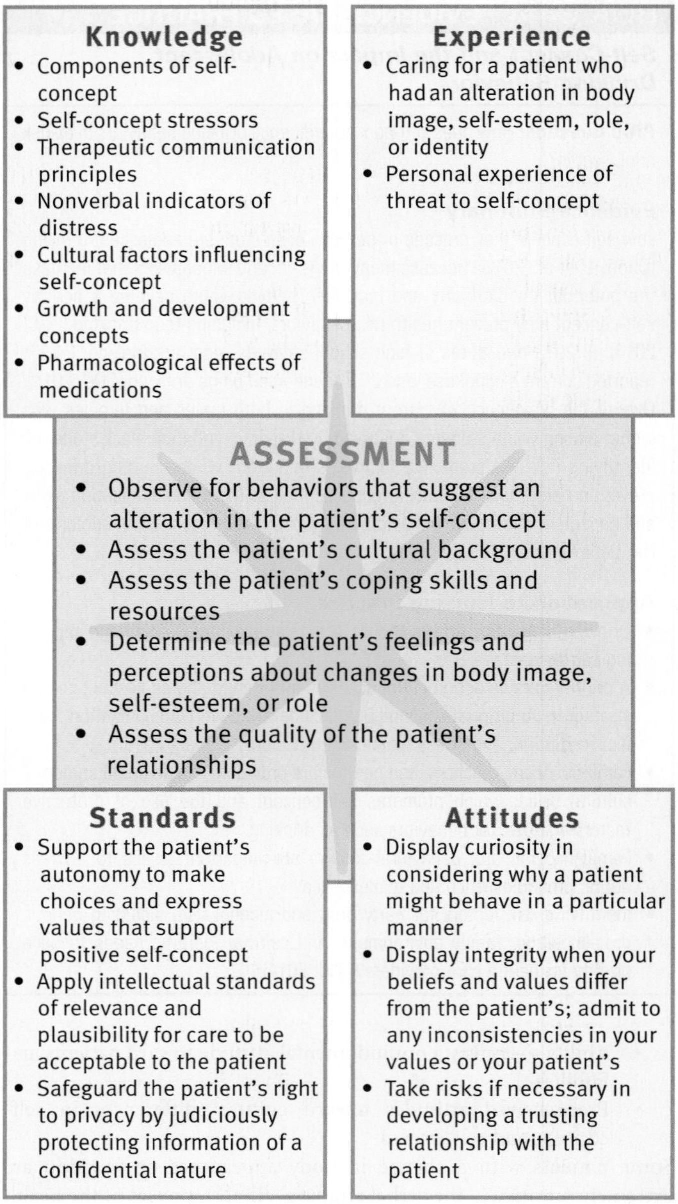

Knowledge
- Components of self-concept
- Self-concept stressors
- Therapeutic communication principles
- Nonverbal indicators of distress
- Cultural factors influencing self-concept
- Growth and development concepts
- Pharmacological effects of medications

Experience
- Caring for a patient who had an alteration in body image, self-esteem, role, or identity
- Personal experience of threat to self-concept

ASSESSMENT
- Observe for behaviors that suggest an alteration in the patient's self-concept
- Assess the patient's cultural background
- Assess the patient's coping skills and resources
- Determine the patient's feelings and perceptions about changes in body image, self-esteem, or role
- Assess the quality of the patient's relationships

Standards
- Support the patient's autonomy to make choices and express values that support positive self-concept
- Apply intellectual standards of relevance and plausibility for care to be acceptable to the patient
- Safeguard the patient's right to privacy by judiciously protecting information of a confidential nature

Attitudes
- Display curiosity in considering why a patient might behave in a particular manner
- Display integrity when your beliefs and values differ from the patient's; admit to any inconsistencies in your values or your patient's
- Take risks if necessary in developing a trusting relationship with the patient

FIGURE 34-4 Critical thinking model for self-concept assessment.

Coping Behaviors. The nursing assessment also includes consideration of previous coping behaviors; the nature, number, and intensity of the stressors; and the patient's internal and external resources. Knowledge of how a patient has dealt with stressors in the past provides insight into his or her style of coping. Patients do not address all issues in the same way, but they often use a familiar coping pattern for newly encountered stressors. Identify previous coping strategies to determine whether these patterns have contributed to healthy functioning or created more problems. For example, the use of drugs or alcohol during times of stress often creates additional stressors (see Chapter 38).

Significant Others. Exploring resources and strengths such as availability of significant others or prior use of community resources is important in formulating a realistic and effective plan of care. Valuable information comes from conversations with family and significant others. Significant others sometimes have insights into the person's way of dealing with stressors. They also have knowledge about what is important to the person's self-concept. The way in which a significant other talks about the patient and the significant other's nonverbal behaviors provide information about which kind of support is available for the patient.

◆ Nursing Diagnosis

Carefully consider the assessment data to identify a patient's actual or potential problem areas. Rely on knowledge and experience, apply appropriate professional standards, and look for clusters of defining characteristics that indicate a nursing diagnosis. The following list (Herdman and Kamitsuru, 2014) provides examples of self-concept–related nursing diagnoses:

- *Disturbed Body Image*
- *Caregiver Role Strain*
- *Disturbed Personal Identity*
- *Ineffective Role Performance*
- *Readiness for Enhanced Self-Concept*
- *Chronic Low Self-Esteem*
- *Situational Low Self-Esteem*
- *Risk for Situational Low Self-Esteem*

Making nursing diagnoses about self-concept is complex. Often isolated data are defining characteristics for more than one nursing diagnosis (Box 34-7). For example, a patient expresses feelings of uncertainty and inadequacy. These are defining characteristics for both *Anxiety* and *Situational Low Self-Esteem.* Realizing that the patient is demonstrating defining characteristics of more than one nursing diagnosis guides you to gather specific data to validate and differentiate the underlying problem. To further assess the possibility of *Anxiety* as the nursing diagnosis, consider whether the person has any of the following defining characteristics: Is the person experiencing increased muscle tension, shakiness, a sense of being "rattled," or restlessness? These symptoms suggest *Anxiety* as the more appropriate diagnosis. On the other hand, if he or she expresses a predominantly negative self-appraisal, including inability to handle situations or events and difficulty making decisions, these characteristics suggest that *Situational Low Self-Esteem* is more appropriate. To further aid in differentiating between the two provisional diagnoses, information regarding recent events in the person's life and how he or she has viewed himself or herself in the past provide insight into the most appropriate nursing diagnosis. As you gather additional data, usually the priority nursing diagnosis becomes evident.

Validate the nursing diagnosis by sharing observations with the patient and allow him or her to verify perceptions. This approach often results in the patient providing additional data, which further clarifies the situation. For example, "I noticed that you jumped when I touched your arm. Are you feeling uneasy today?" allows the patient to verify whether he or she is in fact anxious and describe his or her concerns.

BOX 34-7 Nursing Diagnostic Process

Situational Low Self-Esteem

Assessment Activities	Defining Characteristics
Ask patient to explain thoughts and feelings about self.	Patient is tearful and reports negative thoughts about self. She reports not wanting to have any visitors.
Observe patient's behavior and ask family if she is experiencing emotional or behavior changes.	Spouse describes withdrawal and avoidance of intimacy. He describes wife as unable to make decisions.
Determine if patient has had issues with self-esteem in the past and her plans to improve her self-esteem.	Patient denies any self-esteem issues since adolescence. She is receptive to counseling to discuss ways to return to high self-esteem.

◆ Planning

During planning synthesize knowledge, experience, critical thinking attitudes, and standards (Figure 34-5). Critical thinking ensures that a patient's plan of care integrates information known about the

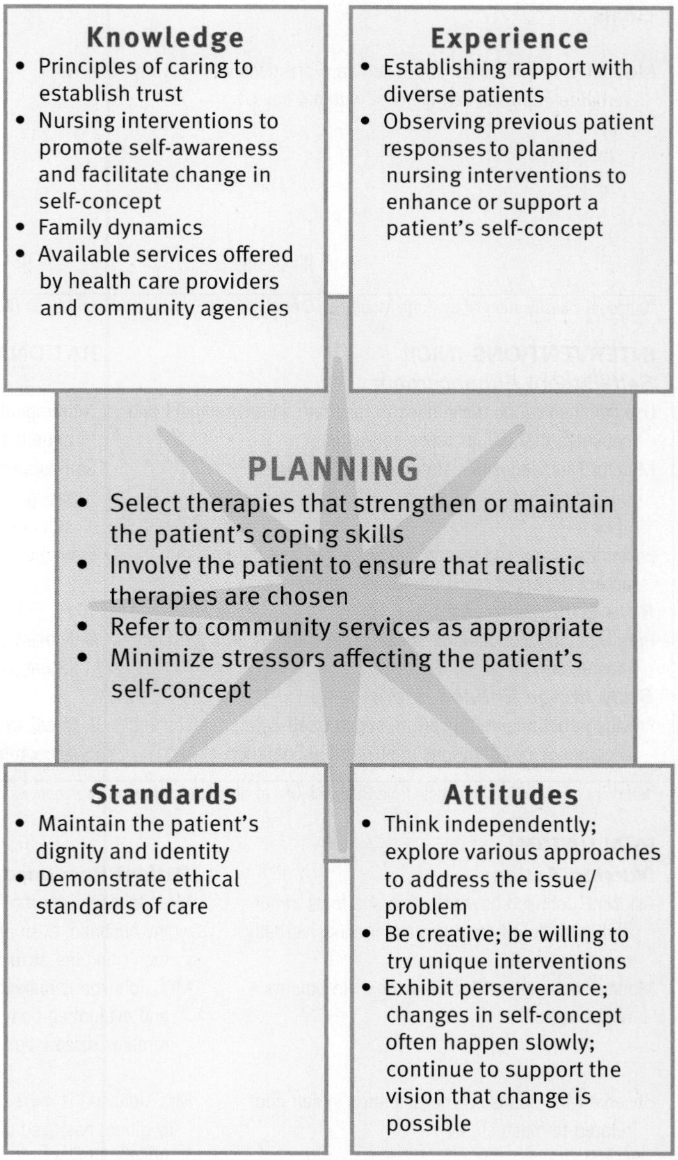

FIGURE 34-5 Critical thinking model for self-concept planning.

NURSING CARE PLAN

Disturbed Body Image

ASSESSMENT

Mrs. Johnson, a 45-year-old married woman who had a bilateral radical mastectomy resulting from malignant breast cancer, has been assigned to Susan Carr, nursing student. Susan completed Mrs. Johnson's physical assessment. After Mrs. Johnson has been medicated adequately for pain, Ms. Carr sits down to discuss how the mastectomy has affected Mrs. Johnson's self-concept and self-esteem.

Assessment Activities	***Findings/Defining Characteristics****
Assess identity and body image concerns (e.g., sexual role, femininity). Ask how the loss of breasts has affected her sense of self.	Mrs. Johnson **looks away, shakes her head**, and states, "**I feel like less of a woman**. My husband says I'm still attractive, but I don't believe him."
Observe Mrs. Johnson's mood and affect and her nonverbal communication and interactions with others.	Mrs. Johnson demonstrates intermittent eye contact, frequent **crying when alone,** pulling hospital gown tightly across chest, and superficial conversations with family members.
Assess Mrs. Johnson's involvement in self-care activities.	Mrs. Johnson is unable to decide when to bathe, comb her hair, or apply typical makeup. She avoids looking in a mirror.
Ask Mrs. Johnson if she would like opportunities to participate in treatment activities.	**Mrs. Johnson avoids** looking at or touching her chest and **does not ask questions** about her condition. "I don't know if I want to do anything right now."

**Defining characteristics* are shown in bold type.

NURSING DIAGNOSIS: Disturbed body image related to negative view of self after mastectomy

PLANNING

Goals	***Expected Outcomes (NOC)***[†]
	Self-Esteem
Mrs. Johnson will demonstrate self-care practices within 2 days and will verbalize improved self-concept within 4 days.	Mrs. Johnson meets basic grooming and hygiene needs within 2 days and verbalizes improved feelings of self-acceptance and self-worth within 4 days.
	Role Performance
	Mrs. Johnson describes role changes associated with mastectomy and verbalizes commitment to accessing community resources by day of discharge.
	Body Image
	Mrs. Johnson demonstrates a positive adjustment to changes in body appearance within 1 week.

[†]Outcome classification labels from Moorhead S et al: *Nursing outcomes classification (NOC)*, ed 5, St Louis, 2013, Mosby.

INTERVENTIONS (NIC)[‡]	**RATIONALE**
Self-Esteem Enhancement	
Use communication techniques to facilitate an environment and activities that will increase self-esteem.	A therapeutic nurse-patient relationship promotes positive patient outcome, including the patient's assuming responsibility for her own care (Stuart, 2013).
Monitor Mrs. Johnson's statements of self-worth.	Self-esteem and body image are strong predictors of depression. The nurse must assess thoughts and feelings, including depression and risk for suicide, to ensure the patient's safety and make appropriate referrals.
Encourage increased responsibility for self and help patient accept dependence on others as appropriate.	Promoting self-care enhances self-concept, including improving role performance (Stuart, 2013).
Role Enhancement	
Help Mrs. Johnson identify specific role changes brought on by mastectomy.	Only after the nurse accurately defines the problem can alternative choices be proposed (Stuart, 2013).
Body Image Enhancement	
Provide patient-centered care to support self-care practices and acceptance of alterations in physical appearance.	A threat to body image and overall self-concept often influences self-care practices and acceptance of changes in physical appearance.

[‡]Intervention classification labels from Bulechek GM et al, editors: *Nursing interventions classification (NIC)*, ed 6, St Louis, 2013, Mosby.

EVALUATION

Nursing Actions	***Patient Response/Finding***	***Achievement of Outcome***
Ask Mrs. Johnson how effective she feels in her ability to identify and express feelings verbally and nonverbally.	Mrs. Johnson reports, "I've been able to talk with my husband, even about my concerns that he won't find me attractive anymore."	Improved verbal and nonverbal communication noted
Monitor changes in Mrs. Johnson's statements about herself.	Mrs. Johnson is making fewer negative comments and evaluating body image more realistically but remains dissatisfied with appearance.	Small improvement in self-esteem; body image more realistic but remains negative Discusses body image with husband and nursing student
Observe Mrs. Johnson's participation in self-care related to mastectomy.	Mrs. Johnson is more assertive in completing basic hygiene; has used a mirror to examine mastectomy scar.	Meeting self-care needs

individual and key critical thinking elements (see the Nursing Care Plan). Professional standards are especially important to consider when developing a plan of care. These standards often establish ethical or evidence-based practice guidelines for selecting effective nursing interventions.

Another method to help plan care is a concept map. An example of an illustrative concept map (Figure 34-6) shows the relationship of a primary health problem (postoperative bilateral radical mastectomy) and four nursing diagnoses and several interventions. The concept map shows how the nursing diagnoses are interrelated. It also helps to show the interrelationships among nursing interventions. A single nursing intervention can be effective for more than one diagnosis.

Goals and Outcomes. Develop an individualized plan of care for each nursing diagnosis. Work collaboratively with the patient to set realistic expectations for care. Make sure that goals are individualized and realistic with measurable outcomes. In establishing goals consult with the patient about whether they are achievable. Consultation with significant others, mental health clinicians, and community resources results in a more comprehensive and workable plan. When you set goals, consider the data necessary to demonstrate that the patient's problem would change if the nursing diagnosis were managed. The outcome criteria should reflect these changes. For example, a patient is diagnosed with *Situational Low Self-Esteem related to a recent job layoff.* Establish a goal: "Patient's self-esteem and self-concept will

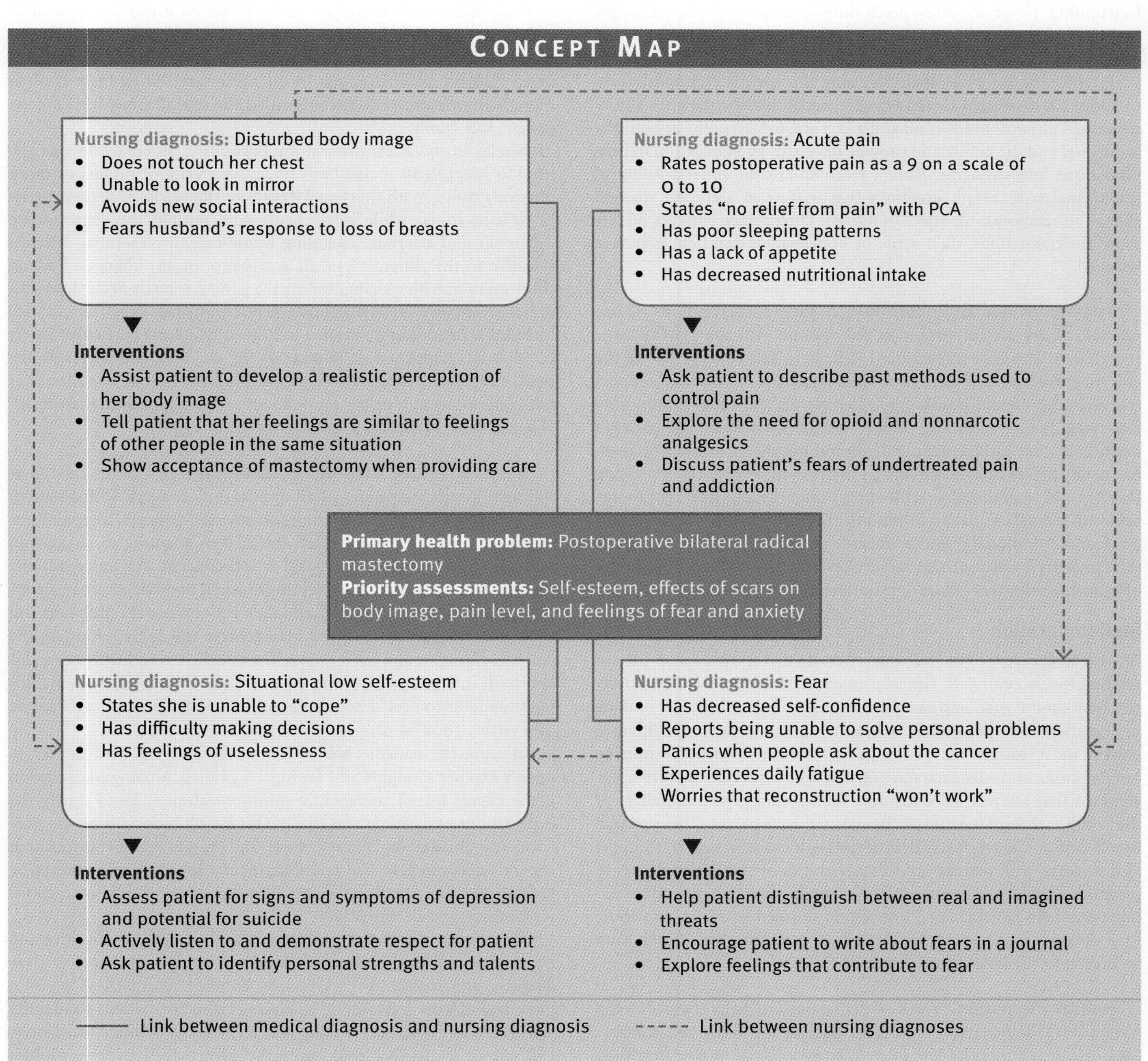

FIGURE 34-6 Concept map for Mrs. Johnson. *PCA,* Patient-controlled analgesia.

improve in 1 week." Examples of expected outcomes directed toward that goal include the following:

- The patient discusses a minimum of three areas of her life in which she is functioning well.
- The patient is able to voice the recognition that losing her job is not reflective of her worth as a person.
- The patient attends a support group and networking session for out-of-work professionals.

Setting Priorities. A care plan presents the goals, expected outcomes, and interventions for a patient with an alteration in self-concept. Interventions help the patient adapt to the stressors that led to the self-concept disturbance and support and reinforce the development of coping methods. Often a patient perceives a situation as overwhelming and feels hopeless about returning to the level of previous functioning. He or she often needs time to adapt to physical changes but can work toward progressive improvement in self-concept and self-esteem.

Establishing priorities includes using therapeutic communication to address self-concept issues, which ensures that the patient's ability to address physical needs is maximized. Look for strengths in both the individual and the family and provide resources and education to turn limitations into strengths. Patient teaching creates understanding of the normalcy of certain situations (e.g., nature of a chronic disease; change in relationships; effect of a loss). Often, once patients understand their situations, their sense of hopelessness and helplessness is lessened.

Teamwork and Collaboration. A patient's perceptions of significant others are important to incorporate into the plan of care. Individuals who have experienced deficits in self-concept before the current episode of treatment have often established a system of support that includes mental health clinicians, clergy, and other community resources. Before including family members, consider the patient's desires for their involvement and cultural norms regarding who most frequently makes decisions in the family. Patients who are experiencing threats to or alterations in self-concept often benefit from collaboration with mental health and community resources to promote increased awareness. Additional resources include physical therapy, occupational therapy, behavioral health, social services, and pastoral care. Knowledge of available resources allows appropriate referrals.

◆ Implementation

As with all the steps of the nursing process, a therapeutic nurse-patient relationship is central to the implementation phase. Collaboratively you develop the goals and outcome criteria and then consider nursing interventions for promoting a healthy self-concept and helping a patient move toward his or her goals. To identify effective nursing interventions, consider each nursing diagnosis and individualize interventions that address the diagnosis. Collaborating with members of the health care team maximizes the comprehensiveness of the approach to self-concept issues. Regardless of the health care setting, it is important to work with patients and their families or significant others to promote a healthy self-concept. For example, select nursing interventions that help patients regain or restore the elements that contribute to a strong and secure sense of self. The approaches chosen vary according to the level of care required.

Health Promotion. Work with patients to help them develop healthy lifestyle behaviors that contribute to a positive self-concept. Measures that support adaptation to stress such as proper nutrition, regular exercise within the patient's capabilities, adequate sleep and rest, and stress-reducing practices contribute to a healthy self-concept. Nurses are in a unique position to identify lifestyle practices that put a person's self-concept at risk or suggest altered self-concepts. For example, a young teacher visits a clinic with complaints of being unable to sleep and experiencing anxiety attacks. In gathering the nursing history, lifestyle practices such as too little rest, a large number of life changes occurring simultaneously, and excessive use of alcohol emerge. These data, when taken together suggest actual or potential self-concept disturbances. Determine how the patient views the various lifestyle elements to facilitate his or her insight into behaviors and make referrals or provide needed health teaching.

Acute Care. In the acute care setting some patients experience potential threats to their self-concept because of the nature of the treatment and/or diagnostic procedures. Threats to a person's self-concept often result in anxiety and/or fear. As a nurse you need to address the patient's numerous stressors, including fear of unknown diagnoses (diagnostic tests), the need to modify lifestyle, and anticipated changes in functioning. In the acute care setting there is often more than one stressor, thus increasing the overall stress level for the patient and family.

Nurses in the acute care setting encounter patients who face the need to adapt to an altered body image as a result of surgery or other physical change. With shortened lengths of stay, addressing these needs is difficult to do while in an acute care setting; thus appropriate follow-up and referrals, including home care, are essential. Remain sensitive to the patient's level of acceptance of any changes. Forcing confrontation with a change before the patient is ready likely delays his or her acceptance. Signs that a person is receptive to accepting a change include asking questions related to how to manage a particular aspect of what has happened or looking at the changed body area. As the patient expresses readiness to integrate the body change into his or her self-concept, let him or her know about support groups that are available and offer to make the initial contact.

Restorative and Continuing Care. Often in a home care environment a nurse has more of an opportunity to work with a patient to reach the goal of attaining a more positive self-concept. Interventions designed to help a patient reach the goal of adapting to changes in self-concept or attaining a positive self-concept are based on the premise that the patient first develops insight and self-awareness concerning problems and stressors and then acts to solve the problems and cope with the stressors. One way to achieve this is by reframing the patient's thoughts and feelings in a more positive way. Incorporate this approach into patient teaching for alterations in self-concept, including situational low self-esteem, that sometimes are present in the home care setting (Box 34-8).

Increase the patient's self-awareness by allowing him or her to openly explore thoughts and feelings. A priority nursing intervention is the expert use of therapeutic communication skills to clarify the expectations of a patient and family. Open exploration makes the situation less threatening for a patient and encourages behaviors that expand self-awareness. Use a nonjudgmental approach when accepting the patient's thoughts and feelings, help the patient clarify interactions with others, and be empathic.

Help the patient define problems clearly and identify positive and negative coping mechanisms. Work closely with him or her to analyze adaptive and maladaptive responses, contrast alternatives, devise a plan, and discuss outcomes. Collaborate with the patient to identify alternative solutions and develop realistic goals to facilitate real change and encourage further goal-setting behaviors. Design opportunities that result in success, reinforce the patient's skills and strengths, and

BOX 34-8 PATIENT TEACHING

Alterations in Self-Concept

Objective

- Situational low self-esteem will be reduced in the home care setting.

Teaching Strategies

- Encourage opportunities for patient to care for self (Stuart, 2013).
- Elicit patient's perceptions of strengths and weaknesses.
- Reaffirm that patient is responsible for behavior.
- Identify stressors with patient and ask for appraisal of them.
- Explore patient's coping responses to problems.
- Incorporate psychiatric co-morbidities (e.g., depression, anxiety, somatoform disorders) and alterations to self-esteem and body image when planning treatment approaches.
- Collaboratively identify alternative solutions and encourage alternatives not previously tried.
- Continue to reinforce strengths and successes.

Evaluation

- Confirm perception and actual use of improved communication skills.
- Observe level of participation in decisions that affect care.
- Observe patient establishing a simple routine.
- Observe patient taking necessary action to use appropriate coping responses (Stuart, 2013).

help him or her find needed assistance. Encourage the patient to commit to decisions and actions to achieve goals by teaching him or her to move away from ineffective coping mechanisms and develop successful coping strategies. Supporting attempts that are helpful is essential because with each success a patient is motivated to make another attempt.

◆ Evaluation

Through the Patient's Eyes. Use critical thinking to evaluate the patient's perceived success in meeting each goal and the established expected outcomes (Figure 34-7). Frequent evaluation of patient progress is necessary. Apply knowledge of behaviors and characteristics of a healthy self-concept when reviewing the actual behaviors that patients display. This determines whether outcomes have been met.

Patient Outcomes. Expected outcomes for a patient with a self-concept disturbance include displaying behaviors indicating a positive self-concept, verbalizing statements of self-acceptance, and validating acceptance of change in appearance or function. Key indicators of a patient's self-concept are nonverbal behaviors. For example, a patient who has had difficulty making eye contact demonstrates a more positive self-concept by making more frequent eye contact during conversation. Social interaction, adequate self-care, acceptance of the use of prosthetic devices, and statements indicating understanding of teaching all indicate progress. Investing in satisfying activities, exerting choices in daily life, understanding their own needs during transitions, and adapting to life circumstances are evidence of self-esteem and self-efficacy in older adults (Touhy and Jett, 2014). A positive attitude toward rehabilitation and increased movement toward independence facilitate a return to preexisting roles at work or at home. Patterns of interacting also reflect changes in self-concept. For example, a patient who has been hesitant to express personal views more readily offers opinions and ideas as self-esteem increases.

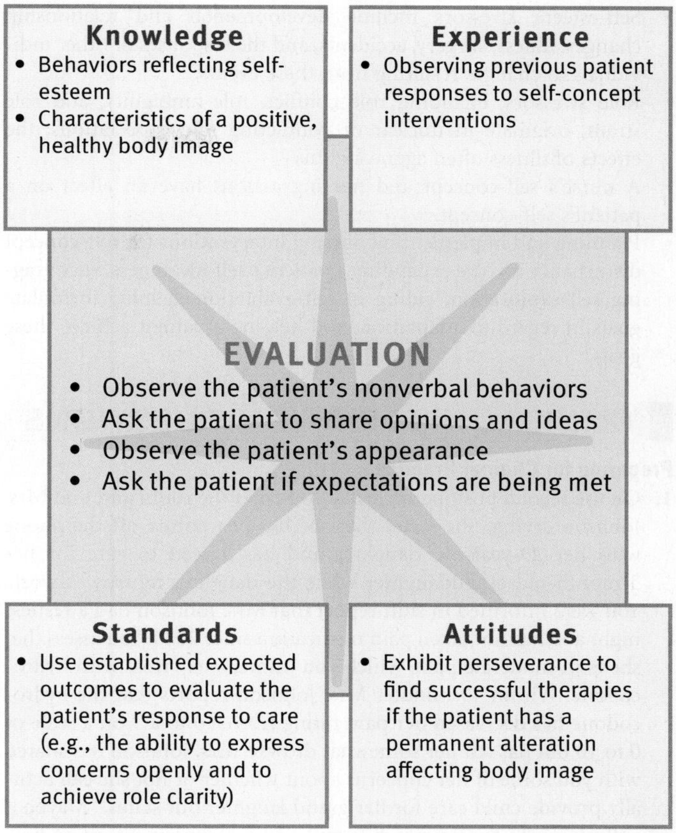

Knowledge
- Behaviors reflecting self-esteem
- Characteristics of a positive, healthy body image

Experience
- Observing previous patient responses to self-concept interventions

EVALUATION
- Observe the patient's nonverbal behaviors
- Ask the patient to share opinions and ideas
- Observe the patient's appearance
- Ask the patient if expectations are being met

Standards
- Use established expected outcomes to evaluate the patient's response to care (e.g., the ability to express concerns openly and to achieve role clarity)

Attitudes
- Exhibit perseverance to find successful therapies if the patient has a permanent alteration affecting body image

FIGURE 34-7 Critical thinking model for self-concept evaluation.

The goals of care sometimes become unrealistic or inappropriate as a patient's condition changes. Revise the plan if needed, reflecting on successful experiences with other patients. Patient adaptation to major changes can take a year or longer, but the fact that this period is long does not suggest problems with adaptation. Look for signs that the patient has reduced some stressors and that some behaviors have become more adaptive. If initial outcomes regarding self-concept are not met, individualize the following questions:

- Tell me what you will do if you are not able to return to work (may substitute school or home) as planned.
- Who will you contact if you are not feeling any better about yourself in 2 weeks?
- What are you doing to actively improve how you view yourself and your perception of how others view you?
- How will you know that your feeling of worth is improving?

Changes in self-concept take time. Although change is often slow, care of a patient with a self-concept disturbance is rewarding.

KEY POINTS

- Self-concept is an integrated set of conscious and unconscious attitudes and perceptions about self.
- Components of self-concept are identity, body image, and role performance.
- Each developmental stage involves factors that are important to the development of a healthy, positive self-concept.
- Identity is particularly vulnerable during adolescence.
- Body image stressors include changes in physical appearance, structure, or functioning caused by normal developmental changes or illness.

- Self-esteem stressors include developmental and relationship changes, illness, surgery, accidents, and the responses of other individuals to changes resulting from these events.
- Role stressors, including role conflict, role ambiguity, and role strain, originate in unclear or conflicting role expectations; the effects of illness often aggravate this.
- A nurse's self-concept and nursing actions have an effect on a patient's self-concept.
- Planning and implementing nursing interventions for self-concept disturbance involve expanding a patient's self-awareness, encouraging self-exploration, aiding in self-evaluation, helping formulate goals in regard to adaptation, and helping a patient achieve these goals.

CLINICAL APPLICATION QUESTIONS

Preparing for Clinical Practice

1. On the second postoperative day you enter the room and find Mrs. Johnson crying. She states that she has just gotten off the phone with her 23-year-old daughter and has agreed to care for her 3-month-old granddaughter while the daughter returns to work. You were informed in shift report that Mrs. Johnson had a restless night and has not taken pain medication since 2030. You assess that she is in moderate pain, which you immediately treat with hydrocodone. Within 40 minutes Mrs. Johnson reports that the hydrocodone has decreased her pain rating from a 6 to a 3 on a scale of 0 to 10 but has left her somewhat drowsy. Mrs. Johnson has shared with you some of her concerns about whether or not she can actually provide child care for her granddaughter but states, "Maybe it will make me feel worthwhile and will take my mind off of how disgusting I look." She continues, "I just want to be normal again." How would you address her comment regarding "being normal again" and her lack of understanding of her physical condition, including pain management, increased fatigue, and limitations regarding lifting?
2. As a part of your home care experience, you are assigned to visit Mrs. Johnson who, in addition to caring for her infant granddaughter, is also caring for her mother, who is increasingly agitated and aggressive secondary to Alzheimer's disease. When you go to the home, you find Mrs. Johnson tearful. She says, "I can't do this anymore. She doesn't like anything I cook. She calls me 2 or 3 times during the night to sit with her; sometimes she doesn't even recognize me. The baby is crying constantly; I think she senses my stress. I feel so overwhelmed." Which additional assessment data would be important to gather? What priority nursing diagnosis could be made for Mrs. Johnson?
3. You suspect that Mrs. Johnson's depressed mood and loss of interest in usual activities exceeds your previous diagnosis of situational low self-esteem. Describe which assessment data are needed to modify your plan of care. Identify your priority actions.

ⓔ *Answers to Clinical Application Questions can be found on the Evolve website.*

REVIEW QUESTIONS

Are You Ready to Test Your Nursing Knowledge?

1. A 50-year-old woman is recovering from a bilateral mastectomy. She refuses to eat, discourages visitors, and pays little attention to her appearance. One morning the nurse enters the room to see the patient with her hair combed and makeup applied. Which of the following is the best response from the nurse?
   1. "What's the special occasion?"
   2. "You must be feeling better today."
   3. "This is the first time I've seen you look this good."
   4. "I see that you've combed your hair and put on makeup."
2. A 30-year-old patient diagnosed with major depressive disorder has a nursing diagnosis of *Chronic Low Self-Esteem related to negative view of self.* Which of the following would be appropriate interventions by the nurse? (Select all that apply.)
   1. Encourage reconnecting with high school friends
   2. Role play to increase assertiveness skills
   3. Focus on identifying strengths and accomplishments
   4. Provide time for journaling to explore underlying thoughts and feelings
   5. Explore new job opportunities
3. Several staff members complain about an adult patient's constant questions such as, "Should I have a cup of coffee or a cup of tea?" and "Should I take a shower now or wait until later?" Which interpretation of the patient's behavior helps the nurses provide optimal care?
   1. Asking questions is attention-seeking behavior.
   2. Inability to make decisions reflects a self-concept issue.
   3. Dependence on staff must be stopped immediately.
   4. Indecisiveness is aimed at testing how the staff reacts.
4. A depressed patient is crying and verbalizes feelings of low self-esteem and self-worth such as, "I'm such a failure … I can't do anything right." What is the nurse's best response?
   1. Remain with the patient until he or she validates feeling more stable.
   2. Tell the patient that is not true and that every person has a purpose in life.
   3. Review recent behaviors or accomplishments that demonstrate skill ability.
   4. Reassure the patient that you know how he is feeling and that things will get better.
5. An adult woman is recovering from a mastectomy for breast cancer and is frequently tearful when left alone. The nurse's approach should be based on an understanding of which of the following?
   1. Patients need support in dealing with the loss of a body part.
   2. The patient's family should take the lead role in providing support.
   3. The nurse should explain that breast tissue is not essential to life.
   4. The patient should focus on the cure of the cancer rather than loss of the breast.
6. When caring for an 87-year-old patient, the nurse needs to understand that which of the following most directly influences the patient's current self-concept?
   1. Attitude and behaviors of relatives providing care
   2. Caring behaviors of the nurse and health care team
   3. Level of education, economic status, and living conditions
   4. Adjustment to role change, loss of loved ones, and physical energy
7. A 20-year-old patient diagnosed with an eating disorder has a nursing diagnosis of *Situational Low Self-Esteem.* Which of the following nursing interventions would be appropriate to address self-esteem? (Select all that apply.)
   1. Offer independent decision-making opportunities.
   2. Review previously successful coping strategies.
   3. Provide a quiet environment with minimal stimuli.
   4. Support a dependent role throughout treatment.
   5. Increase calorie intake to promote weight stabilization.

8. The nurse asks the patient, "How do you feel about yourself?" The nurse is assessing the patient's:
   1. Identity.
   2. Self-esteem.
   3. Body image.
   4. Role performance.
9. The nurse can increase a patient's self-awareness through which of the following actions? (Select all that apply.)
   1. Helping the patient define her problems clearly
   2. Allowing the patient to openly explore thoughts and feelings
   3. Reframing the patient's thoughts and feelings in a more positive way
   4. Having family members assume more responsibility during times of stress
   5. Recommending self-help reading materials
10. When developing an appropriate outcome for a 15-year-old girl, the nurse considers that a primary developmental task of adolescence is to:
   1. Form a sense of identity.
   2. Create intimate relationships.
   3. Separate from parents and live independently.
   4. Achieve positive self-esteem through experimentation.
11. What is an appropriate nursing diagnosis for an individual who experiences confusion in the mental picture of his physical appearance?
   1. Acute Confusion
   2. Disturbed Body Image
   3. Chronic Low Self-Esteem
   4. Situational Low Self-Esteem
12. In planning nursing care for an 85-year-old male, what is the most important basic need that must be met?
   1. Assurance of sexual intimacy
   2. Preservation of self-esteem
   3. Expanded socialization
   4. Increase in monthly income
13. Which of the following assessment findings suggest an altered self-concept? (Select all that apply.)
   1. Uneven gait
   2. Slumped posture and poor personal hygiene
   3. Avoidance of eye contact when answering a question
   4. Requests for visits from the chaplain
   5. Frequent use of the call light
14. The home health nurse is visiting a 90-year-old man who lives with his 89-year-old wife. He is legally blind and is 3 weeks' post right hip replacement. He ambulates with difficulty with a walker. He comments that he is saddened now that his wife has to do more for him and he is doing less for her. Which of the following is the priority nursing diagnosis?
   1. Self-Care Deficit, Toileting
   2. Deficient Knowledge Regarding Resources for the Visually Impaired
   3. Disturbed Body Image
   4. Risk for Situational Low Self-Esteem
15. On the basis of knowledge of the developmental tasks of Erikson's Industry versus Inferiority, the nurse emphasizes proper technique for use of an inhaler with a 10-year-old boy so he will:
   1. Increase his self-esteem with mastery of a new skill.
   2. Accept changes in his appearance and physical endurance.
   3. Experience success in role transitions and increased responsibilities.
   4. Appreciate his body appearance and function.

Answers: 1. 4; **2.** 3, 4; **3.** 2; **4.** 1; **5.** 1; **6.** 4; **7.** 1, 2; **8.** 2; **9.** 1, 2, 3; **10.** 1; **11.** 2; **12.** 2; **13.** 2, 3; **14.** 4; **15.** 1.

Rationales for Review Questions can be found on the Evolve website.

REFERENCES

Centers for Disease Control and Prevention (CDC): Youth risk behavior surveillance—United States, 2013, *MMWR Surveill Summ* 63:1, 2014.

Erikson E: *Childhood and society*, ed 2, New York, 1963, WW Norton.

Herdman TH, Kamitsuru S, editors: *NANDA International: NANDA International nursing diagnoses: definitions and classifications, 2015-2017*, Oxford, UK, 2014, Wiley-Blackwell.

Rosenberg M: *Society and the adolescent self-image*, Princeton, NJ, 1965, Princeton University Press.

Stuart GW: *Principles and practice of psychiatric nursing*, ed 10, St Louis, 2013, Elsevier.

Touhy TA, Jett KF: Ebersole and Hess' *Gerontological nursing and healthy aging*, ed 4, St Louis, 2014, Elsevier.

RESEARCH REFERENCES

Clare L, et al: Self-concept in early stages dementia: profile, course, correlates, predictors and implications for quality of life, *Int J Geriatr Psychiatry* 28:494, 2012.

Diehl M, Hay EL: Self-concept differentiation and self-concept clarity across adulthood: associations with age and psychological well-being, *Int J Aging Hum Dev* 73(2):125, 2011.

Dudovitz RN, et al: Behavioral self-concept as predictor of teen drinking behaviors, *Acad Pediatr* 13(4):316, 2013.

Maldonado L, et al: Impact of early adolescent anxiety disorder on self-esteem development from adolescence to young adulthood, *J Adolesc Health* 53:287, 2013.

Mantilla EF, et al: Self-image and eating disorder symptoms in normal and clinical adolescents, *Eat Behav* 15:125, 2014.

McIntyre K, et al: Workplace self-expansion: implications for job satisfaction, commitment, self-concept clarity, and self-esteem among employed and unemployed, *Basic Appl Soc Psych* 36:59, 2014.

Pai HC, Lee S: Sexual self-concept as influencing intended sexual health behavior of young adolescent Taiwanese girls, *J Clin Nurs* 21:1988, 2012.

Pinquart M: Self-esteem of children and adolescents with chronic illness: a meta-analysis, *Child Care Health Dev* 39(2):153, 2012.

Preckel F, et al: Self-concept in adolescence: a longitudinal study on reciprocal effects of self-perceptions in academic and social domains, *J Adolesc* 36:1165, 2013.

Rhea DJ, Thatcher WG: Ethnicity, ethnic identity, self-esteem, and at-risk eating disordered differences of urban adolescent females, *Eat Disord* 21:223, 2013.

Rissanen M, et al: A systematic literature review: self-mutilation among adolescents as a phenomenon and help for it—what kind of knowledge is lacking?, *Issues Ment Health Nurs* 32:575, 2011.

Schooler D, Daniels EA: "I am not a skinny toothpick and proud of it." Latina adolescents' ethnic identity and responses to mainstream media images, *Body Image* 11:11, 2014.

Ten Hoeve Y, et al: The nursing profession: public image, self-concept and professional identity: a discussion paper, *J Adv Nurs* 70(2):295, 2014.

Thomas JJ, Moring JC: Development of a revised generalized health-related self-concept inventory, *Am J Health Behav* 38(4):614, 2014.

Vartanian LR, Dey S: Self-concept clarity, thin ideal internalization, and appearance-related social comparison as predictors of body dissatisfaction, *Body Image* 10:495, 2013.

Verschueren K, et al: Relationships with mother, teacher, and peers: unique and joint effects on young children's self-concept, *Attach Hum Dev* 14(3):233, 2012.

Wurm S, et al: How do negative self-perceptions of aging become a self-fulfilling prophecy, *Psychol Aging* 28(4):1088, 2013.

35 Sexuality

OBJECTIVES

- Identify personal attitudes, beliefs, and biases related to sexuality.
- Discuss the nurse's role in maintaining or enhancing a patient's sexual health.
- Describe key concepts of sexual development across the life span.
- Identify causes of sexual dysfunction.
- Assess a patient's sexuality.
- Formulate appropriate nursing diagnoses for patients with alterations in sexuality.
- Identify patient risk factors in the area of sexual health.
- Identify and describe nursing interventions to promote sexual health.
- Evaluate patient outcomes related to sexual health needs.
- Identify health care providers and community resources available to help patients resolve sexual concerns that are outside the nurse's level of expertise.
- Use critical thinking skills when helping patients meet their sexual needs.

KEY TERMS

Bisexual, p. 717
Climacteric, p. 728
Condom, p. 718
Contraception, p. 716
Diaphragm, p. 718
Dyspareunia, p. 717
Gay, p. 717
Gender identity, p. 716
Gender roles, p. 716
Hypoactive sexual desire disorder, p. 722
Infertility, p. 721
Lesbian, p. 717
Perimenopausal, p. 717
Sexual dysfunction, p. 721
Sexual health, p. 716
Sexual orientation, p. 716
Sexuality, p. 716
Sexually transmitted infections (STIs), p. 716
Sterilization, p. 718
Transgender, p. 717
Tubal ligation, p. 718
Vasectomy, p. 718

MEDIA RESOURCES

http://evolve.elsevier.com/Potter/fundamentals/

- Review Questions
- Concept Map Creator
- Case Study with Questions
- Audio Glossary
- Content Updates

Sexuality is part of a person's personality and is important for overall health. Even though discussion of sexual topics has increased over the years, many adults lack knowledge regarding **sexuality**. Although patients may be hesitant to bring up their concerns, they often share their feelings when a nurse addresses sexuality in a relaxed, matter-of-fact manner. To feel comfortable addressing sexuality, nurses need therapeutic communication skills and to be knowledgeable about sexual functioning, issues, and assessment. Many values and issues surround sexuality. Religious teachings, cultural influences on **gender roles**, beliefs about **sexual orientation**, and social and environmental climates influence the values systems for both patients and health care providers.

Sexuality has many definitions. Expression of an individual's sexuality is influenced by interaction among biological, sociological, psychological, spiritual, economic, political, religious, and cultural factors (WHO, n.d.). In addition, values, attitudes, behaviors, relationships with others, and the need to establish emotional closeness with others influence sexuality.

Sexuality differs from *sexual health*. According to WHO (n.d.), **sexual health** is "a state of physical, emotional, mental, and social well-being in relation to sexuality; it is not merely the absence of disease, dysfunction, or infirmity." People who are sexually healthy have a positive and respectful approach to sexuality and sexual relationships. They also have a potential for having pleasurable and safe sexual experiences that are free from coercion, discrimination, and violence.

SCIENTIFIC KNOWLEDGE BASE

A sound scientific knowledge base regarding sexuality provides you with the necessary information to help your patients achieve sexual health. A basic understanding of sexual development, sexual orientation, **contraception**, abortion, and **sexually transmitted infections (STIs)** is necessary.

Sexual Development

Sexuality changes as a person grows and develops. Each stage of development brings changes in sexual functioning and the role of sexuality in relationships.

Infancy and Early Childhood. The first 3 years of life are crucial in the development of **gender identity** (Edelman and Mandle, 2014). The child identifies with the parent of the same sex and develops a

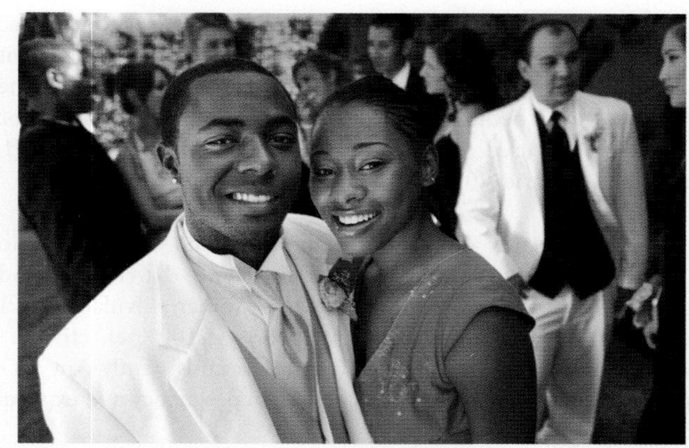

FIGURE 35-1 Adolescents function within a powerful network of peers as they explore their sexual identity. (©bikeriderlondon.)

complementary relationship with the parent of the opposite sex. Children become aware of differences between the sexes, begin to perceive that they are either male or female, and interpret the behaviors of others as behavior appropriate for a female or a male.

School-Age Years. During the school years parents, educators, and peer groups serve as role models and teachers about how men and women act with and relate to one another. School-age children generally have questions regarding the physical and emotional aspects of sex. They need accurate information from home and school about changes in their bodies and emotions during this period and what to expect as they move into puberty (Edelman and Mandle, 2014). Knowledge about normal emotional and physical changes associated with puberty decreases anxiety as these changes begin to happen.

Puberty/Adolescence. The emotional changes during puberty and adolescence are as dramatic as the physical ones. Adolescents function within a powerful peer group, with the almost constant anxiety of "Am I normal?" and "Will I be accepted?" (Figure 35-1). They face many decisions and need accurate information on topics such as body changes, sexual activity, emotional responses within intimate sexual relationships, STIs, contraception, and pregnancy. Adolescence is often a time when individuals explore their primary sexual orientation (Hockenberry and Wilson, 2015; Pascoe, 2013).

Adolescents may identify with a sexual minority group such as **lesbian**, **gay**, **bisexual**, or **transgender** (LGBT) (Young-Bruehl, 2010). A transgender individual's self-recognition as a male or female is in conflict with his or her biological sex characteristics or what is culturally determined as belonging to a male or female (Olson et al., 2011; Rosenthal, 2014). Transgender patients may pursue treatments or modification procedures to promote physical characteristics consistent with their gender identification (Rosenthal, 2014). Adolescents often face significant stress related to sexual identity and benefit from education about sexuality issues (Doty et al., 2010; Johnson and Amella, 2014; Lim et al., 2014). LGBT individuals are at a higher risk for depression; suicide; and abuse of tobacco, alcohol, and drugs than the general population.

In the United States almost 50% of high school students report that they have had sexual intercourse at least 1 time, and 15% of high school students had had four or more sexual partners (Kann et al., 2014; CDC, 2014d). Adolescents who engage in risky sexual behaviors experience negative health outcomes such as STIs and unintended pregnancy (Dunne et al., 2014; Scott et al., 2011). In addition, the pattern of risk-taking behavior tends to be established and continue throughout life. Parents need to understand the importance of providing factual information, sharing their values, and promoting sound decision-making skills. They need to know that, even with the best guidance and information, adolescents make their own decisions and need to be held accountable for them. Support from peers, family, school counselors, clergy, nurses, and other health professionals is important during this time.

Young Adulthood. Although young adults have matured physically, they continue to explore and mature emotionally in relationships. Intimacy and sexuality are issues for all young adults whether they are in a sexual relationship, choose to abstain from sex, remain single by choice, are homosexual, or are widowed. People are sexually healthy in numerous ways. Sexual activity is often defined as a basic need, and healthy sexual desire is channeled into forms of intimacy throughout a lifetime. At times young adults require support and education or therapy to achieve mutually satisfying sexual relationships.

Middle Adulthood. Changes in physical appearance in middle adulthood sometimes lead to concerns about sexual attractiveness. In addition, actual physical changes related to aging affect sexual functioning. Decreasing levels of estrogen in **perimenopausal** woman lead to diminished vaginal lubrication and decreased vaginal elasticity. Both of these changes often lead to **dyspareunia**, or the occurrence of pain during intercourse. Decreasing levels of estrogen may also result in a decreased desire for sexual activity. As men age they are likely to experience changes such as an increase in the postejaculatory refractory period and delayed ejaculation. Anticipatory guidance regarding these normal changes, using vaginal lubrication, and creating time for caressing and tenderness ease concerns regarding sexual functioning. Some aging adults also need to adjust to the impact of chronic illness, medications, aches, pains, and other health concerns about sexuality.

Later in the adult years some individuals have to adjust to the social and emotional changes associated with children moving away from home. This results in either a time of renewed intimacy between partners or a time when formerly intimate partners realize that they no longer care for one another or have common interests. In either case, when children leave home, intimate relationships usually change.

Older Adulthood. Sexuality in older adults is an important aspect of health that often is overlooked by health care providers. Studies show a positive correlation between sexual activity and physical health in older adults (Lindau and Gavrilova, 2010; Stewart and Graham, 2013). Research indicates that many older adults are more sexuality active than previously thought and engage in high-risk sexual encounters, resulting in a steady increase of human immunodeficiency virus (HIV) and STI rates over the past 12 years (Box 35-1).

Factors that determine sexual activity in older adults include present health status, medications, past and present life satisfaction, and the status of marital or intimate relationships. For example, many older women are widowed or divorced and lack available sexual partners, which accounts for their decline in sexual activity. Nurses working with older adults need to assess the sexuality of their patients, sexual interest and functioning, and plan accordingly (Buttaro et al., 2014; Ayaz, 2013). It is essential to maintain a nonjudgmental attitude and convey that sexual activity is normal in later years. Emphasize that it is not essential to maintaining quality of life, especially when patients have decided not to remain sexually active.

To be effective in promoting sexual health, nurses need to understand the normal sexual changes that occur as people age. The excitement phase prolongs in both men and women, and it usually takes longer for them to reach orgasm. The refractory time following orgasm

BOX 35-1 FOCUS ON OLDER ADULTS

Sexuality in Older Adults

- Sexuality and continued interest in sex throughout middle and late life are usually associated with good physical health (Bach et al., 2013; Lindau and Gavrilova, 2010).
- Physiological changes with aging that influence sexual response are multifactorial and related to changes in circulation, hormones, and neurological pathways (Horstman et al., 2012).
- Pathological issues with the aging sexual response are often related to illnesses and side effects from medications (Bach et al., 2013; Buttaro et al., 2014; Syme, 2014).
- Older adults are often reluctant to discuss sexual problems with health care providers (Buttaro et al., 2014).
- Older adults who live in extended care facilities often lose their privacy and experience a decline in physical and cognitive abilities that affects their sexual expression. People who live in assisted living facilities have more privacy and are often able to live as couples (Katz, 2013; Syme, 2014).
- As the population ages and remains healthy, increasing numbers of older lesbian, gay, bisexual, and transgendered (LGBT) people remain sexually active (CDC, 2013b)
- Increased availability of treatments for male and female sexual dysfunction contributes to continued sexual activity throughout the life span (Stewart and Graham, 2013).
- Older sexually active adults are at risk for contracting sexually transmitted infections. Because the risk of pregnancy is not an issue, older adults often do not recognize the need for protected sex when becoming active with new and/or multiple partners (Johnson, 2013; Stewart and Graham, 2013).

is also longer. Both genders experience a reduced availability of sex hormones. Men often have erections that are less firm and shorter acting. Women usually do not have difficulty maintaining sexual function unless they have a medical condition that impairs their sexual activity. Typically the infrequency of sex in older women is related to the age, health, and sexual function of their partner. Women continue to experience changes related to menopause, and those with problems related to urinary incontinence often experience embarrassment during intercourse. Couples who have physically disabling conditions often need information about which positions are more comfortable when having sexual intercourse.

Sexual Orientation

Sexual orientation describes the predominant pattern of a person's sexual attraction over time. Many stereotypical myths remain about people who are LGBT. Current evidence indicates that they experience decreased access to health care and do not readily seek preventive care (Lim et al., 2014; Williamson, 2010). Nonjudgmental nurses who have a solid knowledge base help to discourage these myths and provide nursing care that includes attention to the person's sexual orientation.

Contraception

Numerous contraceptive options are available to sexually active couples today. They provide varying levels of protection against unwanted pregnancies. Some methods do not require a prescription, whereas others require a prescription or some other type of intervention from a health care provider. Methods that are effective for contraception do not always reduce the risk of STIs. For example, the pill and intrauterine contraceptive device (IUD) are effective as birth control but not for protection from STIs. A latex condom should be used during each act of intercourse to reduce the risk of STIs. Effectiveness varies with each contraceptive method and the consistency of use. Unplanned pregnancies occur because contraceptives are not used, are used inconsistently, or are used improperly (Schwartz and Gabelnick, 2011; Trussell and Guthrie, 2011).

Nonprescription Contraceptive Methods. Nonprescription methods for contraception include abstinence, barrier methods, and timing of intercourse with regard to a woman's ovulation cycle. Although abstinence from sexual intercourse is 100% effective, it is often difficult for both men and women to use consistently. Any act of unprotected intercourse potentially results in pregnancy and exposure to STIs.

Barrier methods include over-the-counter spermicidal products and condoms. Spermicidal products (e.g., creams, jellies, foams, and sponges) are put into the vagina before intercourse to create a spermicidal barrier between the uterus and ejaculated sperm. A latex **condom** is a thin rubber sheath that fits over the penis to prevent entrance of sperm into the vagina. A diaphragm is a barrier method, which must be used with a spermicide with each sexual encounter. Vaginal spermicides and condoms are most effective when instructions are followed carefully; their combined use is more effective in preventing pregnancy than the use of either one alone (Cates and Harwood, 2011).

Nonprescription methods of contraception based on the physiological changes of the menstrual cycle include the rhythm, basal body temperature, cervical mucus, and fertility-awareness methods. Couples who use these methods need to understand the reproductive cycle of the woman's body and the subtle signs and signals that her body gives during the cycle. To prevent pregnancy couples abstain from sexual intercourse during designated fertile periods.

Methods That Require a Health Care Provider's Intervention. Contraceptive methods that require the intervention of a health care provider include hormonal contraception, IUDs, the diaphragm, the cervical cap, and **sterilization**. Hormonal contraception is available in several forms: oral contraceptive pills, vaginal contraceptive rings, hormonal injections, subdermal implant, transdermal skin patches, and IUDs. Hormonal contraception alters the hormonal environment to prevent ovulation, thicken cervical mucus, and thin the lining of the uterus.

An IUD is a plastic device inserted by a health care provider into the uterus through the cervical opening. IUDs contain either copper or progesterone. The primary mechanism by which both types of IUDs prevent pregnancy is to stop the sperm from fertilizing an egg (Dean and Schwarz, 2011; Murphy, 2011). The release of progesterone may also increase cervical mucus thickness and alter the lining of the uterus.

The **diaphragm** is a round, rubber dome that has a flexible spring around the edge. It is used with a contraceptive cream or jelly and is inserted in the vagina so it provides a contraceptive barrier over the cervical opening. The woman needs to be refitted after a significant change in weight (10-lb gain or loss) or pregnancy. The cervical cap functions like the diaphragm; however, it covers only the cervix. It may be left in place longer, and some perceive it as more comfortable than the diaphragm.

Sterilization is the most effective contraception method other than abstinence. Female sterilization, or **tubal ligation**, involves cutting, tying, or otherwise ligating the fallopian tubes. In male sterilization, or **vasectomy**, the vas deferens, which carries the sperm away from the testicles, is cut and tied. Both a tubal ligation and a vasectomy usually are considered permanent surgical procedures.

Sexually Transmitted Infections

The incidence of STIs continues to increase. Approximately 20 million people in the United States are diagnosed with an STI each year, with the highest incidence occurring in men who have sex with men, bisexual men, and youths between the ages of 15 and 24 (CDC, 2014a). The prevalence of STIs is a major health concern for several reasons. Black and Hispanic populations are diagnosed with STIs more frequently than whites, and women have more complications associated with STIs than men (Healthy People 2020, n.d.; CDC, 2013a). In addition, race, poverty, access to health care, and sexual practices contribute to disparities in the STI rates.

Treatment of STIs in America costs about $16 million annually (CDC, 2014a). Commonly diagnosed STIs include syphilis, gonorrhea, chlamydia, trichomoniasis, and infection with the human papillomavirus (HPV) and herpes simplex virus (HSV) type II (genital warts and genital herpes, respectively).

As the name implies, STIs are transmitted from infected individuals to partners during intimate sexual contact. The site of transmission is usually genital, but sometimes it is oral-genital or anal-genital. People most likely to be infected share one key characteristic: unprotected sex with multiple partners. Gonorrhea, chlamydia, syphilis, and pelvic inflammatory disease (PID) are caused by bacteria and are usually curable with antibiotics. Patients need to take antibiotics for the full course of treatment. However, an emerging concern is that some of these bacterial infections (e.g., gonorrhea and syphilis) are now developing antibiotic-resistant strains. Infections such as HSV types I and II, HPV, and HIV are caused by viruses and cannot be cured.

A major problem in dealing with STIs is finding and treating the people who have them. Some people do not know that they are infected because symptoms are sometimes absent or go unnoticed. Common symptoms of an STI include discharge from the vagina, penis, anus, or throat; pain during sex or when urinating; and unexplained rash or lesions (Phillippi and Latendresse, 2014). Because sexual behavior often includes the whole body rather than just the genitalia, many parts of the body are potential sites for an STI. The perineum, anus, and rectum frequently are involved in sexual activity. Furthermore, any contact with another person's body fluids around the head or an open lesion on the skin, anus, or genitalia can transmit an STI.

Sometimes people do not seek treatment because they are embarrassed to discuss sexual symptoms or concerns. Often they are hesitant to talk about their sexual behavior if they believe that it is not "normal." Any sexual behavior that embarrasses a patient often hinders the detection of an STI. Develop communication skills and a nonjudgmental attitude to provide effective care for those diagnosed with one. Detect valuable clues about an STI by establishing trust, talking with patients, and asking questions in a caring manner. Assess attitudes toward sexuality and adjust the intervention to make it acceptable to the patient's sexual value system.

Human Immunodeficiency Virus Infection. HIV infection is a bloodborne pathogen and is present in most body fluids. It is sometimes spread through sexual contact. Transmission occurs when there is an exchange of body fluid. Primary routes of transmission include contaminated intravenous (IV) needles, anal intercourse, vaginal intercourse, oral-genital sex, and transfusion of blood and blood products.

The natural history of HIV progresses in three stages. The primary infection stage lasts for about a month after contracting the virus. During this time the person often experiences flulike symptoms. Then he or she enters the clinical latency phase; at this time there are no symptoms of infection. HIV antibodies appear in the blood about 6 weeks to 3 months after infection. If left untreated, people who are infected with HIV live about 10 years. The last stage, acquired immunodeficiency syndrome (AIDS), happens when a person begins to show symptoms of the disease. AIDS is a serious, debilitating, and eventually fatal disease. Highly active antiretroviral therapy (HAART) and having an experienced HIV clinician greatly increase the survival time of people who live with HIV/AIDS (Marrazzo and Cates, 2011).

Human Papillomavirus Infection. HPV is the most common STI in the United States, with approximately 14 million new infections every year (CDC, 2014b). Most HPV infections are asymptomatic and self-limiting. However, certain types can cause cervical cancer in women and anogenital cancers and genital warts in both men and women. HPV is spread through direct contact with warts, semen, and other body fluids from others who have the disease. The textured warts often have a cauliflower appearance and are most common on the penis and scrotum in men and the vagina and cervix in women. A vaccine that protects both men and woman against nine types of HPV that most commonly cause health concerns is now available (ACOG, 2015; CDC, 2015b) (Box 35-2).

Chlamydia. The bacteria *Chlamydia trachomatis* causes chlamydia. It is the most commonly reported infectious disease in the United States, affecting about 3 million Americans each year (CDC, 2014c). Chlamydia is spread by contact with fluids from the infected site. The infection can be transmitted during the birthing process and cause conjunctivitis and pneumonia in newborn babies. It frequently infects the cervix and, if left untreated, can cause PID, ectopic pregnancy, and infertility from damage to the female reproductive organs. Most people do not realize that they are infected with chlamydia because it causes few symptoms (CDC, 2015a). For this reason the CDC recommends annual screening for all sexually active women up to age 25. High-risk populations are people who have multiple sex partners or are infected with other STIs and men who have sex with men.

NURSING KNOWLEDGE BASE

Factors Influencing Sexuality

Use critical thinking skills and basic nursing knowledge when addressing patients' sexual health needs. Draw from the following areas of nursing knowledge: sociocultural dimensions of sexuality, decisional issues, and alterations in sexual health.

Sociocultural Dimensions of Sexuality

People assign different meanings to sexuality on the basis of their culture, gender, education, socioeconomic status, and religion (Giger, 2013). Society plays a powerful role in shaping sexual values and attitudes and supporting specific expression of sexuality in its members.

Each cultural and social group has its own set of rules and norms that guide sexual behavior, sexual health, and the willingness to discuss this private part of life. For example, cultural norms influence how people find partners, whom they choose as partners, how they relate to one another, how often they have sex, and what they do when they have sex. Personal beliefs enable certain practices and prohibit others (Box 35-3).

Impact of Pregnancy and Menstruation on Sexuality. Sexual interest and activity of women and their partners vary during pregnancy and menstruation. Some cultures encourage sexual intercourse or male-female contact during menstruation and pregnancy, but

BOX 35-2 EVIDENCE BASED PRACTICE

Health Risk Behaviors Associated with the Human Papilloma Virus Vaccine

PICO Question: Do youths who receive the human papilloma virus (HPV) vaccine engage in more sexual risk behaviors than youths who do not receive the vaccine?

Evidence Summary

HPV is the most common sexually transmitted infection (STI) in the United States and is associated with development of anogenital cancers and genital warts in males and females (ACOG, 2015; CDC, 2013c; CDC, 2014b). The vaccine targets the specific HPVs linked to cancer and warts. It is recommended for all youths ages 11 to 26 years, but vaccination rates in the United States are low (ACOG, 2015; Dorell et al., 2014; Marchand et al., 2013). Parental acceptance of the vaccine influences vaccination status, and parents have voiced concern that vaccination will promote sexual risk taking in youths despite evidence indicating otherwise (Dorrell et al., 2014; Marchand et al., 2013; Roberts et al., 2010). In a study of females ages 13 to 21, vaccination was not associated with an increase in number of sexual partners or a decrease in the use of condoms (Mayhew et al., 2014). Administration of the HPV vaccine to almost 1400 females ages 11 to 12 did not result in an increase in the occurrence of pregnancy, STIs, or the need for contraception over the next 3 years (Bednarczyk et al., 2012). College-age females who received the vaccine did not differ in age of first intercourse, number of sexual partners, or condom use when compared to nonvaccinated peers (Marchand et al., 2013). Less research has been conducted on male vaccination compliance, but barriers such as lack of knowledge concerning health risks, need for vaccination of males versus females, and provider recommendation to parents have all been shown to impact vaccination rates in males (Donahue et al., 2014; Fontenot et al., 2014). Health care professionals need to consider these findings to encourage vaccine understanding and acceptance among parents and youths.

Application to Nursing Practice

- Vaccine recommendation by health care professionals can increase vaccine acceptance by the public and reduce the incidence of HPV-related cancers (ACOG, 2015; Donahue et al., 2014).
- Nurses need to discuss the benefits of the vaccine with parents and youths ages 11 to 26 years and offer catch-up vaccines as needed (ACOG, 2015; CDC, 2013c).
- Reduce parental concerns by sharing research that indicates that vaccine administration does not increase sexual activity or risk behaviors (Bednarczyk et al., 2012; Marchand et al., 2013; Mayhew et al., 2014).
- Continue to teach safe sex practices.

BOX 35-3 CULTURAL ASPECTS OF CARE

Cultural Factors and Human Immunodeficiency Virus

All sexually active individuals are at risk for HIV; however, some cultures have higher infection rates. For example, Latinos in the United States are 3 times more likely than non-Latino whites to be diagnosed with human immunodeficiency virus (HIV) (Adih et al., 2010). Latino males are 2 times more likely than white males to have HIV, and females are 4 times more likely to be HIV positive than their white counterparts (Peragallo et al., 2012). The majority of HIV cases result from heterosexual activity, and Latino youths are less likely than other ethnic groups to use condoms (Casey and Gomez-Lobo, 2013; Deordorff et al., 2013; Peragallo et al., 2012).

Cultural-specific norms and values that contribute to sexual risk behaviors include gender roles, religion, and sexual communication patterns (Peragallo et al., 2012; Warren et al., 2011). *Marianismo* refers to women who are virtuous and submissive; whereas *machismo* views men as strong, independent, and in a position of authority (Deordorff et al., 2010). In the Latino culture, women are expected to remain virgins before marriage, whereas men are not expected to control sexual desires. Traditional Latino culture maintains that it is not appropriate for men and women to discuss sexual issues, even within families or intimate relationships (Deordorff et al., 2013). Health care providers need to consider cultural values and their influence on sexual practices when working with the Latino population (Lee et al., 2013).

Implications for Patient-Centered Care

- Establish a therapeutic relationship with a patient/family before discussing sexual health.
- Provide both males and females written and verbal information in English and Spanish, or in their native language, regarding contraception, sexually transmitted infections (STIs), and HIV testing and management options (Warren et al., 2011).
- Target adolescents by expanding education on STIs, HIV, and contraception in middle- and high-school curriculum.
- Promote gender neutrality by addressing assertive communication and negotiation strategies among females.
- Increase HIV testing at community clinics and offer combined laboratory work for STIs and HIV to promote acceptance (Adih et al., 2010).
- Promote cultural-specific bilingual multimedia and community education about HIV risk-reduction strategies (Adih et al., 2010).

others strictly forbid it. For example, in the Hindu culture a woman avoids worship, cooking, and other members of the family during menstruation. Research has found no physiological contraindication to intercourse during menstruation or during most pregnancies. Female sexual interest tends to fluctuate during pregnancy, with increased interest during the second trimester and often decreased interest during the first and third trimesters. There is often a decrease in libido during the first trimester because of nausea, fatigue, and breast tenderness. During the second trimester blood flow to the pelvic area increases to supply the placenta, resulting in increased sexual enjoyment and libido. During the third trimester the increased abdominal size often makes finding a comfortable position difficult (Link, 2012).

Discussing Sexual Issues. Sexuality is a significant part of each person's being, yet sexual assessment and interventions are not always included in health care (Ayaz, 2013; Ivarsson et al., 2010; Sobecki et al., 2012; Steinke et al., 2013). The area of sexuality is often emotionally charged for nurses and patients. Sometimes nurses avoid discussing sexual issues with patients because they lack information or have different values than their patients. Nurses who have difficulty discussing topics related to sexuality need to explore their discomfort and develop a plan to address it. If you are uncomfortable with topics related to sexuality, the patient is unlikely to share sexual concerns with you. You need to be aware of your personal beliefs before discussing sexuality with your patients.

Decisional Issues

Individuals make many decisions about their sexuality. Some nurses help patients make decisions about contraception and abortion.

Contraception. Decisions patients make regarding contraception have far-reaching effects on their lives. Pregnancy, whether planned or unplanned, significantly affects the life of the mother and father and often their support network. Effects are physical, interpersonal, social, financial, and societal. The choice to use contraception is multifaceted and not completely understood. Factors that affect the effectiveness of contraception include the type of method used, the couple's understanding of the method, the consistency of use, and compliance with the requirements of the chosen method. Choice of contraception method varies in relation to the age, ethnicity, marital status, income, education, sexual orientation, and previous pregnancies of the woman (Casey and Gomez-Lobo, 2013; Godfrey et al, 2011; Jones et al., 2012). Mobile apps are available to help patients and health professionals monitor reproductive health (e.g., to remind you when to take oral contraceptives, to replace your transdermal patch or vaginal ring, or when your most fertile time is occurring). Some examples of women's health apps include Clue, Period Tracker, Glow, Glow Nurture, Ovia Fertility, and iBreastCheck (Garcia, 2014).

Abortion. Half of all pregnancies in the United States are unplanned; unintended pregnancy rates are highest among low-income women, women ages 18 to 24 and over 40, cohabiting women, and minority women (Finer and Zolna, 2014). Approximately 40% of unintended pregnancies end in abortion. Abortions have been performed since ancient times. The safety and availability of abortions in the United States improved after the 1973 Supreme Court decision *Roe v Wade,* which established the right of every woman to have an abortion. They are safer and less costly when performed in the early weeks of pregnancy.

Abortion is a hotly debated issue. Women and their partners who face an unwanted pregnancy may consider it. If caring for a patient contemplating abortion, provide an environment in which the patient is able to discuss the issue openly, allowing exploration of various options with an unwanted pregnancy. Discuss religious, social, and personal issues in a nonjudgmental manner with patients. Reasons for choosing an abortion vary and include terminating an unwanted pregnancy or aborting a fetus known to have birth defects. When a woman chooses abortion as a way of dealing with an unwanted pregnancy, the woman and often her partner experience a sense of loss, grief, and/or guilt.

Be aware of personal values related to abortion. As a nurse you are entitled to your personal views. You should not be forced to participate in counseling or procedures contrary to your beliefs and values. It is essential to choose specialties or places of employment where personal values are not compromised and the care of a patient in need of health care is not jeopardized.

Prevention of Sexually Transmitted Infections. Responsible sexual behavior includes knowing one's sexual partner and the partner's sexual history, being able to openly discuss drug-use history with the partner, not allowing drugs or alcohol to influence decision making and sexual practices, and using STI and contraceptive protective devices.

Alterations in Sexual Health

Infertility. Infertility is the inability to conceive after 1 year of unprotected intercourse. A couple who wants to conceive but is unable to has special needs. Some experience a sense of failure and think that their bodies are defective. Sometimes the desire to become pregnant grows until it permeates most waking moments. Some individuals become preoccupied with creating just the right circumstances for conception. With advances in reproductive technology, infertile couples face many choices that involve religious and ethical values and financial limitations.

Choices for the infertile couple include pursuit of adoption, medical assistance with fertilization, or adapting to the probability of remaining childless. Organizations such as RESOLVE: The National Organization of Infertility, a national support group for couples with infertility, or international adoption groups provide couples with support and offer referral sources.

Sexual Abuse. Sexual abuse is a widespread health problem. Abuse crosses all gender, socioeconomic, age, and ethnic groups. Most often it is at the hands of a former intimate partner or family member. Sexual abuse has far-ranging effects on physical and psychological functioning (Edelman and Mandle, 2014). Sometimes it begins, continues, or even intensifies during pregnancy. Cues that raise a question of possible sexual abuse include extreme jealousy and refusal to leave a woman's presence. The overall appearance is sometimes that of a very concerned and caring husband or boyfriend, when the underlying reason for this behavior is very different.

Nurses are in an ideal position to assess occurrences of sexual violence, help patients confront these stressors, and educate individuals regarding community services. Nurses are mandated reporters and must report suspected abuse to the proper authorities. When you suspect or recognize abuse, mobilize support for the victim and the family. When abuse is suspected, remember to *not* ask the potential victim about any abusive behaviors in the presence of the suspected abuser. Provide privacy for the abuse victim and obtain information in a protective environment. When there is abuse, all family members usually require therapy to promote healthy interactions and relationships.

Rape victims often need to work through the crisis before feeling comfortable with intimate expressions of affection. The partner needs to know how to help and support the victim. Children who have been molested sexually need to understand that they are not at fault for the incident. The parents need to understand that their response is critical to how the child reacts and adapts.

Personal and Emotional Conflicts. Ideally sex is a natural, spontaneous act that passes easily through a number of recognizable physiological stages and ends in one or more orgasms. In reality this sequence of events is more the exception than the rule. You will care for patients who have problems with one or more of the stages of sexual activity, including the feeling of wanting sex, the physiological processes and emotions of having sex, and the feelings experienced after sex. For example, some women and men who are taking antidepressants report that their ability to reach orgasm is affected negatively.

Sexual Dysfunction. Sexual dysfunction, the absence of complete sexual functioning, is common. The incidence of sexual dysfunction in the general population is estimated to be as high as 40% in men and 60% to 80% in women (Buttaro et al., 2014; Touhy and Jett, 2014). It is more prevalent in men and women with poor emotional and physical health (Box 35-4). Sometimes the exact cause cannot be determined.

The incidence of erectile dysfunction (ED) increases with age but can occur in men under 40 (Capogrosso et al., 2013; Syme, 2014). Risk factors are similar to those for heart disease (i.e., diabetes mellitus, hyperlipidemia, hypertension, hypothyroidism, chronic renal failure, smoking, obesity, alcohol abuse, and lack of exercise). The etiology of ED is often multifactorial. Neurogenic problems, medications, or endocrine or psychogenic factors can cause it. An age-related decrease in testosterone often results in decreased tone of the erectile tissues.

BOX 35-4 Illnesses and Medications That Affect Sexual Functioning of Men and Women

Illnesses
- Diabetes mellitus
- Cancer (e.g., prostate, breast, colon, ovarian, testicular, rectal)
- Neuropathy
- Spina bifida
- Spinal cord injury
- Unstable angina
- Uncontrolled hypertension
- Chronic obstructive pulmonary disease
- Human immunodeficiency virus infection
- Substance abuse
- Depression

Medications
- Antihypertensives
- Antipsychotics
- Antidepressants
- Antianxiety
- Diuretics
- Oncological agents
- Recreational or illicit drugs

Data from Bach LE et al: The association of physical and mental health with sexual activity in older adults in a retirement community, *J Sex Med* 10:2671, 2013; Basson R et al: Sexual function in chronic illness, *J Sex Med* 7:374, 2010; Bispo GS et al: Cardiovascular changes resulting from sexual activity and sexual dysfunction after myocardial infarction: integrative review, *J Clin Nurs* 22:3522, 2013; Buster J: Managing female sexual dysfunction, *Fertil Steril* 100(4):905, 2013; Conaglen HM, Conaglen JV: Drug-induced sexual dysfunction in men and women, *Aust Prescriber* 36(2):42, 2013.

One of the most common problems affecting women of all ages is **hypoactive sexual desire disorder** (HSDD) (Buster, 2013; Buttaro et al., 2014; Kingsberg, 2011; Rosen et al., 2012). Biological, organic, or psychosocial factors can contribute to the incidence of HSDD. Chronic medical conditions such as breast or gynecological cancers and hormonal fluctuations, pain, or depression and anxiety can contribute to a decreased interest in sexual intimacy (Bach et al., 2013).

CRITICAL THINKING

Successful critical thinking requires synthesis of knowledge, experience, information gathered from patients, critical thinking attitudes, and intellectual and professional standards. Nurses use clinical judgment to anticipate information needs, analyze assessment data, and make appropriate decisions regarding patient care. Figure 35-2 shows how to use elements of critical thinking and patient assessment data to develop appropriate nursing diagnoses.

In the case of sexuality, integrate knowledge from nursing and other disciplines. Have a thorough understanding of safe sex practices and the risks and behaviors associated with sexual problems to anticipate how to assess a patient and interpret findings. Use previous experiences to provide care for patients with sexual issues in a more reflective and helpful way. Patients have different customs and values from those of your own. Professional standards require respect for each patient as an individual. Critical thinking attitudes such as integrity require you to recognize when personal opinions and values are in conflict with those

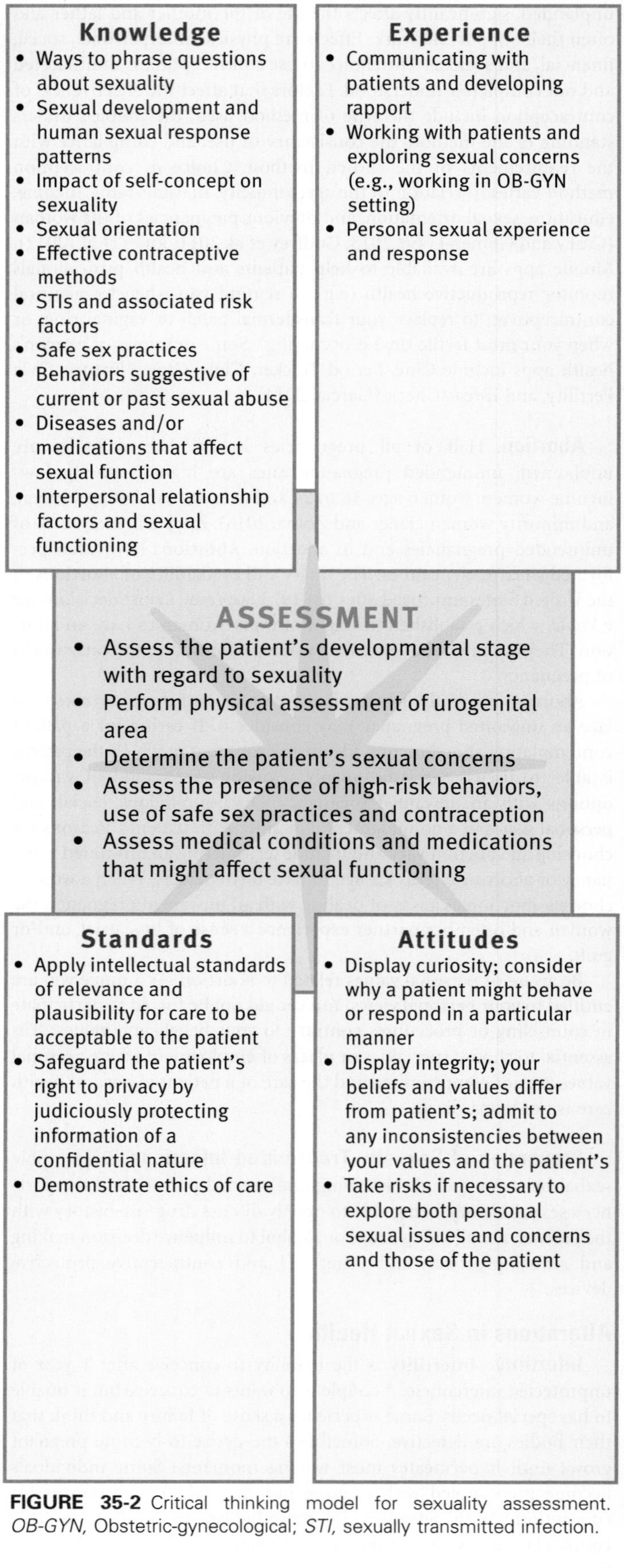

Knowledge
- Ways to phrase questions about sexuality
- Sexual development and human sexual response patterns
- Impact of self-concept on sexuality
- Sexual orientation
- Effective contraceptive methods
- STIs and associated risk factors
- Safe sex practices
- Behaviors suggestive of current or past sexual abuse
- Diseases and/or medications that affect sexual function
- Interpersonal relationship factors and sexual functioning

Experience
- Communicating with patients and developing rapport
- Working with patients and exploring sexual concerns (e.g., working in OB-GYN setting)
- Personal sexual experience and response

ASSESSMENT
- Assess the patient's developmental stage with regard to sexuality
- Perform physical assessment of urogenital area
- Determine the patient's sexual concerns
- Assess the presence of high-risk behaviors, use of safe sex practices and contraception
- Assess medical conditions and medications that might affect sexual functioning

Standards
- Apply intellectual standards of relevance and plausibility for care to be acceptable to the patient
- Safeguard the patient's right to privacy by judiciously protecting information of a confidential nature
- Demonstrate ethics of care

Attitudes
- Display curiosity; consider why a patient might behave or respond in a particular manner
- Display integrity; your beliefs and values differ from patient's; admit to any inconsistencies between your values and the patient's
- Take risks if necessary to explore both personal sexual issues and concerns and those of the patient

FIGURE 35-2 Critical thinking model for sexuality assessment. *OB-GYN*, Obstetric-gynecological; *STI*, sexually transmitted infection.

of the patient and to consider how to proceed in a way that is mutually beneficial.

NURSING PROCESS

Apply the nursing process and use a critical thinking approach in your care of patients. The nursing process provides a clinical decision-making approach to help you develop and implement an individualized plan of care. Assess all relevant factors, including physical, psychological, social, and cultural, to determine a patient's sexual well-being. The nursing role in addressing sexual concerns ranges from ongoing assessment to providing information, counseling, and referral. Keep in mind that nurses are not expected to have answers to all sexual issues and concerns identified.

Assessment

During the assessment process thoroughly assess each patient and critically analyze findings to ensure that you make patient-centered clinical decisions required for safe nursing care.

Through the Patient's Eyes. As in any patient assessment, it is important to understand a patient's expectations regarding care. Questions such as "What would you like to have happen in regard to your sexual health problems?" and "What initial steps might you take?" help a patient identify desired outcomes. It is important to set aside personal views and consider a patient's needs and preferences for care.

Factors Affecting Sexuality. In gathering a sexual history consider physical, functional, relationship, lifestyle, developmental, and self-esteem factors that influence sexual functioning. Sexual desire varies among individuals; some people want and enjoy sex every day, whereas others want sex only once a month, and still others have no sexual desire and are quite comfortable with that fact. Sexual desire becomes an issue if the person wants to satisfy it more often, if he or she believes that it is necessary to measure up to some cultural norm, or if there is a discrepancy between the sexual desires of the partners in a relationship.

Ask patients to describe factors that typically influence their sexual desire. Knowing a patients' medical history and probing for information is helpful. For example, minor illness, medications, and fatigue often decrease sexual desire. Lifestyle factors such as the use or abuse of alcohol, lack of sleep, lack of time, or the demands of caring for a new baby are other influencing factors. For example, working parents sometimes feel so overburdened that they perceive sexual advances from a partner as an additional demand on them. Confirm factors that potentially affect sexual desire and determine with the patient the extent to which sexual function is impaired.

Self-concept issues (see Chapter 34), including identity, body image, role performance, and self-esteem, affect a patient's sexuality. Consider how these factors relate to a patient's condition. For example, poor body image associated with chronic disease magnifies feelings of rejection. This often results in diminished or absent sexual desire.

Issues in a relationship often affect sexual desire. After the initial glow of a new relationship has faded, some couples find that they have major differences in their values or lifestyles. Ask couples to describe how close they feel to each other and how often they interact on an intimate level. Assess communication patterns between sexual partners to determine sexual satisfaction within a relationship.

Sexual Health History. Most patients want to know how medications, treatments, and surgical procedures influence their sexual relationship even though they often do not ask questions. With experience nurses recognize that most patients welcome the opportunity to talk about their sexuality, especially when they are experiencing difficulties. The PLISSIT model provides an approach that nurses can use to assess sexuality in patients (Ayaz, 2013) (Box 35-5).

BOX 35-5 PLISSIT Assessment of Sexuality

Permission to discuss sexuality issues
Limited **I**nformation related to sexual health problems being experienced
Specific **S**uggestions—only when the nurse is clear about the problem
Intensive **T**herapy—referral to professional with advanced training if necessary

Modified from Annon JS: The PLISSIT model: a proposed conceptual scheme for the behavioral treatment of sexual problems, *J Sex Educ Ther* 2(2):1, 1976.

BOX 35-6 Nursing Assessment Questions

- Are you sexually active?
- With whom do you have sex: men, women, or both?
- How many sexual partners do you have (or have you ever had)?
- How do you feel about the sexual aspects of your life?
- Have you noticed any changes in the way you feel about yourself?
- How has your illness, medication, or surgery affected your sex life?
- It is not unusual for people with your condition to be experiencing some sexual changes. Have you noticed any changes, or do you have any concerns?
- Are you in a relationship in which someone is hurting you?
- Has anyone ever forced you to have sex against your will?
- Tell me what you know about safe sex practices, use of contraceptives, or prevention of sexually transmitted infections.
- Tell me the safe sex practices that you follow.

Incorporate assessment questions related to sexuality in the nursing history (Box 35-6). Using an opening statement puts a patient at ease when introducing these questions (e.g., "Sex is an important part of life, and a person's health status often affects sexuality. Many people have questions and concerns about their sexual health. What questions or concerns do you have now?"). Use knowledge of developmental stages to determine which areas are likely to be important for your patient. For example, when gathering a sexual history from an older adult, it is important to keep in mind that some have difficulty discussing intimate details with health care providers.

Nurses who conduct sexual assessments of children and adolescents face special challenges. Use language that is accurate and that the child or adolescent understands. Also promote normal development, avoid minimizing problems, and screen for sexual concerns while making the child or adolescent feel at ease. The sexual counseling of minors raises ethical and legal issues regarding a patient's rights to health care and education on the one hand and a parents' or guardian's right to supervise information on the other. Children and adolescents frequently respond when they know that having questions related to sexuality is normal. Being open, positive, and interested when introducing sexual questions is helpful.

In light of the prevalence of intimate partner violence, questions relating to abusive relationships are important. Address these questions in private. Recognizing both subjective and objective signs and symptoms of abuse in children and adults helps to identify this too-common problem (Table 35-1).

Some individuals are too embarrassed or do not know how to ask sexual questions directly. Look for clues that a person has questions.

TABLE 35-1 Signs and Symptoms That Indicate Possible Current Sexual Abuse or a History of Sexual Abuse

Types of Findings	Symptoms Often Found in Children	Symptoms Often Found in Adults
Injuries and/or physical signs	Bruises, bleeding, soreness, infection, or irritation of external genitalia, anus, mouth, or throat Sexually transmitted infections Recurrent urinary tract infections Unintended pregnancy Chronic pain Difficulty walking or sitting Unusual odor in genital area Penile discharge Torn, stained, or bloody underclothing	Welts, bruising, swelling, scars, burns, or lacerations on arms, legs, breasts, or abdomen Wounds that do not match the patient's "story" Multiple bruises in various stages of healing Vaginal or rectal bleeding Fractures of face, nose, ribs, or arms Trauma to labia, vagina, cervix, or anus Vomiting or abdominal tenderness
Behavior, nonverbal and/or vague somatic complaints	Physical aggression Sexual acting out Excessive masturbation Expressions of low self-esteem Poor school performance Poor peer relationships Sleep disturbances Social withdrawal and excessive daydreaming Running away from home Substance abuse or suicide attempts	Facial grimacing Absence of facial response or flat affect Anxiety Depression Panic attacks Difficulty sleeping Anorexia Slow, unsteady gait

Data from Hockenberry MJ, Wilson D: *Wong's nursing care of infants and children,* ed 10, St Louis, 2015, Elsevier; Touhy TA, Jett K: *Ebersole & Hess' Gerontological nursing and healthy aging,* ed 4, St Louis, 2014, Elsevier.

For example, a patient expresses concern about how his or her partner will respond now or makes a sexual comment or joke. Observing for and listening to concerns about sexuality take practice. With experience you develop skill in clarifying and paraphrasing to help individuals express sexual concerns. By including sexuality in the nursing history, you acknowledge that it is an important component of health and create an opportunity for a person to discuss sexual concerns.

Sexual Dysfunction. Many illnesses, injuries, medications, and aging changes have a negative effect on sexual health. Sexual dysfunction is either temporary or permanent. Apply knowledge about conditions and medications that frequently cause sexual dysfunction while assessing a patient's risks (see Box 35-4). Awareness of the possible effects of physical problems, altered self-concept, medications, and the factors addressed thus far on sexual functioning helps in conducting a thorough assessment. Some patients bring up the topic of sexual dysfunction. Other times issues become evident as the patient answers other nursing history questions.

BOX 35-7 Nursing Diagnostic Process

Sexual Dysfunction

Assessment Activities	Defining Characteristics
Review medical and medication history	History of hypertension History of uncomplicated myocardial infarction (MI) Takes propranolol (Inderal)
Have patient describe sexual problems	Less interested in having intercourse with wife since taking propranolol Rarely has sexual intercourse with wife Sometimes has trouble having an erection
Patient's fears and concerns	Fearful will have chest pain or another MI while having intercourse

Physical Assessment. The physical examination is important in evaluating the cause of sexual concerns or problems and usually provides the best opportunity to teach an individual about sexuality. In examining a woman's breasts and the external and internal genitalia, a nurse has the opportunity to assess the woman's reaction, answer questions, and provide information about the examination of anatomical and physiological structures. For example, a nurse teaches a woman how to perform breast self-examination during physical assessment (see Chapter 31). During physical assessment of the genitalia, he or she teaches men how to perform testicular self-examination (see Chapter 31). Knowledge of normal scrotal anatomical structures helps men detect signs of testicular cancer. Instruct both men and women on signs and symptoms of STIs during the examination when patients' histories suggest risks for them.

◆ Nursing Diagnosis

After completing an assessment, you apply critical thinking to the diagnostic process and select diagnoses applicable to the patient's needs. Assessment data that will include defining characteristics related to sexuality often include history of surgery of reproductive organs, changes in appearance or body image, a history of or current physical or sexual abuse, chronic illness, or developmental milestones such as puberty or menopause. To make a nursing diagnosis related to sexual dysfunction, consider anatomical, physiological, sociocultural, ethical, and situational issues thoroughly. Possible nursing diagnoses related to sexual functioning are listed here:

- *Anxiety*
- *Ineffective Coping*
- *Interrupted Family Processes*
- *Deficient Knowledge (Contraception/STIs)*
- *Sexual Dysfunction*
- *Ineffective Sexuality Pattern*
- *Social Isolation*

Clarify defining characteristics and ensure that the patient perceives a problem or difficulty with regard to sexuality (Box 35-7). Determining the etiological or contributing factors helps to plan effectively and select the appropriate nursing interventions. For example, nursing interventions appropriate for the nursing diagnosis of *Sexual Dysfunction* will differ for different etiological factors. *Sexual Dysfunction related to misinformation about the risk of sexually transmitted infections* requires counseling and education on how to maintain safe sexual practices. In contrast, patients who experience *Sexual Dysfunction related to physical abuse* need counseling and referral to community resources (e.g., crisis services and physical abuse support group).

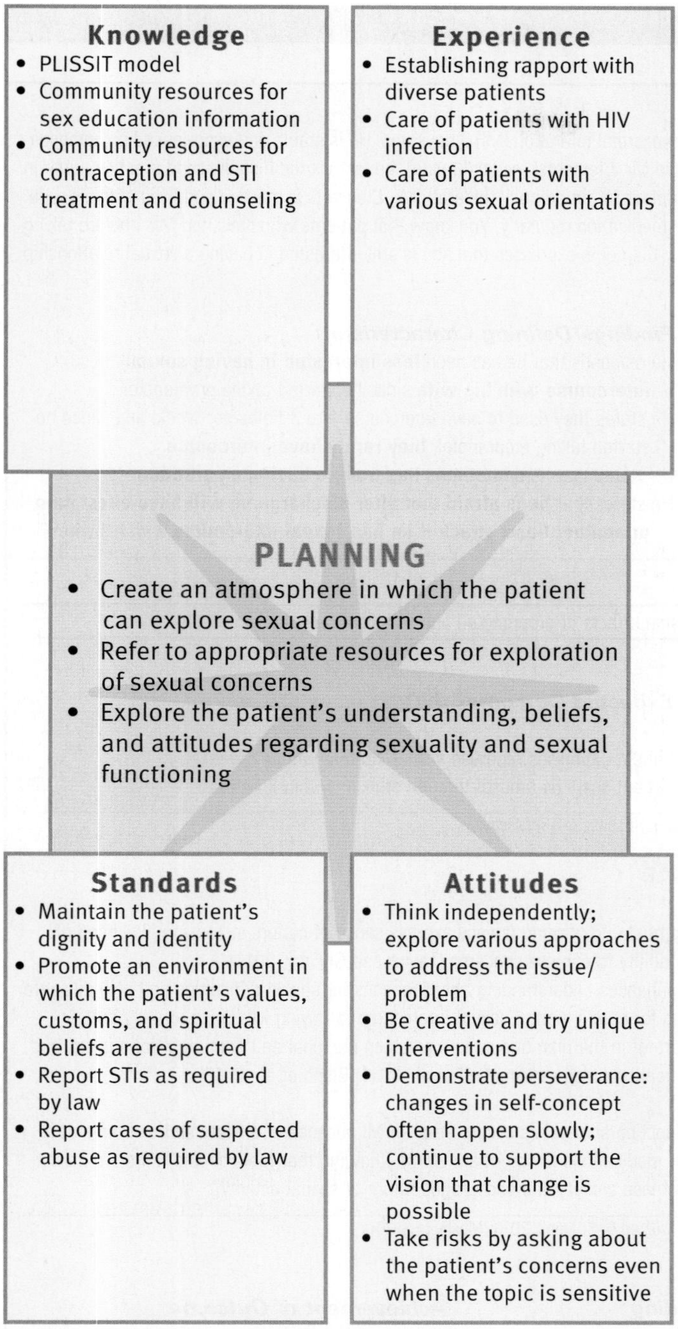

Knowledge
- PLISSIT model
- Community resources for sex education information
- Community resources for contraception and STI treatment and counseling

Experience
- Establishing rapport with diverse patients
- Care of patients with HIV infection
- Care of patients with various sexual orientations

PLANNING
- Create an atmosphere in which the patient can explore sexual concerns
- Refer to appropriate resources for exploration of sexual concerns
- Explore the patient's understanding, beliefs, and attitudes regarding sexuality and sexual functioning

Standards
- Maintain the patient's dignity and identity
- Promote an environment in which the patient's values, customs, and spiritual beliefs are respected
- Report STIs as required by law
- Report cases of suspected abuse as required by law

Attitudes
- Think independently; explore various approaches to address the issue/problem
- Be creative and try unique interventions
- Demonstrate perseverance: changes in self-concept often happen slowly; continue to support the vision that change is possible
- Take risks by asking about the patient's concerns even when the topic is sensitive

FIGURE 35-3 Critical thinking model for sexuality planning. *HIV,* Human immunodeficiency virus; *STI,* sexually transmitted infection.

◆ Planning

Goals and Outcomes. Synthesize information from multiple resources to develop an individualized plan of care (Figure 35-3). Critical thinking ensures that a patient's plan of care integrates all that a nurse knows about an individual's sexuality. Professional standards are especially important to consider when developing a plan of care. Maintain a patient's dignity and identity at all times. For example, to convey respect for the patient's gender preferences, include a lesbian or gay partner in the plan to the degree that the patient wishes.

Develop an individualized plan of care for each nursing diagnosis (see the Nursing Care Plan). Set realistic goals and measurable outcomes with the patient. For example, a patient who has dyspareunia has a nursing diagnosis of *Sexual Dysfunction related to decreased sexual desire.* You and your patient develop a goal to report decreased anxiety and greater satisfaction with sexual activity within 1 month. Expected outcomes include that the patient does the following:

- Discusses stressors that contribute to sexual dysfunction with partner within 2 weeks
- Identifies alternative, satisfying, and acceptable sexual practices for self and partner within 4 weeks

A concept map is another method that is useful in organizing patient care (Figure 35-4). The concept map shows the relationship of a medical diagnosis (decreased libido and depression) to the four nursing diagnoses identified from the patient assessment data. It also shows the links and relationship to the nursing diagnosis and interventions appropriate for each diagnosis. For example, *Ineffective Coping* affects and contributes to social isolation; and, as long as the patient has ineffective coping, the social isolation continues or perhaps worsens.

Setting Priorities. The care plan shows the goals, expected outcomes, and interventions for a patient experiencing sexual dysfunction. Nursing interventions for patients with sexual concerns focus on supporting a patient's need for intimacy and sexual activity. Patients often feel overwhelmed and hopeless about returning to the level of previous sexual functioning. They usually need time to adapt to physical and psychosocial changes that affect their sexuality and sexual health.

The priority in addressing needs related to sexuality includes establishing a therapeutic relationship so the patient feels comfortable in discussing issues related to sexuality. Look for strengths in both the patient and the family while providing education and access to resources to turn limitations into strengths. Patient teaching communicates the normalcy of feelings following certain situations (e.g., the diagnosis of a chronic illness or the loss of a body part). You determine a patient's needs and plan accordingly.

A patient's current problems and needs help you determine the priorities related to his or her sexual health. Priorities for sexual health often include resuming sexual activities. For example, if a patient is recovering from a mastectomy and is having problems resuming an intimate relationship with her spouse because of problems related to body image, you help her adapt to and cope with the changes in her body image associated with the mastectomy. Once the patient's issues related to body image are resolved, she is able to restore intimacy with her spouse and address her sexual health needs.

QSEN QSEN: BUILDING COMPETENCY IN TEAMWORK AND COLLABORATION. Mr. Clements asks what lifestyle changes he will need to make after discharge from the hospital. You know that patients with cardiovascular problems often require an interdisciplinary approach to achieve optimal recovery. Thus you arrange for consultation with different health professionals. You inform Mr. Clements that he will work with a team of experts, including cardiologists, physical therapists, dietitians, and counselors. Discuss how each of these professionals will contribute to Mr. Clements's care during and after hospitalization.

ⓔ *Answers to QSEN Activities can be found on the Evolve website.*

Teamwork and Collaboration. Planning in the area of sexuality often includes collaboration with other health care providers and referrals to community resources (Box 35-8). Nurses generally raise awareness of sexual issues, clarify concerns, and/or provide information. Nurses who have specialized education in sexual functioning and

NURSING CARE PLAN

Sexual Dysfunction

ASSESSMENT

Mr. Clements is a 65-year-old African-American patient who had an uncomplicated myocardial infarction (MI) 3 days ago. He is stable and experienced no complications following his MI. He currently is on a cardiac telemetry nursing unit. According to Mr. Clements' medical record, he last visited his advanced practice nurse in the office 2 months ago and was diagnosed with hypertension. He was given a prescription for propranolol (Inderal). Mr. Clements is married and lives with his wife.

His blood pressure today is 122/82 mm Hg. He reports that he has been taking his medication regularly. You know that patients who have had MIs and are taking antihypertensive medications often experience sexual problems. When assessed, Mrs. Clements expresses that she is still interested in having a sexual relationship with her spouse.

Assessment Activities	*Findings/Defining Characteristics**
Ask Mr. Clements if his interest in sex has changed since he started taking propranolol.	He responds that he has been **less interested in having sexual intercourse with his wife** since he started taking propranolol.
Ask Mr. Clements to compare his sexual relationship with his wife before and after taking propranolol.	He states they used to have intercourse 1 to 3 times per week; and, since he started taking propranolol, **they rarely have intercourse.**
Ask Mr. Clements if he has had difficulties with an erection.	He states that he **sometimes has trouble having an erection.**
Ask Mr. Clements what concerns or fears he has about resuming his sexual relationship with his wife now that he has had an MI.	He states that **he is afraid that after discharge he will have chest pain or another heart attack if he has sexual intercourse** with his wife.

***Defining characteristics** are shown in bold type.

NURSING DIAGNOSIS: Sexual dysfunction related to altered body function (side effects of propranolol) and lack of knowledge

PLANNING

Goal	*Expected Outcomes (NOC)*†
Sexual Functioning	
Patient will express satisfaction with sexual relationship with wife within 1 month.	Patient expresses renewed sexual interest within 2 weeks. Patient sustains arousal through orgasm within 3 weeks.

†Outcome classification labels from Moorhead S et al: *Nursing outcomes classification (NOC),* ed 5, St Louis, 2013, Mosby.

INTERVENTIONS (NIC)‡	**RATIONALE**
Sexual Counseling	
Establish trust and respect with Mr. Clements. Offer privacy during conversations.	Establishing trust and offering privacy express sense of caring, increasing likelihood of patient's ability to express concerns (Taylor and Gosney, 2011).
Discuss possible effects of MI and propranolol on sexual functioning and resumption of sexual activity.	Discussion enhances understanding about reasons for sexual difficulties and provides safe guidelines for resumption of sexual intercourse following MI (Bispo et al., 2013).
Include Mrs. Clements in discussions about sexual issues as frequently as possible and when appropriate.	Including partner in the plan of care can enhance personal and intimate relationships and improve health outcomes (Arenhall et al., 2011; Bispo et al., 2013).
Anxiety Reduction	
Encourage Mr. Clements to express fears about resuming sexual activity and assure him that others who have had MIs experience similar fears.	Sexual dysfunction sometimes occurs after an MI because of anxiety and/or from side effects of medications (Bispo et al., 2013). Knowing that feelings and fears are normal helps decrease anxiety and encourages return of sexual activity.

‡Intervention classification labels from Bulechek GM et al: *Nursing interventions classification (NIC),* ed 6, St Louis, 2013, Mosby.

EVALUATION

Nursing Actions	*Patient Response/Finding*	*Achievement of Outcome*
Ask Mr. Clements if he and his wife are satisfied with their sexual relationship during return office visit.	Mr. Clements reports that his interest in sex is back to normal and he is able to have an erection.	Mr. Clements reports sexual interest and function; he and his wife are satisfied with their relationship.

counseling provide more intensive sex therapy. It is necessary to understand the limits of your knowledge base and include other health care providers such as sex therapists, clinical psychologists, and social workers as appropriate to meet patients' needs for sexual health. For example, conflicts in marriage usually require intensive treatment with a mental health professional or certified sex therapist. For the woman who is currently in an abusive relationship, the nurse collaborates with special women's shelters that provide counseling and serve as a safe place for her while further plans are made.

◆ Implementation

Promote sexual health as a component of overall health and wellness by identifying patients at increased risk, providing appropriate information, helping individuals gain insight into their problems, and exploring methods to deal with them effectively.

Health Promotion. Helping patients maintain or gain sexual health involves consideration of factors that influence sexual satisfaction. Educate patients about sexual health, including measures for

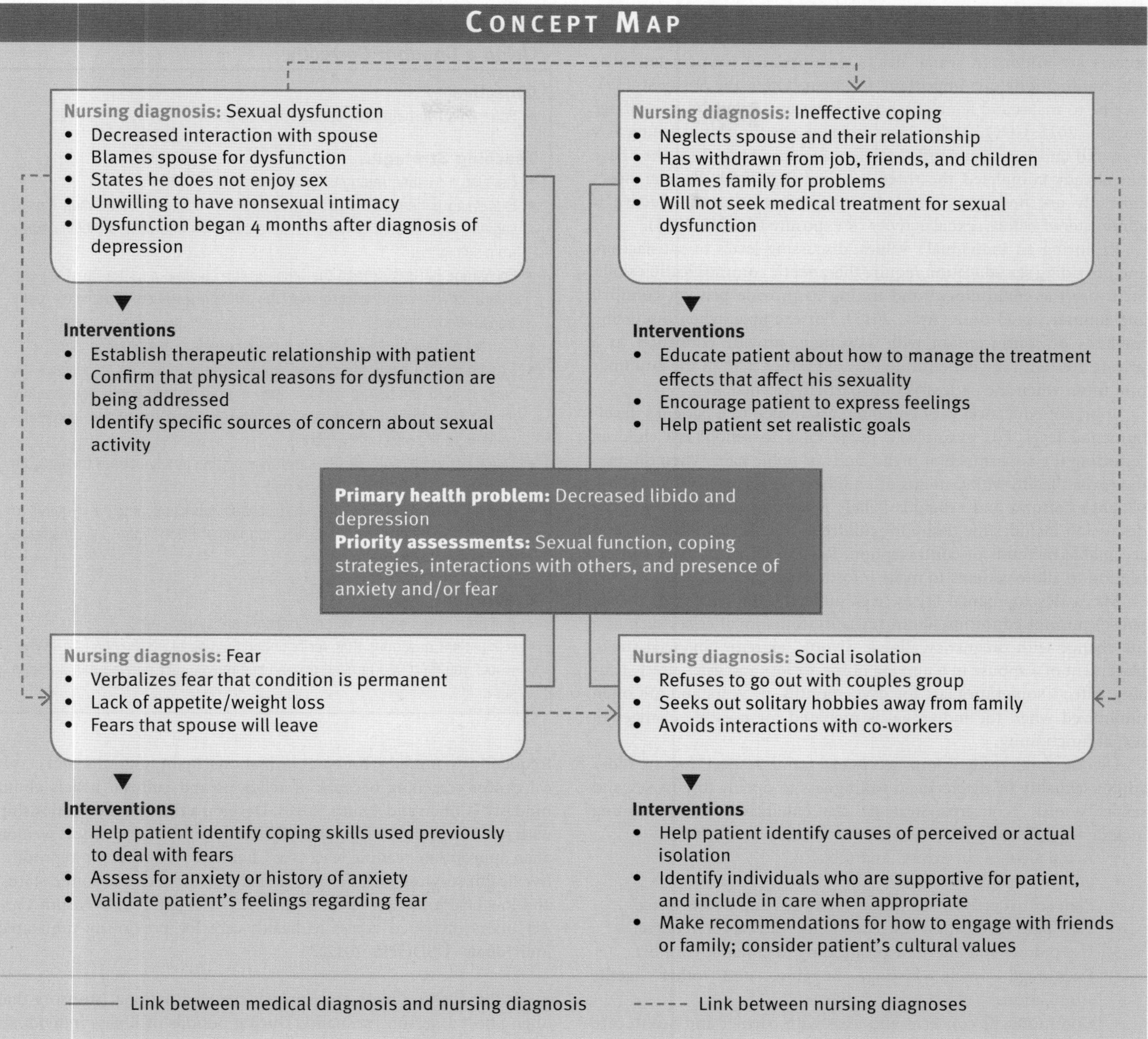

FIGURE 35-4 Concept map for Mr. Clements.

BOX 35-8 Examples of Community Resources Relating to Sexuality

- Community and free clinics offering contraceptive information and resources
- Health department (often for both family planning and sexually transmitted infections)
- Groups that provide education/services for those with particular conditions include the following:
  - American Diabetes Association
  - American Heart Association
  - Muscular Dystrophy Association
  - Muscular Sclerosis Society
- Sexual abuse support groups and hot lines
- Women's shelters (for those who have been physically and/or sexually abused)
- Resolve: The National Infertility Association (http://www.resolve.org)
- North America Menopause Society (http://www.menopause.org)

contraception, safe sex practices, and prevention of STIs. Regular breast self-examinations, mammograms, and Papanicolaou (Pap) smears are important sexual health measures for women; testicular self-examinations are important for men. Offer the 9-valent HPV vaccine to males and females who are between 11 and 26 years of age (ACOG, 2015; CDC 2015b). The vaccine is safe for girls as young as 9 years old and is recommended for females ages 11 to 26 if they have not already completed the three required injections. Booster doses currently are not recommended. The vaccine is most effective if administered before sexual activity or exposure (ACOG, 2015).

Exploring an individual's values, discussing levels of satisfaction, and providing sex education require therapeutic communication skills. Structure the environment and timing to provide privacy, comfort, and uninterrupted time (Ayaz, 2013). For example, when discussing methods of contraception with a woman, provide education in a private area with the patient fully dressed rather than in the examination room when the patient is only partially clothed.

Topics of education vary and often are related to a patient's developmental level. For example, a nurse talks to school-age children regarding the appearance of breast buds or pubic hair. When discussing sexual health with patients of childbearing age, always consider a patient's cultural and religious beliefs regarding contraception. The discussion includes the desire for children, usual sexual practices, and acceptable methods of contraception. Review all methods of contraception to allow patients to make informed decisions.

Major developmental crises (e.g., puberty, climacteric, or menopause) prompt education about sexuality. Situational crises such as a life change with pregnancy, illness, divorce, extreme financial stress, placement of a spouse in a nursing home, or loss and grief affect sexuality. Effects sometimes last for days, months, or years and are often minimized when the individual is prepared for possible changes in sexual functioning.

Demonstrate recognition, acceptance, and respect for an older adult's sexuality by displaying a willingness to openly discuss sex and sexuality-related concerns. Strategies that enhance sexual functioning include the following (Bach et al., 2013; Buttaro et al., 2014):

- Avoid alcohol (in excess) and tobacco.
- Eat well-balanced meals.
- Plan sexual activity for times when the couple feels rested.
- Take pain medication if needed before sexual intercourse.
- Use pillows and alternate positioning to enhance comfort.
- Encourage touch, kissing, hugging, and other tactile stimulation.
- Communicate concerns and fears with partner and health care provider.

Individuals who have more than one sex partner or whose partner has other sexual experiences need to learn about safe sex practices. Provide information about STI symptoms and transmission, use of condoms, and risky sexual activities (e.g., trauma from penile-anal sex). To prevent HIV infection, teach patients to avoid having multiple sex partners and use condoms to reduce the risk of HIV/AIDS. Role play is useful in helping a person learn to say no or negotiate with a partner to use a condom (Box 35-9). Also teach patients to avoid the use of IV drugs. If people do use IV drugs, tell them to avoid sharing needles with others and to always use new needles. When discussing safe sex, consider patients' physical and emotional health.

Encourage patients to have regular health and screening examinations to maintain sexual health. Often asymptomatic STIs are diagnosed during a physical examination with appropriate laboratory work. Annual health examinations provide an opportunity to discuss contraception and safe sex practices. However, some people do not seek annual health examinations routinely. For example, Arab women frequently do not have breast examinations, mammograms, and cervical cancer screening because of religious and cultural beliefs about modesty (Cohen and Azaiza, 2010). Develop a therapeutic relationship with patients and provide culturally sensitive education that is written at an appropriate reading level (see Chapter 25). Barriers to reproductive health services include cultural beliefs, low socioeconomic status, and low health literacy (Hall et al, 2012). The Affordable Health Care Act offers increased access to health care for previously uninsured individuals (USDHHS, 2012).

BOX 35-9 PATIENT TEACHING

Using a Condom Correctly

Objective

- Patient will verbalize correct use of a condom.

Teaching Strategies

- Develop a trusting relationship with patient.
- Explain to patient to always use a latex or rubber condom when having vaginal, oral, or anal sex and to store condoms in a cool, dry place away from sunlight.
- Encourage patient to read the label on the condom package to check the expiration date and ensure that the condom protects against sexually transmitted infections.
- Instruct patient to never reuse a condom or use a damaged condom.
- Explain how to apply the condom correctly (e.g., put it on as soon as the penis is hard and before vaginal, anal, or oral contact; gently squeeze any air out from the tip of the condom, leaving space for semen; unroll the condom to the base of the penis).
- Teach patient to pull out right after ejaculating and hold onto the condom when pulling out.
- Instruct patient to only use water-based lubricants (e.g., K-Y jelly) to prevent the condom from breaking; do not use petroleum jelly, massage oils, body lotions, or cooking oil.

Evaluation

- Ask patient to describe where condoms are stored.
- Ask patient questions that verify understanding of instruction (e.g., What would you do if you noticed that a condom you just opened had an open slit in it?).

Acute Care. Illness and surgery create situational stressors that often affect a person's sexuality. During periods of illness individuals experience major physical changes, the effects of drugs or treatments, the emotional stress of a prognosis, concern about future functioning, and separation from significant others. Never assume that sexual functioning is not a concern merely because of an individual's age or severity of prognosis. After identifying concerns, address them in the context of his or her value system.

When a patient identifies sexual concerns, initiate discussion and education appropriately. Refer to appropriate outpatient resources. Help patients anticipate how their illness or disease will change over time and the adjustments that will be necessary to achieve sexual fulfillment.

Restorative and Continuing Care. You need to establish relationships with couples to encourage honest and open discussions about sexual health during restorative or continuing care. Address needs by taking a sexual health history and implementing a basic model such as PLISSIT to provide options for patients (see Box 35-5). Assessment and management of sexual concerns are important when promoting sexual intimacy and providing closeness and closure between partners at the end of life.

In the home environment it is important to provide information on how an illness limits sexual activity and give ideas for adapting or facilitating sexual activity. Interventions range from giving permission for a partner to lie in bed and hold a patient to coordinating nursing care and medications to provide opportunity for privacy and intimacy. Often nurses help individuals create an environment that is comfortable for sexual activity in the home. This sometimes involves making recommendations for ways to arrange the bedroom to accommodate physical limitations. For example, some individuals who are in a wheelchair prefer being able to move the chair close to the side of the bed at an angle that allows for more ease in touching and caressing. Suggestions regarding how to accommodate barriers such as Foley catheters or drainage tubes contribute to sexual activity.

In the long-term care setting facilities need to make proper arrangements for privacy during residents' sexual experiences (Katz, 2013). The ideal situation is to set up a pleasant room that is used for a variety of activities that the resident is able to reserve for private visits with a spouse or partner. If this is not possible, make arrangements for the roommate of a patient to be somewhere else to allow a couple time alone. Never leave patients alone in a situation in which they can injure themselves.

◆ Evaluation

Through the Patient's Eyes. Evaluate patients' perceptions of nursing interventions to determine if their expectations have been met. Critical thinking ensures that you apply what is known about sexuality and a patient's unique situation.

Have follow-up discussions with the patient or partner to determine if they were satisfied with your approaches. Sexuality is felt more than observed, and sexual expression requires an intimacy that is not amenable to observation.

Patient Outcomes. Evaluate if patient achieved outcomes established in the plan of care (Figure 35-5). Ask patients questions about risk factors, sexual concerns, and their level of satisfaction. Observe behavioral cues such as eye contact, posture, and extraneous hand movements that indicate comfort or suggest continued anxiety or concern as topics are addressed. Anticipate the need to modify expectations with an individual and partner when evaluating outcomes. Sometimes you need to establish more appropriate time frames in which to achieve target goals. Ask patients to define what is acceptable and satisfying while considering the partner's level of sexual satisfaction. When outcomes are not met, begin to ask questions to determine appropriate changes in interventions. Examples of questions include the following:

- What other questions do you have about your sexual health?
- Did you experience less pain during sexual intercourse after taking your pain medication?
- Which positions did you find most comfortable when you had sexual intercourse? Which positions were most awkward?
- What barriers are preventing you from discussing your feelings and fears with your partner?

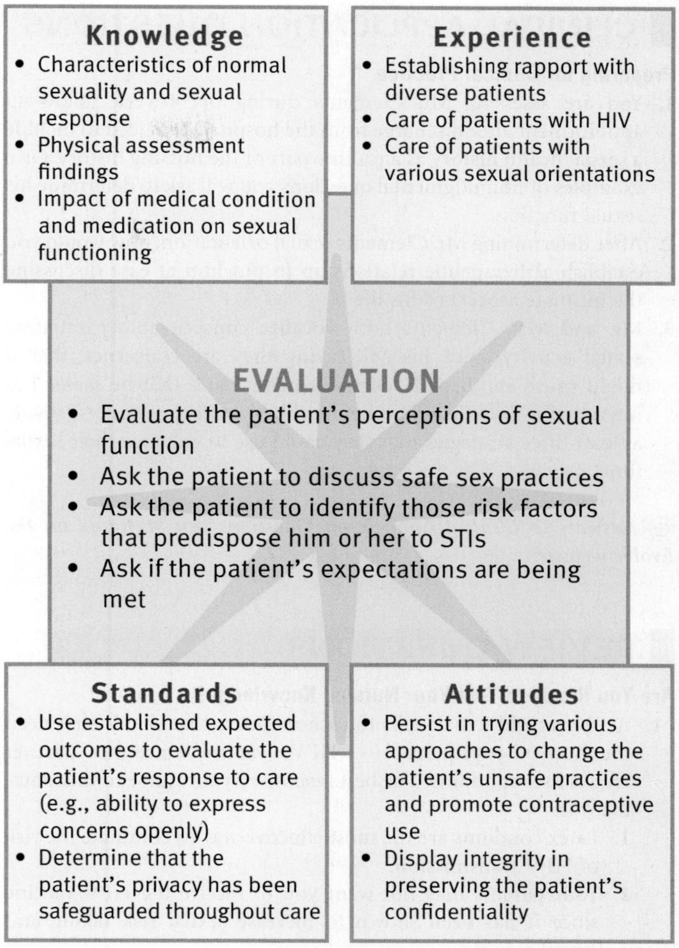

Knowledge
- Characteristics of normal sexuality and sexual response
- Physical assessment findings
- Impact of medical condition and medication on sexual functioning

Experience
- Establishing rapport with diverse patients
- Care of patients with HIV
- Care of patients with various sexual orientations

EVALUATION
- Evaluate the patient's perceptions of sexual function
- Ask the patient to discuss safe sex practices
- Ask the patient to identify those risk factors that predispose him or her to STIs
- Ask if the patient's expectations are being met

Standards
- Use established expected outcomes to evaluate the patient's response to care (e.g., ability to express concerns openly)
- Determine that the patient's privacy has been safeguarded throughout care

Attitudes
- Persist in trying various approaches to change the patient's unsafe practices and promote contraceptive use
- Display integrity in preserving the patient's confidentiality

FIGURE 35-5 Critical thinking model for sexuality evaluation. *HIV,* Human immunodeficiency virus; *STI,* sexually transmitted infection.

KEY POINTS

- Sexuality is related to all dimensions of health, is a part of each individual's identity, and includes biological sex, gender identity, gender role, and sexual partner preference.
- Attitudes toward sexuality vary widely. Religious beliefs, society values, the media, the family, and other factors all influence it.
- Nurses' attitudes toward sexuality vary and often differ from those of patients; be sensitive to patients' sexual preferences and needs.
- Sexual development begins in infancy and involves some level of sexual behavior or growth in all developmental stages.
- The physiological sexual response changes with aging, but aging does not lead to diminished sexuality.
- Sexual health contributes to an individual's sense of self-worth and positive interpersonal relationships.
- Sexual dysfunctions result from varied and complex etiologies.
- Interventions for sexual dysfunctions depend on the condition and the patient; they often include giving information, teaching specific exercises, improving communication between partners, and referral to a knowledgeable professional.
- Sexual biases, comfort with touching genitalia, desire for future fertility, financial status, ability to plan sexual contact, and ability to communicate with the sex partner all affect the choice and use of effective contraceptive methods.
- Include a brief review of sexuality whenever assessing a patient's level of wellness.
- Most nursing interventions that enhance sexual health require providing education.
- Evaluate patient satisfaction with outcomes of care by talking with patients regarding satisfaction with sexual functioning and through observations of nonverbal behaviors that suggest anxiety. Include the partner when appropriate.

CLINICAL APPLICATION QUESTIONS

Preparing for Clinical Practice

1. You are assessing Mr. Clements during his 4-week follow-up appointment after discharge from the hospital. You need to include a sexual health history as a routine part of the nursing history. Give examples of nonjudgmental questions you will ask to determine his sexual function.
2. After determining Mr. Clements sexual orientation, how would you establish a therapeutic relationship to put him at ease discussing the intimate aspects of his life?
3. Mr. and Mrs. Clements both vocalize concern about initiating sexual activity since his MI, saying they are concerned that it might cause another MI. Mrs. Clements states that he seems less interested in intimacy than before the MI and tires easily. Provide at least three strategies that they could use to enhance their sexual functioning.

ⓔ ***Answers to Clinical Application Questions can be found on the Evolve website.***

REVIEW QUESTIONS

Are You Ready to Test Your Nursing Knowledge?

1. A 16-year-old female tells the school nurse that she doesn't need the human papillomavirus (HPV) vaccine since her partner always uses condoms. The best response by the nurse to this statement is:
   1. Latex condoms are the most effective way to eliminate the risk of HPV transmission.
   2. Your parents may not want you to receive the HPV vaccine since it has been shown to increase sexual risk taking and sexual activity.
   3. The HPV 9-valent vaccine is recommended for males and females and targets the specific viruses that cause cancer and genital warts.
   4. You are past the recommended age to receive the vaccine.
2. Place the following in order of sequence for condom application and usage.
   1. Gently squeeze air out from the tip of the condom; leave space at the tip.
   2. Check the condom package for damage, expiration date, and protection from STIs.
   3. After ejaculating, hold onto condom while pulling out.
   4. Place on erect penis and unroll to the base of the penis.
3. An adolescent who is pregnant for the first time is at her initial prenatal visit. The women's health nurse practitioner (NP) informs her that she will be screening her for sexually transmitted infections (STIs). The patient replies, "I know I don't have an STI because I don't have any symptoms." How should the NP respond? (Select all that apply.)
   1. "Untreated STIs can cause serious complications in pregnancy so we routinely screen pregnant women."
   2. "Bacterial STIs don't usually cause symptoms, but you could have an asymptomatic viral STI."
   3. "Chlamydia screening is recommended for all sexually active women up to age 25 even if asymptomatic."
   4. "People between the ages of 15 and 24 have the highest incidence of STIs."
   5. "There is no need to screen for infection since you aren't having any problems or symptoms."
4. A 42-year-old sexually active female is being assessed by a nurse during her annual physical. The woman states that she has not had a period for the last 2 months. The nurse knows that the most likely cause of this occurrence is:
   1. Pregnancy.
   2. Illicit drug use.
   3. Chlamydia infection.
   4. Early-onset menopause.
5. A cardiac nurse who recently graduated from nursing school is providing discharge instructions to a patient who suffered a myocardial infarction (MI). The nurse knows that sexual issues are common after an MI but doesn't feel comfortable bringing up this topic. What is the best way for the nurse to handle this situation? (Select all that apply.)
   1. Instruct the patient to discuss any sexual concerns with his or her partner after discharge
   2. Avoid discussing the topic unless the patient brings it up
   3. Ask a more experienced nurse to cover this with the patient and learn from the example.
   4. Plan to attend conferences or training in the near future on how to discuss such issues
   5. Encourage the patient to discuss any personal concerns with the cardiologist
6. The nurse is gathering a history from a 72-year-old male patient being admitted to a nursing home. The patient requests a private room. The nurse understands that:
   1. The patient cannot be sexually active since he is moving into a nursing home.
   2. The patient may be requesting a private room to facilitate an intimate relationship with his partner.
   3. There is no need to take a sexual history since most older adults are uncomfortable discussing intimate details of their lives.
   4. Older adults in nursing homes usually do not participate in sexual activity.
7. According to *Healthy People 2020*, certain ethnic groups in the United States are disproportionately affected by sexually transmitted infections (STIs) and human immunodeficiency virus (HIV). What are the likely causes of this issue? (Select all that apply.)
   1. The large percentage of lesbian, gay, bisexual, or transgender individuals in the culture
   2. Values and expectations about sexual behavior by the men or women in the culture
   3. Religious beliefs and cultural attitudes toward the use of contraceptives
   4. Educational background and knowledge of health risks associated with sexual behaviors
   5. The higher incidence of sexual abuse in the affected ethnic groups
8. The nurse is completing an admission history on a patient and says, "As a routine part of your medical history, it's important to include the sexual aspects of your life. Would it be alright if we discussed this?" This is an example of the nurse using the PLISSIT model to:
   1. Place the patient in control of the situation.
   2. Ask permission to discuss sexuality issues.
   3. Provide the patent with limited information about sexual issues.
   4. Ask the patient to provide sensitive information.
9. A 17-year-old girl asks for more information about birth control methods and says that she does not want her parents to know she

is using birth control. The nurse informs the patient that the most effective option for her situation would be:
1. An effective long-term method such as a subdermal implant.
2. A hormonal method such as birth control pills or the transdermal patch.
3. A long-acting hormonal injection given every 12 weeks.
4. Abstinence during her most fertile time.

10. The nurse is providing education on sexually transmitted infections (STIs) to a group of older adults. The nurse knows that further teaching is needed when the participants make which statements? (Select all that apply.)
    1. "I don't need to use condoms since there is no risk for pregnancy."
    2. "I should be screened for an STI each time I'm with a new partner."
    3. "I know I'm not infected because I don't have discharge or sores."
    4. "I was tested for STIs last year so I know I'm not infected."
    5. "The infection rate in older adults is low because most are not sexually active."
11. The nurse is providing community education about how the sexual response changes with age. Which statement made by one of the adults indicates the need for further information?
    1. "Health problems such as diabetes, chronic obstructive pulmonary disease, and hypertension have little effect on sexual functioning and desire."
    2. "It usually takes longer for both sexes to reach an orgasm."
    3. "Most of the normal changes in function are related to alteration in circulation and hormone levels."
    4. "Many medications can interfere with sexual function."
12. The nurse is gathering a sexual health history on a patient being admitted to the hospital for surgery. Which question asked by the nurse demonstrates a nonjudgmental attitude?
    1. Can you tell me your sexual orientation?
    2. How do you and your wife feel about intimacy?
    3. Do you have sex with men, women, or both?
    4. Do you have sexual intercourse at your age?
13. The nurse reviews the health history of a 48-year-old man and notes that he was started on medications for elevated blood pressure and depression at his last annual physical. He tells the nurse that over the past 6 months he is having difficulty sustaining an erection. The nurse understands that: (Select all that apply.)
    1. Nurses are not expected to discuss sexual issues with male patients and the physician should address this.
    2. Sexual function can be affected negatively by some medications.
    3. Sexually transmitted infections (STIs) can cause complications such as erectile dysfunction and screening should be done.
    4. It is not unusual for men with health issues to experience erectile dysfunction.
    5. Medications used to treat hypertension and depression seldom interfere with sexual function.
14. The school nurse is counseling an adolescent male who is returning to school after attempting suicide. He denies substance abuse and has no history of treatment for depression. He says he has no friends or family who understand him. Critical thinking encourages the nurse to consider all possibilities, including which of the following? (Select all that apply.)
    1. Adolescents often explore their sexual identity and expose themselves to complications such as sexually transmitted infections (STIs) or unplanned pregnancy.
    2. Peer approval and acceptance are not important in this age-group.
    3. Lesbian, gay, bisexual, and transgender (LGBT) youth often experience stress from identification with a sexual minority group.
    4. Knowledge about normal changes associated with puberty and sexuality can decrease stress and anxiety.
    5. Adolescence is a time of emotional stability and self-acceptance.
15. A 53-year-old female being treated for breast cancer tells the nurse that she has no interest in sex since her surgery 2 months ago. The nurse is aware that: (Select all that apply.)
    1. Sexual issues are expected in a woman this age.
    2. Women experience sexual dysfunction more frequently than men.
    3. Hypoactive sexual desire disorder (HSDD) occurs in women over 65 years of age.
    4. It is not unusual for medical conditions such as cancer to contribute to HSDD.
    5. Disturbances in self-concept affect sexual functioning.

Answers: 1. 3; **2.** 2, 1, 4, 3; **3.** 1, 3, 4; **4.** 1; **5.** 3, 4; **6.** 2; **7.** 2, 3, 4; **8.** 2; **9.** 3; **10.** 1, 3, 4, 5; **11.** 1; **12.** 1; **13.** 2, 4; **14.** 1, 3, 4; **15.** 2, 4, 5.

Rationales for Review Questions can be found on the Evolve website.

REFERENCES

Adih WK, et al: Estimated lifetime risk for diagnosis of HIV infection among Hispanics/Latinos: 37 states and Puerto Rico, 2007, *MMWR Morb Mortal Wkly Rep* 59(40):1297, 2010.

American College of Obstetricians and Gynecologists (ACOG): *Committee Opinion: human papillomavirus vaccination*, Number 641, September 2015, http://www.acog.org/-/media/Committee-Opinions/Committee-on-Adolescent-Health-Care/co641.pdf?dmc=1&ts=20150703T1223246675. Accessed October 2015.

Bispo GS, et al: Cardiovascular changes resulting from sexual activity and sexual dysfunction after myocardial infarction: integrative review, *J Clin Nurs* 22:3522, 2013.

Buster J: Managing female sexual dysfunction, *Fertil Steril* 100(4):905, 2013.

Buttaro TM, et al: Sexuality and quality of life in aging: implications for practice, *J Nurse Pract* 10(7):480, 2014.

Casey F, Gomez-Lobo V: Disparities in contraceptive access and provision, *Semin Reprod Med* 31(5):347, 2013.

Cates W Jr, Harwood B: Vaginal barriers and spermicides. In Hatcher RA, et al, editors: *Contraceptive technology*, ed 20, New York, 2011, Ardent Media.

Centers for Disease Control and Prevention (CDC): *Sexually transmitted disease surveillance 2012*, Atlanta, 2013a, US Department of Health and Human Services.

Centers for Disease Control and Prevention (CDC): *The state of aging and health in America*, 2013b, http://www.cdc.gov/aging/pdf/state-aging-health-in-america-2013.pdf. Accessed October 2015.

Centers for Disease Control and Prevention (CDC): *HPV vaccine Gardasil vaccine information statement*, 2013c, http://www.cdc.gov/vaccines/hcp/vis/vis-statements/hpv-gardasil.pdf. Accessed October 2015.

Centers for Disease Control and Prevention (CDC): *Fact sheet: reported STDs in the United States: 2012 data for chlamydia, gonorrhea and syphilis*, 2014a, http://www.cdc.gov/nchhstp/newsroom/docs/STD-Trends-508.pdf. Accessed October 2015.

Centers for Disease Control and Prevention (CDC): *Genital HPV infection fact sheet*, 2014b, http://www.cdc.gov/std/HPV/STDFact-HPV.htm. Accessed October 2015.

Centers for Disease Control and Prevention (CDC): *Chlamydia: CDC fact sheet*, 2014c, http://www.cdc.gov/std/chlamydia/STDFact-chlamydia-detailed.htm. Accessed October 2015.

Centers for Disease Control and Prevention (CDC): *Adolescent and school health: sexual risk behavior: HIV, STD, & teen pregnancy prevention*, 2014d, http://www.cdc.gov/HealthyYouth/sexualbehaviors/. Accessed October 2015.

Centers for Disease Control and Prevention (CDC): *Chlamydial infections—2015 STD treatment guidelines*, 2015a, http://www.cdc.gov/std/tg2015/chlamydia.htm. Accessed October 2015.

Centers for Disease Control and Prevention (CDC): *Vaccine information statement (interim) HPV vaccine (gardasil-9) (04/15/2015)*, 2015b, http://www.cdc.gov/vaccines/hcp/vis/vis-statements/hpv-gardasil-9.html. Accessed October 2015.

Dean G, Schwarz EB: Intrauterine contraceptives. In Hatcher RA, et al, editors: *Contraceptive technology*, ed 20, New York, 2011, Ardent Media.

Edelman CL, Mandle CL: *Health promotion throughout the life span*, ed 8, St Louis, 2014, Mosby.

Finer LB, Zolna MR: Shifts in intended and unintended pregnancies in the United States, 2001-2008, *Am J Public Health* 104(S1):S43, 2014.

Garcia P: *6 Women's health apps we keep hearing about*, 2014, http://www.vogue.com/946793/period-fertility-pregnancy-health-apps-for-women/. Accessed October 2015.

Giger JN: *Transcultural nursing*, ed 6, St Louis, 2013, Mosby.

Healthy People 2020: *Sexually transmitted disease*, n.d., http://www.healthypeople.gov/2020/topicsobjectives2020/overview.aspx?topicid=37. Accessed October 2015.

Hockenberry MJ, Wilson D: *Wong's nursing care of infants and children*, ed 10, St Louis, 2015, Mosby.

Horstman A, et al: The role of androgens and estrogen on healthy aging and longevity, *J Gerontol A Biol Sci Med Sci* 67(11):1140, 2012.

Johnson BK: Sexually transmitted infections and older adults, *J Gerontol Nurs* 39(11):53, 2013.

Kann L, et al: Youth risk behavior surveillance-United States, 2013, *MMWR Surveill Summ* 63(4):1, 2014.

Katz A: Sexuality in nursing care facilities, *Am J Nurs* 113(3):53, 2013.

Kingsberg SA: Hypoactive sexual desire disorder: understanding the impact on midlife women, *Female Patient* 36(3):39, 2011.

Lim FA, et al: Addressing health care disparities in the lesbian, gay, bisexual, and transgender population: a review of best practices, *Am J Nurs* 114(6):24, 2014.

Link DG: Nursing care of the family during pregnancy. In Lowdermilk D, et al, editors: *Maternity and women's healthcare*, ed 10, St Louis, 2012, Elsevier, p 329.

Marrazzo JM, Cates W Jr: Reproductive tract infections, including HIV and other sexually transmitted infections. In Hatcher RA, et al, editors: *Contraceptive technology*, ed 20, New York, 2011, Ardent Media.

Murphy PA: Contraception and reproductive health. In King TL, Brucker MC, editors: *Pharmacology for women's health*, Sudbury, MA, 2011, Jones & Bartlett.

Olson J, et al: Management of the transgender adolescent, *Arch Pediatr Adolesc Med* 165(2):171, 2011.

Pascoe BHM: Sexuality. In Giddens JF, editor: *Concepts of nursing practice*, St Louis, 2013, Elsevier.

Phillippi JC, Latendresse GA: Sexually transmitted infections. In McCance KL, Huether SE, editors: *Pathophysiology: the biologic basis for disease in adults and children*, ed 7, St Louis, 2014, Elsevier.

Rosenthal SM: Approach to the patient: transgender youth: endocrine considerations, *J Clin Endocrinol Metab* 99(12):4379, 2014.

Schwartz J, Gabelnick HL: Contraceptive research and development. In Hatcher RA, et al, editors: *Contraceptive technology*, ed 20, New York, 2011, Ardent Media.

Steinke EE, et al: Sexual counseling for individuals with cardiovascular disease and their partners: a consensus document from the American Heart Association and the ESC Council on cardiovascular nursing and allied professions (CCNAPP), *Eur Heart J* 34(41):3217, 2013.

Stewart A, Graham S: Sexual risk behavior among older adults, *MMWR Recomm Rep* 52(RR–12):1, 2013.

Syme ML: The evolving context of older adult sexual behavior and its benefits, *J Am Soc Aging* 38(1):35, 2014.

Taylor A, Gosney M: Sexuality in older age: Essential considerations for healthcare professionals, *Age Ageing* 40(5):583, 2011.

Touhy TA, Jett KF: *Ebersole & Hess' gerontological nursing and healthy aging*, ed 4, St Louis, 2014, Elsevier.

Trussell J, Guthrie KA: Choosing a contraceptive: efficacy, safety, and personal considerations. In Hatcher RA, et al, editors: *Contraceptive technology*, ed 20, New York, 2011, Ardent Media.

US Department of Health and Human Services (USDHHS): *Read the law: the affordable care act, section by section*, Washington, DC, 2012, US Department of Health and Human Services. http://www.hhs.gov/healthcare/rights/law/index.html. Accessed October 2015.

Williamson C: Providing care to transgender persons: a clinical approach to primary care, hormones, and HIV management, *J Assoc Nurses AIDS Care* 21(3):221, 2010.

World Health Organization (WHO): *Gender and human rights: sexual health*, n.d., http://www.who.int/reproductivehealth/topics/gender_rights/sexual_health/en/. Accessed October 2015.

Young-Bruehl E: Sexual diversity in cosmopolitan perspective, *Studies Gender Sexuality* 11:1, 2010.

RESEARCH REFERENCES

Arenhall E, et al: The female partners' experiences of intimate relationship after a first myocardial infarction, *J Clin Nurs* 20:1677, 2011.

Ayaz S: Sexuality and nursing process: a literature review, *Sex Disabil* 32:3, 2013.

Bach LE, et al: The association of physical and mental health with sexual activity in older adults in a retirement community, *J Sex Med* 10:2671, 2013.

Bednarczyk RA, et al: Sexual activity-related outcomes after human papilloma-virus vaccination of 11- to 12-year-olds, *Pediatrics* 130(5):798, 2012.

Capogrosso P, et al: One out of four with newly diagnosed erectile dysfunction is a young man-worrisome picture from the everyday clinical practice, *J Sex Med* 10:1833, 2013.

Cohen M, Azaiza F: Increasing breast examinations among Arab women using a tailored culture-based intervention, *Behav Med* 36:92, 2010.

Deordorff J, et al: Sexual values and risky sexual behaviors among Latino youth, *Perspect Sex Reprod Health* 42(1):23, 2010.

Deordorff J, et al: Latino youths' sexual values and condom negotiation strategies, *Perspect Sex Reprod Health* 45(4):182, 2013.

Donahue KL, et al: Acceptability of the human papillomavirus vaccine and reasons for non-vaccination among parents of adolescent sons, *Vaccine* 32:3883, 2014. http://dx.doi.org/10.1016/j.vaccine.2014.05.035. Accessed October 2015.

Dorrell C, et al: Delay and refusal of human papillomavirus vaccine for girls, national immunization survey-teen, 2010, *Clin Pediatr (Phila)* 53(3):261, 2014.

Doty ND, et al: Sexuality-related social support among lesbian, gay, and bisexual youth, *J Youth Adolesc* 39:1134, 2010.

Dunne A, et al: Adolescents, sexually transmitted infections, and education using social media: a review of the literature, *J Nurse Pract* 10(6):401, 2014.

Fontenot HB, et al: Human papillomavirus (HPV) risk factors, vaccination patterns, and vaccine perceptions among a sample of male college students, *J Am Coll Health* 62(3):186, 2014.

Godfrey NP, et al: Contraceptive methods and use by women age 35 and over: a qualitative study of perspectives, *BMC Womens Health* 11(1):5, 2011.

Hall KS, et al: Determinants of and disparities in reproductive health service use among adolescent and young adult women in the United States, 2002-2008, *Am J Public Health* 102(2):359, 2012.

Ivarsson V, et al: Health professionals' views on sexual information following MI, *Br J Nurs* 19(16):1052, 2010.

Johnson MJ, Amella EJ: Isolation of lesbian, gay, bisexual and transgender youth: a dimensional concept analysis, *J Adv Nurs* 70(3):523, 2014.

Jones J, et al: *Current contraceptive use in the United States, 2006-2010, and changes in patterns of use since 1995*, Hyattsville, MD, 2012, National Center for Health Statistics. National health statistics reports No 60.

Lee YM, et al: Factors related to sexual practices and successful sexually transmitted infection/HIV intervention programs for Latino adolescents, *Public Health Nurs* 30(5):390, 2013.

Lindau ST, Gavrilova N: Sex, health and years of sexually active life gained due to good health: evidence from two US population-based cross-sectional surveys of aging, *Br Med J* 340:c810, 2010.

Marchand E, et al: HPV vaccination and sexual behavior in a community college sample, *J Community Health* 38:1010, 2013.

Mayhew A, et al: Risk perceptions and subsequent sexual behaviors after HPV vaccination in adolescents, *Pediatrics* 133(3):401, 2014.

Peragallo N, et al: The efficacy of an HIV risk reduction intervention for Hispanic women, *AIDS Behav* 16(5):1316, 2012.

Roberts ME, et al: Mother-daughter communication and human papillomavirus vaccine uptake by college students, *Pediatrics* 125(5):982, 2010.

Rosen RC, et al: Sexual desire problems in women seeking healthcare: a novel study design for ascertaining prevalence of hypoactive sexual desire disorder in clinic-based samples of US women, *J Women's Health* 215:505, 2012.

Scott ME, et al: Risky adolescent sexual behaviors and reproductive health in young adulthood, *Perspect Sex Reprod Health* 43(2):110, 2011.

Sobecki MA, et al: What we don't talk about when we don't talk about sex: results of a national survey of US obstetrician/gynecologists, *J Sex Med* 9:1285, 2012.

Warren JT, et al: Characteristics related to effective contraceptive use among a sample of nonurban Latinos, *Perspect Sex Reprod Health* 43(4):255, 2011.

36

Spiritual Health

OBJECTIVES

- Discuss the influence of spirituality on patients' health practices.
- Describe the relationship among faith, hope, and spiritual well-being.
- Compare and contrast the concepts of religion and spirituality.
- Assess a patient's spirituality.
- Explain the importance of establishing caring relationships with patients to provide spiritual care.
- Discuss nursing interventions designed to promote a patient's spiritual health.
- Identify approaches for establishing presence with patients.
- Evaluate patient outcomes related to spiritual health.

KEY TERMS

MEDIA RESOURCES

http://evolve.elsevier.com/Potter/fundamentals/

- Review Questions
- Concept Map Creator
- Case Study with Questions
- Audio Glossary
- Content Updates

The word *spirituality* comes from the Latin word *spiritus,* which refers to breath or wind. The spirit gives life to a person. It signifies whatever is at the center of all aspects of a person's life. Florence Nightingale believed that spirituality was a force that provided energy needed to promote a healthy hospital environment and that caring for a person's spiritual needs was just as essential as caring for his or her physical needs (Reinert and Koenig, 2013). Today **spirituality** is often defined as an awareness of one's inner self and a sense of connection to a higher being, nature, or some purpose greater than oneself (McSherry and Jamieson, 2013; Prentis et al., 2014). A person's health depends on a balance of physical, psychological, sociological, cultural, developmental, and spiritual factors. Spirituality helps individuals achieve the balance needed to maintain health and well-being and cope with illness.

Too often nurses and other health care providers fail to recognize the spiritual dimension of their patients because spirituality is not scientific enough, it has many definitions, and it is difficult to measure. In addition, some nurses and health care providers do not believe in God or an ultimate being, some are not comfortable with discussing the topic, and others claim that they do not have time to address patients' spiritual needs (McSherry and Jamieson, 2013; Ronaldson et al., 2012). The concepts of spirituality and religion are often interchanged, but spirituality is a much broader and more unifying concept than religion (Rykkje et al., 2013).

The human spirit is powerful, and spirituality has different meanings for different people. Nurses need to be aware of their own spirituality to provide appropriate and relevant spiritual care to others. They need to care for the whole person and accept a patient's beliefs and experiences (Cockell and McSherry, 2012). Being able to determine the importance that spirituality holds for patients depends on your ability to develop caring relationships (see Chapter 7).

SCIENTIFIC KNOWLEDGE BASE

The relationship between spirituality and healing is not completely understood. However, an individual's intrinsic spirit seems to be an important factor in healing. Healing often takes place because of believing. Research shows that spirituality positively affects and enhances physical and psychological health, quality of life, health promotion behaviors, and disease prevention activities (Conway-Phillips and Janusek, 2014; White, 2013).

Many of the beneficial effects of spirituality are tied to hormonal and neurological function. For example, regular performance of relaxation exercises was found to reduce physiological dysregulation, including inflammation markers in elderly persons (Glei et al., 2012). Integrative body-mind techniques that include relaxation, guided imagery, mindfulness training, and music reduce perceptions of pain and anxiety (Fan et al., 2014). Laughter reduces pain; positively affects depression, life satisfaction, insomnia, and sleep quality; improves blood sugar levels; and elevates self-reports of health (Gilbert, 2014; Hirosaki et al., 2013). A person's inner beliefs and convictions are powerful resources for healing. When you support the spirituality of patients and their families, you help them achieve desirable health outcomes.

NURSING KNOWLEDGE BASE

Nursing research shows the association between spirituality and health. For example, family caregivers of patients with brain tumors who expressed high levels of spirituality experienced less depression and anxiety and better mental health when compared with family caregivers who expressed lower levels of spirituality (Newberry et al., 2013). Research has also shown that prayer often helps African-American women diagnosed with breast cancer cope effectively with cancer-related fatigue (Morgan et al., 2014). The interest in studying the relationship between spirituality and health has greatly contributed to nursing science.

Current Concepts in Spiritual Health

A variety of concepts describing spiritual health are a part of professional nursing practice. To provide meaningful and supportive spiritual care, it is important to understand the concepts of spirituality, spiritual well-being, faith, religion, and hope. Each concept offers direction in understanding the views that individuals have of life and its value.

Spirituality. Spirituality is a complex concept that is unique to each individual; it depends on a person's culture, development, life experiences, beliefs, and ideas about life (Cohen et al., 2012). It is an inherent human characteristic that exists in all people, regardless of their religious beliefs (McSherry and Jamieson, 2013). It gives individuals the *energy* needed to discover themselves, cope with difficult situations, and maintain health. Energy generated by spirituality helps patients feel well and guides choices (e.g., type and extent of health care) made throughout life. Spirituality enables a person to love, have faith and hope, seek meaning in life, and nurture relationships with others. Because it is subjective, multidimensional, and personal, researchers and scholars cannot agree on a universal definition of spirituality (McSherry and Jamieson, 2013). However, five distinct but overlapping constructs are used to define it (Figure 36-1).

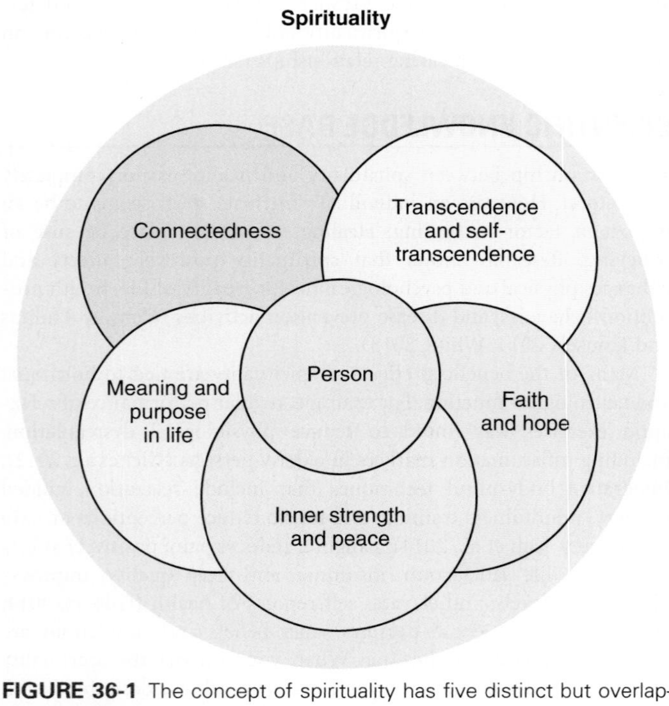

Spirituality

Connectedness

Transcendence and self-transcendence

Person

Meaning and purpose in life

Faith and hope

Inner strength and peace

FIGURE 36-1 The concept of spirituality has five distinct but overlapping constructs.

- Self-transcendence—a sense of authentically connecting to one's inner self (Haugan et al., 2012). This contrasts with transcendence, the belief that a force outside of and greater than the person exists beyond the material world (Hatamipour et al., 2015). Self-transcendence is a positive force. It allows people to have new experiences and develop new perspectives that are beyond ordinary physical boundaries. Examples of transcendent moments include the feeling of awe when holding a new baby or looking at a beautiful sunset.
- Connectedness—being *intrapersonally* connected within oneself; *interpersonally* connected with others and the environment; and *transpersonally* connected with God, or an unseen higher power. Through connectedness patients move beyond the stressors of everyday life and find comfort, faith, hope, and empowerment (Phillips-Salimi et al., 2012).
- Faith—allows people to have firm beliefs despite lack of physical evidence. It enables them to believe in and establish transpersonal connections. Although many people associate faith with religious beliefs, it exists without them (Dyess, 2011).
- Hope—has several meanings that vary on the basis of how it is being experienced; it usually refers to an energizing source that has an orientation to future goals and outcomes (Kavradim et al., 2013; Soundy et al., 2014).

Spirituality gives people the ability to find a dynamic and creative sense of *inner strength* to be used when making difficult decisions. This source of energy helps people stay open to change and life challenges, provides confidence in decision making, and promotes connections with others and a positive outlook on life (Viglund et al., 2014). *Inner peace* fosters calm, positive, and peaceful feelings despite life experiences of chaos, fear, and uncertainty. These feelings help people feel comforted even in times of great distress (Hatamipour et al., 2015). Spirituality also helps people find *meaning and purpose in life* in both positive and negative life events (Hatamipour et al., 2015; White, 2013).

Some people do not believe in the existence of God (atheist), or they believe that there is no known ultimate reality (agnostic). Nonetheless spirituality is important regardless of a person's religious beliefs (Hsiao et al., 2013). Atheists search for meaning in life through their work and their relationships with others. Agnostics discover meaning in what they do or how they live because they find no ultimate meaning for the way things are. They believe that people bring meaning to what they do.

Spirituality is an integrating theme. A person's concept of spirituality begins in childhood and continues to grow throughout adulthood (Bryant-Davis et al, 2012). It represents the totality of one's being, serving as the overriding perspective that unifies the various aspects of an individual. It spreads through all dimensions of a person's life, whether or not the person acknowledges or develops it.

Spiritual Well-Being. The concept of spiritual well-being has two dimensions. One dimension supports the transcendent relationship between a person and God or a higher power. The other dimension describes positive relationships and connections that people have with others (Petersen, 2014). Those who experience spiritual well-being feel connected to others and are able to find meaning or purpose in their lives. Those who are spiritually healthy experience joy, are able to forgive themselves and others, accept hardship and mortality, and report an enhanced quality of life (Haugan et al., 2014).

Faith. In addition to being a component of spirituality, the concept of faith has other definitions. It is a cultural or institutional religion such as Judaism, Buddhism, Islam, or Christianity. It is also a relationship with a divinity, higher power, or spirit that incorporates a reasoning faith (belief) and a trusting faith (action). Reasoning faith provides confidence in something for which there is no proof. It is an acceptance of what reasoning cannot explain. Sometimes faith involves a belief in a higher power, spirit guide, God, or Allah. It is also the manner in which a person chooses to live. It gives purpose and meaning to an individual's life, allowing for action (Dyess, 2011). Patients who are ill often have a positive outlook on life and continue to pursue daily activities rather than resign themselves to the symptoms of their disease. Their faith becomes stronger because they view their illness as an opportunity for personal growth (Granero-Molina et al., 2014).

Religion. Religion is associated with the "state of doing," or a specific system of practices associated with a particular denomination, sect, or form of worship. It is a system of organized beliefs and worship that a person practices to outwardly express spirituality. Many people practice a faith or belief in the doctrines and expressions of a specific religion or sect such as the Lutheran church or Judaism. People from different religions view spirituality differently. For example, a Buddhist believes in Four Noble Truths: life is suffering; suffering is caused by clinging; suffering can be eliminated by eliminating clinging; and to eliminate clinging and suffering, one follows an eightfold path (i.e., right understanding, intention, speech, action, livelihood, effort, mindfulness, and concentration). A Buddhist turns inward, valuing self-control, whereas a Christian looks to the love of God to provide enlightenment and direction in life.

When providing spiritual care, it is important to understand the differences between religion and spirituality. Many people tend to use the terms interchangeably. Although closely associated, they are not synonymous. Religious practices encompass spirituality, but spirituality does not need to include religious practice. Religious care helps patients maintain their faithfulness to their belief systems and worship practices. Spiritual care helps people identify meaning and purpose in life, look beyond the present, and maintain personal relationships and a relationship with a higher being or life force.

Hope. A spiritual person's faith brings hope. When a person has the attitude of something to live for and look forward to, hope is present. It is a multidimensional concept that provides comfort while people endure life-threatening situations, hardships, and other personal challenges. It is closely associated with faith and is energizing. Hope motivates people to achieve such as adopting healthy behaviors. People express hope in all aspects of their lives to help them deal with life stressors. It is a valuable personal resource whenever someone is facing a loss (see Chapter 37) or a difficult challenge (Ruchiwit, 2012).

Spiritual Health

People gain spiritual health by finding a balance between their values, goals, and beliefs and their relationships within themselves and others. Throughout life a person often grows more spiritual, becoming increasingly aware of the meaning, purpose, and values of life. In times of stress, illness, loss, or recovery, a person uses previous ways of responding or adjusting to a situation. Often these coping styles lie within the person's spiritual beliefs.

Spiritual beliefs change as patients grow and develop. Spirituality begins as children learn about themselves and their relationships with others, including a higher power. For example, the attitude of trust in a God actually begins when a baby learns to trust in the dependability of his "God-like" parents' care and love (Neifert, 2011). Nurses who understand a child's spiritual beliefs are able to care for and comfort the child (Petersen, 2014). As children mature into adulthood, they experience spiritual growth by entering into lifelong relationships with people who share similar values and beliefs.

Beliefs among older people vary on the basis of cultural factors such as gender, past experience, religion, ethnicity, and economic status. Healthy spirituality in older adults gives peace and acceptance of the self and is often the result of a lifelong connection with a higher power. A study found that older adult women demonstrate spiritual resilience, expressed by maintaining a purpose in life and expressing gratitude, which promotes spiritual well-being (Manning, 2014). Illness and loss sometimes threaten and challenge the spiritual developmental process. Older adults often express their spirituality by turning to important relationships and giving of themselves to others (Edelman and Mandle, 2014).

Factors Influencing Spirituality

When illness, loss, grief, or a major life change occurs, people either use spiritual resources to help them cope, or spiritual needs and concerns develop. **Spiritual distress** is "a state of suffering related to the impaired ability to experience meaning in life through connections with self, others, the world, or a superior being" (Herdman and Kamitsuru, 2014). It causes people to question their identity and feel doubt, loss of faith, and a sense of being alone or abandoned. Individuals often question their spiritual values, raising questions about their way of life, purpose for living, and source of meaning. Spiritual distress also occurs when there is conflict between a person's beliefs and prescribed health regimens or the inability to practice usual rituals.

Acute Illness. Sudden, unexpected illness often creates spiritual distress. For example, both the 50-year-old patient who has a heart attack and the 20-year-old patient who is in a motor vehicle accident face crises that threaten their spiritual health. The illness or injury creates an unanticipated scramble to integrate and cope with new realities (e.g., disability). People often look for ways to remain faithful to their beliefs and value systems. Some pray, attend religious services more often, or spend time reflecting on the positive aspects of their lives. In an older study that remains relevant today, patients who experienced acute myocardial infarction found spirituality to be a life-giving force that led patients to find meaning and purpose to their lives (Walton, 1999). The researcher found that patients experienced different phases of finding meaning and purpose in life: facing mortality, releasing fear and turmoil, identifying and making lifestyle changes, seeking divine purpose, and making meaning in daily life. Anger and releasing fear are common; patients sometimes express it against God, their families, themselves, or their health care providers. The strength of a patient's spirituality influences how he or she copes with sudden illness and how quickly he or she moves to recovery. Nurses use knowledge of a person's spiritual well-being and implement spiritual interventions to maximize inner peace and healing (Yeager et al., 2010).

Chronic Illness. Many chronic illnesses threaten a person's independence, causing fear, anxiety, and spiritual distress. Dependence on others for routine self-care needs often creates feelings of powerlessness. Powerlessness and the loss of a sense of purpose in life impair the ability to cope with alterations in functioning. Spirituality is an important dimension of how patients live with advanced illness (Asgeirsdottir et al., 2013) (Box 36-1). Successful adaptation provides spiritual growth. Patients who have a sense of spiritual well-being feel connected with a higher power and others, are able to find meaning and purpose in life, and are better able to cope with and accept their chronic illness.

Terminal Illness. Terminal illness causes fears of physical pain, isolation, the unknown, and dying. It creates an uncertainty about

BOX 36-1 EVIDENCE-BASED PRACTICE

Spirituality and Chronic Illness

PICO Question: How do perceptions of spirituality affect well-being and quality of life in patients with chronic illnesses?

Summary of Evidence

All aspects of a patient's life are affected by a chronic illness. Current research supports that spirituality helps patients cope with the effects of their chronic illnesses, leading to enhanced well-being and quality of life (QOL) (Delgado-Guay, 2014). For example, existential well-being (having a purpose in life and being satisfied with life) significantly contributes to the health status of patients living with human immunodeficiency virus (HIV) (Cobb, 2012; Dalmida et al., 2012) and cancer (Delgado-Guay, 2014). Religiosity and closeness to God help patients accept death (Daaleman and Dobbs, 2010). Spiritual care (both religious and nonreligious) is a vital factor in well-being and quality of life at the end of life, and multidisciplinary supportive care is needed (Delgado-Guay, 2014). Nursing interventions, including prayer, establishing presence, establishing a caring relationship, having patients discuss spirituality in groups, and supporting patients within a faith community help patients with chronic illnesses thrive even at the end of life (Dyess and Chase, 2010; Tuck, 2012).

Application to Nursing Practice

- Pay attention to a patient's cultural and spiritual identity throughout the course of their illness (Piotrowski, 2013).
- Listen to a patient's story and angst and provide a compassionate presence (Delgado-Guay, 2014).
- Patients are not looking for answers. What is spoken as a spiritual question is most often an expression of spiritual pain (Delgado-Guay, 2014).
- Pray with your patients if they desire; prayer enhances connectedness to a higher being and often provides a source of strength, enhancing well-being and quality of life (Daaleman and Dobbs, 2010; Dyess and Chase, 2010).
- Patients should agree to interventions, and they should be tailored to their worldly perspectives to help during illness or crisis (Brown et al., 2013).
- Encourage patients with chronic illnesses to maintain connections with others and their faith community (Dyess and Chase, 2010; Tuck, 2012).

what death means, making patients susceptible to spiritual distress. However, some patients have a spiritual sense of peace that enables them to face death without fear. Spirituality helps these patients find peace in themselves and their death. Individuals experiencing a terminal illness find themselves reviewing their life and questioning its meaning. Common questions they ask include, "Why is this happening to me?" or "What have I done?" Terminal illness affects family and friends just as much as the patient. It causes members of the family to ask important questions about its meaning and how it will affect their relationship with the patient (see Chapter 37). When caring for dying patients, help them gain a greater sense of control over their illness, whether they are in a health care setting (e.g., the hospital) or at home. Dying is a holistic process encompassing a patient's physical, social, psychological, and spiritual health (Hayden, 2011; Phelps et al., 2012).

Near-Death Experience. Some nurses care for patients who have had a near-death experience (NDE). An NDE is a psychological phenomenon of people who either have been close to clinical death or have recovered after being declared dead. It is not associated with a mental disorder. Instead experts agree that NDE describes a powerfully close brush with physical, emotional, and spiritual death. For example, people who have an NDE after cardiopulmonary arrest often tell the same story of feeling themselves rising above their bodies and watching caregivers initiate lifesaving measures. Commonly patients who experience an NDE describe feeling totally at peace, having an out-of-body experience, being pulled into a dark tunnel, seeing bright lights, and meeting people who preceded them in death. Instead of moving toward the light, they learn that it is not time for them to die, and they return to life (Agrillo, 2011; Cant et al., 2012).

Patients who have an NDE are often reluctant to discuss it, thinking family or caregivers will not understand. Isolation and depression often occur. Furthermore, not all NDEs are positive experiences. However, individuals experiencing an NDE who discuss it openly with family or caregivers find acceptance and meaning from this powerful experience. They are often no longer afraid of death, and they have a decreased desire to achieve material wealth. They also report increased sensitivity to different chemicals such as alcohol and medications. After patients have survived an NDE, promote spiritual well-being by remaining open, giving patients a chance to explore what happened. and supporting them as they share the experience with significant others (Cant et al., 2012).

CRITICAL THINKING

Successful critical thinking requires a synthesis of knowledge, experience, information gathered from patients, critical thinking attitudes, and intellectual and professional standards. Clinical judgments require you to anticipate information, analyze the data, and make decisions regarding your patient's care. While using the nursing process, apply critical thinking in providing appropriate spiritual care (Figure 36-2).

The helping role is important in nursing practice (Benner, 1984). Patients look to nurses for help that is different than the help they seek from other health care professionals. Expert nurses acquire the ability to anticipate personal issues affecting patients and their spiritual well-being. Critical thinking and the application of knowledge and skills help nurses enhance patients' spiritual well-being and health. Nurses who are comfortable with their own spirituality often are more likely to care for their patients' spiritual needs. Beliefs of a health care provider affect the discussion of treatment options with patients and ultimately their health care choices (Delgado, 2015). Nurses feel strongly about providing spiritual care as part of their holistic practice. Nurses who foster their own personal, emotional, and spiritual health become resources for their patients and use their own spirituality as a tool when caring for themselves and their patients.

After becoming comfortable with your own spirituality, use your nursing knowledge to anticipate your patients' personal issues and the resulting effect on spiritual well-being. Your knowledge about the concept of spirituality, understanding of ethics (see Chapter 22), and knowledge of a patient's faith and belief systems help to provide appropriate spiritual care. Knowledge of a patient's values, beliefs, preferences, and needs provides insight into a person's spiritual practices. Application of therapeutic communication principles (see Chapter 24) and caring (see Chapter 7) helps you establish therapeutic trust with patients. An individual's spiritual beliefs are very personal. When you integrate patient preferences, values, and beliefs into spiritual care, you provide patient-centered care with sensitivity and respect for the diversity of human experience (QSEN Institute, 2014).

Personal experience in caring for patients in spiritual distress is valuable when helping them select coping options. You need to determine if your spirituality is beneficial in assisting patients. Nurses who sense a personal faith and hope regarding life are usually better able to help their patients. A nurse learns from his or her personal faith system and previous professional experiences with dying patients and those

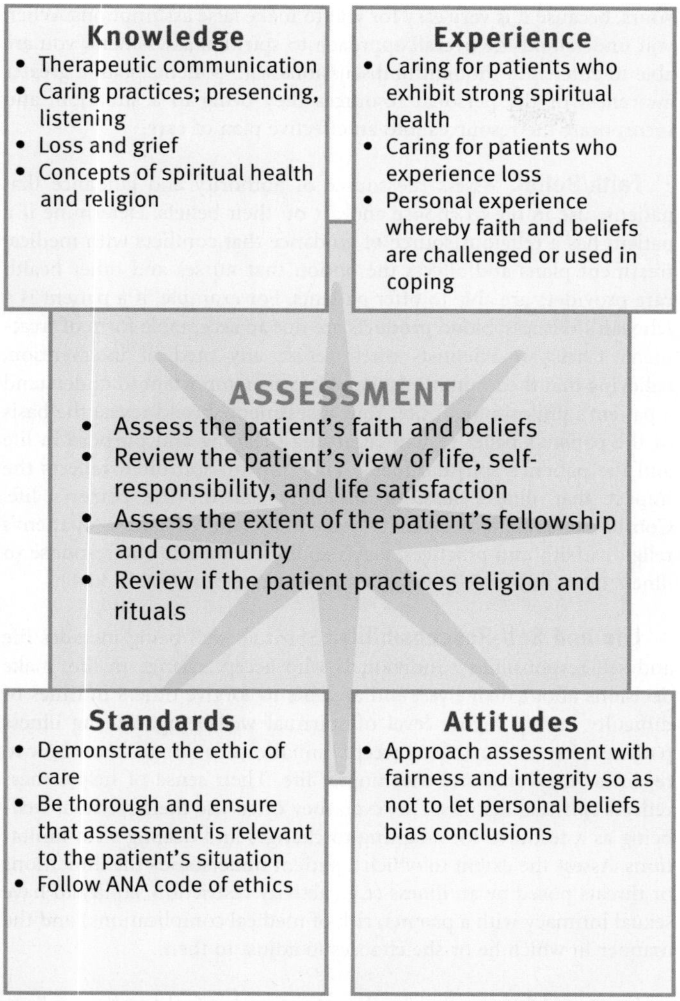

Knowledge
- Therapeutic communication
- Caring practices; presencing, listening
- Loss and grief
- Concepts of spiritual health and religion

Experience
- Caring for patients who exhibit strong spiritual health
- Caring for patients who experience loss
- Personal experience whereby faith and beliefs are challenged or used in coping

ASSESSMENT
- Assess the patient's faith and beliefs
- Review the patient's view of life, self-responsibility, and life satisfaction
- Assess the extent of the patient's fellowship and community
- Review if the patient practices religion and rituals

Standards
- Demonstrate the ethic of care
- Be thorough and ensure that assessment is relevant to the patient's situation
- Follow ANA code of ethics

Attitudes
- Approach assessment with fairness and integrity so as not to let personal beliefs bias conclusions

FIGURE 36-2 Critical thinking model for spiritual health assessment. *ANA*, American Nurses Association.

with chronic disease or severe loss how to provide spiritual care comfortably (Delgado, 2015).

Because each person has a unique spirituality, you need to know your own beliefs so you are able to care for each patient without bias (Tiew and Creedy, 2010). Use critical thinking when assessing each patient's reaction to illness and loss and determining if spiritual intervention is necessary. Humility is essential, especially when caring for patients from diverse cultural backgrounds. Recognize personal limitations in knowledge about patients' spiritual beliefs and religious practices. Effective nurses show genuine concern as they assess their patients' beliefs and determine how spirituality influences their patients' health. You demonstrate integrity by refraining from voicing your opinions about religion or spirituality when your beliefs conflict with those of your patients.

The application of intellectual standards helps you make accurate clinical decisions and helps patients find meaningful and logical ways to acquire spiritual healing. Critical thinking ensures that you obtain significant and relevant information when making decisions about patients' spiritual needs. The nature of a person's spirituality is complex and individualized. Avoid making assumptions about his or her religion and beliefs. Significance and relevance are standards of critical thinking that allow you to explore the issues that are most meaningful to patients and most likely to affect spiritual well-being.

In setting standards for quality health care, The Joint Commission (TJC) (2015) requires health care organizations to assess patients' denomination, beliefs, and spiritual practices and acknowledge their rights to spiritual care. However, TJC does not specify what to include in an assessment. A health care organization must define the content and scope of spiritual assessment and provide for patients' spiritual needs through pastoral care or others who are certified, ordained, or lay individuals.

The American Nurses Association *Code of Ethics for Nurses* (2015) requires nurses to practice nursing with compassion and respect for the inherent dignity, worth, and uniqueness of every person. It is essential to promote an environment that respects patients' values, customs, and spiritual beliefs. Routinely implementing standard nursing interventions such as prayer or meditation is coercive and unethical. Therefore determine which interventions are compatible with your patient's beliefs and values before selecting them. An ethic of caring (see Chapter 7) provides a framework for decision making and places the nurse as the patient's advocate.

❖ NURSING PROCESS

Apply the nursing process and use a critical thinking approach in your care of patients. The nursing process provides a clinical decision-making approach for you to use to develop and implement an individualized plan of care. Understanding a patient's spirituality and then appropriately identifying the level of support and resources needed require a broad perspective and an open mind. As a nurse you make a commitment to meet the spiritual needs of your patients; thus it is essential to respect each patient's personal beliefs. People experience the world and find meaning in life differently. Application of the nursing process from the perspective of a patient's spiritual needs is not simple. It goes beyond assessing his or her religious practices. Caring for your patients' spiritual needs requires you to be compassionate and remove any personal biases or misconceptions. Be willing to share and discover their meaning and purpose in life, illness, and health. Identify common values and respect unique commitments and values with your patients by having quiet conversations, listening effectively, and communicating using presence and touch (Delgado, 2015).

◆ Assessment

During the assessment process thoroughly assess each patient and critically analyze findings to ensure that you make patient-centered clinical decisions required for safe nursing care. Convey caring and openness to successfully promote honest discussion about each patient's spiritual beliefs. Taking a faith history reveals patient's beliefs about life, health, and a Supreme Being.

Through the Patient's Eyes. It is essential to take the time to assess a patient's viewpoints and establish a trusting relationship. As you and your patients reach a point of learning together, spiritual caring occurs. Because completing a spiritual assessment takes time, conduct an ongoing assessment over the course of a patient's stay in the health care setting if possible. Establish trust and rapport and make the opportunity to conduct meaningful discussions with patients a priority. Once you establish a trusting relationship with a patient, you and the patient reach a point of learning together, and spiritual caring occurs (Bailey et al., 2009). Focus your assessment on aspects of spirituality most likely to be influenced by life experiences, events, and questions in the case of illness and hospitalization. Be sure that you discuss what is meaningful and relevant to the patient. Conducting an assessment is therapeutic for you and your patient because it conveys a level of caring and support.

BOX 36-2 Nursing Assessment Questions

Spirituality and Spiritual Health
- Which experiences in the past have been most difficult for you?
- What gives you energy during those difficult times?
- Which aspects of your spirituality have been most helpful to you?
- Which aspects of your spirituality would you like to discuss?

Faith, Belief, Fellowship, and Community
- To what or whom do you look as a source of strength, hope, or faith in times of difficulty?
- How does your faith help you cope?
- Do you use prayer?
- What can I do to support your religious beliefs or faith commitment?
- What gives your life meaning?

Life and Self-Responsibility
- How do you feel about the changes this illness has caused?
- How do these changes affect what you now need to do?

Life Satisfaction
- How happy or satisfied are you with your life?
- Which accomplishments help you feel satisfied with your life?

Connectedness
- What feelings do you have after you pray?
- Who do you feel is the most important person in your life?

Vocation
- How has your illness affected the way you live your life spiritually at home or where you work?
- In what way has your illness affected your ability to express what is important in life to you?

Assessment Tools. Listening to a patient's story is an essential method for obtaining a spiritual assessment. However, you can assess your patients' spiritual health in several different ways, using open-ended questions to prompt them to tell their story or asking them direct questions (Box 36-2). Asking direct questions requires you to feel comfortable asking others about their spirituality. Some health care agencies and researchers have created assessment tools to clarify values and assess spirituality. For example, the spiritual well-being (SWB) scale has 20 questions that assess a patient's relationship with God and his or her sense of life purpose and life satisfaction (Life Advance, 2009). The FICA assessment tool (Borneman et al., 2010) evaluates spirituality and is closely correlated to quality of life. FICA stands for the following criteria:

F—**F**aith or belief
I—**I**mportance and Influence
C—**C**ommunity
A—**A**ddress (Interventions to address)

Effective assessment tools such as the SWB scale and FICA help you remember important areas to assess. Patient responses to the assessment items on the tools indicate areas that you need to investigate further. For example, if, after using the FICA tool with a patient who is having difficulty accepting a new diagnosis of prostate cancer, you find out that he does not want you or his pastor to help him address this issue, you need to spend time understanding how the patient plans to manage this new illness. Remember, when using any spiritual assessment tool, do not impose your personal values on your patient. This is difficult, especially when a patient's values and beliefs are similar to yours, because it is very easy for you to make false assumptions. When you understand the overall approach to spiritual assessment, you are able to enter into thoughtful discussions with patients, gain a greater awareness of the personal resources they bring to a situation, and incorporate the resources into an effective plan of care.

Faith/Belief. Assess the source of authority and guidance that patients use in life to choose and act on their beliefs. Determine if a patient has a religious source of guidance that conflicts with medical treatment plans and affects the option that nurses and other health care providers are able to offer patients. For example, if a patient is a Jehovah's Witness, blood products are not an acceptable form of treatment. Christian Scientists often refuse any medical intervention, believing that their faith heals them. It is also important to understand a patient's philosophy of life. Your assessment should reveal the basis of the patient's belief system regarding meaning and purpose in life and the patient's spiritual focus. This information often reflects the impact that illness, loss, or disability has on the person's life. Considerable religious diversity exists in the United States. A patient's religious faith and practices, views about health, and the response to illness often influence how nurses provide support (Table 36-1).

Life and Self-Responsibility. Spiritual well-being includes life and self-responsibility. Individuals who accept change in life, make decisions about their lives, and are able to forgive others in times of difficulty have a higher level of spiritual well-being. During illness patients often are unable to accept limitations or do not know how to regain a functional and meaningful life. Their sense of helplessness reflects spiritual distress. However, they often use their spiritual well-being as a resource for adapting to changes and dealing with limitations. Assess the extent to which a patient understands the limitations or threats posed by an illness (e.g., activity restriction, ability to have sexual intimacy with a partner, risk of medical complications) and the manner in which he or she chooses to adjust to them.

Connectedness. People who are connected to themselves, others, nature, and God or another Supreme Being cope with the stress brought on by crisis and chronic illness. In a study involving Muslim patients with chronic diabetic foot ulcers, a positive relationship was found between connectedness and health-related quality of life (Alzahrani and Sehlo, 2013). One way patients remain connected with their God is by praying (Figure 36-3). Prayer is personal communication with one's god. It provides a sense of hope, strength, security, and well-being; and it is a part of faith. Help patients become or remain connected by respecting each patient's unique sense of spirituality. Assess whether the patient loses the ability to express a sense of relatedness to something greater than the self.

Life Satisfaction. Spiritual well-being is tied to a person's satisfaction with life and what he or she has accomplished, even in the case of children (Chlan et al., 2011). When people are satisfied with life and how they are using their abilities, more energy is available to deal with new difficulties and resolve problems. You assess a patient's satisfaction with life by asking questions such as, "How happy or satisfied are you with your life?" or "Tell me how satisfied you feel about what you have accomplished in life."

Culture. Spirituality is a personal experience within a cultural context. It is important to know a patient's cultural background and assess his or her values about the health care problem and impending treatment (see Chapter 9). It is common in many cultures for individuals to believe that they have led a worthwhile and purposeful

TABLE 36-1 Religious Beliefs About Health

Religious or Cultural Group	Health Care Beliefs	Response to Illness	Implications for Health and Nursing
Hinduism	Accepts modern medical science.	Past sins cause illness. Prolonging life is discouraged.	Allow time for prayer and purity rituals. Allow use of amulets, rituals, and symbols.
Sikhism	Accepts modern medical science.	Females are to be examined by females. Removing undergarments causes great distress.	Provide time for devotional prayer. Allow use of religious symbols.
Buddhism	Accepts modern medical science.	Followers sometimes refuse treatment on Holy Days. Nonhuman spirits invading body cause illness. Followers may want a Buddhist priest. Followers usually accept death as last stage of life and permit withdrawal of life support. Followers do not practice euthanasia. They often do not take time off from work or family responsibilities when sick.	Health is an important part of life. Good health is maintained by caring for self and others. Medications are not always accepted because of belief that chemical substances in body are harmful.
Islam	Must be able to practice Five Pillars of Islam. Sometimes has fatalistic view of health.	Muslims use faith healing. Family members are comfort. Group prayer is strengthening. They often permit withdrawal of life support. They do not practice euthanasia. They believe that time of death is predetermined and cannot be changed. They maintain sense of hope and often avoid discussions of death.	Women prefer female health care providers. During month of Ramadan Muslims do not eat until after sun goes down. Health and spirituality are connected. Family and friends visit during time of illness. They usually do not consider organ transplantation or donation and postmortem examinations.
Judaism	Believes in sanctity of life. Balance between God and medicine. Observance of Sabbath important. Treatments sometimes refused on Sabbath.	Visiting sick is obligation. There is an obligation to seek care, exercise, sleep, eat well, and avoid drug and alcohol abuse. Euthanasia is forbidden. Life support is discouraged.	They believe that it is important to stay healthy. Jews expect a nurse to provide competent health care. Allow patients to express their feelings. Allow family to stay with dying patient.
Christianity	Accepts modern medical science. Complementary or alternative medicine often followed (see Chapter 33).	Followers use prayer, faith healing. They appreciate visits from clergy. Some use laying on of hands. Holy Communion is sometimes practiced. Anointing of the sick is given when patient is ill or near death (Catholic).	Christians usually in favor of organ donation. Health is important to maintain. Allow time for patients to pray by themselves or with family or friends.
Navajos	Concepts of health have fundamental place in their concept of humans and their place in the universe.	Blessingway is practice that attempts to remove ill health by means of stories, songs, rituals, prayers, symbols, and sand paintings.	Navajos prefer holistic approach to health care. They often are not on time for appointments. Promote physical, mental, spiritual, and social health of people, families, and communities. Allow family members to visit. Provide teaching about wellness, not disease prevention, when possible.
Appalachians	External locus of control. Nature controls life and health. Accept folk healers.	They dislike hospitals. Tend to not follow medical regimens but expect to be helped directly when seeking episodic treatment.	They become anxious in unfamiliar settings. Encourage communication with family and friends when ill.

life. Remaining connected with their cultural heritage often helps patients define their place in the world and express their spirituality. Asking them about their faith and belief systems is a good beginning for understanding the relationship between culture and spirituality (Box 36-3).

Fellowship and Community. Fellowship is one kind of relationship that an individual has with other people, including immediate family, close friends, associates at work or school, fellow members of a church, and neighbors. More specifically this includes the extent of the community of shared faith between people and their support networks. Many times social support from faith-based groups helps patients cope with illness (Heiney et al., 2011) and participate in health promotion behaviors (Newlin et al., 2012). To assess a patient's supportive community, ask questions such as, "With whom do you bond?" "Who do you find to be the greatest source of support in times of difficulty?" or "When you've faced difficult times in the past, who has been your greatest resource?"

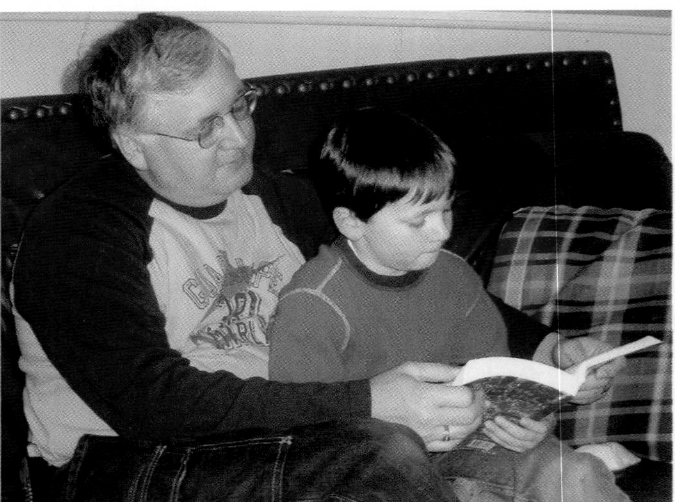

FIGURE 36-3 Praying or reading a bible together enhances the connectedness between parents and their children.

BOX 36-3 CULTURAL ASPECTS OF CARE

Spirituality and Culture

Spirituality and spiritual health vary among cultures. Remember that a person's culture is defined by his or her age, gender, political association, religion, or other variables such as ethnicity and educational background. One way to assess a patient's spirituality through a cultural lens is to first understand his or her definition of health, wellness, and illness. For example, ask questions such as, "What do you call your health problem? What do you think has caused it? What do you think your sickness does to you? How do you find strength to cope with this problem?"

You want to assess how a patient's spirituality is affected by his or her culture. If your focus is on a patient's ethnicity, know the unique characteristics of that ethnic group's spiritual values. For example, spiritual aspects of life are frequently important to Latinos. *Personalismo* is a cultural value that indicates warmth, closeness, and empathy in relationships with other people and a universal being. *Familismo*, another Latino cultural value, indicates commitment and loyalty to immediate and extended family (Campesino et al., 2009).

Implications for Patient–Centered Care

- Explore the spirituality of patients from different cultural backgrounds; assess the meaning of health and how patients achieve balance, stability, peace, or comfort in their lives.
- Offer a universal and holistic approach when assessing patients' needs; demonstrate caring and use therapeutic communication techniques.
- During assessment respect patients' human rights, values, customs, and spiritual beliefs (see Chapter 9).
- Spiritual assessment should be interdisciplinary. If you feel uncomfortable with religion or spirituality, respectfully identify if a patient wishes referral to an appropriate professional chaplain or clergy.
- Avoid use of language that alienates or discriminates among different cultures.

Explore the extent and nature of a person's support networks and their relationship with the patient. It is unwise to assume that a given network offers the kind of support that a patient desires. For example, calling a patient's pastor to request a visit is inappropriate if the patient has little fellowship with the pastor or the pastor's faith community. Does the patient have one significant fellowship or several? What level of support does the community give? Do they visit, say prayers, or support the patient's immediate family? Learn whether openness exists between a patient and the people with whom a fellowship has formed.

Ritual and Practice. Assessing the use of rituals and practices helps you understand a patient's spirituality. Rituals include participation in worship, prayer, sacraments (e.g., baptism, Holy Eucharist), fasting, singing, meditating, scripture reading, and making offerings or sacrifices. Different religions have different rituals for life events. For example, Buddhists practice baptism later in life and find burial or cremation acceptable at death. Muslims wash the body of a dead family member and wrap it in white cloth with the head turned toward the right shoulder. Orthodox and conservative Jews circumcise their newborn sons 8 days after birth. Determine whether illness or hospitalization has interrupted a patient's usual rituals or practices. A ritual often provides the patient with structure and support during difficult times. If rituals are important to a patient, use them as part of nursing intervention.

Vocation. Individuals express their spirituality on a daily basis in life routines, work, play, and relationships. It is often a part of a person's identity and vocation. Determine if illness or hospitalization alters the ability to express some aspect of spirituality as it relates to the person's work or daily activities. Expression of spirituality includes showing an appreciation for life in the variety of things people do, living in the moment and not worrying about tomorrow, appreciating nature, expressing love toward others, and being productive. When illness or loss prevents patients from expressing their spirituality, understand the psychological, social, and spiritual implications and provide appropriate guidance and support.

QSEN QSEN: BUILDING COMPETENCY IN PATIENT-CENTERED CARE. You are caring for Grace, a 52-year-old who experienced multiple fractures following a motor vehicle crash. Grace is experiencing difficulties with mobility, and she is not going to be able to go back to work for at least 6 months. Currently she is having extensive rehabilitation to help her complete activities of daily living. When you walk into Grace's room, she will not look at you. You can tell that she has been crying. She has a flat affect and states, "I just don't know why God did this to me. How am I going to go on from here?"

Identify at least three questions you will ask Grace to assess her spiritual well-being and plan effective, evidence-based care.

Answers to QSEN Activities can be found on the Evolve website.

Nursing Diagnosis

A spiritual assessment allows a nurse to learn a great deal about the patient and the extent that spirituality plays in his or her life. Exploring the patient's spirituality sometimes reveals responses to health problems that require nursing intervention or the existence of a strong set of resources that allow the patient to cope effectively. Analyze data to find risk factors or patterns of defining characteristics and select appropriate nursing diagnoses (Box 36-4). In identifying diagnoses, recognize the significance that spirituality has for all types of health problems. Be sure that each problem-focused nursing diagnosis has an accurate related factor to guide the selection of individualized, purposeful, and goal-directed interventions. Potential nursing diagnoses for spiritual health include the following:

- *Anxiety*
- *Ineffective Coping*

BOX 36-4 Nursing Diagnostic Process

Readiness for Enhanced Spiritual Well-Being

Assessment Activities	Defining Characteristics
Ask patient to describe personal source of faith and hope.	Patient expresses inner strength and source of guidance.
Have patient describe level of satisfaction with life.	Life has purpose and meaning; patient finds satisfaction while providing community service as a volunteer.
Determine who provides greatest source of strength and support to patient during times of difficulty.	Patient pursues interactions with friends and family.

- *Complicated Grieving*
- *Hopelessness*
- *Powerlessness*
- *Readiness for Enhanced Spiritual Well-Being*
- *Spiritual Distress*
- *Risk for Spiritual Distress*
- *Risk for Impaired Religiosity*

Three nursing diagnoses accepted by NANDA International (Herdman and Kamitsuru, 2014) pertain specifically to spirituality. *Readiness for Enhanced Spiritual Well-Being* is based on defining characteristics that show a person's ability to experience and integrate meaning and purpose in life through connectedness with self and others. A patient with this nursing diagnosis has potential resources on which to draw when faced with illness or a threat to well-being.

The nursing diagnoses of *Spiritual Distress* and *Risk for Spiritual Distress* create different clinical pictures. Defining characteristics from a nurse's assessment reveal patterns that reflect a person's actual or potential dispiritedness (e.g., expressing lack of hope, meaning, or purpose in life; anger toward God; or verbalizing conflicts about personal beliefs). Patients likely to be at risk for spiritual distress include those who have poor relationships, have experienced a recent loss, or are suffering some form of mental or physical illness.

Accurate selection of diagnoses requires critical thinking. Review and analyze all concrete data (e.g., religious rituals and sources of fellowship), your assessment of previous patient experiences, your own spirituality, and your appraisal of the patient's spiritual well-being. Commonly patients have multiple nursing diagnoses.

◆ Planning

During the planning step of the nursing process, develop a plan of care for each of the patient's nursing diagnoses. Critical thinking at this step is important because you reflect on previous experiences and apply knowledge and critical thinking attitudes and standards in selecting the most appropriate nursing interventions (Figure 36-4). Prior experience with other patients is valuable when selecting interventions to support spiritual well-being. Integrate assessment data with knowledge about resources and therapies available for spiritual care to develop an individualized plan of care (see the Nursing Care Plan). Match the patient's needs with evidence-based interventions that are supported and recommended in the clinical and research literature. Use a concept map (Figure 36-5) to organize patient care and show how the patient's medical diagnosis, assessment data, and nursing diagnoses are interrelated.

Confidence, an important critical thinking attitude, builds trust, enabling you and a patient to enter into a healing relationship together.

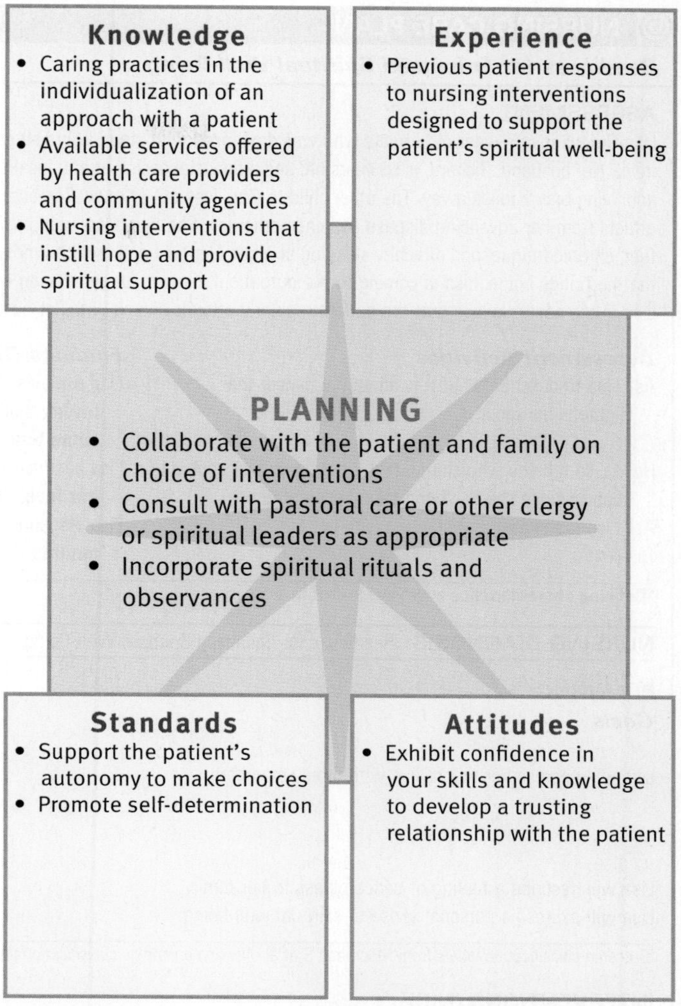

Knowledge
- Caring practices in the individualization of an approach with a patient
- Available services offered by health care providers and community agencies
- Nursing interventions that instill hope and provide spiritual support

Experience
- Previous patient responses to nursing interventions designed to support the patient's spiritual well-being

PLANNING
- Collaborate with the patient and family on choice of interventions
- Consult with pastoral care or other clergy or spiritual leaders as appropriate
- Incorporate spiritual rituals and observances

Standards
- Support the patient's autonomy to make choices
- Promote self-determination

Attitudes
- Exhibit confidence in your skills and knowledge to develop a trusting relationship with the patient

FIGURE 36-4 Critical thinking model for spiritual health planning.

Attempting to meet or support patients' spiritual needs is not simple; frequently you need additional resources. For example, sometimes a nurse's skills in helping patients interpret and understand the meaning of illness and loss are limited. Because spiritual care is so personal, standards of autonomy and self-determination are critical in supporting the patient's decisions about the plan of care.

Goals and Outcomes. A spiritual care plan includes realistic and individualized goals along with relevant outcomes. It is very important to collaborate closely with patients when setting goals for spiritual support and growth and choosing related interventions. Setting realistic goals requires you to know a patient well. When spiritual care requires helping patients adjust to loss or stressful life situations, goals are long term. However, short-term outcomes such as renewing participation in religious practices help patients progressively reach a more spiritually healthy situation. In establishing a plan of care, an example of a goal and associated outcomes follows:

The patient will improve personal harmony and connections with members of his or her support system.

- The patient expresses an acceptance of illness.
- The patient reports the ability to rely on family members for support.
- The patient initiates social interactions with family and friends.

 NURSING CARE PLAN

Readiness for Enhanced Spiritual Well-Being

ASSESSMENT

Lisa Owens is a 61-year-old female who was diagnosed with stage IV breast cancer over 2 years ago. She has undergone numerous rounds of chemotherapy treatment. Her husband, Richard, is 59 years old and a financial assistant at a local bank. The Owens have two children, both adults, with one daughter who is unmarried and living only 2 miles away. The other child, a son, lives out of town. The son is married; he and his wife are about to have their first child. Lisa has numerous side effects from her advancing disease and chemotherapy. She has ongoing hip pain from the cancer having spread to the bone. She also has reduced sensation in her feet, chronic fatigue, and difficulty sleeping at night. Her husband provides most of her support at home, but this sometimes interferes with his ability to do the work that he brings home. Lisa is coming to the outpatient chemotherapy infusion center to begin yet another course of chemotherapy. The nurse who has been seeing Lisa in the center knows that the patient regularly attends church with her husband.

Assessment Activities	*Findings/Defining Characteristics**
Ask Lisa to describe what it is about her cancer that frightens her most.	Lisa explains, "I have found it makes me appreciate what I have with my family. That being said, I worry that I will not see my grandchild born, **but I hope the chemotherapy will give me some time and it will make me feel a bit better."**
Have Lisa tell you who she finds to be the greatest source of support since she has been taking chemotherapy.	Lisa has received support from her husband and daughter. **She wants to be able to show them her love, "I still want to be there for them."**
Ask Lisa if she feels satisfaction with her life.	Lisa responds, "We always want more, don't we? **I have been blessed, but I think God gave me this illness so I can show others what life means**."

***Defining characteristics** are shown in bold type.

NURSING DIAGNOSIS: Readiness for Enhanced Spiritual Well-Being

PLANNING

Goals	*Expected Outcomes (NOC)†*
	Hope
Lisa will express her will to live with family members.	Lisa participates in worship with her family and shares spiritual readings. Lisa connects with members of her church. Lisa interacts with family members and discusses their future.
	Spiritual Health
Lisa will describe a feeling of peacefulness to her family. Lisa will express a personal sense of spiritual well-being.	Lisa engages in regular prayer and meditation. Lisa expresses her feelings through writing.

†Outcome classification labels from Moorhead S et al: *Nursing outcomes classification (NOC)*, ed 5, St Louis, 2013, Mosby.

INTERVENTIONS (NIC)‡	RATIONALE
Spiritual Growth Facilitation	
Plan discussions with Lisa during treatment and listen, allowing her to sort out concerns she might have about her future. Include Lisa's husband if she desires.	Listening provides support or comfort in spiritual care (Delgado, 2015). Family caregivers engage in "meaning making" activities by expressing important values such as hope, dignity, and togetherness (Delgado-Guay, 2014).
Offer to pray with Lisa as she describes what she hopes for.	One study found that cancer patients commonly used prayer and meditation to reduce their side effects (Huebner et al., 2014)
Introduce Lisa to journaling. Encourage her to begin by writing what is meaningful to her about her illness and family	Use of journaling helps individuals facing a crisis deal with the unknown; find meaning and spiritual connection; and physically, emotionally, and spiritually heal (Harvey et al., 2013; Sealy, 2013).
Spiritual Support	
Discuss with Lisa the likely times that her chemotherapy will affect her most and how she can schedule involvement in church activities around those times.	Chemotherapy can cause severe fatigue. Faith communities such as a church play an important role in fostering belief systems of compassion (Delgado-Guay, 2014).
Teach Lisa methods of relaxation, meditation, and guided imagery.	Relaxation methods help promote quality of life and enhance serenity and dignity. Relaxation responses have been associated with improved physiological (blood pressure, exercise capacity, and cardiac symptoms) and psychological (depression and anxiety) outcomes (Horowitz, 2010; Sheeba et al., 2013).

‡Intervention classification labels from Bulechek GM et al: *Nursing interventions classification (NIC)*, ed 6, St Louis, 2013, Mosby.

EVALUATION

Nursing Actions	*Patient Response/Finding*	*Achievement of Outcome*
Ask Lisa to describe in what way relaxation exercises have helped her.	Lisa reported using relaxation daily after being at clinic. She states, "I feel calm. It allows me to connect with God, and know I have my loving family to help me."	Lisa's story reflects spiritual well-being and peacefulness. She needs to share with family.
Have Lisa review her discussions with family and/or church members.	Lisa reports, "We have been talking more. My family knows that I see each day as a blessing and that my hope is to see my son's baby. My church really keeps me connected."	Lisa is connecting with family and church members. She is able to express a sense of hope.

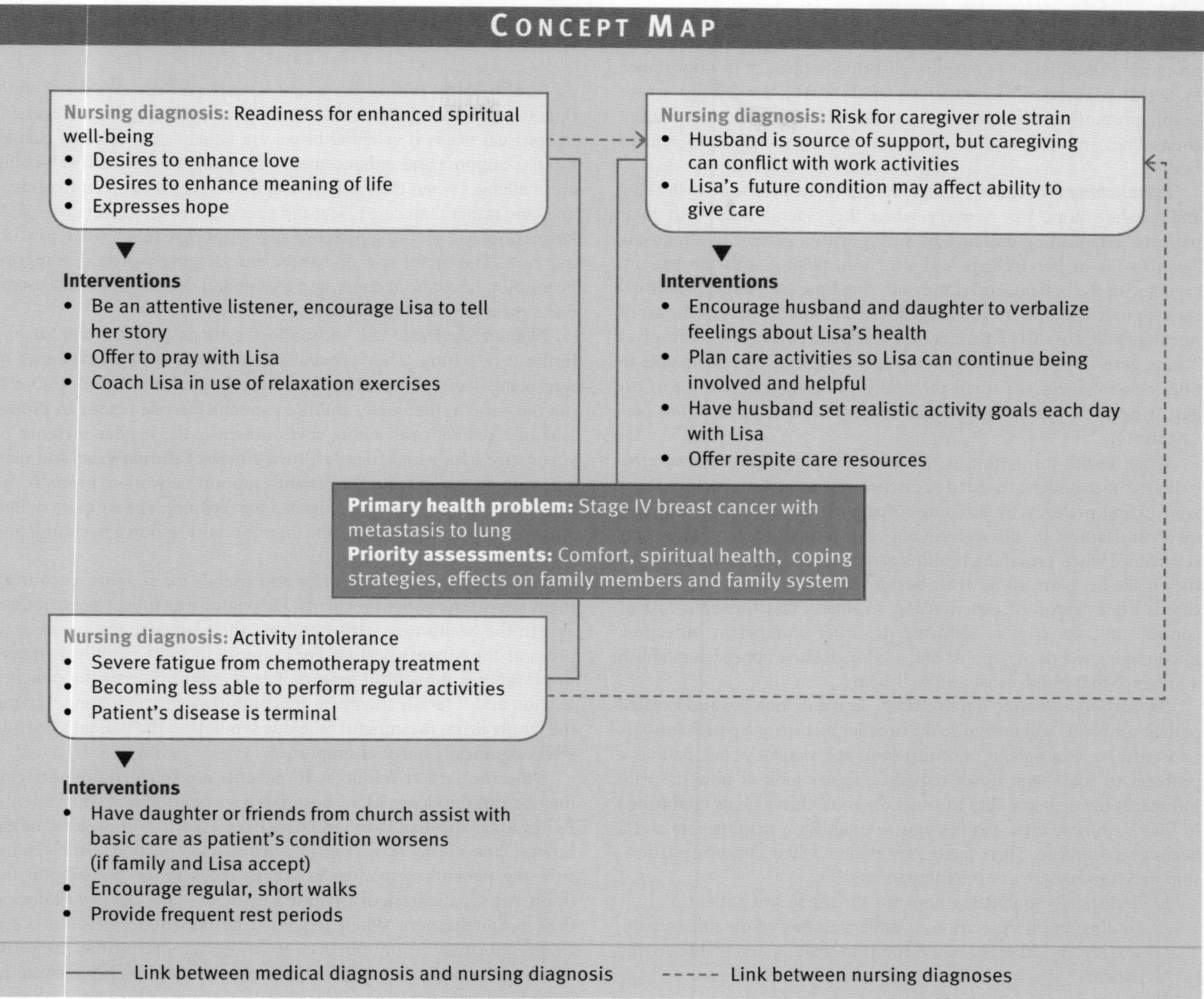

FIGURE 36-5 Concept map for Lisa Owens.

Setting Priorities. Spiritual care is very personalized. Your relationship with a patient allows you to understand the patient's priorities in the context of his or her spiritual life. When establishing a mutually agreed-on plan with the patient, he or she is able to identify what is most important. Spiritual priorities do not need to be sacrificed for physical care priorities. For example, when a patient is in acute distress, focus care to provide him or her a sense of control to minimize powerlessness. When a patient is terminally ill, spiritual care often is the most important nursing intervention (see Chapter 37).

Teamwork and Collaboration. If a patient participates in a formal religion, involve members of the clergy or church, temple, mosque, or synagogue in the plan of care when appropriate. In a hospital setting the pastoral care department is a valuable resource. These spiritual care professionals offer insight about how and when to best support patients and their families. Spiritual care providers provide direct support in the form of actively addressing spiritual or religious needs of a patient and family, having discussions about family members' feelings and patient values, and reminiscing with families about a patient (Johnson et al., 2014). Significant others such as spouses, siblings, parents, and friends need to be involved in the patient's care as appropriate. This means that you learn from an assessment which individuals or groups have formed a relationship with the patient. These individuals sometimes become involved in all levels of the plan of care. They often assist in giving physical care, providing emotional comfort, and sharing spiritual support.

◆ Implementation

Establish caring relationships with patients to discover their beliefs about the meaning of illness or loss and the effects on the meaning and purpose of their lives. This level of understanding enables you to deliver care in a sensitive, creative, and appropriate manner.

Health Promotion. Spiritual care needs to be a central theme in promoting an individual's overall well-being because of its importance in health promotion (Kemppainen et al., 2011). In settings where health promotion activities occur, patients often need information, counseling, and guidance to make the necessary choices to remain healthy.

Establishing Presence. Nurses contribute to a sense of well-being and provide hope for recovery when they spend time with their patients. Establishing presence by sitting with a patient to attentively listen to his or her feelings and situation, talking with the patient, crying with the patient, and simply offering time are powerful spiritual care approaches (Bowers and Rieg, 2014). Presence is part of the art of nursing (Milligan, 2011). Benner (1984) explains that presence involves "being with" a patient versus "doing for" a patient. It is being able to offer closeness with a patient physically, psychologically, and spiritually. It helps to prevent emotional and environmental isolation (see Chapter 7).

When health promotion is the focus of care, your presence gives patients the confidence needed to discuss ways to remain healthy. Show your caring presence by listening to patients' concerns and willingly involving family in discussions about patients' health. Show self-confidence when providing health instruction and support patients as they make decisions about their health. The patient who seeks health care is often fearful of experiencing an illness that threatens loss of control and looks for someone to offer competent direction. Encouraging words of support and a calm, decisive approach establish a presence that builds trust and well-being.

Supporting a Healing Relationship. Learn to look beyond isolated patient problems and recognize the broader picture of a patient's holistic needs. For example, do not just look at a patient's back pain as a problem to solve with quick remedies; rather look at how the pain influences his or her ability to function and achieve goals established in life. A holistic view enables you to establish a helping role and a healing relationship. Three factors are evident when a healing relationship develops between nurse and patient:

1. Realistically mobilizing hope for the nurse and patient
2. Finding an interpretation or understanding of the illness, pain, anxiety, or other stressful emotion that is acceptable to the patient
3. Helping the patient use social, emotional, and spiritual resources (Benner, 1984)

Mobilizing a patient's hope is central to a healing relationship. Hope motivates people with strategies to face challenges in life (Yeager et al., 2010). Help patients find things for which to hope. For example, a patient newly diagnosed with diabetes wants to learn how to manage the disease to continue a productive and satisfying way of life. An adult daughter who has decided to become caregiver to her older adult parent hopes to be able to protect the parent from injury or worsening disability. Hope helps patients work toward recovery. To help patients achieve hope, work together to find an explanation for their situation that is acceptable to them. Help a patient realistically exercise hope by supporting positive attitudes toward life or the desire to be informed and make decisions.

Remain aware of a patient's spiritual resources and needs. It is always important for patients to be able to express and exercise their beliefs and find spiritual comfort. When life stressors or illness create confusion or uncertainty, recognize the possible effect on a patient's well-being. How do you use and strengthen spiritual resources? Begin by encouraging a patient to discuss the effect that illness has had on personal beliefs and faith, thus giving the chance to clarify any misconceptions or inaccuracies in information. Having a clear sense of what illness will be like for an individual helps the person apply all resources toward recovery.

Acute Care. Within acute care settings patients experience multiple stressors that threaten their sense of control. Ongoing assessment of spiritual needs is essential because a patient's needs often change rapidly. Support and enhancement of a patient's spiritual well-being are challenges when the focus of health care seems to be on treatment and cure rather than care (Tiew and Creedy, 2010). To meet these challenges display a soothing presence and supportive touch when providing care. The artful use of hands, encouraging words of support, promotion of connectedness, and a calm and decisive approach establish a presence that builds trust.

Support Systems. Use of support systems is important in any health care setting. They provide patients with the greatest sense of well-being during hospitalization and serve as a human link connecting the patient, the nurse, and the patient's lifestyle before an illness. Part of a patient's caregiving environment is the regular presence of supportive family and friends. Provide privacy during visits and plan care with the patient and the patient's support network to promote the interpersonal bonding that is needed for recovery. The support system is a source of faith and hope and an important resource in conducting meaningful religious rituals.

When patients look to family and friends for support, encourage them to visit the patient regularly. Help family members feel comfortable in the health care setting and use their support and presence to promote the patient's healing. For example, including family members in prayer is a thoughtful gesture if it is appropriate to the patient's religion and if family members are comfortable participating. Having the family bring meaningful religious symbols to the patient's bedside offers significant spiritual support.

Other important resources to patients are spiritual advisors and members of the clergy. Many hospitals have pastoral care departments. Professional spiritual care providers have expertise in understanding how an illness influences a person's beliefs and how these beliefs influence the patient's responses to illness, recovery, or preparation for death. Ask if patients desire to have a member of the clergy visit during their hospitalization. When requested by patients or families, keep clergy informed of any physical, psychosocial, or spiritual concerns affecting the patient. A spiritual care provider is especially helpful in discussing patient and family wishes about end-of-life care (Johnson et al., 2014). Respect patients' spiritual values and needs by allowing time for pastoral care members to provide spiritual care and facilitating the administration of sacraments, rites, and rituals.

Diet Therapies. The intake of food satisfies and promotes a sense of comfort. Food and nutrition are important aspects of patient care and often an important component of some religious observances (Table 36-2). Food and the rituals surrounding the preparation and serving of food are sometimes important to a person's spirituality. Consult with a dietitian to integrate patients' dietary preferences into daily care. In the event that a hospital or other health care agency cannot prepare food in the preferred way, ask the family to bring meals that fit into dietary restrictions posed by the patient's condition.

Supporting Rituals. Nurses provide spiritual care by supporting patients' participation in spiritual rituals and activities. Plan care to allow time for religious readings, spiritual visitations, or attendance at religious services. Allow family members to plan a prayer session or an organized reading of scriptures on a regular basis. Make arrangements with spiritual care professionals for the patient and family to participate in religious practices (e.g., receiving sacraments). Clergy often visit people who are unable to attend religious services. Taped meditations, classical or religious music, and televised religious services

TABLE 36-2 Religious Dietary Regulations Affecting Health Care

Religion	Dietary Practices
Hinduism	Some sects are vegetarians. The belief is not to kill *any* living creature.
Buddhism	Some are vegetarians and do not use alcohol. Many fast on Holy Days.
Islam	Consumption of pork and alcohol is prohibited. Followers fast during the month of Ramadan.
Judaism	Some observe the kosher dietary restrictions (e.g., avoid pork and shellfish, do not prepare and eat milk and meat at same time).
Christianity	Some Baptists, Evangelicals, and Pentecostals discourage use of alcohol and caffeine. Some Roman Catholics fast on Ash Wednesday and Good Friday. Some do not eat meat on Fridays during Lent.
Jehovah's Witnesses	Members avoid food prepared with or containing blood.
Mormonism	Members abstain from alcohol and caffeine.
Russian Orthodox Church	Followers observe fast days and a "no-meat" rule on Wednesdays and Fridays. During Lent all animal products, including dairy products and butter, are forbidden.
Native Americans	Individual tribal beliefs influence food practices.

provide other effective options. Always respect the icons, medals, prayer rugs, or crosses that a patient brings to a health setting and ensure that they are not accidentally lost, damaged, or misplaced. Supporting spiritual rituals is especially important for older adults (Box 36-5).

Restorative and Continuing Care. For patients who are recovering from a long-term illness or disability or who suffer chronic or terminal disease, spiritual care becomes especially important. Many of the nursing interventions applicable in health promotion and acute care apply to this level of health care as well.

Prayer. The act of prayer gives an individual the opportunity to renew personal faith and belief in a higher being in a specific, focused way that is either highly ritualized and formal or quite spontaneous and informal. Prayer is an effective coping resource for physical and psychological symptoms (Oliver and Dutney, 2012). Patients pray in private or participate in group prayer with family, friends, or clergy. Some pray while listening to music. Be supportive of prayer by giving the patient privacy if desired, learning if the patient wishes to have you participate, and suggesting prayer when you know that it is a coping resource for the patient. Delgado (2015) has found that nurses tend to pray for patients rather than with patients; sharing the fact that prayer has been offered gives patients comfort and support. If prayer is not suitable for a patient, alternatives include listening to calming music or reading a book, poetry, or inspirational texts selected by the patient.

Meditation. Meditation creates a relaxation response that reduces daily stress. Patients who meditate often state that they have an increased awareness of their spirituality and of the presence of God or a Supreme Being. Meditation exercises give patients relief from pain, insomnia, anxiety, and depression and increase coping and the ability to relax (Cole et al., 2012; Williams-Orlando, 2012). Meditation involves sitting quietly in a comfortable position with eyes closed and repeating a sound, phrase, or sacred word in rhythm with breathing while disregarding intrusive thoughts. Individuals who meditate regularly (twice a day for 10 or 20 minutes) experience decreased metabolism and heart rate, easier breathing, and slower brain waves (Box 36-6). Chapter 33 addresses relaxation approaches.

Supporting Grief Work. Patients who experience terminal illness or who have suffered permanent loss of body function because of a

BOX 36-5 FOCUS ON OLDER ADULTS

Spirituality and Spiritual Health

- There is an association between an older adult's spirituality and his or her ability to adjust or cope with illness and other life stressors (Manning, 2014).
- Older adults achieve spiritual resilience through frequent expressions of gratitude (e.g., via prayer, meditation, or discussions with friends) and finding ways to maintain purpose in life (e.g., helping family, volunteering) (Manning, 2014).
- Patients use spiritual rituals, exercise, and complementary medicine to cope with pain and chronic illness.
- Feelings of connectedness are important for the older adult (Anderberg and Berglund, 2010). Enhance connectedness by helping older patients find meaning and purpose in life by listening actively to concerns and being present.
- Beliefs in the afterlife increase as adults age. Make visits from clergy, social workers, lawyers, and financial advisors available so patients feel as though they have completed all unfinished business. Leaving a legacy (e.g., oral history, art, photographs) to loved ones prepares an older adult to leave the world with a sense of meaning and maintains a way to continue connection for the one left behind (Touhy and Jett, 2012).
- Older-adult caregivers use their spirituality and spiritual behaviors or practices to help them deal with crisis and conflict (Strudwick and Morris, 2010).

BOX 36-6 PATIENT TEACHING

Meditation Techniques

Objective

- The patient will verbalize feelings of relaxation and self-transcendence after meditation.

Teaching Strategies

- Give patient a brief description of information and a printed teaching guide that describes how to meditate.
- Help patient identify a quiet room in the home that has minimal interruptions.
- Explain that peaceful music or the quiet whirring of a fan blocks out distractions.
- Teach steps of meditation (i.e., sit in a comfortable position with the back straight; breathe slowly; and focus on a sound, prayer, or image).
- Encourage patient to meditate for 10 to 20 minutes twice a day.
- Answer questions and reinforce information as needed.

Evaluation

- Have patient describe feelings following meditation.

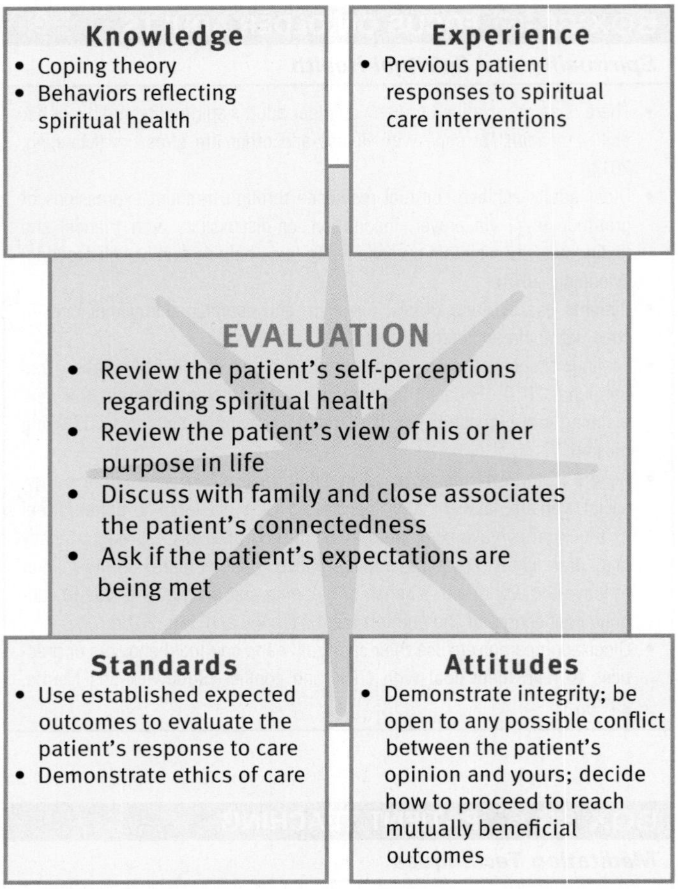

Knowledge
- Coping theory
- Behaviors reflecting spiritual health

Experience
- Previous patient responses to spiritual care interventions

EVALUATION
- Review the patient's self-perceptions regarding spiritual health
- Review the patient's view of his or her purpose in life
- Discuss with family and close associates the patient's connectedness
- Ask if the patient's expectations are being met

Standards
- Use established expected outcomes to evaluate the patient's response to care
- Demonstrate ethics of care

Attitudes
- Demonstrate integrity; be open to any possible conflict between the patient's opinion and yours; decide how to proceed to reach mutually beneficial outcomes

FIGURE 36-6 Critical thinking model for spiritual health evaluation.

disabling disease or injury require a nurse's support in grieving and coping with their loss. Your ability to enter into a caring, therapeutic, and spiritual relationship with patients supports them during times of grief (see Chapter 37).

◆ Evaluation

Through the Patient's Eyes. The evaluation of a patient's spiritual care requires you to think critically in determining if efforts at restoring or maintaining the patient's spiritual health were successful (Figure 36-6). Include the patient in your evaluation of care. Outcomes established during the planning phase serve as the standards to evaluate the patient's progress. Ask him or her if you and the health care team met their expectations and if there is anything else you can do to enhance their spiritual well-being or enable them to practice important religious rituals. In addition, evaluate ethical concerns that arise in the course of the patient's spiritual care and support. Apply critical thinking attitudes and use therapeutic communication techniques to ensure sound nursing judgments.

Patient Outcomes. Attaining spiritual health is a lifelong goal. In evaluating outcomes, compare the patient's level of spiritual health with the behaviors and perceptions noted in the nursing assessment. Evaluation data related to spiritual health are usually subjective. For example, if your assessment finds the patient losing hope, the follow-up evaluation involves asking him or her if feelings of hope have been restored. Include family and friends when gathering evaluative information. Successful outcomes reveal the patient developing an increased or restored sense of connectedness with family; maintaining, renewing, or reforming a sense of purpose in life; and for some a confidence and trust in a Supreme Being or power. When outcomes are not met, ask questions to determine appropriate continuing care. Examples of questions to ask include the following:

- Do you feel the need to forgive someone or to be forgiven by someone?
- Which spiritual activities such as prayer or meditation were helpful to you?
- Would you like for me to ask a friend, family member, or someone from pastoral care to talk with you?
- What can I do to help you feel more at peace?
- Sometimes people need to give themselves permission to feel hope when they experience difficult events. What can you do to allow yourself to feel hope again?

KEY POINTS

- Spirituality is an inherent human characteristic that gives individuals the energy needed to discover themselves, cope with difficult situations, and maintain health.
- Nurses need to be aware of their own spirituality to provide appropriate and relevant spiritual care to others.
- Research shows that spirituality positively affects and enhances physical and psychological health, quality of life, health promotion behaviors, and disease prevention activities.
- Spirituality is important regardless of a person's religious beliefs.
- Spiritual well-being has two dimensions: support of the transcendent relationship between a person and a higher power and the positive relationships and connections that people have with others.
- Nurses who are comfortable with their own spirituality often are more likely to care for their patients' spiritual needs.
- After establishing a trusting relationship with a patient, you and the patient reach a point of learning together, and spiritual caring occurs.
- Nursing assessment of a patient's spiritual needs includes a review of the patient's faith, connectedness, life and self-responsibility, life satisfaction, and fellowship and community.
- It is important to know a patient's cultural background and assess his or her values about his or her health care problem and impending treatment.
- Nurses need to determine if a patient's religious beliefs conflict with medical treatment.
- Establishing presence involves attentive listening, talking with patients and answering questions, crying with patients, and simply offering your time.
- Spiritual care providers provide direct support in the form of actively addressing spiritual or religious needs of a patient and family and having discussions about family members' feelings and patient values.
- Prayer is an effective coping resource for physical and psychological symptoms.
- During evaluation successful outcomes reveal a patient developing an increased or restored sense of connectedness with family and maintaining, renewing, or reforming a sense of purpose in life.

CLINICAL APPLICATION QUESTIONS

Preparing for Clinical Practice

Lisa is coming to the oncology center regularly. Her hip pain is increasing, and she continues having fatigue. Her doctor has told her that this will likely be the last chemotherapy treatment protocol she will be able to have. Magnetic resonance imaging (MRI) shows that the cancer has spread to Lisa's lung. It is 1 month from the time that her son's wife is to have their baby. Her husband has been helping to care for Lisa at home because she is becoming less physically able to do normal daily activities. Her daughter tries to help, but her job sometimes takes her out of town for short trips.

1. The nurse chooses to assess the extent to which Lisa now understands the limitations or threats posed by her cancer. This is an example of which assessment category to cover in a spiritual assessment? Explain its importance.
2. Give three examples of assessment questions the nurse might ask to determine the level of support available to Lisa from members of her church.
3. Because Lisa has a terminal illness, what common reactions might she express in dealing with death?

ⓔ ***Answers to Clinical Application Questions can be found on the Evolve website.***

REVIEW QUESTIONS

1. A student nurse is telling a faculty member that her patient talked about gaining spiritual comfort from being focused on her inner self, including her values and principles. The instructor explains that this is an example of:
   1. Faith.
   2. Community.
   3. Interpersonal connection.
   4. Self-transcendence.
2. Health care agencies often have assessment tools to use in clarifying patient values and assess spirituality. Using the FICA assessment tool, match the criteria on the left with the appropriate assessment question on the right.

1. F—Faith ___	a. Tell me if you have a higher power or authority that helps you act on your beliefs
2. I—Importance of spirituality ___	b. Describe which activities give you comfort spiritually?
3. C—Community ___	c. To whom do you go for support in times of difficulty?
4. A—Interventions to address spiritual needs ___	d. Your illness has kept you from attending church. Is that a problem for you?

3. A nurse is caring for a 78-year-old patient with chronic multiple sclerosis. The patient has severe fatigue, muscle weakness, severe muscle spasms, and difficulties with coordination and balance. Her disease will likely worsen. The nurse has gained the patient's trust and wants to assess her life satisfaction. Which of the following questions should the nurse ask? (Select all that apply.)
   1. How often are you able to attend your synagogue?
   2. What about your family makes you proudest?
   3. What does your husband do for you at home?
   4. Looking back, what is your greatest accomplishment?
   5. How has your illness affected the way you live your life spiritually at home?
4. You are caring for a hospitalized patient who is Muslim and has diabetes. Which of the following items do you need to remove from the meal tray when it is delivered to the patient?
   1. Small container of vanilla ice cream
   2. A dozen red grapes
   3. Bacon and eggs
   4. Garden salad with ranch dressing
5. A 44-year-old male patient has just been told that his wife and child were killed in an auto accident while coming to visit him in the hospital. Which of the following statements are defining characteristics that support a nursing diagnosis of *Spiritual Distress related to loss of family members*? (Select all that apply.)
   1. "I need to call my sister for support."
   2. "I have nothing to live for now."
   3. "Why would my God do this to me?"
   4. "I need to pray for a miracle."
   5. "I want to be more involved in my church."
6. A patient has just learned she has been diagnosed with a malignant brain tumor. She is alone; her family will not be arriving from out of town for an hour. You have cared for her for only 2 hours but have a good relationship with her. What might be the most appropriate intervention for support of her spiritual well-being at this time?
   1. Make a referral to a professional spiritual care advisor
   2. Sit down and talk with the patient; have her discuss her feelings and listen attentively
   3. Move the patient's bible from her bedside cabinet drawer to the top of the over-bed table
   4. Ask the patient if she would like to learn more about the implications of having this type of tumor
7. A nurse is preparing to teach an older adult who has chronic arthritis how to practice meditation. Which of the following strategies are appropriate? (Select all that apply.)
   1. Encourage family members to participate in the exercise.
   2. Have patient identify a quiet room in the home that has minimal interruptions.
   3. Suggest use of a quiet fan running in the room.
   4. Explain that it is best to meditate about 5 minutes 4 times a day.
   5. Show the patient how to sit comfortably with the limitation of his arthritis and focus on a prayer.
8. A student nurse is developing a plan of care for a 74-year-old-female patient who has spiritual distress over losing a spouse. As the nurse develops appropriate interventions, which characteristics of older adults should be considered? (Select all that apply.)
   1. Older adults do not routinely use complementary medicine to cope with illness.
   2. Older adults dislike discussing the afterlife and what might have happened to people who have passed on.
   3. Older adults achieve spiritual resilience through frequent expressions of gratitude.
   4. Have the patient determine if her husband left a legacy behind.
   5. Offer the patient her choice of rituals or participation in exercise.
9. A patient states that he does not believe in a higher power but instead believes that people bring meaning to what they do. This patient most likely is an:
   1. Academic.
   2. Atheist.
   3. Agnostic.
   4. Anarchist.
10. A nurse begins a night shift, assuming care for a critically ill patient who was resuscitated earlier in the day from cardiac arrest. He survived and is physically stable, alert, oriented, and responding appropriately to the nurse's questions. Knowing that the patient experienced a period when his heart stopped beating, what would be the best approach for the nurse to use with him?
    1. Have family come to visit and focus discussion about their gratitude that the patient survived

2. Change the subject when the patient begins talking about entering a dark tunnel when the doctors were resuscitating him
3. Sit and encourage the patient to share what he experienced during resuscitation
4. Provide the patient the opportunity to have passages from the bible read to him

11. A nurse is caring for a patient with a seriously advanced infection who asks to have a spiritual care provider come who can offer Blessingway, a practice that attempts to remove ill health. This patient is likely a member of which religion or culture?
    1. Hinduism
    2. Navajo
    3. Sikhism
    4. Judaism
12. Evaluation of spiritual care is necessary to determine if a patient's level of spiritual health has changed following intervention. If the use of rituals was part of a nurse's care plan, which of the following questions is most appropriate to evaluate its efficacy?
    1. Do you feel the need to forgive your wife over your loss?
    2. What can I do to help you feel more at peace?
    3. Were prayer or meditation helpful to you?
    4. Should we plan on having your family try to visit you more often in the hospital?
13. A patient who is recovering from a bilateral amputation of the legs below the knee shows transcendence when she states:
    1. "My pain medicine helps me feel better."
    2. "I know I'll get better if I just keep trying."
    3. "I see God's grace and become relaxed when I watch the sun set at night."
    4. "I have had a great life and a good marriage. My husband has been so helpful in my healing."
14. The nurse is caring for a 50-year-old woman visiting the outpatient medicine clinic. The patient has had type 1 diabetes since age 13. She has numerous complications from her disease, including reduced vision, heart disease, and severe numbness and tingling of the extremities. Knowing that spirituality helps patients cope with their chronic illness, which of the following principles should the nurse apply in practice? (Select all that apply.)
    1. Pay attention to the patient's spiritual identity throughout the course of her illness
    2. Select interventions that you know scientifically support spiritual well-being
    3. Listen to the patient's story each visit to the clinic and offer a compassionate presence
    4. When the patient questions the reason for her long-time suffering, try to provide answers
    5. Consult with a spiritual care advisor and have the advisor recommend useful interventions
15. Select the three factors that are evident when a healing relationship develops between nurse and patient.
    1. The nurse being able to realistically mobilize hope for the patient
    2. The patient being able to share fears of loss with significant others
    3. Finding an interpretation or understanding of the patient's illness that is acceptable to the patient
    4. Understanding your own beliefs about spirituality
    5. Helping the patient use spiritual resources that he or she chooses

Answers: 1. 4; **2.** 1a, 2d, 3c, 4b; **3.** 2, 4; **4.** 3; **5.** 2, 3; **6.** 2; **7.** 2, 3, 5; **8.** 3, 4, 5; **9.** 3; **10.** 3; **11.** 2; **12.** 3; **13.** 3; **14.** 1, 3; **15.** 1, 3, 5.

Rationales for Review Questions can be found on the Evolve website.

REFERENCES

Agrillo C: Near-death experience: out-of-body and out-of-brain?, *Rev Gen Psychol* 15(1):1, 2011.

American Nurses Association (ANA): *Code of ethics for nurses with interpretive statements*, 2015, http://www.nursingworld.org/MainMenuCategories/EthicsStandards/CodeofEthicsforNurses/Code-of-Ethics-For-Nurses.html. Accessed June 20, 2015.

Benner P: *From novice to expert*, Menlo Park, Calif, 1984, Addison-Wesley.

Bowers H, Rieg LS: Reflections on spiritual care: methods, barriers, recommendations, *J Christian Nurs* 31(1):47, 2014.

Bryant-Davis T, et al: Religiosity, spirituality, and trauma recovery in the lives of children and adolescents, *Prof Psychol Res Pract* 43(4):306, 2012.

Delgado-Guay MO: Spirituality and religiosity in supportive and palliative care, *Curr Opin Support Palliat Care* 8(3):308, 2014.

Edelman CL, Mandle CL: *Health promotion throughout the life span*, ed 8, St Louis, 2014, Mosby.

Gilbert R: Laughter therapy: promoting health and wellbeing, *Nurs Resid Care* 16(7):392, 2014.

Granero-Molina J, et al: Religious faith in coping with terminal cancer: what is the nursing experience? *Eur J Cancer Care* 23(3):300, 2014.

Hayden D: Spirituality in end-of-life care: attending the person on their journey, *Br J Community Nurs* 16(11):546, 2011.

Herdman TH, Kamitsuru S, editors: *NANDA International nursing diagnoses: definitions and classification 2015–2017*, Oxford, 2014, Wiley Blackwell.

Horowitz S: Health benefits of meditation: what the newest research shows, *Altern Complement Ther* 16(4):223, 2010.

Life Advance: *The spiritual well-being scale*, http://www.lifeadvance.com/spiritual-well-being-scale.html, 2009. Accessed October 2015.

Milligan S: Addressing the spiritual care needs of people near the end of life, *Nurs Stand* 26(4):47, 2011.

Neifert M: *Faith development in children: how to instill spiritual beliefs*, 2011, http://www.dr-mom.com/blog/faith-development-children-how-instill-spiritual-beliefs/. Accessed October 2015.

Piotrowski LF: Advocating and educating for spiritual screening assessment and referrals to chaplains, *Omega (Westport)* 67:185, 2013.

QSEN Institute: *Pre-licensure KSAs*, 2014, http://qsen.org/competencies/pre-licensure-ksas/. Accessed October 2015.

Sealy PA: Integrating job, Jesus' passion, and Buddhist Metta to bring meaning to the suffering and recovery from breast cancer, *J Relig Health* 52(4):1162, 2013.

The Joint Commission (TJC): *Standards FAQ details*, 2015, http://www.jointcommission.org/standards_information/jcfaqdetails.aspx?StandardsFaqId=290&ProgramId=1. Accessed October 2015.

Touhy TA, Jett KF: *Ebersole & Hess Toward healthy aging: human needs and nursing response*, ed 8, St Louis, 2012, Mosby.

Williams-Orlando C: Spirituality in integrative medicine, *Integr Med Clin J* 11(4):34, 2012.

Yeager S, et al: Embrace hope: an end-of-life intervention to support neurological critical care patients and their families, *Crit Care Nurs* 30(1):47, 2010.

RESEARCH REFERENCES

Alzahrani HA, Sehlo MG: The impact of religious connectedness on health-related quality of life in patients with diabetic foot ulcers, *J Relig Health* 52(3):840, 2013.

Anderberg P, Berglund A: Elderly persons' experiences of striving to receive care on their own terms in nursing homes, *Int J Nurs Pract* 16(1):64, 2010.

Asgeirsdottir GH, et al: "To cherish each day as it comes": a qualitative study of spirituality among persons receiving palliative care, *Support Care Cancer* 21:1445, 2013.

Bailey ME, et al: Creating a spiritual tapestry: nurses' experiences of delivering spiritual care to patients in an Irish hospice, *Int J Palliat Nurs* 15(9):42, 2009.

Borneman T, et al: Evaluation of the FICA tool for spiritual assessment, *J Pain Symptom Manage* 40(2):163, 2010.

Brown O, et al: The use of religion and spirituality in psychotherapy: enablers and barriers, *J Relig Health* 52:1131, 2013.
Campesino M, et al: Spirituality and cultural identification among Latino and non-Latino college students, *Hispanic Health Care Int* 7(2):72, 2009.
Cant R, et al: The divided self: near-death experiences of resuscitated patients—a review of literature, *Int Emerg Nurs* 20(2):88, 2012.
Chlan KM, et al: Spirituality and life satisfaction with pediatric-onset spinal cord injury, *Spinal Cord* 49(3):371, 2011.
Cobb R: How well does spirituality predict health status in adults living with HIV disease: a Neuman Systems Model study, *Nurs Sci Q* 25(4):347, 2012.
Cockell N, McSherry W: Spiritual care in nursing: an overview of published international research, *J Nurs Manage* 20(8):958, 2012.
Cohen MZ, et al: A platform for nursing research on spirituality and religiosity: definitions and measures, *West J Nurs Res* 34(6):795, 2012.
Cole BS, et al: A randomised clinical trial of the effects of spirituality-focused meditation for people with metastic melanoma, *Ment Health Relig Cult* 15(2):161, 2012.
Conway-Phillips R, Janusek L: Influence of sense of coherence, spirituality, social support and health perception on breast cancer screening motivation and behaviors in African-American women, *ABNF J* 25(3):72, 2014.
Daaleman TP, Dobbs D: Religiosity, spirituality, and death attitudes in chronically ill older adults, *Res Aging* 32(2):224, 2010.
Dalmida SG, et al: The meaning and use of spirituality among African American women living with HIV/AIDS, *Wes J Nurs Res* 34(6):736, 2012.
Delgado C: Nurses' spiritual care practices: becoming less religious?, *J Christian Nurs* 32(2):116, 2015.
Dyess SM: Faith: a concept analysis, *J Adv Nurs* 67(12):2723, 2011.
Dyess S, Chase SK: Caring for adults living with a chronic illness through communities of faith, *Int J Human Caring* 14(4):38, 2010.
Fan Y, et al: Cortisol level modulated by integrative medication in a dose-dependent fashion, *Stress Health* 30(1):65, 2014.
Glei DA, et al: Relaxation practice and physiological regulation in a national sample of older Taiwanese, *J Altern Complement Med* 18(7):653, 2012.
Harvey K, et al: Experiences of mothers of infants with congenital heart disease before, during, and after complex cardiac surgery, *Heart Lung* 42(6):399, 2013.
Hatamipour K, et al: Spiritual needs of cancer patients: a qualitative study, *Indian J Palliat Care* 21(1):61, 2015.
Haugan G, et al: Self-transcendence and nurse-patient interaction in cognitively intact nursing home patients, *J Clin Nurs* 21(23/24):3429, 2012.
Haugan G, et al: The relationships between self-transcendence and spiritual well-being in cognitively intact nursing home patients, *Int J Older People Nurs* 9(1):65, 2014.
Heiney SP, et al: Antecedents and mediators of community connection in African women with breast cancer, *Res Theory Nurs Pract* 25(4):252, 2011.
Hirosaki M, et al: Effects of a laughter and exercise program on physiological and psychological health among community-dwelling elderly in Japan: randomized control trial, *Geriatr Gerontol Int* 13(1):152, 2013.
Hsiao Y, et al: Psychometric testing of the properties of the spiritual health scale short form, *J Clin Nurs* 22(21/22):2981, 2013.
Huebner J, et al: Online survey of cancer patients on complementary and alternative medicine, *Oncol Res Treat* 37(6):304, 2014.
Johnson J, et al: The association of spiritual care providers' activities with family members' satisfaction with care after a death in the ICU, *Crit Care Med* 42(9):1991, 2014.
Kavradim ST, et al: Hope in people with cancer: a multivariate analysis from Turkey, *J Adv Nurs* 69(5):1183, 2013.
Kemppainen J, et al: Health promotion behaviors of residents with hypertension in Iwate, Japan and North Carolina, USA, *Jpn J Nurs Sci* 8(1):20, 2011.
Manning LK: Enduring as lived experience: exploring the essence of spiritual resilience for women later in life, *J Relig Health* 53(2):352, 2014.
McSherry W, Jamieson S: The qualitative findings from an online survey investigating nurses' perceptions of spirituality and spiritual care, *J Clin Nurs* 22(21/22):3170, 2013.
Morgan PD, et al: African-American women share 'real talk' stories about fatigue related to breast cancer treatment, *ABNF J* 25(4):116, 2014.
Newberry AG, et al: Exploring spirituality in family caregivers of patients with primary malignant brain tumors across the disease trajectory, *Oncol Nurs Forum* 40(3):E119, 2013.
Newlin K, et al: A methodological review of faith-based health promotion literature: advancing the science to expand delivery of diabetes education to black Americans, *J Relig Health* 51(4):1075, 2012.
Oliver IN, Dutney A: A randomized, blinded study of the impact of intercessory prayer on spiritual well-being in patients with cancer, *Altern Ther Health Med* 18(5):18, 2012.
Petersen C: Spiritual care of the child with cancer at the end of life: a concept analysis, *J Adv Nurs* 70(6):1243, 2014.
Phelps AC, et al: Addressing spirituality within the care of patients at the end of life: perspectives of patients with advanced cancer, oncologists, and oncology nurses, *J Clin Oncol* 30(20):2538, 2012.
Phillips-Salimi CR, et al: Connectedness in the context of patient-provider relationships: a concept analysis, *J Adv Nurs* 68(1):230, 2012.
Prentis S, et al: Healthcare lecturers' perceptions of spirituality in education, *Nurs Stand* 29(3):44, 2014.
Reinert KG, Koenig HG: Re-examining definitions of spirituality in nursing research, *J Adv Nurs* 69(12):2622, 2013.
Ronaldson S, et al: Spirituality and spiritual caring: nurses' perspectives and practice in palliative and acute care environments, *J Clin Nurs* 21(15/16):2126, 2012.
Ruchiwit M: The effect of the one-to-one interaction process with group supportive psychotherapy on the levels of hope, anxiety and self-care practice for patients that have experienced organ loss: an alternative nursing care model, *Int J Nurs Pract* 18(4):363, 2012.
Rykkje LLR, et al: Spirituality and caring in old age and the significance of religion—a hermeneutical study from Norway, *Scand J Caring Sci* 27(2):275, 2013.
Sheeba N, et al: Current status of spirituality in cardiac rehabilitation programs: a review of literature, *J Cardiopulm Rehabil Prev* 33(3):135, 2013.
Soundy A, et al: Factors influencing patients' hope in stroke and spinal cord injury: a narrative review, *Int J Ther Rehabil* 21(5):210, 2014.
Strudwick A, Morris R: A qualitative study exploring the experiences of African-Caribbean informal stroke caregivers in the UK, *Clin Rehabil* 24(2):159, 2010.
Tiew LH, Creedy DK: Integration of spirituality in nursing practice: a literature review, *Singapore Nurs J* 37(1):15, 2010.
Tuck I: A critical review of a spirituality intervention, *West J Nurs Res* 34(6):712, 2012.
Viglund K, et al: Inner strength as a mediator of the relationship between disease and self-rated health among old people, *J Adv Nurs* 70(1):144, 2014.
Walton J: Spirituality of patients recovering from an acute myocardial infarction: a grounded theory study, *J Holist Nurs* 17(1):34, 1999.
White ML: Spirituality self-care effects on quality of life for patients diagnosed with chronic illness, *Self-Care Depend Care Nurs* 20(1):23, 2013.

37

The Experience of Loss, Death, and Grief

OBJECTIVES

- Identify the nurse's role when caring for patients who are experiencing loss, grief, or death.
- Describe the types of loss experienced throughout life.
- Discuss grief theories.
- Identify types of grief.
- Describe characteristics of a person experiencing grief.
- Discuss variables that influence a person's response to grief.
- Develop a nursing care plan for a patient and family experiencing loss and grief.
- Identify ways to collaborate with family members and the interdisciplinary team to provide palliative care.
- Describe interventions for symptom management in patients at the end of life.
- Discuss the criteria for hospice care.
- Describe care of the body after death.

KEY TERMS

Actual loss, p. 751
Ambiguous loss, p. 752
Anticipatory grief, p. 752
Autopsy, p. 765
Bereavement, p. 751
Complicated grief, p. 752
Disenfranchised grief, p. 752
Grief, p. 751
Hope, p. 754
Hospice, p. 761
Maturational loss, p. 751
Mourning, p. 751
Necessary loss, p. 751
Normal (uncomplicated) grief, p. 752
Organ and tissue donation, p. 765
Palliative care, p. 760
Postmortem care, p. 766
Perceived loss, p. 751
Situational loss, p. 751

MEDIA RESOURCES

http://evolve.elsevier.com/Potter/fundamentals/

- Review Questions
- Concept Map Creator
- Case Study with Questions
- Audio Glossary
- Content Updates

Loss is an inevitable part of life. Accompanying each loss are feelings of grief and sadness. Whether a patient is facing infertility or an amputation, an unwanted diagnosis or impending death, you are in a position to offer both the patient and family support to cope with the loss and provide comfort when continued life is not possible. Regardless of the practice setting, you will provide care for those in grief. Like grief, death is as inescapable in practice as it is in life. Although palliative care and hospice use have increased, nurses in all practice settings and specialties provide care for a majority of the dying.

Although people agree that death is a part of life, many are hesitant to talk about it because of feelings of fear, uncertainty, and not wanting to upset others. Talking openly about death is discouraged in American society (i.e., in our everyday lives, our language, and even our thinking) (Matzo and Sherman, 2015). An example is our avoidance of the word "died" and instead the use of words such as "passed away" or "gone." Many health care professionals feel uncomfortable about discussing and providing end-of-life care (Parker et al., 2012). You need to learn how to become comfortable discussing such sensitive topics and providing patients with the opportunity to express their desires for care at the end of life. Historically health care professionals waited until it was too late to discuss end-of-life wishes. With the Self-Care Determination Act of 1990, nurses and other health care providers are starting these conversations earlier, but there is more work left to do. You have the opportunity to advocate for patients and the high quality of care deserved at the end of life.

As a student you need to know that you are capable of providing what patients and families need most at the end of life: compassion, attentiveness, and patient-centered care. As with other nursing situations, the more experience you have caring for the grieving and the dying, the more confident, courageous, and compassionate you will become when caring for patients and families at this intimate and meaningful time. Your skills and knowledge base will develop quickly if you have the desire and willingness to learn, be present, and seek the help needed to learn how to give excellent care at the end of life. Whether it is educating patients and families about advance directives, managing patients' symptoms, or simply holding a hand, nurses care for the dying every day. It is the caring actions of nursing that help the patient and family during these times (see Chapter 7).

SCIENTIFIC KNOWLEDGE BASE

Loss

Life provides each person with multiple opportunities to grieve a loss or change. Sometimes the change is welcomed (marriage, birth of a child), and sometimes not (divorce, loss of a job, death). The loss can be of tangible things such as a body part or function, relationship, or possession. They can also be intangible such as the loss of self-esteem, confidence, or a dream.

The experience of loss starts early in life and continues until death. Children develop independence from the adults who raise them and as they begin and leave school, change friends, begin careers, and form new relationships. From birth to death people form attachments and experience loss. Illness can also be a source of loss. It can change his or her functioning and therefore his or her job, family role, income level, and overall quality of life (Table 37-1). How one grieves depends on cultural norms, belief systems, support systems, and personal faith (AACN and CHNMC, 2014).

Life changes are normal, expected, and often positive. As people age they learn that change always involves a **necessary loss**. They learn to expect that most necessary losses eventually are replaced by something different or better. However, some losses cause them to undergo permanent changes in their lives that threaten their sense of belonging and security. The death of a loved one, divorce, or loss of independence changes life forever and often significantly disrupts a person's physical, psychological, and spiritual health.

A **maturational loss** is a form of necessary loss and includes all normally expected life changes across the life span. A toddler experiences separation anxiety from mom when starting preschool. A grade school child does not want to lose her favorite teacher and classroom. A college student does not want to leave his campus community. Maturational losses associated with normal life transitions help people develop coping skills to use when they experience unplanned, unwanted, or unexpected loss.

Other losses seem unnecessary and are not part of expected maturation experiences. Sudden, unpredictable external events bring about **situational loss**. For example, a person in an automobile accident sustains an injury with physical changes that make it impossible to return to work or school, leading to loss of function, income, life goals, and self-esteem.

TABLE 37-1 Types of Loss

Definition	Implications of Loss
Loss of possessions or objects (e.g., theft, deterioration, misplacement, or destruction)	Extent of grieving depends on value of object, sentiment attached to it, or its usefulness.
Loss of known environment (e.g., leaving home, hospitalization, new job, moving out of a rehabilitation unit)	Loss occurs through maturational or situational events or by injury/illness. Loneliness in an unfamiliar setting threatens self-esteem, hopefulness, or belonging.
Loss of a significant other (e.g., divorce, loss of friend, trusted caregiver, or pet)	Close friends, family members, and pets fulfill psychological, safety, love, belonging, and self-esteem needs.
Loss of an aspect of self (e.g., body part, job, psychological or physiological function)	Illness, injury, or developmental changes result in loss of a valued aspect of self, altering personal identity and self-concept.
Loss of life (e.g., death of family member, friend, co-worker, or one's own death)	Loss of life grieves those left behind. Dying people also feel sadness or fear pain, loss of control, and dependency on others.

Losses may be actual or perceived. An **actual loss** occurs when a person can no longer feel, hear, see, or know a person or object. Examples include the loss of a body part, death of a family member, or loss of a job. Lost valued objects include those that wear out or are misplaced, stolen, or ruined. A **perceived loss** is uniquely defined by the person experiencing the loss and is less obvious to other people. For example, some people perceive rejection by a friend to be a loss, which creates a loss of confidence or changes their status in the social group. How an individual interprets the meaning of the perceived loss affects the intensity of the grief response. Perceived losses are easy to overlook by others because they are experienced so internally and individually, but they are as painful as an actual loss and grieved in the same way.

Each person responds to loss differently. The type of loss and the person's perception of it influence the depth and duration of the grief response. In addition, a person's previous experience with loss also affects how he or she responds to a new loss. For some individuals the loss of an object (e.g., home or treasured gift) generates the same level of distress as the loss of a person, depending on the value the person places on the object. Chronic illnesses, disabilities, and hospitalization produce multiple losses. When entering an institution for care, patients lose access to familiar people and environments, privacy, and control over body functions and daily routines. A chronic illness or disability adds financial hardships for most people and often brings about changes in lifestyle and dependence on others. Even brief illnesses or hospitalizations cause temporary changes in family role functioning, daily activities, and relationships.

Death is the ultimate loss. Although it is an expected part of life, death represents the unknown and can generate anxiety, fear, and uncertainty for many people. It creates a permanent separation of people and can cause fear, sadness, and regret for the dying person, family members, friends, and caregivers. A person's culture, spirituality, personal beliefs, and values; previous experiences with death; and degree of social support influence the way he or she approaches death.

Grief

Grief is a "normal but bewildering cluster of ordinary human emotions arising in response to a significant loss, intensified and complicated by the relationship to the person or the object lost" (Mitchell and Anderson, 1983) (see Chapters 9 and 36). Grief cannot be prevented (Brohard, 2014). It is very personal. No two people grieve the same loss the same way, nor do they journey through grief in the same way. Grief work is very hard and requires enormous amounts of energy from the griever. It is rarely orderly and predictable. Because objects, memories, and anniversaries can cause a surge in feelings of loss, grief work is never fully completed. However, grief can diminish, and healing can occur when the pain of loss is less (AACN and CHNMC, 2014).

Coping with grief involves a period of **mourning**, the outward, social expressions of grief and the behavior associated with loss (AACN and CHNMC, 2014). Most mourning rituals are culturally influenced, learned behaviors. For example, the Jewish mourning ritual of *Shivah* is a time period when normal life activities come to a stop. Those mourning welcome friends into the home as a way of honoring the dead and receive support during the mourning period.

The term **bereavement** encompasses both grief and mourning and includes the emotional responses and outward behaviors of a person experiencing loss. The bereaved should be encouraged to talk about the loss and reassured that the feelings are normal and that major decisions should be postponed (AACN and CHNMC, 2014). Recognizing that there are different types of grief can help nurses plan and implement appropriate care.

Normal Grief. Normal (uncomplicated) grief is a common and universal reaction characterized by complex emotional, cognitive, social, physical, behavioral, and spiritual responses to loss and death. Some normal feelings of grief are disbelief, yearning, anger, and depression. Although manner of death (violent, unexpected, or traumatic) increases risk to the survivors' normal grief response, it does not always determine how an individual will actually grieve. Helpful coping mechanisms for grieving people include hardiness and resilience, a personal sense of control, and the ability to make sense of and identify positive possibilities after a loss.

Anticipatory Grief. A person experiences anticipatory grief before the actual loss or death occurs, especially in situations of prolonged or predicted loss such as caring for patients diagnosed with dementia or amyotrophic lateral sclerosis (ALS). Family members often grieve the impending loss of companionship, control, and sense of freedom and the mental and physical changes to be experienced by their loved one. Ultimately they grieve the impending death (Chan et al., 2013).

When grief extends over a long period of time, people absorb loss gradually and begin to prepare for its inevitability. They experience intense responses to grief (e.g., shock, denial, and tearfulness) before the actual death occurs and often feel relief when it finally happens. Another way to think about anticipatory grief is that it is a forewarning or cushion that gives people time to prepare or complete the tasks related to the impending death. However, this idea may not apply in every situation. Although forewarning is a buffer for some individuals, it increases stress for others, creating an emotional roller coaster of highs and lows.

Disenfranchised Grief. People experience disenfranchised grief when their relationship to the deceased person is not socially sanctioned, cannot be shared openly, or seems of lesser significance. The person's loss and grief do not meet the norms of grief acknowledged by his or her culture, thereby cutting the grieving person off from social support and the sympathy given to people with more socially acceptable losses. Examples include the death of a former spouse, a married lover, or an incarcerated person or a terminated pregnancy (AACN and CHNMC, 2014).

Ambiguous Loss. Sometimes people experience losses that are marked by uncertainty. Ambiguous loss, a type of disenfranchised grief, can occur when the lost person is physically present but not psychologically available, as in cases of severe dementia or brain injury. Other times the person is gone (e.g., after a kidnapping, prisoner of war, or when there is no body found such as on 9/11/01 or a missing hiker), but the grieving person maintains an ongoing, intense psychological attachment, never sure of the reality of the situation. Ambiguous losses are particularly difficult to process because of the lack of finality and unknown outcomes (Walter and McCoyd, 2009).

Complicated Grief. Some people do not experience a normal grief process. In complicated grief a person has a prolonged or significantly difficult time moving forward after a loss. He or she experiences a chronic and disruptive yearning for the deceased; has trouble accepting the death and trusting others; and/or feels excessively bitter, emotionally numb, or anxious about the future. Complicated grief occurs more often when a person had a conflicted relationship with the deceased, prior or multiple losses or stressors, mental health issues, or lack of social support. Loss associated with homicide, suicide, sudden accidents, or the death of a child has the potential to become complicated. Specific types of complicated grief include chronic, exaggerated, delayed, and masked grief.

Chronic Grief. A person with chronic grief experiences a normal grief response, except that it extends for a longer period of time. This can include years to decades of intense grieving.

Exaggerated Grief. A person with an exaggerated grief response often exhibits self-destructive or maladaptive behavior, obsessions, or psychiatric disorders. Suicide is a risk for these individuals.

Delayed Grief. A person's grief response is unusually delayed or postponed because the loss is so overwhelming that the person must avoid the full realization of the loss. A delayed grief response is frequently triggered by a second loss, sometimes seemingly not as significant as the first loss.

Masked Grief. Sometimes a grieving person behaves in ways that interfere with normal functioning but is unaware that the disruptive behavior is a result of the loss and ineffective grief resolution (AACN and CHNMC, 2014).

Theories of Grief and Mourning

Knowledge of grief theories and normal responses to loss and bereavement helps you to better understand these complex experiences and how to help a grieving person. Grief theorists describe the physical, psychological, and social reactions to loss. Remember that people who vary from expected norms of grief or theoretical descriptions are not abnormal. The variety of theories supports the complexity and individuality of grief responses. Although most grief theories describe how people cope with death, they also help to understand responses to other significant losses (Table 37-2).

Criticism exists for the stages and task theories because they fail to capture the complexity and diversity of the experience (Hall, 2014). The more recent grief theories take into consideration that human beings construct their own experiences and truths differently and make their own meanings when confronted with loss and death. Differences in social and historical context, family structure, and cognitive capacities shape an individual's truths and grief experiences. No one's grief follows a predetermined path, nor is it linear. Grief is cyclical, with movement forward and backward (Figure 37-1). Educating grievers about the cyclical pattern of grief work prepares them for difficult days among the better days. Consider a widow several months after the death of her husband. She may have had several weeks of feeling less sad and depressed. If unprepared for the cyclical nature of grief, she may be taken off guard by her strong grief reaction to a phone call for her husband or a commercial advertising his favorite candy. Knowing that these feelings will come and go help the griever to be prepared for them and allow for the necessary self-care.

NURSING KNOWLEDGE BASE

Nurses develop plans of care to help patients and family members who are undergoing loss, grief, or death experiences. On the basis of nursing research, practice evidence, nursing experience, and patient and family preferences, nurses implement plans of care in acute care, nursing home, hospice, home care, and community settings. Extensive nursing education programs support the improvement of end-of-life care. The End-of-Life Nursing Education Consortium (ELNEC) provides nurses with basic and advanced curricula to care for patients and families experiencing loss, grief, death, and bereavement (AACN and CHNMC, 2014). In conjunction with the Hospice and Palliative Care Nurses Association, the American Nurses Association (ANA) has developed the Scope and Standards of Hospice and Palliative Nursing Practice

TABLE 37-2 Theories of Grief and Mourning

Stages of Dying Kübler-Ross (1969)	**Denial** The person cannot accept the fact of the loss. It is a form of psychological protection from a loss that the person cannot yet bear. **Anger** The person expresses resistance or intense anger at God, other people, or the situation. **Bargaining** The person cushions and postpones awareness of the loss by trying to prevent it from happening. **Depression** The person realizes the full impact of the loss. **Acceptance** The person incorporates the loss into life.
Attachment Theory Bowlby (1980)	**Numbing** Protects the person from the full impact of the loss **Yearning and Searching** Emotional outbursts of tearful sobbing and acute distress; common physical symptoms in this stage: tightness in chest and throat, shortness of breath, a feeling of lethargy, insomnia, and loss of appetite **Disorganization and Despair** Endless examination of how and why the loss occurred or expressions of anger at anyone who seems responsible for the loss **Reorganization** Accepts the change, assumes unfamiliar roles, acquire new skills, builds new relationships, and begins to separate himself or herself from the lost relationship without feeling that he or she is lessening its importance
Grief Tasks Model Worden (2008)	Accepts the reality of the loss Experiences the pain of grief Adjusts to a world in which the deceased is missing Emotionally relocates the deceased and moves on with life
Rando's "R" Process Model Rando (1993)	**Recognizing** the loss **Reacting** to the pain of separation **Reminiscing** **Relinquishing** old attachments **Readjusting** to life after loss **Reminiscence** of the relationship by mentally or verbally anecdotally reliving and remembering the person and past experiences
Dual Process Model Stroebe and Schut (1999)	**Loss-Oriented** activities: (e.g., grief work, dwelling on the loss, breaking connections with the deceased person, and resisting activities to move past the grief) **Restoration-Oriented** activities: attending to life changes, finding new roles or relationships, coping with finances, and participating in distractions, which provide balance to the loss-oriented state
Trajectories of Bereavement Bonanno et al. (2002)	**Common Grief** **Chronic Grief** **Chronic Depression** **Depression Followed by Improvement** **Resilience**

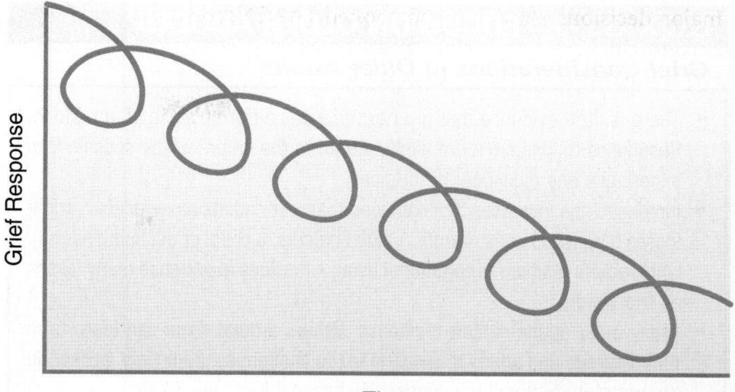

FIGURE 37-1 Cyclical nature of a normal grief response over time.

(ANA, 2014). Professional nursing organizations such as the American Society of Pain Management Nurses and the American Association of Critical Care Nurses offer evidence-based practice guidelines for managing clinical and ethical issues at the end of life in many health care settings.

Factors Influencing Loss and Grief

Multiple factors influence the way a person perceives and responds to loss. They include developmental factors, personal relationships, the nature of the loss, coping strategies, socioeconomic status, and cultural and spiritual influences and beliefs.

Human Development. Patient age and stage of development affect the grief response. For example, toddlers cannot understand loss or death but often feel anxiety over the loss of objects and separation from parents. Common expressions of grief include changes in eating and sleeping patterns, bowel and bladder disturbances, and increased fussiness (AACN, 2014). School-age children understand the concepts of permanence and irreversibility but do not always understand the causes of a loss. Some have intense periods of emotional expression and experience changes in eating, sleeping, and level of social engagement (AACN and CHNMC, 2014).

Young adults undergo many necessary developmental losses related to their evolving future. They leave home, begin school or a work life, or form significant relationships. Illness or death disrupts the young adult's future dreams and establishment of an autonomous sense of self. Midlife adults also experience major life transitions such as caring for aging parents, dealing with changes in marital status, and adapting to new family roles (Walter and McCoyd, 2009). For older adults the aging process leads to necessary and developmental losses. Some older adults experience age discrimination, especially when they become dependent or are near death; but they show resilience after a loss as a result of their prior experiences and developed coping skills (Box 37-1).

Personal Relationships. When loss involves another person, the quality and meaning of the lost relationship influence the grief response. When a relationship between two people was very rewarding and well connected, the survivor often finds it difficult to move forward after the death. Grief work is hampered by regret and a sense of unfinished business, especially when people are closely related but did not have a good relationship at the time of death. Social support and the ability to accept help from others are critical variables in recovery from loss and grief. Grievers experience less depression when they have

BOX 37-1 FOCUS ON OLDER ADULTS

Grief Considerations in Older Adults

- There is little evidence that grief experiences differ because of age alone. Responses to loss are more likely related to the nature of the specific loss experience and individual differences.
- Increased age increases the likelihood that older adults have faced multiple losses (i.e., loved ones, friends, valued objects, a child, or declining health). Older adults residing in communal living situations experience many losses as friends die.
- Many older adults exhibit resilience. Others around them can learn from their courage and ability to respond to life challenges graciously, accepting life with integrity and wholeness (Walter and McCoyd, 2009).
- Older adults are at risk for complicated grieving as a result of multiple losses, potential for cognitive impairment, or decreased physical resources. The risks include depression, loneliness, and accompanying functional decline.
- Physical decline caused by chronic illness sometimes leads to grief over lost health, function, and roles.
- Pain is often undertreated in older adults, particularly in people with dementia or cognitive impairments. Side effects of pain medications are usually more pronounced in older adults (Matzo and Sherman, 2015; Reynolds et al., 2013).
- Older adults benefit from the same therapeutic techniques as people in other age-groups. Evidence indicates that positive reappraisal (cognitive restructuring) helps older adults adapt to significant losses (e.g., seeing a cardiac diagnosis as the opportunity to become healthy by eating nutritiously and exercising regularly) (Brohard, 2014). Relieving depression and maintaining physical function are therapeutic goals for grieving older adults.

highly satisfying personal relationships and friends to support them in their grief (de Vries et al., 2014).

Nature of the Loss. Exploring the nature of a loss will help you understand the effect of the loss on the patient's behavior, health, and well-being. Was the loss avoidable? Is it permanent or temporary? Is it actual or imagined? Encouraging patients to share information about the loss will help you better develop appropriate interventions that meet the individualized needs of your patients.

Highly visible losses generally stimulate a helping response from others. For example, the loss of one's home from a tornado often brings community and governmental support. A more private loss such as a miscarriage brings less support from others. A sudden and unexpected death poses challenges different from those of a person in a debilitating chronic illness. When the death is sudden and unexpected, the survivors do not have time to say good-bye. In chronic illness survivors have memories of prolonged suffering, pain, and loss of function. Death by violence or suicide or multiple losses by their very nature complicate the grieving process in unique ways (Walter and McCoyd, 2009).

Coping Strategies. The losses that patients face from the time they were children formulate the coping skills they will use when faced with larger and more painful losses in adulthood. These coping strategies such as talking, journaling, and sharing their emotions with others may be healthy and effective. They may also be unhealthy and ineffective such as increased use of alcohol, drugs, and violence. Nurses provide support by assessing a patient's coping strategies, educating about new and healthy strategies, and encouraging use of these strategies.

Socioeconomic Status. Socioeconomic status influences a person's grief process in direct and indirect ways. Because of role changes, a newly widowed mom finds herself working several jobs to make ends meet and does not find time to initiate self-care or allow herself to grieve the loss of her husband. With limited resources, activities that support healthy grief work such as buying a tree to plant in honor of the deceased or travel to a support group may be unrealistic. Practical implications also exist when there are limited resources. A patient with limited finances is not able to replace a car demolished in an accident and pay for the associated medical expenses.

Culture. During times of loss and grief patients and families draw on the social and spiritual practices of their culture to find comfort, expressions, and meaning in the experience (Walter and McCoyd, 2009). To provide the best care possible, it is necessary for us to ask about cultural beliefs and practices. Patients and families will rarely offer this information without prompting. Expressions of grief in one culture do not always make sense to people from a different culture (see Chapter 9). Try to understand and appreciate each patient's cultural values related to loss, death, and grieving (Fiorelli and Jenkins, 2012). For example, many people in western European and American cultures hold back their public displays of emotion. In other cultures behaviors such as public wailing and physical demonstrations of grief, including survivor body mutilation, show respect for the dead. Core American cultural values of individualism and self-determination stand in contrast with communal, family, or tribal ways of life. Even urban and rural settings provide a framework of culture in which people draw strength from traditional practices

Culture extends beyond the geographic location of a person. Consider the influence of sexual orientation, socioeconomic status, and family make-up (blended versus nuclear) when assessing cultural influence on grief practices and death rituals.

Spiritual and Religious Beliefs. Like cultural influences, spirituality and/or religious practices and beliefs provide a framework to navigate, understand, and heal from loss, death, and grief (see Chapter 36). Patients' faith may influence the way they respond to an illness, treatment, advanced life-support options, autopsy, organ donation, and what happens to the body and spirit after death. Patients draw on their spiritual beliefs to provide comfort and seek understanding at times of loss. You must remain open to the varying views and beliefs that are in contrast to your own to best support and care for your patients' and their families (Bauer-Wu et al., 2007; Dose et al., 2014). To never offend a patient and to offer high quality care, you must assess your patient's beliefs and practices and encourage expression of them whenever possible. You should encourage patients to draw on their spiritual resources (e.g., faith in a higher power, communities of support, friends, a sense of hope and meaning in life, and religious practices). Spirituality affects the patient's and family members' ability to cope with loss as well. Caring for the patient in a holistic approach, which includes the spirit, ensures that you are providing patients with the best possible individualized care.

Hope, a multidimensional concept considered to be a component of spirituality, energizes and provides comfort to individuals experiencing personal challenges. Hope gives a person the ability to see life as enduring or having meaning or purpose. With hope a patient moves from feelings of weakness and vulnerability to living as fully as possible. Maintaining a sense of hope depends in part on a person having strong relationships and emotional connectedness to others. On the other hand, spiritual distress often arises from a patient's inability to feel hopeful or foresee any favorable outcomes. Spirituality and hope play a vital role in a patient's adjustment to loss and death (see Chapter 36).

CRITICAL THINKING

To provide appropriate and responsive care for the grieving patient and family, use critical thinking skills to synthesize scientific knowledge from nursing and nonnursing disciplines, professional standards, evidence-based practice, patient assessments, previous caregiving experiences, and self-knowledge. Critical thinking informs all steps of the nursing process (see Chapter 15).

During assessment consider all elements that build toward making an appropriate nursing diagnosis (Figure 37-2). To understand a patient's subjective experiences of loss, form assessment questions on the basis of your theoretical and professional knowledge of grief and loss but then listen carefully to the patient's perceptions. A culturally competent nurse also uses culture-specific understanding of grief to explore the meaning of loss with a patient.

Being familiar with commonly experienced responses to loss enables you to better understand a patient's emotions and behaviors. Some patients ignore, lash out, plead with, or withdraw from other people as part of a normal response to loss. Instead of "taking things personally," a critically thinking nurse integrates theory, prior experience, appreciation of subjective experiences, and self-knowledge to respond to the patient's emotions with patience and understanding. In designing plans of care, use professional standards, including the Nursing Code of Ethics (see Chapter 22), the dying person's bill of rights (Box 37-2), the ANA Scope and Standards of Hospice and Palliative Nursing Practice (2014), and the American Society of Pain Management Nurses' position for pain management at the end of life (Reynolds et al., 2013).

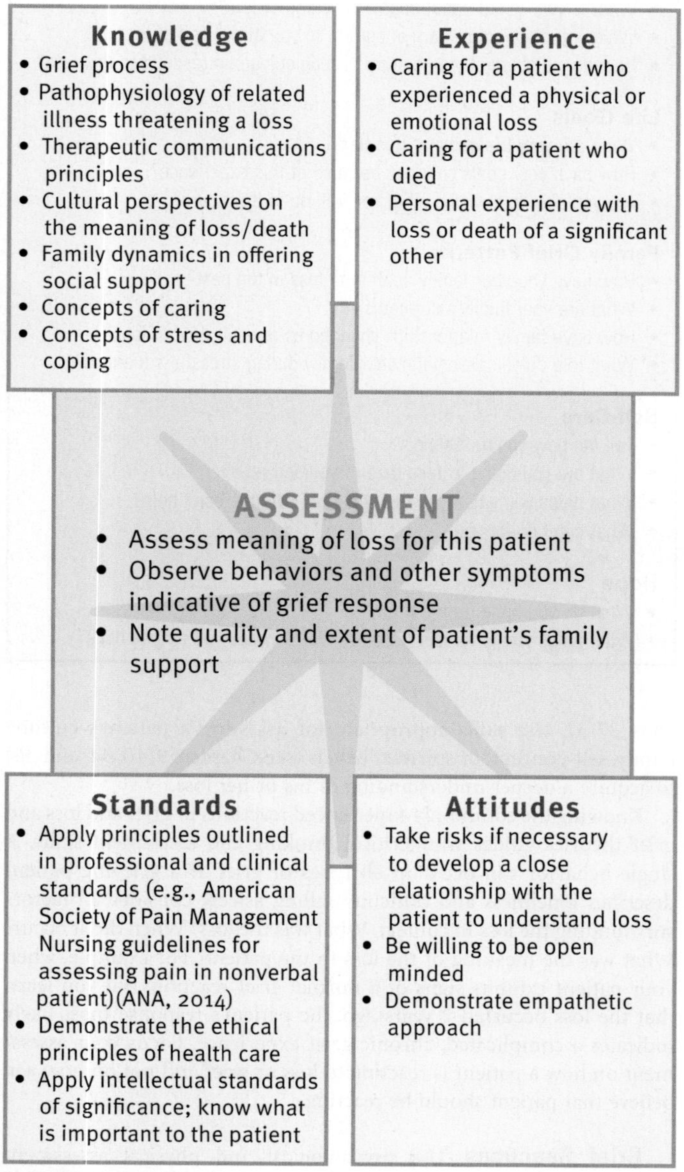

Knowledge
- Grief process
- Pathophysiology of related illness threatening a loss
- Therapeutic communications principles
- Cultural perspectives on the meaning of loss/death
- Family dynamics in offering social support
- Concepts of caring
- Concepts of stress and coping

Experience
- Caring for a patient who experienced a physical or emotional loss
- Caring for a patient who died
- Personal experience with loss or death of a significant other

ASSESSMENT
- Assess meaning of loss for this patient
- Observe behaviors and other symptoms indicative of grief response
- Note quality and extent of patient's family support

Standards
- Apply principles outlined in professional and clinical standards (e.g., American Society of Pain Management Nursing guidelines for assessing pain in nonverbal patient)(ANA, 2014)
- Demonstrate the ethical principles of health care
- Apply intellectual standards of significance; know what is important to the patient

Attitudes
- Take risks if necessary to develop a close relationship with the patient to understand loss
- Be willing to be open minded
- Demonstrate empathetic approach

FIGURE 37-2 Critical thinking model for loss, death, and grieving assessment.

❖ NURSING PROCESS

Apply the nursing process and use a critical thinking approach in your care of patients. The nursing process provides a clinical decision-making approach for you to develop and implement an individualized plan of care.

◆ Assessment

During the assessment process thoroughly assess each patient and critically analyze findings to ensure that you make patient-centered clinical decisions required for safe nursing care. A trusting, helping relationship with grieving patients and family members is essential to the assessment process. A caring nurse encourages a patient to tell his or her story. Look for opportunities to invite patients to share their experiences, being aware that attitudes about self-disclosure; sharing emotions; or talking about illness, fears, and death are shaped by an individual's personality, coping style, and culture. This information is invaluable to understanding the unique and individual needs of each patient.

BOX 37-2 A Dying Person's Bill of Rights

I have the right to be treated as a living human being until I die.

I have the right to maintain a sense of hopefulness, however changing its focus may be.

I have the right to be cared for by those who can maintain a sense of hopefulness, however changing this may be.

I have the right to express my feelings and emotions about my approaching death in my own way.

I have the right to participate in decisions about my care.

I have the right to expect continuing medical and nursing attention even though "cure" goals must be changed to "comfort" goals.

I have the right not to die alone.

I have the right to be free of pain.

I have the right to have my questions answered honestly.

I have the right to retain my individuality and not be judged for my decisions that may be contrary to beliefs of others.

I have a right to expect that the sanctity of my human body will be respected after death.

I have the right to be cared for by caring, sensitive, knowledgeable people who will try to understand my needs and be able to gain some satisfaction in helping me face my death.

Modified from Barbus AJ: The dying person's bill of rights, *Am J Nurs* 75:99, 1975.

Through the Patient's Eyes. One of the best things that you can do for patients and families is to be present. By using the skills of active listening, silence, and therapeutic touch, you can establish a trusting relationship with your patients. This trusting relationship will help you explore with patients their unique responses to grief or their preferences for end-of-life care, which may include advance directives. Patient perceptions and expectations influence how we prioritize our nursing diagnoses. To assess patient perceptions, ask, "What is the most important thing I can do for you right now?" You usually gather information from patients first, but with advanced illness and as death approaches, patients often rely on family members to communicate for them. Encourage family members to share their goals and perceptions with you. Most often they provide valuable information about patient preferences and clarify misunderstandings or identify overlooked information. Assess patients' and family members' understanding of treatment options to implement a mutually developed care plan. Assessment of grief responses extends throughout the course of an illness into the bereavement period following a death. During this time you can work to normalize the grief response (AACN and CHNMC, 2014). Patients with advanced chronic illness and their families eventually face end-of-life care decisions and should discuss the content of any advance directives together. Because most deaths are now "negotiated" among patients, family members, and the health care team, discuss end-of-life care preferences early in the assessment phase of the nursing process. If you feel uncomfortable in assessing a patient's wishes for end-of-life care by yourself, ask a health care provider experienced in discussing these issues to help you. Communicate what you have learned about patient preferences during any registered nurse (RN) hand-off, at health care team conferences, in written care plans, and through ongoing consultation (see Chapter 26).

Speak to patients and family members using honest and open communication, remembering that cultural practices influence how much information the patient shares. Keep an open mind, listen carefully, and observe the patient's verbal and nonverbal responses. Facial expressions, voice tones, and avoided topics often disclose more than words. Anticipate common grief responses, but allow patients to describe their experiences in their own words. Open-ended questions such as, "What do you understand about your diagnosis?" or "You seem sad today. Can you tell me more?" may open the door to a patient-centered discussion. Many people find it difficult to talk about loss, fear, death, or grief. The use of pauses, gentle questioning, and silence honors the patient's privacy and readiness to talk. Talk to patients and family members in a private, quiet setting. Many times a patient wants to have family members present so everyone hears the same thing and has an opportunity to add to the conversation. However, some people want their concerns and questions addressed privately. Ask patients and family members about their preferences. As you gather assessment data, summarize and validate your impressions with the patient or family member. Information from the medical record and other members of the health care team, physicians, social workers, and spiritual care providers contributes to your assessment data.

Because of the importance of symptom management and priority of comfort in end-of-life care, prioritize your initial assessment to encourage patients to identify any distressing symptoms. Completing a thorough assessment is difficult when patients are in pain, anxious, depressed, or short of breath.

Grief Variables. Conversations about the meaning of loss to a patient often leads to other important areas of assessment, including the patient's coping style, the nature of family relationships, social support systems, the nature of the loss, cultural and spiritual beliefs, life goals, family grief patterns, self-care, and sources of hope (Box 37-3). Use skills appropriate for assessing a patient's culture, family, self-concept, or spiritual beliefs (see Chapters 9, 10, 34, and 36) to acquire a deeper understanding of his or her loss.

Knowing the commonly experienced reactions to grief and loss and grief theories guides your critical thinking and assessment skills. A single behavior can occur in all types of grief. If a grieving patient describes loneliness and difficulty falling asleep, consider all factors surrounding the loss in context. What was the loss? When did it occur? What was the meaning of the loss to the patient? For example, when your patient exhibits signs of a normal grief reaction, but you learn that the loss occurred 2 years ago, the patient's response most likely indicates a complicated, chronic grief experience. Focus your assessment on how a patient is reacting to loss or grief and not on how *you* believe that patient should be reacting.

Grief Reactions. Use psychological and physical assessment skills to assess a patient's unique grief responses. Most grieving people show some common outward signs and symptoms (Box 37-4).

BOX 37-3 Nursing Assessment Questions

Nature of Relationships
- How long have you known _______ (the deceased person)?
- What role did (name person) play in your life?
- Tell me about your relationship with (name person).

Social Support Systems
- Who is "there for you?" Absent? Who provides support?
- What do others do for you that is most meaningful or helpful?
- Are family/friends available when needed? Which friends or relatives do you wish were here?

Nature of the Loss
- What does this loss mean to you?
- What other losses have you experienced?
- Was this loss expected or unexpected?

Cultural and Spiritual Beliefs
- What is your belief about death? Meaning of life?
- Which rituals/practices are important to you at the end of life?
- How do members of your culture or religious group respond to this loss?

Life Goals
- What are your life goals at this time?
- How have your goals changed because of this experience?
- Are you able to envision what you will do in the future?

Family Grief Patterns
- How have you/your family dealt with loss in the past?
- What are your family's strengths?
- How have family relationships changed as a result of your loss?
- What role do you assume in your family during stressful situations?

Self-Care
- Tell me how you're feeling.
- What are you doing to take care of yourself now?
- What helps you when you feel this sad? What doesn't help?
- What can I do for you?

Hope
- What do you hope for right now?
- What helps you to remain hopeful? What causes you to lose hope?

BOX 37-4 Symptoms of Normal Grief

Feelings
- Sorrow
- Fear
- Anger
- Guilt or self-reproach
- Anxiety
- Loneliness
- Fatigue
- Helplessness/hopelessness
- Yearning
- Relief

Cognitions (Thought Patterns)
- Disbelief
- Confusion or memory problems
- Problems making decisions
- Inability to concentrate
- Feeling the presence of the deceased

Physical Sensations
- Headaches
- Nausea and appetite disturbances
- Tightness in the chest and throat
- Insomnia
- Oversensitivity to noise
- Sense of depersonalization ("Nothing seems real")
- Feeling short of breath, choking sensation
- Muscle weakness
- Lack of energy
- Dry mouth

Behaviors
- Crying and frequent sighing
- Distancing from people
- Absentmindedness
- Dreams of the deceased
- Keeping the deceased's room intact
- Loss of interest in regular life events
- Wearing objects that belonged to the deceased

Analyze assessment data and identify possible related causes for the signs and symptoms that you observe. For example, after a significant loss a person has a sad affect, withdrawn behaviors, headaches, upset stomach, and decreased ability to concentrate. You associate these symptoms with several potential causes, including anxiety, gastrointestinal disturbances, medication side effects, or impaired memory. Careful analysis of the symptoms in context leads you to an accurate nursing diagnosis. Ask: How are the symptoms related to one another when they occur? When did they begin? Were they present before the loss? To what does the person attribute them?

Loss takes place in a social context; thus family assessment is a vital part of your data gathering. If a father of a young family is dying, he will not be able to fulfill certain roles, causing a change in family structure. When a person develops a disability, the patient and family members realign their roles and responsibilities to meet new demands. Family members also experience a variety of physical and psychological symptoms. Assess the family's response to loss and recognize that sometimes they are dealing with their grief at a different pace.

◆ Nursing Diagnosis

Use critical thinking to cluster assessment data cues, identify defining characteristics, draw conclusions regarding the patient's actual or potential needs or resources, and identify nursing diagnoses applicable to the patient's situation (Box 37-5). In addition to numerous diagnoses related to physical symptoms at the end of life, additional nursing diagnoses relevant for patients experiencing grief, loss, or death include:

- *Compromised Family Coping*
- *Death Anxiety*
- *Grieving*
- *Complicated Grieving*
- *Risk for Complicated Grieving*
- *Hopelessness*
- *Pain (Acute or Chronic)*
- *Spiritual Distress*

BOX 37-5 Nursing Diagnostic Process

Hopelessness Related to Deteriorating Physiological Condition

Assessment Activities	Defining Characteristics
Ask patient to discuss her understanding of her health situation.	Patient sighs and offers a negative view of her future; turns away from health care professionals.
Observe patient's nonverbal behavior.	Patient sighs, keeps eyes closed; decreased verbalization.
Observe patient's responses to care options.	Patient does not want scheduled test. "There is nothing they can do."
Assess activity level.	Patient states that she has no energy and reports pain; can't sleep, wants to stay in bed.
Observe patient's interactions with others.	Patient shows lack of interest, communicates minimally, and does not want to contact daughter yet.

You cannot make accurate nursing diagnoses on the basis of just one or two defining characteristics. Carefully review your patient's assessment data to consider if more than one diagnosis applies. For example, a dying patient who cries often, has angry outbursts, and reports nightmares gives evidence of several possible nursing diagnoses: *Pain (Acute or Chronic), Ineffective Coping, Grieving,* or *Spiritual Distress.* Examine the available data, validate assumptions with the patient, and look for other validating behaviors and symptoms before making a diagnosis.

As part of the diagnostic process, identify the appropriate "related to" factor for each diagnosis. Clarification of the related factors ensures that you select appropriate interventions. For example, a nursing diagnosis of *Complicated Grieving related to the permanent loss of mobility* requires different interventions than a diagnosis of *Complicated Grieving related to infertility after an ectopic pregnancy.*

When identifying nursing diagnoses related to a patient's grief or loss, you sometimes identify other related diagnoses. Some patients experiencing grief or impending death have nursing diagnoses such as *Disturbed Body Image* or *Impaired Physical Mobility.* A patient entering the phase of active dying often has diagnoses related to physical changes, including *Impaired Urinary Elimination, Bowel Incontinence, Acute Pain, Nausea, Disturbed Sensory Perception,* and *Ineffective Breathing Pattern.*

◆ Planning

Nurses provide holistic, physical, emotional, social, and spiritual care to patients experiencing grief, death, or loss. Figure 37-3 illustrates the interrelatedness of critical thinking factors during the planning phase of the nursing process. The use of critical thinking ensures a well-designed care plan that supports a patient's self-esteem and autonomy by including him or her in the planning process. A care plan for the dying patient focuses on comfort; preserving dignity and quality of life; and providing family members with emotional, social, and spiritual support (see the Nursing Care Plan).

Goals and Outcomes. During planning establish realistic goals and expected outcomes on the basis of the nursing diagnoses. Consider a patient's own resources such as physical energy and activity tolerance,

NURSING CARE PLAN

Hopelessness

ASSESSMENT

Mrs. Allison, an 80-year-old woman, was brought to the hospital after a neighbor found her lying on the floor. She was unable to get up after falling down 4 hours earlier. She was admitted to the hospital with low blood pressure, dehydration, and weakness. She reports having severe pain in her back and toes, making it difficult for her to walk. In addition, she has experienced recent weight loss and a poor appetite and reports being too tired to cook or enjoy activities. Blood tests and physical examination reveal that she has a more serious health problem, likely a form of leukemia, for which she needs a bone marrow biopsy to make a medical diagnosis. Mrs. Allison lives alone since her husband's death 2 years earlier. She has the support of her neighbors and church community and one daughter who lives out of town. On entering the room the nurse notes that Mrs. Allison appears withdrawn and tearful. The nurse talks to her to gather more information.

Assessment Activities	*Findings/Defining Characteristics**
Ask open-ended questions. "It looks like you're having a difficult time. What do you understand about your situation right now?"	"The doctors say that **I might have cancer. Shrugging her shoulders,** she states, **"There's nothing they can do. I don't want the test."**
Observe Mrs. Allison's behaviors and nonverbal communication.	Mrs. Allison **appears sad and keeps her eyes closed**. She **cries and sighs frequently**.
Assess Mrs. Allison's pain and energy level.	Mrs. Allison's **great toes are swollen and red** and sore to the touch. Reports **constant back pain**. She has "**no energy for anything."**
Observe Mrs. Allison's interactions and interest in others.	Mrs. Allison **does not look at people and does not want to talk to her daughter yet.**
Assess meaning of recent events with Mrs. Allison and invite her to talk about her situation.	Mrs. Allison states that "**It's time to quit on life and be with my late husband."**

***Defining characteristics** are shown in bold type.

NURSING DIAGNOSIS: Hopelessness related to declining physical condition

PLANNING

Goals	*Expected Outcomes (NOC)†* *Hopelessness*
Mrs. Allison will discuss two care priorities and preferences within 1 day.	Mrs. Allison identifies the concerns causing the greatest amount of suffering or distress.
Mrs. Allison will communicate with one support person within next 12 hours.	Daughter, church community, and neighbors provide supportive care.
Mrs. Allison will identify at least three tasks with which she needs help to live at home by discharge from the hospital.	Mrs. Allison identifies ways she can live at home with the help of others.

†Outcome classification labels from Moorhead S et al: *Nursing outcomes classification (NOC)*, ed 5, St Louis, 2013, Mosby.

INTERVENTIONS (NIC)‡	RATIONALE
Presence	
Develop an open and caring relationship through active listening and emotional support.	Individuals approaching the end of life often experience fragmented care delivery. Therapeutic communication supports patient- and family-centered care at the end of life and helps to ensure that patient needs are communicated among all health care professionals (Meghani et al., 2015).
Provide frequent conversations with patient and family regarding patient's symptom management and grief.	Frequent conversations with patient and family provide opportunity to discuss end-of-life care values, goals, and preferences (Meghani et al., 2015).
Pain Management	
Provide pharmacological and nonpharmacological relief for chronic back and foot pain.	Anxiety, pain, and suffering are reduced with effective pain management; and quality of life is improved (Paice, 2015).
Grief Work Facilitation	
Help Mrs. Allison identify her personal goals, desires, and priorities. Evaluate effectiveness and promote goal achievement as appropriate.	Allowing the patient to direct care decisions helps the patient and family select priority of care and increases patient and family understanding of current and proposed treatments (Brohard, 2014; Coyle, 2015).
Help Mrs. Allison identify available resources. Initiate discussions with interdisciplinary team as appropriate.	Hope is strengthened when one finds realistic possibilities and can adapt to life challenges (McDonald and McCallin, 2010).
Discuss Mrs. Allison's spiritual beliefs, practices, needs, and resources.	Inclusion of spiritual assessment and spiritual care practices at the end of life increases patient's sense of connectedness and overall quality of life (Dose et al., 2014).

‡Intervention classification labels from Bulechek GM et al: *Nursing interventions classification (NIC)*, ed 6, St Louis, 2013, Mosby.

EVALUATION

Nursing Actions	*Patient Response/Finding*	*Achievement of Outcome*
Validate Mrs. Allison's experience: "It must be difficult to face such a big life change."	Mrs. Allison responds, "My life has changed, but I have good friends and a good daughter."	Mrs. Allison shows beginning acceptance of her changed health condition.
Use open-ended question: "Tell me how you're feeling now."	Mrs. Allison explains, "I'm not sure what will happen. I may not be able to take care of myself much longer, but I'll try."	She is able to express normal grieving behaviors and feelings of uncertainty resulting from loss of her life as she knew it.
Observe Mrs. Allison's planning activities and behavior with her daughter and friends.	Mrs. Allison and daughter discuss what they can do so she can stay at home longer.	She indicates ability to make plans for a change of care location. Daughter supports revised plans.

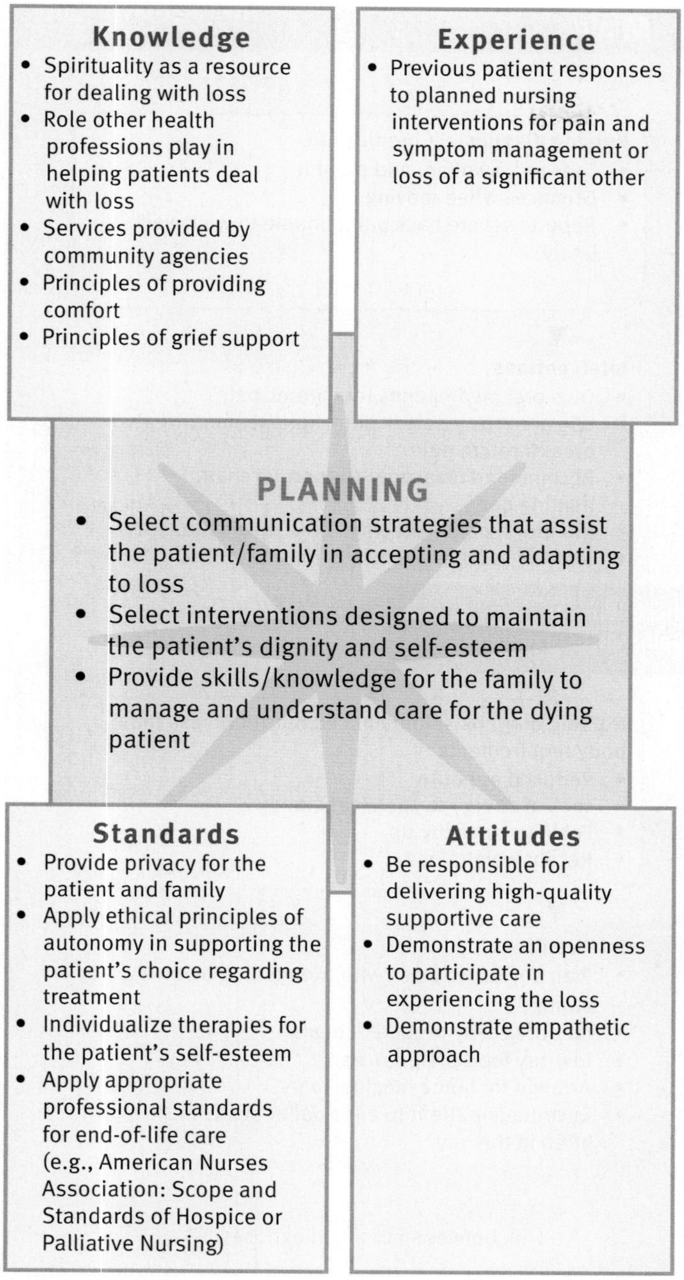

Knowledge
- Spirituality as a resource for dealing with loss
- Role other health professions play in helping patients deal with loss
- Services provided by community agencies
- Principles of providing comfort
- Principles of grief support

Experience
- Previous patient responses to planned nursing interventions for pain and symptom management or loss of a significant other

PLANNING
- Select communication strategies that assist the patient/family in accepting and adapting to loss
- Select interventions designed to maintain the patient's dignity and self-esteem
- Provide skills/knowledge for the family to manage and understand care for the dying patient

Standards
- Provide privacy for the patient and family
- Apply ethical principles of autonomy in supporting the patient's choice regarding treatment
- Individualize therapies for the patient's self-esteem
- Apply appropriate professional standards for end-of-life care (e.g., American Nurses Association: Scope and Standards of Hospice or Palliative Nursing)

Attitudes
- Be responsible for delivering high-quality supportive care
- Demonstrate an openness to participate in experiencing the loss
- Demonstrate empathetic approach

FIGURE 37-3 Critical thinking model for loss, death, and grief planning.

family support, and coping style. A nursing diagnosis of *Powerlessness related to experimental cancer therapy* with a goal of "Patient will be able to describe the expected course of disease" is realistic for a patient who frequently asks for clarification about the treatment plan and participates in educational discussions. In contrast, an expected outcome of "Patient will identify a minimum of three effective coping skills" is appropriate for a patient with the same nursing diagnosis who is experiencing depression from feeling powerless about having experimental cancer treatment.

The goals of care for a patient experiencing loss are either short or long term, depending on the nature of the loss and the patient's condition. Some nursing care goals for patients facing loss or death include accommodating grief, accepting the reality of a loss, or maintaining meaningful relationships. A possible goal for a young woman with advanced breast cancer is "Will maintain a sense of control," with the following potential expected outcomes:

- Patient participates in all treatment decisions.
- Patient identifies a minimum of three ways to maintain a parental role in the care of her young child.
- Patient communicates a minimum of three treatment side effects or concerns to the health care team.

Setting Priorities. Encourage patients and family members to share their priorities for care at the end of life. Patients at the end of life or with advanced chronic illness are more likely to want their comfort, social, or spiritual needs met rather than pursuing medical cures. Give priority to a patient's most urgent physical or psychological needs while also considering his or her expectations and priorities. If a terminally ill patient's goals include pain control and promoting self-esteem, pain control takes priority when the patient experiences acute physical discomfort. When comfort needs have been met, you address other issues important to the patient and family. When it is realistic for the patient to remain independent, strategies that foster his or her sense of autonomy and ability to function independently take priority. A patient's condition at the end of life often changes quickly; therefore maintain an ongoing assessment to revise the plan of care according to patient needs and preferences.

When a patient has multiple nursing diagnoses, it is not possible to address them all simultaneously. Figure 37-4 illustrates a concept map developed for Mrs. Allison, an elderly patient with a medical diagnosis of advanced cancer (leukemia). In conjunction with her recent medical diagnosis, she experiences associated health problems identified in the nursing diagnoses *Chronic Pain, Imbalanced Nutrition: Less Than Body Requirements, Fatigue,* and *Hopelessness.* In such a situation determine which of the four diagnoses should take priority. The chronic pain experienced by the patient is often the first focus. Until her pain is under control, it will not be possible for her to feel more energized, eat well, or regain her sense of hopefulness.

Teamwork and Collaboration. As described previously, grief, loss, and death affect people physically, emotionally, spiritually, and culturally. No one is able to address all of these dimensions alone. A team of nurses, physicians, social workers, spiritual care providers, nutritionists, pharmacists, physical and occupational therapists, patients, and family members works together to provide palliative care, grief care, and care at the end of life. Massage or music/art therapists who provide alternative therapies are sometimes part of the team (see Chapter 33). As a patient's care needs change, team members take a more or less active role, depending on the patient's shifting priorities. Team members communicate with one another on a regular basis to ensure coordination and effectiveness of care.

QSEN QSEN: BUILDING COMPETENCY IN TEAMWORK AND COLLABORATION You are caring for Mrs. Allison, an older patient who has recently been diagnosed with a terminal illness and is preparing for discharge home. She has lost strength as a result of decreased activity, depression, and back pain. Her greatest desire is to be able to attend weekly services at her church; but, because of the weakness, pain, and fatigue, she is afraid that she will be unable to do so. She believes that her feelings of depression will improve if she can again participate in church activities. How can you, with the help of the interprofessional team, help Mrs. Allison respond to her spiritual needs and desire to be involved within her faith community?

ⓔ *Answers to QSEN Activities can be found on the Evolve website.*

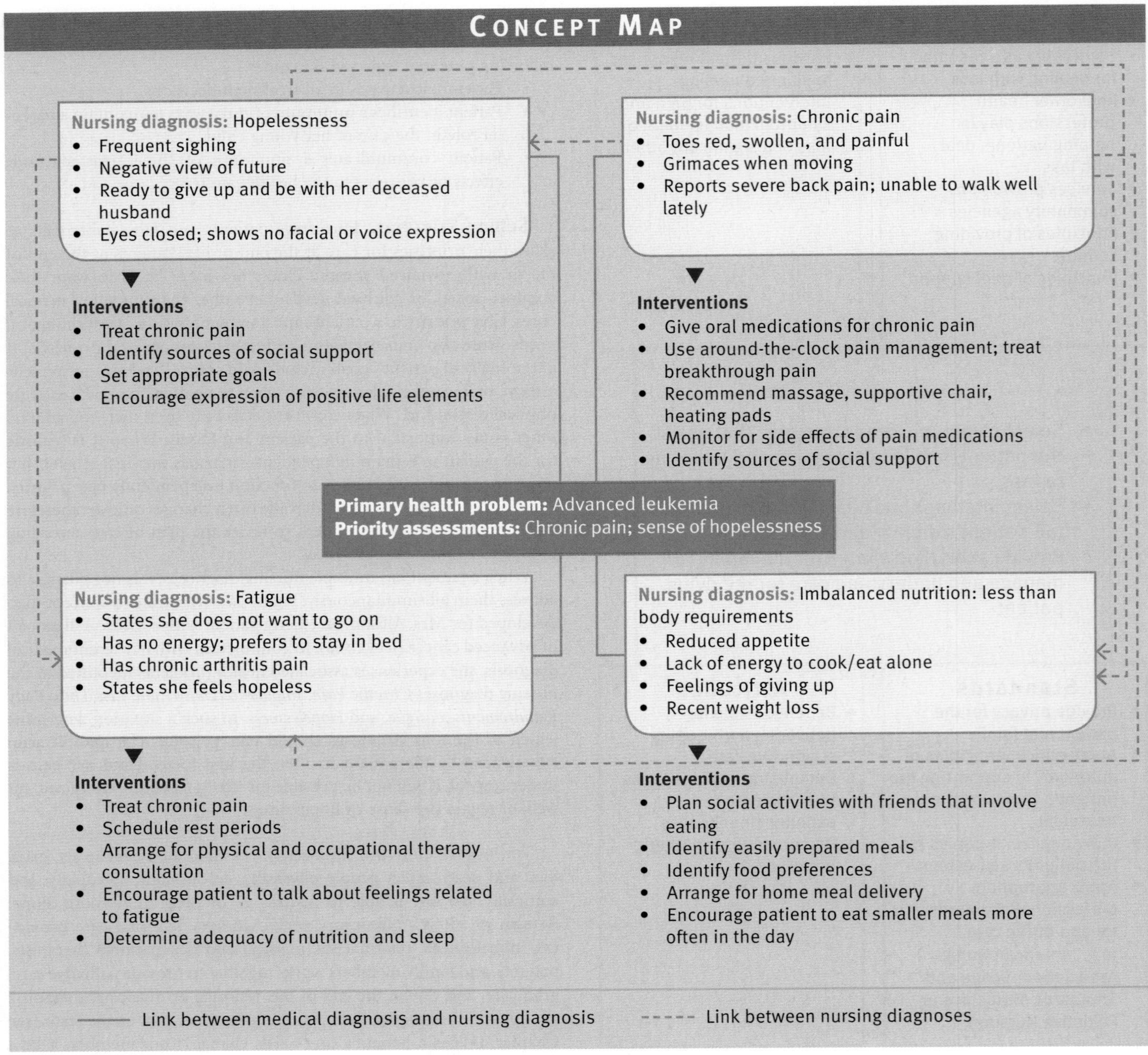

FIGURE 37-4 Concept map for Mrs. Allison.

◆ Implementation

Health Promotion. Health promotion in serious chronic illness or death focuses on facilitating successful coping and optimizing physical, emotional, and spiritual health. Many people continue to look for and find meaning even in difficult life circumstances. They often find personal growth and spiritual insights that they have not previously experienced and need family and nurse support as they strive to maintain a degree of normalcy; live with loss; make health care decisions; prepare for death; and adjust to disappointments, frustration, and anxieties along the way (Box 37-6).

Palliative Care. Patients and families can benefit greatly from the specialized approach of palliative care. This holistic method to prevent and reduce symptoms promotes quality of life and whole-person well-being through care of the mind, body, and spirit.

Palliative care focuses on the prevention, relief, reduction, or soothing of symptoms of disease or disorders throughout the entire course of an illness. It can also include, but is not solely, care of the dying. The primary goal of palliative care is to help patients and families achieve the best possible quality of life (Mariano, 2015). Although it is especially important in advanced or chronic illness, palliative care is appropriate for patients of any age, with any diagnosis, at any time, and in any setting.

A large misconception concerning palliative care is that it is used only when curative treatments are no longer pursued. However, it is appropriate both for patients still receiving aggressive treatment with hope of achieving a cure and for patients who have forgone any life-extending treatment (Coyle, 2015). It is important that you help patients and their families understand the distinction because often

BOX 37-6 PATIENT TEACHING

Maintaining Self-Care

Objective

- The patient will participate in activities to manage symptoms.

Teaching Strategies

- Encourage patient to set realistic goals and identify ways to achieve them.
- Identify ways that patient can maintain usual daily routines that provide comfort and sense of normalcy.
- Demonstrate forms of complementary therapy that patient can use for symptom management.
- Discuss ways that patient can maintain a sense of control over end-of-life planning and maintain a realistic outlook (advance directives, funeral planning, and preferred location of death).
- Discuss patient's needs for presence of particular support people or for solitude.
- Identify methods to facilitate safety and ease in managing activities of daily living as patient's abilities change (assistive devices, in-home caregivers).

Evaluation

- Ask patient to describe symptom-management methods used and rate their effectiveness.

misunderstanding the purpose of palliative care causes patients to refuse it.

The World Health Organization (2015) summarizes palliative care philosophy as follows:

- Affirms life and regards dying as a normal process.
- Neither hastens or postpones death.
- Integrates psychological and spiritual aspects of patient care.
- Offers a support system to help patients live as actively as possible until death.
- Enhances the quality of life.
- Uses a team approach to meet the needs of patients and families.

Because the focus of palliative care is comfort and improved quality of life, it is a valuable approach to caring for patients with a complex illness. A variety of therapies are used to provide patients with a holistic approach to symptom management and ultimately improved quality of life. Kraft (2012) reports that activities such as yoga, acupuncture, massage, and aromatherapies have shown to have a positive effect on feelings of depression. In addition, music therapy, mindfulness-based stress-reduction techniques, and aromatherapy have successfully treated some patient's anxiety. Fatigue, a common symptom reported by the palliative care patient, responds to acupuncture and exercise. Massage has also been shown to reduce the symptoms of pain, anxiety, nausea, shortness of breath, stress and increase relaxation and peacefulness (Trumble et al., 2014).

When the goals of care change and cure for illnesses becomes less likely, the focus shifts to more palliative care strategies and ideally transition to hospice care, a more specialized form of palliative care for the dying.

Hospice Care. Hospice care is a philosophy and model for the care of terminally ill patients and their families at the end of life. It gives priority to managing a patient's pain and other symptoms; comfort; quality of life; and attention to physical, psychological, social, and spiritual needs and resources. Patients accepted into a hospice program usually have less than 6 months to live. Hospice services are available in home, hospital, extended care, and nursing home settings.

The cornerstone of hospice care is a trusting relationship between the hospice team and the patient and family. Knowing expectations, desired location of care, and family dynamics helps the hospice team provide individualized care at the end of life. Unlike traditional care, hospice patients are active participants in all aspects of care, and caregivers prioritize care according to patient wishes. Patient care goals are mutually set, and all participants fully understand the patient's care preferences and try to honor them. Hospice services provide bereavement visits made by the staff after the death of the patient to help the family move through the grieving process. Hospice programs are built on the following core beliefs and services:

- Patient and family are the unit of care
- Coordinated home care with access to inpatient and nursing home beds when needed
- Symptom management
- Physician-directed services
- Provision of an interdisciplinary care team
- Medical and nursing services available at all times
- Bereavement follow-up after patient's death
- Use of trained volunteers for visitation and respite support

To be eligible for home hospice services, a patient must have a family caregiver to provide care when the patient is no longer able to function alone. Home care aides offer help with hygienic needs, and a nurse is available to coordinate and manage symptom relief. Nurses providing hospice care use therapeutic communication, offer psychosocial care and expert symptom management, promote patient dignity and self-esteem, maintain a comfortable and peaceful environment, provide spiritual comfort and hope, protect against abandonment or isolation, offer family support, help with ethical decision making, and facilitate mourning. Hospice team members offer 24-hour accessibility and coordinate care between the home and inpatient setting. A patient receiving home hospice care may enter an inpatient hospice unit for stabilization of symptoms or caregiver respite. As a patient's death comes closer, the hospice team provides intensive support to the patient and family (Hospice Foundation of America, 2014).

Use Therapeutic Communication. The heart of nursing care is the establishment of a caring and trusting relationship with your patient. This patient-focused approach allows you to respond to patients rather than react and encourages the sharing of important information. Open-ended questions invite patients to elaborate on their thoughts and encourage them to tell their stories. Patients usually give short answers (yes or no) when you use closed-ended questions, which limit what we can learn about their situation. Use active listening, learn to be comfortable with silence, and use prompts (e.g., "go on," "tell me more") to encourage continued conversation. Empathizing, touching, and offering self are also effective ways to therapeutically communicate with our patients. Specifically, empathizing allows the patient to see that their feelings are normal and that as the nurse you understand. Sometimes questioning a patient feels uncomfortable; thus stating an observation such as, "You look worried" or "You didn't eat much lunch" invites patients to respond without feeling pressure to answer (see Chapter 24).

Feelings of sadness, numbing, or anger make talking about these situations especially difficult. For example, a patient may experience anger during grief and lash out at caregivers. Some patients even become demanding and accusing. Remain supportive by letting patients and family members know that feelings such as anger are normal by saying, "I see that you're upset right now, and that's understandable. I just want you to know I'm here to talk with you if you want." Encourage patients to share the emotions and concerns of greatest importance to them and then acknowledge their feelings and concerns in a nonjudgmental manner. If a patient chooses not to share feelings or concerns, express a willingness to be available at any time. Some patients do not discuss emotions for personal or cultural reasons, and others hesitate to express their emotions for fear that people will abandon or judge them. If you are reassuring and respectful of a patient's privacy, a therapeutic relationship likely develops. Sometimes patients need to begin resolving their grief privately before they discuss their loss with others, especially strangers.

Do not avoid talking about a topic. When you sense that a patient wants to talk about something, make time to do so as soon as possible. This may be very challenging if you are in a busy acute care setting; however, it is a necessary part of quality nursing care and should be made a priority. Above all, remember that a patient's emotions are not something you can "fix." Instead view emotional expressions as an essential part of the patient's adjustment to significant life changes and development of effective coping skills. Help family members access other professional resources. Social workers, chaplains, and case managers can offer additional information and support to families and patients in grief.

Provide Psychosocial Care. Patients at the end of life experience a range of psychological symptoms, including anxiety, depression, powerlessness, uncertainty, and isolation. They can experience anguish from the unknown surroundings, treatment options, health status, and the dying process. Worry or fear is common in many patients and often heightens their perception of discomfort and suffering. You can alleviate some of it by providing information to them about their condition, the course of their disease, and the benefits and burdens of treatment options.

Manage Symptoms. Managing the multiple symptoms commonly experienced by chronically ill or dying patients remains a primary goal of palliative care nursing. Uncontrolled symptoms cause patients' and families' distress, discomfort, and suffering, which often complicates the dying experience. Despite the availability of effective treatment options for pain, many patients suffer with avoidable pain at the end of life because of misconceptions by the nurse or family (see Chapter 44). Maintain an ongoing assessment of the patient's pain and response to interventions. Reassure the family repeatedly of the need for pain control even if the patient does not appear in pain. Discuss pain control with the family frequently and dispel any myths regarding dependence on narcotics. You are responsible to advocate for change if the patient does not obtain relief from the prescribed regimen. It is imperative that you assess dying patients' nonverbal cues because they often are unable to communicate their intentions. During the dying process patients' renal and liver function decline, decreasing metabolism and rate of drug clearance, which might require modification to the dosage of medication. Also be aware that advancing disease pathology, anxiety, or delirium sometimes requires the use of higher doses or different drug therapies.

Remain alert to the potential side effects of opioid administration: constipation, nausea, sedation, respiratory depression, or myoclonus. Family members often worry about potential addiction to opioid medications. Not only is the incidence of true addiction very low, but a patient's need for pain relief at the end of life takes priority. Education is necessary to help families understand the need for appropriate use of opioid medications. Table 37-3 provides a basic overview of nursing care for common symptoms experienced at the end of life.

Promote Dignity and Self-Esteem. A sense of dignity includes a person's positive self-regard, the ability to find meaning in life and feel valued by others, and treatment by caregivers. Nurses promote a patient's self-esteem and dignity by respecting him or her as a whole person (i.e., as a person with feelings, accomplishments, and passions independent of the illness experience), not just as a diagnosis. Respecting and valuing the things that a patient cares about validates the person and at the same time strengthens communication among the patient, family members, and the nurse. Sharing time with patients as they share their life stories helps you know them and facilitates the development of individualized interventions.

Attending to the patient's physical appearance also promotes dignity and self-esteem. Cleanliness, absence of body odors, and attractive clothing give patients a sense of worth. When caring for a patient's bodily functions, show patience and respect, especially after the patient becomes dependent on others. Remember that patients are directing care at the end of life. Allow them to make decisions such as how and when to administer personal hygiene, diet preferences, and timing of nursing interventions. Keep the patient and family members informed about daily activities, tests, or therapies; their purposes; and anticipated effects. Provide privacy during nursing care procedures and be sensitive to when the patient and family need time alone together.

Maintain a Comfortable and Peaceful Environment. A comfortable, clean, pleasant environment helps patients relax, promotes good sleep patterns, and minimizes symptom severity. Keep a patient comfortable through frequent repositioning, making sure that bed linens are dry, and controlling extraneous environmental noise and offensive odors. Pictures, cherished objects, and cards or letters from family members and friends create a familiar and comforting environment for the patient dying in an institutional setting. When possible, allow patients to wear their own pajamas or lounging clothes to promote a sense of comfort and familiarity. Consider nonpharmacological interventions such as massage therapy to increase patient comfort (Paice, 2015). Family members are often able to provide these interventions, increasing their sense that they are making a positive contribution. Use patient-preferred music in the background, provide guided-imagery exercises, and dim the lights to provide a soothing environment for the patient and family. Patient-preferred forms of complementary therapies offer noninvasive methods to increase comfort and well-being at the end of life (Mariano, 2015) (see Chapter 33).

Promote Spiritual Comfort and Hope. Patients are comforted when they have assurance that some aspect of their lives will transcend death; therefore helping patients make connections to their spiritual practice or cultural community can be a useful intervention. Draw on the resources of spiritual care providers in an institutional setting or collaborate with the patient's own spiritual or religious leaders and communities. Making an audiotape or videotape for the family, writing letters, or keeping a journal assures patients that something of their essence will survive past their death.

The spiritual concept of hope takes on special significance near the end of life. Nursing strategies that promote hope are often quite simple: be present and provide whole-person care. Patients perceive the love of family and friends, faith, goal setting, positive relationships with professional caregivers, humor, and uplifting memories as hope promoting. Circumstances that hinder the preservation of hope include abandonment or isolation, uncontrolled symptoms, or being devalued as a person. Patients and their families hope for different things over the course of their experience with illness and death. Balancing each perspective is imperative to quality patient care at the end of life. Some hope to live for an anniversary, sit outdoors for a meal, see an important person one last time, gain pain relief, or have a peaceful death. Listen for shifts in patients' hopes and find ways to help them meet their desired goals.

Protect Against Abandonment and Isolation. Many patients with terminal illness fear dying alone. Patients feel more hopeful when others are near to help them. Nurses in institutional settings need to answer call lights promptly and check on patients often to reassure them that someone is close at hand. If family members plan to stay

TABLE 37-3 **Promoting Comfort in the Terminally Ill Patient**

Symptoms	Characteristics or Causes	Nursing Implications
Pain	Pain has multiple causes, depending on patient diagnosis.	Collaborate with team members to identify and implement appropriate pharmacological and nonpharmacological interventions to reduce pain and promote comfort (see Chapter 44 for further discussion on pain management).
Skin discomfort	Any source of skin irritation increases discomfort.	Keep skin clean, dry, and moisturized. Monitor for incontinence.
Mucous membrane discomfort	Mouth breathing or dehydration leads to dry mucous membranes; tongue and lips become dry or chapped.	Provide oral care at least every 2 to 4 hours. Apply a light film of lip balm for dryness. Apply topical analgesics to oral lesions prn.
Corneal irritation	Blinking reflexes diminish near death, causing drying of cornea.	Optical lubricants or artificial tears reduce corneal drying.
Fatigue	Metabolic demands, stress, disease states, decreased oral intake, and heart function cause weakness and fatigue.	Provide periods of rest and educate patient about energy conservation.
Anxiety	Physical, social, or spiritual distress causes anxiety; causes may be situational or event specific.	Provide opportunity for patient to express feelings though active listening. Provide calm, supportive environment. Consult members of health care to determine if pharmacological interventions are appropriate.
Nausea	Nausea is caused by medications, pain, or decreased intestinal blood flow with impending death.	Determine the cause of nausea and work to reduce nausea triggers such as strong smells. Administer antiemetics or promotility agents. Encourage patients to lie on their right side. Provide oral care at least every 2 to 4 hours.
Constipation	Opioids, medications, and immobility slow peristalsis. Lack of bulk in diet or reduced fluid is a cause.	Increase fiber in diet if appropriate. Administer stool softeners or laxatives as needed. If possible encourage increased liquid intake and regular periods of ambulation.
Diarrhea	Disease processes, treatment or medications, and gastrointestinal (GI) infections are causes.	Consult with members of the health are to determine the cause and make appropriate changes. Provide skin care and easy accessibility to the toilet or bedside commode.
Urinary incontinence	Progressive disease and decreased level of consciousness are causes.	Provide good skin care and frequent assessment for incontinent urine. Place Foley catheter as appropriate.
Altered nutrition	Medications, depression, decreased activity, and decreased blood flow to GI tract are causes. Nausea produces anorexia.	Encourage patient to eat small, frequent meals of preferred foods. Patients should never be forced to eat.
Dehydration	Patient is less willing or able to maintain oral fluid intake; has fever.	Reduce discomfort from dehydration; give mouth care at least every 2 to 4 hours; offer ice chips or moist cloth to lips. Keep lips and tongue moist.
Ineffective breathing patterns (e.g., dyspnea, shortness of breath)	Anxiety; fever; pain; increased oxygen demand; disease processes; and anemia, which reduces oxygen-carrying capacity, are causes.	Treat or control underlying cause. Use nonpharmacological interventions such as elevating the head of the bed to promote lung expansion. Provide oxygen as needed. Keeping the air cool provides ease and comfort for the terminal patient. Using narcotic to treat tachypnea is sometimes appropriate.
Noisy breathing ("death rattle")	Noisy breathing is the sound of secretions moving in the airway during inspiratory and expiratory phases caused by thick secretions, decreased muscle tone, swallow, and cough.	Elevate head to facilitate postural drainage. Turn patient at least every 2 hours. Provide oral care and maintain hydration as tolerated.

with the patient at all times or if you have assessed high privacy needs for the patient and family, a private room is best.

Some family members who have a difficult time accepting a patient's impending death cope by making fewer visits. When family members do visit, inform them of the patient's status and share meaningful insights or encounters that you have had with the patient. Find simple and appropriate care activities for the family to perform such as offering food, cooling the patient's face, combing hair, or filling out a menu. Nighttime can be particularly lonely for the patient. Suggest that a family member stay through the night if possible. Make exceptions to visiting policies, allowing family members to remain with patients who are dying at any time. Family members appreciate having open access or closeness to their loved one through their experiences at the end of life. Record contact information for them so you can reach them at any time.

Support the Grieving Family. In palliative and hospice care patients and family members constitute the unit of care. When a patient becomes debilitated or approaches the end of life, family members also suffer. They describe caregiving at the end of life as unpredictable, frightening, and anguishing. Yet many family members find meaning in providing practical and simple care to their loved one. In these extremely intimate and emotionally challenging times, offer holistic, family-centered support, compassion, and education that incorporates the uniqueness of each patient. Often family members face challenging and complex situations long before their loved one is actively dying. Family members caring for people with serious life-limiting illness

BOX 37-7 EVIDENCE-BASED PRACTICE

Use of Antimuscarinic Drugs to Control Respiratory Secretions

PICO Question: In patients who are terminally ill, what is the effect of antimuscarinic drugs to reduce excess respiratory secretions compared to no intervention?

Evidence Summary

Many symptoms occur when the body is slowly shutting down. One of the most fearful and troublesome is excess respiratory tract secretions, also known as the *death rattle.* For loved ones and caregivers at the bedside the sound of secretions in the respiratory tract is unnerving and distressing. However, patients most likely are not suffering from these secretions. Because end-of-life care is concerned with the family unit, treatment is often initiated to reduce the amount of secretions and therefore reduce and hopefully eliminate the distressing sound. Health care providers use different antimuscarinic drugs such as scopolamine, glycopyrronium (Robinul), hyoscine butylbromide (Buscopan), atropine, and octreotide (Sandostatin) in hopes of preventing or managing the excess secretions. The question remains if these treatments are effective. A systematic review of the research literature was completed; and 39 studies, published between 1988 and 2012, were identified. The researchers concluded that no evidence exists to support the claim that these drugs are better at reducing the amount of secretions in the terminal patient when compared to no treatment (Lokker et al., 2014).

Application to Nursing Practice

- Provide education about the occurrence of the death rattle to reduce the anxiety and distress often experienced by loved ones (Lokker et al., 2014).
- Help family position loved one to reduce secretion and improve breathing.
- Teach family member how to use oral suction devices to control excess secretions.

BOX 37-8 Physical Changes Hours or Days Before Death

- Increased periods of sleeping/unresponsiveness
- Coolness and color changes in extremities, nose, fingers (cyanosis, pallor, mottling) (see Figure 37-5)
- Bowel or bladder incontinence
- Decreased urine output; dark-colored urine
- Restlessness, confusion, or disorientation
- Decreased intake of food or fluids; inability to swallow
- Congestion/increased pulmonary secretions; noisy respirations (death rattle)
- Altered breathing (apnea, labored or irregular breathing, Cheyne-Stokes pattern)
- Decreased muscle tone, relaxed jaw muscles, sagging mouth
- Weakness and fatigue

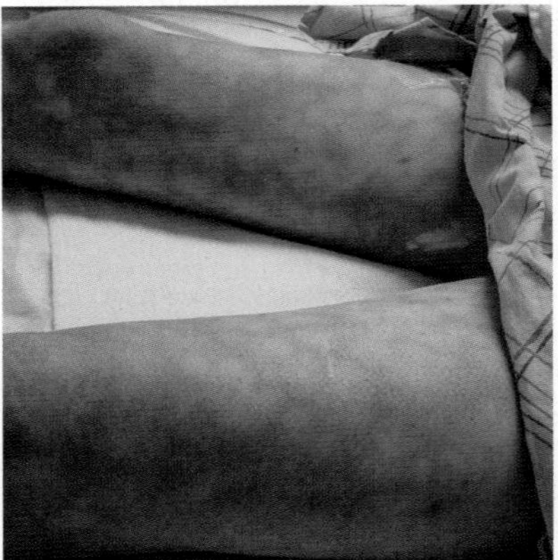

FIGURE 37-5 Skin mottling. (From Adams J et al: *Emergency medicine,* Philadelphia, 2009, Saunders.)

need attention and support early and consistently throughout the experience of illness and death.

Educate family members in all settings about the symptoms that the patient will likely experience and the implications for care (Box 37-7). For example, patients in the last days of life often develop anorexia or feel nauseated by food. Illness, excessive respiratory secretions, decreased activity, treatments, and fatigue decrease a patient's caloric needs and appetite. Family members, distressed with the decline, often believe that they need to encourage the patient to eat. Because the goal of palliative care is comfort, we do not want to force the patient to do anything that is causing discomfort. Eating in the last days of life often causes the patient pain and discomfort. In addition, as the body is shutting down, the nutrients in food are not able to be absorbed. Therefore forcing patients to eat serves no beneficial purpose for the patient. Help families shift their focus to other helping activities during this time.

Family members who have limited prior experience with death do not know what to expect. They may need personal time with the nurse to share their concerns, ask about treatment options, validate perceived changes in the patient's status, or explore the possible meaning of patient behaviors. Whenever possible, communicate news of a patient's declining condition or impending death when family members are together so they can support one another. Provide information privately and stay with the family as long as needed or desired. Reduce family member anxiety, stress, or fear by describing what to expect as death approaches. Become familiar with common manifestations of impending death (Box 37-8), remembering that patients usually experience some but not all of these changes. Do not try to predict the time of death; instead use your assessments to help family members anticipate what is happening. Be compassionate and sensitive in how you share information. "Mottling is an expected sign as a body begins shutting down" instead of "when a person gets closer to death we see mottling" (Figure 37-5). Share your observations and through your role modeling encourage a sense of patience, compassion, and comfort throughout the dying process.

During the dying process check frequently on families, offering support, information, and, if appropriate, encouragement to continue touching and talking with their loved ones. In the time immediately following death determine the family's needs. Some families will want to touch or hold the deceased, others will not. Make the deceased accessible by lowering side rails, having hands exposed, and a chair close to the bedside. Depending on facility policies allow the family the necessary time to be with their loved one.

After death help the family make decisions such as notification of a funeral home, transportation of family members, and collection of the patient's belongings. Nurses are a primary source of family support. Remember that, because of differing responses to grief, some family members prefer to be alone at the time of and after the death, whereas others want to be surrounded by a support community. When uncertain about what a family member prefers for support, pose simple questions and offer suggestions for assistance.

With the death of a patient, family members benefit from the many resources of the health care team. When the patient chooses to die at home, family members provide direct care, which is often emotionally stressful and physically exhausting. In the home setting fatigued family caregivers benefit from respite care. During respite care a patient temporarily receives care from others so family members are able to get away to rest and relax. Hospice program benefits include some days of respite care. Inform family members of home care, hospice, and community service options so they can access the best resources for their situation.

Assist with End-of-Life Decision Making. Patients and family members often face complex treatment decisions at the end of life. Patients and families must decide which treatments to continue and which to forgo; to enroll in hospice or stay in the hospital; or to transfer to a nursing home, in-patient unit, or home. Even after the decision to enroll in hospice, questions arise about symptom management, artificial nutrition and hydration, and the desired location for death. You are able to support and educate patients and families as they identify, contemplate, and ultimately decide how to best journey to the end of life.

Difficult ethical decisions at the end of life complicate a survivor's grief, create family divisions, or increase family uncertainty at the time of death (see Chapter 22). When ethical decisions are handled well, survivors achieve a sense of control and experience a meaningful conclusion to their loved one's death. Suggest to patients that they clearly communicate their wishes for end-of-life care so family members are able to act as faithful surrogates when the patient can no longer speak for himself or herself. Some patients and family members rely on the nurse and other members of the health care team to initiate discussions regarding end-of-life care. Nurses often provide options that family members do not know are available and are advocates for patients and family members making decisions at the end of life in the form of an advanced directive. Over the last decade there has been a 25% increase in completion of advance directives. Although this has increased patients' level of autonomy, it has not reduced the number of deaths that occur in the hospital (Silveira et al., 2014).

Facilitate Mourning. Nurses who work with grieving family members often provide bereavement care after the patient's death. Helpful strategies for assisting grieving persons include the following:

- Help the survivor accept that the loss is real. Discuss how the loss or illness occurred or was discovered, when, under what circumstances, who told him or her about it, and other factual topics to reinforce the reality of the event and put it in perspective.
- Support efforts to adjust to the loss. Use a problem-solving approach. Have survivors make a list of their concerns or needs, help them prioritize, and lead them step-by-step through a discussion of how to proceed. Encourage survivors to ask for help.
- Encourage establishment of new relationships. Reassure people that new relationships do not mean that they are replacing the person who has died. Encourage involvement in nonthreatening group social activities (e.g., volunteer activities or church events).
- Allow time to grieve. "Anniversary reactions" (e.g., renewed grief around the time of the loss in subsequent years) are common. A return to sadness or the pain of grief is often worrisome. Openly acknowledge the loss, provide reassurance that the reaction is normal, and encourage the survivor to reminisce.
- Interpret "normal" behavior. Being distractible, having difficulty sleeping or eating, and thinking that they have heard the deceased's voice are common behaviors following loss. These symptoms do not mean that an individual has an emotional problem or is becoming ill. Reinforce that these behaviors are normal and will resolve over time.
- Provide continuing support. Survivors need the support of a nurse with whom they have bonded for a time following a loss, especially in home care or hospice nursing. The nurse has filled an important role in the deceased's life and death and has helped survivors through some very intimate and memorable times. Attachment for a period of time after the death is appropriate and healing for both the survivor and the nurse. However it is imperative that professional boundaries always be maintained.
- Be alert for signs of ineffective, potentially harmful coping mechanisms such as alcohol and substance abuse or excessive use of over-the-counter analgesics or sleep aids.

Care After Death. Federal and state laws require institutions to develop policies and procedures for certain events that occur after death: requesting organ or tissue donation, performing an autopsy, certifying and documenting the occurrence of a death, and providing safe and appropriate postmortem care. In accordance with federal law, a specially trained professional (e.g., transplant coordinator or social worker) makes requests for **organ and tissue donation** at the time of every death. The person requesting organ or tissue donation provides information about who can give consent legally, which organs or tissues can be donated, associated costs, and how donation affects burial or cremation.

In extremely stressful circumstances created by the loss of a loved one, grieving survivors usually cannot remember all they were told. Nurses provide support and reinforce or clarify explanations given to them during the request process. In addition, understanding the physiology of organ donation is often difficult for family members. Even though a patient who is brain dead is legally declared dead, he or she remains on life support to provide the vital organs with blood and oxygen before transplant. The appearance of a live-looking body confuses the family, and they need help to understand that the life support is only preserving the vital organs. Nonvital tissues such as corneas, skin, long bones, and middle ear bones are taken at the time of death without artificially maintaining vital functions. If the deceased has not left behind instructions concerning organ and tissue donation, the family gives or denies consent at the time of death. Review your state organ retrieval laws and institutional policy and procedure regarding the formal consent process. Be aware that the laws governing who to approach for organ donation may not be acceptable in other cultures.

Family members give consent for an **autopsy** (i.e., the surgical dissection of a body after death) to determine the exact cause and circumstances of death or discover the pathway of a disease (see Chapter 23). In most cases a coroner or medical examiner determines the need to perform an autopsy. Law sometimes requires that an autopsy be performed when death is the result of foul play; homicide; suicide; or accidental causes such as motor vehicle crashes, falls, the ingestion of drugs, or deaths within 24 hours of hospital admission.

Usually the physician or other designated health care provider asks for autopsy permission while the nurse answers questions and supports the family's choices. Inform family members that an autopsy does not deform the body and that all organs are replaced in the body. Family members are often comforted to know that others may be helped by either the gift of organ and tissue donation or autopsy. Respect and honor family wishes and final decisions.

Documentation of a death provides a legal record of the event. Follow agency policies and procedures carefully to provide an accurate and reliable medical record of all assessments and activities surrounding a death. Physicians or coroners sign some medical forms such as a request for autopsy, but the RN gathers and records much of the remaining information surrounding a death. Nurses also usually witness or delegate the signing of forms (e.g., release of body or personal belongings forms). Nursing documentation becomes relevant in risk management or legal investigations into a death, underscoring the importance of accurate, legal reporting. Documentation also validates success in meeting patient goals or provides justification for changes in treatment or expected outcomes. Box 37-9 lists important documentation elements for end-of-life care.

Family members deserve and expect a clear description of what happened to their loved one, especially in cases of sudden, unusual, or unexpected circumstances. Give *only* factual information in a nonjudgmental, objective manner and avoid sharing your opinions. State law and agency policy govern the sharing of the written medical record information, which usually involves a written request. Follow legal guidelines for documentation and sharing of medical records (see Chapter 23).

BOX 37-9 Documentation of End-of-Life Care

- Time and date of death and all actions taken to respond to the impending death
- Name of health care provider certifying the death
- People notified of the death (e.g., health care providers, family members, organ request team, morgue, funeral home, spiritual care providers) and person who comes to declare time of death
- Name of person making request for organ or tissue donation
- Special preparations of the body (e.g., desired or required religious/cultural rituals)
- Medical tubes, devices, or lines left in or on the body
- Personal articles left on and secured to the body
- Personal items given to the family with description, date, time, to whom given
- Location of body identification tags
- Time of body transfer and destination
- Any other relevant information or family requests that help clarify special circumstances
- Verify with health care agency

When a patient dies in an institutional or home care setting, nurses provide or delegate **postmortem care**, the care of a body after death. Above all, a deceased person's body deserves the same respect and dignity as that of a living person and needs to be prepared in a manner consistent with the patient's cultural and religious beliefs. Death produces physical changes in the body quite quickly; thus you need to perform postmortem care as soon as possible to prevent discoloration, tissue damage, or deformities.

Maintaining the integrity of cultural and religious rituals and mourning practices at the time of death gives survivors a sense of fulfilled obligations and promotes acceptance of the patient's death (Box 37-10). The ability of families to mourn in a manner consistent with cultural values helps survivors experience some predictability and control in an otherwise uncertain and confusing time. Some cultures consider "family" as more than a nuclear biological unit. Health care providers need to understand the makeup of a family network and know which individuals to involve in end-of-life decisions and care.

The nurse coordinates patient and family care during and after a death. Become familiar with applicable policies and procedures for postmortem care because they vary across settings or institutions. See the procedural guideline (Box 37-11) for standard activities for care of the body after death.

◆ Evaluation

Through the Patient's Eyes. The success of the evaluation process depends partially on the bond that you have formed with the patient and family. Through a trusting relationship patients are more likely to share personal expectations or their wishes, especially if encouraged through appropriate questioning. Refer back to the goals and expected outcomes established during the planning phase to determine the effectiveness of nursing interventions. A patient's responses and perceptions of the effectiveness of the interventions determine if the existing plan of care is effective or if different strategies are necessary. For example, if the goal is to have the patient communicate a sense of hope to family members, evaluate verbal and nonverbal communication and behaviors for cues related to expressions of hope. Continue

BOX 37-10 CULTURAL ASPECTS OF CARE

Care of the Body After Death

Loved ones use cultural-specific rituals and mourning practices to achieve a sense of acceptance and inner peace and participate in socially accepted expressions of grief. One's culture greatly influences which behaviors and rituals are expected at the time of death. Institutional guidelines and end-of-life care procedures for patients from all cultures provide standards based on compassion, maintaining privacy and dignity, and respect for patients' and family members' cultural beliefs and practices. Expert end-of-life care allows time for patients and their families to make private and public preparations and complete unfinished communication. Understanding the uniqueness of cultural expectations at the end of life helps a nurse know which questions to ask. The following cultural or religious practices are not necessarily exclusive to the culture named but are offered to give you an idea of some cultural-specific concerns that you may encounter in end-of-life care.

Implications for Patient-Centered Care

African-American: Care of the body after death depends on the African-American's country of origin and degree of American acculturation. The presence of large extended family groups, including the church family, is common at time of death. The mourning period is relatively short, with a memorial service and a public viewing of the body or a wake before burial. Organ donation and autopsy are allowed.

Chinese: Death is regarded as a negative life event, and there is no concept of an afterlife. The dead are treated with the same respect as the living and may be buried with food and other artifacts. Members of an extended family usually stay with the deceased for up to 8 hours after death. The oldest son or daughter bathes the body under direction of an older relative or a temple priest. They often believe the body should remain intact; thus organ donation and autopsy are uncommon (Xu, 2007).

Hispanic or Latino: Honoring family values and roles is essential in providing care and making decisions at the end of life. People in Hispanic and Mexican-American cultures often use special objects such as amulets or rosary beads, alternative healing practices (folk medicine), and prayer. Grief is expressed openly. Religious and spiritual rituals (predominantly Catholic) are essential at the end of life. Death is often believed to be the will of God (Owen et al., 2012; Taxis et al., 2008).

Native American: Native Americans encompass diverse tribal groups with differing practices, traditions, and ceremonies. Traditional Navajos do not touch the body after death. Care of the body in the large Navajo tribe includes

BOX 37-10 CULTURAL ASPECTS OF CARE

Care of the Body After Death—cont'd

cleansing the body, painting the deceased's face, dressing in clothing, and attaching an eagle feather to symbolize a return home. Mourners also have a ritual cleansing of their bodies. The dead are buried on the deceased's homeland (Hanley, 2012).

Islamic: The deceased's body is ritualistically washed, wrapped, cried over, prayed for, and buried as soon as possible after death. The eyes and mouth are closed, and the face of the deceased is turned toward Mecca. Muslims of the same gender prepare the body for burial. Bodies are buried, not cremated. Autopsies interfere with a quick burial; make autopsy requests with sensitivity and only if necessary. The proximity of loved ones after death is important since it is believed that the soul stays with the body until it is buried. Organ donation is permissible by some Qur'an interpretations (Gatrad and Sheikh, 2008).

Buddhist: Buddhists believe in an afterlife in which humans manifest in different forms. Death is preferred at home, and a person's state at the time of death is important. Individuals usually minimize emotional expressions and maintain a peaceful, compassionate atmosphere. Male family members prepare the body. Buddhists recommend not touching the body after death to give the deceased a smoother transition to the afterlife. People often say prayers while touching and standing at the head of the deceased. The body is not left alone after death. Family and friends pay respects after death and before cremation of the body (Bauer-Wu et al., 2007).

Hindu: The body is placed on the floor with the head facing north. People of the same gender handle the body after death. There are no general prohibitions against autopsy. Bodies are cremated after death to purify by fire (Gatrad and Sheikh, 2008).

Jewish: If the family practices Orthodox Judaism, determine if members from the Jewish Burial Society are coming to the facility before preparing the body. A family member often stays with the body until burial. Usually the burial occurs within 24 hours but not on the Sabbath. Some but not all types of Judaism avoid cremation, autopsy, and embalming (Bauer-Wu et al., 2007).

BOX 37-11 PROCEDURAL GUIDELINES

Care of the Body After Death

Delegation Considerations

The skill of care of the body after death can be delegated to nursing assistive personnel (NAP). Nurses often find it meaningful to help care for a patient after death and assist the NAP whenever possible. Instruct the NAP to:

- Contact the nurse for all questions and procedures related to organ/tissue donation and autopsy requests.
- Alert nurse to family members' questions related to manner of death or after-death activities.

Equipment

Bath towels, washcloths, washbasin, scissors, shroud kit with name tags, bed linen, documentation forms.

Steps

1. Confirm that the health care provider certified the death and documented the time of death and actions taken.
2. Determine if the health care provider requested an autopsy. An autopsy is required for deaths that occur under certain circumstances.
3. Validate the status of request for organ or tissue donation. Given the complex and sensitive nature of such requests, only specially trained personnel make the requests. Maintain sensitivity to personal, religious, and cultural beliefs in this process.
4. Identify the patient using two identifiers (e.g., name and birthday or name and medical record number according to agency policy).
5. Provide sensitive and dignified nursing care to the patient and family.
   a. Elevate the head of the bed as soon as possible after death to prevent discoloration of the face.
   b. Collect ordered specimens.
   c. Ask if the family wishes to participate in preparation of the body. Offer to make arrangements for supportive company for the family (patient/family religious leader, spiritual care personnel, or bereavement specialist) during body preparation.
   d. Ask about family requests for body preparation such as wearing special clothing or religious artifacts. Be aware that personal, religious, or cultural practices determine whether or not to shave male facial hair. Get permission before shaving a beard.
   e. Remove all equipment, tubes, and indwelling lines. Note that autopsy or organ donation often poses exceptions to removal; thus consult agency policy in these situations.
   f. Cleanse the body thoroughly, maintaining safety standards for body fluids and contamination when indicated. Comb patient's hair or apply personal hairpieces.
   g. Cover body with a clean sheet, place head on a pillow, and leave arms outside covers if possible. Close eyes by gently holding them shut; leave dentures in the mouth to maintain facial shape; cover any signs of body trauma.
   h. Prepare and clean the environment, deodorize room if needed, and lower the lights.
   i. Offer family members the option to view the body and ask if they want you or other support people to accompany them. Honor and respect individual choices.
   j. Encourage grievers to say good-bye in their own way: words, touch, singing, religious rituals, or prayers.
   k. Provide privacy and an unrushed atmosphere. Assess family members' need or desire for your presence at this time. If you leave, tell them how to reach you.
   l. Determine which personal belongings stay with the body (e.g., wedding ring or religious symbol) and give other personal items to family members. Document time, date, description of the items taken, and who received them. Save any items that are left behind accidentally and contact family for further instructions.
   m. Apply identifying name tags and shroud according to agency policy before transporting the body. Follow safety procedures for body fluid precautions or contamination concerns.
   n. Complete documentation in the narrative notes section (see Box 37-9).
   o. Maintain privacy and dignity when transporting the body to another location; cover the body or stretcher with a clean sheet.

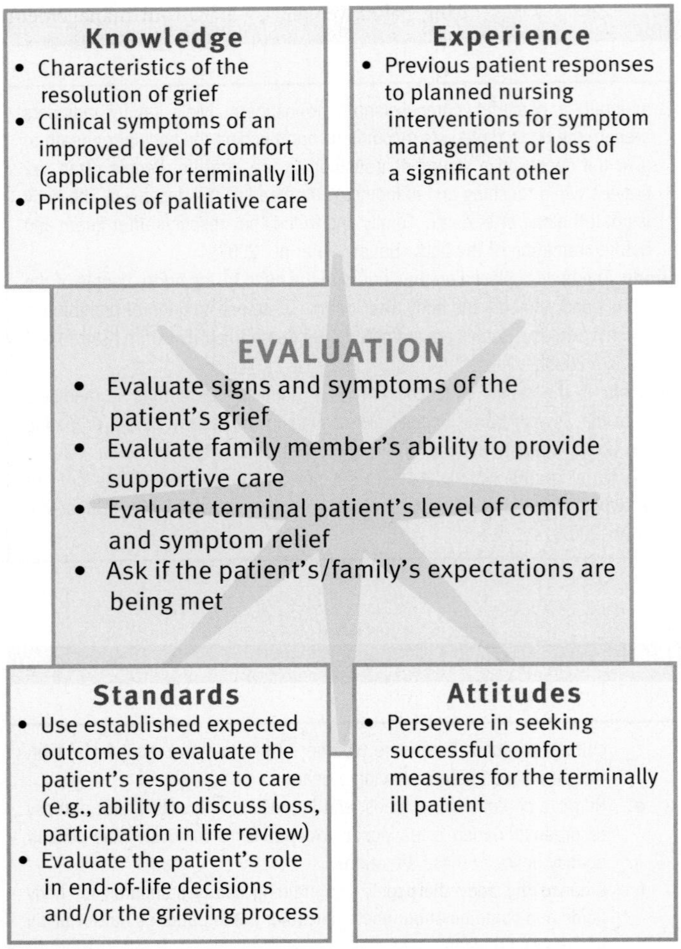

Knowledge
- Characteristics of the resolution of grief
- Clinical symptoms of an improved level of comfort (applicable for terminally ill)
- Principles of palliative care

Experience
- Previous patient responses to planned nursing interventions for symptom management or loss of a significant other

EVALUATION
- Evaluate signs and symptoms of the patient's grief
- Evaluate family member's ability to provide supportive care
- Evaluate terminal patient's level of comfort and symptom relief
- Ask if the patient's/family's expectations are being met

Standards
- Use established expected outcomes to evaluate the patient's response to care (e.g., ability to discuss loss, participation in life review)
- Evaluate the patient's role in end-of-life decisions and/or the grieving process

Attitudes
- Persevere in seeking successful comfort measures for the terminally ill patient

FIGURE 37-6 Critical thinking model for loss, death, and grief evaluation.

to evaluate the patient's progress, the effectiveness of the interventions, and patient and family interactions. Even when a patient is not seeking care specifically related to a loss, be alert for signs and symptoms of grief. They provide the criteria for evaluating whether a patient is coping with a loss and how he or she is moving through the grief process. Critical thinking ensures that the evaluation process accurately reflects the patient's situation and desired outcomes (Figure 37-6).

Patient Outcomes. The following questions help us validate achievement of goals and expectations:

- What is the most important thing I can do for you at this time?
- Are your needs being addressed in a timely manner?
- Are you getting the care for which you hoped?
- Would you like me to help you in a different way?
- Do you have a specific request that I have not met?

Especially in home care settings, include family members in the evaluation process. The short- and long-term outcomes that signal a family's recovery from a loss guide your evaluation. Short-term outcomes indicating effectiveness of grief interventions include talking about the loss without feeling overwhelmed, improved energy level, normalized sleep and dietary patterns, reorganization of life patterns, improved ability to make decisions, and finding it easier to be around other people. Long-term achievements include the return of a sense of humor and normal life patterns, renewed or new personal relationships, and decrease of inner pain.

KEY POINTS

- When caring for patients who have experienced a loss, facilitate the grief process by helping survivors feel the loss, express it, and move through their grief.
- Loss comes in many forms, based on the values and priorities learned within a person's sphere of influence (i.e., family, friends, religion, society, and culture).
- Death is difficult for the dying person and the person's family, friends, and caregivers.
- Survivors move back and forth through a series of stages and/or tasks many times, possibly extending over a long period of time.
- Grieving people use their own unique history, context, and resources to make meaning out of their loss experiences. Listen as patients share the experience in their own way.
- A person's development, coping strategies, socioeconomic status, personal relationships, nature of loss, and cultural and spiritual beliefs influence the way he or she perceives and responds to grief.
- Assess the terminally ill patient and family wishes for end-of-life care, including the preferred place for death, desired level of intervention, and expectations for pain and symptom management.
- Establish a caring presence and use effective communication strategies to encourage patients to share to the degree they are comfortable.
- Palliative care focuses on improving quality of life through an illness or death experience.
- Hospice is a philosophy of family-centered, whole-person care at the end of life.

CLINICAL APPLICATION QUESTIONS

Preparing for Clinical Practice

1. Mrs. Allison is exhibiting signs of grief over her situation and possible cancer diagnosis. In her withdrawn state how might you encourage her to share her feelings? Provide specific statements that would illicit robust responses from Mrs. Allison.
2. Mrs. Allison will be staying in the hospital for the next week until her family can make the necessary arrangements to transfer her home. Describe ways to ensure that Mrs. Allison is comfortable at home and in her hospital room.
3. Before being transferred home, Mrs. Allison changes her mind and is not considering curative treatment; however she would still like to receive hospice care. How could the nurse respond to Mrs. Allison?

ⓔ *Answers to Clinical Application Questions can be found on the Evolve website.*

REVIEW QUESTIONS

Are You Ready to Test Your Nursing Knowledge?

1. To best assist a patient in the grieving process, which of the following is most helpful to determine?
   1. Previous experiences with grief and loss
   2. Religious affiliation and denomination
   3. Ethnic background and cultural practices
   4. Current financial status.
2. Which of the following is the best intervention to help a hospitalized patient maintain some autonomy?
   1. Use therapeutic techniques when communicating with the patient.

2. Allow the patient to determine timing and scheduling of interventions.
3. Encourage family to only visit for short periods of time.
4. Provide the patient with a private room close to the nurse's station.

3. Which factors influence a person's approach to death? (Select all that apply.)
   1. Culture
   2. Age
   3. Spirituality
   4. Personal beliefs
   5. Previous experiences with death
   6. Gender
   7. Level of education
   8. Degree of social support
4. A family member of a dying patient talks casually with the nurse and expresses relief that she will not have to visit at the hospital anymore. Which theoretical description of grief best applies to this family member?
   1. Denial
   2. Anticipatory grief
   3. Yearning and searching
   4. Dysfunctional grief
5. On entering a room the nurse sees the patient crying softly. What is the most therapeutic response?
   1. Using silence
   2. Asking, "Why are you crying today?"
   3. Using therapeutic touch
   4. Stating, "I see that you're crying."
6. A young mother is dying of breast cancer with bone metastasis and tells the nurse, "My body hurts so much. I can hardly move. Why is God making me suffer when I have done nothing bad in my life? I feel like giving up. How can I care for my children when I can't even care for myself?" What is the most appropriate nursing diagnosis for this patient?
   1. *Spiritual Distress related to questioning God*
   2. *Hopelessness related to terminal diagnosis*
   3. *Pain related to disease process*
   4. *Anticipatory Grief related to impending death*
7. A nurse has the responsibility of managing a deceased patient's postmortem care. What is the proper order for postmortem care?
   1. Bathe the body of the deceased.
   2. Collect any needed specimens.
   3. Remove all tubes and indwelling lines.
   4. Position the body for family viewing.
   5. Speak to the family members about their possible participation.
   6. Ensure that the request for organ/tissue donation and/or autopsy was completed.
   7. Notify support person (e.g., spiritual care provider, bereavement specialist) for the family.
   8. Accurately tag the body, including the identity of the deceased and safety issues regarding infection control.
   9. Elevate the head of the bed.
8. Which comment to a patient by a new nurse regarding palliative care needs to be corrected?
   1. "Even though you're continuing treatment, palliative care is something we might want to talk about."
   2. "Palliative care is appropriate for people with any diagnosis."
   3. "Only people who are dying can receive palliative care."
   4. "Children are able to receive palliative care."
9. A patient is receiving palliative care for symptom management related to anxiety and pain. A family member asks if the patient is dying and now in "hospice." What does the nurse tell the family member about palliative care? (Select all that apply.)
   1. Palliative care and hospice are the same thing.
   2. Palliative care is for any patient, any time, any disease, in any setting.
   3. Palliative care strategies are primarily designed to treat the patient's illness.
   4. Palliative care relieves the symptoms of illness and treatment.
   5. Palliative care selects home health care services.
10. A grieving patient complains of confusion, inability to concentrate, and insomnia. What do these symptoms indicate?
    1. These are normal symptoms of grief.
    2. There is a need for pharmacological support for insomnia.
    3. The patient is experiencing complicated grief.
    4. These are common complaints of the admitted patient.
11. When planning care for the dying patient, which interventions promote the patient's dignity? (Select all that apply.)
    1. Providing respect
    2. Viewing patients as a whole
    3. Providing symptom management
    4. Showing interest
    5. Being present
    6. Using a preferred name
12. What are the physical changes that occur as death approaches? (Select all that apply.)
    1. Unresponsiveness
    2. Erythema
    3. Mottling
    4. Restlessness
    5. Increased urine output
    6. Weakness
    7. Incontinence
13. What is the palliative care team's primary obligation for the patient with severe pain?
    1. Providing postmortem care.
    2. Teaching about grief stages.
    3. Enhancing the patient's quality of life.
    4. Supporting the family after the death.
14. A year after her husband's death, a widow visits the unit on which he died. She talks about the anniversary and how much she misses him. Which type of grief is she experiencing?
    1. Normal
    2. Complicated
    3. Chronic
    4. Disenfranchised
15. When providing postmortem care, which action is a priority for the nurse?
    1. Locating the patient's clothing
    2. Providing culturally and religiously sensitive care in body preparation
    3. Transporting the body to the morgue as soon as possible
    4. Providing postmortem care to protect the family of the deceased from having to view the body

Answers: 1. 1; **2.** 2; **3.** 1, 3, 4, 5, 8; **4.** 2; **5.** 4; **6.** 3; **7.** 6, 9, 2, 5, 7, 3, 1, 4, 8; **8.** 3; **9.** 2, 4; **10.** 1; **11.** 1, 2, 4, 5, 6; **12.** 1, 3, 4, 6, 7; **13.** 3; **14.** 1; **15.** 2.

Rationales for Review Questions can be found on the Evolve website.

REFERENCES

American Association of Colleges of Nursing (AACN) and City of Hope National Medical Center (CHNMC): *End-of-Life Nursing Education Consortium (ELNEC)—core*, Duarte, CA, 2014, The Associations.

American Nurses Association (ANA): *Scope and standards of hospice and palliative nursing practice*, Atlanta, 2014, ANA.

Bauer-Wu S, et al: Spiritual perspectives and practices at the end of life: a review of the major world religions and application to palliative care, *Indian J Palliat Care* 13(2):53, 2007.

Bowlby J: *Attachment and loss: loss, sadness, and depression*, vol 3, New York, 1980, Basic Books.

Brohard C: Grief. In Yarbro CH, et al, editors: *Cancer symptom management*, ed 4, Burlington, MA, 2014, Jones & Bartlett Publishers.

Coyle N: Introduction to palliative nursing care. In Ferrell B, Coyle N, editors: *Textbook of palliative nursing*, ed 4, New York, 2015, Oxford University Press.

Fiorelli R, Jenkins W: Cultural competency in grief and loss, *Beginnings* 32(3):11, 2012.

Gatrad R, Sheikh A: Palliative care for Muslims. In Gatrad R, Sheikh A, et al, editors: *Palliative care for South Asians: Muslims, Hindus, & Sikhs*, London, 2008, Quay Books.

Hall C: Bereavement theory: recent developments in our understanding of grief and bereavement, *Bereavement Care* 33(1):7, 2014.

Hanley C: Navajos. In Giger JN, editor: *Transcultural nursing: assessment and intervention*, ed 6, St Louis, 2012, Mosby.

Hospice Foundation of America: *Services*. 2014. http://hospicefoundation.org/End-of-Life-Support-and-Resources/Coping-with-Terminal-Illness/Hospice-Services. Accessed April 20, 2015.

Kübler-Ross E: *On death and dying*, New York, 1969, Macmillan.

Mariano C: Holistic integrative therapies in palliative care. In Matzo M, Sherman D, editors: *Palliative care nursing: quality care to the end-of-life*, ed 4, New York, 2015, Springer.

Matzo M, Sherman D: *Palliative care nursing: quality care to the end of life*, ed 4, New York, 2015, Springer.

McDonald C, McCallin A: Interprofessional collaboration in palliative nursing: what is the patient-family role? *Internat J Palliat Nurs* 16(6):285, 2010.

Meghani S, et al: Policy brief: the Institute of Medicine report: dying in America: improving quality and honoring individual preferences near the end of life, *Nurs Outlook* 63(1):51, 2015.

Mitchell KR, Anderson H: *All our losses all our griefs*, Louisville, 1983, Westminster John Know Press.

Owen DC, et al: Mexican Americans. In Giger JN, editor: *Transcultural nursing: assessment and intervention*, ed 6, St Louis, 2012, Mosby.

Paice JA: Pain at the end of life. In Ferrell B, Coyle N, editors: *Textbook of palliative nursing*, ed 4, New York, 2015, Oxford University Press.

Rando T: *Treatment of complicated mourning*, Champaign, IL, 1993, Research Press.

Reynolds J, et al: American society for pain management nursing position statement: pain management at the end of life, *Pain Manage Nurs* 14(3):172, 2013.

Stroebe M, Schut H: The dual process model of coping with bereavement: rationale and description, *Death Stud* 23(3):197, 1999.

Taxis JC, et al: Mexican Americans and hospice care: culture, control and communication, *J Hospice Palliat Nurs* 10(3):133, 2008.

Walter C, McCoyd J: *Grief and loss across the lifespan: a biopsychosocial perspective*, New York, 2009, Springer.

Worden JW: *Grief counseling and grief therapy: a handbook for the mental health practitioner*, ed 4, New York, 2008, Springer.

World Health Organization (WHO): *Palliative care is an essential part of cancer control*. 2015. http://www.who.int/cancer/palliative/en. Accessed April 20, 2015.

Xu Y: Death and dying in the Chinese culture: implications for health care practice, *Home Health Care Manage Pract* 19:412, 2007.

RESEARCH REFERENCES

Bonanno G, et al: Resilience to loss and chronic grief: a prospective study from pre-loss to 18 month post-loss, *J Pers Soc Psychol* 83:1150, 2002.

Chan D, et al: Grief reactions in dementia carers: a systematic review, *Int J Geriatr Psychiatry* 28(1):1, 2013.

de Vries B, et al: Friend and family contact and support in early widowhood, *J Gerontol B Psychol Sci Soc Sci* 69(1):75, 2014.

Dose AM, et al: The meaning of spirituality at the end of life, *J Hosp Palliat Nurs* 16(3):158, 2014.

Kraft K: CAM for depression, anxiety, grief, and other symptoms in palliative care, *Prog Palliat Care* 20(5):272, 2012.

Lokker ME, et al: Prevalence, impact, and treatment of death rattle: a systematic review, *J Pain Symptom Manage* 47(1):105, 2014.

Parker GD, et al: Assessing attitudinal barriers toward end-of-life care, *Am J Hosp Palliat Care* 29(6):438, 2012.

Silveira MJ, et al: Advance directive completion by elderly Americans: a decade of change, *J Am Geriatr Soc* 62(4):706, 2014.

Trumble EL, et al: Complementary and alternative medicine (CAM) therapies as a means of advancing patient-centered care for veterans receiving palliative care, *J Altern Complement Med* 20(5):A50, 2014.

38

Stress and Coping

OBJECTIVES

- Describe the three stages of the general adaptation syndrome.
- Describe characteristics of post-traumatic stress disorder.
- Discuss the integration of stress theory with nursing theories.
- Describe stress-management techniques beneficial for coping with stress.
- Discuss the process of crisis intervention.
- Develop a care plan for patients who are experiencing stress.
- Discuss how stress in the workplace affects nurses.

KEY TERMS

Adventitious crises, p. 774
Alarm stage, p. 772
Allostasis, p. 772
Allostatic load, p. 772
Appraisal, p. 771
Burnout, p. 781
Coping, p. 773
Crisis, p. 774
Crisis intervention, p. 782
Developmental crises, p. 774
Ego-defense mechanisms, p. 774
Exhaustion stage, p. 772
Fight-or-flight response, p. 771
Flashbacks, p. 774
General adaptation syndrome (GAS), p. 772
Mindfulness, p. 781
Post-traumatic stress disorder (PTSD), p. 774
Primary appraisal, p. 772
Resistance stage, p. 772
Secondary appraisal, p. 773
Situational crises, p. 774
Stress, p. 771
Stressors, p. 771
Trauma, p. 771

MEDIA RESOURCES

http://evolve.elsevier.com/Potter/fundamentals/

- Review Questions
- Concept Map Creator
- Case Study with Questions
- Audio Glossary
- Content Updates

It is important to become familiar with stress to effectively assess and treat your patients and families suffering from the impact of stress. In the presence of physical and/or mental illness, stress affects the entire family, and both the family's and patient's health care needs must be considered in the plan of care. Equally important, health care professionals also experience stressful events in the course of clinical practice and their own lives. Nurses need to recognize the signs and symptoms of stress in the form of compassion fatigue and understand stress-management techniques to aid personal coping and design stress-management interventions for patients and families.

The term **stress** is used in many ways. Most commonly it is a term describing a process beginning with an event that evokes a degree of tension or anxiety. Such events are referred to as stressors. **Stressors** are tension-producing stimuli operating within or on any system (Neuman and Fawcett, 2011). An important element in the perception of a stressor is appraisal. **Appraisal** is how a person interprets the impact of the stressor. It is also a personal evaluation of the meaning of the event to what is happening and a consideration of the resources on hand to help manage the stressor (Lazarus, 2007). Stress emerges when an individual considers the event as a threat and the ability to respond to the demands placed on the individual by the event to be overwhelming. Thus stress is a physical, emotional, or psychological demand that can lead to personal growth or overwhelm a person and lead to illness or worsening of existing acute or chronic illnesses (Okonta, 2012; Santos, 2013). Stress refers to the consequences of the stressor and the person's appraisal of it.

People experience stress as a consequence of daily life events and experiences. It stimulates thinking processes and helps people stay alert to their environment. It can result in personal growth and facilitate development. How people react to stress depends on how they view and evaluate the impact of the stressor, its effect on their situation and support at the time of the stress, and their usual coping mechanisms. When stress overwhelms existing coping mechanisms, patients lose emotional balance, and a crisis results. If symptoms of stress persist beyond the duration of the stressor, a person has experienced a **trauma** (O'Driscoll, 2013; Stevens et al., 2013).

SCIENTIFIC KNOWLEDGE BASE

The initial response to stress involves activation of the sympathetic system, a pattern known as the **fight-or-flight response** (Figure 38-1). Neuroendocrine responses to stress function through negative feedback. The process of negative feedback senses an abnormal state such as lowered body temperature and makes an adaptive response such as

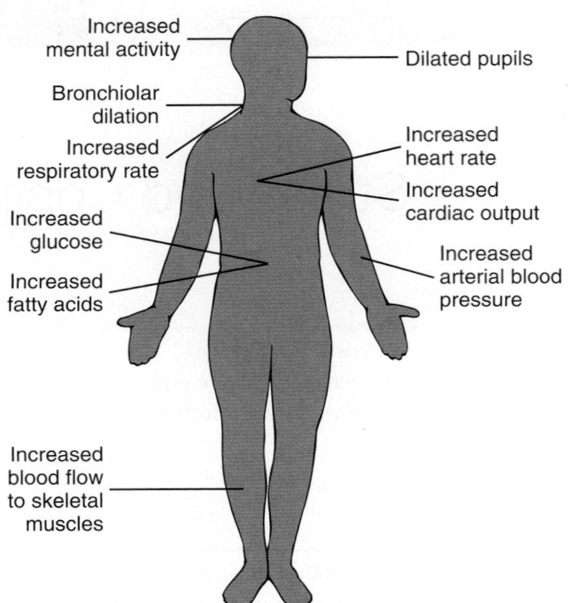

FIGURE 38-1 Fight-or-flight response.

initiating shivering to generate body heat. Three structures, the medulla oblongata, the reticular formation, and the pituitary gland, control the response of the body to a stressor.

Medulla Oblongata

The medulla oblongata located in the lower part of the brainstem controls heart rate, blood pressure, and respirations. Impulses traveling to and from the medulla oblongata increase or decrease these vital functions. For example, sympathetic or parasympathetic nervous system impulses traveling from the medulla oblongata to the heart control regulation of the heartbeat. The heart rate increases in response to impulses from sympathetic fibers and decreases with impulses from parasympathetic fibers.

Reticular Formation

The reticular formation, a small cluster of neurons in the brainstem and spinal cord, continuously monitors the physiological status of the body through connections with sensory and motor tracts. For example, certain cells within the reticular formation cause a sleeping person to regain consciousness or increase the level of consciousness when a need arises.

Pituitary Gland

The pituitary gland is a small gland immediately beneath the hypothalamus. It produces hormones necessary for adaptation to stress such as adrenocorticotropic hormone, which in turn produces cortisol. In addition, the pituitary gland regulates the secretion of thyroid, gonadal, and parathyroid hormones (Santos, 2013). A feedback mechanism continuously monitors hormone levels in the blood and regulates hormone secretion. When hormone levels drop, the pituitary gland receives a message to increase hormone secretion. When they rise, the pituitary gland decreases hormone production.

General Adaptation Syndrome

The general adaptation syndrome (GAS), a three-stage reaction to stress, describes how the body responds physiologically to stressors through stages of alarm, resistance, and exhaustion (Figure 38-2). The GAS is triggered either directly by a physical event or indirectly by a psychological event. It involves several body systems, especially the neuroendocrine feedback, and responds immediately to stress (see Figure 38-2). When the body encounters a physical demand such as an injury, the pituitary gland initiates the GAS. A fundamental concept underlying this reaction is that the body will attempt to return to a state of balance, a process referred to as allostasis (Huether and McCance, 2012).

During the alarm stage the central nervous system is aroused, and body defenses are mobilized; this is the flight-or-fight reaction. During this stage rising hormone levels result in increased blood volume, blood glucose levels, epinephrine and norepinephrine amounts, heart rate, blood flow to muscles, oxygen intake, and mental alertness. In addition, the pupils of the eyes dilate to produce a greater visual field. If the stressor poses an extreme threat to life or remains for a long time, the person progresses to the second stage, resistance.

The resistance stage also contributes to the flight-or-fight response, and the body stabilizes and responds in an attempt to compensate for the changes induced by the alarm stage (Huether and McCance, 2012). Hormone levels, heart rate, blood pressure, and cardiac output should return to normal; and the body tries to repair any damage that occurred. However, these compensation attempts consume energy and other bodily resources.

In the exhaustion stage continuous stress causes progressive breakdown of compensatory mechanisms. This occurs when the body is no longer able to resist the effects of the stressor and has depleted the energy necessary to maintain adaptation. The physiological response has intensified; but the person's ability to adapt to the stressor diminishes (Huether and McCance, 2012). Even in the face of chronic demands, an ongoing state of chronic activation can occur. This chronic arousal with the presence of powerful hormones causes excessive wear and tear on bodily organs and is called allostatic load. A persistent allopathic load can cause long-term physiological problems such as chronic hypertension, depression, sleep deprivation, chronic fatigue syndrome, and autoimmune disorders (Diamond, 2010; Huether and McCance, 2012).

Immune Response. The immune system is integrated with other physiological processes and is sensitive to changes in central nervous system and endocrine functioning that occur during the stress response. The interactions between the neuroendocrine stress response and the immune system are complex. The stress response directly influences the immune system (Huether and McCance, 2012). Stress causes prolonged changes in the immune system, which can result in impaired immune function. As stress increases, the person is more susceptible to changes in health such as increased risk for infection, high-blood pressure, diabetes, and cancers (Janowski et al., 2014; Moreia et al., 2014).

Reaction to Psychological Stress. The GAS is activated indirectly in the face of psychological threats, which are different for each person and produce differing reactions. The intensity and duration of the psychological threat and the number of other stressors that occur at the same time affect the person's response to it. In addition, whether or not the person anticipated the stressor influences its effect. It is often more difficult to cope with an unexpected stressor. Personal characteristics that influence the response to a stressor include the level of personal control, presence of a social support system, and feelings of competence.

One of the many ways of viewing stress is as a transaction between the person and the environment. An event comes along and is appraised or mentally rated in terms of meaning to the person. A person experiences stress only if the event or circumstance is considered significant. Evaluating an event in terms of personal meaning is primary appraisal.

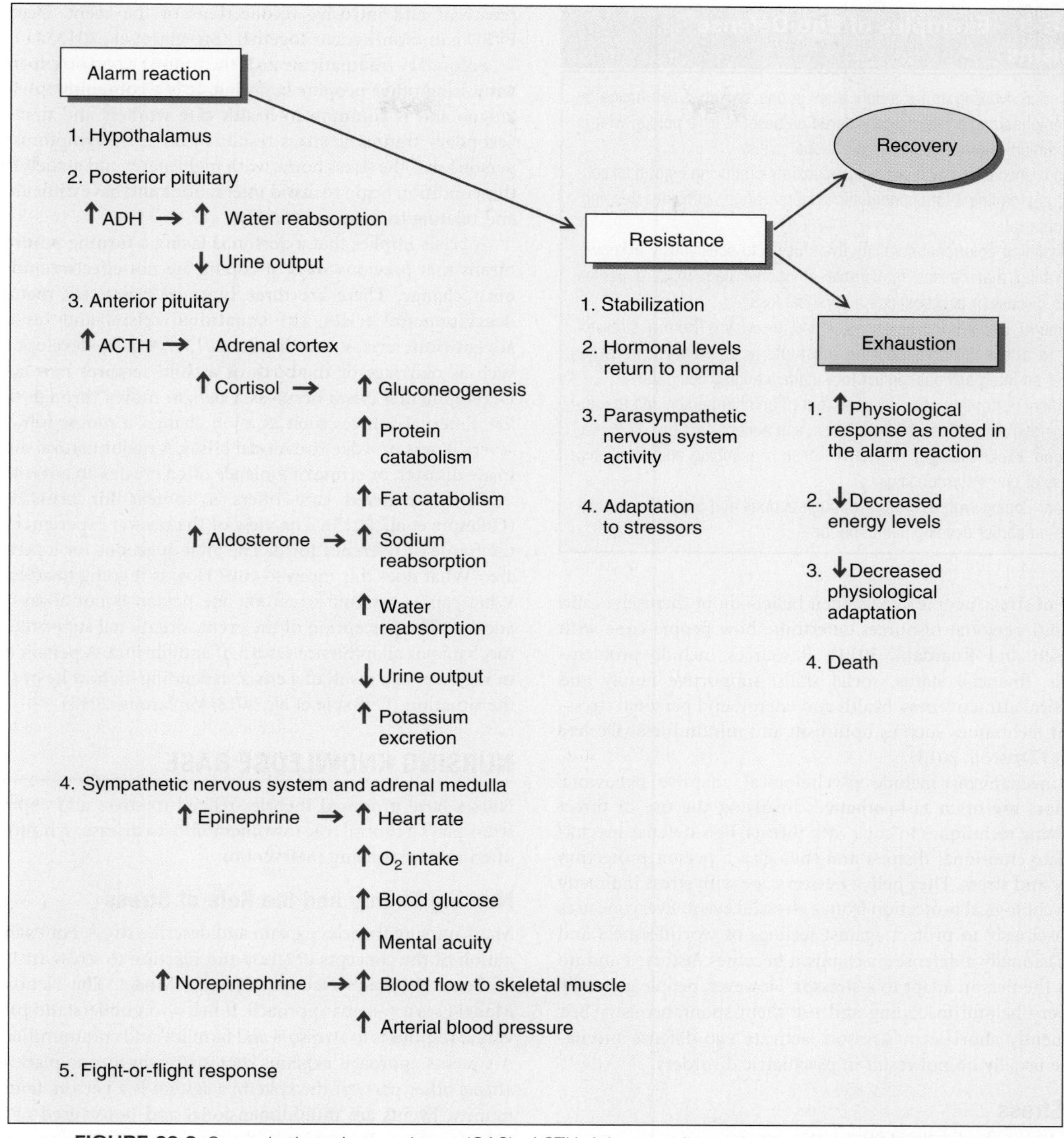

FIGURE 38-2 General adaptation syndrome (GAS). *ACTH,* Adrenocorticotropic hormone; *ADH,* antidiuretic hormone.

Appraisal of an event or circumstance is an ongoing perceptual process. If primary appraisal results in the person identifying the event or circumstance as a harm, loss, threat, or challenge, the person experiences stress. At the same time the person is also considering possible coping strategies or resources available to help deal with the event, a process referred to as **secondary appraisal**. If the demands placed on the person by the event exceed the ability to cope, stress occurs. Balancing factors contribute to restoring equilibrium. According to crisis theory, feedback cues lead to reappraisals of the original perception. Therefore coping behaviors constantly change as individuals perceive new information. Should they prove to be ineffective and the same attempts are repeated over and over, a state of stress can result from ineffective coping. Stress can then emerge either from an event viewed as posing a significant risk of harm or from a realization that the person is not able to cope with the demands placed by an event.

Coping is the person's cognitive and behavioral efforts to manage a stressor (Nielsen and Knardahl, 2014). It is important to physical and psychological health because stress is associated with a range of psychological and health outcomes (Doron et al., 2014). Effectiveness of coping strategies depends on the individual's needs. A person's age and cultural background influence these needs. For this reason no single coping strategy works for everyone or for every stressor. The same person may cope differently from one time to another.

In stressful situations most people use a combination of problem- and emotion-focused coping strategies. In other words, when under stress a person obtains information, takes action to change the situation (problem-focused), and regulates emotions tied to the stress (emotion-focused). In some cases people avoid thinking about the situation or change the way they think about it without changing the actual situation itself.

BOX 38-1 Examples of Ego-Defense Mechanisms

- Compensation: Making up for a deficiency in one aspect of self-image by strongly emphasizing a feature considered an asset (e.g., a person who is a poor communicator relies on organizational skills)
- Conversion: Unconsciously repressing an anxiety-producing emotional conflict and transforming it into nonorganic symptoms (e.g., difficulty sleeping, loss of appetite)
- Denial: Avoiding emotional conflicts by refusing to consciously acknowledge anything that causes intolerable emotional pain (e.g., a person refuses to discuss or acknowledge a personal loss)
- Displacement: Transferring emotions, ideas, or wishes from a stressful situation to a less anxiety-producing substitute (e.g., a person transfers anger over an interpersonal conflict to a malfunctioning computer)
- Identification: Patterning behavior after that of another person and assuming that person's qualities, characteristics, and actions
- Dissociation: Experiencing a subjective sense of numbing and a reduced awareness of one's surroundings
- Regression: Coping with a stressor through actions and behaviors associated with an earlier developmental period

The type of stress, people's goals, their beliefs about themselves and the world, and personal resources determine how people cope with stress (Nielsen and Knardahl, 2014). Resources include problem-solving skills, financial status, social skills, supportive family and friends, physical attractiveness, health and energy, and personal stress-management techniques such as optimism and mindfulness (Desiree et al., 2015; O'Driscoll, 2013).

Coping mechanisms include psychological adaptive behaviors. Such behaviors are often task oriented, involving the use of direct problem-solving techniques to cope with threats. **Ego-defense mechanisms** regulate emotional distress and thus give a person protection from anxiety and stress. They help a person cope with stress indirectly and offer psychological protection from a stressful event. Everyone uses them unconsciously to protect against feelings of worthlessness and anxiety. Occasionally a defense mechanism becomes distorted and no longer helps the person adapt to a stressor. However, people generally find them very helpful in coping and use them spontaneously (Box 38-1). Frequently short-term stressors activate ego-defense mechanisms. These usually do not result in psychiatric disorders.

Types of Stress

Stress includes work, family, daily hassles, trauma, and crisis. Stress may be acute or chronic. One person looks at a stimulus and sees it as a challenge, leading to mastery and growth. Another sees the same stimulus as a threat, leading to stagnation and loss. The individual with family responsibilities and a full-time job outside the home can experience chronic stress. It occurs in stable conditions and from stressful roles. Living with a long-term illness produces chronic stress. Conversely, time-limited events that threaten a person for a relatively brief period provoke acute stress. Recurrent daily hassles such as commuting to work, maintaining a house, dealing with difficult people, and managing money further complicate chronic or acute stress.

Post-traumatic stress disorder (PTSD) begins when a person experiences, witnesses, or is confronted with a traumatic event and responds with intense fear or helplessness. Some examples of traumatic events that lead to PTSD include motor vehicle crashes, natural disasters, violent personal assault, and military combat. Anxiety associated with PTSD is sometimes manifested by nightmares and emotional detachment. Some people with PTSD experience **flashbacks**, or recurrent and intrusive recollections of the event. Depression and PTSD commonly occur together (Stevens et al., 2013).

Secondary traumatic stress is the trauma a person experiences from witnessing other people's suffering. It is a component of compassion fatigue and is common in health care workers and first responders. Secondary traumatic stress results in intrusive symptoms in which a person takes the stress home, with nightmares and anxiety. People with this condition begin to avoid interactions and have difficulties sleeping and relating to friends or family.

A **crisis** implies that a person is facing a turning point in life. This means that previous ways of coping are not effective and the person must change. There are three types of crises: (a) maturational or **developmental crises**, (b) **situational crises**, and (c) disasters or **adventitious crises** (Varcarolis, 2013). A new developmental stage such as marriage or the birth of a child requires new coping styles. Developmental crises occur as a person moves through the stages of life. External sources such as a job change, a motor vehicle crash, or severe illness provoke situational crises. A major natural disaster, man-made disaster, or crime of violence often creates an adventitious crisis.

Patient-centered care offers a context for crisis intervention (Gillespie et al., 2013). The view of the person experiencing a crisis is the frame of reference for it. The vital questions for a person in crisis are, "What does this mean to you? How is it going to affect your life?" What causes extreme stress for one person is not always stressful to another. The perception of the event, situational supports, and coping mechanisms all influence return of equilibrium. A person either grows or regresses as a result of a crisis, depending on how he or she manages the situation (Gillespie et al., 2013; Varcarolis, 2013).

NURSING KNOWLEDGE BASE

Nurses have proposed theories related to stress and coping. Because stress plays a central role in vulnerability to disease, symptoms of stress often require nursing intervention.

Nursing Theory and the Role of Stress

Many nursing theories explain and describe stress. For example, explanation of the concepts of stress and reaction to stress are components of Betty Neuman's Neuman Systems Model. The Neuman Systems Model uses a systems approach. It helps you understand patients' individual responses to stressors and families' and communities' responses. A systems approach explains that a stressor at one place in a system affects other parts of the system; a system is a person, family, or community. Events are multidimensional and not caused or affected by only one thing. Every person develops a set of responses to stress that constitute the "normal line of defense" (Neuman and Fawcett, 2011). This line of defense maintains health and wellness. Physiological, psychological, sociocultural, developmental, or spiritual influences buffer stress. The Neuman Systems Model of nursing views a patient, family, or community as constantly changing in response to the environment and stressors.

On the other hand, Pender's Health Promotion Model focuses on promoting health and managing stress (Pender et al., 2013). In this model people want to live in ways that enable them to be as healthy as possible and capable of assessing their own abilities and assets. Interventions such as increasing physical activity, improving diet and nutrition, and using stress-management strategies help the individual become and remain healthy.

Factors Influencing Stress and Coping

Potential stressors and coping mechanisms vary across the life span (e.g., adolescence, adulthood, and old age bring different stressors).

The appraisal of stressors, the amount and type of social support, and coping strategies all balance when assessing stress and depend on previous life experiences. Furthermore, situational and social stressors place people who are vulnerable at higher risk for prolonged stress.

Situational Factors. Situational stress arises from personal, job, or family changes. Work-related stressors include promotions, transfers, downsizing, and changes in supervisors and responsibilities. Work stress manifests as burnout among health care workers. Burnout is the second component of compassion fatigue. It is defined as a chronic condition in which perceived demands (e.g., workload, difficult patients, insufficient equipment) outweigh perceived resources. It is common in emergency, oncology, and critical care settings but can occur in any setting (Ianello and Balzarotti, 2014; Mealer et al., 2014). Burnout can affect the quality of patient care. Another stressor in the health care workplace is changing work shifts, which increases fatigue. Shift work–related coping strategies vary with individuals and their situations. Some nurses often ease coping with shift work by knowing their own circadian rhythms. People who function best in the morning have the greatest difficulty with night work and changing shifts (Lin et al., 2014).

Other job-related proactive coping strategies such as resilience training for nurses working with trauma and critically ill patients prepare nurses for the critical situations, provide time to practice stress-management techniques, and better manage job-related stress (Gillespie et al., 2013; Mealer et al., 2014).

Chronic illnesses such as cancer, cardiac disease, diabetes, and depression are examples of stress-producing illnesses. Uncertainty associated with treatment and illness triggers stress in patients of all ages. Cancer survivors who made active efforts to control stress changed their physical, psychosocial, and preventive health behaviors during and following cancer treatment (Parelkar et al., 2013). Paying for treatment and limited access to providers also create stress. Although being a family caregiver for someone with a chronic illness such as Alzheimer's disease is associated with stress, the actions of competent health care providers often help minimize the stress for caregivers (see Chapter 10).

Maturational Factors. Stressors vary with life stage. Children identify stressors related to physical appearance, families, friends, and school. Preadolescents experience stress related to self-esteem issues, changing family structure as a result of divorce or death of a parent, or hospitalizations. As adolescents search for identity with peer groups and separate from their families, they experience stress. In addition, they face stressful questions about using mind-altering substances, sex, jobs, school, and career choices. Stress for adults centers around major changes in life circumstances. These include the many milestones of beginning a family and a career, losing parents, seeing children leave home, and accepting physical aging. In old age stressors include the loss of autonomy and mastery resulting from general frailty or health problems that limit stamina, strength, and cognition (Box 38-2).

Sociocultural Factors. Environmental and social stressors often lead to developmental problems. Potential stressors that affect any age-group but are especially stressful for young people include prolonged poverty and physical handicap. Children become vulnerable when they lose parents and caregivers through divorce, imprisonment, or death or when parents have mental illness or substance-abuse disorders. Living under conditions of continuing violence, disintegrated neighborhoods, or homelessness affects people of any age, especially young people (Pender et al., 2013).

BOX 38-2 FOCUS ON OLDER ADULTS

Understanding Differences in Stress and Coping Among Older Adults

- Ordinary hassles of day-to-day living are a source of stress; older people have more hassles with home maintenance and health than do younger people.
- Older adults use more passive, intrapersonal, emotion-focused forms of coping such as distancing, humor, accepting responsibility, and reappraising the stressor in a positive way.
- Life experiences and perspectives of older adults make most problems seem insignificant, especially when older adults have acquired appropriate stress-management techniques (Rayens and Reed, 2014).
- Older adults' coping improves on the basis of earlier experience with coping with traumatic situations (Yancura and Aldwin, 2008).
- Impaired coping affects overall health in older adults more than in younger adults (Rayens and Reed, 2014).
- Because of the high incidence of depression in older adults, you need to assess for suicidal thoughts and intent.
- When marital or partnership dyads are present, the perceived stress of one member has a greater effect on the other member than occurs with middle or young adults (Rayens and Reed, 2014).
- Differentiate signs of stress and crisis in older adults from dementia and acute confusion.

BOX 38-3 CULTURAL ASPECTS OF CARE

Cultural Variations in Stress Appraisal and Coping Strategies

A patient's culture defines what is stressful to the person and ways of coping with stress (Giger, 2012). Cultural context shapes the types of situations that produce stress. Culture affects how a person leaves the parental home, experiences health crises or chronic illness, cares for the family, or becomes disabled or dependent. Furthermore, how a person appraises stress also depends on his or her culture. What is perceived as a major stressor in one culture might be viewed as a minor problem in another. For example, cultures may address developmental transitions and turning points in life differently.

Coping strategies are also influenced by one's cultural background. Cultures vary in their emotion- and problem-focused coping strategies. Some stress that emotions should be controlled, whereas others believe in expressing emotion. Cultures provide different resources for coping with stress (Giger, 2012). These include the legal system for conflict resolution, advice givers or support groups, and rituals.

Implications for Patient-Centered Care

- Realize that stressors and coping styles vary with different cultures.
- Reflect on your own perceptions of stress and coping in a cultural context.
- Assess the influence of culture on a patient's appraisal of stress.
- Identify the presence of individualized cultural practices related to stress management.
- Determine resources in a patient's culture that facilitate coping.

A person's culture also influences stress and coping. Cultural variations produce stress, particularly if a person's values differ from the dominant culture in aspects of gender roles, family relationships, and religious beliefs (Giger, 2012). Other aspects of cultural variations begin with language difference, geographical location, family relationships, time orientation, access to health care programs, and disparities in health care (Box 38-3).

CRITICAL THINKING

When caring for a patient experiencing stress, use critical thinking skills to understand his or her stressor and the stress response. Integrate knowledge from nursing and other disciplines, previous experiences, and information gathered from patients to understand stress and its impact on the patient and family. Know the neurophysiological changes that occur in the patient experiencing the alarm reaction, resistance stage, and exhaustion stage of the GAS. In addition, know communication principles that contribute to assessing patient's behaviors. Give utmost attention to determining the patient's perception of the situation and his or her ability to cope with the stress. If the patient's usual coping skills have not helped or his or her support systems have failed, use crisis intervention counseling.

Experience teaches you to understand the patient's unique perspective and view each person as an individual, recognizing that no two people are exactly alike. Experience with patients also helps you to recognize responses to stress. In addition, personal experiences with stress and coping increase your ability to empathize with a patient temporarily immobilized by stress.

Be confident in the belief that you and your patients can effectively manage stress. Patients who feel overwhelmed and perceive events as beyond their capacity to cope rely on you as an expert. Patients respect your advice and counsel and gain confidence from your belief in their ability to move past the stressful event or illness. Patients overwhelmed by life events are often unable, at least initially, to act on their own behalf and require either direct intervention or guidance. Integrity is an essential attitude through which you respect the patient's perception of the stressor. Make the effort to have the patient explain his or her unique viewpoint and situation.

The practice standards for psychiatric mental health nursing (ANA, 2014) guide assessment of a patient's stress, coping mechanisms, and support system before intervening. Use linguistic and culturally effective communication skills to clearly and precisely understand a patient's perception of stress. Focus on factors relevant to his or her well-being. In addition, the patient expects you to exhibit confidence and integrity when he or she feels vulnerable. Be especially aware of the ethical responsibility in caring for someone who has diminished autonomy as a result of stress.

Knowledge
- Basic stress response
- Factors influencing stress
- Physiological, emotional, and behavioral risks associated with a stressor
- Basic defense mechanisms
- Cultural influences
- Communication principles

Experience
- Caring for patients whose illness, lifestyle, family interactions, and personal/professional demands resulted in stress
- Personal experience in dealing with stressful situations

ASSESSMENT
- Identify actual or potential stressors
- Identify patient's appraisal of stressor
- Obtain data regarding the patient's previous experience with stress
- Determine the impact of illness on the patient's lifestyle

Standards
- Apply intellectual standards of completeness, relevance, precision, and accuracy when assessing the patient's stress response
- Apply ANA Standards of Care for Psychiatric Mental Health Nursing Practice (2014) by using linguistic and culturally effective communication skills and comprehensive assessment

Attitudes
- Exhibit confidence that stress can be managed
- Approach assessment with fairness and integrity to collect data in an unbiased manner and convey that patient information remains confidential

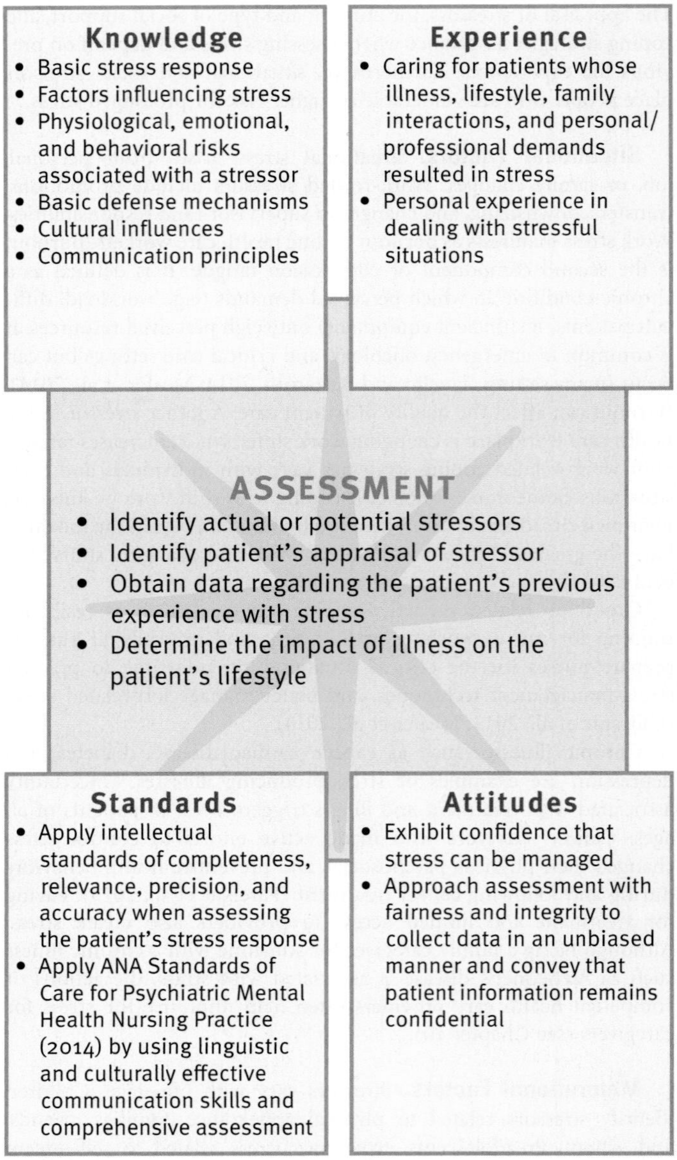

FIGURE 38-3 Critical thinking model for stress and coping assessment. *ANA,* American Nurses Association.

❖ NURSING PROCESS

Apply the nursing process and use a critical thinking approach in your care of patients. The nursing process provides a clinical decision-making approach for you to develop and implement an individualized plan of care.

◆ Assessment

During the assessment process thoroughly assess each patient and critically analyze findings to ensure that you make patient-centered clinical decisions required for safe nursing care.

Through the Patient's Eyes. Assessment of a patient's stress level and coping resources requires that you first establish a trusting nurse-patient relationship because you are asking a patient to share personal and sensitive information. Learn from the patient both by asking questions and by making observations of nonverbal behavior and the patient's environment. Synthesize the information and adopt a critical thinking attitude while observing and analyzing patient behavior (Figure 38-3). Often the patient has difficulty expressing exactly what is most bothersome about the situation until there is an opportunity to discuss it with someone who has time to listen.

Begin your assessment with an open-ended question such as, "What is happening in your life that caused you to come today?" or "What happened in your life that is *different?*" This requires some focusing by the patient. Next assess the patient's perception of the event, available situational supports, and what he or she usually does when there is an unsolvable problem. Determine if a person is suicidal or homicidal by asking directly. For example, ask, "Are you thinking of hurting yourself or someone else?" If so, determine in a caring and concerned manner if the person has a plan and how lethal the means are.

Take time to understand a patient's meaning of the precipitating event and the ways in which stress is affecting his or her life. Allow time for him or her to express priorities for coping with stress. For example, in the case of a woman who has just been told that a breast mass was identified on a routine mammogram, it is important to know what the patient wants and needs most from the nurse. Although some women in this situation identify their need for information about biopsy or mastectomy as their personal priority, others need guidance

BOX 38-4 Nursing Assessment Questions

Patient Safety
- Do you have any thoughts of harming yourself or others?
- Are you having difficulty with sleeping? Falling asleep? Staying awake?
- Is there any change in eating patterns?
- Have you had any accidents at home, in the car, at school, or on the job?

Perception of Stressor
- What do you believe is stressing you right now?
- What impact does this stressor have on your lifestyle?
- How does this stressor impact you now? How will it impact you in the future?

Available Coping Resources
- Which strategies have you used in the past to deal with stress?
- Are you able to confide in friends or family?
- What is relaxing for you?

Maladaptive Coping Used
- Have you started drinking or smoking?
- Do you use any over-the-counter or herbal medications?
- Do you use any street drugs?

Adherence to Healthy Practices
- How long since you saw a health care provider?
- What is your exercise pattern?
- Which type of meals do you eat? Are your meals regular?
- Are you taking your prescribed medications as ordered?

and support in discussing how to share the news with family members. In some cases, when nothing will change or improve the situation, allowing the patient to use denial as a coping mechanism is helpful. Gaining an understanding of patient expectations does not mean excluding certain types of care that are important simply because a patient does not identify them as needs. However, by inquiring about patient expectations and priorities, you are better able to ensure that you address *all* of the patient's needs in some way.

Stress also occurs in a family or a community. Stress in a family is sometimes from a critically ill family member, the sudden loss of a job, a move, or becoming homeless. An example of stress in a community is a natural disaster such as a major flood or the sudden, unexpected death of a beloved teacher or teenager. To develop appropriate and safe nursing care when caring for families or communities, ensure that you understand the meaning stress has for that group.

Subjective Findings. When assessing a patient's level of stress and coping resources, create a nonthreatening physical environment for the interaction. Assume the same height as the patient, arranging the interview environment so you can maintain or avoid eye contact comfortably. You do this by placing chairs at a 90-degree angle or side by side to reduce the intensity of the interaction (Varcarolis, 2013). Gather information about the health status of the patient from his or her perspective and begin the process of developing a trusting relationship with him or her. Use the interview to determine the patient's view of the stress, coping resources, any possible maladaptive coping, and adherence to prescribed medical recommendations such as medication or diet (Box 38-4). If the patient is using denial as a coping mechanism, be alert to whether he or she is overlooking necessary information. As in all interactions with the patient, respect the confidentiality and sensitivity of the information shared.

BOX 38-5 Nursing Diagnostic Process

Ineffective Coping

Assessment Activities	Defining Characteristics
Ask patient about change in sleeping patterns.	Sleep disturbance Difficulty falling asleep at night Sighing
Ask patient to complete a sleep diary for 2 weeks.	Excessive sleeping Poor sleeping
Observe patient's behavior and response to questions during assessment.	Fatigue Inability to concentrate Inaccurate response to questions Inappropriate laugh or crying
Observe patient's appearance.	Poor grooming Lack of eye contact
Ask patient about changes in eating patterns.	Weight gain or loss Lack of interest in food

Objective Findings. Obtain objective findings related to stress and coping through observation of the appearance and nonverbal behavior of a patient. Observe grooming and hygiene, gait, characteristics of the handshake, actions while sitting, quality of speech, eye contact, and the attitude of the patient during the interview. Before the interview begins or at the end of the interview, depending on the anxiety level of the patient, obtain basic vital signs to assess for physiological signs of stress such as elevated blood pressure, heart rate, or respiratory rate. Make certain to incorporate cultural components of interpreting the patient's nonverbal communication behaviors.

◆ Nursing Diagnosis

A review of assessment data leads you to cluster data that indicate a potential or actual stressor and the patient's response. Clustering data, along with the application of your knowledge and experiences with patients in stress, leads to individualized nursing diagnoses (Box 38-5).

Nursing diagnoses for people experiencing stress generally focus on coping. Specifically, major defining characteristics of *Ineffective Coping* include verbalization of an inability to cope and an inability to ask for help. To identify defining characteristics, ask the patient what is of most concern at the time of the interview. It is important to allow him or her sufficient time to answer. Observe for nonverbal signs of anxiety, fear, anger, irritability, and tension in a patient who is experiencing ineffective coping. Other defining characteristics include the presence of life stress, an inability to meet role expectations and basic needs, alteration in societal participation, self-destructive behavior, change in usual communication patterns, high rate of accidents, excessive food intake, drinking, smoking, and sleep disturbances. Stress or the failure of coping often results in multiple nursing diagnoses. Examples of these diagnoses include but are not limited to the following:

- *Anxiety*
- *Denial*
- *Fear*
- *Ineffective Coping*
- *Powerlessness*
- *Risk for Posttrauma Syndrome*
- *Situational Low Self-Esteem*
- *Stress Overload*

◆ Planning

Goals and Outcomes. Desirable goals for people experiencing stress frequently include effective coping, family coping, and caregiver emotional health. Examples of outcomes might include the following: patient engages in support group, family members are able to discuss loss together, caregiver participates in respite care. A nurse often selects interventions for stress and improved coping such as coping enhancement and crisis intervention in addition to individualized interventions after considering the nursing diagnosis, the resources available to the patient, and the goals identified by the patient and nurse (Figure 38-4).

Nursing interventions are designed within the framework of primary, secondary, and tertiary prevention. At the primary level of prevention you direct nursing activities to identifying individuals and populations who may be at risk for stress. Nursing interventions at the secondary level include actions directed at symptoms such as protecting the patient from self-harm. Tertiary-level interventions help the patient readapt and can include relaxation training and time-management training. The nurse and the patient assess the level and source of the existing stress and determine the appropriate points for intervention to reduce it (Pender et al., 2013) (see the Nursing Care Plan).

A tool for planning care is a concept map (Figure 38-5). Concept maps identify multiple nursing diagnoses for a patient from the assessment database and show how they are related. In this example the nursing diagnoses are linked to the patient's medical diagnosis of depression. In addition, the concept map shows the relationship among the nursing diagnoses *Chronic Imbalanced Nutrition: Less Than Body Requirements, Ineffective Coping, Anxiety,* and *Powerlessness*. Use of a concept map requires critical thinking skills to organize patient data and helps to plan for patient-centered care.

Just as the nursing assessment of the patient's stress and coping depends on his or her perception of the problem and coping resources, the interventions focus on a partnership with the patient and support system, usually the family. In the case of a family or community stressor and impaired family or community coping, the view of the situation and resources is broader.

Setting Priorities. Consider the patient's perspective and responses to assessment questions when setting priorities for care (see the Nursing Care Plan). The patient's and family member's physical condition and perception of stressors determine which nursing diagnosis has the greatest priority. As in all areas of nursing, safety of the patient and others in his or her environment is the first priority.

If suicide or homicide is not an issue, examine other potential threats to the safety of vulnerable people who are under the care of the patient. Provide for their temporary care or supervision if necessary. Other potential threats to safety include nutritional deficits; insomnia; self-care deficits; and poor judgment and impulsiveness that may lead to unsafe decisions about sex, drugs, money, or damage to personal relationships that the person might later regret. Determine the degree of work, school, home, and family disruption in the person's life. When you have completed immediate assessment and ensured safety, begin the problem-solving process.

Teamwork and Collaboration. Sometimes nursing practice alone does not meet all of the patient's and family's needs. To effectively plan individualized care, collaborate with occupational therapists, dietitians, pastoral care professionals, and health care professionals from other clinical specialties, depending on the patient's situation.

Patients experiencing stress from medical conditions or psychiatric disorders present needs that make it necessary for you to consult with advanced practice mental health nurses, psychiatrists, psychologists, or psychiatric social workers. An interprofessional approach addresses the holistic needs of the patient. Recognize the need for collaboration and consultation; inform the patient about potential resources; and make arrangements for interventions such as consultations, group sessions, or therapy as needed. A hospital social worker shares ideas for available resources both within the hospital and in the community. A home care nurse knows community services, groups, and appropriate contacts.

In addition to maximizing use of available resources for the patient, collaborative care also benefits the nurse. While working with patients experiencing stress, you gain a broad understanding of the multitude of health care disciplines. Work becomes more satisfying.

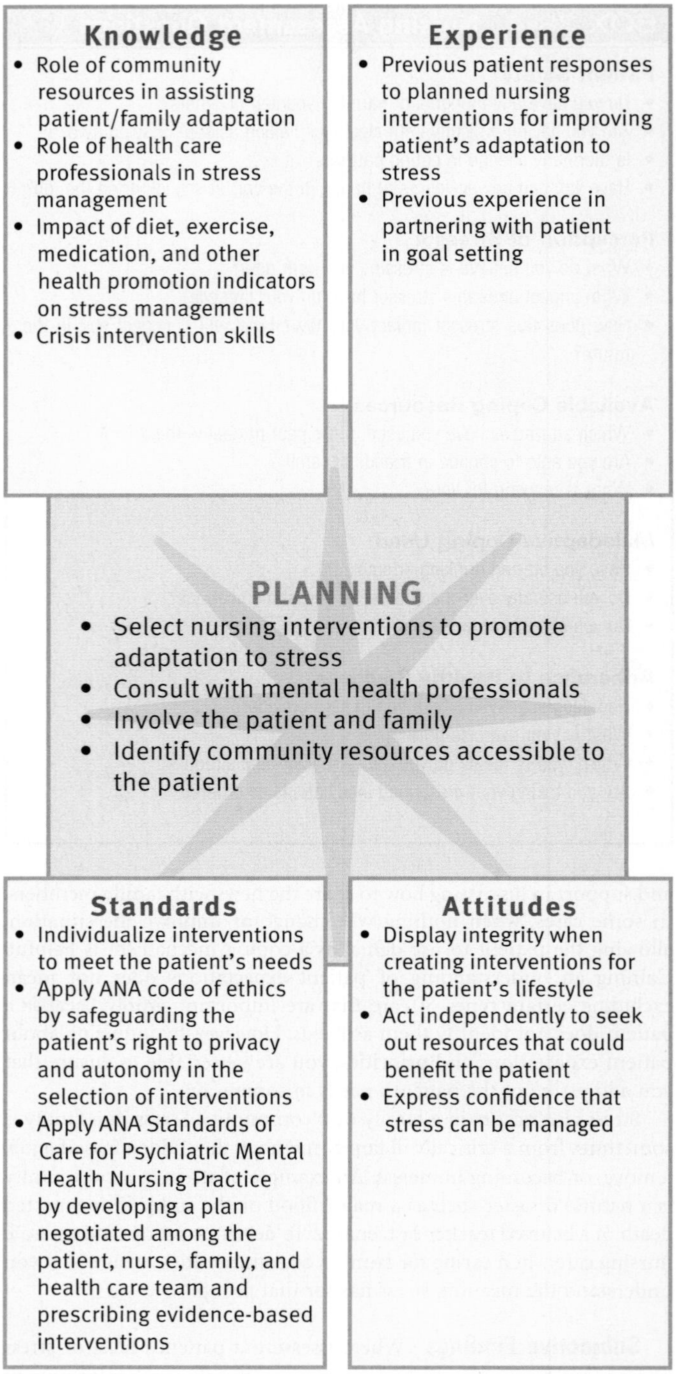

Knowledge
- Role of community resources in assisting patient/family adaptation
- Role of health care professionals in stress management
- Impact of diet, exercise, medication, and other health promotion indicators on stress management
- Crisis intervention skills

Experience
- Previous patient responses to planned nursing interventions for improving patient's adaptation to stress
- Previous experience in partnering with patient in goal setting

PLANNING
- Select nursing interventions to promote adaptation to stress
- Consult with mental health professionals
- Involve the patient and family
- Identify community resources accessible to the patient

Standards
- Individualize interventions to meet the patient's needs
- Apply ANA code of ethics by safeguarding the patient's right to privacy and autonomy in the selection of interventions
- Apply ANA Standards of Care for Psychiatric Mental Health Nursing Practice by developing a plan negotiated among the patient, nurse, family, and health care team and prescribing evidence-based interventions

Attitudes
- Display integrity when creating interventions for the patient's lifestyle
- Act independently to seek out resources that could benefit the patient
- Express confidence that stress can be managed

FIGURE 38-4 Critical thinking model for stress and coping planning. *ANA,* American Nurses Association.

NURSING CARE PLAN

Ineffective Coping

ASSESSMENT

Sandra and John have been married only 3 years; they are both 55 years old. This is a late marriage for both of them; neither was previously married. They both work and plan on retiring at age 66. Last month John was diagnosed with stage 3 pancreatic cancer. Presently John and Sandra are in the early phase of treatment options. At this point in time they are both working. They are at the Cancer Center today to decide on some treatment options. When you greet the couple, you notice that they both look tired, Sandra is disheveled, and John is clean shaven and well groomed. John states that he is worried about Sandra as she appears "just worn out," and he is afraid that she will not be able to help him through this medical crisis.

Assessment Activities	*Findings/Defining Characteristics**
Ask Sandra how she feels about John's diagnosis.	Sandra states, **"There's so much. I just feel inadequate and overwhelmed. I don't even know how I feel. I know I feel very alone."**
Ask Sandra what she remembers about John's treatment options.	She states, "I really **can't remember anything** but stage 3 pancreatic cancer. I got on the Internet so I know this is a bad cancer.
Ask John and Sandy about friends and relatives they have for support.	Both are only children and have **no other family**; they moved to the Northwest 1 year ago for new jobs. They both work for the same company but state that they have **few close friends**.
Ask Sandy to identify people she can turn to for help.	Sandra **sobs** and **feels that she doesn't have anyone locally to whom she can turn**. They are active in their church. On further discussion Sandra mentions a close friend from the Midwest.
Ask Sandra about sleep and nutrition patterns.	She **can't get to sleep easily and awakens 3 to 4 times per night.** States, "Appetite **is poor; I'm just not hungry. I think I've lost weight because my clothes are loose, but I don't know."**
Assess Sandra's mood and affect by asking how she is feeling.	She states, **"I feel very tired. Everything feels overwhelming."**

***Defining characteristics** are shown in bold type.

NURSING DIAGNOSIS: Ineffective coping related to insufficient social support

PLANNING

Goals	*Expected Outcomes (NOC)*[†]
	Social Support
Sandra achieves support from her community in 1 month.	Sandra identifies at least one person in her community who can help support her in this crisis. Sandra participates in a local support group weekly.
	Caregiver Lifestyle Disruption
Sandra achieves a more balanced lifestyle in 1 month.	Sandra reports eating at least 2 meals a day and improved sleep within 1 month. Sandra develops a balanced routine that incorporates time for own rest or relaxation within 1 week.

[†]Outcome classification labels from Moorhead S et al: *Nursing outcomes classification (NOC)*, ed 5, St Louis, 2013, Mosby.

INTERVENTIONS (NIC)[‡]	RATIONALE
Support System Enhancement	
Identify community-based cancer support systems for patients and family for Sandra and John.	Support systems for both patient and family are an effective intervention to cope with the stress of a cancer diagnosis and related therapies and decision making (Parelkar et al., 2013).
Help Sandra identify a person who is willing to come with Sandy and John to some of the early appointments regarding treatment decision and actual treatment.	Having another person hear some of the treatment options and treatment procedures provides opportunities to clarify the discussion. During high-stress times the patient and family may not hear the material provided by health care providers completely (Doron et al., 2014).
Explore community resources for a short-term education group for both Sandra and John for self-care tools to reduce stress.	Education groups help caregivers develop self-care tools to reduce stress, change negative self-talk, communicate more effectively, and make difficult decisions (Oken et al., 2010).
Teach Sandra and John mindfulness meditation strategies.	Mindfulness meditation, a form of cognitive therapy, reduces stress related to cancer diagnosis and treatment in patients and families (Desiree et al., 2015; Lengacher et al., 2014).

[‡]Intervention classification labels from Bulechek GM et al: *Nursing interventions classification (NIC)*, ed 6, St Louis, 2013, Mosby.

EVALUATION

Nursing Actions	*Patient Response/Finding*	*Achievement of Outcome*
Ask Sandra if her fatigue and stress levels have decreased.	Sandra identified two people in her church community. One is a cancer survivor; the second is a spouse of a cancer patient currently in treatment.	Sandra falls asleep within 10 minutes and sleeps for 6 hours. She also has a 30-minute rest period during the day.
Ask Sandra and John to describe modifications they have made in their daily routine.	Both use mindfulness meditation several times a week, and both state that they are feeling much more relaxed.	Meditation is reducing stress and allowing Sandra and John to concentrate on the treatment decision.
Ask Sandra if she attended support group.	Sandra reports she has attended two sessions.	Sandra accepts support from community.

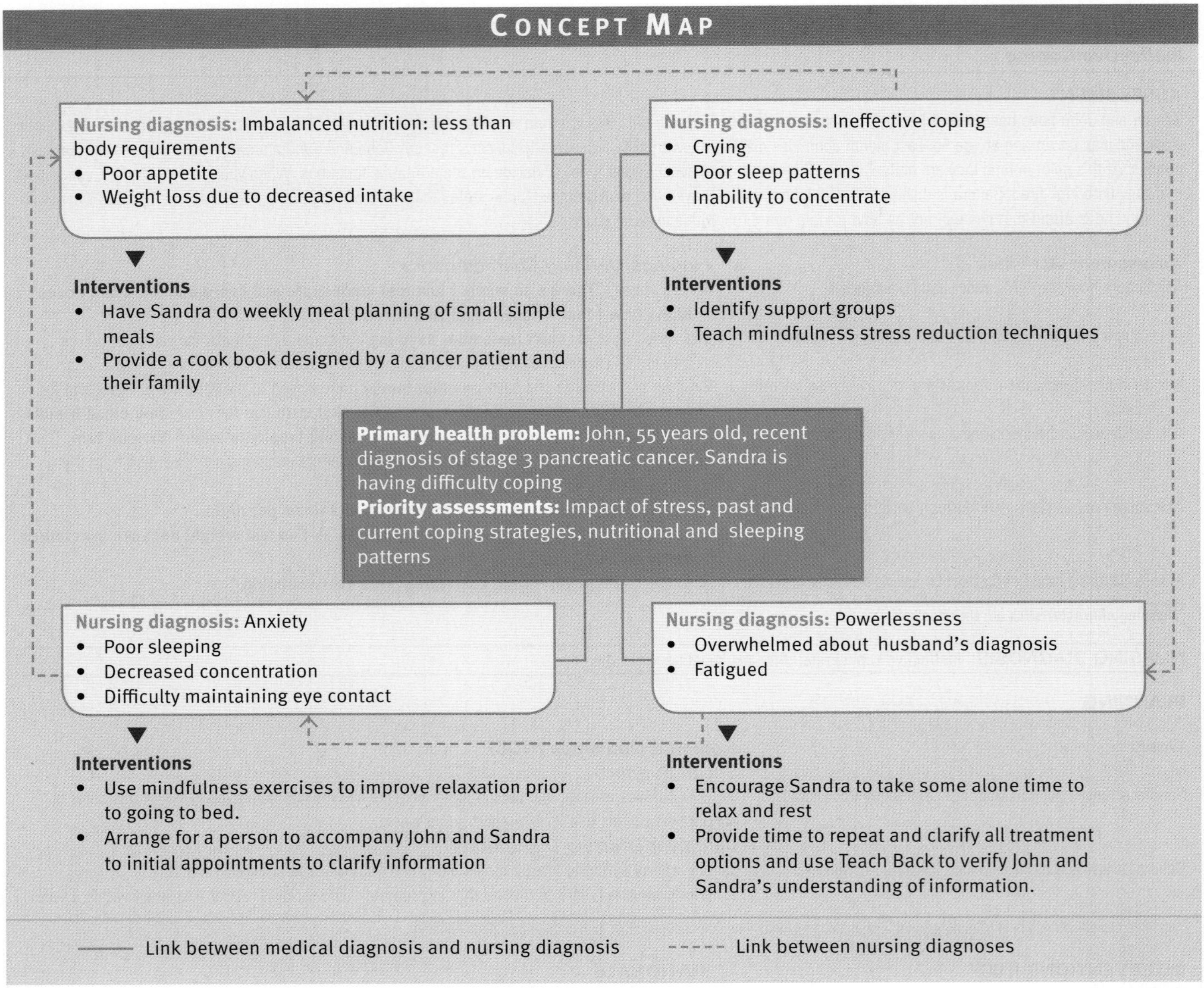

Concept Map

Nursing diagnosis: Imbalanced nutrition: less than body requirements
- Poor appetite
- Weight loss due to decreased intake

Interventions
- Have Sandra do weekly meal planning of small simple meals
- Provide a cook book designed by a cancer patient and their family

Nursing diagnosis: Ineffective coping
- Crying
- Poor sleep patterns
- Inability to concentrate

Interventions
- Identify support groups
- Teach mindfulness stress reduction techniques

Primary health problem: John, 55 years old, recent diagnosis of stage 3 pancreatic cancer. Sandra is having difficulty coping
Priority assessments: Impact of stress, past and current coping strategies, nutritional and sleeping patterns

Nursing diagnosis: Anxiety
- Poor sleeping
- Decreased concentration
- Difficulty maintaining eye contact

Interventions
- Use mindfulness exercises to improve relaxation prior to going to bed.
- Arrange for a person to accompany John and Sandra to initial appointments to clarify information

Nursing diagnosis: Powerlessness
- Overwhelmed about husband's diagnosis
- Fatigued

Interventions
- Encourage Sandra to take some alone time to relax and rest
- Provide time to repeat and clarify all treatment options and use Teach Back to verify John and Sandra's understanding of information.

——— Link between medical diagnosis and nursing diagnosis - - - - - Link between nursing diagnoses

FIGURE 38-5 Concept map for Sandra.

Contacts with other members of the interprofessional team and the community provide a feeling of contributing to the teamwork of providing holistic care.

◆ Implementation

Health Promotion. Three primary modes of intervention for stress are to decrease stress-producing situations, increase resistance to stress, and learn skills that reduce physiological response to stress (Pender et al., 2013). Educate patients and families about the importance of health promotion (Box 38-6).

Regular Exercise and Rest. A regular exercise program improves muscle tone and posture, controls weight, reduces tension, and promotes relaxation. In addition, exercise reduces the risk of cardiovascular disease and improves cardiopulmonary functioning. Patients who have a history of a chronic illness, are at risk for developing an illness, or are older than 35 years of age should begin a physical exercise program only after discussing the plan with a health care provider (Figure 38-6).

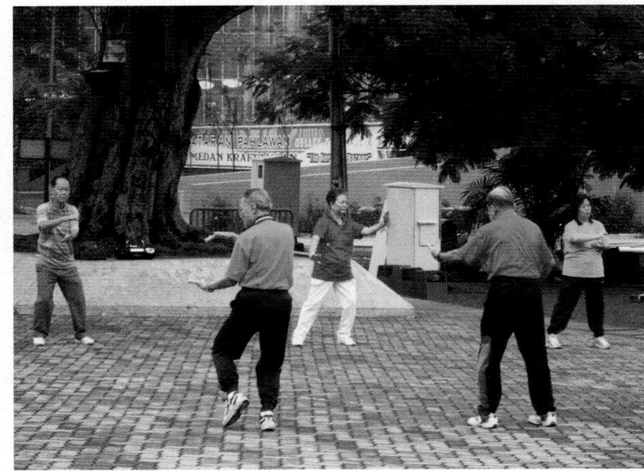

FIGURE 38-6 Regular exercise helps to cope with stress. (Courtesy Rudolph A. Furtado.)

Regular rest and sleep are also effective in reducing stress and stress-related fatigue. When stressful situations are present, encourage

BOX 38-6 PATIENT TEACHING

Stress Management

Objective

- Patient will report less anxiety, depression, and pain related to chronic health problems.

Teaching Strategies

- Familiarize patient with mind-body therapies that will likely benefit patient. Refer to a group or specialized practitioner when necessary (Gillespie and Gates, 2013; Okonta, 2012; Parelkar et al., 2013):
  - Meditation
  - Progressive muscle relaxation
  - Guided imagery
  - Hypnosis
  - Yoga
  - Tai Chi
- Teach patient how to incorporate 15-30 minutes of exercise into daily activities (Doron et al., 2014).
- Instruct patient to identify and use relaxation techniques such as:
  - Listen to music that you enjoy.
  - Keep a journal of your thoughts and feelings.
  - Replace unnecessary time-consuming activities with activities that are pleasurable or interesting.

Evaluation

- Use Teach Back to ask patient to explain how stress-reduction techniques help him or her to cope.
- Ask patient to report effects of the alternative therapy(ies) on anxiety, sleep, and lifestyle.
- Observe patient for signs of stress.

patients and their family members to establish bedtime and sleep routines and try to stick to the schedule (see Chapter 43). Patients and family members who are well rested are able to manage stress, problem solve, and maintain a sense of control over the situation (Akerstedt et al., 2014).

QSEN QSEN: BUILDING COMPETENCY IN EVIDENCE-BASED PRACTICE As a nurse educator for a diabetes rehabilitation program, you recognize the value of exercise for these patients. However, you are not sure about the best way to persuade the patients to increase their exercise. You've located current research articles that support types of interventions that are effective in promoting physical activity among chronically ill adults. Some of these interventions include (1) targeting physical activity exclusively, (2) using behavioral (as opposed to cognitive) strategies, and (3) encouraging self-regulation and monitoring (Park and Iacocca, 2014; Ruppar and Conn, 2010). On the basis of the evidence, which of the following interventions is (are) most likely to be successful? (Select all that apply.)

1. Develop a program that focuses on multiple behaviors, including diet, exercise, and medication compliance.
2. Develop a program that teaches tai chi.
3. Ask patients to keep a written log of the amount of physical activity they have each day.
4. Ask patients to list the ways that exercise helps them.
5. Provide patients with pedometers to record their daily steps.
6. Ask patients to set goals for exercise every day.

Answers to QSEN Activities can be found on the Evolve website.

Support Systems. A support system of family, friends, and colleagues who listen, offer advice, and provide emotional support benefits a patient experiencing stress (Doron et al., 2014). Many support groups are available to individuals (e.g., those sponsored by the American Heart Association and the American Cancer Society, local hospitals and churches, and mental health organizations). Recent research shows that cancer survivors who effectively manage their stress make changes in their physical, psychosocial, and preventive health behaviors (Parelkar et al., 2013).

Time Management. Time-management techniques include developing lists of prioritized tasks. For example, help patients list tasks that require immediate attention, those that are important and can be delayed, and those that are routine and can be accomplished when time becomes available. In many cases setting priorities helps individuals identify tasks that are not necessary or can be delegated to someone else.

Guided Imagery and Visualization. Guided imagery is based on the belief that a person significantly reduces stress with imagination. It is a relaxed state in which a person actively uses imagination in a way that allows visualization of a soothing, peaceful setting. Typically the image created or suggested uses many sensory words to engage the mind and offer distraction and relaxation.

Progressive Muscle Relaxation Therapies. In the presence of anxiety-provoking thoughts and events, a common physiological symptom is muscle tension. Diminish physiological tension through a systematic approach to releasing tension in major muscle groups. Typically an individual achieves a relaxed state through deep breathing. Once the patient is breathing deeply, direct him or her to alternately tighten and relax muscles in specific groupings. Other controlled relaxation exercises such as yoga are effective in regulating stress responses and reducing blood pressure (Doron et al., 2014; Okonta, 2012).

Assertiveness Training. Assertiveness includes skills for helping individuals communicate effectively regarding their needs and desires. The ability to resolve conflict with others through assertiveness training is important for reducing stress. Teaching assertiveness in a group setting increases the benefits of the experience.

Journal Writing. For many people keeping a private, personal journal provides a therapeutic outlet for stress. Suggest that patients keep journals, especially during difficult situations. In a private journal patients are able to express a full range of emotion and vent their honest feelings without hurting anyone else's feelings and without concern for how they appear to others.

Mindfulness-Based Stress Reduction. **Mindfulness** is a moment-to-moment present awareness with an attitude on nonjudgment, acceptance, and openness (Lengacher et al., 2014). Mindfulness-based stress reduction (MBSR) meditative practices are effective in reducing psychological and physical symptoms or perceptions. They are effective in stress management and symptom control with certain chronic conditions (Box 38-7). Through mindfulness exercises people learn to self-regulate awareness and attention to feeling and implement effective changes. Patients use cognitive exercises and subjective experiences to process images or feelings (Desiree et al., 2015). These feelings are then evaluated as pleasant or unpleasant, and the patient learns strategies to enhance the pleasant experiences and replace the unpleasant experiences. Through MBSR patients can control their stress response to illnesses and treatments, employees can manage job-related stress, and students can learn to manage stress anxiety.

Stress Management in the Workplace. Stressors such as rapid changes in health care technology, diversity in the workforce, organizational restructuring, and changing work systems place stress on employees. **Burnout** occurs as a result of chronic stress. In nursing, burnout results when nurses perceive the demands of their work

BOX 38-7 EVIDENCE-BASED PRACTICE

Impact of Meditation Therapies on Illness-Related Stressors

PICO Question: Does the use of meditative training such as yoga and mindfulness-based stress reduction (MBSR) help to reduce illness-related stressors?

Evidence Summary

Prolonged and recurrent stress is associated with multiple psychological and health outcomes. A person's ability to cope with these stressors impacts physical and psychological health (Doron et al., 2014). Proactive coping strategies such as exercise, rest, good nutrition, support systems, meditation, and relaxation activities demonstrate greater stress tolerance when stressors are present (Gillespie and Gates, 2013; Doron et al., 2014).

In addition, coping strategies assist in symptom management in certain chronic illnesses. For example, in hypertension yoga reduces blood pressure, blood glucose, and cholesterol levels and helps with weight control (Doron et al., 2014; Okonta, 2012). In breast cancer survivors MBSR reduced fear of recurrence, which improved physical functioning, which in turn reduced perceived stress and anxiety (Lengacher et al., 2014). Patients with advanced lung cancer and their partners also benefited from MBSR and had reduced psychological stress about the illness; the partners reported decreases in caregiver burden (Desiree et al., 2015).

Cognitive therapies such as mediation and MBSR are important interventions when dealing with illness-related stressors. These therapies are beneficial for managing symptoms and psychological distress associated with chronic conditions. However, it is important that the meditation therapy be individualized to patient needs, patient's ability to learn the therapy, and concurrent treatment.

Application to Nursing Practice

- Perform an assessment on patient's and family's stress-management experiences. This provides a baseline for proactive strategies that have worked in the past (Gillespie and Gates, 2013).
- Identify readiness to begin structured meditation therapies such as yoga or MBSR. Patients must be ready and willing to be active participants in the therapy (Desiree et al., 2015).
- Assess patient's current lifestyle practices regarding exercise, nutrition, and relaxation activities. Determine his or her perception of these activities in managing stress (Doron et al., 2014).
- Reinforce to patient and family that these stress-management techniques are an addition to, not instead of, their current treatment.

exceed perceived resources. It is manifested as emotional exhaustion, poor decision making, loss of a sense of personal identity, and feelings of failure.

It is important that nurses participate in self-care practices. For example, in oncology settings nurses experience compassion fatigue. Effective strategies for compassion fatigue and how to help nurses deal with this phenomenon are available (see Chapter 1). Other clinical settings such as critical care, trauma, and emergency departments use resilience training and clinical debriefing to manage job-related stress and reduce burnout and nursing staff turnover (Ianello and Balzarotti, 2014; Mealer et al., 2014). Recognizing the impact of shift work and changes in schedules enables some managers and nurses to use self-scheduling techniques. This reduces job-related stress and improves sleep quality, collaboration, and teamwork (Lin et al., 2014).

Recognizing the areas over which you have control and can change and those for which you do not have responsibility is a vital insight. Making a clear separation between work and home life is also crucial. Strengthening friendships outside of the workplace, participating in creative activities for personal "recharging" of emotional energy, and spending off-duty hours in interesting activities all help reduce compassion fatigue.

Acute Care

Crisis Intervention. When stress overwhelms a person's usual coping mechanisms and demands mobilization of all available resources, it becomes a crisis. A crisis creates a turning point in a person's life because it changes the direction of his or her life in some way. The precipitating event usually occurs approximately 1 to 2 weeks before the individual seeks help, but sometimes it has occurred within the past 24 hours. Generally a person resolves the crisis in some way within approximately 6 weeks. Crisis intervention aims to return the person to a precrisis level of functioning and promote growth (Figure 38-7).

Because an individual's or family's usual coping strategies are ineffective in managing the stress of the precipitating event, the use of new coping mechanisms is necessary. This experience forces the use of unfamiliar strategies and results in either a heightened awareness of previously unrecognized strengths and resources or deterioration in functioning. Thus a crisis is often referred to as a situation of both danger and opportunity. Some individuals or families emerge from a crisis state functioning more effectively, whereas others find themselves weakened, and still others are completely dysfunctional.

Crisis intervention is a specific type of brief psychotherapy and has two specific goals. First is patient safety. Use external controls to protect the patient and others if the person is suicidal or homicidal. Second is anxiety reduction using techniques so a patient's inner resources are put into effect. It is more directive than traditional psychotherapy or counseling, and any member of the health care team who has been trained in its techniques can use it. The basic approach is problem solving, and it focuses only on the problem presented by the crisis (Varcarolis, 2013).

Help the patient make the mental connection between the stressful event and his or her reaction to it. This is crucial because he or she is sometimes unable to see the whole situation clearly. You also help the person become aware of present feelings such as anger, grief, or guilt to help him or her reduce feelings of tension. In addition, you help the patient explore coping mechanisms, perhaps identifying new methods of coping. Finally you help the person increase social contacts if he or she has been isolated and overly self-focused.

Restorative and Continuing Care. A person under stress recovers when the stress is removed or coping strategies are successful; however, a person who has experienced a crisis has changed, and the effects often last for years or for the rest of the person's life. The final stage of adapting to a crisis is acknowledgment of its long-term implications. If a person has coped with a crisis and its consequences successfully, he or she becomes more mature and healthy. When a person recovers from a stressful situation, the time is right for introducing stress-management skills to reduce the number and intensity of stressful situations in the future.

◆ Evaluation

Through the Patient's Eyes. A patient recovering from acute stress often spontaneously reports feeling better when the stressor is gone. The recovery from chronic stress occurs more gradually as the patient emerges from the strain. In either situation, evaluate the patient for the presence of new or recurring stress-related symptoms (Figure 38-8). Your evaluation must include the patient's perceptions. Ask the patient about sleep patterns, appetite, and ability to concentrate. Ask how the patient feels about coping strategies that are being used and

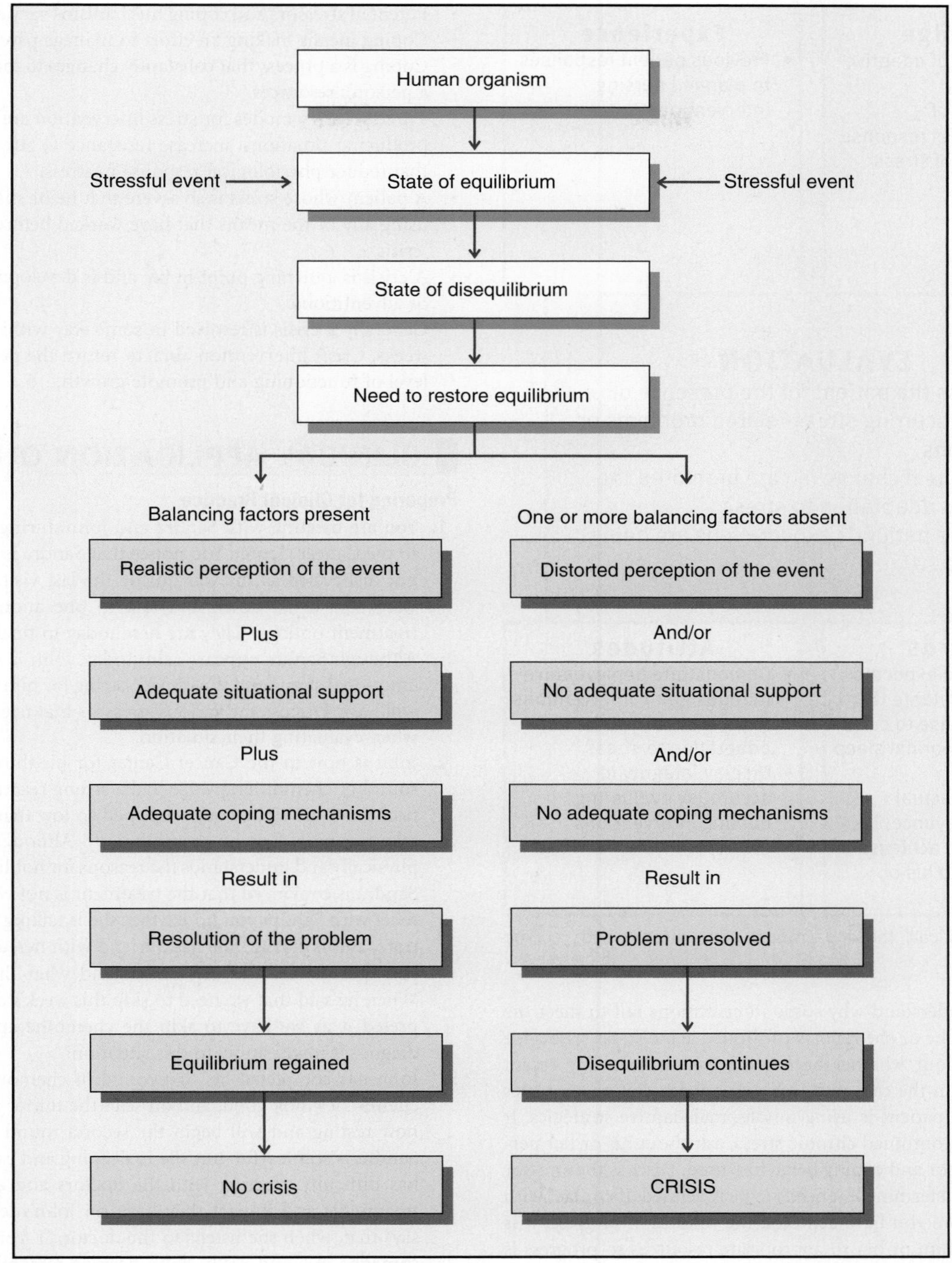

FIGURE 38-7 Crisis intervention model. (Redrawn from Aguilera DC: *Crisis intervention: theory and methodology,* ed 8, St Louis, 1998, Mosby.)

determine their effectiveness. Ask patients to compare current feelings and behaviors with feelings and behaviors 6 months ago. If desired outcomes have been met, the patient reports feeling better now than 6 months ago.

An essential part of the evaluation process is collaborating with patients to determine if their own expectations from nursing have been met. Any revision in the plan of care includes steps to address patient expectations.

Patient Outcomes. Remember that coping with stress takes time. Maintain ongoing communication with patients regarding their coping. Patients under severe stress or trauma often experience feelings of powerlessness, vulnerability, and loss of control. The nurse addresses these feelings by actively involving patients and families in the processes of re-examining problems, prioritizing, goal setting, and revising interventions. Involving patients in these processes gives them an opportunity to direct their energy in a positive way and moves them toward taking greater responsibility for health maintenance and promotion.

Engaging the patient as a partner in health care creates open communication. In such an environment the patient feels freer to give important feedback about interventions that are successful and helps

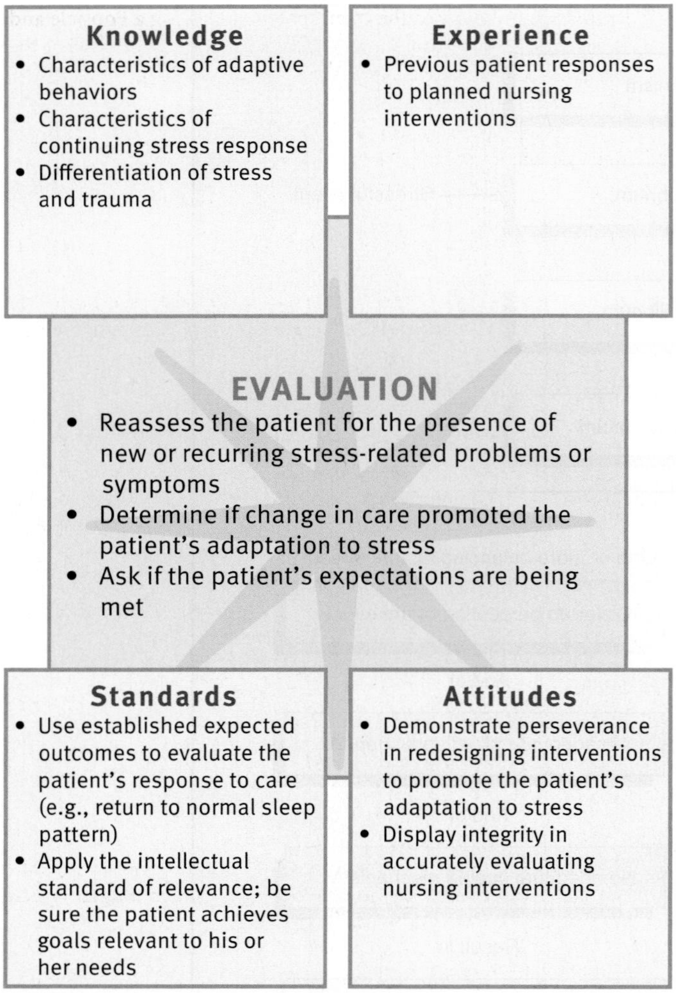

Knowledge
- Characteristics of adaptive behaviors
- Characteristics of continuing stress response
- Differentiation of stress and trauma

Experience
- Previous patient responses to planned nursing interventions

EVALUATION
- Reassess the patient for the presence of new or recurring stress-related problems or symptoms
- Determine if change in care promoted the patient's adaptation to stress
- Ask if the patient's expectations are being met

Standards
- Use established expected outcomes to evaluate the patient's response to care (e.g., return to normal sleep pattern)
- Apply the intellectual standard of relevance; be sure the patient achieves goals relevant to his or her needs

Attitudes
- Demonstrate perseverance in redesigning interventions to promote the patient's adaptation to stress
- Display integrity in accurately evaluating nursing interventions

FIGURE 38-8 Critical thinking model for stress and coping evaluation.

the nurse better understand why some interventions fail to meet the established goals. If he or she reports continued acute stress, assess for safety by asking about whether or not there have been any recent accidents at home, in the car, or at work. Ask about coping strategies to determine if the patient is using unsafe, maladaptive strategies. If the patient reports continued chronic stress, ask about his or her perception of the stressor and coping behaviors used. Discuss the stressor with the patient to determine if it needs to be redefined. If contact with a patient ends before you have achieved the resolution of goals, it is important to refer him or her to appropriate resources so progress is not delayed or interrupted.

KEY POINTS

- The GAS is an immediate physiological response of the whole body to stress and involves several body systems, especially the autonomic nervous and endocrine systems. Physiological responses to stress also include immunological changes.
- Stress can make people ill as a result of increased levels of powerful hormones that change bodily processes.
- A person is under psychological stress only if he or she evaluates the event as a threat or a circumstance as personally significant. Such an evaluation of an event for its personal meaning is called *primary appraisal.*
- Potential stressors and coping mechanisms vary across the life span.
- Coping means making an effort to manage psychological stress.
- Coping is a process that constantly changes to manage demands on a person's resources.
- Three primary modes for stress intervention are to decrease stress-producing situations, increase resistance to stress, and learn skills that reduce physiological response to stress.
- A patient whose stress is so severe that he or she is unable to cope using any of the means that have worked before is experiencing a crisis.
- A crisis is a turning point in life and is developmental, situational, or adventitious.
- Generally a crisis is resolved in some way within approximately 6 weeks. Crisis intervention aims to return the person to a precrisis level of functioning and promote growth.

CLINICAL APPLICATION QUESTIONS

Preparing for Clinical Practice

1. You are meeting with Sandra and John during their second visit to the Cancer Center. You notice that Sandra is well groomed and not disheveled as she was during the last visit. John and Sandra were able to sit down and talk to one another about various treatment options. They are here today to finalize their decision. Although Sandra appears calm today, John is worried about her emotional status and the impact caring for him during treatments will have. Discuss the various stressors that need to be considered when evaluating their situation.
2. John is now in the Cancer Center for his third dose of the first round of chemotherapy. He had a strong reaction to the medications, and his white count dropped so low that he was unable to take the next dose of chemotherapy. Although John feels good physically and understands the reasons for holding the next round, Sandra is convinced that the treatment is not working. When you meet with Sandra you notice that she is talking fast, can't concentrate, and is crying. She has a friend with her, and the friend tells you that Sandra did not understand what the oncologist said. When he said that we need to skip this week's dose, Sandra interpreted it as we have to skip the chemotherapy. Which nursing diagnoses might apply to this situation?
3. John has completed his first round of chemotherapy. His blood chemistries look good, and on scan the tumor is decreased. He is now resting and will begin the second round of chemotherapy. Sandra is still fearful, but she is sleeping and eating well. She still has difficulty meeting with the doctors and understanding the treatments and impact they have on John's level of health. She says that, when she listens to the doctor, "I feel like I'm watching someone else and really don't hear or remember many details." Which approach would be the best to take in planning for Sandra?

ⓔ *Answers to Clinical Application Questions can be found on the Evolve website.*

REVIEW QUESTIONS

Are You Ready to Test Your Nursing Knowledge?

1. When teaching a patient about the negative feedback response to stress, the nurse includes which of the following to describe the benefits of this stress response?
   1. Results in neurophysiological response
   2. Reduces body temperature

3. Causes a person to be hypervigilant
4. Reduces level of consciousness to conserve energy.

2. The nurse is interviewing a patient in the community clinic and gathers the following information about her: she is intermittently homeless, a single parent with two children who have developmental delays, and is suffering from chronic asthma. She does not laugh or smile, does not volunteer any information, and at times appears close to tears. She has no support system and does not work. She is experiencing an allostatic load. As a result, which of the following would be present during complete patient assessment? (Select all that apply.)
   1. Post-traumatic stress disorder
   2. Rising hormone levels
   3. Chronic illness
   4. Return of vital signs to normal
   5. Depression
3. A patient who is having difficulty managing his diabetes mellitus responds to the news that his hemoglobin A1C, a measure of blood sugar control over the past 90 days, has increased by saying, "The hemoglobin A1C is wrong. My blood sugar levels have been excellent for the last 6 months." Which defense mechanism is the patient using?
   1. Denial.
   2. Conversion.
   3. Dissociation.
   4. Displacement.
4. When doing an assessment of a young woman who was a victim of a home invasion 3 months earlier, the nurse learns that the woman has vivid images of the crash whenever she hears loud yelling or a sudden noise. The nurse recognizes this as ____________.
5. A grandfather living in Japan worries about his two young grandsons who disappeared after a tsunami. This is an example of:
   1. A situational crisis.
   2. A maturational crisis.
   3. An adventitious crisis.
   4. A developmental crisis.
6. During the assessment interview of an older woman who is recently widowed, the nurse suspects that this woman is experiencing a developmental crisis. Which of the following questions provide information about the impact of this crisis? (Select all that apply.)
   1. With whom do you talk on a routine basis?
   2. What do you do when you feel lonely?
   3. How is having diabetes affecting your life?
   4. I know this must be hard for you. Let me tell you what might help.
   5. Do you have any changes in lifestyle habits: sleeping, eating, smoking, and drinking?
7. The nurse plans care for a 16-year-old male, taking into consideration that stressors experienced most commonly by adolescents include which of the following?
   1. Loss of autonomy caused by health problems
   2. Physical appearance, family, friends, and school
   3. Self-esteem issues, changing family structure
   4. Search for identity with peer groups and separation from family
8. A 10-year-old girl was playing on a slide at a playground during a summer camp. She fell and broke her arm. The camp notified the parents and took the child to the emergency department according to the camp protocol for injuries. The parents arrive at the emergency department and are stressed and frantic. The 10-year-old is happy in the treatment room, eating a Popsicle and picking out the color of her cast. List in order of priority what the nurse should say to the parents?
   1. "Can I contact someone to help you?"
   2. "Your daughter is happy in the treatment room, eating a Popsicle and picking out the color of her cast."
   3. "I'll have the doctor come out and talk to you as soon as possible."
   4. "Let me help you two calm down a bit so I can take you to your daughter."
9. When assessing an older adult who is showing symptoms of anxiety, insomnia, anorexia, and mild confusion, one of the first assessments includes which of the following?
   1. The amount of family support
   2. A 3-day diet recall
   3. A thorough physical assessment
   4. Threats to safety in her home
10. After a health care provider has informed a patient that he has colon cancer, the nurse enters the room to find the patient gazing out the window in thought. Which of the following are appropriate responses or actions of the nurse? (Select all that apply.)
   1. "I know another patient whose colon cancer was cured by surgery."
   2. Straighten the patient's bed and room
   3. "Have you thought about how you are going to tell your family?"
   4. "Would you like for me to sit down with you for a few minutes so you can talk about this?"
   5. Sit quietly with the patient
11. A 34-year-old single father who is anxious, tearful, and tired from caring for his three young children tells the nurse that he feels depressed and doesn't see how he can go on much longer. Which of the following would be the nurse's best response?
   1. "Are you thinking of suicide?"
   2. "You've been doing a good job raising your children. You can do it!"
   3. "Is there someone who can help you during the evenings and weekends?"
   4. "What do you mean when you say you can't go on any longer?"
12. The nurse is evaluating the coping success of a patient experiencing stress from being newly diagnosed with multiple sclerosis and psychomotor impairment. Which of the following statements indicate that the patient is beginning to cope with the diagnosis? (Select all that apply.)
   1. "I'm going to learn to drive a car so I can be more independent."
   2. "My sister says she feels better when she goes shopping, so I'll go shopping."
   3. "I'm going to let the occupational therapist assess my home to improve efficiency."
   4. "I've always felt better when I go for a long walk. I'll do that when I get home."
   5. "I'm going to attend a support group to learn more about multiple sclerosis."
13. A patient with type 2 diabetes is experiencing a lot of work-related stress and is fearful of losing his job. In addition, his wife is threatening divorce. His blood sugar is elevating, and his doctors want him to attend some stress-management classes. He says, "My blood sugar can't be high because of my work stress." What causes blood glucose to rise during stress? (Select all that apply.)
   1. Increases in antidiuretic hormone (ADH)
   2. Increases in cortisol

3. Increases in aldosterone
4. Increases in adrenocorticotropic hormone (ACTH)
5. Increases in epinephrine

14. A staff nurse is talking with the nursing supervisor about the stress that she feels on the job. Which of the following are true about work-related stress? (Select all that apply.)
1. Job-related stress can affect the quality of patient care.
2. Stress can affect nurses' efficiency and decision making.
3. Nurses who talk about feeling stress are unprofessional and should calm down.
4. Nurses frequently experience stress with the rapid changes in health care technology.
5. Nurses cannot resolve job-related stress.

15. A crisis intervention nurse is working with a mother whose Down syndrome child has been hospitalized with pneumonia and who has lost her child's disability payment while the child is hospitalized. The mother worries that her daughter will fall behind in special-school classes during hospitalization. Which strategies are effective in helping this mother cope with these stressors? (Select all that apply.)
1. Referral to social service process reestablishing the child's disability payment
2. Sending the child home in 72 hours and having the child return to school
3. Coordinating hospital-based and home-based schooling with the child's teacher
4. Teaching the mother signs and symptoms of a respiratory tract infection
5. Telling the mother that the stress will decrease in 6 weeks when everything is back to normal

Answers: 1. 1; **2.** 3, 5; **3.** 1; **4.** Post-traumatic stress disorder (PTSD); **5.** 3; **6.** 1, 2, 5; **7.** 4; **8.** 2, 4, 3, 1; **9.** 3; **10.** 4, 5; **11.** 4; **12.** 3, 5; **13.** 2, 4, 5; **14.** 1, 2, 4; **15.** 1, 3, 4.

Rationales for Review Questions can be found on the Evolve website.

REFERENCES

American Nurses Association (ANA): *Psychiatric–mental health nursing: scope and standards of practice*, ed 2, Silver Spring, MD, 2014, ANA.

Diamond JW: Allostatic medicine: bringing stress, coping, and chronic disease into focus, Part 1, *Integr Med* 8(6):40, 2009/2010.

Giger J: *Transcultural nursing*, ed 6, St Louis, 2012, Mosby.

Huether SE, McCance KL: *Understanding pathophysiology*, ed 5, St Louis, 2012, Mosby.

Ianello P, Balzarotti S: Stress and coping strategies in the emergency room, *Emerg Care J* 10:72, 2014.

Lazarus RS: Stress and emotion: a new synthesis. In Monat A, et al, editors: *The Praeger handbook on stress and coping*, Westport, CN, 2007, Praeger.

Neuman B, Fawcett J, editors: *The Neuman Systems Model*, ed 5, Upper Saddle River, NJ, 2011, Pearson.

O'Driscoll MP: Coping with stress: a challenge for theory, research, and practice, *Stress Health* 29(2):89, 2013.

Pender NJ, et al: *Health promotion in nursing practice*, ed 6, Upper Saddle River, NJ, 2013, Pearson Education.

Santos L: Stress response in critical illness, *Curr Probl Pediatr Adolesc Health Care* 43:264, 2013.

Varcarolis EM: *Essentials of psychiatric mental health nursing*, revised reprint, ed 2, St Louis, 2013, Mosby.

RESEARCH REFERENCES

Akerstedt T, et al: Do sleep, stress, and illness explain daily variations in fatigue? A prospective study, *J Psychosom Res* 76:280, 2014.

Desiree GM, et al: Mindfulness-based stress reduction for lung cancer patients and their partners: results of a mixed methods pilot study, *Palliat Med* 29:652, 2015.

Doron J, et al: Coping profiles, perceived stress and health-related behaviors: a cluster analysis approach, *Health Promot Int* 30:88, 2014.

Gillespie GL, Gates DM: Using proactive coping to manage the stress of trauma patient care, *J Trauma Nurs* 20:44, 2013.

Janowski K, et al: Emotional control, styles of coping with stress and acceptance of illness among patients suffering from chronic somatic disease, *Stress Health* 30:34, 2014.

Lengacher CA, et al: Mindfulness-based stress reduction (MBSR (BC)) in breast cancer: evaluating fear of recurrence (FOR) as a mediator of psychological and physical symptoms in a randomized control trial (RCT), *J Behav Med* 37:185(2), 2014.

Lin SH, et al: The impact of shift work on nurses' job stress, sleep quality and self-perceived health status, *J Nurs Manag* 22(5):604, 2014.

Mealer M, et al: Feasibility and acceptability of a resilience training program for intensive care unit nurses, *Am J Crit Care* 23:97, 2014.

Moreia S, et al: Combined exercise circuit session acutely attenuates stress-induced blood pressure reactivity in health adults, *Braz J Phys Ther* 18:38, 2014.

Nielsen MB, Knardahl S: Coping strategies: a prospective study of patterns, stability, and relationships with physiological distress, *Scand J Psychol* 55:142, 2014.

Oken BS, et al: Pilot controlled trial of mindfulness meditation and education for dementia caregivers, *J Altern Complement Med* 16:1031, 2010.

Okonta NR: Does Yoga therapy reduce blood pressure in patients with hypertension? An integrative review, *Holist Nurs Pract* 26(3):137, 2012.

Parelkar P, et al: Stress coping and changes in health behavior among cancer survivors: a report from the American Cancer Society's study of cancer survivors II (SCS-II), *J Psychosoc Oncol* 31:136, 2013.

Park CL, Iacocca MO: A stress and coping perspective on health behaviors: theoretical and methodological considerations, *Anxiety Stress Coping* 27:123, 2014.

Rayens MK, Reed DB: Predictors of depressive symptoms in older rural couples: the impact of work, stress, and health, *J Rural Health* 30:59, 2014.

Ruppar TM, Conn VS: Interventions to promote physical activity in chronically ill adults, *Am J Nurs* 110(7):30, 2010.

Stevens D, et al: Posttraumatic stress disorder increase risk for suicide attempt in adults with recurrent major depression, *Depress Anxiety* 30:940, 2013.

Yancura LA, Aldwin CM: Coping and health in older adults, *Curr Psychiatry Rep* 10:10, 2008.

Activity and Exercise

OBJECTIVES

- Describe the role of the musculoskeletal and nervous systems in the regulation of activity and exercise.
- Discuss the influence of immobility on body alignment, joint movement, and activity.
- Discuss implications for preventing deconditioning and deep vein thrombosis in hospitalized inpatients.
- Describe the evidence that supports regular activity and exercise in patient care.
- Describe how to maintain and use proper body mechanics.
- Describe important factors to consider when planning an exercise program for patients across the life span and for those with specific chronic illnesses.
- Describe how to assess patients for activity intolerance.
- Formulate nursing diagnoses for patients experiencing problems with activity intolerance.
- Develop an individualized nursing care plan for a patient with activity intolerance.
- Discuss the importance of no-lift policies for patients and health care providers.
- Describe equipment needed for safe patient handling and movement.
- Discuss the impact of national patient safety resources, initiatives, and regulations in relation to patient handling and movement.
- Evaluate the nursing care plan for maintaining activity and exercise for patients across the life span and with specific chronic illnesses.

KEY TERMS

Activities of daily living (ADLs), p. 788
Antagonistic muscles, p. 790
Antigravity muscles, p. 790
Cartilage, p. 789
Cartilaginous joints, p. 789
Center of gravity, p. 788
Concentric tension, p. 789
Crutch gait, p. 807
Deconditioning, p. 787
Eccentric tension, p. 790
Fibrous joints, p. 789
Footboards, p. 788
Isometric contraction, p. 790
Isotonic contraction, p. 790
Joint, p. 789
Ligaments, p. 789
Muscle tone, p. 790
Proprioception, p. 791
Synergistic muscles, p. 790
Synovial joints, p. 789
Tendons, p. 789
Unossified, p. 789

MEDIA RESOURCES

http://evolve.elsevier.com/Potter/fundamentals/

- Review Questions
- Video Clips
- Concept Map Creator
- Case Study with Questions
- Audio Glossary
- Content Updates

Regular physical activity and exercise contribute to patients' physical and emotional well-being (Edelman et al., 2013; Esposito and Fitzpatrick, 2011). This is a principle that you, as a nurse, should apply in the care of patients in all settings. Functional decline (the loss of the ability to perform self-care or activities of daily living) may result not only from illness or adverse treatment effects but also from **deconditioning** associated with inactivity, the negative effects of which can be seen after short periods of time. Deconditioning involves physiological changes following a period of inactivity, bed rest, or sedentary lifestyle. It is a particular risk for hospitalized patients who spend most of their time in bed, even when they are able to walk. As a result, nurses play an important role in increasing the overall activity of inpatients to minimize the risk of deconditioning.

A program of regular physical activity and exercise has the potential to enhance all aspects of a patient's health. This chapter provides you with knowledge of exercise and activity as they relate to health promotion, the acute phase of illness, and the restorative and continuing care of patients. Applying knowledge about exercise and activity will allow you to plan nursing strategies for patients' individualized exercise and activity programs. Knowing the movements and functions of muscles in maintaining posture and movement and implementing evidence-based knowledge about safe patient handling are essential to protecting the safety of both the patient and the nurse (see Chapter 28).

SCIENTIFIC KNOWLEDGE BASE

Regular physical activity and exercise contribute to both physical and emotional well-being (Edelman et al., 2013; Esposito and Fitzpatrick, 2011). Knowing the physiology and regulation of body mechanics, exercise, and activity helps provide individualized patient care.

Overview of Exercise and Activity

The coordinated efforts of the musculoskeletal and nervous systems maintain balance, posture, and body alignment during lifting, bending, moving, and performing activities of daily living (ADLs). Proper balance, posture, and body alignment reduce the risk of injury to the musculoskeletal system and facilitate body movements, allowing physical mobility without muscle strain and excessive use of muscle energy (see Chapter 28).

Body Alignment. Body alignment refers to the relationship of one body part to another along a horizontal or vertical line. Correct alignment involves positioning so no excessive strain is placed on a person's joints, tendons, ligaments, or muscles, thereby maintaining adequate muscle tone and contributing to balance (see Chapter 28).

Body Balance. Body balance occurs when a relatively low center of gravity is balanced over a wide, stable base of support and a vertical line falls from the center of gravity through the base of support. When the vertical line from the center of gravity does not fall through the base of support, the body loses balance. Proper posture or a body position that most favors function, requires the least muscular work to maintain, and places the least strain on muscles, ligaments, and bones to enhance body balance (Patton and Thibodeau, 2012). Nurses rely on balance to maintain proper body alignment and posture through two simple techniques: (1) widening the base of support by separating the feet to a comfortable distance, and (2) increasing balance by bringing the center of gravity closer to the base of support. For example, you raise the height of a hospital bed when performing a procedure such as changing a dressing to prevent bending too far at the waist and shifting the base of support.

Coordinated Body Movement. Coordinated body movement is a result of weight, center of gravity, and balance. Weight is the force exerted on a body by gravity. When an object is lifted, the lifter must overcome the weight of the object and be aware of its center of gravity. In symmetrical objects the center of gravity is located at the exact center of the object. The force of weight is always directed downward. An unbalanced object has its center of gravity away from the midline and falls without support. Because people are not geometrically perfect, their centers of gravity are usually midline, at 55% to 57% of standing height. Like unbalanced objects, patients who are unsteady do not maintain a balance with their center of gravity, which places them at risk for falling. You need to be able to identify these patients and intervene to maintain their safety.

Friction. Friction is a force that occurs in a direction to oppose movement. It increases a patient's risk for skin and tissue damage and potential pressure ulcers (see Chapter 48). Reduce friction by following some basic principles. When you move objects, those with a greater surface area create more friction. To reduce friction, you need to decrease the surface area of the object. For example, when helping patients move up in bed, place their arms across the chest. This decreases surface area and reduces friction (see Chapter 28).

A patient who is passive or immobilized produces greater friction to movement. When possible, use some of your patients' strength and mobility when positioning and transferring them. Explain the procedure and tell your patients when to move. You decrease friction when your patients bend their knees as you help them move up in the bed.

Exercise and Activity. Exercise is physical activity that conditions the body, improves health, and maintains fitness. Sometimes it is also a therapeutic measure. A patient's individualized exercise program depends on any health-related physical limitations, his or her activity tolerance, and the type and amount of exercise or activity that he or she is able to perform. Physiological, emotional, and developmental factors influence a patient's activity tolerance.

An active lifestyle is important for maintaining and promoting health; it is also an essential treatment for chronic illnesses (Combs et al., 2013). Regular physical activity and exercise enhance functioning of all body systems, including cardiopulmonary functioning (endurance), musculoskeletal fitness (flexibility and bone integrity), weight control and maintenance (body image), and psychological well-being (Edelman et al., 2013).

The best program of physical activity includes a combination of exercises that produces different physiological and psychological benefits. Three categories of exercise are isotonic, isometric, and resistive isometric. The type of muscle contraction involved determines the classification of the exercise. Isotonic exercises cause muscle contraction and change in muscle length (isotonic contraction) (see Chapter 28). Examples are walking, swimming, dance aerobics, jogging, bicycling, and moving arms and legs with light resistance. Isotonic exercises enhance circulatory and respiratory functioning; increase muscle mass, tone, and strength; and promote osteoblastic activity (activity by bone-forming cells), thus combating osteoporosis.

Isometric exercises involve tightening or tensing muscles without moving body parts (isometric contraction) (see Chapter 28). Examples are quadriceps set exercises and contraction of the gluteal muscles. This form of exercise is ideal for patients who do not tolerate increased activity. A patient who is immobilized in bed can perform isometric exercises. The benefits are increased muscle mass, tone, and strength, thus decreasing the potential for muscle wasting; increased circulation to the involved body part; and increased osteoblastic activity.

Resistive isometric exercises are those in which an individual contracts the muscle while pushing against a stationary object or resisting the movement of an object (Resnick et al., 2012). A gradual increase in the amount of resistance and length of time that the muscle contraction is held increases muscle strength and endurance. Examples of resistive isometric exercises are push-ups and hip lifting, in which a patient in a sitting position pushes with the hands against a surface such as a chair seat and raises the hips. In some long-term care settings footboards are placed on the end of beds; patients push against them to move up in bed. Resistive isometric exercises help promote muscle strength and provide sufficient stress against bone to promote osteoblastic activity.

Regulation of Movement

Coordinated body movement involves the integrated functioning of the skeletal, muscular, and nervous systems. Because these three systems cooperate so closely in mechanical support of the body, they are often considered as a single functional unit.

Skeletal System. Firmness of the skeleton of the body results from inorganic salts such as calcium and phosphate that are in the bone matrix. It is related to the rigidity of the bone, which is necessary to keep bones straight and enables them to withstand weight bearing. Elasticity and skeletal flexibility change with age. For example, the newborn has a large amount of cartilage and is highly flexible but is unable to support weight. The toddler's bones are more pliable than those of an older person and are better able to withstand falls. Older adults, especially women, are more susceptible to bone loss (resorption) and osteoporosis, which increase the risk of fractures.

Bones perform five functions in the body: support, protection, movement, mineral storage, and hematopoiesis (blood cell formation). In the discussion of body mechanics, two of these functions (i.e.,

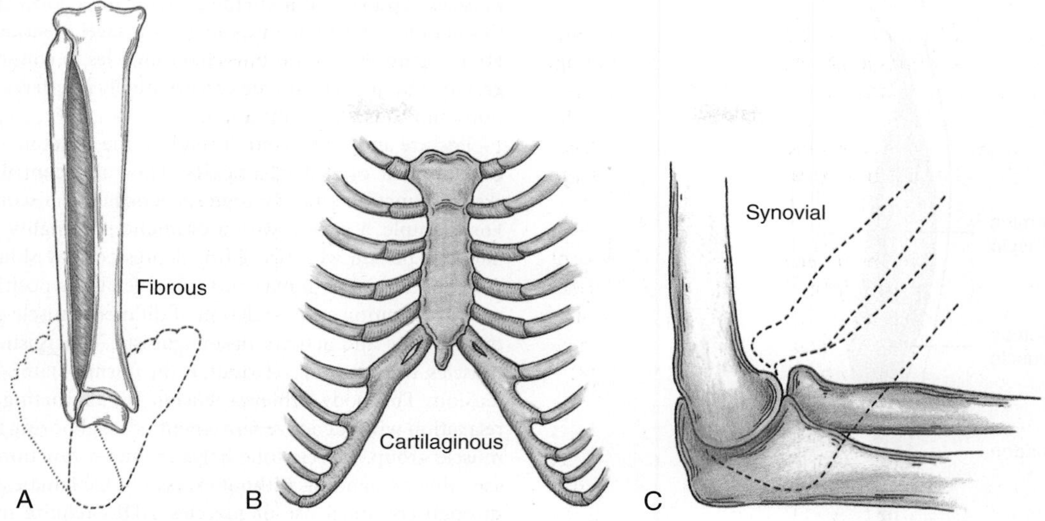

FIGURE 39-1 Joint types. **A,** Fibrous. **B,** Cartilaginous. **C,** Synovial.

support and movement) are most important (see Chapter 28). Bones serve as support by providing the framework and contributing to the shape, alignment, and positioning of the body parts. Bones, together with their joints, constitute levers for muscle attachment to provide movement. As muscles contract and shorten, they pull on bones, producing joint movement (Patton and Thibodeau, 2012).

Joints. An articulation, or joint, is the connection between bones. Each joint is classified according to its structure and degree of mobility. On the basis of connective structures, joints are classified as fibrous, cartilaginous, or synovial (Huether and McCance, 2012). Fibrous joints fit closely together and are fixed, permitting little, if any, movement such as the syndesmosis between the tibia and fibula (Figure 39-1, *A*). Cartilaginous joints have little movement but are elastic and use cartilage to unite separate bony surfaces such as the synchondrosis that attaches the ribs to the costal cartilage. When bone growth is complete, the joints ossify (see Figure 39-1, *B*). Synovial joints, or true joints, such as the hinge type at the elbow, are freely movable and the most mobile, numerous, and anatomically complex body joints (see Figure 39-1, *C*).

Ligaments, Tendons, and Cartilage. Ligaments, tendons, and cartilage support the skeletal system (see Chapter 28). Ligaments are white, shiny, flexible bands of fibrous tissue that bind joints and connect bones and cartilage. They are elastic and aid joint flexibility and support (Figure 39-2).

In addition, some ligaments serve a protective function. For example, ligaments between the vertebral bodies and the ligamentum flavum prevent damage to the spinal cord during movement of the back. Tendons are white, glistening, fibrous bands of tissue that occur in various lengths and thicknesses. They are strong, flexible, and inelastic as they serve to connect muscle to bone. The Achilles tendon (tendo calcaneus) is the thickest and strongest tendon in the body. It begins near the midposterior of the leg and attaches the gastrocnemius and soleus muscles in the calf to the calcaneal bone in the back of the foot (Figure 39-3).

Cartilage is nonvascular, supporting connective tissue with the flexibility of a firm, plastic material. Because of its gristlelike nature, cartilage sustains weight and serves as a shock absorber between articulating bones. Permanent cartilage is unossified (not hardened), except in advanced age and diseases such as osteoarthritis, which impairs mobility.

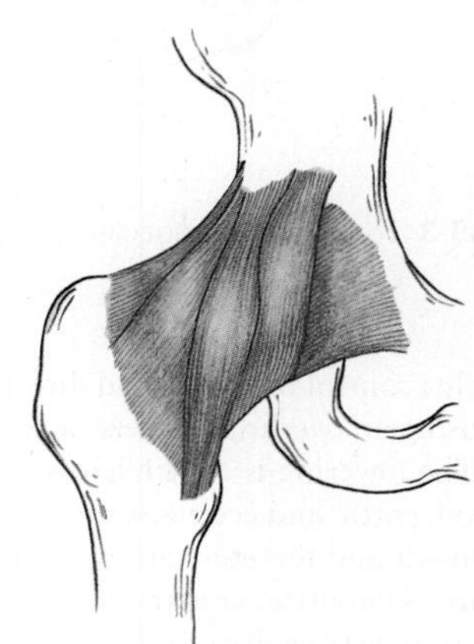

FIGURE 39-2 Ligaments of hip joint.

Strength and flexibility do not result entirely from joints, ligaments, tendons, and cartilage. Adequate skeletal muscle is also necessary.

Skeletal Muscle. Muscles are made of fibers that contract when stimulated by an electrochemical impulse that travels from the nerve to the muscle across the neuromuscular junction. The electrochemical impulse causes the filaments (predominantly protein molecules of myosin and actin) within the fiber to slide past one another, with the filaments changing length.

Contraction of skeletal muscles allows people to walk, talk, run, breathe, or participate in physical activity. There are more than 600 skeletal muscles in the body. In addition to facilitating movement, these muscles determine the form and contour of our bodies. Most of our muscles span at least one joint and attach to both articulating bones. When contraction occurs, one bone is fixed while the other moves. The origin is the point of attachment that remains still; the insertion is the point that moves when the muscle contracts (Patton and Thibodeau, 2012).

Muscle contractions are categorized by functional purpose: moving, resisting, or stabilizing body parts. In concentric tension increased muscle contraction causes muscle shortening, resulting in movement such as when a patient uses an overhead trapeze to pull up in bed.

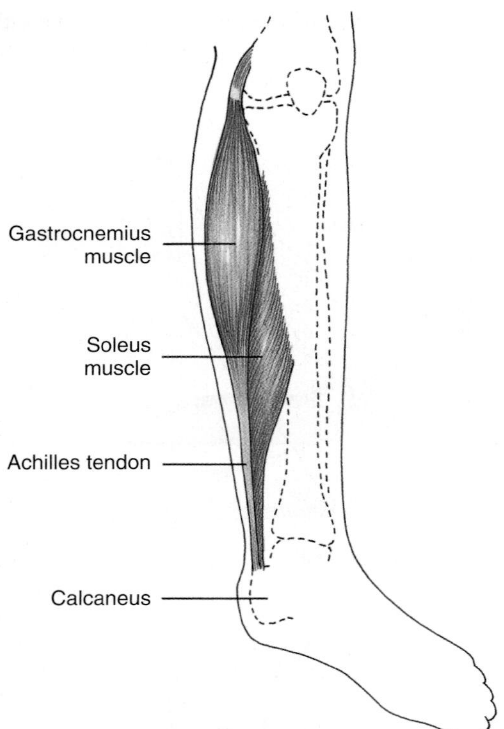

FIGURE 39-3 Tendons and muscles of lower leg.

Eccentric tension helps control the speed and direction of movement. For example, when using an overhead trapeze, a patient slowly lowers himself to the bed. The lowering is controlled when the antagonistic muscles lengthen. Concentric and eccentric muscle actions are necessary for active movement and therefore are referred to as dynamic or isotonic contraction. Isometric contraction (static contraction) causes an increase in muscle tension or muscle work but no shortening or active movement of the muscle (e.g., instructing a patient to tighten and relax a muscle group, as in quadriceps set exercises or pelvic floor exercises). Voluntary movement is a combination of isotonic and isometric contractions.

Although isometric contractions do not result in muscle shortening, energy expenditure increases. This type of muscle work is comparable to having a car in neutral with the driver continually depressing the accelerator and racing the engine. The driver is not going anywhere but expends a large amount of energy. It is important to understand the energy expenditure (increased respiratory rate and increased work on the heart) associated with isometric exercises because the exercises are sometimes contraindicated in certain patients' illnesses (e.g., myocardial infarction [MI] or chronic obstructive pulmonary disease [COPD]).

Muscles Concerned with Movement. The muscles of movement are located near the skeletal region, where a lever system causes movement (Patton and Thibodeau, 2012). The lever system makes the work of moving a weight or load easier. It occurs when specific bones such as the humerus, ulna, and radius and the associated joints such as the elbow act as a lever. Thus the force applied to one end of the bone to lift a weight at another point tends to rotate the bone in the direction opposite that of the applied force. Muscles that attach to bones of leverage provide the necessary strength to move an object.

Muscles Concerned with Posture. Gravity continually pulls on parts of the body; the only way the body is held in position is for muscles to pull on bones in the opposite direction. Muscles accomplish this counterforce by maintaining a low level of sustained contraction. Poor posture places more work on muscles to counteract the force of gravity. This leads to fatigue and eventually interferes with bodily functions and causes deformities.

Posture and movement depend on the skeleton and the shape and development of skeletal muscles. They also contribute to musculoskeletal function and often reflect personality, discomfort, and mood. For example, a person with a dramatic personality gestures with the hands, a person who is tired or depressed may slouch, and a person with abdominal pain may curl into a fetal-like position.

Coordination and regulation of different muscle groups depend on muscle tone and activity of antagonistic, synergistic, and antigravity muscles. Muscle tone, or tonus, is the normal state of balanced muscle tension. The body achieves tension by alternating contraction and relaxation without active movement of neighboring fibers of a specific muscle group. Muscle tone helps maintain functional positions such as sitting or standing without excess muscle fatigue and is maintained through continual use of muscles. ADLs require muscle action and help maintain muscle tone. When a patient is immobile or on prolonged bed rest, activity level, activity tolerance, and muscle tone decrease.

Muscle Groups. The nervous system coordinates the antagonistic, synergistic, and antigravity muscle groups that are responsible for maintaining posture and initiating movement. Antagonistic muscles cause movement at a joint. During movement the active mover muscle contracts while its antagonist relaxes. For example, during flexion of the arm the active mover, the biceps brachii, contracts; and its antagonist, the triceps brachii, relaxes. During extension of the arm the active mover, now the triceps brachii, contracts; and the new antagonist, the biceps brachii, relaxes.

Synergistic muscles contract to accomplish the same movement. When the arm is flexed, the strength of the contraction of the biceps brachii is increased by contraction of the synergistic muscle, the brachialis. Thus with synergistic muscle activity there are now two active movers (i.e., the biceps brachii and the brachialis), which contract while the antagonistic muscle, the triceps brachii, relaxes.

Antigravity muscles stabilize joints. These muscles continuously oppose the effect of gravity on the body and permit a person to maintain an upright or sitting posture. In an adult the antigravity muscles are the extensors of the leg, the gluteus maximus, the quadriceps femoris, the soleus muscles, and the muscles of the back.

Skeletal muscles support posture and carry out voluntary movement. The muscles are attached to the skeleton by tendons, which provide strength and permit motion. The movement of the extremities is voluntary and requires coordination from the nervous system.

Nervous System. The nervous system regulates movement and posture. The major voluntary motor area, located in the cerebral cortex, is the precentral gyrus, or motor strip. A majority of motor fibers descend from the motor strip and cross at the level of the medulla. Thus the motor fibers from the right motor strip initiate voluntary movement for the left side of the body, and motor fibers from the left motor strip initiate voluntary movement for the right side of the body.

Transmission of the impulse from the nervous system to the musculoskeletal system is an electrochemical event and requires a neurotransmitter. Basically neurotransmitters are chemicals (e.g., acetylcholine) that transfer the electrical impulse from the nerve across the myoneural junction to stimulate the muscle, causing movement. Several disorders impair movement. For example, Parkinson's disease alters neurotransmitter production, myasthenia gravis disrupts transfer from the neurotransmitter to the muscle, and multiple sclerosis impairs muscle activity (Huether and McCance, 2012).

Proprioception. Proprioception is the awareness of the position of the body and its parts (Huether and McCance, 2012). Proprioceptors, which monitor body position, are located on nerve endings in muscles, tendons, and joints. The nervous system regulates posture, which requires coordination of proprioception and balance. As a person carries out ADLs, proprioceptors monitor muscle activity and body position. For example, the proprioceptors on the soles of the feet contribute to correct posture while standing or walking. In standing, pressure is continuous on the bottom of the feet. The proprioceptors monitor the pressure, communicating this information through the nervous system to the antigravity muscles. The standing person remains upright until deciding to change position. As a person walks, the proprioceptors on the bottom of the feet monitor pressure changes. Thus, when the bottom of the moving foot comes in contact with the walking surface, the individual automatically moves the stationary foot forward.

Balance. A person needs adequate balance to stand, run, lift, or perform ADLs. The nervous system controls balance specifically through the cerebellum and the inner ear. The cerebellum coordinates all voluntary movement, particularly highly skilled movements such as those required in skiing.

Within the inner ear are the semicircular canals, three fluid-filled structures that help maintain balance. Fluid within the canals has certain inertia; when the head is suddenly rotated in one direction, the fluid remains stationary for a moment, but the canal turns with the head. This allows a person to change position suddenly without losing balance.

Principles of Transfer and Positioning Techniques

Using principles of safe patient transfer and positioning during routine activities decreases work effort and places less strain on musculoskeletal structures (Box 39-1). As a nurse you will teach colleagues and patients' families how to transfer or position patients properly. Teaching a patient's family how to transfer the patient from bed to chair increases and reinforces the family's knowledge about proper transfer and position techniques once the patient returns home.

Whether you are moving a patient who is immobile, helping a patient from the bed to the chair, or teaching a patient to carry out ADLs efficiently, knowledge of safe patient transfer and positioning is crucial. You also incorporate knowledge of physiological and pathological influences on body alignment and mobility.

BOX 39-1 Principles of Safe Patient Transfer and Positioning

- Mechanical lifts and lift teams are essential when a patient is unable to assist.
- When a patient is able to assist, remember the following principles:
  - The wider the base of support, the greater the stability of the nurse.
  - The lower the center of gravity, the greater the stability of the nurse.
  - The equilibrium of an object is maintained as long as the line of gravity passes through its base of support.
  - Facing the direction of movement prevents abnormal twisting of the spine.
  - Dividing balanced activity between arms and legs reduces the risk of back injury.
  - Leverage, rolling, turning, or pivoting requires less work than lifting.
  - When friction is reduced between the object to be moved and the surface on which it is moved, less force is required to move it.

Pathological Influences on Body Alignment, Mobility, and Activity. Many pathological conditions affect body alignment and mobility. These conditions include congenital defects; disorders of bones, joints, and muscles; central nervous system damage; and musculoskeletal trauma.

Congenital Defects. Congenital abnormalities affect the efficiency of the musculoskeletal system in regard to alignment, balance, and appearance. Osteogenesis imperfecta is an inherited disorder that affects bone. Bones are porous, short, bowed, and deformed; as a result, children experience curvature of the spine and shortness of stature (Chapter 28). Scoliosis is a structural curvature of the spine associated with vertebral rotation. Muscles, ligaments, and other soft tissues become shortened. Balance and mobility are affected in proportion to the severity of abnormal spinal curvatures (Hockenberry and Wilson, 2015).

Disorders of Bones, Joints, and Muscles. Osteoporosis, a well-known and well-publicized disorder of aging, results in the reduction of bone density or mass. The bone remains biochemically normal but has difficulty maintaining integrity and support. The cause is uncertain, and theories vary from hormonal imbalances to insufficient intake of nutrients (Huether and McCance, 2012).

Osteomalacia is an uncommon metabolic disease characterized by inadequate and delayed mineralization, resulting in compact and spongy bone (Lewis et al., 2013). Mineral calcification and deposition do not occur. Replaced bone consists of soft material rather than rigid bone.

Joint mobility is altered by inflammatory and noninflammatory joint diseases and articular disruption. Inflammatory joint disease (e.g., arthritis) is characterized by inflammation or destruction of the synovial membrane and articular cartilage and systemic signs of inflammation. Noninflammatory diseases have none of these characteristics, and the synovial fluid is normal (Huether and McCance, 2012). Joint degeneration, which can occur with inflammatory and noninflammatory disease, is marked by changes in articular cartilage combined with overgrowth of bone at the articular ends. Degenerative changes commonly affect weight-bearing joints.

Articular disruption involves trauma to the articular capsules and ranges from mild, such as a tear resulting in a sprain, to severe, such as a separation leading to dislocation. Articular disruption usually results from trauma but sometimes is congenital, as with developmental dysplasia of the hip (Hockenberry and Wilson, 2015).

Central Nervous System Damage. Damage to any part of the central nervous system that regulates voluntary movement causes impaired body alignment and immobility (see Chapter 28). For example, a patient with a traumatic head injury experiences damage in the motor strip in the cerebrum. The amount of voluntary motor impairment is directly related to the amount of destruction of the motor strip. Another patient with a spinal cord injury has permanent damage below the level of the injury and has control of trunk muscles but not the lower-extremity muscles. This patient also experiences reflex and spastic movements.

It is important to understand which type of voluntary and involuntary movement is present after damage to the central nervous system. This information impacts the type of interventions selected to maximize your patient's activity level.

Musculoskeletal Trauma. Musculoskeletal trauma often results in bruises, contusions, sprains, and fractures. A fracture is a disruption of bone tissue continuity. Fractures most commonly result from direct external trauma. They also occur because of some deformity of the bone (e.g., with pathological fractures of osteoporosis) (see Chapter 28).

NURSING KNOWLEDGE BASE

Application of nursing knowledge about activity and exercise allows you to think critically about the holistic needs of patients. Nursing knowledge as it pertains to activity and exercise helps you assess, identify, and intervene when patients have decreased activity tolerance or physical limitation that affects their mobility and/or ability to exercise (Chapter 28).

Deconditioning

Recently concerted effort has been made in hospitals to increase inpatients' activity and mobility levels as soon as possible to prevent deconditioning and other complications of immobilization. The American Association of Critical Care Nurses (2015) now recommends an early progressive mobility protocol for critical care patients (refer to agency policy for protocols used by hospital). However, when patients are transferred out to general nursing units, early mobility protocols should continue. This is often a challenge because staff nurses on general units often have difficulty routinely ambulating patients due to overall patient care demands, access to equipment, or unfamiliarity with transfer skills. Some hospitals have designated special mobility teams or mobility assistants to engage patients in early ambulation and activity.

In a study involving 78 adults who were admitted to a respiratory unit for diagnostic or preoperative evaluation and who were able to walk and were not confined to bed rest, functional capacity decreased over a 5-day period in six assessment areas: upper limb muscle strength, respiratory muscle strength, lung function, chest wall expansion, submaximal exercise tolerance, and spinal and trunk mobility. Longer periods of hospitalization inevitably led to more severe deconditioning (Suesada et al., 2007). These findings support the promotion of early mobility in hospitalized patients.

Safe Patient Handling

Nurses are exposed to the hazards related to lifting and transferring patients in many settings such as inpatient nursing units, long-term care facilities, and the operating room (Griffis, 2012). Manually lifting and transferring patients contributes to the high incidence of work-related musculoskeletal problems and back injuries in nurses and other health care staff. Current evidence shows that many nurses frequently transfer to different positions and leave the profession because of work-related injuries (Griffis, 2012). Implementing evidence-based interventions and programs (e.g., lift teams) reduces the number of work-related injuries, which improves the health of the nurse and reduces indirect costs to the health care agency (e.g., workers' compensation and replacing injured workers).

Today many states have laws that mandate safe patient handling in health care agencies. Health care agencies are implementing comprehensive safe patient–handling programs in all parts of the United States. Comprehensive safe patient–handling programs include the following elements (VISN8, 2015):

- An ergonomics assessment protocol for health care environments
- Patient assessment criteria and algorithms for patient handling and movement
- Special equipment kept in convenient locations to help transfer patients
- Back-injury resource nurses
- An "after-action review" that allows the health care team to apply knowledge about moving patients safely in different settings
- A no-lift policy

Transfer Techniques. Nurses often provide care for immobilized patients whose position must be changed, who must be moved up in bed, or who must be transferred from a bed to a chair or from a bed to a stretcher. As noted earlier, body mechanics alone do not protect nurses from injury to their musculoskeletal systems when moving, lifting, or transferring patients. Although nurses use many transfer techniques, knowledge of ergonomics and safe patient handling is crucial in maintaining caregiver and patient safety.

Assess every situation that involves patient handling and movement to minimize risk of injury. After completing the assessment, you will use an algorithm (Figures 39-4 to 39-6) to guide decisions about safe patient handling (VISN8, 2015). Skill 39-1 on pp. 811-818 describes the steps commonly used in transferring patients safely and effectively. Use a patient's strength when lifting, transferring, or moving when possible. Involving the patient has the added bonus of increasing participation in self-care, thus promoting a sense of accomplishment. In addition to handling patients safely, nurses need to assume an active role in their workplaces to ensure that a culture of safety exists and that appropriate patient-handling equipment is readily available (Hunter et al., 2010).

Factors Influencing Activity and Exercise

Factors influencing activity and exercise include developmental changes, behavioral aspects, environmental issues, family and social support, and cultural and ethnic origin. Consider these areas of knowledge and incorporate into the plan of care whether a patient is seeking health promotion, acute care, or restorative and continuing care.

Developmental Changes. Throughout the life span the appearance and functioning of the body undergo change. The greatest change and effect on the maturational process occur in childhood and old age.

Infants Through School-Age Children. A newborn infant's spine is flexed and lacks the anteroposterior curves of the adult. The first spinal curve occurs when the infant extends the neck from the prone position. As growth and stability increase, the thoracic spine straightens; and the lumbar spinal curve appears, which allows rolling over, sitting, crawling, and standing.

A toddler's posture is awkward because of the slight swayback and protruding abdomen. As the child walks, the legs and feet are usually far apart, and the feet are slightly everted (turned outward). Toward the end of toddlerhood, posture appears less awkward, curves in the cervical and lumbar vertebrae are accentuated, and foot eversion disappears.

By the third year the body is slimmer, taller, and better balanced. Abdominal protrusion decreases, the feet are not as far apart, and the arms and legs have increased in length. The child appears more coordinated. From the third year through the beginning of adolescence, the musculoskeletal system continues to grow and develop (see Chapter 12).

Adolescence. Adolescent growth is often sporadic and uneven. As a result, the adolescent appears awkward and uncoordinated. Adolescent girls usually grow and develop earlier than boys. Hips widen; and fat deposits in the upper arms, thighs, and buttocks. The adolescent boy's changes in shape are usually a result of long-bone growth and increased muscle mass (see Chapter 12).

Young to Middle Adults. An adult with correct posture and body alignment feels good, looks good, and generally appears self-confident.

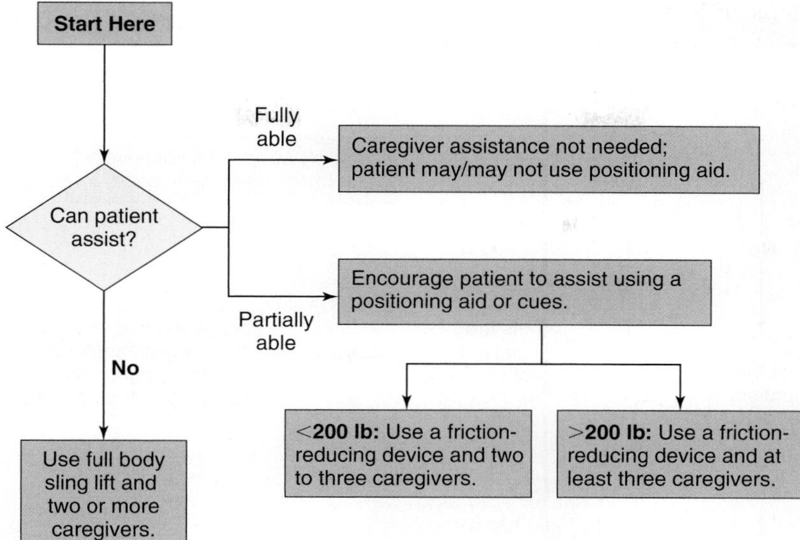

- This is not a one-person task: DO NOT PULL FROM HEAD OF BED.
- When pulling a patient up in bed, the bed should be flat or in a Trendelenburg position (when tolerated) to aid in gravity, with the side rail down.
- For patients with stage III or IV pressure ulcers, care should be taken to avoid shearing force.
- The height of the bed should be appropriate for staff safety (at the elbows).
- If the patient can assist when repositioning "up in bed," ask the patient to flex the knees and push on the count of three.
- During any patient-handling task, if the caregiver is required to lift more than 35 lb of a patient's weight, then the patient should be considered to be fully dependent and assistive devices should be used.

FIGURE 39-4 Algorithm used to reposition patient in bed. (Modified from VISN8 Patient Safety Center (VISN8): *Algorithms for Safe Patient Handling and Movement,* 2015, http://www.visn8.va.gov/patientsafetycenter/safepthandling/. Accessed February 14, 2015.)

The healthy adult also has the necessary musculoskeletal development and coordination to carry out ADLs and physical exercise (see Chapter 13). Normal changes in posture and body alignment in adulthood occur mainly in pregnant women. These changes result from the adaptive response of the body to weight gain and the growing fetus. The center of gravity shifts toward the anterior. The pregnant woman leans back and is slightly swaybacked; as a result, pregnant women often complain of back pain (see Chapter 13).

Older Adults. A progressive loss of total bone mass occurs with older adults. Some of the possible causes of this loss include physical inactivity, hormonal changes, and increased osteoclastic activity (i.e., activity by cells responsible for bone tissue absorption). The effect of bone loss is weaker bones, causing vertebrae to be softer and long shaft bones to be less resistant to bending.

In addition, older adults may walk more slowly and appear less coordinated. They often take smaller steps and keep their feet closer together, which decreases the base of support and thus alters body balance. It is important to encourage or plan physical activities for older adults. These exercises are important for socialization, independence, and maintaining core body strength. Physical exercise can improve endurance, coordination, and muscle stability and reduce the risk for falls and injuries (see Chapter 14).

Behavioral Aspects. Physical activity not only benefits a patient's overall health but also is reported to reduce stress (Childs and deWit, 2014). Patients are more likely to incorporate an exercise program into their daily lives if supported by family, friends, nurses, health care providers, and other members of the health care team. As a nurse, you must consider a patient's knowledge of exercise and activity, their values and beliefs about exercise in relation to health, barriers to a program of exercise and physical activity (e.g., resources or access to a safe area to exercise), and current exercise habits. Patients are more open to developing an exercise program when they are at a stage of readiness to change their behavior. Information about the benefits of regular exercise is often helpful to a patient who is not at the stage of readiness to act. Patients' decisions to change behavior and include a daily exercise routine in their lives sometimes occur gradually with repeated information individualized to patients' needs and lifestyle (Box 39-2). Once a patient is at the stage of readiness, collaborate with him or her to develop an exercise program that fits his or her needs and provide continued follow-up support and assistance until the exercise program becomes a daily routine.

Environmental Issues

Work Site. A common barrier for many patients is the lack of time needed to engage in a daily exercise program. Some work sites help their employees overcome the obstacle of time constraints by offering opportunities, reminders, and rewards for those committed to physical fitness (McGann et al., 2013). Reminders such as signs that encourage employees to use the stairs instead of elevators are useful. Rewards such as free parking or discounted parking fees are also effective for employees who park in distant lots and walk.

Schools. Children today are less active, resulting in an increase in childhood obesity (Bammann et al., 2014; Grossklaus and Marvicsin, 2014). Schools are excellent facilitators of physical fitness and exercise. Strategies for physical activity incorporated early into a child's daily routine often provide a foundation for lifetime commitment to exercise and physical fitness.

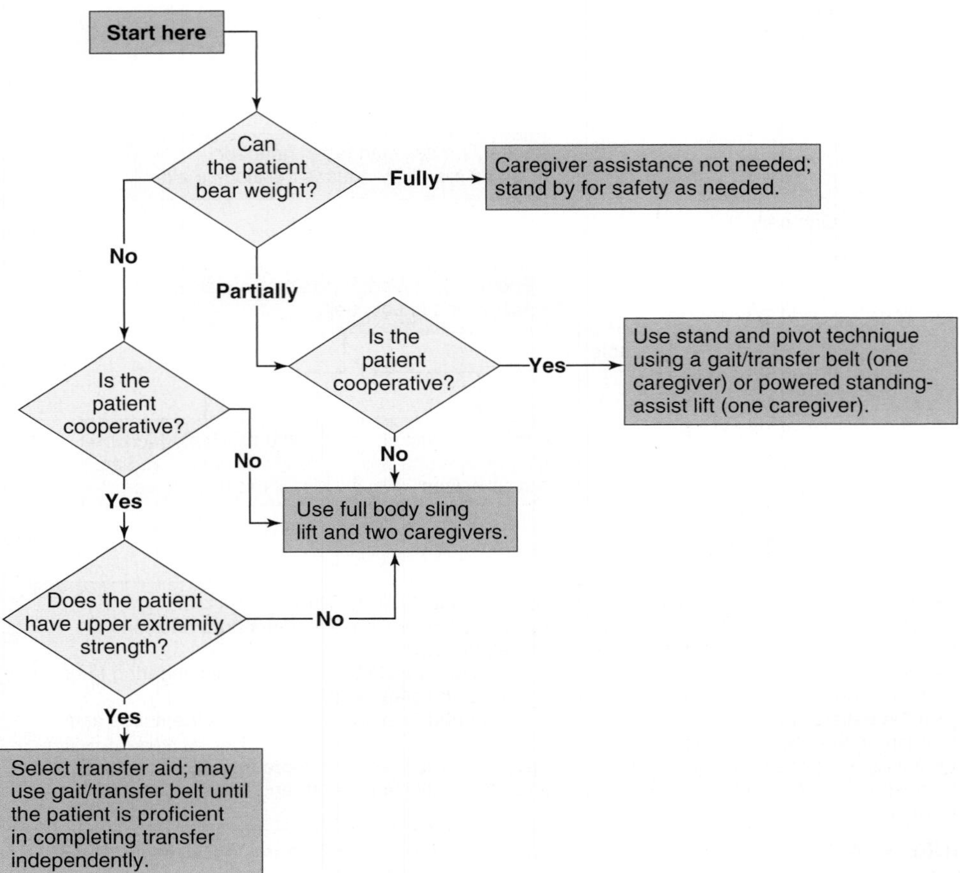

- For seated transfer aid, must have chair with arms that recess or are removable.
- For full body sling lift, select a lift that is specifically designed to access a patient from the car (if the car is the starting or ending destination).
- If patient has partial weight-bearing capacity, transfer toward stronger side.
- Toileting slings are available for toileting.
- Mesh slings are available for bathing.
- During any patient-transferring task, if any caregiver is required to lift more than 35 lb of a patient's weight, then the patient should be considered to be fully dependent and assistive devices should be used for the transfer.

FIGURE 39-5 Algorithm used to transfer patient to and from bed to chair, chair to toilet, chair to chair, or car to chair. (Modified from VISN8 Patient Safety Center (VISN8): *Algorithms for safe patient handling and movement,* 2015, http://www.visn8.va.gov/patientsafetycenter/safepthandling/. Accessed February 14, 2015.)

Community. Community support of physical fitness is instrumental in promoting the health of its members (e.g., providing walking trails and track facilities in parks and physical fitness classes). Success in implementing physical fitness programs depends on a collaborative effort from public health agencies, parks and recreational associations, state and local government agencies, health care agencies, and the members of the community (Combs et al., 2013; Wallace et al., 2014).

Cultural and Ethnic Influences. Exercise and physical fitness are beneficial to all people. When developing a physical fitness program for culturally diverse populations, consider what motivates them for exercise and physical activity and what they see as appropriate, enjoyable, and beneficial. It is also important to know which specific disease entities are associated with different cultural and ethnic origins (Box 39-3).

Family and Social Support. Social support is one motivational tool to encourage and promote exercise and physical fitness. For example, a patient engages a friend or significant other to participate in a "buddy system" (i.e., they walk together each day at a specified time). This companionship provides for socialization, increases the enjoyment, and develops a lifelong commitment to physical fitness. Parents support their children in sports and physical activity by providing encouragement, praise, and transportation (Davison and Jago, 2010; Dunton, 2010). Other parents support physical activity by including their children in family outings such as bicycling or a basketball game in the neighborhood schoolyard.

CRITICAL THINKING

Successful critical thinking requires a synthesis of knowledge, experience, information gathered from patients, critical thinking attitudes,

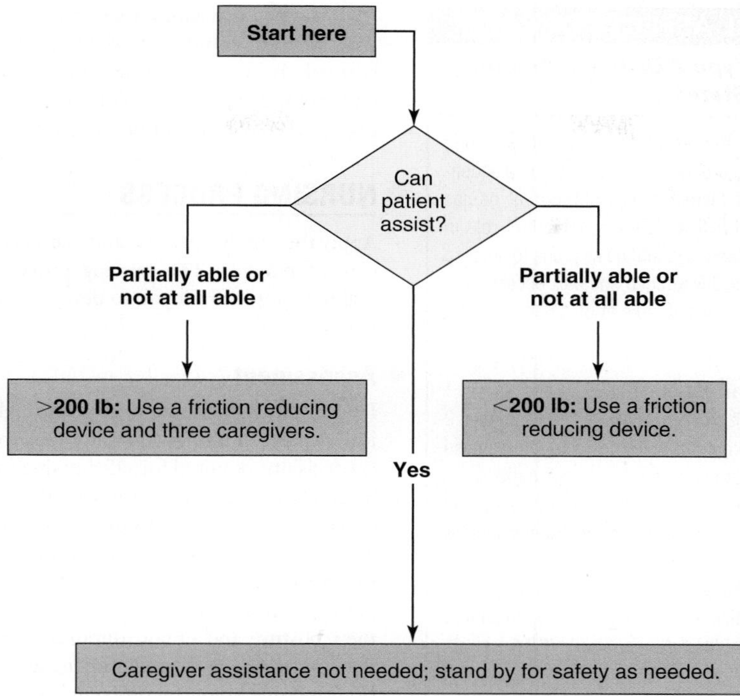

FIGURE 39-6 Algorithm used to complete lateral transfer to and from bed to stretcher, trolley. (Modified from VISN8 Patient Safety Center (VISN8): *Algorithms for safe patient handling and movement*, 2015, http://www.visn8.va.gov/patientsafetycenter/safepthandling/. Accessed February 14, 2015.)

BOX 39-2 General Guidelines for Initiating an Exercise Program

Five steps to beginning an exercise program:

Step 1: Assess Fitness Level

- Seek approval from a health care provider to begin. Are there any limitations to consider before determining the exercises in the fitness program?
- Record baseline fitness scores such as pulse rate before and after walking 1 mile, how long it takes to walk 1 mile, number of pushups that can be done at a time, how far you are able to reach forward while seated on floor with legs outstretched in front, waist circumference, and body mass index.

Step 2: Design the Fitness Program

- Consider fitness goals. Make goals attainable.
- Develop a balanced routine of aerobic activity and strength training.
- Plan a logical progression of activities that goes at your own pace and put it on paper to keep track.
- Build a program that includes different activities into a daily routine.
- Allow time for recovery.

Step 3: Assemble Equipment

- Choose athletic shoes designed for the chosen exercise.
- If choosing to exercise at home, try equipment at a fitness center before purchasing; buy used fitness equipment.
- Try homemade equipment (e.g., half-gallon milk jugs filled with sand for weights).

Step 4: Get Started

- Start slowly and build up a routine gradually.
- Divide exercise time throughout day if time or fatigue is a barrier. Ten minutes of exercise 3 times a day instead of a single 30-minute workout may be better for some patients' schedules and medical conditions.
- Take rest periods as condition warrants.

Step 5: Monitor Progress

- Retake fitness assessment at 6 weeks and then every 3 to 6 months.
- If losing motivation: set new goals, exercise with a friend, or incorporate new activities.

Modified from Mayo Clinic Healthy Living Fitness Program: *5 steps to getting started,* 2014, http://www.mayoclinic.com/healthy-living/fitness/in-depth/fitness/art-20048269?pg=1. Accessed August 12, 2014.

BOX 39-3 CULTURAL ASPECTS OF CARE

Incidence and Challenges of Type 2 Diabetes Among Ethnic Groups in the United States

Recent data in the United States shows the prevalence of diabetes among adults ages 65 years and older to average around 28%. Obesity and a sedentary lifestyle are consistent contributing factors across all cultural groups diagnosed with type 2 diabetes. Physical activity plays an important role in preventing and treating it. However, populations identified as prone to develop type 2 diabetes are also those who are disadvantaged and lack access to or have difficulty navigating the health care system (Clarke et al., 2014; Jain and Paranjape, 2013).

Implications for Patient-Centered Care

- Physical inactivity is a modifiable risk factor for the development of type 2 diabetes. Prevention and treatment programs need to focus on exercise and be tailored to the activity tolerance and interests of each patient.
- Work with patient's community to support promotion of physical activity through formal programs in schools, churches, and government agencies within disadvantaged communities.
- Incorporate motivational factors into the exercise program such as providing a healthy snack or meal for the participants and furnishing each patient with a log to monitor weight loss and blood glucose levels (Clarke et al., 2014).
- Exercise and diabetes-prevention programs need to remove potential barriers such as transportation and cost to facilitate commitment to the program.

and intellectual and professional standards. Clinical judgments require you to anticipate information, analyze the data, and make decisions regarding patient care.

To understand activity tolerance, physical fitness, and the effects on patients, you integrate knowledge from nursing and other disciplines, previous experiences, and information gathered from patients. As you plan patient care, consider the relationship among a variety of concepts to provide the best outcome for your patients. For example, you lay the foundation for planning and decision making by understanding the relationship between the musculoskeletal system and health alterations that may create problems with activity and exercise, positioning, and transferring. Professional standards such as those developed by the American College of Sports Medicine (ACSM) (2011), the ACSM and American Diabetes Association (ADA) (2010), and the Association for Critical Care Nurses (AACN) (2015) provide valuable guidelines for exercise and physical fitness. In addition, the American Nurses Association (ANA) (2010) issued a statement to the committee on Health, Education, Labor and Pensions Subcommittee on Employment and Workplace Safety of the United States Senate. The statement applauded and supports the enactment of the Nurse and Health Care Worker Act of 2009 (H.R. 2381/S.1788).

Your experiences and critical thinking attitude affect the problem-solving approach with patients and are evaluated with each new patient. Remember that some patients have the capacity for recovery in spite of the loss of some physical function. Restoration of function begins early in the care of patients whose ability to perform self-care is disrupted. Encouragement, support, commitment, and perseverance are important attitudes in critical thinking for these patients.

Perseverance is necessary when caring for patients who depend on you for assistance with ambulation or exercise. In addition, responsibility for positioning often becomes repetitive, and some nurses lose sight of its importance (see Chapter 28). Perseverance is especially important in delegating these activities to other personnel and being sure they are completed. Making certain that the task is performed correctly is also an essential nursing function. Problems with activity and mobility are often prolonged; creativity is necessary when designing interventions for improving activity tolerance and mobility skills.

NURSING PROCESS

Apply the nursing process and use a critical thinking approach in your care of patients. The nursing process provides a clinical decision-making approach for you to develop and implement an individualized plan of care.

Assessment

During the assessment process thoroughly assess each patient and critically analyze findings to ensure that you make patient-centered clinical decisions required for safe nursing care. Complete the assessment of body alignment and posture with the patient standing, sitting, or lying down. Use assessment to determine normal physiological changes in growth and development; deviations related to poor posture, trauma, muscle damage, or nerve dysfunction; and any learning needs of patients. In addition, provide opportunities for patients to observe their posture and obtain important information about other factors that contribute to poor alignment such as inactivity, fatigue, malnutrition, and psychological problems. Ask questions related to the patient's exercise and activity tolerance to gather important information (Box 39-4). During assessment (Figure 39-7) consider all of the elements that help you make appropriate nursing diagnoses. The first step in assessing body alignment is to put the patient at ease so he or she does not assume unnatural or rigid positions. When assessing body alignment of a patient who is immobilized or unconscious, remove pillows from the bed if not contraindicated and place the patient in the supine position.

Through the Patient's Eyes. In patient-centered care, assessing a patient's expectations, values, and beliefs concerning activity and exercise and determining individual perceptions of what is normal or acceptable are of utmost importance in developing a plan of care. Perceived self-efficacy is a judgment of capability and applies to a person's willingness to engage in exercise. The outcomes people anticipate, such as from an exercise program, depend on their judgments of how well they will be able to perform in given situations (Bandura, 2006). Ask the patient to what extent he or she enjoys exercising and his or her belief in the ability to exercise. This is a factor positively associated with adult physical activity (*Healthy People 2020,* 2015). Another example of assessing a patient's perceptions of what is acceptable activity is focusing on a patient's pain. One of the factors affecting physical activity is freedom from pain. When patients experience pain or fatigue following exercise, they often lack commitment to desired interventions. When patients are content with their present physical activity and fitness, they do not perceive a need for improvement.

Standing. Assessment of the standing patient includes the following: the head is erect, and midline body parts are symmetrical; the spine is straight with normal curvatures (cervical concave, thoracic convex, lumbar concave); the abdomen is comfortably tucked; the knees are in a straight line between the hips and ankles and slightly flexed; the feet are flat on the floor and pointed directly forward and slightly apart to maintain a wide base of support; and the arms hang comfortably at the sides (Figure 39-8). The patient's center of gravity is in the midline, and the line of gravity is from the middle of the forehead to a midpoint between the feet. Laterally the line of gravity

BOX 39-4 Nursing Assessment Questions

Nature of the Problem

- Tell me about the types of problems you are having with activities and exercise?
- How much do you exercise each day?
- Which type of exercise do you prefer?
- Describe for me your typical day. What type of activities do you do?
- How long do you exercise at any given time?

Signs and Symptoms

- Do you have muscle or joint pain during or after exercise?
- Do you have shortness of breath during any activity?
- Do you ever feel chest discomfort or pain during exercise or activity?

Onset and Duration

- Which activities cause you to become short of breath?
- How long does it take to resume normal breathing after exercise or an activity?

Severity

- How far do you walk before the pain in your legs begins?
- On a scale of 0 to 10 (10 being the worst discomfort), rate your leg pain.
- Do you describe your shortness of breath as minimal, moderate, or severe after activities and/or exercise?

Barriers to Exercise and Activity

- Do you have any chronic illnesses that affect your ability to carry out daily activities such as grocery shopping, washing clothes, or daily walking? Do you have any physical limitations that prevent you from exercising on a daily basis?
- Do you have access to a community walking path and exercise equipment?
- What prevents you from exercising 30 minutes each day?

Patient Values

- Tell me what you believe about the importance of regular exercise.
- How confident are you in being able to perform the exercises your doctor has recommended?

Effect on Patient

- How has the lack of an exercise routine affected your weight?
- Do you feel more tired since you have not been able to exercise routinely?
- Have you noticed any increase in shortness of breath when performing activities that require little exertion?

Knowledge

- Normal activity needs for the patient's developmental stage
- Normal activity patterns
- Effects of therapies on the patient's activity and exercise patterns
- Physiological and emotional effects of exercise
- The influence of patient's culture on preferences for activity

Experience

- Caring for patients who require activity and exercise reconditioning
- Personal experience in beginning an exercise program

ASSESSMENT

- Assess the patient's body alignment, posture, and mobility
- Identify the effect of activity and exercise on the patient's overall level of health
- Assess the patient's routine exercise pattern
- Observe the patient's body systems' response to activity and exercise

Standards

- Apply intellectual standards such as accuracy, relevancy, and specificity when obtaining data related to the patient's activity and exercise status
- Apply professional standards such as those from the ACSM, ADA, and ANA

Attitudes

- Use creativity in observing the patient's activity and exercise patterns
- Carry out your responsibility for collecting appropriate assessment data to assess the patient's activity and exercise pattern

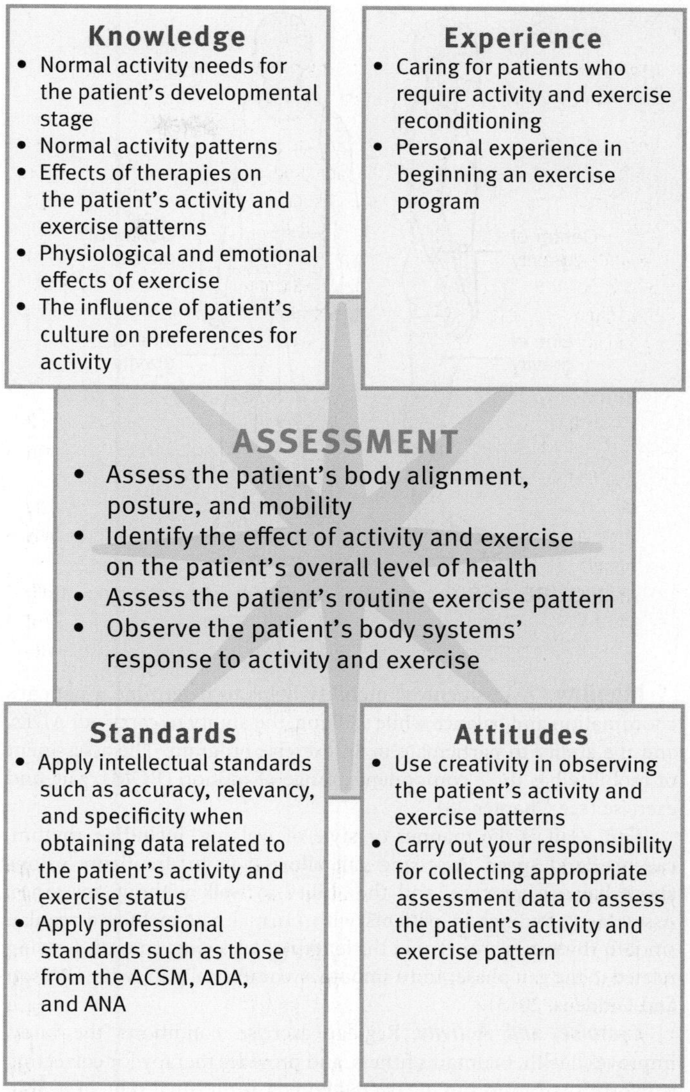

FIGURE 39-7 Critical thinking model for activity and exercise assessment. *ACSM,* American College of Sports Medicine; *ADA,* American Diabetes Association; *ANA,* American Nurses Association.

runs vertically from the middle of the skull to the posterior third of the foot (Wilson and Giddens, 2013).

Sitting. Assessment of a patient in the sitting position includes the following: the head is erect, and the neck and vertebral column are in straight alignment; the body weight is distributed on the buttocks and thighs; the thighs are parallel and in a horizontal plane (be careful to avoid pressure on the popliteal nerve and blood supply); the feet are supported on the floor; and the forearms are supported on the armrest, in the lap, or on a table in front of the chair.

Assessment of alignment in the sitting position is particularly important for the patient with muscle weakness, muscle paralysis, or nerve damage. A patient with these alterations has diminished sensation in affected areas and is unable to perceive pressure or decreased circulation. Proper sitting alignment reduces the risk of musculoskeletal system damage.

Recumbent Position. When assessing a patient in the recumbent position, you place him or her in the lateral position, removing all positioning supports and all but one pillow. The vertebrae are in straight alignment without observable curves. This assessment provides baseline data concerning the patient's body alignment.

Conditions that create a risk of damage to the musculoskeletal system when lying down include impaired mobility (e.g., traction), decreased sensation (e.g., hemiparesis from a stroke), impaired circulation (e.g., diabetes), and lack of voluntary muscle control (e.g., spinal cord injuries) (see Chapter 28).

When a patient is unable to change position voluntarily, assess the position of body parts while he or she is lying down. Make sure that the vertebrae are in straight alignment without any observable curves. Also check that the extremities are in alignment and not crossed over one another. The head and neck need to be aligned without excessive flexion or extension.

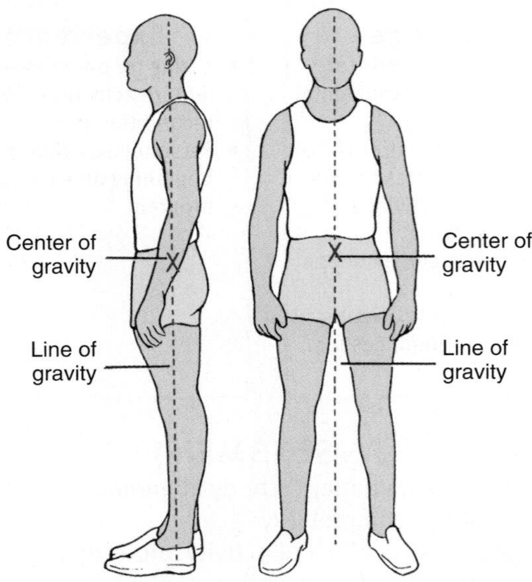

FIGURE 39-8 Correct body alignment when standing.

Mobility. Assessment of mobility helps to determine a patient's coordination and balance while walking, the ability to carry out ADLs, and the ability to participate in an exercise program. The assessment of mobility has three components: range of motion (ROM), gait, and exercise (see Chapter 28).

Gait. Gait is the manner or style of walking, including rhythm, cadence, and speed. Assessing gait allows you to draw conclusions about balance, posture, and the ability to walk without assistance. Assessment findings in patients with normal gait include a regular, smooth rhythm; symmetry in the length of leg swing; smooth swaying related to the gait phase; and a smooth, symmetrical arm swing (Wilson and Giddens, 2013).

Exercise and Activity. Regular exercise conditions the body, improves health, maintains fitness, and provides therapy for correcting a deformity or restoring the overall body to a maximal state of health. Daily activity is a barometer for a patient's functional status. When a person engages in physical activity, physiological changes occur in body systems (Box 39-5). Determine the types of activities a patient engages in normally at home and how much the patient exercises regularly.

Activity Tolerance. Activity tolerance is the response a person has to the type and amount of exercise or activity that he or she performs. Before ambulation, sitting in a chair, or other planned activities, obtain a patient's vital signs, observe skin color, and ask about his or her level of comfort and current energy level or sense of fatigue. Assessment of activity tolerance is necessary when planning physical activity for health promotion and for health maintenance for patients with acute or chronic illness. This assessment provides baseline data about the patient's activity patterns and helps determine which factors (physical, psychological, or motivational) affect activity tolerance (Box 39-6).

BOX 39-5 Effects of Exercise

Cardiovascular System
- Increased cardiac output
- Improved myocardial contraction, thereby strengthening cardiac muscle
- Decreased resting heart rate
- Improved venous return

Pulmonary System
- Increased respiratory rate and depth followed by a quicker return to resting state
- Improved alveolar ventilation
- Decreased work of breathing
- Improved diaphragmatic excursion

Metabolic System
- Increased basal metabolic rate
- Increased use of glucose and fatty acids
- Increased triglyceride breakdown
- Increased gastric motility
- Increased production of body heat

Musculoskeletal System
- Improved muscle tone
- Increased joint mobility
- Improved muscle tolerance to physical exercise
- Possible increase in muscle mass
- Reduced bone loss

Activity Tolerance
- Improved tolerance
- Decreased fatigue

Psychosocial Factors
- Improved tolerance to stress
- Reports of "feeling better"
- Reports of decrease in illness (e.g., colds, influenza)

Data from Huether SE, McCance KL: *Understanding pathophysiology,* ed 5, St Louis, 2012, Mosby.

BOX 39-6 Factors Influencing Activity Tolerance

Physiological Factors
- Skeletal abnormalities
- Muscular impairments
- Endocrine or metabolic illnesses (e.g., diabetes mellitus, thyroid disease)
- Hypoxemia
- Decreased cardiac function
- Decreased endurance
- Impaired physical stability
- Pain
- Sleep pattern disturbance
- Prior exercise patterns
- Infectious processes and fever

Emotional Factors
- Anxiety
- Depression
- Chemical addictions
- Motivation

Developmental Factors
- Age
- Sex

Pregnancy
- Physical growth and development of muscle and skeletal support

Modified from Lewis SL et al: *Medical-surgical nursing assessment and management of clinical problems,* ed 9, St Louis, 2014, Mosby.

◆ Nursing Diagnosis

Assessment of the patient's activity tolerance, physical fitness, body alignment, and joint mobility provides clusters of data or defining characteristics to support a nursing diagnosis. You need to be accurate when identifying diagnoses. For example, you consider nursing diagnoses of *Activity Intolerance* or *Fatigue* in a patient who reports being tired and weak. Further review of assessed defining characteristics (e.g., abnormal heart rate and verbal report of weakness) leads to the definitive diagnosis *(Activity Intolerance).*

When patients have problems with activity and exercise, nursing diagnoses often focus on the ability to move. The diagnostic label and related factors direct nursing interventions. This requires the correct selection of the related factors. For example, *Activity Intolerance related to excess weight gain* requires very different interventions than if the related factor is prolonged bed rest. Box 39-7 provides an example of how the diagnostic process leads to accurate diagnosis selection. The

BOX 39-7 Nursing Diagnostic Process

Impaired Physical Mobility

Assessment Activities	Defining Characteristics
Observe patient's gait.	Shuffled gait Uncoordinated gait Patient report of slower walking speed
Observe patient performing tasks such as feeding, dressing, or recreational activities.	Uncoordinated movements Limited fine-motor coordination
Measure range of joint motion.	Reduced joint motion in lower and/or upper extremities Stiffness in joints
Measure patient's strength.	Has difficulty rising to sitting position or exiting bed

following are examples of nursing diagnoses related to activity and exercise:

- *Activity Intolerance*
- *Ineffective Coping*
- *Impaired Gas Exchange*
- *Risk for Injury*
- *Impaired Bed Mobility*
- *Impaired Physical Mobility*
- *Acute or Chronic Pain*

◆ Planning

During planning synthesize information from multiple resources (Figure 39-9). Critical thinking ensures that the patient's plan of care integrates all patient information. Professional standards are especially important to consider when developing a plan of care. These standards often establish scientifically proven guidelines for selecting effective nursing interventions.

A concept map is a tool to assist in the planning of care. It shows the relationship between multiple nursing diagnoses and planned interventions. Figure 39-10 shows the relationship between a patient's medical diagnosis of heart failure and the identified nursing diagnoses and related nursing interventions.

Goals and Outcomes. Once you identify the nursing diagnoses, you and the patient set goals and expected outcomes to direct interventions. The plan includes consideration of any risks for injury to the patient and preexisting health concerns. It is especially important to have knowledge of the patient's home environment when planning therapies to maintain or improve activity, body alignment, and mobility. Include the patient's family caregiver in the care plan unless the patient prefers no family involvement. Family caregivers play critical roles in the home environment, motivating and coaching patients to stay active. The general goal related to exercise and activity is to improve or maintain the patient's motor function and independence. The following are examples of outcomes for patients with deficits in activity and exercise (Ackley and Ladwig, 2014):

- Participates in prescribed physical activity while maintaining appropriate heart rate, blood pressure, and breathing rate
- Verbalizes an understanding of the need to gradually increase activity on the basis of tolerance and symptoms
- Expresses understanding of balancing rest and activity

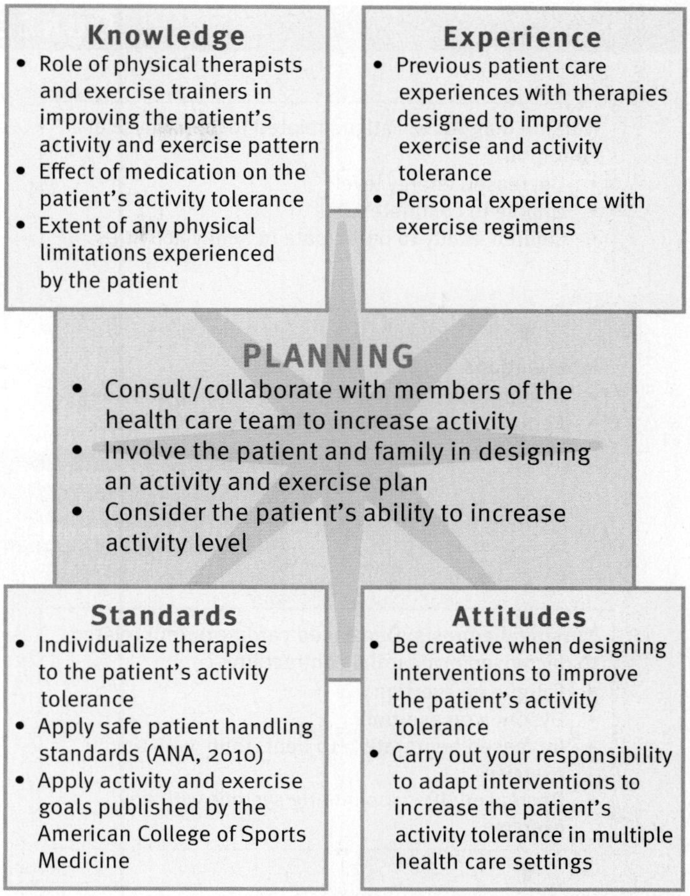

Knowledge
- Role of physical therapists and exercise trainers in improving the patient's activity and exercise pattern
- Effect of medication on the patient's activity tolerance
- Extent of any physical limitations experienced by the patient

Experience
- Previous patient care experiences with therapies designed to improve exercise and activity tolerance
- Personal experience with exercise regimens

PLANNING
- Consult/collaborate with members of the health care team to increase activity
- Involve the patient and family in designing an activity and exercise plan
- Consider the patient's ability to increase activity level

Standards
- Individualize therapies to the patient's activity tolerance
- Apply safe patient handling standards (ANA, 2010)
- Apply activity and exercise goals published by the American College of Sports Medicine

Attitudes
- Be creative when designing interventions to improve the patient's activity tolerance
- Carry out your responsibility to adapt interventions to increase the patient's activity tolerance in multiple health care settings

FIGURE 39-9 Critical thinking model for activity and exercise planning. *ANA,* American Nurses Association.

Setting Priorities. Care planning is patient centered, taking into consideration the patient's most immediate needs. For example, is a patient comfortable enough to participate in exercise, or does the acute occurrence of symptoms require you to delay an exercise session? You determine the immediacy of any problem by its effect on the patient's mental and physical health. Because of the many skills associated with the care of patients who have the diagnoses of activity intolerance and/or impaired mobility, such as turning, transferring, and positioning, it is easy to overlook the complications associated with these health alterations. Therefore be vigilant in monitoring the patient and supervising assistive personnel in carrying out activities to prevent complications and potential injury.

Teamwork and Collaboration. Planning involves understanding a patient's need to maintain function and independence. For example, it is important to collaborate with physicians and physical and occupational therapists. Sometimes long-term rehabilitation is necessary. Discharge planning begins when a patient enters the health care system and involves identifying his or expectations regarding physical activity and what is planned by the health care team. In addition, always individualize a plan of care directed at meeting the actual or potential needs of the patient (see the Nursing Care Plan).

◆ Implementation

Health Promotion. A sedentary lifestyle contributes to the development of health-related problems. You promote health by

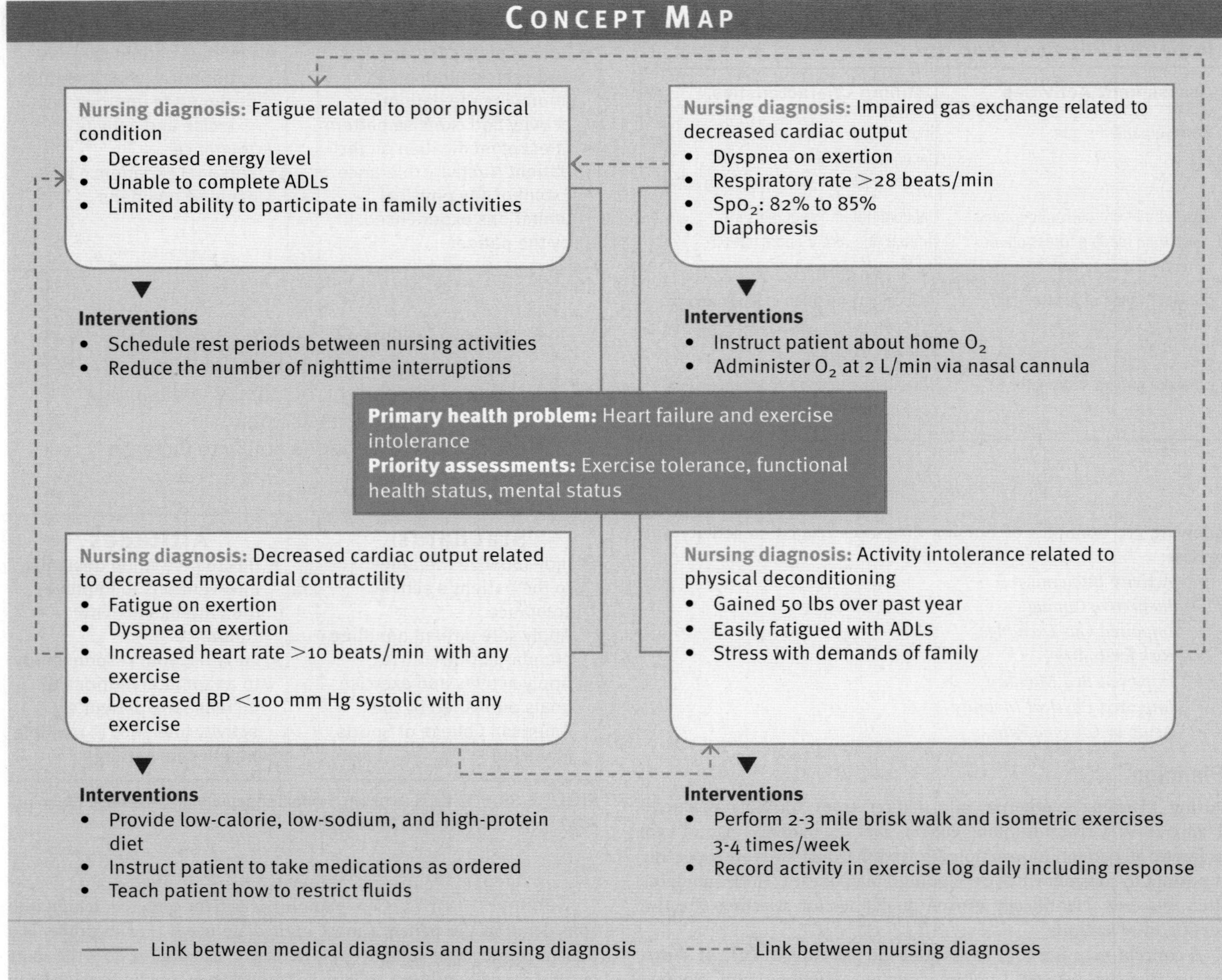

FIGURE 39-10 Concept map for Mrs. Smith. *ADLs,* Activities of daily living; *BP,* blood pressure.

NURSING CARE PLAN

Activity Intolerance

ASSESSMENT

Mrs. Smith is a 45-year-old housewife. She is in a cardiovascular rehabilitation program prescribed by her health care provider and conducted by Erich, a registered nurse. Mrs. Smith has a history of cardiovascular disease with mild heart failure. She expresses feelings of stress caused by excessive demands on her time. Erich's assessment includes a discussion of Mrs. Smith's current health problem and a pertinent physical examination.

Assessment Activities	*Findings/Defining Characteristics**
Ask Mrs. Smith what prompted her health care provider to recommend a cardiovascular rehabilitation program.	She responds, "I **gained 50 lbs** over the past year. I become easily **fatigued** and lack the energy to keep up with even simple household chores. I don't want to leave the house anymore. I don't have extra money to join one of those fancy gyms."
Ask Mrs. Smith about her exercise and eating habits.	She responds, "I want to exercise, but with the demands of child care and taking care of my aging parents, I just don't feel like it. I feel pulled in every direction; that increases my **stress**, and then I want to eat, eat, and eat!"

NURSING CARE PLAN

Activity Intolerance—cont'd

Assessment Activities	*Findings/Defining Characteristics**
Perform baseline assessment.	Height: 5 feet 3 inches Weight: **225 lbs** (102 kg) Blood pressure: **152/90 mm Hg** (at rest) Pulse: 96 beats/min (at rest) Breathing rate: 20 breaths/min (at rest) Blood pressure: **164/96 mm Hg** (after climbing 10 steps) Pulse: **120 beats/min** (after climbing 10 steps) Breathing rate: 36 breaths/min (after climbing 10 steps)

***Defining characteristics** are shown in bold type.

NURSING DIAGNOSIS: Activity intolerance related to inactivity and lack of cardiovascular fitness

PLANNING

Goals	*Expected Outcomes (NOC)*[†]
	Activity Tolerance
Mrs. Smith's activity tolerance will improve above baseline.	Mrs. Smith performs 20-minute exercise two times a week over the next 2 weeks. Mrs. Smith's level of fatigue associated with exercise remains the same or decreases.
	Cardiac Pump Effectiveness
Mrs. Smith's cardiopulmonary response to exercise will improve.	Mrs. Smith's resting diastolic blood pressure remains below 80 mm Hg. Her systolic blood pressure is below 120 mm Hg. Her resting heart rate ranges between 75 and 85 beats/min. Her breathing rate is 16 breaths/min (at rest).

[†]Outcome classification labels from Moorhead S et al, editors: *Nursing outcomes classification (NOC),* ed 5, St Louis, 2013, Mosby.

INTERVENTIONS (NIC)[‡]	**RATIONALE**
Exercise Promotion	
Instruct Mrs. Smith about the physiological benefits of a regular exercise program. Match instruction with her beliefs about the value of exercise.	Physical activity and exercise protect against the further development of cardiovascular disease (CVD) and decrease other risk factors associated with CVD such as obesity, hypertension, and hyperlipidemia (Campos-Outcalt, 2014; Donges et al., 2010).
Develop a progressive plan of exercise with Mrs. Smith such as 2 to 3 miles or 20 minutes of brisk walking and quadriceps, bicep, and gluteal muscle isometric exercises 3 to 4 times per week.	Cross-training (combination of exercise activities) provides variety to combat boredom and increases potential for total-body conditioning (Edelman et al., 2013).
Instruct Mrs. Smith to use an exercise log and record the day, time, duration, and responses (pulse, feelings, shortness of breath, daily weight).	Keeping a log may increase adherence to exercise prescription. Monitoring cardiopulmonary response can indicate potential symptoms of intolerance to activity that may cause harm (Urden L et al., 2014).
Schedule routine visits with Mrs. Smith for follow-up and review of exercise log, progress, and barriers.	Patients are more likely to increase physical activity and remain compliant with an exercise program if they are counseled by a health care professional (Edelman et al., 2013).

[‡]Intervention classification labels from Bulechek GM et al, editors: *Nursing interventions classification (NIC),* ed 6, St Louis, 2013, Mosby.

EVALUATION

Nursing Actions	*Patient Response/Finding*	*Achievement of Outcome*
Review patient's exercise log.	Patient walked 20 minutes twice the first week, 20 minutes three times the next week.	Participation in exercise is increasing.
Record weight, blood pressure, and pulse.	Weight, 210 lbs; resting heart rate remains between 80 and 85 beats/min; blood pressure, 146/86 mm Hg.	15-lb weight loss Improved cardiovascular effects of exercise: • Heart rate is within normal range. • Blood pressure is lower but not at expected range. Monitor blood pressure as patient continues to lose weight.
Ask Mrs. Smith if exercise is helping to lower fatigue level.	"At first, finding time to exercise was hard; but once I started feeling less tired and even less stressed, it was easy to integrate exercise into my daily activities."	Activity tolerance improved with exercise.

BOX 39-8 PROCEDURAL GUIDELINES

Helping Patients to Exercise

Delegation Considerations

The skill of helping patients exercise is a self-care activity. However, in the acute care setting it can be delegated to nursing assistive personnel (NAP). A nurse first must assess the patient's ability and tolerance to exercise. The nurse also teaches patients and their families how to implement exercise programs at home. NAP can prepare patients for exercise (e.g., putting on shoes and clothing, providing hygiene needs and obtaining preexercise and post-exercise vital signs). Instruct NAP to do the following:

- Notify nurse if patient reports pain before, during, or after exercise.
- Notify nurse if patient complains of increased fatigue, dizziness, or lightheadedness when obtaining preexercise and/or post-exercise vital signs.
- Notify nurse of vital sign values.

Steps

1. Identify patient using two identifiers (e.g., name and birthday or name and medical record number according to agency policy).
2. Assess for any medical limitations (e.g., weight-bearing status, untreated fracture, partial paralysis, peripheral neuropathy of feet, current pregnancy, cardiovascular disease).
3. Know patient's mobility level before trauma, illness, or hospitalization.
4. Gather baseline assessment of vital signs and O_2 saturation (if available).
5. Assess patient's pain level. Ask patient to rate pain on a scale of 0 to 10, with 0 being no pain and 10 being the worst pain ever. An analgesic may be needed 30 minutes before exercise but should not have sedative properties.
6. Assess patient's beliefs, values, and perceptions regarding current health status and confidence in being capable of performing exercise.
7. Assess patient's cognitive status and ability to follow instructions while implementing exercise.
8. Assess for joint limitations and do not force a muscle or a joint during exercise.
9. Have patient wear comfortable nonskid shoes. In the home setting, encourage wearing comfortable clothes.
10. Instruct patient to take slow, deep breaths and to focus on relaxation to reduce anxiety and fully oxygenate tissues and expand lungs.
11. When exercising (e.g., ambulating or moving to a chair, walking at home), have the patient move at his or her own pace.
12. Monitor for dizziness, which is an indicator of postural hypotension.
13. Observe for proper posture, body alignment, and body mechanics during exercise.
14. Monitor vital signs before, during, and after exercise.
15. Terminate physical activity if patient's heart rate is greater than 30 beats per minute over baseline; if there is a change in patient's heart rhythm; if the patient is hypotensive (change in systolic BP of 30 mm Hg or change in diastolic BP of 10 mm Hg); if the patient develops dizziness that lasts 60 seconds, fainting, or diaphoresis; if there is a change in patient's breathing pattern with an increase in accessory muscle use; or if patient develops extreme fatigue or severe dyspnea with respiratory rate greater than baseline by more than 20 breaths/min (Perme and Chandrashekar, 2009; Myszenski, 2014).
16. Use ***Teach Back*** to determine patient and family understanding about safe exercise activities. State, "I want to be sure I explained how to safely exercise at home or in your community to prevent the risk for exercise-related injury. Can you explain to me the proper shoes for exercise and how to gradually increase your activity?" Revise your instruction now or develop plan for revised patient teaching if patient is not able to teach back correctly.
17. Document patient's progress and provide feedback as patient exercises.

Data from Edelman CL et al: *Health promotion throughout the life span,* ed 8, St Louis, 2013, Mosby; and Lewis SL et al: *Medical-surgical nursing assessment and management of clinical problems,* ed 9, St Louis, 2014, Mosby.

encouraging patients to engage in a regular exercise program in any setting (Box 39-8). Take a holistic approach to develop and implement a plan that enhances the patient's overall physical fitness. Discuss recommendations for physical activity and fitness and collaborate with the patient to design an exercise program.

Before starting an exercise program, teach patients to calculate their maximum heart rate by subtracting their current age in years from 220 and then obtaining their target heart rate by taking 60% to 90% of the maximum, depending on their health care provider's recommendation. No matter which exercise prescription is implemented for the patient, warm-up and cool-down periods need to be included in the program (Edelman et al., 2013). The warm-up period usually lasts about 5 to 10 minutes and frequently includes stretching, calisthenics, and/or the aerobic activity performed at a lower intensity. It prepares the body and decreases the potential for injury. The cool-down period follows the exercise routine and usually lasts about 5 to 10 minutes. It allows the body to readjust gradually to baseline functioning and provides an opportunity to combine movement such as stretching with relaxation-enhancing mind-body awareness. The American Heart Association (2015) has recommendations for physical activity in adults (http://www.heart.org/HEARTORG/GettingHealthy/PhysicalActivity/FitnessBasics/American-Heart-Association-Recommendations-for-Physical-Activity-in-Adults_UCM_307976_Article.jsp#.VlCR96SFOpo).

QSEN QSEN: BUILDING COMPETENCY IN QUALITY IMPROVEMENT To assess individualized improvement in the patient's tolerance to activity, you need to establish consistent and measurable outcomes for collaborative care. Determine the optimal cardiopulmonary response(s) to exercise for the patient in the nursing care plan, 45-year-old Mary Smith.

Answers to QSEN Activities can be found on the Evolve website.

Many patients find it difficult to incorporate an exercise program into their daily lives because of time constraints or lack of resources (e.g., no open parks or walking paths). For these patients it is beneficial to reinforce that they can use ADLs (e.g., gardening, climbing stairs when doing laundry) to accumulate the recommended 30 minutes or more per day of moderate-intensity physical activity.

Other patients benefit from a prescribed exercise and physical fitness program carefully designed to meet their needs and expectations. An exercise prescription usually includes a combination of aerobic exercises, stretching and flexibility exercises, and resistance training. Aerobic exercise includes walking, running, bicycling, aerobic dance, jumping rope, and cross-country skiing. Recommended frequency of aerobic exercise is 3 to 5 times per week or every other day for approximately 30 minutes. Cross-training is recommended for the patient who prefers to exercise every day. For example, the patient runs one day and does yoga the next day.

Stretching and flexibility exercises include active ROM and stretching of all muscle groups and joints. This form of exercise is ideal for warm-up and cool-down periods. Benefits include increased flexibility, improved circulation and posture, and an opportunity for relaxation.

Resistance training increases muscle strength and endurance and is associated with improved performance of ADLs and avoidance of injuries and disability. Formal resistance training includes weight training; but patients can obtain the same benefits by performing ADLs such as pushing a vacuum cleaner, raking leaves, shoveling snow, and kneading bread. Some patients use weight training to bulk up their muscles. However, its purpose from a health perspective is to develop tone and strength and stimulate and maintain healthy bone (O'Donovan et al., 2010).

Body Mechanics. The U.S. Occupational Safety and Health Administration released federal ergonomic guidelines to prevent musculoskeletal injuries in the workplace (OSHA, 2009). Half of all back pain is associated with manual lifting tasks (Box 39-9). Coordinated musculoskeletal activity is necessary when positioning and transferring patients. The most common back injury is strain on the lumbar muscle group, which includes the muscles around the lumbar vertebrae. Injury to these areas affects the ability to bend forward, backward, and from side to side. The ability to rotate the hips and lower back is also decreased (Lin et al., 2012). Body mechanics alone are not sufficient to prevent musculoskeletal injuries when positioning or transferring patients (Table 39-1).

Before lifting, assess the weight to be lifted, determine the assistance needed, and evaluate available resources. Use safe patient–handling equipment when a patient is unable to assist in transfer. Lift teams, consisting of two physically fit people competent in lifting techniques, reduce the risk of injury to the patient and members of the health care team (Burnfield et al., 2013; Cowley and Leggett, 2010). Use manual lifting only as a last resort when you need to lift a small part of a patient's weight (Tullar et al., 2010). Teaching health care workers about patient-handling equipment, proper body mechanics, and the use of lift teams is most effective in preventing injury (Hunter et al., 2010).

BOX 39-9 EVIDENCE-BASED PRACTICE

Promoting Safe Handling of Patients and Prevention of Injury to Nurses and Their Patients

PICO Question: What is the effect on nurse safety in health care agencies that have safe patient handling policies when compared with agencies that do not have these policies?

Evidence Summary

Musculoskeletal disorders are the most prevalent and debilitating occupational health hazards for nurses. Preventive interventions are needed to avoid the hazards and economic burdens associated with patient-handling tasks. The American Nurses Association (ANA, 2010) position statement calls for the use of assistive equipment and devices to promote a safe health care environment for nurses and their patients. The use of assistive equipment and continued use of proper body mechanics significantly reduce the risk of musculoskeletal injuries. The Occupational Safety and Health Administration (OSHA, 2009) recommends minimizing or eliminating manual lifting of patients. Current evidence supports the benefits of instituting safe patient handling (SPH) programs in health care organizations. However, The U.S. Bureau of Labor Statistics (2010) reported that workers in the health care industry suffered the most loss of time because of general musculoskeletal pain and back pain. As a result, many facilities are implementing limited lift policies to minimize patient handling by nurses and using lift devices. Research shows that these policies effectively reduce on-the-job injuries (Cowley and Leggett, 2010; Tullar et al., 2010).

Application to Nursing Practice

- Be familiar with health care agency safety information and training concerning the transfer, positioning, and lifting of patients.
- Use sufficient personnel along with patient-handling equipment when moving patients who are overweight, confused, or unable to assist (Cowley and Leggett, 2010; VISN8, 2015).
- Use recommended back safety guidelines and appropriate safe patient–handling equipment to reduce the risk for musculoskeletal injuries (Lin et al., 2012).
- Use current research, standards, algorithms, and guidelines regarding safe positioning and transferring of patients (VISN8, 2015).
- Use "lift teams" and patient-handling equipment such as mechanical lifts to prevent injury to yourself and the patient (VISN8, 2015).

Acute Care. Encourage patients who are hospitalized to do stretching exercises, active ROM exercises, and low-intensity walking, depending on their condition. Physical therapists can also assist patients with isometric exercises. When patients cannot participate in active ROM, maintain joint mobility and prevent contractures by implementing passive ROM into the plan of care. If needed, medicate patients for pain 30 minutes before exercise. Do not administer an analgesic that makes the patient feel dizzy.

Musculoskeletal System. Help maintain the musculoskeletal system during acute care by encouraging the use of stretching and isometric exercises. Review the patient's chart and collaborate with physical therapy and the health care provider to identify possible contraindications before initiating isometric exercises. A physical therapist will design an isometric exercise program for the specific needs of a patient. Your role will be to follow that program and assist patients accordingly. For example, an exercise program includes isometric exercises of the biceps and triceps to prepare a patient for crutch walking. Instruct the patient to stop the activity if pain, fatigue, or discomfort is experienced.

During isometrics, a patient tightens or contracts a muscle group for 10 seconds and then completely relaxes for several seconds (Resnick et al., 2012). Repetitions are increased gradually for each muscle group until the isometric exercise is repeated 8 to 10 times. Instruct patients to perform the exercises slowly and increase repetitions as their physical condition improves. A patient needs to do isometric exercise for quadriceps and gluteal muscle groups, which are used for walking, 4 times per day until a patient is ambulatory.

Joint Mobility. The easiest intervention to maintain or improve joint mobility for patients and one that can be coordinated with other activities is the use of ROM exercises (see Chapter 28). In active ROM exercises patients are able to move their joints independently. With passive ROM exercises you move each joint in patients who are unable to perform these exercises themselves. The use of ROM exercises provides data to systematically assess and improve the patient's joint mobility.

Joints that are not moved periodically are at risk for contractures, a permanent shortening of a muscle followed by the eventual shortening of associated ligaments and tendons. Over time the joint becomes fixed in one position, and the patient loses normal use of it. Passive ROM exercises are the exercises of choice for patients who do not have voluntary motor control.

TABLE 39-1 Preventing Lift Injuries in Health Care Workers

Action	Rationale
When planning to move a patient, arrange for adequate help. If your institution has a lift team, use it as a resource (Lin et al., 2012; VISN8, 2015).	A lift team is properly educated in techniques to prevent musculoskeletal injuries.
Use patient-handling equipment and devices such as height-adjustable beds, ceiling-mounted lifts, friction-reducing slide sheets, and air-assisted devices (Hunter et al., 2010; Tullar et al., 2010).	These devices reduce the caregiver's muscular strain during patient handling.
Encourage patient to help as much as possible.	This promotes patient's independence and strength while minimizing workload.
Take position close to patient (or object being lifted).	Keeps object in same plane as lifter and close to caregiver's center of gravity. Reduces horizontal reach and stress on caregiver's back.
Tighten abdominal muscles and keep back, neck, pelvis, and feet aligned. Avoid twisting.	Reduces risk of injury to lumbar vertebrae and muscle groups. Twisting increases risk of injury (Lin et al., 2012).
Bend at knees; keep feet wide apart.	A broad base of support increases stability. Maintains center of gravity.
Use arms and legs (not back).	Leg muscles are stronger, larger muscles capable of greater work without injury.
Slide patient toward your body using pull sheet or slide board. When transferring patient onto a stretcher or bed, a slide board is more appropriate.	Sliding requires less effort than lifting. Pull sheet minimizes shearing forces, which can damage patient's skin.
Person with heaviest load coordinates efforts of team involved by counting to three.	Simultaneous lifting minimizes load for any one lifter.
Perform manual lifting as last resort and only if it does not involve lifting most or all of patient's weight.	Lifting is a high-risk activity that causes significant biochemical and postural stressors (Tullar et al., 2010).

BOX 39-10 FOCUS ON OLDER ADULTS

Helping the Older Adult Initiate and Maintain an Exercise Program

- Encourage older adults to avoid prolonged sitting and get up and stretch. Frequent stretching decreases the risk of developing joint contractures.
- Be sure that the older patient maintains proper body alignment when sitting to minimize joint and muscle stress.
- Teach patients how to use stronger joints or larger muscle groups. Efficient distribution of the workload decreases joint stress and pain.
- Provide resources for planned exercise programs. Weight-bearing and resistance exercise slows bone loss and prevents fractures in older adults with osteoporosis (Roush, 2011).
- Recommend resistance- and agility-training programs. These forms of exercise reduce fear of falling and increase sense of well-being in older adults (Kwun et al., 2012).
- Teach older adults that it is never too late to begin an exercise program (Edelman et al., 2013; Elliott, 2011). Consult a health care provider before beginning an exercise program, particularly in the presence of heart or lung disease and other chronic illnesses.
- Use assessment data and consult with physical therapy to determine when you need to adjust exercise programs for those in advanced age.
- Encourage older adults who are unable to participate in a formal exercise program to improve joint mobility and enhance circulation by simply stretching and exaggerating movements during the performance of routine activities of daily living.

Older adults experiencing a decline in physical activity and changes in joints often have limited mobility and joint flexibility. Use a variety of recommended approaches to help older adults use proper body mechanics and prevent injury (Box 39-10).

The continuous passive motion (CPM) machine is designed to exercise various joints such as the hip, ankle, knee, shoulder, and wrist through repetitive ROM. The CPM machine is most commonly used after knee surgery. However, questions have been raised about CPM benefits (Maniar et al., 2012). A recent review of studies involving knee arthroplastic surgery show that CPM probably improves the ability of a patient to bend the knee slightly but may not improve pain or function (Harvey et al., 2014). It is usually prescribed from the first to fourth day after surgery and is applied for 1.5 to 24 hours a day depending on the surgeon's preference and the patient's condition (Lewis et al., 2013; Harvey et al., 2014). You set the machine to certain degrees of joint mobility based on the health care provider's order, with increasing joint mobility or flexion as the goal.

Unless contraindicated, the nursing care plan includes exercising each joint through as nearly a full ROM as possible. Initiate passive ROM exercises as soon as the patient loses the ability to move the extremity or joint. Chapter 28 details ROM exercises for each area and illustrates the motion of each joint.

Walking. Walking increases joint mobility and can be measured by length of time or distance walked. Measure distances walked in feet or yards instead of charting "ambulated to nurses' station and back." Illness or trauma usually reduces activity tolerance, resulting in the need for help with walking or the use of assistive devices such as crutches, canes, or walkers. Patients who increase their walking distance before discharge improve their ability to independently perform basic ADLs, increase activity tolerance, and have a faster recovery after surgery (AAN, 2015; Pashikanti and Von Ah, 2012)

Helping a Patient Walk. Helping a patient walk requires preparation. Assess the patient's strength, coordination, baseline vital signs, and balance to determine the type of assistance needed. Also assess his or her orientation and determine if there are any signs of distress. Postpone walking if you determine that the patient cannot walk safely. Evaluate the environment for safety before ambulation (e.g., removal of obstacles, a clean and dry floor, and the identification of rest points in case the patient's activity tolerance becomes less than expected or if the patient becomes dizzy). Also have the patient wear supportive, nonskid shoes.

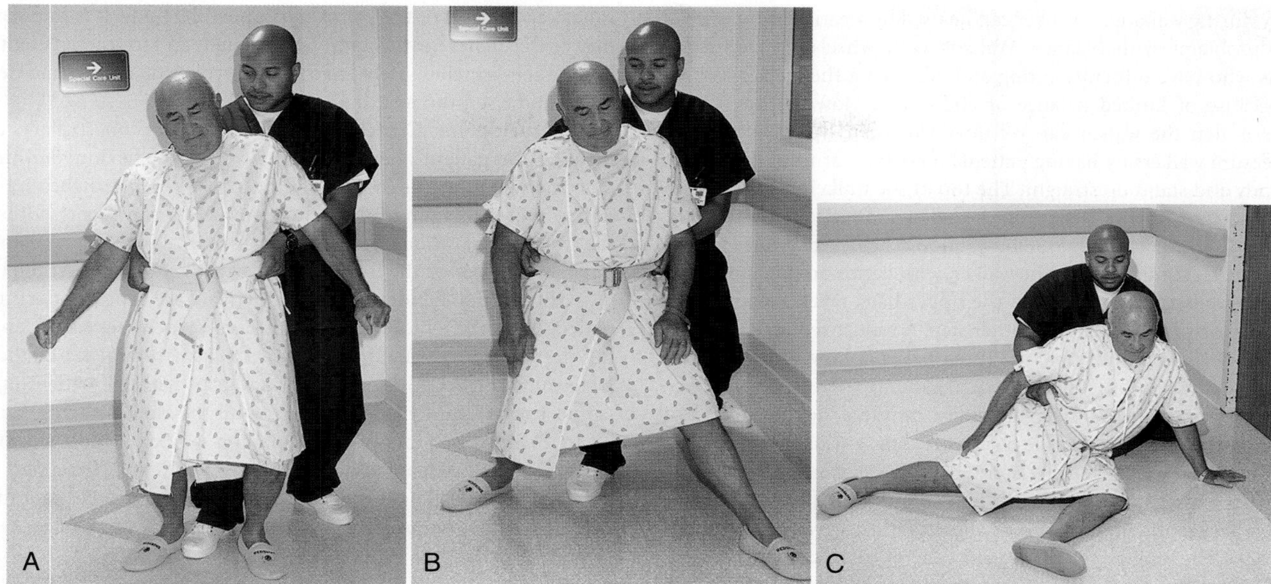

FIGURE 39-11 **A,** Stand with feet apart to provide a broad base of support. **B,** Extend one leg and let patient slide against it to the floor. **C,** Bend knees to lower body as patient slides to the floor.

Help the patient to a position of sitting at the side of the bed and dangling the legs over the side of the bed for 1 to 2 minutes before standing. Some patients experience orthostatic hypotension (i.e., a drop in blood pressure that occurs when they change from a horizontal to a vertical position) (Fedorowski and Melander, 2013; Lewis et al., 2013). Those at higher risk are patients who are immobilized, patients who are on prolonged bed rest, older adults, and patients with chronic illnesses such as diabetes mellitus and cardiovascular disease. Signs and symptoms of orthostatic hypotension include dizziness, light-headedness, nausea, tachycardia, pallor, and even fainting. Orthostatic hypotension usually stabilizes quickly, but if the patient develops dizziness lasting 60 seconds, return the patient to bed (Perme and Chandrashekar, 2009; Myszenski, 2014). Dangling a patient's legs before standing is an intermediate step that allows assessment of the patient before changing positions to maintain safety and prevent injury to the patient. In some instances you need to take the patient's blood pressure while he or she is sitting on the side of the bed.

Several methods are used to help a patient ambulate. Always provide support at the waist with a gait belt so the patient's center of gravity remains midline. A gait belt encircles the patient's waist snugly. You hold the back of the belt behind the patient. Some belts have handles attached for you to hold while the patient ambulates.

If the patient has a fainting (syncope) episode or begins to fall, assume a wide base of support with one foot in front of the other, thus supporting the patient's body weight (Figure 39-11, *A*). Extend one leg, let the patient slide against the leg, and gently lower him or her to the floor, protecting the head (Figure 39-11, *B* and *C*). Practice this technique with a friend or classmate before attempting it in a clinical setting. Use caution to prevent your own injury, especially if the patient is overweight. When the patient attempts to ambulate again, proceed more slowly, monitoring for reports of dizziness; and take the patient's blood pressure before, during, and after ambulation.

Restorative and Continuing Care. Restorative and continuing care involves implementing activity and exercise strategies to help the patient with ADLs after acute care is no longer needed. Restorative and continuing care also includes activities and exercises that restore and promote optimal functioning in patients with specific chronic illnesses such as coronary heart disease (CHD), hypertension, COPD, and diabetes mellitus.

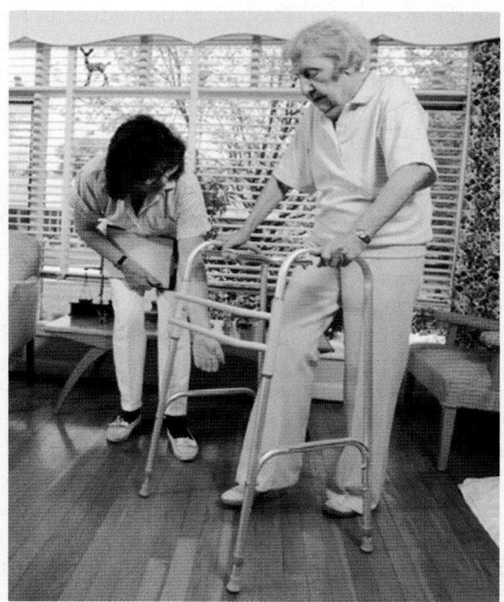

FIGURE 39-12 Patient using a walker.

Assistive Devices for Walking. In collaboration with other health care professionals such as physical therapists, promote activity and exercise by teaching the proper use of canes, walkers, or crutches, depending on the assistive device most appropriate for the patient's condition.

Walkers. A walker is a lightweight, movable device that stands about waist high and consists of a metal frame with handgrips, four widely placed sturdy legs, and one open side (Figure 39-12). Because it has a wide base of support, the walker provides great stability and security during walking. A walker can be used by a patient who is weak or has problems with balance. Walkers with wheels are useful for patients who have difficulty lifting and advancing the walker as they walk because of limited balance or endurance. However, the disadvantage is that the walker can roll forward when weight is applied. You measure walkers by having patients relax their arms at the side of their body and stand up straight. The top of the walker should line up with the crease on the inside of the wrist (American Academy of Orthopaedist Surgeons, 2015). Elbows should be flexed about 15 to 30 degrees when standing inside the walker, with hands on the handgrips. A patient holds the handgrips on the upper bars, takes a step, moves the walker forward, and takes another step. A walker requires a patient to lift the device up and forward. Teach patients how to use walkers safely and avoid risk of falling.

Canes. Canes are lightweight, easily movable devices made of wood or metal. They provide less support than a walker and are less stable. A person's cane length is equal to the distance between the greater trochanter and the floor (Pierson and Fairchild, 2013). Two common types of canes are the single straight-legged cane and the quad cane. The single straight-legged cane is more common and is used to support and balance a patient with decreased leg strength. Have the patient keep the cane on the stronger side of the body. For maximum support when walking, the patient places the cane forward 15 to 25 cm (6 to 10 inches), keeping body weight on both legs. He or she moves the weaker leg forward to the cane so body weight is divided between the cane and the stronger leg. The patient then advances the stronger leg past the cane so the weaker leg and the body weight are supported by the cane and weaker leg. During walking the patient continually repeats these three steps. The patient needs to learn that two points of support such as both feet or one foot and the cane are on the floor at all times.

The quad cane provides the most support and is used when there is partial or complete leg paralysis or some hemiplegia (Figure 39-13). You teach the patient the same three steps that are used with the straight-legged cane.

Crutches. Crutches are often needed to increase mobility. Begin crutch instruction with guidelines for safe use (Box 39-11). The use of crutches is often temporary (e.g., after ligament damage to the knee). However, some patients with paralysis of the lower extremities need them permanently. A crutch is a wooden or metal staff. The two types of crutches are the double adjustable or forearm crutch and the axillary wooden or metal crutch, which is the most common. The forearm crutch has a handgrip and a metal band that fits around the patient's forearm. The metal band and the handgrip are adjusted to fit the patient's height. The axillary crutch has a padded curved surface at the top, which fits under the axilla. A handgrip in the form of a crossbar is held at the level of the palms to support the body. It is important to measure crutches for the appropriate length and to teach patients how to use their crutches safely to achieve a stable gait, ascend and descend stairs, and rise from a sitting position.

Measuring for Crutches. Measurement for an axillary crutch includes the patient's height, the angle of elbow flexion, and the distance between the crutch pad and the axilla. When crutches are fitted, ensure that the length of the crutch is two to three finger widths from the axilla and position the tips approximately 2 inches lateral and 4 to 6 inches anterior to the front of the patient's shoes (Figure 39-14).

Position the handgrips so the axillae are not supporting the patient's body weight. Pressure on the axillae increases risk to underlying nerves, which sometimes results in partial paralysis of the arm. Determine correct position of the handgrips with the patient upright, supporting weight by the handgrips with the elbows slightly flexed at 20 to 25 degrees. Elbow flexion may be verified with a goniometer (Figure 39-15). When you determine the height and placement of the handgrips, verify that the distance between the crutch pad and the patient's axilla is approximately 2 inches (two to three finger widths) (Figure 39-16).

BOX 39-11 PATIENT TEACHING

Crutch Safety

Objective

- Patient will describe and demonstrate safe crutch walking.

Teaching Strategies

- Teach patient not to lean on crutches to support body weight.
- Teach patient with axillary crutches about the dangers of pressure on the axillae, which occurs when patient leans on the crutches to support body weight.
- Explain why patient needs to use only crutches that were measured for him or her.
- Show patient how to routinely inspect crutch tips. Securely attach rubber tips to crutches. Replace worn tips. Rubber crutch tips increase surface friction and help prevent slipping.
- Explain that crutch tips need to remain dry. Water decreases surface friction and increases risk of slipping. Show patient how to dry crutch tips if they become wet; patient may use paper or cloth towels.
- Show patient how to inspect structure of crutches. Cracks in a wooden crutch decrease its ability to support weight. Bends in aluminum crutches alter body alignment.
- Provide patient with list of medical supply companies in the community for obtaining repairs, new rubber tips, handgrips, and crutch pads.
- Instruct patient to have spare crutches and tips readily available.

Evaluation

- Patient states principles of crutch safety.
- Patient correctly demonstrates proper use of crutches.
- Axilla is free of pressure.

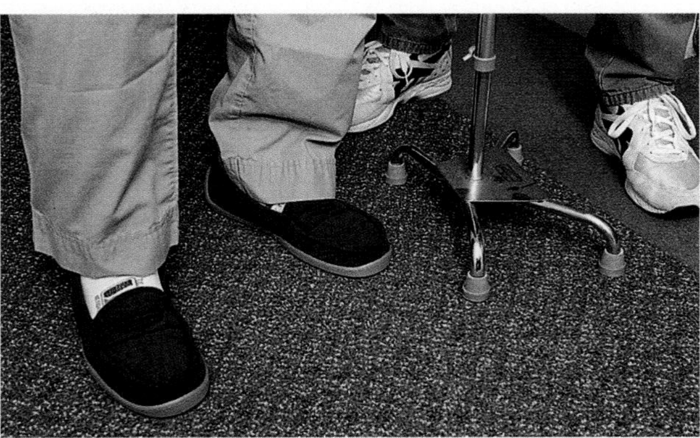

FIGURE 39-13 Bottom of quad cane.

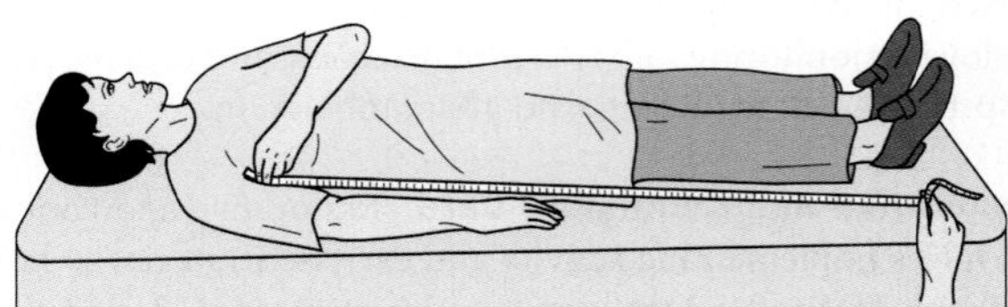

FIGURE 39-14 Measuring crutch length.

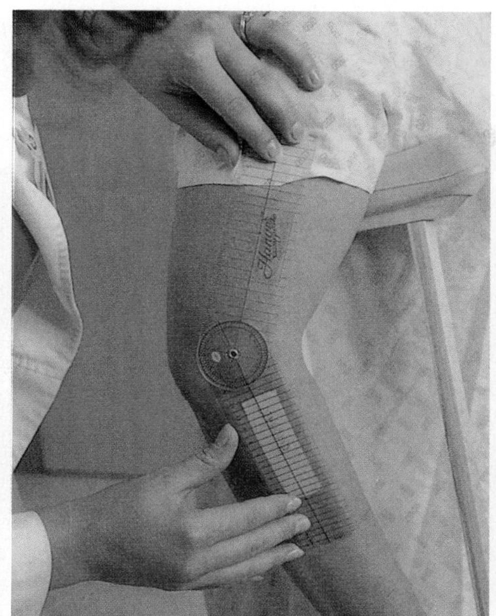

FIGURE 39-15 Using the goniometer to verify correct degree of elbow flexion for crutch use.

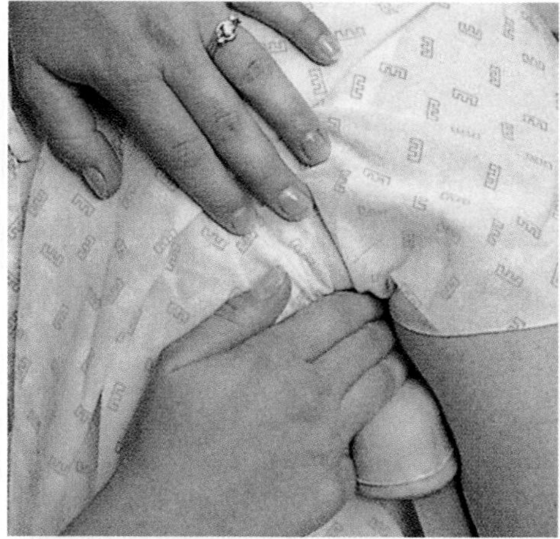

FIGURE 39-16 Verifying correct distance between crutch pads and axilla.

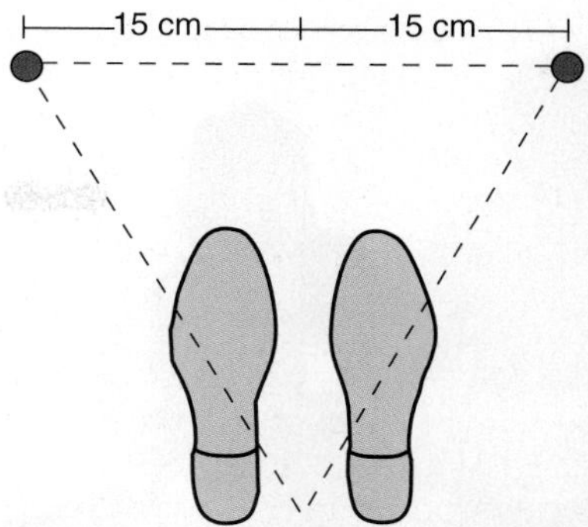

FIGURE 39-17 Tripod position, basic crutch stance.

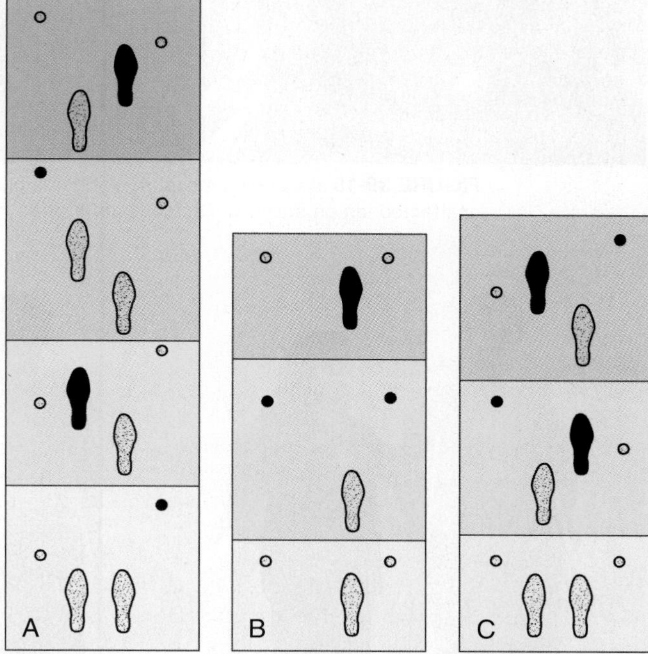

FIGURE 39-18 **A,** Four-point alternating gait. Solid feet and crutch tips show the order of foot and crutch tip movement in each of the four phases. (Read from bottom to top.) **B,** Three-point gait with weight borne on unaffected leg. Solid foot and crutch tips show weight bearing in each phase. (Read from bottom to top.) **C,** Two-point gait with weight borne partially on each foot and each crutch advancing with opposing leg. Solid areas indicate leg and crutch tips bearing weight. (Read from bottom to top.)

Crutch Gait. Patients assume a crutch gait by alternately bearing weight on one or both legs and on the crutches. Determine the gait by assessing the patient's physical and functional abilities and the disease or injury that resulted in the need for crutches. This section summarizes the basic crutch stance and the four standard gaits: four-point alternating gait, three-point alternating gait, two-point gait, and swing-through gait.

The basic crutch stance is the tripod position, formed when the crutches are placed 15 cm (6 inches) in front of and 15 cm (6 inches) to the side of each foot (Figure 39-17). This position improves the patient's balance by providing a wider base of support. The body alignment of the patient in the tripod position includes an erect head and neck, straight vertebrae, and extended hips and knees. The axillae should not bear any weight. The patient assumes the tripod position before crutch walking.

Four-point alternating, or four-point, gait gives stability to the patient but requires weight bearing on both legs. Each leg is moved alternately with each opposing crutch so three points of support are on the floor at all times (Figure 39-18, *A*).

Three-point alternating, or three-point, gait requires the patient to bear all of the weight on one foot. In a three-point gait the patient bears weight on both crutches and then on the uninvolved leg, repeating the sequence (see Figure 39-18, *B*). The affected leg does not touch the ground during the early phase of the three-point gait. Gradually the patient progresses to touchdown and full weight bearing on the affected leg.

The two-point gait requires at least partial weight bearing on each foot (see Figure 39-18, *C*). The patient moves a crutch at the same time as the opposing leg so the crutch movements are similar to arm motion during normal walking.

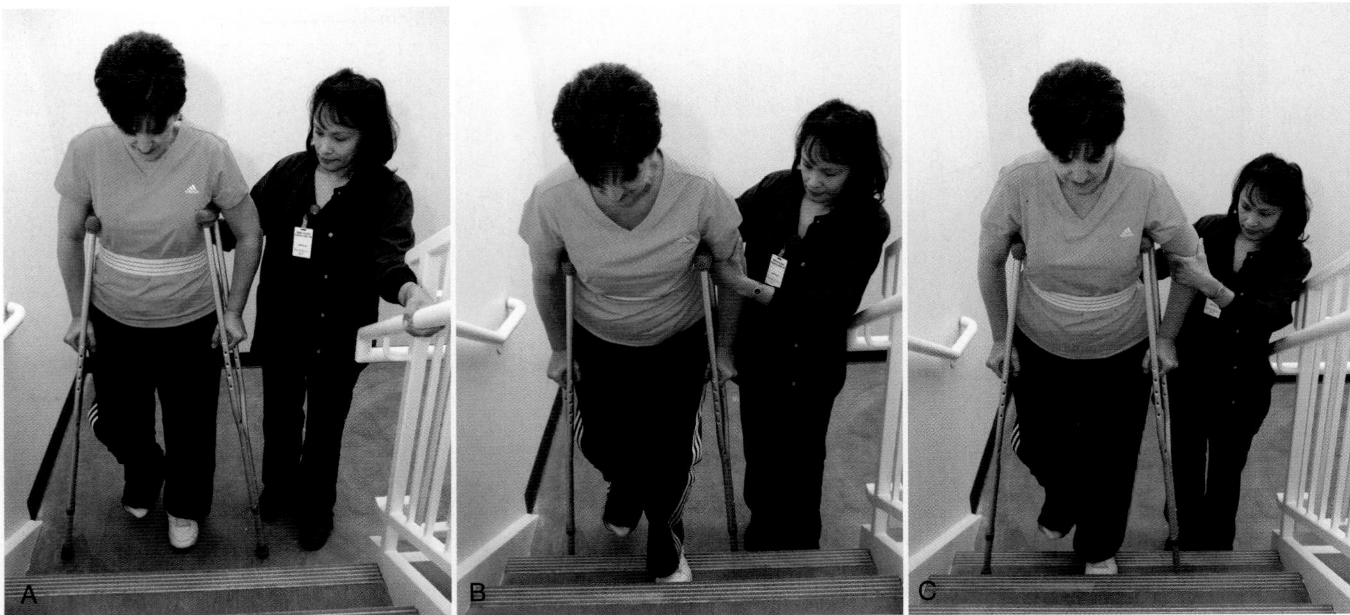

FIGURE 39-19 Ascending stairs. **A,** Weight is placed on crutch. **B,** Weight is transferred from crutches to unaffected leg on stairs. **C,** Crutches are aligned with unaffected leg on stairs.

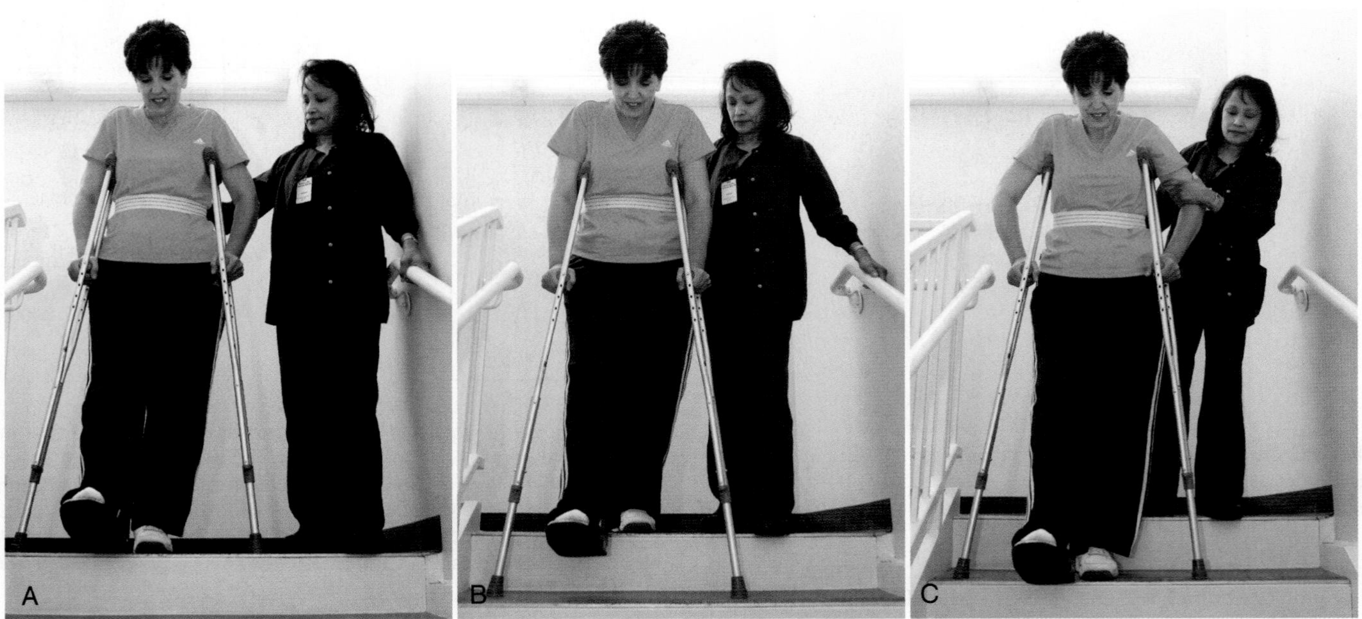

FIGURE 39-20 Descending stairs. **A,** Body weight is on unaffected leg. **B,** Body weight is transferred to crutches. **C,** Unaffected leg is aligned on stairs with crutches.

Individuals with paraplegia who wear weight-supporting braces on their legs frequently use the swing-through gait. With weight placed on the supported legs, the patient places the crutches one stride in front and then swings to or through them while they support his or her weight.

Crutch Walking on Stairs. When ascending stairs on crutches, the patient usually uses a modified three-point gait (Figure 39-19). He or she stands at the bottom of the stairs and transfers body weight to the crutches. He or she advances the unaffected leg between the crutches to the stairs. The patient then shifts weight from the crutches to the unaffected leg. Finally he or she aligns both crutches on the stairs. The patient repeats this sequence until he or she reaches the top of the stairs.

A three-phase sequence is also used to descend the stairs (Figure 39-20). The patient transfers body weight to the unaffected leg. He or she places the crutches on the stairs and begins to transfer body weight to them, moving the affected leg forward. Finally the patient moves the unaffected leg to the stairs with the crutches. The patient repeats the sequence until reaching the bottom of the stairs.

Because in most cases patients need to use crutches for some time, they need to be taught to use them on stairs before discharge. This instruction applies to all patients who are dependent on crutches, not

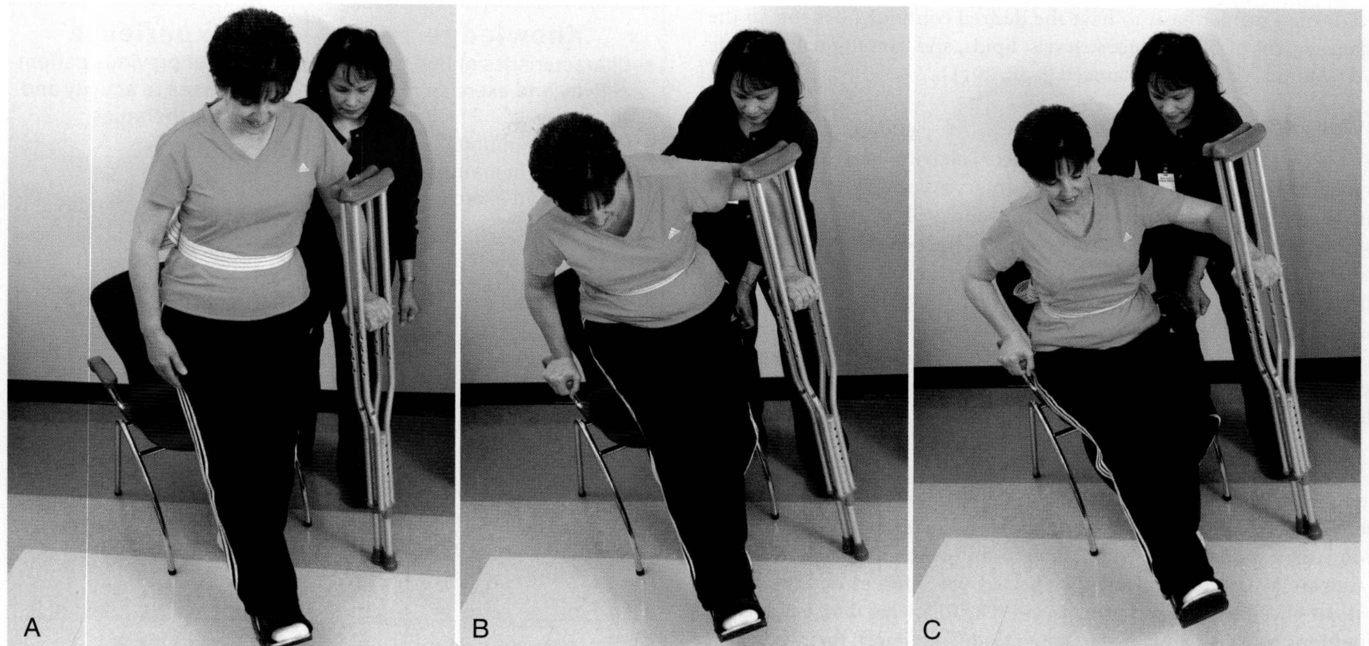

FIGURE 39-21 Sitting in a chair. **A,** Both crutches are held in one hand. Patient transfers weight to crutches and unaffected leg. **B,** Patient grasps arm of chair with free hand and begins to lower herself into chair. **C,** Patient completely lowers herself into chair.

only those who have stairs in their homes. You will frequently collaborate with physical therapists to provide instruction about crutch walking.

Sitting in a Chair with Crutches. As with crutch walking and crutch walking up and down stairs, the procedure for sitting in a chair involves phases and requires the patient to transfer weight (Figure 39-21). First the patient positions himself or herself at the center front of the chair with the posterior aspect of the legs touching the chair. Then the patient holds both crutches in the hand opposite the affected leg. If both legs are affected, as with a person with paraplegia who wears weight-supporting braces, the patient holds the crutches in the hand on his or her stronger side. With both crutches in one hand, the patient supports body weight on the unaffected leg and the crutches. While still holding the crutches, the patient grasps the arm of the chair with the remaining hand and lowers his or her body into it. To stand the procedure is reversed; and the patient, when fully erect, assumes the tripod position before beginning to walk.

Restoration of Activity and Chronic Illness. Nurses design care plans to increase activity and exercise in patients with specific disease conditions and chronic illnesses such as CHD, hypertension, COPD, and diabetes mellitus.

Coronary Heart Disease. Research shows that activity and exercise play a role in secondary prevention or recurrence of CHD. Cardiac rehabilitation is an integral part of comprehensive care of patients diagnosed with CHD. Nurses are involved in many aspects of cardiac rehabilitation and help patients develop a program of exercise that fits their needs and level of functioning. Increased physical activity benefits individuals with MI, angina pectoris, or heart failure and patients who have had a coronary artery bypass graft (CABG) or percutaneous transluminal coronary angioplasty (PTCA). Patients with CHD benefit from exercise and activity in terms of reduced mortality and morbidity, improved quality of life, improved left ventricular function, increased functional capacity, decreased blood lipids and apolipoproteins (protein components of lipoprotein complexes), and psychological well-being (Campos-Outcalt, 2014; Donges et al., 2010).

Hypertension. Exercise reduces systolic and diastolic blood pressure readings. Research shows that low- to moderate-intensity aerobic exercise (brisk walking or bicycling) is the most effective in lowering blood pressure. In addition, a tai chi exercise program has demonstrated a significant reduction in systolic and diastolic blood pressures (Balady et al., 2010; Edelman et al., 2013; Lo et al., 2012).

Chronic Obstructive Pulmonary Disease. Pulmonary rehabilitation helps patients reach an optimal level of functioning. Some patients are fearful of participating in exercise because of the potential of worsening dyspnea (difficulty breathing). This aversion to physical activity sets up a progressive deconditioning in which minimal physical exertion results in dyspnea. Pulmonary rehabilitation provides a safe environment for monitoring patients' progress. In addition, they receive encouragement and support to increase activity and exercise (Berry et al., 2010; Salhi et al., 2010).

Diabetes Mellitus. Along with diet, glucose monitoring, and medication, exercise is an important component in the care of patients with diabetes mellitus. Individuals with type 1 diabetes need to exercise because it leads to improved glucose control, cardiovascular fitness, and psychological well-being. Exercise lowers blood sugar levels, and the effects of exercise on blood sugar levels often last for at least 24 hours. Instruct the patient with type 1 diabetes about the risks and precautions regarding exercise. Instruction includes the need for a physical examination before beginning an exercise program and precautions to monitor blood glucose level immediately before and after exercise. Also instruct patients to perform low- to moderate-intensity exercises, carry a concentrated form of carbohydrates (sugar packets or hard candy), and wear a medical-alert bracelet. Endurance and resistance exercise appear equally effective in improving the control of metabolism in patients with type 2 diabetes. However, exercise must occur on a regular basis to have the desired continued benefits in the management of blood glucose levels, lipids, and overall quality of life (ACSM and ADA, 2010; Hameed et al., 2011).

◆ Evaluation

Through the Patient's Eyes. For activity and exercise you measure the effectiveness of nursing interventions by the success of meeting the patient's expected outcomes and goals of care. The patient is the only one who knows the effectiveness and benefits of activity and exercise (Figure 39-22). Ask the patient questions such as, "How well did you tolerate walking, and is that what you expected?" and "You have been walking regularly for a month now, how has it made you feel?" Continuous evaluation helps to determine whether new or revised therapies are needed and if new nursing diagnoses have developed.

Patient Outcomes. To evaluate the effectiveness of nursing interventions to enhance activity and exercise, make comparisons with baseline measures that include pulse, blood pressure, oxygen saturation (when available), strength, fatigue, and psychological well-being. Compare actual outcomes with expected outcomes to determine the patient's health status and progression. The following is an example of questions you ask when your patients do not meet their expected outcomes:

- The last time we met you planned to walk outside for 20 minutes 3 days a week. However, you report that you are only able to walk twice a week right now. What do you think is preventing you from meeting your goal?
- Your weight is the same this month as it was last month. We were hoping that increasing your activity would lead to a decrease in your weight. Help me understand the factors you believe are preventing you from losing weight right now.
- You state that you experience leg pain after walking short distances. Describe your pain. Which pain-relieving measures have you tried?

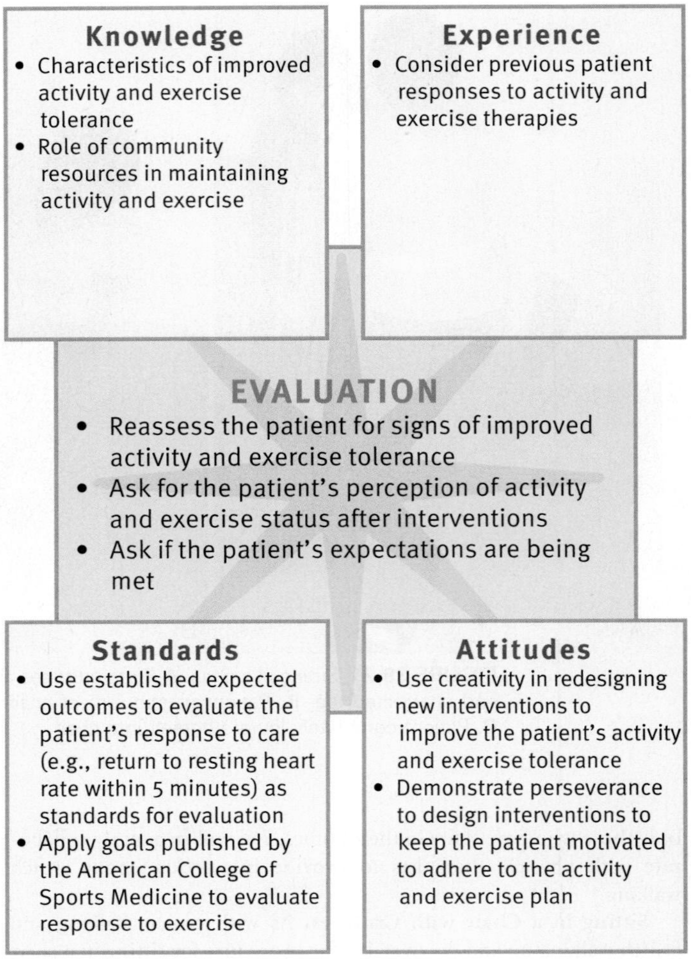

Knowledge
- Characteristics of improved activity and exercise tolerance
- Role of community resources in maintaining activity and exercise

Experience
- Consider previous patient responses to activity and exercise therapies

EVALUATION
- Reassess the patient for signs of improved activity and exercise tolerance
- Ask for the patient's perception of activity and exercise status after interventions
- Ask if the patient's expectations are being met

Standards
- Use established expected outcomes to evaluate the patient's response to care (e.g., return to resting heart rate within 5 minutes) as standards for evaluation
- Apply goals published by the American College of Sports Medicine to evaluate response to exercise

Attitudes
- Use creativity in redesigning new interventions to improve the patient's activity and exercise tolerance
- Demonstrate perseverance to design interventions to keep the patient motivated to adhere to the activity and exercise plan

FIGURE 39-22 Critical thinking model for activity and exercise evaluation.

SAFETY GUIDELINES FOR NURSING SKILLS

Ensuring patient safety is an essential role of the professional nurse. To ensure patient safety, communicate clearly with the members of the health care team, assess and incorporate the patient's priorities of care and preferences, and use the best evidence when making decisions about your patient's care. When performing the skills in this chapter, remember the following points to ensure safe patient handling and individualized patient-centered care.

- Mentally review the transfer steps before beginning the procedure; this ensures both your safety and that of the patient.
- Assess the patient's mobility and strength to determine the assistance that he or she is able to offer during transfer. Stand on patient's weak side when assisting (Pierson and Fairchild, 2013).
- Determine the amount and type of assistance required for transfer, including the type of transfer equipment and the number of personnel to safely transfer and prevent harm to the patient and health care providers.
- Raise the side rail on the side of the bed opposite of where you are standing to prevent the patient from falling out of bed on that side.
- Arrange equipment (e.g., intravenous lines, feeding tube, indwelling catheter) so it does not interfere with the positioning or transfer process.
- Evaluate the patient for correct body alignment and pressure risks after the transfer.
- Make sure that all personnel understand how the equipment functions before it is used.
- Educate patients about how equipment functions to reduce their anxiety and enlist their cooperation.

SKILL 39-1 USING SAFE AND EFFECTIVE TRANSFER TECHNIQUES

DELEGATION CONSIDERATIONS

The skill of effective transfer techniques can be delegated to nursing assistive personnel (NAP). Patients who are transferred for the first time after prolonged bed rest, extensive surgery, critical illness, or spinal cord trauma usually require supervision by the nurse. Instruct NAP about:

- Seeking assistance when moving or lifting a patient (e.g., when the patient is overweight, medicated, or confused).
- Patient limitations (e.g., changes in blood pressure, mobility restrictions) that affect safe transfer techniques.

EQUIPMENT

- Transfer belt, sling, or lapboard (as needed)
- Nonskid shoes, bath blankets, and pillows
- Wheelchair (Position chair at 45- to 60-degree angle to bed, lock brakes, remove footrests, and lock bed brakes.)
- Stretcher (Position next to bed, lock brakes on stretcher, lock brakes on bed.)
- Mechanical/hydraulic lift (Use frame, canvas strips or chains, and hammock or canvas strips.)
- Stand-assist lift device

STEP	RATIONALE
ASSESSMENT	
1. Identify patient using two identifiers (e.g., name and birthday or name and medical record number) according to agency policy. Explain procedure.	Ensures correct patient. Complies with The Joint Commission standards and improves patient safety (TJC, 2016).
2. Assess physiological capacity to transfer:	Provides information relative to patient's abilities, physical status, ability to comprehend, and number of individuals needed to provide safe transferring.
a. Muscle strength (legs and upper arms)	Immobile patients have decreased muscle strength, tone, and mass. Affects ability to bear weight or raise body.
b. Joint mobility (range of motion [ROM]) and contracture formation	Immobility or inflammatory processes (e.g., arthritis) sometimes lead to contracture formation and impaired joint mobility.
c. Paralysis or paresis (spastic or flaccid)	Patient with central nervous system damage often has bilateral paralysis (requiring transfer by swivel bar, sliding bar, or mechanical lift) or unilateral paralysis, which requires belt transfer to "best" side. Weakness (paresis) requires stabilization of knee while transferring. Flaccid arm needs to be supported with sling during transfer.
d. Bone continuity.	Patients with trauma to one leg or hip may be non–weight bearing during transfer. Amputees may use slide board to transfer.
3. Assess for weakness, dizziness, or orthostatic (postural) hypotension or risk for orthostatic hypotension (e.g., previously on bed rest, first time arising from supine position following surgical procedure, history of dizziness when arising)	Determines risk of fainting or falling during transfer. Immobilized patients have decreased ability for autonomic nervous system to equalize blood supply, resulting in drop of 20 mm Hg systolic or more in blood pressure when rising from sitting position (Fedorowski and Melander, 2013; Lewis et al., 2013).
4. Activity tolerance, noting for fatigue during activity	Determines ability of patient to help with transfer.
5. Assess proprioceptive function (awareness of posture and equilibrium), including ability to maintain balance while sitting in bed or on side of bed and tendency to sway toward one side.	Determines stability of patient's balance for transfer and risk for falls.
6. Assess sensory status, including central and peripheral vision, adequacy of hearing, and presence of peripheral sensation loss.	Determines influence of sensory loss on ability to make transfer. Visual field loss decreases patient's ability to see in direction of transfer. Peripheral sensation loss decreases proprioception. Patients with visual and hearing losses need transfer techniques adapted to deficits. Patients with a cerebrovascular accident (CVA) sometimes lose area of visual field, which profoundly affects vision and perception.

CLINICAL DECISION: *Patients with hemiplegia also often "neglect" one side of the body (inattention to or unawareness of one side of body or environment), which distorts perception of the visual field. If patient experiences neglect of one side, instruct him or her to scan all visual fields when transferring.*

STEP	RATIONALE
7. Assess level of comfort (e.g., joint discomfort, muscle spasm) and measure level of pain on a 0-10 scale. Offer prescribed analgesic 30 minutes before transfer.	Pain reduces patient's motivation and ability to be mobile. Pain relief before transfer enhances patient participation (Christo et al., 2011).
8. Assess vital signs.	Vital sign changes such as increased pulse and respiration and drop in BP indicate activity intolerance (see Chapter 30).
9. Assess patient's cognitive status, including ability to follow verbal instructions, short-term memory, and recognition of physical deficits and limitations to movement.	Determines patient's ability to follow directions and learn transfer techniques.

CLINICAL DECISION: *Patients with head trauma or CVA may have perceptual cognitive deficits that create safety risks. If the patient has difficulty comprehending, simplify instructions by providing one step at a time and maintain consistency.*

STEP	RATIONALE
10. Assess patient's level of motivation such as eagerness versus unwillingness to be mobile and perception of value of exercise.	Altered physiological and psychological conditions reduce a patient's desire to engage in activity.

SKILL 39-1 USING SAFE AND EFFECTIVE TRANSFER TECHNIQUES—cont'd

STEP	RATIONALE
11. Assess patient's specific risk for falling or being injured during transfer (e.g., neuromuscular deficits, visual loss, motor weakness, fear of falling, or bone loss).	Causes risk for tripping, losing balance.
12. Assess previous mode of transfer (if applicable).	Determines mode of transfer and assistance required to provide continuity.
13. Assess patient's specific risk of falling or being injured when transferred (e.g., neuromuscular deficits, motor weakness, calcium loss from bones, cognitive and visual dysfunction, altered balance).	Certain conditions increase risk of falling or potential injury.
14. Assess special transfer equipment needed for home setting and previous mode of transfer (if applicable).	Prior teaching of family and support people, assessing home for safety risks and functionality, and providing applicable aids greatly enhance transfer ability at home.

PLANNING

STEP	RATIONALE
1. Gather appropriate equipment.	
2. Determine number of people needed to assist with transfer by referring to proper algorithm. Do not start procedure until all caregivers are available.	Ensures safe patient transfer. Algorithms for safe patient handling and movement are provided at http://www.visn8.va.gov/patientsafetycenter/safepthandling
3. Perform hand hygiene. Verify that bed brakes are locked.	Reduces transmission of microorganisms. Promotes patient and caregiver safety.
4. Explain procedure to patient.	Increases patient participation.

IMPLEMENTATION

1. Transfer patient.

a. Assisting cooperative patient to sitting position in bed:

CLINICAL DECISION: *Careful assessment of your patient's ability to assist in the following position technique is extremely important. Consider the use of a mechanical lift. Your role in helping your patient to a sitting position is to be a guide and instruct. If patient can bear weight and move to a sitting position independently, allow him or her to do so and offer assistance (VISN8, 2015).*

STEP	RATIONALE
(1) Raise bed to waist level. Place patient in supine position.	Enables you to assess patient's body alignment continually.
(2) Face head of bed at 45-degree angle and remove pillows.	Proper positioning reduces twisting of your body when moving patient. Pillows cause interference when patient is sitting up in bed.
(3) Place feet in wide base of support, with foot closer to bed in front of other foot.	Improves balance and allows transfer of body weight as you move patient to sitting position.
(4) Place arm nearer head of bed under patient's shoulders, supporting his or her head and cervical vertebrae.	Maintains alignment of head and cervical vertebrae and allows for even lifting of patient's upper trunk.
(5) Place other hand on bed surface.	Provides support and balance.
(6) Raise patient to sitting position by shifting weight from front to back leg.	Improves balance, overcomes inertia, and transfers weight in direction you move patient.
(7) Push against bed using arm that is placed on bed surface.	Divides activity between arms and legs and protects back from strain. By bracing one hand against mattress and pushing against it as you lift patient, you transfer weight away from your back muscles through your arm onto mattress.

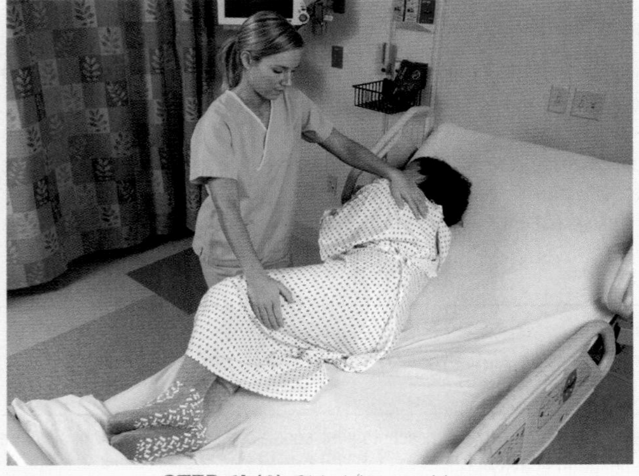

STEP 1b(1) Side-lying position.

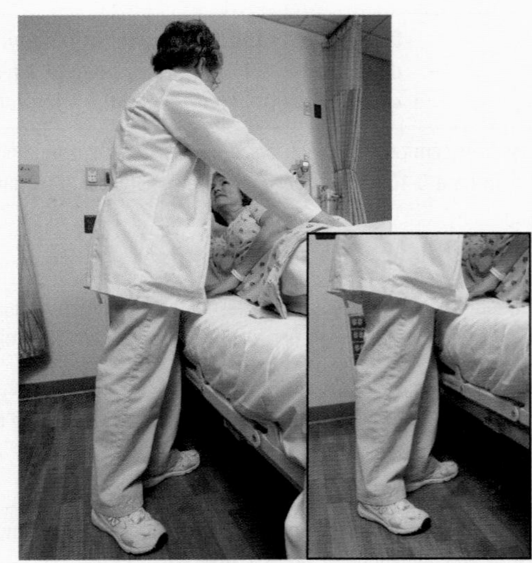

STEP 1b(4) Proper foot placement.

STEP	RATIONALE
b. Assisting cooperative patient who can partially bear weight to sitting position on side of bed:	
(1) With bed flat and waist high, turn patient to a side-lying position with assistance of another caregiver if necessary. Patient needs to face nurse on side of bed that patient will be sitting (see illustration).	Decreases amount of work needed by nurse and patient.
(2) Raise head of bed 30 degrees.	Facilitates raising patient to sitting position and protects him or her from falling.
(3) Stand opposite patient's hips. Turn diagonally so you face patient and far corner of head of bed.	Places your center of gravity nearer patient. Reduces twisting of your body because you are facing direction of movement.
(4) Place feet apart with foot closest to bed in front of other foot (see illustration).	Increases balance and allows transfer of body weight as you move patient to a sitting position.
(5) Place arm nearer head of bed under patient's shoulders, supporting head and cervical vertebrae.	Maintains alignment of head and cervical vertebrae and allows for even lifting of patient's trunk.
(6) Place other arm over patient's thighs (see illustration).	Supports hip and prevents patient from falling backward during procedure.
(7) Move patient's lower legs and feet over side of bed. Pivot toward rear leg, allowing patient's upper legs to swing downward. At same time shift weight to back leg and elevate patient (see illustration).	Decreases friction and resistance. Weight of patient's legs when off bed allows gravity to lower legs, and weight of legs helps to pull to sitting position.
(8) Allow patient to dangle on side of bed for a few minutes. Have patient alternately flex and extend feet and move lower legs. Ask if patient feels dizzy. Have patient relax and take a few deep breaths until dizziness subsides and balance is gained.	Determines ability to tolerate standing. Dizziness that lasts more than 60 seconds may indicate orthostatic hypotension; return patient to bed (Myszenski, 2014). Recheck blood pressure.
c. Transferring cooperative patient who is partially weight bearing from bed to chair:	

CLINICAL DECISION: *Allow patient to transfer independently if able to fully bear weight. Stand by as needed to promote safe transfer (VISN8, 2015). If patient has partial weight bearing with upper-body strength and caregiver must lift more than 35 lbs (115.9 kg) of patient weight, use a stand-assist lift device and follow manufacturer instructions (Figure 39-23).*

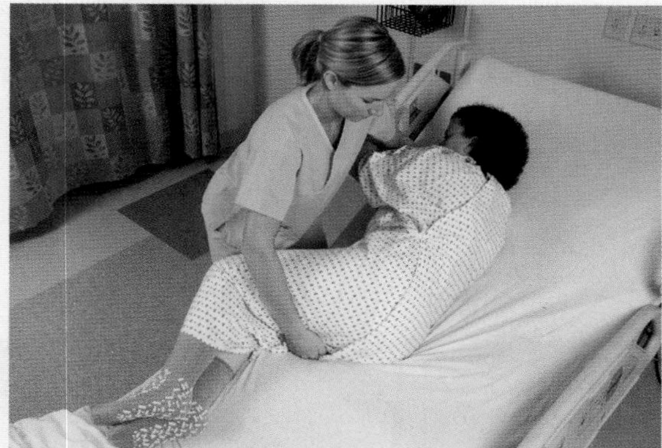

STEP 1b(6) Nurse places arm over patient's thighs.

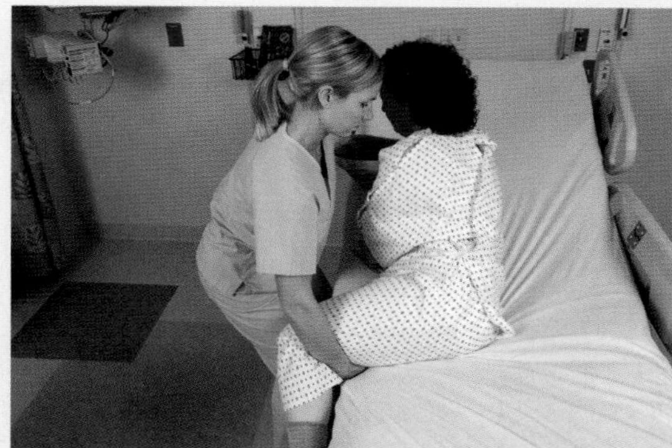

STEP 1b(7) Nurse shifts weight to rear leg and elevates patient.

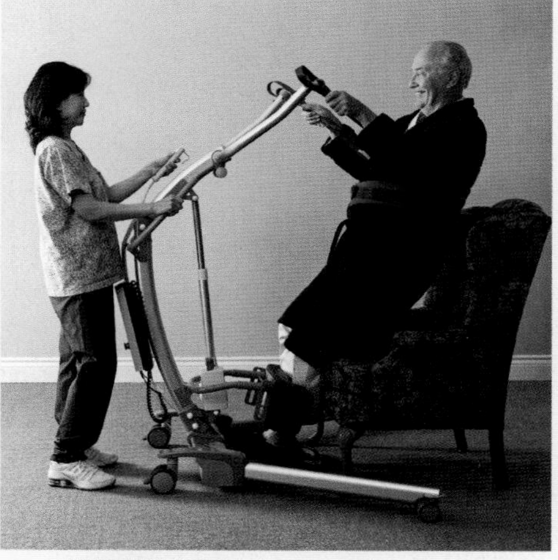

FIGURE 39-23 Stand-assist device.

SKILL 39-1 USING SAFE AND EFFECTIVE TRANSFER TECHNIQUES—cont'd

STEP	RATIONALE
(1) Help patient to sitting position on side of bed (see Step 1b). Have chair placed next to bed at 45-degree angle on patient's strong side. Allow patient to sit on side of bed (dangling) for a few minutes before transferring. Ask if patient feels dizzy. Do not leave unattended while dangling.	Positions chair within easy access for transfer. Placing chair on patient's stronger side allows patient to help with transferring. Dangling helps equilibrate blood pressure, reducing risk for dizziness or fainting when standing.
(2) Apply transfer belt or other transfer aids. Be sure it completely circles patient's waist. Place the belt low and be sure it is snug. You may need to adjust belt once patient stands.	Transfer belt maintains stability of patient during transfer and reduces risk for falling (Pierson and Fairchild, 2013; VISN8, 2015). Patient's arm needs to be in sling if flaccid paralysis is present.
(3) Ensure that patient has stable nonskid shoes. Weight-bearing or strong leg is forward, with weak foot back.	Nonskid soles decrease risk of slipping during transfer. Always have patient wear shoes during transfer; bare feet increase risk of falls. Patient stands on stronger, or weight-bearing, leg.
(4) Spread feet apart.	Ensures balance with wide base of support.
(5) Flex hips and knees, aligning knees with patient's knees (see illustration).	Flexing knees and hips lowers center of gravity to object to be raised; aligning knees with those of patient allows for stabilization of knees when patient stands.
(6) Grasp transfer belt from underneath along patient's sides.	Provides movement of patient at center of gravity. Never lift patients with upper-extremity paralysis or paresis by or under arms (VISN8, 2006).

CLINICAL DECISION: *Use a transfer belt or walking belt with handles in place of the under-axilla technique. The under-axilla technique is physically stressful for nurses and uncomfortable for patients (Pierson and Fairchild, 2013).*

STEP	RATIONALE
(7) Rock patient up to standing position on count of 3 while straightening hips and legs and keeping knees slightly flexed (see illustration). Unless contraindicated, instruct patient to use hands to push up if applicable.	Rocking motion gives patient's body momentum and requires less muscular effort to lift him or her.
(8) Maintain stability of patient's weak or paralyzed leg with knee.	Often patient maintains ability to stand on paralyzed or weak limb with support of knee to stabilize (Pierson and Fairchild, 2013).
(9) Pivot on foot farther from chair.	Maintains support of patient while allowing adequate space for patient to move.
(10) Instruct patient to use armrests on chair for support and ease into chair (see illustration).	Increases patient stability.

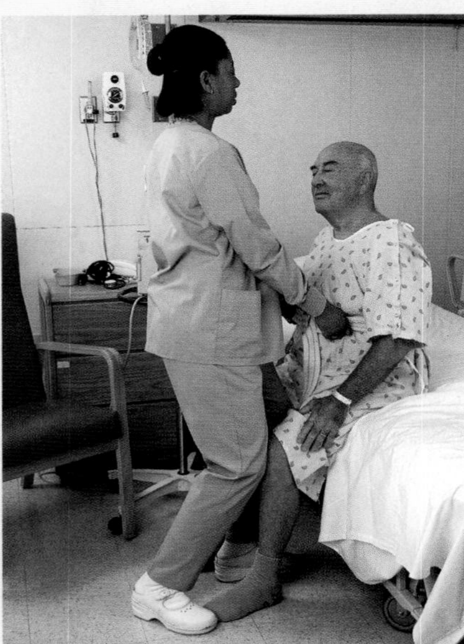

STEP 1c(5) Nurse flexes hips and knees, aligning knees with patient's knees.

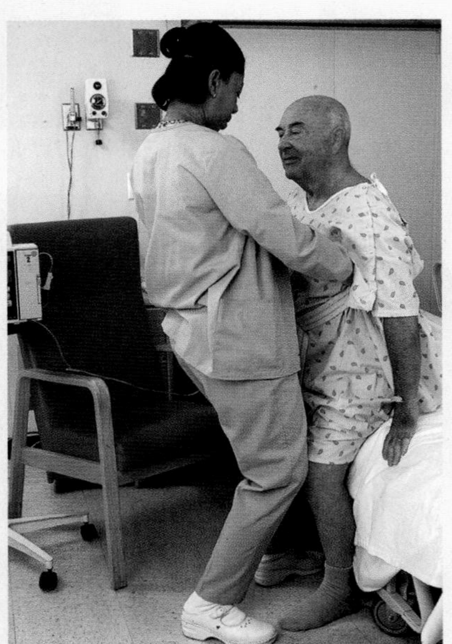

STEP 1c(7) Nurse rocks patient to standing position.

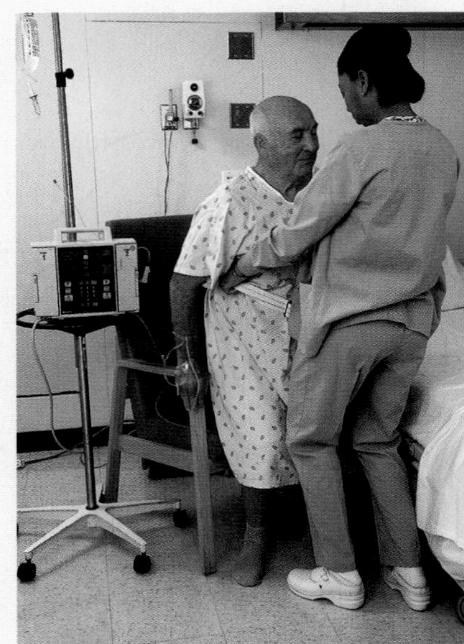

STEP 1c(10) Patient uses armrests for support.

STEP	RATIONALE
(11) Flex hips and knees while lowering patient into chair (see illustration).	Prevents injury to nurse from poor body mechanics.
(12) Assess patient for proper alignment for sitting position. Provide support for paralyzed extremities. Lapboard or sling supports flaccid arm. Stabilize leg with bath blanket or pillow.	Prevents injury to patient from poor body alignment.
(13) Praise patient's progress, effort, or performance.	Continued support and encouragement provide incentive for patient perseverance.
d. Using mechanical lift and full-body sling to transfer uncooperative patient who can bear partial weight or patient who cannot bear weight and is either uncooperative or does not have upper-body strength to move from bed to chair:	Mechanical lift devices prevent musculoskeletal injuries to health care workers (Pelczarski, 2012).
(1) Position lift properly at bedside (see equipment instructions).	Ensures safe elevation of patient off bed. (Before using lift, be thoroughly familiar with its operation.)
(2) Position chair near bed and allow adequate space to maneuver lift.	Prepares environment for safe use of lift and subsequent transfer.
(3) Raise bed to high position with mattress flat. Lower side rail.	Maintains nurses' alignment during transfer.
(4) Keep side rail up on side opposite from you.	Maintains patient safety.
(5) Roll patient away from you.	Positions patient for use of lift sling.
(6) Place sling under patient. Place lower edge under patient's knees (wide piece) and upper edge under patient's shoulders (narrow piece).	Allows positioning of patient on mechanical/hydraulic sling. Places sling under patient's center of gravity and greatest part of body weight.
(7) Roll patient to opposite side and pull body sling through.	Completes positioning of patient on mechanical/hydraulic sling.
(8) Roll patient supine onto canvas seat.	Sling needs to extend from shoulders to knees (hammock) to support patient's body weight equally.
(9) Remove patient's glasses if appropriate.	Swivel bar is close to patient's head and can break eyeglasses.
(10) If using a transportable hydraulic lift, place horseshoe-shaped base of lift under side of bed (on side with chair).	Positions hydraulic lift efficiently and promotes smooth transfer.
(11) Lower upper horizontal bar to sling level following manufacturer directions. Some lifts require valve to be locked.	Positions lift close to patient. Locking valve prevents injury to patient.
(12) Attach hooks on strap to holes in sling. Short straps hook to top holes of sling; longer straps hook to bottom of sling.	Secures hydraulic lift to sling.
(13) Elevate head of bed.	Positions patient in sitting position.
(14) Fold patient's arms over chest.	Prevents injury to paralyzed arms.
(15) Use lift to raise patient off bed (see illustration).	Moves patient off bed.
(16) Use steering handle to pull lift from bed and maneuver to chair.	Moves patient from bed to chair.
(17) Move lift to chair.	Positions lift in front of chair.

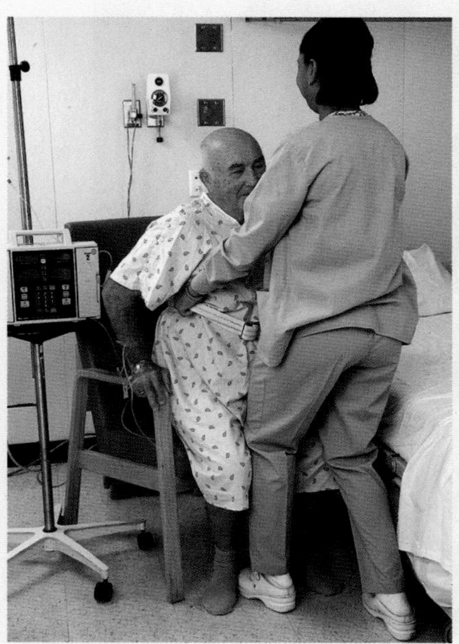
STEP 1c(11) Nurse eases patient into chair.

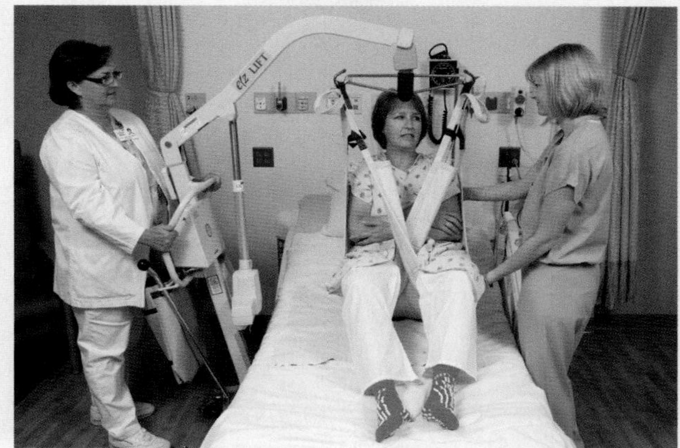
STEP 1d(15) Use mechanical lift to raise patient off bed.

SKILL 39-1 USING SAFE AND EFFECTIVE TRANSFER TECHNIQUES—cont'd

STEP	RATIONALE
(18) Position patient and lower slowly into chair following manufacturer guidelines (see illustration).	Safely guides patient into back of chair as seat descends.
(19) Remove straps and mechanical/hydraulic lift.	Prevents damage to skin and underlying tissues from canvas or hooks.
(20) Check patient's sitting alignment and correct if necessary.	Prevents injury from poor posture.
e. Transferring patient from bed to stretcher (bed at stretcher level):	
(1) Raise bed to height of stretcher.	Bed and stretcher need to be at same level to allow patient to slide from bed to stretcher.
(2) Lower head of bed as much as patient can tolerate. Cross patient's arms on chest. Ensure that bed brakes are locked.	Prevents injury to arms during transfer.
(3) Lower side rails. Two caregivers stand on side where stretcher will be; third caregiver stands on other side.	Minimizes caregivers' stretching. Prevents patient from falling out of bed and promotes safety.
(4) Two caregivers help patient roll onto side toward them (use of drawsheet is optional) with smooth, continuous motion.	Positions patient for placing friction-reducing lateral transfer device.
(5) Place slide board under drawsheet or follow manufacturer guidelines (see illustrations). Gently roll patient back onto slide board.	Patient needs to be placed on transfer device properly to allow safe transfer.
(6) Align stretcher alongside of bed. Lock wheels of stretcher once it is in place. Instruct patient not to move.	Positions stretcher in correct position for transfer and prevents patient from falling out of bed.
(7) All three caregivers place feet widely apart with one slightly in front of the other and grasp friction-reducing device.	Prepares for transfer. Wide base of support allows nurse to shift weight and minimizes back strain.

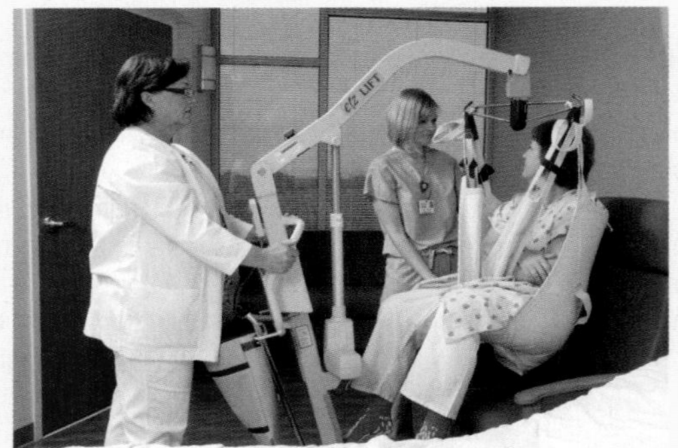

STEP 1d(18) Use mechanical lift to lower patient into chair.

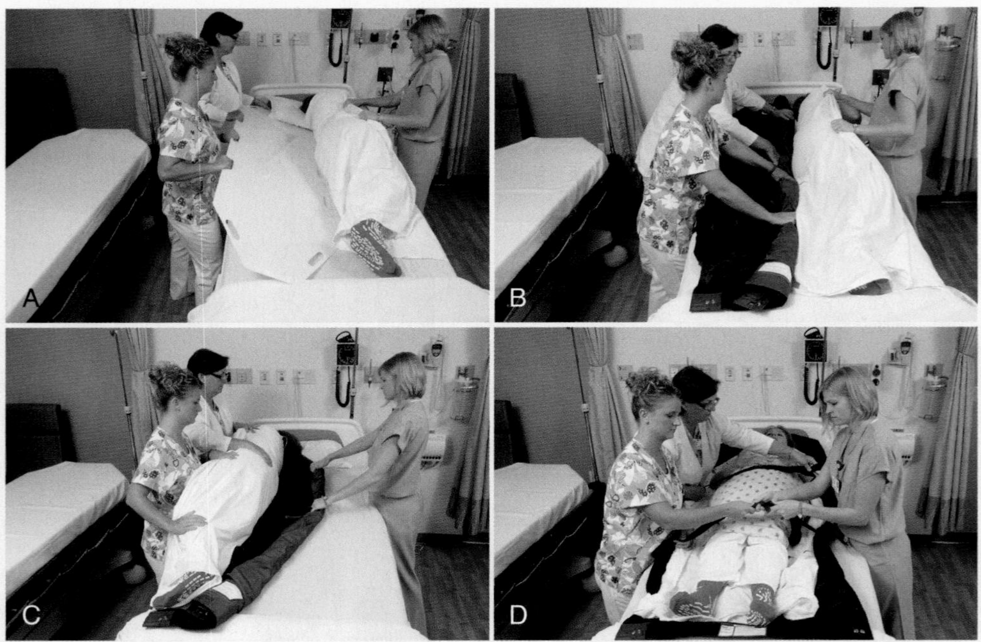

STEP 1e(5) A, Two caregivers position slide board under patient. **B,** Two caregivers place air-assisted device under patient. **C,** Patient rolls to opposite side while other caregiver unrolls air-assisted device. **D,** Secure safety straps.

STEP	RATIONALE
(8) On count of three, two caregivers pull drawsheet or patient from bed onto stretcher while third person holds slide board in place. Using the friction-reducing slide board, shift weight from front to back foot (see illustration). Position patient in center of stretcher.	Transfers patient smoothly and efficiently to the stretcher.
(9) Put up side rail of stretcher on side where caregivers are, roll stretcher away from side of bed, and put side rail up on that side.	Side rails prevent patient from falling off stretcher.
(10) Cover patient with sheet or blanket.	Promotes comfort and preserves patient dignity.
(11) Perform hand hygiene.	Reduces transmission of microorganisms.
(12) Following transfer, evaluate patient's body alignment.	Prompt identification of poor alignment reduces risks to patient's skin and musculoskeletal systems.
2. Perform hand hygiene.	Reduces transmission of microorganisms.

EVALUATION

STEP	RATIONALE
1. Evaluate vital signs. Ask if patient feels tired or dizzy.	Evaluates patient's response to postural changes and activity.
2. Observe for correct body alignment and presence of pressure points on skin.	Minimizes risk for immobility complications.
3. Ask if patient experienced pain during transfer; measure current pain level.	Determines need for additional pain control or alteration of technique of transferring.
4. Use ***Teach Back*** to determine patient and family understanding about safe transfer techniques. State, "I want to be sure I explained how using the slide board prevents the risk for injury while we care for you. Can you explain to me the importance of using the slide board when we transfer you to a stretcher?" Revise your instruction now or develop plan for revised patient teaching if patient is not able to teach back correctly.	Evaluates what patient and family are able to explain or demonstrate.

UNEXPECTED OUTCOMES AND RELATED INTERVENTIONS

1. Patient sustains injury on transfer.
   - Evaluate incident that caused injury (e.g., assessment inadequate, change in patient status, improper use of equipment).
   - Complete occurrence report according to institution policy.
2. Patient's level of weakness does not permit active transfer.
   - Obtain help from additional nursing personnel.
   - Increase bed activity and exercise to heighten tolerance.
3. Patient transfers well on some occasions, poorly on others.
   - Assess patient for factors that affect ability to transfer (e.g., pain, fatigue, confusion) before transfer.
   - Allow for a rest period before transferring, medicate for pain if indicated, or reorient patient.

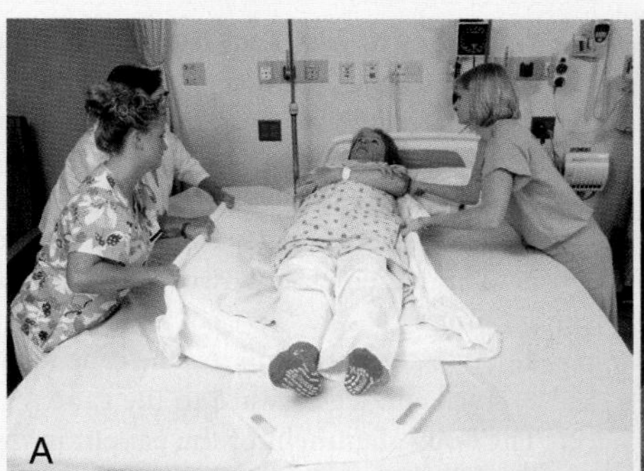
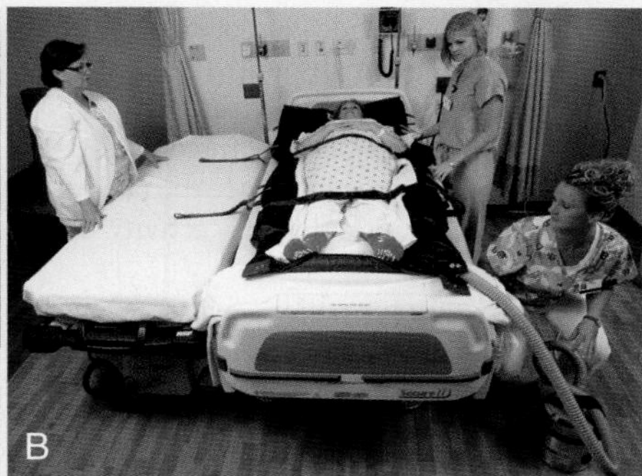
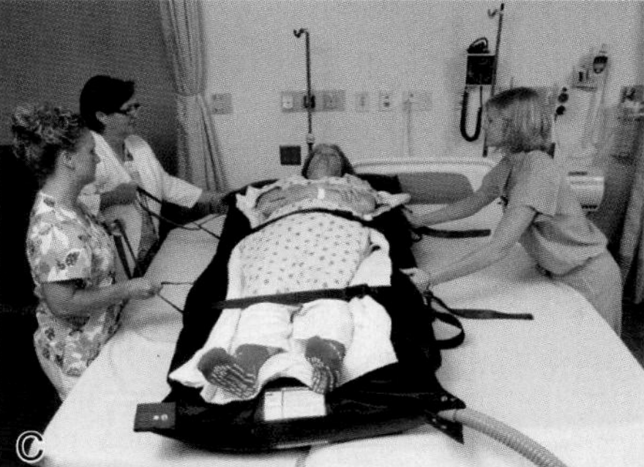

STEP 1e(8) A, Transfer of patient from bed to stretcher using slide board. **B,** Inflating air-assisted transfer device. **C,** Transfer of patient using air-assisted transfer device.

SKILL 39-1 USING SAFE AND EFFECTIVE TRANSFER TECHNIQUES—cont'd

RECORDING AND REPORTING

- Record procedure, including pertinent observations: weakness, ability to follow directions, weight-bearing ability, balance, ability to pivot, number of personnel needed to assist, and amount of assistance (muscle strength) required in nurses' notes.
- Report any unusual occurrence to nurse in charge. Report transfer ability and assistance needed to next shift or other caregivers. Report progress or transfer difficulties to rehabilitation staff (physical therapist or occupational therapist).
- Document your evaluation of patient learning.

HOME CARE CONSIDERATIONS

- Teach family how to use safe patient–handling equipment if necessary.
- Teach patient and family about the importance of safety while helping patients with mobility.

KEY POINTS

- Exercise is physical activity for the purpose of conditioning the body, improving health, and maintaining fitness; it also is a therapeutic measure.
- Deconditioning is a particular risk for hospitalized patients who spend most of their time in bed even when they are able to walk.
- The best program of physical activity includes a combination of exercises that produces different physiological and psychological benefits.
- Body mechanics are the coordinated efforts of the musculoskeletal and nervous systems as the person moves, lifts, bends, stands, sits, lies down, and completes daily activities.
- Coordinated body movement requires integrated functioning of the skeletal system, skeletal muscles, and nervous system.
- Coordination and regulation of muscle groups depend on muscle tone and activity of antagonistic, synergistic, and antigravity muscles.
- The nervous system controls balance through the functions of the cerebellum and inner ear.
- You achieve body balance when there is a wide base of support, the center of gravity falls within the base of support, and a vertical line falls from the center of gravity through the base of support.
- Developmental changes, behavioral aspects, environmental issues, cultural origin, and family and social support influence the patient's perception and motivation to engage in physical activity and exercise.
- Use the nursing process to provide care for patients who are experiencing or are at risk for activity intolerance and impaired physical mobility.
- After identifying nursing diagnoses, plan and implement interventions to increase activity and exercise in collaboration with the patient when possible.
- ROM exercises incorporated into daily activities include one or all of the body joints.
- Apply proper algorithms when you transfer and lift patients.
- Assistive devices to promote walking include canes, walkers, and crutches.

CLINICAL APPLICATION QUESTIONS

Preparing for Clinical Practice

Mrs. Smith has experienced some success in losing weight. She states, "I feel like I should have lost more weight by now." However, she expresses concern about how to incorporate exercise into her daily routine to maintain weight and assist with future weight loss.

1. Mrs. Smith states, "It is hard for me to determine exactly how much exercise I get doing my usual activities." She also expresses feelings of overwhelming stress and excessive demands on her time. Which interventions do you suggest to Mrs. Smith to help assess her current level of exercise?
2. Recognizing the challenges Mrs. Smith has voiced in balancing the excessive demands on her time and incorporating an exercise program. Develop some strategies to help initiate and maintain daily exercise.
3. Develop a feedback method for Mrs. Smith, emphasizing her success in exercise and maintaining a healthy weight.

ⓔ ***Answers to Clinical Application Questions can be found on the Evolve website.***

REVIEW QUESTIONS

Are You Ready to Test Your Nursing Knowledge?

1. A nurse is instructing a patient who has decreased leg strength on the left side how to use a cane. Which action indicates proper cane use by the patient?
   1. The patient keeps the cane on the left side of the body.
   2. The patient slightly leans to one side while walking.
   3. The patient keeps two points of support on the floor at all times.
   4. After the patient places the cane forward, he or she then moves the right leg forward to the cane.
2. The body alignment of the patient in the tripod position includes the following: (Select all that apply.)
   1. An erect head and neck
   2. Straight vertebrae
   3. Extended hips and knees
   4. Axillae resting on the crutch pads
   5. Bent knees and hips
3. A patient is experiencing some problems with joint stability. The doctor has prescribed crutches for the patient to use while still being allowed to bear weight on both legs. Which of the following gaits should the patient be taught to use?
   1. Four-point
   2. Three-point
   3. Two-point
   4. Swing-through

4. Which of the following *most* motivates a patient to participate in an exercise program?
   1. Providing a patient with a pamphlet on exercise
   2. Providing information to the patient when he or she is ready to change behavior
   3. Explaining the importance of exercise at the time of diagnosis of a chronic disease
   4. Providing the patient with a booklet with examples of exercises
   5. Providing the patient with a prescribed exercise program
5. Which of the following is a principle of proper body mechanics when lifting or carrying objects? (Select all that apply.)
   1. Keep the knees in a locked position.
   2. Bend at the waist to maintain a center of gravity.
   3. Maintain a wide base of support.
   4. Hold objects away from the body for improved leverage.
   5. Encourage patient to help as much as possible.
6. The nurse recognizes that the older adult's progressive loss of total bone mass and tendency to take smaller steps with feet kept closer together will most likely:
   1. Increase the patient's risk for falls and injuries.
   2. Result in less stress on the patient's joints.
   3. Decrease the amount of work required for patient movement.
   4. Allow for mobility in spite of the aging effects on the patient's joints.
7. A nurse plans to provide education to the parents of school-age children, which includes the increased prevalence of ________________ as a result of children being less physically active outside of school.
8. A nursing assistive personnel asks for help to transfer a patient who is 125 lbs (56.8 kg) from the bed to a wheelchair. The patient is unable to help. What is the nurse's best response?
   1. "As long as we use proper body mechanics, no one will get hurt."
   2. "The patient only weighs 125 lbs. You don't need my assistance."
   3. "Call the lift team for additional assistance."
   4. "The two of us can lift the patient easily."
9. Which of the following statements made by an older adult reflects the best understanding of the need to exercise regardless of age?
   1. "You are never too old to begin an exercise program."
   2. "My granddaughter and I walk together around the high school track 3 times a week."
   3. "I purchased a subscription to a runner's magazine for my grandson for Christmas."
   4. "When I was a child, I exercised more than I see kids doing today."
10. Which is the correct gait when a patient is ascending stairs on crutches?
    1. A modified two-point gait. (The affected leg is advanced between the crutches to the stairs.)
    2. A modified three-point gait. (The unaffected leg is advanced between the crutches to the stairs.)
    3. A swing-through gait
    4. A modified four-point gait. (Both legs advance between the crutches to the stairs.)
11. Before transferring a patient from the bed to a stretcher, which assessment data do the nurse need to gather? (Select all that apply.)
    1. Patient's weight
    2. Patient's level of cooperation
    3. Patient's ability to assist
    4. Presence of medical equipment
    5. Nutritional intake
12. A patient with a right knee replacement is prescribed no weight bearing on the right leg. You reinforce crutch walking knowing that which of the following crutch gaits is most appropriate for this patient?
    1. Two-point gait
    2. Three-point gait
    3. Four-point gait
    4. Swing-through gait
13. Which of the following indicates that additional assistance is needed to transfer the patient from the bed to the stretcher?
    1. The patient is 5 feet 6 inches and weighs 120 lbs.
    2. The patient speaks and understands English.
    3. The patient is returning to unit from recovery room after a procedure requiring conscious sedation.
    4. The patient received analgesia for pain 30 minutes ago.
14. The nurse encourages a patient with type 2 diabetes to engage in a regular exercise program primarily to improve the patient's:
    1. Gastric motility, thereby facilitating glucose digestion.
    2. Respiratory effort, thereby decreasing activity intolerance.
    3. Overall cardiac output, thereby resuming resting heart rate.
    4. Use of glucose and fatty acids, thereby decreasing blood glucose level.
15. Musculoskeletal disorders are the most prevalent and debilitating occupational health hazards for nurses. To reduce the risk for these injuries, the American Nurses Association advocates which of the following?
    1. Mandate that physical therapists do all patient transfers
    2. Require adequate staffing levels in health care organizations
    3. Require the use of assistive equipment and devices
    4. Require an adequate number of staff to be involved in all patient transfers

Answers: 1. 3; **2.** 1, 2, 3; **3.** 1; **4.** 2; **5.** 3, 5; **6.** 1; **7.** Childhood obesity; **8.** 3; **9.** 2; **10.** 2; **11.** 1, 2, 3, 4; **12.** 2; **13.** 3; **14.** 4; **15.** 3.

Rationales for Review Questions can be found on the Evolve website.

REFERENCES

Ackley BJ, Ladwig GB: *Nursing diagnosis handbook: an evidence-based guide to planning care*, ed 10, St Louis, 2014, Mosby.

American Academy of Orthopaedist Surgeons: *How to use crutches, canes, and walkers*, 2015, http://orthoinfo.aaos.org/topic.cfm?topic=A00181. Accessed December 2015.

American Association of Critical Care Nurses: *Implementing the ABCDE bundle at the bedside: early progressive mobility protocol*, 2015, http://www.aacn.org/wd/practice/content/actionpak/withlinks-ABCDE- ToolKit.content?menu=practice Accessed November 14, 2015.

American College of Sports Medicine (ACSM): *Position stand: the recommended quantity and quality of exercise for developing and maintaining cardiorespiratory, musculoskeletal, and neuromotor fitness in apparently healthy adults: guidance for prescribing exercise*, 2011, http://www.ncbi.nlm.nih.gov/pubmed/21694556. Accessed March 2015.

American College of Sports Medicine (ACSM) and the American Diabetes Association (ADA): *Joint Position Statement: Exercise and type 2 diabetes*, 2010, http://care.diabetesjournals.org/content/33/12/e147.abstract. Accessed March 2015.

American Heart Association: *American Heart Association recommendations for physical activity in adults*, 2015, http://www.heart.org/HEARTORG/GettingHealthy/PhysicalActivity/FitnessBasics/American-Heart-Association-Recommendations-for-Physical-Activity

-in-Adults_UCM_307976_Article.jsp#.VkjC8aSFOpo. Accessed November 15, 2015.

American Nurses Association (ANA): *Statement of the American Nurses Association for the committee on Health, Education, Labor, and Pensions of the United States Senate subcommittee on Employment and Workplace Safety*, 2010, http://www.nursingworld.org/DocumentVault/GOVA/Federal/Testimonies/SPH-Testimony.pdf. Accessed March 2015.

Balady GJ, et al: Clinician's guide to cardiopulmonary exercise testing in adults: a scientific statement from the American Heart Association, *Circulation* 122(2):191, 2010.

Bandura A: Guide for constructing self-efficacy scales. In Pajares F, Urdan T, editors: *Self-efficacy beliefs of adolescents*, Charlotte, NC, 2006, Information Age Publishing.

Campos-Outcalt D: The new cardiovascular disease prevention guidelines: what you need to know, *J Fam Pract* 63(2):89, 2014.

Childs E, deWit H: Regular exercise is associated with emotional resilience to acute stress in healthy adults, *Front Physiol* 5:1, 2014.

Edelman CL, et al: *Health promotion throughout the life span*, ed 8, St Louis, 2013, Mosby.

Elliott M: Taking control of osteoporosis to cut down on risk of fracture, *Nurs Older People* 23(3):30, 2011.

Fedorowski A, Melander O: Syndrome of orthostatic intolerance: a hidden danger, *J Intern Med* 273:322, 2013.

Griffis H: Adverse risk: a dynamic interaction model of patient moving and handling, *J Nurs Manag* 20:713, 2012.

Grossklaus H, Marvicsin D: Parenting efficacy and its relationship to the prevention of childhood obesity, *Pediatr Nurs* 40(2):69, 2014.

Hameed UA: Structured exercise interventions for type 2 diabetes mellitus: strength of current evidence, *J Med Allied Sci* 1(2):61, 2011.

Hockenberry M, Wilson D: *Wong's nursing care of infants and children*, ed 10, St Louis, 2015, Mosby.

Huether SE, McCance KL: *Understanding pathophysiology*, ed 5, St Louis, 2012, Mosby.

Hunter B, et al: Saving costs, saving health care providers' backs, and creating a safe patient environment, *Nurs Econ* 23(2):130, 2010.

Kwun S, et al: Prevention and treatment of postmenopausal osteoporosis, *Obstet Gynaecolt* 14:251, 2012.

Lewis SL, et al: *Medical-surgical nursing assessment and management of clinical problems*, ed 9, St Louis, 2014, Mosby.

Myszenski A: *The essential role of lab values and vital signs in clinical decision making and patient safety for the acutely ill patient*, 2014, http://www.physicaltherapy.com/articles/essential-role-lab-values-and-2336. Accessed November 23, 2015.

Nurse and Health Care Worker Act: *H.R. 2381/S.1788*, 2009, http://www.gpo.gov/fdsys/pkg/BILLS-111s1788is/pdf/BILLS-111s1788is.pdf. Accessed February 15, 2015.

Occupational Safety and Health Administration (OSHA): *Guidelines for nursing homes: ergonomics for the prevention of musculoskeletal disorders*, 2009, http://www.osha.gov/ergonomics/guidelines/nursinghome/final_nh_guidelines.pdf. Accessed March 2015.

O'Donovan G, et al: The ABCs of physical activity for health: a consensus statement from the British association of sport and exercise sciences, *J Sports Sci* 28(6):573, 2010.

Patton KT, Thibodeau GA: *Anatomy and physiology*, ed 8, St Louis, 2012, Mosby.

Pelczarski KM: Back in action, *Health Facil Manag* 55(8):21, 2012.

Perme C, Chandrashekar R: Early mobility and walking program for patients in intensive care units: creating a standard of care, *Am J Crit Care* 18(3):212, 2009.

Pierson F, Fairchild S: *Principles & techniques of patient care*, ed 5, St Louis, 2013, Saunders.

Resnick B, et al: *Restorative care nursing for older adults: a guide for all care settings*, ed 2, New York, 2012, Springer.

The Joint Commission (TJC): *2016 National Patient Safety Goals*, Oakbrook Terrace, IL. 2016, The Commission. Available at http://www.jointcommission.org/standards_information/npsgs.aspx. Accessed November 2015.

Urden L, et al: *Critical care nursing: diagnosis and management*, ed 7, St Louis, 2014, Mosby.

US Bureau of Labor Statistics (BLS) Table R9: *Number of nonfatal occupational injuries and illnesses involving days away from work by occupation and selected natures of injury or illness, private industry*, 2010, http://www.bls.gov/iif/oshwc/osh/case/ostb2833.pdf. Accessed March 2015.

VISN8 Patient Safety Center (VISN8): *Algorithms for safe patient handling and movement*, 2015, http://www.visn8.va.gov/patientsafetycenter/safepthandling/. Accessed March 2015.

Wilson SF, Giddens JF: *Health assessment for nursing practice*, ed 5, St Louis, 2013, Mosby.

RESEARCH REFERENCES

American Academy of Nursing (AAN): Choosing wisely campaign: five things nurses and patients should questions, *Nurs Outlook* 63:96, 2015.

Bammann K, et al: Early life course risk factors for childhood obesity: the IDEFICS case-control study, *PLoS ONE* 9(2):1, 2014.

Berry MJ, et al: A lifestyle activity intervention in patients with chronic obstructive pulmonary disease, *Respir Med* 104(6):829, 2010.

Burnfield J, et al: Comparative kinematic and electromagnetic assessment of clinician- and device-assisted sit-to-stand transfers in patients with stroke, *Phys Ther* 93(10):1331, 2013.

Christo P, et al: Effective treatments for pain in the older patient, *Curr Pain Headache Rep* 15(1):22, 2011.

Clarke DM, et al: The inspired study: a randomized controlled trial of the whole person model of disease self-management for people with type 2 diabetes, *BMC Public Health* 14:134, 2014.

Combs S, et al: Community-based group exercise for persons with Parkinson disease: a randomized controlled trial, *Neurorehabilitation* 32:117, 2013.

Cowley SP, Leggett S: Manual handling risks associated with the care, treatment, and transportation of bariatric patients and clients in Australia, *Int J Nurs Pract* 16:262, 2010.

Davison KK, Jago R: Change in parent and peer support across ages 9 to 15 years and adolescent girls' physical activity, *Med Sci Sports Exercise* 41(9):1816, 2010.

Donges CE, et al: Effects of resistance or aerobic exercise training on interleukin-6, C-reactive protein, and body composition, *Med Sci Sports Exercise* 42(2):304, 2010.

Dunton GF: Adolescents' sports and exercise environments in the US time use survey, *Am J Prevent Med* 39(2):122, 2010.

Esposito E, Fitzpatrick J: Registered nurses' beliefs of the benefits of exercise, their exercise behaviour, and their patient teaching regarding exercise, *Int J Nurs Pract* 17:351, 2011.

Harvey LA, et al: Continuous passive motion following total knee arthroplasty in people with arthritis, *Cochrane Database Syst Rev* (2):Art No.: CD0024260, 2014.

Healthy People 2020: *Physical activity, office of disease prevention and health promotion*, 2015 http://www.healthypeople.gov/2020/topics-objectives/topic/physical-activity Accessed November 14, 2015.

Jain A, Paranjape S: Prevalence of type 2 diabetes mellitus in elderly in primary care facility: an ideal facility, *Indian J Endocrinol Metab* 17(1):S318, 2013.

Lin P, et al: Prevalence, characteristics, and work-related risk factors of low back pain among hospital nurses in Taiwan: a cross-sectional survey, *Int J Occup Environ Health* 25(1):41, 2012.

Lo HM, et al: A tai chi exercise programme improved exercise behavior and reduced blood pressure in outpatients with hypertension, *Int J Nurs Pract* 18:545, 2012.

Maniar RN, et al: To use or not to use continuous passive motion post-total knee arthroplasty: presenting functional assessment results in early recovery, *J Arthroplast* 27(2):193, 2012.

McGann S, et al: Taking the stairs instead: the impact of workplace design standards on health promotion strategies, *Aust Med J* 6(1):23, 2013.

Pashikanti L, Von Ah D: Impact of early mobilization protocol on medical-surgical inpatient population, *Clin Nurse Spec* 26(2):97, 2012.

Roush K: Prevention and treatment of osteoporosis in postmenopausal women: a review, *Am J Nurs* 111(8):26, 2011.

Salhi B, et al: Effects of pulmonary rehabilitation in patients with restrictive lung diseases, *Chest* 137(2):273, 2010.

Suesada MM, et al: Effect of short-term hospitalization on functional capacity in patients not restricted to bed, *Am J Phys Med Rehabil* 86(6):455–462, 2007.

Tullar JM, et al: Occupational safety and health interventions, *J Occup Rehabil* 20(2):199, 2010.

Wallace R, et al: Effects of a 12-week community programme on older people, *Art Sci* 26(1):20, 2014.

40

Hygiene

OBJECTIVES

- Describe factors that influence personal hygiene practices.
- Discuss the role that critical thinking plays in providing hygiene.
- Conduct a comprehensive assessment of a patient's total hygiene needs.
- Discuss conditions that place patients at risk for impaired skin integrity.
- Discuss factors that influence the condition of the nails and feet.
- Explain the importance of foot care for the patient with diabetes.
- Discuss conditions that place patients at risk for impaired oral mucous membranes.
- List common hair and scalp problems and their related interventions.
- Describe how hygiene care for the older adult differs from that for the younger patient.
- Discuss different approaches used in maintaining a patient's comfort and safety during hygiene care.
- Successfully perform hygiene procedures for the care of the skin, perineum, feet and nails, mouth, eyes, ears, and nose.
- Adapt hygiene care for a patient who is cognitively impaired.
- Adapt hygiene care for the bariatric patient.

KEY TERMS

Alopecia, p. 828
Caries, p. 825
Cerumen, p. 830
Cheilitis, p. 828
Complete bed bath, p. 837
Dental caries, p. 823
Edentulous, p. 828
Effleurage, p. 838
Enucleation, p. 844
Epidermis, p. 822
Gingivitis, p. 823
Glossitis, p. 827
Halitosis, p. 828
Maceration, p. 838
Mucositis, p. 832
Partial bed bath, p. 837
Pediculosis capitis, p. 828
Perineal care, p. 838
Stomatitis, p. 841
Xerostomia, p. 823

MEDIA RESOURCES

http://evolve.elsevier.com/Potter/fundamentals/

- Review Questions
- Video Clips
- Concept Map Creator
- Case Study with Questions
- Skills Performance Checklists
- Audio Glossary
- Content Updates

Personal hygiene affects patients' comfort, safety, and well-being. Hygiene care includes cleaning and grooming activities that maintain personal body cleanliness and appearance. Personal hygiene activities such as taking a bath or shower and brushing and flossing the teeth also promote comfort and relaxation, foster a positive self-image, promote healthy skin, and help prevent infection and disease. Healthy people are usually able to meet their own hygiene needs. However, physical or cognitive impairments and emotional challenges often cause individuals to need some degree of assistance with hygiene care. A variety of personal, social, and cultural factors influence hygiene practices.

In agency and home care settings, assess a patient's ability to perform self–hygiene care according to individual needs and preferences. Adaptations may be needed for hygiene techniques and approaches for patient care. Integrate nursing assessments and interventions during hygiene care with nursing activities such as range of motion (ROM), dressing changes, and inspection and care of intravenous (IV) sites. Because hygiene care requires close contact with your patients, use communication skills to build caring, therapeutic relationships. Provide any needed teaching or counseling for patients. During hygiene care ensure privacy, convey respect, and provide safety and comfort.

SCIENTIFIC KNOWLEDGE BASE

Proper hygiene care requires an understanding of the anatomy and physiology of the skin, nails, oral cavity, eyes, ears, and nose. The skin and mucosal cells exchange oxygen, nutrients, and fluids with underlying blood vessels. The cells require adequate nutrition, hydration, and circulation to resist injury and disease. Good hygiene techniques promote the normal structure and function of these tissues.

Apply knowledge of pathophysiology to provide preventive hygiene care. Recognize disease states that create changes in the integument, oral cavity, and sensory organs. For example, diabetes mellitus often results in chronic vascular changes that impair healing of the skin and mucosa. In the early stages of acquired immunodeficiency syndrome (AIDS), fungal infections of the oral cavity are common. Paralysis of the trigeminal nerve (cranial nerve V) eliminates the blink reflex, causing risk of corneal drying. In the presence of conditions such as these, adapt hygiene practices to minimize injury. Use time spent

TABLE 40-1 Function of the Skin and Implications for Care

Function/Description	Implications for Care
Protection	
Epidermis is a relatively impermeable layer that prevents entrance of microorganisms. Although microorganisms reside on skin surface and in hair follicles, relative dryness of surface of skin inhibits bacterial growth. Sebum removes bacteria from hair follicles. Acidic pH of skin further retards bacterial growth.	• Weakening of the epidermis occurs by scraping or stripping its surface (e.g., use of dry razors, tape removal, improper turning or positioning techniques). • Excessive dryness causes cracks and breaks in skin and mucosa that allow bacteria to enter. Emollients soften skin and prevent moisture loss, soaking skin improves moisture retention, and hydrating mucosa prevents dryness. • Constant exposure of skin to moisture causes maceration or softening, interrupting dermal integrity and promoting ulcer formation and bacterial growth. • Keep bed linen and clothing dry. • Misuse of soap, detergents, cosmetics, deodorant, and depilatories cause chemical irritation. Alkaline soaps neutralize the protective acid condition of skin. Cleaning skin removes excess oil, sweat, dead skin cells, and dirt, which promote bacterial growth.
Sensation	
Skin contains sensory organs for touch, pain, heat, cold, and pressure.	• Minimize friction to avoid loss of stratum corneum, which results in development of pressure ulcers. • Smooth linen out to remove sources of mechanical irritation. • Remove rings from fingers to prevent accidentally injuring patient's skin. • Make sure that bath water is not excessively hot or cold.
Temperature Regulation	
Radiation, evaporation, conduction, and convection control body temperature.	• Factors that interfere with heat loss alter temperature control. Wet bed linen or gowns interfere with convection and conduction. Excess blankets or bed coverings interfere with heat loss through radiation and conduction. Coverings promote heat conservation.
Excretion and Secretion	
Sweat promotes heat loss by evaporation. Sebum lubricates skin and hair.	• Perspiration and oil harbor microorganisms. • Bathing removes excess body secretions; although, if excessive, it causes dry skin.

providing hygiene care to identify abnormalities and initiate appropriate actions to prevent further injury to sensitive tissues.

The Skin

The skin serves several functions, including protection, secretion, excretion, body temperature regulation, and cutaneous sensation (Table 40-1). It consists of two primary layers: the epidermis and the dermis. Just beneath the skin lies the subcutaneous tissue (also known as the hypodermis), which shares some of the protective functions of the skin.

Several thin layers of epithelial cells comprise the outer layer, or **epidermis**; these cells shield underlying tissue against water loss and injury and prevent entry of disease-producing microorganisms. The innermost layer of the epidermis generates new cells to replace the dead cells that the outer surface of the skin continuously sheds. Bacteria commonly reside on the outer epidermis. These resident bacteria are normal flora (see Chapter 29) that do not cause disease but instead inhibit the multiplication of disease-causing microorganisms.

Bundles of collagen and elastic fibers form the thicker dermis that underlies and supports the epidermis. Nerve fibers, blood vessels, sweat glands, sebaceous glands, and hair follicles run through the dermal layers. Sebaceous glands secrete sebum, an oily, odorous fluid, into the hair follicles. Sebum softens and lubricates the skin and slows water loss from the skin when the humidity is low. More important, sebum has bactericidal action.

The subcutaneous tissue layer contains blood vessels, nerves, lymph, and loose connective tissue filled with fat cells. The fatty tissue functions as a heat insulator for the body. Subcutaneous tissue also supports upper skin layers to withstand stresses and pressure without injury and anchors the skin loosely to underlying structures such as muscle. Very little subcutaneous tissue underlies the oral mucosa.

The skin often reflects a change in physical condition by alterations in color, thickness, texture, turgor, temperature, and hydration (see Chapter 31). As long as the skin remains intact and healthy, its physiological function remains optimal. Hygiene practices frequently influence skin status and can have beneficial and negative effects on the skin. For example, too-frequent bathing and use of hot water frequently leads to dry, flaky skin and loss of protective oils.

The Feet, Hands, and Nails

The feet, hands, and nails often require special attention to prevent infection, odor, and injury. The condition of a patient's hands and feet influences the ability to perform hygiene care. Without the ability to bear weight, ambulate, or manipulate the hands, the patient is at risk for losing self-care ability.

A wide range of dexterity exists in the hand because of the movement between the thumb and fingers. Any condition (e.g., arthritis, multiple sclerosis, traumatic hand injury) that interferes with hand movement (e.g., superficial or deep pain or joint inflammation) impairs a patient's self-care abilities. Foot pain often changes a patient's gait, causing strain on different joints and muscle groups. Discomfort while standing or walking limits self-care abilities.

The nails grow from the root of the nail bed, which is located in the skin at the nail groove, hidden by the fold of skin called the cuticle. A scalelike modification of the epidermis forms the visible part of the nail (nail body), which has a crescent-shaped white area known as the lunula. Under the nail lies a layer of epithelium called the *nail bed*. A normal healthy nail appears transparent, smooth, and convex, with a pink nail bed and translucent white tip. Disease causes changes in the shape, thickness, and curvature of the nail (see Chapter 31).

The Oral Cavity

The oral cavity consists of the lips surrounding the opening of the mouth, the cheeks running along the sidewalls of the cavity, the tongue and its muscles, and the hard and soft palate. The mucous membrane, continuous with the skin, lines the oral cavity. The floor of the mouth and the undersurface of the tongue are richly supplied with blood vessels. Normal oral mucosa glistens and is pink, soft, moist, smooth, and without lesions. Ulcerations or trauma frequently results in significant bleeding. Several glands within and outside the oral cavity secrete saliva. Saliva cleanses the mouth, dissolves food chemicals to promote taste, moistens food to facilitate bolus formation, and contains enzymes that start breakdown of starchy foods. The effects of medications, exposure to radiation, dehydration, and mouth breathing impair salivary secretion in the mouth. Strong sympathetic nervous system stimulation almost completely inhibits the release of saliva and results in **xerostomia** or dry mouth.

The teeth lie in sockets in the gum-covered mandible and maxilla; they tear and grind ingested food so it can be mixed with saliva and swallowed for digestion. A normal tooth consists of the crown, neck, and root. The enamel-covered crown extends above the gingiva or gum, which normally surrounds the tooth like a tight collar. A constricted part of the tooth called the *neck* connects the crown and the root; the root is embedded in the jawbone. The periodontal membrane lies just below the gum margins, surrounds a tooth, and holds it firmly in place. Healthy teeth are white, smooth, shiny, and properly aligned.

Difficulty in chewing develops when surrounding gum tissues become inflamed or infected or when teeth are lost or become loosened. Regular oral hygiene helps to prevent **gingivitis** (i.e., inflammation of the gums) and **dental caries** (i.e., tooth decay produced by interaction of food with bacteria).

The Hair

Hair growth, distribution, and pattern indicate a person's general health status. Hormonal changes, nutrition, emotional and physical stress, aging, infection, and some illnesses affect hair characteristics. The hair shaft itself is lifeless, and physiological factors do not affect it directly. However, hormonal and nutrient deficiencies of the hair follicle cause changes in hair color or condition.

The Eyes, Ears, and Nose

When providing hygiene, the eyes, ears, and nose require careful attention because of sensitive anatomical structures. For example, the cornea of the eye contains many nerve endings sensitive to irritants such as soap. Chapter 31 describes the structure and function of these organs.

NURSING KNOWLEDGE BASE

A number of factors influence personal preferences for hygiene and the ability to maintain hygiene practices. Since no two individuals perform hygiene care in the same manner, you individualize patient care on the basis of learning about his or her unique hygiene practices and preferences. Individualized hygiene care requires knowing the patient and using therapeutic communication skills to promote a trusting therapeutic relationship. Use the opportunities provided during hygiene care to assess a patient's health promotion practices, emotional status, and health care education needs and then offer educational interventions. Be aware that developmental changes influence the need and preferences for type of hygiene care.

Factors Influencing Hygiene

Social Practices. Social groups influence hygiene preferences and practices, including the type of hygiene products used and the nature and frequency of personal care practices. An example is the choice by adolescent girls of the type of sanitary pads used during menstruation (Kamaljit et al., 2012). Parents and caregivers perform hygiene care for infants and young children. Family customs play a major role during childhood in determining hygiene practices such as the frequency of bathing, the time of day bathing is performed, and even whether certain hygiene practices such as brushing the teeth or flossing are performed. As children enter adolescence, peer groups and media often influence hygiene practices. For example, some young girls become more interested in their personal appearance and begin to wear makeup. During the adult years involvement with friends and work groups shapes the expectations that people have about personal appearance. Some older adults' hygiene practices change because of changes in living conditions and available resources.

Personal Preferences. Patients have individual preferences about when to perform hygiene and grooming care. Some patients prefer to shower, whereas others prefer to bathe. Patients select different hygiene and grooming products according to personal preferences. Knowing patients' personal preferences promotes individualized care. Culture plays a role in sensitivity to personal space and gender (see Box 40-1 and Chapter 9). Help a patient develop new hygiene practices when indicated by an illness or condition. For example, you may need to teach a patient with diabetes proper foot hygiene or a bariatric patient adaptive bathing methods. Safe and effective patient-centered nursing care improves patient satisfaction and health and reduces costs (Burman et al., 2013).

Body Image. Body image is a person's subjective concept of his or her body, including physical appearance, structure, or function (see Chapter 34). Body image affects the way in which individuals maintain personal hygiene. If a patient maintains a neatly groomed appearance, be sure to consider the details of grooming when planning care and consult with the patient before making decisions about how to provide hygiene. Patients who appear unkempt or uninterested in hygiene sometimes need education about its importance or further assessment regarding their ability to participate with daily hygiene.

Surgery, illness, or a change in emotional or functional status often affects a patient's body image. Discomfort and pain, emotional stress, or fatigue diminish the ability or desire to perform hygiene self-care and require extra effort to promote hygiene and grooming.

Socioeconomic Status. A person's economic resources influence the type and extent of hygiene practices used. Be sensitive in considering that a patient's economic status influences the ability to regularly maintain hygiene. He or she may not be able to afford desired basic supplies such as deodorant, shampoo, and toothpaste. A patient may need to modify the home environment by adding safety devices such as nonskid surfaces and grab bars in the bath to perform hygiene self-care safely. When patients lack socioeconomic resources, it becomes difficult for them to participate and take responsible roles in health promotion activities such as basic hygiene.

Health Beliefs and Motivation. Knowledge about the importance of hygiene and its implications for well-being influences hygiene practices. However, knowledge alone is not enough. Motivation also plays a key role in a patient's hygiene practices. Patient teaching is often needed to foster hygiene self-care. Provide information that focuses on a patient's personal health-related issues relevant to the desired hygiene

 BOX 40-1 CULTURAL ASPECTS OF CARE

Hygiene Practices

Patients deserve a culturally congruent plan for hygiene care. For many patients culture influences hygiene practices, and hygiene care becomes a potential source of conflict and stress in the caregiving environment. Patient-centered care mandates that care be based on respect for an individual patient's cultural background (Douglas et al., 2014). A nurse must also consider other aspects of culture such as a patient's educational and developmental levels, extent of any physical disabilities, and geographical location of home when delivering hygiene.

Implications for Patient-Centered Care

- Maintain privacy, especially for women from cultures that value female modesty (e.g., Asian, Muslim, Hispanic, Nigerian) (Giger, 2013).
- Avoid uncovering the lower torso and exposing the arms of Middle Eastern and East Asian women.
- Allow family members to participate in care if desired by adapting the schedule of hygiene activities.
- Provide gender-congruent caregivers as needed or requested.
- Recognize that some cultures prohibit or restrict touching. Incorporate awareness that people from different cultural backgrounds have differing preferences regarding personal space. In some cases touch is considered magical and healing; others view it as evil or anxiety producing (Giger, 2013).
- Do not cut or shave hair without prior discussion with patient or family because of cultural or religious beliefs (e.g., Muslims) (Giger, 2013).
- Be aware that toileting practices vary by culture (Giger, 2013).
- Recognize that different cultures (e.g., Hindu, Asians, Hispanics) have preferences about hot and cold water and their effects on healing or diseases (Giger, 2013).

care behaviors. Patient perceptions of the benefits of hygiene care and the susceptibility to and seriousness of developing a problem affect the motivation to change behavior (Pender et al., 2011). For example, do patients perceive that they are at risk for dental disease, or that dental disease is serious, and that brushing and flossing are effective in reducing risk? When they recognize that there is a risk and that they can take reasonable action without negative consequences, they are more likely to be receptive to nurses' counseling and teaching efforts.

Cultural Variables. Cultural beliefs and personal values influence hygiene care (Box 40-1). People from diverse cultural backgrounds (e.g., level of education, gender preference, geographic location) frequently follow different self-care practices (see Chapter 9). For example, maintaining cleanliness does not hold the same importance for some ethnic or social groups as it does for others (Giger, 2013). In North America many are fortunate to be able to bathe or shower daily and use deodorant to prevent body odors. However, people from some socioeconomic or cultural groups are not sensitive to body odors, prefer to bathe less frequently, and do not use deodorant. Do not express disapproval when caring for patients whose hygiene practices differ from yours. Avoid forcing changes in hygiene practices unless the practices affect a patient's health. In these situations use tact, provide information, and allow choices. Some homeless people may be reluctant to remove shoes for bathing or to check for skin breakdown. Their feet may be edematous or have neuropathic symptoms (Chen et al., 2014).

Religious beliefs associated with culture sometimes influence hygiene practices. Middle Eastern practices encourage one hand to be kept clean at all times. Muslim patients often remove their shoes and assume different positions for prayer. This increases the risk of developing foot pathology such as calluses on the toes and lateral ankles. When caring for Muslim patients who have diabetes mellitus, you need to be supportive of religious practices while also stressing the need to be diligent in inspecting the feet after prayer sessions for any blisters or calluses.

Developmental Stage. The normal process of aging affects the condition of body tissues and structures. A patient's developmental stage affects the ability of a patient to perform hygiene care and the type of care needed.

Skin. The neonate's skin is relatively immature at birth. The epidermis and dermis are bound together loosely, and the skin is very thin. Friction against the skin layers causes bruising. Handle a neonate carefully during bathing. Any break in the skin easily results in an infection.

A toddler's skin layers become more tightly bound together. Thus the child has a greater resistance to infection and skin irritation. However, because of his or her more active play and the absence of established hygiene habits, parents and caregivers need to provide thorough hygiene and teach good hygiene habits.

During adolescence the growth and maturation of the integument increases. In girls estrogen secretion causes the skin to become soft, smooth, and thicker with increased vascularity. In boys male hormones produce an increased thickness of the skin with some darkening in color. Sebaceous glands become more active, predisposing adolescents to acne (i.e., active inflammation of the sebaceous glands accompanied by pimples). Sweat glands become fully functional during puberty. Adolescents usually begin to use antiperspirants. More frequent bathing and shampooing also become necessary to reduce body odors and eliminate oily hair.

The condition of the adult's skin depends on bathing practices and exposure to environmental irritants. Normally the skin is elastic, well hydrated, firm, and smooth. When an adult bathes frequently or is exposed to an environment with low humidity, it becomes dry and flaky. With aging the rate of epidermal cell replacement slows, and the skin thins and loses resiliency. Moisture leaves the skin, increasing the risk for bruising and other types of injury. As the production of lubricating substances from skin glands decreases, the skin becomes dry and itchy (Touhy and Jett, 2014). These changes warrant caution when bathing, turning, and repositioning older adults. Too-frequent bathing and bathing with hot water or harsh soap cause the skin to become excessively dry (American Academy of Dermatology, 2014).

Feet and Nails. With aging and continued exposure to the trauma of walking and weight bearing, a patient is more likely to develop chronic foot problems compounded as a result of poor foot care, improper fit of footwear, and local abnormalities and systemic disease. For example, Morton's neuroma, a common condition in middle-age women, affects health-related quality of life by causing burning, numbness, and pain of the foot on weight bearing (Edwards et al., 2015). Painful feet in older adults result from a variety of congenital deformities, weak structure, and diseases such as diabetes and rheumatoid arthritis (Green, 2014).

Older adults do not always have the strength, flexibility, visual acuity, or manual dexterity to care for their feet and nails. Foot problems may be overlooked and impact a patient's comfort, mobility, and quality of life (Chan et al., 2012). Older adults frequently complain of foot pain. They also often have dry feet because of a decrease in sebaceous gland secretion and dehydration of epidermal cells. Common problems of the feet affecting older adults include corns, calluses, bunions, hammertoes, maceration between toes, and fungal infections (Stolt et al., 2013).

The Mouth. At approximately 6 to 8 months of age, infants begin teething. The first permanent (secondary) teeth erupt at about 6 years of age (Hockenberry and Wilson, 2013). From adolescence, when all of the permanent teeth are in place, through middle adulthood, the teeth and gums remain healthy if a person follows healthy eating patterns and dental care. Avoiding fermentable carbohydrates and sticky sweets helps to keep the teeth free of caries. In addition, regular brushing (twice a day) and flossing reduce caries and periodontal disease.

As a person ages, numerous factors result in poor oral health, including age-related changes of the mouth, chronic disease such as diabetes, physical disabilities involving hand grasp or strength affecting the ability to perform oral care, lack of attention to oral care, and prescribed medications that have oral side effects. Gums lose vascularity and tissue elasticity, which may cause dentures to fit poorly.

Hair. Throughout life changes in the growth, distribution, and condition of the hair influence hair hygiene. As males reach adolescence, shaving becomes a part of routine grooming. Young girls who reach puberty often begin to shave their legs and axillae. With aging, as scalp hair becomes thinner and drier, shampooing is usually performed less frequently.

Eyes, Ears, and Nose. Chapter 49 addresses changes in hearing, vision, and olfaction across the life span as a result of growth and development. Alterations in sensory function often require modifications in hygiene care. Use your knowledge of developmental changes when planning hygiene care.

Physical Condition. Patients with certain types of physical limitations or disabilities associated with disease and injury lack the physical energy and dexterity to perform hygiene self-care safely. A patient whose arm is in a cast or who has an IV line needs help with hygiene care. A weakened grasp resulting from arthritis, stroke, or muscular disorders makes using a toothbrush, washcloth, or hairbrush difficult or ineffective. Sensory deficits not only alter a patient's ability to perform care but also place the patient at risk for injury. Safety is a priority for a patient with a sensory deficit. For example, the inability to feel that the water is too hot can lead to a burn injury during bathing.

Chronic illnesses such as cardiac, pulmonary, and neurological diseases; cancer; dementia; and some mental health illnesses often exhaust or incapacitate patients. Patients who become tired or short of breath frequently need to have complete hygiene care provided. Include periods of rest during care to allow patients who are tired the opportunity to participate in their care. Pain often accompanies illness and injury, limiting a patient's ability to tolerate hygiene and grooming activities or perform self-care. Pain frequently limits ROM, resulting in impaired use of the arms or hands or limited ability to move about in the environment, impairing the ability to perform hygiene self-care. Sedation and drowsiness associated with analgesics used for pain management also limit a patient's ability to safely participate in care.

Limited mobility caused by a variety of factors (e.g., obesity, physical injury, weakness, surgery, pain, prolonged inactivity, medication effect, and presence of medical devices [e.g., indwelling catheter, feeding tube, or IV line]) decreases a patient's ability to perform hygiene self-care activities safely. Individualized care considers a patient's ability to perform care, the amount of assistance needed, and the need for assistive and safety devices to facilitate safe hygiene care.

Acute and chronic cognitive impairments such as stroke, brain injury, psychoses, and dementia often result in the inability to perform self-care independently. When people with cognitive impairments are unaware of their hygiene and grooming needs, they become fearful and agitated during hygiene care, resulting in aggressive behavior (Zimmerman et al., 2014). Safe, effective patient care takes the effect of cognitive impairment on hygiene care into consideration and allows for appropriate modifications.

CRITICAL THINKING

Effective critical thinking requires synthesis of knowledge, experience, information gathered from patients, critical thinking attitudes, and intellectual and professional standards. Clinical judgments require you to anticipate the information necessary to analyze data and make decisions regarding care. A patient's condition is always changing, requiring ongoing critical thinking. During assessment consider all factors to include to make appropriate nursing diagnoses (Figure 40-1). Apply the elements of critical thinking as you use the nursing process to meet patients' hygiene needs.

Integrate nursing knowledge with knowledge from other disciplines. For example, a patient with diabetes mellitus has special needs

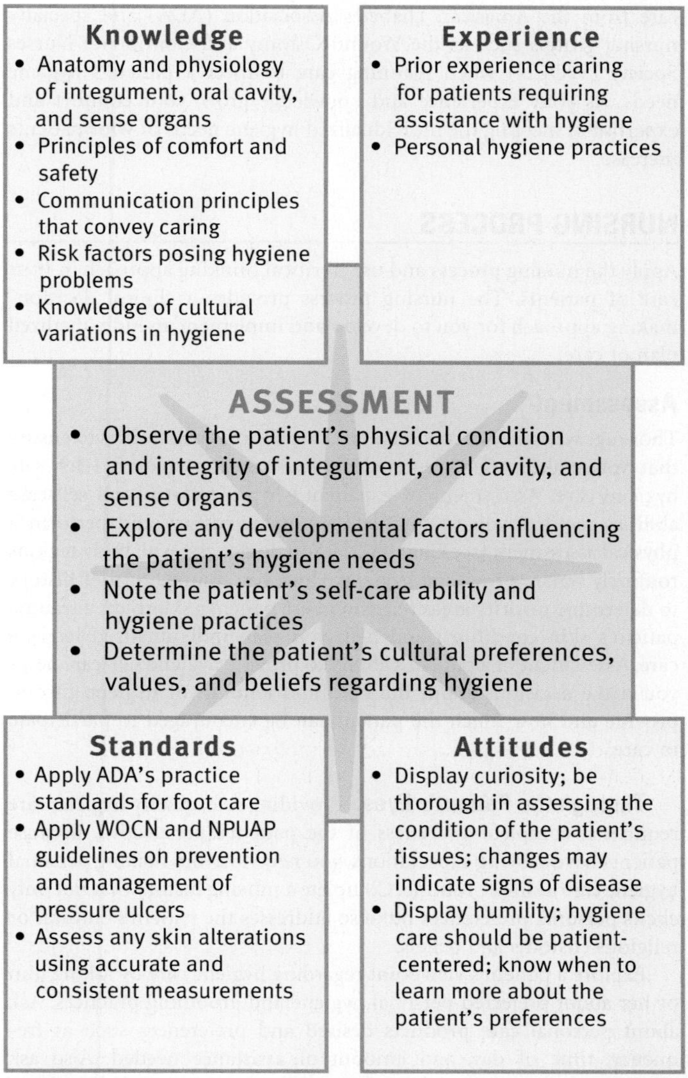

Knowledge
- Anatomy and physiology of integument, oral cavity, and sense organs
- Principles of comfort and safety
- Communication principles that convey caring
- Risk factors posing hygiene problems
- Knowledge of cultural variations in hygiene

Experience
- Prior experience caring for patients requiring assistance with hygiene
- Personal hygiene practices

ASSESSMENT
- Observe the patient's physical condition and integrity of integument, oral cavity, and sense organs
- Explore any developmental factors influencing the patient's hygiene needs
- Note the patient's self-care ability and hygiene practices
- Determine the patient's cultural preferences, values, and beliefs regarding hygiene

Standards
- Apply ADA's practice standards for foot care
- Apply WOCN and NPUAP guidelines on prevention and management of pressure ulcers
- Assess any skin alterations using accurate and consistent measurements

Attitudes
- Display curiosity; be thorough in assessing the condition of the patient's tissues; changes may indicate signs of disease
- Display humility; hygiene care should be patient-centered; know when to learn more about the patient's preferences

FIGURE 40-1 Critical thinking model for hygiene assessment. *ADA,* American Diabetes Association; *NPUAP,* National Pressure Ulcer Advisory Panel; *WOCN,* Wound, Ostomy and Continence Nurses Society.

for nail and foot care. Knowledge about the pathophysiology of diabetes and its potential effects on his or her peripheral circulation and sensory status provides the scientific knowledge base needed to implement safe and effective foot care. In addition, integrate knowledge about developmental and cultural influences as you identify and meet hygiene needs.

Be aware of the impact of critical thinking attitudes as you plan and implement care. For example, think creatively to help patients adapt existing hygiene practices or develop new ones when illness, loss of function, or decreased activity tolerance impairs self-care abilities. Be nonjudgmental and confident when providing care. Because of variations in individual patients' physical status and hygiene practices, you need to approach care with an attitude of flexibility. For example, when caring for a patient who is tired, you pace activities and plan rest periods during bathing to prevent exhaustion.

Draw on your own experiences as you help with your patients' hygiene care. Reflect on times when you helped family members or others close to you with their hygiene. Usually an early clinical experience involves providing or helping with hygiene care for a patient. Finally rely on professional standards such as those for skin and foot care from the American Diabetes Association (ADA) and specialty nursing groups such as the Wound Ostomy and Continence Nurses Society (WOCN) when planning care to meet a patient's hygiene needs. As your experience and knowledge grow, your comfort and expertise in meeting the individualized hygiene needs of your patients increase.

NURSING PROCESS

Apply the nursing process and use a critical thinking approach in your care of patients. The nursing process provides a clinical decision-making approach for you to develop and implement an individualized plan of care.

Assessment

Thoroughly assess each patient and critically analyze findings to ensure that you make patient-centered clinical decisions required for safe hygiene care. Assessment of a patient's hygiene status and self-care abilities requires you to complete a nursing history and perform a physical assessment (see Chapter 31). You do not assess all body regions routinely before providing hygiene. However, conduct a brief history to determine priority areas (e.g., an obese patient's skinfolds, a trauma patient's skin condition) and help you plan individualized hygiene care. Assessment of a patient's ability to provide hygiene self-care helps you make decisions about the kind and amount of hygiene care to provide and how much the patient can be encouraged to participate in care.

Through the Patient's Eyes. Providing safe, quality hygiene care requires a complete awareness of the patient's perspective. Because patients have varying expectations, you need to avoid making personal hygiene care a simple routine. Complete a nursing history that not only elicits personal preferences but also addresses the patient's cultural or religious customs and beliefs.

Explore a patient's viewpoint regarding hygiene care by asking him or her about preferred personal hygiene and grooming practices. Ask about personal care products desired and preferences such as frequency, time of day, and amount of assistance needed. Also ask questions such as, "To make you most comfortable and feel at home, how can I best perform your bath and personal care?" Determine the patient's awareness of any hygiene-related problems and his or her knowledge and ability to perform hygiene care measures (Box 40-2).

BOX 40-2 Nursing Assessment Questions

Cultural and/or Religious Practices
- Do you have preferences for how you bathe or clean your teeth?
- How comfortable are you with someone helping you, with how we care for you?
- In what way can I best help you with your bath, hair care. . . .?

Tolerance of Hygiene Activities
- Does bathing cause any symptoms such as shortness of breath, pain, or fatigue?
- What can I do to minimize these symptoms?
- Which aspects of bathing or toothbrushing cause discomfort or fatigue?

Assistance with Hygiene
- Do you use any aids to help you with your bath such as grab bars in your tub or shower?
- Do you prefer someone of the same gender to help in your hygiene care?
- Which parts of the bath, toothbrushing, and foot care can you do for yourself? With which parts of hygiene care do you need help?

Skin Care
- Which type of bath do you prefer?
- How often and when do you usually bathe?
- What kind of soap and lotion do you use?
- Have you noticed any skin changes or irritation?
- Do you have any known allergies or reactions to soaps, cosmetics, or skin care products?

Mouth Care
- Do you have any mouth pain or toothaches, have you noticed any sores in your mouth, do your gums bleed during brushing or flossing?
- Do you wear dentures or a partial plate?

Foot and Nail Care
- How do you usually care for your feet and nails? Do you soak your feet?
- Do you file or trim your own fingernails and toenails?

Hair and Scalp Care
- Have you recently experienced itching of the scalp or noticed flaking or dandruff?
- Have you noticed any changes in the texture or thickness of your hair?

Learning a patient's expectations and applying them in practice fosters a caring relationship. Fully individualizing hygiene care shows your respect for the patient's needs. As you learn what the patient expects, you incorporate this information into a plan of care.

Assessment of Self-Care Ability. Assess a patient's physical status as it relates to ability to perform or assist with hygiene care safely and efficiently; include assessment of the patient's muscle strength, flexibility, balance, visual acuity, and ability to detect thermal and tactile stimuli. Determine your patient's mental status, including orientation and cognitive function (see Chapter 31). A patient with impaired cognitive function may be unaware of hygiene care needs or less able to follow instructions and help with care. Observe the patient performing hygiene care, noting complaints or physical manifestations that suggest activity intolerance. Assess respiratory rate and effort, skin color, and pulse rate. Ask questions to assess the patient for dizziness, weakness, or fatigue. To determine the amount of assistance the patient needs, observe him or her performing care activities such as brushing teeth or combing hair (Figure 40-2). Patients who have limited

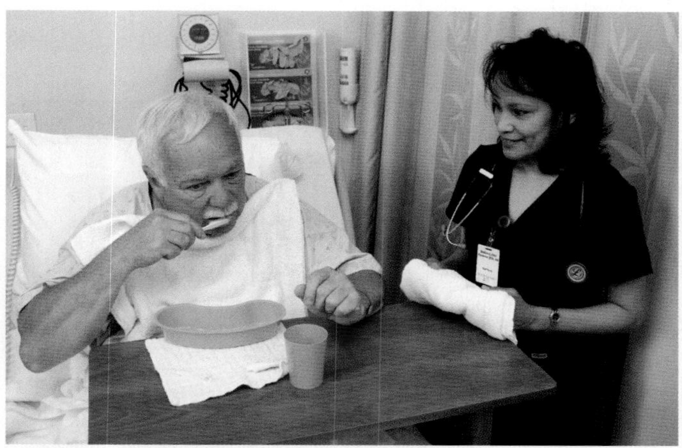

FIGURE 40-2 Nurse observes patient brushing teeth. During such observations the nurse can determine how much assistance the patient may need.

upper-extremity mobility, reduced vision, fatigue, or inability to grasp small objects require help. Patients having difficulty with manual dexterity and cognitive function are likely to show deterioration in physical or oral health (Burns, 2012). Also note the presence of medical devices such as feeding tubes, IV lines, or urinary catheters. These devices require special hygiene measures.

When patients have self-care limitations, family may help with care. Determine how the family can help the patient, how often they can provide this assistance, and their feelings about being caregivers. In addition, assess the home environment and its influence on the patient's hygiene practices. Are there barriers in the home that affect his or her self-care abilities (e.g., water faucets that are too tight to adjust easily, bathtubs with high sides, a bathroom too small to fit a chair in front of a sink, and lack of adjustable bed or adaptive equipment available for assisting with bathing).

Assessment of the Skin. Perform an assessment of the skin (see Chapter 31), noting color, texture, thickness, turgor, temperature, and hydration. In the healthy person the skin is smooth, warm, and supple with good turgor. Pay special attention to the presence and condition of any lesions. Note dryness indicated by flaking, redness, scaling, and cracking. Also carefully inspect the skin in contact with any medical device at least daily (e.g., skin under an oxygen cannula or the nasal mucosa under an endotracheal or feeding tube) (NPUAP, 2013). Look for edema under the sites. Discovering manifestations of common skin problems influences how you administer hygiene care (Table 40-2).

Determine the degree of cleanliness by observing the appearance of the skin and detecting body odors that can indicate inadequate cleansing or excessive perspiration caused by fever or pain. Inspect less obvious or difficult-to-reach skin surfaces such as under the breasts or scrotum, around the female patient's perineum, or in the groin for redness, excessive moisture, and soiling or debris. Separate skinfolds for observation and palpation. Cornstarch may be used to decrease friction and absorb moisture (Cowell and Radley, 2014).

Be attentive to characteristics of skin problems most influenced by hygiene measures. Is the skin dry from too much bathing or from use of hot water or irritating soap? Does the patient have a rash caused by an allergic reaction to a skin care product? Certain conditions place patients at risk for impaired skin integrity (Table 40-3). Because of increased risk be particularly alert when assessing patients with reduced sensation, impaired circulation, nutrition or hydration alterations, body secretions, incontinence, altered cognition, external medical devices, and decreased mobility. Patients may be unaware of skin problems because they are unable to feel pain or pressure or see their skin in some places (e.g., the back or the feet). Carefully assess the skin under orthopedic devices (braces, splints, casts) and beneath items such as antiembolic stockings and tape. Assess the condition and cleanliness of the perineal and anal areas during hygiene care and when the patient requires toileting assistance. When prolonged contact of urine or feces occurs such as with diarrhea or incontinence, skin breakdown often results. Most people consider these areas private; therefore be sensitive in your approach (Touhy and Jett, 2012).

When caring for patients with dark skin pigmentation, be aware of assessment techniques and skin characteristics unique to highly pigmented skin (Ball et al., 2015). Carefully assess the skin in dark-skinned patients at risk for pressure ulcers (see Chapter 48).

Assessment of the Feet and Nails. A variety of common foot and nail problems can be caused by inadequate hygiene and are actually detected during hygiene care. Problems sometimes result from abuse or poor care of the feet and hands such as nail biting or trimming nails improperly, exposure to harsh chemicals, and wearing poorly fitting shoes. Question the patient to determine type of footwear and usual foot and nail care practices.

Examine all skin surfaces of the feet, including the areas between the toes and over the entire sole of the foot. Poorly fitting shoes often irritate the heels, soles, and sides of the feet. Inspection of the feet for lesions includes noting areas of dryness, inflammation, or cracking. Chronic foot problems are common in older adults who often experience dry feet because of a decrease in sebaceous gland secretion, dehydration, or poor condition of footwear.

People are often unaware of foot or nail problems until pain or discomfort occurs. Assess patients with diseases that affect peripheral circulation and sensation for the adequacy of circulation and sensation of the feet. Foot ulceration is the most common single precursor to lower-extremity amputations among people with diabetes (Jarrett, 2013). Daily inspection and preventive foot care help maintain ulcer-free feet. Palpate the dorsalis pedis and posterior tibial pulses and assess for intact sensation to light touch, pinprick, and temperature (Ball et al., 2015).

Observe a patient's gait. Painful foot disorders or decreased sensation cause limping or an unnatural gait. Ask whether the patient has foot discomfort and determine factors that aggravate the pain. Foot problems sometimes result from bone or muscular alterations or wearing poorly fitting footwear.

Inspect the condition of the fingernails and toenails, looking for lesions, dryness, inflammation, or cracking, which are often associated with a variety of common foot and nail problems (Table 40-4). The cuticle that surrounds the nail can grow over it and become inflamed if nail care is not performed correctly and periodically. Ask women whether they polish their nails and use polish remover frequently because chemicals in these products cause excessive nail dryness. Disease changes the shape and curvature of the nails (Ball et al., 2015). Inflammatory lesions and fungus of the nail bed cause thickened, horny nails that separate from the nail bed.

Assessment of the Oral Cavity. The condition of the oral cavity reflects overall health and also indicates oral hygiene needs. Inspect all areas of the mouth carefully for color, hydration, texture, and lesions (see Chapter 31). Patients frequently develop common oral problems as a result of inadequate oral care or disease (e.g., oral malignancy) or as a side effect of treatments such as radiation and chemotherapy. These problems include receding gum tissue, inflamed gums (gingivitis), a coated tongue, **glossitis** (inflamed tongue), discolored teeth

TABLE 40-2 Common Skin Problems

Characteristics	Implications	Interventions
Dry Skin		
Flaky, rough texture on exposed areas such as hands, arms, legs, or face	Skin becomes infected if epidermal layer cracks.	Bathe less frequently. Rinse body of all soap because residue left on skin can cause irritation and breakdown. Add moisture to air with use of humidifier. Increase fluid intake when skin is dry. Use moisturizing cream to aid healing. (Cream forms protective barrier and helps maintain fluid within skin.) Use creams to clean skin that is dry or allergic to soaps and detergents.
Acne		
Inflammatory, papulopustular skin eruption, usually involving bacterial breakdown of sebum; appears on face, neck, shoulders, and back	Infected material within pustule spreads if area is squeezed or picked. Permanent scarring can result.	Wash hair and skin thoroughly each day with warm water and soap to remove oil. Use cosmetics sparingly. Oily cosmetics or creams accumulate in pores and make condition worse. Implement dietary restrictions if necessary. (Eliminate foods that aggravate condition from diet.) Use prescribed topical antibiotics for severe forms of acne.
Skin Rashes		
Skin eruptions that result from overexposure to sun or moisture or from allergic reaction (flat or raised, localized or systemic, pruritic or nonpruritic)	If skin is scratched continually, inflammation and infection may occur. Rashes also cause discomfort.	Wash area thoroughly and apply antiseptic spray or lotion to prevent further itching and aid in healing process. Apply warm or cold soaks to relieve inflammation if indicated.
Contact Dermatitis		
Inflammation of skin characterized by abrupt onset with erythema; pruritus; pain; and appearance of scaly, oozing lesions (seen on face, neck, hands, forearms, and genitalia)	Dermatitis is often difficult to eliminate because person is usually in continual contact with substance causing skin reaction. Substance is often hard to identify.	Avoid causative agents (e.g., cleansers and soaps).
Abrasion		
Scraping or rubbing away of epidermis that results in localized bleeding and later weeping of serous fluid	Infection occurs easily because of loss of protective skin layer.	Be careful not to scratch patient with jewelry or fingernails. Wash abrasions with mild soap and water; dry thoroughly and gently. Observe dressing or bandage for retained moisture because it increases risk of infection.

(particularly along gum margins), **cheilitis** (cracked lips), dental caries, missing teeth, and **halitosis** (foul-smelling breath). Localized pain and infection commonly accompany oral problems. Apply clean gloves to palpate any tender areas or lesions. Observe for cleanliness and use olfaction to detect halitosis. If you identify any oral problems, notify the patient's health care provider. Early identification of poor oral hygiene practices and common oral problems reduces the risk for gum disease and dental caries (USDHHS, 2015). If the older adult becomes **edentulous** (i.e., without teeth) and wears complete or partial dentures, include an assessment of underlying gums and palate.

Assessment of the Hair and Hair Care. Assess the condition of a patient's hair and scalp before performing hair care. Findings help determine the frequency and type of care needed. You can anticipate certain patients who might require a more focused assessment such as a patient who has had head trauma or a homeless patient not able to perform regular hygiene. Normally the hair is clean, shiny, and untangled; and the scalp is clear of lesions. Table 40-5 summarizes hair and scalp problems with implications and interventions.

Observe a patient's ability to perform hair care. A person's appearance and feeling of well-being often are related to the way the hair looks and feels. Illness, disability, and conditions such as arthritis, fatigue, obesity, and the presence of physical barriers (e.g., cast or IV access) alter a patient's ability to maintain daily hair care.

In community health and home care settings it is particularly important to inspect the hair for lice so you can provide appropriate hygienic treatment. If you suspect **pediculosis capitis** (head lice), guard against self-infestations by hand hygiene and using gloves or tongue blades to inspect the patient's hair.

The loss of hair (**alopecia**) results from the effects of chemotherapy medications, hormonal changes, or improper hair care practices. Alopecia often appears as brittle and broken hair in the hair line that progresses to bald patches. If noted, be sure to question the patient about specific hair care practices, especially the use of chemicals and heat application during hair care.

Assessment of the Eyes, Ears, and Nose. Examine the condition and function of the eyes, ears, and nose (see Chapter 31). The

TABLE 40-3 Risk Factors for Hygiene Care

Risks	Hygiene Implications
Oral Problems	
Inability to use upper extremities because of paralysis, weakness, or restriction (e.g., cast, dressing)	Patient lacks upper-extremity strength or dexterity needed to brush teeth (Lewis et al., 2014).
Dehydration, inability to take fluids or food by mouth (NPO)	Dehydration causes excess drying and fragility of mucosa; increases accumulation of secretions on tongue and gums.
Presence of nasogastric or oxygen tubes; mouth breathers	Tubes cause pressure, friction, and drying of mucosa and/or lips.
Chemotherapeutic drugs	Drugs kill rapidly multiplying cells, including normal cells lining oral cavity. Ulcers and inflammation develop.
Lozenges, cough drops, antacids, and chewable over-the-counter vitamins	Medications contain large amounts of sugar. Repeated use increases sugar or acid content in mouth, causing dental caries.
Radiation therapy to head and neck	Radiation therapy reduces salivary flow and lowers pH of saliva; leads to stomatitis and tooth decay (Lewis et al., 2014).
Oral surgery, trauma to mouth, placement of oral airway	These cause trauma to oral cavity with swelling, ulcerations, inflammation, and bleeding.
Immunosuppression; altered blood clotting	These predispose to inflammation and bleeding gums.
Diabetes mellitus	Patients are prone to dryness of mouth, gingivitis, periodontal disease, and loss of teeth.
Endotracheal intubation with mechanical ventilation	Potential for ventilator-associated pneumonia (VAP) exists. Use of chlorhexidine gluconate (CHG) reduces risk of VAP. CHG is an inexpensive effective agent for reducing VAP, especially in patients who have heart surgery (Nicolosi et al., 2014).
Dialysis	Oral problems commonly found in these patients include halitosis, xerostomia (dry mouth), gingivitis, stomatitis, tooth decay, tooth loss, and jaw problems. Causes may include elevated blood sugar, weight control, and smoking (Genco, 2014).
Skin Problems	
Immobilization	Dependent body parts are exposed to pressure from underlying surfaces. The inability to turn or change position increases risk for pressure ulcers.
Bariatric patient	Patient cannot visualize skin properly and keep it clean and dry. Excessive adipose tissue creates pressure from weight, lack of air circulation, and an increase in moisture with poor tissue perfusion (Cowell and Radley, 2014).
Reduced sensation caused by stroke, spinal cord injury, diabetes, local nerve damage	Patient unable to sense skin injury. Does not receive normal transmission of nerve impulses when applying excessive heat or cold, pressure, friction, or chemical irritants to skin.
Altered cognition resulting from dementia, psychological disorders, or temporary delirium	Patient unable to verbalize skin care needs. Does not realize effect of pressure or prolonged contact with excretions or secretions, requiring more vigilant assessment.
Limited protein or caloric intake and reduced hydration (e.g., fever, burns, gastrointestinal alterations, poorly fitting dentures)	Predispose to impaired tissue synthesis. Skin becomes thinner, less elastic, and smoother with loss of subcutaneous tissue. Poor wound healing results. Reduced hydration impairs skin turgor.
Excessive secretions or excretions on skin from perspiration, urine, watery fecal material, and wound drainage	Moisture is medium for bacterial growth and causes local skin irritation, softening of epidermal cells, and skin maceration.
Presence of external medical devices (e.g., cast, restraint, bandage, dressing)	Devices such as casts, cloth restraints, bandages, tubing, and orthopedic devices exert pressure or friction against surface of skin.
Vascular insufficiency	Arterial blood supply to tissues is inadequate, or venous return is impaired, causing decreased circulation to extremities. Tissue ischemia and breakdown often occur. Risk for infection is high.
Foot Problems	
Patient unable to bend over or has reduced visual acuity	Patient is unable to fully visualize entire surface of each foot, impairing ability to adequately assess condition of skin and nails.
Eye Care Problems	
Reduced dexterity and hand coordination	Physical limitations create inability to safely insert or remove contact lenses.

TABLE 40-4 Common Foot and Nail Problems

Characteristics	Implications	Interventions
Callus		
Thickened part of epidermis consists of mass of horny, keratotic cells. Callus is usually flat, painless, and found on undersurface of foot or palm of hand.	Local friction or pressure causes callus formation, which causes discomfort when wearing tight shoes.	Recommend soft-sole shoes with insoles. Advise patient to wear gloves when using tools or objects that create friction on palmar surfaces. Advise patients, especially with callus formation, not to self-treat but seek interventions from a podiatrist.
Corns		
Friction and pressure from ill-fitting or loose shoes cause keratosis. It is seen mainly on or between toes, over bony prominence. Corn is usually cone shaped, round, and raised. Soft corns are macerated.	Compresses the underlying dermis, making it thin and tender. Pain is aggravated when wearing tight shoes. Tissue becomes attached to bone if allowed to grow. Resultant pain causes an alteration in gait.	Surgical removal is necessary, depending on severity of pain and size of corn. Avoid use of oval corn pads, which increase pressure on toes and reduce circulation. Warm water soaks soften corns before gentle rubbing with a callus file or pumice stone. (Consult with health care provider. Not allowed with patients with diabetes.) Wider and softer shoes, with wider toe box, are helpful.
Plantar Warts		
Fungating lesion appears on sole of foot and is caused by papilloma virus.	Some warts are contagious. They are painful and make walking difficult.	Treatment ordered by health care provider often includes applications of salicylic acid, electrodessication (burning with electrical spark), or freezing with solid carbon dioxide.
Athlete's Foot (Tinea Pedis)		
Athlete's foot is fungal infection of foot; scaling and cracking of skin occurs between toes and on soles of feet. Small blisters containing fluid appear.	Athlete's foot spreads to other body parts, especially hands. It is contagious and frequently recurs.	Make sure that feet are well ventilated. Drying feet well after bathing and applying powder help prevent infection. Wearing clean socks or stockings reduces incidence. Health care provider orders application of griseofulvin, miconazole, or tolnaftate.
Ingrown Nails		
Toenail or fingernail grows inward into soft tissue around nail. Ingrown nail often results from improper nail trimming.	Ingrown nails cause localized pain when pressure is applied.	Treatment is frequent warm soaks in antiseptic solution and removal of part of nail that has grown into skin. Instruct patient in proper nail-trimming techniques and refer to podiatrist.
Foot Odors		
Foot odors are result of excess perspiration, promoting microorganism growth.	Condition causes discomfort because of excess perspiration.	Frequent washing, use of foot deodorants and powders, and wearing clean footwear prevent or reduce problem.

healthy eye is not inflamed and is without drainage. The presence of redness indicates allergic or infectious conjunctivitis, which can be highly contagious. The crusty drainage associated with conjunctivitis easily spreads from one eye to the other. Wear clean gloves to examine the eyes and perform proper hand hygiene before and after the examination. Determine if a patient wears contact lenses, especially when he or she enters the health care agency in an unresponsive or confused state. To determine if a contact lens is present, stand to the side of the patient's eyes and observe the corneas for the presence of a soft or rigid lens. Also observe the sclera because the lens may have shifted off the cornea. An undetected contact lens causes corneal injury when left in place too long.

Assessment of the external ear structures includes inspection of the auricle and external ear canal (see Chapter 31). Observe for the presence of accumulated **cerumen** (earwax) or drainage in the ear canal and local inflammation. Question patients about tenderness on palpation or the presence of pain and ask how they usually clean their ears.

Inspect the nares for signs of inflammation, discharge, lesions, edema, and deformity (see Chapter 31). The nasal mucosa is normally pink and clear and has little or no discharge. Allergies cause a clear, watery discharge. If patients have any form of tubing exiting the nose (e.g., nasogastric), observe for edema, skin ulceration, localized tenderness, inflammation, drainage, and bleeding where the tubing comes in contact with the nares.

Use of Sensory Aids. For patients who wear eyeglasses, contact lenses, artificial eyes, or hearing aids, assess their knowledge and methods used for care and have them describe the typical approach used in routine care. When possible observe a patient perform care. Compare information gathered from him or her with the proper care technique for these devices. Any difference between patient and standard practice provides an opportunity for patient education.

Assessment of Hygiene Care Practices. Assessment of hygiene practices reveals a patient's preferences for grooming. For example, a patient chooses to groom the hair in a certain style or trim nails in a certain way. When a patient has a physical disability, special precautions may be necessary to perform grooming without injury. For example, teach patients with loss of sensation to file nails instead of clipping. By observing a patient perform hygiene care, you can detect any needed areas of teaching or assistance while maintaining the patient's maximal level of independence.

TABLE 40-5 Hair and Scalp Problems

Characteristics	Implications	Interventions
Dandruff		
Scaling of scalp is accompanied by itching. In severe cases dandruff is on eyebrows.	Dandruff causes embarrassment. If it enters eyes, conjunctivitis often develops.	Shampoo regularly with medicated shampoo. In severe cases obtain health care provider's advice.
Ticks		
Small, gray-brown parasites burrow into skin and suck blood.	Ticks transmit several diseases to people. Most common are Rocky Mountain spotted fever, tularemia, and Lyme disease.	Using blunt tweezers, grasp tick as close to the head as possible and pull upward with even, steady pressure. Hold until tick pulls out, usually for about 3-4 minutes. Save tick in plastic bag and put in freezer if it is necessary to identify type of tick.
Pediculosis (Lice)		
Pediculosis Capitis (Head Lice)		
Parasite resides on scalp attached to hair strands. Eggs look like oval particles, similar to dandruff. Bites or pustules may be observed behind ears and at hairline.	Head lice are difficult to remove and spread to furniture and other people if not treated. They do not carry disease, cannot fly or jump, and are carried by animals.	Wearing gloves, check entire scalp by using tongue depressor or special lice comb. Use medicated shampoo for eliminating lice. *Caution against use of products containing lindane because the ingredient is toxic and known to cause adverse reactions* (CDC, 2015). Manual removal is best option when treatment has failed. Vacuum infested areas of home.
Pediculosis Corporis (Body Lice)		
Parasites tend to cling to clothing; thus they are not always easy to see. Body lice suck blood and lay eggs on clothing and furniture.	Patient itches constantly. Scratches seen on skin become infected. Hemorrhagic spots appear on skin where lice are sucking blood.	Bathe or shower thoroughly. After skin is dried, apply recommended pediculicide lotion. After 12 to 24 hours take another bath or shower. Bag infested clothing or linen until laundered in hot water. Vacuum rooms thoroughly and throw away bag after completion.
Pediculosis Pubis (Crab Lice)		
Parasites are in pubic hair. Crab lice are gray-white with red legs.	Lice spread through bed linen, clothing, or furniture or between people via sexual contact.	Shave hair off affected area. Clean as for body lice. If lice were sexually transmitted, notify partner.
Hair Loss (Alopecia)		
Alopecia occurs in all races. Balding patches are in periphery of hair line. Hair becomes brittle and broken.	Patches of uneven hair growth and loss alter patient's appearance.	Stop hair care practices that damage hair. Use of hair curlers, hair picks, tight braiding, and hot comb contributes to hair-loss condition.

Assessment of Cultural Influences. Ask what makes a patient feel most comfortable during a bath or other hygiene measures. Perhaps he or she prefers a partial instead of a full bath from a nurse, with a family member completing the bathing of more private body parts. Some patients also defer part of hygiene. If you believe that hygiene is critical to prevent developing or worsening problems such as skin breakdown, take the time to understand the patient's concerns and then offer an explanation that helps him or her accept your intervention. For example, many institutions are using chlorhexidine gluconate (CHG) for daily bathing. CHG can leave the skin feeling sticky. If patients complain about its use, you need to explain their vulnerability to infection and how CHG helps reduce occurrence of health care–associated infection. Consider a patient's level of literacy and be sure that you have adapted your assessment questions to a level the patient can understand.

Patients at Risk for Hygiene Problems. Some patients present risks that require more attentive and rigorous hygiene care (see Table 40-3). These risks result from side effects of medications or other medical therapy; a lack of knowledge; immobilization; an inability to perform hygiene; or a physical condition that potentially injures the skin, mouth, feet and nails, or hair. Anticipate whether a patient is predisposed to risks and follow through with a complete assessment. For example, if a patient is receiving cancer chemotherapy, there is a risk of the medication producing mouth ulcerations, which are painful and create a risk for infection and impaired nutrition because of reluctance to eat and drink. A patient who receives broad-spectrum antibiotics may develop an opportunistic infection when the normal flora of the mouth is disrupted by the antibiotic. Be thorough and detailed during the oral examination, checking all surfaces of the tongue and mucosa. For a bariatric patient or a patient who is diaphoretic, provide special attention to body areas such as beneath the woman's breasts and in the groin, skinfolds, and perineal area, where moisture collects and irritates skin surfaces (Cowell and Radley, 2014). Assessment should include a review of a patient's medical and surgical history, medications, and the specific risk factors that the patient presents.

◆ Nursing Diagnosis

Thorough assessment of a patient's hygiene status and self-care abilities identifies clusters of risk factors or defining characteristics that support actual or at-risk hygiene-related diagnoses. Identification of the defining characteristics or risk factors leads you to select the NANDA

BOX 40-3 Nursing Diagnostic Process

Bathing Self-Care Deficit

Assessment Activities	Findings/Defining Characteristics
Observe patient attempt to bathe self.	Patient is unable to wash lower body, back, or perineal area.
Assess patient's upper-extremity strength and range of motion.	Patient has restricted upper-extremity range of motion and weakness. Patient has difficulty turning in bed by self or reaching items needed. Patient is unable to turn water faucets on and off.
Observe patient's ability to move from bed to bathroom and maneuver in bathroom.	Patient cannot transfer from bed to chair without assistance, cannot ambulate, relies on wheelchair to move around, is unable to maneuver wheelchair in bathroom without help or transfer to shower seat unassisted. Patient may need lift equipment for transfers.

International diagnostic label (Herdman and Kamitsuru, 2014) that best communicates the individual patient's situation. For example, when caring for an older adult with degenerative arthritis, you observe swollen joints, weakness, and limited ROM in the dominant hand along with a generally unkempt appearance. Closer review of data reveals defining characteristics of an inability to wash body parts and difficulty turning and regulating a water faucet. The nursing diagnosis of *Bathing Self-Care Deficit* becomes part of the plan of care. Accurate selection of nursing diagnoses requires critical thinking to identify actual or potential problems. Be thorough in assessment to reveal all appropriate defining characteristics or risk factors so you can make an accurate diagnosis (Box 40-3).

Use a patient's actual alteration (e.g., *Impaired Tissue Integrity*) or the alteration for which the patient is at risk (e.g., *Risk for Infection*) to determine the focus of nursing interventions. A patient with an actual alteration requires extensive hygiene care, often more thorough than routine hygiene. For example, if a patient has skin breakdown, initiate care more frequently to keep skin surfaces clean and dry and eliminate factors such as moisture or drainage. Also provide care to promote healing of injured skin surfaces (see Chapter 48). If a patient is at risk for a problem, take preventive measures. For example, if a patient is at risk for developing an infection in his or her mouth and has the nursing diagnosis *Risk for Infection,* keep the mucosa well hydrated, minimize foods irritating to tissues, and provide cleaning that soothes and reduces tissue inflammation.

Completing a nursing diagnosis requires identification of the related factor (for an actual diagnosis or optional for a risk diagnosis), which will guide your selection of nursing interventions. A diagnosis of *Impaired Oral Mucous Membrane related to malnutrition* and a diagnosis of *Impaired Oral Mucous Membrane related to chemical trauma* require different interventions. When poor nutrition is a causal factor, you need to consult with a dietitian for appropriate dietary supplements and incorporate patient education into the plan. When chemotherapy injures the oral mucosa, you follow cancer nursing guidelines regarding care for oral **mucositis** (i.e., painful inflammation of oral mucous membranes), including frequent gentle brushing with a soft toothbrush, flossing, rinsing with bland rinse, limiting diet to soft foods, and applying water-based moisturizer to lips (USDHHS, 2015). Although many possible nursing diagnoses apply to patients in need of supportive hygiene care, the following list represents examples of diagnoses commonly associated with these problems:

- *Activity Intolerance*
- *Bathing Self-Care Deficit*
- *Dressing Self-Care Deficit*
- *Impaired Physical Mobility*
- *Impaired Oral Mucous Membrane*
- *Ineffective Health Maintenance*
- *Risk for Infection*
- *Risk for Impaired Skin Integrity*

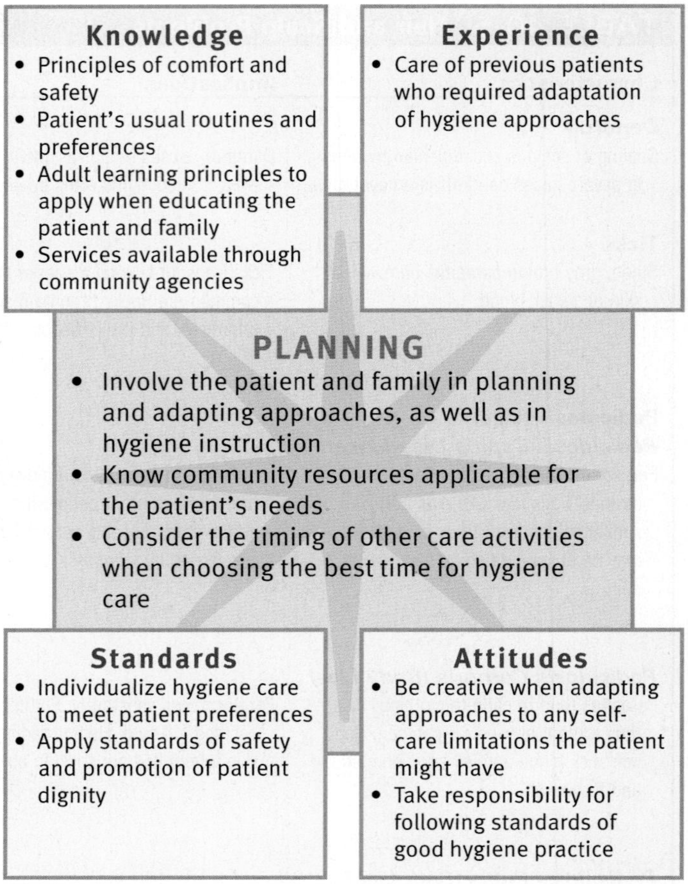

Knowledge
- Principles of comfort and safety
- Patient's usual routines and preferences
- Adult learning principles to apply when educating the patient and family
- Services available through community agencies

Experience
- Care of previous patients who required adaptation of hygiene approaches

PLANNING
- Involve the patient and family in planning and adapting approaches, as well as in hygiene instruction
- Know community resources applicable for the patient's needs
- Consider the timing of other care activities when choosing the best time for hygiene care

Standards
- Individualize hygiene care to meet patient preferences
- Apply standards of safety and promotion of patient dignity

Attitudes
- Be creative when adapting approaches to any self-care limitations the patient might have
- Take responsibility for following standards of good hygiene practice

FIGURE 40-3 Critical thinking model for hygiene planning.

◆ Planning

During planning synthesize information from multiple resources (Figure 40-3). Critical thinking ensures that a patient's plan of care integrates all that is known about the individual patient and key critical thinking elements. In many situations patients present with multiple nursing diagnoses. Use a concept map (Figure 40-4) to visualize and understand how nursing diagnoses interrelate. Rely on knowledge, experience, and established standards of care when developing a care plan. Remember critical thinking attitudes such as creativity when developing a patient-centered plan for hygiene care. Consciously include the patient in this important step of the nursing process. Partner with a patient to identify patient goals and outcomes, set priorities for care, and select evidence-based interventions. Consider continuity of care and involve other health care team members (e.g., occupational or physical therapy) when developing the plan.

Previous experience with other patients is useful in knowing how to adapt hygiene techniques for special needs. Professional standards

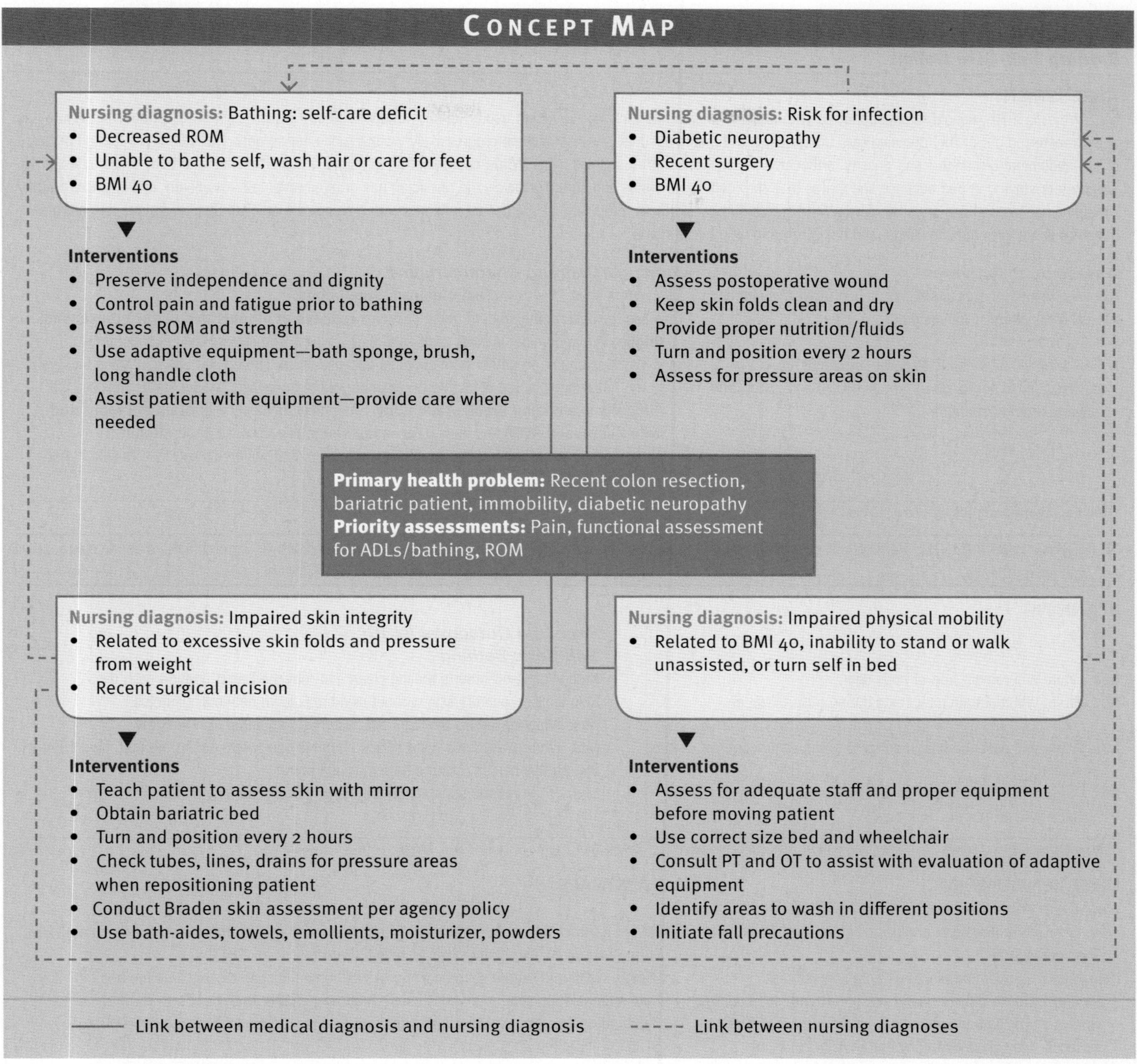

FIGURE 40-4 Concept map for Mrs. White. *ADLs,* Activities of daily living; *BMI,* body mass index; *OT,* occupational therapist; *PT,* physical therapist; *ROM,* range of motion.

guide selection of the most effective nursing interventions. These standards often establish evidence-based guidelines for care.

Goals and Outcomes. Partner with the patient and family to identify goals and expected outcomes to develop a mutually agreed-on plan of care based on the patient's nursing diagnoses (see the Nursing Care Plan). For example, establish goals with the patient's self-care abilities and resources in mind and focus on maintaining or improving the condition of the skin and oral cavity. Make outcomes measurable and achievable within patient limitations. In addition, work with the patient to select individualized hygiene measures.

When providing patient hygiene, you will care for a variety of patients with different self-care abilities and needs. For example, a nurse and a patient who has one-sided paralysis following a cerebral vascular accident develop the following goal: "Patient will be able to groom self (dress and bathe) before discharge." The nurse establishes realistic, individualized expected outcomes to measure the patient's progress toward meeting this goal. These outcomes may include the following:

- Patient is able to bathe in front of sink.
- Patient uses assist devices (bathing mitt and long handled sponge) for bathing.
- Patient dresses self, using dressing stick and sock aid.

Setting Priorities. A patient's condition influences your priorities for hygiene care. Set priorities based on the necessary assistance

NURSING CARE PLAN

Bathing Self-Care Deficit

ASSESSMENT

Mrs. White is a 70-year-old female admitted with abdominal pain and a change in bowel habits. She is now post op day 2 after a colon resection. Mrs. White has been transferred out of the intensive care unit (ICU) onto the surgical unit. She has become progressively weaker since her surgery. Her mobility is limited because of her abdominal discomfort and obesity, although she can walk short distances. Mrs. White has diabetes, a history of hypertension, and body mass index of 40. She prefers staying in bed because she states that she feels tired, weak, and sore. However, the physician has ordered ambulation to begin, and physical therapy is helping her learn to use a walker. Mrs. White states that her buttocks, thigh, and skinfolds feel inflamed with a pain score of 7/10. She lives alone, but her granddaughter is going to nursing school and has offered to help her at home.

Assessment Activities	*Findings/Defining Characteristics**
Ask Mrs. White what hygiene care is important this morning.	Mrs. White says, "I want to **feel clean** and **smell good.**"
Assess Mrs. White's skin condition.	On visual inspection the student nurse observes **redness at elbows and under breasts and thighs.** The abdominal incision is dry and pink, and the sutures are well approximated.
Assess Mrs. White's ability to bathe, including an assessment of her range of motion (ROM) and upper- and lower-extremity strength.	Mrs. White is unable to gather bath supplies because of her immobility. She can stand and walk to the bathroom sink but is unable to wash her entire body. Mrs. White states that she has **difficulty visualizing areas of her body.** She perspires easily. Her **arms are restricted with decreased ROM** and have **decreased sensation** because of her **diabetic neuropathy.** Mrs. White states that her pain level is 7/10 when moving side to side in bed since her surgery.

***Defining characteristics** are shown in bold type.

NURSING DIAGNOSIS: Bathing self-care deficit related to immobility associated with obesity; body mass index (BMI) 40, limited ROM, diabetic neuropathy, and pain score of 7/10

PLANNING

Goals	*Expected Outcomes (NOC)*† *Self-Care: Bathing*
Mrs. White will remain free of body odor.	Mrs. White self-reports feeling clean and refreshed after bathing each day.
Mrs. White will maintain intact skin during hospitalization.	Skin is clean and dry skin without skin breakdown between skinfolds. Mrs. White describes personal risk factors for impaired skin integrity.
Mrs. White will describe best method to bathe using adaptive devices by discharge.	Mrs. White states two ways to use adaptive equipment during her bath by discharge. She bathes herself, using a bath mitt and mirror.
Mrs. White will accept help from a family caregiver to assist with hygiene care within the next week.	Mrs. White reports satisfaction with assistance in bathing by family caregiver.

†Outcome classification labels from Moorhead S et al: *Nursing outcomes classification (NOC),* ed 5, St Louis, 2013, Mosby.

INTERVENTIONS (NIC)‡ *Self-Care Assistance: Bathing/Hygiene*	**RATIONALE**
Administer prn ordered oral analgesic before bath; begin bath 30 minutes later.	Patient participation in bathing or other self-care activities will improve with pain control. Give prn pain medication before pain is severe (Bulechek et al., 2013).
Help patient shower and place her on a shower seat. Demonstrate for patient use of wash mitt with soap pocket. Offer a mirror with long handle to improve view of foot surfaces. Stay close by to prevent an accidental fall.	Using a wash mitt with a soap pocket or a wall-mounted soap dispenser minimizes difficulty of manipulating soap and a washcloth. A shower seat or bath bench makes it easier for patient to focus on washing rather than on balance required for standing (Sokol-McKay, 2013).
Bathing Option: Consider using prepackaged bath/chlorhexidine gluconate (CHG) wipes for bed bath if patient cannot tolerate shower.	Bath wipes are easy to use and disposable and require no rinsing. Skin can air dry. Daily bathing with CHG wipes decreases hospital-acquired infections (Singh and Subhashni, 2013). Keeping skin clean and dry helps to avoid risk of friction and shearing and decreases moisture from sweat glands that become blocked, causing bacteria and fungi infections on skin to occur (Cowell and Radley, 2014).
Teach Mrs. White reasons that she is vulnerable for impaired skin integrity: perspiration, obesity, effects of diabetes, immobility, and changes in skin from aging.	Self-efficacy (i.e., a person's judgment about what one thinks one can accomplish with knowledge and skills) (Bandura, 1997) affects self-care performance, especially if tasks and circumstances are not ambiguous.
Teach patient and granddaughter (as needed) how to use adaptive equipment for bathing and safe patient-handling skills and how to perform skin assessments. Have Mrs. White plan hygiene schedule with granddaughter.	Family members who are taught methods to meet patient's bathing needs increase patient satisfaction, making the experience safe, easy, less stressful. Appropriate assistive devices encourage independence. Return demonstration identifies problem areas and increases self-confidence. Teach Back ensures that patient and family understand the importance of skin integrity and infection control to minimize risks for the obese patient with diabetes (Cowell and Radley, 2014). Individuals in supportive social relationships are happier and healthier than those socially isolated. Providing help that addresses the needs and desires of a patient is uplifting to a caregiver (Schulz and Sherwood, 2008).

‡Intervention classification labels from Bulechek GM et al: *Nursing interventions classifications (NIC),* ed 6, St Louis, 2013, Mosby.

NURSING CARE PLAN

Bathing Self-Care Deficit—cont'd

EVALUATION

Nursing Actions	*Patient Response/Finding*	*Achievement of Outcome*
Ask Mrs. White why it is important for her to inspect skin and have regular bathing.	Mrs. White states that she now knows she is at risk for infection because she is overweight and has diabetes. She also knows her risk for infection is higher in the hospital.	Mrs. White is able to identify her personal risk factors for infection if she does not bathe properly.
Inspect Mrs. White's skin after she bathes in shower and assess for any remaining body odor.	Mrs. White's skin is clear without irritation under breasts and perineum. Had difficulty cleansing back and bottom of feet, but no signs of irritation. No apparent odor. Patient expresses sense of feeling clean.	Mrs. White requires assistance with bathing in areas of body she could not reach. Will refer to occupational therapy for an appropriate assistive device with long handle.
	Because Mrs. White is older, she has learned that she need not bathe daily. She and granddaughter have planned to have a bath every 3 days in the evening after granddaughter returns from work. Granddaughter is able to explain correct technique for helping patient with walker and transferring to and from shower chair.	Mrs. White has a realistic plan for bathing at home. Granddaughter demonstrates knowledge of safe patient handling. Consultation note will be written for home health nurse to check granddaughter's skin assessment skills.

required by the patient, the extent of the hygiene-related problems, and the nature of the patient's nursing diagnoses. For example, a seriously ill patient usually needs a daily bath because body secretions accumulate and the patient is unable to maintain cleanliness independently. Some older patients at home require a visit from a home care aide to help with a tub bath or shower. Patients who are normally inactive during the day and have skin that tends to be dry may need to bathe only twice a week, whereas a patient with urinary and bowel incontinence needs perineal cleaning with each episode of soiling. Plan to help patients who are weakened or possess poor coordination. For example, a patient who is partially paralyzed and has difficulty getting out of a tub needs a tub chair, handrails, or extra personnel available for help.

Timing is also important in planning hygiene care. Being interrupted in the middle of a bath often frustrates and embarrasses a patient. Assess for cultural preferences on time of day or who may help patient with hygiene care.

Teamwork and Collaboration. If a patient is hospitalized, plan care before discharge to home, a rehabilitation facility, or extended care. Provide clear directions for family caregivers or staff who will be assuming the patient's care so the appropriate equipment and hygiene supplies can be used. Be sure that caregivers know any physical or cognitive limitations that will affect their ability to provide safe, effective hygiene care. For example, does the patient require assistance to get into a tub or shower, does the patient have reduced sensation making him or her at risk for burns from hot water, and can the patient remember steps to follow for proper foot care? Collaborate with other health team members as indicated (e.g., work with physical and occupational therapy to enhance the patient's independence with self-care activities).

When a patient needs assistance as a result of a self-care limitation and family members are the ones to provide it, proper education and preparation should be included in the plan of care. Family members also need guidance in adapting techniques to fit patient limitations. Be aware of equipment and procedures used in the agency so the patient and family are knowledgeable about the care, have the skills needed to provide it, and have access to necessary equipment. Depending on a patient's limitations, some insurance plans provide home care assistants to help with basic hygiene needs. Explore this option with the patient and family members.

Collaborate with community agencies as needed. For example, the nurse involved in the care of a homeless patient needs to be aware of the location of clothing distribution centers for basic hygiene supplies, a shelter where bathing facilities are available, and any organization that offers free health care or reduced fees. Partner with social workers or staff in local area churches, not-for-profit organizations, and schools to be sure that patients have the resources they need to maintain hygiene.

◆ Implementation

Hygiene is a part of basic patient care. When you use caring practices to perform hygiene measures, you reduce the patient's anxiety and promote comfort and relaxation. For example, use a gentle approach when giving patients their baths and changing gowns as you turn and reposition them. A soft, gentle voice when conversing with patients relieves fears or concerns. For patients suffering symptoms such as pain or nausea, administering medications to relieve the symptoms before providing hygiene helps to maintain patient comfort during procedures.

Consider the stress that hygiene care can cause and be alert for any cues of embarrassment or anxiety. Some patients fear pain or are frightened about falling or sustaining injury associated with hygiene care.

Implementation also focuses on assisting and preparing patients to be able to perform as much of their hygiene care as they can independently. Teach patients proper hygiene techniques and how their use is associated with better health. Discuss any signs and symptoms of hygiene problems. Inform patients about available resources in the community for dealing with these problems if they arise. Always use Teach Back during instruction to confirm their understanding.

Health Promotion. In primary health care situations educate and counsel patients and caregivers on why proper hygiene techniques are necessary. For example, a new mother needs to learn how to bathe her newborn to reduce risk of skin irritation and infection, whereas an older adult needs information on the importance of regular ear care to avoid accumulated cerumen and hearing impairment. The hygiene skills described throughout this chapter provide standards for excellent physical care. When caring for patients in primary health care settings, maintain these standards and incorporate adaptations as needed to meet the patient's lifestyle, functional status, living arrangements, and preferences. Key points when teaching patients about hygiene include the following:

- Make any instruction relevant on the basis of your assessment of the patient's knowledge, motivation, preferences, and health beliefs. For example, when teaching a patient with diabetes, include how circulation to the feet is impaired and how this causes poor healing and infection, especially when the skin is injured or broken. Use the Teach Back method to ensure that the patient understands skin care.

- Adapt instruction to a patient's personal bathing facilities and resources. Not all patients have the ideal situation that exists in a health care setting (e.g., easily accessible shower or a bedside table to place over a bed). Adapt available resources so the patient can reach and use needed items comfortably and safely. For example, a young mother has more room and believes that bathing her infant is safer if she uses her kitchen sink and counter rather than her bathroom sink.
- Teach patients ways to avoid injury. Almost any hygiene procedure poses risks (e.g., cutting a nail too close to the skin or failing to adjust the water temperature of the bath). Include safety risks and tips with all instructions.
- Reinforce infection control practices. Damage to the skin, mucosa, eyes, or other tissues creates an immediate risk for infection. Determine that a patient understands the relationship among healthy and intact skin and tissues, hand hygiene practices, and the prevention of infection.

Acute, Restorative, and Continuing Care. Nursing knowledge and skills needed for performing hygiene care are consistent across all health care settings. In addition, some of the skills in this section are applicable in areas of health promotion. The variety, frequency, and timing of hygiene measures vary across health care settings and according to individual patient needs. In the acute care setting factors such as more frequent diagnostic and treatment plans and the need for more extensive hygiene care resulting from acute illness or injury affect scheduling. In extended care facilities and nursing homes, bathing may be scheduled less frequently.

Bathing and Skin Care. Consider a patient's normal grooming routines, including type of hygiene products used and the time of day when hygiene is routinely performed. Individualize your care on the basis of the patient's preferences. The extent, type, and timing or frequency of bathing and the methods used depend on a patient's physical abilities, health problems, and the degree of hygiene required (Boxes 40-4 and 40-5). In addition to cleansing baths, the health care provider may prescribe therapeutic baths, including sitz baths. Medicated baths (e.g., oatmeal, cornstarch, or Aveeno) may be recommended in the home setting. A sitz bath cleans and reduces pain and inflammation of perineal and anal areas (see Chapter 48). Medicated baths relieve skin irritation and create an antibacterial and drying effect.

If a patient is physically dependent or cognitively impaired, increase the frequency of skin assessment and provide skin care directed toward reducing the risk for skin breakdown. When bathing patients with cognitive impairments, consider their special needs and challenges. These patients easily become afraid. Patients with dementia often refuse, withdraw, or fight during a bath or shower. It can be difficult managing their physical and verbally aggressive behaviors. If possible, learn the triggers that routinely cause these behaviors (Warchol, 2010). For example, unmanaged pain; being cold; feeling frightened, vulnerable, and exposed; feeling embarrassed; feeling a loss of control; or not understanding what is happening often causes aggressive behavior. Adapt your bathing procedures and the environment to reduce the triggers. For example, administer any ordered analgesic 30 minutes before a bath and be gentle in your approach. Keep the patient's body as warm as possible with warm towels and be sure that the room temperature is comfortable. Reduce fear by making sure that all safety devices (e.g., grab bars in a shower, bath mats) are available. Ask for permission to conduct the bath and give the patient options for making

BOX 40-4 Hygiene Care Schedule in Acute and Long-Term Care Settings

Early Morning Care
Nursing personnel on the night shift provide basic hygiene to patients getting ready for breakfast, scheduled tests, or early morning surgery. "AM care" includes offering a bedpan or urinal if the patient is not ambulatory, washing the patient's hands and face, and helping with oral care.

Routine Morning Care
After breakfast help by offering a bedpan or urinal to patients confined to bed; provide a full or partial bath or a shower, including perineal care and oral, foot, nail, and hair care; give a back rub; change a patient's gown or pajamas; change the bed linens; and straighten a patient's bedside unit and room. This is often referred to as "complete AM care."

Afternoon Care
Hospitalized patients often undergo many exhausting diagnostic tests or procedures in the morning. In rehabilitation centers patients participate in physical therapy in the morning. Afternoon hygiene care includes washing the hands and face, helping with oral care, offering a bedpan or urinal, and straightening bed linen.

Evening, or Hour-before-Sleep, Care
Before bedtime offer personal hygiene care that helps patients relax and promotes sleep. "PM care" often includes changing soiled bed linens, gowns, or pajamas; helping patients wash the face and hands; providing oral hygiene; giving a back massage; and offering the bedpan or urinal to nonambulatory patients. Some patients enjoy a beverage such as juice; check diet to determine which beverages are allowed.

BOX 40-5 Types of Baths

Complete bed bath: Bath administered to totally dependent patient in bed (see Skill 40-1).

Partial bed bath: Bed bath that consists of bathing only body parts that would cause discomfort if left unbathed such as the hands, face, axillae, and perineal area. Partial bath may also include washing back and providing back rub. Provide a partial bath to dependent patients in need of partial hygiene or self-sufficient bedridden patients who are unable to reach all body parts.

Sponge bath at the sink: Involves bathing from a bath basin or sink with patient sitting in a chair. Patient is able to perform part of the bath independently. Assistance is needed for hard-to-reach areas.

Tub bath: Involves immersion in a tub of water that allows more thorough washing and rinsing than a bed bath. Commonly used in long-term care. A patient may require the nurse's help. Some institutions have tubs equipped with lifting devices that facilitate positioning dependent patients in the tub.

Shower: Patient sits or stands under a continuous stream of water. The shower provides more thorough cleaning than a bed bath but can cause fatigue.

Bag bath/travel bath: Contains several soft, nonwoven cotton cloths that are premoistened in a solution of no-rinse surfactant cleanser and emollient. The bag bath offers an alternative because of the ease of use, reduced time bathing, and patient comfort.

Chlorhexidine gluconate (CHG) bath: This antimicrobial bath wipe is used to decrease the frequency of hospital-acquired infections on skin, invasive lines, and catheters.

decisions (e.g., choice of soap, timing of when to wash face). Use comforting words during bathing to enhance a patient's relaxation. Collaborate and communicate to teach family members how to help bathe dependent or cognitively impaired patients for optimal outcomes once the patient is discharged (Hardin, 2012).

Complete Bed Bath. A complete bed bath (see Skill 40-1 on pp. 854-862), tub bath, or shower often exhausts a patient. Turning during a complete bed bath and receiving back care increase oxygen consumption and demand. Getting out of a low tub requires considerable exertion. Assess and be alert for a patient's activity intolerance during hygiene care. Assessing heart rate before, during, and after a bath provides a measure of his her physical tolerance. Provide a partial bed bath (see Skill 40-1) to patients who are aging, dependent, in need of only partial hygiene, or bedridden and unable to reach all body parts. Wear gloves when there is a risk of coming in contact with body fluids. Control environmental factors that alter skin integrity, including moisture, heat, and external sources of pressure such as wrinkled bed linen and improperly placed drainage tubing.

Traditionally baths have been given using soap and warm water. The question of whether to use bath basins with soap and water is an issue because bath basins provide a reservoir for bacteria and are a possible source of transmission of hospital-acquired infections (Johnson et al., 2009). There is a link between waterborne pathogens and the development of biofilm (multiple colonies of microorganisms attached to a surface such as a bath basin). The formation of a biofilm combined with transmission of organisms through contact with unwashed hands can create a reservoir of bacteria. The bacteria can be transferred to and maintained in a patient's bath basin. In contrast, the use of CHG 4% solution in place of standard soap and water in wash basins has been shown to decrease bacterial growth in basins (Powers et al., 2012) and reduce critical care unit–acquired methicillin-resistant *Staphylococcus aureus* (MRSA) (Petlin et al., 2014). It is important to air-dry bath basins completely and not to use a basin for storing supplies.

Another option to using CHG in bath basins is the use of CHG 2% in impregnated washcloths (Box 40-6). The CHG in the cloths is fast acting, has broad-spectrum microorganism coverage, continues antimicrobial activity up to 24 hours after application, and is rinse free and disposable (AHRQ, 2013). Daily bathing with 2% CHG-impregnated cloths versus nonantimicrobial washcloths has been shown to reduce the acquisition of multidrug-resistant organisms (MDROs) (Climo et al., 2013). The cost of implementation of CHG cloths has reduced hospital infection rates and improved outcomes for a shorter patient hospitalization (Rubin et al., 2013). The one factor that may result in health care settings choosing 4% CHG solution versus the 2% CHG cloths is the fact that the 2% cloths are more costly but not any more effective. Daily bathing with some form of CHG is becoming more of a standard practice across hospitals.

- When using CHG solution in bath water or impregnated cloths, use a clean CHG washcloth/cloth for each area of the body. Do not use above a patient's jawline as it can be irritating to the eyes and ears (AHRQ, 2013). Use a regular washcloth moistened in warm water for the face. It is necessary not to rinse the CHG off to maintain its antibacterial effects. Patients often describe their skin as feeling a bit sticky. Be sure to explain to patients the importance of using CHG to protect them against serious infection.
- There are precautions to follow in using CHG. CHG is safe to use on superficial wounds, abrasions, and rashes (AHRQ, 2013). In the case of open or deep wounds such as stage III or IV pressure ulcers, bathe with CHG around a dressing or wound. Do not use CHG on third- or fourth-degree burns (AHRQ, 2013).

BOX 40-6 EVIDENCE-BASED PRACTICE

Reducing Hospital-Acquired Infections Using Bathing Techniques

PICO Question: Do adult hospitalized patients using chlorhexidine gluconate (CHG) wipes for bathing compared to soap and water have a decrease in hospital-acquired infections (HAIs) during their hospital stay?

Evidence Summary

Patient's hospital bath basins are a known source of microorganisms that can lead to infection. These reservoirs for bacteria have been associated with HAI. Research studies have indicated that CHG solutions used for daily bathing decrease the incidence of HAIs. Evidence-based research indicates that use of CHG may also reduce culture growth of bacteria on central line catheters leading to bloodstream infections and decrease multiresistant organisms on skin and at surgical sites (Powers et al., 2012). This is especially important for patients who are immunocompromised or susceptible to infections. Further studies are needed on different types of organisms affected by CHG and water contaminates (Rubin et al., 2013). The long-term effects on neonates and the elderly should also be researched.

Application to Nursing Practice

- The Joint Commission (TJC) has recommended that there is a need for evidence-based practices to help prevent HAIs (Rubin et al., 2013).
- Handwashing and personal protective equipment (PPE) may not be enough to prevent nosocomial infections during hospitalization (TJC, 2016). Check patient for allergies before using on skin. Packaged wipes are convenient and easy to use. They decrease time for bathing. Always check with the patient for sensitivity or allergy. Use wipes as directed on package—one wipe per each area of the body (see Skill 40-1).
- CHG wipes are easy to use and accessible for older patients and bariatric patients, offering a no-rinse or drying procedure. The Centers for Disease Control and Prevention (CDC, 2012; 2009) has suggested using CHG wipes along with proper hand hygiene and isolation precautions to decrease multidrug-resistant HAIs. Reductions in rates of bloodstream infections with the use of CHG wipes are being seen in immunocompromised patients, patients prone to skin infections, patients with central line catheters, and patients in intensive care settings (Climo et al., 2013).

Use a tub bath or shower (see Skill 40-1) to give a more thorough bath than a bed bath. CHG 4% solution can be used in showers, but instruct patients to exit the shower after application and do not rinse the CHG off. Implement safety measures to prevent fall injuries because the surface of the tub or shower stall is slippery. In some settings a health care provider's order for a shower or tub bath is necessary. Place a chair in the shower for patients with weakness or poor balance. Both tubs and showers need to have grab bars for patients to hold during entry and exit and maneuvering during the bath or shower. Patients vary in how much help they need.

Regardless of the type of bath a patient receives, use the following guidelines:

- *Provide privacy.* Close the door and/or pull room curtains around the bathing area. While bathing a patient, expose only the areas being bathed by using proper draping.
- *Maintain safety.* Keep side rails up when away from a patient's bedside when patients are dependent or unconscious. NOTE: When side rails serve as a restraint, you need a health care provider's order (see agency-specific policy for restraint usage) (see Chapter 27). Place the call light in the patient's reach if leaving the bedside even temporarily.

- *Maintain warmth.* Keep the room warm because the patient is partially uncovered and easily chilled. Wet skin causes an excessive loss of heat through evaporation. Control drafts and keep windows closed. Keep the patient covered. Expose only the body part being washed during the bath.
- *Promote independence.* Encourage the patient to participate in as much of the bathing activities as possible. Offer assistance when needed.
- *Anticipate needs.* Bring a new set of clothing and hygiene products to the bedside or bathroom.

Teach patients to follow a few general rules for skin health. Encourage them to routinely inspect their skin for changes in color or texture and report abnormalities to their health care provider. Instruct them to handle the skin gently, avoiding excessive rubbing. Patients with excessively dry skin are predisposed to skin impairment. If patients use bar soap at home, recommend that they choose one that contains emollients to hydrate dry skin. Avoid overly hot water because it can dry the skin by removing natural oils. Lubricate the skin with emollient lotions to reduce dryness.

Also encourage patients to eat nutritious foods from all food groups, including those rich in vitamins and minerals, and to consume adequate fluids. Stress safety concerns such as failing to adjust or check the water temperature, cutting nails too close to the skin, and slipping on wet surfaces. Ensure that patients understand that healthy and intact skin and tissues protect them from infection. Reinforce infection control practices, including proper hand hygiene.

Perineal Care. Cleansing patients' genital and anal areas is called perineal care. It usually occurs as part of a complete bed bath; however, it must be provided at least once a day and more often (see agency policy) if a patient has a urinary catheter (see Skill 40-1). Patients most in need of perineal care include those at greatest risk for acquiring an infection (e.g., uncircumcised males, patients who have indwelling urinary catheters, or those who are recovering from rectal or genital surgery or childbirth). In addition, women who are having a menstrual period require perineal care. CHG is safe to use on the perineum and external mucosa for thorough cleansing (AHRQ, 2013).

When the patient's condition allows, encourage the patient to perform perineal care. Sometimes you are embarrassed about providing perineal care, particularly to patients of the opposite sex. Similarly the patient may feel embarrassed. Do not let embarrassment cause you to overlook the patient's hygiene needs. When staffing levels permit, use a gender-congruent caregiver. A professional, dignified, and sensitive approach reduces embarrassment and helps put the patient at ease.

If a patient performs self-care, various problems such as vaginal and urethral discharge, skin irritation, and unpleasant odors often go unnoticed. Stress the importance of perineal care in preventing skin breakdown and infection. Be alert for complaints of burning during urination or localized soreness, excoriation, or pain in the perineum. Inspect vaginal and perineal areas and the patient's bed linen for signs of discharge and use your sense of smell to detect abnormal odors. Risk factors for skin breakdown in the perineal area include urinary or fecal incontinence, rectal and perineal surgical dressings, indwelling urinary catheters, and morbid obesity.

Back Rub. A back rub or back massage usually follows a patient's bath. It promotes relaxation, relieves muscular tension, and decreases perception of pain. Effleurage (i.e., long, slow, gliding strokes of a massage) is associated with reduced measured anxiety, heart rate, and respiratory rate. Studies show that slow-stroke back massages of 3 minutes and hand massages of 10 minutes significantly improve both physiological and psychological indicators of relaxation in older people (Touhy and Jett, 2012).

When providing a back rub, enhance relaxation by reducing noise and ensuring that the patient is comfortable. It is important to ask whether a patient would like a back rub, because some individuals dislike physical contact. Consult the medical record for any contraindications to a massage (e.g., fractured ribs, burns, heart surgery).

Foot and Nail Care. Incorporate foot and nail care into a person's regular hygiene routine. Routine care involves soaking the hands and feet to soften cuticles and layers of horny cells, thorough cleaning, drying, and proper nail trimming. The one exception is patients with diabetes mellitus or peripheral vascular disease, who are at risk for tissue ulceration or infection because soaking causes skin softening or maceration of tissue.

When providing nail care, have the patient remain in bed or sit in a chair (see Skill 40-2 on pp. 862-865). In some settings or with specific patients such as a person with diabetes mellitus, you need a health care provider's order to trim toenails. Before implementing nail care, check agency policy to determine if an order is necessary.

Take time during the procedure to teach the patient and family proper techniques for cleaning and nail trimming. Stress the importance of how thorough nail care prevents infection and promotes good circulation. Patients must learn to protect the feet from injury, never walk barefoot, keep feet clean and dry, and wear footwear that fits properly. Instruct patients in the proper way to inspect all surfaces of the feet and hands for redness, lesions, dryness, or signs of infection. Teach foot care to family caregivers for patients who need regular foot care and have peripheral vascular disease, visual difficulties, physical constraints preventing movement, or cognitive problems.

Certain conditions place patients with diabetes at increased risk for amputation (ADA, 2015). These factors include peripheral neuropathy, limited joint mobility, bony deformity, peripheral vascular disease, and a history of skin ulcers or previous amputation. Observe for changes that indicate peripheral neuropathy or vascular insufficiency (Box 40-7). Advise patients to use the following guidelines in a routine foot and nail care program (Sheridan, 2012):

- Inspect the feet daily, including the bottoms and tops, heels, and areas between the toes. Use a mirror to help inspect the feet thoroughly or ask a family member to check daily.
- Wash feet daily in lukewarm water. Dry thoroughly, especially between the toes. Avoid harsh chemicals or long soaks, which can cause skin softening or maceration of tissue, causing ulceration or infection.
- Wear well-fitting shoes and clean, dry socks at all times; never go barefoot. Check inside shoes before wearing them for rough areas or objects that may rub against the foot.

BOX 40-7 Signs of Peripheral Neuropathy or Vascular Insufficiency

Peripheral Neuropathy	Vascular Insufficiency
• Muscle wasting of lower extremities	• Decreased hair growth on legs and feet
• Absence of deep tendon reflexes	• Absent or decreased pulses
• Foot deformities	• Infection in the foot
• Infections	• Poor wound healing
• Abnormal gait	• Thickened nails
	• Shiny appearance of the skin
	• Blanching of skin on elevation

Data from Ball J et al: *Seidel's guide to physical examination*, ed 8, St Louis, 2015, Mosby.

- Keep skin soft and smooth by applying an emollient lotion over all surfaces of the feet but not between the toes.
- If you can see and reach your toenails, trim them straight across and square file the edges smooth.
- Keep the blood flowing to your feet by putting them up when sitting and wiggling your toes and moving your ankles up and down for 5 minutes, 2 or 3 times a day. Do not cross your legs for long periods and don't smoke.
- Protect the feet from hot and cold. Do not use heating pads or electric blankets and always wear shoes at the beach or on hot pavement.

Oral Hygiene. Regular oral hygiene, including brushing, flossing, and rinsing, prevents and controls plaque-associated oral diseases. Evidence relates poor oral health to risk of impaired nutrition, stroke, poor blood sugar control in diabetes, and nursing home–acquired pneumonia (Barnes, 2014). Inadequate oral care and some medications diminish salivary production, which in turn reduces the ability of the oral environment to help fight effects of pathogens. Older adults in particular require good oral care (Box 40-8).

Brushing cleans the teeth of food particles, plaque, and bacteria. It also massages the gums and relieves discomfort resulting from unpleasant odors and tastes. Flossing removes tartar that collects at the gum line. Rinsing removes dislodged food particles and excess toothpaste. Complete oral hygiene enhances well-being and comfort and stimulates the appetite.

BOX 40-8 FOCUS ON OLDER ADULTS

Oral Health

- Many older adults are edentulous (without teeth), and the teeth that are present are often diseased or decayed (Touhy and Jett, 2014).
- The periodontal membrane weakens with aging, making it more prone to infection. Periodontal disease predisposes older adults to systemic infection.
- Dentures or partial plates do not always fit properly, causing pain and discomfort, which in turn affects digestive processes, enjoyment of food, and nutritional status.
- An age-related decline in saliva secretion and some medications (e.g., antihypertensives, diuretics, antiinflammatories, antidepressants) cause dry mouth (Touhy and Jett, 2014).
- Financial limitations and the belief that dentures eliminate the need for routine dental care are some of the reasons why older adults do not seek dental care (Touhy and Jett, 2014).

When patients become ill, many factors influence their need for oral hygiene such as their ability to take fluids orally, presence of oral lesions or trauma, and level of consciousness. Patients in hospitals or long-term care facilities do not always receive the aggressive oral care they need. Base the frequency of care on the condition of the oral cavity, risk for aspiration of saliva, and the patient's level of comfort. Some patients (e.g., stroke, trauma to oral cavity, patient with endotracheal tube) require oral care as often as every 1 to 2 hours.

Acidic fruits in a patient's diet reduce plaque formation. A well-balanced diet contributes to the integrity of oral tissues. To prevent tooth decay, patients sometimes need to change eating habits (e.g., reducing intake of carbohydrates, especially sweet snacks between meals). Advise patients of all ages to visit a dentist regularly for checkups. Education about common gum and tooth disorders and methods of prevention may motivate patients to follow good oral hygiene practices.

Brushing. The American Dental Association guidelines (2014) for effective oral hygiene include brushing the teeth at least twice a day with American Dental Association–approved fluoride toothpaste. Fluoride and antimicrobial mouth rinses help prevent tooth decay. Do not use fluoride rinse in children ages 6 or under because of the risk of swallowing the rinse. Use antimicrobial toothpastes and 0.12% CHG oral rinses for patients at increased risk for poor oral hygiene (e.g., older adults and patients with cognitive impairments and who are immunocompromised) (Garcia and Caple, 2014). The toothbrush needs to have a straight handle and a brush small enough to reach all areas of the mouth. Rounded soft bristles stimulate the gums without causing abrasion and bleeding. Any patient who has decreased dexterity as a result of a medical condition or the aging process requires an enlarged handle with an easier grip.

Brush all tooth surfaces thoroughly (Box 40-9). Commercially made foam swabs are ineffective in removing plaque (Garcia and Caple, 2014). Electric or battery-powered toothbrushes improve the quality of cleaning and may be easier to use than manual brushes when nurses provide care for dependent patients. Do not use lemon-glycerin sponges because they dry mucous membranes and erode tooth enamel.

To prevent cross-contamination, teach patients to avoid sharing toothbrushes with family members or drinking directly from a bottle of mouthwash. Disclosure tablets or drops to stain the plaque that collects at the gum line are useful for showing patients how effectively they brush. Instruct patients to obtain a new toothbrush every 3 months or following a cold or upper respiratory infection to minimize growth of microorganisms on the brush surfaces (American Dental Association, 2014).

Flossing. Dental flossing removes plaque and tartar between teeth. Flossing involves inserting waxed or unwaxed dental floss between

BOX 40-9 PROCEDURAL GUIDELINES

Providing Oral Hygiene

Delegation Considerations

The skill of performing oral hygiene can be delegated to nursing assistive personnel (NAP).

However, the nurse is responsible for assessing the patient's gag reflex to determine risk for aspiration. Direct the NAP to:

- Position the patient to avoid aspiration.
- Immediately report to the nurse excessive patient coughing or choking during or after oral hygiene.
- Report bleeding of oral mucosa or gums, patient report of pain, and any types of changes in oral mucosa (e.g., open areas or lesions)

Equipment

Soft-bristle toothbrush; nonabrasive fluoride toothpaste; dental floss; tongue depressor; water glass with cool water, normal saline, or an essential oil-antiseptic mouth rinse *(optional depending on patient preference)*; emesis basin; face towel; paper towels; clean gloves; penlight; linen bag or hamper

Steps

1. Review medical record and identify presence of common oral hygiene problems: dental caries—chalky white discoloration of tooth or presence of brown or black discoloration; gingivitis—inflammation of gums;

Continued

BOX 40-9 PROCEDURAL GUIDELINES

***Providing Oral Hygiene*—cont'd**

periodontitis—receding gum lines, inflammation, gaps between teeth; halitosis—bad breath; cheilitis—cracked lips; dry, cracked, and coated tongue.

2. Perform hand hygiene and apply clean gloves.
3. Identify patient using two identifiers (e.g., name and birthday or name and medical record) according to agency policy.
4. Using tongue depressor and pen light, inspect integrity of lips, teeth, buccal mucosa, gums, palate, and tongue; also assess for gag reflex and ability to swallow (see Chapter 31).
5. Confirm presence of common oral problems.
6. Determine patient's oral hygiene practices such as frequency of brushing and flossing, type of toothpaste and mouthwash used, last and frequency of dental visits.
7. Remove gloves and perform hand hygiene.
8. Explain procedure to patient, discussing preferences and willingness to help with oral care.
9. Assess patient's ability to grasp and manipulate toothbrush.
10. Place paper towels on over-bed table and arrange other equipment within easy reach.
11. Provide privacy by closing room doors and drawing room divider curtain. Raise bed to comfortable working position. Raise head of bed (if allowed) and lower near side rail. Move patient or help him or her move closer to side. Place patient in side-lying position if needed (if aspiration risk). Place towel over patient's chest.
12. Apply clean gloves.
13. Apply enough toothpaste to brush to cover length of bristles. Hold brush over emesis basin. Pour small amount of water over toothpaste.
14. Patient may help with brushing. Hold toothbrush bristles at 45-degree angle to gum line (see illustration). Be sure that tips of bristles rest against and penetrate under gum line. Brush inner and outer surfaces of upper and lower teeth by brushing from gum to crown of each tooth. Clean biting surfaces of teeth by holding top of bristles parallel with teeth and brushing gently back and forth (see illustration). Brush sides of teeth by moving bristles back and forth (see illustration).
15. Have patient lightly brush over surface and sides of tongue. Avoid initiating gag reflex.
16. Allow patient to rinse mouth thoroughly by taking several sips of cool water, swishing water across all tooth surfaces, and spitting into emesis basin. Use this time to observe patient's brushing technique and teach importance of regular hygiene.
17. Have patient rinse mouth with antiseptic rinse for 30 seconds. Then have him or her spit rinse into emesis basin. Help wipe his or her mouth.
18. Floss or allow patient to floss between all teeth (see illustration).
19. Allow patient to rinse mouth thoroughly with cool water and spit into emesis basin. Help wipe his or her mouth.
20. Inspect oral cavity to determine effectiveness of oral hygiene and rinsing. Ask patient if mouth feels clean or if there are any sore or tender areas. Remove towel and place in linen bag.
21. Use ***Teach Back*** to determine patient's and family's understanding about oral care. State, "I want to be sure you know how often to brush your teeth and floss. Can you explain that for me?" Revise your instruction now or develop plan for revised patient teaching if patient is not able to teach back correctly.
22. Remove gloves. Help patient to comfortable position, raise side rail, and lower bed to original position.
23. Perform hand hygiene. Apply clean gloves to clean and dry emesis basin before returning basin and nondisposable supplies.
24. Remove gloves and perform hand hygiene.
25. Record procedure. Note condition of oral cavity, amount of care patient could perform, and whether additional instruction is needed on oral care in nurse's notes.
26. Report bleeding, pain, or presence of lesions to nurse in charge or health care provider.

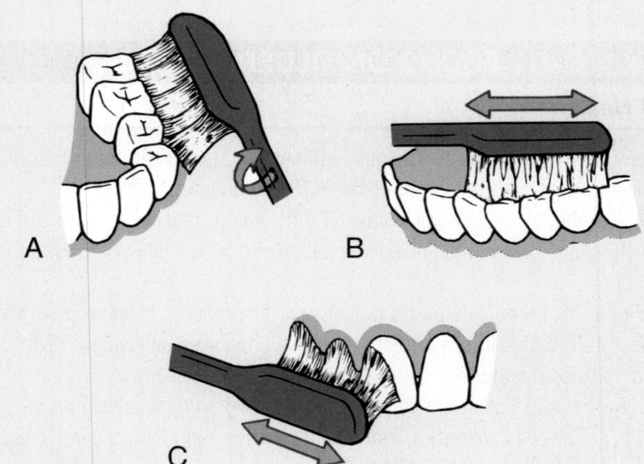

STEP 14 Direction for toothbrush placement. **A,** 45-degree angle brushes gum line. **B,** Parallel position brushes biting surfaces. **C,** Lateral position brushes sides of teeth.

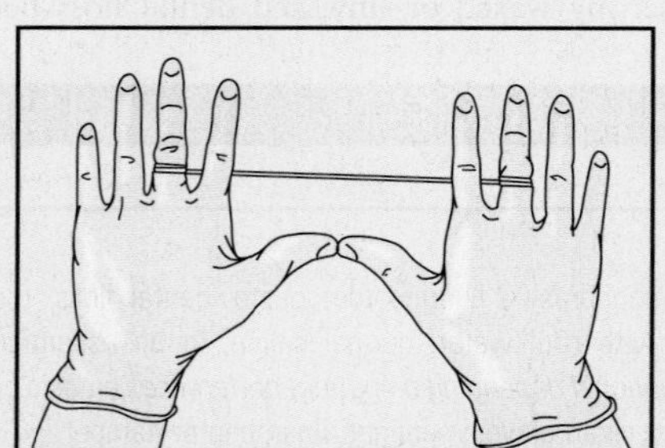

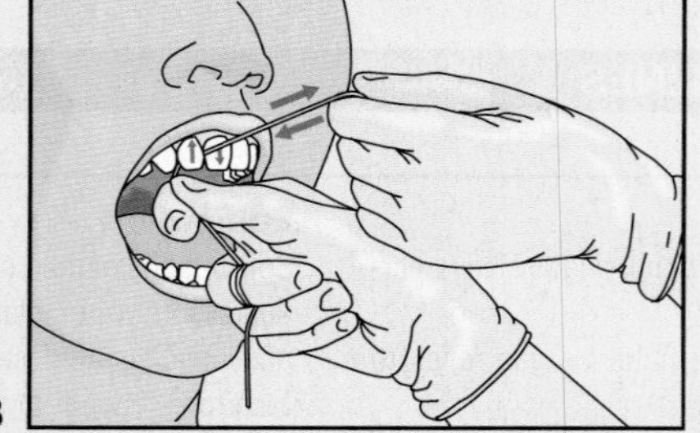

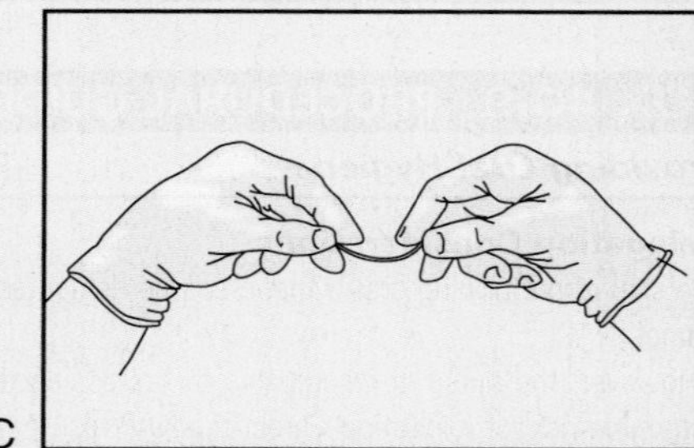

STEP 18 Flossing. **A,** Dental floss held between middle fingers to floss upper teeth. **B,** Floss moved in up-and-down motion between teeth. **C,** Floss held with index fingers to floss lower teeth.

all tooth surfaces, one at a time. The seesaw motion used to pull floss between teeth removes plaque and tartar from tooth enamel. Use unwaxed floss and avoid vigorous flossing near the gum line on patients who are receiving chemotherapy, radiation, or anticoagulant therapy to prevent bleeding. If toothpaste is applied to the teeth before flossing, fluoride comes in direct contact with tooth surfaces, aiding in cavity prevention. According to American Dental Association recommendations (2014), flossing once a day is sufficient. Because it is important to clean all teeth surfaces thoroughly, do not rush to complete flossing. Placing a mirror in front of a patient helps you demonstrate the proper method for holding the floss and cleaning between the teeth. Flossing a patient's teeth is not realistic or appropriate in all care settings.

Patients with Special Needs. Some patients require special oral hygiene methods. For example, patients with diabetes mellitus and who are on chemotherapy frequently experience periodontal disease. Therefore they need to visit a dentist every 3 to 4 months, clean their teeth up to 4 times a day, and handle oral tissues gently with a minimum of trauma. Xerostomia, bruxism, and dental caries may be present with patients who are methamphetamine users. Cravings for sugary sweets may cause decay and gum disease.

Patients may depend on their caregivers for oral care. Being unconscious or having an artificial airway (e.g., endotracheal or tracheal tubes) increases the susceptibility for patients to have drying of salivary secretions because they are unable to eat or drink, unable to swallow, and frequently breathe through the mouth. Unconscious patients cannot swallow salivary secretions that accumulate in the mouth. These secretions often contain gram-negative bacteria that cause pneumonia if aspirated into the lungs. While providing hygiene, protect the patient from choking and aspiration and use topical CHG, especially in ventilated patients (see Skill 40-3 on pp. 865-867). Current evidence shows that use of CHG with oral hygiene reduces the risk for ventilator-associated pneumonia (Wiech et al., 2012).

Patients with decreased levels of consciousness need special attention because they often do not have a gag reflex. Proper oral hygiene requires keeping the mucosa moist and removing secretions that contribute to infection. Pooling of salivary secretions in the back of the throat harbors microorganism growth. When providing oral hygiene to an unconscious patient, you need to protect him or her from choking and aspiration. Have two nurses provide the care; turn the patient's head toward you, and place the bed in semi-Fowler's position. You can delegate nursing assistive personnel to participate. One nurse does the actual cleaning, and the other caregiver removes secretions with suction equipment. Some agencies use equipment that combines a mouth swab with the suction device; you can use this equipment safely by yourself. While cleansing the oral cavity, use a small oral airway or a padded tongue blade to hold the mouth open. Never use your fingers to hold a patient's mouth open. A human bite contains multiple pathogenic microorganisms. Even though the patient is not awake or alert, explain the steps of mouth care and the sensations that he or she will feel. Also tell the patient when the procedure is completed.

Some treatments such as chemotherapy, immunosuppressive agents, head and neck radiation, and nasogastric intubation place patients at higher risk of experiencing stomatitis or inflammation of the oral mucosa. **Stomatitis** causes burning, pain, and change in food and fluid tolerance. When caring for patients with stomatitis, brush with a soft toothbrush and floss gently to prevent bleeding of the gums. In some cases flossing needs to be omitted temporarily from oral care. Advise patients to avoid alcohol and commercial mouthwash and stop smoking. Normal saline rinses (approximately 30 mL) on awaking in the morning, after each meal, and at bedtime help clean the oral cavity. Patients can increase the rinses to every 2 hours if necessary. Consult with the health care provider to obtain topical or oral analgesics for pain control.

Denture Care. Encourage patients to clean their dentures on a regular basis to avoid gingival infection and irritation. When patients become disabled, someone else assumes responsibility for denture care (Box 40-10). Dentures are a patient's personal property and must be handled with care because they break easily. They must be removed at night to rest the gums and prevent bacterial buildup. To prevent warping, keep dentures covered in water when they are not worn and always store them in an enclosed, labeled cup with the cup placed in the patient's bedside stand. Discourage patients from removing their dentures and placing them on a napkin or tissue because they could easily be thrown away.

Implement measures to prevent denture-induced stomatitis when caring for patients who wear dentures. Poorly fitting dentures, wearing dentures while sleeping, and poor dental hygiene habits contribute to denture-induced stomatitis (Martori et al., 2014). Signs and symptoms range from redness and swelling under the dentures to painful red sores on the roof of the mouth and infection with the yeast *Candida albicans*. Some patients deny pain, and others complain of pain worsened by wearing dentures. To prevent denture-induced stomatitis, rinse the mouth and dentures after meals, clean them carefully and regularly, remove and soak them overnight, brush and floss (if appropriate) any remaining teeth, and visit a dentist regularly for examination (American Dental Association, 2014).

Hair and Scalp Care. A person's appearance and feeling of well-being often depend on the way the hair looks and feels. Illness or disability often prevents a patient from maintaining daily hair care. When patients are immobilized, their hair soon becomes tangled. Some dressings or diagnostic procedures leave sticky residue on the hair. Basic hair and scalp care includes brushing, combing, and shampooing.

Brushing and Combing. Frequent brushing helps keep hair clean and distributes oil evenly along hair shafts. Combing prevents hair from tangling. Encourage patients to maintain routine hair care and provide help for patients with limited mobility or weakness and those who are confused or weakened by illness. Patients in a hospital or extended care facility appreciate the opportunity to have their hair brushed and combed before being seen by others.

When caring for patients from different cultures, learn as much as possible from them or their family about preferred hair care practices. For example, the hair of African-Americans tends to be quite dry. Use special lanolin conditioners for conditioning. Cultural preferences also affect how hair is combed and styled and whether it can be cut.

Long hair becomes matted easily when a patient is confined to bed, even for a short period. When lacerations or incisions involve the scalp, blood and topical medications also cause tangling. Frequent brushing and combing keep long hair neatly groomed. Braiding helps to avoid repeated tangles; however, patients need to unbraid hair periodically and comb it to ensure good hygiene. Braids that are too tight lead to bald patches. Obtain permission from the patient before braiding the hair.

To brush hair part it into two sections and separate each section into two more sections. Brushing from the scalp toward the hair ends minimizes pulling. Moistening the hair with water or an alcohol-free detangle product makes it easier to comb. Never cut a patient's hair without consent.

Patients who develop head lice require special considerations in the way combing is performed (Box 40-11). The lice are small, about

BOX 40-10 PROCEDURAL GUIDELINES

Care of Dentures

Delegation Considerations

The skill of denture care can be delegated to nursing assistive personnel (NAP). Instruct the NAP to:

- Inform the nurse if there are cracks in dentures.
- Inform the nurse if the patient complains of oral discomfort.
- Inform the nurse of any lesions in the mouth.

Equipment

Soft-bristle toothbrush or denture toothbrush, denture-cleaning agent or toothpaste, denture adhesive *(optional)*, glass of water, emesis basin or sink, washcloth, clean gloves, denture cup (if dentures are to be stored after cleaning)

Steps

1. Identify patient using two identifiers (e.g., name and birthday or name and medical record number) according to agency policy.
2. Ask patient if dentures fit and if there is any gum or mucous membrane tenderness or irritation.
3. Ask patient about preferences for denture care and products used. If patient is unable to care for own dentures, provide this care. Clean dentures for patient during routine mouth care.
4. Perform hand hygiene. Apply clean gloves. Fill emesis basin with tepid water; or, if using sink, place washcloth in bottom of sink and fill sink with 2.5 cm (1 inch) of water.
5. Remove dentures: If patient is unable to do this independently, grasp upper plate at front with thumb and index finger wrapped in gauze and pull downward. To remove lower denture, gently lift it from jaw and rotate one side downward. Place dentures in emesis basin or sink.
6. Apply cleaning agent to brush and brush surfaces of dentures (see illustration). Hold dentures close to water. Hold brush horizontally and use back-and-forth motion to clean biting surfaces. Use short strokes from top of denture to biting surfaces to clean outer and inner teeth surfaces. Hold brush vertically and use short strokes to clean inner tooth surfaces. Hold brush horizontally and use back-and-forth motion to clean undersurface of dentures.

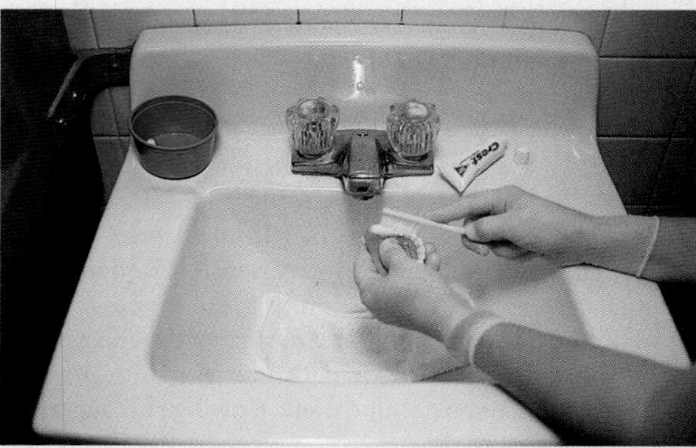

STEP 6 Brushing dentures.

7. Some patients use an adhesive to seal dentures in place. Apply a thin layer to undersurface before inserting.
8. If patient needs help inserting dentures, moisten upper denture and press firmly to seal it in place. Insert moistened lower denture. Ask if dentures feel comfortable.
9. Some patients prefer to have their dentures stored to rest the gums and reduce risk of infection. Keeping dentures moist prevents warping and facilitates easier insertion. Store in secure place to prevent loss.
10. Remove and discard gloves and perform hand hygiene.

BOX 40-11 Hygiene Care for Head Lice

- Perform hand hygiene and apply disposable gown and gloves.
- Use a grooming comb or hairbrush to remove tangles.
- Divide patient's hair in sections and fasten off hair that is not being combed.
- Comb out from scalp to the end of the hair (special combs are available in drug stores).
- Dip comb in a cup of water or use a paper towel to remove lice between each passing.
- After combing look through hair carefully for attached lice; you can catch live lice with a tweezers or comb.
- After combing thoroughly, move to next section of hair.
- Instruct family to clean the comb with an old toothbrush and dental floss. Then boil the comb. The ideal is to discard the comb after each use, but some patients' financial situations prevent purchase of multiple combs.
- Instruct family to comb and screen for lice daily.
- Instruct family to contain patient's clothes and wash them in hot water.
- Instruct family to vacuum the home and patient's room and immediately empty vacuum bag or bagless collection device.
- Instruct caregivers on how to prevent transmission of lice: Do not share bed linens or hair care products. Avoid placing bare hand on patient's head. Immediately wash hands after providing hair care.

the size of a sesame seed; thus you need bright light or natural sunlight to see them. Thorough combing is more effective than use of pediculicidal shampoos, which are often toxic and ineffective against resistant lice.

If a pediculicidal shampoo is ordered, review pertinent information and instruct the patient and caregiver in its proper use. Use with caution because these shampoos may have severe neurological side effects. Make sure to thoroughly rinse shampoo from hair to avoid itching.

Shampooing. Frequency of shampooing depends on a person's daily routines and the condition of the hair. Remind patients in hospitals or extended care facilities that staying in bed, excess perspiration, or treatments that leave blood or solutions in the hair require more frequent shampooing. In some agencies you need a health care provider's order to shampoo a patient who is dependent or has limited mobility because it is challenging to find ways to shampoo the hair without causing injury.

The patient who can shower or tub bathe usually shampoos the hair without difficulty. A shower or tub chair facilitates shampooing for patients who are ambulatory and weight bearing and become tired or faint. Handheld shower nozzles allow patients to easily wash the hair in the tub or shower. Some patients allowed to sit in a chair choose to be shampooed in front of a sink or over a washbasin; however, certain conditions (e.g., eye surgery or neck injury) limit bending. In these situations teach the patient and family the degree of bending allowed.

If a patient is unable to sit but can be moved, transfer him or her to a stretcher for transportation to a sink or shower equipped

BOX 40-12 PROCEDURAL GUIDELINES

Shampooing Hair of Patient Who is Bed Bound

Delegation Considerations

The skill of shampooing hair can be delegated to nursing assistive personnel (NAP). Instruct the NAP:

- About any precautions needed in positioning the patient.
- To inform the nurse if the patient reports neck pain.
- To inform the nurse of any new skin lesions.

Equipment

Brush, comb, shampoo board, shampoo, conditioner *(optional)*, hydrogen peroxide *(optional)*, towels (three or more), waterproof pad, hair dryer, basin of very warm water, clean gloves (if needed) or shampoo cap

Steps

1. Identify patient using two identifiers (e.g., name and birthday or name and medical record number) according to agency policy.
2. Before washing patient's hair, determine that there are no contraindications to procedure (e.g., neck injury).
3. Perform hand hygiene and apply gloves if needed. Inspect hair and scalp before initiating procedure to determine presence of any conditions that require use of special shampoos or treatments (e.g., for dandruff or the removal of dried blood).
4. Place waterproof pad under patient's shoulders, neck, and head. Position patient supine, with head and shoulders at top edge of bed. Place plastic trough under patient's head and washbasin at end of trough (see illustration). Be sure that trough spout extends beyond edge of mattress.

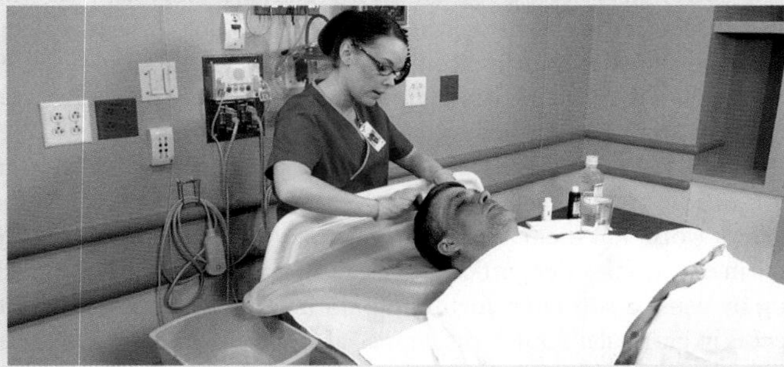

STEP 4 Patient positioned for shampoo. (Copyright © Mosby's Clinical Skills: Essentials Collection.)

5. Place rolled towel under patient's neck and bath towel over patient's shoulders.
6. Brush and comb patient's hair.
7. Obtain warm water.
8. Offer patient the option of holding face towel or washcloth over eyes.
9. Slowly pour water from water pitcher over hair until it is completely wet (see illustration). If hair contains matted blood, put on gloves, apply peroxide to dissolve clots, and rinse hair with saline. Apply small amount of shampoo.

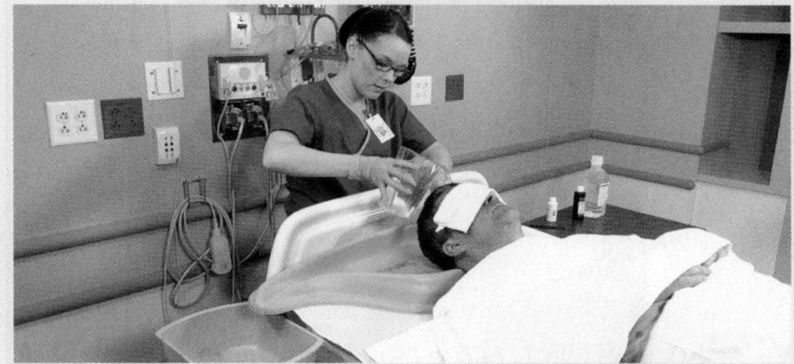

STEP 9 Wetting patient's hair. (Copyright © Mosby's Clinical Skills: Essentials Collection.)

10. Work up lather with both hands. Start at hairline and work toward back of neck. Lift head slightly with one hand to wash back of head. Shampoo sides of head. Massage scalp by applying pressure with fingertips.
11. Rinse hair with water. Make sure that water drains into basin. Repeat rinsing until hair is free of soap.
12. Apply conditioner or cream rinse if requested and rinse hair thoroughly.
13. Wrap patient's head in bath towel. Dry patient's face with cloth used to protect eyes. Dry off any moisture along neck or shoulders.
14. Dry patient's hair and scalp. Use second towel if first becomes saturated.
15. Comb hair to remove tangles and dry with dryer if desired.
16. Apply oil preparation or conditioning product to hair if desired by patient.
17. Help patient to comfortable position and complete styling of hair.

with a handheld nozzle. Use caution when positioning the patient's head and neck, particularly in patients with any form of head or neck injury.

If a patient is unable to sit in a chair or be transferred to a stretcher, shampoo the hair with him or her in bed (Box 40-12). Position a special shampoo trough under his or her head to catch water and suds. After shampooing, patients like having their hair styled and dried. Most health care centers have portable hair dryers. Dry shampoos that reduce the need to wet the patient's hair are also available but are not highly effective. Shampoo caps provide a warm, wet massage to the scalp while cleaning the hair (Box 40-13).

Shaving. Shave a patient's facial hair after the bath or shampoo. Some women prefer to shave their legs or axillae while bathing. When helping a patient, take care to avoid cutting him or her with the razor blade. Patients prone to bleeding (e.g., those receiving anticoagulants or high doses of aspirin or those with low platelet counts) need to use their personal electric razor. Before using an electric razor, check for frayed cords or other electrical hazards. Use razor blades on only one patient because of infection control considerations.

When using a razor blade for shaving, soften the skin to prevent pulling, scraping, or cuts. Moisten the skin with lukewarm water and apply shaving cream. Bar soap may leave a film on the blade, resulting in a poorer-quality shave. You need to shave patients when they are unable to shave themselves independently. To avoid causing discomfort or razor cuts, gently pull the skin taut and use long, firm razor strokes in the direction the hair grows (Figure 40-5). Short downward strokes work best to remove hair over the upper lip or chin. A patient usually explains the best way to move the razor across the skin. Facial hair of African-Americans tends to be curly and becomes ingrown unless shaved close to the skin.

Mustache and Beard Care. Mustaches or beards require daily grooming. Grooming keeps food particles and mucus from collecting in the hair. If a patient is unable to carry out self-care, do so at his or her request. Comb out beards gently and obtain the patient's permission before trimming or shaving off a mustache or beard.

Care of the Eyes, Ears, and Nose. Give special attention to cleaning the eyes, ears, and nose during a routine bath and when

BOX 40-13 Shampooing Using Disposable Shampoo Product

1. Perform hand hygiene; apply gloves as needed.
2. Patient can be sitting on a chair or in bed.
3. Comb hair to remove tangles or debris.
4. Heat package in microwave according to agency policy and instructions.
5. Open package; apply cap with all hair underneath for correct fit (see illustration).

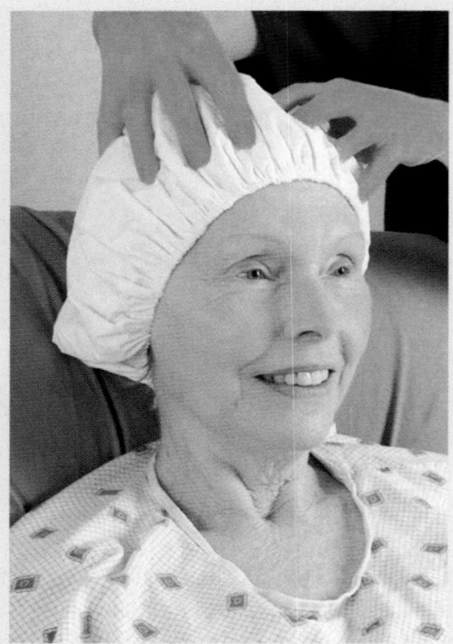

STEP 5 Patient wearing disposable shampoo cap.

6. Massage head through cap 2-4 minutes.
7. Discard cap into garbage; do not dispose in toilet because it may clog plumbing.
8. Towel-dry hair.
9. Brush or comb patient's hair.
10. Remove gloves if applicable; perform hand hygiene.

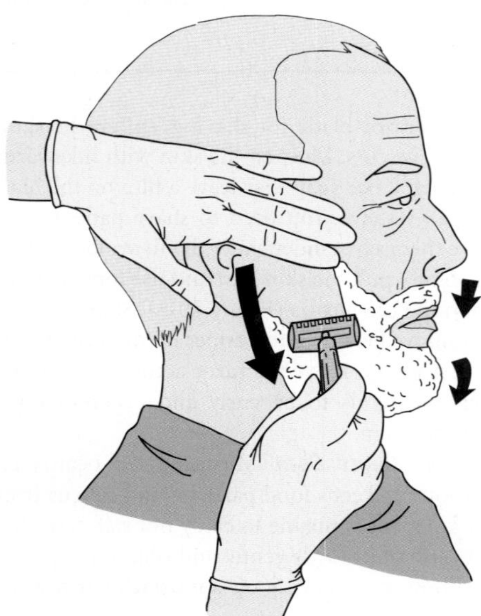

FIGURE 40-5 Shave using short, firm strokes in direction of hair growth.

drainage or discharge accumulates. This aspect of hygiene not only makes a patient more comfortable but also improves sensory reception (see Chapter 49). Care focuses on preventing infection and maintaining normal sensory function. In addition, care of the eyes, ears, and nose requires approaches that consider the patient's special needs.

Medical Devices. If a patient has oxygen tubing, a feeding tube, or a nasotracheal tube, it is essential you care for the area of the skin around the nose or ears underlying the device. The National Pressure Ulcer Advisory Panel (NPUAP, 2013) recommends the following: cushion and protect the skin with dressings in high-risk areas (e.g., nasal bridge) (see Chapter 48); do not place device(s) over sites of prior or existing pressure ulceration; and be sure to gently cleanse a potential area of irritation that underlies a device at least daily.

Basic Eye Care. Cleaning the eyes involves simply washing with a clean washcloth moistened in water (see Skill 40-1). Soap may cause burning and irritation. Never apply direct pressure over the eyeball because it causes serious injury. When cleaning a patient's eyes, obtain a clean washcloth and clean from inner to outer canthus. Use a different section of the washcloth for each eye. Remember, never use CHG solution or cloths to clean the eyes, ears, or face.

Unconscious patients require more frequent eye care. A complication of sedation and coma is that some patients are unable to maintain effective eye closure (Werli-Alvarenga et al., 2013). Thus these patients lose their natural protective mechanisms to protect the cornea. When unprotected, there is an increased risk of corneal dehydration, abrasion, perforation, and infection. Normal protective mechanisms include blinking with lubrication of the eye (Douglas and Berry, 2011). Blinking provides a mechanical barrier to injury and prevents dehydration. Secretions collect along the lid margins and inner canthus when the blink reflex is absent or when the eye does not close completely. When an eye does not close completely, you may need to place an eye patch over it to prevent corneal drying and irritation. Apply lubricating eyedrops according to the health care provider's orders.

Eyeglasses. Eyeglasses are expensive. Be careful when cleaning glasses and protect them from breakage or other damage when they are not worn. Put them in a case in a drawer of the bedside table when not in use. Cool water sufficiently cleans glass lenses. Prevent scratching by using a soft cloth for drying; do not use paper towels. Plastic lenses in particular scratch easily; special cleaning solutions and drying tissues are available.

Contact Lenses. A contact lens is a thin, transparent, circular disk that fits directly over the cornea of the eye. Contact lenses correct refractive errors of the eye or abnormalities in the shape of the cornea. In outpatient or home settings instruct patients on the routines to follow for regular cleansing and care (Box 40-14). Explain that all contact lenses must be removed periodically to prevent ocular infection and corneal ulcers or abrasions from infectious agents such as *Pseudomonas aeruginosa* and staphylococci. Pain, tearing, discomfort, and redness of the conjunctivae indicate lens overwear. Encourage patients to report persistence of these symptoms even after lens removal to their health care provider.

When patients are admitted to the hospital or agency in an unresponsive or confused state, determine if they normally wear contact lenses and if the lenses are in place. If a patient wears contact lenses and no one detects this, severe corneal injury can result. If you find that your patient is wearing contact lenses and cannot remove them, seek help. Once the lenses are removed, document the removal, the condition of the patient's eyes following removal, and the storage of the lenses.

Artificial Eyes. Patients with artificial eyes have had an enucleation (i.e., removal) of an entire eyeball as a result of tumor growth, severe infection, or eye trauma. Some artificial eyes are implanted

BOX 40-14 PATIENT TEACHING

Contact Lens Care

Objective

- Patient verbalizes and/or demonstrates proper care for contact lenses and common warning signs of problems associated with contact lens wear.

Teaching Strategies

- Instruct patients on the following:
  - Do not use fingernail on lens to remove dirt or debris.
  - Do not use tap water to clean soft lenses.
  - Follow recommendations of lens manufacturer or eye care practitioner when inserting, cleaning, and disinfecting lenses.
  - Keep lenses moist or wet when not worn.
  - Use fresh solution daily when storing and disinfecting lenses.
  - Thoroughly wash and rinse lens storage case on a daily basis. Clean periodically with soap or liquid detergent, rinse thoroughly with warm water, and air dry.
  - If lens is dropped, moisten finger with cleaning or wetting solution and gently touch it to pick it up. Then clean, rinse, and disinfect it.
- To avoid mix-up, always start with the same lens when removing or inserting lenses.
- Throw away disposable or planned replacement lenses after prescribed wearing period.
- Encourage patient to remember the acronym RSVP: *R*edness, *S*ensitivity, *V*ision problems, and *P*ain. If one of these problems occurs, remove contact lenses immediately. If problems continue, contact a vision care specialist (Lewis et al., 2014).

Evaluation

- Ask patient to state warning signs of corneal irritation and eye infection.
- Ask patient to describe methods of contact lens care that lead to infection.
- Ask patient to demonstrate cleaning and storing contact lenses.

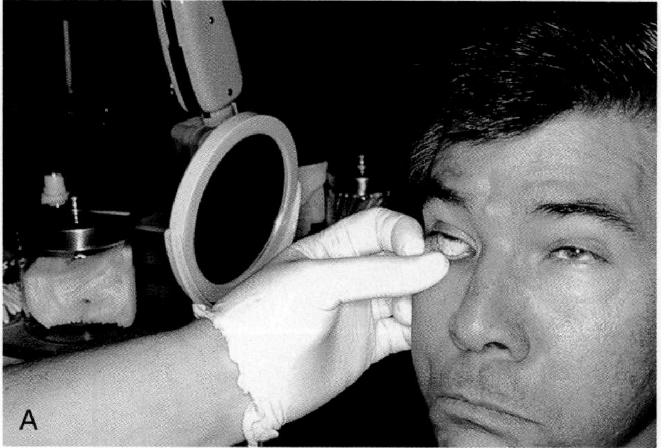

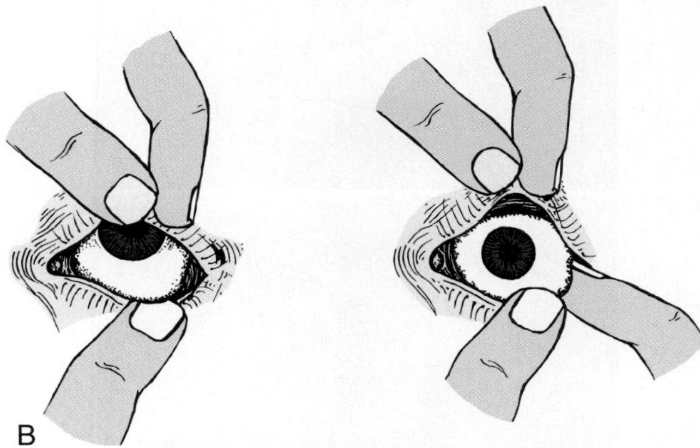

FIGURE 40-6 Removal of prosthetic eye.

permanently, whereas others must be removed for cleaning. Patients with artificial eyes usually prefer to care for their own eyes. Respect the patient's wishes and help by assembling needed equipment.

At times patients require help to remove and clean prosthesis. To remove an artificial eye, retract the lower eyelid and exert slight pressure just below the eye (Figure 40-6). This action causes the artificial eye to rise from the socket because the suction holding the eye in place has been broken. You can also use a small, rubber bulb syringe or medicine-dropper bulb to create a suction effect. Place the bulb tip directly over the eye and squeeze it to create suction needed to lift the eye from the socket.

An artificial eye is usually made of glass or plastic. Warm normal saline cleans the prosthesis effectively. Clean the edges of the eye socket and surrounding tissues with soft gauze moistened in saline or clean tap water. Report signs of infection immediately because bacteria can spread to the neighboring eye, underlying sinuses, or even brain tissue. To reinsert the eye, retract the upper and lower lids and gently slip the eye into the socket, fitting it neatly under the upper eyelid. Store an artificial eye in a labeled container filled with tap water or saline.

Ear Care. Routine ear care involves cleaning the ear with the end of a moistened washcloth rotated gently into the ear canal. Gentle, downward retraction at the entrance of the ear canal usually causes visible cerumen to loosen and slip out. Instruct patients never to use objects such as bobby pins, toothpicks, paper clips, or cotton-tipped applicators to remove earwax. These objects can injure the ear canal and rupture the tympanic membrane. They may also cause cerumen to become impacted within the ear canal.

Children and older adults commonly have impacted cerumen. You can usually remove excessive or impacted cerumen by irrigation, which requires a health care provider's order. Review the order for type of solution and ear(s) to receive the irrigation. Before irrigation question the patient for history of perforated eardrum and inspect his or her tympanic membrane to be sure that it is intact; a perforated tympanic membrane contradicts performing irrigation. Visually inspect the pinna and external meatus for redness, swelling, drainage, and presence of foreign objects. Also determine the patient's ability to hear in the affected ear before irrigation.

To irrigate the ear, have the patient sit or lie on the side with the affected ear up. For adults and children over 3 years of age, gently pull the pinna up and back. In children 3 years of age or younger, the pinna should be pulled down and back. Using a bulb-irrigating syringe or a Water Pik set on No. 2 setting, gently wash the ear canal with warm solution (37° C or 98.6° F), being careful to not occlude the canal, which results in pressure on the tympanic membrane. Direct the fluid slowly and gently toward the superior aspect of the ear canal, maintaining the flow in a steady stream. Periodically during the irrigation ask if the patient is experiencing pain, nausea, or vertigo. These symptoms indicate that the solution is too hot or too cold or is being instilled with too much pressure. After the canal is clear, wipe off any moisture from the ear with cotton balls and inspect the canal for remaining earwax.

Hearing Aid Care. A hearing aid amplifies sounds in a controlled manner; the aid receives normal low-intensity sound inputs and delivers them to a patient's ear as louder outputs. Hearing aids come in a

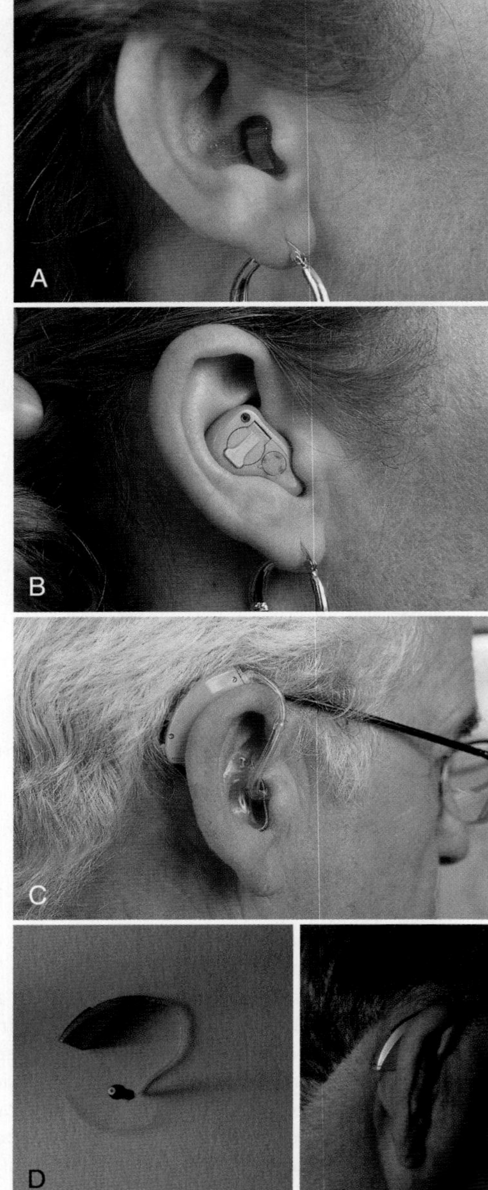

FIGURE 40-7 Common types of hearing aids. **A,** Completely-in-canal (CIC). **B,** In the ear (ITE). **C,** Behind the ear (BTE). **D,** Digital hearing aid.

variety of types. The new class of hearing aids reduces background noise interference. Computer chips placed in the aids allow for fine adjustments to the specific patient's hearing needs.

There are several popular types of hearing aids. A completely-in-canal (CIC) aid (Figure 40-7, *A*) is the newest, smallest, and least visible and fits entirely in the ear canal. It is used for patients with moderately severe hearing loss. It has cosmetic appeal, is easy to manipulate and place in the ear, and does not interfere with wearing eyeglasses or using the telephone; and the patient can wear it during most physical exercise. However, it requires adequate ear diameter and depth for proper fit. It does not accommodate progressive hearing loss; and it requires manual dexterity to operate, insert, remove, and change batteries. In addition, cerumen tends to plug this model more than the others.

An in-the-ear (ITE, or intraaural) aid (Figure 40-7, *B*) fits into the external auditory canal and allows for finer tuning. It is more

BOX 40-15 Care and Use of Hearing Aids

- Initially wear hearing aid 15 to 20 minutes; gradually increase time to 10 to 12 hours.
- Once inserted, turn aid slowly to one-third to one-half volume.
- Whistling sound indicates incorrect earmold insertion, improper fit of aid, or buildup of earwax or fluid.
- Adjust volume to comfortable level for talking at distance of 1 yard.
- Do not wear aid under heat lamps or hair dryer or in very wet, cold weather.
- Batteries last 1 week with daily wearing of 10 to 12 hours.
- Remove or disconnect battery when not in use.
- Replace earmolds every 2 or 3 years.
- Routinely check battery compartment: Is it clean? Are batteries inserted properly? Is compartment shut all the way?
- Make sure that dials on hearing aid are clean and easy to rotate, creating no static during adjusting.
- Keep aid clean. See manufacturer instructions. Aids are usually cleaned with a soft cloth.
- Avoid use of hairspray and perfume while wearing hearing aids; residue from spray causes aid to become oily and greasy.
- Do not submerse in water.
- Routinely check cord or tubing (depending on type of aid) for cracking, fraying, and poor connections.
- Routine follow-up with audiologist is recommended to evaluate effectiveness of current aid.

Data from Touhy T, Jett P: *Toward healthy aging,* ed 8, St Louis, 2012, Mosby.

powerful and stronger and therefore is useful for mild-to-severe hearing loss than the ITC aid. It is easy to position and adjust and does not interfere with wearing eyeglasses. However, it is more noticeable than the ITC aid and is not for people with moisture or skin problems in the ear canal.

A behind-the-ear (BTE, or postaural) aid (Figure 40-7, *C*) hooks around and behind the ear. It is connected by a short, clear, hollow plastic tube to an earmold inserted into the external auditory canal. A BTE aid allows for fine tuning. It is the largest aid and is useful for patients with mild to profound hearing loss or manual dexterity difficulties or for those who find partial ear occlusion intolerable. The larger size of this type of aid can make use of eyeglasses and phones difficult; it is more difficult to keep in place during physical exercise.

Digital hearing aids (Figure 40-7, *D*) analyze sounds to remove background noise. This aid is beneficial for people with mild to severe hearing loss. Digital hearing aids program for low-frequency and high-frequency sounds and must be programmed and adjusted by a licensed audiologist. Box 40-15 reviews guidelines for the care and cleaning of hearing aids.

Nasal Care. A patient usually removes secretions from the nose by gently blowing into a soft tissue. Caution the patient against harsh blowing that creates pressure capable of injuring the eardrum, nasal mucosa, and even sensitive eye structures. Bleeding from the nares is a sign of harsh blowing. If a patient is unable to remove nasal secretions, help by using a wet washcloth or a cotton-tipped applicator moistened in water or saline. Never insert the applicator beyond the length of the cotton tip. You can remove excessive nasal secretions by gentle suctioning.

When nasogastric, feeding, or endotracheal tubes are inserted through a patient's nose, change the tape anchoring the tube at least once a day. When tape becomes moist from nasal secretions, the skin and mucosa easily become macerated. Friction from a tube causes tissue sloughing and eventual ulceration. After carefully removing the tape, maintain hold of the tubing and thoroughly clean and dry the nasal surface.

Patient's Room Environment. Attempt to make a patient's room as comfortable as the home. It needs to be safe and large enough to allow the patient and visitors to move about freely. Removal of barriers along walkways reduces risk of falls. Control room temperature, ventilation, noise, and odors. Keeping the room neat and orderly also contributes to the patient's sense of well-being.

Maintaining Comfort. What makes a comfortable environment depends on a patient's age, severity of illness, and level of normal daily activity. Depending on age and physical condition, maintain the room temperature between 20° and 23° C (68° and 73.4° F). Infants, older adults, and the acutely ill often need a warmer room. However, certain ill patients benefit from cooler room temperatures to lower the metabolic demands of the body.

An effective ventilation system keeps stale air and odors from lingering in a room. Protect the acutely ill, infants, and older adults from drafts by ensuring that they are dressed adequately and covered with a lightweight blanket. Always empty and rinse commodes, bedpans, and urinals promptly. Room deodorizers help remove many unpleasant odors. Before using room deodorizers determine that the patient is not allergic or sensitive to the deodorizer itself. Thorough hygiene measures provide the best control of body or breath odors.

Ill patients seem to be more sensitive to noises and lighting commonly found in health care settings. Try to control the noise level, especially when a patient is trying to sleep. Explain the source of unfamiliar noises such as an IV pump or pulse oximeter alarms. Proper lighting provides for safety and comfort. A brightly lit room usually stimulates, whereas a darkened room promotes rest and sleep. Adjust room lighting by closing or opening drapes, regulating over-bed and floor lights, and closing or opening room doors. When entering a patient's room at night, refrain from abruptly turning on an overhead light unless necessary.

Room Equipment. Although there are variations across health care settings, a typical hospital room contains the following basic pieces of furniture: over-bed table, bedside stand, chairs, and bed (Figure 40-8). Long-term care and rehabilitation facilities often have similar equipment. You can adjust the over-bed table, which rolls on wheels, to various heights over the bed or a chair. The table provides ideal working space for performing procedures. It also provides a surface on which to place meal trays, toiletry items, and objects frequently used by a patient. Clean the top of the over-bed table with an antiseptic cleaner before using it for meals. Do not place the bed pan or urinal on the over-bed table. The bedside stand is for storing the patient's personal possessions and hygiene equipment. The telephone, water pitcher, and drinking cup are usually on top of the bedside stand.

Most hospital rooms contain an armless straight-backed chair or an upholstered lounge chair with arms. Straight-backed chairs are convenient when temporarily transferring patients from a bed such as during bed making. Lounge chairs tend to be more comfortable when a patient is willing and able to sit for an extended period.

Each room usually has an over-bed light and floor level night lighting. Position movable lights that extend over the bed from the wall for easy reach but move them aside when not in use. Additional portable lighting provides extra light during bedside procedures. Some facilities have permanent examination lights mounted in the ceiling or wall.

Other equipment usually found in a patient's room includes a call light, a television set, a wall-mounted blood pressure gauge, oxygen and vacuum wall outlets, and personal care items. Special equipment designed for comfort or positioning patients includes foot boots and special mattresses (see Chapter 48). Whenever you use comfort and positioning equipment, check agency policy and manufacturer directions before application.

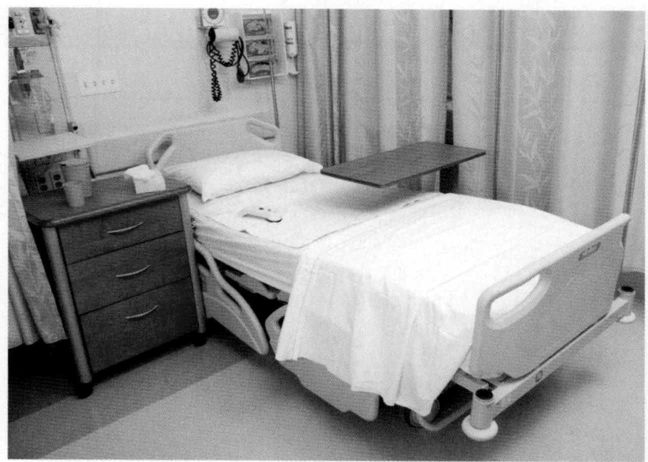

FIGURE 40-8 Typical hospital room.

Beds. Seriously ill patients often remain in bed for a long time. Because a bed is the piece of equipment used most by a hospitalized patient, it is designed for comfort, safety, and adaptability for changing positions. A typical hospital bed has a firm mattress on a metal frame that you can raise and lower horizontally. More and more hospitals are converting the standard hospital bed to one in which the mattress surface can be adjusted electronically for safety and comfort. For example, low beds are being used to prevent falls, and beds that regulate pressure in the mattress help to reduce pressure ulcers. Different bed positions promote patient comfort, minimize symptoms, promote lung expansion, and improve access during certain procedures (Table 40-6).

You usually change the position of a bed by using electrical controls incorporated into the patient's call light and in a panel on the side or foot of the bed (Figure 40-9). Know how to use the bed controls. Ease in raising and lowering a bed and changing position of the head and foot eliminates undue musculoskeletal strain. Also instruct patients and family members in the proper use of controls and caution them against raising the bed to a position that causes the patient harm. Maintain the bed height at the lowest horizontal position when a patient is unattended.

Beds contain safety features such as locks on the wheels or casters. Lock wheels when a bed is stationary to prevent accidental movement. Side rails allow patients to move more easily in bed and prevent accidents. Do not use side rails to restrict a patient from moving in bed. When using side rails as a restraint, you need a health care provider's order (see Chapter 27). You can remove the headboard and footboard from most beds. This is important when the medical team needs to have easy access to the patient such as during cardiopulmonary resuscitation.

Bed Making. Keep a patient's bed clean and comfortable. This requires frequent inspection to be sure that linen is clean, dry, and free of wrinkles. When patients are diaphoretic, have draining wounds, or are incontinent, check more frequently for wet or soiled linen.

Usually you make the bed in the morning after a patient's bath or while he or she is bathing, in a shower, sitting in a chair eating, or out of the room for procedures or tests. Throughout the day straighten linen that is loose or wrinkled. Also check the bed linen for food particles after meals and for wetness or soiling. Change any linen that becomes soiled or wet.

TABLE 40-6 Common Bed Positions

Position	Description	Uses
Fowler's	Head of bed raised to angle of 45 degrees or more; semi-sitting position; foot of bed may also be raised at knee	While patient is eating During nasogastric tube insertion and nasotracheal suction Promotes lung expansion Eases difficult breathing
Semi-Fowler's	Head of bed raised approximately 30 degrees; inclination less than Fowler's position; foot of bed may also be raised at knee	Promotes lung expansion, especially with ventilator-assisted patients Used when patients receive oral care and for gastric feedings to reduce regurgitation and risk of aspiration
Trendelenburg's	Entire bedframe tilted with head of bed down	Used for postural drainage Facilitates venous return in patients with poor peripheral perfusion
Reverse Trendelenburg's	Entire bedframe tilted with foot of bed down	Used infrequently Promotes gastric emptying Prevents esophageal reflux
Flat	Entire bedframe horizontally parallel with floor	Used for patients with vertebral injuries and in cervical traction Used for patients who are hypotensive Patients usually prefer for sleeping

When changing bed linen, follow principles of medical asepsis by keeping soiled linen away from the uniform (Figure 40-10). Place soiled linen in special linen bags before placing in a hamper. To avoid air currents that spread microorganisms, never shake the linen. To avoid transmitting infection, do not place soiled linen on the floor. If clean linen touches the floor or any unclean surface, immediately place it in the dirty-linen container.

During bed making use safe patient-handling procedures (see Chapter 28). Always raise the bed to the appropriate height before changing linen so you do not have to bend or stretch over the mattress. Move back and forth to opposite sides of the bed while applying new linen. Body mechanics and safe handling are important when turning or repositioning a patient in bed.

When patients are confined to bed, you must make an occupied bed. Organize bed-making activities to conserve time and energy (Box 40-16). The patient's privacy, comfort, and safety are all important when making a bed. Using side rails to aid positioning and turning, keeping call lights within the patient's reach, and maintaining the proper bed position help promote comfort and safety. After making a bed, return it to the lowest horizontal position and verify that the wheels are locked to prevent accidental falls when the patient gets in and out alone.

When possible, make the bed while it is unoccupied (Box 40-17). Use judgment to determine the best time for a patient to sit in a chair so you can make the bed. When making an unoccupied bed, follow the same basic principles as for occupied bed making.

An unoccupied bed can be made as an open or closed bed. In an open bed the top covers are folded back so it is easy for a patient to get into bed. Draw up the top sheet, blanket, and bedspread to the head of the mattress and place a pillow at the top to make a closed bed. A closed bed is prepared in a hospital room before a new patient is admitted to that room. A surgical, recovery, or postoperative bed is a modified version of the open bed. The top bed linen is arranged for easy transfer of the patient from a stretcher to the bed. The top sheets and spread are not tucked or mitered at the corners. Instead they are folded to one side or to the bottom third of the bed (Figure 40-12). This makes patient transfer into the bed easier.

Linens. Many agencies have "nurse servers" either within or just outside a patient's room to store a daily supply of linen. Because of the importance of cost control in health care, avoid bringing excess linen into a patient's room. Once you bring linen into a patient's room, if

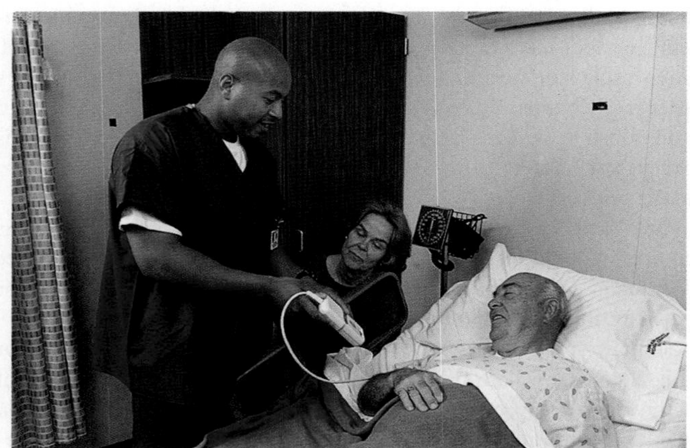

FIGURE 40-9 Nurse instructing patient in use of call light and bed controls.

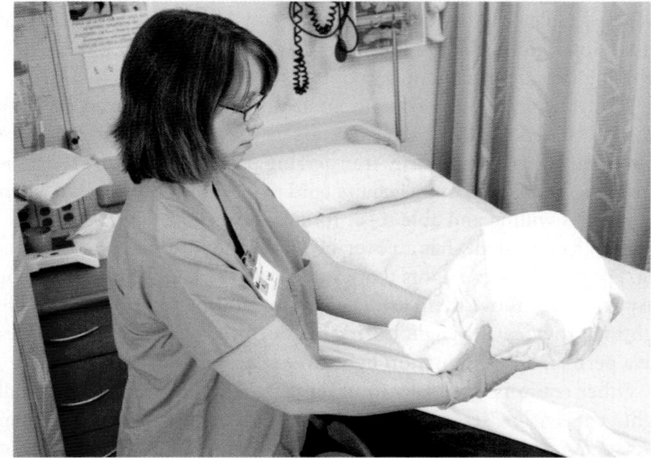

FIGURE 40-10 Holding linen away from uniform prevents contact with microorganisms.

BOX 40-16 PROCEDURAL GUIDELINES

Making an Occupied Bed

Delegation Considerations

The skill of making an occupied bed can be delegated to nursing assistive personnel (NAP). The nurse reviews any precautions or activity restrictions. Instruct the NAP about:

- Any activity or positioning restrictions for the patient, including need to use equipment for lifting and positioning patient.
- Looking for wound drainage, dressing materials, drainage tubes, or intravenous tubing that becomes dislodged or is found in linens.
- What to do if patient becomes tired.

Equipment

Linen bag(s), mattress pad *(optional depending on facility practice;* needs to be changed only when soiled), bottom sheet (flat or fitted), drawsheet, top sheet, blanket *(optional depending on patient preference),* bedspread, waterproof pads and/or bath blankets *(optional),* pillowcases, bedside chair or table, clean gloves *(optional),* paper towels or washcloth, disinfectant (Figure 40-11).

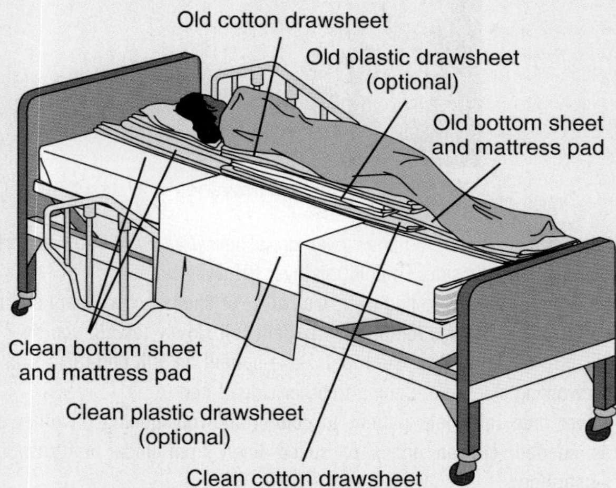

FIGURE 40-11 Equipment for making occupied bed.

Steps

1. Check chart for orders or specific precautions concerning patient movement and positioning.
2. Gather needed supplies, being sure not to let clean linen touch your uniform.
3. Explain procedure to patient, including that he or she will be asked to turn on side and roll over linen.
4. Perform hand hygiene and apply clean gloves (wear gloves only if old linen is soiled or there is risk for contact with body).
5. Assess potential for patient incontinence or excess drainage on bed linen.
6. Arrange equipment on bedside chair or over-bed table. Remove unnecessary equipment such as a dietary tray or items used for hygiene. Pull curtain and close door.
7. Adjust bed height to comfortable working position with bed flat if patient can tolerate. Lower raised side rail on one side of bed. Remove call light.
8. Loosen top linen at foot of bed.
9. Remove bedspread and blanket separately. If spread and blanket are soiled, place them in linen bag. Keep soiled linen away from uniform.
10. If blanket and spread are to be reused, fold them by bringing the top and bottom edges together. Fold farthest side over onto nearer bottom edge. Bring top and bottom edges together again. Place folded linen over back of chair.
11. Cover patient with bath blanket in the following manner: unfold bath blanket over top sheet. Ask patient to hold top edge of bath blanket. If patient is unable to help, tuck top of bath blanket under shoulders. Grasp top sheet under bath blanket at patient's shoulders and bring sheet down to foot of bed. Remove sheet and discard in linen bag.
12. Help patient turn toward far side of bed, turned onto side and facing away from you. Be sure that side rail in front of patient is up. Adjust pillow under patient's head.
13. Loosen bottom linens, moving from head to foot. With seam side down (facing the mattress), fanfold soiled drawsheet and bottom sheet toward patient. Tuck edges of linen just under buttocks, back, and shoulders. Do not fanfold mattress pad if it is to be reused (see illustration).

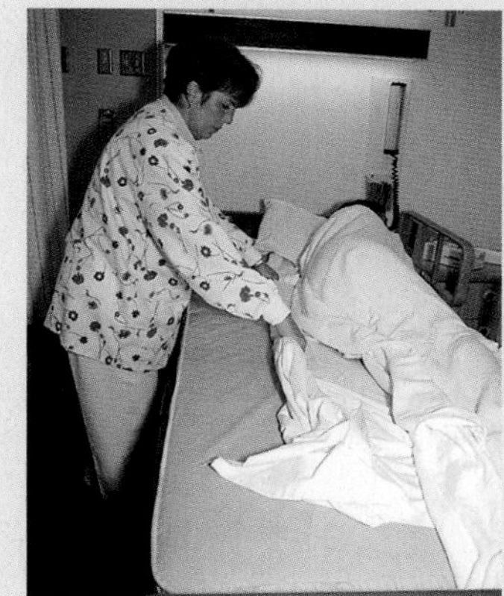

STEP 13 Old linen tucked under patient.

14. Wipe off any moisture on exposed mattress with paper towel and appropriate disinfectant. Make sure that mattress surface is dry before applying linens.
15. Apply clean linen to exposed half of bed:
    a. Place clean mattress pad on bed (if used) by folding it lengthwise with center crease in middle of bed. Fanfold top layer over mattress. (If pad is reused, simply smooth out any wrinkles.)
    b. If using flat sheet for bottom sheet, unfold sheet lengthwise so center crease is situated lengthwise along center of bed. Fanfold top layer of sheet toward center of bed alongside patient (see illustration). Smooth bottom layer of sheet over mattress and bring edge over closest side of mattress. If using fitted sheet, pull sheet smoothly over mattress ends.

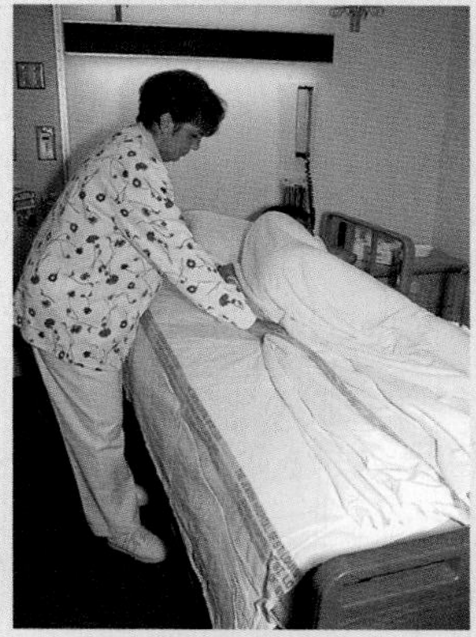

STEP 15b Clean linen applied to bed.

Continued

BOX 40-16 PROCEDURAL GUIDELINES

***Making an Occupied Bed*—cont'd**

c. Allow edge of flat unfitted sheet to hang about 25 cm (10 inches) over mattress edge. Make sure that lower hem of bottom flat sheet lies seam down and even with bottom edge of mattress.

16. If flat sheet is used for bottom sheet, miter bottom flat sheet at head of bed:
    a. Face head of bed diagonally. Place hand away from head of bed under top corner of mattress, near mattress edge, and lift.
    b. With other hand tuck top edge of bottom sheet smoothly under mattress so side edges of sheet above and below mattress meet when brought together.
    c. Face side of bed and pick up top edge of sheet at approximately 45 cm (18 inches) from top of mattress (see illustration).

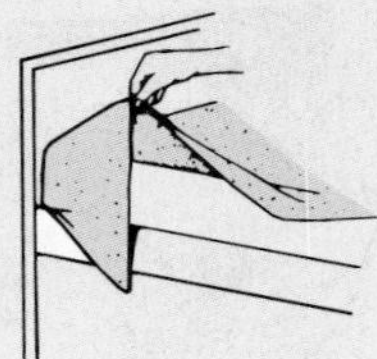

STEP 16c Top edge of sheet picked up.

    d. Lift sheet and lay it on top of mattress to form a neat triangular fold, with lower base of triangle even with mattress side edge (see illustration).

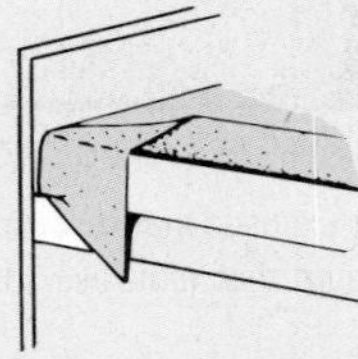

STEP 16d Sheet on top of mattress in a triangular fold.

    e. Tuck lower edge of sheet, which is hanging free below the mattress, under mattress. Tuck with palms down without pulling triangular fold (see illustration).

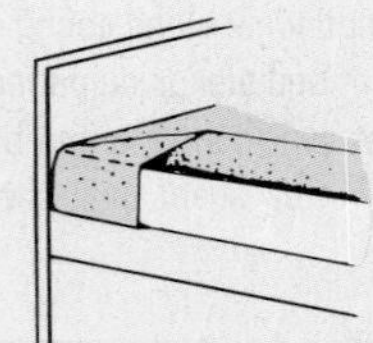

STEP 16e Lower edge of sheet tucked under mattress.

    f. Hold part of sheet covering side of mattress in place with one hand. With the other hand, pick up top of triangular linen fold and bring it down over side of mattress. Tuck this part under mattress (see illustration).

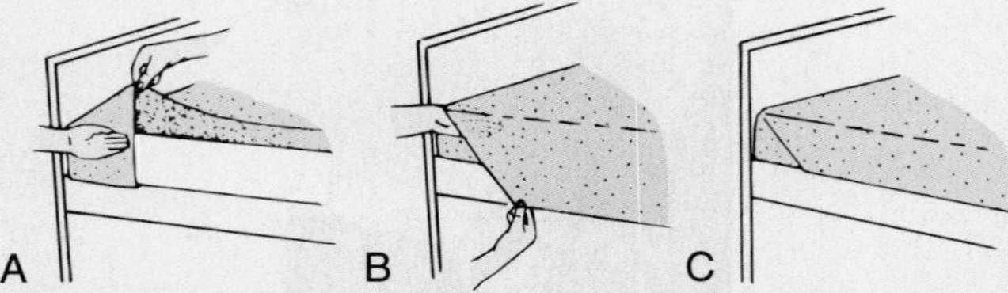

STEP 16f A and B, Triangular fold placed over side of mattress. **C,** Linen tucked under mattress.

    g. Tuck remaining part of sheet under mattress, moving toward foot of bed. Keep linen smooth.

17. *Optional:* Open clean drawsheet so it unfolds in half. Lay centerfold along middle of bed lengthwise and position sheet so it is under patient's buttocks and torso (see illustration). Fanfold top layer of drawsheet toward patient with edge along patient's back. Smooth bottom layer out over mattress and tuck excess edge under mattress (keep palms down).

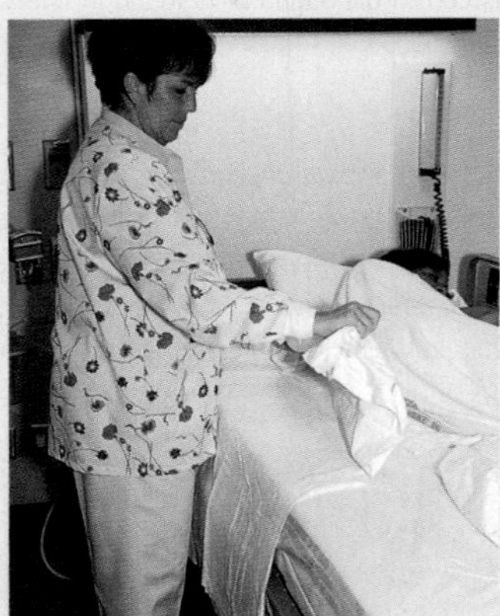

STEP 17 Optional drawsheet.

18. Place single waterproof pad over drawsheet *(optional)* with centerfold against patient's side. Fanfold top layer toward patient.
19. Advise patient that rolling over thick layer of linens is necessary and that he or she will feel a lump. Have patient roll slowly toward you over the layers of linen (rolling like a log). Have patient lie still and raise side rail on working side before going to other side of bed.
20. Lower side rail. Help patient to comfortable positioning on other side as needed. Loosen edges of soiled linen from under mattress (see illustration).

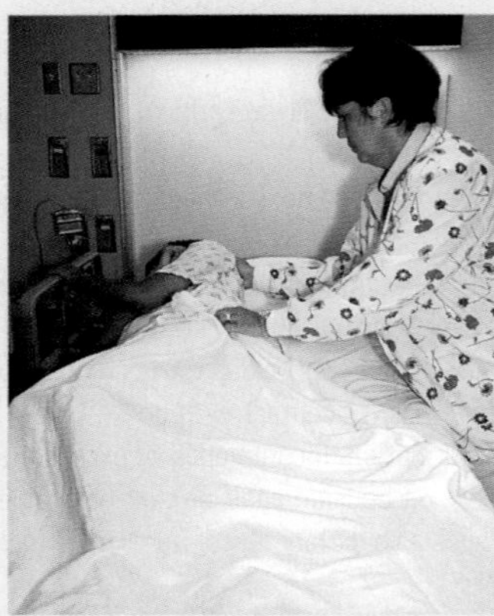

STEP 20 Helping patient to position after rolling over folds of linen.

21. Remove all soiled linen by folding it into a bundle or square with soiled side turned in. Discard in linen bag. If necessary, wipe mattress with antiseptic solution and dry mattress surface before unfolding and applying clean linen.
22. Pull clean, fanfolded linen smoothly over edge of mattress from head to foot of bed. Help patient roll back into supine position (if preferred). Reposition pillow.

BOX 40-16 **PROCEDURAL GUIDELINES**

***Making an Occupied Bed*—cont'd**

23. If using a fitted sheet, pull it smoothly over mattress ends. If using a flat sheet, miter top corner of bottom sheet (see Steps 16 a-g). When tucking corner, be sure that sheet is smooth and free of wrinkles.
24. Facing side of bed, grasp remaining edge of bottom flat sheet. Lean back, keep back straight, and pull while tucking excess linen under mattress. Proceed from head to foot of bed. (Avoid lifting mattress during tucking to ensure fit.)
25. Smooth fanfolded drawsheet out over bottom sheet. Grasp edge of sheet with palms down, lean back, and tuck sheet under mattress. Tuck from middle to top and then to bottom.
26. Place top sheet over patient with centerfold lengthwise down middle of bed. Open sheet from head to foot and unfold over patient. Ask patient to hold clean top sheet or tuck sheet around his or her shoulders. Remove bath blanket and discard in linen bag.
27. Place blanket on bed, unfolding it so crease runs lengthwise along middle of bed. Unfold blanket to cover patient. Make sure that top edge is parallel with edge of top sheet and 15 to 20 cm (6 to 8 inches) from edge of top sheet.
28. Place spread over bed according to Step 27. Be sure that top edge of spread extends about 2.5 cm (1 inch) above edge of blanket. Tuck top edge of spread over and under top edge of blanket.
29. Make cuff by turning edge of top sheet down over top edge of blanket and spread.
30. Standing on one side at foot of bed, lift mattress corner slightly with one hand and tuck sheet and blanket together under mattress. Be sure that lines are loose enough to allow movement of patient's feet. Making a horizontal toe pleat is an option (see illustration).

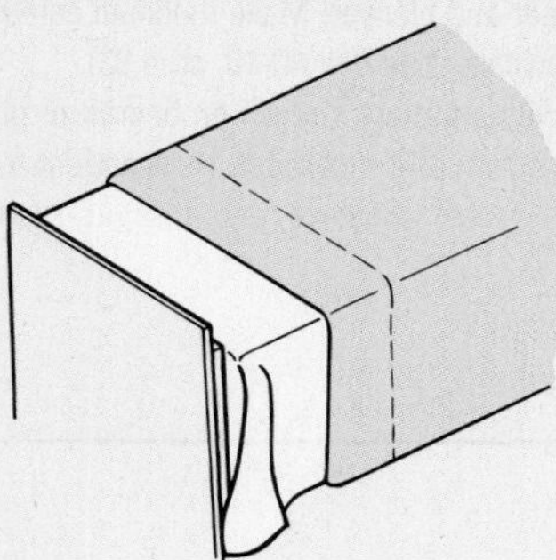

STEP 30 Optional toe pleat.

31. Make modified mitered corner with top sheet, blanket, and spread (follow Steps 16 a-e). After making the triangular fold, do not tuck tip of the triangle (see illustration) under the mattress.

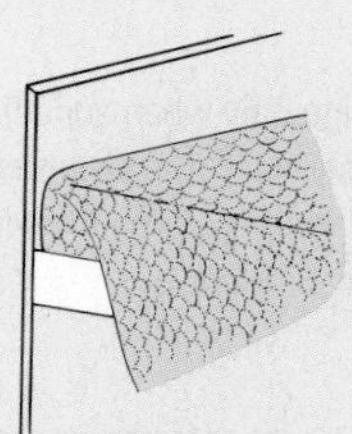

STEP 31 Modified mitered corner.

32. Raise side rail. Make other side of bed; spread sheet, blanket, and bedspread out evenly. Fold top edge of spread over blanket and make cuff with top sheet (see Steps 28 and 29); make modified mitered corner (see Step 31)
33. Change pillowcase:
    a. Have patient raise head. While supporting neck with one hand, remove pillow. Allow patient to lower head.
    b. Remove soiled case by grasping pillow open end with one hand and pulling case back over pillow with other hand. Discard case in linen bag.
    c. Grasp clean pillowcase at center of closed end. Gather case, turning it inside out over the hand holding it. With same hand pick up middle of one end of pillow. Pull pillowcase down over pillow with other hand.
    d. Be sure that pillow corners fit evenly into corners of pillowcase. Place pillow under patient's head.
34. Place call light within patient's reach and return bed to comfortable position and height. Open room curtains and rearrange furniture. Place personal items within easy reach on over-bed table or bedside stand.
35. Place dirty linen in hamper or chute. Remove gloves (if worn); dispose and perform hand hygiene.
36. Ask if patient feels comfortable.
37. Use this time to inspect skin for areas of irritation.

BOX 40-17 PROCEDURAL GUIDELINES

Making an Unoccupied Bed

Delegation Considerations

The skill of making an unoccupied bed can be delegated to nursing assistive personnel (NAP).

Equipment

Linen bag, mattress pad (change only when soiled), bottom sheet (flat or fitted), drawsheet *(optional)*, top sheet, blanket, bedspread, waterproof pads *(optional)*, pillowcases, bedside chair or table, clean gloves (if linen is soiled), washcloth or paper towel, and antiseptic cleanser.

Steps

1. If patient has been incontinent or if excess drainage is on linen, gloves are necessary.
2. Assess activity orders or restrictions in mobility in planning if patient can get out of bed for procedure. Help to bedside chair or recliner.
3. Lower side rails on both sides of bed and raise bed to comfortable working position.
4. Remove soiled linen and place in laundry bag. Avoid shaking or fanning linen.
5. Reposition mattress and wipe off any moisture with a washcloth or paper towel moistened in antiseptic solution. Dry thoroughly.
6. Apply all bottom linen on one side of bed (before moving to opposite side):
   a. Be sure that fitted sheet is placed smoothly over mattress.
   b. To apply a flat unfitted sheet, allow about 25 cm (10 inches) to hang over sides of mattress edges. Make sure that lower hem of sheet lies seam down, even with bottom edge of mattress. Pull remaining top part of sheet over top edge of mattress.
7. While standing at head of bed, miter top corner of bottom sheet (see Box 40-16, Steps 16a-f).
8. Tuck remaining part of unfitted sheet under mattress from head to foot of bed.
9. *Optional:* Apply drawsheet, laying centerfold along middle of bed lengthwise. Smooth drawsheet over mattress and tuck excess edge under mattress, keeping palms down.
10. Move to opposite side of bed and spread bottom sheet smoothly over edge of mattress from head to foot of bed.
11. Apply fitted sheet smoothly over each mattress corner. For an unfitted sheet, miter top corner of bottom sheet (see Step 7), making sure that corner is taut.
12. Grasp remaining edge of unfitted bottom sheet and tuck tightly under mattress while moving from head to foot of bed.
13. Smooth folded drawsheet over bottom sheet and tuck under mattress, first at middle, then at top, and then at bottom.
14. If needed, apply single waterproof pad over bottom sheet or drawsheet.
15. Place top sheet over bed with vertical centerfold lengthwise down middle of bed. Open sheet out from head to foot, being sure that top edge of sheet is even with top edge of mattress.
16. Make horizontal toe pleat: stand at foot of bed and make fanfold in sheet 5 to 10 cm (2 to 4 inches) across bed. Pull sheet up from bottom to make fold approximately 15 cm (6 inches) from bottom edge of mattress.
17. Tuck in remaining part of sheet under foot of mattress. Place blanket over bed with top edge parallel to top edge of sheet and 15 to 20 cm (6 to 8 inches) down from edge of sheet. (*Optional:* Apply additional spread over bed.)
18. Make cuff by turning edge of top sheet down over top edge of blanket and spread.
19. Standing on one side at foot of bed, lift mattress corner slightly with one hand; with other hand tuck top sheet, blanket, and spread under mattress. Be sure that toe pleats are not pulled out.
20. Make modified mitered corner with top sheet, blanket, and spread. After making triangular fold, do not tuck tip of triangle (see Box 40-16, Step 31).
21. Go to other side of bed. Spread sheet, blanket, and spread out evenly. Make cuff with top sheet and blanket. Make modified corner at foot of bed.
22. Apply clean pillowcase (see Box 40-16, step 33).
23. Place call light within patient's reach on bedrail or pillow and return bed to height allowing for patient transfer. Help patient to bed.
24. Arrange patient's room. Remove and discard supplies. Perform hand hygiene.

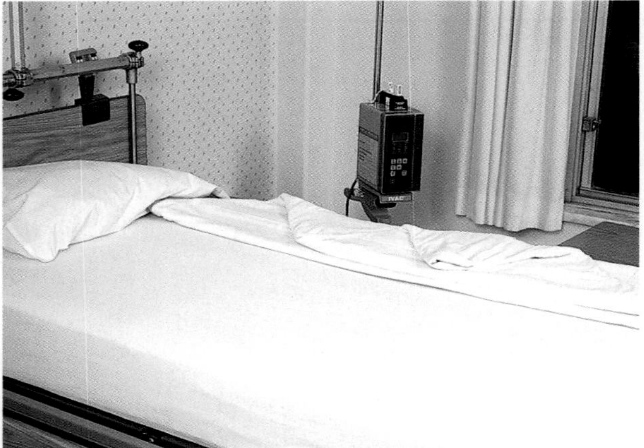

FIGURE 40-12 Surgical or recovery bed.

unused, it must be laundered before being used. Excess linen lying around a patient's room creates clutter and obstacles for patient care activities.

Before making a bed, collect necessary bed linens and the patient's personal items. In this way all equipment is accessible to prepare the bed and room. When fitted sheets are not available, flat sheets usually are pressed with a center crease to be placed down the center of the bed. The linens unfold easily to the sides, with creases often fitting over the mattress edge. Apply clean linens whenever there is soiling.

Handle linen properly to minimize the spread of infection (see Chapter 29). Agency policies provide guidelines for the proper way to bag and dispose of soiled linen. After a patient is discharged, all bed linen goes to the laundry, and housekeeping cleans the mattress and bed before clean linen is applied.

◆ Evaluation

Through the Patient's Eyes. During assessment you collected information about a patient's expectations of care. Both during and after hygiene determine from the patient if care is being provided in an acceptable manner (Figure 40-13). For example, while bathing a

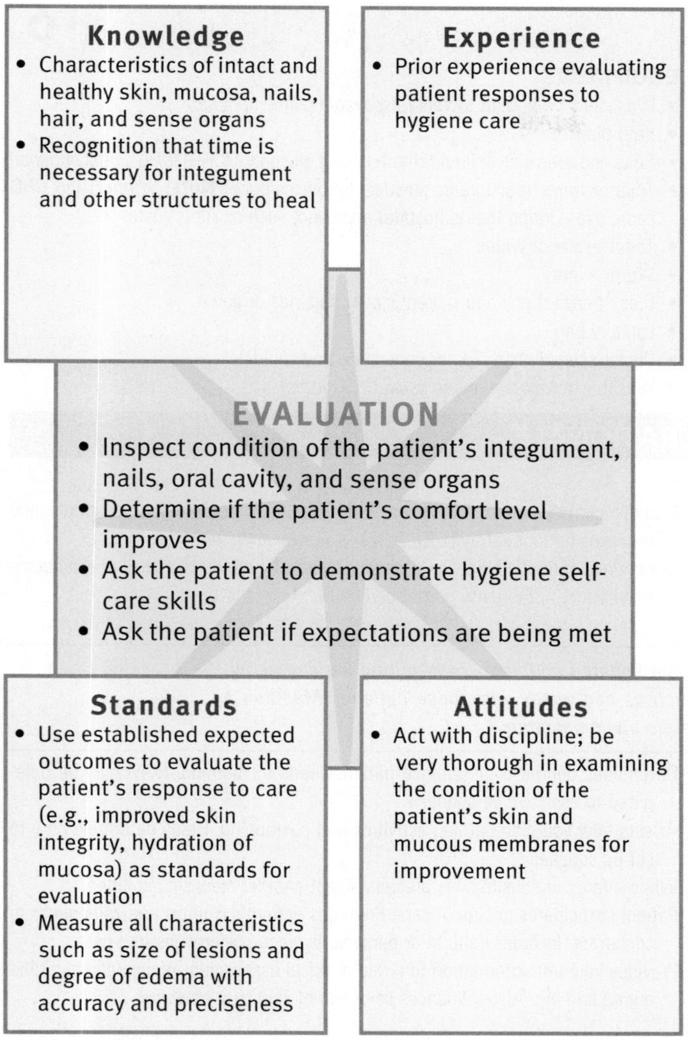

Knowledge
- Characteristics of intact and healthy skin, mucosa, nails, hair, and sense organs
- Recognition that time is necessary for integument and other structures to heal

Experience
- Prior experience evaluating patient responses to hygiene care

EVALUATION
- Inspect condition of the patient's integument, nails, oral cavity, and sense organs
- Determine if the patient's comfort level improves
- Ask the patient to demonstrate hygiene self-care skills
- Ask the patient if expectations are being met

Standards
- Use established expected outcomes to evaluate the patient's response to care (e.g., improved skin integrity, hydration of mucosa) as standards for evaluation
- Measure all characteristics such as size of lesions and degree of edema with accuracy and preciseness

Attitudes
- Act with discipline; be very thorough in examining the condition of the patient's skin and mucous membranes for improvement

FIGURE 40-13 Critical thinking model for hygiene evaluation.

patient, encourage him or her to verbalize any discomfort such as too-cool water or discomfort with movement. To evaluate a patient's satisfaction with your care, ask questions such as, "Do you think your bath helped you feel more comfortable?" "Are there ways we can make you feel less tired during your bath?" "Were you pleased with how we cared for your foot?" Being aware of and addressing a patient's expectations and any concerns foster a caring therapeutic relationship.

Patient Outcomes. Evaluate patient responses to hygiene measures both during and after each particular hygiene intervention. For example, while bathing a patient inspect the skin carefully to see if soiling or drainage is effectively removed. Once a bath is completed, evaluate if the patient feels more comfortable by using a pain scale (see Chapter 44). Frequently it takes time for hygiene care to result in an improvement in a patient's condition. The presence of oral lesions, a scalp infestation, or skin excoriation often requires repeated measures and a combination of nursing interventions. Your knowledge base and experience provide important perspectives when analyzing ongoing evaluation data about a patient. For example, frequent observation of the skin helps to determine the effectiveness of hygiene practices. Does a rash clear or a pressure ulcer heal? Is the patient able to complete hygiene care using adaptive equipment?

To evaluate a patient's or family caregiver's ability to perform self-care hygiene measures use Teach Back. For example, "I want to be sure you are clear about why foot care is so important for you since you have diabetes. Tell me three things you can do to protect your feet from infection?" Another example, "We talked about ways to prevent your skin from drying. Describe them for me."

If outcomes established for the care plan are not met, revise it. Continue to apply critical thinking attitudes when considering all evaluation findings. When outcomes are not met, ask questions by involving the patient to determine appropriate changes in interventions. Examples of questions include:

- What is preventing you from being able to perform your foot care at home?
- Which further measures do you think are necessary to keep your mouth feeling clean?
- What do you think would help you be more independent with your hygiene?

QSEN QSEN: BUILDING COMPETENCY IN PATIENT SAFETY Mrs. White is discharged to her home. Her granddaughter and a home care aide will provide care for her over the next few weeks. Mrs. White is making progress using the walker and bath-adaptive equipment that have been ordered for home care. Which assessments should be made for her following discharge from the hospital? What teaching needs to be provided to the family member to perform safe hygiene care for her grandmother?

Answers to QSEN Activities can be found on the Evolve website.

SAFETY GUIDELINES FOR NURSING SKILLS

Ensuring patient safety is an essential role of the professional nurse. To ensure patient safety, communicate clearly with members of the health care team, assess and incorporate the patient's priorities of care and preferences, and use the best evidence when making decisions about your patient's care. When performing the skills in this chapter, remember the following points to ensure safe, individualized patient care.

- To implement patient safety for the practice setting, identify the patient using two identifiers (TJC, 2016).
- Always perform hygiene measures moving from the cleanest to less clean or dirty areas. This often requires you to change gloves and perform hand hygiene during care activities.
- Use clean gloves when you anticipate contact with nonintact skin or mucous membranes or when there will likely be contact with drainage, secretions, excretions, or blood during hygiene care.
- When using water or solutions for hygiene care, be sure to test the temperature to prevent burn injury.
- Use principles of body mechanics and safe patient handling to avoid injury when performing hygiene care and reduce risk of harm to self or others (QSEN, 2014).
- You are responsible and accountable for the care provided. Give proper direction to nursing assistive personnel to whom you delegate and be sure they are competent with hygiene measures.

SKILL 40-1 BATHING AND PERINEAL CARE

DELEGATION CONSIDERATIONS

The skill of bathing and perineal care can be delegated to nursing assistive personnel (NAP). Direct the NAP to:

- Avoid massaging reddened skin areas.
- Perform range-of-motion (ROM) exercises for patients able to tolerate.
- Report skin changes or early signs of impaired skin integrity, including redness or pale skin, to nurse.
- Properly position patients with musculoskeletal limitations and indwelling catheters or intravenous (IV) lines.
- Report patient fatigue, shortness of breath, or pain during hygiene care.

EQUIPMENT

- Washcloths and bath towels *(disposable cloths optional)*
- Bath blanket
- Soap and soap dish or liquid chlorhexidine gluconate (CHG) *(CHG cloths optional)*
- Toiletry items (deodorant, powder, lotion, cologne) **NOTE:** When using CHG soap, use a lotion that is hospital approved, such as Aloe Vesta.
- Toilet tissue or wipes
- Warm water
- Clean hospital gown or patient's own pajamas or gown
- Laundry bag
- Clean gloves (when risk for contacting body fluids)
- Washbasin *(optional when using CHG cloths)*

STEP	RATIONALE
ASSESSMENT	
1. Identify patient using two identifiers (e.g., name and birthday or name and medical record number, according to agency policy).	Ensures correct patient. Complies with The Joint Commission standards and improves patient safety (TJC, 2016).
2. Assess patient's tolerance for bathing: activity tolerance, comfort level during movement, cognitive ability, musculoskeletal function, and presence of shortness of breath.	Determines patient's ability to perform or tolerate bathing and level of assistance required (e.g., tub bath, partial bed bath).
CLINICAL DECISION: *Patients with dementia may become agitated and aggressive during bathing activities. Consider using alternative bathing procedures such as bag wipes with these patients. Maintain a calm, nonthreatening, quiet environment using therapeutic communication.*	
3. Assess patient's visual status, ability to sit without support, hand grasp, ROM of extremities.	Determines degree of assistance patient needs for bathing. ROM may be delegated to assistive personnel.
4. Assess for presence of equipment (e.g., intravenous [IV] line, oxygen tubing, Foley catheter).	Affects how you plan bathing activities and positioning. Helps determine how to set up supplies.
5. Assess for allergy or sensitivity to CHG.	When allergy or sensitivity is present, select another cleansing solution.
6. Assess patient's bathing preferences: frequency and time of day preferred, type of hygiene products used, and other factors related to patient preferences.	Patient participates in plan of care. Promotes patient's comfort and willingness to cooperate. Includes cultural or personal hygiene preferences into care.
7. Ask if patient has noticed any problems related to condition of skin and genitalia: excess moisture, inflammation, drainage or excretions from lesions or body cavities, rashes or other skin lesions.	Provides you with information to direct physical assessment of skin and genitalia during bathing. Also influences selection of skin care products.
8. Before or during bath assess condition of patient's skin. Note presence of dryness, indicated by flaking, redness, scaling, and cracking.	Provides a baseline for comparison over time in determining if bathing improves condition of skin.
9. Assess patient's knowledge of skin hygiene in terms of its importance, preventive measures to take, and common problems.	Determines patient's learning needs.
PLANNING	
1. Review orders for specific precautions concerning patient's movement or positioning.	Prevents injury to patient during bathing activities. Determines level of assistance required by patient.
2. Check for health care provider's therapeutic bath order; if there is an order, note type of solution, length of time for bath, body part to be attended.	Therapeutic baths are ordered for specific physical effect, which usually includes promotion of healing or soothing effects.
3. Explain procedure and ask patient for suggestions on how to prepare supplies. If partial bath, ask how much of bath patient wishes to complete. If using CHG, explain benefit of reducing infection and that solution leaves a sticky feeling.	Promotes patient's cooperation and participation. Patients who prefer using their own bathing supplies may need to discuss benefits of CHG.
4. Prepare equipment and supplies. If it is necessary to leave room, be sure that call light is within patient's reach.	Avoids interrupting procedure or leaving patient unattended to retrieve missing equipment.
IMPLEMENTATION	
1. Complete or partial bed bath	
a. Assess environment for safety (e.g., check room for spills, make sure that equipment is working properly and that bed is in locked, low position).	Identifies safety hazards that could cause or potentially lead to harm (QSEN, 2014).
b. Close room, door, and windows; draw room divider curtain. Offer patient bedpan or urinal. Provide toilet tissue.	Provides for patient privacy. Helps patient feel more comfortable after voiding. Prevents interruption of bath.
c. Perform hand hygiene. If patient has nonintact skin or skin is soiled with drainage, excretions, or body secretions, apply clean gloves. Ensure that patient is not allergic to latex.	Reduces transmission of microorganisms. Prevents allergic reaction if latex gloves are used.

STEP	RATIONALE
d. Verify that bed is in locked position and raise bed to comfortable working height. Lower side rail closest to you and help patient into comfortable supine position, maintaining body alignment. Bring patient toward side closest to you.	Prevents bed from moving. Helps you reach patient without stretching and reaching across bed, thus minimizing strain on back muscles.
e. Place bath blanket over patient and loosen and remove top covers without exposing him or her. If possible, have patient hold top of bath blanket while you remove linen. Place soiled linen in laundry bag. Take care to not allow linen to touch your uniform. *Optional:* Use top sheet when bath blanket is not available or patient prefers.	Bath blanket provides warmth and privacy during bath.
f. Remove patient's gown or pajamas.	Provides full exposure of body parts during bathing.
(1) If using gown with ties or snaps on sleeves for patient with IV line, upper-extremity injury, or limited ROM, simply unsnap or untie and remove gown.	
(2) If regular gown is used and patient has limited upper-extremity ROM or an IV access, remove gown from *unaffected side first.*	Undressing unaffected side first allows easier manipulation of gown over body part with reduced ROM.
(3) Remove gown from arm with IV line (see illustrations A-C). Remove IV bag and tubing from pole and slide IV container and tubing through arm of patient's gown. Rehang IV container and check flow rate (see illustration D). Regulate if necessary.	Manipulation of IV tubing and container may disrupt flow rate. Do **not** delegate regulation of IV flow rate to NAP.
(4) If IV pump is in use, turn pump off, clamp tubing, remove tubing from pump, and proceed as in Step (3). Reinsert tubing into pump, unclamp tubing, and turn pump on at correct rate. Observe flow rate and regulate if necessary. *Do not disconnect tubing.*	Regulation is necessary to prevent improper infusion of fluids. Do **not** delegate regulation of IV pump to NAP. Disconnecting IV tubing places patient at risk of introduction of microorganisms into the IV line.
g. Pull side rail up. Lower bed temporarily to lowest position and raise to comfortable working height on return after filling washbasin two-thirds full with warm water. (*Option:* if using 4% CHG solution, pour entire single-use container into basin.) Place basin and supplies on over-bed table. Check water temperature and also have patient place fingers in water to test temperature tolerance. Place plastic container of bath lotion in bath water to warm if desired.	Raising side rail and lowering bed position maintain patient's safety while you leave bedside. Keeping bed at working height during bath prevents back strain. Warm water promotes comfort, relaxes muscles, and prevents unnecessary chilling. CHG is most effective at full strength. Testing temperature prevents accidental burns. Bath water warms lotion for application to patient's skin.
h. Lower side rail, remove pillow if tolerated, and raise head of bed 30 to 45 degrees if allowed. Place bath towel under patient's head. Place second bath towel over patient's chest.	Helps your access to patient. You do not have to reach across bed, thus minimizing strain on back muscles. Removal of pillow makes it easier to wash patient's ears and neck. Placing towels prevents bed linen and bath blanket from getting soiled or wet.

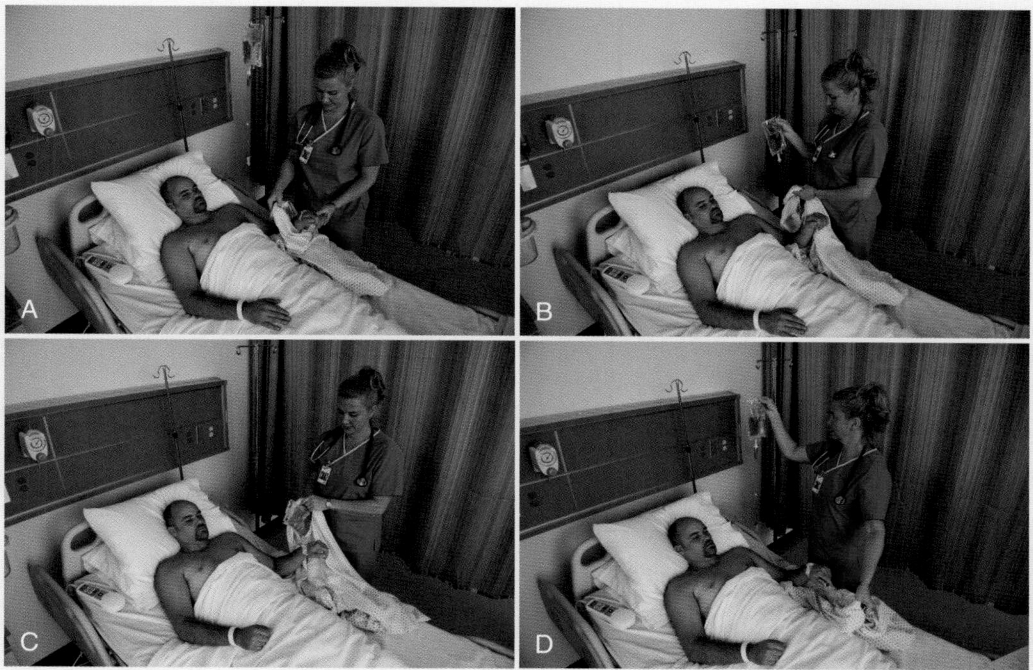

STEP 1f(3) A, Remove patient's gown. **B,** Remove IV tubing from pole. **C,** Slide IV tubing through arm of patient's gown. **D,** Rehang IV bag.

SKILL 40-1 BATHING AND PERINEAL CARE—cont'd

STEP	RATIONALE
i. Wash face.	
CLINICAL DECISION: *If using CHG solution in bath water, do not use to wash face. Only use clear water or mild soap and water on the face.*	
(1) Ask if patient is wearing contact lenses.	Prevents accidental injury to eyes.
(2) Fold washcloth around fingers of your hand to form a mitt (see illustration). Immerse mitt in water and wring thoroughly.	Mitt retains water and heat better than loosely held washcloth; keeps cold edges from brushing against patient and prevents splashing.
(3) Wash patient's eyes with plain warm water. Use different section of mitt for each eye. Move mitt from inner to outer canthus (see illustration). Soak any crusts on eyelid for 2 to 3 minutes with damp cloth before attempting removal. Dry eyes thoroughly but gently.	Soap irritates eyes. Use of separate sections of mitt reduces infection transmission. Bathing eye from inner to outer canthus prevents secretions from entering nasolacrimal duct. Pressure can cause internal injury.
(4) When using soap and water, ask if patient prefers to use soap on face. Otherwise wash, rinse, and dry forehead, cheeks, nose, neck, and ears without using soap. (Men may wish to shave at this point or wait until after bath.)	Soap tends to dry face, which is exposed to air more than other body parts.
j. Wash trunk and upper extremities.	
(1) Remove bath blanket from patient's arm that is closest to you. Place bath towel lengthwise under arm. Bathe arm with soap and water using long, firm strokes from distal to proximal areas (fingers to axilla).	Towel prevents soiling of bed. Soap lowers surface tension and facilitates removal of debris and bacteria when friction is applied during washing. Long, firm strokes stimulate circulation; moving distal to proximal promotes venous return.
(2) Raise and support arm above head (if possible) to wash, rinse, and dry axilla thoroughly (see illustration). Apply deodorant or powder to underarms if desired or needed.	Movement of arm exposes axilla and exercises normal ROM of joint. Alkaline residue from soap discourages growth of normal skin bacteria. Drying prevents excess moisture, which can cause skin maceration or softening. Respect patient's preference for use of hygiene products.
(3) Move to other side of bed and repeat Steps (1) and (2) with other arm.	Provides for better access to patient and helps prevent back strain.
(4) Place bath towel across patient's chest so it covers chest and arms and fold bath blanket down to umbilicus. While lifting edge of towel away from chest with one hand, bathe chest with mitted washcloth on other hand using long, firm strokes. Take special care to wash skinfolds under female's breasts. It is often necessary to lift breast upward while bathing underneath it. Keep patient's chest covered between wash and rinse periods. Rinse and dry well.	Draping prevents unnecessary exposure of body parts. Towel maintains warmth and privacy. Secretions and dirt collect easily in areas of tight skinfolds. Skin under breasts is vulnerable to excoriation if not kept clean and dry.
k. Wash hands and nails.	

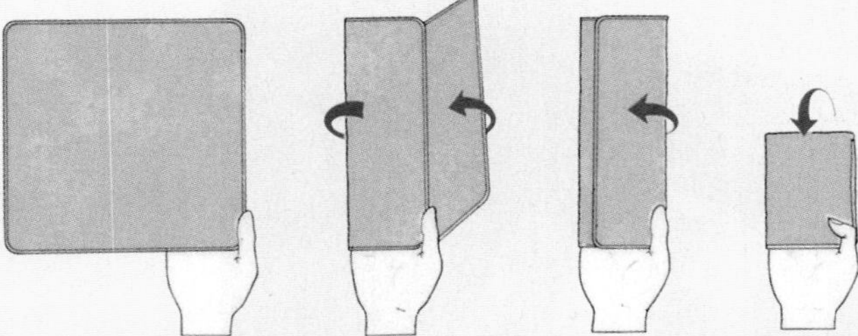

STEP 1i(2) Steps for folding washcloth to form a mitt.

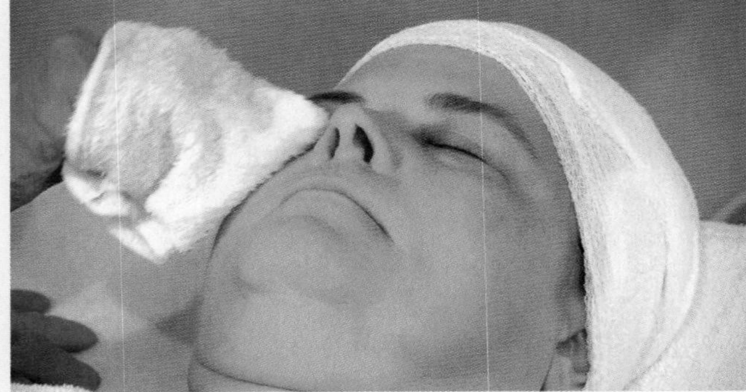

STEP 1i(3) Wash eye from inner to outer canthus.

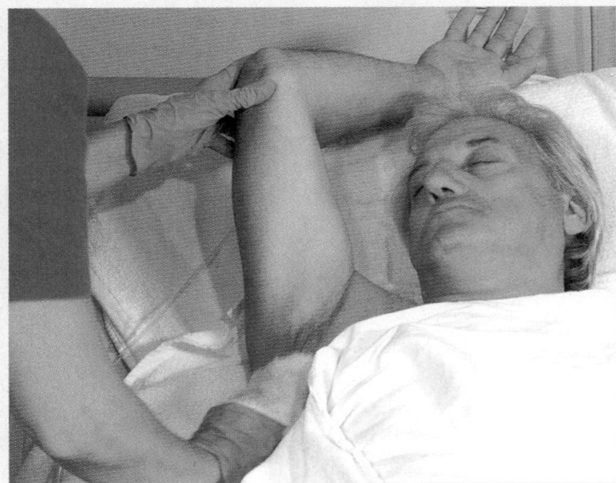

STEP 1j(2) Positioning arm to wash axilla.

STEP	RATIONALE
(1) Fold bath towel in half and lay it on bed beside patient. Place basin on towel. Immerse patient's hand in water. Allow hand to soak for 2 to 3 minutes before washing hand and fingernails. Remove basin and dry hand well. Repeat for other hand.	Soaking softens cuticles and calluses of hand, loosens debris beneath nails, and enhances feeling of cleanliness. Thorough drying removes moisture between fingers.
l. Check temperature of bath water and change water when cool or soapy. (See agency policy regarding changing water when using CHG solution.)	Warm water maintains patient's comfort. Alkaline soap residue is irritating to skin and can decrease the normal protectiveness of acid ph.

CLINICAL DECISION: *If patient is at risk for falling, be sure that two side rails are up before obtaining fresh water. In addition, lower bed when it is necessary to leave bedside. NOTE: Having all side rails raised is considered a restraint. Check agency policy.*

STEP	RATIONALE
m. Wash abdomen.	
(1) Place bath towel lengthwise over chest and abdomen. (Two towels may be needed.) Fold bath blanket down to just above pubic region. With one hand lift bath towel. With mitted hand bathe and rinse abdomen, giving special attention to umbilicus and skinfolds of abdomen and groin. Stroke from side to side. Keep abdomen covered between washing and rinsing. Rinse and dry well.	Draping prevents unnecessary exposure of body parts. Towel maintains warmth and privacy. Keeping skinfolds clean and dry helps prevent odor and skin irritation. Moisture and sediment that collect in skinfolds predispose skin to maceration.
(2) Apply clean gown or pajama top. If an extremity is injured or immobilized, dress affected side first. (This step may be omitted until completion of bath; gown should not become soiled during remainder of bath.)	Maintains patient's warmth and comfort. Dressing affected side first allows easier manipulation of gown over body part with reduced ROM.
n. Wash lower extremities.	
(1) Cover chest and abdomen with top of bath blanket. Cover legs with bottom of blanket. Expose near leg by folding blanket toward midline. Be sure to keep other leg and perineum draped.	Prevents unnecessary exposure.
(2) Place bath towel under leg, supporting leg at knee and ankle. If appropriate, place patient's foot in bath basin to soak while washing and rinsing. (Bend patient's leg at knee; and, while grasping patient's heel, elevate leg from mattress slightly and place bath basin on towel.) If patient is unable to support leg, you can clean by washing feet thoroughly with washcloth.	Towel prevents soiling of bed linen. Support of joint and extremity during lifting prevents strain on musculoskeletal structures. Sudden movement by patient could spill bath water. Soaking softens calluses and rough skin.

CLINICAL DECISION: *If patient has diabetes or peripheral vascular disease with impaired circulation and/or sensation, do not soak feet. Maceration of skin may predispose to infection.*

STEP	RATIONALE
(3) Wash leg using long, firm strokes from ankle to knee and from knee to thigh (see illustration). Do not rub or massage back of calf. Rinse and dry well. Clean foot, making sure to bathe between toes. Rinse and dry toes and feet completely. Clean and clip nails as needed (see Skill 40-2). Remove and discard towel.	Promotes circulation and venous return. Excess massage of calf could loosen deep vein thrombus. Secretions and moisture may be present between toes, predisposing patient to maceration and breakdown. Avoid cutting nails of patient with diabetes. See agency policy for podiatrist care.

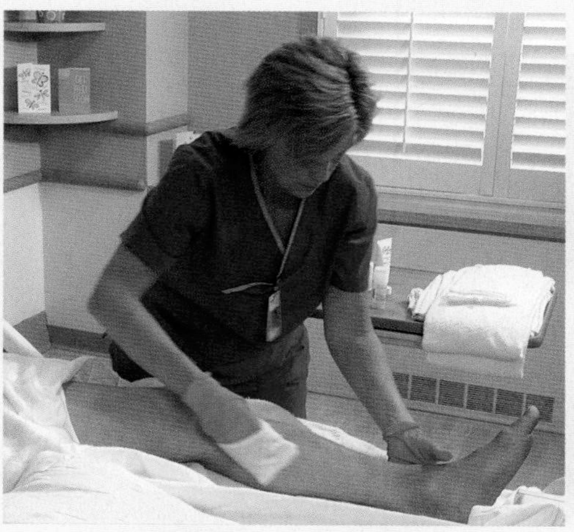

STEP 1n(3) Washing leg.

SKILL 40-1 BATHING AND PERINEAL CARE—cont'd

STEP	RATIONALE
(4) Raise side rail, move to opposite side of bed, lower side rail, and repeat Steps (2) and (3) for other leg and foot. If skin is dry, apply moisturizer. When finished, cover patient with bath blanket.	

CLINICAL DECISION: *Do not use long, firm strokes to wash lower extremities of patients with history of deep vein thrombosis or blood-clotting disorders. Use short, light strokes instead.*

STEP	RATIONALE
o. Cover patient with bath blanket, raise side rail for patient's safety, remove soiled gloves, and/or perform hand hygiene. Change bath water.	Decreased bath water temperature causes chilling. Clean water reduces microorganism transmission to perineal structures.
p. Provide perineal hygiene.	
(1) If patient is able to maneuver and handle washcloth, allow him or her to clean perineum on own.	Maintains patient's dignity and self-care ability.

CLINICAL DECISION: *CHG is safe to use on the perineum and external mucosa (AHRQ, 2013).*

STEP	RATIONALE
(2) Female patient	
(a) Apply pair of clean gloves. Lower side rail. Help patient into dorsal recumbent position. Note restrictions or limitations in patient's positioning. Place waterproof pad under patient's buttocks. Drape patient with bath blanket placed in shape of a diamond. Lift lower edge of bath blanket to expose perineum (see illustration).	Provides full exposure of female genitalia. If patient is totally dependent, provide assistance to support her in side-lying position and raise leg as perineum is bathed. If position causes patient discomfort, reduce degree of abduction in her hips.
(b) Fold lower corner of bath blanket up between patient's legs onto abdomen. Wash and dry patient's upper thighs.	Keeping patient draped until procedure begins minimizes anxiety. Buildup of perineal secretions soils surrounding skin surfaces.
(c) Wash labia majora. Use nondominant hand to gently retract labia from thigh: with dominant hand wash carefully in skinfolds. Wipe in direction from perineum to rectum. Repeat on opposite side with separate section of washcloth. Rinse and dry area thoroughly.	Perineal care involves thorough cleaning of patient's external genitalia and surrounding skin. Skinfolds may contain body secretions that harbor microorganisms. Wiping front to back reduces chance of transmitting fecal organisms to urinary meatus.
(d) Gently separate labia with nondominant hand to expose urethral meatus and vaginal orifice. With dominant hand, wash downward from pubic area toward rectum in one smooth stroke (see illustration). Wash middle and both sides of perineum. Use separate section of cloth for each stroke. Clean thoroughly around labia minora, clitoris, and vaginal orifice. Avoid placing tension on indwelling catheter if present and clean area around it thoroughly.	Cleansing method reduces transfer of microorganisms to urinary meatus. (For menstruating women or patients with indwelling catheters, clean with cotton balls.)
(e) Provide catheter care as needed (see Chapter 46).	Cleaning along catheter from exit site reduces incidence of health care–associated urinary infection.
(f) Rinse area thoroughly. May use bedpan and pour warm water over perineal area. Dry thoroughly from front to back.	Rinsing removes soap and microorganisms more effectively than wiping. Retained moisture harbors microorganisms.
(g) Fold lower corner of bath blanket back between patient's legs and over perineum. Ask patient to lower legs and assume comfortable position.	

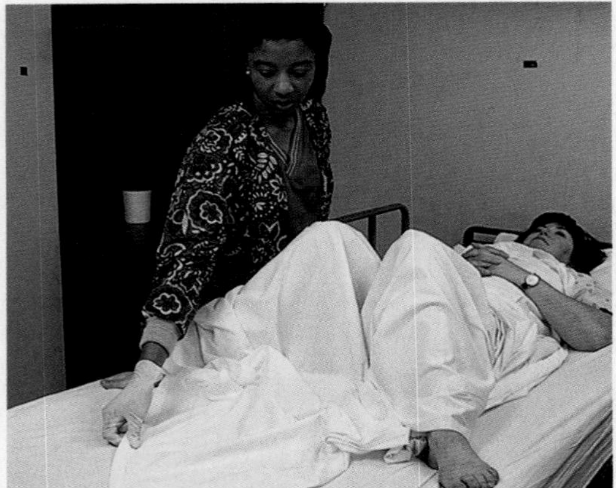

STEP 1p(2)(a) Drape patient for perineal care.

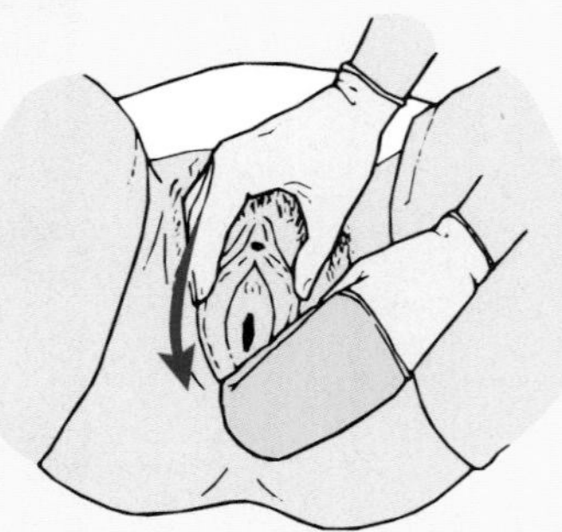

STEP 1p(2)(d) Cleanse from perineum to rectum (front to back).

STEP	RATIONALE
(3) Male patient	
(a) Apply pair of clean gloves. Lower side rail. Help patient to supine position. Note any restriction in mobility.	Provides full exposure of male genitalia. Position patients who are unable to lie supine on their side.
(b) Fold lower half of bath blanket up to expose upper thighs. Wash and dry thighs.	Buildup of perineal secretions soils surrounding skin surfaces.
(c) Cover thighs with bath towels. Raise bath blanket up to expose genitalia. Gently raise penis and place bath towel underneath. Gently grasp shaft of penis. If patient is uncircumcised, retract foreskin (see illustration). If patient has an erection, defer procedure until later.	Draping minimizes patient anxiety. Towel prevents moisture from collecting in inguinal area. Gentle but firm handling of penis reduces chance of an erection. Secretions capable of harboring microorganisms collect underneath foreskin.
(d) Wash tip of penis at urethral meatus first. Using circular motion, clean from meatus outward (see illustration). Discard washcloth and repeat with clean cloth until penis is clean. Rinse and dry gently.	Direction of cleaning moves from area of least contamination to area of most contamination, preventing microorganisms from entering urethra.
(e) Return foreskin to its natural position. This is extremely important in patients with decreased sensation in their lower extremities.	Tightening of foreskin around shaft of penis causes local edema and discomfort. Patients with reduced sensation do not feel tightening of foreskin.
(f) Gently clean shaft of penis and scrotum by having patient abduct legs. Pay special attention to underlying surface of penis. Lift scrotum carefully and wash underlying skinfolds. Rinse and dry thoroughly.	Vigorous massage of penis may cause an erection. Underlying surface of penis is an area where secretions accumulate. Abduction of legs provides easier access to scrotal tissues. Secretions collect easily between skinfolds.
(g) Avoid placing tension on indwelling catheter if present and clean area around it thoroughly. Provide catheter care (see Chapter 46).	Cleaning along catheter from exit site reduces incidence of nosocomial urinary infection.
q. Remove soiled gloves and discard in trash; raise side rail before leaving bedside to dispose of water and obtain fresh water.	Prevents transmission of infection. Protects patient from injury.
r. Wash back. (This follows both female and male perineal care.)	
(1) Perform hand hygiene and apply clean pair of gloves. Lower side rail. Help patient into prone or side-lying position (as applicable). Place towel lengthwise along patient's side and keep him or her covered with bath blanket.	Exposes back and buttocks for bathing while limiting exposure.
(2) Keep patient draped by sliding bath blanket over shoulders and thighs during bathing. Wash, rinse, and dry back from neck to buttocks using long, firm strokes.	Cleaning back before buttocks and anus prevents contamination of water.
(3) Next move from back to buttocks and anus. Have patient remain in prone or side-lying position and keep covered to avoid chilling. Clean anus and buttocks area.	Exposes back and buttocks for bathing while limiting exposure.
(4) If fecal material is present, enclose in fold of underpad or toilet tissue and remove with disposable wipes.	Skinfolds near buttocks and anus may contain fecal secretions that harbor microorganisms.
(5) Clean buttocks and anus, washing front to back (see illustration). Clean, rinse, and dry area thoroughly. If needed, place a clean absorbent pad under patient's buttocks. Remove contaminated gloves. Raise side rail and perform hand hygiene.	Cleaning motion prevents contaminating perineal area with fecal material or microorganisms.
(6) Return to bed and lower side rail; give a back rub.	Promotes patient relaxation. Make sure that back rub is appropriate for your patient. Back rubs are contraindicated in some cardiac patients.

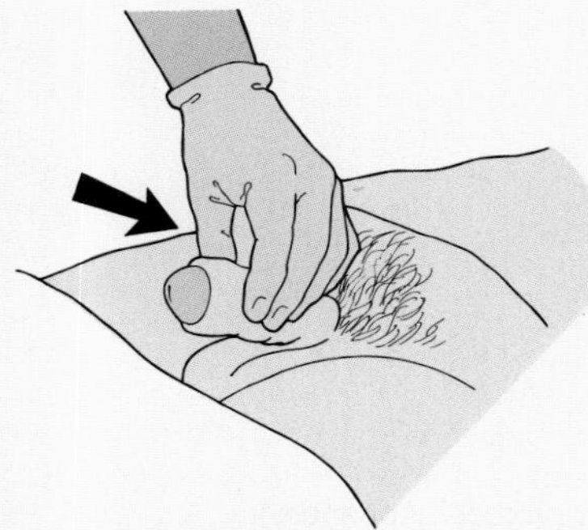

STEP 1p(3)(c) Retract foreskin.

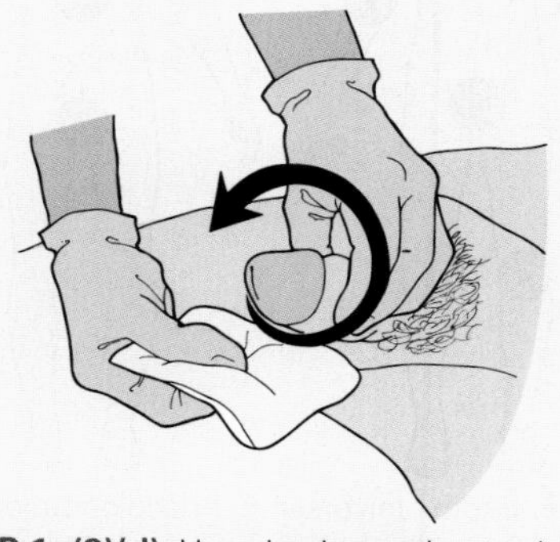

STEP 1p(3)(d) Use circular motion to cleanse tip of penis.

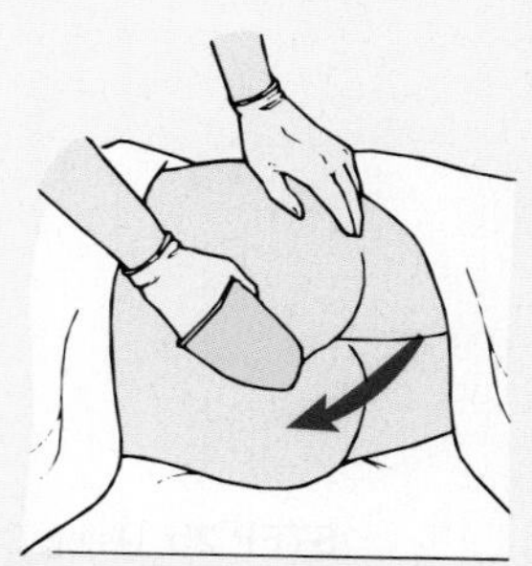

STEP 1r(5) Cleanse buttocks from front to back.

SKILL 40-1 BATHING AND PERINEAL CARE—cont'd

STEP	RATIONALE
s. Apply additional body lotion or oil to patient's skin as needed.	Moisturizing lotion prevents dry, chapped skin.
t. Remove soiled linen and place in dirty-linen bag. Clean and replace bathing equipment. Wash hands.	Reduces transmission of microorganisms.
u. Help patient dress. Comb patient's hair. Women may want to apply makeup. Help as needed.	Promotes patient's body image.
v. Make patient's bed (see Boxes 40-16 and 40-17).	Provides clean, comfortable environment.
w. Check function and position of external devices (e.g., indwelling urethral catheters, nasogastric tubes, IV lines).	Ensures that systems remain functional after bathing activities.
x. Place bed in lowest position.	Maintains patient's safety by decreasing height of bedframe from floor.
y. Replace call light and personal possessions. Leave room as clean and comfortable as possible.	Prevents transmission of infection. Clean environment promotes patient's comfort. Keeping call light and articles of care within reach promotes patient's safety.
z. Perform hand hygiene.	Reduces transmission of microorganisms.
2. Commercial bag bath or CHG cleansing pack	
a. A cleansing pack contains six to eight premoistened towels for cleaning. Warm package contents in microwave following package directions. If you are bathing patient using warm commercial or CHG cloth, check temperature of cloth before use. Gloves diminish sense of heat.	Provides warm, soothing heat. CHG reduces bacteria for up to 24 hours and prevents infection (AHRQ, 2013). Prevents burn to skin.
b. Use all six CHG cloths in the following order (see illustration): • Cloth 1: Neck, shoulders, and chest • Cloth 2: Both arms, both hands, web spaces, and axilla • Cloth 3: Abdomen and then groin/perineum • Cloth 4: Right leg, right foot, and web spaces • Cloth 5: Left leg, left foot, and web spaces • Cloth 6: Back of neck, back, and buttocks	Reduces transmission of microorganisms.
c. Firmly massage skin when using cloth. Allow skin to air dry for 30 seconds. Do not rinse. It is permissible to lightly cover patient with bath towel to prevent chilling.	Drying skin with towel removes emollient that is left behind after water/cleaner solution evaporates.
d. NOTE: If there is excessive soiling (e.g., in perineal region), use an extra cloth or conventional washcloths, soap, water, and towels.	
3. Tub bath or shower	
a. Consider patient's condition and review orders for precautions concerning his or her movement or positioning.	Prevents accidental injury to patient during bathing.
b. Schedule use of shower or tub.	Prevents unnecessary waiting, which causes fatigue.
c. Check tub or shower for cleanliness. Use cleaning techniques outlined in agency policy. Place rubber mat on tub or shower bottom. Place disposable bath mat or towel on floor in front of tub or shower.	Cleaning prevents transmission of microorganisms. Mats prevent slipping and falling.

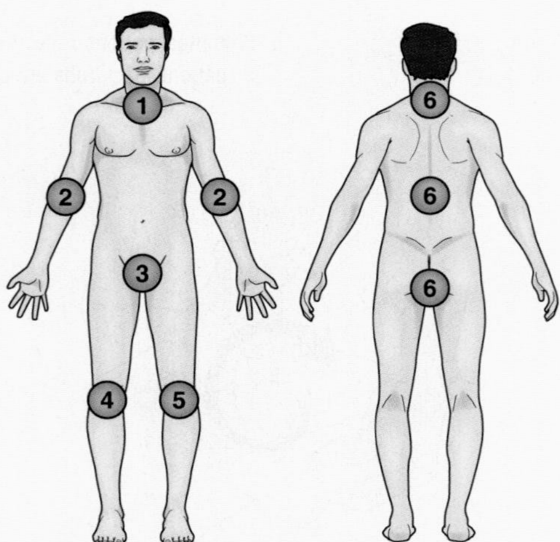

STEP 2b Using CHG bathing cloths. (From Universal ICU decolonization: *An enhanced protocol.* Appendix E: *Training and educational materials,* Rockville, MD, September 2013, Agency for Healthcare Research and Quality.)

STEP	RATIONALE
d. Collect all hygienic aids, toiletry items, and linens requested by patient. Place within easy reach of tub or shower.	Placing items close at hand prevents possible falls when patient reaches for equipment.
e. Help patient to bathroom if necessary. Have him or her wear robe and slippers.	Assistance prevents accidental falls. Wearing robe and slippers prevents chilling.
f. Demonstrate how to use call signal for assistance.	Bathrooms are equipped with signaling devices in case patient feels faint or weak or needs immediate assistance. Patients prefer privacy during bath if safety is not jeopardized.
g. Place "occupied" sign on bathroom door.	Maintains patient's privacy.
h. Fill bath tub halfway with warm water. Check temperature of bath water, have patient test water, and adjust temperature if water is too warm. Explain which faucet controls hot water. If patient is taking shower, turn shower on and adjust water temperature before he or she enters shower stall. Use shower seat or tub chair if needed (see illustration).	Adjusting water temperature prevents accidental burns. Older adults and patients with neurological alterations (e.g., diabetes, spinal cord injury) are at high risk for burn as a result of reduced sensation. Use of assistive devices facilitates bathing and minimizes physical exertion.
i. Instruct patient to use safety bars when getting in and out of tub or shower to pull cord to summon assistance (if available). Caution patient against use of bath oil in tub water.	Prevents slipping and falling. Oil causes tub surfaces to become slippery.
j. Instruct patient not to remain in tub longer than 10 or 15 minutes. Check on him or her every 5 minutes.	Prolonged exposure to warm water causes vasodilation and pooling of blood in some patients, leading to light-headedness or dizziness.
k. Return to bathroom when patient signals and knock before entering.	Provides privacy.
l. For patient who is unsteady, drain tub of water before he or she tries to get out. Place bath towel over patient's shoulders. Help patient out of tub as needed and help with drying.	Prevents accidental falls. Patient may become chilled as water drains.

CLINICAL DECISION: *Weak or unstable patients need extra assistance in getting out of a tub. Planning for additional personnel is essential before attempting to help the patient. Lift equipment may be used for transfer. See agency policy.*

STEP	RATIONALE
m. Help patient as needed with getting dressed in clean gown or pajamas, slippers, and robe. (In home setting patient may put on regular clothing.)	Maintains warmth to prevent chilling.
n. Help patient to room and comfortable position in bed or chair.	Maintains relaxation gained from bathing.
o. Clean tub or shower according to agency policy. Remove soiled linen and place in dirty-linen bag. Discard disposable equipment in proper receptacle. Place "unoccupied" sign on bathroom door. Return supplies to storage area.	Prevents transmission of infection through soiled linen and moisture.
p. Perform hand hygiene.	Reduces transfer of microorganisms.

EVALUATION

STEP	RATIONALE
1. Observe skin, paying particular attention to areas previously soiled, reddened, dry, or showing early signs of breakdown.	Techniques used during bathing leave skin clean and clear. Over time dry skin diminishes. If patient shows areas of redness, use Braden scale to measure risk for pressure ulcers (see Chapter 48).
2. Observe ROM during bath.	Measures joint mobility.

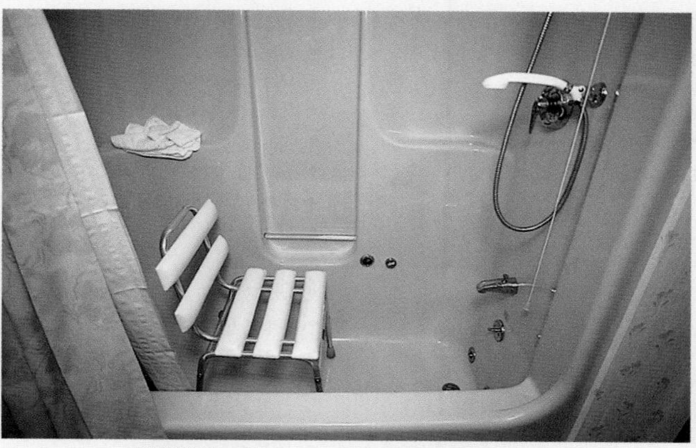

STEP 3h Shower seat for patient safety.

SKILL 40-1 BATHING AND PERINEAL CARE—cont'd

STEP	RATIONALE
3. Ask patient to rate level of comfort.	Determines patient's tolerance of bathing activities.
4. Ask patient to rate level of fatigue.	Determines patient's tolerance of bathing activities.
5. Use ***Teach Back*** to determine patient's and family's understanding of the importance of hygiene care to prevent health care–associated infection (HAI), ask the following, "We talked about why it is important for you to have a daily bath while in the hospital. Can you explain to me why we are using bathing cloths for your bath? Can you explain what you plan to do to be sure the area around your wound is bathed correctly once you get home?" Revise your instruction now or develop plan for revised patient teaching if patient is not able to teach back correctly.	Evaluates what patient and family are able to explain or demonstrate.

UNEXPECTED OUTCOMES AND RELATED INTERVENTIONS

1. Areas of excessive dryness, rashes, or pressure ulcers appear on skin.
   - Complete pressure ulcer assessment (see Chapter 48).
   - Apply moisturizing lotions or topical skin applications per agency policy.
   - Limit frequency of complete baths. It may become necessary (if patient has a sensitivity to CHG) to switch to plain soap and water.
   - Obtain special bed surface if patient is at risk for skin breakdown.
2. Patient becomes excessively tired or unable to cooperate or participate in bathing.
   - Reschedule bathing to a time when patient is more rested.
   - Provide pillow or elevate head of bed during bath for patient with breathing difficulties.
   - Notify health care provider if this is a change in patient's fatigue level.
   - Perform hygiene measures in stages between scheduled rest periods.
3. The rectum, perineum, or genital area is inflamed or swollen or has foul-smelling odor.
   - Bathe perineal area frequently enough to keep clean and dry.
   - Obtain an order for a sitz bath.
   - Apply protective barrier ointment or antiinflammatory cream.
   - Report findings to health care provider.

RECORDING AND REPORTING

- Report any skin irritations, breaks in skin, or ulcerations to nurse in charge or health care provider. These are serious in patients with altered circulation to the lower extremities.
- Report intolerance of activity to patient's nurse.
- Record procedure, amount of assistance provided, patient's participation in care, condition of skin, and any significant findings (e.g., reddened areas, breaks in skin, inflammation, ulcerations).
- Document your evaluation of patient learning.

HOME CARE CONSIDERATIONS

- Assess patient's tub and shower area for need for safety devices (e.g., grab bars, shower chair, handheld shower).
- Assess patient for the need for assistive bathing devices (e.g., long-handle sponge, mirrors, or lift equipment).

SKILL 40-2 PERFORMING NAIL AND FOOT CARE

DELEGATION CONSIDERATIONS

The skill of nail and foot care of patients *without* circulatory problems or diabetes can be delegated to nursing assistive personnel (NAP). Instruct the NAP to:

- Not clip patient's toenails.
- Use warm, not hot, water for soaking nails.
- Not soak feet of patients who have diabetes or peripheral vascular disease.
- Report any changes that may indicate inflammation or injury to tissue.

EQUIPMENT

- Washbasin
- Emesis basin
- Washcloth
- Bath or face towel
- Nail clippers
- Soft cuticle or nail brush
- Plastic orange stick
- Emery board or nail file
- Body lotion
- Disposable bath mat (optional)
- Paper towels
- Clean gloves (if drainage is present)
- Linen bag or hamper

STEP	RATIONALE
ASSESSMENT	
1. Identify patient using two identifiers (e.g., name and birthday or name and medical record number) according to agency policy.	Ensures correct patient. Complies with The Joint Commission standards and improves patient safety (TJC, 2016).
2. Perform hand hygiene. Apply clean gloves if drainage present. Inspect all surfaces of fingers, toes, feet, and nails. Pay particular attention to areas of dryness, inflammation, or cracking. Also inspect areas between toes, heels, and soles of feet.	Integrity of feet and nails determines frequency and level of hygiene required. Heels, soles, and sides of feet are prone to irritation from ill-fitting shoes.
CLINICAL DECISION: *Patients with peripheral vascular diseases or diabetes mellitus, older adults, and patients whose immune system is suppressed often require nail care from a specialist to reduce the risk of tissue injury and infection. Defer care other than washing the feet in these cases until patient has been evaluated.*	
3. Assess color and temperature of toes, feet, and fingers. Assess capillary refill of nails. Palpate radial and ulnar pulse of each hand and dorsalis pedis pulse of foot; note character of pulses (see Chapter 31).	Assesses adequacy of blood flow to extremities. Circulatory alterations often change integrity of nails and increase patient's chance of localized infection when break in skin integrity occurs.
4. Ask female patients whether they use nail polish and polish remover frequently.	Chemicals in these products cause excessive dryness.
5. Assess type of footwear worn by patient: Does patient wear socks? Are shoes tight or ill fitting? Does patient wear garters or knee-high nylons? Is footwear clean?	Types of shoes and footwear predispose patient to foot and nail problems (e.g., infection, areas of friction, ulcerations). These conditions decrease mobility and increase risk for amputation in patient with diabetes.
6. Identify patient's risk for foot or nail problems:	Certain conditions increase likelihood of foot or nail problems.
a. Older adult	Normal physiological changes such as poor vision, lack of coordination, or inability to bend over contribute to difficulty in performing foot and nail care (Touhy and Jett, 2014).
b. Diabetes mellitus, peripheral vascular disease	Vascular changes associated with diabetes mellitus reduce blood flow to peripheral tissues. Break in skin integrity places patient with diabetes at high risk for skin infection.
c. Heart failure, renal disease	Both conditions increase tissue edema, particularly in dependent areas (e.g., feet). Edema reduces blood flow to neighboring tissues.
d. Cerebrovascular accident (stroke)	Presence of residual foot or leg weakness or paralysis results in altered walking patterns. Altered gait pattern causes increased friction and pressure on feet.
7. Assess type of home remedies that patient uses for existing foot problems:	Certain preparations or applications cause more injury to soft tissue than initial foot problem.
a. Over-the-counter liquid preparations to remove corns	Liquid preparations cause burns and ulcerations.
b. Cutting corns or calluses with razor blade or scissors	Cutting corns or calluses sometimes results in infection caused by a break in skin integrity. The patient with diabetes or any patient with decreased peripheral circulation has an increased risk for infection secondary to a break in skin integrity.
c. Use of oval corn pads	Oval pads exert pressure on toes, thereby decreasing circulation to surrounding tissues.
d. Application of adhesive tape	Skin of older adult is thin and delicate and prone to tearing when adhesive tape is removed.
8. Assess patient's ability to care for nails or feet: visual alterations, fatigue, and musculoskeletal weakness.	Determines patient's ability to perform self-care and degree of assistance required from nurse.
9. Assess patient's knowledge of foot and nail care practices.	Determines patient's need for health teaching.
PLANNING	
1. Obtain health care provider's order for cutting nails if agency policy requires it.	Patients with reduced circulation are more at risk for infection. Accidental cutting of skin increases risk for infection for them.
2. Explain procedure, including need to soak feet, which requires several minutes.	Patient needs to be able to place fingers and feet in basin for 10 to 20 minutes. Some patients may become tired.
3. Collect appropriate equipment.	
IMPLEMENTATION	
1. Perform hand hygiene. Apply gloves if lesions or drainage present or anticipated.	Reduces transmission of microorganisms.
2. Arrange equipment on over-bed table.	Easy access to equipment prevents delays.
3. Provide privacy by closing curtains around bed or closing door.	Maintaining privacy reduces embarrassment and anxiety.

SKILL 40-2 PERFORMING NAIL AND FOOT CARE—cont'd

STEP	RATIONALE
4. Help ambulatory patient sit in bedside chair. Help bed-bound patient to supine position with head of bed elevated. Place disposable bath mat or towel on floor under patient's feet or place towel on bed.	Sitting in chair facilitates immersing feet in basin. Bath mat or towel protects feet from exposure to soil or microorganisms on floor; towel lessens chance of splashing water on floor or bed.
5. Fill wash basin with warm water. Test water temperature.	Warm water softens nails and thickened epidermal cells, reduces inflammation of skin, and promotes local circulation. Proper water temperature prevents burns.
6. Place basin on bath mat or towel and help patient place feet in basin. Place call light within patient's reach.	Patients with muscular weakness or tremors often have difficulty positioning feet. Maintains patient's safety.

CLINICAL DECISION: *Soaking the feet of patients with diabetes mellitus or peripheral vascular disease is not recommended. Soaking may lead to maceration (excessive softening of the skin) and drying of the skin (ADA, 2014), leading to tissue breakdown and infection.*

STEP	RATIONALE
7. Adjust over-bed table to low position and place it over patient's lap. (Patient sits in chair or lies in bed.)	Easy access prevents accidental spills.
8. Fill emesis basin with warm water and place basin on paper towels on over-bed table.	Warm water softens nails and thickened epidermal cells.
9. Instruct patient to place fingers in emesis basin and arms in comfortable position.	Prolonged positioning causes discomfort unless normal anatomical alignment is maintained.
10. Allow patient's feet and fingernails to soak for 10 to 20 minutes. Rewarm water after 10 minutes.	Softening corns, calluses, and cuticles ensures easy removal of dead cells and easy manipulation of cuticle. *Do not soak if patient has diabetes.*
11. Clean gently under fingernails with plastic stick while fingers are immersed with water in basin; then dry fingers thoroughly (see illustration).	Plastic stick removes debris under nails that harbors microorganisms. Do not use wood, which could cause splintering. Thorough drying impedes fungal growth and prevents maceration of tissues.
12. Using nail clippers, clip fingernails straight across and even with tops of fingers; check agency policy regarding clipping of nails (see illustration). Using a file, shape nails straight across. If patient has circulatory problems, do not cut nail; file nail only.	Cutting straight across prevents splitting of nail margins and formation of sharp nail spikes that irritate lateral nail margins. Filing prevents cutting nail too close to nail bed.
13. Use soft cuticle brush or nail brush around cuticles. Do not push cuticles back roughly or cut them.	Reduces incidence of inflamed cuticles.
14. Move over-bed table away from patient.	Provides easier access to feet.
15. Put on clean gloves and scrub callused areas of feet with washcloth.	Gloves prevent transmission of fungal infection. Friction removes dead skin layers.
16. Clean gently under nails with plastic orange stick. Remove feet from basin and dry thoroughly.	Nails harbor debris and dirt and are a source of potential infection from poor care habits (Ball et al., 2015).
17. Clean and trim toenails using procedures in Steps 11 and 12. Do not file corners of toenails. Check agency policy for trimming patient's nails.	Shaping corners of toenails damages tissues.
18. Apply lotion to feet and hands and help patient back to bed and into comfortable position.	Lotion lubricates dry skin by helping to retain moisture.
19. Remove clean gloves and place in receptacle. Clean and return equipment and supplies to proper place. Dispose of soiled linen in hamper. Perform hand hygiene.	Reduces transmission of infection.

EVALUATION

STEP	RATIONALE
1. Inspect nails and surrounding skin surfaces after soaking and nail trimming.	Evaluates condition of skin and nails. Allows nurse to note any remaining rough nail edges.

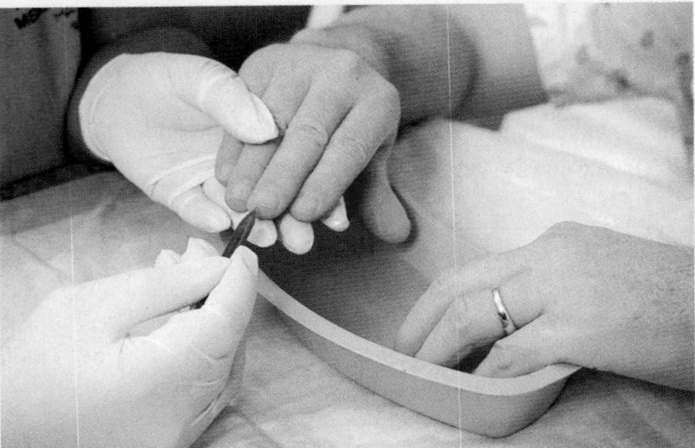

STEP 11 Clean under fingernails.

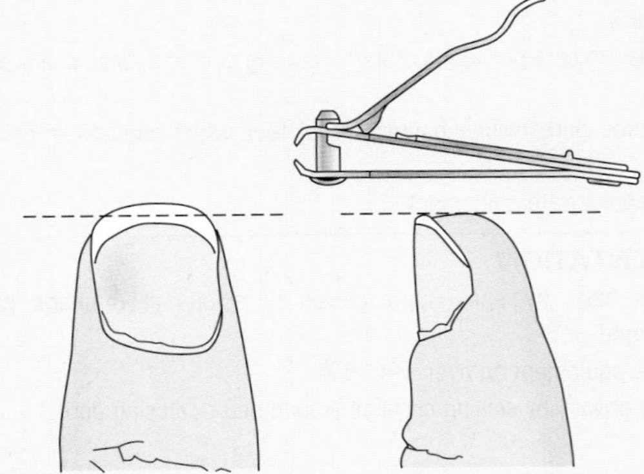

STEP 12 Use nail clippers to clip nails straight across.

STEP	RATIONALE
2. Ask patient to explain or demonstrate nail care.	Evaluates patient's level of learning foot and nail care techniques.
3. Observe patient's walk after toenail care.	Evaluates level of comfort and mobility achieved.
4. Use ***Teach Back*** to determine patient's and family's understanding of risks involved in nail care. State, "I want to be sure you know what problems you can have if you do not take care of nails correctly. Can you tell me how you might get an infection?" Revise your instruction now or develop plan for revised patient teaching if patient is not able to teach back correctly.	Evaluates what patient and family are able to explain or demonstrate.

UNEXPECTED OUTCOMES AND RELATED INTERVENTIONS

1. Cuticles and surrounding tissues are inflamed and tender to touch.
   - Repeated soakings are necessary to relieve inflammation and loosen layers of skin cells.
   - Patients with peripheral vascular disease or diabetes often require referral to a podiatrist.
   - Evaluate need for antifungal cream.
2. Localized areas of tenderness occur on feet with calluses or corns at point of friction.
   - Recommend a change in footwear is necessary.
   - Refer to a podiatrist or nurse in charge.
3. Ulcer appears between toes or other pressure areas in foot.
   - Notify physician or nurse in charge.
   - Implement appropriate pressure ulcer interventions (see Chapter 48).
   - Refer to a podiatrist or nurse certified in foot care.
   - Increase frequency of foot assessment and hygiene.

RECORDING AND REPORTING

- Record procedure and observations (e.g., breaks in skin, inflammation, ulcerations).
- Report any breaks in skin or ulcerations to nurse in charge or physician. These are serious in patients with peripheral vascular disease and illnesses in which patient's circulation is impaired. Special foot-care treatments are often necessary.
- Document your evaluation of patient learning.

HOME CARE CONSIDERATIONS

- If patient has diabetes or decreased peripheral circulation, perform procedure only after consulting with a health care provider.
- Alternative therapies: moleskin applied to areas of feet that are under friction is less likely to cause pressure than corn pads; spot adhesive bandages guard against friction, but they do not have padding to protect against pressure; wrapping small pieces of lamb's wool around toes reduces irritation of soft corns between toes.
- If patient is ambulatory, instruct to soak feet in bathtub. When patient's mobility is limited, use large basin or pan.

SKILL 40-3 PERFORMING MOUTH CARE FOR AN UNCONSCIOUS OR DEBILITATED PATIENT

DELEGATION CONSIDERATIONS

The skill of providing oral hygiene for an unconscious or debilitated patient can be delegated to nursing assistive personnel (NAP). The nurse must assess the patient's risk for aspiration by determining presence of the gag reflex. Instruct the NAP about:

- Proper positioning of patient to lessen chance of aspiration.
- Safe use of oral suction catheter for clearing oral secretions (see Skill 41-1).
- Signs of impaired integrity of oral mucosa to report to nurse.
- Reporting any bleeding of mucosa or gums, painful reaction by patient, or excessive coughing or choking to the nurse.

EQUIPMENT

- Antibacterial solution (e.g., 0.12% chlorhexidine rinse and paste) (requires health care provider's order) (Sedwick et al., 2012)
- Small pediatric soft-bristle toothbrush or toothette sponges for patients for whom brushing is contraindicated
- Tongue blade
- Pen light
- Bath towel
- Small oral airway
- Paper towels
- Emesis basin
- Water glass with cool water
- Water-soluble lip lubricant
- Small-bulb syringe or suction machine equipment (required for patients with poor or absent gag reflex)
- Clean gloves

SKILL 40-3 PERFORMING MOUTH CARE FOR AN UNCONSCIOUS OR DEBILITATED PATIENT—cont'd

STEP	RATIONALE
ASSESSMENT	
1. Identify patient using two identifiers (e.g., name and birthday or name and medical record number) according to agency policy.	Ensures correct patient. Complies with The Joint Commission standards and improves patient safety (TJC, 2016).
2. Perform hand hygiene. Apply clean gloves.	Reduces transmission of microorganisms. Gloves prevent contact with microorganisms in blood or saliva.
3. Assess patient's risk for oral hygiene problems (see Table 40-3).	Impaired level of consciousness increases likelihood of alterations in integrity of oral cavity structures and requires more frequent care. Proper oral care reduces risk of pneumonia (Nicolosi et al., 2014).
4. Test for presence of gag reflex by placing tongue blade on back half of patient's tongue. Do not place fingers in patient's mouth.	Reveals whether patient is at risk for aspiration. Helps determine need for and type of suction apparatus to have available.
5. Use tongue blade and pen light to inspect condition of oral cavity (see Chapter 31).	Determines integrity of gums, teeth, mucosa, and tongue and need for hygiene.
6. Assess patient's respirations	Baseline to determine change. Change in respirations can be early sign of aspiration.
7. Remove gloves. Perform hand hygiene.	Prevents spread of infection.
PLANNING	
1. Explain procedure to patient even if patient is unconscious.	Allows debilitated patient to anticipate procedure without anxiety. Unconscious patient may retain ability to hear.
2. Collect appropriate equipment.	Prevents interruptions during procedure.
3. Place paper towels on over-bed table and arrange equipment. If needed, turn on suction machine and connect tubing to suction catheter.	Prevents soiling of table top. Equipment prepared in advance ensures smooth, safe procedure.
4. Pull curtain around bed or close room door.	Provides privacy.
IMPLEMENTATION	
1. Unless contraindicated (e.g., head injury, neck trauma), raise bed, lower side rail, and position patient close to side of bed with head of bed raised up to 30 degrees; turn patient's head toward mattress. Patient can also be placed on side (Sims' position). (Raise side rail if necessary to leave beside.)	Turning patient's head to side allows secretions to drain from mouth instead of collecting in back of pharynx. Prevents aspiration, which could cause lower respiratory tract infection (pneumonia). Moving patient close to side of bed and raising bed facilitate proper body mechanics during skill and reduce risk for injury to nurse. Proper use of side rail protects caregiver from straining and provides for patient safety.
2. Lower side rail (if needed). Apply clean gloves.	Reduces transfer of microorganism.
3. Place towel under patient's head and emesis basin under chin.	Prevents soiling of bed linen.
4. Remove partial plate or dentures if present (see Box 40-10).	Allows for thorough cleaning of prosthetics later. Provides clearer access to oral cavity.
5. If patient is uncooperative or having difficulty keeping mouth open, insert oral airway. Insert upside down and turn airway sideways and then over tongue to keep teeth apart. Do not use force.	Prevents patient from biting down on your fingers and provides access to oral cavity.

CLINICAL DECISION: *Never place fingers into the mouth of an unconscious or debilitated patient. The normal response of the patient is to bite down.*

STEP	RATIONALE
6. Clean mouth using brush or toothette moistened with water or cleaning agent such as chlorhexidine paste (if prescribed). Clean chewing and inner tooth surfaces first. Clean outer tooth surfaces. Moisten brush with chlorhexidine rinse to rinse. Use toothette to clean roof of mouth, gums, and inside cheeks (see illustration). Gently brush tongue but avoid stimulating gag reflex. Moisten clean brush or toothette with chlorhexidine to rinse. Use bulb syringe or suction as needed to remove excess rinse.	Brushing action removes food particles between teeth and along chewing surfaces. Chlorhexidine 0.12% is an antimicrobial agent effective against dental plaque biofilms (Sedwick et al., 2012). Swabbing helps remove secretions and crusts from mucosa and moistens mucosa. Repeated rinsing removes peroxide, which is irritating to mucosa, and debris.
7. For patients without teeth, use toothette moistened in chlorhexidine rinse to clean oral cavity.	This is less traumatic to mucosa of gums.
8. Suction oral secretions as they accumulate if needed.	Suction removes secretions and fluid that collect in posterior pharynx, which if aspirated could lead to pneumonia.

CLINICAL DECISION: *Do not use a catheter to suction orally and then reuse to suction tracheally. Use separate catheters.*

STEP	RATIONALE
9. Use toothette sponge to apply thin layer of water-soluble jelly to lips (see illustration).	Water-soluble jelly lubricates lips to prevent drying and cracking.

STEP	RATIONALE
10. Inform patient that procedure is completed.	Provides meaningful stimulation to patient.
11. Remove gloves and dispose in proper receptacle. Raise side rail. Perform hand hygiene.	Prevents transmission of microorganisms to environmental surfaces (e.g., side rails, patient's linens). Reduces risk for patient injury.
12. Reposition patient comfortably, raise side rail, and return bed to original position.	Maintains patient's comfort and safety.
13. Apply clean gloves to clean equipment. Return supplies to proper place. Place soiled linen in proper receptacle.	Proper disposal of soiled equipment and handling of soiled linens prevent spread of infection.
14. Remove and discard soiled gloves. Perform hand hygiene.	Reduces transmission of microorganisms.

EVALUATION

1. Apply clean gloves and inspect oral cavity.	Determines efficacy of cleaning. Removing thick secretions reveals any underlying inflammation or lesions.
Remove gloves and dispose in proper receptacle. Perform hand hygiene.	Reduces transmission of microorganisms.
2. Ask patient if mouth feels clean.	Evaluates level of comfort.
3. Assess patient's respirations and auscultate lung sounds on an ongoing basis.	Ensures early recognition of aspiration.
4. Use ***Teach Back*** to determine family caregiver's ability to recognize early signs of aspiration. State, "Your husband is at risk for aspirating fluids down his breathing tube. I want to be sure you know the signs of aspiration. Can you identify them for me?" Revise your instruction now or develop plan for revised teaching if family member is not able to teach back correctly.	Evaluates what family caregiver is able to explain or demonstrate.

UNEXPECTED OUTCOMES AND RELATED INTERVENTIONS

1. Secretions or crusts remain on oral mucosa, tongue, or gums.
   - Increase frequency of oral hygiene.
   - Use a pediatric-size toothbrush to provide better hygiene.
2. Localized inflammation of gums or mucosa is present, or lips are cracked and inflamed.
   - Increase frequency of oral hygiene with a soft-bristle toothbrush.
   - Apply water-soluble moisturizing gel on oral mucosa and massage.
   - Apply water-soluble moisturizing gel or lubricant to lips.
3. Patient aspirates secretions.
   - Turn patient onto side immediately.
   - Suction oral airway as secretions accumulate to maintain patent airway.
   - Perform tracheal bronchial suctioning as needed.
   - Notify health care provider immediately.
   - Elevate patient's head of bed once secretions are clear to facilitate breathing.
   - Be prepared to have chest x-ray film examination ordered by health care provider.

RECORDING AND REPORTING

- Record procedure, including pertinent observations (e.g., presence of bleeding gums, dry mucosa, ulcerations, crusts on tongue) on checklist or nurses' notes.
- Report any unusual findings to nurse in charge or health care provider.
- Document your evaluation of patient learning.

HOME CARE CONSIDERATIONS

- Irrigate oral cavity with bulb syringe; patient can use a gravy baster to remove secretions.
- Give mouth care at least twice a day.
- Have caregivers demonstrate positioning patient to prevent aspiration.

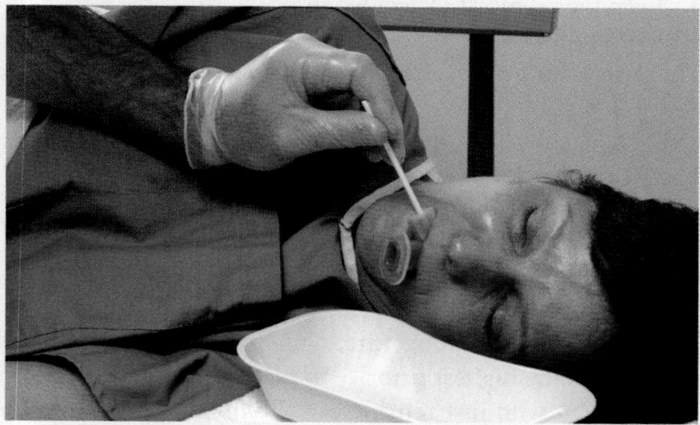

STEP 6 Using moistened toothette to rinse teeth.

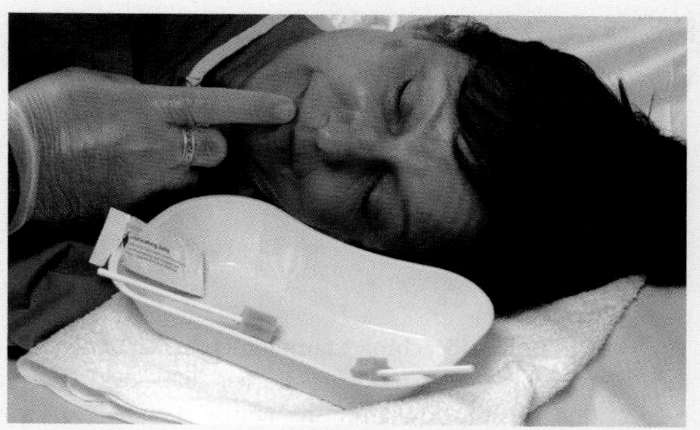

STEP 9 Application of water-soluble moisturizer to lips.

KEY POINTS

- Assess a patient's physical and cognitive ability to perform basic hygiene measures.
- Provide hygiene care according to a patient's needs and preference.
- During hygiene integrate other activities such as physical assessment, wound care, and ROM exercises.
- While providing daily hygiene needs, use teaching and communication skills to develop a caring relationship with the patient.
- Various personal, sociocultural, economic, and developmental factors influence patients' hygiene practices.
- Patients' health beliefs predict the likelihood of assuming health promotion behavior such as maintaining good hygiene.
- Reduced sensation, vascular insufficiency, and immobility place a patient at greater risk for impaired skin integrity.
- Administering symptom-relief therapies before hygiene to patients suffering symptoms such as pain or nausea better prepares them for any procedure.
- When administering oral care to unconscious patients, take measures to prevent aspiration.
- A patient's room needs to be comfortable, safe, and large enough to allow the patient and visitors to move about freely.
- Evaluation of hygiene care is made on the basis of a patient's sense of comfort, relaxation, well-being, and understanding of hygiene techniques.

CLINICAL APPLICATION QUESTIONS

Preparing for Clinical Practice

1. During Mrs. White's stay in the hospital, a student nurse prepares to provide perineal care. Mrs. White has a urinary catheter in place. The patient asks the student nurse why chlorhexidine gluconate (CHG) wipes are being used instead of soap and water. What is the response the student nurse should give Mrs. White?
2. Because the student nurse plans to use chlorhexidine gluconate (CHG) to bathe Mrs. White, list two assessments the student should conduct that are pertinent to using the antiseptic.
3. Given Mrs. White's current condition and medical history, which of the following hygiene activities pose the greatest risk for the patient? Why?
   1. Shampoo
   2. Eye care
   3. Mouth care
   4. Foot care

ⓔ *Answers to Clinical Application Questions can be found on the Evolve website.*

REVIEW QUESTIONS

Are You Ready to Test Your Nursing Knowledge?

1. What is the proper position to use for an unresponsive patient during oral care to prevent aspiration? (Select all that apply.)
   1. Prone position
   2. Sims' position
   3. Semi-Fowler's position with head to side
   4. Trendelenburg position
   5. Supine position
2. The student nurse is teaching a family member the importance of foot care for his or her mother, who has diabetes. Which safety precautions are important for the family member to know to prevent infection? (Select all that apply.)
   1. Cut nails frequently.
   2. Assess skin for redness, abrasions, and open areas daily.
   3. Soak feet in water at least 10 minutes before nail care.
   4. Apply lotion to feet daily.
   5. Clean between toes after bathing.
3. A nurse uses long firm, strokes distal to proximal while bathing a patient's legs because:
   1. It promotes venous circulation.
   2. It covers a larger area of the leg.
   3. It completes care in a timely fashion.
   4. It prevents blood clots in legs.
4. Integrity of the oral mucosa depends on salivary secretion. Which of the following factors impairs salivary secretion? (Select all that apply.)
   1. Use of cough drops
   2. Immunosuppression
   3. Radiation therapy
   4. Dehydration
   5. Presence of oral airway
5. A nurse is assigned to care for the following patients. Which of the patients is most at risk for developing skin problems and thus requiring thorough bathing and skin care?
   1. A 44-year-old female who has had removal of a breast lesion and is having her menstrual period
   2. A 56-year-old male patient who is homeless and admitted to the emergency department with malnutrition and dehydration and who has an intravenous line
   3. A 60-year-old female who experienced a stroke with right-sided paralysis and has an orthopedic brace applied to the left leg.
   4. A 70-year-old patient who has diabetes and dementia and has been incontinent of stool
6. When you are assigned to a patient who has a reduced level of consciousness and requires mouth care, which physical assessment techniques should you perform before the procedure? (Select all that apply.)
   1. Oxygen saturation
   2. Heart rate
   3. Respirations
   4. Gag reflex
   5. Response to painful stimulus
7. A nurse is listening to a student provide instruction to a patient who is having difficulty with activities needed to care for soft contact lenses. Which of the following statements by the nursing student might require some correction by the nurse?
   1. Use tap water to clean soft lenses.
   2. Follow recommendations of lens manufacturer when inserting the lenses.
   3. Keep lenses moist or wet when not worn.
   4. Use fresh solution daily when storing and disinfecting lenses.
8. The American Dental Association suggests that patients who are at risk for poor hygiene use the following interventions for oral care: (Select all that apply.)
   1. Use antimicrobial toothpaste.
   2. Brush teeth 4 times a day.
   3. Use 0.12% chlorhexidine gluconate (CHG) oral rinses.
   4. Use a soft toothbrush for oral care.
   5. Avoid cleaning the gums and tongue.
9. While planning morning care, which of the following patients would have the highest priority to receive his or her bath first?
   1. A patient who just returned to the nursing unit from a diagnostic test

2. A patient who prefers a bath in the evening when his wife visits and can help him
3. A patient who is experiencing frequent incontinent diarrheal stools and urine
4. A patient who has been awake all night because of pain 8/10

10. An 88-year-old patient comes to the medical clinic regularly. During a recent visit the nurse noticed that the patient had lost 10 lbs in 6 weeks without being on a special diet. The patient tells the nurse that he has had trouble chewing his food. Which of the following factors are normal aging changes that can affect an older adult's oral health? (Select all that apply.)
    1. Dentures do not always fit properly.
    2. Most older adults have an increase in saliva secretions.
    3. With aging the periodontal membrane becomes tighter and painful.
    4. Many older adults are edentulous, and remaining teeth are often decayed.
    5. The teeth of elderly patients are more sensitive to hot and cold.
11. A patient with a malignant brain tumor requires oral care. The patient's level of consciousness has declined, with the patient only being able to respond to voice commands. Place the following steps in the correct order for administration of oral care.
    1. If patient is uncooperative or having difficulty keeping mouth open, insert an oral airway.
    2. Raise bed, lower side rail, and position patient close to side of bed with head of bed raised up to 30 degrees.
    3. Using a brush moistened with chlorhexidine paste, clean chewing and inner tooth surfaces first.
    4. For patients without teeth, use a toothette moistened in chlorhexidine rinse to clean oral cavity.
    5. Remove partial plate or dentures if present.
    6. Gently brush tongue but avoid stimulating gag reflex.
12. The nurse delegates needed hygiene care for an elderly stroke patient. Which intervention would be appropriate for the nursing assistive personnel to accomplish during the bath?
    1. Checking distal pulses
    2. Providing range-of-motion (ROM) exercises to extremities
    3. Determining type of treatment for stage 1 pressure ulcer
    4. Changing the dressing over an intravenous site
13. The nurse observes an adult Middle Eastern patient attempting to bathe himself with only his left hand. The nurse recognizes that this behavior likely relates to:
    1. Obsessive compulsive behavior.
    2. Personal preferences.
    3. The patient's cultural norm.
    4. Controlling behaviors.
14. When a nurse delegates hygiene care for a male patient to a nursing assistive personnel, the NAP must use an electric razor to shave the patient with the following diagnosis:
    1. Congestive heart failure
    2. Pneumonia
    3. Arthritis
    4. Thrombocytopenia
15. A patient receiving chemotherapy experiences stomatitis. The nurse advises the patient to use:
    1. Community mouthwash.
    2. Alcohol-based mouth rinse.
    3. Normal saline rinses.
    4. Firm toothbrush.

Answers: 1. 2, 3; **2.** 2, 4, 5; **3.** 1; **4.** 3, 4; **5.** 4; **6.** 3, 4; **7.** 1; **8.** 1, 3, 4; **9.** 3; **10.** 1, 4; **11.** 2, 5, 1, 3, 6, 4; **12.** 2; **13.** 3; **14.** 4; **15.** 3.

Rationales for Review Questions can be found on the Evolve website.

REFERENCES

Agency for Healthcare Research and Quality (AHRQ): *Universal ICU decolonization: an enhanced protocol.* 2013, http://www.ahrq.gov/professionals/systems/hospital/universal_icu_decolonization/universal-icu-ape4.html. Accessed November 2015.

American Academy of Dermatology: *Dry skin tips for relieving.* 2014, http://www.aad.org/dermatology-a-to-z/diseases-and-treatments/a—d/dry-skin/tips. Accessed November 2015.

American Dental Association: *Cleaning teeth and gums.* 2014, http://www.mouthhealthy.org/en/standard-items/search-results?searchStr=cleaning%20teeth%20and%20gums. Accessed November 2015.

American Diabetes Association (ADA): *Foot care.* 2014, http://www.diabetes.org/living-with-diabetes/complications/foot-complications/foot-care.html. Accessed November 2015.

American Diabetes Association (ADA): *Foot complications/neuropathy.* 2015, http://www.diabetes.org/living-with-diabetes/complications/foot-complications/. Accessed November 2015.

Ball J, et al: *Seidel's Guide to physical examination,* ed 8, St Louis, 2015, Mosby.

Bandura A: *Self-efficacy: the exercise of control,* New York, 1997, Freeman.

Barnes C: Dental hygiene intervention to prevent nosocomial pneumonias, *J Evid Based Dent Pract* 14(Suppl):103, 2014.

Bulechek GM, et al: *Nursing Interventions Classification (NIC),* ed 6, St Louis, 2013, Mosby.

Burman M, et al: Linking evidenced-based nursing practice and patient-centered care through patient preferences, *Nurs Adm Q* 37(3):231, 2013.

Burns B: Oral care for older people in residential care, *Nurs Residential Care* 14(1):26, 2012.

Centers for Disease Control and Prevention (CDC): *2009 CAUTI guidelines.* 2009, http://www.cdc.gov/hicpac/cauti/002_cauti_sumORecom.html. Accessed November 2015.

Centers for Disease Control and Prevention (CDC): *Top CDC recommendations to prevent healthcare-associated infections.* 2012, http://www.cdc.gov/HAI/prevent/top-cdc-recs-prevent-hai.html. Accessed November 2015.

Centers for Disease Control and Prevention (CDC): *Parasites-lice-head lice.* 2015, http://www.cdc.gov/parasites/lice/head/treatment.html. Accessed November 2015.

Chen B, et al: Step up for foot care: addressing podiatric care needs in a sample homeless population, *J Am Podiatr Med Assoc* 104(3):269, 2014.

Cowell F, Radley K: What do we know about skin hygiene care for patients with bariatric needs? Implications for nursing practice, *J Adv Nurs* 70(3):543, 2014.

Douglas M, et al: Guidelines for implementing culturally competent nursing care, *J Transcult Nurs* 25(2):109, 2014.

Douglas L, Berry S: Developing clinical guidelines in eye care for intensive care units, *Nurs Child Young People* 23(5):14, 2011.

Garcia M, Caple C: *Evidence-based care sheet: oral care of the hospitalized patient.* Cumulative Index to Nursing and Allied Health Literature (CINAHL) Information Systems, 2014.

Genco R: Common risk factors in the management of periodontal and associated systemic diseases: the dental setting and interprofessional collaboration, *J Evidence-Based Dental Pract* 14(1):4, 2014.

Giger J: *Transcultural nursing assessment and intervention,* ed 6, St Louis, 2013, Mosby.

Green D: Start off on the right foot; provide agreed podiatry support, *Nurs Residential Care* 16(4):225, 2014.

Hardin S: Engaging families to participate in care of older critical care patients, *Crit Care Nurse* 32(3):35, 2012.

Herdman TH, Kamitsuru S, editors: *NANDA International nursing diagnoses: definitions & classification 2015-2017,* Oxford, 2014, Wiley Blackwell.

Hockenberry ML, Wilson D: *Wong's nursing care of infants and children,* ed 9, St Louis, 2013, Mosby.

Jarrett L: Prevention and management of neuropathic diabetic foot ulcers, *Nurs Stand* 28(7):55, 2013.

Kamaljit K, et al: Social beliefs and practices associated with menstrual hygiene among adolescent girls of Amritsar, Punjab, India, *JIMSA* 25(2):69, 2012.

Lewis SL, et al: *Medical-surgical nursing: assessment and management of clinical problems*, ed 9, St Louis, 2014, Mosby.

National Pressure Ulcer Advisory Panel (NPUAP): *Best practices for prevention of medical device pressure ulcers.* 2013, http://www.npuap.org/wp-content/uploads/2013/04/BestPractices-CriticalCare1.pdf. Accessed November 2015.

Pender N, et al: *Health promotion in nursing practice*, Upper Saddle River, NJ, 2011, Pearson Education.

Quality Safety Education for Nurses (QSEN): 2014, http://qsen.org/competencies/pre-licensure-ksas/. Accessed November 2015.

Rubin C, et al: Chlorhexidine gluconate to bathe or not to bathe?, *Crit Care Nurs Q* 36(2):233, 2013.

Sedwick MB, et al: Using evidence-based practice to prevent ventilator-associated pneumonia, *Crit Care Nurse* 32(4):41, 2012.

Sheridan S: The need for a comprehensive foot care model, *Nephrol Nurs J* 39(5):397, 2012.

Sokol-McKay DA: Managing diabetes with physical limitations, *Diabetes Self Manag* 30(6):8, 2013.

The Joint Commission (TJC): *2016 National Patient Safety Goals.* Oakbrook Terrace, IL, 2016, http://www.jointcommission.org/standards_information/npsgs.aspx. Accessed November 2015.

Touhy T, Jett P: *Ebersole & Hess' Toward healthy aging human needs and nursing response*, ed 8, St Louis, 2012, Mosby.

Touhy T, Jett P: *Ebersole & Hess' Gerontological nursing & healthy aging*, ed 4, St Louis, 2014, Mosby.

US Department of Health and Human Services (USDHHS): *Oral health.* 2015, http://www.healthypeople.gov/2020/topics-objectives/topic/oral-health. Accessed November 2015.

Warchol K: *Tips to reduce bathing and showering challenges: a therapist's role.* 2010, Crisis Prevention Institute, http://www.crisisprevention.com/Blog/October-2010/Tips-To-Reduce-Bathing-and-Showering-Challenges-A. Accessed November 2015.

Wiech E, et al: Simple interventions for ventilator associated pneumonia, *Nurs Crit Care* 7(3):18, 2012.

RESEARCH REFERENCES

Chan H, et al: The effects of a foot and toenail care protocol for older adults, *Geriatr Nurs* 33(6):446, 2012.

Climo M, et al: Effect of daily chlorhexidine bathing on hospital-acquired infection, *N Engl J Med* 368(6):533, 2013.

Edwards RT, et al: Cost-effectiveness of steroid (methylprednisolone) injections versus anaesthetic alone for the treatment of Morton's neuroma: economic evaluation alongside a randomised controlled trial (MortISE trial), *J Foot Ankle Res* 8:6, 2015.

Johnson D, et al: Patients' bath basins as potential sources of infection: a multicenter sampling study, *Am J Crit Care* 18(1):31, 2009.

Martori E, et al: Risk factors for denture-related oral mucosal lesions in a geriatric population, *J Prosthet Dent* 111(4):273, 2014.

Nicolosi L, et al: Effect of oral hygiene and 0.12% chlorhexidine gluconate oral rinse in preventing ventilator-associated pneumonia after cardiovascular surgery, *Respir Care* 59(4):504, 2014.

Petlin A, et al: Chlorhexidene gluconate bathing to reduce methicillin-resistant Staphylococcus Aureus, *Crit Care Nurse* 34(5):17, 2014.

Powers J, et al: Chlorhexidine bathing and microbial contamination in patient's bath basins, *Am J Crit Care* 21(5):338, 2012.

Schulz R, Sherwood PR: Physical and mental health effects of family caregiving, *Am J Nurs* 108(9 Suppl):23, 2008.

Singh J, Subhashni D: Chlorhexidine-impregnated bathing cloths reduce risk of infection, *Am J Nurs* 113(8):62, 2013.

Stolt M, et al: Nurses' foot care activities in home health care, *Geriatr Nurs* 34:491, 2013.

Werli-Alvarenga A, et al: Nursing interventions for adult intensive care patients with risk for corneal injury: a systematic review, *Int J Nurs Knowl* 24(1):25, 2013.

Zimmerman S, et al: Changing culture of mouth care: mouth care without a battle, *Gerontologist* 54(S1):25, 2014.

41

Oxygenation

OBJECTIVES

- Describe the structure and function of the cardiopulmonary system.
- Describe the physiological processes of ventilation, perfusion, and exchange of respiratory gases.
- State the process of the neural and chemical regulation of respiration.
- Differentiate among the physiological processes of cardiac output, myocardial blood flow, and coronary artery circulation.
- Describe the relationship of cardiac output, preload, afterload, contractility, and heart rate to the process of oxygenation.
- Identify the clinical outcomes occurring as a result of hyperventilation, hypoventilation, and hypoxemia.
- Identify the clinical outcomes occurring as a result of disturbances in conduction, altered cardiac output, impaired valvular function, myocardial ischemia, and impaired tissue perfusion.
- Discuss the effect of a patient's level of health, age, lifestyle, and environment on oxygenation.
- Assess for the risk factors affecting a patient's oxygenation.
- Assess for the physical manifestations that occur with alterations in oxygenation.
- Develop a plan of care for a patient with altered need for oxygenation.
- Describe nursing care interventions used to promote oxygenation in the primary care, acute care, and restorative and continuing care settings.
- Evaluate a patient's responses to oxygenation therapies.

KEY TERMS

Acute coronary syndrome (ACS), p. 878
Afterload, p. 875
Angina pectoris, p. 878
Apnea, p. 884
Atelectasis, p. 872
Bilevel positive airway pressure (BiPAP), p. 897
Bronchoscopy, p. 882
Capnography, p. 880
Cardiac output, p. 875
Cardiopulmonary rehabilitation, p. 904
Cardiopulmonary resuscitation (CPR), p. 904
Chest physiotherapy (CPT), p. 892
Chest tube, p. 898
Cheyne-Stokes respiration, p. 884
Continuous positive airway pressure (CPAP), p. 897
Diaphragmatic breathing, p. 905
Dyspnea, p. 881
Dysrhythmias, p. 878
Electrocardiogram (ECG), p. 875
Endotracheal (ET) tube, p. 896
Expiration, p. 872
Hematemesis, p. 882
Hemoptysis, p. 882
Hemothorax, p. 898
Humidification, p. 892
Hyperventilation, p. 877
Hypoventilation, p. 877
Hypovolemia, p. 876
Hypoxia, p. 877
Incentive spirometry, p. 896
Inspiration, p. 872
Invasive mechanical ventilation, p. 896
Kussmaul respiration, p. 884
Myocardial infarction (MI), p. 878
Myocardial ischemia, p. 878
Nasal cannula, p. 902
Nebulization, p. 892
Noninvasive positive-pressure ventilation (NPPV), p. 897
Normal sinus rhythm (NSR), p. 875
Orthopnea, p. 882
Perfusion, p. 872
Pneumothorax, p. 898
Postural drainage, p. 892
Preload, p. 875
Pursed-lip breathing, p. 905
Stroke volume, p. 874
Surfactant, p. 872
Tracheostomy, p. 896
Ventilation, p. 872
Ventilator-associated pneumonia (VAP), p. 897
Ventricular fibrillation, p. 878
Ventricular tachycardia, p. 878
Wheezing, p. 882

MEDIA RESOURCES

http://evolve.elsevier.com/Potter/fundamentals/

- Review Questions
- Video Clips
- Concept Map Creator
- Case Study with Questions
- Skills Performance Checklists
- Audio Glossary
- Content Updates

SCIENTIFIC KNOWLEDGE BASE

Oxygen is necessary to sustain life. The cardiac and respiratory systems supply the oxygen demands of the body. Blood is oxygenated through the mechanisms of ventilation, perfusion, and transport of respiratory gases. Neural and chemical regulators control the rate and depth of respiration in response to changing tissue oxygen demands. The cardiovascular system provides the transport mechanisms to distribute oxygen to cells and tissues of the body.

Respiratory Physiology

The exchange of respiratory gases occurs between the environment and the blood. Respiration is the exchange of oxygen and carbon dioxide during cellular metabolism. The airways of the lung transfer oxygen from the atmosphere to the alveoli, where the oxygen is exchanged for carbon dioxide. Through the alveolar capillary membrane, oxygen transfers to the blood, and carbon dioxide transfers from the blood to the alveoli. There are three steps in the process of oxygenation: ventilation, perfusion, and diffusion.

Structure and Function. Conditions or diseases that change the structure and function of the pulmonary system alter respiration. The respiratory muscles, pleural space, lungs, and alveoli (Figure 41-1) are essential for ventilation, perfusion, and exchange of respiratory gases. Gases move into and out of the lungs through pressure changes. Intrapleural pressure is negative, or less than atmospheric pressure, which is 760 mm Hg at sea level. For air to flow into the lungs, intrapleural pressure becomes more negative, setting up a pressure gradient between the atmosphere and the alveoli. The diaphragm and external intercostal muscles contract to create a negative pleural pressure and increase the size of the thorax for inspiration. Relaxation of the diaphragm and contraction of the internal intercostal muscles allow air to escape from the lungs.

Ventilation is the process of moving gases into and out of the lungs. It requires coordination of the muscular and elastic properties of the lung and thorax. The major inspiratory muscle of respiration is the diaphragm. It is innervated by the phrenic nerve, which exits the spinal cord at the fourth cervical vertebra. **Perfusion** relates to the ability of the cardiovascular system to pump oxygenated blood to the tissues and return deoxygenated blood to the lungs. Finally, diffusion is responsible for moving the respiratory gases from one area to another by concentration gradients. For the exchange of respiratory gases to occur, the organs, nerves, and muscles of respiration need to be intact; and the central nervous system needs to be able to regulate the respiratory cycle.

Work of Breathing. Work of breathing (WOB) is the effort required to expand and contract the lungs. In the healthy individual breathing is quiet and accomplished with minimal effort. The amount of energy expended on breathing depends on the rate and depth of breathing, the ease in which the lungs can be expanded (compliance), and airway resistance.

Inspiration is an active process, stimulated by chemical receptors in the aorta. **Expiration** is a passive process that depends on the elastic recoil properties of the lungs, requiring little or no muscle work. **Surfactant** is a chemical produced in the lungs to maintain the surface tension of the alveoli and keep them from collapsing. Patients with advanced chronic obstructive pulmonary disease (COPD) lose the elastic recoil of the lungs and thorax. As a result, the patient's work of breathing increases. In addition, patients with certain pulmonary diseases have decreased surfactant production and sometimes develop atelectasis. **Atelectasis** is a collapse of the alveoli that prevents normal exchange of oxygen and carbon dioxide.

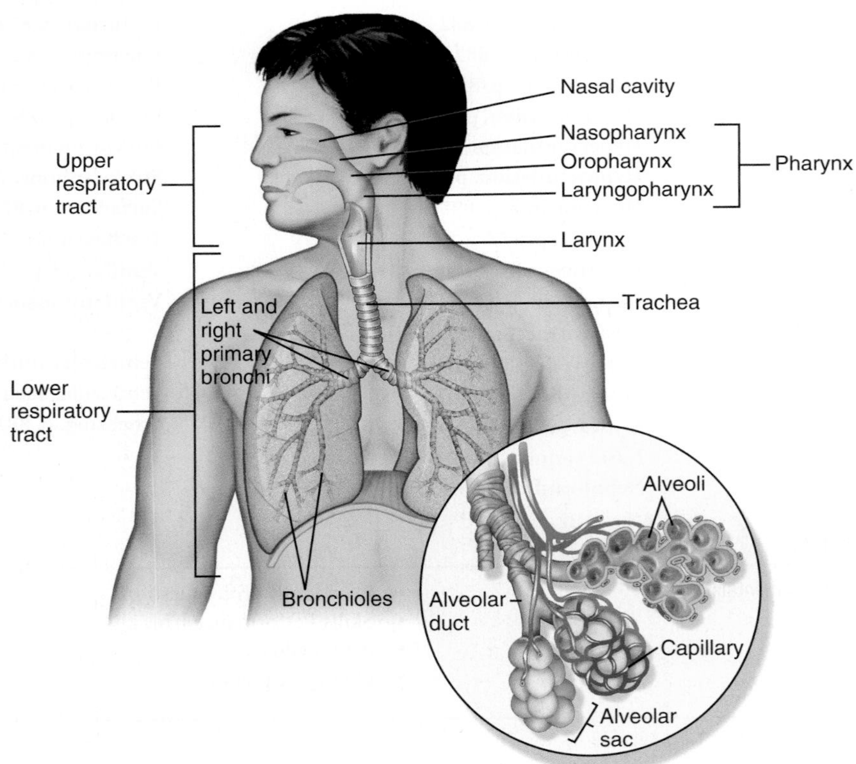

FIGURE 41-1 Structures of pulmonary system. (From Patton KT, Thibodeau GA: *Anatomy & physiology,* ed 9, St Louis, 2016, Mosby.)

Accessory muscles of respiration can increase lung volume during inspiration. Patients with COPD, especially emphysema, frequently use these muscles to increase lung volume. Prolonged use of the accessory muscles does not promote effective ventilation and causes fatigue. During assessment a patient's clavicles may elevate during inspiration, which can indicate ventilatory fatigue, air hunger, or decreased lung expansion.

Compliance is the ability of the lungs to distend or expand in response to increased intraalveolar pressure. Compliance decreases in diseases such as pulmonary edema, interstitial and pleural fibrosis, and congenital or traumatic structural abnormalities such as kyphosis or fractured ribs.

Airway resistance is the increase in pressure that occurs as the diameter of the airways decreases from mouth/nose to alveoli. Any further decrease in airway diameter by bronchoconstriction can increase airway resistance. Diseases causing airway obstruction such as asthma and tracheal edema increase airway resistance. When airway resistance increases, the amount of oxygen delivered to the alveoli decreases.

Decreased lung compliance, increased airway resistance, and the increased use of accessory muscles increase the WOB, resulting in increased energy expenditure. Therefore the body increases its metabolic rate and the need for more oxygen. The need for elimination of carbon dioxide also increases. This sequence is a vicious cycle for a patient with impaired ventilation, causing further deterioration of respiratory status and the ability to oxygenate adequately.

Lung Volumes. The normal lung values are determined by age, gender, and height. Tidal volume is the amount of air exhaled following a normal inspiration. Residual volume is the amount of air left in the alveoli after a full expiration. Forced vital capacity is the maximum amount of air that can be removed from the lungs during forced expiration (McCance and Huether, 2014). Variations in tidal volume and other lung volumes are associated with alterations in patients' health status or activity, such as pregnancy, exercise, obesity, or obstructive and restrictive conditions of the lungs.

Pulmonary Circulation. The primary function of pulmonary circulation is to move blood to and from the alveolar capillary membrane for gas exchange. Pulmonary circulation begins at the pulmonary artery, which receives poorly oxygenated mixed venous blood from the right ventricle. Blood flow through this system depends on the pumping ability of the right ventricle. The flow continues from the pulmonary artery through the pulmonary arterioles to the pulmonary capillaries, where blood comes in contact with the alveolar capillary membrane and the exchange of respiratory gases occurs. The oxygen-rich blood then circulates through the pulmonary venules and pulmonary veins, returning to the left atrium.

Respiratory Gas Exchange. Diffusion is the process for the exchange of respiratory gases in the alveoli of the lungs and the capillaries of the body tissues. Diffusion of respiratory gases occurs at the alveolar capillary membrane (Figure 41-2). The thickness of the membrane affects the rate of diffusion. Increased thickness of the membrane impedes diffusion because gases take longer to transfer across the membrane. Patients with pulmonary edema, pulmonary infiltrates, or pulmonary effusion have a thickened membrane; resulting in slow diffusion, slow exchange of respiratory gases, and decreased delivery of oxygen to tissues. Chronic diseases (e.g., emphysema), acute diseases (e.g., pneumothorax), and surgical processes (e.g., lobectomy) often alter the amount of alveolar capillary membrane surface area.

Oxygen Transport. The oxygen-transport system consists of the lungs and cardiovascular system. Delivery depends on the amount of oxygen entering the lungs (ventilation), blood flow to the lungs and tissues (perfusion), rate of diffusion, and oxygen-carrying capacity. Three things influence the capacity of the blood to carry oxygen: the amount of dissolved oxygen in the plasma, the amount of hemoglobin, and the ability of hemoglobin to bind with oxygen. Hemoglobin, which is a carrier for oxygen and carbon dioxide, transports most oxygen (approximately 97%). The hemoglobin molecule combines with oxygen to form oxyhemoglobin. The formation of oxyhemoglobin is easily reversible, allowing hemoglobin and oxygen to dissociate (deoxyhemoglobin), which frees oxygen to enter tissues.

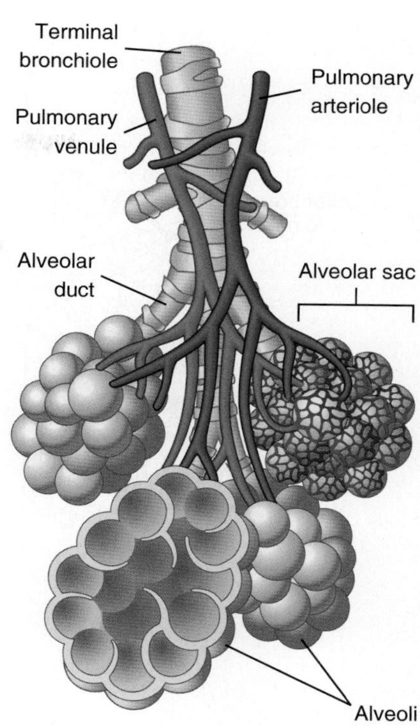

FIGURE 41-2 Alveoli at terminal end of lower airway. (From Patton KT, Thibodeau GA: *Anatomy & physiology,* ed 9, St Louis, 2016, Mosby.)

Carbon Dioxide Transport. Carbon dioxide, a product of cellular metabolism, diffuses into red blood cells and is rapidly hydrated into carbonic acid (H_2CO_3). The carbonic acid then dissociates into hydrogen (H) and bicarbonate (HCO_3^-) ions. Hemoglobin buffers the hydrogen ion, and the HCO_3^- diffuses into the plasma. Reduced hemoglobin (deoxyhemoglobin) combines with carbon dioxide, and the venous blood transports the majority of carbon dioxide back to the lungs to be exhaled.

Regulation of Respiration. Regulation of respiration is necessary to ensure sufficient oxygen intake and carbon dioxide elimination to meet the demands of the body (e.g., during exercise, infection, or pregnancy). Neural and chemical regulators control the process of respiration. Neural regulation includes the central nervous system control of respiratory rate, depth, and rhythm. The cerebral cortex regulates the voluntary control of respiration by delivering impulses to the respiratory motor neurons by way of the spinal cord. Chemical regulation maintains the appropriate rate and depth of respirations based on changes in the carbon dioxide (CO_2), oxygen (O_2), and hydrogen ion (H^+) concentration (pH) in the blood. Changes in levels of O_2, CO_2, and H (pH) stimulate the chemoreceptors located in the medulla, aortic body, and carotid body, which in turn stimulate neural regulators to adjust the rate and depth of ventilation to maintain normal arterial blood gas levels.

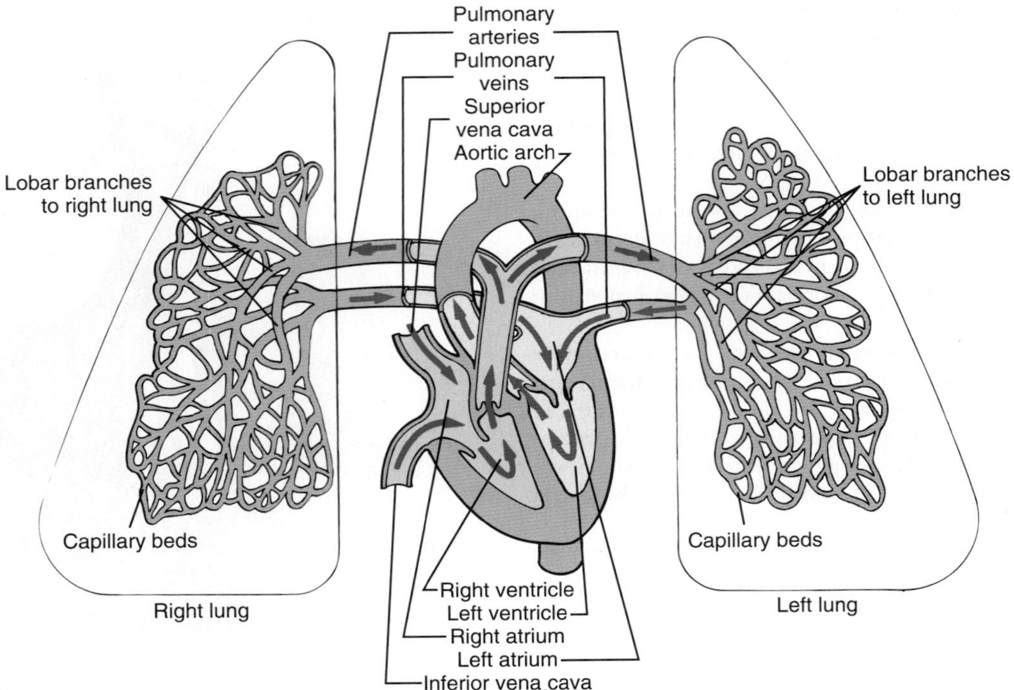

FIGURE 41-3 Schematic representation of blood flow through the heart. *Arrows* indicate direction of flow and pulmonary circulation. (From McCance KL, Huether SE: *Pathophysiology: the biologic basis for disease in adults and children,* ed 7, St Louis, 2014, Mosby.)

Cardiovascular Physiology

Cardiopulmonary physiology involves delivery of deoxygenated blood (blood high in carbon dioxide and low in oxygen) to the right side of the heart and then to the lungs, where it is oxygenated. Oxygenated blood (blood high in oxygen and low in carbon dioxide) then travels from the lungs to the left side of the heart and the tissues. The cardiac system delivers oxygen, nutrients, and other substances to the tissues and facilitates the removal of cellular metabolism waste products by way of blood flow through other body systems such as respiratory, digestive, and renal (McCance and Huether, 2014).

Structure and Function. The right ventricle pumps deoxygenated blood through the pulmonary circulation (Figure 41-3). The left ventricle pumps oxygenated blood through the systemic circulation. As blood passes through the circulatory system, there is an exchange of respiratory gases, nutrients, and waste products between the blood and the tissues.

Myocardial Pump. The pumping action of the heart is essential to oxygen delivery. There are four cardiac chambers: two atria and two ventricles. The ventricles fill with blood during diastole and empty during systole. The volume of blood ejected from the ventricles during systole is the **stroke volume**. Hemorrhage and dehydration cause a decrease in circulating blood volume and a decrease in stroke volume.

Myocardial fibers have contractile properties that allow them to stretch during filling. In a healthy heart this stretch is proportionally related to the strength of contraction. As the myocardium stretches, the strength of the subsequent contraction increases; this is known as the *Frank-Starling (Starling's) law of the heart.* In the diseased heart (cardiomyopathy or myocardial infarction [MI]) Starling's law does not apply because the increased stretch of the myocardium is beyond the physiological limits of the heart. The subsequent contractile response results in insufficient stroke volume, and blood begins to "back up" in the pulmonary (left heart failure) or systemic (right heart failure) circulation.

Myocardial Blood Flow. To maintain adequate blood flow to the pulmonary and systemic circulation, myocardial blood flow must supply sufficient oxygen and nutrients to the myocardium itself. Blood flow through the heart is unidirectional. The four heart valves ensure this forward blood flow (see Figure 41-3). During ventricular diastole the atrioventricular (mitral and tricuspid) valves open, and blood flows from the higher-pressure atria into the relaxed ventricles. As systole begins, ventricular pressure rises and the mitral and tricuspid valves close. Valve closure causes the first heart sound (S_1).

During the systolic phase the semilunar (aortic and pulmonic) valves open, and blood flows from the ventricles into the aorta and pulmonary artery. The mitral and tricuspid valves stay closed during systole so all of the blood is moved forward into the pulmonary artery and aorta. As the ventricles empty, the ventricular pressures decrease, allowing closure of the aortic and pulmonic valves. Valve closure causes the second heart sound (S_2). Some patients with valvular disease have backflow or regurgitation of blood through the incompetent valve, causing a murmur that you can hear on auscultation (see Chapter 31).

Coronary Artery Circulation. The coronary circulation is the branch of the systemic circulation that supplies the myocardium with oxygen and nutrients and removes waste. The coronary arteries fill during ventricular diastole (McCance and Huether, 2014). The left coronary artery has the most abundant blood supply and feeds the more muscular left ventricular myocardium, which does most of the work of the heart.

Systemic Circulation. The arteries of the systemic circulation deliver nutrients and oxygen to tissues, and the veins remove waste from tissues. Oxygenated blood flows from the left ventricle through the aorta and into large systemic arteries. These arteries branch into smaller arteries; then arterioles; and finally the smallest vessels, the capillaries. The exchange of respiratory gases occurs at the capillary level, where the tissues are oxygenated. The waste products exit the capillary network through venules that join to form veins. These veins become larger and form the vena cava, which carry deoxygenated blood back to the right side of the heart, where it then returns to the pulmonary circulation.

Blood Flow Regulation. The amount of blood ejected from the left ventricle each minute is the cardiac output. The normal cardiac output is 4 to 6 L/min in the healthy adult at rest. The circulating volume of blood changes according to the oxygen and metabolic needs of the body. For example, cardiac output increases during exercise, pregnancy, and fever but decreases during sleep. The following formula represents cardiac output:

$$\text{Cardiac output (CO)} = \text{Stroke volume (SV)} \times \text{Heart rate (HR)}$$

Preload, afterload, and myocardial contractility all affect stroke volume.

Preload is the amount of blood in the left ventricle at the end of diastole, often referred to as end-diastolic volume. The ventricles stretch when filling with blood. The more stretch on the ventricular muscle, the greater the contraction and the greater the stroke volume (Starling's law). In certain clinical situations, medical treatment alters preload and subsequent stroke volumes by changing the amount of circulating blood volume. For example, when treating a patient who is hemorrhaging, increased fluid therapy and replacement of blood increase circulating volume, thus increasing the preload and stroke volume, which in turn increases cardiac output. If volume is not replaced, preload, stroke volume and the subsequent cardiac output decrease.

Afterload is the resistance to left ventricular ejection. The heart works harder to overcome the resistance so blood can be fully ejected from the left ventricle. The diastolic aortic pressure is a good clinical measure of afterload. In hypertension the afterload increases, making cardiac workload also increase.

Myocardial contractility also affects stroke volume and cardiac output. Poor ventricular contraction decreases the amount of blood ejected. Injury to the myocardial muscle such as an acute MI causes a decrease in myocardial contractility. The myocardium of the older adult is stiffer with a slower ventricular filling rate and prolonged contraction time (Touhy and Jett, 2014).

Heart rate affects blood flow because of the relationship between rate and diastolic filling time. With a sustained heart rate greater than 160 beats/min, diastolic filling time decreases, decreasing stroke volume and cardiac output. The heart rate of the older adult is slow to increase under stress, but studies have found that this may be caused more by lack of conditioning than age. Exercise is beneficial in maintaining function at any age (Touhy and Jett, 2014).

Conduction System. The rhythmic relaxation and contraction of the atria and ventricles depend on continuous, organized transmission of electrical impulses. The cardiac conduction system generates and transmits these impulses (Figure 41-4).

The conduction system of the heart generates the impulses needed to initiate the electrical chain of events for a normal heartbeat. The autonomic nervous system influences the rate of impulse generation and the speed of transmission through the conductive pathway and the strength of atrial and ventricular contractions. Sympathetic and parasympathetic nerve fibers innervate all parts of the atria and ventricles and the sinoatrial (SA) and atrioventricular (AV) nodes. Sympathetic fibers increase the rate of impulse generation and speed of transmission. The parasympathetic fibers originating from the vagus nerve decrease the rate.

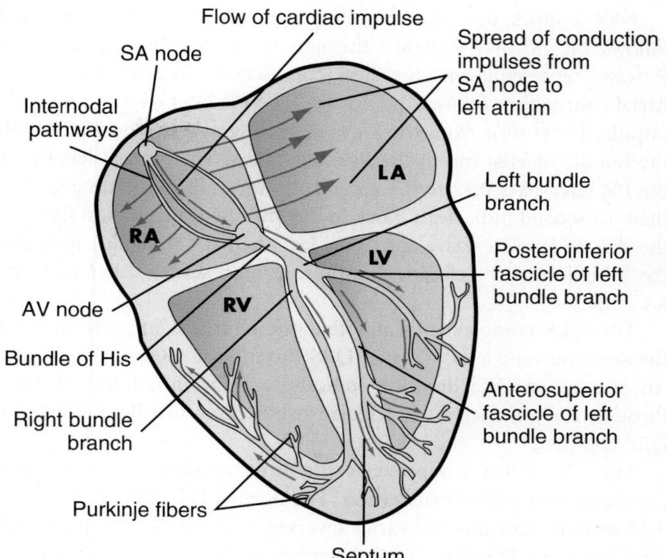

FIGURE 41-4 Conduction system of the heart. *AV,* Atrioventricular; *LA,* left atrium; *LV,* left ventricle; *RA,* right atrium; *RV,* right ventricle; *SA,* sinoatrial. (From Lewis SL et al: *Medical-surgical nursing: assessment and management of clinical problems,* ed 7, St Louis, 2007, Mosby.)

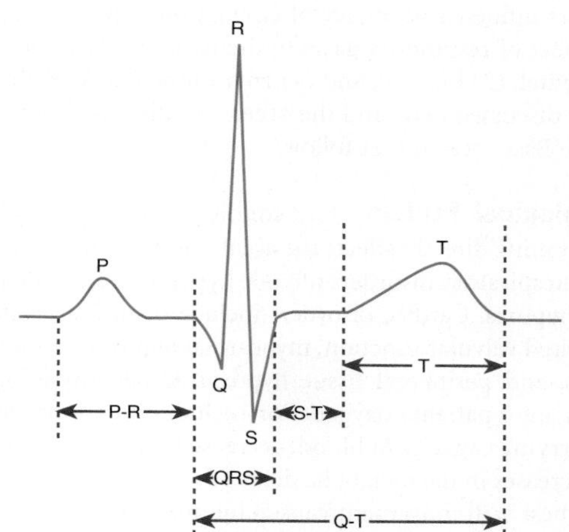

FIGURE 41-5 Normal electrocardiogram waveform.

The conduction system originates with the SA node, the "pacemaker" of the heart. The SA node is in the right atrium next to the entrance of the superior vena cava. Impulses are initiated at the SA node at an intrinsic rate of 60 to 100 cardiac action potentials per minute in an adult at rest (McCance and Huether, 2014).

The electrical impulses are transmitted through the atria along intraatrial pathways to the AV node. The AV node mediates impulses between the atria and the ventricles. It assists atrial emptying by delaying the impulse before transmitting it through the Bundle of His and the ventricular Purkinje network.

An electrocardiogram (ECG) reflects the electrical activity of the conduction system. An ECG monitors the regularity and path of the electrical impulse through the conduction system; however, it does not reflect the muscular work of the heart. The normal sequence on the ECG is called the normal sinus rhythm (NSR) (Figure 41-5).

NSR implies that the impulse originates at the SA node and follows the normal sequence through the conduction system. The P wave represents the electrical conduction through both atria. Atrial contraction follows the P wave. The PR interval represents the impulse travel time from the SA node through the AV node, through the Bundle of His, and to the Purkinje fibers. The normal length for the PR interval is 0.12 to 0.2 second. An increase in the time greater than 0.2 second indicates a block in the impulse transmission through the AV node; whereas a decrease, less than 0.12 second, indicates the initiation of the electrical impulse from a source other than the SA node.

The QRS complex indicates that the electrical impulse traveled through the ventricles. Normal QRS duration is 0.06 to 0.1 second. An increase in QRS duration indicates a delay in conduction time through the ventricles. Ventricular contraction usually follows the QRS complex.

The QT interval represents the time needed for ventricular depolarization and repolarization. The normal QT interval is 0.12 to 0.42 second. This interval varies inversely with changes in heart rate (McCance and Huether, 2014). Changes in electrolyte values such as hypocalcemia or therapy with drugs such as disopyramide (Norpace) or amiodarone (Cordarone) increase the QT interval. Shortening of the QT interval occurs with digitalis therapy, hyperkalemia, and hypercalcemia.

Factors Affecting Oxygenation

Four factors influence adequacy of circulation, ventilation, perfusion, and transport of respiratory gases to the tissues: (1) physiological, (2) developmental, (3) lifestyle, and (4) environmental. The physiological factors are discussed here, and the others are discussed in the Nursing Knowledge Base section that follows.

Physiological Factors. Any condition affecting cardiopulmonary functioning directly affects the ability of the body to meet oxygen demands. Respiratory disorders include hyperventilation, hypoventilation, and hypoxia. Cardiac disorders include disturbances in conduction, impaired valvular function, myocardial hypoxia, cardiomyopathy conditions, and peripheral tissue hypoxia. Other physiological processes affecting a patient's oxygenation include alterations affecting the oxygen-carrying capacity of blood, decreased inspired oxygen concentration, increases in the metabolic demand of the body, and alterations affecting chest wall movement caused by musculoskeletal abnormalities or neuromuscular alterations.

Decreased Oxygen-Carrying Capacity. Hemoglobin carries the majority of oxygen to tissues. Anemia and inhalation of toxic substances decrease the oxygen-carrying capacity of blood by reducing the amount of available hemoglobin to transport oxygen. Anemia (e.g., a lower-than-normal hemoglobin level) is a result of decreased hemoglobin production, increased red blood cell destruction, and/or blood loss. Patients have fatigue, decreased activity tolerance, increased breathlessness, increased heart rate, and pallor (especially seen in the conjunctiva of the eye). Oxygenation decreases as a secondary effect with anemia. The physiological response to chronic hypoxemia is the development of increased red blood cells (polycythemia). This is the adaptive response of the body to increase the amount of hemoglobin and the available oxygen-binding sites.

Carbon monoxide (CO) is the most common toxic inhalant decreasing the oxygen-carrying capacity of blood. In CO toxicity hemoglobin strongly binds with CO, creating a functional anemia. Because of the strength of the bond, CO does not easily dissociate from hemoglobin, making hemoglobin unavailable for oxygen transport.

Hypovolemia. Conditions such as shock and severe dehydration cause extracellular fluid loss and reduced circulating blood volume, or hypovolemia. Decreased circulating blood volume results in hypoxia to body tissues. With significant fluid loss, the body tries to adapt by peripheral vasoconstriction and increasing the heart rate to increase the volume of blood returned to the heart, thus increasing the cardiac output.

Decreased Inspired Oxygen Concentration. With the decline of the concentration of inspired oxygen, the oxygen-carrying capacity of the blood decreases. Decreases in the fraction of inspired oxygen concentration (FiO_2) are caused by upper or lower airway obstruction, which limits delivery of inspired oxygen to alveoli; decreased environmental oxygen (at high altitudes); or hypoventilation (occurs in drug overdoses).

Increased Metabolic Rate. Increased metabolic activity increases oxygen demand. The level of oxygenation declines when body systems are unable to meet this demand. An increased metabolic rate is normal in pregnancy, wound healing, and exercise because the body is using energy or building tissue. Most people are able to meet the increased oxygen demand and do not display signs of oxygen deprivation. Fever increases the need of tissues for oxygen; as a result carbon dioxide production increases. When fever persists, the metabolic rate remains high, and the body begins to break down protein stores. This causes muscle wasting and decreased muscle mass, including respiratory muscles such as the diaphragm and intercostal muscles.

The body attempts to adapt to the increased carbon dioxide levels by increasing the rate and depth of respiration. The patient's WOB increases, and the patient eventually displays signs and symptoms of hypoxemia. Patients with pulmonary diseases are at greater risk for hypoxemia.

Conditions Affecting Chest Wall Movement. Any condition reducing chest wall movement results in decreased ventilation. If the diaphragm does not fully descend with breathing, the volume of inspired air decreases, delivering less oxygen to the alveoli and tissues.

Pregnancy. As the fetus grows during pregnancy, the enlarging uterus pushes abdominal contents upward against the diaphragm. In the last trimester of pregnancy, the inspiratory capacity declines, resulting in dyspnea on exertion and increased fatigue.

Obesity. Patients who are morbidly obese have reduced lung volumes from the heavy lower thorax and abdomen, particularly when in the recumbent and supine positions. Many morbidly obese patients suffer from obstructive sleep apnea. Morbidly obese patients have a reduction in lung and chest wall compliance as a result of encroachment of the abdomen into the chest, increased WOB, and decreased lung volumes. In some patients an obesity-hypoventilation syndrome develops in which oxygenation is decreased and carbon dioxide is retained. The obese patient is also susceptible to atelectasis or pneumonia after surgery because the lungs do not expand fully and the lower lobes retain pulmonary secretions.

Musculoskeletal Abnormalities. Musculoskeletal impairments in the thoracic region reduce oxygenation. Such impairments result from abnormal structural configurations, trauma, muscular diseases, and diseases of the central nervous system. Abnormal structural configurations impairing oxygenation include those affecting the rib cage such as pectus excavatum and the vertebral column such as kyphosis, lordosis, or scoliosis.

Trauma. Flail chest is a condition in which multiple rib fractures cause instability in part of the chest wall. The unstable chest wall allows the lung under the injured area to contract on inspiration and bulge on expiration, resulting in hypoxia. Patients with thoracic or upper abdominal surgical incisions use shallow respirations to avoid pain, which also decreases chest wall movement. Opioids used to treat pain depress the respiratory center, further decreasing respiratory rate and chest wall expansion.

Neuromuscular Diseases. Neuromuscular diseases affect tissue oxygenation by decreasing a patient's ability to expand and contract the chest wall. Ventilation is impaired, resulting in atelectasis, hypercapnia, and hypoxemia. Examples of conditions causing hypoventilation include myasthenia gravis, Guillain-Barré syndrome, and poliomyelitis.

Central Nervous System Alterations. Diseases or trauma of the medulla oblongata and/or spinal cord result in impaired respiration. When the medulla oblongata is affected, neural regulation of respiration is impaired, and abnormal breathing patterns develop. Cervical trauma at C3 to C5 usually results in paralysis of the phrenic nerve. When the phrenic nerve is damaged, the diaphragm does not descend properly, thus reducing inspiratory lung volumes and causing hypoxemia. Spinal cord trauma below the C5 vertebra usually leaves the phrenic nerve intact but damages nerves that innervate the intercostal muscles, preventing anteroposterior chest expansion.

Influences of Chronic Disease. Oxygenation decreases as a direct consequence of chronic lung disease. Changes in the anteroposterior diameter of the chest wall (barrel chest) occur because of overuse of accessory muscles and air trapping in emphysema. The diaphragm is flattened, and the lung fields are overdistended, resulting in varying degrees of hypoxemia and/or hypercapnia (McCance and Huether, 2014).

Alterations in Respiratory Functioning

Illnesses and conditions affecting ventilation or oxygen transport cause alterations in respiratory functioning. The three primary alterations are hypoventilation, hyperventilation, and hypoxia.

The goal of ventilation is to produce a normal arterial carbon dioxide tension ($PaCO_2$) between 35 and 45 mm Hg and a normal arterial oxygen tension (PaO_2) between 80 and 100 mm Hg. Hypoventilation and hyperventilation are often determined by arterial blood gas analysis (McCance and Huether, 2014). Hypoxemia refers to a decrease in the amount of arterial oxygen. Nurses monitor arterial oxygen saturation (SpO_2) using a noninvasive oxygen saturation monitor pulse oximeter. Normally SpO_2 is greater than or equal to 95% (see Chapter 30).

Hypoventilation. Hypoventilation occurs when alveolar ventilation is inadequate to meet the oxygen demand of the body or eliminate sufficient carbon dioxide. As alveolar ventilation decreases, the body retains carbon dioxide. For example, atelectasis, a collapse of the alveoli, prevents normal exchange of oxygen and carbon dioxide. As more alveoli collapse, less of the lung is ventilated, and hypoventilation occurs.

In patients with COPD, the administration of excessive oxygen results in hypoventilation. These patients have adapted to a high carbon dioxide level so their carbon dioxide–sensitive chemoreceptors are not functioning normally. Their peripheral chemoreceptors of the aortic arch and carotid bodies are primarily sensitive to lower oxygen levels, causing increased ventilation. Because the stimulus to breathe is a decreased arterial oxygen (PaO_2) level, administration of oxygen greater than 24% to 28% (1 to 3 L/min) prevents the PaO_2 from falling to a level (60 mm Hg) that stimulates the peripheral receptors, thus destroying the stimulus to breathe (McCance and Huether, 2014). The resulting hypoventilation causes excessive retention of carbon dioxide, which can lead to respiratory acidosis and respiratory arrest.

Signs and symptoms of hypoventilation include mental status changes, dysrhythmias, and potential cardiac arrest. If untreated, the patient's status rapidly declines, leading to convulsions, unconsciousness, and death.

Hyperventilation. Hyperventilation is a state of ventilation in which the lungs remove carbon dioxide faster than it is produced by cellular metabolism. Severe anxiety, infection, drugs, or an acid-base imbalance induces hyperventilation (see Chapter 42). Acute anxiety leads to hyperventilation and exhalation of excessive amounts of carbon dioxide. Increased body temperature (fever) increases the metabolic rate, thereby increasing carbon dioxide production. The increased carbon dioxide level stimulates an increase in the patient's rate and depth of respiration, causing hyperventilation.

Hyperventilation is sometimes chemically induced. Salicylate (aspirin) poisoning and amphetamine use result in excess carbon dioxide production, stimulating the respiratory center to compensate by increasing the rate and depth of respiration. It also occurs as the body tries to compensate for metabolic acidosis. For example, the patient with diabetes in ketoacidosis produces large amounts of metabolic acids. The respiratory system tries to correct the acid-base balance by overbreathing. Ventilation increases to reduce the amount of carbon dioxide available to form carbonic acid (see Chapter 42). This can also result in the patient developing respiratory alkalosis. Signs and symptoms of hyperventilation include rapid respirations, sighing breaths, numbness and tingling of hands/feet, light-headedness, and loss of consciousness.

Hypoxia. Hypoxia is inadequate tissue oxygenation at the cellular level. It results from a deficiency in oxygen delivery or oxygen use at the cellular level. It is a life-threatening condition. Untreated it produces possibly fatal cardiac dysrhythmias.

Causes of hypoxia include (1) a decreased hemoglobin level and lowered oxygen-carrying capacity of the blood; (2) a diminished concentration of inspired oxygen, which occurs at high altitudes; (3) the inability of the tissues to extract oxygen from the blood, as with cyanide poisoning; (4) decreased diffusion of oxygen from the alveoli to the blood, as in pneumonia; (5) poor tissue perfusion with oxygenated blood, as with shock; and (6) impaired ventilation, as with multiple rib fractures or chest trauma.

The clinical signs and symptoms of hypoxia include apprehension, restlessness, inability to concentrate, decreased level of consciousness, dizziness, and behavioral changes. The patient with hypoxia is unable to lie flat and appears both fatigued and agitated. Vital sign changes include an increased pulse rate and increased rate and depth of respiration. During early stages of hypoxia the blood pressure is elevated unless the condition is caused by shock. As the hypoxia worsens, the respiratory rate declines as a result of respiratory muscle fatigue.

Cyanosis, blue discoloration of the skin and mucous membranes caused by the presence of desaturated hemoglobin in capillaries, is a late sign of hypoxia. The presence or absence of cyanosis is not a reliable measure of oxygen status. Central cyanosis, observed in the tongue, soft palate, and conjunctiva of the eye where blood flow is high, indicates hypoxemia. Peripheral cyanosis, seen in the extremities, nail beds, and earlobes, is often a result of vasoconstriction and stagnant blood flow.

Alterations in Cardiac Functioning

Illnesses and conditions affecting cardiac rhythm, strength of contraction, blood flow through the heart or to the heart muscle, and decreased peripheral circulation cause alterations in cardiac functioning. Older adults experience alterations in cardiac function as a result of calcification of the conduction pathways, thicker and stiffer heart valves caused by lipid accumulation and fibrosis, and a decrease in the number of pacemaker cells in the SA node (Touhy and Jett, 2014; Meiner, 2011).

Disturbances in Conduction. Electrical impulses that do not originate from the SA node cause conduction disturbances. These rhythm disturbances are called **dysrhythmias**, meaning a deviation from the normal sinus heart rhythm. Dysrhythmias occur as a primary conduction disturbance such as in response to ischemia; valvular abnormality; anxiety; drug toxicity; caffeine, alcohol, or tobacco use; or a complication of acid-base or electrolyte imbalance (see Chapter 42).

Dysrhythmias are classified by cardiac response and site of impulse origin. Cardiac response is tachycardia (greater than 100 beats/min), bradycardia (less than 60 beats/min), a premature (early) beat, or a blocked (delayed or absent) beat. Tachydysrhythmias and bradydysrhythmias lower cardiac output and blood pressure. Tachydysrhythmias reduce cardiac output by decreasing diastolic filling time. Bradydysrhythmias lower cardiac output because of the decreased heart rate.

Atrial fibrillation is a common dysrhythmia in older adults. The electrical impulse in the atria is chaotic and originates from multiple sites. The rhythm is irregular because of the multiple pacemaker sites and the unpredictable conduction to the ventricles. The QRS complex is normal; however, it occurs at irregular intervals. Atrial fibrillation is often described as an irregularly irregular rhythm.

Abnormal impulses originating above the ventricles are supraventricular dysrhythmias. The abnormality on the waveform is the configuration and placement of the P wave. Ventricular conduction usually remains normal, and there is a normal QRS complex.

Paroxysmal supraventricular tachycardia is a sudden, rapid onset of tachycardia originating above the AV node. It often begins and ends spontaneously. Sometimes excitement, fatigue, caffeine, smoking, or alcohol use precipitates paroxysmal supraventricular tachycardia.

Ventricular dysrhythmias represent an ectopic site of impulse formation within the ventricles. It is ectopic in that the impulse originates in the ventricle, not the SA node. The configuration of the QRS complex is usually widened and bizarre. P waves are not always present; often they are buried in the QRS complex. **Ventricular tachycardia** and **ventricular fibrillation** are life-threatening rhythms that require immediate intervention. Ventricular tachycardia is a life-threatening dysrhythmia because of the decreased cardiac output and the potential to deteriorate into ventricular fibrillation or sudden cardiac death (AHA, 2010b).

Altered Cardiac Output. Failure of the myocardium to eject sufficient volume to the systemic and pulmonary circulations occurs in heart failure. Primary coronary artery disease, cardiomyopathy, valvular disorders, and pulmonary disease lead to myocardial pump failure.

Left-Sided Heart Failure. Left-sided heart failure is an abnormal condition characterized by decreased functioning of the left ventricle. If left ventricular failure is significant, the amount of blood ejected from the left ventricle drops greatly, resulting in decreased cardiac output. Signs and symptoms include fatigue, breathlessness, dizziness, and confusion as a result of tissue hypoxia from the diminished cardiac output. As the left ventricle continues to fail, blood begins to pool in the pulmonary circulation, causing pulmonary congestion. Clinical findings include crackles in the bases of the lungs on auscultation, hypoxia, shortness of breath on exertion, cough, and paroxysmal nocturnal dyspnea.

Right-Sided Heart Failure. Right-sided heart failure results from impaired functioning of the right ventricle. It more commonly results from pulmonary disease or as a result of long-term left-sided failure. The primary pathological factor in right-sided failure is elevated pulmonary vascular resistance (PVR). As the PVR continues to rise, the right ventricle works harder, and the oxygen demand of the heart increases. As the failure continues, the amount of blood ejected from the right ventricle declines, and blood begins to "back up" in the systemic circulation. Clinically the patient has weight gain, distended neck veins, hepatomegaly and splenomegaly, and dependent peripheral edema.

Impaired Valvular Function. Valvular heart disease is an acquired or congenital disorder of a cardiac valve that causes either hardening (stenosis) or impaired closure (regurgitation) of the valves. When stenosis occurs, the flow of blood through the valves is obstructed. For example, when stenosis occurs in the semilunar valves (aortic and pulmonic valves), the adjacent ventricles have to work harder to move the ventricular blood volume beyond the stenotic valve. Over time the stenosis causes the ventricle to hypertrophy (enlarge); and, if the condition is untreated, left- or right-sided heart failure occurs. When regurgitation occurs, there is a backflow of blood into an adjacent chamber. For example, in mitral regurgitation the mitral leaflets do not close completely. When the ventricles contract, blood escapes back into the atria, causing a murmur, or "whooshing" sound (see Chapter 31).

Myocardial Ischemia. **Myocardial ischemia** results when the supply of blood to the myocardium from the coronary arteries is insufficient to meet myocardial oxygen demands. Two common outcomes of this ischemia are angina pectoris and MI.

Angina. **Angina pectoris** is a transient imbalance between myocardial oxygen supply and demand. The condition results in chest pain that is aching, sharp, tingling, or burning or that feels like pressure. Typically chest pain is left sided or substernal and often radiates to the left or both arms, the jaw, neck, and back. In some patients angina pain does not radiate. It usually lasts from 3 to 5 minutes (McCance and Huether, 2014). Patients report that it is often precipitated by activities that increase myocardial oxygen demand (e.g., eating heavy meals, exercise, or stress). It is usually relieved with rest and coronary vasodilators, the most common being a nitroglycerin preparation.

Myocardial Infarction. **Myocardial infarction (MI)** or **acute coronary syndrome (ACS)** results from sudden decreases in coronary blood flow or an increase in myocardial oxygen demand without adequate coronary perfusion. Infarction occurs because ischemia is not reversed. Cellular death occurs after 20 minutes of myocardial ischemia (McCance and Huether, 2014).

Chest pain associated with MI in men is usually described as crushing, squeezing, or stabbing. The pain is often in the left chest and sternal area; may be felt in the back; and radiates down the left arm to the neck, jaws, teeth, epigastric area, and back. It occurs at rest or exertion and lasts more than 20 minutes. Rest, position change, or sublingual nitroglycerin administration does not relieve the pain.

There is a significant difference between men and women in relation to coronary artery disease. As women get older, their risk of heart disease begins to rise (AHA, 2015). Women on average have greater blood cholesterol and triglyceride levels than men. Obesity in women is more prevalent, which also increases risk for diabetes and cardiac disease (Najafi et al., 2013). Women's symptoms differ from those of men. The most common initial symptom in women is angina, but they also present with atypical symptoms such as fatigue, indigestion, shortness of breath, and back or jaw pain. Women have twice the risk of dying within the first year after a heart attack than men (Najafi et al., 2013).

NURSING KNOWLEDGE BASE

Factors Influencing Oxygenation

In addition to physiological factors, multiple developmental, lifestyle, and environmental factors affect patients' oxygenation status. It is important to recognize these as possible risks or factors that impact their health care goals.

Developmental Factors. The developmental stage of a patient and the normal aging process affect tissue oxygenation.

Infants and Toddlers. Infants and toddlers are at risk for upper respiratory tract infections as a result of frequent exposure to other children, an immature immune system, and exposure to secondhand smoke. In addition, during the teething process some infants develop nasal congestion, which encourages bacterial growth and increases the potential for respiratory tract infection. Upper respiratory tract infections are usually not dangerous, and infants or toddlers recover with little difficulty.

School-Age Children and Adolescents. School-age children and adolescents are exposed to respiratory infections and respiratory risk factors such as cigarette smoking or secondhand smoke. A healthy child usually does not have adverse pulmonary effects from respiratory infections. The CDC (2013b) reported that 6.7% of middle school–age children and 23.3% of high school–age children currently used tobacco products, which include cigarettes, cigars, hookahs, snus, smokeless tobacco pipes, bidis, keteks, dissolvable tobacco, and electronic cigarettes (CDC, 2013b). Current cigarette smoking among middle school– and high school–age children has declined. Nine out of ten smokers started smoking by the age of 18, and 99% started by the age of 26 (CDC, 2014c). A person who starts smoking in adolescence and continues to smoke into middle age has an increased risk for cardiopulmonary disease and lung cancer.

Young and Middle-Age Adults. Young and middle-age adults are exposed to multiple cardiopulmonary risk factors: an unhealthy diet, lack of exercise, stress, over-the-counter and prescription drugs not used as intended, illegal substances, and smoking. Reducing these modifiable factors decreases a patient's risk for cardiac or pulmonary diseases. This is also the time when individuals establish lifelong habits and lifestyles. It is important to help your patients make good choices and informed decisions about their health care practices. The increased cost of cigarettes plus the state smoke-free air policies and laws that reduce smoking in public places have proven to be helpful in smoking cessation (CDC, 2012).

Older Adults. The cardiac and respiratory systems undergo changes throughout the aging process (Box 41-1). The changes are associated with calcification of the heart valves, SA node, and costal cartilages. The arterial system develops atherosclerotic plaques.

Osteoporosis leads to changes in the size and shape of the thorax. The trachea and large bronchi become enlarged from calcification of the airways. The alveoli enlarge, decreasing the surface area available for gas exchange. The number of functional cilia is reduced, causing a decrease in the effectiveness of the cough mechanism, putting the older adult at increased risk for respiratory infections (Touhy and Jett, 2014).

Lifestyle Factors. Lifestyle modifications are difficult for patients because they often have to change an enjoyable habit such as cigarette smoking or eating certain foods. Risk-factor modification is important and includes smoking cessation, weight reduction, a low-cholesterol and low-sodium diet, management of hypertension, and moderate exercise (see Chapter 6). Although it is difficult to change long-term behavior, helping patients acquire healthy behaviors reduces the risk for or slows or halts the progression of cardiopulmonary diseases.

Nutrition. Nutrition affects cardiopulmonary function in several ways. Severe obesity decreases lung expansion, and increased body weight increases tissue oxygen demands. The malnourished patient experiences respiratory muscle wasting, resulting in decreased muscle strength and respiratory excursion. Cough efficiency is reduced secondary to respiratory muscle weakness, putting a patient at risk for retention of pulmonary secretions.

Patients who are morbidly obese and/or malnourished are at risk for anemia. Diets high in carbohydrates play a role in increasing the carbon dioxide load for patients with carbon dioxide retention. As carbohydrates are metabolized, an increased load of carbon dioxide is created and excreted via the lungs.

Dietary practices also influence the prevalence of cardiovascular diseases. Cardioprotective nutrition includes diets rich in fiber; whole grains; fresh fruits and vegetables; nuts; antioxidants; lean meats, fish, and chicken; and omega-3 fatty acids. Restriction of sodium, controlling arterial pressure, and weight loss independently facilitate the regression of left ventricular hypertrophy (Katholi and Couri, 2011). Diets high in potassium prevent hypertension and help improve control in patients with hypertension. A 2000-calorie diet of fruits; vegetables; and low-fat dairy foods that are high in fiber, potassium,

BOX 41-1 FOCUS ON OLDER ADULTS

Cardiopulmonary Implication in Older Adults

- The tuberculin skin test is an unreliable indicator of tuberculosis in older patients. They frequently display false-positive or false-negative skin test reactions.
- Older patients are at an increased risk for reactivation of dormant organisms that were present for decades as a result of age-related changes in the immune system.
- The standard 5-TU Mantoux test is given and repeated or repeated with the 250-TU strength to create a booster effect. If the older patient has a positive reaction, a complete history is necessary to determine any risk factors.
- Cardiac problems differ from other chronic conditions in that, when they become acute, symptoms worsen rapidly and necessitate hospitalization, whereas other chronic conditions can be managed in the home (Touhy and Jett, 2014).
- Controlling blood pressure in older adults results in 30% fewer strokes, 64% heart failure, 23% fewer fatal cardiac events, and 21% fewer cardiac related deaths (Touhy and Jett, 2014).
- Mental status changes are often the first signs of cardiac and/or respiratory problems and often include forgetfulness and irritability.
- Changes in the older adult's cough mechanism lead to retention of pulmonary secretions, airway plugging, and atelectasis if patients do not use cough suppressants with caution.
- Age-related changes in the immune system lead to a decline of both cell-mediated and humoral immunity, resulting in an increased risk of respiratory infections (McCance and Huether, 2014).
- Changes in the thorax that occur from ossification of costal cartilage, decreased space between vertebrae, and diminished respiratory muscle strength lead to problems with chest expansion and oxygenation (Touhy and Jett, 2014).

calcium, and magnesium and low in saturated and total fat helps prevent and reduce the effects of hypertension.

Exercise. Exercise increases the metabolic activity and oxygen demand of the body. The rate and depth of respiration increase, enabling the person to inhale more oxygen and exhale excess carbon dioxide. A physical exercise program has many benefits (see Chapter 39). People who exercise for 30 to 60 minutes daily have a lower pulse rate and blood pressure, decreased cholesterol level, increased blood flow, and greater oxygen extraction by working muscles. Fully conditioned people increase oxygen consumption by 10% to 20% because of increased cardiac output and increased efficiency of the myocardial muscle (James et al, 2014).

Smoking. Cigarette smoking and secondhand smoke are associated with a number of diseases, including heart disease, COPD, and lung cancer. Cigarette smoking worsens peripheral vascular and coronary artery diseases (McCance and Huether, 2014). Inhaled nicotine causes vasoconstriction of peripheral and coronary blood vessels, increasing blood pressure and decreasing blood flow to peripheral vessels.

Women who take birth control pills and smoke cigarettes have an increased risk for thrombophlebitis and pulmonary emboli. Smoking during pregnancy can result in low-birth-weight babies, preterm delivery, and babies with reduced lung function (CDC, 2014f). Even exposure to secondhand smoke can be a risk for low-birth-weight babies, preterm delivery, and miscarriages (CDC, 2014f).

The risk of lung cancer is 10 times greater for a person who smokes than for a nonsmoker. In the United States the use of tobacco accounts for 30% of all cancer deaths. This includes 87% of the deaths from lung cancer and cancer of the larynx, mouth, pharynx, esophagus, and bladder. Smoking has been linked to the development of other cancers, including kidney, cervix, and leukemia (ACS, 2014a). Nicotine patches, gum, and lozenges are available over the counter, and nicotine nasal spray and inhalers can be obtained by prescription. Prescription drugs such as bupropion (Zyban) and varenicline (Chantix) are also available to help people quit smoking (ACS, 2014b).

Exposure to environmental tobacco smoke (secondhand smoke) increases the risk of lung cancer and cardiovascular disease in the nonsmoker. Children with parents who smoke have a higher incidence of asthma, pneumonia, and ear infections. Babies exposed to secondhand smoke are at higher risk for sudden infant death syndrome (ACS, 2014a).

Substance Abuse. Excessive use of alcohol and other drugs impairs tissue oxygenation in two ways. First, the person who chronically abuses substances often has a poor nutritional intake. With the resultant decrease in intake of iron-rich foods, hemoglobin production declines. Second, excessive use of alcohol and certain other drugs depresses the respiratory center, reducing the rate and depth of respiration and the amount of inhaled oxygen. Substance abuse by either smoking or inhaling substances such as crack cocaine or fumes from paint or glue cans causes direct injury to lung tissue that leads to permanent lung damage (Stoppler, 2013). The report on inhalant abuse (huffing) by teenagers to get a euphoric effect includes use of a wide variety of substances such as paint thinner, nail polish remover, glue, spray paint, nitrous oxide, and other common household products. Sudden death can occur from cardiac arrhythmias; or chronic abuse can cause damage to heart, lungs, and kidneys (Stoppler, 2013).

Stress. A continuous state of stress or severe anxiety increases the metabolic rate and oxygen demands of the body. The body responds to anxiety and other stresses with an increased rate and depth of respiration. Most people adapt; but some, particularly those with chronic illnesses or acute life-threatening illnesses such as an MI, cannot tolerate the oxygen demands associated with anxiety (see Chapter 38).

Environmental Factors. The environment influences oxygenation. The incidence of pulmonary disease is higher in smoggy, urban areas than in rural areas. In addition, a patient's workplace sometimes increases the risk for pulmonary disease. Occupational pollutants include asbestos, talcum powder, dust, and airborne fibers. For example, farm workers in dry regions of the southwestern United States are at risk for coccidioidomycosis, a fungal disease caused by inhalation of spores of the airborne bacterium *Coccidioides immitis.* Asbestosis is an occupational lung disease that develops after exposure to asbestos. The lung with asbestosis often has diffuse interstitial fibrosis, creating a restrictive lung disease. Patients exposed to asbestos are at risk for developing lung cancer, and this risk increases with exposure to tobacco smoke.

CRITICAL THINKING

Successful critical thinking requires a synthesis of knowledge, experience, information gathered from patients, critical thinking attitudes, and intellectual and professional standards. Clinical judgments require you to anticipate information, analyze the data, and make decisions regarding your patient's care. During assessment consider all elements that build toward making an appropriate nursing diagnosis (Figure 41-6).

To understand how alterations in oxygenation affect patients and your selection of appropriate interventions, you need to integrate knowledge from nursing and other disciplines and information gathered from patients. Critical thinking attitudes ensure that you approach patient care in a methodical and logical way. The use of professional standards such as those developed by the Centers for Disease Control and Prevention (CDC), the American Cancer Society (ACS), the American Heart Association (AHA), the American Lung Association (ALA), the American Thoracic Society (ATS), and the American Nurses Association (ANA) provide valuable guidelines for care and management of patients.

❖ NURSING PROCESS

Apply the nursing process and use a critical thinking approach in your care of patients. The nursing process provides a clinical decision-making approach for you to develop and implement an individualized plan of care.

◆ Assessment

During the assessment process, thoroughly assess each patient and critically analyze findings to ensure that you make patient-centered clinical decisions required for safe nursing care. Nursing assessment of cardiopulmonary functioning includes an in-depth history of a patient's normal and present cardiopulmonary function, past impairments in circulatory or respiratory functioning, and methods that a patient uses to optimize oxygenation. The nursing history includes a review of drug, food, and other allergies. Physical examination of a patient's cardiopulmonary status reveals the extent of existing signs and symptoms. Utilizing assessment values of pulse oximetry and capnography aids in the assessment of patients with spontaneous breathing, intubated patients, and patients requiring oxygen therapy or mechanical ventilation. Pulse oximetry provides an instant feedback about the patient's level of oxygenation. **Capnography**, also known as *end-tidal CO_2 monitoring,* provides instant information about the patient's ventilation (how effectively CO_2 is being eliminated by the pulmonary system), perfusion (how effectively CO_2 is being transported through the vascular system), and how effectively CO_2 is produced by cellular metabolism (Urden et al., 2014). Capnography is

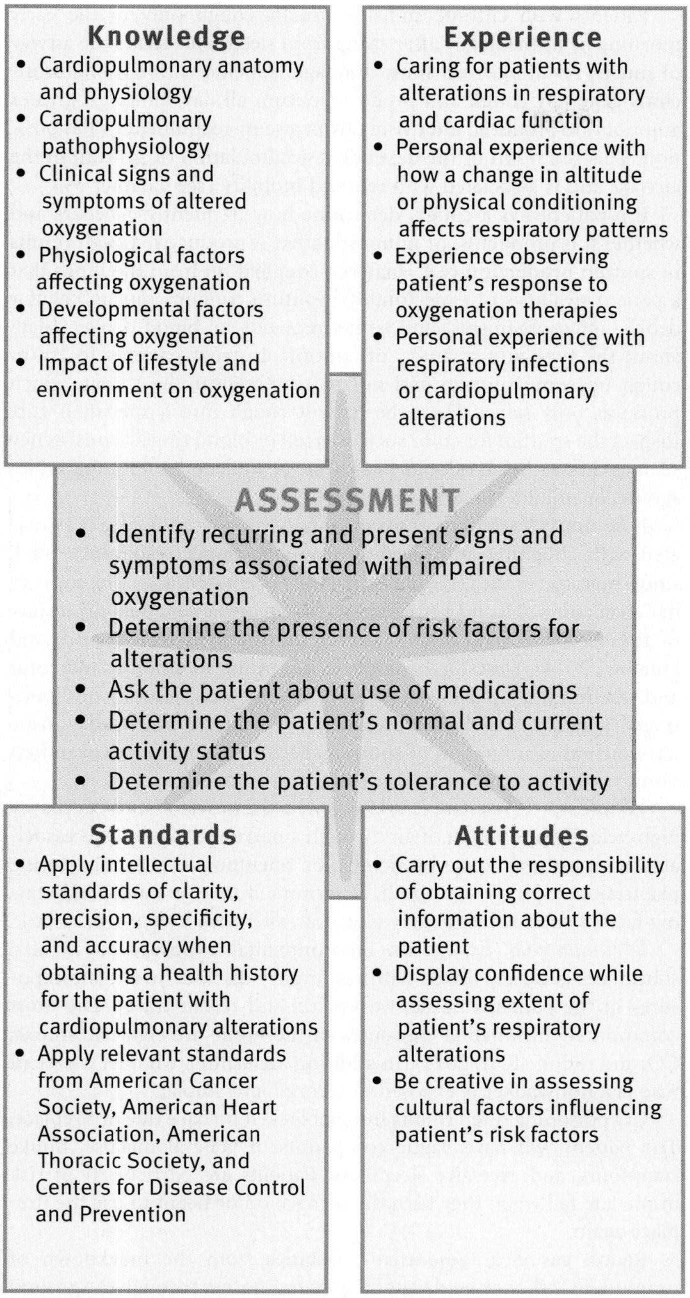

Knowledge
- Cardiopulmonary anatomy and physiology
- Cardiopulmonary pathophysiology
- Clinical signs and symptoms of altered oxygenation
- Physiological factors affecting oxygenation
- Developmental factors affecting oxygenation
- Impact of lifestyle and environment on oxygenation

Experience
- Caring for patients with alterations in respiratory and cardiac function
- Personal experience with how a change in altitude or physical conditioning affects respiratory patterns
- Experience observing patient's response to oxygenation therapies
- Personal experience with respiratory infections or cardiopulmonary alterations

ASSESSMENT
- Identify recurring and present signs and symptoms associated with impaired oxygenation
- Determine the presence of risk factors for alterations
- Ask the patient about use of medications
- Determine the patient's normal and current activity status
- Determine the patient's tolerance to activity

Standards
- Apply intellectual standards of clarity, precision, specificity, and accuracy when obtaining a health history for the patient with cardiopulmonary alterations
- Apply relevant standards from American Cancer Society, American Heart Association, American Thoracic Society, and Centers for Disease Control and Prevention

Attitudes
- Carry out the responsibility of obtaining correct information about the patient
- Display confidence while assessing extent of patient's respiratory alterations
- Be creative in assessing cultural factors influencing patient's risk factors

FIGURE 41-6 Critical thinking model for oxygenation assessment.

measured near the end of exhalation. Finally, a review of laboratory and diagnostic test results provides valuable assessment data.

Through the Patient's Eyes. Ask patients about their priorities and what they expect from their health care visit. Identifying their expectations involves patients in the decision-making process and helps them participate in their care. For example, planning a smoking cessation program for a patient who is not ready for the change is frustrating for both the patient and the nurse. Establish realistic, short-term outcomes that build to a larger goal. For example, tobacco cessation treatments are effective, but a patient needs to be willing to participate in the program and may need to use several strategies to be successful. Educating the patient on the opportunities for individual, group, or telephone counseling and identifying a social support system give more individual choices when developing the cessation plan. After this is determined, the various nicotine and nonnicotine medications for treatment of tobacco dependence can be discussed to find one that may fit the patient's lifestyle. A combination of counseling and medication is more effective than either one alone (CDC, 2014c).

Remember that your goals and expectations do not always coincide with those of your patient. By addressing a patient's concerns and expectations, you establish a relationship that addresses other health care goals and expected outcomes. Knowing your patients' mindsets and respecting their wishes goes a long way in helping them make significant beneficial lifestyle changes.

Nursing History. The nursing history focuses on the patient's ability to meet oxygen needs. The nursing history for respiratory function includes the presence of a cough, shortness of breath, dyspnea, wheezing, pain, environmental exposures, frequency of respiratory tract infections, pulmonary risk factors, past respiratory problems, current medication use, and smoking history or secondhand smoke exposure. The nursing history for cardiac function includes pain and characteristics of pain, fatigue, peripheral circulation, cardiac risk factors, and the presence of past or concurrent cardiac conditions. Ask specific questions related to cardiopulmonary disease (Box 41-2).

Pain. The presence of chest pain requires an immediate thorough assessment, including location, duration, radiation, and frequency. In addition, it is important to note any other symptoms associated with chest pain, such as nausea, diaphoresis, extreme fatigue, or weakness. Cardiac pain does not occur with respiratory variations. Chest pain in men is most often on the left side of the chest and radiates to the left arm. Chest pain in women is much less definitive and is often a sensation of breathlessness, jaw or back pain, nausea, and fatigue (AHA, 2015). Pericardial pain results from inflammation of the pericardial sac, occurs on inspiration, and does not usually radiate.

Pleuritic chest pain results from inflammation of the pleural space of the lungs; the pain is peripheral and radiates to the scapular regions. Inspiratory maneuvers such as coughing, yawning, and sighing worsen pleuritic chest pain. Patients usually describe it as knifelike, lasting from a minute to hours and always in association with inspiration.

Musculoskeletal pain is often present following exercise, rib trauma, and prolonged coughing episodes. Inspiration worsens this pain, and patients often confuse it with pleuritic chest pain.

Fatigue. Fatigue is a subjective sensation in which a patient reports a loss of endurance. Fatigue in the patient with cardiopulmonary alterations is often an early sign of a worsening of the chronic underlying process. To provide an objective measure of fatigue, ask the patient to rate it on a scale of 0 to 10, with 10 being the worst level and 0 representing no fatigue.

Dyspnea. Dyspnea is associated with hypoxia. It is the subjective sensation of difficult or uncomfortable breathing. Dyspnea is shortness of breath usually associated with exercise or excitement, but in some patients it is present without any relation to activity or exercise. It is associated with many conditions such as pulmonary diseases, cardiovascular diseases, neuromuscular conditions, and anemia. In addition, it occurs in the pregnant woman in the final months of pregnancy. Finally, environmental factors such as pollution, cold air, and smoking also cause or worsen dyspnea.

Dyspnea is associated with exaggerated respiratory effort, use of the accessory muscles of respiration, nasal flaring, and marked increases in the rate and depth of respirations. The use of a visual analogue scale (VAS) helps patients objectively assess their dyspnea. The VAS is a 100-mm vertical line. Have patients rate their dyspnea on a scale of

BOX 41-2 Nursing Assessment Questions

Nature of the Cardiopulmonary Problem
- What types of breathing problems are you having?
- Describe the problem that you're having with your heart.
- Does the problem (e.g., chest pain, rapid heart rate) occur at a specific time of the day, during or after exercise, or all the time?
- If you have chest pain, what relieves or makes the pain worse?

Signs and Symptoms
- How has your breathing pattern changed?
- Do you have sputum with coughing? Is this different in color, volume or thickness?
- If you have chest pain, does the pain occur with breathing?

Onset and Duration
- If you are having chest pain, what causes the pain and how long does it last? Is this a different type of pain?
- When did you notice your sputum change in color and amount?
- When did your coughing increase? How does this differ from your usual pattern of coughing?

Severity
- On a scale of 0 to 10, with 10 being the most severe, rate your shortness of breath.
- What helps relieve your shortness of breath?
- On a scale of 0 to 10, with 0 being no pain and 10 the most severe pain, rate your chest pain. Is the severity of your pain different today?
- What do you do for this pain?

Predisposing Factors
- Have you been exposed to a cold or flu?
- Are you taking your prescribed medications?
- Do you smoke? Have you been exposed to secondhand smoke?
- Have you been doing any unusual exercises?

Effect of Symptoms
- Do any of your symptoms affect your daily activities? If so, how?
- How do your symptoms affect your appetite, sleeping habits, and activity status?

0 to 10, with 0 equated with no dyspnea and 10 equated with the worst breathlessness a patient has experienced. The use of the VAS to assess the level of a patient's dyspnea is helpful in later evaluating interventions designed to reduce dyspnea (Pang et al., 2014).

When gathering information about a patient's sensation of dyspnea, ask the patient when the dyspnea occurs (such as with exertion, stress, or respiratory tract infection) and what improves the dyspnea (e.g., rest, inhaled medication, or position change). Determine whether the patient's dyspnea affects the ability to lie flat. **Orthopnea** is an abnormal condition in which a patient uses multiple pillows when reclining to breathe easier or sits leaning forward with arms elevated. The number of pillows used usually helps to quantify the orthopnea (e.g., two- or three-pillow orthopnea). Also ask if the patient must sleep in a recliner chair to breathe easier.

Cough. Cough is a sudden, audible expulsion of air from the lungs. The person breathes in, the glottis is partially closed, and the accessory muscles of expiration contract to expel the air forcibly. Coughing is a protective reflex to clear the trachea, bronchi, and lungs of irritants and secretions. Patients with a chronic cough tend to deny, underestimate, or minimize their coughing, often because they are so accustomed to it that they are unaware of its frequency.

Patients with chronic sinusitis usually cough only in the early morning or immediately after rising from sleep. This clears the airway of mucus resulting from sinus drainage. Patients with chronic bronchitis generally cough and produce sputum all day, although greater amounts are produced after rising from a semi-recumbent or flat position. This is a result of the dependent accumulation of sputum in the airways and is associated with reduced mobility (see Chapter 39).

If a patient has a cough, determine how frequently it occurs and whether it is productive or nonproductive. A productive cough results in sputum production (e.g., material coughed up from the lungs that a patient swallows or expectorates). Sputum contains mucus, cellular debris, microorganisms, and sometimes pus or blood. Collect data about the type and quantity of sputum. Instruct patients to try to cough up some sputum and not to simply clear the throat, which produces only saliva. Have the patient cough into a specimen cup. Inspect the sputum for color such as green or blood tinged, consistency such as thin or thick, odor such as none or foul, and amount in tablespoons or milliliters.

If **hemoptysis** (bloody sputum) is present, determine if it is associated with coughing and bleeding from the upper respiratory tract, sinus drainage, or the gastrointestinal tract (**hematemesis**). Hemoptysis has an alkaline pH, and hematemesis has an acidic pH; thus pH testing of the specimen may help to determine the source (McCance and Huether, 2014). Describe hemoptysis according to amount and color and whether it is mixed with sputum. When there is bloody or blood-tinged sputum, health care providers frequently perform diagnostic tests such as examination of sputum specimens, chest x-ray examinations, **bronchoscopy**, and other x-ray film studies.

Wheezing. **Wheezing** is a high-pitched musical sound caused by high-velocity movement of air through a narrowed airway. It is associated with asthma, acute bronchitis, or pneumonia. It occurs during inspiration, expiration, or both. Determine if there are any precipitating factors such as respiratory infection, allergens, exercise, or stress.

Environmental Exposures. Environmental exposure to inhaled substances is closely linked with respiratory disease. Investigate exposures in the patient's home, workplace, and recent travel. The most common environmental exposures in the home are cigarette smoke, CO, and radon (EPA, 2014). In addition, determine whether a patient who is a nonsmoker is exposed to secondhand smoke.

CO poisoning often results from a blocked furnace flue or fireplace. The patient will have vague complaints of general malaise, flulike symptoms, and excessive sleepiness. Patients are particularly at risk in the late fall when they turn the furnace on or begin to use the fireplace again.

Radon gas is a radioactive substance from the breakdown of uranium in soil, rock, and water that enters homes through the ground or well water. When homes are poorly ventilated, this gas is unable to escape and becomes trapped. If a patient who smokes also lives in a home with a high radon level, the risk for lung cancer is very high (EPA, 2014). Ask if there are any CO or radon detectors in the home.

Smoking. It is important to determine patients' direct and secondary exposure to tobacco. Ask about any history of smoking; include the number of years smoked and the number of packages smoked per day. This is recorded as pack-year history (packages per day × years smoked). For example, if a patient smoked two packs a day for 20 years, the patient has a 40 pack-year history. Determine exposure to secondhand smoke, because any form of tobacco exposure increases a patient's risk for cardiopulmonary diseases.

Respiratory Infections. Obtain information about a patient's frequency and duration of respiratory tract infections. Although everyone occasionally has a cold, for some people it results in bronchitis or pneumonia. On average patients have four colds per year. Determine if and when a patient has had a pneumococcal or influenza (flu) vaccine. This is especially important when assessing older adults because of their increased risk for respiratory disease (Touhy and Jett, 2014). Ask about any known exposure to tuberculosis (TB) and the date and results of the last tuberculin skin test.

Determine a patient's risk for human immunodeficiency virus (HIV) infection. Patients with a history of intravenous (IV) drug use and multiple unprotected sex partners are at risk of developing HIV infection. Patients do not always display symptoms of HIV infection until they present with *Pneumocystis carinii* pneumonia (PCP) or *Mycoplasma* pneumonia.

Allergies. Inquire about your patient's exposure to airborne allergens (e.g., pet dander or mold). The allergic response is often watery eyes, sneezing, runny nose, or respiratory symptoms such as cough or wheezing. When obtaining information, ask specific questions about the type of allergens, response to these allergens, and successful and unsuccessful relief measures. In addition, determine the effect of environmental air quality and secondhand smoke exposure on the patient's allergy and symptoms.

Safe nursing practice also includes obtaining information about food, drug, or insect sting allergies on the initial history and physical. However, always double-check this information with the patient on any subsequent assessment, especially concerning respiratory allergens.

Health Risks. Determine familial risk factors such as a family history of lung cancer or cardiovascular disease. Documentation includes blood relatives who had cardiopulmonary disease and their present level of health or age at time of death. Other family risk factors include the presence of infectious diseases, particularly TB.

Medications. Another component of the nursing history describes all medications that a patient is using. These include prescribed medications, over-the-counter medications, folk medicine, herbal medicines, alternative therapies, and illicit drugs and substances. Some of these preparations have adverse effects by themselves or because of interactions with other drugs. For example, a person using a prescribed bronchodilator drug decides to use an over-the-counter inhalant as well. Many of these contain ephedrine or *ma huang,* a natural ephedrine, which acts like epinephrine. This product reacts with the prescribed medication by potentiating or decreasing the effect of the prescribed medication. Patients taking warfarin (Coumadin) for blood thinning prolong the prothrombin time (PT)/international normalized ratio (INR) results if they are taking gingko biloba, garlic, or ginseng with the anticoagulant. The drug interaction can precipitate a life-threatening bleed.

It is important to determine if a patient uses illicit drugs. Illicit drugs, particularly inhaled opioids, which are often diluted with talcum powder, cause pulmonary disorders resulting from the irritant effect of the powder on lung tissues. Marijuana is usually smoked in the form of a joint or pipe. Marijuana smoke contains carcinogens and is an irritant to the lungs, putting users at higher risk for lung cancer and respiratory illnesses (NIDA, 2014). Cocaine is snorted through the nose, smoked, or injected. Cocaine abusers can have acute cardiovascular changes such as constricted blood vessels and increased heart rate and blood pressure, which increases the risk for heart attack or stroke. Cocaine deaths are caused by cardiac arrest and respiratory failure (NIDA, 2013).

As with all medications, assess the patient's knowledge and ability to self-administer medications correctly (see Chapter 32). Of particular importance is the assessment that the patient understands the potential side effects of medications. Patients need to recognize adverse reactions and be aware of the dangers in combining prescribed medications with over-the-counter drugs.

TABLE 41-1 Effects of Aging on Assessment Findings of the Cardiopulmonary System

Function	Pathophysiological Change	Key Clinical Findings
Heart		
Muscle contraction	Thickening of the ventricular wall, increased collagen and decreased elastin in the heart muscle	Decreased cardiac output Diminished cardiac reserve
Blood flow	Heart valves become thicker and stiffer, more often in the mitral and aortic valves	Systolic murmur
Conduction system	SA node becomes fibrotic from calcification; decrease of number of pacemaker cells in SA node	Increased PR, QRS, and Q-T intervals, decreased amplitude of QRS complex Irregular heart rhythm
Arterial vessel compliance	Calcified vessels, loss of arterial distensibility, decreased elastin in vessel walls, more tortuous vessels	Hypertension with an increase in systolic blood pressure.
Lungs		
Breathing mechanics	Decreased chest wall compliance, loss of elastic recoil Decreased respiratory muscle mass/strength	Prolonged exhalation phase Decreased vital capacity
Oxygenation	Increased ventilation/perfusion mismatch Decreased alveolar surface area Decreased carbon dioxide diffusion capacity	Decreased PaO_2 Decreased cardiac output Slightly increased $PaCO_2$
Breathing control/breathing pattern	Decreased responsiveness of central and peripheral chemoreceptors to hypoxemia and hypercapnia	Increased respiratory rate Decreased tidal volume
Lung defense mechanisms	Decreased number of cilia Decreased IgA production and humoral and cellular immunity	Decreased airway clearance Diminished cough reflex Increased risk for infection
Sleep and breathing	Decreased respiratory drive Decreased tone of upper airway muscles	Increased risk of aspiration and respiratory infection Decreased PaO_2 Snoring, obstructive sleep apnea

IgA, Immunoglobulin A; *$PaCO_2$,* arterial carbon dioxide tension; *PaO_2,* arterial oxygen tension; SA, sinoatrial.

Physical Examination. The physical examination includes assessment of the cardiopulmonary system (see Chapter 31). Give special consideration when assessing an older adult patient for changes that occur with the aging process (Table 41-1). These changes affect the patient's activity tolerance and level of fatigue or cause transient

TABLE 41-2 Inspection of Cardiopulmonary Status

Abnormality	Cause
Eyes	
Xanthelasma (yellow lipid lesions on eyelids)	Hyperlipidemia
Corneal arcus (whitish opaque ring around junction of cornea and sclera)	Abnormal finding in young to middle-age adults with hyperlipidemia (normal finding in older adults with arcus senilis)
Pale conjunctivae	Anemia
Cyanotic conjunctivae	Hypoxemia
Petechiae on conjunctivae	Fat embolus or bacterial endocarditis
Mouth and Lips	
Cyanotic mucous membranes	Decreased oxygenation (hypoxia)
Pursed-lip breathing	Associated with chronic lung disease
Neck Veins	
Distention	Associated with right-sided heart failure
Nose	
Flaring nares	Air hunger, dyspnea
Chest	
Retractions	Increased work of breathing, dyspnea
Asymmetry	Chest wall injury
Skin	
Peripheral cyanosis	Vasoconstriction and diminished blood flow
Central cyanosis	Hypoxemia
Decreased skin turgor	Dehydration (normal finding in older adults as a result of decreased skin elasticity)
Dependent edema	Associated with right- and left-sided heart failure
Periorbital edema	Associated with kidney disease
Fingertips and Nail Beds	
Cyanosis	Decreased cardiac output or hypoxia
Splinter hemorrhages	Bacterial endocarditis
Clubbing	Chronic hypoxemia

From Ball JW et al: *Seidel's Physical examination handbook,* ed 8, St Louis, 2015, Elsevier.

changes in vital signs and are not always associated with a specific cardiopulmonary disease.

Inspection. Using inspection techniques, perform a head-to-toe observation of the patient for skin and mucous membrane color, general appearance, level of consciousness, adequacy of systemic circulation, breathing patterns, and chest wall movement (Table 41-2). Investigate any abnormalities further during palpation, percussion, and auscultation.

Inspection includes observations of the nails for clubbing (see Chapter 31). Clubbed nails often occur in patients with prolonged oxygen deficiency, endocarditis, and congenital heart defects.

Observe chest wall movement for retraction (e.g., sinking in of soft tissues of the chest between the intercostal spaces) and use of accessory muscles. Elevation of a patient's clavicles reveals increased work of breathing. Also observe the patient's breathing pattern and assess for paradoxical breathing (the chest wall contracts during inspiration and expands during exhalation) or asynchronous breathing. At rest the normal adult rate is 12 to 20 regular breaths/min. Bradypnea is less than 12 breaths/min, and tachypnea is greater than 20 breaths/min (see Chapter 30). In some conditions, such as metabolic acidosis, the acidic pH stimulates an increase in rate, usually greater than 35 breaths/min, and depth of respirations (**Kussmaul respiration**) to compensate by decreasing carbon dioxide levels. **Apnea** is the absence of respirations lasting for 15 seconds or longer. **Cheyne-Stokes respiration** occurs when there is decreased blood flow or injury to the brainstem. This is an abnormal respiratory pattern with periods of apnea followed by periods of deep breathing and then shallow breathing followed by more apnea (McCance and Huether, 2014). Also note the shape of the chest wall. Conditions such as emphysema, advancing age, and COPD cause the chest to assume a rounded "barrel" shape.

Palpation. Palpation of the chest provides assessment data in several areas. It documents the type and amount of thoracic excursion; elicits any areas of tenderness; and helps to identify tactile fremitus, thrills, heaves, and the cardiac point of maximal impulse (PMI). Palpation of the extremities provides data about the peripheral circulation (e.g., the presence and quality of peripheral pulses, skin temperature, color, and capillary refill) (see Chapter 31).

Palpation of the feet and legs determines the presence or absence of peripheral edema. Patients with alterations in cardiac function such as those with heart failure or hypertension often have pedal or lower-extremity edema. Edema is graded from 1+ to 4+ depending on the depth of visible indentation after firm finger pressure (see Chapter 31).

Palpate the pulses in the neck and extremities to assess arterial blood flow (see Chapter 31). Use a scale of 0 (absent pulse) to 4 (full, bounding pulse) to describe what you feel. The normal pulse is 2; and a weak, thready pulse is 1.

Percussion. Percussion detects the presence of abnormal fluid or air in the lungs. It also determines diaphragmatic excursion.

Auscultation. Auscultation helps identify normal and abnormal heart and lung sounds (see Chapter 31). Auscultation of the cardiovascular system includes assessment for normal S_1 and S_2 sounds and the presence of abnormal S_3 and S_4 sounds (gallops), murmurs, or rubs. Identify the location, intensity, pitch, and quality of a murmur. Auscultation also identifies any bruit over the carotid, abdominal aorta, and femoral arteries.

Auscultation of lung sounds involves listening for movement of air throughout all lung fields: anterior, posterior, and lateral. Adventitious, or abnormal, breath sounds occur with collapse of a lung segment, fluid in a lung segment, or narrowing or obstruction of an airway.

Diagnostic Tests. A variety of diagnostic tests monitor cardiopulmonary functioning. Some of these screening tests involve simple blood specimens, x-ray films, or other noninvasive means. One screening mechanism is TB skin testing (Box 41-3). This is a simple test and is required for health care workers; restaurant employees; students on entry to school, teachers, and other school employees; prisoners and correctional facility employees; and residents of long-term care facilities (CDC, 2014a, 2014b).

Diagnostic testing used in the assessment and evaluation of the patient with cardiopulmonary alterations is summarized in Tables 41-3 through 41-5. When reviewing results of pulmonary function studies, be aware of expected variations in patients from different cultures.

BOX 41-3 Tuberculosis Skin Testing

- Skin testing determines whether a person is infected with *Mycobacterium tuberculosis*.
- Tuberculosis (TB) skin testing (TST) is performed by an intradermal injection of 0.1 mL of tuberculin purified protein derivative (PPD) on the inner surface of the forearm (see Chapter 32). The injection produces a pale elevation of the skin (a wheal) 6 to 10 mm in diameter. Afterward the injection site is circled, and the patient is instructed not to wash the circle off.
- Read tuberculin skin tests between 48 to 72 hours after the test. If the site is not read within 72 hours, a patient must have another skin test.
- *Positive results:* A palpable, elevated, hardened area around the injection site, caused by edema and inflammation from the antigen-antibody reaction, measured in millimeters. (See Chapter 32 for evaluation of positive results by millimeters.) People born outside the United States may have had bacille Calmette-Guérin (BCG) vaccine for TB disease, which results in a positive reaction to the TST and may complicate the treatment plan. The positive skin reaction does not indicate that the BCG vaccine provided protection against the disease (CDC, 2014e).
- Reddened flat areas are *not* positive reactions and are not measured.
- TST is less reliable in older adults (see Box 41-1) and those with an altered immune function such as a human immunodeficiency virus (HIV)–positive patient or someone receiving chemotherapy.

TABLE 41-3 Cardiopulmonary Diagnostic Blood Studies

Test and Normal Values	Interpretation
Complete Blood Count	
Normal values for a complete blood count (CBC) vary with age and gender	A CBC determines the number and type of red and white blood cells per cubic millimeter of blood.
Cardiac Enzymes	
Creatine kinase (CK): A serial CK with 50% increase between two samples 3-6 hours apart, peaking 12-24 hours after chest pain or a single CK elevation twofold is diagnostic for an acute myocardial infarction. Male normal: 55-170 units/L; female normal: 30-135 units/L	Providers use cardiac enzymes to diagnose acute myocardial infarcts.
Cardiac Troponins	
Plasma cardiac troponin I <0.03 ng/mL	Value elevates as early as 3 hours after myocardial injury. Value often remains elevated for 7-10 days.
Plasma cardiac troponin T <0.1 ng/mL	Value often remains elevated for 10-14 days.
Serum Electrolytes	
Potassium (K^+) 3.5-5 mEq/L or 3.5-5 mmol/L	Patients on diuretic therapy are at risk for hypokalemia (low potassium). Patients receiving angiotensin-converting enzyme (ACE) inhibitors are at risk for hyperkalemia (elevated potassium).
Cholesterol	
Fasting cholesterol less than 200 mg/dL or less than 5.2 mmol/L (SI units)	Contributing factors include sedentary lifestyle with intake of saturated fatty acids, familial hypercholesterolemia.
Low-density lipoproteins (LDLs) (bad cholesterol) <130 mg/dL Very low–density lipoproteins (VLDLs) 7-32 mg/dl	High LDL cholesterol (hypercholesterolemia) is caused by excessive intake of saturated fatty acids, dietary cholesterol intake, and obesity. Familial hypercholesterolemia and hyperlipidemia, hypothyroidism, nephrotic syndrome, and diabetes mellitus are also contributing factors. VLDLs are predominant carriers of triglycerides and can be converted to LDL by lipoprotein lipase. Levels in excess of 25%-50% indicate increased risk of cardiac disease.
High-density lipoproteins (HDLs) (good cholesterol) Male: >45 mg/dL; female: >55 mg/dL	Factors such as cigarette smoking, obesity, lack of regular exercise, beta-adrenergic blocking agents, genetic disorders of HDL metabolism, hypertriglyceridemia, and type 2 diabetes cause low HDL cholesterol.
Triglycerides Male: 40-160 mg/dL; female: 35-135 mg/dL	Obesity, excessive alcohol intake, diabetes mellitus, beta-adrenergic blocking agents, and familial hypertriglyceridemia cause hypertriglyceridemia.
Additional Tests	
Brain natriuretic peptide <100 pg/mL	Increased levels may be used to help determine severity of congestive heart failure.
C-reactive protein <0.1/dL or <10 mg/L	Test used by clinicians to detect inflammation if there is a high suspicion of tissue injury or infection somewhere in the body. It can also be used to evaluate a patient's risk of developing coronary artery disease and stroke.

Data from Pagana KD et al: *Mosby's diagnostic and laboratory test reference,* ed 12, St Louis, 2015, Mosby.

TABLE 41-4 Cardiac Function Diagnostic Tests

Test	Significance
Holter monitor	Portable ECG worn by a patient. The test produces a continuous ECG tracing over a period of time. Patients keep a diary of activity, noting when they experience rapid heartbeats or dizziness. Evaluation of the ECG recording along with the diary provides information about the electrical activity of the heart during activities of daily living.
ECG exercise stress test	ECG is monitored while a patient walks on a treadmill at a specified speed and duration of time. Test evaluates the cardiac response to physical stress. It is not a valuable tool for evaluation of cardiac response in women because of an increased false-positive finding.
Thallium stress test	ECG stress test with the addition of thallium-201 injected intravenously. It determines coronary blood flow changes with increased activity.
Electrophysiological study (EPS)	EPS is an invasive measure of intracardiac electrical pathways. It provides more specific information about difficult-to-treat dysrhythmias and assesses adequacy of antidysrhythmic medication.
Echocardiography	This is a noninvasive measure of heart structure and heart wall motion. It graphically demonstrates overall cardiac performance.
Scintigraphy	Scintigraphy is radionuclide angiography; used to evaluate cardiac structure, myocardial perfusion, and contractility.
Cardiac catheterization and angiography	These are used to visualize cardiac chambers, valves, the great vessels, and coronary arteries. Pressures and volumes within the four chambers of the heart are also measured.

Data from Pagana KD et al: *Mosby's diagnostic and laboratory test reference,* ed 12, St Louis, 2015, Mosby.
ECG, Electrocardiogram.

These changes are caused by structural variations in chest wall size (Box 41-4).

Invasive diagnostic tests such as a thoracentesis are painful. How painful a diagnostic procedure is depends on the patient's tolerance for pain (see Chapter 44). Reduce the patient's anxiety by explaining the thoracentesis procedure and telling him or her what to expect. Be sure that he or she understands the importance of following instructions such as taking a deep breath and holding it when requested and not coughing during the procedure. Provide appropriate pain management 30 to 60 minutes before the procedure to reduce the perception of pain. After any procedure monitor the patient for signs of changes in cardiopulmonary functioning such as sudden shortness of breath, pain, oxygen desaturation, and anxiety.

◆ Nursing Diagnosis

Based upon your assessment, you develop nursing diagnoses for patients with oxygenation alterations by clustering specific defining characteristics and identifying the related etiology (Box 41-5). The defining characteristics for diagnoses related to oxygenation can be similar. For example, both *Impaired Gas Exchange* and *Ineffective Breathing Pattern* have the defining characteristics of dyspnea and nasal flaring. A closer review of assessment findings as well as an analysis of the patient's history will help you clarify and select the correct diagnosis. For example, a patient who is a victim of trauma and has rib pain and is showing an increased respiratory rate is more likely to be suffering *Ineffective Breathing Pattern.* The clustered defining characteristics and related factor will support a problem nursing diagnosis. The clustering of risk factors will support a risk nursing diagnosis.

These nursing diagnosis examples are appropriate for the patient with alterations in oxygenation:

- *Activity Intolerance*
- *Decreased Cardiac Output*
- *Fatigue*
- *Impaired Gas Exchange*
- *Impaired Verbal Communication*
- *Ineffective Airway Clearance*
- *Ineffective Breathing Pattern*
- *Risk for Aspiration*

BOX 41-4 CULTURAL ASPECTS OF CARE

Cultural Impact on Pulmonary Diseases

The impact of pulmonary diseases on patients and their families varies among cultures. It is important to understand these variations in terms of assessing for and providing care in patients with lung diseases. In 2010, 84% of all TB reported cases occurred in racial and ethnic minorities (CDC, 2013a). Major countries of origin for foreign-born TB cases are the Philippines, Vietnam, India, and China (American Lung Association, 2010).

The cigarette smoking prevalence rate in America's youth is highest in Alaskan Natives (23.1%), followed by Caucasians (14.9%), Hispanics (9.3%), African-Americans (6.5%), and Asian Americans (4.3%). This puts them at risk for lung cancer, chronic obstructive pulmonary disease (COPD), and heart disease. African-Americans have higher mortality rates from lung cancer despite the lower smoking prevalence (American Lung Association, 2010).

Immigrant families are more likely to live in urban areas, which have high level of toxins and heavy vehicle traffic. Air pollution has been linked to cancer, asthma, and heart disease. African-American women have the highest mortality rates from asthma among all ethnic/gender groups (American Lung Association, 2010). A recent report on health care disparities found that Asian Americans over the age of 65 had the highest rates of never having received a pneumococcal vaccine, which explains why influenza and pneumonia are the fourth leading cause of death in this group (American Lung Association, 2010). Community Health Departments need to target these groups during education programs for their flu and pneumonia vaccine clinics.

Implications for Patient-Centered Care

- If your patients are foreign born, ask if they have had the bacille Calmette-Guérin (BCG) vaccine, which can cause a positive reaction to the TB skin test.
- Immunization clinics should concentrate on the underserved urban communities, especially those with large numbers of older adults. Provide TB skin testing, flu vaccines, pneumonia vaccines as needed.
- Community Health Departments need to target at risk population for flu and pneumonia vaccine clinics.
- Public health programs for those at highest risk for pulmonary diseases should focus on pollution prevention, immunizations, and smoking cessation programs.

TABLE 41-5 Ventilation and Oxygenation Diagnostic Studies

Measurement and Normal Values	Interpretation/Purpose
Arterial Blood Gases	
pH 7.35-7.45 PCO_2 35-45 mm Hg HCO_3 21-28 mEq/L PO_2 80-100 mm Hg SaO_2 saturation 95%-100% Older adult: 95% Base excess 0 ± 2 mEq/L	Provides important information for assessment of patient's respiratory and metabolic acid/base balance and adequacy of oxygenation (see Chapter 42)
Pulmonary Function Tests	
Basic ventilation studies (Pulmonary functions vary by ethnic group.)	Determines ability of the lungs to efficiently exchange oxygen and carbon dioxide Used to differentiate pulmonary obstructive from restrictive disease
Peak Expiratory Flow Rate (PEFR)	
The point of highest flow during maximal expiration (Normal in adults is based on age and body weight.)	Reflects changes in large airway sizes; an excellent predictor of overall airway resistance in a patient with asthma Daily measurement for early detection of asthma exacerbations
Bronchoscopy	
Normal airways without masses, pus, or foreign bodies	Visual examination of the tracheobronchial tree through a narrow, flexible fiberoptic bronchoscope Performed to obtain fluid, sputum, or biopsy samples; remove mucus plugs or foreign bodies
Lung Scan	
Normal lung structure without masses	Nuclear scanning test used to identify abnormal masses by size and location Identification of masses used in planning therapy and treatments Also used to find a blood clot preventing normal perfusion or ventilation ($\dot{V}/\dot{Q}$ scan)
Thoracentesis	
Surgical perforation of chest wall and pleural space with a needle to aspirate fluid for diagnostic or therapeutic purposes or to remove a specimen for biopsy; performed using aseptic technique and local anesthetic (Patient usually sits upright with the anterior thorax supported by pillows or an over-bed table.)	Specimen of plural fluid obtained for cytological examination Results may indicate an infection or neoplastic disease Identification of infection or a type of cancer important in determining a plan of care
Sputum Specimens Normal: negative	Nasal aspirate/swabs for respiratory syncytial virus, influenza
Sputum culture and sensitivity	Obtained to identify a specific microorganism or organism growing in sputum Identifies drug resistance and sensitivities to determine appropriate antibiotic therapy
Sputum for acid-fast bacillus (AFB)	Screens for presence of AFB for detection of tuberculosis by early-morning specimens on 3 consecutive days
Sputum for cytology	Obtained to identify lung cancer Differentiates type of cancer cells (small cell, oat cell, large cell)

Data from Pagana KD et al: *Mosby's diagnostic and laboratory test reference,* ed 12, St Louis, 2015, Mosby.

◆ Planning

During planning, use critical thinking skills to synthesize information from multiple sources (Figure 41-7). Critical thinking ensures that your plan of care integrates individualized patient needs. Professional standards are especially important to consider when developing a plan of care. These standards often establish scientifically proven guidelines for selecting effective nursing interventions.

Goals and Outcomes. Develop an individualized plan of care for each nursing diagnosis (see the Nursing Care Plan). Together with your patient set realistic expectations, goals, and measurable outcomes of care.

Patients with impaired oxygenation require a nursing care plan directed toward meeting actual or potential oxygenation needs. Allow patients to collaborate in setting relevant goals of care. Develop individual outcomes based on patient-centered goals. For example, for the goal of maintaining a patent airway, select specific expected outcomes for the patient, such as the following:

- Patient's lungs are clear to auscultation.
- Patient achieves bilateral lung expansion.

BOX 41-5 Nursing Diagnostic Process

Impaired Gas Exchange Related to Decreased Lung Expansion

Assessment Activities	Defining Characteristics
Ask patient or family about patient's mood, attentiveness, memory, and activity level.	Confusion Decreased activity Fatigue Irritability Restlessness Sleepiness
Observe patient's respirations for rate, rhythm, depth.	Dyspnea Nasal flaring Tachypnea Use of accessory muscles
Inspect skin and mucous membranes.	Diaphoresis Pallor Cyanosis
Auscultate chest.	Decreased respiratory excursion Abnormal, distant lung sounds

- Patient coughs productively.
- Pulse oximetry (SpO_2) is maintained or improved.

Often a patient with cardiopulmonary disease has multiple nursing diagnoses (Figure 41-8). In this case identify when goals or outcomes apply to more than one diagnosis. The presence of multiple diagnoses also makes priority setting a critical activity.

Setting Priorities. A patient's level of health, age, lifestyle, and environmental risks affect the level of tissue oxygenation. Patients with severe impairments in oxygenation frequently require nursing interventions in multiple areas. Consider which goal is the most important to achieve while the patient is in the hospital or primary care setting. For example, in an acute care setting maintaining a patent airway has a higher priority than improving the patient's exercise tolerance. The need for a patent airway is immediate; and, as the patient's level of oxygen improves, activity tolerance increases. In a second example, when caring for a patient who has an abdominal incision, pain control is a priority. In this situation controlling the patient's pain facilitates coughing and deep breathing and activity.

However, in a community-based or primary care setting, priorities often focus on smoking cessation, exercise, and/or diet modifications. Both you and the patient need to focus on the same goal and expected outcomes. In addition to individualizing each goal, be sure that the goals are realistic, have a reasonable time frame, and are attainable for the patient. In addition, be sure to respect the patient's preferences for his or her degree of active engagement in the care process. Some will choose to be very active and desire to make day-to-day decisions. Others may choose to assume a more passive role, preferring you to choose a course of action while keeping them informed.

Teamwork and Collaboration. The time spent with a patient in any setting is limited. Therefore collaborate with family members, colleagues, and other health care specialists to achieve the established goals and expected outcomes. Some patients need to improve their exercise and activity tolerance; for other patients continuing care involves participating in a community-based cardiopulmonary rehabilitation program. Finally, some patients need home physical therapy.

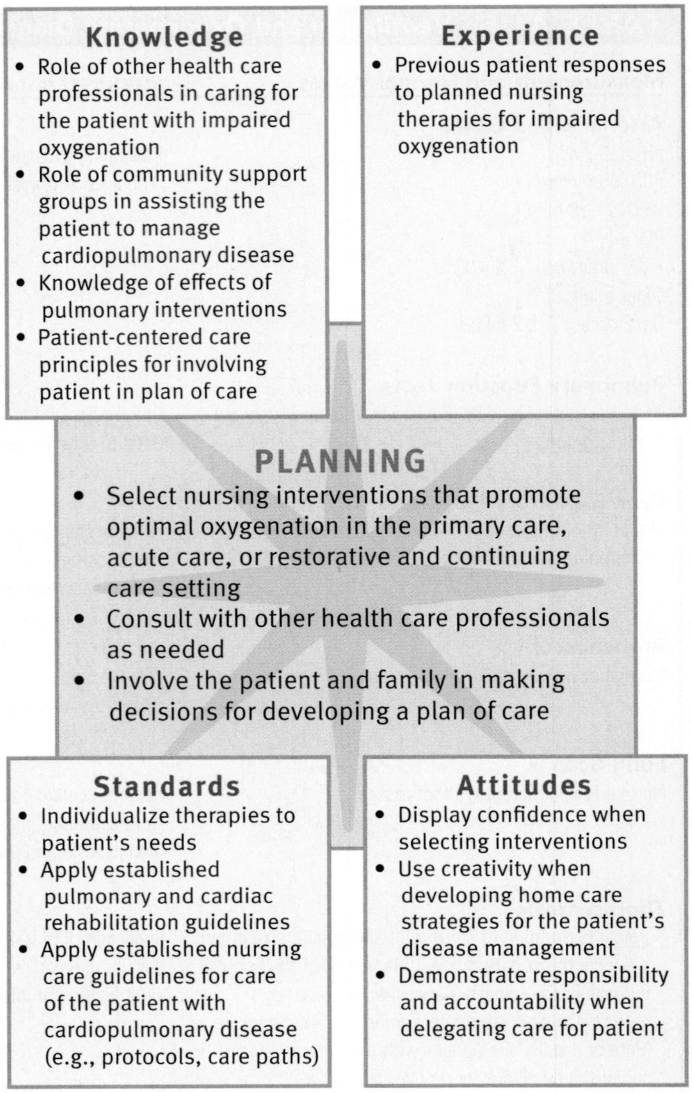

Knowledge
- Role of other health care professionals in caring for the patient with impaired oxygenation
- Role of community support groups in assisting the patient to manage cardiopulmonary disease
- Knowledge of effects of pulmonary interventions
- Patient-centered care principles for involving patient in plan of care

Experience
- Previous patient responses to planned nursing therapies for impaired oxygenation

PLANNING
- Select nursing interventions that promote optimal oxygenation in the primary care, acute care, or restorative and continuing care setting
- Consult with other health care professionals as needed
- Involve the patient and family in making decisions for developing a plan of care

Standards
- Individualize therapies to patient's needs
- Apply established pulmonary and cardiac rehabilitation guidelines
- Apply established nursing care guidelines for care of the patient with cardiopulmonary disease (e.g., protocols, care paths)

Attitudes
- Display confidence when selecting interventions
- Use creativity when developing home care strategies for the patient's disease management
- Demonstrate responsibility and accountability when delegating care for patient

FIGURE 41-7 Critical thinking model for oxygenation planning.

Collaboration with physical therapists, nutritionists, and community-based nurses is valuable for patients with heart failure or chronic lung conditions. These professionals work with patients and use resources in the community to assist them in attaining and maintaining the highest possible level of wellness. In addition, professionals identify community resources and support systems for both the patient and family in preventing and managing symptoms related to cardiopulmonary diseases. Communicating among everyone on the patient's health care team and recognizing everyone's contributions in achieving the health care goals for the patient are imperative.

◆ Implementation

There are interventions for promoting and maintaining adequate oxygenation across the continuum of care. As a nurse, you will be responsible for independent interventions such as positioning, coughing techniques, and health education for disease prevention. In addition, you will provide physician-initiated interventions such as oxygen therapy, lung inflation techniques, and chest physiotherapy.

Health Promotion. Maintaining a patient's optimal level of health is important in reducing the number and/or severity of

NURSING CARE PLAN

Ineffective Airway Clearance

ASSESSMENT

Mr. Edwards is a 75-year-old currently lying in a semi-Fowler's position in bed talking with his wife. Kathy Allen is a nursing student completing a respiratory assessment. Mr. Edwards has a history of chronic obstructive pulmonary disease for 2 years. He continues to smoke ½ pack of cigarettes a day and does not participate in any exercise. He does not "see any reason" to increase his fluid intake. His SpO_2 ranges from 78% to 84%. On ambulation is SpO_2 falls to 78%-80%. He must do his self-care activities slowly because of fatigue. Presently he is admitted for right upper lobe pneumonia. He reports having an intermittent productive cough that occasionally produces thick, yellow sputum. He has more episodes of coughing when lying flat. His vital signs are temperature, 101.4° F (38.5° C); pulse, 102 beats/min; respirations, 30 breaths/min; blood pressure, 130/90 mm Hg; and SpO_2, 84%. He has episodes of chilling and diaphoresis. His health care provider has told him that, if he gradually increases his exercise, drinks more fluids, and stops smoking, his respiratory status will improve.

Assessment Activities	*Findings/Defining Characteristics**
Ask Mr. Edwards how long he has had this cough.	He replies, "I have a morning **cough** every day, but this cough is different. It started about a week ago. It is **worse when I lie flat**."
Ask Mr. Edwards what is different about this cough.	He replies, "My ribs are getting sore. It is difficult to cough up anything, my **mouth** is **dry**, and I have become more **fatigued**."
Observe Mr. Edwards' skin and mucous membranes.	**Skin and mucous membranes** are **dry.**
Auscultate lung fields.	**Abnormal lung sounds** (crackles) are heard in the right upper lobe and left and right lower lobes.
Ask Mr. Edwards to produce a sputum sample.	Sputum is **thick** and **discolored** yellow to yellow-green and difficult to cough up and expectorate.

***Defining characteristics** are shown in bold type.

NURSING DIAGNOSIS: Ineffective airway clearance related to retained thick pulmonary secretions

PLANNING

Goals	*Expected Outcomes (NOC)*[†]
	Respiratory Status: Airway Patency
Mr. Edwards will be able to effectively clear secretions by discharge.	Lung sounds will improve in 48 hours. Mr. Edwards will notice increased ease in coughing within 48 hours. Sputum will be thin and white within 3 days. Respiratory rate will be within 12 to 20 breaths/min in 48 hours.
Mr. Edwards will increase oral hydration within 48 hours.	Mr. Edwards will drink 2500 mL of water or preferred liquids every 24 hours starting today. Mr. Edwards will verbalize that his mouth is not dry in 48 hours.

[†]Outcome classification labels from Moorhead S et al.: *Nursing outcomes classification (NOC)*, ed 5, St Louis, 2013, Elsevier.

INTERVENTIONS (NIC)[‡]	RATIONALE
Airway Management	
Position Mr. Edwards with head elevated at least 45 degrees.	Maintaining a semi-Fowler's position allows for thoracic expansion. This position prevents the abdominal organs from pushing up against the diaphragm, compromising inspiration. This position improves respiratory gas exchange.
Ambulate in room or hall as tolerated at least 2 times a day. If unable to ambulate, reposition from side to side every 2 hours or more.	Body movement helps patients take bigger breaths, increasing their tidal volume and preventing atelectasis (Atkins and Kautz, 2014).
Have Mr. Edwards deep breathe and cough every hour. Teach him to take a deep breath, hold it for several seconds, open his mouth, tighten his abdominal muscles, and cough 2 to 3 times with his mouth open.	Retained secretions predispose patient to atelectasis and pneumonia. Controlled coughing improves effectiveness of cough and removal of airway secretions (AARC, 1993, 2011, Borge et al., 2014).
Increase fluids to 2500 mL in 24 hours if not contraindicated by cardiac or renal status. Offer fluids Mr. Edwards prefers.	Fluids help may help promote secretion removal and relieve oral mucosa and skin dryness (Hong et al., 2013).

[‡]Intervention classification labels from Bulechek GM et al: *Nursing interventions classification (NIC)*, ed 6, St Louis, 2013, Elsevier.

EVALUATION

Nursing Actions	*Patient Response/Finding*	*Achievement of Outcome*
Auscultate the chest.	Lung sounds are clear in left lung, crackles present in right lower lobe.	Improving lung sounds
Ask Mr. Edwards if he can deep breathe and cough. Measure SpO_2.	Mr. Edwards reports that it is easier to cough up his secretions. SpO_2 is 95%.	Airway clears with coughing. SpO_2 is within normal levels.
Observe sputum.	"Sputum is thinner and white."	Sputum is thin and white.
Monitor respiratory rate.	Rate is between 12 and 20 breaths/min.	Mr. Edwards verifies it is easier to breathe.
Assess Mr. Edwards' level of hydration: Assess skin turgor and observe oral mucosa and calculate 20 hour fluid intake.	Skin turgor is normal. Mucous membranes are moist. Fluid intake in previous 24 hours was 2600 mL.	Oral membranes are pink and moist. Minimum fluid intake of 2500 mL was achieved.

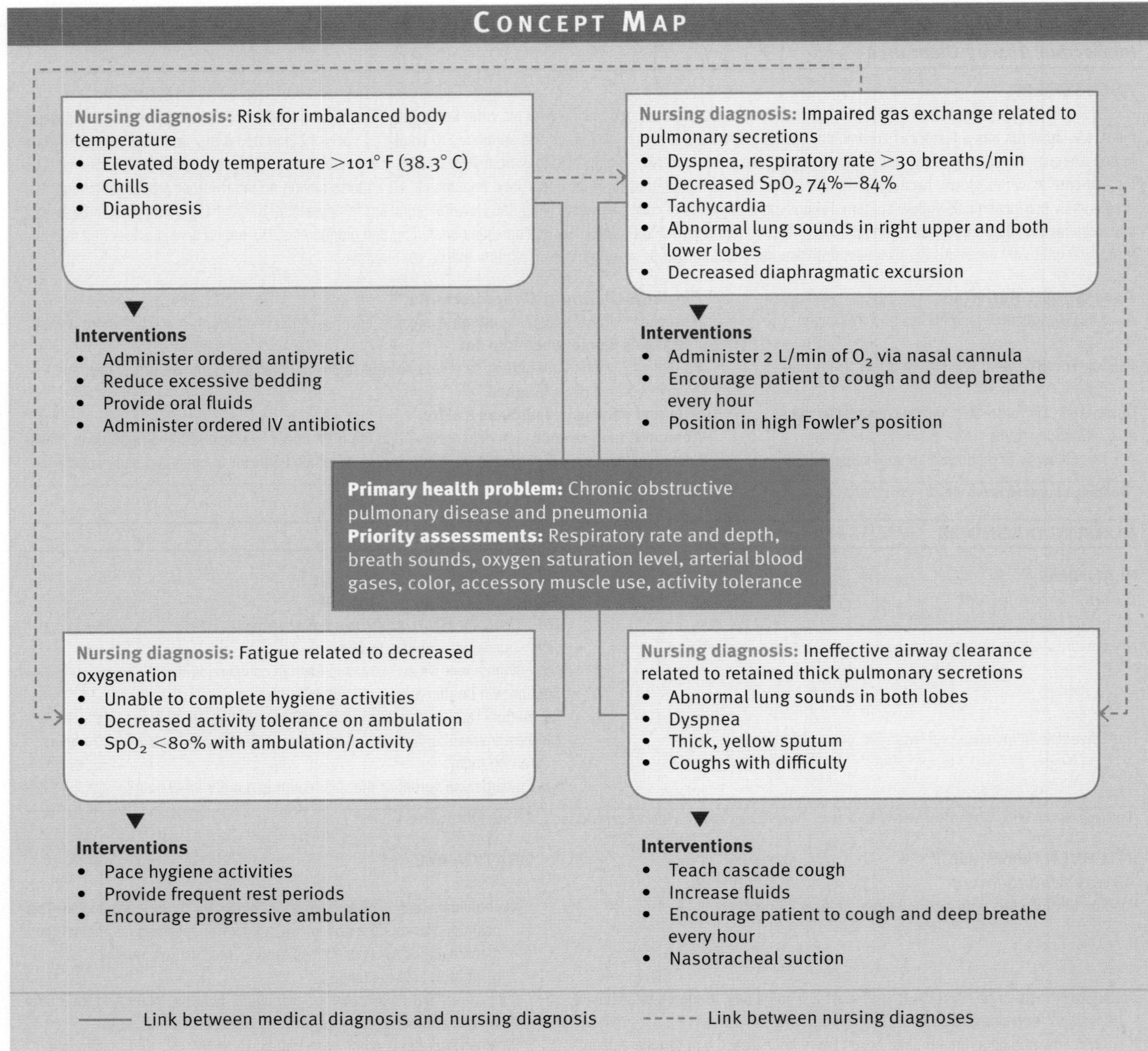

FIGURE 41-8 Concept map for Mr. Edwards.

respiratory symptoms. Prevention of respiratory infections is foremost in maintaining optimal health. Providing cardiopulmonary-related health information (Box 41-6) is an important nursing responsibility.

The health information that your patients and their families bring to the situation varies. Some patients have a lot of exposure to health care information and understand their treatment plans. Other families might have a lot of exposure to health care information but are unable to understand and follow treatment plans. Last, you might encounter families who are experiencing their first exposure to health care information and are very unsure of their interpretation of the information. When providing health information, be sure that the patient's health literacy levels are assessed and addressed through individualized patient education sessions (see Chapter 25).

Vaccinations. Annual flu vaccines are recommended for all people 6 months and older (CDC, 2014e). Patients with chronic illnesses (heart, lung, kidney, or immunocompromised), infants, older adults, and pregnant women can get very sick; thus they should be immunized (CDC, 2014g). Close contacts of infants under 6 months should also be immunized. Seasonal flu vaccine protects against influenza viruses that research indicates will be the most common during that year. The vaccine is also recommended for people in close or frequent contact with anyone in the high-risk groups. It is effective in reducing the severity of illness and the risk of serious complications and death. Researchers do not fully understand the value of vaccination in immune-compromised patients. HIV-positive patients receive the flu vaccine; however, they often require a second vaccine to gain protection. It is important to assess patient's allergies and any allergic response

BOX 41-6 PATIENT TEACHING

Prevention of Recurrent Respiratory Infections

Objective

- The patient will be able to verbalize the methods to reduce the risk factors for recurring respiratory infections.

Teaching Strategies

- Assess the patient's health literacy, educational background, reading level, and cultural preferences to determine appropriate educational approaches.
- Communicate with patient and family to identify collaborative goals for reducing risk factors.
- Explain the link between smoking and increase risk for respiratory infections (CDC, 2014c).
- Refer to smoking cessation programs and discuss appropriate medication to support smoking cessation from the primary health provider (ACS, 2014b).
- If a patient does not smoke, teach the importance of avoiding secondhand smoke and areas of high air pollution.
- Instruct patient and family about appropriate hand hygiene techniques to reduce transmission of microorganisms.
- Explain to patient and family why annual influenza vaccines and appropriate pneumonia vaccines are needed (CDC, 2014c, e, g).
- Instruct patient and family about signs and symptoms of respiratory infection that should be reported to health care provider such as increased coughing, shortness of breath, change of color of sputum, fever, and fatigue.

Evaluation

- Ask patient to state benefits of smoking cessation and the risks for secondhand smoke.
- Ask patient about plans for flu and pneumonia vaccines.
- Ask patient to describe in simple terms the symptoms of respiratory infection and when to call the health care provider.

to vaccines or any components. People with a known hypersensitivity to eggs or other components of the vaccine should consult their physician before being vaccinated. There is a flu vaccine made without egg proteins that is approved for adults 18 years of age and older (Li, 2013). Adults with an acute febrile illness should schedule the vaccination after they have recovered. The vaccines are formulated annually based on worldwide surveillance data. The live, attenuated nasal spray vaccine is given to people from 2 through 49 years of age if they are not pregnant or do not have certain long-term health problems such as asthma; heart, lung or kidney disease; diabetes; or anemia. The inactivated flu vaccine should be given to these individuals and those 50 and older (CDC, 2014e).

Pneumococcal vaccine (PCV13) is routinely given to infants in a series of four doses and is recommended for patients at increased risk of developing pneumonia. This includes all adults over 65 years of age, those with chronic illnesses or who are immunocompromised (such as HIV/AIDS), any adult who smokes or has asthma, and those living in special environments such as nursing homes or long-term care facilities (CDC, 2013c).

Healthy Lifestyle. Identification and elimination of risk factors for cardiopulmonary disease are important parts of primary care. Encourage patients to eat a healthy low-fat, high-fiber diet; monitor their cholesterol, triglyceride, high-density lipoprotein (HDL), and low-density lipoprotein (LDL) levels; reduce stress; exercise; and maintain a body weight in proportion to their height. Eliminating cigarettes and other tobacco, reducing exposure to pollutants, monitoring air quality, and adequately hydrating are additional healthy behaviors. Encourage patients to examine their habits and make appropriate changes. Patients with cardiopulmonary alterations need to minimize their risk for infection, especially during the winter months (see Box 41-6).

Exercise is a key factor in promoting and maintaining a healthy heart and lungs. Encourage patients to exercise at least 3 to 4 times a week for 30 to 60 minutes. Aerobic exercise is necessary to improve lung and heart function and strengthen muscles. Walking is an efficient way to achieve a good aerobic workout. Many shopping malls have programs allowing people to walk in the enclosed mall before the shops open. During the hot summer months teach patients to limit activities to early in the day or late in the evening, when temperatures are lower. Teach them how to maintain adequate hydration and sodium intake, especially if they are taking diuretics. Patients with known cardiac disease and those with multiple risk factors are cautioned to avoid exertion in cold weather. Shoveling snow is especially risky and often precipitates a cardiac event. Other activities such as hanging holiday lights and decorations in the extreme cold can precipitate chest pain and bronchospasm.

Environmental Pollutants. Avoiding exposure to secondhand smoke is essential to maintaining optimal cardiopulmonary function. Most businesses and restaurants now ban smoking or have separate areas designated as smoking areas. If patients are exposed to secondhand smoke in their home environments, counseling and support for all family members are necessary. Family members need to support the smoker in successful smoking cessation.

Consider if a patient is exposed to chemicals and pollutants in the work environment. Farmers, painters, carpenters, and others benefit from the use of particulate filter masks to reduce the inhalation of particles.

Acute Care. Patients with acute pulmonary illnesses require nursing interventions directed toward halting the pathological process (e.g., respiratory tract infection); shortening the duration and severity of an illness (e.g., hospitalization with pneumonia); and preventing complications from the illness or treatments (e.g., hospital-acquired infection resulting from invasive procedures).

Dyspnea Management. Dyspnea is difficult to treat. Health care providers individualize treatments for each patient and usually implement more than one therapy. Treatment of the underlying process causing dyspnea is then followed with other therapies (e.g., pharmacological measures, oxygen therapy, physical techniques, and psychosocial techniques). Pharmacological agents include bronchodilators, inhaled steroids, mucolytics, and low-dose antianxiety medications. Oxygen therapy reduces dyspnea associated with exercise and hypoxemia. Physical techniques such as cardiopulmonary reconditioning (e.g., exercise, breathing techniques, and cough control), relaxation techniques, biofeedback, and meditation are also beneficial.

Airway Maintenance. The airway is patent when the trachea, bronchi, and large airways are free from obstructions. Airway maintenance requires adequate hydration to prevent thick, tenacious secretions. Proper coughing techniques remove secretions and keep the airway open. A variety of interventions such as suctioning, chest physiotherapy, and nebulizer therapy assist patients in managing alterations in airway clearance.

Mobilization of Pulmonary Secretions. The ability of a patient to mobilize pulmonary secretions makes the difference between a short-term illness and a long recovery involving complications. Nursing interventions promoting removal of pulmonary secretions assist in achieving and maintaining a clear airway and help to promote lung expansion and gas exchange.

Hydration. Maintenance of adequate systemic hydration keeps mucociliary clearance normal. In patients with adequate hydration, pulmonary secretions are thin, white, watery, and easily removable with minimal coughing. Excessive coughing to clear thick, tenacious secretions is fatiguing and energy depleting. The best way to maintain thin secretions is to provide a fluid intake of 1500 to 2500 mL/day unless contraindicated by cardiac or renal status. The color, consistency, and ease of mucus expectoration determine adequacy of hydration.

Humidification. Humidification is the process of adding water to gas. Temperature is the most important factor affecting the amount of water vapor a gas can hold. Relative humidity is the percentage of water in the gas. Air or oxygen with a high relative humidity keeps the airways moist and loosens and mobilizes pulmonary secretions. Humidification is necessary for patients receiving oxygen therapy at greater than 4 L/min (check agency protocol). It might be necessary to add humidification at lower oxygen concentrations if the environment is dry and arid. Bubbling oxygen through water adds humidity to the oxygen delivered to the upper airways (see Skill 41-4).

An oxygen hood is used for infants, and a humidity tent is used for children with illnesses such as croup and tracheitis to liquefy secretions and help reduce fever (Hockenberry and Wilson, 2015). The nebulizer at the top of the humidity tent remains filled with water to prevent nonhumidified air or oxygen from entering the tent. Air in the humidity tent sometimes becomes cool and falls below 20° C (68° F), causing the child to become chilled. Children in humidity tents require frequent changes of clothing and bed linen to remain warm and dry.

Nebulization. Nebulization adds moisture or medications to inspired air by mixing particles of varying sizes with the air. Aerosolization suspends the maximum number of water drops or particles of the desired size in inspired air. The moisture added through nebulization improves clearance of pulmonary secretions. Nebulization delivers bronchodilators and mucolytic agents.

When the thin layer of fluid supporting the mucous layer over the cilia dries, the cilia are damaged and unable to adequately clear the airway. Humidification through nebulization enhances mucociliary clearance, the natural mechanism of the body for removing mucus and cellular debris from the respiratory tract.

Coughing and Deep-Breathing Techniques. Coughing is effective for maintaining a patent airway. Directed coughing is a deliberate maneuver that is effective when spontaneous coughing is not adequate (AARC, 1993; Borge et al., 2014). Directed coughing permits a patient to remove secretions from both the upper and lower airways. The normal series of events in the cough mechanism are deep inhalation, closure of the glottis, active contraction of the expiratory muscles, and glottis opening. Deep inhalation increases the lung volume and airway diameter, allowing the air to pass through partially obstructing mucus plugs or other foreign matter. Contraction of the expiratory muscles against the closed glottis causes a high intrathoracic pressure to develop. When the glottis opens, a large flow of air is expelled at a high speed, providing momentum for mucus to move to the upper airways where the patient can expectorate or swallow it.

Diaphragmatic breathing/belly breathing is a technique that encourages deep breathing to increase air to the lower lungs. The diaphragm descends (belly moves out) when breathing in and ascends (belly sinks in) when breathing out (CFF, 2012). Deep breathing also opens the pores of Kohn between alveoli to allow sharing of oxygen between alveoli. This is especially important if the airway of the alveoli is plugged with mucus. The neighboring alveoli can share the air distribution through the pores of Kohn.

Evaluate the effectiveness of coughing by sputum expectoration, the patient's report of swallowed sputum, or clearing of adventitious sounds by auscultation. Encourage patients with chronic pulmonary diseases, upper respiratory tract infections, and lower respiratory tract infections to deep breathe and cough at least every 2 hours while awake. Encourage patients with a large amount of sputum to cough every hour while awake and then awaken them at night to cough every 2 to 3 hours. This is necessary until the acute phase of mucus production has ended. After surgery it is recommended that patients perform directed cough every 2 to 4 hours while awake to prevent accumulation of secretions. Offer postoperative patients support devices (folded blanket, pillow, or palmed hands) to splint an abdominal or thoracic incision to minimize pain during directed coughing. Cough is a source of droplet transmission of pulmonary pathogens; thus the health care provider should follow Standard Precautions. Coughing techniques include deep breathing and coughing for the postoperative patient, cascade, huff, and quad coughing (Borge et al., 2014).

With the *cascade cough* the patient takes a slow, deep breath and holds it for 2 seconds while contracting expiratory muscles. Then he or she opens the mouth and performs a series of coughs throughout exhalation, thereby coughing at progressively lowered lung volumes. This technique promotes airway clearance and a patent airway in patients with large volumes of sputum.

The *huff cough* stimulates a natural cough reflex and is generally effective only for clearing central airways. While exhaling, the patient opens the glottis by saying the word *huff.* With practice he or she inhales more air and is able to progress to the cascade cough.

The *quad cough* technique is for patients without abdominal muscle control such as those with spinal cord injuries. While the patient breathes out with a maximal expiratory effort, the patient or nurse pushes inward and upward on the abdominal muscles toward the diaphragm, causing the cough.

Chest Physiotherapy. Chest physiotherapy (CPT) is a group of therapies for mobilizing pulmonary secretions. These therapies include postural drainage, chest percussion, and vibration. CPT is followed by productive coughing or suctioning of a patient who has a decreased ability to cough. It is recommended for patients who produce greater than 30 mL of sputum per day or have evidence of atelectasis on chest x-ray examination (AARC, 2012). The procedure is safe for infants and young children; however, at times conditions and diseases unique to children contraindicate it. CPT is for a select group of patients. Box 41-7 describes the guidelines to determine if CPT is indicated.

Postural drainage is a component of pulmonary hygiene; it consists of drainage, positioning, and turning and is sometimes accompanied by chest percussion and vibration (CFF, 2012). It improves secretion clearance and oxygenation. Positioning involves draining affected lung segments (Table 41-6) and helps to drain secretions from those segments of the lungs and bronchi into the trachea. Some patients do not require postural drainage of all lung segments, and clinical assessment is crucial in identifying specific lung segments requiring it. For example, patients with left lower lobe atelectasis require postural drainage of only the affected region, whereas a child with cystic fibrosis often requires postural drainage of all lung segments.

Chest percussion involves rhythmically clapping on the chest wall over the area being drained to force secretions into larger airways for expectoration (AARC, 2012). It is commonly performed by respiratory therapists in larger health care settings. Position your hand so the fingers and thumb touch and the hands are cupped. The cupping makes the hand conform to the chest wall while trapping a cushion of air to soften the intensity of the clapping. The procedure should produce a hollow sound and should not be painful (CFF, 2012). Perform chest percussion by vigorously striking the chest wall

BOX 41-7 Guidelines for Chest Physiotherapy

Nursing and respiratory therapy collaborate with the health care provider to determine if chest physiotherapy (CPT) is best for the patient. The following guidelines help in physical assessment and subsequent decision making:

- Know a patient's normal range of vital signs. The degree of change is related to the level of hypoxia, overall cardiopulmonary status, and tolerance to activity.
- Conditions requiring CPT such as atelectasis and complicated pneumonia affect vital signs. Conduct a respiratory assessment to confirm need for CPT, including sputum production, effectiveness of cough, history of pulmonary problems successfully relieved with CPT, abnormal lung sounds, documented conditions such as atelectasis, complicated pneumonia, and changes in oxygenation status (AARC, 2012).
- Know the patient's medications. Certain medications, particularly diuretics and antihypertensives, cause fluid and hemodynamic changes. These decrease a patient's tolerance to positional changes and postural drainage. Long-term steroid use increases a patient's risk of pathological rib fractures and often contraindicates vibration.
- Know the patient's medical history. Certain conditions such as increased intracranial pressure, spinal cord injuries, and abdominal aneurysm resection contraindicate the positional changes of postural drainage. Thoracic trauma or surgery contraindicates percussion and vibration.
- Know the patient's level of cognitive function. Participation in controlled coughing techniques requires him or her to follow instructions. Congenital or acquired cognitive limitations alter a patient's ability to learn and participate in these techniques.
- Be aware of the patient's exercise tolerance. CPT maneuvers are fatiguing.

TABLE 41-6 Positions for Postural Drainage

Lung Segment	Position of Patient	Lung Segment	Position of Patient
Adult			
Bilateral 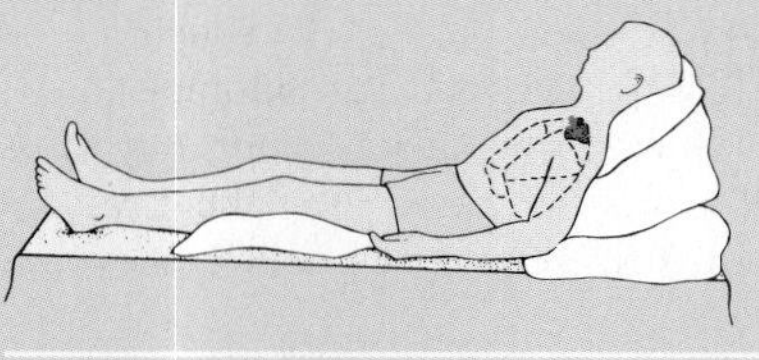	High-Fowler's	Left lower lobe—lateral segment 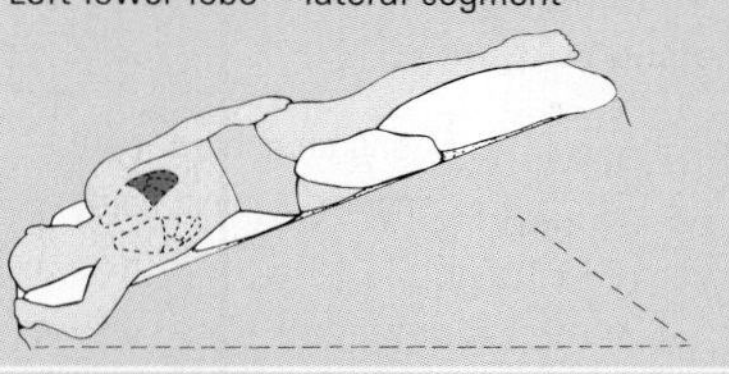	Right side-lying in Trendelenburg's position
Apical segments	Sitting on side of bed	Right lower lobe—lateral segment 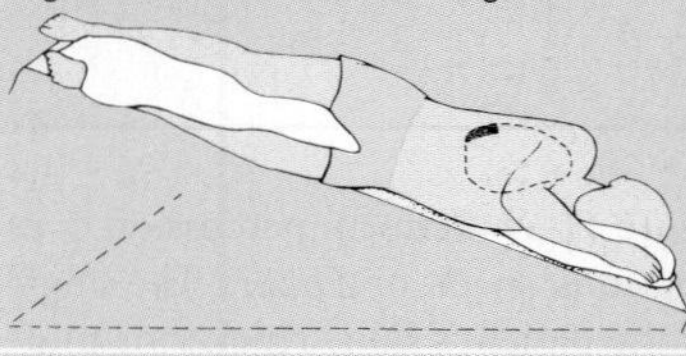	Left side-lying in Trendelenburg's position
Right upper lobe—anterior segment 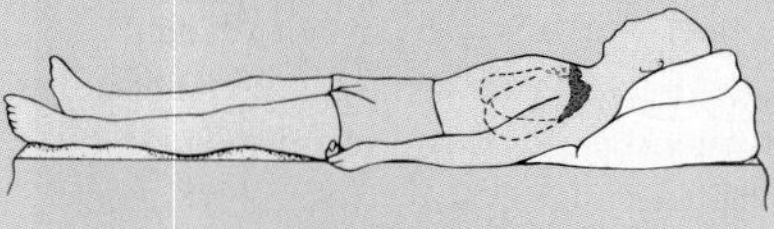	Supine with head elevated	Right lower lobe—posterior segment 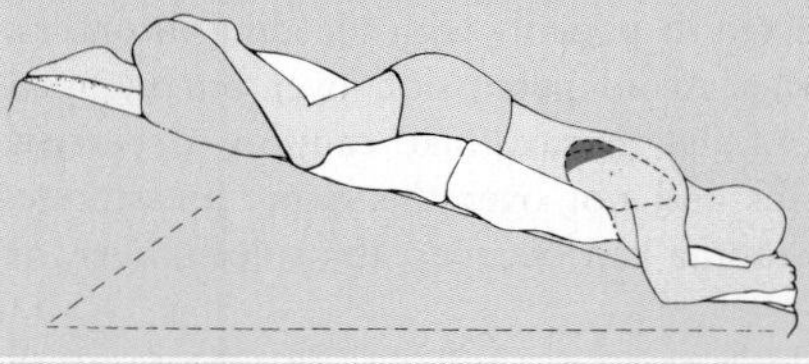	Prone with right side of chest elevated in Trendelenburg's position
Left upper lobe—anterior segment 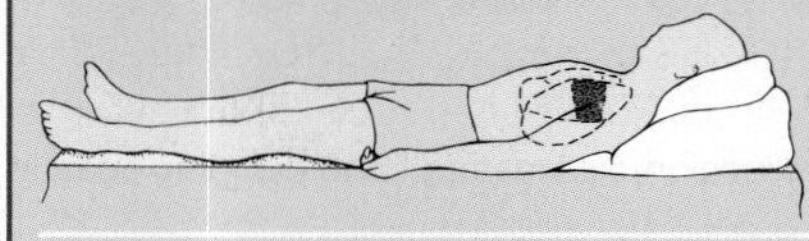	Supine with head elevated	Right middle lobe—posterior segment 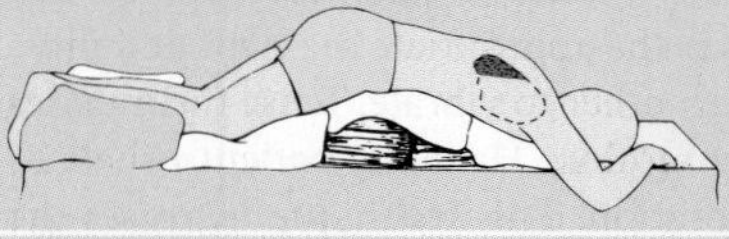	Prone with thorax and abdomen elevated
Right upper lobe—posterior segment 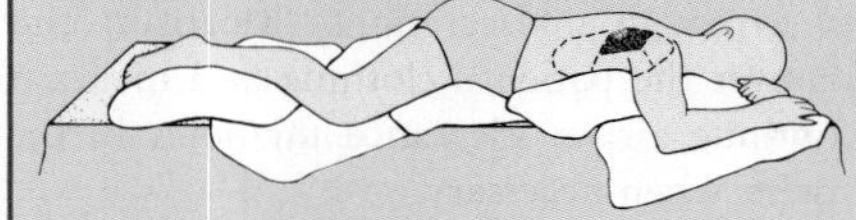	Side-lying with right side of chest elevated on pillows	Both lower lobes—anterior segments 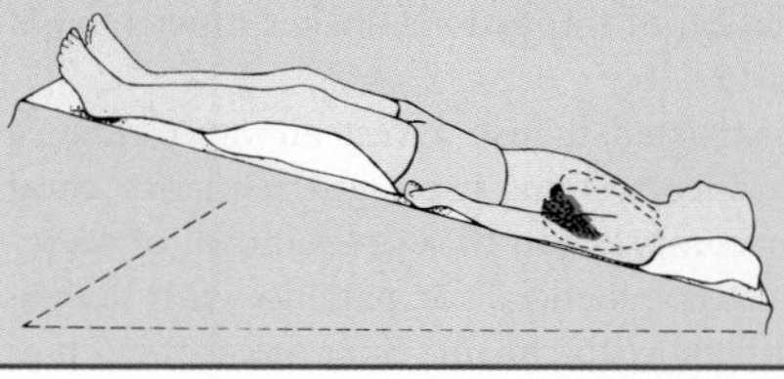	Supine in Trendelenburg's position

Continued

TABLE 41-6 Positions for Postural Drainage—cont'd

Lung Segment	Position of Patient	Lung Segment	Position of Patient
Left upper lobe—posterior segment 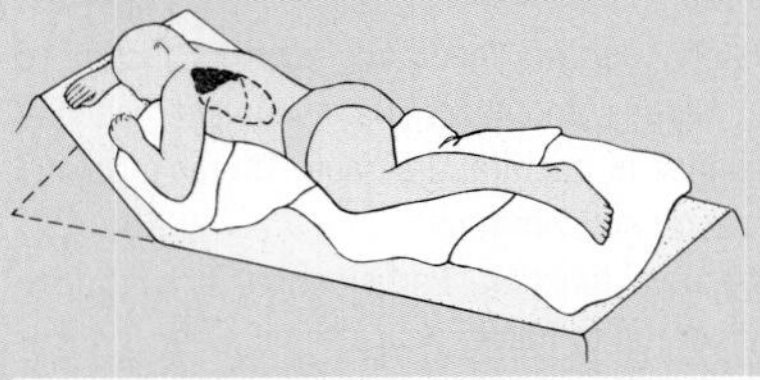	Side-lying with left side of chest elevated on pillows	Both lower lobes—posterior segments 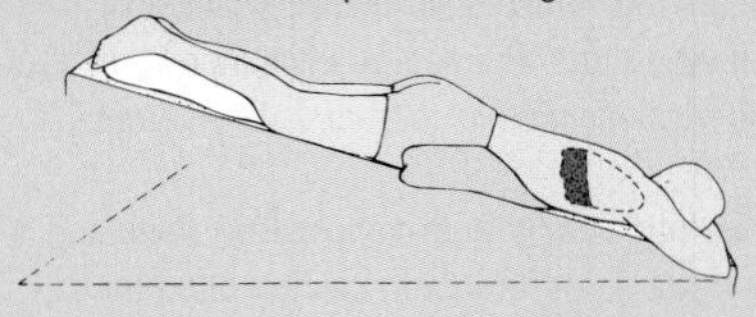	Prone in Trendelenburg's position
Right middle lobe—anterior segment 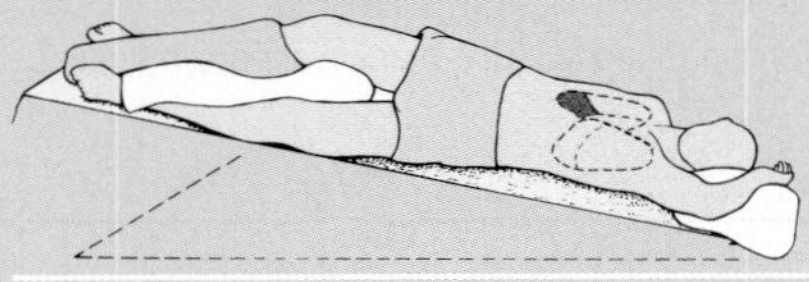	Three-fourths supine position with dependent lung in Trendelenburg's position		
Child			
Bilateral—apical segments 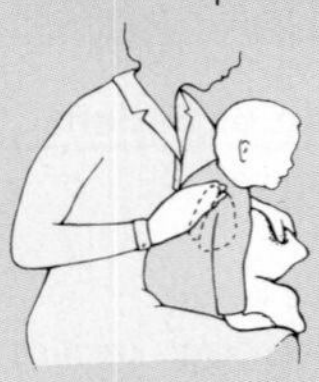	Sitting on nurse's lap, leaning slightly forward flexed over pillow	Bilateral lobes—anterior segments 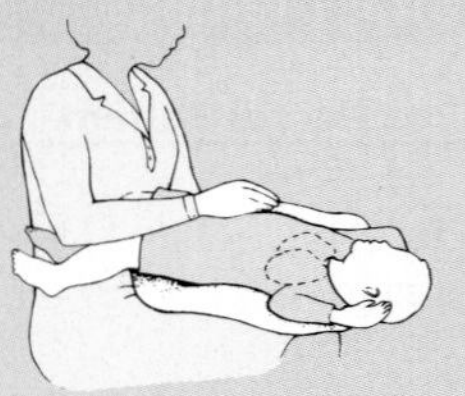	Lying supine on nurse's lap, back supported with pillow
Bilateral—middle anterior segments 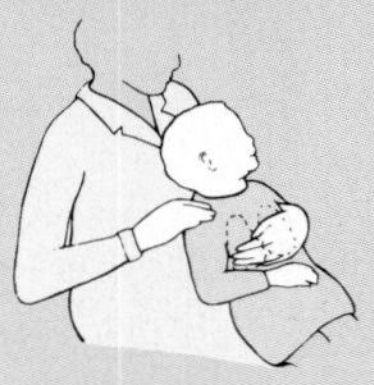	Sitting on nurse's lap, leaning against nurse		

alternately with cupped hands (Figure 41-9). Perform percussion over a single layer of clothing, not over buttons, snaps, or zippers. The single layer of clothing prevents slapping the patient's skin. Thicker or multiple layers of material dampen the vibrations.

Percussion is contraindicated in patients with bleeding disorders, osteoporosis, or fractured ribs. Avoid percussion over burns, open wounds, or skin infections of the thorax. Take caution to percuss the lung fields under the ribs and not over the spine, breastbone, stomach, or lower back or trauma can occur to the spleen, liver, or kidneys (CFF, 2012).

Vibration is a gentle, shaking pressure applied to the chest wall to shake secretions into larger airways. Place a flattened hand or two hands firmly on the chest wall over the appropriate segment and press the top and bottom hand into each other to vibrate. Tense the muscles of the arm to provide a shaking motion. Have the patient exhale as slowly as possible during the vibration. This technique increases the velocity and turbulence of exhaled air, facilitating secretion removal. Vibration increases the exhalation of trapped air, shakes mucus loose, and induces a cough (CFF, 2012).

A patient may also be instructed to use a vest airway clearance system. The vest airway clearance systems use high-frequency chest wall oscillation (HFCWO) or compression to assist removal of secretions from the lungs. This vest is beneficial for patients with neuromuscular diseases and for patients with chronic lung diseases, such as cystic fibrosis. The goals of oscillating vests are (1) to clear the airways of excessive secretions to reduce the work of breathing, and (2) to improve a patient's ability to cough up secretions (Morrison and Agnew, 2014). The vest fits over the patient's clothing and makes it possible for patients to continue airway clearance therapies in the home and school environments when necessary.

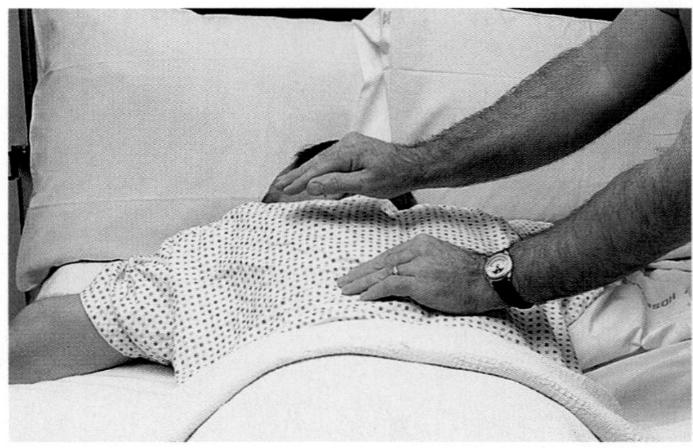

FIGURE 41-9 Chest wall percussion, alternating hand clapping against patient's chest wall.

Suctioning Techniques. Suctioning is necessary when patients are unable to clear respiratory secretions from the airways by coughing or other less invasive procedures. Suctioning techniques include oropharyngeal and nasopharyngeal suctioning, orotracheal and nasotracheal suctioning, and suctioning an artificial airway.

In most cases use sterile technique for suctioning because the oropharynx and trachea are considered sterile. The mouth is considered clean; therefore you suction oral secretions after suctioning the oropharynx and trachea. In the home setting, use a "clean" versus "sterile" technique because the patient is not exposed to pathogens common to health care settings. Teach patients appropriate measures for disinfecting equipment (AARC, 2004, 2010a).

Each type of suctioning requires the use of a round-tipped, flexible catheter with holes on the sides and end of the catheter. When suctioning, you apply negative pressures (100-150 mm Hg for adults) during withdrawal of the catheter, never on insertion (AARC, 2010a). Patient assessment determines the frequency of suctioning. It is indicated when rhonchi, gurgling breath sounds, and diminished breath sounds are audible on auscultation or visible secretions are present after other methods to remove airway secretions have failed. You may also use suctioning to obtain a sputum specimen for culture or cytology if the patient is not able to cough productively. Too-frequent suctioning puts patients at risk for development of hypoxemia, hypotension, arrhythmias, and possible trauma to the mucosa of the lungs (AARC, 2010a; Lynn-McHale, 2011).

Oropharyngeal and Nasopharyngeal Suctioning. Oropharyngeal or nasopharyngeal suctioning is used when a patient is able to cough effectively but unable to clear secretions by expectorating. Apply suction after a patient has coughed (see Skill 41-1 on pp. 907-914). Once the pulmonary secretions decrease and a patient is less fatigued, he or she is then able to expectorate or swallow the mucus, and suctioning is no longer necessary.

Orotracheal and Nasotracheal Suctioning. Orotracheal or nasotracheal suctioning is necessary when a patient with pulmonary secretions is unable to manage secretions by coughing and does not have an artificial airway present (see Skill 41-1). You pass a sterile catheter through the mouth or nose into the trachea. The nose is the preferred route because stimulation of the gag reflex is minimal. The procedure is similar to nasopharyngeal suctioning, but you advance the catheter tip farther into the patient's trachea. The entire procedure from catheter passage to its removal is done quickly, lasting no longer than 10 seconds (AARC, 2010a). Allow the patient to rest between passes of the catheter. If the patient develops respiratory distress, stop suctioning unless the collection of secretions is causing distress. If the patient is using supplemental oxygen, replace the oxygen cannula or mask during rest periods.

Tracheal Suctioning. Perform tracheal suctioning through an artificial airway such as an endotracheal (ET) or tracheostomy tube. The size of a catheter should be as small as possible but large enough to remove secretions. Recommendation is about half the internal diameter of the ET tube (AARC, 2010a). Never apply suction pressure while inserting the catheter to avoid traumatizing the lung mucosa. Once you insert a catheter the necessary distance, maintain suction pressure between 120 and 150 mm Hg (AARC, 2010a) as you withdraw. Apply suction intermittently ***only*** while withdrawing the catheter. Rotating the catheter enhances removal of secretions that have adhered to the sides of the airway.

The practice of normal saline instillation (NSI) into artificial airways to improve secretion removal may be harmful and is not recommended. Clinical studies comparing the results of suctioning following NSI with standard suctioning have not shown any clinical or significant results (AARC, 2010a).

The two current methods of suctioning are the open and closed methods. Open suctioning involves using a new sterile catheter for each suction session (AARC, 2010a). Wear sterile gloves and follow Standard Precautions during the suction procedure. Closed suctioning involves using a reusable sterile suction catheter that is encased in a plastic sheath to protect it between suction sessions (Figure 41-10).

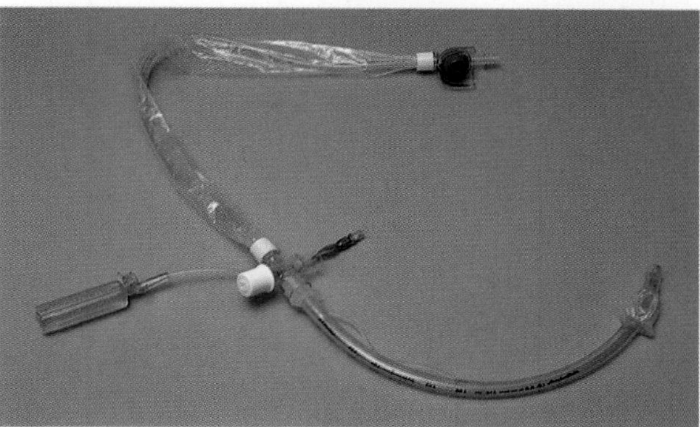

FIGURE 41-10 Ballard tracheal care, closed suction catheter.

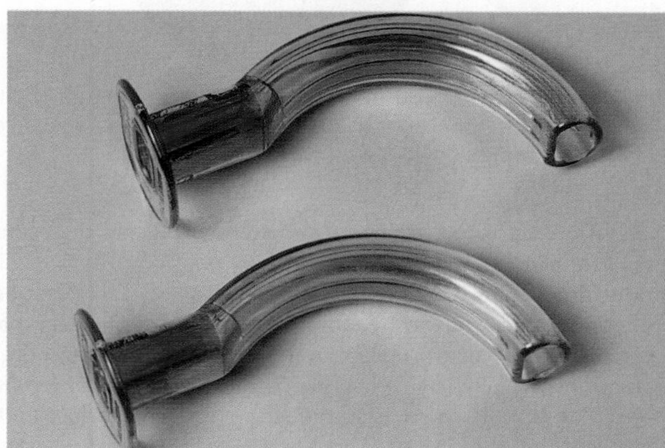

FIGURE 41-11 Artificial oral airways.

Closed suctioning is most often used on patients who require invasive mechanical ventilation to support their respiratory efforts because it permits continuous delivery of oxygen while suction is performed and reduces the risk of oxygen desaturation. Although sterile gloves are not used in this procedure, nonsterile gloves are recommended to prevent contact with splashes from body fluids (see Skill 41-1).

Artificial Airways. An artificial airway is for a patient with a decreased level of consciousness or airway obstruction and aids in removal of tracheobronchial secretions. The presence of an artificial airway places a patient at high risk for infection and airway injury. Use clean technique for oral airways, but use sterile technique in caring for and maintaining endotracheal and tracheal airways to prevent health care–associated infections (HAIs). Artificial airways need to stay in the correct position to prevent airway damage (see Skill 41-2 on pp. 915-922).

Oral Airway. The oral airway, the simplest type of artificial airway, prevents obstruction of the trachea by displacement of the tongue into the oropharynx (Figure 41-11). The oral airway extends from the teeth to the oropharynx, maintaining the tongue in the normal position. Use the correct-size airway. Determine the proper oral airway size by measuring the distance from the corner of the mouth to the angle of the jaw just below the ear. The length is equal to the distance from the flange of the airway to the tip. If the airway is too small, the tongue does not stay in the anterior portion of the mouth; if the airway is too large, it forces the tongue toward the epiglottis and obstructs the airway.

Insert the airway upside down, then turn to the curve of the airway toward the cheek and place it over the tongue. When the airway is in the oropharynx, turn it so the opening points downward. Correctly placed, the airway moves the tongue forward away from the oropharynx, and the flange (e.g., the flat portion of the airway) rests against

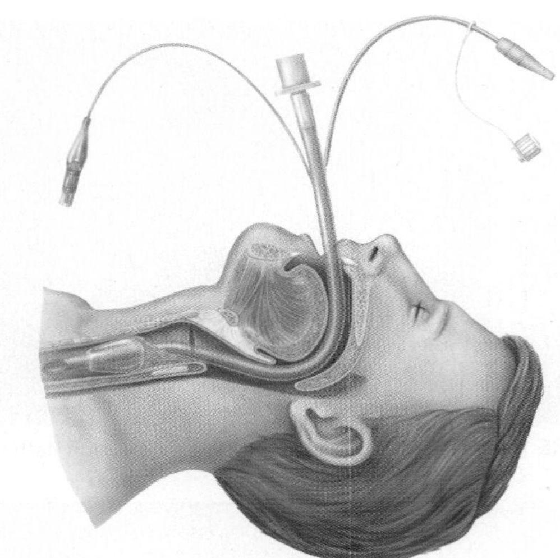

FIGURE 41-12 Endotracheal tube inserted into trachea. Cuff inflated to maintain position. (Copyright © 2015 Medtronic. All rights reserved. Used with the permission of Medtronic.)

the patient's teeth. Incorrect insertion merely forces the tongue back into the oropharynx.

Endotracheal and Tracheal Airway. An endotracheal (ET) tube is a short-term artificial airway to administer invasive mechanical ventilation, relieve upper airway obstruction, protect against aspiration, or clear secretions. A physician or specially trained clinician inserts the ET tube. The tube is passed through the patient's mouth, past the pharynx, and into the trachea (Figure 41-12). It is generally removed within 14 days; however, it is sometimes used for a longer period of time if the patient is still showing progress toward weaning from invasive mechanical ventilation and extubation.

If a patient requires long-term assistance from an artificial airway, a tracheostomy is considered. A surgical incision is made into the inferior border of the cricoid cartilage of the trachea, and a short tracheostomy tube is inserted. Most tracheostomies have a small plastic inner tube that fits inside a larger one (the inner cannula). The most common complication of a tracheostomy tube is partial or total airway obstruction caused by buildup of respiratory secretions. If this occurs, the inner tube can be removed and cleaned or replaced with a temporary spare inner tube that should be kept at the patient's bedside. Keep tracheal dilators at the bedside to have available for emergency tube replacement or reinsertion. Humidification from air humidifiers or humidified oxygen tracheostomy collars can help prevent drying of secretions that cause occlusion. Tracheostomy suctioning should be done as often as necessary to clear secretions. The majority of patients with a tracheostomy tube cannot speak because the tube is inserted below the vocal cords. It is important to use written or nonverbal communication (lip reading) strategies to help patients communicate. Be sure to assess patients for anxiety caused by the inability to speak. Care and cleaning of the tracheostomy tube is discussed in Skill 41-2.

Maintenance and Promotion of Lung Expansion. Nursing interventions to maintain or promote lung expansion include noninvasive techniques such as ambulation, positioning, incentive spirometry, and noninvasive ventilation. Invasive medical interventions such as chest tube insertion and management assist in restoring lung expansion.

Ambulation. Immobility is a major factor in developing atelectasis, ventilator-associated pneumonia (VAP), and functional limitations. The research has shown that, after 1 week of bed rest, muscle strength declines by as much as 20%, which results in an increased oxygen demand, weakened respiratory muscles, and a decline of functional status. Early ambulation studies indicate that the therapeutic benefits of activity include an increase in general strength and lung expansion. Even the patient who requires invasive mechanical ventilation benefits by an early mobility program. Such mobility programs should include input from both respiratory and physical therapists in the treatment plan (Atkins and Kautz, 2014). Progressive mobilization from dangling the legs to standing and then walking is safe for intubated patients (Atkins and Kautz, 2014).

Positioning. The healthy, completely mobile person maintains adequate ventilation and oxygenation by frequent position changes during daily activities. However, when a person's illness or injury restricts mobility, the risk for respiratory impairment is increased. Frequent changes of position are simple and cost-effective methods for reducing stasis of pulmonary secretions and decreased chest wall expansion, both of which increase the risk of pneumonia. Research has shown that turning critically ill patients every 2 hours is not often enough to prevent pneumonia (Rauen et al., 2008).

The 45-degree semi-Fowler's is the most effective position to promote lung expansion and reduce pressure from the abdomen on the diaphragm. When a patient is in this position, be sure that he or she does not slide down in bed, which can reduce lung expansion. Sliding also increases the risk of pressure ulcers. A patient with unilateral lung disease such as pneumothorax, atelectasis, or pneumonia of one lung should be positioned in a manner to promote perfusion of the healthy lung and improve oxygenation. In most cases, position the patient with the good lung down (Rauen et al., 2008). In the presence of pulmonary abscess or hemorrhage, position the patient with the affected lung down to prevent drainage toward the healthy lung. For bilateral lung disease the best position depends on the severity of the disease.

Incentive Spirometry. Incentive spirometry encourages voluntary deep breathing by providing visual feedback to patients about inspiratory volume. It promotes deep breathing and prevents or treats atelectasis in the postoperative patient. There is solid evidence to support the use of lung expansion with incentive spirometry in preventing postoperative pulmonary complications following surgery (AARC, 2011; Cassidy et al., 2013).

Flow-oriented incentive spirometers consist of one or more plastic chambers that contain freely moving colored balls. A patient inhales slowly and with an even flow to elevate the balls and keep them floating as long as possible to ensure a maximally sustained inhalation.

Volume-oriented incentive spirometry devices have a bellows that is raised to a predetermined volume by an inhaled breath (Figure 41-13). An achievement light or counter is used to provide feedback. Some devices are constructed so the light does not turn on unless the bellows is held at a minimum desired volume for a specified period to enhance lung expansion (see Chapter 50).

Incentive spirometry encourages patients to use visual feedback to maximally inflate their lungs and sustain that inflation (AARC, 2011). A postoperative inspiratory capacity one half to three fourths of the preoperative volume is acceptable because of postoperative pain. The AARC guidelines (2011) recommend 5 to 10 breaths per session every hour while awake. Administration of pain medications before incentive spirometry helps a patient achieve deep breathing by reducing pain and splinting.

Invasive Mechanical Ventilation. Invasive mechanical ventilation, also referred to as positive-pressure ventilation, is a lifesaving technique used with artificial airways (ET or tracheostomy) for various physiological and clinical indications. Physiological indications for invasive mechanical ventilation include supporting cardiopulmonary gas exchange (alveolar ventilation and arterial oxygenation), increasing lung volume, and reducing the work of breathing (Urden et al., 2014).

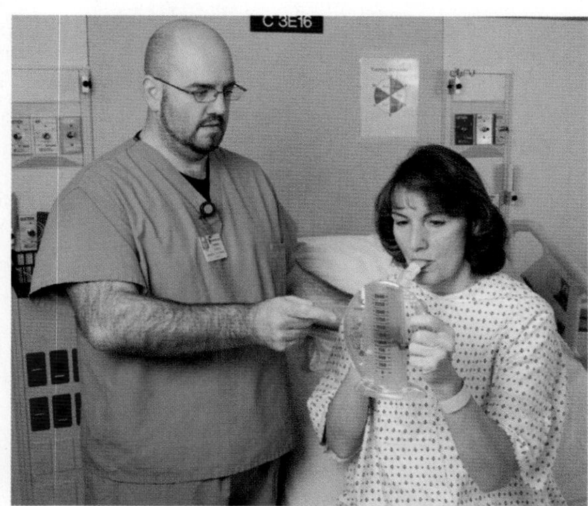

FIGURE 41-13 Volume-oriented incentive spirometer.

Clinical indications for invasive mechanical ventilation include reversing hypoxia and acute respiratory acidosis, relieving respiratory distress, preventing or reversing atelectasis and respiratory muscle fatigue, allowing for sedation and/or other neuromuscular blockade, decreasing oxygen consumption, reducing intracranial pressure and stabilizing the chest wall (Urden et al., 2014). It can be used to either fully or partially replace spontaneous breathing depending on the need of the patient. Invasive mechanical ventilation also redistributes blood flow from working respiratory muscles to other vital organs. Following an inspiratory trigger, invasive mechanical ventilation forces a preset mixture of air (oxygen and other gases) into the central airways and then flows into the alveoli, causing the intraalveolar pressure to increase as the lungs inflate. A termination signal triggers the ventilator to cease forcing air into the central airways, causing the central airway pressure to decrease. Expiration then follows passively, the air flowing from the higher alveoli pressure to the lower pressure of the central airways.

There are a variety of ventilator modes; the choice depends on the patient's situation and goals of treatment. Many of the modes are used in conjunction with each other. There are numerous brands of ventilators and they vary in their ability to perform certain functions; not all modes are available on all ventilators. The most commonly used modes include assist-control (AC), synchronized intermittent mandatory ventilation (SIMV) and pressure support ventilation (PSV). Assist control delivers a set tidal volume (VT) with each breath, regardless if the breath was triggered by the patient or the ventilator. Synchronized intermittent mandatory ventilation, like AC, delivers a minimum number of fully assisted breaths per minute that are synchronized with the patient's respiratory effort. Any breaths taken between volume-cycled breaths are not assisted; the volume of these breaths is determined by the patient's strength, effort, and lung mechanics. Pressure Support mode is often combined with SIMV mode, inspiratory pressure is added to spontaneous breaths to overcome the resistance of the endotracheal tube or to help increase the volume of the patient's spontaneous breaths.

Although invasive mechanical ventilation is often lifesaving, it is not without complications. Some complications are preventable and others can be minimized. Physiological complications associated with invasive mechanical ventilation include volutrauma, cardiovascular compromise, gastrointestinal disturbances, and ventilator assisted pneumonia (Urden et al., 2014).

Volutrauma occurs as a result of alveolar overdistention secondary to the mechanical ventilation. Cardiovascular compromise occurs as a result of the increased intrathoracic pressure. It is caused by positive-pressure ventilation that decreases venous return to the right side of the heart, decreasing preload and resulting in a decreased cardiac output. Gastrointestinal (GI) disturbances commonly occur. They are related to gastric distention, vomiting related to pharyngeal stimulation from the artificial airway, constipation, and hypomotility (due to immobility and the administration of analgesics, sedatives and paralytic agents).

Ventilator-associated pneumonia (VAP) is a significant potential complication because the artificial airway tube bypasses many of the lung's normal defense mechanisms. Ventilator associated pneumonia (VAP) is a health care–acquired infection (HAI) that develops in a person requiring invasive mechanical ventilation (via endotracheal intubation or tracheotomy tube) for at least 48 hours (Shi et al., 2013). It is a potentially serious complication in patients who are already critically ill. VAP mortality rates ranges from 20% to 50% among ventilated patients and is estimated to add an additional $40,000 to the cost of a hospital admission (Monaco et al., 2014) (Box 41-8). Hospitals are not reimbursed for costs associated with VAP.

Noninvasive Ventilation. **Noninvasive positive-pressure ventilation (NPPV)** is used to prevent using invasive artificial airways (ET tube or tracheostomy) in patients with acute respiratory failure, cardiogenic pulmonary edema, or exacerbation of COPD. It has also been used following extubation of an ET tube (Luo et al., 2014). The purpose of NPPV is to maintain a positive airway pressure and improve alveolar ventilation. This prevents or treats atelectasis by inflating the alveoli, reducing pulmonary edema by forcing fluid out of the lungs back into circulation, and improving oxygenation in those with sleep apnea. Ventilatory support is achieved using a variety of modes, including **continuous positive airway pressure (CPAP)** and **bilevel positive airway pressure (BiPAP)**.

CPAP treats patients with obstructive sleep apnea, patients with heart failure, and preterm infants with underdeveloped lungs. In obstructive sleep apnea, airways collapse, causing shallow or absent breathing. Any air moving past the obstruction results in loud snoring. An overnight sleep study may be needed to determine the correct settings for a CPAP machine (see Chapter 43). Equipment includes a mask (Figure 41-14) that fits over the nose or both nose and mouth and a CPAP machine that delivers air to the mask (National Heart Lung and Blood Institute, 2011). The smallest mask with the proper fit is the most effective. Because straps hold the mask in place, it is important to assess for excess pressure on the patient's face or nose that could cause skin breakdown or necrosis. The mask should have enough slack to allow one to two fingers between the straps and the face (Soo Hoo et al., 2014). However, it must also be tight enough to form a tight seal on the face so the air does not escape. With higher pressures escape of some air may be avoidable.

The most common mode of support is BiPAP that provides both inspiratory positive airway pressure (IPAP) and expiratory airway pressure (EPAP), also known as *positive end-expiratory pressure (PEEP)*. The difference between these two pressures indicates the amount of pressure support a patient needs (Soo Hoo et al., 2014). During inhalation the positive pressure increases the patient's tidal volume and alveolar ventilation. The pressure support decreases when the patient exhales, allowing for easier exhalation.

Complications of noninvasive ventilation include facial and nasal injury and skin breakdown, dry mucous membranes and thick secretions, and aspiration of gastric contents if vomiting occurs. Complications avoided by noninvasive ventilation are VAP, sinusitis, and effects of large-dose sedative agents. Use of noninvasive ventilation

BOX 41-8 EVIDENCE-BASED PRACTICE

Adherence to a Ventilator Care Bundle on Reducing Ventilator-Associated Pneumonia

PICO Question: In patients requiring invasive mechanical ventilation, does adhering to an evidenced-based ventilator care bundle contribute to a reduction of ventilator-associated pneumonia (VAP)?

Evidence Summary

Ventilator associated pneumonia (VAP) is a health care–acquired infection (HAI) that develops in a person requiring invasive mechanical ventilation (via endotracheal intubation or tracheostomy tube) for at least 48 hours (Shi et al., 2013). *Pseudomonas aeruginosa* and *Staphylococcus aureus* are considered major causes of endotracheal tube–associated VAP, 41.7% and 36.7% respectively. *Streptococcus pneumonia, Acinetobacter baumannii, Enterobacteriacea* and other gram-negative aerobic bacteria are the other microorganisms that contribute to VAP (Loo et al., 2015). Patients with VAP have increased fever, increased secretions, and pulmonary infiltrates seen on chest radiograph. Over time these infiltrates progressively increase, and the patient's lung functions decline. VAP is also highly correlated with sepsis, and interventions to reduce the risk of VAP also assist in reducing the risk for sepsis (O'Leary, 2014). The incidence of VAP increases with the duration of invasive mechanical ventilation.

In 2001, The Institute for Health Care Improvement identified four interventions to prevent complications in high-risk ventilated patients. The Ventilator Bundle (IHCI, 2012) as it came to be known, is a series of evidenced-based interventions related to ventilator care that, when implemented together, achieve significantly better outcomes than when implemented individually (Monaco et al., 2014). In 2010, components of the IHI Ventilator Bundle were revised to add an intervention. The key components of the IHI Ventilator Bundle are (IHCI, 2012):

- Elevation of the head of the bed (HOB) 45 degrees
- Daily "sedation vacations" and assessment of readiness to extubate
- Peptic ulcer disease prophylaxis
- Deep venous thrombosis prophylaxis
- Daily oral care with chlorhexidine

Increased compliance with the IHI's recommended Ventilator Bundle reduces the incidence of VAP in ICU settings (Morris et al., 2011; Monaco et al., 2014).

Application to Nursing Practice

- Follow ICHI bundle.
- Avoid prolonged supine positioning. Pulmonary aspiration is increased by supine positioning and pooling of secretions above the ET tube cuff (Sedwick et al., 2012).
- Compared to supine positioning, studies have shown that with simple positioning with HOB elevation to 30 degrees or higher significantly reduces gastric reflux and VAP. Keep the patient's HOB raised between 30 and 45 degrees unless other medical conditions do not allow this to occur.
- Orotracheal and orogastric tubes are preferred over nasal devices to reduce the risk of VAP (Lacherade et al., 2010).
- Suction frequently to remove oropharyngeal and subglottic secretions to reduce the risk of early-onset VAP.
- Monitor cuff pressure frequently to ensure that there is an adequate seal to prevent aspiration of secretions (Lacherade et al., 2010).
- Provide daily oral care with chlorhexidine (IHCI, 2012; Labeau et al., 2011).
- Always drain ventilator circuit condensation away from patient and into the appropriate receptacle (AARC, 2010a). Drain the tubing hourly to prevent accumulation.

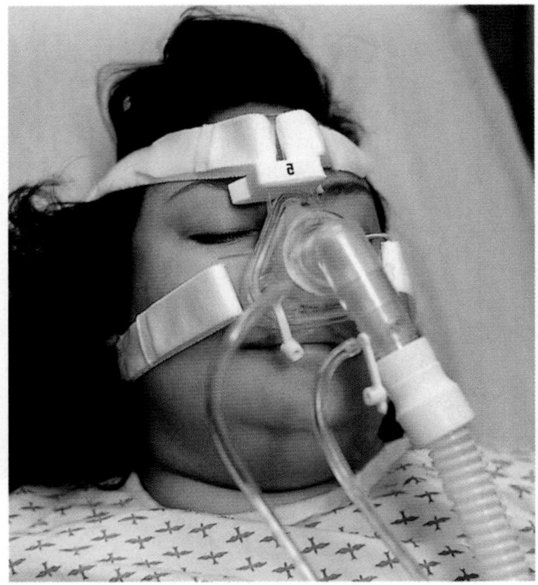

FIGURE 41-14 CPAP mask.

results in shorter intensive care unit (ICU) and hospital stays (Soo Hoo et al., 2014). Perform good oral hygiene every few hours while a patient is on BiPAP to relieve dryness.

Chest Tubes. A **chest tube** (Figure 41-15) is a catheter inserted through the thorax to remove air and fluids from the pleural space, to prevent air or fluid from reentering the pleural space, or to reestablish normal intrapleural and intrapulmonic pressures (Bauman et al., 2011). Chest tubes are common after chest surgery and chest trauma and are used for treatment of pneumothorax or hemothorax to promote lung reexpansion (see Skill 41-3 on pp. 922-926).

A **pneumothorax** is a collection of air in the pleural space. The loss of negative intrapleural pressure causes the lung to collapse. There are a variety of causes for a pneumothorax. A secondary pneumothorax can occur as a result of chest trauma (e.g., stabbing, gunshot wound, or rib fracture from striking the chest against the steering wheel in an automobile accident). Other causes of secondary pneumothorax are the rupture of an emphysematous bleb on the surface of the lung (the destruction caused by emphysema), tearing of the pleura from an invasive procedure such as surgery, insertion of a subclavian IV line, and invasive mechanical ventilation, including PEEP. Spontaneous (primary) pneumothorax is a genetic condition that occurs unexpectedly in healthy individuals who develop blisterlike formations (blebs) on the visceral pleura, usually on the apex of the lungs. The blebs can rupture during sleep or exercise (McCance and Huether, 2014). A patient with a pneumothorax usually feels pain as atmospheric air irritates the parietal pleura. The pain is sharp and pleuritic and worsens on inspiration. Dyspnea is common and worsens as the size of the pneumothorax increases.

A **hemothorax** is an accumulation of blood and fluid in the pleural cavity between the parietal and visceral pleura, usually as a result of trauma. It produces a counter pressure and prevents the lung from full expansion. A rupture of small blood vessels from inflammatory processes such as pneumonia or TB can cause a hemothorax. In addition to pain and dyspnea, signs and symptoms of shock develop if blood loss is severe.

A variety of chest tubes are available to drain air or excess fluid from the pleural space to relieve respiratory distress. A small-bore chest tube (12 to 20 Fr) is used to remove a small amount of air, and a

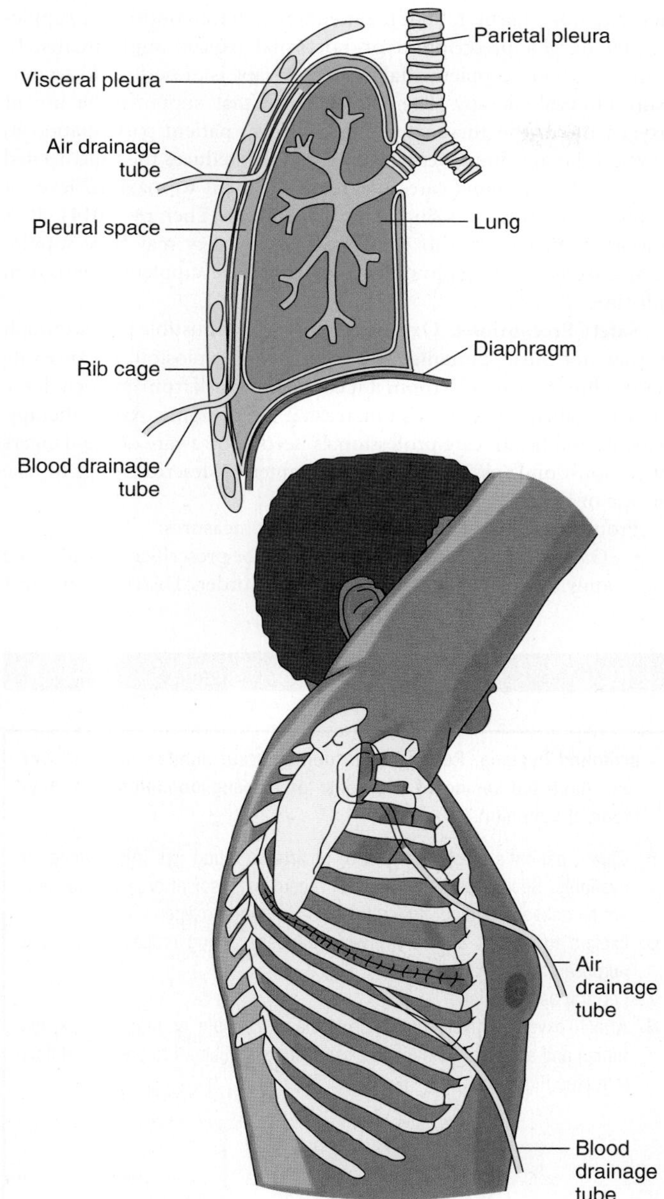

FIGURE 41-15 Chest tube placement.

larger-bore chest tube is used to remove large amounts of fluid or blood and large amounts of air (Carroll, 2015).

After a chest tube is inserted, it is attached to a drainage system. A traditional chest drainage unit (CDU) has three chambers for collection, water seal, and suction control. This unit can drain a large amount of both fluid and air (Carroll, 2015). Mobile systems rely on gravity, not suction, for drainage. In selected patients these mobile drains reduce the length of time needed for the chest tube, improve ambulation, and decrease the length of time in the hospital (Carroll, 2015). Nonventilated patients and patients who had thoracoscopic lung surgery or minimally invasive cardiac surgery do well with these mobile chest drains. They are lighter and smaller; thus patients are able to move more easily. As a result this reduces the risks of deep vein thrombosis and pulmonary embolism.

The simplest closed drainage system is the single chamber unit. The chamber serves as a fluid collector and a water seal. During normal respiration the fluid in the chamber ascends with inspiration and descends with expiration. A single chamber is used for smaller amounts of drainage such as an empyema (e.g., a collection of infected fluid or pus in the pleural space).

The use of two chambers permits any fluid to flow into the collection chamber as air flows into the water-seal chamber. Fluctuations in the water-seal tube are still anticipated. Two chambers allow for more accurate measurement of chest drainage and are used when larger amounts of drainage are expected.

When a volume of air or fluid needs to be evacuated with controlled suction, all three chambers are used. Mark the suction control with centimeter readings to adjust the amount of suction. Usually 15 to 20 cm of water is used for adults (Carroll, 2015). This means that the chamber is filled with sterile water to the 15- or 20-cm water level.

There is a new dry chest drainage system that does not use water in the suction chamber. An automatic control valve (ACV) is located inside the regulator and continuously balances the force of the suction with the atmospheres. As a result, the ACV responds and adjusts to changes in patient air leaks and fluctuations in suction source vacuum to deliver accurate suction. Set the pressure between −10 cm H_2O and −40 cm H_2O (RTC, 2011). Regardless of the system used, the principles of patient management are the same.

Special Considerations. Keep a chest tube system closed and below the chest (see Skill 41-3). The tube should be secured to the chest wall. Watch for slow, steady bubbling in the suction-control chamber and keep it filled with sterile water at the prescribed level. Make sure that the water-seal chamber is filled to the manufacturer-specified level and watch for fluctuation (tidaling) of the fluid level to ensure that the chest tube and system are working. A constant or intermittent bubbling in the water-seal chamber indicates a leak in the drainage system, and the health care provider must be notified immediately. Mark the level on the outside of the collection chambers every shift. Report any unexpected cloudy or bloody drainage. Do not let the tubing kink or loop, and ideally it should lie horizontally across the bed or chair before dropping vertically into the drainage device. Encourage your patient to cough, deep breath, and use the incentive spirometer. Make sure that he or she is frequently repositioned and ambulated if not contraindicated. Routinely evaluate respiratory rate, breath sounds, SpO_2 levels, and the insertion site for subcutaneous emphysema (RTC, 2011; Carroll, 2015).

Clamping a chest tube is contraindicated when ambulating or transporting a patient. Clamping can result in a tension pneumothorax. Air pressure builds in the pleural space, collapsing the lung and creating a life-threatening event. A chest tube is only clamped when replacing the chest drainage system, assessing for an air leak, or during removal (Bauman et al., 2011).

Chest tubes are not routinely stripped or milked to move clots or increase chest tube drainage (Bauman et al., 2011). Stripping or milking chest tubes is based on nursing assessment (see Skill 41-3).

Handle the chest drainage unit carefully and maintain the drainage device below the patient's chest. If the tubing disconnects from the drainage unit, instruct the patient to exhale as much as possible and to cough. This maneuver rids the pleural space of as much air as possible. Temporarily reestablish a water seal by immersing the open end of the chest tube into a container of sterile water (Bauman et al., 2011).

Removal of chest tubes requires patient preparation. The most frequent sensations reported by patients during chest tube removal include burning, pain, and a pulling sensation. Make sure that the patient is given pain medication at least 30 minutes before removal.

The nurse assists the health care provider in removing the chest tube and monitors the dressing placed over the insertion site and the patient's respiratory status after tube removal.

Maintenance and Promotion of Oxygenation. Promotion of lung expansion, mobilization of secretions, and maintenance of a patent airway assist patients in meeting their oxygenation needs. However, some patients also require oxygen therapy to keep a healthy level of tissue oxygenation.

Oxygen Therapy. Oxygen therapy is widely available and used in a variety of settings to relieve or prevent tissue hypoxia. The goal of oxygen therapy (AARC, 2007) is to prevent or relieve hypoxia by delivering oxygen at concentrations greater than ambient air (21%). Oxygen has dangerous side effects such as oxygen toxicity. The dosage or concentration of oxygen is monitored continuously. Routinely check the health care provider's orders to verify that the patient is receiving the prescribed oxygen concentration. The six rights of medication administration also pertain to oxygen administration (see Chapter 32).

Supplemental oxygen therapy offers many benefits to patients with chronic cardiopulmonary diseases. This therapy reduces mortality, improves self-reported sleep quality and general comfort, increases exercise tolerance, and reduces polycythemia and pulmonary hypertension (Earnest, 2002). Patients may have continuous supplemental oxygen prescription or nocturnal oxygen supplements. In some situations, supplemental oxygen therapy is prescribed to accompany physical therapy. There is evidence that supports the use of oxygen therapy in these situations improves patient participation in physical therapy, improves activity tolerance, reduces the time needed for extended or home care, and returns patient to maximal level of health (Task Force on Supplemental Oxygen Therapy, 2014). It is important to reinforce to your patients why they may have supplemental oxygen during physical therapy but have supplemental oxygen full-time (Box 41-9).

Safety Precautions. Oxygen is a highly combustible gas. Although it does not burn spontaneously or cause an explosion, it can easily cause a fire in a patient's room if it contacts a spark from an open flame or electrical equipment. With increasing use of home oxygen therapy, patients and health care professionals need to be aware of the dangers of combustion (Kassis et al., 2014). Chapter 27 describes steps to take in case of fire.

Promote oxygen safety by the following measures:

- Oxygen is a therapeutic gas and must be prescribed and adjusted only with a health care provider's order. Distribution must

BOX 41-9 PROCEDURAL GUIDELINES 

Applying a Nasal Cannula or Oxygen Mask

Delegation Considerations

The skill of applying (not adjusting oxygen flow) a nasal cannula or oxygen mask can be delegated to nursing assistive personnel (NAP). You are responsible for assessing patient's respiratory system; response to oxygen therapy; and setup of oxygen therapy, including adjustment of oxygen flow rate. Direct the NAP by:

- Informing how to safely position and adjust the device (e.g., loosening the strap on oxygen mask) and clarifying its correct placement and positioning.
- Instructing to inform the nurse immediately about any vital sign changes; skin irritation from the cannula, mask, or straps; if patient reports pain or breathlessness; or if patient presents with decreased level of consciousness or increased confusion.
- Having personnel provide skin care around patient's ears and nose

Equipment

NOTE: When device is used in the home, the home care equipment vendor provides the equipment. Oxygen-delivery device as ordered by patient's health care provider. Oxygen tubing (consider extension tubing), humidifier if indicated, sterile water for humidifier, oxygen source, oxygen flowmeter, stethoscope, pulse oximeter, appropriate room signs

Steps

1. Identify patient using two identifiers (e.g., name and birth date or name and medical record number) according to agency policy. Compare identifiers with information on patient's MAR or medical record.
2. Review patient's medical record for medical order for oxygen, noting delivery method, flow rate, duration of oxygen therapy, and parameters for titration of oxygen settings.
3. Assess patient's respiratory status, including symmetry of chest wall expansion, chest wall abnormalities (e.g., kyphosis), temporary conditions (e.g., pregnancy, trauma) affecting ventilation, respiratory rate and depth, sputum production, and lung sounds.
4. Observe for patent airway and remove secretions by having patient cough and expectorate mucus or by suctioning.

   CLINICAL DECISION: Patients with sudden changes in their vital signs, level of consciousness, or behavior are often experiencing profound hypoxia. Patients who demonstrate subtle changes over time have worsening of a chronic or existing condition or a new medical condition.
5. Obtain patient's most recent SpO_2 or arterial blood gas (ABG) values if available. Review patient's medical record for medical order for oxygen, noting delivery method, flow rate, and duration of oxygen therapy.
6. Explain to patient and family what happens during procedure and the purpose of oxygen therapy.
7. Perform hand hygiene.
8. Attach oxygen-delivery device (e.g., nasal cannula or mask) to oxygen tubing and attach to humidified oxygen source adjusted to prescribed flow rate (see illustration).

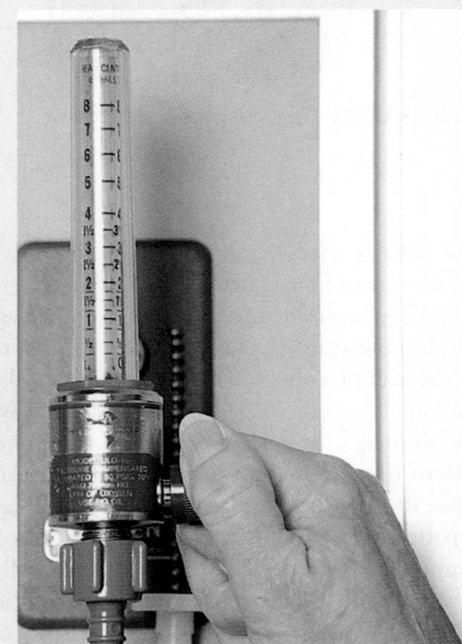

STEP 8 Adjusting flowmeter to prescribed oxygen flow rate.

BOX 41-9 PROCEDURAL GUIDELINES

Applying a Nasal Cannula or Oxygen Mask—cont'd

9. Position tips of nasal cannula properly in patient's nares and adjust elastic headband or plastic slide on cannula so it is snug and comfortable (see illustration). If using an oxygen face mask, adjust elastic band over ears until mask fits comfortably over patient's face and mouth.
10. Maintain sufficient slack on oxygen tubing and secure to patient's clothes.
11. Observe for proper functioning of oxygen-delivery device.
    a. *Nasal cannula:* Cannula is positioned properly in nares with humidification functioning.
    b. *Reservoir nasal cannula Oxymizer:* Fit as for nasal cannula. Reservoir is positioned under patient's nose or worn as a pendant (see illustration).
    c. *Nonrebreathing mask:* Apply mask over patient's mouth and nose to form tight seal. Valves on mask close so exhaled air does not enter reservoir bag (see illustration).
    d. *Partial rebreathing mask:* Apply mask over patient's mouth and nose to form tight seal. Ensure that bag remains partially inflated.
    e. *Venturi mask:* Apply mask over patient's mouth and nose to form a tight seal. Select appropriate flow rate (see illustration).

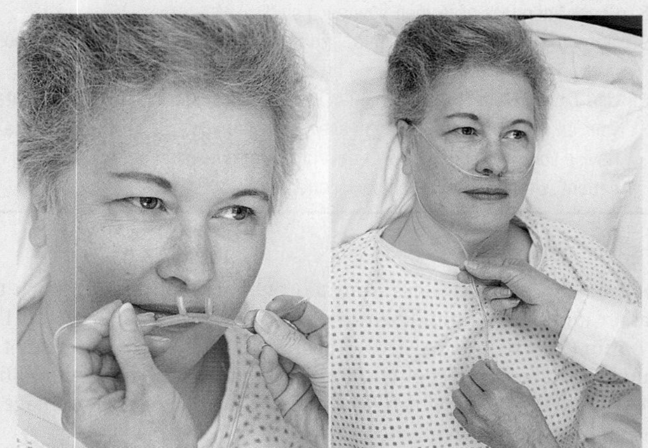

STEP 9 Applying nasal cannula and adjusting fit to patient comfort.

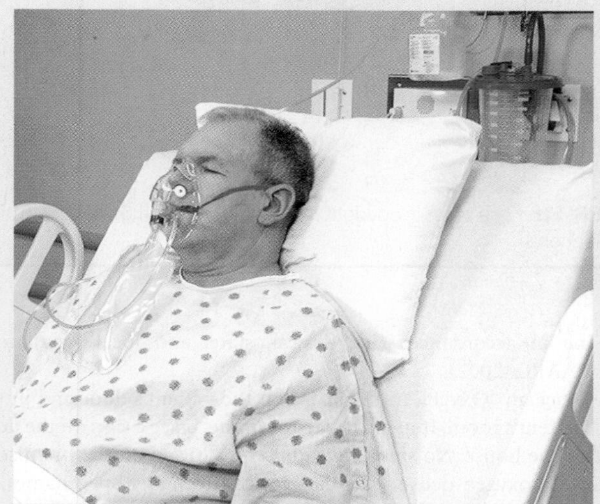

STEP 11c Nonrebreathing mask. (Copyright © Mosby's Clinical Skills: Essentials Collection.)

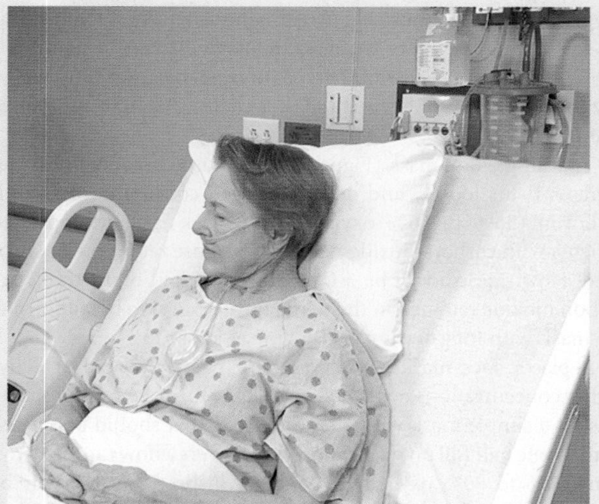

STEP 11b Reservoir nasal cannula/Oxymizer. (Copyright © Mosby's Clinical Skills: Essentials Collection.)

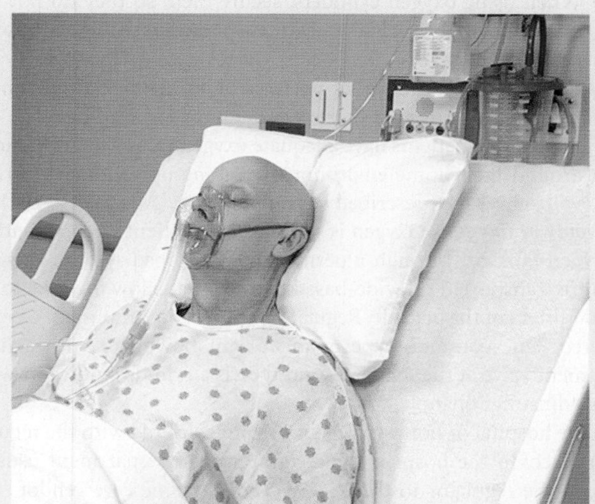

STEP 11e Venturi mask. (Copyright © Mosby's Clinical Skills: Essentials Collection.)

Continued

BOX 41-9 PROCEDURAL GUIDELINES

Applying a Nasal Cannula or Oxygen Mask—cont'd

f. *Face tent:* Apply tent under patient's chin and over mouth and nose. It will be loose, and a mist is always present (see illustration).

12. Verify setting on flowmeter and oxygen source for proper setup and prescribed flow rate.

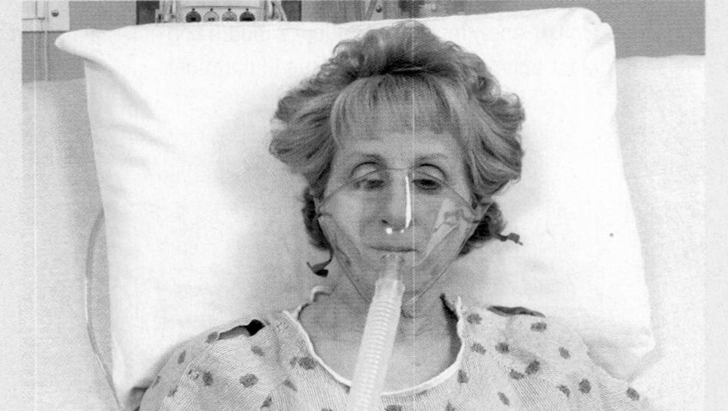

STEP 11f Face tent. (Copyright © Mosby's Clinical Skills: Essentials Collection.)

13. Check cannula/mask every 8 hours. Keep humidification container filled at all times.
14. Post "Oxygen in use" signs on wall behind bed and at entrance to room.
15. Properly dispose of gloves (if used) and perform hand hygiene.
16. Monitor patient's response to changes in oxygen flow rate with pulse oximetry. **Note:** Monitor ABGs when ordered; however, obtaining ABG measurement is an invasive procedure, and ABGs are not measured frequently.
17. Observe for decreased anxiety, improved level of consciousness and cognitive abilities, decreased fatigue, absence of dizziness, decreased respiratory rate, improved color, improved oxygen saturation, and return to patient's baseline vital signs.
18. Check adequacy of oxygen flow each shift.
19. Observe patient's external ears, bridge of nose, nares, and nasal mucous membranes for evidence of skin breakdown.
20. Use ***Teach Back:*** State, "I want to be sure that I explained how to regulate your oxygen flow rate. Can you show me how you will set the flow rate? Revise your instruction now or develop plan for revised patient teaching if patient is not able to teach back correctly.

be in accordance with federal, state, and local regulations (AARC, 2007).

- Place an "Oxygen in Use" sign on the patient's door and in the patient's room. If using oxygen at home, place a sign on the door of the house. No smoking should be allowed on the premises.
- Keep oxygen-delivery systems 10 feet from any open flames.
- Determine that all electrical equipment in the room is functioning correctly and properly grounded (see Chapter 27). An electrical spark in the presence of oxygen can result in a serious fire.
- When using oxygen cylinders, secure them so they do not fall over. Store them upright and either chained or secured in appropriate holders.
- Check the oxygen level of portable tanks before transporting a patient to ensure that there is enough oxygen in the tank.
- Ensure that patients have adequate oxygen tubing to safely move around their home environment. Tubing up to 98 feet (30 m) will deliver the prescribed oxygen flow rate (Aguiar et al., 2015).

Supply of Oxygen. Oxygen is supplied to a patient's bedside either by oxygen tanks or through a permanent wall-piped system. Oxygen tanks are transported on wide-based carriers that allow the tank to be placed upright at the bedside. Regulators control the amount of oxygen delivered. One common type is an upright flowmeter with a flow adjustment valve at the top. A second type is a cylinder indicator with a flow adjustment handle.

In the hospital or home oxygen tanks are delivered with the regulator in place. In the hospital the respiratory care department usually connects the regulator to the oxygen source. Home care vendors are usually responsible for connecting the oxygen tank to the regulator for home use.

Methods of Oxygen Delivery. The nasal cannula and oxygen masks are the most common devices to deliver oxygen to patients. These devices deliver different levels of oxygen to patients (Table 41-7).

Nasal Cannula. A nasal cannula is a simple, comfortable device used for precise oxygen delivery. The two nasal prongs are slightly curved and inserted in a patient's nostrils. To keep the nasal prongs in place, fit the attached tubing over the patient's ears and secure it under the chin using the sliding connector. Be alert for skin breakdown over the ears and in the nostrils from too tight an application. Attach the nasal cannula to a humidified oxygen source with a flow rate up 1 to 6 L/min (24% to 44% oxygen). Flow rates equal to or greater than 4 L/min have a drying effect on the mucosa and thus need to be humidified (AARC, 2007). Know which flow rate produces a given percentage of inspired oxygen concentration (FiO_2).

Oxygen Masks. An oxygen mask is a plastic device that fits snugly over the mouth and nose and is secured in place with a strap. It delivers oxygen as the patient breathes through either the mouth or nose by way of a plastic tubing at the base of the mask that is attached to an oxygen source. An adjustable elastic band is attached to either side of the mask that slides over the head to above the ears to hold the mask in place. There are two primary types of oxygen masks: those delivering low concentrations of oxygen and those delivering high concentrations (see Box 41-9).

The simple face mask (Figure 41-16) is used for short-term oxygen therapy. It fits loosely and delivers oxygen concentrations from 6 to 12 L/min (35% to 50% oxygen). The mask is contraindicated for patients with carbon dioxide retention because retention can be worsened. Flow rates should be 5 L or more to avoid rebreathing exhaled carbon dioxide retained in the mask. Be alert to skin breakdown under the mask with long-term use (Downie et al., 2013).

A plastic face mask with a reservoir bag is capable of delivering higher concentrations of oxygen. A partial rebreather or nonrebreather mask is a simple mask with a reservoir bag that should be at least one third to one half full on inspiration and delivers a flow rate of 10 to 15 L/min (60% to 90% oxygen). Frequently inspect the reservoir bag to make sure that it is inflated. If it is deflated, the patient is breathing large amounts of exhaled carbon dioxide. High-flow oxygen systems should be humidified (AARC, 2007).

The Venturi mask delivers higher oxygen concentrations of 24% to 60% and usually requires oxygen flow rates of 4 to 12 L/min, depending on the flow-control meter selected.

Home Oxygen Therapy. Indications for home oxygen therapy include an arterial partial pressure (PaO_2) of 55 mm Hg or less or an arterial oxygen saturation (SaO_2) of 88% or less on room air at rest, on exertion, or with exercise (American Thoracic Society, 2011). Home

TABLE 41-7 Oxygen Delivery Systems

Delivery System	FiO_2 Delivered	Advantages	Disadvantages
Low-Flow Delivery Devices			
Nasal cannula	1-6 L/min: 24%-44%	Safe and simple Easily tolerated Effective for low concentrations Does not impede eating or talking Inexpensive, disposable	Unable to use with nasal obstruction Drying to mucous membranes Can dislodge easily May cause skin irritation or breakdown around ears or nares Patient's breathing pattern (mouth or nasal) affects exact FiO_2
Simple face mask	6-12 L/min: 35%-50%	Useful for short periods such as patient transportation	Contraindicated for patients who retain CO_2 May induce feelings of claustrophobia Therapy interrupted with eating and drinking Increased risk of aspiration
Partial and nonrebreather masks	10-15 L/min: 60%-90%	Useful for short periods Delivers increased FiO_2 Easily humidifies O_2 Does not dry mucous membranes	Hot and confining; may irritate skin; tight seal necessary Interferes with eating and talking Bag may twist or kink; should not totally deflate
Oxygen-conserving cannula *(Oxymizer)*	8 L/min: up to 30%-50%	Indicated for long-term O_2 use in the home Allows increased O_2 concentration and lower flow	Cannula cannot be cleaned More expensive than standard cannula
High-Flow Delivery Devices			
Venturi mask	24%-50%	Provides specific amount of oxygen with humidity added Administers low, constant O_2	Mask and added humidity may irritate skin Therapy interrupted with eating and drinking Specific flow rate must be followed

CO_2, Carbon dioxide; *FiO_2,* fraction of inspired oxygen concentration.

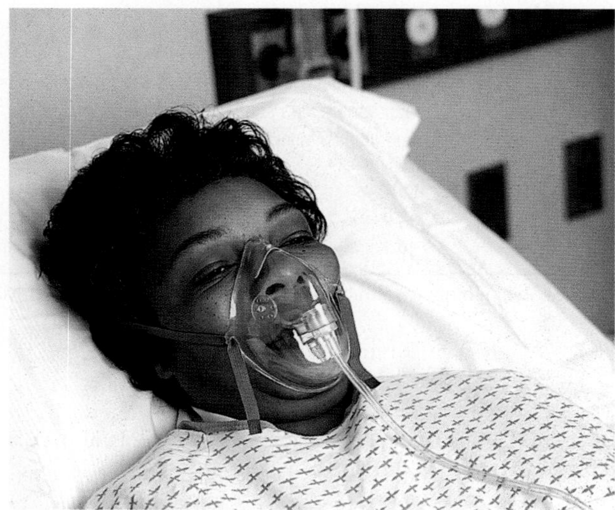

FIGURE 41-16 Simple face mask.

oxygen therapy is administered via nasal cannula or face mask. Patients with permanent tracheostomies use either a T tube or tracheostomy collar (AARC, 2007). Home oxygen therapy has beneficial effects for patients with chronic cardiopulmonary diseases. This therapy improves patients' exercise tolerance and fatigue levels and in some situations assists in the management of dyspnea (see Skill 41-4).

There are three types of oxygen delivery systems: compressed gas cylinders, liquid oxygen, and oxygen concentrators. Before placing a certain delivery system in a home, assess the advantages and disadvantages (Table 41-8) of each type, along with the patient's needs and community resources. In the home the major consideration is the oxygen-delivery source.

Patients and their family caregivers need extensive teaching to be able to manage oxygen therapy efficiently and safely (see Skill 41-4 on pp. 927-929). Teach the patient and family about home oxygen delivery (e.g., oxygen safety, regulation of the amount of oxygen, and how to use the prescribed home oxygen-delivery system) to ensure their ability to maintain the oxygen-delivery system. The home health nurse coordinates the efforts of the patient and family, home respiratory therapist, and home oxygen equipment vendor. The social worker usually assists initially with arranging for the home care nurse and oxygen vendor.

QSEN QSEN: BUILDING COMPETENCY IN SAFETY Mr. Jackson, a 68-year-old has a history of chronic obstructive pulmonary disease for 2 years. His SpO_2 ranges from 75% to 82%. Upon reviewing the care plan of your patient Mr. Edwards; you note that the plan is to send him home on oxygen. How do you promote safe oxygen delivery in his home?

Answers to QSEN Activities can be found on the Evolve website.

Restoration of Cardiopulmonary Functioning. If a patient's hypoxia is severe and prolonged, cardiac arrest results. A cardiac arrest is a sudden cessation of cardiac output and circulation. When this occurs, oxygen is not delivered to tissues, carbon dioxide is not transported from tissues, tissue metabolism becomes anaerobic, and metabolic and respiratory acidosis occurs. Permanent heart, brain, and other tissue damage occur within 4 to 6 minutes.

Cardiopulmonary Resuscitation. During cardiac arrest there is an absence of pulse and respiration. The American Heart Association continues to research cardiac arrest treatment and outcomes. The 2010 Consensus Conference reviewed the most current and comprehensive resuscitation literature/research to develop the *2010 AHA Guidelines for Cardiopulmonary Resuscitation (CPR) and Emergency Cardiac Care (ECC),* thus simplifying the basic life support (BLS) steps (AHA, 2010b).

TABLE 41-8 Home Oxygen Storage Systems

Primary Use	Advantages	Disadvantages
Compressed Gas Cylinders		
Stationary and portable systems designed for intermittent therapy such as for exercise or sleep or as a back-up system for a concentrator only.	100% oxygen stored in steel or aluminum cylinders; relatively inexpensive, no loss of gas during storage, relatively portable, delivery of up to 15 L/min; does not require electrical source; smaller tanks available for portability.	Bulky and heavy; must be secured safely to prevent them from falling over; frequent refilling necessary with continuous use; patient must know how to read regulator and understand when to call supplier; portable cylinders weigh 15 lbs.
Liquid Oxygen Systems		
Stationary and portable system of choice for high-volume users and active patients.	100% oxygen; more oxygen occupies a smaller space; patient carries convenient ambulatory units refilled at home as shoulder bag, backpack, or wheeled luggage cart; delivery of up to 6 L/min; they come with a battery pack or electrical connections for cars; patient can safely refill ambulatory units from larger reservoir; quiet and easy operation; minimal maintenance; does not require electricity for operation; requires relatively fewer deliveries of oxygen.	Evaporates, especially in warmer temperatures and when not in use; potential for connections to freeze together or form frost at connections if tight connection not maintained during filling; costly setup and delivery fees. The liquid oxygen is very cold and can harm the skin instantly upon contact.
Oxygen Concentrators		
Stationary system; cost-effective for patients requiring low-flow continuous oxygen and patients with limited mobility inside or outside the home.	Provide a large source of oxygen, inexpensive, fixed monthly costs; most units with delivery of 1 to 5 L/min; good choice for people who do not leave their homes frequently; no cylinders or tanks to refill; delivery up to 10 L/min with specific makes and models. They must be placed in an open, well-ventilated area away from heat and flames. They work by removing nitrogen from room air to make the air 94% to 98% oxygen. They can be small and can weigh from 22 to 70 pounds.	Oxygen concentration decreases as liter flow increases; power supply needed; increased electric costs; is not an ambulatory unit, therefore requires second system for portability; requires regular maintenance and backup system.
Compressed Gas		
Small cylinders with compressed gas that allow for portability.	Different models allow from 1 to 5 hours of portable oxygen. Cylinders can be easily wheeled on a cart or a stroller. Smaller tanks can be carried in backpacks, fanny packs, or shoulder bags. Each cylinder is fitted with a regulator used for adjusting the flow rate. At a rate of 2 L/min, they last only a few hours. The most common cylinder used is the E-cylinder; it lasts about 5 hours at a rate of 2 L/min.	They only last a few hours. E-cylinders are not appropriate as a sole source of oxygen for continuous, long-term therapy.

National Heart, Lung, and Blood Institute: What is oxygen therapy? 2012, http://www.nhlbi.nih.gov/health/health-topics/topics/oxt. Accessed May 2015.
The COPD Foundation: *COPD oxygen therapy systems: container/storage and delivery system,* Web MD Medical Reference from the COPD Foundation, 2010, http://www.webmd.com/lung/copd/deciding-which-oxygen-system-meets-your-needs. Accessed May 2015.

The previous ABC (establish an ***A***irway, initiate ***B***reathing, and maintain ***C***irculation) of cardiopulmonary resuscitation (CPR) is changed to CAB (***C***hest compression, ***A***irway, ***B***reathing) for adults and pediatric patients (excluding newborns). In adults (the majority of cardiac arrests) the critical initial elements found to be essential for survival were chest compressions and early defibrillation. Ventilation is done after the first cycle of 30 chest compressions. In addition the AHA (2014) has set a goal for hospitals to deliver the first electrical shock to patients in ventricular fibrillation in less than 2 minutes.

Another issue is that bystander CPR may increase if those not comfortable with doing ventilations would at least perform chest compression. For most adults with out-of-the-hospital arrest, hands-only CPR by bystanders has had similar outcomes to conventional CPR. A lone health care provider who sees an adult in cardiac arrest should activate the emergency response system, get and use an automatic external defibrillator (AED) if available, and give CPR. Defibrillation by AED (Box 41-10) is needed to stop an abnormal heart rhythm, and AEDs are now available in public places such as schools, airports, and workplaces (AHA, 2006, 2010a, b).

Restorative and Continuing Care. Restorative and continuing care emphasizes cardiopulmonary reconditioning as a structured rehabilitation program. Cardiopulmonary rehabilitation helps patients achieve and maintain an optimal level of health through controlled physical exercise, nutrition counseling, relaxation and stress-management techniques, and prescribed medications and oxygen. As physical reconditioning occurs, a patient's complaints of dyspnea, chest pain, fatigue, and activity intolerance decrease. In addition, the patient's anxiety, depression, or somatic concerns often decrease. The patient and the rehabilitation team define the goals of rehabilitation.

Respiratory Muscle Training. Respiratory muscle training improves muscle strength and endurance, resulting in improved activity tolerance. Respiratory muscle training prevents respiratory failure in patients with COPD. One method for respiratory muscle training is the incentive spirometer resistive breathing device (ISRBD). Patients

BOX 41-10 Automated External Defibrillator

- The automated external defibrillator (AED) is a device used to administer an electrical shock through the chest wall to the heart to stop the abnormal rhythm and restore a normal heart rhythm.
- The AED has built-in computers that assess patient's heart rhythm and determine if defibrillation is necessary. New technology has made them user friendly with audio and visual cues telling users what to do when using them (AHA, 2010b, 2011). The AED analyzes the patient's heart rhythm and determines if a shock is needed. It delivers a shock to the patient after announcing, "Everyone stand clear of patient." A shock is only delivered if the patient needs it.
- Lay rescuer AED programs train lay personnel (security guards, police, and firefighters) on the use of the AED (AHA, 2006, 2010b, 2011).
- The AED is used to strengthen the chain of survival. Every minute of a sudden cardiac arrest without defibrillation decreases the survival rate by 7% to 10% (AHA, 2011).

For witnessed ventricular fibrillation, early cardiopulmonary resuscitation with defibrillation within the first 3 to 5 minutes can result in greater than 50% long-term survival (AHA, 2010a).

achieve resistive breathing by placing a resistive breathing device into a volume-dependent incentive spirometer. Patients achieve muscle training when they use the ISRBD on a scheduled routine (e.g., twice a day for 15 minutes or 4 times a day for 15 minutes).

Breathing Exercises. Breathing exercises include techniques to improve ventilation and oxygenation. The three basic techniques are deep-breathing and coughing exercises, pursed-lip breathing, and diaphragmatic breathing. Deep-breathing and coughing exercises, previously discussed, are routine interventions used by postoperative patients (see Chapter 50).

Pursed-Lip Breathing. Pursed-lip breathing involves deep inspiration and prolonged expiration through pursed lips to prevent alveolar collapse. While sitting up, instruct the patient to take a deep breath and exhale slowly through pursed lips as if blowing through a straw. Have him or her blow through a straw into a glass of water to learn the technique. Patients need to gain control of the exhalation phase so it is longer than inhalation. The patient is usually able to perfect this technique by counting the inhalation time and gradually increasing the count during exhalation. In studies using pursed-lip breathing as a method to improve exercise tolerance in patients with COPD, patients were able to demonstrate increases in their exercise tolerance, breathing pattern, and arterial oxygen saturation (Cabral et al., 2014).

Diaphragmatic Breathing. Diaphragmatic breathing is useful for patients with pulmonary disease, postoperative patients, and women in labor to promote relaxation and provide pain control. The exercise improves efficiency of breathing by decreasing air trapping and reducing the WOB.

Diaphragmatic breathing is more difficult than other breathing methods because it requires a patient to relax intercostal and accessory respiratory muscles while taking deep inspirations, which takes practice. The patient places one hand flat below the breastbone (upper hand) and the other hand (lower hand) flat on the abdomen. Ask him or her to inhale slowly, making the abdomen push out (as the diaphragm flattens, the abdomen should extend out) and moving the lower hand outward. When the patient exhales, the abdomen goes in (the diaphragm ascends and pushes on lungs to help expel trapped air). The patient practices these exercises initially in the supine position and then while sitting and standing. The exercise is often used with the pursed-lip breathing technique.

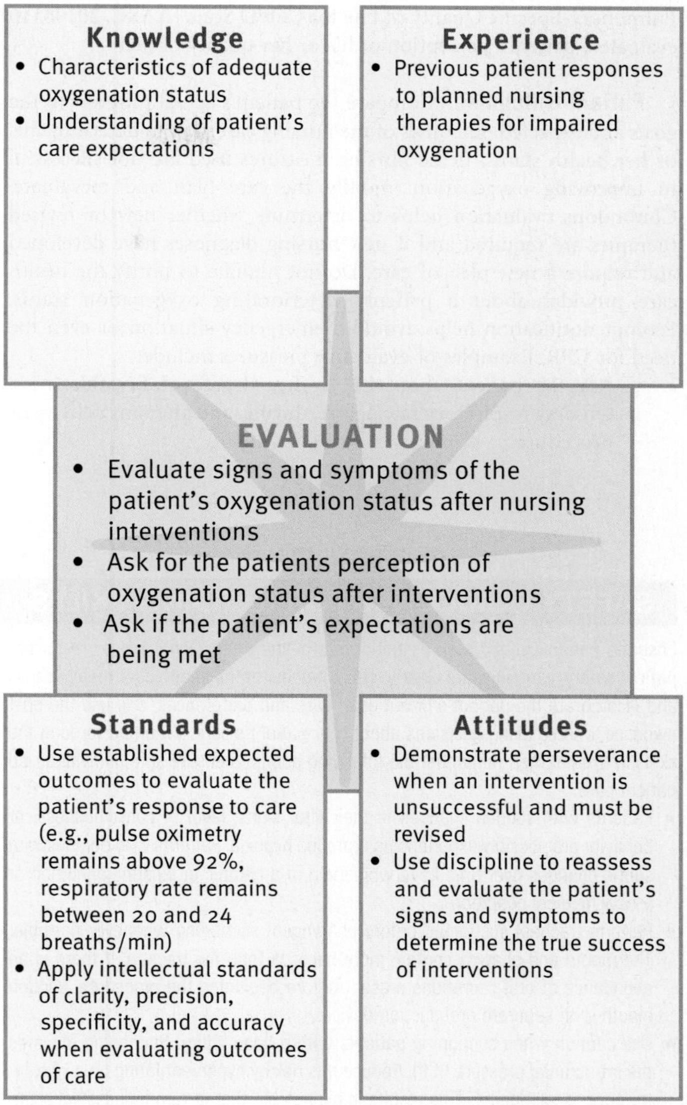

Knowledge
- Characteristics of adequate oxygenation status
- Understanding of patient's care expectations

Experience
- Previous patient responses to planned nursing therapies for impaired oxygenation

EVALUATION
- Evaluate signs and symptoms of the patient's oxygenation status after nursing interventions
- Ask for the patients perception of oxygenation status after interventions
- Ask if the patient's expectations are being met

Standards
- Use established expected outcomes to evaluate the patient's response to care (e.g., pulse oximetry remains above 92%, respiratory rate remains between 20 and 24 breaths/min)
- Apply intellectual standards of clarity, precision, specificity, and accuracy when evaluating outcomes of care

Attitudes
- Demonstrate perseverance when an intervention is unsuccessful and must be revised
- Use discipline to reassess and evaluate the patient's signs and symptoms to determine the true success of interventions

FIGURE 41-17 Critical thinking model for oxygenation evaluation.

◆ Evaluation

Evaluate nursing interventions and therapies by evaluating if patient expectations have been met and by comparing the patient's progress with the goals and expected outcomes of the nursing care plan (Figure 41-17).

Through the Patient's Eyes. It is important to determine a patient's perceptions of his or her care. Does the patient feel that interventions have improved the ability to maintain a more normal lifestyle? Focus on evaluating how the disease is affecting day-to-day activities and how the patient believes he or she is responding to treatment. Patients who have chronic lung problems often must be motivated to participate in necessary therapies. Evaluate the patient's motivation and emotional readiness to adhere to treatments provided. Be aware of the need to change a treatment plan to be culturally sensitive to improve adherence. Determine if the patient and family/caregiver feel more in control of their health situation after you have provided instruction. Consider the use of survey tools such as the COPD Self-Efficacy Scale, Chronic Respiratory Disease Questionnaire, and

Pulmonary-Specific Quality of Life for COPD Scale (AARC, 2010b) to evaluate a patient's perception of his or her quality of life.

Patient Outcomes. Compare the patient's actual progress to the goals and expected outcomes of the nursing care plan to determine his or her health status. If the nursing measures used are not successful in improving oxygenation, modify the care plan and reevaluate. Continuous evaluation helps to determine whether new or revised therapies are required and if new nursing diagnoses have developed and require a new plan of care. Do not hesitate to notify the health care provider about a patient's deteriorating oxygenation status. Prompt notification helps avoid an emergency situation or even the need for CPR. Examples of evaluative measures include:

- Ask the patient about his or her degree of breathlessness. Observe respiratory rate before, during, and after any activity or procedure.
- Ask the patient if the distance ambulated without fatigue has increased.
- Ask the patient to rate breathlessness on a scale of 0 to 10, with 0 being no shortness of breath and 10 being severe shortness of breath.
- Ask the patient which interventions help reduce dyspnea.
- Ask the patient about frequency of cough and sputum production and assess any sputum produced.
- Auscultate lung sounds for improvement in adventitious sounds.
- Evaluate pulse oximetry changes to decreases in oxygen delivery.
- Monitor arterial blood gas levels, pulmonary function tests, chest x-ray films, ECG tracings, and physical assessment data to provide objective measurement of the success of therapies and treatments.

SAFETY GUIDELINES FOR NURSING SKILLS

Ensuring patient safety is an essential role of the professional nurse. To ensure patient safety, communicate clearly with members of the health care team, assess and incorporate the patient's priorities of care and preferences, and use the best evidence when making decisions about your patient's care. When performing the skills in this chapter, remember the following points to ensure safe, individualized patient care.

- Patients with sudden changes in their vital signs, level of consciousness, or behavior are possibly experiencing profound hypoxia. Patients who demonstrate subtle changes over time have worsening of a chronic or existing condition or a new medical condition.
- Perform tracheal suctioning before pharyngeal suctioning whenever possible. The mouth and pharynx contain more bacteria than the trachea. If there is an abundance of oral secretions present before beginning the procedure, suction mouth with separate oral suction device.
- Use caution when suctioning patients with a head injury. Suctioning elevates the intracranial pressure (ICP). Reduce this risk by hyperventilating on a ventilator prior to suctioning. This results in hypocarbia that in turn induces vasoconstriction. Vasoconstriction reduces the potential increase in ICP. It is recommended that you limit the introduction of the catheter to 2 times with each suctioning procedure (Kaiser et al., 2011).
- The routine use of normal saline instillation into the airway before endotracheal and tracheostomy suctioning is not recommended. Use of NSI is associated with the adverse effects of excessive coughing, bronchospasm, spread of organisms to the lower respiratory tract, and decreased oxygen saturation (AARC, 2010b). In certain circumstances, if it is necessary to simulate a cough, normal saline may be indicated. This requires collaboration with the health care team.
- Check your institutional policy before stripping or milking chest tubes. Most institutions have stopped using this practice because stripping the tube greatly increases intrapleural pressure, which can damage the pleural tissue and cause pneumothorax or worsen an existing pneumothorax.
- The most serious tracheostomy complication is airway obstruction, which can result in cardiac arrest. Most tracheostomy tubes are designed with a small plastic inner tube that sits inside the larger one. If the airway becomes occluded, the smaller one can be removed and replaced with a temporary spare. It is important to always have a spare at the bedside for emergency replacement.
- Patients with COPD who are breathing spontaneously should never receive high levels of oxygen therapy because it results in a decreased stimulus to breathe. Do not administer oxygen more than 2 L/min unless a health care provider's order is obtained (AARC, 2007).

SKILL 41-1 SUCTIONING

DELEGATION CONSIDERATIONS

The skill of nasotracheal suctioning and suctioning a new artificial airway cannot be delegated to nursing assistive personnel (NAP). However, when a patient has been assessed by the nurse to be stable, oropharyngeal and permanent tracheostomy tube suctioning can be delegated to NAP. Instruct NAP about:

- Any modifications of the skill such as the need to reapply any supplemental oxygen equipment following the procedure.
- Appropriate suction limits and risk of applying excessive or inadequate suction pressure.
- Reporting any change in patient's respiratory status, level of consciousness, secretion color or volume, or unresolved coughing or gagging.
- Reporting any change in patient's color, vital signs, or complaints of pain.

EQUIPMENT

- Stethoscope
- Pulse oximeter
- Portable or wall suction machine
- Connecting tubing (6 feet)
- Bedside table
- Mask, goggles, gown, or face shield, if indicated

Oropharyngeal (Nonsterile) and Nasotracheal (Sterile) Suctioning

- Oropharyngeal suctioning: Clean, nonsterile suction catheter or Yankauer suction tip catheter
    - One sterile and one clean glove
- Nasotracheal suctioning: Sterile suction catheter (12 to 16 Fr) (smallest diameter that effectively removes secretions)
    - Two sterile gloves
- Sterile basin (e.g., sterile disposable cup)
- Sterile water or normal saline (about 100 mL)
- Clean towel or paper drape

Endotracheal or Tracheostomy Suctioning

- 12- to 16-Fr catheter (approximate; size of the suction catheter in an adult patient should be no more than half of the internal diameter of the artificial airway to minimize decrease in PaO_2) (AARC, 2010a). Formula for suction tracheostomy catheter size: divide internal diameter of the tube by 2 and multiply by 3 (Freeman, 2011).
- Two sterile gloves or one sterile and one clean glove
- Sterile basin
- Sterile normal saline (about 100 mL)
- Clean towel or sterile drape

Closed System or In-Line Suctioning

- Closed-system or in-line suction catheter
- 5- to 10-mL normal saline in syringe or vials
- Two clean gloves

STEP	RATIONALE
ASSESSMENT	
1. Identify patient using two identifiers (e.g., name and birth date or name and medical record number) according to agency policy.	Ensures correct patient. Complies with The Joint Commission standards and improves patient safety (TJC, 2016).
2. Assess for signs and symptoms of upper and lower airway obstruction requiring suctioning: abnormal respiratory rate, adventitious sounds on inspiration or expiration, nasal secretions, gurgling, drooling, restlessness, gastric secretions or vomitus in mouth, and coughing without clearing secretions from airway.	Physical signs and symptoms result from decreased oxygen to tissues and pooling of secretions in upper and lower airways. Complete these assessment measures before and after suction procedure (AARC, 2004).
3. Assess signs and symptoms associated with hypoxia and hypercapnia: decreased SpO_2, increased pulse and blood pressure, increased respiratory rate, apprehension, anxiety, decreased ability to concentrate, lethargy, decreased level of consciousness (especially acute), increased fatigue, dizziness, behavioral changes (especially irritability), dysrhythmias, pallor, and cyanosis.	Physical signs and symptoms resulting from decreased oxygen to tissues indicate need for suctioning (AARC, 2004).
4. Assess for risk factors for upper or lower airway obstruction, including chronic obstructive pulmonary disease, pulmonary infection, fluid imbalance, lack of humidity, impaired mobility, decreased level of consciousness, decreased gag or cough reflex, dysphagia, presence of feeding tube.	The presence of these risk factors impairs a patient's ability to clear secretions from the airway, thickens secretions, or increases risk for retaining secretions and thus requires suctioning.
5. Assess for neuromuscular disease or anatomical factors that influence upper or lower airway function, such as recent surgery; head, chest, or neck trauma; tumors.	Abnormal anatomy or head and neck trauma impairs normal drainage of secretions. Tumors in or around the lower airway impair secretion removal by occluding or externally compressing lumen of airway.

SKILL 41-1 SUCTIONING—cont'd

STEP	RATIONALE
6. Identify **contraindications to nasotracheal suctioning** (AARC, 2004): occluded nasal passages; nasal bleeding, epiglottitis, or croup; acute head, facial, or neck injury or surgery; coagulopathy or bleeding disorder; irritable airway; laryngospasm or bronchospasm; gastric surgery with high anastomosis; myocardial infarction.	These conditions are **contraindicated because the passage of a catheter through the nasal route** causes trauma to existing facial trauma or surgery, increases nasal bleeding, or causes severe bleeding in the presence of bleeding disorders. In the presence of epiglottitis, croup, laryngospasm, or irritable airway, the entrance of a suction catheter via the nasal route causes intractable coughing, hypoxemia, and severe bronchospasm, necessitating emergency intubation or tracheostomy. Hypoxemia could worsen cardiac damage in myocardial infarction (AARC, 2004).
7. Review sputum microbiology data.	Certain bacteria are easier to transmit or require isolation because of virulence or antibiotic resistance.
8. Assess patient's understanding of procedure.	Reveals need for patient instruction.
PLANNING	
1. Explain to patient how procedure will help clear airway and relieve breathing problems and that temporary coughing, sneezing, gagging, or shortness of breath is normal. Encourage patient to cough out secretions.	Encourages cooperation and minimizes risks, anxiety, and pain.
2. Explain importance of and encourage coughing when catheter is introduced. Have patient practice coughing if able and splint surgical incisions (if present).	Facilitates secretion removal and reduces frequency and duration of future suctioning.
3. Assist patient with assuming comfortable position (usually semi-Fowler's or sitting upright with head hyperextended, unless contraindicated). Stand on patient's right if you are right-handed or on patient's left if you are left-handed.	Reduces stimulation of gag reflex, promotes patient comfort and secretion drainage, and prevents aspiration. Hyperextension facilitates insertion of catheter into trachea. Position facilitates catheter insertion.
4. If not already in place, position pulse oximeter on patient's finger. Take reading and leave pulse oximeter in place.	Provides baseline SpO_2 to determine patient's response to suctioning.
5. Place towel across patient's chest.	Reduces transmission of microorganisms by protecting gown from secretions.
IMPLEMENTATION	
1. Perform hand hygiene. Apply mask, gown, goggles, or face shield if splashing is likely.	Reduces transmission of microorganisms.
2. Connect one end of connecting tubing to suction machine and place other end in convenient location near patient. Turn suction device on and set vacuum regulator to appropriate negative pressure: 120 to 150 mm Hg for adults (AARC, 2010a), 40 to 60 mm Hg for infants, and 60 to 100 mm Hg for children (Hockenberry and Wilson, 2015).	Excessive negative pressure damages nasal, pharyngeal, and tracheal mucosa and induces greater hypoxia. Negative pressures should not exceed 150 mm Hg because higher pressure increases risk for airway trauma, hypoxemia, and atelectasis (AARC, 2010a).
3. If indicated, increase supplemental oxygen therapy to 100% or as ordered by health care provider. Encourage patient to deep breathe.	Hyperoxygenation provides some protection from suction-induced decline in oxygenation. It is most effective in the presence of hyperinflation such as encouraging patient to deep breathe or increase ventilator tidal volume settings (Sole et al., 2014; AARC, 2010a).
4. Preparation for all types of suctioning (except in-line).	
a. Open appropriate suction kit or catheter, using aseptic technique and leaving catheter in sterile wrapper or kit. If sterile drape is available, place it across patient's chest or on over-bed table. Do not allow suction catheter to touch any nonsterile surfaces.	Prepares catheter and prevents transmission of microorganisms. Provides sterile surface on which to lay suction catheter between passes, if needed.
b. Unwrap or open sterile basin and place on bedside table. Fill basin or cup with approximately 100 mL of sterile normal saline solution or water (see illustration).	Solution is used to flush catheter after each suction pass.
c. Open lubricant. Squeeze small amount onto open sterile wrapper or kit without touching it. **NOTE:** Lubricant is not necessary for oropharyngeal or artificial airway suctioning.	Prepares lubricant while maintaining sterility. Use water-soluble lubricant to avoid lipoid aspiration pneumonia. Excessive lubricant application can occlude catheter.

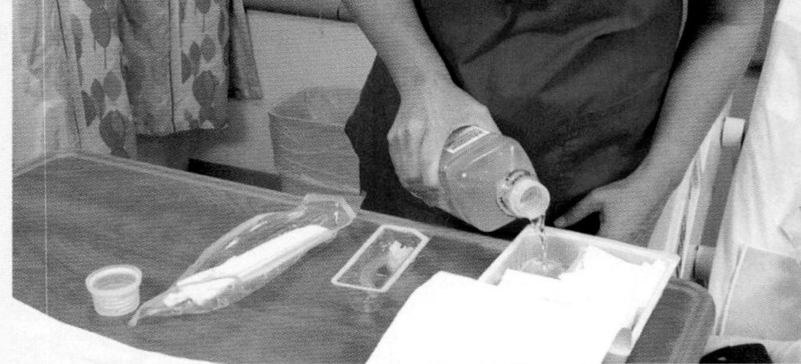

STEP 4b Pouring saline into tray. (Copyright © Mosby's Clinical Skills: Essentials Collection.)

STEP	RATIONALE
5. Apply gloves:	
a. Apply clean glove to each hand or dominant hand for oropharyngeal suctioning.	Suction of oral cavity does not require sterile glove use.
b. Apply sterile glove to each hand or nonsterile glove to nondominant hand and sterile glove to dominant hand for nasopharyngeal, nasotracheal, and artificial airway suctioning.	Reduces transmission of microorganisms and allows nurse to maintain sterility of suction catheter.
6. Pick up suction catheter with dominant hand without touching nonsterile surface. Pick up connecting tubing with nondominant hand. Secure catheter to tubing (see illustration).	
7. Place tip of catheter into sterile basin and suction a small amount of normal saline by occluding suction vent.	Ensures suction is functioning. Lubricates internal catheter and tubing.
8. Suction airway.	
a. Oropharyngeal suctioning	
(1) Remove oxygen mask if present. Keep oxygen mask near patient's face. If patient has a nasal cannula, it may remain in place.	Allows access to patient's mouth while having access to oxygen-delivery system.

CLINICAL DECISION: *Be prepared to quickly reapply oxygen mask if* SpO_2 *falls or respiratory distress develops during or at the end of suctioning.*

STEP	RATIONALE
(2) Insert Yankauer catheter into patient's mouth. Apply suction once the catheter is in patient's mouth, move catheter around mouth along gum line to pharynx. Then apply suction and move catheter around mouth until secretions are cleared.	If catheter does not have a suction control to apply intermittent suction, take care not to allow suction tip to irritate oral mucosal surfaces with continuous suction.
(3) Encourage patient to cough and repeat suctioning if needed. Replace oxygen mask if used.	Coughing moves secretions from lower to upper airways into mouth.
(4) Suction water or saline through catheter until catheter is cleared of secretions.	Clearing secretions before they dry reduces probability of transmission of microorganisms and enhances delivery of preset suction pressures.
(5) Place catheter in a clean, dry area for reuse with suction turned off. If patient is capable of self-oral suctioning, place catheter within reach.	Provides for prompt removal of future oral secretions.
b. Nasopharyngeal and nasotracheal suctioning	
(1) Lightly coat distal 6-8 cm (2-3 inches) of catheter tip with water-soluble lubricant.	Lubricates catheter for easier insertion of catheter and reduces mucosal surface trauma.
(2) If indicated increase supplemental oxygen therapy as ordered by health care provider. Have patient deep breathe with oxygen delivery device or hyperoxygenate with ventilation bag as ordered.	Hyperoxygenation before suctioning can minimize hypoxemia after suctioning (AARC, 2010a).
(3) Remove oxygen-delivery device, if applicable, with nondominant hand. Without applying suction and using dominant thumb and forefinger, gently insert catheter into naris during inhalation. ***Never apply suction during insertion.***	Application of suction pressure while introducing catheter into nasopharyngeal tissues increases risk of damage to mucosa. When advanced into trachea, suction could damage mucosa and increase risk of hypoxia.

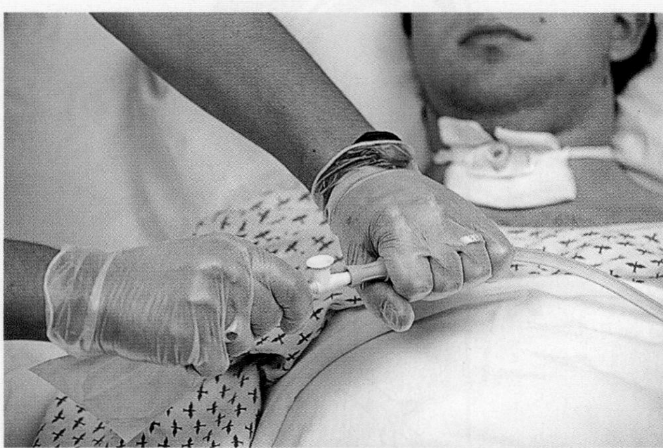

STEP 6 Attaching catheter to suction.

SKILL 41-1 SUCTIONING—cont'd

STEP	RATIONALE
CLINICAL DECISION: *Be sure to insert catheter during patient inhalation. This closes epiglottis, making it easier to pass catheter through larynx into trachea. Do not insert during swallowing, or catheter will most likely enter the esophagus. If patient gags or becomes nauseated, the catheter is most likely in the esophagus and must be removed.*	
(4) *Nasopharyngeal:* As patient takes a deep breath, insert catheter, following natural course of naris; slightly slant catheter downward and advance to back of pharynx. Do not force through naris. In adults insert catheter about 20 cm (6 to 8 inches); in older children, 16 to 20 cm (6 to 8 inches); in infants and young children, 4 to 14 cm (3 to 5½ inches) into trachea until resistance is met or patient coughs; then pull back 1 to 2 cm (½ inch).	Proper placement ensures removal of pharyngeal secretions. Pulling back on catheter before initiating suctioning prevents invagination of the tracheal membrane (AARC, 2010a).
(a) Apply intermittent suction for no more than 10 seconds by placing and releasing nondominant thumb over catheter vent (AARC, 2010a). Slowly withdraw catheter while rotating it back and forth between thumb and forefinger.	Intermittent suction up to 10 seconds safely removes pharyngeal secretions. Suction time greater than 10 seconds increases risk for suction-induced hypoxemia (AARC, 2010a).
(5) *Nasotracheal:* As patient takes deep breath, advance catheter following natural course of naris. Advance catheter slightly slanted and downward to just above entrance into larynx and then the trachea. While patient takes a deep breath, quickly insert catheter about 15 to 20 cm (6 to 8 inches in adult) into trachea (see illustration). Patient will begin to cough, then pull back catheter 1 to 2 cm (½ inch) before applying suction.	Ensures that catheter is inserted into trachea with minimum stress to patient. In young children and infants, shallow suctioning is recommended instead of deep tracheal suctioning, which increases the risk of tracheal edema and inflammation (AARC, 2010a).
NOTE: In older children advance the catheter 16 to 20 cm (6 to 8 inches), and in young children and infants, 8 to 14 cm (3 to 5½ inches).	Premeasured suction catheters are used in some pediatric settings to avoid deep suctioning (Hockenberry and Wilson, 2015).
CLINICAL DECISION: *When there is difficulty passing the catheter, ask patient to cough or say "ahh" or try to advance during inspiration. Both these measures assist in opening the glottis to permit passage of the catheter into the trachea.*	
(a) *Positioning option:* In some instances turning patient's head to right helps suction the left mainstem bronchus; turning head to left helps suction the right mainstem bronchus.	Turning patient's head to the side elevates the bronchial passage on the opposite side and facilitates passage of the catheter.
(b) If you feel resistance after insertion of catheter to maximum recommended distance, catheter has probably hit carina. Pull it back 1 to 2 cm (½ inch) before applying suction.	
CLINICAL DECISION: *Use nasotracheal suctioning before pharyngeal suctioning whenever possible. The mouth and pharynx contain more bacteria than the trachea. If copious oral secretions are present before beginning the procedure, suction mouth with oral suction device.*	

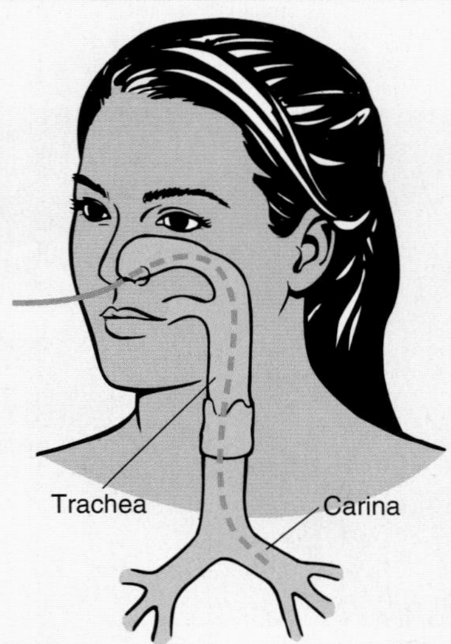

STEP 8b(5) Distance of insertion of nasotracheal catheter.

STEP	RATIONALE
(c) Apply intermittent suction for no more than 10 seconds by placing and releasing nondominant thumb over vent of catheter. Slowly withdraw catheter while rotating it back and forth between the dominant thumb and forefinger. Encourage patient to cough. Replace oxygen device if applicable.	Intermittent suction and rotation of catheter prevent injury to mucosa. If catheter "grabs" mucosa, remove thumb to release suction. Suctioning longer than 10 seconds causes cardiopulmonary compromise, usually from hypoxemia or vagal overload.

CLINICAL DECISION: *Monitor patient's vital signs and oxygen saturation during procedure; note whether there is a change of 20 beats/min (either increase or decrease) or if pulse oximetry falls below 90% or 5% from baseline. If this occurs, stop suctioning.*

STEP	RATIONALE
(6) Rinse catheter and connecting tubing with normal saline or water until cleared.	Removes secretions from catheter. Secretions that remain in suction catheter or connecting tubing decrease suctioning efficiency.
(7) Assess for need to repeat suctioning procedure. Do not perform more than two passes with catheter. Allow at least 1 minute between passes for ventilation and oxygenation (AARC, 2010a). Ask patient to deep breathe and cough.	Observe for alterations in cardiopulmonary status. Suctioning induces hypoxemia, dysrhythmias, laryngospasm, and bronchospasm (AARC, 2010a). Hyperoxygenation is recommended before, during, and after open suctioning to reduce risk for suction-induced hypoxemia (Yazdannik et al., 2013). Repeated passes clear the airway of excessive secretions but also remove oxygen and can induce laryngospasm.
c. Artificial airway (tracheostomy or endotracheal [ET] tube) suctioning	

CLINICAL DECISION: *Reduces transmission of microorganisms.* **NOTE:** *If risk for splash is present or patient is on respiratory precautions, gown, face shield or mask, and goggles may be needed.*

STEP	RATIONALE
(1) Check that equipment is functioning properly by placing tip of catheter into basin and suctioning small amount of saline by occluding suction vent.	Ensures equipment function; lubricates catheter and tubing.
(2) Hyperoxygenate patient before suctioning using manual resuscitation bag and increasing FiO_2 for several minutes; or, if mechanically ventillated, use the ventilator to provide additional breaths without increasing tidal volume. Some mechanical ventilators have a button that, when pushed, delivers 100% oxygen for a few minutes and then resets to the previous value.	Hyperoxygenation for 30-60 seconds decreases suction-induced hypoxemia. Most sources recommend hyperoxygenation with 100% oxygen in the adult patient (AARC, 2010a).
(3) If patient is receiving invasive mechanical ventilation, open swivel adapter or, if necessary, remove oxygen- or humidity-delivery device with nondominant hand.	Exposes artificial airway.
(4) Advise patient that you are about to begin suctioning and, without applying suction, gently but quickly insert catheter using dominant thumb and forefinger into artificial airway (see illustration). Insert catheter during inspiration until you meet resistance or patient coughs; then pull back 1 cm (½ inch) (Ozden and Gorgulu, 2012).	Prepares patient for procedure. Application of suction pressure while introducing catheter into trachea increases risk of damage to tracheal mucosa and increased hypoxia related to removal of entrained oxygen present in airways. Pulling back stimulates cough and removes catheter from mucosal wall so catheter is not resting against tracheal mucosa during suctioning.

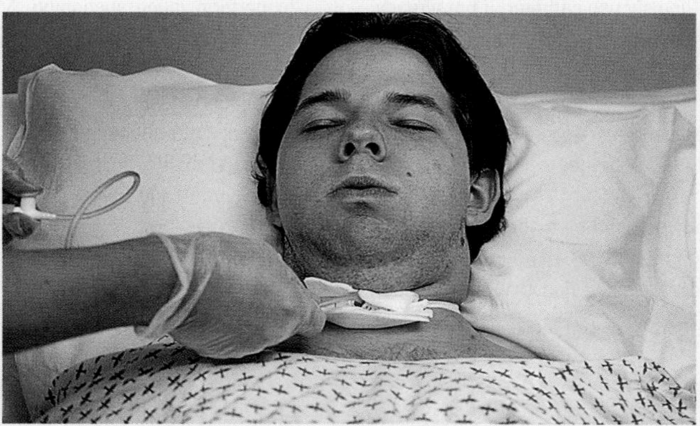

STEP 8c(4) Suctioning tracheostomy.

SKILL 41-1 SUCTIONING—cont'd

STEP	RATIONALE
CLINICAL DECISION: *If unable to insert catheter past the end of the ET tube, it is probably caught in the Murphy eye (e.g., side hole at the distal end of the ET tube that allows for collateral airflow in the event of mainstem intubation). If this happens, rotate the catheter to reposition it away from the Murphy eye or withdraw it slightly and reinsert with the next inhalation. Usually the catheter meets resistance at the carina. One indication that the catheter is at the carina is acute onset of coughing because the carina contains many cough receptors. Pull the catheter back 1 cm (½ inch).*	
(5) Apply intermittent suction no longer than 10 seconds (Ozden and Gorgulu, 2012). Apply intermittent suction by placing and releasing nondominant thumb over vent of catheter; slowly withdraw catheter while rotating it back and forth between dominant thumb and forefinger (AARC, 2010a). Encourage patient to cough. Watch for respiratory distress.	Intermittent suction and rotation of catheter prevent injury to tracheal mucosal lining. If catheter "grabs" mucosa, remove thumb to release suction.
CLINICAL DECISION: *If patient develops respiratory distress, immediately withdraw catheter and supply additional oxygen and breaths as needed. In an emergency administer oxygen directly through the catheter. Disconnect suction and give 100% oxygen through the catheter.*	
(6) If patient is receiving invasive mechanical ventilation, close swivel adapter or replace oxygen-delivery device.	Reestablishes the artificial airway.
(7) Encourage patient to deep breathe if able. Some patients respond well to several manual breaths from the mechanical ventilator or bag-valve mask.	Reoxygenates and expands alveoli. Suctioning sometimes causes hypoxemia and atelectasis.
(8) Rinse catheter and connecting tubing with normal saline until clear. Use continuous suction.	Removes catheter secretions. Secretions left in tubing decrease suction and provide environment for microorganism growth. Secretions left in connecting tube decrease suctioning efficiency.
(9) Assess patient's cardiopulmonary status for secretion clearance and complications. Repeat Steps (2) through (5) once or twice more to clear secretions. Allow adequate time (at least 1 full minute) between suction passes for ventilation and hyperoxygenation. Do not perform more than two passes with the catheter (AARC, 2010a).	Suctioning sometimes induces dysrhythmias, hypoxia, and bronchospasm and impairs cerebral circulation or adversely affects hemodynamics (AARC, 2010a). Repeated passes with suction catheter clear airway of excessive secretions and promote improved oxygenation.
(10) Perform nasopharyngeal and oropharyngeal suctioning if necessary. After performing nasopharyngeal and oropharyngeal suctioning, catheter is contaminated; do not reinsert into ET or tracheostomy tube.	Upper airway is "clean," and lower airway is "sterile." Therefore you can use the same catheter to suction from sterile to clean areas but not from clean to sterile areas.
d. Artificial airway (tracheostomy or endotracheal [ET] tube) using inline suctioning	
(1) In many facilities a respiratory therapist attaches catheter to mechanical ventilator circuit. If the catheter is not already in place, open closed-suction catheter package using aseptic technique, attach catheter to ventilator circuit by removing swivel adapter, and place catheter apparatus on endotracheal or tracheostomy tube. Connect Y on mechanical ventilator circuit to closed-suction catheter with flex tubing (see Fig. 41-10).	Attaches suction catheter to the ET or tracheostomy if not already done in order to perform inline suctioning. In some settings the catheter is attached to the closed ventilator circuit by a respiratory therapist.
(2) Connect one end of connecting tubing to suction machine and the other to the end of a closed system or in-line suction catheter, if not already done. Turn suction device on and set vacuum regulator to appropriate negative pressure (see manufacturer directions).	Attaches inline suction catheter to the suction machine if not already done in order to perform inline suctioning. Many closed-system suction catheters require slightly higher suction; consult manufacturer guidelines.
(3) Hyperoxygenate patient (increase FiO_2) with bag-valve mask or manual breathing mechanism on mechanical ventilator according to institution protocol and clinical status (usually 100% oxygen).	Hyperinflation along with hyperoxygenation decreases risk for a decrease in oxygenation saturation. Routine use of hyperinflation is not recommended because of the possibility of trauma resulting from large volumes and high peak pressures (Ozden and Gorgulu, 2012; AARC, 2010a).
(4) Unlock suction control mechanism if required by manufacturer. Open saline port and attach saline syringe or vial.	
(5) Pick up suction catheter enclosed in plastic sleeve with dominant hand.	

STEP	RATIONALE
(6) Wait until patient inhales, then insert catheter using a repeating maneuver of pushing catheter and sliding (or pulling) plastic sleeve back between thumb and forefinger until you feel resistance or patient coughs. Pull back 1 cm (½ inch) before applying suction to avoid tissue damage to carina.	Pushing and sliding the catheter in helps the patient to cough, which aids in bringing up secretions that can then be removed with the inline suction catheter.
(7) Encourage patient to cough and apply suction by squeezing on suction-control mechanism while withdrawing catheter. It is difficult to apply intermittent pulses of suction and nearly impossible to rotate the catheter compared with a standard catheter. Be sure to withdraw catheter completely into plastic sheath so it does not obstruct airflow (AARC, 2004).	Having patient cough helps to bring up additional secretions that can then be suctioned and removed with the inline suction catheter.
(8) Evaluate cardiopulmonary status, including pulse oximetry, to determine need for subsequent suctioning or complications. Repeat Steps (3) through (7) one to two more times to clear secretions. Allow adequate time (at least 1 full minute) between suction passes for ventilation and reoxygenation.	Suctioning sometimes induces dysrhythmias, hypoxia, and bronchospasm and impairs cerebral circulation or adversely affects hemodynamics (AARC, 2010a). Repeated passes with suction catheter clear airway of excessive secretions and promote improved oxygenation.
(9) When airway is clear, withdraw catheter completely into sheath. Be sure that colored indicator line on catheter is visible in the sheath. Squeeze vial or push syringe while applying suction to rinse inner lumen of catheter. Use at least 5 to 10 mL of saline to rinse catheter until it is clear of retained secretions, which cause bacterial growth and increase the risk of infection (AARC, 2004). Lock suction mechanism, if applicable, and turn off suction.	Removes catheter secretions. Secretions left in tubing decrease suction and provide environment for microorganism growth. Secretions left in connecting tube decrease suctioning efficiency.
(10) If patient requires oral or nasal suctioning, perform Skill 41-1 with separate standard suction catheter.	Oral and nasal suctioning require the use of a separate suction catheter in order to maintain the sterility of the inline suction catheter.
(11) Rinse catheter and connecting tubing with normal saline until clear. Use continuous suction.	Removes catheter secretions. Secretions left in tubing decrease suction and provide environment for microorganism growth. Secretions left in connecting tube decrease suctioning efficiency.
9. Complete procedure.	
a. Place Yankauer catheter in a clean, dry area for reuse with suction turned off or within patient's reach with suction on if patient is capable of suctioning self.	Facilitates prompt removal of airway secretions when suctioning is necessary in the future.
b. Disconnect nasal and artificial airway catheters from connecting tubing. Turn off suction. Roll catheter around fingers of dominant hand. Pull glove off inside out so catheter remains in glove. Pull off other glove over first glove in same way to contain contaminants. Discard into appropriate receptacle. Turn off suction device.	Reduces transmission of microorganisms. Do not touch clean equipment with contaminated gloves.
(1) When discarding the inline suction catheter, disconnect by removing it from the ventilator circuit. Dispose of catheter by pulling glove off inside out so catheter remains contained in glove. Before leaving patient's bedside, replace with a new inline catheter as in Step 8d(1).	
c. Remove towel and place in laundry or remove drape and discard in appropriate receptacle.	Reduces transmission of organisms.
d. Reposition patient as indicated by condition. Reapply clean gloves for patient's personal care (e.g., oral hygiene).	Proper positioning based on patient's condition promotes comfort, encourages secretion drainage, and reduces risk of aspiration.
e. If indicated, readjust oxygen to original level.	Helps patient's blood oxygen level return to baseline.

CLINICAL DECISION: *If patient develops respiratory distress during the suctioning procedure, immediately withdraw catheter and supply additional oxygen and breaths as needed. In an emergency administer oxygen directly through the catheter. Disconnect suction and attach oxygen at prescribed flow rate through the catheter.*

STEP	RATIONALE
f. Discard remainder of normal saline into appropriate receptacle. If basin is disposable, discard into appropriate receptacle. If basin is reusable, rinse and place in soiled utility room.	Solution is contaminated; this reduces transmission of microorganisms.
g. Remove and discard goggles, mask, or face shield and perform hand hygiene.	Reduces transmission of microorganisms.
h. Place unopened suction kit on suction machine table or at head of bed according to institution preference.	Provides for immediate access of suction catheter and equipment in event of an emergency or for next suctioning procedure.

SKILL 41-1 SUCTIONING—cont'd

STEP	RATIONALE
EVALUATION	
1. Compare patient's vital signs and SpO_2 saturation before and after suctioning.	Provides objective data about any physiological effects of suctioning.
2. Ask patient if breathing is easier and congestion is decreased.	Provides subjective confirmation that airway obstruction is relieved with suctioning procedure.
3. Auscultate lungs and compare patient's respiratory assessment before and after suctioning.	Provides objective information about any improvement in lung sounds.
4. Observe airway secretions.	Provides data to document presence or absence of respiratory tract infection.
5. Observe patient perform oropharyngeal suctioning.	Documents patient's ability to correctly perform oral suctioning.
6. Use ***Teach Back:*** State, "I want to be sure that I explained the suctioning procedure correctly. Squeeze my hand if you understand the steps that we discussed." (You can also use the communication board for a patient with an ETT.) Revise your instruction now or develop plan for revised patient teaching if patient is not able to teach back correctly.	Evaluates what the patient is able to explain or demonstrate.

UNEXPECTED OUTCOMES AND RELATED INTERVENTIONS

1. Worsening cardiopulmonary status
   - Limit length of suctioning.
   - Determine need for presuctioning hyperoxygenation and hyperinflation.
   - Determine need for more frequent suctioning, possibly shorter duration.
   - Notify health care provider of changes.
2. Return of bloody secretions
   - Determine amount of suction pressure used and adjust accordingly.
   - Evaluate suctioning frequency and reduce if appropriate.
   - Determine other factors that lead to bloody secretions (e.g., prolonged bleeding time).
   - Provide more frequent oral hygiene.
3. Unable to pass suction catheter through first naris attempted
   - Try other naris or oral route.
   - Insert nasal airway, especially if suctioning through patient naris frequently.
   - Guide catheter along naris floor to avoid turbinates.
   - If obstruction is mucus, apply suction to relieve obstruction but do not apply suction to mucosa. If you think obstruction is a blood clot, consult health care provider.
   - Increase lubrication of catheter.

RECORDING AND REPORTING

- Record amount, consistency, color, and odor of secretions and patient's response to procedure in EHR or chart.
- Record and report patient's presuctioning and postsuctioning cardiopulmonary status.
- Document your evaluation of patient learning.

HOME CARE CONSIDERATIONS

- Adhere to best practices for infection control while weighing cost-effectiveness in the presence of a chronic situation. If a patient has an established tracheostomy or requires long-term nasotracheal suctioning and infection is not present, clean suction technique is appropriate.
- Although most patients with airway clearance problems at home have a tracheostomy, some also require nasal pharyngeal suctioning. Catheters are often used for a 24-hour period and then cleaned and disinfected; or they are cleaned with soapy water after each use and discarded after 24 hours.
- Stress to family caregivers the importance of brief intervals of applying suction pressure. Instruct those performing suction to hold their breath during the application of negative suction pressure to help them remember to not suction too long.
- Instruct patient to clean and disinfect or change the secretion collection container every 24 hours according to home care or institutional protocol.
- Teach patient and family how to practice infection-control measures when emptying the suction container jar. These secretions are emptied in the toilet but have a splash risk. Instruct caregiver to apply mask (shield if available) and gloves and bring the jar as close to the toilet bowel as possible to decrease the risk of splash.

SKILL 41-2 CARE OF AN ARTIFICIAL AIRWAY

DELEGATION CONSIDERATIONS

The skill of performing artificial airway care in an acute care setting cannot be delegated to nursing assistive personnel (NAP). In long-term care settings, patients who have well-established tracheostomy tubes may have their care delegated to the NAP. Instruct the NAP to:

- Report any changes in patient's respiratory status, change in level of consciousness, confusion, restlessness or irritability, change in vital signs (range to report), decreased pulse oximetry level (values to report), or change in level of comfort.
- Report if the endotracheal (ET) tube or tracheostomy tube appears to have becomes dislodged, obstructed, or moved.
- Report any unexpected drainage or secretions from tracheostomy or change in color of stoma.

EQUIPMENT

- Stethoscope
- Face shield, if indicated for splash risk
- Bedside table
- Towel

Endotracheal Tube Care

- ET and oropharyngeal suction equipment
- 1- to 1½-inch (2.5- to 4-cm) adhesive or waterproof tape (not paper or silk tape) or commercial ET holder and mouth guard (follow manufacturer instructions for securing)
- Clean gloves (two pairs)
- Adhesive remover swab
- Mouth care supplies: pediatric toothbrush, toothette for edentulous patients; toothpaste
- 0.12% to 0.20% chlorhexidine mouthwash, rinse, or gel
- Face cleaner (e.g., wet washcloth, towel, soap, shaving supplies)
- Clean 2 × 2 gauze
- Tincture of benzoin, liquid adhesive, or skin preparation pad
- Oral airway

Tracheostomy Care

- Tracheostomy suction supplies
- Sterile tracheostomy care kit, if available, or:
  - Three sterile 4 × 4 gauze pads
  - Sterile cotton-tipped applicators
  - Sterile tracheostomy dressing (precut and sewn surgical dressing)
  - Sterile basin
  - Small sterile brush (or disposable inner cannula)
  - Tracheostomy ties (e.g., twill tape, manufactured tracheostomy ties, Velcro tracheostomy ties)
  - Normal saline (NS)
  - Scissors
  - Pair of sterile and clean gloves

STEP	RATIONALE
ASSESSMENT	
1. Identify patient using two identifiers (e.g., name and birth date or name and medical record number) according to agency policy.	Ensures correct patient. Complies with The Joint Commission standards and improves patient safety (TJC, 2016).
2. Auscultate lung sounds and observe respiratory rate and depth.	Provides baseline measure of ventilation and ease of breathing.
3. Observe condition of tissues surrounding airway insertion site and condition of airway (soiled or loose tape, ties, or dressing; pressure sores on nares, lips, or corner of mouth; excess nasal, oral, or peristomal secretions; patient moving endotracheal tube with tongue; biting tube or tongue; or foul-smelling mouth).	Patient is at risk for potential impaired skin integrity and infection due to inability to control secretions and pressure on skin/mucosa from airway devices (Zaratkiewicz et al., 2012).
4. Observe patency of airway. Excess intratracheal or endotracheal secretions, diminished airflow through airway, signs and symptoms of airway obstruction.	Buildup of secretions in airways impairs oxygenation.
5. Observe for factors that increase risk for complications from ET tube: type and size of tube, movement of tube up and down trachea, cuff size and overinflation or underinflation, duration of tube placement, facial trauma, malnutrition, and neck or thoracic radiation.	Movement of tube predisposes patient to tracheal trauma or tube dislodgement and indicates the need for another size airway. Cuff size indicates the amount of air needed to properly inflate cuff. An underinflated cuff increases patient's risk for aspiration. Cuff overly inflated may cause ischemia or necrosis of tracheal tissue (Hamilton et al., 2012). Longer duration of intubation increases risk for complications. Tissue is prone to breakdown in the presence of malnutrition and radiation.
6. Determine proper ET tube depth, noted by centimeters at lip or gum line. Line is marked on tube and recorded in medical record at time of intubation.	Confirms ET tube position.
7. Assess patient's knowledge of procedure, comfort with procedure, and ability to perform trach care at home, and answer any questions of family.	Reinforces information given to patient and family caregiver and provides opportunity to ask additional questions. Encourages cooperation and minimizes anxiety.
PLANNING	
1. Obtain assistance from available staff for this procedure.	Reduces risk for accidental extubation of artificial airway.
2. Assist patient with assuming comfortable position for both patient and you (usually supine or semi-Fowlers).	Provides access to site and facilitates completion of procedure without causing you to have muscle strain or patient discomfort.

SKILL 41-2 CARE OF AN ARTIFICIAL AIRWAY—cont'd

STEP	RATIONALE
3. Place towel across patient's chest.	Reduces transmission of microorganisms to linens and bedclothes.
4. Explain importance of patient's participation, including importance of not biting or moving ET tube with tongue, trying not to cough when tape is temporarily removed from the airway, not pulling on tube with hand.	Reduces anxiety, encourages cooperation, and reduces risks. Removal of tape can be uncomfortable.
IMPLEMENTATION	
1. Perform hand hygiene. Apply mask, goggles, gown, or face shield if indicated.	Reduces transmission of microorganisms.
2. Perform tracheal (tracheostomy), endotracheal (endotracheal tube), nasopharyngeal, or oropharyngeal suction (see Skill 41-1). (After suctioning tracheostomy, remove soiled dressing and discard in glove with coiled catheter.)	Removes secretions and diminishes patient's need to cough during procedure.
3. Connect Yankauer suction catheter to suction source.	Prepares for oropharyngeal suctioning.
4. Care of artificial airways	
a. Endotracheal (ET) tube care	
(1) Prepare equipment at bedside: oral care supplies, securement devices. Then prepare method to secure ET tube (check agency policy).	
(a) **Commercially available ET tube holder:** Open package per manufacturer instructions. Set device aside with head guard in place and Velcro strips open.	Commercial devices are latex free, fast, and convenient. These devices avoid need for tape and resultant skin breakdown and are easily applied in presence of facial hair.
(b) **Tape method:** Cut piece of tape long enough to go completely around patient's head from naris to naris plus 15 cm (6 inches): adult, about 30 to 60 cm (1 to 2 feet). Lay adhesive side up on bedside table. Cut and lay 8 to 15 cm (3 to 6 inches) of tape, adhesive sides together, in center of long strip to prevent tape from sticking to hair. Smaller strip of tape covers area between ears around back of head.	Preparing tape ahead will allow you to have one hand positioned on ET tube throughout procedure. Adhesive tape needs to be placed around head from cheek to cheek below ears. Avoid over ears because this results in a pressure sore.
(2) Apply clean gloves and instruct NAP or another RN to apply gloves and hold ET tube firmly at patients' lips or naris throughout the procedure. Note the number marking on ET tube at gum line or lips.	Reduces transmission of microorganisms. Maintains proper tube position and prevents accidental extubation or pushing tube further into airway.
(3) Remove device or old tape.	Provides access to underlying skin for assessment and hygiene. Reduces transmission of microorganisms.
(a) **Commercially available device:** Remove Velcro strips from ET tube and remove ET tube holder from patient.	Velcro strips secure ET tube in place and provide a marker to measure distance to patient's lips or gums. These devices are latex free and permit access to patient's mouth and lips for ease in oropharyngeal suctioning and oral hygiene.
(b) **Tape:** Carefully remove tape from ET tube and patient's face. If tape is difficult to remove, moisten with soapy water or adhesive tape remover. Discard tape in appropriate receptacle if nearby.	Adhesive can cause damage to skin and prevent adhesion of new tape.

CLINICAL DECISION: *Do not allow helper to hold the tube away from the lips or naris. Doing so allows too much "play" in the tube and increases the risk for tube movement and accidental extubation. Never let go of the ET tube because it could become dislodged.*

STEP	RATIONALE
(4) Remove excess secretions or adhesive left on patient's face. Use adhesive remover swab to remove excess adhesive left on face after tape removal. Wash adhesive remover from face.	Promotes hygiene. Retained adhesive causes damage to skin and makes it difficult for new tape to adhere.
(5) Remove oral airway or bite block if present and place on towel.	Provides access and complete observation of patient's oral cavity.

CLINICAL DECISION: *Do not remove oral airway if patient is actively biting. Wait until tape or device is partially or completely secured to ET tube.*

STEP	RATIONALE
(6) Keep ET tube cuff inflated. Have assistant continue to hold tube and not let go.	Inflated cuff and securing tube reduces risk for aspiration and accidental extubation or pushing tube further into airway.
Provide oral care. (Have Yankauer suction catheter on and at hand.) Assess oral cavity on side exposed. Brush oral mucosa, gums, and teeth with powdered toothbrush, or brush with nonfoaming antiseptic paste for 3 to 4 minutes (Booker et al., 2013; Needleman et al., 2011). Rinse carefully using sterile water. Suction orally as needed during brushing and rinsing. Moisten brush with sterile water to rinse, then use brush or a clean toothette to apply chlorhexidine rinse or gel (Labeau et al., 2011; Morris et al., 2011; Booker et al., 2013). Perform oral care twice daily at 12-hour intervals minimally (Booker et al., 2013).	The use of an oral antiseptic for oral care of intubated patients has a beneficial effect in preventing ventilator-associated pneumonia (Labeau et al., 2011; Shi et al., 2013; Morris et al., 2011, Booker et al., 2013).

STEP	RATIONALE
(7) Oral ET tube only: Note "cm" ET tube marking at lips or gums. With help of assistant, move ET tube to opposite side or center of mouth. Do not change tube depth.	Prevents pressure sore formation at sides of patient's mouth. Ensures correct position of tube and allows for quick visual of displaced tube (Cooper, 2013). Measuring tube at lip line can be distorted because of edema, trauma, or disease process.
(8) Repeat oral cleaning as in Step 4a(6) on opposite side of mouth.	Cleanses oral cavity and removes secretions from mouth and oropharynx.
(9) Clean face and neck with soapy washcloth; rinse and dry. Shave male patient as necessary.	Moisture and beard growth prevent adhesive tape adherence.
(10) Secure ET tube (assistant continues to hold ET tube).	
(a) Tape method	
[1] Pour a small amount of skin protectant or liquid adhesive on clean 2 × 2 gauze and dot on upper lip (oral ET tube) or across nose (nasal ET tube) and cheeks to ear. Allow tincture to dry completely.	Protects and makes skin more receptive to tape.
[2] Slip tape under patient's head and neck, adhesive side up. Take care not to twist tape or catch hair. Do not allow tape to stick to itself. It helps to stick tape gently to a tongue blade, which serves as a guide as tape is passed behind patient's head. Center tape so double-faced tape extends around back of neck from ear to ear.	Positions tape to secure ET tube in proper position.
[3] On one side of face, secure tape from ear to naris (nasal ET tube) or over lip to edge of mouth (oral ET tube). Tear remaining tape in half lengthwise, forming two pieces that are ½- to ¼-inch (1 to 1.5 cm) wide. Secure bottom half of tape across upper lip (oral ET tube) or across top of nose (nasal ET tube) to opposite ear (see illustration *A*). Wrap top half of tape around tube (see illustration *B*). Tape should encircle main part of tube at least 2 times for security.	Secures tape to face. Using top tape to wrap prevents downward drag on ET tube.
[4] Gently pull other side of tape firmly to pick up slack and secure to remaining side of face (see illustration). Have assistant release hold when tube is secure.	Secures tape to face and tube. ET tube should be at same depth as the lips. Check earlier assessment for verification of tube depth in centimeters.

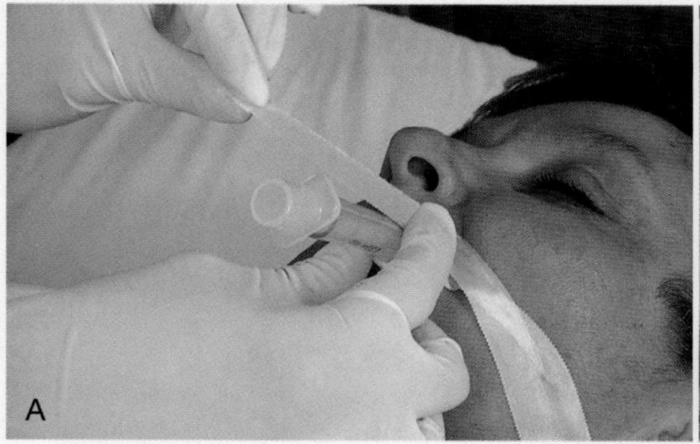

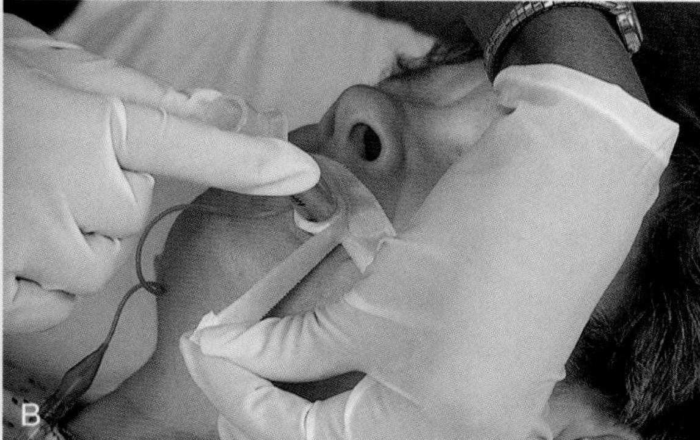

STEP 4a(10)(a)[3] **A,** Securing bottom half of tape across patient's upper lip. **B,** Securing top half of tape around tube.

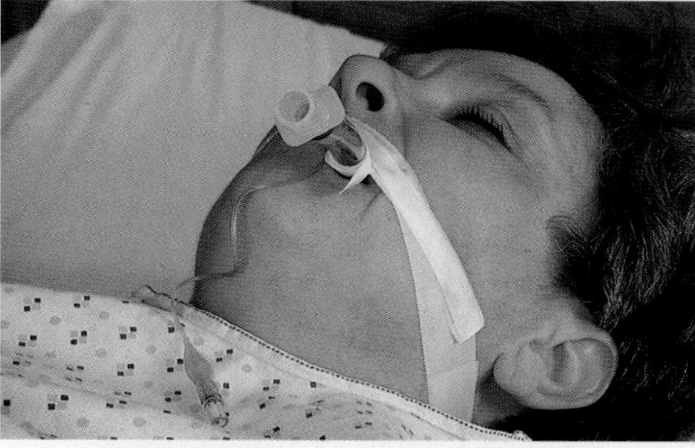

STEP 4a(10)(a)[4] Tape securing ET tube.

SKILL 41-2 CARE OF AN ARTIFICIAL AIRWAY—cont'd

STEP	RATIONALE
(b) Commercially available device	
[1] Thread ET tube through opening designed to secure it. Be sure that pilot balloon tube is accessible.	Commercially available holders have a slit in front of holder designed to secure the ET tube.
[2] Place Velcro strips of ET holder under patient at occipital region of the head.	
[3] Verify that ET tube is at established depth, using lip or gum line marker as guide.	Ensures that ET tube remains at correct depth as determined during assessment.
[4] Secure Velcro strips at base of patient's head. Leave 1 cm (½ inch) slack in strips.	
[5] Verify that tube is secure, it does not move forward from patient's mouth or backward down into patient's throat, and there are no pressure areas on the oral mucosa or occipital region of the head (see illustration).	Tube needs to be secure so its position remains at correct depth. It can be secured without being tight and causing pressure.
(11) Remove and clean oral airway in warm soapy water and rinse well. Then rinse in chlorhexidine rinse. Shake excess solution from oral airway. **Option:** Insert new oral airway if secretions are difficult to remove.	Promotes hygiene. Reduces transmission of microorganisms.
(12) For unconscious patient reinsert oral airway without pushing tongue into oropharynx and secure with tape.	Prevents patient from biting ET tube and allows access for oropharyngeal suctioning. An oral airway in a conscious, cooperative patient causes excessive gagging and pressure ulcers to mouth and tongue.
b. Tracheostomy care	Tracheostomy stoma care should be performed a minimum of two times a day to prevent odor, irritation, and infection (Johns Hopkins Medicine, 2015).
(1) Preoxygenate patient for a minimum of 30 seconds, by asking patient to take 5-6 deep breaths or use a manual resuscitation bag connected to 100% oxygen.	Replenishes oxygen lost in suctioning (AARC, 2010a).
(2) Prepare equipment on bedside table.	Preparation and organization of equipment allows completion of tracheostomy care procedure efficiently and reconnection of patient to oxygen source in timely manner.
(a) Open tracheostomy kit. Open two 4 × 4 gauze packages using aseptic technique and pour saline on one package. Leave second package dry. Do not recap NS.	Tracheostomy tube has multiple components (see illustration). Some of these components might be used during tracheostomy care.
(b) Open two packages of cotton-tipped swabs. Keeping contents sterile, pour NS onto one of the packages.	
(c) Open sterile tracheostomy dressing package.	

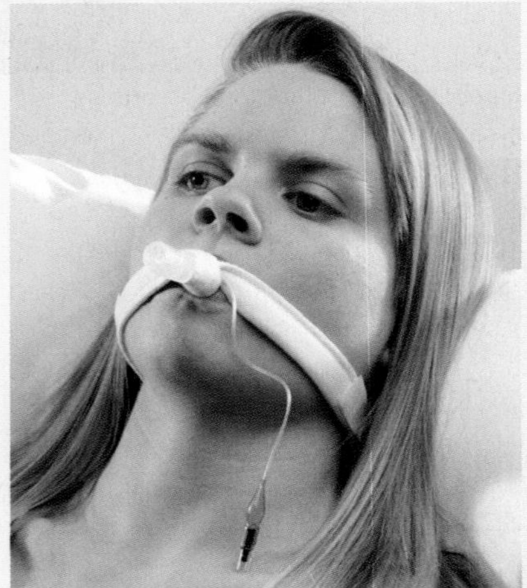

STEP 4a(10)(b)[5] ET holder in place. (Courtesy Dale Medical Products, Plainesville, Mass.)

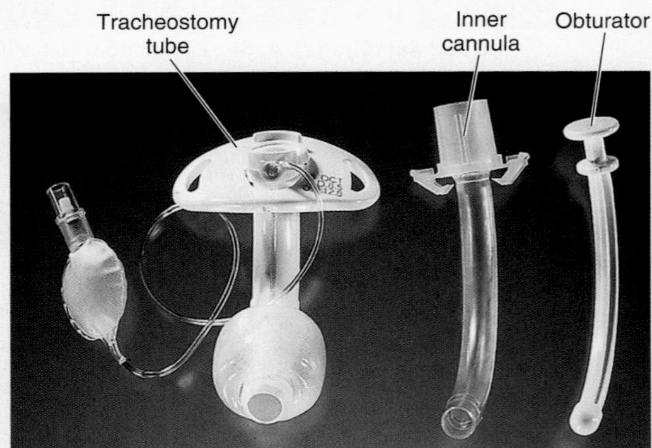

STEP 4b(2)(a) Tracheostomy tube. (Courtesy Mallinckrodt Inc. Shiley Tracheostomy Products, St Louis.)

STEP	RATIONALE
(d) Unwrap sterile basin and pour about 2 cm (1 inch) of NS into it. Open small sterile brush package and place aseptically into sterile basin.	
(e) Prepare fixation equipment.	
[1] Prepare length of twill tape long enough to go around patient's neck two times, about 60 to 75 cm (25 to 30 inches) for an adult. Cut ends on the diagonal. Lay aside in dry area.	Cutting ends of tie on a diagonal aids in inserting tie through eyelet.
[2] If using commercial tracheostomy tube holder, open package according to manufacturer's directions.	
(3) Apply sterile gloves. Keep dominant hand sterile throughout procedure.	Reduces transmission of microorganisms.
(4) Remove oxygen source if present.	

CLINICAL DECISION: *It is important to stabilize the tracheostomy tube at all times during tracheostomy care to prevent injury and unnecessary discomfort. Have another nurse or NAP assist during procedure wearing clean gloves.*

STEP	RATIONALE
(5) Tracheostomy with **inner cannula** care.	
(a) While touching only the outer aspect of tube, unlock and remove inner cannula with nondominant hand. Drop inner cannula into NS basin.	Removes inner cannula for cleaning. Hydrogen peroxide loosens secretions from inner cannula; but, if it is too irritating, use NS only (Morris et al., 2013).
(b) Place tracheostomy collar or T tube and ventilator oxygen source over or near outer cannula. (**Note:** T tube and ventilator oxygen devices cannot be attached to all outer cannulas when inner cannula is removed.)	Maintains supply of oxygen to patient.
(c) To prevent oxygen desaturation in affected patients, quickly pick up inner cannula and use small brush to remove secretions inside and outside cannula (see illustration).	Tracheostomy brush provides mechanical force to remove thick or dried secretions.
(d) Hold inner cannula over basin and rinse with NS, using nondominant hand to pour.	Removes secretions from inner cannula (Cleveland Clinic, 2014).
(e) Replace inner cannula (see illustration) and secure "locking" mechanism. Hyperventilate patient if needed. Reapply ventilator or oxygen sources.	Secures inner cannula and reestablishes oxygen supply.
(6) Disposable inner cannula care	
(a) Remove new cannula from manufacturer packaging.	
(b) While touching only the outer aspect of tube, withdraw old inner cannula and replace with new cannula. Lock into position.	Reestablishes airway quickly.
(c) Dispose of contaminated cannula in appropriate receptacle and apply oxygen source or ventilator.	Prevents unnecessary oxygen desaturation.

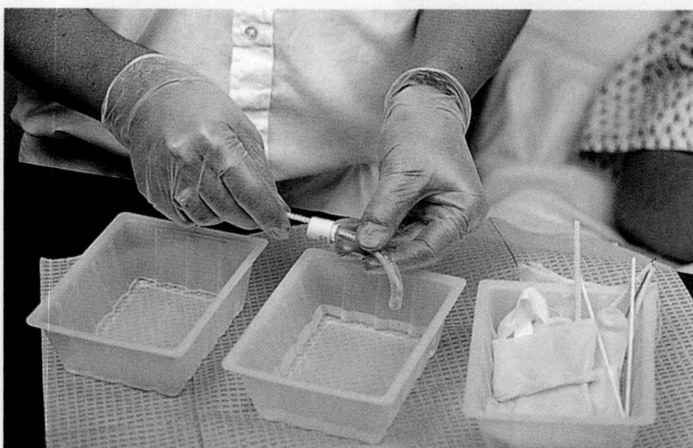

STEP 4b(5)(c) Cleaning tracheostomy inner cannula.

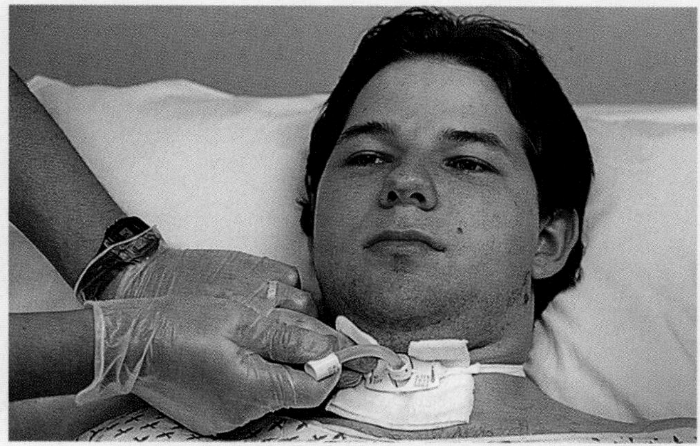

STEP 4b(5)(e) Reinserting inner cannula.

SKILL 41-2 CARE OF AN ARTIFICIAL AIRWAY—cont'd

STEP	RATIONALE
(7) Using NS-saturated cotton-tipped sterile swabs and 4 × 4 gauze, clean exposed outer cannula surfaces and stoma under faceplate, extending 5 to 10 cm (2 to 4 inches) in all directions from stoma (see illustration). Clean in circular motion from stoma site outward using dominant hand to handle sterile supplies.	Aseptically removes secretions from stoma site. Moving in outward circle pulls mucus and other contaminants from stoma to periphery.
(8) Using NS-prepared cotton-tipped swabs and 4 × 4 gauze, clean outer tracheostomy tube flange and skin surfaces.	Removes secretions that can be source of infection.
(9) Using dry 4 × 4 gauze, pat lightly at skin and exposed outer cannula surfaces.	Dry surfaces prohibit formation of moist environment for microorganism growth and skin excoriation.
(10) Securing tracheostomy	
(a) Tracheostomy tie method	
[1] Instruct assistant to securely hold tracheostomy tube in place, then cut old ties.	Secures tracheostomy tube to prevent accidental extubation.

CLINICAL DECISION: *Assistant must not release hold on tracheostomy tube until new ties are firmly tied to reduce risk of accidental extubation. If no assistant is present, do not cut old ties until new ties are in place and securely tied.*

STEP	RATIONALE
[2] Take prepared twill tape, insert one end of tie through faceplate eyelet, and pull ends even (see illustration).	
[3] Slide both ends of ties behind head and around neck to other eyelet and insert one tie through second eyelet.	
[4] Pull snugly.	Secures tracheostomy tube in place.

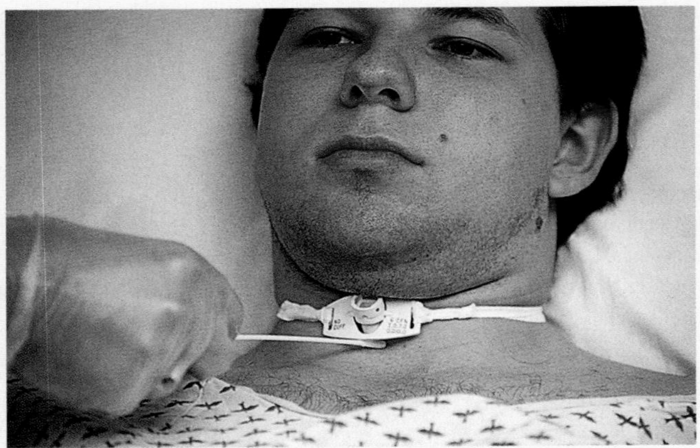

STEP 4b(7) Cleaning around stoma.

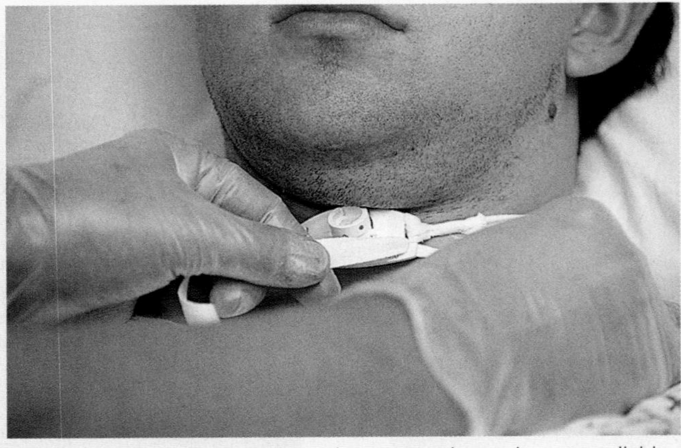

STEP 4b(10)(a)[2] Replacing tracheostomy ties when an assistant is not available. Do not remove old tracheostomy ties until new ones are secure.

STEP	RATIONALE
[5] Tie ends securely in double square knot, allowing space for only one loose or two snug finger widths in tie.	One-finger slack prevents ties from being too tight when tracheostomy dressing is in place and also prevents movement of tracheostomy into lower airway.
(b) Tracheostomy tube holder method (see illustration).	
[1] While wearing gloves, maintain secure hold on tracheostomy tube. This can be done with an assistant or, when an assistant is not available, leave old tracheostomy tube holder in place until new device is secure.	Prevents incidental displacement of tube.
[2] Align strap under patient's neck. Be sure that Velcro attachments are positioned on either side of tracheostomy tube.	
[3] Place narrow end of ties under and through faceplate eyelets. Pull ends even and secure with Velcro closures.	
[4] Verify that there is space for only one loose or two snug finger width(s) under neck strap.	Prevents skin necrosis.
(11) Insert fresh tracheostomy dressing under clean ties/holder and faceplate (see illustration).	Absorbs drainage. Dressing prevents pressure on clavicle heads.
5. Position patient comfortably and evaluate respiratory status.	Promotes comfort. Some patients require post-tracheostomy care suctioning.
6. Replace any oxygen-delivery devices.	Maintains oxygen therapy.
7. Remove and discard gloves. Perform hand hygiene.	Prevents transmission of microorganisms.

CLINICAL DECISION: *Keep tracheostomy obturator at bedside with a fresh tracheostomy to facilitate reinsertion of the outer cannula if dislodged. Keep an additional tracheostomy tube of the same size and shape on hand for emergency replacement (Morris et al., 2013).*

EVALUATON

STEP	RATIONALE
1. Compare respiratory assessments before and after procedure.	Identifies any changes in presence and quality of breath sounds after procedure. Determines effectiveness of artificial airway care.
2. Observe depth and position of ET tubes according to health care provider's recommendation.	Verifies that position of tube is correct and not altered.
3. Evaluate security of tape/holder securing ET tube by gently tugging at tube.	Artificial airway (ET tube) should not move. Patient may cough.
4. Check fit of new tracheostomy ties and ask patient if tube feels comfortable.	If tracheostomy ties are uncomfortable, ties that are too loose or tight place patient at risk for injury.
5. Evaluate skin around mouth, oral mucosa (ET tube), and tracheostomy stoma for drainage, pressure, irritation, or signs of infection.	Skin breakdown and/or irritation should not be present. Broken skin places patient at risk for infection.
6. Use ***Teach Back:*** State,"I want to be sure that I explained the importance of changing your family member's tracheostomy tube dressing. Can you tell me why this is important?" Revise your instruction now or develop plan for revised family caregiver education if unable to teach back correctly.	Evaluates what the family caregiver is able to explain or demonstrate.

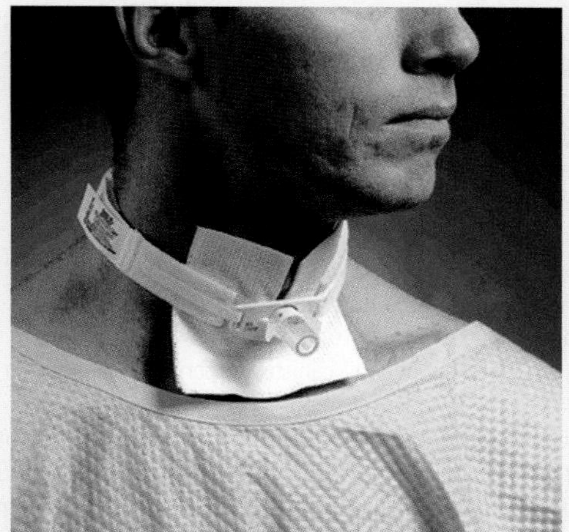

STEP 4b(10)(b) Tracheostomy tube holder in place. (Courtesy Dale Medical Products, Plainesville, Mass.)

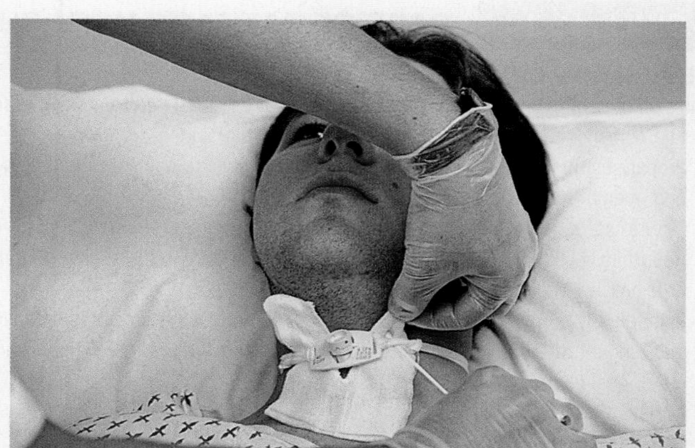

STEP 4b(11) Applying tracheostomy dressing.

SKILL 41-2 CARE OF AN ARTIFICIAL AIRWAY—cont'd

UNEXPECTED OUTCOMES AND RELATED INTERVENTIONS

1. Unexpected extubation of ET tube
   - Call for assistance while remaining with patient.
   - Assist respirations with bag-valve mask as needed.
   - Assess patient for airway patency, spontaneous breathing, and vital signs.
   - Prepare for reintubation.
2. Accidental decannulation of tracheostomy tube
   - Call for assistance while remaining with patient.
   - Replace old tracheostomy tube with new spare tube of same size and kind kept at the bedside. Some experienced nurses or respiratory therapists may be able to quickly reinsert tracheostomy tube (Morris et al., 2013).
   - Same-size ET tube can be inserted in stoma in an emergency.
   - Be prepared to manually ventilate patient who develops respiratory distress.
3. Movement of ET tube
   - Repeat taping or securing procedure. **Note:** Chest x-ray may be needed to confirm placement.
   - In very active patients without facial injury who are at risk for self-extubation, consider applying a second piece of tape around back of head.
4. Pressure area around tracheostomy tube
   - Increase frequency of tracheostomy care. Keep dressing under faceplate at all times.
   - Consider using double dressing or applying hydrocolloid or stoma adhesive dressing around stoma.

RECORDING AND REPORTING

- Record respiratory assessment measures before and after care.
- Record ET tube care: depth of ET tube, frequency and extent of care, patient tolerance of procedure, and special care of any unexpected outcomes related to presence of the tube.
- Record tracheostomy care: type and size of tracheostomy tube, frequency and extent of care, patient tolerance of procedure, and special care of any unexpected outcomes related to presence of the tube.
- Document your evaluation of family caregiver learning.

HOME CARE CONSIDERATIONS TRACHEOSTOMY ONLY (CLEVELAND CLINIC, 2014).

- Instruct family caregivers in how to obtain supplies. Routine tracheostomy care should be done at least once a day after discharge from hospital. At home clean technique is used with nonsterile gloves.
- Immediately after tracheostomy insertion, patients must communicate with others by writing or use of computer.
- Instruct caregivers in signs and symptoms of respiratory distress, tube dysfunction, and respiratory and stoma infections. Call health care provider if patient feels pain or discomfort longer than a week after insertion, if breathing does not improve after usual method of clearing secretions, or if secretions become thick or mucus plugs are present.
- When outside, use tracheostomy covers to protect from dust or cold air.
- Never remove the outer cannula unless instructed by health care provider to do so.

SKILL 41-3 CARE OF PATIENTS WITH CHEST TUBES

DELEGATION CONSIDERATIONS

The skill of care of chest tube management cannot be delegated to nursing assistive personnel (NAP). The nurse instructs the NAP about:

- Proper positioning of patient with chest tubes to facilitate chest tube drainage and optimal function of the system.
- How to safely ambulate and transfer patient with chest drainage.
- Reporting changes in vital signs or SpO_2, chest pain, sudden shortness of breath, or excessive bubbling in water-seal chamber.
- Immediately notifying nurse if there is disconnection of system, change in type and amount of drainage, sudden bleeding, or sudden cessation of bubbling in water-seal chamber.

EQUIPMENT

- Stethoscope
- Pulse oximeter
- Clean gloves
- Two rubber-tipped (also called *shodded*) hemostats for each tube
- 2-inch (5-cm) adhesive tape for taping connections
- Sterile gauze sponges
- Suction source and setup (wall canister or portable) if physician is inserting chest tube
- Water suction system: Add sterile water or normal saline (NS) solution to cover the lower 2.5 cm (1 inch) of water-seal U tube, sterile water or NS solution to put into the suction-control chamber if suction is to be used (see manufacturer directions)
- Waterless system: Add vial of 30-mL injectable sodium chloride or water, 20-mL syringe, 21-gauge needle, and antiseptic swab

STEP	RATIONALE
ASSESSMENT	
1. Identify patient using two identifiers (e.g., name and birthday or name and medical record number) according to agency policy.	Ensures correct patient. Complies with The Joint Commission Standards and improves patient safety (TJC, 2016).
2. Assess pulmonary status.	Baseline measures allow you to determine if signs and symptoms of respiratory distress improve after insertion of chest tube. If respiratory distress is not relieved or worsens or if there is sharp stabbing chest pain with or without decreased blood pressure and increased heart rate, notify health care provider immediately. These symptoms indicate a pneumothorax.
a. Signs and symptoms of increased respiratory distress (displaced trachea, decreased breath sounds over affected and nonaffected lungs, marked cyanosis, asymmetrical chest movements).	
b. Assess for sharp, stabbing chest pain or chest pain on inspiration; hypotension; and tachycardia. Ask patient to rate level of comfort on a scale of 0 to 10.	Symptoms may indicate a tension pneumothorax. Presence of a pneumothorax or hemothorax is painful, often causing sharp inspiratory pain.
3. Obtain baseline and serial vital signs, level of cognition, and SpO_2.	Changes in pulse, SpO_2, and blood pressure often indicate infection, respiratory distress, or pain. Cognitive changes indicate hypoxia.
4. Assess patient's current hemoglobin and hematocrit levels.	Provides measure reflecting blood loss and subsequent levels of oxygenation.
5. Observe chest tube status:	
a. Chest tube dressing and site surrounding tube insertion. Apply clean gloves if drainage is present.	Ensures that dressing is intact, without air or fluid leaks, and that area surrounding insertion site is free of drainage or skin irritation.
b. Tubing for kinks, dependent loops, or clots.	Maintains patent, freely draining system, preventing fluid accumulation in chest cavity. Presence of kinks, dependent loops, or clotted drainage increases patient's risk for infection, atelectasis, and tension pneumothorax (Carroll, 2015).
c. Check existing drainage system to ensure that it is upright and below level of tube insertion. Note amount of drainage in system (see illustration).	Facilitates drainage. Ensures that system is in this position to function properly.

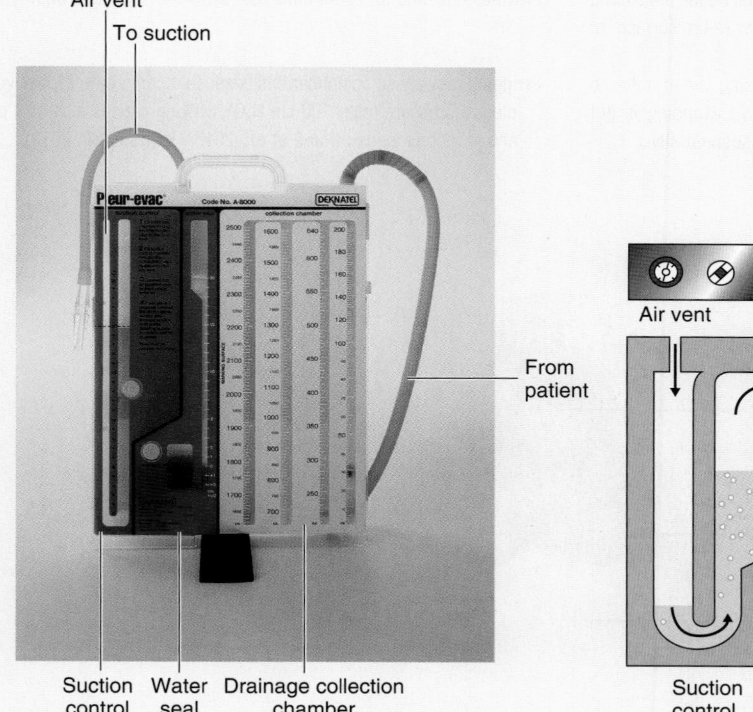

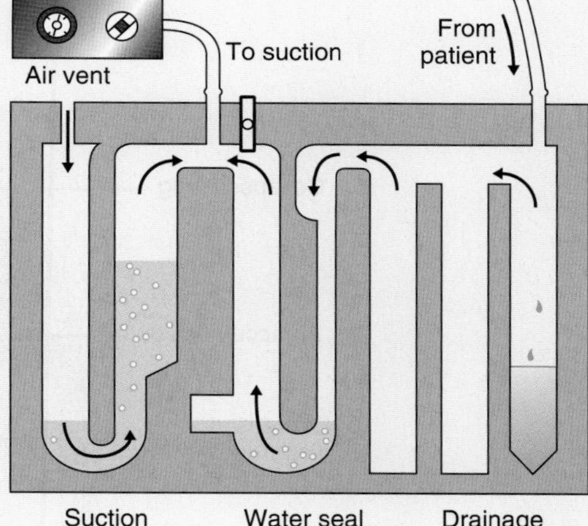

STEP 5c *Left,* Pleur-Evac drainage system, a commercial three-bottle chest drainage device. *Right,* Schematic of drainage device.

SKILL 41-3 CARE OF PATIENTS WITH CHEST TUBES—cont'd

STEP	RATIONALE
PLANNING	
1. Provide two rubber-tipped hemostats or approved clamps for each chest tube, attached to top of patient's bed with adhesive tape. Chest tubes are only clamped under specific circumstances per health care provider's order or nursing policy and procedure:	Hemostat has a covering to prevent it from penetrating chest tube. Use of these rubber-tipped hemostats or other clamps prevents air from reentering pleural space in emergencies (Bauman et al., 2011).
a. To assess air leak.	
b. To quickly empty or change disposable systems; performed by a nurse who has received education in the procedure.	
c. To assess if patient is ready to have chest tube removed (which is done by health care provider's order); monitor patient for recurrent pneumothorax (see illustration).	
2. Position patient.	Permits optimal drainage of fluid and/or air.
a. Semi-Fowler's position to evacuate air (pneumothorax)	Air rises to highest point in chest. Pneumothorax tubes are usually placed on anterior aspect at midclavicular line, second or third intercostal space.
b. High-Fowler's position to drain fluid (hemothorax, effusion)	Permits optimal drainage of fluid. Posterior tubes are placed on midaxillary line, eighth or ninth intercostal space.
3. Explain to patient steps for tube management.	Promotes understanding and minimizes patient anxiety.
IMPLEMENTATION	
1. Perform hand hygiene. Apply clean gloves.	Reduces transmission of microorganisms.
2. Be sure that tube connection between chest and drainage tube is intact and taped.	Secures chest tube to drainage system and reduces risk of air leak causing breaks in airtight system.
a. Make sure that water-seal vent on drainage system is not occluded.	Permits displaced air to pass into atmosphere.
b. Make sure that suction-control chamber vent is not occluded when using suction. Waterless systems have relief valves without caps.	Provides safety factor of releasing excess negative pressure into atmosphere.
3. Coil excess drainage tubing on mattress next to patient. Secure with rubber band, safety pin, or plastic clamp. Allow enough room for patient to reposition.	Prevents excess tubing from hanging over edge of mattress in dependent loop. It is possible for drainage to collect in loop and occlude drainage system (Carroll, 2015).
4. Adjust tubing to hang in straight line from top of mattress to drainage chamber.	Promotes drainage and prevents fluid or blood from accumulating in pleural cavity (Carroll, 2015).
5. If chest tube is draining fluid, indicate time (e.g., 0900) that you began measuring drainage on adhesive tape on drainage bottle or on write-on surface of disposable commercial system.	Provides baseline for continuous assessment of type and quality of drainage.
6. Milk chest tube only if indicated (this means compressing along tube to encourage clots to pass through tube) (see agency policy.) Stripping is not recommended. Milking is compressing and releasing tube sequentially.	Stripping may cause complications because it can create excessive negative intrapleural pressure (over 100 cm H_2O). Milking causes less of a pressure change and is recommended (Kane et al., 2013; Dango et al., 2010).

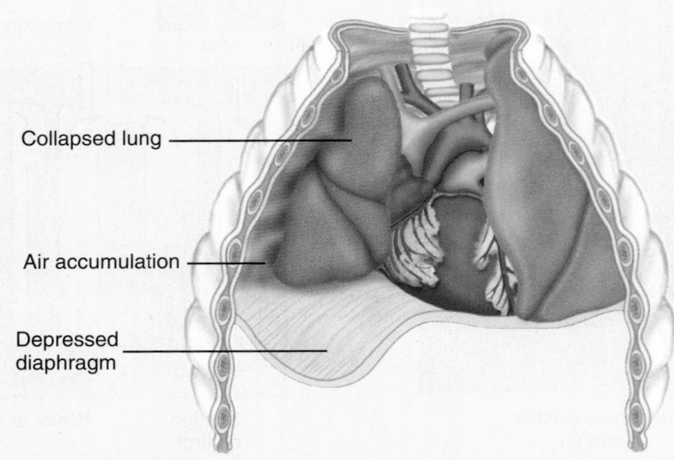

STEP 1c Pneumothorax. (From Ball JW et al: *Seidel's guide to physical examination*, ed 8, St Louis, 2015, Mosby).

STEP	RATIONALE
a. Milk postoperative mediastinal chest tubes if assessment indicates an obstruction or decreased drainage from clots or debris in tubing. Order is necessary (see agency policy).	Stripping is not recommended. There is evidence that milking is associated with a significant increase of pleural fluid drainage; however, it does not improve postoperative morbidity and mortality and therefore cannot be recommended as a routine postoperative procedure (Dango et al., 2010).
7. Remove and discard gloves. Perform hand hygiene.	Reduces transmission of infection.

EVALUATION

STEP	RATIONALE
1. Monitor vital signs and pulse oximetry as ordered or if patient's condition changes.	Provides ongoing data about patient's level of oxygenation.
2. Evaluate patient for decreased respiratory distress and chest pain and monitor SpO_2.	Increasing respiratory distress, decreased breath sounds, marked cyanosis, asymmetrical chest wall movements, presence of subcutaneous emphysema around insertion site or neck, hypotension, tachycardia, and/or mediastinal shift are critical and indicate a severe change in patient status such as excessive blood loss or tension pneumothorax. Notify health care provider immediately.
3. Auscultate lungs for breath sounds.	Decreased breath sounds indicate lung area is not aerating and can be a sign of respiratory distress.
4. Observe:	
a. Appearance of chest tube dressing.	Drainage is often caused by tube occlusion, causing drainage to exit around tube.

CLINICAL DECISION: *Check the dressing carefully because it needs to remain occlusive. It can come loose from the skin, although this is not readily apparent. Assess for drainage and reinforce to maintain seal. Follow hospital policy as needed.*

STEP	RATIONALE
b. Make sure that tubing is free of kinks and dependent loops.	Straight and coiled drainage tube positions are optimal for pleural drainage. However, when a dependent loop is unavoidable, periodic lifting and draining the tube promote pleural drainage.
c. Make sure that chest drainage system is upright and below level of tube insertion. Note presence of clots or debris in tubing. Monitor position of system relative to chest tube carefully, especially during patient transport.	System must be in the upright position to function and facilitate proper drainage.
d. Observe water seal for fluctuations with patient's inspiration and expiration.	Indicates appropriate function of negative pressure system.
(1) *Waterless system:* Diagnostic indicator for fluctuations with patient's inspirations and expirations	In nonmechanically ventilated patient, fluid rises in water seal or diagnostic indicator with inspiration and falls with expiration. Opposite occurs in a patient who is mechanically ventilated. This indicates that system is functioning properly (Lewis et al., 2014).
(2) *Water-seal system:* Bubbling in water-seal chamber	When system is initially connected to patient, expect bubbles from the chamber. These are from air present in system and from patient's intrapleural space. After a short time bubbling stops. Fluid continues to fluctuate in water seal on inspiration and expiration until lung reexpands or system is occluded.
(3) *Water-seal system:* Bubbling in suction-control chamber (when using suction)	Suction-control chamber has constant gentle bubbling. Tubing remains free of obstruction, and suction source is turned to appropriate setting.
e. Observe type and amount of fluid drainage: note color of drainage and skin color. Look at fluid in drainage tubing and not just in collection chamber. What is the normal amount of drainage? Is it bright red, dark red, or pink? Is it opaque, or can you see through it?	Character of drainage indicates if it is as expected or if infection or hemorrhage is developing.
(1) *In adult:* less than 50 to 200 mL/hr immediately after surgery in a mediastinal chest tube; approximately 500 mL in first 24 hours.	Dark-red drainage is normal only in postoperative period, turning serous with time.
(2) Between 100 and 300 mL of fluid drains in a pleural chest tube in an adult during first 3 hours after insertion. Rate decreases after 2 hours; expect 500 to 1000 mL in first 24 hours. Drainage is grossly bloody during first several hours after surgery and then changes to serous. Sudden gush of drainage is often retained blood and not active bleeding and is usually the result of patient repositioning (Lewis et al., 2014).	Reexpansion of lungs forces drainage into tube. Coughing also causes large gushes of drainage or air. Report excessive amounts and/or continued presence of frank, bloody drainage the first several hours after surgery to health care provider, along with patient's vital signs and respiratory status.

CLINICAL DECISION: *If drainage increases suddenly or is bright red or if there is more than 100 mL/hr of bloody drainage (except for the first 3 hours after surgery), notify the health care provider, remain with the patient, and assess vital signs and cardiopulmonary status. This may indicate hemorrhage or perforation of the lung.*

SKILL 41-3 CARE OF PATIENTS WITH CHEST TUBES—cont'd

STEP	RATIONALE
f. *Waterless system:* Suction control (float ball) indicates amount of suction that patient's intrapleural space is receiving.	Suction float ball dictates amount of suction in system. Float ball allows no more suction than dictated by its setting. If suction source is set too low, suction float ball cannot reach prescribed setting. In this case increase suction for float ball to reach prescribed setting.
g. Ask patient to rate level of comfort on a scale of 0 to 10.	Indicates need for analgesia. Patient with chest tube discomfort hesitates to take deep breaths and as a result is at risk for pneumonia and atelectasis.
5. Use ***Teach Back:*** State, "I want to go over what we discussed about keeping your chest tubes open and clear. Tell me how you can help keep the tubes open." Revise your instruction now or develop a plan for revised patient teaching if patient or family is not able to teach back correctly.	Evaluates what the patient is able to explain or demonstrate.

UNEXPECTED OUTCOMES AND RELATED INTERVENTIONS

1. Air leak unrelated to patient respirations
   - Assess all connections between patient and drainage system to find source and tighten any loose connections (Carroll, 2015).
   - If air leak persists, notify health care provider to change drainage system.
2. Tension pneumothorax present
   - Determine that chest tubes are not clamped, kinked, or occluded. Obstructed chest tubes trap air in intrapleural space when air leak originates within patient and can cause a tension pneumothorax.
   - Notify patient's health care provider immediately.
   - Prepare immediately for another chest tube insertion; obtain a flutter (Heimlich) valve or large-gauge needle for short-term emergency release of air in intrapleural space; have emergency equipment (e.g., oxygen, code cart) near patient.
3. Continuous bubbling in water-seal chamber, indicating that leak is between patient and water seal
   - Tighten loose connections between patient and water-seal system.
   - Check agency policy and, if instructed, cross-clamp chest tube closer to patient's chest using hemostat clamps. If bubbling stops, the air leak is inside patient's thorax or at chest tube insertion site.
   - Unclamp chest tube.
   - Reinforce dressing.
   - Notify health care provider.

RECORDING AND REPORTING

- Record and report patency of chest tube; presence, type, and amount of drainage; presence of fluctuations; patient's vital signs; chest dressing status; amount of suction and/or water seal; and patient's level of comfort.
- Document your evaluation of patient learning.

HOME CARE CONSIDERATIONS

- Patients with chronic conditions (e.g., uncomplicated pneumothorax, effusions, empyema) that require long-term chest tube may be discharged with smaller mobile drains. These systems do not have a suction-control chamber and use a mechanical one-way valve instead of a water-seal chamber.
- Instruct patient in how to ambulate and remain active with a mobile chest tube drainage system.
- Provide patient with information as to when to contact health care professionals regarding changes in health status or drainage system (e.g., chest pain, breathlessness, change in drainage).

SKILL 41-4 USING HOME OXYGEN EQUIPMENT

DELEGATION CONSIDERATIONS

The skill of administering home oxygen equipment cannot be delegated to nursing assistive personnel (NAP). Instruct the NAP about:

- The unique needs of patient (e.g., amount of assistance in applying nasal cannula or mask) and any assistance needed in filling liquid canisters.
- The type of equipment patient should have in the home and the oxygen flow rate.
- Immediately reporting to the nurse increased rate of breathing, decreased level of consciousness, increased confusion, and pain.

EQUIPMENT

- Nasal cannula equipment (see Procedural Guideline Box 41-9)
- Humidification device if oxygen delivery greater than 4 L/min
- Oxygen tubing available in lengths of 50 feet
- Home low-flow oxygen-delivery system with appropriate equipment

STEP	RATIONALE
ASSESSMENT	
1. Identify patient using two identifiers (e.g., name and birth date or name and medical record number) according to agency policy. Compare identifiers with information on patient's MAR or medical record.	Ensures correct patient. Complies with The Joint Commission Standards and improves patient safety (TJC, 2016).
2. While patient is still in the hospital, determine patient's or family caregiver's ability to use oxygen equipment correctly. In home setting reassess for access to and appropriate use of equipment.	Physical or cognitive impairments necessitate instructing family member or significant other how to operate home oxygen equipment. Ongoing assessment enables nurse to determine specific components of skill that patient or family can complete easily.
3. Assess home environment for adequate electrical service if oxygen concentrator is ordered.	Oxygen concentrators require electricity to work. Continuous oxygen therapy must not be interrupted.
4. Assess patient's and family's ability to observe for signs and symptoms of hypoxia: apprehension, anxiety, decreased ability to concentrate, decreased level of consciousness, increased fatigue, dizziness, behavioral changes, increased pulse, increased respiratory rate, pallor, or cyanosis of the mucous membranes.	Hypoxia occurs at home despite use of oxygen therapy. Worsening of patient's physical condition or another underlying condition such as change in the respiratory status can cause hypoxia.
PLANNING	
1. Determine appropriate resources in community for equipment and assistance, including maintenance and repair services and medical equipment supplier.	Ensures readily available assistance for patients with home oxygen systems. Delivery and setup with basic instruction on how to use and maintain home oxygen equipment must be in accordance with federal, state, and local laws (AARC, 2007).
2. Instruct family to investigate municipal requirements for home medical equipment, especially oxygen.	Many municipalities require that patients with home oxygen equipment notify emergency medical service (EMS) before bringing equipment home. When there is a power outage, EMS calls the home, and in some cases the home is on a priority list for power restoration.
3. Obtain appropriate referrals to determine if patient meets standards for third-party reimbursement.	Indications include (1) a PaO_2 less than or equal to 55 mm Hg or SaO_2 less than or equal to 88% breathing room air; (2) PaO_2 less than or equal to 56-59 mm Hg or SaO_2 less than or equal to 89% with conditions such as cor pulmonale, heart failure, or hematocrit greater than 56%; (3) oxygen therapy is needed during activities that cause hypoxia such as ambulation, sleep, or exercise causing an SaO_2 of less than or equal to 88% (CMS, 2015; AARC, 2007).
IMPLEMENTATION	
1. Perform hand hygiene.	Reduces transmission of infection.
2. Place oxygen-delivery system in clutter-free environment that is well ventilated; away from walls, drapes, bedding, and combustible materials; and at least 8 feet from heat source.	Prevents injury from improper placement of oxygen equipment.
3. Demonstrate each step for preparation and completion of oxygen therapy.	Teaches psychomotor skills and enables patient to ask questions. When patients and family members are adequately informed about supplemental oxygen therapy, the patient consistent use of the therapy is enhanced (Earnest, 2002).
a. **Compressed oxygen system**—available in large cylinders as stationary units or smaller, lightweight cylinders in carrying bags and/or wheel carts.	Smaller units are used for ambulation and as a backup of stationary unit if there is power failure or equipment malfunction (AARC, 2007).
(1) Turn cylinder valve counterclockwise two or three turns with wrench. Store wrench with oxygen tank.	Turns on oxygen. Keeps wrench available.

SKILL 41-4 USING HOME OXYGEN EQUIPMENT—cont'd

STEP	RATIONALE
(2) Check cylinders by reading amount on pressure gauge (see illustration).	Verifies adequate oxygen supply for patient use.
b. **Oxygen concentrator system**—available as stationary unit or portable device.	Extracts oxygen from other gases in atmospheric air (AARC, 2007).
(1) Plug concentrator into appropriate outlet.	Provides power source. Make sure that it is in an open area and never in a closet or other closed space
(2) Turn on power switch.	Starts concentrator motor.
(3) Alarm sounds for a few seconds.	Alarm turns off when desired pressure inside concentrator is reached.
c. **Liquid oxygen systems**—available in large-reservoir canisters that can be used to refill a smaller portable unit (AARC, 2007). Portable unit weighs 5 to 13 lbs and can be carried with a shoulder strap or pulled on a cart.	When liquid oxygen is warmed, it goes from liquid to gas. More oxygen can be stored as a liquid than gas.
d. Refill oxygen tank	
(1) Check for amount of oxygen in tank.	If not in use, evaporation empties portable canister; thus always check it before use.
(2) Wipe both filling connectors with clean, dry, lint-free cloth.	Removes dust and moisture from system.
(3) Turn off flow selector of ambulatory unit.	
(4) Attach ambulatory unit to stationary reservoir by inserting adapter from ambulatory tank into adapter of stationary reservoir.	
(5) Open fill valve on ambulatory tank and apply firm pressure to top of stationary reservoir (see illustration). Stay with unit while it is filling. You will hear a loud hissing noise. Tank fills in about 2 minutes.	Prevents leaking of oxygen during filling process. If oxygen leaks during filling process, connection between ambulatory tank and reservoir ices up and valves stick together.
(6) Disengage ambulatory unit from stationary reservoir when hissing noise changes and vapor cloud begins to form from stationary unit.	Overfilling causes ambulatory unit to malfunction caused by high pressure in tank.
(7) Wipe both filling connectors with clean, dry, lint-free cloth.	Ice sometimes forms during filling. Removes moisture from oxygen system.

CLINICAL DECISION: *If ambulatory unit does not separate easily, valves from reservoir and ambulatory unit may be frozen together. Wait until valves warm to disengage (about 5 to 10 minutes). Do not touch any frosted areas because contact with skin causes skin damage from frostbite.*

STEP	RATIONALE
4. Connect oxygen-delivery device to oxygen system.	Connects oxygen source to delivery system.
5. Adjust to prescribed flow rate (L/min).	Ensures appropriate oxygen prescription.
6. Place oxygen-delivery device on patient.	Delivers oxygen to patient.
7. Perform hand hygiene.	Reduces transmission of microorganisms.

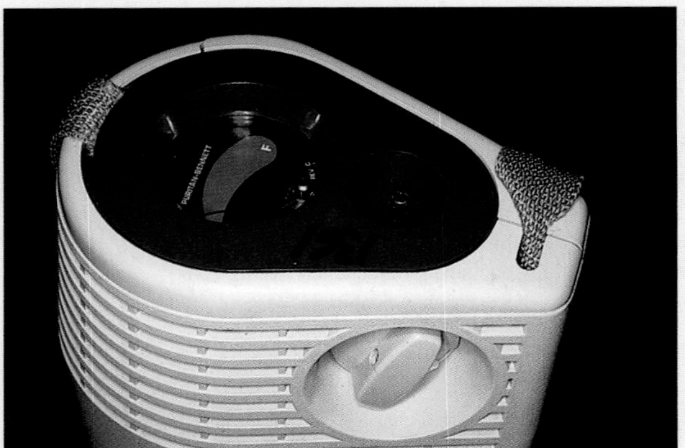

STEP 3a(2) Verify oxygen level by reading gauge on top of canister.

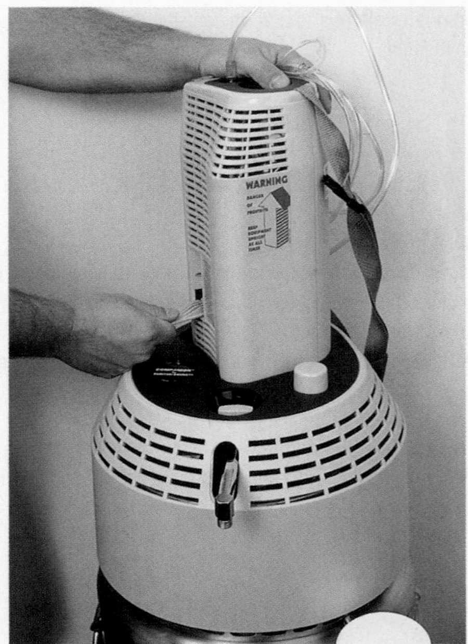

STEP 3d(5) Open fill valve on ambulatory tank while applying firm pressure to top of ambulatory unit.

STEP	RATIONALE
8. Instruct patient and family not to change oxygen flow rate.	Can lead to serious oxygenation alterations.
9. Guide patient and family caregiver as they perform each step. Provide written material for reinforcement and review.	Allows you to correct for errors in technique and discuss their implications.
10. Instruct patient and family caregiver to notify health care provider if signs or symptoms of hypoxia or respiratory tract infection (e.g., fever, increased sputum, change in color of sputum, or odor) occur.	Respiratory tract infections increase oxygen demand and affect oxygen transfer from lungs to blood. Can create severe exacerbation of patient's pulmonary disease.
11. Discuss emergency plan for power loss, natural disaster, and acute respiratory distress. Have patient or family/caregiver call 911 and notify health care provider and home care agency.	Ensures appropriate response and prevents worsening of patient's condition.
12. Instruct patient and family caregiver in safe home oxygen practices, including not allowing smoking in the house, keeping oxygen tanks away from open flame, and storing tanks upright.	Ensures safe use of oxygen in the home and prevents injury to patient and family.
13. Monitor oxygen-delivery rate. All oxygen-delivery equipment should be checked at least daily by patient or caregiver.	Determines if patient is using oxygen at prescribed rate.
14. Oxygen-delivery equipment must be maintained and serviced routinely according to manufacturer's guidelines (AARC, 2007).	Routine maintenance ensures proper function of equipment.
EVALUATION	
1. Ask patient and family about ease of administering or any problems with the home oxygen delivery system.	Determines ability of patient and family to deal with stressors associated with home oxygen use.
2. Ask patient and family to state safety guidelines, emergency precautions, and emergency plan.	Determines patient's knowledge of what to do if power fails, there is a failure in equipment, or patient's status worsens.
3. Use ***Teach Back*** to determine patient's and family's ability to use home oxygen equipment. State, "I want to be sure I explained how to administer the home oxygen equipment. Can you show me how to apply your nasal cannula and regulate the oxygen source?" Revise your instruction now or develop a plan for revised patient teaching if patient or family is not able to teach back correctly.	Evaluates what the patient and family are able to explain or demonstrate.

UNEXPECTED OUTCOMES AND RELATED INTERVENTIONS

1. Patient reports no oxygen flow.
   - Check tank pressure gauge. If level of oxygen is low, refill tank if portable or provide alternate source of oxygen such as concentrator.
   - Notify home oxygen supplier of need for refill.
   - Reassure patient and family.
2. Patient or family caregiver is unable to fill portable liquid oxygen from main source.
   - Check to see that portable tank is connected correctly.
   - Determine if valve is frozen.
   - Contact home oxygen supplier for service visit.
   - Provide alternate oxygen source if necessary.

RECORDING AND REPORTING

- Record teaching plan and describe patient's and family caregiver's ability to safely use home oxygen equipment.
- Record type of home oxygen equipment being used and oxygen flow rate, knowledge of safety guidelines, how to use equipment, unexpected outcomes to observe, and ability to return demonstrate proper use of oxygen-delivery device.

KEY POINTS

- The primary function of the lungs is to transfer oxygen from the atmosphere into the alveoli and carbon dioxide out of the body as a waste product.
- Changes in intrapleural and intraalveolar pressures and lung volumes cause the process of inspiration (active process) and expiration (passive process).
- The primary functions of the heart are to deliver deoxygenated blood to the lungs for oxygenation and oxygen and nutrients to the tissues.
- The nursing history includes information about the patient's cough, dyspnea, fatigue, wheezing, chest pain, environmental exposures, respiratory infection, cardiopulmonary risk factors, and use of medications.
- Nursing assessment includes respiratory pattern, thoracic inspection, palpation, and auscultation for deviations from normal.
- Diagnostic and laboratory tests complete the database for a patient with decreased oxygenation.
- Health promotion includes vaccinations against flu and pneumonia, exercise programs, nutrition support, smoking cessation, and environmental assessment for pollutants and air quality.

- Airway maintenance requires mobilization of secretions by increased fluid intake, humidification, or nebulization.
- Breathing exercises improve ventilation, oxygenation, and sensations of dyspnea.
- Chest physiotherapy includes postural drainage, percussion, and vibration to mobilize pulmonary secretions.
- Airway maintenance may require use of artificial airways and suctioning.
- Promotion of lung expansion can be achieved by mobility, positioning, incentive spirometry, and chest tube insertion.
- Nasal cannulas and oxygen masks deliver oxygen therapy, which improves the levels of tissue oxygenation.
- Learning breathing exercises, including pursed-lip breathing and diaphragmatic breathing, benefits patients with chronic pulmonary diseases.

CLINICAL APPLICATION QUESTIONS

Preparing for Clinical Practice

Forty-eight hours after admission to the hospital, Mr. Edwards had abnormal lung sounds (crackles) in the left base and both upper lobes; he was dyspneic and coughing up thick yellow sputum. His vital signs were as follows: temperature, 102.4° F (39.1° C); blood pressure, 88/42 mm Hg; pulse, 110 beats/min; respirations, 32 breaths/min; and SpO_2, 82%. He could not lie flat, and it was difficult for him to speak because of dyspnea. He was placed on a nonrebreather mask at an oxygen concentration of 60%. He was also unable to cough up any sputum.

Mr. Edwards's health care provider determined that his pneumonia had worsened. A chest x-ray film and arterial blood gas levels were obtained. His chest x-ray film indicated that both upper lobes and the left lower lobe had infiltrates. The arterial blood gas levels indicated respiratory acidosis (see Chapter 42). His PaO_2 was 55 mm Hg, $PaCO_2$ was 65 mm Hg, pH was 7.30, and SpO_2 was 80%. His WBC count had risen from 7 to 15. He spent 5 days in an intensive care unit (ICU) and 2 weeks in a transitional care unit. He is being discharged on home oxygen therapy. His discharge plan includes an outpatient rehabilitation program to begin 1 month after discharge.

1. Given the acute change in Mr. Edward's condition in the beginning of the case scenario, noting his vital signs and lab level results, along with a diagnosis of pneumonia as the source of infection, what interventions/orders/treatment might you anticipate are needed to care for Mr. Edwards?
2. Based on the initial description of Mr. Edwards condition in the case scenario, determine two priority nursing diagnoses and list two or three appropriate interventions or nursing activities for each that you must implement.
3. What do you need to do to prepare Mr. and Mrs. Edwards for home oxygen therapy? (Refer to the Nursing Care Plan.)

ⓔ *Answers to Clinical Application Questions can be found on the Evolve website.*

REVIEW QUESTIONS

Are You Ready to Test Your Nursing Knowledge?

1. For which of the following health problems is a patient who has a 40-year history of smoking at risk?
   1. Alcoholism and hypertension
   2. Obesity and diabetes
   3. Stress-related illnesses
   4. Cardiopulmonary disease and lung cancer
2. A patient has been diagnosed with severe iron deficiency anemia. During physical assessment, which of the following symptoms are associated with decreased oxygenation as a result of the anemia?
   1. Increased breathlessness but increased activity tolerance
   2. Decreased breathlessness and decreased activity tolerance
   3. Increased activity tolerance and decreased breathlessness
   4. Decreased activity tolerance and increased breathlessness
3. A patient is admitted to the emergency department with suspected carbon monoxide poisoning. Even though the patient's color is ruddy and not cyanotic, the nurse understands the patient is at a risk for decreased oxygen-carrying capacity of blood because carbon monoxide does which of the following:
   1. Stimulates hyperventilation, causing respiratory alkalosis
   2. Forms a strong bond with hemoglobin, thus preventing oxygen binding in the lungs
   3. Stimulates hypoventilation, causing respiratory acidosis
   4. Causes alveoli to overinflate, leading to atelectasis
4. An 86-year-old woman is admitted to the unit with chills and a fever of 104° F. What physiological process explains why she is at risk for dyspnea?
   1. Fever increases metabolic demands, requiring increased oxygen need.
   2. Blood glucose stores are depleted and the cells do not have energy to use oxygen.
   3. Carbon dioxide production increases due to hyperventilation.
   4. Carbon dioxide production decreases due to hypoventilation.
5. A patient is admitted with the diagnosis of severe left-sided heart failure. What adventitious lung sounds are expected on auscultation?
   1. Sonorous wheezes in the left lower lung
   2. Rhonchi mid sternum
   3. Crackles only in apex of lungs
   4. Inspiratory crackles in lung bases
6. The nurse is caring for a patient who has decreased mobility. Which intervention is a simple and cost-effective method for reducing the risks of pulmonary complication?
   1. Antibiotics
   2. Frequent change of position
   3. Oxygen humidification
   4. Chest physiotherapy
7. A patient is admitted with severe lobar pneumonia. Which of the following assessment findings would indicate that the patient needs airway suctioning?
   1. Coughing up sputum occasionally
   2. Coughing up thin, watery sputum after nebulization
   3. Decreased ability to clear airway through coughing
   4. Lung sounds clear only after coughing
8. A patient was admitted following a motor vehicle accident with multiple fractured ribs. Respiratory assessment includes signs/symptoms of secondary pneumothorax. Which are the most common assessment findings associated with a pneumothorax? (Select all that apply.)
   1. Sharp pleuritic pain that worsens on inspiration
   2. Crackles over lung bases of affected lung
   3. Tracheal deviation toward the affected lung
   4. Worsening dyspnea
   5. Absent lung sounds to auscultation on affected side
9. A patient has been newly diagnosed with chronic lung disease. In discussing the lung disease with the nurse, which of the patient's statements would indicate a need for further education?

1. "I'll make sure that I rest between activities so I don't get so short of breath."
2. "I'll practice the pursed-lip breathing technique to improve my exercise tolerance."
3. "If I have trouble breathing at night, I'll use two or three pillows to prop up."
4. "If I get short of breath, I'll turn up my oxygen level to 6 L/min."

10. The nurse assesses a new patient and finds the patient short of breath with a respiratory rate of 32 and lying supine in bed. What is the priority nursing action?

1. Raise the head of the bed to 45 degrees or higher.
2. Get the oxygen saturation with a pulse oximeter.
3. Take the blood pressure and respiratory rate.
4. Notify the health care provider of the shortness of breath.

11. The nurse is caring for a patient who exhibits labored breathing, is using accessory muscles, and is coughing up pink frothy sputum. The patient has diminished breath sounds in bilateral lung bases. What are the priority nursing assessments for the nurse to perform prior to notifying the patient's health care provider? (Select all that apply.)

1. SpO_2 levels
2. Amount, color, and consistency of sputum production
3. Fluid status
4. Change in respiratory rate and pattern
5. Pain in lower leg

12. Place the following in correct sequence for suctioning a patient.

1. Open kit and basin
2. Apply gloves
3. Lubricate catheter
4. Verify functioning of suction device and pressure
5. Connect suction tubing to suction catheter
6. Increase supplemental oxygen
7. Reapply oxygen
8. Suction airway

13. Which of the following skills can the nurse delegate to nursing assistive personnel (NAP)? (Select all that apply.)

1. Nasotracheal suctioning
2. Oropharyngeal suctioning of a stable patient
3. Suctioning a new artificial airway
4. Permanent tracheostomy tube suctioning
5. Care of an endotracheal tube

14. Two hours after surgery, the nurse assesses a patient who had a chest tube inserted during surgery. There is 200 ml of dark red drainage in the chest tube at this time. What is the appropriate action for the nurse to perform?

1. Record the amount and continue to monitor drainage.
2. Notify the physician.
3. Strip the chest tube starting at the chest.
4. Increase the suction by 10 mm Hg.

15. The nurse is reviewing the results of the patient's diagnostic testing. Of the following results, the finding that falls within expected or normal limits is:

1. Palpable, elevated hardened area around a tuberculosis skin testing site
2. Sputum for culture and sensitivity identifies mycobacterium tuberculosis
3. Presence of acid-fast bacilli in sputum
4. Arterial oxygen tension (PaO_2) of 95 mm Hg

Answers: 1. 4; **2.** 4; **3.** 2; **4.** 1; **5.** 4; **6.** 2; **7.** 3; **8.** 1, 4, 5; **9.** 4; **10.** 1; **11.** 1, 2, 4; **12.** 4, 6, 1, 3, 2, 5, 8, 7; **13.** 2, 4; **14.** 1; **15.** 4.

Rationales for Review Questions can be found on the Evolve website.

REFERENCES

Ackley BJ, Ladwig GB: *Nursing diagnosis handbook: an evidence-based guide to planning care*, ed 9, St Louis, 2011, Mosby.

American Association of Respiratory Care (AARC): AARC clinical practice guideline, directed cough, *Respir Care* 38(5):495, 1993.

American Association of Respiratory Care (AARC): AARC clinical practice guideline, nasotracheal suction—2004 revision and update, *Respir Care* 49:1080, 2004.

American Association of Respiratory Care (AARC): AARC clinical practice guideline, oxygen therapy in the home or alternate site health care facility—2007 revision and update, *Respir Care* 52(1):1063, 2007.

American Association of Respiratory Care (AARC): AARC clinical practice guideline, endotracheal suctioning of mechanically ventilated patients with artificial airways—2010 update, *Respir Care* 55(60):758, 2010a.

American Association of Respiratory Care (AARC): AARC clinical practice guideline, providing patient and caregiver training—2010, *Respir Care* 55:765, 2010b.

American Association of Respiratory Care (AARC): Clinical practice guideline: incentive spirometry, *Respir Care* 56(10):1600, 2011.

American Association of Respiratory Care (AARC): AARC clinical practice guidelines: incentive spirometry-2011, *Respir Care* 56(10):1600, 2011.

American Association of Respiratory Care (AARC): Effectiveness of nonpharmacologic airway clearance therapies in hospitalized patients, *Respir Care* 58:2187, 2012.

American Cancer Society (ACS): *Questions about smoking, tobacco, and health*, 2014a, http://www.cancer.org/cancer/cancercauses/tobaccocancer/questionsaboutsmokingtobaccoandhealth/index Accessed September 4, 2014.

American Cancer Society (ACS): *Guide to quitting smoking*, 2014b, http://www.cancer.org/healthy/stayawayfromtobacco/guidetoquittingsmoking/index Accessed September 4, 2014.

American Heart Association (AHA): Community lay rescuer automated external defibrillator programs, *Circulation* 113:1260, 2006.

American Heart Association (AHA): 2010 American heart association guidelines for cardiopulmonary resuscitation and emergency cardiovascular care science, *Circulation* 122:S685, 2010a.

American Heart Association (AHA): Part 1: Executive Summary: 2010 American Heart Association guidelines for cardiopulmonary resuscitation and emergency cardiovascular care, *Circulation* 122(Suppl):S640–S656, 2010b.

American Heart Association (AHA): Importance and implementation of training in cardiopulmonary resuscitation and automated external defibrillation in schools: a science advisory from American heart association, *Circulation* 123:691, 2011.

American Heart Association (AHA): *Get with the guidelines-resuscitation recognition criteria*, 2014, http://my.americanheart.org/professional/ScienceNews/New-Recommendations-to-Improve-Outcomes-After-In-Hospital-Cardiac-Arrest_UCM_450078_Article.jsp Accessed May 2015.

American Heart Association: *Heart attack symptoms in women*, 2015, http://www.heart.org/HEARTORG/Conditions/HeartAttack/WarningSignsofaHeartAttack/Heart-Attack-Symptoms-in-Women_UCM_436448_Article.jsp#.VkYLs8ZzOUk. Accessed November 2015.

American Lung Association: *State of the lung disease in diverse communities 2010*, 2010, http://www.lung.org/finding-cures/our-research/solddc-index.html. Accessed May 2015.

American Thoracic Society (ATS): *Diagnosis and management of stable chronic obstructive pulmonary disease: a clinical practice guideline update from the American College of Physicians, American College of Chest Physicians, American Thoracic Society, and Europena Respiratory Society*, 2011, http://www.thoracic.org/statements/resources/copd/179full.pdf. Accessed November 2015.

Bauman M, et al: Chest tube care, the more you know, the easier it gets, *Am Nurse Today* 9:2011. http://www.americannursetoday.com/chest-tube-care-the-more-you-know-the-easier-it-gets. Accessed May 2015.

Carroll P: *Chest tube and drainage management*, 2015, http://www.rn.org/courses/coursematerial-98.pdf. Accessed November 2015.

Centers for Disease Control and Prevention (CDC): Current cigarette smoking among adults-United

States, 2011, *MMWR Morb Mortal Wkly Rep* 61(44):889, 2012.

Centers for Disease Control and Prevention (CDC): *Tuberculosis, African-American community*, Atlanta, 2013a, Centers for Disease Control and Prevention, Division of Tuberculosis Elimination. http://www.cdc.gov/tb/topic/populations/TbinAfricanAmericans/default.htm. Accessed May 2015.

Centers for Disease Control and Prevention (CDC): Tobacco product use among middle and high school students- United States, 2011 and 2012, *MMWR Morb Mortal Wkly Rep* 62(45):893, 2013b. http://www.cdc.gov/mmwr/preview/mmwrhtml/mm6245a2.htm. Accessed May 2015.

Centers for Disease Control and Prevention (CDC): *Vaccines & immunizations: pneumococcal vaccination*, 2013c, Centers for Disease Control and Prevention, National Center for Immunization and Respiratory Diseases. http://www.cdc.gov/vaccines/vpd-vac/pneumo/default.htm. Accessed May 2015.

Centers for Disease Control and Prevention (CDC): *Testing for TB infection*, Atlanta, 2014a, Centers for Disease Control and Prevention, Division of Tuberculosis Elimination. http://www.cdc.gov/tb/topic/testing/default.htm. Accessed May 2015.

Centers for Disease Control and Prevention (CDC): *Diagnosis of TB disease*, Atlanta, 2014b, Centers for Disease Control and Prevention, Division of Tuberculosis Elimination. http://www.cdc.gov/tb/topic/testing/default.htm#diagnosis. Accessed May 2015.

Centers for Disease Control and Prevention (CDC): *Smoking and tobacco use, quitting smoking*, Atlanta, 2014c, Centers for Disease Control and Prevention, Office on Smoking and Health, National Center for Chronic Disease Prevention and Health. http://www.cdc.gov/tobacco/data_statistics/fact_sheets/cessation/quitting/index.htm. Accessed May 2015.

Centers for Disease Control and Prevention (CDC): *Fact Sheet: Adult cigarette smoking in the United States: current estimates*, 2014d, Centers for Disease Control and Prevention, Smoking and Tobacco Use. http://www.cdc.gov/tobacco/data_statistics/fact_sheets/adult_data/cig_smoking/index.htm. Accessed May 2015.

Centers for Disease Control and Prevention (CDC): *Recommended adult immunization schedule—United States*, Atlanta, 2014e, Centers for Disease Control and Prevention, Morbidity and Mortality Weekly. http://www.cdc.gov/vaccines/schedules/downloads/adult/adult-combined-schedule.pdf. Accessed May 2015.

Centers for Disease Control and Prevention (CDC): *Smoking and tobacco use, smoking during pregnancy*, 2014f, Centers for Disease Control and Prevention Office on Smoking and Health, National Center for Disease Prevention and Health Promotion. http://www.cdc.gov/tobacco/basic_information/health_effects/pregnancy. Accessed May 2015.

Centers for Disease Control (CDC): *Key facts about seasonal flu vaccine*, 2014g, Centers for Disease Control and Prevention. http://www.cdc.gov/flu/protect/keyfacts.htm. Accessed May 2015.

Centers for Medicare and Medicaid Services (CMS): *Home oxygen therapy*, 2015, https://www.cms.gov/Outreach-and-Education/Medicare-Learning-Network-MLN/MLNProducts/Downloads/Home-Oxygen-Therapy-ICN908804.pdf. Accessed January 2016.

Cleveland Clinic: *Information for patients: tracheostomy care*, 2014, Cleveland Clinic Head and Neck Institute. http://my.clevelandclinic.org/head_neck/patients/head_neck_cancer/tracheostomy_care.aspx. Accessed May 2015.

Cooper KLL: Evidence-based prevention of pressure ulcers in the intensive care unit, *Crit Care Nurse* 33(6):57, 2013.

Cystic Fibrosis Foundation (CFF): *An introduction to postural drainage & percussion—consumer fact sheet*, Bethesda, Md, 2012, Cystic Fibrosis Foundation.

Downie F, et al: Opsite flexifit gentle: preventing skin breakdown in vulnerable skin, *Br J Nurs* 22(12):S20, 2013.

Environmental Protection Agency (EPA): *A citizen's guide to radon*, 2014. http://www.epa.gov/radon/pubs/citguide.html. Accessed May 2015.

Freeman S: Care of adult patients with a temporary tracheostomy, *Nurs Stand* 26(20):49, 2011.

Hamilton VA, et al: The role of the endotracheal tube cuff in microaspiration, *Heart Lung* 41(2):2012.

Hockenberry MJ, Wilson D: *Wong's nursing care of infants and children multimedia enhanced version*, ed 10, St Louis, 2015, Mosby.

Johns Hopkins Medicine: *Stoma care*, 2015. http://www.hopkinsmedicine.org/tracheostomy/living/stoma.html. Accessed May 2015.

Kane C, et al: Chest tubes in the critically ills patient, *Dimens Crit Care Nurs* 32(3):112, 2013.

Katholi RE, Couri DM: Left ventricular hypertrophy: major risk factor in patients with hypertension: update and practical clinical applications, *Int J Hypertens* 2011:Article ID 495349, 2011. http://www.hindawi.com/journals/ijhy/2011/495349/. Accessed May 2015.

Lewis SL, et al: *Medical surgical nursing, assessment and management of clinical problems*, ed 9, St Louis, 2014, Mosby.

Li TC: *Can I get the flu vaccine if I am allergic to eggs? Mayo Clinic*, 2013, http://www.mayoclinic.org/diseases-conditions/swine-flu/expert-answers/flu-vaccine-egg-allergy/faq-20057773. Accessed May 2015.

McCance KL, Huether SE: *Pathophysiology: the biologic basis for disease in adults and children*, ed 7, St Louis, 2014, Mosby Elsevier.

Meiner S: *Gerontologic nursing*, ed 4, St Louis, 2011, Mosby.

Morris LL, et al: Tracheostomy care and complications in the intensive care unit, *Crit Care Nurse* 33(5):18, 2013.

Morrison L, Agnew J: *Oscillating devices for airway clearance in people with cystic fibrosis (Review)*, 2014, The Cochrane Library, http://onlinelibrary.wiley.com/doi/10.1002/14651858.CD006842.pub3/abstract. Accessed January 2016.

National Heart Lung and Blood Institute: *What is CPAP?* 2011, National Institutes of Health. http://www.nhlbi.nih.gov/health/health-topics/topics/cpap. Accessed May 2015.

National Institute on Drug Abuse (NIDA): *NIDA Drugfacts: marijuana*, 2014, National Institutes of Health. http://www.drugabuse.gov/publications/drugfacts/marijuana. Accessed May 2015.

National Institute on Drug Abuse (NIDA): *Drugfacts: cocaine*, 2013, National Institutes of Health. http://www.drugabuse.gov/publications/drugfacts/cocaine. Accessed May 2015.

Respiratory Therapy Cave (RTC), *Chest tubes and pleural drainage*, 2011. http://respiratorytherapycave.blogspot.com/2011/10/chest-tubes-and-pleural-drainage.html. Accessed May 2015.

Soo Hoo GW, et al: *Noninvasive ventilation*, 2014, http://emedicine.medscape.com/article/304235-overview. Accessed May 2015.

Stoppler MC: *Is your child or teen "huffing"*, MedicineNet.com, 2013, http://www.medicinenet.com/script/main/art.asp?articlekey=47975 Accessed September 4, 2014.

Task Force on Supplemental Oxygen Therapy: Supplemental oxygen utilization during physical therapy intervention, *Cardiopulm Phys Ther J* 25(2):38, 2014.

The Joint Commission (TJC): *2016 National Patient Safety Goals*, Oakbrook Terrace, IL, 2016, The Commission. Available at: http://www.jointcommission.org/standards_information/npsgs.aspx. Accessed November 2015.

Touhy TA, Jett KF: *Ebersole and Hess' gerontological nursing and healthy aging*, ed 4, St Louis, 2014, Elsevier.

Urden LD, et al: *Thelan's critical care nursing diagnosis and management*, ed 7, St Louis, 2014, Elsevier.

RESEARCH REFERENCES

Aguiar C, et al: Tubing length for long-term oxygen therapy, *Respir Care* 60(2):178, 2015.

Atkins JR, Kautz DD: Move to improve: progressive mobilization in the intensive care unit, *Dimens Crit Care Nurs* 33(5):275, 2014.

Booker S, et al: Mouth care to reduce ventilator-associated pneumonia, *Am J Nurs* 113(10):24, 2013.

Borge CR, et al: Effects of controlled breathing exercises and respiratory muscle training in people with chronic obstructive pulmonary disease: results from evaluating the quality of evidence in systematic reviews, *BMC Pulm Med* 14:184, 2014.

Cabral LF, et al: Pursed lip breathing improves exercise tolerance in COPD: a randomized crossover study, *Eur J Phys Rehabil Med* 2014. [Epub ahead of print].

Cassidy MR, et al: I cough: reducing postoperative pulmonary complications with a multidisciplinary patient care program, *JAMA Surg* 148(8):740–5745, 2013.

Dango S, et al: Impact of chest tube clearance on postoperative morbidity after thoracotomy: results of a prospective, randomized trial, *Eur J Cardiothorac Surg* 37(1):51, 2010.

Earnest MA: Explaining adherence to supplemental oxygen therapy, *J Gen Intern Med* 17:749, 2002.

Hong CM, et al: Patients with chronic obstructive pulmonary disorder, *Med Clin North Am* 97(6): 1095, 2013.

Institute for Health Care Improvement (IHCI): *Implement the IHI ventilator bundle*, 2012, http://www.ihi.org/resources/Pages/Tools/HowtoGuidePreventVAP.aspx. Accessed May 2015.

James PA, et al: 2014 evidence-based guideline for the management of high blood pressure in adults: report from the panel members appointed to the Eighth Joint National Committee (JNC 8), *JAMA* 311(5):507, 2014.

Kaiser JR, et al: The effects of closed tracheal suctioning plus volume guarantee on cerebral hemodynamics, *J Perinatol* 31(10):671, 2011.

Kassis A, et al: Characteristics of patients with injury secondary to smoking on home oxygen therapy transferred intubated to a burn center, *J Am Coll Surg* 8(6):1182, 2014.

Labeau SO, et al: Prevention of ventilator-associated pneumonia with oral antiseptics: a systematic review and meta-analysis, *Lancet Infect Dis* 11(11):845, 2011.

Lacherade JC, et al: Intermittent subglottic secretion drainage and ventilator associated pneumonia: a multicenter trial, *Am J Respir Crit Care Med* 182(7):910, 2010.

Loo CY, et al: Implications and emerging control strategies for ventilator associated infections, *Expert Rev Anti Infect Ther* 13(3):379, 2015.

Luo Z, et al: Noninvasive positive pressure ventilation is required following extubation at the pulmonary infection control window: a prospective observational study, *Clin Respir J* 8(3):338, 2014.

Lynn-McHale DJ: *AACN procedural manual for critical care*, St Louis, ed 6, 2011, Saunders.

Monaco SS, et al: Preventing ventilator-associated events, complying with evidence-based practice, *Crit Care Nurs Q* 37(4):384, 2014.

Morris AC, et al: Reducing ventilator-associated pneumonia in intensive care: impact of implementing a care bundle, *Crit Care Med* 39(10):2218, 2011.

Najafi M, et al: Gender differences in coronary artery disease: correlational study on dietary pattern and known cardiovascular risk factors, *Int Cardiovasc Res J* 7(4):124, 2013.

Needleman M, et al: Randomized controlled trial of tooth-brushing to reduce ventilator-associated pneumonia pathogens and dental plaque in a critical care unit, *J Clin Periodontol* 38(3):246, 2011.

O'Leary C: Evidenced-based management of sepsis, *Clin J Oncol Nurs* 18(3):280, 2014.

Ozden D, Gorgulu S: Development of standard practice guidelines for open and closed system suctioning, *J Clin Nurs* 21(9–10):1327, 2012.

Pang PS, et al: Assessment of dyspnea early in acute heart failure: patient characteristics and response differences between Likert and visual analog scales, *Acad Emerg Med* 21(6):659, 2014.

Pedersen CM, et al: Endotracheal suctioning of the adult intubated patient—what is the evidence? *Intensive Crit Care Nurs* 25:21, 2009.

Rauen CA, et al: Seven evidenced-based practice habits: putting some sacred cows out to pasture, *Crit Care Nurse* 28(2):98, 2008.

Sedwick MB, et al: Using evidence-based practice to prevent ventilator-associated pneumonia, *Crit Care Nurse* 32(4):41, 2012.

Shi Z, et al: Oral hygiene care for critically ill patients to prevent ventilator-associated pneumonia, *Cochrane Database Syst Rev* (8):CD008367, 2013. http://onlinelibrary.wiley.com/doi/10.1002/14651858.CD008367.pub2/abstract. Accessed May 2015.

Sole ML, et al: Comparison of airway management practices between registered nurses and respiratory care practitioners, *Am J Crit Care* 23(3):191, 2014.

Yazdannik AR, et al: Comparing two levels of closed system suction pressure in ICU patients: evaluating the relative safety of higher values of suction pressure, *Iran J Nurs Midwifery Res* 18(2):117, 2013.

Zaratkiewicz S, et al: Retrospective review of the reduction of oral pressure ulcers in mechanically ventilated patients: a change in practice, *Crit Care Nurs Q* 35(3):247, 2012.

42

Fluid, Electrolyte, and Acid-Base Balance

OBJECTIVES

- Describe the processes involved in regulating extracellular fluid volume, body fluid osmolality, and fluid distribution.
- Describe the processes involved in regulating plasma concentrations of potassium, calcium, magnesium, and phosphate ions.
- Describe the processes involved in regulating acid-base balance.
- Describe common fluid, electrolyte, and acid-base imbalances.
- Identify risk factors for fluid, electrolyte, and acid-base imbalances.
- Choose appropriate clinical assessments for specific fluid, electrolyte, and acid-base imbalances.
- Interpret basic fluid, electrolyte, and acid-base laboratory values.
- Apply the nursing process when caring for patients with fluid, electrolyte, and acid-base imbalances.
- Discuss purpose and procedure for initiation and maintenance of intravenous therapy.
- Calculate an intravenous flow rate.
- Describe how to measure and record fluid intake and output.
- Explain how to change intravenous solutions and tubing and discontinue an infusion.
- Describe potential complications of intravenous therapy and what to do if they occur.
- Discuss the procedure for initiating a blood transfusion and interventions to manage a transfusion reaction.

KEY TERMS

Acidosis, p. 944
Active transport, p. 936
Alkalosis, p. 944
Anion gap, p. 944
Anions, p. 935
Arterial blood gases (ABGs), p. 943
Autologous transfusion, p. 962
Buffers, p. 943
Cations, p. 935
Colloid osmotic pressure, p. 936
Colloids, p. 936
Crystalloids, p. 955
Dehydration, p. 939
Electrolytes, p. 935
Electronic infusion devices (EIDs), p. 958
Extracellular fluid (ECF), p. 935
Extracellular fluid volume deficit (ECV deficit), p. 939
Extracellular fluid volume excess (ECV excess), p. 939
Extravasation, p. 961
Filtration, p. 936
Fluid, p. 935
Hydrostatic pressure, p. 936
Hypercalcemia, p. 941
Hyperkalemia, p. 941
Hypermagnesemia, p. 941
Hypernatremia, p. 939
Hypertonic, p. 936
Hypocalcemia, p. 941
Hypokalemia, p. 940
Hypomagnesemia, p. 941
Hyponatremia, p. 939
Hypotonic, p. 936
Hypovolemia, p. 939
Infiltration, p. 961
Interstitial fluid, p. 935
Intracellular fluid (ICF), p. 935
Intravascular fluid, p. 935
Ions, p. 935
Isotonic, p. 936
Metabolic acidosis, p. 944
Metabolic alkalosis, p. 944
Oncotic pressure, p. 936
Osmolality, p. 936
Osmosis, p. 936
Osmotic pressure, p. 936
Phlebitis, p. 961
Respiratory acidosis, p. 944
Respiratory alkalosis, p. 944
Transcellular fluids, p. 935
Transfusion reaction, p. 962
Vascular access devices (VADs), p. 956
Venipuncture, p. 957

MEDIA RESOURCES

http://evolve.elsevier.com/Potter/fundamentals/

- Review Questions
- Video Clips
- Case Study with Questions
- Skills Performance Checklists
- Audio Glossary
- Calculations Tutorial
- Butterfield's Fluids and Electrolytes Tutorial
- Content Updates

Fluid surrounds all the cells in the body and is also inside cells. Body fluids contain electrolytes such as sodium and potassium and also have a degree of acidity. Fluid, electrolyte, and acid-base balances within the body maintain the health and function of all body systems. The characteristics of body fluids influence body system function because of their effects on cell function. These characteristics include the fluid amount (volume), concentration (osmolality), composition (electrolyte concentration), and degree of acidity (pH). All of these characteristics have regulatory mechanisms that keep them in balance for normal function. In this chapter you learn how the body normally maintains fluid, electrolyte, and acid-base balance. You also learn how imbalances develop; how various fluid, electrolyte, and acid-base imbalances affect patients; and ways to help patients maintain or restore balance safely.

SCIENTIFIC KNOWLEDGE BASE

This section provides the foundation for your critical thinking regarding patients who have or are at risk of having fluid, electrolyte, or acid-base imbalances.

Location and Movement of Water and Electrolytes

Water is a substantial proportion of body weight. In fact, about 60% of the body weight of an adult man is water. This proportion decreases with age; approximately 50% of an older man's weight is water. Women typically have less water content than men. Obese people have less water in their bodies than lean people because fat contains less water than muscle (Hall, 2016). The term **fluid** means water that contains dissolved or suspended substances such as glucose, mineral salts, and proteins.

Fluid Distribution. Body fluids are located in two distinct compartments: **extracellular fluid (ECF)** outside the cells, and **intracellular fluid (ICF)** inside the cells (Figure 42-1). In adults ICF is approximately two thirds of total body water. ECF is approximately one third of total body water. ECF has two major divisions (**intravascular fluid** and **interstitial fluid**) and a minor division (**transcellular fluids**). Intravascular fluid is the liquid part of the blood (i.e., the plasma). Interstitial fluid is located between the cells and outside the blood vessels. Transcellular fluids such as cerebrospinal, pleural, peritoneal, and synovial fluids are secreted by epithelial cells (Hall, 2016).

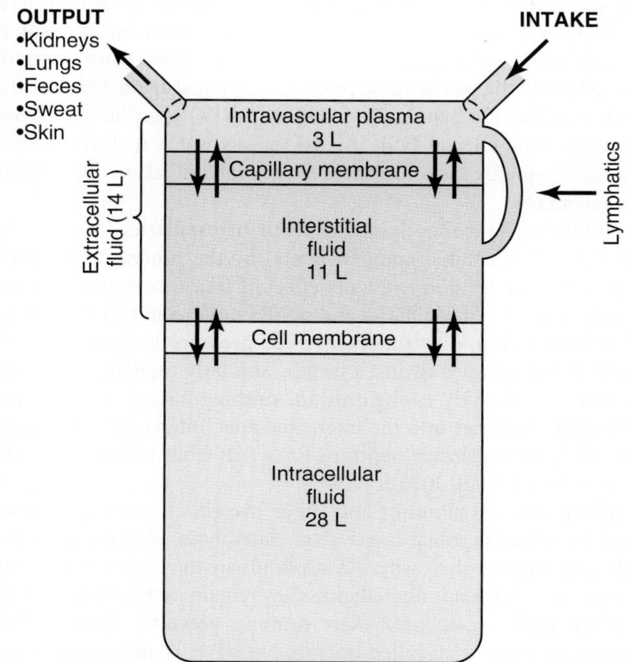

FIGURE 42-1 Body fluid compartments. (From Hall JE: *Guyton and Hall textbook of medical physiology*, ed 13, Philadelphia, 2016, Saunders.)

Composition of Body Fluids. Fluid in the body compartments contains mineral salts known technically as **electrolytes**. An electrolyte is a compound that separates into **ions** (charged particles) when it dissolves in water. Ions that are positively charged are called **cations**; ions that are negatively charged are called **anions**. Cations in body fluids are sodium (Na^+), potassium (K^+), calcium (Ca^{2+}), and magnesium ions (Mg^{2+}). Anions in body fluids are chloride (Cl^-) and bicarbonate (HCO_3^-). Anions and cations combine to make salts. If you put table salt (NaCl) in water, it separates into Na^+ and Cl^-. Other combinations of anions and cations do the same. Clinical laboratories usually report electrolyte measurements in milliequivalents per liter (mEq/L) or millimoles per liter (mmol/L), which are two different units of concentration (Table 42-1). Millimoles per liter represent the number of milligrams of the electrolyte divided by its molecular weight that are contained in a liter of the fluid being measured (usually blood plasma or serum). Milliequivalents per liter are the millimoles per liter multiplied by the electrolyte charge (e.g., 1 for Na^+, 2 for Ca^{2+}). A milliequivalent of one electrolyte can combine with a milliequivalent of another electrolyte, which is why this measurement unit is used.

Fluid that contains a large number of dissolved particles is more concentrated than the same amount of fluid that contains only a few

TABLE 42-1 Laboratory Normal Values for Adults

Item Measured	Normal Value in Serum or Blood
Osmolality	280-300 mOsm/kg H_2O (280-300 mmol/kg H_2O)
Electrolytes	
Sodium (Na^+)	136-145 mEq/L (136-145 mmol/L)
Potassium (K^+)	3.5-5.0 mEq/L (3.5-5 mmol/L)
Chloride (Cl^-)	98-106 mEq/L (98-106 mmol/L)
Total CO_2 (CO_2 total content)	22-30 mEq/L (22-30 mmol/L)
Bicarbonate (HCO_3^-)	Arterial 22-26 mEq/L (22-26 mmol/L) Venous 24-30 mEq/L (24-30 mmol/L)
Total calcium (Ca^{2+})	8.4-10.5 mg/dL (2.1-2.6 mmol/L)
Ionized calcium (Ca^{2+})	4.5-5.3 mg/dL (1.1-1.3 mmol/L)
Magnesium (Mg^{2+})	1.5-2.5 mEq/L (0.75-1.25 mmol/L)
Phosphate	2.7-4.5 mg/dL (0.87-1.45 mmol/L)
Anion gap	5-11 mEq/L (5-11 mmol/L)
Arterial Blood Gases	
pH	7.35-7.45
$PaCO_2$	35-45 mm Hg (4.7-6 kPa)
PaO_2	80-100 mm Hg (10.7-133.3 kPa)
O_2 saturation	95%-100% (0.95-1.00)
Base excess	−2 to +2 mm Eq/L (mmol/L)

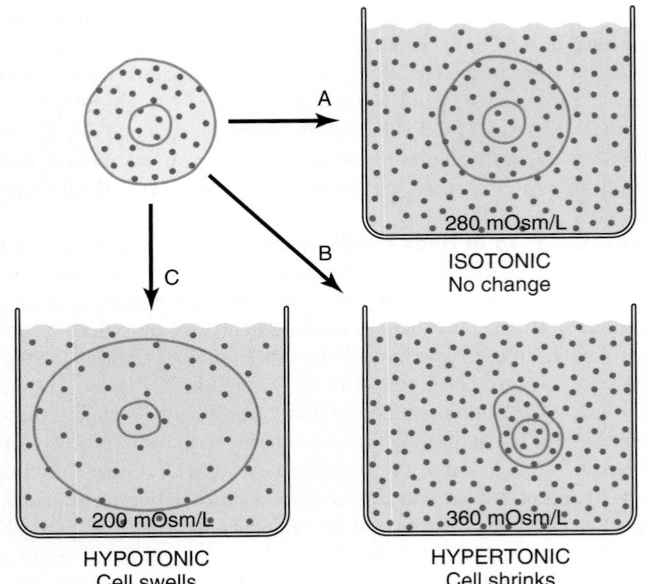

FIGURE 42-2 Effects of isotonic, hypotonic, and hypertonic solutions. (From Hall JE: *Guyton and Hall textbook of medical physiology*, ed 13, Philadelphia, 2016, Saunders.)

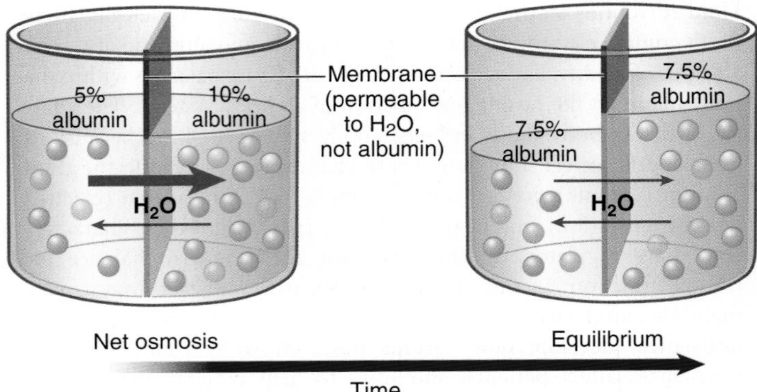

FIGURE 42-3 Osmosis moves water through semi-permeable membrane. (From Patton KT, Thibodeau GA: *Anatomy and physiology*, ed 9, St Louis, 2016, Mosby.)

particles. Osmolality of a fluid is a measure of the number of particles per kilogram of water. Some particles (e.g., urea) pass easily through cell membranes; others such as Na^+ cannot cross easily. The particles that cannot cross cell membranes easily determine the tonicity (effective concentration) of a fluid (Davison et al., 2014). A fluid with the same tonicity as normal blood is called isotonic. A hypotonic solution is more dilute than the blood, and a hypertonic solution is more concentrated than normal blood (Figure 42-2).

Movement of Water and Electrolytes. Active transport, diffusion, osmosis, and filtration are processes that move water and electrolytes between body compartments. These processes maintain equal osmolality in all compartments while allowing for different electrolyte concentrations.

Active Transport. Fluids in different body compartments have different concentrations of electrolytes that are necessary for normal function. For example, concentrations of Na^+, Cl^-, and HCO_3^- are higher in the ECF, whereas the concentrations of K^+, Mg^{2+}, and phosphate are higher in the ICF. Cells maintain their high intracellular electrolyte concentration by active transport. Active transport requires energy in the form of adenosine triphosphate (ATP) to move electrolytes across cell membranes against the concentration gradient (from areas of lower concentration to areas of higher concentration). One example of active transport is the sodium-potassium pump, which moves Na^+ out of a cell and K^+ into it, keeping ICF lower in Na^+ and higher in K^+ than the ECF.

Diffusion. Diffusion is passive movement of electrolytes or other particles down a concentration gradient (from areas of higher concentration to areas of lower concentration). Within a body compartment electrolytes diffuse easily by random movements until the concentration is the same in all areas. However, diffusion of electrolytes across cell membranes requires proteins that serve as ion channels. For example, when a sodium channel in a cell membrane is open, Na^+ diffuses passively across the cell membrane into the ICF because concentration is lower in the ICF. Opening of ion channels is tightly controlled and plays an important part in muscle and nerve function.

Osmosis. Water moves across cell membranes by osmosis, a process by which water moves through a membrane that separates fluids with different particle concentrations (Figure 42-3). Cell membranes are semi-permeable, which means that water crosses them easily but they are not freely permeable to many types of particles, including electrolytes such as sodium and potassium. These semi-permeable cell membranes separate interstitial fluid from ICF. The fluid in each of these compartments exerts osmotic pressure, an inward-pulling force caused by particles in the fluid. The particles already inside the cell exert ICF osmotic pressure, which tends to pull water into the cell. The particles in the interstitial fluid exert interstitial fluid osmotic pressure, which tends to pull water out of the cell. Water moves into the compartment that has a higher osmotic pressure (inward-pulling force) until the particle concentration is equal in the two compartments.

If the particle concentration in the interstitial compartment changes, osmosis occurs rapidly and moves water into or out of cells to equalize the osmotic pressures. For example, when a hypotonic solution (more dilute than normal body fluids) is administered intravenously, it dilutes the interstitial fluid, decreasing its osmotic pressure below intracellular osmotic pressure. Water moves rapidly into cells until the two osmotic pressures are equal again. On the other hand, infusion of a hypertonic intravenous (IV) solution (more concentrated than normal body fluids) causes water to leave cells by osmosis to equalize the osmolality between interstitial and intracellular compartments.

Filtration. Fluid moves into and out of capillaries (between the vascular and interstitial compartments) by the process of filtration (Figure 42-4). Filtration is the net effect of four forces, two that tend to move fluid out of capillaries and small venules and two that tend to move fluid back into them. Hydrostatic pressure is the force of the fluid pressing outward against a surface. Similarly, capillary hydrostatic pressure is a relatively strong outward-pushing force that helps move fluid from capillaries into the interstitial area. Interstitial fluid hydrostatic pressure is a weaker opposing force that tends to push fluid back into capillaries (Hall, 2016).

Blood contains albumin and other proteins known as colloids. These proteins are much larger than electrolytes, glucose, and other molecules that dissolve easily. Most colloids are too large to leave capillaries in the fluid that is filtered; thus they remain in the blood. Because they are particles, colloids exert osmotic pressure. Blood colloid osmotic pressure, also called oncotic pressure, is an inward-pulling force caused by blood proteins that helps move fluid from the interstitial area back into capillaries. Interstitial fluid colloid osmotic pressure normally is a very small opposing force.

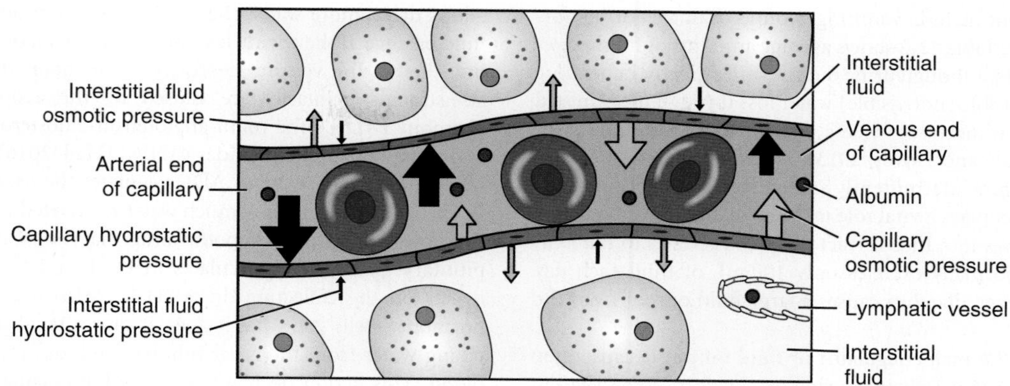

FIGURE 42-4 Capillary filtration moves fluid between vascular and interstitial compartments. (From Copstead LC, Banasik JL: *Pathophysiology*, ed 5, St Louis, 2013, Saunders.)

At the arterial end of a normal capillary, capillary hydrostatic pressure is strongest; and fluid moves from the capillary into the interstitial area, bringing nutrients to cells. At the venous end capillary hydrostatic pressure is weaker, and the colloid osmotic pressure of the blood is stronger. Thus fluid moves into the capillary at the venous end, removing waste products from cellular metabolism. Lymph vessels remove any extra fluid and proteins that have leaked into the interstitial fluid.

Disease processes and other factors that alter these forces may cause accumulation of excess fluid in the interstitial space, known as *edema*. For example, people with heart failure develop edema. In this situation venous congestion from a weakened heart that no longer pumps effectively increases capillary hydrostatic pressure, causing edema by moving excessive fluid into the interstitial space. Inflammation is another cause of edema. It increases capillary blood flow and allows capillaries to leak colloids into the interstitial space. The resulting increased capillary hydrostatic pressure and increased interstitial colloid osmotic pressure produce localized edema in the inflamed tissues.

Fluid Balance

Fluid homeostasis is the dynamic interplay of three processes: fluid intake and absorption, fluid distribution, and fluid output (Felver, 2013d). To maintain fluid balance, fluid intake must equal output. Because some of the normal daily fluid output (e.g., urine, sweat) is a hypotonic salt solution, people must have an equivalent fluid intake of hypotonic sodium-containing fluid (or water plus foods with some salt) to maintain fluid balance (intake equal to output).

Fluid Intake. Fluid intake occurs orally through drinking but also through eating because most foods contain some water. Food metabolism creates additional water. Average fluid intake from these routes for healthy adults is about 2300 mL, although this amount can vary widely, depending on exercise habits, preferences, and the environment (Table 42-2). Other routes of fluid intake include IV, rectal (e.g., enemas), and irrigation of body cavities that can absorb fluid.

Although you might think that the major regulator of oral fluid intake is thirst, habit and social reasons also play major roles in fluid intake. Thirst, the conscious desire for water, is an important regulator of fluid intake when plasma osmolality increases (osmoreceptor-mediated thirst) or the blood volume decreases (baroreceptor-mediated thirst and angiotensin II– and III–mediated thirst) (Arai et al., 2013). The thirst-control mechanism is located within the hypothalamus in the brain (Figure 42-5). Osmoreceptors continually monitor plasma osmolality; when it increases, they cause thirst by stimulating neurons in the hypothalamus. People who are alert can obtain fluid or communicate their thirst to others, and fluid intake restores fluid balance. Infants, patients with neurological or psychological problems, and some older adults who are unable to perceive or communicate their thirst are at risk for dehydration.

TABLE 42-2 Healthy Adult Average Fluid Intake and Output

	Normal (per Day)	Prolonged Heavy Exercise (per Hour)
Fluid Intake		
Fluids Ingested		
Oral	1100-1400 mL	280-1100 mL/hr
Foods	800-1000 mL	Highly variable
Metabolism	300 mL	16-50 mL/hr
TOTAL	2200-2700 mL	300-1150 mL/hr
Fluid Output		
Skin (insensible and sweat)	500-600 mL	300-2100 mL/hour
Insensible lungs	400 mL	20 mL/hr
Gastrointestinal	100-200 mL	Negligible, unless diarrhea during exercise
Urine	1200-1500 mL	20-1000 mL/hr, depending on hydration status
TOTAL	2200-2700 mL	340-3120 mL/hr Rehydration with Na^+-containing fluid necessary after prolonged vigorous exercise

Data from Hall JE: *Guyton and Hall textbook of medical physiology*, ed 13, Philadelphia, 2016, Saunders; American College of Sports Medicine (ACSM): Position stand on exercise and fluid replacement, *Med Sci Sports Exerc* 39(2):377, 2007.

Fluid Distribution. The term *fluid distribution* means the movement of fluid among its various compartments. Fluid distribution between the extracellular and intracellular compartments occurs by osmosis. Fluid distribution between the vascular and interstitial parts of the ECF occurs by filtration.

Fluid Output. Fluid output normally occurs through four organs: the skin, lungs, gastrointestinal (GI) tract, and kidneys. Examples of abnormal fluid output include vomiting, wound drainage, or hemorrhage (Felver, 2013d). Table 42-2 shows average amounts of fluid excretion for healthy adults, although urine output varies greatly, depending on fluid intake. Insensible (not visible) water loss through the skin and lungs is continuous. It increases when a person has a fever or a recent burn to the skin (Hale and Hovey, 2013). Sweat, which is visible and contains sodium, occurs intermittently and increases fluid output substantially. The GI tract plays a vital role in fluid balance. Approximately 3 to 6 L of fluid moves into the GI tract daily and returns to the ECF. The average adult normally excretes only 100 mL of fluid each day through feces. However, diarrhea causes a large fluid output from the GI tract.

The kidneys are the major regulator of fluid output because they respond to hormones that influence urine production. When healthy

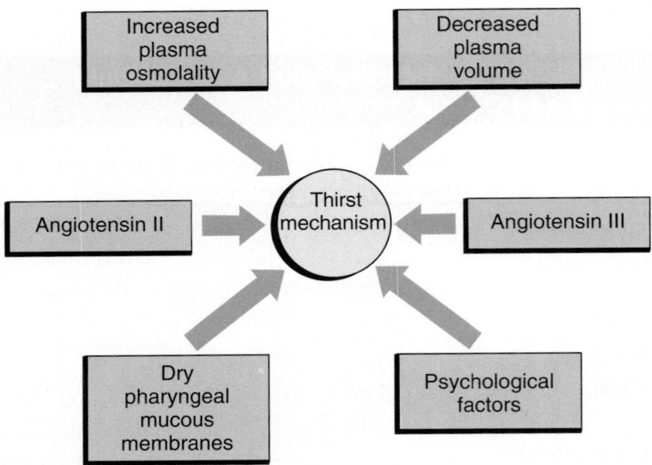

FIGURE 42-5 Stimuli affecting thirst mechanism.

adults drink more water, they increase urine production to maintain fluid balance. If they drink less water, sweat a lot, or lose fluid by vomiting, their urine volume decreases to maintain fluid balance. These adjustments primarily are caused by the actions of antidiuretic hormone (ADH), the renin-angiotensin-aldosterone system (RAAS), and atrial natriuretic peptides (ANPs) (Hall, 2016) (Figure 42-6).

Antidiuretic Hormone. ADH regulates the osmolality of the body fluids by influencing how much water is excreted in urine. It is synthesized by neurons in the hypothalamus that release it from the posterior pituitary gland. ADH circulates in the blood to the kidneys, where it acts on the collecting ducts (Hall, 2016). Its name—antidiuretic hormone—tells you what it does. It causes renal cells to resorb water, taking water from the renal tubular fluid and putting it back in the blood. This action decreases urine volume, concentrating the urine while diluting the blood by adding water to it (see Figure 42-6, *A*).

People normally have some ADH release to maintain fluid balance. More ADH is released if body fluids become more concentrated. Factors that increase ADH levels include severely decreased blood volume (e.g., dehydration, hemorrhage), pain, stressors, and some medications.

ADH levels decrease if body fluids become too dilute. This allows more water to be excreted in urine, creating a larger volume of dilute urine and concentrating the body fluids back to normal osmolality. For example, ethyl alcohol decreases ADH release, which causes people to urinate frequently when they drink alcoholic beverages.

Renin-Angiotensin-Aldosterone System. The RAAS regulates ECF volume by influencing how much sodium and water are excreted in urine. It also contributes to regulation of blood pressure. Specialized cells in the kidneys release the enzyme renin, which acts on angiotensinogen, an inactive protein secreted by the liver that circulates in the blood. Renin converts angiotensinogen to angiotensin I, which is converted to angiotensin II by other enzymes in the lung capillaries (Hall, 2016). Angiotensin II has several functions, one of which is

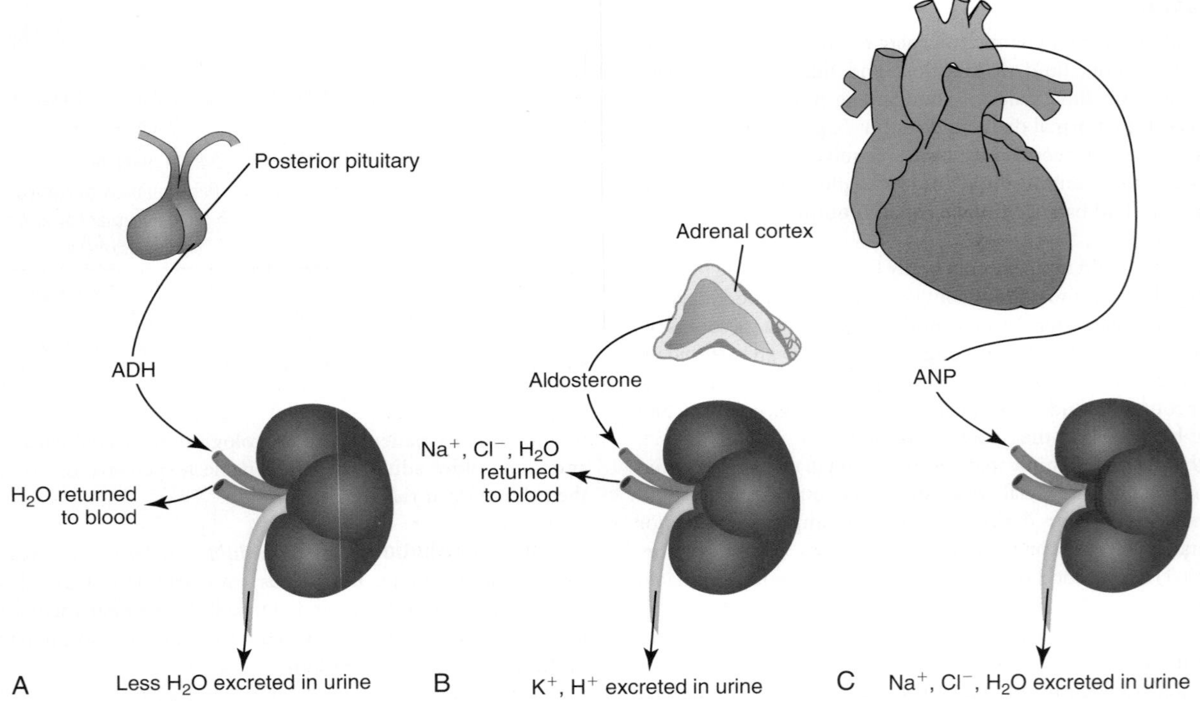

FIGURE 42-6 Major hormones that influence renal fluid excretion. **A,** Antidiuretic hormone (ADH). **B,** Aldosterone. **C,** Atrial natriuretic peptide (ANP).

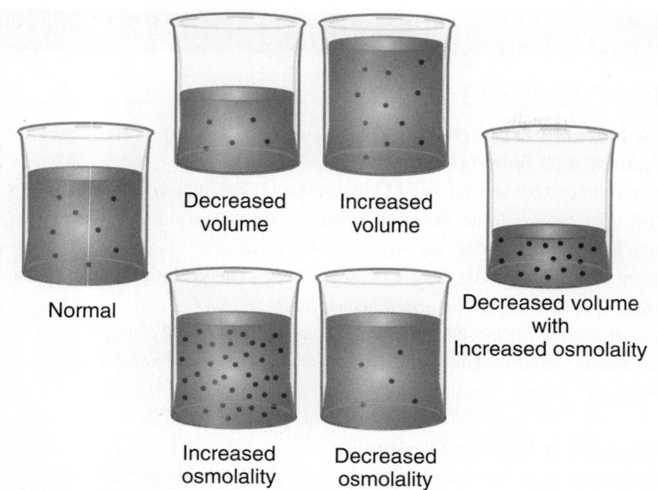

FIGURE 42-7 Fluid volume and osmolality imbalances. (From Copstead LC, Banasik JL: *Pathophysiology online for pathophysiology*, ed 4, St Louis, 2013, Mosby.)

vasoconstriction in some vascular beds. The important fluid homeostasis functions of angiotensin II include stimulation of aldosterone release from the adrenal cortex.

Aldosterone circulates to the kidneys, where it causes resorption of sodium and water in isotonic proportion in the distal renal tubules. Removing sodium and water from the renal tubules and returning it to the blood increases the volume of the ECF (see Figure 42-6, *B*). Aldosterone also contributes to electrolyte and acid-base balance by increasing urinary excretion of potassium and hydrogen ions.

To maintain fluid balance, normally some action of the RAAS occurs. Certain stimuli increase or decrease the activity of this system to restore fluid balance. For example, if hemorrhage or vomiting decreases the extracellular fluid volume (ECV), blood flow decreases through the renal arteries, and more renin is released. This increased RAAS activity causes more sodium and water retention, helping to restore ECV.

Atrial Natriuretic Peptide. ANP also regulates ECV by influencing how much sodium and water are excreted in urine. Cells in the atria of the heart release ANP when they are stretched (e.g., by an increased ECV). ANP is a weak hormone that inhibits ADH by increasing the loss of sodium and water in the urine (see Figure 42-6, *C*). Thus ANP opposes the effect of aldosterone (Hall, 2016).

Fluid Imbalances

If disease processes, medications, or other factors disrupt fluid intake or output, imbalances sometimes occur (Felver, 2013d). For example, with diarrhea there is an increase in fluid output, and a fluid imbalance (dehydration) occurs if fluid intake does not increase appropriately. There are two major types of fluid imbalances: volume imbalances and osmolality imbalances (Figure 42-7). Volume imbalances are disturbances of the *amount of fluid in the extracellular compartment.* Osmolality imbalances are disturbances of the *concentration of body fluids.* Volume and osmolality imbalances occur separately or in combination.

Extracellular Fluid Volume Imbalances. In an ECV imbalance there is either too little (ECV deficit) or too much (ECV excess) isotonic fluid. ECV deficit is present when there is insufficient isotonic fluid in the extracellular compartment. Remember that there is a lot of sodium in normal ECF. With ECV deficit, output of isotonic fluid exceeds intake of sodium-containing fluid. Because ECF is both vascular and interstitial, signs and symptoms arise from lack of volume in both of these compartments. Table 42-3 lists specific causes and signs and symptoms of ECV deficit. The term hypovolemia means decreased vascular volume and often is used when discussing ECV deficit (Hale and Hovey, 2013).

ECV excess occurs when there is too much isotonic fluid in the extracellular compartment. Intake of sodium-containing isotonic fluid has exceeded fluid output. For example, when you eat more salty foods than usual and drink water, you may notice that your ankles swell or rings on your fingers feel tight and you gain 2 lbs (1 kg) or more overnight. These are manifestations of mild ECV excess. See Table 42-3 for other specific causes and signs and symptoms.

Osmolality Imbalances. In an osmolality imbalance body fluids become hypertonic or hypotonic, which causes osmotic shifts of water across cell membranes. The osmolality imbalances are called *hypernatremia* and *hyponatremia.*

Hypernatremia, also called *water deficit,* is a hypertonic condition. Two general causes make body fluids too concentrated: loss of relatively more water than salt or gain of relatively more salt than water (Felver, 2013d). Table 42-3 lists specific causes under these categories. When the interstitial fluid becomes hypertonic, water leaves cells by osmosis, and they shrivel. Signs and symptoms of hypernatremia are those of cerebral dysfunction, which arise when brain cells shrivel. Hypernatremia may occur in combination with ECV deficit; this combined disorder is called clinical dehydration.

Hyponatremia, also called *water excess* or *water intoxication,* is a hypotonic condition. It arises from gain of relatively more water than salt or loss of relatively more salt than water (Felver, 2013d) (see Table 42-3). The excessively dilute condition of interstitial fluid causes water to enter cells by osmosis, causing the cells to swell. Signs and symptoms of cerebral dysfunction occur when brain cells swell.

Clinical Dehydration. ECV deficit and hypernatremia often occur at the same time; this combination is called *clinical dehydration.* The ECV is too low, and the body fluids are too concentrated. Clinical dehydration is common with gastroenteritis or other causes of severe vomiting and diarrhea when people are not able to replace their fluid output with enough intake of dilute sodium-containing fluids. Signs and symptoms of clinical dehydration are those of both ECV deficit and hypernatremia (see Table 42-3).

Electrolyte Balance

You can best understand electrolyte balance by considering the three processes involved in electrolyte homeostasis: electrolyte intake and absorption, electrolyte distribution, and electrolyte output (Table 42-4) (Felver, 2013d). Although sodium is an electrolyte, it is not included here because serum sodium imbalances are the osmolality imbalances discussed previously.

Electrolyte distribution is an important issue. Plasma concentrations of K^+, Ca^{2+}, Mg^{2+}, and phosphate are very low compared with their concentrations in cells and bone (Hall, 2016). These concentration differences are necessary for normal muscle and nerve function. The electrolyte values that you review from laboratory reports are measured in blood serum and do not measure intracellular levels.

Electrolyte output occurs through normal excretion in urine, feces, and sweat. Output also occurs through vomiting, drainage tubes, or fistulas. When electrolyte output increases, electrolyte intake must increase to maintain electrolyte balance. Similarly, if electrolyte output decreases such as with oliguria, electrolyte intake must also decrease to maintain balance (Felver, 2013c).

TABLE 42-3 Fluid Imbalances

Imbalance and Related Causes	Signs and Symptoms
Isotonic Imbalances—Water and Sodium Lost or Gained in Equal or Isotonic Proportions	
Extracellular Fluid Volume Deficit—Body Fluids Have Decreased Volume but Normal Osmolality	
Sodium and Water Intake Less Than Output, Causing Isotonic Loss: Severely decreased oral intake of water and salt Increased GI output: vomiting, diarrhea, laxative overuse, drainage from fistulas or tubes Increased renal output: use of diuretics, adrenal insufficiency (deficit of cortisol and aldosterone) Loss of blood or plasma: hemorrhage, burns Massive sweating without water and salt intake	*Physical examination:* Sudden weight loss (overnight), postural hypotension, tachycardia, thready pulse, dry mucous membranes, poor skin turgor, slow vein filling, flat neck veins when supine, dark yellow urine If severe: thirst, restlessness, confusion, hypotension; oliguria (urine output *below* 30 mL/hr); cold, clammy skin; hypovolemic shock *Laboratory findings:* Increased hematocrit; increased BUN *above* 25 mg/dL (8.9 mmol/L) (hemoconcentration); urine specific gravity usually *above* 1.030, unless renal cause
Extracellular Fluid Volume Excess—Body Fluids Have Increased Volume but Normal Osmolality	
Sodium and Water Intake Greater Than Output, Causing Isotonic Gain: Excessive administration of Na^+-containing isotonic IV fluids or oral intake of salty foods and water Renal retention of Na^+ and water: heart failure, cirrhosis, aldosterone or glucocorticoid excess, acute or chronic oliguric renal disease	*Physical examination:* Sudden weight gain (overnight), edema (especially in dependent areas), full neck veins when upright or semi-upright, crackles in lungs If severe: confusion, pulmonary edema *Laboratory findings:* Decreased hematocrit, decreased BUN *below* 10 mg/dL (3.6 mmol/L) (hemodilution)
Osmolality Imbalances	
Hypernatremia (Water Deficit; Hyperosmolar Imbalance)—Body Fluids Too Concentrated	
Loss of Relatively More Water Than Salt: Diabetes insipidus (ADH deficiency) Osmotic diuresis Large insensible perspiration and respiratory water output without increased water intake **Gain of Relatively More Salt Than Water:** Administration of tube feedings, hypertonic parenteral fluids, or salt tablets Lack of access to water, deliberate water deprivation, inability to respond to thirst (e.g., immobility, aphasia) Dysfunction of osmoreceptor-driven thirst drive	*Physical examination:* Decreased level of consciousness (confusion, lethargy, coma), perhaps thirst, seizures if develops rapidly or is very severe *Laboratory findings:* Serum Na^+ level *above* 145 mEq/L (145 mmol/L), serum osmolality *above* 300 mOsm/kg (300 mmol/kg)
Hyponatremia (Water Excess; Water Intoxication; Hypo-osmolar Imbalance)—Body Fluids Too Dilute	
Gain of Relatively More Water Than Salt: Excessive ADH (SIADH) Psychogenic polydipsia or forced excessive water intake Excessive IV administration of D_5W Use of hypotonic irrigating solutions Tap-water enemas **Loss of Relatively More Salt Than Water:** Replacement of large body fluid output (e.g., diarrhea, vomiting) with water but no salt	*Physical examination:* Decreased level of consciousness (confusion, lethargy, coma), seizures if develops rapidly or is very severe *Laboratory findings:* Serum Na^+ level *below* 135 mEq/L (135 mmol/L), serum osmolality *below* 280 mOsm/kg (280 mmol/kg)
Combined Volume and Osmolality Imbalance	
Clinical Dehydration (ECV Deficit plus Hypernatremia)—Body Fluids Have Decreased Volume and Are Too Concentrated	
Sodium and Water Intake Less Than Output, With Loss of Relatively More Water Than Salt: All of the causes of ECV deficit (see previous causes) plus poor or no water intake, often with fever causing increased insensible water output	*Physical examination and laboratory findings:* Combination of those for ECV deficit plus those for hypernatremia (see previous signs)

ADH, Antidiuretic hormone; *BUN*, blood urea nitrogen; *ECV*, extracellular fluid volume; *GI*, gastrointestinal; *D_5W*, 5% dextrose in water; *IV*, intravenous; *SIADH*, syndrome of inappropriate secretion of antidiuretic hormone.

Electrolyte Imbalances

Factors such as diarrhea, endocrine disorders, and medications that disrupt electrolyte homeostasis cause electrolyte imbalances. Electrolyte intake greater than electrolyte output or a shift of electrolytes from cells or bone into the ECF causes plasma electrolyte excess. Electrolyte intake less than electrolyte output or shift of electrolyte from the ECF into cells or bone causes plasma electrolyte deficit (Felver, 2013c).

Potassium Imbalances. Hypokalemia is abnormally low potassium concentration in the blood. It results from decreased potassium intake and absorption, a shift of potassium from the ECF into cells,

TABLE 42-4 Electrolyte Intake and Absorption, Distribution, and Output

Electrolyte	Intake and Absorption	Distribution	Output/Loss	Important Function
Potassium (K^+)	Fruits Potatoes Instant coffee Molasses Brazil nuts Absorbs easily	Low in ECF, high in ICF. Insulin, epinephrine, and alkalosis shift K^+ into cells. Some types of acidosis shift K^+ out of cells.	Aldosterone, black licorice, hypomagnesemia, and polyuria increase renal excretion; oliguria decreases renal excretion. Acute or chronic diarrhea increases fecal excretion.	Maintains resting membrane potential of skeletal, smooth, and cardiac muscle, allowing normal muscle function
Calcium (Ca^{2+})	Dairy products Canned fish with bones Broccoli Oranges Requires vitamin D for best absorption Undigested fat prevents absorption	Ca^{2+} is low in ECF, mostly in bones and intracellular. Some Ca^{2+} in blood is bound and inactive; only ionized Ca^{2+} is active. Parathyroid hormone shifts Ca^{2+} out of bone; calcitonin shifts Ca^{2+} into bone. Ca^{2+} decreases in blood if phosphate rises and vice versa.	Thiazide diuretics decrease renal excretion. Chronic diarrhea and undigested fat increase fecal excretion.	Influences excitability of nerve and muscle cells; necessary for muscle contraction
Magnesium (Mg^{2+})	Dark green leafy vegetables Whole grains Mg^{2+}-containing laxatives and antacids Undigested fat prevents absorption	Mg^{2+} is low in ECF, mostly in bones and intracellular. Some Mg^{2+} in blood is bound and inactive; only free Mg^{2+} is active.	Rising blood ethanol increases renal excretion; oliguria decreases renal excretion. Chronic diarrhea and undigested fat increase fecal excretion.	Influences function of neuromuscular junctions; is a cofactor for numerous enzymes
Phosphate	Milk Processed foods Aluminum antacids prevent absorption	Phosphate is low in ECF; it is higher in ICF and in bones. Insulin and epinephrine shift phosphate into cells. Decreases in blood if calcium rises and vice versa.	Oliguria decreases renal excretion.	Necessary for production of ATP, the energy source for cellular metabolism

ATP, Adenosine triphosphate; *ECF*, extracellular fluid volume; *ICF*, intracellular fluid.

and an increased potassium output (Table 42-5). Common causes of hypokalemia from increased potassium output include diarrhea, repeated vomiting, and use of potassium-wasting diuretics. People who have these conditions need to increase their potassium intake to reduce their risk of hypokalemia. Hypokalemia causes muscle weakness, which becomes life threatening if it includes respiratory muscles and potentially life-threatening cardiac dysrhythmias.

Hyperkalemia is abnormally high potassium ion concentration in the blood. Its general causes are increased potassium intake and absorption, shift of potassium from cells into the ECF, and decreased potassium output (see Table 42-5). People who have oliguria (decreased urine output) are at high risk of hyperkalemia from the resultant decreased potassium output unless their potassium intake also decreases substantially. Understanding this principle helps you remember to check urine output before you administer IV solutions containing potassium. Hyperkalemia can cause muscle weakness, potentially life-threatening cardiac dysrhythmias, and cardiac arrest.

Calcium Imbalances. **Hypocalcemia** is abnormally low calcium concentration in the blood. The physiologically active form of calcium in the blood is ionized calcium. Total blood calcium also contains inactive forms that are bound to plasma proteins and small anions such as citrate. Factors that cause too much ionized calcium to shift to the bound forms cause symptomatic *ionized hypocalcemia*. Table 42-5 summarizes general causes. People who have acute pancreatitis frequently develop hypocalcemia because calcium binds to undigested fat in their feces and is excreted. This process decreases absorption of dietary calcium and also increases calcium output by preventing resorption of calcium contained in GI fluids. Hypocalcemia increases neuromuscular excitability, the basis for its signs and symptoms.

Hypercalcemia is abnormally high calcium concentration in the blood. Hypercalcemia results from increased calcium intake and absorption, shift of calcium from bones into the ECF, and decreased calcium output (see Table 42-5). Patients with some types of cancers such as lung and breast cancers often develop hypercalcemia because some cancer cells secrete chemicals into the blood that are related to parathyroid hormone. When these chemicals reach the bones, they cause shift of calcium from bones into the ECF. This weakens bones, and the person sometimes develops pathological fractures (i.e., bone breakage caused by forces that would not break a healthy bone). Hypercalcemia decreases neuromuscular excitability, the basis for its other signs and symptoms, the most common of which is lethargy.

Magnesium Imbalances. **Hypomagnesemia** is abnormally low magnesium concentration in the blood. Its general causes are decreased magnesium intake and absorption, shift of plasma magnesium to its inactive bound form, and increased magnesium output (see Table 42-5). Signs and symptoms are similar to those of hypocalcemia because hypomagnesemia also increases neuromuscular excitability.

Hypermagnesemia is abnormally high magnesium concentration in the blood (see Table 42-5). End-stage renal disease causes hypermagnesemia unless the person decreases magnesium intake to match the decreased output. Signs and symptoms are caused by decreased neuromuscular excitability, with lethargy and decreased deep tendon reflexes being most common.

TABLE 42-5 Electrolyte Imbalances

Imbalance and Related Causes	Signs and Symptoms
Hypokalemia—Low Serum Potassium (K^+) Concentration	
Decreased K^+ Intake: Excessive use of K^+-free IV solutions **Shift of K^+ into Cells:** Alkalosis; treatment of diabetic ketoacidosis with insulin **Increased K^+ Output:** Acute or chronic diarrhea; vomiting; other GI losses (e.g., nasogastric or fistula drainage); use of potassium-wasting diuretics; aldosterone excess; polyuria; glucocorticoid therapy	*Physical examination:* Bilateral muscle weakness that begins in quadriceps and may ascend to respiratory muscles, abdominal distention, decreased bowel sounds, constipation, dysrhythmias *Laboratory findings:* Serum K^+ level *below* 3.5 mEq/L (3.5 mmol/L); ECG abnormalities: U waves, flattened or inverted T waves; ST segment depression
Hyperkalemia—High Serum Potassium (K^+) Concentration	
Increased K^+ Intake: Iatrogenic administration of large amounts of IV K^+; rapid infusion of stored blood; excess ingestion of K^+ salt substitutes **Shift of K^+ out of Cells:** Massive cellular damage (e.g., crushing trauma, cytotoxic chemotherapy); insufficient insulin (e.g., diabetic ketoacidosis); some types of acidosis **Decreased K^+ Output:** Acute or chronic oliguria (e.g., severe ECV deficit, end-stage renal disease); use of potassium-sparing diuretics; adrenal insufficiency (deficit of cortisol and aldosterone)	*Physical examination:* Bilateral muscle weakness in quadriceps, transient abdominal cramps, diarrhea, dysrhythmias, cardiac arrest if severe *Laboratory findings:* Serum K^+ level *above* 5 mEq/L (5 mmol/L); ECG abnormalities: peaked T waves; widened QRS complex; PR prolongation; terminal sine-wave pattern
Hypocalcemia—Low Serum Calcium (Ca^{2+}) Concentration	
Decreased Ca^{2+} Intake and Absorption: Calcium-deficient diet; vitamin D deficiency (includes end-stage renal disease); chronic diarrhea; laxative misuse; steatorrhea **Shift of Ca^{2+} into Bone or Inactive Form:** Hypoparathyroidism; rapid administration of citrated blood; hypoalbuminemia; alkalosis; pancreatitis; hyperphosphatemia (includes end-stage renal disease) **Increased Ca^{2+} Output:** Chronic diarrhea; steatorrhea	*Physical examination:* Numbness and tingling of fingers, toes, and circumoral (around mouth) region, positive Chvostek's sign (contraction of facial muscles when facial nerve is tapped), hyperactive reflexes, muscle twitching and cramping; carpal and pedal spasms, tetany, seizures, laryngospasm, dysrhythmias *Laboratory findings:* Total serum Ca^{2+} level *below* 8.4 mg/dL (2.1 mmol/L) or serum ionized Ca^{2+} level *below* 4.5 mg/dL (1.1 mmol/L); ECG abnormalities: prolonged ST segments
Hypercalcemia—High Serum Calcium (Ca^{2+}) Concentration	
Increased Ca^{2+} Intake and Absorption: Milk-alkali syndrome **Shift of Ca^{2+} out of Bone:** Prolonged immobilization; hyperparathyroidism; bone tumors; nonosseous cancers that secrete bone-resorbing factors **Decreased Ca^{2+} Output:** Use of thiazide diuretics	*Physical examination:* Anorexia, nausea and vomiting, constipation, fatigue, diminished reflexes, lethargy, decreased level of consciousness, confusion, personality change, cardiac arrest if severe *Laboratory findings:* Total serum Ca^{2+} level *above* 10.5 mg/dL (2.6 mmol/L) or serum ionized Ca^{2+} level *above* 5.3 mg/dL (1.3 mmol/L); ECG abnormalities: heart block, shortened ST segments
Hypomagnesemia—Low Serum Magnesium (Mg^{2+}) Concentration	
Decreased Mg^{2+} Intake and Absorption: Malnutrition; chronic alcoholism; chronic diarrhea; laxative misuse; steatorrhea **Shift of Mg^{2+} Into Inactive Form:** Rapid administration of citrated blood **Increased Mg^{2+} Output:** Chronic diarrhea; steatorrhea; other GI losses (e.g., vomiting, nasogastric or fistula drainage); use of thiazide or loop diuretics; aldosterone excess	*Physical examination:* Positive Chvostek's sign, hyperactive deep tendon reflexes, muscle cramps and twitching, grimacing, dysphagia, tetany, seizures, insomnia, tachycardia, hypertension, dysrhythmias *Laboratory findings:* Serum Mg^{2+} level *below* 1.5 mEq/L (0.75 mmol/L); ECG abnormalities: prolonged QT interval
Hypermagnesemia—High Serum Magnesium (Mg^{2+}) Concentration	
Increased Mg^{2+} Intake and Absorption: Excessive use of Mg^{2+}-containing laxatives and antacids; parenteral overload of magnesium **Decreased Mg^{2+} Output:** Oliguric end-stage renal disease; adrenal insufficiency	*Physical examination:* Lethargy, hypoactive deep tendon reflexes, bradycardia, hypotension Acute elevation in Mg^{2+} levels: Flushing, sensation of warmth Severe acute hypermagnesemia: Decreased rate and depth of respirations, dysrhythmias, cardiac arrest *Laboratory findings:* Serum Mg^{2+} level *above* 2.5 mEq/L (1.25 mmol/L); ECG abnormalities: prolonged PR interval

Data from Felver L: Fluid and electrolyte homeostasis and imbalances. In Copstead LC, Banasik JL: *Pathophysiology,* ed 5, St Louis, 2013, Saunders.

ECG, electrocardiogram, *ECV,* extracellular fluid volume, *GI,* gastrointestinal, *IV,* intravenous.

TABLE 42-6 Arterial Blood Gas Measures

Laboratory Measure	Normal Range in Adult Arterial Blood	Definition and Interpretation
pH	7.35-7.45	pH is a negative logarithm of the free H^+ concentration, a measure of how acid or alkaline the blood is. Values below 7.35 indicate abnormally acid; above 7.45 they indicate abnormally alkaline. Small changes in pH denote large changes in H^+ concentration and are clinically important.
$PaCO_2$	35-45 mm Hg (4.7-6 kPa)	$PaCO_2$ is partial pressure of carbon dioxide (CO_2), a measure of how well the lungs are excreting CO_2 produced by cells. Increased $PaCO_2$ indicates CO_2 accumulation in blood (more carbonic acid) caused by hypoventilation; decreased $PaCO_2$ indicates excessive CO_2 excretion (less carbonic acid) through hyperventilation.
HCO_3^-	22-26 mEq/L (22-26 mmol/L)	HCO_3^- is concentration of the base (alkaline substance) bicarbonate, a measure of how well the kidneys are excreting metabolic acids. Increased HCO_3^- indicates that the blood has too few metabolic acids; decreased HCO_3^- indicates that the blood has too many metabolic acids.
PaO_2	80-100 mm Hg (10-13.3 kPa)	PaO_2 is partial pressure of oxygen (O_2), a measure of how well gas exchange is occurring in the alveoli of the lungs. Values below normal indicate poor oxygenation of the blood.
SaO_2	95%-100%	SaO_2 is oxygen saturation, the percentage of hemoglobin that is carrying as much O_2 as possible. It is influenced by pH, $PaCO_2$, and body temperature. It drops rapidly when PaO_2 falls below 60 mm Hg (8 kPa).
Base excess	−2 to +2 mEq/L (mmol/L)	Base excess is observed buffering capacity minus the normal buffering capacity, a measure of how well the blood buffers are managing metabolic acids. Values below −2 (negative base excess) indicate excessive metabolic acids; values above +2 indicate excessive amounts of bicarbonate.

Acid-Base Balance

For optimal cell function the body maintains a balance between acids and bases. Acid-base homeostasis is the dynamic interplay of three processes: acid production, acid buffering, and acid excretion (Felver, 2013a). Normal acid-base balance is maintained with acid excretion equal to acid production. Acids release hydrogen (H^+) ions; bases (alkaline substances) take up H^+ ions. The more H^+ ions that are present, the more acidic is the solution.

The degree of acidity in blood and other body fluids is reported from the clinical laboratory as pH. The pH scale goes from 1.0 (very acid) to 14.0 (very alkaline; basic). A pH of 7.0 is considered neutral. The normal pH range of adult arterial blood is 7.35 to 7.45. Maintaining pH within this normal range is very important for optimal cell function. If the pH goes outside the normal range, enzymes within cells do not function properly; hemoglobin does not manage oxygen properly; and serious physiological problems occur, including death. Laboratory tests of a sample of arterial blood called **arterial blood gases (ABGs)** are used to monitor a patient's acid-base balance (Ayers and Dixon, 2012) (Table 42-6).

Acid Production. Cellular metabolism constantly creates two types of acids: carbonic acid and metabolic acids (Figure 42-8). Cells produce carbon dioxide (CO_2), which acts like an acid in the body by converting to carbonic acid (H_2CO_3):

$$CO_2 + H_2O \leftrightarrow H_2CO_3 \leftrightarrow H^+ + HCO_3^-$$
$$\text{Carbon dioxide} + \text{Water} \leftrightarrow \text{Carbonic acid} \leftrightarrow \text{Hydrogen ion} + \text{Bicarbonate}$$

Metabolic acids are any acids that are not carbonic acid. They include citric acid, lactic acid, and many others.

Acid Buffering. **Buffers** are pairs of chemicals that work together to maintain normal pH of body fluids. If there are too many free H^+ ions, a buffer takes them up so they no longer are free. If there are too few, a buffer can release H^+ ions to prevent an acid-base imbalance. Buffers work rapidly, within seconds.

All body fluids contain buffers. The major buffer in the ECF is the bicarbonate (HCO_3^-) buffer system, which buffers metabolic acids. It consists of a lot of bicarbonate and a small amount of carbonic acid (normally a 20 to 1 ratio). Addition of H^+ released by a metabolic acid to a bicarbonate ion makes more carbonic acid. Now the H^+ is no longer free and will not decrease the blood pH:

$$HCO_3^- + H^+ \leftrightarrow H_2CO_3$$
$$\text{Bicarbonate ion} + \text{Hydrogen ion} \leftrightarrow \text{Carbonic acid}$$

If there are too few H^+ ions, the carbonic acid part of the buffer pair releases some, increasing the bicarbonate, again returning pH to normal.

$$H_2CO_3 \leftrightarrow HCO_3^- + H^+$$
$$\text{Carbonic acid} \leftrightarrow \text{Bicarbonate ion} + \text{Hydrogen ion}$$

Other buffers include hemoglobin, protein buffers, and phosphate buffers. Cellular and bone buffers also contribute. Buffers normally keep the blood from becoming too acid when acids that are produced by cells circulate to the lungs and kidneys for excretion.

Acid Excretion. The body has two acid-excretion systems: lungs and kidneys. The lungs excrete carbonic acid; the kidneys excrete metabolic acids (see Figure 42-8).

Excretion of Carbonic Acid. When you exhale, you excrete carbonic acid in the form of CO_2 and water. If the $PaCO_2$ (i.e., level of CO_2 in the blood) rises, the chemoreceptors trigger faster and deeper respirations to excrete the excess. If the $PaCO_2$ falls, the chemoreceptors trigger slower and shallower respirations so more of the CO_2 produced by cells remains in the blood and makes up the deficit. These alterations in respiratory rate and depth maintain the carbonic acid part of acid-base balance (Hale and Hovey, 2013). People who have respiratory disease may be unable to excrete enough carbonic acid, which causes the blood to become more acidic and blood CO_2 to increase. If an increased respiratory rate is unable to correct the problem, the kidneys begin some compensatory excretion of metabolic acid.

Excretion of Metabolic Acids. The kidneys excrete all acids except carbonic acid. They secrete H^+ into the renal tubular fluid, putting

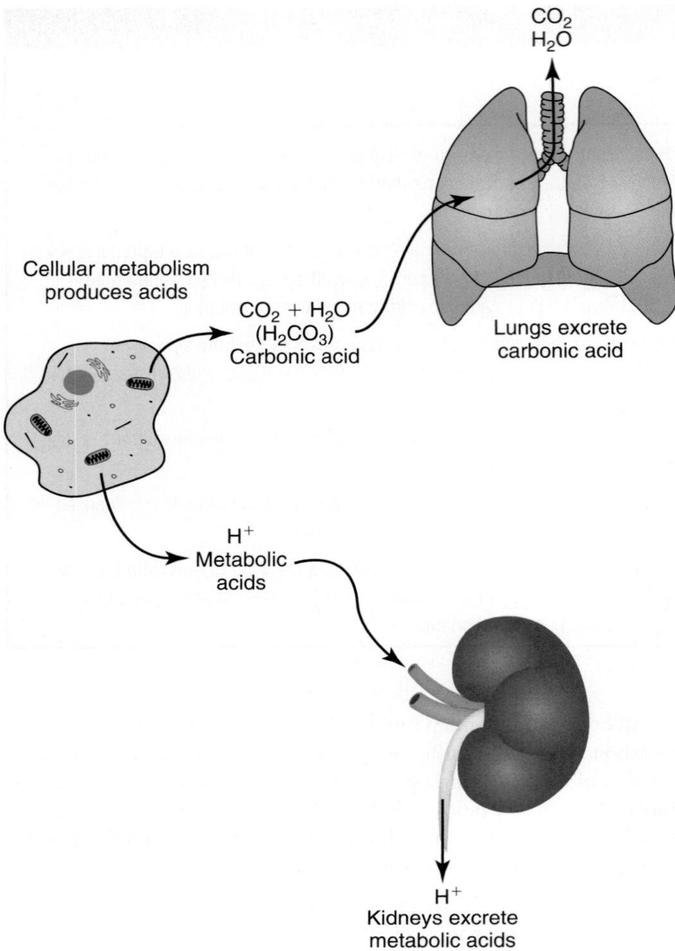

FIGURE 42-8 Acid production and excretion.

HCO_3^- back into the blood at the same time. If there are too many H^+ ions in the blood, renal cells move more H^+ ions into the renal tubules for excretion, retaining more HCO_3^- in the process. If there are too few H^+ ions in the blood, renal cells secrete fewer H^+ ions.

Phosphate buffers in the renal tubular fluid keep the urine from becoming too acidic when the kidneys excrete H^+ ions. If the kidneys need to excrete a lot of H^+, renal tubular cells secrete ammonia, which combines with the H^+ ions in the tubules to make NH_4^+, ammonium ions. Buffering by phosphate and the creation of NH_4^+ turn free H^+ ions into other molecules in the renal tubular fluid (Hale and Hovey, 2013). This process enables metabolic acid excretion in urine without making urine too acidic. People who have oliguric kidney disease often are unable to excrete metabolic acids normally; and these acids accumulate, making the blood too acidic. If the kidneys are unable to correct this problem, respiratory rate and depth increase, causing compensatory excretion of carbonic acid.

Acid-Base Imbalances

People develop acid-base imbalances when their normal homeostatic mechanisms are dysfunctional or overwhelmed. The term acidosis describes a condition that tends to make the blood relatively too acidic. Because our cells produce two types of acid, there are two different types of acidosis: respiratory acidosis and metabolic acidosis. The term alkalosis describes a condition that tends to make the blood relatively too basic (alkaline). There are two types of alkalosis: respiratory alkalosis and metabolic alkalosis.

The body has compensatory mechanisms that limit the extent of pH change with acid-base imbalances (Berend et al., 2014). Compensation involves physiological changes that help normalize the pH but do not correct the cause of the problem. If the problem is a respiratory acid-base imbalance, only the lungs can correct the problem, but the kidneys can compensate by changing the amount of metabolic acid in the blood. If the problem is a metabolic acid-base imbalance, only the kidneys can correct the problem, but the lungs can compensate by changing the amount of carbonic acid in the blood. Thus the kidneys compensate for respiratory acid-base imbalances; the respiratory system compensates for metabolic acid-base imbalances. These compensatory mechanisms do not correct the problem, but they help the body survive by moving the blood pH toward normal. However, if the underlying condition is not corrected, these compensatory mechanisms eventually will fail.

Respiratory Acidosis. Respiratory acidosis arises from alveolar hypoventilation; the lungs are unable to excrete enough CO_2. The $PaCO_2$ rises, creating an excess of carbonic acid in the blood, which decreases pH (Table 42-7). The kidneys compensate by increasing excretion of metabolic acids in the urine, which increases blood bicarbonate. This compensatory process is slow, often taking 24 hours to show clinical effect and 3 to 5 days to reach steady state. Decreased cerebrospinal fluid (CSF) pH and intracellular pH of brain cells cause decreased level of consciousness.

Respiratory Alkalosis. Respiratory alkalosis arises from alveolar hyperventilation; the lungs excrete too much carbonic acid (CO_2 and water). The $PaCO_2$ falls, creating a deficit of carbonic acid in the blood, which increases pH (see Table 42-7). Respiratory alkalosis usually is short lived; thus the kidneys do not have time to compensate. When the pH of blood, CSF, and ICF increases acutely, cell membrane excitability also increases, which can cause neurological symptoms such as excitement, confusion, and paresthesias. If the pH rises high enough, central nervous system (CNS) depression can occur.

Metabolic Acidosis. Metabolic acidosis occurs from an increase of metabolic acid or a decrease of base (bicarbonate). The kidneys are unable to excrete enough metabolic acids, which accumulate in the blood, or bicarbonate is removed from the body directly as with diarrhea (see Table 42-7). In either case the blood HCO_3^- decreases, and the pH falls. With an increase of metabolic acids, blood HCO_3^- decreases because it is used to buffer metabolic acids. Similarly, when patients have conditions that cause the removal of HCO_3^-, the amount of HCO_3^- in the blood decreases. To help identify the specific cause, health care providers and the laboratory calculate the anion gap, a reflection of unmeasured anions in plasma. You calculate anion gap by subtracting the sum of plasma concentrations of the anions Cl^- and HCO_3^- from the plasma concentration of the cation Na^+ (Berend et al., 2014). When reviewing laboratory reports, check the reference values from the laboratory that measured the electrolyte concentrations (Table 42-8).

The abnormally low pH in metabolic acidosis stimulates the chemoreceptors so the respiratory system compensates for the acidosis by hyperventilation. Compensatory hyperventilation begins in a few minutes and removes carbonic acid from the body. This process does not correct the problem, but it helps limit the pH decrease. Metabolic acidosis decreases one's level of consciousness (see Table 42-7).

Metabolic Alkalosis. Metabolic alkalosis occurs from a direct increase of base (HCO_3^-) or a decrease of metabolic acid, which increases blood HCO_3^- by releasing it from its buffering function.

TABLE 42-7 Acid-Base Imbalances

Imbalance and Related Causes	Signs and Symptoms
Respiratory Acidosis—Excessive Carbonic Acid Caused by Alveolar Hypoventilation	
Impaired Gas Exchange: Type B COPD (chronic bronchitis) or end-stage type A COPD (emphysema) Bacterial pneumonia Airway obstruction Extensive atelectasis (collapsed alveoli) Severe acute asthma episode **Impaired Neuromuscular Function:** Respiratory muscle weakness or paralysis from hypokalemia or neurological dysfunction Respiratory muscle fatigue, respiratory failure Chest wall injury or surgery causing pain with respiration **Dysfunction of Brainstem Respiratory Control:** Drug overdose with a respiratory depressant Some types of head injury	*Physical examination:* Headache, light-headedness, decreased level of consciousness (confusion, lethargy, coma), dysrhythmias *Laboratory findings:* Arterial blood gas alterations: pH *below* 7.35, $PaCO_2$ *above* 45 mm Hg (6 kPa), HCO_3^- level normal if uncompensated or *above* 26 mEq/L (26 mmol/L) if compensated
Respiratory Alkalosis—Deficient Carbonic Acid Caused by Alveolar Hyperventilation	
Hypoxemia from any cause (e.g., initial part of asthma episode, pneumonia) Acute pain Anxiety, psychological distress, sobbing Inappropriate mechanical ventilator settings Stimulation of brainstem respiratory control (e.g., meningitis, gram-negative sepsis, head injury, aspirin overdose)	*Physical examination:* Light-headedness, numbness and tingling of fingers, toes, and circumoral region, increased rate and depth of respirations, excitement and confusion possibly followed by decreased level of consciousness, dysrhythmias *Laboratory findings:* Arterial blood gas alterations: pH *above* 7.45, $PaCO_2$ *below* 35 mm Hg (4.7 kPa), HCO_3^- level normal if short lived or uncompensated or *below* 22 mEq/L (22 mmol/L) if compensated
Metabolic Acidosis—Excessive Metabolic Acids	
Increase of Metabolic Acids (High Anion Gap): Ketoacidosis (diabetes, starvation, alcoholism) Hypermetabolic state (severe hyperthyroidism, burns, severe infection) Oliguric renal disease (acute kidney injury, end-stage renal disease) Circulatory shock (lactic acidosis) Ingestion of acid or acid precursors (e.g., methanol, ethylene glycol, boric acid, aspirin overdose) **Loss of Bicarbonate (Normal Anion Gap):** Diarrhea Pancreatic fistula or intestinal decompression Renal tubular acidosis	*Physical examination:* Decreased level of consciousness (lethargy, confusion, coma), abdominal pain, dysrhythmias, increased rate and depth of respirations (compensatory hyperventilation) *Laboratory findings:* Arterial blood gas alterations: pH *below* 7.35, $PaCO_2$ normal if uncompensated or *below* 35 mm Hg (4.7 kPa) if compensated, HCO_3^- level *below* 22 mEq/L (22 mmol/L)
Metabolic Alkalosis—Deficient Metabolic Acids	
Increase of Bicarbonate: Excessive administration of sodium bicarbonate Massive blood transfusion (liver converts citrate to HCO_3^-) Mild or moderate ECV deficit (contraction alkalosis) **Loss of Metabolic Acid:** Excessive vomiting or gastric suctioning Hypokalemia Excess aldosterone	*Physical examination:* Light-headedness, numbness and tingling of fingers, toes, and circumoral region; muscle cramps; possible excitement and confusion followed by decreased level of consciousness, dysrhythmias (may be caused by concurrent hypokalemia) *Laboratory findings:* Arterial blood gas alterations: pH *above* 7.45, $PaCO_2$ normal if uncompensated or *above* 45 mm Hg (6.0 kPa) if compensated, HCO_3^- *above* 26 mEq/L (26 mmol/L)

Data from Felver L: Acid-base homeostasis and imbalances. In Copstead LC, Banasik JL: *Pathophysiology,* ed 5, St Louis, 2013, Saunders.
COPD, Chronic obstructive pulmonary disease, *ECV,* extracellular fluid volume.

Common causes include vomiting and gastric suction (see Table 42-7). The respiratory compensation for metabolic alkalosis is hypoventilation. The decreased rate and depth of respiration allow carbonic acid to increase in the blood, as seen by an increased $PaCO_2$. The need for oxygen may limit the degree of respiratory compensation for metabolic alkalosis. Because HCO_3^- crosses the blood-brain barrier with difficulty, neurological signs and symptoms are less severe or even absent with metabolic alkalosis (Hale and Hovey, 2013).

NURSING KNOWLEDGE BASE

You will apply knowledge about fluid, electrolyte, and acid-base imbalance in many clinical settings. Use the scientific knowledge base in clinical decision making to provide safe, optimal fluid therapy. For example, apply knowledge of risk factors for fluid imbalances and physiology of normal aging when assessing older adults, knowing that this age-group has high risk of fluid imbalances (Touhy and Jett, 2014).

TABLE 42-8 Anion Gap in Metabolic Acidosis

Anion Gap Type	Values (Without K^+)	Causes
Normal anion gap	3-12 mEq/L (3-12 mmol/L) Varies, depending on laboratory	*Excess output of bicarbonate:* Diarrhea, pancreatic fistula, intestinal decompression, renal tubular acidosis Increase of chloride-containing acid: Parenteral HCl therapy
High anion gap	Greater than 5 mEq/L (5 mmol/L) above the laboratory reference range	*Increase of any acid except HCl:* Ketoacids (DKA, starvation, alcoholism), lactic acid (circulatory shock, extreme exercise), excessive normal metabolic acids (oliguric acute kidney injury, end-stage renal disease, severe hyperthyroidism, burns, severe infection), unusual organic acids (salicylate overdose, acids metabolized from methanol, ethylene glycol, paraldehyde)

Data from Berend K, deVries A, Gans, R: Physiological approach to assessment of acid-base disturbances, *New Engl J Med* 371(15): 1434, 2014.
DKA, Diabetic ketoacidosis.

Nursing knowledge includes questions to ask to elicit risk factors for fluid, electrolyte, and acid-base imbalance; specific clinical assessments for signs and symptoms of these imbalances; and nursing and collaborative interventions to maintain or restore fluid and electrolyte and acid-base balance (Felver 2013a,b,c). Skills and techniques for safe IV therapy are a vital area of the nursing knowledge base and the focus of much nursing research to support evidence-based practice.

CRITICAL THINKING

Successful critical thinking requires a synthesis of knowledge, experience, information gathered from patients, critical thinking attitudes, and intellectual and professional standards. Clinical judgments require you to anticipate the information necessary to analyze the data and make decisions regarding patient care. During assessment consider all elements that build toward making an appropriate nursing diagnosis (Figure 42-9).

In the case of fluid, electrolyte, and acid-base balance, you integrate knowledge of physiology, pathophysiology, and pharmacology and previous experiences and information gathered from patients. Critical analysis of data enables an understanding of how fluid, electrolyte, and acid-base imbalances affect a specific patient and his or her family. In addition, critical thinking attitudes such as accountability, discipline, and integrity, applied during assessment, help you identify appropriate nursing diagnoses and plan successful interventions. Professional standards such as the Infusion Nurses Society (INS) standards of practice (INS, 2011) provide valuable guidance for appropriate assessment.

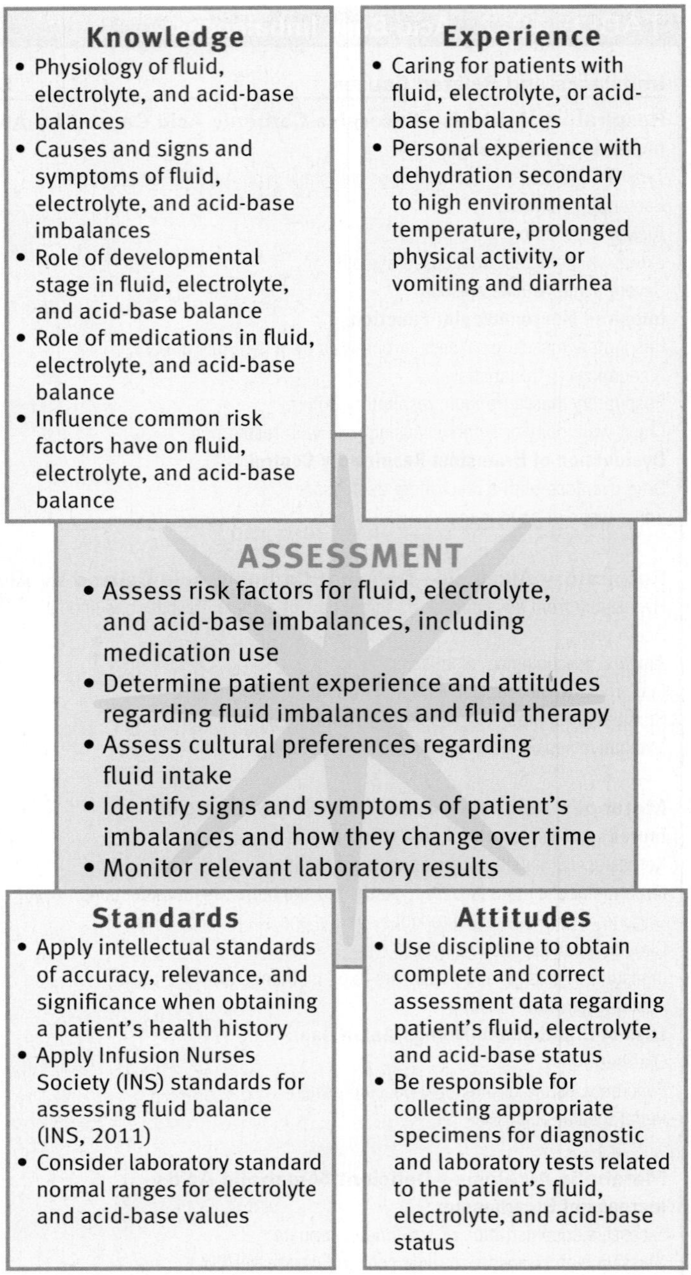

Knowledge
- Physiology of fluid, electrolyte, and acid-base balances
- Causes and signs and symptoms of fluid, electrolyte, and acid-base imbalances
- Role of developmental stage in fluid, electrolyte, and acid-base balance
- Role of medications in fluid, electrolyte, and acid-base balance
- Influence common risk factors have on fluid, electrolyte, and acid-base balance

Experience
- Caring for patients with fluid, electrolyte, or acid-base imbalances
- Personal experience with dehydration secondary to high environmental temperature, prolonged physical activity, or vomiting and diarrhea

ASSESSMENT
- Assess risk factors for fluid, electrolyte, and acid-base imbalances, including medication use
- Determine patient experience and attitudes regarding fluid imbalances and fluid therapy
- Assess cultural preferences regarding fluid intake
- Identify signs and symptoms of patient's imbalances and how they change over time
- Monitor relevant laboratory results

Standards
- Apply intellectual standards of accuracy, relevance, and significance when obtaining a patient's health history
- Apply Infusion Nurses Society (INS) standards for assessing fluid balance (INS, 2011)
- Consider laboratory standard normal ranges for electrolyte and acid-base values

Attitudes
- Use discipline to obtain complete and correct assessment data regarding patient's fluid, electrolyte, and acid-base status
- Be responsible for collecting appropriate specimens for diagnostic and laboratory tests related to the patient's fluid, electrolyte, and acid-base status

FIGURE 42-9 Critical thinking model for fluid, electrolyte, and acid-base balance assessment.

❖ NURSING PROCESS

Apply the nursing process and use a critical thinking approach in your care of patients. The nursing process provides a clinical decision-making approach for you to develop and implement an individualized plan of care. For patients at high risk for fluid, electrolyte, and/or acid-base imbalances or those who already have these imbalances, an individualized approach is the foundation for safe and effective patient-centered nursing care.

◆ Assessment

During the assessment process thoroughly assess each patient and critically analyze findings to ensure that you make patient-centered clinical decisions required for safe nursing care. Using a systematic approach in assessment enables you to help patients maintain or restore fluid, electrolyte, and acid-base balances safely (see Figure 42-9).

Through the Patient's Eyes. A patient's fluid, electrolyte, or acid-base imbalance is sometimes so severe that it prevents initial discussion of his or her expressed needs, values, and preferences. However, when a patient is alert enough to discuss care, you need to elicit this information through a patient-centered assessment. Focus on the patient's experience with fluid, electrolyte, or acid-base alterations and his or her perceptions of the illness. For example, for a patient who is hospitalized for clinical dehydration from diarrhea, ask if he or she has experienced dehydration previously and assess his or her interpretation of the signs and symptoms experienced and possible causes. Also ask how the person has managed diarrhea at home to assess his or her understanding of how to prevent the imbalances from occurring in the future. Assess potential barriers to rehydration such as concerns regarding IV therapy or lack of availability of favorite fluids at the preferred fluid temperature. Ask about the patient's greatest concerns regarding fluid status to build the basis for active partnership in planning, implementing, and evaluating patient-centered care.

Nursing History. Clinical assessment begins with a patient history designed to reveal risk factors that cause or contribute to fluid, electrolyte, and acid-base imbalances (Table 42-9). Ask specific, focused questions to identify factors that contribute to a patient's potential imbalances (Box 42-1).

Age. First assess a patient's age. An infant's proportion of total body water (70% to 80% total body weight) is greater than that of children or adults. Infants and young children have greater water needs and immature kidneys (Hockenberry and Wilson, 2015). They are at greater risk for ECV deficit and hypernatremia because body water loss is proportionately greater per kilogram of weight.

Children who are between the ages of 2 and 12 frequently respond to illnesses with fevers of higher temperatures and longer duration than those of adults (Hockenberry and Wilson, 2015). At any age fever increases the rate of insensible water loss. Adolescents have increased metabolism and water production because of their rapid growth changes. Fluctuations in fluid balance are greater in adolescent girls because of hormonal changes associated with the menstrual cycle.

Older adults experience a number of age-related changes that potentially affect fluid, electrolyte, and acid-base balances (Box 42-2). They often have more difficulty recovering from imbalances resulting from the combined effects of normal aging, various disease conditions, and multiple medications.

Environment. Hot environments increase fluid output through sweating. Sweat is a hypotonic sodium-containing fluid. Excessive sweating without adequate replacement of salt and water can lead to ECV deficit, hypernatremia, or clinical dehydration. Ask patients about their normal level of physical work and whether they engage in vigorous exercise in hot environments. Do the patients have fluid replacements containing salt available during exercise and activity?

Dietary Intake. Assess dietary intake of fluids; salt; and foods rich in potassium, calcium, and magnesium (see Table 42-4). Ask patients if they follow weight-loss diets. Starvation diets or those with high fat and no carbohydrate content often lead to metabolic acidosis (see Table 42-7). In addition, assess the patient's ability to chew and swallow, which, if altered, interferes with adequate intake of electrolyte-rich foods and fluids.

Lifestyle. Take an alcohol intake history. How many days does a person have an alcoholic drink each week, and how many drinks does he or she have at any one time? Chronic alcohol abuse commonly causes hypomagnesemia, in part because it increases renal magnesium excretion.

Medications. Obtain a complete list of your patient's current medications, including over-the-counter (OTC) and herbal preparations, to assess the risk for fluid, electrolyte, and acid-base imbalances (Box 42-3). Use a drug reference book or reputable online database to check the potential effects of other medications. Ask specifically about the use of baking soda as an antacid, which can cause ECV excess because of its high sodium content that holds water in the extracellular compartments. For an individual who uses laxatives, ask about the type of laxative, the frequency of use, and the consistency and frequency of stools. Multiple loose stools remove fluid and electrolytes from the body, thus causing numerous imbalances.

TABLE 42-9 Risk Factors for Fluid, Electrolyte, and Acid-Base Imbalances

Age	*Very young:* ECV deficit, osmolality imbalances, clinical dehydration *Very old:* ECV excess or deficit, osmolality imbalances
Environment	Sodium-rich diet: ECV excess Electrolyte-poor diet: Electrolyte deficits *Hot weather:* Clinical dehydration
Gastrointestinal output	*Diarrhea:* ECV deficit, clinical dehydration, hypokalemia, hypocalcemia (if chronic), hypomagnesemia (if chronic), metabolic acidosis *Drainage (e.g., nasogastric suctioning, fistulas):* ECV deficit, hypokalemia; metabolic acidosis if intestinal or pancreatic drainage *Vomiting:* ECV deficit, clinical dehydration, hypokalemia, hypomagnesemia, metabolic alkalosis
Chronic diseases	*Cancer:* Hypercalcemia; with tumor lysis syndrome: hyperkalemia, hypocalcemia, hyperphosphatemia; other imbalances, depending on side effects of therapy *Chronic obstructive pulmonary disease:* Respiratory acidosis *Cirrhosis:* ECV excess, hypokalemia *Heart failure:* ECV excess; other imbalances, depending on therapy *Oliguric renal disease:* ECV excess, hyperkalemia, hypermagnesemia, hyperphosphatemia, metabolic acidosis
Trauma	*Burns:* ECV deficit, metabolic acidosis Crush injuries: Hyperkalemia *Head injuries:* Hyponatremia or hypernatremia, depending on ADH response *Hemorrhage:* ECV deficit, hyperkalemia if circulatory shock
Therapies	Diuretics and other medications (see Box 42-3) *IV therapy:* ECV excess, osmolality imbalances, electrolyte excesses *PN:* Any fluid or electrolyte imbalance, depending on components of solution

ADH, Antidiuretic hormone; *ECV,* extracellular fluid volume; *IV,* intravenous; *PN,* parenteral nutrition.

Medical History

Recent Surgery. Surgery causes a physiological stress response, which increases with extensive surgery and blood loss. In the first 24 to 48 hours after surgery, increased secretion of aldosterone, glucocorticoids, and ADH cause increased ECV, decreased osmolality, and increased potassium excretion (Lewis et al., 2014). In otherwise healthy patients these imbalances resolve without difficulty, but patients who

BOX 42-1 Nursing Assessment Questions

Environment

- Do you work or exercise in a hot environment?
- If so, which type of fluid do you drink during that time?

Dietary Intake

- About how many glasses of fluids do you usually drink every day? Which type of fluids do you normally drink?
- Tell me what you usually eat in a day.
- Which snacks do you usually eat?
- Are you on a special diet because of a medical problem? How does that work for you?
- Are you following any weight loss program?
- Do you use a salt substitute?
- Do you take calcium, magnesium, or potassium supplements? If so, how often?
- Do you have any difficulties chewing or swallowing?

Lifestyle

- How much alcohol do you drink in a typical week?

Gastrointestinal Output

- Have you had recent vomiting or diarrhea? If so, for how long? How many times per day?

Medications and Other Therapies

- Which medicines/herbal remedies do you use regularly? Occasionally?
- Do you take diuretics? Drugs for high blood pressure?
- Do you use antacids? If so, which ones? How often? Do you ever use baking soda as an antacid? Do you use fizzy (effervescent) medications for colds?
- Do you use laxatives? If so, how often? Which type of stool do you get when you use them?
- What do you use for an upset stomach?

Signs and Symptoms

- If you weigh yourself every day, how has your weight changed over the past few days?
- Do you get light-headed when you stand up?
- Do you feel thirsty, have a dry mouth, or notice a lack of tears?
- Have you noticed a change in your urine output: decreased volume, dark color, or concentrated appearance?
- Are you experiencing swelling of your fingers, feet, or ankles?
- Do you have difficulty breathing when you lie down at night?
- Are you having difficulty concentrating, or do you feel confused? What is normal for you?
- Are you having more difficulty than usual standing up from a sofa or soft chair? Do your legs feel unusually heavy when you climb stairs? Do you have muscle weakness that is unusual for you?
- Have you noticed any muscle cramps or unusual sensations such as numbness or tingling fingers?

have preexisting illnesses or additional risk factors often need treatment during this time period.

Gastrointestinal Output. Increased output of fluid through the GI tract is a common and important cause of fluid, electrolyte, and acid-base imbalances that requires careful assessment. Vomiting and diarrhea, either acute or chronic, can cause ECV deficit, hypernatremia, clinical dehydration, and hypokalemia by increasing the output of fluid, Na^+, and K^+. In addition, chronic diarrhea can cause hypocalcemia and hypomagnesemia by decreasing electrolyte absorption. Removal of gastric acid from the body through vomiting or nasogastric suction

BOX 42-2 FOCUS ON OLDER ADULTS

Factors Affecting Fluid, Electrolyte, and Acid-Base Balance

- Body composition changes, causing a decreased percentage of body weight as water (50%), which increases risk of extracellular fluid volume (ECV) deficit and dehydration (Felver, 2013d).
- Some older adults restrict fluid intake because of impaired mobility or concerns about bladder control; this increases their risk of hypernatremia and ECV deficit.
- Decreased elasticity of skin alters skin turgor even with normal fluid balance; do not rely on skin turgor to assess ECV deficit or dehydration in older adults.
- Decreased thirst sensation increases risk of hypernatremia and dehydration; do not rely on thirst to assess hypernatremia, ECV deficit, or dehydration in older adults (Touhy and Jett, 2014).
- Baroreceptors become sluggish with age, often causing brief postural hypotension; have older adults arise slowly when you take orthostatic blood pressure measurements.
- Cardiovascular changes with aging often decrease the ability to adapt to a sudden increase in vascular volume, increasing risk of pulmonary edema with rapid infusion of isotonic intravenous fluids.
- Older-adult kidneys are less able to concentrate urine, making them less able to conserve fluid when needed; this increases the risk of hypernatremia, ECV deficit, and dehydration (Touhy and Jett, 2014).
- Kidney changes of normal aging make it more difficult to excrete a large acid load, increasing the risk of metabolic acidosis.
- Increased sensitivity to anticholinergic effects of medications causes dry mouth; use several different assessments for ECV deficit and dehydration rather than relying solely on dry mouth (Burchum and Rosenthal, 2016).
- The combined effects of normal aging, chronic diseases, and multiple medications often pose challenges to maintaining fluid and electrolyte balance.

BOX 42-3 Commonly Used Medications That Cause Fluid, Electrolyte, and Acid-Base Imbalances

- *ACE inhibitors (e.g., captopril [Capoten]) and angiotensin II receptor blockers (e.g., Losartan [Cozaar]):* Hyperkalemia
- *Antidepressants, SSRI (e.g., fluoxetine [Prozac]):* Hyponatremia
- *Calcium carbonate antacids:* Hypercalcemia, mild metabolic alkalosis
- *Corticosteroids (e.g., prednisone):* Hypokalemia, metabolic alkalosis
- *Diuretics, potassium-wasting (e.g., furosemide [Lasix], thiazides):* ECV deficit, hyponatremia (thiazides), hypokalemia, hypomagnesemia, mild metabolic alkalosis
- *Diuretics, potassium-sparing (e.g., spironolactone [Aldactone]):* Hyperkalemia, mild metabolic acidosis
- *Effervescent (fizzy) antacids and cold medications (high Na^+ content):* ECV excess
- *Laxatives:* ECV deficit, hypokalemia, hypocalcemia, hypomagnesemia, metabolic acidosis
- *Magnesium hydroxide (e.g., Milk of Magnesia):* Hypermagnesemia
- *Nonsteroidal antiinflammatory drugs (e.g., ibuprofen [Advil]):* Mild ECV excess, hyponatremia
- *Penicillins, high-dose (e.g., carbenicillin):* Hypokalemia, metabolic alkalosis; hyperkalemia with penicillin G (contains K^+)

Data from Burchum JR, Rosenthal LD: *Lehne's pharmacology for nursing care*, ed 9, St Louis, 2016, Elsevier.
ACE, Angiotensin-converting enzyme; *ECV*, extracellular fluid volume; *SSRI*, selective serotonin reuptake inhibitor.

can cause metabolic alkalosis. In contrast, removal of the bicarbonate-rich intestinal or pancreatic fluids through diarrhea, intestinal suction, or fistula can cause metabolic acidosis.

Acute Illness or Trauma. Acute conditions that place patients at high risk for fluid, electrolyte, and acid-base alterations include respiratory diseases, burns, trauma, GI alterations, and acute oliguric renal disease.

Respiratory Disorders. Many acute respiratory disorders predispose patients to respiratory acidosis. For example, bacterial pneumonia causes alveoli to fill with exudate that impairs gas exchange, causing the patient to retain carbon dioxide, which leads to increased $PaCO_2$ and respiratory acidosis.

Burns. Burns place patients at high risk for ECV deficit from numerous mechanisms, including plasma-to-interstitial fluid shift and increased evaporative and exudate output. The greater the body surface burned, the greater is the fluid loss (Lewis et al., 2014). Patients with burns have cellular damage that releases potassium into the blood, and they may become hyperkalemic. In addition, these patients often develop metabolic acidosis because of greatly increased cellular metabolism, which produces more metabolic acids than their kidneys are able to excrete.

Trauma. Hemorrhage from any type of trauma causes ECV deficit from blood loss. Some types of trauma create additional risks. For example, crush injuries destroy cellular structure, causing hyperkalemia by massive release of intracellular K^+ into the blood.

Head injury typically alters ADH secretion. It may cause diabetes insipidus (deficit of ADH), in which patients excrete large volumes of very dilute urine and develop hypernatremia. In contrast, head injury may cause the syndrome of inappropriate antidiuretic hormone (SIADH), in which excess secretion of ADH causes hyponatremia by retaining too much water and concentrating the urine (Lewis et al., 2014).

Chronic Illness. Many chronic diseases create ongoing risk of fluid, electrolyte, and acid-base imbalances. For example, type B chronic obstructive pulmonary disease (COPD) often causes chronic respiratory acidosis. In addition, the treatment regimens for chronic disease often cause imbalances. Assess patients for the presence of these conditions.

Cancer. The specific fluid and electrolyte imbalances that occur with cancer depend on the type and progression of the cancer and treatment regimen. Many patients with cancer develop hypercalcemia when their cancer cells secrete chemicals that circulate to bones and cause calcium to enter the blood. Other fluid and electrolyte imbalances occur in cancer because some types of tumors cause metabolic and endocrine abnormalities. In addition, patients with cancer are at risk for fluid and electrolyte imbalances as a result of the side effects (e.g., anorexia, diarrhea) of chemotherapy, biological response modifiers, or radiation (Lewis et al., 2014).

Heart Failure. Patients who have chronic heart failure have diminished cardiac output, which reduces kidney perfusion and activates the RAAS. The action of aldosterone on the kidneys causes ECV excess and risk of hypokalemia. Most diuretics used to treat heart failure increase the risk of hypokalemia while reducing the ECV excess. Dietary sodium restriction is important with heart failure because Na^+ holds water in the ECF, making the ECV excess worse. In severe heart failure restriction of both fluid and sodium is prescribed to decrease the workload of the heart by reducing excess circulating fluid volume (Lewis et al., 2014).

Oliguric Renal Disease. Oliguria occurs when the kidneys have a reduced capacity to make urine. Some conditions such as acute nephritis cause sudden onset of oliguria, whereas other problems such as chronic kidney disease lead to chronic oliguria. Oliguric renal disease prevents normal excretion of fluid, electrolytes, and metabolic acids, resulting in ECV excess, hyperkalemia, hypermagnesemia, hyperphosphatemia, and metabolic acidosis. The severity of these imbalances is proportional to the degree of renal failure. Although chronic kidney disease is progressive, successful management of imbalances is possible with dietary restriction of sodium and other electrolytes, fluid restriction in severe cases, and eventually dialysis or renal transplant (Lewis et al., 2014).

Physical Assessment. Data gathered through a focused physical assessment validates and extends the information collected in the patient history. Table 42-10 summarizes focused assessments for patients with fluid, electrolyte, and acid-base imbalances. Focus your assessment on the areas pertinent to each patient situation. For example, for patients at risk of fluid imbalances, focus your assessment on body weight changes, clinical markers of vascular and interstitial volume, thirst, behavior changes, and level of consciousness. Additional focused assessments for patients at high risk of electrolyte and acid-base imbalances include specific cardiac, respiratory, neuromuscular, and GI markers. Grouping your assessments under these categories helps you know which assessments to prioritize and enables you to assess effectively.

Daily Weights and Fluid Intake and Output Measurement. Daily weights are an important indicator of fluid status (Felver, 2013c). Each kilogram (2.2 lbs) of weight gained or lost overnight is equal to 1 L of fluid retained or lost. These fluid gains or losses indicate changes in the amount of total body fluid, usually ECF, but do not indicate shift between body compartments. Weigh patients with heart failure and those who are at high risk for or actually have ECV excess daily. Daily weights are also useful for patients with clinical dehydration or other causes or risks for ECV deficit. Weigh the patient at the same time each day with the same scale after a patient voids. Calibrate the scale each day or routinely. The patient needs to wear the same clothes or clothes that weigh the same; if using a bed scale, use the same number of sheets on the scale with each weighing. Compare the weight of each day with that of the previous day to determine fluid gains or losses. Look at the weights over several days to recognize trends. Interpretation of daily weights guides medical therapy and nursing care. Teach patients with heart failure to take and record their daily weights at home and to contact their health care provider if their weight increases suddenly by a set amount (obtain parameters from their health care providers). Recognizing trends in daily weights taken at home is important. Patients who are hospitalized for decompensated heart failure often experience steady increases in daily weights during the week before hospitalization.

Measuring and recording all liquid intake and output (I&O) during a 24-hour period is an important aspect of fluid balance assessment. Compare a patient's 24-hour intake with his or her 24-hour output. The two measures should be approximately equal if the person has normal fluid balance (Felver, 2013c). To interpret situations in which I&O are substantially different, consider the individual patient. For example, if intake is substantially greater than output, there are two possibilities: the patient may be gaining excessive fluid or returning to normal fluid status by replacing fluid lost previously from the body. Similarly, if intake is substantially smaller than output, there are also two possibilities: the patient may be losing needed fluid from the body and developing ECV deficit and/or hypernatremia or returning to normal fluid status by excreting excessive fluid gained previously.

In most health care settings I&O measurement is a nursing assessment. Some agencies require a health care provider's order for I&O. If you want to measure I&O for a patient with compromised fluid status,

TABLE 42-10 Focused Nursing Assessments for Patients with Fluid, Electrolyte, and Acid-Base Imbalances

Assessment	Imbalances
Body Weight Changes from Previous Day	
Loss of 2.2 lbs (1 kg) or more in 24 hours for adults	ECV deficit
Gain of 2.2 lbs (1 kg) or more in 24 hours for adults	ECV excess
Clinical Markers of Vascular Volume	
Blood pressure:	
Hypotension or orthostatic hypotension	ECV deficit
Light-headedness on sitting upright or standing	ECV deficit
Pulse rate and character:	
Rapid, thready	ECV deficit
Bounding	ECV excess
Fullness of neck veins:	
Flat or collapsing with inhalation when supine	ECV deficit
Full or distended when upright or semi-upright	ECV excess
Other assessments of vascular volume:	
Capillary refill: Sluggish	ECV deficit
Lung auscultation, dependent lobe: Crackles or rhonchi with progressive dyspnea	ECV excess
Urine output: Small volume of dark yellow urine	ECV deficit
Clinical Markers of Interstitial Volume	
Presence of edema: Present in dependent areas (ankles or sacrum) and possibly fingers or around eyes	ECV excess
Mucous membranes: Dry between cheek and gum, decreased or absent tearing	ECV deficit
Skin turgor: Pinched skin fails to return to normal position within 3 seconds	ECV deficit
Presence of thirst: Thirst present	Hypernatremia, severe ECV deficit
Behavior and level of consciousness	
Restlessness and mild confusion	Severe ECV deficit
Decreased level of consciousness (lethargy, confusion, coma)	Hyponatremia, hypernatremia, hypercalcemia, acid-base imbalances
Cardiac and Respiratory Signs of Electrolyte or Acid-Base Imbalances	
Pulse rhythm and ECG: Irregular pulse and ECG changes	K^+, Ca^{2+}, Mg^{2+}, and/or acid-base imbalances
Rate and depth of respirations:	
Increased rate and depth	Metabolic acidosis (compensatory mechanism); respiratory alkalosis (cause)
Decreased rate and depth	Metabolic alkalosis (compensatory mechanism); respiratory acidosis (cause)
Neuromuscular Markers of Electrolyte or Acid-Base Imbalances	
Muscle strength bilaterally, especially quadriceps muscles:	
Muscle weakness	Hypokalemia, hyperkalemia
Reflexes and sensations:	
Decreased deep tendon reflexes	Hypercalcemia, hypermagnesemia
Hyperactive reflexes, muscle twitching and cramps, tetany	Hypocalcemia, hypomagnesemia
Numbness, tingling in fingertips, around mouth	Hypocalcemia, hypomagnesemia, respiratory alkalosis
Muscle cramps, tetany	Hypocalcemia, hypomagnesemia, respiratory alkalosis
Tremors	Hypomagnesemia
Gastrointestinal Signs of Electrolyte Imbalances	
Inspection and auscultation:	
Abdominal distention	Hypokalemia, third-spacing of fluid
Decreased bowel sounds	Hypokalemia
Motility: Constipation	Hypokalemia, hypercalcemia

ECG, Electrocardiogram; *ECV*, extracellular fluid volume.

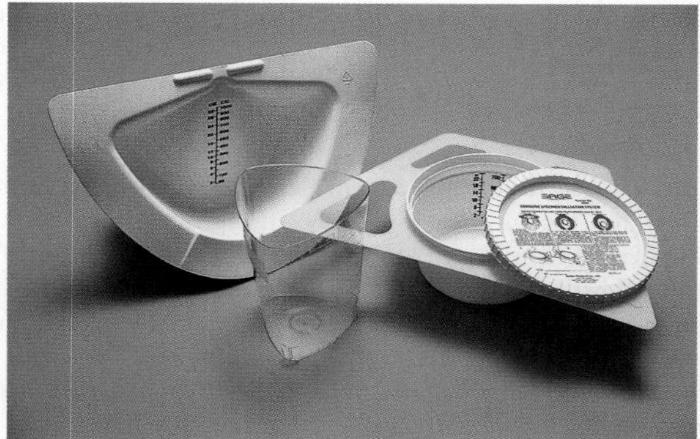

FIGURE 42-10 Containers for measuring urine output.

check your agency policies to determine whether you can set it up or if you need a health care provider's order.

Fluid intake includes all liquids that a person eats (e.g., gelatin, ice cream, soup), drinks, (e.g., water, coffee, juice), or receives through nasogastric or jejunostomy feeding tubes (see Chapter 45). IV fluids (continuous infusions and intermittent IV piggybacks) and blood components also are sources of intake. Water swallowed while taking pills and liquid medications counts as intake. A patient receiving tube feedings often receives numerous liquid medications, and water is used to flush the tube before and/or after medications. Over a 24-hour period these liquids amount to significant intake and always are recorded on the I&O record. Ask patients who are alert and oriented to help with measuring their oral intake and explain to families why they should not drink or eat from the patient's meal trays or water pitcher.

Fluid output includes urine, diarrhea, vomitus, gastric suction, and drainage from postsurgical wounds or other tubes (see Chapter 50). Record a patient's urinary output after each voiding. Instruct patients who are alert, oriented, and ambulatory to save their urine in a calibrated insert, which attaches to the rim of the toilet bowl (Figure 42-10). Teach patients and families the purpose of I&O measurements. Also teach them to notify the nurse or nursing assistive personnel (NAP) to empty any container with voided fluid or how to measure and empty the container themselves and report the result appropriately. Patients need to have good vision and motor skills to perform these measurements. Active involvement of patient and family is an aspect of patient-centered care that is essential to maintaining accurate I&O measurements. When a patient has an indwelling urinary catheter, drainage tube, or suction, record output (e.g., at the end of each nursing shift or every hour) as the patient's condition requires.

You can delegate parts of I&O measurement and recording to NAP with competent skills in measurement. Actual measurement of fluid volumes is more accurate than visual estimates. In many institutions NAP record oral intake but not intake through feeding or IV tubes, which are nursing responsibilities. Similarly NAP often record urine, diarrhea, and vomitus output but not drainage through tubes. The responsible registered nurse (RN) or licensed practical nurse/licensed vocational nurse (LPN/LVN) and the NAP work as a team to record measurements in the designated location in the electronic health record (EHR), often on a flow sheet with other information. The EHR program usually calculates the 24-hour totals. If an EHR is not used, record I&O on paper forms attached to the bedside chart or room door. You or the NAP calculates the 24-hour totals (see agency policy). Accurate I&O facilitates ongoing evaluation of a patient's hydration status.

BOX 42-4 Nursing Diagnostic Process

Deficient Fluid Volume Related to Loss of Gastrointestinal Fluids via Vomiting

Assessment Activities	Defining Characteristics
Assess postural blood pressure and pulse.	Patient has postural hypotension with increased heart rate; pulse is weak.
Inspect oral mucous membranes for degree of moisture.	Oral mucous membranes between cheek and gum are dry.
Obtain daily weight measurements.	Adult patient loses 2.2 lbs (1 kg) or more in 24 hours.
Measure urine output and observe color; if available, measure specific gravity of urine.	Patient produces small volume of dark yellow urine; urine specific gravity is increased.
Test skin turgor (not reliable for older adults).	Decreased skin turgor noted.

Laboratory Values. Review the patient's laboratory test results and compare them with the normal ranges to obtain further objective data about fluid, electrolyte, and acid-base balances. Normal and abnormal test results are summarized in Tables 42-1, 42-3, and 42-5 to 42-7. The frequency of electrolyte level measurements depends on the severity of a patient's illness. Analysis of laboratory results requires a good medical clinician, especially if a person develops an acute imbalance while also having a chronic disease. Serum electrolyte tests usually are performed routinely on patients entering a hospital to screen for imbalances and serve as a baseline for future comparisons.

◆ Nursing Diagnosis

When caring for patients with suspected fluid, electrolyte, and acid-base imbalances, it is particularly important to use critical thinking to formulate nursing diagnoses. The assessment data that establish the risk for or the actual presence of a nursing diagnosis in these areas may be subtle, and patterns and trends emerge only when there has been astute assessment. Multiple body systems often are involved; careful clustering of defining characteristics leads to selection of the appropriate diagnoses (Box 42-4).

In addition to the accurate clustering of assessment data, an important part of formulating nursing diagnoses is identifying the relevant causative or related factor (when a diagnosis is problem focused) or risk factors (when a diagnosis is a risk diagnosis). You choose interventions that treat or modify the related factor for the diagnosis to be resolved. For example, *Deficient Fluid Volume related to loss of GI fluids from vomiting* requires therapies that manage the patients' emesis and restore fluid volume with IV therapy. In contrast, the diagnosis of *Deficient Fluid Volume related to elevated body temperature* requires therapies to lower the patient's body temperature and replace lost body fluids through oral fluid replacement or possibly IV therapy. Possible nursing diagnoses for patients with fluid, electrolyte, and acid-base alterations include the following:

- *Decreased Cardiac Output*
- *Acute Confusion*
- *Risk for Electrolyte Imbalance*
- *Deficient Fluid Volume*
- *Excess Fluid Volume*
- *Impaired Gas Exchange*
- *Risk for Injury*
- *Deficient Knowledge Regarding Disease Management*

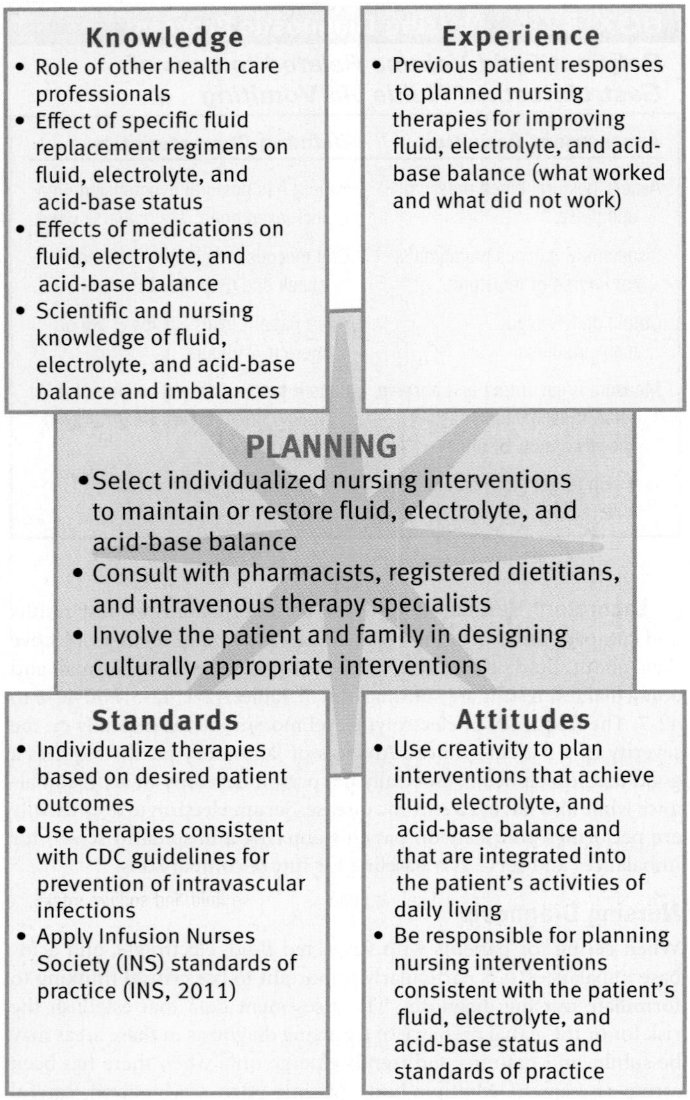

Knowledge
- Role of other health care professionals
- Effect of specific fluid replacement regimens on fluid, electrolyte, and acid-base status
- Effects of medications on fluid, electrolyte, and acid-base balance
- Scientific and nursing knowledge of fluid, electrolyte, and acid-base balance and imbalances

Experience
- Previous patient responses to planned nursing therapies for improving fluid, electrolyte, and acid-base balance (what worked and what did not work)

PLANNING
- Select individualized nursing interventions to maintain or restore fluid, electrolyte, and acid-base balance
- Consult with pharmacists, registered dietitians, and intravenous therapy specialists
- Involve the patient and family in designing culturally appropriate interventions

Standards
- Individualize therapies based on desired patient outcomes
- Use therapies consistent with CDC guidelines for prevention of intravascular infections
- Apply Infusion Nurses Society (INS) standards of practice (INS, 2011)

Attitudes
- Use creativity to plan interventions that achieve fluid, electrolyte, and acid-base balance and that are integrated into the patient's activities of daily living
- Be responsible for planning nursing interventions consistent with the patient's fluid, electrolyte, and acid-base status and standards of practice

FIGURE 42-11 Critical thinking model for fluid, electrolyte, and acid-base balance planning. *CDC,* Centers for Disease Control and Prevention.

◆ Planning

During the planning process use critical thinking to synthesize information from multiple resources (Figure 42-11). Ensure that the patient's plan of care integrates both scientific and nursing knowledge and all of the information that you collected about the individual patient.

Goals and Outcomes. Establish an individual patient plan of care for each nursing diagnosis (see the Nursing Care Plan) that includes mutually established patient goals for each diagnosis. Collaborate with and inform patients as you individualize goals with realistic, measurable outcomes. For example, with a nursing diagnosis of *Deficient Fluid Volume,* the following related outcomes might be established for the goal, "The patient achieves normal hydration status at discharge":

- The patient is free of complications associated with the IV device throughout the duration of IV therapy.
- The patient demonstrates balanced I&O measurements within 48 hours.
- The patient has serum electrolytes within the normal range within 48 hours.

Setting Priorities. The patient's clinical condition determines which of the nursing diagnoses takes the greatest priority. Many nursing diagnoses in the area of fluid, electrolyte, and acid-base balances are of highest priority because the consequences for the patient can be serious or even life threatening. For example, in the concept map (Figure 42-12) for Mrs. Beck, the occurrence of vomiting and diarrhea created a high-priority nursing diagnosis of *Deficient Fluid Volume.* The priority for Mrs. Beck is to restore her fluid balance. To achieve this priority, her vomiting and diarrhea must be controlled and resolved, and her fluid volume replaced. If these goals are unmet, Mrs. Beck's fluid imbalance likely will worsen.

Teamwork and Collaboration. Consultation with a patient's health care provider helps to set realistic time frames for the goals of care, particularly when the patient's physiological status is unstable. Ongoing communication and consultation are important because the patient's condition can change quickly. Collaboration with the patient and family and other members of the interprofessional health care team such as IV therapist and pharmacist helps in achieving patient outcomes. Patient and family are very helpful in identifying approaches for successful therapies such as ways to increase fluid intake. Incorporate patient preferences and resources into the plan of care. Do not delegate administration of IV fluid and hemodynamic assessment to NAP. When the patient is stable, you can delegate daily weights, I&O, and direct physical care to NAP.

Begin discharge planning early for patients with acute or chronic fluid and electrolyte disturbances by anticipating the needs of the patient and family as they transition to another setting. In the hospital collaboration with other members of the health care team ensures that care will continue in the home or long-term care setting with few disruptions. You ensure that therapeutic regimens established in one setting continue through completion at the next setting. For example, for a patient who is discharged on IV therapy, you assess the knowledge and skills of the family member or friend who is to assume caregiving responsibilities and initiate a referral to home IV therapy as soon as possible. Close collaboration with members of the health care team such as the patient's health care provider, registered dietitian, and pharmacist is essential to ensure positive patient outcomes. A registered dietitian is a valuable resource in recommending food sources to increase or reduce intake of specific electrolytes, incorporating the patient's preferences when possible (see Chapter 45). A pharmacist helps identify medications or combinations of medications likely to cause electrolyte or acid-base disturbances and offers information regarding patient education about side effects to anticipate for prescribed drugs. The patient's health care provider directs the treatment of fluid, electrolyte, or acid-base imbalances.

◆ Implementation

Health Promotion. Health promotion activities focus primarily on patient education on the basis of your assessment of patient and family health literacy. Use plain language to teach patients and caregivers to recognize risk factors for developing imbalances and implement appropriate preventive measures. For example, parents of infants need to understand that GI losses quickly lead to serious imbalances; therefore, when vomiting or diarrhea occurs in an infant, they need to promptly rehydrate with sodium-containing fluid or seek health care

NURSING CARE PLAN

Deficient Fluid Volume

ASSESSMENT

Mrs. Hilda Beck is a 72-year-old seen by her health care provider this morning after falling at home and telephoning a neighbor for assistance. She lives alone in an apartment and has no chronic disease except for osteoarthritis of her hands. She has had diarrhea and vomiting for over 24 hours and has not eaten anything. Despite feeling slightly nauseated, she tried to drink a little water, because she knew she needed fluid. Mrs. Beck is admitted for intravenous (IV) fluid therapy. X-ray films indicate that she has no broken bones. Review of laboratory findings: hematocrit 55% (hemoconcentration caused by hypovolemia); sodium 148 mEq/L, and potassium 3 mEq/L. (NOTE: Mrs. Beck has hypokalemia in addition to extracellular fluid volume [ECV] deficit and hypernatremia [clinical dehydration].)

Assessment Activities	*Findings/Defining Characteristics**
Ask Mrs. Beck to describe when her vomiting and diarrhea began and any accompanying signs and symptoms.	She states that her gastrointestinal (GI) problems began suddenly yesterday and that she **gets weak and light-headed when she stands or sits upright,** which is why she fell. She feels **weak** and has a **dry mouth.**
Ask her about current status of vomiting and diarrhea.	Says she still was vomiting earlier this morning. Has not done so for the past 3 hours. Feels slightly nauseated. Had three episodes of watery diarrhea this morning and more than six yesterday.
Assess Mrs. Beck's vital signs.	**Heart rate 110** beats/min with regular rhythm and a **weak pulse; supine blood pressure (BP) is 90/58.** Temperature and respirations within normal limits. Postural BP measurement not taken since patient says that she **gets light-headed when she sits upright.**
Evaluate physical signs of extracellular fluid volume (ECV).	Neck veins flat when she is supine; **100 mL of dark yellow urine** in past 4 hours; dry mucous membranes between cheek and gum; prolonged capillary refill time of 5 seconds.
Weigh Mrs. Beck using a bed scale.	Weight 120 lbs (54.5 kg). States usual weight at home is 127 lbs (46.27 kg) **(7 lbs [3.17 kg] weight loss).**

***Defining characteristics** are shown in bold type.

NURSING DIAGNOSIS: Deficient fluid volume related to increased output of GI fluids from vomiting and diarrhea

PLANNING

Goals	*Expected Outcomes (NOC)*[†]
Fluid Balance	
Mrs. Beck's fluid volume will return to normal by hospital discharge.	Heart rate and BP return to normal within 24 hours. Mrs. Beck does not report light-headedness when sitting or standing within 24 hours. Urine color becomes light yellow within 24 hours. Daily urine output equals intake of at least 1500 mL by discharge.
Mrs. Beck will describe how to manage fluid balance at home before hospital discharge.	Mrs. Beck describes how to replace GI fluid loss with fluids that contain sodium. She describes signs and symptoms indicating need to increase fluid and sodium intake.

[†]Outcome classification labels from Moorhead S et al: *Nursing outcomes classification (NOC)*, ed 5, St Louis, 2013, Mosby.

INTERVENTIONS[‡] (NIC)	RATIONALE
Fluid/Electrolyte Management	
Provide Mrs. Beck her favorite fluids at her preferred temperature.	Patient-centered care takes individual preferences into account. Offer cultural preferences regarding temperature of oral fluid influence fluid intake (Giger, 2013). In contrast to popular belief, moderate amounts of caffeinated beverages are not likely to have excessive diuretic effect (Killer et al., 2014).
Provide pitcher and glass of water at Mrs. Beck's preferred temperature at her bedside; ensure that she can access and pour from it easily; provide straw if she wishes.	Weakness or chronic disease such as osteoarthritis of hands may make it difficult to manipulate a full water pitcher. Make fluid available in form that is easy for patient to access (Felver, 2013c).
Administer IV therapy as prescribed, monitoring closely for early side effects of complications.	IV fluid replacement augments oral replacement when ECV deficit exists. Age-appropriate care is needed because of older adult's anatomical and physiological changes that affect volume delivery (INS, 2011).
Discuss different ways to prevent and treat dehydration at home. Provide written handout of information.	Patient education is enhanced in older adults when you use multiple senses during teaching sessions (Touhy and Jett, 2014).

[‡]Intervention classification labels from Bulechek GM et al.: *Nursing interventions classification (NIC)*, ed 6, St Louis, 2013, Mosby.

EVALUATION

Nursing Actions	*Patient Response/Finding*	*Achievement of Outcome*
Monitor vital signs, intake and output (I&O), daily weight, and postural BP when no longer light-headed.	T 37° C (98.6° F), RR 10, HR 72 beats/min, BP 120/78 sitting, 122/78 standing, denies light-headedness Intake 2000 mL, output 2000 mL of light yellow urine Today's weight 129 lbs (58.5 kg)	Vital signs returned to normal range. No postural hypotension. I&O measurements are balanced, urine is light yellow. Daily weight returned to Mrs. Beck's normal.
Assess neck vein fullness when supine, mucous membranes.	Neck veins full when supine; mucous membranes moist	Additional markers of ECV are normal.
Evaluate effectiveness of teaching regarding maintaining fluid balance at home.	Mrs. Beck identified salty broth and commercial electrolyte replacement fluids for replacing GI fluid loss and indicated need to increase her intake if her urine becomes dark yellow or she becomes light-headed when sitting upright.	Mrs. Beck describes effective home management of fluid balance.

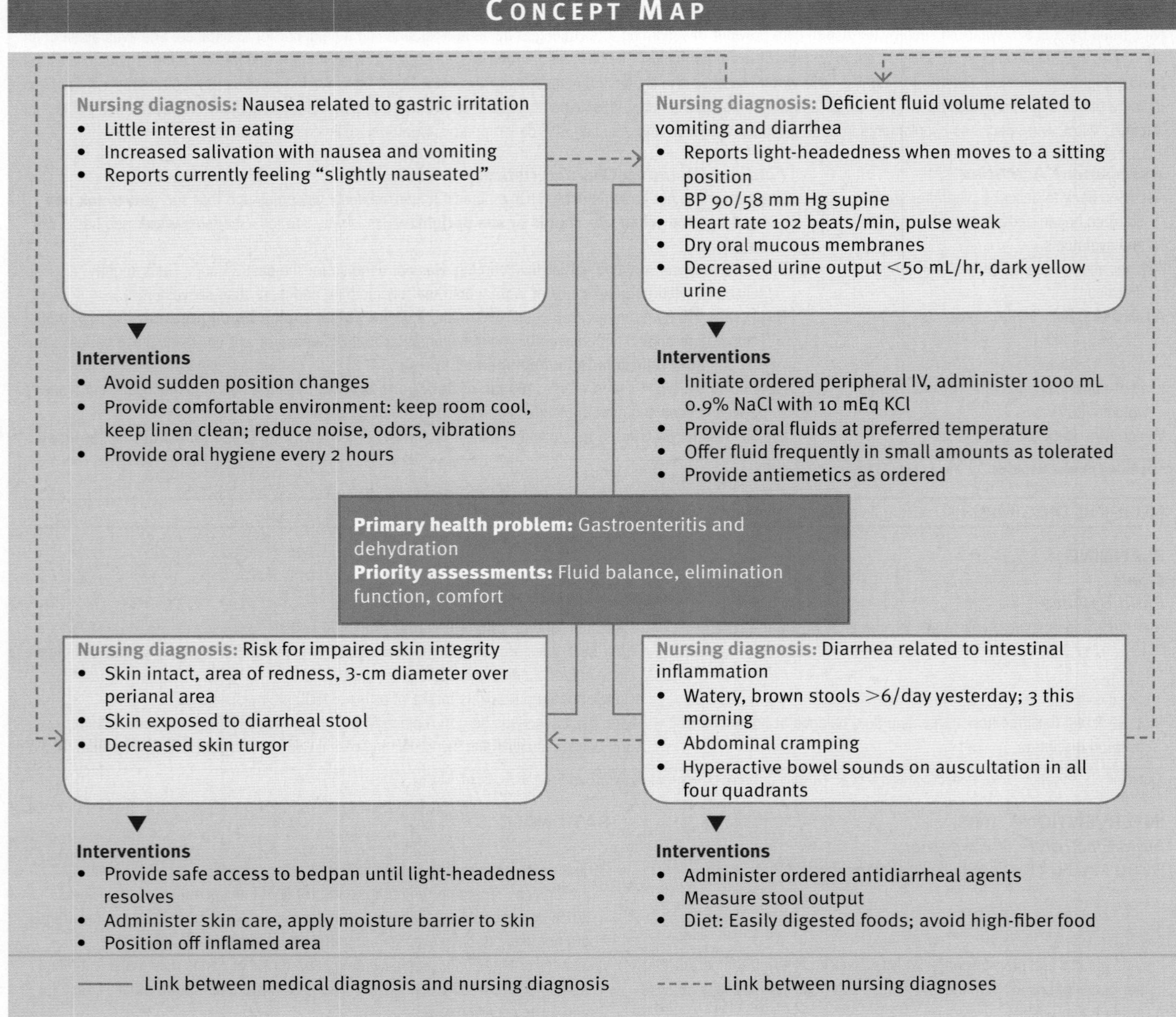

FIGURE 42-12 Concept map for Mrs. Beck.

to restore normal balance. People of any age need to learn to replace body fluid losses with sodium-containing fluid and water.

Patients with chronic health alterations often are at risk for developing fluid, electrolyte, and acid-base imbalances. They need to understand their own risk factors and the measures to be taken to avoid imbalances. For example, patients with end-stage renal disease often need to restrict intake of fluid, sodium, potassium, magnesium, and phosphate. Through diet education these patients learn the types of foods to avoid and the suitable volume of fluid that they are permitted daily (see Chapter 45). Teach patients with chronic diseases and their family caregivers the early signs and symptoms of the fluid, electrolyte, and acid-base imbalances for which they are at risk and what to do if these occur.

Acute Care. Although fluid, electrolyte, and/or acid-base imbalances occur in all settings, they are common in acute care. Acute care

BOX 42-5 CULTURAL ASPECTS OF CARE

Fluid Therapy

Cultural and religious beliefs influence how you manage fluid therapy and how patients communicate their needs. For example, a family elder may be the person who receives explanations and makes health care decisions rather than the patient. A person's cultural and religious beliefs may cause refusal of therapies. For example, hot-cold beliefs often cause patients to refuse cold oral fluids when they have certain illnesses because they believe that hot fluids are needed to restore balance (Giger, 2013). Religious practices may require modifications of intravenous (IV) tubing length (e.g., when patients need to kneel on the floor and pray several times daily).

Implications for Patient-Centered Care

- Establish communication. If appropriate, determine who makes decisions for the patient and explain fluid restriction or IV therapy procedures.
- Elicit patient/family values and preferences in your clinical interview. Ask specifically about preferred temperature of oral fluids and provide (if oral intake is allowed).
- Determine needed length of IV tubing and incorporate one or more segments of long extension tubing into the IV setup if patient kneels on the floor to pray.
- Determine acceptance of or abstinence from therapeutic regimens and respect patients/family choices regarding therapy.
- Know patient's beliefs regarding blood therapy. Although some patients refuse whole blood or packed red blood cells because of religious or personal beliefs, they may accept other blood products or alternatives.
- When the patient has dark-colored skin, assess carefully for subtle color changes at vascular access device site that might indicate phlebitis, which may be more difficult to recognize.

nurses administer medications and oral and IV fluids to replace fluid and electrolyte deficits or maintain normal homeostasis; they also help with restricting intake as part of therapy for excesses.

Enteral Replacement of Fluids. Oral replacement of fluids and electrolytes is appropriate as long as the patient is not so physiologically unstable that they cannot be replaced rapidly. Oral replacement of fluids is contraindicated when a patient has a mechanical obstruction of the GI tract, is at high risk for aspiration, or has impaired swallowing. Some patients unable to tolerate solid foods are still able to ingest fluids. Strategies to encourage fluid intake include offering frequent small sips of fluid, popsicles, and ice chips. Record one half the volume of the ice chips in I&O measurement. For example, if a patient ingests 240 mL of ice chips, you record 120 mL of intake. Encourage patients to keep their own record of intake to involve them actively. Family members who are properly instructed can also help. Pay attention to each patient's preferred temperature of oral fluids. Cultural beliefs regarding appropriate fluids and fluid temperature may become a barrier to achieving adequate fluid intake unless the fluid with the preferred temperature is available (Box 42-5).

When replacing fluids by mouth in a patient with ECV deficit, choose fluids that contain sodium (e.g., Pedialyte and Gastrolyte). Liquids that contain lactose or have low-sodium content are not appropriate when a patient has diarrhea.

A feeding tube is appropriate when a patient's GI tract is healthy but he or she cannot ingest fluids (e.g., after oral surgery or with impaired swallowing). Options for administering fluids include gastrostomy or jejunostomy instillations or infusions through small-bore nasogastric feeding tubes (see Chapter 45).

Restriction of Fluids. Patients who have hyponatremia usually require restricted water intake. Patients who have very severe ECV

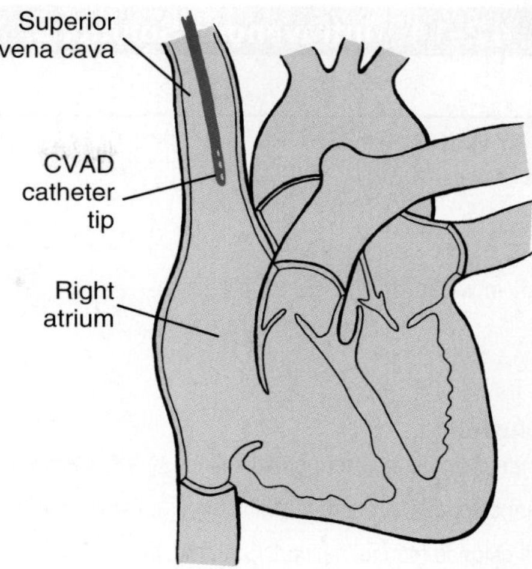

FIGURE 42-13 Central venous lines deliver intravenous fluid into superior vena cava near heart. *CVAD,* Central venous access device.

excess sometimes have both sodium and fluid restrictions. Fluid restriction often is difficult for patients, particularly if they take medications that dry the oral mucous membranes or if they are mouth breathers. Explain the reason that fluids are restricted. Make sure that the patient, family, and visitors know the amount of fluid permitted orally and understand that ice chips, gelatin, and ice cream are fluids. Help the patient decide the amount of fluid to drink with each meal, between meals, before bed, and with medications. It is important to allow patients to choose preferred fluids unless contraindicated. Frequently patients on fluid restriction can swallow a number of pills with as little as 1 oz (30 mL) of liquid.

In acute care settings fluid restrictions usually allot half the total oral fluids between 7 AM and 3 PM (i.e., the period when patients are more active, receive two meals, and take most of their oral medications). Offer the remainder of the fluids during the evening and night shifts. Patients on fluid restriction need frequent mouth care to moisten mucous membranes, decrease the chance of mucosal drying and cracking, and maintain comfort (see Chapter 40).

Parenteral Replacement of Fluids and Electrolytes. Fluid and electrolytes may be replaced through infusion of fluids directly into veins (intravenously) rather than via the digestive system. Parenteral replacement includes parenteral nutrition (PN), IV fluid and electrolyte therapy (**crystalloids**), and blood and blood component (colloids) administration. IV devices are called *peripheral IVs* when the catheter tip lies in a vein in one of the extremities; they are called *central venous IVs* when the catheter tip lies in the central circulatory system (e.g., in the vena cava close to the right atrium of the heart) (Figure 42-13).

Practice standard body fluid precautions when preparing and administering parenteral fluids (see Chapter 29) to minimize your own risk for exposure to bloodborne pathogens. Read and understand the policy and procedures for parenteral infusions at the agency for which you work.

Parenteral Nutrition. PN, also called *total PN (TPN),* is IV administration of a complex, highly concentrated solution containing nutrients and electrolytes that is formulated to meet a patient's needs. Depending on their osmolality, PN solutions are administered through a central IV catheter (high osmolality) or peripherally (lower osmolality). Chapter 45 reviews principles and guidelines for PN administration, which is used when patients are unable to receive enough nutrition orally or through enteral feeding.

Intravenous Therapy (Crystalloids). The goal of IV fluid administration is to correct or prevent fluid and electrolyte disturbances. It

TABLE 42-11 Intravenous Solutions

Solution	Concentration	Comments
Dextrose in Water Solutions		**Dextrose is another name for glucose.**
Dextrose 5% in water (D_5W)	Isotonic	Isotonic when first enters vein; dextrose enters cells rapidly, leaving free water, which dilutes ECF; most of water then enters cells by osmosis.
Dextrose 10% in water ($D_{10}W$)	Hypertonic	Hypertonic when first enters vein, dextrose enters cells rapidly, leaving free water, which dilutes ECF; most of water then enters cells by osmosis.
Saline Solutions		**Saline is sodium chloride in water.**
0.225% sodium chloride (quarter normal saline; ¼ NS; 0.225% NaCl)	Hypotonic	Expands ECV (vascular and interstitial) and rehydrates cells.
0.45% sodium chloride (half normal saline; ½ NS; 0.45% NaCl)	Hypotonic	Expands ECV (vascular and interstitial) and rehydrates cells.
0.9% sodium chloride (normal saline; NS; 0.9% NaCl)	Isotonic	Expands ECV (vascular and interstitial); does not enter cells.
3% or 5% sodium chloride (hypertonic saline; 3% or 5% NaCl)	Hypertonic	Draws water from cells into ECF by osmosis.
Dextrose in Saline Solutions		
Dextrose 5% in 0.45% NaCl sodium chloride (D_5 ½ NS; $D_5$0.45% NaCl)	Hypertonic	Dextrose enters cells rapidly, leaving 0.45% sodium chloride.
Dextrose 5% in 0.9% sodium chloride (D_5NS; $D_5$0.9% NaCl)	Hypertonic	Dextrose enters cells rapidly, leaving 0.9% sodium chloride.
Balanced Electrolyte Solutions		
Lactated Ringer's (LR)	Isotonic	Contains Na^+, K^+, Ca^{2+}, Cl^-, and lactate, which liver metabolizes to HCO_3^-. Expands ECV (vascular and interstitial); does not enter cells.
Dextrose 5% in lactated Ringer's (D_5LR)	Hypertonic	Dextrose enters cells rapidly, leaving lactated Ringer's.

ECF, Extracellular fluid; *ECV,* extracellular fluid volume.

allows for direct access to the vascular system, permitting the continuous infusion of fluids over a period of time. IV therapy requires a health care provider's order for type, amount, and speed of administration of the solution. You regulate IV fluid therapy continuously because of ongoing changes in a patient's fluid and electrolyte balance. To provide safe and appropriate therapy to patients who require IV fluids, you need knowledge of the correct ordered solution, the reason the solution was ordered, the equipment needed, the procedures required to initiate an infusion, how to regulate the infusion rate and maintain the system, how to identify and correct problems, and how to discontinue the infusion.

Types of Solutions. Many prepared IV solutions are available for use (Table 42-11). An IV solution is isotonic, hypotonic, or hypertonic. Isotonic solutions have the same effective osmolality as body fluids. Sodium-containing isotonic solutions such as normal saline are indicated for ECV replacement to prevent or treat ECV deficit. Hypotonic solutions have an effective osmolality less than body fluids, thus decreasing osmolality by diluting body fluids and moving water into cells. Hypertonic solutions have an effective osmolality greater than body fluids. If they are hypertonic sodium-containing solutions, they increase osmolality rapidly and pull water out of cells, causing them to shrivel (Wunderlich, 2013). The decision to use a hypotonic or hypertonic solution is made on the basis of a patient's specific fluid and electrolyte imbalance. For example, a patient with hypernatremia that cannot be treated with oral water generally receives a hypotonic IV solution to dilute the ECF and rehydrate cells. Too-rapid or excessive infusion of any IV fluid has the potential to cause serious patient problems.

Additives such as potassium chloride (KCl) are common in IV solutions (e.g., 1000 mL D_5 ½ NS with 20 mEq KCl at 125 mL/hr). Administer KCl carefully because hyperkalemia can cause fatal cardiac dysrhythmias. *Under no circumstances should KCl be administered by IV push* (directly through a port in IV tubing). Verify that a patient has adequate kidney function and urine output before administering an IV solution containing potassium. Patients with normal renal function who are receiving nothing by mouth should have potassium added to IV solutions. The body cannot conserve potassium, and the kidneys continue to excrete it even when the plasma level falls. Without potassium intake, hypokalemia develops quickly.

Vascular Access Devices. Vascular access devices (VADs) are catheters or infusion ports designed for repeated access to the vascular system. Peripheral catheters are for short-term use (e.g., fluid restoration after surgery and short-term antibiotic administration). Devices for long-term use include central catheters and implanted ports, which empty into a central vein. Remember that the term *central* applies to the location of the catheter tip, not to the insertion site. Peripherally inserted central catheters (PICC lines) enter a peripheral arm vein and extend through the venous system to the superior vena cava where they terminate. Other central lines enter a central vein such as the subclavian or jugular vein or are tunneled through subcutaneous tissue before entering a central vein. Central lines are more effective than peripheral catheters for administering large volumes of fluid, PN, and medications or fluids that irritate veins. Proper care of central line insertion sites is critical for the prevention of central line–associated bloodstream infection (CLABSI). The National Quality Forum (NQF) (2015) emphasized prevention of CLABSIs with evidence-based interventions as an important patient safety measure. The Centers for Medicare and Medicaid Services (CMS) does not reimburse hospitals for the added costs and hospital days needed to treat a CLABSI (Hadaway, 2012b). Nurses require specialized education regarding care

BOX 42-6 EVIDENCE-BASED PRACTICE

Preventing Central Line–Associated Bloodstream Infections (CLABSI)

PICO Question: In hospitalized adult patients, which interventions for central IV site care are best to prevent central line–associated bloodstream infection (CLABSI)?

Evidence Summary

CLABSI is a serious complication of intravenous (IV) therapy that increases morbidity, hospital length of stay, and health care costs. Research shows that effective strategies for prevention of CLABSI include the use of several evidence-based practices together as a "bundle" or "checklist" (Chopra et al., 2013). Such bundles are effective in reducing CLABSIs at the time of insertion of central lines and also during their maintenance (TJC, 2012). For example, a recommended bundle at *insertion* of a central line is hand hygiene before catheter insertion; use of maximum sterile barrier precautions on insertion; chlorhexidine skin antisepsis before insertion and during dressing changes; avoidance of the femoral vein for central venous access for adults; and daily evaluation of line necessity, with prompt removal of nonessential lines (Chopra et al., 2013). Maintenance bundles are similar, with attention to hand hygiene, catheter hub asepsis, dressing and line change, and continued daily evaluation of line necessity. For the most effective reduction of CLABSIs, research demonstrates the necessity for organized educational strategies and attention to institutional support and culture in addition to the use of bundled central line insertion and maintenance practices. One hospital had instituted the central line insertion bundle but still had not achieved zero CLABSI rate in the intensive care unit (ICU); with addition of a collaborative program involving staff education, daily surveillance, single-use line insertion kits, and updated policies and protocols, a zero CLABSI rate was achieved (Matocha, 2013). Dumyati et al. (2014) reduced CLABSI rate by 50% with a multimodal intervention that included involvement of nursing leadership and staff, education on the central line maintenance bundle components, competency evaluation, and line care audits. Zingg et al. (2014) achieved a hospital-wide clinically relevant reduction of CLABSIs with an interdisciplinary multimodal program that included educational components, single-use insertion kits, catheter insertion checklist, and catheter maintenance bundle.

Application to Nursing Practice

- If CLABSI prevention bundles are not used for central line insertion and maintenance at your agency, review the current research in a nursing practice committee or with your IV therapy team to influence policy and procedures and implement these bundles.
- Extend use of central line maintenance bundles to hospital units outside the ICU where patients have central lines.
- Work with infection control personnel and medical and nursing administration to establish a multidisciplinary CLABSI prevention program that includes institutional support for education, competency demonstration, use of insertion and maintenance bundles, and daily line audits.

of central venous catheters and implanted infusion ports. Nursing responsibilities for central lines include careful monitoring, flushing to keep the line patent, and site care and dressing changes to prevent CLABSIs (Box 42-6).

Equipment. Correct selection and preparation of IV equipment helps in safe and rapid placement of an IV line. Because fluids infuse directly into the bloodstream, sterile technique is necessary. Organize all equipment at the bedside for an efficient insertion. IV equipment includes VADs; tourniquet; clean gloves; dressings; IV fluid containers; various types of tubing; and electronic infusion devices (EIDs), also called *infusion pumps*. VADs that are short, peripheral IV catheters are

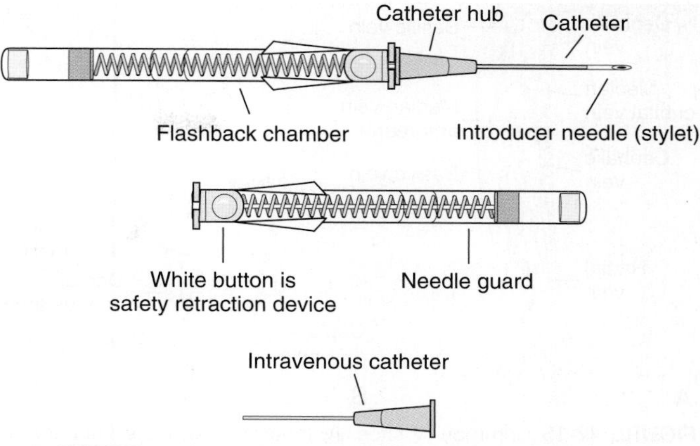

FIGURE 42-14 Over-the-needle catheter for venipuncture.

available in a variety of gauges such as the commonly used 20 and 22 gauges. A larger gauge indicates a smaller-diameter catheter. A peripheral VAD is called an over-the-needle catheter; it consists of a small plastic tube or catheter threaded over a sharp stylet (needle). Once you insert a stylet and advance the catheter into the vein, you withdraw the stylet, leaving the catheter in place. These devices have a safety mechanism that covers the sharp stylet when withdrawing it to reduce the risk of needlestick injury (Figure 42-14). Needleless systems allow you to make connections without using needles, which reduces needlestick injuries (Hadaway, 2012a).

The main IV fluid used in a continuous infusion flows through tubing called the *primary line.* The primary line connects to the IV catheter. Injectable medications such as antibiotics are usually added to a small IV solution bag and "piggybacked" as a secondary set into the primary line or as a primary intermittent infusion to be administered over a 30- to 60-minute period (see Chapter 32). The type and amount of solution are prescribed by the patient's health care provider and depend on the medication added and the patient's physiological status. If an IV infusion is connected to an EID, use the tubing designated for that EID. For gravity-flow IVs (not using an EID), select tubing as described in the equipment list of Skill 42-1 on pp. 967-977. Add IV extension tubing to increase the length of the primary line, which reduces pulling of the tubing and increases a patient's mobility when changing positions.

Initiating the Intravenous Line. After you collect the equipment at the patient's bedside, prepare to insert the IV line by assessing the patient for a venipuncture site (see Skill 42-1). The most common IV sites are on the inner arm (Figure 42-15). Do not use hand veins on older adults or ambulatory patients. IV insertion in a foot vein is common with children, but avoid these sites in adults because of the increased risk of thrombophlebitis (INS, 2011).

As you assess a patient for potential venipuncture sites, consider conditions that exclude certain sites. Venipuncture is contraindicated in a site that has signs of infection, infiltration, or thrombosis. An infected site is red, tender, swollen, and possibly warm to the touch. Exudate may be present. Do not use an infected site because of the danger of introducing bacteria from the skin surface into the bloodstream. Avoid using an extremity with a vascular (dialysis) graft/fistula or on the same side as a mastectomy. Avoid areas of flexion if possible (INS, 2011; Wallis et al., 2014). Choose the most distal appropriate site (INS, 2011). Using a distal site first allows for the use of proximal sites later if the patient needs a venipuncture site change.

Venipuncture is a technique in which a vein is punctured through the skin by a sharp rigid stylet (e.g., metal needle). The stylet is partially

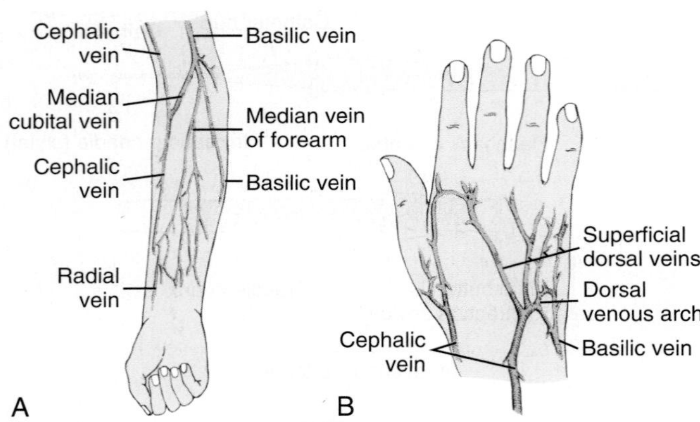

FIGURE 42-15 Common IV sites. **A,** Inner arm. **B,** Dorsal surface of hand.

BOX 42-7 FOCUS ON OLDER ADULTS

Protection of Skin and Veins During Intravenous Therapy

- Use the smallest-gauge catheter or needle possible (e.g., 22 to 24 gauge). Veins are very fragile, and a smaller gauge allows better blood flow to provide increased hemodilution of the intravenous (IV) fluids or medications (Gresser, 2014).
- Avoid the back of the hand, which may compromise a patient's need for independence and mobility.
- Avoid placement of IV line in veins that are easily bumped because older adults have less subcutaneous support tissue (Gresser, 2014).
- Avoid vigorous friction while cleaning a site to prevent tearing fragile skin.
- If a patient has fragile skin and veins, use minimal or no tourniquet pressure (Gresser, 2014).
- If using a tourniquet, place it over the patient's sleeve or use a blood pressure cuff.
- With loss of supportive tissue, veins tend to lie more superficially; lower the insertion angle for venipuncture to 10 to 15 degrees after penetrating the skin (Gresser, 2014).
- Veins roll away from the needle easily because of loss of subcutaneous tissue. To stabilize a vein, apply traction to the skin below the projected insertion site (Gresser, 2014).
- Secure IV site with a catheter stabilization device, avoiding excessive use of tape on fragile skin; consider covering the site additionally with surgical stretch mesh (Gresser, 2014).
- Numerous medications and supplements (e.g., anticoagulants, antibiotics, glucocorticoids, and garlic) increase the likelihood of bruising and bleeding (Burchum and Rosenthal, 2016).

covered either with a plastic catheter or a needle attached to a syringe. General purposes of venipuncture are to collect a blood specimen, start an IV infusion, provide vascular access for later use, instill a medication, or inject a radiopaque or other tracer for special diagnostic examinations. Skill 42-1 on pp. 967-977 describes venipuncture for peripheral IV fluid infusion, incorporating INS (2011) standards of practice. It takes practice to become proficient in venipuncture. Only experienced practitioners perform it for patients whose veins are fragile or collapse easily such as older adults. Box 42-7 describes principles to follow for venipuncture in older adults.

Nurses require specialized knowledge and education to place PICCs. Some central lines and implanted ports require insertion by physicians or advanced practice nurses. Both types of central catheters require close monitoring and maintenance. This chapter focuses on peripheral catheters.

Regulating the Infusion Flow Rate. After initiating a peripheral IV infusion and checking it for patency, regulate the rate of infusion according to the health care provider's orders (see Skill 42-2 on pp. 977-980). For patient safety avoid uncontrolled flow of IV fluid into a patient. You are responsible for calculating the flow rate (mL/hr) that delivers the IV fluid in the prescribed time frame. The correct IV infusion rate ensures patient safety by preventing too-slow or too-rapid administration of IV fluids. An infusion rate that is too slow often leads to further physiological compromise in a patient who is dehydrated, in circulatory shock, or critically ill. An infusion rate that is too rapid overloads the patient with IV fluid, causing fluid and electrolyte imbalances and cardiac complications in vulnerable patients (e.g., older adults or patients with preexisting heart disease).

Electronic infusion devices (EIDs), also called *IV pumps* or *infusion pumps,* deliver an accurate hourly IV infusion rate. EIDs use positive pressure to deliver a measured amount of fluid during a specified unit of time (e.g., 125 mL/hr). Familiarize yourself with the brand of EID in use at your agency so you are able to set the flow rate accurately. Many EIDs have capabilities that allow for single- and multiple-solution infusions at different rates. Electronic detectors and alarms respond to air in IV lines, occlusion, completion of infusion, high and low pressure, and low battery power.

When you open a roller clamp or other type of clamp on an infusion tubing that is not yet properly inserted in an EID or on a gravity-flow IV system, the IV fluid infuses very rapidly. Nonelectronic volume-control devices are used occasionally with an IV solution infused by gravity to prevent accidental infusion of a large fluid volume. These devices hang between the IV bag and the patient and hold only a small volume of fluid that can infuse into the patient. Regardless of the device in use, monitor the patient regularly to verify correct infusion of IV fluids. Patency of an IV catheter means that IV fluid flows easily through it. For patency there must be no clots at the tip of the catheter, and the catheter tip must not be against the vein wall. A blocked catheter slows or stops the rate of infusion of the IV fluids. IV flow rate also can be slowed by infiltration, vasospasm, a knot or kink in the tubing, external pressure on the tubing, and position changes of the patient's extremity. If the flow decreases or stops and the EID is working correctly, inspect the tubing. Sometimes the patient is lying or sitting on it. The tubing may be kinked or caught in or under equipment. Also inspect the area around the insertion site for anything that obstructs the flow of IV fluids. For gravity flow, the height of the container influences flow rate. Raising the container usually increases the rate because of increased driving pressure.

Flexion of an extremity, particularly at the wrist or elbow, can decrease IV flow rate by compressing the vein. Although VAD placement in areas of flexion is discouraged, occasionally it becomes necessary. In that case INS standards specify use of an arm board or other joint stabilization device to protect the IV site by keeping the joint extended (INS, 2011). Use padding with arm boards because they may cause skin or nerve damage from pressure. Starting an infusion in a new location rather than relying on a site that causes problems may be more comfortable for a patient. Before discontinuing the current infusion, choose another site and start the infusion to verify that the patient has other accessible veins.

Maintaining the System. After placing an IV line and regulating the flow rate, maintain the IV system. Line maintenance involves (1) keeping the system sterile and intact; (2) changing IV fluid containers, tubing, and contaminated site dressings; (3) helping a patient with self-care activities so as not to disrupt the system; and (4) monitoring

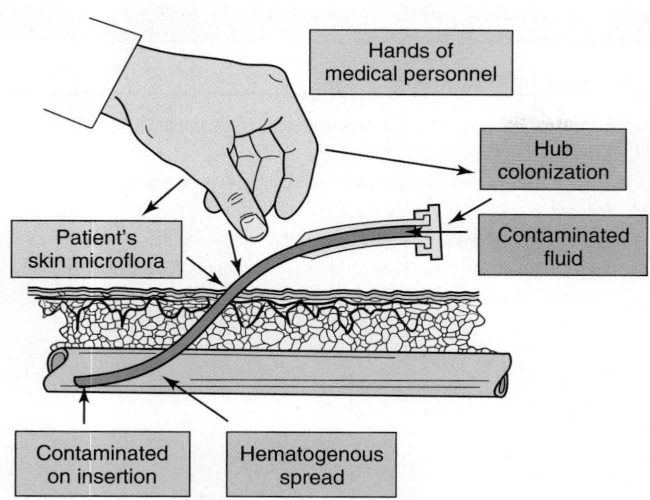

FIGURE 42-16 Potential sites for contamination of vascular access device.

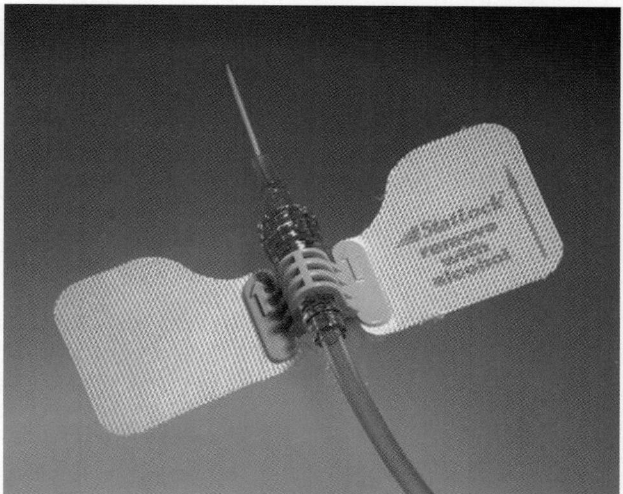

FIGURE 42-17 Catheter stabilization device. (Copyright © C.R. Bard, Inc. Used with permission.)

for complications of IV therapy. The frequency and options for maintaining the system are identified in agency policies.

An important component of patient care is maintaining the integrity of an IV line to prevent infection. Potential sites for contamination of a VAD are shown in Figure 42-16. Inserting an IV line under appropriate aseptic technique reduces the chances of contamination from the patient's skin. After insertion, prevent infection by the conscientious use of infection control principles such as thorough hand hygiene before and after handling any part of the IV system and maintaining sterility of the system during tubing and fluid container changes.

Always maintain the integrity of an IV system. Never disconnect tubing because it becomes tangled or it might seem more convenient for positioning or moving a patient or applying a gown. If a patient needs more room to maneuver, use aseptic technique to add extension tubing to an IV line. However, keep the use of extension tubing to a minimum because each connection of tubing provides opportunity for contamination. *Never let IV tubing touch the floor.* Do not use stopcocks for connecting more than one solution to a single IV site because they are sources of contamination (INS, 2011). IV tubing contains needleless injection ports through which syringes or other adaptors can be inserted for medication administration. Clean an injection port thoroughly with 2% chlorhexidine (preferred), 70% alcohol, or povidone-iodine solution and let it dry before accessing the system (INS, 2011).

Protective devices designed to prevent movement or accidental dislodgement of a VAD are called *catheter stabilization devices* (Figure 42-17). These devices are available in many hospitals, and nurses decide whether or not to use them when starting an IV line. This is a patient safety issue (Billingsley and Kinchen, 2014). Movement of the VAD in a vein can cause phlebitis and infiltration; VAD dislodgement requires using another VAD at a new IV infusion site. INS standards indicate that use of these devices is preferable over taping when feasible (INS, 2011).

Changing Intravenous Fluid Containers, Tubing, and Dressings. Patients receiving IV therapy over several days require periodic changes of IV fluid containers (see Skill 42-3 on pp. 981-986). It is important to organize tasks so you can change containers rapidly before a thrombus forms in the catheter.

Recommended frequency of IV tubing change depends on whether it is used for continuous or intermittent infusion. INS (2011) standards specify that continuous infusion tubing changes occur *no more frequently* than every 96 hours unless the tubing has been compromised or become contaminated, which requires immediate tubing change (Ullman et al., 2013). In contrast, change tubing for *intermittent* infusion every 24 hours because of the increased risk of contamination from opening the IV system (INS, 2011). Blood, blood components, and lipids are likely to promote bacterial growth in tubing. INS standards (2011) specify tubing changes every 4 hours for blood and blood components and every 24 hours for continuous IV lipids. For lipids use tubing that is free of diethylhexyl-phthalate (DEHP), a toxin that leaches into lipid solutions (INS, 2011). Whenever possible, schedule tubing changes when it is time to hang a new IV container to decrease risk of infection (INS, 2011). To prevent entry of bacteria into the bloodstream, maintain sterility during tubing and IV fluid container changes (INS, 2011).

A sterile dressing over an IV site reduces the entrance of bacteria into the insertion site. Transparent dressings, the most common type, help secure the VAD, allow continuous visual inspection of the IV site, and are less easily soiled or moistened than gauze dressings (Bernatchez, 2014). Leave transparent dressings in place until the IV tubing is replaced (INS, 2011). If a gauze dressing is used, change it every 48 hours (INS, 2011). Both types of dressings must be changed when the IV device is removed or replaced or when the dressing becomes damp, loosened, or soiled (INS, 2011) (see Skill 42-4 on pp. 987-989).

Helping Patients to Protect Intravenous Integrity. To prevent the accidental disruption of an IV system, a patient often needs help with hygiene, comfort measures, meals, and ambulation. Changing gowns is difficult for a patient with an IV in the arm. Teach NAP and patients that they must not break the integrity of an IV line to change a gown because it leads to contamination. It helps to use a gown with snaps along the top sleeve seam to facilitate changing the gown without disturbing the venipuncture site. Change regular gowns by following these steps for maximum speed and arm mobility:

1. *To remove a gown,* remove the sleeve of the gown from the arm without the IV line, maintaining the patient's privacy.
2. Remove the sleeve of the gown from the arm with the IV line.
3. Remove the IV solution container from its stand and pass it and the tubing through the sleeve. (If this involves removing the tubing from an EID, use the roller clamp to slow the infusion to prevent the accidental infusion of a large volume of solution or medication).
4. *To apply a gown,* place the IV solution container and tubing through the sleeve of the clean gown and hang it on its stand.

TABLE 42-12 Complications of Intravenous Therapy with Nursing Interventions

Complication	Description	Assessment Findings	Nursing Interventions
Circulatory overload of IV solution	IV solution infused too rapidly or in too great an amount	Depends on type of solution ECV excess with Na^+-containing isotonic fluid (crackles in dependent parts of lungs, shortness of breath, dependent edema) Hyponatremia with hypotonic fluid (confusion, seizures) Hypernatremia with Na^+-containing hypertonic fluid (confusion, seizures) Hyperkalemia from K^+-containing fluid (cardiac dysrhythmias, muscle weakness, abdominal distention)	If symptoms appear, reduce IV flow rate and notify patient's health care provider. With ECV excess raise head of bed; administer oxygen and diuretics if ordered. Monitor vital signs and laboratory reports of serum levels. Health care provider may adjust additives in IV solution or type of IV fluid; watch for and implement order.
Infiltration or extravasation	IV fluid entering subcutaneous tissue around venipuncture site Extravasation: technical term used when a vesicant (tissue-damaging) drug (e.g., chemotherapy) enters tissues (Coyle et al., 2014)	Skin around catheter site taut, blanched, cool to touch, edematous; may be painful as infiltration or extravasation increases; infusion may slow or stop	Stop infusion. Discontinue IV infusion if no vesicant drug (see Skill 42-3). If vesicant drug, disconnect IV tubing and aspirate drug from catheter (Dychter et al., 2012). Agency policy and procedures may require delivery of antidote through catheter before removal. Elevate extremity. Contact health care provider if solution contained KCl, a vasoconstrictor, or other potential vesicant. Apply warm, moist or cold compress according to procedure for type of solution infiltrated. Start new IV line in other extremity.
Phlebitis	Inflammation of inner layer of a vein	Redness, tenderness, pain, warmth along course of vein starting at access site; possible red streak and/or palpable cord along vein	Stop infusion and discontinue IV line (see Skill 42-3). Start new IV line in other extremity or proximal to previous insertion site if continued IV therapy is necessary. Apply warm, moist compress or contact IV therapy team or health care provider if area needs additional treatment.
Local infection	Infection at catheter-skin entry point during infusion or after removal of IV catheter	Redness, heat, swelling at catheter-skin entry point; possible purulent drainage	Culture any drainage (if ordered). Clean skin with alcohol; remove catheter and save for culture; apply sterile dressing. Notify health care provider. Start new IV line in other extremity. Initiate appropriate wound care (see Chapter 48) if needed.
Bleeding at venipuncture site	Oozing or slow, continuous seepage of blood from venipuncture site	Fresh blood evident at venipuncture site, sometimes pooling under extremity	Assess if IV system is intact. If catheter is within vein, apply pressure dressing over site or change dressing. Start new IV line in other extremity or proximal to previous insertion site if VAD is dislodged, IV is disconnected, or bleeding from site does not stop.

ECV, Extracellular volume; *IV,* intravenous; *VAD,* vascular access device.

(If the IV line is controlled by an EID, reassemble, turn on the pump, and open the roller clamp.)

5. Place the arm with the IV line through the gown sleeve.
6. Place the arm without the IV line through the gown sleeve.

A patient with an arm or a hand infusion is able to walk unless contraindicated. Offer a rolling IV pole on wheels. Help the patient get out of bed and place the IV pole next to the involved arm. Teach him or her to hold the pole with the involved hand and push it while walking. Check that the IV container is at the proper height, there is no tension on the tubing, and the flow rate is correct. Instruct the patient to report any blood in the tubing, a stoppage in the flow, or increased discomfort.

Complications of Intravenous Therapy. Table 42-12 presents complications of IV therapy, with assessments and nursing interventions. A potentially dangerous complication of IV therapy is circulatory overload with IV solution, which occurs when a patient receives too-rapid administration or an excessive amount of fluids. Assessment findings depend on the type of IV solution that infuses in excess (see Table 42-12). The signs and symptoms often arise rapidly, which highlights the importance of frequent assessment of patients receiving IV therapy.

QSEN QSEN: BUILDING COMPETENCY IN SAFETY

You have an order to change an intravenous (IV) fluid container for Mrs. Jamison, age 48, who has no oral intake. The new IV fluid is 1000 mL NS with 20 mEq KCl; the previous IV fluid was 1000 mL NS and did not contain KCl. Which nursing assessments related to fluid and electrolyte imbalances do you need to make before you hang the new IV fluid container? Why?

Answers to QSEN Activities can be found on the Evolve website.

TABLE 42-13 Infiltration Scale

Grade	Clinical Criteria
0	No symptoms
1	Skin blanched Edema <2.54 cm (1 inch) in any direction Cool to touch With or without pain
2	Skin blanched Edema 2.54-15.2 cm (1-6 inches) in any direction Cool to touch With or without pain
3	Skin blanched, translucent Gross edema >15.2 cm (6 inches) in any direction Cool to touch Mild-moderate pain Possible numbness
4	Skin blanched, translucent Skin tight, leaking Skin discolored, bruised, swollen Gross edema >15.2 cm (6 inches) in any direction Deep pitting tissue edema Circulatory impairment Moderate-to-severe pain Infiltration of any amount of blood product, irritant, or vesicant

From Groll D et al: Evaluation of the psychometric properties of the phlebitis and infiltration scales for the assessment of complications of peripheral vascular access devices, *J Infus Nurs* 33(6):385, 2010.

Infiltration occurs when an IV catheter becomes dislodged or a vein ruptures and IV fluids inadvertently enter subcutaneous tissue around the venipuncture site. When the IV fluid contains additives that damage tissue, **extravasation** occurs (Dychter et al., 2012). Infiltration or extravasation causes coolness, paleness, and swelling of the area. When infiltration occurs, immediately assess for any additives in the infiltrated fluid to determine the type of action necessary to prevent local tissue damage and sloughing. Vasoconstrictors, high-dose potassium, and other IV additives in subcutaneous tissue need different treatments from those needed for an infiltrated additive-free IV (Dychter et al., 2012) (see Table 42-12). Although the INS removed their previous infiltration scale from their 2011 standards because of insufficient research validation, the society does recommend use of an infiltration scale to provide objectivity in infiltration measurement (Table 42-13).

Phlebitis (i.e., inflammation of a vein) results from chemical, mechanical, or bacterial causes. Risk factors for phlebitis include acidic or hypertonic IV solutions; rapid IV rate; IV drugs such as KCl, vancomycin, and penicillin; VAD inserted in area of flexion, poorly secured catheter; poor hand hygiene; and lack of aseptic technique (Wallis et al., 2014). The typical signs of inflammation (i.e., heat, erythema [redness], tenderness) occur along the course of a vein (Table 42-14). Phlebitis can be dangerous because blood clots (thrombophlebitis) form along the vein and in some cases cause emboli. This may cause permanent damage to veins. Routine changes of peripheral IV catheters to reduce infection are not recommended (O'Grady et al., 2011). The INS Standards of Practice (2011) recommend avoiding routine replacement of peripheral IV catheters in infants and children and replacement of a peripheral IV catheter in adults only if clinically indicated (Rickard et al., 2012; Webster et al., 2013). An INS position

TABLE 42-14 Phlebitis Scale

Grade	Clinical Criteria
0	No symptoms
1	Erythema at access site with or without pain
2	Pain at access site with erythema and/or edema
3	Pain at access site with erythema and/or edema; streak formation; palpable venous cord
4	Pain at access site with erythema and/or edema; streak formation; palpable venous cord >2.54 cm (1 inch) in length; purulent drainage

From Infusion Nurses Society: Infusion nursing standards of practice, *J Infus Nurs* 34(1S):S1, 2011.

paper provides the following guidelines for how frequently to assess the peripheral VAD site to see if its replacement is clinically indicated (Gorski et al., 2012):

- At least every 4 hours for alert, oriented adults who are able to report problems at the VAD site and are not receiving vesicant (tissue-damaging) infusions
- At least every 1 to 2 hours for critically ill patients and adults who are receiving sedatives, are unable to report problems at the VAD site, or have VADs in high-risk locations such as areas of flexion
- At least every hour for neonates and children
- Every 5 to 10 minutes during infusions of vesicants or vasoconstrictors
- During every home or outpatient visit

In the absence of phlebitis, local infection at the venipuncture site is usually caused by poor aseptic technique during catheter insertion, daily monitoring, or catheter removal. Early recognition of local infection and treatment is important to prevent bacteria from entering the bloodstream (see Table 42-12). Bloodstream infections may arise from short peripheral IV catheter sites (Hadaway, 2012b).

Bleeding can occur around the venipuncture site during the infusion or through the catheter or tubing if these become disconnected inadvertently (see Table 42-12). Bleeding is more common in patients who receive heparin or other anticoagulants or who have a bleeding disorder (e.g., hemophilia or thrombocytopenia).

Discontinuing Peripheral Intravenous Access. Discontinue IV access after infusion of the prescribed amount of fluid; when infiltration, phlebitis, or local infection occurs; or if the IV infusion slows or stops, indicating the catheter has developed a thrombus at its tip. Skill 42-3 presents the steps for discontinuing peripheral IV access. You help patients and families understand that moving from IV infusion to oral fluid intake is a sign of progress toward recovery.

Blood Transfusion. Blood transfusion, or blood component therapy, is the IV administration of whole blood or a blood component such as packed red blood cells (RBCs), platelets, or plasma. Objectives for administering blood transfusions include (1) increasing circulating blood volume after surgery, trauma, or hemorrhage; (2) increasing the number of RBCs and maintaining hemoglobin levels in patients with severe anemia; and (3) providing selected cellular components as replacement therapy (e.g., clotting factors, platelets, albumin).

Caring for patients receiving blood or blood-product transfusion is a nursing responsibility. You must be thorough in patient assessment, checking the blood product against prescriber's orders, checking it against patient identifiers, and monitoring for any adverse reactions. Blood transfusions are never regarded as routine; overlooking any

TABLE 42-15 ABO Compatibilities for Transfusion Therapy

Component	Compatibilities	
Whole Blood	**Give Type-Specific Blood Only**	
Packed red cells (stored, washed, or frozen/washed)	**Donor**	**Recipient**
	0	0, A, B, AB
	A	A, AB
	B	B, AB
	AB	AB
Fresh-frozen plasma	**Donor**	**Recipient**
	0	0
	A	A, 0
	B	B, 0
	AB	AB, B, A, 0
Platelets	RBC: ABO and Rh compatible *preferred*	
	Donor	**Recipient**
	0	0, A, B, AB
	A	A, AB
	B	B, AB
	AB	AB

Data from Alexander M et al: *Core curriculum for infusion nursing,* ed 4, Philadelphia, 2014, Lippincott.
ABO, Blood group consisting of groups A, AB, B, and O.

minor detail can have dangerous and life-threatening events for a patient (AABB, 2014a,b).

Blood Groups and Types. Blood transfusions must be matched to each patient to avoid incompatibility. RBCs have antigens in their membranes; the plasma contains antibodies against specific RBC antigens. If incompatible blood is transfused (i.e., a patient's RBC antigens differ from those transfused), the patient's antibodies trigger RBC destruction in a potentially dangerous **transfusion reaction** (i.e., an immune response to the transfused blood components).

The most important grouping for transfusion purposes is the ABO system, which identifies A, B, O, and AB blood types. Determination of blood type is made on the basis of the presence or absence of A and B RBC antigens. Individuals with type A blood have A antigens on their RBCs and anti-B antibodies in their plasma. Individuals with type B blood have B antigens on their RBCs and anti-A antibodies in their plasma. A person who has type AB blood has both A and B antigens on the RBCs and no antibodies against either antigen in the plasma. A type O individual has neither A nor B antigens on RBCs but has both anti-A and anti-B antibodies in the plasma (Alexander et al., 2014). Table 42-15 shows the compatibilities between blood types of donors and recipients. People with type O blood are considered universal blood donors because they can donate packed RBCs and platelets to people with any ABO blood type. People with type AB blood are called *universal blood recipients* because they can receive packed RBCs and platelets of any ABO type.

Another consideration when matching blood components for transfusions is the Rh factor, which refers to another antigen in RBC membranes. Most people have this antigen and are Rh positive; a person without it is Rh negative. People who are Rh negative receive only Rh-negative blood components.

Autologous Transfusion. **Autologous transfusion** (autotransfusion) is the collection and reinfusion of a patient's own blood. Blood for an autologous transfusion most commonly is obtained by preoperative donation up to 6 weeks before a scheduled surgery (e.g., heart, orthopedic, plastic, or gynecological). A patient can donate several units of blood, depending on the type of surgery and his or her ability to maintain an acceptable hematocrit. Blood for autologous transfusion is also obtained at the time of surgery by normovolemic hemodilution or through blood salvage (e.g., during surgery for liver transplantation, trauma, or vascular and orthopedic conditions). After surgery blood is salvaged from drainage from chest tubes or joint cavities. Autologous transfusions are safer for patients because they decrease the risk of mismatched blood and exposure to bloodborne infectious agents (Alexander et al., 2014).

Transfusing Blood. Transfusion of blood or blood components is a nursing procedure that requires an order from a health care provider. Patient safety is a nursing priority; and patient assessment, verification of health care provider's order, and verification of correct blood products for the correct patient are imperative (AABB, 2014a,b).

Perform a thorough patient assessment before initiating a transfusion and monitor carefully during and after the transfusion. Assessment is critical because of the risk of transfusion reactions. Pretransfusion assessment includes establishing whether a patient knows the reason for the blood transfusion and whether he or she has ever had a previous transfusion or transfusion reaction. A patient who has had a transfusion reaction is usually at no greater risk for a reaction with a subsequent transfusion. However, he or she may be anxious about the transfusion, requiring nursing intervention. Before beginning a transfusion, explain the procedure and instruct the patient (if alert) to report any side effects (e.g., chills, dizziness, or fever) once the transfusion begins. Have a professional translator available if the patient does not speak English. Ensure that he or she has signed an informed consent. Patients with certain cultural or religious backgrounds may refuse blood transfusions (see Box 42-5).

Because of the danger of transfusion reactions, your pretransfusion assessment always includes the patient's baseline vital signs. These data allow you to identify when vital sign changes occur as a result of a transfusion reaction.

Always check agency policy and procedures before initiating any blood therapy. For patient safety always verify three things: (1) that blood components delivered are the ones that were ordered, (2) that blood delivered to a patient is compatible with the blood type listed in the medical record, and (3) that the right patient receives the blood. Together two RNs or one RN and an LPN (check agency policy and procedures) must check the label on the blood product against the medical record and the patient's identification number, blood group, and complete name. If even a minor discrepancy exists, do not give the blood; notify the blood bank immediately to prevent infusion errors.

When administering a transfusion, you need an appropriate-size IV catheter and blood administration tubing that has a special in-line filter (Figure 42-18). Adults require a large catheter (e.g., 18- or 20-gauge) because blood is more viscous than crystalloid IV fluids. Children with small veins need a smaller catheter. Prime the tubing with 0.9% sodium chloride (normal saline) to prevent hemolysis or breakdown of RBCs. Initiate a transfusion slowly to allow for the early detection of a transfusion reaction. Maintain the ordered infusion rate, monitor for side effects, assess vital signs, and promptly record all findings. It is important to stay with the patient during the first 15 minutes because this is the time when a reaction is most likely to occur. After the initial time period, continue to monitor the patient and obtain vital signs periodically during the transfusion as directed by agency policy. If a transfusion reaction is anticipated or suspected, obtain vital signs more frequently (Table 42-16).

The transfusion rate usually is specified in the health care provider's orders. Ideally a unit of whole blood or packed RBCs is transfused in 2 hours. This time can be lengthened to 4 hours if the patient is at risk

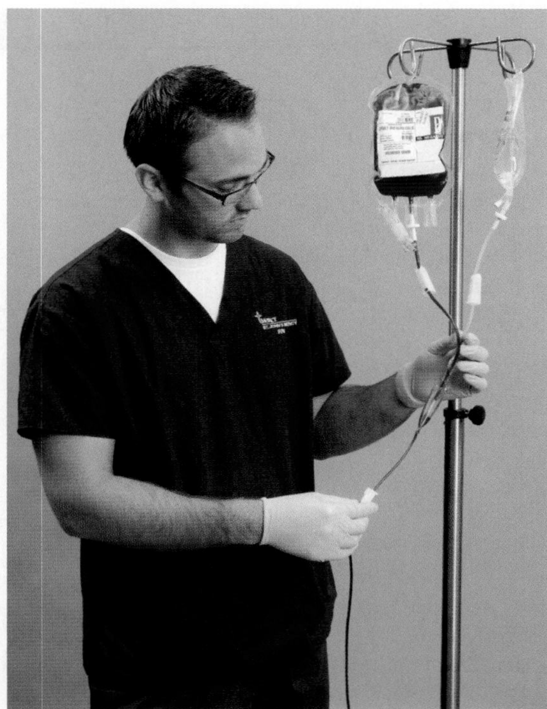

FIGURE 42-18 Filling tubing for blood administration.

for ECV excess. Beyond 4 hours there is a risk for bacterial contamination of the blood.

When patients have a severe blood loss such as with hemorrhage, they often receive rapid transfusions through a central venous catheter. A blood-warming device often is necessary because the tip of the central venous catheter lies in the superior vena cava, above the right atrium. Rapid administration of cold blood can cause cardiac dysrhythmias. Patients who receive large-volume transfusion of citrated blood have high risk of hyperkalemia, hypocalcemia, hypomagnesemia, and metabolic alkalosis; therefore they need careful monitoring.

Transfusion Reactions and Other Adverse Effects. A transfusion reaction is an immune system reaction to the transfusion that ranges from a mild response to severe anaphylactic shock or acute intravascular hemolysis, both of which can be fatal (Clark, 2011). Table 42-16 presents the causes, manifestations, management, and prevention of transfusion reactions. Prompt intervention when a transfusion reaction occurs maintains or restores a patient's physiological stability. When you suspect acute intravascular hemolysis, do the following (Alexander et al., 2014):

- Stop the transfusion immediately.
- Keep the IV line open by replacing the IV tubing down to the catheter hub with new tubing and running 0.9% sodium chloride (normal saline).
- ***Do not*** turn off the blood and simply turn on the 0.9% sodium chloride (normal saline) that is connected to the Y-tubing infusion set. This would cause blood remaining in the IV tubing to infuse into the patient. Even a small amount of mismatched blood can cause a major reaction.
- Immediately notify the health care provider or emergency response team.
- Remain with the patient, observing signs and symptoms and monitoring vital signs as often as every 5 minutes.
- Prepare to administer emergency drugs such as antihistamines, vasopressors, fluids, and corticosteroids per health care provider order or protocol.
- Prepare to perform cardiopulmonary resuscitation.
- Save the blood container, tubing, attached labels, and transfusion record for return to the blood bank.
- Obtain blood and urine specimens per health care provider order or protocol.

Acute adverse effects that do not involve an immune response to the blood components also can occur during a transfusion (see Table 42-16). Circulatory overload is a risk when a patient receives massive whole blood or packed RBC transfusions for massive hemorrhagic shock or when a patient with normal blood volume receives blood. Patients particularly at risk for circulatory overload are older adults and those with cardiopulmonary diseases. Transfusion of blood components that are contaminated with bacteria, especially gram-negative bacteria, can cause sepsis.

Another category of adverse transfusion effects is diseases transmitted by blood from infected donors who are asymptomatic. Symptoms of these conditions may arise long after the transfusion. Diseases transmitted through transfusions include hepatitis B and C, human immunodeficiency virus (HIV) infection and acquired immunodeficiency syndrome (AIDS), and cytomegalovirus infection. In the United States all units of blood for blood banks undergo screening for HIV, hepatitis B and C viruses, syphilis, and West Nile virus, which reduces the risk of acquiring these bloodborne infections (CDC, 2013).

Interventions for Electrolyte Imbalances. In addition to the administration of prescribed medical therapies, there are nursing interventions for preserving or restoring electrolyte imbalance (Felver, 2013c). For example, people who have hypokalemia or hypercalcemia often need bowel management for constipation. Patient safety interventions to prevent falls (see Chapter 27) are vital for patients who become lethargic from hypercalcemia and those with muscle weakness. Patients who have hypercalcemia need an increased fluid intake to prevent renal damage; nurses can help them meet the oral fluid intake goals. Teach patients the reasons for their therapies and the importance of balancing electrolyte I&O to prevent imbalances in the future.

Interventions for Acid-Base Imbalances. Nursing interventions to promote acid-base balance support prescribed medical therapies and aim at reversing the existing acid-base imbalance while providing for patient safety (Felver, 2013b). When these imbalances are life threatening, they require rapid treatment. Maintain a functional IV line and check the health care provider's orders frequently for new medications or fluids. Give fluid and electrolyte replacement and prescribed drugs such as insulin promptly. In addition, monitor patients closely for changes in their status. Use protective measures such as side rails for patients with decreased level of consciousness. Support compensatory hyperventilation for patients with metabolic acidosis by keeping their oral mucous membranes moist and positioning them to facilitate chest expansion. Chapter 41 reviews appropriate therapies for patients with respiratory acidosis. Patients with acid-base imbalances often require repeated ABG analysis.

Arterial Blood Gases. Determination of a patient's acid-base status requires obtaining a sample of arterial blood for laboratory testing. ABG analysis reveals acid-base status and the adequacy of ventilation and oxygenation. A qualified RN or other health care provider draws arterial blood from a peripheral artery (usually the radial) or from an existing arterial line (see agency policy and procedures). Before an arterial blood draw, perform an Allen test, which assesses arterial circulation in the hand (Pagana et al., 2015). When performing the Allen test, apply pressure to both the ulnar and radial arteries in the selected hand. The fingers to the hand should be pale and blanched,

TABLE 42-16 Acute Adverse Effects of Transfusions

Adverse Effect	Cause	Clinical Manifestations	Management	Prevention
Transfusion Reactions—Caused by Immune Response to Blood Components				
Acute intravascular hemolytic	Infusion of ABO-incompatible whole blood, RBCs, or components containing 10 mL or more of RBCs Antibodies in recipient's plasma attach to antigens on transfused RBCs, causing RBC destruction	Chills, fever, low back pain, flushing, tachycardia, tachypnea, hypotension, hemoglobinuria, hemoglobinemia, sudden oliguria (acute kidney injury), circulatory shock, cardiac arrest, death	Stop transfusion and save blood bag and administration set for follow-up. Keep IV site open with normal saline infused through new tubing. Maintain BP and treat shock as ordered, if present. Obtain blood samples **slowly** to avoid hemolysis; send for serological testing. Send urine specimen to laboratory. Give diuretics as prescribed to maintain urine flow. Insert indwelling urinary catheter or measure each voiding to monitor hourly urine output. Dialysis may be required if acute kidney injury occurs. ***Patient safety alert:*** Do not transfuse additional RBC-containing components until transfusion service provides newly cross-matched units.	Meticulously verify and document patient identification from sample collection to component infusion.
Febrile nonhemolytic (most common)	Antibodies against donor white blood cells	Sudden shaking chills (rigors), fever (rise in temperature 0.5° C [1° F] or more from start), headache, flushing, anxiety, muscle pain	Stop transfusion. Give antipyretics as prescribed; avoid aspirin in thrombocytopenic patients. ***Patient safety alert:*** Do not restart transfusion.	Consider leukocyte-poor blood products (filtered, washed, or frozen). Pretreat with antipyretics if prior history.
Mild allergic	Antibodies against donor plasma proteins	Flushing, itching, urticaria (hives)	Stop transfusion temporarily. Give antihistamine as directed. If symptoms are mild and transient, restart transfusion slowly. ***Patient safety alert:*** Do not restart transfusion if fever, pulmonary symptoms, or hypotension develop.	Treat prophylactically with antihistamines.
Anaphylactic	Antibodies to donor plasma, especially anti-IgA	Anxiety, urticaria, dyspnea, wheezing progressing to cyanosis, severe hypotension, circulatory shock, possible cardiac arrest	Stop transfusion. Have epinephrine ready for injection (0.4 mL of 1 : 1000 solution subcutaneously or 0.1 mL of 1 : 1000 solution diluted to 10 mL with saline for IV use). Provide blood pressure support as ordered. Initiate CPR if indicated. ***Patient safety alert:*** Do not restart transfusion.	Transfuse extensively washed RBC products from which all plasma has been removed. Alternately use blood from IgA-deficient donor.
Other Acute Adverse Effects				
Circulatory overload	Blood administered faster than circulation can accommodate	*Dyspnea,* cough, crackles, or rales in dependent lobes of lungs; distended neck veins when upright	Turn down transfusion rate or stop transfusion. Place patient upright with feet in dependent position. Administer prescribed diuretics, oxygen, morphine. Phlebotomy may be indicated.	Adjust transfusion volume and flow rate on basis of patient size and clinical status. Have transfusion service divide unit into smaller aliquots for better spacing of fluid input.
Sepsis	Bacterial contamination of transfused blood components	Rapid onset of chills, high fever, severe hypotension, and circulatory shock *May occur:* Vomiting, diarrhea, sudden oliguria (acute kidney injury), disseminated intravascular coagulation (DIC)	Stop transfusion. Obtain culture of patient's blood and send bag with remaining blood to transfusion service for further study. Treat as ordered: antibiotics, IV fluids, vasopressors, glucocorticoids.	Collect, process, store, and transfuse blood products according to blood-banking standards and infuse within 4 hours of starting time.

Data from Alexander et al: *Core curriculum for infusion nursing,* ed 4, Philadelphia, 2014, Lippincott.
ABO, Blood group consisting of groups A, AB, B, and O; *BP,* blood pressure; *CPR,* cardiopulmonary resuscitation; *DIC,* disseminated intravascular coagulation; *IgA,* immunoglobulin A; *IV,* intravenous; *RBC,* red blood cell.

indicating a lack of arterial blood flow. Release the pressure on the ulnar artery and observe for color to return to the fingers and hand, which indicates that there is adequate circulation to the hand and fingers via the ulnar artery. The Allen test ensures that a patient will have adequate blood flow to the hand if the radial artery is damaged. If color does not return, do not perform radial artery puncture on that arm. After the ABG puncture, apply pressure to the puncture site for at least 5 minutes to reduce the risk of hematoma formation. A longer time is necessary if the patient takes anticoagulant medications. Reassess the radial pulse after removing the pressure. After obtaining the specimen, take care to prevent air from entering the syringe because this alters the blood gas values. To reduce oxygen usage by blood cells, submerge the syringe in crushed ice and transport it immediately to the laboratory.

Restorative Care. After experiencing acute alterations in fluid, electrolyte, or acid-base balance, patients often require ongoing maintenance to prevent a recurrence of health alterations. Older adults require special considerations to prevent complications from developing (see Box 42-2).

Home Intravenous Therapy. IV therapy often continues in the home setting for patients requiring long-term hydration, PN, or long-term medication administration. Initiate patient referral for discharge planning to social services, counselors, or a home care coordinator for assessment of patient and community resources (Petroulias et al., 2013). A home IV therapy nurse works closely with a patient to ensure that a sterile IV system is maintained and complications can be avoided or recognized promptly. Box 42-8 summarizes patient education guidelines for home IV therapy.

Nutritional Support. Most patients who have had electrolyte disorders or metabolic acid-base imbalances require ongoing nutritional support. Depending on the type of disorder, fluid or food intake may be encouraged or restricted (see Chapter 45). Patients or family members who are responsible for meal preparation need to learn to understand nutritional content of foods and read the labels of commercially prepared foods.

Medication Safety. Numerous medications, OTC drugs, and herbal preparations contain components or create potential side effects that can alter fluid and electrolyte balance. Patients with chronic disease who are receiving multiple medications and those with renal disorders are at significant risk for imbalances. Once patients return to restorative care settings, whether in the home, long-term care, or other setting, drug safety is very important. Patient and family education regarding potential side effects and drug interactions that can alter fluid, electrolyte, or acid-base balance is essential. Review all medications with patients and encourage them to consult with their local pharmacist, especially if they wish to try a new OTC drug or herbal preparation (Chapter 32).

◆ Evaluation

Through the Patient's Eyes. Review with patients how well their major concerns and expectations regarding fluid, electrolyte, or acid-base situations were alleviated or addressed. For example, ask a person admitted with dehydration who was concerned about falling because of light-headedness, "How confident are you in your ability to stand without getting light-headed now?" If the patient's concern was feeling uncomfortable with very dry mouth, ask, "How does your mouth feel now?" If the patient's concerns involved having a better understanding of a chronic problem, focus the evaluation on his or her view of the patient education provided. A patient's perspectives regarding care often depend in part on involvement of family and friends. If patients have concerns about returning home or to a different care setting, it is important to evaluate how well prepared they feel for the transition from acute care.

Patient Outcomes. Evaluate the effectiveness of interventions using the goals and outcomes established for the patient's nursing diagnoses. Evaluation of a patient's clinical status is especially important if acute fluid, electrolyte, and/or acid-base imbalances exist. A patient's condition can change very quickly, and it is important to recognize impending problems by integrating information about his or her presenting risk factors, clinical status, effects of the present

BOX 42-8 PATIENT TEACHING

Home Intravenous Therapy

Objective

- The patient and/or family caregiver will demonstrate competence with administering intravenous (IV) therapy safely in the home.

Teaching Strategies

- Explain the importance of IV therapy in maintaining hydration and access for the delivery of medications.
- Emphasize the risks involved when the IV system is not kept sterile.
- Be sure that the patient and/or family caregiver is able to manipulate the required equipment.
- Instruct in aseptic technique and hand hygiene in the handling of all IV equipment.
- Teach how to change IV solutions, tubing, and dressing when they become soiled or dislodged (Alexander et al., 2014). (NOTE: As the home care nurse, you may be able to visit frequently enough to perform scheduled tubing changes.)
- Teach procedures for safe disposal in appropriate containers of all sharps and IV materials exposed to blood. Keep sharps containers away from children (see Chapter 29).
- Instruct to apply pressure with sterile gauze if catheter falls out and, if patient is on anticoagulants, to tape pieces of sterile gauze in place for at least 20 minutes with pressure or until bleeding stops.
- Instruct about signs and symptoms of infiltration, phlebitis, and infection and reporting symptoms immediately.
- Instruct patient and/or family caregiver to report if the infusion slows or stops or if blood is seen in the tubing.
- Teach patient with family caregiver's assistance how to ambulate, perform hygiene, and participate in other activities of daily living without dislodging or disconnecting catheter and tubing:
  - For showering, protect the IV site and dressing from getting wet by covering it completely with plastic. If using an electronic infusion device, unplug around water.
  - Wear clothes that avoid pressure on the IV site and avoid trauma to the site when changing clothes.
  - Have patient avoid strenuous exercise of the arm with the IV line.

Evaluation

- Ask patient and family caregiver why it is necessary to maintain hydration and IV access for the delivery of medications.
- Ask what to do if the IV infusion stops.
- Ask patient and family caregiver to describe signs and symptoms of complications and the action they should take.
- Observe the patient or family caregiver changing the IV container, tubing, and dressing.
- Observe the patient ambulating and participating in activities of daily living to see how he or she protects and manipulates the IV catheter and apparatus.

treatment regimen, and potential causative agent. For evaluation, apply knowledge of how various pathophysiological conditions affect fluid, electrolyte, and acid-base balance; the effects of medications and fluids; and the patient's presenting clinical status when making clinical decisions (Figure 42-19).

Compare your current evaluation findings with the previous patient assessment. For example, a patient's hypokalemia demonstrates improvement when the serum potassium is increasing toward normal and the physical signs and symptoms of hypokalemia begin to disappear or lessen in intensity. Specifically the patient's heart rhythm becomes more regular, and normal bowel function returns.

For patients with less acute alterations, evaluation likely occurs over a longer period of time. In this situation evaluation may be more focused on behavioral changes (e.g., the patient's adherence to dietary restrictions and medication schedules). Another important element of evaluation is the family's ability to anticipate alterations and prevent problems from recurring.

The patient's level of progress determines whether the plan of care needs to continue or be revised. If goals are not met, you may need to consult a health care provider to discuss additional methods such as increasing the frequency of an intervention (e.g., providing more fluids to a dehydrated patient), introducing a new therapy (e.g., initiating insertion of an IV line), or discontinuing a particular therapy. Once outcomes are met, the nursing diagnosis is resolved, and you are able to focus on other priorities, including maintaining normal fluid, electrolyte, and acid-base balance. If established outcomes are not achieved, explore factors that contributed to why the planned outcomes were not met. Modification of the care plan occurs after this evaluation. If outcomes are not achieved, the questions asked may include the following:

- "What difficulties are you having with measuring your I&O daily and keeping a record?"
- "What barriers are you experiencing to obtaining the potassium-rich foods you need?"
- "Are you continuing to have frequent loose stools or diarrhea?"
- "Have you purchased an antacid, or are you still using baking soda as an antacid?"

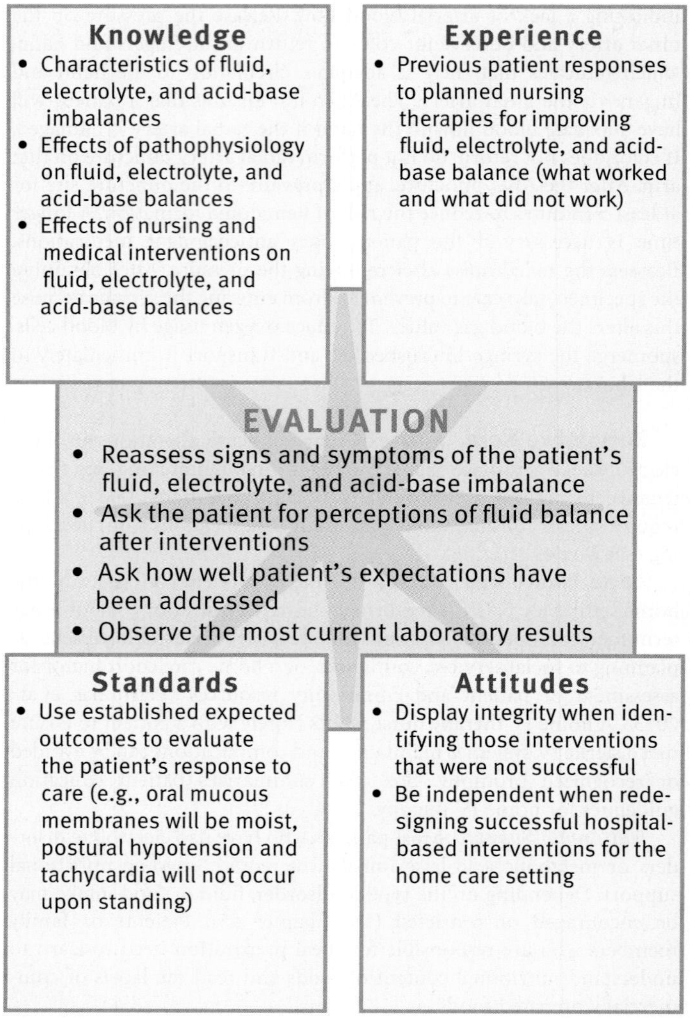

Knowledge
- Characteristics of fluid, electrolyte, and acid-base imbalances
- Effects of pathophysiology on fluid, electrolyte, and acid-base balances
- Effects of nursing and medical interventions on fluid, electrolyte, and acid-base balances

Experience
- Previous patient responses to planned nursing therapies for improving fluid, electrolyte, and acid-base balance (what worked and what did not work)

EVALUATION
- Reassess signs and symptoms of the patient's fluid, electrolyte, and acid-base imbalance
- Ask the patient for perceptions of fluid balance after interventions
- Ask how well patient's expectations have been addressed
- Observe the most current laboratory results

Standards
- Use established expected outcomes to evaluate the patient's response to care (e.g., oral mucous membranes will be moist, postural hypotension and tachycardia will not occur upon standing)

Attitudes
- Display integrity when identifying those interventions that were not successful
- Be independent when redesigning successful hospital-based interventions for the home care setting

FIGURE 42-19 Critical thinking model for fluid, electrolyte, and acid-base balances evaluation.

SAFETY GUIDELINES FOR NURSING SKILLS

Ensuring patient safety is an essential role of the professional nurse. To ensure patient safety, communicate clearly with members of the health care team, assess and incorporate the patient's priorities of care and preferences, and use the best evidence when making decisions about your patient's care. When performing the skills in this chapter, remember the following points to ensure safe, individualized patient care:

- Check that you have the necessary information, a health care provider's order if required, and equipment available for the procedure before beginning.
- Before initiation of therapy, check patient identification using two patient identifiers (TJC, 2016) and assess the appropriate route and rate of infusion and potential incompatibilities between infusing fluids and medications (INS, 2011).
- Determine if the patient has a latex allergy and use nonlatex items if allergy is present (INS, 2011).
- Use special designated tubing for the brand of EID and for blood transfusions and some medications.
- Review the steps of the procedure mentally before entering a patient's room (i.e., consider modifications that you may need to make for this specific patient and verify that the type of IV solution is appropriate for this patient).
- Maintain strict aseptic and sterile techniques when required and sterility and integrity of the IV system to prevent bloodstream infections (INS, 2011).
- If you contaminate a sterile object during the procedure, do not use it. Use a new sterile one.
- Use standard body fluid precautions during procedures and place all disposable blood-contaminated items and sharp items in designated puncture-resistant biohazard containers (INS, 2011).

SKILL 42-1 INITIATING INTRAVENOUS THERAPY

DELEGATION CONSIDERATIONS

The skill of initiating peripheral intravenous (IV) therapy cannot be delegated to nursing assistive personnel (NAP). Delegation to licensed practical nurses (LPNs) varies by state Nurse Practice Act. Instruct the NAP to inform you if:

- Patient indicates burning, bleeding, swelling, or coolness at the catheter insertion site.
- An intravenous (IV) dressing becomes wet or loose.
- Electronic infusion device (EID) alarm signals.
- Fluid container is almost empty.

EQUIPMENT

- Agency-approved vascular access device (VAD) for venipuncture such as an over-the-needle catheter of appropriate gauge, depending on vein size; for continuous fluid infusions: peripheral 20-gauge catheter for an adult, 22-gauge for older adults and children (Alexander et al., 2014)
- IV start kit (available in some agencies)—contains a sterile drape to place under patient's arm, tourniquet, cleaning and antiseptic preparations, sterile dressings, and a small roll of sterile tape
- If IV kit not available:
  - Disposable drape or towel
  - Tourniquet (Determine type of tourniquet on basis of patient assessment [e.g., blood pressure [BP] cuff—older adult, rubber band—infants]. Use single-use tourniquets to prevent transfer of microorganisms between patients.) (Alexander et al., 2014)
  - Antiseptic swabs (2% chlorhexidine preferred) (INS, 2011)]
  - Transparent dressing or, less commonly, 2 × 2 or 4 × 4 gauze sponge
  - Nonallergenic tape and sterile tape
- Local anesthetic (e.g., intradermal lidocaine, topical transdermal anesthetic, vapocoolant) *(optional)*
- Short extension tubing with fused or separate needleless connector (also called *saline lock, heparin lock, IV plug, injection cap, prn adapter, buff cap,* or *buffalo cap)*
- Prefilled 5-mL syringe with flush agent (preservative-free sterile 0.9% sodium chloride (normal saline) for adults) (INS, 2011)
- Manufactured catheter stabilization device (e.g., STATLOCK), if available (INS, 2011). (see Figure 42-17)
- Personal protective equipment: clean gloves, goggles, mask *(optional,* check agency policy)
- Patient gown with snaps at shoulder seams if available
- Needle disposal container (sharps container) **For continuous IV fluid infusion, in addition to previous equipment:**
  - Correct type and amount of IV fluid
  - EID
- IV tubing administration set with tubing specific for type of EID
- If using gravity-flow, use microdrip tubing for small or very precise volumes and macrodrip tubing to infuse fluid more rapidly.
  - In-line filter if particulate matter is likely or long-term or high-volume IV therapy is expected or required by agency policy; size appropriate to type of solution (e.g., 0.22 micron for nonlipid solution, 1.2 microns for lipid solution)
  - Long extension tubing if desired for patient mobility
  - IV pole, rolling, ceiling mounted, or attached to bed
  - Bar-code scanner, if using bar-code system

STEP	RATIONALE
ASSESSMENT	
1. Review accuracy and completeness of health care provider's order for patient name, type and amount of IV fluid, medication additives, infusion time, and purpose of infusion. Follow six rights of medication administration (see Chapter 32).	Ensures that correct IV fluid is administered.

CLINICAL DECISION: *In most institutions health care providers do not write orders to "initiate peripheral access" or "perform venipuncture." The statement "Start IV" usually is written followed by the exact IV therapy order. The order to perform the venipuncture is implied. If the order is confusing or in question, clarify with the health care provider before proceeding.*

STEP	RATIONALE
2. Identify patient using two identifiers (e.g., name and birthday or name and medical record number) according to agency policy. Compare identifiers with information on patient's MAR or medical record.	Ensures correct patient. Complies with The Joint Commission standards and improves patient safety (TJC, 2016).
3. Assess for clinical variables that respond to or are affected by IV fluid administration:	Provides baseline to determine effect that IV fluids have on patient's fluid and electrolyte balance.

SKILL 42-1 INITIATING INTRAVENOUS THERAPY—cont'd

STEP	RATIONALE
a. Body weight	Daily weights reflect fluid retention or loss. A 1-L amount of fluid weighs 2.2 lbs (1 kg). Compare with previous day's weight if available. Gain or loss of 2 lbs (1 kg) in 24 hours indicates gain or loss of 1 L of fluid. Body fat gain or loss takes longer.
b. Clinical markers of vascular volume:	Assess signs and symptoms as a group to interpret them accurately. Infusion of Na^+-containing IV fluid expands extracellular fluid volume (ECV) (vascular and interstitial).
(1) BP	Decreased BP or orthostatic hypotension may indicate ECV deficit caused by decreased stroke volume. Increased BP may indicate ECV excess.
(2) Pulse	Baroreceptor response causes rapid, thready pulse with ECV deficit; bounding, full pulse with ECV excess.
(3) Fullness of neck veins (normally neck veins are full when person is supine and flat when person is upright or semi-upright)	Indicator of fluid volume status: flat or collapsing with inhalation when supine with ECV deficit; full or distended when upright or semi-upright with ECV excess.
(4) Capillary refill	Provides an indirect measure of tissue perfusion. Can indicate poor tissue perfusion (sluggish with ECV deficit).
(5) Auscultation of lungs	Crackles or rhonchi in dependent lobes of lung may signal fluid buildup in lungs caused by ECV excess.
(6) Urine output (decreased; dark yellow with ECV deficit)	Kidneys respond to ECV deficit by reducing urine production and concentrating the urine. Average daily adult urine output is 1500 mL; oliguria is urine output of less than 400 mL/24 hr. Kidney disease and syndrome of inappropriate antidiuretic hormone (SIADH) also can cause oliguria. Dark yellow indicates concentrated urine.
c. Clinical markers of interstitial volume:	Assess signs and symptoms as a group to interpret them accurately. Infusion of Na^+-containing IV fluid expands ECV (vascular and interstitial).
(1) Dependent edema (rate severity by assessing pitting over bony prominences (i.e., 1+ indicates barely detectable edema; 4+ indicates deep persistent pitting) (see Chapter 31).	Edema, indicating expanded interstitial fluid volume, is most evident in dependent areas bilaterally (i.e., feet and ankles if sitting) or sacrum if bedfast.
(2) Oral mucous membranes between cheek and gum	More reliable indicator than dry lips or skin. Dry between cheek and gums indicates ECV deficit.
(3) Skin turgor (pinch skin over sternum or inside of forearm) (Failure of skin to return to normal position within 3 seconds indicates ECV deficit.)	Pinched skin that stays elevated for several seconds is called *poor skin turgor* or *"tenting."* May occur from ECV deficit, rapid weight loss, or normal aging.
d. Thirst	Occurs with hypernatremia and severe ECV deficit. Not a reliable indicator for older adults because thirst sensation decreases with age (Touhy and Jett, 2014).
e. Behavior and level of consciousness	
(1) Restlessness and mild confusion	Occurs with severe ECV deficit caused by lack of blood flow to brain.
(2) Decreased level of consciousness (lethargy, confusion, coma)	May occur with osmolality imbalances (hyponatremia and hypernatremia) and acid-base imbalances.
f. Cardiac signs of electrolyte or acid-base imbalances (e.g., irregular pulse and electrocardiogram [ECG] changes)	Rhythm and ECG changes may occur with K^+, Ca^{2+}, Mg^{2+}, and/or acid-base imbalances. Should improve as IV fluid replaces deficient electrolytes or occur if electrolyte infusion is excessive.
4. Assess patient's previous experience with and perceptions of IV therapy, understanding of purpose of IV therapy, and arm placement preference.	Provides patient-centered care by determining level of emotional support and instruction necessary. If patient is apprehensive about venipuncture, use a local anesthetic.
5. Obtain information from approved online database, drug reference book, or pharmacist about composition of IV fluids, purposes of administration, potential incompatibilities, side effects, monitoring guidelines, and need for special catheter or tubing for administration.	Allows detection of an inadvisable IV fluid order and helps to determine priority assessments.
6. Determine if patient is to undergo any planned surgeries or procedures.	Allows anticipation and placement of appropriate VAD and gauge for fluid infusion and avoids placement in an area that will interfere with medical procedures.
7. Assess for following risk factors: child or older adult; presence of heart failure or oliguric renal disease; skin lesions or infection near potential venipuncture sites; low platelet count or patient receiving anticoagulants.	Older adults have proportionately less body water; people with heart failure cannot adapt to sudden increases in vascular volume; and people with oliguria cannot eliminate excess extracellular fluid, K^+, or Mg^{2+}. Skin lesions or infection influence choice of access site. Low platelet count or anticoagulant use increases patient's risk for bleeding from VAD site and seepage of blood from puncture site during venipuncture.
8. Assess laboratory electrolyte or acid base balance data.	Helps determine priority assessments, establishes baseline for determining if therapy is effective, and may allow detection of an inadvisable fluid order.

STEP	RATIONALE
CLINICAL DECISION: *If the current K^+, Ca^{2+}, or Mg^{2+} serum values are high, clarify order with health care provider before administering an IV solution containing the elevated electrolyte to avoid worsening the electrolyte excess.*	
9. Assess patient's history of allergies, especially to iodine, adhesive, or latex.	Equipment used during insertion of VAD may contain substances to which patient is allergic. Use alternatives if patient has allergy.
10. Assess patient's medical history for chronic illnesses and all prescribed and over-the-counter medications.	Reveals background information that might cause adverse effects on patient (e.g., heart failure may require slower infusion rate) or conflict with prescribed therapy such as drug-drug interactions.
PLANNING	
1. Collect appropriate equipment. Be sure that you have the correct infusion set for the EID that will be used. If the IV container is rigid rather than collapsible, you need a vented spike on the IV tubing.	Provides patient safety.
2. Explain to patient and family the rationale for IV fluids and medications, procedure for initiating an IV infusion, signs and symptoms of complications, what is expected of patient, and which sensations patient should expect.	Cognitive and sensory information decreases anxiety and helps promote cooperation.
3. Help patient to comfortable sitting or supine position. Position a chair so you are level with patient. Provide adequate lighting.	Promotes comfort and relaxation for patient. Provides proper body mechanics for nurse. Aids in successful vein location.
IMPLEMENTATION	
1. Perform hand hygiene. Organize equipment on clean, clutter-free bedside stand or over-bed table.	Reduces transmission of infection and risk of accidents.
2. Change patient's gown to more easily removable gown with snaps at shoulder if available.	Use of a special IV gown makes gown removal easier and protects VAD site from trauma during gown changes.
3. Open sterile packages using sterile aseptic technique (see Chapter 29).	Maintains sterility of equipment and reduces spread of microorganisms.
4. *Option:* Prepare short extension tubing with needleless connector or stand-alone saline lock (check agency policy and procedures) to attach to VAD catheter hub.	Short extension tubing prevents traction on VAD. Many agencies use short extension tubing for continuous infusions and stand-alone saline locks (capped catheters). Continuous infusion attaches to needleless connector on short extension tubing. Saline locks provide IV access when continuous IV infusions are not needed.
a. Remove protective cap from needleless connector and attach syringe with 1 to 3 mL 0.9% sodium chloride (normal saline), maintaining sterility. Slowly inject enough saline to prime (fill) short extension tubing and connector, removing all air. Leave syringe attached to tubing (see illustration).	Replaces air with normal saline, preventing air from entering patient's vein later during VAD insertion.
b. Maintain sterility of end of connector by reapplying end caps, and set aside for attaching to catheter hub after successful venipuncture.	Prevents touch contamination, which allows microorganisms to enter infusion equipment and bloodstream.
5. ***For continuous infusion:*** Prepare IV tubing and solution	
a. Check IV solution, using six rights of medication administration (see Chapter 32). If using bar-code system, scan bar code on patient's wristband and then on IV fluid container. Be sure that prescribed additives such as potassium or vitamins are included and noted on bag label. Check solution for color, clarity, and expiration date. Check bag for leaks.	IV solutions are medications and need to be checked carefully to reduce risk of error. Bar-code systems reduce medication errors by verifying right patient, medication, dose, route, and time with the electronic health record (EHR) (FitzHenry et al., 2013). Do not use solutions that are discolored, contain particles, or are expired. Do not use leaky bags because they present an opportunity for infection (INS, 2011).

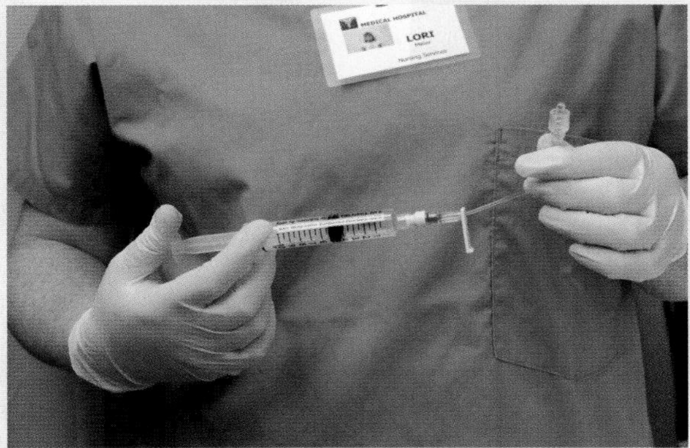

STEP 4a Prime short extension tubing, leaving syringe attached.

SKILL 42-1 INITIATING INTRAVENOUS THERAPY—cont'd

STEP	RATIONALE
b. Open infusion set, maintaining sterility of both ends of tubing. **NOTE:** EIDs sometimes have a special dedicated administration set; follow manufacturer instructions.	Prevents touch contamination, which allows microorganisms to enter infusion equipment and bloodstream.
c. Removing appropriate end caps, attach extension tubing with injection port to distal end of infusion set, maintaining sterility of the connection. Do not touch point of entry of connection. Leave end cap on distal end of extension tubing.	Distal end of extension tubing with injection port attaches to IV catheter hub after venipuncture, providing greater ease of access and ability to change easily between continuous and intermittent IV infusion. Prevents touch contamination, which allows microorganisms to enter infusion equipment and bloodstream.
d. Place roller clamp of IV tubing approximately 2 to 5 cm (1 to 2 inches) below drip chamber and move it to closed position (see illustrations).	Close proximity of roller clamp to drip chamber allows more accurate regulation of flow rate. Closing clamp prevents accidental spillage of IV fluid on patient, nurse, bed, or floor.
e. Remove protective sheath from IV tubing port on plastic IV solution bag or top of IV solution bottle while maintaining sterility (see illustration).	Provides access for insertion of infusion tubing into solution while preventing touch contamination.
f. *Insert infusion set into fluid bag or bottle:* Remove protective cap from tubing insertion spike, not touching spike, and insert it into port of IV bag, using a twisting motion (see illustration). Cleanse rubber stopper on glass-bottled solution with single-use antiseptic and insert spike into rubber stopper of IV bottle.	Prevents contamination of IV solution during insertion of spike. Flat surface on top of bottled solution may contain contaminants, whereas opening to plastic bag is recessed.

CLINICAL DECISION: *Do not touch spike (it is sterile). If contamination occurs (e.g., you accidentally touch outside of bag with the spike or drop spike), discard that IV tubing and obtain a new one.*

STEP	RATIONALE
g. Compress drip chamber and release, allowing it to fill one-half full with infusion fluid (see illustration).	Creates suction effect; fluid enters drip chamber, which prevents air from entering tubing.
h. Prime tubing by filling with IV solution: Remove protector cap on end of tubing if necessary (you can prime some tubing without removing cap) and slowly open roller clamp to allow fluid to travel from drip chamber through tubing to distal end. Maintain sterility of the end. Return roller clamp to closed position after tubing is filled with IV fluid. Replace protective cap on end of tubing if you removed it.	Priming replaces air in tubing with IV solution so air does not enter patient's vein. Slow fill of tubing decreases turbulence and chance of bubble formation. Closing clamp prevents continued flow of IV fluid. Cap on end of tubing maintains system sterility.

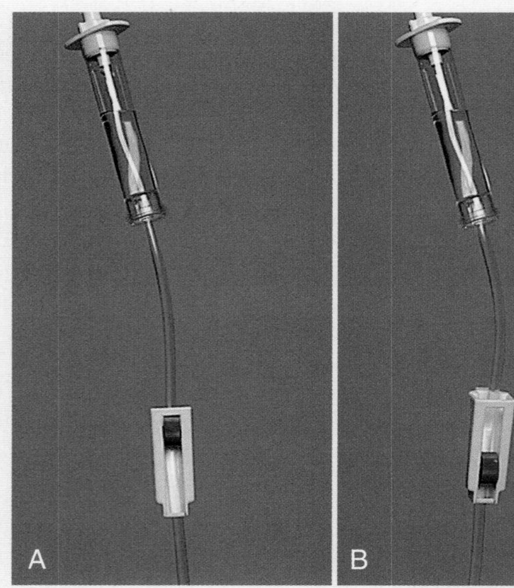

STEP 5d A, Roller clamp in open position. **B,** Roller clamp in off or closed position.

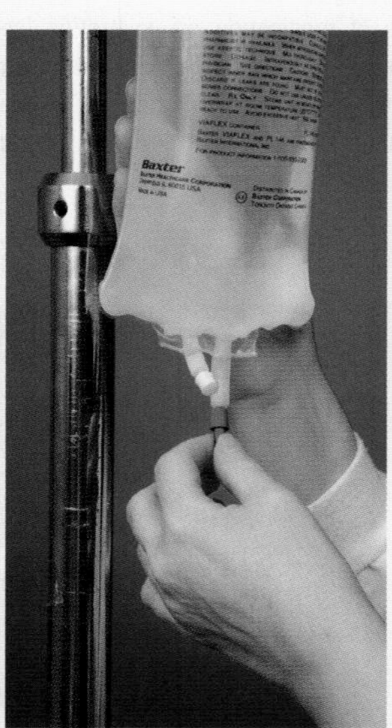

STEP 5e Remove protective covering from IV solution tubing port.

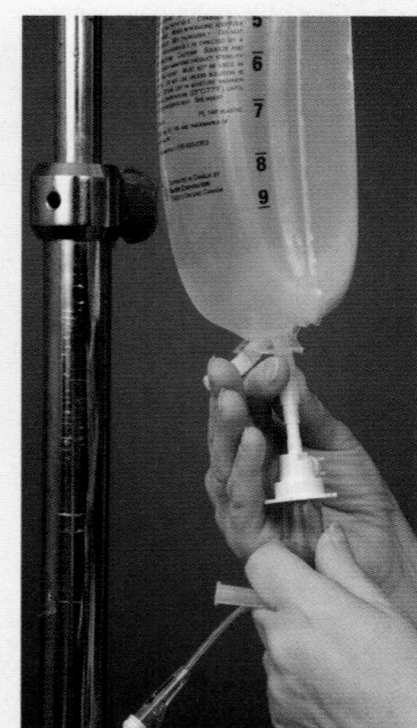

STEP 5f Insert tubing spike into IV container.

STEP	RATIONALE
i. Be certain that tubing is clear of air and air bubbles. To remove small air bubbles, firmly tap tubing where they are located (see illustration). Check entire length of tubing to ensure that all air bubbles are removed. If using multiple-port tubing, turn ports upside down and tap to fill and remove air.	Tapping causes air bubbles to rise up to drip chamber. Large air bubbles may act as emboli (Cook, 2013).
CLINICAL DECISION: *Add long extension tubing to IV tubing to provide more length, which enables patient to move much more freely while still keeping IV line stable.*	
j. If using optional long extension tubing (not short extension tubing in Step 4), remove protective cap and attach it to distal end of IV tubing, maintaining sterility. Then prime the long extension tubing.	Priming replaces air in tubing with IV solution so air does not enter patient's vascular system.
k. Insert primed tubing into EID with power off.	Facilitates starting infusion as soon as IV site is ready.
CLINICAL DECISION: *You can apply gloves before or after assessing veins. You must apply them before VAD insertion.*	
6. Perform hand hygiene and apply clean gloves. Wear eye protection and mask (check agency policy) if splash or spray of blood is possible.	Reduces transmission of microorganisms. Prevents spraying of blood on nurse's mucous membranes.
CLINICAL DECISION: *According to INS (2011), the use of visualization technologies (ultrasound) aids in vein identification and selection. Use an ultrasound device if veins are difficult to visualize or palpate.*	
7. Apply tourniquet to begin vein selection around arm above antecubital fossa or 10 to 15 cm (4 to 6 inches) above proposed insertion site (see illustration). Do not apply it too tightly to avoid injury, bruising the skin, or occluding arterial flow. Check for presence of radial pulse.	Tourniquet needs to be tight enough to decrease venous return but not occlude arterial flow. If patient has fragile veins, apply tourniquet loosely or not at all to prevent damage to veins or bruising. Avoid using antecubital fossa for IV insertion because a VAD at this site limits mobility.
Option a: You may apply tourniquet on top of thin layer of clothing such as a gown sleeve to protect fragile or hairy skin.	
Option b: Use BP cuff instead of tourniquet. Inflate it to a level just below patient's normal diastolic pressure (less than 50 mm Hg).	Use of BP cuff reduces trauma to skin and underlying tissues.
8. Select vein for VAD insertion. Veins on dorsal and ventral surfaces of upper extremities (e.g., cephalic, basilic, and median veins) are preferred in adults (see Figure 42-15).	Ensures adequate vein that is easy to puncture and less likely to rupture.
a. Use most distal site in nondominant arm if possible.	Patients with VAD placement in their dominant hand have decreased ability to perform activities of daily living (ADLs). Performing venipuncture distal to proximal increases availability of other sites for future IV therapy (INS, 2011).

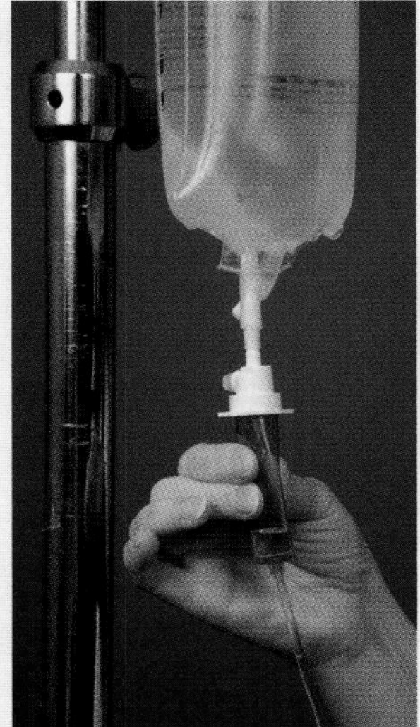

STEP 5g Squeeze drip chamber to fill with fluid.

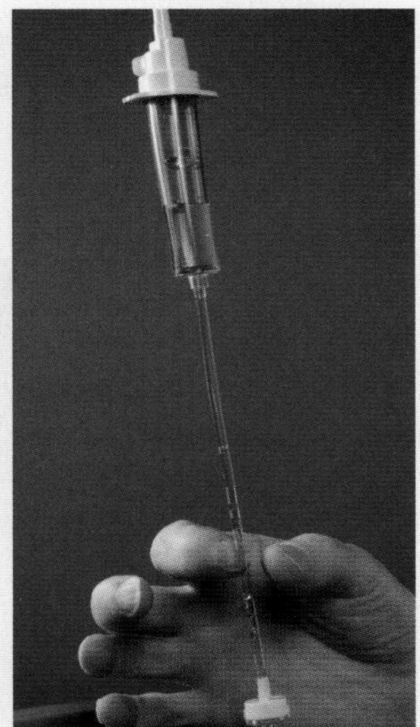

STEP 5i Remove air bubbles from tubing.

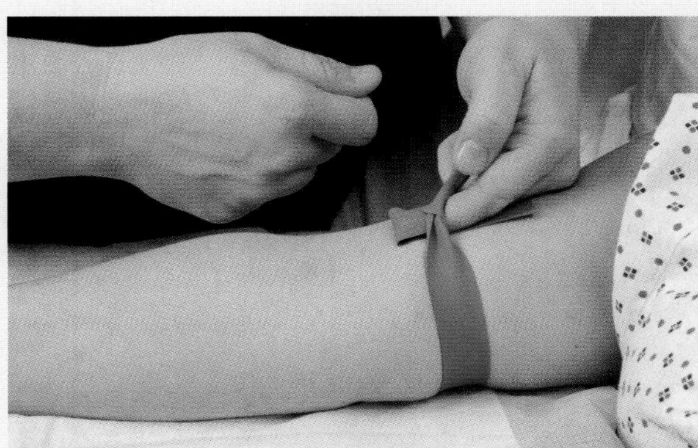

STEP 7 Tourniquet placed on arm for initial vein selection.

SKILL 42-1 INITIATING INTRAVENOUS THERAPY—cont'd

STEP	RATIONALE
b. Select a well-dilated vein. Methods to foster venous distention include:	Increased volume of blood in vein at venipuncture site makes vein more visible.
(1) Place extremity in dependent position.	Gravity promotes venous dilation.
(2) Apply warmth to extremity for several minutes (e.g., with a warm washcloth).	Increases blood in vein by causing dilation.

CLINICAL DECISION: *Vigorous friction and multiple tapping of a vein, especially in older adults, causes hematoma and/or venous constriction. Choose appropriate dilation method.*

STEP	RATIONALE
c. Select vein large enough for a VAD. NOTE: Sometimes you need to remove gloves to palpate vein.	Prevents interruption of venous flow while allowing adequate blood flow around catheter.
d. With your index finger, palpate vein by pressing downward. Note resilient, soft, bouncy feeling while releasing pressure (see illustration).	Fingertip is more sensitive and better for assessing vein location and condition.
e. Avoid vein selection in:	
(1) Area with tenderness, pain, infection, or wound.	May indicate inflamed vein or increase risk of infection.
(2) Extremity affected by previous stroke (cerebrovascular accident [CVA]), paralysis, mastectomy, or dialysis graft.	Increases risk of complications such as lymphedema or vessel damage.
(3) Site distal to previous venipuncture site, sclerosed or hardened veins, infiltrate site or phlebotic vessels, bruised areas, or areas of venous valves.	Such sites cause infiltration around newly placed VAD site and excessive vessel damage.
(4) Fragile dorsal veins in older-adult patients and vessels in an extremity with compromised circulation.	Small, fragile veins have increased risk of infiltration, hematoma from vessel rupture, and phlebitis from vessel damage.
f. Choose a site that does not interfere with patient's ADLs, use of mobility aids such as a cane, or planned procedures. Clip arm hair with scissors if necessary (explain to patient).	Keeps patient as mobile and independent as possible. Hair impedes venipuncture or adherence of dressing.

CLINICAL DECISION: *If hair removal is needed, do not shave area with a razor. Shaving may cause microabrasions that increase risk of infection (INS, 2011).*

STEP	RATIONALE
9. Release tourniquet temporarily and carefully. *Option:* At this point in procedure you may apply a local anesthetic to the planned insertion site; wait several minutes for it to take effect (see product directions). Monitor for allergic reaction.	Restores blood flow and prevents venospasm while preparing for venipuncture. Local anesthetic reduces insertion pain (Ganter-Ritz et al., 2012).
10. Apply clean gloves if not done in Step 6.	Reduces transmission of microorganisms.
11. Place distal end of short infusion tubing (prepared in Step 4) or adaptor end of saline lock nearby on sterile gauze, avoiding touch contamination.	Permits smooth, quick connection to VAD after accessing vein. Prevents microorganisms from entering infusion equipment and bloodstream.
12. If area of insertion needs cleaning, use soap and water first and dry. Use antiseptic swab or applicator to clean insertion site, using friction in a horizontal plane with first swab, in a vertical plane with second swab, and in a circular motion moving outward with third swab (see illustration). Allow to dry completely. Refrain from touching clean site unless using sterile technique.	Mechanical friction penetrates antiseptic solution into cracks and fissures of the skin. Allowing antiseptic solution to air-dry completely reduces microbial counts and risk of phlebitis. Chlorhexidine 2% preparation is preferred (INS, 2011; O'Grady et al., 2011). If your fingers touch clean area, you have introduced microorganisms from your gloves, and you must clean it again (Alexander et al., 2014).

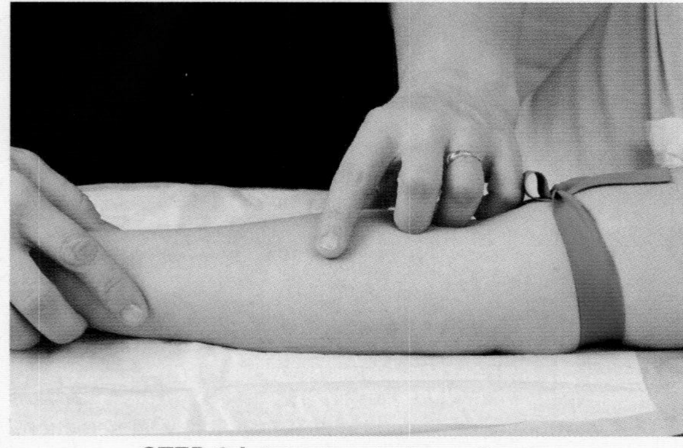

STEP 8d Palpate vein for resilience.

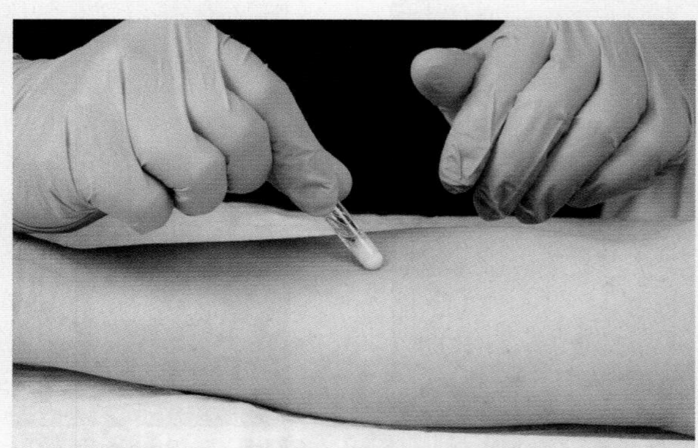

STEP 12 Cleanse site with chlorhexidine.

STEP	RATIONALE
13. Reapply tourniquet or BP cuff 10 to 12 cm (4 to 6 inches) above anticipated insertion site or keep BP cuff inflated <50 mm Hg until venipuncture completed. Check presence of distal pulse.	Diminished arterial flow prevents venous filling. The pressure of the tourniquet causes vein to fill and dilate.
14. Perform venipuncture. Anchor vein by placing thumb over it and stretching skin against direction of insertion 4 to 5 cm (1½ to 2 inches) distal to site (see illustration).	Stabilizes vein for needle insertion. Places VAD parallel to vein.
a. Warn patient of sharp, quick stick.	Prepares patient to avoid movement of extremity during venipuncture.
b. Insert VAD with bevel up at 10- to 30-degree angle slightly distal to actual site of venipuncture in direction of vein (see illustration).	Places needle at optimal angle to vein to reduce risk of puncturing posterior vein wall when entering vein. Superficial veins require smaller insertion angle. Deeper veins require greater angle.

CLINICAL DECISION: *Use each VAD only once for each insertion attempt. If you need to try again, use a new VAD for patient safety and protection from infection.*

STEP	RATIONALE
15. Observe for blood return in flashback chamber of catheter, indicating that needle has entered vein (see illustration A). Lower catheter until almost flush with skin. Advance catheter approximately ¼ inch (0.6 cm) into vein and loosen stylet. Continue to hold skin taut and advance catheter into vein until hub is near venipuncture site (see illustration B). *Do not reinsert stylet once it is loosened.* Advance catheter while safety device automatically retracts stylet. (Techniques for retracting stylet vary with different VADs.) Follow manufacturer guidelines for specific safety catheter use. Place stylet directly into sharps container.	Increased venous pressure caused by tourniquet increases backflow of blood into catheter or tubing. Allows for full penetration of vein wall, placement of catheter in vein lumen, and advancement of catheter off stylet. Reduces risk of introduction of infectious microorganisms along catheter. Advancing entire stylet into vein may penetrate posterior vein wall, causing hematoma. Reinsertion of stylet can cause catheter shearing and potential catheter embolization (INS, 2011). Proper sharps disposal prevents needlestick injury (OSHA, 2012).

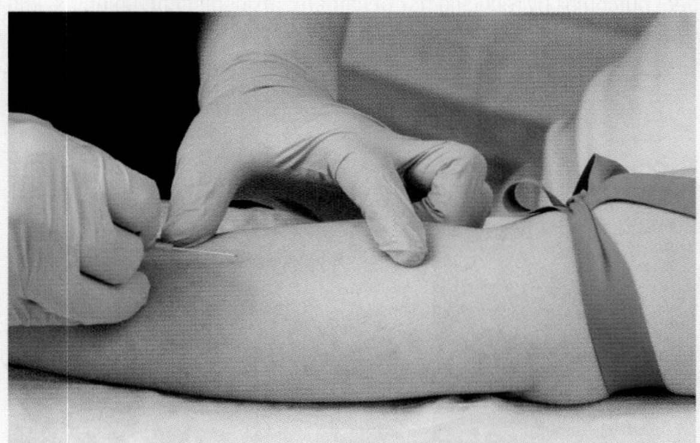

STEP 14 Stabilize vein below insertion site.

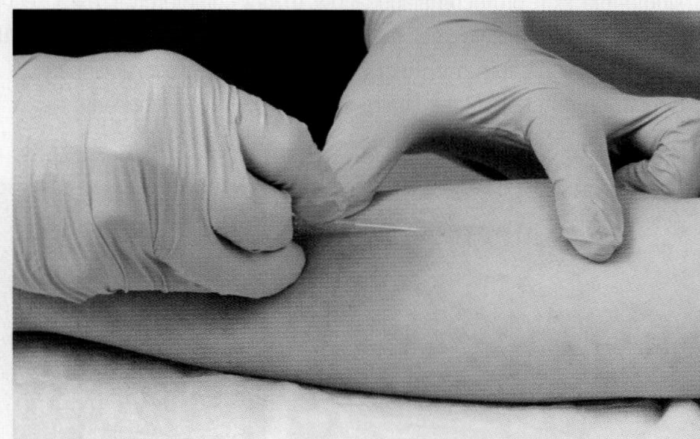

STEP 14b Puncture vein with catheter at a 10- to 30-degree angle. Catheter enters vein.

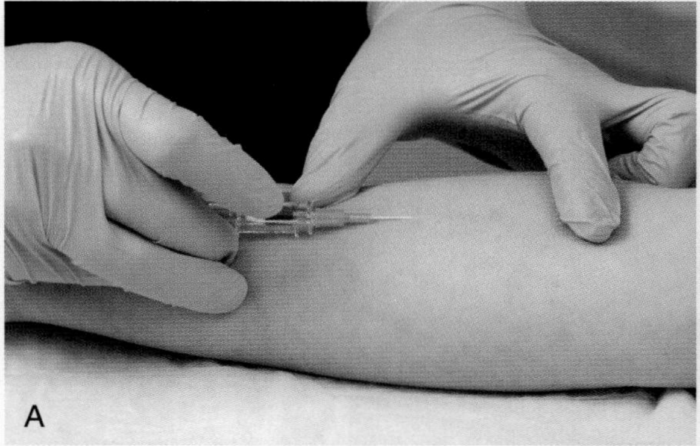

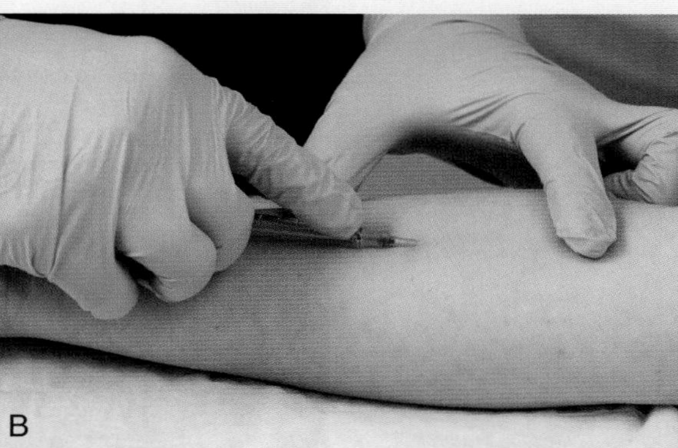

STEP 15 A, Look for blood return in flashback chamber. **B,** Advance catheter into vein until hub is near insertion site.

SKILL 42-1 INITIATING INTRAVENOUS THERAPY—cont'd

STEP	RATIONALE
CLINICAL DECISION: *Each nurse should make no more than two attempts at initiating IV access (INS, 2011). If you are not successful with two attempts, have another nurse attempt the insertion.*	
16. Stabilize catheter with nondominant hand and release tourniquet or BP cuff with other. Apply gentle but firm pressure with middle finger of nondominant hand 3 cm (1¼ inches) above insertion site. Keep catheter stable with index finger.	Permits venous flow. Pressure with finger on vein reduces backflow of blood and allows connection with short extension tubing or saline lock with minimal blood loss (INS, 2011).
17. Quickly connect distal end of primed short extension tubing from Step 11 or end of a prepared saline lock from Step 4 to catheter. Do not touch point of entry of connection. Secure connection.	Prompt connection of infusion set maintains patency of vein and prevents risk for exposure to blood. Maintains sterility.
18. If saline lock is attached, gently flush catheter with attached saline syringe to ensure that site is patent (see illustration). Observe for swelling at site while flushing. Then remove syringe.	Provides patient safety by not beginning infusion if site is not patent. Swelling during flush indicates infiltration, and site must be discontinued.
19. For continuous infusion, attach distal end of IV tubing to needleless connector on short extension tubing that is attached to catheter (see illustration). Turn on EID, program it, and begin infusion at correct rate (see Skill 42-2). If using gravity flow instead of EID, begin infusion by slowly opening roller clamp to regulate rate.	Initiates flow of fluid through IV catheter, preventing clotting of device.
CLINICAL DECISION: *Be sure to calculate rate (see Skill 42-2) and set EID correctly to infuse IV solution at prescribed rate.*	
20. Observe insertion site for swelling.	Swelling indicates infiltration, which requires immediate catheter removal.
21. Secure catheter and apply sterile dressing over site (procedures differ; follow agency policy).	Prevents accidental dislodgement of catheter and protects site from infection.
a. *Manufactured catheter stabilization device:* Wipe selected area with single-use skin protectant and allow to dry completely (10-15 seconds). Apply sterile adhesive strip over catheter hub. Place retainer over tubing end just behind spin nut. Peel off half of liner; press to adhere to skin. Repeat on other side (see Figure 42-17). Then apply dressing.	A manufactured catheter stabilization device holds the catheter in place, improving patient outcomes by reducing risk of catheter dislodgement, phlebitis, and other complications (INS, 2011).

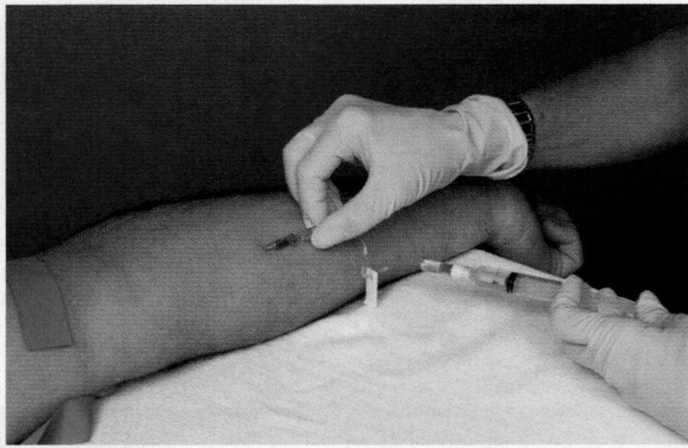

STEP 18 Flush catheter gently to ensure patency.

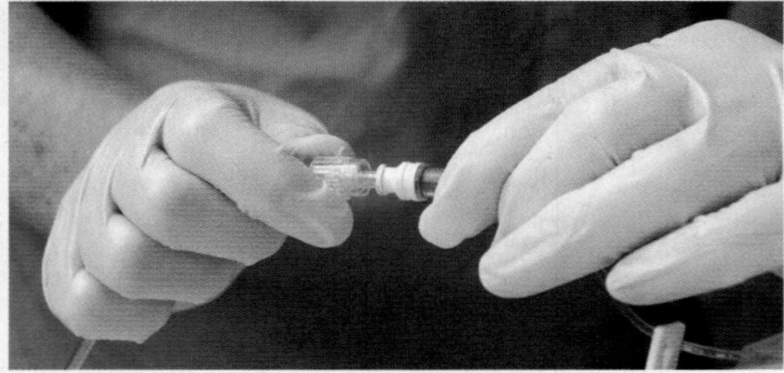

STEP 19 Connect IV tubing to short extension set that is attached to catheter.

STEP	RATIONALE
b. *Transparent dressing:* Continue to secure catheter with nondominant hand.	Prevents accidental dislodgement of catheter.
(1) Remove adherent backing. Apply one edge of dressing and gently smooth remaining dressing over IV site, leaving connection between IV tubing and catheter hub uncovered. Remove outer covering and smooth dressing gently over site (see illustration).	Occlusive dressing protects site from bacterial contamination. Connection between administration set and hub needs to be uncovered to facilitate changing tubing if necessary.
(2) After applying the transparent dressing, secure catheter by placing a 2.5-cm (1-inch) piece of transparent tape over extension tubing or administration set. Do not apply tape on top of transparent dressing.	Removal of tape from transparent dressing might cause accidental dislodgement of catheter. Tape on top of transparent dressing prevents moisture from being carried away from skin.
c. *Sterile gauze dressing:* If manufactured catheter stabilization device is not used, secure catheter by placing a narrow piece ($\frac{1}{2}$ inch) of sterile tape over catheter hub (see illustration). Place sterile tape only on hub, *never* over insertion site. Secure site for easy visualization. Avoid applying tape or gauze around arm.	Less frequently used than transparent dressing. Prevents accidental removal of catheter from vein. Prevents back-and-forth motion, which can irritate vein and introduce microorganisms on skin into vein. Sterile tape prevents site contamination. Wrapping anything around arm compresses veins or prevents visualization of insertion site.
(1) Place 2 × 2 gauze pad over insertion site and catheter hub. Secure all edges with tape (see illustration). Do not cover connection between IV tubing and catheter hub.	Secure dressing is less likely to allow entrance of microorganisms.
(2) *Option:* Fold 2 × 2 gauze pad in half and cover with a 2.5 cm (1 inch)–wide tape extending about an inch from each side. Place under tubing/catheter hub junction.	Tape on top of gauze makes it easier to access hub/tubing junction. Gauze pad elevates hub off skin to prevent pressure area.

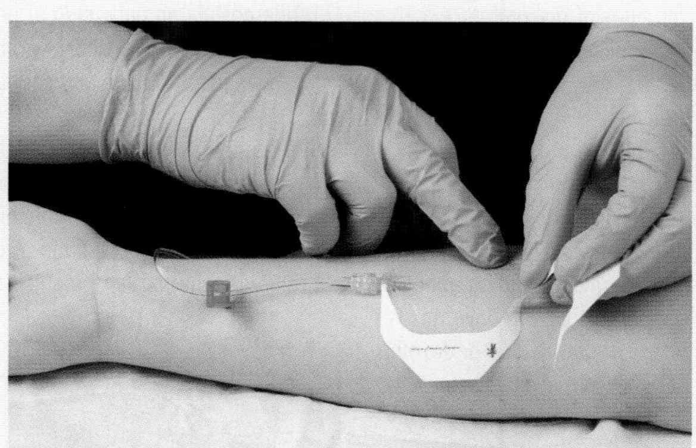

STEP 21b(1) Apply transparent dressing.

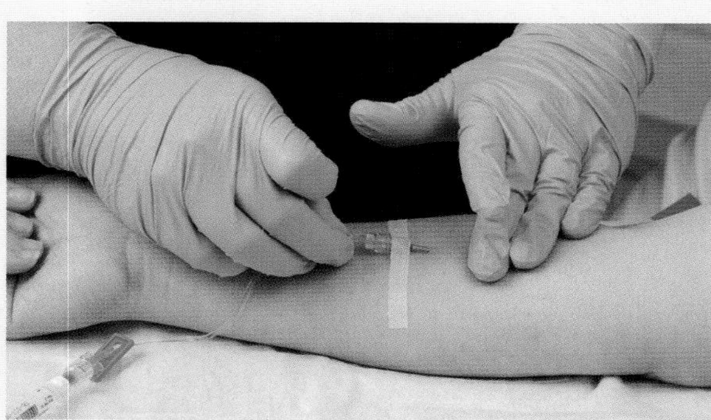

STEP 21c Apply tape over catheter hub.

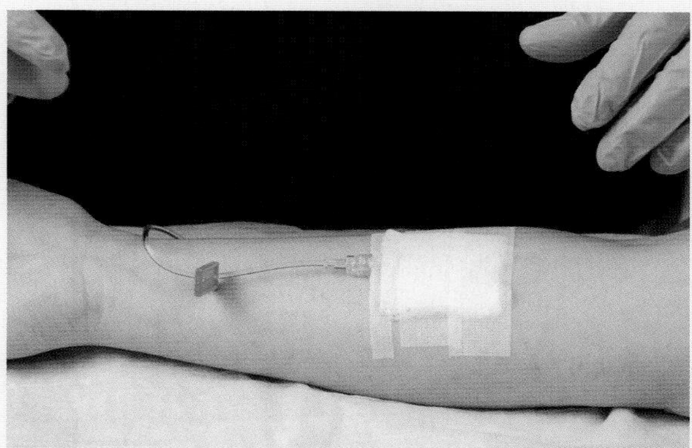

STEP 21c(1) Place 2 × 2–inch gauze over insertion site and catheter hub.

SKILL 42-1 INITIATING INTRAVENOUS THERAPY—cont'd

STEP	RATIONALE
CLINICAL DECISION: *Think carefully about where you place tape. Do not apply it over the catheter insertion site, over the connection between the tubing or port and the IV catheter hub, or on top of the transparent dressing.*	
22. Curl loop of tubing alongside arm and place second piece of tape directly over tubing to secure it (see illustration).	Securing loop of tubing reduces risk of dislodging catheter if IV tubing is pulled (i.e., loop comes apart before catheter dislodges).
23. For continuous infusion, check ordered rate of infusion programmed into EID and be sure that it is functioning properly. If using gravity-flow IV infusion, recheck flow rate to correct drops per minute (see Skill 42-2).	Manipulation of catheter during dressing application may alter flow rate. Check flow rate to maintain accurate administration of IV fluids. Flow can fluctuate; thus it must be checked at intervals for accuracy.
24. Label dressing per agency policy. Include date and time of IV insertion, VAD gauge and length, and your initials (see illustration).	Provides immediate access to data regarding when IV was inserted and when to rotate site.
25. Dispose of used stylet or other sharps in appropriate sharps container if not done previously. Discard supplies. Remove gloves and perform hand hygiene.	Reduces transmission of microorganisms, prevents accidental injuries, and follows guidelines for disposal of sharps (OSHA, 2012).
26. Teach patient how to move or turn without dislodging VAD.	Prevents accidental dislodgement of catheter.
EVALUATION	
1. Observe patient every 1 to 2 hours.	Allows you to confirm integrity of IV site and system.
a. Check that correct amount of IV fluid has infused by observing fluid level in IV container.	Administration of prescribed amount of fluid maintains or restores fluid balance.
b. Check rate on EID or count drip rate (if gravity drip).	Accurate monitoring of rate further ensures administration of correct amount of fluid.
c. Check patency of VAD.	Flow rate slows or stops if catheter becomes partially occluded or obstructed.
CLINICAL DECISION: *If IV line is positional, fluid runs quickly, slowly, or stops, depending on position of patient's arm. Instruct patient to position arm to maintain flow; if this continues, consider restarting IV in another site.*	
d. Observe patient during palpation of vessel for signs of discomfort.	Tenderness is an early sign of phlebitis.
e. Inspect insertion site, note skin color (e.g., redness, pallor). Inspect for presence of swelling, infiltration (see Table 42-13), and phlebitis (see Table 42-14). Palpate temperature of skin above dressing.	Redness, tenderness, and warmth indicate vein inflammation or phlebitis. Swelling above insertion site and cool temperature often indicate infiltration of fluid into tissues.
2. Change peripheral IV access per agency policy, per health care provider's orders, or immediately on suspected contamination or complication.	INS standards recommend VAD replacement and site rotation when clinically indicated rather than at set intervals (INS, 2011).
3. Observe patient to determine response to therapy (e.g., measure intake and output [I&O], daily weights, vital signs).	IV fluids and additives are administered to maintain or restore fluid and electrolyte balance. Early recognition of complications leads to prompt treatment.
4. Use ***Teach Back*** to determine patient's and family's understanding about IV therapy. State, "I want to be sure I explained the reason that you have this IV. Can you explain why you have the IV?" Revise your instruction now or develop plan for revised teaching if patient or family is not able to teach back correctly.	Evaluates what patient is able to explain or demonstrate.

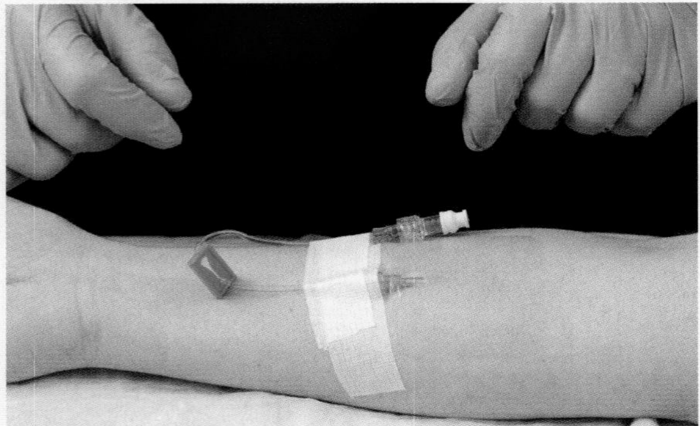

STEP 22 Curl a loop of the short or long intravenous tubing alongside the arm. Secure tubing.

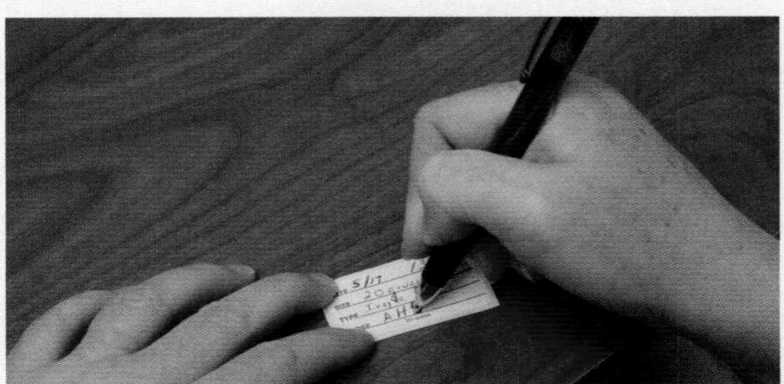

STEP 24 Label IV dressing.

UNEXPECTED OUTCOMES AND RELATED INTERVENTIONS

1. Overload of IV solution, infiltration, phlebitis, local infection, and bleeding at venipuncture site
   - See Table 42-12.
2. Lack of effectiveness of IV therapy for ECV
   - Notify patient's health care provider, providing baseline and current heart rate and BP and length of time IV has been infusing; adjust infusion rate or type of IV solution as ordered.
   - Be prepared to draw blood for laboratory testing.

RECORDING AND REPORTING

- Document in nurses' notes or other designated location in an electronic health record (EHR) date and time of insertion; number and sites of attempts, precise description of insertion site (e.g., cephalic vein on dorsal surface of right lower arm, 2.5 cm above wrist); catheter gauge, type, length, and brand; type of dressing and catheter stabilization; flow rate; type of infusion, EID use, and your identity (INS, 2011). If using bar-code system, fluid type and time record automatically.
- Record patient's status, IV fluid, amount infused, and integrity and patency of system.
- Document your evaluation of patient learning.
- Report to oncoming nursing staff: type of fluid, flow rate, status of VAD, amount of fluid remaining in present container, expected time to hang subsequent IV container, and patient condition.
- Report to health care provider any adverse reactions.

HOME CARE CONSIDERATIONS

- Ensure that patient is able and willing to self-administer IV therapy or that a reliable family caregiver will provide IV therapy at home.
- Teach patient and family caregiver information needed to administer IV therapy safely (see Box 42-8). Consider their cultural norms (e.g., health beliefs and comfort with caregivers using touch) (Petroulias et al., 2013).

SKILL 42-2 REGULATING INTRAVENOUS FLOW RATE

DELEGATION CONSIDERATIONS

The skill of regulating intravenous (IV) flow rate cannot be delegated to nursing assistive personnel (NAP). Instruct the NAP to inform you if:

- Patient indicates burning, bleeding, swelling, or coolness at catheter insertion site.
- Electronic infusion device (EID) alarm signals.
- Fluid container is almost empty.

EQUIPMENT

- EID, IV pump
- Watch with second hand
- Calculator or paper and pen/pencil
- Tape
- Label
- Clean gloves

STEP	RATIONALE
ASSESSMENT	
1. Review accuracy and completeness of health care provider's order for patient name, type, and amount of IV fluid, medication additives, infusion time, and purpose of infusion. Follow six rights of medication administration (see Chapter 32).	Ensures administration of correct IV fluid at proper rate. IV fluids are medications. The six rights prevent medication administration error.
2. Perform hand hygiene and apply clean gloves.	Prevents transmission of microorganisms.
3. Observe for patency of IV tubing and vascular access device (VAD).	For fluid to infuse at proper rate, IV line and VAD must be free of kinks, knots, and clots.
4. Identify patient using two identifiers (e.g., name and birthday or name and medical record number) according to agency policy. Compare identifiers with information on the patient's MAR or medical record.	Ensures correct patient. Complies with The Joint Commission standards and improves patient safety (TJC, 2016).
5. Inspect IV site and verify with patient how existing IV feels (e.g., determine if any tenderness, pain, or burning exists).	Tenderness, pain, or burning may be early indication of phlebitis. Includes patient in own care.
6. Assess patient's knowledge of how positioning of IV site affects flow rate.	Fosters patient participation in maintaining most effective position of arm with IV equipment.
7. Assess patient risk for fluid and electrolyte imbalance, given type of IV fluid (e.g., neonate, cardiac or kidney disease)	Helps prioritize nursing assessments.

SKILL 42-2 REGULATING INTRAVENOUS FLOW RATE—cont'd

STEP	RATIONALE
PLANNING	
1. Gather paper and pencil or calculator to calculate flow rate.	Use accurate mathematical calculations to obtain correct rate for patient safety.
2. Check order to see how long each liter of fluid should infuse. If hourly rate (mL/hr) is not provided in order, calculate it by dividing volume by hours. For example: $\text{mL/hr} = \frac{\text{Total infusion volume (mL)}}{\text{Hours of infusion}}$ 1000 mL/8 hr = 125 mL/hr or if 3 L is ordered for 24 hours, 3000 mL/24 hr = 125 mL/hr	Provides even infusion of fluid over prescribed hourly rate. A volume of 1 L = 1000 mL.

CLINICAL DECISION: *It is common for health care providers to write an abbreviated IV order such as "D_5W with 20 mEq KCl 125 mL/hr continuous." This order implies that IV infusion should be maintained at this rate until an order has been written for IV infusion to be discontinued. Occasionally an IV order calls for 1 L "TKO" (to keep open) or "KVO (keep vein open)," either of which means at a slow rate to keep vein open. Clarify with the provider if any part of the order is unclear.*

STEP	RATIONALE
3. If KVO (or TKO) rate is ordered, check agency policy regarding flow rate. KVO often falls in the range of 10 to 25 mL/hr.	KVO rate prevents catheter clotting, thus preserving venous access while infusing a minimal amount of fluid.
4. Use hourly rate to program electronic infusion device (EID) (see Implementation) or, if gravity-flow infusion, use to calculate minute flow rate (gtt/min).	EID automatically delivers correct minute flow rate. Gravity infusion requires nurse calculation.
5. Calculate minute flow rate for gravity-flow infusion:	Use microdrip tubing when infusing small or very precise volumes. Use macrodrip tubing to infuse fluid more rapidly.
a. Determine drop factor (calibration) in drops per milliliter (gtt/mL) of infusion set currently in use: *Microdrip:* 60 gtt/mL *Macrodrip:* 10 or 15 gtt/mL; see label on administration set packaging.	Drop factor for macrodrip tubing varies with manufacturer.
b. Select one of the following formulas to calculate minute flow rate (drops/min) based on drop factor of infusion set: **(1)** mL/hr/60 min = mL/min Drop factor × mL/min = gtt/min Or **(2)** mL/hr × drop factor/60 min = gtt/min Using formula (2) above, calculate minute flow rate for an IV solution that should infuse at 125 mL/hr:	Formulas compute correct flow rate over a minute.
Microdrip: 125 mL/hr × 60 gtt/mL = 7500 gtt/hr 7500 gtt ÷ 60 minutes = 125 gtt/min	When using microdrip, mL/hr always equals gtt/min.
Macrodrip: 125 mL/hr × 15 gtt/mL = 1875 gtt/hr 1875 gtt ÷ 60 minutes = 31-32 gtt/min	Multiply hourly rate (mL/hr) by drop factor and divide product by 60 to convert hours to minutes.
IMPLEMENTATION	
1. Using an EID (infusion pump or smart pump):	Smart pumps with medication safety software are designed for administration of IV fluid that contains medications.
a. Consult manufacturer directions for setup of infusion. Use tubing compatible with EID.	Special infusion tubing is required for most EIDs. It is designed to prevent free flow of fluid when tubing is removed from device. Check agency equipment and associated policies and procedures.

STEP	RATIONALE
b. Close roller clamp on primed IV tubing and insert tubing into chamber of EID control mechanism or pump module per manufacturer directions (see illustration). Roller clamp on IV tubing goes between EID and patient.	Most electronic infusion pumps use positive pressure to infuse. They move fluid through IV tubing by compressing and milking tubing.
c. Turn on EID power; test alarm; select required volume per hour, volume to be infused (VTBI), and any other information required. Close control chamber door if not already done and press run/start button. If smart pump alarms immediately and shuts down, your settings were outside unit parameters. Recalculate infusion rate and set EID again.	Program EID per manufacturer instructions for patient safety. Smart pumps require additional information such as patient unit and medication. They contain a computer that matches pump setting against a drug dose database (Harding, 2013). If your setting does not match database, pump alarms and automatically shuts down for patient safety.
d. Open roller clamp completely while EID is in use.	Ensures that EID regulates infusion rate.
e. Check intermittently (hourly for adults, more frequently for pediatric patients) to see that correct amount of IV fluid has infused by observing fluid level in IV container.	EIDs do not replace frequent, accurate nursing evaluation. They may continue to infuse IV fluids even after an infiltration or other complication.
f. Assess patency of system if EID alarm signals.	Alarm indicates problem in system. An empty solution container, kinked tubing, air in tubing, closed clamp, infiltration, clotted catheter, and/or low battery all trigger EID alarm.
2. Using gravity flow:	
a. Ensure that IV container is 36 inches above IV site for adults.	Pressure caused by gravity is necessary to overcome venous pressure and resistance from tubing and catheter.
b. Slowly open roller clamp on tubing until you can see drops in drip chamber. Hold a watch with second hand at same level as drip chamber and count drip rate for 1 minute (see illustration). Adjust roller clamp to increase or decrease drip rate until you obtain desired number of drops per minute.	Regulate to prescribed rate of fluid infusion.
c. Monitor drip rate at least hourly.	Many factors influence drip rate; frequent monitoring ensures IV fluid administration as prescribed.
3. Attach piece of tape or label to IV fluid container with date and time of container change (check agency policy). If using polyvinylchloride (PVC) container, mark only on label and not container.	Provides reference to determine next time for container change, especially with KVO rate. Ink may leak into IV fluid through PVC container.
4. Instruct patient to avoid raising arm with IV line because it can affect flow rate; to avoid touching control clamp or other equipment; and about purpose of EID alarms.	Provides information so patient does not alter infusion rate. Ask patient to instruct family if appropriate.
5. Remove and discard gloves, perform hand hygiene.	Reduces transmission of microorganisms.

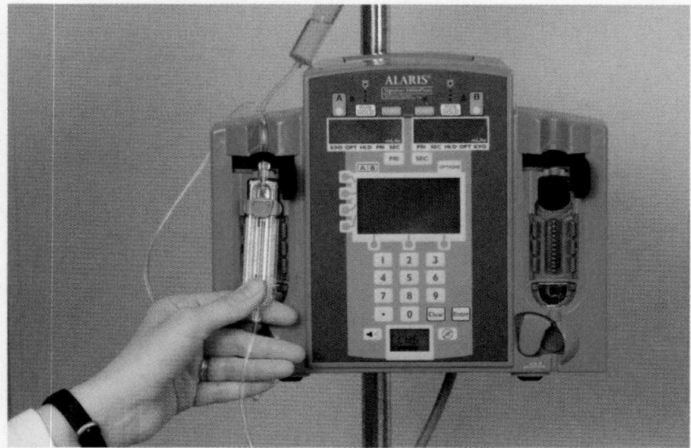

STEP 1b Insert IV tubing into chamber of control mechanism of electronic infusion device.

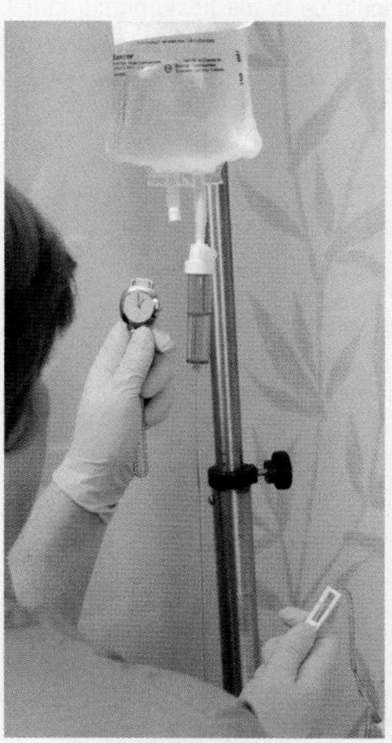
STEP 2b Nurse counting drip rate on gravity-flow infusion.

SKILL 42-2 REGULATING INTRAVENOUS FLOW RATE—cont'd

STEP	RATIONALE
EVALUATION	
1. Monitor IV infusion at least every hour, noting volume of IV fluid infused and rate.	Ensures that correct volume infuses over prescribed time period.
2. Observe patient for signs of overhydration or dehydration to determine response to therapy and restoration of fluid balance.	Signs and symptoms of new overhydration or continued dehydration warrant changing rate of fluid infused. Contact health care provider for new infusion rate order.
3. Evaluate for signs of infiltration, inflammation at site, kink or knot in infusion tubing, or occluded VAD.	Prevents or identifies conditions that decrease or stop flow rate.
4. Use ***Teach Back*** to determine patient's and family's understanding about arm position. State, "I want to be sure I explained how your arm position can affect the IV flow. Can you show me a correct arm position?" Revise your instructions now or develop a plan for revised patient teaching if patient is not able to teach back correctly.	Evaluates what patient is able to explain or demonstrate.

UNEXPECTED OUTCOMES AND RELATED INTERVENTIONS

1. Sudden infusion of large fluid volume of solution. Patient has symptoms of dyspnea, crackles in lungs, and increased urinary output, indicating fluid overload.
   - Temporarily slow infusion rate to 10 gtt/min; notify health care provider.
   - Place patient in high-Fowler's position.
   - See Table 42-12.
2. IV fluid container empties with subsequent loss of VAD patency.
   - Discontinue present IV infusion and start new IV line in other extremity or proximal to previous insertion site.
3. IV fluid infuses slower than prescribed.
   - Check for positional change that might affect rate, EID malfunction (or insufficient height of IV fluid container with gravity flow), kinking or obstruction of tubing, infiltration, or other complications at VAD site.
   - Consult health care provider for new order to provide necessary fluid volume.

RECORDING AND REPORTING

- Record rate of infusion in milliliters per hour (or drops per minute with gravity flow) in designated location in patient's medical record.
- Document use of EID.
- Immediately record any new IV fluid rate.
- At change of shift or when leaving on break, report rate and volume left of infusion to nurse in charge or next nurse assigned to care for patient.
- Document your evaluation of patient learning.

HOME CARE CONSIDERATIONS

- Ensure that patient or family caregiver is able and willing to operate infusion pump and administer IV therapy. Assess for any visual or physical limitations with ability to connect and disconnect infusion therapy and problem solve infusion pump malfunction (Alexander et al., 2014).
- Home care nurse should be in the home during initiation of infusion therapy to ensure correct pump settings for solution, rate, time, and alarms. The nurse ensures that EID functions properly before use and that patient's electrical outlets are properly grounded.
- Provide a 24-hour access telephone number for patient to call for assistance.

SKILL 42-3 MAINTENANCE OF INTRAVENOUS SYSTEM

DELEGATION CONSIDERATIONS

The skills of changing an intravenous (IV) fluid container and tubing cannot be delegated to nursing assistive personnel (NAP). Instruct the NAP to:

- Watch for appropriate position of patient to avoid kinking of intravenous IV tubing and injury at insertion site.
- Report when the IV fluid container is nearly empty.
- Report any leakage that occurs from or around the IV site.
- Report observations of changes in patient's temperature or signs and symptoms of IV-related complications such as pain or tenderness around IV site.

EQUIPMENT

Changing an IV fluid container and tubing (continuous infusion)

- Clean gloves
- Correct type and volume of IV solution
- Infusion tubing
- Tape or tubing label
- Pen
- Filter (size appropriate to solution) and extension tubing (if necessary)
- Manufactured catheter stabilization device if available
- Handheld bar-code scanner if using bar-code system

Changing an IV fluid container and tubing (intermittent infusion or saline lock)

- Correct type and volume of IV solution
- Infusion tubing
- Tape or tubing label
- Pen
- Prefilled 5-mL syringe with flush agent (preservative-free sterile 0.9% sodium chloride (normal saline) for adults) (INS, 2011).
- Sterile 2 × 2 gauze pads (optional)
- Clean gloves
- Antiseptic swab (chlorhexidine 2% preferred [INS, 2011])
- Handheld bar-code scanner if using bar-code system

Discontinuing peripheral IV access

- Clean gloves
- Sterile 2 × 2 or 4 × 4 gauze pad
- Antiseptic swab (chlorhexidine 2% preferred [INS, 2011])
- Tape

STEP	RATIONALE
ASSESSMENT	
1. Changing IV fluid container:	
a. Review accuracy and completeness of health care provider's order for patient name, type and amount of IV fluid, medication additives, infusion time, and purpose of infusion. Follow six rights of medication administration (see Chapter 32). If order is written for KVO (keep vein open) or TKO (to keep open), note date and time of last fluid container change and refer to agency policy to determine need for IV fluid container change.	Provides patient safety by preventing medication errors. Agency policy determines how often IV fluid container change is required for KVO infusion rate.
b. Determine compatibility of all IV fluids and additives by consulting approved online database, drug reference book, or pharmacist.	Incompatibilities cause physical and chemical changes with adverse patient outcomes.
2. Changing IV tubing:	
a. Assess current tubing for puncture, contamination, or occlusion, which requires immediate tubing change.	Compromised tubing allows fluid leakage, bacterial contamination, and entry of pathogens into patient's bloodstream. Whole blood, blood component products, or incompatible mixtures can occlude or partially occlude tubing because viscous solutions adhere to walls of tubing, decreasing size of lumen.
b. Note date and time of last IV tubing change. Agency policy indicates frequency of routine change for IV administration sets and saline/heparin locks.	INS recommends changing continuous IV tubing no more often than 96-hour intervals unless tubing becomes compromised. Change primary intermittent tubing set every 24 hours (INS, 2011).
3. Discontinuing peripheral IV access: Review accuracy and completeness of health care provider's order for discontinuing IV therapy.	Order required for discontinuing IV therapy.
4. Identify patient using two identifiers (e.g., name and birthday or name and medical record number) according to agency policy. Compare identifiers with information on patient's MAR or medical record. If using bar-code system, scan bar code on patient's wristband and then on IV fluid container.	Ensures correct patient. Complies with The Joint Commission standards and improves patient safety (TJC, 2016). Bar-code systems reduce medication errors by verifying right patient, medication, dose, and time with EHR (FitzHenry et al., 2013).
5. Determine patient's/family member's understanding of need for IV therapy or reason for discontinuing it.	Reveals need for patient teaching.

SKILL 42-3 MAINTENANCE OF INTRAVENOUS SYSTEM—cont'd

STEP	RATIONALE
PLANNING	
1. Collect appropriate equipment, perform hand hygiene, and arrange equipment at patient's bedside.	Keeps procedure organized and provides patient safety. Hand hygiene reduces transmission of microorganisms.
For changing IV fluid container: Have next solution prepared at least 1 hour before needed. If prepared in pharmacy, ensure that it has been delivered to patient care unit. Check that solution is correct and properly labeled. Allow solution to warm to room temperature if refrigerated. Follow six rights of medication administration and verify solution expiration date. Observe for precipitate, discoloration, and leakage.	Adequate planning for changing solution reduces risk of clot formation at catheter tip caused by lack of flow from empty IV container. Checking that solution is correct prevents medication error (Alexander et al., 2014).
2. Coordinate tubing changes with IV fluid container changes if possible.	Promotes patient safety by reducing number of times IV system is open.
3. Explain to patient/family member procedure, its purpose, and what is expected of patient.	Promotes patient cooperation and decreases anxiety.
For discontinuing peripheral IV access: Explain that patient must hold extremity still; that he or she may feel burning sensation when you remove catheter; and that procedure will take about 5 minutes.	
IMPLEMENTATION	
1. Changing IV fluid container:	
a. Determine patency of current vascular access device (VAD) site: Look for swelling, coolness to touch, or tenderness around VAD site. With EID use, VAD should be patent if site is not infiltrated and EID functions without alarm signals. If not using EID, carefully adjust roller clamp to see an increase in flow rate and then regulate back to prescribed rate.	New IV access site is necessary if infiltration or phlebitis is present, IV tubing is compromised, or VAD site is not patent. EID alarm signals when system is occluded. In absence of EID, adjusting roller clamp increases flow rate if there is no obstruction.

CLINICAL DECISION: *Lowering IV container below level of IV site for presence of blood return (retrograde) is an unreliable indicator of patency.*

STEP	RATIONALE
b. Prepare to change solution when approximately 50 mL of fluid remains in container. Be sure that drip chamber is at least half full.	Prevents air from entering tubing and vein from clotting from lack of flow.
c. Prepare new IV fluid container for changing. If using plastic bag, hang on IV pole and remove protective cover from IV tubing port. If using glass bottle, remove metal cap and disks.	Permits quick, smooth, and organized change from old to new IV fluid container.
d. Close roller clamp to stop flow of existing infusion. Remove tubing from EID. Then remove old IV fluid container from IV pole and hold it with tubing port pointing upward.	Prevents solution remaining in drip chamber from emptying while changing IV fluid container. Port held upward prevents IV fluid from spilling.
e. Quickly remove spike from old solution container (see illustration) and, without touching tip, insert it into new container (see illustration).	Reduces risk of solution in drip chamber running dry and maintains sterility.

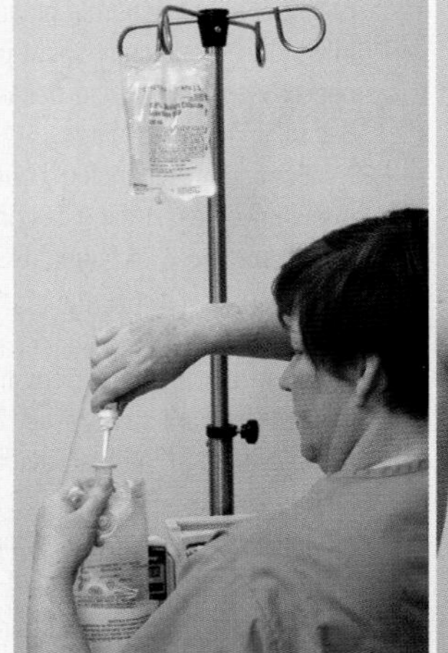
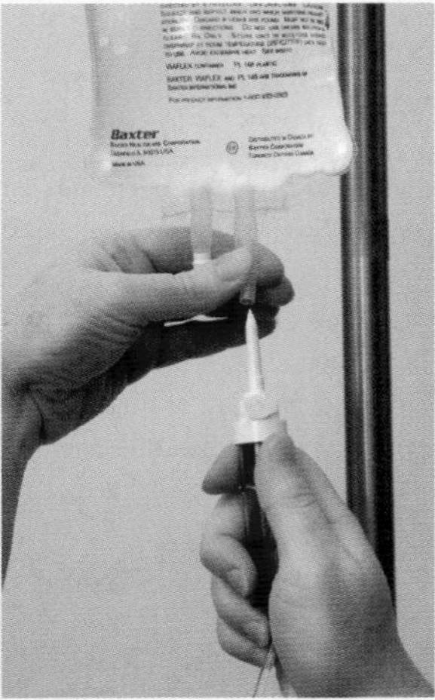

STEP 1e A, Quickly remove spike from old solution container. **B,** Without touching tip, insert spike into new container.

STEP	RATIONALE
CLINICAL DECISION: *If you contaminate the spike, discard that IV tubing and use a new one.*	
f. Hang new fluid container on IV pole.	Gravity helps delivery of fluid into drip chamber.
g. Check for air in tubing. If bubbles form, remove them by closing roller clamp below them, stretching tubing downward, and tapping tubing with finger (bubbles rise in fluid to drip chamber) (see illustration). For larger amount of air, swab the port below the air with alcohol and allow to dry; insert needleless syringe into port and aspirate air into syringe.	Reduces risk of air descending the tubing. Use of air-eliminating filter also reduces this risk.
h. Make sure that drip chamber is one-third to one-half full. If it is too full, pinch off tubing below it, invert container, squeeze drip chamber (see illustration) to push fluid into container, release tubing, and hang container.	Reduces risk of air entering tubing. If chamber is completely filled, you cannot observe drips.
i. Insert tubing into EID and restart pump. If no EID, regulate flow to prescribed rate with roller clamp.	Delivers IV fluid as ordered.
j. Attach piece of tape or label to IV fluid container with date and time of container change (check agency policy). If using polyvinylchloride (PVC) container, mark only on label and not container.	Provides reference to determine next time for container change, especially with KVO rate. Ink may leak into IV fluid through PVC container.
2. Changing IV tubing:	
a. Open new infusion set and connect add-on pieces (e.g., filter, extension tubing). Keep protective coverings over infusion spike and distal connector for VAD. Secure all connections.	Protective covers maintain sterility of IV system. Securing connections reduces risk of contamination, infection, and hemorrhage.
b. Apply clean gloves.	Reduces transmission of microorganisms (OSHA, 2012).
c. If catheter hub is not accessible, remove IV dressing as directed in Skill 42-4. Do not remove catheter-securing device, transparent dressing, or tape that secures catheter hub to skin.	Catheter hub must be accessible to provide smooth transition when removing old and inserting new tubing.

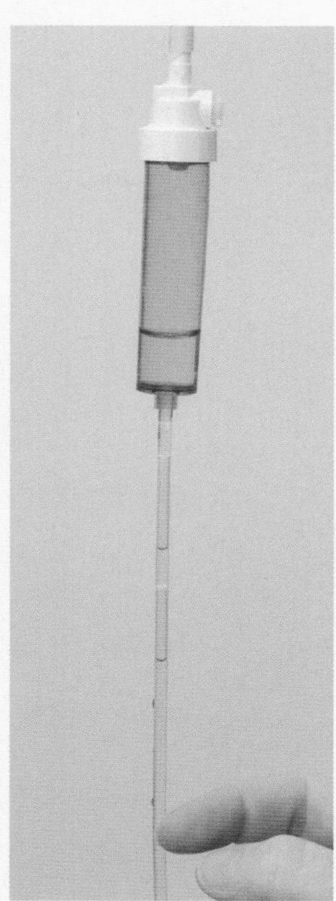

STEP 1g Nurse taps tubing to cause air bubbles to rise up to drip chamber.

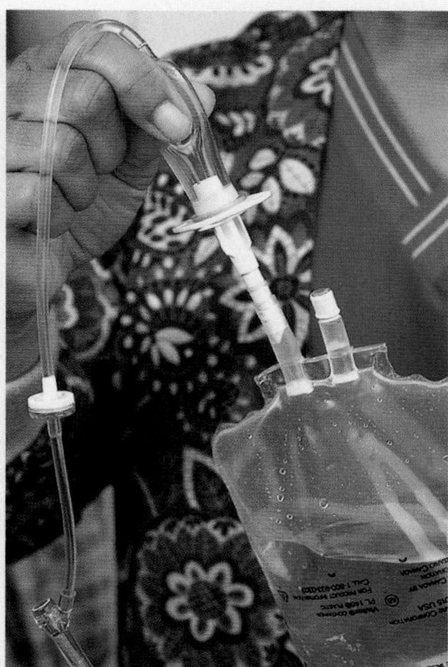

STEP 1h Remove excess fluid from drip chamber.

SKILL 42-3 MAINTENANCE OF INTRAVENOUS SYSTEM—cont'd

STEP	RATIONALE
d. *Prepare tubing, using existing continuous IV infusion:*	
(1) Close roller clamp on new IV tubing.	Prevents spillage of fluid after spiking container.
(2) Slow rate of infusion through old tubing to KVO rate, using EID or roller clamp if no EID.	Prevents complete infusion of fluid remaining in tubing, thus decreasing risk of VAD clotting.
(3) Compress and fill drip chamber of old tubing.	Ensures that drip chamber contains enough fluid to maintain IV patency while changing tubing.
(4) Invert IV fluid container and remove old tubing. Keep spike sterile and upright. *Optional:* Tape old drip chamber to IV pole without contaminating spike.	Allows fluid to continue to flow through IV catheter while new tubing is prepared.
(5) Place insertion spike of new tubing into IV fluid container. Hang container on IV pole, compress and release drip chamber on new tubing, and fill drip chamber one-third to one-half full.	Permits flow of fluid from solution into new infusion tubing.

CLINICAL DECISION: *If you contaminate the spike, discard that IV tubing and use a new one.*

STEP	RATIONALE
(6) Slowly open roller clamp, remove protective cap from adapter (if necessary), and flush new tubing with solution. Close roller clamp when full. Replace cap. Place capped end of adapter near patient's IV site.	Priming slowly instead of allowing a wide-open flow reduces formation of air in tubing. Removes air from tubing and replaces it with fluid. Positions equipment for quick, smooth connection of new tubing.
(7) Stop EID if used and close roller clamp on old tubing.	Prevents spillage of fluid as tubing is removed from catheter.
e. *Prepare tubing, using existing saline lock:*	
(1) If loop or short extension tubing is needed, use sterile technique to connect new injection cap to new loop or tubing.	Sterile technique prevents transmission of infection.
(2) Swab injection cap with antiseptic swab and let dry. Insert syringe with 1 to 3 mL saline solution and inject through injection cap into loop of extension tubing (see illustration). Place capped end of tubing near patient's IV site.	Maintains patency of VAD.

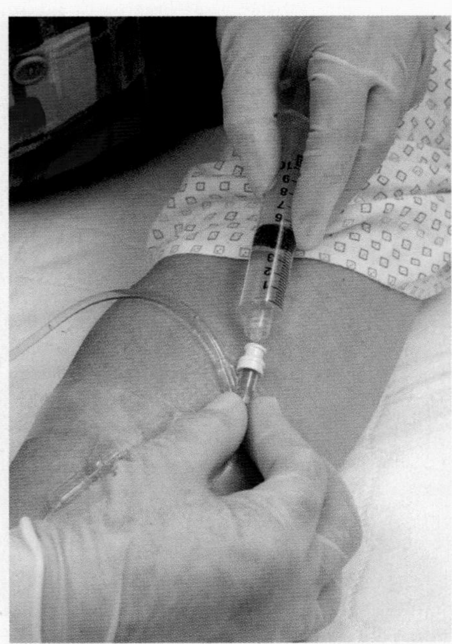

STEP 2e(2) Flush injection port slowly.

STEP	RATIONALE
f. *Reestablish infusion:*	
(1) Remove manufactured catheter stabilization device or tape from tubing. Gently disconnect old tubing from catheter hub (see illustration A) and quickly insert adapter of new tubing into catheter hub, being sure that it is secure, thus maintaining sterility of point of entry of connection (see illustration B).	Allows smooth transition from old to new tubing, minimizing time that system is open to infection. Careful technique prevents VAD dislodgement or vein trauma during tubing change and transmission of microorganisms.
(2) *For continuous infusion:* Open roller clamp on new tubing, allowing solution to run rapidly for 30 to 60 seconds; then regulate drip rate using EID or roller clamp if gravity drip.	Brief rapid flow ensures catheter patency and prevents occlusion. Regulation restores infusion rate to deliver IV fluid as prescribed.
(3) Attach piece of tape or label with date and time of tubing change onto tubing below drip chamber.	Provides reference to determine next time for tubing change.
(4) Apply new manufactured catheter stabilization device or tape if used (see Skill 42-1, Step 21). Form loop of tubing and secure it to patient's arm with strip of tape.	Avoids accidental pulling against site and stabilizes catheter.
g. Remove and discard old IV tubing. If necessary, apply new dressing (see Skill 42-4). Remove and dispose of gloves. Perform hand hygiene.	Reduces transmission of microorganisms.
3. Discontinuing peripheral IV access:	
a. Perform hand hygiene. Apply clean gloves.	Reduces transmission of microorganisms.
b. Turn off EID and close roller clamp or, if no EID, close roller clamp that controls rate.	Prevents spillage of IV fluid.
c. Remove IV site dressing and manufactured catheter stabilization device (see Skill 42-4). Remove any tape that secures catheter. Do not use scissors.	Exposes catheter with minimal discomfort. Scissors might accidentally damage catheter or injure patient (INS, 2011).
d. Hold catheter hub and clean site with antiseptic swab. Allow to dry completely.	Removes secretions around skin puncture site.
e. Place sterile gauze over venipuncture site and apply light pressure while withdrawing catheter, using slow, steady motion. Keep hub parallel to skin (see illustration). Do not raise or lift catheter before it is completely out of vein. Inspect end of catheter, being sure it is intact after removal.	Dry pad causes less irritation to puncture site. Removal technique avoids trauma to vein or hematoma formation. Inspection determines if catheter tip is intact. Tip of catheter can break off and embolize, which is an emergency situation.

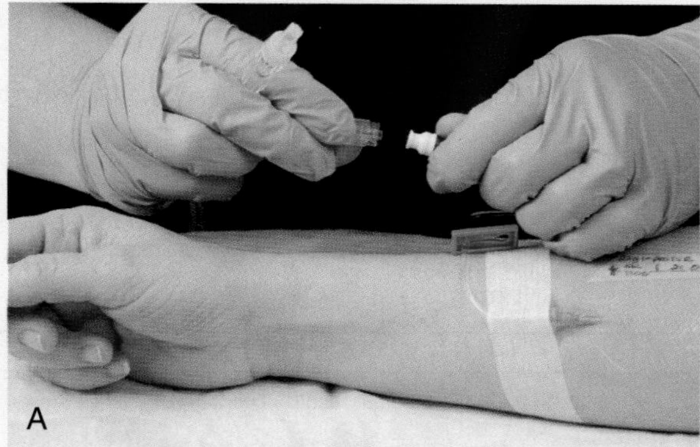

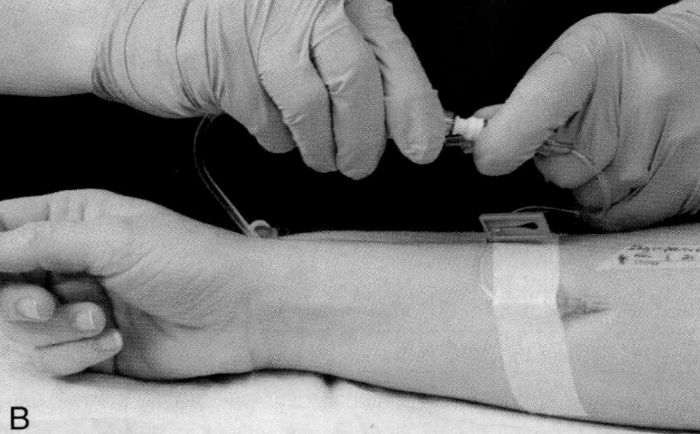

STEP 2f(1) A, Disconnect old intravenous tubing. **B,** Connect Luer-Lok adapter of new IV tubing.

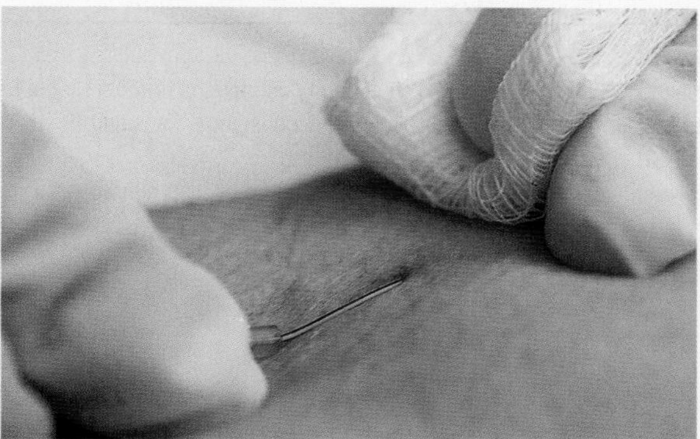

STEP 3e Remove IV catheter slowly, keeping catheter parallel to vein.

SKILL 42-3 MAINTENANCE OF INTRAVENOUS SYSTEM—cont'd

STEP	RATIONALE
f. Keep gauze in place and apply continuous pressure to site for 2 to 3 minutes and assess bleeding.	Controls bleeding and hematoma formation. Pressure should be applied until hemostasis occurs (INS, 2011).

CLINICAL DECISION: *If patient receives anticoagulants or platelet inhibitors (e.g., low-dose aspirin, warfarin sodium [Coumadin], heparin) or has a low platelet count, apply steady pressure longer (for 5 to 10 minutes) and assess bleeding.*

STEP	RATIONALE
g. Apply sterile folded gauze dressing over insertion site and secure with tape.	Maintains pressure to prevent bleeding and reduces bacterial entry into puncture site.
h. Discard used supplies, remove gloves, and perform hand hygiene.	Reduces transmission of microorganisms.

EVALUATION

STEP	RATIONALE
1. *For changing IV fluid container and/or tubing:*	
a. Evaluate IV flow rate hourly; observe connections for leaking and patency of system.	Ensures proper fluid administration.
b. Observe patient for signs of overhydration or dehydration to determine response to therapy and restoration of fluid balance.	Signs and symptoms of overhydration or continued dehydration warrant changing rate of fluid infused. Contact health care provider for new infusion rate order.
2. *For discontinuing peripheral IV access:*	
a. Observe site for bleeding soon after procedure and assess for redness, tenderness, drainage, or swelling daily.	Detects bleeding after catheter removal. Detects local infection or postinfusion phlebitis (INS, 2011). Postinfusion phlebitis may occur 48 to 96 hours after catheter removal.
b. Use ***Teach Back*** to determine patient's and family's understanding about discontinuing IV therapy. State, "I want to be sure I explained what may happen to your arm after removing the IV. Can you tell me what to look for and tell the RN?" Revise your instruction now or develop plan for revised teaching if patient or family is not able to teach back correctly.	Evaluates what patient or family is able to explain or demonstrate.

UNEXPECTED OUTCOMES AND RELATED INTERVENTIONS

1. Flow rate is incorrect; patient receives too little or too much fluid.
   - Readjust infusion rate to ordered rate.
   - Evaluate patient for adverse effects; notify health care provider if apparent.
   - Determine and correct cause of incorrect flow rate (e.g., positional change that might affect rate, EID malfunction [or poor height of IV container with gravity flow], kinking or obstruction of tubing, infiltration or other complications of VAD site).
   - Notify health care provider if patient's anticipated infusion is 100 to 200 mL less than or greater than expected (check agency policy).
2. Catheter tip is missing after withdrawal.
   - Apply tourniquet high on extremity to restrict mobility of catheter embolus.
   - Immediately notify health care provider.
3. See Table 42-12 for infiltration, phlebitis, and local infection.

RECORDING AND REPORTING

- Record amount and type of fluid infused, amount and type of fluid started, and tubing change on patient's medical record according to agency policy. If using bar-code system, fluid type and time record automatically in an electronic health record (EHR).
- Record time that peripheral IV access was discontinued on patient's record according to agency policy. Include site assessment information and status of catheter, including gauge, length, and catheter tip integrity.
- Document your evaluation of patient learning.

HOME CARE CONSIDERATIONS

- Ensure that patient is able and willing to self-manage IV therapy (including changing IV containers) or that reliable family caregiver is at home to provide IV care.
- Instruct patient or family caregiver in procedure for performing an IV solution and tubing change. Consider their cultural norms (e.g., health beliefs and comfort with caregivers using touch) (Petroulias et al., 2013).
- Instruct patient or caregiver to notify health care provider if bleeding or drainage is noted at insertion site or if pain or tenderness occurs up to 4 days after catheter removal.

SKILL 42-4 CHANGING A PERIPHERAL INTRAVENOUS DRESSING

DELEGATION CONSIDERATIONS

The skill of changing a peripheral intravenous (IV) dressing cannot be delegated to nursing assistive personnel (NAP). Delegation to licensed practical nurses (LPNs) varies by state Nurse Practice Act. Instruct the NAP to inform you if:

- Patient indicates moistness or loosening of an IV dressing.

EQUIPMENT

- Antiseptic swabs (chlorhexidine 2% preferred [INS, 2011])
- Adhesive remover *(optional)*
- Skin protectant swab
- Clean gloves
- Strips of nonallergenic tape
- Manufactured catheter stabilization device if available
- Dressing: Sterile transparent dressing (preferred) or sterile 2 × 2- or 4 × 4-inch gauze pad

STEP	RATIONALE
ASSESSMENT	
1. Determine agency policy regarding peripheral IV dressing changes. Transparent dressings usually remain in place until IV site is changed unless dressing becomes wet, soiled, or loose.	Dressing change increases risk of catheter displacement and is performed only if dressing is compromised.
2. Perform hand hygiene. Observe present dressing for moisture and intactness. Determine whether moisture is from site leakage or external source.	Moisture is a medium for bacterial growth and renders dressing contaminated. Loose dressing increases risk for bacterial contamination of venipuncture site or displacement of vascular access device (VAD).
3. Observe IV system for proper functioning or complications. Apply clean gloves if dressing is moist. Palpate VAD site through intact dressing, assessing for pain or burning.	Unexplained decrease in flow rate requires investigating VAD placement and patency. Pain is associated with both phlebitis and infiltration.
4. Identify patient using two identifiers (e.g., name and birthday or name and medical record number) according to agency policy.	Ensures correct patient. Complies with The Joint Commission standards and improves patient safety (TJC, 2016).
5. Assess patient's understanding of need for continued IV infusion.	Determines need for patient teaching.
PLANNING	
1. Explain procedure and purpose to patient and family. Explain that patient must hold affected extremity still and how long procedure will take.	Decreases anxiety, promotes cooperation, and gives patient time frame around which to plan personal activities.
2. Collect equipment, perform hand hygiene and arrange equipment at bedside.	Ensures organized procedure.
IMPLEMENTATION	
1. Apply clean gloves.	Reduces transmission of microorganisms.
2. Remove transparent dressing by pulling up one corner and pulling dressing laterally while holding catheter hub and tubing with nondominant hand (see illustration). Leave tape or catheter stabilization device that secures IV catheter in place. *For gauze dressing:* Stabilize catheter hub while removing old dressing one layer at a time. Be cautious if catheter tubing becomes tangled between two layers of dressing.	Prevents accidental displacement of VAD.
3. Observe insertion site for signs and symptoms of infiltration, phlebitis (see Tables 42-12 to 42-14), and local infection (inflammation and exudate). Discontinue infusion if complication exists (see Skill 42-3).	Presence of infiltration, phlebitis, or local infection requires removal of VAD and new IV start in other extremity or proximal to previous insertion site if continued therapy is necessary.
4. If IV is infusing properly, gently remove any tape or stabilization device that secures catheter. Stabilize catheter with one hand. Use adhesive remover to clean skin and remove adhesive residue if needed.	Exposes venipuncture site. Stabilization prevents accidental displacement of catheter. Adhesive residue decreases ability of new tape to adhere securely to skin.

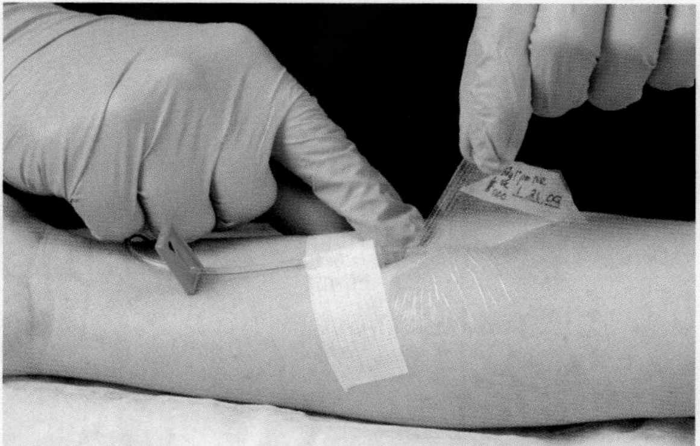

STEP 2 Remove transparent dressing while pulling it laterally.

SKILL 42-4 CHANGING A PERIPHERAL INTRAVENOUS DRESSING—cont'd

STEP	RATIONALE
CLINICAL DECISION: *Keep one finger stabilizing VAD at all times until dressing is applied. This requires careful advance planning regarding placing and opening supplies and how to work with one hand. If patient is restless or uncooperative, ask another nurse to help with dressing change.*	
5. While stabilizing VAD, clean insertion site with antiseptic swab using friction in a horizontal plane and then a vertical plane, followed by a circular motion moving from insertion site outward (see illustration). Allow antiseptic to dry completely.	Friction penetrates antiseptic into epidermal layer of skin. Antimicrobial solutions should be allowed to air-dry completely to reduce microbial counts effectively (Alexander et al, 2014; INS, 2011).
6. *Optional:* Apply skin protectant solution (e.g., skin preparation, no-sting barrier film) to area where you will apply tape or dressing. Allow to dry.	Coats skin with protective solution to maintain skin integrity, prevents irritation from adhesive, and promotes adherence of dressing.
7. Secure catheter with new stabilization device or tape (see Skill 42-1, Step 21) and apply sterile dressing over site (procedures differ; follow agency policy).	Prevents accidental dislodgement of catheter and protects site from infection (INS, 2011; Vizcarra et al, 2014).
a. *Transparent dressing:* Apply as directed in Skill 42-1, Step 21b.	Occlusive dressing protects site from bacterial contamination (Bernatchez, 2014).
b. *Gauze dressing:* Apply as directed in Skill 42-1, Step 21c.	Less frequently used than transparent dressing.
CLINICAL DECISION: *Think carefully about where you place tape. Do not apply it over catheter insertion site, over connection between tubing or port and IV catheter hub, or on top of transparent dressing.*	
8. Remove and discard gloves.	Reduces transmission of microorganisms.
9. *Optional:* Apply protective device over area if patient may pick at or bump dressing (see illustration).	Site protection devices include vented plastic or stretch netting coverings and mitts for hands. Designed to reduce risk of phlebitis, infiltration, or catheter displacement from mechanical motion.
10. Anchor IV tubing with additional pieces of tape if necessary.	Prevents accidental displacement of IV catheter.
11. Label dressing per agency policy. Label information should include date and time of original IV insertion and VAD gauge and length.	Labeling with IV insertion date and VAD length facilitates appropriate site rotation and safe discontinuation of IV access.
12. Discard equipment and perform hand hygiene.	Reduces transmission of microorganisms.
EVALUATION	
1. Observe new dressing to be sure that it is applied, taped, and labeled properly.	Validates quality of completed dressing change.
2. Ensure that flow rate is accurate.	Validates that IV line is patent and functioning correctly. Manipulation of catheter and tubing may affect rate of infusion.
3. Use ***Teach Back*** to determine patient's and family's understanding about dressing change. State, "I want to be sure I explained why I changed your IV dressing. Can you explain why I changed the dressing?" Revise your instruction now or develop plan for revised teaching if patient or family is not able to teach back correctly.	Evaluates what patient or family is able to explain or demonstrate.

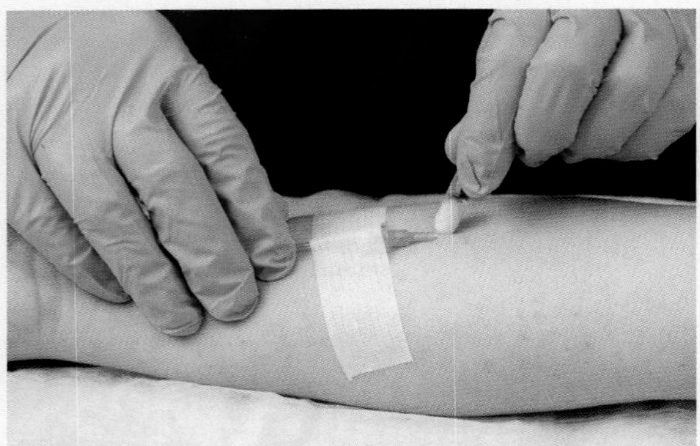

STEP 5 Cleanse peripheral insertion site with antiseptic swab.

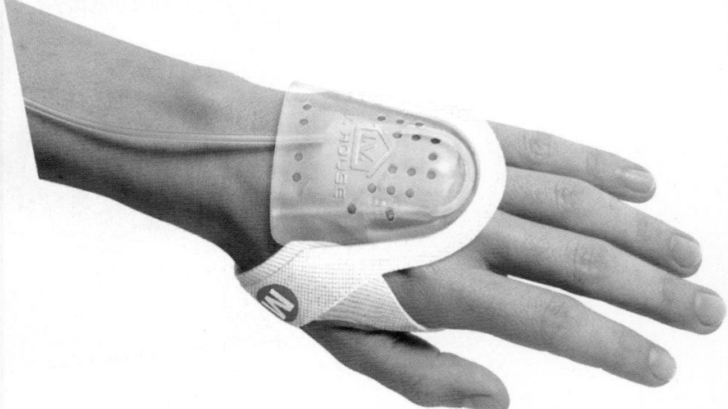

STEP 9 IV House protective device. (Courtesy IV House, St Louis, MO)

UNEXPECTED OUTCOMES AND RELATED INTERVENTIONS

1. VAD is accidentally dislodged or removed.
   - Start new IV line in other extremity or proximal to previous insertion site if continued therapy is necessary.
2. IV site develops infiltration, phlebitis, and local infection.
   - See Table 42-12.

RECORDING AND REPORTING

- Record time that peripheral dressing was changed, reason for change, type of dressing material used, patency of system, and description of venipuncture site.
- Document your evaluation of patient learning.
- Report to charge nurse or oncoming nursing shift that dressing was changed and any significant information about integrity of system.
- Report any complications to health care provider and document them.

KEY POINTS

- Body fluids containing water, Na^+, and other electrolytes are distributed between ECF and ICF compartments.
- A dynamic interplay of fluid and electrolyte intake and absorption, distribution, and output determines fluid and electrolyte balance.
- Fluid moves between blood vessels and interstitial fluid by filtration; water moves between ECF and ICF by osmosis.
- ECV deficit and excess are abnormal *volumes* of isotonic fluid, manifested as sudden changes in body weight and changes in markers of vascular and interstitial volume.
- Osmolality imbalances are abnormal *concentrations* of body fluids, manifested as altered serum Na^+ levels and decreased level of consciousness.
- Interplay of acid production, acid buffering, and acid excretion determines acid-base balance.
- Acid-base imbalances are excesses or deficits of carbonic or metabolic acids, manifested as changes in level of consciousness and abnormalities of $PaCO_2$, HCO_3^-, and pH.
- Patients who are very young or very old, whose I&O of fluid and/or electrolytes are not equal, or who have various chronic diseases or trauma are at high risk for fluid, electrolyte, and acid-base imbalances.
- Treatment for ECV excess is Na^+ restriction and fluid restriction if severe; treatment for hyponatremia usually is water restriction. Prevention and treatment of ECV deficit, hypernatremia, and electrolyte deficits involve oral or parenteral administration of appropriate fluid.
- Initiation and maintenance of IV therapy require clinical decision making, skill, and organized procedures to maintain sterility and patency of the system and periodic updating of procedures on the basis of current research evidence.
- Nurses monitor vigilantly for complications of IV therapy, which include fluid overload, infiltration, phlebitis, local infection, and bleeding at the infusion site.
- Administration of blood or blood products requires a specific procedure for correctly identifying patient and blood product and responding to transfusion reactions quickly.
- Patient and family teaching is important for preventing fluid, electrolyte, and acid-base imbalances and effective restorative care.

CLINICAL APPLICATION QUESTIONS

Preparing for Clinical Practice

Mrs. Hilda Beck, age 72, fell at home because she became light-headed after vomiting and diarrhea that lasted over 24 hours. Even though she was nauseated, she drank some water because she knew she needed fluid. She was admitted for oral and intravenous (IV) fluid therapy.

1. What was problematic about Mrs. Beck's oral fluid replacement at home when she had vomiting and diarrhea?
2. Mrs. Beck's intravenous (IV) fluid order is 1000 mL 0.9% sodium chloride to run over 5 hours. Calculate the mL/hr that you should program into her infusion pump.
3. Mrs. Beck says, "When I get diarrhea, I should drink sodium-containing fluid when I'm thirsty." She needs what additional teaching?

Answers to Clinical Application Questions can be found on the Evolve website.

REVIEW QUESTIONS

Are You Ready to Test Your Nursing Knowledge?

1. An intravenous (IV) fluid is infusing more slowly than ordered. The infusion pump is set correctly. Which factors could cause this slowing? (Select all that apply.)
   1. Infiltration at vascular access device (VAD) site
   2. Patient lying on tubing
   3. Roller clamp wide open
   4. Tubing kinked in bedrails
   5. Circulatory overload
2. Which patients does a nurse plan to teach regarding water restriction?
   1. A 23-year-old with extracellular fluid volume (ECV) deficit
   2. A 34-year-old with hyponatremia
   3. A 47-year-old with hypercalcemia
   4. A 69-year-old with metabolic acidosis
3. A nurse assesses pain and redness at a vascular access device (VAD) site. Which action is taken first?
   1. Apply a warm, moist compress
   2. Monitor the patient's blood pressure

3. Aspirate the infusing fluid from the VAD
4. Stop the infusion and discontinue the intravenous infusion

4. When delegating input and output (I&O) measurement to nursing assistive personnel, a nurse instructs them to record what information for ice chips?
   1. The total volume
   2. Two-thirds of the volume
   3. One-half of the volume
   4. One-quarter of the volume
5. A nurse assesses four patients. Which patient has greatest risk for hypomagnesemia?
   1. A 72-year-old with chronic alcoholism
   2. A 79-year-old with bone cancer
   3. A 41-year-old with hypernatremia
   4. A 46-year-old with respiratory acidosis
6. Which assessment does a nurse interpret as a transfusion reaction?
   1. Crackles in dependent lobes of lungs
   2. High fever, severe hypotension
   3. Anxiety, itching, confusion
   4. Chills, tachycardia, and flushing
7. What assessment does a nurse make before hanging an intravenous (IV) fluid that contains potassium?
   1. Urine output
   2. Arterial blood gases
   3. Fullness of neck veins
   4. Level of consciousness
8. The health care provider's order is 500 mL 0.9% NaCl intravenously over 4 hours. Which rate does a nurse program into the infusion pump?
   1. 125 mL/hr
   2. 167 mL/hr
   3. 200 mL/hr
   4. 1000 mL/hr
9. An older-adult patient is receiving intravenous (IV) 0.9% NaCl. A nurse detects new onset of crackles in the lung bases. What is the priority action?
   1. Notify a health care provider
   2. Record in medical record
   3. Decrease the IV flow rate
   4. Discontinue the IV site
10. Place the following steps for discontinuing intravenous (IV) access in the correct order:
    1. Perform hand hygiene and apply gloves.
    2. Explain procedure to patient.
    3. Remove IV site dressing and tape.
    4. Use two identifiers to ensure correct patient.
    5. Stop the infusion and clamp the tubing.
    6. Carefully check the health care provider's order.
    7. Clean the site, withdraw the catheter, and apply pressure.
11. A patient has severe hypercalcemia. What are the priority nursing interventions? (Select all that apply.)
    1. Fall prevention interventions
    2. Teaching regarding sodium restriction
    3. Encouraging increased fluid intake
    4. Monitoring for constipation
    5. Explaining how to take daily weights
12. A patient has hypokalemia with stable cardiac function. What are the priority nursing interventions? (Select all that apply.)
    1. Fall prevention interventions
    2. Teaching regarding sodium restriction
    3. Encouraging increased fluid intake
    4. Monitoring for constipation
    5. Explaining how to take daily weights
13. A patient is admitted to the hospital with severe dyspnea and wheezing. Arterial blood gas levels on admission are pH 7.26; $PaCO_2$, 55 mm Hg; PaO_2, 68 mm Hg; and HCO_3^-, 24. The nurse interprets these laboratory values to indicate:
    1. Metabolic acidosis.
    2. Metabolic alkalosis.
    3. Respiratory acidosis.
    4. Respiratory alkalosis.
14. Which assessment does a nurse use as a clinical marker of vascular volume in a patient at high risk of extracellular fluid volume (ECV) deficit?
    1. Dryness of mucous membranes
    2. Presence or absence of edema
    3. Fullness of neck veins when supine
    4. Fullness of neck veins when upright
15. A patient is hyperventilating from acute pain and hypoxia. Interventions to manage his pain and oxygenation will decrease his risk of which acid-base imbalance?
    1. Metabolic acidosis
    2. Metabolic alkalosis
    3. Respiratory acidosis
    4. Respiratory alkalosis

Answers: 1. 1, 2, 4; **2.** 2; **3.** 4; **4.** 3; **5.** 1; **6.** 4; **7.** 1; **8.** 1; **9.** 3; **10.** 6, 4, 2, 1, 5, 3, 7; **11.** 1, 3, 4; **12.** 1, 4; **13.** 3; **14.** 3; **15.** 4.

Rationales for Review Questions can be found on the Evolve website.

REFERENCES

Alexander M, et al: *Core curriculum for infusion nursing*, ed 4, Philadelphia, 2014, Lippincott, Williams & Wilkins.

American Association of Blood Banks (AABB): *Technical manual*, ed 18, Bethesda, MD, 2014a, AABB.

American Association of Blood Banks (AABB): *Standards for blood banks and transfusion services*, ed 29, Bethesda, MD, 2014b, AABB.

Arai S, et al: Thirst in critically ill patients: from physiology to sensation, *Am J Crit Care* 22(4):328, 2013.

Ayers P, Dixon C: Simple acid-base tutorial, *JPEN J Parenter Enteral Nutr* 36(1):18, 2012.

Berend K, et al: Physiological approach to assessment of acid-base disturbances, *N Engl J Med* 371(15):1434, 2014.

Bernatchez S: Care of peripheral venous catheter sites: advantages of transparent film dressings over tape and gauze, *J Vasc Access* 19(4):256, 2014.

Billingsley L, Kinchen L: Peripheral intravenous catheter protection: are we using best practice? *J Contin Educ Nurs* 45(8):338, 2014.

Burchum JR, Rosenthal LD: *Lehne's pharmacology for nursing care*, ed 9, St Louis, 2016, Elsevier.

Centers for Disease Control and Prevention (CDC): *Blood safety*, 2013, http://www.cdc.gov/bloodsafety/bbp/diseases_organisms.html. Accessed April 24, 2015.

Chopra V, et al: Prevention of central line–associated bloodstream infections: brief update review. In Shakelle PG, et al, editors: *Making health care safer II: an updated critical analysis of the evidence for patient safety practices*, AHRQ publication no. 13-E001-EF, Rockville, MD, 2013, Agency for Healthcare Research and Quality. http://www.ncbi.nlm.nih.gov/books/NBK133364/. Accessed December 9, 2015.

Clark CT: Recent efforts and available technologies for safety in delivery of blood products, *J Infus Nurs* 34(1):23, 2011.

Cook LS: Infusion-related air embolism, *J Infus Nurs* 36(1):26, 2013.

Coyle CE, et al: Eliminating extravasation events: a multidisciplinary approach, *J Infus Nurs* 37(3):157, 2014.

Davison D, et al: Fluid management in adults and children: core curriculum 2014, *Am J Kidney Dis* 63(4):700, 2014.

Dychter SS, et al: Intravenous therapy: a review of complications and economic considerations of peripheral access, *J Infus Nurs* 35(2):85, 2012.

Felver L: Acid-base balance. In Giddens JF, editor: *Concepts for nursing practice*, St Louis, 2013a, Mosby.

Felver L: Acid-base homeostasis and imbalances. In Copstead LC, Banasik JL, editors: *Pathophysiology*, ed 5, St Louis, 2013b, Saunders.

Felver L: Fluid and electrolyte balance. In Giddens JF, editor: *Concepts for nursing practice*, St Louis, 2013c, Mosby.

Felver L: Fluid and electrolyte homeostasis and imbalances. In Copstead LC, Banasik JL, editors: *Pathophysiology*, ed 5, St Louis, 2013d, Saunders.

FitzHenry F, et al: Applying bar-code medication administration to make a difference in adverse drug events with potential for harm: lessons learned, *Comput Inform Nurs* 31(10):457, 2013.

Giger JN: *Transcultural nursing: assessment and intervention*, ed 6, St Louis, 2013, Mosby.

Gorski LA, et al: INS position paper: Recommendations for frequency of assessment of the short peripheral catheter site, *J Infus Nurs* 35(5):290, 2012.

Gresser S: Infusion therapy in an older adult. In Weinstein SM, Hagle ME, editors: *Plumer's principles and practice of infusion therapy*, ed 9, Philadelphia, 2014, Lippincott, Williams & Wilkins.

Hadaway L: Needlestick injuries, short peripheral catheters, and health care worker risks, *J Infus Nurs* 35(3):164, 2012a.

Hadaway L: Short peripheral intravenous catheters and infections, *J Infus Nurs* 35(4):230, 2012b.

Hale A, Hovey MJ: *Fluid, electrolyte, and acid-base imbalances*, Philadelphia, 2013, FA Davis.

Hall JE: *Guyton and Hall textbook of medical physiology*, ed 13, Philadelphia, 2016, Saunders.

Harding AD: Smart pumps, *J Infus Nurs* 36(5):191, 2013.

Hockenberry MJ, Wilson D: *Wong's nursing care of infants and children*, ed 10, St Louis, 2015, Mosby.

Infusion Nurses Society (INS): Infusion nursing standards of practice, *J Infus Nurs* 34(1S):S1, 2011.

Lewis SL, et al: *Medical-surgical nursing: assessment and management of clinical problems*, ed 9, St Louis, 2014, Mosby.

National Quality Forum (NQF): *NQF-endorsed measures for patient safety: technical report*, Washington, DC, 2015, NQF.

Occupational Safety and Health Administration (OSHA): *Bloodborne pathogens standard,* United States Department of Labor, last amended April 3, 2012, https://www.osha.gov/pls/oshaweb/owadisp.show_document?p_table=STANDARDS&p_id=10051. Accessed April 24, 2015.

O'Grady N, et al: *Centers for Disease Control and Prevention Guidelines for the Prevention of Intravascular Catheter-Related Infections*, 2011, http://www.cdc.gov/hicpac/pdf/guidelines/bsi-guidelines-2011.pdf. Accessed April 24, 2015.

Pagana KD, et al: *Mosby's diagnostic & laboratory test reference*, ed 12, St Louis, 2015, Mosby.

Petroulias P, et al: Providing culturally competent care in home infusion nursing, *J Infus Nurs* 36(2):108, 2013.

The Joint Commission (TJC): *Preventing central line–associated bloodstream infections: a global challenge, a global perspective*, 2012, TJC, http://www.PreventingCLABSIs.pdf. Accessed April 25, 2015.

The Joint Commission (TJC): *2016 National Patient Safety Goals*, Oakbrook Terrace, IL, 2016, The Commission. Available at http://www.jointcommission.org/standards_information/npsgs.aspx. Accessed November 2015.

Touhy TA, Jett KF: *Ebersole and Hess's gerontological nursing & healthy aging*, ed 4, St Louis, 2014, Mosby.

Vizcarra C, et al: INS position paper: recommendations for improving safety practices with short peripheral catheters, *J Infus Nurs* 37(2):121, 2014.

Wunderlich R: Principles in the selection of intravenous solutions replacement: sodium and water, *J Infus Nurs* 36(2):126, 2013.

RESEARCH REFERENCES

Dumyati G, et al: Sustained reduction of central line–associated bloodstream infections outside the intensive care unit with a multimodal intervention focusing on central line maintenance, *Am J Infect Control* 42:723, 2014.

Ganter-Ritz V, et al: A randomized double-blind study comparing intradermal anesthetic tolerability, efficacy, and cost-effectiveness of lidocaine, buffered lidocaine, and bacteriostatic normal saline for peripheral intravenous insertion, *J Infus Nurs* 35(2):93, 2012.

Killer SC, et al: No evidence of dehydration with moderate daily coffee intake: a counterbalanced cross-over study in a free-living population, *PLoS ONE* 9(1):e84154, 2014.

Matocha D: Achieving near-zero and zero: who said interventions and controls don't matter? *J Vasc Access* 18(3):157, 2013.

Rickard CM, et al: Routine versus clinically indicated replacement of peripheral intravenous catheters: a randomised controlled equivalence trial, *Lancet* 380(9847):1066, 2012.

Ullman AJ, et al: Optimal timing for intravascular administration set replacement, *Cochrane Database Syst Rev* 4:CD003588, 2013.

Wallis MC, et al: Risk factors for peripheral intravenous catheter failure: a multivariate analysis of data from a randomized controlled trial, *Infect Control Hosp Epidemiol* 35(1):63, 2014.

Webster J, et al: Clinically indicated replacement versus routine replacement of peripheral venous catheters, *Cochrane Database Syst Rev* 4:CD007798, 2013.

Zingg W, et al: Hospital-wide multidisciplinary, multimodal intervention programme to reduce central catheter-associated bloodstream infection, *PLoS ONE* 9(4):e93898, 2014.

43

Sleep

OBJECTIVES

- Explain the effect that the 24-hour sleep-wake cycle has on biological function.
- Discuss mechanisms that regulate sleep.
- Describe the stages of a normal sleep cycle.
- Explain the functions of sleep.
- Compare and contrast the sleep requirements of different age-groups.
- Identify factors that normally promote and disrupt sleep.
- Discuss characteristics of common sleep disorders.
- Conduct a sleep history for a patient.
- Identify nursing diagnoses appropriate for patients with sleep alterations.
- Identify nursing interventions designed to promote normal sleep cycles for patients of all ages.
- Describe ways to evaluate the effects of sleep therapies.

KEY TERMS

Biological clocks, p. 992
Cataplexy, p. 996
Circadian rhythm, p. 992
Excessive daytime sleepiness (EDS), p. 996
Hypersomnolence, p. 995
Hypnotics, p. 1010
Insomnia, p. 996
Narcolepsy, p. 996
Nocturia, p. 995
Nonrapid eye movement (NREM) sleep, p. 993
Polysomnogram, p. 996
Rapid eye movement (REM) sleep, p. 993
Rest, p. 997
Sedatives, p. 1010
Sleep, p. 992
Sleep apnea, p. 996
Sleep deprivation, p. 997
Sleep hygiene, p. 996

MEDIA RESOURCES

http://evolve.elsevier.com/Potter/fundamentals/

- Review Questions
- Concept Map Creator
- Case Study with Questions
- Audio Glossary
- Content Updates

Proper rest and sleep are as important to health as good nutrition and adequate exercise. Physical and emotional health depends on the ability to fulfill these basic human needs. Individuals need different amounts of sleep and rest. Without proper amounts, the ability to concentrate, make judgments, and participate in daily activities decreases; and irritability increases.

Identifying and treating patients' sleep pattern disturbances are important goals. To help patients you need to understand the nature of sleep, the factors influencing it, and patients' sleep habits. Patients require individualized approaches on the basis of their personal habits, patterns of sleep, and the particular problem influencing sleep. Nursing interventions are often effective in resolving short- and long-term sleep disturbances.

Sleep provides healing and restoration (Huether et al., 2012). Achieving the best possible sleep quality is important for the promotion of good health and recovery from illness. Ill patients often require more sleep and rest than healthy patients. However, the nature of illness often prevents some patients from getting adequate rest and sleep. The environment of a hospital or long-term care facility and the activities of health care personnel often make sleep difficult. Some patients have preexisting sleep disturbances; others develop sleep problems as a result of an illness or hospitalization.

SCIENTIFIC KNOWLEDGE BASE

Physiology of Sleep

Sleep is a cyclical physiological process that alternates with longer periods of wakefulness. The sleep-wake cycle influences and regulates physiological function and behavioral responses.

Circadian Rhythms. People experience cyclical rhythms as part of their everyday lives. The most familiar rhythm is the 24-hour, day-night cycle known as the diurnal or **circadian rhythm** (derived from Latin: *circa,* "about," and *dies,* "day"). The suprachiasmatic nucleus (SCN) nerve cells in the hypothalamus control the rhythm of the sleep-wake cycle and coordinate this cycle with other circadian rhythms (Huether et al., 2012). Circadian rhythms influence the pattern of major biological and behavioral functions. The predictable changing of body temperature, heart rate, blood pressure, hormone secretion, sensory acuity, and mood depend on the maintenance of the 24-hour circadian cycle (Kryger et al., 2011).

Factors such as light, temperature, social activities, and work routines affect circadian rhythms and daily sleep-wake cycles. All people have **biological clocks** that synchronize their sleep cycles. This explains why some people fall asleep at 8 PM, whereas others go to bed at midnight or early in the morning. Different people also function best at different times of the day.

Hospitals or extended care facilities usually do not adapt care to an individual's sleep-wake cycle preferences. Typical hospital routines interrupt sleep or prevent patients from falling asleep at their usual time. Poor quality of sleep results when a person's sleep-wake cycle changes. Reversals in the sleep-wake cycle, such as when a person who is normally awake during the day falls asleep during the day, often indicate a serious illness.

The biological rhythm of sleep frequently becomes synchronized with other body functions. For example, changes in body temperature correlate with sleep patterns. Normally body temperature peaks in the afternoon, decreases gradually, and drops sharply after a person falls asleep. When the sleep-wake cycle becomes disrupted (e.g., by working rotating shifts), other physiological functions usually change as well. For example, a new nurse who starts working the night shift experiences a decreased appetite and loses weight. Anxiety, restlessness, irritability, and impaired judgment are other common symptoms of sleep cycle disturbances. Failure to maintain an individual's usual sleep-wake cycle negatively influences the patient's overall health.

Sleep Regulation. Sleep involves a sequence of physiological states maintained by highly integrated central nervous system (CNS) activity. It is associated with changes in the peripheral nervous, endocrine, cardiovascular, respiratory, and muscular systems (Huether et al., 2012). Specific physiological responses and patterns of brain activity identify each sequence. Instruments such as the electroencephalogram (EEG), which measures electrical activity in the cerebral cortex; the electromyogram (EMG), which measures muscle tone; and the electrooculogram (EOG), which measures eye movements provide information about some structural physiological aspects of sleep.

The major sleep center in the body is the hypothalamus. It secretes hypocretins (orexins) that promote wakefulness and rapid eye movement (REM) sleep. Prostaglandin D_2, L-tryptophan, and growth factors control sleep (Huether et al., 2012).

Researchers believe that the ascending reticular activating system (RAS) located in the upper brainstem contains special cells that maintain alertness and wakefulness. The RAS receives visual, auditory, pain, and tactile sensory stimuli. Activity from the cerebral cortex (e.g., emotions or thought processes) also stimulates the RAS. Arousal, wakefulness, and maintenance of consciousness result from neurons in the RAS releasing catecholamines such as norepinephrine (Kryger et al., 2011).

The homeostatic process (Process S), which primarily regulates the length and depth of sleep; and the circadian rhythms (Process C: "biological time clocks"), which influence the internal organization of sleep and the timing and duration of sleep-wake cycles, operate simultaneously to regulate sleep and wakefulness (Daroff et al., 2012). Time of wake up is defined by the intersection of Process S and Process C (Figure 43-1).

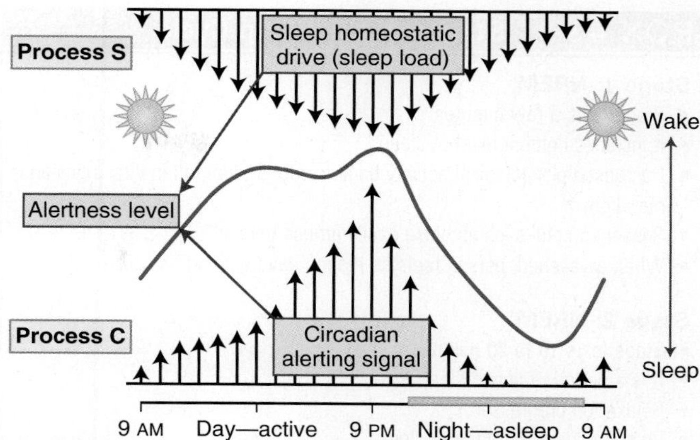

FIGURE 43-1 Two-process model of sleep regulation shows the time course of the homeostatic process *(Process S)* and the circadian process *(Process C)*. Process S rises during waking and declines during sleep. The intersection of Process S and Process C defines the time of wake-up. (From Daroff RB et al: *Bradley's neurology in clinical practice,* ed 6, Philadelphia, 2012, Saunders.)

Stages of Sleep. Current theory suggests that sleep is an active multiphase process. Different brain-wave, muscle, and eye activity is associated with different stages of sleep (Chase, 2013). Normal sleep involves two phases: **nonrapid eye movement (NREM) sleep** and **rapid eye movement (REM) sleep** (Box 43-1). During NREM a sleeper progresses through four stages during a typical 90-minute sleep cycle. The quality of sleep from stage 1 through stage 4 becomes increasingly deep. Lighter sleep is characteristic of stages 1 and 2, during which a person is more easily aroused. Stages 3 and 4 involve a deeper sleep, called *slow-wave sleep*. REM sleep is the phase at the end of each sleep cycle. Different factors promote or interfere with various stages of the sleep cycle.

Sleep Cycle. The normal sleep pattern for an adult begins with a presleep period during which the person is aware only of a gradually developing sleepiness. This period normally lasts 10 to 30 minutes; however, if a person has difficulty falling asleep, it lasts an hour or more.

Once asleep, the person usually passes through four or five complete sleep cycles per night, each consisting of four stages of NREM sleep and a period of REM sleep (Huether et al., 2012). Each cycle lasts approximately 90 to 100 minutes. The cyclical pattern usually progresses from stage 1 through stage 4 of NREM, followed by a reversal from stages 4 to 3 to 2, ending with a period of REM sleep (Figure 43-2). A person usually reaches REM sleep about 90 minutes into the sleep cycle. Seventy-five to eighty percent of sleep time is spent in NREM sleep.

With each successive cycle stages 3 and 4 shorten, and the period of REM lengthens. REM sleep lasts up to 60 minutes during the last sleep cycle. Not all people progress consistently through the stages of sleep. For example, a sleeper moves back and forth for short intervals between NREM stages 2, 3, and 4 before entering REM stage. The amount of time spent in each stage varies over the life span. Newborns and children spend more time in deep sleep. Sleep becomes more fragmented with aging, and a person spends more time in lighter stages (National Sleep Foundation, 2014a). Shifts from stage to stage of sleep tend to accompany body movements. Shifts to light sleep or wakefulness tend to occur suddenly, whereas shifts to deep sleep tend to be gradual (Kryger et al., 2011). The number of sleep cycles depends on the total amount of time that the person spends sleeping.

Functions of Sleep

The primary function of sleep is unclear (Gilsenan, 2012). It contributes to physiological and psychological restoration. NREM sleep contributes to body tissue restoration (Huether et al., 2012). During NREM sleep biological functions slow. A healthy adult's normal heart rate throughout the day averages 70 to 80 beats/min or less if the individual is in excellent physical condition. However, during sleep the heart rate falls to 60 beats/min or less, which benefits cardiac function.

BOX 43-1 Stages of the Sleep Cycle

Stage 1: NREM
- Stage lasts a few minutes.
- It includes lightest level of sleep.
- Decreased physiological activity begins with gradual fall in vital signs and metabolism.
- Sensory stimuli such as noise easily arouse person.
- When awakened, person feels as though daydreaming has occurred.

Stage 2: NREM
- Stage lasts 10 to 20 minutes.
- It is a period of sound sleep.
- Relaxation progresses.
- Body functions continue to slow.
- Arousal remains relatively easy.

Stage 3: NREM
- Stage lasts 15 to 30 minutes.
- It involves initial stages of deep sleep.
- Muscles are completely relaxed.
- Vital signs decline but remain regular.
- Sleeper is difficult to arouse and rarely moves.

Stage 4: NREM
- Stage lasts approximately 15 to 30 minutes.
- It is the deepest stage of sleep.
- If sleep loss has occurred, sleeper spends considerable part of night in this stage.
- Vital signs are significantly lower than during waking hours.
- Sleepwalking and enuresis (bed-wetting) sometimes occur.
- It is very difficult to arouse sleeper.

REM Sleep
- Stage usually begins about 90 minutes after sleep has begun.
- Duration increases with each sleep cycle and averages 20 minutes.
- Vivid, full-color dreaming occurs; less vivid dreaming occurs in other stages.
- Stage is typified by rapidly moving eyes, fluctuating heart and respiratory rates, increased or fluctuating blood pressure, loss of skeletal muscle tone, and increase of gastric secretions.
- It is very difficult to arouse sleeper.

NREM, Nonrapid eye movement; *REM,* rapid eye movement.

FIGURE 43-2 Stages of adult sleep cycle. *NREM,* Nonrapid eye movement; *REM,* rapid eye movement.

Other biological functions decreased during sleep are respirations, blood pressure, and muscle tone (Huether et al., 2012).

The body needs sleep to routinely restore biological processes. During deep slow-wave (NREM stage 4) sleep, the body releases human growth hormone for the repair and renewal of epithelial and specialized cells such as brain cells (Huether et al., 2012). Protein synthesis and cell division for renewal of tissues such as the skin, bone marrow, gastric mucosa, or brain occur during rest and sleep. NREM sleep is especially important in children, who experience more stage 4 sleep.

Another theory about the purpose of sleep is that the body conserves energy during sleep. The skeletal muscles relax progressively, and the absence of muscular contraction preserves chemical energy for cellular processes. Lowering of the basal metabolic rate further conserves body energy supply (Redeker and McEnany, 2011).

REM sleep is necessary for brain tissue restoration and appears to be important for cognitive restoration and memory (Conte and Ficca, 2013). It is associated with changes in cerebral blood flow, increased cortical activity, increased oxygen consumption, and epinephrine release. This association helps with memory storage and learning (Huether et al., 2012).

The benefits of sleep on behavior often go unnoticed until a person develops a problem resulting from sleep deprivation. A loss of REM sleep leads to feelings of confusion and suspicion. Various body functions (e.g., mood, motor performance, memory, and equilibrium) are altered when prolonged sleep loss occurs (National Sleep Foundation, 2014e). Changes in the natural and cellular immune function also occur with moderate-to-severe sleep deprivation. The annual direct cost of sleep-related problems in this country is 16 billion dollars. An additional 50 to 100 billion dollars are spent on indirect costs related to accidents, litigation, property damage, hospitalization, and death (University of Maryland Medical Center Sleep Disorders Center, 2015).

Dreams. Although dreams occur during both NREM and REM sleep, the dreams of REM sleep are more vivid and elaborate; and some believe that they are functionally important to learning, memory processing, and adaptation to stress (Kryger et al., 2011). REM dreams progress in content throughout the night from dreams about current events to emotional dreams of childhood or the past. Personality influences the quality of dreams (e.g., a creative person has elaborate and complex dreams, whereas a depressed person dreams of helplessness).

Most people dream about immediate concerns such as an argument with a spouse or worries over work. Sometimes a person is unaware of fears represented in bizarre dreams. Clinical psychologists try to analyze the symbolic nature of dreams as part of a patient's psychotherapy. The ability to describe a dream and interpret its significance sometimes helps resolve personal concerns or fears.

Another theory suggests that dreams erase certain fantasies or nonsensical memories. Because most people forget their dreams, few have dream recall or do not believe they dream at all. To remember a dream, a person has to consciously think about it on awakening. People who recall dreams vividly usually awake just after a period of REM sleep.

Physical Illness

Any illness that causes pain, physical discomfort, or mood problems such as anxiety or depression often results in sleep problems. People with such alterations frequently have trouble falling or staying asleep. Illnesses also force patients to sleep in unfamiliar positions. For example, it is difficult for a patient with an arm or leg in traction to rest comfortably.

Respiratory disease often interferes with sleep. Patients with chronic lung disease such as emphysema are short of breath and frequently cannot sleep without two or three pillows to raise their heads. Asthma, bronchitis, and allergic rhinitis alter the rhythm of breathing and disturb sleep. A person with a common cold has nasal congestion, sinus drainage, and a sore throat, which impair breathing and the ability to relax.

Connections among heart disease, sleep, and sleep disorders exist. Sleep-related breathing disorders are linked to increased incidence of nocturnal angina (chest pain), increased heart rate, electrocardiogram changes, high blood pressure, and risk of heart diseases and stroke (Huether et al., 2012). Hypertension often causes early-morning awakening and fatigue. Research also identifies an increased risk of sudden cardiac death in the first hours after awakening. Sleep disruptions and frequent arousals occur in people with heart failure as a result of the apnea, hypercapnia, and hypoxemia that develops as the disease progresses (Kryger et al., 2011). Hypothyroidism decreases stage 4 sleep, whereas hyperthyroidism causes people to take more time to fall asleep.

Nocturia, or urination during the night, disrupts sleep and the sleep cycle. After repeated awakenings to urinate, returning to sleep is difficult, and the sleep cycle is not complete. Although this condition is most common in older people with reduced bladder tone or people with cardiac disease, diabetes, urethritis, or prostatic disease, it also occurs in a significant number of younger people (Van Kerrebroeck, 2011).

Many people experience restless legs syndrome (RLS), which occurs before sleep onset. More common in women, older people, and those with iron deficiency anemia, RLS symptoms include recurrent, rhythmical movements of the feet and legs. Patients feel an itching sensation deep in the muscles. Relief comes only from moving the legs, which prevents relaxation and subsequent sleep. RLS is sometimes a relatively benign condition, depending on how severely sleep is disrupted. Primary RLS is a CNS disorder. Researchers associate secondary RLS with lower levels of iron, pregnancy, renal failure, stress, diet, Parkinson's disease, or a side effect of drugs (Chasens and Umlauf, 2012).

People with peptic ulcer disease often awaken in the middle of the night. Studies showing a relationship between gastric acid secretion and stages of sleep are conflicting. One consistent finding is that people with duodenal ulcers fail to suppress acid secretion in the first 2 hours of sleep (Kryger et al., 2011). Many patients experience gastroesophageal reflux as a result of the acid production, which disrupts sleep (Kryger et al., 2011).

Sleep Disorders

Sleep disorders are conditions that, if untreated, generally cause disturbed nighttime sleep that results in one of three problems: insomnia, abnormal movements or sensation during sleep or when waking up at night, or excessive daytime sleepiness (EDS) (Kryger et al., 2011). Many adults in the United States have significant sleep problems from inadequacies in either the quantity or quality of their nighttime sleep and experience **hypersomnolence** on a daily basis (National Sleep Foundation, 2014e). The American Academy of Sleep Medicine developed the International Classification of Sleep Disorders version 2 (ICSD-2), which classifies sleep disorders into eight major categories (Box 43-2).

Insomnia disorders are related to difficulty falling asleep, frequently awaking from sleep, short periods of sleep, or sleep that is nonrestorative (Kryger et al., 2011). Individuals with sleep-related breathing disorders have changes in respirations during sleep. Hypersomnias are sleep disturbances that result in daytime sleepiness and are not caused by disturbed sleep or alterations in circadian rhythms (Kryger et al., 2011). The circadian rhythm sleep disorders are caused by a misalignment between the timing of sleep and individual desires or the societal norm. The parasomnias are undesirable behaviors that occur usually during sleep. Sleep and wake disturbances are associated with many medical and psychiatric sleep disorders, including psychiatric, neurological, or other medical disorders. In sleep-related movement disorders the person experiences simple stereotyped movements

BOX 43-2 Classification of Select Sleep Disorders

Insomnias
- Adjustment sleep disorder (acute insomnia)
- Inadequate sleep hygiene
- Behavioral insomnia of childhood
- Insomnia caused by medical condition

Sleep-Related Breathing Disorder

Central Sleep Apnea Syndromes
- Primary central sleep apnea
- Central sleep apnea caused by medical condition
- Obstructive sleep apnea syndromes

Hypersomnias Not Caused by a Sleep-Related Breathing Disorder
- Narcolepsy (four specified types)
- Menstrual-related hypersomnia
- Hypersomnia caused by a medical condition

Parasomnias

Disorders of Arousal
- Sleepwalking
- Sleep terrors

Parasomnias Usually Associated with REM Sleep
- Nightmare disorder
- REM sleep-behavior disorder

Other Parasomnias
- Sleep-related hallucinations
- Sleep-related eating disorder
- Sleep-related enuresis (bed-wetting)

Circadian Rhythm Sleep Disorders

Primary Circadian Rhythm Sleep Disorders
- Delayed–sleep phase type
- Advanced–sleep phase type

Behaviorally Induced Circadian Rhythm Sleep Disorders
- Jet lag type
- Shift work type
- Drug or substance use

Sleep-Related Movement Disorders
- Restless legs syndrome
- Periodic limb movements
- Sleep-related bruxism (teeth grinding)

Isolated Symptoms, Apparently Normal Variants, and Unresolved Issues
- Long sleeper
- Short sleeper
- Sleep talking

Other Sleep Disorders
- Physiological (organic) sleep disorders
- Environmental sleep disorder

Data from American Academy of Sleep Medicine: International classes of diseases and international classification of sleep disorders. In Kryger HM et al: *Principles and practice of sleep medicine,* ed 5, St Louis, 2011, Saunders.
REM, Rapid eye movement.

that disturb sleep. The category of isolated symptoms, apparently normal variants, and unresolved issues includes sleep-related symptoms that fall between normal and abnormal sleep. The "other" sleep disorders category contains sleep problems that do not fit into other categories.

Sleep laboratory studies diagnose a sleep disorder. A **polysomnogram** involves the use of EEG, EMG, and EOG to monitor stages of sleep and wakefulness during nighttime sleep. The Multiple Sleep Latency Test (MSLT) provides objective information about sleepiness and selected aspects of sleep structure by measuring eye movements, muscle-tone changes, and brain electrical activity during at least four napping opportunities spread throughout the day. The MSLT takes 8 to 10 hours to complete. Patients wear an Actigraph device on the wrist to measure sleep-wake patterns over an extended period of time. Actigraphy data provide information about sleep time, sleep efficiency, number and duration of awakenings, and levels of activity and rest.

Insomnia. **Insomnia** is a symptom that patients experience when they have chronic difficulty falling asleep, frequent awakenings from sleep, and/or a short sleep or nonrestorative sleep (Kryger et al., 2011). It is the most common sleep-related complaint. People with insomnia experience EDS and insufficient sleep quantity and quality. However, frequently a patient gets more sleep than he or she realizes. Insomnia often signals an underlying physical or psychological disorder. It occurs more frequently in and is the most common sleep problem for women.

People experience transient insomnia as a result of situational stresses such as family, work, or school problems; jet lag; illness; or loss of a loved one. Insomnia sometimes recurs, but between episodes a patient is able to sleep well. However, a temporary case of insomnia caused by a stressful situation can lead to chronic difficulty in getting enough sleep, perhaps because of the worry and anxiety that develop about getting it.

Insomnia is often associated with poor **sleep hygiene**, or practices that a patient associates with sleep. If the condition continues, the fear of not being able to sleep is enough to cause wakefulness. During the day people with chronic insomnia feel sleepy, fatigued, depressed, and anxious. Treatment is symptomatic, including improved sleep-hygiene measures, biofeedback, cognitive techniques, and relaxation techniques. Behavioral and cognitive therapies have few adverse effects and show evidence of sustained improvement in sleep over time (Babson et al., 2010).

Sleep Apnea. **Sleep apnea** is a disorder characterized by the lack of airflow through the nose and mouth for periods of 10 seconds or longer during sleep. There are three types of sleep apnea: central, obstructive, and mixed apnea. The most common form is obstructive sleep apnea (OSA). Research estimates that 2% to 4% of the adults in the United States meet the diagnostic criteria for OSA (Adult Obstructive Sleep Apnea Task Force, 2009). The two major risk factors for OSA are obesity and hypertension. Smoking, heart failure, type II diabetes, alcohol, and a positive family history of OSA also greatly increase the risk of developing the problem (Adult Obstructive Sleep Apnea Task Force, 2009). It occurs in up to 2% of middle-age women and up to 4% of middle-age men, with occurrence higher in the older-adult population and African-Americans (Malhotra and Desai, 2010).

OSA occurs when muscles or structures of the oral cavity or throat relax during sleep. The upper airway becomes partially or completely blocked, diminishing nasal airflow (hypopnea) or stopping it (apnea) for as long as 30 seconds (Kryger et al., 2011). The person still attempts to breathe because chest and abdominal movement continue, which often results in loud snoring and snorting sounds. When breathing is partially or completely diminished, each successive diaphragmatic movement becomes stronger until the obstruction is relieved. Structural abnormalities such as a deviated septum, nasal polyps, certain jaw configurations, larger neck circumference, or enlarged tonsils predispose a patient to OSA (Pinto and Caple, 2010). The effort to breathe during sleep results in arousals from deep sleep often to the stage 2 cycle. In severe cases hundreds of hypopnea/apnea episodes occur every hour, resulting in severe interference with deep sleep.

Excessive daytime sleepiness (EDS) and fatigue are the most common complaints of people with OSA. People with severe OSA often report taking daytime naps and experience a disruption in their daily activities because of sleepiness (Adult Obstructive Sleep Apnea Task Force, 2009). Feelings of sleepiness are usually most intense on waking, right before going to sleep, and about 12 hours after the mid-sleep period. EDS often results in impaired waking function, poor work or school performance, accidents while driving or using equipment, and behavioral or emotional problems. In general, OSA has the potential to contribute to high blood pressure and increased risk for heart attack and stroke (National Sleep Foundation, 2014c).

OSA causes a serious decline in arterial oxygen saturation level. Patients are at risk for cardiac dysrhythmias, right heart failure, pulmonary hypertension, angina attacks, stroke, and hypertension.

Central sleep apnea (CSA) involves dysfunction in the respiratory control center of the brain. The impulse to breathe fails temporarily, and nasal airflow and chest wall movement cease. The oxygen saturation of the blood falls. The condition is common in patients with brainstem injury, muscular dystrophy, and encephalitis. Less than 10% of sleep apnea is predominantly central in origin. People with CSA tend to awaken during sleep and therefore complain of insomnia and EDS. Mild and intermittent snoring is also present.

Patients with sleep apnea rarely achieve deep sleep. In addition to complaints of EDS, sleep attacks, fatigue, morning headaches, irritability, depression, difficulty concentrating, and decreased sex drive are common (Kryger et al., 2011). OSA affects quality-of-life issues such as marital relationships and interactions within and outside the family and often is an embarrassment to a patient (Adult Obstructive Sleep Apnea Task Force, 2009). Treatment includes therapy for underlying cardiac or respiratory complications and emotional problems that occur as a result of the symptoms of this disorder.

Narcolepsy. **Narcolepsy** is a dysfunction of mechanisms that regulate sleep and wake states. Excessive daytime sleepiness is the most common complaint associated with this disorder. During the day a person suddenly feels an overwhelming wave of sleepiness and falls asleep; REM sleep occurs within 15 minutes of falling asleep. **Cataplexy**, or sudden muscle weakness during intense emotions such as anger, sadness, or laughter, occurs at any time during the day. If the cataplectic attack is severe, a patient loses voluntary muscle control and falls to the floor. A person with narcolepsy often has vivid dreams that occur as he or she is falling asleep. These dreams are difficult to distinguish from reality. Sleep paralysis, or the feeling of being unable to move or talk just before waking or falling asleep, is another symptom. Some studies show a genetic link for narcolepsy (Ahmed and Thorpy, 2010).

A person with narcolepsy falls asleep uncontrollably at inappropriate times. When individuals do not understand this disorder, a sleep attack is easily mistaken for laziness, lack of interest in activities, or drunkenness. Typically the symptoms first begin to appear in adolescence and are often confused with the EDS that commonly occurs in teens. Narcoleptic patients are treated with stimulants or wakefulness-promoting agents such as sodium oxybate, modafinil (Provigil) or armodafinil (Nuvigil) that only partially increase wakefulness and reduce sleep attacks. Patients also receive antidepressant medications that suppress cataplexy and the other REM-related symptoms. Brief daytime naps no longer than 20 minutes help reduce subjective feelings of sleepiness. Other management methods that help are following a regular exercise program, practicing good sleep habits, avoiding shifts in sleep, strategically timing daytime naps if possible, eating light meals high in protein, practicing deep breathing, chewing gum, and taking vitamins (Kryger et al., 2011). Patients with narcolepsy need to avoid factors that increase drowsiness (e.g., alcohol; heavy meals; exhausting activities; long-distance driving; and long periods of sitting in hot, stuffy rooms).

Sleep Deprivation. Sleep deprivation is a problem many patients experience as a result of dyssomnia. Causes include symptoms (e.g., fever, difficulty breathing, or pain) caused by illnesses, emotional stress, medications, environmental disturbances (e.g., frequent nursing care), and variability in the timing of sleep because of shift work. Physicians and nurses are particularly prone to sleep deprivation as a result of long work schedules and rotating shifts. Chronic sleep deprivation is associated with development of cardiovascular disease, weight gain, type II diabetes, poor memory, depression, and digestive problems (Redeker and McEnany, 2011).

Hospitalization, especially in intensive care units (ICUs), makes patients particularly vulnerable to the extrinsic and circadian sleep disorders that cause the "ICU syndrome of sleep deprivation" (Fontana and Pittiglio, 2010). Constant environmental stimuli within the ICU such as strange noises from equipment, the frequent monitoring and care given by nurses, and ever-present lights confuse patients. Repeated environmental stimuli and the patient's poor physical status lead to sleep deprivation (Fontana and Pittiglio, 2010).

A person's response to sleep deprivation is highly variable. Patients experience a variety of physiological and psychological symptoms (Box 43-3). The severity of symptoms is often related to the duration of sleep deprivation.

Parasomnias. The parasomnias are sleep problems that are more common in children than adults. Some have hypothesized that sudden infant death syndrome (SIDS) is thought to be related to apnea, hypoxia, and cardiac arrhythmias caused by abnormalities in the autonomic nervous system that are manifested during sleep (Kryger et al., 2011). Because of an association between the prone position and the occurrence of SIDS, the American Academy of Pediatrics recommends that parents place apparently healthy infants in the supine position during sleep (Koren et al., 2010).

Parasomnias that occur among older children include somnambulism (sleepwalking), night terrors, nightmares, nocturnal enuresis (bed-wetting), body rocking, and bruxism (teeth grinding). When adults have these problems, it often indicates more serious disorders. Specific treatment varies. However, in all cases it is important to support patients and maintain their safety.

BOX 43-3 Sleep-Deprivation Symptoms

Physiological Symptoms
- Ptosis, blurred vision
- Fine-motor clumsiness
- Decreased reflexes
- Slowed response time
- Decreased reasoning and judgment
- Decreased auditory and visual alertness
- Cardiac arrhythmias

Psychological Symptoms
- Confused and disoriented
- Increased sensitivity to pain
- Irritable, withdrawn, apathetic
- Agitated
- Hyperactive
- Decreased motivation
- Excessive sleepiness

NURSING KNOWLEDGE BASE

Sleep and Rest

When people are at rest, they usually feel mentally relaxed, free from anxiety, and physically calm. Rest does not imply inactivity, although everyone often thinks of it as settling down in a comfortable chair or lying in bed. When people are at rest, they are in a state of mental, physical, and spiritual activity that leaves them feeling refreshed, rejuvenated, and ready to resume the activities of the day. People have their own habits for obtaining rest and can find ways to adjust to new environments or conditions that affect the ability to rest. They rest by reading a book, practicing a relaxation exercise, listening to music, taking a long walk, or sitting quietly.

Illness and unfamiliar health care routines easily affect the usual rest and sleep patterns of people entering a hospital or other health care facility. Nurses frequently care for patients who are on bed rest to reduce physical and psychological demands on the body in a variety of health care settings. However, these people do not necessarily feel rested. Some still have emotional worries that prevent complete relaxation. For example, concern over physical limitations or a fear of being unable to return to their usual lifestyle causes such patients to feel stressed and unable to relax. You must always be aware of a patient's need for rest. A lack of rest for long periods causes illness or worsening of existing illness.

Normal Sleep Requirements and Patterns

Sleep duration and quality vary among people of all age-groups. For example, one person feels adequately rested with 4 hours of sleep, whereas another requires 10 hours. Nurses play an important role in identifying treatable sleep-deprivation problems.

Neonates. The neonate up to the age of 3 months averages about 16 hours of sleep a day, sleeping almost constantly during the first week. The sleep cycle is generally 40 to 50 minutes with wakening occurring after one to two sleep cycles. Approximately 50% of this sleep is REM sleep, which stimulates the higher brain centers. This is essential for development because the neonate is not awake long enough for significant external stimulation.

Infants. Infants usually develop a nighttime pattern of sleep by 3 months of age. The infant normally takes several naps during the day but usually sleeps an average of 8 to 10 hours during the night for a total daily sleep time of 15 hours. About 30% of sleep time is in the REM cycle. Awakening commonly occurs early in the morning, although it is not unusual for an infant to wake up during the night.

Toddlers. By the age of 2 children usually sleep through the night and take daily naps. Total sleep averages 12 hours a day. After 3 years of age children often give up daytime naps (Hockenberry and Wilson, 2015). It is common for toddlers to awaken during the night. The percentage of REM sleep continues to fall. During this period toddlers may be unwilling to go to bed at night because they need autonomy or fear separation from their parents.

Preschoolers. On average a preschooler sleeps about 12 hours a night (about 20% is REM). By the age of 5 he or she rarely takes daytime naps except in cultures in which a siesta is the custom (Hockenberry and Wilson, 2015). The preschooler usually has difficulty relaxing or quieting down after long, active days and has bedtime fears, awakens during the night, or has nightmares. Partial awakening followed by normal return to sleep is frequent (Hockenberry and

Wilson, 2015). In the awake period the child exhibits brief crying, walking around, unintelligible speech, sleepwalking, or bed-wetting.

School-Age Children. The amount of sleep needed varies during the school years. A 6-year-old averages 11 to 12 hours of sleep nightly, whereas an 11-year-old sleeps about 9 to 10 hours (Hockenberry and Wilson, 2015). The 6- or 7-year-old usually goes to bed with some encouragement or by doing quiet activities. The older child often resists sleeping because he or she is unaware of fatigue or has a need to be independent.

Adolescents. On average the majority of teenagers get about 7 hours or less of sleep per night (National Sleep Foundation, 2014d). The typical adolescent is subject to a number of changes such as school demands, after-school social activities, and part-time jobs, which reduce the time spent sleeping (Wiggins and Freeman, 2014). Adolescents typically have electronic devices such as televisions, computers, smartphones, or video games in their rooms, which further contribute to sleep disruption, poor sleep quality, and decreased amount of sleep (National Sleep Foundation, 2014d). Shortened sleep time often results in EDS, which frequently leads to reduced performance in school, vulnerability to accidents, behavior and mood problems, and increased use of alcohol (Wiggins and Freeman, 2014).

Young Adults. Most young adults average 6 to 8½ hours of sleep a night. Approximately 20% of sleep time is REM sleep, which remains consistent throughout life. It is common for the stresses of jobs, family relationships, and social activities to frequently lead to insomnia and the use of sleep medication. Daytime sleepiness contributes to an increased number of accidents, decreased productivity, and interpersonal problems in this age-group.

Pregnancy increases the need for sleep and rest. However, a majority of pregnant women describe variations in sleep habits (Redeker and McEnany, 2011). Increases in estrogen and progesterone during pregnancy affect sleep. Estrogen has been shown to decrease REM sleep (Redeker and McEnany, 2011). First-trimester sleep disturbances include a reduction in overall sleep time and quality. Daytime drowsiness, insomnia, and nighttime awakenings also increase because of frequent nocturnal voiding. These disturbances level off in the second trimester (Redeker and McEnany, 2011). Insomnia, periodic limb movements, RLS, and sleep-disordered breathing are common problems during the third trimester of pregnancy (Kryger et al., 2011).

Middle Adults. During middle adulthood the total time spent sleeping at night begins to decline. The amount of stage 4 sleep begins to fall, a decline that continues with advancing age. Insomnia is particularly common, probably because of the changes and stresses of middle age. Anxiety, depression, or certain physical illnesses cause sleep disturbances. Women experiencing menopausal symptoms often experience insomnia.

Older Adults. Complaints of sleeping difficulties increase with age. Older adults experience weakening, desynchronized circadian rhythms that alter the sleep-wake cycle (Neikrug and Ancoli-Israel, 2010). Episodes of REM sleep tend to shorten. Stages 3 and 4 NREM sleep progressively decrease; some older adults have almost no stage 4, or deep sleep. An older adult awakens more often during the night, and it takes more time for him or her to fall asleep. The tendency to nap seems to increase progressively with age because of the frequent awakenings experienced at night.

The presence of chronic illness often results in sleep disturbances for the older adult. For example, an older adult with arthritis frequently has difficulty sleeping because of painful joints. Changes in sleep pattern are often caused by changes in the CNS that affect the regulation of sleep. Many older adults with insomnia have co-morbid psychiatric illness or medical conditions, take medications that disrupt sleep patterns, or use drugs or alcohol (Fiorentino and Martin, 2010). Sensory impairment reduces an older person's sensitivity to time cues that maintain circadian rhythms.

Factors Influencing Sleep

A number of factors affect the quantity and quality of sleep. Often a single factor is not the only cause for a sleep problem. Physiological, psychological, and environmental factors frequently alter the quality and quantity of sleep.

Drugs and Substances. Sleepiness, insomnia, and fatigue often result as a direct effect of commonly prescribed medications (Box 43-4). These medications alter sleep and weaken daytime alertness, which is problematic (Kryger et al., 2011). Medications prescribed for sleep often cause more problems than benefits. Older adults take a variety of drugs to control or treat chronic illness, and the combined effects of their drugs often seriously disrupt sleep. Some substances such as L-tryptophan, a natural protein found in foods such as milk, cheese, and meats, promote sleep.

Lifestyle. A person's daily routine influences sleep patterns. An individual working a rotating shift (e.g., 2 weeks of days followed by a

BOX 43-4 Drugs and Their Effects on Sleep

Hypnotics
- Interfere with reaching deeper sleep stages
- Provide only temporary (1-week) increase in quantity of sleep
- Eventually cause "hangover" during day; excess drowsiness, confusion, decreased energy
- Sometimes worsen sleep apnea in older adults

Antidepressants and Stimulants
- Suppress REM sleep
- Decrease total sleep time

Alcohol
- Speeds onset of sleep
- Reduces REM sleep
- Awakens person during night and causes difficulty returning to sleep

Caffeine
- Prevents person from falling asleep
- Causes person to awaken during night
- Interferes with REM sleep

Diuretics
- Nighttime awakenings caused by nocturia

Beta-Adrenergic Blockers
- Cause nightmares
- Cause insomnia
- Cause awakening from sleep

Benzodiazepines
- Alter REM sleep
- Increase sleep time
- Increase daytime sleepiness

Nicotine
- Decreases total sleep time
- Decreases REM sleep time
- Causes awakening from sleep
- Causes difficulty staying asleep

Opiates
- Suppress REM sleep
- Cause increased daytime drowsiness

Anticonvulsants
- Decrease REM sleep time
- Cause daytime drowsiness

REM, Rapid eye movement.

week of nights) often has difficulty adjusting to the altered sleep schedule. For example, the body's internal clock is set at 11 PM, but the work schedule forces sleep at 9 AM instead. The individual is able to sleep only 3 or 4 hours because his or her body clock perceives that it is time to be awake and active. Difficulties maintaining alertness during work time result in decreased and even hazardous performance. After several weeks of working a night shift, a person's biological clock usually does adjust. Other alterations in routines that disrupt sleep patterns include performing unaccustomed heavy work, engaging in late-night social activities, and changing evening mealtime.

Usual Sleep Patterns. In the past century the amount of sleep obtained nightly by U.S. citizens has decreased, causing many Americans to be sleep deprived and experience excessive sleepiness during the day. Sleepiness becomes pathological when it occurs at times when individuals need or want to be awake. People who experience temporary sleep deprivation as a result of an active social evening or lengthened work schedule usually feel sleepy the next day. However, they are able to overcome these feelings even though they have difficulty performing tasks and remaining attentive. Chronic lack of sleep is much more serious and causes serious alterations in the ability to perform daily functions. Sleepiness tends to be most difficult to overcome during sedentary (inactive) tasks such as driving.

Emotional Stress. Worry over personal problems or a situation frequently disrupts sleep. Emotional stress causes a person to be tense and often leads to frustration when sleep does not occur. Stress also causes a person to try too hard to fall asleep, to awaken frequently during the sleep cycle, or to oversleep. Continued stress causes poor sleep habits.

Older patients frequently experience losses that lead to emotional stress such as retirement, physical impairment, or the death of a loved one. Older adults and other individuals who experience depressive mood problems experience delays in falling asleep, earlier appearance of REM sleep, frequent or early waking, feelings of sleeping poorly, and daytime sleepiness (National Sleep Foundation, 2014c).

Environment. The physical environment in which a person sleeps significantly influences the ability to fall and remain asleep. Good ventilation is essential for restful sleep. The size, firmness, and position of the bed affect the quality of sleep. If a person usually sleeps with another individual, sleeping alone often causes wakefulness. On the other hand, sleeping with a restless or snoring bed partner disrupts sleep.

In hospitals and other inpatient facilities, noise creates a problem for patients. Noise in hospitals is usually new or strange and often loud. Thus patients wake easily. This problem is greatest the first night of hospitalization, when patients often experience increased total wake time, increased awakenings, and decreased REM sleep and total sleep time. People-induced noises (e.g., nursing activities) are sources of increased sound levels. ICUs are sources of high noise levels because of staff, monitor alarms, and equipment. Close proximity of patients, noise from confused and ill patients, ringing alarm systems and telephones, and disturbances caused by emergencies make the environment unpleasant. Noise causes increased agitation; delayed healing; impaired immune function; and increased blood pressure, heart rate, and stress (Dennis et al., 2010).

Light levels affect the ability to fall asleep. Some patients prefer a dark room, whereas others such as children or older adults prefer keeping a soft light on during sleep. Patients also have trouble sleeping because of the room temperature. A room that is too warm or too cold often causes a patient to become restless.

Exercise and Fatigue. A person who is moderately fatigued usually achieves restful sleep, especially if the fatigue is the result of enjoyable work or exercise. Exercising 2 hours or more before bedtime allows the body to cool down and maintain a state of fatigue that promotes relaxation. However, excess fatigue resulting from exhausting or stressful work makes falling asleep difficult. This is often seen in grade-school children and adolescents who keep stressful, long schedules because of school, social activities, and work.

Food and Caloric Intake. Following good eating habits is important for proper sleep. Eating a large, heavy, and/or spicy meal at night often results in indigestion that interferes with sleep. Caffeine, alcohol, and nicotine consumed in the evening produce insomnia. Coffee, tea, cola, and chocolate contain caffeine and xanthines that cause sleeplessness. Thus drastically reducing or avoiding these substances can improve sleep. Some food allergies cause insomnia. A milk allergy sometimes causes nighttime waking and crying or colic in infants.

Weight loss or gain influences sleep patterns. Weight gain contributes to OSA because of increased size of the soft tissue structures in the upper airway (Kryger et al., 2011). Weight loss causes insomnia and decreased amounts of sleep (Ross et al., 2011). Certain sleep disorders are the result of the semi-starvation diets popular in a weight-conscious society.

CRITICAL THINKING

Successful critical thinking requires a synthesis of knowledge, including information gathered from patients, experience, critical thinking attitudes, and intellectual and professional standards. Clinical judgments require you to anticipate the information necessary, analyze the data, and make decisions regarding patient care. You adapt critical thinking to the changing needs of the patient. During assessment consider all elements to make appropriate nursing diagnoses (Figure 43-3).

In the case of sleep, integrate knowledge from nursing and disciplines such as pharmacology and psychology. Personal experience with a sleep problem and experience with patients prepares you to know effective forms of sleep therapies. You use critical thinking attitudes such as perseverance, confidence, and discipline to complete a comprehensive assessment and develop a plan of care to provide successful management of the sleep problem. Professional standards such as the *Nursing Scope and Standards of Practice* (American Nurses Association, 2010), *Clinical Guidelines for the Treatment of Primary Insomnia* (National Guideline Clearinghouse, 2014), and "Excessive Sleepiness" in *Evidence-based Geriatrics Nursing Protocols for Best Practice* (Chasens and Umlauf., 2012) provide valuable guidelines to assess and address the needs of patients with sleep disorders.

❖ NURSING PROCESS

Apply the nursing process and use a critical thinking approach in the care of patients. The nursing process provides a clinical decision-making approach for you to develop and implement an individualized plan of care.

◆ Assessment

During the assessment process thoroughly assess each patient and critically analyze findings to ensure that you make patient-centered clinical decisions required for safe nursing care.

Through the Patient's Eyes. Sleep is a subjective experience. Only the patient is able to report whether or not it is sufficient and

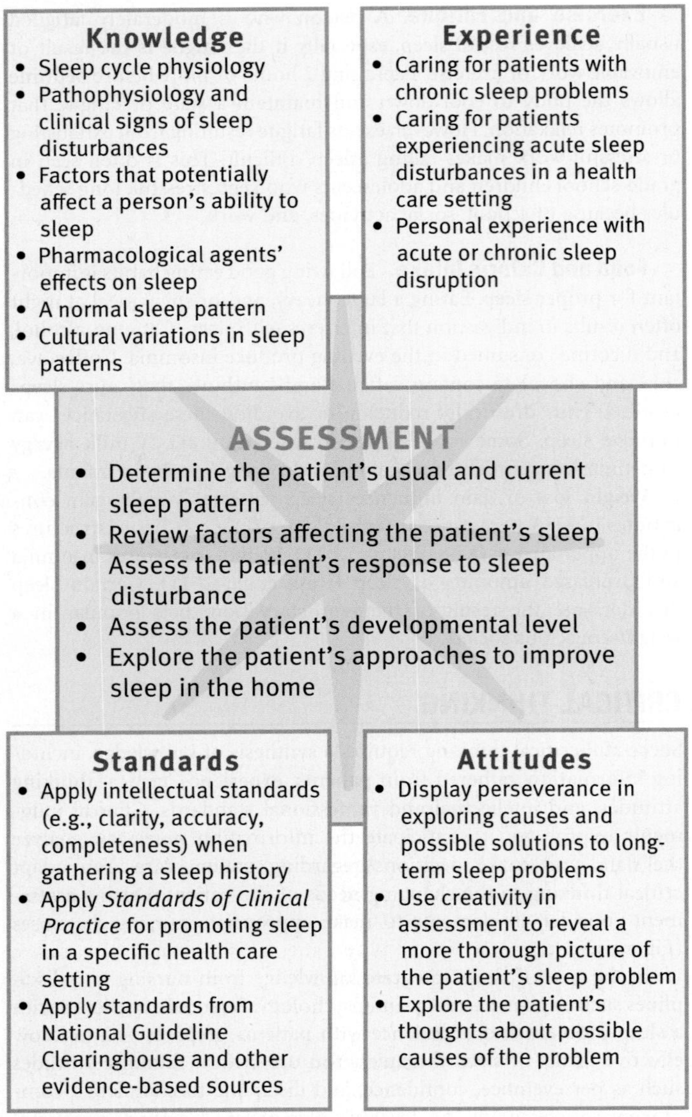

Knowledge
- Sleep cycle physiology
- Pathophysiology and clinical signs of sleep disturbances
- Factors that potentially affect a person's ability to sleep
- Pharmacological agents' effects on sleep
- A normal sleep pattern
- Cultural variations in sleep patterns

Experience
- Caring for patients with chronic sleep problems
- Caring for patients experiencing acute sleep disturbances in a health care setting
- Personal experience with acute or chronic sleep disruption

ASSESSMENT
- Determine the patient's usual and current sleep pattern
- Review factors affecting the patient's sleep
- Assess the patient's response to sleep disturbance
- Assess the patient's developmental level
- Explore the patient's approaches to improve sleep in the home

Standards
- Apply intellectual standards (e.g., clarity, accuracy, completeness) when gathering a sleep history
- Apply *Standards of Clinical Practice* for promoting sleep in a specific health care setting
- Apply standards from National Guideline Clearinghouse and other evidence-based sources

Attitudes
- Display perseverance in exploring causes and possible solutions to long-term sleep problems
- Use creativity in assessment to reveal a more thorough picture of the patient's sleep problem
- Explore the patient's thoughts about possible causes of the problem

FIGURE 43-3 Critical thinking model for sleep assessment.

restful. If the patient is satisfied with the quantity and quality of sleep received, you consider it normal, and the nursing history that you will collect is brief. If a patient admits to or suspects a sleep problem, you will need a detailed history and assessment. If a patient has an obvious sleep problem, consider asking if his or her sleep partner can be approached for further assessment data.

A poor night's sleep for a patient often starts a vicious cycle of anticipatory anxiety. The patient fears that sleep will again be disturbed while trying harder and harder to sleep. Use a skilled and caring approach to assess the patient's sleep needs. A caring nurse individualizes care for each patient. Always ask patients what they expect regarding sleep. This includes asking about the interventions that they currently use and how successful they are. It is important to understand patients' expectations regarding their sleep pattern. When they ask for help because of sleep disturbances, they typically expect a nurse to respond promptly to help them improve the quantity and quality of their sleep.

Sleep Assessment. Most people are able to provide a reasonably accurate estimate of their sleep patterns, particularly if any changes have occurred. Aim your assessment at first understanding the characteristics of the patient's sleep problem and usual sleep habits so you incorporate ways for promoting sleep into nursing care. For example, if the nursing history reveals that a patient always reads before falling asleep, it makes sense to offer reading material at bedtime.

Sources for Sleep Assessment. Usually patients are the best resource for describing sleep problems and how they are a change from their usual sleep and waking patterns. Often the patient knows the cause for sleep problems such as a noisy environment or worry over a relationship.

In addition, bed partners are able to provide information about patients' sleep patterns that help reveal the nature of certain sleep disorders. For example, partners of patients with sleep apnea often complain that the patient's snoring disturbs their sleep. Ask bed partners (if the patient agrees) whether patients have breathing pauses during sleep and how frequently the apneic attacks occur. Some partners mention becoming fearful when patients apparently stop breathing for periods.

When caring for children, seek information about sleep patterns from parents or guardians because they are usually a reliable source of information. Hunger, excessive warmth, and separation anxiety often contribute to an infant's difficulty going to sleep or frequent awakenings during the night. Parents of infants need to keep a 24-hour log of their infant's waking and sleeping behavior for several days to determine the cause of the problem. They also need to describe the infant's eating pattern and sleeping environment because these influence sleeping behavior. Older children often are able to relate fears or worries that inhibit their ability to fall asleep. If children frequently awaken in the middle of bad dreams, parents are able to identify the problem but perhaps do not understand the meaning of the dreams. Ask parents to describe the typical behavior patterns that foster or impair sleep. For example, excessive stimulation from active play or visiting friends predictably impairs sleep. With chronic sleep problems, parents need to relate the duration of the problem, its progression, and children's responses.

Tools for Sleep Assessment. Two effective subjective measures of sleep are the Epworth Sleepiness Scale and the Pittsburgh Sleep Quality Index. The Epworth Sleepiness Scale evaluates the severity of EDS (Chasens and Umlauf, 2012). The Pittsburgh Sleep Quality Index assesses sleep quality and patterns (Redeker and McEnany, 2011). Another effective, brief method for assessing sleep quality is the use of a visual analog scale. Draw a straight horizontal line 100 mm (4 inches) long. Opposing statements such as "best night's sleep" and "worst night's sleep" are at opposite ends of the line. Ask patients to place a mark on the horizontal line at the point corresponding to their perceptions of the previous night's sleep. Measuring the distances of the mark along the line in millimeters offers a numerical value for satisfaction with sleep. Use the scale repeatedly to show change over time. Such a scale is useful to assess an individual patient, not to compare patients.

Another brief subjective method to assess sleep is a numeric scale with a 0-to-10 sleep rating. Ask individuals to separately rate the quantity and quality of their sleep on the scale. Instruct them to indicate with a number between 0 and 10 their sleep quantity and then their quality of sleep, with 0 being the worst sleep and 10 being the best.

Sleep History. When suspecting a patient has a sleep problem, assess the quality and characteristics of sleep in greater depth by asking the patient to describe the problem. This includes recent changes in sleep pattern, sleep symptoms experienced during waking hours, use of sleep and other prescribed or over-the-counter medications, diet

BOX 43-5 Nursing Assessment Questions

Nature of the Problem

- Describe for me the type of sleep problem you're having.
- Why do you think you're not getting enough sleep?
- Describe a recent night's sleep. How is this sleep different from your usual sleep?

Signs and Symptoms

- Do you have difficulty falling asleep, staying asleep, or waking up?
- Have you been told that you snore loudly?
- Do you have headaches when awakening?

Onset and Duration of Signs and Symptoms

- When did you notice the problem?
- What do you do to relieve the symptom?
- How long has this problem lasted?

Severity

- How long does it take you to fall asleep?
- How often during the week do you have trouble falling asleep?
- How many hours of sleep a night did you get this week?
- How does this compare to your usual amount of sleep?
- What do you do when you awaken during the night or too early in the morning?

Predisposing Factors

- What do you do just before you go to bed?
- Have you recently had any changes at work or at home?
- How is your mood? Have you noticed any changes recently?
- Which medications or recreational drugs do you take on a regular basis?
- Are you taking any new prescriptions or over-the-counter medications?
- Do you eat food (spicy or greasy foods) or drink substances (alcohol or caffeinated beverages) that affect your sleep?
- Do you have a physical illness that affects your sleep?
- Does anyone in your family have a history of sleep problems?

Effect on Patient

- How has the loss of sleep affected you?
- Do you feel excessively sleepy or irritable or have trouble concentrating during waking hours?
- Do you have trouble staying awake? Have you fallen asleep at the wrong times (e.g., while driving, sitting quietly in a meeting)?

and intake of substances such as caffeine or alcohol that influence sleep, and recent life events that have affected the patient's mental and emotional status.

Description of Sleeping Problems. Conduct a more detailed history when a patient has a persistent or what appears to be a serious sleep problem. Open-ended questions help a patient describe a problem more fully. A general description of the problem followed by more focused questions usually reveals specific characteristics that are useful in planning therapies. To begin, you need to understand the nature of the sleep problem, its signs and symptoms, its onset and duration, its severity, any predisposing factors or causes, and the overall effect on the patient. Ask specific questions related to the sleep problem (Box 43-5).

Proper questioning helps to determine the type of sleep disturbance and the nature of the problem. Box 43-6 gives examples of additional questions for you to ask a patient when you suspect specific sleep disorders. The questions help to select specific sleep therapies and the best time for implementation.

BOX 43-6 Questions to Ask to Assess for Specific Sleep Disorders

Insomnia

- How easily do you fall asleep?
- Do you fall asleep and have difficulty staying asleep? How many times do you awaken?
- What time do you awaken in the morning? What causes you to awaken early?
- What do you do to prepare for sleep? To improve your sleep?
- What do you think about as you try to fall asleep?
- How often do you have trouble sleeping?

Sleep Apnea

- Do you snore loudly? Does anyone else in your family snore loudly?
- Has anyone ever told you that you often stop breathing for short periods during sleep? (Spouse or bed partner/roommate may report this.)
- Do you experience headaches after awakening?
- Do you have difficulty staying awake during the day?

Narcolepsy

- Do you fall asleep at the wrong times? (Friends or relatives may report this.)
- Do you have episodes of losing muscle control or falling to the floor?
- Have you ever had the feeling of being unable to move or talk just before waking or falling asleep?
- Do you have vivid, lifelike dreams when going to sleep or awakening?

As an adjunct to the sleep history, have the patient and bed partner keep a sleep-wake log for 1 to 4 weeks. The patient completes the sleep-wake log daily to provide information on day-to-day variations in sleep-wake patterns over extended periods. Entries in the log often include 24-hour information about various waking and sleeping health behaviors such as physical activities, mealtimes, type and amount of intake (alcohol and caffeine), time and length of daytime naps, evening and bedtime routines, the time the patient tries to fall asleep, nighttime awakenings, and the time of morning awakening. A partner helps record the estimated times the patient falls asleep or awakens. Although the log is helpful, the patient needs to be motivated to participate in its completion.

Usual Sleep Pattern. Normal sleep is difficult to define because individuals vary in their perception of adequate quantity and quality of sleep. However, it is important to have patients describe their usual sleep pattern to determine the significance of the changes caused by a sleep disorder. Knowing a patient's usual, preferred sleep pattern allows you to try to match sleeping conditions in a health care setting with those in the home. Ask the following questions to determine a patient's sleep pattern:

1. What time do you usually get in bed each night?
2. How much time does it usually take to fall asleep? Do you do anything special to help you fall asleep?
3. How many times do you wake up during the night? Why?
4. What time do you typically wake up in the morning?
5. On average, how many hours do you sleep each night?

Compare patient data with their pattern before the sleep problem or with the predominant pattern usually found for other patients of the same age. On the basis of this comparison, you begin to assess for identifiable patterns such as insomnia.

Patients with sleep problems frequently show patterns drastically different from their usual one, or sometimes the change is relatively minor. Hospitalized patients usually need or want more sleep as a result of illness. However, some require less sleep because they are less active. Some patients who are ill think that it is important to try to sleep more than usual, eventually making sleeping difficult.

Physical and Psychological Illness. Determine whether the patient has any preexisting health problems that interfere with sleep. A history of psychiatric problems also makes a difference. For example, a patient who is living with bipolar disorder sleeps more when depressed than when manic. A patient who is depressed often experiences an inadequate amount of fragmented sleep. Chronic diseases such as chronic obstructive pulmonary disease and painful disorders such as arthritis interfere with sleep. Also assess the patient's medication history, including a description of over-the-counter and prescribed drugs. If a patient takes medications to aid sleep, gather information about the type and amount of medication and frequency used. Also assess the patient's daily caffeine intake.

If the patient has recently had surgery, expect him or her to experience some sleep disturbance. Patients usually awaken frequently during the first night after surgery and receive little deep or REM sleep. Depending on the type of surgery, it takes several days to months for a normal sleep cycle to return.

Current Life Events. In your assessment learn if the patient is experiencing any changes in lifestyle that disrupt sleep. A person's occupation often offers a clue to the nature of the sleep problem. Changes in job responsibilities, rotating shifts, or long hours contribute to a sleep disturbance. Questions about social activities, recent travel, or mealtime schedules help clarify the assessment.

Emotional and Mental Status. A patient's emotions and mental status affect the ability to sleep. For example, if a patient is experiencing anxiety, emotional stress related to illness, or situational crises such as loss of job or a loved one, he or she often experiences insomnia. When a sleep disturbance is related to an emotional problem, the key is to treat the primary problem; its resolution often improves sleep (Chasens and Umlauf, 2012). Patients with mental illnesses may need mild sedation for adequate rest. Assess the effectiveness of any medication and its effect on daytime function.

Bedtime Routines. Ask patients what they do to prepare for sleep. For example, some patients drink a glass of milk, take a sleeping pill, eat a snack, or watch television. Assess habits that are beneficial compared with those that disturb sleep. For example, watching television promotes sleep for one person, whereas it stimulates another to stay awake. Sometimes pointing out that a particular habit is interfering with sleep helps patients find ways to change or eliminate habits that are disrupting sleep.

Pay special attention to a child's bedtime rituals. For example, the parents need to report whether it is necessary to read a bedtime story, rock the child to sleep, or engage in quiet play. Some young children need a special blanket or stuffed animal when going to sleep.

Bedtime Environment. During assessment ask the patient to describe preferred bedroom conditions, including preferences for lighting in the room, music or television in the background, or needing to have the door open versus closed. Include questions about the presence of electronic devices in the bedroom (e.g., phones, televisions), all of which have small lights that remain on or have a light that blinks when the battery is low. Patients are often surprised how many of these devices are in the sleeping environment.

In addition, some children need the company of a parent to fall asleep. In a health care environment environmental distractions such as a roommate's television, an electronic monitor in the hallway, a noisy nurses' station, or another patient who cries out at night often interfere with sleep. Identify those factors to reduce or control the environment.

Behaviors of Sleep Deprivation. Some patients are unaware of how their sleep problems are affecting their behavior. Observe for behaviors such as irritability, disorientation (similar to a drunken state), frequent yawning, and slurred speech. If sleep deprivation has lasted a long time, psychotic behavior such as delusions and paranoia sometimes develop. For example, a patient reports seeing strange objects or colors in the room, or he or she acts afraid when the nurse enters the room.

BOX 43-7 Nursing Diagnostic Process

Insomnia

Assessment Activities	Defining Characteristics
Ask patient to explain nature of sleep problem.	Patient reports difficulty falling asleep, taking up to 1 hour. Patient reports waking up two to three times nightly with difficulty returning to sleep.
Observe patient's behavior and ask spouse if patient is experiencing behavior changes.	Patient admits to not feeling well rested. Spouse describes times when patient was lethargic and irritable.
Determine if patient has had recent lifestyle changes.	Spouse reports that patient recently lost job and is concerned about finding new position.

◆ Nursing Diagnosis

Review your assessment data, looking for clusters that include defining characteristics for a sleep pattern disturbance or other health problem. If you identify a sleep problem, specify the condition such as insomnia or sleep deprivation. By specifying the sleep disturbance diagnosis, you are able to design more effective interventions. For example, you choose different therapies for patients with insomnia who are unable to fall asleep than for those with sleep deprivation. Box 43-7 demonstrates how to use nursing assessment activities to identify and cluster defining characteristics to make an accurate nursing diagnosis.

Assessment also identifies the related factor or probable cause of a sleep disturbance such as a noisy environment or a high intake of caffeinated beverages in the evening. These causes become the focus of interventions for minimizing or eliminating a problem-focused diagnosis. For example, if a patient is experiencing insomnia as a result of a noisy health care environment, offer some basic recommendations for helping sleep such as controlling the noise of hospital equipment, reducing interruptions, or keeping doors closed. If the insomnia is related to worry over a threatened marital separation, introduce coping strategies and create an environment for sleep. If you incorrectly define the probable cause or related factors, the patient does not benefit from care.

Sleep problems affect patients in other ways. For example, you find that a patient with sleep apnea has problems with a spouse who is tired and frustrated over the patient's snoring. In addition, the spouse is concerned that the patient is breathing improperly and thus is in danger. The nursing diagnosis of *Compromised Family Coping* indicates that you need to provide support to the patient and spouse so they understand sleep apnea and obtain the medical treatment needed. Examples of nursing diagnoses for patients with sleep problems include the following:

- *Anxiety*
- *Ineffective Breathing Pattern*
- *Acute Confusion*
- *Ineffective Coping*

- *Insomnia*
- *Fatigue*
- *Disturbed Sleep Pattern*
- *Sleep Deprivation*
- *Readiness for Enhanced Sleep*

◆ Planning

Goals and Outcomes. During planning you again synthesize information from multiple resources to develop an individualized plan of care (Figure 43-4) (see the Nursing Care Plan). Professional standards are especially important to consider in developing a care plan. These standards often offer evidence-based guidelines for effective nursing interventions. For example, the *Evidence-based Geriatrics Nursing Protocols for Best Practice,* titled "Excessive Sleepiness" (Chasens and Umlauf, 2012), recommends individualized nursing interventions that maintain and support an older adult's normal sleep pattern and bedtime ritual. It is important for a plan of care for sleep promotion to include strategies appropriate to the patient's sleep routines, living environment, and lifestyle.

As you plan care for a patient with sleep disturbances, creation of a concept map is another method for developing holistic patient-centered care (Figure 43-5). Create the map after identifying relevant nursing diagnoses from the assessment database. In this example the nursing diagnoses are linked to the patient's medical diagnosis of depression and situational stress. The concept map shows the relationships among the nursing diagnoses *Insomnia, Stress Overload, Sedentary Lifestyle,* and *Readiness for Enhanced Sleep.* This approach to planning care helps the nurse recognize relationships among planned interventions. For this patient, interventions and successful outcomes for one nursing diagnosis affect the resolution of another.

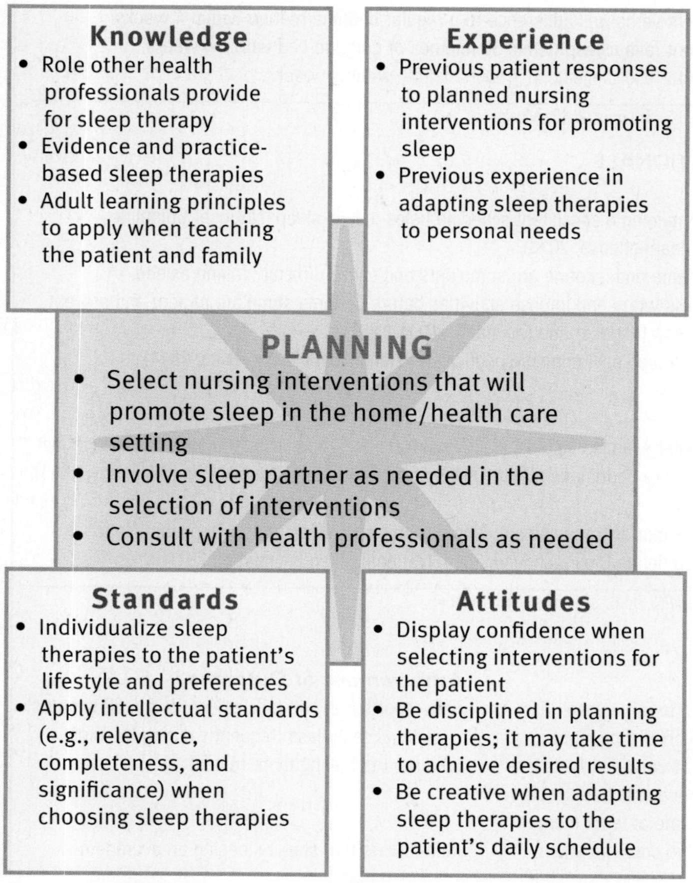

When developing goals and outcomes, it is important for a nurse and patient to collaborate. As a result, you are more likely to set realistic goals and measurable outcomes with your patients. An effective plan includes outcomes established over a realistic time frame that focus on the goal of improving the quantity and quality of sleep in the home. Often family members are very helpful in contributing to the plan. A sleep-promotion plan frequently requires many weeks to accomplish. The following is an example of a goal with patient outcomes:

Goal: The patient will control environmental sources disrupting sleep within 1 month.

Outcomes:

- Patient identifies factors in the immediate home environment that disrupt sleep in 2 weeks.
- Patient reports having a discussion with family members about environmental barriers to sleep in 2 weeks.
- Patient reports changes made in the bedroom to promote sleep within 4 weeks.
- Patient reports having fewer than two awakenings per night within 4 weeks.

Setting Priorities. Work with patients to establish priority outcomes and interventions. Frequently sleep disturbances are the result of other health problems. For example, when physical symptoms are interfering with sleep, managing the symptoms is your first priority. After symptoms are relieved, focus on sleep therapies. Patients are a helpful resource in determining which interventions hold priority. For example, once patients understand the factors that disrupt sleep, they make choices about the types of changes they would like to make in their lifestyle or sleeping environment.

Teamwork and Collaboration. Partner closely with the patient and sleep partner to ensure that any therapies such as a change in the sleep schedule or changes to the bedroom environment are realistic and achievable. In a health care setting plan treatments or routines so the patient is able to rest. For example, in the ICU use available electronic monitors to track trends in vital signs without waking a patient each hour. Other staff members need to be aware of the care plan so they can cluster activities at certain times to reduce awakenings. In a nursing home the focus of the plan involves better planning of rest periods around the activities of the other residents. Roommates often have very different schedules.

When patients have chronic sleep problems, the initial referral for a patient is often to a comprehensive sleep center for assessment of the problem. The nature of the sleep disturbance then determines whether referrals to additional health care providers are necessary. For example, if a sleep problem is related to a situational crisis or emotional problem, refer the patient to a mental health clinical nurse specialist or clinical psychologist for counseling. If the nurse works in an inpatient setting and the patient needs a referral for continued care after discharge, offering information about the sleep problem is useful to the home care nurse. The success of sleep therapy depends on an approach that fits the patient's lifestyle and the nature of the sleep disorder.

Knowledge
- Role other health professionals provide for sleep therapy
- Evidence and practice-based sleep therapies
- Adult learning principles to apply when teaching the patient and family

Experience
- Previous patient responses to planned nursing interventions for promoting sleep
- Previous experience in adapting sleep therapies to personal needs

PLANNING
- Select nursing interventions that will promote sleep in the home/health care setting
- Involve sleep partner as needed in the selection of interventions
- Consult with health professionals as needed

Standards
- Individualize sleep therapies to the patient's lifestyle and preferences
- Apply intellectual standards (e.g., relevance, completeness, and significance) when choosing sleep therapies

Attitudes
- Display confidence when selecting interventions for the patient
- Be disciplined in planning therapies; it may take time to achieve desired results
- Be creative when adapting sleep therapies to the patient's daily schedule

FIGURE 43-4 Critical thinking model for sleep planning.

◆ Implementation

Nursing interventions designed to improve the quality of a person's rest and sleep are largely focused on health promotion. Patients need adequate sleep and rest to maintain active and productive lifestyles. During times of illness rest and sleep promotion are important for recovery. Nursing care in an acute, restorative, or continuing care

NURSING CARE PLAN

Insomnia

ASSESSMENT

Julie Arnold, a 43-year-old attorney, is the first patient of the morning at the neighborhood health clinic where you work. When you ask her how she's doing, she tells you that she's having difficulty sleeping. Her physician has diagnosed that she's suffering from depression. Julie is married and has two school-age children. She also tells you that she is caring for her mother, who is staying with them currently after she was discharged from the hospital following an exacerbation of her heart failure. Julie's assessment includes a thorough sleep history and a discussion of how the sleep problem has affected her life. You also conduct a physical examination.

Assessment Activities	*Findings/Defining Characteristics**
Ask Julie to explain the nature of her sleep problem.	Julie explains that she **wakes up once or twice a night.** She states, "I feel tired when I wake up, and I have trouble concentrating at work in the afternoon." She also reports that she has less patience with her children at home and no energy in the evenings.
Ask Julie if there have been any recent changes in her life.	Julie says that she is feeling pressured at work to complete an important case that she started 2 weeks ago and because of this she is working longer hours. She also reports that, because of her heavy work schedule, she has stopped her routine of walking 1 to 2 miles daily. She reports that she has no time for any exercise when she gets home because **she needs to take care of her mother and the children.**
Ask Julie to describe her bedtime routine.	Julie responds that she is **going to bed** between 12 AM and 1 AM, which is **2 hours later than her usual bedtime. It takes her an hour to fall asleep.** She says that she used to get 7 to 8 hours of sleep a night and now **it is more like 5 to 6 hours.** She drinks two to three cups of coffee after dinner while she is working on her case before bedtime.
Assess Julie for physical signs of sleep problems.	During the examination you note that Julie has dark circles under her eyes; she shifts her position in the chair multiple times and yawns frequently. She admits to **fatigue.**

***Defining characteristics** are shown in bold type.

NURSING DIAGNOSIS: Insomnia related to psychological stress from job pressures

PLANNING

Goals	*Expected Outcomes (NOC)*† *Sleep*
Patient will achieve an improved sense of adequate sleep within 4 weeks.	Patient reports waking up less frequently during the night and feeling rested within 4 weeks. Patient verbalizes adherence to a regular bedtime routine within 4 weeks.
Patient will achieve a more normal sleep pattern within 4 weeks.	Patient falls asleep within 30 minutes of going to bed within 4 weeks. Patient reports sleeping 7 hours nightly within 4 weeks.

†Outcome classification labels from Moorhead S et al: *Nursing outcomes classification (NOC)*, ed 5, St Louis, 2013, Mosby.

INTERVENTIONS (NIC)‡	RATIONALE
Sleep Enhancement	
Encourage patient to establish a bedtime routine and a regular sleep pattern.	Maintaining a consistent schedule helps induce sleep (National Guideline Clearinghouse, 2014).
Instruct patient to avoid caffeine and nicotine before bedtime.	Caffeine and nicotine are stimulants and cause difficulty falling asleep.
Help patient identify ways to eliminate stressful concerns about work before bedtime (e.g., taking time before actual sleep to read a light novel).	Excess worry and intense activities before bedtime stimulate patient and prevent sleep (Redeker and McEnany, 2011).
Adjust environment; have patient control noise, temperature, and light in the bedroom.	Develop an environment conducive to sleep (Flynn Makic et al., 2014).
Exercise Promotion	
Encourage patient to begin walking routinely during the day but not 2 to 3 hours before bedtime.	Regular exercise increases activity levels and improves sleep quality. Exercise just before bedtime is a stimulant that prevents sleep (Redeker and McEnany, 2011).
Relaxation Therapy	
Teach patient how to perform muscle relaxation before bedtime; include demonstration.	Relaxation therapy helps reduce anxiety, which interferes with sleep (National Guideline Clearinghouse, 2014; National Sleep Foundation 2014b).

‡Intervention classification labels from Bulechek GM, et al: *Nursing interventions classification (NIC)*, ed 6, St Louis, 2013, Mosby.

EVALUATION

Nursing Actions	*Patient Response/Finding*	*Achievement of Outcome*
Ask Julie if she is able to fall asleep and stay asleep.	Julie responds, "It usually takes 15 to 20 minutes to fall asleep; last week, on two separate nights, I only woke up once each night."	Julie reports that she falls asleep within 30 minutes and wakes up less frequently during the night.
Ask Julie to describe her waking behaviors at work and home during the day.	Julie responds that she has completed her case at work and feels less pressure. She has restarted her walking routine and is better able to cope with her children. She is able to concentrate at work more.	Julie reports feeling more rested.
Observe Julie's waking nonverbal expressions and behavior.	Julie sits in the chair without shifting position. She does not yawn during the conversation. The dark circles under her eyes are almost gone.	Julie reports that she is sleeping an average of 7 hours a night.

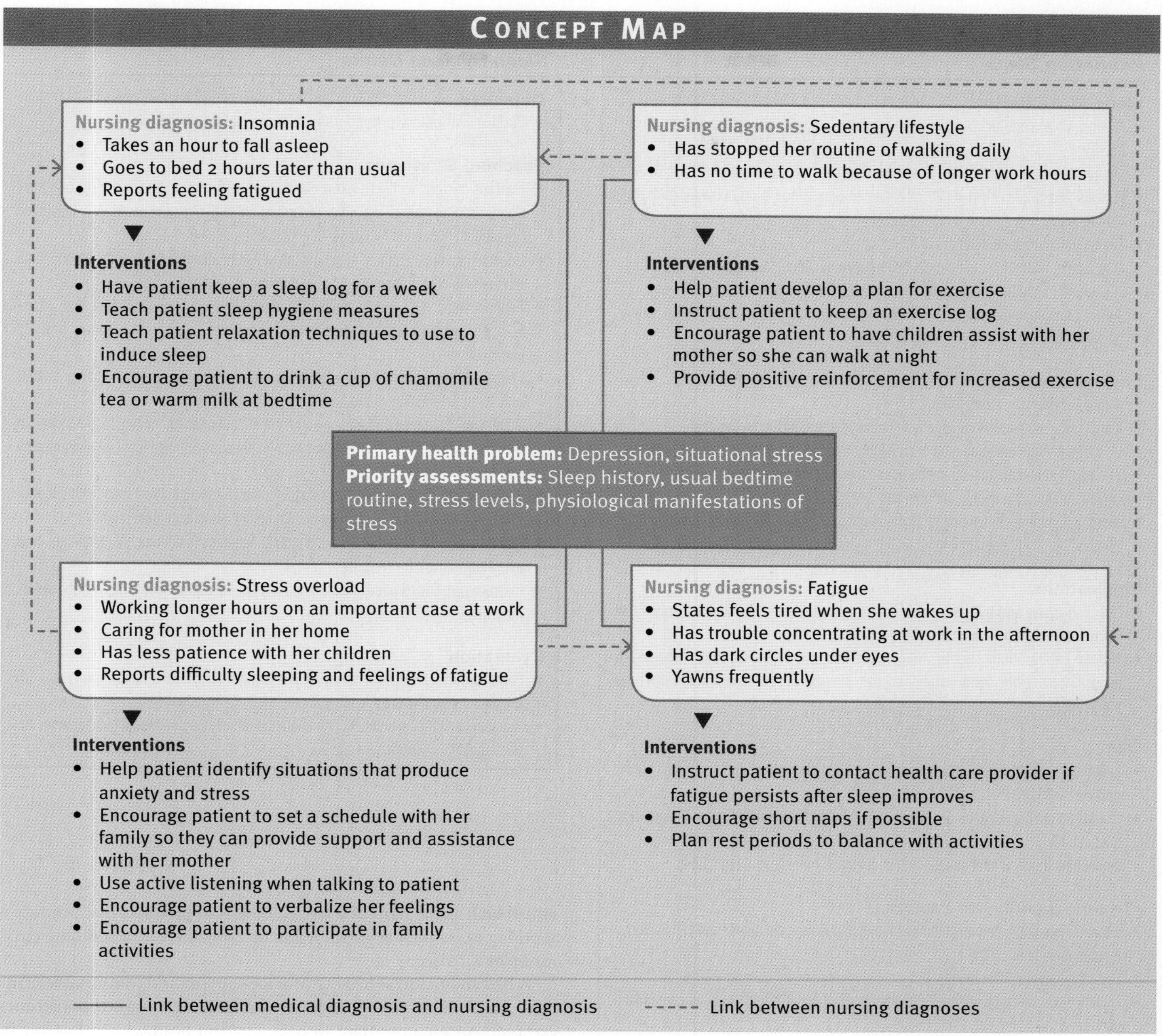

FIGURE 43-5 Concept map for Julie Arnold.

setting differs from that provided in a patient's home. The primary differences are in the environment and the nurse's ability to support normal rest and sleep habits. A patient's age also influences the types of therapies that are most effective. Box 43-8 provides principles for promoting sleep in older patients.

Health Promotion. In community health and home settings help patients develop behaviors conducive to rest and relaxation. To develop good sleep habits at home, patients and their bed partners need to learn techniques that promote sleep and conditions that interfere with it (Kryger et al., 2011) (Box 43-9). Parents also learn how to promote good sleep habits for their children. Patients benefit most from instructions based on information about their homes and lifestyles such as which type of activities promote sleep in a night-shift worker or how to make the home environment more conducive to sleep. They will more likely apply information that is useful and valued.

Environmental Controls. All patients require a sleeping environment with a comfortable room temperature and proper ventilation, minimal sources of noise, a comfortable bed, and proper lighting (National Heart, Lung, and Blood Institute, 2011). Children and adults

BOX 43-8 FOCUS ON OLDER ADULTS

Promoting Sleep

Sleep-Wake Pattern

- Maintain a regular bedtime and wake-up schedule (Rybarczyk et al., 2013).
- Eliminate naps unless they are a routine part of the schedule.
- If naps are taken, limit to 20 minutes or less twice a day (Touhy and Jett, 2014).
- Go to bed when sleepy.
- Use warm bath and relaxation techniques (Touhy and Jett, 2014).
- If unable to sleep in 15 to 30 minutes, get out of bed.
- Avoid stimulating activities such as exercise or watching television before bedtime (Chasens and Umlauf, 2012).

Environment

- Sleep where you sleep best.
- Keep noise to minimum; use soft music to mask it if necessary.
- Use night-light and keep path to bathroom free of obstacles.
- Set room temperature to preference; use socks to promote warmth.
- Listen to relaxing music (Touhy and Jett, 2014).
- Increase exposure to bright light during the day (Chasens and Umlauf, 2012).

Medications

- Use sedatives and hypnotics with caution as last resort and then only short term if absolutely necessary (Kryger et al., 2011).
- Adjust medications being taken for other conditions and assess for drug interactions that may cause insomnia or excessive daytime sleepiness.

Diet

- Limit alcohol, caffeine, and nicotine in late afternoon and evening (Touhy and Jett, 2014).
- Consume carbohydrates or milk as a light snack before bedtime (Touhy and Jett, 2014).
- Decrease fluids 2 to 4 hours before sleep (Touhy and Jett, 2014).

Physiological/Illness Factors

- Elevate head of bed and provide extra pillows as preferred (Townsend-Roccichelli et al., 2010).
- Use analgesics 30 minutes before bed to ease aches and pains.
- Use therapeutics to control symptoms of chronic conditions as prescribed (Chasens and Umlauf, 2012).

BOX 43-9 PATIENT TEACHING

Sleep-Hygiene Habits

Objective

- Patient will follow proper sleep-hygiene habits at home.

Teaching Strategies

- Instruct patient to try to exercise daily, preferably in the morning or afternoon, and to avoid vigorous exercise in the evening within 2 hours of bedtime.
- Caution patient against sleeping long hours during weekends or holidays to prevent disturbance of normal sleep-wake cycle.
- Explain that, if possible, patients should not use the bedroom for intensive studying, snacking, television watching, or other nonsleep activity besides sex.
- Encourage patients to try to avoid worrisome thinking when going to bed and to use relaxation exercises.
- If patient does not fall asleep within 30 minutes of going to bed, advise him or her to get out of bed and do some quiet activity until feeling sleepy enough to go back to bed.
- Recommend that patient limit caffeine to morning coffee and limit alcohol intake (more than one to two drinks a day interrupts sleep cycle).
- Ask patient to examine environment. Instruct that use of earplugs and eyeshades may be helpful.
- Instruct patient to avoid heavy meals 3 hours before bedtime; a light snack may help.

Evaluation

- Have patient complete sleep-wake log for 1 week and compare it with previous sleep-wake log.
- Ask patient to periodically complete visual analog or sleep-rating scale for perceptions of quality of sleep.

vary more in regard to comfortable room temperature. Instruct parents to place the infant on a firm mattress that is covered by a fitted sheet that meets current safety standards; to clothe the baby in a sleeper for warmth; to not place pillows, quilts, toys, or anything in the crib; and to position the crib away from open windows or drafts (AAP, 2012). Older adults often require extra blankets or covers.

Eliminate distracting noise so the bedroom is as quiet as possible. In the home the television, telephone, or intermittent chiming of a clock often disrupts a patient's sleep. Involve the family in identifying approaches for reducing noise in the home, especially if there are several family members, all with different sleep schedules. It is also important to remember that some patients sleep with familiar inside noises such as the hum of a fan. Commercial products that produce a soothing noise such as ocean waves or rainfall create a soothing environment for sleep.

A bed and mattress need to provide support and comfortable firmness. Bed boards placed under mattresses add support. Sometimes extra pillows are important to help a person position comfortably in bed. The position of the bed in the room also makes a difference for some patients.

Patients vary in regard to the amount of light that they prefer at night. Infants and older adults sleep best in softly lit rooms. Light should not shine directly on their eyes. Small table lamps prevent total darkness. For older adults light reduces the chance of confusion and prevents falls when walking to the bathroom. If streetlights shine through windows or when patients nap during the day, heavy shades, drapes, or slatted blinds are helpful.

Promoting Bedtime Routines. Bedtime routines relax patients in preparation for sleep (Bulechek et al., 2013). It is always important for people to go to sleep when they feel tired or sleepy. Going to bed while fully awake and thinking about other things often causes insomnia and interferes with the bed as a stimulus for sleep. Newborns and infants sleep through so much of the day that a specific routine is hardly necessary. However, quiet activities such as holding them snugly in blankets, singing or talking softly, and gentle rocking help them fall asleep.

A bedtime routine (e.g., same hour for bedtime, snack, or quiet activity) used consistently helps young children avoid delaying sleep. Parents need to reinforce patterns of preparing for bedtime. Quiet activities such as reading stories, coloring, allowing children to sit in a parent's lap while listening to music or listening to a prayer are routines that are often associated with preparing for bed.

Adults need to avoid excessive mental stimulation just before bedtime. Reading a light novel, watching an enjoyable television program, or listening to music helps a person relax. Relaxation exercises such as slow, deep breathing for 1 or 2 minutes relieve tension and prepare the body for rest (see Chapter 44). Guided imagery and praying also promote sleep for some patients.

At home discourage patients from trying to finish office work or resolve family problems before bedtime. The bedroom is not a place to work, and patients need to always associate it with sleep. Working toward a consistent time for sleep and awakening helps most patients gain a healthy sleep pattern and strengthens the rhythm of the sleep-wake cycle.

Promoting Safety. For any patient prone to confusion or falls, safety is critical. A small night-light helps a patient orient to the room environment before going to the bathroom. Beds set lower to the floor can lessen the chance of a person falling when first standing. Instruct patients to remove clutter and throw rugs from the path used to walk from the bed to the bathroom. If a patient needs help to ambulate from a bed to the bathroom, place a small bell at the bedside to call family members. Sleepwalkers are unaware of their surroundings and are slow to react, increasing the risk of falls. Do not startle sleepwalkers but instead gently wake them and lead them back to bed.

Infants' beds need to be safe. To reduce the chance of suffocation, do not place pillows, stuffed toys, or the ends of loose blankets in cribs (AAP, 2012). Loose-fitting plastic mattress covers are dangerous because infants pull them over their faces and suffocate. Parents need to place an infant on his or her back to prevent suffocation (Meadows-Oliver and Hendrie, 2013).

Promoting Comfort. People fall asleep only after feeling comfortable and relaxed (Bulechek et al., 2013). Minor irritants often keep patients awake. Soft cotton nightclothes keep infants or small children warm and comfortable. Instruct patients to wear loose-fitting nightwear. An extra blanket is sometimes all that is necessary to prevent a person from feeling chilled and being unable to fall asleep. Patients need to void before retiring so they are not kept awake by a full bladder.

Establishing Periods of Rest and Sleep. In the home it helps to encourage patients to stay physically active during the day so they are more likely to sleep at night. Increasing daytime activity lessens problems falling asleep. In a home setting you frequently care for patients with chronic debilitating disease. The nursing care plan includes having patients set aside afternoons for rest to promote optimal health. Help adjust medication schedules, instruct patients to regularly void before rest periods, and suggest silencing the telephone ringer so rest periods are uninterrupted.

Stress Reduction. The inability to sleep because of emotional stress also makes a person feel irritable and tense. When patients are emotionally upset, encourage them to try not to force sleep. Otherwise insomnia frequently develops, and soon bedtime is associated with the inability to relax. Encourage a patient who has difficulty falling asleep to get up and pursue a relaxing activity such as sewing or reading rather than staying in bed and thinking about sleep.

Preschoolers have bedtime fears (fear of the dark or strange noises), awaken during the night, or have nightmares. After nightmares the parent enters the child's room immediately and talks to him or her briefly about fears to provide a cooling-down period. One approach is to comfort children and leave them in their own beds so their fears are not used as excuses to delay bedtime. Keeping a light on in the room also helps some children. Cultural tradition causes families to approach sleep practices differently (Box 43-10). Always respect those that differ from traditional recommendations.

Bedtime Snacks. Some people enjoy bedtime snacks, whereas others cannot sleep after eating. A dairy product such as warm milk or cocoa that contains L-tryptophan is often helpful in promoting sleep. A full meal before bedtime often causes gastrointestinal upset or reflux and interferes with the ability to fall asleep.

Warn patients against drinking or eating foods with caffeine before bedtime. Coffee, tea, colas, and chocolate act as stimulants, causing a person to stay awake or to awaken throughout the night. Caffeinated foods and liquids and alcohol act as diuretics and cause a person to awaken in the night to void (National Heart, Lung, and Blood Institute, 2011).

BOX 43-10 CULTURAL ASPECTS OF CARE

Co-sleeping

Practices and patterns of sleep and rest vary among cultures. Culture and biology influence the development of sleep problems in children. Sleep patterns, bedtime routines, sleep aids, and sleep arrangements are components of cultural practices related to the use of space and interaction distances (Giger, 2013). Traditionally experts recommend having infants and children sleep in their own beds. Co-sleeping, in which infants and children sleep with their parents, is a culturally preferred habit; and the practice varies among cultures (Jain et al., 2011). It is more common in nonindustrialized countries. Reasons for co-sleeping practices are breastfeeding, comfort, tradition, better or more sleep, and environmental for warmth and protection for an infant (i.e., against the cold) (Ward, 2014). This practice is also common in the United States with some Asian, Hispanic, and African-American families (Jain et al., 2011). Health care providers in the United States discourage it because of safety issues, even though research does not show that the practice is unsafe. American culture promotes independence in childhood. One belief is that co-sleeping does not promote this independence; thus health care providers discourage it (Getter and McKenna, 2010). Research results related to co-sleeping and the incidence of sudden infant death syndrome (SIDS) are mixed (Blair et al., 2014). Sofa sharing is not a safe practice. Bed should not be shared if the infant was born preterm or the parents use alcohol or drugs or smoke (Blair et al., 2014). As a nurse be culturally sensitive when discussing co-sleeping practices with parents and developing sleeping plans for children.

Implications for Patient-Centered Care

- Complete a thorough sleep assessment of the child and family.
- Discuss the risks of co-sleeping with parents. During the discussion remain culturally sensitive and respectful of the parents' views (Jain et al., 2011).
- Co-sleeping has been linked to increased risk of SIDS under certain conditions such as parental smoking and alcohol or drug use (Getter and McKenna, 2010).
- Instruct parents who practice co-sleeping to avoid using alcohol or drugs that impair arousal. Decreased arousal prevents the parents from waking if the child is having problems (Ward, 2014).
- Co-sleeping should occur on a firm mattress (never on a water bed, sofa, or couch) (Ward, 2014).
- Encourage parents to use light sleeping clothes, keep room temperature comfortable, and not bundle the child tightly or in too many clothes.

Infants require special measures to minimize nighttime awakenings for feeding. It is common for children to need middle-of-the-night bottle-feeding or breastfeeding. Hockenberry and Wilson (2015) recommend offering the last feeding as late as possible. Tell parents not to give infants bottles in bed.

QSEN QSEN: BUILDING COMPETENCY IN EVIDENCE-BASED PRACTICE At her annual checkup, Julie Arnold tells you that she continues to have trouble falling asleep so she drinks 1 to 2 glasses of wine before bedtime to make her sleepy. On the basis of the current evidence, what is your best response?

Answers to QSEN Activities can be found on the Evolve website.

Pharmacological Approaches. Melatonin is a neurohormone produced in the brain that helps control circadian rhythms and promote sleep (Kryger et al., 2011). It is a popular nutritional supplement that is found to be helpful in improving sleep efficiency and decreasing nighttime awakenings. The recommended dose is 0.3 to 1 mg taken 2 hours before bedtime. Older adults who have decreased levels of melatonin find it beneficial as a sleep aid (Kryger et al., 2011). Short-term use of melatonin has been found to be safe, with mild side effects of nausea, headache, and dizziness being infrequent (Redeker and McEnany, 2011). Ramelteon (Rozerem), a melatonin receptor agonist, is well tolerated and appears to be effective in improving sleep by improving the circadian rhythm and shortening time-to-sleep onset (National Guideline Clearinghouse, 2014; Redeker and McEnany, 2011). It is safe for long- and short-term use, particularly in older adults.

Several other herbal products help in sleep. Valerian is effective in mild insomnia and RLS. It affects the release of neurotransmitters and produces very mild sedation (Redeker and McEnany, 2011). Kava helps promote sleep in patients with anxiety. It should be used cautiously because of its potential toxic effects on the liver (Larzelere et al., 2010). Chamomile, an herbal tea, has a mild sedative effect that may be beneficial in promoting sleep (Redeker and McEnany, 2011). Caution patients about the dosage and use of herbal compounds because the U.S. Food and Drug Administration (FDA) does not regulate them. Herbal compounds may interact with prescribed medication, and patients need to avoid using these together (Meiner, 2015).

The use of nonprescription sleeping medications is not advisable. Patients need to learn the risks of such drugs. Over the long term these drugs lead to further sleep disruption, even when they initially seemed effective. Caution older adults about using over-the-counter antihistamines because of their long duration of action, which can cause confusion, constipation, urinary retention, and increased risk of falls (Redeker and McEnany, 2011). Help patients use behavioral and proper sleep-hygiene measures to establish sleep patterns that do not require the use of drugs.

Acute Care. Patients in acute care settings have their normal rest and sleep routine disrupted, which generally leads to sleep problems. In this setting nursing interventions focus on controlling factors in the environment that disrupt sleep, relieving physiological or psychological disruptions to sleep, and providing for uninterrupted rest and sleep periods for patients. "Excessive Sleepiness" in the *Evidence-based Geriatric Nursing Protocols for Best Practice* is based on the principle that nurses need to individualize an effective strategy on the basis of patient needs and that sleep medications are a last-resort intervention (Chasens and Umlauf, 2012).

BOX 43-11 EVIDENCE-BASED PRACTICE

Sleep Hygiene in Hospitalized Patients

PICO Question: Does the use of a sleep-hygiene protocol versus routine care in hospitalized patients improve sleep?

Evidence Summary

Sleep disruption commonly occurs in hospitalized patients because of disruption of normal routines, anxiety and stress, noise, pain, medical treatments, and environmental factors (Faraklas et al., 2013; Flynn Makic et al., 2014). Sleep deprivation impacts physical and psychological healing and often causes delirium (Brand, 2014; Faraklas et al., 2013). Implementation of nurse-driven sleep-hygiene protocols has been shown to be effective in improving sleep in hospitalized patients (Brand, 2014; Faraklas et al., 2013; Flynn Makic et al., 2014). Effective strategies in the protocols focused on education of staff nurses on protocol and interventions to decrease environmental stimuli and limit patient disruptions (Brand, 2014: Faraklas et al., 2013). After implementation of sleep-hygiene protocols, noise levels decreased on the nursing unit (Brand, 2014). Patients also reported that they were able to fall asleep more quickly and had fewer sleep disruptions (Faraklas et al., 2013).

Application to Nursing Practice

- Work with nurses on the unit to develop a sleep-hygiene protocol (Brand, 2014; Faraklas et al., 2013).
- Cluster nursing activities to provide uninterrupted periods of sleep (Murphy et al., 2013).
- Ask patients about sleep-hygiene measures used at home and work to use these in the hospital (Faraklas et al., 2013).
- Provide programs for staff on the effects of noise and noise-reduction strategies (Brand, 2014).
- Reduce lighting, telephone volumes, and staff conversations in the halls during quiet time and nighttime (Flynn Makic et al., 2014).
- Use sleep-hygiene measures with patients such as personal hygiene, adjusting room temperature, and relaxation methods.

Environmental Controls. In a hospital the nurse controls the environment in several ways (Box 43-11). Close the curtains between patients in semiprivate rooms. Dim lights on a hospital nursing unit at night. One of the biggest problems for patients in the hospital is noise. Important ways to reduce noise are to conduct conversations and reports in a private area away from patient rooms and keep necessary conversations to a minimum, especially at night (Flynn Makic et al., 2014). Additional ways to control noise in the hospital are listed in Box 43-12.

Promoting Comfort. Compared with beds at home, hospital beds are often harder and of a different height, length, or width. Keeping them clean and dry and in a comfortable position helps patients relax. Some patients suffer painful illnesses requiring special comfort measures such as the application of dry or moist heat, the use of supportive dressings or splints, and the use of pillows to assist in proper positioning before retiring (Figure 43-6).

Establishing Periods of Rest and Sleep. In a hospital or extended care setting it is difficult to provide patients with the time needed to rest and sleep. The most effective treatment for sleep disturbances is elimination or correction of factors that disrupt the sleep pattern. You need to plan care to avoid waking patients for nonessential tasks. Do this by scheduling assessments, treatments, procedures, and routines for times when patients are awake. For example, if a patient's physical condition has been stable, avoid waking him or her to check vital signs.

BOX 43-12 Control of Noise in the Hospital

- Close doors to patients' room when possible.
- Keep doors to work areas on unit closed when in use.
- Reduce volume of nearby telephone and paging equipment.
- Wear rubber-soled shoes. Avoid clogs.
- Turn off bedside oxygen and other equipment that is not in use.
- Turn down alarms and beeps on bedside monitoring equipment.
- Turn off room television and radio unless patient prefers soft music.
- Avoid abrupt loud noise such as flushing a toilet or moving a bed.
- Keep necessary conversations at low levels, particularly at night.
- Conduct conversations and reports in a private area away from patient rooms.
- Designate a time period during the day for "quiet time" for patients.

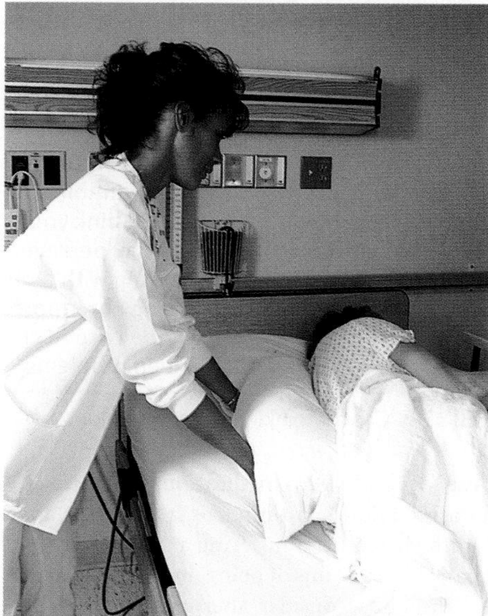

FIGURE 43-6 Positioning patient for sleep.

Allowing patients to determine the timing and methods of delivery of basic care measures promotes rest. Do not give baths and routine hygiene measures during the night for nursing convenience. Draw blood samples at a time when the patient is awake. Unless maintaining the therapeutic blood level of a drug is essential, give medications during waking hours. Work with the radiology department and other support services to schedule diagnostic studies and therapies at intervals that allow patients time for rest. Always try to provide the patient with 2 to 3 hours of uninterrupted sleep during the night.

When the patient's condition demands more frequent monitoring, plan activities to allow extended rest periods. A nurse instructs assistive personnel in the coordination of patient care to reduce patient disturbances. This means planning activities so the patient has as long as an hour or more to rest quietly rather than having a nurse or other personnel return to the room every few minutes. For example, if a patient needs frequent dressing changes, is receiving intravenous therapy, and has drainage tubes from several sites, do not make a separate trip into the room to check each problem. Instead use a single visit to perform all three tasks. Become the patient's advocate for promoting optimal sleep. This means becoming a gatekeeper by postponing or rescheduling visits by family or by questioning the frequency of certain procedures.

Promoting Safety. Patients with OSA are at risk for complications while in the hospital. Surgery and anesthesia disrupt normal sleep patterns. After surgery patients reach deep levels of REM sleep. This deep sleep causes muscle relaxation that leads to OSA. Patients with OSA who are given opioid analgesics after surgery have an increased risk of developing airway obstruction because the medications suppress normal arousal mechanisms (Redeker and McEnany, 2011). These patients often need ventilator support in the postoperative period because of the increased risk of respiratory complications. Monitor the patient's airway, respiratory rate and depth, and breath sounds frequently after surgery.

Recommend lifestyle changes to patients with OSA that include sleep hygiene, alcohol moderation, smoking cessation, and a weight-loss program (Freedman, 2010). Teach the patient to elevate the head of the bed and use a side or prone position for sleep. Use pillows to prevent a supine position (Pinto and Caple, 2010).

One of the most effective therapies is use of a nasal continuous positive airway pressure (CPAP) device at night, which requires a patient to wear a mask over the nose. A mask delivers room air at a high pressure. The air pressure prevents airway collapse. The CPAP device is portable and effective particularly for OSA. Another treatment option is the use of an oral appliance. These appliances advance the mandible or tongue to relieve pharyngeal obstruction (Wickwire and Collop, 2010). In cases of severe sleep apnea the tonsils, uvula, or parts of the soft palate are removed surgically. The success of surgical procedures to correct OSA varies.

Stress Reduction. Patients who are hospitalized for extensive diagnostic testing often have difficulty resting or sleeping because of uncertainty about the state of their health. Giving patients control over their health care minimizes uncertainty and anxiety. Providing information about the purpose of procedures and routines and answering questions gives patients the peace of mind needed to rest or fall asleep. A nurse on the night shift needs to take time to sit and talk with patients unable to sleep. This helps to determine the factors keeping patients awake. Back rubs also help patients relax more thoroughly. If a sedative is indicated, confer with the patient's health care provider to be sure that the lowest dose is used initially. Discontinuing a sedative as soon as possible prevents a dependence that seriously disrupts the normal sleep cycle. Older adults' metabolism of drugs is slow, making them more vulnerable to the side effects of sedatives, hypnotics, antianxiety drugs, or analgesics.

Restorative or Continuing Care. The nursing interventions implemented in the acute care setting are also used in the restorative or continuing care environment. Controlling the environment, especially noise; establishing periods of rest and sleep; and promoting comfort are important considerations. Nursing interventions related to stress reduction and controlling physiological disturbances are also implemented in these settings. Helping a patient achieve restful sleep in this environment sometimes takes time.

Promoting Comfort. Providing for personal hygiene improves a patient's sense of comfort. A warm bath or shower before bedtime is relaxing. Offer patients restricted to bed the opportunity to void and wash their face and hands. Toothbrushing and care of dentures also help to prepare patients for sleep. Position patients to support their dependent body parts and protect pressure points. Offer a back or hand massage to aid in muscle relaxation just before a patient goes to sleep (Harris and Richards, 2010) (see Chapter 44).

Controlling Physiological Disturbances. As a nurse you learn to control symptoms of physical illness that disrupt sleep. For example, a patient with respiratory abnormalities sleeps with two pillows or in a semi-sitting position to ease the effort to breathe. He or she benefits from taking prescribed bronchodilators before sleep to prevent airway obstruction. A patient with a hiatal hernia also needs special care. After meals he or she often experiences a burning sensation as a result of gastric reflux. To prevent sleep disturbances have the patient eat a small meal several hours before bedtime and sleep in a semi-sitting position. Patients with pain, nausea, or other recurrent symptoms receive any symptom-relieving medication timed so the drug takes effect at bedtime. Remove or change any irritants against the patient's skin such as moist dressings or drainage tubes.

Pharmacological Approaches. The liberal use of drugs to manage insomnia is quite common in American culture. CNS stimulants such as amphetamines, caffeine, nicotine, terbutaline, theophylline, and modafinil need to be used sparingly and under medical management (Burchum and Rosenthal, 2016). In addition, withdrawal from CNS depressants such as alcohol, barbiturates, tricyclic antidepressants (amitriptyline, imipramine, and doxepin), and triazolam causes insomnia. Consult with pharmacist and health care provider about managing doses.

Medications that induce sleep are called **hypnotics**. **Sedatives** are medications that produce a calming or soothing effect (Burchum and Rosenthal, 2016). A patient who takes sleep medications needs to know about their proper use and their risks and possible side effects. Long-term use of antianxiety, sedative, or hypnotic agents disrupts sleep and leads to more serious problems. The FDA requires that the product labels of all sleep medications contain safety information related to the potential adverse effects of severe allergic reactions; severe facial swelling; and complex sleep behaviors such as sleep-driving, making phone calls, and preparing and eating food while asleep (USFDA, 2015).

Benzodiazepines and benzodiazepine-like drugs are common classifications of drugs used to treat sleep problems. The benzodiazepine-like drugs have become the treatment of choice for insomnia because of improved efficacy and safety of use (Burchum and Rosenthal, 2016). Experts recommend a low dose of a short-acting medication such as zolpidem (Ambien) for short-term use (no longer than 2 to 3 weeks) (Burchum and Rosenthal, 2016). These drugs cause fewer problems with dependence and abuse and fewer rebound insomnia and hangover effects than benzodiazepines.

The benzodiazepines cause relaxation, antianxiety, and hypnotic effects by facilitating the action of neurons in the CNS that suppress responsiveness to stimulation, thereby decreasing levels of arousal (Burchum and Rosenthal, 2016). Short-acting benzodiazepines (e.g., oxazepam, lorazepam, or temazepam) at the lowest possible dose for short-term treatment of insomnia are recommended. Initial doses are small; and increments are added gradually, on the basis of patient response, for a limited time. Warn patients not to take more than the prescribed dose, especially if the medication seems to become less effective after initial use. The use of benzodiazepines in older adults is potentially dangerous because of the tendency of the drugs to remain active in the body for a longer time. As a result, they also cause respiratory depression; next-day sedation; amnesia; rebound insomnia; and impaired motor functioning and coordination, which leads to increased risk of falls (Burchum and Rosenthal, 2016). If older patients who were recently continent, ambulatory, and alert become incontinent or confused and/or demonstrate impaired mobility, the use of benzodiazepines needs to be considered as a possible cause.

Administer benzodiazepines cautiously to children under 12 years of age. These medications are contraindicated in infants less than 6 months. Pregnant patients need to avoid them because their use is associated with risk of congenital anomalies. Nursing mothers do not receive the drugs because they are excreted in breast milk. Raise these issues with patients' health care providers.

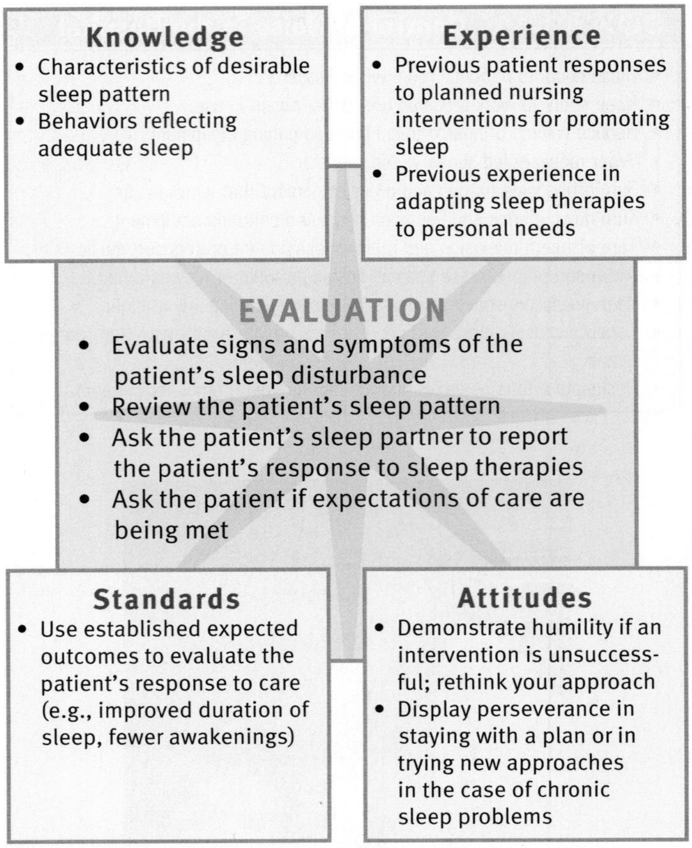

Knowledge
- Characteristics of desirable sleep pattern
- Behaviors reflecting adequate sleep

Experience
- Previous patient responses to planned nursing interventions for promoting sleep
- Previous experience in adapting sleep therapies to personal needs

EVALUATION
- Evaluate signs and symptoms of the patient's sleep disturbance
- Review the patient's sleep pattern
- Ask the patient's sleep partner to report the patient's response to sleep therapies
- Ask the patient if expectations of care are being met

Standards
- Use established expected outcomes to evaluate the patient's response to care (e.g., improved duration of sleep, fewer awakenings)

Attitudes
- Demonstrate humility if an intervention is unsuccessful; rethink your approach
- Display perseverance in staying with a plan or in trying new approaches in the case of chronic sleep problems

FIGURE 43-7 Critical thinking model for sleep evaluation.

Regular use of any sleep medication often leads to tolerance and withdrawal. Rebound insomnia is a problem after stopping a medication. Immediately administering a sleeping medication when a hospitalized patient complains of being unable to sleep does the patient more harm than good. Consider alternative approaches to promote sleep. Routine monitoring of patient response to sleep medications is important.

◆ Evaluation

Through the Patient's Eyes. With regard to problems with sleep, the patient is the source for evaluating if expectations are met. Each patient has a unique need for sleep and rest. He or she is the only one who knows if sleep problems are improved and which interventions or therapies are most successful in promoting sleep (Figure 43-7). It is important to ask the patient if his or her sleep needs have been met. For example, ask the patient, "Are you feeling more rested?"; "Can you tell me if you believe that we've done all we can to help improve your sleep?" or "Which interventions have been most effective in helping you sleep?" If expectations have not been met, you need to spend more time trying to understand the patient's needs and preferences. Working closely with the patient and bed partner enables you to redefine expectations that can be met realistically within the limits of the patient's condition and treatment.

Patient Outcomes. To evaluate the effectiveness of nursing interventions, make comparisons with baseline assessment data to evaluate if sleep has improved. Determine whether expected outcomes have been met. Use evaluative measures shortly after a therapy has been tried (e.g., observing whether a patient falls asleep after reducing noise and darkening a room). Use other evaluative measures after a patient wakes from sleep (e.g., asking him or her to describe the number of awakenings during the previous night). The patient and bed partner usually provide accurate evaluative information. Over longer periods use assessment tools such as the visual analog or sleep-rating scale to determine whether sleep has progressively improved or changed.

Also evaluate the level of understanding that patients or family members gain after receiving instruction in sleep habits. You measure compliance with these practices during a home visit, when you are able to observe the environment. When expected outcomes are not met, revise the nursing measures or expected outcomes on the basis of the patient's needs or preferences. When outcomes are not met, ask questions such as:

- Are you able to fall asleep within 20 minutes of getting in bed?
- Describe how well you sleep when you exercise.
- Does the use of quiet music at bedtime help you to relax?
- Do you feel rested when you wake up?

If a nurse has successfully developed a good relationship with a patient and a therapeutic plan of care, subtle behaviors often indicate the level of the patient's satisfaction. Note the absence of signs of sleep problems such as lethargy, frequent yawning, or position changes in the patient. You are effective in promoting rest and sleep if the patient's goals and expectations are met.

KEY POINTS

- Sleep provides physiological and psychological restoration.
- The 24-hour sleep-wake cycle is a circadian rhythm that influences physiological function and behavior.
- The control and regulation of sleep depends on a balance among regulators within the CNS.
- During a typical night's sleep a person passes through four to five complete sleep cycles. Each sleep cycle contains three NREM stages of sleep and a period of REM sleep.
- The most common type of sleep disorder is insomnia.
- The hectic pace of a person's lifestyle, emotional and psychological stress, and alcohol ingestion frequently disrupt the sleep pattern.
- If a patient's sleep is adequate, assess his or her usual bedtime, normal bedtime ritual, preferred environment for sleeping, and usual preferred rising time.
- When a patient has a sleep problem, conduct a complete sleep history. Identifying nursing diagnoses for sleep problems depends on identifying factors that impair sleep.
- When planning interventions to promote sleep, consider the usual characteristics of the patient's home environment and normal lifestyle.
- A regular bedtime routine of relaxing activities prepares a person physically and mentally for sleep.
- An environment with a darkened room, reduced noise, comfortable bed, and good ventilation promotes sleep.
- Important nursing interventions for promoting sleep in the hospitalized patient are establishing periods for uninterrupted sleep and rest and controlling noise levels.
- Pain or other disease symptom control is essential to promoting the ability to sleep.
- Long-term use of sleeping pills often leads to difficulty initiating and maintaining sleep.

CLINICAL APPLICATION QUESTIONS

Preparing for Clinical Practice

Julie returns to the neighborhood health clinic for a follow-up visit. She tells you that, since she started her sleep-hygiene plan, she feels more rested. She tells you that she is concerned because her husband says that she has started snoring loudly when she's sleeping.

1. On the basis of Julie's husband's report of her snoring, which additional assessment data should you gather from her?
2. Julie tells you that her 76-year-old mother is having trouble sleeping after being in the hospital. Julie asks you about a prescription for a sleeping pill for her mother. What is your best response?
3. Julie and David tell you that they are concerned about their 14-year-old daughter. She just started high school and is having sleep problems. List at least three interventions for Julie and David to use to improve their teenage daughter's sleep patterns.

ⓔ ***Answers to Clinical Application Questions can be found on the Evolve website.***

REVIEW QUESTIONS

Are You Ready to Test Your Nursing Knowledge?

1. The nurse is developing a plan for a patient who was diagnosed with narcolepsy. Which interventions should the nurse include on the plan? (Select all that apply.)
   1. Take brief, 20-minute naps no more than twice a day.
   2. Drink a glass of wine with dinner.
   3. Eat the large meal at lunch rather than dinner.
   4. Establish a regular exercise program.
   5. Teach the patient about the side effects of modafinil (Provigil).
2. The nurse incorporates which priority nursing intervention into a plan of care to promote sleep for a hospitalized patient?
   1. Have patient follow hospital routines.
   2. Avoid waking patient for nonessential tasks.
   3. Give prescribed sleeping medications at dinner.
   4. Turn television on low to late-night programming.
3. A 72-year-old patient asks the nurse about using an over-the-counter antihistamine as a sleeping pill to help her get to sleep. What is the nurse's best response?
   1. "Antihistamines are better than prescription medications because these can cause a lot of problems."
   2. "Antihistamines should not be used because they can cause confusion and increase your risk of falls."
   3. "Antihistamines are effective sleep aids because they do not have many side effects."
   4. "Over-the-counter medications when combined with sleep-hygiene measures are a good plan for sleep."
4. The nurse is providing health teaching for a patient using herbal compounds such as kava for sleep. Which points need to be included? (Select all that apply.)
   1. Can cause urinary retention
   2. Should not be used indefinitely
   3. May have toxic effects on the liver
   4. May cause diarrhea and anxiety
   5. Are not regulated by the U.S. Food and Drug Administration (FDA)
5. The patient reports episodes of sleepwalking to the nurse. Through understanding of the sleep cycle, the nurse recognizes that sleepwalking occurs during which sleep phase?
   1. Rapid eye movement (REM) sleep
   2. Stage 1 nonrapid eye movement (NREM) sleep
   3. Stage 4 NREM sleep
   4. Transition period from NREM to REM sleep
6. The nurse is administering a benzodiazepine sleep aid to an older adult. What should be the priority assessment for the patient?

1. Incontinence
2. Nausea and vomiting
3. Bradycardia
4. Respiratory depression

7. The nurse is contacting the health care provider about a patient's sleep problem. Place the steps of the SBAR (*s*ituation, *b*ackground, *a*ssessment, *r*ecommendation) in the correct order.
   1. Mrs. Dodd, 46 years old, was admitted 3 days ago following a motor vehicle accident. She is in balanced skeletal traction for a fractured left femur. She is having difficulty falling asleep.
   2. "Dr. Smithson, this is Pam, the nurse caring for Mrs. Dodd. I'm calling because Mrs. Dodd is having difficulty sleeping."
   3. "I'm calling to ask if you would order a hypnotic such as zolpidem (Ambien) to use on a prn basis."
   4. Mrs. Dodd is taking her pain medication every 4 hours as ordered and rates her pain as 2 out of 10. Last night she was still awake at 0100. She states that she is comfortable but just can't fall asleep. Her vital signs are BP 124/76, P 78, R 12 and T 37.1° C (98.8° F).
8. Which statement made by a mother being discharged to home with her newborn infant indicates that she understands the discharge teaching related to best sleep practices?
   1. "I'll give the baby a bottle to help her fall asleep."
   2. "We'll place the baby on her back to sleep."
   3. "We put the baby's stuffed animals in the crib to make her feel safe."
   4. "I know the baby will not need to be fed until morning."
9. The nurse is developing a plan of care for a patient experiencing obstructive sleep apnea (OSA). Which intervention is appropriate to include on the plan?
   1. Instruct the patient to sleep in a supine position.
   2. Have patient limit fluid intake 2 hours before bedtime.
   3. Elevate head of bed and assume a side or prone position.
   4. Encourage patient to take an over-the-counter sleep aid.
10. Which statement made by the parent of a school-age child requires follow-up by the nurse?
    1. "I encourage evening exercise about an hour before bedtime."
    2. "I offer my daughter a glass warm milk before bedtime."
    3. "I make sure that the room is dark and quiet at bedtime."
    4. "We use quiet activities such as reading a book before bedtime."
11. Which sleep-hygiene actions at bedtime can the nurse delegate to the nursing assistant? (Select all that apply.)
    1. Giving the patient a backrub
    2. Turning on quiet music
    3. Dimming the lights in the patient's room
    4. Giving a patient a cup of coffee
    5. Monitoring for the effect of the sleeping medication that was given
12. Which statement made by the patient indicates a need for further teaching on sleep hygiene?
    1. "I'm going to do my exercises before I eat dinner."
    2. "I'm going to go to bed every night at about the same time."
    3. "I set my alarm to get up at the same time every morning."
    4. "I moved my computer to the bedroom so I could work before I go to sleep."
13. Which statement made by an older adult best demonstrates understanding of taking a sleep medication?
    1. "I'll take the sleep medicine for 4 or 5 weeks until my sleep problems disappear."
    2. "Sleep medicines won't cause any sleep problems once I stop taking them."
    3. "I'll talk to my health care provider before I use an over-the-counter sleep medication."
    4. "I'll contact my health care provider if I feel extremely sleepy in the mornings."
14. The school nurse is teaching health-promoting behaviors that improve sleep to a group of high-school students. Which points should be included in the education? (Select all that apply.)
    1. Go to bed at the same time each night.
    2. Study in your bedroom to have a quiet place.
    3. Turn on the television to help you fall asleep.
    4. Avoid drinking coffee or soda before bedtime.
    5. Turn off your cell phone at bedtime.
15. The nurse is taking a sleep history from a patient. Which statement made by the patient needs further follow-up?
    1. "I feel refreshed when I wake up in the morning."
    2. "I use soft music at night to help me relax."
    3. "It takes me about 45 to 60 minutes to fall asleep."
    4. "I take the pain medication for my leg pain about 30 minutes before I go to bed."

Answers: 1. 1, 4, 5; **2.** 2; **3.** 2; **4.** 2, 3, 5; **5.** 3; **6.** 4; **7.** 2, 1, 4, 3; **8.** 2; **9.** 3; **10.** 1; **11.** 1, 2, 3; **12.** 4; **13.** 3; **14.** 1, 4, 5; **15.** 3.

ⓔ ***Rationales for Review Questions can be found on the Evolve website.***

REFERENCES

Adult Obstructive Sleep Apnea Task Force of the American Academy of Sleep Medicine: Clinical guideline for the evaluation, management and long-term care of obstructive sleep apnea in adults, *J Clin Sleep Med* 5(3):263, 2009.

Ahmed I, Thorpy M: Clinical features, diagnosis and treatment of narcolepsy, *Clin Chest Med* 31(2):371, 2010.

American Academy of Pediatrics: *A parent's guide to safe sleep*, 2012, http://www.healthychildcare.org/PDF/SIDSparentsafesleep.pdf. Accessed November 2015.

American Nurses Association (ANA): *Nursing scope and standards of practice*, Washington, DC, 2010, The Association.

Babson KA, et al: Cognitive behavioral therapy for sleep disorders, *Psychiatr Clin North Am* 33(3):629, 2010.

Bulechek GM, et al: *Nursing interventions classification (NIC)*, ed 6, St Louis, 2013, Mosby.

Burchum JR, Rosenthal LD: *Lehne's Pharmacology for nurses*, ed 9, St Louis, 2016, Elsevier.

Chase MH: Motor control during sleep and wakefulness: clarifying controversies and resolving paradoxes, *Sleep Med Rev* 17:299, 2013.

Chasens ER, Umlauf MG: Excessive sleepiness. In Boltz M, et al, editors: *Evidence-based geriatric nursing protocols for best practice*, ed 4, New York, 2012, Springer.

Conte F, Ficca G: Caveats on psychological models of sleep and memory: a compass in an overgrown scenario, *Sleep Med Rev* 17:105, 2013.

Daroff RB, et al, editors: *Bradley's neurology in clinical practice*, ed 6, Philadelphia, 2012, Saunders.

Fiorentino L, Martin JL: Awake at 4 AM: treatment of insomnia with early-morning awakenings among older adults, *Clin Psychol J* 66(11):1161, 2010.

Freedman N: Treatment of obstructive sleep apnea, *Clin Chest Med* 31:187, 2010.

Getter LT, McKenna JJ: Never sleep with baby? Or keep me close but keep me safe; eliminating inappropriate "safe infant sleep" rhetoric in the United States, *Curr Pediatr Rev* 6(1):71, 2010.

Giger JN: *Transcultural nursing: assessment and intervention*, ed 6, St Louis, 2013, Mosby.

Gilsenan I: Nursing interventions to alleviate insomnia, *Nurs Older People* 24(4):14, 2012.

Hockenberry MJ, Wilson D: *Wong's nursing care of infants and children*, ed 10, St Louis, 2015, Elsevier.

Huether SE, et al: *Understanding pathophysiology*, ed 5, St Louis, 2012, Elsevier.

Kryger MH, et al: *Principles and practice of sleep medicine*, ed 5, St Louis, 2011, Saunders.

Larzelere MM, et al: Complementary and alternative medicine usage for behavioral health indicators, *Prim Care Clin Office Pract* 37(2):213, 2010.

Malhotra RK, Desai AK: Healthy brain aging: what has sleep got to do with it? *Clin Geriatr Med* 26:45, 2010.

Meadows-Oliver M, Hendrie J: Expanded back to sleep guidelines, *Pediatr Nurs* 39(1):40, 2013.

Meiner SE: *Gerontologic nursing*, ed 5, St Louis, 2015, Mosby.

National Guideline Clearinghouse: *Clinical guidelines for the treatment of primary insomnia in middle-aged and older adults*, NCG10414, 2014, http://www.guideline.gov/content.aspx?id=48218&search=insomnia. Accessed November 2015.

National Heart, Lung, and Blood Institute: *How is insomnia treated?* 2011, http://www.nhlbi.nih.gov/health/health-topics/topics/inso/treatment.html. Accessed November 2015.

National Sleep Foundation: *Aging and sleep*, Washington, DC, 2014a, http://www.sleepfoundation.org/article/sleep-topics/aging-and-sleep. Accessed November 2015.

National Sleep Foundation: *Depression and sleep*, 2014b, http://sleepfoundation.org/sleep-disorders-problems/depression-and-sleep. Accessed November 2015.

National Sleep Foundation: *Sleep apnea*, Washington, DC, 2014c, http://sleepfoundation.org/sleep-disorders-problems/sleep-apnea. Accessed November 2015.

National Sleep Foundation: *2014 Sleep in American poll: sleep in the modern family*, Washington, DC, 2014d, http://sleepfoundation.org/sites/default/files/2014-NSF-Sleep-in-America-poll-summary-of-findings---FINAL-Updated-3-26-14-.pdf. Accessed November 2015.

National Sleep Foundation: *The ABCs of ZZZs—When you can't sleep*, Washington, DC, 2014e, http://sleepfoundation.org/how-sleep-works/abcs-zzzzs-when-you-cant-sleep. Accessed November 2015.

Neikrug AB, Ancoli-Israel S: Sleep disorders in the older adult—a mini review, *Gerontology* 56:181, 2010.

Pinto S, Caple C: Obstructive sleep apnea in adults, *CINAHL Information Systems*, April 23, 2010.

Redeker NS, McEnany GP, editors: *Sleep disorders and sleep promotion in nursing practice*, New York, 2011, Springer.

Rybarczyk B, et al: Cognitive behavioral therapy for insomnia in older adults: background, evidence, and overview of treatment protocol, *Clin Gerontol* 36:70, 2013.

Touhy TA, Jett KF: *Ebersole and Hess' gerontological nursing healthy aging*, ed 4, St Louis, 2014, Mosby.

Townsend-Rocchichelli J, et al: Managing sleep disorders in the elderly, *Nurse Pract* 35(5):30, 2010.

University of Maryland Medical Center Sleep Disorders Center: *Sleep disorders-overview*, 2015, http://umm.edu/health/medical/ency/articles/sleep-disorders-overview. Accessed November 2015.

US Food and Drug Administration (USFDA): *Side effects of sleep drugs*, 2015, http://www.fda.gov/ForConsumers/ConsumerUpdates/ucm107757.htm. Accessed November 2015.

Van Kerrebroeck P: Nocturia: current status and future perspectives, *Curr Opin Obstet Gynecol* 23(5):376, 2011.

Wickwire EM, Collop NA: Insomnia and sleep-related breathing disorders, *Chest* 137(6):1449, 2010.

RESEARCH REFERENCES

Blair PS, et al: Bed-sharing in the absence of hazardous circumstances: is there a risk of sudden infant death syndrome? An analysis from two case studies conducted in the UD, *PLoS ONE* 9(9):e107799, 2014.

Brand H: EB67 Sleep hygiene in hospitals for patient healing, *Crit Care Nurse* 334(2):e10, 2014.

Dennis CM, et al: Benefits of quiet time for neurointensive care patients, *J Neurosci Nurs* 43(4):217, 2010.

Faraklas I, et al: Impact of a nursing-driven sleep hygiene protocol on sleep quality, *J Burn Care Res* 34:249, 2013.

Flynn Makic MB, et al: Examining the evidence to guide practice: challenging practice habits, *Crit Care Nurse* 34(2):28, 2014.

Fontana CJ, Pittiglio LI: Sleep deprivation among critical care patients, *Crit Care Nurs Q* 33(1):75, 2010.

Harris M, Richards KC: The physiological and psychological effect of slow-stroke back massage and hand massage on relaxation in older people, *J Clin Nurs* 19:197, 2010.

Jain S, et al: Bed sharing in school-age children—clinical and social implications, *J Child Adolesc Psychiatr Nurs* 24:185, 2011.

Koren A, et al: Parental information and behaviors and provider practices related to tummy time and back to sleep, *J Pediatr Health Care* 24(4):222, 2010.

Murphy G, et al: Quiet at night: implementing a Nightingale principle, *Am J Nurs* 113(12):43, 2013.

Ross C, et al: Association between insomnia symptoms and weight change in older women: caregiver osteoporotic fractures study, *J Am Geriatr Soc* 59(9):1697, 2011.

Ward TC: Reasons for mother-infant bed sharing: a systematic narrative synthesis of the literature and implications for future research, *Matern Child Health J* 19(3):675, 2014.

Wiggins SA, Freeman JL: Understanding sleep during adolescence, *Pediatr Nurs* 40(2):91, 2014.

44

Pain Management

OBJECTIVES

- Discuss common misconceptions about pain.
- Describe the physiology of pain.
- Identify components of the pain experience. Explain how the physiology of pain relates to selecting interventions for pain relief.
- Assess a patient experiencing pain.
- Explain how cultural factors influence the pain experience.
- Describe guidelines for selecting and individualizing pain therapies.
- Explain various pharmacological approaches to treating pain.
- Describe applications for use of nonpharmacological pain interventions.
- Discuss nursing implications for administering analgesics.
- Identify barriers to effective pain management.
- Evaluate a patient's response to pain interventions.

KEY TERMS

Acupressure, p. 1033
Acute pain, p. 1017
Addiction, p. 1044
Adjuvants, p. 1035
Analgesics, p. 1035
Biofeedback, p. 1031
Breakthrough pain, p. 1041
Chronic pain, p. 1017
Cutaneous stimulation, p. 1033
Drug tolerance, p. 1044
Epidural analgesia, p. 1039
Guided imagery, p. 1032
Idiopathic pain, p. 1018
Local anesthesia, p. 1039
Modulation, p. 1016
Multimodal analgesia, p. 1036
Neurotransmitters, p. 1015
Nociceptor, p. 1015
Opioids, p. 1035
Pain threshold, p. 1016
Pain tolerance, p. 1017
Patient-controlled analgesia (PCA), p. 1038
Perception, p. 1016
Perineural infusions, p. 1039
Physical dependence, p. 1044
Placebos, p. 1044
Prostaglandins, p. 1015
Pseudoaddiction, p. 1043
Regional anesthesia, p. 1039
Relaxation, p. 1032
Transcutaneous electrical nerve stimulation (TENS), p. 1033
Transduction, p. 1015
Transmission, p. 1015

MEDIA RESOURCES

http://evolve.elsevier.com/Potter/fundamentals/

- Review Questions
- Video Clips
- Concept Map Creator
- Case Study with Questions
- Skills Performance Checklists
- Audio Glossary
- Content Updates

Pain is a universal but individual experience and a condition that nurses encounter among patients in all settings. It is the most common reason that people seek health care; yet it is often underrecognized, misunderstood, and inadequately treated. A person in pain often feels distress or suffering and seeks relief. One of the major challenges of pain is that as a nurse you cannot see or feel a patient's pain. It is purely subjective. No two people experience pain in the same way, and no two painful events create identical responses or feelings in a person. The International Association for the Study of Pain (IASP) defines it as "an unpleasant, subjective sensory *and* emotional experience associated with actual or potential tissue damage, or described in terms of such damage" (IASP, 2014b).

Recently there has been a call to increase research efforts related to pain. Congress declared 2000 to 2010 the Decade of Pain Control and Research; and, although the body of evidence has grown, pain continues to be a leading public health problem in the United States. The 2010 Patient Protection and Affordable Care Act required the Department of Health and Human Services to obtain the support of the Institute of Medicine (IOM) in conducting an extensive examination of pain as a public health problem. The results of the IOM study were released in the 2011 report, *Relieving Pain in America: a Blueprint for Transforming Prevention, Care, Education, and Research.* This report acknowledges the tragic epidemic of pain in the United States and calls for major coordinated efforts to develop safe, effective, preventive, and management strategies (IOM, 2011). The IASP, in the "Declaration of Montreal," declared that access to pain management is a fundamental human right (IASP, 2015). Nurses are legally and ethically responsible for managing pain and relieving suffering.

Pain management should be patient centered, with nurses practicing patient advocacy, empowerment, compassion, and respect. Caring for patients in pain requires recognition that pain can and should be relieved. Effective communication among the patient, family, and professional caregivers is essential to achieve adequate pain management. Recognition of the subjective nature of pain and respect for the patient in pain is demonstrated when a nurse accepts McCaffery's classic definition: "Pain is whatever the experiencing person says it is, existing whenever he says it does" (Pasero and McCaffery, 2011). Effective pain management improves quality of life; reduces physical discomfort; promotes earlier mobilization and return to previous baseline functional activity levels; results in fewer hospital and clinic visits; and decreases hospital lengths of stay, resulting in lower health care costs.

SCIENTIFIC KNOWLEDGE BASE

Nature of Pain

The pain experience is complex, involving more than a single physiological sensation caused by a specific stimulus. It has physical, emotional, and cognitive components. It is subjective and highly individualized. It depletes a person's energy and may contribute to chronic fatigue. It interferes with interpersonal relationships and influences the meaning of life. Left untreated, it may lead to serious physical, psychological, social, and financial consequences. Pain itself cannot be measured objectively. Only the patient knows whether pain is present and how the experience feels. However, careful assessment is critical as you assess the effects (e.g., behaviors and physiological changes) associated with pain. It is not the responsibility of a patient to prove that he or she is in pain; it is a nurse's responsibility to assess a patient's condition and accept his or her subjective report (APS, 2009).

Physiology of Pain

There are four physiological processes of normal pain: transduction, transmission, perception, and modulation (Pasero and McCaffery, 2011). A patient in pain cannot discriminate among the processes. Understanding each process helps you recognize factors that cause pain, symptoms that accompany it, and the rationale for selected therapies.

Transduction. Thermal, chemical, or mechanical stimuli usually cause pain. Transduction converts energy produced by these stimuli into electrical energy. It begins in the periphery when a pain-producing stimulus (e.g., exposure to pressure or a hot surface) sends an impulse across a sensory peripheral pain nerve fiber (nociceptor), initiating an action potential. Once transduction is complete, transmission of the pain impulse begins.

Transmission. Cellular damage caused by thermal, mechanical, or chemical stimuli results in the release of excitatory neurotransmitters such as prostaglandins, bradykinin, substance P, and histamine (Box 44-1). The neurotransmitters affect the sending of nerve stimuli. They either excite during transmission or inhibit during modulation. Excitatory neurotransmitters send electrical impulses across the synaptic cleft between two nerve fibers, enhancing transmission of the pain impulse. These pain-sensitizing substances surround the pain fibers in the extracellular fluid, spreading the pain message and causing an inflammatory response (Pasero and McCaffery, 2011). The pain stimulus enters the spinal cord via the dorsal horn and travels one of several routes until ending within the gray matter of the spinal cord. At the dorsal horn substance P is released, causing a synaptic transmission from the afferent (sensory) peripheral nerve to spinothalamic tract nerves, which cross to the opposite side (Pasero and McCaffery, 2011) (Figure 44-1).

Nerve impulses resulting from the painful stimulus travel along afferent (sensory) peripheral nerve fibers. Two types of peripheral nerve fibers conduct painful stimuli: the fast, myelinated A–delta fibers and the very small, slow, unmyelinated C fibers. The A fibers send

BOX 44-1 Neurophysiology of Pain: Neuroregulators

Neurotransmitters (Excitatory)

Prostaglandins
- Generated from the breakdown of phospholipids in cell membranes
- Thought to increase sensitivity to pain

Bradykinin
- Released from plasma that leaks from surrounding blood vessels at the site of tissue injury
- Binds to receptors on peripheral nerves, increasing pain stimuli
- Binds to cells that cause the chain reaction producing prostaglandins

Substance P
- Found in pain neurons of dorsal horn (excitatory peptide)
- Needed to transmit pain impulses from periphery to higher brain centers
- Causes vasodilation and edema

Histamine
- Produced by mast cells causing capillary dilation and increased capillary permeability

Serotonin
- Released from the brainstem and dorsal horn to inhibit pain transmission

Neuromodulators (Inhibitory)
- Are the natural supply of morphinelike substances in the body
- Activated by stress and pain
- Located within the brain, spinal cord, and gastrointestinal tract
- Cause analgesia when they attach to opiate receptors in the brain
- Present in higher levels in people who have less pain than others with a similar injury

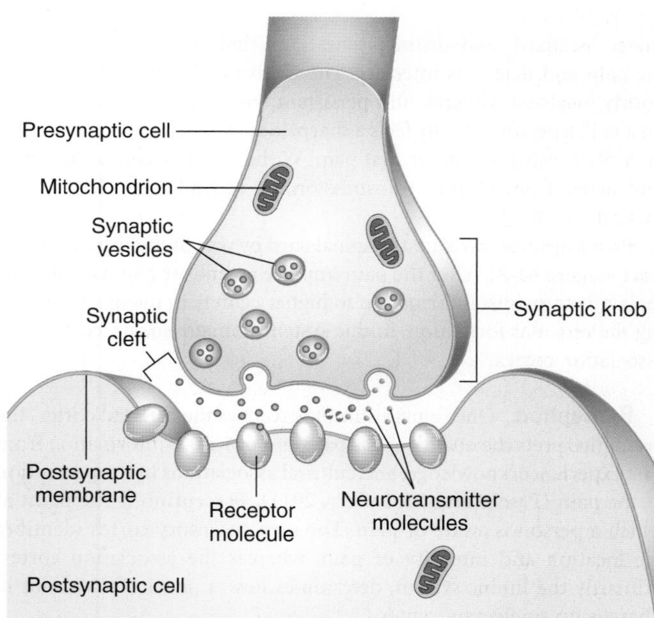

FIGURE 44-1 Chemical synapses involve transmitter chemicals (neurotransmitters) that signal postsynaptic cells. (From Patton KT, Thibodeau GA: *Anatomy & physiology*, ed 9, St Louis, 2016, Mosby.)

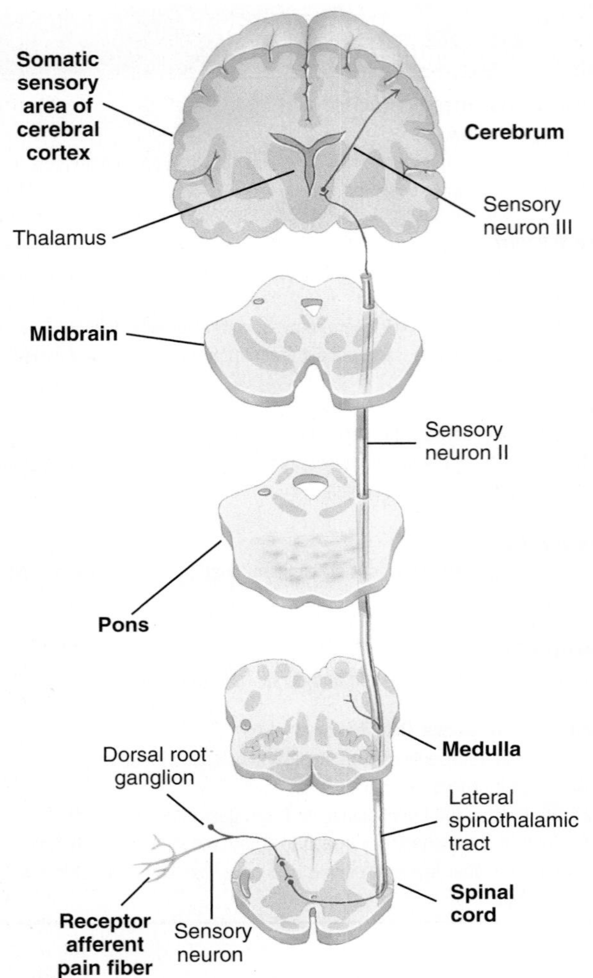

FIGURE 44-2 Spinothalamic pathway that conducts pain stimuli to the brain.

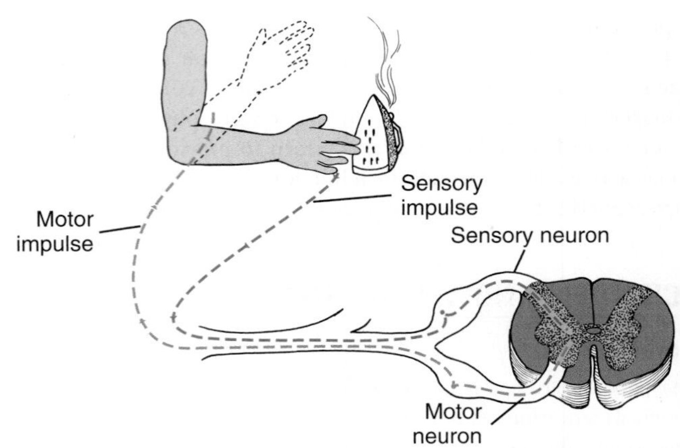

FIGURE 44-3 Protective reflex to pain stimulus.

sharp, localized, and distinct sensations that specify the source of the pain and detect its intensity. The C fibers relay impulses that are poorly localized, visceral, and persistent. For example, after stepping on a nail, a person initially feels a sharp, localized pain, which is a result of A-fiber transmission, or first pain. Within a few seconds the whole foot aches from C-fiber transmission, or second pain (Pasero and McCaffery, 2011).

Pain impulses travel up the spinal cord by way of the spinothalamic tract (Figure 44-2). After the pain impulse ascends the spinal cord, the thalamus transmits information to higher centers in the brain, including the reticular formation, limbic system, somatosensory cortex, and association cortex.

Perception. Once a pain stimulus reaches the cerebral cortex, the brain interprets the quality of the pain and processes information from past experience, knowledge, and cultural associations in the perception of the pain (Pasero and McCaffery, 2011). **Perception** is the point at which a person is aware of pain. The somatosensory cortex identifies the location and intensity of pain, whereas the association cortex, primarily the limbic system, determines how a person feels about it. There is no single pain center.

As a person becomes aware of pain, a complex reaction occurs. Psychological and cognitive factors interact with neurophysiological ones. Perception gives awareness and meaning to pain, resulting in a reaction. The reaction to pain includes the physiological and behavioral responses that occur after an individual perceives pain (Pasero and McCaffery, 2011).

Modulation. Once the brain perceives pain, there is a release of inhibitory neurotransmitters (see Box 44-1) such as endorphins (endogenous opioids), serotonin, norepinephrine, and gamma-aminobutyric acid (GABA), which hinder the transmission of pain and help produce an analgesic effect (Pasero and McCaffery, 2011). The neurotransmitters decrease neuron activity without directly transferring a nerve signal through a synapse. This inhibition of the pain impulse is the fourth and last phase of the normal pain process known as **modulation** (Pasero and McCaffery, 2011).

A protective reflex response also occurs with pain reception (Figure 44-3). A–delta fibers send sensory impulses to the spinal cord, where they synapse with spinal motor neurons. The motor impulses travel via a reflex arc along efferent (motor) nerve fibers back to a peripheral muscle near the site of stimulation, thus bypassing the brain. Contraction of the muscle leads to a protective withdrawal from the source of pain. For example, when you accidentally touch a hot iron, you feel a burning sensation, but your hand also reflexively withdraws from the surface of the iron. Pain processes require an intact nervous system and spinal cord. Common factors that disrupt the pain process include trauma, drugs, tumor growth, and metabolic disorders.

Gate-Control Theory of Pain

Melzack and Wall's gate-control theory (1965) was the first to suggest that pain has emotional and cognitive components in addition to physical sensations. According to this theory, gating mechanisms located along the central nervous system regulate or block pain impulses. Pain impulses pass through when a gate is open and are blocked when a gate is closed. Closing the gate is the basis for nonpharmacological pain-relief interventions. You gain a useful conceptual framework for pain management by understanding the physiological, emotional, and cognitive influences on the gates. For example, factors such as stress and exercise increase the release of endorphins, often raising an individual's **pain threshold** (the point at which a person feels pain). Because the amount of circulating substances varies with every individual, the response to pain varies.

Physiological Responses. As pain impulses ascend the spinal cord toward the brainstem and thalamus, the stress response stimulates the autonomic nervous system (ANS). Pain of low-to-moderate intensity and superficial pain elicit the fight-or-flight reaction of the general adaptation syndrome (see Chapter 38). Stimulation of the sympathetic

TABLE 44-1 Physiological Reactions to Pain

Response	Cause or Effect
Sympathetic Stimulation*	
Dilation of bronchial tubes and increased respiratory rate	Provides increased oxygen intake
Increased heart rate	Provides increased oxygen transport
Peripheral vasoconstriction (pallor, elevation in blood pressure)	Elevates blood pressure with shift of blood supply from periphery and viscera to skeletal muscles and brain
Increased blood glucose level	Provides additional energy
Increased cortisol level (short term)	Heightened memory functions, a burst of increased immunity, and lower sensitivity to pain
Diaphoresis	Controls body temperature during stress
Increased muscle tension	Prepares muscles for action
Dilation of pupils	Affords better vision
Decreased gastrointestinal motility	Frees energy for more immediate activity
Parasympathetic Stimulation†	
Pallor	Causes blood supply to shift away from periphery
Nausea and vomiting	Vagus nerve sends impulses to chemoreceptor trigger zone in the brain
Decreased heart rate and blood pressure	Results from vagal stimulation
Rapid, irregular breathing	Causes body defenses to fail under prolonged stress of pain

*Pain of low-to-moderate intensity and superficial pain.
†Severe or deep pain.

branch of the ANS results in physiological responses (Table 44-1). Continuous, severe, or deep pain typically involving the visceral organs (e.g., with a myocardial infarction or colic from gallbladder or renal stones) activates the parasympathetic nervous system. Sustained physiological responses to pain sometimes seriously harm individuals. Except in cases of severe traumatic pain, which cause a person to go into shock, most people adapt to their pain reflexively, and their physical signs return to normal baseline. Note that normal is not the same for each individual. Thus patients in pain do *not* always have changes in their vital signs. Changes in vital signs more often indicate problems other than pain.

Behavioral Responses. The pain response is complex, influenced by a person's culture, pain experiences, perception of pain, and ability to manage stress. If left untreated or unrelieved, pain significantly alters quality of life with physical and psychological consequences. The widespread effects of pain support why effective pain management is essential. Some patients choose not to report pain if they believe that it inconveniences others or if it signals loss of self-control. Others endure severe pain without asking for assistance. Be familiar with behavioral responses to pain. Clenching the teeth, facial grimacing, holding or guarding the painful part, and bent posture are common indications of acute pain. Chronic pain affects a patient's activity (eating, sleeping, socialization), thinking (confusion, forgetfulness), or emotions (anger, depression, irritability) and quality of life and productivity (IOM, 2011). You soon learn to recognize patterns of behavior that reflect pain even when there is no verbal report. This ability becomes especially important in patients who are unable to report their pain such as individuals who are cognitively impaired or unable to communicate (e.g., intubated with artificial airway). However, lack of pain expression does not indicate that a patient is not experiencing it (Pasero and McCaffery, 2011). Critically analyze the conditions that cause pain and advocate for appropriate management even if a patient cannot.

Recognizing a patient's unique response to pain is important in assessing success of pain-management therapies. Encourage your patients to accept pain-relieving measures so they remain active and continue to maintain daily activities. A patient's ability to tolerate pain significantly influences your perceptions of the degree of his or her discomfort. Patients who have a low **pain tolerance** (level of pain a person is willing to accept) are sometimes inaccurately perceived as complainers. Teach patients the importance of reporting their pain sooner rather than later to facilitate better control and optimal functional status.

Acute and Chronic Pain

Pain is categorized by duration (acute or chronic) or pathological condition (e.g., cancer or neuropathic). The two types of pain that you observe in patients are acute (transient) and chronic (persistent), which includes cancer and noncancer pain.

Acute/Transient Pain. **Acute pain** is protective, usually has an identifiable cause, is of short duration, and has limited tissue damage and emotional response. It is common after acute injury, disease, or surgery. Acute pain warns people of injury or disease; thus it is protective. It eventually resolves, with or without treatment, after an injured area heals. Patients in acute pain are frightened and anxious and expect relief quickly. It is self-limiting; therefore a patient knows than an end is in sight. Because acute pain has a predictable ending (healing) and an identifiable cause, health team members are usually willing to treat it aggressively.

Acute pain seriously threatens a patient's recovery by hampering his or her ability to become active and involved in self-care. This results in prolonged hospitalization from complications such as physical and emotional exhaustion, immobility, sleep deprivation, and pulmonary complications. Physical and psychological progress is delayed as long as acute pain persists because a patient focuses all energy on pain relief. Efforts aimed at teaching and motivating a patient toward self-care can be hindered until the pain is managed successfully. Complete pain relief is not always achievable, but reducing pain to a tolerable level is a realistic goal. A primary nursing goal is to provide pain relief that allows patients to participate in their recovery, prevent complications, and improve functional status. Unrelieved acute pain can progress to chronic pain (Althaus et al., 2014).

Chronic/Persistent Noncancer Pain. The IOM (2011) estimates that chronic pain affects approximately 100 million American adults, more than the total affected by heart disease, cancer, and diabetes combined. Unlike acute pain, **chronic pain** is not protective and thus serves no purpose, but it has a dramatic effect on a person's quality of life. Chronic noncancer pain is prolonged, varies in intensity, and usually lasts longer (typically at least 6 months) than is expected or predicted (IOM, 2011). It does not always have an identifiable cause and leads to great personal suffering. Examples of chronic noncancer pain include arthritis, low back pain, headache, fibromyalgia, and peripheral neuropathy. It may result from an initial injury such as a

TABLE 44-2 Classification of Pain by Inferred Pathology

Nociceptive Pain	Neuropathic Pain
I. *Nociceptive pain:* Normal stimulation of special peripheral nerve endings—called *nociceptors;* usually responsive to nonopioids and/or opioids A. *Somatic pain:* Comes from bone, joint, muscle, skin, or connective tissue; is usually aching or throbbing in quality and well localized B. *Visceral pain:* Arises from visceral organs such as the gastrointestinal tract and pancreas; is sometimes subdivided: 1. Tumor involvement of organ capsule that causes aching and fairly well-localized pain 2. Obstruction of hollow viscus, which causes intermittent cramping and poorly localized pain	II. *Neuropathic pain:* Abnormal processing of sensory input by the peripheral or central nervous system; treatment usually includes adjuvant analgesics. A. Centrally generated pain 1. *Deafferentation pain:* Injury to either the peripheral or central nervous system. *Examples:* Phantom pain indicates injury to the peripheral nervous system; burning pain below the level of a spinal cord lesion reflects injury to the central nervous system. 2. *Sympathetically maintained pain:* Associated with impaired regulation of the autonomic nervous system. *Examples:* Pain is associated with complex regional pain syndrome, type I, type II. B. Peripherally generated pain 1. *Painful polyneuropathies:* Pain felt along the distribution of many peripheral nerves. *Examples:* Diabetic neuropathy, alcohol-nutritional neuropathy, and Guillain-Barré syndrome. 2. *Painful mononeuropathies:* Usually associated with a known peripheral nerve injury; pain is felt at least partly along the distribution of the damaged nerve. *Examples:* Nerve root compression, nerve entrapment, trigeminal neuralgia.

From Pasero C, McCaffery M: *Pain assessment and pharmacologic management,* St Louis, 2011, Mosby.

back sprain, or there may be an ongoing cause such as illness. Chronic noncancer pain may be viewed as a disease since it has a distinct pathology that causes changes throughout the nervous system that may worsen over time (IOM, 2011). It has significant psychological and cognitive effects and can constitute a serious, separate disease entity itself. Chronic noncancer pain is usually non–life threatening. In some cases an injured area healed long ago, yet the pain is ongoing and does not respond to treatment.

The possible unknown cause of chronic pain, combined with ineffective treatments and the unrelenting nature and uncertainty of its duration, frustrates a patient, frequently leading to psychological depression and even suicide. Chronic pain is a major cause of psychological and physical disability, leading to problems such as job loss, inability to perform simple daily activities, sexual dysfunction, and social isolation. The goal of treating chronic noncancer pain is to improve functional status with a multimodality plan.

The person with chronic noncancer pain often experiences pain that may not have the same physiological response as acute pain; however, the subjective reports and interference with activities of daily living (ADLs), socialization, and ability to perform work duties is very real. Patients often suffer more with time because of physical and mental exhaustion. Associated symptoms of chronic pain include fatigue, insomnia, anorexia, weight loss, apathy, hopelessness, depression, and anger. Chronic pain creates the uncertainty of how one will feel from day to day. A person with chronic noncancer pain often does not show obvious symptoms and does not adapt to the pain. Health care providers are usually less willing to treat chronic pain with opioids, although there are guidelines that support their use (Chou et al., 2009). In addition, the American Society of Anesthesiologists (2010) released *Practice Guidelines for Chronic Pain Management*, which includes opioid use. Often a person with chronic pain who consults with numerous health care providers is labeled a drug seeker, when he or she is actually seeking adequate pain relief. Nurses need to discourage patients from having multiple health care providers for treating pain and refer them to specialists. Pain centers offer nonpharmacological and pharmacological strategies for a holistic approach to pain management.

Chronic Episodic Pain. Pain that occurs sporadically over an extended period of time is episodic pain. Pain episodes last for hours, days, or weeks. An example of chronic episodic pain is the migraine headache that occurs up to 14 days per month compared to chronic migraine that occurs more than 15 days per month (Katsarava et al., 2012).

Cancer Pain. Not all patients with cancer experience pain. For those who do, many are able to have their pain managed with relatively simple means (Burchum and Rosenthal, 2016). Some patients with cancer experience acute and/or chronic pain. The pain is normal (nociceptive), resulting from stimulus of an undamaged nerve and/or neuropathic, arising from abnormal or damaged pain nerves (Table 44-2). Cancer pain is usually caused by tumor progression and related pathological processes, invasive procedures, toxicities of chemotherapy, infection, and physical limitations. A patient senses pain at the actual site of the tumor or distant to the site, called *referred pain.* Always completely assess reports of new pain by a patient with existing pain. Despite the availability and wide use of opioids and updated guidelines from reliable leading professional societies, undertreatment of cancer pain is still frequent. More than 75% of patients with advanced cancer experience pain, yet research shows that approximately one third of patients still do not receive pain medication proportional to their pain intensity (Greco et al., 2014; Paice and Ferrell, 2011).

Idiopathic Pain. Idiopathic pain is chronic pain in the absence of an identifiable physical or psychological cause or pain perceived as excessive for the extent of an organic pathological condition. An example of idiopathic pain is complex regional pain syndrome (CRPS). Research is needed to better identify the causes of idiopathic pain to identify more effective treatment (Pasero and McCaffery, 2011).

NURSING KNOWLEDGE BASE

Nursing knowledge of pain mechanisms and interventions continues to grow through nursing research. This section explores factors that influence the pain experience.

Knowledge, Attitudes, and Beliefs

Attitudes of nurses and other health care providers affect pain management. The traditional medical model of illness generates attitudes about pain. This model suggests that physical problems result from

BOX 44-2 Common Biases and Misconceptions About Pain

The following statements are *false:*
- Patients who abuse substances (e.g., use drugs or alcohol) overreact to discomforts.
- Patients with minor illnesses have less pain than those with severe physical alteration.
- Administering analgesics regularly leads to drug addiction.
- The amount of tissue damage in an injury accurately indicates pain intensity.
- Health care personnel are the best authorities on the nature of a patient's pain.
- Psychogenic pain is not real.
- Chronic pain is psychological.
- Patients who are hospitalized experience pain.
- Patients who cannot speak do not feel pain.

physical causes. Thus pain is a physical response to organic dysfunction. When there is no obvious source of pain (e.g., the patient with chronic low back pain or neuropathies), health care providers sometimes stereotype pain sufferers as malingerers, complainers, or difficult patients.

Studies of nurses' attitudes regarding pain management show that a nurse's personal opinion about a patient's report of pain affects pain assessment and titration of opioid doses. It has been shown that nurses' assessment of pain intensity underestimates patients' pain reports (Goulet et al., 2013). A number of nurse and patient variables, including cultural (e.g., gender, age, education), knowledge, and patient diagnosis, may contribute to the differences in pain ratings. The amount of analgesia administered may vary on the basis of whether a patient is grimacing or smiling during the nurse's assessment (Pasero and McCaffery, 2011). Nurses with more than 6 years of work experience, higher job motivation, and perceived higher levels of pain-care skills in themselves often use more patient advocacy skills in providing pain management for patients (Vaartio et al., 2009).

Nurses' assumptions about patients in pain seriously limit their ability to offer pain relief. Biases based on culture, education, and experience influence everyone. Too often nurses allow misconceptions about pain (Box 44-2) to affect their willingness to intervene. Some nurses avoid acknowledging a patient's pain because of their own fear and denial. They do not believe a patient's report of pain if he or she does not look in pain. A nurse is entitled to personal beliefs; however, he or she must *accept* a patient's report of pain and act according to professional guidelines, standards, position statements, policies and procedures, and evidence-based research findings (Pasero and McCaffery, 2011).

To help a patient gain pain relief, it is important to view the experience through the patient's eyes. Acknowledging a personal prejudice or misconception helps to address patient problems more professionally. When one becomes an active, knowledgeable observer of a patient in pain, it is possible to more objectively analyze the pain experience. The patient makes the diagnosis that pain is present, and the nurse provides interventions that ultimately offer relief.

Factors Influencing Pain

Pain is a complex process, involving physiological, social, spiritual, psychological, and cultural influences. Thus each individual's pain experience is different. Consider all factors that affect a patient in pain to ensure a holistic approach to the assessment and care of the patient.

BOX 44-3 FOCUS ON OLDER ADULTS

Factors Influencing Pain in Older Adults

- With aging, muscle mass decreases, body fat increases, and percentage of body water decreases. This increases the concentration of water-soluble drugs such as morphine given in normal doses. The volume of distribution for fat-soluble drugs such as fentanyl increases (Burchum and Rosenthal, 2016; Tracy and Morrison, 2013).
- Older adults frequently eat poorly, resulting in low serum albumin levels. Many drugs are highly protein bound. In the presence of low serum albumin, more free drug (active form) is available, thus increasing the risk for side and/or toxic effects (Burchum and Rosenthal, 2016; Tracy and Morrison, 2013.
- A decline of liver and renal function naturally occurs with aging. This results in reduced metabolism and excretion of drugs. Thus older adults often experience a greater peak effect and longer duration of analgesics (Arnstein, 2010).
- Age-related changes in the skin such as thinning and loss of elasticity affect the absorption rate of topical analgesics.

Physiological Factors

Age. Age influences the pain experience. It is important to consider how a painful event affects a patient developmentally. For example pain may prevent an adolescent from engaging socially with friends. A middle-age adult may be unable to continue work in cases when it is severe. It is particularly important to recognize how developmental differences affect how infants and older adults react to pain. Young children have trouble understanding pain, its meaning, and the procedures that cause it. If they have not developed full vocabularies, they have difficulty verbally describing and expressing pain to parents or caregivers. Toddlers and preschoolers are unable to recall explanations about pain or associate it with experiences that may not be related to the painful condition. With these developmental considerations in mind, it is necessary to adapt approaches for assessing a child's pain (e.g., what to ask, including parents), the behaviors to observe, and how to prepare a child for a painful medical procedure.

Pain is not an inevitable part of aging. Likewise pain perception does not decrease with age. However, older adults have a greater likelihood of developing pathological conditions, which are accompanied by pain. In addition, age-related changes and increased frailty may lead to a less predictable response to analgesics, increased sensitivity to medications, and potential harmful drug effects (van Ojik et al., 2012). The person in pain, his or her family, and health care providers frequently take their chronic medical conditions for granted and underestimate the pain. Serious impairment of functional status often accompanies pain in older patients. It potentially reduces mobility, ADLs, social activities, and activity tolerance. The presence of pain in an older adult requires aggressive assessment, diagnosis, and management (Box 44-3).

The ability of older patients to interpret pain is sometimes complicated. They often suffer from multiple diseases with symptoms that affect similar parts of the body. The nurse must make detailed assessments when the source of pain is not clear. Different diseases sometimes cause similar symptoms. For example, chest pain does not always indicate a heart attack; it also is a symptom of arthritis of the spine or an abdominal disorder. When older adults experience cognitive impairment and confusion, they have difficulty recalling pain experiences and providing detailed explanations of their pain (Pasero and McCaffery, 2011). It is necessary to address misconceptions about pain

TABLE 44-3 Pain in Infants

Misconception	Correction
Infants cannot feel pain.	Infants have the anatomical and functional requirements for pain processing by mid-to-late gestation.
Infants are less sensitive to pain than older children and adults.	Term neonates have the same sensitivity to pain as older infants and children. Preterm neonates have a greater sensitivity to pain than term neonates or older children.
Infants cannot express pain.	Although infants cannot verbalize pain, they respond with behavioral cues and physiological indicators that are observable.
Infants must learn about pain from previous painful experiences.	Pain requires no prior experience; infants do not need to learn it from earlier painful experience. It occurs with the first insult.
You cannot accurately assess pain in infants.	You use behavioral cues (e.g., facial expressions, cry, body movements) and physiological indicators of pain (e.g., changes in vital signs) to reliably and validly assess pain in infants.
You cannot safely give analgesics and anesthetics to infants and neonates because of their immature capacity to metabolize and eliminate drugs and their sensitivity to opioid-induced respiratory depression.	Infants are very sensitive to drugs. Response to drugs is often intense and prolonged. Absorption is faster than expected. Dosages of drugs excreted by the kidneys need to be reduced (Burchum and Rosenthal, 2016). Prescribers carefully select the medication, dosage, administration route, and time. Nurses monitor frequently for desired and undesired effects. They also follow medication orders to titrate and wean medications to minimize adverse effects.

TABLE 44-4 Misconceptions About Pain in Older Adults

Misconception	Correction
Pain is a natural outcome of growing old.	Older adults are at greater risk (as much as twofold) than younger adults for many painful conditions; however, pain is not an inevitable result of aging.
Pain perception, or sensitivity, decreases with age.	This assumption is unsafe. Although there is evidence that emotional suffering specifically related to pain may be less in older than in younger patients, no scientific basis exists for the claim that a decrease in perception of pain occurs with age or that age dulls sensitivity to pain.
If the older patient does not report pain, he or she does not have pain.	Older patients commonly underreport pain. Reasons include expecting to have pain with increasing age; not wanting to alarm loved ones; being fearful of losing their independence; not wanting to distract, anger, or bother caregivers; and believing that caregivers know they have pain and are doing all they can to relieve it. The absence of a report of pain does not mean the absence of pain.
If an older patient appears to be occupied, asleep, or otherwise distracted from pain, he or she does not have pain.	Older patients often believe that it is unacceptable to show pain and have learned to use a variety of ways to cope with it (e.g., many patients use distraction successfully for short periods of time). Sleeping is sometimes a coping strategy; alternately, it indicates exhaustion, not pain relief. Do not make assumptions about the presence or absence of pain solely on the basis of a patient's behavior.
The potential side effects of opioids make them too dangerous to use to relieve pain in older adults.	Opioids are safe to use in older adults with moderate-to-severe pain (Arnstein, 2010). Although the opioid-naive older adult is usually more sensitive to opioids, this does not justify withholding their use in pain management. Slow titration prevents potentially dangerous opioid-induced side effects. Regular, frequent monitoring and assessment of a patient's response are necessary. Adjust dose and the interval between doses when you detect side effects. If necessary, administer an opioid antagonist drug to reverse clinically significant respiratory depression.
Patients with Alzheimer's disease and other cognitive impairments do not feel pain, and their reports of pain are most likely invalid.	No evidence exists that cognitively impaired older adults experience less pain or that their reports of pain are less valid than those of individuals with intact cognitive function (Herr, 2010). Patients with dementia or other deficits of cognition most likely suffer significant unrelieved pain and discomfort. Assessment of pain in these patients is challenging but possible. The best approach is to accept a patient's report of pain and treat it as you would treat it in an individual with intact cognitive function.
Older patients report more pain as they age.	Even though older patients experience a higher incidence of painful conditions such as arthritis, osteoporosis, peripheral vascular disease, and cancer than younger patients, studies show that they underreport pain. Many older adults grew up valuing the ability to "grin and bear it" (Pasero and McCaffery, 2011).

management in the very young and in older adults before intervening for a patient (Tables 44-3 and 44-4).

Fatigue. Fatigue heightens the perception of pain and decreases coping abilities. If it occurs along with sleeplessness, the perception of pain is even greater. Pain is often experienced less after a restful sleep than at the end of a long day.

Genes. Research on healthy human subjects suggests that genetic information passed on by parents possibly increases or decreases a person's sensitivity to pain and determines pain threshold or tolerance. Recent advances in the study of genetics and pain have shown that even slight changes in deoxyribonucleic acid (DNA) could partially explain individual differences in pain. Genetic influences have been shown to play a role in sensitivity, perception, and expression of pain (James, 2013).

Neurological Function. A patient's neurological function influences the pain experience. Any factor that interrupts or influences normal pain reception or perception (e.g., spinal cord injury, peripheral neuropathy, or neurological disease) affects a patient's awareness of and response to pain. Some pharmacological agents (analgesics, sedatives, and anesthetics) influence pain perception and response because of the manner in which they affect the nervous system.

Social Factors

Attention. The degree to which a patient focuses attention on pain influences its perception. Increased attention is associated with increased pain, whereas distraction is associated with a diminished pain response. This concept is one that nurses apply in various pain-relief interventions such as relaxation, guided imagery, and massage. By focusing patients' attention and concentration on other stimuli, their perception of pain declines (see Chapter 33).

Previous Experience. Each person learns from painful experiences. Prior experience does not mean that a person accepts pain more easily in the future. Previous frequent episodes of pain without relief or bouts of severe pain cause anxiety or fear. In contrast, if a person repeatedly experiences the same type of pain that was relieved successfully in the past, he or she finds it easier to interpret the pain sensation. As a result, the patient is better prepared to take necessary actions to relieve the pain.

When a patient has no experience with a painful condition, the first perception of pain often impairs the ability to cope. For example, after abdominal surgery patients often experience severe incisional pain for several days. Unless a patient knows that this is a common occurrence following surgery, the onset of pain seems like a serious complication. Rather than participate actively in postoperative breathing exercises (see Chapter 50), the patient lies immobile in bed and breathes shallowly because of fear that something is not right. In the anticipatory phase of the pain experience, you need to prepare a patient with a clear explanation of the type of pain to expect and methods to reduce it. This usually results in a reduced perception of pain.

Family and Social Support. People in pain often depend on family members or close friends for support, assistance, or protection. Although pain still exists, the presence of family or friends can often make the experience less stressful. Conversation with family is a useful distraction. The presence of parents is especially important for children experiencing pain.

Spiritual Factors. Spirituality is an active searching for meaning in situations in which one finds oneself (Chapter 36). Spiritual beliefs affect the way patients view or cope with pain. Research studies have demonstrated that spiritual beliefs and preferences for spiritual interventions have been useful in pain management (Dezutter et al., 2011; Weinstein et al., 2014). Patients often ask spiritually based questions such as, "Why has this happened to me?" "Why am I suffering?" Spiritual pain goes beyond what we can see. "Why has God done this to me?" "Is this suffering teaching me something?" Other spiritual concerns include loss of independence and becoming a burden to family. Consider making a referral to pastoral care for patients in pain. Recall that pain is an experience that has physical *and* emotional components. Thus providing interventions designed to treat both aspects is essential for the best possible pain management.

Psychological Factors

Anxiety. A person perceives pain differently if it suggests a threat, loss, punishment, or challenge. For example, a woman in labor perceives pain differently than a woman with a history of cancer who is experiencing a new pain and fearing recurrence. In addition, the degree and quality of pain perceived by a patient influences its meaning. The relationship between pain and anxiety is complex. Anxiety often increases the perception of pain, and pain causes feelings of anxiety. It is difficult to separate the two sensations.

Critically ill or injured patients who perceive a lack of control over their environment and care have high anxiety levels. This anxiety leads to serious pain-management problems. Pharmacological and nonpharmacological approaches to the management of anxiety are appropriate; however, anxiolytic medications are not a substitute for analgesia (Pasero and McCaffery, 2011).

Coping Style. Pain is a lonely experience that often causes patients to feel a loss of control. Coping style influences the ability to deal with it. People with internal loci of control perceive themselves as having control over events in their life and the outcomes such as pain. They ask questions, desire information, and make choices about treatment. In contrast, people with external loci of control perceive that other factors in their life such as nurses are responsible for the outcome of events. These patients follow directions and are more passive in managing their pain. Learn to understand patients' coping resources during painful experiences so you can incorporate these into your plan of care. For example, a patient who does not ask for pain medication but shows behavioral signs of discomfort might require you to be more responsive in offering prn medications on time (see Chapter 38).

Cultural Factors. The meaning that a person associates with pain affects the experience of pain and how one adapts to it. This is often closely associated with a person's cultural background, including age, education, race, and familial factors. Cultural beliefs and values affect how individuals cope with pain. They learn what is expected and accepted by their culture, including how to react to pain. Health care providers often mistakenly assume that everyone responds to pain in the same way. Different meanings and attitudes are associated with pain across various cultural groups. An understanding of the cultural meaning of pain helps you design culturally sensitive care for people with pain (Pasero and McCaffery, 2011).

Culture affects pain expression. Some people believe that it is natural to be demonstrative about pain. Others tend to be more introverted. When a person moves to another country, it is important to know to what extent the individual has assimilated into his or her new home. For example, if several generations of a Hispanic patient's family have lived in the United States, the influence of the Spanish culture may be limited, whereas newly immigrated patients still often embrace their cultural norms.

As a nurse explore the impact of cultural differences on a patient's pain experience and make adjustments to the plan of care (Box 44-4). Ask if the patient has had any previous bad experiences with pain management. Work with a patient and family to learn their cultural beliefs, values, and preferences to adequately assess and manage pain (Chapter 9). Find a culturally appropriate assessment tool and communicate use of that tool to other health care providers.

CRITICAL THINKING

Successful critical thinking requires a synthesis of knowledge, experience, information gathered from patients, critical thinking attitudes, and intellectual and professional standards. To make clinical judgments, you anticipate the information you need, analyze the data, and make decisions regarding patient care. A patient's condition or situation is always changing. During assessment consider all critical thinking elements that lead to appropriate nursing diagnoses.

BOX 44-4 CULTURAL ASPECTS OF CARE

Assessing Pain in Culturally Diverse Patients

Pain is a biopsychosocial phenomenon. Culture shapes the experience of pain, including its expression and a patient's behaviors, or coping responses. For example, an individual from a higher socioeconomic group has more resources for managing pain and is more likely to adapt behaviors that will lessen pain. One research study showed that people in the lowest as compared to the highest socioeconomic class were 2 to 3 times more likely to feel disabled through pain (Dorner et al., 2011). Culture also affects a person's choice of lay remedies, help-seeking activities, and receptivity to medical treatment. Some health care providers undertreat pain because they do not understand the cultural effects on the perception of pain intensity. Nurses care for patients with pain from a variety of cultural backgrounds; thus you need to develop strategies to assess and manage pain in culturally diverse patients.

Implications for Patient-Centered Care

- Use culturally appropriate assessment tools such as tools written in the patient's native language to assess pain (Pasero and McCaffery, 2011).
- Assess the patient's health literacy level because this affects your ability to provide appropriate education about pain management and therapies.
- Recognize variations in subjective responses to pain. Some patients are stoic and less expressive, whereas others are emotive and more likely to verbalize pain.
- Be sensitive to variations in communication styles. Some cultures believe that nonverbal expression of pain is sufficient to describe the pain experience, whereas others assume that, if pain medication is appropriate, the nurse will bring it; thus asking is inappropriate.
- Understand that expression of pain is unacceptable within certain cultures. Some patients believe that asking for help indicates a lack of respect, whereas others believe acknowledging pain is a sign of weakness.
- The meaning of pain varies among cultures. Pain is personal and related to religious beliefs. Some cultures consider suffering a part of life to be endured to enter heaven.
- Use knowledge of biological variations of pain. Significant differences in drug metabolism, dosing requirements, therapeutic response, and adverse effects occur in cultural groups. A wide range of responses is also possible within this group. Therefore assess each patient's response to pain medication carefully.
- Develop a personal awareness of your own values and beliefs that affect your responses to patients' reports of pain.

Knowledge of pain physiology and the many factors that influence pain help you manage a patient's pain. Previous experience in caring for patients with pain sharpens your assessment skills and ability to choose effective therapies. Critical thinking attitudes and intellectual standards ensure the aggressive assessment, creative planning, and thorough evaluation needed to obtain an acceptable level of patient pain relief while balancing treatment benefits with treatment-associated risks. Successful pain management does not necessarily mean pain elimination but rather attainment of a mutually agreed-on pain-relief goal that allows patients to control their pain instead of the pain controlling them.

NURSING PROCESS

Apply the nursing process and use a critical thinking approach in your care of patients. The nursing process provides a clinical decision-making approach for you to develop and implement an individualized plan of care.

Nurses approach pain management systematically to understand and treat a patient's pain. Successful management of pain depends on establishing a relationship of trust among health care providers, patient, and family. Pain management extends beyond relief, encompassing the patient's quality of life and ability to work productively, enjoy recreation, and function normally in the family and society.

The American Nurses Association (ANA, 2005) upholds that pain assessment and management is within the scope of every nurse's practice. Thus the ANA offers a certification examination in pain management to staff nurses (http://www.aspmn.org/certification). Several clinical guidelines are available for managing pain in specific disorders. Guidelines are available through the American Pain Society (APS) on the management of pain in the primary care setting; sickle cell pain; cancer pain in adults and children; and pain in osteoarthritis, rheumatoid arthritis, and juvenile chronic arthritis. Sigma Theta Tau International offers guidelines for the older adult on its website (www.geriatricpain.org). In addition, the National Guidelines Clearinghouse (www.guideline.gov) posts a variety of pain-management guidelines.

Assessment

During the assessment process thoroughly assess each patient and critically analyze findings to ensure that you make patient-centered clinical decisions required for safe nursing care. A comprehensive assessment of pain aims to gather information about the cause of a person's pain and determine its effect on his or her ability to function.

Through the Patient's Eyes. Many people view pain as a part of life. Some patients experience it for hours or days before seeking health care assistance. They often expect and even accept a certain amount of pain while being hospitalized. It is important to learn a patient's own values and beliefs about the management of pain and recognize that patient expectations will influence your ability to achieve outcomes in its management (QSEN, 2014). Asking a patient about his or her tolerable pain level is a first step in helping a patient regain control. Assessing previous pain experiences and effective home interventions provides a foundation on which you can build. Patients expect nurses to accept their reports of pain and be prompt in meeting their pain needs.

When assessing pain, be sensitive to the level of discomfort and determine which level will allow your patient to function. For example, when caring for a patient with pain, ask, "Which level of pain will allow you to walk down the hall?" The patient answers that walking is possible when pain is at a level of 2 on a scale of 0 to 10, with 0 being no pain and 10 being worst pain imaginable. You then plan therapies to decrease the patient's pain to that level. Be sure that he or she is a partner in making decisions about the best approaches for managing pain.

Another aspect of assessing pain through the patient's eyes is determining his or her health literacy. People who struggle to find a range of words to talk about their pain lack the ability to use language for symptom relief. Psychologists suggest that having a wide vocabulary with which to describe pain symptoms helps equip a person to better manage pain and reduce distress. Many agencies have assessment tools that allow you to get a more accurate measure of a patient's literacy skills.

If pain is acute or severe, it is unlikely that a patient is able to provide a detailed description of the entire experience. During an episode of acute pain, streamline your assessment and assess its location, severity, and quality. Collect a more detailed acute pain assessment when the patient is more comfortable (Box 44-5). For patients with chronic pain, a thorough pain assessment includes affective,

BOX 44-5 Nursing Assessment Questions

Current Pain: (Modify Assessment for Patient's Age, Cognitive Ability, Culture, Language, and Other Factors)

Palliative or Provocative factors: What makes your pain worse? What makes it better?
Quality: How do you describe your pain?
Relief measures: What do you take at home to gain pain relief?
Region (location): Show me where you hurt.
Severity: On a scale of 0 to 10, how bad is your pain now?
- What is the worst pain you have had in the past 24 hours?
- What is the average pain you have had in the past 24 hours?

Timing: Is your pain constant, intermittent, or both?
U: Effect of pain: What are you not able to do because of your pain?
- With whom do you live, and how do they help you when you have pain?

Current Medications
- Which medications/herbs are you taking now?
- Are these medications and herbs effective in relieving the pain?
- Which nonpharmacological treatments have you tried to relieve the pain?
- Which medications have you tried in the past that worked to stop your pain?
- Have you ever used recreational drugs or alcohol to alleviate pain?

Activity
- What level of daily exercise can you maintain with your pain?
- Which type of movement increases or relieves your pain?
- Which type of activities do you now avoid because of your pain?

BOX 44-6 Routine Clinical Approach to Pain Assessment and Management: ABCDE

A: ***Ask*** about pain regularly. Assess pain systematically.
B: ***Believe*** patient and family in their report of pain and what relieves it.
C: ***Choose*** pain control options appropriate for the patient, family, and setting.
D: ***Deliver*** interventions in a timely, logical, and coordinated fashion.
E: ***Empower*** patients and their families. Enable them to control their course to the greatest extent possible.

From Jacox A et al: *Management of cancer pain,* Clinical Practice Guideline No. 9, AHCPR Publication No. 94-0592, Rockville, MD, 1994, Agency for Health Care Policy and Research, Public Health Service, US Department of Health and Human Services.

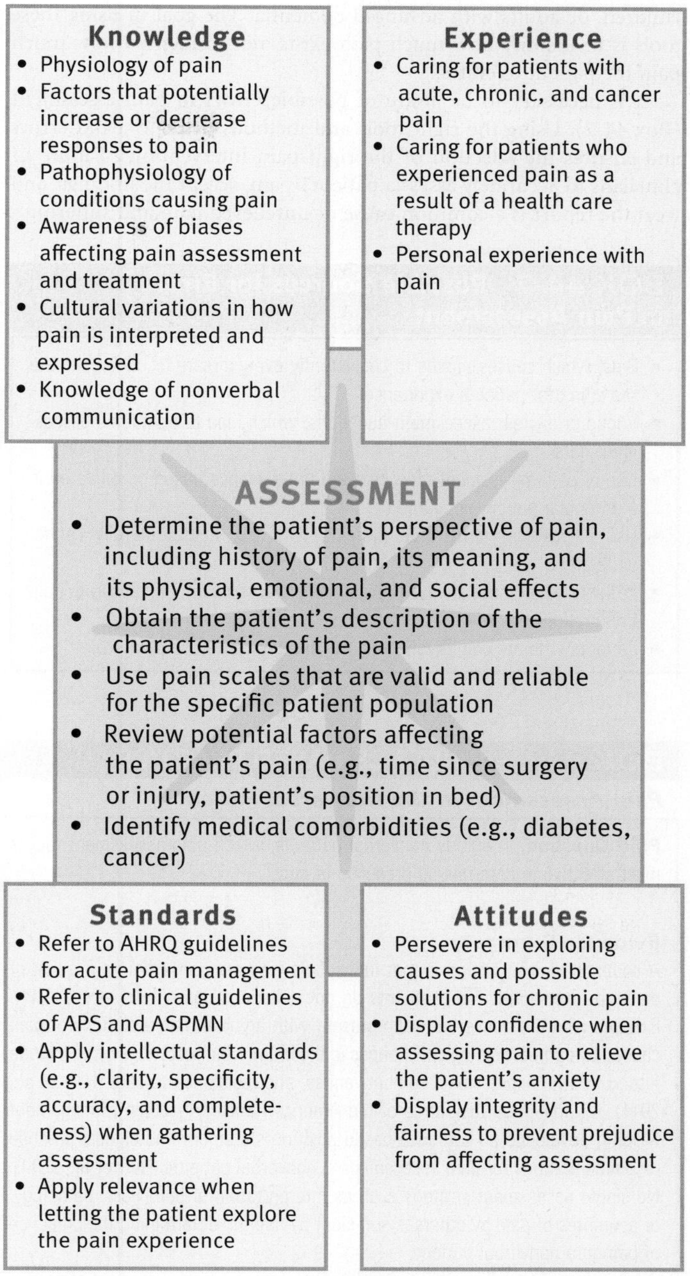

Knowledge
- Physiology of pain
- Factors that potentially increase or decrease responses to pain
- Pathophysiology of conditions causing pain
- Awareness of biases affecting pain assessment and treatment
- Cultural variations in how pain is interpreted and expressed
- Knowledge of nonverbal communication

Experience
- Caring for patients with acute, chronic, and cancer pain
- Caring for patients who experienced pain as a result of a health care therapy
- Personal experience with pain

ASSESSMENT
- Determine the patient's perspective of pain, including history of pain, its meaning, and its physical, emotional, and social effects
- Obtain the patient's description of the characteristics of the pain
- Use pain scales that are valid and reliable for the specific patient population
- Review potential factors affecting the patient's pain (e.g., time since surgery or injury, patient's position in bed)
- Identify medical comorbidities (e.g., diabetes, cancer)

Standards
- Refer to AHRQ guidelines for acute pain management
- Refer to clinical guidelines of APS and ASPMN
- Apply intellectual standards (e.g., clarity, specificity, accuracy, and completeness) when gathering assessment
- Apply relevance when letting the patient explore the pain experience

Attitudes
- Persevere in exploring causes and possible solutions for chronic pain
- Display confidence when assessing pain to relieve the patient's anxiety
- Display integrity and fairness to prevent prejudice from affecting assessment

FIGURE 44-4 Critical thinking model for pain assessment. *AHRQ,* Agency for Healthcare Research and Quality; *APS,* American Pain Society; *ASPMN,* American Society for Pain Management Nursing.

cognitive, behavioral, spiritual, and social dimensions. In the home care setting family members assess pain. Using the ABCs of pain management is an effective way to manage pain (Box 44-6).

Because pain is dynamic, accurate assessment requires you to monitor it on a regular basis along with other vital signs. Some institutions treat it as the fifth vital sign. Pain assessment is *not* simply a number. Relying solely on a number fails to capture the multidimensionality of pain and may be unsafe, particularly when the number fails to reflect the entire pain experience or when the patient does not understand the use of the selected pain-rating scale. Pain assessment is a nursing function. However, nursing assistive personnel (NAP), physical therapists, social workers, and others also screen for pain by asking patients if they are having pain. When pain is noted by any care provider, it is essential that a nurse be informed immediately so he or she can make a thorough assessment to confirm the patient's discomfort and provide appropriate treatment.

The ability to establish a nursing diagnosis, decide on appropriate interventions, and evaluate a patient's response (outcomes) to interventions depends on the fundamental activity of a factual, timely, accurate pain assessment (Figure 44-4). The core of this complex activity is the exploration of the pain experience through the eyes of the patient. Nurses use a variety of tools to assess nociceptive and neuropathic pain. In selecting a tool to be used with a patient, be aware of the clinical usefulness, reliability, and validity of the tool in that specific patient population. For example, a tool that has been validated for use with preverbal children may not have validity or reliability for use with adults. Assessment tools (or scales) are available for use with a number of different patient populations, including critically ill adults, young children, or adults with advanced dementia. The goal in using these tools is to identify how much pain exists, not to identify how much pain the patient tolerates.

It is necessary to be aware of possible errors in pain assessment (Box 44-7). Using the right tools and methods helps to avoid errors and ensures the selection of the right pain interventions. Failure of clinicians to accurately assess a patient's pain, accept the findings, and treat the report is a common cause of unrelieved pain and suffering.

BOX 44-7 Possible Sources for Error in Pain Assessment

- Bias, which causes nurses to consistently overestimate or underestimate the pain that patients experience
- Vague or unclear assessment questions, which lead to unreliable assessment data
- Use of pain assessment tools that are not evidence based or validated in a particular patient population
- Use of medical terms that patients with low health literacy cannot understand
- Patients who do not always provide complete, relevant, and accurate pain information
- Patients who are cognitively impaired and unable to use pain scales

Patient's Expression of Pain. A patient's self-report of pain is the single most reliable indicator of its existence and intensity (APS, 2009; Pasero and McCaffery, 2011). Pain is individualistic. Many patients fail to report or discuss discomfort. At the same time many nurses believe that patients report pain if they have it. If patients sense that you doubt that pain exists, they share little information about their pain experience or minimize their report. A caring therapeutic relationship must be established with the patient that allows for open communication. Simple measures such as sitting when talking to patients about pain lets them know that you are sincerely concerned about their pain.

Patients unable to communicate effectively often require special attention during assessment. Infants and children, people who are developmentally delayed, patients who are psychotic, the patient who is critically ill or at end of life, patients with dementia, and patients who are aphasic or do not speak English all require different approaches. Herr et al. (2011) examined various pain behavior-assessment tools used with patients who were cognitively impaired. Although no one tool had sufficient reliability and validity, there are clinical practice recommendations (Box 44-8). However, you need to understand that "the number obtained when using a pain-behavior scale is a pain-behavior score, not a pain-intensity rating" (Pasero and McCaffery, 2011). These tools identify the presence of pain but do not determine its intensity.

BOX 44-8 EVIDENCE-BASED PRACTICE

Pain Assessment in the Nonverbal Patient

PICO Question: In elderly nonverbal patients, which pain-assessment tool is most effective in determining presence of pain?

Evidence Summary

A common misconception is that individuals who are nonverbal as a result of dementia or cognitive impairments do not experience pain (Herr et al., 2011). Patients who are nonverbal often present with atypical manifestations of pain caused by pathophysiological changes in the brain. Manifestations often include hitting, fearful expressions, combativeness, and resistance to care (Herr et al., 2011). An appointed task force of the American Society for Pain Management Nursing developed an evidence-based position statement and clinical practice recommendations for pain assessment in nonverbal patients (Herr et al., 2011). No single assessment strategy such as interpretation of behaviors, pathology, or estimates of pain by others is sufficient by itself in determining the presence of pain in a nonverbal patient.

A number of tools have been developed to assess for the presence of pain in cognitively impaired adults. Although research studies have demonstrated that these tools can be used to determine the presence of pain, there has been little evidence to determine whether they can be used to identify pain intensity. In a study by Lukas et al (2013), the Abbey Pain Scale, Pain Assessment in Advanced Dementia Scale (PAINAD), and Noncommunicative Patient's Pain Assessment Instrument (NOPPAIN) were shown to enable observers to recognize the presence or absence of pain and provide a rating of pain severity in older people with impaired cognition.

Application to Nursing Practice

- Recommended assessment considerations:
  - Attempt a self-report of pain using simple yes/no responses or vocalizations or a numerical rating scale (Herr et al., 2011).
  - Search for potential causes of pain (Herr et al., 2011). Examples include pain associated with intravenous insertion site infiltrations, abdominal cramping and fullness, urinary retention, muscle spasm, and prolonged pressure on body parts associated with immobility.
  - Assume that pain is present (APP) after ruling out other problems (infection, constipation) that cause pain.
  - Identify pathological conditions or procedures that cause pain.
  - Observe patient behaviors and list behaviors (e.g., facial expressions, vocalizations, body movements, changes in interactions or mental status) that indicate pain. These vary, depending on patient's developmental level (Herr et al., 2011).
  - Ask family members, parents, or caregivers for a surrogate report.
- Use behavioral pain assessment tools.
  - Use evidence-based tools to ensure appropriate pain assessment (Herr et al., 2011).
  - Evidence supports use of the PAINAD for assessment of pain in patients with advanced dementia (Mosele et al., 2012).
  - Determine the appropriate scale on the basis of individual patient needs; no one scale measures pain accurately for all groups of patients.
- Vital signs are not sensitive indicators for the presence of pain.
- Choose analgesic, dose, and titration on the basis of estimated intensity of pain.
- For mild-to-moderate pain, confer with health care provider to give nonopioid analgesics around the clock.
- After 24 hours reassess. If behaviors improve, assume that pain was the cause.
- If behaviors persist, consult with physician about giving a single, low-dose short-acting opioid (e.g., morphine). Observe effect.
- If behaviors continue, obtain order to titrate dose upward by 25% to 50% and observe effect.
- Continue to titrate up until a therapeutic effect or bothersome adverse effects occur or if there is no benefit.
- If behaviors continue after a reasonable analgesic trial, explore other potential causes.

TABLE 44-5 Classification of Pain by Location

Location	Characteristics	Examples of Causes
Superficial or Cutaneous		
Pain resulting from stimulation of skin	Pain is of short duration and localized. It usually is a sharp sensation.	Needlestick; small cut or laceration
Deep or Visceral		
Pain resulting from stimulation of internal organs	Pain is diffuse and radiates in several directions. Duration varies, but it usually lasts longer than superficial pain. Pain is sharp, dull, or unique to organ involved.	Crushing sensation (e.g., angina pectoris); burning sensation (e.g., gastric ulcer)
Referred		
Common in visceral pain because many organs themselves have no pain receptors (The entrance of sensory neurons from affected organ into same spinal cord segment as neurons from areas where individual feels pain causes perception of pain in unaffected areas.)	Pain is in part of body separate from source of pain and assumes any characteristic.	Myocardial infarction, which causes referred pain to the jaw, left arm, and left shoulder; kidney stones, which refer pain to groin
Radiating		
Sensation of pain extending from initial site of injury to another body part	Pain feels as though it travels down or along body part. It is intermittent or constant.	Low back pain from ruptured intravertebral disk accompanied by pain radiating down leg from sciatic nerve irritation

Patients with cognitive impairments often require insightful assessment approaches involving close observation of vocal response, facial movements (e.g., grimacing, clenched teeth), and body movements (e.g., restlessness, pacing). Also assess social interaction (e.g., does the patient avoid conversation?). Patients who are critically ill and have a clouded sensorium or the presence of nasogastric tubes or artificial airways require specific questions that they can answer with a nod of the head or by writing out a response. If the patient speaks a different language, pain assessment is difficult. A professional interpreter is often necessary (Pasero and McCaffery, 2011).

When a patient is in pain, conduct a focused physical and neurological examination and observe for nonverbal responses to pain (e.g., grimacing, rigid body posture, limping, frowning, or crying) (Pasero and McCaffery, 2011). Examine the painful area to see if palpation or manipulation of the site increases pain.

Characteristics of Pain. Assessment of the characteristics of pain allows you to understand the type of pain, its pattern, and the types of interventions that bring relief. Use of instruments to quantify the extent and degree of pain depends on a patient being cognitively alert enough to be able to understand and follow instructions.

Timing (Onset, Duration, and Pattern). Ask questions to determine the onset, duration, and time sequence of pain. When did it begin? How long has it lasted? Does it occur at the same time each day? Is it intermittent, constant, or a combination? How often does it recur? It is sometimes easier to diagnose the nature of pain by identifying time factors. Knowing the time cycle or pattern of pain helps you intervene before the pain occurs or worsens.

Location. Ask a patient to describe or point to all areas of discomfort to assess pain location. To localize the pain specifically, have him or her trace the area from the most severe point outward. This is difficult to do if pain is diffuse or involves several sites or parts of the body. Do not assume that your patient's pain always occurs in the same location. When describing pain location to other health care providers, use anatomical landmarks and descriptive terminology. The statement "Pain is localized in the upper right abdominal quadrant" is more specific than "The patient states the pain is in the abdomen." Pain classified by location is superficial or cutaneous, deep or visceral, referred, or radiating (Table 44-5).

Severity. One of the most subjective and therefore most useful characteristics for reporting pain is its severity. Nurses teach patients how to use pain scales to help them communicate pain severity or intensity. Many scales are available in several languages to aid nurses when a professional interpreter is not present (Pasero and McCaffery, 2011). The purpose of using a pain scale is to identify pain intensity over time so the effectiveness of interventions can be evaluated (Pasero and McCaffery, 2011). It is important to select the scale that is appropriate for a patient's age, language, and ability and to ensure that the patient understands how to use it. Examples of pain-intensity scales include numerical rating scales (NRSs), verbal descriptor scales (VDSs), and visual analog scales (VASs) (Figure 44-5).

An NRS requires patients to rate pain on a line scale of 0 to 10, with 0 representing no pain and 10 representing the worst pain the patient can imagine. These scales work best when assessing pain intensity before and after therapeutic interventions. A VDS consists of a line with three to six word descriptors equally spaced along the line. Show a patient the scale and ask him or her to choose the descriptor that best represents the severity of pain. A VAS consists of a straight line without labeled subdivisions. The straight line shows a continuum of intensity and has labeled end points. A patient indicates pain by marking the appropriate point on the line. Use a scale to measure the current severity of a patient's pain. Also ask patients to rate their average pain and the worst pain they have had in the past 24 hours. This information allows you to see trends in pain severity.

A good pain scale is easy to use, understandable, and not time consuming. If a patient is able to read and understand a scale easily, the pain description is more accurate. If patients use a hearing aid or glasses, be sure that they are using them when answering pain-assessment questions or marking a pain scale. Once you select a scale that works for a patient, be sure to use it consistently. Do not use a pain scale to compare the pain of one patient to that of another.

Assessing pain intensity in children requires special techniques. Children's verbal statements are most important (Hockenberry and Wilson, 2015). Young children do not always know what the word *pain* means; therefore assessment requires you to use words such as *owie, boo-boo,* or *hurt.* Some unique tools are available to measure pain intensity in children. Faces Pain Scales are commonly used, with four having undergone extensive psychometric testing for reliability and validity: Faces Pain Scale (FPS) (scored 0-6); Faces Pain Scale—revised (FPS-R) (0-10); Oucher pain scale (0-10); and Wong-Baker Faces Pain-Rating Scale (WBFPRS) (0-10) (Tomlinson et al., 2010). The "Oucher" (Beyer et al., 1992) uses photographs of the face of a child (in increasing levels of discomfort) to cue children into understanding pain and its severity. A child points to a face on the tool, thus simplifying the task of describing the pain. There are cultural versions of the tool (Figure 44-6). The WBFPRS (Wong and Baker, 1988) assesses pain in verbal children (Figure 44-7). The scale consists of six cartoon faces ranging from a smiling face ("no hurt") to increasingly less happy faces; to a final sad, tearful face ("hurts worst"). Children as young as 3 years of age use the scale. The FPS was adapted by the IASP in 2001 to facilitate a rating score from 0-10. This version, known as the FPS-R (Figure 44-8) has the advantage of not displaying emotion such as smiles or tears and may be used with children ages 4 to 16 years (IASP, 2014a). Nurses use a variety of other tools to assess pain in neonates, infants, nonverbal toddlers, and children with cognitive impairments.

Quality. There is no common or specific pain vocabulary in general use. Patients describe pain in their own way. A study conducted in 1990 showed that Hispanics, American Indians, blacks, and whites all rated pain as the most intense term, followed by hurt; ache was the least intense (Gaston-Johansson et al., 1990). The research is dated, but it

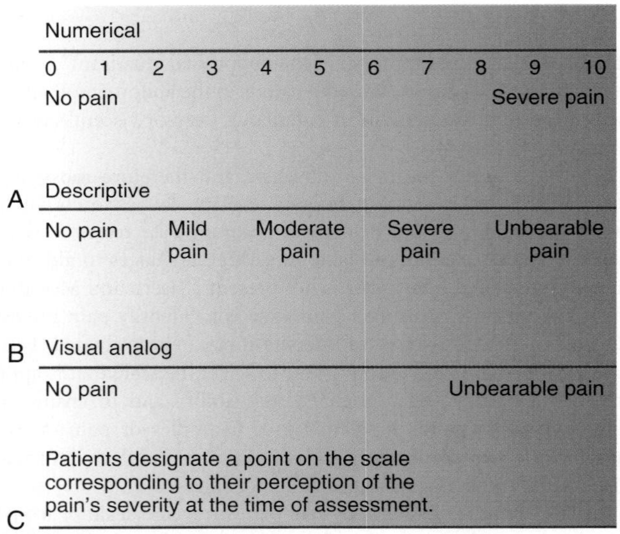

Numerical

0 1 2 3 4 5 6 7 8 9 10

No pain Severe pain

A

Descriptive

No pain | Mild pain | Moderate pain | Severe pain | Unbearable pain

B

Visual analog

No pain Unbearable pain

Patients designate a point on the scale corresponding to their perception of the pain's severity at the time of assessment.

C

FIGURE 44-5 Sample pain scales. **A,** Numerical. **B,** Verbal descriptive. **C,** Visual analog.

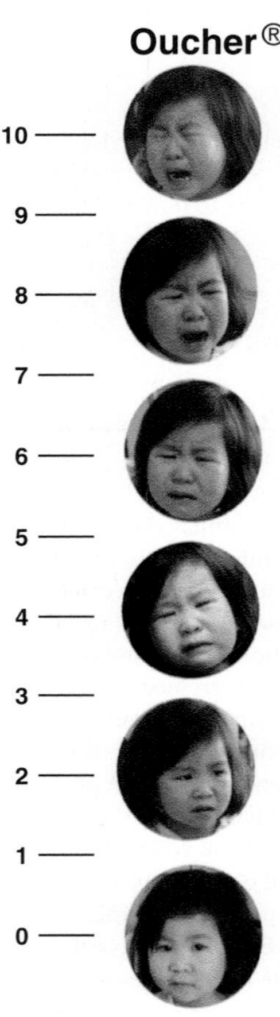

FIGURE 44-6 Asian girl version of the Oucher pain scale. (The Asian versions of the Oucher scale [male and female] were developed and copyrighted in 2003 by CH Yeh [University of Pittsburgh] and CH Wang, Taiwan.)

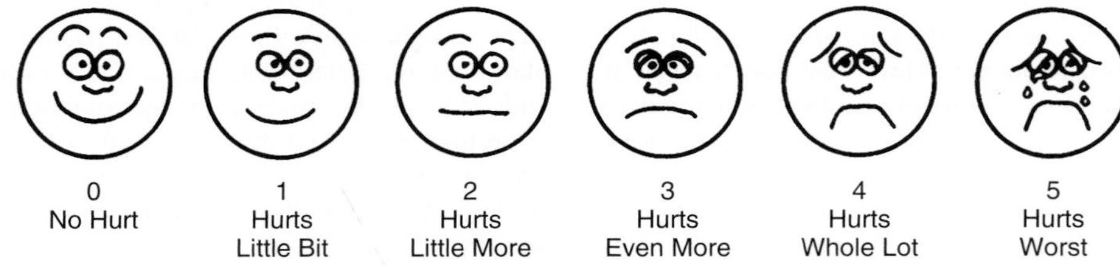

Brief word instructions: Point to each face using the words to describe the pain intensity. Ask the child to choose face that best describes own pain and record the appropriate number.

FIGURE 44-7 Wong-Baker Faces Pain Scale. (From Hockenberry MJ, Wilson D: *Wong's nursing care of infants and children,* ed 10, St Louis, 2015, Mosby.)

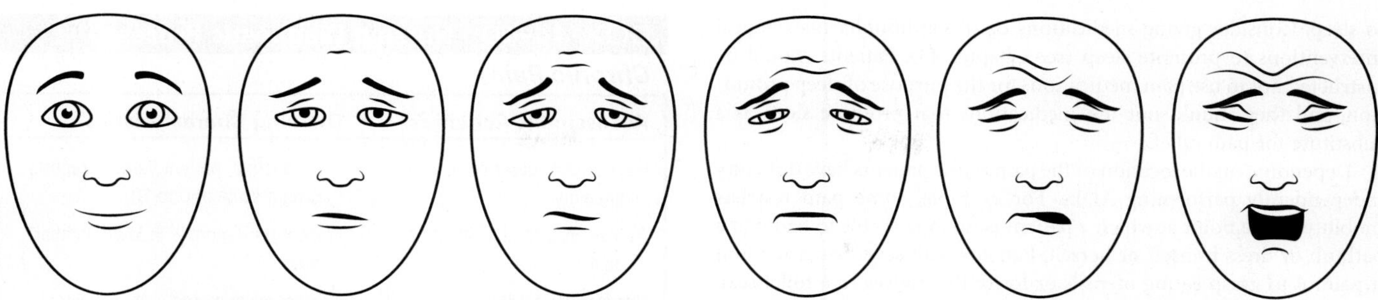

FIGURE 44-8 Faces Pain Scale-revised (FPS-R). (From the International Association for the Study of Pain.)

shows the importance of not assuming that one patient perceives pain differently than another only on the basis of cultural background. Assess the terms that patients use to describe their discomfort and then always use these words consistently to obtain an accurate report. For example, say, "Tell me what your discomfort feels like." The patient may describe the pain as crushing, throbbing, sharp, or dull. For example, if it is dull, when you return to the patient, ask if it is still "dull." It is always more accurate to have patients describe the pain in their own words whenever possible.

There is some consistency in the way people describe certain types of pain. The pain associated with a myocardial infarction is often described as crushing or viselike; whereas the pain of a surgical incision is often described as dull, aching, and throbbing, indicating nociceptive pain. Neuropathic pain is usually burning, shooting, or electric-like (Sadler, 2013). When a patient's descriptions fit the pattern forming in the assessment, you then make a clearer analysis of the nature and type of pain. This leads to more appropriate pain management because you treat nociceptive and neuropathic pain differently.

Aggravating and Precipitating Factors. Various factors or conditions precipitate or aggravate pain. Ask a patient to describe activities that cause or aggravate pain such as physical movement, positions, drinking coffee or alcohol, urination, swallowing, eating food, or psychological stress. Also ask them to demonstrate actions that cause a painful response such as coughing or turning a certain way. Some symptoms (depression, anxiety, fatigue, sedation, anorexia, sleep disruption, spiritual distress, and guilt) cause worsening of pain or may be aggravated by it. Assess for these associated symptoms and evaluate their effects on the patient's pain perception. After identifying specific aggravating or precipitating factors, it is easier to plan interventions to avoid worsening the pain.

Relief Measures. It is useful to know whether a patient has an effective way of relieving pain such as changing position, using ritualistic behavior (pacing, rocking, or rubbing), eating, meditating, praying, or applying heat or cold to the painful site. The patient's methods are ones that can often be used for treatment if appropriate to the cause of pain. Patients gain trust when they know that nurses are willing to try their relief measures. This is particularly the case in home settings. Patients gain a sense of control over the pain instead of the pain controlling them. Assessment of relieving factors also includes identification of all the patient's health care providers (e.g., internist, orthopedist, acupuncturist, chiropractor, or dentist).

Effects of Pain on the Patient. Pain alters a person's lifestyle and psychological well-being. For example, chronic/persistent pain causes suffering, loss of control, loneliness, exhaustion, and an impaired quality of life. To understand a pain experience, ask the patient what the pain prevents him or her from doing.

BOX 44-9 Behavioral Indicators of Effects of Pain

Vocalizations
- Moaning
- Crying
- Gasping
- Grunting

Facial Expressions
- Grimace
- Clenched teeth
- Wrinkled forehead
- Tightly closed or widely opened eyes or mouth
- Lip biting

Body Movement
- Restlessness
- Immobilization
- Muscle tension
- Increased hand and finger movements
- Pacing activities
- Rhythmic or rubbing motions
- Protective movement of body parts
- Grabbing or holding a body part

Social Interaction
- Avoidance of conversation
- Focus only on activities for pain relief
- Avoidance of social contacts
- Reduced attention span
- Reduced interaction with environment

Behavioral Effects. When a patient has pain, assess verbalization, vocal response, facial and body movements, and social interaction. A verbal report of pain is a vital part of assessment. You need to be willing to listen and understand. When a patient is unable to communicate pain, it is especially important for you to be alert for behaviors that indicate it (Box 44-9).

The nonverbal expression of pain either supports or contradicts other information about it. If a woman in labor reports that her labor pains are occurring more frequently and if she begins to massage her abdomen more often, this confirms her report. If a patient reports severe abdominal pain but continues to grasp the chest, a more detailed assessment is likely needed.

Influence on Activities of Daily Living. Patients who live with daily pain or have prolonged pain during a hospitalization are less able to participate in routine activities, which results in physical deconditioning. This deconditioning can slow recovery of hospitalized patients. Assessment of these changes reveals the extent of the patients' disabilities and adjustments necessary to help them participate in self-care. The primary goal of the nurse is to improve patient function.

Ask a patient whether pain interferes with sleep. Some patients experience difficulty in falling asleep and/or staying asleep. The pain may awaken the patient during the night and make it hard to fall back to sleep. Consider giving medications or trying nonpharmacological interventions to promote sleep (see Chapter 43). Patients should be instructed not to use pain medications for the purpose of sleep promotion, and they should not use medications that promote sleep as a substitute for pain relief.

Depending on the location of the pain, some patients have difficulty independently performing ADLs. For example, some pain restricts mobility to the point at which a patient is no longer able to bathe in a bathtub or dress himself or herself. Patients with severe arthritis find it painful to grasp eating utensils or lower themselves to a toilet seat. Assess the patient's need for help with self-care activities, determine if a family caregiver provides assistance at home, and collaborate with members of the health care team (e.g., physical and occupational therapy).

Pain sometimes impairs the ability to maintain normal sexual relations. Physical conditions such as arthritis or back pain may prevent patients from assuming usual positions during intercourse. Pain or fatigue may reduce a patient's desire for sex. An assessment should include the extent to which pain affects the patient's usual sexual activity (i.e., physically unable or reduced desire). Pain threatens a person's ability to work. The more physical activity required in a job, the greater the risk of discomfort when the pain is associated with movement. Pain related to emotional stress increases in individuals whose jobs involve stressful decision making. Assess the work that patients do and their abilities to function in their jobs. Assess the daily chores of homemakers in the same manner as the duties involved in jobs outside the home. Also assess whether it is necessary for patients to stop activity occasionally because of pain and help them select ways to minimize or control it so they are able to remain productive.

Include an assessment of the effect of pain on social activities. Some pain is so debilitating that the patient becomes too exhausted to socialize. Identify a patient's normal social activities, the extent to which activities have been disrupted, and the desire to participate in these activities.

Concomitant Symptoms. Concomitant symptoms, including nausea, headache, dizziness, urge to urinate, constipation, depression and restlessness, occur with pain and usually increase a patient's pain severity. Certain types of pain have predictable concomitant symptoms. For example, severe rectal pain often leads to constipation. These symptoms are as much a problem to a patient as the pain itself.

◆ Nursing Diagnosis

An accurate nursing diagnosis may be made only after you perform a complete assessment. The development of accurate nursing diagnoses for a patient in pain results from thorough data collection and analysis (Box 44-10). Careful assessment reveals the presence or potential for pain. Be sure that your assessment includes the patient's history of recent procedures or preexisting painful conditions.

The nursing diagnosis focuses on the specific nature of a patient's pain to identify the most useful types of interventions for alleviating it and improving the patient's function. *Acute Pain related to physical trauma* and *Acute Pain related to natural childbirth processes* require very different nursing interventions. Accurate identification of related factors is necessary in choosing appropriate nursing interventions. For example, interventions for *Acute Pain related to physical trauma* usually require pharmacological intervention, whereas *Acute Pain related to natural childbirth processes* is sometimes managed more appropriately with nonpharmacological interventions such as controlled breathing techniques.

A pain assessment often directs you to identify additional diagnoses other than that of *Acute* or *Chronic Pain.* The extent to which pain affects a patient's function and general state of health determines whether other nursing diagnoses are relevant. For example, your assessment reveals that a patient reports having pain of the hands and shoulders and has difficulty removing or fastening necessary items of clothing. The patient has had osteoarthritis for over 3 years with persistent discomfort and weakness of the upper extremities. The nursing diagnoses for this patient are *Dressing Self-Care Deficit* and *Chronic Pain.* The diagnosis of *Dressing Self-Care Deficit* requires involvement by members of the interdisciplinary health care team to provide the patient with assistive devices for performing self-care. Examples of other diagnoses that may be related to pain follow:

- *Activity Intolerance*
- *Anxiety*
- *Bathing Self-Care Deficit*
- *Ineffective Coping*
- *Fatigue*
- *Impaired Physical Mobility*
- *Insomnia*
- *Impaired Social Interaction*

BOX 44-10 Nursing Diagnostic Process

Chronic Pain

Assessment Activities	Defining Characteristics
Have patient describe pain intensity.	Pain constant; patient verbally reports 5 on a scale of 0 to 10
Assess onset and location of pain.	Present for 7 months in lower lumbar area
Observe patient behaviors.	Grimaces and grunts with movement, rubs flanks frequently; reduced movement
Assess effect of pain on activities of daily living (ADLs).	Appetite poor; gets little sleep; difficulty dressing
Review medical history.	Previous trauma; effectiveness of past pain control measures

◆ Planning

During the planning step of the nursing process, analyze information from multiple sources. Critical thinking ensures that a patient's plan of care (see the Nursing Care Plan) integrates all that is known about the individual and key critical thinking elements (Figure 44-9). Professional standards are especially important to consider when developing a plan of care. These standards establish evidence-based guidelines for selecting effective nursing interventions. Professional standards of care regarding pain management are available as agency policies or through professional organizations such as the American Society for Pain Management Nursing (ASPMN).

Another strategy for planning care is using a concept map. Patients who are in pain frequently have interrelated problems. As one problem gets worse, other aspects of a patient's level of health also change. A concept map helps you determine how the nursing diagnoses are interrelated with one another and linked to the patient's medical diagnosis. This eventually allows you to also see how interventions are related for different diagnoses. Using the example for Mrs. Mays, the patient with osteoarthritis, note the relationships among *Acute Pain, Impaired Physical Mobility, Dressing and Feeding Self-Care Deficit,* and *Fatigue* (Figure 44-10). Identifying these relationships helps you develop a holistic and patient-centered plan of care.

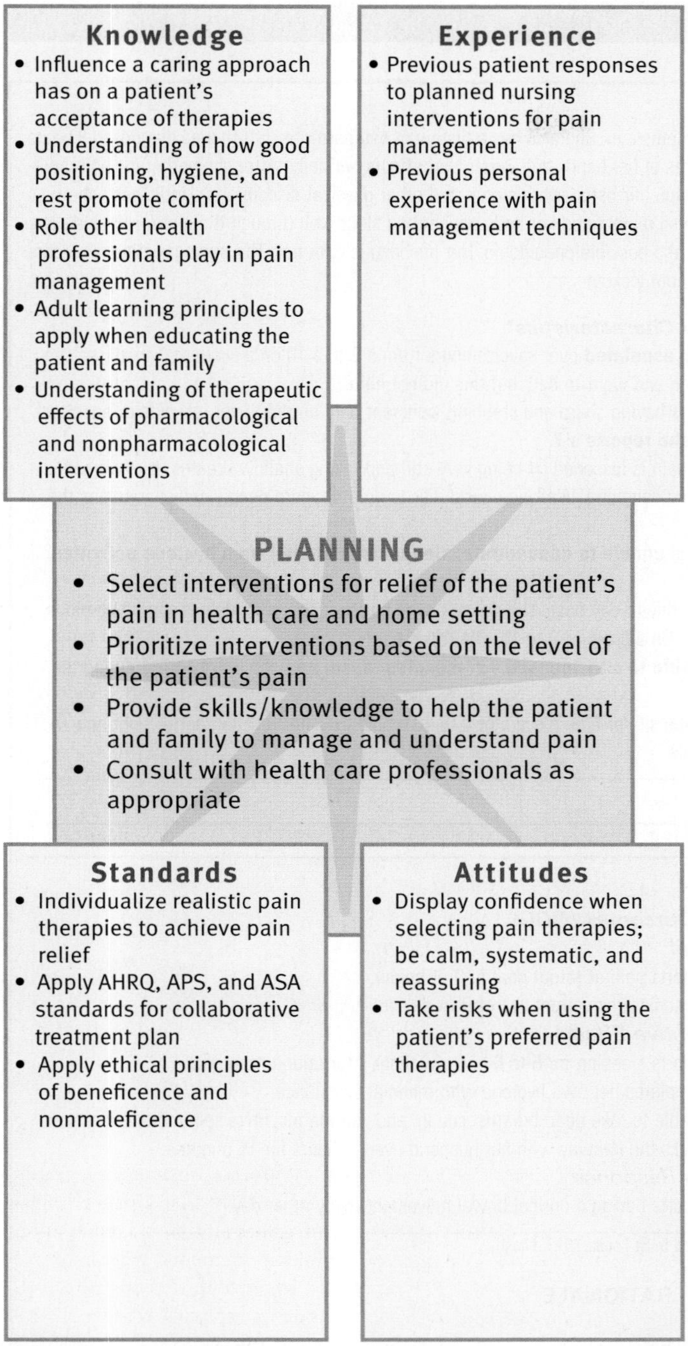

Knowledge
- Influence a caring approach has on a patient's acceptance of therapies
- Understanding of how good positioning, hygiene, and rest promote comfort
- Role other health professionals play in pain management
- Adult learning principles to apply when educating the patient and family
- Understanding of therapeutic effects of pharmacological and nonpharmacological interventions

Experience
- Previous patient responses to planned nursing interventions for pain management
- Previous personal experience with pain management techniques

PLANNING
- Select interventions for relief of the patient's pain in health care and home setting
- Prioritize interventions based on the level of the patient's pain
- Provide skills/knowledge to help the patient and family to manage and understand pain
- Consult with health care professionals as appropriate

Standards
- Individualize realistic pain therapies to achieve pain relief
- Apply AHRQ, APS, and ASA standards for collaborative treatment plan
- Apply ethical principles of beneficence and nonmaleficence

Attitudes
- Display confidence when selecting pain therapies; be calm, systematic, and reassuring
- Take risks when using the patient's preferred pain therapies

FIGURE 44-9 Critical thinking model for pain management planning. *AHRQ,* Agency for Healthcare Research and Quality; *APS,* American Pain Society; *ASA,* American Society of Anesthesiologists.

Goals and Outcomes. When managing pain, goals of care promote a patient's optimal function. Along with the patient, determine the realistic expectations for pain relief. Decide on a mutually acceptable level of pain that allows return of function. Make sure that the patient understands that complete pain relief is probably not possible but that every effort will be made to allow him or her to safely reach a pain level that allows for maximum function.

It is important to remember that a successful plan of care requires a therapeutic relationship with a patient and family to focus on a relevant education plan. Helping patients learn how to manage their pain is always a goal of care. You help best by listening to the patient's concerns, needs, and understanding of available pain relief measures. A patient knows the most about his or her pain and is an important partner in selecting successful pain therapies.

An indication of the success of a plan of care is determined through attainment of goals and outcomes. For example, for the goal "the patient will achieve a satisfactory level of pain relief within 24 hours," the following are possible outcomes:

- Reports that pain is a 3 or less on a scale of 0 to 10
- Avoids factors that intensify pain
- Uses pain-relief measures safely
- Level of discomfort does not interfere with dressing self

Setting Priorities. When setting priorities in pain management, consider the type of pain the patient is experiencing and the effect that it has on various body functions. Work with the patient to select interventions that are appropriate. For example, if an analgesic is relieving acute pain, turn your attention to how the pain is affecting the patient's activity, appetite, and sleep. In contrast, when a patient's pain continues to be severe, preventing implementation of other interventions, immediate pain relief is the obvious priority. Priorities change as a patient's pain experience changes.

Teamwork and Collaboration. A comprehensive plan includes a variety of resources from the health care team such as advanced practice nurses, doctors of pharmacology (PharmDs), physical therapists, occupational therapists, physicians, social workers, psychologists, and clergy. An oncology or pain clinical nurse specialist is very familiar with pharmacological and nonpharmacological interventions that are most effective for chronic/persistent pain. PharmDs are knowledgeable about pharmacological treatments of pain. Physical therapists plan exercises that strengthen muscle groups and lessen pain in affected areas. Occupational therapists devise splints to support painful body parts. Physicians are familiar with pharmacological interventions, and some are skilled in interventional pain procedures such as nerve blocks and spinal cord stimulator implantations. Social workers and psychologists may offer nonpharmacological approaches to pain management such as cognitive behavioral therapy or mindfulness training. Clergy members help patients focus on spiritual health. It is important to also involve family caregivers in the plan of care. They will often administer care in the home after discharge. If the pain-management plan is not successful in achieving the identified pain-relief goal, talk with the patient's health care provider about revising it. Consultation with a pain expert is sometimes necessary.

◆ Implementation

Pain therapy requires an individualized approach, perhaps more so than any other patient problem. The nurse, patient, and frequently the family are partners in pain management. You are responsible for administering and monitoring therapies ordered by health care providers for pain relief and independently providing measures that complement those prescribed. Generally try the least invasive or safest therapy first along with previously used successful patient remedies. If you question a medical therapy, consult with the health care provider.

Regardless of the therapies chosen, your ability to show compassionate care toward patients has the potential for maximizing their pain control. You can help the patient minimize pain through caring behaviors such as listening, offering a gentle touch, and responding promptly to a pain request.

 NURSING CARE PLAN

Acute Pain

ASSESSMENT

Mrs. Mays, 72 years old, was diagnosed with a cancerous tumor in her left lung 2 months ago. She also has a history of osteoarthritis, which was diagnosed 8 years ago. The arthritis causes chronic inflammation with mild-to-moderate pain in the joints of her hands and wrists that affects her daily. After chemotherapy and radiation therapy, she took ibuprofen (Advil) 200 mg on an as-needed (prn) basis to manage her osteoarthritis pain and other physical discomforts. Until today she was able to clean her home and climb the stairs to her bedroom without difficulty. She also maintained her body weight and slept well through the night. However, she is now admitted to the hospital with uncontrollable chest pain, shortness of breath, and possible pneumonia. Her husband is with her. The nurse practitioner orders a patient-controlled analgesia (PCA) of morphine 0.5 mg demand dose with a 10-minute lockout.

Assessment Activities	*Findings/Defining Characteristics**
Ask Mrs. Mays what she did at home to control her acute onset of chest pain.	Her chest **pain rapidly escalated** over several hours from a 3 to a 10 on a scale of 0 to 10, so she doubled her ibuprofen and went to bed; but this did not help.
Ask Mrs. Mays to describe the pain she is having now.	She responds that she is having sharp and stabbing, constant pain on the lower left side of her chest.
Ask Mrs. Mays what her chest pain intensity is now.	On a scale of 0 to 10, **she reports a 7.**
Ask Mrs. Mays what has helped and worsened her chest pain.	She responds that her pain is lessened by being very still and taking shallow breaths. It is worsened by deeper breaths and coughing. Walking causes her to breathe more deeply, which worsens the pain.
Ask Mrs. Mays what her pain has prevented her from doing.	She responds that she is **unable to concentrate, sleep, complete her own hygiene activities, or eat.**
Ask Mrs. Mays what her joint pain intensity is now.	She responds that on a day-to-day basis she doesn't even notice it anymore, unless she has periods of increased activity. On a scale of 0 to 10, she reports a 1.
Observe Mrs. Mays's nonverbal behavior.	She is **restless,** is **unable to stay focused,** her **muscles tense, and** she is **frowning** during the history taking.
Ask Mrs. Mays what her pain-intensity goal (on a scale of 0 to 10) is?	She says that a pain intensity of 5 on a scale of 0 to 10 would help her function better right now. A goal of 3 is preferable.

*__Defining characteristics__ are shown in bold type.

NURSING DIAGNOSIS: Acute pain related to abrupt onset of inflammation

PLANNING

Goals	*Expected Outcomes (NOC)*[†]
	Pain Control
Mrs. Mays will reach a tolerable level of pain before discharge.	Mrs. Mays reports pain at target goal of 3 or below.
	Mrs. Mays demonstrates correct use of PCA device.
	Pain: Disruptive Effects
Mrs. Mays will actively participate in activities of daily living (ADLs).	Mrs. Mays reports sleeping for 5 to 6 hours without interruption from pain.
	Mrs. Mays completes her own hygiene with minimal assistance.
	Mrs. Mays is able to take deep breaths, cough, and use the incentive spirometer every hour.
	Mrs. Mays walks the hallway with her husband every 4 hours for 15 minutes.
	Medication Response
Mrs. Mays will be free of opioid side effects.	Mrs. Mays reports having a normal bowel movement every other day.

[†]Outcome classification labels from Moorhead S et al: *Nursing outcomes classification (NOC),* ed 5, St Louis, 2013, Mosby.

INTERVENTIONS (NIC)[‡]	RATIONALE
Pain Management	
Begin PCA at ordered dose. Explain to patient how to use the PCA. Explain to patient and spouse the purpose of the pump and emphasize the importance of only the patient pushing the button, not the husband.	Severe acute pain requires immediate-release opioid. Discouraging the husband from pushing the button prevents unnecessary doses and reduces potential dangerous effects of the opioid. Patient needs to be awake to perceive the pain and push the button (Pasero and McCaffery, 2011).
Monitor intravenous (IV) PCA morphine use. Explain to patient and spouse the action of the medication, potential side effects, and the importance of reporting unrelieved pain.	Pain is easier to prevent than to treat. Side effects are usually transient, except for constipation. Calculating 24-hour dosage of opioid helps determine appropriate oral dose (Pasero and McCaffery, 2011).
Have patient select nonpharmacological interventions that have relieved her pain in the past (e.g., distraction, music, simple relaxation therapy) or that are acceptable to her.	Nonpharmacological approaches augment pharmacological therapy and help patients improve quality of life and decrease anxiety and depression (Kolanowski, 2013).
Teach spouse how to perform slow-stroke back massage.	Slow-stroke back massage is easy to do, takes a short time, and induces relaxation (Buyukyilmaz and Asti, 2013).

[‡]Intervention classification labels from Bulechek GM et al: *Nursing interventions classification (NIC),* ed 6, St Louis, 2013, Mosby.

NURSING CARE PLAN

***Acute Pain*—cont'd**

EVALUATION

Nursing Actions	*Patient Response/Finding*	*Achievement of Outcome*
Ask Mrs. Mays if she has attained her pain-relief goal most of the time.	She responds, "My pain usually runs around a 3, except when I start coughing or walking."	Mrs. Mays reports an acceptable level of pain. Instruct her to push her button before ambulating or when she feels the pain intensity rising above 3 out of 10.
Observe Mrs. Mays while using the incentive spirometer.	Mrs. Mays is using the incentive spirometer and is able to cough and take deep breaths without splinting every hour.	Ability to cough, breathe deeply, and use the incentive spirometer has improved. Encourage her to continue pulmonary exercises hourly.
Observe Mrs. Mays performing ADLs, walking, and during sleep.	Mrs. Mays is dressed for breakfast, walking the hallway every 4 hours with her husband. The night nurse's notes indicate that she slept through the night.	Ability to perform ADLs and sleep has improved. Continue to monitor.
Observe Mrs. Mays as she ambulates in the hallway.	Mrs. Mays successfully ambulated in the hallway with her husband twice during the shift with minimal increase in pain intensity.	Improved pain control has increased her activity, a nonverbal indicator of pain. Continue to monitor.
Ask Mr. Mays if he was able to give his wife a backrub.	Mr. Mays reported that she did not want a backrub but preferred to have her feet rubbed, which he was happy to do. "She said it made her feel more relaxed."	Nonpharmacological intervention was successful but needs to be changed from backrub to footrub in the nursing care plan.
Ask Mrs. Mays when she last had a bowel movement and its consistency.	She has not had a bowel movement in 3 days (since starting the morphine PCA).	Assess her abdomen for bowel sounds and distention and return of flatus. Consult with health care provider about starting a stimulant laxative once intestinal obstruction is ruled out (Pasero and McCaffery, 2011).
Observe Mrs. Mays for excessive drowsiness.	Mrs. Mays is awake and alert during conversations and interacts frequently with her husband.	Sedation, an indicator of too much opioid, is not identified. Continue to monitor.

Health Promotion. When providing pain-relief measures, choose therapies suited to a patient's unique pain experience. Apply guidelines for individualizing pain therapy, including the following:

- Use different types of pain-relief measures.
- Use measures that patient believes are effective.
- Keep an open mind about ways to relieve pain.
- Keep trying. When efforts at pain relief fail, do not abandon the patient but reassess the situation.

Maintaining Wellness. Patients are better prepared to handle almost any situation when they understand it. The experience of pain and related therapies are no exception. However, patients with moderate-to-severe pain are not always able to participate in decision making until the pain is controlled at an acceptable level. Once you accomplish this, you can begin teaching.

Health literacy significantly affects a patient's pain experience and understanding of pain-management strategies. Low health literacy poses significant barriers to optimal pain management. In a study of patients with chronic pain, patients with low health literacy were found to have low overall pain medication knowledge and did not know where to find health care professionals to help them with their pain (Devraj et al., 2013). The patients in the study also lacked knowledge about nonpharmacological approaches to pain management and did not know which nonprescription pain medications could provide pain relief. Research conducted with patients with chronic back pain and other patient groups provides evidence for why educational materials and approaches must be adapted so they are suited for low–health literacy patients. In addition, combat any cultural norms that may stop patients from talking about pain at all. Stoicism not only potentially obscures dangerous signs about which you should know, but it also denies people the opportunity to use labels as a tool to cope with pain. Help patients who don't have the words to describe their pain find them (Bucher, 2014). Because pain affects physical and mental functioning, holistic health approaches are important interventions for maintaining wellness. Holistic health is an ongoing state of wellness that involves taking care of the whole person: body, mind, spirit, and emotions. To achieve optimal health and well-being, it is necessary to have balance of all of the interdependent elements of the whole person (Matthews-Kozanecka, 2014).

Patients actively participate in their own well-being whenever possible. Common holistic health approaches include wellness education, regular exercise, rest, attention to good hygiene practices and nutrition, and management of interpersonal relationships. When a person develops pain, you can offer nonpharmacological and pharmacological strategies. Several nonpharmacological interventions are nurse initiated.

Nonpharmacological Pain-Relief Interventions. A number of nonpharmacological interventions are available for lessening pain. However, more research is needed to truly know the best approach, intensity, duration, and content of these interventions, especially for the treatment of chronic pain (Park and Hughes, 2012). The researchers suggest that nonpharmacological interventions may be useful for patients who cannot tolerate pain medications, those who wish to reduce multiple medications, and those who are seeking alternative methods of relieving chronic pain.

Nonpharmacological interventions can be used alone or in combination with pharmacological measures. However, in the case of acute pain, they should never be used in place of pharmacological therapies. Nonpharmacological interventions include cognitive-behavioral and physical approaches. Cognitive-behavioral interventions change patients' perceptions of pain, alter pain behavior, and provide patients with a greater sense of control. Distraction, prayer, relaxation, guided imagery, music, and **biofeedback** are examples.

Physical approaches aim to provide pain relief, correct physical dysfunction, alter physiological responses, and reduce fears associated with pain-related immobility. Complementary and alternative medicine (CAM) therapies such as therapeutic touch and mindfulness meditation help to alleviate pain in some patients (see Chapter 33). An evidence-based practice protocol for pain management in older

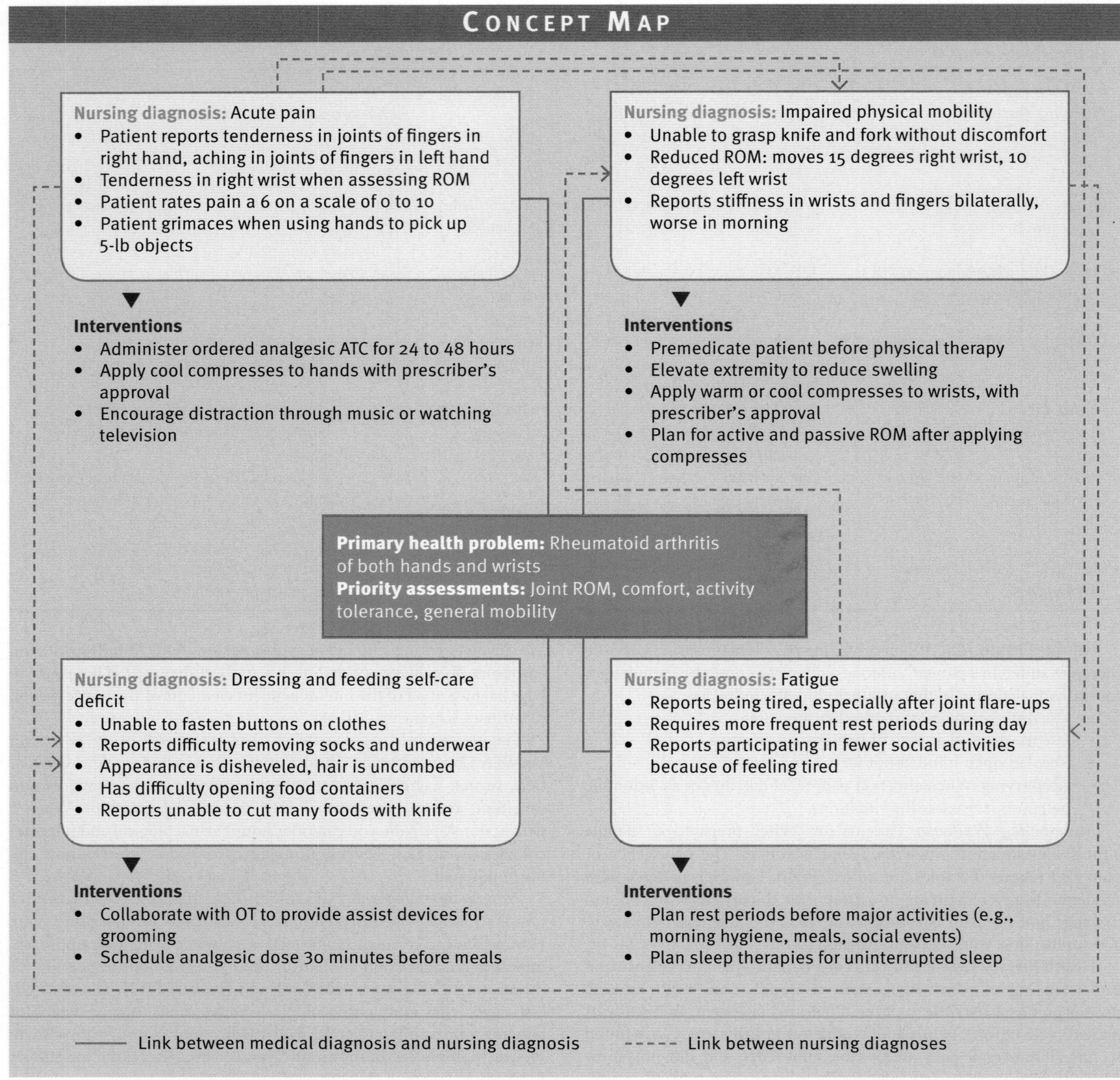

FIGURE 44-10 Concept map for Mrs. Mays. *ATC,* Around the clock; *OT,* occupational therapist; *ROM,* range of motion.

adults recommends these guidelines for nonpharmacological therapies (Horgas et al., 2012):

- Tailor nonpharmacological techniques to the individual.
- Cognitive behavioral strategies may not be appropriate for the cognitively impaired.
- Physical pain-relief strategies focus on promoting comfort and altering physiological responses to pain and are generally safe and effective.

Relaxation and Guided Imagery. Relaxation and guided imagery allow patients to alter affective-motivational and cognitive pain perception. Relaxation is mental and physical freedom from tension or stress that provides individuals a sense of self-control. You use relaxation techniques at any phase of health or illness. Physiological and behavioral changes associated with relaxation include the following: decreased pulse, blood pressure, and respirations; heightened awareness; decreased oxygen consumption; a sense of peace; and decreased muscle tension and metabolic rate (Topcu and Findik, 2012). Relaxation techniques include meditation, yoga, Zen, guided imagery, and progressive relaxation exercises (see Chapter 33). For effective relaxation, teach techniques only when a patient is not distracted by acute discomfort. Sometimes a combination of these techniques is needed to achieve optimal pain relief. With practice the patient performs relaxation exercises independently.

Distraction. The reticular activating system inhibits painful stimuli if a person receives sufficient or excessive sensory input. With sufficient sensory stimuli, a person ignores or becomes unaware of pain. People who are bored or in isolation have only their pain to think about and thus perceive it more acutely. Distraction directs a patient's attention to something other than pain and thus reduces awareness of it. A disadvantage of distraction is that, if it works, health care providers or family members may question the existence or severity of the pain. Distraction works best for short, intense pain lasting a few minutes such as during an invasive procedure or while waiting for an analgesic to work. Use activities enjoyed by the patient as distractions (e.g., singing, praying, listening to music, or playing games).

Music. Music therapy may be useful in treating acute or chronic pain, stress, anxiety, and depression (Allred et al., 2010; Korhan et al., 2014). It diverts a person's attention away from the pain and creates a relaxation response. Music creates positive changes in mood and emotional states and allows patients to actively participate in treatment. Music therapy uses all kinds of music. It is important to let patients select the type of music they prefer. Music produces an altered state of consciousness through sound, silence, space, and time. Therapeutic sessions usually last 20 to 30 minutes (Hughes, 2008). Patients may use earphones to enhance their concentration on the music. This allows them to adjust the volume without interrupting other patients or staff. Evidence shows that music contributes to the pain relief of hospitalized patients and may decrease the use of analgesics in some postoperative patients (Cole and LoBiondo-Wood, 2014).

Cutaneous Stimulation. Stimulation of the skin through a massage, warm bath, cold application, and **transcutaneous electrical nerve stimulation (TENS)** may be helpful in reducing pain perception. How **cutaneous stimulation** works is unclear. One suggestion is that it causes release of endorphins, thus blocking the transmission of painful stimuli. The gate-control theory suggests that cutaneous stimulation activates larger, faster-transmitting A-beta sensory nerve fibers. This closes the gate, thus decreasing pain transmission through small-diameter C fibers (Melzack and Wall, 1965).

Cutaneous stimulation gives patients and families some control over pain symptoms and treatment in the home. Using it properly helps to reduce muscle tension, resulting in less pain. When using cutaneous stimulation, eliminate sources of environmental noise, help the patient to assume a comfortable position, and explain the purpose of the therapy. Do not use it directly on sensitive skin areas (e.g., burns, bruises, skin rashes, inflammation, and underlying bone fractures).

Massage is effective for producing physical and mental relaxation, reducing pain, and enhancing the effectiveness of pain medication. Massaging the back, shoulders, hands, and/or feet for 3 to 5 minutes relaxes muscles and promotes sleep and comfort. Cutshall et al. (2010) reported a significant decrease in pain, anxiety, and tension in patients with cardiac problems who received a 20-minute massage. In older adults slow back massage and a 20-minute hand massage improved pain, anxiety, tension, and insomnia (Harris and Richards, 2010). Massages communicate caring and are easy for family members or other health care personnel to learn (Box 44-11).

Cold and heat applications (see Chapter 48) relieve pain and promote healing. The selection of heat-versus-cold interventions varies with patients' conditions (Guild, 2012). For example, moist heat helps to relieve the pain from a tension headache, and cold applications reduce the acute pain from inflamed joints. When using any form of heat or cold application, instruct the patient to avoid injury to the skin by checking the temperature and not applying cold or heat directly to the skin. Especially at risk for injury are patients with diabetic neuropathies, spinal cord or other neurological disorders, older adults, and patients who are confused.

Cold therapies are particularly effective for acute pain relief. Ice massage involves the use of a large ice cube or a small paper cup filled with water and frozen (water rises out of the cup as it freezes to create a smooth surface of ice for massage). A nurse or the patient applies the ice with firm pressure to the skin, which is covered with a lightweight cloth. Then use a slow, steady, circular massage over the area. Apply cold within a 6-inch circular area near the pain site or on the opposite side of the body corresponding to the pain site. Limit application to 5 minutes or when the patient feels numbness (Spine Health, 2006). Each patient responds differently to the site of application. Application near the actual site of pain tends to work best. A patient feels cold, burning, and aching sensations and numbness. You can apply ice 2 to 5 times a day (Spine Health, 2006). Cold is effective for tooth or mouth pain when you place the ice on the web of the hand between the thumb and index finger. This point on the hand is an **acupressure** point that influences nerve pathways to the face and head. Cold applications are also effective before invasive needle punctures.

Heat application is more effective for some patients, especially those with chronic pain. Chapter 48 discusses in detail the type of heat devices (e.g., warm compresses and commercial heat packs) that are safe to use. Never place a heat application in a microwave unless it is directed by the manufacturer. Then follow directions carefully. Teach patients to check the temperature of the compress carefully and not to lie on the heating element because burning can occur.

Another form of cutaneous stimulation is TENS, involving stimulation of the skin with a mild electrical current passed through external electrodes. A TENS unit consists of a battery-powered transmitter, lead wires, and electrodes. TENS works both peripherally and centrally: centrally it acts by activating sites in the spinal cord and brainstem that use opioid and serotonin receptors; peripherally neuroreceptors at the site of the TENs application produce analgesia (DeSantana et al., 2008). It can be applied at various frequencies (<10 Hz to >50 Hz) and intensity (sensory versus motor) (DeSantana et al., 2008). Stimulation intensity has been shown to be the critical factor in TENS efficacy. A TENS unit requires a health care provider's order that identifies the site for the TENS electrode placement. Remove any hair or skin preparations before attaching the electrodes. Then place the electrodes directly over or near the pain site. Turn the transmitter on to the ordered level when the patient feels pain. The TENS creates a buzzing or tingling sensation. After assessing the patient's tolerance, he or she can then turn on the transmitter and adjust the intensity and quality of skin stimulation until pain relief occurs. TENS is effective for acute, emergent, and postsurgical and procedural pain control (DeSantana et al., 2008).

Herbals. Many patients use herbals and dietary supplements such as echinacea, ginseng, ginkgo biloba, and garlic despite conflicting research evidence supporting their use in pain relief. Significant attention has been paid to the potential benefits of glucosamine and chondroitin in the treatment of osteoarthritis, but the evidence is inconclusive (Fouladbakhsh, 2012). Herbal supplements may interact with prescribed analgesics; thus it is important to ask patients to report to their health care provider all of the substances they take to relieve pain (see Chapter 33).

Reducing Pain Perception and Reception. One simple way to promote comfort is to remove or prevent painful stimuli (Box 44-12). This is especially important for patients who are immobilized or have difficulty expressing themselves. For example, your patient becomes constipated and has abdominal distention and cramping. You should

BOX 44-11 PROCEDURAL GUIDELINES

Massage

Delegation Considerations

The skill of administering a massage may be delegated to nursing assistive personnel (NAP). However, the nurse must first assess for any possible contraindication and evaluate the patient's response to massage. Direct the NAP to:

- Use massage techniques that are effective for patient.
- Massage specific body parts.
- Avoid massaging reddened skin areas.
- Notify the nurse of early signs of impaired skin integrity or changes in skin appearance.
- Report worsening in patient's pain.

Equipment

Bath towel, lotion, blanket

Steps

1. On the basis of patient assessment, decide on performing massage on one or more body parts.
2. Assess skin areas for reddened areas or impaired skin integrity.
3. Collect appropriate equipment.
4. Explain procedure to the patient.
5. Identify patient using two identifiers (e.g., name and birthday or name and medical record) according to agency policy.
6. Perform hand hygiene.
7. Help patient assume a comfortable lying or sitting position.
8. Dim room lights and/or turn on soft music according to patient preference.
9. Use warm body lotion as lubricant.

   CLINICAL DECISION: Do not give back or neck massages to patients who have had neck or spinal trauma and/or surgery without an order from their health care provider.

10. Massage each body part at least 10 minutes.
    a. *Back:* Begin at the sacral area and massage in a circular motion (see illustration) while moving upward from buttocks to shoulders. Use a firm, smooth stroke over scapula. Continue in one smooth stroke to upper arms and laterally along sides of back down to iliac crests. Use long, gliding strokes along muscles of spine. Knead any muscles that feel tense or tight. Knead skin by gently grasping tissue between thumb and fingers. Knead upward along one side of spine from buttocks to shoulders around nape of neck. Knead or stroke downward toward sacrum. Repeat along other side of back.

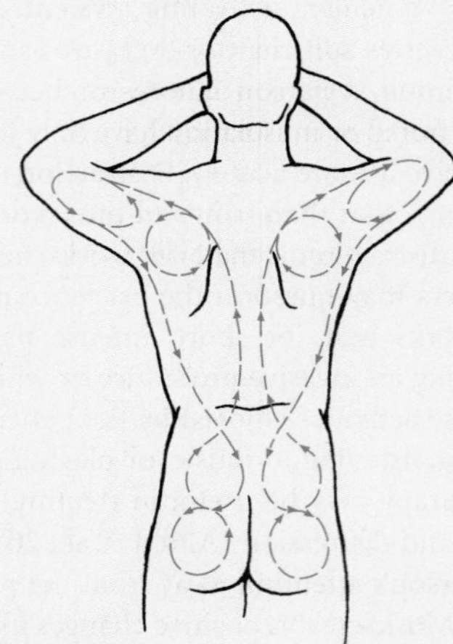

STEP 10a Back massage pattern.

    b. *Neck:* Support neck at hairline with one hand and massage up with a gliding stroke. Knead muscles on one side. Switch hands to support neck and knead other side. Stretch neck slightly, with one hand at top and the other at bottom.
    c. *Arms:* Use gliding stroke to massage from patient's wrist or forearm. With thumb and forefinger of both hands, knead muscles from forearm to shoulder. Continue kneading biceps, deltoid, and triceps muscles. Finish with gliding strokes from wrists to shoulder.
    d. *Hands:* Using both hands, slowly open patient's palm; glide fingers over palmar surface. While supporting patient's hand, use both thumbs to apply friction to palm and move them in a circular motion to stretch palm outward. Massage each finger with a corkscrew-like motion from base of finger to tip. With thumb and forefinger gently knead each muscle in patient's fingers. Glide hands smoothly from fingertips to wrists. Repeat for other hand.
    e. *Feet:* Gently massage top and bottom of each foot. Using gliding motion, massage from heel to toe. Gently massage dorsal surface of foot and each toe. Repeat for other foot.

   CLINICAL DECISION: Do not massage patient's legs or calf muscles because of the risk of dislodging a vascular clot.

11. At end of massage have patient relax, taking slow, deep breaths.
12. Ask patient to rate level of pain.
13. Note any areas of muscle pain or tension.
14. Note any areas of redness or impairment.
15. Report any areas of skin breakdown to the health care team.

BOX 44-12 Controlling Painful Stimuli in Patient's Environment

- Tighten and smooth wrinkled bed linen.
- Reposition patient anatomically to relieve any pressure points.
- Reposition patient to avoid lying on tubing (e.g., intravenous tubing, chest tubes).
- Loosen constricting bandages (unless specifically applied as a pressure dressing).
- Change wet dressings and linens.
- Position patient in anatomical alignment according to individual preference or requirements.
- Check temperature of hot or cold applications, including bath water.
- Lift patient in bed—do not pull. Use safe patient–handling lift devices.
- Position patient correctly on a bedpan.
- Avoid exposing skin or mucous membranes to irritants (e.g., urine, stool, wound drainage).
- Keep patients clean, dry, and turned if needed. Use urinary incontinence pads if indicated.
- Prevent urinary retention by keeping Foley catheters patent and free flowing if in use, while also monitoring urinary output.
- Prevent constipation with fluids, diet, exercise, and stimulant laxatives if needed.

intervene to ensure that the normal elimination process continues: increasing fluids, ambulating the patient, and/or requesting stool softeners or laxatives. Another example involves reducing pain perception during procedures using techniques such as proper patient positioning and coaching to perform progressive muscle relaxation. Always consider the patient's condition, aspects of the procedure that are uncomfortable, and techniques to avoid causing pain. In a patient with severe arthritic knee pain who has severe discomfort during any extreme flexion of the knee, take precautions before walking the patient to the bathroom. Use an elevated toilet seat to allow him or her to sit and rise with minimal discomfort.

Acute Care. Nurses often care for patients who have acute pain resulting from invasive procedures (e.g., surgery) or trauma. Many professional organizations such as the APS, American Society of Anesthesiologists (ASA), ASPMN, and the American Society of PeriAnesthesia Nurses (ASPAN), have published guidelines and position papers related to acute pain management. The key to success is ongoing pain assessment and evaluation of the efficacy of interventions. Does the patient feel relief? Are there any unacceptable side effects from the medications? It is the responsibility of the health care team to collaborate to find the combination of therapy that works best for a patient.

Pharmacological Pain Therapies. Many pharmacological agents are available to provide pain relief. Your judgment in the use and management of analgesics with or without other pain therapies ensures the best pain relief possible. Unfortunately the ideal analgesic (i.e., one that provides highly effective pain relief without significant risks or side effects) has yet to be developed.

Analgesics. Analgesics are the most common and effective method of pain relief. However, health care providers and nurses still tend to undertreat patients because of insufficient knowledge about pain management, incorrect drug information, concerns about addiction, exaggerated concerns about opioid analgesic safety, and administration of less medication than was ordered (D'Arcy, 2008; Gordon et al., 2008). You need to understand the medications available for pain relief, their indications for use, and their pharmacological effects. Reassure patients that treatment of pain is necessary to aid recovery and that addiction is highly unlikely when analgesics are taken correctly.

There are three types of analgesics: (1) nonopioids, including acetaminophen and nonsteroidal antiinflammatory drugs (NSAIDs); (2) opioids (traditionally called *narcotics*); and (3) adjuvants or co-analgesics, a variety of medications that enhance analgesics or have analgesic properties that were originally unknown (Pasero and McCaffery, 2011).

Acetaminophen (Tylenol), considered one of the most tolerated and safest analgesics available, is available in a variety of over-the-counter (OTC) oral medications (e.g., cold and flu remedies) or rectal forms and in an intravenous (IV) preparation (Ofirmev). The analgesic effect of acetaminophen is not entirely clear, but it is believed to have a direct effect on the central nervous system. It has no antiinflammatory effects. IV acetaminophen (Ofirmev) is an effective analgesic agent because it crosses the blood-brain barrier rapidly, thus providing nonopioid analgesia for postoperative patients, especially those who cannot take oral medications. The maximum 24-hour dose is 4 g (the same limitation as aspirin). Acetaminophen is often combined with opioids (e.g., oxycodone [Percocet], hydrocodone [Lortab], tramadol [Ultracet]) because it reduces the dose of opioid needed to achieve successful pain control. When acetaminophen is combined with an opioid in these products, it is important to recognize the abbreviations that describe the contents of the product. The order and package label often state "name of opioid/acetaminophen (abbreviated as APAP) 5/325" which means that the opioid is 5 mg and the acetaminophen (APAP) is 325 mg per tablet. For example, oxycodone/APAP 5/325 indicates that each tablet contains 5 mg of oxycodone and 325 mg of acetaminophen. Similar abbreviations are used for combination products of hydrocodone and tramadol.

The major adverse effect of acetaminophen is hepatotoxicity; and, because the drug is so widely used, the Food and Drug Administration (USFDA, 2014) issued an order to limit the amount of acetaminophen in prescription combination products to 325 mg per tablet, capsule, or other dosage unit. Instructions for acetaminophen-containing products such as 1 to 2 tablets every 4 to 6 hours, were not required to change in the order. Higher dosing units continue to be available in OTC products, but the products are required to include dosage labeling information about safety risks, including liver injury and the risks of serious skin rashes. Although some manufacturers have voluntarily reduced the maximum daily acetaminophen dose labeling on their OTC products, the FDA has not reduced the maximum daily dose limit of 4 g for adults. Reduced doses are necessary for inadequate liver function and are recommended to prevent accidental overdose in the outpatient setting. It is important to read and understand these warning labels. Dangerous hepatotoxic overdoses of acetaminophen are treated with acetylcysteine (Mucomyst) (Pasero and McCaffery, 2011).

Nonselective NSAIDs such as aspirin, ibuprofen, and naproxen relieve mild-to-moderate acute intermittent pain such as that from headache or muscle strain. Treatment of mild-to-moderate postoperative pain begins with an NSAID unless contraindicated (Pasero and McCaffery, 2011). NSAIDs likely act by inhibiting the synthesis of prostaglandins (Day and Graham, 2013) and thus inhibit cellular responses to inflammation. Most NSAIDs act on peripheral nerve receptors to reduce transmission of pain stimuli and inflammation. Unlike opioids, NSAIDs do not depress the central nervous system, nor do they interfere with bowel or bladder function (Pasero and McCaffery, 2011). However, NSAID use in the older patient is not recommended because it is associated with more frequent adverse effects (gastrointestinal bleeding and renal insufficiency) (AGS, 2009). Mild-to-moderate musculoskeletal pain in older adults is managed effectively with acetaminophen (AGS, 2009; Pasero and McCaffery, 2011). Some patients with asthma or an allergy to aspirin are also allergic to other NSAIDs (Morales et al., 2015). As with all OTC medications, patients should be advised to discuss their use of NSAIDs and their pain with their health care provider.

Opioid or opioid-like analgesics are prescribed for moderate-to-severe pain. These analgesics act on higher centers of the brain and spinal cord by binding with opiate receptors to modify perceptions of pain. Examples of opioids include morphine, codeine, hydromorphone (Dilaudid), fentanyl, oxycodone, and hydrocodone (Vicodin, Lortab). Some are available in IV and oral preparations (morphine and hydromorphone), whereas others are only available in oral formulations (oxycodone and hydrocodone). Most are available in a short-acting form, which provides relief for about 4 hours; some are also available in longer-acting preparations (oral morphine, oxycodone, hydromorphone, and a transdermal fentanyl patch).

Opioids can cause numerous common side effects (Box 44-13). Except for constipation and central nervous system changes, patients usually become tolerant to many of them. Other side effects associated with long-term use include depression, impaired sleep patterns, endocrine effects (decreased testosterone levels, decreased libido), and immune system suppression. To reduce side effects, patients should take the lowest dose of an opioid needed to manage pain. For example, if the prescriber initially ordered oxycodone 10 mg PO every 4 hours and the patient has nausea and is very drowsy, the nurse might suggest

BOX 44-13 Common Opioid Side Effects

Central Nervous System (CNS) Toxicity
- Drowsiness
- Cognitive impairment
- Confusion
- Hallucinations
- Myoclonic jerks
- Euphoria
- Sedation
- Sleep disturbances
- Dizziness

Ocular
- Pupil constriction

Respiratory
- Bradypnea
- Hypoventilation

Cardiac
- Hypotension
- Bradycardia
- Peripheral edema

Gastrointestinal
- Constipation
- Nausea
- Vomiting
- Delayed gastric emptying

Genitourinary
- Urinary retention

Endocrine
- Hormonal and sexual dysfunction

Skin
- Pruritus

Immunological
- Immune system impairment possible with chronic use

Tolerance
- Over time, increased doses needed to obtain analgesic effect

Withdrawal Syndrome
- Rapid or sudden cessation or marked dose reduction may cause rhinitis, chills, pupil dilatation, diarrhea, "gooseflesh"

Adapted from American Chronic Pain Association (ACPA): *ACPA resource guide to chronic pain medication & treatment,* 2014 edition, 2014, http://www.theacpa.org/uploads/ACPA_Resource_Guide_2014_FINAL.pdf. Accessed April 27, 2015.

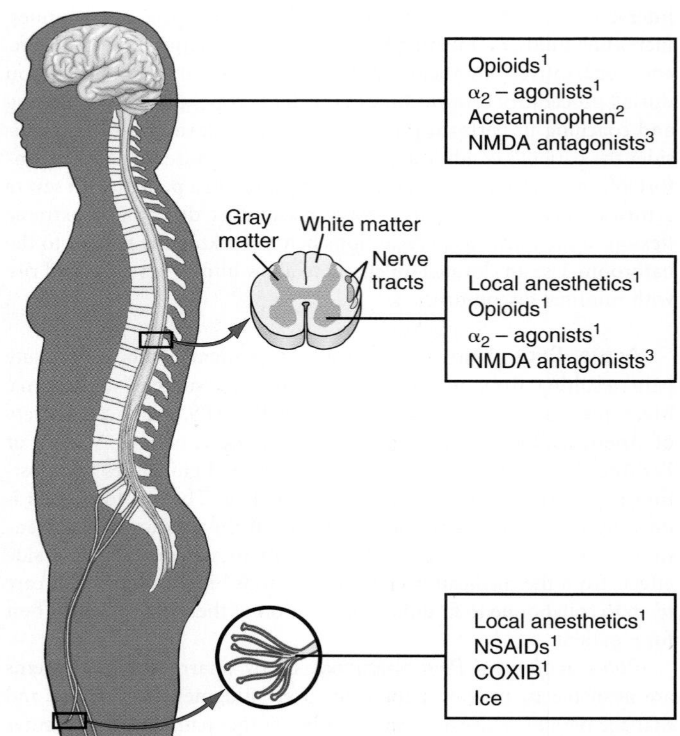

FIGURE 44-11 Multimodal analgesia sites of action. (© Elsevier collections.) *COXIB,* Cox-2 inhibitor; *NMDA, N*-methyl-d-aspartate; *NSAID,* nonsteroidal antiinflammatory drug. 1. Gottschalk A, Smith DS. New concepts in acute pain therapy: preemptive analgesia. *Am Fam Physician* 2001; 63(10):1979-1984. (http://www.aafp.org/afp/2001/0515/p1979.html). 2. Smith HS. Potential analgesic mechanisms of acetaminophen. *Pain Physician* 2009; 12:269-280. (http://www.painphysicianjournal.com/current/pdf?article=MTE4NA%3D%3D&journal=47). 3. Sinatra RS, Jahr JS, eds. The Essence of Analgesia and Analgesics. New York, NY: Cambridge University Press; 2011.

that the prescriber reduce the dose to 5 mg. After administration, reassess a patient for the effect of the lowered dose on pain level and side effects. If reducing a dose does not relieve a side effect, confer with the prescriber about a change in the type of opioid. If side effects persist, it may be necessary to prevent or treat them by administering other medications (antihistamines, antiemetics, stimulants). Constipation should always be anticipated and prevented through diet, hydration, and the use of stool softeners and stimulants as needed.

A rare adverse effect of opioids in opioid-naïve patients (patients who have used opioid around the clock (ATC) *less* than approximately 1 week) is respiratory depression. Respiratory depression is only clinically significant if there is a decrease in the rate and depth of respirations from a patient's baseline assessment (Pasero and McCaffery, 2011). All patients who receive opioids are at risk, but patients who are opioid naïve (new or restarting opioids) are at greater risk than those who have been taking them daily on a regular basis (TJC, 2012). It is important for nurses to obtain a complete opioid medication history, including dose, frequency, and duration of use to determine whether patients are opioid naïve or tolerant. Patients who breathe deeply rarely have clinical respiratory depression. Sedation always occurs before respiratory depression. Closely monitor for sedation in opioid-naïve patients (Pasero and McCaffery, 2011). If an adult patient experiences respiratory depression, administer naloxone (Narcan) (0.4 mg diluted with 9 mL saline) IV push (IVP) at a rate of 0.5 mL every 2 minutes until the respiratory rate is greater than 8 breaths/min with good depth (Pasero and McCaffery, 2011). Administering naloxone faster than recommended may cause severe pain and serious complications such as hypotension and hypertension, cardiac arrhythmias, dyspnea, and pulmonary edema (Pasero and McCaffery, 2011). Evaluate patients who receive naloxone every 15 minutes for 2 hours following drug administration because its duration may be less than that of the opioid and respiratory depression sometimes returns.

One way to maximize pain relief while potentially decreasing opioid use is to administer analgesics ATC rather than a prn basis. This approach ensures a more constant therapeutic blood level of an analgesic. The APS (2009) supports ATC administration if pain is anticipated for the majority of the day. There are also a variety of extended- or controlled-release oral opioid formulations (dosing intervals of 8, 10, 12 or 24 hours) and transdermal patches (72 hours). These formulations maintain constant serum opioid concentration, minimizing toxic and subtherapeutic concentrations (Burchum and Rosenthal, 2016). An ATC medication lessens the severity of end-of-dose pain, allowing a patient to sleep through the night and reduce "clock watching" for the next dose.

Careful assessment and critical thinking are required to safely administer analgesics (Box 44-14). The current pharmacological approach to acute and chronic pain management is to provide **multimodal analgesia**. Multimodal analgesia combines drugs with at least two different mechanisms of action so pain control can be optimized. Medications are combined to target different sites in the peripheral or central pain pathways (Figure 44-11). A main benefit of multimodal analgesia is that the use of different agents allows for lower-than-usual

BOX 44-14 Nursing Principles for Administering Analgesics

Know Patient's Previous Response to Analgesics

- Determine whether patient has allergies.
- Know whether patient is at risk for using NSAIDs (e.g., history of GI bleeding or renal insufficiency) or opioids (e.g., history of obstructive or central sleep apnea).
- Identify previous doses and routes of analgesic administration to avoid undertreatment.
- Determine whether patient obtained relief.
- Ask whether a nonopioid was as effective as an opioid.

Select Proper Medications When More Than One Is Ordered

- Use nonopioid analgesics or opioid combination drugs for mild-to-moderate pain.
- Give opioids with nonopioids to provide a multimodal analgesia approach.
- Avoid using multiple opioids with the same duration and mechanism of action.
- Intravenous medications act more quickly and usually relieve severe, acute pain within 1 hour; whereas oral medications take as long as 2 hours to relieve pain.
- Avoid intramuscular analgesics, especially in older adults.
- Use an opioid with a nonopioid analgesic for severe pain because such combinations treat pain peripherally and centrally.
- For chronic pain give sustained-release oral formulations ATC.

Know Accurate Dosage

- Recall that 4 g is considered the maximum 24-hour dosage for acetaminophen and acetylsalicylic acid (ASA); 3200 mg for ibuprofen.
- Adjust doses as appropriate for children and older patients.
- Large doses of opioids are acceptable in opioid-tolerant patients but not in opioid-naive patients.
- When titrating opioid, it is important to titrate to effect or to uncontrollable side effects.

Assess Right Time and Interval for Administration

- Administer analgesics as soon as pain occurs and before it increases in severity.
- An ATC administration schedule is usually best.
- Give analgesics before pain-producing procedures or activities.
- Know the average duration of action for a drug and the time of administration so the peak effect occurs when the pain is most intense.
- Use extended-release opioid formulations to treat chronic pain.
- Avoid stopping opioids abruptly in patients who are opioid tolerant.

Modified from Pasero, C. McCaffery M: *Pain assessment and pharmacological management,* St Louis, 2011, Mosby.
ATC, Around the clock; *GI,* gastrointestinal; *NSAIDs,* nonsteroidal antiinflammatory drugs.

doses of each medication, therefore lowering the risk of side effects while providing pain relief that is as good as or even better than could be obtained from each of the medications alone.

A person's response to an analgesic is highly individualized. If the pain is caused by inflammation, an NSAID is sometimes as effective as, or more effective than, an opioid. An orally administered analgesic usually has a longer onset and duration of action than an injectable form. In addition, for pain that persists for most of the day, controlled- or extended-release opioid formulations (morphine [MS Contin, Kadian, Avinza], oxycodone [OxyContin], and methadone) are available for administration every 8 to 12 hours ATC; they are not ordered prn.

BOX 44-15 Patient Characteristics Associated with Higher Risk for Opioid-Related Adverse Drug Events

- Sleep apnea or sleep disordered breathing
- Morbid obesity with high risk of sleep apnea
- Snoring
- Older age
- Significant co-morbidities (cardiac, pulmonary, or major organ failure)
- No recent opioid use
- Increased opioid dose requirement
- Receiving other sedating medications (e.g., antihistamines, antipsychotics)
- Recent surgery, especially thoracic or upper abdominal
- Prolonged general anesthesia
- Smoker

Modified from The Joint Commission: 2013, *Sentinel Event Alert: safe use of opioids in hospitals,* Issue 49; August 8, 2012. http://www.jointcommission.org/assets/1/18/SEA_49_opioids_8_2_12_final.pdf. Accessed August 12, 2014.

When you convert a patient from an IV to an oral form of the same opioid, understand that the dose of the oral opioid is usually much higher than the IV dose because of the first-pass effect (Pasero and McCaffery, 2011). When a patient takes oral opioids, the opioid first goes to the liver, where most (but not all) of the medication is inactivated. Thus the body needs larger doses of oral opioids to achieve the same level of pain relief as with IV opioids. Know the comparative potencies of analgesics in oral and injectable form. In addition, know the route of administration most effective for a patient so controlled, sustained pain relief is achieved. The intramuscular (IM) route for analgesic administration should not be used because the IM injection is painful and drug absorption is inconsistent and erratic (Pasero and McCaffery, 2011). When comparing opioids, equianalgesic charts (i.e., charts converting one opioid to another or parenteral forms of opioids [e.g., morphine to hydromorphone] to oral forms [or vice versa]) should be available on nursing units or by contacting pharmacy staff. There are "smartphone apps" for opioid dosing conversions, but check with the pharmacy staff to ensure accuracy before using these electronic conversion tools.

Opioids are usually necessary and effective for acute pain and cancer pain of moderate or severe intensity. The goal of opioid therapy is a reduction in pain intensity to a level of acceptable comfort. In both types of pain, progress toward pain relief is measured by changes in pain-intensity scores. Opioid doses often need to be adjusted up or down according to individual patient circumstances and conditions. A prescriber must carefully individualize drug selection, dosing, and schedule. Many patients are at higher risk for opioid-related adverse drug events (Box 44-15).

According to the American Geriatrics Society (AGS, 2009), opioids are probably not used enough with older people. The AGS suggests a "start-low" (dose) and "go-slow" (upward dose titration) philosophy. Careful use of multiple drugs together can be seen as potentially helpful. Combining smaller doses of more than one medication may minimize the dose-limiting adverse effects of using a particular single drug (ACPA, 2014). The elderly require special consideration because age-related changes and increased frailty lead to less predictable drug responses, including increased drug sensitivity and severity of side effects (van Ojik et al., 2012). Opioids may place the elderly at increased risk for falls and other injuries. Many elderly patients have multiple co-morbidities and require various medications, placing them at risk for polypharmacy and drug-drug interactions. Dizziness, confusion, and changes in vision are opioid-related side effects that pose increased safety risks for the elderly; special care must be taken to ensure that the environment is safe and patients are educated about the need for caution. Despite these concerns, elderly patients should not be deprived of opioid therapy when needed to treat pain. Carefully selected opioids and doses, along with patient education and monitoring, are important in providing safe and effective pain management. Most opioids present similar risks and benefits; but methadone, because of its long half-life, drug-drug interactions, and risk for cardiac abnormalities, is generally avoided in the elderly (van Ojik et al., 2012).

TJC requires health care agencies, where permissible, to have range-order policies in place to guide nurses in selecting the most appropriate dose of a medication. "Range orders are medication orders in which the dose varies over a prescribed range depending on the situation or a patient's status" (Drew et al., 2013). Range orders enable needed and safe adjustments in doses on the basis of individual patient responses to treatment (Drew et al., 2013). However, improperly written orders can lead to problems in pain management and patient safety. Review the following order, "Administer 5 to 10 mg morphine sulfate IVP q3h prn for acute pain." Such an order is dangerous when there are no clinical guidelines to use for selecting the exact dose. Follow these guidelines from the ASPMN (Drew et al., 2013):

- Avoid administration of partial doses at more frequent intervals so as to not underdose a patient with small, frequent, ineffective doses from within a range (e.g., giving oxycodone 10 mg q2h when the order reads oxycodone 10 to 20 mg q3h prn).
- Avoid making a patient wait a full time interval after giving a partial dose within the allowed range.
- Wait until peak effect of the first dose has been reached before giving a subsequent dose.

A proper range order offers specifics for when a range of doses can be given and gives nurses the flexibility needed to treat patients' pain in a timely way while allowing for differences in patient response to pain and analgesia. Safe and effective range orders consider the patient's age, pain intensity, and co-morbidities and prescribe a maximum dose that is at least 2 times but not more than 4 times the minimum dose in the range (Drew et al., 2013; Pasero and McCaffery, 2011).

Co-analgesics or adjuvants are drugs originally developed to treat conditions other than pain but also have analgesic properties. For example, tricyclic antidepressants (e.g., nortriptyline [Pamelor]), anticonvulsants (e.g., gabapentin [Neurontin]), and infusional lidocaine successfully treat chronic pain, especially neuropathic pain. Corticosteroids relieve the pain from inflammation and bone metastasis. Other examples of co-analgesics are bisphosphonates and calcitonin for bone pain (Pasero and McCaffery, 2011). Adjuvants have analgesic properties, enhance pain control, or relieve other symptoms associated with neuropathic pain. You give adjuvants alone or with analgesics. Sedatives, antianxiety agents, and muscle relaxants have *no* analgesic effect, although they may be effective for their specific indications.

Patient-Controlled Analgesia. When patients depend on nurses for prn analgesia, an erratic cycle of alternating pain and analgesia often occurs. A patient feels pain and asks for medication; but the patient first must be assessed, and then the medication must be obtained and prepared. Under this circumstance analgesia finally occurs in about an hour, but pain relief may last only 30 minutes. Gradually the patient again feels discomfort, and the cycle begins again. The patient is constantly going in and out of analgesic therapeutic range.

A drug delivery system called **patient-controlled analgesia (PCA)** is a method for pain management that many patients prefer (see Skill 44-1 on pp. 1046-1049). It is a drug delivery system that allows patients to self-administer opioids (usually morphine, hydromorphone, or fentanyl) with minimal risk of overdose. The goal is to maintain a constant plasma level of analgesic to avoid the problems of prn dosing. Systemic PCA traditionally involves IV or subcutaneous drug administration; however, a controlled analgesia device for oral medications is available. This device allows patients access to their own oral prn mediations, including opioids and other analgesics, antiemetics, and anxiolytics, at the bedside.

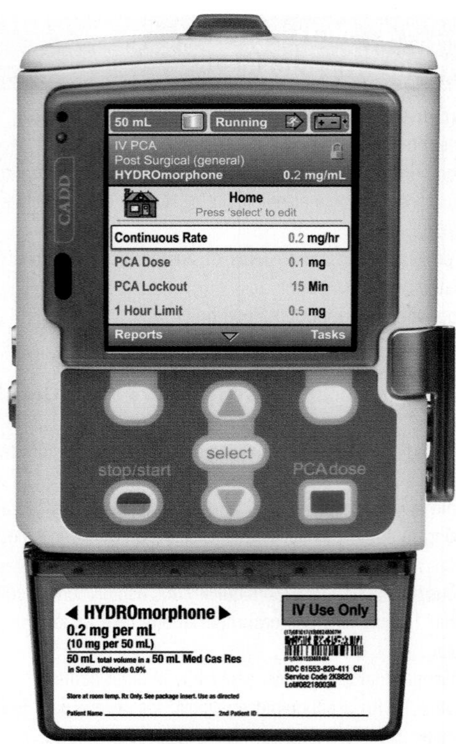

FIGURE 44-12 Patient-controlled analgesia pump with cassette. (Courtesy Smiths Medical ASD, Inc., St Paul, MN.)

PCA infusion pumps are portable and computerized and contain a chamber for a syringe or bag that delivers a small, preset dose of opioid (Figure 44-12). To receive a demand dose, a patient pushes a button attached to the PCA device. The PCA infusion pumps are designed to deliver a specific dose, which is programmed to be available at specific time intervals (usually in the range of 8 to 15 minutes) when the patient activates the delivery button. A limit on the number of doses per hour or a 4-hour interval may also be set. Most pumps have locked safety systems that prevent tampering by patients or family members and are generally safe to be managed in the home. For opioid-tolerant patients such as those with cancer pain, a low-dose continuous infusion (basal rate) is sometimes programmed to deliver a steady dose of continuous medication (Pasero and McCaffery, 2011).

There are many benefits to PCA use. The patient gains control over pain, and pain relief does not depend on nurse availability. Patients also have access to medication when they need it. This decreases anxiety and leads to decreased medication use. Small doses of medications are delivered at short intervals, stabilizing serum drug concentrations for sustained pain relief.

Patient preparation and teaching are critical to the safe and effective use of PCA devices (Box 44-16). A patient needs to understand PCA and be physically able to locate and press the button to deliver a dose. Family members and visitors must be instructed not to "push the button" for the patient (a dangerous action known as "PCA by Proxy"),

BOX 44-16 PATIENT TEACHING

Patient-Controlled Analgesia

Objective

- Patient will achieve pain control with proper use of the patient-controlled analgesia (PCA) device.

Teaching Strategies

- Teach how to use the PCA before procedures so patient understands how to use it after awakening from anesthesia or sedation. Reinforce as needed with Teach Back.
- Instruct patient in the purpose of PCA, emphasizing that patient controls medication delivery.
- Explain that the pump reduces risk of overdose.
- Tell family members or friends *not* to operate the PCA device for patient.

Evaluation

- Ask patient to tell you the purpose of the PCA device and when the button should be activated.
- Observe patient administering a dose.
- Evaluate the severity of patient's pain while using the PCA device.

as this bypasses the safety feature of PCA, which requires an awake patient to activate the device. In particular situations, when patients are unable to activate the PCA device, a carefully selected family member or nurse may be authorized to activate the device based on specific criteria. The authorized agent–controlled analgesia (AACA) guidelines should be used to guide this practice when appropriate (Cooney et al., 2013).

An established and properly functioning IV catheter is needed for IV PCA. Check the IV line and PCA device per institutional policy to ensure proper functioning (see Chapter 42). Programming of settings usually requires independent verification by two nurses to ensure accuracy. Even though patients control administration of analgesics, a nurse's diligence is needed to prevent errors related to programmable PCA devices. In opioid-naive patients, do not increase demand or basal dose *and* shorten the interval time simultaneously because this increases the risk for oversedation and respiratory depression. Document drug dosages and track medication wastes according to agency policy (Pasero and McCaffery, 2011). PCA basal doses are *not* recommended for opioid-naive patients following surgery because of the possibility for respiratory depression.

Topical Analgesics. Topical analgesics include prescription and OTC creams, ointments, and patches that are applied to a painful area. Commonly used topical agents include NSAID products (ketoprofen patch) and capsaicin (Pasero and McCaffery, 2011). Other topical analgesics contain local anesthetics. Products such as ELA-Max/LMX and eutectic mixture of local anesthetics (EMLA) are available for children. Apply EMLA via a disk or thick cream to the skin 30 to 60 minutes before minor procedures (e.g., IV start, intramuscular injection) or anesthetic infiltration of soft tissue. Do not place EMLA around the eyes, the tympanic membrane, or over large skin surfaces. The Lidoderm patch is a topical analgesic effective for cutaneous neuropathic pain such as postherpetic neuralgia in adults. Place three patches, cut to size, on and around the pain site using a 12-hour on, 12-hour off schedule (Pasero and McCaffery, 2011).

Local Anesthesia. Local anesthesia is the local infiltration of an anesthetic medication to induce loss of sensation to a body part. Health care providers often use local anesthesia during brief surgical procedures such as removing a skin lesion or suturing a wound by applying local anesthetics topically on skin and mucous membranes or injecting them subcutaneously or intradermally to anesthetize a body part. Regional anesthesia is the injection or infusion of local anesthetics to block a group of sensory nerve fibers. The anesthetics produce temporary loss of sensation by inhibiting nerve conduction. Local anesthetics also block motor and autonomic functions, depending on the amount used and the location and depth of administration. Smaller sensory nerve fibers are more sensitive to local anesthetics than are large motor fibers. As a result, the patient loses sensation before losing motor function, and conversely motor activity returns before sensation.

Perineural Local Anesthetic Infusion. A type of regional anesthesia is the use of perineural injections and infusions of local anesthetic agents to relieve pain. This technique is used for a variety of inpatient and outpatient adult and pediatric surgical procedures. A surgeon places the tip of an unsutured catheter near a nerve or groups of nerves, and the catheter exits from the surgical wound. Infusions of local anesthetics (bupivacaine or ropivacaine) may be run on a pump similar to those used for IV infusions, on ambulatory pumps, or on disposable systems (e.g., On-Q). The pump may be set on demand or continuous mode, and the catheter is usually left in place for 48 hours. Some patients have pump systems that are left in place even after discharge. Patients learn how to discontinue the pump at home and bring the catheter to the next health care provider visit. Some patients still need oral analgesics, but perineural infusions often reduce the total dosage (Pasero and McCaffery, 2011).

Local anesthetics cause side effects, depending on their absorption into the circulation. Pruritus or burning of the skin or a localized rash is common after topical applications. Application to vascular mucous membranes increases the chance of systemic effects such as a change in heart rate. The use of local anesthetics in peripheral nerve and epidural infusions (see following paragraph) may block both motor nerves and sensory nerves. This effect resolves within hours of the reduction or discontinuation of an infusion.

Epidural Analgesia. Another pain therapy that often involves the administration of anesthetic agents is epidural analgesia, a form of regional anesthesia. Preservative-free opioids are often administered as single agents or in combination with local anesthetics into a patient's epidural space. Epidural analgesia effectively treats acute postoperative pain, rib fracture pain, labor and delivery pain, and chronic cancer pain. Research has shown that adults having surgery under general anesthesia experience fewer postoperative cardiovascular, respiratory, and gastrointestinal complications when receiving epidural analgesia compared with patients receiving systemic analgesia (IV analgesics) (Pöpping et al., 2014). Epidural analgesia controls or reduces severe pain and reduces a patient's overall opioid requirement, thus minimizing adverse effects. It is short or long term, depending on a patient's condition and life expectancy.

The health care provider administers epidural analgesia into the spinal epidural space (Figure 44-13) by inserting a blunt-tip needle into the level of the vertebral interspace nearest to the area requiring analgesia. He or she advances the catheter into the epidural space, removes the needle, and secures the remainder of the catheter with a dressing while ensuring that the catheter is taped securely. The end of the catheter is capped or, if a continuous infusion is prescribed, it is connected to special tubing and an infusion pump that is designated for epidural infusion. Nurse anesthetists, anesthesiologists, and certified nurses control epidural analgesia, depending on agency policy. Some patients are able to use a technique known as *patient-controlled epidural analgesia (PCEA),* which allows them to self-administer demand doses of epidural solution when connected to a special administration pump (Pasero and McCaffery, 2011).

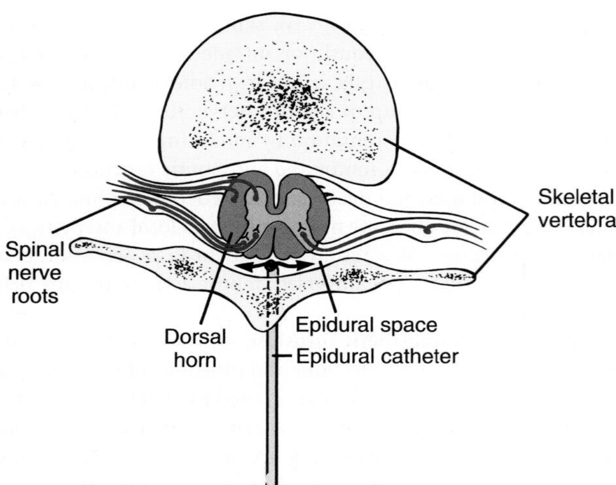

FIGURE 44-13 Anatomical drawing of epidural space.

One of the concerns related to the use of peripheral and epidural anesthetic techniques is the risk of bleeding and subsequent hematoma formation near the injection/insertion site. Although relatively uncommon, the risk is increased when patients receive anticoagulant or antiplatelet medications. Safe placement or removal of these injections and catheters is made on the basis of knowledge of the patients' coagulation status and the timing of administration of anticoagulant or antiplatelet medications. Guidelines for the use of anticoagulation in patients with regional anesthesia are available (Narouze et al., 2015) Because the epidural space is a highly vascular area, patients with epidural catheters are at risk for the development of epidural hematomas, which may lead to ischemia of the spinal cord, and if unaddressed, serious neurological complications.

Nursing Implications for Local and Regional Anesthesia. Provide emotional support to patients receiving local or regional anesthesia by explaining the insertion technique and warning patients that they will temporarily lose sensory function within minutes of injection. Motor and autonomic (bowel and bladder control) function may also be lost quickly, depending on the area anesthetized. It is common for patients to fear paralysis because epidural and spinal injections come close to the spinal cord. To reassure the patient, explain that numbness, tingling, and coldness are common. Catheter insertion should be comfortable because the health care provider should first numb the injection site. Prepare patients for possible discomfort. Before a patient receives an analgesic, check for allergies. Also check to be sure that the drugs (e.g., morphine [Duramorph] and fentanyl [Sublimaze]) administered via the epidural catheter are free of potentially neurotoxic substances such as preservatives and additives. Assess vital signs to monitor systemic effects.

After administration of a local or regional anesthetic, protect the patient from injury until full sensory and motor function return. Patients are at risk for injuring an anesthetized body part without knowing it. For patients with topical anesthesia, avoid applying heat or cold to numb areas. After an injection into the knee joint, warn the patient to avoid standing without assistance because there is a high risk of falling. With peripheral nerve or epidural local anesthetics, patients may experience sensory loss along with significant motor weakness. Assess patients for sensory and motor nerve blockade and notify the prescriber when motor blockade is unintended. Protect patients from injury and educate about necessary precautions until full sensory and motor function return. During and after epidural anesthesia a patient stays in bed until motor function returns. Help the patient the first time he or she tries to get out of bed.

TABLE 44-6 Nursing Care for Patients with Epidural Infusions

Goal	Actions
Prevent catheter displacement.	Secure catheter (if not connected to implanted reservoir) carefully to outside skin.
Maintain catheter function.	Check external dressing around catheter site for dampness or discharge. (Leakage of epidural solution may occur if catheter is dislodged.) Use transparent dressing to secure catheter and aid inspection. Inspect catheter for breaks.
Prevent infection.	Use strict aseptic technique when caring for catheter (see Chapter 29). Do not change dressing routinely over site. Inspect insertions site for signs of infection. Follow institutional policies for tubing change.
Monitor for respiratory depression.	Monitor vital signs, especially respirations, per policy. Use pulse oximetry, end-tidal carbon dioxide, and apnea monitoring.
Prevent undesirable complications.	Assess for hemodynamic changes associated with use of local anesthetics that may cause vasodilation and subsequent hypotension: • Ensure adequate hydration and administer prescribed intravenous fluids. • Notify prescriber if significant change in vital signs occurs and reduce or stop epidural infusion. • Anticipate need for change in epidural solution. Assess for pruritus (itching) and nausea and vomiting associated with use of epidural opioids: • Notify prescriber for dose reduction or epidural solution change. • Administer antihistamines and antiemetics as ordered. Assess sensation and motor strength; notify health provider if deviation from baseline.
Maintain urinary and bowel function.	Monitor intake and output. Assess for bladder and bowel distention. Assess for discomfort, frequency, and urgency.

When managing epidural infusions, if agency policy allows, connect the catheter to an infusion pump, a port, or a reservoir or cap it off for bolus injections. To reduce the risk of accidental epidural injection of drugs intended for IV use, clearly label the catheter *epidural catheter*. Always administer continuous infusions through appropriately labeled electronic infusion devices for proper control. Because of the catheter location, use surgical asepsis to prevent a serious and potentially fatal infection. Notify a patient's health care provider immediately of any signs or symptoms of infection or pain at the insertion site. Thorough hygiene is necessary during nursing procedures to keep the catheter system clean and dry. Maintain a closed system and prevent catheter disconnection by ensuring tight connections.

Nursing implications for managing epidural analgesia are numerous (Table 44-6). Do not administer supplemental doses of opioids or sedative/hypnotics because of possible additive central nervous system adverse effects. Monitoring for effects of medications differs, depending on medication used and whether infusions are intermittent or continuous. Complications of epidural opioid use include nausea and vomiting, urinary retention, constipation, respiratory depression, and pruritus (Pasero and McCaffery, 2011). When patients receive epidural analgesia, initially monitor them as often as every 15 minutes, including assessment of vital signs, respiratory effort, and skin color. Once stabilized, monitoring occurs every hour in the first 12 to 24 hours and then with less frequency if the patient is stable (refer to agency policy).

To minimize bleeding risks and the potential for hematoma formation, anticoagulant and antiplatelet medications should not be administered until a pain specialist can verify safe use. To detect development of a possible epidural hematoma, notify the health care provider or pain specialist if the patient develops severe pain at the epidural insertion site or unexplained sensory or motor loss. The provider who performs the procedure should also be notified when patients with peripheral nerve injections/catheter have similar signs and symptoms.

The patient needs to receive thorough education about epidural analgesia in terms of the action of the medication and its advantages and disadvantages. Instruct patients about the potential for side effects and to notify their health care provider if side effects develop. If the patient requires long-term epidural use, the health care provider tunnels a permanent catheter through the skin. The catheter exits at the patient's side. Teach a patient on long-term therapy how to safely administer home infusions with minimal ongoing nursing intervention and coordinate with the case manager or social worker to ensure that appropriate home care services will be provided.

Invasive Interventions for Pain Relief. When severe pain persists despite medical treatment, available invasive interventions include intrathecal implantable pumps or injections, spinal cord and deep brain stimulation, neuroablative procedures (cordotomy, rhizotomy), trigger point injections, cryoablation, and intraspinal medications (e.g., opioids, steroids, local anesthetics). These techniques are useful for chronic pain. It is not acceptable to tell a patient with severe unrelieved pain that there is "nothing more we can do for you." Patients with severe chronic pain should be referred to comprehensive pain-management programs whenever possible. These programs offer many different interventional strategies, pharmacological options, physical medicine, and rehabilitation therapies to address the complex needs of patients with chronic pain. When comprehensive pain programs are not available, referral to a chronic pain-management program may be the best available option.

Procedure Pain Management. Diagnostic and treatment procedures potentially produce pain and anxiety, both of which should be assessed and treated before a procedure begins (Czarnecki et al., 2011). Barriers to successful pain control include numerous patient-specific factors, but perhaps more influential is the lack of acknowledgment by health care providers that pain may occur during or after a procedure. Without this acknowledgment, the necessary anticipation, prevention, and management of potential or actual procedural pain cannot occur (Czarnecki et al., 2011). The Thunder Project II (Puntillo et al., 2001) identified several procedures causing pain in critical care patients: turning, wound drain removal, tracheal suctioning, femoral catheter removal, placement of a central line, and changing of nonburn wound dressings. Common pharmacological agents for managing procedural comfort include local anesthetics, NSAIDs, acetaminophen, opioids, anxiolytics, and sedatives (Czarnecki et al., 2011). Premedicating patients before painful procedures allows them to cooperate more fully and reduces the experience of pain. Using nonpharmacological therapies such as relaxation techniques, meditation, imagery, and music, in addition to medications, has been effective in select situations (Czarnecki et al., 2011). When you premedicate a patient before a procedure, keep in mind the time to onset and time to peak effect of the analgesic to properly time the beginning of the painful procedure.

Cancer Pain and Chronic Noncancer Pain Management. Cancer pain is either chronic or acute. The prevalence of pain varies among cancer patients. A review of research spanning 40 years shows the prevalence ranging from 64% in patients with metastatic, advanced, or terminal phases of the disease, 59% in patients on anticancer treatment, and 33% in patients after curative treatment (van den Beuken-van Everdingen et al., 2007). Experts and consensus panels agree that cancer pain is still not adequately treated (Ripamonti et al., 2011). Organizations such as the APS and the National Comprehensive Cancer Network (NCCN) have published guidelines for assessing and treating cancer-related pain. The guidelines support comprehensive and aggressive treatment, including many options for pain relief. The best choice of pain treatment often changes as a patient's condition and the characteristics of pain change. You can use nonpharmacological interventions with pharmacological interventions to optimize care.

Similar recommendations are made for the treatment of pain in patients with chronic noncancer pain. In 2009 the APS and the American Academy of Pain Medicine jointly recommended that chronic opioid therapy can be an effective therapy for carefully selected and monitored patients with chronic noncancer pain (Chou et al., 2009). Analgesics for chronic pain should be prescribed on a regular basis and not on "as required" schedule (Ripamonti et al., 2011). However, chronic pain is complex and requires the careful selection of patients, identification of their risks, use of different treatments (often in combination), and ongoing monitoring to offer patients the best possible outcomes. Treatment options are continuously expanding and include a variety of pharmacological agents, physical therapies, behavioral medicine, surgical interventions, neuromodulation, complementary, and alternative approaches (Turk et al., 2011). No one approach has demonstrated superiority, and overall treatment effectiveness is poor and inconsistent (Turk et al., 2011). Patients are often desperate, frustrated, and anxious when presenting for treatment. It is important to provide emotional support and educate them about taking an active role in their pain management with realistic goals and expectations. Co-morbidities such as anxiety and depression can worsen pain and require separate assessment and treatment.

Many patients with cancer experience breakthrough cancer pain (BTCP), a transient worsening of pain that occurs either spontaneously or in relation to a specific predictable or unpredictable trigger, despite relatively stable and adequately controlled background pain (European Oncology Nursing Society, 2013). BTCP is a challenging aspect of cancer because, even though it is self-limiting in nature, its presence has a significant, negative impact on the quality of life of patients and family caregivers (European Oncology Nursing Society, 2013). Individualized assessment is critical for understanding how BTCP affects a patient's life. A holistic approach to care is often needed (Box 44-17) There is evidence for the proper treatment of **breakthrough pain** in cancer patients; however, there is little evidence for how to treat it in patients with chronic noncancer pain (Manchikanti et al., 2011). Multiple issues related to the concept of breakthrough pain in chronic noncancer pain evolve around extensive use, overuse, misuse, and abuse of opioids. In the era of eliminating opioids or significantly curtailing their use to only appropriate indications, the concept of breakthrough pain raises multiple questions without any scientific evidence.

BOX 44-17 Types of Breakthrough Pain and Treatment

Types of Breakthrough Pain

Incident pain: Pain that is predictable and elicited by specific behaviors or triggers such as a voluntary act (walking), involuntary act (coughing) or treatments (e.g., wound dressing changes)

End-of-dose failure pain: Pain that occurs toward the end of the usual dosing interval of a regularly scheduled analgesic

Spontaneous pain: Pain that is unpredictable and not associated with any activity or event

Treatment

- Lifestyle changes
- Management of reversible causes
- Modification of pathological processes
- Nonpharmacological management
- Pharmacological management—rescue dose of medication
- Interventional techniques

From Haugen DF et al: Assessment and classification of cancer breakthrough pain: a systematic literature review, *Pain* 149(3):476, 2010; European Oncology Nursing Society: *Breakthrough cancer pain guidelines,* European Oncology Nursing Society guidelines, 2013, http://www.cancernurse.eu/documents/EONSBreakthroughCancerPainGuidelines.pdf. Accessed August 17, 2015.

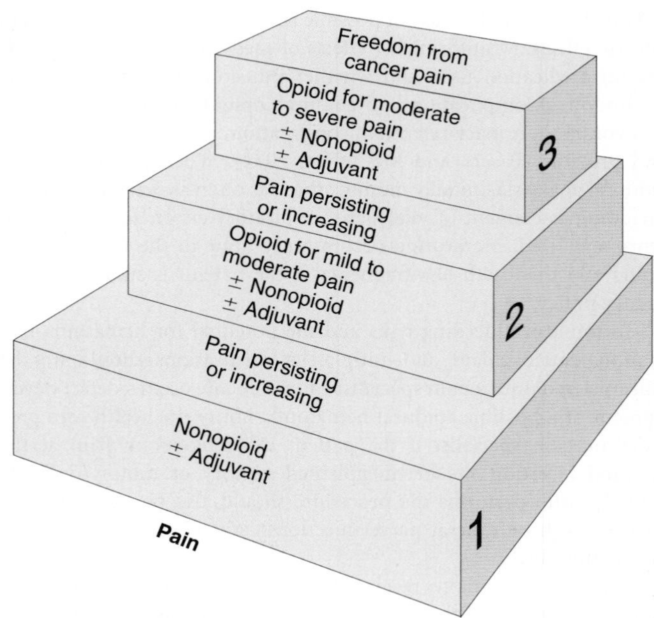

FIGURE 44-14 WHO analgesic ladder is a three-step approach in treating cancer pain. (Accessed September 27, 2010 from http://www.who.int/cancer/palliative/painladder/en/.)

The APS reports that the primary goal in treating chronic noncancer pain with opioids is to increase patients' level of function rather than just to provide pain relief (ACPA, 2014). The use of opioid therapy in patients with chronic pain requires careful patient selection and consideration of the risks and benefits of opioids. For example, to determine whether opioids are beneficial for a patient, it is necessary to assess his or her level of participation in ADLs, physical therapies, family activities, and work-related functions. Family members are often included in office visits to provide input about a patient's functional level. Research has not yet provided clear evidence to support or guide the use of chronic opioid therapy for patients with chronic noncancer pain (Chou et al., 2015). It is recommended that each person with chronic noncancer pain be medically managed individually; medication use should be determined by weighing benefit compared to other alternatives, cost, potential side effects, and the person's other medical problems (ACPA, 2014). Concerns about long-term opioid use are related to loss of beneficial effect over time, increasing tolerance, and escalating use with decreasing function (ACPA, 2014).

The World Health Organization (WHO) in 1986 introduced the WHO three-step analgesic ladder as a recommended approach for the management of cancer pain (Figure 44-14). This approach has been used worldwide and has been praised for its simplicity and ease of use. However, the ladder has been the object of criticism (Vargas-Schaffer, 2010). The three-step approach recommends that therapy begin at the first step with the use of nonopioid analgesics and/or adjuvants and progress to the next higher step as pain intensity increases. Weak opioids alone or in combination with the nonopioid analgesics and/or adjuvants are recommended at step two; and, if pain persists, strong opioids are recommended at step three. There have been efforts to modify the steps to facilitate use of the ladder for different pain presentations. A bidirectional approach has been suggested in which, in addition to the original step-up approach, a step-down approach would be used for patients with intense acute pain, uncontrolled cancer pain, and breakthrough pain (Thapa et al., 2011). With this modification, therapy would begin at the third step with the strong opioids and descend down the ladder with improvement in pain. Another modification includes the addition of a fourth step, which recommends neurosurgical and other invasive procedures and also includes management of pediatric and acute pain in emergency departments and postoperative situations (Vargas-Schaffer, 2010) (Figure 44-15). The new fourth step is recommended for the treatment of crises of chronic pain. Many other modifications of the ladder have been proposed, including those that recommend the use of a multimodal approach at each level.

Long-acting or controlled-release medications may provide relief for all types of chronic pain, including cancer pain. These controlled-release medications (e.g., morphine [MS Contin, Roxanol SR], and oxycodone [OxyContin]) relieve pain for 8 to 12 hours. Long-acting or sustained-release opioids are dosed on a scheduled basis, not prn or "as needed." Transdermal fentanyl, which is 100 times more potent than morphine, is available for opioid-tolerant patients with cancer or chronic pain. It delivers predetermined doses that provide analgesia for up to 72 hours. The transdermal route is useful when patients are unable to take drugs orally. Patients find the transdermal patch easy to use because it allows for continuous opioid administration without needles or pumps. Self-adhesive patches release the medication slowly over time, achieving effective analgesia. Transdermal fentanyl is not for adult patients who weigh less than 100 lbs (too little subcutaneous tissue for absorption) or who are hyperthermic (increases drug absorption). *Do not place heating pads over a patch and never cut it.* To dispose of a patch, fold in half, adhesive side onto itself, and flush down the toilet (Pasero and McCaffery, 2011).

All patients on chronic opioid therapy require monitoring and follow-up. Side effects should be anticipated, prevented when possible, and treated when necessary. Over time, tolerance develops to the analgesic effect of opioids, necessitating dose escalation to achieve pain relief. The higher opioid dose is usually not lethal because patients also develop a tolerance to respiratory depression. Less commonly, chronic

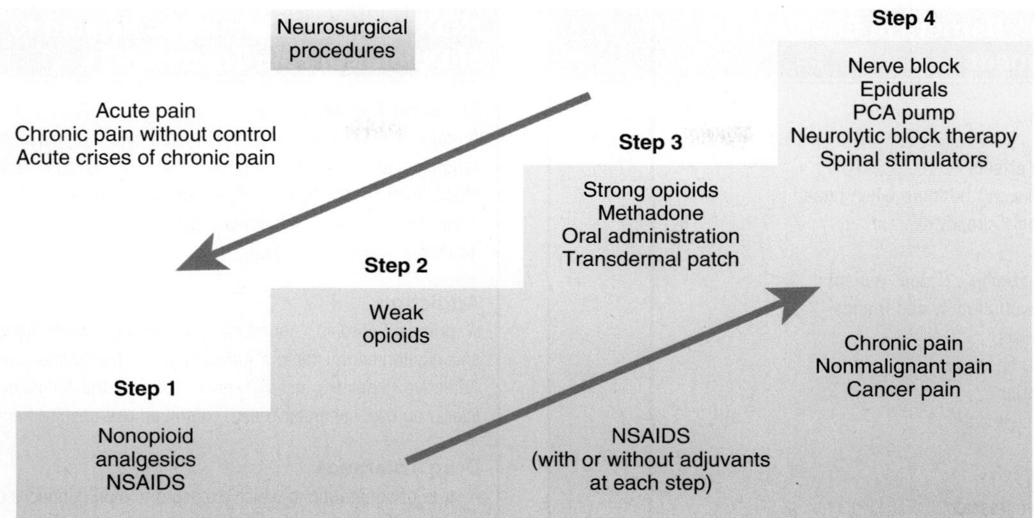

FIGURE 44-15 Adaptation of the WHO analgesic ladder. *NSAID,* Nonsteroidal antiinflammatory drug; *PCA,* patient-controlled analgesia. (From Vargas-Schaffer G: Is the WHO analgesic ladder still valid?: Twenty-four years of experience, *Can Fam Physician* 56:514, 2010.)

opioid use may lead to hyperalgesia (increased pain sensitivity). Especially in the case of noncancer pain, patients should be closely monitored for signs of aberrant opioid-related behaviors such as misuse, abuse, and addiction. A transmucosal fentanyl "unit" now exists to treat breakthrough pain in opioid-tolerant patients. Swab the fentanyl unit in the mouth over the buccal mucosa and gums. The unit remains intact to dissolve in the mouth, not chewed. Allow to absorb over a 15-minute period, delaying swallowing as long as possible. Use no more than 2 units per breakthrough pain episode. If the patient's pain is not relieved after 2 units, notify the patient's health care provider (Pasero and McCaffery, 2011).

Many patients, family members, and health care providers have concerns about the risks of addiction associated with opioid use. Estimates of addiction in patients with chronic persistent pain range from 6% to 10% (Pasero and McCaffery, 2011). Often a person with chronic pain who consults with numerous health care providers is labeled a drug seeker, when he or she is actually seeking adequate pain relief. This situation may be associated with behaviors that are indicative of pseudoaddiction. Nurses need to discourage patients from "doctor shopping" and having multiple health care providers for treating pain and refer them to pain specialists. Pain centers offer a holistic approach to chronic pain, using both nonpharmacological and pharmacological strategies for chronic pain management (Pasero and McCaffery, 2011).

As with constant acute pain, it is necessary to give patients with chronic pain required analgesics on a regular basis. The oral route of administration of analgesic drugs should be advocated as the first choice (Ripamonti et al., 2011). Prescribing analgesics on a prn basis for chronic pain is ineffective and causes more suffering. The patient with chronic pain needs to take an analgesic ATC, even when the pain subsides. Regular administration maintains therapeutic drug blood levels for ongoing pain control.

Administer analgesics rectally when patients are unable to swallow, have nausea or vomiting, or are near death. This route is contraindicated for patients with diarrhea or cancerous lesions involving the anus or rectum. Morphine, hydromorphone, and oxymorphone are available in suppositories (Pasero and McCaffery, 2011).

Some patients use PCA devices to treat severe cancer pain in the home. PCA devices provide improved, uniform pain control with fewer peaks and valleys in plasma concentration, more effective drug action, and lower drug dosages overall. Patients who usually benefit from continuous infusions include those with severe pain for whom oral and injectable medications provide minimal relief, those with severe nausea and vomiting, and those unable to swallow oral medications.

When a patient first receives continuous-drip opioids, the IV access needs to be patent and without complications (see Chapter 42). A central venous catheter, an implanted venous access port, or a peripherally inserted central catheter is usually best for long-term IV infusion. When IV access is poor, the subcutaneous route with a concentrated dose is possible. When an infusion begins, monitor a patient's sedation level and respiratory status closely during the first 24 hours and with any increases in the infusion rate (follow agency policy). Patients who are placed on continuous analgesic infusions are opioid tolerant; thus respiratory depression is rare.

> **QSEN QSEN: BUILDING COMPETENCY IN PATIENT-CENTERED CARE** Mrs. Mays in the care plan continues to have issues with uncontrollable pain. During your assessment you learn that she is reluctant to take medication to relieve the pain because it is a sign of weakness. Mrs. Mays usually takes as little medication as possible and prefers to shop in the organic market for her foods and dietary supplements, which do more for her health than any prescription medication. How would you initiate effective interventions to relieve her pain and suffering in light of her values, preferences, and expressed needs?
>
> *Answers to QSEN Activities can be found on the Evolve website.*

Barriers to Effective Pain Management. Barriers to effective pain management are complex, involving the patient, the patient's family caregivers, health care providers, and the health care system (Box 44-18). Lack of knowledge and misconceptions about pain and appropriate pain management present significant barriers. Various cultural

BOX 44-18 Barriers to Effective Pain Management

Patient Barriers
- Fear of addiction
- Worry about side effects
- Fear of tolerance (won't be there when I need it)
- Takes too many pills already
- Fear of injections
- Concern about not being a "good" patient
- Doesn't want to worry family and friends
- May need more tests
- Needs to suffer to be cured
- Inadequate education
- Reluctance to discuss pain
- Pain inevitable
- Pain part of aging
- Fear of disease progression
- Believes health care providers and nurses are doing all they can
- Just forgets to take analgesics
- Fear of distracting health care providers from treating illness
- Believes health care providers have more important or sicker patients to see
- Suffering in silence noble and expected

Health Care Provider Barriers
- Inadequate pain-assessment skills
- Concern with addiction or accidental overdose (could also use opioid-related adverse effect)
- Concern with co-morbid mental health conditions
- Opiophobia, fear of opioids
- Fear of legal repercussions
- No visible cause of pain
- Belief that patients need to learn to live with pain
- Reluctance to deal with side effects of analgesics
- Not believing patient's report of pain
- Fear that giving a dose will kill patient
- Time constraints
- Inadequate reimbursement
- Belief that opioids "mask" symptoms
- Belief that pain is part of aging
- Overestimation of rates of respiratory depression

Health Care System Barriers
- Concern with creating "addicts"
- Difficulty in filling prescriptions
- Absolute dollar restriction on amount reimbursed for prescriptions
- Mail-order pharmacy restrictions
- Advanced practice nurses not used efficiently
- Extensive documentation requirements
- Poor pain policies and procedures regarding pain management
- Lack of money
- Inadequate access to pain clinics
- Poor understanding of economic impact of unrelieved pain

beliefs about the meaning of pain and pain interventions also pose challenges to effective pain management. Controversy among health care providers exists related to the use of opioid therapy, particularly for treatment of patients with chronic noncancer pain.

Patients and health care providers often do not understand the differences among physical dependence, addiction, and drug tolerance (Box 44-19). Experiencing a physical dependency does not imply addiction, and drug tolerance in and of itself is not the same as addiction. That is not to say that addiction does not occur or that patients who suffer from addiction should not be treated for pain. "Patients with addictive disease and pain have the right to be treated with dignity, respect, and the same quality of pain assessment and management as all other patients" (Oliver et al., 2012). An interdisciplinary team approach ensures a more effective pain-management plan for a patient with acute pain who also suffers from addiction. Nurses and health care providers need to avoid labeling patients as *drug seeking* because this term is poorly defined and can cause bias and prejudice. If there are concerns that a patient is abusing opioids, they should be voiced to the patient, and the patient's health care provider should be advised of the concerns. Many patients on long-term opioid medications have pain contracts with expected responsibilities of both the patient and health care provider. If the agreement is violated or other assessments dictate, additional resources may be identified to aid the patient in addressing the addictive illness.

BOX 44-19 Definitions Related to the Use of Opioids in Pain Treatment*

Physical Dependence
A state of adaptation that is manifested by a drug class–specific withdrawal syndrome produced by abrupt cessation, rapid dose reduction, decreasing blood level of the drug, and/or administration of an antagonist. Common symptoms of opioid withdrawal include shaking, chills, abdominal cramps, excessive yawning, and joint pain.

Addiction
A primary, chronic, neurobiological disease with genetic, psychosocial, and environmental factors influencing its development and manifestations. Addictive behaviors include one or more of the following: impaired control over drug use, compulsive use, continued use despite harm, and craving.

Drug Tolerance
A state of adaptation in which exposure to a drug induces changes that result in a diminution of one or more effects of the drug over time.

*Approved by the Boards of Directors of the American Academy of Pain Medicine, the American Pain Society, and the American Society of Addiction Medicine, February 2001 (American Pain Society, 2011).

Placebos. There are many different definitions and interpretations of the terms *placebo* and *placebo effect*. It is generally accepted that placebos are pharmacologically inactive preparations or procedures that produce no beneficial or therapeutic effect. Professional organizations discourage the use of placebos to treat pain. It is considered unethical and deceitful to administer them. Placebo use jeopardizes the trust between patients and their caregivers. If a placebo is ordered, question the order. Many health care agencies have policies that limit the use of placebos to research only (Pasero and McCaffery, 2011).

Restorative and Continuing Care

Pain Clinics, Palliative Care, and Hospices. Health professionals recognize pain as a significant health problem. Growth of pain centers, palliative care departments, and hospices designed to manage pain and suffering has increased. The Commission on Accreditation of Rehabilitation Facilities (CARF) accredits chronic pain treatment programs and sets standards for chronic pain management. A comprehensive pain center treats people on an inpatient or outpatient basis. Staff members representing all health care disciplines (e.g., nursing, medicine, physical therapy, psychology, pastoral care, and dietetics) work with patients to find the most effective pain-relief measures. A comprehensive clinic provides not only diverse therapy but also research into new treatments and training for professionals.

Many hospitals have palliative-care departments to help patients and their family members successfully manage their life-limiting conditions. The goal of palliative care is to help patients manage disease-related symptoms while living life fully with an incurable condition (see Chapter 37). Patients and their family members need ongoing assistance in managing pain at home. Teaching pain management during discharge and ensuring continuation of pain management after discharge is essential.

Hospices are programs that care for patients at the end of life (see Chapter 37). Hospice provides support and care for people in the last stages of incurable disease, with an emphasis on enhancing the quality of remaining life (National Hospice and Palliative Care Organization, 2010). It helps patients who are nearing the end of life to continue to live at home or in a health care setting in comfort and privacy. Pain control is a priority for hospices. Under the guidance of hospice nurses, families learn to monitor patients' symptoms and become the primary caregivers. Some hospice patients become hospitalized such as in the event of a brief acute care crisis or family problem.

Hospice programs help nurses overcome their fears of contributing to a patient's death when administering large doses of opioids. The ANA supports aggressive treatment of pain and suffering even if it hastens a patient's death (Fowler, 2015). The ANA position is supported by the ethical principle of double effect, which, when applied to pain at end of life, supports the use of opioids for the purpose of pain relief, despite the risk that a secondary effect may be the hastening of the patient's death from respiratory depression. Recent research suggests that moderate opioid dose increases in patients who are terminally ill do not hasten death (Bengoechea et al., 2010). The disease, not the opioid, is killing the patient.

◆ Evaluation

Through the Patient's Eyes. Evaluate patients' perceptions of the effectiveness of interventions used to relieve pain. Patients help decide the best times to attempt pain treatments. Essentially they are the best judge of whether a pain-relief intervention works. Often the family is another valuable resource, particularly in the case of a patient with pain who is not able to express discomfort. For patients with chronic pain, the effect of the pain intervention on the patient's function should be considered when evaluating the patient's perception of his or her response to treatment. If the intervention results in the patient feeling an improvement in the participation in self-care or activities such as physical therapy, the pain intervention should be viewed positively. Also ask patients about tolerance to therapy and the overall amount of relief obtained. If patients state that an intervention is not helpful or even aggravates the discomfort, stop it immediately and seek an alternative. Time and patience are necessary to maximize the effectiveness of pain management. Educate patients about what to expect. For a patient in acute pain, reassure him or her that you will check back frequently to assess for changes in pain level. Continually assess if the character of the patient's pain changes and whether individual interventions are effective.

Patient Outcomes. Evaluation of pain is one of many nursing responsibilities that require effective critical thinking (Figure 44-16). Evaluate your success in achieving the outcomes of the plan of care. A patient's behavioral responses to pain-relief interventions are not always obvious. Evaluating the effectiveness of a pain intervention requires you to evaluate for change in the severity and quality of the pain. Also be sure to evaluate after an appropriate period of time. For instance, oral medications usually peak in about 1 hour; whereas IVP medications peak in 15 to 30 minutes. Ask a patient if a medication alleviates the pain when it is peaking. Do not expect the patient to volunteer the information. Evaluate psychological and physiological responses to pain (e.g., vital sign changes and asking questions such as, "Do you feel more at ease or less anxious since we administered the medication?" It is also important to evaluate if the patient has any adverse effects from pain therapies.

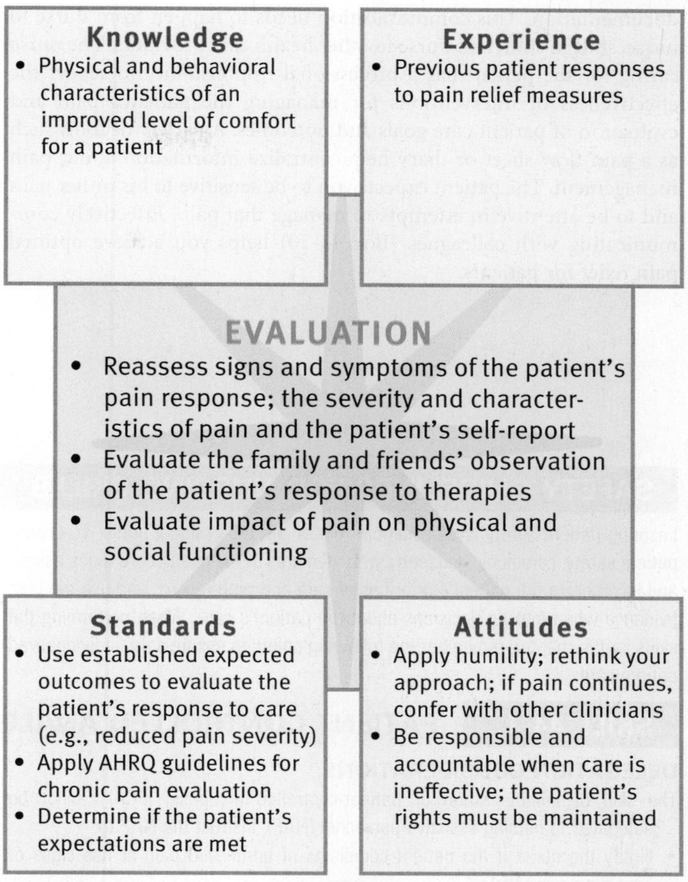

If a patient continues to have discomfort after an intervention, try a different approach. For example, if an analgesic provides only partial relief, add relaxation exercises or guided-imagery exercises. Consult with the patient's health care provider about increasing the dose, decreasing the interval between doses, or trying different analgesics. If patient outcomes are not met, ask the patient:

- What is your current pain level?
- How far away is your pain level from your goal?
- Which side effects are you experiencing from your pain medication?
- What have you done to help manage your pain?
- Describe limitations in function that you are experiencing related to uncontrolled pain.
- How is your pain limiting or altering your rest and sleep?

Effective communication of the assessment of a patient's pain and the response to intervention is facilitated by accurate and thorough

Knowledge
- Physical and behavioral characteristics of an improved level of comfort for a patient

Experience
- Previous patient responses to pain relief measures

EVALUATION
- Reassess signs and symptoms of the patient's pain response; the severity and characteristics of pain and the patient's self-report
- Evaluate the family and friends' observation of the patient's response to therapies
- Evaluate impact of pain on physical and social functioning

Standards
- Use established expected outcomes to evaluate the patient's response to care (e.g., reduced pain severity)
- Apply AHRQ guidelines for chronic pain evaluation
- Determine if the patient's expectations are met

Attitudes
- Apply humility; rethink your approach; if pain continues, confer with other clinicians
- Be responsible and accountable when care is ineffective; the patient's rights must be maintained

FIGURE 44-16 Critical thinking model for pain-management evaluation. *AHRQ,* Agency for Healthcare Research and Quality.

documentation. This communication needs to happen from nurse to nurse, shift to shift, and nurse to other health care providers. The nurse caring for the patient has a professional responsibility to report the effectiveness of interventions for managing the patient's pain and evaluation of patient care goals and outcomes. A variety of tools such as a pain flow sheet or diary help centralize information about pain management. The patient expects you to be sensitive to his or her pain and to be attentive in attempts to manage that pain. Effectively communicating with colleagues (Box 44-20) helps you achieve optimal pain relief for patients.

BOX 44-20 Checklist for Communicating Patients' Unrelieved Pain to Colleagues

- What is the pain rating now? Over the past period of time?
- Which pain rating is acceptable to the patient?
- How do you recommend that the patient's treatment be changed to reduce the pain rating?
- Which professional reference can be used, if needed, to support this recommendation?

From Pasero C, McCaffery M: *Pain assessment and pharmacologic management,* St Louis, 2011, Mosby.

SAFETY GUIDELINES FOR NURSING SKILLS

Ensuring patient safety is an essential role of the professional nurse. To ensure patient safety, communicate clearly with members of the health care team, assess and incorporate the patient's priorities of care and preferences, and use the best evidence when making decisions about the patient's care. When performing the skills in this chapter, remember the following points to ensure safe, individualized patient care:

- The patient is the only person who should press the PCA button to administer the pain medication.
- Monitor the patient for signs and symptoms of oversedation and respiratory depression.
- Monitor for potential side effects of opioid analgesics.

SKILL 44-1 PATIENT-CONTROLLED ANALGESIA

DELEGATION CONSIDERATIONS

The skill of administration of patient-controlled analgesia (PCA) cannot be delegated to nursing assistive personnel (NAP). Instruct the NAP to:

- Notify the nurse if the patient complains of unrelieved pain or has signs of becoming oversedated.
- Notify the nurse if the patient has questions about the PCA process or equipment.
- Never administer a PCA dose for the patient and notify the nurse if anyone other than the patient is observed administering a dose for the patient.

EQUIPMENT

- PCA system
- Identification label and time tape (may already be attached and completed by pharmacy)
- Alcohol swab
- Adhesive tape
- Clean gloves, when applicable
- Equipment for vital signs and pulse oximeter

STEP	RATIONALE
ASSESSMENT	
1. Check accuracy and completeness of medical administration record (MAR) or computer printout with health care provider's order for patient's name, name of medication, dose, frequency of medication (continuous or demand or both), and lockout period.	Health care provider order required for administration of opioid medication. Ensures that patient receives right medications.
2. Review medication information in drug reference manual or consult with pharmacist if uncertain about any medications to be administered.	Understanding medications before administering them prevents medication errors (Adhikari et al., 2014).
3. Assess severity and character of patient's pain. Use standard pain scale. If patient is unable to provide a self-report, select an appropriate scale for assessing pain in patients who are nonverbal or not cognitively alert.	Reveals source and nature of pain and factors that may increase it.
4. Assess environment for factors that could contribute to pain (e.g., noise, room temperature).	Elimination of irritating stimuli may help to reduce pain perception.
5. Assess for conditions that predispose patients to unwanted effects from opioids. Known, untreated, or unknown obstructive sleep apnea (OSA) poses a significant risk for respiratory depression (Craft, 2010). Use the STOP-BANG questionnaire to assess for OSA (Chung et al., 2008) (see agency policy).	Assessment should be completed before surgery by anesthesia. Identification allows treatment teams (surgeon, respiratory therapy, anesthesia) to take appropriate precautions such as making continuous positive airway pressure or bilevel positive airway pressure ventilation devices available.
6. Perform hand hygiene. Assess patency of intravenous (IV) access and surrounding tissue for inflammation or swelling (see Chapter 42).	IV line needs to be patent for safe administration of pain medication. Confirmation of placement of IV catheter and integrity of surrounding tissues ensures that medication is administered safely.
7. If patient has had surgery, inspect incision while wearing clean gloves. Gently palpate around area for tenderness. Use sterile gloves if necessary to place hand directly on incision. Remove gloves and perform hand hygiene.	Reveals evidence of tissue trauma or damage, which stimulates peripheral pain receptors to transmit impulses to cortex to create conscious awareness of pain (Drew and St. Marie, 2011).
8. Check medical record for patient's history for drug allergies and typical reactions.	Avoids placing patient at risk for allergic reaction.

STEP	RATIONALE
CLINICAL DECISION POINT: *Be aware that nausea is not an allergic reaction and it can be treated; pruritus alone is not an allergic reaction and is common to opioid use. Pruritus is treatable and does not rule out the use of PCA.*	
9. Assess patient's knowledge and perceived effectiveness of previous pain-management strategies, especially previous PCA use.	Response to pain-control strategies helps identify learning needs and affects patient's willingness to try therapy.
PLANNING	
1. Collect appropriate equipment.	Aids in organization.
2. Draw curtains around patient's bed or close door to room.	Maintains patient privacy.
IMPLEMENTATION	
1. Perform hand hygiene.	Reduces transmission of infection.
2. Obtain PCA analgesic in module prepared by pharmacy. Check medication label 2 times: when removing from storage and when preparing for assembly.	Follows the six rights of medication administration to be sure of correct medication. *This is the first and second check for accuracy.*
3. At bedside, identify patient using two identifiers (e.g., name and birthday or name and medical record number) according to agency policy. Compare identifiers with information on patient's MAR or medical record.	Ensures correct patient. Complies with The Joint Commission standards and improves patient safety (TJC, 2016).
4. At bedside compare the MAR or computer printout with name of medication on the drug cartridge. Have second registered nurse (RN) confirm health care provider's order and the correct setup of the PCA. Second RN should check order and device independently and not just look at existing setup.	Ensures that correct patient receives right medication. *This is the third check for accuracy*
5. Before initiating analgesia, explain purpose and demonstrate function of PCA to patient and family as follows: a. Explain type of medication in device. b. Explain that device safely administers self-initiated small but frequent amounts of medication when needed to provide comfort and minimizes side effects from analgesia. c. Explain that self-dosing aids in repositioning, walking, or coughing and deep breathing. d. Explain that device is programmed to deliver ordered type and dose of pain medication, lockout interval, and 1- to 4-hour dosage limits. Explain how lockout time prevents overdose. e. Demonstrate to patient how to push medication demand button (see illustration). f. Instruct patient to notify nurse for possible side effects, problems in gaining pain relief, changes in severity or location of pain, alarm sounding, or questions.	Allows patient participation in care and independence in pain control. Preoperative education about PCA therapy improves postoperative pain relief (D'Arcy, 2011; Pasero and McCaffery, 2011).
6. Apply clean gloves. Check infuser and patient-controlled module for accurate labeling or evidence of leaking.	Avoids medication error and injury to patient.
7. Position patient comfortably to be sure venipuncture or central line site is accessible.	Ensures unimpeded flow of infusion.

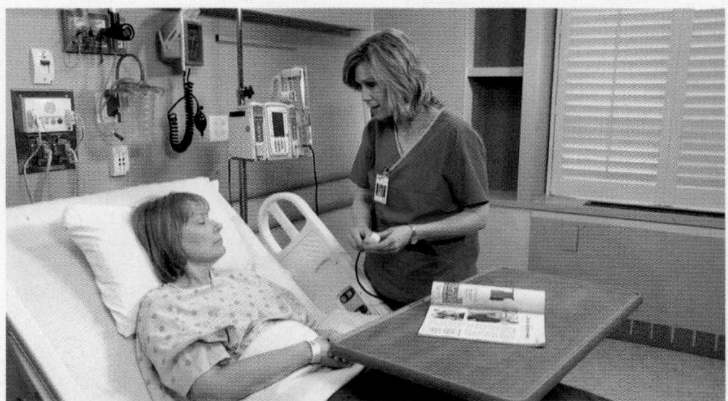

STEP 5e Explain purpose and demonstrate function of PCA.

SKILL 44-1 PATIENT-CONTROLLED ANALGESIA—cont'd

STEP	RATIONALE
8. Insert drug cartridge into infusion device (see illustration) and prime tubing.	Locks system and prevents air from infusing into IV tubing.
9. Attach needleless adapter to tubing adapter of patient-controlled module.	Needed to connect with IV line.
10. Wipe injection port of maintenance IV line vigorously with alcohol or antiseptic for 15 seconds and allow to dry.	Minimizes entry of surface microorganisms during needle insertion, reducing risk of catheter-related bloodstream infection.
11. Insert needleless adapter into injection port nearest patient (at Y-site of peripheral IV or central line, or connect to its own IV site). There should not be a chance to use PCA tubing for administering an IV push with another drug.	Establishes route for medication to enter main IV line. Needleless systems prevent needlestick injuries. Prevents medication interaction and incompatibility.
12. Secure connection and anchor PCA tubing with tape. Label PCA tubing.	Prevents dislodging of needleless adapter from port. Facilitates patient's ability to ambulate. Label prevents error from connecting tubing from different device to PCA.
13. Program computerized PCA pump as ordered to deliver prescribed medication dose and lockout interval. Have second RN check setting. (**NOTE:** Recheck with oncoming RN during shift hand-off to ensure line reconciliation.)	Ensures safe, therapeutic drug administration. With appropriate dose intervals (e.g., 10 minutes), usually an appreciable analgesic effect and/or mild sedation is achieved before the patient can access the next dose; thus there is a lower chance for oversedation and respiratory depression (Craft, 2010).
14. Administer loading dose of analgesia as prescribed. Manually give a 1-time dose or turn on pump and program dose into pump.	Establishes initial level of analgesia.
15. Discard gloves and supplies in appropriate containers. Dispose of empty cassette or syringe in compliance with institutional policy. Perform hand hygiene.	Reduces transmission of microorganisms. The Federal Controlled Substances Act regulates the control and dispensation of opioids for all institutions.
16. If experiencing pain, have patient demonstrate use of PCA system; if not, have patient repeat instructions given earlier.	Repeating instructions reinforces learning. Checking patient's understanding through return demonstration helps you determine patient's level of understanding and ability to manipulate device.
17. Be sure that venipuncture or central line site is protected and recheck before leaving patient.	Ensures patency of IV line.
18. To Discontinue PCA	
a. Check health care provider order for discontinuation. Obtain necessary PCA information from pump for documentation; note date, time, amount infused, amount of drug wasted, and reason for waste.	Ensures correct documentation of a schedule II drug.
b. Perform hand hygiene and apply clean gloves. Turn pump off. Disconnect PCA tubing from primary IV line but maintain IV access.	Reduces transmission of infection. Ensures continuation of IV line.
c. Dispose of empty cartridge according to agency policy.	Two RNs must witness wastage of opioids (narcotics) and sign record to meet requirements of Controlled Substances Act for scheduled drugs.

EVALUATION

STEP	RATIONALE
1. Use pain-rating scale to evaluate patient's pain intensity following treatments and procedures according to agency policy.	Determines response to PCA dosing. Documenting "PCA in use" or "PCA effective" is not an adequate record of the patient's pain level.
2. Observe patient for nausea or pruritus.	Common side effects of opioid.
3. Monitor patient's level of sedation, vital signs, and pulse oximetry or capnography every 1 to 2 hours for the first 12 hours (APS and AAPM, 2009). Monitor more often at the start, during first 24 hours, and at night when hypoventilation and hypoxia tend to occur. Follow agency policy.	Patient is at highest risk the first 24 hours of use. Excess sedation (difficult to arouse) precedes respiratory depression.

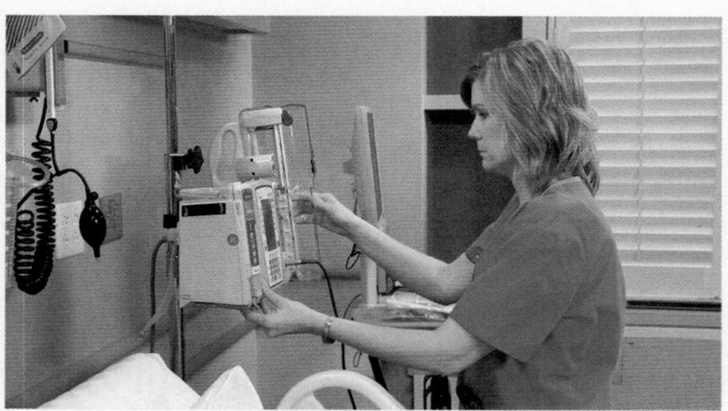

STEP 8 Programming PCA pump.

STEP	RATIONALE
4. Have patient demonstrate dose delivery.	Evaluates skill in use of PCA.
5. According to agency policy, evaluate number of attempts (number of times patient pushed button), delivery of demand doses (number of times drug actually given and total amount of medication delivered in particular time frame), and basal dose if ordered.	Helps to evaluate effectiveness of PCA dose and frequency in relieving pain. Maintains compliance with Controlled Substances Act.
6. Observe patient initiate self-care.	Demonstrates pain relief.
7. Use ***Teach Back*** to determine patient's and family's understanding about PCA. For example, state, "I want to be sure I explained how PCA will help with your pain and how you should use the device. Can you explain to me how you should use the PCA?" Revise your instruction now or develop plan for revised patient teaching if patient is not able to teach back correctly.	Evaluates what patient and family are able to explain or demonstrate.

UNEXPECTED OUTCOMES AND RELATED INTERVENTIONS

1. Patient verbalizes continued or worsening discomfort or displays nonverbal behaviors indicative of pain, suggesting that underlying condition has changed or patient is undermedicated.
   - Perform complete pain assessment.
   - Check function of PCA device to ensure that the patient is receiving the medication.
   - Inspect IV site for possible catheter occlusion or infiltration.
   - Consult with health care provider.
2. Patient is not readily arousable.
   - Stop PCA; elevate head of bed unless contraindicated; and assess vital signs, including pulse oximetry (and end-tidal CO_2 if available). *Do not* leave patient's bedside and continue to try to arouse patient.
   - Notify health care provider and/or call for help.
   - Prepare to administer an opioid-reversing agent (naloxone [Narcan]).
3. Patient unable to manipulate PCA device to maintain pain control.
   - Consult with health care provider regarding alternative medication route or possible basal (continuous) dose if patient is opioid tolerant.
   - If agency allows, assess for feasibility of authorized agent–controlled analgesia if nurse (nurse-controlled analgesia) or patient's significant other (family-controlled analgesia) is available to responsibly manipulate analgesic pump (Cooney et al., 2013).

RECORDING AND REPORTING

- Record drug, dose, and time begun on MAR. Note lockout time, demand, and basal dose.
- Record regular assessments of patient's pain, vital signs, and oxygen saturation.
- Record amount of drug delivered and amount wasted.
- Document your evaluation of patient learning.

KEY POINTS

- Pain is a purely subjective physical and psychosocial experience.
- Misconceptions about pain often result in doubt about the degree of the patient's suffering and unwillingness to provide relief.
- Knowledge of the nociceptive pain processes of the pain experience (i.e., transmission, transduction, perception, and modulation) provides guidelines for selecting pain-relief measures.
- A person's cultural background influences the meaning of pain and how it is expressed.
- Older patients commonly underreport pain and believe that it is unacceptable to show or express pain.
- Cancer pain is still not adequately treated, despite clinical guidelines for the effective use of opioids and other pharmacological alternatives.
- The difference between acute and chronic pain involves the concept of harm. Acute pain is protective, thus preventing harm; chronic pain is no longer protective and does not provide any benefit.
- Do not collect an in-depth pain history when the patient is experiencing severe discomfort. Wait until the pain is better controlled.
- Pain often causes physical signs and symptoms similar to those of other diseases.
- Individualize pain interventions by collaborating closely with patient, using assessment findings and trying a variety of interventions.
- Eliminating sources of painful stimuli is a basic nursing measure for promoting comfort.
- Prescribing analgesics on a prn basis for chronic pain is ineffective and causes more suffering; thus patients with chronic pain need to take analgesics ATC, even when their pain subsides.
- Sedation is an adverse effect of opioids that always precedes respiratory depression.
- A PCA device (without a basal infusion) gives patients pain control with lower risk of overdose.
- While caring for a patient who receives local anesthesia, protect him or her from injury.

- Nursing implications for administering epidural analgesia include preventing infection, assessing sensation and motor function, and monitoring closely for respiratory depression.
- Addiction rarely occurs in patients who take opioids to relieve pain.
- Breakthrough pain is a challenging aspect of cancer because it can impact the quality of life of patients and family caregivers; thus it requires a holistic approach to treatment.
- Pain evaluation includes measuring the changing character of pain, the patient's response to interventions, and his or her perceptions of the effectiveness of a therapy.

CLINICAL APPLICATION QUESTIONS

Preparing for Clinical Practice

After three doses (0.5 mg each) of morphine from the patient-controlled analgesia (PCA) device, Mrs. Mays started vomiting and stated that she was feeling "out of her head." She rated her chest pain as 3 on a scale of 0 to 10. She is breathing comfortably on 2 L of nasal cannula oxygen, and her lung sounds are clear to auscultation. Her husband is very concerned and anxious about his wife and wants the morphine stopped so she will not become "addicted."

1. Do you think that Mrs. Mays is allergic to morphine? Support your answer.
2. What do you need to tell Mr. and Mrs. Mays about the adverse effects of morphine?
3. Which interventions do you need to complete before consulting the health care provider?

ⓔ *Answers to Clinical Application Questions can be found on the Evolve website.*

REVIEW QUESTIONS

Are You Ready to Test Your Nursing Knowledge?

1. Which of the following signs or symptoms in a patient who is opioid-naïve is of greatest concern to the nurse when assessing the patient 1 hour after administering an opioid?
   1. Oxygen saturation of 95%
   2. Difficulty arousing the patient
   3. Respiratory rate of 10 breaths/min
   4. Pain intensity rating of 5 on a scale of 0 to 10
2. A health care provider writes the following order for a patient who is opioid-naïve who returned from the operating room following a total hip replacement: "Fentanyl patch 100 mcg, change every 3 days." On the basis of this order, the nurse takes the following action:
   1. Calls the health care provider and questions the order
   2. Applies the patch the third postoperative day
   3. Applies the patch as soon as the patient reports pain
   4. Places the patch as close to the hip dressing as possible
3. A patient is being discharged home on an around-the-clock (ATC) opioid for chronic back pain. Because of this order, the nurse anticipates an order for which class of medication?
   1. Opioid antagonists
   2. Antiemetics
   3. Stool softeners
   4. Muscle relaxants
4. A new medical resident writes an order for oxycodone CR (Oxy Contin) 10 mg PO q2h prn. Which part of the order does the nurse question?
   1. The drug
   2. The time interval
   3. The dose
   4. The route
5. The nurse reviews a patient's medical administration record (MAR) and finds that the patient has received oxycodone/acetaminophen (Percocet) (5/325), two tablets PO every 3 hours for the past 3 days. What concerns the nurse the most?
   1. The patient's level of pain
   2. The potential for addiction
   3. The amount of daily acetaminophen
   4. The risk for gastrointestinal bleeding
6. A patient with chronic low back pain who took an opioid around-the-clock (ATC) for the past year decided to abruptly stop the medication for fear of addiction. He is now experiencing shaking chills, abdominal cramps, and joint pain. The nurse recognizes that this patient is experiencing symptoms of:
   1. Opioid toxicity.
   2. Opioid tolerance.
   3. Opioid addiction.
   4. Opioid withdrawal.
7. A patient has returned from the operating room, recovering from repair of a fractured elbow, and states that her pain level is 6 on a 0-to-10 pain scale. She received a dose of hydromorphone just 15 minutes ago. Which interventions may be beneficial for this patient at this time? (Select all that apply.)
   1. Transcutaneous electrical nerve stimulation (TENS)
   2. Administer naloxone (Narcan) 2 mg intravenously
   3. Provide back massage
   4. Reposition the patient
   5. Withhold any pain medication and tell the patient that she is at risk for addiction
8. Which of the following instructions is crucial for the nurse to give to both family members and the patient who is about to be started on a patient-controlled analgesia (PCA) of morphine? (Select all that apply.)
   1. Only the patient should push the button.
   2. Do not use the PCA until the pain is severe.
   3. The PCA system can set limits to prevent overdoses from occurring.
   4. Notify the nurse when the button is pushed.
   5. Do not push the button to go to sleep.
9. A patient with a 3-day history of a stroke that left her confused and unable to communicate returns from interventional radiology following placement of a gastrostomy tube. The patient has been taking hydrocodone/APAP 5/325 up to four tablets/day before her stroke for arthritic pain. The health care provider's order reads as follows: "Hydrocodone/APAP 5/325 1 tab, per gastrostomy tube, q4h, prn." Which action by the nurse is most appropriate?
   1. No action is required by the nurse because the order is appropriate.
   2. Request to have the order changed to around the clock (ATC) for the first 48 hours.
   3. Ask for a change of medication to meperidine (Demerol) 50 mg IVP, q3 hours, prn.
   4. Begin the hydrocodone/APAP when the patient shows nonverbal symptoms of pain.
10. A patient is prescribed morphine patient-controlled analgesia (PCA). Arrange the following steps for administering PCA in the correct order.
    1. Program computerized PCA pump to deliver prescribed medication dose and lockout interval.
    2. Check label of medication 3 times: when removed from storage, when brought to bedside, when preparing for assembly.

3. Administer loading dose of analgesia as prescribed.
4. Attach drug reservoir to infusion device, prime tubing, and attach needleless adapter to end of tubing.
5. Identify patient using two identifiers.
6. Insert and secure needleless adapter into injection port nearest patient.

11. A patient rates his pain as a 6 on a scale of 0 to 10, with 0 being no pain and 10 being the worst pain. The patient's wife says that he can't be in that much pain since he has been sleeping for 30 minutes. Which is the most accurate resource for assessing the pain?
    1. Patient's self-report
    2. Behaviors
    3. Surrogate (wife) report
    4. Vital sign changes
12. When using ice massage for pain relief, which of the following is correct? (Select all that apply.)
    1. Apply ice using firm pressure over skin.
    2. Apply ice for 5 minutes or until numbness occurs.
    3. Apply ice no more than 3 times a day.
    4. Limit application of ice to no longer than 10 minutes.
    5. Use a slow, circular steady massage.
13. When teaching a patient about transcutaneous electrical nerve stimulation (TENS), which information do you include?
    1. TENS works by causing distraction.
    2. TENS therapy does not require a health care provider's order.
    3. TENS requires an electrical source for use.
    4. TENS electrodes are applied near or directly on the site of pain.
14. While caring for a patient with cancer pain, the nurse knows that a multimodal analgesia plan includes: (Select all that apply.)
    1. Using analgesics such as nonsteroidal antiinflammatory drugs (NSAIDs) along with opioids.
    2. Stopping acetaminophen when the pain becomes very severe.
    3. Avoiding polypharmacy by limiting the use of medication to one agent at a time.
    4. Avoiding total sedation, regardless of the severity of the pain.
    5. The use of adjuvants (co-analgesics) such as gabapentin (Neurontin) to manage neuropathic type pain.
15. A postoperative patient currently is asleep. Therefore the nurse knows that:
    1. The sedative administered may have helped him sleep, but it is still necessary to assess pain.
    2. The intravenous (IV) pain medication given in recovery is relieving his pain effectively.
    3. Pain assessment is not necessary.
    4. The patient can be switched to the same amount of medication by the oral route.

Answers: 1. 2; **2.** 1; **3.** 3; **4.** 2; **5.** 3; **6.** 4; **7.** 1, 3, 4; **8.** 1, 3, 5; **9.** 2; **10.** 2, 5, 1, 4, 6, 3; **11.** 1; **12.** 1, 2, 5; **13.** 4; **14.** 1, 5; **15.** 1.

Rationales for Review Questions can be found on the Evolve website.

REFERENCES

Adhikari RJ, et al: A multi-disciplinary approach to medication safety and the implication for nursing education and practice, *Nurse Educ Today* 34(2):185, 2014.

American Chronic Pain Association (ACPA): *ACPA Resource guide to chronic pain medication & treatment*, 2014 edition, 2014, http://www.theacpa.org/uploads/ACPA_Resource_Guide_2014_FINAL.pdf. Accessed April 27, 2015.

American Geriatrics Society (AGS): Pharmacological management of persistent pain in older persons, *J Am Geriatr Soc* 57(8):1331, 2009.

American Nurses Association (ANA): *Pain management nursing: scope and standards of practice*, Silver Spring, MD, 2005, The Association.

American Pain Society (APS) and American Association of Pain Medicine (AAPM): Opioids guideline panel-Part 1, *J Pain* 10(2):113–e22, 2009.

American Pain Society (APS): *Principles of analgesic use in the treatment of acute and cancer pain*, ed 6, Glenview, IL, 2009, The Society.

American Society of Anesthesiologists (ASA): Practice guidelines for chronic pain management, *Anesthesiology* 112:1, 2010.

Arnstein P: Balancing analgesic efficacy with safety concerns in the older adult, *Pain Manag Nurs* 11(2):S11, 2010.

Bucher A: *Health literacy & communicating about pain*, 2014, http://engagingthepatient.com/2014/10/06/health-literacy-communicating-about-pain/. Accessed May 8, 2015.

Burchum JR, Rosenthal LD: *Lehne's pharmacology for nursing care*, ed 9, St Louis, 2016, Elsevier.

Chou R, et al: Clinical guidelines for the use of chronic opioid therapy in chronic noncancer pain, *J Pain* 10(2):113, 2009.

Chung F, et al: High STOP-Bang score indicates a high probability of obstructive sleep apnoea, *Br J Anaest* 108(5):768, 2008.

Cooney MF, et al: American Society for Pain Management Nursing position statement with clinical practice guidelines: authorized agent–controlled analgesia, *Pain Manag Nurs* 14(3):178, 2013.

Craft J: Patient-controlled analgesia: is it worth the painful prescribing process? *Proc (Bayl Univ Med Cent)* 23(4):434, 2010.

Czarnecki ML, et al: Procedural pain management: a position statement with clinical practice recommendations, *Pain Manag Nurs* 12(2):95, 2011.

D'Arcy Y: *Meeting the challenges of acute pain management*, Medscape Multispecialty, 2008, http://www.medscape.org/viewarticle/574105_3. Accessed August 15, 2015.

D'Arcy Y: New thinking about postoperative pain management, *OR Nurse* 5(6):29, 2011.

Day R, Graham G: Non-steroidal anti-inflammatory drugs (NSAIDs), *Br J Sports Med* 47(17):1127, 2013.

Devraj R, et al: Pain awareness and medication knowledge: a health literacy evaluation, *J Pain Palliat Care Pharmacother* 27(1):19, 2013.

Dezutter J, et al: Prayer and pain: the mediating role of positive re-appraisal, *J Behav Med* 34(6):542, 2011.

Drew DJ, St Marie BJ: Pain in critically ill patients with substance abuse disorder or long-term opioid use for chronic pain, *AACN Adv Crit Care* 22(3):238, 2011.

Drew D, et al: The use of "as-needed" range orders for opioid analgesics in the management of pain: a consensus statement of the American Society for Pain Management Nurses and the American Pain Society, *Pain Manag Nurs* 15(2):551, 2013.

European Oncology Nursing Society: *Breakthrough cancer pain guidelines*, 2013, European Oncology Nursing Society guidelines. http://www.cancernurse.eu/documents/EONSBreakthroughCancerPainGuidelines.pdf. Accessed August 17, 2015.

Fouladbakhsh J: Complementary and alternative modalities to relieve osteoarthritis symptoms, *Am J Nurs* 112(3):S44, 2012.

Fowler MDM: *Guide to the code of ethics for nurses with interpretive statements*, ed 2, Silver Spring, MD, 2015, American Nurses Association.

Guild DG: Mechanical therapy for low back pain, *Prim Care* 39(3):511, 2012.

Herr K: Pain in the older adult: an imperative across all health care settings, *Pain Manag Nurs* 11(2):S1, 2010.

Herr K, et al: Pain assessment in the patient unable to self-report: position statement with clinical practice recommendations, *Pain Manag Nurs* 12(4):230, 2011.

Hockenberry MJ, Wilson D: *Wong's nursing care of infants and children*, ed 10, St Louis, 2015, Mosby.

Horgas AL, et al: Pain management. In Boltz M, et al, editors: *Evidence-based geriatric nursing protocols for best practice*, ed 4, New York, 2012, Springer, p 246.

Hughes RG, editor: *Patient safety and quality: an evidence-based handbook for nurses*, prepared with support from the Robert Wood Johnson Foundation, AHRQ Publication No. 08-0043. Rockville, MD, 2008, Agency for Healthcare Research and Quality.

Institute of Medicine (IOM): *Relieving pain in America: a blueprint for transforming prevention, care, education, and research*, Washington, DC, 2011, National Academies Press.

International Association for the Study of Pain (IASP): *Faces Pain Scale—revised home*, 2014a, http://www.iasp-pain.org/Education/Content.aspx?ItemNumber=1519. Accessed December 28, 2014.

International Association for the Study of Pain (IASP): *Pain taxonomy*, 2014b, http://www.iasp-pain.org/Taxonomy#Pain. Accessed July 10, 2015.

International Association for the Study of Pain (IASP): *Declaration of Montreal*, 2015, http://www.iasp-pain.org/DeclarationofMontreal. Accessed April 27, 2015.

James S: Human pain and genetics: some basics, *Br J Pain* 7(4):171, 2013.

Katsarava Z, et al: Defining the differences between episodic migraine and chronic migraine, *Curr Pain Headache Rep* 16(1):86, 2012.

Manchikanti L, et al: Breakthrough pain in chronic non-cancer pain: fact, fiction, or abuse, *Pain Physician* 14(2):E103, 2011.

Matthews-Kozanecka M: Holistic approach to treatment in the context of bioethics, *Dev Period Med* 18(1):13, 2014.

Melzack R, Wall PD: Pain mechanisms: a new theory, *Science* 150:971, 1965.

Narouze S, et al: Interventional spine and pain procedures in patients on antiplatelet and anticoagulant medications: guidelines from the American Society of Regional Anesthesia and Pain Medicine, the European Society of Regional Anaesthesia and Pain Therapy, the American Academy of Pain Medicine, the International Neuromodulation Society, the North American Neuromodulation Society, and the World Institute of Pain, *Reg Anesth Pain Med* 40(3):182, 2015.

National Hospice and Palliative Care Organization (NHPCO): *Preamble and philosophy*, 2010, http://www.nhpco.org/ethical-and-position-statements/preamble-and-philosophy. Accessed December 12, 2014.

Oliver J, et al: American Society for Pain Management Nursing Position Statement: Pain management in patients with substance use disorders, *Pain Manag Nurs* 13(3):169, 2012.

Paice J, Ferrell B: The management of cancer pain, *CA Cancer J Clin* 61:157, 2011.

Pasero C, McCaffery M: *Pain assessment and pharmacologic management*, St Louis, 2011, Mosby.

QSEN Institute: *Pre-licensure KSAS*, 2014, http://qsen.org/competencies/pre-licensure-ksas/. Accessed May 9, 2015.

Ripamonti CI, et al: Management of cancer pain: ESMO Clinical Practice Guidelines, *Ann Oncol* 22(Suppl 6): vi69, 2011.

Sadler A: Acute and chronic neuropathic pain in the hospital setting: use of screening tools, *Clin J Pain* 29(6):507, 2013.

Spine Health: *How to use ice massage therapy for back pain*, 2006, http://www.spine-health.com/treatment/heat-therapy-cold-therapy/how-use-ice-massage-therapy-back-pain. Accessed 8/10/15.

Thapa D, et al: Cancer pain management-current status, *J Anaesthesiol Clin Pharmacol* 27(2):162, 2011.

The Joint Commission (TJC): *Sentinel event alert issue 49: Safe use of opioids in hospitals*, 2012, http://www.jointcommission.org/assets/1/18/SEA_49_opioids_8_2_12_final.pdf. Accessed August 12, 2014.

The Joint Commission (TJC): *2016 National Patient Safety Goals*, Oakbrook Terrace, IL, 2016, The Commission. Available at http://www.jointcommission.org/standards_information/npsgs.aspx. Accessed November 2015.

Topcu SY, Findik UY: Effect of relaxation exercises on controlling postoperative pain, *Pain Manag Nurs* 13(1):11, 2012.

Tracy B, Morrison RS: Pain management in older adults, *Clin Ther* 35(11):1659, 2013.

Turk DC, et al: Treatment of chronic non-cancer pain, *Lancet* 377(9784):2226, 2011.

US Food and Drug Administration (USFDA): FDA Drug Safety Communication: *Prescription acetaminophen products to be limited to 325 mg per dosage unit; boxed warning will highlight potential for severe liver failure*, 2014, http://www.fda.gov/Drugs/DrugSafety/ucm239821.htm. Accessed May 10, 2015.

van Ojik AL, et al: Treatment of chronic pain in older people: evidence-based choice of strong acting opioids, *Drugs Aging* 29(8):615, 2012.

Vargas-Schaffer G: Is the WHO analgesic ladder still valid? *Can Fam Physician* 56(6):514, 2010.

Weinstein F, et al: *Spirituality assessments and interventions in pain management*, 2014, Pract Pain Manag, http://www.practicalpainmanagement.com/treatments/psychological/spirituality-assessments-interventions-pain-medicine. Accessed November 18, 2015.

Wong DL, Baker CM: Pain in children: comparison of assessment scales, *Okla Nurse* 33(1):8, 1988.

RESEARCH REFERENCES

Allred K, et al: The effect of music on postoperative pain and anxiety, *Pain Manag Nurs* 11(1):15, 2010.

Althaus A, et al: Distinguishing between pain intensity and pain resolution: using acute post-surgical pain trajectories to predict chronic post-surgical pain, *Eur J Pain* 18(4):513, 2014.

Bengoechea I, et al: Opioid use at the end of life and survival in a hospital at home unit, *J Palliat Med* 13(9):1079, 2010.

Beyer JE, et al: The creation, validation, and continuing development of the Oucher: a measure of pain intensity in children, *J Pediatr Nurs* 7(5):335, 1992.

Buyukyilmaz F, Asti T: The effect of relaxation techniques and back massage on pain and anxiety in Turkish total hip or knee arthroplasty patients, *Pain Manag Nurs* 14(3):143, 2013.

Chou R, et al: The effectiveness and risks of long-term opioid therapy for chronic pain: a systematic review for a National Institutes of Health Pathways to Prevention Workshop, *Ann Intern Med* 162(4):276, 2015.

Cole LC, LoBiondo-Wood G: Music as an adjuvant therapy in control of pain and symptoms in hospitalized adults: a systematic review, *Pain Manag Nurs* 15(1):406, 2014.

Cutshall SM, et al: Effect of massage therapy on pain, anxiety, and tension in cardiac surgical patients: a pilot study, *Complement Ther Clin Pract* 16(2):92, 2010.

DeSantana JM, et al: Effectiveness of transcutaneous electrical nerve stimulation for treatment of hyperalgesia and pain, *Curr Rheumatol Rep* 10(6):492, 2008.

Dorner TE, et al: The impact of socio-economic status on pain and the perception of disability due to pain, *Eur J Pain* 15(1):103, 2011.

Gaston-Johansson F, et al: Similarities in pain descriptions of four different ethnic-culture groups, *J Pain Symptom Manage* 5(2):94, 1990.

Gordon DB, et al: Nurses' opinions on appropriate administration of prn range opioid analgesic orders for acute pain, *Pain Manage Nurs* 3:131, 2008.

Goulet JL, et al: Agreement between electronic medical-based and self-administered pain numeric rating scale: clinical and research implications, *Med Care* 51(3):245, 2013.

Greco TM, et al: Quality of cancer pain management: an update of a systematic review of undertreatment of patients with cancer, *J Clin Oncol* epub November 17, 2014, http://jco.ascopubs.org/content/early/2014/11/20/JCO.2014.56.0383.full. Accessed April 27, 2015.

Harris M, Richards KC: The physiological and psychological effects of slow-stroke back massage and hand massage on relaxation in older people, *J Clin Nurs* 19(7–8):917, 2010.

Kolanowski A: Advances in nonpharmacological interventions, 2011–2012, *Res Gerontol Nurs* 6(1):5, 2013.

Korhan E, et al: The effects of music therapy on pain in patients with neuropathic pain, *Pain Manag Nurs* 15(1):306, 2014.

Lukas A, et al: Observer-rated pain assessment instruments improve both the detection of pain and the evaluation of pain intensity in people with dementia, *Eur J Pain* 17(10):1558, 2013.

Morales DR, et al: NSAID-exacerbated respiratory disease: a meta-analysis evaluating prevalence, mean provocative dose of aspirin and increased asthma morbidity, *Allergy* 70(7):828, 2015.

Mosele M, et al: Psychometric properties of the pain assessment in advanced dementia scale compared to self assessment of pain in elderly patients, *Dement Geriatr Cogn Disord* 34(1):38, 2012.

Park J, Hughes AK: Nonpharmacological approaches to the management of chronic pain in community-dwelling older adults: a review of empirical evidence, *J Am Geriatr Soc* 60(3):555, 2012, http://www.ncbi.nlm.nih.gov/pubmedhealth/PMH0046585/. Accessed May 10, 2015.

Pöpping DM, et al: Impact of epidural analgesia on mortality and morbidity after surgery: systematic review and meta-analysis of randomized controlled trials, *Ann Surg* 259(6):1056, 2014.

Puntillo K, et al: Patients' perceptions and responses to procedural pain: results from Thunder Project II, *Am J Crit Care* 10(4):238, 2001.

Tomlinson D, et al: A systematic review of faces scales for the self-report of pain intensity in children, *Pediatrics* 126:e1168, 2010.

Vaartio H, et al: Nursing advocacy in procedural pain care, *Nurs Ethics* 16(3):340, 2009.

van den Beuken-van Everdingen MHJ, et al: Prevalence of pain in patients with cancer: a systematic review of the past 40 years, *Ann Oncol* 18:1437, 2007.

45

Nutrition

OBJECTIVES

- Explain the importance of a balance between energy intake and energy requirements.
- List the end products of carbohydrate, protein, and fat metabolism.
- Explain the significance of saturated, unsaturated, and polyunsaturated fats.
- Describe the ChooseMyPlate and discuss its value in planning meals for good nutrition.
- List the current dietary guidelines for the general population.
- Explain the variance in nutritional requirements throughout growth and development.
- Discuss the major methods of nutritional assessment.
- Identify three major nutritional problems and describe patients at risk.
- Establish a plan of care to meet the nutritional needs of a patient.
- Describe the procedure for initiating and maintaining enteral feedings.
- Describe the methods for avoiding complications of enteral feedings.
- Describe the methods for avoiding complications of parenteral nutrition.
- Discuss medical nutrition therapy in relation to three medical conditions.
- Discuss how to implement diet counseling and patient teaching in relation to patient expectations.

KEY TERMS

Amino acid, p. 1055
Anabolism, p. 1057
Anorexia nervosa, p. 1060
Anthropometry, p. 1064
Basal metabolic rate (BMR), p. 1054
Body mass index (BMI), p. 1064
Bulimia nervosa, p. 1060
Carbohydrates, p. 1054
Catabolism, p. 1057
Chyme, p. 1057
Daily values, p. 1058
Dietary reference intakes (DRIs), p. 1058
Dispensable amino acids, p. 1055
Dysphagia, p. 1066
Enteral nutrition (EN), p. 1074
Enzymes, p. 1056
Fat-soluble vitamins, p. 1055
Fatty acids, p. 1055
Fiber, p. 1054
Food security, p. 1054
Gluconeogenesis, p. 1058
Glycogenesis, p. 1058
Glycogenolysis, p. 1058
Hypervitaminosis, p. 1055
Ideal body weight (IBW), p. 1064
Indispensable amino acids, p. 1055
Intravenous fat emulsions, p. 1078
Ketones, p. 1058
Kilocalories (kcal), p. 1054
Lipids, p. 1055
Macrominerals, p. 1055
Malabsorption, p. 1081
Malnutrition, p. 1064
Medical nutrition therapy (MNT), p. 1080
Metabolism, p. 1057
Minerals, p. 1055
Monounsaturated fatty acids, p. 1055
Nitrogen balance, p. 1055
Nutrient density, p. 1054
Nutrients, p. 1054
Parenteral nutrition (PN), p. 1076
Peristalsis, p. 1057
Polyunsaturated fatty acids, p. 1055
Resting energy expenditure (REE), p. 1054
Saccharides, p. 1054
Saturated fatty acids, p. 1055
Simple carbohydrates, p. 1054
Trace elements, p. 1055
Triglycerides, p. 1055
Unsaturated fatty acids, p. 1055
Vegetarianism, p. 1061
Vitamins, p. 1055
Water-soluble vitamins, p. 1055

MEDIA RESOURCES

http://evolve.elsevier.com/Potter/fundamentals/

- Review Questions
- Video Clips
- Concept Map Creator
- Case Study with Questions
- Skills Performance Checklists
- Audio Glossary
- Content Updates

Nutrition is a basic component of health and is essential for normal growth and development, tissue maintenance and repair, cellular metabolism, and organ function. The human body needs an adequate supply of nutrients for essential functions of cells. Food security is critical for all members of a household. This means that all household members have access to sufficient, safe, and nutritious food to maintain a healthy lifestyle. Household members have sufficient food available on a consistent basis and the resources to obtain appropriate food for a nutritious diet. Food also holds symbolic meaning. Giving or taking food is part of ceremonies, social gatherings, holiday traditions, religious events, the celebration of birth, and the mourning of death. The difficulty of the decision to withdraw food in a terminal illness, even in the form of intravenous (IV) nutrients, is a testament to the symbolic power of food and feeding.

Florence Nightingale understood the importance of nutrition, stressing a nurse's role in the science and art of feeding during the mid-1800s. Since then the nurse's role in nutrition and diet therapy has changed. Medical nutrition therapy (MNT) uses nutrition therapy and counseling to manage diseases (American Dietetic Association, 2010b). In some illnesses such as type 1 diabetes mellitus (DM) or mild hypertension, diet therapy is often the major treatment for disease control (ADA, 2012; AHA, 2010). Other conditions such as severe inflammatory bowel disease require specialized nutrition support such as enteral nutrition (EN) or parenteral nutrition (PN). Current standards of care promote optimal nutrition in all patients, including a low-fat diet and limiting red meat specifically (ACS, 2015; AHA, 2010).

The U.S. Department of Health and Human Services (USDHHS) and the Public Health Service established nutritional goals and objectives for *Healthy People 2020* (USDHHS, 2015). *Healthy People 2020* is the United States' contribution to the "Health for All" strategy of the World Health Organization (WHO, 2015). *Healthy People 2020* (Box 45-1) continues the objectives initiated in *Healthy People 2000* and *Healthy People 2010,* with overall goals of promoting health and reducing chronic disease. All nutrition-related objectives include baseline data from which progress is measured. The challenge remains to motivate consumers to put these dietary recommendations into practice.

BOX 45-1 Examples of Nutrition Objectives for *Healthy People 2020*

Weight and Growth

- Increase proportion of adults who are at a healthy weight (body mass index [BMI] 18.5 to 24.9).
- Reduce the proportion of adults who are obese.
- Reduce the proportion of children (2 to 11 years) who are overweight or obese.

Food and Nutrient Consumption

- Decrease saturated fat intake in population 2 years and older.
- Increase the variety of vegetables and fruit intake in the population 2 years and older.
- Increase grain product intake and consumption of calcium in the population 2 years and older.
- Reduce sodium daily intake in the population 2 years and older.

Iron Deficiency and Anemia

- Reduce prevalence of iron deficiency in children and childbearing women.
- Reduce prevalence of anemia in pregnant women in third trimester to 20%.

Schools, Work Sites, and Nutrition Counseling

- Increase work-site nutrition-education and weight-management program offerings.
- Offer nutrition assessment and individualized planning at primary care sites.
- Increase the percentage of schools that offer nutritious foods and beverages outside of school meals.
- Increase the number of states with nutrition standards for food and beverages provided to preschool-age children in child care.

Food Security

- Increase food security to 94% of households.

Data from U.S. Department of Health and Human Services: *Healthy people 2020,* 2010, http://www.healthypeople.gov/hp2020/objectives.

SCIENTIFIC KNOWLEDGE BASE

Nutrients: The Biochemical Units of Nutrition

The body requires fuel to provide energy for cellular metabolism and repair, organ function, growth, and body movement. The basal metabolic rate (BMR) is the energy needed at rest to maintain life-sustaining activities (breathing, circulation, heart rate, and temperature) for a specific amount of time. Factors such as age, body mass, gender, fever, starvation, menstruation, illness, injury, infection, activity level, and thyroid function affect energy requirements. The resting energy expenditure (REE), or resting metabolic rate, is the amount of energy you need to consume over a 24-hour period for your body to maintain all of its internal working activities while at rest. Factors that affect metabolism include illness, pregnancy, lactation, and activity level.

When the kilocalories (kcal) of the food we eat meets our energy requirements, our weight does not change (Nix, 2012). When the kilocalories ingested exceed our energy demands, we gain weight. Likewise, if the kilocalories ingested fail to meet our energy requirements, we lose weight.

Nutrients are the elements necessary for the normal function of numerous body processes. We meet energy needs through the intake of a variety of nutrients: carbohydrates, proteins, fats, water, vitamins, and minerals. The nutrient density of food refers to the proportion of essential nutrients to the number of kilocalories. High–nutrient dense foods such as fruits and vegetables provide a large number of nutrients in relationship to kilocalories. Low–nutrient dense foods such as alcohol or sugar are high in kilocalories but nutrient poor.

Carbohydrates. Carbohydrates, composed of carbon, hydrogen, and oxygen, are the main source of energy in the diet. Each gram of carbohydrate produces 4 kcal/g and serves as the main source of fuel (glucose) for the brain, skeletal muscles during exercise, erythrocyte and leukocyte production, and cell function of the renal medulla. We obtain carbohydrates primarily from plant foods, except for lactose (milk sugar). Carbohydrate classification occurs according to their carbohydrate units, or saccharides.

Monosaccharides such as glucose (dextrose) or fructose do not break down into a more basic carbohydrate unit. Disaccharides such as sucrose, lactose, and maltose are composed of two monosaccharides and water. Simple carbohydrates is the classification for both monosaccharides and disaccharides; they are found primarily in sugars. Polysaccharides such as glycogen make up carbohydrate units too (i.e., complex carbohydrates). They are insoluble in water and digested to varying degrees. Starches are polysaccharides.

The body is unable to digest some polysaccharides because we do not have enzymes capable of breaking them down. Fiber, a polysaccharide, is the structural part of plants that is not broken down by our digestive enzymes. The inability to break down fiber means that it does not contribute calories to the diet. Therefore insoluble fibers, including cellulose, hemicellulose, and lignin, are not digestible. Soluble fibers dissolve in water and include barley, cereal grains, cornmeal, and oats.

Proteins. Proteins provide a source of energy (4 kcal/g); they are essential for the growth, maintenance, and repair of body tissue. Collagen, hormones, enzymes, immune cells, deoxyribonucleic acid (DNA), and ribonucleic acid (RNA) are all made of protein. In addition, blood clotting, fluid regulation, and acid-base balance require proteins. Proteins transport nutrients and many drugs in the blood. Ingestion of proteins maintains nitrogen balance.

The simplest form of protein is the amino acid, consisting of hydrogen, oxygen, carbon, and nitrogen. Because the body does not synthesize indispensable amino acids, we need these to be provided in our diet. Examples of indispensable amino acids are histidine, lysine, and phenylalanine. The body synthesizes dispensable amino acids. Examples of amino acids synthesized in the body are alanine, asparagine, and glutamic acid. Amino acids can link together. Albumin and insulin are simple proteins because they contain only amino acids or their derivatives. The combination of a simple protein with a nonprotein substance produces a complex protein such as lipoprotein, formed by a combination of a lipid and a simple protein.

A complete protein, also called a *high-quality protein,* contains all essential amino acids in sufficient quantity to support growth and maintain nitrogen balance. Examples of foods that contain complete proteins are fish, chicken, soybeans, turkey, and cheese. Incomplete proteins are missing one or more of the nine indispensable amino acids and include cereals, legumes (beans, peas), and vegetables. Complementary proteins are pairs of incomplete proteins that, when combined, supply the total amount of protein provided by complete protein sources.

Achieving nitrogen balance means that the intake and output of nitrogen are equal. When the intake of nitrogen is greater than the output, the body is in positive nitrogen balance. Positive nitrogen balance is required for growth, normal pregnancy, maintenance of lean muscle mass and vital organs, and wound healing. The body uses nitrogen to build, repair, and replace body tissues. Negative nitrogen balance occurs when the body loses more nitrogen than it gains (e.g., with infection, burns, fever, starvation, head injury, and trauma). The increased nitrogen loss is the result of body tissue destruction or loss of nitrogen-containing body fluids. Nutrition during this period needs to provide nutrients to put patients into positive balance for healing.

Protein provides energy but, because its essential role is to promote growth, maintenance, and repair, a diet needs to provide adequate kilocalories from nonprotein sources. When there is sufficient carbohydrate in the diet to meet the energy needs of the body, protein is spared as an energy source.

Fats. Fats (lipids) are the most calorie-dense nutrient, providing 9 kcal/g. Fats are composed of triglycerides and fatty acids. Triglycerides circulate in the blood and are composed of three fatty acids attached to a glycerol. Fatty acids are composed of chains of carbon and hydrogen atoms with an acid group on one end of the chain and a methyl group at the other. Fatty acids can be *saturated,* in which each carbon in the chain has two attached hydrogen atoms; or *unsaturated,* in which an unequal number of hydrogen atoms are attached and the carbon atoms attach to one another with a double bond. Monounsaturated fatty acids have one double bond, whereas polyunsaturated fatty acids have two or more double carbon bonds. The various types of fatty acids referred to in the dietary guidelines have significance for health and the incidence of disease.

We also classify fatty acids as essential or nonessential. Linoleic acid, an unsaturated fatty acid, is the only essential fatty acid in humans. Linolenic acid and arachidonic acid, another type of unsaturated fatty acids, are important for metabolic processes. The body manufactures them when linoleic acid is available. Deficiency occurs when fat intake falls below 10% of daily nutrition. Most animal fats have high proportions of saturated fatty acids, whereas vegetable fats have higher amounts of unsaturated and polyunsaturated fatty acids.

Water. Water is critical because cell function depends on a fluid environment. Water makes up 60% to 70% of total body weight. Lean people have a greater percent of total body water than obese people do because muscle contains more water than any other tissue except blood. Infants have the greatest percentage of total body water because of greater surface area, and older people have the least. When deprived of water, a person usually cannot survive for more than a few days.

We meet our fluid needs by drinking liquids and eating solid foods high in water content such as fresh fruits and vegetables. Digestion produces fluid during food oxidation. In a healthy individual fluid intake from all sources equals fluid output through elimination, respiration, and sweating (see Chapters 41 and 45). An ill person has an increased need for fluid (e.g., with fever or gastrointestinal [GI] losses). By contrast, he or she also has a decreased ability to excrete fluid (e.g., with cardiopulmonary or renal disease), which often leads to the need for fluid restriction.

Vitamins. Vitamins are organic substances present in small amounts in foods that are essential to normal metabolism. They are chemicals that act as catalysts in biochemical reactions. When there is enough of any specific vitamin to meet the catalytic demands of the body, the rest of the vitamin supply acts as a free chemical and is often toxic to the body. Certain vitamins are currently of interest in their role as antioxidants. These vitamins neutralize substances called *free radicals,* which produce oxidative damage to body cells and tissues. Researchers think that oxidative damage increases a person's risk for various cancers. Antioxidant vitamins include beta-carotene and vitamins A, C, and E (Nix, 2012).

The body is unable to synthesize vitamins in the required amounts. Vitamin synthesis depends on dietary intake. Vitamin content is usually highest in fresh foods that have minimal exposure to heat, air, or water before their use. Vitamin classifications include fat soluble or water soluble.

Fat-Soluble Vitamins. The fat-soluble vitamins (A, D, E, and K) are stored in the fatty compartments of the body. With the exception of vitamin D, people acquire vitamins through dietary intake. Because the body has a high storage capacity for these vitamins, toxicity is possible when a person takes large doses of them. Hypervitaminosis of fat-soluble vitamins results from megadoses (intentional or unintentional) of supplemental vitamins, excessive amounts in fortified food, and large intake of fish oils.

Water-Soluble Vitamins. The water-soluble vitamins are vitamin C and the B complex (which is eight vitamins). The body does not store water-soluble vitamins; thus we need them provided in our daily food intake. Water-soluble vitamins absorb easily from the GI tract. Although they are not stored, toxicity can still occur.

Minerals. Minerals are inorganic elements essential to the body as catalysts in biochemical reactions. They are classified as macrominerals when the daily requirement is 100 mg or more and microminerals or trace elements when less than 100 mg is needed daily. Macrominerals help to balance the pH of the body, and specific amounts are necessary in the blood and cells to promote acid-base balance. Interactions occur among trace minerals. For example, excess of one trace mineral sometimes causes deficiency of another. Selenium

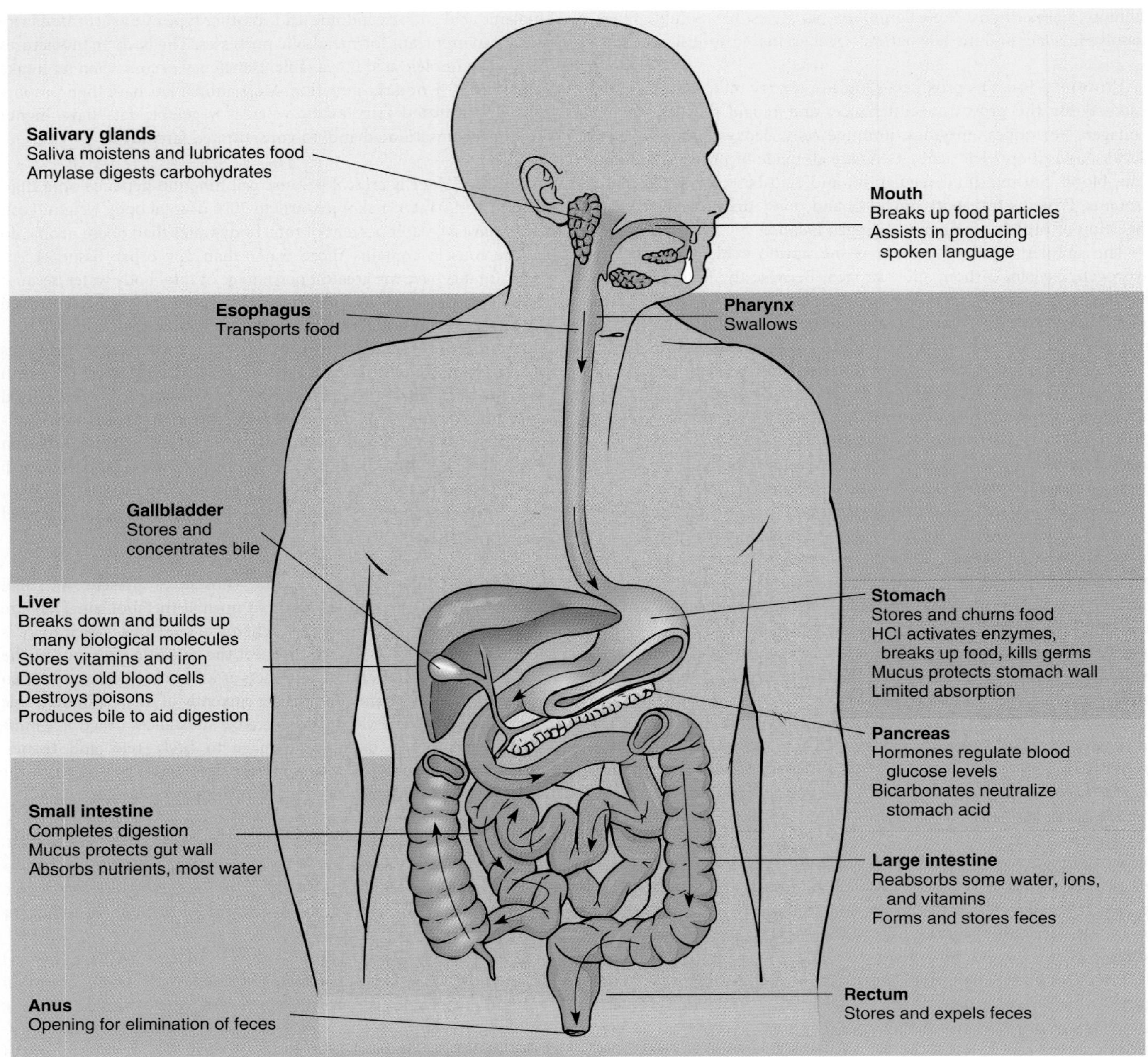

FIGURE 45-1 Summary of digestive system anatomy/organ function. *HCl,* Hydrochloric acid.

is a trace element that also has antioxidant properties. Silicon, vanadium, nickel, tin, cadmium, arsenic, aluminum, and boron play an unidentified role in nutrition. Arsenic, aluminum, and cadmium have toxic effects.

Anatomy and Physiology of the Digestive System

Digestion. Digestion of food is the mechanical breakdown that results from chewing, churning, and mixing with fluid and chemical reactions in which food reduces to its simplest form. Each part of the GI system has an important digestive or absorptive function (Figure 45-1). **Enzymes** are the protein-like substances that act as catalysts to speed up chemical reactions. They are an essential part of the chemistry of digestion.

Most enzymes have one specific function. Each enzyme works best at a specific pH. For example, the enzyme amylase in the saliva breaks down starches into sugars. The secretions of the GI tract have very different pH levels. Saliva is relatively neutral, gastric juice is highly acidic, and the secretions of the small intestine are alkaline.

The mechanical, chemical, and hormonal activities of digestion are interdependent. Enzyme activity depends on the mechanical breakdown of food to increase its surface area for chemical action. Hormones regulate the flow of digestive secretions needed for enzyme supply. Physical, chemical, and hormonal factors regulate the secretion of digestive juices and the motility of the GI tract. Nerve stimulation from the parasympathetic nervous system (e.g., the vagus nerve) increases GI tract action.

Digestion begins in the mouth, where chewing mechanically breaks down food. The food mixes with saliva, which contains ptyalin (salivary amylase), an enzyme that acts on cooked starch to begin its conversion to maltose. The longer an individual chews food, the more starch digestion occurs in the mouth. Proteins and fats are broken down physically but remain unchanged chemically because enzymes in the mouth do not react with these nutrients. Chewing reduces food particles to a size suitable for swallowing, and saliva provides lubrication to ease swallowing of the food. The epiglottis is a flap of skin that closes over the trachea as a person swallows to prevent aspiration. Swallowed food enters the esophagus, and wavelike muscular contractions (**peristalsis**) move the food to the base of the esophagus, above the cardiac sphincter. Pressure from a bolus of food at the cardiac sphincter causes it to relax, allowing the food to enter the fundus, or uppermost part, of the stomach.

The chief cells in the stomach secrete pepsinogen; and the pyloric glands secrete gastrin, a hormone that triggers parietal cells to secrete hydrochloric acid (HCl). The parietal cells also secrete HCl and intrinsic factor (IF), which is necessary for absorption of vitamin B_{12} in the ileum. HCl turns pepsinogen into pepsin, a protein-splitting enzyme. The body produces gastric lipase and amylase to begin fat and starch digestion, respectively. A thick layer of mucus protects the lining of the stomach from autodigestion. Alcohol and aspirin are two substances directly absorbed through the lining of the stomach. The stomach acts as a reservoir where food remains for approximately 3 hours, with a range of 1 to 7 hours.

Food leaves the antrum, or distal stomach, through the pyloric sphincter and enters the duodenum. Food is now an acidic, liquefied mass called **chyme**. Chyme flows into the duodenum and quickly mixes with bile, intestinal juices, and pancreatic secretions. The small intestine secretes the hormones secretin and cholecystokinin (CCK). Secretin activates release of bicarbonate from the pancreas, raising the pH of chyme. CCK inhibits further gastrin secretion and initiates release of additional digestive enzymes from the pancreas and gallbladder.

Manufactured in the liver, bile is then concentrated and stored in the gallbladder. It acts as a detergent because it emulsifies fat to permit enzyme action while suspending fatty acids in solution. Pancreatic secretions contain six enzymes: amylase to digest starch; lipase to break down emulsified fats; and trypsin, elastase, chymotrypsin, and carboxypeptidase to break down proteins.

Peristalsis continues in the small intestine, mixing the secretions with chyme. The mixture becomes increasingly alkaline, inhibiting the action of the gastric enzymes and promoting the action of the duodenal secretions. Epithelial cells in the small intestinal villi secrete enzymes (e.g., sucrase, lactase, maltase, lipase, and peptidase) to facilitate digestion. The major part of digestion occurs in the small intestine, producing glucose, fructose, and galactose from carbohydrates; amino acids and dipeptides from proteins; and fatty acids, glycerides, and glycerol from lipids. Peristalsis usually takes approximately 5 hours to pass food through the small intestine.

Absorption. The small intestine, lined with fingerlike projections called *villi*, is the primary absorption site for nutrients. Villi increase the surface area available for absorption. The body absorbs nutrients by means of passive diffusion, osmosis, active transport, and pinocytosis (Table 45-1).

Absorption of carbohydrates, protein, minerals, and water-soluble vitamins occurs in the small intestine and are then processed in the liver and released into the portal vein circulation. Fatty acids are absorbed in the lymphatic circulatory systems through lacteal ducts at the center of each microvilli in the small intestine.

TABLE 45-1 Mechanisms for Intestinal Absorption of Nutrients

Mechanism	Definition
Active transport	An energy-dependent process whereby particles move from an area of lesser concentration to an area of greater concentration. A special "carrier" moves the particle across the cell membrane.
Passive diffusion	The force by which particles move outward from an area of greater concentration to one of lesser concentration. The particles do not need a special "carrier" to move outward in all directions.
Osmosis	Movement of water through a semipermeable membrane that separates solutions of different concentrations. Water moves to equalize the concentration pressures on both sides of the membrane.
Pinocytosis	Engulfing of large molecules of nutrients by the absorbing cell when the molecule attaches to the absorbing cell membrane.

Data from Nix S: *Williams' basic nutrition and diet therapy*, ed 14, St Louis, 2012, Mosby.

Approximately 85% to 90% of water is absorbed in the small intestine (McCance et al., 2013). The GI tract manages approximately 8.5 L of GI secretions and 1.5 L of oral intake daily. The small intestine resorbs 9.5 L, and the colon absorbs approximately 0.4 L. Elimination of the remaining 0.1 L occurs via feces. In addition, electrolytes and minerals are absorbed in the colon, and bacteria synthesize vitamin K and some B-complex vitamins. Finally, feces form for elimination.

Metabolism and Storage of Nutrients. **Metabolism** refers to all of the biochemical reactions within the cells of the body. Metabolic processes are anabolic (building) or catabolic (breaking down). **Anabolism** is the building of more complex biochemical substances by synthesis of nutrients. It occurs when an individual adds lean muscle through diet and exercise. Amino acids are anabolized into tissues, hormones, and enzymes. Normal metabolism and anabolism are physiologically possible when the body is in positive nitrogen balance. **Catabolism** is the breakdown of biochemical substances into simpler substances and occurs during physiological states of negative nitrogen balance. Starvation is an example of catabolism when wasting of body tissues occurs.

Nutrients absorbed in the intestines, including water, transport through the circulatory system to the body tissues. Through the chemical changes of metabolism, the body converts nutrients into a number of required substances. Carbohydrates, protein, and fat metabolism produce chemical energy and maintain a balance between anabolism and catabolism. To carry out the work of the body, the chemical energy produced by metabolism converts to other types of energy by different tissues. Muscle contraction involves mechanical energy, nervous system function involves electrical energy, and the mechanisms of heat production involve thermal energy.

Some of the nutrients required by the body are stored in tissues. The major form of body reserve energy is fat, stored as adipose tissue. Protein is stored in muscle mass. When the energy requirements of the body exceed the energy supplied by ingested nutrients, stored energy is used. Monoglycerides from the digested part of fats convert to glucose by gluconeogenesis. Amino acids are also converted to fat and stored or catabolized into energy through gluconeogenesis. All body cells except red blood cells and neurons oxidize fatty acids into **ketones** for energy when dietary carbohydrates (glucose) are not adequate. Glycogen, synthesized from glucose, provides energy during brief periods of fasting (e.g., during sleep). It is stored in small reserves in liver and muscle tissue. Nutrient metabolism consists of three main processes:

1. Catabolism of glycogen into glucose, carbon dioxide, and water (**glycogenolysis**)
2. Anabolism of glucose into glycogen for storage (**glycogenesis**)
3. Catabolism of amino acids and glycerol into glucose for energy (**gluconeogenesis**)

Elimination. Chyme moves by peristaltic action through the ileocecal valve into the large intestine, where it becomes feces (see Chapter 47). Water absorbs in the mucosa as feces move toward the rectum. The longer the material stays in the large intestine, the more water is absorbed, causing the feces to become firmer. Exercise and fiber stimulate peristalsis, and water maintains consistency. Feces contain cellulose and similar indigestible substances, sloughed epithelial cells from the GI tract, digestive secretions, water, and microbes.

Dietary Guidelines

Dietary Reference Intakes. **Dietary reference intakes (DRIs)** present evidence-based criteria for an acceptable range of amounts of vitamins and nutrients for each gender and age-group (IOM, 2015). There are four components to the DRIs. The estimated average requirement (EAR) is the recommended amount of a nutrient that appears sufficient to maintain a specific body function for 50% of the population on the basis of age and gender. The recommended dietary allowance (RDA) is the average needs of 98% of the population, not the exact needs of the individual. The adequate intake (AI) is the suggested intake for individuals based on observed or experimentally determined estimates of nutrient intakes and used when there is not enough evidence to set the RDA. The tolerable upper intake level (UL) is the highest level that likely poses no risk of adverse health events. It is not a recommended level of intake (Tolerable upper-level intake, 2010).

Food Guidelines. The U.S. Department of Health and Human Services (USDHHS) and the U.S. Department of Agriculture (USDA) published the *Dietary Guidelines for Americans 2015-2020* and provide average daily consumption guidelines for the five food groups: grains, vegetables, fruits, dairy products, and meats (Box 45-2). These guidelines are for Americans over the age of 2 years. As a nurse, consider the food preferences of patients from different cultural groups, vegetarians, and others when planning diets. The U.S. Department of Agriculture developed the *ChooseMyPlate* program to replace the *My Food Pyramid* program. *ChooseMyPlate* provides a basic guide for making food choices for a healthy lifestyle (Figure 45-2). It includes guidelines for balancing calories; decreasing portion size; increasing healthy foods; increasing water consumption; and decreasing fats, sodium, and sugars (USDA, 2011).

Daily Values. The U.S. Food and Drug Administration (FDA) created **daily values** for food labels in response to the 1990 Nutrition Labeling and Education Act (NLEA). The FDA first established two sets of reference values. The referenced daily intakes (RDIs) are the first set, comprising protein, vitamins, and minerals based on the RDA. The daily reference values (DRVs) make up the second set and consist of nutrients such as total fat, saturated fat, cholesterol, carbohydrates, fiber, sodium, and potassium. Combined, both sets make up the daily values used on food labels. Daily values did not replace RDAs but provided a separate, more understandable format for the public. Daily values are based on percentages of a diet consisting of 2000 kcal/day for adults and children 4 years or older.

BOX 45-2 2015-2020 Dietary Guidelines for Americans: Key Recommendations for the General Population

- Adopt a healthy eating pattern at an appropriate calorie level with a variety of nutrient-dense food and beverages among all the food groups.
- Maintain body weight in a healthy range.
- Encourage physical activity and decrease sedentary activities.
- Encourage fruits, vegetables, whole-grain products, seafood, and fat-free or low-fat milk.
- Eat a variety of proteins, including lean meats, seafood, poultry, eggs, legumes, nuts, seeds, and soy products.
- Limit saturated fats and trans fats, consuming less than 10% of calories per day from saturated fats.
- Limit added sugar or sweeteners so that less than 10% of calories are from added sugars.
- Consume less than 2300 milligrams (mg) of sodium per day.
- Choose and prepare foods with little salt and eat potassium-rich foods.
- Limit intake of alcohol to moderate use (i.e., one drink daily for women and two drinks daily for men).
- Practice food safety to prevent bacterial foodborne illness. Use food-safety principles of *C*lean, *S*eparate, *C*ook, and *C*hill.

Data from US Department of Health and Human Services and US Department of Agriculture: *Dietary guidelines for Americans 2015-2020,* 8e, http://health.gov/dietaryguidelines/2015/guidelines. Accessed January 11, 2016.

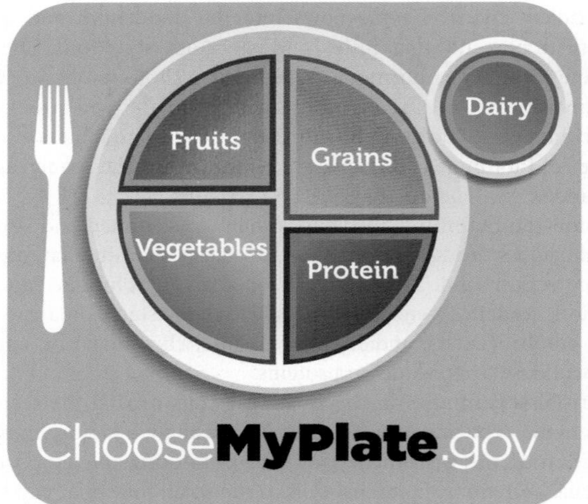

FIGURE 45-2 ChooseMyPlate. (From US Department of Agriculture: ChooseMyPlate, 2011, http://www.choosemyplate.gov).

NURSING KNOWLEDGE BASE

Sociological, cultural, psychological, and emotional factors are associated with eating and drinking in all societies. We celebrate holidays and events with food, bring it to those who are grieving, and use it for medicinal purposes. We incorporate it into family traditions and rituals and often associate food with eating behaviors. You need to understand patients' values, beliefs, and attitudes about food and how these values affect food purchase, preparation, and intake to affect eating patterns.

Nutritional requirements depend on many factors. Individual caloric and nutrient requirements vary by stage of development, body composition, activity levels, pregnancy and lactation, and the presence of disease. Registered dietitians (RDs) use predictive equations that take into account some of these factors to estimate patients' nutritional requirements.

Factors Influencing Nutrition

Environmental Factors. Environmental factors beyond the control of individuals contribute to the development of obesity. Obesity is an epidemic in the United States. Presently 68.7% of Americans are overweight or obese (CDC, 2015). In the annual "F is for Fat" report, authored by the Robert Woods Johnson Foundation and the Trust for America's Health (2013), the adult obesity rate, which consistently increased for three decades, now has leveled off. Proposed contributing factors for obesity are sedentary lifestyle, work schedules, and poor meal choices often related to the increasing frequency of eating away from home and eating fast food (Wang et al., 2013). Environmental factors can limit a person's likelihood of healthy eating and participation in exercise or other activities of healthy living. Lack of access to full-service grocery stores, high cost of healthy food, widespread availability of less healthy foods in fast-food restaurants, widespread advertising of less healthy food, and lack of access to safe places to play and exercise are environmental factors that contribute to obesity (Hedwig et al., 2013).

Developmental Needs

Infants Through School-Age. Rapid growth and high protein, vitamin, mineral, and energy requirements mark the developmental stage of infancy. The average birth weight of an American baby is 7 to 7½ lbs. (3.2 to 3.4 kg). An infant usually doubles birth weight at 4 to 5 months and triples it at 1 year. Infants need an energy intake of approximately 90 to 110 kcal/kg of body weight per day, with premature infants needing 105 to 130 kcal/kg per day (Nix, 2012). Commercial formulas and human breast milk both provide approximately 20 kcal/oz. A full-term newborn is able to digest and absorb simple carbohydrates, proteins, and a moderate amount of emulsified fat. Infants need about 100 to 120 mL/kg/day of fluid because a large part of total body weight is water.

Breastfeeding. The American Academy of Pediatrics strongly supports breastfeeding for the first 6 months of life and breastfeeding with complementary foods from 6 to 12 months (AAP, 2012). Breastfeeding has multiple benefits for both infant and mother, including fewer food allergies and intolerances; fewer infant infections; easier digestion; convenience, availability, and freshness; temperature always correct; economical because it is less expensive than formula; and increased time for mother and infant interaction.

Formula. Infant formulas contain the approximate nutrient composition of human milk. Protein in the formula is typically whey, soy, cow's milk base, casein hydrolysate, or elemental amino acids. Infants with allergies or intolerant to cow's milk should consume soy protein–based formulas instead (Nix, 2012).

Infants should not have regular cow's milk during the first year of life. It is too concentrated for an infant's kidneys to manage, increases the risk of milk-product allergies, and is a poor source of iron and vitamins C and E (Nix, 2012). Furthermore, children under 1 year of age should never ingest honey and corn syrup products because they are potential sources of the botulism toxin, which increases the risk of infant death.

Introduction to Solid Food. Breast milk or formula provides sufficient nutrition for the first 4 to 6 months of life. The development of fine-motor skills of the hand and fingers parallels an infant's interest in food and self-feeding. Iron-fortified cereals are typically the first semisolid food to be introduced. For infants 4 to 11 months, cereals are the most important nonmilk source of protein (Dunne, 2012).

Adding foods to an infant's diet depends on the infant's nutrient needs, physical readiness to handle different forms of foods, and the need to detect and control allergic reactions. Introducing foods that have a high incidence of causing allergic reaction such as wheat, egg white, nuts, citrus juice, and chocolate should happen later in the infant's life (Nix, 2012). In addition, caregivers should introduce new foods one at a time, approximately 4 to 7 days apart to identify allergies. It is best to introduce new foods before milk or other foods to avoid satiety (Hockenberry and Wilson, 2015).

The growth rate slows during toddler years (1 to 3 years). A toddler needs fewer kilocalories but an increased amount of protein in relation to body weight; consequently, appetite often decreases at 18 months of age. Toddlers exhibit strong food preferences and become picky eaters. Small, frequent meals consisting of breakfast, lunch, and dinner with three interspersed high nutrient–dense snacks help improve nutritional intake (Hockenberry and Wilson, 2015). Calcium and phosphorus are important for healthy bone growth.

Toddlers who consume more than 24 ounces of milk daily in place of other foods sometimes develop milk anemia because milk is a poor source of iron. Toddlers need to drink whole milk until the age of 2 years to make sure that there is adequate intake of fatty acids necessary for brain and neurological development. Avoid certain foods such as hot dogs, candy, nuts, grapes, raw vegetables, and popcorn because they present a choking hazard. Dietary requirements for preschoolers (3 to 5 years) are similar to those for toddlers. They consume slightly more than toddlers, and nutrient density is more important than quantity.

School-age children, 6 to 12 years old, grow at a slower and steadier rate, with a gradual decline in energy requirements per unit of body weight. Despite better appetites and more varied food intake, you need to assess school-age children's diets carefully for adequate protein and vitamins A and C. They often fail to eat a proper breakfast and have unsupervised intake at school. High fat, sugar, and salt result from too-liberal intake of snack foods. Physical activity level decreases consistently; and high-calorie, readily available food increases in consumption, leading to an increase in childhood obesity (Hedwig et al., 2013).

In the last 20 years the prevalence of overweight children has risen. The percent of obesity in children ages 6 to 11 years has doubled to 17%, and the percent of overweight adolescents has more than tripled to 17.6% (Li and Hooker, 2010). A combination of factors contributes to the problem, including a diet rich in high-calorie foods, food advertising targeting children, inactivity, genetic predisposition, use of food as a coping mechanism for stress or boredom or as a reward or celebration, and family and socioeconomic factors (Tuan et al., 2012). Childhood obesity contributes to medical problems related to the cardiovascular system, endocrine system, and mental health. With the increase in obesity, the incidence of type 2 diabetes in children is also increasing. Prevention of childhood obesity is critical because of its long-term effects. Family education is an important component in decreasing the prevalence of this problem. Promote healthy food choices and eating in moderation along with increased physical activity.

Adolescents. During adolescence physiological age is a better guide to nutritional needs than chronological age. Energy needs increase to meet greater metabolic demands of growth. Daily requirement of protein also increases. Calcium is essential for the rapid bone growth of adolescence, and girls need a continuous source of iron to replace menstrual losses. Boys also need adequate iron for muscle development. Iodine supports increased thyroid activity, and use of iodized table salt ensures availability. B-complex vitamins are necessary to support heightened metabolic activity.

Many factors other than nutritional needs influence the adolescent's diet, including concern about body image and appearance, desire for independence, eating at fast-food restaurants, peer pressure, and fad diets. Nutritional deficiencies often occur in adolescent girls because of dieting and use of oral contraceptives. An adolescent boy's diet is often inadequate in total kilocalories, protein, iron, folic acid, B vitamins, and iodine. Snacks provide approximately 25% of a teenager's total dietary intake. Fast food, particularly value-size or super-size meals, is common and adds extra salt, fat, and kilocalories. Skipping meals or eating meals with unhealthy choices of snacks contributes to nutrient deficiency and obesity (Hockenberry and Wilson, 2015). Furthermore, research on public school lunch programs demonstrates that adolescents have higher body mass indexes (BMIs) than students enrolled in private school lunch programs (Li and Hooker, 2010).

Fortified foods (nutrients added) are important sources of vitamins and minerals. Snack food from the dairy, fruit, and vegetable groups are good choices. To counter obesity, increasing physical activity is often more important than curbing intake. The onset of eating disorders such as anorexia nervosa or bulimia nervosa often occurs during adolescence. Recognition of eating disorders is essential for early intervention (Box 45-3).

Sports and regular moderate-to-intense exercise necessitate dietary modification to meet increased energy needs for adolescents. Carbohydrates, both simple and complex, are the main source of energy, providing 55% to 60% of total daily kilocalories. Protein needs increase to 1 to 1.5 g/kg/day. Fat needs do not increase. Adequate hydration is very important. Adolescents need to ingest water before and after exercise to prevent dehydration, especially in hot, humid environments.

BOX 45-3 Diagnostic Criteria for Eating Disorders

Anorexia Nervosa

- Restriction of energy intake relative to requirements, leading to a significantly low body weight in relation to age, sex, developmental trajectory, and physical health
- Intense fear of gaining weight or of becoming fat, or persistent behavior that interferes with weight gain, even though at a significantly low weight
- Disturbance in the way in which one's body weight, size, or shape is experienced; undue influence of body weight or shape on self-evaluation; or persistent lack of recognition of the seriousness of the current low body weight (e.g., the person claims to "feel fat" even when emaciated, believes that one area of the body is "too fat" even when obviously underweight)

Bulimia Nervosa

- Recurrent episodes of binge eating (rapid consumption of a large amount of food in a discrete period of time)
- A feeling of lack of control over eating behavior during eating binges
- Recurrent inappropriate compensatory behaviors to prevent weight gain, such as self-induced vomiting, use of laxatives or diuretics, strict dieting or fasting, or vigorous exercise
- Binge eating and inappropriate compensatory behaviors that both occur, on average, at least once a week for 3 months
- Self-evaluation unduly influenced by body shape and weight

Vitamin and mineral supplements are not required, but intake of iron-rich foods is required to prevent anemia.

Parents have more influence on adolescents' diets than they believe. Effective strategies include limiting the amount of unhealthy food choices kept at home; encouraging smart snacks such as fruits, vegetables, or string cheese; and enhancing the appearance and taste of healthy foods (Mayo Clinic Staff, 2015). Some ways to promote healthy eating include making healthy food choices more convenient at home and at fast-food restaurants and discouraging adolescents from eating while watching television or using the computer.

Pregnancy occurring within 4 years of menarche places a mother and fetus at risk because of anatomical and physiological immaturity. Malnutrition at the time of conception increases risk to the adolescent and her fetus. Most teenage girls do not want to gain weight. Counseling related to nutritional needs of pregnancy is often difficult, and teens tolerate suggestions better than rigid directions. The diet of pregnant adolescents is often deficient in calcium, iron, and vitamins A and C. The American College of Obstetricians and Gynecologists recommends prenatal vitamin and mineral supplements.

Young and Middle Adults. There is a reduction in nutrient demands as the growth period ends. Mature adults need nutrients for energy, maintenance, and repair. Energy needs usually decline over the years. Obesity becomes a problem because of decreased physical exercise, dining out more often, and increased ability to afford more luxury foods. Adult women who use oral contraceptives often need extra vitamins. Iron and calcium intake continues to be important.

Pregnancy. Poor nutrition during pregnancy causes low birth weight in infants and decreases chances of survival. Generally meeting the needs of a fetus is at the expense of the mother. However, if nutrient sources are not available, both suffer. The nutritional status of the mother at the time of conception is important. Significant aspects of fetal growth and development often occur before the mother suspects the pregnancy. The energy requirements of pregnancy relate to the mother's body weight and activity. The quality of nutrition during pregnancy is important, and food intake in the first trimester includes balanced parts of essential nutrients with emphasis on quality. Protein intake throughout pregnancy needs to increase to 60 g daily. Calcium intake is especially critical in the third trimester, when fetal bones mineralize. Providing iron supplements to meet the mother's increased blood volume, fetal blood storage, and blood loss during delivery is important.

Folic acid intake is particularly important for DNA synthesis and the growth of red blood cells. Inadequate intake can lead to fetal neural tube defects, anencephaly, or maternal megaloblastic anemia (Nix, 2012). Women of childbearing age need to consume 400 mcg of folic acid daily, increasing to 600 mcg daily during pregnancy. Prenatal care usually includes vitamin and mineral supplementation to ensure daily intakes; however, pregnant women should not take additional supplements beyond prescribed amounts.

Lactation. The lactating woman needs 500 kcal/day above the usual allowance because the production of milk increases energy requirements. Protein requirements during lactation are greater than those required during pregnancy. The need for calcium remains the same as during pregnancy. There is an increased need for vitamins A and C. Daily intake of water-soluble vitamins (B and C) is necessary to ensure adequate levels in breast milk. Fluid intake needs to be adequate but not excessive. Excretion of caffeine, alcohol, and drugs occurs through breast milk. Therefore lactating mothers need to avoid their ingestion.

Older Adults. Adults 65 years and older have a decreased need for energy because their metabolic rate slows with age. However, vitamin and mineral requirements remain unchanged from middle adulthood.

BOX 45-4 FOCUS ON OLDER ADULTS

Factors Affecting Nutritional Status

- Age-related gastrointestinal changes that affect digestion of food and maintenance of nutrition include changes in the teeth and gums, reduced saliva production, atrophy of oral mucosal epithelial cells, increased taste threshold, decreased thirst sensation, reduced gag reflex, and decreased esophageal and colonic peristalsis (Touhy and Jett, 2010).
- The presence of chronic illnesses (e.g., diabetes mellitus, end-stage renal disease, cancer) often affects nutrition intake (CDC, 2015).
- Adequate nutrition in older adults is affected by multiple causes such as lifelong eating habits, culture, socialization, income, educational level, physical functional level to meet activities of daily living (ADLs), loss, dentition, and transportation (Touhy and Jett, 2010).
- Adverse effects of medications cause problems such as anorexia, gastrointestinal bleeding, xerostomia, early satiety, and impaired smell and taste perception (Burcham and Rosenthal, 2016).
- Cognitive impairments such as delirium, dementia, and depression affect ability to obtain, prepare, and eat healthy foods.

Numerous factors influence the nutritional status of the older adult (Box 45-4). Age-related changes in appetite, taste, smell, and the digestive system affect nutrition (Touhy and Jett, 2010). For example, older adults often experience a decrease in taste cells that alters food flavor and may decrease intake. Multiple factors contribute to the risk of food insecurity in the older adult. Income is significant because living on a fixed income often reduces the amount of money available to buy food. Health is another important influence that affects a person's desire and ability to eat. Lack of transportation or ability to get to the grocery store because of mobility problems contributes to inability to purchase adequate and nutritious food. Often availability of nutritionally adequate and safe foods is limited or uncertain.

Maintaining good oral health is significant throughout adulthood, particularly as an individual ages. Difficulty chewing, missing teeth, having teeth in poor condition, and oral pain result from poor oral health. These often contribute to malnutrition and dehydration in older adults (Touhy and Jett, 2010). Poor oral hygiene and periodontal disease are potential risk factors for systemic diseases such as joint infections, ischemic stroke, cardiovascular disease, DM, and aspiration pneumonia (Borrelli and Talih, 2012).

The older adult is often on a therapeutic diet; has difficulty eating because of physical symptoms, lack of teeth, or dentures; or is at risk for drug-nutrient interactions (Table 45-2). Caution older adults to avoid grapefruit and grapefruit juice because they alter absorption of many drugs. Thirst sensation diminishes, leading to inadequate fluid intake or dehydration (see Chapter 42). Symptoms of dehydration in older adults include confusion; weakness; hot, dry skin; furrowed tongue; rapid pulse; and high urinary sodium. Some older adults avoid meats because of cost or because they are difficult to chew. Cream soups and meat-based vegetable soups are nutrient-dense sources of protein. Cheese, eggs, and peanut butter are also useful high-protein alternatives. Milk continues to be an important food for older women and men who need adequate calcium to protect against osteoporosis (a decrease of bone mass density). Screening and treatment are necessary for both older men and women. Vitamin D supplements are important for improving strength and balance, strengthening bone health, and preventing bone fractures and falls. The diet of older adults needs to contain choices from all food groups and often requires a vitamin and mineral supplement. MyPlate for Older Adults addresses the specific nutritional needs for older adults and encourages physical activity (Tufts University, 2011).

The USDHHS Administration on Aging (AOA) requires states to provide nutritional screening services to older adults who benefit from home-delivered or congregate meal services. This program requires meals to provide at least one third of the DRI for an older adult and meet the Dietary Guidelines for Americans (American Dietetic Association, 2010a). Homebound older adults with chronic illnesses have additional nutritional risks. They frequently live alone with little or no social or financial resources to help obtain or prepare nutritionally sound meals, contributing to the risk for food insecurity. Approximately 19% of older adults experience some degree of food insecurity resulting from low income or poverty (American Dietetic Association, 2010a). Increased nutrition screening by the nurse results in early recognition and treatment of nutritional deficiencies. Undernourishment of older adults often results in health problems that lead to admission to acute care hospitals or long-term care facilities.

Alternative Food Patterns

Long before the FDA issued recommended allowances and guidelines, many people followed special patterns of food intake on the basis of religion (Table 45-3), cultural background (Box 45-5), health beliefs, personal preference, or concern for the efficient use of land to produce food. Such special diets are not necessarily more or less nutritious than diets based on the MyPlate or other nutritional guidelines because good nutrition depends on a balanced intake of all required nutrients.

Vegetarian Diet. A common alternative dietary pattern is the vegetarian diet. **Vegetarianism** is the consumption of a diet consisting predominantly of plant foods. Some vegetarians are ovolactovegetarian (avoid meat, fish, and poultry but eat eggs and milk), lactovegetarians (drink milk but avoid eggs), or vegans (consume only plant foods). Through careful selection of foods, individuals following a vegetarian diet can meet recommendations for proteins and essential nutrients (Nix, 2012). Zen macrobiotic (primarily brown rice, other grains, and herb teas) and fruitarian (only fruit, nuts, honey, and olive oil) diets are nutrient poor and frequently result in malnutrition. Knowledge related to complementary use of high and low biological value proteins is necessary. Children who follow a vegetarian diet are especially at risk for protein and vitamin deficiencies such as vitamin B_{12}. Careful planning helps to ensure a balanced, healthy diet.

CRITICAL THINKING

Successful critical thinking requires a synthesis of knowledge, experience, information gathered from patients, critical thinking attitudes, and intellectual and professional standards. Clinical judgments require you to anticipate information, analyze the data, and make decisions regarding your patient's care. During assessment consider all elements that build toward making an appropriate nursing diagnosis (Figure 45-3).

Integrate knowledge from nursing and other disciplines, previous experiences, and information gathered from patients and families regarding customary food preferences and recent diet history. Use of professional standards such as the DRIs, the USDA MyPlate dietary guidelines, and *Healthy People 2020* objectives provide guidelines to assess and maintain patients' nutritional status. Other professional standards by the AHA (2010), the American Diabetes Association (ADA, 2012), The ACS (2015), and the American Society for Parenteral and Enteral Nutrition (National Guideline Clearinghouse, 2013) are

TABLE 45-2 Sample of Drug-Nutrient Interactions*

Drug	Effect
Analgesic	
Acetaminophen	Decreased drug absorption with food; overdose associated with liver failure
Aspirin	Absorbed directly through stomach; decreased drug absorption with food; decreased folic acid, vitamins C and K, and iron absorption
Antacid	
Aluminum hydroxide	Decreased phosphate absorption
Sodium bicarbonate	Decreased folic acid absorption
Antiarrhythmic	
Amiodarone (Cordarone)	Taste alteration
Digitalis	Anorexia, decreased renal clearance in older people
Antibiotic	
Penicillin	Decreased drug absorption with food, taste alteration
Cephalosporin	Decreased vitamin K
Rifampin (Rifadin)	Decreased vitamin B_6, niacin, vitamin D
Tetracycline	Decreased drug absorption with milk and antacids; decreased nutrient absorption of calcium, riboflavin, vitamin C caused by binding
Trimethoprim/sulfamethoxazole	Decreased folic acid
Anticoagulant	
Warfarin (Coumadin)	Acts as antagonist to vitamin K
Anticonvulsant	
Carbamazepine (Tegretol)	Increased drug absorption with food
Phenytoin (Dilantin)	Decreased calcium absorption; decreased vitamins D and K and folic acid; taste alteration; decreased drug absorption with food
Antidepressant	
Amitriptyline	Appetite stimulant
Clomipramine (Anafranil)	Taste alteration, appetite stimulant
Fluoxetine (Prozac) (selective serotonin reuptake inhibitors [SSRIs])	Taste alteration, anorexia
Antihypertensive	
Captopril (Capoten)	Taste alteration, anorexia
Hydralazine	Enhanced drug absorption with food, decreased vitamin B_6
Labetalol (Normodyne)	Taste alteration (weight gain for all beta-blockers)
Methyldopa	Decreased vitamin B_{12}, folic acid, iron
Antiinflammatory	
All steroids	Increased appetite and weight, increased folic acid, decreased calcium (osteoporosis with long-term use); promotes gluconeogenesis of protein
Antiparkinson	
Levodopa (Dopar)	Taste alteration, decreased vitamin B_6 and drug absorption with food
Antipsychotic	
Chlorpromazine	Increased appetite
Thiothixene	Decreased riboflavin, increased need
Bronchodilator	
Albuterol sulfate	Appetite stimulant
Theophylline	Anorexia
Cholesterol Lowering	
Cholestyramine (Prevalite)	Decreased fat-soluble vitamins (A, D, E, K); vitamin B_{12}; iron
Diuretic	
Furosemide (Lasix)	Decreased drug absorption with food
Spironolactone (Aldactone)	Increased drug absorption with food
Thiazides	Decreased magnesium, zinc, and potassium
Laxative	
Mineral oil	Decreased absorption of fat-soluble vitamins (A, D, E, K), carotene
Platelet Aggregate Inhibitor	
Dipyridamole (Persantine)	Decreased drug absorption with food
Potassium Replacement	
Potassium chloride	Decreased vitamin B_{12}
Tranquilizer	
Benzodiazepines	Increased appetite

Data from Hermann J: *Nutrient and drug interactions,* http://pods.dasnr.okstate.edu/docushare/dsweb/Get/Document-2458/T-3120web.pdf. Accessed August 20, 2014; Burcham and Rosenthal: *Lehne's pharmacology for nursing care,* ed 9, St Louis, 2016, Elsevier.

*Not intended to be an exhaustive or all-inclusive list. Always check pharmacology references before administering medications.

TABLE 45-3 Religious Dietary Restrictions

Muslim	Christianity	Hinduism	Judaism	Church of Jesus Christ of Latter-Day Saints (Mormons)	Seventh-Day Adventists Church
Pork Alcohol Caffeine Ramadan fasting sunrise to sunset for a month Ritualized methods of animal slaughter required for meat ingestion	Some faiths such as Baptists have minimal or no alcohol Some meatless days may be observed during the calendar year, commonly during Lent	All meats Fish, shellfish with some restrictions Alcohol	Pork Predatory fowl Shellfish (eat only fish with scales) Rare meats Blood (e.g., blood sausage) Mixing of milk or dairy products with meat dishes Must adhere to kosher food preparation methods 24 hr of fasting on Yom Kippur, a day of atonement No leavened bread eaten during Passover (8 days) No cooking on the Sabbath from sundown Friday to sundown Saturday	Alcohol Tobacco Caffeine such as teas, coffees, and sodas	Pork Shellfish Fish Alcohol Caffeine Vegetarian or ovolactovegetarian diets encouraged

BOX 45-5 CULTURAL ASPECTS OF CARE

Nutrition

Food patterns developed as a child, habits, and culture interact to influence food intake. Culture also influences the meaning of food not related to nutrition. Eating is associated with sentiments and feelings such as "good" and "bad." For example, children are often rewarded for "being good" with a treat such as candy. They then associate candy with "being good." Food frequently enhances interpersonal relationships and demonstrates love and caring.

The incidence of lactose intolerance around the world occurs in the following ethnic or racial groups: Asian-Pacific, African and African-American, Native American, Mexican American, Middle Eastern, and Caucasians. The incidence is highest in Asian-Pacific populations and lowest in Caucasians. It affects nutrient absorption. Calcium deficiency often results, causing decreased bone mass density.

The theory of hot and cold foods predominates in many cultures. The origin appears to be from Hippocratic beliefs concerning health and the four humors. Arabs were keepers of this knowledge during the Dark Ages and later influenced the Spanish to adopt this belief system in the later Middle Ages. The foundation of the theory is keeping harmony with nature by balancing "cold," "hot," "wet," and "dry." Some cultures believe that hot is warmth, strength, and reassurance; whereas cold is menacing and weak. Classification has nothing to do with spiciness but is a symbolic representation of temperature (Giger and Davidhizar, 2012). Different cultures also have beliefs about food and special dishes that should be eaten when sick (e.g., chicken soup during illness).

Implications for Patient-Centered Care

- Ask patient or family caregiver to identify the meaning that types of food have for each patient.
- Lactose and other food intolerances unique to specific cultures require diet adaptation to meet nutrient, mineral, and vitamin daily intake requirements.
- When patients use hot and cold foods as part of their cultural health practices, dietary modifications are necessary. Hot foods include rice, grain cereals, alcohol, beef, lamb, chili peppers, chocolate, cheese, temperate zone fruits, eggs, peas, goat's milk, cornhusks, oils, onions, pork, radishes, and tamales. By contrast, cold foods are beans, citrus fruits, tropical fruits, dairy products, most vegetables, honey, raisins, chicken, fish, and goat.
- Ask patient or family caregiver if there are:
  - Specific conditions such as menstruation, cancer, pneumonia, earache, colds, paralysis, headache, and rheumatism, which are cold illnesses and require hot foods.
  - Other conditions such as pregnancy, fever, infections, diarrhea, rashes, ulcers, liver problems, constipation, kidney problems, and sore throats, which are hot conditions and require cold foods.

available. These standards are evidence based and regularly updated for optimal patient care.

❖ NURSING PROCESS

Apply the nursing process and use a critical thinking approach in your care of patients. The nursing process provides a clinical decision-making approach for you to develop and implement an individualized plan of care.

◆ Assessment

During the assessment process thoroughly assess each patient and critically analyze findings to ensure that you make patient-centered clinical decisions required for safe nursing care. Early recognition of malnourished or at-risk patients has a strong positive influence on both short- and long-term health outcomes. Studies demonstrate a link between malnutrition in adult hospitalized patients and readmission rates, higher mortality rates, and increased cost (Tappenden et al., 2013). Patients who are malnourished on admission are at greater risk of life-threatening complications such as arrhythmia, sepsis, or hemorrhage during hospitalization.

Through the Patient's Eyes. Assess patients' nutritional status by using the nursing history to gather information about factors that usually influence nutrition. You are in an excellent position to recognize signs of poor nutrition and take steps to initiate change. Close contact with patients and their families enables you to observe physical status, food intake, food preferences, weight changes, and response to therapy. Always ask patients about their food preferences, values regarding nutrition, and expectations from nutritional therapy. In attempting to affect eating patterns, you need to understand patients' values, beliefs, and attitudes about food. Also assess family traditions

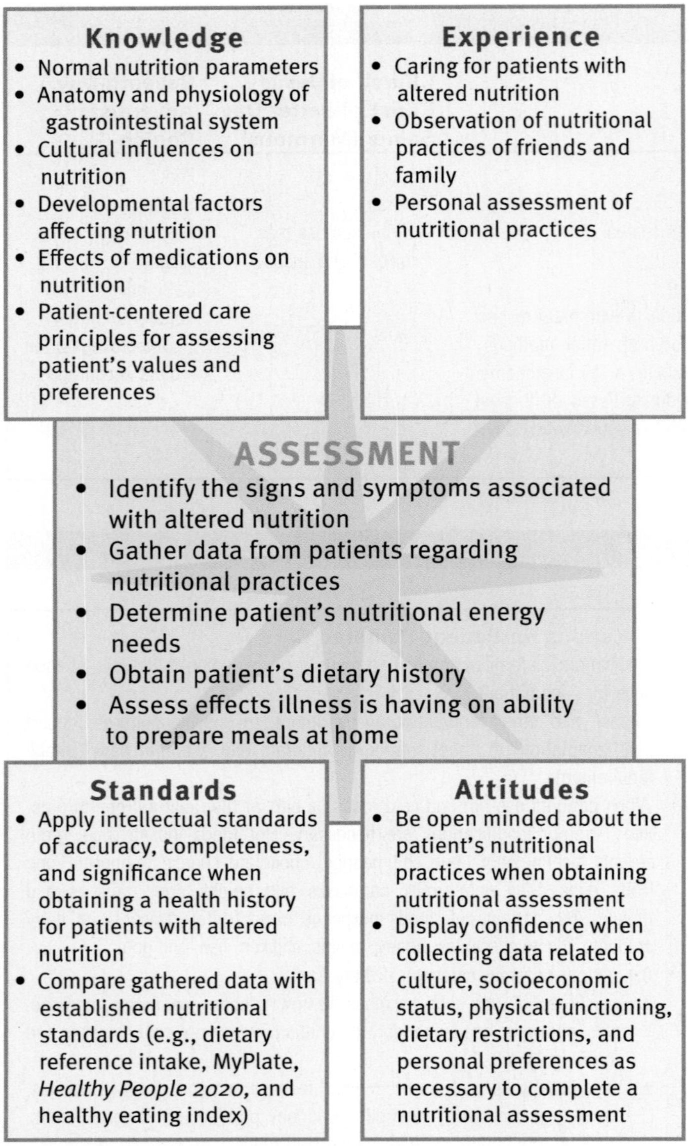

Knowledge
- Normal nutrition parameters
- Anatomy and physiology of gastrointestinal system
- Cultural influences on nutrition
- Developmental factors affecting nutrition
- Effects of medications on nutrition
- Patient-centered care principles for assessing patient's values and preferences

Experience
- Caring for patients with altered nutrition
- Observation of nutritional practices of friends and family
- Personal assessment of nutritional practices

ASSESSMENT
- Identify the signs and symptoms associated with altered nutrition
- Gather data from patients regarding nutritional practices
- Determine patient's nutritional energy needs
- Obtain patient's dietary history
- Assess effects illness is having on ability to prepare meals at home

Standards
- Apply intellectual standards of accuracy, completeness, and significance when obtaining a health history for patients with altered nutrition
- Compare gathered data with established nutritional standards (e.g., dietary reference intake, MyPlate, *Healthy People 2020*, and healthy eating index)

Attitudes
- Be open minded about the patient's nutritional practices when obtaining nutritional assessment
- Display confidence when collecting data related to culture, socioeconomic status, physical functioning, dietary restrictions, and personal preferences as necessary to complete a nutritional assessment

FIGURE 45-3 Critical thinking model for nutrition assessment.

and rituals related to food, cultural values and beliefs, and nutritional needs. Determine how these factors affect food purchase, preparation, and intake.

Screening. Nutrition screening is an essential part of an initial assessment. Screening a patient is a quick method of identifying malnutrition or risk of malnutrition using simple tools (Holst et al., 2013). Nutrition screening tools gather data on the current condition, stability of the condition, assessment of whether it will worsen, and if the disease process accelerates. These tools typically include objective measures such as height, weight, weight change, primary diagnosis, and the presence of other co-morbidities (Holst et al., 2013). Combine multiple objective measures with subjective measures related to nutrition to adequately screen for nutritional problems. Identification of risk factors such as unintentional weight loss, presence of a modified diet, or the presence of altered nutritional symptoms (i.e., nausea, vomiting, diarrhea, and constipation) requires nutritional consultation.

Several standardized nutritional screening tools are available for use in outpatient and inpatient settings. The Subjective Global Assessment (SGA) uses the patient history, weight, and physical assessment data to assess nutritional status (Tsai et al., 2013). The SGA is a simple, inexpensive technique that is able to predict nutrition-related complications. The Mini Nutritional Assessment (MNA) (Figure 45-4) screens older adults in home care programs, nursing homes, and hospitals. The tool has 18 items divided into screening and assessment. If a patient scores 11 or less on the screening part, the health care provider completes the assessment part. A total score of less than 17 indicates protein-energy malnutrition (Guigoz and Vellas, 1999; Guigoz et al., 1996). In conclusion, malnutrition screening tools (MSTs) are an effective way to measure nutritional problems for patients in a variety of health care settings.

Assess patients for malnutrition when they have conditions that interfere with their ability to ingest, digest, or absorb adequate nutrients. Use standardized tools to assess nutrition risks when possible. Congenital anomalies and surgical revisions of the GI tract interfere with normal function. Patients receiving only an IV infusion of 5% or 10% dextrose are at risk for nutritional deficiencies. Chronic diseases or increased metabolic requirements are risk factors for development of nutritional problems. Infants and older adults are at greatest risk.

Anthropometry. Anthropometry is a measurement system of the size and makeup of the body. Nurses obtain height and weight for each patient on hospital admission or entry into any health care setting. If you are not able to measure height with the patient standing, position him or her lying flat in bed as straight as possible with arms folded on the chest and measure him or her lengthwise. Serial measures of weight over time provide more useful information than one measurement. Weigh the patient at the same time each day, on the same scale, and with the same type of clothing or linen. Document the patient's actual weight and compare height and weight to standards for height-weight relationships. An ideal body weight (IBW) provides an estimate of what a person should weigh. Rapid weight gain or loss is important to note because it usually reflects fluid shifts. One pint or 500 mL of fluid equals 1 lb (0.45 kg). For example, for a patient with renal failure, a weight increase of 2 lbs (0.90 kg) in 24 hours is significant because it usually indicates that the patient has retained 1 L (1000 mL) of fluid.

Other anthropometric measurements often obtained by RDs help identify nutritional problems. These include the ratio of height-to-wrist circumference, mid–upper arm circumference (MAC), triceps skinfold (TSF), and mid–upper arm muscle circumference (MAMC). An RD compares values for MAC, TSF, and MAMC to standards and calculates them as a percentage of the standard. Changes in values for an individual over time are of greater significance than isolated measurements (Nix, 2012).

Body mass index (BMI) measures weight corrected for height and serves as an alternative to traditional height-weight relationships. Calculate BMI by dividing a patient's weight in kilograms by height in meters squared: weight (kg) divided by height^2 (m^2). For example, a patient who weighs 165 lbs (75 kg) and is 1.8 m (5 feet 9 inches) tall has a BMI of 23.15 ($75 \div 1.8^2 = 23.15$). The website for the National Heart Lung and Blood Institute (http://www.nhlbi.nih.gov/) provides an easy way to calculate BMI. A patient is overweight if his or her BMI is 25 to 30. Obesity, defined by a BMI of greater than 30, places a patient at higher medical risk of coronary heart disease, some cancers, DM, and hypertension.

Laboratory and Biochemical Tests. No single laboratory or biochemical test is diagnostic for malnutrition. Factors that frequently alter test results include fluid balance, liver function, kidney function,

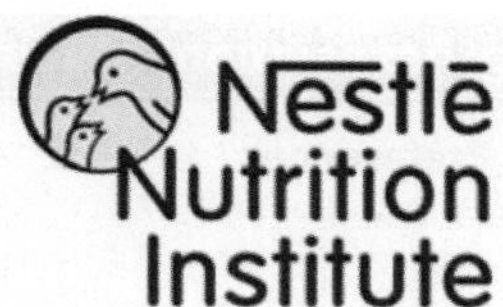

Mini Nutritional Assessment
MNA®

Last name: First name:

Sex: Age: Weight, kg: Height, cm: Date:

Complete the screen by filling in the boxes with the appropriate numbers. Total the numbers for the final screening score.

Screening

A Has food intake declined over the past 3 months due to loss of appetite, digestive problems, chewing or swallowing difficulties?
0 = severe decrease in food intake
1 = moderate decrease in food intake
2 = no decrease in food intake

B Weight loss during the last 3 months
0 = weight loss greater than 3 kg (6.6 lbs)
1 = does not know
2 = weight loss between 1 and 3 kg (2.2 and 6.6 lbs)
3 = no weight loss

C Mobility
0 = bed or chair bound
1 = able to get out of bed / chair but does not go out
2 = goes out

D Has suffered psychological stress or acute disease in the past 3 months?
0 = yes 2 = no

E Neuropsychological problems
0 = severe dementia or depression
1 = mild dementia
2 = no psychological problems

F1 Body Mass Index (BMI) (weight in kg) / (height in m^2)
0 = BMI less than 19
1 = BMI 19 to less than 21
2 = BMI 21 to less than 23
3 = BMI 23 or greater

IF BMI IS NOT AVAILABLE, REPLACE QUESTION F1 WITH QUESTION F2.
DO NOT ANSWER QUESTION F2 IF QUESTION F1 IS ALREADY COMPLETED.

F2 Calf circumference (CC) in cm
0 = CC less than 31
3 = CC 31 or greater

Screening score
(max. 14 points)

12-14 points: Normal nutritional status
8-11 points: At risk of malnutrition
0-7 points: Malnourished

Ref. Vellas B, Villars H, Abellan G, et al. *Overview of the MNA® - Its History and Challenges.* J Nutr Health Aging 2006;10:456-465.
Rubenstein LZ, Harker JO, Salva A, Guigoz Y, Vellas B. *Screening for Undernutrition in Geriatric Practice: Developing the Short-Form Mini Nutritional Assessment (MNA-SF).* J. Geront 2001;56A: M366-377.
Guigoz Y. *The Mini-Nutritional Assessment (MNA®) Review of the Literature - What does it tell us?* J Nutr Health Aging 2006; 10:466-487.
Kaiser MJ, Bauer JM, Ramsch C, et al. *Validation of the Mini Nutritional Assessment Short-Form (MNA®-SF): A practical tool for identification of nutritional status.* J Nutr Health Aging 2009; 13:782-788.

For more information: www.mna-elderly.com

FIGURE 45-4 Mini Nutritional Assessment (MNA). (Copyright ©Nestlé, 1994, Revision 2009. N67200 12/99 10M.)

and the presence of disease. Common laboratory tests used to study nutritional status include measures of plasma proteins such as albumin, transferrin, prealbumin, retinol-binding protein, total iron-binding capacity, and hemoglobin. After feeding, the response time for changes in these proteins ranges from hours to weeks. The metabolic half-life of albumin is 21 days, transferrin is 8 days, prealbumin is 2 days, and retinol-binding protein is 12 hours. Use this information to determine the most effective measure of plasma proteins for your patients. Factors that affect serum albumin levels include hydration; hemorrhage; renal or hepatic disease; large amounts of drainage from wounds, drains, burns, or the GI tract; steroid administration; exogenous albumin infusions; age; and trauma, burns, stress, or surgery. Albumin level is a better indicator for chronic illnesses, whereas prealbumin level is preferred for acute conditions (Jensen et al., 2013).

Nitrogen balance is important in determining serum protein status (see discussion of protein in this chapter). Calculate nitrogen balance by dividing 6.25 into the total grams of protein ingested in a day (24 hours). Use laboratory analysis of a 24-hour urine urea nitrogen (UUN) to determine nitrogen output. For patients with diarrhea or fistula drainage, estimate a further addition of 2 to 4 g of nitrogen output. Calculate nitrogen balance by subtracting the nitrogen output from the nitrogen intake. A positive 2- to 3-g nitrogen balance is necessary for anabolism. By contrast, negative nitrogen balance is present when catabolic states exist.

Diet History and Health History. In addition to the general nursing history, use data from a more specific diet history to assess a patient's actual or potential nutritional needs. Box 45-6 lists some specific assessment questions to ask in the diet history. The diet history focuses on a patient's habitual intake of foods and liquids and includes information about preferences, allergies, and other relevant areas such as the patient's ability to obtain food. Gather information about the patient's illness/activity level to determine energy needs and compare food intake. Your nursing assessment of nutrition includes health status; age; cultural background (see Box 45-5); religious food patterns (see Table 45-3); socioeconomic status; personal food preferences; psychological factors; use of alcohol or illegal drugs; use of vitamin, mineral, or herbal supplements; prescription or over-the-counter (OTC) drugs (see Table 45-2); and the patient's general nutrition knowledge.

In an outpatient setting, have a patient keep a 3- to 7-day food diary. This allows you to calculate nutritional intake and to compare it with DRI to see if the patient's dietary habits are adequate. Use food questionnaires to establish patterns over time. In a health care setting nurses collaborate with RDs to complete calorie counts for patients.

Physical Examination. The physical examination is one of the most important aspects of a nutritional assessment. Because improper nutrition affects all body systems, observe for malnutrition during physical assessment (see Chapter 31). Complete the general physical assessment of body systems and recheck relevant areas to evaluate a patient's nutritional status. The clinical signs of nutritional status (Table 45-4) serve as guidelines for observation during physical assessment.

Dysphagia. Dysphagia refers to difficulty swallowing. The causes (Box 45-7) and complications of dysphagia vary. Complications include aspiration pneumonia, dehydration, decreased nutritional status, and weight loss. Dysphagia leads to disability or decreased functional status, increased length of stay and cost of care, increased likelihood of discharge to institutionalized care, and increased mortality (Ellis and Hannibal, 2013).

BOX 45-6 Nursing Assessment Questions

Dietary Intake and Food Preferences
- What type of food do you like?
- How many meals a day do you eat?
- What times do you normally eat meals and snacks?
- What portion sizes do you eat at each meal?
- Are you on a special diet because of a medical problem?
- Do you have any dietary religious or cultural food preferences?
- Who prepares the food at home?
- Who purchases the food?
- How do you cook your food (e.g., fried, broiled, baked, grilled)?

Unpleasant Symptoms
- Which foods cause indigestion, gas, or heartburn?
- Does this occur each time you have the food?
- What relieves the symptoms?

Allergies
- Are you allergic to any foods?
- Which types of problems do you have with these foods?
- How are these food allergies treated (e.g., EpiPen, oral antihistamines)?

Taste, Chewing, and Swallowing
- Have you noticed any changes in taste?
- Did these changes occur with medications or following an illness?
- Do you wear dentures? Are the dentures comfortable?
- Do you have any mouth pain or sores (e.g., cold sore, canker sores)?
- Do you have difficulty swallowing?
- Do you cough or gag when you swallow?

Appetite and Weight
- Have you had a change in appetite?
- Have you noticed a change in your weight?
- Was this change anticipated (e.g., were you on a weight-reduction diet)?

Use of Medications
- Which medications do you take?
- Do you take any over-the-counter medications that your doctor does not prescribe?
- Do you take any nutritional or herbal supplements?

Be aware of warning signs for dysphagia. They include cough during eating; change in voice tone or quality after swallowing; abnormal movements of the mouth, tongue, or lips; and slow, weak, imprecise, or uncoordinated speech. Abnormal gag, delayed swallowing, incomplete oral clearance or pocketing, regurgitation, pharyngeal pooling, delayed or absent trigger of swallow, and inability to speak consistently are other signs of dysphagia. Patients with dysphagia often do not show overt signs such as coughing when food enters the airway. *Silent aspiration* is aspiration that occurs in patients with neurological problems that lead to decreased sensation. It often occurs without a cough, and symptoms usually do not appear for 24 hour. Silent aspiration accounts for most of the 51% to 78% of aspiration in patients with dysphagia following stroke (Sorensen et al., 2013).

Dysphagia often leads to an inadequate amount of food intake, which results in malnutrition. Frequently patients with dysphagia become frustrated with eating and show changes in skinfold thickness and albumin. During the rehabilitation period patients experience longer adjustment periods regarding new dietary restrictions. Furthermore, malnutrition significantly slows swallowing recovery and may increase mortality (Jensen et al., 2013).

TABLE 45-4 Physical Signs of Nutritional Status

Body Area	Signs of Good Nutrition	Signs of Poor Nutrition
General appearance	Alert: responsive	Listless, apathetic, cachectic
Weight	Weight normal for height, age, body build	Obesity (usually 10% above ideal body weight [IBW]) or underweight (special concern for underweight)
Posture	Erect posture; straight arms and legs	Sagging shoulders; sunken chest; humped back
Muscles	Well-developed, firm; good tone; some fat under skin	Flaccid, poor tone, underdeveloped tone; "wasted" appearance; impaired ability to walk properly
Nerve conduction and mental status	Good attention span; not irritable or restless; normal reflexes; psychological stability	Inattention; irritability; confusion; burning and tingling of hands and feet (paresthesia); loss of position and vibratory sense; weakness and tenderness of muscles (may result in inability to walk); decrease or loss of ankle and knee reflexes
Gastrointestinal function	Good appetite and digestion; normal regular elimination; no palpable organs or masses	Anorexia; indigestion; constipation or diarrhea; liver or spleen enlargement
Cardiovascular function	Normal heart rate and rhythm; lack of murmurs; normal blood pressure for age	Rapid heart rate (above 100 beats/min), enlarged heart; abnormal rhythm; elevated blood pressure
General vitality	Endurance; energy; sleeps well; vigorous	Easily fatigued; no energy; falls asleep easily; tired and apathetic
Hair	Shiny, lustrous; firm; not easily plucked; healthy scalp	Stringy, dull, brittle, dry, thin, and sparse, depigmented; easily plucked
Skin (general)	Smooth and slightly moist skin with good color	Rough, dry, scaly, pale, pigmented, irritated; bruises; petechiae; subcutaneous fat loss
Face and neck	Uniform color; smooth, pink, healthy appearance; not swollen	Greasy, discolored, scaly, swollen; dark skin over cheeks and under eyes; lumpiness or flakiness of skin around nose and mouth
Lips	Smooth; good color; moist; not chapped or swollen	Dry, scaly, swollen; redness and swelling (cheilosis); angular lesions at corners of mouth; fissures or scars (stomatitis)
Mouth, oral membranes	Reddish-pink mucous membranes in oral cavity	Swollen, boggy oral mucous membranes
Gums	Good pink color; healthy and red; no swelling or bleeding	Spongy gums that bleed easily; marginal redness, inflammation; receding
Tongue	Good pink or deep reddish color; no swelling; smooth, presence of surface papillae; lack of lesions	Swelling, scarlet and raw; magenta, beefiness (glossitis); hyperemic and hypertrophic papillae; atrophic papillae
Teeth	No cavities; no pain; bright, straight; no crowding; well-shaped jaw; clean with no discoloration	Unfilled caries; missing teeth; worn surfaces; mottled (fluorosis), malocclusion
Eyes	Bright, clear, shiny; no sores at corner of eyelids; moist and healthy pink conjunctivae; prominent blood vessels; no fatigue circles beneath eyes	Eye membranes pale (pale conjunctivas); redness of membrane (conjunctival injection); dryness; signs of infection; Bitot's spots; redness and fissuring of eyelid corners (angular palpebritis); dryness of eye membrane (conjunctival xerosis); dull appearance of cornea (corneal xerosis); soft cornea (keratomalacia)
Neck (glands)	No enlargement	Thyroid or lymph node enlargement
Nails	Firm, pink	Spoon shape (koilonychia); brittleness; ridges
Legs, feet	No tenderness, weakness, or swelling; good color	Edema; tender calf; tingling; weakness
Skeleton	No malformations	Bowlegs; knock-knees; chest deformity at diaphragm; prominent scapulae and ribs

From Nix S: *Williams' basic nutrition and diet therapy,* ed 14, St Louis, 2012, Mosby.

Dysphagia screening quickly identifies problems with swallowing and helps you initiate referrals for more in-depth assessment by an RD or a speech-language pathologist (SLP) (see Skill 45-1 on pp. 1083-1085). Early and ongoing assessment of patients with dysphagia using a valid dysphagia-screening tool increases quality of care and decreases incidence of aspiration pneumonia. Dysphagia screening includes medical record review; observation of a patient at a meal for change in voice quality, posture, and head control; percentage of meal consumed; eating time; drooling or leakage of liquids and solids; cough during/after a swallow; facial or tongue weakness; palatal movement; difficulty with secretions; pocketing; choking; and a spontaneous dry cough. A number of validated screening tools are available such as the Bedside Swallowing Assessment, Burke Dysphagia Screening Test, Acute Stroke Dysphagia Screen, and Standardized Swallowing Assessment (Edmiaston et al., 2010). The Acute Stroke Dysphagia screen is an easily administered and reliable tool for health care professionals who are not speech-language pathologists (SLPs). Screening for and treatment of dysphagia requires a multidisciplinary team approach of nurses, RDs, health care providers, and SLPs (Sorensen et al., 2013).

BOX 45-7 Causes of Dysphagia

Myogenic
- Myasthenia gravis
- Aging
- Muscular dystrophy
- Polymyositis

Neurogenic
- Stroke
- Cerebral palsy
- Guillain-Barré syndrome
- Multiple sclerosis
- Amyotrophic lateral sclerosis (Lou Gehrig disease)
- Diabetic neuropathy
- Parkinson's disease

Obstructive
- Benign peptic stricture
- Lower esophageal ring
- Candidiasis
- Head and neck cancer
- Inflammatory masses
- Trauma/surgical resection
- Anterior mediastinal masses
- Cervical spondylosis

Other
- Gastrointestinal or esophageal resection
- Rheumatological disorders
- Connective tissue disorders
- Vagotomy

BOX 45-8 Nursing Diagnostic Process

Imbalanced Nutrition: Less Than Body Requirements

Assessment Activities	Defining Characteristics
Body mass index (BMI)	Body mass index (BMI) = 17
Obtain weight	68-year-old woman 24-lb (10.8-kg) weight loss Weight is 20% below her ideal body weight
Obtain 24-hour food and fluid history	Lack of satiety Lack of interest in food Fluid intake is juice and coffee Eats sandwich in afternoon
Physical assessment	Poor muscle tone Fatigue Hair loss Dry scaly skin Pale conjunctiva and mucous membranes
Medication	Takes sertraline for depression
Social	Husband died 6 months ago Has quit attending monthly quilting club Started counseling 3 months ago

◆ Nursing Diagnosis

Cluster all assessment data to identify appropriate nursing diagnoses (Box 45-8). A nutritional problem occurs when overall intake is significantly decreased or increased or when one or more nutrients are not ingested, completely digested, or completely absorbed. When identifying a problem-focused nursing diagnosis, you select the appropriate related factors (e.g., inability to digest food or reduced daily activity). Related factors need to be accurate so you select the right interventions. For example, *Imbalanced Nutrition: Less Than Body Requirements* related to economic disadvantage will require very different interventions than *Imbalanced Nutrition: Less Than Body Requirements* related to an inability to ingest food.

A patient will have a risk nursing diagnosis when assessment reveals risk factors. For example, *Risk for Overweight* can be identified by the presence of risk factors such as excessive alcohol consumption or high frequency of eating restaurant food and adult BMI approaching 25 kg/m^2. Be specific so you can direct interventions toward risk factors.

Defining characteristics may also point to a health promotion diagnosis such as *Readiness for Enhanced Nutrition*. The following are nursing diagnoses applicable to nutritional problems:

- *Risk for Aspiration*
- *Diarrhea*
- *Overweight*
- *Imbalanced Nutrition: Less Than Body Requirements*
- *Readiness for Enhanced Nutrition*
- *Feeding Self-Care Deficit*
- *Impaired Swallowing*
- *Obesity*

In addition, there are clinical situations in which patients have multiple related nursing diagnoses. The concept map in Figure 45-5 shows the relationship of nursing diagnoses for Mrs. Cooper.

◆ Planning

Planning to maintain patients' optimal nutritional status requires a higher level of care than simply correcting nutritional problems. Often there is a need for patients to make long-term changes for nutrition to improve. Synthesis of patient information from multiple sources is necessary to create an individualized approach of care that is relevant to a patient's needs and situation (Figure 45-6). Apply critical thinking to ensure that you consider all data sources in developing a patient's plan of care. The accurate identification of nursing diagnoses related to patients' nutritional problems results in a care plan that is relevant and appropriate (see the Nursing Care Plan). Referring to professional standards for nutrition is especially important during this step, because scientific findings support current published standards.

Goals and Outcomes. Goals and outcomes of care reflect a patient's physiological, therapeutic, and individualized needs. Nutrition education and counseling are important to prevent disease and promote health. Educate your patients about the therapeutic diet prescribed, specifically on how it controls their illnesses and if there are any implications. When planning care, be aware of all factors that influence a patient's food intake. For example, patients with heart failure experience decreased hunger, dietary restrictions, fatigue, shortness of breath, and sadness, which influence their food intake.

Individualized planning is essential. Explore patients' feelings about their weight and diet and help them set realistic and achievable goals. Mutually planned goals negotiated among the patient, RD, and nurse ensure success. For the patient with heart failure described previously, an overall goal is "Patient will achieve appropriate BMI height-weight range or be within 10% of IBW." The following outcomes help to achieve this goal:

- Patient's daily nutritional intake meets the minimal DRIs.
- Patient's daily nutritional fat intake is less than 30%.
- Patient removes sugared beverages and high carbohydrate foods from diet.
- Patient refrains from eating unhealthy foods between meals and after dinner.
- Patient loses at least ½ to 1 lb (0.2 to 0.45 kg) per week.

Meeting nutritional goals requires input from the patient and the interprofessional team. Knowledge of the role of each discipline in providing nutrition support is necessary to maximize nutritional outcomes. For example, collaboration with an RD helps develop appropriate nutrition treatment plans. Calorie counts are frequently ordered, and help is necessary to obtain accurate data. An effective plan of care requires accurate exchange of information among disciplines.

Setting Priorities. After identifying patients' nursing diagnoses, determine priorities to plan timely and successful interventions. For

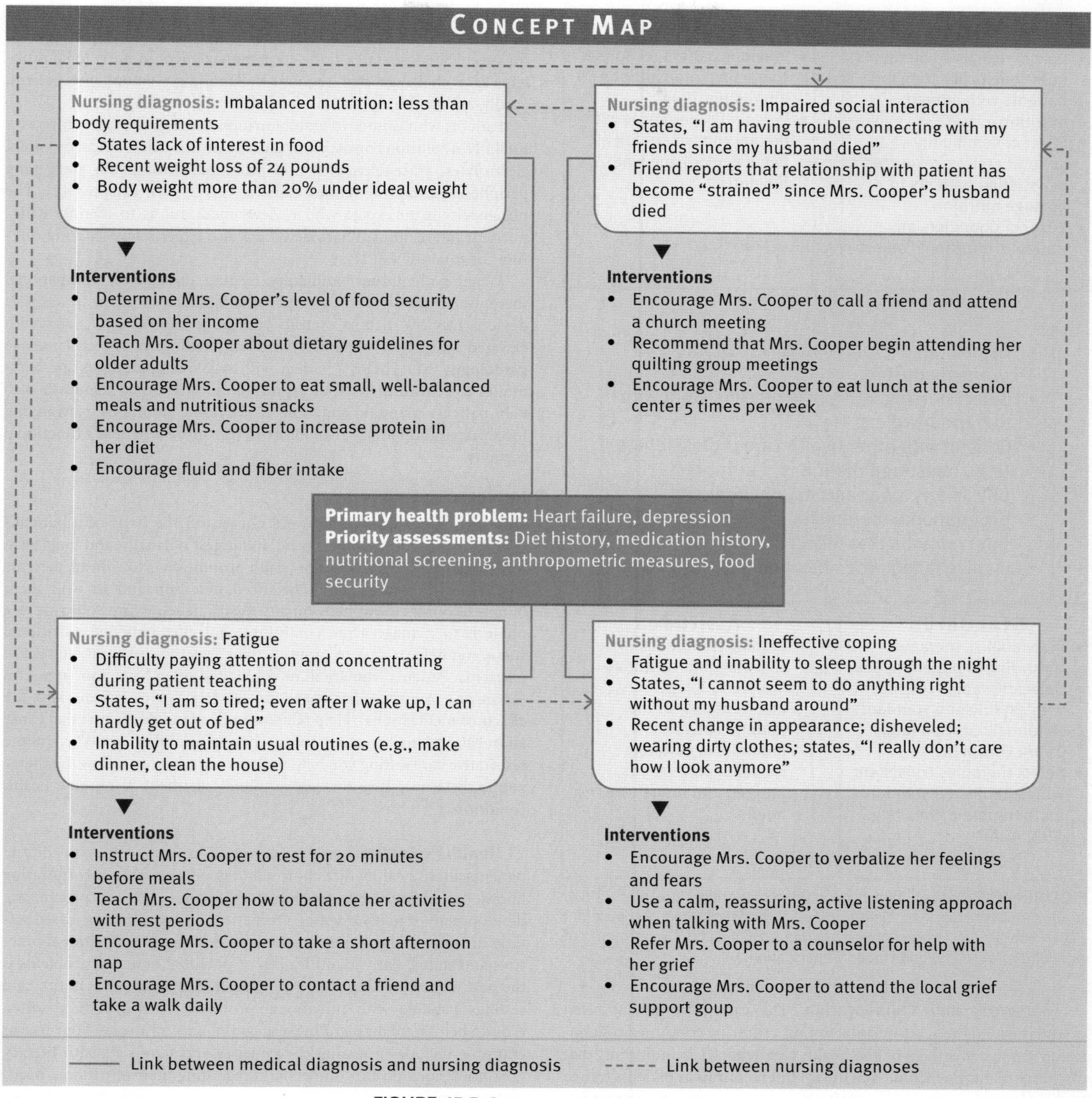

FIGURE 45-5 Concept map for Mrs. Cooper.

example, managing a patient's oral pain will be a priority over the intervention of diet education to improve nutrition if the patient is unable to swallow and maintain adequate food intake. *Deficient Knowledge* regarding diet therapy will become a priority if it is necessary to promote long-term and effective weight loss for a patient being discharged from a hospital.

During acute illness and surgery, food intake varies in the perioperative period. The priority of care is to provide optimal preoperative nutrition support in patients with malnutrition. The priority for the resumption of food intake after surgery depends on the return of bowel function, the extent of the surgical procedure, and the presence of any complications (see Chapter 50). For example, when patients have oral and throat surgery, they chew and swallow food in the presence of excision sites, sutures, or tissue manipulated during surgery. The priority of care is to first provide comfort and pain control. Then address nutritional priorities and plan care to maintain nutrition that does not cause pain or injury to the healing tissues.

The patient and family must collaborate with the nurse in planning care and setting priorities. This is important because food preferences, food purchases, and preparation involve the entire family. The plan of care cannot succeed without their commitment to, involvement in, and understanding of the nutritional priorities.

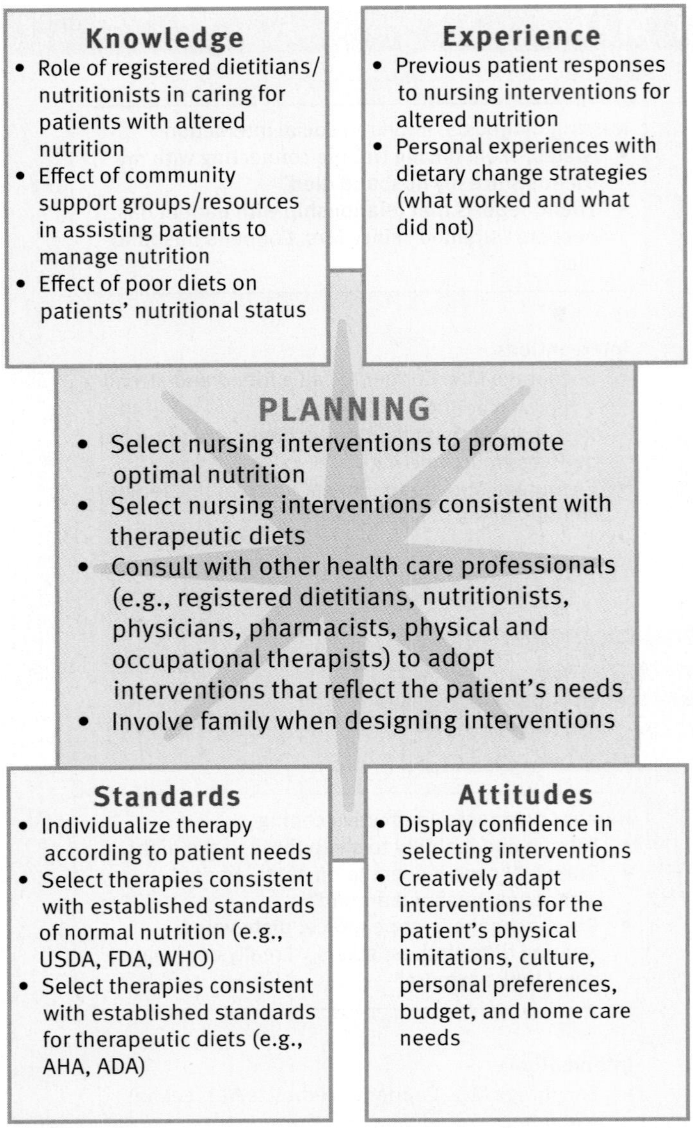

Knowledge
- Role of registered dietitians/nutritionists in caring for patients with altered nutrition
- Effect of community support groups/resources in assisting patients to manage nutrition
- Effect of poor diets on patients' nutritional status

Experience
- Previous patient responses to nursing interventions for altered nutrition
- Personal experiences with dietary change strategies (what worked and what did not)

PLANNING
- Select nursing interventions to promote optimal nutrition
- Select nursing interventions consistent with therapeutic diets
- Consult with other health care professionals (e.g., registered dietitians, nutritionists, physicians, pharmacists, physical and occupational therapists) to adopt interventions that reflect the patient's needs
- Involve family when designing interventions

Standards
- Individualize therapy according to patient needs
- Select therapies consistent with established standards of normal nutrition (e.g., USDA, FDA, WHO)
- Select therapies consistent with established standards for therapeutic diets (e.g., AHA, ADA)

Attitudes
- Display confidence in selecting interventions
- Creatively adapt interventions for the patient's physical limitations, culture, personal preferences, budget, and home care needs

FIGURE 45-6 Critical thinking model for nutrition planning. *ADA,* American Diabetes Association; *AHA,* American Heart Association; *FDA,* Food and Drug Administration; *USDA,* US Department of Agriculture; *WHO,* World Health Organization.

Teamwork and Collaboration. The care of a patient often extends beyond the acute hospital setting, requiring continued collaboration among members of the health care team. It is important that discharge planning include nutritional interventions as patients return to their homes or extended care facilities. Communicate patient goals and planned interventions to all team members to achieve expected patient outcomes. In addition, as nurses, consult with an SLP, RD, pharmacist, and/or occupational therapist about patients with dysphagia and those who need ongoing nutritional assessment and interventions to meet their nutritional needs.

Administration of enteral tube feedings typically enters through the stomach or intestines via a tube inserted through the nose or a percutaneous access (see Skills 45-2 and 45-3 on pp. 1085-1094). These enteral feedings supplement a patient's oral nutritional intake in the home, acute care, extended care, or rehabilitation setting when they cannot meet their nutritional needs by mouth. Regardless of the setting, the RD assesses and monitors the patient's nutritional status and intake and makes recommendations for changes. RDs are expert in the choice of enteral formulas and dietary modifications required for specific disease states. Long-term management of nutritional problems is a challenge that requires collaboration among the patient, family, and health care team members.

Patients who cannot tolerate nutrition through the GI tract receive total PN, a solution consisting of glucose, amino acids, lipids, minerals, electrolytes, trace elements, and vitamins, through an indwelling peripheral or central venous catheter (CVC) (see Chapter 42). The pharmacist is an expert who reviews medications to identify drug-nutrient interactions. Pharmacists are also experts in preparing mixtures of total PN (TPN).

When patients have difficulty feeding themselves, occupational therapists work with them and their families to identify assistive devices. Devices such as utensils with large handles and plates with elevated sides help a patient with self-feeding. A speech-language pathologist (SLP) helps a patient with swallowing exercises and techniques to reduce the risk of aspiration. Occupational therapists also help patients maintain function in the home setting by rearranging food preparation areas in an effort to maximize a patient's functional capacity.

◆ Implementation

Diet therapies are numerous and chosen on the basis of a patient's overall health status, ability to eat and digest normally, and long-term nutritional needs. The focus of health promotion is to educate patients and family caregivers about balanced nutrition and to help them obtain resources to eat high-quality meals. In acute care your role as a nurse is to manage acute conditions that alter patients' nutritional status and help in ways to promote their appetite and ability to take in nutrients. Patients who are ill or debilitated often have poor appetites (anorexia). Anorexia has many causes (e.g., pain, fatigue, and the effects of medications). Help patients understand the factors that cause anorexia and use creative approaches to stimulate appetite. In the restorative care setting you help patients learn how to follow the therapeutic diets necessary for recovery and treatment of chronic health conditions.

Health Promotion. As a nurse you are in a key position to educate patients about healthy diet choices and good nutrition. Incorporating knowledge of nutrition into patients' lifestyles serves to prevent the development of many diseases. Outpatient and community-based settings are optimal locations for nursing assessment of nutritional practices and status. Early identification of potential or actual problems is the best way to avoid serious problems. Similarly, in other health care settings patients with nutritional problems such as obesity often require help in menu planning and compliance strategies. Your role as educator includes assessing the patient's and family's health literacy (i.e., how much do they understand regarding their nutritional need) and providing nutritional education and information about community resources. Telephone numbers of an RD or nurse for follow-up questions are always a part of counseling.

Meal planning takes into account a family's budget and different preferences of family members. Choose specific foods on the basis of the dietary prescription and recommended food groups. For families on limited budgets, use substitutes. For example, bean or cheese dishes often replace meat in a meal, and the use of evaporated milk or dry skim milk when cooking is a low-cost nutritional supplement. Have patients modify the method of preparation when it is necessary to minimize certain substances. Baking rather than frying reduces fat intake, and patients can use lemon juice or spices to add flavor to low-sodium diets.

NURSING CARE PLAN

Imbalanced Nutrition: Less Than Body Requirements

ASSESSMENT

A nurse practitioner in a senior citizens' center is seeing Mrs. Cooper, who is 68 years old and has a history of heart failure. Recently Mrs. Cooper experienced an unexpected 15% weight loss. Three months have passed since she started taking sertraline (Zoloft) for depression related to the loss of her husband 6 months ago. She no longer participates in her monthly quilting club. Mrs. Cooper started receiving counseling 3 months ago for help with grief and depression through a local senior service agency. When the nurse inquires about her financial situation, Mrs. Cooper responds by saying that it was tight living on a small pension and Social Security but she was able to manage.

Assessment Activities	*Findings/Defining Characteristics**
Ask Mrs. Cooper about her food intake during the last 2 days.	She responds that she drinks some juice in the morning and two or three cups of coffee. In addition, she often has a sandwich in the late afternoon. She often skips dinner. "**I'm just not interested in food.** It has no taste."
Ask Mrs. Cooper about social interaction.	Mrs. Cooper complains of loneliness and says that she does not get out much, although her psychologist recommended more socializing. Her friends at church call her to come back to meetings, but she is just not ready. She says that she tires easily and no longer attends the monthly meetings of her quilt club.
Weigh patient and assess posture.	Her **weight is 20% below her ideal body weight (IBW)** and her body mass index (BMI) is 17. This weight loss has happened over the past 6 months, and she has **lost 24 lbs.** Stooped posture
Observe Mrs. Cooper for signs of poor nutrition.	**Hair loss** **Sore oral mucous membranes** **Pale mucous membranes**

***Defining characteristics** are shown in bold type.

NURSING DIAGNOSIS: Imbalanced nutrition: less than body requirements related to a decreased ability to ingest food as a result of depression and insufficient intake

PLANNING

Goals	*Expected Outcomes (NOC)*[†]
	Weight Gain Behavior
Mrs. Cooper will progressively gain weight.	Mrs. Cooper gains 1 to 2 lbs per month until reaching a goal of 130 lbs.
	Nutritional Status
Mrs. Cooper will consume adequate nourishment each day.	Mrs. Cooper ingests 1900 kcal/day, including 50 g of protein per day.
	Nutritional Status: Biochemical Measures
Mrs. Cooper will exhibit no signs of malnutrition.	Physical assessment findings are within normal limits. Laboratory values are within normal limits.

[†]Outcome classification labels from Moorhead S et al: *Nursing outcomes classification (NOC),* ed 5, St Louis, 2013, Mosby.

INTERVENTIONS (NIC)[‡]	**RATIONALE**
Nutritional Counseling	
Coordinate plan of care with health care provider, psychologist, Mrs. Cooper, and registered dietitian.	Successful nutrition care planning is a multidisciplinary approach throughout the continuum of care (Jensen et al., 2013).
Individualize menu plans according to Mrs. Cooper's preferences.	Incorporating her food preferences into the meal plans encourages the patient to eat (Jensen et al., 2013).
Teach Mrs. Cooper about MyPlate for Older Adults.	MyPlate for Older Adults is adapted to meet the nutritional requirements for older adults (Tufts University, 2011).
Nutrition Management	
Encourage Mrs. Cooper to eat small nutritious meals and snacks and increase dietary intake to help offset anorexia secondary to sertraline.	Sertraline is a selective serotonin reuptake inhibitor (SSRI) antidepressant medication that causes diminished taste and anorexia. Frequent small nutritious meals and snacks help to reduce anorexia-associated weight loss.
Encourage fluid intake.	Older adults need eight 8-oz (240 mL) glasses per day of fluid from beverage and food sources. Concentrating intake in the morning and early afternoon is acceptable to prevent nocturia (Meiner, 2011).
Encourage fiber intake.	Deters constipation and enhances appetite.
Encourage Mrs. Cooper to eat lunch at the senior center 5 times per week.	Eating with others encourages good nutrition and promotes socialization with peers (American Dietetic Association, 2010a; Nix, 2012).

[‡]Intervention classification labels from Bulechek GM et al: *Nursing interventions classification (NIC),* ed 6, St Louis, 2013, Mosby.

Continued

NURSING CARE PLAN

Imbalanced Nutrition: Less Than Body Requirements—cont'd

EVALUATION

Nursing Actions	*Patient Response/Finding*	*Achievement of Outcome*
Monitor Mrs. Cooper monthly for weight gain, anemia, serum albumin level, and transferrin levels.	After 2 weeks Mrs. Cooper has gained 3 lbs, and her hemoglobin B level is 12.	Mrs. Cooper is making progress with weight gain; her hemoglobin level still reflects mild anemia.
Ask Mrs. Cooper to keep a food diary for 3 days.	Food diary reflects that she ate her main meal at the senior center, has fruit and bran flakes for breakfast, and in the evening either has soup or a sandwich with fruit.	Mrs. Cooper is selecting more nutritionally rich foods, consistent with current guidelines.
Observe Mrs. Cooper's physical appearance.	At 2 weeks her mucous membranes are less pale, and her hair appears to be in better condition and styled.	Mrs. Cooper has improved physical parameters of nutrition; still needs follow-up.
Ask Mrs. Cooper about appetite and energy level.	Mrs. Cooper responds that on days that she eats at the senior center her appetite seems better and she "wants to do more things." She notes that weekends are very lonely.	Weekday support for nutritional status appears effective; needs to increase patient's activity status and nutritional intake during weekends.

TABLE 45-5 Food Safety

Foodborne Disease	Organism	Food Source	Symptoms*
Botulism	*Clostridium botulinum*	Improperly home-canned foods, smoked and salted fish, ham, sausage, shellfish	Symptoms varied from mild discomfort to death in 24 hours; initially nausea, vomiting, dizziness, and weakness progressing to motor (respiratory) paralysis
Escherichia coli	*E. coli*	Undercooked meat (ground beef)	Severe cramps, nausea, vomiting, diarrhea (may be bloody), renal failure; appears 1-8 days after eating; lasts 1-7 days
Listeriosis	*Listeria* *L. monocytogenes*	Soft cheese, meat (hot dogs, pâté, lunch meats), unpasteurized milk, poultry, seafood	Severe diarrhea, fever, headache, pneumonia, meningitis, endocarditis; appears 3-21 days after infection
Perfringens enteritis	*Clostridium* *C. perfringens*	Cooked meats, meat dishes held at room or warm temperature	Mild diarrhea, vomiting; appears 8-24 hours after eating; lasts 1-2 days
Salmonellosis	*Salmonella* *S. typhi* *S. paratyphi*	Milk, custards, egg dishes, salad dressings, sandwich fillings, polluted shellfish	Mild-to-severe diarrhea, cramps, vomiting; appears up to 72 hours after ingestion; lasts 4-7 days
Shigellosis	*Shigella* *S. dysenteriae*	Milk, milk products, seafood, salads	Cramps, diarrhea to fatal dysentery; appears 12-50 hours after ingestion; lasts 3-14 days
Staphylococcus	*Staphylococcus* *S. aureus*	Custards, cream fillings, processed meats, ham, cheese, ice cream, potato salad, sauces, casseroles	Severe abdominal cramps, pain, vomiting, diarrhea, perspiration, headache, fever, prostration; appears 1-6 hours after ingestion; lasts 1-2 days

From Nix S: *Williams' basic nutrition and diet therapy*, ed 14, St Louis, 2012, Mosby.
*Symptoms are generally most severe for youngest and oldest age-groups.

Planning menus a week in advance has several benefits. It helps ensure good nutrition or compliance with a specific diet and helps a family stay within their allotted budget. Nurses or RDs need to check menus for content. Often a simple tip is helpful in meal planning such as avoiding grocery shopping when hungry, which can lead to impulsive purchases of more expensive or less nutritious foods that are not included in meal plans. The U.S. Department of Agriculture (USDA, 2011) provides sample weekly meal-planning services for a range of budgets on its website.

Support individuals who are interested in losing weight. A high percentage of those who attempt to lose weight are unsuccessful, regaining lost weight over time. Diet and exercise compliance affects success with weight loss. Information on weight loss is available from multiple sources. Help patients develop a successful weight-loss plan that considers their preferences and resources and includes awareness of portion sizes and knowledge of energy content of food (AHA, 2010).

Food safety is an important public health issue. Foodborne bacteria can occur from improper food cleaning, preparation, or poor hygiene practices of food workers. Health care professionals not only need to be aware of the factors related to food safety but also should provide patient education to reduce the risks for foodborne illnesses (Table 45-5; Box 45-9).

Acute Care. The nutritional care of acutely ill patients requires a nurse to consider a variety of factors that influence nutritional intake. Diagnostic testing and procedures in the acute care setting disrupt food intake. Often a patient must refrain from eating or drinking anything by mouth (NPO) as he or she prepares for or recovers from a

BOX 45-9 PATIENT TEACHING

Food Safety

Objective

- Patient is able to verbalize measures to protect from foodborne illness.

Teaching Strategies

- Explain that food safety is an important public health issue. Populations particularly at risk are older and younger people and immunosuppressed individuals.
- Instruct patients using the following four principles:
  1. CLEAN
     - Wash hands with warm, soapy water before touching or eating food.
     - Wash fresh fruits and vegetables thoroughly.
     - Clean the inside of refrigerator and microwave regularly to prevent microbial growth.
     - Clean cutting surfaces after each use.
     - When possible, use separate surfaces for fruit, meat, poultry, fish
  2. SEPARATE
     - Wash cooking utensils and cutting boards with hot soapy water.
     - Wash hands after handling foods, especially meats, poultry, and eggs.
     - Clean vegetables and lettuce used in salads thoroughly.
     - Wash dishrags, towels, and sponges regularly or use paper towels.
  3. COOK
     - Use a food thermometer to verify that meat, poultry, and fish are cooked properly.
     - Do not eat raw meats or unpasteurized milk.
  4. CHILL
     - Keep foods properly refrigerated at 40° F (4.4° C) and frozen at 0° F (−17.8° C).
     - Do not save leftovers for more than 2 days in refrigerator.

Evaluation

- Ask patient to verbalize measures to prevent foodborne illnesses.
- Observe patient at home for safe practices if making home visit.

Data from US Department of Agriculture and US Department of Health and Human Services: *Report of the dietary guidelines advisory committee dietary guidelines for Americans 2010,* 2010, http://www.cnpp.usda.gov/dietaryguidelines.htm. Accessed November 2015.

QSEN QSEN: BUILDING COMPETENCY IN TEAMWORK AND COLLABORATION You are the nurse in charge of developing an interdisciplinary team to help senior citizens with heart failure manage their diet at home. Knowing that it is important to have heart-failure patients lower their sodium content, cholesterol, and saturated fat to preserve their cardiac function, you bring your nursing knowledge to the team. Which strengths and limitations do you bring to the interdisciplinary team? Who would be on the team to help prepare the care plan for the heart-failure patients? How would you promote effective teamwork?

Answers to QSEN Activities can be found on the Evolve website.

diagnostic test. Frequent interruptions during mealtimes occur in the health care setting, or patients have poor appetites. Patients often are too tired or uncomfortable to eat. It is important to assess a patient's nutritional status continuously and adopt interventions that promote normal intake, digestion, and metabolism of nutrients. Patients who are NPO and receive only standard IV fluids for more than 4 to 7 days are at nutritional risk.

Advancing Diets. Acute and chronic conditions affect a patient's immune system and nutritional status. Patients with decreased immune function (e.g., from cancer, chemotherapy, human immunodeficiency virus/acquired immunodeficiency syndrome [HIV/AIDS], or organ transplants) require special diets that decrease exposure to microorganisms and are higher in selected nutrients. Table 45-6 provides an overview of the immune system, the impact of malnutrition, and beneficial nutrients. In addition, patients who are ill, who have had surgical procedures, or who were NPO for an extended time have specialized dietary needs. Health care providers order a gradual progression of dietary intake or therapeutic diet to manage patients' illness (Box 45-10).

Promoting Appetite. Providing an environment that promotes nutritional intake includes keeping a patient's environment free of odors, providing oral hygiene as needed to remove unpleasant tastes, and maintaining patient comfort. Offering smaller, more frequent meals often helps. In addition, certain medications affect dietary intake and nutrient use. For example, medications such as insulin, glucocorticoids, and thyroid hormones affect metabolism. Other medications such as antifungal agents frequently affect taste. Some of the

TABLE 45-6 Nutrition and the Immune System

Immune/Physiological Component	Malnutrition Effect	Vital Nutrient
Antibodies	Decreased amount	Protein, vitamins A, B_6, B_{12}, C, folic acid, thiamin, biotin, riboflavin, niacin
GI tract	Systemic movement of bacteria	Arginine, glutamine, omega-3 fatty acids
Granulocytes and macrocytes	Longer time for phagocytosis kill time and lymphocyte activation	Protein, vitamins A, B_6, B_{12}, C, folic acid, thiamin, riboflavin, niacin, zinc, iron
Mucus	Flat microvilli in GI tract, decreased antibody secretion	Vitamins B_6, B_{12}, C, biotin
Skin	Integrity compromised, density reduced, wound healing slowed	Protein, vitamins A, B_{12}, C, niacin, copper, zinc
T-lymphocytes	Depressed T-cell distribution	Protein, arginine, iron, zinc, omega-3 fatty acids, vitamins A, B_6, B_{12}, folic acid, thiamin, riboflavin, niacin, pantothenic acid

Modified from Grodner M, et al: *Foundations and clinical applications of nutrition: a nursing approach,* ed 5, St Louis, 2012, Mosby.
GI, Gastrointestinal.

BOX 45-10 Diet Progression and Therapeutic Diets

Clear Liquid
Clear fat-free broth, bouillon, coffee, tea, carbonated beverages, clear fruit juices, gelatin, fruit ices, popsicles

Full Liquid
As for clear liquid, with addition of smooth-textured dairy products (e.g., ice cream), strained or blended cream soups, custards, refined cooked cereals, vegetable juice, pureed vegetables, all fruit juices, sherbets, puddings, frozen yogurt

Dysphagia Stages, Thickened Liquids, Pureed
As for clear and full liquid, with addition of scrambled eggs; pureed meats, vegetables, and fruits; mashed potatoes and gravy

Mechanical Soft
As for clear and full liquid and pureed, with addition of all cream soups, ground or finely diced meats, flaked fish, cottage cheese, cheese, rice, potatoes, pancakes, light breads, cooked vegetables, cooked or canned fruits, bananas, soups, peanut butter, eggs (not fried)

Soft/Low Residue
Addition of low-fiber, easily digested foods such as pastas, casseroles, moist tender meats, and canned cooked fruits and vegetables; desserts, cakes, and cookies without nuts or coconut

High Fiber
Addition of fresh uncooked fruits, steamed vegetables, bran, oatmeal, and dried fruits

Low Sodium
4-g (no added salt), 2-g, 1-g, or 500-mg sodium diets; vary from no-added-salt to severe sodium restriction (500-mg sodium diet), which requires selective food purchases

Low Cholesterol
300 mg/day cholesterol, in keeping with American Heart Association guidelines for serum lipid reduction

Diabetic
Nutrition recommendations by the American Diabetes Association: focus on total energy, nutrient and food distribution; include a balanced intake of carbohydrates, fats, and proteins; varied caloric recommendations to accommodate patient's metabolic demands

Gluten Free
Eliminates wheat, oats, rye, barley and their derivatives

Regular
No restrictions unless specified

psychotropic medications affect appetite, cause nausea, and alter taste. You and the RD help patients select foods that reduce the altered taste sensations or nausea. Consult with an RD regarding using seasonings that improve food taste. In other situations medications need to be changed. Assessing patients for the need for pharmacological agents to stimulate appetite such as cyproheptadine, megestro, or dronabinol or to manage symptoms that interfere with nutrition requires health care provider consultation.

Mealtime is usually a social activity. If appropriate, encourage visitors to eat with a patient. When patients experience anorexia, encourage other nurses or care providers to converse and engage them in conversation. Mealtime is also an excellent opportunity for patient education. Instruct a patient about any therapeutic diets, medications, energy conservation measures, or adaptive devices to help with independent feeding.

Assisting Patients with Oral Feeding. When a patient needs help with eating, it is important to protect his or her safety, independence, and dignity. Clear the table or over-bed tray of clutter. Assess his or her risk of aspiration (see Skill 45-1). Patients at high risk for aspiration have decreased level of alertness, decreased gag and/or cough reflexes, and difficulty managing saliva (see Assessment section of this chapter).

Patients with dysphagia are at risk for aspiration and need more help with feeding and swallowing. A speech-language pathologist (SLP) identifies patients at risk and provides recommendations for therapy (Ellis and Hannibal, 2013). Provide a 30-minute rest period before eating and position the patient in an upright, seated position in a chair or raise the head of the bed to 90 degrees. Have the patient flex the head slightly to a chin-down position to help prevent aspiration. If the patient has unilateral weakness, teach him or her and the caregiver to place food in the stronger side of the mouth. With the help of an SLP, determine the viscosity of foods that the patient tolerates best using trials of different consistencies of foods and fluids. Thicker fluids are generally easier to swallow. The American Dietetic Association published the National Dysphagia Diet Task Force National Dysphagia Diet in 2010 to provide uniformity of diets provided to patients with dysphagia (NDDTF, 2010). There are four levels of diet: dysphagia puree, dysphagia mechanically altered, dysphagia advanced, and regular. The four levels of liquid include thin liquids (low viscosity), nectarlike liquids (medium viscosity), honeylike liquids (viscosity of honey), and spoon-thick liquids (viscosity of pudding) (NDDTF, 2010).

Feed a patient with dysphagia slowly, providing smaller-size bites. Allow him or her to chew thoroughly and swallow the bite before taking another. More frequent chewing and swallowing assessments throughout the meal are necessary. Allow the patient time to empty the mouth after each spoonful, matching the speed of feeding to the patient's readiness (see Skill 45-1). If he or she begins to cough or choke, remove the food immediately (Ellis and Hannibal, 2013). Sometimes it is necessary to have oral suction equipment available at the patient's bedside.

Provide opportunities for patients to direct the order in which they want to eat the food items and how fast they wish to eat. Determine a patient's food preferences and, unless contraindicated, try to have these items included on his or her dietary tray. Ask the patient if the food is the right temperature. These seem like small acts, but they go a long way in maintaining the patient's sense of independence.

Patients with visual deficits also need special assistance. Patients with decreased vision are able to feed themselves when given adequate information. For example, identify the food location on a meal plate as if it were a clock (e.g., meat at 9 o'clock and vegetable at 3 o'clock). Tell the patient where the beverages are located in relation to the plate. Be sure that other care providers set the meal tray and plate in the same manner. Patients with impaired vision and those with decreased motor skills are more independent during mealtimes with the use of large-handled adaptive utensils (Figure 45-7). These are easier to grip and manipulate.

Enteral Tube Feeding. **Enteral nutrition (EN)** provides nutrients into the GI tract. It is the preferred method of meeting nutritional needs if a patient is unable to swallow or take in nutrients orally yet has a functioning GI tract. EN provides physiological, safe, and economical nutritional support. Patients with enteral feedings receive formula via nasogastric, jejunal, or gastric tubes. Patients with a low

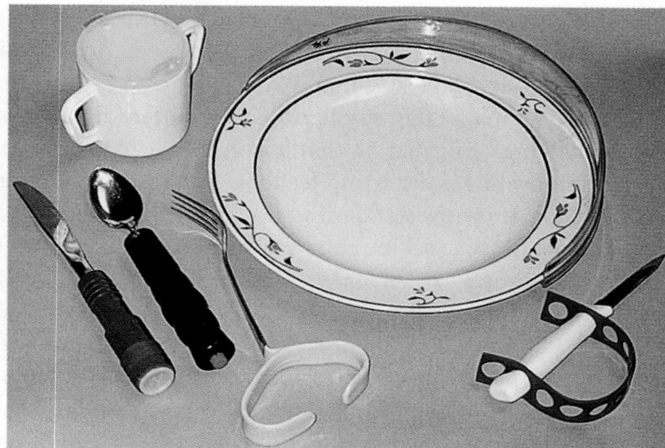

FIGURE 45-7 Adaptive equipment. Clockwise from upper left: Two-handled cup with lid, plate with plate guard, utensils with splints, and utensils with enlarged handles.

risk of gastric reflux receive gastric feedings; however, if there is a risk of gastric reflux, which leads to aspiration, jejunal feeding is preferred. Box 45-11 lists indications for tube feeding. Either the nurse or a family caregiver can easily give enteral tube feedings in the home setting. After insertion of an enteral tube, it is necessary to verify tube placement by x-ray film examination. Confirmation of placement is needed before a patient receives the first enteral feeding (see Skill 45-2 on pp. 1085-1089).

An enteral formula is usually one of four types. Polymeric (1 to 2 kcal/mL) includes milk-based blenderized foods prepared by hospital dietary staff or in a patient's home. The polymeric classification also includes commercially prepared whole-nutrient formulas. For this type of formula to be effective, a patient's GI tract needs to be able to absorb whole nutrients. The second type, modular formulas (3.8 to 4 kcal/mL), are single macronutrient (e.g., protein, glucose, polymers, or lipids) preparations and are not nutritionally complete. You can add this type of formula to other foods to meet your patient's individual nutritional needs. The third type, elemental formulas (1 to 3 kcal/mL), contain predigested nutrients that are easier for a partially dysfunctional GI tract to absorb. Finally, specialty formulas (1 to 2 kcal/mL) are designed to meet specific nutritional needs in certain illness (e.g., liver failure, pulmonary disease, or HIV infection).

Typically tube feedings start at full strength at slow rates (see Skill 45-3 on pp. 1090-1094; Box 45-12). Increase the hourly rate every 8 to 12 hours per health care provider's order if no signs of intolerance appear (high gastric residuals, nausea, cramping, vomiting, and diarrhea). Studies have demonstrated a beneficial effect of enteral feedings compared with PN. Feeding by the enteral route reduces sepsis, minimizes the hypermetabolic response to trauma, decreases hospital mortality, and maintains intestinal structure and function (Khalid et al., 2010). EN is successful within 24 to 48 hours after surgery or trauma to provide fluids, electrolytes, and nutritional support. If the patient develops a gastric ileus, it prevents instituting nasogastric feedings. Nasointestinal or jejunal tubes allow successful postpyloric feeding because the formula instills directly into the small intestine or jejunum or beyond the pyloric sphincter of the stomach (Hodin et al., 2014).

A serious complication associated with enteral feedings is aspiration of formula into the tracheobronchial tree. Aspiration of enteral formula into the lungs irritates the bronchial mucosa, resulting in decreased blood supply to affected pulmonary tissue (McCance et al., 2014). This leads to necrotizing infection, pneumonia, and potential abscess formation. The high glucose content of a feeding serves as a bacterial medium for growth, promoting infection. Acute respiratory distress syndrome (ARDS) is also an outcome frequently associated with pulmonary aspiration. Some of the common conditions that increase the risk of aspiration include coughing, gastroesophageal reflux disease (GERD), nasotracheal suctioning, an artificial airway, decreased level of consciousness, and lying flat. Prokinetic medications such as metoclopramide, erythromycin, or cisapride promote gastric emptying and decrease the risk of aspiration (Metheny et al., 2012). Keep the head of the bed elevated a minimum of 30 degrees, preferably 45 degrees, unless medically contraindicated (Hodin et al., 2014). You need to measure gastric residual volumes (GRVs) every 4 to 6 hours in patients receiving continuous feedings and immediately before the feeding in patients receiving intermittent feedings (Metheny et al., 2012). Delayed gastric emptying is a concern if 250 mL or more remains in a patient's stomach on two consecutive assessments (1 hour apart) or if a single GRV measurement exceeds 500 mL (Stewart, 2014). There is a lack of consensus for recommendations for stopping feedings; decisions to stop feedings must include assessment of patient's condition (Metheny et al., 2012). The North American Summit on Aspiration in the Critically Ill Patient recommends the following: (1) stop feedings immediately if aspiration occurs; (2) withhold feedings and reassess patient tolerance to feedings if GRV is over 500 mL; (3) routinely evaluate the patient for aspiration; and (4) use nursing measures to reduce the risk of aspiration if GRV is between 250 and 500 mL (Stewart, 2014).

BOX 45-11 Indications for Enteral and Parenteral Nutrition

Enteral Nutrition
(Used with patients who have a functional gastrointestinal tract)

- Cancer
  - Head and neck
  - Upper GI
- Critical illness/trauma
- Neurological and muscular disorders
  - Brain neoplasm
  - Cerebrovascular accident
  - Dementia
  - Myopathy
- Parkinson's disease
- GI disorders
  - Enterocutaneous fistula
  - Inflammatory bowel disease
  - Mild pancreatitis
- Respiratory failure with prolonged intubation
- Inadequate oral intake
  - Anorexia nervosa
  - Difficulty chewing, swallowing
  - Severe depression

Parenteral Nutrition

- Nonfunctional GI tract
  - Massive small bowel resection/GI surgery/massive GI bleed
  - Paralytic ileus
  - Intestinal obstruction
  - Trauma to abdomen, head, or neck
  - Severe malabsorption
  - Intolerance to enteral feeding (established by trial)
  - Chemotherapy, radiation therapy, bone marrow transplantation
- Extended bowel rest
  - Enterocutaneous fistula
  - Inflammatory bowel disease exacerbation
  - Severe diarrhea
  - Moderate-to-severe pancreatitis
- Preoperative total parenteral nutrition
  - Preoperative bowel rest
  - Treatment for co-morbid severe malnutrition in patients with nonfunctional GI tracts
- Severely catabolic patients when GI tract not usable for more than 4 to 5 days

GI, Gastrointestinal.

Enteral Access Tubes. The inability of patients to ingest food but still able to digest and absorb nutrients supports the use of enteral tube feeding. Feeding tubes are inserted through the nose (nasogastric or nasointestinal), surgically (gastrostomy or jejunostomy), or endoscopically (percutaneous endoscopic gastrostomy or jejunostomy [PEG or PEJ]). If EN therapy is for less than 4 weeks, total, nasogastric, or nasojejunal feeding tubes may be used. Surgical or endoscopically placed tubes are preferred for long-term feeding (more than 6 weeks) to reduce the discomfort of a nasal tube and provide a more secure, reliable access (Yantis and Velander, 2011). Some patients such as those with gastroparesis (decreased or absent innervation to the stomach that results in delayed gastric emptying), esophageal reflux, or a history of aspiration pneumonia require placement of tubes beyond the stomach into the intestine (Metheny et al., 2012; Yantis and Velander, 2011).

BOX 45-12 Advancing the Rate of Tube Feeding

Protocols for advancing tube feedings are commonly institution specific. Most of these protocols are untested for validity. There does not appear to be a benefit to slow initiation of enteral nutrition over days. Most patients are able to tolerate feeding 24 to 48 hours after initiation. Do not dilute formulas with water; this increases the risk of bacterial contamination (Stewart, 2014).

Intermittent

1. Start formula at full strength for isotonic formulas (300 to 400 mOsm) or at ordered concentration.
2. Infuse bolus of formula over at least 20 to 30 minutes via syringe or feeding container.
3. Begin feedings with a volume of 2.5-5 mL/kg 5 to 8 times per day. Increase by 60-120 mL per feeding every 8-12 hours to achieve needed volume and calories in four to six feedings (Stewart, 2014).

Continuous

1. Start formula at full strength for isotonic formulas (300 to 400 mOsm) or at ordered concentration.
2. Begin infusion rate at designated rate typically at 10 to 40 mL/hr (Stewart, 2014).
3. Advance rate slowly (e.g., 10 to 20 mL/hr every 8 to 12 hours) to target rate if tolerated (tolerance indicated by absence of nausea and diarrhea and low gastric residuals) (Stewart, 2014).

Most health care settings use small-bore feeding tubes because they create less discomfort for a patient (Figure 45-8, *A*). Adult patients typically have an 8- to 12-Fr tube that is 36 to 44 inches (90 to 110 cm) long. Using a stylet makes the very flexible tube stiffer for easier insertion. Once receiving confirmation that it is in the correct location, the stylet needs removal before starting feedings and should not be reinserted in the tube. It is now standard to use an enteral-only connector (ENFit) designed for the specific enteral tube. Standardization of connector tubing improves patient safety (Figure 45-8, *B*). Tubing standards are designed to reduce tubing misconnections that result in patient injury (TJC, 2014). Skill 45-3 describes the procedure for initiating beginning nasogastric, gastrostomy, and jejunostomy enteral feedings.

Historically nurses verified feeding tube placement by injecting air through the tube while auscultating the stomach for a gurgling or bubbling sound or asking the patient to speak. However, evidence-based research repeatedly demonstrates that auscultation is ineffective in detecting tubes accidentally placed in the lung (Yantis and Velander, 2011). Some patients are able to speak despite placement of feeding tubes in the lung. Furthermore, auscultation is not effective in distinguishing between gastric and intestinal placement for feeding tubes. The measurement of pH of secretions withdrawn from the feeding tube helps to differentiate the location of a tube (Box 45-13). At present the most reliable method for verification of placement of small-bore feeding tubes is x-ray film examination (Box 45-14).

Table 45-7 outlines major complications of EN. Of special note, severely malnourished patients are at risk for electrolyte disturbances from refeeding syndrome during EN or PN therapy. In refeeding syndrome, potassium, magnesium, and phosphate move intracellularly, resulting in low serum (extracellular) levels and edema. These changes may cause cardiac dysrhythmias, heart failure, respiratory distress, convulsions, coma, or death.

Parenteral Nutrition. Parenteral nutrition (PN) is a form of specialized nutrition support provided intravenously. A basic PN formula is a combination of crystalline amino acids, hypertonic dextrose, electrolytes, vitamins, and trace elements. Total PN (TPN), administered through a central line, is a 2-in-1 formula in which administration of fat emulsions occurs separately from the protein and dextrose solution (Krzywda and Meyer, 2010). Safe administration depends on appropriate assessment of nutrition needs, meticulous management of the CVC, and careful monitoring to prevent or treat metabolic complications. Administration of PN happens in a variety of settings, including a patient's home. Regardless of the setting, adhere to

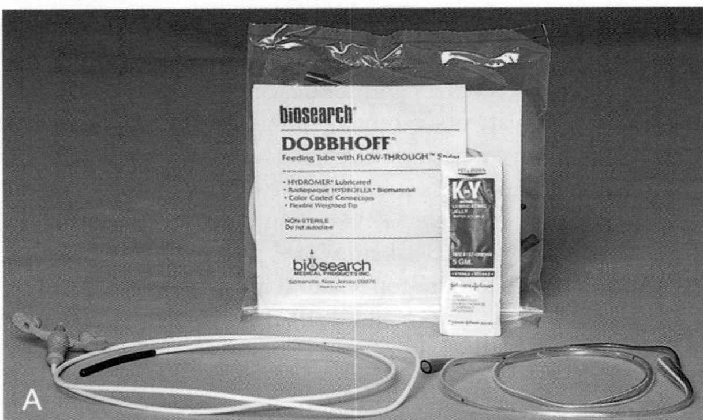

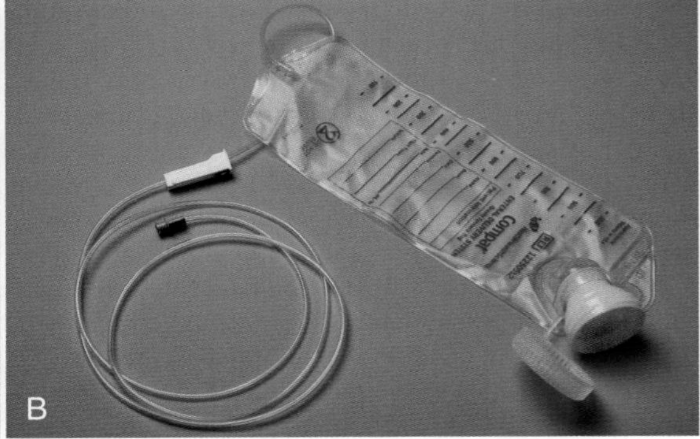

FIGURE 45-8 A, Enteral tubes, small-bore. **B,** Enteral-only connector (ENFit) designed to fit the specific enteral tube.

BOX 45-13 PROCEDURAL GUIDELINES

Obtaining Gastrointestinal Aspirate for pH Measurement, Large-Bore, and Small-Bore Feeding Tubes: Intermittent and Continuous Feeding

Delegation Considerations

Do not delegate the skill of measuring pH in gastrointestinal (GI) aspirate to nursing assistive personnel.

Equipment

Cone-tipped or Asepto syringe, pH test paper (scale of 1.0 to 11.0 or greater), paper towel, small medication cup, clean gloves

Steps

1. Perform measures to verify placement of tube:
   a. For intermittently fed patients, test placement immediately before feeding (usually a period of at least 4 hours has elapsed since previous feeding). More frequent checking has been associated with increased clogging of small-bore tubes. To avoid clogging, flush tube with 30 mL water after aspirating for the gastric residual volume (Yantis and Velander, 2011).
   b. For continuously tube-fed patients, test placement every 4 to 6 hours (Yantis and Velander, 2011). If patient is tolerating the feedings without incident and other indicators of correct location are present (i.e., the mark on the tube at the exit site has remained in its original position, and the most recent x-ray films confirm correct position of tube), it is reasonable to continue feedings. If risk of tube displacement is high, and the tube has moved, consider the need for an x-ray film to verify placement (Stewart, 2014). Plan pH testing at times when feeding may be withheld (e.g., during diagnostic testing or chest physiotherapy or to avoid medication interaction).
   c. Wait at least 1 hour after medication administration by tube or mouth.
2. Perform hand hygiene and apply clean gloves.
3. Draw up 30 mL of air into syringe and attach to end of feeding tube. Flush tube with 30 mL of air before attempting to aspirate fluid. It is likely to be more difficult to aspirate fluid from the small intestine than from the stomach. Repositioning patient from side to side is helpful. More than one bolus of air through the tube is necessary in some cases. Burst of air aids in aspirating fluid more easily.
4. Draw back on syringe and obtain 5 to 10 mL of gastric aspirate.
   a. Observe appearance of aspirate (see illustration).

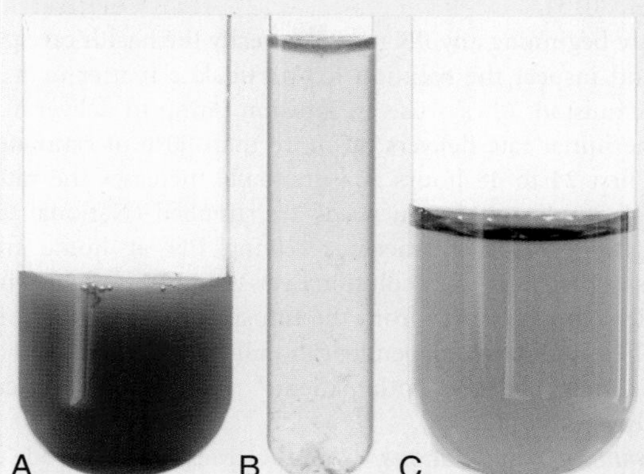

STEP 4a Gastrointestinal contents. **A,** Stomach. **B,** Stomach. **C,** Intestinal. (Courtesy Dr. Norma Metheny, Professor, St Louis University School of Nursing.)

   b. Gently mix aspirate in syringe. Expel a few drops into a clean medicine cup. Dip the pH strip into the fluid or apply a few drops of the fluid to the strip (see illustration). Compare the color of the strip with the color on the chart provided by the manufacturer (Yantis and Velander, 2011).

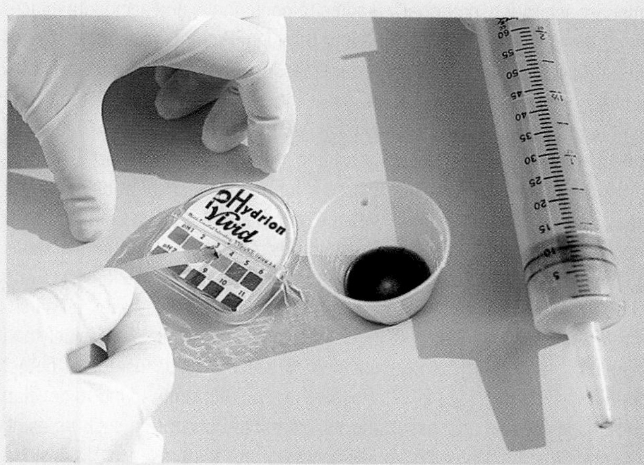

STEP 4b Comparing pH strip with color chart.

- Gastric fluid from patient who has fasted for at least 4 hours usually has pH range of 1.0 to 4.0.
- Fluid from nasointestinal tube of fasting patient usually has pH greater than or equal to 6.0 (Stewart, 2014).
- Patient with continuous tube feeding often has pH of 5.0 or higher.
- pH of pleural fluid from tracheobronchial tree is generally greater than 6.0.

5. Remove gloves and discard supplies. Perform hand hygiene.

CLINICAL DECISION: If after repeated attempts you cannot aspirate fluid from a tube that was originally established by x-ray film examination to be in desired position and (a) there are no risk factors for tube dislocation, (b) there is no change in external marked tube length, and (c) patient is not experiencing difficulty, assume that tube is placed correctly (Yantis and Velander, 2011).

BOX 45-14 EVIDENCE-BASED PRACTICE

Accuracy in Determining Placement of Feeding Tubes

PICO Question: In adult patients which method of assessment provides the most accurate information that an enteral feeding tube is in the correct location?

Evidence Summary

Two of the most frequent complications associated with tube feedings are pulmonary aspiration, potentially leading to pneumonia, and accidental placement of a nasoenteric feeding tube into the lung. Patients at highest risk for aspiration present with dysphagia, decreased level of consciousness, confusion, uncooperativeness, agitation, presence of an endotracheal tube, and absent or poor gag reflex (Metheny et al., 2012). Gastric residual volume has not been found to be consistently related to aspiration (Stewart, 2014). A traditional bedside method used to assess for pulmonary aspiration of enteral feeding into the respiratory tract was the glucose method. The premise of the glucose method was that normal tracheal secretions contain minimal levels of glucose. Therefore, if aspiration of glucose-rich enteral formula occurs into the airway, glucose levels of tracheal secretions increase. However, researchers have shown that the glucose levels of tracheal secretions vary widely and this method is not sufficiently sensitive or specific to be useful to detect aspiration (Metheny et al., 2012). Researchers are currently trying to develop new bedside methods for assessing for pulmonary aspiration such as using electromagnetic tracking devices and assessing for the presence of pepsin, a substance produced in the stomach in tracheal secretions (Stewart, 2014).

Traditionally nurses have used the auscultatory method of assessing placement, which is unreliable. Auscultation does not detect when a feeding tube has inadvertently been placed into the respiratory tract and does not distinguish between placement in the stomach versus the intestine. The most accurate method for checking feeding tube placement is x-ray film examination (Kenny and Goodman, 2010; Stewart, 2014). The most effective nonradiological methods include aspirating fluid from the feeding tube, measuring its pH, and describing its appearance (Stewart, 2014). However, gastric aspirate may not be accurate if the patient is being administered medication to suppress gastric acid (Yantis and Velander, 2011).

Application to Nursing Practice

- X-ray film verification of feeding tube placement is the most reliable method available to confirm correct tube location. It is required in most acute care facilities immediately after insertion of a small-bore tube.
- Verify the placement of the feeding tube every 4 to 6 hours by aspirating gastric contents, observing its appearance, and testing pH. A properly obtained pH of 0 to 4.0 is a good indication of gastric placement. A pH of 6.0 or higher likely indicates placement in the lung, intestine, or even the stomach when gastric pH is unusually high. Intestinal fluid is usually bile stained (dark golden yellow). Gastric fluid is usually grassy green, off-white to tan, or clear and colorless (Stewart, 2014).
- Do not use the auscultatory method to determine tube location.
- Do not use the glucose detection method to determine if aspiration has occurred.
- Check gastric residual volumes every 4 hours in patients at high risk for aspiration (Stewart, 2014).

principles of asepsis and infusion management to ensure safe nutrition support.

Patients who are unable to digest or absorb EN benefit from PN. Patients in highly stressed physiological states such as sepsis, head injury, or burns are candidates for PN therapy (see Box 45-11).

PN therapy requires clinical and laboratory monitoring by a multidisciplinary team. Consistent reevaluation for the continuation of PN is required. The goal to move toward use of the GI tract is constant (Fletcher, 2013). Disuse of the GI tract has been associated with villus atrophy and generalized cell shrinkage. Furthermore, the disuse of the GI tract may cause bacteria to move from the unused gut into the bloodstream, resulting in gram-negative septicemia.

Sometimes adding **intravenous fat emulsions** to PN supports the patient's need for supplemental kilocalories to prevent essential fatty-acid deficiencies and help control hyperglycemia during periods of stress (Phillips, 2010). Administer these emulsions through a separate peripheral line, through the central line by using Y-connector tubing (see Chapter 42), or as an admixture to the PN solution. The addition of fat emulsion to a PN solution is called a *3-in-1 admixture* or *total nutrient admixture*. The patient receives it over a 24-hour period. Do not use the admixture if you observe oil droplets or an oily or creamy layer on the surface of the admixture. This observation indicates that the emulsion has broken into large lipid droplets that cause fat emboli if administered. IV fat emulsions are white and opaque. Take care to avoid confusing enteral formula with parenteral lipids.

Initiating Parenteral Nutrition. Patients with short-term nutritional needs often receive IV solutions of less than 10% dextrose via a peripheral vein in combination with amino acids and lipids. TPN is more calorically dense than peripheral solutions; therefore peripheral solutions are usually temporary. PN with greater than 10% dextrose requires a CVC that a health care provider places into a high-flow central vein such as the superior vena cava under sterile conditions (see Chapter 41). If you are using a CVC that has multiple lumens, use a port exclusively dedicated for the TPN. Label the port for TPN and do not infuse other solutions or medications through it (Krzywda and Meyer, 2010). Nurses with special training insert peripherally inserted central catheters (PICCs) that start in a vein of the arm and then thread into the subclavian or superior vena cava vein.

After catheter placement wait to flush and use the catheter until position confirmation by radiology. The health care provider secures the CVC with a securement device and covers the site with a sterile bio-occlusive dressing. Before applying the sterile dressing, stabilize the PICC with sterile strips of tape. A chest x-ray film verifies catheter tip placement for a CVC or PICC before starting a PN infusion (Fletcher, 2013).

Before beginning any PN infusion, verify the health care provider's order and inspect the solution for particulate matter or a break in the fat emulsion. Always use an infusion pump to deliver a constant rate. The initial rate delivers no more than 50% of estimated needs for the first 24 to 48 hours and gradually increases the rate until a patient's complete nutrition needs are supplied (National Guideline Clearinghouse, 2013). Patients receiving PN at home frequently administer the entire daily solution over 12 hours at night. This allows the patient to disconnect from the infusion each morning, flush the central line, and have independent mobility during the day. Home PN therapy often interferes with patients' normal activities, causing a poorer quality of life.

Preventing Complications. Complications of PN include catheter-related problems and metabolic alterations (Table 45-8). Pneumothorax results from a puncture insult to the pulmonary system and involves the accumulation of air in the pleural cavity with subsequent collapse of the lung and impaired breathing. The clinical symptoms of a pneumothorax include sudden sharp chest pain, dyspnea, and coughing. In relation to PN, pneumothorax most often occurs during CVC placement. Monitor a patient with a CVC for the first 24 hours for signs and symptoms of pulmonary distress.

TABLE 45-7 Enteral Tube-Feeding Complications

Problem	Possible Cause	Intervention*
Pulmonary aspiration	Regurgitation of formula	Verify tube placement. Place patient in high-Fowler's position or elevate head of bed a minimum of 30 (preferably 45) degrees during feedings and for 2 hours afterward.
	Feeding tube displaced	Reposition tube and verify tube placement.
	Deficient gag reflex	Reassess for return of normal gag reflex; until then place patient on aspiration precautions and in semi-Fowler's position.
	Delayed gastric emptying	See delayed gastric emptying that follows.
Diarrhea	Hyperosmolar formula or medications	Deliver formula continuously, lower rate, dilute, or change to isotonic enteral nutrition.
	Antibiotic therapy	Antibiotics destroy normal intestinal flora; consult with health care provider to consider changing medication; treat symptoms with antidiarrheal agents; culture stool for *Clostridium difficile.*
	Bacterial contamination	Do not hang formula longer than 4-8 hours in bag, wash bag out well when refilling, change tube-feeding bags and tubing q24h and use aseptic practices. Check expiration dates.
	Malabsorption	Check for pancreatic insufficiency; use low-fat, lactose-free formula and continuous feedings.
Constipation	Lack of fiber	Consult with a dietitian to select a formula containing fiber.
	Lack of free water	Add water during tube flushes.*
	Inactivity	Monitor patient's ability to ambulate; collaborate with health care provider and/or physical therapist for activity order.
Tube occlusion	Pulverized medications given per tube	Irrigate with 30 mL water before and after each medication per tube.* Use liquid medications when available. Completely dissolve crushed medications in liquid if liquid medication is not available.
	Sedimentation of formula	Shake cans well before administering (read label).
	Reaction of incompatible medications or formula	Read pharmacological information on compatibility of drugs and formula.
Tube displacement	Coughing, vomiting	Replace tube and confirm placement before restarting tube feeding.
	Not taped securely	With placement verification check that tape is secure (nasoenteric).
Abdominal cramping, nausea/vomiting	High osmolality of formula	Suggest an isotonic formula or dilution of current formula to health care provider.
	Rapid increase in rate/volume	Lower rate of delivery to increase tolerance. Maintain head of bed at least 45 degrees.
	Lactose intolerance	Suggest use of lactose-free formula.
	Intestinal obstruction	Stop feeding with GI obstruction.
	High-fat formula used	Use greater proportion of carbohydrate.
	Cold formula used	Warm formula to room temperature.
Delayed gastric emptying	Diabetic gastroparesis	Consult with health care provider regarding prokinetic medication for increasing gastric motility.
	Serious illnesses	Consult health care provider regarding advancing tube to intestinal placement.
	Inactivity	Monitor medications and pathological conditions that affect GI motility.
Serum electrolyte imbalance	Excess GI losses	Monitor serum electrolyte levels daily. Provide free water per registered dietitian recommendation.
	Dehydration	
	Presence of disease states such as cirrhosis, renal insufficiency, heart failure, or diabetes mellitus	
Fluid overload	Refeeding syndrome in malnutrition	Restrict fluids if necessary and use either a specialized formula or a diluted enteral formula at first.
	Excess free water or diluted (hypotonic) formula	Monitor levels of serum proteins and electrolytes. Use more concentrated formula with fluid volume excess without risk of refeeding syndrome.
Hyperosmolar dehydration	Hypertonic formula with insufficient free water	Slow rate of delivery, dilute, or change to isotonic formula.

*First check for fluid-restricted conditions that affect how much water can be given safely.
GI, Gastrointestinal.

An air embolus possibly occurs during insertion of the catheter or when changing the tubing or cap. Turn the patient into a left lateral decubitus position and have him or her perform a Valsalva maneuver (holding the breath and "bearing down") during catheter insertion to help prevent air embolus. The increased venous pressure created by the maneuver prevents air from entering the bloodstream. Maintaining integrity of the closed IV system also helps prevent air embolus.

Catheter occlusion is present when there is sluggish or no flow through the catheter. Temporarily stop the infusion and flush with saline or heparin per protocol or orders. If this is unsuccessful, attempt to aspirate a clot. If still unsuccessful, follow institution protocol for use of a thrombolytic agent (e.g., urokinase).

Suspect catheter sepsis if a patient develops fever, chills, or glucose intolerance and has a positive blood culture. To prevent infection,

TABLE 45-8 **Metabolic Complications of Parenteral Nutrition**

Problem	Signs/Symptoms	Intervention
Electrolyte imbalance	See Chapter 42 for signs of deficiency/toxicity	Check TPN for supplemental electrolyte levels. Notify health care provider of imbalances. Maintain steady rate of infusion. Monitor intake and output.
Hypercapnia	Increased oxygen consumption, CO_2, respiratory quotient (>1), and minute ventilation	Ventilator-dependent patients are at risk; provide 30% to 60% of energy requirements per health care provider's order.
Hypoglycemia	Diaphoresis, shakiness, confusion, loss of consciousness	To prevent hypoglycemia, do not abruptly discontinue TPN but taper rate down to within 10% of infusion rate 1 to 2 hours before stopping. If you suspect hypoglycemia, test blood glucose and administer IV bolus of 50% dextrose or glucagon per order or protocol if necessary.
Hyperglycemia	Thirst, headache, lethargy, increased urination	Monitor blood glucose level every 6 hours. Initiate TPN slowly and taper up to maximal infusion rate to prevent hyperglycemia. Additional insulin may be required during therapy if problem persists or patient has diabetes mellitus.
Hyperglycemic hyperosmolar nonketotic coma (HHNKC) or hyperosmolar hyperglycemic nonketotic syndrome (HHNS)	Hyperglycemia (>500 mg/dL), glycosuria, serum osmolarity >350 mOsm/L, confusion, azotemia, headache, severe signs of dehydration (see Chapter 41), hypernatremia, metabolic acidosis, convulsions, coma	Monitor blood glucose, BUN, serum osmolarity, glucose in urine, and fluid losses; administer insulin as ordered; replace fluids as ordered; maintain constant infusion rate; and provide 30% of daily energy needs as fat. Patients at risk are those receiving steroids; older adults diagnosed with diabetes who have impaired renal or pancreatic function or increased metabolism or who are septic.

BUN, Blood urea nitrogen; *IV,* intravenous; *TPN,* total parenteral nutrition.

change the TPN infusion tubing every 24 hours. Do not hang a single container of PN for more than 24 hours or lipids more than 12 hours. Change the administration system every 72 hours when infusing a 2-in-1 solution and every 24 hours for a 3-in-1 solution (Phillips, 2010). During CVC dressing changes always use a sterile mask and gloves and assess insertion sites for signs and symptoms of infection (see Chapter 42). Change the CVC dressing per institution policy and anytime it becomes wet or contaminated. Use either alcohol or an alcoholic solution of chlorhexidine gluconate to clean the injection port or catheter hub 15 seconds before and after each time it is used (National Guideline Clearinghouse, 2013). Use a 1.2-micron filter for 3-in-1 formulas and an inline 0.22-micron filter for PN solutions that do not include IV fat emulsions.

PN solutions contain most of the major electrolytes, vitamins, and minerals. Patients also need supplemental vitamin K as ordered throughout therapy. Synthesis of vitamin K occurs by the microflora found in the jejunum and ileum with normal use of the GI tract; however, because PN circumvents GI use, patients need to receive exogenous vitamin K.

Electrolyte and mineral imbalances often occur. Administration of concentrated glucose accompanies an increase in endogenous insulin production, which causes cations (potassium, magnesium, and phosphorus) to move intracellularly. Monitor blood glucose levels every 6 hours to assess for hyperglycemia and administer supplemental insulin as needed (Phillips, 2010) (see Skill 45-4 on pp. 1094-1097).

Too-rapid administration of hypertonic dextrose can result in an osmotic diuresis and dehydration (see Chapter 42). If an infusion falls behind schedule, do not increase the rate in an attempt to catch up. Sudden discontinuation of a solution can cause hypoglycemia. Usually it is recommended to infuse 10% dextrose when discontinuing PN solution suddenly. Patients with diabetes are more at risk.

The goal is to move patients from PN to EN and/or oral feeding. Once patients are meeting one third to one half of their kilocalorie needs per day, health care providers usually decrease PN by half the original volume and increase EN feedings to meet the patient's nutritional needs. Patients who make the transition from PN to oral feedings typically have early satiety and decreased appetite. Gradually decrease PN in response to increased oral intake. If oral intake is inadequate, small frequent meals are helpful. Recommend calorie/protein counts when patients begin taking soft foods. When meeting 75% of nutritional needs by enteral feedings or reliable dietary intake, it is usually safe to discontinue PN therapy. Discontinuation of PN may also happen if complications occur or the health care provider determines that it is not benefiting the patient (Krzywda and Meyer, 2010).

Restorative and Continuing Care. Patients discharged from a hospital with diet prescriptions often need dietary education to plan meals that meet specific therapeutic requirements. Restorative care includes both immediate postsurgical care and routine medical care and therefore includes patients in the hospital and at home. The following sections address nutritional interventions for some common disease states.

Medical Nutrition Therapy. Optimal nutrition is just as important in illness as it is in health. As a result, dietary modifications and intake are often needed to maintain the nutritional requirements of patients with certain illnesses. Medical nutrition therapy (MNT) is the use of specific nutritional therapies to treat an illness, injury, or condition. It is necessary to help the body metabolize certain nutrients, correct nutritional deficiencies related to the disease, and eliminate foods that may exacerbate disease symptoms. It is most effective using a team approach that promotes collaboration between the health care team and an RD (American Dietetic Association, 2010b).

Gastrointestinal Diseases. Control peptic ulcers with regular meals and medications such as histamine receptor antagonists that block secretion of HCl or proton pump inhibitors. Marshall and Warren first identified *Helicobacter pylori* in 1984. *H. pylori,* a bacterium that causes up to 85% of peptic ulcers, is confirmed by laboratory tests or a biopsy during endoscopy (Nix, 2012). Antibiotics treat and control the bacterial infection. Stress and overproduction of gastric HCl also irritate a preexisting ulcer. Encourage patients to avoid foods that increase stomach acidity and pain such as caffeine, decaffeinated coffee, frequent milk intake, citric acid juices, and certain seasonings (hot chili peppers, chili powder, black pepper). Discourage smoking, alcohol, aspirin, and nonsteroidal antiinflammatory drugs (NSAIDs). Teach patients to eat a well-balanced, healthy diet; avoid eating large meals; and eat three regular meals (or several small meals) without snacks, especially at bedtime (Nix, 2012). Family members of the patient with *H. pylori* infection also need to be tested and, if indicated, treated.

Inflammatory bowel disease includes Crohn's disease and idiopathic ulcerative colitis. Treatment of acute inflammatory bowel disease includes elemental diets (formula with the nutrients in their simplest form ready for absorption) or PN when symptoms such as diarrhea and weight loss are prevalent. In the chronic stage of the disease, a regular highly-nourishing diet is appropriate. Vitamins and iron supplements are often required to correct or prevent anemia. Patients manage irritable bowel syndrome by increasing fiber, reducing fat, avoiding large meals, and avoiding lactose or sorbitol-containing foods for susceptible individuals.

The treatment of malabsorption syndromes such as celiac disease includes a gluten-free diet. Gluten is present in wheat, rye, barley, and oats. Short-bowel syndrome results from extensive resection of bowel, after which patients suffer from malabsorption caused by lack of intestinal surface area. These patients require lifetime feeding with either elemental enteral formulas or PN.

Diverticulitis is a condition that results from an inflammation of diverticula, which are abnormal but common pouchlike herniations that occur in the bowel lining. Nutritional treatment for diverticulitis includes a moderate- or low-residue diet until the infection subsides. Afterward prescribing a high-fiber diet for chronic diverticula problems ensues.

Diabetes Mellitus. Type 1 DM requires both insulin and dietary restrictions for optimal control, with treatment beginning at diagnosis (ADA, 2012). By contrast, patients often control type 2 DM initially with exercise and diet therapy. If these measures prove ineffective, it is common to add oral medications. Insulin injections often follow if type 2 DM worsens or fails to respond to these initial interventions.

Individualize the diet according to a patient's age, build, weight, and activity level. Maintaining a prescribed carbohydrate intake is the key in diabetes management. The ADA recommends a diet that includes carbohydrates from fruits, vegetables, whole grains, legumes, and low-fat milk (American Dietetic Association, 2010b). Monitoring carbohydrate consumption is a key strategy in achieving glycemic control (ADA, 2012). Limit saturated fat to less than 7% of the total calories and cholesterol intake to less than 200 mg/day. In addition, varieties of foods containing fiber are recommended. Patients are able to substitute sucrose-containing foods for carbohydrates but need to make sure to avoid excess energy intake. Patients with diabetes can eat sugar alcohols and nonnutritive sweeteners as long as they follow the recommended daily intake level (ADA, 2012). Patients with diabetes and normal renal function should continue to consume usual amounts of protein (15% to 20% of energy) (ADA, 2012).

The goal of MNT treatment is to have glycemic levels that are normal or as close to normal as safely possible; lipid and lipoprotein profiles that decrease the risk of microvascular (e.g., renal and eye disease), cardiovascular, neurological, and peripheral vascular complications; and blood pressure in the normal or near-normal range (ADA, 2012). Be aware of signs and symptoms of hypoglycemia and hyperglycemia.

Cardiovascular Diseases. The goal of the American Heart Association (AHA) dietary guidelines (AHA, 2010) is to reduce risk factors for the development of hypertension and coronary artery disease. Diet therapy for reducing the risk of cardiovascular disease includes balancing calorie intake with exercise to maintain a healthy body weight; eating a diet high in fruits, vegetables, and whole-grain high-fiber foods; eating fish at least 2 times per week; and limiting food and beverages that are high in added sugar and salt. The AHA guidelines also recommend limiting saturated fat to less than 7%, trans-fat to less than 1%, and cholesterol to less than 300 mg/day. To accomplish this goal, patients choose lean meats and vegetables, use fat-free dairy products, and limit intake of fats and sodium (Nix, 2012).

Cancer and Cancer Treatment. Malignant cells compete with normal cells for nutrients, increasing a patient's metabolic needs. Most cancer treatments cause nutritional problems. Patients with cancer often experience anorexia, nausea, vomiting, and taste distortions. The goal of nutrition therapy is to meet the increased metabolic needs of a patient (Nix, 2012). Malnutrition in cancer is associated with increased morbidity and mortality. Enhanced nutritional status often improves a patient's quality of life.

Radiation therapy destroys rapidly dividing malignant cells; however, normal rapidly dividing cells such as the epithelial lining of the GI tract are often affected. Radiation therapy causes anorexia, stomatitis, severe diarrhea, strictures of the intestine, and pain. Radiation treatment of the head and neck region causes taste and smell disturbances, decreased salivation, and dysphagia. Nutrition management of a patient with cancer focuses on maximizing intake of nutrients and fluids. Individualize diet choices to a patient's needs, symptoms, and situation (Nix, 2012). Use creative approaches to manage alterations in taste and smell. For example, patients with altered taste often prefer chilled foods or foods that are spicy. Encourage patients to eat small frequent meals and snacks that are nutritious and easy to digest.

Human Immunodeficiency Virus/Acquired Immunodeficiency Syndrome. Patients with HIV/AIDS typically experience body wasting and severe weight loss related to anorexia, stomatitis, oral thrush infection, nausea, or recurrent vomiting, all resulting in inadequate intake. Factors associated with weight loss and malnutrition include severe diarrhea, GI malabsorption, and altered metabolism of nutrients. Systemic infection results in hypermetabolism from cytokine elevation. The medications that treat HIV infection often cause side effects that alter patients' nutritional status.

Restorative care of malnutrition resulting from AIDS focuses on maximizing kilocalories and nutrients. Diagnose and address each cause of nutritional depletion in the care plan. The progression of individually tailored nutrition support begins with administering oral, to enteral, and finally to parenteral. Good hand hygiene and food safety are essential because of a patient's reduced resistance to infection. For example, minimization of exposure to *Cryptosporidium* in drinking water, lakes, or swimming pools is important. Small, frequent, nutrient-dense meals that limit fatty and overly sweet foods are easier to tolerate. Patients benefit from eating cold foods and drier or saltier foods with fluid in between (Nix, 2012).

◆ Evaluation

Through the Patient's Eyes. Patients expect competent and accurate care. If ongoing nutrition therapies do not result in successful outcomes, patients expect nurses to recognize this and alter the plan of care accordingly. Expectations and health care values held by nurses frequently differ from those held by patients. Successful interventions and outcomes require nurses to know what patients expect in addition to nursing knowledge and skill. Work closely with patients to define their expectations and talk with them about their concerns if their expectations are not realistic. Consider the limits of their conditions and treatment, their dietary preferences, and their cultural beliefs when evaluating outcomes.

Patient Outcomes. Care plans need to reflect achievable goals and outcomes. Evaluate the actual outcomes of nursing actions and compare them with expected outcomes to determine if the goals were met (Figure 45-9). Interprofessional collaboration remains essential in providing nutritional support. Nutrition therapy does not always produce rapid results. You need to evaluate a patient's current weight in comparison with his or her baseline weight, serum albumin or prealbumin, and protein and kilocalorie intake routinely. If you do not observe gradual weight gain or if weight loss continues, evaluate the dietary EN prescription and determine if the patient is experiencing any adverse effects from medications that are affecting his or her nutritional status. Changes in condition also indicate a need to change the nutritional plan of care. Consult multidisciplinary members of the health care team in an effort to better individualize this plan. The patient is an active participant whenever possible. In the end a patient's ability to incorporate dietary changes into his or her lifestyle with the least amount of stress or disruption facilitates attainment of outcome measures. Failing to meet expected outcomes requires revising the nursing interventions or expected outcomes on the basis of the patient's needs or preferences. When not meeting outcomes, ask questions such as, "How has your appetite been?" "Have you noticed a change in your weight?" "How much would you like to weigh?" or "Have you changed your exercise pattern?"

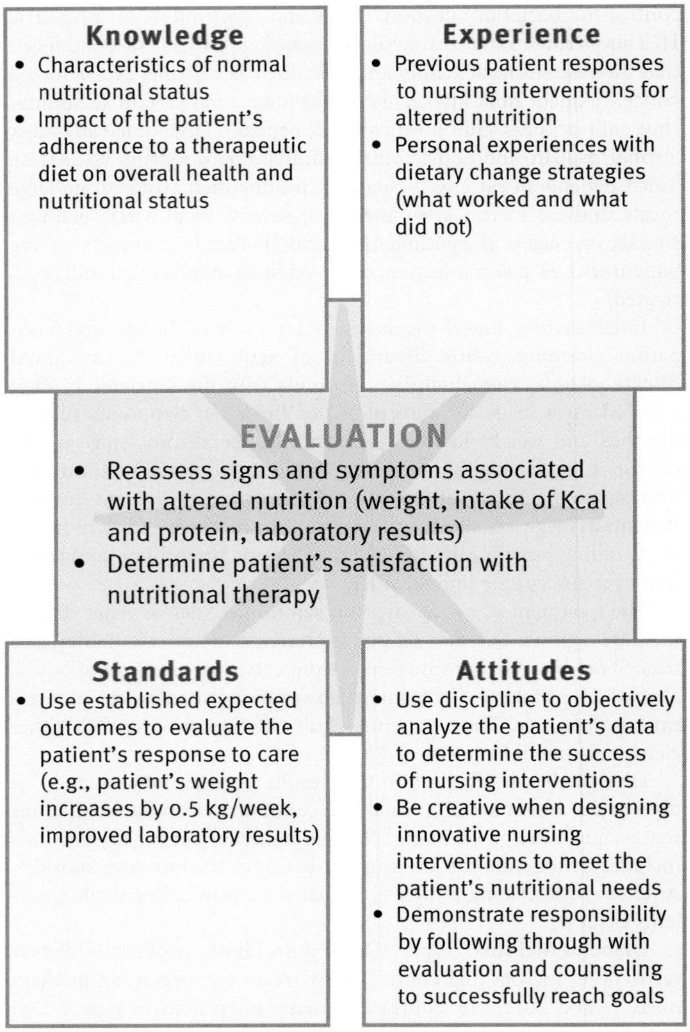

Knowledge
- Characteristics of normal nutritional status
- Impact of the patient's adherence to a therapeutic diet on overall health and nutritional status

Experience
- Previous patient responses to nursing interventions for altered nutrition
- Personal experiences with dietary change strategies (what worked and what did not)

EVALUATION
- Reassess signs and symptoms associated with altered nutrition (weight, intake of Kcal and protein, laboratory results)
- Determine patient's satisfaction with nutritional therapy

Standards
- Use established expected outcomes to evaluate the patient's response to care (e.g., patient's weight increases by 0.5 kg/week, improved laboratory results)

Attitudes
- Use discipline to objectively analyze the patient's data to determine the success of nursing interventions
- Be creative when designing innovative nursing interventions to meet the patient's nutritional needs
- Demonstrate responsibility by following through with evaluation and counseling to successfully reach goals

FIGURE 45-9 Critical thinking model for nutrition evaluation.

SAFETY GUIDELINES FOR NURSING SKILLS

Ensuring patient safety is an essential role of the professional nurse. To ensure patient safety, communicate clearly with members of the health care team, assess and incorporate a patient's priorities of care and preferences, and use the best evidence when making decisions about your patient's care. When performing the skills in this chapter, remember the following points to ensure safe, individualized patient care.

- Verify that the appropriate ENFit connector is attached to the enteral tube when administering tube feedings (TJC, 2014).
- Use aseptic technique when preparing and delivering enteral feedings. Check agency policy for wearing gloves when handling feedings (Stewart, 2014).
- Label enteral equipment with patient name and room number; formula name, rate, and date and time of initiation; and nurse initials (Stewart, 2014).
- Practice "right patient, right formula, right tube, right ENFit adaptor" by matching formula and rate to feeding order and verifying that enteral tubing set connects formula to a feeding tube (Stewart, 2014).
- Position the patient upright or elevate the head of the bed a minimum of 30 (preferably 45) degrees unless medically contraindicated for patients receiving enteral feedings (Stewart, 2014).
- Trace all lines and tubing back to the patient to ensure only enteral-to-enteral connections (Stewart, 2014).
- Do not add food coloring or dye to EN because the use of dye has been linked to hypotension, metabolic acidosis, and death (Metheny, 2009).
- Refer to manufacturer guidelines to determine hang time for enteral feedings. Maximum hang time for formula is 8 hours in an open system and 24 to 48 hours in a closed, ready-to-hang system (if it remains closed). There is increased risk of bacterial growth in feedings that exceed the recommended hang time.
- Always use an infusion pump for continuous enteral feedings and PN.

SKILL 45-1 ASPIRATION PRECAUTIONS

DELEGATION CONSIDERATIONS

The skill of assessing a patient's risk for aspiration and determining positioning cannot be delegated to nursing assistive personnel (NAP). NAP may feed patients after receiving instructions in aspiration precautions. Instruct NAP to:

- Position patient upright (45 to 90 degrees preferred) or according to medical restrictions.
- Follow aspiration precautions while feeding patient.
- Report any onset of coughing, gagging, or pocketing of food in the mouth.

EQUIPMENT

- Chair or electric bed (to allow patient to sit upright)
- Thickening agents as designated by RD or SLP (rice, cereal, yogurt, gelatin, commercial thickening agent)
- Tongue blade
- Oral-hygiene supplies (see Chapter 40)
- Penlight
- Suction equipment
- Clean gloves
- *Option:* Pulse oximeter

STEP	RATIONALE
ASSESSMENT	
1. Identify patient using two identifiers (e.g., name and birthday or name and medical record number) according to agency policy.	Ensures correct patient. Complies with The Joint Commission standards and improves patient safety (TJC, 2016).
2. Perform hand hygiene. Perform nutrition screening.	Patients at risk for aspiration from dysphagia often alter their eating patterns or choose foods that do not provide adequate nutrition (Ochoa, 2012).
3. Perform dysphagia screening or review results of dysphagia screen by an SLP. Note symptoms such as cough, pharyngeal pooling, change in voice after swallowing. Use a validated screening tool (when available).	Patients at risk for dysphagia include those who have neurological or neuromuscular diseases and those who have had trauma to or surgical procedures of the oral cavity or throat (see Box 45-7).
4. *Option:* Measure patient's oxygen saturation.	Provides baseline to help determine if aspiration develops. However, changes in oxygen saturation may not be related to aspiration; further research is needed (ASHA, 2014).
5. Assess mental status: alertness, orientation, ability to follow simple commands.	Determines patient's ability to participate in feeding.
6. Observe patient during previous mealtime for signs of dysphagia and allow him or her to attempt to feed self. Observe patient eat various consistencies of foods and liquids. Note at end of meal if patient becomes tired.	Helps detect abnormal eating patterns such as frequent clearing of throat or prolonged eating time. Fatigue increases risk of aspiration and may reveal a need to plan smaller, more frequent meals.
7. Assess patient's oral cavity (apply gloves as needed) for level of hygiene, missing teeth, or poorly fitting dentures.	Poor oral hygiene (decayed teeth, plaque) causes growth of bacteria in the mouth, which can be aspirated.
8. Ask patient and or family caregiver about any difficulties with chewing or swallowing various textures of food.	Certain types of foods are easier to aspirate than others.
9. Assess patient's swallowing reflex before initial feeding by placing fingers on patient's throat at level of larynx and asking patient to swallow saliva. Feel for movement of larynx.	Movement of larynx can be palpated.
10. Take tongue blade and, while asking patient to say "Ah," observe movement of the tongue. Then gently elicit gag reflex. This should be done on initial assessment or if there is a change in patient's swallowing ability.	Tongue movement may reveal weakness on one side of the mouth, impairing swallowing.
PLANNING	
1. Arrange equipment and supplies at bedside.	
2. Explain to patient what you will be doing while he or she eats.	Increases patient cooperation.
3. Provide a 30-minute rest period before meals.	Swallowing difficulty is less likely in a well-rested patient (Metheny et al., 2012).
IMPLEMENTATION	
1. Perform hand hygiene. Apply clean gloves, then have patient perform hand hygiene.	Reduces transmission of microorganisms.
2. Perform oral hygiene, including brushing of tongue, before meal. Remove and dispose of gloves. Perform hand hygiene.	Risk of aspiration pneumonia is associated with poor oral hygiene (Borrelli and Talih, 2012).
3. Position patient upright in a chair or elevate head of patient's bed to a 45- to 90-degree angle or to the highest position allowed by patient's medical condition during feeding.	Positions aim to prevent gastric reflux and reduces occurrence of aspiration (Grodner et al., 2012; Metheny and Frantz, 2013).
4. Using penlight and tongue blade, gently inspect mouth for pockets of food.	Pockets of food in mouth often indicate difficulty swallowing (Remig and Weeden, 2012).
5. Have patient assume a chin-tuck position. Begin by having patient try sips of water. Monitor for swallowing and respiratory difficulties continuously. If patient tolerates water, offer a larger volume of water and then different consistencies of foods and liquids.	Chin-tuck or chin-down position may help reduce aspiration (Terré and Mearin, 2012). Supine position increases probability of aspiration (Metheny et al., 2012).
6. Add thickener to thin liquids to create consistency of mashed potatoes or serve patient pureed foods per SLP evaluation.	Thin liquids such as water and fruit juice are difficult to control in mouth and are more easily aspirated (Ellis and Hannibal, 2013).
7. Encourage patient to feed self.	

SKILL 45-1 ASPIRATION PRECAUTIONS—cont'd

STEP	RATIONALE
8. If patient is unable to feed self, place ½ to 1 teaspoon of food on unaffected side of mouth, allowing utensil to touch mouth or tongue.	Provides tactile cue to begin eating. Placement of food on affected (or weakened) side increases risk for aspiration.
9. Place hand on throat and gently palpate swallowing event as it occurs. Swallowing twice is often necessary to clear pharynx.	Helps evaluate swallowing effort.
10. Provide verbal coaching while feeding patient and give positive reinforcement, as follows: **a.** Open your mouth. **b.** Feel the food in your mouth. **c.** Chew and taste the food. **d.** Raise your tongue to the roof of your mouth. **e.** Think about swallowing. **f.** Close your mouth and swallow. **g.** Swallow again. **h.** Cough to clear airway.	Verbal cueing keeps patient focused on swallowing. Positive reinforcement enhances patient's confidence in ability to swallow (Metheny et al., 2012).
11. Avoid mixing food of different textures in same mouthful.	Single textures are easier to swallow than multiple textures.
12. Observe for coughing, choking, gagging, and drooling food; suction airway as necessary.	These are indications of dysphagia and risk for aspiration (National Stroke Association, 2013).
13. Do not rush patient, and avoid distractions. Provide rest periods as necessary during meal.	Avoiding fatigue decreases risk of aspiration (Metheny et al., 2012). Environmental distractions and conversation during meal increases risk for aspiration (Chang and Roberts, 2011).
14. Use tongue blade to inspect patient's mouth for pocketed food. (Apply gloves if needed.)	Checking for pocketed food provides information on patient's swallowing ability and prevents aspiration.
15. Have patient remain sitting upright for at least 30 to 60 minutes after meal.	Requiring patients to remain upright after meals or snacks reduces chance of aspiration by allowing food particles remaining in pharynx to clear (Frey and Ramsberger, 2011).
16. Help patient perform hand hygiene and mouth care. (Apply gloves if necessary.)	Mouth care after meals helps prevent dental caries and reduces colonization of bacteria, which reduces risk of pneumonia (Metheny et al., 2012).
17. Consult with registered dietician (RD) or speech-language pathologist to advance diet to thicker foods that require more chewing and, finally, to thin liquids.	RD or speech-language pathologist develop a safe patient-centered plan to advance the diet.
18. Return patient's tray to appropriate place and perform hand hygiene.	Reduces spread of microorganisms.
EVALUATION	
1. Observe patient's ability to swallow foods of various textures and thickness.	Indicates whether aspiration risk increases with thin liquids.
2. Observe patient for signs of choking, coughing, and wet voice.	Provides continual data about patient's ability to effectively swallow and if the aspiration risk increases.
3. Inspect patient's oral cavity after meal to detect pockets of food.	Determines patient's ability to completely swallow food.
4. Monitor patient's intake and output, calorie count, food intake, and weight.	Aids in prompt detection of nutritional deficits, decreased caloric intake, or dehydration.
5. *Option:* For high-risk patients, monitor pulse oximetry readings throughout the feeding session.	Deteriorating oxygen saturation levels may help indicate aspiration, but currently more research is needed to determine efficacy (ASHA, 2014).
6. Use ***Teach Back*** to determine patient's and family's understanding about dysphagia. State, "I want to be sure I explained what dysphagia is and how to prevent choking. Can you explain to me the steps you can take to protect yourself from choking?" Revise your instruction now or develop plan for revised patient teaching if patient is not able to teach back correctly.	Evaluates what the patient is able to explain or demonstrate.

UNEXPECTED OUTCOMES AND RELATED INTERVENTIONS

1. Patient coughs, gags, complains of food "stuck in throat," or has pockets of food in mouth.
   - Stop feeding. If choking persists, suction oral cavity and place patient on NPO.
   - Notify health care provider.
   - Patient may require a swallowing evaluation.
   - Initiate consultation with health care provider so that a referral to a speech-language pathologist (SLP) can be made for different swallowing exercises and techniques to improve swallowing and reduce risk of aspiration.
2. Patient avoids certain textures of food.
   - Change consistency and texture of food.
3. Patient experiences weight loss.
   - Discuss findings with health care provider, SLP, and/or registered dietitian.

RECORDING AND REPORTING

- Record assessment findings, patient's tolerance of various food textures, amount of help required, position during meal, absence or presence of any symptoms of dysphagia, and amount eaten on flow sheet or nurses' notes in EHR or chart.
- Place information in patient's medical record indicating aspiration precautions.
- Document your evaluation of patient learning.
- Report any coughing, gagging, choking, or swallowing difficulties to health care provider.

SKILL 45-2 INSERTING AND REMOVING A SMALL-BORE NASOENTERIC TUBE FOR ENTERAL FEEDINGS

DELEGATION CONSIDERATIONS

The skill of inserting a small-bore feeding tube cannot be delegated to nursing assistive personnel (NAP). The nurse guides the NAP to assist with patient positioning during tube insertion.

EQUIPMENT

Insertion

- Small bore nasogastric or nasoenteric feeding tube with or without stylet (select smallest diameter possible to enhance patient comfort)
- Stethoscope and pulse oximeter/capnography device
- Water-soluble lubricant
- 60-mL or larger Luer-Lok or catheter-tip syringe
- Hypoallergenic tape and tincture of benzoin or tube fixation device
- pH indicator strip (scale 1.0 to 11.0 or greater)
- Glass of water and straw
- Emesis basin
- Towel
- Facial tissues
- Clean gloves
- Suction equipment in case of aspiration
- Penlight to check placement in nasopharynx
- Tongue blade

Removal

- Towel
- Facial tissue
- Oral hygiene supplies
- 30-mL Luer-Lok catheter-tip syringe

STEP	RATIONALE
ASSESSMENT	
1. Verify health care provider's order for type of tube and enteric feeding schedule. Order should indicate delivery site and device, patient's name and identifying information (see agency policy), formula type, and administration method and rate.	Health care provider's order is needed to intubate patients with feeding tubes.
2. Review patient's medical history for basilar skull fracture, nosebleeds, oral facial surgery, facial trauma, nasal septum deviation, past history of aspiration, anticoagulation therapy, or coagulopathy.	A history of these problems may contraindicate tube placement and require you to consult with health care provider to change route of nutrition support. Passage of tube intracranially can cause neurological injury.
3. Identify patient using two identifiers (e.g., name and birthday or name and medical record number) according to agency policy.	Ensures correct patient. Complies with The Joint Commission standards and improves patient safety (TJC, 2016).
4. Assess patient's knowledge of procedure.	Encourages cooperation, reduces anxiety, and minimizes risks. Identifies patient teaching needs.
5. Assess data on patient's height, weight, hydration status and I&O, electrolyte balance, and caloric needs in medical record.	Provides baseline information to measure nutritional improvement after enteral feedings are initiated.
6. Perform hand hygiene. Have patient close each nostril alternately and breathe. Examine each naris for patency and skin breakdown.	Sometimes nares are obstructed or irritated, or a septal defect or facial fractures are present. Place tube in most patent nostril.
7. Assess patient's mental status (ability to cooperate with procedure, sedation level), presence of cough and gag reflex, ability to swallow, presence of an artificial airway.	These are risk factors for inadvertent feeding tube placement into the tracheobronchial tree (Krenitsky, 2011). Patients with impaired level of consciousness often have impaired gag reflex; their risk of aspiration increases during insertion of feeding tubes and subsequent tube feedings (Altman et al., 2013).

CLINICAL DECISION: *Recognize situations in which blind placement of a feeding tube poses an unacceptable risk for patient. Devices for detecting accidental insertion of a tube into the airway, such as carbon dioxide sensors or electromagnetic tracking devices, enhance patient safety. Electromagnetically guided nasointestinal (NI) tubes enhance placement with real-time tip tracking to verify tube placement (Taylor et al., 2010). Only clinicians trained in the use of visualization or imaging techniques should perform blind placement of tubes (AACN, 2012; Krenitsky, 2011).*

SKILL 45-2 INSERTING AND REMOVING A SMALL-BORE NASOENTERIC TUBE FOR ENTERAL FEEDINGS—cont'd

STEP	RATIONALE
8. Perform physical assessment of abdomen.	Absence of bowel sounds or presence of abdominal pain, tenderness, or distention may indicate GI problem, contraindicating feeding.
9. Check medical record to determine if health care provider wants prokinetic agent administered before tube placement.	Prokinetic agents such as metoclopramide given before tube placement help advance tube into intestine (Metheny, 2006).
PLANNING	
1. Explain procedure to patient, including sensations anticipated during insertion (burning in nasal passages) and to raise index finger to indicate gagging or discomfort during insertion.	Reduces anxiety and helps patient assist in insertion.
2. Perform hand hygiene. Organize supplies at bedside.	
3. Stand on same side of bed as naris chosen for insertion and help patient to high-Fowler's position unless contraindicated. Place pillow behind head and shoulders. If patient is comatose, raise HOB as tolerated in semi-Fowler's position with head tipped forward, using a pillow chin to chest. If necessary, have NAP assist. If patient is forced to lie supine, place in reverse Trendelenburg's position.	Allows easier manipulation of tube. Fowler's position reduces risk of aspiration and promotes effective swallowing.
4. Place bath towel over patient's chest. Keep facial tissues within reach.	Prevents soiling of gown. Insertion of tube frequently produces tearing.
5. Determine length of tube to be inserted and mark with tape.	
a. Measure distance from tip of nose to earlobe to xiphoid process of sternum (see illustration).	Length approximates distance from nose to stomach. The NEX (nose-earlobe-xiphoid) method is commonly used in clinical settings.
b. Measure distance from tip of nose to earlobe to mid-umbilicus for pediatric patients.	
c. Add additional 20 to 30 cm (8 to 12 inches) for nasointestinal (NI) tubes.	Length approximates distance from nose to intestine.
6. Prepare nasogastric or nasointestinal tube for insertion: **Note:** Do not ice plastic tubes.	Tubes becomes stiff and inflexible, causing trauma to mucous membranes.
a. If tube has guidewire or stylet, inject 10 mL of water from the Luer-Lok or catheter-tip syringe into tube.	Ensures tube is patent. Activates lubrication of tube for easier passage and ensures the tube is patent. Aids in guidewire or stylet removal once the tube is placed.
b. If using stylet, ensure that is it securely positioned within tube and that both Luer-Lok connections are snugly fit.	Promotes smooth passage of tube into GI tract. Improperly positioned stylet induces serious trauma.
7. Prepare materials for tube fixation. Tear off a 3- to 4-inch length of hypoallergenic tape or open membrane dressing or other fixation device). (See Step 13a in Implementation.)	Fixation devices allow the tube to float free of the nares, thus reducing pressure on the nares and preventing device-related pressure ulcer (DRPU).
IMPLEMENTATION	
1. Perform hand hygiene. Apply clean gloves.	Reduces transmission of microorganisms.
2. Apply pulse oximeter/capnography device and measure vital signs.	Provides objective assessment of respiratory status during tube insertion.
3. *Option:* Dip tube with surface lubricant into glass of room temperature water or apply water soluble lubricant (see manufacturer's directions).	Activates lubricant to facilitate passage of tube into naris to GI tract.

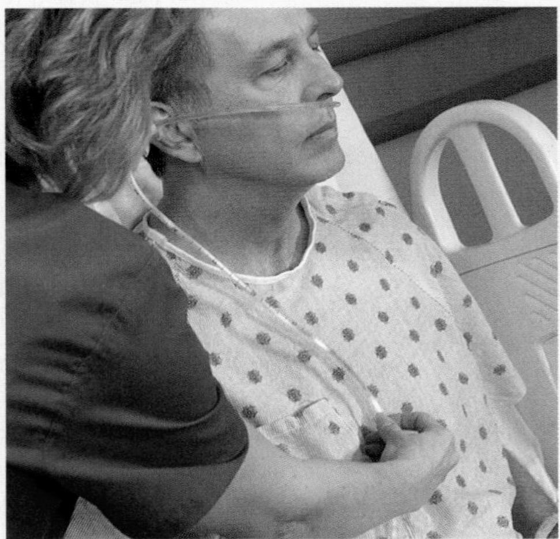

STEP 5a Determine length of tube to be inserted. (Copyright © Mosby's Clinical Skills: Essentials Collection.)

STEP	RATIONALE
4. Hand an alert patient a cup of water if able to hold cup and swallow. Explain that you are about to insert tube.	Swallowing water facilitates tube passage.
5. Explain next steps. Insert tube gently through nostril to back of throat (posterior nasopharynx). Aim back and down toward ear.	Natural contour facilitates passage of tube into GI tract and reduces gagging by patient.
6. Have patient relax and flex head toward chest after tube has passed through nasopharynx.	Closes off glottis and reduces risk of tube entering trachea.
7. Encourage patient to swallow by taking small sips of water when possible. Advance tube as patient swallows. Rotate tube gently 180 degrees while inserting.	Swallowing facilitates passage of tube past oropharynx. A tug may be felt as patient swallows, indicating tube is following desired path.
8. Emphasize need to mouth breathe and swallow during procedure.	Helps facilitate passage of tube and alleviates patient's fears during procedure.
9. Do not advance tube during inspiration or coughing becuase it will likely enter respiratory tract. Monitor oximetry/capnography.	Can cause tube to inadvertently enter patient's airway, which will be reflected in changes in O_2 saturation or end tidal CO_2.
10. Advance tube each time patient swallows until you have reached desired length (see illustration).	Reduces discomfort and trauma to patient.

CLINICAL DECISION: *Do not force the tube. If patient starts to cough or has a drop in oxygen saturation or an increased CO_2, withdraw tube into the posterior nasopharynx until normal breathing resumes.*

STEP	RATIONALE
11. Using penlight and tongue blade, check to be sure tube is not positioned in back of throat.	Tube could become coiled, kinked, or enter the trachea.
12. Temporarily anchor tube to nose with a small piece of tape.	Movement of tube stimulates gagging. Allow for assessment of tube position before anchoring the tube securely.
13. Keep tube secure. Attach syringe to end of feeding tube and obtain gastric aspirate; assess amount, color, and quality of return. Measure gastric pH.	Proper tube position is essential before initiating feeding. Properly obtained pH of 1.0 to 4.0 is good indication of gastric placement (Fernandez et al., 2010).

CLINICAL DECISION: *Auscultation of the insufflation of air is not a reliable method for verification of tube placement because a tube inadvertently placed in the lungs, pharynx, or esophagus also transmits a sound similar to that of air entering the stomach (Kenny and Goodman, 2010; Stewart, 2014).*

STEP	RATIONALE
14. Anchor tube to nose with a fixation device. Avoid pressure on nares. Mark tube at exit site with indelible ink. Select one of the following fixation methods.	Properly secured tube allows patient more mobility and prevents trauma to nasal mucosa.
a. Apply tape.	
(1) Apply tincture of benzoin or other skin adhesive on tip of patient's nose and tube and allow it to become "tacky."	Helps tape adhere better. Protects skin.
(2) Remove gloves. Tear small horizontal slits at ⅓ and ⅔ length of tape without splitting tape (see illustration). Fold middle sections forward and seal.	
(3) Place top end of tape over bridge of patient's nose. Print date and time on the tape.	

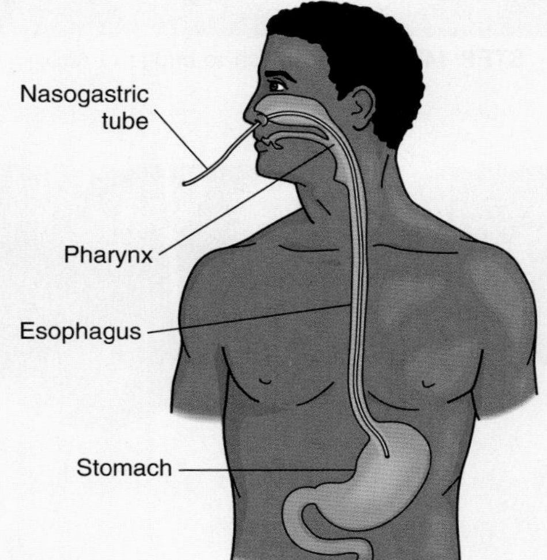

STEP 10 Insert NG tube through nose and esophagus into stomach.

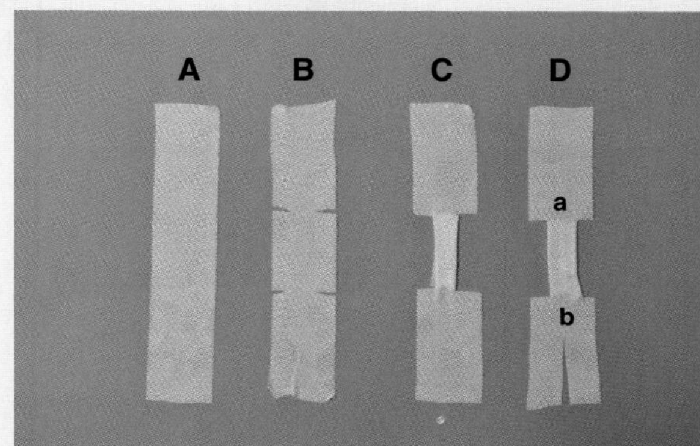

STEP 14a(2) Taping method. **A,** Start with a piece of tape. **B,** Make two slits on both sides of tape. **C,** Fold middle section inward. **D,** Tear a new slit in bottom of tape. The top part (*a*) should attach to the patient's nose and the bottom part (*b*) should be wrapped around the tube.

SKILL 45-2 INSERTING AND REMOVING A SMALL-BORE NASOENTERIC TUBE FOR ENTERAL FEEDINGS—cont'd

STEP	RATIONALE
(4) Wrap bottom end of tape around tube as it exits nose (see illustration).	Securing tape to nares in this method reduces pressure on nares and reduces the risk for device-related pressure ulcer (AACN, 2014).
b. Apply tube fixation device using shaped adhesive patch (see manufacturer directions).. **(1)** Apply wide end of patch to bridge of nose (see illustration). **(2)** Slip connector around tube as it exits nose (see illustration).	Secures tube and reduces friction on naris.
15. Fasten end of nasogastric tube to patient's gown with piece of tape (see illustration). Do not use safety pins to fasten tube to gown.	Reduces traction on naris if tube moves. Safety pins become unfastened and possibly cause injury to patient.
16. Keep head of bed elevated at least 30 degrees (preferably 45 degrees) unless contraindicated (Metheny and Frantz, 2013). For intestinal tube placement, place patient on right side when possible until radiographic confirmation of correct placement.	Positioning patient on right side promotes passage of tube into small intestine.
17. Remove gloves, perform hand hygiene, and help patient to comfortable position.	Prevents transmission of infection.

CLINICAL DECISION: *Leave guidewire or stylet in place until a radiologist verifies correct position by x-ray film. Never attempt to reinsert partially or fully removed guidewire or stylet while feeding tube is in place.*

STEP	RATIONALE
18. Obtain ordered x-ray film of chest/abdomen.	X-ray film examination is gold standard for verifying tube placement (Stewart, 2014).

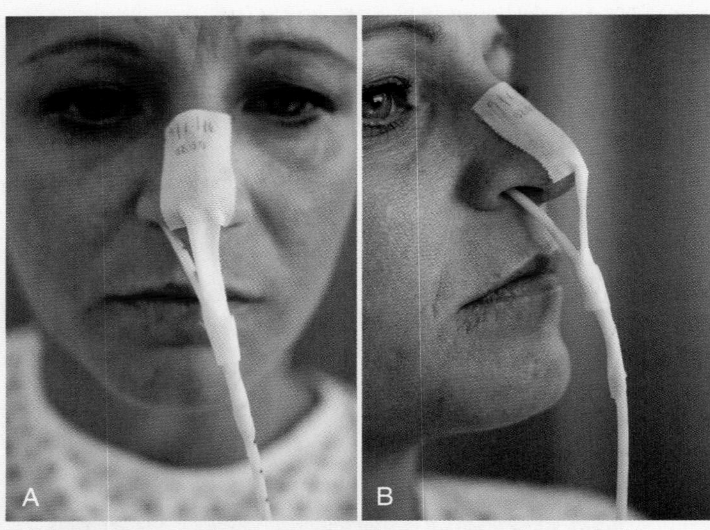

STEP 14a(4) A, Applying tape to anchor nasoenteral tube. **B,** Nares are free of pressure from tape and feeding tube.

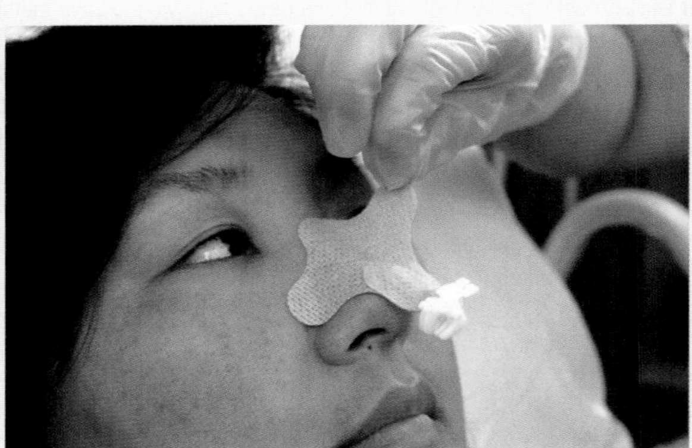

STEP 14b(1) Apply patch to bridge of nose.

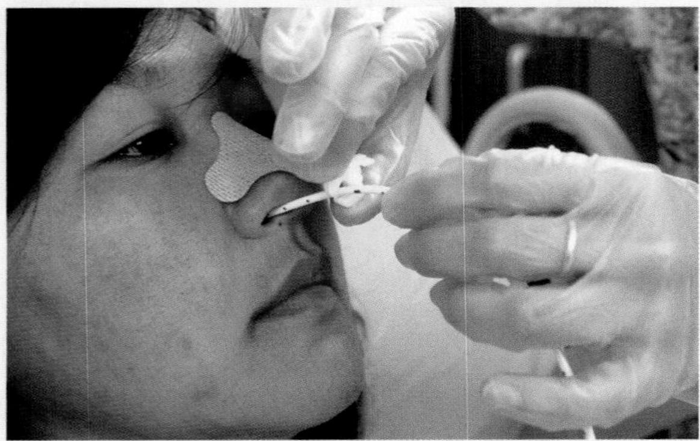

STEP 14b(2) Slip connector around feeding tube.

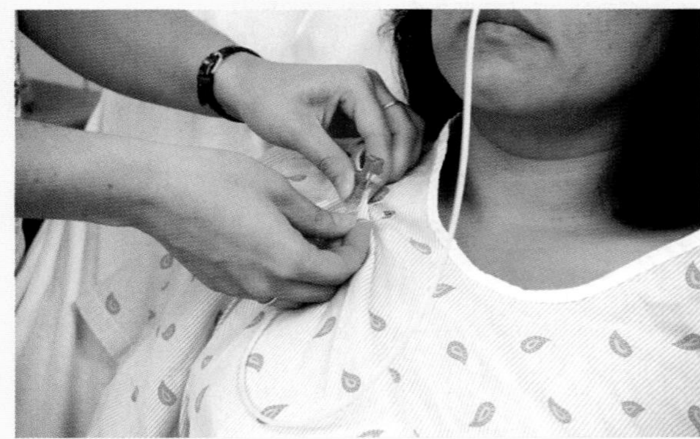

STEP 15 Fasten feeding tube to patient's gown.

STEP	RATIONALE
19. After proper tube placement is verified, measure the amount of tube that is external and mark the exit of the tube at the nares with indelible marker as a guide for displacement.	The mark alert nurses to possible tube displacement, which will require confirmation of tube placement before further use.
20. Apply clean gloves and administer oral hygiene (see Chapter 40). Clean tubing at nostril.	Promotes patient comfort and integrity of oral mucous membranes.
21. Remove gloves, dispose of equipment, and perform hand hygiene.	Reduces transmission of microorganisms.
TUBE REMOVAL	
22. Verify health care provider's order for tube removal.	
23. Gather equipment and explain procedure to patient.	Informs patient and enhances cooperation.
24. Perform hand hygiene and apply clean gloves.	Reduces transmission of microorganisms.
25. Position patient upright in high-Fowler's unless contraindicated.	Reduces risk of aspiration in the event the patient vomits.
26. Place disposable pad or towel on patient's chest. If present, disconnect tube from feeding administration set and cap end..	Prevents mucus and secretions from soiling patient's gown.
27. Remove tape or tube fixation device from patient's nose and gown.	Allows for easy tube removal.
28. Instruct patient to take a deep breath and hold it.	Prevents inadvertent aspiration of gastric contents during tube removal.
29. Kink end of tubing securely by folding it over on itself. Then completely withdraw tube by pulling it out steadily and smoothly. Dispose of tubing in proper receptacle.	Prevents residual leakage of fluid from tube. Minimizes patient discomfort. Reduces transmission of microorganisms.
30. Offer tissues to patient to blow nose. Clean nares and provide oral care.	Provides patient comfort.
31. Remove gloves and perform hand hygiene.	Reduces transmission of microorganisms.
EVALUATION	
1. Inspect naris and oropharynx for any irritation after insertion.	If insertion was difficult, irritation of naris or oropharynx may have occurred.
2. Ask if patient feels comfortable.	Evaluates patient's level of comfort.
3. Observe patient for any difficulty breathing, coughing, or gagging.	Malposition of tube causes these symptoms.
4. Auscultate lung sounds.	Abnormal lung sounds are early sign of aspiration.
5. Confirm x-ray film results.	Verifies position of tube before initiating enteral feeding.
6. Routinely check location of external exit site marking on the tube as well as color and pH of fluid withdrawn from the feeding tube.	Routine checking ensures correct tube placement and reduces the risk of aspiration.
7. Use ***Teach Back*** to determine patient's and family's understanding about feeding tube. State, "I want to be sure I explained the feeding tube and its purpose. Can you explain to me why I placed this tube?" Revise your instruction now or develop plan for revised patient teaching if patient is not able to teach back correctly.	Evaluates what patient and family are able to explain or demonstrate.

UNEXPECTED OUTCOMES AND RELATED INTERVENTIONS

1. Suspected aspiration of stomach contents into the respiratory tract
   - Position patient on side.
   - Suction nasotracheally and orotracheally.
   - Consult health care provider immediately to order chest x-ray film examination.
   - Prepare for possible initiation of antibiotics.
2. Displacement of feeding tube to another site (e.g., from duodenum to stomach, mark at exit site if tube is moved); possibly occurs when patient coughs or vomits
   - Aspirate GI contents and measure pH.
   - Remove displaced tube; insert and verify placement of new tube.
   - If there is a question of aspiration, obtain order for chest x-ray film.

RECORDING AND REPORTING

- Record the type and size of tube placed, location of distal tip of tube, patient's tolerance of procedure, pH value, and confirmation of tube position by x-ray film examination on flow sheet or nurses' notes in EHR or chart.
- Document your evaluation of patient learning.
- If patient develops signs of aspiration, notify health care provider immediately.

SKILL 45-3 ADMINISTERING ENTERAL FEEDINGS VIA NASOENTERIC, GASTROSTOMY, OR JEJUNOSTOMY TUBES

DELEGATION CONSIDERATIONS

The skill of administering enteral tube feeding via a NG, NI, gastrostomy, or jejunostomy tube can be delegated to nursing assistive personnel (NAP) after the tube placement is verified by the nurse (refer to agency policy). However, the nurse must verify tube placement and patency and that the feeding formula and fluid (water) to be administered are correct. The nurse must monitor the patient for effectiveness and tolerance of the feeding being delivered. The nurse directs the NAP to:

- Elevate the head of the bed to a minimum of 30 degrees (45 degrees is preferred) or sit patient up in bed or in a chair.
- Infuse feeding as ordered.
- Report any difficulty infusing feeding or any discomfort voiced by patient.
- Report any gagging, paroxysms of coughing, or choking.

EQUIPMENT

- Disposable feeding bag and tubing or ready-to-hang system. **NOTE:** Feeding tubes must have ENFit adapter (see Figure 45-8, *B*).
- 30-mL or larger Luer-Lok or catheter-tip syringe
- Stethoscope
- pH indicator strip (scale 1.0 to 11.0 or greater)
- Infusion pump (required for continuous or intestinal feedings): use pump designed for tube feedings
- Prescribed enteral feedings
- Clean gloves
- Equipment to obtain blood glucose by fingerstick

STEP	RATIONALE
ASSESSMENT	
1. Verify health care provider's order for formula, rate, route, and frequency. Health care provider also orders laboratory data and bedside assessments such as fingerstick blood glucose measurement.	Tube feedings, laboratory tests, and bedside tests must be ordered by health care provider.
2. Review medical record to assess patient's need for enteral tube feedings: impaired swallowing, decreased level of consciousness, head or neck surgery, facial trauma, surgeries of upper alimentary canal.	Identify patients who need tube feedings before they become nutritionally depleted.
3. Identify patient using two identifiers (e.g., name and birthday or name and medical record number) according to agency policy.	Ensures correct patient. Complies with The Joint Commission standards and improves patient safety (TJC, 2016).
4. Assess patient's nutritional status (see Table 45-4). Obtain baseline weight and review laboratory values (e.g., electrolytes, capillary blood glucose measurement). Assess patient for fluid volume excess or deficit, electrolyte abnormalities, and metabolic abnormalities such as hyperglycemia.	Enteral feedings are to restore or maintain a patient's nutritional status. Provides objective data to measure effectiveness of feedings.
5. Assess patient for food allergies or intolerances.	Prevents patient from developing localized or systemic allergic responses to feeding.
6. Perform physical assessment of abdomen.	Absent bowel sounds are not a contraindication to feeding, but you need to report a change from baseline abdominal assessment. If tenderness or distention develop, determine if feeding can proceed safely (Bankhead et al., 2009). May need to hold tube feeding (see agency policy).
7. For feedings administered through abdominal wall, assess insertion site for breakdown, irritation, drainage, discomfort, or presence of an external disk that is not excessively snug. Monitor that length of external tube remains the same as when originally placed.	Infection, pressure from tube, or drainage of gastric secretions causes skin breakdown. A disk that is too snug may cause skin breakdown. Internal tube migration may block pylorus and cause patient distress.
PLANNING	
1. Explain procedure to patient.	Well-informed patient is more cooperative and at ease.
2. Perform hand hygiene and apply clean gloves.	Reduces transmission of microorganisms.
3. Prepare feeding container and formula:	Tube feedings administered within designated shelf life from container without cracks or breaks reduce patient's risk of obtaining tube feeding–borne GI infections. In addition, container without cracks or breaks prevents leakage of tube feeding.
a. Check expiration date on formula and integrity of container.	
b. Have tube feeding at room temperature.	Cold formula causes gastric cramping and discomfort because mouth and esophagus do not warm liquid.
c. Connect tubing to container as needed or prepare ready-to-hang container. Use proper ENFit connector and aseptic technique and avoid handling feeding system or touching can tops, container openings, spike, and spike port.	Correct enteral access connector designed for the specific of enteral tube reduces enteral tube misconnections and medication errors (TJC, 2016). These devices are not compatible with Luer-Lok or needleless connectors. Ensures that feeding system, including bag, connections, and tubing, is free of contamination to prevent bacterial growth (Stewart, 2014).
d. Shake formula container well. Cleanse top of canned formula with alcohol swab before opening it. Fill container with formula (see illustration). Open roller clamp on tubing and fill with formula to remove air. Reclamp tubing. Hang on intravenous (IV) pole.	Filling tubing with formula prevents excess air from entering GI tract.

STEP	RATIONALE
4. For intermittent feeding have syringe ready and be sure that formula is at room temperature.	Cold formula causes gastric cramping.

IMPLEMENTATION

STEP	RATIONALE
1. Place patient in high-Fowler's position or elevate head of bed at least 30 (preferably 45) degrees. For patients forced to remain supine, place in reverse Trendelenburg's position.	Elevated head helps prevent aspiration (Kenny and Goodman, 2010).
2. Verify tube placement: (see Skill 45-2)	
a. *Nasogastric tube* (see Box 45-14): Attach syringe and aspirate 5 mL of gastric contents. Observe appearance of aspirate and note pH. b. *Gastrostomy tube:* Attach syringe and aspirate 5 mL of gastric contents. Observe appearance of aspirate and note pH.	Verifies if tip of feeding tube is in stomach or intestine. Feedings instilled in misplaced tube can cause serious injury or death. Gastric fluid of patient who has fasted for at least 4 hours usually has a pH of 5 or less, especially when patient is not receiving gastric-acid inhibitor. Continuous administration of tube feedings elevates pH (Stewart, 2014). A pH greater than 6 indicates intestinal or pulmonary placement. (Bourgault et al., 2015).
c. *Jejunostomy tube:* Aspirate intestinal secretions, observe their appearance, and check pH.	Presence of intestinal fluid indicates that end of tube is in small intestine.

CLINICAL DECISION: *Auscultation of insufflated air is not a reliable method for verification of placement of a tube because a tube inadvertently placed in lungs, pharynx, or esophagus transmits sound similar to that of air entering the stomach (Kenny and Goodman, 2010; Stewart, 2014).*

STEP	RATIONALE
3. Check for gastric residual volume (GRV) before each feeding for bolus and intermittent feedings, every 4 hours in critically ill patients, and every 4 to 6 hours in non–critically ill patients for continuous feedings.	GRV indicates if there is delayed gastric emptying.
a. Draw up 10 to 30 mL of air into syringe. Connect to end of feeding tube. Flush tube with air. Pull back slowly to aspirate total amount of gastric contents and measure (see illustration).	
b. Return aspirated contents to stomach unless volume exceeds 250 mL (check agency policy). Some questions exist regarding safety of returning high volumes of fluid into the stomach (Delegge, 2011; Stewart, 2014).	Return of aspirate prevents fluid and electrolyte imbalance (Stewart, 2014).

CLINICAL DECISION: *Numerous factors affect measurement accuracy of GRV, including size of gastric tube, position of the tube port in the gastric atrium, patient's position, and whether tube location is near the gastroesophageal junction. Best evidence suggests that a single high GRV should be monitored for the following hour but that the enteral feeding should not be stopped or withheld for an isolated high GRV (Makic et al., 2011).*

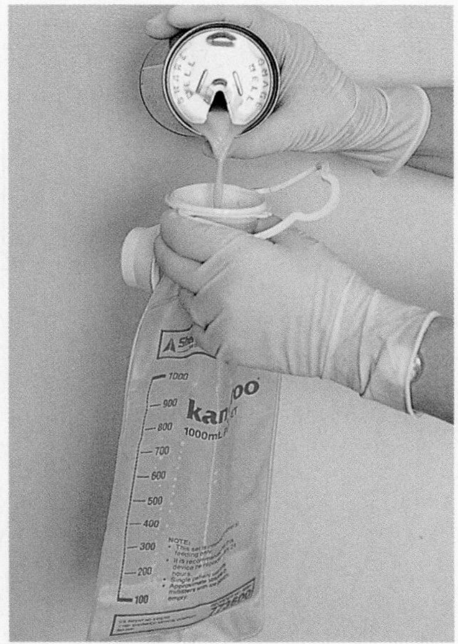

STEP 3d Pour formula into feeding container.

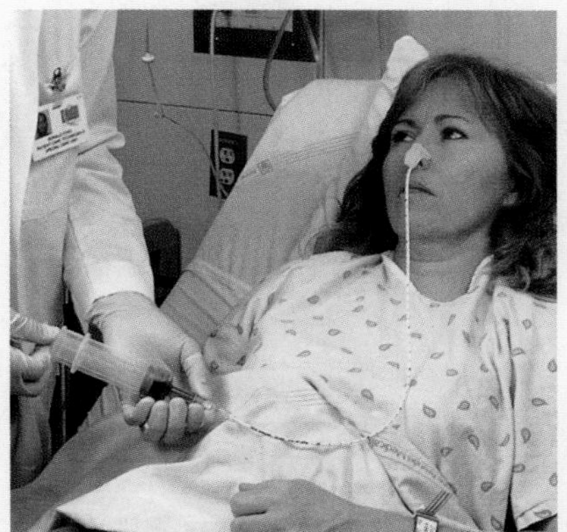

STEP 3a Check for gastric residual (small-bore tube).

SKILL 45-3 ADMINISTERING ENTERAL FEEDINGS VIA NASOENTERIC, GASTROSTOMY, OR JEJUNOSTOMY TUBES—cont'd

STEP	RATIONALE
c. Do not administer feeding when a single GRV exceeds 500 mL or when two consecutive measurements (taken 1 hour apart) each exceed 250 mL (Stewart, 2014; Yantis and Velander, 2011) (check agency policy).	Some controversy exists regarding ability of elevated GRVs to identify risk for pulmonary aspiration. However, frequent interruptions of feeding on the basis of GRV levels is a well-recognized reason for failure to meet nutritional goals (Delegge, 2011; Metheny et al., 2012; Stewart, 2014).
d. GRV in the range of 250 to 500 mL should raise concern and lead to implementation of measures to reduce aspiration risk. Automatic cessation of feeding should not occur for GRV less than 500 mL in the absence of other signs of intolerance (McCarthy et al., 2015).	Raising the cutoff value for GRV from a lower number to a higher number does not increase the risk for aspiration or pneumonia. Elevated GRV should raise concern and lead to measures to reduce the risk of aspiration.
4. Flush tubing with 30 mL water. Before attaching feeding administration set to feeding tube, trace tube to origin and label "Tube feeding only."	Ensures that tube is clear and patent (Metheny et al., 2012). Usually patients receive enteral feedings continuously. Avoids misconnections (Stewart, 2014). However, they often receive initial feedings by bolus to assess formula tolerance. See Box 45-12 for guidelines to advance enteral feedings.
5. Initiate feeding:	
a. Syringe for intermittent feeding	
(1) Pinch proximal end of feeding tube.	Prevents excessive air from entering patient's stomach/intestine or leaking of contents.
(2) Remove plunger from syringe and attach tip of syringe to end of tube.	
(3) Fill syringe with measured amount of formula (see illustration). Release tube, elevate syringe to no more than 45 cm (18 inches) above insertion site, and allow it to empty gradually by gravity. Repeat Steps (1) to (3) until you have delivered prescribed amount to patient.	Height of syringe allows for safe, slow, gravity drainage of formula. This gradual emptying of tube feeding by gravity reduces risk of abdominal discomfort, vomiting, or diarrhea induced by bolus or too-rapid infusion of tube feedings.
b. Feeding bag for intermittent feeding	

CLINICAL DECISION: *Before attaching feeding administration set to a feeding tube, trace the tube to its point of origin. Label the administration set "Tube Feeding Only." This prevents misconnections between feeding set and intravenous systems or other medical tubing or devices (Stewart, 2014).*

STEP	RATIONALE
(1) Pinch proximal end of feeding tube and remove bag. Connect distal end of administration set tubing to end of feeding tube. Set rate by adjusting roller clamp on tubing or placing on feeding pump.	Prevents excess air from entering stomach and leakage of gastric contents.
(2) Allow bag to empty gradually over 30 to 45 minutes (see illustration). Label bag with tube-feeding type, strength, and amount (include date, time, and initials). Change bag every 24 hours.	Gradual emptying of tube feeding by gravity reduces risk for abdominal discomfort, vomiting, or diarrhea induced by bolus or too-rapid infusion of tube feedings. Helps decrease bacterial colonization.
(3) Immediately follow feeding with water (per health care provider's order). Cover end of bag with cap.	Cleans bag and feeding tube, prevents tube from clogging, and provides patient with adequate water.
(4) Keep bag as clean as possible, and change bag every 24 hours.	Helps decrease bacterial growth in feeding tube system.

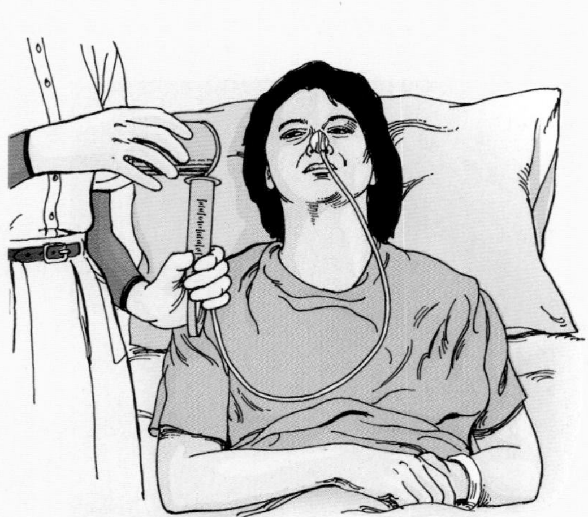

STEP 5a(3) Fill syringe with formula.

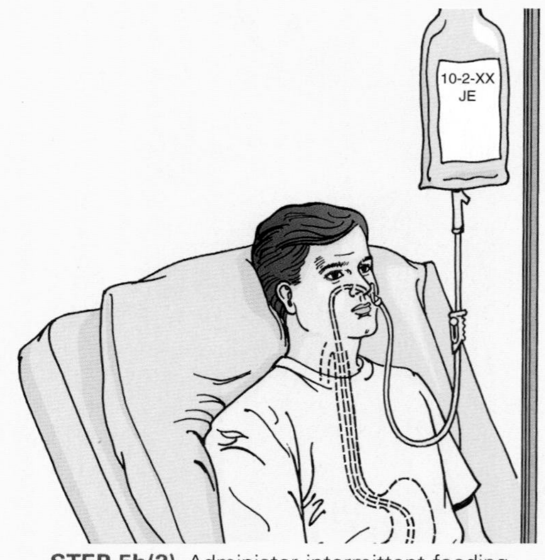

STEP 5b(2) Administer intermittent feeding.

STEP	RATIONALE
c. Continuous-drip method	
(1) Remove cap and connect feeding tube to distal end of administration set tubing.	Prevents excess air from entering stomach and leakage of gastric contents.
(2) Insert tubing through infusion pump and set rate (see illustration). Use pump designated for tube feeding and not one for IV fluids.	Delivers continuous feeding at steady rate and pressure. Pump alarms for increased resistance.
6. Advance rate of tube feeding gradually as ordered (see Box 45-12).	Advancing tube feedings gradually helps prevent diarrhea and gastric intolerance to formula.
7. Flush with 30 mL water every 4 hours during continuous feeding, before and after an intermittent feeding (check agency policy). Collaborate with registered dietitian and health care provider regarding recommended total free water requirement per day and obtain order.	Clears tubing of formula and prevents clogging of tube (Stewart, 2014). Also provides water source for patient to help maintain fluid and electrolyte balance.

CLINICAL DECISION: *Flush tube with 30 mL sterile water in immunocompromised or critically ill patients (Stewart, 2014).*

STEP	RATIONALE
8. When patient is receiving intermittent tube feeding, cap or clamp proximal end of feeding tube when not in use.	Prevents air from entering stomach between feedings.
9. Rinse bag and tubing with warm water whenever feedings are interrupted.	Clears old tube feedings and reduces bacterial growth.
10. Change bag and use new administration set every 24 hours.	Reduces patient's exposure to bacterial growth occurring in bag and tubing.
11. For abdominally placed feeding tubes, clean insertion site daily and as needed. A small breathable dressing may be used to protect the insertion site. However, the site is usually left open to air.	Decreases risk for infection.
12. Dispose of supplies and perform hand hygiene.	Reduces transmission of microorganisms.
EVALUATION	
1. Measure GRV per agency policy, usually every 4 to 6 hours. Ask patient if nausea is present.	Evaluates tolerance of tube feeding.
2. Monitor fingerstick blood glucose every 6 hours until patient reaches maximum administration rate and maintains it for 24 hours (see Skill 45-4).	Alerts nurse to patient's tolerance of glucose. If blood glucose levels are elevated, glucose testing will continue.
3. Monitor intake and output every 8 hours and calculate daily totals every 24 hours.	Intake and output are indications of fluid balance, fluid volume excess or deficit.
4. Weigh patient daily until maximum administration rate is reached and maintained for 24 hours; then weigh patient 3 times per week at same time using same scale.	Weight gain is indicator of improved nutritional status; however, sudden gain of more than 2 lbs in 24 hours usually indicates fluid retention.
5. Monitor laboratory values.	Improving laboratory values (e.g., albumin, transferrin, and prealbumin) indicate an improved nutritional status (Stewart, 2014).

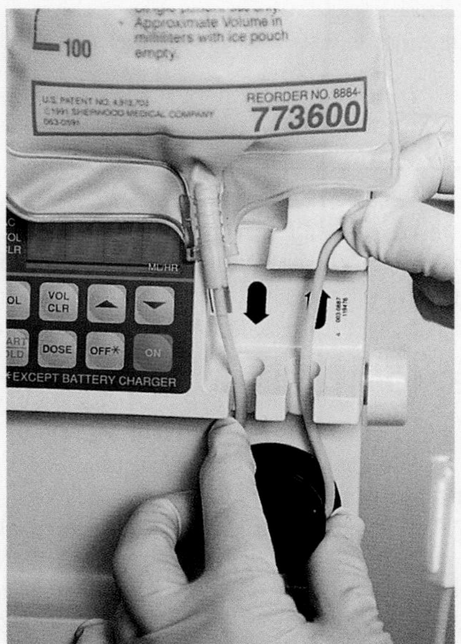

STEP 5c(2) Connect tubing through infusion pump.

SKILL 45-3 ADMINISTERING ENTERAL FEEDINGS VIA NASOENTERIC, GASTROSTOMY, OR JEJUNOSTOMY TUBES—cont'd

STEP	RATIONALE
6. Observe patient's respiratory status.	Change in respiratory status (e.g., increased rate, declining SpO_2) may indicate aspiration of tube feeding.
7. Examine abdomen and auscultate bowel sounds.	Evaluates GI function.
8. Observe nasoenteral tube insertion site for impaired skin integrity. For tubes placed through abdominal wall, inspect insertion site for signs of impaired skin integrity and signs of infection, injury, or tightness of tube.	Enteral tubes often cause pressure and excoriation at insertion site. Gastric secretions also cause irritation to skin.
9. Use ***Teach Back*** to determine patient's and family's understanding about tube feedings. State, "I want to be sure I explained why we are giving tube feedings. Can you explain to me why tube feedings are necessary?" Revise your instruction now or develop plan for revised patient teaching if patient is not able to teach back correctly.	Evaluates what patient and family are able to explain or demonstrate.

UNEXPECTED OUTCOMES AND RELATED INTERVENTIONS (IN ADDITION TO THOSE IN SKILL 45-1)

1. Feeding tube is clogged.
    - Attempt to flush the tube with water
    - Special products, such as pancreatic enzymes, are available for unclogging feeding tubes.
    - Hold feeding and notify health care provider.
    - Maintain patient in semi-Fowler's position.
2. GRV exceeds 250 mL for each of two consecutive assessments (see agency policy).
    - Hold feeding and notify health care provider.
    - Maintain patient in upright position in chair/bed or elevate head of bed at least 30 (preferably 45) degrees.
    - Recheck residual in 1 hour.
3. Patient develops diarrhea 3 times or more in 24 hours.
    - Notify health care provider.
    - Confer with dietitian.
    - Institute skin-care measures.
    - Consider change in antibiotics, only for patients receiving antibiotics.
4. Patient develops nausea, vomits, and aspirates formula when gastric emptying is delayed or formula is administered too rapidly and produces vomiting.
    - Position patient in side-lying position.
    - Suction airway.
    - Notify health care provider.
    - Obtain chest x-ray film.
    - Check patency of tube.
    - Aspirate for GRV.

RECORDING AND REPORTING

- Record amount and type of feeding instilled, patient's response to tube feeding, patency of tube, condition of naris or skin at tube site for tubes placed in abdominal wall, and any side effects.
- Report patient's tolerance and adverse effects.
- Document your evaluation of patient learning.

HOME CARE CONSIDERATIONS

- Teach patient or family caregiver how to determine correct placement of feeding tube.
- Inform patient or family caregiver of signs associated with pulmonary aspiration, delayed gastric emptying.
- Reinforce signs and symptoms associated with feeding tube complications and when to call health care provider.
- Explain and demonstrate how to do skin care around gastrostomy or jejunostomy tube and explain signs and symptoms of infection at the insertion site.

SKILL 45-4 BLOOD GLUCOSE MONITORING

DELEGATION CONSIDERATIONS

When the patient is stable, the skill of measuring blood glucose level can be delegated to nursing assistive personnel (NAP). When the patient's condition changes frequently, you should not delegate this skill to NAP. The nurse directs the NAP by:

- Explaining appropriate sites to use for puncture and when to obtain glucose levels.
- Reviewing expected level and when to report unexpected glucose levels to the nurse.

EQUIPMENT

- Antiseptic swab
- Cotton ball
- Sterile lancet or blood-letting device
- Paper towel
- Blood glucose meter (e.g., OneTouch, Freestyle) (Figure 45-10)
- Blood glucose reagent strips (brand determined by meter used)
- Clean gloves

STEP	RATIONALE
ASSESSMENT	
1. Identify patient using two identifiers (e.g., name and birthday or name and medical record number) according to agency policy.	Ensures correct patient. Complies with The Joint Commission standards and improves patient safety (TJC, 2016).
2. Assess patient's understanding of procedure and purpose of glucose monitoring. Determine if patient with diabetes mellitus performs test at home and, if so, confirm his or her competency.	Data set guidelines for nurse to develop teaching plan.
3. Determine if specific conditions need to be met before or after sample collection (e.g., with fasting, after meals, after certain medications, before insulin doses).	Dietary intake of carbohydrates and ingestion of concentrated glucose preparations alter blood glucose levels.
4. Determine if risks exist for performing skin puncture (e.g., low platelet count, anticoagulant therapy, bleeding disorders).	Abnormal clotting mechanisms increase risk for local ecchymosis and bleeding.
5. Assess area of skin that you will use as puncture site (e.g., fingers or heel). Alternative sites are palm, arm, or thigh. Avoid areas of bruising and open lesions.	Sides of fingers and heels are commonly selected because they have fewer nerve endings. If the patient has diabetes mellitus, do not do a heelstick. Measurements from alternative sites are meter specific and may differ from traditional sites (ADA, 2012). Puncture site should not be edematous, inflamed, or recently punctured because these factors cause increased interstitial fluid and blood to mix and increase risk for infection.
6. Review health care provider's order for time of frequency of measurement.	Health care provider determines test schedule on basis of patient's physiological status and risk for glucose imbalance.
7. For patient with diabetes who performs test at home, assess knowledge about procedure and ability to handle skin-puncturing device. If patient chooses, he or she may wish to continue self-testing while in hospital.	Patient's physical health may change (e.g., vision disturbance, fatigue, pain, disease process), preventing him or her from performing test.
PLANNING	
1. Explain procedure and purpose to inexperienced or uninformed patient and/or family. Offer patient and family opportunity to practice testing procedures. Provide resources/teaching aids for patient.	Promotes understanding and cooperation.
IMPLEMENTATION	
1. Perform hand hygiene.	Reduces transfer of microorganisms.
2. Instruct adult to perform hand hygiene with soap and warm water. Rinse and dry.	Reduces presence of microorganisms and any food residue on patient's hand. Food residue can contaminate blood drop and cause a false reading. Warmth promotes vasodilation at selected puncture site. Handwashing establishes practice for patient when performing test at home.
3. Position patient comfortably in chair or in semi-Fowler's position in bed.	Ensures easy accessibility to puncture site. Patient assumes position when self-testing.

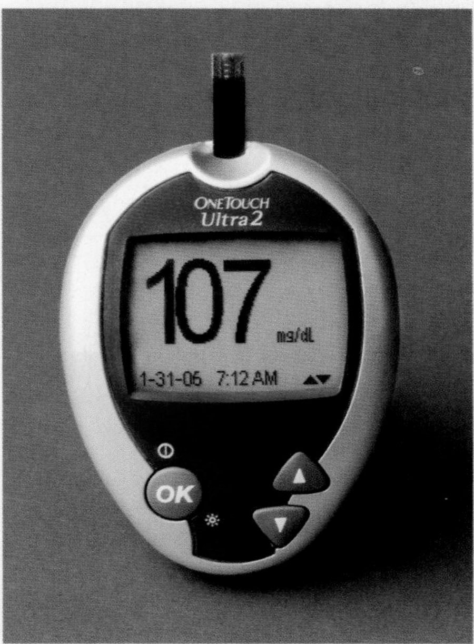

FIGURE 45-10 Blood glucose monitor. (Courtesy LifeScan, Inc., Milpitas, Calif.)

SKILL 45-4 BLOOD GLUCOSE MONITORING—cont'd

STEP	RATIONALE
4. Remove reagent strip from container; tightly seal cap. Check code on test strip vial.	Protects strips from accidental discoloration caused by exposure to air or light. Code on test strip vial must match code entered into glucose meter.
5. Turn on glucose meter if necessary.	Activates meter.
CLINICAL DECISION: *Some monitors activate when the reagent strip is inserted and therefore do not have a specific on/off switch.*	
6. Insert reagent strip into glucose meter (refer to manufacturer directions) and make necessary adjustments (see illustration).	Some machines need calibration; others require zeroing of timer. Each meter is adjusted differently.
7. Apply clean gloves.	Reduces risk for contamination by blood.
8. Choose puncture site. Puncture site should be vascular. In stable adults select lateral side of finger; be sure to avoid central tip of finger, which has more dense nerve supply.	Ensures free flow of blood following puncture. Lateral sides of fingers are less sensitive to pain.
9. Hold area to be punctured in dependent position. Do not milk or massage site.	Increases blood flow to area before puncture. Milking or messaging may hemolyze specimen and introduce excess tissue fluid, causing inaccurate readings (Pagana et al., 2015).
10. Wipe site with antiseptic swab and *allow it to dry completely*.	Removes resident microorganisms. Too much alcohol can cause blood to hemolyze.
11. Remove cover of lancet or bloodletting device. Hold lancet perpendicular to puncture site and pierce finger or heel quickly in one continuous motion (do not force lancet).	Placement ensures that lancet enters skin properly.
12. Some agencies use lancet devices with an automatic blade retraction system. This reduces possibility of self-sticks, preventing exposure to bloodborne pathogens. Place bloodletting device firmly against side of finger and push release button, causing needle to pierce skin (see illustration).	Bloodletting devices pierce skin to specific depth, ensuring adequate blood flow. Perpendicular position ensures proper skin penetration.
13. Wipe away first drop of blood with cotton ball. (See manufacturer directions for meter used.)	First drop of blood may contain more serous fluid than blood cells.
14. Lightly squeeze puncture site (without touching) until large drop of blood has formed (see illustration). Repuncturing is necessary if large-enough drop does not form to ensure accurate test results. (See manufacturer directions regarding how blood is applied.)	You need an adequate-size drop to activate monitor and obtain accurate results. Excessive squeezing of tissues during blood sample collection may contribute to pain, bruising, scarring, and hematoma formation.
CLINICAL DECISION: *Patients with diabetes frequently have peripheral vascular disease, making it difficult to produce a large drop of blood after a fingerstick. Be sure to hold finger in dependent position before puncturing to improve blood flow.*	
15. Obtain test results.	Exposure of blood to test strip for prescribed time ensures proper results.
CLINICAL DECISION: *Some meters (e.g., OneTouch [LifeScan]) require application of blood sample to a test strip already in the meter. Once the drop of blood is applied, the meter automatically calculates the reading.*	

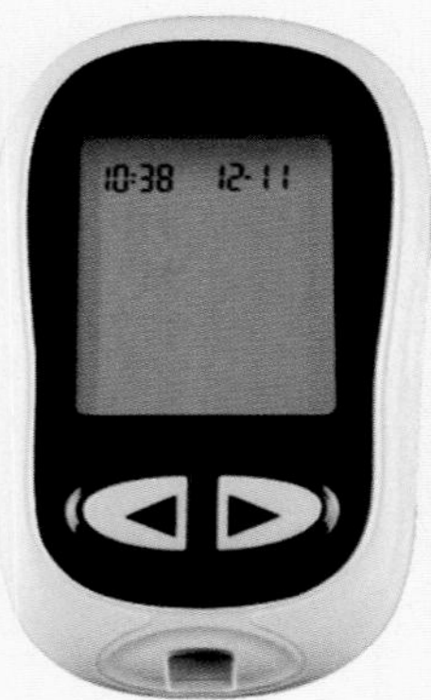

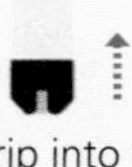

STEP 6 Load test strip into meter. (Courtesy of the manufacturer.)

STEP 12 Prick side of finger with lancet.

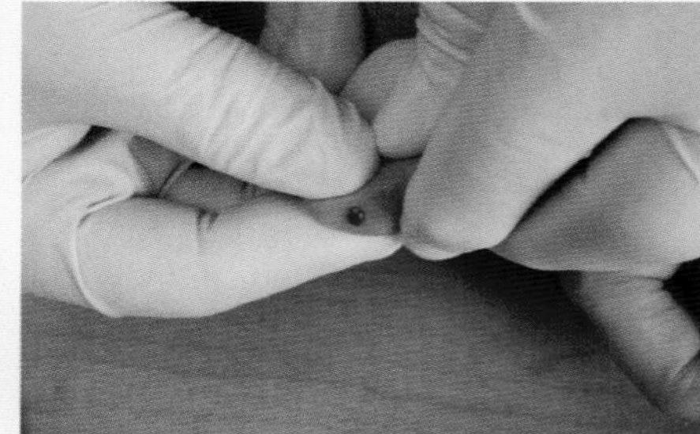

STEP 14 Squeeze puncture site until large droplet of blood forms.

STEP	RATIONALE
a. Be sure that meter is still powered on. Bring test strip in meter to drop of blood. The blood is wicked onto test strip (see manufacturer instructions).	Blood enters strip, and glucose device shows message on screen to signal that you have obtained enough blood.

CLINICAL DECISION: *Do not scrape blood onto the test strips or apply it to the wrong side of the test strip. This prevents accurate glucose measurement.*

STEP	RATIONALE
b. Blood glucose test result appears on screen (see illustration). Some devices "beep" when completed.	
16. Turn off meter. Dispose of test strip, lancet, and gloves in proper receptacles. Perform hand hygiene.	Meter is battery powered. Proper disposal reduces risk for needlestick injury and spread of infection.
17. Discuss test results with patient.	Promotes participation and compliance with therapy.

EVALUATION

STEP	RATIONALE
1. Observe puncture site for bleeding or tissue injury.	Site is a possible source of discomfort and infection.
2. Compare glucose meter reading with normal blood glucose levels and previous test results.	Determines if glucose level is normal.
3. Ask patient to explain test results.	Results of test may cause anxiety. Patient needs to understand range of glucose values to maintain blood glucose management.
4. Use ***Teach Back*** to determine patient's and family's understanding of how to monitor blood glucose. State, "It is important that you understand how to monitor your blood glucose. Can you explain why you need to monitor blood glucose? Can you explain to me the steps in performing a fingerstick?" Revise your instruction now or develop plan for revised patient teaching if patient is not able to teach back correctly.	Evaluates what patient and family are able to explain or demonstrate.

UNEXPECTED OUTCOMES AND RELATED INTERVENTIONS

1. Puncture site continues to bleed or bruised.
   - Apply pressure to site.
   - Notify health care provider if bleeding lasts more than 5 minutes.
2. Glucose meter malfunctions.
   - Repeat test, following directions.
   - Follow manufacturer directions for malfunctions.
3. Blood glucose level is above or below target range.
   - Check medical record to see if there is a medication order for deviations in glucose level; if not, notify health care provider.
   - Continue to monitor patient.
   - Follow agency protocol for laboratory confirmation testing of very high or very low results. Generally laboratory testing is considered more accurate.
   - Administer insulin or carbohydrate source as ordered (depending on glucose level).
   - Notify health care provider of patient's response.

RECORDING AND REPORTING

- Record glucose results on flow sheet or nurses' notes in EHR or chart, including presence or absence of pain or excessive oozing of blood at puncture site.
- Document your evaluation of patient learning.
- Report blood glucose levels out of target range and take appropriate action for hypoglycemia or hyperglycemia.

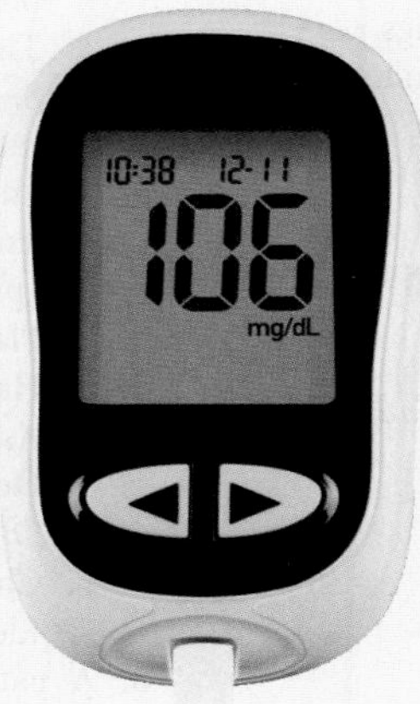

STEP 15b Results appear on meter screen. (Courtesy of the manufacturer.)

KEY POINTS

- Ingestion of a diet balanced with carbohydrates, fats, proteins, vitamin, and minerals provides the essential nutrients to carry out the normal physiological functioning of the body throughout the life span.
- Through digestion food is broken down into its simplest form for absorption. Digestion and absorption occur mainly in the small intestine.
- Guidelines for dietary change recommend reduced fat, saturated fat, sodium, refined sugar, and cholesterol and increased intake of complex carbohydrates and fiber.
- Because improper nutrition affects all body systems, nutritional assessment includes a review of total physical assessment.
- Enteral feedings are for patients who are unable to ingest food but are able to digest and absorb food in the gastrointestinal tract.
- EN protects intestinal structure and function and enhances immunity.
- TPN supplies essential nutrients in appropriate amounts to support life through the administration of a concentrated nutrient solution into the superior vena cava near the right atrium of the heart.
- MNT is a recognized treatment modality for both acute and chronic disease states.
- One of the most important responsibilities of a nurse administering enteral feedings is to take precautions to prevent patients from aspirating feeding formula.
- Special diets alter the composition, texture, digestibility, and residue of foods to suit the patient's particular needs.

CLINICAL APPLICATION QUESTIONS

Preparing for Clinical Practice

1. Knowing that Mrs. Cooper is on a fixed income, you need to develop a plan to help her decrease her risk for complicating her present disease processes. Using your knowledge of medical nutrition therapy (MNT), summarize three points that you will include in a plan to help her meet her nutritional needs while living on a budget.
2. Six months later, Mrs. Cooper is admitted to the hospital for an exacerbation of her heart failure. She is diagnosed with a viral infection. She has increased weight gain because of fluid retention and decreased urinary output because her kidneys are starting to fail. Her appetite is poor; she has frequent nausea and vomiting. Her abdomen is soft and nontender, and bowel sounds are present. The health care provider orders the starting of enteral feedings.
   a. Which type of tube would be most appropriate for you to select?
   b. How would you verify tube placement?
   c. Which measures would you take to make sure that the tube stays in the correct position?
   d. Which tube-feeding complications would be appropriate for you to include in your patient assessment?

ⓔ *Answers to Clinical Application Questions can be found on the Evolve website.*

REVIEW QUESTIONS

Are You Ready to Test Your Nursing Knowledge?

1. The nurse is caring for a patient with pneumonia who has severe malnutrition. The nurse recognizes that, because of the nutritional status, the patient is at increased risk for: (Select all that apply.)
   1. Heart disease.
   2. Sepsis.
   3. Pleural effusion.
   4. Cardiac arrhythmias.
   5. Diarrhea.
2. The nurse evaluates which laboratory values to assess a patient's potential for wound healing?
   1. Fluid status
   2. Potassium
   3. Lipids
   4. Nitrogen balance
3. The nurse is caring for a patient with dysphagia and is feeding her a pureed chicken diet when she begins to choke. What is the priority nursing intervention?
   1. Suction her mouth and throat
   2. Turn her on their side
   3. Put on oxygen at 2-L nasal cannula
   4. Stop feeding her and place on NPO
4. A patient who is receiving parenteral nutrition (PN) through a central venous catheter (CVC) has an air embolus. What would the nurse do first?
   1. Have the patient perform a Valsalva maneuver
   2. Clamp the intravenous (IV) tubing to prevent more air from entering the line
   3. Have the patient take a deep breath and hold it
   4. Notify the health care provider immediately
5. A patient is receiving both parenteral (PN) and enteral nutrition (EN). When would the nurse collaborate with the health care provider and request discontinuing parenteral nutrition?
   1. When 25% of the patient's nutritional needs are met by the tube feedings
   2. When bowel sounds return
   3. When central line has been in for 10 days
   4. When 75% of the patient's nutritional needs are met by the tube feedings
6. The nurse is educating the patient and his family about the parenteral nutrition. Which aspect related to this form of nutrition would be appropriate to include? (Select all that apply.)
   1. The purpose of the fat emulsion in parenteral nutrition is to prevent a deficiency in essential fatty acids.
   2. We can give you parenteral nutrition through your peripheral intravenous line to prevent further infection.
   3. The fat emulsion will help control hyperglycemia during periods of stress.
   4. The parenteral nutrition will help your wounds heal.
   5. Since we just started the parenteral nutrition, we will only infuse it at 50% of your daily needs for the next 6 hours.
7. The nurse is inserting a small-bore nasoenteric tube before starting enteral feedings. Place the following steps in order to perform this procedure.
   1. Place patient in high-Fowler's position.
   2. Have patient flex head toward chest.
   3. Assess patient's gag reflex.
   4. Determine length of the tube to be inserted.
   5. Obtain radiological confirmation of tube placement.
   6. Check pH of gastric aspirate for verifying placement.
   7. Identify patient with two identifiers.
8. A patient's gastric residual volume was 250 mL at 0800 and 350 mL at 0900. What is the appropriate nursing action?
   1. Assess bowel sounds
   2. Raise the head of the bed to at least 45 degrees

3. Position the patient on his or her right side to promote stomach emptying
4. Do not reinstall aspirate and hold the feeding until you talk to the primary care provider

9. The nurse would delegate which of the following to nursing assistive personnel (NAP)? (Select all that apply.)
   1. Repositioning and retaping a patient's nasogastric tube
   2. Performing glucose monitoring every 6 hours on a patient
   3. Documenting PO intake on a patient who is on a calorie count for 72 hours
   4. Administering enteral feeding bolus after tube placement has been verified
   5. Hanging a new bag of enteral feeding
10. The patient's blood glucose level is 330 mg/dL. What is the priority nursing intervention?
   1. Recheck by performing another blood glucose test.
   2. Call the primary health care provider.
   3. Check the medical record to see if there is a medication order for abnormal glucose levels.
   4. Monitor and recheck in 2 hours.
11. Which statement made by a patient of a 2-month-old infant requires further education?
   1. I'll continue to use formula for the baby until he is a least a year old.
   2. I'll make sure that I purchase iron-fortified formula.
   3. I'll start feeding the baby cereal at 4 months.
   4. I'm going to alternate formula with whole milk starting next month.
12. The nurse is teaching a program on healthy nutrition at the senior community center. Which points should be included in the program for older adults? (Select all that apply.)
   1. Avoid grapefruit and grapefruit juice, which impair drug absorption.
   2. Increase the amount of carbohydrates for energy.
   3. Take a multivitamin that includes vitamin D for bone health.
   4. Cheese and eggs are good sources of protein.
   5. Limit fluids to decrease the risk of edema.
13. The nurse sees the nursing assistive personnel (NAP) perform the following intervention for a patient receiving continuous enteral feedings. Which action would require immediate attention?
   1. Fastening tube to the gown with new tape
   2. Placing patient supine while giving a bath
   3. Hanging a new container of enteral feeding
   4. Ambulating patient with enteral feedings still infusing
14. A patient is receiving total parenteral nutrition (TPN). What is the primary intervention the nurse should follow to prevent a central line infection?
   1. Institute isolation precautions
   2. Clean the central line port through which the TPN is infusing with antiseptic
   3. Change the TPN tubing every 24 hours
   4. Monitor glucose levels to watch and assess for glucose intolerance
15. Which patients are at high risk for nutritional deficits? (Select all that apply.)
   1. The divorced computer programmer who eats precooked food from the local restaurant
   2. The middle-age female with celiac disease who does not follow her gluten-free diet
   3. The 45-year-old patient with type II diabetes who monitors her carbohydrate intake and exercises regularly
   4. The 25-year-old patient with Crohn's disease who follows a strict diet but does not take vitamins or iron supplements
   5. The 65-year-old patient with gallbladder disease whose electrolyte, albumin, and protein levels are normal

Answers: 1. 2, 3, 4; **2.** 4; **3.** 4; **4.** 1; **5.** 4; **6.** 1, 3, 4; **7.** 1, 3, 4, 2, 5, 6; **8.** 4; **9.** 2, 3; **10.** 3; **11.** 4; **12.** 1, 3, 4; **13.** 2; **14.** 2; **15.** 2, 4.

ⓔ ***Rationales for Review Questions can be found on the Evolve website.***

REFERENCES

Altman KW, et al: Dysphagia in stroke, neurodegenerative disease, and advanced dementia, *Otolaryngol Clin North Am* 46(6):1137, 2013.

American Academy of Pediatrics (AAP): Policy statement: breast feeding and the use of human milk, *Pediatrics* 129(3):496, 2012.

American Association of Critical Care Nurses (AACN): *Verification of feeding tube placement (blindly inserted), AACN Practice Alert*, 2012, http://www.aacn.org/wd/practice/content/feeding-tube-practice-alert.pcms?menu=practice. Accessed November 2015.

American Association of Critical Care Nurses (AACN): *Try a new taping method: preventing DRPU, Acute and Critical Care Webinar Series*, The Association, Aliso Viejo, Calif, 2014, The Association.

American Cancer Society (ACS): *American Cancer Society guidelines on nutrition and physical activity for cancer prevention*, 2015, http://www.cancer.org/healthy/eathealthygetactive/acsguidelinesonnutritionphysicalactivityforcancerprevention/acs-guidelines-on-nutrition-and-physical-activity-for-cancer-prevention-intro. Accessed November 2015.

American Diabetes Association (ADA): Management of hyperglycemia in type 2 diabetes: a patient centered approach, *Diabetes Care* 35(6):1364, 2012.

American Dietetic Association: Position of the American Dietetic Association, American Society for Nutrition, and Society for Nutrition Education: Food and nutrition programs for community-residing older adults, *J Am Diet Assoc* 110(3):463, 2010a.

American Dietetic Association: Position of the American Dietetic Association: Integration of medical nutrition therapy and pharmacotherapy, *J Am Diet Assoc* 110(6):950, 2010b.

American Heart Association (AHA): *Diet and lifestyle recommendations revision*, 2010, http://www.heart.org/HEARTORG/GettingHealthy/Diet-and-Lifestyle-Recommendations_UCM_305855_Article.jsp. Accessed November 2015.

Bankhead R, et al: ASPEN Enteral nutrition practice recommendations, *J Parenter Enteral Nutr* 33(2):122, 2009.

Borrelli LN, Talih M: Examining periodontal disease disparities among US adults 20 years of age and older: NHANESIII (1988-1994) and NHANES 1999-2004, *Public Health Rep* 127:497, 2012.

Burcham JR, Rosenthal LD: *Lehne's pharmacology for nursing care*, ed 9, St Louis, 2016, Elsevier.

Centers for Disease Control and Prevention (CDC): *Childhood obesity facts*, 2015, http://www.cdc.gov/HealthyYouth/obesity/facts.htm. Accessed November 2015.

Chang C, Roberts B: Strategies for feeding patients with dementia, *Am J Nurs* 111(4):36, 2011.

Delegge DH: Managing gastric residual volumes in the critically ill patient: an update, *Curr Opin Nutr Metab Care* 14:193, 2011.

Dunne A: Early infant nutrition: the importance of getting it right, *Br J Nurs* 21(7):390, 2012.

Ellis AL, Hannibal RR: Nursing swallowing screening: why is testing water not enough?, *J Neurosci Nurs* 45(5):244, 2013.

Fernandez RS, et al: Accuracy of biochemical markers for predicting nasogastric tube placement in adults: a systematic review of diagnostic studies, *Int J Nurs Stud* 47:1037, 2010.

Fletcher J: Parental nutrition: indication, risk and nursing care, *Nurs Stand* 27(46):50, 2013.

Giger JN, Davidhizar RE: *Transcultural nursing: assessment and intervention*, ed 6, St Louis, 2012, Mosby.

Grodner M, et al: *Nutritional foundations and clinical applications: a nursing approach*, ed 5, St Louis, 2012, Mosby.

Hockenberry MJ, Wilson D: *Wong's nursing care of infants and children*, ed 10, St Louis, 2015, Mosby.

Hodin RA, et al: *Nasogastric and nasoenteric tubes*, 2014, http://www.uptodate.com/contents/nasogastric-and-nasoenteric-tubes. Accessed August 20, 2014.

Institute of Medicine (IOM): *Dietary reference intakes: essential nutrient guide*, 2015, http://www.cdc.gov/

healthyschools/obesity/facts.htm. Accessed November 2015.

Krzywda EA, Meyer D: Parenteral nutrition. In Alexander M, et al, editors: *Infusion nursing society infusion nursing: an evidence-based approach*, ed 3, St Louis, 2010, Saunders.

Mayo Clinic Staff: *Teen weight loss: healthy habits count*, 2015, http://www.mayoclinic.org/healthy-living/tween-and-teen-health/in-depth/teen-weight-loss/art-20045224. Accessed November 2015.

McCance KL, et al: *Pathophysiology: the biologic basis for disease in adults and children*, ed 7, St Louis, 2013, Mosby.

McCarthy MS, et al: What's on the menu? Delivering evidence-based nutritional therapy, *Nursing* 45:8, 2015.

Meiner SE: *Gerontologic nursing*, ed 4, St Louis, 2011, Mosby.

Metheny NA: *Practice Alert: Dye in enteral feedings*, 2009, American Association of Critical Care Nurses. http://www.aacn.org/wd/practice/content/dye-enteral-feedings-practice-alert.pcms?menu=practice. Accessed November 2015.

National Dysphagia Diet Task Force (NDDTF): *National Dysphagia Diet: standardization for optimal care*, Chicago, 2010, American Dietetic Association.

National Guideline Clearinghouse: ASPEN Clinical Guidelines: *Parenteral nutrition ordering, ordering review, compounding, labeling and dispensing*, 2013, http://elbiruniblogspotcom.blogspot.com/2014/08/national-guideline-clearinghouse-aspen.html. Accessed November 2015.

National Stroke Association: *Dysphagia symptoms*, 2013, http://www.stroke.org. Retrieved November 2015.

Nix S: *Williams' basic nutrition and diet therapy*, ed 14, St Louis, 2012, Mosby.

Ochoa JB: Nutrition assessment and intervention in the patient with dysphagia: challenges for quality improvement, *Nestle Nutr Inst Workshop Ser* 72:77–83, 2012.

Pagana KD, et al: *Mosby's diagnostic and laboratory test reference*, ed 12, St Louis, 2015, Mosby.

Phillips LD: *Manual of IV therapeutics: evidence-based practice for infusion therapy*, ed 5, Philadelphia, 2010, FA Davis.

Remig V, Weeden A: Medical nutrition therapy for neurologic disorders. In Mahan LK, et al, editors: *Krause's food and the nutrition care process*, ed 13, St Louis, 2012, Saunders.

Robert Woods Johnson Foundation: *F as in fat: how obesity threatens America's future*, 2013, http://www.rwjf.org/en/research-publications/find-rwjf-research/2013/08/f-as-in-fat–how-obesity-threatens-america-s-future-2013.html. Accessed November 2015.

Stewart ML: Interruptions in enteral nutrition delivery in the critically ill patients and recommendations for clinical practice, *Crit Care Nurse* 34:14, 2014.

Tappenden KA, et al: Critical role of nutrition in improving quality of care: an interdisciplinary call to action to address adult hospital malnutrition, *Medsurg Nurs* 22(3):147, 2013.

The Joint Commission (TJC): *Sentinel alert event: managing risk during transition to new ISO connector standards*, 2014, http://www.jointcommission.org/assets/1/6/SEA_53_Connectors_8_19_14_final.pdf. Accessed November 2015.

The Joint Commission (TJC): *2016 National Patient Safety Goals*, Oakbrook Terrace, IL, 2016, The Commission. Available at http://www.jointcommission.org/standards_information/npsgs.aspx. Accessed November 2015.

Tolerable upper-level intake, 2010, National Institutes of Health, http://ods.od.nih.gov/pubs/conferences/tolerable_upper_intake.pdf. Accessed November 2015.

Touhy TA, Jett KF: *Ebersole and Hess' gerontological nursing healthy aging*, St Louis, 2010, Mosby.

Tuan NT, et al: Demographics and socioeconomic correlates of adiposity assessed with dual-energy x-ray absorptiometry in US children and adolescents, *Am J Clin Nutr* 96:1104, 2012.

Tufts University: *MyPlate for older adults*, 2011, http://nutrition.tufts.edu/research/myplate-older-adults. Accessed November 2015.

US Department of Agriculture (USDA): *Choose MyPlate*, 2011, http://www.choosemyplate.gov. Accessed November 2015.

US Department of Health and Human Services (USDHHS): *Healthy people 2020*, 2015, http://www.healthypeople.gov/. Accessed November 2015.

World Health Organization (WHO): *Food security*, 2015, http://www.who.int/trade/glossary/story028/en. Accessed November 2015.

Yantis MA, Velander R: Untangling enteral nutrition guidelines, *Nursing* 41(9):32, 2011.

RESEARCH REFERENCES

American Speech-Language-Hearing Association (ASHA): *ASHA's evidence maps: adult dysphagia in non-imaging assessment instruments*, September 2014, http://ncepmaps.org/adultdysp/assess/non-image/. Accessed December 28, 2015.

Edmiaston J, et al: Validation of a dysphagia screening tool in acute stroke patients, *Am J Crit Care* 19(4):357, 2010.

Frey K, Ramsberger G: Comparison of outcomes before and after implementation of a water protocol for patients with cerebrovascular accident and dysphagia, *J Neurosci Nurs* 43(3):165, 2011.

Guigoz Y, Vellas B: The Mini Nutritional Assessment (MNA) for grading the nutritional state of elderly patients: presentation of the MNA, history and validation, *Nestle Nutr Workshop Ser Clin Perform Programme* 1:3, 1999.

Guigoz YB, et al: Assessing the nutritional status of the elderly: the Mini Nutritional Assessment as part of the geriatric evaluation, *Nutr Rev* 54(1 Pt 2):S59, 1996.

Hedwig L, et al: Multiple levels of social disadvantage and links to obesity in adolescence and young adults, *J School Health* 83:139, 2013.

Holst M, et al: Nutritional screening and risk factors in elderly hospitalized patients: association to clinical outcomes?, *Scand J Caring Sci* 27:953, 2013.

Jensen GL, et al: Recognizing malnutrition in adults: definitions and characteristics, screening, assessment and team approach, *ASPEN* 37:802, 2013.

Kenny DJ, Goodman P: Care of the patient with enteral tube feeding: an evidence-based practice protocol, *Nurs Res* 59(1S):S22, 2010.

Khalid I, et al: Early enteral nutrition and outcomes of critically ill patients treated with vasopressors and mechanical ventilation, *Am J Crit Care* 19(3):261, 2010.

Krenitsky J: Blind bedside placement of feeding tubes: treatment of threat?, *Prac Gastroenterol* XXXV(3):32, 2011.

Li J, Hooker NH: Childhood obesity and schools: evidence from the national survey of children's health, *J School Health* 80(2):96, 2010.

Makic MB, et al: Evidence-based practice habits: putting more sacred cows out to pasture, *Crit Care Nurse* 31(2):38, 2011.

Metheny NA: Preventing respiratory complications of tube feedings: evidence-based practice, *Am J Crit Care* 15(4):360, 2006.

Metheny NA, et al: Monitoring for intolerance to gastric tube feedings: a national survey, *Am J Crit Care* 21(2):e33, 2012.

Metheny NA, Frantz RA: Head-of-bed elevation in critically ill patients: a review, *Crit Care Nurse* 33(3):53, 2013.

Sorensen RT, et al: Dysphagia screening and intensified oral hygiene reduce pneumonia after stroke, *J Neurosci Nurs* 45(3):139, 2013.

Taylor SJ, et al: Treating delayed gastric emptying in critical illness: metoclopramide, erythromycin, and bedside (cortrak) nasointestinal tube placement, *J Parenter Enteral Nutr* 34(3):289, 2010.

Tierré R, Mearin F: Effectiveness of chin-down posture to prevent tracheal aspiration in dysphagia secondary to acquired brain injury. a videofluoroscopy study, *Neurogastroenterol Motil* 24(5):414–419, 2012.

Tsai AC, et al: A comparison of the full Mini Nutritional Assessment, short-form Mini Nutritional Assessment, and Subjective Global Assessment to predict the risk of protein energy malnutrition in patients on peritoneal dialysis: a cross-sectional study, *Int J Student Nurses* 50(1):83, 2013.

Wang J, et al: Factors associated with health-related quality of life among overweight or obese adults, *J Clin Nurs* 22:2172, 2013.

Urinary Elimination

OBJECTIVES

- Explain the function and role of urinary system structures in urine formation and elimination.
- Identify factors that commonly impact urinary elimination.
- Compare and contrast common alterations associated with urinary elimination.
- Obtain a nursing history from a patient with an alteration in urinary elimination.
- Perform a physical assessment focused on urinary elimination.
- Describe characteristics of normal and abnormal urine.
- Describe nursing implications of common diagnostic tests of the urinary system.
- Identify nursing diagnoses associated with alterations in urinary elimination.
- Discuss nursing measures to promote normal micturition and improve bladder control.
- Discuss nursing measures to reduce risk for urinary tract infections.
- Apply an external catheter and insert a urinary catheter.
- Perform closed catheter irrigation correctly.
- Measure postvoid residual with a bladder scanner.

KEY TERMS

Bacteremia, p. 1103
Bacteriuria, p. 1103
Catheter-associated UTI (CAUTI), p. 1105
Catheterization, p. 1119
Cystitis, p. 1103
Dysuria, p. 1103
Hematuria, p. 1102
Micturition, p. 1101
Nephrostomy, p. 1106
Pelvic floor muscle training, p. 1126
Postvoid residual (PVR), p. 1103
Pyelonephritis, p. 1103
Renin, p. 1102
Suprapubic catheter, p. 1122
Urinary incontinence (UI), p. 1105
Urinary retention, p. 1103
Ureterostomy, p. 1106

MEDIA RESOURCES

http://evolve.elsevier.com/Potter/fundamentals/

- Review Questions
- Video Clips
- Concept Map Creator
- Case Study with Questions
- Skills Performance Checklists
- Audio Glossary
- Content Updates

A basic human function is urinary elimination. This function can be compromised by a wide variety of illnesses and conditions. Nurses are key members of the health care team when treating patients with urinary problems. It is your role to assess patients' urinary tract function and provide support for bladder emptying. During acute illness a patient may require urinary catheterization for close monitoring of urine output or to facilitate bladder emptying when bladder function is compromised. Some patients require long-term indwelling catheters, urethral or suprapubic, when the bladder fails to empty effectively. You also implement measures to minimize risk for infection when bladder function is impaired or urinary drainage tubes are required. Nurses in all health care settings play an important role in teaching patients about bladder health and supporting them to improve or obtain continence.

SCIENTIFIC KNOWLEDGE BASE

Urinary elimination is the last step in the removal and elimination of excess water and by-products of body metabolism. Adequate elimination depends on the coordinated function of the kidneys, ureters, bladder, and urethra (Figure 46-1). The kidneys filter waste products of metabolism from the blood. The ureters transport urine from the kidneys to the bladder. The bladder holds urine until the volume in the bladder triggers a sensation of urge, indicating the need to pass urine. **Micturition** occurs when the brain gives the bladder permission to empty, the bladder contracts, the urinary sphincter relaxes, and urine leaves the body through the urethra.

Kidneys

The kidneys lie on either side of the vertebral column behind the peritoneum and against the deep muscles of the back. Normally the left kidney is higher than the right because of the anatomical position of the liver.

Nephrons, the functional unit of the kidneys, remove waste products from the blood and play a major role in the regulation of fluid and electrolyte balance. Each nephron contains a cluster of capillaries called the *glomerulus*. The glomerulus filters water, glucose, amino acids, urea, uric acid, creatinine, and major electrolytes. Large proteins

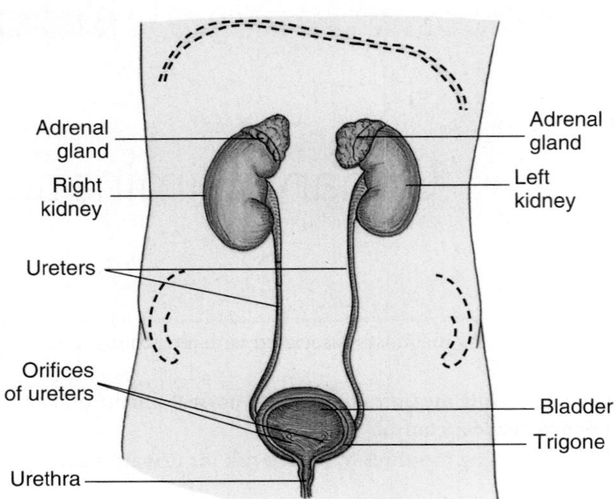

FIGURE 46-1 Organs of urinary system.

and blood cells do not normally filter through the glomerulus. When protein (proteinuria) or blood (**hematuria**) is found in the urine, glomerular injury is suspected.

Not all glomerular filtrate is excreted as urine. Approximately 99% is resorbed into the plasma by the proximal convoluted tubule of the nephron, the loop of Henle, and the distal tubule. The remaining 1% is excreted as urine. It is in the resorption process that the delicate balance of fluid and electrolytes is maintained (Huether and McCance, 2012). The normal range of urine production is 1 to 2 L/day (Huether and McCance, 2012). Many factors can influence the production of urine such as fluid intake and body temperature (Box 46-1).

The kidneys have essential functions other than elimination of body wastes. Erythropoietin, produced by the kidneys, stimulates red blood cell production and maturation in bone marrow. Patients with chronic kidney conditions cannot produce sufficient quantities of this hormone; therefore they are prone to anemia.

The kidneys play a major role in blood pressure control via the renin-angiotensin system (i.e., release of aldosterone and prostacyclin) (Huether and McCance, 2012). In times of renal ischemia (decreased blood supply), **renin** is released from juxtaglomerular cells. Renin

BOX 46-1 Factors Influencing Urinary Elimination

Growth and Development

- Children cannot voluntarily control voiding until 18 to 24 months.
- Readiness for toilet training includes the ability to recognize the feeling of bladder fullness, hold urine for 1 to 2 hours, and communicate the sense of urgency.
- Older adults may experience a decrease in bladder capacity, increased bladder irritability, and an increased frequency of bladder contractions during bladder filling.
- In older adults the ability to hold urine between the initial desire to void and an urgent need to void decreases.
- Older adults are at increased risk for urinary incontinence because of chronic illnesses and factors that interfere with mobility, cognition, and manual dexterity.

Sociocultural Factors

- Cultural and gender norms vary. North Americans expect toilet facilities to be private, whereas some cultures accept communal toilet facilities.
- Religious or cultural norms may dictate who is acceptable to help with elimination practices.
- Social expectations (e.g., school recesses, work breaks) can interfere with timely voiding.

Psychological Factors

- Anxiety and stress sometimes affect a sense of urgency and increase the frequency of voiding.
- Anxiety can impact bladder emptying because of inadequate relaxation of the pelvic floor muscles and urinary sphincter.
- Depression can decrease the desire for urinary continence.

Personal Habits

- The need for privacy and adequate time to void can influence the ability to empty the bladder adequately.

Fluid Intake

- If fluids, electrolytes, and solutes are balanced, increased fluid intake increases urine production.
- Alcohol decreases the release of antidiuretic hormones, thus increasing urine production.
- Fluids containing caffeine and other bladder irritants can prompt unsolicited bladder contractions, resulting in frequency, urgency, and incontinence.

Pathological Conditions

- Diabetes mellitus, multiple sclerosis, and stroke can alter bladder contractility and the ability to sense bladder filling. Patients experience either bladder overactivity or deficient bladder emptying.
- Arthritis, Parkinson's disease, dementia, and chronic pain syndromes can interfere with timely access to a toilet.
- Spinal cord injury or intervertebral disk disease (above S-1) can cause the loss of urine control because of bladder overactivity and impaired coordination between the contracting bladder and urinary sphincter.
- Prostatic enlargement (e.g., benign prostatic hyperplasia [BPH]) can cause obstruction of the bladder outlet, causing urinary retention.

Surgical Procedures

- Local trauma during lower abdominal and pelvic surgery sometimes obstructs urine flow, requiring temporary use of an indwelling urinary catheter.
- Anesthetic agents and other agents given during surgery can decrease bladder contractility and/or sensation of bladder fullness, causing urinary retention (Elsamara and Ellsworth, 2012).

Medications

- Diuretics increase urinary output by preventing resorption of water and certain electrolytes.
- Some drugs change the color of urine (e.g., phenazopyridine-orange, riboflavin–intense yellow).
- Anitcholinergics (e.g., atropine, overactive agents) may increase the risk for urinary retention by inhibiting bladder contractility (Burchum and Rosenthal, 2016).
- Hypnotics and sedatives (e.g., analgesics, antianxiety agents) may reduce the ability to recognize and act on the urge to void.

Diagnostic Examinations

- Cystoscopy may cause localized trauma of the urethra, resulting in transient (1 to 2 days) dysuria and hematuria.
- Whenever the sterile urinary tract is catheterized, there is a risk for infection.

functions as an enzyme to convert angiotensinogen (a substance synthesized by the liver) into angiotensin I. Angiotensin I is converted to angiotensin II in the lungs. Angiotensin II causes vasoconstriction and stimulates aldosterone release from the adrenal cortex. Aldosterone causes retention of water, which increases blood volume. The kidneys also produce prostaglandin E_2 and prostacyclin, which help maintain renal blood flow through vasodilation. These mechanisms increase arterial blood pressure and renal blood flow (Huether and McCance, 2012).

The kidneys affect calcium and phosphate regulation by producing a substance that converts vitamin D into its active form. Patients with kidney impairment can have problems such as anemia, hypertension, and electrolyte imbalances.

Ureters

A ureter is attached to each kidney pelvis and carries urinary waste to the bladder. Urine draining from the ureters to the bladder is sterile. Peristaltic waves cause the urine to enter the bladder in spurts rather than steadily. Contractions of the bladder during micturition compress the lower part of the ureters to prevent urine from backflowing into the ureters (Huether and McCance, 2012). Obstruction of urine flow through the ureters such as by a kidney stone can cause a backflow of urine (urinary reflux) into the ureters and pelvis of the kidney, causing distention (hydroureter/hydronephrosis) and in some cases permanent damage to sensitive kidney structures and function.

Bladder

The urinary bladder is a hollow, distensible, muscular organ that holds urine. When empty, the bladder lies in the pelvic cavity behind the symphysis pubis. In males the bladder rests against the rectum, and in females it rests against the anterior wall of the uterus and vagina. The bladder has two parts, a fixed base called the *trigone* and a distensible body called the *detrusor*. The bladder expands as it fills with urine. Normally the pressure in the bladder during filling remains low, and this prevents the dangerous backward flow of urine into the ureters and kidneys. Backflow can cause infection. In a pregnant woman the developing fetus pushes against the bladder, reducing capacity and causing a feeling of fullness.

Urethra

Urine travels from the bladder through the urethra and passes to the outside of the body through the urethral meatus. The urethra passes through a thick layer of skeletal muscles called the *pelvic floor muscles.* These muscles stabilize the urethra and contribute to urinary continence. The external urethral sphincter, made up of striated muscles, contributes to voluntary control over the flow of urine (Huether and McCance, 2012). The female urethra is approximately 3 to 4 cm (1 to 1.5 inch) long, and the male urethra is about 18 to 20 cm (7 to 8 inches) long (Huether and McCance, 2012). The shorter length of the female urethra increases risk for urinary tract infection (UTI) because of close access to the bacteria-contaminated perineal area.

Act of Urination

Urination, micturition, and voiding are all terms that describe the process of bladder emptying. Micturition is a complex interaction among the bladder, urinary sphincter, and central nervous system. Several areas in the brain are involved in bladder control: cerebral cortex, thalamus, hypothalamus, and brainstem. There are two micturition centers in the spinal cord: one that coordinates inhibition of bladder contraction, and the other that coordinates bladder contractility. As the bladder fills and stretches, bladder contractions are inhibited by sympathetic stimulation from the thoracic micturition center. When the bladder fills to approximately 400 to 600 mL, most people experience a strong sensation of urgency. When in the appropriate place to void, the central nervous system sends a message to the micturition centers, stopping sympathetic stimulation and starting parasympathetic stimulation from the sacral micturition center. The urinary sphincter relaxes, and the bladder contracts. When the time and place are inappropriate, the brain sends messages to the micturition centers to contract the urinary sphincter and relax the bladder muscle.

Factors Influencing Urination. Physiological factors, psychosocial conditions, and diagnostic or treatment-induced factors can all affect normal urinary elimination (see Box 46-1). Knowledge of these factors enables you to anticipate possible elimination problems and intervene when problems develop.

Common Urinary Elimination Problems. The most common urinary elimination problems involve the inability to store urine or fully empty urine from the bladder. Problems can result from infection; irritable or overactive bladder; obstruction of urine flow; impaired bladder contractility; or issues that impair innervation to the bladder, resulting in sensory or motor dysfunction.

Urinary Retention. Urinary retention is the inability to partially or completely empty the bladder. Acute or rapid-onset urinary retention stretches the bladder, causing feelings of pressure, discomfort/pain, tenderness over the symphysis pubis, restlessness, and sometimes diaphoresis. Patients may have no urine output over several hours and in some cases experience frequency, urgency, small-volume voiding, or incontinence of small volumes of urine. Chronic urinary retention has a slow, gradual onset during which patients may experience a decrease in voiding volumes, straining to void, frequency, urgency, incontinence, and sensations of incomplete emptying. Postvoid residual (PVR) is the amount of urine left in the bladder after voiding and is measured either by ultrasound or straight catheterization. Incontinence caused by urinary retention is called *overflow incontinence* or *incontinence associated with chronic retention of urine.* The pressure in the bladder exceeds the ability of the sphincter to prevent the passage of urine, and the patient will dribble urine (see Table 46-1).

Urinary Tract Infections. UTIs are one of the most common health care–acquired infections, with almost all caused by instrumentation of the urinary tract (CDC, 2015). *Escherichia coli,* a bacterium commonly found in the colon, is the most common causative pathogen (Gupta and Hooton, 2011; Nicolle, 2014). The risk for a UTI increases in the presence of an indwelling catheter, any instrumentation of the urinary tract, urinary retention, urinary and fecal incontinence, and poor perineal hygiene practices.

UTIs are characterized by location (i.e., upper urinary tract [kidney] or lower urinary tract [bladder, urethra]) and have signs and symptoms of infection. Bacteriuria, or bacteria in the urine, does not always mean that there is a UTI. In the absence of symptoms, the presence of bacteria in the urine as found on a urine culture is called *asymptomatic bacteriuria* and is not considered an infection and should not be treated with antibiotics (Mody and Juthani-Mehta, 2014). Symptomatic infection of the bladder can lead to a serious upper UTI (pyelonephritis) and life-threatening bloodstream infection (bacteremia or urosepsis) and should be treated with antibiotics. Symptoms of a lower UTI (bladder) can include burning or pain with urination (dysuria); irritation of the bladder (cystitis) characterized by urgency, frequency, incontinence, suprapubic tenderness; and foul-smelling cloudy urine. Older adults may experience a change in mental status called *delirium.* In some cases there will be obvious blood in the urine (hematuria). If infection spreads to the upper urinary tract (pyelonephritis), patients

TABLE 46-1 Urinary Incontinence

Definition	Characteristics	Selected Nursing Interventions
Transient Incontinence		
Incontinence caused by medical conditions that in many cases are treatable and reversible	Common reversible causes include: • Delirium and/or acute confusion. • Inflammation (e.g., urinary tract infection [UTI], urethritis). • Medications (e.g., diuretics) (Hall et al., 2012). • Excessive urine output (e.g., hyperglycemia, congestive heart failure). • Mobility impairment from any cause. • Fecal impaction. • Depression. • Acute urinary retention.	With new-onset or increased incontinence look for reversible causes. Notify health care provider of any suspected reversible causes.
Functional Incontinence		
Loss of continence because of causes outside the urinary tract Usually related to functional deficits such as altered mobility and manual dexterity, cognitive impairment, poor motivation, or environmental barriers Direct result of caregivers not responding in a timely manner to requests for help with toileting	Toilet access restricted by: • Sensory impairments (e.g., vision). • Cognitive impairments (e.g., delirium, dementia, severe retardation). • Altered mobility (e.g., hip fracture, arthritis, chronic pain, spastic paralysis associated with multiple sclerosis, slow movements associated with Parkinson's disease, hemiparesis). • Altered manual dexterity (e.g., arthritis, upper extremity fracture) • Environmental barriers (e.g., caregiver not available to help with transfers, pathway to bathroom not maneuverable with a walker, tight clothing that is difficult to remove, incontinence briefs).	Adequate lighting in the bathroom Individualized toileting program designed for the degree of cognitive impairment: habit training program, scheduled toileting program, prompted voiding program Mobility aides (e.g., raised toilet seats, toilet grab bars) Toilet area cleared to allow access for a walker or wheelchair Elastic-waist pants without buttons or zippers Call bell always within reach Use of incontinence containment product patient can easily remove such as a pull-up–type pant or a pad that can be moved aside easily for voiding
Urinary Incontinence Associated with Chronic Retention of Urine (Overflow Urinary Incontinence)		
Involuntary loss of urine caused by an overdistended bladder often related to bladder outlet obstruction or poor bladder emptying because of weak or absent bladder contractions	Distended bladder on palpation High postvoid residual Frequency Involuntary leakage of small volumes of urine Nocturia	Interventions are individualized related to the severity of the urinary retention, ability of bladder to contract, existing kidney damage. Mild retention with some bladder function: • Timed voiding • Double voiding • Monitor postvoid residual per health care provider's direction • Intermittent catheterization Severe retention, no bladder function: • Intermittent catheterization • Indwelling catheterization
Stress Urinary Incontinence		
Involuntary leakage of small volumes of urine associated with increased intraabdominal pressure related to either urethral hypermobility or an incompetent urinary sphincter (e.g., weak pelvic floor muscles, trauma after childbirth, radical prostatectomy) Result of weakness or injury to the urinary sphincter or pelvic floor muscles Underlying result: urethra cannot stay closed as pressure increases in the bladder as a result of increased abdominal pressure (e.g., a sneeze or cough)	Small-volume loss of urine with coughing, laughing, exercise, walking, getting up from a chair Usually does not leak urine at night when sleeping	As directed by the health care provider, instruct patient in pelvic muscle exercises.

TABLE 46-1 Urinary Incontinence—cont'd

Definition	Characteristics	Selected Nursing Interventions
Urge or Urgency Urinary Incontinence		
Involuntary passage of urine often associated with strong sense of urgency related to an overactive bladder caused by neurological problems, bladder inflammation, or bladder outlet obstruction In many cases bladder overactivity is idiopathic; cause is not known Caused by involuntary contractions of the bladder associated with an urge to void that causes leakage of urine	May experience one or all of the following symptoms: • Urgency • Frequency • Nocturia • Difficulty or unable to hold urine once the urge to void occurs • Leaks on the way to the bathroom • Leaks larger volumes of urine, sometimes enough to wet outer clothing • Dribbles small amounts on the way to the bathroom • Strong urge/leaks when one hears water running, washes hands, drinks fluids	Ask patient about symptoms of a UTI Avoid bladder irritants (e.g., caffeine, artificial sweeteners, alcohol). As directed by the health care provider, instruct patient in pelvic muscle exercises, in urge-inhibition exercises, and/or in bladder training. If ordered by the health care provider, monitor patient symptoms and for the presence of side effects of antimuscarinic medications.
Reflex Urinary Incontinence		
Involuntary loss of urine occurring at somewhat predictable intervals when patient reaches specific bladder volume related to spinal cord damage between C1 to S2	Diminished or absent awareness of bladder filling and the urge to void Leakage of urine without awareness May not completely empty the bladder because of dyssynergia of the urinary sphincter; inappropriate contraction of the sphincter when the bladder contracts, causing obstruction to urine flow **CAUTION:** At risk for developing autonomic dysreflexia, a life-threatening condition that causes severe elevation of blood pressure and pulse rate and diaphoresis	Follow the prescribed schedule for emptying the bladder either through voiding or by intermittent catheterization. Supply urine-containment products: condom catheter, undergarments, pads, briefs. Monitor for signs and symptoms of urinary retention and UTI. Monitor for autonomic dysreflexia; this is a medical emergency requiring immediate intervention. Notify the health care provider immediately.

may also experience fever, chills, diaphoresis, and flank pain (Schaeffer and Schaeffer, 2012).

Catheter-associated UTIs (CAUTIs) are an ongoing problem for hospitals because they are associated with increased hospitalizations, increased morbidity and mortality, longer hospital stays, and increased hospital costs (Gould et al., 2009; Hooton and Bradley, 2010). Because a CAUTI is common, costly, and believed to be reasonably preventable, as of October 1, 2008, the Centers for Medicare and Medicaid Services (CMS) chose it as one of the complications for which hospitals no longer receive additional payment to compensate for the extra cost of treatment. Consequently there has been a shift in clinical care practices from the traditional focus on early recognition and prompt treatment to one of prevention. CAUTI needs to be defined with some caution. Urine sampling for a microbiological workup needs to be done carefully to avoid contamination. For critically ill patients, urine sampling must be done either routinely once a week or at the beginning of a new episode of sepsis. CAUTI is usually deemed present if at least 10^3 colony-forming units (CFU)/mL of 1 or 2 microorganisms are identified by urine culture (Maki and Tambyah, 2001; Mnatzaganian et al., 2005).

Urinary Incontinence. Urinary incontinence (UI) is defined as the "complaint of any involuntary loss of urine" (Staskin et al., 2013) (Table 46-1). UI is a common problem affecting 27% of men and 43% women over the age of 40 (Coyne and Kvasz, 2012), 20% to 40% of older adults (Aguilar-Navarro et al., 2012), and over 70% of elderly nursing home patients (Coyne and Wein, 2014). Common forms of UI are urge or urgency UI (involuntary leakage associated with urgency) and stress UI (involuntary loss of urine associated with effort or exertion on sneezing or coughing (Staskin et al., 2013). Mixed UI is when stress- and urgency-type symptoms are both present. Overactive bladder is defined as urinary urgency, often accompanied by increased urinary frequency and nocturia that may or may not be associated with urgency incontinence and is present without obvious bladder pathology or infection (Staskin et al., 2013). UI associated with chronic retention of urine (formally called *overflow UI*) is urine leakage caused by an overfull bladder (Staskin et al., 2013). Functional UI is caused by factors that prohibit or interfere with a patient's access to the toilet or other acceptable receptacle for urine. In most cases there is no bladder pathology. It is a significant problem for older adults who experience problems with mobility or the dexterity to manage their clothing and toileting behaviors. Patients with other types of incontinence can also have a functional aspect to their incontinence. A recently added category of incontinence is identified as multifactorial incontinence. This describes incontinence that has multiple interacting risk factors, some within the urinary tract and others not, such as multiple chronic illnesses, medications, age-related factors, and environmental factors (Staskin et al., 2013).

Urinary Diversions. Patients who have had the bladder removed (cystectomy) because of cancer or significant bladder dysfunction related to radiation injury or neurogenic dysfunction with frequent UTI require surgical procedures that divert urine to the outside of the body through an opening in the abdominal wall called a *stoma.* Urinary diversions are constructed from a section of intestine to create a storage reservoir or conduit for urine. Diversions can be temporary or permanent, continent or incontinent.

There are two types of continent urinary diversions. The first is called a *continent urinary reservoir* (Figure 46-2, *A*) which is created from a distal part of the ileum and proximal part of the colon. The ureters are embedded into the reservoir. This reservoir is situated under the abdominal wall and has a narrow ileal segment brought out

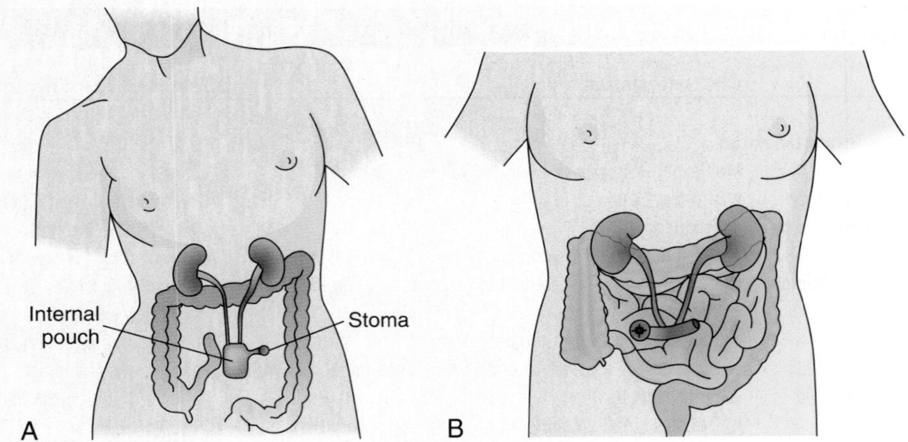

FIGURE 46-2 Types of urinary diversions. **A,** Continent urinary reservoir. **B,** Urostomy (ileal conduit).

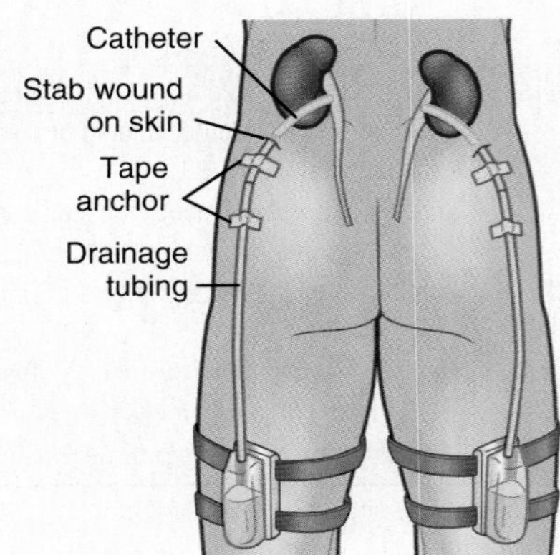

FIGURE 46-3 Nephrostomy tubes. (From Lewis SL et al: *Medical-surgical nursing,* ed 9, St Louis, 2014, Mosby.)

through the abdominal wall to form a small stoma. The ileocecal valve creates a one-way valve in the pouch through which a catheter is inserted through the stoma to empty the urine from the pouch. Patients must be willing and able to catheterize the pouch 4 to 6 times a day for the rest of their lives.

The second type of continent urinary diversion is called an *orthotopic neobladder,* which uses an ileal pouch to replace the bladder. Anatomically the pouch is in the same position as the bladder was before removal, allowing a patient to void through the urethra using a Valsalva technique.

A **ureterostomy** or ileal conduit is a permanent incontinent urinary diversion created by transplanting the ureters into a closed-off part of the intestinal ileum and bringing the other end out onto the abdominal wall forming a stoma (Figure 46-2, *B*). The patient has no sensation or control over the continuous flow of urine through the ileal conduit, requiring the effluent (drainage) to be collected in a pouch.

Nephrostomy tubes are small tubes that are tunneled through the skin into the renal pelvis. These tubes are placed to drain the renal pelvis when the ureter is obstructed. Patients do go home with these tubes and need careful teaching about site care and signs of infection (Figure 46-3).

NURSING KNOWLEDGE BASE

Urinary elimination is a basic body function and carries with it a variety of psychological and physiological needs. When illness or disability interferes with meeting these needs, nursing care that addresses both the physiological and the psychological is essential. You need an understanding beyond anatomy and physiology of the urinary system to give appropriate care.

Infection Control and Hygiene

The urinary tract is sterile. Use infection control principles to help prevent the development and spread of UTIs. You need to follow the principles of medical asepsis when carrying out procedures involving the urinary tract or external genitalia. Perineal hygiene is an essential component of care (see Chapter 40) when there is an alteration in the usual pattern of urinary elimination. Perineal care or examination of the genitalia requires medical asepsis, including proper hand hygiene. Any invasive procedure such as catheterization requires sterile aseptic technique.

Growth and Development

It is important to apply knowledge of normal growth and development when caring for the patient with urinary problems. A patient's ability to control micturition changes during the life span. The neurological system is not well developed until 2 to 3 years of age. Until this stage of development, the small child is not able to associate the sensation of filling and urge with urination. When the child recognizes feelings of urge, can hold urine for 1 to 2 hour, and is able to communicate his or her needs, toilet training becomes successful. Continence starts during daytime hours. Children who wet the bed at night without waking from sleep have what is called *nocturnal enuresis.* In some cases they can experience this nighttime incontinence until late in childhood. Infants and young children cannot effectively concentrate urine. Their urine appears light yellow or clear. In relation to their small body size, infants and children excrete large volumes of urine. For example, a 6-month-old infant who weighs 13 to 18 lbs (6 to 8 kg) excretes 400 to 500 mL of urine daily.

Pregnancy causes many changes in the body, including the urinary tract. In early and late pregnancy urinary frequency is common. Hormonal changes and the pressure of the growing fetus on the bladder cause increased urine production and shrinking bladder capacity.

Normal aging causes changes in the urinary tract and the rest of the body. These changes are not the cause of bladder dysfunction, but age does increase risk and incidence (Box 46-2).

BOX 46-2 FOCUS ON OLDER ADULTS

Urinary Incontinence

A number of normal aging changes impact urinary continence. Prostatic enlargement in older men can cause obstruction of urine flow from the bladder, resulting in incomplete bladder emptying, urgency, frequency, urinary tract infections, and damage to the upper urinary tract from urinary retention. Patterns of urine production may change as a result of a shift in circadian rhythm of water secretion, causing increased urine production at night and nocturia (Varilla et al., 2011). Nocturia disturbs sleep and increases risk for falls (Foley et al., 2012; Gomelsky and Dmochowski, 2011). Older adults have a decreased ability to delay voiding; an increased incidence of overactive bladder; and possibly a loss of bladder contractility, increasing the risk for urinary retention. Older women have a decrease in estrogenization of perineal tissue that increases the risk of urinary tract infection (Mody and Juthani-Mehta, 2014).

Advancing age is associated with increased prevalence of chronic illnesses such as stroke, diabetes, degenerative joint disease, Parkinson's disease, heart disease, and voiding dysfunction (Harris and Smith, 2010; Nobili et al., 2011). These illnesses and the problems associated with them such as cognitive impairment, mobility limitation, and other functional impairments can impact continence and increase the risk for urinary incontinence (Erekson et al., 2015; Gomelsky and Dmochowski, 2011). The use of multiple medications, called *polypharmacology,* is more common in older adults (Touhy and Jett, 2014). Many of these medications have the potential to impact normal elimination by affecting the ability of the bladder to hold urine or adequately empty (antihypertensives, cholinesterase inhibitors, antidepressants, sedatives) (Burchum and Rosenthal, 2016).

Implications for Practice

- Older adults with cognitive impairment may need to be reminded to void more frequently to improve continence.
- Evaluate all possible causes of new-onset incontinence, which should include taking note of any new medications that might impact cognition, alertness, mobility, or voiding.
- Older adults newly started on an antimuscarinic medication should be assessed carefully for mental status changes. This class of medications has the potential to cause cognitive impairment in older adults (American Geriatrics Society, 2012).
- Older adults with impaired mobility and incontinence should have interventions put in place to maximize self-care and continence (e.g., toileting program, mobility aids, help with hygiene).
- Teach older women with stress incontinence about pelvic muscle exercises. There is no age limit on their effectiveness.
- The sensation of thirst decreases with aging. Adequate hydration promotes bladder health. Older adults may need to be reminded to drink adequate amounts of water (Touhy and Jett, 2014).
- To decrease nocturia, instruct patients to restrict fluid intake for the 2 hours before bedtime.
- Older men with voiding pattern changes (e.g., urgency, frequency, slow stream, decreased output, dribbling) should be assessed for urinary retention because of age-related prostate enlargement.

Psychosocial Implications

Self-concept, culture, and sexuality are all closely related concepts that are affected when patients have elimination problems. Self-concept changes over one's life span and includes body image; self-esteem, roles, and identity (see Chapters 34 and 35). When children begin to achieve bladder control and learn the appropriate toileting skills, they sometimes resist urinating on the toilet and associate their urine and feces as extensions of self and thus do not want to flush them away. The process of micturition is often a culturally private event and requires you to be sensitive to a need for privacy. Incontinence can be devastating to self-image and self-esteem. When your patient asks for help for such a private and personal activity, it can be perceived as embarrassing or being treated like a child, or it may threaten the patient's sense of self-determination. When a patient has a urinary diversion, it will influence his or her sense of body image, resulting in a perceived threat in being able to maintain a healthy sexual relationship with a partner. As a nurse, be aware of how elimination disorders affect patients psychosocially so that you can understand the full impact of the patient's elimination problem.

CRITICAL THINKING

Successful critical thinking requires synthesis of knowledge, experience, information gathered from patients, critical thinking attitudes, and intellectual and professional standards. Clinical judgments require you to anticipate and collect necessary information, analyze the data, and make decisions regarding your patient's care.

When applying the nursing process, take into consideration the knowledge you have learned about the urinary system. Integrate the knowledge from nursing and other disciplines, previous experiences, and patients to understand the process of urinary elimination and the impact on a patient and family. The urinary system is affected by many factors, both as part of or outside the urinary tract. As a result you are able to identify the unique impact of these problems on patients and families. For example, men after prostate cancer surgery may experience stress UI because of trauma to the urinary sphincter, people with high caffeine intake or those who take a diuretic may experience increased urinary urgency and frequency, and patients who are normally continent and become immobile may become incontinent.

Urinary elimination problems are common in all health care settings. Reflect on previous and personal experiences to help you determine a patient's elimination needs. If you have personally had a UTI, the experience helps you to understand a patient's frustration and embarrassment as a result of frequency, urgency, and dysuria. Caring for other older adults with functional disabilities helps you to anticipate patient needs related to toileting.

In addition, use critical thinking attitudes such as perseverance to find a plan of care to provide successful management of urinary elimination problems. Professional standards also provide valuable directions. You are in a key position to serve as a patient advocate by suggesting noninvasive alternatives to catheterization use (e.g., the use of a bladder scanner to evaluate urine volume without invasive instrumentation or implementation of a voiding schedule for the incontinent patient).

Practice standards and guidelines prepared by nursing specialty organizations and those developed by national and international professional organizations are valuable tools to use when critically assessing patient problems and developing a plan of care. Box 46-3 lists some of these resources. The professional nurse incorporates such evidence-based guidelines into the plan of care. There are two nursing organizations, the Society for Urological Nurses and Associates (http://www.suna.org) and the Wound, Ostomy, Continence Nurses Society (http://www.wocn.org), that offer many resources related to continence care. Both organizations have specialty certification agencies offering entry level and advanced practice specialty certification

❖ NURSING PROCESS

Apply the nursing process and use a critical thinking approach in the care of patients. The nursing process provides a clinical

BOX 46-3 Resources for Urology/Continence Nurses

1. Association for Professionals in Infection Control and Epidemiology (APIC): *Guide to preventing catheter-associated urinary tract infections,* http://www.apic.org/Professional-Practice/Implementation-guides
2. Centers for Disease Control and Prevention (CDC): *Health care–associated infections (HAIs); catheter-associated urinary tract infections (CAUTI),* http://www.cdc.gov/HAI/ca_uti/uti.html
3. European Association of Urology Nurses (EAUN): http://www.uroweb.org/nurses/nursing-guidelines/
4. International Continence Society (ICS): http://www.ics.org/
5. National Association For Continence (NAFC): http://www.nafc.org/
6. Society of Urologic Nurses and Associates (SUNA): https://www.suna.org/
7. The Simon Foundation for Continence: http://www.simonfoundation.org/index.html
8. The Wound Ostomy and Continence Nurses Society™ (WOCN): http://www.wocn.org/

decision-making approach for you to develop and implement an individualized plan of care.

◆ Assessment

During the assessment process, critically analyze assessment findings to ensure that you make patient-centered clinical decisions required for safe nursing care (Figure 46-4).

Through the Patient's Eyes. Throughout the nursing assessment it is important for you to consider a patient's frame of reference related to his or her illness or urinary problem. Assess the patient's understanding of the urinary problem and expectations of treatment. Because urination is a private matter, some patients find it difficult to talk about their voiding habits. Approach patients in a professional manner and assure them that their problems will be kept confidential. Postoperative patients or patients receiving medications that affect bladder function may become concerned that something is wrong when you assess voiding amount and frequency. Patients receiving intravenous (IV) fluids do not always realize that they have an increased need for urination. Sensitivity to patient misconceptions will allow you to quickly identify areas for patient education. Always ask what he or she expects from care. For example, does the patient expect that the UTI will be resolved? Does the patient expect the colostomy to be only temporary?

Self-Care Ability. It is very important to thoroughly assess patients' ability to perform necessary behaviors associated with voiding. Investigate their expectations of what the nurses will do and what they can do independently. Do not assume that because a patient has a diagnosis of cognitive impairment that he or she cannot understand or participate in care. Balancing patient safety and supporting self-care are sometimes challenges and should be discussed with the patient. For example, a patient with poor balance will need nursing assistance with transfers to a toilet and may need continued nursing supervision while on the toilet, something the patient may find embarrassing or demeaning.

Cultural Considerations. Be aware of cultural and gender differences related to the very private act of voiding and how they affect nursing assessment and care. Be sensitive and ask questions in a straightforward manner. Be aware of gender preferences in positioning

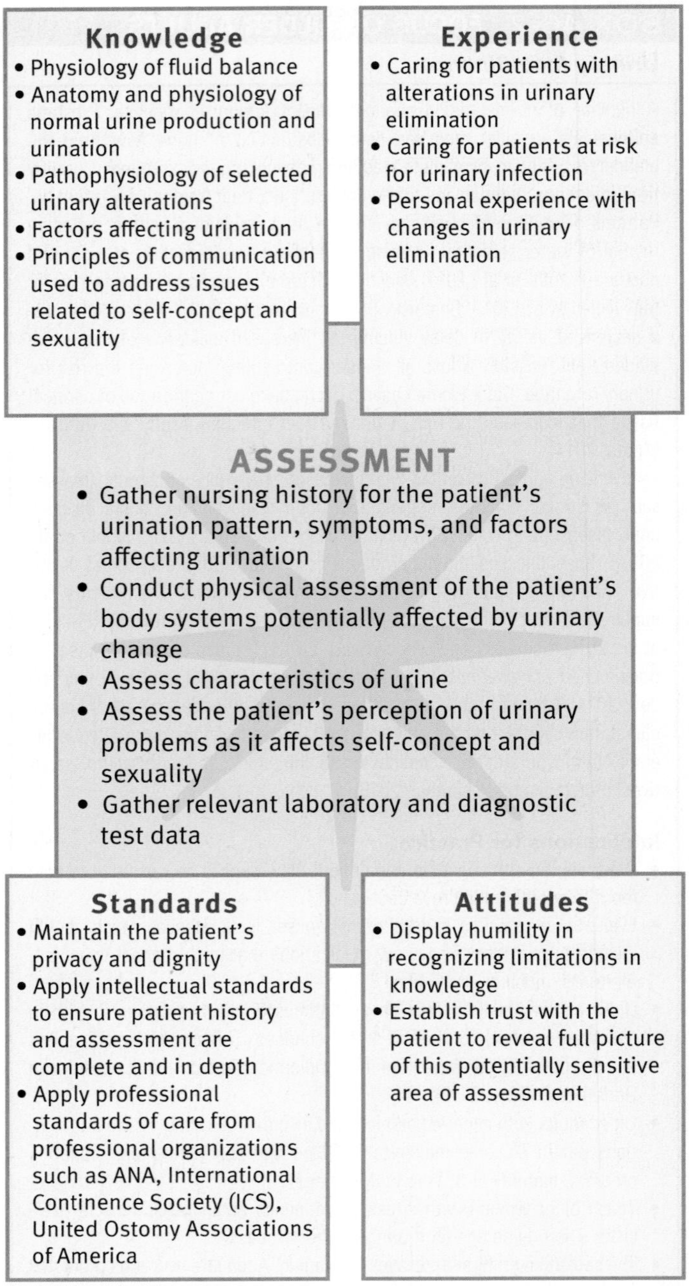

Knowledge
- Physiology of fluid balance
- Anatomy and physiology of normal urine production and urination
- Pathophysiology of selected urinary alterations
- Factors affecting urination
- Principles of communication used to address issues related to self-concept and sexuality

Experience
- Caring for patients with alterations in urinary elimination
- Caring for patients at risk for urinary infection
- Personal experience with changes in urinary elimination

ASSESSMENT
- Gather nursing history for the patient's urination pattern, symptoms, and factors affecting urination
- Conduct physical assessment of the patient's body systems potentially affected by urinary change
- Assess characteristics of urine
- Assess the patient's perception of urinary problems as it affects self-concept and sexuality
- Gather relevant laboratory and diagnostic test data

Standards
- Maintain the patient's privacy and dignity
- Apply intellectual standards to ensure patient history and assessment are complete and in depth
- Apply professional standards of care from professional organizations such as ANA, International Continence Society (ICS), United Ostomy Associations of America

Attitudes
- Display humility in recognizing limitations in knowledge
- Establish trust with the patient to reveal full picture of this potentially sensitive area of assessment

FIGURE 46-4 Critical thinking model for urinary elimination assessment. *ANA,* American Nurses Association.

for urination: many men stand to void, whereas women sit. There are gender-linked urinary alterations such as prostate enlargement in men and pelvic organ prolapse in women. Culture often dictates gender-specific roles when it comes to care of elimination issues. It may be inappropriate for a male to touch or even talk about elimination matters with a woman (Box 46-4).

Health Literacy. When taking a nursing history, you should be careful to assess a patient's understanding of his or her urinary tract problem. Urinary tract problems are not common topics of conversation in families and other settings. Limited knowledge of basic anatomy and how the urinary tract functions can contribute to poor understanding and outcomes of treatment (Anger et al., 2012). Assess

BOX 46-4 CULTURAL ASPECTS OF CARE

Urinary Elimination

Urinary elimination is a private human activity. It is important when caring for patients from diverse cultures and religions to incorporate into the plan of care sensitivity and awareness of factors that may impact care when dealing with urinary elimination problems. Many cultures have specific beliefs and practices related to elimination, privacy, and gender-specific care. Because of the personal nature of the problem and cultural practices surrounding elimination, urinary problems such as incontinence often are not discussed with medical professionals (Beji et al., 2010; Gemmill and Wells, 2010). Variations within a cultural group are common; thus each patient must be assessed and cared for as an individual.

Implications for Patient-Centered Care

- Each patient is unique. As a professional nurse you must determine the extent to which a patient's cultural background, such as age-group, geographic location, ethnicity, or race, affect their elimination problems.
- Whenever possible, provide for a same-gender caregiver for individuals whose cultural preferences emphasize female modesty and prohibit non-related males and females from touching (Beji et al., 2010). Patients from the Iranian, Jewish Orthodox, Korean, Hindu, and Vietnamese cultures may prefer same-gender care.
- Privacy is important in many cultures; thus careful attention to closing doors, bedside curtains, and draping is important.
- Pay special attention that the patient understands instructions and patient education when English is not the primary language (see Chapter 10). If available, provide written materials in patient's primary language. Provide a professional interpreter as needed.
- Certain cultures such as Hindus and Muslims observe meticulous hygiene practices that designate the left hand to perform unclean procedures such as genitourinary hygiene. Perform hand hygiene before touching the patient and use your right hand when possible. Use the left hand to handle the urinal and/or secretions.
- Some cultures (e.g., African, Western, and Southeastern Asia) continue to practice female genital cutting or female genital circumcision, which can include removal of all or part of the clitoris and part or complete removal of the labia minora or, in its most severe form, the total removal of the clitoris and labia and sewing together the labia majora, leaving only a small opening for urine and menses (American Academy of Pediatrics, 2010). Some long-term consequences include recurrent urinary tract infections, incontinence, pelvic infections, fistulas, scarring, and sexual dysfunction (Odemerho and Baier, 2012).
- Cultural practices dictate the level of involvement of family in a patient's care. This source of strength is important to the health of the patient, and family must be included in the plan of care.

BOX 46-5 Nursing Assessment Questions

Nature of the Problem

- Which problems are you having with passing urine?

Signs and Symptoms

- Does it hurt or burn when you pass your urine?
- Are you having abdominal pain/flank pain/fevers/chills?
- Has there been a change in the color or odor of your urine? Please describe that change.
- Do you feel like you are emptying your bladder completely?
- Are you passing urine more frequently than normal during the day?
- Do you need to strain and/or wait before your urine stream starts?
- Do you need to get up at night to pass urine?
- Do you leak urine when feeling a strong desire to void?
- Do you ever leak urine when you cough, sneeze, and/or exercise?
- Are you ever wet with urine and do not know when it happened?
- Do you dribble urine before you void, after you void, or at other times?

Onset and Duration

- When did you first notice a problem?
- How long has this problem lasted?

Severity

- How many times a day do you pass urine?
- How many times a day and how many times at night do you leak urine?
- How many times are you wet/need to change a pad in a day and at night?
- How often are you awakened with the urge to void and get up to use the bathroom?
- How does this pattern compare with the pattern you last remember?

Predisposing Factors

- Have you noticed any patterns to your urinary problem?
- Tell me what you usually eat/drink in a day. Does it include such things as caffeinated beverages, chocolate, citrus, or alcohol?
- Which medicines do you take routinely, and have any recently changed?
- Have you been hospitalized or diagnosed with a new medical problem recently?

Effect on Patient

- How have these symptoms affected your life?
- Does your urinary problem interfere with any of your usual activities?
- Have you ever tried any treatment for this problem (self-help, complementary therapies, over-the-counter remedies, medical professional, and specialist)?

the patient's health literacy level before engaging in education (see Chapter 25).

Nursing History. The nursing history includes a review of the patient's elimination patterns, symptoms of urinary alterations, and assessment of factors that are affecting the ability to urinate normally. Box 46-5 lists nursing history questions that will help direct the patient to focus on urinary problems.

Pattern of Urination. Ask the patient about daily voiding patterns, including frequency and times of day, normal volume at each voiding, and history of recent changes. Frequency of voiding varies among individuals depending on fluid intake, medications such as diuretics, and the intake of bladder irritants such as caffeine or other caffeinated beverages. The common times for urination are on awakening, after meals, and before bedtime. Most people void an average of 5 or more times a day. Be sure to ask if the patient is awakened from sleep with an urge to void and how many times this occurs. It is normal for patients who wake at night because of noise, pain, or nighttime treatments to experience an urge to void. Information about the pattern of urination is necessary to establish a baseline for comparison.

Symptoms of Urinary Alterations. Certain symptoms specific to urinary alterations may occur in more than one type of disorder. During assessment ask the patient about the presence of symptoms related to urination (Table 46-2). Also determine whether the patient is aware of conditions or factors that precipitate or aggravate the symptoms and determine what he or she does if any of these symptoms occur.

TABLE 46-2 Common Symptoms of Urinary Alterations

Description	Common Causes
Urgency	
An immediate and strong desire to void that is not easily deferred	Full bladder Urinary tract infection Inflammation or irritation of the bladder Overactive bladder
Dysuria	
Pain or discomfort associated with voiding	Urinary tract infection Inflammation of the prostate Urethritis Trauma to the lower urinary tract Urinary tract tumors
Frequency	
Voiding more than 8 times during waking hours and/or at decreased intervals such as less than every 2 hours.	High volumes of fluid intake Bladder irritants (e.g., caffeine) Urinary tract infection Increased pressure on bladder (e.g., pregnancy) Bladder outlet obstruction (e.g., prostate enlargement, pelvic organ prolapse) Overactive bladder
Hesitancy	
Delay in start of urinary stream when voiding	Anxiety (e.g., voiding in public restroom) Bladder outlet obstruction (e.g., prostate enlargement, urethral stricture)
Polyuria	
Voiding excessive amounts of urine	High volumes of fluid intake Uncontrolled diabetes mellitus Diabetes insipidus Diuretic therapy
Oliguria	
Diminished urinary output in relation to fluid intake	Fluid and electrolyte imbalance (e.g., dehydration) Kidney dysfunction or failure Increased secretion of antidiuretic hormone (ADH) Urinary tract obstruction
Nocturia	
Awakened from sleep because of the urge to void	Excess intake of fluids (especially coffee or alcohol before bedtime) Bladder outlet obstruction (e.g., prostate enlargement) Overactive bladder Medications (e.g., diuretic taken in the evening) Cardiovascular disease (e.g., hypertension) Urinary tract infection
Dribbling	
Leakage of small amounts of urine despite voluntary control of micturition	Bladder outlet obstruction (e.g., prostatic enlargement) Incomplete bladder emptying Stress incontinence
Hematuria	
Presence of blood in urine Gross hematuria (blood is easily seen in urine) Microscopic hematuria (blood not visualized but measured on urinalysis)	Tumors (e.g., kidney, bladder) Infection (e.g., glomerular nephritis, cystitis) Urinary tract calculi Trauma to the urinary tract
Retention	
Acute retention: Suddenly unable to void when bladder is adequately full or overfull Chronic retention: Bladder does not empty completely during voiding, and urine is retained in the bladder	Bladder outlet obstruction (e.g., prostatic enlargement, urethral obstruction) Absent or weak bladder contractility (e.g., neurological dysfunction such as caused by diabetes, multiple sclerosis, lower spinal cord injury) Side effects of certain medications (e.g., anesthesia, anticholinergics, antispasmodics, antidepressants)

Physical Assessment. A physical examination (see Chapter 31) provides you with data to determine the presence and severity of urinary elimination problems. The primary areas to assess include the kidneys, bladder, external genitalia, urethral meatus, and perineal skin. Fluid intake and the pattern and amounts provides additional objective data.

Kidneys. When the kidneys become infected or inflamed, they can become tender, resulting in flank pain. You assess for tenderness by gently percussing the costovertebral angle (the angle formed by the spine and twelfth rib). Auscultation is sometimes performed to detect the presence of a renal artery bruit (sound resulting from turbulent blood flow through a narrowed artery), but this skill is usually performed by an advanced practice nurse.

Bladder. In adults the bladder rests below the symphysis pubis. When distended with urine, the bladder will rise above the symphysis pubis along the midline of the abdomen. A very full bladder can extend as far as the umbilicus. On inspection you may observe a swelling or convex curvature of the lower abdomen. On gentle palpation of the lower abdomen, a full bladder may be felt as a smooth and rounded mass. When a full bladder is palpated, patients report a sensation of urinary urge tenderness or even pain. If an overfull bladder is suspected, further assessment with an ultrasound device or a bladder scanner is recommended if available.

External Genitalia and Urethral Meatus. Careful and sensitive inspection of the external genitalia and urethral meatus yield important data that may indicate inflammation and infection. Normally there should be no drainage or inflammation. To best examine the female patient, position her in the dorsal recumbent position to provide full exposure of the genitalia. Observe the labia majora for swelling, redness, tenderness, rashes, lesions, or evidence of scratching. Using a gloved hand, retract the labial folds. The labia minora is normally pink and moist. The urethral meatus will appear as an irregular or slitlike opening below the clitoris and above the vaginal orifice. Look for drainage and lesions and ask the patient if there is discomfort. If there is drainage, note the color and consistency and any odor. The vaginal tissue of a postmenopausal woman may be dryer and less pink than that of younger women.

Examine the penis. Look for any redness or irritation. If the man is uncircumcised, retract the foreskin or ask the patient to do so. The foreskin should move back easily to expose the glans penis. In some cases the foreskin will become tight and cannot be retracted (phimosis), increasing risk for inflammation and infection. The urethral meatus is a slitlike opening just below the tip of the penis. Inspect the glans penis and meatus for discharge, lesions, and inflammation. Following inspection, return the foreskin to the unretracted position. Retracted foreskins can cause dangerous swelling (paraphimosis) of the penis (Ball and Dains, 2015).

All patients with an indwelling catheter should have the urinary meatus assessed for catheter-related damage and for the presence of inflammation and discharge that can indicate infection. Pulling and traction on catheters can damage the urinary meatus by creating pressure on the urethra and meatus. In some severe cases the catheter will erode through the meatus to the vagina or in men through the glans and shaft of the penis. Early detection of trauma means that a plan of prevention for further damage can be implemented.

Perineal Skin. Assessment of skin exposed to moisture, especially urine, needs to occur at least daily (and more often if incontinence is ongoing) to pick up early signs of skin damage related to the moisture. Observe for erythema in areas exposed to moisture, skin erosion, and patient complaints of a burning itching pain (Gray et al., 2012).

Assessment of Urine. The assessment of urine includes measuring the patient's fluid intake and urinary output (I&O) and observing the characteristics of the urine.

Intake and Output. Assessment of I&O is a way to evaluate bladder emptying, renal function, and fluid and electrolyte balance. Although often written as part of a health care provider's order, placing a patient on I&O is also a nursing judgment. Obtaining accurate I&O measurement often requires cooperation and assistance from the patient and family. Intake measurements need to include all oral liquids and semiliquids, enteral feedings, and any parenteral fluids (see Chapter 42). Output measurement includes not only urine but any fluid that leaves the body that can be measured such as vomitus, gastric drainage tubes, and wound drains.

Urinary output is a key indicator of kidney and bladder function. A change in urine volume can be a significant indicator of fluid imbalance, kidney dysfunction, or decreased blood volume. For example, a postoperative catheterized patient's hourly urinary output provides an indirect measure of circulating blood volume. If the urinary output falls below 30 mL/hr, the nurse should immediately assess for signs of blood loss and notify the health care provider. Urinary output is also an indicator of bladder function. Patients who have not voided for longer than 3 to 6 hours and have had fluid intake recorded should be evaluated for urinary retention. Just helping some patients to a normal position to void prompts voiding. Assess for any extreme increase or decrease in urine volume. Urine output less than 30 mL per hour for more than two consecutive hours or excessive urine output (polyuria) is a cause for concern and should prompt further assessment and notification of the health care provider.

Urine volume is measured using receptacles with volume-measurement markings. After a patient voids in a bedside commode, bedpan, or urinal, or when urine is emptied from a catheter drainage bag, urine can be measured using a graduated measuring container. For patients who void in a toilet, a urine hat (Figure 46-5) collects urine, allowing for patient privacy in the bathroom. Catheterized patients may have a specialized drainage bag with a urometer (Figure 46-6) attached between the drainage tubing and drainage bag that allows for accurate hourly urine measurement. When emptying catheter drainage bags, follow Standard Precautions (Chapter 29) and make sure that the drainage tube is reclamped and secured. Each patient needs to have a graduated receptacle for individual use to prevent potential cross-contamination. Label each container with the patient's name. The container needs to be rinsed after each use to minimize odor and bacterial growth.

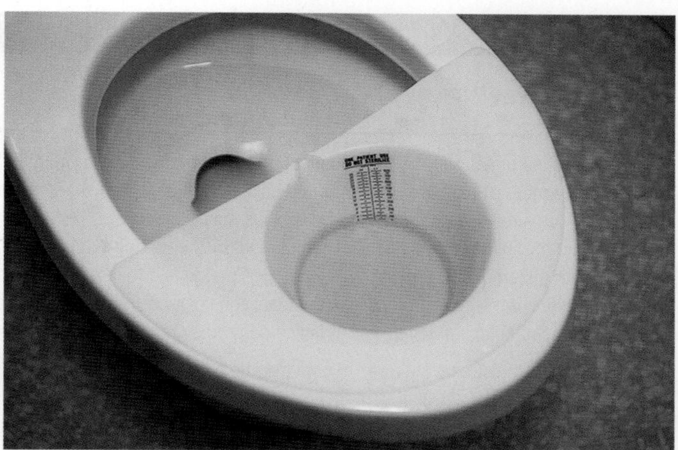

FIGURE 46-5 Urine hat.

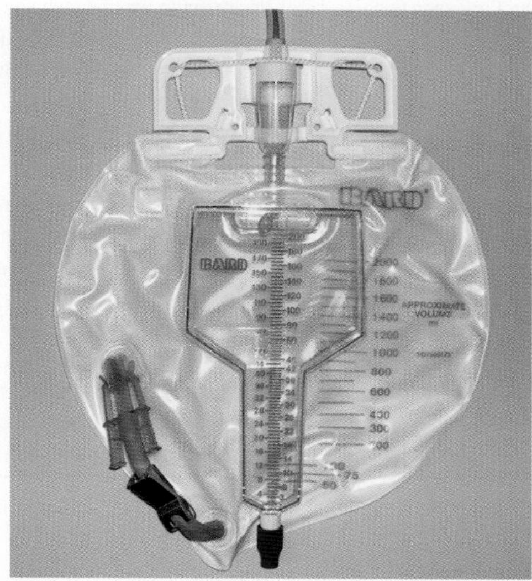

FIGURE 46-6 Urometer. (Courtesy Michael Gallager, RN, BSN, OSF Saint Francis Medical Center, Peoria, IL.)

Characteristics of Urine. Inspect the patient's urine for color, clarity, and odor. Monitor and document any changes.

Color. Normal urine ranges in color from a pale straw color to amber, depending on its concentration. Urine is usually more concentrated in the morning or with fluid volume deficits. As the patient drinks more fluids, urine becomes less concentrated, and the color lightens. Patients taking diuretics commonly void dilute urine while the medication is active.

TABLE 46-3 Urine Testing

Collection Type/Use of Specimen	Nursing Considerations
Random (routine urinalysis) Includes a number of tests that are used for screening and are diagnostic for fluid and electrolyte disturbances, urinary tract infection, presence of blood and other metabolic problems	Collect during normal voiding or from an indwelling catheter or urinary diversion collection bag. Do not collect from an indwelling catheter drainage bag (urine is not freshly voided). Use a clean specimen cup. In some health care settings you may be responsible for testing urine with reagent strips. Follow manufacturer instructions when performing and reading the strips. Dip the reagent strip into fresh urine, then observe color changes on the strip. Compare the color on the strip with the color chart on the reagent strip container. Each color is examined at the exact time indicated on the container.
Clean-voided or midstream (culture and sensitivity)	Urine may be collected by the patient after detailed instruction on proper cleansing and collection technique (see Skill 46-1 on pp. 1128-1131). Always use a sterile specimen cup.
Sterile specimen for culture and sensitivity Determines the presence of bacteria and to which antibiotic the bacteria are sensitive	If the patient has an indwelling catheter, collect a specimen by using sterile aseptic technique through the special sampling port (see Figure 46-12) found on the side of the catheter. Never collect the specimen from the drainage bag. Clamp the tubing below the port, allowing fresh, uncontaminated urine to collect in the tube. After wiping the port with an antimicrobial swab, insert a sterile syringe hub and withdraw at least 3 to 5 mL of urine (check agency policy). Using sterile aseptic technique, transfer the urine to a sterile container (see Chapter 28). Patients with a urinary diversion need to have the stoma catheterized to obtain an accurate specimen. A preliminary report will be available in 24 hours; but usually 48 to 72 hours are needed for bacterial growth and sensitivity testing.
Timed urine specimens Measure bodily substances that may be excreted at higher levels at specific times of the day or over a specific time period	Requires urine collection and testing either at specific time of day or urine collected over a specific time period (e.g., 2-, 12-, or 24-hour collections). The timed period begins after the patient urinates and ends with a final voiding at the end of the time period. In most 24-hour specimen collections discard the first voided specimen and then start collecting urine. Patient voids into a clean receptacle; and the urine is transferred to the special collection container, which often contains special preservatives. Depending on the test, the urine container may need to be kept cool by setting it in a container of ice. Each specimen must be free of feces and toilet tissue. Missed specimens make the whole collection inaccurate. Check with agency policy and the laboratory for specific instructions. Patients' education should include an explanation of the test, an emphasis on the need to collect all urine voided during the prescribed time period, and urine collection procedure.

Blood in the urine (hematuria) is never a normal finding. Bleeding from the kidneys or ureters usually causes urine to become dark red; bleeding from the bladder or urethra usually causes bright red urine. Hematuria and blood clots are a common cause of urinary catheter blockage.

Various medications and foods change the color of the urine. For example, patients taking phenazopyridine, a urinary analgesic, void urine that is bright orange. Eating beets, rhubarb, and blackberries causes red urine. The kidneys excrete special dyes used in IV diagnostic studies, and this discolors the urine. Dark amber urine is the result of high concentrations of bilirubin (urobilinogen) in patients with liver disease. Report unexpected color changes to the health care provider.

Clarity. Normal urine appears transparent at the time of voiding. Urine that stands several minutes in a container becomes cloudy. In patients with renal disease, freshly voided urine appears cloudy because of protein concentration. Urine may also appear thick and cloudy as a result of bacteria and white blood cells. Early-morning voided urine may be cloudy because of urine held in the bladder overnight but will be clear on the next voiding.

Odor. Urine has a characteristic ammonia odor. The more concentrated the urine, the stronger the odor. As urine remains standing (e.g., in a collection device), more ammonia breakdown occurs, and the odor becomes stronger. A foul odor may indicate a UTI. Some foods such as asparagus and garlic can change the odor of urine.

Laboratory and Diagnostic Testing. You are often responsible for collecting urine specimens for laboratory testing. The type of test determines the method of collection. Label all specimens with the patient's name, date, time, and type of collection. Most urine specimens need to reach the laboratory within 2 hours of collection or must be preserved according to the laboratory protocol (Pagana and Pagana, 2013). Urine that stands in a container at room temperature without the required preservative will grow bacteria resulting in changes that will affect the accuracy of the test. Agency infection control policies require the adherence to standard precautions during the handling of urine specimens (see Chapter 29). To obtain urine that is fresh or new you need to ask the patient to double void. The second voided specimen is the one sent to the laboratory. To obtain urine as free of bacterial contamination as possible, a midstream clean-catch urine specimen may be required. Table 46-3 describes nursing considerations for a variety of common tests. Table 46-4 describes the components of the most common of the urinary tests, urinalysis.

Diagnostic Examinations. The urinary system is one of the few organ systems accessible to accurate diagnostic study by radiographic techniques. Studies can be simple and noninvasive or complex and invasive. See Table 46-5 for a review of some common diagnostic testing of the urinary tract.

TABLE 46-4 Routine Urinalysis

Measurement (Normal Value)	Interpretation
pH (4.6 to 8.0)	pH level indicates acid-base balance. Acid pH helps protect against bacterial growth. Urine that stands for several hours becomes alkaline from bacterial growth.
Protein (up to 8 mg/100 mL)	Protein is normally not present in urine. The presence of protein is a very sensitive indicator of kidney function. Damage to the glomerular membrane (such as in glomerulonephritis) allows for the filtration of larger molecules such as protein to seep through.
Glucose (not normally present)	Patients with poorly controlled diabetes have glucose in the urine because of inability of tubules to resorb high serum glucose concentrations (>180 mg/100 mL). Ingestion of high concentrations of glucose causes some to appear in urine of healthy people.
Ketones (not normally present)	With poor control of diabetes, patients experience breakdown of fatty acids. End products of fatty acid metabolism are ketones. Patients with dehydration, starvation, or excessive aspirin ingestion also have ketonuria.
Blood	A positive test for occult blood occurs when intact erythrocytes, hemoglobin, or myoglobin is present. Damage to the glomerulus or tubules causes blood cells to enter urine. Trauma or disease of the lower urinary tract also causes hematuria.
Specific gravity (1.0053 to 1.030)	Specific gravity tests measure concentration of particles in urine. High specific gravity reflects concentrated urine, and low specific gravity reflects diluted urine. Dehydration, reduced renal blood flow, and increase in ADH secretion elevate specific gravity. Overhydration, early renal disease, and inadequate ADH secretion reduce specific gravity.
Microscopic examination RBC (up to 2)	Damage to glomeruli or tubules allows RBCs to enter the urine. Trauma, disease, presence of urethral catheters, or surgery of the lower urinary tract also causes RBCs to be present.
WBCs (0-4 per low-power field)	Elevated numbers indicate inflammation or infection.
Bacteria (not normally present)	Bacteria in the urine can mean infection or colonization (if the patient shows no symptoms).
Casts (cylindrical bodies not normally present, the shapes of which take on the likeness of objects within the renal tubule)	Types include hyaline, WBCs, RBCs, granular cells, and epithelial cells. Their presence indicates renal disease.
Crystals (not normally present)	Crystals indicate increased risk for the development of renal calculi (stone). Patients with high uric acid levels (gout) may develop uric acid crystals.

Data from Pagana KD, Pagana TJ: *Mosby's diagnostic and laboratory test reference*, ed 11, St Louis, 2013, Mosby.
ADH, Antidiuretic hormone; *RBC*, red blood cell; *WBC*, white blood cell.

Many of the nursing responsibilities related to diagnostic testing of the urinary tract are common to most studies. Those responsibilities before testing include the following:

- Ensure that a signed consent is completed (check agency policy).
- Assess the patient for any allergies and if he or she has experienced a previous reaction to a contrast agent (Pagana and Pagana, 2013).
- Administer bowel-cleansing agents as ordered (check agency policy).
- Ensure that the patient adheres to the appropriate pretest diet (clear liquids) or nothing by mouth (NPO).
- Responsibilities after testing include:
  - Assessing I&O.
  - Assessing voiding and urine (color, clarity, presence of blood, dysuria, problems emptying.)
- Encouraging fluid intake, especially if using radiopaque dye.

◆ Nursing Diagnosis

A thorough assessment of a patient's urinary elimination function reveals patterns of data that allow a nurse to make relevant and accurate nursing diagnoses. Use critical thinking to reflect on knowledge of previous patients, apply knowledge of urinary function and the effects of disorders, review defining characteristics, and make a specific nursing diagnosis. Data from questions about the urinary system are important in identifying nursing diagnoses. The diagnosis focuses on a specific urinary elimination alteration or an associated problem such as *Impaired Skin Integrity related to UI.* Identification of defining characteristics leads to selection of an appropriate problem-focused diagnosis. Identification of risk factors leads to section of a risk diagnosis (see Chapter 17).

An important part of formulating problem-focused nursing diagnoses is identifying the relevant causative or related factor. In the case of risk diagnoses, you select correct risk factors. You will choose interventions that treat or modify the related factor or risk factor for the diagnosis to be resolved. Specifying related factors for a diagnosis allows selection of individualized nursing interventions (Ackley and Ladwig, 2011). For example, *Toileting Self-Care Deficit related to impaired transfer ability* or *impaired mobility* status guides the selection of nursing interventions that remove barriers to toilet access. *Toileting Self-Care Deficit related to cognitive impairment* guides the selection of nursing interventions such as a prompted voiding program or habit training program. Box 46-6 provides an example of diagnostic reasoning. Some nursing diagnoses common to patients with urinary elimination problems include the following:

- *Functional Urinary Incontinence*
- *Stress Urinary Incontinence*
- *Urge Urinary Incontinence*
- *Reflex Incontinence*
- *Risk For Infection*
- *Toileting Self-Care Deficit*

TABLE 46-5 Common Diagnostic Tests of Urinary Tract

Procedure	Description	Special Nursing Considerations
Noninvasive Procedures		
Abdominal roentgenogram (plain film; kidney, ureter, bladder (KUB) or flat plate)	X-ray film of the abdomen to determine the size, shape, symmetry, and location of the structures of the lower urinary tract Common uses: Detect and measure the size of urinary calculi	No special preparation
Computerized axial tomography (CT) scan	Detailed imagery of the abdominal structures provided by computerized reconstruction of cross-sectional images. Common uses: Identify anatomical abnormalities, renal tumors and cysts, calculi, and obstruction of the ureters	Preparation: Cleanse bowel (see agency or health care provider protocol). Assess for presence of any allergies and previous reaction to contrast media. All patients with allergies are at increased risk for anaphylactoid reactions to radiocontrast. Adverse reactions to contrast media are anaphylactoid, not true allergies (Kaufman et al., 2013). **Note:** The myth that anyone allergic to contrast media is allergic to shellfish or iodine is untrue. Iodine is an essential trace element and not an allergen (Schabelman and Witting, 2010). The allergens in shellfish are proteins that do not contain iodine. Restrict food and fluid up to 4 hours before test (see agency or health care provider protocol). After procedure: Encourage fluids to promote dye excretion. Assess for delayed hypersensitivity reaction to the contrast media. Patient teaching: Explain that he or she will be placed on a special bed that will move through a tunnel-like imaging chamber. He or she will need to lie still when instructed by the technician; some patients may feel claustrophobic.
Intravenous pyelogram (IVP)	Imaging of the urinary tract that views the collecting ducts and renal pelvis and outlines the ureters, bladder, and urethra (After intravenous injection of contrast media [iodine based that converts to a dye], a series of x-ray films are taken to observe the passage of urine from the renal pelvis to the bladder.) Common uses: Detect and measure urinary calculi, tumors, hematuria, obstruction of the urinary tract	Preparation: Assess for allergies. Assess for dehydration. Cleanse bowel (see agency or health care provider protocol). Restrict food and fluid up to 4 hours before test (see agency or health care provider protocol). After procedure: Assess for delayed hypersensitivity to the contrast media. Encourage fluids after the test to dilute and flush dye from the patient. Assess urine output. Less than 30/mL hr increases risk for contrast-induced nephropathy. Patient teaching: Facial flushing is a normal response during dye injection, and patients may feel dizzy or warm or feel some nausea.
Ultrasound: Renal bladder	Imaging of the kidneys, ureters, and bladder using sound waves Identifies gross structural abnormalities and estimates the volume of urine in the bladder Common uses: Detect masses, obstruction, presence of hydronephrosis or hydroureter, abnormalities of the bladder wall, and calculi; measure postvoid residual	Patients need to come to the study with a full bladder.
Invasive Procedures		
Endoscopy-cystoscopy	Introduction of a cystoscope through the urethra into the bladder to provide direct visualization, specimen collection, and/or treatment of the bladder and urethra (In most cases the procedure is performed using local anesthesia, but under certain circumstances general anesthesia or conscious sedation may be used.) Common uses: Microscopic hematuria, detect bladder tumors and obstruction of the bladder outlet and urethra	When applicable, follow agency protocol for preoperative preparation (see Chapter 39). Patient teaching: Urine may be pink tinged after the test; signs and symptoms of urinary tract infection.

Data from Pagana KD, Pagana TJ: *Mosby's diagnostic and laboratory test reference*, ed 11, St Louis, 2013, Mosby.

BOX 46-6 Nursing Diagnostic Process

Urge Urinary Incontinence Related to Bladder infection

Assessment Activities	Defining Characteristics
Ask patient to describe voiding problems/incontinence.	Patient complains of urine leakage associated with a strong urge to void.
Assess patient's voiding pattern.	Bladder record shows episodes of urinary incontinence. Patient describes or is observed to leak urine on the way to or at the toilet. Patient describes or is observed to rush or hurry to the toilet.

- *Impaired Skin Integrity*
- *Impaired Urinary Elimination*
- *Urinary Retention*

◆ Planning

During planning integrate the knowledge from assessment and information about available resources and therapies to develop an individualized plan of care (see the Nursing Care Plan). Match the patient's needs with clinical and professional standards recommended in the literature (Figure 46-7). Building a relationship of trust with patients is important because the implementation of care involves interaction of a very personal nature.

Goals and Outcomes. The plan of care for urinary elimination alterations must include realistic and individualized goals along with relevant outcomes. The nurse and the patient need to collaborate in setting goals and outcomes and ultimately in choosing nursing interventions. A general goal is often normal urinary elimination; but sometimes the individual goal differs, depending on the problem. The goals are short or long term.

For example, a realistic short-term goal for a patient with *Toileting Self-Care Deficit related to impaired mobility status* would be that the patient will be able to independently use the toilet. An appropriate outcome would be that the "patient is observed to safely transfer to the toilet." To achieve this outcome you identify a number of interventions such as ensuring that the call bell is within reach, providing assistive devices such as a raised toilet seat, and providing easy access to the urinal when in bed. Conversely, the patient with stress incontinence often has a long-term goal that depends on weeks of pelvic floor muscle exercise to improve urinary control: Patient will experience normal continence. An outcome for this goal would be to "decrease the number of incontinence pads by 1 to 2 within 8 weeks after start of Kegel exercise program." Interventions will include daily Kegel exercises. Make sure that goals and outcomes are reasonably achievable and relevant to the patient's situation (see Box 46-8).

Setting Priorities. It is important to establish priorities of care on the basis of a patient's immediate physical and safety needs, patient expectations, and readiness to perform some self-care activities. Establish a relationship with the patient that allows discussion and intervention. While you are collaborating with the patient, priorities become apparent, enhancing patient understanding of all the goals. When a patient has multiple nursing diagnoses (Figure 46-8), it is important to recognize the primary health problem and its influence on other problems. For example, a patient with a long-term indwelling catheter is admitted to acute care with a severe UTI. The patient expects to resume self-care of the catheter. However, because of the severity of the infection and the patient's condition, the nurse needs to perform all care for the patient's catheter. In this case the priorities are to treat the infection, prevent reinfection, and teach the patient how to resume care of the catheter using techniques to prevent infection.

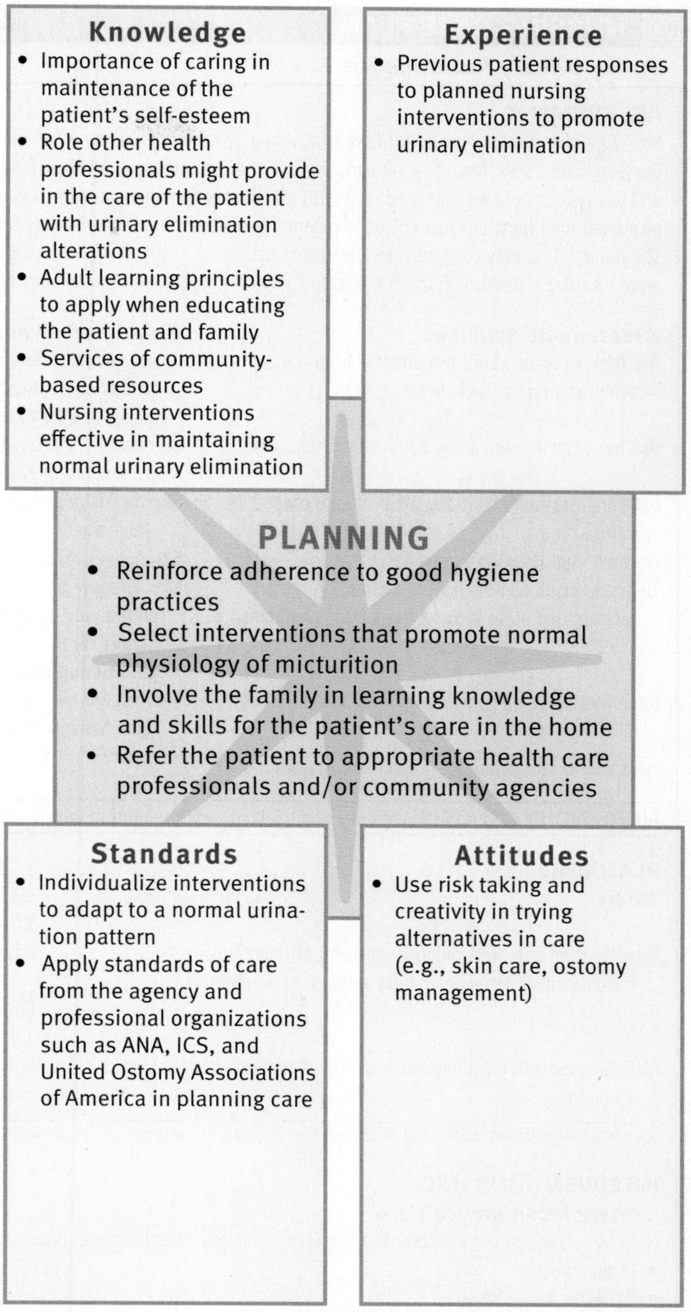

Knowledge
- Importance of caring in maintenance of the patient's self-esteem
- Role other health professionals might provide in the care of the patient with urinary elimination alterations
- Adult learning principles to apply when educating the patient and family
- Services of community-based resources
- Nursing interventions effective in maintaining normal urinary elimination

Experience
- Previous patient responses to planned nursing interventions to promote urinary elimination

PLANNING
- Reinforce adherence to good hygiene practices
- Select interventions that promote normal physiology of micturition
- Involve the family in learning knowledge and skills for the patient's care in the home
- Refer the patient to appropriate health care professionals and/or community agencies

Standards
- Individualize interventions to adapt to a normal urination pattern
- Apply standards of care from the agency and professional organizations such as ANA, ICS, and United Ostomy Associations of America in planning care

Attitudes
- Use risk taking and creativity in trying alternatives in care (e.g., skin care, ostomy management)

FIGURE 46-7 Critical thinking model for urinary elimination planning. *ANA*, American Nurses Association; *ICS*, International Continence Society.

Teamwork and Collaboration. When planning individualized care, it is essential to use the expertise of the health care team and incorporate them into the plan. For example, when planning care for a patient with urge UI, incorporate the expertise of a continence nurse

NURSING CARE PLAN

Stress Urinary Incontinence

ASSESSMENT

Mrs. Kay, the nurse, is caring for Mrs. Grayson, a 75-year-old woman, who has recently been seen in the emergency department for a urinary tract infection. Mrs. Grayson shares with Mrs. Kay her concerns over her incontinence. Medical history includes: postmenopausal, has a history of three vaginal births, is "overweight," and has type 2 diabetes managed well with oral medication and diet. She lives with her husband, and her three grown children live nearby. Mrs. Grayson volunteers at a local food bank but had not gone recently because of her incontinence. She confides to the nurse that her uncontrollable urine leakage has affected her life. The patient's primary care provider has prescribed for Mrs. Grayson pelvic muscle exercise and lifestyle modifications to treat her incontinence. Mrs. Kay's assessment includes a discussion of Mrs. Grayson's current health status with emphasis on her urinary concerns.

Assessment Activities	*Findings/Defining Characteristics**
Ask Mrs. Grayson about the effects of her urinary symptoms on her daily life.	She responds, "I find myself being embarrassed and frustrated for **losing control.** I **dribble** when I'm on the way to the bathroom. I'm afraid to cough, sneeze, or laugh because I **leak urine.** I don't go places and try to avoid being close to other people because I'm afraid I might have an odor."
Ask her what she has been doing about her condition.	She states, "I've been wearing a pad and will go to the bathroom every hour just in case. I try to limit the amount of water I drink so I will not have to go to the bathroom."
Ask Mrs. Grayson about any other effects caused by her leakage.	She begins to cry and states, "I don't even like to go to the movies or visit my grandchildren. It's safer to stay home."
Observe Mrs. Grayson's behavior.	She appears anxious and sad.
Take a focused nursing history addressing urinary leakage and other lower urinary tract symptoms.	Mrs. Grayson's report of **urine leakage on physical exertion, sneezing, and laughing** and leakage on the way to the bathroom increases the likelihood of a diagnosis of mixed incontinence. Her risk factors for this condition include a **history of type 2 diabetes, three pregnancies,** being **postmenopausal,** and being **overweight.** The history helps to define the proper interventions.
Have Mrs. Grayson complete a 3-day bladder diary.	The bladder diary provides objective verification of fluid intake, urine elimination pattern, and patterns of urine leakage. The record also is a baseline for evaluation of the effectiveness of the treatment plan.

***Defining characteristics** are shown in bold type.

NURSING DIAGNOSIS: Stress urinary incontinence related to weakened pelvic musculature

PLANNING

Goals	*Expected Outcomes (NOC)†*
	Urinary Continence
Mrs. Grayson will have reduced episodes of urine leakage (incontinence) between voiding within 6 to 8 weeks.	Patient reports fewer than two episodes of daily incontinence following the start of daily pelvic muscle–strengthening exercises (Kegel) and urge-suppression strategies. Patient states decreased anxiety about her incontinence.
	Urinary Elimination
Mrs. Grayson will have improved urinary elimination pattern within 2 months.	Patient remains free of urinary tract infection. Patient is able to resist the urge to void for 15 or more minutes without leaking.

†Outcome classification labels from Moorhead S et al: *Nursing outcomes classification (NOC),* ed 5, St Louis, 2013, Mosby.

INTERVENTIONS (NIC)‡	RATIONALE
Urinary Incontinence Care	
Help Mrs. Grayson with supportive measures to reduce intraabdominal pressure by: • Losing weight. • Avoiding heavy lifting.	These measures reduce intraabdominal and bladder pressure, which increase leakage.
Teach Mrs. Grayson about how to keep her bladder healthy (see Box 46-7): • Avoid bladder irritants. • Keep blood sugars controlled by adherence to her diabetic diet. • Drink adequate amounts of water; avoid drinking large amounts at one time.	Fluids that contain caffeine and other irritants can prompt unwanted bladder contractions, resulting in frequency, urgency, and incontinence.
Pelvic Muscle Exercise	
Teach Mrs. Grayson how to perform pelvic muscle exercises (see Box 46-8): • Instruct her how to identify and contract the muscle. • Help her set up a daily schedule for performing the exercises. • Instruct her to squeeze the muscle immediately before coughing and sneezing.	Pelvic muscle training is effective in treating stress urinary incontinence (Dumoulin et al., 2011).
Bladder retraining (behavioral therapy) • Teach her how to inhibit strong sensations of urinary urgency by taking slow and deep breaths to relax and performing 5 to 6 quick, strong pelvic muscle exercises (flicks) in quick succession, followed by focusing the attention away from the bladder sensations. • Once successful with inhibiting the urge to void and avoiding incontinence, instruct her to gradually increase the time period between trips to the bathroom.	Behavioral therapy that includes pelvic muscle training should be offered as first-line treatment for stress, urge, and mixed incontinence in women of all ages (Moore et al., 2013).

‡Intervention classification labels from Bulechek GM et al: *Nursing interventions classifications (NIC),* ed 6, St Louis, 2013, Mosby.

NURSING CARE PLAN

Stress Urinary Incontinence—cont'd

EVALUATION

Nursing Actions	Patient Response/Finding	Achievement of Outcomes
Ask Mrs. Grayson about frequency of incontinence since starting pelvic muscle exercises and urge-suppression strategies.	She responds, "I'm dry most of the time now. I'm now babysitting my grandchildren and have returned to my volunteer job."	Mrs. Grayson reports increasing success with bladder control and with this sense of increased control is less anxious and more socially active.
Ask Mrs. Grayson to keep a 3-day bladder diary.	Bladder diary revealed one small-volume loss of urine with a strong cough and voiding every 3 to 4 hours.	Mrs. Grayson has been free of urinary tract infection. Mrs. Grayson is able to resist the urge to void for 15 or more minutes without leaking as seen in her ability to void every 3 to 4 hours.

CONCEPT MAP

Primary health problem: Stress urinary incontinence
Priority assessments: Voiding patterns, bladder diary, skin integrity

Nursing diagnosis: Stress urinary incontinence related to weakened pelvic musculature
- Leakage of urine on the way to the bathroom
- Leakage of urine associated with sneezing and coughing
- Obese
- Three pregnancies

Interventions
- Encourage Mrs. Grayson to decrease intra-abdominal pressure: weight loss, avoid heavy lifting
- Avoid caffeine and other bladder irritants
- Encourage adequate hydration
- Teach Mrs. Grayson pelvic muscle exercises
- Initiate a bladder retraining

Nursing diagnosis: Risk for infection
- Recent UTI
- Urinary incontinence
- Diabetes

Interventions
- Instruct Mrs. Grayson to maintain adequate fluid intake
- Teach good perineal hygiene
- Reinforce teaching related to type 2 diabetes to maintain normal blood sugars (diet, take medication as ordered)
- Teach about signs and symptoms of UTI

Nursing diagnosis: Risk for impaired skin integrity
- Wet skin due to dribbling/incontinence
- 75 years old with diabetes

Interventions
- Teach Mrs. Grayson to change pads frequently
- Teach Mrs. Grayson to inspect skin daily
- Instruct Mrs. Grayson to gently cleanse after each incontinent episode
- Teach Mrs. Grayson to apply moisture barrier product as needed

Nursing diagnosis: Deficient knowledge—treatment of urinary incontinence
- Lifestyle modifications
- Pelvic muscle exercises
- Bladder retraining

Interventions
- Use written and verbal instructions
- Use pictures to teach about pelvic anatomy
- Evaluate learning

—— Link between medical diagnosis and nursing diagnosis
- - - - Link between nursing diagnoses

FIGURE 46-8 Concept map for Mrs. Grayson.

BOX 46-7 Health Promotion/Restoration: Patient Education for a Healthy Bladder

1. Maintain adequate hydration.
   - Drink six to eight glasses of water a day. Spread it out evenly throughout the day.
   - Avoid or limit drinking beverages that contain caffeine (coffee, tea, chocolate drinks, soft drinks).
   - To decrease nocturia, avoid drinking fluids 2 hours before bedtime.
   - Do not limit fluids if you experience incontinence. Concentrated urine may irritate the bladder and increase bladder symptoms.
2. Keep good voiding habits,
   - Women: sit well back on the toilet seat, avoid "hovering over the toilet," and make sure that the feet are flat on the floor.
   - Void at regular intervals, usually every 3 to 4 hours, depending on fluid intake.
   - Avoid straining when voiding or moving the bowels.
   - Take enough time to empty the bladder completely.
3. Keep the bowels regular. A rectum full of stool may irritate the bladder, causing urgency and frequency.
4. Prevent urinary tract infections.
   - Women: Cleanse the perineum from front to back after each voiding and bowel movement; wear cotton undergarments
   - Drink enough water to pass pale yellow urine.
   - Shower or bathe regularly
5. Stop smoking to reduce your risk for bladder cancer and reduce risk of developing a cough which can contribute to stress urinary incontinence.
6. Report to your health care provider any changes in bladder habits, frequency, urgency, pain when voiding, or blood in the urine.

specialist to help the patient learn techniques to inhibit the urinary urge, strengthen pelvic floor muscles, and learn fluid and food modifications; the occupational therapist to help the patient learn efficient and safe toilet transfers; the physical therapist to help with strengthening exercises of the lower extremities; and the social worker to facilitate obtaining assistive devices in the home that are covered by insurance. The family caregiver is included in planning when applicable. When a patient requires an indwelling urinary catheter because of acute illness and a need to measure accurate urinary output, the nurse is a key member of the team by monitoring patient progress and ensuring that the catheter is removed in a timely manner. Your active and thoughtful role in planning these interventions will result in the patient's progress toward improved urinary elimination.

◆ Implementation

Complete independent and collaborative interventions to help the patient achieve the desired outcomes and goals. The independent activities are those in which nurses use their own judgment. An example of this is teaching self-care activities to the patient. Collaborative activities are those prescribed by the health care provider and carried out by the nurse such as medication administration.

Health Promotion. Health promotion helps the patient understand and participate in self-care practices to preserve and protect healthy urinary system function (Box 46-7). You can achieve this focus using several means.

Patient Education. Success of therapies aimed at eliminating or minimizing urinary elimination problems depends in part on successful patient education (see Box 46-7). Although many patients need to learn about all aspects of healthy urinary elimination, it is best to focus on a specific elimination problem first. For example, a patient who has a UTI would greatly benefit from learning about the significance of symptoms that might indicate another UTI and learning to seek early treatment, which potentially can prevent serious illness. You can easily incorporate teaching when giving nursing care. For example, teach about common bladder irritants such as caffeine when helping a patient with his or her meal. Include in your teaching sensitivity to the patient's health literacy. Pictures are helpful when teaching about urinary tract anatomy and the relationship with UTI. If a patient speaks a different language, involve a professional interpreter.

BOX 46-8 PATIENT TEACHING

Teaching Patients About Pelvic Muscle Exercises (Kegel Exercises)

Objective

- Patient will verbalize and/or demonstrate how to perform pelvic muscle exercises (Kegel exercises).

Teaching Strategies

- Use pictures and plain language to teach the patient pelvic anatomy and the location of the pelvic muscles (see Fig 46-16).
- Teach patient how to identify and contract the correct muscle.
  - Women: Instruct the patient to squeeze the anus as if to hold in gas or to insert a finger into the vagina and feel the muscle squeeze around her finger. The woman can also observe the perineum pulling in by using a mirror.
  - Men: Instruct the patient to stand in front of a mirror, squeeze the anus as if to hold in gas, and watch to see if the penis moves up and down as he contracts the pelvic floor muscles.
  - Instruct to not contract the abdomen, buttocks, or thighs when contracting the pelvic muscles.
- Teach patients pelvic muscle contraction exercises.
  - Quick flicks: Squeeze the muscle for 2 to 3 seconds and relax.
  - Sustained contractions: Squeeze the muscle for 10 seconds and relax after each contraction for 10 seconds.
  - Counting out loud prevents breath holding during exercises.
- Teach patient to maintain a daily exercise schedule.
  - Perform three to five quick flicks followed by 10 sustained contractions.
  - Do these exercises 3 to 4 times a day.

Evaluation

- Use open-ended questions to determine level of learning.
- Ask the patient to describe how to correctly identify the pelvic floor muscles.
- Ask the patient to demonstrate and/or explain how to perform pelvic muscle exercises.

Promoting Normal Micturition. Maintaining normal urinary elimination helps to prevent many problems. Many measures that promote normal voiding are independent nursing interventions.

Maintaining Elimination Habits. Many patients follow routines to promote normal voiding. When in a hospital or long-term care facility, institutional routines often conflict with those of the patient. Integrating the patient's habits into the care plan fosters a more normal voiding pattern. Elimination is a very private act. Create as much privacy as possible by closing the door and bedside curtain; asking visitors to leave a room when a bedside commode, bedpan or urinal is used; and masking the sounds of voiding with running water. Respond to requests for help with toileting as quickly as possible. Embarrassing accidents are easily avoided when help comes in time. Avoid the use of

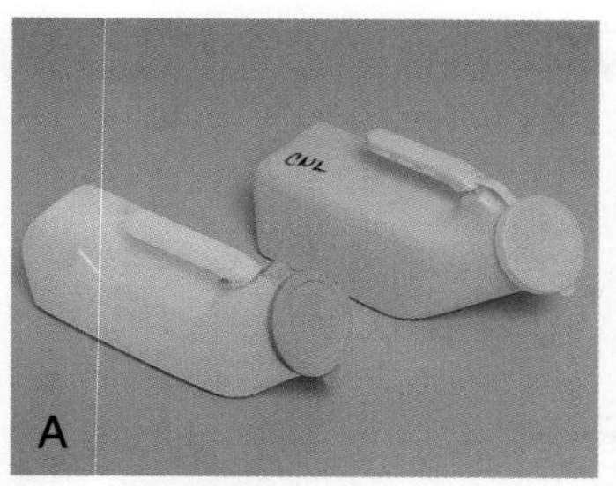
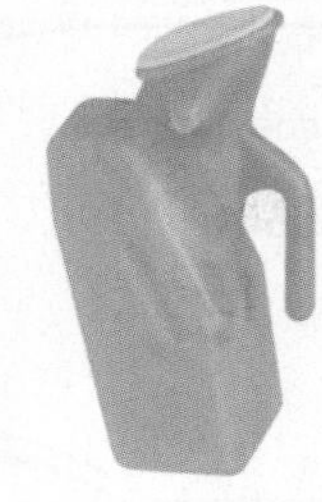

FIGURE 46-9 Types of male **(A)** and female **(B)** urinals. (**B** Courtesy Briggs Medical Service Co.)

incontinence-containment products unless needed for uncontrolled urine leakage. Some containment products may be difficult to remove and interfere with prompt toilet access.

Maintaining Adequate Fluid Intake. A simple method to promote normal micturition is maintaining optimal fluid intake. A patient with normal renal function who does not have heart disease or alterations requiring fluid restriction should have approximately 30 mL/kg of body weight or 0.5 ounces/lb/day (Gray, 2011). Adequate fluid intake will help flush out solutes or particles that collect in the urinary system and decrease bladder irritability. Help patients change their fluid intake by teaching the importance of adequate hydration. If a patient needs to increase fluid intake, set a schedule for drinking extra fluids, identify fluid preferences, increase high fluid foods such as fruits, and encourage fluid intake in small volumes frequently. Excessive fluid intake should be avoided. To prevent nocturia, suggest that the patient avoid drinking fluids 2 hours before bedtime.

Promoting Complete Bladder Emptying. It is normal for a small volume of urine to remain in the bladder after micturition. When the bladder does not empty completely and residual urine volumes are high, there is risk for incontinence and dangerous urinary retention. Urinary retention increases the risk for UTI and damage to the kidneys. Adequate bladder emptying depends on feeling an urge to urinate, contraction of the bladder, and the ability to relax the urethral sphincter. A strategy to promote relaxation and stimulate bladder contractions is to help patients assume the normal position for voiding. The normal anatomical position for female voiding is in the squatting position. Women empty the bladder better when sitting on the toilet or bedside commode with the feet on the floor. If the patient cannot use a toilet, position her on a bedpan (see Chapter 47). After bedpan use help the patient perform perineal hygiene (see Chapter 40). A man voids more easily in the standing position. If the patient is unable to reach a toilet, have him stand at the bedside and void into a urinal (a plastic or metal receptacle for urine) (Figure 46-9, *A*). Always assess mobility status and determine if he can stand safely. At times it is necessary for one or more nurses to help a male patient stand. If the patient is unable to stand at the bedside, you will need to help him use the urinal in bed. Some patients need the nurse to position the penis completely within the urinal and hold the urinal in place or help them hold the urinal. Once the patient has finished voiding, carefully remove the urinal and perform perineal hygiene (see Chapter 40). Most urinals are used by men, but there are specially designed urinals for women (see Figure 46-9, *B*). The female urinal has a larger opening at the top with a defined rim, which helps position the urinal closely against the genitalia.

There are other measures that improve bladder emptying. To promote relaxation and stimulate bladder contractions, use sensory stimuli (e.g., turning on running water, putting a patient's hand in a pan of warm water) and provide privacy. In addition, bladder exercises help to improve pelvic muscles, which reduces stress incontinence and improves bladder emptying (Box 46-8). To improve bladder emptying, encourage patients to wait until the urine flow completely stops when voiding and encourage them to attempt a second void (double voiding). Timed voiding is voiding according to the clock, not the urge to void, and is a helpful strategy when the bladder does not fully empty. The Credé method or manual compression of the bladder (i.e., placing the hands over the bladder and compressing it to help in emptying) should not be implemented until consultation with the health care provider. In the presence of high PVRs or a complete inability of the bladder to empty, urinary catheterization, either intermittent or indwelling, is needed.

Preventing Infection. UTIs are one of the most common bacterial infections encountered by health care providers (Gupta and Hooton 2011; Schaeffer and Schaeffer, 2012). Nurses play a key role in implementing evidence-based practices to avoid this common and potentially dangerous infection. Some key interventions include promoting adequate fluid intake, promoting perineal hygiene, and having patients void at regular intervals. Encourage women to wipe front to back after voiding and defecation and teach them to avoid perfumed perineal washes and sprays, bubble baths, and tight clothing. If a patient has a problem with urine leakage, hygiene should be especially stressed. Patients should use containment products that are designed for urine and wick wetness away from the body. Prolonged periods of urine wetness should be avoided.

Acute Care. Patients with acute illness, surgery, or impaired function of the urinary tract may require more invasive interventions that support urinary elimination.

Catheterization. Urinary catheterization is the placement of a tube through the urethra into the bladder to drain urine. This is an invasive procedure that requires a medical order and, in institutional settings, aseptic technique (Gould et al., 2009; Lo et al., 2014). Skill 46-2 on pp. 1131-1140 lists steps for performing female and male urethral catheterization.

Urinary catheterization can be intermittent (one-time catheterization for bladder emptying) or indwelling (remains in place over a period of time). Indwelling catheterization may be short term (2 weeks or less) or long term (more than 1 month) (Cottenden et al., 2013). Conditions requiring the use of a short- or long-term urinary catheter include the need for accurate monitoring of urine output either perioperative or postoperative after urologic or gynecological procedures and when the bladder inadequately empties because of obstruction or a neurological condition. Excessive accumulation of urine in the bladder is painful for a patient; increases the risk for UTI; and can cause backward flow of urine up the ureters, increasing risk for kidney damage. UI may require indwelling catheterization if the leaking urine interferes with wound healing or in the presence of terminal illness when incontinence care is overly burdensome for the patient (Cottenden et al., 2013). Intermittent catheterization is used to measure PVR when ultrasound or a bladder scanner is not available or as a way to manage chronic urinary retention.

Types of Catheters. The difference among urinary catheters is related to the number of catheter lumens, the presence of a balloon to keep the indwelling catheter in place, the shape of the catheter, and a closed drainage system. Urinary catheters are made with one to three lumens (Figure 46-10). Single-lumen catheters (see Figure 46-10, *A*) are used for intermittent/straight catheterization. Double-lumen catheters, designed for indwelling catheters, provides one lumen for urinary drainage while a second lumen is used to inflate a balloon that keeps the catheter in place (see Figure 46-10, *B*). Triple-lumen catheters (see Figure 46-10, *C*) are used for continuous bladder irrigation (CBI) or when it becomes necessary to instill medications into the bladder.

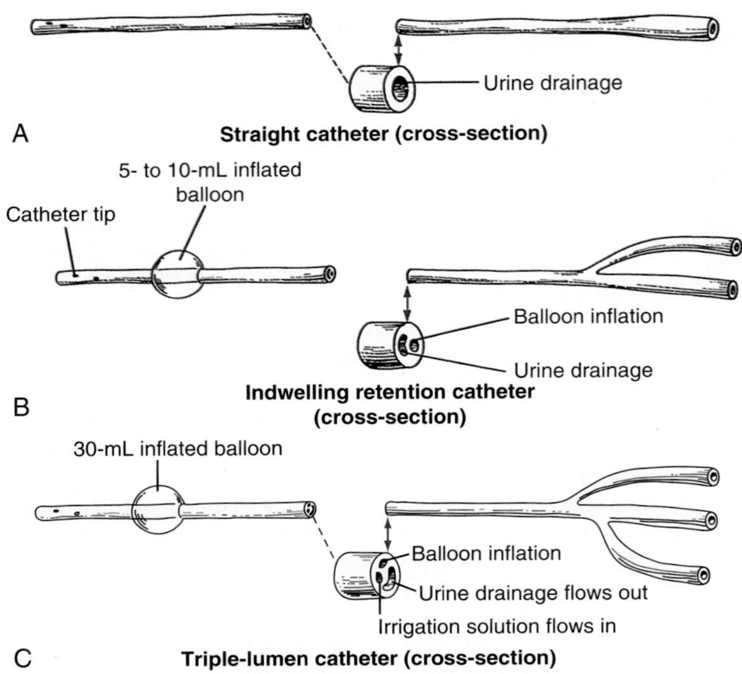

FIGURE 46-10 **A,** Straight catheter (cross-section). **B,** Indwelling (Foley) retention catheter (cross-section). **C,** Triple-lumen catheter (cross-section.)

One lumen drains the bladder, a second lumen is used to inflate the balloon, and a third lumen delivers irrigation fluid into the bladder.

A health care provider chooses a catheter on the basis of factors such as latex allergy, history of catheter encrustation, anatomical factors, and susceptibility to infection. Indwelling catheters are made of latex or silicone. Latex catheters with special coatings reduce urethral irritation (Cottenden et al., 2013). All silicone catheters have a larger internal diameter and may be helpful in patients who require frequent catheter changes as a result of encrustation. Intermittent/straight catheters are made of rubber (softer and more flexible) or polyvinyl chloride (PVC). Patients who self-catheterize have a large selection of catheters, some with special coatings that do not require lubrication and others that are self-contained systems consisting of a prelubricated catheter and packaged with a preconnected drainage bag. Catheter shape can differ; shape chosen is based on anatomical differences in patients. One such catheter is a coudé-tip catheter. This catheter has a curvature at the end that helps it maneuver through the prostatic urethra in the presence of a large prostate. Nurses need special training to use this type of catheter.

Catheter Sizes. The size of a urinary catheter is based on the French (FR) scale, which reflects the internal diameter of the catheter. Most adults with an indwelling catheter should use a size 14 to 16 Fr to minimize trauma and risk for infection. Larger catheter diameters increase the risk for urethral trauma (Cottenden et al., 2013). However, larger sizes are used in special circumstances such as after urological surgery or in the presence of gross hematuria. Smaller sizes are needed for children such as a 5 to 6 Fr for infants, 8 to 10 Fr for children, and 12 Fr for young girls.

Indwelling catheters come in a variety of balloon sizes from 3 mL (for a child) to 30 mL for CBI. The size of the balloon is usually printed on the catheter port (Figure 46-11). The recommended balloon size for an adult is a 10-mL balloon (the balloon is 5 ml and requires 10 mL to fill completely). Long-term use of larger balloons (30 mL) has been associated with increased patient discomfort, irritation and trauma to the urethra, increased risk of catheter expulsion, and incomplete emptying of the bladder resulting from urine that pools below the level of the catheter drainage eyes (Cottenden et al., 2013).

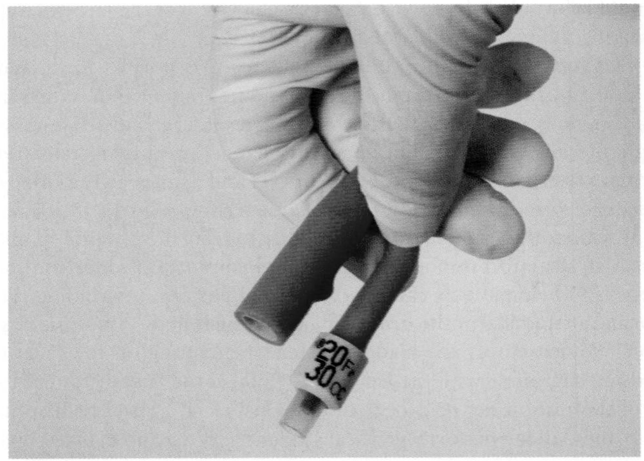

FIGURE 46-11 Size of catheter and balloon printed on catheter.

Catheter Drainage Systems. An indwelling catheter is attached to a urinary drainage bag to collect the continuous flow of urine. The drainage system should not be separated unless absolutely necessary to avoid introducing pathogens. In patients with indwelling catheters specimens are collected without opening the drainage system using a special port in the tubing (Figure 46-12). Always hang the drainage bag below the level of the bladder on the bedframe or a chair so urine will drain down out of the bladder. The bag should never touch the floor to prevent accidental contamination during emptying. When a patient ambulates, carry the bag below the level of the patient's bladder. Ambulatory patients may use a leg bag. This is a bag that attaches to the leg with straps. Leg bags are usually worn during the day and replaced at night with a standard drainage bag. The only drainage bag that does not need to be kept dependent to the bladder is a specially

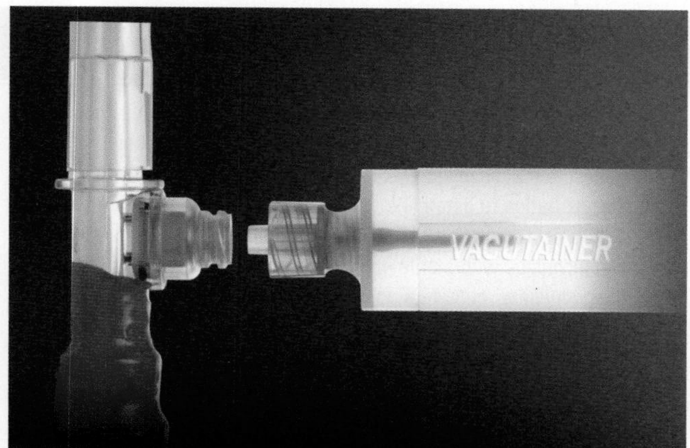

FIGURE 46-12 Urine specimen collection: aspiration from a collection port in drainage tubing of indwelling catheter (needleless technique). (Courtesy and © Becton, Dickinson and Company.)

designed drainage bag (belly bag) that is worn across the abdomen. A one-way valve prevents the back flow of urine into the bladder. To keep the drainage system patent, check for kinks or bends in the tubing, avoid positioning the patient on drainage tubing, prevent tubing from becoming dependent, and observe for clots or sediment that may block the catheter or tubing.

Routine Catheter Care. Patients with indwelling catheters require regular perineal hygiene, especially after a bowel movement, to reduce the risk for catheter-associated UTI (CAUTI) (Gould et al., 2009; Lo et al., 2014). In many institutions patients receive catheter care every 8 hours as the minimal standard of care. See Chapter 40 for routine perineal care and Skill 46-3 on pp. 1140-1142 for catheter care. Empty drainage bags when ½ full (Figure 46-13). An overfull drainage bag can create tension and pulling on the catheter, resulting in trauma to the urethra and/or urinary meatus, and increase risk for CAUTI (Cipa-Tatum and Kelly-Signs, 2011; Rassin and Markovski, 2013). Expect continuous drainage of urine into the drainage bag. In the presence of no urine drainage, first check to make sure that there are no kinks or obvious occlusion of the drainage tubing or catheter.

Preventing Catheter-Associated Infection. A critical part of routine catheter care is reducing the risk for CAUTI (Box 46-9). Box 46-10 includes some important interventions included in the CDC *Guideline for Prevention of Catheter-Associated Urinary Tract Infections* (Gould et al., 2009; Lo et al., 2014). A key intervention to prevent infection is maintaining a closed urinary drainage system. Portals for entry of bacteria into the system are illustrated in Figure 46-14. Another key intervention is prevention of urine backflow from the tubing and bag into the bladder. Many urine drainage systems are equipped with an antireflux valve, but the nurse should monitor the system to prevent pooling of urine within the tubing and to keep the drainage bag below the level of the bladder.

> **QSEN QSEN: BUILDING COMPETENCY IN EVIDENCE-BASED PRACTICE** A nursing unit is experiencing an increase in catheter-associated urinary tract infection (CAUTIs). A team of staff nurses are investigating this problem and discover that some nurses are resistant to implementing new evidence-based practice (EBP) guidelines in CAUTI prevention. What can you do to decrease resistance and enhance EBP care on this unit?
>
> *Answers to QSEN Activities can be found on the Evolve website.*

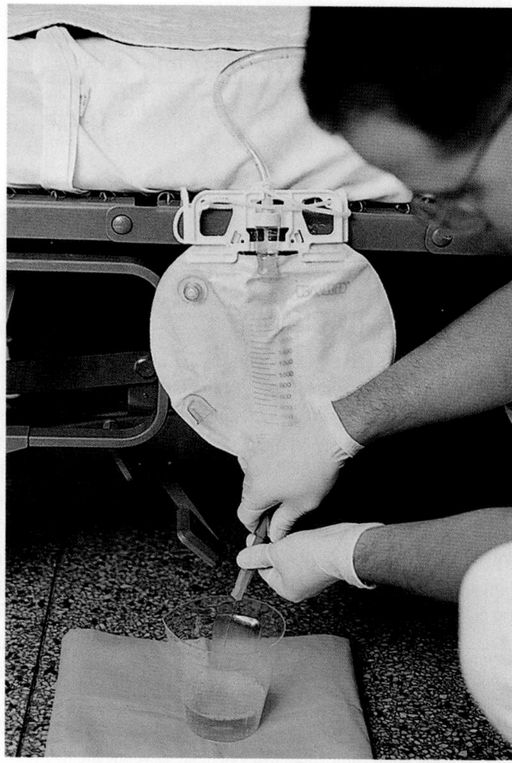

FIGURE 46-13 Urine drainage bag.

Catheter Irrigations and Instillations. To maintain the patency of indwelling urinary catheters, it is sometimes necessary to irrigate or flush a catheter with sterile solution. However, irrigation poses the risk for causing a UTI and thus must be done maintaining a closed urinary drainage system. Generally, if a catheter becomes occluded, it is best to change it rather than risk flushing debris into the bladder. In some instances the health care provider will determine that irrigations are needed to keep a catheter patent such as after genitourinary surgery when there is high risk for catheter occlusion from blood clots. Bladder instillations are used to instill medication into the bladder. Refer to specific instructions for these medications in terms of how long the medication needs to stay in the bladder.

Closed catheter irrigation provides intermittent or continuous irrigation of a urinary catheter without disrupting the sterile connection between the catheter and the drainage system (see Skill 46-4 on pp. 1142-1145). CBI is an example of a continuous infusion of a sterile solution into the bladder, usually using a three-way irrigation closed system with a triple-lumen catheter. CBI is frequently used following genitourinary surgery to keep the bladder clear and free of blood clots or sediment.

Removal of Indwelling Catheter. Prompt removal of an indwelling catheter after it is no longer needed is a key intervention that has proven to decrease the incidence and prevalence of hospital-acquired UTIs (HAUTIs), one of the "never events" identified by the Centers for Medicare and Medicaid Services (CMS) (APIC, 2014) (see Skill 46-2). All patients should have their voiding monitored after catheter removal for at least 24 to 48 hours by using a voiding record or bladder diary. The bladder diary should record the time and amount of each voiding, including any incontinence. The use of ultrasound or a bladder scanner can monitor bladder function by measuring PVR (Box 46-11). The first few times a patient voids after catheter removal may be accompanied by some discomfort, but continued complaints of painful urination indicate possible infection. Abdominal pain and

BOX 46-9 EVIDENCE-BASED PRACTICE

Factors to Decrease Urinary Tract Infections

PICO Question: Which factors decrease the risk of urinary tract infections (UTIs) in hospitalized patients with indwelling urinary catheters?

Evidence Summary

Catheter-associated UTI (CAUTI) is responsible for 30% or more infections in the acute care setting, with increased length of hospital stay, morbidity, mortality, and cost (Bernard et al., 2012). In 2009 the Centers for Disease Control and Prevention (CDC) published a long-awaited update for their Guideline for Prevention of Catheter-Associated Urinary Tract Infections (Gould et al., 2009). Measures to reduce CAUTI are organized into: criteria for appropriate use, proper insertion and maintenance techniques, quality improvement programs, and ongoing surveillance for CAUTI and related causative factors. Current research continues to reinforce the validity of these guidelines and successful reduction in CAUTI when implemented in the acute care setting. A review of current evidence found that nurse-led interventions reduced the duration of indwelling catheter use and incidence of CAUTI (Bernard et al., 2012). Oman et al. (2012) showed how a hospital-wide strategy that included reeducation of nurses about CAUTI prevention and infusing best practice into current practice nursing care also decreased CAUTI rates. Purvis et al. (2014) showed that a nurse-managed program that included evidence-based best practices, staff education, data reporting, and using an icon in the electronic health record as a catheter reminder decreased the CAUTI rate in an academic medical center. A systematic review and meta-analysis of studies regarding measures to use to reduce catheter use and decrease CAUTI showed that CAUTI rates can be reduced when reminders to evaluate catheter need and stop orders are in place (Meddings et al., 2014). Nurses play a key role in this strategy of catheter awareness.

Application to Nursing Practice

- Become familiar with guidelines related to CAUTI prevention and care.
- Be aware of indications for catheter insertion and be prepared to advocate for the patient if the indications do not meet accepted guidelines.
- Collaborate with health care providers to remove catheters early when medical indications no longer exist.
- Become a patient advocate in your institution through careful adherence to CAUTI preventive practices.

BOX 46-10 Preventing Catheter-Associated Urinary Tract Infection (CAUTI)

- Prevention of CAUTI often requires use of an evidence based "bundle" to perform all elements of care at one time along with completion of a checklist to ensure that each element is included in that care. Know the policies of your institution to determine which components are in a care bundle.
- Patients in acute care hospital should have urinary catheters inserted using aseptic technique with sterile equipment.
- Secure indwelling catheters to prevent movement and pulling on the catheter.
- Maintain a closed urinary drainage system.
- Maintain an unobstructed flow of urine through the catheter, drainage tubing, and drainage bag.
- Keep the urinary drainage bag below the level of the bladder at all times.
- Avoid dependent loops in urinary drainage tubing.
- Prevent the urinary drainage bag from touching or dragging on the floor.
- When emptying the urinary drainage bag, use a separate measuring receptacle for each patient. Do not let the drainage spigot touch the receptacle.
- Before transfers or activity, drain all urine from the tubing into bag and empty the drainage bag.
- Empty the drainage bag when ½ full.
- Perform routine perineal hygiene daily and after soiling using antiseptic wipes. Be sure to use a wipe to clean the length of the exposed catheter.
- Obtain urine samples using the sampling port. Cleanse the port with disinfectant. Use a sterile syringe/cannula.
- Quality improvement programs should be in place that alert providers that a catheter is in place and include regular educational programming about catheter care.

Data from Gould CV et al: *Guideline for prevention of catheter-associated urinary tract infections,* 2009, http://www.cdc.gov/hicpac/cauti/001_cauti.html. Accessed October 4, 2014.

distention, a sensation of incomplete emptying, incontinence, constant dribbling of urine, and voiding in very small amounts can indicate inadequate bladder emptying requiring intervention.

The risk of UTI increases with the use of an indwelling catheter (APIC, 2014; Lo et al., 2014). Symptoms of infection can develop 2 to 3 or more days after catheter removal. Patients need to be informed of the risk for infection, prevention measures, and signs and symptoms that need to be reported to the nurse and health care provider.

Alternative to Catheterization. To avoid the risks associated with urethral catheters, two alternatives are available for urinary drainage.

Suprapubic Catheterization. A suprapubic catheter is a urinary drainage tube inserted surgically into the bladder through the abdominal wall above the symphysis pubis (Figure 46-15). The catheter may be sutured to the skin, secured with an adhesive material, or retained in the bladder with a fluid-filled balloon similar to an indwelling catheter. Suprapubic catheters are placed when there is blockage of the urethra (e.g., enlarged prostate, urethral stricture, after urological surgery) and in situations when a long-term urethral catheter causes irritation or discomfort or interferes with sexual functioning.

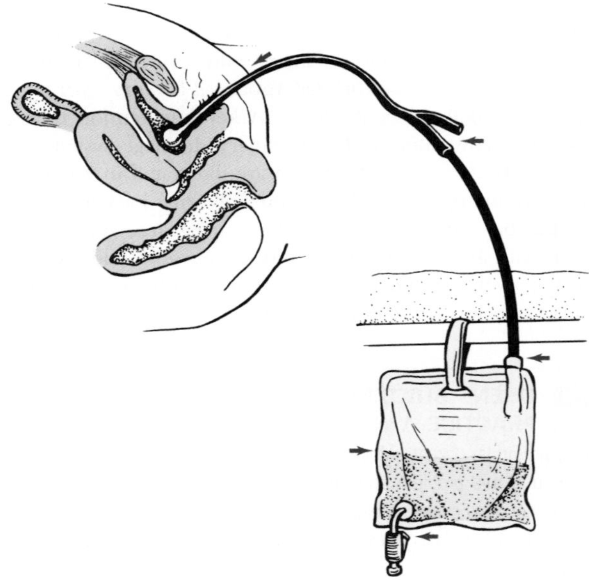

FIGURE 46-14 Potential sites for introduction of infectious organisms into urinary drainage system.

BOX 46-11 PROCEDURAL GUIDELINES

Using a Bladder Scanner to Measure Postvoid Residual

Delegation Considerations

The skill of measuring bladder volume by bladder scan can be delegated to nursing assistive personnel (NAP). However, it is important to establish competency in bladder scan measurements because reliability between different care provider readings can be poor. An RN must first determine the timing and frequency of the bladder scan measurement and interpret the measurements obtained. The nurse is also responsible for assessing the patient's ability to toilet before measurement of postvoid residual (PVR) and assessing the abdomen for distention if urinary retention is suspected. The nurse directs the NAP to:

- Follow manufacturer recommendations for the use of the device.
- Measure PVR volumes 10 minutes after helping the patient to void.
- Report and record bladder scan volumes.

Equipment

Bladder scanner, ultrasound gel, cleaning agent for scanner head such as an alcohol pad, clean gloves (optional)

Steps

1. Identify patient using two identifiers (e.g., name and birthday or name and medical record number, according to agency policy) (TJC, 2016).
2. Perform hand hygiene. Discuss procedure with patient. If the measurement is for PVR, ask him or her to void and measure and record voided urine volume. (apply gloves if patient requires assistance with voiding). The scan measurement should be within 10 minutes of voiding.
3. Help patient to the supine position with the head slightly elevated. Raise bed to appropriate working height. If side rails are raised, lower side rail on working side.
4. Expose patient's lower abdomen.
5. Turn on the scanner per manufacturer guidelines.
6. Set the gender designation per manufacturer guidelines. Women who have had a hysterectomy should be designated as male.
7. Wipe the scanner head with an alcohol pad or other cleanser and allow to air dry.
8. Palpate the patient's symphysis pubis (pubic bone). Apply a generous amount of ultrasound gel (or if available a bladder scan gel pad) to the midline abdomen 2.5 to 4 cm (1 to 1.5 inches) above the symphysis pubis. The ultrasound gel ensures adequate transmission and thus accurate measurement.
9. Place the scanner head on the gel, ensuring that the scanner head is oriented per manufacturer guidelines (see illustration).

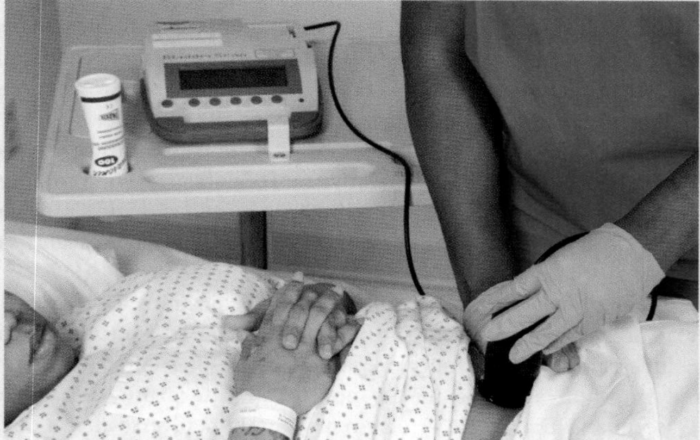

STEP 9 Point scanner head slightly downward toward bladder.

10. Apply light pressure, keep the scanner head steady, and point it slightly downward toward the bladder. Press and release the scan button.
11. Verify accurate aim (refer to manufacturer guidelines). Complete the scan and print the image (if needed) (see illustration).

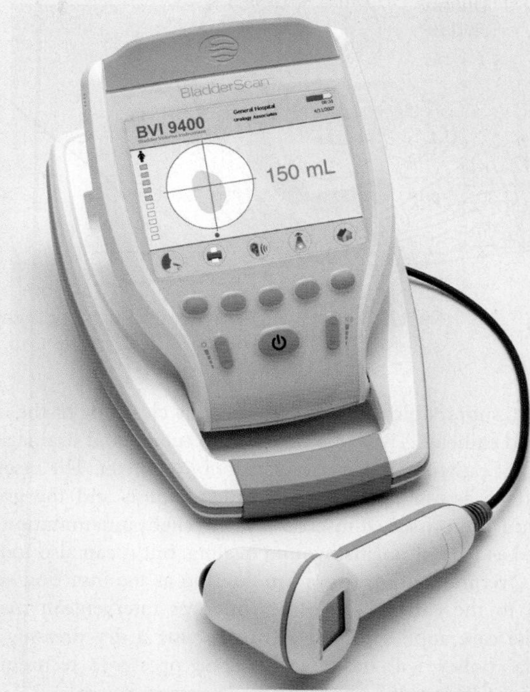

STEP 11 Bladder scan image. (Courtesy Verathon Inc.)

12. Remove ultrasound gel from patient's abdomen with a paper towel.
13. Remove ultrasound gel from scanner head and wipe with alcohol pad or other cleanser; let air dry.
14. Help patient to a comfortable position. Lower bed and place side rails accordingly.
15. Dispose of soiled towels and pad. Perform hand hygiene.

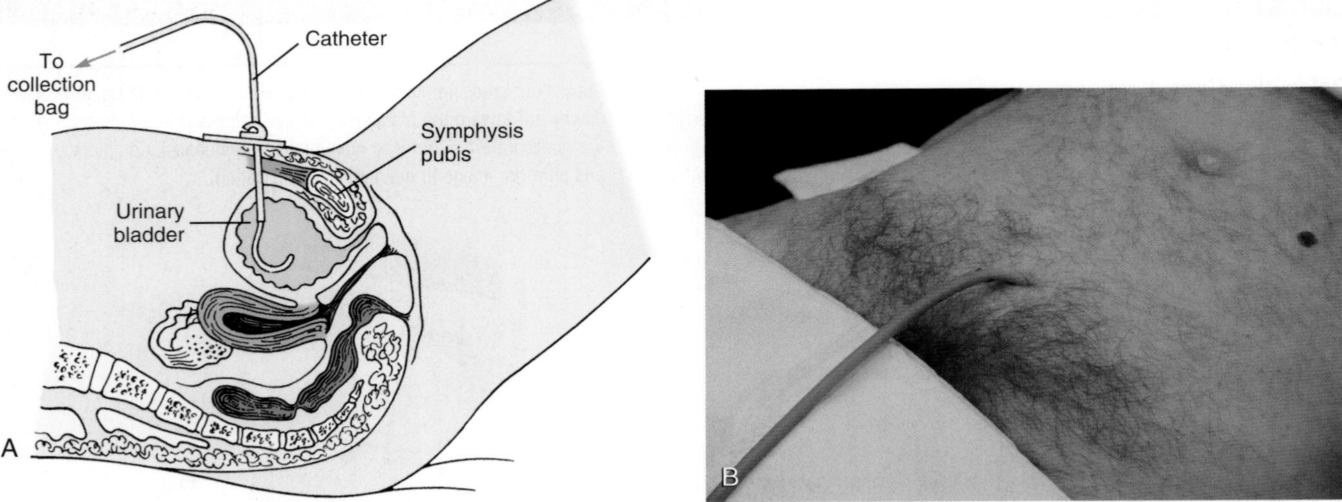

FIGURE 46-15 **A**, Placement of suprapubic catheter above symphysis pubis. **B**, Suprapubic catheter without a dressing.

Care of a suprapubic catheter involves daily cleansing of the insertion site and catheter. The same care for the tubing and drainage bag for a urethral catheter applies to a suprapubic catheter. The insertion site should be assessed for signs of inflammation and the growth of overgranulation tissue. If insertion is new, slight inflammation may be expected as part of normal wound healing, but it can also indicate infection. Overgranulation tissue can develop at the insertion site as a reaction to the catheter. In some instances intervention may be needed. Site care applies principles of applying a dry dressing, and institutional policy will indicate if aseptic or sterile technique is required (see Chapter 48).

External Catheter. The external catheter, also called a *condom catheter* or *penile sheath,* is a soft, pliable condom-like sheath that fits over the penis, providing a safe and noninvasive way to contain urine. Most external catheters are made of soft silicone that aids in reducing friction and are clear to allow for easy visualization of skin under the catheter. Latex catheters are still available and used by some patients. It is important to verify that a patient does not have a latex allergy before applying this type of catheter. Condom-type external catheters are held in place by an adhesive coating of the internal lining of the sheath, a double-sided self-adhesive strip, brush-on adhesive applied to the penile shaft, or in rare cases an external strap or tape. They may be attached to a small-volume (leg) drainage bag or a large-volume (bedside) urinary drainage bag, both of which need to be kept lower than the level of the bladder. The condom-type external catheter is suitable for incontinent patients who have complete and spontaneous bladder emptying. Condom-type external catheters come in a variety of styles and sizes. For the best fit and correct application it is important to refer to manufacturer guidelines. See Box 46-12 for the steps in applying a condom catheter. Condom-type external catheters are associated with less risk for UTI than indwelling catheters; thus they are an excellent option for the male with UI. For men who cannot be fitted for a condom-type external catheter, there are other externally applied catheters. One type attaches to the glans penis using hydrocolloid strips that stay in place for multiple days and allow intermittent/straight catheterization (Kyle, 2011). Another available option is a reusable condom-like device that is held in place by specially designed underwear.

Urinary Diversions. Immediately after surgery the patient with an incontinent urinary diversion must wear a pouch to collect the effluent (drainage). The pouch will keep the patient clean and dry, protect the skin from damage, and provide a barrier against odor. Urinary pouches with an antireflux flap can be opaque or clear, drainable one-piece or two-piece pouches, with cut-to-fit or precut wafers. The pouch should be changed every 4 to 6 days. Each pouch may be connected to a bedside drainage bag for use at night.

When changing a pouch, gently cleanse the skin surrounding the stoma with warm tap water using a washcloth and pat dry. Do not use soap because it can leave a residue on the skin. Measure the stoma and cut the opening in the pouch. Then apply the pouch after removing the protective backing from the adhesive surface. Press firmly into place over the stoma. Observe the appearance of the stoma and surrounding skin. The stoma is normally red and moist and is located in the right lower quadrant of the abdomen. It is important for the patient to have the correct type and fit of an ostomy pouch. A specialty ostomy nurse is an essential resource when selecting the right appliance so the pouch fits snugly against the surface of the skin around the stoma, preventing damaging leakage of urine (see Chapter 47).

Patients with continent urinary diversions do not have to wear an external pouch. However, if the patient has a continent urinary reservoir, he or she must be taught how to intermittently catheterize the pouch. Patients need to be able and willing to do this 4 to 6 times a day for the rest of their lives. After creation of an orthopic neobladder, patients will have frequent episodes of incontinence until the neobladder slowly stretches and the urinary sphincter is strong enough to contain the urine. To achieve continence the patient will need to follow a bladder-training schedule and perform pelvic muscle exercises (Geng et al., 2010). The postoperative care of patients having continent urinary diversions varies widely with the surgical techniques used, and it is important to learn the surgeon's preferred routine or health care facility procedures before caring for these patients.

Medications. A small number of medications are used to treat urgency, frequency, nocturia, and urgency UI. Antimuscarinics include darifenacin, oxybutynin, solifenacin, fesoterodine, tolterodine, and tropsium and one that is not an antimuscarinic, mirabegron (Qaseem and Dallas, 2014). The most common adverse effects of the antimuscarinics are dry mouth, constipation, and blurred vision. In some cases these medications can cause a change in mental status in older adults (Burchum and Rosenthal, 2016). Patients taking mirabegron should have their blood pressure monitored because of possible

BOX 46-12 PROCEDURAL GUIDELINES

Applying a Condom Catheter

Delegation Considerations

The skill of applying condom catheters can be delegated to nursing assistive personnel (NAP). Before delegation instruct the NAP to:

- Inform the nurse if there is any redness, swelling, or skin irritations or breakdown of glans penis or penile shaft.
- Be sensitive to privacy needs of patients.
- Follow manufacturer directions for applying the condom catheter and securing the device.

Equipment

Condom catheter (includes securing device such as internal adhesive, strap, or tape), collection bag, basin with warm water, towel and washcloth, clean gloves, scissors, hair guard or paper towel, bath blanket and sheet

Steps

1. Identify patient using two identifiers (e.g., name and birthday or name and medical record number, according to agency policy) (TJC, 2016).
2. Perform hand hygiene.
3. Assess urinary elimination patterns, patient's ability to empty bladder effectively, and degree of continence.
4. Assess patient's mental status, knowledge about the procedure, and ability to self-apply device. Explain procedure.
5. Provide for privacy by closing room door or bedside curtain. Raise bed to working height and lower side rail on working side.
6. Prepare condom catheter (prescribed size and type), drainage bag, and tubing (see manufacturer directions). Most manufacturers provide a measuring guide and instructions.
7. Help patient to a supine or sitting position. Place bath blanket over upper torso; fold a sheet over lower torso so only penis is exposed.
8. Apply clean gloves; provide perineal care (see Chapter 40), and dry thoroughly. If patient is uncircumcised, ensure that the foreskin is in the normal nonretracted position. Do not apply barrier cream and make sure that any remaining adhesive is removed (Cottenden et al., 2013).
9. Assess penis for erythema, rashes, and/or open areas. Condom catheters can only be applied to intact skin.
10. Clip hair at base of penile shaft as necessary. Do not shave the pubic area. Some manufacturers provide a hair guard, which is placed over the penis before applying the device. An alternative to a hair guard is to tear a hole in a paper towel, place it over the penis, and remove after application of the device (Cottenden et al., 2013; Kyle, 2011).
11. Apply condom catheter. With nondominant hand, grasp penis along shaft. With dominant hand, hold condom sheath at tip of penis and smoothly roll sheath onto penis. Allow 2.5 to 5 cm (1 to 2 inches) of space between tip of penis and end of catheter (see illustration).

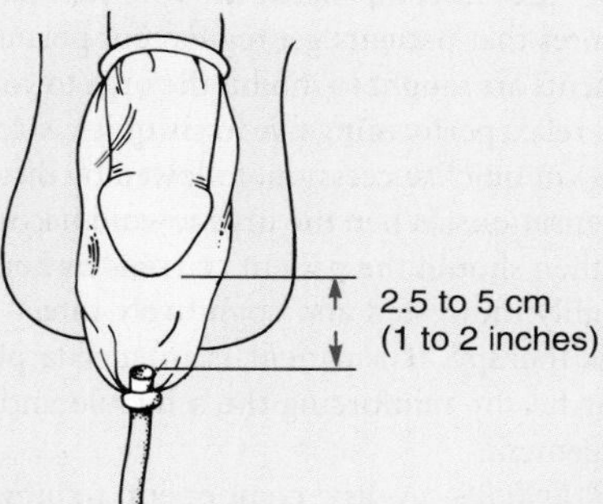

STEP 11 Distance between end of penis and tip of condom.

12. Secure condom catheter according to manufacturer directions:
    a. Outer-securing strip-type catheter: Spiral wrap the penile shaft with supplied elastic adhesive. Strip should not overlap. The elastic strip should be snug, not tight (see illustration). **NOTE: Never use adhesive tape.**

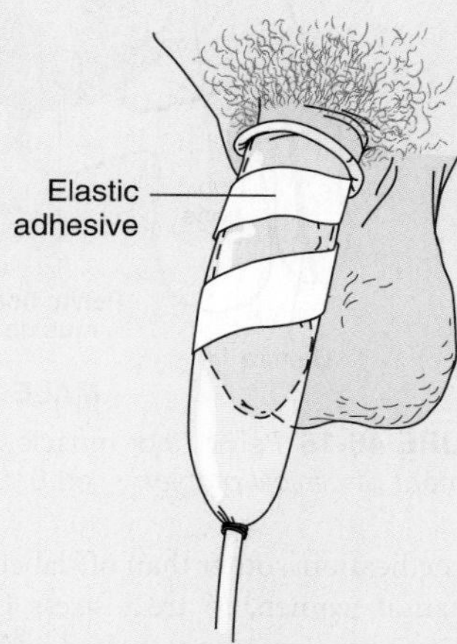

STEP 12a Apply elastic adhesive in spiral fashion to secure condom catheter to penis.

    b. For self-adhesive catheter, apply gentle pressure on penile shaft for 10 to 15 seconds to secure.
13. Connect drainage tubing to end of condom catheter. Be sure that condom is not twisted. Connect catheter to large-volume drainage bag or leg (see illustration).

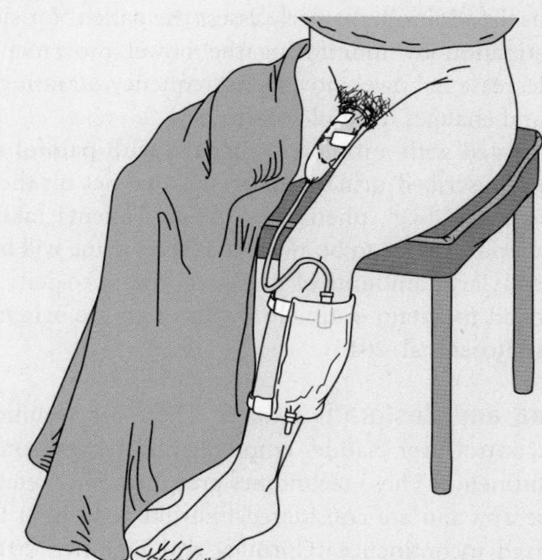

STEP 13 Attach condom catheter to leg bag.

14. Help patient to a safe, comfortable position, lower bed, and place side rails accordingly.
15. Dispose of contaminated supplies, remove gloves, and perform hand hygiene.
16. Inspect penis with condom catheter in place within 15 to 30 minutes after application for any swelling, discoloration, or discomfort. Observe for patency of urinary drainage system, characteristics of urine, condition of penis, and proper placement of condom catheter.
17. Remove and reapply daily following the previous steps unless an extended-wear device is used. For removal, wash the penis with warm, soapy water and gently roll the sheathe and adhesive off the penile shaft (Kyle, 2011).
18. Perform ***Teach Back*** to determine patient's understanding about the catheter. State, "We talked about what you need to do to prevent the drainage tube from blocking urine flow. Can you tell me what you need to do?"

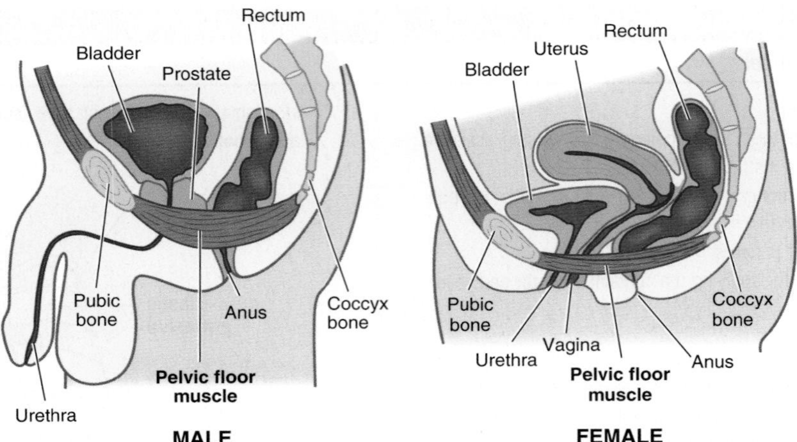

FIGURE 46-16 Pelvic floor muscles. (From Lewis S et al: *Medical-surgical nursing: assessment and management of clinical problems*, ed 9, St Louis, 2014, Mosby.)

increases. There are no medications, other than off-label use of vaginal estrogen in postmenopausal women, to treat stress UI (Shamliyan et al., 2012). Urinary retention is sometimes treated with bethanechol, and men with outlet obstruction caused by an enlarged prostate are treated with agents that relax the smooth muscle of the prostatic urethra such as tamsulosin and silodosin and agents that shrink the prostate such as finasteride and dutasteride. Know the medications and indications for all medications your patient is taking.

When a patient is newly started on an antimuscarinic, monitor for effectiveness, watching for a decrease in symptoms such as urgency, frequency, and urgency UI episodes. A bladder diary is one of the best ways to do this. In addition, regularly assess the patient for side effects such as constipation by monitoring the bowel movement record. Watch for a decrease in bowel movement frequency, straining at bowel movements, and changes in stool consistency.

UTIs are treated with antibiotics. Patients with painful urination are sometimes prescribed urinary analgesics that act on the urethral and bladder mucosa (e.g., phenazopyridine). Patients taking drugs with phenazopyridine need to be aware that their urine will be orange. They must drink large amounts of fluids to prevent toxicity from the sulfonamides and maintain optimal flow through the urinary system (Burchum and Rosenthal, 2016).

Continuing and Restorative Care. There are techniques that can improve control over bladder emptying and restore some degree of urinary continence. These techniques are commonly referred to as behavioral therapy and are considered first-line treatment for stress, urge, and mixed incontinence (Gormley and Lightner, 2012). They include lifestyle changes, pelvic floor muscle training (PFMT), bladder retraining, and a variety of toileting schedules (see Table 46-1). In some cases, when the bladder does not empty, patients or caregivers learn to intermittently catheterize. Whenever there is a risk for urine leakage, skin care is an essential component of the plan of care. Adequate urine containment and skin protection promotes patient comfort and dignity.

Lifestyle Changes. A number of lifestyle modifications can improve bladder function and decrease incontinence. In addition to interventions listed earlier in this chapter under health promotion and in Box 46-7, you can teach patients about foods and fluids that cause bladder irritation and increase symptoms such as frequency, urgency, and incontinence. Teach patients to avoid common irritants such as artificial sweeteners, spicy foods, citrus products, and especially caffeine (Jura et al., 2011; Lohsiriwat, 2011). Discourage patients from drinking large volumes of fluid at one time. Constipation can also impact bladder symptoms, and measures to promote bowel regularity should be implemented (see Chapter 47). Encourage patients with edema to elevate the feet for a minimum of a few hours in the afternoon to help diminish nighttime voiding frequency.

Pelvic Floor Muscle Training. Evidence has shown that patients with urgency, stress, and mixed UI experience improvement and can eventually achieve continence when treated with pelvic floor muscle training (Bettez et al., 2012 Lucas et al., 2013; Shamliyan et al., 2012). Pelvic floor muscle training involves teaching patients how to identify and contract the pelvic floor muscles in a structured exercise program. This exercise program is commonly called *Kegel exercises* and is based on therapy first developed by obstetrician gynecologist Dr. Arnold Kegel in the 1940s. The exercises work by increasing the pressure within the urethra by strengthening the pelvic floor muscles and inhibiting unwanted bladder contractions (Figure 46-16). Many patients benefit from verbal instructions on how to do the exercises (see Box 46-8). Patients who have difficulty correctly identifying and contracting the pelvic floor muscles can be sent to a continence specialist for biofeedback. Biofeedback involves intensive instruction augmented by computerized measurement of muscle activity that is displayed on a monitor. The visual feedback helps the patient learn to contract the muscles correctly.

Bladder Retraining. Bladder retraining is a behavioral therapy designed to help patients control bothersome urinary urgency and frequency. Patients are taught about their bladder and techniques to suppress urgency. They are given a schedule of toileting on the basis of their diary of voiding and leaking, and a schedule is designed to slowly increase the interval between voiding. Successful bladder retraining requires that patients get regular support and positive reinforcement. Patients are taught to inhibit the urge to void by taking slow, deep breaths to relax, performing five to six quick, strong pelvic muscle exercises (flicks) in quick succession, followed by distracting attention from bladder sensations. When the urge to void becomes less severe or subsides, only then should the patient start his or her trip to the bathroom. Only highly motivated and cognitively intact patients are candidates for this therapy. If a patient is in such a program, you can support him or her by reinforcing the schedule and providing emotional encouragement.

Toileting Schedules. A key component to any treatment plan for UI is regular toilet access. Toileting schedules should be individualized based on the type of incontinence and functional disability (e.g., cognitive impairment). Toileting can be implemented in any care setting and should be the first plan of action when you assess a patient to be incontinent. Timed voiding or scheduled toileting is toileting based on a fixed schedule, not the patient's urge to void. The schedule may be set by a time interval, every 2 to 3 hours or at times of day such as before and after meals. It is very successful with moderate-to-severe cognitively- and mobility-impaired adults. Habit training is a toileting schedule based on the patient's usual voiding pattern. Using a bladder diary, the usual times a patient voids are identified. It is at these times that the patient is then toileted. Prompted voiding is a program of toileting designed for patients with mild or moderately cognitive impairment. Patients are toileted based on their usual voiding pattern. Caregivers ask the patient if they are wet or dry, give positive feedback for dryness, prompt the patient to toilet, and reward the patient for desired behavior. This is a very successful toileting program; but it does require a consistent motivated caregiver, a cooperative patient, and evidence that the patient will void when toileted at least 50% of the time or more.

Intermittent Catheterization. Some patients experience chronic inability to completely empty the bladder as a result of neuromuscular damage related to multiple sclerosis, diabetes, spinal cord injury, and urinary retention caused by outlet obstruction. To minimize the risk of UTI, patients or family caregivers are taught to catheterize the bladder. It is important they follow the principles of asepsis as discussed earlier in the chapter. Teach patients and caregivers about the importance of adequate fluid intake, signs of infection, and their individualized catheterization schedule. The goal for intermittent catheterization is drainage of 400 mL of urine with the schedule individualized to meet this goal.

Skin Care. Incontinence-associated dermatitis (IAD) is defined as "erythema and edema of the surface of the skin, sometimes accompanied by bullae with serous exudates, erosion or secondary cutaneous infection" (Gray et al., 2012). It is caused by irritation of the skin by urine caused by skin overhydration, increased pH, and friction injury during movement (Gray et al., 2012). Exposure to stool and urine increases the risk for skin injury. Key components for IAD prevention and treatment include gentle skin cleansing with a no-rinse pH balanced cleanser, using a skin moisturizer, and applying a moisture barrier product (Doughty et al., 2012). In some cases patients may develop a topical fungal infection that requires treatment with a steroid/antifungal cream or ointment. Typically these patients present with erythema with raised red spots located near the edge. Patients may complain of intense itchiness.

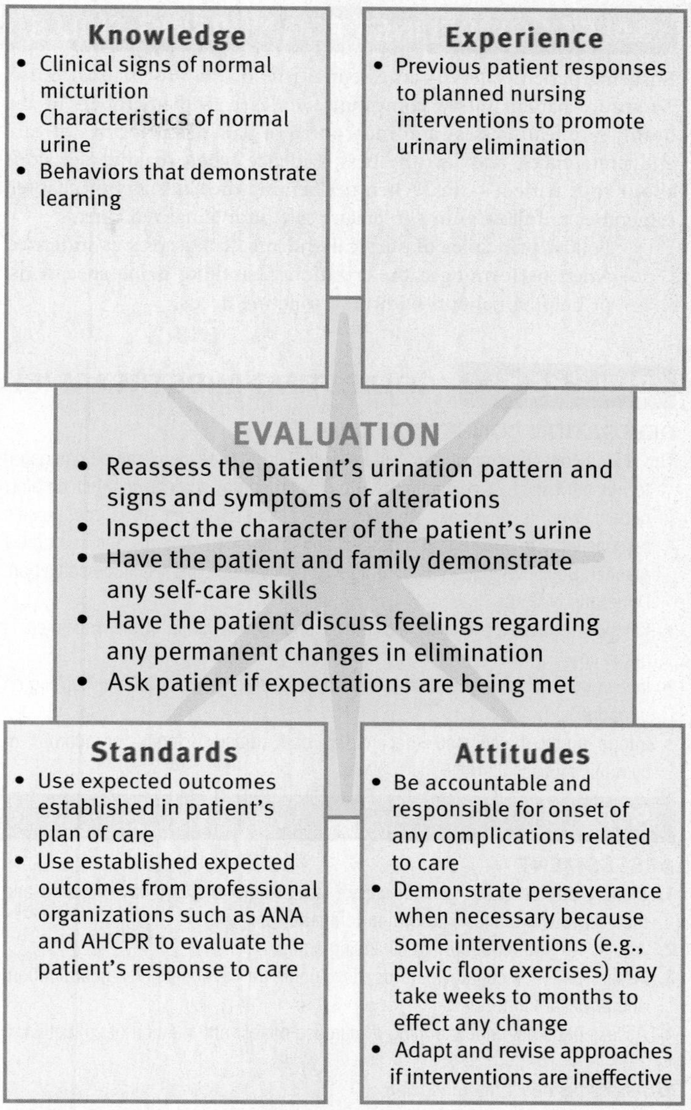

Knowledge
- Clinical signs of normal micturition
- Characteristics of normal urine
- Behaviors that demonstrate learning

Experience
- Previous patient responses to planned nursing interventions to promote urinary elimination

EVALUATION
- Reassess the patient's urination pattern and signs and symptoms of alterations
- Inspect the character of the patient's urine
- Have the patient and family demonstrate any self-care skills
- Have the patient discuss feelings regarding any permanent changes in elimination
- Ask patient if expectations are being met

Standards
- Use expected outcomes established in patient's plan of care
- Use established expected outcomes from professional organizations such as ANA and AHCPR to evaluate the patient's response to care

Attitudes
- Be accountable and responsible for onset of any complications related to care
- Demonstrate perseverance when necessary because some interventions (e.g., pelvic floor exercises) may take weeks to months to effect any change
- Adapt and revise approaches if interventions are ineffective

FIGURE 46-17 Critical thinking model for urinary elimination evaluation. *AHCPR*, Agency for Health Care Policy and Research; *ANA*, American Nurses Association.

◆ Evaluation

Through the Patient's Eyes. The patient is the best source of evaluation of outcomes and responses to nursing care. Include patients in the planning of nursing care and revision of the plan based on their perception of its success. It is important to remember that urinary problems impact the patient not only physically but emotionally, psychologically, spiritually, and socially. Carefully assess the patient's self-image, social interactions, sexuality, and emotional status as impacted by the urinary problem (Figure 46-17).

Patient Outcomes. To evaluate the care plan use the expected outcomes developed during planning to determine whether interventions were effective. This evaluation process is dynamic. Information gathered is used to modify the plan of care to meet expected outcomes. Evaluate for changes in the patient's voiding pattern and/or presence of symptoms such as dysuria, urinary retention, and UI. If a behavioral plan is in effect, evaluate patient/caregiver compliance with the plan such as toileting according to the schedule or the number of incontinent episodes. Actual outcomes are compared with expected outcomes to determine success or partial success in achieving these outcomes. Examples of questions to ask for evaluation include:

- "Tell me, how frequently are you voiding now?"
- "How many times are you awakened from sleep with a strong urge to void?"
- "Do you continue to experience that sensation of urgency or need to rush to the toilet?"
- "How many episodes of urine leakage have you experienced over the past week?"
- "Do you have pain or burning when you pass urine?

Evaluation of an intervention may take place within a day or two, or it may take weeks or months to fully evaluate effectiveness. Evaluate initial compliance with dietary changes, understanding of instructions for pelvic muscle exercise, or effectiveness of antibiotic treatment for UTI in 1 to 2 days. Evaluation of the effectiveness of pelvic muscle exercises in decreasing urgency and incontinence will need to be weeks or months after therapy is started. Continuous evaluation, when possible, allows you to determine progress toward goals, encourage compliance, and revise the diagnosis and/or plan as needed.

SAFETY GUIDELINES FOR NURSING SKILLS

Ensuring patient safety is an essential role of the professional nurse. To ensure patient safety, communicate clearly with members of the health care team, assess and incorporate a patient's priorities of care and preferences, and use the best evidence when making decisions about your patient's care. When performing the skills in this chapter, remember to follow points to ensure safe, individualized care:

- Follow principles of surgical and medical asepsis as indicated when performing catheterizations, handling urine specimens, or helping patients with their toileting needs.
- Identify patients at risk for latex allergies (i.e., patient history of hay fever; asthma; and allergies to certain foods such as bananas, grapes, apricots, kiwi fruit, and hazelnuts).
- Identify patients with allergies to povidone-iodine (Betadine). Provide alternatives such as chlorhexidine.

SKILL 46-1 COLLECTING MIDSTREAM (CLEAN-VOIDED) URINE SPECIMEN 

DELEGATION CONSIDERATIONS

The skill of collecting midstream (clean-voided) urine specimens can be delegated to nursing assistive personnel (NAP). If appropriate, you can instruct an alert patient who is physically able to collect the specimen. It is the nurse's responsibility to ensure that this specimen is obtained correctly and in a timely manner. Be knowledgeable about agency policy regarding specimen collection. Direct the NAP to:

- Consider patient's mobility restrictions and inform nurse when specimen is obtained.
- Inform nurse if patient is unable to initiate a stream or has pain or burning on urination.
- Inform nurse if collected specimen is dark, bloody, cloudy, or odorous or contains mucus.

EQUIPMENT

- Soap or cleaning solution, washcloth, and towel
- Commercial kit for clean-voided specimen (Figure 46-18) or individual supplies as listed
  - Antiseptic towelettes or
  - Antiseptic solution (e.g., chlorhexidine [Hibiclens] or povidone-iodine [Betadine]) and sterile cotton balls or sterile 2 × 2 or 4 × 4 gauze pads
  - Sterile specimen container
- Clean gloves
- Bedpan, bedside commode, or specimen hat
- Completed specimen label and laboratory requisition form with proper patient identifiers

STEP	RATIONALE
ASSESSMENT	
1. Identify patient using two identifiers (e.g., name and birthday or name and medical record number) according to agency policy.	Ensures correct patient. Complies with The Joint Commission standards and improves patient safety (TJC, 2016).
2. Assess for patient allergy to cleansing agent.	If allergic to iodine, provide cleansing alternative such as chlorhexidine.
3. Assess patient's cognitive status, developmental level, mobility, coordination, and physical limitations.	Identifies patient's needs for help and ability to cooperate during procedure
4. Assess patient's understanding of purpose of test and method of collection.	Allows you to clarify misunderstandings, promotes patient cooperation, and improves accuracy of specimen collection.
5. Assess perineal area for soiling.	Cleansing of genitourinary and perianal areas can be completed before obtaining specimen.

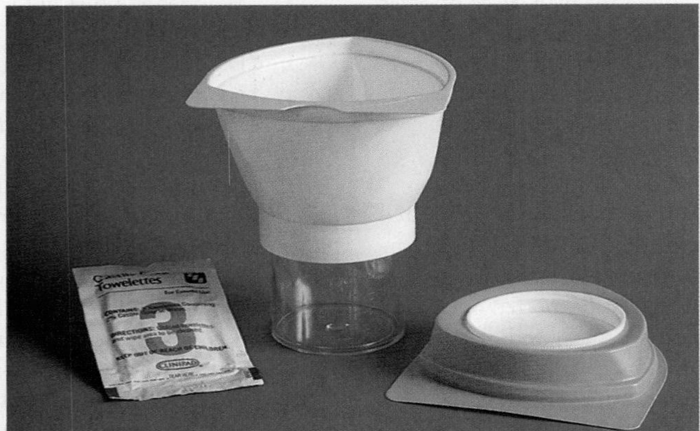

FIGURE 46-18 Commercial midstream urine collection kit.

STEP	RATIONALE
PLANNING	
1. Provide fluids to drink ½ hour before collection unless contraindicated (i.e., fluid restriction) if patient does not feel urge to void.	Improves likelihood of patient being able to void.
2. Explain procedure to patient:	Helps patient understand procedure.
a. Reason midstream specimen is necessary	
b. Ways for patient and family to help	
c. Ways to obtain specimen free of feces	Feces change characteristics of urine and cause abnormal values.
d. Use plain language and visual aids (if applicable) to explain procedure	Illustrations demonstrating midstream collection techniques help to clarify a complex procedure, especially with patients for whom English is a second language.
3. If female patient is menstruating, record this on laboratory requisition form.	
IMPLEMENTATION	
1. Perform hand hygiene and apply gloves.	Reduces transmissions of microorganisms.
2. Provide privacy for patient by closing door or bed curtain.	Privacy allows patient to relax and produce specimen more quickly.
3. Help patient as needed to toilet or onto bedpan or position the urinal. If on a bedpan, raise the head of the bed.	Semi-sitting position may ease voiding.
4. Prepare sterile specimen container.	
a. Remove lid from sterile urine cup and place lid with sterile inside surface up nearby. Do not touch inside of container	Maintains inside of container sterile.
b. Open antiseptic towelette package or prepare cotton balls/gauze sponges with antiseptic solution.	
c. If helping patient, apply clean pair of gloves.	
5. Collect specimen.	
a. **Female**	
(1) Spread labia with thumb and forefinger of nondominant hand.	Provides access to urethral meatus.
(2) Clean area with towelette/cotton ball/gauze, moving from front (above urethral orifice) to back (toward anus). Using a fresh towelette/cotton ball/gauze each time, repeat front-to-back motion 3 times (begin with left side, then right side, then center) (see illustration).	Clean from area of least contamination to area of greatest contamination to decrease bacterial levels.
(3) While continuing to hold labia apart, have patient initiate stream. After patient starts urine stream, pass container into stream and collect 30 to 60 mL (see illustration)	Initial stream flushes out microorganisms that accumulate at urethral meatus and prevents transfer into specimen.
b. **Male**	
(1) Hold penis with one hand and cleanse glans penis using circular motion with antiseptic towelette/cotton ball/gauze; clean moving from center to outside (see illustration). In uncircumcised men retract foreskin before cleaning.	Clean from area of least contamination to area of greatest contamination to decrease bacterial levels.
(2) After patient has initiated urine stream, pass specimen collection container into stream and collect 30 to 60 mL (see illustration).	Initial stream flushes out microorganisms that accumulate at urethral meatus and prevents transfer into specimen.

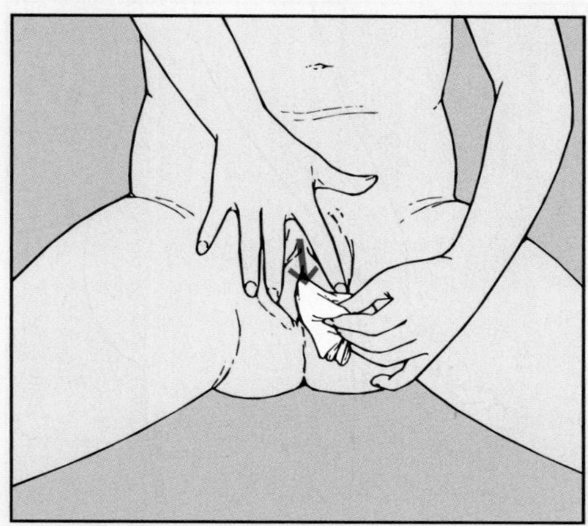

STEP 5a(2) Cleaning technique (female).

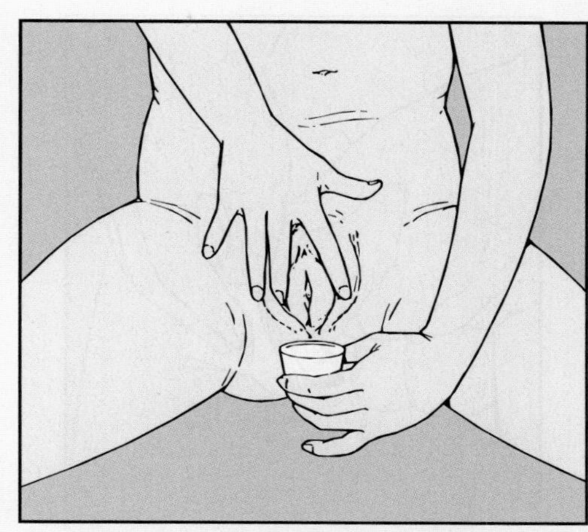

STEP 5a(3) Specimen collection (female).

SKILL 46-1 COLLECTING MIDSTREAM (CLEAN-VOIDED) URINE SPECIMEN—cont'd

STEP	RATIONALE
6. Remove specimen container before flow of urine stops and before releasing labia or penis. Patient finishes voiding in bedpan/toilet/urinal.	Prevents contamination of specimen with skin flora.

CLINICAL DECISION: *If foreskin was retracted for specimen collection, replace it over the glans. If foreskin is not replaced, swelling and constriction occur, causing pain and possible obstruction to urine flow.*

STEP	RATIONALE
7. Replace cap securely on specimen container (touch outside only).	Retains sterility of inside of container and prevents spillage of urine.
8. Clean any urine from exterior surface of container. Attach label on side of container (not lid) in front of patient. Be sure label is complete with two identifiers, specimen source, and date and time. Place in plastic specimen biohazard bag as required by agency.	Prevents transfer of microorganisms to others.
9. Remove and empty bedpan/urinal (if applicable) and help patient to comfortable position.	Promotes relaxing environment.
10. Attach laboratory requisition to specimen bag.	Prevents inaccurate identification and minimizes errors in diagnosis or treatment.
11. Remove gloves, dispose of them in proper receptacle, and perform hand hygiene.	Reduces transmission of infection.
12. Transport specimen to laboratory within 15 to 30 minutes or refrigerate immediately.	Because bacteria grow quickly in urine, urine not received by laboratory within 30 minutes should be refrigerated. However, refrigeration should not exceed 2 hours (Pagana and Pagana, 2013).

EVALUATION

STEP	RATIONALE
1. Observe characteristics of urine and look for any contaminants such as feces.	Contaminants prevent specimen from being used.
2. Evaluate laboratory results of urine test.	Determines presence of bacteria and kidney function.
3. Use ***Teach Back*** to determine patient's and family's understanding about the correct steps in obtaining a clean-catch urine specimen. State, "I want to be sure I explained the steps in obtaining the urine specimen. Can you repeat those steps for me?" Revise your instruction now or develop a plan for revised patient teaching if patient is not able to teach back correctly.	Evaluates what patient and family are able to explain or demonstrate.

UNEXPECTED OUTCOMES AND RELATED INTERVENTIONS

1. Urine specimen is contaminated with feces or toilet paper.
   - Repeat instruction to patient or help patient obtain specimen.
   - Obtain a new specimen.
   - Request an order for using a straight catheterization to obtain specimen.
2. Specimen is spilled or accidentally discarded.
   - Repeat specimen collection.

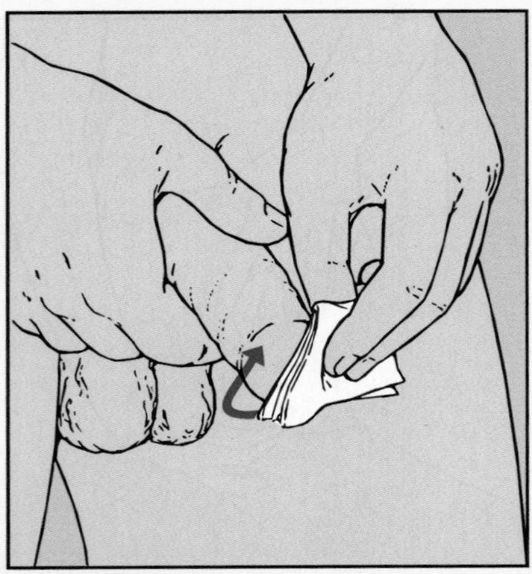

STEP 5b(1) Cleaning technique (male).

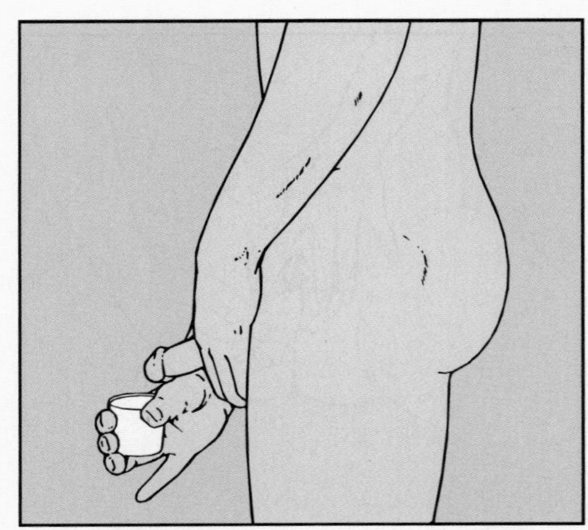

STEP 5b(2) Specimen collection (male).

RECORDING AND REPORTING

- Record date and time urine specimen was obtained in nurses' notes.
- Notify health care provider of any significant abnormalities.
- Document your evaluation of patient learning.

HOME CARE CONSIDERATIONS

- If patient is to collect specimen as outpatient, a clean technique may be used. Provide instruction for collection and appropriate equipment.
- Provide information about storing specimen until time for delivery to health care provider's office or hospital laboratory.

SKILL 46-2 INSERTING AND REMOVING A STRAIGHT (INTERMITTENT) OR INDWELLING CATHETER

DELEGATION CONSIDERATIONS

The skill of inserting a straight or an indwelling catheter cannot be delegated. The nurse is responsible for assessing the need for and evaluation of catheterization. The nurse directs nursing assistive personnel (NAP) to:

- Help with patient positioning, focus lighting for the procedure, empty urine from collection bag, and help with perineal care.
- Report postprocedure patient discomfort, fever, or catheter leakage to the nurse.
- Report abnormal color, odor, or amount of urine to the nurse.

EQUIPMENT

Catheter insertion

- Sterile drainage tubing and bag (if not included in the kit)
- Device to secure catheter (catheter strap or other device)
- Extra sterile gloves and catheter (optional)
- Bath blanket
- Waterproof absorbent pad
- Clean gloves, basin with warm water, soap or perineal cleanser, washcloth, and towel for perineal care
- Additional lighting as needed (such as a flashlight or procedure light)
- Measuring container for urine
- Bladder scanner (if available)
- Catheter kit containing the following sterile items: (Catheter kits vary; thus it is important to check the list of contents on the package.)

Straight/intermittent catheterization kit

- Single-lumen catheter (commonly 12-14 Fr)
- Drapes (one fenestrated—has an opening in the center)
- Sterile gloves
- Lubricant
- Cleansing solution incorporated in an applicator or to be added to cotton balls (forceps to pick up cotton balls)
- Specimen container

Indwelling catheterization kit

- Double-lumen catheter (Some kits contain a catheter with attached drainage bag; others contain only a catheter; others with no catheter.)
- Drapes (one fenestrated—has an opening in the center)
- Lubricant
- Cleansing solution incorporated in an applicator or to be added to cotton balls (forceps to pick up cotton balls)
- Prefilled syringe with sterile water for balloon inflation
- Sterile drainage tubing and bag (some kits come preconnected; others do not, and a separate package is required)
- Sterile gloves
- Specimen container

Catheter removal

- Clean gloves
- Waterproof pad
- Bath blanket
- Soap, washcloth, towel, and basin filled with warm water
- 10-mL or larger syringe without needle—information on balloon size (mL) is printed directly on balloon inflation valve (see Figure 46-11)
- Graduated cylinder to measure urine
- Toilet, bedside commode, urine "hat," urinal, or bedpan
- Bladder scanner (if available and indicated)

SKILL 46-2 INSERTING AND REMOVING A STRAIGHT (INTERMITTENT) OR INDWELLING CATHETER—cont'd

STEP	RATIONALE
ASSESSMENT	
1. Review patient's medical record, including health care provider's order and nurses' notes. Note previous catheterizations, including catheter size, response of patient, and time of catheterization.	Identifies purpose of inserting catheter such as for measurement of residual urine or specimen collection, previous catheter size, and potential difficulty with catheter insertion.
2. Review medical record for any pathological condition that may impair passage of catheter (e.g., enlarged prostate gland in men, urethral strictures).	Obstruction of urethra may prevent passage of catheter into bladder. Men with enlarged prostates may require the use of a coudé-tip catheter.
3. Identify patient using two identifiers (e.g., name and birthday or name and medical record number) according to agency policy.	Ensures correct patient. Complies with The Joint Commission standards and improves patient safety (TJC, 2016).
4. Ask patient and check medical record for allergies.	Identifies allergy to components of catheterization kit and/or catheter (e.g., antiseptic, tape, latex).
5. Assess patient's weight, level of consciousness, developmental level, ability to cooperate, and mobility.	Determines positioning for catheterization and indicates how much help is needed to properly position patient, ability of patient to cooperate during procedure, and level of explanation needed.
6. Review patient's gender and age.	Determines catheter size.

CLINICAL DECISION: *Large catheters can damage the urethra and urinary meatus, increase bladder irritability, and cause urine to leak around the catheter because of spasm (Cottenden et al., 2013). Use the smallest size catheter possible to minimize trauma and patient discomfort (Gould et al., 2009).*

STEP	RATIONALE
7. Assess bladder for fullness by palpation of bladder over symphysis pubis or by use of bladder scanner (if available).	Palpation of full bladder causes pain and/or urge to void, indicating full or overfull bladder.
8. Perform hand hygiene and apply clean gloves. Inspect the perineal area for anatomical landmarks, erythema, drainage or discharge, and odor. Remove gloves and perform hand hygiene.	Assessment of female perineum landmarks improves accuracy and speed of catheter insertion.
9. Assess patient's knowledge and prior experience with catheterization.	Reveals extent of instruction or support needed by patient.
PLANNING	
1. Collect appropriate equipment.	
2. Arrange for extra nursing personnel to help as necessary.	More than one person is needed to help position patients who are weak, frail, obese, or confused.
3. Explain procedure to patient and why catheter is necessary. Describe sensations patient will feel (e.g., liquid cleansing of perineum, burning during catheter insertion).	Promotes cooperation and facilitates anxiety reduction.
IMPLEMENTATION	
1. Perform hand hygiene.	Reduces transmission of microorganisms.
2. Provide privacy by closing room door and bedside curtain.	Protects patient confidentiality.
3. Raise bed to appropriate working height. If side rails in use, raise side rail on opposite side of bed and lower side rail on working side.	Promotes good body mechanics. Use of side rails in this manner promotes patient safety.
4. Place waterproof pad under patient.	Prevents soiling of bed linen.
5. Provide perineal hygiene if needed (apply clean gloves, complete cleansing, discard gloves and perform hand hygiene).	Hygiene before catheter insertion removes secretions, urine, and feces that could contaminate the sterile field and increase risk for catheter-associated urinary tract infection (CAUTI).

CLINICAL DECISION: *Obtain help to position and support weak, frail, or confused patients.*

STEP	RATIONALE
6. Position and drape patient:	
a. Female Patient	
(1) Help to dorsal recumbent position (supine with knees flexed). Ask patient to relax thighs to externally rotate hip joints (see illustration).	Provides good visualization of structures of perineum and decreases risk for fecal contamination.
(2) Alternate female position: Position side-lying (Sims') position with upper leg flexed at knee and hip. Ensure that rectal area is covered with drape to reduce risk of contamination. Support patient with pillows if necessary to maintain position.	Alternate position is more comfortable if patient cannot abduct leg at hip joint (e.g., patient has arthritic joints or contractures).
b. Male Patient	
(1) Position supine with legs extended and thighs slightly abducted.	Comfortable position for patient that aids in visualization of penis.
c. Drape Patient: Cover upper part of body with small sheet or blanket. Cover lower extremities with sheet or blanket, exposing only genitalia. In women it is helpful to place blanket diamond fashion over patient, with one corner at patient's neck, side corners over each arm and side, and last corner over perineum (see illustration).	Protects patient dignity by avoiding unnecessary exposure of body parts.
7. Position light to illuminate genitals or have assistant available to hold light source to visualize urinary meatus.	Adequate visualization of urinary meatus helps with speed and accuracy of catheter insertion.
8. Perform hand hygiene.	
9. Open catheterization kit (some products have a double wrapping requiring removal of outer wrapper or plastic covering; others require peeling back a paper top). Place opened kit on clean bedside table or, if possible, between patient's open legs. Patient size and positioning will dictate exact placement.	Provides easy access to supplies during catheter insertion.
10. If present, open inner sterile wrap covering box using sterile technique (see Chapter 29).	Inner sterile wrap serves as sterile field. Straight catheterization trays do not routinely come with double wrapping.
a. Straight/intermittent catheterization: All needed supplies are in sterile tray. Tray that contains supplies can be used for urine collection.	
b. Indwelling catheterization open system: Open separate package containing drainage bag, check to make sure that clamp on drainage port is closed, and place drainage bag and tubing easily accessible. Open outer package of sterile catheter, maintaining sterility of inner wrapper.	An open drainage bag system requires separate sterile packaging for sterile catheter, drainage bag, and tubing and insertion kit.

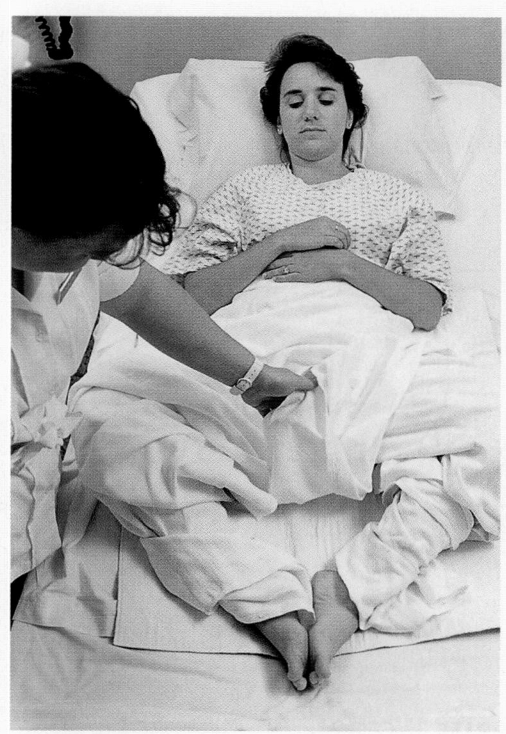

STEP 6a(1) Draping female for catheterization.

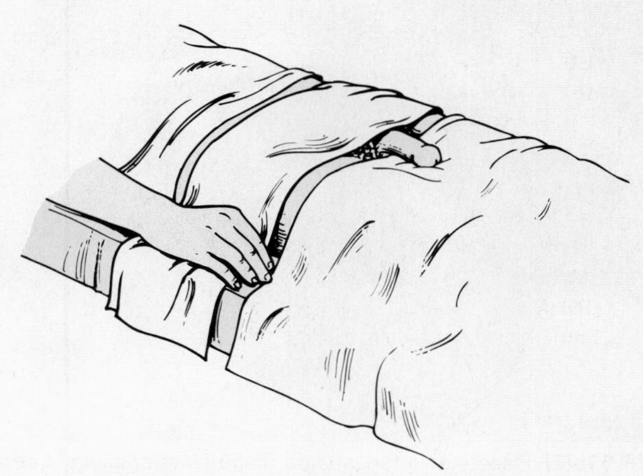

STEP 6c Draping male for catheterization.

SKILL 46-2 INSERTING AND REMOVING A STRAIGHT (INTERMITTENT) OR INDWELLING CATHETER—cont'd

STEP	RATIONALE
CLINICAL DECISION: *Some companies are now inserting CDC guidelines lists inside sterile packages to outline indications for indwelling catheterization. Simply discard after reviewing.*	
c. Indwelling catheterization closed system: All supplies are in sterile tray. Once sterile gloves are put on, check to make sure clamp on drainage bag is closed.	Closed drainage bag systems have catheter preattached to drainage tubing and bag.
11. Apply sterile gloves. Drape perineum, keeping gloves and working surface of drape sterile.	Sterile drapes provide sterile field over which nurse will work during catheterization.
a. **Sterile Drape Female**	
(1) Pick up square drape and allow unfolding without touching unsterile surfaces. Allow top edge of drape to form cuff over both hands. Place drape with shiny side down on bed between patient's thighs. Slip cuffed edge just under buttocks as you ask patient to lift hips. Take care not to touch contaminated surfaces with sterile gloves.	When creating cuff over sterile gloved hands, sterility of gloves and workspace is maintained. If gloves are contaminated, remove and apply new pair.
(2) Pick up fenestrated sterile drape. Allow drape to unfold without touching unsterile surfaces. Allow top edge of drape to form cuff over both hands. Drape over perineum, exposing labia (see illustration).	Opening in drape creates sterile field around labia.
b. **Sterile Drape Male:** Pick up square drape and allow unfolding without touching unsterile surfaces. Place over thighs with shiny side down, just below penis. Place fenestrated drape with opening centered over penis (see illustration).	
c. In some kits sterile gloves may be below square sterile drape. In this case, pick up the square drape from tray by edges and allow it to unfold without touching unsterile surfaces. The top edge is then folded away (sterile side up, hands on shiny underside) from patient to form cuff over both hands and carefully placed. Then put on sterile gloves and place fenestrated drape.	Sequence of supplies in kit varies. Use supplies in order to prevent contamination of underlying supplies.
12. Arrange supplies on sterile field, maintaining sterility of gloves. Place sterile tray with cleaning medium (premoistened swab sticks or cotton balls, forceps, and solution), lubricant, catheter, and prefilled balloon inflation syringe (indwelling catheterization only) on sterile drape.	Provides easy access to supplies during catheter insertion and helps to maintain aseptic technique. Appropriate placement is determined by size of patient and position during catheterization.
a. Open package of sterile antiseptic solution. Open end of package for easy access. Pour solution over sterile cotton balls. Some kits may contain a package of premoistened swab sticks or sticks that will be in the tray in which you pour antiseptic.	Use of sterile supplies and antiseptic solution will reduce risk of CAUTI (Geng et al., 2012; Gould et al., 2009).
b. Open sterile specimen container if urine specimen required.	Makes container accessible to receive urine from catheter if specimen is needed.

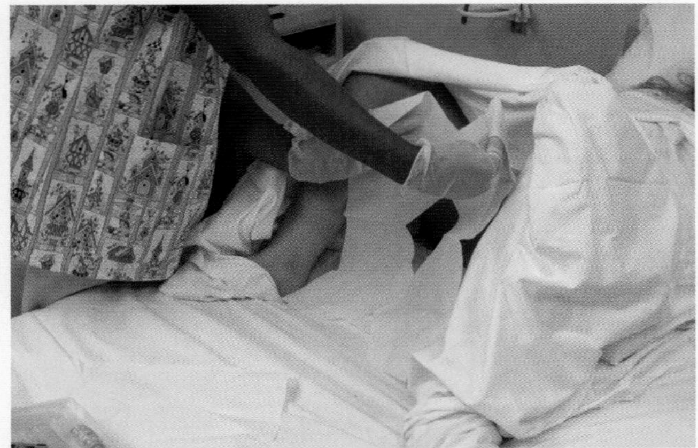

STEP 11a(2) Place sterile fenestrated drape (with opening in center) over perineum with labia exposed.

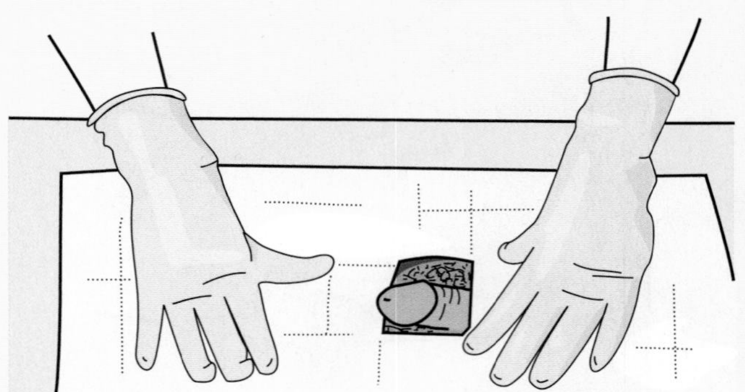

STEP 11b Draping male with fenestrated drape.

STEP	RATIONALE
c. Indwelling catheterization: Open inner sterile wrapper of catheter. If part of kit, remove tray with catheter and attached drainage bag and place on sterile drape. Make sure that clamp on drainage port of bag is closed.	
d. Open packet of lubricant (some kit lubricant comes in a syringe) and squeeze out on sterile field. Lubricate catheter by dipping catheter into water-soluble gel 2.5 cm to 5 cm (1 to 2 inches) for women and 12.5 to 17.5 cm (5 to 7 inches) for men.	Lubrication minimizes trauma to urethra and discomfort during catheter insertion. Male catheter needs enough lubricant to cover length of catheter inserted.

CLINICAL DECISION: *It is essential to check manufacturer instructions before inserting an indwelling catheter. Some manufacturers do not recommend pretesting the inflation balloon. Pretesting by inflation/deflation of the balloon may lead to formation of ridges in the balloon, potentially causing trauma on insertion.*

STEP	RATIONALE
13. Cleanse urethral meatus:	
a. Female Patient	
(1) Gently separate labia with fingers of nondominant hand (now contaminated) to fully expose urinary meatus.	Optimal visualization of urethral meatus is possible. Closure of labia during cleansing means that area is now contaminated and requires cleaning procedure to be repeated.
(2) Maintain position of nondominant hand throughout remainder of procedure.	
(3) Use forceps to hold one cotton ball or hold one swab stick at a time. Clean labia and urinary meatus from clitoris toward anus. Use new cotton ball or swab for each area you cleanse. Cleanse by wiping far labial fold, near labial fold, and directly over center of urethral meatus (see illustration).	Front-to-back cleansing is cleaning from area of least contamination toward highly contaminated area (see Chapter 29). Dominant gloved hand remains sterile.
b. Male Patient	
(1) With nondominant hand (now contaminated) retract foreskin (if uncircumcised) and gently grasp penis at shaft just below glans. Hold shaft of penis at right angle to body. This hand remains in this position for remainder of procedure.	When grasping shaft of penis, avoid pressure on dorsal surface to prevent compression of urethra. Positioning penis at this 90-degree angle to patient straightens out curvature of male urethra and eases insertion (Geng et al., 2012; Mendez-Probst et al., 2012).
(2) With uncontaminated dominant hand cleanse meatus with cotton balls/swab sticks, using circular strokes, beginning at meatus and working outward in spiral motion. Repeat 3 times using clean cotton ball/stick each time (see illustration).	Circular cleansing pattern follows principles of medical asepsis (see Chapter 29).

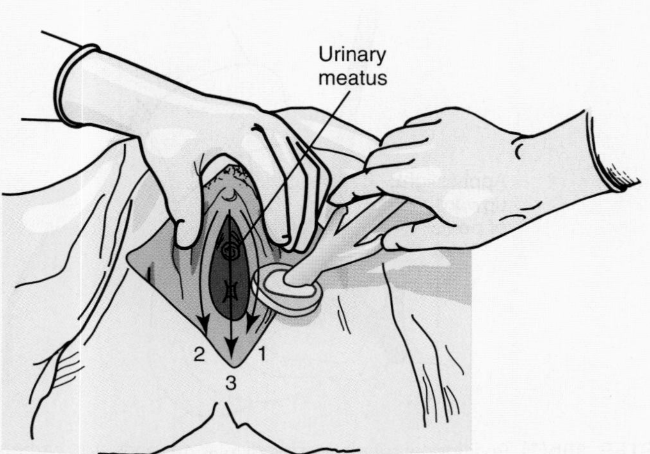

STEP 13a(3) Cleansing female perineum.

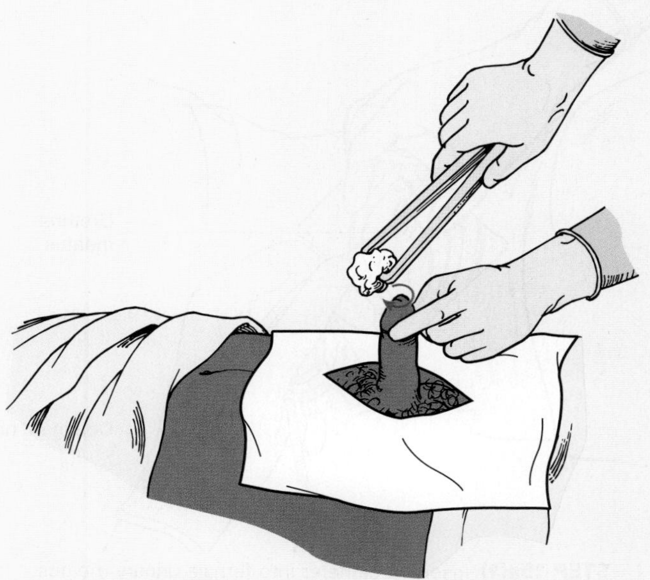
STEP 13b(2) Cleansing male urinary meatus.

SKILL 46-2 INSERTING AND REMOVING A STRAIGHT (INTERMITTENT) OR INDWELLING CATHETER—cont'd

STEP	RATIONALE
14. Pick up and hold catheter 7.5 to 10 cm (3 to 4 inches) from catheter tip with catheter loosely coiled in palm of hand. If catheter is not attached to drainage bag, make sure to position urine tray so end of catheter can be placed there once insertion begins.	Holding catheter near tip allows for easier manipulation of catheter during insertion. Coiling catheter in palm prevents distal end from striking nonsterile surface.
15. Insert catheter:	
a. **Female Patient**	
(1) Ask patient to bear down gently and slowly insert catheter through urethral meatus (see illustration).	Bearing down may help visualize urinary meatus and promotes relaxation of external urinary sphincter, aiding in catheter insertion.
(2) Advance catheter total of 5 to 7.5 cm (2 to 3 inches) in an adult **or until urine flows out end of catheter.** Release labia but maintain secure hold on catheter.	Urine flow indicates that catheter tip is in bladder. Prevents accidental dislodgement of catheter.

CLINICAL DECISION: *If no urine appears, catheter may be in vagina. If misplaced, leave catheter in vagina as landmark indicating where not to insert and insert another sterile catheter.*

STEP	RATIONALE
b. **Male Patient**	
(1) Gently apply upward traction to penis as it is held in 90-degree angle from body (see illustration).	Straightens urethra to ease catheter insertion.
(2) Ask patient to bear down as if to void and slowly insert catheter through urethral meatus.	Relaxation of external sphincter aids in insertion of catheter (Geng et al., 2012).
(3) Advance catheter 17 to 22.5 cm (7 to 9 inches) or until urine flows out end of catheter.	Length of male urethra varies. Flow of urine indicates that tip of catheter is in bladder but not necessarily the balloon part of an indwelling catheter.

CLINICAL DECISION: *If there is resistance or pain when advancing the catheter, DO NOT USE FORCE and stop catheter advancement. Ask the patient to take slow, deep breaths to promote relaxation. Hold catheter gently in place without forcing. After a few seconds the sphincter may relax, and catheter can be advanced. An inability to advance a catheter may mean an enlarged prostate or some other obstruction of the urethra.*

STEP	RATIONALE
(4) Lower penis and hold catheter securely in nondominant hand.	Prevents accidental dislodgement of catheter.
16. Allow bladder to empty fully unless institution policy restricts maximum volume of urine drained (see agency policy).	There is no definitive evidence regarding whether there is benefit in limiting maximal volume drained.

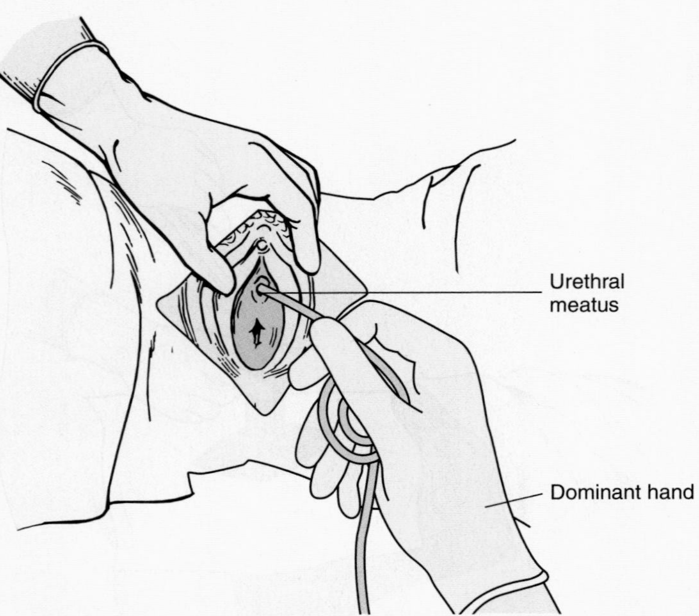

STEP 15a(1) Inserting catheter into female urinary meatus.

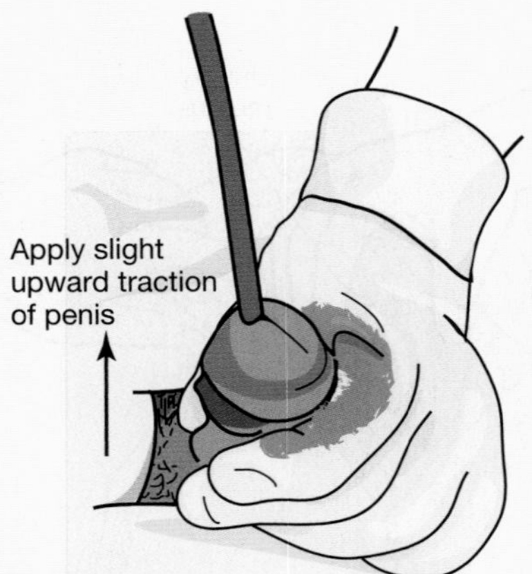

STEP 15b(1) Position of penis perpendicular to body for catheter insertion.

STEP	RATIONALE

CLINICAL DECISION: *In the case of acute urinary retention (rapid onset) when the volume of urine is known to be excessive (greater than 1 L), notify the health care provider for guidance related to gradual bladder decompression to avoid possible decompression-induced hematuria (Mendez-Probst et al., 2012).*

STEP	RATIONALE
17. Collect urine specimen as needed by holding end of catheter over cup. Fill to desired level. Label and bag specimen according to agency policy. Send specimen to laboratory as soon as possible.	A sterile specimen for culture analysis can be obtained. Fresh urine specimen ensures more accurate findings (Pagana and Pagana, 2013).
18. Straight/intermittent catheterization: when urine flow stops, withdraw catheter slowly and smoothly until removed.	
19. Indwelling catheterization: inflate catheter balloon.	
a. Female patient	
(1) As soon as urine appears, advance catheter another 2.5 to 5 cm (1 to 2 inches). Do not force catheter if resistance is met.	Ensures catheter tip is completely inside bladder.
(2) Release labia but maintain secure hold of catheter with nondominant hand.	Prevents accidental removal.
b. Male patient	
(1) After catheter is inserted through meatus and urine appears, advance catheter to bifurcation of drainage and balloon inflation port (see illustration).	There is natural resistance as the catheter passes through the U-shaped bulbar urethra. Further advancement of catheter to bifurcation of drainage and balloon inflation port ensures that balloon part of catheter is not still in prostatic urethra (Geng et al., 2012; Mendez-Probst et al., 2012).
(2) Lower penis and hold catheter securely in nondominant hand.	
c. With free dominant hand, connect prefilled syringe in injection port at end of catheter. Slowly inject amount of solution required to fill balloon as designated by manufacturer (see illustration).	Indwelling catheter balloons should not be overinflated or underinflated to prevent occlusion of catheter drainage holes, balloon distortion, and bladder irritation (Geng et al., 2012). Catheter balloons are only filled with sterile water. Other solutions might precipitate and occlude the fill tubing and catheter balloon fill valve (Mendez-Probst et al., 2012).

CLINICAL DECISION: *If the patient complains of sudden pain during inflation of a catheter balloon or resistance is felt when inflating the balloon, stop inflation, allow the fluid from the balloon to flow back into the syringe, advance catheter further, and reinflate balloon. The balloon may have been inflating in the urethra.*

STEP	RATIONALE
d. After inflating catheter balloon, release catheter from nondominant hand. Gently withdraw catheter until resistance is felt. Then advance catheter slightly.	Withdrawing catheter places catheter balloon at base of bladder; slight advancement reduces risk of excessive pressure (Geng et al., 2012).
e. Male patient: If retracted, replace foreskin over glans penis.	Leaving foreskin retracted can cause discomfort and dangerous edema.
f. Connect drainage tubing to catheter if it is not already preconnected.	Ensures proper drainage by gravity. Placement on side rails increases risk for tension applied to catheter, and bag can be raised above level of bladder.

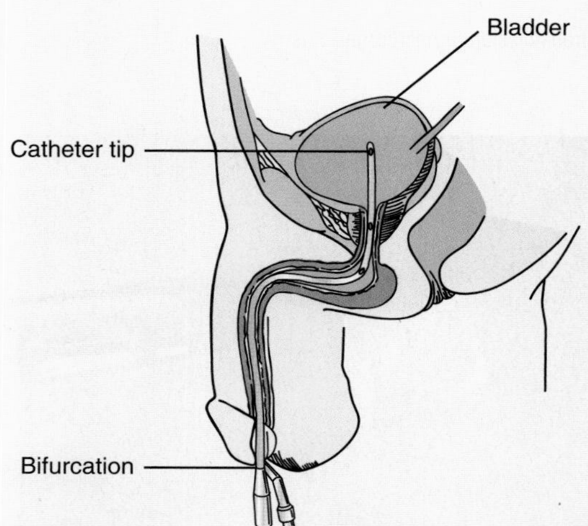

STEP 19b(1) Male anatomy with correct catheter insertion to bifurcation of drainage and balloon inflation port.

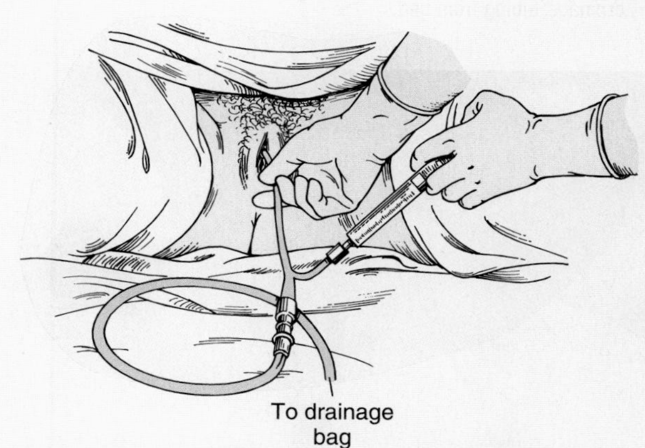

STEP 19c Inflating balloon (indwelling catheter).

SKILL 46-2 INSERTING AND REMOVING A STRAIGHT (INTERMITTENT) OR INDWELLING CATHETER—cont'd

STEP	RATIONALE
20. Secure catheter with catheter securement device at catheter bifurcation (see manufacturer directions). Allow enough slack to allow leg movement and avoid any traction on catheter (see illustration).	Securing indwelling catheters reduces risk of urethral trauma, urethral erosion, CAUTI, or accidental removal (Callan et al., 2012; Cipa-Tatum and Kelly-Signs, 2011; Gould et al., 2009).
a. Female Patient: Secure catheter tubing to inner thigh.	
b. Male Patient: Secure catheter tubing to top of thigh or lower abdomen (with penis directed toward chest).	
21. Clip drainage tubing to edge of mattress. Position drainage bag lower than bladder by attaching to bedframe. Do not attach to side rails of bed (see illustration).	Drainage bags that are below level of bladder ensure free flow of urine, thus decreasing risk for CAUTI (Gould et al., 2009). Bags attached to movable objects such as a side rail increase risk for urethral trauma because of pulling or accidental dislodgement (Gould et al., 2009).
22. Check to make sure that there is no obstruction to urine flow. Coil excess tubing on bed and fasten to bottom sheet with clip or other securement device.	Obstruction prevents free flow of urine and increases risk for CAUTI (Geng et al., 2012; Gould et al., 2009).
23. Provide hygiene as needed. Help patient to comfortable position.	
24. Dispose of used equipment in appropriate receptacles.	Reduces transmission of microorganisms.
25. Label specimen container correctly for culture with patient present, place in biohazard container, and send to laboratory with completed requisition.	Ensures prompt diagnostic analysis.
26. Measure urine and record.	
27. Remove gloves and perform hand hygiene.	
28. Removal of indwelling Foley catheter:	
a. Review medical order for removal of catheter. In cases of genitourinary surgery, it is especially important to obtain an order.	Premature removal of catheter inpatients who have undergone GU surgery could injure patient.
b. Perform hand hygiene, put on clean gloves, and provide privacy.	Procedure requires use of medical asepsis.
c. Prepare the patient:	
(1) Provide an explanation of procedure.	Prepares patient to minimize anxiety.
(2) Position patient with waterproof pad under buttocks and cover with bath blanket, exposing only genital area and catheter. Position females in dorsal recumbent position and male patients in supine position.	Shows respect for patient dignity by only exposing genital area and catheter.
(3) Remove catheter securement device and free drainage tubing.	
d. If needed provide hygiene of genital area with soap and water.	Antiseptic cleaners have not been proven to decrease risk for CAUTI (Geng et al., 2012; Gould et al., 2009).
e. Move syringe plunger up and down to loosen and then withdraw plunger to 0.5 mL. Insert hub of syringe into inflation valve (balloon port). Allow balloon fluid to drain into syringe by gravity. Make sure that entire amount of fluid is removed by comparing removed amount to volume needed for inflation.	Partially inflated balloon can traumatize urethral wall during removal. Passive drainage of catheter balloon will prevent formation of ridges in balloon. These ridges can cause discomfort or trauma during removal.
f. Pull catheter out smoothly and slowly. Examine it to ensure that it is whole. Catheter should slide out easily. Do not use force. If you note any resistance, repeat Step 28e to remove remaining water. Notify health care provider if balloon does not deflate completely.	Promotes patient comfort and safety.
g. Wrap contaminated catheter in waterproof pad. Unhook collection bag and drainage tubing from bed.	Prevents transmission of microorganisms.

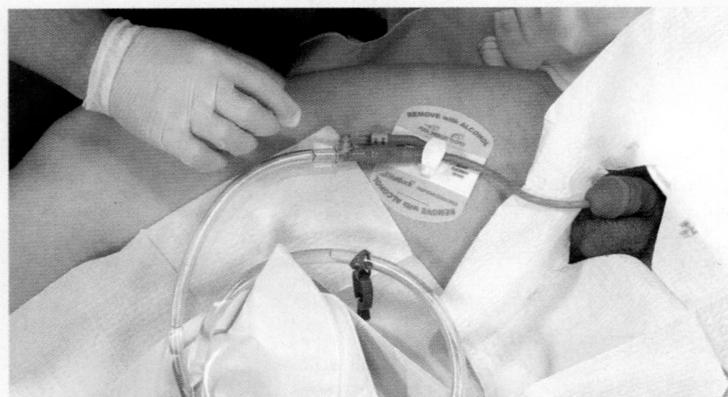

STEP 20 Catheter securement device. (Copyright © Mosby's Clinical Skills: Essentials Collection.)

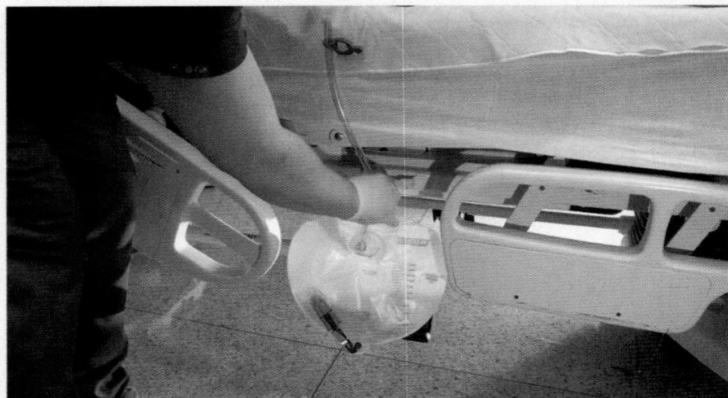

STEP 21 Drainage bag below level of bladder, connected to bedframe. (Copyright © Mosby's Clinical Skills: Essentials Collection.)

STEP	RATIONALE
h. Reposition patient as necessary. Provide hygiene as needed. Lower level of bed and position side rails accordingly	
i. Empty, measure, and record urine present in drainage bag. Discard in appropriate receptacle. Remove and discard gloves. Perform hand hygiene.	Records urinary output. Reduces transmission of microorganisms.
j. Encourage patient to maintain or increase fluid intake (unless contraindicated).	Maintains normal urine output.
k. Initiate voiding record or bladder diary. Instruct patient to report when urge to void occurs and that all urine needs to be measured. Make sure that patient understands how to use collection container.	Evaluates bladder function.
l. Ensure easy access to toilet, commode, bedpan, or urinal. Place urine "hat" on toilet seat if patient is using toilet. Place call bell within easy reach.	
EVALUATION	
1. Intermittent catheter:	
a. Palpate bladder for distention.	Determines if distention is relieved.
b. Ask patient to describe level of comfort.	Determines if patient's sensation of discomfort or bladder fullness has been relieved.
2. Indwelling catheter:	
a. Observe character and amount of urine in drainage system.	Determines if urine is flowing adequately.
b. Determine that no urine is leaking from catheter or tubing connections.	Prevents injury to patient's skin and ensures closed sterile system.
3. Observe time and measure amount of first voiding after catheter removal.	Indicates return of bladder function after catheter removal.
4. Evaluate patient for signs and symptoms of urinary tract infection.	Any patient with an indwelling catheter, who has recently had a catheter removed, or who has been catheterized recently is at risk for infection.
5. Use ***Teach Back*** to determine patient's and family's understanding about catheterization. State, "I want to be sure that I explained to you how you can help keep this catheter draining correctly. Can you explain to me the ways you can keep the catheter draining so urine can flow out the catheter?" Revise your instruction now or develop plan for revised patient teaching if patient is not able to teach back correctly.	Evaluates what patient and family are able to explain or demonstrate.

UNEXPECTED OUTCOMES AND RELATED INTERVENTIONS

1. Patient complains of bladder discomfort and/or catheter leaking.
   - Check catheter for kinking or bending causing occlusion of flow.
   - Check catheter to ensure that there is no traction/pulling on it.
   - Assess for signs of infection.
   - Notify health care provider. Patient may be experiencing bladder spasms or symptoms of a urinary tract infection.
2. Adult patient exhibits one or more of the following: fever, chills, burning sensation, flank pain, back pain, hematuria, painful urination, urgency, frequency, lower abdominal pain, change in mental status, lethargy (Gupta and Hooton, 2011; Hooton and Bradley, 2010).
   - Monitor vital signs and urine output.
   - Report findings to health care provider; signs and symptoms may indicate a urinary tract infection.
3. Older adults, particularly those with underlying cognitive impairments, may exhibit one or more of the following: cognitive changes, lethargy, anorexia, and more generalized symptoms (Matthews and Lancaster, 2011).
   - Monitor vital signs and urine output.
   - Report findings to health care provider; signs and symptoms may indicate a urinary tract infection.
4. Patient is unable to void after catheter removal, has a sensation of not emptying, strains to void, or experiences small voiding amounts with increasing frequency.
   - Assess for bladder distention.
   - Help to a normal position for voiding.
   - Provide privacy for voiding.
   - Perform bladder scan or ultrasound (if available) to assess for excessive urine volume in bladder.
   - If patient unable to void within 6 to 8 hours of catheter removal and/or experiences abdominal pain, notify health care provider.

RECORDING AND REPORTING

- Report and record type and size of catheter inserted, amount of fluid used to inflate the balloon, characteristics and amount of urine, and reasons for catheterization and specimen collection if appropriate.
- Document your evaluation of patient learning.
- Initiate intake and output (I&O) record.
- Report and record time of catheter removal and time, amount, and characteristics of first voiding.
- Report hematuria, dysuria, inability or difficulty voiding, or incontinence after catheter removal.

SKILL 46-2 INSERTING AND REMOVING A STRAIGHT (INTERMITTENT) OR INDWELLING CATHETER—cont'd

HOME CARE CONSIDERATIONS

- Patients who are at home may use a leg bag during the day and switch to a larger-volume bag at night. If a patient changes from a large-volume bag to a leg bag, instruct in the importance of handwashing and cleansing the connection ports with alcohol before changing bags.
- Teach patients and family caregivers how to properly position the drainage bag, empty a urinary drainage bag, and observe urine color, clarity, odor, and amount.
- Educate patients and/or caregivers about the signs of UTI and troubleshooting techniques for a leaking catheter.
- Arrange for home delivery of catheter supplies, always ensuring that there is at least one extra catheter, insertion kit, and drainage bag in the home.

SKILL 46-3 INDWELLING CATHETER CARE

DELEGATION CONSIDERATIONS

The skill of perineal care is often part of routine hygiene care that can be delegated to nursing assistive personnel (NAP). Proper assessment and care of the perineal area is the responsibility of the nurse. If patient has had trauma or surgical procedures that involve the perineal area, do not delegate this care.

The nurse instructs the NAP to:

- Report patient discomfort and perineal pain, discharge, perineal rash, and/or odor.
- Report condition of the catheter and drainage tubing (e.g., leaks, encrustations).
- Report any discolored or foul-smelling urine.

EQUIPMENT

- Clean gloves
- Clean washcloth and towel
- Warm water and soap
- Bath blanket
- Waterproof absorbent pad
- Antiseptic swab or cloth (e.g., chlorhexidine) (optional)

STEP	RATIONALE
ASSESSMENT	
1. Identify patient using two identifiers (e.g., name and birthday or name and medical record number) according to agency policy.	Ensures correct patient. Complies with The Joint Commission standards and improves patient safety (TJC, 2016).
2. Perform hand hygiene and apply gloves (**NOTE:** This assessment can be completed just prior to cleansing). Assess urethral meatus and surrounding tissues for inflammation, swelling, secretions, and tissue trauma. Assess catheter for presence of debris or crusting. Remove gloves and perform hand hygiene.	Redness, swelling, and inflammation may indicate that there is urine leakage around catheter. Tissue trauma, especially near the meatus, indicates trauma from catheter pulling and rubbing. Debris or crusting on catheter indicates need for more frequent catheter hygiene.
3. Assess urine for color, clarity, and odor.	Cloudy and foul-smelling urine may indicate infection.
4. Assess for presence of fever, chills, burning, flank pain, back pain, blood in urine, lower abdominal pain, change in mental status and/or lethargy (Gupta et al., 2011; Hooton et al., 2010).	Signs and symptoms indicate catheter-associated urinary tract infection (CAUTI):
5. Assess patient's knowledge of and experience with catheter care.	Patients who perform their own catheter care may be uncomfortable or unsure of touching catheter. Assesses patient's ability and knowledge to provide instruction as needed.
PLANNING	
1. Explain procedure to patient. Offer patient opportunity to perform self-care.	Reduces anxiety and promotes cooperation.
2. Gather supplies.	Ensures organized procedure.
IMPLEMENTATION	
1. Perform hand hygiene and apply clean gloves.	Reduces transmission of microorganisms.
2. Provide privacy by closing curtains around bed and closing door.	Reduces embarrassment for patient.
3. Position patient:	Ensures easy access and visualization of perineal tissues.
a. **Female**	
(1) Dorsal recumbent position	
b. **Male**	
(1) Supine or Fowler's position	
4. Place waterproof pad under patient.	Protects bed linens from soiling.
5. Drape bath blanket on patient so only perineal area is exposed.	Prevents unnecessary exposure of body parts.
6. Provide perineal care (see Chapter 40). Dispose of gloves and perform hand hygiene.	Cleans area surrounding catheter of secretions, soiling.
7. Apply clean gloves.	Reduces transmission of microorganisms.
8. Remove catheter tubing from securing device.	Allows access of tubing for cleansing.

STEP	RATIONALE
9. With nondominant hand:	
a. Female	
(1) Gently retract labia to fully expose urethral meatus and catheter; maintain position of hand throughout procedure.	Provides full visualization of urethral meatus. Full retraction of labia prevents contamination of meatus during cleaning.
b. Male	
(1) Retract foreskin if not circumcised and hold penis at shaft just below glans; maintain position throughout procedure.	Retraction of foreskin provides full visualization of urethral meatus.
c. Grasp catheter with two fingers to stabilize it near meatus.	Secures catheter during cleaning.
10. Using clean washcloth, soap, and water, with your dominant hand wipe in a circular motion along length of catheter for about 10 cm (4 inches), starting at meatus and moving away (see illustration). Avoid placing tension on or pulling on exposed catheter tubing. Make sure to remove all traces of soap. If applicable, return the foreskin to down position.	Reduces presence of secretions, drainage, and bacteria on exterior of catheter surface. Formation of biofilms by urinary pathogens is common on the surfaces of catheters and collecting systems (CDC, 2015).

CLINICAL DECISION: *Some hospitals use antiseptic cloths or pads containing chlorhexidine to wipe off catheter tubing. Check agency policy.*

STEP	RATIONALE
11. Reapply catheter securement device at area of catheter bifurcation (see manufacturer instructions). Catheter should not slide, and there should be some slack in it.	Catheter movement and traction (pulling) increases risk for local trauma to urethra, urinary meatus, and bladder (Cipa-Tatum and Kelly-Signs, 2011; Geng et al., 2012; Gould et al., 2009). In long-term catheter use, catheter traction can lead to formation of pressure ulcer in urinary meatus (Rassin and Markovski, 2013).
12. Place patient in safe, comfortable position.	Promotes comfort.
13. Dispose of contaminated supplies, remove gloves, and perform hand hygiene.	Prevents spread of infection.

EVALUATION

STEP	RATIONALE
1. Check drainage tubing and bag to ensure that drainage bag is positioned below level of bladder and that there are no kinks in drainage tubing.	Prevents CAUTI (Cipa-Tatum and Kelly-Signs, 2011).
2. Use ***Teach Back*** to determine patient's understanding about peri-care. State, "We talked about the importance of preventing infection while you have a catheter. Can you tell me ways we try to prevent you from getting a urine infection?" Revise your instruction now or develop plan for revised patient teaching if patient is not able to teach back correctly	Evaluates what the patient is able to explain or demonstrate.

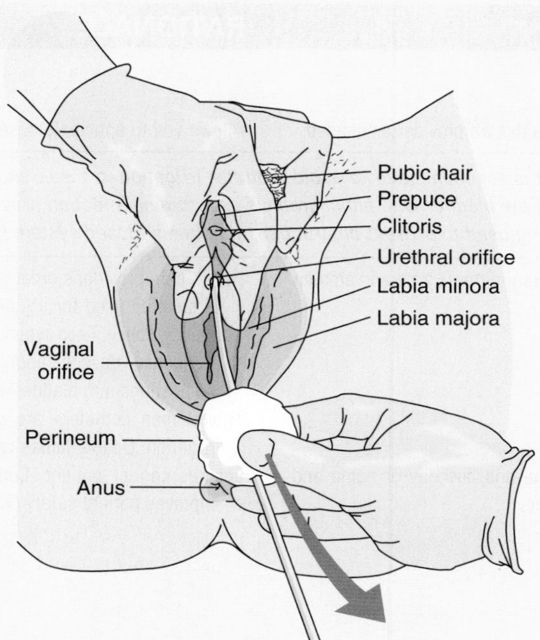

STEP 10 Cleaning catheter during catheter care. (From Sorrentino S: *Mosby's textbook for nursing assistants*, St Louis, 2007, Mosby.)

SKILL 46-3 INDWELLING CATHETER CARE—cont'd

UNEXPECTED OUTCOMES AND RELATED INTERVENTIONS

1. Urethral discharge or perineal irritation is present.
   - Observe for leaking from around catheter; catheter may need replacing.
   - Increase frequency of indwelling catheter care.
   - Notify health care provider.
2. Catheter is dislodged accidentally.
   - Notify health care provider.
   - Assess for urethral trauma.
   - Monitor urine output.

RECORDING AND REPORTING

- Report and record presence and characteristics of drainage, condition of perineal tissue, and any discomfort reported by patient.
- If infection is suspected, report findings to health care provider.
- Document your evaluation of patient learning.

HOME CARE CONSIDERATIONS

- If patient is discharged with indwelling catheter, teach patient and family catheter care and signs and symptoms to report to nurse or health care provider.

SKILL 46-4 CLOSED CATHETER IRRIGATION

DELEGATION CONSIDERATIONS

The skill of catheter irrigation or instillation cannot be delegated to nursing assistive personnel (NAP). Direct the NAP to:

- Report patient complaints of abdominal pain or discomfort, fever, chills, and leakage of urine around catheter.
- Report presence of blood clots or change in color of urine.
- Monitor and record intake and output (I&O); immediately report any decrease or absence of urinary output.

EQUIPMENT

Closed Intermittent Irrigation

- Antiseptic swabs
- Sterile irrigation solution at room temperature as prescribed
- Sterile container
- Syringe to access system: Luer-Lok syringe without needle for needleless access port (per manufacturer directions)
- Screw clamp or rubber band (used to temporarily occlude catheter as irrigant is instilled)

Closed Continuous Irrigation

- Antiseptic swabs
- Sterile irrigation solution at room temperature (as prescribed)
- Irrigation tubing with clamp to regulate irrigation flow rate
- Y connector (optional) to connect irrigation tubing to double-lumen catheter
- Intravenous (IV) pole (closed continuous or intermittent)

STEP	RATIONALE
ASSESSMENT	
1. Review patient's record to determine:	
a. Purpose of bladder irrigation. Confer with health care provider as needed.	Allows you to anticipate observations to make (e.g., blood or mucus in urine).

CLINICAL DECISION: *It is recommended to avoid catheter irrigation in these situations: Do not perform continuous irrigation of the bladder with antimicrobials as a routine infection prevention measure. If continuous irrigation is being used to prevent obstruction, maintain a closed system (Lo et al., 2014).*

STEP	RATIONALE
b. Prescriber's order for method (continuous or intermittent), type and amount of irrigant (e.g., saline, medicated solutions).	Health care provider's order is required to initiate therapy. Frequency and volume of solution used for irrigation may be in the order or standardized as part of agency policy. Each type of irrigation requires different equipment. Procedure (frequency, dosage, and duration of time dwelling in bladder) for instilling medications into bladder are specific to medication.
c. Type of catheter used (see Figure 46-10).	Triple-lumen catheters are used for both intermittent and continuous closed irrigation. Double-lumen catheters can only be used for intermittent irrigation.
2. Identify patient using two identifiers (e.g., name and birthday or name and medical record number) according to agency policy.	Ensures correct patient. Complies with The Joint Commission standards and improves patient safety (TJC, 2016).

STEP	RATIONALE
3. Assess patient:	
a. Perform hand hygiene and apply gloves.	Reduces transmission of microorganisms.
b. Inspect urine for color, amount, and clarity and presence of mucus, blood clots, or sediment.	Indicates if patient is bleeding or sloughing tissue, which would require increased irrigation rate or frequency of catheter irrigation.
c. Palpate bladder for distention and tenderness.	Bladder distention and tenderness may indicate that urine is not draining freely from bladder. Make sure there is free flow of urine through catheter drainage tubing (e.g., tubing kinked, occlusion with mucus or blood clots).
d. Observe patient for abdominal pain, spasms, sensation of bladder fullness or catheter bypassing (leaking).	May indicate overdistention of bladder caused by blockage of catheter. Offers baseline to determine if therapy is successful.
4. Review input and I&O record.	If continuous bladder irrigation (CBI) is being used, amount of fluid draining from bladder should exceed amount of fluid infused into bladder. If output does not exceed irrigant infused, catheter obstruction (i.e., blood clots, kinked tubing) should be suspected, irrigation stopped, and prescriber notified.
5. Remove gloves and perform hand hygiene.	Reduces transmission of microorganisms.
6. Assess patient's knowledge and experience regarding purpose of performing catheter irrigations.	Reveals extent of patient instruction needed.
PLANNING	
1. Gather supplies needed for catheter irrigation.	Type of irrigation indicates supplies needed to take into patient's room.
2. Explain procedure to patient.	Reduces anxiety and promotes cooperation.
IMPLEMENTATION	
1. Perform hand hygiene and apply clean gloves.	Reduces transmission of microorganisms.
2. Provide privacy by closing room door and bed curtains.	Protects patient confidentiality.
3. Raise bed to appropriate working height. If side rails are raised, lower side rail on working side.	Promotes use of good body mechanics and patient safety.
4. Position patient in dorsal recumbent or supine position and expose catheter junctions (catheter and drainage tubing).	Position provides access to catheter and promotes patient dignity as much as possible.
5. Remove catheter securement device.	Eases access to catheter irrigation ports.
6. Organize supplies according to type of irrigation prescribed.	Ensures easy access to supplies during procedure.
7. Closed intermittent irrigation or instillation with double-lumen catheter:	

CLINICAL DECISION: *Closed intermittent irrigation should be done only in cases in which catheter is occluded and health care provider deems that removal of catheter can injure patient.*

STEP	RATIONALE
a. Draw up in syringe prescribed amount of medication or sterile solution. Place sterile cap on tip of needleless syringe.	Ensures that irrigation or instillation fluid remains sterile.
b. Clamp indwelling retention catheter just below specimen port.	Occlusion of catheter ensures that irrigation solution goes into bladder not down into drainage tubing.

CLINICAL DECISION: *Avoid irrigating with or instilling cold solution because it results in bladder spasm and discomfort.*

STEP	RATIONALE
c. Using circular motion, thoroughly clean injection port with antiseptic swab (same port used for specimen collection). Allow to dry.	Reduces transmission of infection. Drying achieves full antimicrobial properties.
d. Insert tip of needleless syringe with twisting motion into irrigation port (see manufacturer instructions for possible variation).	Ensures that hub enters lumen of catheter and flow is directed into bladder.
e. Slowly and evenly inject fluid into catheter and bladder.	Slow injection minimizes potential trauma to bladder mucosa.

CLINICAL DECISION: *If catheter does not irrigate easily, stop the irrigation. The catheter may be totally occluded, or the end of the catheter may have been displaced into the urethra. Contact the prescriber; the catheter may need to be removed and replaced.*

STEP	RATIONALE
f. Withdraw syringe, cleanse port with antiseptic swab, remove clamp, and allow solution to drain into drainage bag. Some medicated irrigants may need to dwell in bladder for a prescribed period of time, requiring catheter to be clamped temporarily.	Allows drainage by gravity. Some irrigation solutions require time in catheter and bladder to exert therapeutic effect. Clamped catheters should not be left unattended.

SKILL 46-4 CLOSED CATHETER IRRIGATION—cont'd

STEP	RATIONALE
8. Closed continuous irrigation (see illustration).	
a. Close clamp on tubing and hang bag of solution on intravenous (IV) pole. Insert (spike) tip of sterile irrigation tubing into designated port of irrigation solution bag using aseptic technique.	Closing clamp on tubing allows tubing drip chamber to fill after tip of tubing is inserted into port of irrigation solution bag.
b. Fill drip chamber half full by squeezing chamber; then open clamp and allow solution to flow (prime) through tubing, keeping end of tubing sterile. Once fluid has completely filled tubing, close clamp and recap end of tubing.	Priming tubing with fluid prevents introduction of air into bladder.
c. Use aseptic technique to wipe off irrigation port of triple-lumen catheter and attach to irrigation tubing.	Third lumen provides means for irrigation solution to enter bladder.
d. Be sure that drainage bag and tubing are securely connected to drainage port of triple-lumen catheter.	Ensures that urine and irrigation solution drain from bladder without leaking.
e. Calculate drip rate and adjust rate at roller clamp. If urine is bright red or has clots, increase irrigation rate until drainage appears pink (according to ordered rate or agency protocol).	Continuous drainage is expected. It helps with prevention of clotting in presence of active bleeding in bladder and flushes blood clots out of bladder.
f. Observe for outflow of fluid into drainage bag. Empty catheter drainage bag as needed.	Discomfort, bladder distention, and possibly injury can occur from overdistention of bladder when bladder irrigant cannot adequately flow from bladder. Bag will fill rapidly and may need to be emptied every 1 to 2 hours.
g. Compare urine output with infusion of irrigation solution every hour.	Determines urinary output and ensures that irrigant is draining freely.
9. When procedure is completed, dispose of contaminated supplies in appropriate receptacle, replace catheter securement device if removed, remove gloves, help patient to safe and comfortable position with bed in low position, and perform hand hygiene.	Promotes patient comfort and safety and reduces transmission of microorganisms.

EVALUATION

STEP	RATIONALE
1. Measure actual urine output by subtracting total amount of irrigation fluid infused from total volume drained.	Determines accurate urinary output.
2. Review I&O flow sheet to verify that hourly output into drainage bag is in appropriate proportion to irrigating solution entering bladder. Expect more output than fluid instilled because of urine production.	Determines urinary output in relation to irrigation.

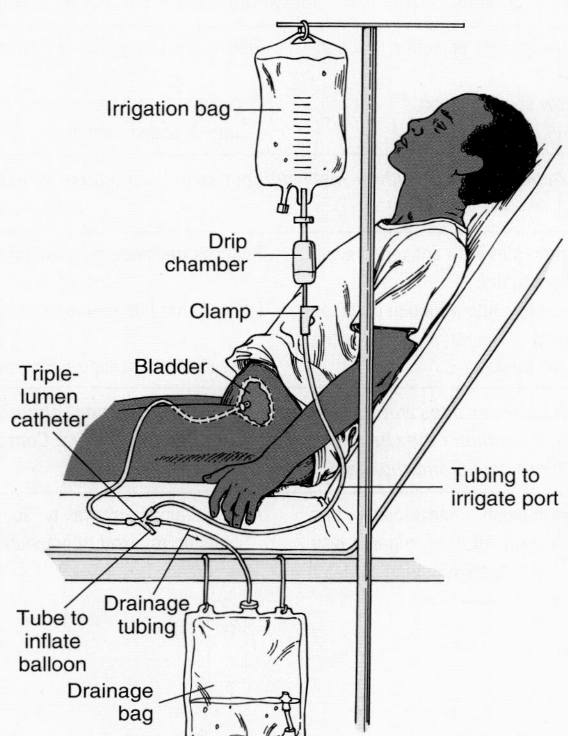

STEP 8 Closed continuous bladder irrigation.

STEP	RATIONALE
3. Observe for catheter patency, inspect urine for blood clots and sediment, and ensure that tubing is not kinked or occluded.	Decrease in blood clots means that therapy is successful in maintaining catheter patency. Ensures that bladder is emptying freely.
4. Assess patient comfort.	An indicator of catheter patency by absence of symptoms of bladder distention.
5. Assess for signs and symptoms of infection.	Evaluates for presence of infection.
6. Use ***Teach Back*** to determine patient's understanding about irrigation. State, "I want to go over the reason we discussed about why we are irrigating your urinary catheter. Can you tell me the reason we need to irrigate it?" Revise your instruction now or develop plan for revised patient teaching if patient is not able to teach back correctly.	Evaluates what the patient is able to explain or demonstrate.

UNEXPECTED OUTCOMES AND RELATED INTERVENTIONS

1. Irrigating solution does not return (intermittent irrigation); drainage is less than amount of irrigation solution infused or is not flowing at prescribed rate (CBI).
   - Examine tubing for clots, sediment, and kinks.
   - Inspect urine for presence of or increase in blood clots and sediment.
   - Evaluate patient for pain and distended bladder.
   - Notify health care provider if irrigant does not flow freely from the bladder, patient complains of pain, or bladder distention occurs.
2. Bright-red bleeding with irrigation (CBI) drip is wide open.
   - Assess for hypovolemic shock (vital signs, skin color and moisture, anxiety level).
   - Leave irrigation drip wide open and notify health care provider.
3. Patient experiences pain with irrigation.
   - Examine drainage tubing for clots, sediment, or kinks.
   - Evaluate urine for presence of or increase in blood clots and sediment.
   - Evaluate for distended bladder.
   - Notify health care provider.

RECORDING AND REPORTING

- Record irrigation method, amount of and type of irrigation solution, amount returned as drainage, characteristics of output, and urine output.
- Report catheter occlusion, sudden bleeding, infection, or increased pain.
- Record I&O.
- Document your evaluation of patient learning.

HOME CARE CONSIDERATIONS

- Patients and/or family caregivers can be taught to perform catheter irrigations with adequate support, demonstration/return demonstration, and written instructions.
- Teach patients and/or family caregivers to observe urine color, clarity, odor, and amount.
- Arrange for home delivery and storage of catheter/irrigation supplies.
- Teach patients and/or family caregivers signs of catheter obstruction or urinary tract infection.

KEY POINTS

- Micturition involves complex interactions between the central nervous system, bladder, and urinary sphincter.
- Common urinary tract symptoms include urgency, dysuria, frequency, hesitancy, polyuria, oliguria, nocturia, dribbling, hematuria, and urinary retention.
- Nursing care for patients with urinary dysfunction needs to take into account multiple factors that affect urinary function such as fluid intake, medications, functional ability, environment, medical problems outside the urinary tract, and dysfunction within the urinary tract.
- The most common size for an indwelling catheter in adults is 14-16 Fr and a 10-mL balloon.
- The presence or recent history of an indwelling catheter increases risk for a UTI.
- Prevention of catheter associated urinary tract infection (CAUTI) requires use of an evidence based "bundle" to perform all elements of care at one time.
- To minimize the risk for infection when caring for a patient with a closed bladder drainage system, nursing care must include careful attention to aseptic technique.
- Planning care for an incontinent patient requires selecting interventions specific to the type of incontinence.
- A key intervention when caring for an incontinent patient is to ensure regular toilet access.

CLINICAL APPLICATION QUESTIONS

Preparing for Clinical Practice

Mrs. Grayson is a 75-year-old woman who has had problems with urge incontinence for the past 2 years. She has not spoken to anyone about her problems because she is embarrassed. She finally confides to her health care practitioner that the problem is causing her to avoid social situations and she would like help to regain urinary control. Mrs. Grayson has type 2 diabetes and is obese. She has been referred to a continence specialist. A plan of care was developed after a thorough assessment of her urinary pattern and symptoms.

1. She has recently begun pelvic muscle exercises (Kegel) and bladder retraining. She shares her concern that the exercises are not working and that she is still wet multiple times a day. Which additional teaching does Mrs. Grayson need?
2. Two months after your first encounter with Mrs. Grayson, she has been seen by her primary health care provider for burning on urination associated with increased incontinence, frequency, and urgency. She was treated with an antibiotic. Which health teaching does Mrs. Grayson need now?
3. Mrs. Grayson is seen in the emergency department for a fever, hematuria, and elevated postvoid residual (PVR). She is treated for a urinary tract infection (UTI). Which ongoing assessment is needed?

ⓔ ***Answers to Clinical Application Questions can be found on the Evolve website.***

REVIEW QUESTIONS

Are You Ready to Test Your Nursing Knowledge?

1. A patient is scheduled to have an intravenous pyelogram (IVP) the next morning. Which nursing measures should be implemented before the test? (Select all that apply.)
   1. Ask the patient about any allergies and reactions.
   2. Instruct the patient that a full bladder is required for the test.
   3. Instruct the patient to save all urine in a special container.
   4. Ensure that informed consent has been obtained.
   5. Explain that the test includes instrumentation of the urinary tract.
2. When assessing a patient's first voided urine of the day, which finding should be reported to the health care provider?
   1. Pale yellow urine
   2. Slightly cloudy urine
   3. Light pink urine
   4. Dark amber urine
3. What is a critical step when inserting an indwelling catheter into a male patient?
   1. Slowly inflate the catheter balloon with sterile saline.
   2. Secure the catheter drainage tubing to the bed sheets.
   3. Advance the catheter to the bifurcation of the drainage and balloon ports.
   4. Advance the catheter until urine flows, then insert ¼ inch more.
4. Which nursing intervention minimizes the risk for trauma and infection when applying an external/condom catheter?
   1. Leaving a gap of 3 to 5 inches between the tip of the penis and drainage tube
   2. Shaving the pubic area so hair does not adhere
   3. Washing with soap and water before applying the condom-type catheter
   4. Applying tape to the condom sheath to keep it securely in place
5. Which instructions should the nurse give the nursing assistive personnel (NAP) concerning a patient who has had an indwelling urinary catheter removed that day?
   1. Limit oral fluid intake to avoid possible urinary incontinence.
   2. Expect patient complaints of suprapubic fullness and discomfort.
   3. Report the time and amount of first voiding.
   4. Instruct patient to stay in bed and use a urinal or bedpan.
6. A postoperative patient with a three-way indwelling urinary catheter and continuous bladder irrigation (CBI) complains of lower abdominal pain and distention. What should be the nurse's *initial* intervention?
   1. Increase the rate of the CBI
   2. Assess the intake and output from system
   3. Decrease the rate of the CBI
   4. Assess vital signs
7. An ambulatory elderly woman with dementia is incontinent of urine. She has poor short-term memory and has not been seen toileting independently. What is the *best* nursing intervention for this patient?
   1. Recommend that she be evaluated for an overactive bladder (OAB) medication
   2. Start a scheduled toileting program
   3. Recommend that she be evaluated for an indwelling catheter
   4. Start a bladder-retraining program
8. What should the nurse teach a young woman with a history of urinary tract infections (UTIs) about UTI prevention? (Select all that apply.)
   1. Keep the bowels regular.
   2. Limit water intake to 1 to 2 glasses a day.
   3. Wear cotton underwear.
   4. Cleanse the perineum from front to back.
   5. Practice pelvic muscle exercise (Kegel) daily.
9. Which nursing assessment question would *best* indicate that an incontinent man with a history of prostate enlargement might not be emptying his bladder adequately?
   1. Do you leak urine when you cough or sneeze?
   2. Do you need help getting to the toilet?
   3. Do you dribble urine constantly?
   4. Does it burn when you pass your urine?
10. Place the following steps for insertion of an indwelling catheter in a female patient in appropriate order.
    1. Insert and advance catheter.
    2. Lubricate catheter.
    3. Inflate catheter balloon.
    4. Cleanse urethral meatus with antiseptic solution.
    5. Drape patient with the sterile square and fenestrated drapes.
    6. When urine appears, advance another 2.5 to 5 cm.
    7. Prepare sterile field and supplies.
    8. Gently pull catheter until resistance is felt.
    9. Attach drainage tubing.
11. The nursing assistive personnel (NAP) reports to the nurse that a patient's catheter drainage bag has been empty for 4 hours. What is a priority nursing intervention?
    1. Implement the "as-needed" order to irrigate the catheter
    2. Assess the catheter and drainage tubing for obvious occlusion
    3. Notify the health care provider immediately
    4. Assess the vital signs and intake and output record
12. Which nursing interventions should a nurse implement when removing an indwelling urinary catheter in an adult patient? (Select all that apply.)
    1. Attach a 3-mL syringe to the inflation port
    2. Allow the balloon to drain into the syringe by gravity
    3. Initiate a voiding record/bladder diary
    4. Pull the catheter quickly
    5. Clamp the catheter before removal
13. What best describes measurement of postvoid residual (PVR)?
    1. Bladder scan the patient immediately after voiding.
    2. Catheterize the patient 30 minutes after voiding.
    3. Bladder scan the patient when he or she reports a strong urge to void.
    4. Catheterize the patient with a 16 Fr/10 mL catheter.

14. Which nursing intervention decreases the risk for catheter-associated urinary tract infection (CAUTI)?
    1. Cleansing the urinary meatus 3 to 4 times daily with antiseptic solution
    2. Hanging the urinary drainage bag below the level of the bladder
    3. Emptying the urinary drainage bag daily
    4. Irrigating the urinary catheter with sterile water
15. There is no urine when a catheter is inserted 3 inches into a female's urethra. What should the nurse do next?
    1. Remove the catheter and start all over with a new kit and catheter
    2. Leave the catheter there and start over with a new catheter
    3. Pull the catheter back and reinsert at a different angle
    4. Ask the patient to bear down and insert the catheter further

Answers: 1. 1, 4; **2.** 3; **3.** 3; **4.** 3; **5.** 3; **6.** 2; **7.** 2; **8.** 1, 3, 4; **9.** 3; **10.** 5, 7, 2, 4, 1, 6, 3, 8, 9; **11.** 2; **12.** 2, 3; **13.** 1; **14.** 2; **15.** 2.

ⓔ ***Rationales for Review Questions can be found on the Evolve website.***

REFERENCES

Ackley BJ, Ladwig GB: *Nursing diagnosis handbook: a guide for planning care*, ed 9, St Louis, 2011, Mosby.

American Academy of Pediatrics: Ritual genital cutting of female minors, *Pediatrics* 125(5):1088, 2010.

American Geriatrics Society 2012 Beers Criteria Update Expert Panel: American Geriatrics Society updated Beers criteria for potentially inappropriate medication use in older adults, *J Am Geriatr Soc* 60(4):616, 2012.

Association for Professionals in Infection Control and Epidemiology (APIC): *APIC Implementation Guide: Guide to preventing catheter-associated urinary tract infections*, 2014, http://apic.org/Resource_/EliminationGuideForm/6473ab9b-e75c-457a-8d0f-d57d32bc242b/File/APIC_CAUTI_web_0603.pdf. Accessed December 2015.

Ball JW, Dains J: *Seidel's Guide to physical examination*, ed 8, St Louis, 2015, Mosby.

Beji NK, et al: Overview of the social impact of urinary incontinence with a focus on Turkish women, *Urol Nurs* 30(6):327, 2010.

Bettez M, et al: 2012 Update: Guidelines for adult urinary incontinence collaborative consensus document for the Canadian urological association, *Can Urol Assoc J* 6(35):354, 2012.

Burchum JR, Rosenthal LD: *Lehne's Pharmacology for nursing care*, ed 9, St Louis, 2016, Elsevier.

Callan L, et al: *Indwelling urinary catheter securement: best practice for clinicians*, Mount Laurel, NJ, 2012, Wound, Ostomy and Continence Nurses Society.

Centers for Disease Control and Prevention (CDC): *Catheter-associated urinary tract infection (CAUTI) toolkit*, 2015 http://www.cdc.gov/HAI/prevent/prevention_tools.html. Accessed December 6, 2015.

Cipa-Tatum J, Kelly-Signs M: Urethral erosion: a case for prevention, *J Wound Ostomy Continence Nurs* 38(5):581, 2011.

Cottenden A, et al: Management using continence products. In Abrams P, et al, editors: *Incontinence, 2013*, ed 5, Paris, France, 2013, ICUD-EAU, p 1661.

Doughty D, et al: Incontinence-associated dermatitis: consensus statements, evidence-based guidelines for preventions and treatment, and current challenges, *J Wound Ostomy Continence Nurs* 39(3):303, 2012.

Dumoulin C, et al: Determining the optimal pelvic floor muscle training regimen for women with stress urinary incontinence, *Neurourol Urodynam* 30:746, 2011.

Elsamara SE, Ellsworth P: Effects of analgesic and anesthetic medications on lower urinary tract function, *Urol Nurs* 32(2):67, 2012.

Gemmill R, Wells A: Promotion of urinary continence worldwide, *Urol Nurs* 30(6):336, 2010.

Geng V, et al: *Good practice in health care continent urinary diversion*, European Association of Urology Nurses, 2010, http://nurses.uroweb/wp-content/uploads/0628EAUN_Guideline_2010_HR.pdf. Accessed December 2015.

Geng V, et al: *Catheterisation: indwelling catheters in adults: urethral and suprapubic*, Arnhern (The Netherlands): European Association of Urology Nurses (EAUN), 2012, http://www.guideline.gov/content.aspx?id=36631. Accessed December 2015.

Gomelsky A, Dmochowski RR: Urinary incontinence in the aging female, *Aging Health* 7(1):79, 2011.

Gormley EA, Lightner DJ: Diagnosis and treatment of overactive bladder (non-neurogenic) in adults: AUA/SUFU Guideline, *J Urol* 18:2455, 2012.

Gould CV, et al: *Guideline for prevention of catheter-associated urinary tract infections*, 2009, http://www.cdc.gov/hicpac/cauti/001_cauti.html. Accessed December 2015.

Gray M: Urinary retention. In Ackley BJ, Ladwig GB, editors: *Nursing diagnosis handbook: a guide for planning care*, ed 9, St Louis, 2011, Mosby.

Gray M, et al: Incontinence-associated dermatitis: a comprehensive review and update, *J Wound Ostomy Continence Nurs* 39(1):61, 2012.

Gupta K, Hooton TM: International clinical practice guidelines for the treatment of acute uncomplicated cystitis and pyelonephritis in women: a 2010 update by the Infectious Disease Society of America and the European Society for Microbiology and Infectious Diseases, *Clin Infect Dis* 52(5):e103, 2011. http://cid.oxfordjournals.org/content/52/5/561.full. Accessed December 2015.

Harris C, Smith PP: Overactive bladder in the older woman, *Clin Geriatr* 18(9):41, 2010.

Hooton TM, Bradley SF: Diagnosis, prevention, and treatment of catheter-associated urinary tract infection in adults: 2009 international clinical practice guidelines from the Infectious Diseases Society of America, *Clin Infect Dis* 50:625, 2010.

Huether SE, McCance KL: *Understanding pathophysiology*, ed 5, St Louis, 2012, Mosby.

Kaufman E, et al: Mythmaking in medical education and medical practice, *Eur J Int Med* 24:222–226, 2013.

Kyle G: The use of urinary sheaths in male incontinence, *Br J Nurs* 20(6):338, 2011.

Lucas MG, et al: *Guidelines on urinary incontinence*, European Association of Urology, 2013, http://www.uroweb.org/gls/pdf/19_Urinary_Incontinence_LR.pdf. Accessed December 2015.

Matthews SJ, Lancaster JW: Urinary tract infections in the elderly population, *Am J Geriatr Pharmacother* 9:286, 2011.

Mendez-Probst C, et al: Fundamentals of instrumentation and urinary tract drainage. In Wein A, et al, editors: *Campbell-Walsh urology*, ed 10, Philadelphia, 2012, Elsevier.

Mody L, Juthani-Mehta M: Urinary tract infections in older women: a clinical review, *JAMA* 311(8):844, 2014.

Moore K, et al: Adult conservative management. In Abrams P, et al, editors: *Incontinence, 2013*, ed 5, Paris, France, 2013, ICUD-EAU, p 1103.

Nicolle LE: Catheter-associated urinary tract infections, *Antimicrob Resist Infect Control* 3(23):2014.

Nobili A, et al: Multiple diseases and polypharmacy in the elderly: challenges for the internist of the third millennium, *J Comorbidity* 1:28, 2011.

Odemerho BI, Baier M: Female genital cutting and the need for culturally competent communication, *J Nurse Pract* 8(6):452, 2012.

Pagana KD, Pagana TJ: *Mosby's diagnostic and laboratory test reference*, ed 11, St Louis, 2013, Mosby.

Qaseem A, Dallas P: Nonsurgical management of urinary incontinence in women: a clinical practice guideline from the American College of Physicians, *Ann Intern Med* 161:429, 2014.

Rassin M, Markovski I: Preventing pressure ulcers in the urinary meatus, *Dimens Crit Care Nurs* 32(2):95, 2013.

Schaeffer AJ, Schaeffer EM: Infections of the urinary tract. In Wein A, et al, editors: *Campbell-Walsh urology*, ed 10, Philadelphia, 2012, Elsevier.

Shamliyan T, et al: *Nonsurgical treatments for urinary incontinence in adult women: diagnosis and comparative effectiveness*, Comparative Effectiveness Review No. 36, Prepared by the University of Minnesota Evidence-Based Practice Center under Contract No. HHSA 290-2007-10064-I, AHRQ Publication No. 11(12)-EHC074-EF, Rockville, MD, 2012, Agency for Healthcare Research and Quality.

Staskin D, et al: Initial assessment of urinary incontinence in adult male and female patients. In Abrams P, et al, editors: *Incontinence, 2013*, ed 5, Paris, France, 2013, ICUD-EAU, p 361.

The Joint Commission (TJC): *2016 National Patient Safety Goals*, Oakbrook Terrace, IL, 2016, The Commission. Available at http://www.jointcommission.org/standards_information/npsgs.aspx. Accessed November 2015.

Touhy TA, Jett KF: *Ebersole and Hess' Gerontological nursing and healthy aging*, ed 4, St Louis, 2014, Elsevier.

Varilla V, et al: Nocturia in the elderly: a wake-up call, *Cleve Clin J Med* 78(11):757, 2011.

RESEARCH REFERENCES

Aguilar-Navarro S, et al: The severity of urinary incontinence decreases health-related quality of life among community-dwelling elderly, *J Gerontol A Biol Sci Med Sci* 67(11):1266, 2012.

Anger JT, et al: Health literacy and disease understanding among aging women with pelvic floor disorders, *Female Pelvic Med Reconstr Surg* 18(6):340, 2012.

Bernard MS, et al: A review of strategies to decrease the duration of indwelling urethral catheters and potentially reduce the incidence of catheter-associated urinary tract infections, *Urol Nurs* 32(1):29, 2012.

Coyne KS, Kvasz M: Urinary incontinence and its relationship to mental health and health-related quality of life in men and women in Sweden, the United Kingdom, and the United States, *Eur Urol* 61(1):88, 2012.

Coyne KS, Wein A: Economic burden of urgency urinary incontinence in the United States: a systemic review, *J Manag Care Pharm* 20(2):130, 2014.

Erekson EA, et al: Functional disability and compromised mobility among older women with urinary incontinence, *Female Pelvic Med Reconstr Surg* 21(3):170, 2015.

Foley AL, et al: Association between the geriatric giants of urinary incontinence and falls in older people using data from the Leicestershire MRC Incontinence Study, *Age Aging* 41:35, 2012.

Hall SA, et al: Associations of commonly used medications with urinary incontinence in a community-based sample, *J Urol* 188(1):183, 2012.

Jura YH, et al: Caffeine intake, and the risk of stress, urgency, and mixed urinary incontinence, *J Urol* 185(5):1775, 2011.

Lo E, et al: Strategies to prevent catheter-associated urinary tract infections in acute care hospitals, *Infect Control Hosp Epidemiol* 35(5):464, 2014.

Lohsiriwat S: Effect of caffeine on bladder function in patients with overactive bladder symptoms, *Urol Ann* 3(1):14, 2011.

Maki DG, Tambyah PA: Engineering out the risk for infection with urinary catheters, *Emerg Infect Dis* 7:342, 2001.

Meddings J, et al: Reducing unnecessary urinary catheter use and other strategies to prevent catheter-associated urinary tract infection: an integrative review, *BMJ Qual Saf* 23:277, 2014.

Mnatzaganian G, et al: Increased risk of bloodstream and urinary infections in intensive care unit (ICU) patients compared with patients fitting ICU admission criteria treated in regular wards, *J Hosp Infect* 59:331, 2005.

Oman KS, et al: Nurse-directed interventions to reduce catheter-associated urinary tract infections, *Am J Infect Control* 40:548, 2012.

Purvis S, et al: Catheter-associated urinary tract infection: a successful prevention effort employing a multipronged initiative at an academic medical center, *J Nurs Care Qual* 29(2):141, 2014.

Schabelman E, Witting M: The relationship of radiocontrast, iodine and seafood allergies, a medical myth exposed, *J Emerg Med* 39(5):701, 2010.

47

Bowel Elimination

OBJECTIVES

- Discuss the role of gastrointestinal organs in digestion and elimination.
- Explain the physiological aspects of normal defecation.
- Discuss psychological and physiological factors that influence the elimination process.
- Describe common physiological alterations in elimination.
- Assess a patient's elimination pattern.
- List nursing diagnoses related to alterations in elimination.
- Describe nursing implications for common diagnostic examinations of the gastrointestinal tract.
- List nursing interventions that promote normal elimination.
- List nursing interventions included in bowel training.
- Discuss nursing care measures required for patients with a bowel diversion.
- Use critical thinking in providing care to patients with alterations in bowel elimination.

KEY TERMS

Bowel training, p. 1168
Cathartics, p. 1151
Chyme, p. 1150
***Clostridium difficile*, p. 1152**
Colonoscopy, p. 1156
Colostomy, p. 1153
Constipation, p. 1150
Diarrhea, p. 1152
Effluent, p. 1153
Endoscopy, p. 1158
Enema, p. 1151
Fecal occult blood test (FOBT), p. 1156
Flatulence, p. 1153
Hemorrhoids, p. 1150
Ileostomy, p. 1153
Ileus, p. 1151
Impaction, p. 1152
Incontinence, p. 1152
Laxatives, p. 1151
Peristalsis, p. 1149
Polyps, p. 1158
Stoma, p. 1153
Wound, ostomy and continence nurse (WOCN), p. 1168

MEDIA RESOURCES

http://evolve.elsevier.com/Potter/fundamentals/
- Review Questions
- Video Clips
- Concept Map Creator
- Case Study with Questions
- Skills Performance Checklists
- Audio Glossary
- Content Updates

Regular elimination of bowel waste products is essential for normal body functioning. Alterations in bowel elimination are often early signs or symptoms of problems within either the gastrointestinal (GI) tract or other body systems. Because bowel function depends on the balance of several factors, elimination patterns and habits vary among individuals.

Understanding normal bowel elimination and factors that promote, impede, or cause alterations in elimination help a nurse manage patients' elimination problems. Supportive nursing care respects a patient's privacy and emotional needs. Measures designed to promote normal elimination also need to minimize a patient's discomfort and embarrassment.

SCIENTIFIC KNOWLEDGE BASE

The GI tract is a series of hollow mucous membrane–lined muscular organs. These organs absorb fluid and nutrients, prepare food for absorption and use by body cells, and provide for temporary storage of feces (Figure 47-1). The GI tract absorbs high volumes of fluids, making fluid and electrolyte balance a key function of the GI system. In addition to ingested fluids and foods, the GI tract also receives secretions from the gallbladder and pancreas.

Mouth

The mouth mechanically and chemically breaks down nutrients into usable size and form. The teeth chew food, breaking it down into a size suitable for swallowing. Saliva, produced by the salivary glands in the mouth, dilutes and softens the food in the mouth for easier swallowing.

Esophagus

As food enters the upper esophagus, it passes through the upper esophageal sphincter, a circular muscle that prevents air from entering the esophagus and food from refluxing into the throat. The bolus of food travels down the esophagus with the aid of **peristalsis**, which is a contraction that propels food through the length of the GI tract. The food moves down the esophagus and reaches the cardiac sphincter, which lies between the esophagus and the upper end of the stomach. The sphincter prevents reflux of stomach contents back into the esophagus.

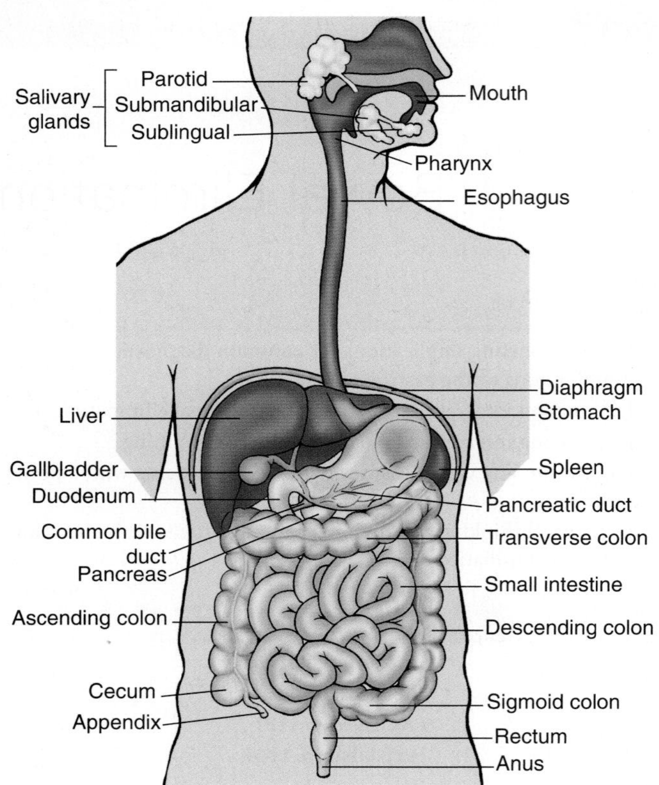

FIGURE 47-1 Organs of gastrointestinal tract. (From Monahan FD, Neighbors M: *Medical-surgical nursing,* ed 2, Philadelphia, 1998, Saunders.)

Stomach

The stomach performs three tasks: storage of swallowed food and liquid; mixing of food with digestive juices into a substance called chyme; and regulated emptying of its contents into the small intestine. The stomach produces and secretes hydrochloric acid (HCl), mucus, the enzyme pepsin, and intrinsic factor. Pepsin and HCl help to digest protein. Mucus protects the stomach mucosa from acidity and enzyme activity. Intrinsic factor is essential in the absorption of vitamin B_{12}.

Small Intestine

Movement within the small intestine, occurring by peristalsis, facilitates both digestion and absorption. Chyme comes into the small intestine as a liquid material and mixes with digestive enzymes. Resorption in the small intestine is so efficient that, by the time the fluid reaches the end of the small intestine, it is a thick liquid with semisolid particles in consistency. The small intestine is divided into three sections: the duodenum, the jejunum, and the ileum.

The duodenum is approximately 20 to 28 cm (8 to 11 inches) long and continues to process fluid from the stomach. The second section, the jejunum, is approximately 2.5 m (8 feet) long and absorbs carbohydrates and proteins. The ileum is approximately 3.7 m (12 feet) long and absorbs water, fats, and bile salts. The duodenum and jejunum absorb most nutrients and electrolytes in the small intestine. The ileum absorbs certain vitamins, iron, and bile salts. Digestive enzymes and bile enter into the small intestine from the pancreas and the liver to further break down nutrients into a form usable by the body.

The digestive process is greatly altered when small intestine function is impaired. Conditions such as inflammation, infection, surgical resection, or obstruction disrupt peristalsis, reduce absorption, or block the passage of fluid, resulting in electrolyte and nutrient deficiencies.

Large Intestine

The lower GI tract is called *the large intestine* or *colon* because it is larger in diameter than the small intestine. However, its length, 1.5 to 1.8 m (5 to 6 feet), is much shorter. The large intestine is divided into the cecum, ascending colon, transverse colon, descending colon, sigmoid colon, and rectum. The large intestine is the primary organ of bowel elimination.

Digestive fluid enters the large intestine by waves of peristalsis through the ileocecal valve (i.e., a circular muscle layer that prevents regurgitation back into the small intestine). The muscular tissue of the colon allows it to accommodate and eliminate large quantities of waste and gas (flatus). The colon has three functions: absorption, secretion, and elimination. The colon resorbs a large volume of water (up to 1.5 L) and significant amounts of sodium and chloride daily. The amount of water absorbed depends on the speed at which colonic contents move. Normally the fecal matter becomes a soft, formed solid or semisolid mass. If peristalsis is abnormally fast, there is less time for water to be absorbed, and the stool will be watery. If peristaltic contractions slow down, water continues to be absorbed, and a hard mass of stool forms, resulting in constipation.

Peristaltic contractions move contents through the colon. Intestinal content is the main stimulus for contraction. Mass peristalsis pushes undigested food toward the rectum. These mass movements occur only 3 or 4 times daily, with the strongest during the hour after mealtime.

The rectum is the final part of the large intestine. Normally the rectum is empty of fecal matter until just before defecation. It contains vertical and transverse folds of tissue that help to control expulsion of fecal contents during defecation. Each fold contains veins that can become distended from pressure during straining. This distention results in hemorrhoid formation.

Anus

The body expels feces and flatus from the rectum through the anus. Contraction and relaxation of the internal and external sphincters, which are innervated by sympathetic and parasympathetic nerves, aid in the control of defecation. The anal canal contains a rich supply of sensory nerves that allow people to tell when there is solid, liquid, or gas that needs to be expelled and aids in maintaining continence.

Defecation

The physiological factors essential to bowel function and defecation include normal GI tract function, sensory awareness of rectal distention and rectal contents, voluntary sphincter control, and adequate rectal capacity and compliance. Normal defecation begins with movement in the left colon, moving stool toward the anus. When stool reaches the rectum, the distention causes relaxation of the internal sphincter and an awareness of the need to defecate. At the time of defecation, the external sphincter relaxes, and abdominal muscles contract, increasing intrarectal pressure and forcing the stool out. Normally defecation is painless, resulting in passage of soft, formed stool. Straining while having a bowel movement indicates that the patient may need changes in diet or fluid intake or that there is an underlying disorder in GI function.

NURSING KNOWLEDGE BASE

Factors Influencing Bowel Elimination

Many factors influence the process of bowel elimination. Knowledge of these factors helps to anticipate measures required to maintain a normal elimination pattern.

Age. Infants have a smaller stomach capacity, less secretion of digestive enzymes, and more rapid intestinal peristalsis. The ability to control defecation does not occur until 2 to 3 years of age. Adolescents experience rapid growth and increased metabolic rate. There is also rapid growth of the large intestine and increased secretion of gastric acids to digest food fibers and act as a bactericide against swallowed organisms. Older adults may have decreased chewing ability. Partially chewed food is not digested as easily. Peristalsis declines, and esophageal emptying slows. This impairs absorption by the intestinal mucosa. Muscle tone in the perineal floor and anal sphincter weakens, which sometimes causes difficulty in controlling defecation (Constipation, n.d.).

Diet. Regular daily food intake helps maintain a regular pattern of peristalsis in the colon. Fiber in the diet provides the bulk in the fecal material. Bulk-forming foods such as whole grains, fresh fruits, and vegetables help remove the fats and waste products from the body with more efficiency. Some of these foods such as cabbage, broccoli, or beans may also produce gas, which distends the intestinal walls and increases colonic motility. The bowel walls stretch, creating peristalsis and initiating the defecation reflex.

Fluid Intake. Although individual fluid needs vary with the person, a fluid intake of 3L per day for men and 2.2 L per day for women is recommended (Mayo Clinic, 2014). Some fluid needs are met by drinking fluids, but there is also fluid in foods that are ingested such as fruits. An inadequate fluid intake or disturbances resulting in fluid loss (such as vomiting) affect the character of feces. Fluid liquefies intestinal contents by absorbing into the fiber from the diet and creating a larger, softer stool mass. This increases peristalsis and promotes movement of stool through the colon. Reduced fluid and fiber intake slows passage of food through the intestine and results in hardening of stool contents, causing constipation.

Physical Activity. Physical activity promotes peristalsis, whereas immobilization depresses it. Encourage early ambulation as illness begins to resolve or as soon as possible after surgery to promote maintenance of peristalsis and normal elimination. Maintaining tone of skeletal muscles used during defecation is important. Weakened abdominal and pelvic floor muscles impair the ability to increase intraabdominal pressure and control the external sphincter. Muscle tone is sometimes weakened or lost as a result of long-term illness, spinal cord injury, or neurological diseases that impair nerve transmission. As a result of these changes in the abdominal and pelvic floor muscles, there is an increased risk for constipation.

Psychological Factors. Prolonged emotional stress impairs the function of almost all body systems (see Chapter 38). During emotional stress the digestive process is accelerated, and peristalsis is increased. Side effects of increased peristalsis include diarrhea and gaseous distention. A number of diseases of the GI tract are exacerbated by stress, including ulcerative colitis, irritable bowel syndrome, certain gastric and duodenal ulcers, and Crohn's disease. If a person becomes depressed, the autonomic nervous system may slow impulses that decrease peristalsis, resulting in constipation.

Personal Habits. Personal elimination habits influence bowel function. Most people benefit from being able to use their own toilet facilities at a time that is most effective and convenient for them. A busy work schedule sometimes prevents the individual from responding appropriately to the urge to defecate, disrupting regular habits and causing possible alterations such as constipation. Individuals need to recognize the best time for elimination.

Position During Defecation. Squatting is the normal position during defecation. Modern toilets facilitate this posture, allowing a person to lean forward, exert intraabdominal pressure, and contract the gluteal muscles. For a patient immobilized in bed, defecation is often difficult. In a supine position it is hard to effectively contract the muscles used during defecation. If a patient's condition permits, raise the head of the bed to help him or her to a more normal sitting position on a bedpan, enhancing the ability to defecate.

Pain. Normally the act of defecation is painless. However, a number of conditions such as hemorrhoids; rectal surgery; anal fissures, which are painful linear splits in the perianal area; and abdominal surgery result in discomfort. In these instances the patient often suppresses the urge to defecate to avoid pain, contributing to the development of constipation.

Pregnancy. As pregnancy advances, the size of the fetus increases, and pressure is exerted on the rectum. A temporary obstruction created by the fetus impairs passage of feces. Slowing of peristalsis during the third trimester often leads to constipation. A pregnant woman's frequent straining during defecation or delivery may result in formation of hemorrhoids.

Surgery and Anesthesia. General anesthetic agents used during surgery cause temporary cessation of peristalsis (see Chapter 50). Inhaled anesthetic agents block parasympathetic impulses to the intestinal musculature. The action of the anesthetic slows or stops peristaltic waves. A patient who receives a local or regional anesthetic is less at risk for elimination alterations because this type of anesthesia generally affects bowel activity minimally or not at all.

Any surgery that involves direct manipulation of the bowel temporarily stops peristalsis. This condition, called an **ileus,** usually lasts about 24 to 48 hours. If a patient remains inactive or is unable to eat after surgery, return of normal bowel elimination is further delayed.

Medications. Many medications prescribed for acute and chronic conditions have secondary effects on a patient's bowel elimination patterns. For example, opioid analgesics slow peristalsis and contractions, often resulting in constipation; and antibiotics decrease intestinal bacterial flora, often resulting in diarrhea (Burchum and Rosenthal, 2016). It is important for the nurse and patient to be aware of these possible side effects and use appropriate measures to promote healthy bowel elimination. Some medications are used primarily for their action on the bowel and will promote defecation such as **laxatives** or **cathartics** or control diarrhea. If laxatives are needed for regular evacuation of the rectum, a fiber laxative is the first type used. If this is not sufficient to relieve constipation, the next one tried should be an osmotic laxative. Patients need to avoid regular use of a stimulant laxative because the intestine often becomes dependent on it.

Diagnostic Tests. Diagnostic examinations involving visualization of GI structures often require a prescribed bowel preparation (e.g., laxatives and/or **enemas**) to ensure that the bowel is empty. Usually patients cannot eat or drink several hours before examinations such as an endoscopy, colonoscopy, or other testing that requires visualization of the GI tract. Following the diagnostic procedure, changes in elimination such as increased gas or loose stools often occur until the patient resumes a normal eating pattern.

BOX 47-1 Common Causes of Constipation

- Irregular bowel habits and ignoring the urge to defecate
- Chronic illnesses (e.g., Parkinson's disease, multiple sclerosis, rheumatoid arthritis, chronic bowel diseases, depression, eating disorders)
- Low-fiber diet high in animal fats (e.g., meats and carbohydrates); low fluid intake
- Stress (e.g., illness of a family member, death of a loved one, divorce)
- Physical inactivity
- Medications, especially use of opiates
- Changes in life or routine such as pregnancy, aging, and travel
- Neurological conditions that block nerve impulses to the colon (e.g., stroke, spinal cord injury, tumor)
- Chronic bowel dysfunction (e.g., colonic inertia, irritable bowel)

BOX 47-2 Signs of Dehydration

- Signs of dehydration in adults include:
  - Thirst
  - Less frequent urination than usual
  - Dark-colored urine
  - Dry skin
  - Fatigue
  - Dizziness
  - Light-headedness
- Signs of dehydration in infants and young children include:
  - Dry mouth and tongue
  - No tears when crying
  - No wet diapers for 3 hours or more
  - Sunken eyes or cheeks or soft spot in the skull
  - High fever
  - Listlessness or irritability

Common Bowel Elimination Problems

You will frequently care for patients who have or are at risk for elimination problems because of physiological changes in the GI tract such as abdominal surgery, inflammatory diseases, medications, emotional stress, environmental factors, or disorders impairing defecation is common in the practice of nursing.

Constipation. Constipation is a symptom, not a disease, and there are many possible causes (Box 47-1). Improper diet, reduced fluid intake, lack of exercise, and certain medications can cause constipation. For example, patients receiving opiates for pain after surgery often require a stool softener or laxative to prevent constipation. A recent integrative review of the literature revealed that female gender and older age were the highest risk factors for constipation (Schmidt and Santos, 2014). Signs of constipation include infrequent bowel movements (less than three per week) and hard, dry stools that are difficult to pass (Constipation, n.d.). When intestinal motility slows, the fecal mass becomes exposed to the intestinal walls over time, and most of the fecal water content is absorbed. Little water is left to soften and lubricate the stool. Passage of a dry, hard stool often causes rectal pain. Constipation is a significant source of discomfort. Assess the need for intervention before defecation becomes painful or the stool is impacted.

Impaction. Fecal impaction results when a patient has unrelieved constipation and is unable to expel the hardened feces retained in the rectum. In cases of severe impaction the mass extends up into the sigmoid colon. If not resolved or removed, severe impaction results in intestinal obstruction. Patients who are debilitated, confused, or unconscious are most at risk for impaction. They are dehydrated or too weak or unaware of the need to defecate, and the stool becomes too hard and dry to pass.

An obvious sign of impaction is the inability to pass a stool for several days, despite the repeated urge to defecate. Suspect an impaction when a continuous oozing of liquid stool occurs. The liquid part of feces located higher in the colon seeps around the impacted mass. Loss of appetite (anorexia), nausea and/or vomiting, abdominal distention and cramping, and rectal pain may accompany the condition. If you suspect an impaction, gently perform a digital examination of the rectum and palpate for the impacted mass (Hussain et al., 2014).

Diarrhea. Diarrhea is an increase in the number of stools and the passage of liquid, unformed feces. It is associated with disorders affecting digestion, absorption, and secretion in the GI tract. Intestinal contents pass through the small and large intestine too quickly to allow for the usual absorption of fluid and nutrients. Irritation within the colon results in increased mucus secretion. As a result, feces become watery, and the patient often has difficulty controlling the urge to defecate.

Excess loss of colonic fluid results in dehydration (Box 47-2) with fluid and electrolyte or acid-base imbalances if the fluid is not replaced. Infants and older adults are particularly susceptible to associated complications (see Chapter 42). Because repeated passage of diarrhea stools exposes the skin of the perineum and buttocks to irritating intestinal contents, meticulous skin care and containment of fecal drainage is necessary to prevent skin breakdown (see Chapter 48).

Incontinence. Fecal incontinence is the inability to control passage of feces and gas from the anus. Incontinence harms a patient's body image (see Chapter 34). The embarrassment of soiling clothes often leads to social isolation. Physical conditions that impair anal sphincter function or large-volume liquid stools cause incontinence. Impaired cognitive function often leads to incontinence of both urine and stool.

Many conditions cause fecal incontinence or diarrhea. You need to identify precipitating conditions and refer patients to health care providers for medication management. Antibiotic use alters the normal flora in the GI tract. A common causative agent of diarrhea is *Clostridium difficile (C. difficile),* which produces symptoms ranging from mild diarrhea to severe colitis. Patients acquire *C. difficile* infection in one of two ways: by antibiotic therapy that causes an overgrowth of *C. difficile* and by contact with the *C. difficile* organism. A newly identified strain of *C. difficile* is more virulent with more toxic effects (Grossman and Mager, 2010). Patients are exposed to the organism from a health care worker's hands or direct contact with environmental surfaces contaminated with it. Only hand hygiene with soap and water is effective to physically remove *C. difficile* spores from the hands. The most common diagnostic test for the bacteria is the enzyme-linked immunosorbent assay (ELISA) test, which detects *C. difficile* A and B in the stool. Elderly patients are especially vulnerable to *C. difficile* infection when exposed to antibiotics, and higher mortality and morbidity are observed in this age-group (Daniel and Rapose, 2015).

Communicable foodborne pathogens also cause diarrhea. Hand hygiene following the use of the bathroom, before and after preparing foods, and when cleaning and storing fresh produce and meats greatly reduces the risk of foodborne illnesses. When diarrhea results from a foodborne pathogen, the goal usually is to rid the GI system of the pathogen rather than slow peristalsis.

Surgeries or diagnostic testing of the lower GI tract may also cause diarrhea. Patients receiving enteral nutrition are also at risk for diarrhea and need a dietary consult to find the right formula for the feeding (Chapter 45). Food intolerances can increase peristalsis and cause diarrhea. Food intolerance is not an allergy; rather, a particular food causes the body distress within a few hours of ingestion. The result is diarrhea, cramps, or **flatulence**. For example, people who drink cow's milk and have these symptoms are not allergic to milk but lack the enzyme needed to digest the milk sugar lactase and therefore are lactose intolerant. Another condition called *celiac disease* is a syndrome in which a patient has a hypersensitivity to protein in certain cereal grains and gluten. Food allergies are less common but do occur, and people with these allergies need to know how to read labels on foods carefully. True food allergies may be life threatening and lead to anaphylaxis (Food Allergies, 2015).

Flatulence. As gas accumulates in the lumen of the intestines, the bowel wall stretches and distends. **Flatulence** is a common cause of abdominal fullness, pain, and cramping. Normally intestinal gas escapes through the mouth (belching) or the anus (passing of flatus). However, flatulence causes abdominal distention and severe, sharp pain if intestinal motility is reduced because of opiates, general anesthetics, abdominal surgery, or immobilization.

Hemorrhoids. Hemorrhoids are dilated, engorged veins in the lining of the rectum. They are either external or internal. External hemorrhoids are clearly visible as protrusions of skin. There is usually a purplish discoloration (thrombosis) if the underlying vein is hardened. This causes increased pain and sometimes requires excision. Internal hemorrhoids occur in the anal canal and may be inflamed and distended. Increased venous pressure from straining at defecation, pregnancy, heart failure, and chronic liver disease causes hemorrhoids.

Bowel Diversions

Certain diseases or surgical alterations make the normal passage of intestinal contents throughout the small and large intestine difficult or inadvisable. When these conditions are present, a temporary or permanent opening (**stoma**) is created surgically by bringing part of the intestine out through the abdominal wall. These surgical openings are called an **ileostomy** or **colostomy**, depending on which part of the intestinal tract is used to create the stoma (Figures 47-2 and 47-3). Newer surgical techniques allow more patients to have parts of their small and large intestine removed and the remaining parts reconnected so they will continue to defecate through the anal canal.

Ostomies. The location of an ostomy determines stool consistency. A person with a sigmoid colostomy will have a more formed stool. The output from a transverse colostomy will be thick liquid to soft consistency. These ostomies are the easiest to perform surgically and are done as a temporary means to divert stool from an area of trauma or perianal wounds. They may also be a palliative diversion if obstruction from a tumor is present. With an ileostomy the fecal effluent leaves the body before it enters the colon, creating frequent, liquid stools.

Loop colostomies are reversible stomas that a surgeon constructs in the ileum or the colon. The surgeon pulls a loop of intestine onto the abdomen and often places a plastic rod, bridge, or rubber catheter temporarily under the bowel loop to keep it from slipping back. The surgeon then opens the bowel and sutures it to the skin of the abdomen. The loop ostomy has two openings through the stoma. The proximal end drains fecal effluent, and the distal part drains mucus.

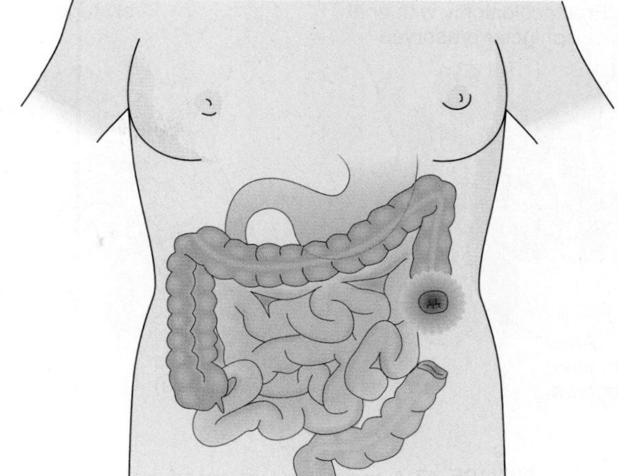

FIGURE 47-2 Sigmoid colostomy.

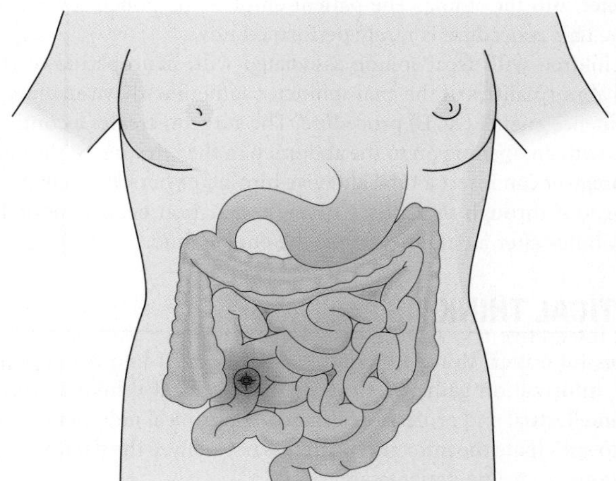

FIGURE 47-3 Ileostomy.

The end colostomy consists of a stoma formed by bringing a piece of intestine out through a surgically created opening in the abdominal wall, turning it down like a turtleneck and suturing it to the abdominal wall. The intestine distal to the stoma is either removed or sewn closed (called *Hartmann's pouch;* see Figure 47-2) and left in the abdominal cavity. End ostomies are permanent or reversible. The rectum is either left intact or removed.

Other Procedures

Ileoanal Pouch Anastomosis. The ileoanal pouch anastomosis is a surgical procedure for patients who need to have a colectomy for treatment of ulcerative colitis or familial adenopolyposis (FAP) (Goldberg et al., 2010). In this procedure the surgeon removes the colon, creates a pouch from the end of the small intestine, and attaches the pouch to the patient's anus (Figure 47-4). This pouch provides for the collection of fecal material, which simulates the function of the rectum. The patient is continent of stool because stool is evacuated via the anus. When the ileal pouch is created, the patient has a temporary ileostomy to divert the fecal stream or **effluent** and allow the suture lines in the pouch to heal.

A continent ileostomy involves creating a pouch from the small intestine. The pouch has a continent stoma on the abdomen created with a valve that can be drained only when the patient places a large

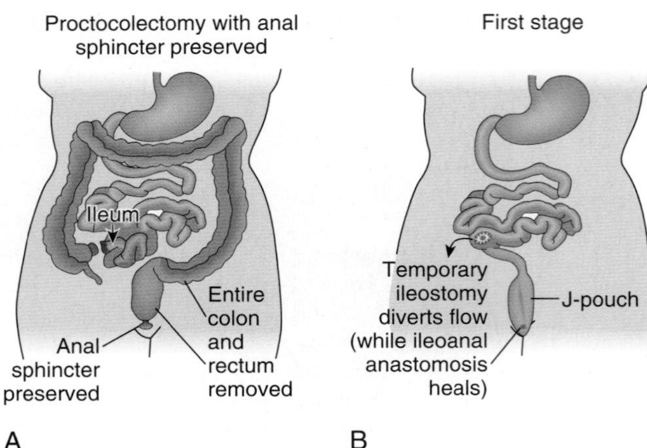

FIGURE 47-4 Ileoanal pouch anastomosis.

catheter into the stoma. The patient empties the pouch several times a day. This procedure is rarely performed now.

Children with fecal soiling associated with neuropathic or structural abnormalities of the anal sphincter sometimes have an antegrade continence enema (ACE) procedure. The surgeon creates a continence valve with an opening on to the abdomen in the intestine so the patient or caregiver can insert a tube and give himself or herself an enema that comes out through the anus. Colonic evacuation begins about 10 to 20 minutes after a patient receives the enema fluid.

CRITICAL THINKING

Successful critical thinking requires a synthesis of knowledge, experience, information gathered from patients, critical thinking attitudes, and intellectual and professional standards. Clinical judgments require you to anticipate the information necessary, analyze the data, and make decisions regarding patient care.

In the case of bowel elimination, integrate knowledge from nursing and other disciplines to understand a patient's response to bowel elimination alterations. Experience in caring for patients with elimination alterations helps you provide an appropriate plan of care. Use critical thinking attitudes such as fairness, confidence, and discipline when listening to and exploring a patient's nursing history. Apply relevant standards of practice when selecting nursing measures.

❖ NURSING PROCESS

Apply the nursing process and use a critical thinking approach in your care of patients. The nursing process provides a clinical decision-making approach for you to develop and implement an individualized plan of care.

◆ Assessment

During the assessment process thoroughly assess each patient and critically analyze findings to ensure that you make patient-centered clinical decisions required for safe nursing care. Consider all critical thinking elements that build toward making appropriate diagnoses (Figure 47-5).

Assessment for bowel elimination patterns and abnormalities includes a nursing history, physical assessment of the abdomen, inspection of fecal characteristics, and review of relevant test results. In addition, determine the patient's medical history, pattern and types of fluid and food intake, mobility, chewing ability, medications, recent illnesses and/or stressors, and environmental situation.

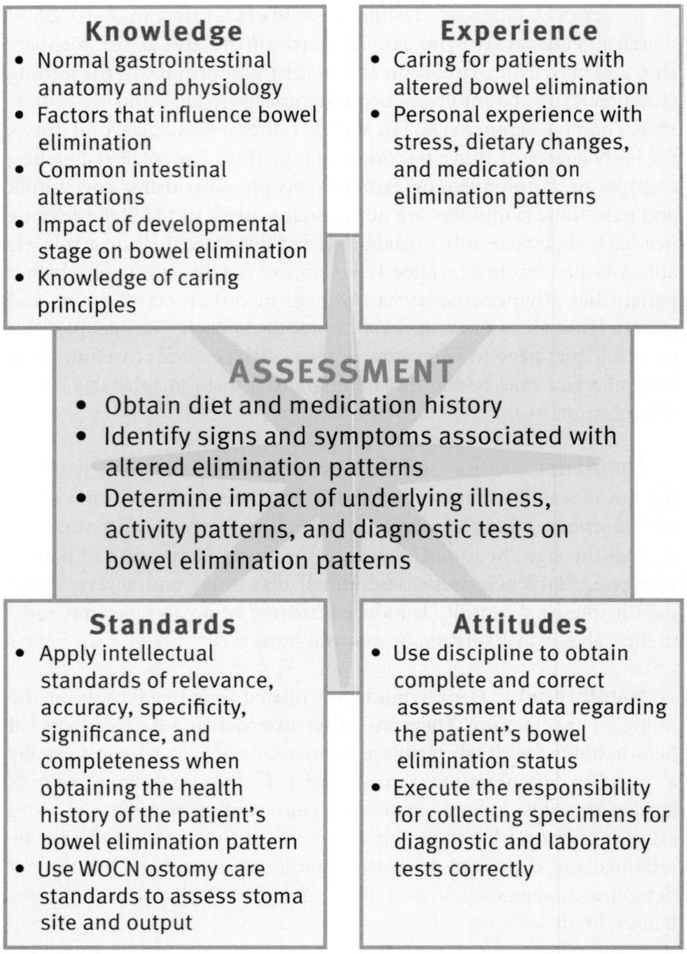

Knowledge
- Normal gastrointestinal anatomy and physiology
- Factors that influence bowel elimination
- Common intestinal alterations
- Impact of developmental stage on bowel elimination
- Knowledge of caring principles

Experience
- Caring for patients with altered bowel elimination
- Personal experience with stress, dietary changes, and medication on elimination patterns

ASSESSMENT
- Obtain diet and medication history
- Identify signs and symptoms associated with altered elimination patterns
- Determine impact of underlying illness, activity patterns, and diagnostic tests on bowel elimination patterns

Standards
- Apply intellectual standards of relevance, accuracy, specificity, significance, and completeness when obtaining the health history of the patient's bowel elimination pattern
- Use WOCN ostomy care standards to assess stoma site and output

Attitudes
- Use discipline to obtain complete and correct assessment data regarding the patient's bowel elimination status
- Execute the responsibility for collecting specimens for diagnostic and laboratory tests correctly

FIGURE 47-5 Critical thinking model for elimination assessment. *WOCN,* Wound, Ostomy and Continence Nurses Society.

Through the Patient's Eyes. Patients expect nurses to answer all of their questions regarding diagnostic tests and the preparation for these tests. They are concerned about discomfort and exposure of their perineal area. Bowel problems are often a source of discomfort and embarrassment for the patient and their families. Fecal and urinary incontinence in older people is the second most common reason for admission to a long-term care facility (Long, 2010). Some older patients who fail to recognize their elimination needs need monitoring for elimination patterns so negative consequences do not occur. Remember that each patient has a unique situation and a perception of what is "right" for him or her. Patients expect a knowledgeable nurse with the ability to teach methods of promoting and maintaining normal bowel elimination patterns or means of managing altered elimination. Encourage the patient and/or caregiver to describe cultural practices and use this information when providing care to enhance the patient's comfort.

Nursing History. The nursing history provides information about a patient's usual bowel pattern and habits. What a patient describes as normal or abnormal is often different from factors and conditions that tend to promote normal elimination. Identifying normal and abnormal patterns, habits, and the patient's perception of normal and abnormal in regard to bowel elimination allows you to better determine a patient's problems. Organize the nursing history around factors that affect elimination.

- *Determination of the usual elimination pattern:* Include frequency and time of day. Having a patient or caregiver complete a bowel elimination diary provides an accurate assessment of a patient's current bowel elimination pattern.
- *Patient's description of usual stool characteristics:* Determine if the stool is normally watery or formed, soft or hard, and the typical color. Ask the patient to describe the shape of a normal stool and the number of stools per day. Use a scale such as the Bristol Stool Form Scale to get an objective measure of stool characteristics (Figure 47-6).
- *Identification of routines followed to promote bowel elimination:* Examples are drinking hot liquids, eating specific foods, or taking time to defecate during a certain part of the day or use of laxatives, enemas, or bulk-forming fiber additives.
- *Presence and status of bowel diversions:* If a patient has an ostomy, assess frequency of emptying the ostomy pouch, character of feces, appearance and condition of the stoma (color, height at or above skin level), condition of peristomal skin, type of pouching system device used, and methods used to maintain the function of the ostomy.
- *Changes in appetite:* Include changes in eating patterns and a change in weight (amount of loss or gain). If a loss of weight is present, ask if the patient intended to lose weight (e.g., a diet or exercise routine) or if it happened unexpectedly.
- *Diet history:* Determine the patient's dietary preferences. Determine the intake of fruits, vegetables, and whole grains and if mealtimes are regular or irregular.
- *Description of daily fluid intake:* This includes the type and amount of fluid. Patients often estimate the amount using common household measurements.
- *History of surgery or illnesses affecting the GI tract:* This information helps explain symptoms, the potential for maintaining or restoring normal bowel elimination pattern, and whether there is a family history of GI cancer.
- *Medication history:* Ask patients for a list of all the medications they take and assess whether they take medications such as laxatives, antacids, iron supplements, and analgesics that alter defecation or fecal characteristics.
- *Emotional state:* A patient's emotional status may alter frequency of defecation. Ask the patient if he or she has experienced unusual stress and if he or she thinks that this may have caused a change in bowel movements.
- *History of exercise:* Ask the patient to specifically describe the type and amount of daily exercise.
- *History of pain or discomfort:* Ask the patient whether there is a history of abdominal or anal pain. The type, frequency, and location of pain help identify the source of the problem. For instance, cramping pain, nausea, and the absence of bowel movements sometimes indicate there is an intestinal obstruction.
- *Social history:* Patients have many different living arrangements. Where patients live affects their toileting habits. If the patient lives with other people, ask how many bathrooms there are. Find out if the patient has to share a bathroom, creating a need to adjust the time that he or she uses the bathroom to accommodate others. If the patient lives alone, can he or she ambulate to the toilet safely? When patients are not independent in bowel management, determine who helps them and how.
- *Mobility and dexterity:* Evaluate patients' mobility and dexterity to determine if they need assistive devices or help from personnel.

See Box 47-3 for a summary of the types of assessment questions to use for gathering a detailed nursing history.

Type 1 Separate hard lumps like nuts (difficult to pass)

Type 2 Sausage shaped but lumpy

Type 3 Like a sausage but with cracks on surface

Type 4 Like a sausage or snake, smooth and soft

Type 5 Soft blobs with clear-cut edges (passed easily)

Type 6 Fluffy pieces with ragged edges, a mushy stool

Type 7 Watery, no solid pieces (entirely liquid)

FIGURE 47-6 Bristol stool form scale. (Used with permission. Bristol Stool Form Guideline, http://www.aboutconstipation.org/bristol.)

Physical Assessment. Conduct a physical assessment of body systems and functions likely to be influenced by the presence of elimination problems (see Chapter 31).

Mouth. Inspect the patient's teeth, tongue, and gums. Poor dentition or poorly fitting dentures influence the ability to chew. Sores in the mouth make eating not only difficult but also painful.

Abdomen. Inspect all four abdominal quadrants for contour, shape, symmetry, and skin color. Note masses, peristaltic waves, scars, venous patterns, stomas, and lesions. Normally you do not see peristaltic waves. Observable peristalsis is often a sign of intestinal obstruction.

Abdominal distention appears as an overall outward protuberance of the abdomen. Intestinal gas, large tumors, or fluid in the peritoneal cavity causes distention. A distended abdomen feels tight like a drum; the skin is taut and appears stretched.

Auscultate the abdomen with a stethoscope to assess bowel sounds in each quadrant (see Chapter 31). Normal bowel sounds occur every 5 to 15 seconds and last a second to several seconds. Absent (no auscultated bowel sounds) or hypoactive sounds occur with an ileus such as after abdominal surgery but may also mean that you did not capture the bowel sounds when you were assessing them. High-pitched and hyperactive bowel sounds occur with small intestine obstruction and inflammatory disorders. Although auscultating bowel sounds during assessment is standard nursing practice, some current research questions its validity. A recent study found that only 11.4% of nurses and 47.6% of doctors could make correct clinical judgments on the basis of their auscultatory findings (Li et al., 2014). Another study comparing surgical and internal medicine clinicians' interpretation of bowel sounds concluded that auscultation of bowel sounds is not a useful clinical practice when differentiating patients with normal versus pathological bowel sounds (Felder et al., 2014).

Percussion identifies underlying abdominal structures and detects lesions, fluid, or gas within the abdomen. Gas or flatulence creates a tympanic note. Masses, tumors, and fluid are dull to percussion.

Gently palpate the abdomen for masses or areas of tenderness. It is important for your patient to relax. Tensing abdominal muscles interferes with palpating underlying organs or masses.

BOX 47-3 Nursing Assessment Questions

Signs and Symptoms

Nausea or Vomiting: Onset, Duration, Associated Symptoms, Character, Exposures

- When did the nausea/vomiting start?
- Is it related to particular stimuli (odors, after eating specific food)?
- How does the emesis look (mucus, blood, coffee-ground appearance, undigested food) and what is the color?
- Do you have other symptoms such as fever, dizziness, headaches, abdominal pain, or weight loss?
- Do you have family members who are experiencing the same symptoms?

Indigestion: Onset, Character, Location, Associated Symptoms, Alleviating Factors

- Is the indigestion related to meals, types or quantity of food, time of day or night?
- Does the discomfort from indigestion radiate to the shoulders or arms?
- Do you feel bloated after eating?
- Do you have any other symptoms (vomiting, headaches, diarrhea, belching, flatulence, heartburn, or pain)?
- Does the indigestion respond to antacids or other self-care measures?

Diarrhea: Onset, Duration, Character, Associated Symptoms, Alleviating Factors, Exposure

- When did the diarrhea start? Was it gradual or sudden?
- How many stools do you have per day? Is it watery or explosive? What is the color and consistency?
- Have you had fever, chills, weight loss, or abdominal pain?
- Have you taken antibiotics recently?
- Have you been under stress?
- What have you used to try to alleviate the diarrhea? Was it successful?
- Have you been out of the country recently?

Constipation: Onset, Character, Symptoms, Alleviating Factors

- When was your last bowel movement? How many bowel movements do you have in a typical week?
- Is this a recent occurrence or a long-standing problem?
- Describe your bowel movements.
- Do you have to strain to have a bowel movement?
- Do you have abdominal or rectal pain when you have a bowel movement?
- Do you feel as though your bowel movements are incomplete?
- Have you recently changed your diet or fluid intake?
- Do you use stool softeners, laxatives, or enemas?
- Has it ever been necessary to manually remove the bowel movements?

Medical History

- Do you have a previous history of gastrointestinal problems or disease? If yes, explain.
- Have you had abdominal surgery or trauma?
- Do you have a history of major illnesses such as cancer; arthritis; or respiratory, kidney, or cardiac disease?
- Which medications do you take?

Effect on the Patient

- How do these symptoms affect you?
- Have you missed work or social engagements because of these symptoms?

Rectum. Inspect the area around the anus for lesions, discoloration, inflammation, and hemorrhoids. Pain results when hemorrhoid tissues are irritated. The primary goal for a patient with hemorrhoids is to have soft-formed, painless bowel movements. Proper diet, fluids, and regular exercise improve the likelihood of stools being soft. If the patient becomes constipated, passage of hard stools causes bleeding and irritation. An ice pack or a warm sitz bath (see Chapter 48) provides temporary relief of swollen hemorrhoids. A health care provider sometimes prescribes topical medication to relieve the swelling and pain.

Laboratory Tests. There are no blood tests to specifically diagnose most GI disorders, but hemoglobin and hematocrit help determine if anemia from GI bleeding is present. Other laboratory tests often ordered by the health care provider include liver function tests, serum amylase, and serum lipase, which are used to assess for hepatobiliary diseases and pancreatitis.

Fecal Specimens. You need to ensure that specimens are obtained accurately, labeled properly in appropriate containers, and transported to the laboratory on time. Laboratories provide special containers for fecal specimens. Some tests require that specimens are placed in chemical preservatives, and some require that they are refrigerated or placed on ice after collection and before delivery to the laboratory. Use medical aseptic technique during collection of stool specimens (see Chapter 29).

Hand hygiene is necessary for anyone who comes in contact with the specimen. Often the patient is able to obtain the specimen if properly instructed. Teach the patient to avoid mixing feces with urine or water. He or she defecates into a clean, dry bedpan or a special container under the toilet seat. Observe the stool characteristics when collecting a specimen (Table 47-1).

Tests performed by the laboratory for occult (microscopic) blood in the stool and stool cultures require only a small sample. Collect about a 3-cm (1-inch) mass of formed stool or 15 to 30 mL of liquid stool. Tests for measuring the output of fecal fat require a 3- to 5-day collection of stool. You need to save all fecal material throughout the test period.

After obtaining a specimen, label and tightly seal the container and complete all laboratory requisition forms. Record specimen collections in the patient's medical record. It is important to avoid delays in sending specimens to the laboratory. Some tests such as measurement for ova and parasites require the stool to be warm. When stool specimens remain at room temperature, bacteriological changes that alter test results occur.

A common stool test is the fecal occult blood test (FOBT), which measures microscopic amounts of blood in the feces. It is a useful screening test for colon cancer as recommended by the American Cancer Society. There are two types of tests, the guaiac fecal occult blood test (gFOBT) and the fecal immunochemical test (FIT). The FIT test requires no preparation or dietary restrictions and is a more sensitive test, but it is more expensive; thus the gFOBT is more commonly used. The nurse or the patient needs to repeat the test at least 3 times on three separate bowel movements. The FOBT is done in a patient's home or health care provider's office (Box 47-4). All positive tests are followed up with flexible sigmoidoscopy or colonoscopy (ACS, 2015).

When your patients are going to have a gFOBT, it is important to instruct them to avoid eating red meat for 3 days before testing. If there are no contraindications and it is approved by the health care provider, instruct your patient to stop taking aspirin, ibuprofen, naproxen, or other nonsteroidal antiinflammatory drugs for 7 days because these could cause a false-positive test result. Patients also need to avoid vitamin C supplements and citrus fruits and juices for 3 days before the test because they can cause a false-negative result (ACS, 2015).

Diagnostic Examinations. For patients experiencing alterations in the GI system, various radiological and diagnostic examinations such as a colonoscopy require bowel preparation (bowel prep) for the test to be completed successfully. A bowel-cleansing program is sometimes difficult or unpleasant for patients. You provide education and support to ensure an optimal test result (Box 47-5).

◆ Nursing Diagnosis

Nursing assessment of a patient's bowel function sometimes reveals data that indicate an actual or potential elimination problem or a problem resulting from elimination alterations. In the examples discussed in the Nursing Care Plan, a patient has constipation as a result of pain medications and decreased fiber intake. Examples of diagnoses that apply to patients with elimination problems include the following:

- *Disturbed Body Image*
- *Bowel Incontinence*
- *Constipation*
- *Perceived Constipation*
- *Risk for Constipation*
- *Diarrhea*
- *Nausea*
- *Deficient Knowledge (Nutrition)*
- *Acute Pain*
- *Toileting Self-Care Deficit*

TABLE 47-1 Fecal Characteristics

Characteristic	Normal	Abnormal	Abnormal Cause
Color	Infant: yellow; adult: brown	White or clay	Absence of bile
		Black or tarry (melena)	Iron ingestion or gastrointestinal (GI) bleeding
		Red	GI bleeding, hemorrhoids, ingestion of beets
		Pale and oily	Malabsorption of fat
Odor	Malodorous; may be affected by certain foods	Noxious change	Blood in feces or infection
Consistency	Soft, formed	Liquid	Diarrhea, reduced absorption
		Hard	Constipation
Frequency	Varies: infant 4 to 6 times daily (breastfed) or 1 to 3 times daily (bottle-fed); adult twice daily to 3 times a week	Infant more than 6 times daily or less than once every 1 to 2 days; adult more than 3 times a day or less than once a week	Hypermotility or hypomotility
Shape	Resembles diameter of rectum	Narrow, pencil shaped	Obstruction, increased peristalsis
Constituents	Undigested food, dead bacteria, fat, bile pigment, cells lining intestinal mucosa, water	Blood, pus, foreign bodies, mucus, worms	Internal bleeding, infection, swallowed objects, irritation, inflammation, infestation of parasites
		Oily stool	Malabsorption syndrome, enteritis, pancreatic disease, surgical resection of intestine
		Mucus	Intestinal irritation, inflammation, infection, or injury

BOX 47-4 PROCEDURAL GUIDELINES

Performing a Guaiac Fecal Occult Blood Test

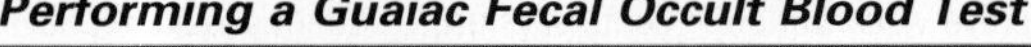

Delegation Considerations

The skill of fecal occult blood test (FOBT) can be delegated to nursing assistive personnel (NAP). However, the nurse is responsible for assessing the significance of the findings. You may need to send the specimen to the laboratory. Refer to your agency policies. The nurse instructs the NAP to:

Notify the nurse if frank bleeding occurs after obtaining the sample.

Equipment

Hemoccult test paper, Hemoccult developer, wooden applicator, and clean gloves (Check the expiration dates on the developer and the test paper before using.)

Steps

1. Identify patient using two identifiers (e.g., name and birthday or name and account number) according to agency policy.
2. Explain purpose of test and ways patient can help. Patient can collect own specimen if possible.
3. Perform hand hygiene and apply clean gloves.
4. Use tip of wooden applicator (see illustration) to obtain a small part of stool specimen. Be sure that specimen is free of toilet paper and not contaminated with urine.

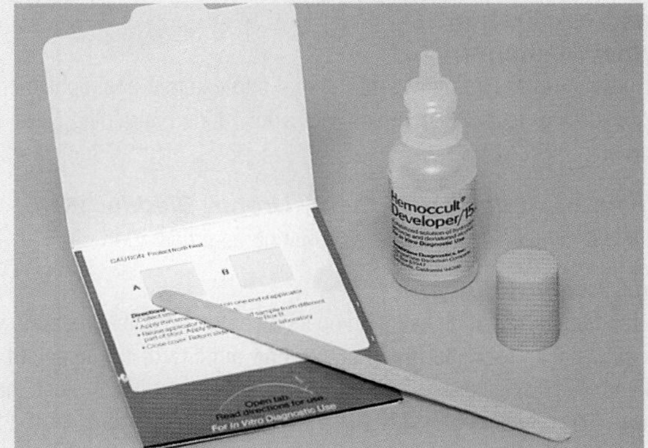

STEP 4 Equipment needed for fecal occult blood testing.

Continued

BOX 47-4 PROCEDURAL GUIDELINES

Performing a Guaiac Fecal Occult Blood Test—cont'd

5. Perform Hemoccult slide test:
   a. Open flap of slide and, using a wooden applicator, thinly smear stool in first box of the guaiac paper. Apply a second fecal specimen from a different part of the stool to second box of slide (see illustration).
   b. Close slide cover and turn the packet over to reverse side (see illustration). After waiting 3 to 5 minutes, open cardboard flap and apply 2 drops of developing solution on each box of guaiac paper. A blue color indicates a positive guaiac or presence of fecal occult blood.
   c. Interpret the color of the guaiac paper after 30 to 60 seconds.
   d. After determining if the patient's specimen is positive or negative, apply 1 drop of developer to the quality control section and interpret within 10 seconds.
   e. Dispose of test slide in proper receptacle.
6. Wrap wooden applicator in paper towel, remove gloves, and discard in proper receptacle.
7. Perform hand hygiene.
8. Record results of test; note any unusual fecal characteristics. (Submit only one sample per day.)

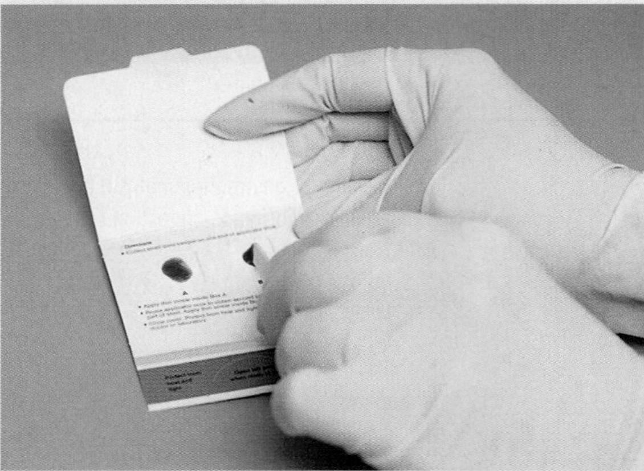

STEP 5a Application of fecal specimen on guaiac paper.

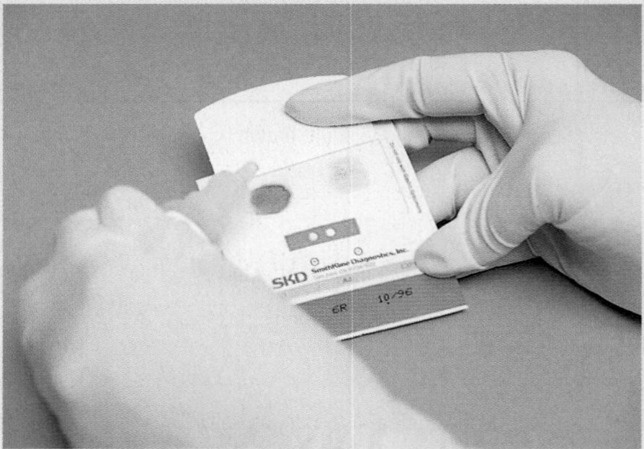

STEP 5b Application of Hemoccult developing solution on guaiac paper on reverse side of test kit.

BOX 47-5 Radiological and Diagnostic Tests

Direct Visualization

Endoscopy

- Examinations such as a gastroscopy or colonoscopy use a lighted fiberoptic tube to gain direct visualization of the upper gastrointestinal (GI) tract (upper **endoscopy**) or large intestine (colonoscopy). The fiberoptic tube contains a lens, forceps, and brushes for biopsy. If an endoscopy identifies a lesion such as a polyp, the polyp can be removed, and a biopsy will be done.
- These tests are done under sedation, usually in outpatient centers.
- Patients receive instruction about the preparation needed for the tests at the time they are scheduled for the procedure. Patients are usually on a clear liquid diet the day before the test. Bowel preparation is necessary before a colonoscopy can be performed successfully.

Indirect Visualization

Anorectal Manometry

- Measures the pressure activity of internal and external anal sphincters and reflexes during rectal distention, relaxation during straining, and rectal sensation.

Plain Film of Abdomen/Kidneys, Ureter, Bladder (KUB)

- A simple x-ray film of the abdomen requiring no preparation.

Barium Swallow/Enema

- An x-ray film examination using an opaque contrast medium (barium, which is swallowed) to examine the structure and motility of the upper GI tract, including pharynx, esophagus, and stomach. Barium instilled through the anal opening via an enema provides visualization of the structures of the lower GI tract.
- Preparation required varies by physician and agency doing the procedure but usually includes a clear liquid diet, laxatives the day before the procedure, and in some instances enemas to empty out any remaining stool particles.

Ultrasound Imaging

- A technique that uses high-frequency sound waves to echo off body organs, creating a picture of the GI tract.

Computed Tomography Scan (Virtual Colonoscopy)

- An x-ray examination of the body from many angles using a scanner analyzed by a computer. An oral contrast solution for the patient to drink may be ordered before the test. Intravenous contrast solution may be injected during the test to improve visualization. If contrast is used, patient should not have food or fluids for 4 to 6 hours before the examination.
- Virtual colonoscopy or computerized tomography (CT) colonography requires bowel preparation before the test. This does not replace the colonoscopy because it does not allow for removal of **polyps** and biopsies to be obtained.

Colonic Transit Study

- The patient swallows a capsule containing radiopaque markers.
- The patient maintains their normal diet and fluid intake for 5 days and refrains from medications that affect bowel function. On the fifth day x-ray film examination is performed.

Magnetic Resonance Imaging

- A noninvasive examination that uses magnet and radio waves to produce a picture of the inside of the body.
- Preparation is NPO 4 to 6 hours before examination.
- The patient needs to lie very still. If claustrophobia is a problem, light sedation may be ordered.
- No metallic objects, including metal objects on clothes, are allowed in the room. If the patient has a pacemaker or a metal implanted in his or her body, he or she may not be able to have magnetic resonance imaging (MRI).

NURSING CARE PLAN

Constipation

ASSESSMENT

Javier, a home care nurse, is visiting Mr. Johnson at his home. Mr. Johnson lives alone in a suburban community and has two grown children who reside in another state. They came to visit while he was hospitalized and helped him get settled back at home, but now they have returned to their homes and families. He is 76 years old and had surgery 10 days ago for a total knee replacement after suffering from osteoarthritis for many years. Mr. Johnson tells Javier that he is trying to follow the exercise program that the physical therapist has recommended but is having difficulty because of pain from the surgery. His past history includes hypertension, which has been controlled with medication for the last 10 years. He had some edema of both feet in the hospital and took a mild diuretic for 5 days for relief. Javier knows that immobility from the surgery, recent use of a diuretic, and opioid pain medication are factors that can cause constipation.

Assessment Activities	*Findings/Defining Characteristics**
Ask Mr. Johnson about his bowel elimination patterns since his surgery.	Mr. Johnson tells Javier that **he had one small hard bowel movement in the hospital but has not had one in the 7 days since he has been home.**
Review patient's medication.	Mr. Johnson says he is taking his blood pressure medication, a daily multivitamin with **iron**, a stool softener once a day, and 1 or 2 **oxycodone** 4 times a day.
Review dietary and fluid intake over last day.	Diet included **whole grain cereal**, a banana, and toast for breakfast; a sandwich for lunch; and a frozen dinner in the evening, which has a small serving of meat, potatoes or rice, and corn or green beans. He says he is **trying to drink fluids but has started feeling a little nauseated when he drinks very much.** He also isn't sure if too much fluid would make his feet swell again. He has a cup of coffee and a small glass of orange juice in the morning. He drinks a small glass of iced tea with lunch and dinner.
Assess which foods and fluids Mr. Johnson likes, can obtain, and will prepare.	He reports that a friend will shop for him for groceries. Occasionally a friend brings him dinner, but he relies on frozen dinners because they are easy to get and to heat. **He hates prune juice but will drink apple or orange juice. He agrees that he can drink more water but prefers iced tea with sugar. He likes lettuce and tomato salads; most fruits; and frozen peas, corn or green beans. He'll try whole-grain bread but prefers white bread.**
Ask about any nausea or vomiting.	Complains of **mild nausea** when he eats and a constant **feeling of fullness** but no vomiting.
Palpate abdomen.	While Javier is palpating Mr. Johnson's abdomen, Mr. Johnson tells him, "It really feels full," and he winces with very little pressure applied. Abdomen feels taut and mildly distended.

***Defining characteristics** are shown in bold type.

NURSING DIAGNOSIS: Constipation related to opiate-containing pain medication, decreased mobility, and decreased food and fluid intake

PLANNING

Goals	*Expected Outcomes (NOC)*[†]
	Bowel Elimination
Mr. Johnson will establish normal defecation.	Mr. Johnson reports passage of soft, formed stool without straining in next 24 hours.
	Nutritional Status: Food and Fluid Intake
Mr. Johnson will make changes to his diet to prevent constipation.	Mr. Johnson drinks at least 1500 mL of fluid over the next 24 hours.
	Mr. Johnson increases the fiber content of his diet by eating an apple with his breakfast, lettuce and tomato on his sandwich, and some carrots with his dinner.

[†]Outcome classification labels from Moorhead S et al: *Nursing outcomes classification (NOC)*, ed 5, St Louis, 2013, Mosby.

INTERVENTIONS (NIC)[‡]	RATIONALE
Constipation/Impaction Management	
Encourage fluid intake of appropriate fluids, fruit juice, and water.	At least 1500 mL fluid intake daily will help to soften the stool.
Encourage activity within patient's mobility regimen.	Minimal activity (such as leg lifts) increases peristalsis.
Instruct Mr. Johnson to eat more fruits and vegetables and have a bran cereal for breakfast.	Added fiber in food relieves constipation.
Provide stimulant laxative and stool softeners as ordered.	Stimulant laxatives increase peristalsis and are an effective way to relieve constipation and promote normal bowel function when used on a short-term basis.
Encourage Mr. Johnson to try to have a bowel movement at the same time each day.	A regular time for bowel movements encourages normal bowel function.

[‡]Intervention classification labels from Bulechek GM et al: *Nursing interventions classification (NIC)*, ed 6, St Louis, 2013, Mosby.

EVALUATION

Nursing Actions	*Patient Response/Finding*	*Achievement of Outcomes*
Ask Mr. Johnson to identify foods high in fiber and fluid intake.	Able to state appropriate foods and fluids, but still has little appetite and feels full soon after eating.	Mr. Johnson verbalizes understanding of teaching.
Get medication history for last 2 days.	Patient has taken a stimulant laxative and stool softener twice a day for last 2 days.	Patient has not had a bowel movement.
Ask Mr. Johnson about physical activity.	Mr. Johnson states that he has not changed his activity pattern.	Mr. Johnson did not increase activity pattern and needs to continue to work on this intervention.
Inquire about bowel movements.	Mr. Johnson still has not had a bowel movement.	Mr. Johnson did not achieve passage of regular, formed stool.

BOX 47-6 Nursing Diagnostic Process

Constipation

Assessment Activities	Defining Characteristics
Ask patient about bowel elimination patterns.	Patient reports no bowel movement for 4 days.
Ask patient about other gastrointestinal symptoms.	Patient denies any feeling of nausea, abdominal cramping, or loss of appetite.
Ask patient to describe recent food and fluid intake.	Patient reports drinking two cups of coffee and one glass of iced tea each day; eating one serving of cooked vegetables and a banana every other day; having peanut butter and jelly sandwiches, meat, potatoes, and white bread every day.
Palpate abdomen.	Patient reports feeling of fullness. Left lower quadrant is firm.

Associated problems such as age, body-image changes, or skin breakdown require interventions unrelated to bowel function impairment. It is important to establish the correct "related to" factor for a diagnosis. This depends on the thoroughness of your assessment and your recognition of the defining characteristics and factors that impair elimination (Box 47-6). For example, with the diagnosis of *Constipation* you distinguish between related factors of *nutritional imbalance, exercise, medications,* and *emotional problems.* Selection of the correct related factors for each diagnosis ensures that you will implement the appropriate nursing interventions.

◆ Planning

When planning care, synthesize information from multiple resources (Figure 47-7). Critical thinking ensures that the plan of care integrates everything known about a patient and current clinical problems. Rely on professional standards when possible. For example, the Wound, Ostomy and Continence Nurse guidelines (WOCN, 2013) on fecal incontinence help to protect a patient's skin, promote continence, and reduce the embarrassment associated with incontinence.

Goals and Outcomes. Help patients establish goals and outcomes by incorporating their elimination habits or routines as much as possible and reinforcing the routines that promote health (see the Nursing Care Plan). In addition, consider preexisting health concerns. For example, if a patient's diet, activity, and irregular bowel habits caused the elimination problem, help him or her learn to make lifestyle changes to improve bowel function. The overall goal of returning a patient to a normal bowel elimination pattern includes the following outcomes:

- Patient establishes a regular defecation schedule.
- Patient lists proper fluid and food intake needed to soften stool and promote regular bowel elimination.
- Patient implements a regular exercise program.
- Patient reports daily passage of soft, formed brown stool.
- Patient does not report straining or discomfort associated with defecation.

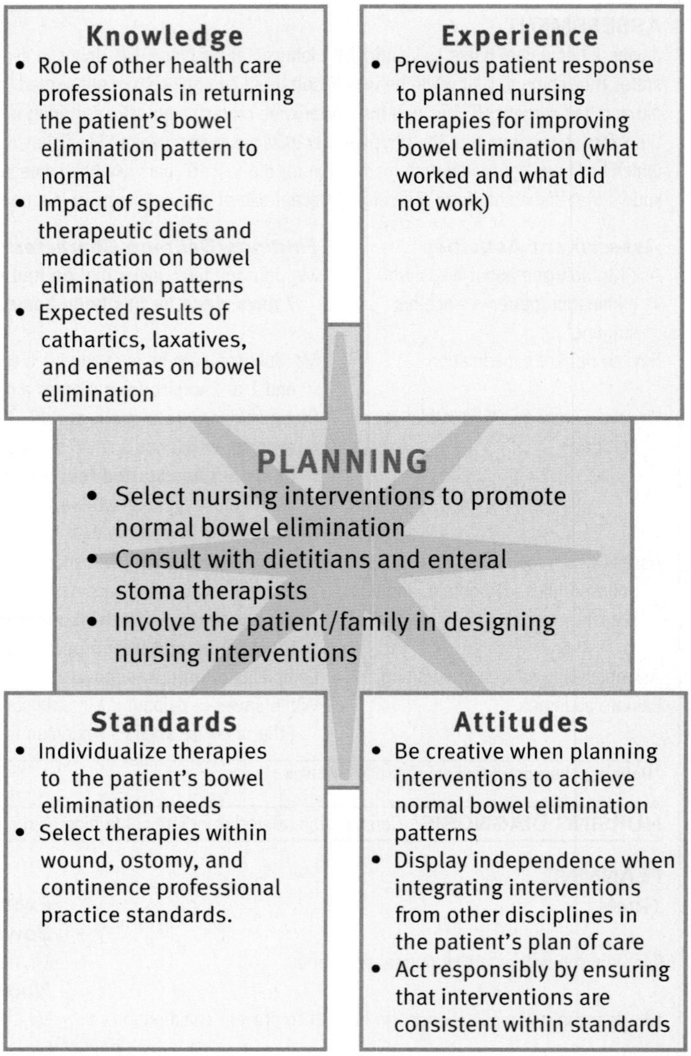

Knowledge
- Role of other health care professionals in returning the patient's bowel elimination pattern to normal
- Impact of specific therapeutic diets and medication on bowel elimination patterns
- Expected results of cathartics, laxatives, and enemas on bowel elimination

Experience
- Previous patient response to planned nursing therapies for improving bowel elimination (what worked and what did not work)

PLANNING
- Select nursing interventions to promote normal bowel elimination
- Consult with dietitians and enteral stoma therapists
- Involve the patient/family in designing nursing interventions

Standards
- Individualize therapies to the patient's bowel elimination needs
- Select therapies within wound, ostomy, and continence professional practice standards.

Attitudes
- Be creative when planning interventions to achieve normal bowel elimination patterns
- Display independence when integrating interventions from other disciplines in the patient's plan of care
- Act responsibly by ensuring that interventions are consistent within standards

FIGURE 47-7 Critical thinking model for elimination planning. *AHRQ,* Agency for Healthcare Research and Quality; *WOCN,* Wound, Ostomy and Continence Nurses Society.

QSEN QSEN: BUILDING COMPETENCY IN PATIENT-CENTERED CARE Mr. Johnson started taking a stimulant laxative every day to avoid constipation after he had a fecal impaction removed. He drank more fluids, especially water, and began adding more fruits and vegetables to his diet. On the day after the impaction was removed, he had a formed, firm bowel movement with some straining required. Then he began having daily bowel movements with soft, formed stool. Now it is 1 month later, and he is still taking laxatives but not continuing with the fluid and dietary modifications that were recommended for him. The physical therapist is ready to discharge him from home care but asks the nurse to make another visit when Mr. Johnson states he is having trouble moving his bowels. Which assessment questions and teaching strategies, approaches, and tools does the nurse use to enhance Mr. Johnson's learning and ability to prevent constipation?

ⓔ*Answers to QSEN Activities can be found on the Evolve website.*

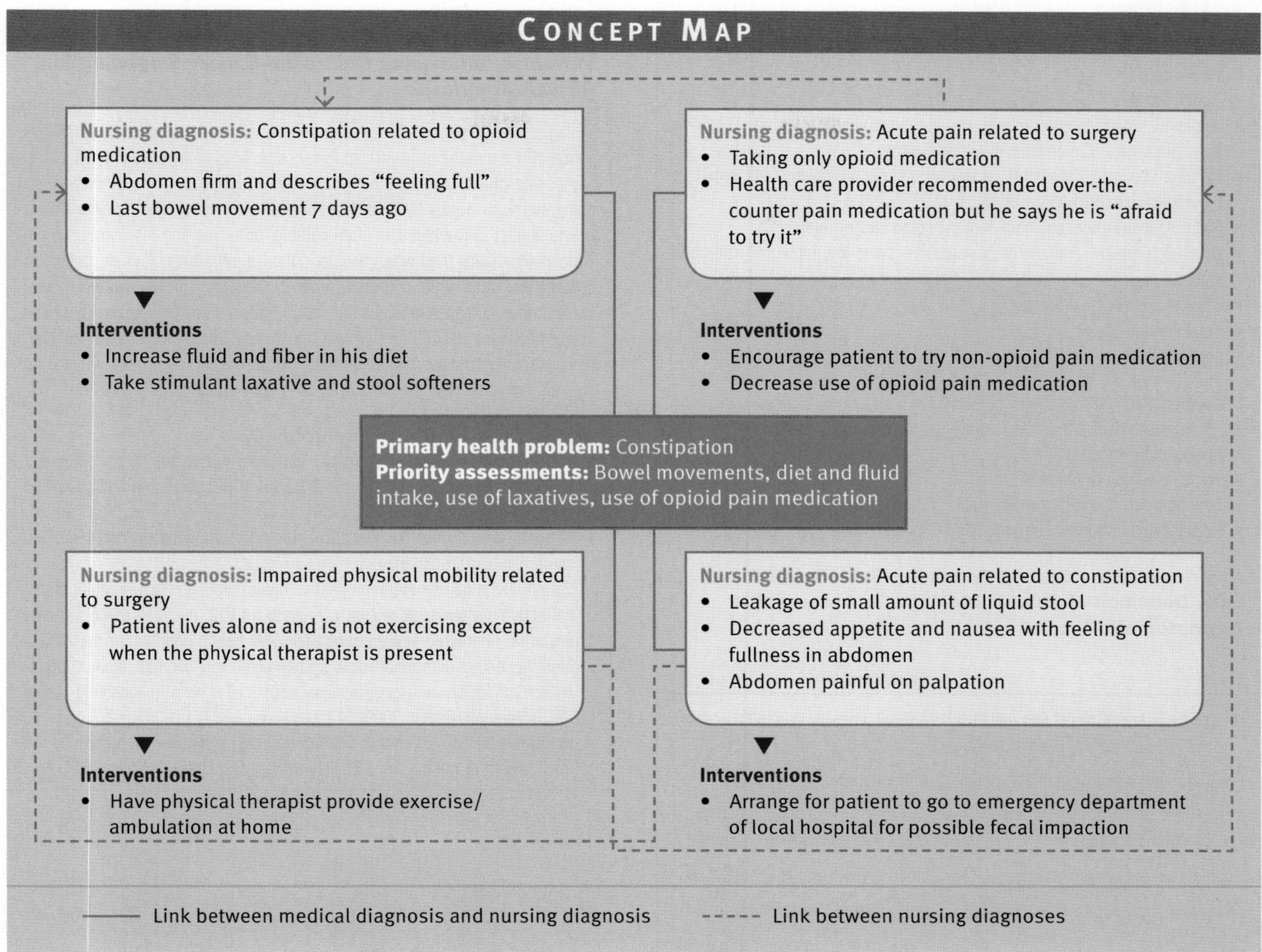

FIGURE 47-8 Concept map for Mr. Johnson.

Setting Priorities. Defecation patterns vary among individuals. For this reason a nurse and patient work together closely to plan effective interventions. Patients often have multiple diagnoses. The concept map (Figure 47-8) shows an example of how the nursing diagnosis of constipation is related to three other diagnoses and their respective interventions. A realistic time frame to establish a normal defecation pattern for one patient is sometimes very different for another. In the patient with recent abdominal surgery, the priorities of pain management and the avoidance of constipation through increasing fluids in the diet and encouraging early ambulation help in the recovery process.

Teamwork and Collaboration. When patients are disabled or debilitated by illness, you need to include the family in the plan of care. In some situations family members have the same ineffective elimination habits as the patient. Thus patient and family teaching is an important part of the care plan. Other health team members such as dietitians and WOCNs are often valuable resources. You coordinate activities of the multidisciplinary health care team.

A patient with alterations in bowel elimination sometimes requires intervention from several members of the health care team. Certain tasks such as assisting patients onto the bedpan or bedside commode are appropriate to delegate to nursing assistive personnel (NAP). It is important to remind the NAP to report any abnormal findings or difficulties encountered during the elimination process. Many of the diagnostic tests for evaluation of the GI system are performed by nonnursing personnel. Maintaining ongoing communication with these caregivers will ensure that you provide safe and effective patient-centered care and address a patient's needs, wants, and concerns.

◆ Implementation

Successful nursing interventions improve patients' and family members' understanding of bowel elimination. Teach them about proper diet, adequate fluid intake, and factors that stimulate or slow peristalsis such as emotional stress. This is often best done during a patient's mealtime. Patients also need to learn the importance of establishing regular bowel routines, exercising regularly, and taking appropriate measures when elimination problems develop.

Health Promotion. One of the most important habits to teach regarding bowel habits is to take time for defecation. To establish regular bowel habits, a patient needs to know when the urge to defecate normally occurs. Advise the patient to begin establishing a routine

BOX 47-7 Screening for Colorectal Cancer

Risk Factors

- Age: Over 50
- Family history: Colorectal cancer, familial adenomatous polyposis, hereditary nonpolyposis colon cancer (Lynch syndrome)
- Personal history: Colorectal cancer or colorectal polyps, inflammatory bowel disease (IBD)
- Race: African-Americans have highest colon cancer rates
- Diet: High intake of animal fats or red meat and low intake of fruits and vegetables
- Obesity and physical inactivity
- Smoking and heavy alcohol consumption
- Type 2 diabetes

Warning Signs

- Change in bowel habits (e.g., diarrhea, constipation, narrowing of stool lasting more than few days)
- Rectal bleeding or blood in stool
- Sensation of incomplete evacuation
- Unexplained abdominal or back pain

American Cancer Society Screening Guidelines for the Early Detection of Colorectal Cancer in Average-Risk Asymptomatic People

Test	Frequency
Guaiac fecal occult blood test (gFOBT) done on multiple samples at home	Annual, starting at age 50
Fecal immunochemical test (FIT) done on multiple samples at home	Annual, starting at age 50
Flexible sigmoidoscopy	Every 5 years, starting at age 50
Double-contrast barium enema	Every 5 years, starting at age 50
Computed tomography, colonography	Every 5 years, starting at age 50
Colonoscopy	Every 10 years, starting at age 50

Data from American Cancer Society, 2015, www.cancer.gov. These procedures will be ordered by a health care provider, depending on availability of resources and patient needs. If positive findings result from the flexible sigmoidoscopy, barium enema, or colonography, follow-up with a colonoscopy should be done.

BOX 47-8 CULTURAL ASPECTS OF CARE

Variables Influencing Colorectal Cancer Screening in African-Americans

Biological, psychological, behavioral, and social variables influence colorectal cancer (CRC) screenings in African-Americans. African-Americans have a 20% higher rate of CRC and 40% higher incidence of disease-related death when compared with whites (ACS, 2015). Prevention resulting in early detection is key to finding CRC when it is often curable, but screening rates are lower in African-Americans than white people in the United States. A study looking at compliance rates with colorectal cancer screening in the United States showed that African-Americans and Asians were more compliant with a fecal occult blood test (FOBT) and whites and Asians were more compliant with having a colonoscopy. When barriers to care were removed, the rate of colonoscopy screening was higher in all groups (Inadomi et al., 2012).

Implications for Patient-Centered Care

- Lack of routine visits to a primary care provider is one of the strongest predictors for inadequate colorectal cancer (CRC) screening and advanced stage at presentation (Griffin, 2009).
- Patients who do not have health insurance frequently do not seek CRC screening (Griffin, 2009).
- Patients who participate in preventive health practices (e.g., regular physical activity) often seek regular screening for CRC because these patients are often interested in promoting their own health (Inadomi et al., 2012).
- Identification of additional social system predictors such as family support, church affiliation, and geographical access also help in receiving timely CRC screening (Griffin, 2009).
- Removing barriers of safety, quality, and cost-effectiveness improves the involvement of patients in CRC screening (ACS, 2015).

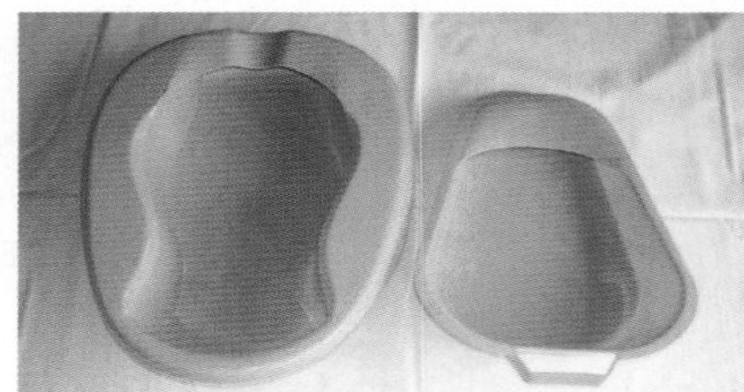

FIGURE 47-9 Types of bedpans. From left, Regular bedpan and fracture bedpan.

during a time when defecation is most likely to occur, usually an hour after a meal. When patients are restricted to bed or need help to ambulate, offer a bedpan or help them reach the bathroom in a timely manner.

Colorectal cancer is the third most common cancer to occur in the United States (ACS, 2015). When diagnosed early, it can be treated and eliminated. Following the guidelines for prevention, knowing the early symptoms, and seeking medical help if these symptoms occur are the most effective ways to prevent death from this disease (Box 47-7).

African-Americans have the highest rates of cancer and highest death rates from cancer of any cultural group. The death rates have dropped for lung and oropharyngeal cancers, but the rates for colorectal cancer continue to be 33% higher for African-American men and 16% higher for African-American women than for non-Hispanic white men and women. There still is a lower rate of colorectal cancer screening among African-Americans, but this disparity is decreasing (Box 47-8).

Promotion of Normal Defecation. A number of interventions stimulate the defecation reflex, affect the character of feces, or increase peristalsis to help patients evacuate bowel contents normally and without discomfort.

Sitting Position. Help patients who have difficulty sitting because of muscular weakness and mobility problems. Place an elevated seat on the toilet or a bedside commode when patients are unable to lower themselves to a sitting position because of pain or weakness. These seats require patients to use less effort to sit or stand.

Positioning on Bedpan. Patients restricted to bed use bedpans for defecation. Women use bedpans to pass both urine and feces, whereas men use bedpans only for defecation. Sitting on a bedpan is often uncomfortable. Help position patients comfortably. Two types of bedpans are available (Figure 47-9). The regular bedpan, made of plastic, has a curved smooth upper end and a sharper-edged lower end and is about 5 cm (2 inches) deep. The smaller fracture pan, designed for patients with lower-extremity fractures, has a shallow upper end

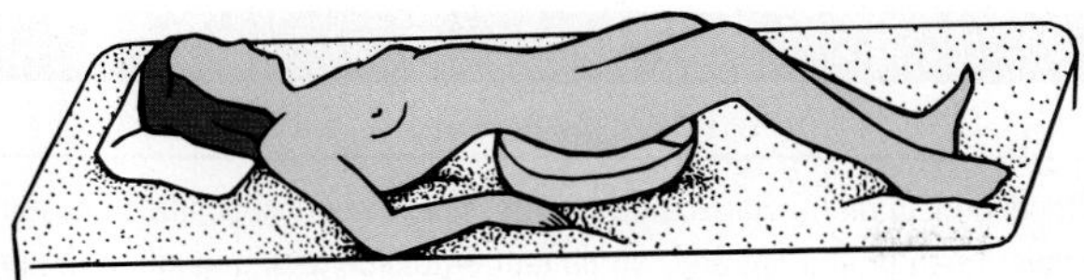

FIGURE 47-10 Improper positioning of patient on bedpan.

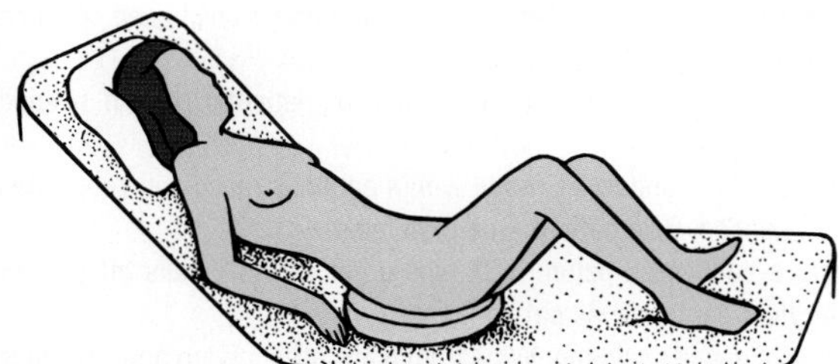

FIGURE 47-11 Proper position reduces patient's back strain.

about 2.5 cm (1 inch) deep. The shallow end of the pan fits under the buttocks toward the sacrum; the deeper end, which has a handle, goes just under the upper thighs. The pan needs to be high enough so feces enter it.

When positioning a patient, it is important to prevent muscle strain and discomfort. Never try to lift a patient onto a bedpan. Never place a patient on a bedpan and then leave with the bed flat unless activity restrictions demand it because it forces the patient to hyperextend the back to lift the hips on the pan. The proper position for the patient on a bedpan is with the head of the bed elevated 30 to 45 degrees (Figures 47-10 and 47-11). When patients are immobile or it is unsafe to allow them to raise their hips, it is safest for both caregivers and patients to roll them on to the bedpan (Box 47-9). Always wear gloves when handling a bedpan.

Acute Care. With some acute illnesses the GI system becomes affected. Changes in a patient's fluid status, mobility patterns, nutrition, and sleep cycle affect regular bowel habits. Surgical interventions on the GI tract obviously affect bowel elimination. However, surgery on other systems (e.g., the musculoskeletal and cardiovascular systems) also sometimes affects it.

Chronically ill and hospitalized patients are not always able to maintain privacy during defecation. In a hospital or extended care setting, patients sometimes share bathroom facilities with a roommate. In addition, chronic illness may limit a patient's mobility and activity tolerance and require the use of a bedpan or bedside commode. The sights, sounds, and odors associated with sharing toilet facilities or using bedpans are often embarrassing. This embarrassment often causes patients to ignore the urge to defecate, which leads to constipation and discomfort. Remain sensitive to patients' elimination needs and intervene to help them maintain as normal bowel elimination habits as possible.

Cathartics and Laxatives. Some medications initiate and facilitate stool passage. Laxatives and cathartics have the short-term action of emptying the bowel. These agents are also used to cleanse the bowel for patients undergoing GI tests and abdominal surgery. Although the terms *laxative* and *cathartic* are often used interchangeably, cathartics generally have a stronger and more rapid effect on the intestines. Teach patients about the potential harmful effects of overuse of laxatives such as impaired bowel motility and decreased response to sensory stimulus. Make sure patients understand that laxatives are not to be used long term for maintenance of bowel function.

Although patients usually take medications orally, laxatives prepared as suppositories may act more quickly because of their stimulant effect on the rectal mucosa. Suppositories such as bisacodyl act within 30 minutes. Give the suppository shortly before a patient's usual time to defecate or immediately after a meal.

Laxatives are classified by the method by which the agent promotes defecation (Table 47-2). Some newer drugs are being used now for chronic constipation or motility disorders. It is too soon to tell if these medications will be effective and safe for long-term treatment, but they are not used for the relief of occasional constipation.

Antidiarrheal Agents. Antidiarrheal agents decrease intestinal muscle tone to slow the passage of feces. As a result, the body absorbs more water through the intestinal walls. However, the cause of diarrhea must be determined before effective treatment can be ordered by a health care provider. For example, if an infection is the causative factor, an antibiotic may be used for treatment; or if inflammation is the cause, steroids may be given. The most commonly used antidiarrheal agents are loperamide or diphenoxylate with atropine. Codeine or tincture of opium may be used for management of chronic severe diarrhea in patients with diseases such as Crohn's disease, ulcerative colitis, and acquired immunodeficiency syndrome (AIDS). Patients need to use antidiarrheal agents that contain opiates with caution because opiates are habit forming.

Enemas. An enema is the instillation of a solution into the rectum and sigmoid colon. The primary reason for an enema is to promote defecation by stimulating peristalsis. The volume of fluid instilled breaks up the fecal mass, stretches the rectal wall, and initiates the defecation reflex. Enemas are also a vehicle for medications that exert a local effect on rectal mucosa. They are used most commonly for the immediate relief of constipation, emptying the bowel before diagnostic tests or surgery, and beginning a program of bowel training.

Cleansing Enemas. Cleansing enemas promote the complete evacuation of feces from the colon. They act by stimulating peristalsis through the infusion of a large volume of solution or through local irritation of the mucosa of the colon. They include tap water, normal saline, soapsuds solution, and low-volume hypertonic saline. Each solution has a different osmotic effect, influencing the movement of fluids between the colon and interstitial spaces beyond the intestinal wall. Infants and children receive only normal saline because they are at greater risk for fluid imbalance.

Tap Water. Tap water is hypotonic and exerts an osmotic pressure lower than fluid in interstitial spaces. After infusion into the colon, tap water escapes from the bowel lumen into interstitial spaces. The net movement of water is low. The infused volume stimulates defecation before large amounts of water leave the bowel. Use caution if ordered to repeat tap-water enemas because water toxicity or circulatory overload develops if the body absorbs large amounts of water.

Normal Saline. Physiologically normal saline is the safest solution to use because it exerts the same osmotic pressure as fluids in interstitial spaces surrounding the bowel. The volume of infused saline stimulates peristalsis. Giving saline enemas lessens the danger of excess fluid absorption.

Hypertonic Solutions. Hypertonic solutions infused into the bowel exert osmotic pressure that pulls fluids out of interstitial spaces. The colon fills with fluid, and the resultant distention promotes defecation. Patients unable to tolerate large volumes of fluid benefit most from this type of enema, which is by design low volume. This type of enema is contraindicated for patients who are dehydrated and young infants. A hypertonic solution of 120 to 180 mL (4 to 6 ounces) is

BOX 47-9 PROCEDURAL GUIDELINES

Assisting Patient On and Off a Bedpan

Delegation Considerations

The skill of assisting a patient onto a bedpan can be delegated to nursing assistive personnel (NAP). The nurse guides and assists the NAP in the proper way to position patients who have mobility restrictions. The nurse also instructs the NAP in how to position patients who have therapeutic equipment present such as drains, intravenous catheters, or traction.

Equipment

Appropriate type of clean bedpan; toilet tissue; specimen container (if necessary); washbasin; washcloths; towels; soap; waterproof, absorbent pads; clean drawsheet *(optional)*; clean gloves

Steps

1. Assess the patient's level of mobility, strength, ability to help, and presence of any condition (e.g., orthopedic) that interferes with the use of a bedpan.
2. Explain the technique you will use in turning and positioning to the patient.
3. Offer the bedpan after meals because the patient may have an urge to defecate at that time.
4. Perform hand hygiene and apply clean gloves.
5. Close the room curtain for privacy.
6. Raise bed to a comfortable working height. Position patient high in bed with head elevated 30 degrees (unless contraindicated).
7. Fold back top linen to patient's knees.
8. Help with positioning an independent patient: Raise side rails. Instruct patient to bend knees, place weight on feet, grasp side rails, and lift hips while you slip bedpan into place.
9. Dependent patient: Raise side rail on side of bed opposite from nurse. Lower head of bed flat and roll patient onto side facing away from nurse. Apply powder lightly to lower back and buttocks *(optional)*. Place bedpan firmly against buttocks (see illustration *A*). Push bedpan down into mattress with open rim toward patient's feet (see illustration *B*). Keeping one hand against bedpan, place other hand on patient's hip (see illustration *C*). Ask patient to roll onto pan, flat on bed. With patient positioned comfortably, raise head of bed 30 degrees.
10. Place rolled towel under lumbar curve of patient's back if needed for support.
11. Place call light and toilet tissue within patient's reach and keep side rails up as needed. Give patient time to defecate.
12. Remove bedpan as patient lifts hips up or carefully rolls off pan and to side. Hold pan firmly as patient moves.
13. Help to cleanse anal area. Wipe from pubic area toward anus. Replace top covers.
14. If you are collecting a specimen or recording urine output, do not dispose of tissue in bedpan.
15. Have patient wash and dry hands.
16. Empty contents of pan and rinse pan, dispose of gloves, and perform hand hygiene.
17. Inspect stool for color, amount, consistency, odor, or presence of abnormal substances. Document findings.

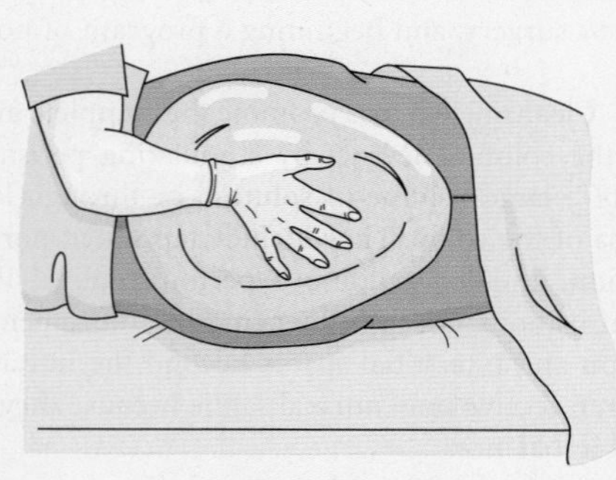

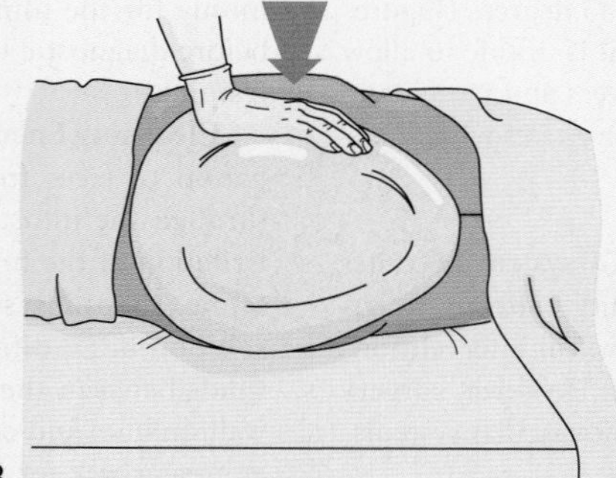

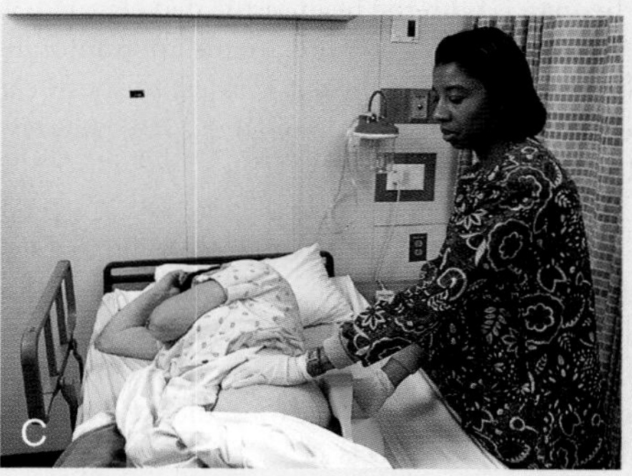

STEP 9 Positioning immobilized patient on bedpan. **A,** Place bedpan firmly against buttocks. **B,** Push buttocks down into mattress with open rim toward feet. **C,** Place one hand against bedpan; place other hand around patient's fore hip.

usually effective. The commercially prepared Fleet enema is the most common.

Soapsuds. You add soapsuds to tap water or saline to create the effect of intestinal irritation to stimulate peristalsis. Use only pure castile soap that comes in a liquid form included in most soapsuds enema kits. Use soapsuds enemas with caution in pregnant women and older adults because they could cause electrolyte imbalance or damage to the intestinal mucosa.

A health care provider sometimes orders a high- or low-cleansing enema. The terms *high* and *low* refer to the height from which, and hence the pressure with which, the fluid is delivered. High enemas cleanse more of the colon. After the enema is infused, ask the patient to turn from the left lateral to the dorsal recumbent, over to the right lateral position. The position change ensures that fluid reaches the large intestine. A low enema cleanses only the rectum and sigmoid colon.

Oil Retention. Oil-retention enemas lubricate the feces in the rectum and colon. The feces absorb the oil and become softer and easier to pass. To enhance action of the oil, the patient retains the enema for several hours if possible.

Other Types of Enemas. Carminative enemas provide relief from gaseous distention. They improve the ability to pass flatus. An example

TABLE 47-2 Common Types of Laxatives and Cathartics

Agent/Brand Name	Action	Indications	Risks
Bulk Forming			
Methylcellulose (Citrucel) Psyllium (Metamucil, Naturacil) Polycarbophil (Fibercon)	High-fiber content absorbs water and increases solid intestinal bulk, which will stretch intestinal wall to stimulate peristalsis. Passage of stool will occur in 12 to 24 hours. These agents must be taken with water and should be used with patients who have an adequate food and fluid intake. Patients may note increased gas formation and flatus when they first start taking these laxatives, but this will abate after 4-5 days.	Agents are least irritating, most natural, and safest type of laxatives. Agents are drugs of choice for chronic constipation (e.g., pregnancy, low-residue diet). They also relieve mild diarrhea. If treating diarrhea, administer less water.	Agents that are in powder form could cause constipation if not mixed with at least 240 mL of water or juice and swallowed quickly. Caution is necessary with bulk-forming laxatives that also contain stimulants. Agents are not for patients for whom large fluid intake is contraindicated.
Emollient or Wetting			
Docusate sodium (Colace) Docusate calcium (Surfak) Docusate potassium (Dialose)	Stool softeners are detergents that lower surface tension of feces, allowing water and fat to penetrate. They increase secretion of water by intestine.	Agents are for short-term therapy to relieve straining on defecation (e.g., hemorrhoids, perianal surgery, pregnancy, recovery from myocardial infarction).	Agents are of little value for treatment of chronic constipation.
Osmotic			
Saline-based Magnesium citrate or citrate of magnesia Magnesium hydroxide (Milk of Magnesia) Sodium phosphate (Fleet Phospho-Soda) Polyethylene glycol, lactulose, sorbitol based, Lactulose, Miralax	Osmotic effect increases pressure in bowel to act as stimulant for peristalsis. Osmotic laxatives are any agents that pull fluid into the bowel to soften the stool and distend the bowel to stimulate peristalsis.	Saline-based agents are only for acute emptying of bowel (e.g., endoscopic examination, suspected poisoning, acute constipation). Agents may be used to treat chronic constipation.	Saline-based agents are not for long-term management of constipation or for patients with kidney dysfunction. They may cause toxic buildup of magnesium. Phosphate salts are not recommended for patients on fluid restriction.
Stimulant Cathartics			
Bisacodyl (Dulcolax) Castor oil Casanthranol (Peri-Colace) Correctol Senna (Ex-Lax, Senokot)	Agents cause local irritation to the intestinal mucosa, increase intestinal motility, and inhibit resorption of water in the large intestine. The rapid movement of feces causes retention of water in the stool. The drugs cause formation of a soft-to-liquid stool in 6 to 8 hours and usually contain bisacodyl or senna. These laxatives should be used occasionally because regular use of a stimulant laxative can lead to dependence on the stimulus for defecation.	Agents prepare bowel for diagnostic procedures or may be needed for those with constipation from frequent opioid use	Agents cause severe cramping. Agents are not for long-term use. Chronic use could cause fluid and electrolyte imbalances.

of a carminative enema is MGW solution, which contains 30 mL of magnesium, 60 mL of glycerin, and 90 mL of water.

Medicated enemas contain drugs. An example is sodium polystyrene sulfonate (Kayexalate), used to treat patients with dangerously high serum potassium levels. This drug contains a resin that exchanges sodium ions for potassium ions in the large intestine. Another medicated enema is neomycin solution, an antibiotic used to reduce bacteria in the colon before bowel surgery. An enema containing steroid medication may be used for acute inflammation in the lower colon.

Enema Administration. Enemas are available in commercially packaged, disposable units or with reusable equipment prepared before use. Sterile technique is unnecessary because the colon normally contains bacteria. However, wear gloves to prevent the transmission of fecal microorganisms.

Explain the procedure, including the position to assume, precautions to take to avoid discomfort, and length of time necessary to retain the solution before defecation. If a patient needs to take the enema at home, explain the procedure to a family member.

Giving an enema to a patient who is unable to contract the external sphincter poses difficulties. Give the enema with the patient positioned on the bedpan. Giving the enema with a patient sitting on the toilet is unsafe because the position of the rectal tubing could injure the rectal wall. Skill 47-1 on pp. 1170–1173 outlines the steps for an enema administration.

Digital Removal of Stool. For a patient with an impaction, the fecal mass is sometimes too large to pass voluntarily. If a digital rectal examination reveals a hard stool mass in the rectum, it may be necessary to manually remove it by breaking it up and bringing out a section at a time. Digital removal is the last resort in the management of severe constipation, but it may be necessary if the fecal mass is too large to pass through the anal canal. The procedure (Box 47-10) is very uncomfortable for the patient. Excess rectal manipulation causes irritation to the mucosa, bleeding, and stimulation of the vagus nerve, which sometimes results in a reflex slowing of the heart rate (Hussain et al., 2014).

Inserting and Maintaining a Nasogastric Tube. A patient's condition or situation sometimes requires special interventions to decompress the GI tract. Such conditions include surgery (see Chapter 50), obstruction of the GI tract often caused by tumors, trauma to the GI tract, and conditions in which peristalsis is absent.

A nasogastric (NG) tube is a pliable hollow tube that is inserted through the patient's nasopharynx into the stomach. NG intubation has several purposes (Table 47-3). There are two main categories of NG tubes: fine- or small-bore tubes and large-bore tubes. Small-bore tubes are frequently used for medication administration and enteral feedings (see Chapter 45 for enteral feedings). Large-bore tubes, 12-Fr and above, are usually used for gastric decompression or removal of gastric secretions. The Levin and Salem sump tubes are the most common for stomach decompression. The Levin tube is a single-lumen tube with holes near the tip. It is connected to a drainage bag or an intermittent suction device to drain stomach secretions.

The Salem sump tube is preferable for stomach decompression. The tube has two lumina: one for removal of gastric contents and one to provide an air vent. A blue "pigtail" is the air vent that connects with the second lumen. When the main lumen of the sump tube is connected to suction, the air vent permits free, continuous drainage of secretions. Do not clamp off the air vent if the tube is connected to suction.

NG tube insertion does not require sterile technique. Instead you use clean technique. The procedure is uncomfortable. Patients experience a burning sensation as the tube passes through the sensitive nasal mucosa. When it reaches the back of the pharynx, patients sometimes begin to gag. Help them relax to make tube insertion easier. Some institutions allow the use of Xylocaine jelly or atomized lidocaine when inserting the tube because it decreases patient discomfort during the procedure. The procedure for inserting an NG tube is described in Skill 47-2 on pp. 1174–1179.

One of the greatest problems in caring for a patient with a NG tube is maintaining comfort. Because the tube irritates the nasal and pharyngeal mucosa, you assess the condition of the patient's nares and throat for inflammation. The tape or fixation device used to anchor the tube often becomes soiled or loosened. Change it as needed to prevent migration of the tube. Frequent lubrication of the nares may minimize discomfort. With one nostril occluded, the patient breathes through the mouth. Frequent mouth care helps minimize discomfort from a dry mouth. Water-moistened swabs or lozenges for the patient to suck may provide some relief of mouth and throat dryness. Often patients complain of a sore throat. A health care provider may order gargles with topical Xylocaine jelly to minimize the irritation.

After you insert the tube, you need to maintain its patency. Sometimes the tip of the tubing rests against the stomach wall, or the tube becomes blocked with thick secretions. Flushing the tube regularly with a catheter-tipped syringe filled with normal saline or warm water helps to prevent blockage of the tube. If a NG tube does not drain properly after flushing, reposition it by advancing or withdrawing it slightly. Any change in tube position requires you to verify its placement in the patient's GI tract.

BOX 47-10 PROCEDURAL GUIDELINES

Digital Removal of Stool

Delegation Considerations

The skill of digitally removing stool cannot be delegated to nursing assistive personnel (NAP). In some institutions only health care providers perform this procedure. The nurse instructs the NAP:

- To provide perineal care and other necessary hygiene following each bowel movement.
- To observe any evacuated stool for color and consistency.

Equipment

Bedpan, waterproof pad, water-soluble lubricant, washcloths, towels, soap, and clean gloves

Steps

1. Identify patient using two identifiers (e.g., name and birthday or name and medical record number) according to agency policy.
2. Perform hand hygiene, pull curtains around bed, obtain patient's baseline vital signs and assess level of comfort, and palpate for abdominal distention before the procedure.
3. Explain the procedure and help patient lie on left side in Sims' position with knees flexed and back toward you.
4. Drape trunk and lower extremities with a bath blanket and place a waterproof pad under buttocks. Keep a bedpan next to patient.
5. Perform hand hygiene and apply clean gloves; lubricate index finger of dominant hand with water-soluble lubricant.
6. Instruct patient to take slow, deep breaths. Gradually and gently insert index finger into the rectum, and advance the finger slowly along the rectal wall.
7. Gently loosen the fecal mass by massaging around it. Work the finger into the hardened mass.
8. Work the feces downward toward the end of the rectum. Remove small pieces one at a time and discard into bedpan.
9. Periodically reassess patient's pulse and look for signs of fatigue. Stop the procedure if pulse rate drops significantly (check agency policy) or rhythm changes.
10. Continue to clear rectum of feces and allow patient to rest at intervals.
11. After completion, wash and dry buttocks and anal area.
12. Remove bedpan; inspect feces for color and consistency. Dispose of feces. Remove gloves by turning them inside out and then discard.
13. Help patient to toilet or on a bedpan if urge to defecate develops.
14. Perform hand hygiene. Record results of procedure by describing fecal characteristics and amount.
15. Follow procedure with enemas or cathartics as ordered by health care provider.
16. Reassess patient's vital signs and level of comfort and observe status of abdominal distention.

Continuing and Restorative Care. Regular elimination patterns should begin before a patient goes home or to an extended care facility. With a new ostomy, a patient and/or a caregiver need to learn to manage the care that is required (Box 47-11). Other patients require bowel retraining. It is important to remember that you initiate ostomy

TABLE 47-3 Purposes of Nasogastric Intubation

Purpose	Description	Type of Tube
Decompression	Removal of secretions and gaseous substances from gastrointestinal (GI) tract; prevention or relief of abdominal distention (Lewis et al., 2014)	Salem sump, Levin, Miller-Abbott
Enteral feeding (see Chapter 45)	Instillation of liquid nutritional supplements or feedings into stomach or small intestine for patients with impaired swallowing (Lewis et al., 2014)	Duo, Dobhoff, Levin
Compression	Internal application of pressure by means of inflated balloon to prevent internal esophageal or GI hemorrhage (Lewis et al., 2014)	Sengstaken-Blakemore
Lavage	Irrigation of stomach in cases of active bleeding, poisoning, or gastric dilation (Lewis et al., 2014)	Levin, Ewald, Salem sump

BOX 47-11 PATIENT TEACHING

Teaching Patients How to Provide Ostomy Care

Objective

- Patient/caregiver will demonstrate how to empty and change an ostomy pouch.

Teaching Strategies

- Provide a comprehensive list of the products needed to care for the ostomy (Prinz et al., 2015)
- Provide patient/caregiver with supplies to last 1 to 2 weeks and the contact number information for a medical supply company (Prinz et al., 2015)
- Show patient/caregiver the step-by-step approach for changing an ostomy pouch.
- Provide at least one opportunity for patient/caregiver to empty and change the ostomy pouch while patient is in the hospital (Prinz et al., 2015)
- Provide detailed instructions for diet, fluids, peristomal skin care, restrictions on lifting, resuming exercise, intimacy, and when to contact the health care provider (Prinz et al., 2015).
- Arrange follow-up with an ostomy nurse if possible.

Evaluation

- Observe patient/caregiver change ostomy pouch.
- Ask patient/caregiver to teach back instructions given.

care and bowel retraining in acute care settings. However, because these are long-term care needs, teaching usually continues in restorative care or home settings.

Care of Ostomies. Patients with temporary or permanent bowel diversions have unique elimination needs. An individual with an ostomy wears a pouch to collect effluent or output from the stoma. The pouches are odor proof and have a protective skin barrier surrounding the stoma. Empty the pouch when it is $\frac{1}{3}$ to $\frac{1}{2}$ full. Change the pouching system approximately every 3 to 7 days, depending on a patient's individual needs (Goldberg et al., 2010). Assess the stoma color. It should be pink or red. You observe the skin at each pouch change for signs of irritation or skin breakdown. Skin protection is important because the effluent has digestive enzymes that cause irritant dermatitis if there is leakage on the peristomal skin. Other peristomal skin problems are fungal rashes, folliculitis, or ulcerations. Refer patients with these problems to an ostomy care nurse (Goldberg et al., 2010) (Box 47-12).

BOX 47-12 EVIDENCE-BASED PRACTICE

Recognition of Peristomal Skin Problems

PICO Question: In patients with ostomies, what is the effect of patient education and knowledge on the prevention of peristomal skin breakdown?

Evidence Summary

Patients with an ostomy are at risk for development of peristomal skin problems. In a study looking at patients with an ostomy in the first 3 months after surgery, 63% developed peristomal skin breakdown (Salvadena, 2013). Maintenance of healthy peristomal skin, with the skin around the stoma being clean, dry, and intact, is a priority following ostomy surgery (Goldberg et al., 2010). The most common cause of peristomal skin disorders is effluent, which causes skin irritation, ulceration, or erosion. Reasons for effluent leakage include poor-fitting stoma pouches, poor adhesive adherence, peristomal hernia, and surgical complications (Williams et al., 2010). With shorter postoperative hospital stays, it is challenging for nurses to provide the extensive patient education on pouching systems, ostomy care, and problem-solving techniques needed to prevent peristomal skin problems (Pittman et al., 2014). Patients often failed to recognize early signs of skin irritation and did not report a skin problem (Erwin-Toth et al., 2012). This lack of knowledge resulted in patients delaying to seek health care to treat the skin problem. Patient education is an important factor in preventing complications following ostomy surgery. Nurses need to provide education to patients before discharge and follow up with them after discharge to prevent peristomal skin problems (Prinz et al., 2015).

Application to Nursing Practice

- Evaluate patients' knowledge and ability to assess their peristomal skin changes for early recognition and treatment of skin disorders.
- Provide patient education about signs and symptoms of skin disorders to ensure early identification of skin problems.
- Refer patients to an ostomy nurse if assistance is needed to manage the ostomy (Erwin-Toth et al., 2012)

Irrigating a Colostomy. Although this practice is not as common because of improved odor-proof pouches, some patients irrigate their sigmoid colostomies to regulate colon emptying. This process takes about an hour a day to complete but usually means that a patient wears only a mini-pouch afterward to absorb mucus from the stoma and contain gas. Specific equipment designed for ostomies is used. The equipment has a silicone cone attached by plastic tubing to a bag that will hold the irrigation fluid, which is usually warm water. Follow the routine that the patient has established for this care. Occasionally a patient with a colostomy who has constipation will have an irrigation or enema ordered. Use equipment that is designed specifically for the irrigation rather than an enema administration set used by patients without a stoma.

Pouching Ostomies. An ostomy requires a pouch to collect fecal material. An effective pouching system protects the skin, contains fecal material, remains odor free, and is comfortable and inconspicuous. A person wearing a pouch needs to feel secure enough to participate in any activity (Goldberg et al., 2010).

Many pouching systems are available. To ensure that a pouch fits well and meets a patient's needs, consider the location of the ostomy, type and size of the stoma, type and amount of ostomy drainage, size

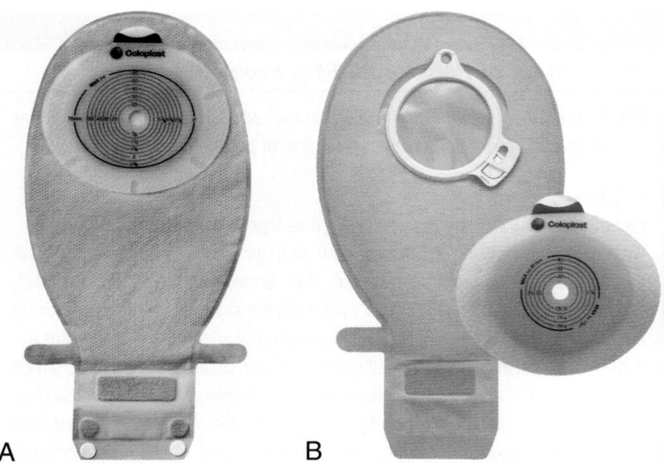

FIGURE 47-12 Ostomy pouches and skin barriers. **A,** SenSura® one-piece pouch with Velcro closure. **B,** SenSura® two-piece pouching system with separate skin barrier and attachable pouch. NOTE: Skin barriers need to be custom cut according to stoma size. (Courtesy Coloplast, Minneapolis, Minn.)

BOX 47-13 FOCUS ON OLDER ADULTS

Bowel Retraining

- Older age is a risk factor for having constipation.
- Increase fiber in diet with whole grains, legumes, fruits, and vegetables.
- A minimum of 1500 mL of fluid per day reduces the risk of constipation, with increased fluid needs during summer months and for those on diuretics with stable cardiovascular status.
- If holding a drinking cup is a problem, consider using a lighter plastic cup and filling half full, refilling frequently.
- Encourage regular exercise within the limitations imposed by other conditions.
- Patients need to feel at ease during elimination. Lack of privacy leads a patient to ignore the urge to defecate.
- Review all medications with a patient's health care provider to substitute medications that are less likely to cause constipation whenever possible.
- Behavioral interventions such as timed toileting helps establish a scheduled time for bowel elimination. Try to maintain the same schedule each day for toileting.

and contour of the abdomen, condition of the skin around the stoma, physical activities of the patient, patient's personal preference, age and dexterity, and cost of equipment. A **wound, ostomy and continence nurse (WOCN)** is a nurse specially educated to care for ostomy patients. A WOCN collaborates with staff nurses and patients to be sure that the patients have the best pouching system for their individual needs. A pouching system consists of a pouch and skin barrier (Figure 47-12). Pouches come in one- and two-piece systems and are flat or convex. Some pouches have the opening precut by the manufacturer; others require the stoma opening to be custom cut to a patient's specific stoma size. Newer pouches have an integrated closure; older ones use a clip to close the pouch. One of the first skills to teach a patient with a new ostomy is how to open and close the pouch. Skill 47-3 on pp. 1179–1181 describes steps for applying an ostomy pouch.

Nutritional Considerations. After surgery it usually takes a few days for patients with new ostomies to feel that their appetite has returned to normal. Small servings of soft foods are typically more appetizing as they would be for any patient who has had an abdominal surgery.

Patients with colostomies have no diet restrictions other than the diet discussed for normal healthy bowel function, with adequate fiber and fluid to keep the stool softly formed. Patients with ileostomies digest their food completely but lose both fluid and salt through their stoma and need to be sure to replace this to avoid dehydration. A good reminder for patients is to encourage drinking an 8-ounce glass of fluid when they empty their pouch. This helps them remember that they have greater fluid needs than they did before having an ileostomy. A condition that occurs infrequently with people with ileostomies is called a *food blockage*. Foods with indigestible fiber such as sweet corn, popcorn, raw mushrooms, fresh pineapple, and Chinese cabbage can cause this problem. However, if patients eat these foods in small quantities, drink fluids with the food and chew it well, they are unlikely to experience any difficulty.

Psychological Considerations. After ostomy surgery patients face a variety of anxieties and concerns, from learning how to manage their stoma to coping with conflicts of self-esteem, body image, and sexuality. Provide emotional support before and after surgery (Goldberg et al., 2010). Adjustment to a stoma takes time and is a very individual matter. A study of patients with colorectal cancer and a colostomy showed that the lowest quality of life after ostomy surgery occurred at 2 months, with improvement at 6 months and return to almost preoperative levels at 12 months (Li, 2014). Important factors affecting adjustment to the stoma include the ability to successfully assume care of the ostomy, including emptying the pouch and changing the pouching system so unexpected odor and leakage of stool does not occur. Inability to resume self-care sometimes causes a loss of self-esteem. The aging process often affects the ability to manage stomas, even in people who have had them for years. You need to recognize and intervene when problems resulting from advanced age such as skin changes, weight loss or gain, visual impairments, or changes in diet occur. If possible, consult with an ostomy nurse. The Wound, Ostomy and Continence Nurses Society (http://www.wocn.org) provides information and helps patients locate a WOCN. Consider referral to local ostomy groups such as those affiliated with the United Ostomy Associations of America at http://www.uoaa.org.

Bowel Training. A patient with chronic constipation or fecal incontinence secondary to cognitive impairment may benefit from **bowel training**, also called *habit training*. The training program involves setting up a daily routine. By attempting to defecate at the same time each day and using measures that promote defecation, a patient may establish a normal defecation pattern. The program requires time, patience, and consistency. A patient with cognitive impairment needs to have a caregiver able to devote the time to the training program. A successful program includes the following:

- Assessing the normal elimination pattern and recording times when a patient is incontinent
- Incorporating principles of gerontological nursing when providing bowel retraining programs for an older adult (Box 47-13)
- Choosing a time based on the patient's pattern to initiate defecation-control measures
- Offering a hot drink (hot tea) or fruit juice (prune juice) (or whatever fluids normally stimulate peristalsis for the patient) before the defecation time
- Helping the patient to the toilet at the designated time
- Providing privacy
- Instructing the patient to lean forward at the hips while sitting on the toilet, apply manual pressure with the hands over the abdomen, and bear down but not strain to stimulate colon emptying
- An unhurried environment and a nonjudgmental caregiver
- Maintaining normal exercise within the patient's physical ability

Maintenance of Proper Fluid and Food Intake. In choosing a diet for promoting normal elimination, consider the frequency of defecation, characteristics of feces, and types of foods that impair or promote defecation. A well-balanced diet with whole grains, legumes, fresh fruits, and vegetables eaten regularly promotes normal elimination. Fiber adds bulk to the stool, eliminates excess fluids, and promotes more frequent and regular movements. With increasing fiber it is important to drink enough fluids. If fluid intake is inadequate, the stool becomes hard because less water is retained in the large intestine to soften it. The amount of fiber and fluids necessary for optimal bowel function varies among individuals. Consulting a dietitian may be helpful if a patient has chronic problems with constipation.

When a patient has diarrhea, low-residue foods such as white rice, potatoes, bread, bananas, and cooked cereals are recommended until the diarrhea is controlled. Discourage foods that typically cause gastric upset or abdominal cramping. Diarrhea caused by illness is sometimes debilitating. If the patient cannot tolerate foods or liquids orally, intravenous therapy with electrolyte replacement is necessary. The patient returns to a normal diet slowly, often beginning with fluids.

Promotion of Regular Exercise. A daily exercise program helps prevent elimination problems. Walking, riding a stationary bicycle, or swimming stimulates peristalsis. It is recommended by the American Heart Association and the Centers for Disease Control and Prevention that adults get at least 150 minutes of exercise each week.

For a patient temporarily immobilized, attempt ambulation as soon as possible. If the condition permits, help the patient walk to a chair on the evening of the day of surgery and encourage him or her to walk a little more each day.

Management of the Patient with Fecal Incontinence or Diarrhea. You may apply a fecal collector around the anal opening if the skin is intact. These can be difficult to apply when there is a deep fold between the buttocks and there is hair in the area; but it may be considered if a patient is having very frequent liquid stools. There are also fecal-management systems available for short-term use with high-volume diarrhea. They are intended for use primarily in acute care settings. The devices have an intra-anal soft silicone catheter with a retention balloon much like a Foley catheter for insertion into the rectal vault to divert liquid stool away from the skin in immobilized patients. The catheter is connected to a drainage bag for collection of the liquid fecal effluent (Bliss and Norton, 2010). Refer to package insertion instructions and agency policies for appropriate use.

Maintenance of Skin Integrity. A patient with diarrhea, fecal incontinence, or an ileostomy is at risk for skin breakdown when fecal contents remain on the skin. Liquid stool usually contains digestive enzymes, which causes rapid skin breakdown. Irritation from repeated wiping with toilet tissue or frequent ostomy pouch changes further irritate the skin. Meticulous perianal skin care and frequent removal of fecal drainage is necessary to prevent skin breakdown (see Chapter 48). Clean the skin with a no-rinse cleanser and apply a barrier ointment after each episode of diarrhea. If a patient is incontinent, check on the patient frequently and change absorbent products immediately after providing thorough but gentle skin cleansing. Patients with ostomies are often unaware of the skin irritation under their ostomy wafer or think that this is a normal part of having an ostomy. Education about skin breakdown and its management are important roles for the ostomy nurse (see Box 47-12).

◆ Evaluation

Through the Patient's Eyes. The effectiveness of care depends on success in meeting the expected outcomes of self-care. Optimally a patient will be able to have regular, pain-free defecation of soft-formed stools. The patient or caregiver is the only one who is able to determine if the bowel elimination problems have been relieved and which therapies were the most effective (Figure 47-13).

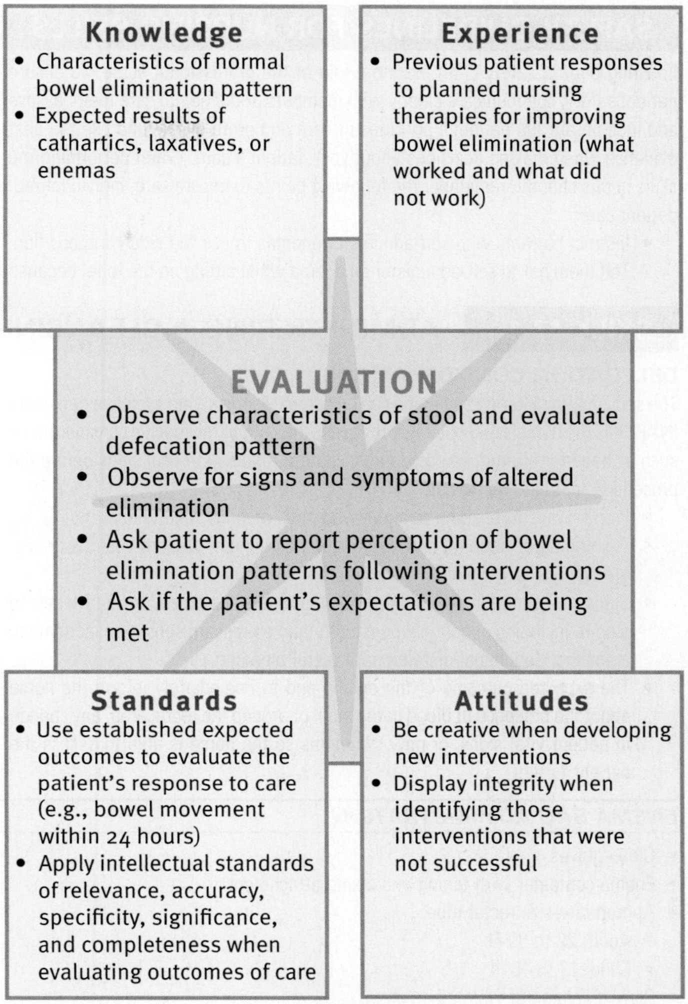

Knowledge
- Characteristics of normal bowel elimination pattern
- Expected results of cathartics, laxatives, or enemas

Experience
- Previous patient responses to planned nursing therapies for improving bowel elimination (what worked and what did not work)

EVALUATION
- Observe characteristics of stool and evaluate defecation pattern
- Observe for signs and symptoms of altered elimination
- Ask patient to report perception of bowel elimination patterns following interventions
- Ask if the patient's expectations are being met

Standards
- Use established expected outcomes to evaluate the patient's response to care (e.g., bowel movement within 24 hours)
- Apply intellectual standards of relevance, accuracy, specificity, significance, and completeness when evaluating outcomes of care

Attitudes
- Be creative when developing new interventions
- Display integrity when identifying those interventions that were not successful

FIGURE 47-13 Critical thinking model for elimination evaluation.

Patient Outcomes. When you establish a therapeutic relationship with a patient, the patient feels comfortable to discuss the intimate details often associated with bowel elimination. Patients are less embarrassed as you help them with elimination needs. Patients relate feelings of comfort and freedom from pain as elimination needs are met within the limits of their condition and treatment. Evaluate a patient's level of knowledge regarding establishing a normal elimination pattern, caring for an ostomy, and promoting skin integrity. Also determine the extent to which the patient accomplishes normal defection. Ask the patient to describe changes in diet, fluid intake, and activity to promote bowel health. Ask the following questions when the patient's expected outcome has not been achieved:

- Do you use medications such as laxatives or enemas to help you defecate? How often?
- Which barriers prevent you from eating a diet high in fiber and participating in regular exercise?
- How much fluid do you drink in a typical day? Which types of fluids do you normally drink?
- What challenges do you encounter when you change your ostomy pouch?

SAFETY GUIDELINES FOR NURSING SKILLS

Ensuring patient safety is an essential role of the professional nurse. To ensure patient safety, communicate clearly with members of the health care team, assess and incorporate the patient's priorities of care and preferences, and use the best evidence when making decisions about your patient's care. When performing the skills in this chapter, remember the following points to ensure safe, individualized, patient care:

- Instruct patients who self-administer enemas to use the side-lying position. Tell them not to self-administer an enema while sitting on the toilet because this position results in the rectal tubing causing friction that could injure the rectal wall.
- If a patient has cardiac disease or is taking cardiac or hypertensive medication, obtain a pulse rate, because manipulation of rectal tissue stimulates the vagus nerve and sometimes causes a sudden decline in pulse rate, which increases the patient's risk of fainting while on the bedpan, bedside commode, or toilet.

SKILL 47-1 ADMINISTERING A CLEANSING ENEMA

DELEGATION CONSIDERATIONS

The skill of administering an enema can be delegated to nursing assistive personnel (NAP). It is the nurse's responsibility to assess the patient for specific considerations such as need for alternative positioning, comfort, and stable vital signs before the procedure. Instruct NAP about:

- Proper ways to position patients who have mobility restrictions.
- Positioning of patients with therapeutic equipment present such as drains, intravenous (IV) catheters, or traction.
- Signs and symptoms of patient not tolerating the procedure and when to stop it, including abdominal pain more than a pressure sensation, abdominal cramping, abdominal distention, or rectal bleeding.
- The expected outcome of the enema and to immediately inform the nurse about the presence of blood in the stool or around the rectal area, any change in patient vital signs, or new symptoms so the nurse is able to assess the patient further.

EQUIPMENT

- Clean gloves
- Water-soluble lubricant
- Waterproof, absorbent pads
- Bath blanket
- Toilet tissue
- Bedpan, bedside commode, or access to toilet
- Basin, washcloths, towel, and soap
- IV pole

ENEMA BAG ADMINISTRATION

- Clean gloves
- Enema container with tubing and clamp attachment
- Appropriate-size rectal tube:
  - Adult: 22 to 30 Fr
  - Child: 12 to 18 Fr
- Correct volume of warmed solution:
  - Adult: 750 to 1000 mL
  - Child:
    - 150 to 250 mL, infant
    - 250 to 350 mL, toddler
    - 300 to 500 mL, school-age child
    - 500 to 700 mL, adolescent

ENEMA ADMINISTRATION

An enema container with rectal tip (Figure 47-14).

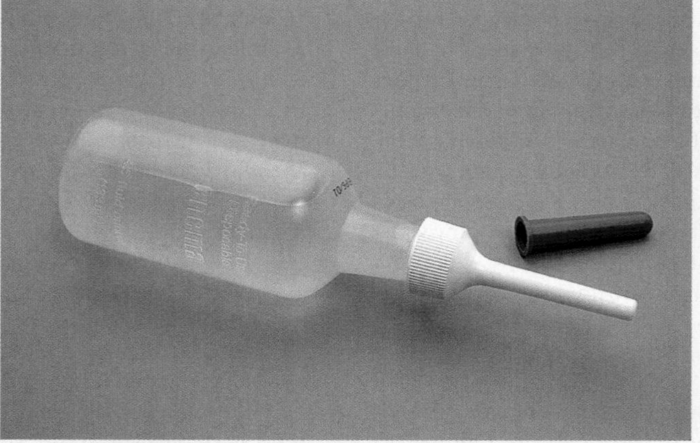

FIGURE 47-14 Prepackaged enema container with rectal tip.

STEP	RATIONALE
ASSESSMENT	
1. Assess status of patient: last bowel movement, normal versus most recent bowel pattern, presence of hemorrhoids, mobility, and presence of abdominal pain.	Determines factors indicating need for enema and influencing type of enema used. Also establishes a baseline for bowel function.
2. Review medical record for presence of increased intracranial pressure, glaucoma, or recent abdominal, rectal, or prostate surgery.	These conditions contraindicate use of enemas.
3. Inspect abdomen for presence of distention.	Provides a baseline for determining effectiveness of the enema.
4. Determine patient's level of understanding of purpose of enema.	Allows you to plan for appropriate teaching measures.
5. Review the health care provider's order for type of enema and number to administer.	Enemas require a health care provider's order. Determines number and type of enema you will give.

CLINICAL DECISION: *"Enemas until clear" order means that you repeat enemas until patient passes fluid that is clear of fecal matter. Check agency policy, but usually patients receive no more than three consecutive enemas to avoid disruption of fluid and electrolyte balance. It is essential to observe contents of solution passed. Consider the results "clear" when no solid fecal material exists but the solution is sometimes colored.*

STEP	RATIONALE
PLANNING	
1. Collect appropriate equipment.	
2. Identify patient using two identifiers (e.g., name and birthday or name and medical record number) according to agency policy.	Ensures correct patient. Complies with The Joint Commission standards and improves patient safety (TJC, 2016).
3. Assemble enema bag with appropriate solution and rectal tube if enema administration set does not have tube integrated into kit.	The proper equipment promotes the best outcome from the procedure.
IMPLEMENTATION	
1. Perform hand hygiene and apply clean gloves.	Reduces transmission of microorganisms.
2. Provide privacy by closing curtains around bed or closing door.	Reduces embarrassment for patient.
3. Raise bed to appropriate working height for nurse: Stand on right side of bed and raise side rail on opposite side.	Promotes good body mechanics and patient safety.
4. Help patient into left side-lying (Sims') position with right knee flexed. Children may also be placed in dorsal recumbent position.	Positioning allows enema solution to flow downward by gravity along natural curve of sigmoid colon and rectum, thus improving retention of solution.

CLINICAL DECISION: *If you suspect the patient has poor sphincter control, position on bedpan in a comfortable dorsal recumbent position. Patients with poor sphincter control are unable to retain all of the enema solution. Administering an enema with the patient sitting on the toilet is unsafe because it is impossible to safely guide the tubing into the rectum, and it will be difficult for the patient to retain the fluid as he or she is in the position used for emptying the bowel.*

STEP	RATIONALE
5. Place waterproof pad under hips and buttocks.	Prevents soiling of linen.
6. Cover patient with bath blanket, exposing only rectal area, clearly visualizing anus. Separate buttocks and examine perianal region for abnormalities, including hemorrhoids, anal fissure, and rectal prolapse (protrusion of the colon through the anal opening).	Provides warmth, reduces exposure of body parts, and allows patient to feel more relaxed and comfortable. Findings will influence approach to insert enema tip. An enema is contraindicated if there is a prolapse.
7. Place bedpan or commode in easily accessible position. If patient will be expelling contents in toilet, ensure that toilet is free. (If patient will be getting up to go to bathroom to expel enema, place his or her slippers and bathrobe in easily accessible position.)	Try to avoid incontinence of the stool and enema fluid to avoid discomfort and psychological stress.
8. Administer enema:	
a. Enema bag	
(1) Add warmed solution to enema bag: warm tap water as it flows from faucet, place saline container in basin of hot water before adding saline to enema bag, and check temperature of solution by pouring small amount of solution over inner wrist. If soapsuds enema is ordered, add castile soap.	Hot water will burn intestinal mucosa. Cold water causes abdominal cramping and is difficult to retain.
(2) Raise container, release clamp, and allow solution to flow long enough to fill tubing.	Removes air from tubing.
(3) Reclamp tubing.	Prevents further loss of solution.
(4) Lubricate 6 to 8 cm (2½ to 3 inches) of tip of rectal tube with water-soluble lubricating jelly.	Allows smooth insertion of rectal tube without risk for irritation or trauma to mucosa.
(5) Gently separate buttocks and locate anus. Instruct patient to relax by breathing out slowly through mouth.	Breathing out promotes relaxation of external anal sphincter.

SKILL 47-1 ADMINISTERING A CLEANSING ENEMA—cont'd

STEP	RATIONALE
(6) Insert tip of enema tube slowly by pointing tip in direction of patient's umbilicus. Length of insertion varies: adult and adolescent: 7.5 to 10 cm (3 to 4 inches); child: 5 to 7.5 cm (2 to 3 inches); infant: 2.5 to 3.75 cm (1 to 1½ inch).	Careful insertion prevents trauma to rectal mucosa from accidental lodging of tube against rectal wall. Insertion beyond proper limit causes bowel damage.

CLINICAL DECISION: *If pain occurs or resistance is felt during the procedure, stop the instillation of the fluid and confer with health care provider. Do not force tube into rectum.*

STEP	RATIONALE
(7) Hold tubing in rectum constantly until end of fluid instillation.	Bowel contraction causes expulsion of rectal tube.
(8) Open regulating clamp and allow solution to enter slowly while holding container at patient's hip level.	Rapid instillation stimulates evacuation of rectal tube.
(9) Raise height of enema container slowly to appropriate level above anus: 30 to 45 cm (12 to 18 inches) for high enema, 30 cm (12 inches) for regular enema, 7.5 cm (3 inches) for low enema. Instillation time varies, depending on volume of solution you administer (e.g., 1 L/10 min) (see illustration).	Allows for continuous, slow instillation of solution; raising container too high causes rapid instillation and possible painful distention of colon.
(10) Lower container or clamp tubing if patient complains of cramping or if fluid escapes around rectal tube.	Temporarily stopping instillation prevents cramping, which prevents patient from retaining all fluid, altering the effectiveness of enema.
(11) Clamp tubing after you instill all solution.	Prevents air from entering rectum.
b. Prepackaged disposable container	
(1) Remove plastic cap from rectal tip. Apply more jelly as needed to the prelubricated tip.	Lubrication provides for smooth insertion of rectal tube without causing rectal irritation or trauma.
(2) Gently separate buttocks and locate rectum. Instruct patient to relax by breathing out slowly through mouth.	Breathing out promotes relaxation of external rectal sphincter.
(3) Expel air from the enema container.	Introducing air into colon causes further distention and discomfort.
(4) Insert tip of bottle gently into rectum toward the umbilicus (see illustration). *Adult/adolescent:* 7.5 to 10 cm (3 to 4 inches) *Child:* 5 to 7.5 cm (2 to 3 inches) *Infant:* 2.5 to 3.75 cm (1 to 1½ inches)	Gentle insertion prevents trauma to rectal mucosa.
(5) Squeeze bottle until all solution has entered rectum and colon. Instruct patient to retain solution until urge to defecate occurs, usually 2 to 5 minutes.	Hypertonic solutions require only small volumes to stimulate defecation.

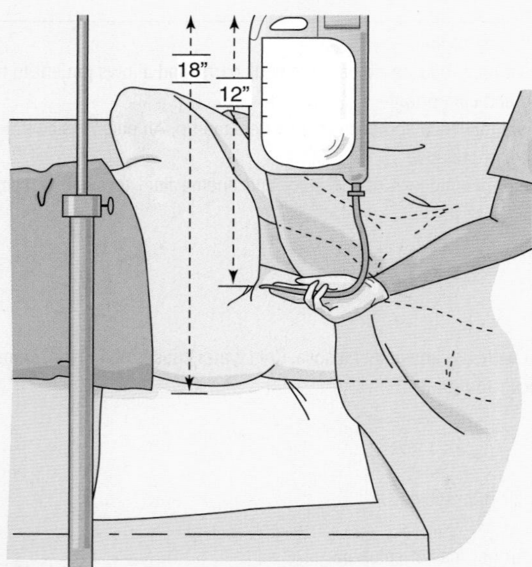

STEP 8a(9) An enema is given in the Sims' position. The IV pole is positioned so the enema bag is 12 inches above the anus and approximately 18 inches above the mattress (depending on patient's size). (From Sorrentino SA: *Mosby's textbook for nursing assistants*, ed 8, St Louis, 2012, Mosby.)

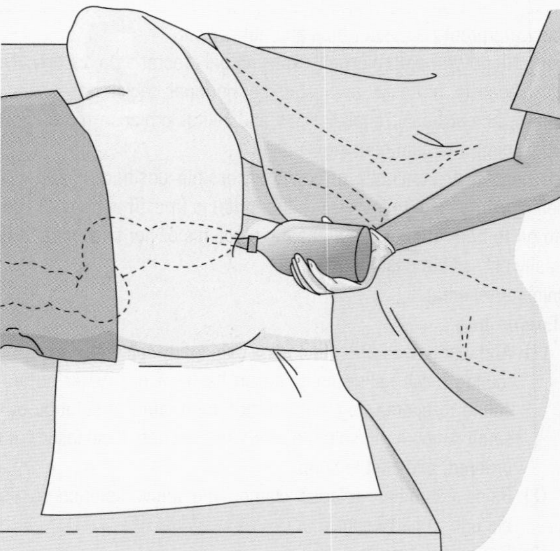

STEP 8b(4) Insertion of enema tube into rectum. (From Sorrentino SA: *Mosby's textbook for nursing assistants*, ed 8, St Louis, 2012, Mosby.)

STEP	RATIONALE
9. Place layers of toilet tissue around tube at anus and gently withdraw rectal tube.	Provides for patient's comfort and cleanliness.
10. Explain to patient that a feeling of distention and some abdominal cramping are normal. Ask patient to retain solution as long as possible while lying quietly in bed. (For infant or young child, gently hold buttocks together for few minutes.)	Solution distends bowel. Length of retention varies with type of enema and patient's ability to contract rectal sphincter. Longer retention promotes more effective stimulation of peristalsis and defecation.
11. Discard enema container and tubing in proper receptacle or rinse bag out thoroughly with warm soap and water if container is reusable.	Reduces transmission and growth of microorganisms.
12. Help patient to bathroom or help to position patient on bedpan.	Normal sitting position promotes defecation.
13. Help patient as needed to wash anal area with warm water, premoistened perineal wipe, or no-rinse perineal cleanser. (If you administer perineal care, use clean gloves.)	Fecal contents irritate skin. Hygiene promotes patient's comfort.
14. Remove and discard gloves and perform hand hygiene.	Reduces transmission of microorganisms.

EVALUATION

STEP	RATIONALE
1. Observe character of feces and solution evacuated. (Caution patient against flushing toilet before inspection.) Inspect color, consistency, amount of stool, odor, and fluid passed.	Determines if stool is evacuated or fluid is retained. Note abnormalities such as presence of blood or mucus.
2. Assess condition of abdomen; cramping, rigidity, or distention indicates a serious problem.	Determines if distention is relieved. Excess volume distends or damages the bowel.
3. Use ***Teach Back*** to determine patient's and family's understanding about the reason for the enema. State, "I want to be sure I explained how the enema works to clean your bowel. Can you explain to me why the enema is being given to you?" Revise your instruction now or develop plan for revised patient teaching if patient is not able to teach back correctly.	Evaluates what patient is able to explain or demonstrate.

UNEXPECTED OUTCOMES AND RELATED INTERVENTIONS

1. Abdomen becomes rigid and distended, and patient complains of severe pain.
   - Stop enema.
   - Notify health care provider.
   - Obtain vital signs.
2. Abdominal pain or cramping develops.
   - Slow rate of instillation; have patient take slow, deep breaths.
3. Bleeding develops.
   - Stop enema.
   - Notify health care provider.
   - Remain with patient and obtain vital signs.

RECORDING AND REPORTING

- Record type and volume of enema given, time administered, characteristics of results, and patient's tolerance to the procedure in nurses' notes.
- Report failure of patient to defecate and any adverse effects to health care provider.
- Document your evaluation of patient learning.

HOME CARE CONSIDERATIONS

- For patients who require enemas at home, instruct family not to exceed recommended fluid volume levels or number of enemas. Instruct family about need for slow administration of warmed fluid.
- Place waterproof padding on the bed.
- Instruct family members not to give the enema on the toilet.

SKILL 47-2 INSERTING AND MAINTAINING A NASOGASTRIC TUBE FOR GASTRIC DECOMPRESSION

DELEGATION CONSIDERATIONS

The skill of inserting and maintaining a nasogastric (NG) tube cannot be delegated to nursing assistive personnel (NAP). Instruct the NAP to:

- Measure and record the drainage.
- Provide oral and nasal hygiene.
- Perform selected comfort measures such as positioning and offering ice chips if allowed.
- Correctly anchor NG tube to patient's gown after changing gown or repositioning patient.

EQUIPMENT

- Inserting large-bore tube
  - 14- or 16-Fr NG tube (smaller lumens are not used for decompression in adults because the tube must be able to remove thick secretions)
  - Water-soluble lubricating jelly
  - Clean gloves
  - pH test strips (measure gastric aspirate acidity)
  - Tongue blade
  - Flashlight
  - Emesis basin
  - Asepto bulb or catheter-tipped syringe
  - Normal saline
  - 2.5 cm (1 inch)–wide hypoallergenic tape or commercial fixation device
  - Tincture of benzoin (optional)
  - Safety pin and rubber band
  - Clamp of suction machine and pressure gauge if wall suction is used
  - Towel, facial tissues
  - Glass of water with straw
- Irrigating NG tube
  - Asepto bulb or catheter-tipped syringe
  - Normal saline and basin
  - Clean gloves
- Discontinuing NG tube
  - Towel, facial tissue
  - Clean gloves
  - Soap and water

STEP	RATIONALE
ASSESSMENT	
1. Perform hand hygiene.	Good hygiene reduces transmission of organisms.
2. Inspect condition of patient's nasal and oral cavity.	Baseline condition of nasal and oral cavity determines need for special nursing measures for oral hygiene after tube placement.
3. Ask if patient has had history of nasal surgery and note if deviated nasal septum is present.	Insert tube into uninvolved nasal passage. Procedure is often contraindicated if surgery is recent.
4. Auscultate for bowel sounds. Palpate patient's abdomen for distention, pain, and rigidity.	Baseline determination of level of abdominal distention later serves as comparison once tube is inserted. In presence of diminished or absent bowel sounds, auscultate each quadrant for 5 minutes.
5. Assess patient's level of consciousness and ability to follow instructions.	Assessment determines patient's ability to help in procedure.

CLINICAL DECISION: *If patient is confused, disoriented, or unable to follow commands, obtain assistance from another staff member to insert the tube.*

STEP	RATIONALE
PLANNING	
1. Identify patient using two identifiers (e.g., name and birthday or name and medical record number) according to agency policy.	Ensures correct patient. Complies with The Joint Commission standards and improves patient safety (TJC, 2016).
2. Explain procedure.	Explanation gains patient's cooperation and lessens possibility that patient will remove tube.
3. Determine if patient had an NG tube insertion in the past and, if so, which naris was used.	Previous experience complements explanations and helps you determine which naris to use.
4. Check medical record for health care provider's order; type of NG tube to be placed; and whether tube is to be attached to suction, gravity, or feeding solution.	Procedure requires health care provider's order. Adequate decompression depends on NG suction.
5. Prepare equipment at bedside. Cut a piece of tape about 10 cm (4 inches) long and split one end in half to form a V or have NG tube fixator device available.	Ensures well-organized procedure. Tape or fixator device is used to hold tube in place after insertion.
IMPLEMENTATION	
1. Position patient in high-Fowler's position with pillows behind head and shoulders. Raise bed to horizontal level comfortable for nurse.	Promotes patient's ability to swallow during procedure. Positioning of bed prevents strain on nurse.

STEP	RATIONALE
2. Have patient blow nose. Place bath towel over his or her chest; give him or her facial tissues. Place emesis basin within reach.	Removes existing nasal secretions. Prevents soiling of patient's gown. Tube insertion through nasal passages sometimes causes tearing and coughing with increased salivation.
3. Pull curtain around bed or close room door.	Provides privacy.
4. Stand on patient's right side if right-handed, left side if left-handed.	Allows easiest manipulation of tubing.
5. Perform hand hygiene and apply clean gloves.	Reduces transmission of microorganisms.
6. Instruct patient to relax and breathe normally while occluding one naris. Repeat this action for other naris. Select nostril with greater airflow.	Tube passes more easily through naris that is more patent. Ensures that tube insertion does not obstruct nasal airflow.
7. Measure distance to insert tube:	Approximates distance from naris to stomach. Distance varies with each patient.
a. Traditional method*:* Measure distance from tip of nose to earlobe to xiphoid process (see illustration).	
b. Hanson method*:* Mark 50-cm (20-inch) point on tube and measure traditionally. Tube insertion is at midway point between 50 cm (20 inches) and traditional mark.	
8. Mark length of tube to be inserted by placing small piece of tape so it can be removed easily.	Marks amount of tube to be inserted from nares to stomach (Miller et al., 2014).
9. Curve 10 to 15 cm (4 to 6 inches) of end of tube tightly around index finger and release.	Curving tube tip aids insertion and decreases tube stiffness.
10. Lubricate 7.5 to 10 cm (3 to 4 inches) of end of tube with water-soluble lubricating jelly.	Minimizes friction against nasal mucosa and aids insertion of tube. Water-soluble lubricant is less toxic than oil-based if aspirated.
11. Initially instruct patient to extend neck back against pillow (see illustration); insert tube gently and slowly through naris, aiming end of tube downward.	Facilitates initial passage of tube through naris and maintains clear airway for open naris.
12. Continue to pass tube along floor of nasal passage, aiming downward toward patient's ear. If resistance is met, apply gentle downward pressure to advance tube. (Do not force past resistance.)	Minimizes discomfort of tube rubbing against upper nasal turbinates. Resistance is caused by posterior nasopharynx. Downward pressure helps tube curl around corner of nasopharynx.
13. If you meet resistance, try to rotate tube and see if it advances. If still resistant, withdraw tube, allow patient to rest, re-lubricate tube, and insert into other naris.	Forcing against resistance causes trauma to mucosa. Helps relieve patient's anxiety.

CLINICAL DECISION: *If unable to insert tube in either naris, stop procedure and notify health care provider.*

STEP	RATIONALE
14. Continue inserting tube until just past nasopharynx by gently rotating it toward opposite nostril and passing it just above oropharynx.	Helps prevent coiling of tube in oropharynx.
a. Stop tube advancement, allow patient to relax, and provide tissues.	Relieves patient's anxiety; tearing is natural response to mucosal irritation, and excessive salivation often occurs because of oral stimulation.
b. Explain to patient that next step requires that he or she swallow. Give patient glass of water unless contraindicated.	Sipping water aids passage of NG tube into esophagus.

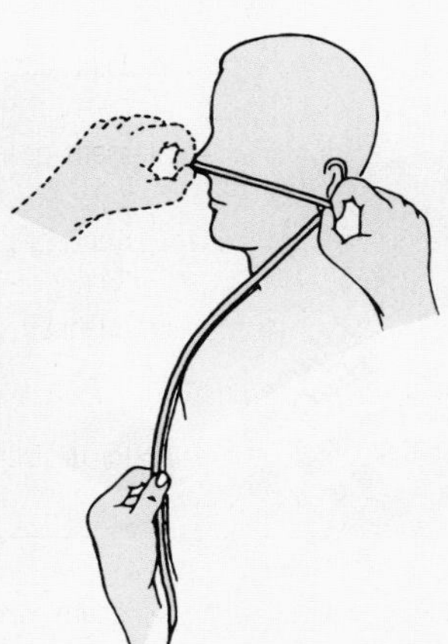

STEP 7a Technique for measuring distance to insert NG tube.

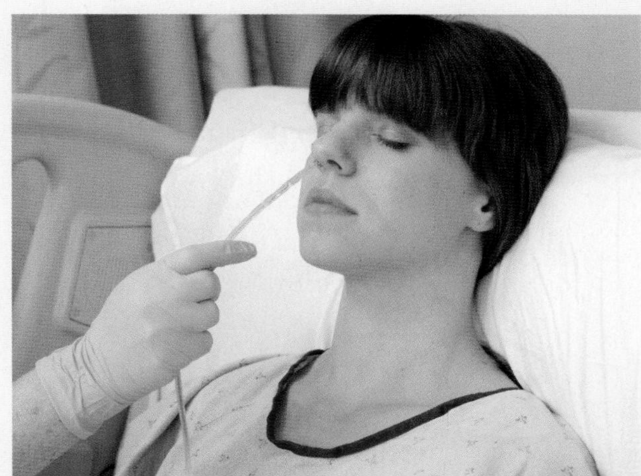

STEP 11 Insert nasogastric tube with curved end pointing downward.

SKILL 47-2 INSERTING AND MAINTAINING A NASOGASTRIC TUBE FOR GASTRIC DECOMPRESSION—cont'd

STEP	RATIONALE
15. With tube just above oropharynx, instruct patient to flex head forward, take a small sip of water, and swallow. Advance tube 2.5 to 5 cm (1 to 2 inches) with each swallow of water. If patient is not allowed fluids, instruct to dry swallow or suck air through straw.	Flexed position closes off upper airway to trachea and opens esophagus. Swallowing closes epiglottis over trachea and helps move tube into esophagus. Swallowing water reduces gagging or choking. Suction removes water from stomach once it is connected.
16. If patient begins to cough, gag, or choke, withdraw tube slightly (do not remove it) and stop tube advancement. Instruct patient to breathe easily and take sips of water.	Sometimes tube accidentally enters larynx and produces coughing; withdrawal of tube reduces risk of laryngeal entry. Swallowing water eases gagging. Give water cautiously to reduce risk of aspiration.

CLINICAL DECISION: *If vomiting occurs, help patient clear airway; use oral suctioning if needed. Do not proceed until airway is cleared.*

STEP	RATIONALE
17. If patient continues to gag and cough or complains that tube feels as though it is coiling in back of throat, check back of oropharynx with tongue blade. If tube has coiled, withdraw it until tip is back in oropharynx. Reinsert with patient swallowing.	When tube coils around itself in back of throat, it stimulates gag reflex.
18. After patient relaxes, continue to advance tube with swallowing until tape or mark is reached. Temporarily anchor tube to patient's cheek with piece of tape until tube placement is verified.	Tip of tube needs to be well within stomach for adequate decompression. Anchor tube before verifying placement.
19. Verify tube placement. Check agency policy for preferred methods for checking NG tube placement.	
a. Inspect posterior pharynx for presence of coiled tube.	Tube is pliable and can coil up in back of pharynx instead of advancing into esophagus.
b. Attach Asepto or catheter-tipped syringe to end of tube and aspirate gently back on syringe to obtain gastric contents, observing color (see illustration).	Gastric contents are usually cloudy and green but may be off-white, tan, bloody, or brown in color. Aspiration of contents provides means to measure fluid pH and thus determine tube tip placement in gastrointestinal tract. Other common aspirate colors include the following: duodenal placement (yellow or bile stained), esophagus (may or may not have saliva-appearing aspirate).
c. Measure pH of aspirate with color-coded pH paper with range of whole numbers from 1.0 to 11.0 or greater (see illustration).	Gastric aspirates have decidedly acidic pH values, preferably 5.5 or less, compared with intestinal aspirates, which are usually 6.0 or greater, or respiratory secretions, which are usually alkaline at 7.0 or greater. Use only gastric (Gastroccult) pH test and not Hemoccult test.
d. Have ordered x-ray film examination performed of chest/abdomen.	X-ray film is best verification of initial placement of tube (Miller et al., 2014).
e. If tube is not in stomach, advance another 2.5-5 cm (1-2 inches) and repeat Steps 19a-e to check tube position.	Tube must be in stomach to provide decompression.
20. Anchoring tube:	
a. After tube is properly inserted and positioned, either clamp end or connect it to drainage bag or suction source.	Drainage bag is used for gravity drainage. Intermittent low suction is most effective for decompression. Patient going to operating room or for diagnostic test often has tube clamped.

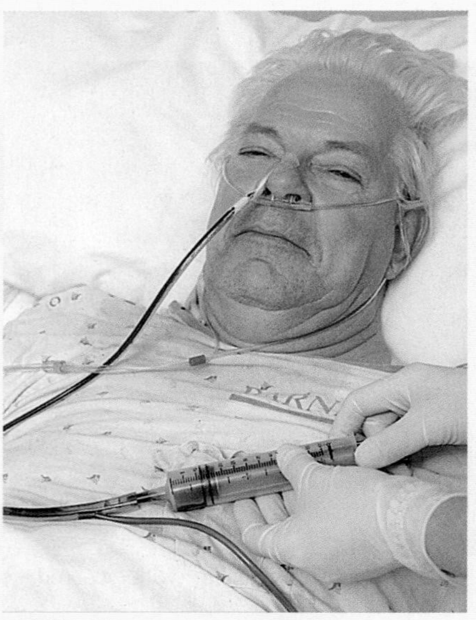

STEP 19b Aspiration of gastric contents.

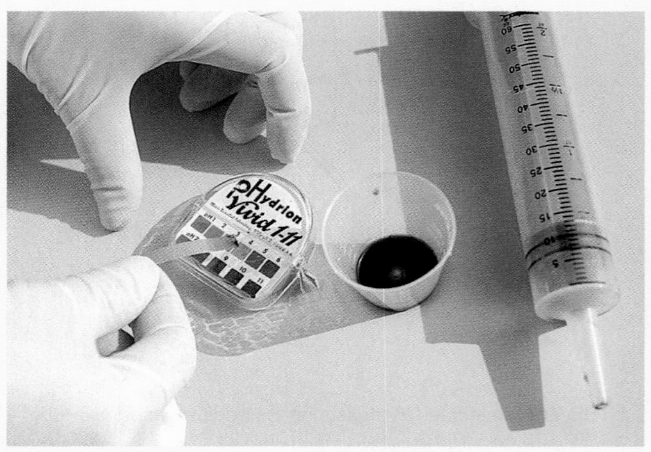

STEP 19c Checking pH of gastric aspirate.

STEP	RATIONALE
b. Tape tube to nose; avoid putting pressure on nares.	Prevents tissue necrosis. Tape anchors tube securely.
(1) Apply small amount of tincture of benzoin to lower end of nose and allow to dry (optional).	Benzoin prevents loosening of tape if patient perspires.
(2) Apply tape to nose, leaving split ends free. Be sure that top end of tape over nose is secure.	
(3) Carefully wrap two split ends of tape around tube (see illustration).	
(4) Alternative: Apply tube fixation device using shaped adhesive patch (see illustration).	
c. Fasten end of NG tube to patient's gown by looping rubber band around tube in slipknot. Pin rubber band to gown (provides slack for movement).	Reduces pressure on nares if tube moves.
21. Unless health care provider orders otherwise, elevate head of bed 30 degrees.	Helps prevent esophageal reflux and minimizes irritation of tube against posterior pharynx.
22. Once placement is confirmed: **a.** Place red mark on tube to indicate where it exits nose. **b.** Measure tube length from nares to connector as an alternate method. **c.** Document tube length in patient record.	The mark or tube length is to be used as a guide to indicate whether displacement may have occurred.
23. Remove gloves and perform hand hygiene.	Reduces transmission of microorganisms.
24. Tube irrigation:	
a. Perform hand hygiene and apply gloves.	Reduces transmission of microorganisms.
b. Check for tube placement in stomach (see Step 19). Reconnect NG tube to connecting tube.	Prevents accidental entrance of irrigating solution into lungs.
c. Draw up 30 mL of normal saline into Asepto or catheter-tipped syringe.	Use of saline minimizes loss of electrolytes from stomach fluids.
d. Clamp NG tube. Disconnect from connection tubing and lay end of connection tubing on towel.	Reduces soiling of patient's gown and bed linen.
e. Insert tip of irrigating syringe into end of NG tube. Remove clamp. Hold syringe with tip pointed at floor and inject saline slowly and evenly. Do not force solution.	Position of syringe prevents introduction of air into vent tubing, which could cause gastric distention. Solution introduced under pressure causes gastric trauma. Do not introduce saline through blue "pigtail" air vent of Salem sump tube.
f. If resistance occurs, check for kinks in tubing. Turn patient onto left side. Report repeated resistance to health care provider.	Tip of tube may be against stomach lining. Repositioning on left side helps to dislodge tube away from stomach lining. Buildup of secretions causes distention.
g. After instilling saline, immediately aspirate or pull back slowly on syringe to withdraw fluid. If amount aspirated is greater than amount instilled, record difference as output. If amount aspirated is less than amount instilled, record difference as intake.	Irrigation clears tubing; thus stomach remains empty. Fluid remaining in stomach is measured as intake.
h. Reconnect NG tube to drainage or suction. (If solution does not return, repeat irrigation.)	Reestablishes drainage collection; repeat irrigation or repositioning of tube until NG tube drains properly.
i. Remove gloves and perform hand hygiene.	Reduces transmission of microorganisms.
EVALUATION	
1. Determine amount and character of contents draining from NG tube. Ask if patient feels nauseated.	Determines if tube is decompressing stomach of contents.
2. After palpating patient's abdomen, note any distention, pain, and rigidity and auscultate for presence of bowel sounds. Turn off suction while auscultating.	Determines success of abdominal decompression and return of peristalsis. The sound of suction apparatus is transmitted to abdomen and misinterpreted as bowel sounds.
3. Evaluate condition of nares and nose.	Evaluates onset of skin and tissue irritation.
4. Observe position of tubing.	Determines if tension is being applied to nasal structures.
5. Ask if patient feels sore throat or irritation in pharynx.	Evaluates level of patient's discomfort.

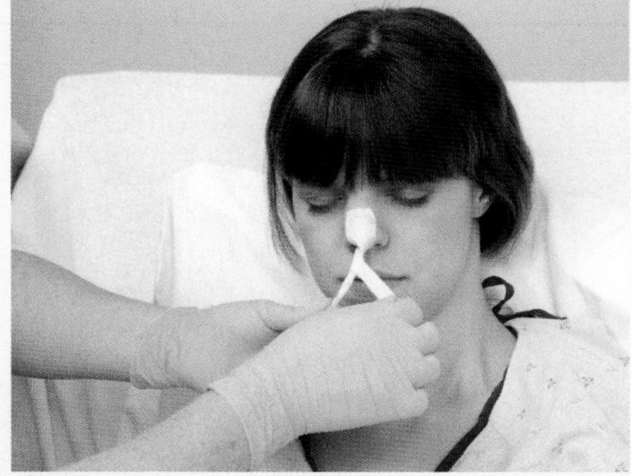

STEP 20b(3) Tape is crossed over and around NG tube.

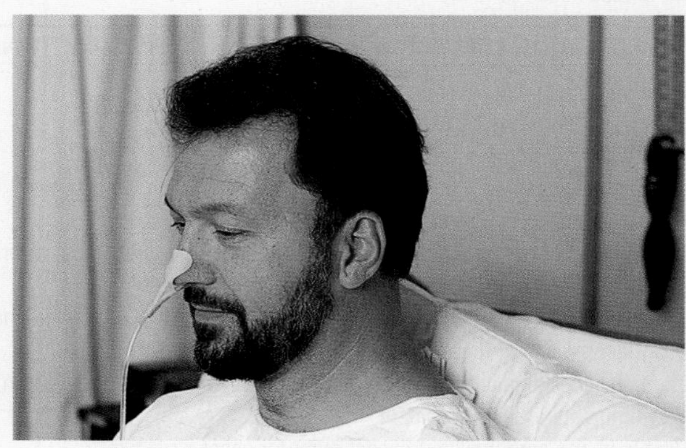

STEP 20b(4) Patient with tube fixation device.

SKILL 47-2 INSERTING AND MAINTAINING A NASOGASTRIC TUBE FOR GASTRIC DECOMPRESSION—cont'd

STEP	RATIONALE
6. Use ***Teach Back*** to determine patient's and family's understanding about the nasogastric tube. State, "I want to be sure I explained the reason for the nasogastric tube and the care of the tube. Can you explain to me why you need the nasogastric tube after surgery?" Revise your instruction now or develop plan for revised patient teaching if patient is not able to teach back correctly.	Evaluates what the patient is able to explain or demonstrate.

DISCONTINUATION OF NASOGASTRIC TUBE

STEP	RATIONALE
ASSESSMENT	
1. Auscultate for presence of bowel sounds.	Serves as baseline for when tube is removed.
PLANNING	
1. Verify order to discontinue NG tube.	Health care provider's order required for procedure.
2. Identify patient using two identifiers (e.g., name and birthday or name and medical record number) according to agency policy.	Ensures correct patient. Complies with The Joint Commission standards and improves patient safety (TJC, 2016).
3. Explain procedure to patient and reassure that removal is less distressing than insertion.	Minimizes anxiety and increases patient cooperation.
IMPLEMENTATION	
1. Perform hand hygiene and apply clean gloves.	Reduces transmission of microorganisms.
2. Turn off suction and disconnect NG tube from drainage bag or suction. Remove tape or fixation device from bridge of nose and unpin tube from gown.	Have tube free of all connections before removal.
3. Stand on patient's right side if right-handed, left side if left-handed.	Allows easiest manipulation of tube.
4. Hand patient facial tissue; place clean towel across chest. Instruct patient to take and hold deep breath.	Patient sometimes needs to blow nose after removal of tube. Towel prevents gown from getting soiled. Airway is temporarily obstructed during tube removal.
5. Clamp or kink tubing securely and pull tube out steadily and smoothly into towel held in other hand while patient holds breath.	Clamping prevents tube contents from draining into oropharynx. Reduces trauma to mucosa and minimizes patient's discomfort. Towel covers tube, which is usually an unpleasant sight. Holding breath prevents aspiration.
6. Clean nares and provide mouth care.	Promotes comfort.
7. Dispose of tube and drainage equipment into proper container.	Reduces transmission of microorganisms.
8. Remove gloves and perform hand hygiene.	Reduces transmission of microorganisms.
EVALUATION	
1. After tube removal, auscultate patient's bowel sounds and periodically check for abdominal distention.	Confirms that peristalsis has returned.
2. Measure amount of drainage in container and note character of content.	Provides accurate measure of fluid output.
3. Explain procedure for drinking fluids if not contraindicated.	Requires health care provider's order. Once fluids are allowed, the order usually begins with small amount of ice chips; amount increases as patient is able to tolerate more.
4. Use ***Teach Back*** to determine patient's and family's understanding about the procedure for removing the nasogastric tube. State, "I want to be sure I explained to you what to expect as the nasogastric tube is removed. Can you explain to me how the nasogastric tube will be removed?" Revise your instructions now or develop plan for revised patient teaching if patient is not able to teach back correctly.	Evaluates what patient is able to explain or demonstrate.

UNEXPECTED OUTCOMES AND RELATED INTERVENTIONS

1. Patient's abdomen becomes distended and/or painful.
   - Assess patency of tube and irrigate as needed.
   - Verify that suction is on as ordered.
2. Patient complains of sore throat from dry, irritated mucous membranes.
   - Increase frequency of oral hygiene.
   - Ask health care provider if patient can suck on ice chips or throat lozenges.
3. Patient develops irritation of skin around nares.
   - Provide skin care to nares and retape so tube does not press against nares.
   - Consider switching tube to other naris.
4. Patient develops signs of pulmonary aspiration: fever, shortness of breath, pulmonary congestion.
   - Perform respiratory assessment.
   - Notify health care provider; expect order for chest x-ray film.

RECORDING AND REPORTING

- Record in nurses' notes time, type, and size of NG tube inserted; patient's tolerance of procedure; confirmation of placement; character of gastric contents; pH value; whether tube is clamped or connected to drainage device; and amount of suction applied.
- Record in nurses' notes and/or flow sheet placement checks and amount and character of contents draining from NG tube every shift, unless ordered more often by health care provider.
- Record in nurse's notes time and date that NG tube was removed, patient's tolerance of procedure, and his or her status following procedure.
- Document your evaluation of patient learning.

SKILL 47-3 POUCHING AN OSTOMY

DELEGATION CONSIDERATIONS

The skill of pouching an ostomy can be delegated to nursing assistive personnel (NAP) who have been trained to do this procedure. Whether this skill can be delegated depends on agency policy. The nurse should do the first postoperative pouch change. The nurse informs the NAP about:

- Expected amount, color, and consistency of drainage from ostomy.
- Expected appearance of the stoma.
- Special equipment needed to complete procedure.
- When to report changes in patient's stoma and surrounding skin integrity.

EQUIPMENT

- Clear drainable one-piece or two-piece, cut-to-fit or precut ostomy wafer/pouch
- Pouch closure device such as a clip if needed
- Ostomy measuring guide
- Adhesive remover *(optional)*
- Clean gloves
- Washcloth
- Towel or disposable waterproof barrier
- Basin with warm tap water
- Scissors

STEP	RATIONALE
ASSESSMENT	
1. Perform hand hygiene and apply gloves (e.g., if there is drainage). Observe existing skin barrier and pouch for leakage and length of time in place. Pouch should be changed every 3 to 7 days, not daily (Goldberg et al., 2010). Depending on type of pouching system used (such as opaque pouch), you may have to remove pouch to fully observe stoma. Clear pouches permit viewing of stoma without their removal.	Assesses effectiveness of pouching system and allows for early detection of potential problems. To minimize skin irritation, avoid unnecessary changing of entire pouching system; but, if effluent is leaking under wafer, change it because skin damage from effluent will cause more skin trauma than early removal of wafer. Repeated leaking sometimes indicates the need for a different type of pouch.

CLINICAL DECISION: *If the ostomy pouch is leaking, change it. Taping or patching it to contain effluent leaves the skin exposed to chemical or enzymatic irritation.*

STEP	RATIONALE
2. Observe amount of effluent in pouch and empty pouch if it is more than one-third to one-half full by opening clip and draining it into a container for measurement of the output. Note consistency of effluent and record intake and output.	Empty pouches when they are one-third to one-half full because weight of pouch disrupts seal of adhesive on skin. Monitors fluid balance, return of bowel function after surgery.
3. Observe stoma for location, color, swelling, trauma, and healing or irritation of peristomal skin. Assess type of stoma. Determine if it is budded, flush with the skin level, or retracted below skin level (see illustrations). Remove gloves.	Stoma characteristics are a factor to consider in selecting an appropriate pouching system. Convexity in skin barrier is often necessary with a flush or retracted stoma.
4. Observe abdomen for best type of pouching system. Consider: **a.** Abdominal contour. **b.** Presence of scars or incisions.	Determines pouching system selection. Abdominal contours, scars, or incisions affect type of system and adhesion to skin surface.

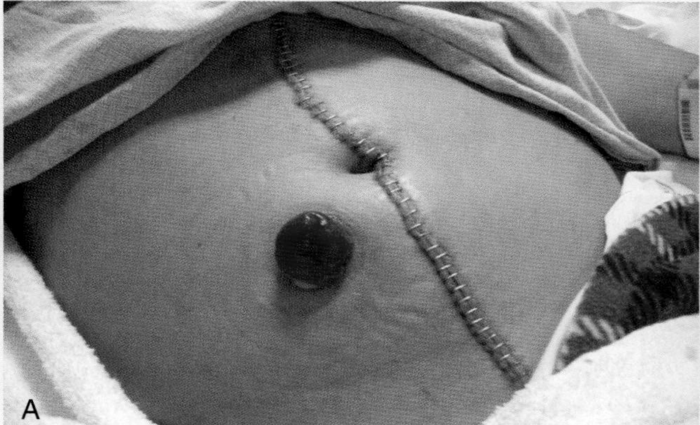

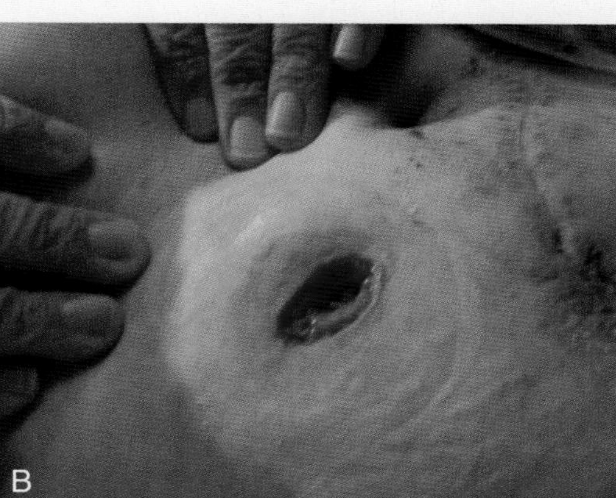

STEP 3 A, Budded stoma. **B,** Retracted stoma. (Courtesy Jane Fellows.)

SKILL 47-3 POUCHING AN OSTOMY—cont'd

STEP	RATIONALE
5. Explore patient's attitude toward learning self-care and identify others who will be helping patient after leaving hospital.	Facilitates teaching plan and timing of care to coincide with availability of caregivers.
PLANNING	
1. Identify patient using two identifiers (e.g., name and birthday or name and medical record number) according to agency policy.	Ensures correct patient. Complies with The Joint Commission standards and improves patient safety (TJC, 2016).
2. Explain procedure to patient; encourage patient's interaction and questions.	Lessens patient's anxiety and promotes his or her participation.
3. Assemble equipment and close room curtains or door.	Optimizes use of time; provides privacy.
IMPLEMENTATION	
1. Position patient in semireclining position. If possible, provide patient a mirror for observation.	When patient is semireclining, there are fewer skin wrinkles, which allows for ease of application of pouching system.
2. Perform hand hygiene and apply clean gloves.	Reduces transmission of microorganisms.
3. Place towel or disposable waterproof barrier across patient's lower abdomen.	Protects bed linen; maintains patient's dignity.
4. If not done during assessment, remove used pouch and skin barrier gently by pushing skin away from barrier. An adhesive remover may be used to facilitate removal of skin barrier.	Reduces skin trauma. Improper removal of pouch and barrier can cause peristomal skin irritation or breakdown.
5. Cleanse peristomal skin gently with warm tap water using washcloth; do not scrub skin. Pat the skin dry.	Avoid soap. It leaves residue on skin, which may irritate skin (Wound, Ostomy, and Continence Nurses Society et al., 2016). Pouch does not adhere to wet skin.
6. Measure stoma (see illustration). Size of stoma may change in the 2-4 weeks after surgery; thus measurement may change during this time.	Allows for proper fit of pouch that will protect peristomal skin. Pouch opening should fit around stoma and cover peristomal skin to prevent contact with effluent.
7. Trace pattern on pouch/skin barrier (see illustration).	Prepares for cutting opening in the pouch.
8. Cut opening on skin barrier wafer (see illustration).	Customizes pouch to provide appropriate fit over stoma.
9. Remove protective backing from adhesive (see illustration).	Prepares skin barrier for placement.
10. Apply pouch over stoma (see illustration). Press firmly into place around stoma and outside edges. Have patient hold hand over pouch to apply heat to secure seal.	Pouch adhesives are heat and pressure sensitive and will hold more securely at body temperature.
11. Close end of pouch with clip or integrated closure.	Contains effluent.
12. Properly dispose of used pouch and remove drape from patient.	Avoids odor in room.
13. Remove gloves. Perform hand hygiene.	Reduces transmission of microorganisms.
EVALUATION	
1. Observe condition of skin barrier and adherence to abdominal surface.	Determines presence of leaks.
2. Observe appearance of stoma, peristomal skin, abdominal contours, and suture line during pouch change.	Provides information if another type of pouching system or additional skin care products are needed.

CLINICAL DECISION: *If peristomal skin is raw, blistered, or weeping, the skin surface will be moist, and the pouch will not adhere, making the patient vulnerable to more severe skin breakdown. Consult the ostomy care nurse before proceeding with placing a pouch over moist, damaged skin.*

STEP	RATIONALE
3. Observe patient's, family caregiver's or significant other's willingness to view stoma and ask questions about procedure.	Determines level of adjustment and understanding of stoma care and pouch application. Allows planning for future education needs and progress toward acceptance of altered body image.

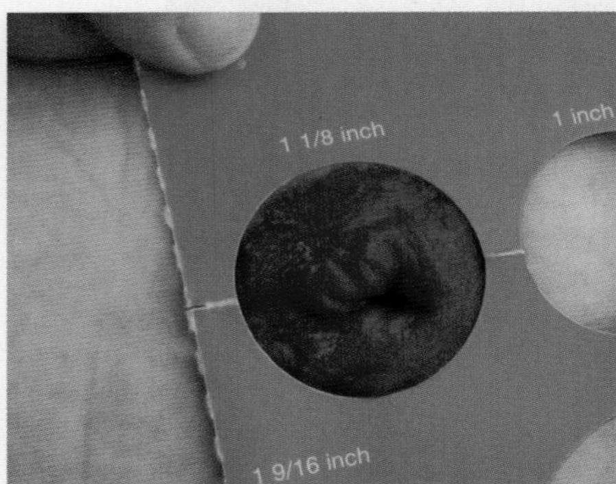

STEP 6 Measure stoma. (Courtesy Coloplast, Minneapolis, MN.)

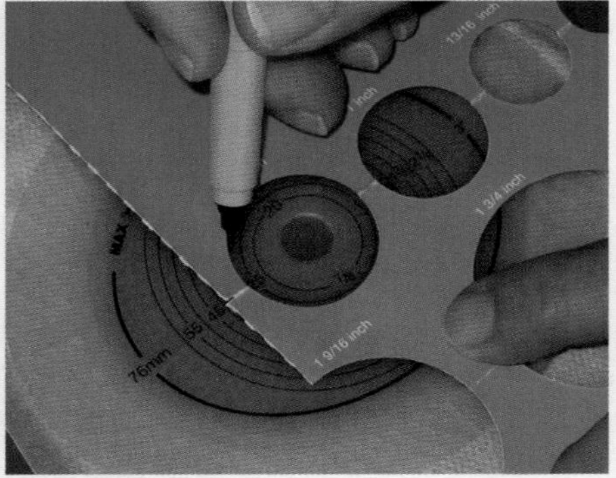

STEP 7 Trace measurement on skin barrier. (Courtesy Coloplast, Minneapolis, MN.)

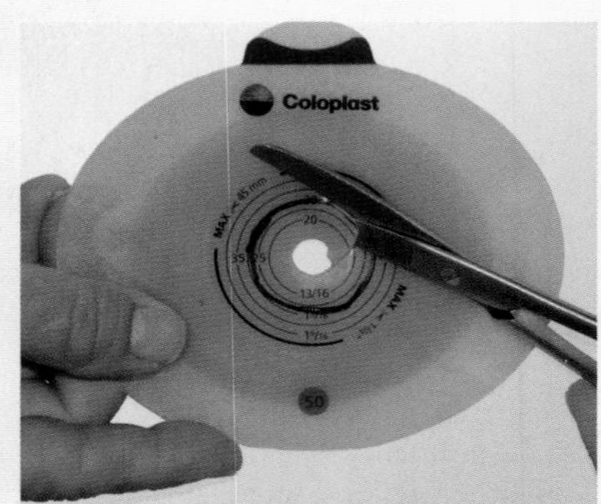

STEP 8 Cut opening in wafer. (Courtesy Coloplast, Minneapolis, MN.)

STEP	RATIONALE
4. Use ***Teach Back*** to determine patient's and family's understanding about caring for the ostomy. State, "I want to be sure I explained how to pouch the ostomy to protect your skin. Can demonstrate to me how to change the pouch on your ostomy?" Revise your instruction now or develop plan for revised patient teaching if patient is not able to teach back correctly.	Evaluates what patient and family are able to explain or demonstrate.

UNEXPECTED OUTCOMES AND RELATED INTERVENTIONS

1. Skin around stoma is irritated, blistered, or bleeding; or a rash is noted. May be caused by undermining of pouch seal by fecal contents, allergic reaction, or fungal skin eruption.
   - Remove pouch more carefully.
   - Change pouch more frequently or use a different type of pouching system.
   - Consult ostomy care nurse.
2. Necrotic stoma is manifested by purple or black color, dry instead of moist texture, or failure to bleed when washed gently or tissue sloughing.
   - Report to health care provider.
   - Document appearance.
3. Patient refuses to view stoma or participate in care.
   - Obtain referral for ostomy care nurse.
   - Allow patient to express feelings.
   - Encourage family support.

RECORDING AND REPORTING

- Record type of pouch and skin barrier used, amount and appearance of effluent in pouch, size and appearance of stoma, and condition of peristomal skin.
- Record patient/family level of participation, teaching performed, and response to teaching.
- Report abnormal appearance of stoma, suture line, peristomal skin, or character of output to health care provider.
- Document your evaluation of patient learning.

HOME CARE CONSIDERATIONS

- Evaluate patient's home toileting facilities and help patient develop an ostomy care routine that is compatible with available facilities. Ostomy pouches are not flushable.
- Encourage patient to stand in front of a mirror when changing pouch to increase visibility and avoid abdominal creases that might be present in the sitting position.

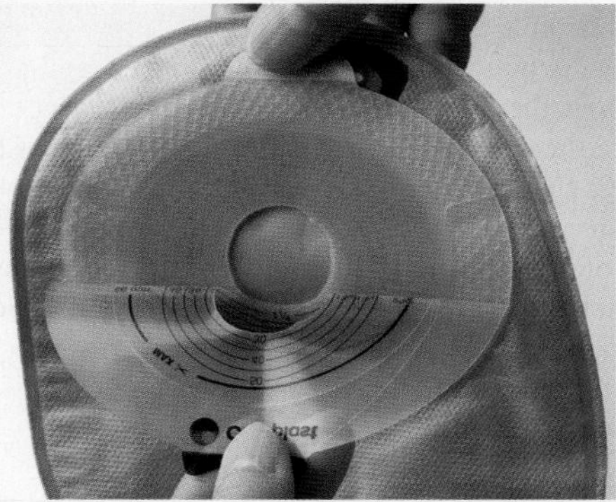

STEP 9 Remove protective backing. (Courtesy Coloplast, Minneapolis, MN.)

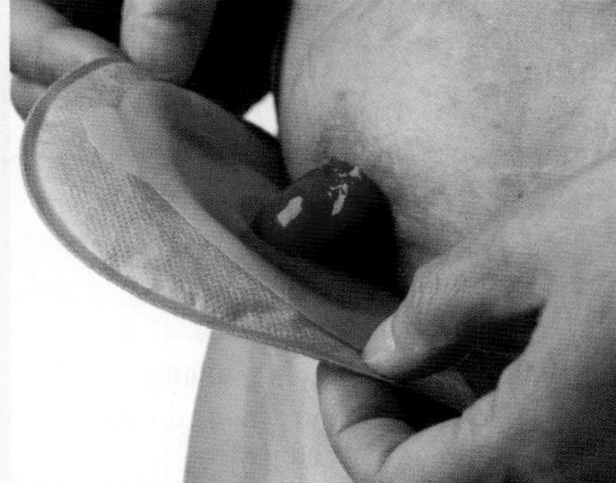

STEP 10 Apply pouch over stoma. (Courtesy Coloplast, Minneapolis, MN.)

KEY POINTS

- Mechanical breakdown of food elements, GI motility, and selective absorption and secretion of substances by the large intestine influence the character of feces.
- Food high in fiber content and an increased fluid intake normalize stool consistency.
- Use of cathartics, laxative, and enemas are short-term solutions to constipation; long-term management includes lifestyle changes in diet, activity, and defecation schedule.
- Fecal incontinence is a source of physical and psychological distress and frequently leads to the need for agency-based care in the elderly.
- The greatest risk from diarrhea is development of fluid and electrolyte imbalance.
- The location of an ostomy influences consistency of the stool.
- Focus assessment of elimination patterns on bowel habits, factors that normally influence defecation, recent changes in elimination, and a physical examination.
- Endoscopic procedures for diagnostic testing of the GI tract may require cleansing of the bowel before the procedure.

- Consider frequency of defecation and fecal characteristics when instructing a patient on establishing a bowel-elimination routine.
- NG intubation decompresses the stomach by removing gastric contents until GI motility returns and decreases the risk of vomiting and aspiration.
- Proper selection and use of an ostomy-pouching system are necessary to prevent damage to the skin around the stoma.
- Digital removal of stool relieves the obstruction and discomfort of a fecal impaction but causes trauma to the rectal mucosa and vagal nerve stimulation.
- Skin breakdown occurs after repeated exposure to liquid stool.

CLINICAL APPLICATION QUESTIONS

Preparing for Clinical Practice

On his next visit to Mr. Johnson 2 days later, Javier, the home care nurse, found that Mr. Johnson still had not had a normal bowel movement and his blood pressure is 160/92. He had tried to increase his intake of fruits and vegetables but had very little appetite and felt mildly nauseous after eating even a small meal. Mr. Johnson took a laxative with a stool softener each evening, but reported only small, liquid bowel movements 2 to 3 times a day. He feels pressure in his rectum that is not relieved when he takes his pain medication. Because of his elevated blood pressure, increasing discomfort, and his lack of bowel movement for at least 9 days, Javier thinks that Mr. Johnson should go to the emergency department of his local hospital.

1. Mr. Johnson arrives in the emergency department of the hospital with rectal pressure and a lack of appetite. Which nursing assessment questions do you ask?
2. The emergency medicine health care provider does a digital rectal examination and feels a hard stool mass. You receive an order to remove a fecal impaction. Describe what you need to do to prepare the patient for this procedure.
3. After successfully removing the impaction, what do you need to teach Mr. Johnson before he is discharged from the emergency department?

ⓔ ***Answers to Clinical Application Questions can be found on the Evolve website.***

REVIEW QUESTIONS

Are You Ready to Test Your Nursing Knowledge?

1. Which of the following nursing actions do you take after placing a bedpan under an immobilized patient?
   1. Lift the patient's hips off the bed and slide the bedpan under the patient
   2. After positioning the patient on the bedpan, elevate the head of the bed to a 45-degree angle
   3. Adjust the head of the bed so it is lower than the feet and use gentle but firm pressure to push the bedpan under the patient
   4. Have the patient stand beside the bed and then have him or her sit on the bedpan on the edge of the bed
2. A patient has not had a bowel movement for 4 days. Now she has nausea and severe cramping throughout her abdomen. On the basis of these findings, what do you suspect is wrong with the patient?
   1. An intestinal obstruction
   2. Irritation of the intestinal mucosa
   3. Gastroenteritis
   4. A fecal impaction
3. During the administration of a warm tap-water enema, a patient complains of cramping abdominal pain that he rates 6 out of 10. What is your priority nursing intervention?
   1. Stop the instillation
   2. Ask the patient to take deep breaths to decrease the pain
   3. Add soapsuds to the enema
   4. Tell the patient to bear down as he would when having a bowel movement
4. Which instructions do you include when educating a person with chronic constipation? (Select all that apply.)
   1. Increase fiber and fluids in the diet
   2. Use a low-volume enema daily
   3. Avoid gluten in the diet
   4. Take laxatives twice a day
   5. Exercise for 30 minutes every day
   6. Schedule time to use the toilet at the same time every day
   7. Take probiotics 5 times a week
5. Which skills do you teach a patient with a new colostomy before discharge from the hospital? (Select all that apply.)
   1. How to change the pouch
   2. How to empty the pouch
   3. How to open and close the pouch
   4. How to irrigate the colostomy
   5. How to determine if the ostomy is healing appropriately
6. Which of the following cause *Clostridium difficile* infection? (Select all that apply.)
   1. Chronic laxative use
   2. Contact with *C. difficile* bacteria
   3. Overuse of antibiotics
   4. Frequent episodes of diarrhea caused by food intolerance
   5. Inflammation of the bowel
7. Place the steps for an ostomy pouch change in the correct order.
   1. Close the end of the pouch.
   2. Measure the stoma.
   3. Cut the hole in the wafer.
   4. Press the pouch in place over the stoma.
   5. Remove the old pouch.
   6. Trace the correct measurement onto the back of the wafer.
   7. Assess the stoma and the skin around it.
   8. Cleanse and dry the peristomal skin.
8. Which of the following symptoms are warning signs of possible colorectal cancer according to the American Cancer Society guidelines? (Select all that apply.)
   1. Change in bowel habits
   2. Blood in the stool
   3. A larger-than-normal bowel movement
   4. Fecal impaction
   5. Muscle aches
   6. Incomplete emptying of the colon
   7. Food particles in the stool
   8. Unexplained abdominal or back pain
9. A nurse is teaching a patient to obtain a specimen for fecal occult blood testing using fecal immunochemical (FIT) testing at home. How does the nurse instruct the patient to collect the specimen?
   1. Get three fecal smears from one bowel movement.
   2. Obtain one fecal smear from an early-morning bowel movement.
   3. Collect one fecal smear from three separate bowel movements.
   4. Get three fecal smears when you see blood in your bowel movement.
10. What do you need to teach family caregivers when a patient has fecal incontinence as a result of cognitive impairment?

1. Cleanse the skin with antibacterial soap and apply talcum powder to the buttocks
2. Use diapers and heavy padding on the bed
3. Initiate bowel or habit training program to promote continence
4. Help the patient to toilet once every hour

11. Your patient states, "I have diarrhea and cramping every time I have ice cream. I am sure this is because the food is cold." Based on this assessment data, which health problem do you suspect the patient has?
    1. A food allergy
    2. Irritable bowel syndrome
    3. Increased peristalsis
    4. Lactose intolerance
12. Place the steps to administering a prepackaged enema the correct order.
    1. Insert enema tip gently in the rectum.
    2. Help patient to bathroom when he or she feels urge to defecate.
    3. Position patient on side.
    4. Perform hand hygiene and apply clean gloves.
    5. Squeeze contents of container into rectum.
    6. Explain procedure to the patient.
13. Which nursing intervention is most important when caring for a patient with an ileostomy?
    1. Cleansing the stoma with hot water
    2. Inserting a deodorant tablet in the stoma bag
    3. Selecting or cutting a pouch with an appropriate-size stoma opening
    4. Wearing sterile gloves while caring for the stoma
14. A nurse is taking a health history of a newly admitted patient with a diagnosis of possible fecal impaction. Which of the following is the priority question to ask the patient or caregiver?
    1. Have you eaten more high-fiber foods lately?
    2. Are your bowel movements soft and formed?
    3. Have you experienced frequent, small liquid stools recently?
    4. Have you taken antibiotics recently?
15. An elderly patient comes to the hospital with a complaint of severe weakness and diarrhea for several days. Of the following problems, which is the most important to assess initially?
    1. Malnutrition
    2. Dehydration
    3. Skin breakdown
    4. Incontinence

Answers: 1. 2; **2.** 1; **3.** 1; **4.** 1, 5, 6; **5.** 1, 2, 3, 5; **6.** 2, 3; **7.** 5, 8, 7, 2, 6, 3, 4, 1; **8.** 1, 2, 6; **9.** 3; **10.** 3; **11.** 4; **12.** 6, 4, 3, 1, 5, 2; **13.** 3; **14.** 3; **15.** 2.

Rationales for Review Questions can be found on the Evolve website.

REFERENCES

American Cancer Society (ACS): *Colorectal cancer*, 2015, http://www.cancer.org/Cancer/ColonandRectumCancer/DetailedGuide/index. Accessed November 19, 2015.

Bliss DZ, Norton C: Conservative management of fecal incontinence, *Am J Nurs* 110(9):30, 2010.

Burchum JR, Rosenthal LD: *Lehne's pharmacology for nursing care*, ed 9, St Louis, 2016, Elsevier.

Constipation: http://www.niddk.nih.gov/health-information/health-topics/digestive-diseases/constipation/Pages/overview.aspx. n.d. Accessed November 19, 2015.

Food allergies: what you need to know, 2015, http://www.fda.gov/Food/IngredientsPackagingLabeling/FoodAllergens/ucm079311.htm. Accessed November 19, 2015.

Goldberg M, et al: *Management of the patient with a fecal ostomy: best practice guideline for clinicians*, Mount Laurel, NJ, 2010, Wound, Ostomy, and Continence Nurses Society.

Grossman S, Mager D: *Clostridium difficile*: implications for nursing, *Medsurg Nurs* 19(3):155, 2010.

Hussain Z, et al: Fecal impaction, *Curr Gastroenterol Rep* 16(9):404, 2014.

Lewis S, et al: *Medical-surgical nursing: assessment and management of clinical problems*, ed 9, St Louis, 2014, Mosby.

Long MA: Fecal incontinence, 2010, *Long-Term Living* 59(10):50, 2010.

Mayo Clinic: *Water: how much should you drink every day?* 2014, http://www.mayoclinic.org/healthy-living/nutrition-and-healthy-eating/in-depth/water/art-20044256. Accessed November 19, 2015.

Miller KR, et al: A tutorial on enteral access in adult patients in the hospitalized setting, *JPEN J Parenter Enteral Nutr* 38(3):282, 2014.

Prinz A, et al: Discharge planning for a patient with a new ostomy: best practice for clinicians, *J Wound Ostomy Continence Nurs* 42(1):79, 2015.

The Joint Commission (TJC): *2016 National Patient Safety Goals*, Oakbrook Terrace, IL, 2016, The Commission. Available at http://www.jointcommission.org/standards_information/npsgs.aspx. Accessed November 2015.

Wound, Ostomy and Continence Nurses Society (WOCN): *Continence committee: quick management guide for fecal incontinence*, 2013, www.wocn.org, http://c.ymcdn.com/sites/www.wocn.org/resource/resmgr/Publications/A_Quick_Ref_Guide_FI_(2013).pdf. Accessed November 19, 2015.

Wound, Ostomy, and Continence Nurses Society, et al: *Ostomy management*, Philadelphia, 2016, Wolters Kluwer.

RESEARCH REFERENCES

Daniel A, Rapose A: The evaluation of *Clostridium difficile* infection (CDI) in a community hospital, *J Infect Public Health* 8(2):155, 2015.

Erwin-Toth P, et al: Factors impacting the quality of life of people with ostomies in North America, *J WOCN* 39(4):417, 2012.

Felder S, et al: Usefulness of bowel sound auscultation: a prospective evaluation, *J Surg Educ* 71(5):768, 2014.

Griffin K: Biological, psychological and behavioral, and social variables influencing colorectal cancer screening in African Americans, *Nurs Res* 58(5):312, 2009.

Inadomi JM, et al: Adherence to colorectal cancer screening: a randomized clinical trial of competing strategies, *Arch Intern Med* 172(7):575, 2012.

Li B, et al: Analysis of bowel sounds application status for gastrointestinal function monitoring in the intensive care unit, *Crit Care Nurs Q* 37(2):199, 2014.

Pittman J, et al: Psychometric evaluation of the ostomy complication severity index, *JWOCN* 41(2):147, 2014.

Salvadena G: The incidence of stomal and peristomal complications during the first 3 months after ostomy creation, *JWOCN* 40(4):400, 2013.

Schmidt FM, Santos VL: Prevalence of constipation in the general adult population: an integrative review, *JWOCN* 41(1):70, 2014.

Williams J, et al: Evaluating skin care problems in people with stomas, *Br J Nurs* 19(17):S6, 2010.

48

Skin Integrity and Wound Care

OBJECTIVES

- Discuss the risk factors that contribute to pressure ulcer formation.
- Describe the pressure ulcer staging system.
- Discuss the normal process of wound healing.
- Describe the differences in wound healing by primary and secondary intention.
- Describe complications of wound healing.
- Explain the factors that impede or promote wound healing.
- Describe the differences between nursing care of acute and chronic wounds.
- Complete an assessment for a patient with impaired skin integrity.
- List nursing diagnoses associated with impaired skin integrity.
- Develop a nursing care plan for a patient with impaired skin integrity.
- List appropriate nursing interventions for a patient with impaired skin integrity.
- State evaluation criteria for a patient with impaired skin integrity.

KEY TERMS

Abrasion, p. 1198
Approximated, p. 1190
Blanching, p. 1186
Blanchable hyperemia, p. 1186
Collagen, p. 1185
Debridement, p. 1206
Dehiscence, p. 1191
Drainage evacuators, p. 1215
Epithelialization, p. 1191
Eschar, p. 1188
Evisceration, p. 1192
Exudate, p. 1189
Fibrin, p. 1191
Fluctuance, p. 1187
Friction, p. 1187
Granulation tissue, p. 1188
Hematoma, p. 1191
Hemorrhage, p. 1191
Hemostasis, p. 1191
Induration, p. 1186
Laceration, p. 1198
Negative pressure wound therapy, p. 1233
Nonblanchable erythema, p. 1186
Pressure ulcer, p. 1185
Primary intention, p. 1190
Puncture, p. 1198
Purulent, p. 1191
Reactive hyperemia, p. 1205
Sanguineous, p. 1198
Secondary intention, p. 1190
Serosanguineous, p. 1198
Serous, p. 1198
Shearing force, p. 1204
Slough, p. 1188
Sutures, p. 1214
Tissue ischemia, p. 1186
Vacuum-assisted closure (V.A.C.), p. 1212
Wound, p. 1189

MEDIA RESOURCES

http://evolve.elsevier.com/Potter/fundamentals/

- Review Questions
- Video Clips
- Concept Map Creator
- Case Study with Questions
- Skills Performance Checklists
- Audio Glossary
- Content Updates

Skin, the largest organ in the body, constitutes 15% of the total adult body weight (Wysocki, 2016). It is a protective barrier against disease-causing organisms and a sensory organ for pain, temperature, and touch; and it synthesizes vitamin D. Injury to the skin poses risks to safety and triggers a complex healing response. Your most important responsibilities include assessing and monitoring skin integrity, identifying patient risks for skin problems, identifying actual problems, and planning, implementing, and evaluating interventions to maintain skin integrity. Once a wound occurs, it is critical to know the process of normal wound healing to identify the appropriate nursing interventions.

SCIENTIFIC KNOWLEDGE BASE

Skin

The skin has two layers: the epidermis and the dermis (Figure 48-1). They are separated by a membrane, often referred to as the *dermal-epidermal junction*. The epidermis, or the top layer, has several layers. The stratum corneum is the thin, outermost layer of the epidermis. It consists of flattened, dead, keratinized cells. The cells originate from the innermost epidermal layer, commonly called the *basal layer*. Cells in the basal layer divide, proliferate, and migrate toward the epidermal surface. After they reach the stratum corneum, they flatten and die.

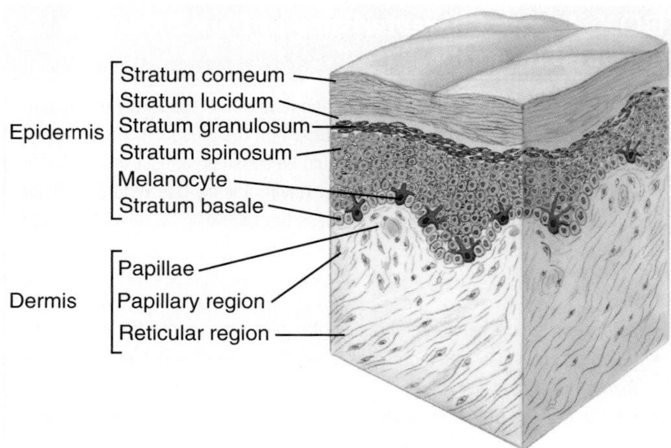

FIGURE 48-1 Layers of skin. (From Applegate E: *The anatomy and physiology learning system*, ed 3, St Louis, 2006, Saunders.)

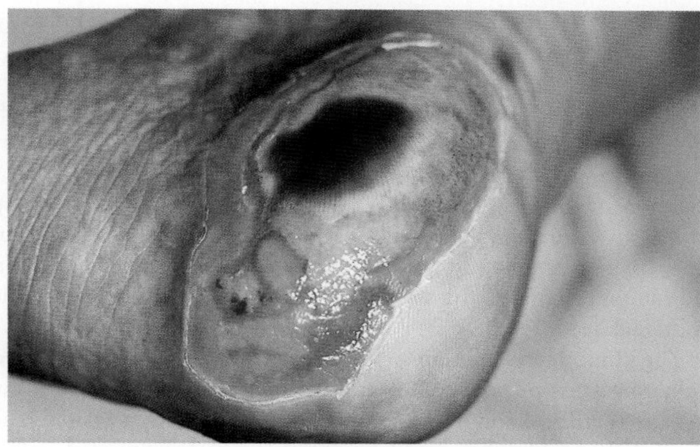

FIGURE 48-2 Pressure ulcer with tissue necrosis.

This constant movement ensures replacement of surface cells sloughed during normal desquamation or shedding. The thin stratum corneum protects underlying cells and tissues from dehydration and prevents entrance of certain chemical agents. The stratum corneum allows evaporation of water from the skin and permits absorption of certain topical medications.

The dermis, the inner layer of the skin, provides tensile strength; mechanical support; and protection for the underlying muscles, bones, and organs. It differs from the epidermis in that it contains mostly connective tissue and few skin cells. Collagen (a tough, fibrous protein), blood vessels, and nerves are found in the dermal layer. Fibroblasts, which are responsible for collagen formation, are the only distinctive cell type within the dermis.

Understanding skin structure helps you maintain skin integrity and promote wound healing. Intact skin protects the patient from chemical and mechanical injury. When the skin is injured, the epidermis functions to resurface the wound and restore the barrier against invading organisms, and the dermis responds to restore the structural integrity (collagen) and the physical properties of the skin. The normal aging process alters skin characteristics and makes skin more vulnerable to damage. Box 48-1 provides a summary of the changes in aging skin.

Pressure Ulcers

Pressure ulcer, pressure sore, decubitus ulcer, and *bedsore* are terms used to describe impaired skin integrity related to unrelieved, prolonged pressure. The most current terminology is pressure ulcer (Figure 48-2), which is consistent with the recommendations of the pressure ulcer guidelines written by the Wound, Ostomy and Continence Nurses Society (WOCN, 2010). A pressure ulcer is localized injury to the skin and other underlying tissue, usually over a bony prominence (e.g., sacrum, greater trochanter), as a result of pressure or pressure in combination with shear and/or friction. A number of contributing factors are also associated with pressure ulcers; the significance of these factors is not yet clear (NPUAP, EPUAP, PPPIA, 2014). Any patient experiencing decreased mobility, decreased sensory perception, fecal or urinary incontinence, and/or poor nutrition is at risk for pressure ulcer development. Examples of patients who are at risk for development of pressure ulcers include the following:

- Older adults, those who have experienced trauma
- Those with spinal-cord injuries (SCI)
- Those who have sustained a fractured hip
- Those in long-term homes or community care, the acutely ill
- Individuals with diabetes
- Patients in critical care settings (NPUAP, EPUAP, PPPIA, 2014)

Many factors contribute to the formation of a pressure ulcer. Pressure is the major cause. Tissue receives oxygen and nutrients and eliminates metabolic wastes via the blood. Any factor that interferes with blood flow in turn interferes with cellular metabolism and the function or life of the cells. Prolonged, intense pressure affects cellular metabolism by decreasing or obliterating blood flow, resulting in tissue ischemia and ultimately tissue death.

Pathogenesis of Pressure Ulcers. Pressure is the major element in the cause of pressure ulcers. Three pressure-related factors

BOX 48-1 FOCUS ON OLDER ADULTS

Skin-Associated Issues

The older adult has several skin-related issues that should be considered when assessing skin and skin breakdown. Age-related changes such as reduced skin elasticity, decreased collagen, and thinning of underlying muscle and tissues can cause the older adult's skin to be easily torn in response to mechanical trauma, especially shearing forces (Wysocki, 2016). The attachment between the epidermis and dermis becomes flattened in older adults, allowing the skin to be easily torn in response to mechanical trauma (e.g., tape removal). Concomitant medical conditions and polypharmacy, which are common in the older adult, are factors that interfere with wound healing. Aging causes a diminished inflammatory response, resulting in slow epithelialization and wound healing (Doughty and Sparks-Defriese, 2016). The hypodermis decreases in size with age. Older patients have little subcutaneous padding over bony prominences; thus they are more prone to skin breakdown (Wysocki, 2016).

Implications for Practice

1. When removing any adhesive dressings or tapes, gently release the skin from the tape; do not pull the tape away from the skin. Release the skin from the adhesive by pushing the skin from the adhesive.
2. To help an elder patient reposition in bed consider the use of a repositioning device and teach the patient or family caregiver how to reposition without sliding on the sheets.
3. Be diligent about assessing bony prominences where impaired skin integrity and injury to other tissues are most likely to occur.
4. Assess the medications that a patient may be taking for effect on delayed wound healing and revise outcomes in the plan of care to reflect that possibility.

contribute to pressure ulcer development: (1) pressure intensity, (2) pressure duration, and (3) tissue tolerance.

Pressure Intensity. A classic research study identified capillary closing pressure as the minimal amount of pressure required to collapse a capillary (e.g., when the pressure exceeds the normal capillary pressure range of 15 to 32 mm Hg) (Burton and Yamada, 1951). Therefore, if the pressure applied over a capillary exceeds the normal capillary pressure and the vessel is occluded for a prolonged period of time, **tissue ischemia** can occur. If the patient has reduced sensation and cannot respond to the discomfort of the ischemia, tissue ischemia and tissue death result.

The clinical presentation of obstructed blood flow occurs when evaluating areas of pressure. After a period of tissue ischemia, if the pressure is relieved and the blood flow returns, the skin turns red. The effect of this redness is vasodilation (blood vessel expansion), called *hyperemia* (redness). You assess an area of hyperemia by pressing a finger over the affected area. If it blanches (turns lighter in color) and the erythema returns when you remove your finger, the hyperemia is transient and is an attempt to overcome the ischemic episode, thus called **blanchable hyperemia**. However, if the erythematous area does not blanch (**nonblanchable erythema**) when you apply pressure, deep tissue damage is probable.

Blanching occurs when the normal red tones of the light-skinned patient are absent. When checking for pressure ulcers in dark-skinned patients, dark skin may not show the blanch response. Instead, after applying light pressure, look for an area darker than the surrounding skin or one that is taut, shiny, or indurated (hardened). The light from a camera flash can be used to enhance visualization of dark skin. Check for localized changes in skin texture and temperature. Early signs of skin damage include **induration**, bogginess (less-than-normal stiffness), and increased warmth at the injury site compared to nearby areas. Over time, as tissues become more damaged, the area becomes cooler to the touch (Sommers, 2011). There are characteristics of intact dark skin that alert nurses to the potential for pressure ulcers Box 48-2.

Pressure Duration. Low pressure over a prolonged period and high-intensity pressure over a short period are two concerns related to duration of pressure. Both types of pressure cause tissue damage. Extended pressure occludes blood flow and nutrients and contributes to cell death (Pieper, 2016). Clinical implications of pressure duration include evaluating the amount of pressure (checking skin for nonblanching hyperemia) and determining the amount of time that a patient tolerates pressure (checking to be sure after relieving pressure that the affected area blanches).

Tissue Tolerance. The ability of tissue to endure pressure depends on the integrity of the tissue and the supporting structures. The extrinsic factors of shear, friction, and moisture affect the ability of the skin to tolerate pressure: the greater the degree to which the factors of shear, friction, and moisture are present, the more susceptible the skin will be to damage from pressure. The second factor related to tissue tolerance is the ability of the underlying skin structures (blood vessels, collagen) to help redistribute pressure. Systemic factors such as poor nutrition, increased aging, hydration status, and low blood pressure affect the tolerance of the tissue to externally applied pressure.

Risk Factors for Pressure Ulcer Development. A variety of factors predispose a patient to pressure ulcer formation. These factors are often directly related to disease such as decreased level of consciousness, the presence of a cast, or secondary to an illness (e.g., decreased sensation following a cerebrovascular accident).

Impaired Sensory Perception. Patients with altered sensory perception for pain and pressure are more at risk for impaired skin integrity than those with normal sensation. Patients with impaired sensory perception of pain and pressure are unable to feel when a part of their body undergoes increased, prolonged pressure or pain. Thus a patient who can't feel or sense that there is pain or pressure is at risk for the development of pressure ulcers.

Impaired Mobility. Patients unable to independently change positions are at risk for pressure ulcer development. For example, a morbidly obese patient who is seriously ill will be weakened and less likely to turn independently. Patients with spinal cord injuries have decreased or absent motor and sensory impairment and are unable to reposition off bony prominences.

Alteration in Level of Consciousness. Patients who are confused or disoriented, those who have expressive aphasia or the inability to verbalize, or those with changing levels of consciousness are unable to protect themselves from pressure ulcer development. Patients who are confused or disoriented are sometimes able to feel pressure but are not always able to understand how to relieve it or communicate their discomfort. A patient in a coma cannot perceive pressure and is unable to move voluntarily to relieve pressure.

Shear. Shear force is the sliding movement of skin and subcutaneous tissue while the underlying muscle and bone are stationary (Bryant, 2016). For example, shear force occurs when the head of the bed is elevated and the sliding of the skeleton starts but the skin is fixed because of friction with the bed (Figure 48-3). It also occurs when transferring a patient from bed to stretcher and the patient's skin is pulled across the bed. When shear is present, the skin and subcutaneous layers adhere to the surface of the bed, and the layers

BOX 48-2 Characteristics of Dark Skin with Impaired Integrity

Dark skin tones may not demonstrate change in color, especially darkly pigmented skin. To assess a dark-skinned patient for the presence of a category/stage I pressure ulcer, the following should be considered: assess the skin in a well-illuminated setting (i.e., a well-lit environment). Use natural light or halogen light. Avoid florescent light. Assess the following (assess noninjured skin areas first):

Color

- Color remains unchanged and does not blanch when pressure is applied.
- If patient previously had a pressure ulcer, that area of skin might be lighter than original color.
- Localized areas of inflammation may take on an eggplant (purplish-blue or violet) color rather than appearing reddened.

Temperature

- Circumscribed area of intact skin may be warm to touch. As tissue changes color, intact skin feels cool to touch.
- Inflammation is detected by making comparisons to surrounding skin.

Appearance

- Edema may occur with induration and appear taut and shiny.
- Injured skin with a stage I pressure ulcer might show low resilience. Document tissue resilience: tissue on palpation is boggy or mushy when compared to surrounding skin.

Palpation

- Surrounding area may be sensitive or tender to touch or may be hard or lumpy on palpation.

Adapted from Nix DP: Skin and wound inspection and assessment. In Bryant RA, Nix DP, editors: *Acute and chronic wounds: current management concepts*, ed 5, St Louis, 2016, Elsevier.

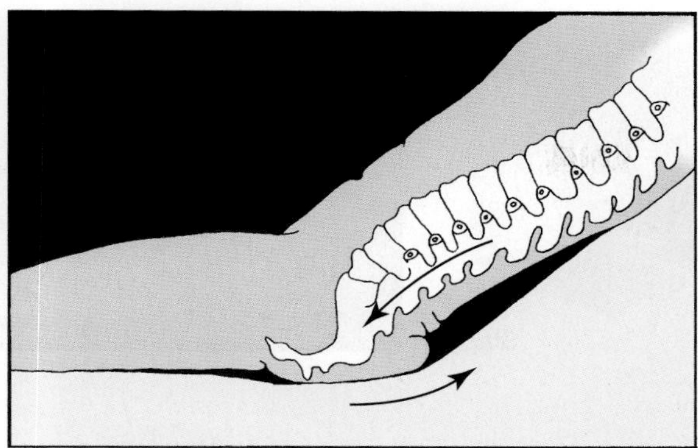

FIGURE 48-3 Shear exerted in sacral area.

of muscle and the bones slide in the direction of body movement. The underlying tissue capillaries are stretched and angulated by the shear force. As a result, necrosis occurs deep within the tissue layers. The tissue damage is deep in the tissues and causes undermining of the dermis.

Friction. The force of two surfaces moving across one another such as the mechanical force exerted when skin is dragged across a coarse surface such as bed linens is called friction (WOCN, 2010). Unlike shear injuries, friction injuries affect the epidermis or top layer of the skin. The denuded skin appears red and painful and is sometimes referred to as a *sheet burn.* A friction injury occurs in patients who are restless, in those who have uncontrollable movements such as spastic conditions, and in those whose skin is dragged rather than lifted from the bed surface during position changes or transfer to a stretcher.

Moisture. The presence and duration of moisture on the skin increases the risk of ulcer formation. Moisture reduces the resistance of the skin to other physical factors such as pressure and/or shear force. Prolonged moisture softens skin, making it more susceptible to damage. Immobilized patients who are unable to perform their own hygiene needs depend on nurses to keep the skin dry and intact. Skin moisture originates from wound drainage, excessive perspiration, and fecal or urinary incontinence.

Classification of Pressure Ulcers

As a nurse, you need to perform an initial assessment of a pressure ulcer using systematic parameters. Then you will evaluate at regular intervals to determine the status and progress toward wound healing and to plan appropriate interventions.. Assessment includes wound location, depth of tissue involvement (staging), type and approximate percentage of tissue in wound bed, wound dimensions (if present, include sinus tracts and tunneling), exudate description (if present, odor), and condition of surrounding skin.

One method for assessment of a pressure ulcer is the use of a staging system. Staging systems for pressure ulcers are based on describing the depth of tissue loss. Accurate staging requires knowledge of the skin layers. A major drawback of a staging system is that you cannot stage an ulcer covered with necrotic tissue because the necrotic tissue is covering the depth of the ulcer. The necrotic tissue must be debrided or removed to expose the wound base to allow for assessment.

Pressure ulcer staging describes the pressure ulcer depth at the point of assessment. Thus, once you have staged the pressure ulcer, this stage endures even as it heals. Pressure ulcers do not progress from a stage III to a stage I; rather, a stage III ulcer demonstrating signs of healing is described as a healing stage III pressure ulcer (Pieper, 2016). The NPUAP, EPUAP, and PPPIA (2014) have developed clinical practice guidelines for pressure ulcers and have advanced the following classification/staging system. The NPUAP uses the term *staging* and the European group uses the term *category,* both describing the same assessment parameter.

Category/Stage I: Nonblanchable Redness. Intact skin presents with nonblanchable redness of a localized area, usually over a bony prominence. Discoloration of the skin, warmth, edema, hardness, or pain may also be present. Darkly pigmented skin may not have visible blanching but its coloring may differ from the surrounding area. The area may be painful, firm, soft, warmer, or cooler compared to adjacent tissue. Category I may be difficult to detect in individuals with dark skin tones. It may indicate "at risk" people (Figure 48-4, *A*).

Category/Stage II: Partial-Thickness. Partial thickness loss of dermis presents as a shallow, open ulcer with a red-pink wound bed without slough. It may also present as an intact or open/ruptured serum-filled or serosanguineous-filled blister. It presents as a shiny or dry shallow ulcer without slough or bruising (see Figure 48-4, *B*). The presence of bruising indicates deep tissue injury. This category should not be used to describe skin tears, tape burns, incontinence-associated dermatitis, maceration, or excoriation.

Category/Stage III: Full-Thickness Skin Loss. In full-thickness tissue loss subcutaneous fat may be visible; but bone, tendon, and muscle are *not* exposed. Slough may be present but does not obscure the depth of tissue loss. It *may* include undermining and tunneling. The depth of a category/stage III pressure ulcer varies by anatomical location. The bridge of the nose, ear, occiput, and malleolus do not have (adipose) subcutaneous tissue; and category/stage III ulcers can be shallow. In contrast, areas of significant adiposity can develop extremely deep category/stage III pressure ulcers. Bone/tendon is not visible or directly palpable (see Figure 48-4, *C*).

Category/Stage IV: Full-Thickness Tissue Loss. In full-thickness tissue loss with exposed bone, tendon, or muscle, subcutaneous fat may be visible; but bone, tendon, and muscle *are* exposed. Slough or eschar may be present. It often includes undermining and tunneling. The depth of a category/stage IV pressure ulcer varies by anatomical location. The bridge of the nose, ear, occiput, and malleolus do not have (adipose) subcutaneous tissue; and these ulcers can be shallow. Category/stage IV ulcers can extend into muscle and/or supporting structures (e.g., fascia, tendon, or joint capsule), making osteomyelitis or osteitis likely to occur. Exposed bone/muscle is visible or directly palpable (see Figure 48-4, *D*).

Unstageable/Unclassified: Full-Thickness Skin or Tissue Loss—Depth Unknown. Full-thickness tissue loss in which actual depth of an ulcer is completely obscured by slough (yellow, tan, gray, green or brown) and/or eschar (tan, brown or black) in the wound bed is unstageable. Until enough slough and/or eschar are removed to expose the base of a wound, the true depth cannot be determined; but it will be either a category/stage III or IV. Stable (dry, adherent, intact without erythema or fluctuance) eschar on the heels serves as "the natural (biological) cover of the body" and should not be removed (see Figure 48-4, *E*).

Suspected Deep-Tissue Injury—Depth Unknown. Suspected deep-tissue injury is a purple or maroon localized area of discolored intact skin or a blood-filled blister caused by damage of underlying soft tissue from pressure and/or shear. The area may be preceded by tissue that is painful, firm, mushy, boggy, warmer, or cooler compared

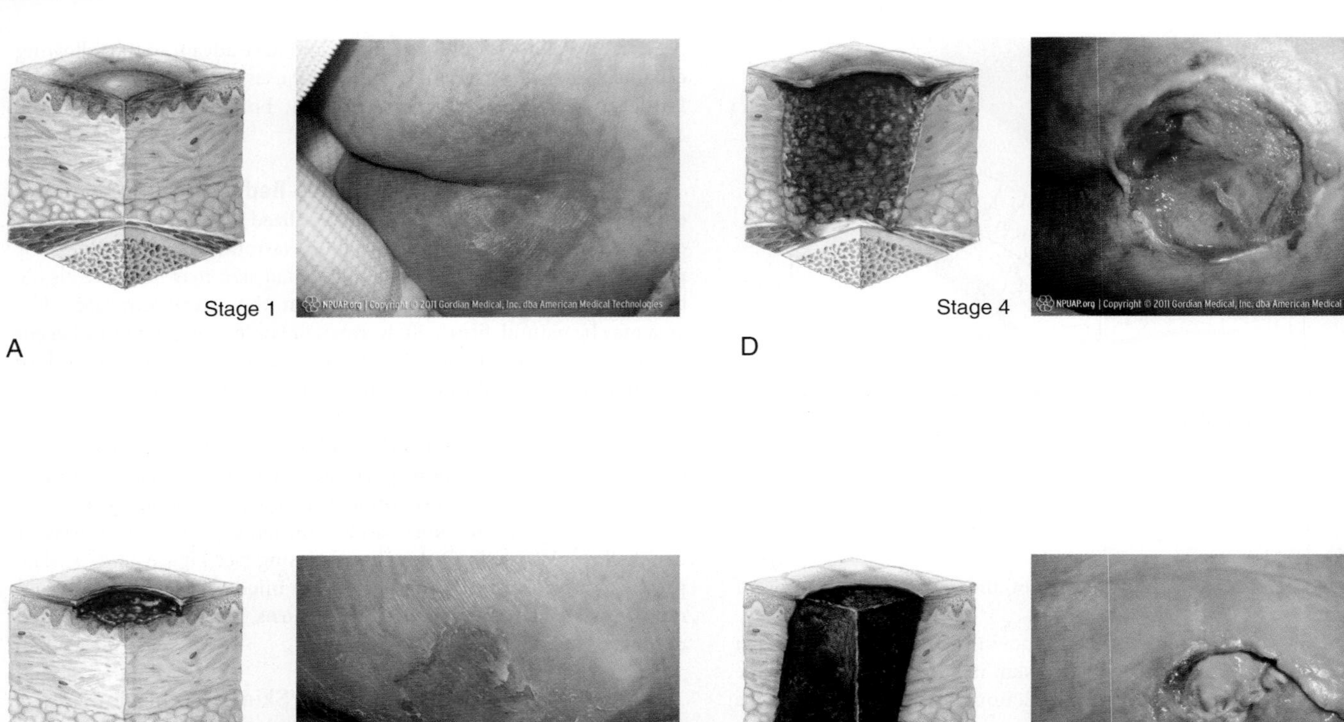

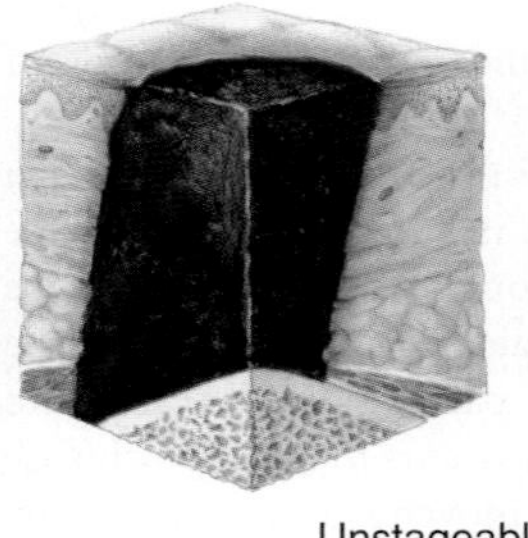

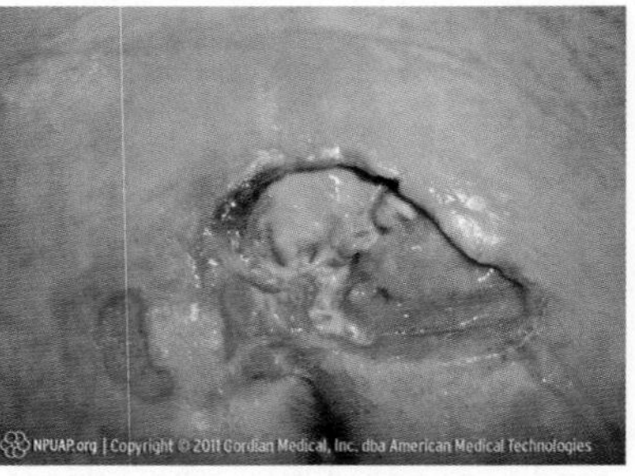

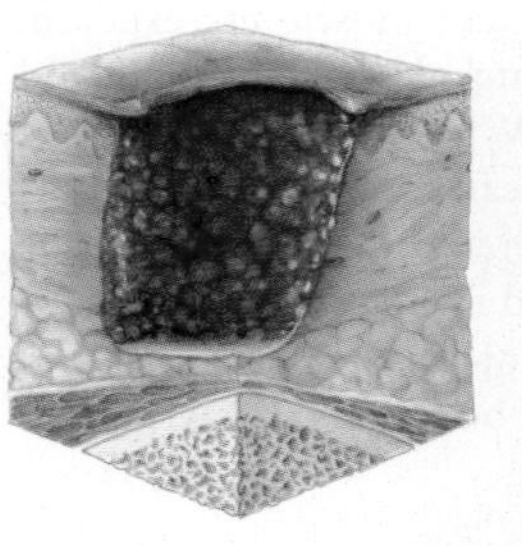

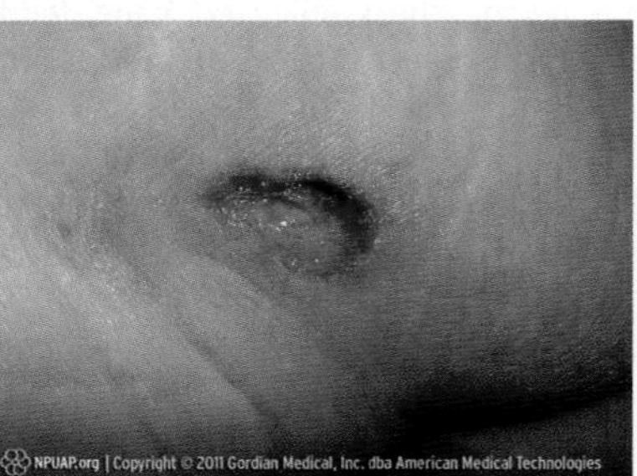

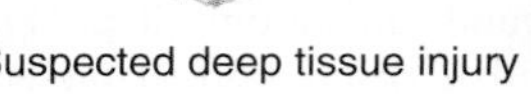

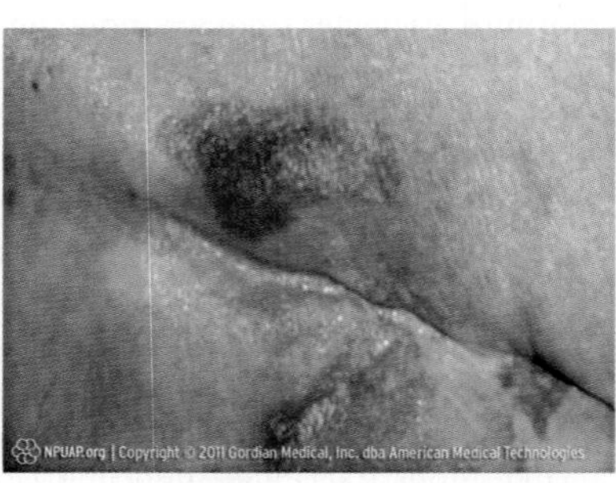

FIGURE 48-4 Diagram of stages. **A,** Stage I pressure ulcer. **B,** Stage II pressure ulcer. **C,** Stage III pressure ulcer. **D,** Stage IV pressure ulcer. **E,** Unstageable wound. **F,** Suspected deep-tissue injury. (Used with permission of the National Pressure Ulcer Advisory Panel. Copyright ©NPUAP.)

to adjacent tissue. Deep-tissue injury may be difficult to detect in individuals with dark skin tones. It may begin as a thin blister over a dark wound bed. The wound may further evolve and become covered by thin eschar. Evolution may be rapid, exposing additional layers of tissue even with optimal treatment (see Figure 48-4, *F*).

The NPUAP, EPUAP, PPPIA (2014) guidelines suggest that, when conducting a skin assessment on an individual with darkly pigmented skin, prioritize assessment of skin temperature, edema, and change in tissue consistency in relation to surrounding tissue. Additional aspects of assessing dark skin are in Box 48-3.

You need to assess the type of tissue in a wound base; then use this information to plan appropriate interventions. The assessment includes the amount (percentage) and appearance (color) of viable and nonviable tissue. **Granulation tissue** is red, moist tissue composed of new blood vessels, the presence of which indicates progression toward healing. Soft yellow or white tissue is characteristic of **slough** (stringy substance attached to wound bed), and it must be removed by a skilled clinician or with the use of an appropriate wound dressing before the wound is able to heal. Black, brown, tan, or necrotic tissue is **eschar,** which needs to be removed before healing can proceed.

BOX 48-3 CULTURAL ASPECTS OF CARE

Impact of Skin Color

Detecting cyanosis and other changes in skin color in patients is an important clinical skill. However, this detection becomes a challenge in dark-skinned patients (Nix, 2016). There are concerns about the inability of practitioners to describe early pressure ulcer or pressure injury in people with darkly pigmented skin accurately (Henderson et al., 1997). Cyanosis is "a slightly bluish-grayish slatelike or dark purple discoloration of the skin caused by the presence of at least 5 g of reduced hemoglobin in arterial blood." Color differentiation of cyanosis varies according to skin pigmentation. In dark-skinned patients you need to know the individual's baseline skin tone. You should not confuse the normal hyperpigmentation of Mongolian spots that are seen on the sacrum of African, Native American, and Asian patients with cyanosis. Observe the patient's skin in nonglare daylight. The Gaskin Nursing Assessment of Skin Color (GNASC) is a useful tool for assessment for identifying changes in skin color that increase the patient's risk for pressure ulcers (Gaskin, 1986).

Implications for Patient-Centered Care

- It is difficult but possible to detect cyanosis in the dark-skinned patient.
- Be aware of situations that produce changes in skin tone such as inadequate lighting.
- Examine body sites with the least melanin such as under the arm for underlying color identification (Nix, 2016).
- When conducting a skin assessment in an individual with darkly pigmented skin, prioritize assessment of skin temperature, edema, and change in tissue consistency in relation to surrounding tissues (NPUAP, EPUAP, PPPIA, 2014).

The measurement of the wound size provides overall changes in dimensions, which is an indicator for wound healing progress (Nix, 2016). This includes measuring the length and width of a wound as well as determining its depth.

Wound **exudate** should describe the amount, color, consistency, and odor of wound drainage and is part of the wound assessment. Excessive exudate indicates the presence of infection. The skin around the wound (periwound) should be assessed. Examine the periwound area for redness, warmth, and signs of maceration and palpate the area for signs of pain or induration. The presence of any of these factors on the periwound skin indicates wound deterioration.

Wound Classifications

A **wound** is a disruption of the integrity and function of tissues in the body (Baranoski, 2012). It is imperative for the nurse to know that *all wounds are not created equal.* Understanding the etiology of a wound is important because the treatment for it varies, depending on the underlying disease process.

There are many ways to classify wounds. Wound classification systems describe the status of skin integrity, cause of the wound, severity or extent of tissue injury or damage, cleanliness of the wound (Table 48-1), and descriptive qualities of the wound tissue such as color (Figure 48-5). Wound classification enables a nurse to understand the risks associated with a wound and implications for healing.

Process of Wound Healing. Wound healing involves integrated physiological processes. The tissue layers involved and their capacity for regeneration determine the mechanism for repair for any wound (Doughty and Sparks-Defriese, 2016).

Wounds can be classified by the extent of tissue loss: partial-thickness wounds that involve only a partial loss of skin layers (the epidermis and superficial dermal layers) and full-thickness wounds

TABLE 48-1 Wound Classification

Description	Causes	Implications for Healing
Onset and Duration		
Acute		
Wound that proceeds through an orderly and timely reparative process that results in sustained restoration of anatomical and functional integrity	Trauma Surgical incision	Wound edges are clean and intact.
Chronic		
Wound that fails to proceed through an orderly and timely process to produce anatomical and functional integrity	Vascular compromise, chronic inflammation, or repetitive insults to tissue (Doughty and Sparks-Defriese, 2016)	Continued exposure to insult impedes wound healing.
Healing Process		
Primary Intention		
Wound that is closed	Surgical incision Wound that is sutured or stapled	Healing occurs by epithelialization; heals quickly with minimal scar formation.
Secondary Intention		
Wound edges not approximated	Pressure ulcers, surgical wounds that have tissue loss or contamination	Wound heals by granulation tissue formation, wound contraction, and epithelialization.
Tertiary Intention		
Wound that is left open for several days; then wound edges are approximated (see Figure 48-4,*C*)	Wounds that are contaminated and require observation for signs of inflammation	Closure of wound is delayed until risk of infection is resolved (Doughty and Sparks-Defriese, 2016).

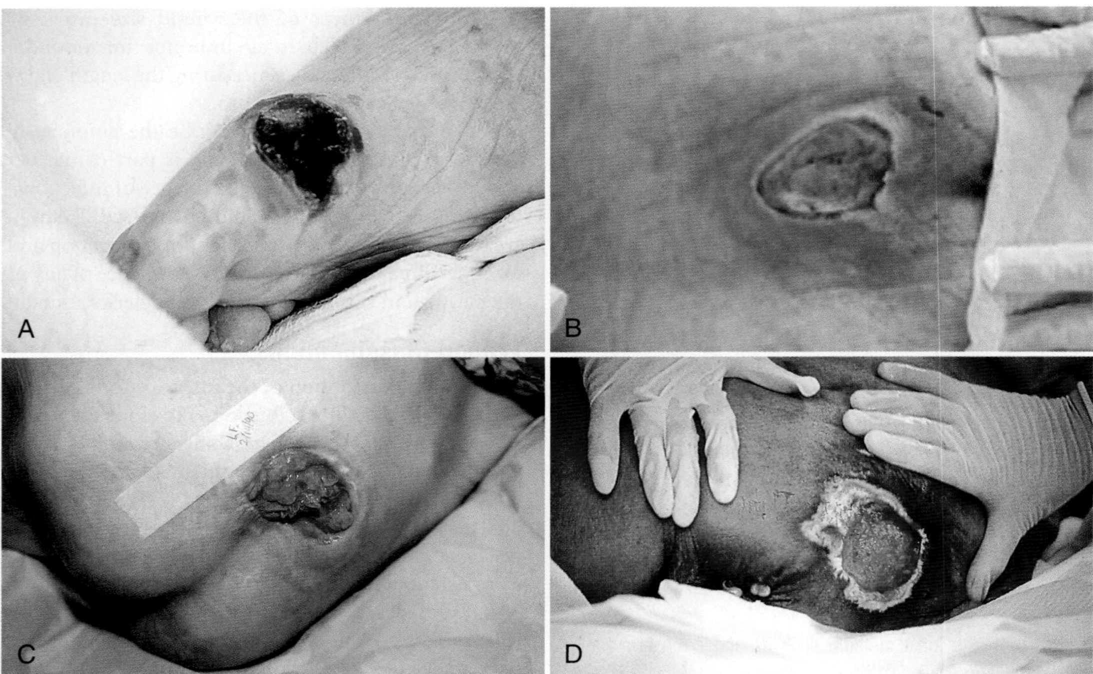

FIGURE 48-5 Wounds classified by color assessment. **A,** Black wound. **B,** Yellow wound. **C,** Red wound. **D,** Mixed-color wound. (**A** and **D** Courtesy Scott Health Care—A Mölnlycke Company, Philadelphia, PA; **B** and **C** from Bryant RA, Nix DP, editors: *Acute and chronic wounds: current management concepts,* ed 5, St Louis, 2016, Elsevier.)

that involve total loss of the skin layers (epidermis and dermis) (Doughty and Sparks-DeFriese, 2016). Partial-thickness wounds are shallow in depth, moist, and painful; and the wound base generally appears red. A full-thickness wound extends into the subcutaneous layer, and the depth and tissue type varies, depending on body location. The significance of determining if a wound is a partial or full thickness lies in the mechanism of healing. A partial-thickness wound heals by regeneration; and a full-thickness wound heals by forming new tissue, a process that can take longer than the healing of a partial-thickness wound.

A clean surgical incision is an example of a wound with little tissue loss. The surgical incision heals by primary intention (Figure 48-6, *A*). The skin edges are approximated, or closed, and the risk of infection is low. Healing occurs quickly, with minimal scar formation, as long as infection and secondary breakdown are prevented (Doughty and Sparks-Defriese, 2016). In contrast, a wound involving loss of tissue such as a burn, pressure ulcer, or severe laceration heals by secondary intention. The wound is left open until it becomes filled by scar tissue. It takes longer for a wound to heal by secondary intention; thus the chance of infection is greater. If scarring from secondary intention is severe, loss of tissue function is often permanent (see Figure 48-6, *B*).

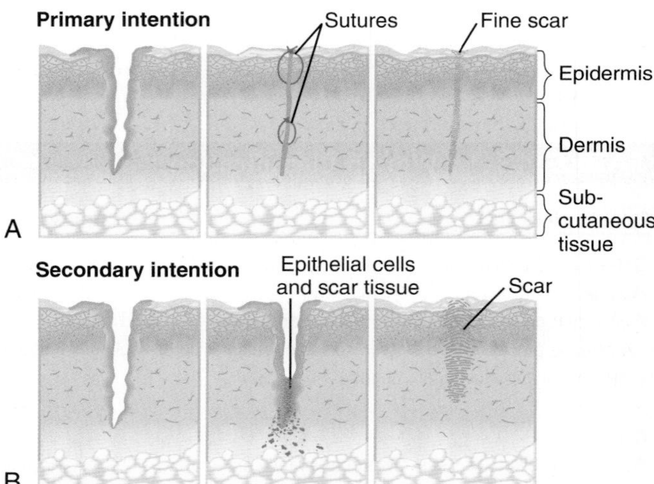

FIGURE 48-6 **A,** Wound healing by primary intention such as a surgical incision. Wound healing edges are pulled together and approximated with sutures or staples, and healing occurs by connective tissue deposition. **B,** Wound healing by secondary intention. Wound edges are not approximated, and healing occurs by granulation tissue formation and contraction of the wound edges. (From Black JM, Hawks JH: *Medical-surgical nursing: clinical management for positive outcomes,* ed 8, St Louis, 2009, Mosby.)

Wound Repair. Partial-thickness wounds are shallow, involving loss of epidermis and possible loss of dermis. These wounds heal by regeneration because epidermis regenerates. An example of a partial-thickness wound is a scrape or an abrasion. Full-thickness wounds extend into the dermis and heal by scar formation because deeper structures do not regenerate. Pressure ulcers are an example of full-thickness wounds.

Partial-Thickness Wound Repair. Three components are involved in the healing process of a partial-thickness wound: inflammatory response, epithelial proliferation (reproduction) and migration, and reestablishment of the epidermal layers.

Tissue trauma causes the *inflammatory response,* which in turn causes redness and swelling to the area with a moderate amount of serous exudate. This response generally is limited to the first 24 hours after wounding. The epithelial cells begin to regenerate, providing new cells to replace the lost cells. The *epithelial proliferation and migration* start at both the wound edges and the epidermal cells lining the epidermal appendages, allowing for quick resurfacing. Epithelial cells begin to migrate across a wound bed soon after the wound occurs. A wound left open to air can resurface within 6 to 7 days, whereas one that is kept moist can resurface in 4 days. The difference in the healing rate is related to the fact that epidermal cells only migrate across a moist surface. In a dry wound the cells migrate down into a moist level before migration can occur (Doughty and Sparks-Defriese, 2016). New epithelium is only a few cells thick and must undergo *reestablishment of the epidermal layers.* The cells slowly reestablish normal thickness and appear as dry, pink tissue.

Full-Thickness Wound Repair. The four phases involved in the healing process of a full-thickness wound are hemostasis, inflammatory, proliferative, and maturation.

Hemostasis. A series of events designed to control blood loss, establish bacterial control, and seal the defect occurs when there is an injury. During **hemostasis** injured blood vessels constrict, and platelets gather to stop bleeding. Clots form a **fibrin** matrix that later provides a framework for cellular repair.

Inflammatory Phase. In the inflammatory stage damaged tissue and mast cells secrete histamine, resulting in vasodilation of surrounding capillaries and movement/migration of serum and white blood cells into the damaged tissues. This results in localized redness, edema, warmth, and throbbing. The inflammatory response is beneficial, and there is no value in attempting to cool the area or reduce the swelling unless the swelling occurs within a closed compartment (e.g., ankle or neck).

Leukocytes (white blood cells) reach a wound within a few hours. The primary-acting white blood cell is the neutrophil, which begins to ingest bacteria and small debris. The second important leukocyte is the monocyte, which transforms into macrophages. The macrophages are the "garbage cells" that clean a wound of bacteria, dead cells, and debris by phagocytosis. Macrophages continue the process of clearing a wound of debris and release growth factors that attract fibroblasts, the cells that synthesize collagen (connective tissue). Collagen appears as early as the second day and is the main component of scar tissue.

In a clean wound the inflammatory phase establishes a clean wound bed. The inflammatory phase is prolonged if too little inflammation occurs, as in a debilitating disease such as cancer or after administration of steroids. Too much inflammation also prolongs healing because arriving cells compete for available nutrients. An example is a wound infection in which the increased metabolic energy requirements present in an infected wound compete for the available calorie intake.

Proliferative Phase. With the appearance of new blood vessels as reconstruction progresses, the proliferative phase begins and lasts from 3 to 24 days. The main activities during this phase are the filling of a wound with granulation tissue, wound contraction, and wound resurfacing by **epithelialization**. Fibroblasts are present in this phase and are the cells that synthesize collagen, providing the matrix for granulation. Collagen mixes with the granulation tissue to form a matrix that supports the reepithelialization. Collagen provides strength and structural integrity to a wound. During this period a wound contracts to reduce the area that requires healing. Finally the epithelial cells migrate from the wound edges to resurface. In a clean wound the proliferative phase accomplishes the following: the vascular bed is reestablished (granulation tissue), the area is filled with replacement tissue (collagen, contraction, and granulation tissue), and the surface is repaired (epithelialization). Impairment of healing during this stage usually results from systemic factors such as age, anemia, hypoproteinemia, and zinc deficiency.

Maturation. Maturation, the final stage of healing, sometimes takes place for more than a year, depending on the depth and extent of the wound. The collagen scar continues to reorganize and gain strength for several months. However, a healed wound usually does not have the tensile strength of the tissue it replaces. Collagen fibers undergo remodeling or reorganization before assuming their normal appearance. Usually scar tissue contains fewer pigmented cells (melanocytes) and has a lighter color than normal skin. In dark-skinned individuals the scar tissue may be more highly pigmented than surrounding skin.

Complications of Wound Healing

Hemorrhage. **Hemorrhage**, or bleeding from a wound site, is normal during and immediately after initial trauma. Hemostasis occurs within several minutes unless large blood vessels are involved or a patient has poor clotting function. Hemorrhage occurring after hemostasis indicates a slipped surgical suture, a dislodged clot, infection, or erosion of a blood vessel by a foreign object (e.g., a drain). Hemorrhage occurs externally or internally. For example, if a surgical suture slips from a blood vessel, bleeding occurs internally within the tissues, and there are no visible signs of blood unless a surgical drain is present. A surgical drain may be inserted into tissues beneath a wound to remove fluid that collects in underlying tissues.

You detect internal bleeding by looking for distention or swelling of the affected body part, a change in the type and amount of drainage from a surgical drain, or signs of hypovolemic shock. A **hematoma** is a localized collection of blood underneath the tissues. It appears as a swelling, change in color, sensation, or warmth that often takes on a bluish discoloration. A hematoma near a major artery or vein is dangerous because pressure from the expanding hematoma obstructs blood flow.

External hemorrhaging is obvious. You observe dressings covering a wound for bloody drainage. If bleeding is extensive, the dressing soon becomes saturated, and frequently blood drains from under the dressing and pools beneath the patient. Observe all wounds closely, particularly surgical wounds, in which the risk of hemorrhage is great during the first 24 to 48 hours after surgery or injury.

Infection. Wound infection is the second most common health care–associated infection (nosocomial) (see Chapter 29). All wounds have some level of bacterial burden; few wounds are infected (Stotts, 2016b). Wound infection is present when the microorganisms invade the wound tissues. The local clinical signs of wound infection can include erythema; increased amount of wound drainage; change in appearance of the wound drainage (thick, color change, presence of odor); and periwound warmth, pain, or edema. A patient may have a fever and an increase in white blood cell count. Laboratory tests such as a wound culture, tissue biopsy, or swab culture can be done to evaluate the wound for infection. Bacterial infections inhibit wound healing.

Some contaminated or traumatic wounds show signs of infection early, within 2 to 3 days. A surgical wound infection usually does not develop until the fourth or fifth postoperative day. A patient will have a fever, tenderness and pain at the wound site, and an elevated white blood cell count. The edges of the wound will appear inflamed. If drainage is present, it is odorous and **purulent**, which causes a yellow, green, or brown color, depending on the causative organism (Table 48-2).

Dehiscence. When an incision fails to heal properly, the layers of skin and tissue separate. This most commonly occurs before collagen formation (3 to 11 days after injury). **Dehiscence** is the partial or total separation of wound layers. A patient who is at risk for poor wound healing (e.g., poor nutritional status, infection) is at risk for dehiscence. Obese patients have a higher risk of wound dehiscence because of the

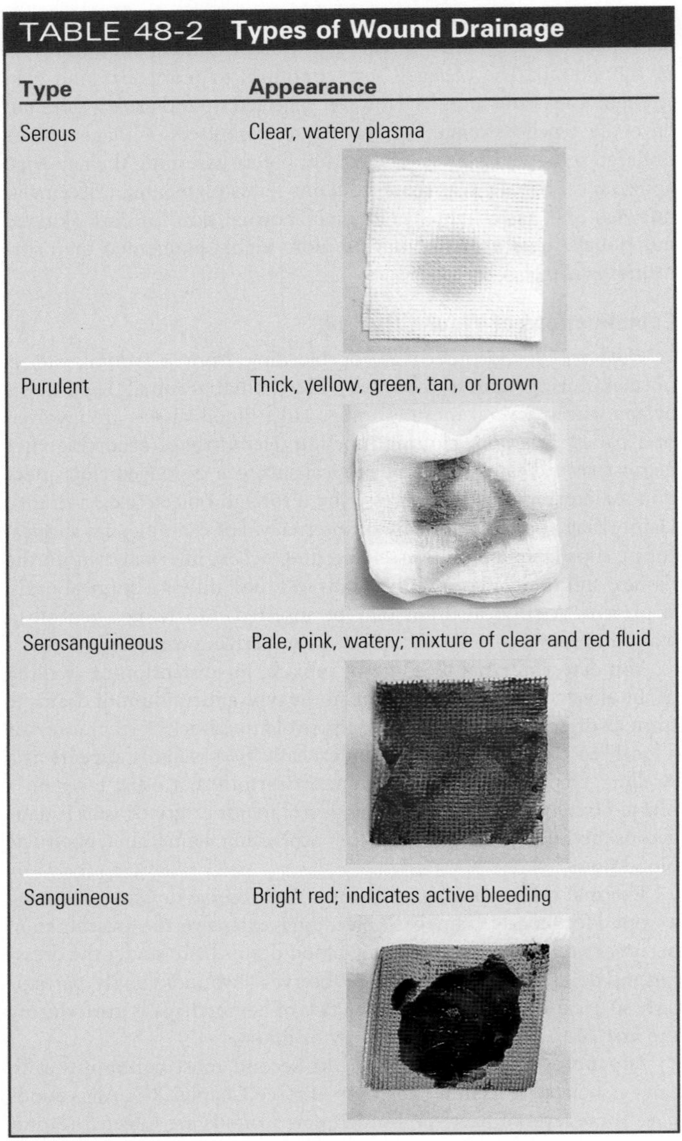

TABLE 48-2 Types of Wound Drainage

Type	Appearance
Serous	Clear, watery plasma
Purulent	Thick, yellow, green, tan, or brown
Serosanguineous	Pale, pink, watery; mixture of clear and red fluid
Sanguineous	Bright red; indicates active bleeding

constant strain placed on their wounds and the poor healing qualities of fat tissue (Pierpont et al., 2014). Dehiscence can happen in abdominal surgical wounds and occurs after a sudden strain such as coughing, vomiting, or sitting up in bed. Patients often report feeling as though something has given way. When there is an increase in serosanguineous drainage from a wound in the first few days after surgery, be alert for the potential for dehiscence.

Evisceration. With total separation of wound layers, evisceration (protrusion of visceral organs through a wound opening) occurs. The condition is an emergency that requires surgical repair. When evisceration occurs, a nurse places sterile gauzed soaked in sterile saline over the extruding tissues to reduce chances of bacterial invasion and drying of the tissues. If the organs protrude through the wound, blood supply to the tissues can be compromised. The presence of an evisceration is a surgical emergency. Immediately place damp sterile gauze over the site, contact the surgical team, do not allow the patient anything by mouth (NPO), observe for signs and symptoms of shock, and prepare the patient for emergency surgery.

NURSING KNOWLEDGE BASE

Prediction and Prevention of Pressure Ulcers

A major aspect of nursing care is the maintenance of skin integrity. Consistent, planned skin-care interventions are critical to ensuring high-quality care. Whenever you are in direct contact with a patient, observe the skin for breaks or impaired skin integrity. Impaired skin integrity occurs from prolonged pressure (e.g., from lying in one position, or from rubbing of external devices), fecal or urinary incontinence, and/or immobility, leading to the development of pressure ulcers.

A pressure ulcer is localized injury to the skin and/or underlying tissue, usually over a bony prominence, as a result of pressure or pressure in combination with shear. A number of contributing or confounding factors are also associated with pressure ulcers; the significance of these factors is yet to be explained (NPUAP, EPUAP, PPPIA, 2014).

Risk Assessment. Several instruments are available for assessing patients who are at risk for developing a pressure ulcer. By identifying at-risk patients, you are able to put interventions into place and spare patients with little risk for pressure ulcer development the unnecessary and sometimes costly preventive treatment. Prevention and treatment of pressure ulcers are major nursing priorities. The incidence of pressure ulcers in a facility or agency is an important indicator of quality of care. Evidence exists that a program of prevention guided by risk assessment simultaneously reduces the institutional incidence of pressure ulcers by as much as 60% and brings down the costs of prevention at the same time (Berry et al., 2013). Several risk-assessment scales developed by nurses enable systematic risk assessment of patients. The Braden Scale is the most widely used risk-assessment tool for pressure ulcers and is in the WOCN guidelines (2010) as being a valid tool to use for pressure ulcer risk assessment. The Braden Scale (Table 48-3) was developed on the basis of risk factors in a nursing home population (Braden and Bergstrom, 1994) and is widely used on general patient care units in hospitals. However, the Braden Scale has shown insufficient predictive validity and poor accuracy in discriminating intensive care patients at risk for developing pressure ulcers (Hyun et al., 2013). Research involving critical care patients continues. The Braden Scale contains six subscales: sensory perception, moisture, activity, mobility, nutrition, and friction/shear. The total score ranges from 6 to 23; a lower total score indicates a higher risk for pressure ulcer development (Braden and Bergstrom, 1989). The cutoff score for onset of pressure ulcer risk with the Braden Scale in the general adult population is 18 (Ayello et al., 2012). Research has shown that the cutoff score for onset of risk in intensive care patients is 13 (Hyun et al., 2013).

Prevention. Preventing pressure ulcers is a priority in caring for patients and is not limited to patients with restrictions in mobility. Impaired skin integrity usually is not a problem in healthy, immobilized individuals but is a serious and potentially devastating problem in ill or debilitated patients (WOCN, 2010).

Economic Consequences of Pressure Ulcers. Pressure ulcers are a continual problem in acute and restorative care settings. For adult patients with pressure ulcers, 56.5% were 65 years and older (WOCN, 2010). Paralysis and spinal cord injury are common preexisting conditions among younger adults with primary diagnosis of pressure ulcers. Older adults admitted to acute and long-term facilities are a vulnerable population. In a study examining early intervention of high-risk patients admitted to the emergency department in an acute care facility, early prevention was 81% likely to be cost-effective (Pham, 2011).

TABLE 48-3 Braden Scale for Predicting Pressure Ulcer Risk

Patient's Name __________ Evaluator's Name ___________ Date of Assessment __________

	1	2	3	4
Sensory Perception Ability to respond meaningfully to pressure-related discomfort	1. Completely limited Unresponsive (does not moan, flinch, or grasp) to painful stimuli caused by diminished level of consciousness or sedation *or* Limited ability to feel pain over most of body surface	2. Very limited Responds only to painful stimuli Cannot communicate discomfort except by moaning or restlessness *or* Has sensory impairment that limits ability to feel pain or discomfort over ½ of body	3. Slightly limited Responds to verbal commands but cannot always communicate discomfort or need to be turned *or* Has some sensory impairment that limits ability to feel pain or discomfort in one or two extremities	4. No impairment Responds to verbal commands Has no sensory deficit that would limit ability to feel or voice pain or discomfort
Moisture Degree to which skin is exposed to moisture	1. Constantly moist Skin kept moist almost constantly by bodily elimination such as perspiration or urine Dampness detected every time patient is moved or turned	2. Moist Skin often, but not always, moist Necessary to change linen at least once a shift	3. Occasionally moist Skin occasionally moist, requiring an extra linen change approximately once a day	4. Rarely moist Skin usually dry Required linen changing only at routine intervals
Activity Degree of physical activity	1. Bedfast Confined to bed	2. Chairfast Ability to walk severely limited or nonexistent Cannot bear own weight and/or must be helped into chair or wheelchair	3. Walks occasionally during day but for very short distances, with or without help Spends majority of each shift in bed or chair	4. Walks frequently Walks outside room at least twice a day and inside room at least once every 2 hours during waking hours
Mobility Ability to change and control body position	1. Completely immobile Does not make even slight changes in body or extremity position without help	2. Very limited Makes occasional slight changes in body or extremity position but unable to make frequent or significant changes independently	3. Slightly limited Makes frequent, although slight, changes in body or extremity position independently	4. No limitations Makes major and frequent changes in position without help
Nutrition *Usual* food intake pattern	1. Very poor Never eats a complete meal; rarely eats more than ⅓ of any food offered; eats two servings or less of protein (meat or dairy products) per day Takes fluids poorly; does not take a liquid dietary supplement *or* Is NPO and/or maintained on clear liquids or IV for more than 5 days	2. Probably inadequate Rarely eats a complete meal and generally eats only about ½ of any food offered Protein intake includes only 3 servings of meat or dairy products per day; occasionally takes a dietary supplement *or* Receives less than optimum amount of liquid diet or tube feeding	3. Adequate Eats over half of most meals; eats a total of four servings of protein (meat, dairy products) each day Occasionally refuses a meal but usually takes a supplement if offered *or* Is on tube feeding or total parenteral nutrition regimen that probably meets most of nutritional needs	4. Excellent Eats most of every meal; never refuses a meal; usually eats a total of four or more servings of meat and dairy products Occasionally eats between meals Does not require supplementation
Friction and Shear	1. Problem Requires moderate-to-maximum help to move; complete lifting without sliding against sheets impossible Frequently slides down in bed or chair, requiring frequent repositioning with maximum assistance Spasticity, contractures, or agitation leads to almost constant friction	2. Potential problem Moves feebly or requires minimum assistance; during a move skin probably slides to some extent against sheets, chair, restraints, or other devices Maintains relatively good position in chair or bed most of the time but occasionally slides down	3. No apparent problem Moves in bed and in chair independently and has sufficient muscle strength to lift up completely during move Maintains good position in bed or chair at all times	**TOTAL SCORE**

TABLE 48-4 Role of Selected Nutrients in Wound Healing

Nutrient	Role in Healing	Recommendations	Sources
Calories	Fuel for cell energy "Protein protection"	30-35 kcal/kg/day (Individuals who are underweight or have significant unintentional weight loss may need additional calories.)	
Protein	Fibroplasia, angiogenesis, collagen formation and wound remodeling, immune function	1.25-1.5 g protein/kg body weight	Poultry, fish, eggs, beef
Vitamin C (ascorbic acid)	Collagen synthesis, capillary wall integrity, fibroblast function, immunological function, antioxidant	1000 mg/day	Citrus fruits, tomatoes, potatoes, fortified fruit juices
Vitamin A	Epithelialization, wound closure, inflammatory response, angiogenesis, collagen formation Can reverse steroid effects on skin and delayed healing	1600-2000 retinol equivalents per day	Green leafy vegetables (spinach), broccoli, carrots, sweet potatoes, liver
Zinc	Collagen formation, protein synthesis, cell membrane and host defenses	15-30 mg Correct deficiencies No improvement in wound healing with supplementation unless zinc deficient Use with caution—large doses can be toxic May inhibit copper metabolism and impair immune function	Vegetables, meats, legumes
Fluid	Essential fluid environment for all cell function	30-35 mL/kg/day	Use noncaffeinated, nonalcoholic fluids without sugar Water is best—6-8 glasses/day

Adapted from Stotts NA: Nutritional assessment and support. In Bryant RA, Nix DP, editors: *Acute and chronic wounds: current management concepts,* ed 5, St Louis, 2016a, Elsevier.

When a pressure ulcer occurs, the length of stay in a hospital and the overall cost of health care increase. The actual cost of treatment is difficult to estimate. About 1.6 million patients each year in acute care settings develop pressure ulcers, representing a cost of $11 to $17.2 billion to the U.S. health care system (Pieper, 2016). Although it is difficult to identify the exact numbers of pressure ulcers and the number of patients with pressure ulcers, the occurrence of pressure ulcers is costly to patients in terms of disability, pain, and suffering. The occurrence of pressure ulcers is also costly for health care institutions and third-party payers. The Centers for Medicare and Medicaid Services (CMS) implemented a policy effective October 1, 2008 whereby hospitals no longer receive additional reimbursement for care related to eight conditions, including stage III and IV pressure ulcers that occur during a hospitalization. This policy was put in place to provide additional incentives for hospitals to improve quality of care. Using guidelines such as the WOCN Guidelines (WOCN, 2010) helps reduce or eliminate the occurrence of pressure ulcers and prevent the expenses that will not be reimbursed.

Factors Influencing Pressure Ulcer Formation and Wound Healing

Impaired skin integrity resulting in pressure ulcers is primarily the result of pressure. However, additional factors, including shear force, friction, moisture, nutrition, tissue perfusion, infection, and age, increase the patient's risk for pressure ulcer development and poor wound healing.

Nutrition. For patients weakened or debilitated by illness, nutritional therapy is especially important. A patient who has undergone surgery (see Chapter 50) and is well nourished still requires at least 1500 kcal/day for nutritional maintenance. Alternatives such as enteral feedings (see Chapter 45) and parenteral nutrition (see Chapter 45) are available for patients unable to maintain normal food intake.

Normal wound healing requires proper nutrition (Table 48-4). Deficiencies in any of the nutrients result in impaired or delayed healing (Stotts, 2016a). Physiological processes of wound healing depend on the availability of protein, vitamins (especially A and C), and the trace minerals zinc and copper. Collagen is a protein formed from amino acids acquired by fibroblasts from protein ingested in food. Vitamin C is necessary for synthesis of collagen. Vitamin A reduces the negative effects of steroids on wound healing. Trace elements are also necessary; (i.e., zinc for epithelialization and collagen synthesis and copper for collagen fiber linking).

Calories provide the energy source needed to support the cellular activity of wound healing. Protein needs especially are increased and are essential for tissue repair and growth. A balanced intake of various nutrients (i.e., protein, fat, carbohydrates, vitamins, and minerals) is critical to support wound healing. Provide 30 to 35 kcal/kg of body weight for adults with a pressure ulcer who are assessed as being at risk of malnutrition (NPUAP, EPUAP, PPPIA, 2014).

Serum proteins are biochemical indicators of malnutrition (Stotts, 2016a). Serum albumin is probably the most frequently measured of these laboratory parameters. Albumin alone is not sensitive to rapid changes in nutritional status. Transferrin also evaluates protein status, but alone it does not determine malnutrition. The best measure of nutritional status is prealbumin because it reflects not only what the patient has ingested but also what the body has absorbed, digested, and metabolized (Stotts, 2016a).

Tissue Perfusion. Oxygen fuels the cellular functions essential to the healing process; therefore the ability to perfuse the tissues with adequate amounts of oxygenated blood is critical to wound healing (Doughty and Sparks-Defriese, 2016). Patients with peripheral vascular disease are at risk for poor tissue perfusion because of poor circulation. Oxygen requirements depend on the phase of wound healing (e.g., chronic tissue hypoxia is associated with impaired collagen synthesis and reduced tissue resistance to infection).

Infection. Wound infection prolongs the inflammatory phase; delays collagen synthesis; prevents epithelialization; and increases the production of proinflammatory cytokines, which leads to additional tissue destruction (Stotts, 2016b). Indications that a wound infection is present include the presence of purulent drainage; change in odor, volume, or character of wound drainage; redness in the surrounding tissue; fever; or pain.

Age. Increased age affects all phases of wound healing. A decrease in the functioning of the macrophage leads to a delayed inflammatory response, delayed collagen synthesis, and slower epithelialization.

Psychosocial Impact of Wounds. The psychosocial impact of wounds on the physiological process of healing is unknown. Body image changes often impose a great stress on a patient's adaptive mechanisms. They also influence self-concept (see Chapter 34) and sexuality (see Chapter 35). Factors that affect a patient's perception of a wound include the presence of scars, stitches, drains (often needed for weeks or months), odor from drainage, and temporary or permanent prosthetic devices.

CRITICAL THINKING

Successful critical thinking requires a synthesis of knowledge, experience, information gathered from patients, critical thinking attitudes, and intellectual and professional standards. Clinical judgments require a nurse to anticipate the information necessary, analyze the data, and make decisions regarding patient care. Critical thinking is always changing. During assessment (Figure 48-7) consider all elements that build toward making appropriate nursing diagnoses.

When caring for patients who have impaired skin integrity and chronic wounds, integrate knowledge from nursing and other disciplines, previous experiences, and information gathered from patients to understand the risk to skin integrity and wound healing. Knowledge of normal musculoskeletal physiology, the pathogenesis of pressure ulcers, pressure ulcer stages, normal wound healing, and the pathophysiology of underlying diseases enables you to have a scientific basis for care. The WOCN (2010) has guidelines for assessment of risk for impaired skin integrity, prevention measures, interventions to promote wound healing, and other standards of practice, which you should use in planning care. Past experience with patients at risk for impaired skin integrity or patients with wounds increases the experiential knowledge base, helping you to identify interventions. Finally you need to be disciplined during assessment to obtain comprehensive and correct data. You also need to be creative. Because chronic wounds are difficult to heal, be diligent in evaluating nursing interventions and determining which interventions are effective and which need modification.

Knowledge
- Pathogenesis of pressure ulcers
- Factors contributing to pressure ulcer formation or poor wound healing
- Factors contributing to wound healing
- Impact of underlying disease process on skin integrity
- Impact of medication on skin integrity and wound healing

Experience
- Caring for patients with impaired skin integrity or wounds
- Observation of normal wound healing

ASSESSMENT
- Identify the patient's risk for developing impaired skin integrity or poor wound healing
- Identify signs and symptoms associated with impaired skin integrity or poor wound healing
- Examine patient's skin for actual impairment in skin integrity

Standards
- Apply intellectual standards of accuracy, relevance, completeness, and precision when obtaining health history regarding skin integrity and wound management
- Knowledge of WOCN (2010), NPUAP, EPUAP, and PPPIA 2014 Clinical Practice Guidelines standards for prevention of pressure ulcers
- Knowledge of standards for assessment of risk for impaired skin integrity and for prevention and treatment

Attitudes
- Use discipline to obtain complete and correct assessment data regarding patient's skin and/or wound integrity
- Demonstrate responsibility for collecting appropriate specimens for diagnostic and laboratory tests related to wound management

FIGURE 48-7 Critical thinking model for skin integrity and wound-care assessment. *WOCN,* Wound, Ostomy, and Continence Nurses Society.

❖ NURSING PROCESS

Apply the nursing process and use a critical thinking approach in your care of patients. The nursing process provides a clinical decision-making approach for you to develop and implement an individualized plan of care.

◆ Assessment

During the assessment process, thoroughly assess each patient and critically analyze findings to ensure that you make patient-centered clinical decisions required for safe nursing care. Baseline and continual assessment data provide critical information about a patient's skin integrity and the increased risk for pressure ulcer development. Focusing on specific elements such as a patient's level of sensation, movement, and continence status helps guide the skin assessment (Box 48-4).

BOX 48-4 Nursing Assessment Questions

Sensation
- Do you have tingling, decreased feeling, or absent feeling in your extremities or any other region?
- Is your skin sensitive to heat or cold?

Mobility
- Do you have any physical limitations, injury, or paralysis that limits your ability to move on your own?
- Can you change your position easily?
- Is movement painful?

Continence
- Do you have any problems or accidents leaking urine or stool?
- What help do you need when using the toilet? In what way?
- How often do you need to use the toilet? During the day? At night?

Presence of Wound
- What caused the wound?
- When did the wound occur? Where is it located?
- When did you receive a tetanus shot?
- What has happened to this wound since it occurred? What were the changes and what caused them?
- Which treatments, activities, or care have slowed or helped the wound to heal? Are there special needs for this wound to heal?
- Do you have any pain, itching, or other symptoms with the wound? How are you managing the itching, and what works best for you?
- Who helps you care for your wound?

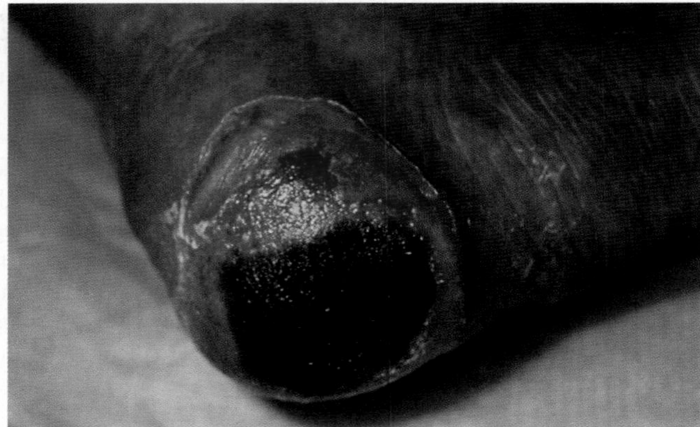

FIGURE 48-8 Formation of pressure ulcer on heel resulting from external pressure from bed mattress. (Courtesy Janice Colwell, RN, MS, CWOCN, FAAN, Clinical Nurse Specialist, University of Chicago Medicine.)

Through the Patient's Eyes. When patients have acute surgical or traumatic wounds, the wounds sometimes heal promptly and without complications. However, when pressure ulcers or chronic wounds develop, the course of treatments is lengthy and costly. Because a patient and family need to be involved with wound-care management, it is important to know a patient's expectations. Does the patient expect to have home care? Is there the expectation the patient will heal to allow a quick return to work? A patient who has realistic goals and is informed about the length of time for wound healing is more likely to adhere to the specific therapies designed to promote healing and prevent further skin breakdown. Therefore it is important to assess each patient's perception of what is occurring with the wound-healing interventions. For example, why are certain dressings being used and how do they work? As a nurse, you want to determine a patient's and family's understanding of wound assessment; wound interventions; and supportive interventions such as positioning, nutrition, and ambulation.

Skin. Perform skin assessment of a patient when you initiate care and then at a minimum of once a shift (see agency policies). However, high-risk patients have more frequent skin assessments such as every 4 hours. Assess the skin for signs of skin breakdown and/or ulcer development (see Skill 48-1). The neurologically impaired patient; the chronically ill patient in long-term care; the patient with altered mental status; those in the intensive care unit (ICU), oncology, hospice, or orthopedic units; and patients with medical devices have increased potential for developing pressure ulcers.

Assessment for tissue pressure damage includes visual and tactile inspection of the skin. Perform a baseline assessment to determine a patient's normal skin characteristics and any actual or potential areas of breakdown. Individualize assessment characteristics of a patient's skin, depending on his or her skin tone (NPUAP, EUPAP, PPPIA, 2014, Sommers, 2011). Accurate assessment of patients with darker skin pigmentation is an essential skill for all health care providers (Nix, 2016). Assessment characteristics of darkly pigmented skin are in Boxes 48-2 and 48-3.

Pay particular attention to areas located over bony prominences; next to medical devices; and under casts, traction, splints, braces, collars, or other orthopedic devices. The frequency of pressure checks depends on the schedule of appliance application and the response of the skin to the external pressure (Figure 48-8). Consider adults with medical devices (e.g., tubes, drainage systems, and oxygen devices) to be at risk for pressure ulcers (Black et al., 2010; 2015). Avoid positioning the individual directly onto medical devices (NPUAP, EUPAP, PPPIA, 2014). In addition, carefully assess skin exposed to adhesive tape or other adhesive devices, which cause skin and tissue injury and increase risk for pressure ulcer development (McNichol et al., 2013).

When you note hyperemia, gently palpate the reddened tissue; differentiate whether the skin redness is blanchable or nonblanchable. Blanchable erythema is visible skin redness that becomes white when pressure is applied and reddens when pressure is relieved. It may result from normal reactive hyperemia that should disappear within several hours or from inflammatory erythema with an intact capillary bed. Nonblanchable erythema is visible skin redness that persists with the application of pressure. It indicates structural damage to the capillary bed/microcirculation. This is an indication for a category/stage I pressure ulcer (NPUAP, EUPAP, PPPIA, 2014).

Use visual and tactile inspection over the body areas most frequently at risk for pressure ulcer development (Figure 48-9). For example, when a patient lies in bed or sits in a chair, he or she places body weight heavily on certain bony prominences. Turn the patient in bed to inspect the skin and, once you return a patient to bed from a chair, look at all areas exposed to pressure. Body surfaces subjected to the greatest weight or pressure are at greatest risk for pressure ulcer formation.

Pressure Ulcers. Pressure ulcers have multiple etiological factors. Review the previous section on pp. 1187-1189 for assessment of pressure ulcer staging when one is identified. Assessment for pressure ulcer risk includes using an appropriate predictive measure and assessing a patient's mobility, nutrition, presence of body fluids, and comfort level (see Skill 48-1 on pp. 1221-1223).

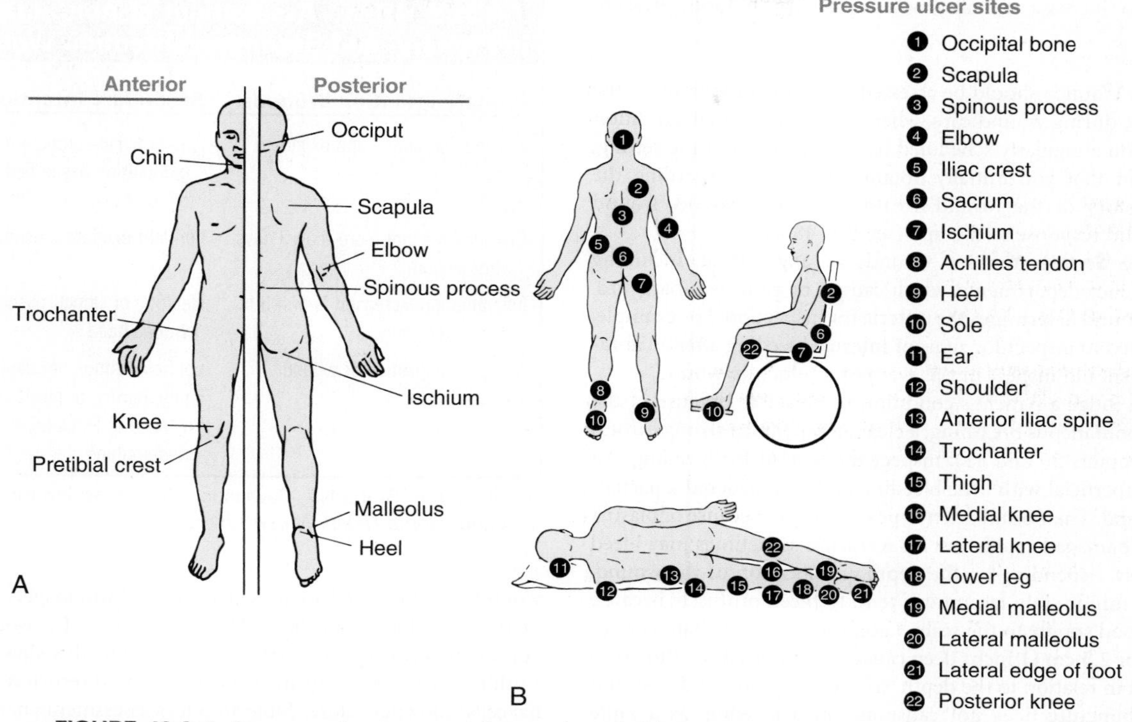

FIGURE 48-9 A, Bony prominences most frequently underlying pressure ulcer. **B,** Pressure ulcer sites. (Modified from Trelease CC: Developing standards for wound care, *Ostomy Wound Manage* 20:46, 1988.)

Predictive Measures. On admission to acute care, rehabilitation hospitals, nursing homes, home care, and other health care facilities, individuals need to be assessed for risk of pressure ulcer development (WOCN, 2010). Perform pressure ulcer risk assessment systematically (WOCN, 2010). Use an assessment tool such as the Braden Scale (see Table 48-3) or a tool preferred by your agency. The interpretation of the meaning of the total numerical scores differs with each risk-assessment scale relevant to their population. Lower numerical scores on the Braden Scale indicate that the patient is at high risk for skin breakdown. A benefit of the predictive instruments is to increase a nurse's early detection of patients at greater risk for ulcer development. Once you identify these patients, institute appropriate interventions to maintain skin integrity and implement prevention strategies (WOCN, 2010). Perform reassessment for pressure ulcer risk on a scheduled basis.

Mobility. Assessment includes documenting the level of mobility and the potential effects of impaired mobility on skin integrity. Documenting assessment of mobility includes obtaining data regarding the quality of muscle tone and strength. For example, determine whether the patient is able to lift his or her weight off of the sacral area and roll the body to a side-lying position. Some patients have inadequate range of motion to move independently into a more protective position. Finally, assess a patient's activity tolerance to determine if the patient can be transferred to a chair or ambulated more often to relieve pressure from lying down (see Chapter 39).

You must assess mobility as part of baseline data. If a patient has some degree of mobility independence, reinforce the frequency of position changes and measures to relieve pressure. The frequency of position changes is based on ongoing skin assessment and is revised as data change.

Nutritional Status. An assessment of patients' nutritional status is an integral part of the initial assessment data for all patients, especially those at risk for impaired skin integrity (Stotts, 2016a). The Joint Commission (2008, 2015) recommends nutritional assessment within 24 hours of admission. Malnutrition is a risk factor for pressure ulcer development (Litchford et al., 2014). Weigh the patient, and perform this measure more often for at-risk patients. A loss of 5% of usual weight, weight less than 90% of ideal body weight, and a decrease of 10 lbs in a brief period are all signs of actual or potential nutritional problems (Stotts, 2016a). Also assess the patient's appetite and food preferences to determine what food choices might be added to better supplement the diet. Assess the patient's mouth and skin for signs of nutritional deficiencies (see Chapter 45).

Body Fluids. Continual exposure of the skin to body fluids increases a patient's risk for skin breakdown and pressure ulcer formation. Some body fluids such as saliva and serosanguineous drainage are not as caustic to the skin, and the risk of skin breakdown from exposure to these fluids is low. However, exposure to urine, bile, stool, ascitic fluid, and purulent wound exudate carries a moderate risk for skin breakdown, especially in patients who have other risk factors such as chronic illness or poor nutrition. Exposure to gastric and pancreatic drainage has the highest risk for skin breakdown. These fluids have digestive qualities that can irritate and break down the skin quickly. It is important to prevent and reduce the patient's exposure to body fluids; when exposure occurs, provide meticulous hygiene and skin care.

Pain. Significant research has been conducted in the study of pain in surgical patients with wounds. The routine assessment of pain in surgical patients is critical to selecting appropriate pain management therapies and to determine a patient's ability to progress towards recovery (see Chapter 50). Until recently there has been little research about pain and pressure ulcers. The WOCN (2010) has recommended that assessment and management of pain be included in the care of patients with pressure ulcers (NPUAP, EUPAP, PPPIA, 2014). Use standard pain assessment tools to measure pain acuity, and be thorough in assessing the character of a patient's pain (Chapter 44). Maintaining adequate pain control and patient comfort increases the patient's willingness and ability to increase mobility, which in turn reduces pressure ulcer risk.

Wounds. Wounds should be assessed on an ongoing basis: at the time of injury, during wound care, when a patient's overall condition changes, and on a regularly scheduled basis. Regardless of the setting, it is important that you initially obtain information regarding the cause and history of the wound, treatment of the wound, wound description, and response to therapy (see Box 48-4).

Emergency Setting. You see wounds in any setting, including clinics, emergency departments, youth camps, or your own backyard. The type of wound determines the criteria for inspection. For example, you do not need to inspect for signs of internal bleeding after an abrasion, but you should inspect in the event of a puncture wound.

When you judge a patient's condition to be stable because of the presence of spontaneous breathing, a clear airway, and a strong carotid pulse (see Chapters 30 and 41), inspect the wound for bleeding. An **abrasion** is superficial with little bleeding and is considered a partial-thickness wound. The wound often appears "weepy" because of plasma leakage from damaged capillaries. A **laceration** sometimes may bleed more profusely, depending on the depth and location of the wound. For example, minor scalp lacerations tend to bleed profusely because of the rich blood supply to the scalp. Lacerations greater than 5 cm (2 inches) long or 2.5 cm (1 inch) deep cause serious bleeding. **Puncture** wounds bleed in relation to the depth, size, and location of the wound (e.g., a nail puncture does not cause as much bleeding as a knife wound). The primary dangers of puncture wounds are internal bleeding and infection.

Inspect wounds for foreign bodies or contaminant material. Most traumatic wounds are dirty. Soil, broken glass, shreds of cloth, and foreign substances clinging to penetrating objects sometimes become embedded in a wound.

The size and depth of a wound are the next steps in assessment. Use a disposable wound-measuring device to measure wound width and length. This approach offers a uniform, consistent method for measuring wound length and width to facilitate meaningful comparisons of wound status across time (EPUAP, NPUAP PPPIA, 2014). Measure depth by using a cotton-tipped applicator in the wound bed (see Skill 48-2). A deep laceration requires suturing. A large, open wound may expose bone or tissue that needs to be protected.

When an injury is a result of trauma from a dirty penetrating object, determine when the patient last received a tetanus toxoid injection. Tetanus bacteria reside in soil and in the gut of humans and animals. A tetanus antitoxin injection is necessary if the patient has not had one within 10 years.

Stable Setting. When a patient's condition is stabilized (e.g., after surgery or treatment), assess the wound to determine progress toward healing. If the wound is covered by a dressing and the health care provider has not ordered it changed, do not inspect it directly unless you suspect serious complications such as a large volume of bright red bleeding, excessive odor, or severe pain under the dressing. In such a situation inspect only the dressing and any external drains. If the health care provider prefers to change the dressing, he or she should assess the wound at least daily. When removing dressings, take care to avoid accidental removal or displacement of underlying drains. Because removal of dressings can be painful, consider giving an analgesic at least 30 minutes before exposing a wound. Assess the wound thoroughly using standard measurements.

Wound Appearance. A surgical incision healing by primary intention should have clean, well-approximated edges. Crusts often form along wound edges from exudate. A puncture wound is usually a small, circular wound with the edges coming together toward the center. If a wound is open, the edges are separated, and you inspect the condition of tissue at the wound base. The outer edges of a wound normally appear inflamed for the first 2 to 3 days, but this slowly disappears. Within 7 to 10 days a normally healing wound resurfaces with epithelial cells, and edges close. Table 48-5 lists assessment characteristics for abnormal wound healing in primary and secondary wounds. If infection develops, the area directly surrounding the wound becomes brightly inflamed and swollen.

TABLE 48-5 Assessment of Abnormal Healing in Primary- and Secondary-Intention Wounds

Primary Intention Wounds	Secondary Intention Wounds
Incision line poorly approximated	Pale or fragile granulation tissue, granulation tissue bed excessively dry or moist
Drainage present more than 3 days after closure	Purulent exudate present
Inflammation increased in first 3-5 days after injury	Necrotic or slough tissue present in wound base
No epithelialization of wound edges by day 4	Epithelialization not continuous Fruity, earthy, or putrid odor present Presence of fistula(s), tunneling, undermining

Modified from Stotts NA, Cavanaugh CE: Assessing the patient with a wound, *Home Health Nurse* 17(1):27, 1999.

Skin discoloration usually results from bruising of interstitial tissues or hematoma formation. Blood collecting beneath the skin first takes on a bluish or purplish appearance. Gradually, as the clotted blood is broken down, shades of brown and yellow appear.

Character of Wound Drainage. Note the amount, color, odor, and consistency of wound drainage. The amount of drainage depends on the type of wound. For example, drainage is minimal after a simple appendectomy. In contrast, it is moderate for 1 to 2 days after drainage of a large abscess. When you need an accurate measurement of the amount of drainage within a dressing, weigh the dressing and compare it with the weight of the same dressing that is clean and dry. The general rule is that 1 g of drainage equals 1 mL of volume of drainage. Another method of quantifying wound drainage is to chart the number of dressings used and the frequency of change. An increase or decrease in the number or frequency of dressings indicates a relative increase or decrease in wound drainage.

The color and consistency of drainage vary, depending on the components. Types of drainage include: **serous**, **sanguineous**, **serosanguineous**, and purulent (see Table 48-2). If the drainage has a pungent or strong odor, you should suspect an infection. Describe the appearance of the wound according to characteristics observed. An example of an accurate recording follows:

> Abdominal incision in the RLQ is 5 cm in length; edges well approximated without inflammation or exudate. 1.2 cm diameter circle of serous drainage present on one 4 × 4 gauze changed every 8 hours.

Drains. The surgeon inserts a drain into or near a surgical wound if there is a large amount of drainage. Some drains are sutured in place. Exercise caution when changing a dressing around drains that are not sutured in place to prevent accidental removal. A Penrose drain lies under a dressing; at the time of placement a pin or clip is placed through the drain to prevent it from slipping farther into a wound

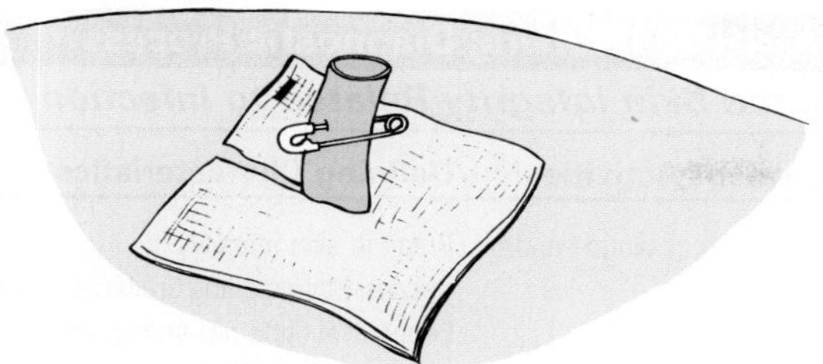

FIGURE 48-10 Penrose drain with dressing.

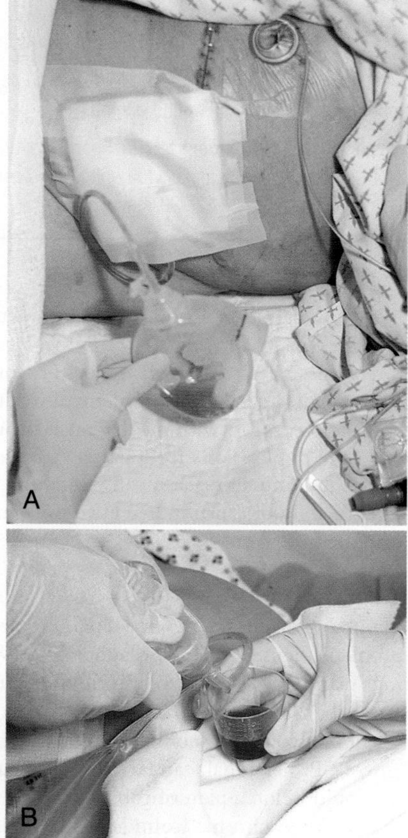

FIGURE 48-11 Jackson-Pratt drainage device. **A,** Drainage tube and reservoir. **B,** Emptying drainage reservoir.

(Figure 48-10). It is usually the health care provider's responsibility to pull or advance the drain as drainage decreases to permit healing deep within the drain site. The wound will heal from the inside out.

Assess the number and type of drains, drain placement, character of drainage, and condition of collecting equipment. Observe the security of the drain and its location with respect to the wound. Next note the character of drainage. If there is a collecting device, measure the drainage volume. Because a drainage system needs to be patent, look for drainage flow through and around the tubing. A sudden decrease in drainage through the tubing may indicate a blocked drain, and you need to notify the health care provider. When a drain is connected to suction, assess the system to be sure that the pressure ordered is being exerted. Evacuator units such as a Hemovac or Jackson-Pratt (Figure 48-11) exert a constant low pressure as long as the suction device (bladder or container) is fully compressed. These types of drainage devices are often referred to as *self-suction*. When the evacuator device is unable to maintain a vacuum on its own, notify the surgeon, who then orders a secondary vacuum system (such as wall suction). If fluid accumulates within the tissues, wound healing does not progress at an optimal rate, and this increases the risk of infection.

Wound Closures. Surgical wounds are closed with staples, sutures, or wound adhesives. A frequent skin closure is the stainless-steel staple. The staple provides more strength than nylon or silk sutures and tends to cause less irritation to tissue. Look for irritation with redness around staple or suture sites, and note whether closures are intact. Normally for the first 2 to 3 days after surgery the skin around sutures or staples is edematous because of the normal inflammatory response.

Dermabond is a liquid tissue adhesive that forms a strong bond across approximated wound edges, allowing normal healing to occur below. It can be used to replace small sutures for incisional repair. A vial containing the Dermabond solution is used to apply the product to approximated tissue. The wound edges are held together until the solution dries, providing an adhesive closure. Tissue adhesives take less time to apply, have lower risk of infection, have comparable tensile strength as sutures, and also provide less pain and anxiety (Januchowski and Ferguson, 2014).

Palpation of Wound. When inspecting a wound, observe for swelling or separation of wound edges. While wearing gloves, lightly press the wound edges, detecting localized areas of tenderness or drainage collection. If pressure causes fluid to be expressed, note the character of the drainage. The patient is normally sensitive to palpation of wound edges. Extreme tenderness indicates infection.

Wound Cultures. If you detect purulent or suspicious-looking drainage, report to the health care provider because a specimen of the drainage may need to be obtained for culture. Never collect a wound culture sample from old drainage. Resident colonies of bacteria flora from the skin grow within exudate and are not always the true causative organisms of a wound infection. Clean a wound first with normal saline to remove skin flora. Aerobic organisms grow in superficial wounds exposed to the air, and anaerobic organisms tend to grow within body cavities. Use a different method of specimen collection for each type of organism per agency policy (Box 48-5).

Gram stains of drainage are often performed as well. This test allows the health care provider to order appropriate treatment earlier than when only cultures are done. No additional specimens are usually required. The microbiology laboratory needs only to be notified to perform the additional test.

The gold standard of wound culture is tissue biopsy. A health care provider or wound-care specialist with special training obtains the biopsy (Stotts, 2016b).

Psychosocial. Assess how the wound is influencing the patient's self-perception and socialization. Ask the patient to describe how the wound affects his or her view of self. Does the patient have unwarranted fears that the wound will not heal? Does a chronic wound interfere with the patient's willingness to participate in social activities at home? Does it affect the patient's ability to continue working? Make sure that the patient's personal and social resources for adaptation are a part of your assessment. Is there a family caregiver who is able to assist with wound care in the home?

◆ Nursing Diagnosis

Assessment reveals clusters of data to indicate whether a problem-focused diagnosis of *Impaired Skin Integrity* or a risk diagnosis of *Risk for Impaired Skin Integrity* exists. In addition, the assessment data provides information about the related factor. For example, a postoperative patient has purulent drainage from a surgical wound and reports tenderness around the area of the wound. These data support a nursing diagnosis of *Impaired Skin Integrity* related to infection (Box 48-6).

BOX 48-5 Recommendations for Standardized Techniques for Wound Cultures*

Needle Aspiration Procedure

- Clean intact skin with a disinfectant solution to remove skin flora. Allow to dry.
- Use a 10-mL disposable syringe with a 22-gauge needle, pulling 0.5 mL of air into the syringe.
- Insert the needle through intact skin next to the wound; withdraw plunger and apply suction to the 10-mL mark.
- Move the needle back and forward at different angles for two to four explorations.
- Remove and safely discard the needle, expel the excess air from the syringe, and cap and prepare the syringe for the laboratory (Stotts, 2016b).

Quantitative Swab Procedure

- Clean the wound surface with a nonantiseptic solution to remove skin flora. Allow to dry.
- Use a sterile swab from a culturette tube (Figure 48-12).
- Moisten the swab with normal saline.
- Rotate the swab in 1 cm^2 (0.4 in^2) of clean tissue in the open wound. Apply pressure to the swab to elicit tissue fluid (Stotts, 2016b). Insert the tip of the swab into the appropriate sterile container, label, and transport to the laboratory.

Modified from Stotts NA: Wound infection: diagnosis and management. In Bryant RA, Nix DP, editors: *Acute and chronic wounds: current management concepts,* ed 5, St Louis, 2016, Elsevier.

*Check agency policy to determine need to obtain health care provider order.

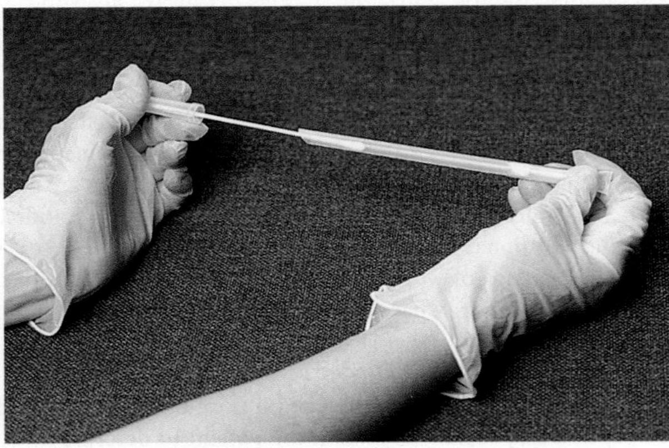

FIGURE 48-12 Wound culturette tube.

After completing an assessment of a patient's wound, the nurse identifies nursing diagnoses that direct the interventions that will be needed to support wound healing and prevent complications. Multiple nursing diagnoses are associated with impaired skin integrity and wounds:

- *Risk for Infection*
- *Imbalanced Nutrition: Less Than Body Requirements*
- *Acute or Chronic Pain*
- *Impaired Physical Mobility*
- *Impaired Skin Integrity*
- *Risk for Impaired Skin Integrity*
- *Ineffective Peripheral Tissue Perfusion*
- *Impaired Tissue Integrity*

Some patients are at risk for poor wound healing because of the presence of previously defined conditions that impair healing. Thus, even though a patient's wound appears normal, the nurse identifies nursing diagnoses such as *Impaired Nutrition* or *Ineffective Peripheral Tissue Perfusion* that direct nursing care toward support of wound repair.

The nature of a wound can cause problems unrelated to wound healing. An alteration in comfort with the diagnosis of *Acute Pain* and *Impaired Mobility* have implications for a patient's eventual recovery. For example, a large abdominal incision causes enough pain to interfere with the patient's ability to turn in bed effectively, making him or her at risk for impaired skin integrity.

BOX 48-6 Nursing Diagnostic Process

Impaired Skin Integrity Related to Infection

Assessment Activities	Defining Characteristics
Inspect surface of wound and periwound skin.	Break in skin integrity Yellow, foul-smelling drainage from wound Edges of wound red and warm, not approximated Macerated periwound area
Inspect wound for signs of healing.	Brown-red or beige drainage 5 days after surgery Edges of wound not approximated
Palpate wound and ask patient if there is tenderness.	Patient expresses pain on palpitation Periwound edema
Obtain patient's temperature, heart rate, white blood cell count.	Patient febrile, heart rate 125 beats/min, leukocyte (white blood cell) count 12,000/mm^3

◆ Planning

After identifying nursing diagnoses, develop a plan of care for a patient who has the problem-focused or risk diagnosis for *Impaired Skin Integrity*. During planning synthesize information from multiple resources (Figure 48-13). Critical thinking ensures that a patient's plan of care integrates all that you know about the individual and key critical thinking elements. Professional standards are especially important to consider when you develop a plan of care.

Patients who have large, chronic wounds or infected wounds have multiple nursing care needs. A concept map helps to individualize care for a patient who has multiple health problems and related nursing diagnoses (Figure 48-14). This map helps you use critical thinking skills to organize complex patient assessment data into related nursing diagnoses with the patient's chief medical diagnosis. As you identify links between the nursing diagnoses and the chief medical diagnosis, the concept map also links potential interventions that apply to the patient's health care needs.

Goals and Outcomes. Nursing care is based on a patient's identified needs and priorities. You establish goals and expected outcomes, and from the goals you plan interventions according to the risk for pressure ulcers or the type and severity of the wound and the presence of any complications such as infection, poor nutrition, peripheral vascular diseases, or immunosuppression that can affect wound healing (see the Nursing Care Plan). A goal frequently identified when working with a patient with a wound is to see the wound progressing toward healing within a 2-week period. The outcomes of this goal can include the following:

- Increase in the percentage of granulation tissue in the wound base

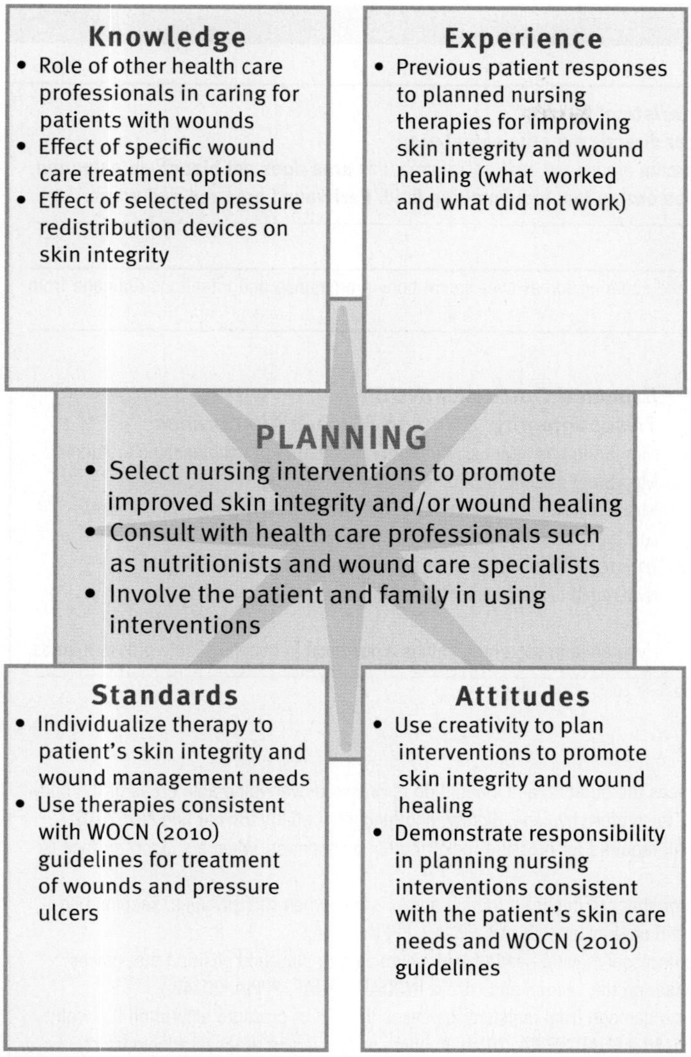

Knowledge
- Role of other health care professionals in caring for patients with wounds
- Effect of specific wound care treatment options
- Effect of selected pressure redistribution devices on skin integrity

Experience
- Previous patient responses to planned nursing therapies for improving skin integrity and wound healing (what worked and what did not work)

PLANNING
- Select nursing interventions to promote improved skin integrity and/or wound healing
- Consult with health care professionals such as nutritionists and wound care specialists
- Involve the patient and family in using interventions

Standards
- Individualize therapy to patient's skin integrity and wound management needs
- Use therapies consistent with WOCN (2010) guidelines for treatment of wounds and pressure ulcers

Attitudes
- Use creativity to plan interventions to promote skin integrity and wound healing
- Demonstrate responsibility in planning nursing interventions consistent with the patient's skin care needs and WOCN (2010) guidelines

FIGURE 48-13 Critical thinking model for skin integrity and wound-care planning. *WOCN,* Wound, Ostomy, and Continence Nurses Society.

- No further skin breakdown
- Increase in caloric intake by 10%

These outcomes are reasonable if the overall goal for the patient is to heal the wound. Plan therapies according to the severity and type of wound and the presence of any complicating conditions (e.g., infection, poor nutrition, immunosuppression, and diabetes) that affect wound healing. Other goals of care for patients with wounds include the following: promoting wound hemostasis, preventing infection, promoting wound healing, maintaining skin integrity, gaining comfort, and promoting health.

Setting Priorities. Establish nursing care priorities in wound care on the basis of the comprehensive patient assessment and goals and established outcomes. These priorities also depend on whether the patient's condition is stable or emergent. An acute wound needs immediate intervention; whereas in the presence of a chronic, stable wound, the patient's hygiene and education on wound care is more important. When there is a risk for pressure ulcer development, preventive interventions such as skin-care practices, elimination of shear, and positioning are high priorities. Promotion of wound healing is a major nursing priority; and the type of wound care administered depends on the type, size, and location of the wound and overall treatment goals.

Other patient factors to consider when establishing priorities include patient preferences, daily activities, and family factors. These factors are important, regardless of the setting for health care. The priorities of care may not vary from outpatient, home, acute care, or restorative care settings.

Teamwork and Collaboration. With early discharge from health care settings, it is important to consider a patient's plan for discharge. Anticipating the patient's discharge wound-care needs and related equipment and resources such as referral to a home care agency or outpatient wound-care clinic helps to improve not only wound healing but also the patient's level of independence. Patients and their family caregivers often need to continue the objectives of wound management after discharge (Box 48-7). Carefully consider the ability of a family caregiver and the amount of time needed to change a particular dressing when selecting a dressing for the patient to use after discharge. For example, in the home setting a patient's spouse may choose more expensive dressing materials to reduce the frequency of dressing

NURSING CARE PLAN

Impaired Skin Integrity

ASSESSMENT

Mrs. Stein, who is 76 years of age, is 7 days postoperative for an elective total hip replacement. She developed redness and oozing of foul-smelling tan-colored drainage from the hip incision on postoperative day 4. Significant medical history includes osteoarthritis and mild hypertension. Her hospital stay has been prolonged because of the development of a lower-extremity blood clot. Because of surgical pain at the incision site and her lower extremity, she does not turn on her own or transfer easily from her bed to the chair. On day 7 she notes pain at the incision and complains of a painful, burning sensation in the sacral region. She is continent of urine and stool but continues to "scoot" over to the side of the bed when preparing for bed-to-chair transfers.

Assessment Activities	***Findings/Defining Characteristics****
Obtain an oral temperature.	Patient has elevated temperature and is diaphoretic.
Ask Mrs. Stein how the surgical site or anything else limits her mobility.	She relates that her hip always aches **limiting movement** and her lower leg is sore and the pain increases on movement. She tells you that she prefers to **keep the hip and leg immobile** to keep the pain level down. Position of comfort is supine, and **Mrs. Stein resists position changes.**
Perform a total body skin assessment, paying special attention to the surgical incision, lower extremities, and sacral area.	

Continued

NURSING CARE PLAN

Impaired Skin Integrity—cont'd

Assessment Activities	*Findings/Defining Characteristics**
Sacral area.	There is a **partial-thickness ulcer directly over the sacral area.** Patient has **nonblanchable erythema** around the open sacral area; this **area does not blanch on palpation.**
Left hip, surgical incision.	**Small openings between staples oozing tan, foul-smelling fluid. Periwound area red and warm.**

*__Defining characteristics__ are shown in bold type.

NURSING DIAGNOSIS: Impaired skin integrity related to pressure, friction, and shearing forces over sacral bony prominence and infectious drainage from surgical site

PLANNING

Goals	*Expected Outcomes (NOC)*†
	Tissue Integrity: Skin and Mucous Membranes
Injury to Mrs. Stein's skin and underlying tissue resulting from pressure, friction, and shear over the bony prominence will be reduced within 2 to 4 weeks.	Mrs. Stein has intact skin integrity in the area of nonblanching erythema. Mrs. Stein's sacral ulcer shows signs of healing. Mrs. Stein maintains intact skin over other pressure points.
Red area around hip wound and tan-colored drainage will be absent within 5 days.	Left hip wound demonstrates signs of healing.
	Immobility Consequences: Physiological
Mrs. Stein's ability to tolerate position changes and correctly change positions will improve within 2 to 4 weeks.	Hyperemia is not present at any pressure points. Hyperemia in sacral region has a decrease in nonblanchable pressure areas.

†Outcome classification labels from Moorhead S et al: *Nursing outcomes classification (NOC)*, ed 5, St Louis, 2013, Mosby.

INTERVENTIONS (NIC)‡	RATIONALE
Pressure Management	
Order and place on Mrs. Stein's bed a pressure redistribution surface. Help Mrs. Stein with repositioning every 90 minutes as her condition allows. Use a drawsheet when helping to reposition.	Repositioning reduces the duration and magnitude of pressure over vulnerable areas of the body and contributes to comfort, hygiene, dignity, and functional ability (Bryant and Nix, 2016). Repositioning is still required for pressure redistribution and comfort when a support surface is in use. Use a lift or transfer sheet to minimize friction and/or shear when repositioning, keeping bed linens smooth and unwrinkled (NPUAP, EPUAP, PPPIA, 2014).
Elevate head of bed no more than 30 degrees. Hip patient may not be allowed to turn in to 30-degree lateral position.	If sitting in bed is necessary, avoid head-of-bed elevation or a slouched position that places pressure and shear on the sacrum and coccyx (NPUAP, EPUAP, PPPIA, 2014).
Keep skin dry and clean; avoid rubbing or massaging around the open area.	The presence of skin damage from moisture increases the risk of pressure ulceration (Colwell et al., 2011; NPUAP, EPUAP, PPPIA, 2014). Rubbing or massaging areas of nonblanching erythema causes further tissue damage (WOCN, 2010).
Use moisture barrier ointment over the ulcer at least 3 times a day to decrease friction and provide moisture to the open tissue.	An ointment covers the area, providing base of ulcer with moisture, which encourages healing. Ointment prevents sheets from rubbing on area, thus decreasing the friction (Rolstad et al., 2016).
Wound Care	
Irrigate wound with saline solution twice per day per wound-care provider's order.	Cleanse wound and surrounding area of wound debris and exudate.
Apply dressing (i.e., gauze moistened with solution twice a day after irrigation) according to wound-care provider's order.	Provides appropriate topical therapy to wound, placing wound in best environment for healing (Rolstad et al., 2016).
At frequent intervals evaluate patient's pain level and offer pain medication as indicated by assessment.	Provides patient with pain reduction/relief, allowing for greater mobility and comfort (Krazner, 2016).

‡Intervention classification labels from Bulechek GM et al: *Nursing interventions classification (NIC)*, ed 6, St Louis, 2013, Mosby.

EVALUATION

Nursing Actions	*Patient Response/Findings*	*Achievement of Outcome*
Perform daily total body skin and wound assessments. Chart results.	No new skin breakdown noted.	No other areas of pain or discomfort are reported.
	Decreased redness at the sacral area.	Decreased or absence of pain at sacral site is reported.
	Presence of reepithelialization in sacral area.	Ulcer in sacral area is healed.
	Reduction in hip wound, periwound redness, and amount of wound drainage.	Surgical incision is no longer open; no drainage and no periwound redness.
Palpate reddened area around sacrum.	Sacral area begins to show signs of reactive hyperemia and blanching following palpation.	Sacral region is improving; no break in epidermis.
	Other pressure points have reactive hyperemia and blanching.	Other pressure points remain intact.

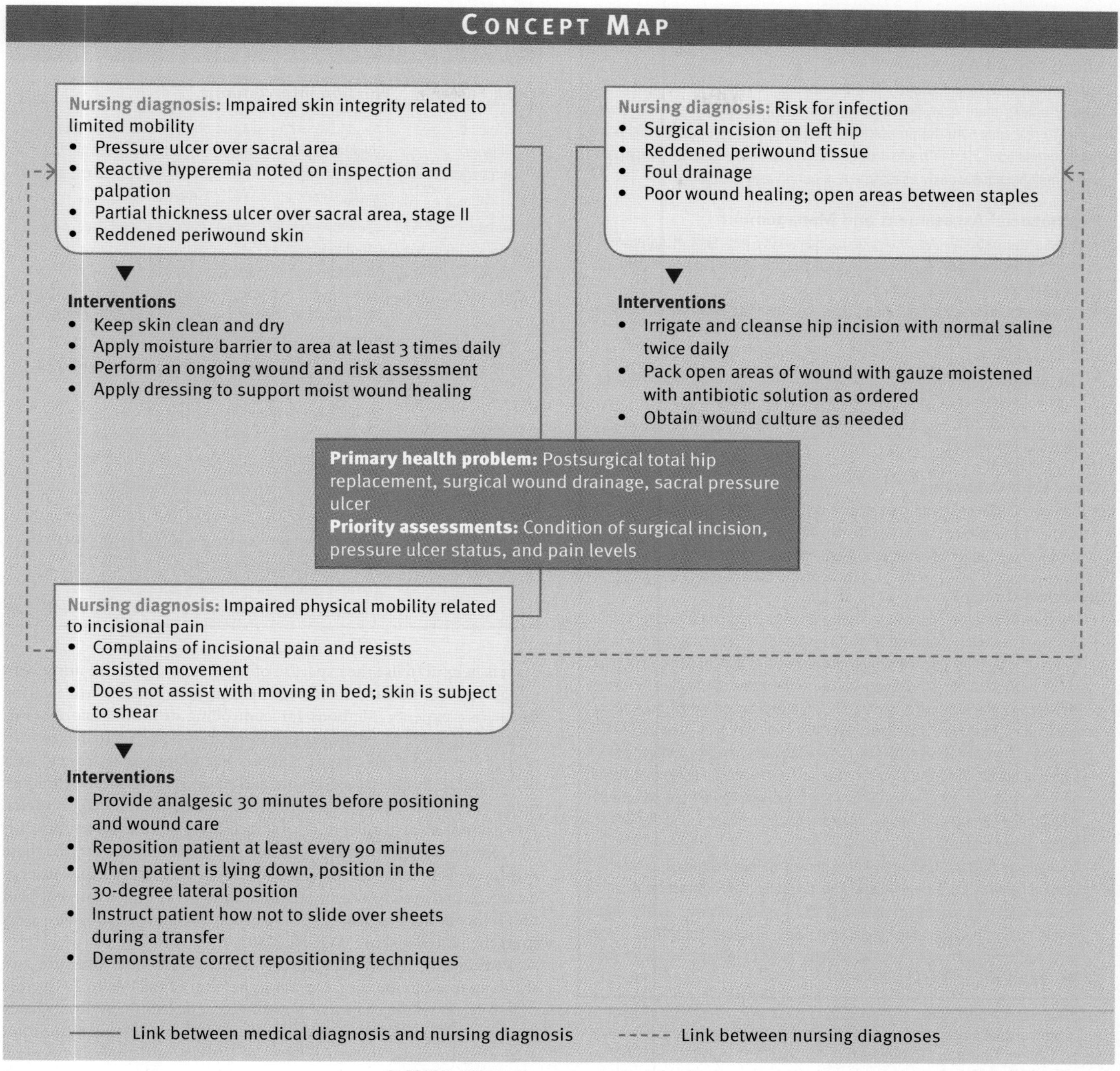

FIGURE 48-14 Concept map for Mrs. Stein.

changes. It is important that you and the patient work together to establish ways of maintaining patient involvement in nursing care to promote wound healing, whether the patient is in the hospital or at home.

◆ Implementation

Health Promotion. Perhaps the most effective intervention for problems with skin integrity and wound care is prevention. Prompt identification of high-risk patients and their risk factors helps to identify the interventions needed to prevent pressure ulcers.

Prevention of Pressure Ulcers. Nursing interventions for patients who are immobile or have other risk factors for pressure ulcers focus on prevention. Table 48-6 describes basic nursing care measures for preventing ulcers based on a patient's risk factors.

Prevention minimizes the impact that risk factors or contributing factors have on pressure ulcer development. Three major areas of nursing interventions for prevention of pressure ulcers are: (1) skin care and management of incontinence; (2) mechanical loading and support devices, which include proper positioning and the use of therapeutic surfaces; and (3) education (WOCN, 2010).

Topical Skin Care and Incontinence Management. When you clean the skin, avoid soap and hot water. Use cleaners with nonionic surfactants that are gentle to the skin (WOCN, 2010). Many types of products are available for skin care, and you need to match their use

BOX 48-7 Home Care Recommendations

Ulcer/Wound Assessment

Assessment and documentation of a pressure ulcer needs to occur at least weekly unless there is evidence of deterioration, in which case the nurse needs to reassess both the pressure ulcer and the patient's overall management immediately. In the home setting this requires the help of the patient and family because weekly assessment is not always feasible.

Psychosocial Assessment and Management

- Assess the patient's resources (e.g., availability and skill of caregivers, finances, equipment). A successful treatment program requires adequate caregiver and equipment resources.
- Assess family caregivers for their ability to comprehend and implement the treatment requirements.
- Assess family caregivers for their level of strength and endurance.
- Consider economic factors because they often limit the supply and availability of equipment and opportunities to relieve caregivers.
- Use an approach that focuses on the psychosocial and physical factors affecting wound care.

Ulcer Care Dressings

- Consider family caregiver time and ability when selecting a dressing.
- In the home setting some family caregivers choose dressing materials manufactured to reduce the frequency of dressing changes.

Infection Control

- Clean dressings, as opposed to sterile ones, are recommended for home use until research demonstrates otherwise. This recommendation is in keeping with principles regarding nosocomial infections and with past success of clean urinary catheterization in the home setting, and it takes into account the expense of sterile dressings and the dexterity required for application. The family caregiver can use the "no-touch" technique for dressing changes. This technique is a method of changing surface dressings without touching the wound or the surface of any dressing that might be in contact with the wound. Adherent dressings should be grasped by the corner and removed slowly, whereas gauze dressings can be pinched in the center and lifted off.
- Contaminated dressings in the home should be disposed of in a manner consistent with local regulations. The Environmental Protection Agency recommends placing soiled dressings in securely fastened plastic bags before adding them to other household trash. However, local regulations vary, and home care agencies and patients need to follow procedures that are consistent with local laws.

Modified from Agency for Health Care Policy and Research, Panel for the Treatment of Pressure Ulcers in Adults: *Treatment of pressure ulcers,* Clinical Practice Guideline No. 15, AHCPR Pub No. 95-0653, Rockville, MD, 1994, Agency for Health Care Policy and Research, Public Health Service, US Department of Health and Human Services.

to the specific needs of the patient. After you clean the skin and make sure that it is completely dry, apply moisturizer to keep the epidermis well lubricated but not oversaturated.

Make an effort to control, contain, or correct incontinence, perspiration, or wound drainage (see Chapters 46 and 47). Patients who have fecal incontinence and who are also receiving enteral tube feeding provide a management challenge. Often the feedings can result in diarrhea. When patients have an incontinent episode, gently clean the area, dry, and apply a thick layer of moisture barrier to the exposed areas. A moisture barrier protects the skin from excessive moisture and bacteria found in the urine or stool.

TABLE 48-6 Quick Guide to Pressure Ulcer Prevention

Risk Factor	Nursing Interventions
Decreased sensory perception	Provide pressure-redistribution surface. Be sure to include protection for pressure points from medical devices such as oxygen tubing, feeding tubes, and casts (Black et al., 2015; Fletcher, 2012).
Moisture	Following each incontinent episode, clean area with no-rinse perineal cleaner and protect skin with moisture-barrier ointment (Rolstad et al., 2016). Keep skin dry and free of maceration (Gray et al., 2011; Colwell et al., 2011). Turn patient off of at-risk areas often.
Friction and shear	Reposition patient using drawsheet or a transfer board surface. Provide trapeze to facilitate movement in bed. Position patient at a 30-degree lateral turn and limit head elevation to 30 degrees (see Figure 48-15).
Decreased activity/mobility	Establish and post individualized turning schedule.
Poor nutrition	Provide adequate nutritional and fluid intake; help with intake as necessary. Consult dietitian for nutritional assessment and recommended nutrients.

It is helpful to use the expertise of an advanced practice nurse with a focus on wound care or management of incontinence while caring for at-risk patients. Methods for controlling or containing incontinence vary. Bowel incontinence can sometimes be better managed with proper diet and medications. Urinary incontinence is treated with behavioral techniques, medication, and surgery. Behavioral techniques help patients learn ways to control their bladder and sphincter muscles. Two examples are bladder and habit training, also called *timed voiding.*

Consider using absorbent pads and garments only after trying these measures. Although controversial, absorbent products such as absorptive underpads and garments are sometimes part of the treatment plan for an incontinent patient. Use only products that wick moisture away from the patient's skin (WOCN, 2010).

Positioning. Positioning interventions redistribute pressure and shearing force to the skin. Elevating the head of the bed to 30 degrees or less decreases the chance of pressure ulcer development from shearing forces (WOCN, 2010). Change the immobilized patient's position according to tissue tolerance, level of activity and mobility, general medical condition, overall treatment objectives, skin condition, and comfort (NPUPA, EUPAP, PPPIA, 2014). A standard turning interval of 1½ to 2 hours does not always prevent pressure ulcer development. Consider repositioning the patient at least every 2 hours if allowed by his or her overall condition. When repositioning, use positioning devices to protect bony prominences (WOCN, 2010). The WOCN guidelines (2010) recommend a 30-degree lateral position (Figure 48-15), which should prevent positioning directly over the bony prominence. To prevent shear and friction injuries, use a transfer device to lift rather than drag the patient when changing positions (see Chapter 39).

For patients at risk for skin breakdown who are able to sit in a chair, limit the amount of time they sit to 2 hours or less at any given time. In the sitting position the pressure on the ischial tuberosities is greater than in the supine position. In addition, teach the patient to shift weight every 15 minutes while sitting (WOCN, 2010). Shifting weight

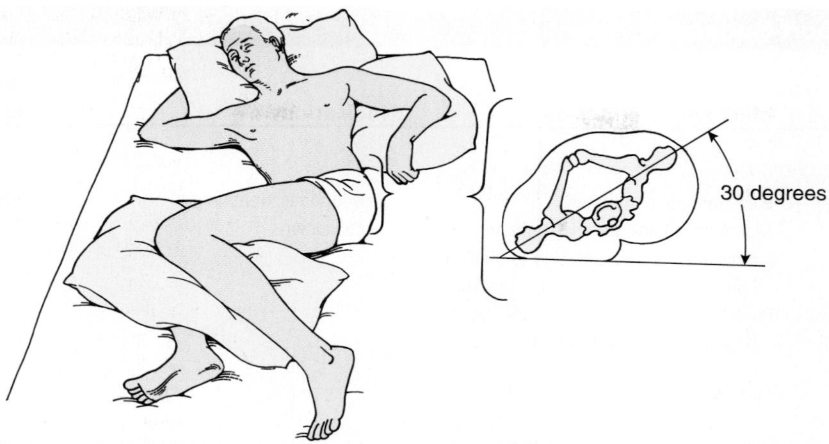

FIGURE 48-15 Thirty-degree lateral position at which pressure points are avoided. (Adapted from Bryant RA, Nix DP, editors: *Acute and chronic wounds: current management concepts,* ed 5, St Louis, 2016, Elsevier.)

QSEN QSEN: BUILDING COMPETENCY IN EVIDENCE-BASED PRACTICE The nurses on an orthopedic unit are concerned about patients who develop skin breakdown after hip-replacement surgery. The nurses would like to implement a new evidence-based postoperative positioning protocol with the goal of preventing pressure ulcer development. What is the nurses' PICO question, and what topics should the nurses include in the evidence-based literature review?

Answers to QSEN Activities can be found on the Evolve website.

provides short-term relief on the ischial tuberosities. Also have him or her sit on foam, gel, or an air cushion to redistribute weight away from the ischial areas. Rigid and donut-shaped cushions are contraindicated because they reduce blood supply to the area, resulting in wider areas of ischemia (WOCN, 2010).

After repositioning the patient, reassess the skin. Remember to use caution when evaluating early signs of tissue ischemia in darkly pigmented skin. For patients with light-toned skin, observe for reactive hyperemia and blanching. Never massage reddened areas. Massaging reddened areas increases the breakdown of the capillaries in the underlying tissues and leads to the risk of tissue injury and pressure ulcer formation (WOCN, 2010).

Support Surfaces (Therapeutic Beds and Mattresses). Support surfaces are "specialized devices for pressure redistribution designed for management of tissue loads, microclimate, and/or other therapeutic functions (i.e., any mattress, integrated bed system, mattress replacement, overlay, seat cushion, or seat cushion overlay)" (NPUAP, EUPAP, PPPIA, 2014). Support surfaces reduce the hazards of immobility to the skin and musculoskeletal system. However, none eliminates the need for meticulous nursing care. No single device completely eliminates the effects of pressure on the skin.

When selecting support surfaces, consider a patient's unique needs. Knowledge about support-surface characteristics (Table 48-7) helps you in clinical decision making. In selecting a support surface, know the patient's risks and the purpose for the support surface; a flow chart is often helpful (Figure 48-16). Teach patients and families the reason for and proper use of the devices (Box 48-8). Some common errors with support surfaces are placing the wrong side of the support surface toward the patient, not plugging powered support surfaces into the electrical source, not turning on the power source for powered support surfaces, failing to place a hand between the metal bedframe and the mattress to determine if the patient sinks to the point of touching the bedframe for some support surfaces, and improperly inflating some support surfaces. When used correctly, these support services help redistribute pressure to the patients skin who are at risk for or have skin breakdown.

Acute Care

Management of Pressure Ulcers. Treatment of patients with pressure ulcers requires a holistic approach that uses the expertise of several multidisciplinary health care professionals (WOCN, 2010). In addition to the nurse, the health care provider, the wound-care nurse specialist, physical therapist, occupational therapist, nutritionist, and pharmacist are involved. Aspects of pressure ulcer treatment include local care of the wound and supportive measures such as adequate nutrients and redistribution of pressure (see Skill 48-2 on pp. 1224-1226).

Before treating a pressure ulcer, reassess the wound for location, stage, size, tissue type and amount, exudate, and surrounding skin condition (Nix, 2016). Acute wounds require close monitoring (every 8 hours). Chronic wound assessment occurs less frequently. Depending on the topical management system, evaluate the wound with every dressing change, usually not more than 1 time per day.

The use and documentation of a systematic approach to monitor progress of an actual pressure ulcer leads to better decision making and optimum outcomes (Nix, 2016). Several healing and documentation tools are available to document wound assessments over time. Using a tool helps link assessment to outcomes so an evaluation of the plan of care follows objective criteria (Nix, 2016). For example, the Bates-Jensen Wound Assessment Tool (Harris et al., 2010) addresses 15 wound characteristics. You score individual items and calculate the sum total, providing an overall indication of wound status. The scoring helps to evaluate whether the goals of the wound management are effective.

Wound Management. Maintenance of a physiological local wound environment is the goal of effective wound management (Rolstad et al., 2016). To maintain a healthy wound environment, you need to address the following objectives: prevent and manage infection, clean the wound, remove nonviable tissue, maintain the wound in a moist environment, eliminate dead space, control odor, eliminate or minimize pain, and protect the wound and periwound skin (Ramundo, 2016).

A wound does not move through the phases of healing if infected. Preventing wound infection includes cleaning and removing nonviable tissue. Clean pressure ulcers *only with noncytotoxic wound cleaners* such

TABLE 48-7 Support Surfaces

Categories and Definitions	Mechanism of Action	Indications	Examples of Manufacturers' and Product Names
Low-Air-Loss			
Air circulated through a mattress/overlay that is covered by a water-vapor permeable cover Available as a mattress placed directly on the existing bedframe or an overlay placed directly on top of an existing surface	Pressure redistribution Maintains a constant and slight air movement against the skin to prevent buildup of moisture and skin breakdown Provides a flow of air to help manage the heat and humidity of the skin	Prevention or treatment of skin breakdown	Hill Rom/Synergy Air Elite
Nonpowered			
Any support surface not requiring or using external sources of energy for operation *Examples:* Foam, interconnected air-filled cells	Reduces pressure by lowering mean interface pressure between patient's tissue and mattress Pressure redistribution Air moves to and from cells as body position changes	Prevention or treatment of skin breakdown	ROHO/ Dry Flotation Mattress, Gaymar Industries/Sof-Care
Air-Fluidized Beds			
Surfaces that change load distribution properties when powered and when patient is in contact with the surface	Uses air and fluid support to provide pressure redistribution via a fluidlike medium created by forcing air through beads as characterized by immersion and envelopment (NPUAP, EPUAP, PPPIA, 2014)	Prevention or treatment of skin breakdown May also be used to protect newly flapped or grafted surgical sites and for patients with excessive moisture	Hill Rom/Clinitron
Lateral Rotation			
Provides passive motion turning the patient from side to side on a low–air loss surface	Passive motion provides pressure relief and mobilization of respiratory secretions A feature of a support surface that provides rotation about a longitudinal axis as characterized by degree of patient turn, duration, and frequency	Treatment and prevention of pulmonary, venous stasis, and urinary complications associated with immobility	Hill Rom/TotalCare SpO2RT

as normal saline or commercial wound cleaners. Noncytotoxic cleaners do not damage or kill fibroblasts and healing tissue (Rolstad et al., 2016). Some commonly used cytotoxic solutions are Dakin's solution (sodium hypochlorite solution), acetic acid, povidone-iodine, and hydrogen peroxide. These are not to be used in clean, granulating wounds.

Irrigation is a common method of delivering a wound-cleansing solution to the wound. Wound irrigation debrides necrotic tissue with pressure that can remove debris from the wound bed without damaging healthy issues (Ramundo, 2016). One method to ensure an irrigation pressure within the correct range is to use a 19-gauge angiocatheter and a 35-mL syringe that delivers saline to a pressure ulcer at 8 psi (Figure 48-17).

Debridement is the removal of nonviable, necrotic tissue. Removal of necrotic tissue is necessary to rid the wound of a source of infection, enable visualization of the wound bed, and provide a clean base necessary for healing.

The method of debridement depends on which is most appropriate for a patient's condition and goals of care (WOCN, 2010). It is important to remember that during the debridement process some normal wound observations include an increase in wound exudate, odor, and size. You need to assess and prevent or effectively manage pain that occurs with debridement (WOCN, 2010). Plan to administer an ordered analgesic 30 minutes before debridement.

Methods of debridement include mechanical, autolytic, chemical, and sharp/surgical. Autolytic debridement is the removal of dead tissue via lysis of necrotic tissue by the white blood cells and natural enzymes of the body (Ramundo, 2016). You accomplish this by using dressings that support moisture at the wound surface. If the wound base is dry, use a dressing that adds moisture; if there is excessive exudate, use a dressing that absorbs the excessive moisture while maintaining moisture at the wound bed. Some examples of these dressings are transparent film and hydrocolloid dressings.

You can accomplish chemical debridement with the use of a topical enzyme preparation, Dakin's solution, or sterile maggots. Topical enzymes induce changes in the substrate, resulting in the breakdown of necrotic tissue (Ramundo, 2016). Depending on the type of enzyme used, the preparation either digests or dissolves the tissue. These preparations require a health care provider's order. Dakin's solution breaks down and loosens dead tissue in a wound. Apply the solution to gauze and apply to the wound. Sterile maggots are used in a wound because it is thought that they ingest the dead tissue.

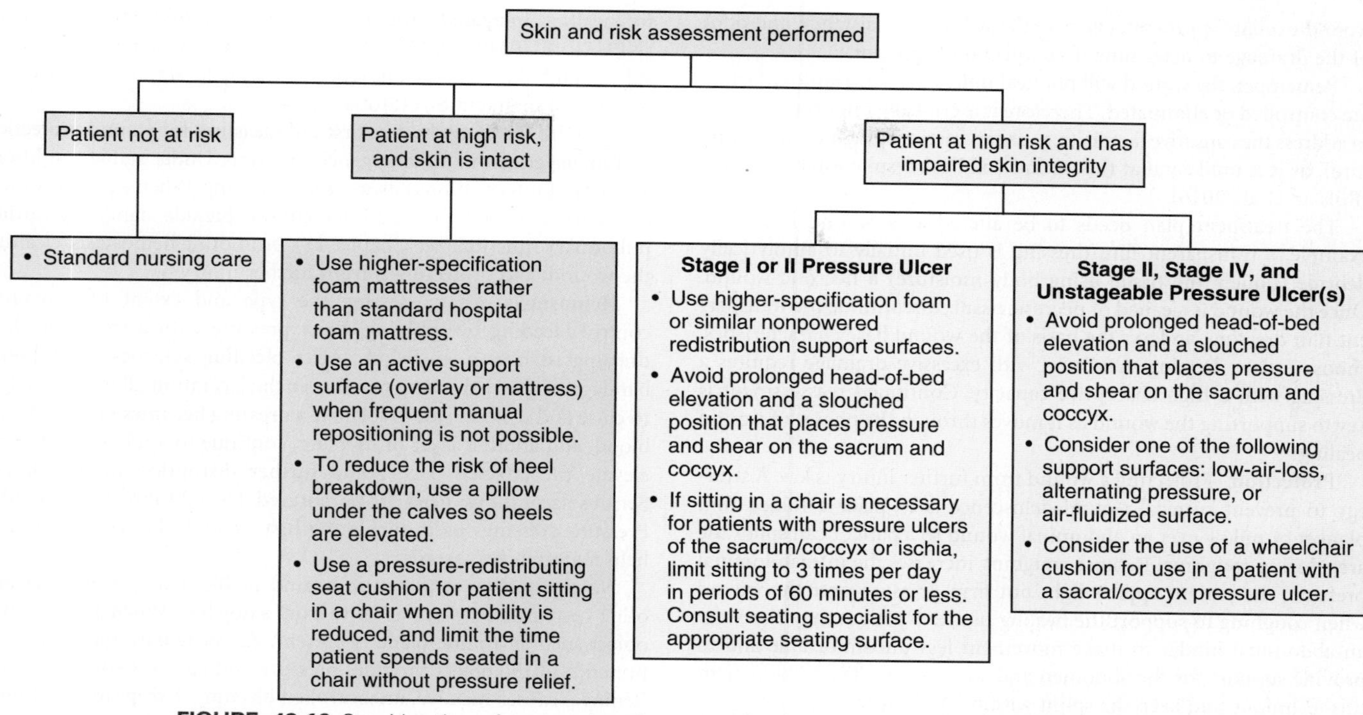

FIGURE 48-16 Considerations for choosing the appropriate support surface. (Modified from WOCN: *Guideline for prevention and management of pressure ulcers,* 2010, Mt Laurel, NJ; and National Pressure Ulcer Advisory Panel (NPUAP) and European Pressure Ulcer Advisory Panel (EPUAP): *International guideline for prevention and treatment of pressure ulcers,* Washington DC, 2009, National Pressure Ulcer Advisory Panel.)

BOX 48-8 PATIENT TEACHING

Pressure-Redistribution Surfaces

Objective

- Patient and family caregiver will describe understanding of the purposes and basic operations of the pressure-redistribution surface.

Teaching Strategies

- Explain the reasons for the pressure-redistribution surface.
- Explain the need to maintain proper body mechanics while using the pressure-redistribution surface. Demonstrate technique.
- Discuss possible patient sensations associated with the device.
- Instruct that minimal layers of linens should be placed over the pressure redistribution surface.
- Educate in the use and care of the pressure-redistribution surface (WOCN, 2010) (based on manufacturer guidelines).
- Explain common errors in use of support surfaces.
- Explain additional pressure-redistribution measures (e.g., turning, avoidance of friction, 30-degree lateral position.

Evaluation

- Patient and family caregiver will state basic purposes for the pressure-redistribution surface.
- Patient and family caregiver will discuss possible sensations associated with the support surface.
- Patient and family caregiver will be able to describe the function of the pressure-redistribution surface.
- Patient and family caregiver will be able to demonstrate turning/repositioning techniques and proper use of the pressure-redistribution surface.

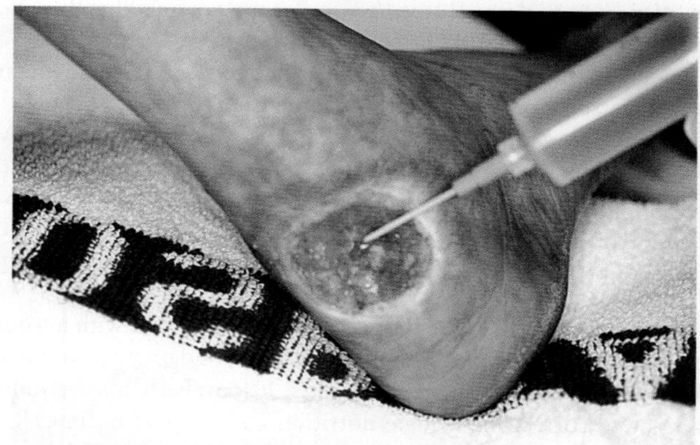

FIGURE 48-17 Wound irrigation.

Surgical debridement is the removal of devitalized tissue with a scalpel, scissors, or other sharp instrument. Physicians and, in some states, trained advanced practice nurses perform surgical debridement of an ulcer or wound. Nurses should check the Nurse Practice Act for their state to see if surgical debridement is a nursing function. It is the quickest method of debridement. It is usually indicated when the patient has signs of cellulitis or sepsis. Other methods of mechanical debridement are wound irrigation (high-pressure irrigation and pulsatile high-pressure lavage) and whirlpool treatments (Ramundo, 2016).

A moist environment supports the movement of epithelial cells and facilitates wound closure. A wound that has excessive exudate (drainage) provides an environment that supports bacterial growth, macerates the periwound skin, and slows the healing process. If excessive wound exudate is present, evaluate the volume, consistency, and odor of the drainage to determine if an infection is present.

Remember, the wound will not heal unless the contributory factors are controlled or eliminated. Therefore it is critically important for you to address the causative factors (e.g., shear, friction, pressure, and moisture), or it is unlikely that the wound will heal despite topical therapy (Rolstad et al., 2016).

The treatment plan needs to be altered as a wound heals. For example, a transparent film dressing is used initially to autolytically debride (liquefy the tissue using body moisture) a necrotic wound. Once the wound is cleaned of necrotic tissue, discontinue the transparent film dressing; and, on the basis of the wound base characteristics, choose a new dressing. A wound with excessive drainage requires a dressing with a high absorptive capacity. Continued reassessment is key to supporting the wound as it moves through the phases of wound healing.

Protection. Protecting a wound from further injury is key. A strategy to prevent surgical wound dehiscence is to place a folded thin blanket or pillow over an abdominal wound so a patient can splint the area during coughing. Because coughing increases the intraabdominal pressure, the patient applies light but firm pressure over the wound when coughing to support the healing tissue. A patient may also wear an abdominal binder to make movement less uncomfortable and to provide support for the abdomen and surgical site. Teach the patient this technique and keep the splint within hand's reach.

Education. Education of the patient and caregivers is an important nursing function (Rolstad et al., 2016). A variety of educational tools, including videotapes and written materials, are available for you to use when teaching patients and caregivers/family to prevent and treat pressure ulcers and care for wounds. The U.S. National Library of Medicine has an excellent website with information on the prevention of pressure ulcers (https://www.nlm.nih.gov/medlineplus/ency/patientinstructions/000147.htm).

Understanding and assessing the experience of the patient and support person are also important dimensions in the treatment of people with pressure ulcers (WOCN, 2010). Clinicians are only just now exploring through research the caregiver's perspective of the concerns and issues faced by frail older spouses caring for their loved ones with pressure ulcers. You need to plan interventions to meet the identified psychosocial needs of patients and their support people (WOCN, 2010).

Nutritional Status. Nutritional support of a patient with a wound is based on the appreciation that nutrition is fundamental to normal cellular integrity and tissue repair (Stotts, 2016a). Early intervention is necessary to correct inadequate nutrition and support healing. Refer patients with pressure ulcers to a registered dietitian for early intervention involving therapeutic diets or enteral or parenteral nutrition (see Chapter 45). If a patient's oral intake is inadequate, enteral nutrition is a likely choice. The dietitian will recommend an individualized energy intake (calories) on the basis of underlying medical condition and level of activity. You will provide 30 to 35 calories/kg of body weight for individuals with a pressure ulcer who are assessed to be at risk for malnutrition. Increased caloric intake helps replace subcutaneous tissue. Patients will also receive vitamin and mineral supplements if suspected or known deficiencies exist. Vitamin C promotes collagen synthesis, capillary wall integrity, fibroblast function, and immunological function.

Patients with pressure ulcers who are underweight or losing weight need enhanced protein supplementation (WOCN, 2010). A patient can lose as much as 50 g of protein per day from an open, high exudative pressure ulcer. Although the recommended intake of protein for adults is 0.8 g/kg/day, a higher intake up to 1.8 g/kg/day is necessary for healing. Increased protein intake helps rebuild epidermal tissue (NPUAP, EUPAP, PPPIA, 2014). Evaluation of weight, laboratory values, and skin parameters reflect changes in status and effects of nutritional interventions (Stotts, 2016a).

First Aid for Wounds. Use first-aid measures for wound protection and management in an emergency situation. Under stable conditions a variety of interventions ensure wound healing. When a patient suffers a traumatic wound, first-aid interventions include stabilizing cardiopulmonary function (see Chapter 41), promoting hemostasis, cleaning the wound, and protecting it from further injury.

Hemostasis. After assessing the type and extent of a wound, control bleeding by applying direct pressure with a sterile or clean dressing such as a washcloth. After bleeding subsides, an adhesive bandage or gauze dressing taped over the laceration allows skin edges to close and a blood clot to form. If a dressing becomes saturated with blood, add another layer of dressing, continue to apply pressure, and elevate the affected part. Avoid further disruption of skin layers. Serious lacerations need to be sutured by a health care provider. Pressure dressings used during the first 24 to 48 hours after trauma help maintain hemostasis.

Normally allow a puncture wound to bleed to remove dirt and other contaminants such as saliva from a dog bite. When a penetrating object such as a knife blade is present, *do not remove the object.* The presence of the object provides pressure and controls some bleeding. Removal causes massive, uncontrolled bleeding. Except for skull injuries, apply pressure around the penetrating object but not on it and transport the patient to an emergency facility.

Cleaning. The process of cleaning a wound involves selecting an appropriate cleaning solution and using a mechanical means of delivering that solution without causing injury to the healing wound tissue (WOCN, 2010). Gently cleaning a wound removes contaminants that serve as sources of infection. However, vigorous cleaning using a method with too much mechanical force causes bleeding or further injury. For abrasions, minor lacerations, and small puncture wounds, first rinse the wound with normal saline and lightly cover the area with a dressing. When a laceration is bleeding profusely, only brush away surface contaminants and concentrate on hemostasis until the patient can be cared for in a clinic or hospital.

According to the WOCN guidelines (2010), normal saline is the preferred cleaning agent. It is physiologically neutral and does not harm tissue. Normal saline keeps the wound surface moist to promote the development and migration of epithelial tissue. Gentle cleansing with normal saline and application of moist saline dressings are commonly used for healing wounds.

Protection. Regardless of whether bleeding has stopped, protect a traumatic wound from further injury by applying sterile or clean dressings and immobilizing the body part. A light dressing applied over minor wounds prevents entrance of microorganisms.

Dressings. The more extensive a wound, the larger the dressing required. For example, a bulky dressing applied with pressure minimizes movement of underlying tissues and helps immobilize the entire body part. A bandage or cloth wrapped around a penetrating object should immobilize it adequately.

Alternative dressings are available to cover and protect certain types of wounds such as large wounds, wounds with drainage tubes or suction catheters in the wound, and wounds that need frequent changing because of excessive drainage. In the home setting a clean towel or diaper is often the best secondary dressing. Pouches or special wound collection systems cover wounds with excessive drainage and collect the drainage. Some of the collection systems have a plastic window on the front of the wound pouch, allowing you to change the packing without removing the pouch from the skin.

The use of dressings requires an understanding of wound healing. A variety of dressing materials are available commercially. The correct dressing selection facilitates wound healing (Rolstad et al., 2016). The dressing type depends on the assessment of the wound and the phase of wound healing. When you identify the objectives for the wound care, the dressing choice becomes clear. A wound that requires infection management requires a different set of dressings than one requiring the removal of nonviable tissue.

For surgical wounds that heal by primary intention, it is common to remove dressings as soon as drainage stops. In contrast, when dressing a wound healing by secondary intention, the dressing material becomes a means for providing moisture to the wound or helping in debridement.

Purposes of Dressings. A dressing serves several purposes:

- Protects a wound from microorganism contamination
- Aids in hemostasis
- Promotes healing by absorbing drainage and debriding a wound
- Supports or splints a wound site
- Promotes thermal insulation of a wound surface
- Provides a moist environment

When the skin is broken, a dressing helps reduce exposure to microorganisms. However, when drainage is minimal, the healing process forms a natural fibrin seal that eliminates the need for a dressing. Wounds with extensive tissue loss always need a dressing.

Pressure dressings promote hemostasis. Applied with elastic bandages, a pressure dressing exerts localized downward pressure over an actual or potential bleeding site. It eliminates dead space in underlying tissues so wound healing progresses normally. Check pressure dressings to be sure that they do not interfere with circulation to a body part. Assess skin color, pulses in distal extremities, the patient's comfort, and changes in sensation. Pressure dressings are not removed routinely.

The primary function of a dressing on a healing wound is to absorb drainage. Most surgical gauze dressings have three layers: a contact or primary layer, an absorbent layer, and an outer protective or secondary layer. The contact dressing covers the incision and then overlaps and covers part of the adjacent skin. Fibrin, blood products, and debris adhere to its surface. A problem occurs if wound drainage dries, causing the dressing to stick to the suture line. Improperly removing a dressing disrupts the healing epidermal surface. If a gauze dressing sticks to a surgical incision, lightly moisten it with saline solution. This saturates the dressing and loosens it from the incisional area, thus preventing trauma to the incisional area during removal.

The dressing technique varies, depending on the goal of the treatment plan for a wound. For example, if the goal is to maintain a moist environment to promote wound healing, it is important to not let the saline-moistened gauze dressing become dry and stick to the wound. This is in direct contrast to the dressing technique that you use if the goal of care is to mechanically debride the wound using a saline moist-to-dry dressing. When wounds such as a necrotic wound require debriding, a moist-to-dry dressing technique can be considered. You place the moist dressing (contact dressing) over the wound bed, cover with a clean gauze and allow the contact layer to dry. In this case the contact dressing is allowed to dry so it sticks to underlying tissue and debrides the wound during removal. This type of debridement is nonselective and can remove viable tissue; it is recommended for debridement in a necrotic wound (Ramundo, 2016).

Dressings applied to a draining wound require frequent changing to prevent microorganism growth and skin breakdown. Bacteria grow readily in the dark, warm, moist environment under a dressing. Skin surfaces become macerated and irritated. Minimize periwound skin breakdown by keeping the skin clean and dry and reducing the use of tape. The absorbent dressing inner layer serves as a reservoir for secretions. The wicking action of woven gauze dressings pulls excess drainage into the dressing and away from the wound. The final outer layer of the dressing helps prevent bacteria and other external contaminants from reaching the wound surface. Usually the outer dressing is made of a thicker dressing material. Apply adhesives to this layer to secure the dressings.

BOX 48-9 Dressing Considerations

- Clean the wound and periwound area at each dressing change, minimizing trauma to the wound (WOCN, 2010).
- Use a dressing that continuously provides a moist environment.
- Perform wound care using topical dressings as determined by a thorough assessment.
- No specific studies have proven an optimal dressing type for pressure ulcers (WOCN, 2010).
- Choose a dressing that keeps the periwound skin dry while keeping the ulcer bed moist.
- Choose a dressing that controls exudate but does not desiccate the ulcer bed.
- The type of dressing may change over time as the pressure ulcer heals or deteriorates. The wound should be monitored at every dressing change and regularly assessed to determine whether modifications in the dressing type are needed (WOCN, 2010).
- Consider caregiver time, ease of use, availability, and cost when selecting a dressing.

A dressing needs to support a moist wound environment if the wound is healing by secondary intention. A moist wound base facilitates the movement of epithelialization, thus allowing the wound to resurface as quickly as possible.

Types of Dressings. Dressings vary by type of material and mode of application (moist or dry) (see Skill 48-3 on pp. 1226-1230). They need to be easy to apply, comfortable, and made of materials that promote wound healing. The WOCN guidelines (2010) are helpful when selecting dressings based on the goal of wound treatment (Box 48-9). To avoid causing damage to the periwound skin, it is important that the dressing technique that you use to treat pressure ulcers and other wounds is not excessively moist (Box 48-10).

Most pressure ulcers require dressings. The type of dressing is usually based on the stage of the pressure ulcer, the type of tissue in the wound, and the function of the dressing (Table 48-8). Before placing a dressing on a pressure ulcer, it is important based on the nursing diagnosis to understand the goal of the treatment, the mechanism of action of the dressing, and principles of wound care.

Gauze sponges are the oldest and most common dressing. They are absorbent and are especially useful in wounds to wick away wound exudate. Gauze is available in different textures and various lengths and sizes; the 4 × 4 is the most common size. Gauze can be saturated with solutions and used to clean and pack a wound. When used to pack a wound, the gauze is saturated with the solution (usually normal saline), wrung out (leaving the gauze only moist), unfolded, and lightly packed into the wound. Unfolding the dressing allows easy wicking action. The purpose of this type of dressing is to provide moisture to the wound yet to allow wound drainage to be wicked into the dry cover gauze pad.

Another type of dressing is a self-adhesive, transparent film that traps moisture over a wound, providing a moist environment (Figure 48-18). The transparent film dressing is ideal for small superficial wounds such as a Stage I pressure ulcer or a partial-thickness wound.

BOX 48-10 EVIDENCE-BASED PRACTICE

Moisture-Associated Skin Damage

PICO Question: In patients with pressure ulcers or chronic wounds, which wound care interventions prevent moisture-associated skin damage in the periwound area?

Evidence Summary

Appropriate wound management to support healing is critical for patients with pressure ulcers and other chronic wounds. Advances in wound healing document the benefit of a moist wound environment and the accepted practice of moist wound healing. But when moisture is present in excess and allowed to sit on the periwound skin, it leads to damaging maceration. Maceration is defined as a softening of tissues by soaking until connective fibers can be teased apart (Colwell et al., 2011). This condition is classified as moisture-associated skin damage (MASD)—the inflammation and erosion of the skin caused by prolonged exposure to various sources of moisture and its contents, including urine, stool, perspiration, wound exudate, mucus, or saliva. Exudate is created by the normal inflammatory process of wound healing. However, when high volumes of exudate occur, it poses clinical difficulties, and healing may be affected as the overhydrated skin becomes macerated, potentially leading to skin breakdown.

Interventions that focus on preventive steps include use of a dressing that absorbs excessive moisture while maintaining a moist wound bed (Colwell et al., 2011), selection of the right dressing and size to absorb the wound exudate, the appropriate frequency of dressing change, and use of a skin protectant on the periwound skin (Guest et al., 2011)

Application to Nursing Practice

- Use of a skin protectant (no-sting film barrier, petrolatum-based or zinc-based protectant) helps to prevent periwound skin maceration (Gray and Weir, 2007; Guest et al., 2011).
- Enzymatic debridement is the topical application of enzymes over the necrotic tissue. The only enzyme available in the United States is collagenase. Collagenase digests the necrotic tissue by dissolving the collagen in the dead tissue (NPUAP, EPUAP, PPPIA, 2014).
- Assess the wound and surrounding skin for irritation, itching, burning, or drainage amount. These symptoms are exacerbated during dressing changes or stomal pouching (Gray et al., 2013).
- Prevent peristomal MASD by selecting a pouching system with an effective seal between peristomal skin and fecal material (Gray et al., 2013).
- Make changes in dressing material and frequency of dressing change on the basis of the amount of wound drainage (Rolstad et al., 2016).
- Assess perineal skin for incontinence-related dermatitis, which is an early sign of MASD. When needed, use a moisture barrier in addition to frequent perineal hygiene (Voegeli, 2012).

Use a film dressing as a secondary dressing and for autolytic debridement of small wounds. It has the following advantages:

- Adheres to undamaged skin
- Serves as a barrier to external fluids and bacteria but still allows the wound surface to "breathe" because oxygen passes through the transparent dressing (Guest et al., 2011)
- Promotes a moist environment that speeds epithelial cell growth
- Can be removed without damaging underlying tissues
- Permits viewing a wound
- Does not require a secondary dressing

Hydrocolloid dressings are dressings with complex formulations of colloids and adhesive components. They are adhesive and occlusive. The wound contact layer of this dressing forms a gel as wound exudate is absorbed and maintains a moist healing environment. Hydrocolloids support healing in clean granulating wounds and autolytically debride necrotic wounds; they are available in a variety of sizes and shapes. This type of dressing has the following functions:

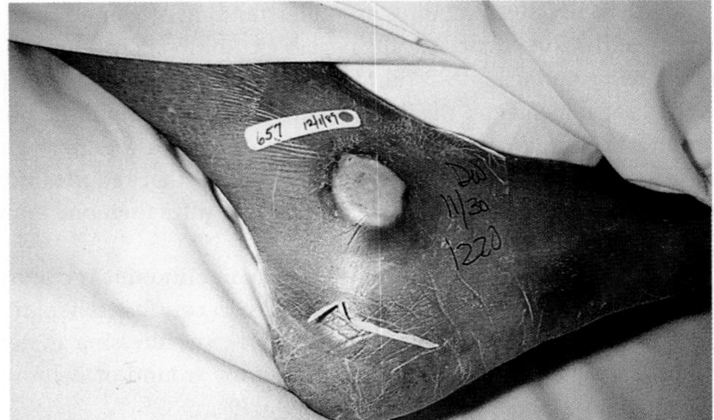

FIGURE 48-18 Transparent film dressing.

- Absorbs drainage through the use of exudate absorbers in the dressing
- Maintains wound moisture
- Slowly liquefies necrotic debris
- Is impermeable to bacteria and other contaminants
- Is self-adhesive and molds well
- Acts as a preventive dressing for high-risk friction areas
- May be left in place for 3 to 5 days, minimizing skin trauma and disruption of healing

The hydrocolloid dressing is useful on shallow-to–moderately deep dermal ulcers. Hydrocolloid dressings cannot absorb the amount of drainage from heavily draining wounds, and some are contraindicated for use in full-thickness and infected wounds. Most hydrocolloids leave a residue in the wound bed that is easy to confuse with purulent drainage.

Hydrogel dressings are gauze or sheet dressings impregnated with water or glycerin-based amorphous gel. This type of dressing hydrates wounds and absorbs small amounts of exudate. Hydrogel dressings are for partial-thickness and full-thickness wounds, deep wounds with some exudate, necrotic wounds, burns, and radiation-damaged skin. They can be very useful in painful wounds because they are very soothing to a patient and do not adhere to the wound bed and thus cause little trauma during removal. A disadvantage is that some hydrogels require a secondary dressing and you must take care to prevent periwound maceration. Hydrogels come in a sheet dressing or a tube; thus you are able to squirt the gel directly into the wound base. Hydrogel has the following advantages:

- Is soothing and can reduce wound pain
- Provides a moist environment
- Debrides necrotic tissue (by softening the necrotic tissue)
- Does not adhere to the wound base and is easy to remove

Many other types of dressings are available. Foam and alginate dressings are for wounds with large amounts of exudate and those that need packing. Foam dressings are also used around drainage tubes to absorb drainage. Calcium alginate dressings are manufactured from seaweed and come in sheet and rope form. The alginate forms a soft gel when in contact with wound fluid. These highly absorbent dressings are for wounds with an excessive amount of drainage and do not cause trauma when removed from the wound. *Do not use these in dry wounds, and they require a secondary dressing.* Several manufacturers produce composite dressings, which combine two different dressing types into one dressing. Research is ongoing regarding which type of dressing is best for which type of wound.

Changing Dressings. To prepare for changing a dressing, you need to know the type of dressing, the presence of underlying drains or

TABLE 48-8 **Dressings by Pressure Ulcer Stage**

Pressure Ulcer Category/Stage	Pressure Ulcer Status	Dressing	Comments*	Expected Change	Adjuvants
I	Intact	None	Allows visual assessment	Resolves slowly without epidermal loss over 7-14 days	Turning schedule Support hydration Nutritional support
		Transparent dressing	Protects from shear and friction		
		Hydrocolloid	Does not always allow visual assessment		Pressure-redistribution surface or chair cushion
II	Clean	Composite film	Limits shear	Heals through reepithelialization	Turning schedule Support hydration Nutritional support Manage incontinence
		Hydrocolloid	Change when seal of dressing breaks; maximal wear time 7 days		
		Hydrogel	Provides a moist environment		
III	Clean	Hydrocolloid	Must change when seal of dressing breaks; maximal wear time 7 days	Heals through granulation and reepithelialization	See previous stages; evaluate pressure-redistribution needs
		Hydrogel covered with foam dressing	Applied over wound to protect and absorb moisture		
		Calcium alginate	Used with significant exudate; must cover with secondary dressing		
		Gauze	Used with normal saline or other prescribed solution; must unfold to make contact with wound		
IV	Clean	Hydrogel covered with foam dressing	Applied over wound to protect and absorb moisture	Heals through granulation and reepithelialization	Surgical consultation often necessary for closure
		Calcium alginate	Used with significant exudate; must cover with secondary dressing		
		Gauze	Used with normal saline or other prescribed solution; must unfold to make contact with wound; fill all dead space with gauze		
Unstageable	Wound covered with eschar	Adherent film	Facilitates softening of eschar	Eschar lifts at edges as debridement progresses	See previous stages; surgical consultation sometimes considered for debridement
		Gauze plus ordered solution	Delivers solution and softens eschar	Eschar softens	
		Enzymes	Facilitate debridement	Eschar softens	
		None	If eschar is dry and intact, no dressing used, allowing eschar to act as physiological cover; may be indicated for treatment of heel eschar		

*As with all occlusive dressings, wound should *not* be clinically infected.

tubing, and the type of supplies needed for wound care. Poor preparation causes a break in aseptic technique (see Chapter 29) or accidental dislodging of a drain. Your judgment in modifying a dressing-change procedure is important during wound care, particularly if the character of a wound changes. Notifying the health care provider of any change is essential.

Sometimes (e.g., with chronic nonsurgical wounds) you will use clean medical aseptic technique for a dressing change. The clean technique refers to the fact that the nurse maintains medical versus sterile asepsis (Chapter 29). You will wear clean gloves, but the dressing materials are in sterile packages and are carefully placed over the wound. Deep wounds that require irrigation are usually irrigated with a sterile solution. A complete patient and wound history is essential in determining when a clean dressing technique is appropriate. For example, chronic pressure ulcer wounds use a clean technique. On the other hand, a fresh surgical wound may require sterile technique, which requires the use of sterile gloves so as not to introduce microorganisms into a healing wound.

A health care provider's order for changing a dressing indicates the dressing type, the frequency of changing, and any solutions or ointments to be applied to the wound. An order to "reinforce dressing prn" (add dressings without removing the original one) is common right after surgery, when the health care provider does not want accidental disruption of the suture line or bleeding. The medical or operating

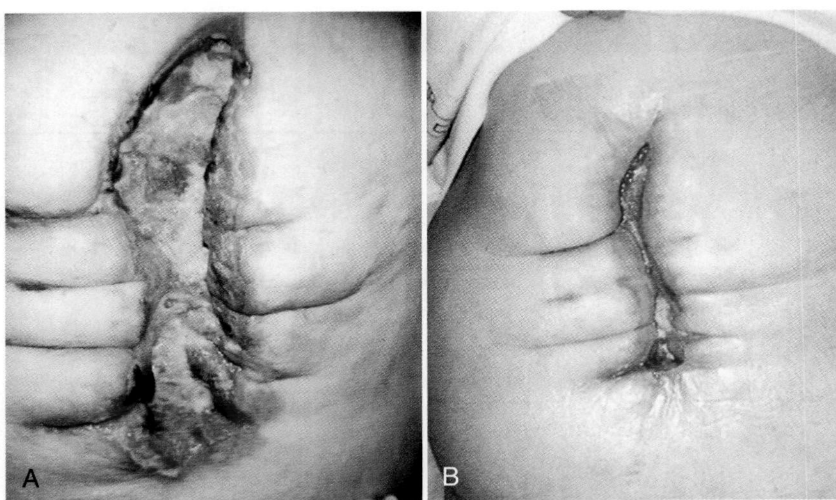

FIGURE 48-19 A, Dehisced wound before wound V.A.C. therapy. **B,** Dehisced wound after wound V.A.C. therapy. *V.A.C.,* Vacuum-assisted closure. (Courtesy Kinetic Concepts, [KCI], San Antonio, TX.)

room record usually indicates whether drains are present and from which body cavity they drain. After the first dressing change, describe the location of drains and the type of dressing materials and solutions to use in the patient's care plan. See Skill 48-3 for guidelines to use during a dressing change procedure.

Often it is necessary to teach patients how to change dressings in preparation for home care. In this situation, demonstrate dressing changes to a patient and family and then provide an opportunity for them to practice. Usually wound healing has progressed to the point that risks of complications such as dehiscence or evisceration are minimal. A patient needs to be able to change a dressing independently or with help from a family caregiver before discharge. Contaminated dressings in the home should be disposed of in a manner consistent with local regulations. Skill 48-3 outlines the steps for changing dry and moist dressings.

Packing a Wound. The first step in packing a wound is to assess its size, depth, and shape. These characteristics are important in determining the size and type of dressing used to pack a wound. The dressing needs to be flexible and in contact with the entire wound surface. Make sure that the type of material used to pack the wound is appropriate. Many new dressing materials such as alginates are also used for packing. If gauze is the appropriate dressing material, saturate with the ordered solution, wring out, unfold, and lightly pack into the wound. The entire wound surface needs to be in contact with part of the moist gauze dressing (see Skill 48-3).

It is important to remember not to pack a wound too tightly. Overpacking causes pressure on the wound bed tissue. Pack the wound only until the packing material reaches the surface of the wound; there should never be so much packing material that it extends higher than the wound surface. Packing that overlaps onto the wound edges causes maceration of the skin surrounding the wound.

A treatment modality for wounds is negative-pressure wound therapy (NPWT) or vacuum-assisted closure (one brand name is V.A.C.). NPWT is the application of subatmospheric (negative) pressure to a wound through suction to facilitate healing and collect wound fluid (Netsch, 2016). The **vacuum-assisted closure (V.A.C.)** is a device that helps in wound closure by applying localized negative pressure to draw the edges of a wound together (Figure 48-19, *A* and *B*). NPWT supports wound healing by edema reduction and fluid removal, macro deformation and wound contraction, and micro deformation and mechanical stretch perfusion. Secondary effects include angiogenesis, granulation tissue formation, and reduction in bacterial bioburden (Netsch, 2016) (Figure 48-20). There have been modifications to the V.A.C. The V.A.C. Instill allows intermittent instillation of fluids into a wound, especially wounds not responding to traditional NPWT (Wolvos, 2013).

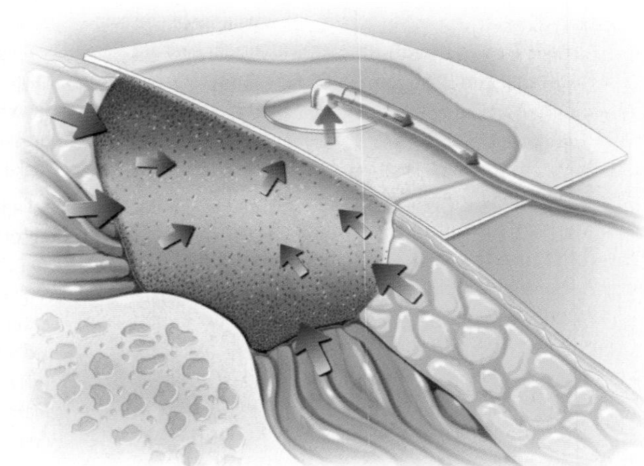

FIGURE 48-20 V.A.C. system using negative pressure to remove fluid from area surrounding wound, reducing edema and improving circulation to area. *V.A.C.,* Vacuum-assisted closure. (Courtesy Kinetic Concepts [KCI], San Antonio, TX.)

NPWT treats acute and chronic wounds (see Skill 48-4 on pp. 1231-1234). The schedule for changing NPWT dressings varies, depending on the type of wound and amount of drainage. Wear time for the dressing is anywhere from 24 hours to 5 days. As a wound heals, granulation tissue lines its surface. The wound has a stippled or granulated appearance. The surface area sometimes increases or decreases, depending on wound location and the amount of drainage removed by the NPWT system. NPWT also enhances the adherence of split-thickness skin grafts. It is placed over a graft intraoperatively, decreasing the ability of the graft to shift and evacuating fluids that build up under it (Netsch, 2016; Xie et al., 2010). An airtight seal must be maintained (Box 48-11).

BOX 48-11 Negative-Pressure Wound Therapy: Maintaining an Airtight Seal

To avoid wound desiccation, the wound needs to remain sealed once therapy is initiated. Problem seal areas include wounds around joints, uneven areas, and near the sacrum. The following interventions help maintain an airtight seal:

- Clip hair around wound.
- Dry periwound thoroughly.
- Frame periwound area with skin sealant; skin barrier, hydrocolloid, or transparent film to extend 3 to 5 cm (1.2 to 2 in) beyond wound parameter.
- Fill uneven skin surfaces with a skin-barrier product or hydrocolloid.
- Protect skin near or under suction from contact dermatitis with a hydrocolloid or transparent filmed dressing framed under the vulnerable area.
- Avoid adhesive remover because it leaves a residue that hinders film adherence.

From Netsch DS: Negative-pressure wound therapy, In Bryant RS, Mix DP, editors: *Acute and chronic wounds: current management concepts,* ed 5, St Louis, 2016, Elsevier.

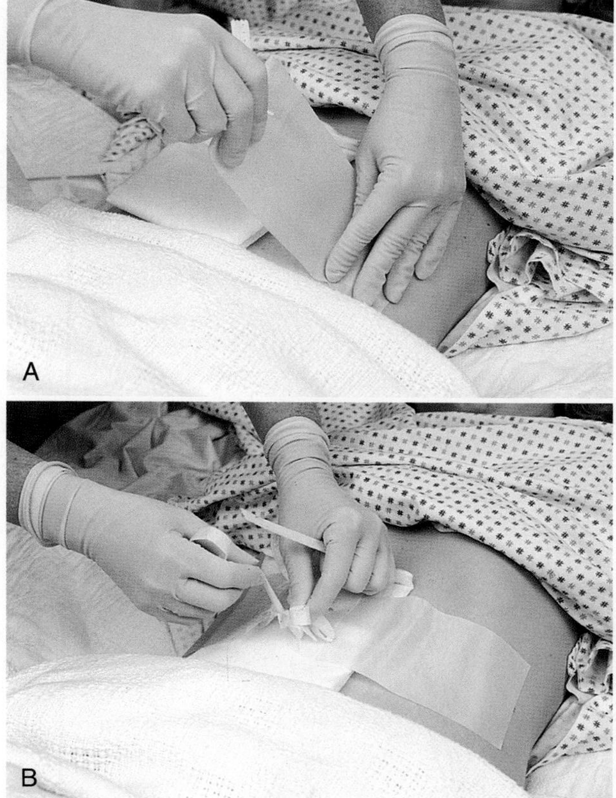

FIGURE 48-21 Montgomery ties. **A,** Each tie is placed at side of dressing. **B,** Securing ties encloses dressing.

Securing Dressings. Use tape, ties, or a secondary dressing to secure a dressing over a wound site. The choice of anchoring depends on the wound size and location, the presence of drainage, the frequency of dressing changes, and the patient's level of activity.

You will most often use strips of tape to secure dressings. Nonallergenic paper and silicone tapes minimize skin reactions. Common adhesive tape adheres well to the surface of the skin, whereas elastic adhesive tape compresses closely around pressure bandages and permits more movement of a body part. Skin sensitive to adhesive tape becomes severely inflamed and denuded and in some cases even sloughs when the tape is removed. It is important to assess skin under tape at each dressing change.

Tape is available in various widths such as 1.3, 2.5, 5 and 7.5 cm (½, 1, 2, and 3 inches). Choose the size that secures a dressing sufficiently. For example, a large abdominal wound dressing needs to remain secure over a large area despite frequent stress from movement, respiratory effort, and possibly abdominal distention. Strips of 7.5-cm (3-inch) adhesive better stabilize such a large dressing so it does not continually slip off. When applying tape, ensure that it adheres to several inches of skin on both sides of the dressing and that it is placed across the middle of the dressing. When securing a dressing, press the tape gently. Make sure to exert pressure away from a wound so that tension occurs in both directions away from the wound, minimizing skin distortion and irritation. Never apply tape over irritated or broken skin. Protect irritated skin by using a solid skin barrier and applying the tape over the barrier.

To remove tape safely, loosen the ends and gently pull the outer end parallel with the skin surface toward the wound. Apply light traction to the skin away from the wound as the tape is loosened and removed. The traction minimizes pulling of the skin. Adhesive remover also loosens the tape from the skin. If tape covers an area of hair growth, a patient experiences less discomfort if you pull it in the direction of the hair growth.

To avoid repeated removal of tape from sensitive skin, secure dressings with pairs of reusable Montgomery ties (Figure 48-21). Each section consists of a long strip; half contains an adhesive backing to apply to the skin, and the other half folds back and contains a cloth tie or a safety pin/rubber band combination that you fasten across a dressing and untie at dressing changes. A large, bulky dressing often requires two or more sets of Montgomery ties. Another method to protect the surrounding skin on wounds that need frequent dressing changes is to place strips of hydrocolloid dressings on either side of the wound edges, cover the wound with a dressing, and apply the tape to the dressing. To provide even support to a wound and immobilize a body part, apply elastic gauze, elastic stretch net, or binders over a dressing.

Comfort Measures. A wound is often painful, depending on the extent of tissue injury; and wound care often requires the use of well-timed analgesia before any wound procedure (Krazner, 2016). Administer analgesic medications 30 to 60 minutes before dressing changes (depending on the time of peak action of a drug). In addition, several techniques are useful in minimizing discomfort during wound care. Carefully removing tape, gently cleaning wound edges, and carefully manipulating dressings and drains minimize stress on sensitive tissues. Careful turning and positioning also reduce strain on a wound.

Cleaning Skin and Drain Sites. Although a moderate amount of wound exudate promotes epithelial cell growth, some health care providers order cleaning a wound or drain site if a dressing does not absorb drainage properly or if an open drain deposits drainage onto the skin. Wound cleaning requires good hand hygiene and aseptic techniques (see Chapter 29). You sometimes use irrigation to remove debris from a wound.

Basic Skin Cleaning. Clean surgical or traumatic wounds by applying noncytotoxic solutions with sterile gauze or by irrigation. The following three principles are important when cleaning an incision or the area surrounding a drain:

1. Clean in a direction from the least contaminated area such as from a wound or incision to the surrounding skin (Figure 48-22) or from an isolated drain site to the surrounding skin (Figure 48-23).

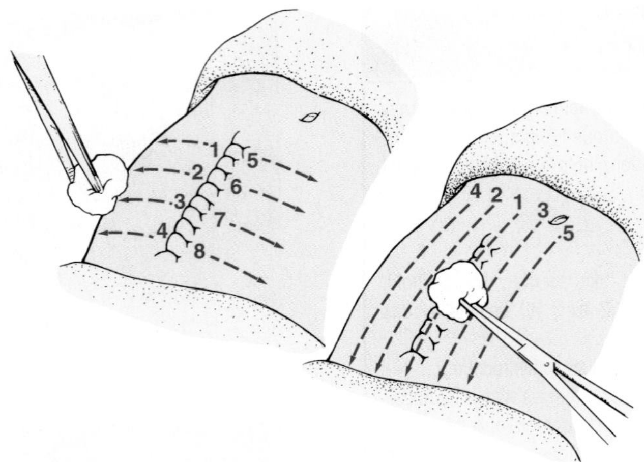

FIGURE 48-22 Methods for cleaning wound site.

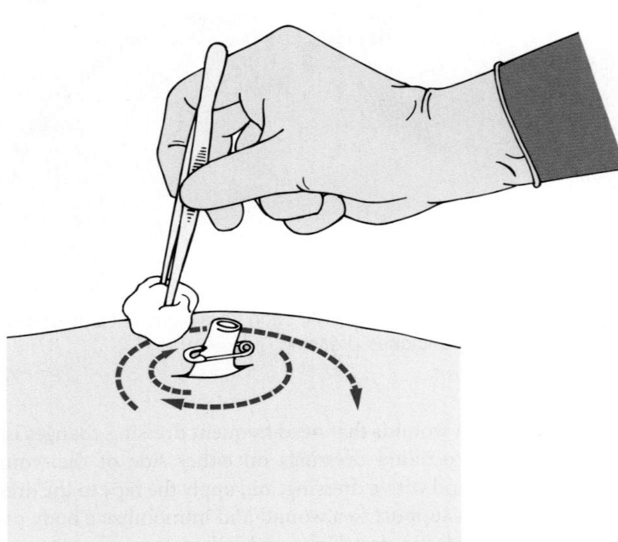

FIGURE 48-23 Cleaning drain site.

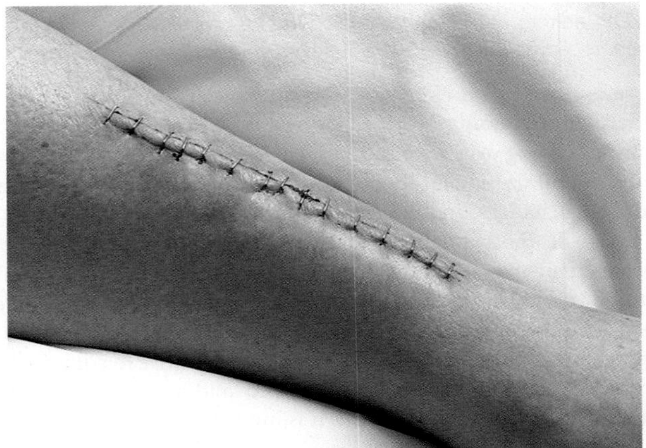

FIGURE 48-24 Incision closed with metal staples.

2. Use gentle friction when applying solutions locally to the skin.
3. When irrigating, allow the solution to flow from the least to most contaminated area (see Skill 48-5).

After applying a solution to sterile gauze, clean away from the wound. Never use the same piece of gauze to clean across an incision or wound twice.

Drain sites are a source of contamination because moist drainage harbors microorganisms. If a wound has a dry incisional area and a moist drain site, cleaning moves from the incisional area toward the drain. Use two separate swabs or gauze pads, one to clean from the top of the incision toward the drain and one to clean from the bottom of the incision toward the drain. To clean the area of an isolated drain site, clean around the drain, moving in circular rotations outward from a point closest to the drain. In this situation the skin near the site is more contaminated than the site itself. To clean circular wounds, use the same technique as in cleaning around a drain.

Irrigation. Irrigation is a way of cleaning wounds. Use an irrigating syringe to flush the area with a constant low-pressure flow of solution. The gentle washing action of the irrigation cleanses a wound of exudate and debris. Irrigation is particularly useful for open, deep wounds; wounds involving an inaccessible body part such as the ear canal; or when cleaning sensitive body parts such as the conjunctival lining of the eye.

Wound Irrigations. Typically the irrigation of an open wound involves use of clean gloves. Review the health care provider's order to determine if a sterile solution is required. Sterile solutions may be necessary with new traumatic wounds (Graybill et al., 2016). Use a 35-mL syringe with a 19-gauge soft angiocatheter (Rolstad et al., 2016) to irrigate an open wound. Deliver the solution. This irrigation system has a safe pressure and does not damage healing wound tissue. It is important to never occlude a wound opening with a syringe because this results in the introduction of irrigating fluid into a closed space. The pressure of the fluid causes tissue damage, discomfort, and possibly forcing infection or debris into the wound bed. Always irrigate a wound with the syringe tip over but not in the drainage site. Make sure that fluid flows directly into the wound and not over a contaminated area before entering the wound. Skill 48-5 on pp. 1234-1236 lists steps for wound irrigation.

Suture Care. A surgeon closes a wound by bringing the wound edges as close together as possible to reduce scar formation. Proper wound closure involves minimal trauma and tension to tissues with control of bleeding.

Sutures are threads or metal used to sew body tissues together (Figure 48-24). A patient's history of wound healing, the site of surgery, the tissues involved, and the purpose of the sutures determine the suture material used. For example, if a patient has had repeated surgery for an abdominal hernia, the health care provider can choose wire sutures to provide greater strength for wound closure. In contrast, a small laceration of the face calls for the use of very fine Dacron (polyester) sutures to minimize scar formation.

Sutures are available in a variety of materials, including silk, steel, cotton, linen, wire, nylon, and Dacron. They come with or without sharp surgical needles attached. Steel staples are a common type of outer skin closure that traumatizes tissue less than sutures while providing extra strength.

Sutures are placed within tissue layers in deep wounds and superficially as the final means for wound closure. Deep sutures are usually composed of an absorbable material that disappears over time. Sutures are foreign bodies and thus are capable of causing local inflammation. A surgeon tries to minimize tissue injury by using the finest suture possible and the smallest number necessary.

Policies vary within institutions as to who is able to remove sutures. If it is appropriate that the nurse remove them, a health care provider's order is required. An order for suture removal is not written until the health care provider believes that the wound has closed (usually in 7 days). Special scissors with curved cutting tips or special staple removers slide under the skin closures for suture removal (Figure 48-25). The health care provider usually specifies the number of sutures or staples to remove. If the suture line appears to be healing in certain locations better than in others, some health care providers choose to have only some sutures removed (e.g., every other one).

To remove staples, insert the tips of the staple remover under each wire staple. While slowly closing the ends of the staple remover together, squeeze the center of the staple with the tips, freeing it from the skin (see Figure 48-25).

To remove sutures, first check the type of suturing used (Figure 48-26). With intermittent suturing the surgeon ties each individual suture made in the skin. Continuous suturing, as the name implies, is a series of sutures with only two knots, one at the beginning and one at the end of the suture line. Retention sutures are placed more deeply than skin sutures, and nurses may or may not remove them, depending on agency policy. The manner in which the suture crosses and penetrates the skin determines the method for removal. *Never pull the visible part of a suture through underlying tissue.* Sutures on the surface of the skin harbor microorganisms and debris. The part of the suture beneath the skin is sterile. Pulling the contaminated part of the suture through tissues can lead to infection. Before taking out the sutures, cleanse the suture line with normal saline. Clip suture materials as close to the skin edge on one side as possible and pull the suture through from the other side (Figure 48-27).

Drainage Evacuation. When drainage interferes with healing, evacuation is achieved by using either a drain alone or a drainage tube with continuous suction. You may apply special skin barriers, including hydrocolloid dressings similar to those used with ostomies (see Chapter 47), around drain sites with significant drainage. The skin barriers are soft material applied to the skin with adhesive. Drainage flows on the barrier but not directly on the skin. **Drainage evacuators** (Figure 48-28) are convenient portable units that connect to tubular drains lying within a wound bed and exert a safe, constant, low-pressure vacuum to remove and collect drainage. Ensure that suction is exerted and that connection points between the evacuator and tubing are intact. The evacuator collects drainage. Assess for volume and character every shift and as needed. When the evacuator fills, measure output by emptying the contents into a graduated cylinder and immediately reset the evacuator to apply suction.

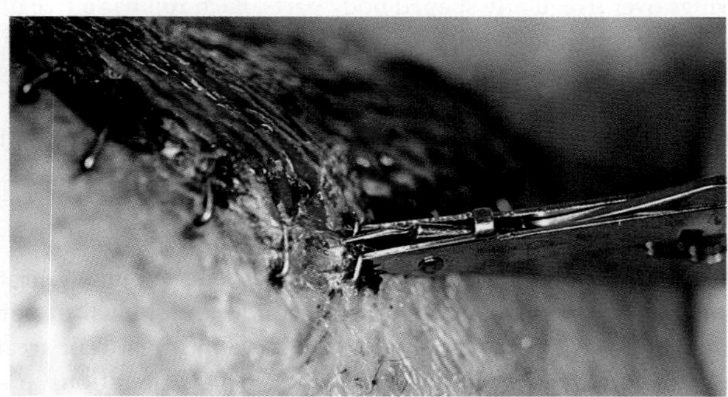

FIGURE 48-25 Staple remover.

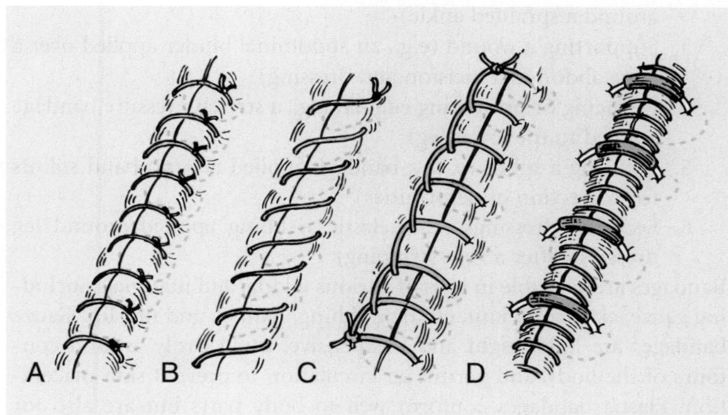

FIGURE 48-26 Examples of suturing methods. **A,** Intermittent. **B,** Continuous. **C,** Blanket continuous. **D,** Retention.

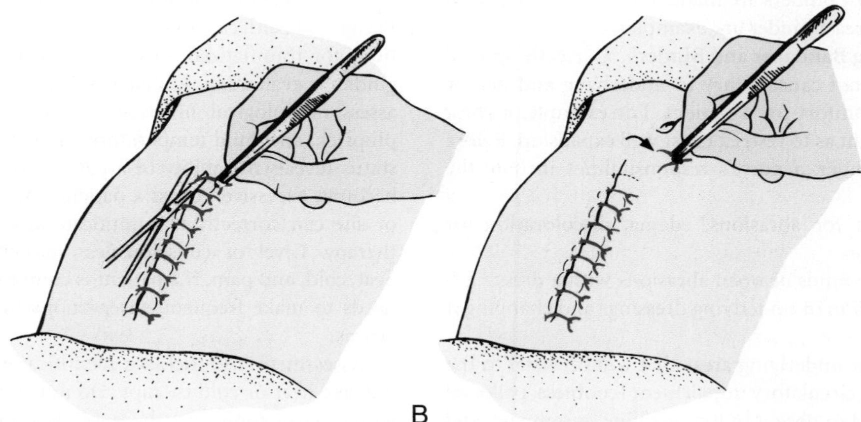

FIGURE 48-27 Removal of intermittent suture. **A,** Cut suture as close to skin as possible, away from knot. **B,** Remove suture and never pull contaminated stitch through tissues.

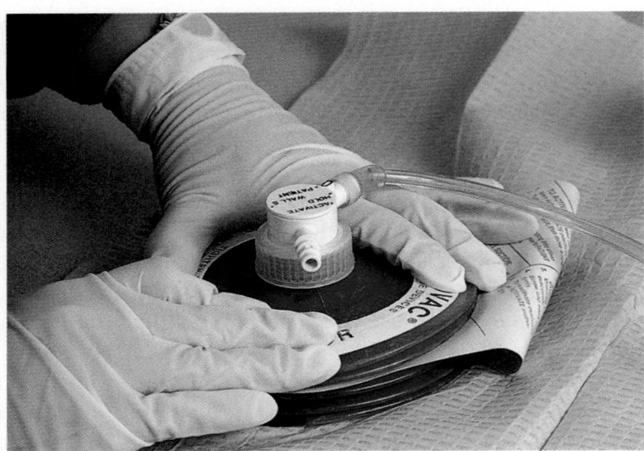

FIGURE 48-28 Setting suction on drainage evacuator. *1,* With drainage port open, raise level on diaphragm. *2,* Push straight down on lever to lower diaphragm. *3,* Closure of port prevents escape of air and creates vacuum pressure.

Bandages and Binders. A simple gauze dressing is often not enough to immobilize or provide support to a wound. Binders and bandages applied over or around dressings provide extra protection and therapeutic benefits by the following:

1. Creating pressure over a body part (e.g., an elastic pressure bandage applied over an arterial puncture site)
2. Immobilizing a body part (e.g., an elastic bandage applied around a sprained ankle)
3. Supporting a wound (e.g., an abdominal binder applied over a large abdominal incision and dressing)
4. Reducing or preventing edema (e.g., a stretch pressure bandage applied to the lower leg)
5. Securing a splint (e.g., a bandage applied around hand splints for correction of deformities)
6. Securing dressings (e.g., elastic webbing applied around leg dressings after a vein stripping)

Bandages are available in rolls of various widths and materials, including gauze, elasticized knit, elastic webbing, flannel, and muslin. Gauze bandages are lightweight and inexpensive, mold easily around contours of the body, and permit air circulation to prevent skin maceration. Elastic bandages conform well to body parts but are also for exerting pressure.

Binders are bandages that are made of large pieces of material to fit a specific body part. Most binders are made of elastic or cotton. An abdominal binder and a breast binder are examples.

Principles for Applying Bandages and Binders. Correctly applied bandages and binders do not cause injury to underlying and nearby body parts or create discomfort for a patient. For example, a chest binder should not be so tight as to restrict chest wall expansion. Before applying a bandage or binder, a nurse's responsibilities include the following:

- Inspecting the skin for abrasions, edema, discoloration, or exposed wound edges
- Covering exposed wounds or open abrasions with a dressing
- Assessing the condition of underlying dressings and changing if soiled
- Assessing the skin of underlying areas that will be distal to the bandage for signs of circulatory impairment (coolness, pallor or cyanosis, diminished or absent pulses, swelling, numbness, and tingling) to provide a means for comparing changes in circulation after bandage application

After applying a bandage, the nurse assesses, documents, and immediately reports changes in circulation, skin integrity, comfort level, and body function (e.g., ventilation or movement). The nurse who applies a bandage loosens or readjusts it as necessary. He or she needs a health care provider's order before loosening or removing a bandage applied by the health care provider. The nurse explains to the patient that any bandage or binder feels relatively firm or tight. Carefully assess a bandage to be sure that it is applied properly and providing therapeutic benefit and replace any soiled bandages.

Binder Application. Binders are especially designed for the body part to be supported. The most common type of binder is the abdominal binder (Box 48-12). An abdominal binder supports large abdominal incisions that are vulnerable to tension or stress as a patient moves or coughs (Figure 48-29). Secure an abdominal binder with safety pins or Velcro strips.

Slings. Slings support arms with muscular sprains or fractures. A commercially manufactured sling consists of a long sleeve that extends above the elbow with a strap that fits around the neck. In the home patients can use a large triangular piece of cloth. The patient sits or lies supine during sling application (Figure 48-30). Instruct him or her to bend the affected arm, bringing the forearm straight across the chest. The open sling fits under the patient's arm and over the chest, with the base of the triangle under the wrist and the point of the triangle at his or her elbow. One end of the sling fits around the back of the patient's neck. Bring the other end up and over the affected arm while supporting the extremity. Tie the two ends at the side of the neck so the knot does not press against the cervical spine. Fold the loose material at the elbow evenly around the elbow and then pin to secure. Always support the lower arm and hand at a level above the elbow to prevent the formation of dependent edema.

Roll Bandage Application. Rolls of bandage secure or support dressings over irregularly shaped body parts. Each roll has a free outer end and a terminal end at the center of the roll. The rolled part of the bandage is its body, and its outer surface is placed against the patient's skin or dressing. Skill 48-6 on pp. 1236-1237 describes the steps for applying an elastic bandage. Use a variety of bandage turns, depending on the body part to be bandaged.

Heat and Cold Therapy

Assessment for Temperature Tolerance. Before applying heat or cold therapies, assess a patient's physical condition for signs of potential intolerance to heat and cold. First observe the area to be treated. Assess the skin, looking for any open areas such as alterations in skin integrity (e.g., abrasions, open wounds, edema, bruising, bleeding, or localized areas of inflammation) that increase a patient's risk for injury. Because a health care provider commonly orders heat and cold applications for traumatized areas, the baseline skin assessment provides a guide for evaluating skin changes that can occur during therapy. Also assess neurological function, testing for sensation to light touch, pinprick, and mild temperature variations (see Chapter 31). Sensory status reveals the ability of a patient to recognize when heat or cold becomes excessive. Assess a patient's mental status to be sure that he or she can correctly communicate any issues with the hot or cold therapy. Level of consciousness influences the ability to perceive heat, cold, and pain. If a patient is confused or unresponsive, the nurse needs to make frequent observations of skin integrity after therapy begins.

Assessment also includes identification of conditions that contraindicate heat or cold therapy. Do not cover an active area of bleeding with a warm application because bleeding will continue. Warm applications are contraindicated when a patient has an acute, localized inflammation such as appendicitis because the heat could cause the

BOX 48-12 PROCEDURAL GUIDELINES

Applying a Binder

Delegation Considerations

The skill of applying an abdominal binder can be delegated to nursing assistive personnel (NAP). The nurse is responsible for wound assessment; the evaluation of wound-care interventions and assessment of the patient's ability to breathe deeply, cough effectively, and move independently; and assessment of skin for irritation/abrasion, of incision/wound and dressing, and of comfort level before a binder or sling is applied for the first time. Direct the NAP to:

- Immediately notify the nurse of any change in patient's respiratory status.
- Report any increase in wound drainage to the nurse.
- Report any changes in skin integrity under or adjacent to the binder to the nurse.
- Remove the binder at prescribed intervals.

Equipment

Gloves if wound drainage is present; abdominal binder; correct size cloth/elastic straight binder; safety pins (unless Velcro closure or metal fasteners are attached): six to eight safety pins are usually adequate for abdominal binders

Steps

1. Identify patient using two identifiers (e.g., name and birthday or name and medical record number) according to agency policy.
2. Observe patient with need for support of abdomen. Observe ability to breathe deeply and cough effectively.
3. Review medical record if medical order for binder is required and reasons for application.
4. Inspect skin for actual or potential alterations in integrity. Observe for irritation, abrasion, skin surfaces that rub against one another, or allergic response to adhesive tape used to secure dressing.
5. Inspect any surgical dressing.
6. Assess patient's comfort level, using analog scale of 0 to 10 and noting any objective signs and symptoms.
7. Explain procedure to patient and family.
8. Perform hand hygiene and apply gloves (if likely to contact wound drainage).
9. Apply abdominal binder.
   a. Position patient in supine position with head slightly elevated and knees slightly flexed.
   b. Fanfold far side of binder toward midline of binder.
   c. Instruct and help patient to roll onto side away from you and toward raised side rail while firmly supporting abdominal incision and dressing with hands.
   d. Place fan-folded ends of binder under patient.
   e. Instruct or help patient to roll back over folded ends.
   f. Unfold and stretch ends out smoothly on far side of bed.
   g. Instruct patient to roll back into supine position.
   h. Adjust binder so supine patient is centered over it, using symphysis pubis and costal margins as lower and upper landmarks.
   i. Close binder. Pull one end of binder over center of patient's abdomen. While maintaining tension on that end of binder, pull opposite end over center and secure with Velcro closure tabs, metal fasteners, or horizontally placed safety pins.
   j. Adjust binder as necessary.
10. ***Apply mastectomy sports bra:***
    a. Protect surgical incision with prescribed dressing.
    b. Slip arms in bra strap openings (same as putting on a blouse) opening to the front.
    c. Fasten bra.
    d. If using a bra with additional support straps or binder, follow manufacturer instructions in application.

CLINICAL DECISION: Assess patient's ability to breathe deeply and cough effectively.

11. Remove and dispose of gloves and perform hand hygiene.
12. Observe site for skin integrity, circulation, and characteristics of wound. (Periodically remove binder and surgical dressing to assess wound characteristics.)
13. Evaluate comfort level of patient, using analog scale of 0 to 10 and noting any objective signs and symptoms.
14. Evaluate patient's ability to ventilate properly, including deep breathing and coughing.
15. Use ***Teach Back*** to determine if the patient understands about binder application. State, "I want to be sure that you understand how to correctly apply the binder. Can you demonstrate how to apply the binder?" Revise your instruction now or develop plan for revised patient teaching if patient is not able to correctly demonstrate bandage application.

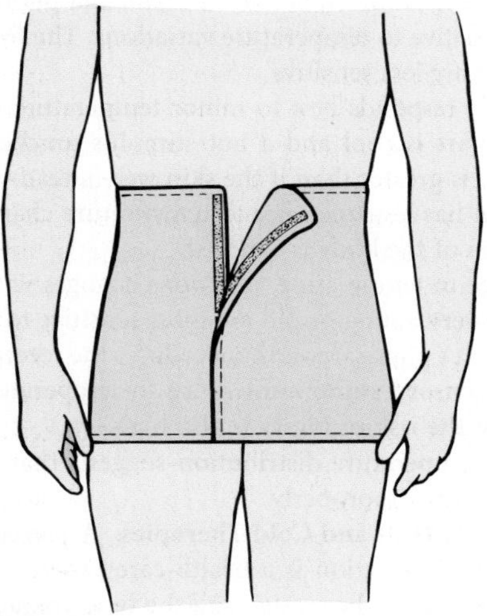

FIGURE 48-29 Securing abdominal binder with Velcro.

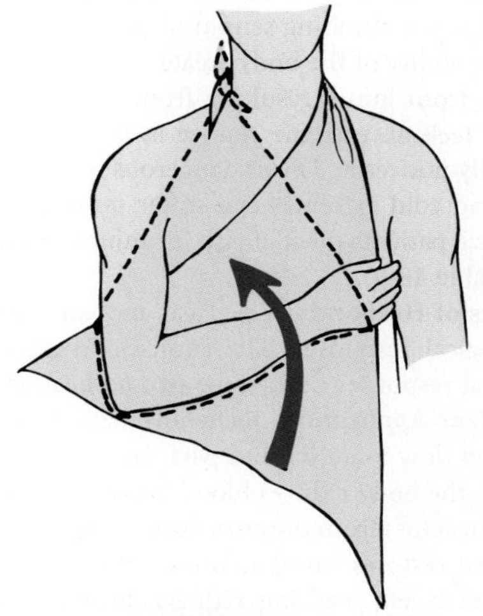

FIGURE 48-30 Application of sling.

appendix to rupture. If a patient has cardiovascular problems, it is unwise to apply heat to large parts of the body because the resulting massive vasodilation disrupts blood supply to vital organs.

Cold is contraindicated if the site of injury is already edematous. It further retards circulation to the area and prevents absorption of the interstitial fluid. If a patient has impaired circulation (e.g., arteriosclerosis), it further reduces blood supply to the affected area. Cold therapy is also contraindicated in the presence of neuropathy, because the patient is unable to perceive temperature change and damage resulting from temperature extremes. One other contraindication for cold therapy is shivering. Cold applications sometimes intensify shivering and dangerously increase body temperature.

If a patient has peripheral vascular disease, pay particular attention to the integrity of extremities. For example, if the health care provider's order is to apply a cold compress to a lower extremity, assess circulation to the leg by assessing for capillary refill; observing skin color; and palpating skin temperatures, distal pulses, and edematous areas. If signs of circulatory inadequacy are present, it is important for you to question the order.

When applying heat or cold pads, check electrical equipment for cracked cords, frayed wires, damaged insulation, and exposed heating components. Make sure that equipment containing circulating fluids does not have leaks. Check equipment for evenness of temperature distribution.

Local application of heat and cold to an injured body part is sometimes therapeutic. You are legally responsible to perform necessary assessments for safe administration of heat and cold applications.

Bodily Responses to Heat and Cold. Exposure to heat and cold causes systemic and local responses. Systemic responses occur through heat-loss mechanisms (sweating and vasodilation) or mechanisms promoting heat conservation (vasoconstriction and piloerection) and heat production (shivering) (see Chapter 30). Local responses to heat and cold occur through stimulation of temperature-sensitive nerve endings within the skin. This stimulation sends impulses from the periphery to the hypothalamus, which becomes aware of local temperature sensations and triggers adaptive responses for maintenance of normal body temperature. If alterations occur along temperature sensation pathways, the reception and eventual perception of stimuli are altered.

The body is able to tolerate wide variations in temperature. The normal temperature of the surface of the skin is 34°C (93.2°F), but temperature receptors usually adapt quickly to local temperatures between 15° and 45°C (59° and 113°F). Pain develops when local temperatures exceed this range. Excessive heat causes a burning sensation. Cold produces a numbing sensation before pain.

The adaptive ability of the body creates the major problem in protecting patients from injury resulting from temperature extremes. A person initially feels an extreme change in temperature but within a short time hardly notices it. This is dangerous because a person insensitive to heat and cold extremes can suffer serious tissue injury. You need to recognize patients most at risk for injuries from heat and cold applications (Table 48-9).

Local Effects of Heat and Cold. Heat and cold stimuli create different physiological responses. The choice of heat or cold therapy depends on local responses desired for wound healing (Table 48-10).

Effects of Heat Application. Generally heat is quite therapeutic, improving blood flow to an injured part. However, if it is applied for 1 hour or more, the body reduces blood flow by a reflex vasoconstriction to control heat loss from the area. Periodic removal and reapplication of local heat restores vasodilation. Continuous exposure to heat damages epithelial cells, causing redness, localized tenderness, and even blistering.

TABLE 48-9 Conditions That Increase Risk of Injury from Heat and Cold Application

Condition	Risk Factors
Very young or older patients	Thinner skin layers in children increase risk of burns. Older patients have reduced sensitivity to pain and may not perceive any pain associated with heat or cold applications.
Open wounds, broken skin, stomas	Subcutaneous and visceral tissues are more sensitive to temperature variations. They also contain no temperature and fewer pain receptors.
Areas of edema or scar formation	Reduced sensation to temperature stimuli occurs because of thickening of skin layers from fluid buildup or scar formation.
Peripheral vascular disease (e.g., diabetes, arteriosclerosis)	As a result of decreased peripheral circulation, extremities are less sensitive to temperature and pain stimuli because of circulatory impairment and local tissue injury. Cold application further compromises blood flow.
Confusion or unconsciousness	Perception of sensory or painful stimuli is reduced.
Spinal cord injury	Alterations in nerve pathways prevent reception of sensory or painful stimuli.
Abscessed tooth or appendix	Infection is highly localized. Application of heat causes rupture, with spread of microorganisms systemically.

Effects of Cold Application. The application of cold initially diminishes swelling and pain. Prolonged exposure of the skin to cold results in a reflex vasodilation. The inability of the cells to receive adequate blood flow and nutrients results in tissue ischemia. The skin initially takes on a reddened appearance, followed by a bluish-purple mottling, with numbness and a burning type of pain. Skin tissues freeze from exposure to extreme cold.

Factors Influencing Heat and Cold Tolerance. The response of the body to heat and cold therapies depends on the following factors:

- A person is better able to tolerate short exposure to temperature extremes than prolonged exposure.
- Exposed skin layers and certain areas of the skin (e.g., the neck, inner aspect of the wrist and forearm, and perineal region) are more sensitive to temperature variations. The foot and palm of the hand are less sensitive.
- The body responds best to minor temperature adjustments. If a body part is cool and a hot stimulus touches the skin, the response is greater than if the skin were already warm.
- A person has less tolerance to temperature changes to which a large area of the body is exposed.
- Tolerance to temperature variations changes with age. Patients who are very young or old are most sensitive to heat and cold.
- If a patient's physical condition reduces the reception or perception of sensory stimuli, tolerance to temperature extremes is high, but the risk of injury is also high.
- Uneven temperature distribution suggests that the equipment is functioning improperly.

Application of Heat and Cold Therapies. A prerequisite to using any heat or cold application is a health care provider's order, which includes the body site to be treated and the type, frequency, and duration of application. Safety guidelines for the use of heat and cold are

TABLE 48-10 Therapeutic Effects of Heat and Cold Applications

Physiological Response	Therapeutic Benefit	Examples of Conditions Treated
Heat		
Vasodilation	Improves blood flow to injured body part; promotes delivery of nutrients and removal of wastes; lessens venous congestion in injured tissues (Ebbinghaus and Kobayashi, 2010)	Open wounds, rectal surgery, episiotomy, painful hemorrhoids, muscle tension, vaginal inflammation, wound debridement
Reduced blood viscosity	Improves delivery of leukocytes and antibiotics to wound site	
Reduced muscle tension	Promotes muscle relaxation and reduces pain from spasm or stiffness (Bleakley and Costello, 2013)	
Increased tissue metabolism	Increases blood flow; provides local warmth	
Increased capillary permeability	Promotes movement of waste products and nutrients	
Cold		
Vasoconstriction	Reduces blood flow to injured body part, preventing edema formation; reduces inflammation	Direct trauma (sprains, strains, fractures, muscle spasms), superficial laceration or puncture wound, minor burn, suspected malignancy in area of injury or pain, injections, arthritis, and joint trauma
Local anesthesia	Reduces localized pain (Maxwell and Sterling, 2013)	
Reduced cell metabolism	Reduces oxygen needs of tissues	
Increased blood viscosity	Promotes blood coagulation at injury site	
Decreased muscle tension	Relieves pain	

summarized in Box 48-13. Consult agency procedure manual for correct temperatures to use.

You can administer heat and cold applications in dry or moist forms. The type of wound or injury, the location of the body part, and the presence of drainage or inflammation are factors to consider in selecting dry or moist applications. Box 48-14 summarizes advantages and disadvantages of both.

Warm, Moist Compresses. Warm, moist compresses improve circulation, relieve edema, and promote consolidation of purulent drainage. A compress is a piece of gauze dressing moistened in a prescribed warmed solution. A pack is a larger cloth or dressing applied to a larger body area.

Heat from warm compresses dissipates quickly. To maintain a constant temperature, you need to change the compress often. You can use a layer of plastic wrap or a dry towel to insulate the compress and retain heat. Moist heat promotes vasodilation and evaporation of heat from the surface of the skin. For this reason a patient can feel chilly. Always try to control drafts within the room and keep the patient covered with a blanket or robe.

Warm Soaks. Immersion of a body part in a warmed solution promotes circulation, lessens edema, increases muscle relaxation, and provides a means to apply medicated solution. Sometimes a soak is also accompanied by wrapping the body part in dressings and saturating them with the warmed solution.

Position the patient comfortably, place waterproof pads under the area to be treated, and heat the solution to about 40.5° to 43°C (105°

BOX 48-13 Safety Suggestions for Applying Heat or Cold Therapy

- *Explain* to patient sensations to be felt during the procedure.
- *Prevention:* Injuries from heat and cold therapies are preventable (NQF, 2011).
- *Instruct* patient that exposed layers of skin are more sensitive to heat and cold application than intact skin. Therefore instruct patient and family to protect skin when applying heat or cold therapy.
- *Instruct* patient to report changes in sensation or discomfort immediately.
- *Provide* a timer, clock, or watch so patient can help the nurse time the application.
- *Check* patient and skin frequently every 20 minutes during therapy. Observe for excess redness, pain, tingling.
- *Keep* the call light within patient's reach.
- *Refer* to the policy and procedure manual of the institution for safe temperatures.
- *Do not* allow patient to adjust temperature settings.
- *Do not* allow patient to move an application or place hands on the wound site.
- *Do not* place patient in a position that prevents movement away from the temperature source.
- *Do not* leave unattended a patient who is unable to sense temperature changes or move from the temperature source.

BOX 48-14 Choice of Dry or Moist Applications

Advantages

Moist Applications

- Moist application reduces drying of skin and softens wound exudate.
- Moist compresses conform well to most body areas.
- Moist heat penetrates deeply into tissue layers.
- Warm moist heat does not promote sweating and insensible fluid loss.

Dry Applications

- Dry heat has less risk of burns to skin than moist applications.
- Dry application does not cause skin maceration.
- Dry heat retains temperature longer because evaporation does not occur.

Disadvantages

Moist Applications

- Prolonged exposure causes maceration of skin.
- Moist heat cools rapidly because of moisture evaporation.
- Moist heat creates greater risk for burns to skin because moisture conducts heat.

Dry Applications

- Dry heat increases body fluid loss through sweating.
- Dry applications do not penetrate deep into tissues.
- Dry heat causes increased drying of skin.

to 110°F). After immersing the body part, cover the container and extremity with a towel to reduce heat loss. It is usually necessary to remove the cooled solution and add heated solution after about 10 minutes. The challenge is to keep the solution at a constant temperature. Never add a hotter solution while the body part remains immersed. After any soak dry the body part thoroughly to prevent maceration.

Sitz Baths. A patient who has had rectal surgery, an episiotomy during childbirth, painful hemorrhoids, or vaginal inflammation benefits from a sitz bath, a bath in which only the pelvic area is immersed in warm or, in some situations, cool fluid. The patient sits in a special tub or chair or a basin that fits on the toilet seat so the legs and feet remain out of the water. Immersing the entire body causes widespread vasodilation and nullifies the effect of local heat application to the pelvic area.

The desired temperature for a sitz bath depends on whether the purpose is to promote relaxation or to clean a wound. It is often necessary to add warm or cool water during the procedure, which normally lasts 20 minutes, to maintain a constant temperature. Agency procedure manuals recommend safe water temperatures. A disposable sitz basin contains an attachment resembling an enema bag that allows gradual introduction of additional water.

Prevent overexposure of patients by draping bath blankets around their shoulders and thighs and controlling drafts. A patient should be able to sit in the basin or tub with feet flat on the floor and without pressure on the sacrum or thighs. Because exposure of a large part of the body to heat causes extensive vasodilation, assess the pulse and facial color and ask whether the patient feels light-headed or nauseated.

Commercial Hot and Cold Packs. Commercially prepared disposable hot packs apply warm, dry heat to an injured area. The chemicals mix and release heat when you strike, knead, or squeeze the pack. Package directions recommend the time for heat application.

Commercially prepared cold packs that are similar to the disposable hot packs for dry applications are available. They come in various shapes and sizes to fit different body parts. When using cold compresses, observe for adverse reactions such as burning or numbness, mottling of the skin, redness, extreme paleness, and a bluish skin discoloration.

Cold, Moist, and Dry Compresses. The procedure for applying cold, moist compresses is the same as that for warm compresses. Apply cold compresses for 20 minutes at a temperature of 15°C (59°F) to relieve inflammation and swelling. You can use clean or sterile compresses.

Cold Soaks. The procedure for preparing cold soaks and immersing a body part is the same as for warm soaks. The desired temperature for a 20-minute cold soak is 15°C (59°F). Control drafts and use outer coverings to protect the patient from chilling. It is often necessary to add cold water during the procedure to maintain a constant temperature.

Ice Bags or Collars. For a patient who has a muscle sprain, localized hemorrhage, or hematoma or who has undergone dental surgery, an ice bag is ideal to prevent edema formation, control bleeding, and anesthetize the body part. Proper use of the bag requires the following steps:

1. Fill the bag with water, secure the cap, invert to check for leaks, and pour out the water.
2. Fill the bag two-thirds full with crushed ice so you are able to easily mold it over a body part.
3. Release any air from the bag by squeezing its sides before securing the cap because excess air interferes with conduction of cold.
4. Wipe off excess moisture.
5. Cover the bag with a flannel cover, towel, or pillowcase.
6. Apply the bag to the injury site for 30 minutes; you can reapply the bag in an hour.

◆ Evaluation

You evaluate nursing interventions for reducing and treating pressure ulcers by determining the patient's response to nursing therapies and whether he or she achieved each goal. To evaluate outcomes and responses to care, you measure the effectiveness of interventions. The optimal outcomes are to prevent injury to the skin, to reduce injury to the skin and underlying tissues, and possible wound healing with restoration of skin integrity.

Through the Patient's Eyes. It is important to include the patient and family caregiver in the evaluation process. Review whether their expectations of care were met. For example, is the patient satisfied with the level of comfort achieved during wound care? Chronic wounds such as pressure ulcers take time to heal, so home care is likely. Does the patient feel comfortable or confident in being able to perform wound care at home? Does the family caregiver feel she or she has the information needed to know when to report a problem with a wound? If patient and family caregiver expectations are unmet, revise your plan of care to select the best ways to support and re-educate.

Patient Outcomes. The outcomes selected for a patient in the plan of care are the milestones you hope to achieve in order to meet goals of care. Each patient will have unique outcomes depending on whether he or she has an actual wound or is at risk to develop a wound. You evaluate nursing interventions for reducing and treating pressure ulcers by determining the patient's response to nursing therapies and whether he or she achieved each goal (Figure 48-31).

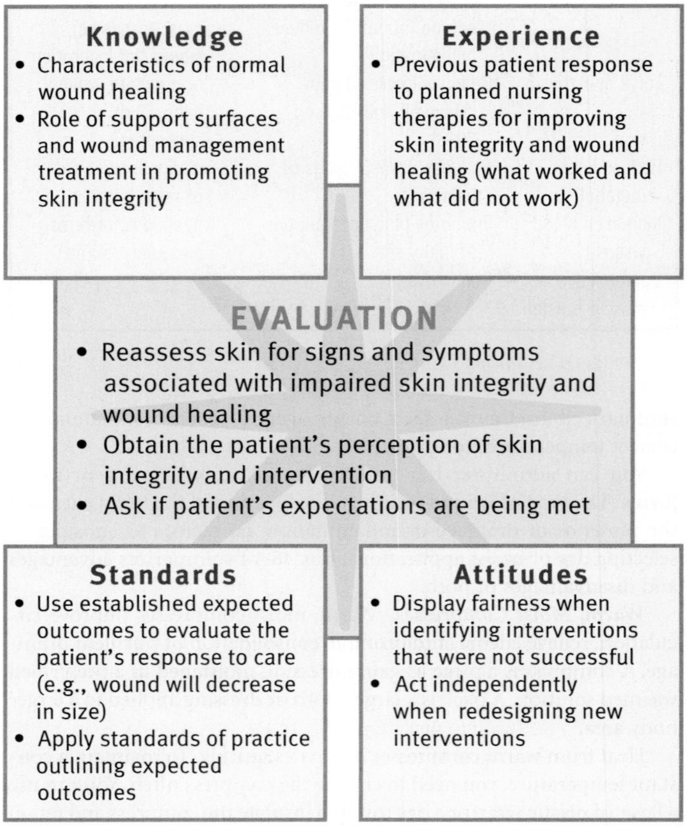

Knowledge
- Characteristics of normal wound healing
- Role of support surfaces and wound management treatment in promoting skin integrity

Experience
- Previous patient response to planned nursing therapies for improving skin integrity and wound healing (what worked and what did not work)

EVALUATION
- Reassess skin for signs and symptoms associated with impaired skin integrity and wound healing
- Obtain the patient's perception of skin integrity and intervention
- Ask if patient's expectations are being met

Standards
- Use established expected outcomes to evaluate the patient's response to care (e.g., wound will decrease in size)
- Apply standards of practice outlining expected outcomes

Attitudes
- Display fairness when identifying interventions that were not successful
- Act independently when redesigning new interventions

FIGURE 48-31 Critical thinking model for skin integrity and wound-care evaluation.

You will evaluate patients with impaired skin integrity on an ongoing basis for factors that contribute to skin breakdown and wound status. For example, during direct patient contact, if a patient continues to be diaphoretic or incontinent, apply wound assessment skills to note the condition of the skin and decide if additional therapies are needed. Your evaluation will include elements of a comprehensive skin reassessment. Use a validated wound assessment tool when appropriate. Evaluation provides information regarding the patient's progress toward wound healing or maintenance of skin integrity.

If the identified outcomes are not met for a patient with impaired skin integrity, questions to ask include the following:

- Was the etiology of the skin impairment addressed? Were the pressure, friction, shear, and moisture components identified; and did the plan of care decrease the contribution of each of these components?
- Was wound healing supported by providing the wound base with a moist protected environment?
- Were issues such as nutrition assessed and a plan of care developed that provided the patient with the calories to support healing?

Finally evaluate the need for additional referrals to other experts in wound care and pressure ulcers such as nurses certified in wound care. Care of patients with a pressure ulcer or wound requires a multidisciplinary team approach.

SAFETY GUIDELINES FOR NURSING SKILLS

Ensuring patient safety is an essential role of the professional nurse. To ensure patient safety, communicate clearly with all members of the health care team, assess and incorporate a patient's priorities of care and preferences, and use the best evidence when making decisions about care. When performing the skills in this chapter, remember the following points to ensure safe, individualized patient-centered care:

- When changing wound dressings, follow proper aseptic technique. Keep a plastic bag within reach to discard dressings and prevent cross-contamination. Keep extra gloves within reach to allow a change of gloves if the gloves become soiled.
- If irrigating a wound, use goggles and other personal protective equipment when the risk for splash exists.
- When applying an elastic bandage, check the extremity where the bandage is applied for temperature or sensation changes.

SKILL 48-1 ASSESSMENT FOR PRESSURE ULCER DEVELOPMENT

DELEGATION CONSIDERATIONS

The skill of assessing patients for risk of pressure ulcers cannot be delegated to nursing assistive personnel (NAP). Instruct the NAP to:

- Report any changes to patient's skin such as redness, blistering, abrasion, or cuts to nurse for further nursing assessment.
- Keep patient's skin dry and provide hygiene following fecal or urinary incontinence or exposure to other body fluids.
- Reposition patient according to frequency established on nursing care plan or agency policy.
- Avoid trauma to patient's skin from tape, pressure, friction, or shear.

EQUIPMENT

- Risk assessment tool, Braden Scale
- Documentation record
- Clean gloves when open wound is present

STEP	RATIONALE
ASSESSMENT	
1. Identify patient using two identifiers (e.g., name and birthday or name and medical record number) according to agency policy.	Ensures correct patient. Complies with The Joint Commission standards and improves patient safety (TJC, 2016).
2. Inspect skin during the patient admission process and at least each shift for at-risk individuals needing prevention and for specific factors placing them at risk.	Determines factors that increase patient's risk for developing pressure ulcers (Bryant and Nix, 2016).
a. Use validated risk assessment tool such as Braden Scale. Assess patient and obtain risk score on admission to acute care, critical care rehabilitation hospitals, nursing homes, home care programs, and other health care facilities.	Pressure ulcer assessment scale provides objective baseline assessment. It should be used for all patients with one of more risk factors for pressure ulcer development: restricted mobility, moisture, impaired sensation, impaired nutrition, and medical devices such as casts or drainage tubes (Bryant and Nix, 2016).
3. Assess patient's level of consciousness and ability to respond meaningfully (e.g., move away) to pressure-related discomfort (sensory perception).	Patient with complete or partial limited ability to respond to pressure-related discomfort cannot communicate discomfort, has a limitation in ability to feel pain, and thus is at risk for developing pressure ulcers.
4. Perform hand hygiene. Apply clean gloves and conduct a systematic skin assessment from head to toe with special attention to the areas over bony prominences.	Bony prominences are at high risk of skin breakdown because of high pressures exerted on the area. If a patient has restricted mobility or other risk factor, risk for skin breakdown over bony prominences increases (Bryant and Nix, 2016).
a. Observe at-risk areas, including back of head, shoulders, ribs, hips, sacral region, ischium, inner and outer knees, inner and outer ankles, heels, and feet (see Figure 48-9).	The presence of redness or impairment in skin integrity necessitates planning appropriate interventions.

SKILL 48-1 ASSESSMENT FOR PRESSURE ULCER DEVELOPMENT—cont'd

STEP	RATIONALE
5. Assess the following potential sites for skin breakdown related to medical devices:	Pressure from medical devices or how the device is secured increases a patient's risk for tissue injury and skin breakdown under and around the device (Fletcher, 2012; McNichol et al., 2013).
a. Ears and nares	Cartilage that nasal cannulas or tubing compresses develops pressure necrosis.
b. Lips	Oral airway and endotracheal tubes exert pressure if left in place for prolonged time periods.
c. Tube sites (e.g., gastrostomy or nasogastric tubes, Foley catheters, Jackson-Pratt drains)	Tubes exert pressure if taped snugly against skin or if there is stress at insertion site (Black et al., 2015). If moisture is present around tube insertion sites, leakage of bodily fluids compromises skin integrity.
d. Orthopedic and positioning devices (e.g., casts, braces, cervical collar)	Improperly fitted or applied devices have potential to cause pressure on adjacent skin and underlying tissue (Black et al., 2010, 2015).
6. Assess all skin surfaces for the following:	
a. Absence of superficial skin layers	Damage of superficial skin layers indicates injury from friction or moisture. The area is moist and sore to the touch.
b. Blisters	Suggests skin damage from friction and/or inappropriate tape removal (McNichol et al., 2013). Blisters occur when top layer of skin is pulled or rubbed, separating epidermis from dermis.
c. Any loss of epidermis and dermis	Indicates damage to skin. Determine cause of this damage in order to select interventions to prevent further damage.
7. Assess degree to which patient's skin is exposed to moisture. If necessary, remove gloves to palpate skin surface. Then dispose of gloves and perform hand hygiene.	Exposure to excessive moisture increases risk for maceration and skin breakdown (Bryant, 2016; Colwell et al., 2011).
8. Assess patient's activity level.	Patient who is bedfast or chairfast or only walks occasionally is at risk for developing pressure areas because of the degree of physical inactivity (WOCN, 2010).
a. Determine patient's ability to change and control body position (mobility).	Potential for friction and shear increases when patient is completely dependent on others for position change.
b. Determine patient's preferred positions.	Weight of body is on certain bony prominences, and patient resists repositioning off these areas.
9. Assess patient's usual food intake pattern (nutrition).	Patient who rarely or never eats a complete meal is at risk for pressure ulcer formation.
a. Review recent weight pattern over last month, daily calorie intake, and nutritional laboratory values.	Decreased nutrition status is linked with pressure ulcer formation and poor wound healing (WOCN, 2010).
b. Complete fluid intake assessment.	Fluid imbalance, either dehydration or edema, increases patient's risk for pressure ulcers (Stotts, 2016a).
10. Assess presence of friction and/or shear.	Patient who has a problem moving, requires maximum assistance in moving, or slides against sheets when moved is at an increased risk of skin damage (Bryant, 2016).
PLANNING	
1. Explain procedures for reducing pressure ulcer risk patient.	Promotes patient cooperation and reduces anxiety.
IMPLEMENTATION	
1. Note score on Braden risk assessment scale.	Documentation provides a baseline for comparison of increased or decreased risk for development of pressure ulcers and allows planning of interventions.
a. As Braden Scale scores become lower, predicted risk becomes higher.	*Scores:* 15 to 18, at risk general population, 13 at risk ICU patients 13 to 14, moderate risk 10 to 12, high risk 9 or below, very high risk
b. Link risk assessment to preventive protocols. Perform hand hygiene and apply gloves.	Protocols target the problem areas to help prevent skin breakdown.
(1) Institute at-risk interventions (score of 15 to 18). Consider instituting frequent turning, protecting patient's heels, using a pressure-redistribution surface, and managing moisture.	Decreases risk of skin breakdown.
(2) Institute moderate-risk interventions (score of 13 to 14). Consider protocol of frequent turning; protecting patient's heels; providing pressure-redistribution surface; providing foam wedges for 30-degree lateral positioning; and managing moisture, shear, and friction.	Decreases pressure on bony prominences and reduces increased risk of skin breakdown.

STEP	RATIONALE
(3) Institute high-risk interventions (score of 10 to 12). Consider protocol that increases frequency of turning; supplements turning with small shifts in position; facilitates maximal remobilization; protects patient's heels; provides pressure-redistribution surface; provides foam wedges for 30-degree lateral positioning; and manages moisture, friction, and shear. If needed, institute nutritional interventions to reduce risk of pressure ulcer development.	Addresses factors that contribute to skin breakdown and plans for interventions to address causative factors (Bryant, 2016). Nutrition therapy promotes skin healing (Stotts, 2016a).
(4) Institute very high–risk interventions (score of 9 or below). Consider protocol that incorporates points for high-risk patients and uses pressure-redistribution surface if patient has intractable pain or severe pain exacerbated by turning.	Plans interventions to decrease effects of immobility, decreased sensory perception, moisture, friction, shear, decreased activity, and nutritional issues in high-risk individual.
2. When you note a reddened area, check for the following:	
a. Skin discoloration (e.g., redness in light-tone skin; purplish or bluish in darkly pigmented skin) (see Box 48-3)	May indicate that tissue was under pressure.
b. Blanchable erythema	Blanchable erythema is an early indication of pressure and usually resolves without tissue loss if pressure is eliminated. Blanching erythema is an area of erythema that turns white (blanches) under application of pressure (Pieper, 2016).
c. Nonblanchable erythema	Indicates potential damage to blood vessels and tissue damage. Once blood vessels are damaged, red area will not lighten in color because tissue and blood vessels are inflamed. Color of skin can be intense bright red to dark red or purple (Pieper, 2016). Position patient off area.
d. Pallor or mottling	Persistent hypoxia in tissues alters circulation, and pallor or mottling may occur.
3. Remove gloves and perform hand hygiene. Reposition patient in 30-degree lateral position (see Figure 48-15).	Reduces transmission of infection. Positions patient off bony prominences.
4. Educate patient and family regarding specific pressure ulcer risk factors and prevention.	Helps patients and family understand and adhere to interventions designed to reduce pressure ulcer risk (Berlowitz, 2014a).
EVALUATION	
1. Observe condition of patient's skin each shift, especially areas at risk (check agency policy).	Determines over time patient's response to risk-redistribution interventions.
2. Observe tolerance of patient for positioning.	Frequent change in position further reduces patient's risk for pressure ulcer development.
3. Compare current risk assessment with previous scores.	Documents effectiveness of interventions and helps provide individualized plan of care.
4. Evaluate food intake and nutrition laboratory values.	Determines success of nutritional supplements in improving nutritional status.
5. Use ***Teach Back*** to determine patient's and family's understanding about pressure ulcer risk and prevention. State, "I want to be sure I explained the reasons why you are at risk to get a pressure ulcer. Can you explain to me the pressure ulcer risk factors that affect you?" Revise your instruction now or develop plan for revised patient teaching if patient is not able to teach back correctly.	Evaluates what patient and family are able to explain or demonstrate.

UNEXPECTED OUTCOMES AND RELATED INTERVENTIONS

1. Skin does not blanch when firmly pressed, has purple discoloration, or has significant color change.
   - Reassess frequency of turning schedule.
   - Implement agency skin-care protocols.
   - Consider use of pressure-redistribution surface to reduce pressure ulcer risk.

RECORDING AND REPORTING

- Record patient's risk score and appearance of skin under pressure in progress notes in EHR or chart.
- Record position, turning intervals, pressure-redistribution devices, and other prevention strategies used and patient response in EHR or chart.
- Report any need for additional consultations for the high-risk patient.
- Document your evaluation of patient learning.

HOME CARE CONSIDERATIONS

- Instruct family caregiver in use of the 30-degree lateral position and how to assist patient into the position. This position prolongs the time between position changes, resulting in fewer sleep interruptions for patient and caregiver.
- Individualize pressure-redistribution maneuvers for patient needs and home environment.
- Provide family with community resources for hospital equipment.

SKILL 48-2 TREATING PRESSURE ULCERS

DELEGATION CONSIDERATIONS

The skill of treating pressure ulcers cannot be delegated to nursing assistive personnel (NAP). In some practice settings you can delegate *nonsterile* dressing application for chronic, established wounds when a nurse has evaluated and designated a protocol. The nurse is responsible for *assessment* of the wound, even if the dressing change is delegated. Instruct the NAP to:

- Report changes in skin integrity to the nurse immediately.
- Report pain, fever, or wound drainage to the nurse immediately.
- Report any potential contamination to existing dressing (e.g., patient incontinence or other bodily fluids; dressing becomes dislodged).

EQUIPMENT

- Clean gloves
  - Sterile gloves (check agency policy)
- Goggles and personal protective equipment if splash risk is present
- Plastic bag for dressing disposal
- Measuring device
- Cotton-tipped applicators
- Topical cleaning agent
- Dressing of choice (see Table 48-8)
- Hypoallergenic tape (if needed)
- Documentation record
- Scale for assessing wound healing

STEP	RATIONALE
ASSESSMENT	
1. Identify patient using two identifiers (e.g., name and birthday or name and medical record number) according to agency policy.	Ensures correct patient. Complies with The Joint Commission standards and improves patient safety (TJC, 2016).
2. Assess patient's level of comfort using a scale of 0 to 10 and determine need for pain medication.	Patients tolerate dressing change procedure better if pain is controlled. Some dressings may also contain a foam preparation of an analgesic such as ibuprofen to help in patient comfort (Berlowitz, 2014b).
3. Determine if patient has allergies to topical agents.	Topical agents cause localized skin reactions.
4. Review order for topical agent or dressing and location.	Ensures that you administer proper medication and treatment.
5. Close room door or bedside curtains. Describe to patient what will be done. Position patient to allow for access to ulcer and dressing removal.	Provides privacy and ensures that area is accessible for dressing change. Decreases patient's anxiety.
6. Perform hand hygiene and apply clean gloves. Remove dressing and place in plastic bag. If glove is soiled with drainage, remove, perform hand hygiene, and then reglove.	Reduces transmission of microorganisms and prevents accidental exposure to body fluids.
7. Assess pressure ulcer(s).	Consistent assessment provides basis for evaluating wound progress (Nix, 2016).
a. Note color, type, and percentage of tissue type present in wound base.	Tissue type helps in choice of dressing.
b. Measure width and length of ulcer(s). Determine width by measuring from left to right and length from top to bottom using a measuring device (see illustration).	Ulcer size changes as healing progresses; therefore the longest and widest areas of the wound change over time. Measuring width and length by measuring consistent areas provides a consistent measurement (Nix, 2016).
c. Measure depth of pressure ulcer with sterile cotton-tipped applicator or other device that allows measurement of wound depth.	Depth measure is important for determining wound volume. Although surface area adequately represents tissue loss in stage II ulcers, volume more adequately represents tissue loss in stage III and IV wounds.
d. Measure depth of undermining by using a cotton-tipped applicator and gently probing under skin edges.	Undermining represents the loss of underlying tissue (subcutaneous and muscle). It indicates progressive tissue loss and needs to be accommodated with an appropriate dressing.
8. Assess periwound skin; check for maceration, redness, denuded area.	
9. Remove and discard gloves. Perform hand hygiene. Assist patient to comfortable position.	Reduces transmission of microorganisms.
10. Review medical record to assess for significant weight loss (>5% change in 30 days or > 10% in 180 days).	Patients who are underweight or losing weight need increased caloric and protein supplements (Berlowitz, 2014b; WOCN, 2010).

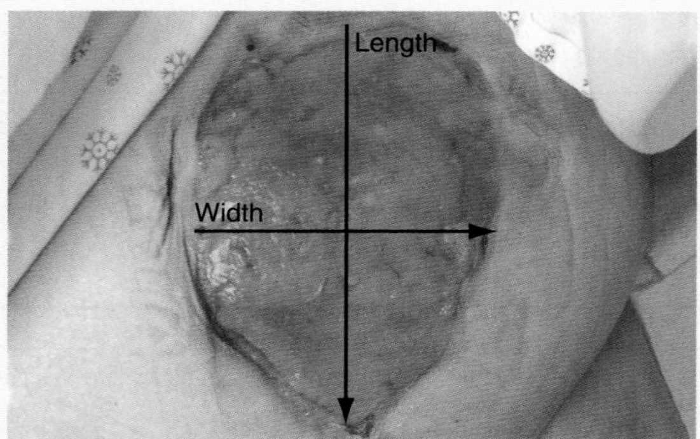

STEP 7b Measuring wound width, length, and undermining. (From Bryant RA, Nix DP, editors: *Acute and chronic wounds: current management concepts*, ed 5, St Louis, 2016, Elsevier.)

STEP	RATIONALE
PLANNING	
1. Explain procedure to patient and family.	Preparatory explanations relieve anxiety, correct any misconceptions about ulcer and its treatment, and offer opportunity for patient and family education.
2. Prepare the following necessary equipment and supplies:	
a. Washbasin, warm water, soap, washcloth, and bath towel	
b. Normal saline or other wound-cleaning agent in sterile-solution container	Ulcer surface must be cleaned before application of topical agents and new dressing.

CLINICAL DECISION: *Use only noncytotoxic agents such as normal saline or commercially available wound cleansers to clean ulcers.*

STEP	RATIONALE
c. Prescribed topical agent (e.g., enzymatic agents, topical antibiotic). Follow manufacturer instruction on package insert carefully.	Enzymes debride dead tissue to clean ulcer surface. Topical antibiotics are used to decrease bioburden of wound and should be considered for use if no healing is noted after 2 to 4 weeks of optimal care (WOCN, 2010).

CLINICAL DECISION: *If using enzymatic debriding agent, do not use wound-cleaning agents with metals.*

STEP	RATIONALE
d. Select appropriate dressing and tape on the basis of pressure ulcer characteristics, purpose for which dressing is intended, and patient care setting (see Table 48-8).	Dressing should maintain moist environment for wound while keeping surrounding skin dry.
3. Position patient to allow dressing removal and position plastic bag for dressing disposal.	Area should be accessible for dressing change. Proper disposal of old dressing promotes proper handling of contaminated waste.
IMPLEMENTATION	
1. Perform hand hygiene. Open sterile packages and topical solution containers as necessary.	Reduces transmission of microorganisms. Provides organized access to supplies.
2. Remove bed linen and patient's gown as necessary to expose ulcer and surrounding skin. Keep remaining parts covered and apply clean gloves.	Prevents unnecessary exposure of body parts. Reduces transmission of microorganisms.
3. Clean ulcer thoroughly with normal saline or cleaning agent. Clean with irrigating syringe for deep ulcers.	Removes wound debris.
4. Remove gloves, perform hand hygiene, and apply clean or sterile gloves.	Aseptic technique must be maintained during cleaning and all phases of pressure ulcer treatment. Check agency policy regarding use of clean or sterile gloves.
5. Apply topical agents as prescribed:	
a. **Debriding enzymes**	
(1) Apply thin, even layer of ointment over necrotic areas of ulcer only. Do not apply enzyme to surrounding skin. Check manufacturer directions for frequency of application.	Thin layer absorbs and acts more effectively than thick layer. Excess medication irritates surrounding skin (Rolstad et al., 2016). Some enzymes cause burning, paresthesia, and dermatitis to surrounding skin.
(2) Apply gauze dressing directly over ulcer.	Protects wound and keeps enzymes in place. Prevents bacteria from entering wound.
(3) Tape securely in place.	Keeps dressing in place.
b. **Hydrogel**	
(1) Cover surface of ulcer with hydrogel using applicator or gloved hand.	Hydrogel dressings are designed to hydrate and donate moisture to wound, thus facilitating moist wound healing (Rolstad et al., 2016).
(2) Apply dry gauze, hydrocolloid, or transparent film dressing over wound and adhere to intact skin.	Covers wound base, maintaining hydrogel wound interface.
c. **Calcium alginate**	Alginate dressings absorb serous fluid or exudate, forming a nonadhesive hydrophilic gel, which conforms to the shape of the wound (Rolstad et al., 2016).
(1) Pack wound with alginate using applicator or gloved hand.	Provides maintenance of wound moisture while absorbing excess drainage.
(2) Apply dry gauze or foam over alginate. Tape in place.	Holds alginate against wound surface.
6. Reposition patient comfortably off pressure area and other pressure points.	Reduces pressure on existing wound and decreases pressure on at-risk areas.
7. Remove gloves and dispose of soiled supplies. Perform hand hygiene.	Reduces transmission of microorganisms.
EVALUATION	
1. Evaluate condition of pressure ulcer at each dressing change or sooner if wound or patient's condition deteriorates (Nix, 2016). Use agency tool for wound assessment.	Not all patients with wounds demonstrate quick wound healing because of other health care issues. Wound evaluation provides a report of wound-healing progress or lack of it.
2. Compare wound findings (e.g., type and amount of drainage, wound size, appearance of tissue) to previous findings.	Evaluates progress of wound healing.

CLINICAL DECISION: *A clean pressure ulcer should show evidence of some healing within 2 to 4 weeks. Do not use the pressure ulcer staging system to measure healing. System measures depth of wound, not healing (WOCN, 2010).*

SKILL 48-2 TREATING PRESSURE ULCERS—cont'd

STEP	RATIONALE
3. Use ***Teach Back*** to determine patient's and family's understanding about pressure ulcer treatment. State, "I want to be sure I explained how to pack the pressure ulcer wound. Can you show me how you will use the applicator to pack your wound?" Revise your instruction now or develop plan for revised patient teaching if patient is not able to teach back correctly.	Evaluates what patient and family are able to explain or demonstrate.

UNEXPECTED OUTCOMES AND RELATED INTERVENTIONS

1. Skin surrounding ulcer becomes macerated.
   - Reduce exposure of surrounding skin to topical agents and moisture.
   - Consider the use of a liquid skin barrier on periwound skin.
2. Ulcer becomes deeper with increased or foul-smelling drainage and pain.
   - Notify health care provider about possible change in pressure ulcer status.
   - Obtain necessary wound cultures.
   - Consult with health care provider about possible change in analgesic.
   - Obtain additional consults (e.g., wound-care specialist).

RECORDING AND REPORTING

- Complete wound documentation required for the wound-assessment instrument per agency protocol.
- Record assessment of ulcer; describe type of topical agent, dressing applied, and patient response.
- Report any deterioration in ulcer assessment to nurse in charge or health care provider.
- Document your evaluation of patient learning.

HOME CARE CONSIDERATIONS

- Patients need to dispose of contaminated dressings in the home in a manner consistent with local regulations for contaminated waste.
- Educate patient and family caregiver about signs of wound infection.
- Discuss need for home pressure-redistribution surface or bed and whether it will fit in a room within the home.

SKILL 48-3 APPLYING DRY AND MOIST DRESSINGS

DELEGATION CONSIDERATIONS

The skill of applying dry and moist dressings to a new acute wound cannot be delegated to nursing assistive personnel (NAP). In some settings aspects of wound care such as changing dressings using *clean* technique for chronic wounds are delegated. The nurse's responsibility is *assessment* of the wound, even if the dressing change is delegated. Direct the NAP to:

- Report pain, fever, bleeding, or wound drainage to the nurse immediately.
- Report any potential contamination to existing dressing (e.g., patient incontinence or other bodily fluids, dressing becomes dislodged).
- Adapt the skill (e.g., need for special tape or devices to secure dressing.

EQUIPMENT

- Sterile gloves
- Variety of gauze dressings and pads
- Irrigation kit
- Cleaning solution
- Sterile solution: water, normal saline, sodium hypochlorite (Dakin's solution).
- Clean, disposable gloves
- Tape, ties, or bandage as needed
- Waterproof pad and bag
- Extra gauze dressings, or topper dressing (ABD pads)
- Montgomery ties; elastic net
- Mask, goggles, or gown for risk of splashing

STEP	RATIONALE
ASSESSMENT	
1. Identify patient using two identifiers (e.g., name and birthday or name and medical record number) according to agency policy.	Ensures correct patient. Complies with The Joint Commission standards and improves patient safety (TJC, 2016).
2. Review medical record for information about size and location of wound.	Provides baseline to compare your findings. Helps to plan for proper type and amount of supplies needed. Alerts you when help is needed to hold dressings in place.
3. Assess patient's level of comfort using a scale of 0 to 10.	Removal of dry dressing is painful; some patients require pain medication. Superficial wounds with multiple exposed nerves may be intensely painful, whereas deeper wounds with destruction of nerves should be less painful (Krazner, 2016).
4. Review orders for dressing change procedure.	Indicates type of dressing or applications to use.
5. Assess patient for allergies to wound cleansing agents or tape.	Prevents adverse reactions.
6. Assess patient's and family's knowledge of purpose and steps of dressing change.	Determine specific areas for patient and family teaching.

STEP	RATIONALE
7. Assess for risk of delayed or poor wound healing (e.g., age, obesity, diabetes, peripheral vascular diseases, poor nutritional status, steroid medications, stress, immunosuppression medications, and radiation therapy).	Physiological changes and effects of disease and treatment conditions can affect wound healing (Doughty and Sparks-DeFriese, 2016).
PLANNING	
1. Explain procedure to patient and instruct him or her not to touch wound area or sterile supplies.	Decreases anxiety. Sudden, unexpected movement on patient's part results in contamination of wound and supplies.
2. Position patient comfortably and drape with bath blanket to expose only wound site.	Provides access to wound yet minimizes unnecessary exposure.
3. Plan dressing change 30 to 60 minutes following administration of analgesia.	Allows for peak action of medication so patient has optimal level of comfort during dressing change. Patients tolerate dressing changes when their pain is controlled.
IMPLEMENTATION	
1. Close room door or pull bedside curtains. Perform hand hygiene and apply gloves.	Provides privacy and reduces transmission of microorganisms.
2. Position patient comfortably and drape only to expose wound site.	Draping provides access to wound while minimizing unnecessary exposure.
3. Place disposable bag within reach of work area. Fold top of bag to make cuff (see illustration).	Ensures easy disposal of soiled dressings. Prevents soiling of outer surface of bag.
4. *Remove tape:* Gently push skin away from tape while pulling adhesive from skin.	Push-pull technique releases tape from skin, reducing chance of skin damage.
5. With gloved hand carefully remove gauze dressings one layer at a time, taking care not to dislodge drains or tubes.	Removal of one layer at a time reduces chance of accidental removal of underlying drains.
a. If dressing sticks on dry dressing, moisten with saline and then remove.	Prevents damage to wound tissue.

CLINICAL DECISION: *Never use a moist-to-dry dressing in a clean granulating wound. Use only for debridement. For highly colonized wounds, use sodium hypochlorite (Dakin's solution) instead of water or normal saline (Ramundo, 2016).*

STEP	RATIONALE
6. Observe wound for color, edema, drains, and exudates and amount of drainage on dressing.	Provides estimate of drainage amount and assessment of condition of wound.
7. Fold dressings with drainage contained inside and remove gloves inside out. With small dressings remove gloves inside out over dressing (see illustration). Dispose of gloves and soiled dressings in disposable bag. Perform hand hygiene.	Reduces transmission of microorganisms. Prevents contact of hands with material on gloves.

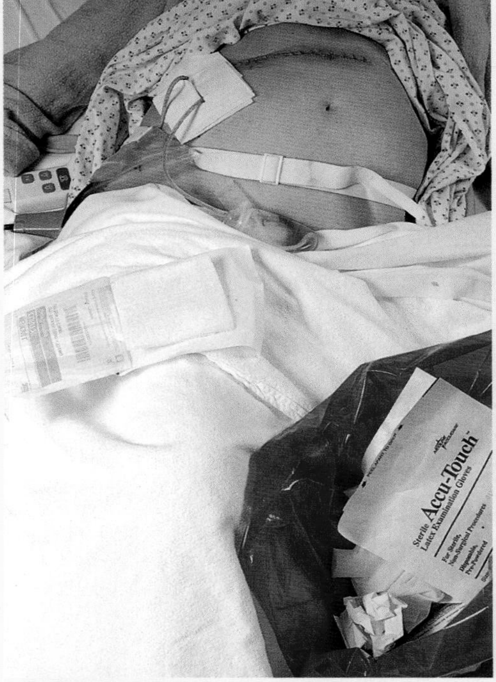

STEP 3 Disposable waterproof bag placed near dressing site.

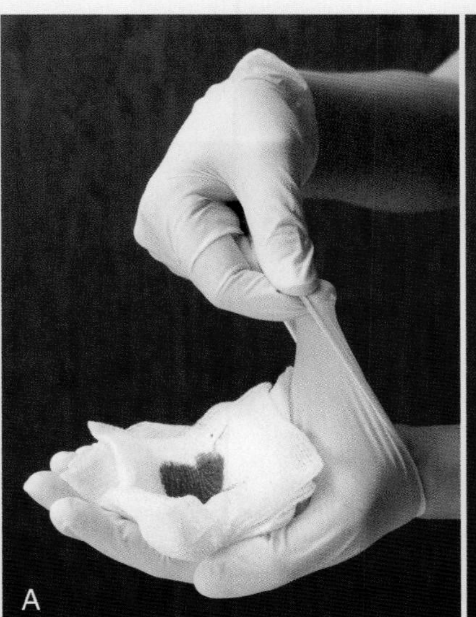

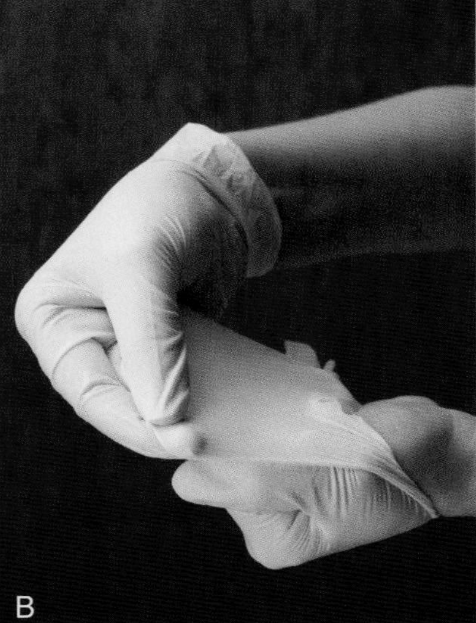

STEP 7 Removing disposable gloves over contaminated dressing.

SKILL 48-3 APPLYING DRY AND MOIST DRESSINGS—cont'd

STEP	RATIONALE
8. Open sterile dressing tray or individually wrapped sterile supplies. Place on bedside table and apply clean gloves.	Sterile dressings remain sterile while on or within sterile surface. Preparation of supplies prevents break in technique during dressing change.
9. Clean wound with solution. Using gauze or antiseptic swab, clean from least-contaminated area, which is the incision or center of wound, to most-contaminated area, which is outside of incision and surrounding skin (see Chapter 29). Dry area. Remove and dispose of gloves and perform hand hygiene.	Prevents contamination of previously cleaned area. Reduces transmission of infection.
10. If ordered irrigate wound:	Removes drainage containing microorganisms.
a. Pour ordered solution into sterile irrigation container.	
b. Apply clean gloves, protective eyewear, mask, and protective gown if needed. Place waterproof pad under patient. Using syringe, gently allow solution to flow over wound. (Some commercial cleaners come in a spray bottle. Spray wound to loosen debris.)	Protects you from splash and reduces transmission of microorganisms.
c. Continue until irrigation creates a clear flow of solution.	Indicates debris is removed.
d. Dry surrounding skin with gauze pads.	
e. Measure wound (see Skill 48-1). Then remove and dispose of gloves. Perform hand hygiene.	Measurement of wound size with each dressing change provides data about progression of wound healing. Reduces transmission of microorganisms.
11. Apply dressing:	
a. Dry dressing	
(1) Apply clean or sterile gloves. Check agency policy.	Some agencies or condition of wound requires sterile gloves. Allows handling of sterile supplies without contamination.
(2) Inspect wound for appearance, drains, drainage, and integrity.	Once wound is clean you are able to better inspect wound condition. Indicates status of wound healing.
(3) Apply sterile, loose woven gauze (4 × 4, 2 × 2) dry dressing, covering wound. Apply additional gauze as needed.	Protects wound from external environment.

CLINICAL DECISION: *When a drain is present, use a precut, split gauze. Never cut gauze to fit around a drain because the cut edges will fray and enter the wound or irritate the periwound tissue.*

STEP	RATIONALE
(4) Apply topper dressing (e.g., ABD) if indicated.	Topper dressing is a thicker dressing that prevents strike-through of wound drainage and provides a surface to tape the dressing in place.
b. Moist to dry dressing	
(1) Apply sterile gloves (see agency policy).	Allows handling of sterile supplies without contamination.
(2) Assess appearance of surrounding skin (see illustration). Look for maceration.	Surrounding skin assessment provides evaluation of wound management.
(3) Moisten gauze with prescribed solution. Gently wring out excess solution. Unfold.	Gauze needs to be moist to allow for absorption of wound debris.

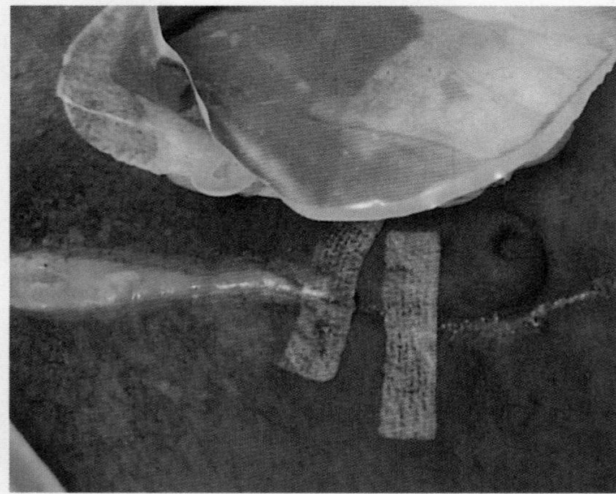

STEP 11b(2) Exposure of wound facilitates assessment of wound and surrounding skin.

STEP	RATIONALE
(4) Apply gauze as single layer directly onto wound surface (see illustration). If wound is deep, gently pack dressing into wound base by hand until all wound surfaces are in contact with gauze. If tunneling is present, use cotton-tipped applicator to place gauze into tunneled area. Be sure that gauze does not touch surrounding skin.	Inner gauze needs to be moist, not dripping wet, to absorb drainage and adhere to debris. Excessively moist dressings result in moisture-associated skin damage (maceration) in periwound skin (Gray et al., 2011). Wound needs to be packed loosely to facilitate wicking of drainage into absorbent outer layer of dressing.
(5) Cover with sterile dry gauze and topper dressing.	Dry dressing wicks drainage out of moist gauze. Topper dressing is thicker; it prevents strike-through of wound drainage and provides surface to tape dressing in place.
12. Secure dressing.	Goal for securing a dressing is to keep dressing in place and intact without causing damage to underlying and surrounding skin.
a. *Tape:* Apply tape 2.5-5 cm (1 to 2 inches) beyond dressing. Use nonallergenic tape to secure dressing in place.	Secures dressing. Reduces sensitivity reaction to tape.
b. Montgomery ties (see Figure 48-21)	Ties allow for repeated dressing changes without the need for tape removal and subsequent skin and tissue damage.
(1) Open by exposing adhesive surface of tape on end of each tie.	
(2) Place ties on opposite sides of dressing.	
(3) Place adhesive directly on skin or apply a solid skin barrier to skin and secure end of tape on skin barrier.	Solid skin barrier protects intact skin from stretch and tension of adhesive tape.
(4) Secure dressing by lacing ties across it.	
c. For dressings on an extremity, secure dressing with rolled gauze or elastic net (see illustration).	Prevents slipping of dressing.

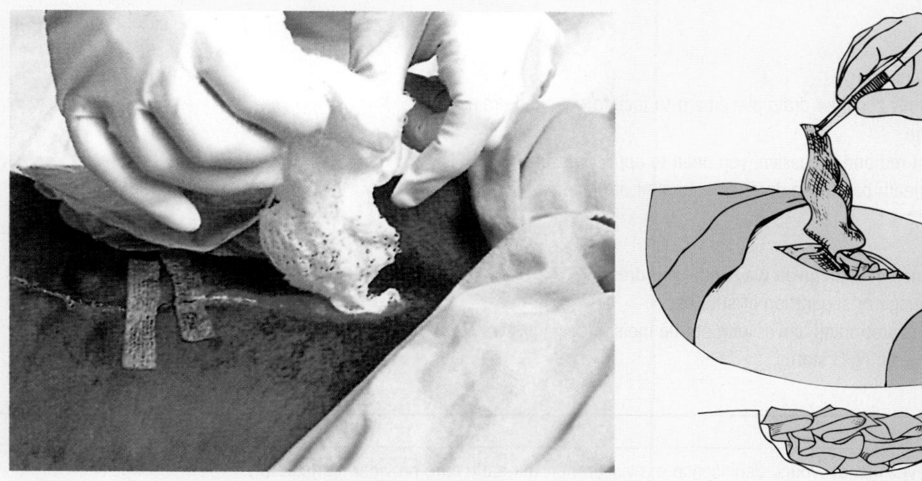
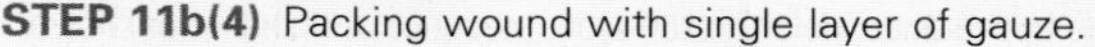

STEP 11b(4) Packing wound with single layer of gauze.

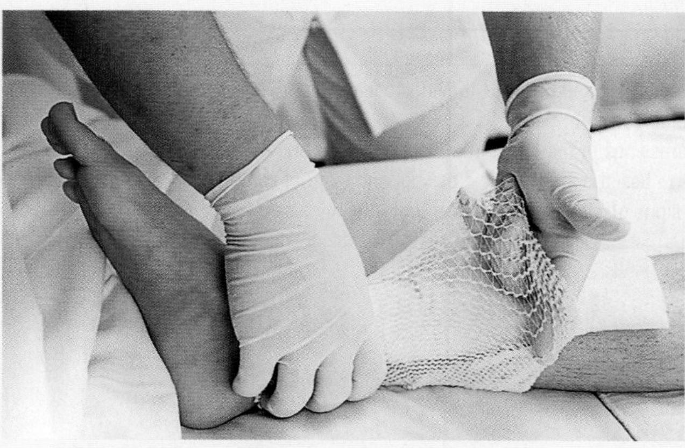

STEP 12c Elastic net securing lower-extremity dressing.

SKILL 48-3 APPLYING DRY AND MOIST DRESSINGS—cont'd

STEP	RATIONALE
13. Remove gloves and dispose of them in bag. Remove any mask, eyewear, or gown.	Reduces transmission of infection.
14. Write date and time dressing applied in ink on tape securing dressing (not marker).	Provides guide for when to perform next dressing change.
15. Help patient to comfortable position.	Improves patient comfort.
16. Dispose of supplies and perform hand hygiene.	Reduces transmission of infection.
EVALUATION	
1. Inspect condition of wound and any drainage.	Determines rate of healing.
2. Ask patient to rate level of pain during and after procedure.	Pain is early indicator of wound complications or result of dressing material pulling underlying tissue.
3. Inspect condition of dressing and note any observable drainage every shift.	Determines status of wound drainage.
4. Use ***Teach Back*** to determine patient's and family's understanding of dressing change procedure. State, "We talked about how to apply a gauze dressing at home. Can you show me now how to apply the dressing?" Revise your instruction now or develop plan for revised patient teaching if patient is not able to teach back correctly.	Evaluates what patient and family are able to explain or demonstrate.

UNEXPECTED OUTCOMES AND RELATED INTERVENTIONS

1. Wound appears inflamed, tender, with or without drainage.
   - Monitor patient for signs of infection (e.g., increased temperature, white blood cell count).
   - Obtain wound culture per order.
   - Notify health care provider.
2. Wound drainage increases.
   - Increase frequency of dressing changes.
   - Notify health care provider, who may consider drain placement to facilitate wound drainage.
3. Wound bleeds during dressing change.
   - Observe color. If drainage is bright red and excessive, you need to apply pressure.
   - Inspect along dressing and underneath patient to determine amount of bleeding.
   - Obtain vital signs as needed.
   - Notify health care provider.
4. Patient reports a sensation that "something has given way under the dressing."
   - Observe wound for increased drainage or separation of sutures.
   - Protect wound. If underlying organs protruding, cover with sterile moist dressing.
   - Instruct patient to lie still and place on NPO status.
   - Notify health care provider.

RECORDING AND REPORTING

- Report brisk, bright red bleeding or evidence of wound dehiscence or evisceration to health care provider immediately.
- Record condition of wound and periwound tissue appearance, color, tissue type, presence and characteristics of exudate, type and amount of dressings used, and tolerance of patient to procedure in EHR or chart.
- Record patient's level of comfort and response to analgesic.
- Document your evaluation of patient learning.

HOME CARE CONSIDERATIONS

- More expensive specialty dressings are sometimes used because they decrease the frequency of dressing changes.
- Clean dressings may also be used in the home setting.
- Patients need to dispose of contaminated dressings in the home in a manner consistent with local regulations.
- Be sure patient has a family caregiver able to assist and/or apply dressing, and instruct caregiver on dressing procedure.
- Be sure patient and family caregiver know signs of infection and when to notify physician.

SKILL 48-4 IMPLEMENTATION OF NEGATIVE-PRESSURE WOUND THERAPY

DELEGATION CONSIDERATIONS

The skill of negative-pressure wound therapy (NPWT) cannot be delegated to nursing assistive personnel (NAP). Instruct the NAP to:

- Use caution in positioning and turning patient to avoid tubing displacement.
- Report to the nurse any change in patient's temperature, level of comfort.
- Report change in pressure in NPWT unit.
- Report any change in the integrity of the dressing.

EQUIPMENT

- NPWT unit (For this skill the vacuum-assisted closure (V.A.C.) unit is used for illustration; several other systems are available, and their application may be slightly different; refer to manufacturer directions; requires health care provider order.)
- NPWT dressing (gauze or foam dressing and transparent dressing) (check manufacturer instructions)
- NPWT suction device
- Tubing for connection between NPWT unit and dressing
- Gloves, clean and sterile
- Sterile scissors
- Skin preparation/skin barrier
- Moist washcloth
- Waterproof, disposable biohazard bag
- Linen bag
- Protective gown, mask, goggles if risk of splashing wound drainage

STEP	RATIONALE
ASSESSMENT	
1. Identify patient using two identifiers (e.g., name and birthday or name and medical record number) according to agency policy.	Ensures correct patient. Complies with The Joint Commission standards and improves patient safety (TJC, 2016).
2. Review medical record for signs and symptoms related to condition of patient's wound.	Provides you a baseline to compare with your findings, which will reflect if progress is occurring.
3. Assess location, appearance, and size of wound to be dressed (see Skill 48-2).	Allows you to gather information regarding status of wound healing, presence of complications, and type of supplies and help needed to apply NPWT dressing.
4. Review health care provider's orders for frequency of dressing change, type of foam to use, and amount of negative pressure to be used.	Health care provider orders frequency of dressing changes and special instructions.
5. Assess patient's level of comfort using a scale of 0 to 10.	Patient who is comfortable during procedure is less likely to move suddenly, causing wound or supply contamination.
6. Assess patient's and family member's knowledge of purpose of dressing.	Identifies patient's learning needs. Prepares patient and family if dressing needs to be changed at home.
PLANNING	
1. Explain to patient what dressing change involves, including sensations to be felt.	Provides patient with rationale for dressing change and reduces fears. Maintaining patient comfort helps to complete skill smoothly.
2. Administer ordered analgesic 30 minutes before dressing change.	Pain has been reported with NPWT removal and application; pain medication given before dressing change can reduce procedural pain (Upton and Andrews, 2015).
3. Perform hand hygiene. Assemble supplies.	Reduces transmission of microorganisms. Organizes procedure.
IMPLEMENTATION	
1. Close room door or cubicle curtains.	Provides privacy.
2. Position patient comfortably and drape to expose only wound site. Instruct patient not to touch wound or sterile supplies.	Draping provides access to wound while minimizing unnecessary exposure.
3. Place disposable waterproof bag within reach of work area with top folded to make a cuff.	Facilitates safe disposal of soiled dressings.
4. Apply clean gloves. If there is risk for splash or spray, apply protective gown, goggles, and mask.	Reduces exposure to infectious microorganisms.
5. Keep system in "de vac" mode for 30 to 60 minutes before changing dressing.	Loosens foam dressing for easier, less painful removal.
6. When NPWT is in place, push therapy on/off button (follow manufacturer directions).	
a. Keeping tube connectors with NPWT unit, raise tubing connectors above level of NPWT unit; disconnect tubes from one another to drain fluids into canister.	Deactivates therapy and allows for proper drainage of fluid in drainage tubing.
b. Before lowering, tighten clamp on canister tube and disconnect canister and dressing tubing at connection points.	
7. Remove transparent film by gently stretching transparent film horizontally and slowly pull away from skin.	Prevents skin breakdown from adhesive.
8. Remove old dressing, observing drainage on dressing. Use caution to avoid tension on any drains that are present. Discard dressing and remove gloves. Perform hand hygiene.	Determines dressings needed for replacement. Avoids accidental removal of drains because they are sometimes sutured in place.

SKILL 48-4 IMPLEMENTATION OF NEGATIVE-PRESSURE WOUND THERAPY—cont'd

STEP	RATIONALE
CLINICAL DECISION: *Verify that all prior dressing foam is removed. Infections from retained pieces of foam filer can result in further surgery, antibiotic use, and resistant wound infections (Netsch, 2016).*	
9. Apply sterile or clean gloves (see agency policy). Irrigate wound with normal saline or other solution ordered by health care provider (see Skill 48-3). Blot dry with gauze.	Irrigation removes wound debris.
CLINICAL DECISION: *When drainage looks purulent, amount or color changes, or it has a foul odor, obtain wound cultures even when they are not ordered for that particular dressing change (Netsch, 2016; Stotts 2016b).*	
10. Measure wound as ordered: at baseline, first dressing change, weekly; discharge from therapy. Remove and discard gloves. Perform hand hygiene.	Objectively documents wound-healing process in response to NPWT (Nix, 2016).
11. Depending on type of wound, apply new sterile or clean gloves.	Fresh sterile wounds require sterile gloves. Chronic wounds may require clean technique. Never wear same gloves worn to remove old dressing or irrigate wound because cross-contamination may occur.
12. Prepare periwound skin by applying skin protectant/barrier film to protect and enhance adherence of adhesive drape.	Maintains air-tight seal needed for NPWT and protects periwound skin from maceration.
13. Prepare foam dressing.	
a. Select appropriate foam (follow manufacturer directions).	Black, polyurethane (PU) foam has larger pores and is most effective in stimulating granulation tissue and wound contraction. White, polyvinyl alcohol (PVA) soft foam is denser with smaller pores and is used when growth of granulation tissue needs to be restricted (Netsch, 2016).
CLINICAL DECISION: *The brand of NPWT or specific wound filler dressing may need to be adjusted on the basis of undermining, tunneling, or sinus tracts (Netsch, 2016).*	
b. Using sterile scissors, cut foam to exact wound size with foam height extending 1-2 cm (½ inch) above skin surface. Dressing must fit size and shape of wound, including tunnels and undermined areas.	Foam will contract to level of skin.
CLINICAL DECISION: *Some patients experience more pain with the black foam because of excessive wound contraction. If this occurs, change wound filler to one that causes less contraction and is less likely to allow granulation growth into the dressing (Netsch, 2016).*	
14. Gently place foam in wound; be sure that foam is in contact with entire wound base, margins, and tunneled and undermined areas (see illustration).	Achieves even distribution of negative pressure to entire wound.
15. Apply wrinkle-free transparent dressing over foam and to 3-5 cm (1.2-2 inches) of surrounding healthy skin. Secure tubing to unit (see illustration).	Ensures that wound is properly covered and helps achieve negative-pressure seal (see Box 48-12). Connects negative pressure from NPWT unit to wound foam.
16. Secure tubing to transparent film, aligning drainage holes to ensure occlusive seal. Do not apply tension to drape and tubing.	Excessive tension compresses foam dressing and impedes wound healing. Tension also produces shear force on periwound area (KCI, 2007).
17. Secure tubing several centimeters away from dressing, avoiding pressure points.	Drainage tubes over bony prominences can cause pressure ulcers (Netsch, 2016).
CLINICAL DECISION: *Prevent medical device–related pressure ulcers (MD PUs) by avoiding placement of drainage tubing and suction device over bony prominences and other areas at risk for pressure ulcer development (Black et al., 2015; Netsch, 2016).*	

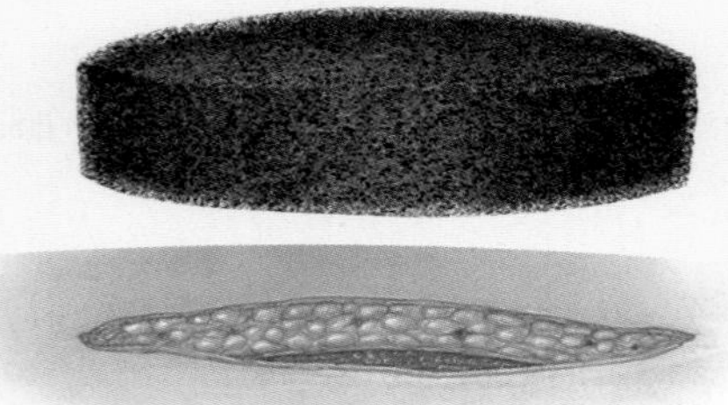

STEP 14 Dressing application. Properly sized foam to cover wound.

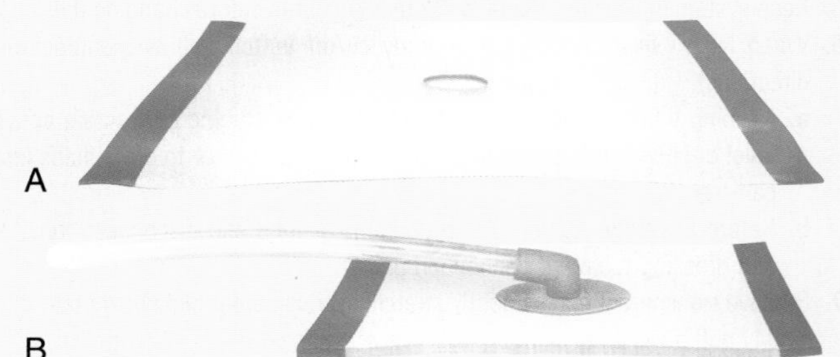

STEP 15 A, Wrinkle-free transparent dressing applied over foam. **B,** Secure tubing to foam and transparent dressing. (Courtesy Kinetic Concepts, Inc [KCI], San Antonio, Tex.)

STEP	RATIONALE
18. Once you have completely covered the wound (see illustration), connect tubing from dressing to tubing from canister and NPWT unit.	Intermittent or continuous negative pressure can be administered at 50 to 175 mm Hg, according to health care provider's order and patient comfort. Continuous therapy is most routinely used. Average is 125 mm Hg (Netsch, 2016).
a. Remove canister from sterile packaging and push into unit until you hear a click. NOTE: An alarm sounds if canister is not engaged properly.	
b. Connect dressing tubing to canister tubing. Make sure that both clamps are open.	
c. Place unit on level surface or hang from foot of bed. NOTE: Unit alarms and deactivates therapy if it is tilted beyond 45 degrees.	
d. Press in green-lit power button and set pressure as ordered.	
19. Discard old dressing materials; remove gloves, discard, and perform hand hygiene.	Reduces transmission of microorganisms.
20. Inspect NPWT system to verify that negative pressure is achieved.	Negative pressure is achieved when there is an airtight seal.
a. Verify that display screen reads THERAPY ON.	
b. Be sure that clamps are open and tubing is patent.	
c. Listen for air leaks.	
d. If leak is present, use strips of transparent film to patch areas around edges of wound.	

EVALUATION

1. Inspect condition of wound on ongoing basis; note drainage and odor.	Determines status of wound healing.
2. Ask patient to rate pain using a scale of 0 to 10.	Determines patient's level of comfort following procedure.
3. Compare wound size and condition with baseline wound assessment.	Provides objective documentation of wound healing.
4. Verify airtight dressing seal and proper negative pressure.	To achieve prescribed vacuum level, wound must be covered with airtight seal. This airtight seal and negative pressure promote wound drainage, circulation, and healing.
5. Measure wound drainage in canister on regular basis per agency policy.	Monitors fluid balance and wound drainage.
6. Use ***Teach Back*** to determine patient's and family's understanding about **negative pressure wound therapy**. State, "I want to be sure I explained why you have this suction device attached to your dressing. Can you tell me what this suction does to help heal your wound?" Revise your instruction now or develop plan for revised patient teaching if patient is not able to teach back correctly.	Evaluates what patient and family are able to explain or demonstrate.

UNEXPECTED OUTCOMES AND RELATED INTERVENTIONS

1. Wound appears inflamed and tender, drainage has increased, and an odor is present.
   - Notify health care provider.
   - Obtain wound culture per order.
   - Increase frequency of dressing changes.
2. Patient reports increase in pain.
   - If using black foam, switch to the PVA foam product.
   - Patient sometimes needs more analgesic support when NPWT is initiated.
   - Reduce suction.
3. Negative pressure seal has broken.
   - *Take preventive measures:* Shave hair around wound, avoid wrinkles in transparent dressing, and avoid use of adhesive remover because it leaves residue that hinders film adherence.
   - Reinforce with transparent dressing strips.

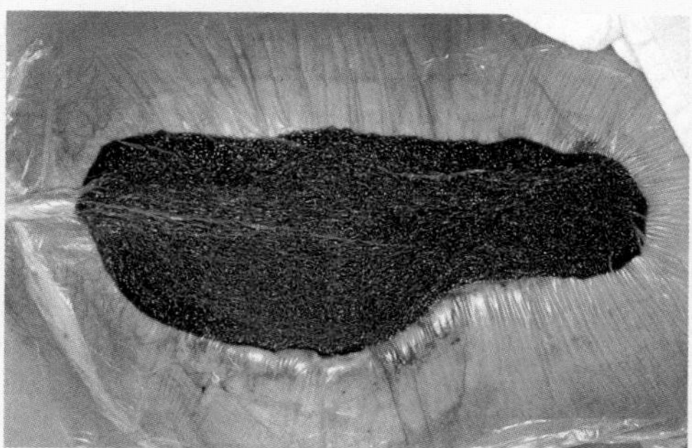

STEP 18 Foam, transparent dressing, and tubing secured over existing wound. (Courtesy Kinetic Concepts, Inc [KCI], San Antonio, Tex.)

SKILL 48-4 IMPLEMENTATION OF NEGATIVE-PRESSURE WOUND THERAPY—cont'd

RECORDING AND REPORTING

- Record appearance of wound, size, color, characteristics of any drainage, presence of wound healing, and patient's response to dressing change in progress notes in EHR or chart.
- Record pressure setting of NPWT.
- Record date and time of dressing change.
- Report brisk, bright bleeding; evidence of poor wound healing; and possible wound infection to health care provider.
- Document your evaluation of patient learning.

HOME CARE CONSIDERATIONS

- Patients can use NPWT in the home safely. Some patients need clinic or home care nursing visits to change and monitor wound healing.
- Provide resources to patient for supplies for NPWT.
- Instruct family and family caregiver regarding proper disposal of contaminated product.

SKILL 48-5 PERFORMING WOUND IRRIGATION

DELEGATION CONSIDERATIONS

The skill of wound irrigation cannot be delegated to nursing assistive personnel. Direct the NAP to:

- Report any change in wound appearance or increased wound drainage to the nurse.
- Report patient pain.

EQUIPMENT

- Irrigant/cleaning solution (volume 1.2 to 2 times the estimated wound volume)
- Irrigation delivery system, depending on amount of pressure desired:
- 35-mL irrigation syringe with soft 19-gauge angiocatheter (Rolstad et al., 2016)
- Clean gloves
- Waterproof under pad, if needed
- Gauze dressing supplies
- Disposable waterproof bag
- Gown, goggles, or mask, if risk of spray

STEP	RATIONALE
ASSESSMENT	
1. Identify patient using two identifiers (e.g., name and birthday or name and medical record number) according to agency policy.	Ensures correct patient. Complies with The Joint Commission standards and improves patient safety (TJC, 2016).
2. Assess patient's level of pain.	Provides baseline to measure patient's response to therapy. Discomfort is related directly to wound or indirectly to muscle tension or immobility.
3. Review medical record for health care provider's prescription for irrigation of open wound and type of solution to be used.	Open-wound irrigation requires medical order, including type of solution to use.
4. Review medical record for signs and symptoms related to patient's open wound.	Data provide baseline to indicate change in condition of wound (Nix, 2016).
a. Extent of impairment of skin integrity, including size of wound (Measure length, width, and depth in centimeters in the following order: length, width, and depth.)	Assesses volume of irrigation solution needed. Data also used as baseline to indicate change in condition of wound.
b. Verify number and types of drains present.	Awareness of drain placement facilitates safe dressing removal and identifies type and quantity of new dressings needed.
c. Drainage from wound (amount and color) (Amount can be measured by part of dressing saturated or in terms of quantity [e.g., scant, moderate, copious].)	Expect amount to decrease as healing takes place. Serous drainage is clear like plasma; sanguineous or bright red drainage indicates fresh bleeding; serosanguineous drainage is pink; purulent drainage is thick and yellow, pale green, or white.
d. Odor (must state whether or not there is odor)	Strong odor indicates infectious process.
e. Wound tissue color	Color represents balance between necrotic tissue and new scar tissue. Proper selection of wound products on the basis of color of wound facilitates removal of necrotic tissue and promotes new tissue growth (Nix, 2016).
f. Consistency of drainage	Type and color of drainage depend on moisture of wound and type of organisms present.
g. Culture reports	Chronic wounds heal by secondary intention, and they are often colonized with bacteria.
h. Condition of dressing: dry and clean; evidence of bleeding, profuse drainage	Provides initial assessment of present wound drainage.
PLANNING	
1. Explain procedure of wound irrigation and cleaning and how you will prepare patient.	Information reduces patient's anxiety.

STEP	RATIONALE
2. Administer prescribed analgesic 30 to 60 minutes before starting wound irrigation procedure.	Promotes pain control and permits patient to move more easily and be positioned to facilitate wound irrigation.
3. Position patient to access wound for easy irrigation.	
a. Position comfortably so wound is vertical to collection basin, which permits gravitational flow of irrigating solution through wound and into collection receptacle.	Directing solution from top to bottom of wound and from clean to contaminated area reduces spread of infection. Position patient, keeping in mind bed surfaces needed for later preparation of equipment.
b. Place container of irrigant/cleaning solution in basin of hot water to warm solution to body temperature.	Warmed solution increases comfort and reduces vascular constriction response in tissues.
c. Place padding or extra towel in bed.	Protects bedding.

IMPLEMENTATION

STEP	RATIONALE
1. Perform hand hygiene.	Reduces transmission of microorganisms.
2. Form cuff on waterproof bag and place it near bed.	Cuffing helps to maintain large opening, thereby permitting placement of contaminated dressing without touching refuse bag itself.
3. Close room door or bed curtains.	Maintains privacy.
4. Apply gown, mask, or goggles if needed.	Protects nurse from splashes or sprays of blood and body fluids.
5. Apply clean gloves and remove soiled dressing and discard in waterproof bag. Discard gloves and perform hand hygiene.	Reduces transmission of microorganisms.
6. Prepare equipment; open supplies.	
7. Apply clean gloves.	Reduces transmission of microorganisms.
8. To irrigate wound with wide opening:	
a. Fill 35-mL syringe with irrigation solution.	Flushing wound helps remove debris and facilitates healing by secondary intention.
b. Attach soft 19-gauge angiocatheter (see Figure 48-17).	Provides ideal pressure for cleaning and removing debris (Ramundo, 2016).
c. Hold syringe tip 2.5 cm (1 inch) above upper end of wound and over area being cleaned.	Prevents syringe contamination. Careful placement of syringe prevents unsafe pressure of flowing solution.
d. Using continuous pressure, flush wound; repeat Steps 8a, b, and c until solution draining into basin is clear.	Clear solution indicates that you have removed all debris.
9. To irrigate deep wound with very small opening:	
a. Attach soft 19-gauge angiocatheter to filled irrigating syringe.	Catheter permits direct flow of irrigant into wound. Expect wound to take longer to empty when opening is small.
b. Gently insert tip of catheter into wound and pull out about 1 cm (½ inch).	Removes tip from fragile inner wall of wound.
c. Using slow, continuous pressure, flush wound. *Caution:* Splashing sometimes occurs during this step.	Cleans all wound surfaces.
d. Pinch off catheter just below syringe while keeping catheter in place.	Avoids contamination of solution.
e. Remove and refill syringe. Reconnect to catheter and repeat until solution draining into basin is clear.	Indicates wound clear of debris.

CLINICAL DECISION: *Pulsatile high-pressure lavage may be the irrigation of choice for necrotic wounds. The amount of irrigant depends on the size of the wound. Pressure settings on the device should remain between 8 and 15 psi. Do not use pulsatile high-pressure lavage on exposed blood vessels, muscle, tendon, and bone. This type of irrigation should not be used with graft sites and should be used with caution in patients receiving anticoagulant therapy (Ramundo, 2016).*

STEP	RATIONALE
10. Obtain cultures, if ordered, after cleaning with nonbacteriostatic saline.	Type of wound culture obtained depends on resources available in facility. The three most common types of wound specimens are tissue biopsy, needle aspirated wound fluid, and swab technique (Stotts, 2016b).

CLINICAL DECISION: *Consider culturing a wound if it has a foul, purulent odor; inflammation surrounds the wound; a nondraining wound begins to drain; or patient is febrile.*

STEP	RATIONALE
11. Assess type of tissue in wound bed and periwound skin.	Identifies wound-healing progress and determines if wound has increased in size.
12. Dry wound edges with gauze.	Prevents maceration of surrounding tissue caused by excess moisture.
13. Apply appropriate dressing (see Skills 48-2 and 48-3).	Maintains protective barrier and healing environment for wound.
14. Remove gloves and, if worn, mask, goggles, and gown.	Prevents transfer of microorganisms.
15. Dispose of equipment and soiled supplies. Perform hand hygiene.	Reduces transmission of microorganisms.
16. Help patient to comfortable position.	

EVALUATION

STEP	RATIONALE
1. Inspect dressing periodically.	Determines patient's response to wound irrigation and need to modify plan of care.
2. Determine patient's level of pain.	Patient's pain should not increase as result of wound irrigation.
3. Observe for presence of retained irrigant.	Retained irrigant is medium for bacterial growth and subsequent infection.

SKILL 48-5 PERFORMING WOUND IRRIGATION—cont'd

STEP	RATIONALE
4. Use ***Teach Back*** to determine patient's and family's understanding about the need for the wound to be irrigated. State, "I want to be sure I explained why we irrigate your abdominal wound. Can you tell me why irrigation is important?" Revise your instruction now or develop plan for revised patient teaching if patient is not able to teach back correctly.	Evaluates what patient and family are able to explain or demonstrate.

UNEXPECTED OUTCOMES AND RELATED INTERVENTIONS

1. Wound does not appear to heal.
   - Obtain wound culture per order.
   - Notify health care provider, who may change dressing and/or irrigation frequency.
2. Wound drainage increases.
   - Apply more absorbent gauze; consider more observant dressing such as an alginate.
   - Increase the frequency of irrigation.

RECORDING AND REPORTING

- Record wound irrigation, patient response, and appearance of wound in progress notes in EHR or chart.
- Immediately report any evidence of fresh bleeding, sharp increase in pain, retention of irrigant, or signs of shock to attending health care provider.
- Document your evaluation of patient learning.

HOME CARE CONSIDERATIONS

- Teach patient and family caregiver how to make normal saline, especially if cost is an issue. You make normal saline by using 8 tsp of salt in 1 gallon of distilled water.
- Instruct family caregiver on irrigation technique and have caregiver demonstrate.
- Be sure patient and family know signs of infection and when to notify health care provider.
- Solutions to use for irrigation in the home includes: Potable tap water, distilled water, cooled boiled water, and normal saline (WOCN, 2016).

SKILL 48-6 APPLYING AN ELASTIC BANDAGE

DELEGATION CONSIDERATIONS

The skill of applying an elastic bandage can be delegated to nursing assistive personnel (NAP). The nurse is responsible for assessing the wound and the adequacy of circulation to the extremity distal to the bandage. Direct the NAP to:

- Report any restrictions that patient has (e.g., unable to independently raise leg or roll over).
- Report any change in skin color of patient's injured extremity.
- Report any increases in patient's pain.

EQUIPMENT

- Correct width and number of bandages
- Safety pins, clips, or adhesive tape
- Clean gloves if wound drainage is present

STEP	RATIONALE
ASSESSMENT	
1. Identify patient using two identifiers (e.g., name and birthday or name and medical record number) according to agency policy.	Ensures correct patient. Complies with The Joint Commission standards and improves patient safety (TJC, 2016).
2. Review medical record for specific orders related to application of elastic bandage. Note area to be covered, type of bandage required, frequency of change, and previous response to treatment.	Specific orders sometimes direct procedure, including factors such as extent of application (e.g., toe to knee, toe to groin) and duration of treatment.
3. Perform hand hygiene and apply gloves if needed. Inspect skin for alterations in integrity as indicated by abrasions, discoloration, chafing, or edema. (Look carefully at bony prominences.)	Altered skin integrity contraindicates use of elastic bandages.
4. Inspect surgical dressing if present. Remove gloves and perform hand hygiene.	Surgical dressing replacement or reinforcement precedes application of any bandage. Reduces transmission of microorganisms.
5. Observe adequacy of circulation (distal to bandage) by noting surface temperature, skin color, and sensation in body parts to be wrapped.	Comparison of area before and after application of bandage is necessary to ensure continued adequate circulation. Impairment of circulation can result in coolness to touch when compared with opposite side of body, cyanosis, pallor of skin, diminished or absent pulses, edema or localized pooling, and numbness or tingling of part.
PLANNING	
1. Explain each step of procedure to patient.	Increased knowledge promotes cooperation and reduces anxiety.
2. Demonstrate skill to patient and family caregiver during bandage application.	Helps to ensure continuity of care after discharge.

CLINICAL DECISION: *Apply bandages to lower extremities before patient sits or stands. Elevate dependent extremities for 20 minutes before bandage application to enhance venous return.*

STEP	RATIONALE
IMPLEMENTATION	
1. Close room door or curtains.	Maintains patient's comfort and dignity.
2. Help patient assume comfortable, anatomically correct position.	Maintains alignment. Prevents musculoskeletal deformity.
3. Perform hand hygiene and apply gloves if drainage is present.	Reduces transmission of microorganisms.
4. Hold roll of elastic bandage in dominant hand and use other hand to lightly hold beginning of bandage at distal body part. Continue transferring roll to dominant hand as bandage is wrapped.	Maintains appropriate and consistent bandage tension.

CLINICAL DECISION: *Toes or fingertips need to be visible for follow-up circulatory assessment.*

STEP	RATIONALE
5. Apply bandage from distal point toward proximal boundary using variety of turns to cover various shapes of body parts.	Bandage is applied in manner that conforms evenly to body part and promotes venous return.
a. Spiral dressing is often used to cover cylindrical body parts such as wrist or upper arms. To apply bandage in an ascending motion, overlap previous bandage by one-half to two-thirds width of bandage.	
b. Use figure-eight dressing to cover joint because snug fit provides excellent immobilization. *To apply:* Overlap turns, alternately ascending and descending over bandaged part; each turn crossing previous one to form figure eight.	
6. Unroll and very slightly stretch bandage.	Maintains uniform bandage tension.
7. Overlap turns by one-half to two-thirds width of bandage roll.	Prevents uneven bandage tension and circulatory impairment.
8. Secure first bandage with clip or tape before applying additional rolls.	
9. Apply additional rolls without leaving any skin surface uncovered. Secure last bandage applied.	Prevents wrinkling or loose ends.
10. Remove gloves if worn and perform hand hygiene.	Reduces transmission of microorganisms.
EVALUATION	
1. Assess distal circulation when bandage application is complete and at least twice during 8-hour period.	Early detection and management of circulatory impairment ensures healthy neurovascular status.
a. Observe skin color for pallor or cyanosis.	
b. Palpate skin for warmth.	
c. Palpate pulses and compare bilaterally.	
d. Ask if patient is aware of pain, numbness, tingling, or other discomfort.	Neurovascular changes indicate impaired venous return.
e. Observe mobility of extremity.	Determines if bandage is too tight, which restricts movement, or if joint immobility is attained.
2. Use ***Teach Back*** to determine patient's and family's understanding about bandage application. State, "I want to be sure that you can correctly apply the bandage. Can you demonstrate how to apply the elastic bandage for me now?" Revise your instruction now or develop plan for revised patient teaching if patient is not able to teach back correctly.	Evaluates what patient and family are able to demonstrate.

UNEXPECTED OUTCOMES AND RELATED INTERVENTIONS

1. Impaired circulation distal to elastic bandage
   - Release bandage.
   - Palpate extremity and assess pulse, temperature, and capillary refill.
   - Reapply dressing with less pressure.
2. Break in skin under elastic bandage
   - Remove bandage.
   - Reapply bandage over different area of skin with less pressure.
3. Patient unable to perform dressing change
   - Reinstruct patient or family caregiver on bandage application.
   - Observe patient or family caregiver apply bandage.

RECORDING AND REPORTING

- Document condition of wound, integrity of dressing, application of bandage, circulation, and patient's comfort level in progress notes in EHR or chart.
- Report any changes in neurological or circulatory status to nurse in charge or health care provider.
- Document your evaluation of patient learning.

HOME CARE CONSIDERATIONS

- Instruct patient or caregiver not to make bandages too tight, which interferes with circulation.
- Elastic bandages that reduce swelling are best applied to the feet and ankles in the morning, before getting out of bed.
- Always remove an elastic bandage daily and inspect skin beneath it.
- Be sure patient has two sets of bandages to alternate; making it easy to clean one set while other is in place.

KEY POINTS

- Pressure ulcers contribute to patient discomfort and decreased functional status, increased length of stay in acute and extended care settings, and increased cost of care.
- Wound assessment determines progress toward pressure ulcer healing; do not use the staging system for this purpose.
- Assess all patients on an ongoing basis for risk factors that contribute to development of any type of impaired skin integrity such as blistering or burning sensation.
- Alterations in mobility, sensory perception, level of consciousness, and nutrition and the presence of moisture increase the risk for pressure ulcer development.
- Pressure, shearing force, and friction are contributing factors to the development of pressure ulcers.
- Meticulous ongoing assessment of the skin and identification of risk factors are important in decreasing the opportunity for pressure ulcer development.
- Preventive skin care is aimed at controlling external pressure on bony prominences and keeping the skin clean, well lubricated and hydrated, and free of excess moisture.
- Proper positioning reduces the effects of pressure and guards against the shearing force.
- Therapeutic beds and mattresses redistribute the effects of pressure; however, base selection on assessment data to identify the best support surface for individual needs.
- Cleaning and topical agents used to treat pressure ulcers vary according to the stage of the pressure ulcer and condition of the wound bed. Assessment of the ulcer enables the nurse to select proper skin-care agents.
- Direct nutritional interventions at improving wound healing through increasing protein and calorie levels.
- Wound assessment requires a description of the appearance of the wound base, size, presence of exudate, and periwound skin condition.
- The chances of wound infection are greater when a wound contains dead or necrotic tissue, when foreign bodies lie on or near the wound, and when the blood supply is reduced.
- The principles of wound first aid include control of bleeding, cleaning, and protection.
- A moist environment supports wound healing.
- An acute sprain, closed fracture, or bruise responds best to cold applications.
- The selection of the type of dressing is determined by the type and condition of a wound.
- Use medical versus surgical asepsis when applying dressings on a clean chronic wound versus a new surgical wound.

CLINICAL APPLICATION QUESTIONS

Preparing for Clinical Practice

1. Because of the foul-smelling tan-colored drainage from Mrs. Stein's hip incision, the staples were removed by the health care provider, and an order was written for moist saline gauze dressing to the area 3 times a day. When the dressing is removed, which factors are critical to assess?
2. A head-to-toe skin assessment is done per institutional policy each shift or on a daily basis. At the most recent assessment of Mrs. Stein's skin, blistering was noted over the sacral area; on direct examination it was a small area of denuded tissue with redness around the blistered area. The area was found to have minimal depth and a red, moist base. How would you describe the impairment in skin integrity in your charting?
3. What will you include in your plan of care for Mrs. Stein to address the impairment in skin integrity in the sacral area?

ⓔ ***Answers to Clinical Application Questions can be found on the Evolve website.***

REVIEW QUESTIONS

Are You Ready to Test Your Nursing Knowledge?

1. When repositioning an immobile patient, the nurse notices redness over the hip bone. What is indicated when a reddened area blanches on fingertip touch?
   1. A local skin infection requiring antibiotics
   2. Sensitive skin that requires special bed linen
   3. A stage III pressure ulcer needing the appropriate dressing
   4. Blanching hyperemia, indicating the attempt by the body to overcome the ischemic episode
2. Match the pressure ulcer categories/stages with the correct definition.
   1. Category/stage I
   2. Category/stage II
   3. Category/stage III
   4. Category/stage IV

   a. Nonblanchable redness of intact skin. Discoloration, warmth, edema, or pain may also be present.
   b. Full-thickness skin loss; subcutaneous fat may be visible. May include undermining.
   c. Full thickness tissue loss; muscle and bone visible. May include undermining.
   d. Partial-thickness skin loss or intact blister with serosanguinous fluid.
3. When obtaining a wound culture to determine the presence of a wound infection, from where should the specimen be taken?
   1. Necrotic tissue
   2. Wound drainage
   3. Wound circumference
   4. Cleansed wound
4. After surgery the patient with a closed abdominal wound reports a sudden "pop" after coughing. When the nurse examines the surgical wound site, the sutures are open, and pieces of small bowel are noted at the bottom of the now-opened wound. Which are the priority nursing interventions? (Select all that apply.)
   1. Notify the surgeon.
   2. Allow the area to be exposed to air until all drainage has stopped.
   3. Place several cold packs over the area, protecting the skin around the wound
   4. Cover the area with sterile, saline-soaked towels immediately.
   5. Cover the area with sterile gauze and apply an abdominal binder.
5. What is the correct sequence of steps when performing wound irrigation to a large open wound?
   1. Use slow, continuous pressure to irrigate wound.
   2. Attach 19-gauge angiocatheter to syringe.
   3. Fill syringe with irrigation fluid.
   4. Place waterproof bag near bed.
   5. Position angiocatheter over wound.
6. For a patient who has a muscle sprain, localized hemorrhage, or hematoma, which wound-care product helps prevent edema formation, control bleeding, and anesthetize the body part?

1. Binder
2. Ice bag
3. Elastic bandage
4. Absorptive dressing

7. Which skin-care measures are used to manage a patient who is experiencing fecal and/or urinary incontinence? (Select all that apply.)
   1. Frequent position changes
   2. Keeping the buttocks exposed to air at all times
   3. Using a large absorbent diaper, changing when saturated
   4. Using an incontinence cleaner
   5. Frequent cleaning, applying an ointment, and covering the areas with a thick absorbent towel
   6. Applying a moisture barrier ointment
8. Which of the following describes a hydrocolloid dressing?
   1. A seaweed derivative that is highly absorptive
   2. Premoistened gauze placed over a granulating wound
   3. A debriding enzyme that is used to remove necrotic tissue
   4. A dressing that forms a gel that interacts with the wound surface
9. Which of the following is an indication for a binder to be placed around a surgical patient with a new abdominal wound? (Select all that apply.)
   1. Collection of wound drainage
   2. Providing support to abdominal tissues when coughing or walking
   3. Reduction of abdominal swelling
   4. Reduction of stress on the abdominal incision
   5. Stimulation of peristalsis (return of bowel function) from direct pressure
10. When is an application of a warm compress to an ankle muscle sprain indicated? (Select all that apply.)
   1. To relieve edema
   2. To reduce shivering
   3. To improve blood flow to an injured part
   4. To protect bony prominences from pressure ulcers
   5. To immobilize area
11. What is the removal of devitalized tissue from a wound called?
   1. Debridement
   2. Pressure reduction
   3. Negative pressure wound therapy
   4. Sanitization
12. Name the three important dimensions to consistently measure to determine wound healing.
13. What does the Braden Scale evaluate?
   1. Skin integrity at bony prominences, including any wounds
   2. Risk factors that place the patient at risk for skin breakdown
   3. The amount of repositioning that the patient can tolerate
   4. The factors that place the patient at risk for poor healing
14. On assessing your patient's sacral pressure ulcer, you note that the tissue over the sacrum is dark, hard, and adherent to the wound edge. What is the correct category/stage for this patient's pressure ulcer?
   1. Category/stage II
   2. Category/stage IV
   3. Unstageable
   4. Suspected deep-tissue damage
15. Which of the following are measures to reduce tissue damage from shear? (Select all that apply.)
   1. Use a transfer device (e.g., transfer board)
   2. Have head of bed elevated when transferring patient
   3. Have head of bed flat when repositioning patient
   4. Raise head of bed 60 degrees when patient positioned supine
   5. Raise head of bed 30 degrees when patient positioned supine

Answers: 1. 4; **2.** 1a, 2d, 3b, 4c; **3.** 4; **4.** 1, 4; **5.** 4, 3, 2, 5, 1; **6.** 2; **7.** 1, 4, 6; **8.** 4; **9.** 2, 4; **10.** 1, 3; **11.** 1; **12.** Width, length, and depth; **13.** 2; **14.** 3; **15.** 1, 3, 5

Rationales for Review Questions can be found on the Evolve website.

REFERENCES

Ayello EA, et al: Pressure ulcers. In Baranoski S, Ayello AE, editors: *Wound care essentials: practice principles*, ed 3, Philadelphia, 2012, Lippincott Williams & Wilkins.

Baranoski S, et al: Wound assessment. In Baranoski S, Ayello AE, editors: *Wound care essentials: practice principles*, ed 3, Philadelphia, 2012, Lippincott, Williams & Wilkins.

Berlowitz D: Prevention of pressure ulcers, *UpToDate* 2014a. http://www.uptodate.com/contents/prevention-of-pressure-ulcers. Accessed January 2016.

Berlowitz D: Clinical staging and management of pressure ulcers, *UpToDate* 2014b. http://www.uptodate.com/contents/clinical-staging-and-management-of-pressure-ulcers. Accessed January 2016.

Bryant RA: Types of skin damage and differential diagnosis. In Bryant RA, Nix DP, editors: *Acute and chronic wounds: current management concepts*, ed 5, St Louis, 2016, Elsevier.

Bryant RA, Nix DP: Developing and maintaining a pressure ulcer prevention program. In Bryant RA, Nix DP, editors: *Acute and chronic wounds: current management concepts*, ed 5, St Louis, 2016, Elsevier.

Colwell JC, et al: MASD Part 3: Peristomal moisture–associated dermatitis and periwound moisture–associated dermatitis a consensus, *J Wound Ostomy Continence Nurs* 38(5):541, 2011.

Doughty DB, Sparks-Defriese B: Wound-healing physiology. In Bryant RA, Nix DP, editors: *Acute and chronic wounds: current management concepts*, ed 6, St Louis, 2016, Elsevier.

Ebbinghaus S, Kobayashi A: Safe heat application for pediatric patients, *J Nurs Care Qual* 25(2):168, 2010.

Fletcher J: Device-related pressure ulcers made easy, *Wounds UK* 8(2):1, 2012.

Gaskin FC: Detection of cyanosis in the person with dark skin, *J Natl Black Nurses Assoc* 1:52, 1986.

Gray M, et al: Moisture-associated skin damage: overview and pathophysiology, *J Wound Ostomy Continence Nurs* 38(3):233, 2011.

Graybill JC, et al: Traumatic wounds: bullets, blasts, and vehicle crashes. In Bryant RS, Nix DP, editors: *Acute and chronic wounds: current management concepts*, ed 5, St Louis, 2016, Elsevier.

Harris C, et al: Bates Jensen wound assessment tool: pictorial guide validation project, *J Wound Ostomy Continence Nurs* 37(3):253, 2010.

Henderson CT, et al: Draft definition of stage I pressure ulcers: inclusion of persons with darkly pigmented skin, *Adv Wound Care* 10(5):16, 1997.

KCI USA: *The VAC: therapy safety information, product information*, San Antonio, 2007, Author.

Krazner DL: Wound pain: impact and assessment. In Bryant RA, Nix DP, editors: *Acute and chronic wounds: nursing management*, ed 5, St Louis, 2016, Elsevier.

Litchford MD, et al: Malnutrition as a precursor of pressure ulcers, *Adv Wound Care* 3(1):54, 2014.

McNichol L, et al: Medical adhesives and patient safety: state of the science: consensus statements for the assessment, prevention, and treatment of adhesive-related skin injuries, *J Wound Ostomy Continence Nurs* 40(4):365, 2013.

National Pressure Ulcer Advisory Panel, European Pressure Ulcer Advisory Panel and Pan Pacific Pressure Injury Alliance. Prevention and Treatment of Pressure Ulcers (NPUAP, EPUAP, PPPIA): Haesler Emily, editor: *Clinical Practice Guideline*, Osborne Park, Western Australia, 2014, Cambridge Media.

National Quality Forum (NQF): *National Voluntary Consensus Standards for Public Reporting of Patient Safety Event Information*, National Quality Forum, 2011, http://www.qualityforum.org/Publications/2011/02/National_Voluntary_Consensus_Standards_for_Public_Reporting_of_Patient_Safety_Event_Information.aspx. Accessed July 15, 2015.

Netsch DS: Negative-pressure wound therapy. In Bryant RA, Nix DP, editors: *Acute and chronic wounds:*

current management concepts, ed 5, St Louis, 2016, Elsevier.

Nix D: Skin and wound inspection and assessment. In Bryant RA, Nix DP, editors: *Acute and chronic wounds: current management concepts*, ed 5, St Louis, 2016, Elsevier.

Pieper B: Pressure ulcers: impact, etiology, and classification. In Bryant RA, Nix DP, editors: *Acute and chronic wounds: current management concepts*, ed 5, St Louis, 2016, Elsevier.

Ramundo JM: Wound debridement. In Bryant RA, Nix DP, editors: *Acute and chronic wounds: current management concepts*, ed 5, St Louis, 2016, Elsevier.

Rolstad BS, et al: Topical management. In Bryant RA, Nix DP, editors: *Acute and chronic wounds: current management concepts*, ed 5, St Louis, 2016, Elsevier.

Sommers MS: Color awareness: a must for patient assessment, *Am Nurs Today* 6(1):6, 2011.

Stotts NA: Nutritional assessment and support. In Bryant RA, Nix DP, editors: *Acute and chronic wounds: current management concepts*, ed 5, St Louis, 2016a, Elsevier.

Stotts NA: Wound infection: diagnosis and management. In Bryant RA, Nix DP, editors: *Acute and chronic wounds: current management concepts*, ed 5, St Louis, 2016b, Elsevier.

The Joint Commission (TJC): *Nutritional, functional and pain assessments and screens*, 2008, http://www.jointcommission.org/standards_information/jcfaqdetails.aspx?StandardsFAQId=471. Accessed September 2015.

The Joint Commission (TJC): *Pain management*, 2015. Available at http://www.jointcommission.org/topics/pain_management.aspx. Accessed December 2015.

The Joint Commission (TJC): *2016 National Patient Safety Goals*, Oakbrook Terrace, IL, 2016, The Commission. Available at, http://www.jointcommission.org/standards_information/npsgs.aspx. Accessed November 2015.

Wolvos T: The use of negative pressure wound therapy with an automated volumetric fluid administration, *Wounds* 25(2):75, 2013.

Wound, Ostomy and Continence Nurses Society (WOCN): *Guideline for prevention and management of pressure ulcers, WOCN* Clinical Practice Guideline Series, Mount Laurel, NJ, 2010, WOCN.

Wound, Ostomy and Continence Nurses Society (WOCN): *Guideline for prevention and management of pressure injuries (ulcers): An executive summary, WOCN* Clinical Practice Guideline Series, Mount Laurel, NJ, 2016, WOCN.

Wysocki AB: Wound-healing physiology. In Bryant RA, Nix DP, editors: *Acute and chronic wounds: current management concepts*, ed 5, St Louis, 2016, Elsevier.

RESEARCH REFERENCES

Berry KM, et al: Implementation of a pressure ulcer prevention program (PUPP) at two urban hospitals, *J Wound Ostomy Continence Nurs* 40(S1):2013.

Black JM, et al: Medical device related pressures in hospitalized patients, *Int Wound J* 7(5):358, 2010.

Black JM, et al: Use of wound dressings to enhance prevention of pressure ulcers caused by medical devices, *Int Wound J* 12:322, 2015.

Bleakley CM, Costello JT: Do thermal agents affect range of movement and mechanical properties in soft tissues? A systematic review, *Arch Phys Med Rehabil* 94:140, 2013.

Braden BJ, Bergstrom N: Clinical utility of the Braden Scale for predicting pressure sore risk, *Decubitus* 2(3):50, 1989.

Braden BJ, Bergstrom N: Predictive validity of the Braden Scale for pressure sore risk in a nursing home population, *Res Nurs Health* 17(6):459, 1994.

Burton AC, Yamada S: Relation between blood pressure and flow in the human forearm, *J Appl Physiol* 4(5):329, 1951.

Gray M, Weir D: Prevention and treatment of moisture-associated skin damage (maceration) in the periwound skin, *J Wound Ostomy Continence Nurs* 34(2):153, 2007.

Gray M, et al: Peristomal moisture-associated skin damage with fecal ostomies: a comprehensive review and consensus, *J Wound Ostomy Continence Nurs* 40(4):389, 2013.

Guest JF, et al: Clinical and economic evidence supporting a transparent barrier film dressing in incontinence-associated dermatitis and peri-wound skin protection, *J Wound Care* 20(2):76, 2011.

Hyun S, et al: Predictive validity of the Braden scale for patients in intensive care units, *Am J Crit Care* 22(6):514, 2013.

Januchowski R, Ferguson WJ: The clinical use of tissue adhesives: a review of the literature, *Osteopath Fam Phys* 2:25, 2014.

Maxwell S, Sterling M: An investigation of the use of a numeric pain rating scale with ice application to the neck to determine cold hyperalgesia, *Man Ther* 18:172, 2013.

Pham B, et al: Early prevention of pressure ulcers among elderly patients admitted through emergency departments: a cost-effectiveness analysis, *Ann Emerg Med* 58(5):468, 2011.

Pierpont VN, et al: Obesity and surgical wound healing: a current review, *ISRN Obes* 2014. http://dx.doi.org/10.1155/2014/638936.

Upton D, Andrews A: Pain and trauma in negative pressure wound therapy: a review, *Int Wound J* 12(1):100, 2015.

Voegeli D: Moisture-associated skin damage: aetiology, prevention and treatment, *Br J Nurs* 21(9):517, 2012.

Xie X, et al: The clinical effectiveness of negative-pressure wound therapy: a systematic review, *J Wound Care* 19(11):490, 2010.

49

Sensory Alterations

OBJECTIVES

- Differentiate among the processes of reception, perception, and reaction to sensory stimuli.
- Discuss the relationship of sensory function to an individual's level of wellness.
- Discuss common causes and effects of sensory alterations.
- Discuss common sensory changes that normally occur with aging.
- Assess a patient's sensory status.
- Identify nursing diagnoses relevant to patients with sensory alterations.
- Develop a plan of care for patients with sensory deficits.
- List interventions for preventing sensory deprivation and controlling sensory overload.
- Describe conditions in a health care agency or patient's home that you can modify to promote meaningful sensory stimulation.
- Discuss ways to maintain a safe environment for patients with sensory deficits.

KEY TERMS

Aphasia, p. 1248
Auditory, p. 1241
Conductive hearing loss, p. 1253
Expressive aphasia, p. 1248
Gustatory, p. 1241
Hyperesthesia, p. 1253
Kinesthetic, p. 1241
Olfactory, p. 1241
Otolaryngologist, p. 1246
Ototoxic, p. 1248
Proprioceptive, p. 1244
Receptive aphasia, p. 1248
Refractive error, p. 1252
Sensory deficit, p. 1242
Sensory deprivation, p. 1242
Sensory overload, p. 1243
Stereognosis, p. 1241
Strabismus, p. 1252
Tactile, p. 1241

MEDIA RESOURCES

http://evolve.elsevier.com/Potter/fundamentals/

- Review Questions
- Concept Map Creator
- Case Study with Questions
- Audio Glossary
- Content Updates

Imagine the world without sight, hearing, the ability to feel objects, or the ability to sense aromas around you. People rely on a variety of sensory stimuli to give meaning and order to events occurring in their environment. The senses form the perceptual base of our world. Stimulation comes from many sources in and outside the body, particularly through the senses of sight (visual), hearing (**auditory**), touch (**tactile**), smell (**olfactory**), and taste (**gustatory**). The body also has a **kinesthetic** sense that enables a person to be aware of the position and movement of body parts without seeing them. **Stereognosis** is a sense that allows a person to recognize the size, shape, and texture of an object. The ability to speak is not a sense, but it is similar in that some patients lose the ability to interact meaningfully with other human beings. Meaningful stimuli allow a person to learn about the environment and are necessary for healthy functioning and normal development. When sensory function is altered, a person's ability to relate to and function within the environment changes drastically.

Many patients seeking health care have preexisting sensory alterations. Others develop them as a result of medical treatment (e.g., hearing loss from antibiotic use or hearing or visual loss from brain tumor removal) or hospitalization. The health care environment is a place of unfamiliar sights, sounds, and smells and minimal contact with family and friends. If patients feel depersonalized and are unable to receive meaningful stimuli, serious sensory alterations sometimes develop.

As a nurse you meet the needs of patients with existing sensory alterations and recognize those most at risk for developing sensory problems. You also help patients who have partial or complete loss of a major sense to find alternate ways to function safely within their environment.

SCIENTIFIC KNOWLEDGE BASE

Normal Sensation

The nervous system continually receives thousands of bits of information from sensory nerve organs, relays the information through appropriate neurological channels, and integrates the information into a meaningful response. Sensory stimuli reach the sensory organs to elicit an immediate reaction or store information in the brain for future use. The nervous system must be intact for sensory stimuli to reach appropriate brain centers and for an individual to perceive the sensation. After interpreting the significance of a sensation, the person is

TABLE 49-1 Normal Hearing and Vision

Function	Anatomy and Physiology
Ear	
Transmits to brain a pattern of all sounds received from the environment, the relative intensity of these sounds, and the direction from which they originate	Two ears provide stereophonic hearing to judge sound direction. The external ear canal shelters the eardrum and maintains relatively constant temperature and humidity to maintain elasticity. The middle ear is an air-containing space between the eardrum and oval window. It contains three small bones (ossicles). The eardrum and ossicles transfer sound to the fluid-filled inner ear. Movement of the stapes in the oval window creates vibrations in the fluid that bathes the membranous labyrinth, which contains the end organs of hearing and balance. The union of the vestibular (balance) and cochlear (hearing) parts of the labyrinth explains the combination of hearing and balance symptoms that occur with inner ear disorders. Vibration of the eardrum transmits through the bony ossicles. Vibrations at the oval window transmit in perilymph within the inner ear to stimulate hair cells that send impulses along the eighth cranial nerve to the brain.
Eye	
Transmits a pattern of light to the brain that is reflected from solid objects in the environment and becomes transformed into color and hue	Light rays enter the convex cornea and begin to converge. An adjustment of light rays occurs as they pass through the pupil and lens. Change in the shape of the lens focuses light on the retina. The retina has a pigmented layer of cells to enhance visual acuity. The sensory retina contains the rods and cones (i.e., photoreceptor cells sensitive to stimulation from light). Photoreceptor cells send electrical potentials by way of the optic nerve to the brain.

then able to react to the stimulus. Table 49-1 summarizes normal hearing and vision.

Reception, perception, and reaction are the three components of any sensory experience. Reception begins with stimulation of a nerve cell called a *receptor,* which is usually for only one type of stimulus such as light, touch, taste, or sound. In the case of special senses, the receptors are grouped close together or located in specialized organs such as the taste buds of the tongue or the retina of the eye. When a nerve impulse is created, it travels along pathways to the spinal cord or directly to the brain. For example, sound waves stimulate hair cell receptors within the organ of Corti in the ear, which causes impulses to travel along the eighth cranial nerve to the acoustic area of the temporal lobe. Sensory nerve pathways usually cross over to send stimuli to opposite sides of the brain.

The actual perception or awareness of unique sensations depends on the receiving region of the cerebral cortex, where specialized neurons interpret the quality and nature of sensory stimuli. When a person becomes conscious of a stimulus and receives the information, perception takes place. Perception includes integration and interpretation of stimuli on the basis of the person's experiences. A person's level of consciousness influences perception and interpretation of stimuli. Any factors lowering consciousness impair sensory perception. If sensation is incomplete such as blurred vision or if past experience is inadequate for understanding stimuli such as pain, the person can react inappropriately to the sensory stimulus.

It is impossible to react to all stimuli entering the nervous system. The brain prevents sensory bombardment by discarding or storing sensory information. A person usually reacts to stimuli that are most meaningful or significant at the time. After continued reception of the same stimulus, a person stops responding, and the sensory experience goes unnoticed. For example, a person concentrating on reading a good book is not aware of background music. This adaptability phenomenon occurs with most sensory stimuli except for those of pain.

The balance between sensory stimuli entering the brain and those actually reaching a person's conscious awareness maintains a person's well-being. If an individual attempts to react to every stimulus within the environment or if the variety and quality of stimuli are insufficient, sensory alterations occur.

Sensory Alterations

The most common types of sensory alterations are sensory deficits, sensory deprivation, and sensory overload. When a patient suffers from more than one sensory alteration, the ability to function and relate effectively within the environment is seriously impaired.

Sensory Deficits. A deficit in the normal function of sensory reception and perception is a **sensory deficit**. When a person loses visual or hearing acuity, he or she withdraws by avoiding communication or socialization with others in an attempt to cope with the sensory loss. It becomes difficult for the person to interact safely with the environment until he or she learns new skills. When a deficit develops gradually or when considerable time has passed since the onset of an acute sensory loss, a person learns to rely on unaffected senses. Some senses may even become more acute to compensate for an alteration. For example, a blind patient develops an acute sense of hearing to compensate for visual loss.

Patients with sensory deficits often change behavior in adaptive or maladaptive ways. For example, a patient with a hearing impairment turns the unaffected ear toward the speaker to hear better, whereas another patient avoids people because he or she is embarrassed about not being able to understand what other people say. Box 49-1 summarizes common sensory deficits and their influence on those affected.

Sensory Deprivation. The reticular activating system in the brainstem mediates all sensory stimuli to the cerebral cortex; thus patients are able to receive stimuli even while sleeping deeply. Sensory stimulation must be of sufficient quality and quantity to maintain a person's awareness. Three types of **sensory deprivation** are reduced sensory input (sensory deficit from visual or hearing loss), the elimination of patterns or meaning from input (e.g., exposure to strange environments), and restrictive environments (e.g., bed rest) that produce monotony and boredom (Touhy and Jett, 2014).

BOX 49-1 Common Sensory Deficits

Visual Deficits

Presbyopia: A gradual decline in the ability of the lens to accommodate or focus on close objects. Individual is unable to see near objects clearly.

Cataract: Cloudy or opaque areas in part of the lens or the entire lens that interfere with passage of light through the lens, causing problems with glare and blurred vision. Cataracts usually develop gradually, without pain, redness, or tearing in the eye.

Dry eyes: Result when tear glands produce too few tears, resulting in itching, burning, or even reduced vision.

Glaucoma: A slowly progressive increase in intraocular pressure that, if left untreated, causes progressive pressure against the optic nerve, resulting in peripheral visual loss, decreased visual acuity with difficulty adapting to darkness, and a halo effect around lights.

Diabetic retinopathy: Pathological changes occur in the blood vessels of the retina, resulting in decreased vision or vision loss caused by hemorrhage and macular edema.

Macular degeneration: Condition in which the macula (specialized part of the retina responsible for central vision) loses its ability to function efficiently. First signs include blurring of reading matter, distortion or loss of central vision, and distortion of vertical lines.

Hearing Deficits

Presbycusis: A common progressive hearing disorder in older adults.

Cerumen accumulation: Buildup of earwax in the external auditory canal. Cerumen becomes hard and collects in the canal and causes conduction deafness.

Balance Deficit

Dizziness and disequilibrium: Common condition in older adulthood, usually resulting from vestibular dysfunction. Frequently a change in position of the head precipitates an episode of vertigo or disequilibrium.

Taste Deficit

Xerostomia: Decrease in salivary production that leads to thicker mucus and a dry mouth. Often interferes with the ability to eat and leads to appetite and nutritional problems.

Neurological Deficits

Peripheral neuropathy: Disorder of the peripheral nervous system, characterized by symptoms that include numbness and tingling of the affected area and stumbling gait.

Stroke: Cerebrovascular accident caused by clot, hemorrhage, or emboli disrupting blood flow to the brain. Creates altered proprioception with marked incoordination and imbalance. Loss of sensation and motor function in extremities controlled by the affected area of the brain also occurs. A stroke affecting the left hemisphere of the brain results in symptoms on the right side such as difficulty with speech. A stroke on the right hemisphere has symptoms on the left side, which includes visual spatial alterations such as loss of half of a visual field or inattention and neglect, especially to the left side.

There are many effects of sensory deprivation (Box 49-2). In adults the symptoms are similar to those of psychological illness, confusion, symptoms of severe electrolyte imbalance, or the influence of psychotropic drugs. Therefore always be aware of a patient's existing sensory function and the quality of stimuli within the environment.

Sensory Overload. When a person receives multiple sensory stimuli and cannot perceptually disregard or selectively ignore some stimuli, sensory overload occurs. Excessive sensory stimulation prevents the brain from responding appropriately to or ignoring certain stimuli. Because of the multitude of stimuli leading to overload, a person no longer perceives the environment in a way that makes sense. Overload prevents meaningful response by the brain; the patient's thoughts race, attention scatters in many directions, and anxiety and restlessness occur. As a result, overload causes a state similar to that produced by sensory deprivation. However, in contrast to deprivation, overload is individualized. The amount of stimuli necessary for healthy function varies with each individual. People are often subject to environmental overload more at one time than another. A person's tolerance to sensory overload varies with level of fatigue, attitude, and emotional and physical well-being.

BOX 49-2 Effects of Sensory Deprivation

Cognitive

- Reduced capacity to learn
- Inability to think or problem solve
- Poor task performance
- Disorientation/confusion
- Bizarre thinking
- Increased need for socialization, altered mechanisms of attention

Affective

- Boredom
- Restlessness
- Increased anxiety
- Emotional lability
- Panic
- Increased need for physical stimulation

Perceptual

- Changes in visual/motor coordination
- Reduced color perception
- Less tactile accuracy
- Changes in ability to perceive size and shape
- Changes in spatial and time judgment

A patient who is acutely ill, especially one in a critical care unit, experiences sensory overload easily. A patient in constant pain or who undergoes frequent monitoring of vital signs is also at risk. Multiple stimuli combine to cause overload even if you offer a comforting word or provide a gentle backrub. Some patients do not benefit from nursing intervention because their attention and energy are focused on more stressful stimuli. In a critical care unit where the activity is constant, the lights are frequently on. Patients can hear sounds from monitoring equipment, staff conversations, equipment alarms, and the activities of people entering the unit.

It is easy to confuse the behavioral changes associated with sensory overload with mood swings or simple disorientation. Look for symptoms such as racing thoughts, scattered attention, restlessness, and anxiety. Patients in intensive care units (ICUs) sometimes constantly play with tubes and dressings. Constant reorientation and control of excessive stimuli become an important part of a patient's care.

NURSING KNOWLEDGE BASE

Factors Influencing Sensory Function

Many factors influence the capacity to receive or perceive stimuli. You manage all of these conditions or situations when delivering patient care.

Age. Infants and children are at risk for visual and hearing impairment because of a number of genetic, prenatal, and postnatal conditions. A concern with high-risk neonates is that early intense visual and auditory stimulation can adversely affect visual and auditory pathways and alter the developmental course of other sensory organs (Hockenberry and Wilson, 2015). Visual changes during adulthood include presbyopia and the need for glasses for reading. These changes usually occur from ages 40 to 50. In addition, the cornea, which assists with light refraction to the retina, becomes flatter and thicker, which often leads to astigmatism. Pigment is lost from the iris; and collagen fibers build up in the anterior chamber, which increases the risk of glaucoma by decreasing the resorption of intraocular fluid. Other normal visual changes associated with aging include reduced visual fields, increased glare sensitivity, impaired night vision, reduced depth perception, and reduced color discrimination.

Hearing changes begin at the age of 30. Changes associated with aging include decreased hearing acuity, speech intelligibility, and pitch discrimination. Low-pitched sounds are easiest to hear, but it is difficult to hear conversation over background noise. It is also difficult to discriminate the consonants *(z, t, f, g)* and high-frequency sounds *(s, sh, ph, k)*. Vowels that have a low pitch are easiest to hear. Speech sounds are distorted, and there is a delayed reception and reaction to speech. A concern with normal age-related sensory changes is that older adults with a deficit are sometimes inappropriately diagnosed with dementia (Touhy and Jett, 2014).

Gustatory and olfactory changes begin around age 50 and include a decrease in the number of taste buds and sensory cells in the nasal lining. Reduced taste discrimination and sensitivity to odors are common.

Proprioceptive changes common after age 60 include increased difficulty with balance, spatial orientation, and coordination. The person cannot avoid obstacles as quickly, and the automatic response to protect and brace oneself when falling is slower. There are also tactile changes, including declining sensitivity to pain, pressure, and temperature secondary to peripheral vascular disease and neuropathies.

Meaningful Stimuli. Meaningful stimuli reduce the incidence of sensory deprivation. In the home meaningful stimuli include pets, music, television, pictures of family members, and a calendar and clock. The same stimuli need to be present in health care settings. Note whether patients have roommates or visitors. The presence of others offers positive stimulation. However, a roommate who constantly watches television, persistently tries to talk, or continuously keeps lights on contributes to sensory overload. The presence or absence of meaningful stimuli influences alertness and the ability to participate in care.

Amount of Stimuli. Excessive stimuli in an environment causes sensory overload. The frequency of observations and procedures performed in an acute health care setting are often stressful. If a patient is in pain or restricted by a cast or traction, overstimulation frequently is a problem. In addition, a room that is near repetitive or loud noises (e.g., an elevator, stairwell, or nurses' station) contributes to sensory overload.

Social Interaction. The amount and quality of social contact with supportive family members and significant others influence sensory function. The absence of visitors during hospitalization or residency in an extended care facility influences the degree of isolation a patient feels. This is a common problem in hospital intensive care settings, where visitation is often restricted. The ability to discuss concerns with loved ones is an important coping mechanism for most people. Therefore the absence of meaningful conversation results in feelings of isolation, loneliness, anxiety, and depression for a patient. Often this is not apparent until behavioral changes occur.

Environmental Factors. A person's occupation places him or her at risk for hearing, visual, and peripheral nerve alterations. Individuals who have occupations involving exposure to high noise levels (e.g., factory or airport workers) are at risk for noise-induced hearing loss and need to be screened for hearing impairments. Hazardous noise is common in work settings and recreational activities. Noisy recreational activities that weaken hearing ability include target shooting and hunting, woodworking, and listening to loud music. Individuals who have occupations involving risk of exposure to chemicals or flying objects (e.g., welders) are at risk for eye injuries and need to be screened for visual impairments. Sports activities and consumer fireworks also place individuals at risk for visual alterations. Occupations that involve repetitive wrist or finger movements (e.g., heavy assembly line work, long periods of computer use) cause pressure on the median nerve, resulting in carpal tunnel syndrome. Carpal tunnel syndrome alters tactile sensation and is one of the most common industrial or work-related injuries. Patients at risk for carpal tunnel need to be carefully assessed for numbness, tingling, weakness, and pain.

A patient who is hospitalized is sometimes at risk for sensory alterations as a result of exposure to environmental stimuli or a change in sensory input. Patients who are immobilized by bed rest or who have a chronic disability are unable to experience all of the normal sensations of free movement. Another group at risk includes patients isolated in a health care setting or at home because of conditions such as active tuberculosis (see Chapter 29). These patients stay in private rooms and are often unable to enjoy normal interactions with visitors.

Cultural Factors. Certain sensory alterations occur more commonly in select cultural groups. Analysis of data from the National Health and Nutrition Examination Survey (NHANES) and the National Health Interview Survey (NHIS) showed that non-Hispanic whites had a higher prevalence of age-related macular degeneration than non-Hispanic African-Americans but a lower prevalence of diabetic retinopathy and glaucoma (Zhang et al., 2012). Cultural disparities in vision impairment are significant, in part because vision loss has a significant impact on activities of daily living, symptoms of depression, and feelings of anxiety (Box 49-3) (Kempen et al., 2012). Changes in hearing and visual acuity also impact a person's health literacy and his or her ability to understand medications, procedures, and restorative and home care interventions, which are further complicated when English is a second language.

CRITICAL THINKING

Successful critical thinking requires a synthesis of knowledge and information gathered from patients, experience, critical thinking attitudes, and intellectual and professional standards. Clinical judgments require you to anticipate the information necessary, analyze the data, and make decisions regarding patient care. Patients' conditions are always changing. During assessment (Figure 49-1) consider all critical thinking elements that help you make appropriate nursing diagnoses. In the case of sensory alterations, integrate knowledge of the pathophysiology of sensory deficits, factors that affect sensory function, and therapeutic communication principles. This knowledge enables you to conduct appropriate assessments, anticipate what to recognize when a patient describes a sensory problem, and make judgments of abnormalities. For example, knowing the typical symptoms caused by a cataract helps you recognize the pattern of visual changes that a patient with cataracts reports.

Previous experiences in caring for patients with sensory deficits help you recognize limitations in a patient's functioning and how these limitations affect the ability to carry out daily activities. For example, after caring for one patient with a hearing impairment, you are able to conduct a more effective assessment of the next patient by using

BOX 49-3 CULTURAL ASPECTS OF CARE

Disparities in Eye Care Practices

The early diagnosis and treatment of visual impairments in people from other cultures could improve their quality of life (Wang et al., 2014). However, some individuals, especially older adults, do not always volunteer information about impairments or seek professional advice because of cultural reasons or language difficulties (Higginbottom et al., 2014). A lack of awareness of existing services also contributes to disparities in using eye care resources. Findings from the Behavioral Risk Factor Surveillance System data revealed state-level disparities in eye care use by culture, annual income, and education level (Chou et al., 2012). In some states Hispanics and non-Hispanic African-Americans were less likely to have visited an eye doctor in the previous year than non-Hispanic whites. In nearly all states a lack of awareness regarding vision health was greater among people at lower income and education levels (Chou et al., 2012).

Implications for Patient-Centered Care

- Encourage patients to discuss changes in visual acuity or other eye or vision issues by asking a few focused questions.
- Enhance your knowledge of the eye care services available to patients.
- Facilitate access to services to promote the early detection and treatment of visual impairments.
- When English is a second language, identify the patient's preferred method of communication; use an interpreter service if needed.
- Ensure that written eye care information is available in the appropriate language and format (e.g., large print).

previously successful approaches that promote the patient's ability to hear your questions.

When critical thinking attitudes and standards are applied during assessment, they ensure a thorough and accurate database from which to make decisions. For example, perseverance is necessary to learn details about how visual changes influence a patient's ability to socialize. Evidence-based standards of care and practice such as those from the American Academy of Ophthalmology and the American Speech-Language-Hearing Association provide criteria for screening sensory problems and establishing standards for competent, safe, effective care and practice. Use critical thinking to conduct a thorough assessment and then plan, implement, and evaluate care that enables a patient to function safely and effectively (Box 49-4).

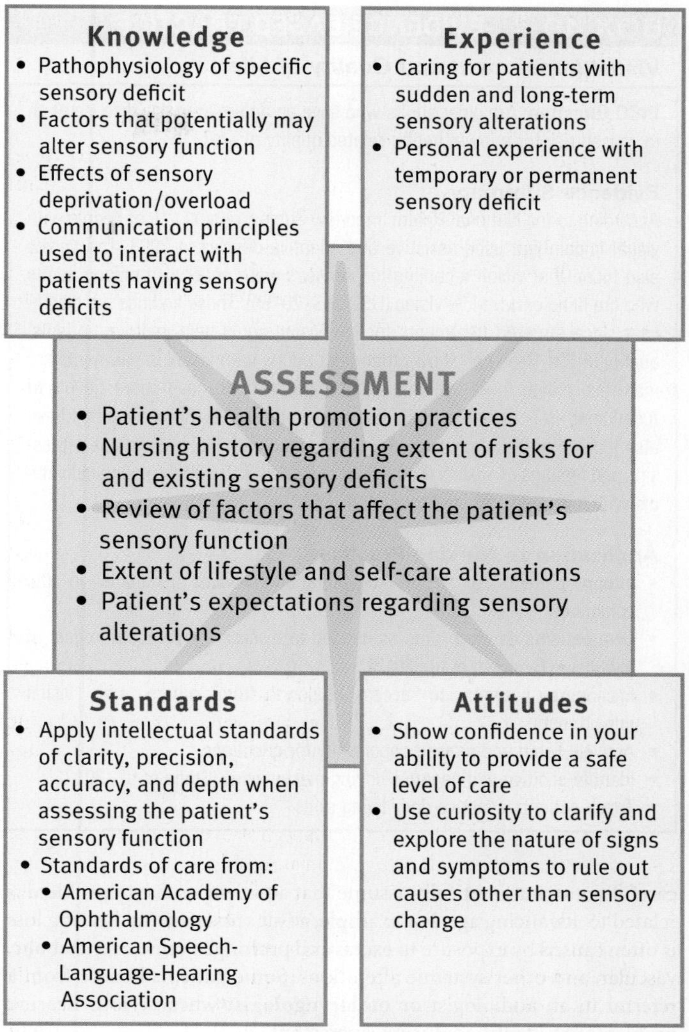

Knowledge
- Pathophysiology of specific sensory deficit
- Factors that potentially may alter sensory function
- Effects of sensory deprivation/overload
- Communication principles used to interact with patients having sensory deficits

Experience
- Caring for patients with sudden and long-term sensory alterations
- Personal experience with temporary or permanent sensory deficit

ASSESSMENT
- Patient's health promotion practices
- Nursing history regarding extent of risks for and existing sensory deficits
- Review of factors that affect the patient's sensory function
- Extent of lifestyle and self-care alterations
- Patient's expectations regarding sensory alterations

Standards
- Apply intellectual standards of clarity, precision, accuracy, and depth when assessing the patient's sensory function
- Standards of care from:
  - American Academy of Ophthalmology
  - American Speech-Language-Hearing Association

Attitudes
- Show confidence in your ability to provide a safe level of care
- Use curiosity to clarify and explore the nature of signs and symptoms to rule out causes other than sensory change

FIGURE 49-1 Critical thinking model for sensory alterations assessment.

NURSING PROCESS

Apply the nursing process and use a critical thinking approach in your care of patients. The nursing process provides a clinical decision-making approach for you to develop and implement an individualized plan of care for your patients.

Assessment

During the assessment process, thoroughly assess each patient and critically analyze findings to ensure that you make patient-centered clinical decisions required for safe nursing care.

Through the Patient's Eyes. When conducting an assessment, value the patient as a full partner in planning, implementing, and evaluating care. Patients are often hesitant to admit sensory losses. Therefore start gathering information by establishing a therapeutic rapport with the patient. Elicit his or her values, preferences, and expectations with regard to his or her sensory impairment. Many patients have a definite plan as to how they want their care delivered. Some patients expect caregivers to recognize and appropriately manage and adjust their environment to meet their sensory needs. This includes helping the family and patient learn and adapt to a changed lifestyle on the basis of the specific sensory impairment. Determine from the patient which interventions were helpful in the past in the management of limitations. Assess the patient's expertise with his or her own health and symptoms. Always remember that patients with sensory alterations have strengthened their other senses and expect caregivers to anticipate their needs (e.g., for safety and security).

When assessing a patient with or at risk for sensory alteration, first consider the pathophysiology of existing deficits and the factors influencing sensory function to anticipate how to approach his or her assessment. For example, if a patient has a hearing disorder, adjust your communication style and focus the assessment on relevant criteria related to hearing deficits. Collect a history that also assesses the patient's current sensory status and the degree to which a sensory deficit affects the patient's lifestyle, psychosocial adjustment, developmental status, self-care ability, health promotion habits, and safety. Also focus the assessment on the quality and quantity of stimuli within the patient's environment.

People at Risk. Older adults are a high-risk group because of normal physiological changes involving sensory organs. However, be

BOX 49-4 EVIDENCE-BASED PRACTICE

Visual Impairment and Quality of Life

PICO Question: Are older adults who have an age-related eye disease at an increased risk for a lower health-related quality of life?

Evidence Summary

According to the National Health Interview Survey, only 11.2% of people with visual impairment used assistive and adaptive devices in 2008. The survey also found that vision rehabilitation services were underused among adults who are blind or have low vision (USDHHS, 2015b). These findings are significant since targeted treatments for low vision could help improve patients' quality of life. Research shows that older adults with visual impairments are more likely than those without visual impairment to have poorer levels of functioning in activities of daily (Kempen et al., 2012). Recent studies have also found that visual impairment is associated with higher levels of depression and feelings of anxiety (Kempen et al., 2012), particularly among individuals with low coping skills (Stone et al., 2012)

Application to Nursing Practice

- Inform patients of vision rehabilitation services available in the community.
- Give patients as much time as needed to discuss the personal impact of low vision (Kempen et al., 2012).
- Encourage patients to access support from others with visual impairments.
- Actively listen and provide opportunity for questions.
- Identify positive and negative coping mechanisms (Stone et al., 2012).
- Teach patients adaptive daily living skills.

careful not to automatically assume that a patient's sensory problem is related to advancing age. For example, adult sensorineural hearing loss is often caused by exposure to excess and prolonged noise or metabolic, vascular, and other systemic alterations. Some patients benefit from a referral to an audiologist or **otolaryngologist** when serious hearing problems are identified during assessment.

Other individuals at risk for sensory alterations include those living in a confined environment such as a nursing home. Although most quality nursing homes or centers offer meaningful stimulation through group activities, environmental design, and mealtime gatherings, there are exceptions. An individual who is confined to a wheelchair, suffers from poor hearing and/or vision, has decreased energy, and avoids contact with others is at significant risk for sensory deprivation.

Patients who are acutely ill are also at risk because of an unfamiliar and unresponsive environment. This does not mean that all hospitalized patients have sensory alterations. However, you need to carefully assess patients subjected to continued sensory stimulation (e.g., ICU settings, long-term hospitalization, or multiple therapies). Assess a patient's environment within both the health care setting and the home, looking for factors that pose risks or need adjustment to provide safety and more appropriate sensory stimulation.

Sensory Alterations History. The nursing history includes assessment of the nature and characteristics of sensory alterations or any problem related to an alteration (Box 49-5). When taking the history, consider the ethnic or cultural background of the patient because certain alterations are higher in some cultural groups.

During the history it is useful to have a patient self-rate his or her sensory deficit by asking, "Rate your hearing as excellent, good, fair, poor, or bad." Then, on the basis of the patient's self-rating, explore his or her perception of a sensory loss more fully. This provides an in-depth look at how the sensory loss influences the patient's quality of life. In the case of hearing problems, a screening tool such as the Hearing Handicap Inventory for the Elderly (HHIE-S) effectively identifies patients needing audiological intervention (Tomioka et al., 2013). The HHIE-S is a 5-minute, 10-item questionnaire that assesses how the individual perceives the social and emotional effects of hearing loss. The higher the HHIE-S score, the greater the handicapping effect of a hearing impairment.

BOX 49-5 Nursing Assessment Questions

Nature of the Problem

- Which type of problem are you having with your vision/hearing?
- What have you tried to correct the vision/hearing difficulty?
- Do you use any devices to improve your vision/hearing?
- How effective are your glasses or hearing aids?

Signs and Symptoms

- Ask a patient with visual alterations: Do you require books with large print or on audiotape? Are you able to prepare a meal or write a check? Do you notice any eye irritation or drainage?
- Ask a patient with hearing alterations: Which types of sounds or tones do you have difficulty hearing? Do people tell you that they have to "shout" for you to hear them? Do people ask you not to talk so loud? Do you have a ringing, crackling, or buzzing in your ears? Is there pain: sharp, dull, burning, itching? Have you noticed any redness, swelling, or drainage? Any signs of infection?

Onset and Duration

- When did you notice the problem? How long has it lasted?
- Does it come and go, or is it constant?
- What makes the problem better or worse?

Predisposing Factors

- Do you work or participate in any activities that have the potential for vision/hearing injury? If so, how do you protect your hearing and vision?
- Do you have a family history of cataracts, glaucoma, macular degeneration, or hearing loss?
- When was your last vision/hearing examination?

Effect on Patient

- What effect has your vision/hearing problem had on your work, family, or social life?
- Have changes in your vision/hearing affected your feelings of independence?
- How does your vision/hearing problem make you feel about yourself?
- Do you have problems with routine care of glasses, contact lenses, or hearing aids?

A nursing history also reveals any recent changes in a patient's behavior. Frequently friends or family are the best resources for this information. Ask the family the following questions:

- Has your family member shown any recent mood swings (e.g., outbursts of anger, nervousness, fear, or irritability)?
- Have you noticed the family member avoiding social activities?

Mental Status. Assessment of mental status is valuable when you suspect sensory deprivation or overload. Observation of a patient during history taking, during the physical examination (see Chapter 31), and while providing nursing care offers valuable data about a patient's behaviors and mental status. Observe the patient's physical appearance and behavior, measure cognitive ability, and assess his or her emotional status. The Mini-Mental State Examination (MMSE) is

TABLE 49-2 Assessment of Sensory Function

Assessment Activities	Behavior Indicating Deficit (Children)	Behavior Indicating Deficit (Adults)
Vision		
Ask patient to read newspaper, magazine, or lettering on menu. Ask patient to identify colors on color chart or crayons. Observe patients performing ADLs.	Self-stimulation, including eye rubbing, body rocking, sniffing or smelling, arm twirling; hitching (using legs to propel while in sitting position) instead of crawling	Poor coordination, squinting, underreaching or overreaching for objects, persistent repositioning of objects, impaired night vision, accidental falls
Hearing		
Assess patient's hearing acuity (see Chapter 31) using spoken word and tuning fork tests. Assess for history of tinnitus. Observe patient conversing with others. Inspect ear canal for hardened cerumen. Observe patient behaviors in a group.	Frightened when unfamiliar people approach, no reflex or purposeful response to sounds, failure to be awakened by loud noise, slow or absent development of speech, greater response to movement than to sound, avoidance of social interaction with other children	Blank looks, decreased attention span, lack of reaction to loud noises, increased volume of speech, positioning of head toward sound, smiling and nodding of head in approval when someone speaks, use of other means of communication such as lip-reading or writing, complaints of ringing in ears
Touch		
Check patient's ability to discriminate between sharp and dull stimuli. Assess whether patient is able to distinguish objects (coin or safety pin) in the hand with eyes closed. Ask whether patient feels unusual sensations.	Inability to perform developmental tasks related to grasping objects or drawing, repeated injury from handling of harmful objects (e.g., hot stove, sharp knife)	Clumsiness, overreaction or underreaction to painful stimulus, failure to respond when touched, avoidance of touch, sensation of pins and needles, numbness Unable to identify object placed in hand
Smell		
Have patient close eyes and identify several nonirritating odors (e.g., coffee, vanilla).	Difficult to assess until child is 6 or 7 years old, difficulty discriminating noxious odors	Failure to react to noxious or strong odor, increased body odor, decreased sensitivity to odors
Taste		
Ask patient to sample and distinguish different tastes (e.g., lemon, sugar, salt). (Have patient drink or sip water and wait 1 minute between each taste.)	Inability to tell whether food is salty or sweet, possible ingestion of strange-tasting things	Change in appetite, excessive use of seasoning and sugar, complaints about taste of food, weight change

ADLs, Activities of daily living.

a tool you can use to measure disorientation, change in problem-solving abilities, and altered conceptualization and abstract thinking (see Chapter 31). For example, a patient with severe sensory deprivation is not always able to carry on a conversation, remain attentive, or display recent or past memory. An important step toward preventing cognition-related disability is education by nurses about disease process, available services, and assistive devices.

Physical Assessment. To identify sensory deficits and their severity, use physical assessment techniques to assess vision; hearing; olfaction; taste; and the ability to discriminate light touch, temperature, pain, and position (see Chapter 31). Table 49-2 summarizes specific assessment techniques for identifying sensory deficits. You gather more accurate data when the examination room is private, quiet, and comfortable for the patient. In addition, rely on personal observation to detect sensory alterations. Patients with a hearing impairment may seem inattentive to others, respond with inappropriate anger when spoken to, believe people are talking about them, answer questions inappropriately, have trouble following clear directions, and have monotonous voice quality and speak unusually loud or soft.

Ability to Perform Self-Care. Assess patients' functional abilities in their home environment or health care setting, including the ability to perform feeding, dressing, grooming, and toileting activities. For example, assess whether a patient with altered vision is able to find items on a meal tray and read directions on a prescription. Also determine a patient's ability to perform instrumental activities of daily living (IADLs) such as reading bills and writing checks, differentiating money denominations, and driving a vehicle at night. If a patient seems to have a sensory deficit, does he or she show concern for grooming? Does a patient's loss of balance prevent rising from a toilet seat safely? Can a patient recovering from a stroke manipulate buttons or zippers for dressing? If a sensory alteration impairs a patient's functional ability, providing resources within the home is a necessary part of discharge planning. Your findings may indicate the need for an occupational therapy consultation.

Health Promotion Habits. Assess the daily routines that patients follow to maintain sensory function. Which type of eye and ear care is a part of a patient's daily hygiene? For individuals who participate in sports (e.g., racquetball) or recreational activities (e.g., motorcycle riding) or who work in a setting in which ear or eye injury is a possibility (e.g., chemical exposure, welding, glass or stone polishing, or constant exposure to loud noise), determine if they wear safety glasses or hearing-protective devices (HPDs). Do patients who use assistive devices such as eyeglasses, contact lenses, or hearing aids know how to provide daily care (see Chapter 40)? Do patients use the devices, and are they in proper working order?

It is also important to assess a patient's adherence with routine health screening. When was the last time the patient had an eye examination or hearing evaluation? For adults routine screening of visual and hearing function is imperative to detect problems early. This is especially true in the case of glaucoma, which, if undetected, leads to permanent visual loss. Recommended screening guidelines usually occur on the basis of age. When a patient begins to show a hearing deficit, incorporate routine screening in regular examinations.

Environmental Hazards. Patients with sensory alterations are at risk for injury if their living environments are unsafe. For example, a patient with reduced vision cannot see potential hazards clearly. A patient with proprioceptive problems loses balance easily. A patient with reduced sensation cannot perceive hot-versus-cold temperatures. The condition of the home, the rooms, and the front and back entrances is often problematic to the patient with sensory alterations. Assess his or her home for common hazards, including the following:

- Uneven, cracked walkways leading to front/back door
- Extension and phone cords in the main route of walking traffic
- Loose area rugs and runners placed over carpeting
- Bathrooms without shower or tub grab bars
- Water faucets unmarked to designate hot and cold
- Unlit stairways, lack of handrails
- Poor lighting in stairways, halls, and entrance doors

In the hospital environment caregivers often forget to rearrange furniture and equipment to keep pathways from the bed and chair to the bathroom and entrance clear. It is helpful to walk into a patient's room and look for safety hazards:

- Is the call light within easy, safe reach?
- Are intravenous (IV) poles on wheels and easy to move?
- Are suction machines, IV pumps, or drainage bags positioned so a patient can rise from a bed or chair easily?
- Are bedside tables and areas clutter free?

An additional problem faced by patients who are visually impaired is the inability to read medication labels and syringe markings. Ask the patient to read a label to determine if he or she is able to read the dosage and frequency. If a patient has a hearing impairment, check to see whether the sounds of a doorbell, telephone, smoke alarm, and alarm clock are easy to discriminate.

Communication Methods. To understand the nature of a communication problem, you need to know whether a patient has trouble speaking, understanding, naming, reading, or writing. Patients with existing sensory deficits often develop alternate ways of communicating. To interact with a patient and promote interaction with others, understand his or her method of communication (Figure 49-2). Vision becomes almost a primary sense for people with hearing impairments. As a result, face-to-face communication is essential.

Patients with visual impairments are unable to observe facial expressions and other nonverbal behaviors to clarify the content of spoken communication. Instead they rely on voice tones and inflections to detect the emotional tone of communication. Some patients with visual deficits learn to read Braille. Patients with aphasia have varied degrees of inability to speak, interpret, or understand language. Expressive aphasia, a motor type of aphasia, is the inability to name common objects or express simple ideas in words or writing. For example, a patient understands a question but is unable to express an answer. Sensory or receptive aphasia is the inability to understand written or spoken language. A patient is able to express words but is unable to understand questions or comments of others. Global aphasia is the inability to understand language or communicate orally.

The temporary or permanent loss of the ability to speak is extremely traumatic to an individual. Assess for alternate communication methods and whether they cause anxiety. Patients who have undergone laryngectomies often write notes, use communication boards or laptop computers, speak with mechanical vibrators, or use esophageal speech. Patients with endotracheal or tracheostomy tubes have a temporary loss of speech. Most use a notepad to write their questions and requests. However, some patients become incapacitated and unable to write messages. Determine whether the patient has developed a sign-language system or symbols to communicate needs.

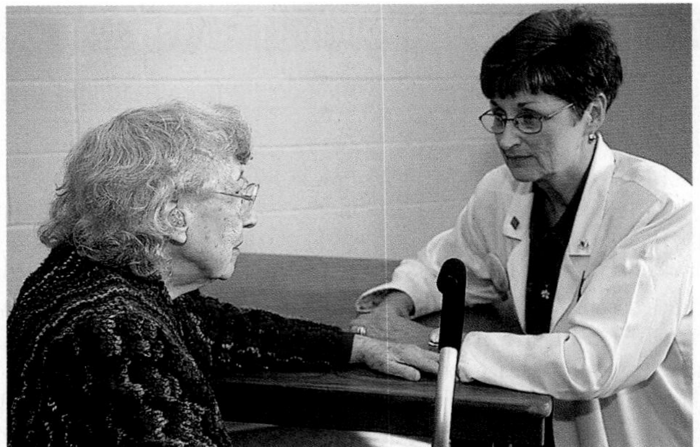

FIGURE 49-2 Nurse sits at eye level so patient with hearing impairment can communicate.

Social Support. Determine if a patient lives alone and whether family or friends visit frequently. Assess the patient's social skills and level of satisfaction with the support given by family and friends. Is the patient satisfied with the support available? Is he or she able to solve problems with family members? Is there a family caregiver who offers support when the patient requires assistance as a result of a sensory loss? The long-term effects of sensory alterations influence family dynamics and a patient's willingness to remain active in society.

Use of Assistive Devices. Assess the use of assistive devices (e.g., use of a hearing aid or glasses). Assess if the patient thinks that these devices are beneficial. This includes learning how often the patient uses the devices daily, the patient's or family caregiver's method of caring for and cleaning the devices, and the patient's knowledge of what to do when a problem develops. When you identify that a patient has an assistive device, remember that, just because the individual has the device, it does not mean that it works or that the patient uses it or benefits from it.

Other Factors Affecting Perception. Factors other than sensory deprivation or overload cause impaired perception (e.g., medications or pain). Assess the patient's medication history, which includes prescribed and over-the-counter medications and herbal products. Also gather information regarding the frequency, dose, method of administration, and last time these medications were taken. Some antibiotics (e.g., streptomycin, gentamicin, and tobramycin) are ototoxic and permanently damage the auditory nerve, whereas chloramphenicol sometimes irritates the optic nerve. Opioid analgesics, sedatives, and antidepressant medications often alter the perception of stimuli. Conduct a thorough pain assessment (see Chapter 44) when you suspect that pain is causing perceptual problems.

◆ Nursing Diagnosis

After assessment review all available data and look critically for patterns and trends suggestive of a health problem relating to sensory alterations (e.g., visual problems [Box 49-6]). Validate findings to ensure accuracy of the diagnosis. Determine the factor that likely causes a patient's health problem. The etiology or related factor of a nursing diagnosis is a condition that nursing interventions can affect. The etiology needs to be accurate; otherwise nursing therapies are ineffective.

Some patients have health care problems for which sensory alteration is the etiology such as with the diagnosis of *Risk for Injury.* You select nursing diagnoses by recognizing the way that sensory alterations affect a patient's ability to function (e.g., *Self-Care Deficit*). In addition, most patients present themselves to health care professionals with multiple diagnoses (Figure 49-3). In the concept map example, a patient with a cataract has the nursing diagnoses of *Risk for Injury, Anxiety, Fear,* and *Risk for Falls.* The sensory alteration caused by the cataract is an etiology for both risk for injury and risk for falls. Furthermore, fear occurs as a response to a perceived risk of falling. You need to recognize patterns of data that reveal health problems created by a patient's sensory alteration. Examples of nursing diagnoses that apply to patients with sensory alterations include the following:

- *Risk-Prone Health Behavior*
- *Impaired Verbal Communication*
- *Risk for Injury*
- *Impaired Physical Mobility*
- *Bathing Self-Care Deficit*
- *Situational Low Self-Esteem*
- *Risk for Falls*
- *Social Isolation*

BOX 49-6 Nursing Diagnostic Process

Risk for Injury

Assessment Activities	Defining Characteristics
Assess patient's visual acuity.	Has reduced ability to see objects clearly; needs brighter light to read; has trouble distinguishing edges of stairs
Visit home setting and inspect for hazards that pose risks to patient.	Lighting in rooms, hallways, and stairwells very dim; carpet in living room old, edges curled up; steps leading up to front entrance of home
Review medical record from clinic visit.	Bilateral cataracts

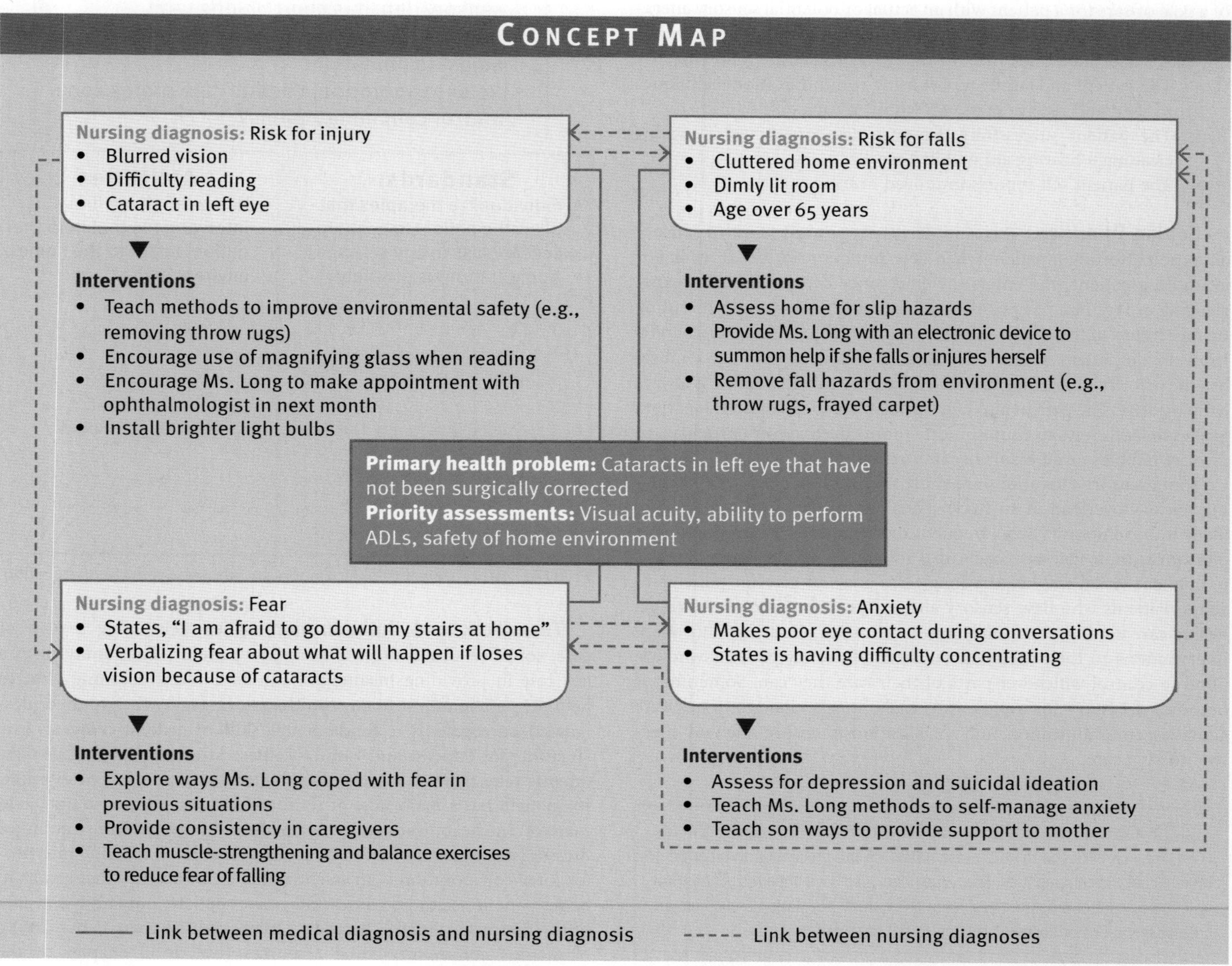

FIGURE 49-3 Concept map for Ms. Long.

◆ Planning

During planning synthesize information from multiple resources (Figure 49-4). Reflect on knowledge gained from the assessment and knowledge of how sensory deficits affect normal functioning. In this way you are able to recognize the extent of a patient's deficit and know the type of interventions most likely to be helpful. Also consider the role that health professionals play in planning care and the available community resources that will be useful. Previous experience in caring for patients with sensory alterations is invaluable.

When applying critical thinking to planning care, professional standards are particularly useful. These standards recommend evidence-based interventions for the patient's condition. For example, patients who have visual deficits and are hospitalized are often placed on a fall-prevention protocol that incorporates research-based precautions to ensure patient safety.

Goals and Outcomes. During planning develop an individualized plan of care for each nursing diagnosis (see the Nursing Care Plan). Partner with your patient to develop a realistic plan that incorporates what you know about his or her sensory problems and the extent to which he or she can maintain or improve sensory function. Goals and outcomes need to be realistic and measurable. An example of a goal of care for a patient with an actual or potential sensory alteration is, "The patient will achieve improvement in hearing acuity within 2 weeks." Associated outcomes for this goal include the following:

- The patient and family report using communication techniques to send and receive messages within 2 days.
- The patient successfully demonstrates correct technique for cleaning a hearing aid within 1 week.
- The patient self-reports improved hearing acuity.

Setting Priorities. You consider the type and extent of sensory alteration affecting a patient when determining priorities of care. For example, a patient who enters the emergency department after experiencing eye trauma has priorities of reducing anxiety and preventing further injury to the eye. In contrast, a patient who is being discharged from an outpatient surgery department following cataract removal has the priority of learning about self-care restrictions. Safety is always a top priority. The patient also helps prioritize aspects of care. A patient wishes to learn ways to communicate more effectively or participate in favorite hobbies given his or her limitation.

Some sensory alterations are short term (e.g., a patient experiencing sensory overload in an ICU). Thus appropriate interventions are likely to be temporary (e.g., frequent reorientation or introduction of pleasant stimuli such as a backrub). Some sensory alterations such as permanent visual loss require long-term goals of care for patients to adapt. Patients who have sensory alterations at the time of entering a health care setting are usually most informed about how to adapt interventions to their lifestyles. For example, allow patients who are blind to control whichever parts of their care they can. Sometimes it becomes necessary for a patient to make major changes in self-care activities, communication, and socialization to ensure safe and effective nursing care.

> **QSEN QSEN: BUILDING COMPETENCY IN SAFETY** Ms. Long's church asks you to do a presentation on fall prevention to older adult members of the congregation. Many members also have impaired vision. How will you develop a program to educate this elderly population and communicate observations or concerns related to fall hazards to them?
>
> *Answers to QSEN Activities can be found on the Evolve website.*

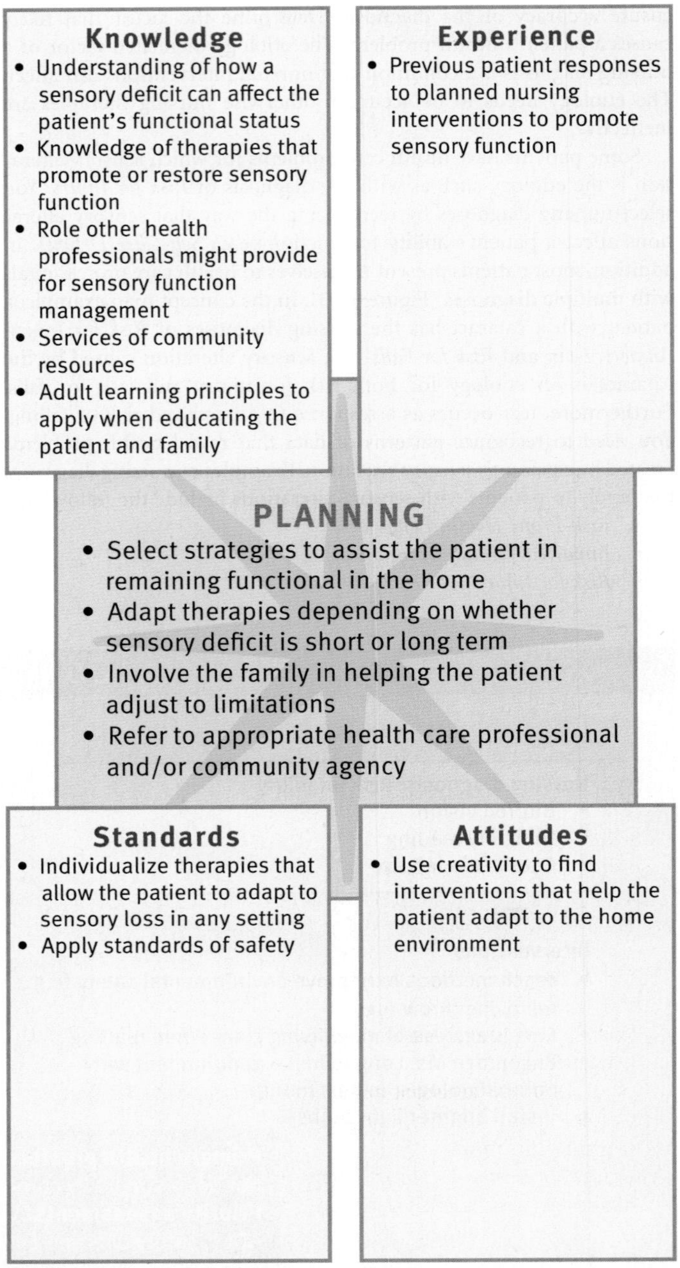

Knowledge
- Understanding of how a sensory deficit can affect the patient's functional status
- Knowledge of therapies that promote or restore sensory function
- Role other health professionals might provide for sensory function management
- Services of community resources
- Adult learning principles to apply when educating the patient and family

Experience
- Previous patient responses to planned nursing interventions to promote sensory function

PLANNING
- Select strategies to assist the patient in remaining functional in the home
- Adapt therapies depending on whether sensory deficit is short or long term
- Involve the family in helping the patient adjust to limitations
- Refer to appropriate health care professional and/or community agency

Standards
- Individualize therapies that allow the patient to adapt to sensory loss in any setting
- Apply standards of safety

Attitudes
- Use creativity to find interventions that help the patient adapt to the home environment

FIGURE 49-4 Critical thinking model for sensory alterations planning.

Teamwork and Collaboration. When developing a plan of care, consider all resources available to patients. The family plays a key role in providing meaningful stimulation and learning ways to help the patient adjust to any limitations. Engaging the family or designated surrogate is a fundamental skill of patient-centered care (Institute for Patient- and Family-Centered Care, 2015). You also frequently refer patients to other health care professionals. For example, if a patient has a major loss of sensory function and is also unable to manage medical needs such as medication self-administration or dressing changes, referral to home care is an option. Valuing interprofessional collaboration is an essential nurse competency that results in better patient health outcomes and greater patient and family satisfaction (Interprofessional Education Collaborative Expert Panel, 2011). Numerous community-based resources (e.g., local chapter of the Society for the Blind and Visually Impaired and the Area Agency on

NURSING CARE PLAN

Risk for Injury

ASSESSMENT

Ms. Judy Long is a 70-year-old retired widow who resides in a ranch-style home with her son. The family and craft room is located in a walkout basement area. She tells the community health nurse that she is having increased difficulty with night driving and blurry vision. She enjoys reading and sewing; however, her reduced vision limits her ability to participate in these activities. Ms. Long reports that her vision is blurred even with glasses and she is afraid that she will fall. She visited an ophthalmologist 1 year ago but didn't follow up with the recommended treatment.

Assessment Activities	*Findings/Defining Characteristics**
Ask Ms. Long to describe her vision changes.	Ms. Long states, "My left eye seems to have a film over it that makes my **vision blurred.** I am having **difficulty reading.** I also have **difficulty with night driving."**
Ask Ms. Long to describe life changes that have occurred since the change in vision.	Ms. Long states, "I've lost my independence because I can no longer drive at night. **I'm afraid to use the stairs at home because I can't judge steps clearly**."
Assess Ms. Long's visual acuity.	Ms. Long states she can't read the Snellen chart with her left eye.
Ask Ms. Long the results of the visit to the ophthalmologist.	Ms. Long states, "I was told I had a **cataract of the left eye,** and surgery was recommended."
Conduct a home hazard assessment.	There is **clutter in the home, dim lighting,** and stairs with **poor lighting and a broken handrail.**

*__Defining characteristics__ are shown in bold type.

NURSING DIAGNOSIS: Risk for injury

PLANNING

Goal	*Expected Outcomes (NOC)†* *Safe Home Environment*
Ms. Long will maintain independence in a safe home environment.	Ms. Long and her son make recommended changes in lighting, handrail, and clutter in the home environment within 4 weeks. Ms. Long reports an increased sense of home safety and independence within 4 weeks.

†Outcome classification labels from Moorhead S et al: *Nursing outcomes classification (NOC),* ed 5, St Louis, 2013, Mosby.

INTERVENTIONS (NIC)‡	RATIONALE
Environmental Management	
Teach Ms. Long and her son methods to improve environmental safety such as installing handrails along stairs, securing carpeting, removing throw rugs, and painting stairs.	Home environmental and health-related factors place a patient at risk for falls. Environmental safety modifications reduce the risk of falls and injury (Lim and Sung, 2012).
Teach Ms. Long to use a light over the shoulder for reading and sewing.	Adequate lighting with an adjustable lamp helps reduce eye strain and increase enjoyment (Perlmutter et al., 2013).
Explain use of a pocket magnifier and offer list of locations where Ms. Long can purchase one.	Magnifier enlarges visual images when reading or doing close work (Touhy and Jett, 2014).
Have Ms. Long make appointment with ophthalmologist within the next 4 weeks.	Older adults need a routine eye examination annually or as recommended (Touhy and Jett, 2014).
Emotional Support	
Encourage Ms. Long to discuss with family and friends how a loss of vision affects her independence and lifestyle.	Visual impairment may lead to depression, social isolation, and some functional disabilities, which can have adverse effects on a person's quality of life (Higginbottom et al., 2014).

‡Intervention classification labels from Bulechek GM et al: *Nursing interventions classification (NIC),* ed 6, St Louis, 2013, Mosby.

EVALUATION

Nursing Actions	*Patient Response/Finding*	*Achievement of Outcome*
Ask Ms. Long to describe the changes made in the home to reduce environmental hazards.	Ms. Long responds that she removed the clutter and placed handrails at the entryway. She also placed lighting behind her chair, and there are 100-watt lights in the living room. She has a specific craft light that provides additional "over-the-shoulder" lighting.	Ms. Long reports feeling safer walking the stairs and moving about in her home. She reduced the home hazards. She is now able to enjoy her craft activities.
Ask Ms. Long to read a medication label using her magnifier.	Ms. Long is able to read name of medication and dosage correctly.	Visual acuity has not been further compromised.
Ask Ms. Long if she is able to maintain a degree of independence with the environmental and lifestyle modifications.	Ms. Long states, "I'm more independent at home, and until surgery I don't mind having someone drive for me."	Ms. Long has attained some degree of independence.

Aging) are also available. Try to arrange for a volunteer to visit a patient or have printed materials made available that describe ways to cope with sensory problems.

◆ Implementation

Nursing interventions involve a patient and family so the patient is able to maintain a safe, pleasant, and stimulating sensory environment. The most effective interventions enable a patient with sensory alterations to function safely with existing deficits and continue a normal lifestyle. Patients can learn to adjust to sensory impairments at any age with the proper support and resources. Use measures to maintain a patient's sensory function at the highest level possible.

Health Promotion. Good sensory function begins with prevention. When a patient seeks health care, provide education about interventions that reduce the risk for sensory losses. Also recommend relevant visual and hearing guidelines. Remember to assess a patient's capacity to process and understand the health information to ensure that the patient makes appropriate decisions regarding his or her health.

Screening. An estimated 285 million people in the world are visually impaired (WHO, 2010). Preventable blindness is a worldwide health issue that begins with children and requires appropriate screening. Four recommended interventions are: (1) screening for rubella, syphilis, chlamydia, and gonorrhea in women who are considering pregnancy; (2) advocating adequate prenatal care to prevent premature birth (with the danger of exposure of the infant to excessive oxygen); (3) administering eye prophylaxis in the form of erythromycin ointment approximately 1 hour after an infant's birth; and (4) periodic screening of all children, especially newborns through preschoolers, for congenital blindness and visual impairment caused by refractive errors and strabismus (Hockenberry and Wilson, 2015).

Visual impairments are common during childhood. The most common visual problem is a refractive error such as nearsightedness. The nurse's role is one of detection, education, and referral. Parents need to know the signs of visual impairment (e.g., failure to react to light and reduced eye contact from the infant). Instruct parents to report these signs to their health care provider immediately. Vision screening of school-age children and adolescents helps detect problems early (USDHHS, 2015b). School nurses are usually responsible for vision testing.

In the United States glaucoma is the second leading cause of blindness in the general population and the primary cause of blindness in African-Americans. If left undetected and untreated, it leads to permanent visual loss. The American Optometric Association (2014) recommends a regular medical eye examination annually for those over 60 years old. Screening every 1 or 2 years is also recommended for individuals between 18 and 60 years of age who are at risk for developing eye and vision problems. Individuals at risk include the following: those with diabetes, hypertension, or a family history of ocular disease; working in occupations that are highly demanding visually or eye hazardous; taking prescription or nonprescription drugs with ocular side effects; or wearing contact lenses. Individuals who have had eye surgery or who have other health concerns or conditions are also at risk for the development of vision problems.

Hearing impairment is one of the most common disabilities in the United States. The prevalence of hearing loss is nearly 50% in those older than 75 years of age (NIDCD, 2014). Deafness or hearing impairment affects not only older adults but also children. Children at risk include those with a family history of childhood hearing impairment, perinatal infection (rubella, herpes, or cytomegalovirus), low birth weight, chronic ear infection, and Down syndrome. Advise pregnant women of the importance of early prenatal care, avoidance of ototoxic drugs, and testing for syphilis or rubella.

Children with chronic middle ear infections, a common cause of impaired hearing, need to receive periodic auditory testing. Warn parents of the risks and to seek medical care when a child has symptoms of earache or respiratory infection.

Because aging is associated with degenerative changes in the ear, patients need to have hearing screenings at least every decade through age 50 and every 3 years thereafter (American Speech-Language-Hearing Association, 2014). Once a patient reports a hearing loss, regular testing also becomes necessary. In addition, a patient who works or lives in a high–noise level environment requires annual screening. Occupational health nurses play a key role in the assessment of the auditory system and the initiation of prompt referrals. The early identification and treatment of problems help older adults be more active and healthy.

Preventive Measures. Trauma is a common cause of blindness in children. Penetrating injury from propulsive objects such as firecrackers or slingshots or from penetrating wounds from sticks, scissors, or toy weapons are just a few examples. Parents and children require counseling on ways to avoid eye trauma such as avoiding use of toys with long, pointed projections and instructing children not to walk or run while carrying pointed objects. Instruct patients that they can find safety equipment in most sports shops and large department stores.

Adults are at risk for eye injury while playing sports and working in jobs involving exposure to chemicals or flying objects. The Occupational Safety and Health Administration (OSHA, n.d.) has guidelines for workplace safety. Employers are required to have eyewash stations and to have employees wear eye goggles and/or use equipment such as HPDs to reduce the risk of injury. *Healthy People 2020* (USDHHS, 2015a) identifies goals that include reducing new cases of work-related, noise-induced hearing loss. Occupational health nurses reinforce the use of protective devices. In addition, nurses need to routinely assess patients for noise exposure and participate in providing hearing conservation classes for teachers, students, and patients.

Another means of prevention involves regular immunization of children against diseases capable of causing hearing loss (e.g., rubella, mumps, and measles). Nurses who work in health care providers' offices, schools, and community clinics instruct patients about the importance of early and timely immunization. Use caution when administering ototoxic drugs in all populations.

Use of Assistive Devices. Patients who wear corrective contact lenses, eyeglasses, or hearing aids need to make sure that they are clean, accessible, and functional (see Chapter 40). It is helpful to have a family member or friend who also knows how to care for and clean an assistive aid. A contact lens wearer must clean lenses frequently (see Chapter 40) and use the appropriate solutions for cleaning and disinfection. Contact lens wearers are subject to serious eye infections caused by infrequent lens disinfection, contamination of lens storage cases or contact lens solutions, and use of homemade saline. Swimming while wearing lenses also creates a serious risk of infection. Reinforce proper lens care in any health maintenance discussion.

Older adults are often reluctant to use hearing aids. Reasons cited most often include cost, appearance, insufficient knowledge about hearing aids, amplification of competing noise, and unrealistic expectations. Neuromuscular changes in the older adult such as stiff fingers, enlarged joints, and decreased sensory perception also make the handling and care of a hearing aid difficult. Fortunately today there are a wide variety of aids that not only enhance a person's hearing but also are cosmetically acceptable and useful for people with manual dexterity issues. Chapter 40 summarizes the types of hearing aids available and tips for proper care and use.

BOX 49-7 PATIENT TEACHING

Effective Use of a Hearing Aid

Objective

- Patient and family member will describe how to use a hearing aid correctly.

Teaching Strategies

- Show patient and family member locations on hearing aid device where damage (e.g., cracks, fraying) is likely to occur: earmold or case, earphone, dials, cord, and connection plugs.
- Instruct patient and family how to assess integrity of aid each day.
- Demonstrate battery replacement: Have extra set of unused batteries available.
- Instruct patient to store batteries in a dry, secure place away from pets and children.
- Instruct patient to clean ear canal daily.
- Instruct patient not to use hair spray and other hair products when hearing aid is in place
- Review method to check volume: Turn dial to maximum gain and check. Is voice clear?
- Review factors to report to hearing aid laboratory: static, distortion of sound, poor volume quality.

Evaluation

- Have patient and family demonstrate how to assess for hearing aid damage.
- Have patient and family demonstrate battery removal and cleaning.
- Have patient describe where to safely store battery.

Acknowledging a need to improve hearing is a person's first step. Give patients useful information on the benefits of hearing aid use. A person who understands the need for good hearing will likely be influenced to wear hearing aids. It is also important to have a significant other available to assist with hearing aid adjustment (Box 49-7). Federal regulations require prospective hearing aid users to either have a medical examination or sign a waiver saying they do not want it. The purpose of the examination is to rule out a medical reason for the hearing loss before hearing aids are purchased (U.S. Food and Drug Administration, 2014). Hearing aid dispensers should have prospective users consult their health care provider or an otolaryngologist for the following conditions: visible congenital or traumatic deformity of the ear, active drainage in the last 90 days, sudden or progressive hearing loss within the last 90 days, acute or chronic dizziness, unilateral sudden hearing loss within the last 90 days, visible cerumen accumulation or a foreign body in the ear canal, pain or discomfort in the ear, or an audiometric air-bone gap of 15 decibels or greater (U.S. Food and Drug Administration, 2015).

Promoting Meaningful Stimulation. Life becomes more enriching and satisfying when meaningful and pleasant stimuli exist within the environment. You can help patients adjust to their environment in many ways so it becomes more stimulating. You do this best by considering the normal physiological changes that accompany sensory deficits.

Vision. The pupil's ability to adjust to light diminishes as a result of the normal changes of aging; thus older adults are often very sensitive to glare. Suggest the use of yellow or amber lenses and shades or blinds on windows to minimize glare. Wearing sunglasses outside obviously reduces the glare of direct sunlight. Other interventions to enhance vision for patients with visual impairment include warm incandescent lighting and colors with sharp contrast and intensity.

The ability to read is important. Therefore allow patients to use their glasses whenever possible (e.g., during procedures and instruction). Some patients with reduced visual acuity need more than corrective lenses. A pocket magnifier helps a patient read most printed material. Telescopic-lens eyeglasses are smaller, easier to focus, and have a greater range. Books and other publications are also available in larger print. If a patient has a legal or another important document that he or she wishes to read, standard copying machines have enlarging capabilities. Software is also available that converts text into artificial voice output (Touhy and Jett, 2014).

With aging a person experiences a change in color perception. Perception of the colors blue, violet, and green usually declines. Brighter colors such as red, orange, and yellow are easier to see. Offer suggestions of ways to decorate a room and paint hallways or stairwells so the patient is able to differentiate surfaces and objects in a room.

Hearing. To maximize residual hearing function, work closely with a patient to suggest ways to modify the environment. Patients can amplify the sound of telephones and televisions. An innovative way to enrich the lives of patients with hearing impairments is recorded music. Some patients with severe hearing loss are able to hear music recorded in the low-frequency sound cycles.

One way to help an individual with a hearing loss is to ensure that the problem is not impacted cerumen. With aging cerumen thickens and builds up in the ear canal. Excessive cerumen occluding the ear canal causes **conductive hearing loss**. Instilling a softening agent such as 0.5 to 1 mL of warm mineral oil into the ear canal followed by irrigation of a solution of 3% hydrogen peroxide in a quart of warmed water removes cerumen and significantly improves a patient's hearing ability (Touhy and Jett, 2014).

Taste and Smell. Promote the sense of taste by using measures to enhance remaining taste perception. Good oral hygiene keeps the taste buds well hydrated. Well-seasoned, differently textured food eaten separately heightens taste perception. Flavored vinegar or lemon juice adds tartness to food. Always ask a patient which foods are most appealing. Improving taste perception improves food intake and appetite as well.

Stimulation of the sense of smell with aromas such as brewed coffee, cooked garlic, and baked bread heightens taste sensation. Patients need to avoid blending or mixing foods because these actions make it difficult to identify tastes. Older people need to chew food thoroughly to allow more food to contact remaining taste buds.

Improve smell by strengthening pleasant olfactory stimulation. Make a patient's environment more pleasant with smells such as cologne, mild room deodorizers, fragrant flowers, and sachets. Consult with patients to find out which scents they can tolerate. The removal of unpleasant odors (e.g., bedpans or soiled dressings) also improves the quality of a patient's environment.

Touch. Patients with reduced tactile sensation usually have the impairment over a limited part of their bodies. Providing touch therapy stimulates existing function. If a patient is willing to be touched, hair brushing and combing, a backrub, and touching the arms or shoulders are ways of increasing tactile contact. When sensation is reduced, a firm pressure is often necessary for a patient to feel a nurse's hand. Turning and repositioning also improves the quality of tactile sensation.

If a patient is overly sensitive to tactile stimuli (**hyperesthesia**), minimize irritating stimuli. Keeping bed linens loose to minimize direct contact with a patient and protecting the skin from exposure to irritants are helpful measures. Physical therapists can recommend special wrist splints for patients to wear to dorsiflex their wrists and relieve nerve pressure when they have numbness and tingling or pain in the hands, as with carpal tunnel syndrome. For patients who use computers, special keyboards and wrist pads are available to decrease the pressure on the median nerve, aid in pain relief, and promote healing.

Establishing Safe Environments. When sensory function becomes impaired, individuals become less secure within their home and workplace. Security is necessary for a person to feel independent. Make recommendations for improving safety within a patient's living environment without restricting independence. During a home visit or while completing an examination in the clinic, offer several useful suggestions for home safety. The nature of the actual or potential sensory loss determines the safety precautions you take.

Adaptations for Visual Loss. When a patient experiences a decrease in visual acuity, peripheral vision, adaptation to the dark, or depth perception, safety is a concern. With reduced peripheral vision a patient cannot see panoramically because the outer visual field is less discrete. With reduced depth perception a person is unable to judge how far away objects are located. This is a special danger when he or she walks down stairs or over uneven surfaces.

Driving is a particular safety hazard for older adults with visual alterations. Reduced peripheral vision prevents a driver from seeing a car in an adjacent lane. A sensitivity to glare creates a problem for driving at night with headlights. Vision is a primary consideration for safety, but there are other factors as well. In the case of older adults, decreased reaction time, reduced hearing, and decreased strength in the legs and arms further compromise driving skills. Some safety tips to share with those who continue to drive include the following: drive in familiar areas, do not drive during rush hour, avoid interstate highways for local drives, drive defensively, use rear-view and side-view mirrors when changing lanes, avoid driving at dusk or night, go slow but not too slow, keep the car in good working condition, and carry a preprogrammed cellular phone.

The presence of visual alterations makes it difficult for a person to conduct normal activities of living within the home. Because of reduced depth perception, patients can trip on throw rugs, runners, or the edge of stairs. Teach patients and family members to keep all flooring in good condition, and advise them to use low-pile carpeting. Thresholds between rooms need to be level with the floor. Recommend the removal of clutter to ensure clear pathways for walking and arrangement of furniture so a patient can move about easily without fear of tripping or running into objects. Suggest that stairwells have a securely fastened banister or handrail extending the full length of the stairs.

Front and back entrances to the home, work areas, and stairwells need to be lighted properly. Light fixtures need high-wattage bulbs with wider illumination. There needs to be a light switch at the top and bottom of stairwells. It is also important to be sure that lighting on the stairs does not cast shadows. Have a family member paint the edge of steps so the patient can see each step, especially the first and last, clearly. When possible have patients replace steps inside and outside the home with ramps.

An added consideration is to administer eye medications safely (see Chapter 32). Patients need to closely adhere to regular medication schedules for conditions such as glaucoma. Labels on medication containers need to be in large print. Make sure that a friend or spouse is familiar with dosage schedules in case a patient is unable to self-administer a medication. Patients with visual impairments often have difficulty manipulating eyedroppers.

Adaptations for Reduced Hearing. Patients hear important environmental sounds (e.g., doorbells and alarm clocks) best if they are amplified or changed to a lower-pitched, buzzer-like sound. Lamps designed to turn on in response to sounds such as doorbells, burglar alarms, smoke detectors, and babies crying are also available. Family members and anyone who calls the patient regularly need to learn to let the phone ring for a longer period. Amplified receivers for telephones and telephone communication devices (TCDs) are available that use a computer and printer to transfer words over the telephone for the hearing impaired. Both sender and receiver need to have the special device to complete a call.

Adaptations for Reduced Olfaction. The patient with a reduced sensitivity to odors is often unable to smell leaking gas, a smoldering cigarette, fire, or spoiled food. Advise patients to use smoke detectors and take precautions such as checking ashtrays or placing cigarette butts in water. In addition, teach patients to check food package dates, inspect the appearance of food, and keep leftovers in labeled containers with the preparation date. Pilot gas flames need to be checked visually.

Adaptations for Reduced Tactile Sensation. When patients have reduced sensation in their extremities, they are at risk for impaired skin integrity and injury from exposure to temperature extremes. Always caution these patients about the use of heating and cooling devices (see Chapter 48). The temperature setting on the home water heater should be no higher than 48.8° C (120° F). If a patient also has a visual impairment, it is important to be sure that water faucets are clearly marked "hot" and "cold" or use color codes (i.e., red for hot and blue for cold). Discourage the use of heating pads in this population.

Communication. A sensory deficit often causes a person to feel isolated because of an inability to communicate with others. It is important for individuals to be able to interact with people around them. The nature of the sensory loss influences the methods and styles of communication that nurses use during interactions with patients (Box 49-8). You also teach communication methods to family members and significant others. For patients with visual deficits or blindness, speak normally, not from a distance, and be sure to have sufficient lighting.

The patient with a hearing impairment is often able to speak normally. To more clearly hear what a person communicates, family and friends need to learn to move away from background noise, rephrase rather than repeat sentences, be positive, and have patience. In a group setting it is better to form a semicircle in front of the patient so he or she can see who is speaking next; this helps foster group involvement. On the other hand, some patients who are deaf have serious speech alterations. Some use sign language or lip reading, wear special hearing aids, write with a pad and pencil, or learn to use a computer for communication. Special communication boards that contain common terms (e.g., *pain, bathroom, dizzy*, or *walk*) help patients express their needs.

Patient education is one aspect of communication. Teaching booklets are available in large print for patients with visual loss. The patient who is blind often requires more frequent and detailed verbal descriptions of information. This is particularly true if there are no instructional booklets written in Braille. Patients with visual impairments can also learn by listening to audiotapes or the sound part of a televised teaching session. Patients with hearing impairments often benefit from written instructional materials and visual teaching aids (e.g., posters and graphs). Demonstrations by the nurse are very useful. Hospitals are required to make professional interpreters available to read sign language for patients who are deaf.

BOX 49-8 Communication Methods

Patients with Aphasia

- Listen to patient and provide sufficient time for him or her to communicate.
- Do not shout or speak loudly (hearing loss is not the problem).
- If patient has problems with comprehension, use simple, short questions and facial gestures to give additional clues.
- Speak of things familiar and of interest to patient.
- If patient has problems speaking, ask questions that require simple yes or no answers or blinking of the eyes. Offer pictures or a communication board so patient can point.
- Speak slowly and give patient time to understand; be calm and patient; do not pressure or tire him or her.
- Avoid patronizing and childish phrases.

Patients with an Artificial Airway

- Use pictures, objects, or word cards so patient can point.
- Offer a pad and pencil or Magic Slate for patient to write messages.
- Do not shout or speak loudly.
- Give patient time to write messages because patients tire easily.
- Provide an artificial voice box (vibrator) for patient with a laryngectomy to use to speak.

Patients with Hearing Impairment

- Get patient's attention. Do not startle him or her when entering the room. Do not approach patient from behind. Be sure that he or she knows that you want to speak.
- Face patient and stand or sit on the same level. Be sure that your face and lips are illuminated to promote lip reading. Keep hands away from mouth.
- Be sure that the environment is not noisy.
- Be sure that patients keep eyeglasses clean so they are able to see your gestures and face.
- If patient wears a hearing aid, make sure that it is in place and working.
- Speak slowly and articulate clearly. Sometimes people with hearing loss take longer to process verbal messages.
- Use a normal tone of voice and inflections of speech. Do not speak with something in your mouth.
- When you are not understood, rephrase rather than repeat the conversation.
- Use visible expressions. Speak with your hands, face, and eyes.
- Do not shout. Loud sounds are usually higher pitched and often impede hearing by accentuating vowel sounds and concealing consonants. If you need to raise your voice, speak in lower tones.
- Talk toward patient's best or normal ear.
- Use written information to enhance the spoken word.
- Do not restrict the hands of patient who is deaf. Never have intravenous lines in both of patient's hands if the preferred method of communication is sign language.
- Avoid eating, chewing, or smoking while speaking.
- Avoid speaking from another room or while walking away.

Acute Care. When patients enter acute care settings for therapeutic management of sensory deficits or as a result of traumatic injury, use different approaches to maximize sensory function existing at the time. Safety is an obvious priority until a patient's sensory status is either stabilized or improved. For example, patients with sensory deficits have a high risk for falls in the acute care environment. It is very important to know the extent of any existing sensory impairment before the acute episode of illness so you are able to reinforce what the patient already knows about self-care or plan for more instruction before and after discharge.

Orientation to the Environment. A patient with a sensory impairment requires a complete orientation to the immediate environment. Provide reorientation as needed to the institutional environment by ensuring that name tags on uniforms are visible, addressing the patient by name, explaining where the patient is (especially if patients are transported to different areas for treatment), and using conversational cues to time or location. Reduce the tendency for patients to become confused by offering short, simple, repeated explanations and reassurance. Encourage family members and visitors to help orient patients to the hospital surroundings.

Patients with serious visual impairment need to feel comfortable in knowing the boundaries of the immediate environment. Normally people see physical boundaries within a room. Patients who are blind or severely visually impaired often touch the boundaries or objects to gain a sense of their surroundings. The patient needs to walk through a room and feel the walls to establish a sense of direction. Help patients by explaining objects within the hospital room such as furniture or equipment. It takes time for a patient to absorb room arrangement. He or she often needs to reorient again as you explain the location of key items (e.g., call light, telephone, and chair). Remember to approach the patient from the front to avoid startling him or her.

It is important to keep all objects in the same position and place. After an object is moved even a short distance, it no longer exists for a person who is blind. Simply moving a chair creates a safety hazard. Ask the patient if any item needs to be rearranged to make ambulation easier. Clear traffic patterns to the bathroom. Give the patient extra time to perform tasks. He or she needs a detailed description of how to perform an activity and moves slowly to remain safe.

Patients confined to bed are at risk for sensory deprivation. Normally movement gives an awareness of self through vestibular and tactile stimulation. Movement patterns influence sensory perception. The limited movement of bed rest changes how a person interprets the environment; surroundings seem different, and objects seem to assume shapes different from normal. A person who is on bed rest requires routine stimulation through range-of-motion exercises, positioning, and participation in self-care activities (as appropriate). Comfort measures such as washing the face and hands and providing backrubs improve the quality of stimulation and lessen the chance of sensory deprivation. Planning time to talk with patients is also essential. Explain unfamiliar environmental noises and sensations. A calm, unhurried approach gives you quality time to help reorient and familiarize the patient with care activities. The patient who is well enough to read will benefit from a variety of reading material.

Communication. The most common language disorder following a stroke is aphasia. Depending on the type of aphasia, the inability to communicate is often frustrating and frightening (see Box 49-8). Initially you need to establish very basic communication and recognize that it does not indicate intellectual impairment or degeneration of personality. Explain situations and treatments that are pertinent to the patient because he or she is able to understand the speaker's words. Because a stroke often causes partial or complete paralysis of one side of a patient's body, the patient needs special assistive devices. A variety of communication boards for different levels of disability are available. Sensitive pressure switches activated by the touch of an ear, nose, or chin control electronic communication boards (Touhy and Jett, 2014). Make referrals to speech therapists to develop appropriate rehabilitation plans.

In acute care hospitals or long-term care facilities, nurses often care for patients with artificial airways (such as an endotracheal tube) (see Chapter 41). The placement of an endotracheal tube prevents a patient from speaking. In this case the nurse uses special communication methods to facilitate his or her ability to express needs. The patient is sometimes completely alert and able to hear and see the nurse normally. Giving him or her time to convey any needs or requests is very important. Use creative communication techniques (e.g., a communication board or electronic tablet) to foster and strengthen a patient's interactions with health care personnel, family, and friends.

Controlling Sensory Stimuli. Patients need time for rest and freedom from stress caused by frequent monitoring and repeated tests. Reduce sensory overload by organizing the patient's plan of care. Combine activities such as dressing changes, bathing, and vital sign measurement in one visit to conserve a patient's energy and prevent fatigue. A patient also needs scheduled time for rest and quiet. Planning for rest periods often requires cooperation from family, visitors, and health care colleagues. Coordination with laboratory and radiology departments minimizes the number of interruptions for procedures. A creative solution to decrease excessive environmental stimuli that prevents restful, healing sleep is to institute "quiet time" in ICUs. Quiet time means dimming the lights throughout the unit, closing the shades, and shutting the doors. Data collected from one hospital that implemented 1 hour of quiet time daily found decreased staff and unit noise and improved patient satisfaction (Haupt, 2012).

When patients experience sensory overload or deprivation, their behavior is often difficult for family or friends to accept. Encourage the family not to argue with or contradict the patient but to calmly explain location, identity, and time of day. Engaging a patient in a normal discussion about familiar topics helps in reorientation. Anticipating patient needs such as voiding helps reduce uncomfortable stimuli.

Try to control extraneous noise in and around a patient's room. It is often necessary to ask a roommate to lower the volume on a television or to move the patient to a quieter room. Keep equipment noise to a minimum. Turn off bedside equipment not in use such as suction and oxygen equipment. Avoid making abrupt loud noises such as dropping objects or causing the over-bed table to suddenly adjust to the lowest level. Nursing staff also need to control laughter or conversation outside the patients' rooms. Allow patients to close their room doors.

When a patient leaves an acute care setting for the home environment, communicate with colleagues in the home care setting about the patient's existing sensory deficits and the interventions that helped the patient adapt to sensory problems. You achieve continuity of care when the patient has to make only minimal changes in the home setting.

Safety Measures. A patient with recent visual impairment often requires help with walking. The presence of an eye patch, frequently instilled eyedrops, and the swelling of eyelid structures following surgery are just a few factors that cause a patient to need more help than usual. A sighted guide gives confidence to patients with visual impairments and ensures safe mobility. The American Foundation for the Blind (2015) lists several suggestions for a sighted guide:

1. Ask the patient if he or she wants a "sighted guide." If assistance is accepted, offer your arm. Tap the back of your hand against his or her hand. The person will then grasp your arm directly above the elbow (Figure 49-5).
2. Relax and walk at a comfortable pace. Walk one step ahead of the person you are guiding, except at the top and bottom of stairs and streets. At these places pause and stand alongside the person. Be sure that the person has a strong grasp on your arm.
3. While walking with a patient, describe the surroundings and ensure that obstacles have been removed. Never leave a patient with a visual impairment standing alone in an unfamiliar area.
4. To guide a person to a seat, place his or her hand on the back of the seat. The person you are guiding will find the seat by following along your arm.

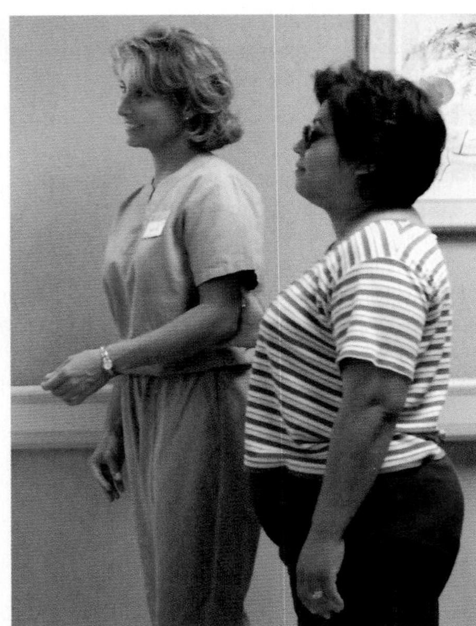

FIGURE 49-5 Nurse helps to ambulate patient with visual impairment. (From Sorrentino SA, Remmert LN: *Mosby's textbook for nursing assistants,* ed 8, St Louis, 2012, Mosby.)

It is important to teach family members techniques for helping with ambulation. Nursing staff also need to ensure that the patient knows where the call light is before leaving him or her alone. Place necessary objects in front of the patient to prevent falls caused by reaching over the bedside. Appropriate use of side rails is also an option.

Nurses often rely on patients in health care settings to report unusual sounds such as a suction apparatus running improperly or an IV pump alarm. However, a patient with a hearing loss does not always hear these sounds and thus requires more frequent visits by nurses. The patient also benefits from learning to use vision to discover sources of danger. It is wise to note on the intercom system at the nurse's station and in the medical record if the patient is deaf and/or blind. A patient lacking the ability to speak cannot call out for assistance. Patients need to have message boards and call lights close at hand.

Patients with reduced tactile sensation risk injury when their conditions confine them to bed because they are unable to sense pressure on bony prominences or the need to change position. These patients rely on nurses for timely repositioning, moving tubes or devices on which the patient is lying, and turning to avoid skin breakdown. When a patient is less able to sense temperature variations, use extra caution in applying heat and cold therapies (see Chapter 48) and preparing bath water. Check the condition of the patient's skin frequently.

Restorative and Continuing Care

Maintaining Healthy Lifestyles. After a patient has experienced a sensory loss, it becomes important to understand the implications of the loss and make adjustments needed to continue a normal lifestyle. Sensory impairments need not prevent a person from leading an active, rewarding life. Many of the interventions applicable to health promotion such as adapting the home environment are useful after a patient leaves an acute care setting.

Understanding Sensory Loss. Patients who have experienced a recent sensory loss need to understand how to adapt so their living environments are safe and appropriately stimulating. All family members need to understand how a patient's sensory impairment affects normal daily activities. Family and friends are more supportive when they understand sensory deficits and factors that worsen or

BOX 49-9 FOCUS ON OLDER ADULTS

Principles for Reducing Loneliness in Patients with Sensory Impairments

- Spend time with a person in silence or conversation.
- When it is culturally appropriate, use physical contact (e.g., holding a hand, embracing a shoulder) to convey caring.
- Recommend alterations in living arrangements if physical isolation is a factor.
- Help patients keep contact with people important to them.
- Provide information about support groups or groups that provide assistive services.
- Arrange for security escort services as needed.
- Introduce the idea of bringing a companion such as a pet into the home when appropriate.
- Link a person with organizations attuned to the social needs of older adults.

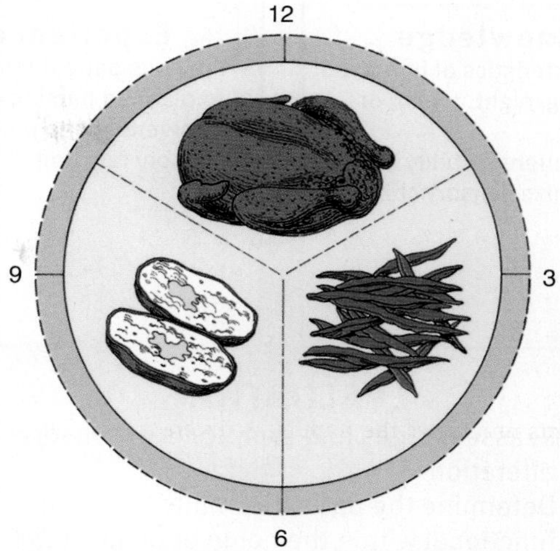

FIGURE 49-6 Location of food using clock as frame of reference.

lessen sensory problems. For example, they need to learn how to communicate with someone who has a hearing loss. Community resources are available to provide information to help patients with personal management needs. The American Foundation for the Blind, American Red Cross, and National Association for Speech and Hearing offer resource materials and product information.

Socialization. The ability to communicate is gratifying. It tests a person's intellect, opens opportunities, and allows him or her to exchange the feelings that he or she has about others. When sensory alterations hinder interactions, a person feels ineffective and loses self-esteem. When patients feel socially unaccepted, they perceive sensory losses as seriously impairing their quality of life.

Interacting with others becomes a burden for many patients with sensory alterations. They lose the motivation to engage in social situations, resulting in a deep sense of loneliness. Use therapies to reduce loneliness, particularly in older adults (Box 49-9). These principles support the *Healthy People 2020* objective to increase the proportion of adults with disabilities reporting sufficient emotional support. In addition, family members need to learn to focus on a person's ability to interact rather than on his or her disability. For example, do not assume that a person who is hard of hearing does not want to speak. A person who is blind can still enjoy a walk through a park with a companion describing the sights around them.

Promoting Self-Care. The ability to perform self-care is essential for self-esteem. Frequently family members and nurses believe that people with sensory impairments require assistance, when in fact they are able to help themselves. To help with meals, arrange food on the plate and condiments, salad, or drinks according to numbers on the face of a clock (Figure 49-6). A patient can also use this method to place personal care items on the bedside or on the bathroom vanity. It is easy for a patient to become oriented to the items after a nurse or family member explains the location of each item.

Help patients reach toilet facilities safely. Safety bars need to be installed near the toilet. It is often helpful to have the bar a different color than the wall for easier visibility. Never place towels on a safety bar because they interfere with a person's grasp. Toilet paper needs to be within easy reach. Sharply contrasting colors within the room help the partially sighted and promote functional independence. General principles for promoting self-care in older adults also include using warm incandescent lighting and controlling glare by using shades and blinds (Touhy and Jett, 2014).

If the sense of touch is diminished, a patient can dress more easily with zippers or Velcro strips, pullover sweaters or blouses, and elasticized waists. If a patient has partial paralysis and reduced sensation, he or she dresses the affected side first. Encourage family members responsible for selecting clothing for patients with visual impairments to follow the patient's preferences. Any sensory impairment has a significant influence on body image, and it is important for the patient to feel well groomed and attractive. Some patients need assistance with basic grooming such as brushing, combing, and shampooing hair. Others need assistance with medication administration, clothing identification, and learning to manage routine procedures such as blood pressure and glucose monitoring. An assortment of low-vision devices is now available. It is important for you to make appropriate referrals to allow the patient to maintain a maximum degree of independence.

Patients with proprioceptive problems often lose their balance easily. Make sure that bathrooms have nonskid surfaces in the tub and shower. Install grab bars either vertically or horizontally in tubs and showers, depending on how a patient is able to grasp or hold onto the bar. Instruct family members to supervise ambulation and sitting, make frequent checks to prevent falls, and caution the patient against leaning forward.

◆ Evaluation

Through the Patient's Eyes. It is important to evaluate whether care measures maintain or improve a patient's ability to interact and function within the environment. The patient is the source for evaluating outcomes. He or she is the only one who knows if sensory abilities are improved and which specific interventions or therapies are most successful in facilitating a change in his or her performance (Figure 49-7). Collaborate with family members to determine if a patient's ability to function within the home has improved.

If you have developed a positive relationship with a patient successfully, notice that subtle behaviors often indicate the level of his or her satisfaction. You may notice that the patient responds appropriately such as by smiling. However, it is important for you to ask the patient if his or her sensory needs have been met. For example, ask, "Have we done all we can do to help improve your ability to hear?" If the patient's expectations have not been met, ask him or her, "How can the health care team better meet your needs?" Working closely with the patient and family enables you to redefine expectations that can be met realistically within the limits of the patient's condition and therapies. You have been effective when the patient's goals and expectations have been met.

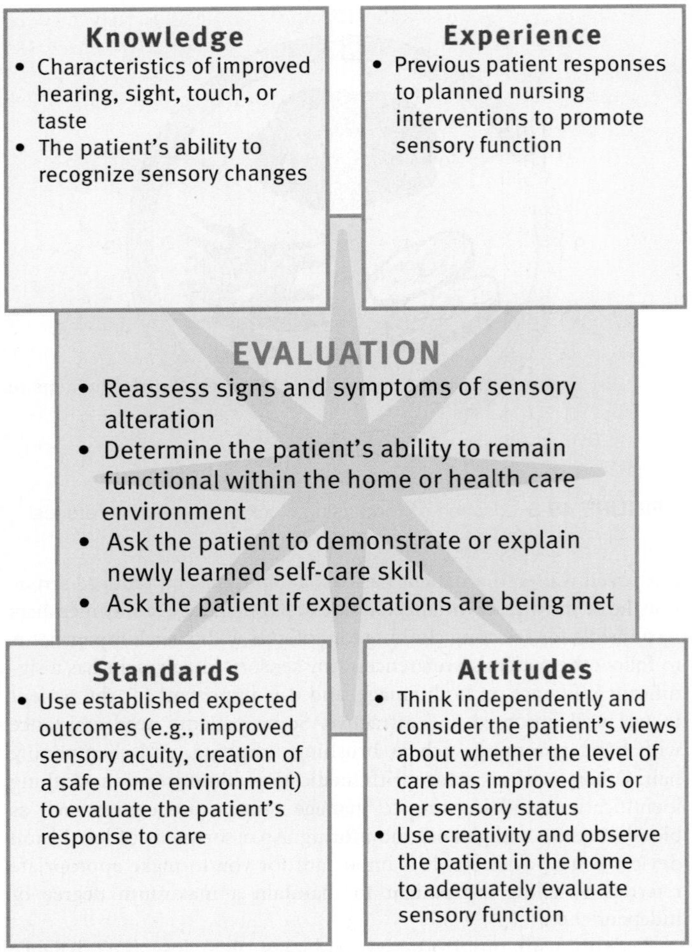

Knowledge
- Characteristics of improved hearing, sight, touch, or taste
- The patient's ability to recognize sensory changes

Experience
- Previous patient responses to planned nursing interventions to promote sensory function

EVALUATION
- Reassess signs and symptoms of sensory alteration
- Determine the patient's ability to remain functional within the home or health care environment
- Ask the patient to demonstrate or explain newly learned self-care skill
- Ask the patient if expectations are being met

Standards
- Use established expected outcomes (e.g., improved sensory acuity, creation of a safe home environment) to evaluate the patient's response to care

Attitudes
- Think independently and consider the patient's views about whether the level of care has improved his or her sensory status
- Use creativity and observe the patient in the home to adequately evaluate sensory function

FIGURE 49-7 Critical thinking model for sensory alterations evaluation.

Patient Outcomes. To evaluate the effectiveness of specific nursing interventions, use critical thinking and make comparisons with baseline sensory assessment data to evaluate if sensory alterations have changed. It is your responsibility to determine if expected outcomes have been met. For example, use evaluative data to determine whether care measures improve or at least maintain a patient's ability to interact and function within the environment. The nature of a patient's sensory alterations influences how you evaluate the outcome of care. When caring for a patient with a hearing deficit, use proper communication techniques and then evaluate whether he or she has gained the ability to hear or interact more effectively. When expected outcomes have not been achieved, there is a need to change interventions or alter the patient's environment. If outcomes are not met, it is important to ask questions such as, "How are you feeling emotionally?" "Do you feel that you are at risk for injury?"

If you have directed nursing care at improving or maintaining sensory acuity, evaluate the integrity of the sensory organs and the patient's ability to perceive stimuli. Evaluate interventions designed to relieve problems associated with sensory alterations on the basis of a patient's ability to function normally without injury. When you directly or indirectly (through education) alter a patient's environment, evaluate by observing whether the patient makes environmental changes. When designing patient teaching to improve sensory function, it is important to determine whether the patient is following recommended therapies and meeting mutually set goals. Asking a patient to explain or demonstrate self-care skills is an effective evaluative measure. It is often necessary to reinforce previous instruction if learning has not taken place. If outcomes are not met, these are examples of questions to ask:

- "How often do you wear your hearing aids/corrective lenses?"
- "Are you able to participate in a small group discussion?"
- "Are you able to read the newspaper without squinting?"

The results of your evaluation will determine whether to continue the existing plan of care, make modifications, or end the use of select interventions.

KEY POINTS

- Sensory reception involves the stimulation of sensory nerve fibers and the transmission of impulses to higher centers within the brain.
- Sensory deprivation results from an inadequate quality or quantity of sensory stimuli.
- Aging results in a gradual decline of acuity in all senses.
- Patients who are older, immobilized, or confined in isolated environments are at risk for sensory alterations.
- Assessment of a patient's health promotion habits reveals risks for sensory impairment.
- An assessment of hazards in the environment requires the nurse to tour living areas in the home and look for conditions that increase the chances of injury such as falls.
- The plan of care for patients with sensory alterations needs to include participation by family members. The extent of support from family members and significant others influences the quality of sensory experiences.
- Patients with sensory deficits often develop alternate ways of communicating that rely on other senses.
- Care of patients at risk for sensory deprivation includes introducing meaningful and pleasant stimuli for all senses.
- To prevent sensory overload, control stimuli and orient the patient to the environment.
- Patients with artificial airways are able to communicate effectively with communication boards, laptop computers, and written messages.

CRITICAL APPLICATION QUESTIONS

Preparing for Clinical Practice

Ms. Long made an informed decision to have cataract surgery 1 month ago. After surgery she reported improved vision and ability to participate in activities of daily living. Today the community health nurse visits, and Ms. Long reports shortness of breath with activity. After the nurse consults with Ms. Long's health care provider, Ms. Long is admitted from the emergency department to a telemetry heart monitoring unit with a diagnosis of heart failure.

1. Three days after being admitted, Ms. Long reports less shortness of breath; however, she is restless, tired, and irritable. She is on a cardiac monitor and continues to receive oxygen. The staff nurse reports that Ms. Long has slept very little since her admission. Her semiprivate room is directly across from a busy central nurses' station, and she frequently calls out for assistance. Identify the sensory alteration Ms. Long is experiencing and three strategies that will ensure that she gets enough sleep.
2. Ms. Long was released from the hospital in good health 1 week after admission. Following the recommendation of her health care provider, she regularly attends a heart-failure support group. She asks you to speak with the group regarding age-related visual changes

and signs and symptoms that may indicate problems. What information will you share with them to promote healthy vision?

3. Ms. Long is worried about how to communicate with her sister who had a stroke and developed aphasia. What would you teach her to help her communicate more effectively with her sister?

Answers to Clinical Application Questions can be found on the Evolve website.

REVIEW QUESTIONS

Are You Ready to Test Your Nursing Knowledge?

1. A patient has been on contact isolation for 4 days because of a hospital-acquired infection. He has had few visitors and few opportunities to leave his room. His ambulation is also still limited. Which are the correct nursing interventions to reduce sensory deprivation? (Select all that apply.)
   1. Teaching how activities such as reading and using crossword puzzles provide stimulation
   2. Moving him to a room away from the nurse's station
   3. Turning on the lights and opening the room blinds
   4. Sitting down, speaking, touching, and listening to his feelings and perceptions
   5. Providing auditory stimulation for the patient by keeping the television on continuously
2. The home care nurse is instructing a nursing assistant about interventions to facilitate location of items for patients with vision impairment. Which are effective strategies for enhancing a patient's impaired vision? (Select all that apply.)
   1. Use of fluorescent lighting
   2. Use of warm, incandescent lighting
   3. Use of yellow or amber lenses to decrease glare
   4. Use of adjustable blinds, sheer curtains, or draperies
   5. Indirect lighting to reduce glare
3. An elderly patient with bilateral hearing loss wears a hearing aid in her left ear. Which of the following approaches best facilitates communication with her?
   1. Talk to the patient at a distance so he or she may read your lips.
   2. Keep your arms at your side; speak directly into the patient's left ear.
   3. Face the patient when speaking; demonstrate ideas you wish to convey.
   4. Position the patient so the light is on his or her face when speaking.
4. The nurse is caring for a patient with glaucoma. When developing a discharge plan, which priority intervention enables the patient to function safely with existing deficits and continue a normal lifestyle?
   1. Encourage the patient to rearrange her home furnishings regularly to keep active.
   2. Suggest to the patient that he or she consider either moving to a smaller home or long-term care facility.
   3. Say nothing because it is most appropriate that the patient identify personal interventions to compensate for a sensory alteration.
   4. Work closely with the patient and family to identify in-home modifications to create a comfortable and accessible environment.
5. A patient is returning to an assisted-living apartment following a diagnosis of declining, progressive visual loss. Although she is familiar with her apartment and residence, she reports feeling a little uncertain about walking alone. There is one step into her apartment. Her children are scheduling themselves to be available to their mom for the next 2 weeks. Which of the following approaches will you teach the children to assist ambulation? (Select all that apply.)
   1. Walk one-half step behind and slightly to her side.
   2. Have her grasp your arm just above the elbow and walk at a comfortable pace.
   3. Stand next to your mom at the top and bottom of stairs.
   4. Stand one step ahead of mom at the top of the stairs.
   5. Place yourself alongside your mom and hold onto her waist.
6. A new nurse is going to help a patient walk down the corridor and sit in a chair. The patient has an eye patch over the left eye and poor vision in the right eye. What is the correct order of steps to help the patient safely walk down the hall and sit in the chair?
   1. Tell patient when you are approaching the chair.
   2. Walk at a relaxed pace.
   3. Guide patient's hand to nurse's arm, resting just above the elbow.
   4. Position yourself one-half step in front of patient.
   5. Position patient's hand on back of chair.
7. Because hearing impairment is one of the most common disabilities among children, a health promotion intervention is to teach parents and children to:
   1. Avoid activities in which there may be crowds.
   2. Delay childhood immunizations until hearing can be verified.
   3. Take precautions when involved in activities associated with high-intensity noises.
   4. Prophylactically administer antibiotics to reduce the incidence of infections.
8. A nurse is conducting discharge teaching for a patient with diminished tactile sensation. Which of the following statements made by the patient indicates that additional teaching is needed?
   1. "I am at risk for injury from temperature extremes."
   2. "I may be able to dress more easily with zippers or pullover sweaters."
   3. "A home care nurse may help me figure out how to be more independent."
   4. "I have right-sided partial paralysis and reduced sensation; so I should dress the left side of my body first."
9. Which of the following is the best nursing intervention when communicating with a patient who has expressive aphasia?
   1. Ask open-ended questions
   2. Speak to the patient as if he or she is a child
   3. Use a dry-erase board or paper and pen for writing messages
   4. Avoid the use of gestures and other nonverbal forms of communication
10. A patient with progressive vision impairments had to surrender his driver's license 6 months ago. He comes to the medical clinic for a routine checkup. He is accompanied by his son. His wife died 2 years ago, and he admits to feeling lonely much of the time. Which of the following interventions reduce loneliness? (Select all that apply.)
    1. Sharing information about senior transportation services
    2. Reassuring the patient that loneliness is a normal part of aging
    3. Maintaining distance while talking to avoid overstimulating the patient
    4. Providing information about local social groups in the patient's neighborhood
    5. Recommending that the patient consider making living arrangements that will put him closer to family or friends

11. A nurse is performing an assessment on a patient admitted to the unit following treatment in the emergency department for severe bilateral eye trauma. During patient admission the nurse's priority interventions include which of the following? (Select all that apply.)
    1. Conducting a home-safety assessment and identifying hazards in the patient's living environment
    2. Reinforcing eye safety at work and in activities that place the patient at risk for eye injury
    3. Placing necessary objects such as the call light and water in front of the patient to prevent falls caused by reaching
    4. Orienting the patient to the environment to reduce anxiety and prevent further injury to the eye
    5. Placing signage on the patient's room door and over the bed to alert health care providers about patient's visual status
12. Which patient is most likely to experience sensory overload?
    1. A patient in the intensive care unit whose pain is not well controlled
    2. A patient with a protective patch on her right eye following cataract surgery
    3. A woman whose hearing aids were lost when she transferred to a long-term care facility
    4. A visually impaired resident of a nursing home who enjoys taking part in different hobbies and activities
13. An older adult is admitted from a skilled nursing home to a medical unit with pneumonia. A review of the medical record reveals that he had a stroke affecting the right hemisphere of the brain 6 months ago and was placed in the skilled nursing home because he was unable to care for himself. Which of these assessment findings does the nurse expect to find? (Select all that apply.)
    1. Slow, cautious behavioral style
    2. Inattention and neglect, especially to the left side
    3. Cloudy or opaque areas in part of the lens or the entire lens
    4. Visual spatial alterations such as loss of half of a visual field
    5. Loss of sensation and motor function on the right side of the body
14. A nurse is performing a home care assessment on a patient with a hearing impairment. The patient reports, "I think my hearing aid is broken. I can't hear anything." Which of the following teaching strategies does the nurse implement? (Select all that apply.)
    1. Demonstrate hearing aid battery replacement.
    2. Review method to check volume on hearing aid.
    3. Demonstrate how to wash the earmold and microphone with hot water.
    4. Discuss the importance of having wax buildup in the ear canal removed.
    5. Recommend a chemical cleaner to remove difficult buildup.
15. Identify the measures to ensure safety for a patient who has no sensation on one side of the body.

Answers: **1.** 1, 3, 4; **2.** 2, 3, 4; **3.** 3; **4.** 4; **5.** 2, 3; **6.** 3, 4, 2, 1, 5; **7.** 3; **8.** 4; **9.** 3; **10.** 1, 4, 5; **11.** 3, 4, 5; **12.** 1; **13.** 2, 4; **14.** 1, 2, 4; **15.** See Evolve.

Rationales for Review Questions can be found on the Evolve website.

REFERENCES

American Foundation for the Blind: *Being a sighted guide,* 2015, http://www.afb.org/info/friends-and-family/etiquette/being-a-sighted-guide/235. Accessed November 22, 2015.

American Optometric Association: *Recommended eye examination frequency for pediatric patients and adults,* 2014, http://www.aoa.org/patients-and-public/caring-for-your-vision/comprehensive-eye-and-vision-examination/recommended-examination-frequency-for-pediatric-patients-and-adults?sso=y. Accessed November 22, 2015.

American Speech-Language-Hearing Association: *Who should be screened for hearing loss?* 2014, http://www.asha.org/public/hearing/Who-Should-be-Screened/. Accessed November 22, 2015.

Haupt B: Instituting quiet hour improves patient satisfaction, *Nursing2012* 42(4):14, 2012.

Hockenberry MJ, Wilson D: *Wong's nursing care of infants and children,* ed 10, St Louis, 2015, Mosby.

Interprofessional Education Collaborative Expert Panel: *Core competencies for interprofessional collaborative practice: report of an expert panel,* 2011, http://www.aacn.nche.edu/education-resources/ipecreport.pdf. Accessed November 22, 2015.

Institute for Patient- and Family-Centered Care: *Institute for patient- and family-centered care,* 2015, http://www.ipfcc.org/. Accessed November 20, 2015.

National Institute on Deafness and other Communication Disorders (NIDCD): *Hearing loss and older adults,* 2014, http://www.nidcd.nih.gov/health/hearing/Pages/older.aspx. Accessed November 22, 2015.

Occupational Safety and Health Administration (OSHA): *Eye and face protection,* n.d., https://www.osha.gov/SLTC/eyefaceprotection/index.html. Accessed November 22, 2015.

Touhy T, Jett P: *Ebersole and Hess' Gerontological nursing & healthy aging,* ed 4, St Louis, 2014, Mosby.

US Food and Drug Administration: *How to get hearing aids,* 2014, http://www.fda.gov/MedicalDevices/ProductsandMedicalProcedures/HomeHealthandConsumer/ConsumerProducts/HearingAids/ucm181479.htm. Accessed November 22, 2015.

US Food and Drug Administration: *CFR Code of Federal Regulations Title 21,* 2015, http://www.accessdata.fda.gov/scripts/cdrh/cfdocs/cfcfr/CFRSearch.cfm?fr=801.420. Accessed November 22, 2015.

US Department of Health and Human Services (USDHHS): *Healthy People 2020, Occupational Safety and Health,* 2015a, http://www.healthypeople.gov/2020/topics-objectives/topic/occupational-safety-and-health. Accessed November 22, 2015.

US Department of Health and Human Services (USDHHS): *Vison,* 2015b, http://www.healthypeople.gov/2020/topics-objectives/topic/vision. Accessed November 22, 2015.

World Health Organization (WHO): *Global data on visual impairments,* 2010, http://www.who.int/blindness/publications/globaldata/en/. Accessed November 22, 2015.

RESEARCH REFERENCES

Chou CF, et al: Disparities in eye care utilization among the United States adults with visual impairment: findings from the Behavioral Risk Factor Surveillance System 2006-2009, *Am J Ophthalmol* 154(6):S45, 2012.

Higginbottom G, et al: Health and social care needs of Somali refugees with visual impairment (VIP) living in the United Kingdom: a focused ethnography with Somali people with VIP, their caregivers, service providers, and members of the Horn of Africa Blind Society, *J Transcult Nurs* 25(2):192, 2014.

Kempen GI, et al: The impact of low vision on activities of daily living, symptoms of depression, feelings of anxiety and social support in community-living older adults seeking vision rehabilitation services, *Qual Life Res* 21:1405, 2012.

Lim YM, Sung MH: Home environmental and health-related factors among home fallers and recurrent fallers in community dwelling older Korean women, *Int J Nurs Pract* 18:481, 2012.

Perlmutter M, et al: Home lighting assessment for clients with low vision, *Am J Occup Ther* 67(6):674, 2013.

Stone T, et al: Mediating and moderating effects on the association between vision loss and depression among an older population, *Insight: Res Pract Visual Impairment Blindness* 5(1):30, 2012.

Tomioka K, et al: The Hearing Handicap Inventory for Elderly-Screening (HHIE-S) versus a single question: reliability, validity, and relations with quality of life measures in the elderly community, Japan, *Qual Life Res 22*(5):1151, 2013.

Wang X, et al: Health burden associated with visual impairment in Singapore: the Singapore epidemiology of eye disease study, *Ophthalmology* 121(9):1837, 2014.

Zhang X, et al: Vision health disparities in the United States by race/ethnicity, education, and economic status: findings from two nationally representative surveys, *Am J Ophthalmol* 154:S53, 2012.

50

Care of Surgical Patients

OBJECTIVES

- Explain the concept of perioperative nursing care.
- Discuss common surgical risk factors and related nursing implications.
- Describe preoperative assessment data to collect for a surgical patient.
- Explain the elements of a typical preoperative teaching plan.
- Explain the components of an effective perioperative communication hand-off.
- Demonstrate postoperative exercises.
- Prepare a patient physically and psychologically for surgery.
- Discuss the benefits of preoperative warming.
- Explain the registered nurse's role in the operating room.
- Describe factors to assess in a patient during postoperative recovery.
- Describe the rationale for nursing interventions designed to prevent postoperative complications.
- Describe patients at risk for postoperative complications.

KEY TERMS

MEDIA RESOURCES

http://evolve.elsevier.com/Potter/fundamentals/

- Review Questions
- Video Clips
- Concept Map Creator
- Case Study with Questions
- Skills Performance Checklists
- Audio Glossary
- Content Updates

Perioperative nursing includes activities performed by a professional registered nurse (RN) before (preoperative), during (intraoperative) and after (postoperative) surgery. Nurses provide this care in many settings, including hospitals, surgical centers attached to hospitals, free-standing surgical centers, or health care providers' offices. Perioperative nursing is a fast-paced, changing, and challenging field. It is based on a nurse's understanding of several important principles, including:

- High-quality and patient safety–focused care, including a safe environment of care.
- Evidence-based practices and participation in generation of new knowledge through research.
- Multidisciplinary teamwork.
- Effective therapeutic communication and collaboration with a patient, the patient's family, and the surgical team.
- Effective and efficient assessment and intervention in all phases of surgery.
- Advocacy for a patient and the patient's family.
- Understanding of cost containment.

Perioperative nursing is a dynamic process guided by theoretical knowledge, ethical principles, ongoing research, specialized clinical skills, and caring practices (Operating Room Nurses Association of Canada (ORNAC, 2015). A nurse working within the perioperative setting responds to complex and changing clinical needs during a crucial period of a patient's surgical experience. When you work in any perioperative setting, you need to use critical thinking, practice competently using strict surgical asepsis, communicate effectively with members of the surgical team, and emphasize patient safety in all phases of care. Effective teaching and discharge planning involving patients and their family members prevent or minimize complications and ensure quality outcomes. The nursing process provides a basis for perioperative nursing, allowing you to individualize strategies throughout the perioperative period. A patient's smooth transition from admission into the health care system through convalescence is the aim of quality perioperative care.

Care of a patient having surgery has shifted from a hospital- to home-based focus. Often convalescence occurs in the home or in rehabilitation sites within long-term care facilities. When care is in the home, responsibility shifts to the patient and/or family. As the length of hospital stay decreases, the educational needs of a patient undergoing a surgical procedure increase. Patients return home with complex medical/surgical conditions that require education and follow-up. Proper patient and family education is essential to ensuring positive surgical outcomes.

SCIENTIFIC KNOWLEDGE BASE

Classification of Surgery

The types of surgical procedures are classified according to seriousness, urgency, and purpose (Table 50-1). Some procedures fall into more than one classification. For example, surgical removal of a disfiguring scar is minor in seriousness, elective in urgency, and reconstructive in purpose. Frequently the classes overlap. An urgent procedure is also major in seriousness. Sometimes the same operation is performed for different reasons on different patients. For example, a gastrectomy may be performed as an emergency procedure to resect a bleeding ulcer or as an urgent procedure to remove a cancerous growth. Knowing the classifications helps you plan appropriate intraoperative care.

The surgical classification indicates the level of care a patient requires. The American Society of Anesthesiologists (ASA) assigns classification on the basis of a patient's physiological condition independent of the proposed surgical procedure (Table 50-2). Anesthesia always involves risks even in healthy patients, but certain patients are at higher risk, including those with metabolic and cardiac dysfunction.

Surgical Risk Factors

Numerous factors create risks for patients facing surgery. Risk factors can affect patients at any point in the perioperative experience. Knowledge of the physiology of the stress response (Chapter 38) and risk factors that affect patients' responses to surgery is necessary to anticipate patient needs and the type of preparation required.

Smoking. Cigarette smoking by surgical patients is associated with increased perioperative complications, particularly respiratory problems (e.g., pneumonia and atelectasis) and poor wound healing

TABLE 50-1 Classification of Surgical Procedures

Classification Type	Description	Example
Seriousness		
Major	Involves extensive reconstruction or alteration in body parts; poses great risks to well-being	Coronary artery bypass, colon resection, removal of larynx, resection of lung lobe
Minor	Involves minimal alteration in body parts; often designed to correct deformities; involves minimal risks compared with major procedures	Cataract extraction, facial plastic surgery, tooth extraction
Urgency		
Elective	Performed on basis of patient's choice; is not essential and is not always necessary for health	Bunionectomy, facial plastic surgery; hernia repair; breast reconstruction
Urgent	Necessary for patient's health; often prevents development of additional problems (e.g., tissue destruction or impaired organ function); not necessarily emergency	Excision of cancerous tumor; removal of gallbladder for stones; vascular repair for obstructed artery (e.g., coronary artery bypass)
Emergency	Must be done immediately to save life or preserve function of body part	Repair of perforated appendix or traumatic amputation; control of internal hemorrhaging
Purpose		
Diagnostic	Surgical exploration that allows health care providers to confirm diagnosis; often involves removal of tissue for further diagnostic testing	Exploratory laparotomy (incision into peritoneal cavity to inspect abdominal organs); breast mass biopsy
Ablative	Excision or removal of diseased body part	Amputation; removal of appendix or an organ such as gallbladder (cholecystectomy)
Palliative	Relieves or reduces intensity of disease symptoms; does not produce cure	Colostomy; debridement of necrotic tissue; resection of nerve roots
Reconstructive/restorative	Restores function or appearance to traumatized or malfunctioning tissues	Internal fixation of fractures; scar revision
Procurement for transplant	Removal of organs and/or tissues from a person pronounced brain dead for transplantation into another person	Kidney, heart, or liver transplant
Constructive	Restores function lost or reduced as result of congenital anomalies	Repair of cleft palate; closure of atrial septal defect in heart
Cosmetic	Performed to improve personal appearance	Blepharoplasty for eyelid deformities; rhinoplasty to reshape nose

TABLE 50-2 ASA Physical Status (PS) Classification

ASA PS Class	Definition	Characteristics
ASA I	A normal healthy patient	No physiological, biological, organic disturbance; healthy, nonsmoking; no or minimal alcohol use
ASA II	A patient with mild systemic disease	Mild diseases only without substantive functional changes (e.g., current smoker, social alcohol drinker, pregnancy, obesity [BMI 30-39], well-controlled DM/HTN, mild lung disease)
ASA III	A patient with severe systemic disease	Substantive functional changes with one or more moderate-to-severe diseases (e.g., poorly controlled DM or HTN, COPD, morbid obesity [BMI 40 or greater], active hepatitis, alcohol dependence or abuse, implanted pacemaker, or moderate reduction of cardiac ejection fraction)
ASA IV	A patient with severe systemic disease that is a constant threat to life	Examples include: recent (less than 3 months) MI, CVA, TIA, ongoing cardiac ischemia or severe valve dysfunction, sepsis, disseminated intravascular coagulation, end-stage renal disease not undergoing regularly scheduled dialysis
ASA V	A **moribund** patient who is not expected to survive without the operation	Examples include ruptured abdominal/thoracic aneurysm, massive trauma, intracranial bleed with mass effect, ischemic bowel with significant cardiac pathology
ASA VI	A patient declared brain dead whose organs are being removed for donor purpose	Wide variety of dysfunctions that are being managed to optimize blood flow to the heart and organs (e.g., aggressive fluid replacement and blood pressure medications)

Modified from American Society of Anesthesiologists: *ASA Physical Status Classification System,* October 15, 2014, http://www.asahq.org/resources/clinical-information/asa-physical-status-classification-system. Accessed May 17, 2015.
BMI, Body mass index; *CVA,* cardiovascular accident; *COPD,* chronic obstructive pulmonary disease; *DM,* diabetes mellitus; *HTN,* hypertension; *MI,* myocardial infarction; *TIA,* transient ischemic attack.

(Lee et al., 2013). Chronic smoking increases the amount and thickness of airway secretions. After surgery a patient who smokes has greater difficulty clearing the airways of mucus. When patients have elective surgery, encourage them to stop smoking as early as possible. There has been limited research showing that a simple perioperative smoking cessation intervention for a busy preadmission surgery clinic has success in reducing patients' smoking rates and intraoperative and immediate postoperative complications (Lee et al., 2013).

Age. Very young and older patients are at greater surgical risk as a result of an immature or a declining physiological status. These patients often present problems in temperature control during surgery. General anesthetics inhibit shivering and cause vasodilation, which results in heat loss. These anesthetic changes coupled with age-related physiological factors increase the risk for unintended hypothermia. Infants also have difficulty maintaining normal circulatory blood volume, causing a risk for dehydration and overhydration.

Older adults account for 55% of all those who undergo operative procedures (Kotthoff-Burrell et al., 2012). With advancing age patients have less physical capacity to adapt to the stress of surgery (Table 50-3). Thus the risk for surgical complications increases due to the physiological, cognitive/psychological, and sociological changes associated with aging (AORN, 2010; Nelson & Carrington, 2011).

Nutrition. Normal tissue repair and resistance to infection depend on adequate nutrition. Surgery increases the need for nutrients. Patients who are thin or obese are often deficient in protein and vitamins, putting them at greater risk for complications following surgery (Lewis et al., 2014). After surgery a patient requires at least 1500 kcal/day to maintain energy reserves. This intake is difficult to attain when a patient's food or fluid intake is limited after surgery or if a patient experiences postoperative nausea and vomiting (PONV). Traditionally patients gradually increase their dietary intake over 3 to 5 days after surgery until they can tolerate normal meals. Patients who enter surgery malnourished are more likely to have poor tolerance for anesthesia, negative nitrogen balance, delayed postoperative recovery, infection, and delayed wound healing. Current recommendations suggest replacing iron, vitamin B_{12}, and folate at least 28 days before scheduled elective surgery (Goodnough et al., 2011). Some studies show that recovery is enhanced in several ways: regulating the metabolic status of a patient before surgery (e.g., minimizing metabolic stress and insulin resistance by giving carbohydrate-based drinks and fluid loading) and after surgery (e.g., early oral feeding and giving prokinetic medications to enhance gastric motility, resulting in improved enteral feeding tolerance) (Awad and Lobo, 2011; Fearon and Luff, 2003).

Obesity. Patients who are morbidly obese typically live up to 20 years less than their average-weight counterparts (Dunham, 2013). According to the CDC (2015a), more than one third (34.9% or 78.6 million) of U.S. adults are obese, but the prevalence of morbid obesity isn't limited to adults. Approximately 17% (or 12.7 million) of children and adolescents ages 2 to 19 years are also obese (CDC, 2015b). As a patient's weight increases, his or her ventilatory and cardiac function reduces, increasing the risk for postoperative **atelectasis**, pneumonia, and death. Obstructive sleep apnea (OSA), hypertension, coronary artery disease, diabetes mellitus, and heart failure are **co-morbid** conditions in the **bariatric** (obese) population. Patients who are obese often have difficulty resuming normal physical activity after surgery because of the pain and fatigue caused by surgery in addition to preexisting impaired physical mobility. This combination of factors increases the risk of developing venous thromboembolism (VTE).

Excess weight placed on skin over bony prominences restricts blood flow and poses risks for pressure ulcers to form on the operating table. Obesity increases the risk of poor wound healing, wound infection, dehiscence, and evisceration because fatty tissue contains a poor blood supply, slowing the delivery of essential nutrients and antibodies needed for wound healing (see Chapter 48). In addition, surgeons

TABLE 50-3 Physiological Factors That Place the Older Adult at Risk During Surgery

Alterations	Risks	Nursing Implications
Cardiovascular System		
Degenerative change in myocardium and valves	Decreased cardiac reserve puts older adults at risk for decreased cardiac output, especially during times of stress (AORN, 2010)	Assess baseline vital signs for tachycardia, fatigue, and arrhythmias (AORN, 2010).
Rigidity of arterial walls and reduction in sympathetic and parasympathetic innervation to the heart	Alterations predispose patient to postoperative hemorrhage and rise in systolic and diastolic blood pressure	Maintain adequate fluid balance to minimize stress to the heart. Ensure that blood pressure level is adequate to meet circulatory demands.
Increased calcium and cholesterol deposits within small arteries; thickened arterial walls	Predispose patient to clot formation in lower extremities	Instruct patient in techniques of leg exercises and proper turning. Apply elastic stockings or intermittent pneumatic compression (IPC) devices. Administer anticoagulants as ordered by health care provider. Provide education regarding effects, side effects, and dietary considerations.
Integumentary System		
Decreased subcutaneous tissue and increased fragility of skin	Prone to pressure ulcers and skin tears	Assess skin every 4 hours; pad all bony prominences during surgery. Turn or reposition at least every 2 hours.
Pulmonary System		
Decreased respiratory muscle strength and cough reflex (AORN, 2010)	Increased risk for atelectasis	Instruct patient in proper technique for coughing, deep breathing, and use of spirometer. Ensure adequate pain control to allow for participation in exercises.
Reduced range of movement in diaphragm	Residual capacity (volume of air left in lung after normal breath) increased, reducing amount of new air brought into lungs with each inspiration	When possible, have patient ambulate and sit in chair frequently.
Stiffened lung tissue and enlarged air spaces	Blood oxygenation reduced	Obtain baseline oxygen saturation; measure throughout perioperative period.
Gastrointestinal System		
Gastric emptying delayed	Increases risk for reflux and indigestion (AORN, 2010)	Position patient with head of bed elevated at least 45 degrees. Reduce size of meals in accordance with ordered diet.
Renal System		
Decreased renal function, with reduced blood flow to kidneys	Increased risk of shock when blood loss occurs; increased risk for fluid and electrolyte imbalance (AORN, 2010)	For patients hospitalized before surgery, determine baseline urinary output for 24 hours.
Reduced glomerular filtration rate and excretory times	Limited ability to eliminate drugs or toxic substances	Assess for adverse response to drugs.
Decreased bladder capacity	Increased risk for urgency, incontinence, and urinary tract infections (AORN, 2010) (Sensation of need to void often does not occur until bladder is filled.)	Instruct patient to notify nurse immediately when sensation of bladder fullness develops. Keep call light and bedpan within easy reach. Toilet every 2 hours or more frequently if indicated.
Neurological System		
Sensory losses, including reduced tactile sense and increased pain tolerance	Decreased ability to respond to early warning signs of surgical complications	Inspect bony prominences for signs of pressure that patient is unable to sense. Orient patient to surrounding environment. Observe for nonverbal signs of pain.
Blunted febrile response during infection (AORN, 2010)	Increased risk of undiagnosed infection	Ensure careful, close monitoring of patient temperature; provide warm blankets; monitor heart function; warm intravenous fluids (AORN, 2010).
Decreased reaction time	Confusion and delirium after anesthesia; increased risk for falls	Allow adequate time to respond, process information, and perform tasks. Perform fall-risk screening and institute fall precautions. Screen for delirium with validated tools. Orient frequently to reality and surroundings.

TABLE 50-3 Physiological Factors That Place the Older Adult at Risk During Surgery—cont'd

Alterations	Risks	Nursing Implications
Metabolic System		
Lower basal metabolic rate	Reduced total oxygen consumption	Ensure adequate nutritional intake when diet is resumed but avoid intake of excess calories.
Reduced number of red blood cells and hemoglobin levels	Reduced ability to carry adequate oxygen to tissues	Administer necessary blood products. Monitor blood test results and oxygen saturation.
Change in total amounts of body potassium and water volume	Greater risk for fluid or electrolyte imbalance	Monitor electrolyte levels and supplement as necessary. Provide cardiac monitoring (telemetry) as needed.

often have difficulty closing surgical wounds because of the thick adipose layer.

Obstructive Sleep Apnea. Obstructive sleep apnea (OSA) is a disorder of sleep and wakefulness resulting from periodic, partial, or complete obstruction of the upper airway during sleep. An individual's throat muscles intermittently relax and block the airway. The disorder is a combination of structural and neuromuscular dysfunction. Patients with OSA experience periodic episodes of apnea (stops breathing), resulting in significant oxygen desaturation, also referred to as intermittent hypoxia. During the apnea there is increasing negative intrathoracic pressure (down to −80 mm Hg), which makes it difficult for the heart to pump effectively against such a negative pressure; thus cardiac output decreases. In response to the oxygen desaturation, there is an arousal, which ends the apnea. The arousal is accompanied by a huge increase in sympathetic output, which causes a significant increase in blood pressure.

The disorder hinders daily functioning because of chronic fatigue and sleepiness and adversely affects health and longevity. Patients who suffer from OSA develop numerous complications, including hypertension, heart disease, vascular disease, neurological disease, and diabetes. Approximately 75% of adults with OSA are unaware they have OSA (Simpson et al., 2013). In addition, perioperative health care providers often fail to screen for OSA, resulting in a high prevalence of undiagnosed patients (Lockhart et al., 2013).

Patients with OSA who are to undergo surgery present a significant risk. Receiving sedatives, opioid analgesics, and general anesthesia causes relaxation of the upper airway and may worsen OSA. The risk is higher when a patient is sedated and lying on his or her back. Patients have experienced severe apnea and hypoxemia leading to death following surgical and diagnostic procedures under conscious sedation. Careful screening of patients for OSA is essential before surgery.

Immunosuppression. Patients with conditions that alter immune function (e.g., primary immune deficiency, acquired immunodeficiency syndrome (AIDS), cancer, bone marrow alterations, and organ transplants) are at an increased risk for developing infection after surgery. The risk for infection increases when patients receive radiation or chemotherapy for cancer treatment, take immunosuppressive medications to treat AIDS or prevent rejection after organ transplant, and require steroids to treat a variety of inflammatory or autoimmune conditions. Radiation sometimes is given before surgery to reduce the size of a cancerous tumor so it can be removed surgically. Ideally a surgeon waits to perform surgery 4 to 6 weeks after completion of radiation treatments because of the unavoidable effects that radiation has on normal tissue. Radiation thins the layers of the skin, destroys collagen, and impairs tissue perfusion. Otherwise the patient may face serious wound-healing problems.

Fluid and Electrolyte Imbalance. The body responds to surgery as a form of trauma. Severe protein breakdown causes a negative nitrogen balance (see Chapter 42) and hyperglycemia. Both of these effects decrease tissue healing and increase the risk of infection. As a result of the adrenocortical stress response, the body retains sodium and water and loses potassium in the first 2 to 5 days after surgery. The severity of the stress response influences the degree of fluid and electrolyte imbalance. Extensive surgery results in a greater stress response. A patient who is hypovolemic before surgery or who has serious electrolyte alterations is at significant risk during and after surgery. For example, an excess or depletion of potassium increases the chance of dysrhythmias during or after surgery. The risk of fluid and electrolyte alterations is even greater in patients with preexisting diabetes mellitus, renal disease, gastrointestinal (GI), or cardiovascular abnormalities.

Postoperative Nausea and Vomiting. The experience of having nausea and vomiting after surgery is uncomfortable and often immobilizing. PONV affects approximately 30% of patients in recovery rooms after surgery (Fetzer, 2015). It can lead to serious complications, including pulmonary aspiration, dehydration, and arrhythmias resulting from fluid and electrolyte imbalance. A patient who vomits frequently after surgery runs the risk of pulling apart surgical sutures. Patients predisposed to developing PONV include females, nonsmokers, those who have had a history of PONV or motion sickness, use of volatile anesthetics or nitrous oxide, and those who receive intraoperative or postoperative opioids (Kapoor et al., 2008). Patients with four or more risk factors have a higher incidence of PONV (Rothrock, 2015). Management of PONV begins before surgery.

Venous Thromboembolism. The Centers for Medicare and Medicaid Services (CMS, 2010) ruled deep vein thrombosis (DVT) (clot formed in the deep veins) after total knee and hip surgery as a never event. If a patient develops a DVT after surgery, Medicare and some private insurance companies withhold payment to the hospital because DVTs are typically preventable. The Joint Commission (TJC, 2015) has a set of accountability measures (i.e., quality measures that produce the greatest positive impact on patient outcomes when hospitals demonstrate improvement in them). One of the accountability measures is treatment and prevention of VTE. Some VTEs are subclinical (without symptoms), whereas others present as sudden pulmonary embolus or symptomatic DVT. Patients most at risk for developing VTE are those who undergo surgical procedures with a total anesthetic and surgical time of more than 90 minutes, or 60 minutes if the surgery involves the pelvis or lower limb; acute surgical admissions with inflammatory or intraabdominal conditions; and those expected to have significant reduction in mobility after surgery. In addition, patients are at higher risk if they have one or more risk factors (National Institute for Health and Clinical Excellence [NICE], 2010):

- Active cancer or cancer treatment
- Age over 60 years
- Critical care admission
- Dehydration
- Known clotting disorders
- Obesity (body mass index [BMI] of 30 kg/m^2 or greater)

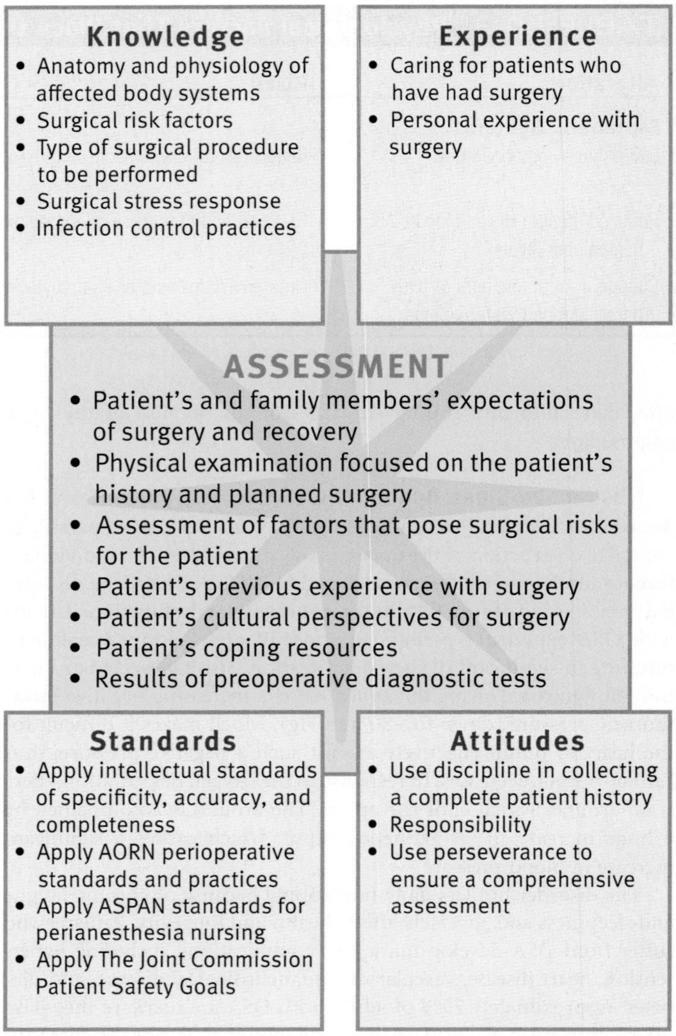

NURSING KNOWLEDGE BASE

Perioperative Communication

Perioperative nurses recognize the importance of providing continuity of care for surgical patients. In some settings perioperative nurses follow patients throughout the operative experience, assessing a patient's health status before surgery, identifying specific patient needs, teaching and counseling, preparing for the operating room (OR), and following a patient's recovery. However, different nurses and other health care providers usually care for a patient during each phase of the surgical experience. A smooth communication "hand-off" between caregivers is needed to ensure continuity of care and reduce risk of medical errors. Transitions from one care provider to another place patients at risk for injuries, missed care, and errors in translating information. TJC National Patient Safety Goals address the importance of accurate patient identification and communication (TJC, 2016). Nursing research shows that having a standardized checklist or protocol for hand-off communication between perioperative health care providers minimizes these risks (Boat and Spaeth, 2013; Petrovic et al., 2012).

Glycemic Control and Infection Prevention

Evidence supports a relationship between wound and tissue infection and surgical patients' blood glucose levels. Poor control of blood glucose levels (specifically hyperglycemia) during and after surgery increases patients' risks for adverse outcomes such as wound infection and mortality. Controlling blood sugars perioperatively reduces mortality in patients with or without diabetes who have general surgery and in patients who have cardiac surgery (Giakoumidakis et al., 2013; Kwon et al., 2013). Perioperative evaluation of patients coupled with appropriate insulin administration is a critical standard of care.

Pressure Ulcer Prevention

Patients who have surgery pose a unique challenge in pressure ulcer prevention. Patients are at risk intraoperatively for pressure ulcers as a result of sustained pressure from positioning on OR tables, changes in hemodynamics (blood pressure and perfusion) from anesthesia, use of multiple layers of drapes, and exposure of the skin to fluids used to irrigate wounds during surgery (Bulfone et al., 2012). You prevent pressure ulcers intraoperatively by carefully positioning patients and using pressure-relieving surfaces. After surgery, perform careful skin assessment and use appropriate pressure reduction strategies (see Chapter 48).

CRITICAL THINKING

Successful critical thinking requires a synthesis of knowledge, experience, information gathered from patients, critical thinking attitudes, and intellectual and professional standards. Clinical judgments require you to anticipate information, analyze the data, and make decisions regarding your patient's care. During assessment, consider all elements that build toward making an appropriate nursing diagnosis (Figure 50-1).

Knowledge
- Anatomy and physiology of affected body systems
- Surgical risk factors
- Type of surgical procedure to be performed
- Surgical stress response
- Infection control practices

Experience
- Caring for patients who have had surgery
- Personal experience with surgery

ASSESSMENT
- Patient's and family members' expectations of surgery and recovery
- Physical examination focused on the patient's history and planned surgery
- Assessment of factors that pose surgical risks for the patient
- Patient's previous experience with surgery
- Patient's cultural perspectives for surgery
- Patient's coping resources
- Results of preoperative diagnostic tests

Standards
- Apply intellectual standards of specificity, accuracy, and completeness
- Apply AORN perioperative standards and practices
- Apply ASPAN standards for perianesthesia nursing
- Apply The Joint Commission Patient Safety Goals

Attitudes
- Use discipline in collecting a complete patient history
- Responsibility
- Use perseverance to ensure a comprehensive assessment

FIGURE 50-1 Critical thinking model for surgical patient assessment. *AORN,* Association of periOperative Registered Nurses; *ASPAN,* American Society of PeriAnesthesia Nurses.

When caring for a patient having surgery, integrate knowledge regarding the patient's specific clinical situation along with previous experiences in caring for surgical patients. Apply this knowledge using a patient-centered care approach, partnering with your patient to make clinical decisions. Using critical thinking attitudes (see Chapter 15) ensures that a plan of care is comprehensive and incorporates evidence-based principles for successful perioperative care. A key attitude for a perioperative nurse is responsibility (i.e., being responsible not only for standards of care but being a patient advocate as well). The use of professional perioperative standards developed by the Agency for Health Care Research and Quality (AHRQ) (http://www.ahrq.gov), the Association of periOperative Registered Nurses (AORN) (http://www.aorn.org), and the American Society of PeriAnesthesia Nurses (ASPAN) (http://www.aspan.org/) provides valuable guidelines for perioperative management and evaluation of process and outcomes. TJC Hospital National Patient Safety Goals include two sets of recommendations for perioperative care: prevent infection and prevent mistakes in surgery (TJC, 2016). Always review these guidelines within the context of new emerging evidence-based practice, agency policies, and the scope of practice of the state in which you practice.

PREOPERATIVE SURGICAL PHASE

❖ NURSING PROCESS

Apply the nursing process and use a critical thinking approach in your care of patients. The nursing process provides a clinical decision-making approach for you to develop and implement an individualized plan of care.

Patients having surgery enter the health care setting in different stages of health. For example, a patient enters the hospital or ambulatory surgery center (ASC) on a predetermined day feeling relatively healthy and prepared to face elective surgery, while another person in a motor vehicle crash faces emergency surgery with no time to prepare. The ability to establish rapport and maintain a professional relationship with a patient is essential during the preoperative phase. Patients having surgery meet many health care personnel, including surgeons, nurse anesthetists, anesthesiologists, surgical technologists, and nurses. All play a role in a patient's care and recovery. Family members attempt to provide support through their presence but face many of the same stressors as the patient. You need to form a caring relationship (see Chapter 7) and effectively communicate (see Chapter 24) with the patient and family to gain a patient's trust. This helps you to learn the depth of information needed to provide a relevant and appropriate plan of care. Be culturally sensitive when you assess a patient's physical, psychological, emotional, sociocultural, and spiritual well-being; recognize the degree of surgical risk; coordinate diagnostic tests; identify nursing diagnoses and nursing interventions; and establish outcomes in collaboration with patients and their families. Communicate pertinent data and the plan of care to surgical team members.

◆ Assessment

During the assessment process, thoroughly assess each patient and critically analyze findings to ensure you make patient-centered clinical decisions required for safe nursing care. The goal of the preoperative assessment is to identify a patient's normal preoperative function and the presence of any risks to recognize, prevent, and minimize possible postoperative complications. The thoroughness of your assessment will depend on the surgical setting, the time you have with a patient, and the urgency of a procedure. Ambulatory and same-day surgical programs offer challenges in gathering a complete assessment in a short time. A multidisciplinary team approach is essential. Patients are admitted only hours before surgery; thus it is important for you to organize and verify data obtained before surgery and implement a perioperative plan of care. This occurs both in ASCs and with patients who require a hospital stay.

Most assessments begin before admission for surgery in a health care provider's office, preadmission clinic, or anesthesia clinic or by telephone. Some patients answer a self-report inventory before arriving to a center. Other times a health care provider performs a physical examination or orders laboratory tests. Nurses begin teaching, answering questions, and completing paperwork before surgery to streamline patient care on the day of surgery. When surgery is emergent, often little time is available; thus assessment must be prioritized to a patient's presenting clinical condition and risk factors.

Through the Patient's Eyes. When there is time to conduct a thorough assessment, begin by determining a patient's expectations of surgery and the road to recovery. Is the patient able to identify or describe the type of surgery scheduled? Does he or she understand the expected care and anticipated length of stay after surgery? If not, what does the patient or family want to know? Does the patient expect full pain relief or simply to have his or her pain reduced after surgery? Does the patient expect to be independent immediately after surgery, or does he or she expect to be fully dependent on the nurse or family? These are only a few of the questions that you need to ask to establish a plan of care that matches a patient's needs and expectations. Listen to the patient's explanation, be attentive, and begin to explain what surgery will involve. You need to form a relationship with the patient so shared decision making will occur. By opening an assessment with these types of questions, the patient will become your partner and share the details you need to learn about his or her health.

Nursing History. A preoperative nursing history includes information similar to that described in Chapter 31. If a patient is unable to relay all of the necessary information, rely on family members (if appropriate) as resources. As with any admission to a health care agency, include information about advance directives. Ask if a patient has a durable power of attorney for health care or a living will (see Chapter 23) and include a copy in the patient's medical record. The law requires advance directive identification for patients of all ages and for all surgical procedures. Often directives are modified before surgery but are reestablished after postoperative stabilization. To help ensure a thorough and accurate nursing assessment, electronic health records provide standardized documentation forms for preoperative assessment. Be sure to use all drop-down menus to most clearly portray a patient's history but also be willing to enter full text descriptions as needed.

Medical History. A review of a patient's medical history includes past illnesses and surgeries and the primary reason for seeking medical care. A history screens candidates for surgery for major medical conditions that increase the risk for complications during or after surgery (Table 50-4). For example, a patient who has a history of heart failure is at risk for a further decline in cardiac function during and after surgery. The patient with heart failure in the preoperative period often requires beta-blocker medications, intravenous (IV) fluids infused at a slower rate, or administration of a diuretic after blood transfusions. Box 50-1 provides a list of assessment questions for a patient with a cardiac history. If a patient has any surgical risk from a medical condition, surgery as an outpatient may not be advisable, or it will be necessary to take special precautions. Also ask about a family history for anesthetic complications such as malignant hyperthermia (an inherited disorder). Malignant hyperthermia is a life-threatening condition that can occur during surgery.

Surgical History. A review of a patient's past experience with surgery reveals physical and psychological responses that may occur during the current planned procedure. Complications such as anaphylaxis or malignant hyperthermia during previous surgery alert you to the need for preventive measures and availability of appropriate emergency equipment. A history of postoperative complications such as persistent vomiting or uncontrolled pain helps in the selection of appropriate medications (as ordered by the medical team). Reports of severe anxiety before a previous surgery identify the need for additional emotional support, medications, and preoperative teaching. Inform the surgeon or anesthesiologist of your findings, especially when you believe that medications are indicated.

Risk Factors. Your knowledge of potential surgical risk factors allows you to focus your assessment and screen patients carefully so you can take necessary precautions in planning perioperative care.

TABLE 50-4 Medical Conditions That Increase Risks of Surgery

Type of Condition	Reason for Risk
Bleeding disorders (thrombocytopenia, hemophilia)	Increases risk of hemorrhage during and after surgery.
Diabetes mellitus	Increases susceptibility to infection and impairs wound healing from altered glucose metabolism and associated circulatory impairment. Stress of surgery often results in hyperglycemia (Lewis et al., 2014).
Heart disease (recent myocardial infarction, dysrhythmias, heart failure) and peripheral vascular disease	Stress of surgery causes increased demands on myocardium to maintain cardiac output. General anesthetic agents depress cardiac function.
Hypertension	Increases risk for cardiovascular complications during anesthesia (e.g., stroke, inadequate tissue oxygenation).
Obstructive sleep apnea	Administration of opioids increases risk of airway obstruction after surgery. Patients desaturate as revealed by drop in oxygen saturation by pulse oximetry.
Upper respiratory infection	Increases risk of respiratory complications during anesthesia (e.g., pneumonia and spasm of laryngeal muscles).
Renal disease	Alters excretion of anesthetic drugs and their metabolites, increasing risk for acid-base imbalance and other complications.
Liver disease	Alters metabolism and elimination of drugs administered during surgery and impairs wound healing and clotting time because of alterations in protein metabolism.
Fever	Predisposes patient to fluid and electrolyte imbalances and sometimes indicates underlying infection.
Chronic respiratory disease (emphysema, bronchitis, asthma)	Reduces patient's means to compensate for acid-base alterations (see Chapter 41). Anesthetic agents reduce respiratory function, increasing risk for severe hypoventilation.
Immunological disorders (leukemia, acquired immunodeficiency syndrome [AIDS], bone marrow depression, and use of chemotherapeutic drugs or immunosuppressive agents)	Increases risk of infection and delayed wound healing after surgery.
Abuse of alcohol, street drugs	People abusing drugs sometimes have underlying disease (human immunodeficiency virus [HIV], hepatitis) that affects healing. Alcohol addiction causes unpredictable reactions to anesthesia. People go into withdrawal during and after surgery.
Chronic pain	Regular use of pain medications often results in higher tolerance. Increased doses of analgesics are sometimes necessary to achieve postoperative pain control.

BOX 50-1 Nursing Assessment Questions: Cardiac History

Nature of the Problem

- Do you have a history of heart attack, heart failure, angina (chest pain), irregular heartbeat, or valve disease?
- Which medications do you take?
- Are you taking any vitamins or other supplements?
- Have you had any recent medical testing or procedures on your heart (e.g., cardiac catheterization or echocardiogram)?

Signs and Symptoms

- Are you having any chest pain?
- How do you sleep at night (position, use of pillows, awakened with chest pain)?
- Do your feet swell?
- Are you short of breath, or do you have any difficulty breathing?

Onset and Duration

- How often do you have chest pain, when does it start, how long does it last, what alleviates it?
- When do your feet swell (all the time, end of the day, only after a busy day)?
- When do you become short of breath?

Severity

- On a scale of 0 to 10 (with 0 being no pain and 10 the worst pain), what number do you give your chest pain?
- Describe your usual activity level. Can you climb stairs; can you do housework?
- Do you exercise regularly? What exercise?

Self-Management and Culture

- Have you changed your activity level, sleep amount, diet, or fluid intake recently?
- Are you taking any herbal or over-the-counter medications?

Through the Patient's Eyes

- How are you feeling about your upcoming surgery? Has it affected your symptoms?
- Are you having any additional stress currently?

BOX 50-2 The STOP-BANG Questionnaire

Height _____ cm /inches Weight _____ lbs/kg
Age _____
Male/Female
BMI _____
Collar size of shirt: S, M, L, XL, or _____ cm /inches
Neck circumference* _____ cm

1. ***S*noring**
   Do you *s*nore loudly (louder than talking or loud enough to be heard through closed doors)?
   Yes No
2. ***T*ired**
   Do you often feel *t*ired, fatigued, or sleepy during daytime?
   Yes No
3. ***O*bserved**
   Has anyone *o*bserved you stop breathing during your sleep?
   Yes No
4. **Blood *P*ressure**
   Do you have or are you being treated for high blood *p*ressure?
   Yes No
5. ***B*MI**
   *B*MI more than 35 kg/m^2?
   Yes No
6. ***A*ge**
   *A*ge over 50 years old?
   Yes No
7. ***N*eck circumference (measure with approved measuring tape)***
   *N*eck circumference greater than 40 cm?
   Yes No
8. ***G*ender**
   *G*ender male?
   Yes No

Score of 4—High sensitivity of 88% for identifying severe obstructive sleep apnea (OSA)
Score of 5 or more—High risk of OSA; a score of 6 is more specific

Modified from Chung F et al: Predictive performance of the STOP-BANG score for identifying obstructive sleep apnea in obese patients, *Obes Surg* 23(12):2050, 2013.
BMI, Body mass index.
*Neck circumference is measured by staff.

Consider if any of the risk factors described earlier affect your patient. Collaborate closely with the health care provider when you identify a risk factor that requires therapy. For example, some patients need to stop taking estrogen-containing oral contraceptives or hormone-replacement therapy 4 weeks before elective surgery to reduce risk of thromboembolism (NICE, 2010). Carefully screen patients who have signs and symptoms of suspected OSA. Include the patient's sleeping partner as appropriate to assess for signs of OSA such as snoring. Also determine if the patient uses a continuous positive airway pressure (CPAP), noninvasive positive-pressure ventilation (NIPPV), or apnea monitoring at home. Instruct patients who use CPAP or NIPPV to bring their machine to the hospital or surgery center. Many hospitals are now making OSA screening mandatory using evidence-based tools, such as the STOP-BANG sleep apnea assessment tool (Box 50-2) (Chung et al., 2013).

Some patients need a detailed nutritional assessment to determine surgical risk. If a patient presents with signs of malnourishment, perform a nutritional screening using your agency's tool or confer with a clinical dietitian (see Chapter 45). If a patient has a smoking history, use the information to plan aggressive postoperative pulmonary hygiene, including more frequent turning, use of incentive spirometry, deep breathing, and coughing. Smoking causes hypercoagulability of the blood and increased risk for clot formation. Provide preventive measures to decrease the risk for clots such as pneumatic compression stockings, leg exercises, and early ambulation.

Medications. Review whether a patient is taking any medications that increase the risk for surgical complications (Table 50-5). Many medications interact unpredictably with anesthetic agents during surgery (Lehne, 2016). Sometimes surgeons temporarily discontinue or adjust doses of a patient's prescription or over-the-counter (OTC) medications or herbal supplements before surgery. If you are in an outpatient setting, instruct patients to ask their surgeons whether they should take their usual medications the morning of surgery. Often preprinted instruction sheets given to patients in physician offices contain this information. If you are in an acute care setting, determine if your patient discontinued medications appropriately. If a patient is having inpatient surgery, all prescription medications taken before surgery are discontinued automatically after surgery unless reordered. Be vigilant in reviewing a surgeon's preoperative orders so you administer the correct medications and hold those not to be given. It is important that, as a patient moves through different areas (e.g., holding area to the OR), a complete list of medications is communicated accurately during hand-off report (TJC, 2016).

Allergies. Allergies to medications, latex, and topical agents used to prepare the skin for surgery create significant risks for patients during surgery. An allergic response to any agent is potentially fatal, depending on severity. Latex allergies are on the rise, with 1% to 6% of the general population and 8% to 12% of the health care workforce sensitive to latex (CDC, 2011). Patients most at risk for a latex allergy include people with genetic predisposition to latex allergy, children with spina bifida, patients with urogenital abnormalities or spinal cord injury (because of a long history of urinary catheter use), patients with a history of multiple surgeries, health care professionals, and workers who manufacture rubber products. Patients with an allergy to certain foods such as bananas, chestnuts, kiwi fruit, avocadoes, potatoes, strawberries, nectarine, tomatoes, and wheat often have a cross-sensitivity to latex (Cleveland Clinic, 2014). Symptoms of a latex allergy vary in severity (e.g., contact dermatitis with redness, inflammation, and blisters; contact urticaria with pruritus, redness, and swelling; hay fever–like symptoms; and anaphylaxis).

If you identify that a patient has an allergy, provide an allergy identification band at the time of admission that remains on until discharge. List all allergies in the patient's medical record. It is also common to list allergies on the front of paper charts.

Smoking Habits. Screen all patients for a history of smoking, including cigarettes, cigars, and pipes. This is usually included in the nursing health history. Ask how long a patient has smoked and the number of cigarettes/cigars smoked daily. Use this information to plan for aggressive pulmonary hygiene, including more frequent turning, deep breathing, coughing, and use of incentive spirometry after surgery.

Alcohol Ingestion and Substance Use and Abuse. Habitual use of alcohol and illegal drugs predisposes patients to adverse reactions to anesthetic agents. Some patients experience a cross-tolerance to anesthetic agents and analgesics, resulting in the need for

TABLE 50-5 Medications with Special Implications for the Surgical Patient

Drug Class	Effects During Surgery
Antibiotics	Potentiate (enhance action of) anesthetic agents. If taken within 2 weeks before surgery, aminoglycosides (gentamicin, neomycin, tobramycin) may cause mild respiratory depression from depressed neuromuscular transmission.
Antidysrhythmics	Medications (e.g., beta blockers) can reduce cardiac contractility and impair cardiac conduction during anesthesia.
Anticoagulants	Medications such as warfarin (Coumadin) or aspirin alter normal clotting factors and thus increase risk of hemorrhaging. Discontinue at least 48 hours before surgery.
Anticonvulsants	Long-term use of certain anticonvulsants (e.g., phenytoin [Dilantin] and phenobarbital) alters metabolism of anesthetic agents.
Antihypertensives	Medications such as beta blockers and calcium channel blockers interact with anesthetic agents to cause bradycardia, hypotension, and impaired circulation. They inhibit synthesis and storage of norepinephrine in sympathetic nerve endings.
Corticosteroids	With prolonged use, corticosteroids such as prednisone cause adrenal atrophy, reducing the ability of the body to withstand stress. Before and during surgery, dosages are often increased temporarily.
Insulin	A patient's insulin requirements fluctuate after surgery. For example, some patients need increased doses due to the stress response from surgery. Other patients need less insulin due to decreased nutritional intake following surgery.
Diuretics	Diuretics such as furosemide (Lasix) potentiate electrolyte imbalances (particularly potassium) after surgery.
Nonsteroidal antiinflammatory drugs (NSAIDs)	NSAIDs (e.g., ibuprofen) inhibit platelet aggregation and prolong bleeding time, increasing susceptibility to postoperative bleeding.
Herbal therapies: ginger, gingko, ginseng	These herbal therapies have the ability to affect platelet activity and increase susceptibility to postoperative bleeding. Ginseng increases hypoglycemia with insulin therapy.

higher-than-normal doses. Patients with a history of excessive alcohol ingestion are often malnourished, which delays wound healing. These patients are also at risk for liver disease, portal hypertension, and esophageal varices (which increase the risk of bleeding). A patient who habitually uses alcohol and is required to remain in the hospital longer than 24 hours is also at risk for acute alcohol withdrawal and its more severe form, delirium tremens (DTs). It is important to assess all age-groups because there is a high prevalence of at-risk drinking and binge drinking (17% overall) in adults ages 18 years and older (CDC, 2012b). The CDC further reports that individuals with household incomes greater than $75,000 have the highest binge-drinking prevalence (20.2%), but those with household incomes less than $25,000 had the highest frequency (5 episodes per month) and intensity (8.5 drinks on occasion).

Pregnancy. During preoperative assessment routinely ask women of childbearing age who are scheduled for surgery about their last menstrual period and if it was "typical" for them. Also ask if they have had unprotected sex in the last month. Because many women do not know they are pregnant early in the first trimester, many institutions require a pregnancy test when a patient is scheduled for surgery. The perioperative plan of care addresses not one, but two patients: the mother and the developing fetus. A pregnant patient has surgery only on an emergent or urgent basis. Because all of the mother's major systems are affected during pregnancy, the risk for intraoperative complications is increased. General anesthesia is administered with caution because of the increased risk of fetal death and preterm labor. Regional anesthesia is used in preference to general anesthesia when appropriate (Reitman and Flood, 2011). Psychological assessment of mother and family is also essential.

Perceptions and Knowledge Regarding Surgery. A patient's past experience with surgery influences physical and psychological responses to a procedure. Assess the patient's previous experiences with surgery as a foundation for anticipating his or her needs, providing teaching, addressing fears, and clarifying concerns. Ask him or her to discuss the previous type of surgery, level of discomfort, extent of disability, and overall level of care required. Address any complications that the patient experienced. Prior anesthesia records are a useful source of information if previous surgical problems occurred.

The surgical experience affects the family unit as a whole. Therefore prepare both the patient and the family for the surgical experience. Understanding a patient's and family's knowledge and expectations (during recovery and convalescence and following discharge) allows you to plan teaching and provide individualized emotional support measures.

Each patient fears surgery. Some fears are the result of past hospital experiences, warnings from friends and family, or lack of knowledge. Assess the patient's understanding of the planned surgery, its implications, and planned postoperative activities. Ask questions such as, "Tell me what you think will happen before and after surgery" or "Explain what you know about surgery." Nurses face ethical dilemmas when patients are misinformed or unaware of the reason for surgery. Confer with the surgeon if a patient has an inaccurate perception or knowledge of the surgical procedure before the patient is sent to the surgical suite. Also determine whether the health care provider explained routine preoperative and postoperative procedures and assess the patient's readiness and willingness to learn. When a patient is well prepared and knows what to expect, reinforce his or her knowledge.

Support Sources. Always assess who comprises a patient's family and their level of support. The patient usually cannot immediately assume the same level of physical activity enjoyed before surgery. With **ambulatory surgery**, patients and/or family caregivers assume responsibility for postoperative care. The family caregiver frequently is an important resource for a patient with physical limitations and provides the emotional support needed to motivate the patient to return to his or her previous state of health. Ask the family caregiver if he or she is able to provide support. Sometimes the caregiver remembers preoperative and postoperative teaching better than the patient. Patients having ambulatory surgery will receive a postdischarge phone call to evaluate their recovery. Because patients, especially older adults, are unable to hear or reach a phone after surgery, identify if a family member will be staying with the patient to answer the phone. Your responsibility is to fully prepare a patient and any family caregiver for patient self-care if the patient returns home. This includes providing information so the patient can anticipate any problems, know how to act, and be able to perform care measures (e.g., medication administration, dressing changes, exercises). Often a family member becomes the patient's coach, offering valuable support after surgery when a patient's participation in care is vital.

Occupation. Surgery often results in physical changes and limits that prevent a person from immediately returning to work. Assess the patient's occupational history to anticipate the possible effects of surgery on recovery, return to work, and eventual work performance. Explain postoperative restrictions such as lifting, walking, or climbing stairs before a patient returns to work. When a patient is unable to return to a job, refer to a social worker and/or occupational therapist for job-training programs or to seek economic assistance.

Preoperative Pain Assessment. Surgical manipulation of tissues, treatments, and positioning on the OR table contribute to postoperative pain. Conduct a comprehensive pain assessment before surgery (see Chapter 44), including the patient's and family's expectations for pain management following surgery. Ask patients to describe their perceived tolerance to pain, past experiences, and prior successful interventions. Providing patient education about pain reduces preoperative anxiety, which is frequently associated with postoperative pain (Alanazi, 2014). Teach patients before surgery how to use a pain scale so they are prepared to rate their pain after surgery (see Chapter 44).

Review of Emotional Health. Surgery is psychologically stressful and often creates anxiety in patients and their families. Patients often feel powerless over their situation. Potential disruptions in lifestyle, a lengthy recovery period at home, and uncertainty about the long-term effects of surgery on a patient's life place stress on patients and their families. When a patient has a chronic illness, the family is either fearful that surgery will result in further disability or hopeful that it will improve the patient's lifestyle. To understand the effect of surgery on a patient's and family's emotional health, assess the patient's feelings about surgery, self-concept, body image, and coping resources.

It is difficult to assess a patient's feelings thoroughly when ambulatory surgery is scheduled because you do not have much time to establish a therapeutic relationship with the patient. You can address these concerns initially with the patient during a home visit or on the telephone before surgery. In a hospital room choose a private time for discussion after completing admitting procedures or diagnostic tests. Explain that it is normal to have fears and concerns. A patient's ability to share feelings partially depends on your willingness to listen, be supportive, and clarify misconceptions. Assure patients of their right to ask questions and seek information.

Self-Concept. Patients with a positive self-concept are more likely to approach surgical experiences appropriately. Assess self-concept by asking patients to identify personal strengths and weaknesses (see Chapter 34). Patients who quickly criticize or scorn their own personal characteristics may have little self-regard or may be testing your opinion of their character. Poor self-concept hinders the ability to adapt to the stress of surgery and aggravates feelings of guilt or inadequacy.

Body Image. Surgery or surgical removal of any body part often leaves permanent scars, alteration in body function, or concern over mutilation. Loss of body functions (e.g., with a colostomy or amputation) compound a patient's fears. Assess patients' perceptions of body image alterations from surgery. Individuals respond differently depending on their culture, self-concept, and self-esteem (see Chapter 34).

Surgery, such as removal of a breast, an ostomy, or removal of the prostate gland, sometimes changes the physical or psychological aspects of a patients' sexuality. Some surgeries, such as a hernia repair or cataract extraction, require patients to temporarily refrain from sexual intercourse until they return to normal physical activity. Encourage patients to express concerns about their sexuality. A patient facing even temporary sexual dysfunction requires understanding and support. Hold discussions about the patient's sexuality with his or her sexual partner so the partner gains a shared understanding of how to cope with limitations in sexual function (see Chapter 35).

Coping Resources. Assessment of patients' feelings and self-concept reveals whether they have the ability to cope with the stress of surgery. Thus you need to ask patients about stress management and how they typically cope with stress. Physiologically, stress causes activation of the endocrine system, resulting in the release of hormones and catecholamines, which increases blood pressure, heart rate, and respiration. Platelet aggregation also occurs, along with many other physiological responses. Be aware of these responses and help with stress management by offering healthy coping strategies, such as relaxation exercises (see Chapters 33 and 38). Involve social work or clergy as needed.

Cultural and Spiritual Factors. Culture is a system of beliefs and values developed over time and passed on through many generations. Patients come from diverse cultural, educational, geographical, and spiritual backgrounds that affect the way each patient perceives and reacts to the surgical experience. A recent study shows that sometimes there is a discrepancy between the information provided before surgery and a patient's expectation, which highlights why nurses need to listen to patients to identify their expectations (Tocher, 2014). If you do not acknowledge and plan for cultural and spiritual differences in the perioperative plan of care, your patient may not achieve desired surgical outcomes (Box 50-3). To bridge cultural differences, you explore and respect your patients' beliefs as well as their meaning of illness, preferences, and needs. Understanding a patient's cultural and ethnic heritage helps you better care for a patient having surgery. Although it is important to recognize and plan for differences on the basis of culture, it is also necessary to recognize that members of the same culture are individuals and do not always hold these shared beliefs.

Physical Examination. Conduct a partial or complete physical examination, depending on the amount of time available and the patient's preoperative condition. Chapter 31 describes physical assessment techniques. Assessment focuses on a patient's medical history and on body systems that the surgery is likely to affect. While completing a nursing assessment, you validate existing information, reinforce preoperative teaching, and review discharge instructions.

General Survey. Observe a patient's general appearance. Gestures and body movements (gait, posture, purposeful movement) may reflect decreased energy or weakness caused by illness. Height, body weight, and history of recent weight loss are important indicators of nutritional status and are used to calculate medication dosages. Preoperative vital signs, including blood pressure while sitting and standing, and pulse oximetry provide important baseline data with which to compare alterations that occur during and after surgery, including response to anesthetics and medications and fluid and electrolyte abnormalities (see Chapter 42). An elevated temperature is cause for concern. If a patient has an underlying infection, elective surgery is often postponed until the infection is treated or resolved. An elevated body temperature also alters drug metabolism and increases the risk for fluid and electrolyte changes. Notify the surgeon immediately if a patient has an elevated temperature.

Head and Neck. To determine if your patient is dehydrated, you assess your patient's oral mucous membranes. Dehydration increases the risk for serious fluid and electrolyte imbalances during surgery. Inspect the area between the gums and cheek, the soft palate, and the nasal sinuses. Sinus drainage that is yellow or greenish may indicate respiratory or sinus infection. To rule out the presence of local or systemic infection, palpate the cervical lymph nodes and note any enlargement, which indicates systemic disease.

During the examination of the oral mucosa, identify any loose or capped teeth because they can become dislodged during endotracheal intubation. Note the presence of dentures, prosthetic devices, or piercings so they can be removed before surgery, especially if the patient receives general anesthesia.

Integument. The overall condition of the skin reveals a patient's level of hydration. Carefully inspect the skin, especially over bony prominences such as the heels, elbows, sacrum, back of head, and scapula. In patients who are obese, separate the body folds to ensure that you examine the skin thoroughly. During surgery patients often lie in a fixed position for several hours, placing them at increased risk for pressure ulcers (see Chapter 48). Although physiological blood and lymphatic flow rates vary among patients, capillary pressures may increase to as much as 150 mm Hg during prolonged, unrelieved pressure without a position change (AORN, 2015). The normal pressure needed to keep capillaries open (12 to 32 mm Hg) was identified in classic research (Landis, 1930; Williams et al., 1988). When the intensity of pressure exerted on capillaries exceeds 12 to 32 mm Hg, ischemic injury to the skin can develop. Consider the type of surgery a patient will undergo and the position that is required on the OR table (Figure 50-2) to identify areas at risk for pressure ulcer formation.

Multiple factors affect skin integrity during and after surgery. For example, chronic use of steroids increases a patient's susceptibility to skin tears. Older adults are at high risk for alteration in skin integrity from decrease in epidermis, positioning (pressure forces), and repositioning on the OR table (shearing forces).

Thorax and Lungs. Assess a patient's breathing pattern and chest excursion to detect presence of a decline in ventilation. When ventilation is reduced, a patient is at increased risk for respiratory complications (e.g., atelectasis) following surgery. Auscultation of breath sounds indicates whether the patient has pulmonary congestion or narrowing of airways, which can postpone a surgery. Breath sounds provide an important baseline for a patient's condition. Certain anesthetics potentially cause laryngeal muscle spasm. If you auscultate wheezing in the airways before surgery, a patient is at risk for further airway narrowing during surgery and after extubation (removal of the endotracheal tube); therefore notify health care providers immediately.

Heart and Vascular System. If a patient has a history of heart disease, assess the character of the apical pulse and listen to heart sounds. Assessment of peripheral pulses, capillary refill, and color and

BOX 50-3 CULTURAL ASPECTS OF CARE

Providing Culturally Sensitive Care for the Patient Having Surgery

Patients' culture, religious group, and country of origin influence their health care beliefs. Your approach to perioperative care needs to respect patients' cultural values and incorporate them to improve adherence to the care plan (Galanti, 2008). The use of a wide variety of resources within a health care agency, in the literature, and from the Internet helps nurses provide culturally sensitive care.

Implications for Patient-Centered Care

- Preoperative assessment needs to include a cultural assessment with questions such as primary language spoken, feelings regarding surgery and pain, pain management, expectations, support system, and feelings toward self-care with postoperative implications (e.g., Does patient relate to concept of pain? Does patient have feelings about gender of caregiver? Does patient follow custom of giving family members control over decisions? Does patient have religious convictions that affect perioperative care such as opposition to the administration of blood products?).
- Be sensitive about when and who to use as professional interpreters to communicate with non–English-speaking patients because some patients may have difficulty sharing personal health information with people who are younger or of a specific gender.
- Use materials and teaching techniques that are culturally relevant and language appropriate to communicate and assess the non–English-speaking patient regarding factors such as pain, general comfort, temperature, and need to void.
- Provide preoperative and postoperative educational materials in a variety of languages.

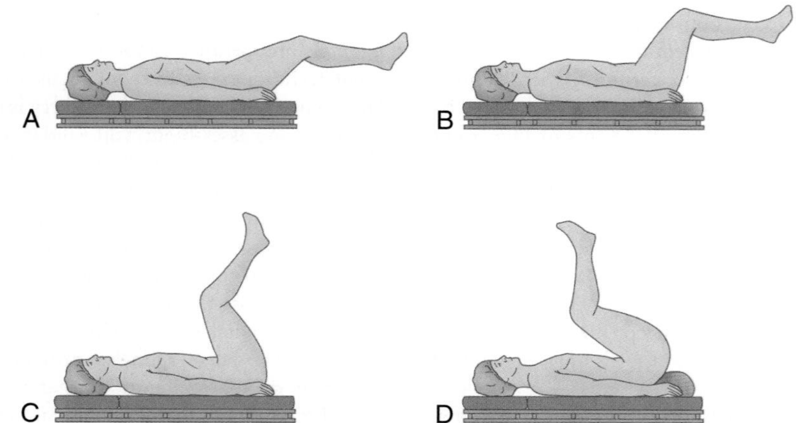

FIGURE 50-2 Examples of patient positions requiring a lithotomy position during surgery. **A,** Low. **B,** Standard. **C,** High. **D,** Exaggerated. (From Rothrock J: *Alexander's care of the patient in surgery,* ed 15, St Louis, 2015, Mosby.)

temperature of extremities is particularly important for patients undergoing vascular or orthopedic surgery and when you know that a patient will have constricting bandages or casts on an extremity after surgery. Screen a patient for one or more of the three primary causative factors of DVT formation (Virchow's triad: venous stasis, vessel wall injury, and hypercoagulability [noted in coagulation laboratory tests]) (AORN, 2015). If peripheral pulses are not palpable, use a Doppler instrument for assessment of their presence. Acceptable capillary refill occurs in less than 2 seconds. Postoperative changes in circulatory status in a patient who had adequate circulation before surgery indicates impaired circulation.

Abdomen. Alterations in GI function after surgery often result in decreased or absent bowel sounds and abdominal distention. Assess the patient's usual abdominal anatomy for size, shape, symmetry, and presence of distention before surgery. Ask how often the patient has bowel movements and inquire about the color and consistency of stools. Auscultate bowel sounds over all four abdominal quadrants.

Neurological Status. A surgical patient's level of consciousness changes as a result of anesthesia, sedatives, and complications that may develop during surgery. Preoperative assessment of baseline neurological status is important for all patients. The baseline neurological status helps with the assessment of ascent (awakening) from anesthesia. Observe a patient's level of orientation, alertness, mood, and ease of speech, noting whether he or she answers questions appropriately and is able to recall recent and past events. Patients who have surgery for neurological disease (e.g., brain tumor or aneurysm) may demonstrate an impaired level of consciousness or altered behavior. If a patient is scheduled for spinal or regional anesthesia, preoperative assessment of gross motor function and strength is important. Spinal anesthesia causes temporary paralysis of the lower extremities (see Chapter 44). Be aware of a patient entering surgery with weakness or impaired mobility of the lower extremities and communicate this to the perioperative team so care providers do not become alarmed when full motor function does not return as the anesthetic wears off.

Diagnostic Screening. Patients undergo diagnostic tests and procedures for preexisting abnormalities before surgery. Patients scheduled for elective or ambulatory surgery usually have tests done several days before surgery. Testing done the day of surgery is usually limited to tests such as glucose monitoring for a patient with diabetes, or an electrocardiogram (ECG) for patients with heart disease. If tests reveal severe problems, a surgeon or anesthesiologist will postpone surgery until the condition stabilizes. As a preoperative nurse you coordinate the completion of tests and verify that a patient is properly prepared. Be familiar with the purpose of diagnostic tests, know a patient's results, and alert a surgeon or anesthesiologist when findings are abnormal.

A patient's medical history, physical assessment findings, and surgical procedure determine the type of tests ordered. For example, a type and cross-match for blood are indicated before surgery for procedures in which blood loss is expected (e.g., hip and knee replacements) in case a patient needs a blood transfusion during surgery. The surgeon designates the number of blood units to have available during surgery. Table 50-6 gives the purpose and normal values for common blood tests.

Maintenance of circulating blood volume is critical for any patient undergoing surgery and is accomplished with administration of whole blood or blood components. Patients undergoing elective surgery who will most likely need blood products will have a pretransfusion type and screen sample taken 1 to 7 days before surgery (see agency policy) (Rothrock, 2015). This test ensures blood compatibility (if a transfusion is needed) and avoids antibodies that may emerge in response to exposure through transfusions or a patient's disease. Autotransfusion (i.e., the reinfusion of a patient's own blood intraoperatively), is more common today (Rothrock, 2015). During intraoperative autotransfusion (cell salvage) blood is collected as it is lost during the surgery and reinfused to the patient after it is filtered and washed. Predated (up to 1 month before surgery) autologous blood donation is in decreasing use (Rothrock, 2015).

◆ Nursing Diagnosis

Cluster the patterns of defining characteristics from your assessment to identify nursing diagnoses relevant for a surgical patient (Box 50-4). A patient with preexisting health problems is likely to have a variety of risk diagnoses. For example, a patient with preexisting bronchitis who has abnormal breath sounds and a productive cough is at risk for *Ineffective Airway Clearance.* The nature of the surgery and assessment of the patient's health status provide defining characteristics and risk factors for a number of nursing diagnoses. For example, because a patient will have a surgical incision and an IV infusion, there is a risk for developing infection at the surgical site, in the bloodstream (sepsis), or phlebitis. A diagnosis of *Risk for Infection* requires attention from admission through recovery.

The related factors for each diagnosis establish directions for nursing care that is provided during one or all surgical phases. For example, the diagnosis of *Ineffective Airway Clearance related to abdominal pain* requires different interventions than the diagnosis *Ineffective Airway Clearance related to excess mucus.* Preoperative nursing diagnoses allow nursing staff to take precautions and actions so care provided during the intraoperative and postoperative phases is consistent with the patient's needs.

Nursing diagnoses made before surgery also focus on the potential risks a patient may face after surgery. Preventive care is essential to manage the surgical patient effectively. The following are common nursing diagnoses relevant to the patient having surgery:

- *Ineffective Airway Clearance*
- *Anxiety*
- *Ineffective Coping*
- *Impaired Skin Integrity*
- *Risk for Aspiration*
- *Risk for Perioperative Positioning Injury*
- *Risk for Infection*
- *Deficient Knowledge (Specify)*
- *Impaired Physical Mobility*
- *Ineffective Thermoregulation*
- *Nausea*
- *Acute Pain*
- *Delayed Surgical Recovery*

◆ Planning

During planning synthesize information to establish a plan of care based on a patient's nursing diagnoses (see the Nursing Care Plan). Apply critical thinking in the selection of nursing interventions (Figure 50-3). For example, apply knowledge of adult learning principles, standards for preoperative education (AORN, 2014), and a patient's unique learning needs and anticipated needs following discharge to formulate a well-designed **preoperative teaching plan** for the diagnosis of *Deficient Knowledge.* Critical thinking ensures that a patient's plan of care integrates knowledge, previous experiences, critical thinking attitudes, and established standards of practice. Previous experience in caring for surgical patients helps establish approaches to patient care (e.g., complications to prevent and anticipate and methods to reduce anxiety). Use professional standards when selecting interventions for

TABLE 50-6 Common Laboratory Tests for Surgical Patients

		SIGNIFICANCE	
Test	**Normal Values***	**Low**	**High**
Complete Blood Count (CBC)			
Hemoglobin (Hgb)	Female: 12-16 g/dL; male: 14-18 g/dL	Anemia	Polycythemia (elevated red blood cell count)
Hematocrit (Hct)	Female: 37%-47%; male: 42%-52%	Fluid overload	Dehydration
Platelet count	150,000-400,000/mm^3	Decreased clotting	Increased risk of blood clot
White blood cell count	5000-10,000/mm^3	Decreased ability to fight infection	Infection
Blood Chemistry			
Sodium (Na)	136-145 mEq/L	Fluid overload	Dehydration
Potassium (K)	3.5-5.0 mEq/L	Cardiac rhythm irregularities	Cardiac rhythm irregularities
Chloride (Cl)	98-106 mEq/L	Follows shifts in sodium blood levels	Follows shifts in sodium blood levels
Carbon dioxide (CO_2)	23-30 mEq/L	Affects acid base balance in blood	Affects acid base balance in blood
Blood urea nitrogen (BUN)	10-20 mg/dL	Liver disease/fluid overload	Renal disease/dehydration
Glucose	70-110 mg/dL fasting	Insulin reaction, inadequate glucose intake	Diabetes mellitus and stress of surgery
Creatinine	Female: 0.5-1.1 mg/dL; male: 0.6-1.2 mg/dL	Malnutrition	Renal disease
Coagulation Studies			
International Normalized Ratio (INR)	0.76-1.27	Risk of clot	Risk of bleeding
Prothrombin time (PT)	11-12.5 sec; 85%-100%	Risk of clot	Risk of bleeding
Partial thromboplastin time (PTT)	60-70 sec	Risk of clot	Risk of bleeding
Activated PTT	30-40 sec	Risk of clot	Excess heparin; risk of spontaneous bleeding (activated PTT)

From Pagana KD, Pagana TJ: *Mosby's diagnostic and laboratory test reference*, ed 11, St Louis, 2013, Mosby.
*Normal ranges vary slightly among laboratories.

BOX 50-4 Nursing Diagnostic Process

Fear Related to Knowledge Deficit and Previous Surgical Experience

Assessment Activities	Defining Characteristics
Ask patient to describe previous surgical experiences.	Apprehension over anesthesia and postoperative pain
Ask patient about understanding of preoperative education/ preparation before admission.	Expresses feeling of dread, worry over complications that may result; unaware of preoperative testing
Observe patient's nonverbal behavior.	Has trouble making decisions about including family member in discussion

the nursing plan of care. These standards often use evidence-based guidelines for preferred nursing interventions.

Successful planning requires a patient-centered approach involving the patient and family to set realistic expectations for care. Early involvement of a patient and family caregiver when developing the surgical care plan minimizes surgical risks and postoperative complications and improves transition of care through discharge. A patient informed about the planned surgical experience is less likely to be fearful and is better able to participate in the postoperative recovery phase so expected outcomes are met. Establish diagnosis, interventions, and outcomes to ensure recovery or maintenance of the preoperative state.

Goals and Outcomes. Base the goals and outcomes of care on the individualized nursing diagnoses. Review and modify the plan during the intraoperative and postoperative periods. Outcomes established for each goal of care provide measurable evidence to gauge a patient's progress toward meeting stated goals. As an example, the goal "Patient will be able to perform postoperative exercises during postoperative recovery" is measured through the following expected outcomes:

- Patient performs deep-breathing and coughing exercises on awakening from anesthesia.
- Patient performs postoperative leg exercises and early ambulation 12 hours after surgery.
- Patient performs incentive spirometry on return to patient care unit after surgery.
- Patient verbalizes rationale for early ambulation 24 hours after surgery.

Setting Priorities. Use clinical judgment to prioritize nursing diagnoses and interventions based on the unique needs of each patient. Patients requiring emergent surgery often experience changes in their physiological status that require urgent reprioritizations. For example,

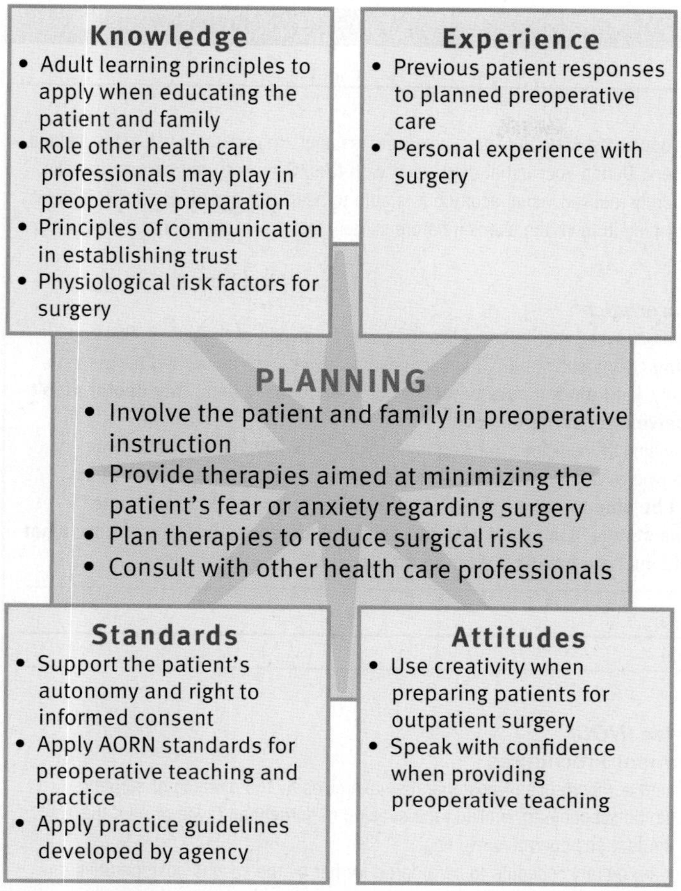

Knowledge
- Adult learning principles to apply when educating the patient and family
- Role other health care professionals may play in preoperative preparation
- Principles of communication in establishing trust
- Physiological risk factors for surgery

Experience
- Previous patient responses to planned preoperative care
- Personal experience with surgery

PLANNING
- Involve the patient and family in preoperative instruction
- Provide therapies aimed at minimizing the patient's fear or anxiety regarding surgery
- Plan therapies to reduce surgical risks
- Consult with other health care professionals

Standards
- Support the patient's autonomy and right to informed consent
- Apply AORN standards for preoperative teaching and practice
- Apply practice guidelines developed by agency

Attitudes
- Use creativity when preparing patients for outpatient surgery
- Speak with confidence when providing preoperative teaching

FIGURE 50-3 Critical thinking model for surgical patient planning. *AORN,* Association of periOperative Registered Nurses.

if a patient's blood pressure begins to drop, hemodynamic stabilization becomes a priority over education and stress management. Ensure that the approach to each patient is thorough and reflects an understanding of the implications of a patient's age, physical and psychological health, educational level, cultural and religious practices, and stated and/or written wishes concerning advance medical directives.

Teamwork and Collaboration. For patients having ambulatory surgery, those admitted the day of their scheduled surgery, and those with special issues (e.g., morbid obesity), the health care team needs to collaborate to ensure continuity of care. Preoperative planning ideally occurs days before admission to a hospital or surgical center. The collaboration between the health care provider's office and the surgical center is crucial to prepare a patient for a procedure and ensure that the proper equipment/supplies are available. Preoperative instruction gives patients time to think about their surgical experience, make necessary physical preparations (e.g., altering diet or discontinuing medication use), and ask questions about postoperative procedures. A patient having ambulatory surgery usually returns home on the day of surgery. Thus well-planned preoperative care ensures that he or she is well informed and able to be an active participant during recovery. The family or significant others also play an active supportive role for a patient.

◆ Implementation

Preoperative nursing interventions provide patients (and families) with a complete understanding of the surgery and anticipated postoperative activities and prepare them physically and psychologically for surgical intervention and recovery.

Informed Consent. Except in emergencies, surgery cannot be performed legally or ethically until a patient fully understands a surgical procedure and all implications. Surgical procedures are not performed without documentation of a patient's consent in the medical record. Chapter 23 discusses a nurse's responsibilities for **informed consent**. It is the surgeon's responsibility to explain the procedure, associated risks, benefits, alternatives, and possible complications before obtaining the patient's oral and documented informed consent (Rothrock, 2015). The patient also needs to know who will perform the procedure. To ensure that a patient understands information about surgery, TJC (2014) recommends that consent materials be written at a fifth-grade or lower reading level. After the patient or power of attorney signs the consent form, place it in the medical record. The record goes to the OR with the patient. As a nurse, if you have concerns about a patient's understanding of surgery, report them to the operating surgeon or anesthesia provider before the patient goes to surgery (Rothrock, 2015).

Privacy and Social Media. Although patients can now access their medical records electronically, confidentiality risks exist. Inappropriate discussions of a patient and any planned surgery in elevators, cafeterias, or social settings after work can end up being communicated "worldwide" (Rothrock, 2015). You have an obligation to protect each patient's privacy by avoiding inappropriate discussions and not using social media to convey information. Posting patient information and photos on websites is prohibited; 26 state boards of nursing have taken disciplinary action against nurses who practice such behavior (Rothrock, 2015). In addition, you are violating federal and state patient privacy laws.

Health Promotion. Health promotion activities during the preoperative phase focus on health maintenance, patient safety, prevention of complications, and anticipation of continued care needed after surgery.

Preoperative Teaching. Patient education is an important aspect of a patient's surgical experience (see Chapter 25). The topics and principles discussed depend on the type of surgery scheduled, whether a procedure is inpatient or outpatient, and the ability of a patient to attend to and learn content provided. Research shows that patient education often reduces patients' preoperative anxiety, which often leads to an increase in postoperative pain, poor outcomes, and prolonged hospital stays (Alanazi, 2014). In addition, education about the surgical experience increases patient satisfaction and knowledge, speeds up the recovery process, and facilitates a return to functioning (Lewis et al., 2014). Structured teaching throughout the perioperative period influences the following:

- *Ventilatory function*: Teaching improves the ability and willingness to deep breathe and cough effectively.
- *Physical functional capacity*: Teaching increases understanding and willingness to ambulate and resume activities of daily living.
- *Sense of well-being*: Patients who are prepared for surgery have less anxiety and report a greater sense of psychological well-being (Haufler and Harrington, 2011).
- *Length of hospital stay*: Being informed reduces a patient's length of hospital stay by preventing or minimizing complications.
- *Anxiety about pain and its management*: Patients who learn about pain and ways to relieve it before surgery are less anxious about it, ask for what they need, and require less analgesia after surgery (Grawe et al., 2010).

NURSING CARE PLAN

Deficient Knowledge

ASSESSMENT

Mrs. Campana is an 80-year-old patient scheduled for admission in 5 days for elective bowel resection to remove a cancerous tumor. You are the nurse in the ambulatory surgery center (ASC) preoperative testing area assigned to prepare her for surgery. During your initial discussion with Mrs. Campana, you assess that she is alert and oriented to person, place, time, and situation. She states that she has severely reduced visual acuity but is able to hear your questions clearly. The last time she had surgery was 10 years ago. She lives alone but has a daughter who is coming in town the evening before surgery and will stay with her 2 weeks after surgery.

Assessment Activities	*Findings/Defining Characteristics**
Ask Mrs. Campana what she has been told by her surgeon regarding her surgery.	She states that her surgeon explained where her tumor is located using a drawing of the bowel. She had **difficulty seeing the drawing** clearly and states, "I know I have a cancer in my colon, and the surgeon said I might require a colostomy, but **I am not sure what that is.**" She further states, **"My doctor didn't explain the care I will receive after surgery is over."**
Ask Mrs. Campana what she understands about preoperative preparation and what to expect after surgery.	She correctly verbalizes understanding of medicines to take the morning of surgery, her diet before surgery and when to stop eating, and who to call for questions. **She cannot explain what to expect after surgery. She states, "Will I be able to eat anything? And what do I need to do to go home?"**
Assess Mrs. Campana's concerns about surgery.	She appears slightly anxious. **She states, "I'm afraid how this might change my life. I don't know what to expect. My neighbor told me I am having a dangerous surgery."**

***Defining characteristics** are shown in bold type.

NURSING DIAGNOSIS: Deficient knowledge related to insufficient information

PLANNING

Goals	*Expected Outcomes (NOC)*[†]
	Knowledge: Treatment Procedures
Mrs. Campana will express understanding of expected postoperative care by the morning of surgery.	Mrs. Campana describes the importance of postoperative exercises by the morning of surgery. Mrs. Campana describes the schedule for walking the evening of surgery and type of pain therapy she will receive by the first postoperative evening. Mrs. Campana explains the dietary schedule to be ordered for her by the second postoperative day.
Mrs. Campana will participate actively in postoperative recovery activities by postoperative day 1.	Mrs. Campana successfully performs postoperative exercises (turning, coughing, and deep breathing [TCDB], diaphragmatic breathing [DB], incentive spirometry [IS], and leg exercises) on the evening of surgery.
Mrs. Campana and daughter will describe expectations regarding home care by postoperative day 2.	Mrs. Campana and daughter explain expected activity restrictions, diet schedule, and wound care for home care guidelines by day 2 after surgery.

[†]Outcome classification labels from Moorhead S et al: *Nursing outcomes classification (NOC)*, ed 5, St Louis, 2013, Mosby.

INTERVENTIONS (NIC)[‡] *Preoperative Teaching*	**RATIONALE**
Before admission to the hospital, provide Mrs. Campana with audiotape program that explains preoperative and postoperative routines. Supply instruction booklet designed for patients with visual impairments. Make a follow-up call 24 hours before surgery to patient encouraging her to ask questions and voice concerns.	Preoperative education is effective in reducing patients' postoperative fatigue and pain and improving their knowledge (Ronco et al., 2012).
On admission to hospital, demonstrate to Mrs. Campana and daughter how patient is to perform postoperative exercises and how to get out of bed with assistance.	Demonstration is an effective method to reinforce instruction.
Coach Mrs. Campana during a return demonstration of postoperative exercises before surgery.	Learning occurs when a patient is actively involved in an education session (Edelman and Mandle, 2014). When possible, have patient perform return demonstration of use of incentive spirometer (Rothrock, 2015).
Using audiotape and information sheets, explain to patient and daughter the activity restrictions likely to be followed at home, expected diet schedule, and wound care guidelines.	Influential factors in patient satisfaction for surgery are receiving information at admission and being given home care information (Mira et al., 2009).

[‡]Intervention classification labels from Bulechek GM, et al: *Nursing interventions classification (NIC)*, ed 6, St Louis, 2013, Mosby.

NURSING CARE PLAN

Deficient Knowledge—cont'd

EVALUATION

Nursing Actions	Patient Response/Finding	Achievement of Outcome
Ask Mrs. Campana to describe activity and diet therapies to expect while in hospital after surgery.	She verbalizes understanding of diet progression from NPO to full liquids but is not sure how quickly she will be expected to ambulate.	Mrs. Campana requires additional discussion of activity and long-term diet plan.
Observe Mrs. Campana demonstrate postoperative exercises.	She correctly demonstrates leg exercises and turning, coughing, and deep breathing (TCDB) but is having difficulty using incentive spirometer.	Mrs. Campana demonstrates most postoperative exercises but needs further teaching and practice on incentive spirometer use.
Have Mrs. Campana and daughter describe activity limits following surgery and pain-management expectations or concerns.	Both Mrs. Campana and her daughter are able to describe safety of taking analgesics after surgery and importance of pain control. Both are able to describe limits on lifting objects but are unsure of other restrictions.	Patient and daughter show understanding of pain management. Require reinforcement of all activity restrictions to expect once returning home.
Ask Mrs. Campana and her daughter to describe signs of a wound infection.	Mrs. Campana's daughter is able to describe tenderness, drainage, and fever as signs of wound infection. Patient is unclear of signs of wound complications.	Patient requires further education and reinforcement.

The health care provider's office or hospital often provide preoperative information and instructions by telephone calls and home mailings. Instructions are available as preprinted teaching guidelines and checklists or in the form of videotapes or educational websites. The American College of Surgeons developed a patient education website titled *Surgical Patient Education Program,* which provides patient information and education materials on types of surgeries, health resources, insurance information, and even some home care skills training (American College of Surgeons, 2015). When a patient is scheduled for surgery (outpatient or inpatient), preadmission nurses call patients up to 1 week before the surgery to clarify questions and reinforce explanations (Rothrock, 2015) For example, they:

- Describe time for a patient to arrive at facility and time of surgery (approximately).
- Explain extent and purpose of food and fluid restrictions.
- Teach about physical preparation (e.g., bowel preparation, bathing or showering with antiseptic).
- Explain procedures performed in preanesthesia (holding area) just before transport to the OR (IV line insertion, preoperative medications).

Including family members in preoperative instruction is advisable. Often a family member is the coach for postoperative exercises when a patient returns from surgery. A family often has better retention of preoperative teaching and will be with the patient and able to help him or her in recovery. If anxious relatives do not understand routine postoperative events, it is likely that their anxiety heightens the patient's fears and concerns. Preoperative preparation of family members lessens anxiety and misunderstanding. To ensure comprehensive preoperative instruction, include the following topics (AORN, 2015).

Reasons for Preoperative Instructions and Exercises. When given a rationale for preoperative and postoperative procedures, patients are better prepared to participate in care. Patients who undergo ambulatory surgery need to learn how their instructions and exercises will promote healthy recovery, prevent complications, and allow them to return to a normal lifestyle as soon as possible. For example, a patient needs to know how recommended care activities (e.g., regular antibiotics, wound care) in the home will prevent wound infection, avoid complications (e.g., activity restrictions prevent wound stress), and maintain a level of health (e.g., diet and progressive exercise allowed). Patients having ambulatory surgery also need to know the signs of complications and when to call their surgeon.

Patients who have inpatient surgery need to understand what is required to facilitate their recovery, including pain control, anticipated activity level, diet progression, wound care, and postoperative exercises (e.g., diaphragmatic breathing, incentive spirometry, coughing, turning, and leg exercises). Postoperative exercises help to prevent pulmonary and vascular complications (see Skill 50-1 on pp. 1297-1302). After you explain each exercise, demonstrate it for the patient and use Teach Back to confirm his or her understanding. Guide your patient through each exercise. Ask your patient to perform a return demonstration of the skill to reinforce it and increase the confidence in performing it.

Changes in the circulatory system, a patient's immobility during surgery, and a patient's underlying health condition create risks for development of DVT. Patients need to know which precautions are taken after surgery to avoid DVT (e.g., leg exercises and use of compression hose or intermittent pneumatic compression [IPC] devices). Teach about the purposes and the specific nursing care associated with the device (see Chapter 28).

Preoperative Routines. Explain the preoperative routines that a patient can expect. Knowing which tests and procedures are planned and why increase a patient's sense of control. Explain that an anesthesiologist will visit a patient to complete a preanesthesia assessment either during the preoperative admission process or in the presurgical care unit of a hospital.

A patient usually takes nothing by mouth for several hours before surgery to reduce risks for vomiting and aspirating emesis during surgery. Instruct a patient to eat and drink sufficient amounts during the week before surgery to ensure an adequate fluid and nutrient intake. Recommend foods high in protein with sufficient amounts of carbohydrates, fat, and vitamins in the diet. Explain to a patient and family the importance of following oral intake instructions for food and liquids before surgery.

Surgical Procedure. After the surgeon explains the basic purpose of a surgical procedure and its steps, some patients ask you additional questions. First clarify with the patient what was discussed with the surgeon. Avoid using technical medical terms because this adds to a patient's confusion. Avoid saying anything that contradicts the surgeon's explanation. If a patient has little or no understanding about the surgery, notify the surgeon that the patient requires further explanation. You can augment the surgeon's explanations.

Time of Surgery. The scheduled operative time is only an anticipated time. Unanticipated delays occur for many reasons that often have nothing to do with the patient. Emphasize that the scheduled time is a rough estimate and the actual time can be sooner or later. Make the family aware that delays occur for various reasons and do not necessarily indicate a problem. Communicate excessive delays when they do occur.

Postoperative Unit and Location of Family During Surgery and Recovery. Few patients are admitted to a hospital unit before surgery unless their case is emergent or a complication develops during hospitalization. When surgery is elective, patients and families will come to the surgical center admission area first. During the admission process, the patient and family will find out which unit the patient most likely will be admitted to after surgery. Be sure to explain where the family can wait and where the surgeon will come to find family members after surgery. In many institutions the circulating nurse gives periodic reports to the family in the waiting room for surgeries that are expected to be prolonged. If a patient will be taken to a special unit, it helps to orient the patient and family members to the environment of the unit before surgery.

Anticipated Postoperative Monitoring and Therapies. A patient and family need to know about routine postoperative monitoring and therapies (e.g., frequency of vital signs, IV therapy, dressings and drains, planned activity, and physical therapy). If they understand the frequency of anticipated monitoring and procedures, they are less apprehensive when nurses perform care activities. Try not to overprepare or underprepare a patient. It is easier to prepare a patient appropriately in elective cases when a surgeon has care guidelines for a specific procedure and you have adequate time for patient education. You cannot predict all of a patient's care requirements. Contradictions between your explanations and reality cause anxiety.

Sensory Preparation. Provide patients with information about the sensations typically experienced after surgery. Preparatory information helps them anticipate the steps of a procedure and thus form realistic images of the surgical experience. For example, warn that the OR is very bright and cold. Patients often undergo prewarming or are given warm blankets. A patient will have a cuff for a noninvasive blood pressure monitor placed around his or her arm. The monitor makes a hum and a beep, and the cuff tightens to take a reading. Informing a patient about these and other sensations in the OR reduces anxiety before the patient is anesthetized, which helps reduce the amount of anesthetic needed for induction. Postoperative sensations to describe include blurred vision from ophthalmic ointment in the eyes, expected pain at the surgical site and in areas of the body affected by prolonged positioning, the tightness of dressings, dryness of the mouth, and the sensation of a sore throat resulting from an endotracheal tube.

Postoperative Activity Resumption. The type of surgery determines how quickly patients can resume normal physical activity and regular eating habits. Explain what to expect after surgery. It is normal in most surgical cases for patients to progress gradually in activity and eating.

Pain-Relief Measures. Pain following surgery is one of a patient's most common fears. The family is also concerned for the patient's comfort. Pain after surgery is expected. Inform the patient and family of the need to manage pain so patients can resume activity and the type of therapies likely to be used for pain relief (e.g., splinting, and relaxation exercises). Patient-controlled analgesia (PCA) is common and provides patients with control over pain. Explain and demonstrate to a patient how to operate a pump and the importance of administering medication as soon as pain becomes persistent (see Chapter 44). Patients who receive epidural analgesia need a thorough understanding of how it will affect their movement and sensation after surgery.

Some patients avoid taking pain-relief drugs after surgery for fear of the negative side effects or becoming dependent on the drugs. Encourage a patient to use analgesics as ordered. Unless pain is controlled, it is difficult for a patient to participate in postoperative therapy. Encourage the patient to take pain medications at the ordered intervals. Pain relief has been shown to be more effective when analgesics are given around the clock (ATC) rather than as needed (prn) (Paice et al., 2005), especially if pain is expected throughout the day. However, prn administration of analgesics after surgery is still very common. When pain is not addressed regularly, it often becomes excruciating, and the analgesic does not provide relief at the dose ordered. Explain to a patient the length of time it takes for a drug to begin working. Information from preoperative pain assessment is helpful when teaching about pain-relief measures (such as positioning and splinting). Remember that pain is a subjective experience of a patient, and you must accept his or her perception of pain.

Rest. Rest is essential for normal healing. Anxiety about surgery interferes with the ability to relax and sleep. Meet each patient's individual needs.. If a patient is in the hospital, make the environment quiet and comfortable. The surgeon often orders a sedative-hypnotic or antianxiety agent for the night before surgery. Sedative-hypnotics promote sleep. Antianxiety agents (e.g., alprazolam [Xanax]) act on the cerebral cortex and limbic system to relieve anxiety. The advantage of ambulatory surgery is that a patient is able to sleep at home the night before surgery.

Feelings Regarding Surgery. Some patients feel like part of an assembly line before surgery. Frequent visits by staff, diagnostic testing, and physical preparation for surgery consume time; and the patient has few opportunities to reflect on the experience. Recognize the patient as a unique individual. The patient and family need time to express feelings about surgery and ask questions. The patient's level of anxiety influences the frequency of discussions. While delivering preoperative instruction, encourage expression of concerns, be patient, and listen attentively. The family may wish to discuss concerns without the patient present so their fears do not frighten the patient and vice versa. Establishing a trusting and therapeutic relationship with the patient and family allows this process to happen.

Acute Care. Acute care activities in the preoperative phase focus on the preparation of a patient on the morning of surgery or before an emergent surgery.

Minimizing Risk for Surgical Wound Infection. A surgical site infection (SSI) is one of the National Quality Forum (NQF)–endorsed patient safety measures that hospitals are encouraged to report (NQF, 2010). As of 2008 the CMS (2010) no longer pays a higher reimbursement for hospitalizations complicated by certain types of surgical site infections (e.g., mediastinitis after heart surgery, select orthopedic procedures, and certain bariatric procedures for obesity) if they were not present on admission. Thus there is great emphasis within hospitals on preventing the occurrence of SSIs. Antibiotics are sometimes ordered in the preoperative period. A reduction in wound infection rates occurs when an antibiotic is administered 60 minutes before the surgical incision is made and the antibiotics are stopped within 24 hours after surgery (CDC, 2012a). The surgeon orders a specific time before surgery for the patient to have an oral or IV antibiotic.

Preoperative care involves skin antisepsis (i.e., removing soil and transient microorganisms at the surgical site) to reduce the risk of a patient developing an SSI (Dumville et al., 2013). Routine components of skin antisepsis include preoperative bathing (showers or baths) and hair management, both of which reduce the number of microorganisms on the skin. Research has not confirmed that preoperative bathing reduces SSI (AORN, 2015), but the benefits outweigh harm. Most patients bathe the evening before surgery or that morning. There is no one antiseptic agent found to be most effective, although 2%

chlorhexidine gluconate is becoming a preferred solution (AORN, 2015). Whatever product is recommended, it is very important for patients to follow package directions. Patients who have head and neck surgery typically shampoo the hair before surgery to reduce resident flora on the scalp.

The AORN (2015) recommends that you remove hair at the surgical site only in select clinical situations. The current evidence supports leaving hair at the surgical site in place unless it interferes with exposure, closure, or dressing of the surgical site. When hair removal is required, clipping it is likely to result in less SSI than removal with a razor (AORN, 2015). Use single-use clipper heads for each patient and remove hair as close to the time of surgery as possible.

Maintaining Normal Fluid and Electrolyte Balance. A patient having surgery is vulnerable to fluid and electrolyte imbalance as a result of the stress of surgery, inadequate preoperative intake, and the potential for excessive fluid losses during surgery (see Chapter 42). The American Society of Anesthesiologists (ASA) recommendations for fluid and food intake before nonemergent procedures requiring general and regional anesthesia or sedation/analgesia, including fasting from intake of clear liquids for 2 or more hours, breast milk for 4 hours, formula and nonhuman milk for 6 hours, and a light meal of toast and clear liquids for 6 hours. A patient also cannot have any meat or fried foods 8 hours before surgery, unless explicitly specified by the anesthesiologist or surgeon (ASA, 2011). When a patient is hospitalized before surgery, remove all fluids and solid foods as ordered from the bedside and post a sign over the bed to alert personnel to fasting restrictions.

Despite the ASA standards, many surgeons still have patients maintain nothing by mouth after midnight. Ensure that you follow the health care provider's orders. During general anesthesia the muscles relax, and gastric contents can reflux into the esophagus. The anesthetic alters the patient's gag reflex. Therefore a patient is at risk for aspiration of food or fluids from the stomach into the lungs. The surgeon's orders will provide additional guidance for routines (e.g., IV line placement and preoperative medications). Some patients are allowed to take specific medications (e.g., anticoagulants, cardiovascular medications, anticonvulsants, and antibiotics) with a sip of water as ordered by their health care providers. Allow patients time to rinse their mouths with water or mouthwash and brush their teeth immediately before surgery as long as they do not swallow water. Notify the surgeon and anesthesia provider if a patient eats or drinks during the fasting period.

If a patient cannot eat because of GI alterations or impairments in consciousness, you will probably start an IV route for fluid replacement. The health care provider assesses serum electrolyte levels to determine the type of IV fluids and electrolyte additives to administer before and during surgery. Patients with severe nutritional imbalances sometimes require supplements with concentrated protein and glucose such as total parenteral nutrition (see Chapter 45).

Preventing Bowel Incontinence and Contamination. Some patients receive a bowel preparation (e.g., a cathartic or enema) if the surgery involves the lower GI system. Manipulation of parts of the GI tract during surgery results in absence of peristalsis for 24 hours and sometimes longer. Enemas and cathartics (see Chapter 47) such as a polyethylene glycol electrolyte solution (e.g., GoLytely®, NuLytely®) clean the GI tract to prevent intraoperative incontinence. An empty bowel reduces risk of injury to the intestines and minimizes contamination of the operative wound if colon surgery is planned or a part of the bowel is incised or opened accidentally. In addition, bowel cleansing reduces postoperative constipation. If a surgeon's order reads "give enemas until clear," this means that you administer enemas until the enema return solution contains no solid fecal material (see Chapter 47). Too many enemas given over a short time can cause serious fluid and electrolyte imbalances (see Chapter 42). Most agencies limit the number of enemas (usually three) that a nurse may administer successively. Verify a patient's potassium level following bowel preparation. Diarrhea may cause hypokalemia.

Preparation on the Day of Surgery. Complete several routine procedures before releasing patients for surgery.

Hygiene. Basic hygiene measures provide additional comfort before surgery. If a patient is unwilling to take a complete bath, a partial bath is refreshing and removes irritating secretions or drainage from the skin. A patient cannot wear personal nightwear to the OR because it is restrictive and is a flammable hazard. Thus you provide a clean hospital gown. When a patient is NPO for the last several hours, his or her mouth is often very dry. Offer the patient mouthwash and toothpaste, again cautioning the patient not to swallow water.

Preparation of Hair and Removal of Cosmetics. During major surgery an anesthesiologist positions a patient's head to place an endotracheal tube into the airway (see Chapter 41). This involves manipulation of the hair and scalp. To avoid injury ask the patient to remove hairpins or clips before leaving for surgery. Electrocautery is frequently used during surgery. Hairpins and clips can become an exit source for the electricity and cause burns. Remove hairpieces or wigs as well. Patients can braid long hair and wear disposable hats to contain hair before entering the OR.

During and after surgery the anesthesia provider and nurse assess skin and mucous membranes to determine a patient's level of oxygenation, circulation, and fluid balance. A pulse oximeter is often applied to a finger to monitor oxygen saturation (see Chapter 31). Anesthesia providers also use end-tidal carbon dioxide, by way of capnography, to assess patients' physical status. When using a pulse oximeter, have patients remove all makeup (lipstick, powder, blush, nail polish) and at least one artificial fingernail to expose normal skin and nail color. Anything in or around the eye irritates or injures the eye during surgery. Have patients remove contact lenses, false eyelashes, and eye makeup. Give the patient's eyeglasses to the family immediately before the patient leaves for the OR. Document all valuables per agency policy.

Removal of Prostheses. It is easy for any type of prosthetic device to become lost or damaged during surgery. Have patients remove all removable prosthetics (e.g., artificial limbs, partial or complete dentures, artificial eyes, and hearing aids) for safekeeping just before leaving for surgery. If a patient has a brace or splint, check with the health care provider to determine whether it should remain in place. For many patients it is embarrassing to remove dentures, wigs, or other devices that enhance personal appearance. Always offer privacy as a patient removes personal items. Patients are sometimes allowed to keep these until they reach the preoperative holding area. Place dentures in special containers labeled with the patient's name and other identification required by the agency for safekeeping to prevent loss or breakage. In many agencies you complete an inventory of all prosthetic devices or personal items and place them in a secured area. It is also common practice for nurses to give prostheses to family members or to keep the devices at the patient's bedside. Document these actions in the nursing notes, surgical checklist, or per agency policy.

Safeguarding Valuables. If a patient has valuables, give them to family members or place in a secure designated location. Many hospitals require patients to sign a release to free the facility of responsibility for lost valuables. Prepare a list with a description of items, place a copy with a patient's medical record (see agency policy), and give a copy to a designated family member. Patients are often reluctant to remove wedding rings or religious medals. A wedding band can be taped in place, but this is not the preferred practice. If there is a risk that the patient will experience swelling of the hand or fingers (mastectomy, hand surgery, fluid shifts), remove the band. Many hospitals allow patients to pin religious medals to their gowns, although the risk of loss increases. Remove other metal items such as piercings to reduce risk of burns.

Preparing the Bowel and Bladder. Some patients receive an enema or cathartic the morning of surgery (see Chapter 47). If so, give at least 1 hour before a patient leaves for surgery, allowing time for him or her to defecate without rushing. Instruct a patient to void just before leaving for the OR and before giving preoperative medications. An empty bladder reduces discomfort and the risk of incontinence during surgery and makes abdominal organs more accessible to the surgeon. If a patient is unable to void, record this information on the preoperative checklist. The surgeon may order insertion of an indwelling catheter if the surgery is to be long or the incision is in the lower abdomen (see Chapter 46).

Vital Signs. Monitor preoperative vital signs before surgery. The anesthesia provider uses these values as a baseline for intraoperative vital signs. If preoperative vital signs are abnormal, surgery is sometimes postponed. Notify the surgeon of any abnormalities before sending a patient to surgery. In addition, assess the patient for presence and character of pain (see Chapter 44). Many patients have pain before surgery caused by the condition requiring surgery.

Prevention of Deep Vein Thrombosis—Antiembolism Devices. Preventing DVTs is a priority quality measure. The AORN (2015) recommends that each health care organization implement a DVT prevention protocol. A patient's condition and type of surgery determine the preventive measures you take before surgery. For example, patients who have cardiac, GI, genitourinary (GU), gynecological (GYN), neurological, and orthopedic surgeries will likely have mechanical VTE prophylaxis applied the morning of surgery. This includes application of one of the following devices: antiembolism stockings (thigh or knee length), foot-impulse devices, or IPC devices (thigh or knee length) (NICE, 2010). In addition, some patients receive pharmacological VTE prophylaxis, which includes medications such as low-molecular-weight heparin (LMWH) (NICE, 2010). The health care provider needs to screen patients carefully for the risk of bleeding before ordering pharmacological VTE prophylaxis.

When correctly sized and applied, antiembolism devices reduce the risk for DVT. Antiembolic stockings maintain compression of small veins and capillaries of the legs. The constant compression forces blood into larger vessels, thus promoting venous return and preventing venous stasis. You attach **intermittent pneumatic compression (IPC) stockings** to an air pump that inflates and deflates the stockings, allowing intermittent pressure sequentially from the ankle to the knee and alternating calves, mimicking normal venous return when walking. Foot-inflation devices simulate natural walking by compressing the plantar venous plexus (AORN, 2015). See Chapter 28 for the correct procedure for applying antiembolism devices. Do not use antiembolism devices when patients have an allergy to the material (e.g., latex) or an unusual leg size or shape or a history of peripheral arterial disease, peripheral arterial bypass grafting, or peripheral neuropathy (NICE, 2010).

Administering Preoperative Medications. The increase in ambulatory surgeries has reduced the use of preoperative medications. However, the anesthesia provider or surgeon may order preanesthetic drugs ("on-call medications," "preops") to reduce patient anxiety; the amount of general anesthesia required; respiratory tract secretions; and the risk of nausea, vomiting, and possible aspiration. Typically you administer preoperative medications before a patient leaves for the OR. Complete all nursing care measures first. Preoperative drugs such as benzodiazepines, opioids, antiemetics, and anticholinergics usually cause dry mouth, drowsiness, and dizziness but do not induce sleep. To maintain patient safety, keep side rails in the up position, the bed in the low position, and the call light within easy reach. Instruct the patient to stay in bed until the surgical nursing assistant or transporter arrives to take him or her to the OR. If the patient needs to get out of bed to void, explain the importance of using the call light to ask for assistance. A patient can easily fall, thinking nothing is wrong. Be sure that the patient has signed surgical consent before administering drugs that will alter consciousness.

Documentation and Hand-Off. Before the patient goes to the OR, an accurate medical record is essential to ensure safe and appropriate patient care. Check the contents of the medical record for presence of ordered laboratory and imaging test results, accuracy and completeness of consent forms, and the preoperative checklist that agencies use as a tool to document all preoperative preparation activities. Check your nurses' notes to be sure your documentation is current. Also have a current medication administration record prepared for the OR. Once a patient is ready to go to the OR, a written (or electronic) record is inadequate to communicate information to the receiving health care team. The transfer of information about the patient from one health care provider to another requires an effective hand-off (Rothrock, 2015). Box 50-5 lists critical elements for hand-offs from preoperative to intraoperative providers. The AORN (2015) and TJC (2015) recommend hand-off reports occur in person to ensure that the right patient receives the right surgery at the right surgical site.

Eliminating Wrong Site and Wrong Procedure Surgery. Because of errors made in the past with patients undergoing the wrong surgery or having surgery performed on the wrong site, TJC instituted Universal Protocol guidelines for preventing such mishaps. The

BOX 50-5 Example of Elements of a Preoperative-to-Intraoperative Hand-Off Using SBAR Communication

Situation

- Name of patient, date of birth
- Name of operative procedure to be performed, including site and modifiers
- Pertinent documents present and consistent

Background

- Elements of patient history pertinent to surgery
- Medical clearance
- Patient allergies and NPO status
- Patient's vital signs and pain level
- Medication profile and medications taken today; laboratory results; imaging results
- Code status of patient

Assessment

- Patient's current level of understanding of the surgery
- Special patient needs or precautions
- Pertinent cultural or emotional factors
- Anesthesia requests

Recommendations

- State whether patient has been seen before surgery by a surgeon and anesthesia care provider.
- Determine if patient is ready for surgery.
- Allow chance for all staff members to ask questions and voice concerns.

Adapted from Amato-Vealey EJ et al: Hand-off communication: a requisite for patient safety, *AORN J* 88(5):766, 2008.

Universal Protocol is part of TJC ongoing National Patient Safety Goals (TJC, 2016). The preoperative-to-intraoperative hand-off described previously is an example of part of the protocol. Implement the Universal Protocol whenever an invasive surgical procedure is to be performed no matter the location (e.g., hospital, ASC, or health care provider office). The three principles of the protocol are: (1) a preoperative verification that ensures all relevant documents (e.g., consent forms, allergies, medical history, physical assessment findings) and results of laboratory tests and diagnostic studies are available before the start of the procedure and that the type of surgery scheduled is consistent with the patient's expectations; (2) marking the operative site with indelible ink to mark left and right distinction, multiple structures (e.g., fingers), and levels of the spine; and (3) a "time-out" just before starting the procedure for final verification of the correct patient, procedure, site, and any implants (TJC, 2016). The marking and "time-out" most commonly occur in the holding area, just before the patient enters the OR. The individual performing surgery and who is accountable for it must personally mark the site and involves the patient if possible (Rothrock, 2015). All members of the surgical/procedure team perform the time-out. This protocol includes the patient or a legally designated representative in the entire process. If the patient refuses a mark, document this on the procedure checklist.

QSEN BUILDING COMPETENCY IN SAFETY You are the nurse in the preoperative holding area and are preparing a patient for the operating room. You completed all preliminary procedures (i.e., storing valuables, checking the preoperative checklist, and assisting the patient to the bathroom). You are preparing to perform the Universal Protocol with patient verification. When is the right time to administer the preoperative sedative?

Answers to QSEN Activities can be found on the Evolve website.

◆ Evaluation

The nurse caring for a patient in the preoperative area evaluates initial patient outcomes (Figure 50-4). Although limited time is available to evaluate outcomes before surgery, compare the patient's current status with expected outcomes to determine whether new or revised interventions and/or nursing diagnoses need to be implemented intraoperatively.

Through the Patient's Eyes. Evaluate whether the patient's expectations were met with respect to surgical preparation. For example, ask patients if they require additional information, if they desire to have their family members more involved, and if they have any unidentified needs. During evaluation include a discussion of any misunderstandings so patient concerns can be clarified. When patients have expectations about pain control, this is a good time to reinforce how it will be managed after surgery.

Patient Outcomes. Evaluate a patient's response to interventions designed for preoperative nursing diagnoses such as *Deficient Knowledge* or *Anxiety*. For example, ask the patient to describe the reason for postoperative exercises and the type of care activities to expect when he or she returns from surgery. Observe the patient's behaviors and discuss concerns to see if anxiety remains. Be thorough in your evaluation to determine if further instruction or emotional support is needed after surgery. Interventions continue during and after surgery; thus the evaluation of many goals and outcomes does not occur until after surgery.

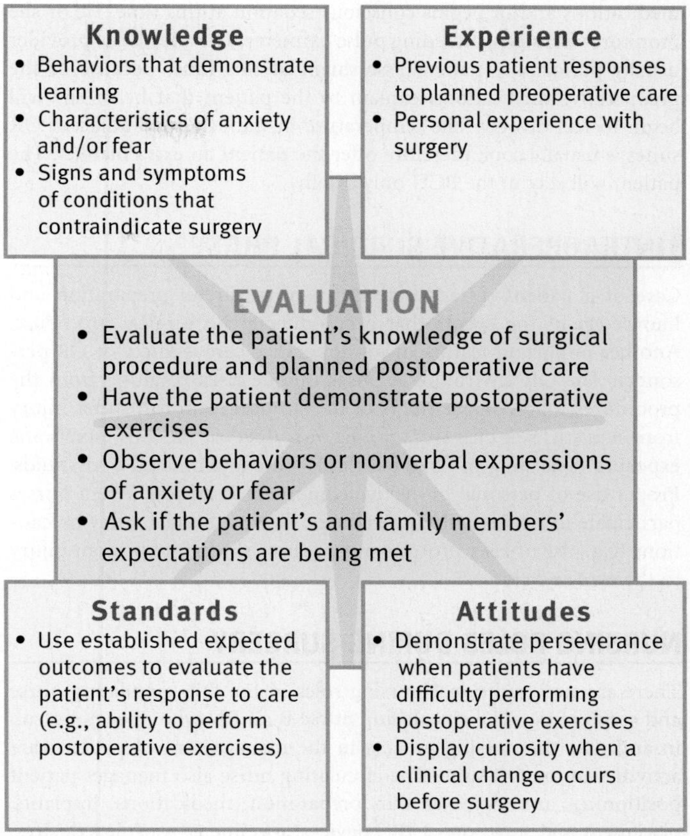

Knowledge
- Behaviors that demonstrate learning
- Characteristics of anxiety and/or fear
- Signs and symptoms of conditions that contraindicate surgery

Experience
- Previous patient responses to planned preoperative care
- Personal experience with surgery

EVALUATION
- Evaluate the patient's knowledge of surgical procedure and planned postoperative care
- Have the patient demonstrate postoperative exercises
- Observe behaviors or nonverbal expressions of anxiety or fear
- Ask if the patient's and family members' expectations are being met

Standards
- Use established expected outcomes to evaluate the patient's response to care (e.g., ability to perform postoperative exercises)

Attitudes
- Demonstrate perseverance when patients have difficulty performing postoperative exercises
- Display curiosity when a clinical change occurs before surgery

FIGURE 50-4 Critical thinking model for surgical patient evaluation.

TRANSPORT TO THE OPERATING ROOM

Personnel in the OR notify the nursing unit or ambulatory surgery area when it is time for surgery. In many facilities a transporter brings a stretcher to transport the patient to surgery. The transporter checks the patient's identification bracelet for two identifiers (name, birthday, or hospital number) (refer to institutional or agency policy) against the patient's medical record to ensure that the correct person is going to surgery. Because some patients receive preoperative sedatives, the nurses, nursing assistive personnel, and transporter help the patient transfer from bed to stretcher to prevent falls. A patient in ambulatory surgery ambulates to the OR if able and not medicated. Provide the family an opportunity to visit before the patient is transported to the OR. Direct the family to the appropriate waiting area. If a patient has been hospitalized before surgery and will be returning to the same nursing unit, prepare the bed and room for his or her return.

Preanesthesia Care Unit

In most hospitals a patient enters a **preanesthesia care unit** (PCU) or presurgical care unit (PSCU) (sometimes called the *holding area*) outside the OR where preoperative preparations are completed. Nurses in the PCU are members of the OR staff and wear surgical scrub suits, hats, and footwear in accordance with infection control policies. In some ambulatory surgical settings a perioperative primary nurse admits the patient, circulates during the operative procedure, and manages the patient's recovery and discharge.

If an IV catheter is not present already, a nurse or anesthesia provider inserts one into a vein to establish a route for fluid replacement, IV drugs, or blood products. The nurse also administers preoperative medications and/or begins conscious sedation at this time. He or she monitors vital signs, including pulse oximetry. The anesthesia provider usually performs a patient assessment at this time. Because of the preoperative medications, explain to the patient that he or she will begin to feel drowsy. The temperature in the PCU and adjacent OR suites is usually cool; therefore offer the patient an extra blanket. The patient will stay in the PCU only briefly.

INTRAOPERATIVE SURGICAL PHASE

Care of a patient intraoperatively requires careful preparation and knowledge of the events that occur during the surgical procedure. Another important feature of intraoperative care is safety of OR personnel. The OR environment poses unique risks resulting from the procedures followed. Members of the surgical team can suffer injury from skin sticks or cuts (e.g., needle or scalpel) or mucous membrane exposure (splashing of irrigated fluids) to contaminated body fluids. Proper use of personal protective equipment is critical. When nurses participate in laser surgical procedures, they use special safety precautions (e.g., use of laser protective eyewear or shields) to prevent injury to the eyes and skin.

NURSING ROLES DURING SURGERY

There are two traditional nursing roles in the OR: circulating nurse and scrub nurse. The **circulating nurse** is an RN who does not scrub in and uses the nursing process in the management of patient care activities in the OR suite. The circulating nurse also manages patient positioning, antimicrobial skin preparation, medications, implants, placement and function of IPC devices, specimens, warming devices, and surgical counts of instruments and dressings (AORN, 2015; Rothrock, 2015). The **scrub nurse** is either an RN or surgical technologist who is often certified (CST). The scrub nurse must have a thorough knowledge of each step of a surgical procedure and the ability to anticipate each and every instrument and supply needed by the surgeons (Rothrock, 2015). A circulating nurse and scrub nurse partner together to ensure patient safety by minimizing risk of error. The team also works together to ensure cost-efficient use of supplies.

A new role in the OR includes the RN first assistant (RNFA). This is an expanded role that requires formal academic education (AORN, 2012). The RNFA collaborates with the surgeon by handling and cutting tissue, using instruments and medical devices, providing exposure of the surgical area and hemostasis, and suturing (Rothrock, 2015).

❖ NURSING PROCESS

Apply the nursing process and use a critical thinking approach in your care of patients. The nursing process provides a clinical decision making approach for you to develop and implement an individualized plan of care.

◆ Assessment

During the assessment process in the OR, the circulating nurse thoroughly assesses the patient and critically analyzes findings to make patient-centered clinical decisions required for safe nursing care. Assessment focuses on a patient's immediate clinical status, skin integrity (over surgical site and dependent areas where patient will lay on operating table bed), and joint function (when unusual positions on the OR table are required). This allows the nurse to anticipate problems that predispose the patient to injury if he or she is not positioned on the OR table correctly. Because patients are not able to speak for themselves while under general anesthesia, this assessment in the OR is very important for their safety. As the nurse, review the preoperative care plan to establish or revise the intraoperative care plan as indicated.

◆ Nursing Diagnosis

Review preoperative nursing diagnoses and modify them to individualize the care plan in the OR. The following are common nursing diagnoses relevant to the patient intraoperatively:

- *Ineffective Airway Clearance*
- *Risk for Deficient Fluid Volume*
- *Risk for Perioperative Positioning Injury*
- *Impaired Skin Integrity*
- *Risk for Thermal Injury*
- *Risk for Injury*

◆ Planning

Goals and Outcomes. Patient-centered goals and outcomes of preoperative nursing diagnoses extend into the intraoperative phase. For example, a goal for the nursing diagnosis of *Risk for Thermal Injury* is "Skin will remain free of burn injury through surgical procedure." An expected outcome for this goal is:

- Patient is free of burns from the grounding pad at end of surgery.

Setting Priorities. The circulating nurse uses judgment to provide a safe operative experience for the patient. Ensuring an aseptic environment, conducting instrument and sponge counts according to policy, managing tissue and specimens correctly, and ensuring proper use of equipment and instruments are top priorities. If an unsafe practice occurs (e.g., break in sterility, missing sponge in wound), the circulating nurse is integral in ensuring the safety of the patient and operative personnel.

Teamwork and Collaboration. For optimal patient safety the preoperative health care team communicates assessment findings and patient problems via a formal hand-off with the surgical team to ensure a smooth transition in care (see Box 50-5). For example, alerting the operative team of a latex allergy or risk factors for complications during surgery (smoker) requires collaboration and timely communication among all team members.

◆ Implementation

A primary focus of intraoperative care is to prevent injury and complications related to anesthesia, surgery, positioning, and equipment use. The perioperative nurse is an advocate for the patient during surgery and protects his or her dignity and rights at all times.

Acute Care

Physical Preparation. A patient is usually still awake and notices health care providers in their surgical attire and masks when entering the OR. You transfer a patient to the OR bed by being sure that the stretcher and bed are locked in place. Explain to the patient all the activities you are completing. After safely securing the patient on the OR table with safety straps, you apply monitoring devices such as continuous ECG electrodes, a pulse oximeter sensor, and blood pressure cuff. For ECG, place electrodes on the chest and extremities correctly to record electrical activity of the heart accurately. The anesthesia provider will use the cuff to monitor the patient's blood pressure. An electronic monitor in the OR will display the patient's heart rate, vital signs, and pulse oximetry continuously. Capnography is also used frequently to measure the patient's ongoing end-tidal carbon dioxide values. Apply an electrical cautery grounding pad to the skin so cauterizing instruments can be used safely. If not applied before surgery, now is the time to apply antiembolism devices. You help insert temperature probes via the bladder, esophagus, or rectum if required to continuously measure a patient's body temperature.

Intraoperative Warming. The unplanned occurrence of perioperative hypothermia is now minimized with the use of active intraoperative warming. Prevention of hypothermia (core temperature less than 36° C [96.8° F]) helps to reduce complications such as shivering, cardiac arrest, blood loss, SSI, pressure ulcers, and mortality (Hart et al., 2011; Seamon et al., 2012). Evidence suggests that prewarming for a minimum of 30 minutes may reduce occurrence of hypothermia (Hart et al., 2011; Stuart et al., 2011). The nurse in the OR applies warm cotton blankets, forced-air warmers, or circulating-water mattresses to patients. Forced-air warmers tend to be the most effective when used before surgery or intraoperatively (Hart et al., 2011).

Latex Sensitivity/Allergy. As the incidence and prevalence of latex sensitivity and allergy increase, the need for recognition of potential sources of latex is extremely critical. All medical supplies contain a label notifying the consumer of the latex content. The OR and PCU have many products that contain latex (e.g., gloves, IV tubing, syringes, and rubber stoppers on bottles and vials). It is also present in common objects such as adhesive tape, disposable electrodes, endotracheal tube cuffs, protective sheets, and ventilator equipment. Signs and symptoms of a latex reaction include local effects ranging from urticaria and flat or raised red patches to vesicular, scaling, or bleeding eruptions. Acute dermatitis is sometimes present. Rhinitis and/or rhinorrhea are other common reactions to mild and severe latex allergy. Immediate hypersensitivity reactions are life threatening, with the patient exhibiting focal or generalized urticaria and edema, bronchospasm, and mucus hypersecretion, all of which can compromise respiratory status. Vasodilation compounded by increased capillary permeability sometimes lead to circulatory collapse and eventual death. The draping of a patient during surgery blocks your ability to visualize the skin. Thus be prepared to investigate any unexplained acute deterioration in a previously healthy patient for possible latex allergy.

A latex-free cart needs to be available at all times in the OR to create a latex-safe environment. All of the contents must be latex free. The American Association of Nurse Anesthetists (AANA, 2015) recommends that, when facilities are not latex safe, you need to take steps to prepare an OR the night before to avoid the release of latex particles. Any patient with a latex allergy needs to receive scheduling priority and be the first case in the morning. It is important to know that patients may develop anaphylaxis 30 to 60 minutes after being exposed to latex. Box 50-6 lists latex precautions.

Introduction of Anesthesia. The nature and extent of a patient's surgery and current physical status influence the type of anesthesia administered during surgery. Know the complications to anticipate after surgery for each type (Table 50-7).

General Anesthesia. Under general anesthesia a patient loses all sensation, consciousness, and reflexes, including gag and blink reflexes. The patient's muscles relax, and the patient experiences amnesia. Amnesia is a protective measure from the unpleasant events of the procedure. An anesthesia provider gives general anesthetics by IV infusion and inhalation routes through the three phases of anesthesia: induction, maintenance, and emergence. Surgery requiring general anesthesia involves major procedures with extensive tissue manipulation. During emergence anesthetics are decreased, and the patient begins to awaken. Because of the short half-life of today's medications, emergence often occurs in the OR. The duration of anesthesia depends on the length of surgery.

Regional Anesthesia. Regional anesthesia results in loss of sensation in an area of the body by anesthetizing sensory pathways. This

BOX 50-6 Latex Avoidance Precautions

1. Health care workers can transmit the allergen by hand to patients after touching any object with latex. *Caution:* Keep the powder from the gloves away from patients because the powder acts as a carrier for the latex protein. Do not snap gloves on and off.
2. Identify patients who are latex sensitive. The operating room (OR) needs to be labeled latex free to prevent personnel from bringing rubber products (e.g., wristbands, chart labels) into the room.
3. Develop programs to educate health care workers in the care of latex-sensitive patients.

Recommendations for Patient Care (Patients with Latex Allergy or Latex Risk)

The Operating Room

- Notify the OR of patients who have potential latex allergies. Remove all latex products from the OR and bring a latex-free cart (if available) into the room.
- Use a latex-free reservoir bag, airways and endotracheal tubes, and laryngeal mask airways.
- Use a nonlatex anesthesia breathing circuit with plastic mask and bag.
- Place all monitoring devices and cords/tubes (oximeter, blood pressure, electrocardiograph wires) in stockinette and secure with tape to prevent direct skin contact. Rinse items sterilized in ethylene oxide before use. Residual ethylene oxide reacts and can cause an allergic response in a patient with a latex allergy.

Intravenous Line Preparation

- Use intravenous (IV) tubing without latex ports; use stopcocks if available.
- If unable to obtain IV tubing without latex ports, cover latex ports with tape.
- Cover all rubber injection ports on IV bags with tape and label as follows: *Do not inject or withdraw fluid through the latex port. Note: Pulmonary artery catheters (especially the balloon), central venous catheters, and arterial lines may contain latex components.*

Operating Room Patient Care

- Use nonlatex gloves. (*Caution:* Not all substitutes are equally impermeable to bloodborne pathogens; ensure that you select substitute gloves that provide appropriate protection.)
- Use nonlatex tourniquets or nonlatex examination gloves or polyvinyl chloride tubing.
- Draw medication directly from opened multidose vials (remove stoppers) if medications are not available in ampules.
- The rubber allergen can possibly move from the plunger of a syringe into the medication, which sometimes causes an allergic reaction. The intensity of this reaction increases over time. Therefore you draw up medications immediately before the beginning of the surgery or just before administration.
- Use latex-free or glass syringes.
- Use stopcocks to inject drugs rather than latex ports.
- Notify pharmacy and central supply that your patient is latex sensitive so these departments can use appropriate procedures when preparing medications and instruments. Also notify radiology, respiratory therapy, housekeeping, food service, and postoperative care units so they will take appropriate precautions to protect the patient.
- Place clear and readily visible signs on the doors of the OR to inform all who enter that the patient has a latex allergy.

Modified from *Perioperative Standards and Recommended Practices: AORN latex guideline*, Denver, 2011, AORN.

TABLE 50-7 Examples of Complications of Anesthesia

Type	Complications
General	Aspiration of vomitus, cardiac irregularities, decreased cardiac output, hypotension, hypothermia, hypoxemia, laryngospasm, malignant hyperthermia, nephrotoxicity, and respiratory depression
Regional: epidural, spinal and caudal blocks	Hypotension, hypothermia, injury to spinal cord, respiratory paralysis, spinal headache
Local	Hives, rash, anaphylaxis
Conscious sedation	Aspiration, decreased level of consciousness, hypoxemia, respiratory depression

type of anesthesia is accomplished by injecting a local anesthetic along the pathway of a nerve from the spinal cord. A patient requires careful monitoring during and immediately after regional anesthesia for return of sensation and movement distal to the point of anesthetic injection. As the nurse, you protect a patient's limbs from injury until sensation returns. Serious complications such as respiratory paralysis occur if the level of anesthesia rises, moving upward in the spinal cord. Elevation of the upper body helps prevents respiratory paralysis. Some patients have a sudden fall in blood pressure, which results from extensive vasodilation caused by the anesthetic block to sympathetic vasomotor nerves and pain, and motor nerve fibers. Remember that burns and other trauma can occur on the anesthetized part of the body without the patient being aware of the injury. It is necessary to observe the position of extremities and the condition of the skin frequently.

Local Anesthesia. Local anesthesia involves loss of sensation at the desired site (e.g., a skin growth or the cornea of the eye) by inhibiting peripheral nerve conduction. It is commonly used in ambulatory surgery. A local can also be used in addition to general or regional anesthesia. The anesthetic agent (e.g., lidocaine [Xylocaine]) inhibits nerve conduction until the drug diffuses into the circulation. It is injected locally or applied topically. The patient experiences a loss in pain and touch sensation and motor and autonomic activities (e.g., bladder emptying). It is necessary to monitor patients continually during a local procedure. The frequency of observation and monitoring of patients are tailored to the patient, procedure, and the medications used (Rothrock, 2015).

Moderate (Conscious) Sedation. IV moderate sedation (i.e., conscious sedation) is used routinely for short-term surgical, diagnostic, and therapeutic procedures that do not require complete anesthesia but rather a depressed level of consciousness. A patient maintains spontaneous ventilation and a patent airway and requires no interventions during conscious sedation (Rothrock, 2015). In addition, the patient responds appropriately to physical (light touch) and verbal stimuli. The preferred sedative for conscious sedation is short-acting IV sedatives such as midazolam (Versed).

Advantages of conscious sedation include adequate sedation, reduction of fear and anxiety, amnesia, relief of pain and noxious stimuli, mood alteration, elevation of pain threshold, enhanced patient cooperation, stable vital signs, and rapid recovery. Nurses assisting with the administration of conscious sedation need to demonstrate competency in the care of these patients. Knowledge of anatomy, physiology, cardiac dysrhythmias, procedural complications, and pharmacological principles related to the administration of individual agents is essential. You also need to assess, diagnose, and intervene in the event of unexpected reactions, such as an adverse reaction to a medication, and demonstrate skill in airway management and oxygen delivery. Resuscitation equipment must be readily available when using conscious sedation The AORN (2014) publishes recommendations for managing patients undergoing conscious sedation.

Positioning the Patient for Surgery. Prevention of positioning injuries requires anticipation of the position and surgical approach to be used during a surgical procedure, the positioning equipment to be used, and whether a patient has conditions causing risk for injury (AORN, 2015). During general anesthesia the nursing personnel and surgeon often wait to position a patient until the full stage of relaxation so an injury is less likely to be caused by moving and lifting the patient's body parts. Ideally a patient's position provides clear access to the operative site; sustains adequate circulatory and respiratory function; and ensures the patient's safety, comfort, and skin integrity. If a patient has conditions such as morbid obesity, malnourishment, existing pressure ulcers, or chronic disease, special considerations are needed in positioning. It is important for the circulating nurse to assess circulatory, respiratory, integumentary, musculoskeletal, and neurological structures during surgery (AORN, 2015).

An alert person maintains normal range of joint motion by pain and pressure receptors. If a joint is extended too far, pain stimuli provide a warning that muscle and joint strain is too great. In a patient who is anesthetized, normal defense mechanisms cannot guard against joint damage, muscle stretch, and strain. The muscles are so relaxed that it is relatively easy to place the patient in a position that the individual normally could not assume while awake. He or she often remains in a given position for several hours. Although it is sometimes necessary to place a patient in an unusual position, try to maintain correct alignment and protect skin from pressure, abrasion, and other injuries. Special mattresses, use of foam padding, and attachments to the OR table provide protection to extremities and bony prominences. Positioning should not impede normal movement of the diaphragm or interfere with circulation to body parts. If restraints are necessary, pad the skin to prevent trauma.

Documentation of Intraoperative Care. Throughout the surgical procedure, the circulating nurse keeps an accurate record of patient care activities and procedures performed by OR personnel (e.g., surgical count status, special equipment, IV and irrigation fluids, specimens, and medications). A standardized documentation format helps practitioners ensure continuity of information from the OR to the postanesthesia care unit (PACU) or recovery area (AORN, 2015). The AORN recommends the use of verbal and standardized forms to transfer patient information between care providers.

◆ Evaluation

The circulating nurse conducts an ongoing evaluation to ensure that interventions such as patient position are implemented correctly during the intraoperative phase of surgery.

Through the Patient's Eyes. While a patient is undergoing surgery, it is important to keep the family informed. Hospitals vary on their policies for when and how often families are given updates of the patient's condition. Families expect an estimate of when surgery begins and the length of time it will likely last. When you give an update to family members, ask if they have further questions or concerns and if their needs are being met.

Patient Outcomes. Evaluate a patient's ongoing clinical status during surgery. The anesthesia provider continuously monitors vital signs. The circulating nurse monitors and records intake and output (I&O), specimens obtained, medications and irrigations, type of dressing packing, and other treatments. Measure the patient's body temperature during and at completion of the surgery, with the goal of keeping the patient normothermic. Inspect the skin under the grounding pad and at areas where positioning exerts pressure.

POSTOPERATIVE SURGICAL PHASE

A patient's surgical recovery is divided into three phases: immediately after surgery, an intermediate time period in which a patient is hospitalized, and a convalescent phase, which occurs while a patient transitions from hospital discharge to full recovery. After surgery a patient's care is often complex as a result of physiological changes. The type of anesthesia, nature of surgery, and the patient's previous condition determine the phases of recovery and the length of time spent on an acute care nursing unit. Typically at the end of surgery the anesthesia provider and the circulating nurse accompany the patient to the PACU and provide a thorough hand-off report to the nursing staff.

For a patient following ambulatory surgery, the immediate recovery period normally lasts only 1 or 2 hours in phase II recovery, and convalescence occurs at home. However, phase I recovery may be necessary, depending on a patient's condition and anesthesia. For a patient in the hospital, the immediate postoperative recovery (phase I) period often lasts a few hours in the PACU, and phase II recovery occurs on a surgical unit. The patient typically remains on the surgical unit for 1 or more days to recover before going home.

IMMEDIATE POSTOPERATIVE RECOVERY (PHASE I)

When a PACU nurse receives a patient during hand-off, he or she obtains data from the surgical team to prepare for proper support of a patient's recovery status. This includes anticipating possible clinical problems on the basis of assessment and being sure that special equipment needed for nursing care is available. Careful planning allows the nursing staff to consider placement of patients in the PACU. For example, patients who undergo spinal anesthesia are aware of their surroundings and benefit from being in a quieter part of the PACU, away from patients needing frequent monitoring. You isolate patients with a serious infection such as tuberculosis from other patients. Use standard precautions for infection control (see Chapter 29) for all patients.

When a patient is admitted to phase I recovery, personnel notify the nurses on the acute care nursing unit of his or her arrival. This allows the nursing staff to inform family members. Family members usually remain in the designated waiting area so they can be found when the surgeon arrives to explain the patient's condition. *It is the surgeon's responsibility to describe the patient's status, the results of surgery, and any complications that occurred.* You are a valuable resource to the family if complications occurred in the operative phase and clarifying explanations are necessary.

When a patient enters the PACU, the nurse and members of the surgical team discuss his or her status. A standardized approach or tool for "hand-off" communications helps to provide accurate information about a patient's care, treatment and services, current condition, and any recent or anticipated changes (Rothrock, 2015). The hand-off is interactive, multidisciplinary, and done at the patient's bedside, allowing for a communication exchange that gives caregivers the chance to dialogue and ask questions. The surgical team's report includes topics such as the type of anesthesia provided, vital sign trends, intraoperative medications, IV fluids, estimated blood and urine loss, and pertinent information about the surgical wound (e.g., dressings, tubes, drains) (Rothrock, 2015). The information obtained from hand-off report allows a recovery nurse to anticipate how quickly a patient should regain consciousness, any likely complications, and what his or her analgesic needs will be. A report on IV fluids or blood products administered during surgery from the anesthesia provider or perfusionist alerts the nurse to the patient's fluid and electrolyte balance. The surgeon or anesthesia provider often reports special concerns (e.g., whether the patient is at risk for hemorrhaging or infection) and whether there were complications during surgery such as excessive blood loss or cardiac irregularities. The circulating nurse also reports intraoperative patient positioning and condition of the skin. Frequently this report takes place while PACU nurses are admitting the patient. The PACU nurse attaches the patient to monitoring equipment such as the noninvasive blood pressure monitor, ECG monitor, and pulse oximeter. Patients often receive some form of oxygen in this immediate recovery period.

BOX 50-7 Initial Postanesthesia Care Assessment: Parameters to Assess

Initial assessment in the PACU includes documentation of the following:

- Integration of data received at hand-off for transfer of care
- Vital signs
  - Respiratory status—airway patent, breath sounds, type of artificial airway, mechanical ventilator settings, oxygen saturation, and end-tidal CO_2 values
- Intake and output
- Pain/sedation/comfort assessment (including psychoemotional status), presence of nausea or vomiting
- Neurological function: level of consciousness (may use Glascow Coma scale), pupillary response (if indicated)
- Position of patient
- Condition and color of skin, status of any suspected pressure areas
- Patient safety needs
- Neurovascular status: peripheral pulses and sensation of extremity or extremities
- Condition of surgical dressings or suture line, drains, tubes, receptacles
- Amount, appearance, and type of drainage
- Muscular response and strength/mobility
- Fluid therapy—location of intravenous (IV) lines, patency of IV lines, amount and type of solution (crystalloids or blood products) infused, next fluid to be administered
- Procedure-specific assessments, such as expected drainage amount, specific positioning aids for orthopedic surgery

Adapted from Rothrock JC: *Alexander's care of the patient in surgery,* ed 15, St Louis, 2015, Mosby.

After receiving hand-off communication from the OR, the PACU nurse conducts a complete systems assessment during the first few minutes of PACU care (Rothrock, 2015) (Box 50-7). You perform assessments at least every 15 minutes or more frequently, depending on the patient's condition and unit policy. This assessment usually continues until discharge from the PACU. Perform assessments quickly and thoroughly and target them to a patient's unique needs and type of surgery.

Evaluate the patient's status and eventual readiness for discharge from the PACU on the basis of vital sign stability compared with the preoperative data. Other outcomes for discharge include body temperature control, good ventilation and oxygenation status, orientation to surroundings, absence of complications, minimal pain and nausea, controlled wound drainage, adequate urine output, and fluid and electrolyte balance. Patients with more extensive surgery requiring anesthesia of longer duration usually recover more slowly. It is common for hospitals and ambulatory care centers to use objective scoring systems to identify when patients are ready for discharge.

Standard tools include the modified Aldrete score (Aldrete, 1998) or the modified postanesthesia recovery score (PARS) and the DASAIM discharge assessment tool (Gärtner et al., 2010). Each tool has criteria assessed at select time intervals (e.g., 5, 15, 30, 45, and 60 minutes) and on discharge from the PACU (see agency policy). A patient must receive a predetermined score before discharge from the PACU. If the patient's condition is still poor after 2 or 3 hours or the stay lengthens, the surgeon may transfer him or her to an intensive care unit (ICU).

When the patient is discharged from the PACU, another hand-off communication occurs at the patient's bedside between the PACU nurse and the nurse on the acute nursing unit or in the ICU. The nurses verify the patient's identification using two identifiers. The hand-off includes review of vital signs, the type of surgery and anesthesia performed, blood loss, level of consciousness, general physical condition, medications administered during surgery and in PACU, and the presence of IV lines, drainage tubes, and dressings. The PACU nurse's report helps the receiving nurse anticipate special patient needs and obtain necessary equipment. It is important to have uninterrupted time to review the recent pertinent events and ask questions. It is also important at this time for patient's family members to be informed as soon as possible of the patient's transfer plan.

The PACU staff transport the patient on a stretcher to the nursing unit. Staff members from the unit help to safely transfer the patient to a bed (see Chapter 39). The PACU nurse shows the receiving nurse the recovery room record and reviews the patient's condition and course of care. The PACU nurse also reviews the surgeon's orders that require attention. *Before the PACU nurse leaves the acute care area, the staff nurse assuming care for the patient takes a complete set of vital signs to compare with PACU findings.* Minor vital sign variations normally occur after transporting the patient.

RECOVERY IN AMBULATORY SURGERY (PHASE II)

The thoroughness and extent of postoperative recovery after ambulatory surgery depends on a patient's condition, type of surgery, and anesthesia. In some cases a patient goes through both phase I (PACU) and phase II recovery. Assess and care for patients in need of close monitoring in the same fashion as inpatients in phase I. It is common to assess patients using an objective recovery score tool. After patients stabilize and no longer require close monitoring, transfer them to phase II recovery. With new anesthetic agents and minimally invasive surgical techniques, *fast-track surgery* is becoming more common, with patients experiencing a more rapid awakening in the OR, quicker recovery, and reduced morbidity (Kehlet and Wilmore, 2008). Many ambulatory surgery patients are able to bypass phase I.

Phase II recovery is performed in a room equipped with medical recliner chairs, side tables, and foot rests. Kitchen facilities for preparing light snacks and beverages are usually located in the area, along with bathrooms. The phase II environment promotes a patient's and family's comfort and well-being until discharge. Monitor patients but not at the same intensity as during phase I. In phase II recovery initiate postoperative teaching with patients and family members (Box 50-8).

Patients are discharged to home following ambulatory surgery after they meet certain criteria. When you are using a tool for assessing a patient's recovery score such as the PARS, the patient must achieve a certain score before being discharged. Patients with known OSA or at high risk for the condition are not discharged from the recovery area to home until they are no longer at risk for postoperative respiratory depression, which may require a longer stay (ASA, 2014). Postoperative nausea and vomiting (PONV) sometimes occurs once the patient is home, even if the symptoms were not present in the surgery center. Options for therapy include the prophylactic use of drugs such as ondansetron (Zofran) aprepitant, dolasetron and transcutaneous AccuPoint electrical stimulation, or a transdermal scopolamine patch (McCaffrey, 2007; Rothrock, 2015).

BOX 50-8 PATIENT TEACHING

Postoperative Instructions for an Ambulatory Surgical Patient

Objective

- Patient will describe signs and symptoms of postoperative problems to report to health care provider.

Teaching Strategies

- Give instruction sheet with contact information, including health care provider's telephone number, number of surgery center, and follow-up appointment date and time. Allow patient and family to ask questions.
- Explain to family member the signs and symptoms of infection.
- Explain name, dose, schedule, and purpose of medications and possible side effects. Provide printed drug information.
- Explain activity restrictions, diet progression, wound care guidelines, and the signs of any associated problems. Provide instruction sheet with clear, focused explanations.

Evaluation

- Have patient explain when and how to call health care provider with problems.
- Have patient recite date for follow-up appointment.
- Have patient and family member describe signs and symptoms of infection.
- Have patient verbalize name of drug, dose, when to take, and common side effects.
- Have patient demonstrate proper activity/movement and wound care.

Review written postoperative instructions and prescriptions with the patient and family before releasing the patient and ensure that they verbalize understanding of these instructions. Always discharge the patient to a responsible adult.

POSTOPERATIVE RECOVERY AND CONVALESCENCE

Inpatients remain in the PACU until their condition stabilizes; they then return to the postoperative nursing unit. Nursing care in both settings focuses on returning the patient to a relatively functional level of wellness as soon as possible. The speed of recovery depends on the type or extent of surgery, risk factors, pain management, and postoperative complications.

❖ NURSING PROCESS

Apply the nursing process and use a critical thinking approach in your care of patients. The nursing process provides a clinical decision making approach for you to develop and implement an individualized plan of care. Once a surgical patient is transferred to an acute care nursing unit, ongoing postoperative care is essential to support recovery.

◆ Assessment

During the assessment process, thoroughly assess each patient and critically analyze findings to ensure you make patient-centered clinical decisions required for safe nursing care. During a postoperative assessment, apply critical thinking while relying on information from the preoperative nursing assessment, knowledge regarding the surgical procedure performed, and events occurring during surgery. This analysis will help you focus your postoperative assessment. A variation from the patient's norm possibly indicates the onset of surgically related complications.

Before a patient arrives on the nursing unit, prepare the bed and room for his or her return if he or she is returning to the same nursing unit. You are better prepared to care for the patient after surgery if the room is readied before the patient's return. A postoperative bedside unit includes the following:

1. Sphygmomanometer and/or automated noninvasive blood pressure monitor, stethoscope, and thermometer
2. Emesis basin
3. Incentive spirometer
4. Clean gown, washcloth, towel, and facial tissues
5. IV pole and infusion pump (if needed)
6. Suction equipment (if needed)
7. Oxygen equipment and oximetry monitor (if needed)
8. Extra pillows for positioning the patient comfortably
9. Bed pads to protect bed linen from drainage
10. Bed raised to stretcher height with bed linens pulled back and furniture moved to accommodate the stretcher and equipment (such as IV lines)

When a patient arrives on the acute care unit, monitor vital signs according to institution policy. Generally you check vital signs every 15 minutes twice, every 30 minutes twice, hourly for 2 hours, and then every 4 hours or per orders. As the patient's condition stabilizes, you usually assess the patient at least once a shift until discharge. Always base the frequency of assessment on a patient's current condition. *Do not assume that further monitoring is unnecessary if the patient appears normal during the initial assessment.* A patient's condition can change rapidly, especially during the postoperative period.

Thoroughly document the initial nursing assessment, including vital signs, level of consciousness, airway status, condition of dressings and drains, pulses distal to site of surgery, comfort level, IV fluid status, and urinary output measurements. Enter patient data into the medical record on flow sheets, surgical assessment drop-down menus, or written progress notes. The initial findings provide a baseline for comparing postoperative changes.

Through the Patient's Eyes. When a patient initially returns to the acute care nursing unit, the family and patient have expectations of receiving prompt and attentive care. There is also the expectation that a nurse will explain the patient's immediate status and the plan of care for the next few hours. Seeing the patient return from surgery is a relief in many ways; but, if the patient has had complications or is not responding well, anxiety easily returns. As a patient stabilizes it is important to assess the patient's and family's expectations for recovery and convalescence once he or she returns home. Be sure to review their expectations for management of pain and other symptoms. What do they expect from staff during the hospitalization? What are their expectations after the patient is discharged from the hospital? Are family members prepared to assume care at discharge? Make the patient and family partners in your assessment so you can gather information necessary to develop a relevant plan of care. For example, determine a patient's and family's values and beliefs as they pertain to the meaning of the surgical condition and how it will affect the patient's ability to reassume his or her role in the family.

Airway and Respiration. The first priority in the care of a patient after anesthesia is to establish a patent airway. Assess airway patency, respiratory rate, rhythm, depth of ventilation, symmetry of chest wall movement, breath sounds, and color of mucous membranes. Also know that certain anesthetic agents cause respiratory depression. A patient may present with snoring, little or no air movement on auscultation of the lungs, retraction of intercostal muscles, asynchronous movements of the chest, and decreased oxygen saturation. Be alert for shallow, slow breathing and a weak cough. If breathing is unusually shallow, place your hand near the patient's nose or mouth to feel exhaled air. Normal pulse oximetry values range between 92% and 100% saturation. Postoperative confusion is frequently secondary to hypoxia, especially in older adults.

An oral or nasal airway (see Chapter 41) is sometimes inserted in the OR or PACU after removal of the endotracheal tube. It maintains a patent airway until patients can protect their airway. However, aspiration or the passage of regurgitated material into the lungs occurs most often with removal of endotracheal tubes (Rothrock, 2015). As patients awaken they spit out the airway, or you ask them to spit it out. The ability to do so signifies the return of a normal gag reflex. Be alert for nausea and vomiting, which may precipitate regurgitation, avoid any rapid movement of the patient, and keep his or her head elevated while lying on the side.

One of your greatest concerns is airway obstruction. A number of factors contribute to obstruction, including history of OSA; weak pharyngeal/laryngeal muscle tone from anesthetics; secretions in the pharynx, bronchial tree, or trachea; and laryngeal or subglottic edema. After anesthesia, a patient's tongue causes the majority of airway obstructions. Ongoing assessment of airway patency is crucial. Patients remain in a side-lying position until airways are clear. Continue to assess respiratory status and breath sounds. Older patients, smokers, and patients with a history of respiratory disease are prone to developing complications such as atelectasis or pneumonia. Patients with OSA are often required to have continuous pulse oximetry while receiving IV opioids to detect oxygen desaturation quickly. Use of the Pasero Opioid-Induced Sedation Scale (POSS) in the PACU helps assess patients more accurately and meets the pain needs of the patient, while preventing oversedation (Kobelt et al., 2014).

Circulation. The patient is at risk for cardiovascular complications resulting from actual or potential blood loss from the surgical site, side effects of anesthesia, electrolyte imbalances, and depression of normal circulatory-regulating mechanisms and ischemia. Careful assessment of heart rate and rhythm, along with blood pressure, reveals a patient's cardiovascular status. Compare preoperative vital signs with postoperative values. If a patient's blood pressure drops progressively with each check or if the heart rate changes or becomes irregular, notify the health care provider. A rhythm strip of the heart is obtained after surgery, compared with preoperative ECG tracings, and placed in the medical record.

Assess circulatory perfusion by noting capillary refill, pulses, and the color and temperature of the nail beds and skin. If a patient had vascular surgery or has casts or constricting devices that may impair circulation, assess peripheral pulses and capillary refill distal to the site of surgery. For example, after surgery to the femoral artery, assess posterior tibial and dorsalis pedis pulses. In addition, compare pulses in the affected extremity with those in the nonaffected extremity.

A common early circulatory problem is bleeding or hemorrhage. Blood loss may occur internally or externally through a drain or incision. Either type of hemorrhage results in a fall in blood pressure; elevated heart and respiratory rates; thready pulse; cool, clammy, pale skin; and restlessness. Notify the surgeon if these changes occur. Maintain IV fluid infusion. Monitor the patient's vital signs every 15 minutes or more frequently until the patient's condition stabilizes. Continue oxygen therapy. The surgeon may consider medications or volume replacement and order blood counts and coagulation studies.

Temperature Control. The OR and recovery room environments are extremely cool. A patient's anesthetically depressed level of body function results in a lowering of metabolism and fall in body temperature. When patients begin to awaken more fully, they complain of feeling cold and uncomfortable. Older adults and pediatric patients are at higher risk for developing problems associated with postoperative hypothermia (temperature less than 36° C [96.8° F]). Also closely assess body temperature of other at-risk patients, including those of female gender, patients with burns, patients who received general anesthesia, patients who are cachexic or had low temperatures intraoperatively, and those whose surgery involved use of cold irrigants (Rothrock, 2015).

In rare instances a genetic disorder known as **malignant hyperthermia**, a life-threatening complication of anesthesia, develops. Malignant hyperthermia causes hypercarbia (elevated carbon dioxide), tachypnea, tachycardia, premature ventricular contractions (PVCs), unstable blood pressure, cyanosis, skin mottling, and muscular rigidity. Despite the name, an elevated temperature occurs late. The increased expired carbon dioxide is one of the first signs. Although it often occurs during the induction phase of anesthesia, symptoms can occur after surgery or with repeated exposures to anesthesia (Rothrock, 2015). Without prompt detection and treatment, it is potentially fatal.

Monitor temperature closely in the acute care area. Because an elevated temperature may be the first indication of an infection, assess the patient for a potential source of infection, including the IV site (if present), the surgical incision/wound, and the respiratory and urinary tracts. Notify the health care provider because further evaluation is often necessary.

Fluid and Electrolyte Balance. Because of the risk for fluid and electrolyte abnormalities after surgery, assess the patient's hydration status and monitor for signs of electrolyte alterations (see Chapter 42). Monitor and compare laboratory values with the patient's baseline. An important responsibility of the nurse is maintaining patency of IV infusions. The patient's only source of fluid intake immediately after surgery is through IV catheters until the gag reflex and bowel sounds resume. Inspect the patient's catheter insertion site to ensure that the catheter is properly positioned within a vein, fluid flows freely, and the site is free of phlebitis or infiltration. Accurate recording of I&O assesses renal and circulatory function. Measure all sources of output, including urine, surgically placed drains, and gastric and wound drainage; note any insensible loss from diaphoresis. Assess daily weight for the first several days after surgery and compare with the preoperative weight. If the patient has a known cardiac history such as heart failure, continue daily weights. It is important to use a consistent scale, amount of clothing, and time of day to obtain accurate weight measurement.

Neurological Functions. In the PACU the patient is often drowsy. As anesthetic agents begin to metabolize, his or her reflexes return, muscle strength is regained, and a normal level of orientation returns. Continue monitoring neurological status on the nursing unit. Ensure that the patient is oriented to self and the hospital and responds to questions appropriately. Assess pupil and gag reflexes, hand grips, and movement of extremities (see Chapter 31). If a patient had surgery involving part of the neurological system, conduct a more thorough neurological assessment. For example, if the patient had low-back surgery, assess leg movement, sensation, and strength.

Patients with regional anesthesia experience a return in motor function before tactile sensation returns. Check the patient's sensation to touch (see Chapter 31). Knowing where regional anesthesia was introduced helps you check the distribution of the spinal nerves affected. Typically assess sensation by touching the patient bilaterally in the same area (e.g., lower arm on both sides or leg on both sides) and note where the patient feels touch. Test the sense of touch using hand pressure or a gentle pinch of the skin. Extremity strength assessment is important if a patient had spinal or epidural anesthesia. Patients remain in the PACU until sensation and voluntary movement of the lower extremities are reestablished.

Skin Integrity and Condition of the Wound. During recovery and acute postoperative care assess the condition of the skin, noting pressure areas, rashes, petechiae, abrasions, or burns. A rash often indicates a drug sensitivity or allergy. Abrasions or petechiae sometimes result from a clotting disorder or inappropriate positioning or restraining that injures skin layers. Burns may indicate that an electrical cautery grounding pad was placed incorrectly on the patient's skin. Document burns or serious injury to the skin on an occurrence or adverse-event report according to agency policy (see Chapter 23). Note if the patient is complaining of any burning or pain in the eye, which could indicate a corneal abrasion.

After surgery a patient may only have butterfly tape, skin staples, or even glue to close small wounds. Look at the incision carefully and notice any drainage or swelling. Most surgical wounds that are larger have dressings that protect the wound site and collect drainage. Observe the amount, color, odor, and consistency of drainage on dressings. It is most common to see serosanguineous drainage immediately after surgery. Estimate the amount of drainage by noting the number of saturated gauze sponges. If drainage appears on the outer surface of a dressing, another way of assessing it is marking the outer perimeter of the drainage with tape or marking and dating it with the time noted. This way you can easily note if drainage is increasing (see Chapter 48). However, this is not the most accurate measure of volume of fluid lost. Reinforce the dressing as needed and call the surgeon if wound drainage is leaking through the dressing.

Many surgeons prefer to change surgical dressings the first time so they can inspect the incisional area. This applies to both outpatients and inpatients. You have the opportunity on the acute care nursing unit to view and thoroughly assess and document the status of the incision/wound at the time of this initial dressing change. Assess if wound edges are approximated and whether bleeding or drainage is present. It is also important to assess the patient's mobility level. If he or she is unable or unwilling to turn because of pain from the incisional area, pressure ulcer development is a concern. Institute the use of the Braden Scale or another assessment tool to determine a patient's risk of developing pressure ulcers.

Metabolism. Research over the past decade shows postoperative hyperglycemia (blood glucose greater than 180 mg/dL) is associated with surgical wound infection and longer hospital stays in surgical patients. Normoglycemia or a glucose level less than 150 mg/dL and reducing blood glucose variability is usually both safe and effective for patient management and are now recommended as an evidenced-based practice (Lipshutz and Gropper, 2009). Nurses need to monitor blood glucose levels routinely on the basis of surgeon order or hospital policy.

Genitourinary Function. Depending on the surgery, some patients do not regain voluntary control over urinary function for 6 to 8 hours after anesthesia. An epidural or spinal anesthetic often prevents a patient from feeling bladder fullness. Palpate the lower abdomen just above the symphysis pubis for bladder distention. Another option is to use a bladder scan or ultrasound to assess bladder volume. If the patient has a urinary catheter, there should be a continuous flow of urine of approximately 30 to 50 mL/hr in adults (see agency policy). Observe the color and odor of urine. Surgery involving parts of the urinary tract normally causes bloody urine for at least 12 to 24 hours, depending on the type of surgery. A urine output of less than 0.5 mL/kg/hr is reported to the surgeon or health care provider (Lewis et al., 2014).

Gastrointestinal Function. General anesthetics slow GI motility and often cause nausea. In addition, manipulation of the intestines during abdominal surgery further impairs peristalsis. Faint or absent bowel sounds are typical immediately after surgery. Normally patients who undergo abdominal or pelvic surgery have decreased peristalsis for at least 24 hours or longer (Rothrock, 2015). Paralytic ileus (i.e., loss of function of the intestine), which causes abdominal distention, is always possible after surgery. Auscultate bowel sounds in all four quadrants, noting faint or absent bowel sounds. Inspect the abdomen for distention caused by accumulation of gas. Ask whether a patient is passing flatus, an important sign indicating return of normal bowel function. The return of flatus is usually more indicative of normal bowel function return than the return of bowel sounds (Massey, 2012). If a nasogastric (NG) tube is in place for decompression, assess the patency of the tube and the color and amount of drainage (see Chapter 47).

Comfort. As patients awaken from general anesthesia, the sensation of pain becomes prominent. They perceive pain before regaining full consciousness. Acute incisional pain causes them to become restless and is often responsible for temporary changes in vital signs. It is difficult for patients to begin coughing and deep-breathing exercises when they experience incisional pain. The patient who had regional or local anesthesia usually does not experience pain initially because the incisional area is still anesthetized. Ongoing assessment of the patient's discomfort and evaluation of pain-relief therapies are essential throughout the postoperative course. Pain scales are effective for assessing postoperative pain, evaluating the response to analgesics, and objectively documenting pain severity (see Chapter 44). Using preoperative pain assessments as a baseline, evaluate the effectiveness of interventions throughout the patient's recovery.

◆ Nursing Diagnosis

Determine the status of preoperative nursing diagnoses by clustering new postoperative assessment data. Then either revise or resolve preoperative diagnoses and identify relevant new diagnoses after surgery. A previously defined diagnosis such as *Impaired Skin Integrity* may continue as a postoperative problem, particularly if your assessment reveals continued risks such as reduced mobility or excess diaphoresis. It is common to identify new nursing diagnoses after surgery because of the risks or problems associated with it. Also consider the assessed needs of a patient's family when you identify nursing diagnoses. In the formulation of nursing diagnoses, be accurate in identifying a related factor (when appropriate). For example, *Impaired Physical Mobility related to reduced lower-extremity strength* compared with *Impaired Physical Mobility related to exercise intolerance* requires different nursing interventions. Potential nursing diagnoses for the postoperative patient include the following:

- *Ineffective Airway Clearance*
- *Anxiety*
- *Fear*
- *Risk for Infection*
- *Deficient Knowledge (specify)*
- *Impaired Physical Mobility*
- *Impaired Skin Integrity*
- *Nausea*
- *Acute Pain*
- *Delayed Surgical Recovery*

◆ Planning

During the convalescent phase use current physical assessment data and analysis of the preoperative nursing history to plan the patient's care. The surgeon's postoperative orders and surgical team's report of the patient's operative condition also provide valuable data. Typical postoperative orders include:

- Frequency of vital sign monitoring and special assessments.
- Types of IV fluids and rates of infusion.
- Postoperative medications (especially those for pain and nausea).
- Resumption of preoperative medications as condition allows (some oral medications are converted to the IV route with appropriate dose adjustment).
- Fluids and food allowed by mouth.
- Level of activity that the patient is allowed to resume.
- Position that the patient is to maintain while in bed.
- I&O and daily weights.
- Laboratory tests and x-ray film studies.
- Special directions (e.g., surgical drains to suction, tube irrigations, dressing changes).

Goals and Outcomes. Review nursing diagnoses when establishing goals, expected outcomes, and interventions for your patient. Measurable outcomes provide specific guidelines for determining a patient's progress toward recovery from surgery. For example, a patient recovering from hip replacement surgery with the diagnosis of *Impaired Physical Mobility related to pain and lower-extremity weakness* has specific outcomes that include targeted ambulation (e.g., steps to take and distance down hallway), pain relief, and improved range of joint movement. After meeting each outcome, a patient ultimately achieves the goal of independent ambulation at a preoperative level or better. At times goals and outcomes extend from the convalescent period into the home setting. Also consider all goals of care established during the preoperative surgical phase that are still relevant. For example, a goal for the diagnosis of *Risk for Infection* would be "Patient will remain free of infection after surgery." Expected outcomes for this goal include:

- Patient's incision remains closed and intact.
- Patient's incision remains free of infectious drainage.
- Patient remains afebrile.

Setting Priorities. During the convalescent phase of recovery from general anesthesia, priorities for the first 24 hours continue to include maintenance of respiratory, circulatory, and neurological status; wound management; and pain control. In addition, most surgeons are aggressive in increasing a patient's activity as soon as possible. As a patient progresses, focus priorities on advancement of patient activity (e.g., mobility, diet tolerance) to return the patient to preoperative functioning or better. A patient generally has multiple nursing diagnoses (Figure 50-5). Reestablish priorities as the status of the patient's health problems change.

Teamwork and Collaboration. During recovery collaborate on the plan of care with respiratory therapy, physical therapy, occupational therapy, dietary, social work, home care, and others. Include family members as much as possible, especially if they will be assuming care responsibilities in the home. The goal of an interdisciplinary approach to care is to help the patient return to the best possible level of functioning with a smooth transition to home, rehabilitation, or long-term care. Acute care settings often have a nurse or social worker in a case-manager role to coordinate interdisciplinary care so the most appropriate resources are available to patients.

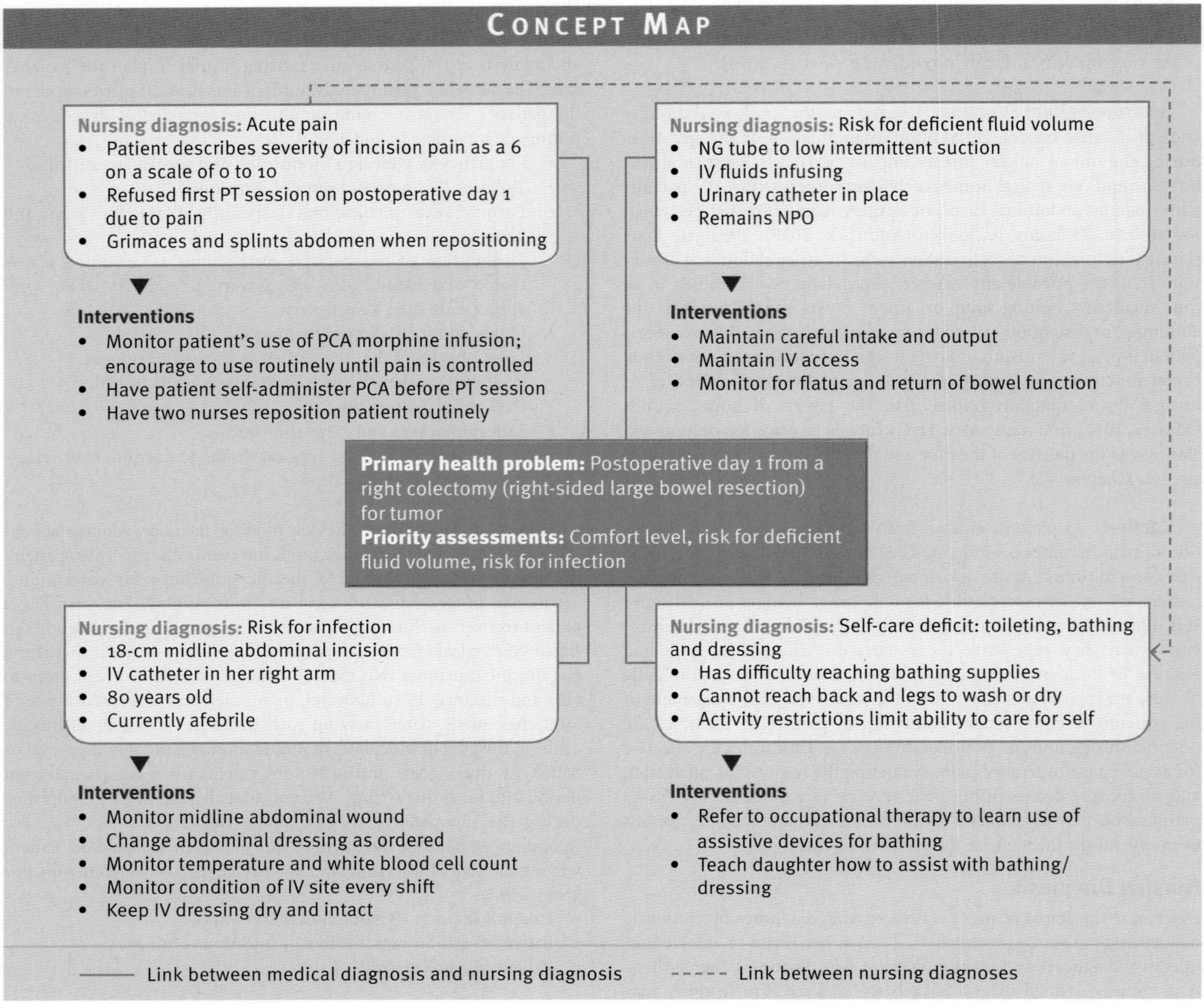

CONCEPT MAP

Nursing diagnosis: Acute pain
- Patient describes severity of incision pain as a 6 on a scale of 0 to 10
- Refused first PT session on postoperative day 1 due to pain
- Grimaces and splints abdomen when repositioning

Interventions
- Monitor patient's use of PCA morphine infusion; encourage to use routinely until pain is controlled
- Have patient self-administer PCA before PT session
- Have two nurses reposition patient routinely

Nursing diagnosis: Risk for deficient fluid volume
- NG tube to low intermittent suction
- IV fluids infusing
- Urinary catheter in place
- Remains NPO

Interventions
- Maintain careful intake and output
- Maintain IV access
- Monitor for flatus and return of bowel function

Primary health problem: Postoperative day 1 from a right colectomy (right-sided large bowel resection) for tumor
Priority assessments: Comfort level, risk for deficient fluid volume, risk for infection

Nursing diagnosis: Risk for infection
- 18-cm midline abdominal incision
- IV catheter in her right arm
- 80 years old
- Currently afebrile

Interventions
- Monitor midline abdominal wound
- Change abdominal dressing as ordered
- Monitor temperature and white blood cell count
- Monitor condition of IV site every shift
- Keep IV dressing dry and intact

Nursing diagnosis: Self-care deficit: toileting, bathing and dressing
- Has difficulty reaching bathing supplies
- Cannot reach back and legs to wash or dry
- Activity restrictions limit ability to care for self

Interventions
- Refer to occupational therapy to learn use of assistive devices for bathing
- Teach daughter how to assist with bathing/dressing

——— Link between medical diagnosis and nursing diagnosis - - - - - Link between nursing diagnoses

FIGURE 50-5 Concept map for Mrs. Campana. *IV,* Intravenous; *NG,* nasogastric; *PCA,* patient-controlled analgesia; *PT,* physical therapy.

◆ Implementation

Acute Care. Primary causes for postoperative complications include impaired healing of the surgical wound, the effects of prolonged immobilization during surgery, recovery, and convalescence, and the influence of anesthesia and analgesics. If a patient has surgical risks before surgery (e.g., increased age, OSA, history of smoking, history of diabetes), the likelihood of complications is greater (Box 50-9). Direct your postoperative nursing interventions at preventing complications so the patient returns to the highest level of functioning possible. Failure of a patient to become actively involved in recovery adds to the risk of complications (Table 50-8). Virtually any body system can be affected. Consider the interrelationship of all systems and therapies provided. Purposeful hourly rounds meet patient needs and increase patient satisfaction. Rounds include the 4 *P*s (i.e., *p*ain, *p*otty, *p*ositioning, and *p*eriphery). Nursing staff ask patients about their pain and if they need to toilet, the patients are positioned for comfort, and an environmental check is done of the periphery to ensure that possessions such as a phone and call light are in reach (Olrich et al., 2012).

Maintaining Respiratory Function. To prevent respiratory complications begin pulmonary interventions early. The benefits of thorough preoperative teaching are reached when patients are able to participate actively in postoperative exercises. When patients awaken from anesthesia, help them maintain a patent airway. Position the patient on one side with the face downward and the neck slightly extended to facilitate a forward movement of the tongue and the flow of mucus secretions out of the mouth. A small folded towel supports the head. Another positioning technique to promote a patent airway involves elevating the head of the bed slightly and extending the patient's neck slightly, with the head turned to the side. In the PACU you sometimes need to perform a jaw-thrust maneuver and/or chin lift continuously to maintain the patient's airway. Never position a patient with arms over or across the chest because this reduces maximum chest expansion.

Place patients with known OSA or at risk for OSA in the lateral, prone, or upright position throughout the perioperative period, never

BOX 50-9 FOCUS ON OLDER ADULTS

Care of the Older Adult After Surgery

- Many older adults tolerate elective surgery well with effective preoperative and postoperative care. However, they do not tolerate emergency or long, complicated surgeries as well because of a decrease in physiological reserves (Clayton, 2008).
- Co-morbidities (preexisting medical conditions) and reduction in physiological reserve consistently predict poor postoperative outcomes in older adults. Adverse postoperative outcomes, particularly medical complications, are more common in older people when compared with young adults (Partridge et al., 2012).
- During the perioperative period assess for changes that occur as a result of infection, hemorrhage, alterations in blood pressure, and fluid/electrolyte abnormalities. Ongoing, focused assessments are necessary.
- Older patients are at greater risk for postoperative delirium associated with an acute onset. Reduced level of consciousness, reduced ability to maintain attention, perceptual disturbances, and memory impairment characterize the typical presentation (Meiner, 2015).
- Implement individualized measures to help the older adult achieve rest, sleep, and orientation in the postoperative period to reduce the risk of delirium development.
- Altered and unexpected drug responses are often related to different pharmacokinetics in the older adult. Thus be alert to the possibility of a high risk for adverse medication events with the administration of anesthetic agents and postoperative analgesics, especially narcotics (Meiner, 2015). "Start low and go slow" is the guiding principle when medicating older adults because of their slow drug-clearance capability.

TABLE 50-8 Postoperative Complications

Complication	Cause
Respiratory System	
Atelectasis: Collapse of alveoli with retained mucus secretions. Signs and symptoms include elevated respiratory rate, dyspnea, fever, crackles auscultated over involved lobes of lungs, and productive cough.	Inadequate lung expansion. Anesthesia, analgesia, and immobilized position prevent full lung expansion. There is greater risk in patients with upper abdominal surgery who have pain during inspiration and repress deep breathing.
Pneumonia: Inflammation of alveoli involving one or several lobes of lung. Development in lower dependent lobes of lung is common in patient who is immobilized after surgery. Signs and symptoms include fever, chills, productive cough, chest pain, purulent mucus, and dyspnea.	Poor lung expansion with retained secretions or aspirated secretions. Common resident bacterium in respiratory tract is *Diplococcus pneumoniae,* which causes most cases of pneumonia.
Hypoxemia: Inadequate concentration of oxygen in arterial blood. Signs and symptoms include restlessness, confusion, dyspnea, high or low blood pressure, tachycardia or bradycardia, diaphoresis, and cyanosis.	Anesthetics and analgesics depress respirations. Increased retention of mucus with impaired ventilation occurs because of pain or poor positioning. Patients with obstructive sleep apnea are at increased risk for hypoxemia.
Pulmonary embolism: Embolus blocking pulmonary arterial blood flow to one or more lobes of lung. Signs and symptoms include dyspnea, sudden chest pain, cyanosis, tachycardia, and drop in blood pressure.	Same factors lead to formation of thrombus or embolus. Patients with preexisting circulatory or coagulation disorders and who are immobile are at risk.
Circulatory System	
Hemorrhage: Loss of large amount of blood externally or internally in short period of time. Signs and symptoms include hypotension, weak and rapid pulse, cool and clammy skin, rapid breathing, restlessness, and reduced urine output.	Slipping of suture or dislodged clot at incisional site. Patients with coagulation disorders are at greater risk.
Hypovolemic shock: Inadequate perfusion of tissues and cells from loss of circulatory fluid volume. Signs and symptoms are same as for hemorrhage.	Hemorrhage usually causes hypovolemic shock after surgery.
Thrombophlebitis: Inflammation of vein often accompanied by clot formation. Veins in legs are most commonly affected. Signs and symptoms include swelling and inflammation of involved site and aching or cramping pain. Vein feels hard, cordlike, and sensitive to touch.	Prolonged sitting or immobilization aggravates venous stasis. Trauma to vessel wall and hypercoagulability of blood increase risk of vessel inflammation.
Thrombus: Formation of clot attached to interior wall of a vein or artery, which can occlude the vessel lumen. Symptoms include localized tenderness along distribution of the venous system, swollen calf or thigh, calf swelling >3 cm (1.2 inches) compared to asymptomatic leg, pitting edema in symptomatic leg, and decrease in pulse below location of thrombus (if arterial).	Venous stasis (see discussion of thrombophlebitis) and vessel trauma. Venous injury is common after surgery of hips and legs, abdomen, pelvis, and major vessels. Patients with pelvic and abdominal cancer or traumatic injuries to the pelvis or lower extremities are at high risk for thrombus formation.

Continued

TABLE 50-8 Postoperative Complications—cont'd

Complication	Cause
Embolus: Piece of thrombus that has dislodged and circulates in bloodstream until it lodges in another vessel (commonly lungs, heart, brain, or mesentery).	Thrombi form from increased coagulability of blood (e.g., polycythemia and use of birth-control pills containing estrogen).
Gastrointestinal System	
Paralytic ileus: Nonmechanical obstruction of the bowel caused by physiological, neurogenic, or chemical imbalance associated with decreased peristalsis. Common in initial hours after abdominal surgery.	Handling of intestines during surgery leads to loss of peristalsis for a few hours to several days.
Abdominal distention: Retention of air within intestines and abdominal cavity during gastrointestinal surgery. Signs and symptoms include increased abdominal girth, patient complaints of fullness, and "gas pains."	Slowed peristalsis from anesthesia, bowel manipulation, or immobilization. During laparoscopic surgeries influx of air for procedure causes distention and pain up to shoulders.
Nausea and vomiting: Symptoms of improper gastric emptying or chemical stimulation of vomiting center. Patient complains of gagging or feeling full or sick to stomach.	Abdominal distention, fear, severe pain, medications, eating or drinking before peristalsis returns, and initiation of gag reflex.
Genitourinary System	
Urinary retention: Involuntary accumulation of urine in bladder as result of loss of muscle tone. Signs and symptoms include inability to void, restlessness, and bladder distention. It appears 6-8 hours after surgery.	Effects of anesthesia and narcotic analgesics. Local manipulation of tissues surrounding bladder and edema interfere with bladder tone. Poor positioning of patient impairs voiding reflexes.
Urinary tract infection: Infection of the urinary tract as a result of bacterial or yeast contamination. Signs and symptoms include dysuria, itching, abdominal pain, possible fever, cloudy urine, presence of white blood cells, and leukocyte esterase positive on urinalysis.	Most frequently a result of catheterization of the bladder.
Integumentary System	
Wound infection: Invasion of deep or superficial wound tissues by pathogenic microorganisms; signs and symptoms include warm, red, and tender skin around incision; fever and chills; purulent material exiting from drains or from separated wound edges. Infection usually appears 3-6 days after surgery.	Infection is caused by poor aseptic technique or contaminated wound or surgical site before surgical exploration. For example, with a bowel perforation patient is at increased risk for a wound infection because of bacterial contamination from the large intestine.
Wound dehiscence: Separation of wound edges at suture line. Signs and symptoms include increased drainage and appearance of underlying tissues. This usually occurs 6-8 days after surgery.	Malnutrition, obesity, preoperative radiation to surgical site, old age, poor circulation to tissues, and unusual strain on suture line from coughing or positioning.
Wound evisceration: Protrusion of internal organs and tissues through incision. Incidence usually occurs 6-8 days after surgery.	See discussion of wound dehiscence. Patient with dehiscence is at risk for developing evisceration.
Skin breakdown: Result of pressure or shearing forces. Patients are at increased risk if alterations in nutrition and circulation are present, resulting in edema and delayed healing.	Prolonged periods on the operating room (OR) table and in the bed after surgery lead to pressure breakdown. Skin breakdown results from shearing during positioning on the OR table and improperly pulling patient up in bed.
Nervous System	
Intractable pain: Pain that is not amenable to analgesics and pain-alleviating interventions.	Intractable pain may be related to the wound or dressing, anxiety, or positioning.
Malignant hyperthermia: Severe hypermetabolic state and rigidity of the skeletal muscles caused by an increase in intracellular calcium ion concentration.	Rare genetic condition triggered with exposure to inhaled anesthetic agents and the depolarizing muscle relaxant succinylcholine.

the supine position (ASA, 2014). Suction artificial airways and the oral cavity for mucus secretions (see Chapter 41). Avoid continually eliciting the gag reflex, which might cause vomiting. Before you remove an artificial airway (or the patient removes it), suction the back of the airway so secretions are not retained. The following interventions promote expansion of the lungs:

- Encourage diaphragmatic breathing exercises every hour while patients are awake.
- Administer CPAP or NIPPV to patients who use this modality at home (ASA, 2014).
- Instruct patients to use an incentive spirometer for maximum inspiration. The patient should try to reach the inspiratory target volume achieved before surgery on the spirometer.
- Encourage early ambulation. Walking causes patients to assume a position that does not restrict chest wall expansion and stimulates an increased respiratory rate.

- Help patients who are restricted to bed to turn on their side every 1 to 2 hours while awake and to sit when possible.
- Keep the patient comfortable. A patient who is comfortable is able to participate in deep breathing and coughing. Administer analgesics on time so pain does not become severe.

The following measures promote removal of pulmonary secretions if they are present:

- Encourage coughing exercises every 1 to 2 hours while patients are awake and maintain pain control to promote a deep, productive cough. *For patients who have had eye, intracranial, or spinal surgery, coughing may be contraindicated because of the potential increase in intraocular or intracranial pressure.*
- Provide oral hygiene to facilitate expectoration of mucus. The oral mucosa becomes dry when patients are NPO or placed on limited fluid intake.
- Initiate orotracheal or nasotracheal suction for patients who are too weak or unable to cough (see Chapter 41).
- Administer oxygen as ordered and monitor oxygen saturation with a pulse oximeter. Continue monitoring oxygen saturation after discharge from the PACU for patients at risk for respiratory compromise from OSA (ASA, 2014). Administer oxygen to patients at risk for or diagnosed with OSA until they are able to maintain their baseline oxygen saturation while breathing room air.

Preventing Circulatory Complications. Interventions to prevent circulatory complications also prevent venous stasis and thrombus formation (Box 50-10). Some patients are at greater risk of venous stasis because of the nature of their surgery or medical history. The following interventions promote normal venous return and circulatory blood flow:

- Encourage patients to perform leg exercises at least every hour while awake. Exercise may be contraindicated in an extremity with a vascular repair or realignment of fractured bones and torn cartilage.
- Apply graded compression stockings or IPC devices as ordered by the health care provider. Remove the stockings or device at least once per shift. Perform a thorough reassessment of the skin of the lower extremities at this time.
- Encourage early ambulation. Most patients ambulate the evening of surgery, depending on the severity of the surgery and their condition. The degree of activity allowed progresses as the patient's condition improves. Encourage ambulation even if a patient has an epidural catheter or PCA device.
- Before ambulation, assess the patient's vital signs. Abnormalities such as hypotension or certain arrhythmias may contraindicate ambulation. If vital signs are at baseline, first help the patient sit on the side of the bed. Patient complaints of dizziness are a sign of postural hypotension. A recheck of blood pressure determines whether ambulation is safe. Assist with ambulation by standing on the patient's strong side and making sure that he or she is able to walk steadily. Patients may be able to walk only a few feet the first few times out of bed. This usually improves each time. Evaluate tolerance to activity by periodically assessing the pulse rate as the patient ambulates and note the rhythm and increase in rate. Know the patient's maximum heart rate achieved during maximum exercise. One simple method to calculate a predicted maximum heart rate is by using this formula (Cleveland Clinic, 2015):

$$220 - \text{Patient's age} = \text{Predicted maximum heart rate}$$

Example: A 60-year-old's predicted maximum heart rate is 160 beats/min. However, remember that a patient's acute surgical condition may

BOX 50-10 EVIDENCE-BASED PRACTICE

Prevention of Venous Thromboembolism in the Postsurgical Patient

PICO Question: Is mechanical prophylaxis compared with pharmacological prophylaxis the best method to prevent a venous thromboembolism (VTE) in the postsurgical patient?

Evidence Summary

VTE is a high-risk concern for almost all hospitalized patients. A VTE can lead to stroke, myocardial infarction, and death. It is the most common cause of preventable death in patients who are hospitalized (American College of Chest Physicians, 2012). Treatment targets two of the three components of Virchow's triad (stasis and hypercoagulability). Mechanical treatment measures focus on prevention of stasis, whereas pharmacological measures prevent hypercoagulability.

Mechanical prevention includes early ambulation, graded compression stockings, intermittent pneumatic compression devices, or venous foot pumps (Gould et al., 2012; AORN, 2015). Perioperative pharmacological antithrombotic management is based on risk assessment for thromboembolism and bleeding. Recommended approaches simplify patient management and minimize adverse clinical outcomes (Douketis et al., 2012). Guidelines for the use of antithrombotic medications and mechanical prophylaxis follow (Gould et al., 2012):

- When the risk for VTE is very low (less than 0.5%), no specific pharmacological or mechanical prophylaxis is used other than early ambulation.
- For patients at low risk for VTE, mechanical prophylaxis, preferably with intermittent pneumatic compression (IPC), is recommended.
- For patients having general or abdominal-pelvic surgery and at moderate risk for VTE who are not at high risk for major bleeding complications, low-molecular-weight heparin (LMWH), low-dose unfractionated heparin (LDUH), or mechanical prophylaxis, preferably with IPC, is recommended.
- For patients having general or abdominal-pelvic surgery and at high risk for VTE who are not at high risk for major bleeding complications, the same prophylaxis as moderate-risk patients is needed, with mechanical prophylaxis with elastic stockings or IPC added.
- For patients at moderate-to-high risk for VTE who are at high risk for major bleeding complications or those in whom the consequences of bleeding are believed to be particularly severe, mechanical prophylaxis, preferably with IPC, is recommended until the risk of bleeding diminishes and pharmacological prophylaxis may be initiated.

Application to Nursing Practice

- Monitor patients' INR levels: when using LMWH or LDUH, the target international normalized ratio (INR) is 2.5 with a range of 2-3, and dosing is based on renal function and manufacturer recommendations. Notify surgeon or health care provider of abnormal values.
- Check all orders or antithrombotic medications closely.
- Perform ongoing assessments of patient's lower extremities for signs of deep vein thrombosis: swelling in one or both legs; pain or tenderness in one or both legs, which may occur only while standing or walking; warmth in the skin of the affected leg; red or discolored skin in the affected leg.
- Early ambulation and the use of mechanical prophylaxis are recommended in all patients following surgery.

not allow him or her to reach this rate. *Confer with the patient's surgeon or physical therapist about a safe heart rate target.* Always ask patients how they feel during exercise and whether they note chest pain or shortness of breath.

- Avoid positioning patients in a manner that interrupts blood flow to extremities. Do not place pillows or rolled blankets under a patient's knees while in bed. Compression of the popliteal vessels can cause thrombi. When patients sit in chairs, elevate their legs on footstools. Never allow a patient to sit with one leg crossed over the other.
- Administer anticoagulant drugs as ordered. Patients at greatest risk for thrombus formation often receive prophylactic doses of anticoagulants such as LMWH (e.g., enoxaparin [e.g., Lovenox, Fragmin, Arixtra]) or low-dose unfractionated heparin (LDUH) for anticoagulation.
- Promote adequate fluid intake orally or intravenously. Adequate hydration prevents concentrated accumulation of formed blood elements such as platelets and red blood cells. When the plasma volume is low, these elements gather and form small clots within blood vessels.

Achieving Rest and Comfort. Pain control is a priority to facilitate a patient's recovery. Without pain control a patient will not move or ambulate as readily or initiate coughing exercises after surgery. The anesthesia provider orders medications for pain management in the PACU. IV opioid analgesics such as morphine sulfate are the drugs of choice for the immediate postoperative period. Advances have been made in the use of multimodal analgesia (more than one analgesic), which combines different drug classes delivered through various routes, including use of local anesthetics alone or in combination with other nerve blocks or therapies such as PCA. The goal is to enhance the efficacy of pain control while minimizing side effects of each modality (Costantini et al., 2011).

A patient's pain increases following surgery as the effects of anesthesia diminish. The patient becomes more aware of the surroundings and more perceptive of discomfort. The incisional area is only one source of pain. Irritation from drainage tubes, tight dressings, or casts and the muscular strains caused from positioning on the OR table also cause discomfort. Even in local procedures (e.g., laparoscopy), air inflation causes significant discomfort in the area of surgery.

When a patient requests pain medication or shows signs of discomfort, assess the nature and character of his or her pain thoroughly (see Chapter 44). Also determine if the ordered dose of analgesic is within the recommended range. Patients have the most surgical pain the first 24 to 48 hours after surgery. IV PCA or epidural analgesia may be ordered. A PCA device delivers analgesic medications by IV or subcutaneous infusion. The PCA system allows patients to administer their own IV analgesics from a specially prepared pump (see Chapter 44). If patients gain a sense of control over their pain, they usually have fewer postoperative problems. Many patients receive regional analgesia such as epidural analgesia continuously throughout the recovery period, especially for thoracic and abdominal surgery. Studies show that continuous epidural analgesia provides superior pain relief in terms of less analgesic use, better postoperative pain relief (especially first 24 hours), less sedation, and faster return of GI function (Hazem and Mokbel, 2014). Epidural techniques are especially useful in patients with OSA who are at increased risk of airway compromise and postoperative complications with the use of systemic opioids after surgery. Nonsteroidal antiinflammatory agents are an alternative to systemic opioids in patients with OSA (ASA, 2014). You care for patients with a variety of pain-control techniques. Monitor closely for side effects and educate the patient and family regarding the pain-management therapy and expected response.

As the patient begins to tolerate oral fluids, facilitate changing his or her pain medication from IV or epidural to oral administration. Do not overlook the importance of nonpharmacological interventions (see Chapter 44). Assess which care routines contribute to pain and use nonpharmacological measures to treat them. An example is to lower the head of the bed and use a pillow for incisional splinting while turning a patient with recent abdominal surgery. Use other methods of promoting pain relief such as positioning, back rubs, distraction, or imagery. Remember, *do not assume that a patient's pain is incisional.* When a patient without PCA or epidural analgesic asks for pain medication, provide analgesics as often as allowed ATC the first 24 to 48 hours after surgery to improve pain control. If pain medications are not relieving discomfort, notify the health care provider for additional orders. You need to recognize potential complications of analgesics and know what to do if they occur.

Temperature Regulation. Unless intraoperative warming is used, patients are usually cool when arriving in the PACU as a result of the cool temperature in the OR and evaporative heat loss. When a patient comes to the PACU or surgical unit, provide warmed blankets or heated air blankets if no other warming device is available. Increasing a patient's body temperature raises metabolism and improves circulatory and respiratory function.

Sometimes shivering is a side effect of certain anesthetic agents instead of hypothermia. Clonidine (Catapres) in small increments can decrease shivering as prescribed by the health care provider. When this happens, encourage your patient to use deep breathing and coughing to help to expel retained anesthetic gases.

Malignant hyperthermia is a hypermetabolic state occurring within skeletal muscle cells that become triggered by anesthesia. It results in an increase in intracellular calcium ion concentration. It is a potentially lethal condition that can occur in patients receiving various inhaled anesthetic agents and succinylcholine. The hyperthermic condition results in high carbon dioxide levels, metabolic and respiratory acidosis, increased oxygen consumption, production of heat, activation of the sympathetic nervous system, high serum potassium levels, and multiple organ dysfunction and failure. Early signs of malignant hyperthermia include tachypnea, tachycardia, heart arrhythmias, hyperkalemia, and muscular rigidity. Later signs include elevated temperature, myoglobinuria, and multiple organ failure (Johns et al., 2012; Chapin and Geibel, 2015). Monitor a patient's end-tidal carbon dioxide and anticipate clinical changes in patients at risk. When malignant hyperthermia develops, immediately administer dantrolene sodium as ordered by the health care provider (Malignant Hyperthermia Association of the United States, 2015).

Patients are at risk for infection following surgery for various reasons. If a patient becomes febrile, be aggressive in providing routine postoperative nursing interventions. For example, deep breathing and coughing, early ambulation, prompt removal of indwelling urinary and IV catheters, and aseptic care of the surgical wound decrease the risk of postoperative infections. Since microorganisms require time to incubate, infections are rare within the first 48 hours after surgery. If the health care provider suspects an infection, he or she orders wound and or blood cultures.

Maintaining Neurological Function. Deep breathing and coughing expel retained anesthetic gases and facilitate a patient's return to consciousness. Try to arouse a patient by calling his or her name in a moderate tone of voice. If that is not successful, waken him or her by using touch or gently moving a body part. If painful stimulation is needed to arouse a patient, notify anesthesia immediately. When patients are elderly, know the status of their renal function because delayed renal clearance of operatively administered anesthetic agents slows awakening. Orientation to the environment is important in maintaining the patient's mental status. Reorient the patient, explain that surgery is completed, and describe procedures and nursing measures.

Maintaining Fluid and Electrolyte Balance. Immediately after surgery, patients receive fluids only intravenously. It is important to maintain patency of IV infusions in the postoperative period (see Chapter 42). You typically remove an IV catheter once a patient awakens after ambulatory surgery and is able to tolerate water without GI upset. A more seriously ill patient requires IV fluids for a longer period of time to achieve hydration and electrolyte balance. Some patients require blood products after surgery, depending on the amount of blood loss during surgery. A surgeon orders a prescribed solution and rate for each IV infusion. As a patient begins to take and tolerate oral fluids, you decrease the IV rate. When patients no longer need a continuous IV infusion, you will most likely saline lock the IV line to preserve the site for the administration of medications such as antibiotics or other types of intravenous therapy (see Chapter 42).

Promoting Normal Gastrointestinal Function and Adequate Nutrition. Normally a patient who received general anesthesia does not drink fluids in the PACU because of reduced peristalsis, risk of nausea and vomiting, and grogginess from general anesthesia. For patients at high risk for the development of nausea and vomiting or those who must not vomit, you administer a combination of antiemetics to block multiple receptors. A combination of antiemtic medications is often more effective than a single agent (Kovac, 2013). If a patient has a NG tube, keep it patent by irrigating it as ordered (see Chapter 47). Occlusion of a NG tube results in accumulation of gastric contents within the stomach.

Recent research provides a simple remedy for promoting return of GI peristalsis. Studies show that patients who chew gum after surgery experience a faster return of bowel function (bowel sounds), pass flatus significantly sooner, and have their first bowel movement significantly sooner (Jang et al., 2012; Marwah et al., 2012). Research also shows that patients who are fed soon after surgery are more likely to vomit than those who chew gum (Askarpour, 2010).

A patient likely begins taking ice chips or sips of fluids when arriving on an acute surgical care unit. If fluids are tolerated, the diet progresses with clear liquids next. Interventions for preventing GI complications promote return of normal elimination and faster return of normal nutritional intake. It takes several days for a patient who has had GI surgery (e.g., a colon resection) to resume a normal diet. Normal peristalsis often does not return for 2 to 3 days. In contrast, the patient whose GI tract is unaffected directly by surgery can resume dietary intake after recovering from the effects of anesthesia. The following measures promote return of normal elimination:

- Advance a patient's dietary intake gradually. One study showed that the return of flatus and the first postoperative bowel movement are more reliable than a return of bowel sounds in determining when to begin a normal diet in patients who have undergone abdominal surgery (Madsen et al., 2005). Most surgeons rely on the return of flatus or bowel sounds to order a normal diet. Patients usually receive a normal diet the first evening after surgery unless they had surgery on GI structures. Use patient assessment data to determine how quickly to advance your patient's diet. For example, provide clear liquids such as water, apple juice, broth, or tea after nausea subsides. Ingesting large amounts of fluids leads to distention and vomiting. If a patient tolerates liquids without nausea, advance the diet as ordered. Patients who had abdominal surgery are usually NPO the first 24 to 48 hours. As flatus and peristalsis return, provide clear liquids, followed by full liquids, a light diet of solid foods, and finally a patient's usual diet. Encourage intake of foods high in protein and vitamin C.
- Promote ambulation and exercise. Physical activity stimulates a return of peristalsis. A patient who has abdominal distention and "gas pain" may obtain relief when walking.
- Maintain an adequate fluid intake. Fluids keep fecal material soft for easy passage. Fruit juices and warm liquids are especially effective.
- Promote adequate food intake by stimulating a patient's appetite; remove sources of noxious odors and provide small servings of nonspicy foods.
- Avoid moving a patient suddenly to minimize nausea.
- Help the patient get into a comfortable position during mealtime. If possible, have him or her sit to minimize pressure on the abdomen.
- Provide desired servings of food. For example, some patients are more willing to eat the first meal when servings are not large.
- Provide frequent oral hygiene. Adequate hydration and cleaning of the oral cavity eliminate dryness and bad tastes.
- Administer fiber supplements, stool softeners, and rectal suppositories as ordered. If constipation or distention develops, the health care provider orders cathartics or enemas to stimulate peristalsis.
- Provide meals when the patient is rested and free from pain. Often a patient loses interest in eating if mealtime follows exhausting activities such as ambulation, coughing and deep-breathing exercises, or extensive dressing changes. When a patient has pain, the associated nausea often causes a loss of appetite.

Promoting Urinary Elimination. The depressant effects of anesthetics and analgesics impair the sensation of bladder fullness. A full bladder is painful and causes a patient awakening from surgery to be restless or agitated. Patients who have abdominal surgery or surgery of the urinary system often have indwelling catheters inserted until voluntary urination returns. However, patients without a catheter need to void within 8 to 12 hours after surgery. Sometimes it is necessary to insert a straight catheter. If a patient has an indwelling urinary catheter, the goal is to remove it as soon as possible because of the high risk for the development of a health care–associated bladder or urinary tract infection (HAI). Use evidence-based protocols to ensure prompt removal of urinary catheters (Willson et al., 2009). The following measures promote normal urinary elimination (see Chapter 46):

- Help patients assume their normal position to void if possible.
- Check a patient frequently for the need to void when a catheter is not in place. The feeling of bladder fullness is often sudden, and you need to respond promptly when a patient calls for assistance.
- Assess for bladder distention. If a patient does not void within 8 hours of surgery or bladder distention is present, you will insert a straight urinary catheter if you have an order from a health care provider. Continued difficulty in voiding sometimes requires an indwelling catheter, which increases the risk for a urinary tract infection. Although the evidence is inconclusive, some agencies use bladder ultrasound to assess bladder volume and assist in the decision to place a urinary catheter.
- Monitor I&O. If a patient has an indwelling catheter, expect an output of about 30 to 50 mL/hr. Another way to gauge adequacy of output is by determining a patient's weight. An accepted level of urinary output is at least 1 mL/kg/hr for adults (Lewis et al., 2014). If the urine is dark, concentrated, and low in volume, notify a health care provider. Patients easily become dehydrated as a result of fluid loss from surgical wounds and inadequate fluid intake. Measure I&O for several days after surgery until a patient achieves normal fluid intake and urinary output.

Skin and Wound Care. A wound undergoes considerable stress after surgery from inadequate nutrition, impaired circulation, and metabolic alterations (see Chapter 48). A wound also undergoes considerable physical stress. Strain on sutures from coughing, vomiting, distention, and movement of body parts can disrupt wound layers. Protect a wound and promote healing. A critical time for wound healing is 24 to 72 hours after surgery, after which a seal is established. If infection of a clean surgical wound occurs, you will usually find symptoms of infection 4 to 5 days after surgery. Thus you monitor patients on an ongoing basis for fever, tenderness at a wound site, and presence of local drainage on dressings (i.e., yellow, green or brown, and odorous). A clean surgical wound usually does not regain strength against normal stress for 15 to 20 days after surgery.

Surgical dressings (if present) remain in place the first 24 hours after surgery to reduce risk of infection. During this time add an extra layer of gauze on top of the original dressing if drainage develops. After that, use aseptic technique during dressing changes and wound care (see Chapter 48). Time any dressing change to begin 5 to 30 minutes after you give a patient pain medication (depending on route: 5 minutes intravenously, 30 minutes oral). Keep surgical drains patent so accumulated secretions can escape from the wound bed.

Maintaining/Enhancing Self-Concept. The appearance of wounds, bulky dressings, drains, and tubes threatens a patient's self-concept. The effects of surgery such as disfiguring scars often create permanent changes in a patient's body image. If surgery leads to impairment in body function, a patient's role within the family can change significantly. Observe patients for behaviors reflecting alterations in self-concept (see Chapter 34). Some patients show revulsion toward their appearance by refusing to look at incisions, carefully covering dressings with bed clothes, or refusing to get out of bed because of tubes and devices. The fear of not being able to return to a functional family role causes some patients to avoid participating in the plan of care.

A family often plays an important role in efforts to improve a patient's self-concept. Explain the patient's appearance to the family and ways to avoid nonverbal expressions of revulsion or surprise. Encourage the family to accept the patient's needs and support his or her independence. The following measures help to maintain a patient's self-concept:

- Provide privacy during dressing changes or inspection of the wound. Keep room curtains closed around the bed and drape the patient to expose only the dressing or incisional area.
- Maintain the patient's hygiene. Wound drainage and antiseptic solutions from the surgical skin preparation dry on the surface of the skin, causing foul odor and skin irritation. A complete bath the first day after surgery renews the patient. Offer a clean gown and washcloth if a gown becomes soiled. Keep the patient's hair neatly combed and offer frequent oral hygiene every 2 hours while awake, especially if patient is NPO.
- Prevent drainage devices from overflowing. Measure contents of drainage collection devices every 8 hours for output recording. Measure and empty more often if drainage is excessive.
- Maintain a pleasant environment. Being in pleasant, comfortable surroundings heightens self-concept. Store or remove unused supplies. Keep the patient's bedside orderly and clean.
- Offer opportunities for the patient to discuss feelings about appearance. A patient who avoids looking at an incision possibly needs to discuss fears or concerns. A patient having surgery for the first time is often more anxious than one who has had multiple surgeries. When a patient looks at an incision for the first time, make sure that the area is clean. Eventually he or she will be able to care for the incision site by applying simple dressings or bathing the affected area.
- Provide the family with opportunities to discuss ways to promote the patient's self-concept. Encouraging independence is sometimes difficult for a family member who has a strong desire to help the patient in any way. Family members are more able to be supportive during dressing changes when they know about the appearance of a wound or incision. Help family members know when it is appropriate to discuss future plans. This allows the patient and family to discuss realistic plans for a patient's return home.

Restorative and Continuing Care. In the postoperative period, the nurse, patient, and family collaborate to prepare the patient for discharge. Patients often have to continue wound care, follow activity or diet restrictions, continue medication therapy, and observe for signs and symptoms of complications at home. Education regarding these activities is specific to the type of surgery and is an ongoing process throughout hospitalization. It is important to provide specific, culturally appropriate, and accurate verbal and written discharge instructions to enhance the ability of patients to care for themselves at home (Williams, 2008).

When caring for a patient who had ambulatory surgery, you need to prioritize education because of the limited time you have with the patient. Including the family or support system provides a resource for the patient once home. Provide a wide variety of written educational materials for all patients after surgery. For example, offer materials with more pictures and illustrations for patients who do not speak English or have limited reading ability. Ensure that all materials are sensitive to various cultures and religions. Patients receive a copy of signed discharge instructions, and one copy remains in the medical or electronic record.

Surgical recovery is slowed if patients are deconditioned and then fail to exercise regularly. Recent research shows the importance of keeping frail older adults active after surgery (Liu and Fielding, 2011). A person is considered frail if they have three of the following: unintentional weight loss, low physical activity, slowed motor performance, weakness, and fatigue or exercise intolerance. Aerobic exercise and physical resistance training sometimes improve patients' gait speed and ability to perform ADLs (Liu and Fielding, 2011). You need to find strategies to help patients adhere to recommended exercise programs. Involve family caregivers if a patient has dementia or mental alterations.

Some patients need home care assistance after discharge. For example, nurses make referrals to home care for skilled nursing requirements when patients need ongoing wound care, IV therapy, or drain management. In addition, patients who are more physically dependent often require assistance from nursing assistive personnel to provide bathing and hygiene needs. The case coordinator or social worker at the hospital helps with discharge coordination. Encourage patients to show their discharge instructions to home care providers.

Other patients, especially older adults, sometimes require discharge to a rehabilitation or skilled nursing facility after their hospital recovery. During their convalescence patients work to gain mobility and recovery of their independent living skills. In addition, nurses provide wound care and other specialized services. A case coordinator or social worker works with the patient, family, and nurse to coordinate transfer to the skilled facility.

◆ Evaluation

Through the Patient's Eyes. Consult with a patient and family to gather evaluation data and remember that evaluation is ongoing. Ask specific questions that evaluate patient expectations and perceptions during your hourly rounds. For example you ask, "Is your pain being managed well?" "How well are you sleeping?" and "Is there anything I can for you at this time?" Evaluate your patient's level of comfort and ensure that the patient understands all aspects of nursing care. Resolve any concerns or issues and answer the patient's questions before discharge.

Patient Outcomes. Evaluate the effectiveness of your care on the basis of the patient-centered expected outcomes established after surgery for each nursing diagnosis. If a patient fails to progress as expected, revise his or her care plan on the basis of evaluation findings and the patient's needs.

Make sure to evaluate for pain relief, using a pain scale. Determine the efficacy of both pharmacological and nonpharmacological measures. Use appropriate evaluative measures; inspect the condition of a wound, monitor usage of the incentive spirometer, measure the distance or number of times that a patient is able to ambulate, and monitor the amount of fluid and food intake.

Part of your evaluation is determining the extent to which a patient and family caregiver learn self-care measures. Use the Teach Back method of patient education by having the patient restate information you taught in his or own words (Tamura-Lis, 2013). If a patient must perform any skill at home such as a dressing change or exercise, evaluate through return demonstration (see Chapter 25).

Many agencies call patients at home 24 hours after discharge to help evaluate patient outcomes. This allows you to monitor the progress of a patient's recovery and to identify the development of complications. This also allows you to evaluate and reinforce a patient's understanding of restrictions, wound care, medications, and necessary follow-up.

SAFETY GUIDELINES FOR NURSING SKILLS

Ensuring patient safety is an essential role of the professional nurse. To ensure patient safety, communicate clearly with the members of the health care team, assess and incorporate the patient's priorities of care and preferences, and use the best evidence when making decisions about your patient's care. When performing the skill in this chapter, remember the following points to ensure safe, individualized patient-centered care:

- Coughing and deep breathing is sometimes contraindicated after brain, spinal, head, neck, or eye surgery.
- Patients who are severely obese sometimes have more improved lung function and vital capacity in the reverse Trendelenburg or side-lying position.
- Report any signs of VTE such as pain, tenderness, redness, warmth, or swelling in the upper or lower extremities to the medical team immediately.

SKILL 50-1 DEMONSTRATING POSTOPERATIVE EXERCISES 

DELEGATION CONSIDERATIONS

The skill of teaching postoperative exercises cannot be delegated to nursing assistive personnel (NAP). Direct the NAP to:

- Encourage patients to practice postoperative exercises regularly following instruction.
- Inform the nurse if patient is unwilling to perform these exercises.

EQUIPMENT

- Pillow or wrapped blanket (used to splint surgical incision during coughing)
- Incentive spirometer
- Positive expiratory pressure device

STEP	RATIONALE
ASSESSMENT	
1. Identify patient using two identifiers (e.g., name and birthday or name and medical record number) according to agency policy.	Ensures correct patient. Complies with The Joint Commission standards and improves patient safety (TJC, 2016).
2. Assess patient's risk for postoperative respiratory complications. Review medical history to identify presence of chronic pulmonary conditions (e.g., emphysema, asthma), any condition that affects chest wall movement, history of smoking, and presence of reduced hemoglobin.	General anesthesia predisposes patient to respiratory problems because lungs do not inflate fully during surgery, cough reflex is suppressed, and mucus collects within airway passages. After surgery some patients have reduced lung volume and require greater efforts to cough and deep breathe; inadequate lung expansion commonly leads to atelectasis and pneumonia. Patient is at greater risk for developing respiratory complications if chronic lung conditions are present (Sifain and Papadakos, 2011). Smoking damages ciliary clearance and increases mucus. Reduced hemoglobin leads to inadequate oxygenation.
3. Auscultate lungs.	Establishes baseline for postoperative comparison.
4. Assess patient's ability to cough and deep breathe by having him or her take a deep breath and observing movement of shoulders, abdomen, and chest wall. Palpate chest excursion during deep breath. Ask patient to cough after taking deep breath.	Reveals maximum potential for chest expansion and ability to cough forcefully; serves as baseline to measure ability to perform exercises after surgery.
5. Assess patient's risk for postoperative thrombus formation (e.g., older patients, primary admitting diagnosis [e.g., trauma, orthopedic fracture, burn], patient's medical history [e.g., active cancer, atrial fibrillation, stroke, dehydration, previous clots], immobilization, women over 35 years who smoke and are taking oral contraceptives, position assumed on operating room table) (AORN, 2014).	Venous stasis, hypercoagulability, and vein trauma are the Virchow's triad for thrombus formation to occur (Lewis et al., 2014). After general anesthesia circulation slows, causing a greater tendency for clot formation. Immobilization results in decreased muscular contraction in lower extremities, which promotes venous stasis. Manipulation and positioning during surgery sometimes cause trauma to leg veins.
6. Observe calves for redness, warmth, and tenderness; swollen calf or thigh; calf swelling more than 3 cm (1.2 inches) compared with asymptomatic leg; pitting edema in symptomatic leg; and collateral superficial veins. Compare legs for bilateral equality (Lewis et al., 2014).	Signs of phlebitis and thrombus formation.

SKILL 50-1 DEMONSTRATING POSTOPERATIVE EXERCISES—cont'd

STEP	RATIONALE
CLINICAL DECISION: *If any of the signs of thrombus formation is present, notify the health care provider immediately and do not manipulate extremity further. Surgery will usually be postponed. Graduated compression stockings, intermittent pneumatic compression stockings, and/or coagulation may be ordered.*	
7. Assess patient's ability to move independently while in bed. Have patient turn, sit up in bed, and move all extremities.	Determines existence of mobility restrictions.
8. Assess patient's willingness and capability to learn exercises: note attention span, anxiety, level of consciousness, language level. Also assess family members' willingness to learn and support patient after surgery.	Determines ability of patient to learn exercises successfully. Prepares family member to encourage or coach patient in performing exercises after surgery.
9. Assess patient's medical orders before and after surgery.	Some patients require adaptations to perform exercises. In some cases certain exercises are contraindicated.
PLANNING	
1. Explain postoperative exercises to patient and family caregiver, including importance to recovery and physiological benefits.	Information allows patient to understand significance of exercises and can motivate learning. People tend to learn new skills when they know their benefits.
2. Plan exercises when patient is not in pain.	Decreased pain enhances patient's ability to practice exercises.
3. Prepare equipment and room for instruction and demonstration.	Makes environment conducive to learning.
IMPLEMENTATION	
1. Demonstrate exercises.	
a. Diaphragmatic breathing	
(1) Help patient to comfortable semi-Fowler's position or to sit on side of bed or in chair.	Upright position facilitates diaphragmatic excursion.
(2) Stand or sit facing patient.	Allows patient to observe breathing exercise.
(3) Instruct patient to place palms of hands across from one another, down and along lower borders of anterior rib cage. Place tips of fingers lightly together (see illustration). Demonstrate for patient.	Position of hands allows patient to feel movement of chest and abdomen as diaphragm descends and lungs expand.
(4) Show patient how to take slow, deep breaths, inhaling through nose and pushing abdomen against hands. Have patient feel middle fingers separate during inhalation. Explain that he or she will feel normal downward movement of diaphragm while inhaling and that abdominal organs descend and chest wall expands. Demonstrate again.	Taking slow, deep breaths prevents panting or hyperventilation. Inhaling through nose warms, humidifies, and filters air. Diaphragmatic breathing allows air to pass by, partially obstructing mucus plug, increasing force to expel mucus. Explanation and demonstration focus on normal ventilatory movement of chest wall. Patient learns how diaphragmatic breathing feels.
(5) Instruct patient to avoid using chest and shoulders while inhaling.	Using auxiliary chest and shoulder muscles during breathing wastes energy and does not promote full lung expansion.
(6) Have patient hold slow, deep breath for count of three and then slowly exhale through mouth as if blowing out a candle (through pursed lips). Demonstrate for patient. Tell patient that middle fingertips will touch as chest wall contracts during exhalation.	Pursed-lip exhalation allows for gradual expulsion of all air.
(7) Repeat complete breathing exercise 3 to 5 times.	Allows patient to observe slow, rhythmic breathing pattern. Repetition of exercise reinforces learning.
(8) Have patient practice exercise. Instruct him or her to take 10 slow, deep breaths every hour while awake during postoperative period.	Regular deep breathing prevents postoperative complications of atelectasis.

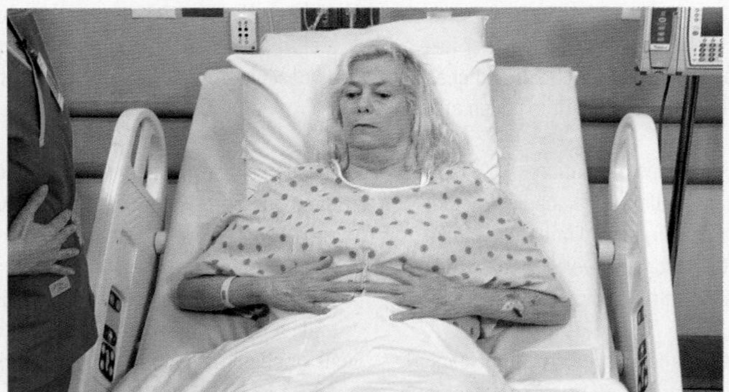

STEP 1a(3) Deep-breathing exercise—placement of hands during inhalation.

STEP	RATIONALE
b. Incentive spirometry	
(1) Perform hand hygiene.	Reduces transmission of microorganisms.
(2) Instruct patient to assume semi-Fowler's or high-Fowler's position.	Promotes optimal lung expansion during respiratory maneuver.
(3) For a patient who is severely obese, consider reverse Trendelenburg or side-lying position.	Patients who are severely obese are often able to move their diaphragm better in the reverse Trendelenburg or side-lying position than in a Fowler's position.
(4) Either set or indicate to patient on the incentive spirometer (IS) device scale the volume level to be attained with each breath (a targeted tidal volume). Use manufacturer guidelines to set volume.	Establishes goal of volume level necessary for adequate lung expansion. Package insert helps determine target on the basis of patient height and age (Pruitt, 2006).
(5) Explain to patient how to place mouthpiece of IS so lips completely cover mouthpiece (see illustration). Have patient demonstrate until position is correct.	Return demonstration is a reliable technique to validate patient's understanding of instructions, evaluate psychomotor skills, and enable patient to ask questions.
(6) Instruct patient to inhale slowly while maintaining constant flow through unit until reaching goal volume. Once maximal inspiration is reached, have patient hold breath for 2 to 3 seconds (see illustration) and exhale slowly (Davis, 2012). Ensure that number of breaths does not exceed 10 to 12 per minute.	Maintains maximal inspiration and reduces risk of progressive collapse of individual alveoli. Slow breath (less than 12 breaths/min) prevents or minimizes pain from sudden pressure changes in chest.
(7) Instruct patient to breathe normally for short period between each of the 10 breaths on IS.	Prevents hyperventilation and fatigue.
(8) Have patient repeat breaths until goals are achieved.	Ensures correct use of IS.
(9) Have patient end with two coughs after end of 10 IS breaths hourly while awake.	Cough helps with lung secretion mobilization (Pruitt, 2006).
(10) Perform hand hygiene.	Reduces transmission of microorganisms.
c. Positive expiratory pressure therapy and "huff" coughing	
(1) Perform hand hygiene.	Reduces transmission of microorganisms.
(2) Set positive expiratory pressure (PEP) device for setting ordered.	Higher settings require more ventilatory effort.
(3) Instruct patient to assume semi-Fowler's or high-Fowler's position and place nose clip on nose (see illustration).	Promotes optimum lung expansion, enabling patient to expectorate mucus. Clip prevents release of air through nose.

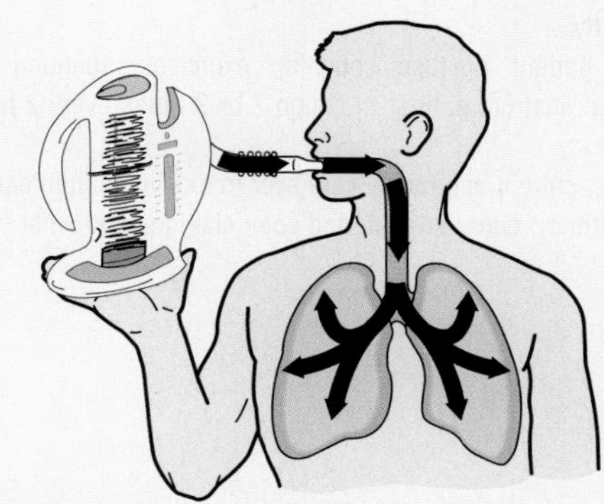

STEP 1b(6) Diagram of use of incentive spirometer.

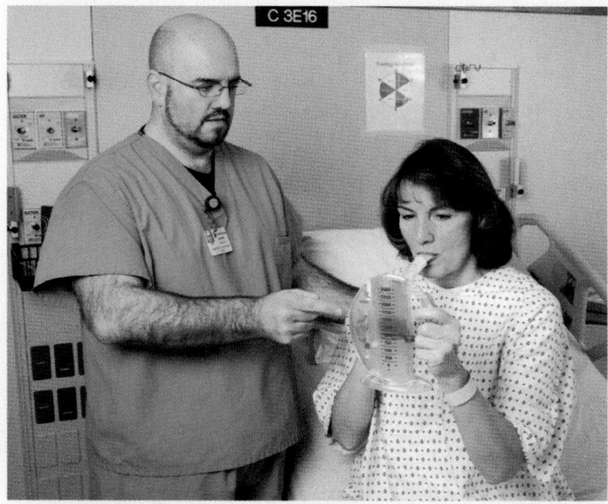

STEP 1b(5) Patient demonstrating incentive spirometry.

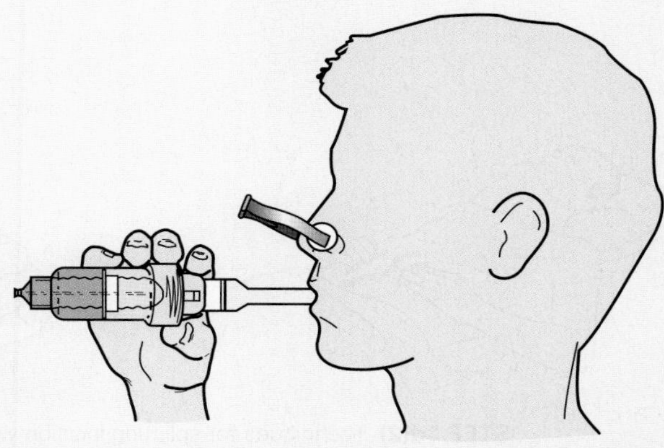

STEP 1c(3) Diagram of use of positive expiratory pressure device.

SKILL 50-1 DEMONSTRATING POSTOPERATIVE EXERCISES—cont'd

STEP	RATIONALE
(4) Instruct patient to place lips around mouthpiece or demonstrate placement. Instruct patient to take a full breath and exhale through device 2 or 3 times longer than inhalation. Repeat pattern for 10 to 20 breaths.	Ensures that patient does all breathing through mouth and uses device properly.
(5) Have patient remove device from mouth; take a slow, deep breath; and hold for 3 seconds.	Promotes lung expansion before coughing.
(6) Have patient exhale in quick, short, forced "huffs."	"Huff" coughing or forced expiratory technique promotes bronchial hygiene by increasing expectoration of secretions (Fink, 2007).
d. Controlled coughing	
(1) Explain importance of maintaining an upright semi-Fowler's or sitting position.	Position facilitates diaphragm excursion and enhances thorax expansion.
(2) If surgical incision will be either abdominal or thoracic, teach patient to place pillow (or bath blanket) over incisional area and place hands over pillow to splint incision. During breathing and coughing exercises, have patient press gently against incisional area for splinting or support (see illustration).	Surgical incision cuts through muscles, tissues, and nerve endings. Deep breathing and coughing place additional stress on suture line and cause discomfort. Splinting incision with hands or pillow provides firm support and reduces pulling.
(3) Demonstrate coughing. Instruct patient to take two slow, deep breaths, inhaling through nose and exhaling through mouth.	Deep breaths expand lungs fully so air moves behind mucus and facilitates effects of coughing.
(4) Instruct and show how to inhale deeply a third time and hold breath to count of three. Cough fully for two or three consecutive coughs without inhaling between coughs. (Tell patient to push all air out of lungs.)	Consecutive coughs help remove mucus more effectively and completely than one forceful cough.

CLINICAL DECISION: *Coughing is often contraindicated after brain, spinal, head, neck, or eye surgery because of potential increase in intracranial or intraocular pressure.*

STEP	RATIONALE
(5) Caution patient against just clearing throat instead of coughing. Explain that coughing does not cause injury to incision when done correctly.	Clearing throat does not remove mucus from deeper airways. Postoperative incisional pain makes it harder for patient to cough effectively.
(6) Have patient practice coughing exercises, splinting imaginary incision. Instruct patient to cough 2 or 3 times every 2 hours while awake.	Stresses value of deep coughing with splinting to effectively expectorate mucus with less discomfort.
(7) Instruct patient and family caregiver to look at sputum each time for consistency, odor, amount, and color changes and what to report to nurse.	Sputum characteristics indicate presence of pulmonary complication such as pneumonia.

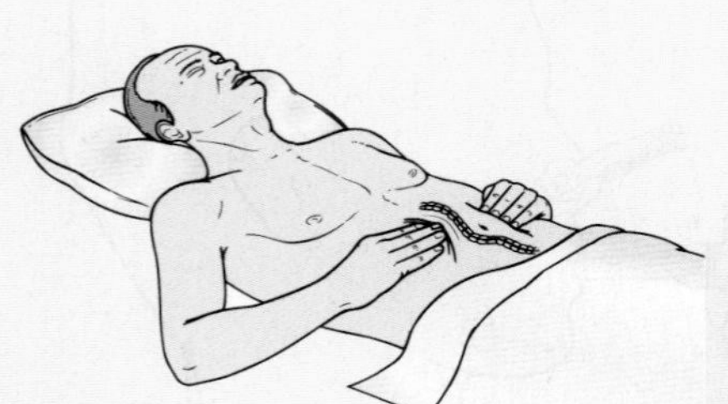
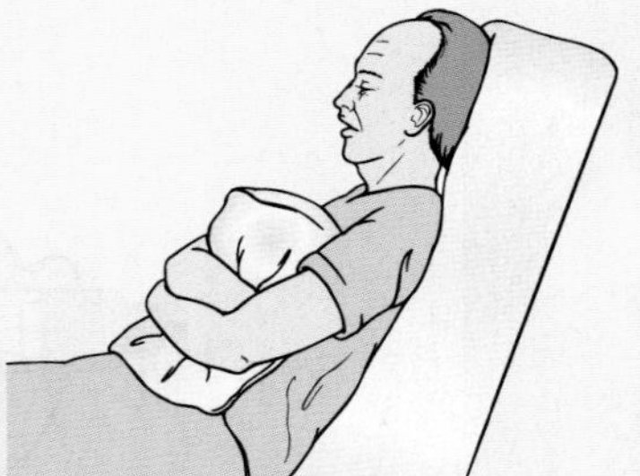
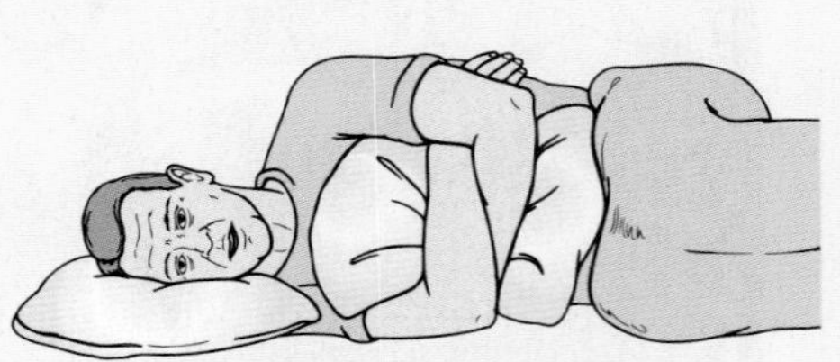

STEP 1d(2) Techniques for splinting incision when coughing. (From Lewis S et al: *Medical-surgical nursing: assessment and management of clinical problems,* ed 9, St Louis, 2014, Mosby.)

STEP	RATIONALE
e. Turning (example shows turning to right side)	
(1) Instruct patient to assume supine position and move to side of bed (in this case left side) if permitted by surgery. Instruct patient to move by bending knees and pressing heels against mattress to raise and move buttocks (see illustration). Top side rails on both sides of bed should be in up position.	Positioning begins on side of bed so turning to other side does not cause patient to roll toward edge of bed. Buttocks lift prevents shearing force from body movement against sheets. If patient bed has a turn-assist feature, use it to help positon him or her.
(2) Instruct patient to place right hand over incisional area to splint it *(optional)*	Supports and minimizes pulling on suture line during turning.
(3) Instruct patient to keep right leg straight and flex left knee up (see illustration). If back or vascular surgery was performed, patient needs to logroll (see Chapter 47) or requires assistance with turning.	Straight leg stabilizes patient's position. Flexed left leg shifts weight for easier turning.
(4) Have patient grab right side rail with left hand, pull toward right, and roll onto right side.	Pulling toward side rail reduces effort needed for turning.
(5) Instruct patient to turn every 2 hours while awake. Often patients require assistance with turning after surgery.	Reduces risk of vascular and pulmonary complications.
f. Leg exercises	
(1) Have patient assume supine position in bed. Demonstrate leg exercises by performing passive range-of-motion exercises while simultaneously explaining exercise.	Provides normal anatomical position of lower extremities.

CLINICAL DECISION: *If patient's surgery involves one or both lower extremities, surgeon must order leg exercises in postoperative period. Leg unaffected by surgery can be exercised safely unless patient has preexisting thrombosis or thrombophlebitis.*

STEP	RATIONALE
(2) Rotate each ankle in complete circle. Instruct patient to draw imaginary circles with big toe (see illustration). Repeat 5 times.	Maintains joint mobility and promotes venous return to prevent thrombi.
(3) Alternate dorsiflexion and plantar flexion of both feet. Direct patient to feel calf muscles contract and relax alternately (see illustrations *A* and *B*). Repeat 5 times.	Stretches and contracts gastrocnemius muscles, improving venous return.

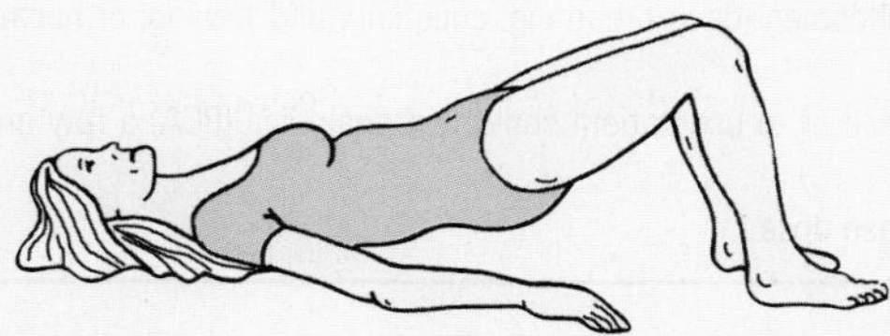

STEP 1e(1) Buttocks lift for moving to side of bed. (From Lowdermilk D, Perry SE: *Maternity and women's health care,* ed 9, St Louis, 2007, Mosby.)

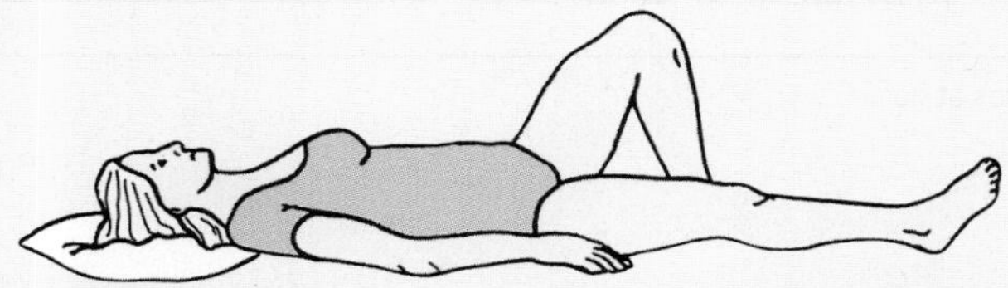

STEP 1e(3) Leg position for turning. (From Lowdermilk D, Perry SE: *Maternity and women's health care,* ed 9, St Louis, 2007, Mosby.)

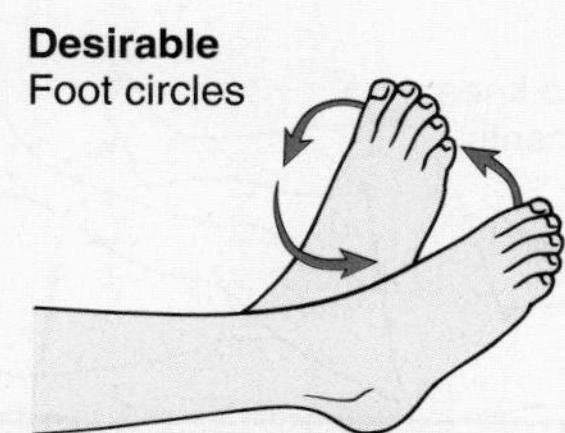

STEP 1f(2) Foot circles. (From Lewis S et al: *Medical-surgical nursing: assessment and management of clinical problems,* ed 7, St Louis, 2007, Mosby.)

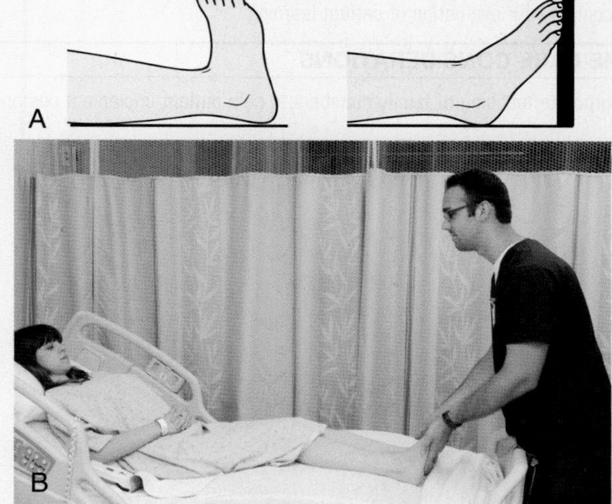

STEP 1f(3) A, Alternate dorsiflexion and plantar flexion. **B,** Patient pushes feet to perform plantar flexion. (**A** From Lewis S et al: *Medical-surgical nursing: assessment and management of clinical problems,* ed 7, St Louis, 2007, Mosby.)

SKILL 50-1 DEMONSTRATING POSTOPERATIVE EXERCISES—cont'd

STEP	RATIONALE
(4) Perform quadriceps setting by tightening thigh and bringing knee down toward mattress, then relaxing (see illustration). Repeat 5 times.	Contracts muscles of upper legs, maintains knee mobility, and enhances venous return.
(5) Have patient alternately raise each leg straight up from bed surface, keeping knees flexed; have patient bend leg at hip and knee (see illustration). Repeat 5 times.	Promotes contraction and relaxation of quadriceps muscles and prevents venous pulling. Bending reduces strain on back.
2. Have patient continue to practice exercises before surgery at least every 2 hours while awake. Teach patient to coordinate turning and leg exercises with diaphragmatic breathing, IS, and coughing exercises.	Repetition of exercise sequence reinforces learning and establishes routine for exercises that develops habit for performance. Sequence of exercises is leg exercises, turning, breathing, and coughing.

EVALUATION

STEP	RATIONALE
1. Observe patient perform all five exercises (only IS or PEP, not both) independently.	Provides opportunity for practice and return demonstration. Ensures that patient has learned correct technique.
2. Observe family member coach patient through steps of exercise.	Determines if family member can help in a positive, appropriate way.
3. After surgery measure patient's chest excursion and auscultate lungs	Determines extent of lung expansion and reveals presence of secretions or narrowed airways.
4. After surgery palpate calves gently for redness, warmth, and tenderness. Assess pedal pulses.	Absent signs and normal pulses indicate that no venous thrombosis is present.
5. Use ***Teach Back.*** State to patient, "I want to be sure that you understand why I want you to sit upright and take deep breaths every hour. Tell me how that helps you." Revise your instruction now or develop plan for revised patient teaching to be implemented at an appropriate time if patient is not able to teach back correctly.	Evaluates what patient is able to explain or demonstrate.

UNEXPECTED OUTCOMES AND RELATED INTERVENTIONS

1. Patient is unable to perform exercises correctly before surgery.
   - Assess for presence of anxiety, pain, and fatigue.
   - Repeat teaching using more demonstration or redemonstration at time when family or friends are present.
2. Patient is unwilling to perform exercises after surgery because of incisional pain of thorax or abdomen (deep breathing, coughing, and turning) or because of surgery involving lower abdomen, groin, buttocks, or legs (leg exercises, turning).
   - Instruct patient to ask for pain medication 30 minutes before performing postoperative exercise or to use patient-controlled analgesia (PCA) a few minutes before exercising.
   - Report to surgeon or pain team inadequate pain relief and need to change analgesic or increase dose.

RECORDING AND REPORTING

- Record exercises demonstrated and whether patient is able to perform them independently.
- Report any problems patient has in completing exercises to nurse assigned to patient on next shift for follow-up.
- Document your evaluation of patient learning.

HOME CARE CONSIDERATIONS

- Incorporate teaching of family members to help patient implement postoperative exercises at home.

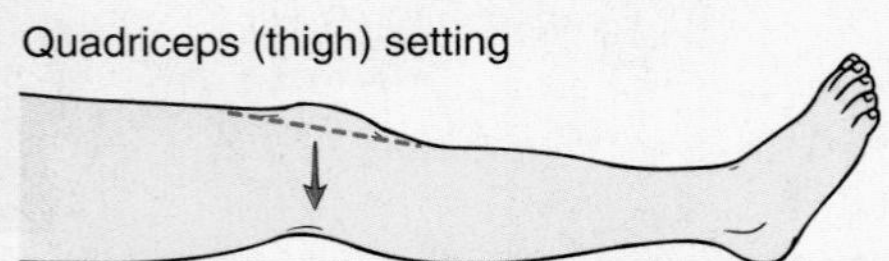

STEP 1f(4) Quadriceps (thigh) setting. (From Lewis S et al: *Medical-surgical nursing: assessment and management of clinical problems,* ed 7, St Louis, 2007, Mosby.)

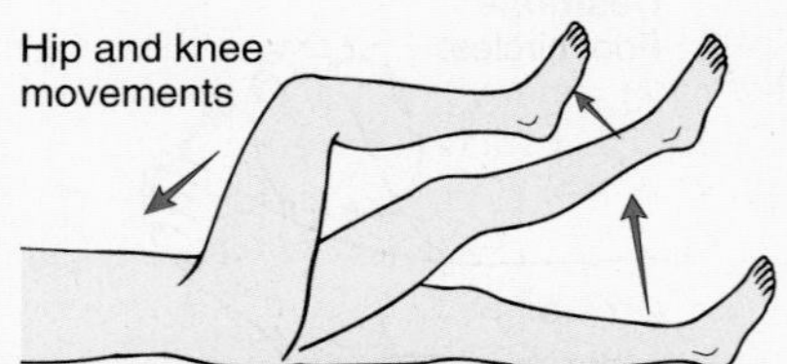

STEP 1f(5) Hip and knee movements. (From Lewis S et al: *Medical-surgical nursing: assessment and management of clinical problems,* ed 7, St Louis, 2007, Mosby.)

KEY POINTS

- The preoperative period ranges from hours to days, with some patients assessed in the health care provider's office, preadmission clinic, anesthesia clinic, or by telephone.
- The goal of the preoperative assessment is to identify a patient's normal preoperative function and the presence of any risks to recognize, prevent, and minimize possible postoperative complications.
- Physical examination of a patient before surgery focuses on findings from the patient's medical history and on body systems that the surgery is likely to affect.
- Nursing diagnoses for a surgical patient apply to nursing care during one or all phases of surgery.
- All medications taken before surgery are discontinued automatically after surgery unless a health care provider reorders the drugs.
- Having a standardized checklist or protocol for hand-off communication between perioperative health care providers minimizes risks of injuries, missed care, and errors in translating information.
- Primary responsibility for informed consent rests with a patient's surgeon.
- Preoperative patient education increases patient satisfaction and knowledge and reduces patients' preoperative anxiety, which often leads to an increase in postoperative pain, poor outcomes, and prolonged hospital stays.
- Include family members in preoperative instruction when appropriate, since a family member often is the coach for postoperative exercises when a patient returns from surgery.
- Avoid inappropriate discussions about a surgical patient's condition and do not use social media to convey information.
- The circulating nurses' responsibilities within the OR focus on protecting a patient from potential harm.
- The information obtained from OR to PACU hand-off report allows a recovery nurse to anticipate how quickly to expect a patient to regain consciousness and what his or her analgesic needs will be.
- Postoperative nursing care aims to reduce the primary causes for postoperative complications, including impaired healing of the surgical wound, the effects of prolonged immobilization during surgery and convalescence, and the influence of anesthesia and analgesics.
- Pain relief is necessary for a patient to ambulate frequently and increase participation in care activities following surgery.

CLINICAL APPLICATION QUESTIONS

Preparing for Clinical Practice

Mrs. Campana has just been transported to your surgical nursing division from the PACU. She is 80 years old and had a right colectomy (right-sided large bowel resection) for removal of a tumor. Her vital signs were stable in the PACU, and her temperature was 36.8° C (98° F). She has an intravenous (IV) line in her right arm, a Foley catheter, a nasogastric (NG) tube, and oxygen at 4 L/min per nasal cannula. She received a total of 5 mg of morphine sulfate intravenously in the PACU and now has morphine patient-controlled analgesia (PCA) with a demand dose of 1 mg every 10 minutes connected to her IV line. When you assess her, she is slow to respond to your verbal questions.

1. Why may Mrs. Campana be slow to respond?
2. What are your priority assessments at this time considering Mrs. Campana's current decreased responsiveness? What do you need to do if you discover any unexpected or abnormal assessment findings?
3. Mrs. Campana's daughter enters the room and is very concerned about her mother's slowness to awaken. What do you tell her?

ⓔ***Answers to Clinical Application Questions can be found on the Evolve website.***

REVIEW QUESTIONS

Are You Ready to Test Your Nursing Knowledge?

1. Obesity places patients at an increased surgical risk because of which of the following factors? (Select all that apply.)
   1. Risk for bleeding is increased.
   2. Ventilatory capacity is reduced.
   3. Fatty tissue has a poor blood supply.
   4. Metabolic demands are increased.
   5. Physical mobility is often impaired.
2. The primary reason that you need to include family members when you teach a patient preoperative exercises is so they can:
   1. Coach and encourage the patient after surgery.
   2. Demonstrate to the patient at home.
   3. Relieve the nurse by getting the patient to do the exercises every 2 hours.
   4. Practice with the patient while he or she is waiting to be taken to the operating room.
3. In the postanesthesia care unit (PACU) a nurse notes that a patient is having difficulty breathing and suspects an upper-airway obstruction. The nurse's priority intervention at this time is:
   1. Suction the pharynx and bronchial tree.
   2. Give oxygen through a mask at 4 L/min.
   3. Ask the patient to use an incentive spirometer.
   4. Position the patient on one side with the face down and the neck slightly extended so the tongue falls forward.
4. Because an older adult is at increased risk for respiratory complications after surgery, the nurse needs to:
   1. Withhold pain medications and ambulate the patient every 2 hours.
   2. Monitor fluid and electrolyte status every shift and vital signs with temperature every 4 hours.
   3. Orient the patient to the surrounding environment frequently and ambulate him or her every 2 hours.
   4. Encourage the patient to turn, deep breathe, and cough frequently and ensure adequate pain control.
5. You are caring for a patient after surgery who had a liver resection. His prothrombin time (PT) is greater than normal. He has low blood pressure; tachycardia; thready pulse; and cool, clammy, pale skin, and he is restless. You assess his surgical wound, and the dressing is saturated with blood. Which immediate interventions do you perform? (Select all that apply.)
   1. Notify the surgeon.
   2. Maintain intravenous (IV) fluid infusion and prepare to give volume replacement.
   3. Monitor the patient's vital signs every 15 minutes or more frequently until his condition stabilizes.
   4. Wean oxygen therapy.
   5. Provide comfort through bathing.
6. You are a nurse in the postanesthesia care unit (PACU), and you note that your patient has a heart rate of 130 beats/min and a respiratory rate of 32 breaths/min; you also assess jaw muscle rigidity and rigidity of limbs, abdomen, and chest. What do you suspect, and which intervention is indicated?
   1. *Infection:* Notify surgeon and anticipate administration of antibiotics.

2. *Pneumonia:* Listen to breath sounds, notify surgeon, and anticipate order for chest radiography.
3. *Hypertension:* Check blood pressure, notify surgeon, and anticipate administration of antihypertensives.
4. *Malignant hyperthermia:* Notify surgeon/anesthesia provider immediately, prepare to administer dantrolene sodium (Dantrium), and monitor vital signs frequently.

7. After a patient has been given preoperative sedatives, which safety precaution do you take?
    1. Reinforce to patient to remain in bed or on the stretcher
    2. Raise the side rails and keep the bed or stretcher in the high position
    3. Determine if patient has any allergies to latex
    4. Obtain informed consent immediately after sedative administration
8. The operating room (OR) and postanesthesia care unit (PACU) are high-risk environments for patients with a latex allergy. Which safety measures do nurses in these areas implement to prevent a latex reaction? (Select all that apply.)
    1. Screen patients about food allergies known to have cross-reactivity to latex.
    2. Have a latex allergy cart available at all times.
    3. Communicate with the operating room (OR) team as soon as 24 to 48 hours in advance of the surgery when a patient with latex sensitivity is identified.
    4. Schedule the patient with a latex allergy for the last operative case of the day.
    5. Plan for the patient to be admitted to a private room after surgery.
9. A nurse is recovering a patient who received conscious sedation for cosmetic surgery. Which of the following is an advantage that conscious sedation has over general anesthesia? (Select all that apply.)
    1. Loss of sensation at the surgical site
    2. Reduction of fear and anxiety
    3. Amnesia about procedure
    4. Monitoring in phase I recovery
    5. Close monitoring for airway patency
10. You are assigned to care for the following patients on your surgical unit. On the basis of the information provided, which patient do you need to see first?
    1. A 75-year-old following hip replacement surgery who is complaining of moderate pain in the surgical site, with a heart rate of 92
    2. A 57-year-old following hip replacement 6 hours earlier who is receiving intravenous patient-controlled analgesia (PCA) with a history of obstructive sleep apnea (OSA) (The pulse oximeter has been alarming and reading 85%.)
    3. A 36-year-old following bladder neck suspension who is 30 minutes late to receive her postoperative dose of antibiotic
    4. A 48-year-old following total knee replacement who needs help repositioning in bed
11. Hand-off communications that occur between the postanesthesia care unit (PACU) nurse and the nurse on the postoperative nursing unit need to be done when a patient returns to the nursing unit. Which are appropriate components of a safe and effective hand-off? (Select all that apply.)
    1. Vital signs, type of anesthesia provided, blood loss, and level of consciousness
    2. Uninterrupted time to review the recent pertinent events and ask questions
    3. Verification of the patient using one identifier and the type of surgery performed
    4. Review of pertinent events occurring in the operating room (OR) while at the nurses' station
    5. Location of patient's family members
12. A nurse is working in the preoperative holding area and is assigned to care for a patient who is having a prosthetic aortic valve placed. The nurse inserts an intravenous (IV) line and obtains vital signs. The patient has a temperature of 39° C (102° F), heart rate of 120, blood pressure (BP) of 84/50, and an elevated white blood cell (WBC) count. The nurse immediately notifies the surgeon of the patient's vital signs because:
    1. He or she needs to get the patient into the operating room (OR) quickly to start the surgery because of the low BP.
    2. The surgery may need to be delayed to recheck the patient's WBC count and investigate the source of fever before surgery.
    3. The nurse anticipates the need for a fluid bolus to increase the patient's BP.
    4. The nurse anticipates an order for a sedative to help calm the patient and decrease the heart rate.
13. A nurse is preparing to provide a patient with instructions for how to perform incentive spirometry. The patient will likely have incisional pain after returning from an elective colon resection. Which of the following steps for incentive spirometry is the patient likely to have the most difficulty performing? (Select all that apply.)
    1. Assuming semi-Fowler's or high-Fowler's position
    2. Setting the incentive spirometer device scale at the volume level to be attained
    3. Placing the mouthpiece of the incentive spirometer so lips completely cover the mouthpiece
    4. Inhaling slowly while maintaining constant flow through unit until it reaches goal volume
    5. Breathing normally for a short period between each of the 10 breaths on incentive spirometry
    6. Ending with two coughs after the end of 10 incentive spirometry breaths hourly
14. A patient is admitted through the emergency department following a motorcycle crash with multiple orthopedic injuries. He goes to surgery for repair of fractures. He is postoperative day 3 from an open-reduction internal fixation of bilateral femur fractures and external fixator to his unstable pelvic fracture. Interventions that are necessary for prevention of venous thromboembolism in this patient include: (Select all that apply.)
    1. Intermittent pneumatic compression stockings.
    2. Vitamin K therapy.
    3. Passive range-of-motion exercises every 4 hours.
    4. Subcutaneous heparin or enoxaparin (Lovenox).
    5. Continuous heparin drip with a goal of an international normalized ratio (INR) 5 times higher than baseline.
15. You are caring for a 65-year-old patient 2 days after surgery and helping him ambulate down the hallway. The surgeon ordered exercise as tolerated. Your assessment indicates that the patient's heart rate at baseline is 88. After walking approximately 30 yards down the hallway, his heart rate is 110. What is your next action?
    1. Stop exercise immediately and have him sit in a nearby chair.
    2. Ask him how he feels; determine if there is any discomfort or shortness of breath; and, if not, continue exercise.
    3. Tell him that he needs to walk further to reach a heart rate of 120.
    4. Have him walk slower; he has reached his maximum.

Answers: 1. 2, 3, 5; **2.** 1; **3.** 4; **4.** 4; **5.** 1, 2, 3; **6.** 4; **7.** 1; **8.** 1, 2, 3; **9.** 2, 3; **10.** 2; **11.** 1, 2, 5; **12.** 2; **13.** 1, 4, 6; **14.** 1, 4; **15.** 2.

Rationales for Review Questions can be found on the Evolve website.

REFERENCES

Aldrete JA: Modifications to the post anesthesia score for use in ambulatory surgery, *J Perianesth Nurs* 13(3):148, 1998.

American Association of Nurse Anesthetists (AANA): *Latex allergy management (guidelines)*, 2015, http://www.aana.com/resources2/professionalpractice/Pages/Latex-Allergy-Protocol.aspx. Accessed December 7, 2015.

American College of Chest Physicians: Methodology for the development of antithrombotic therapy and prevention of thrombosis guidelines: antithrombotic therapy and prevention of thrombosis, 9th ed: American College of Chest Physicians evidence-based clinical practice guidelines, *Chest* 141(2 Suppl):53S, 2012.

American College of Surgeons: *Surgical patient education program*, 2015, https://www.facs.org/education/patient-education. Accessed December 7, 2015.

American Society of Anesthesiologists (ASA): Practice guidelines for preoperative fasting and the use of pharmacologic agents to reduce the risk of pulmonary aspiration: application to healthy patients undergoing elective procedures: an updated report by the American Society of Anesthesiologists Committee on Standards and Practice Parameters, *Anesthesiology* 114:495, 2011.

American Society of Anesthesiologists (ASA): Practice guidelines for the perioperative management of patients with obstructive sleep apnea: an updated report by the American Society of Anesthesiologists Task Force on Perioperative Management of Patients With Obstructive Sleep Apnea, *Anesthesiology* 120(2):268, 2014.

Association of periOperative Registered Nurses (AORN): *AORN Position statement on care of the older adult in perioperative settings, AORN*, Denver, 2010, AORN. https://www.aorn.org/guidelines/clinical-resources/position-statements. Accessed December 7, 2015.

Association of periOperative Registered Nurses (AORN): *Position statement: registered nurse*, Denver, 2012, the Association.

Association of periOperative Registered Nurses (AORN): *Perioperative standards and recommended practices for inpatient and ambulatory setting*, Denver, 2014, AORN.

Association of periOperative Registered Nurses (AORN): *Guidelines for perioperative practice*, Denver, 2015, AORN.

Boat AC, Spaeth JP: Handoff checklists improve the reliability of patient handoffs in the operating room and postanesthesia care unit, *Paediatr Anaesth* 23(7):647, 2013.

Centers for Disease Control and Prevention (CDC): *Latex allergy: what's the problem?*, 2011, http://www.cdc.gov/healthcommunication/toolstemplates/entertainmented/tips/latexallergy.html. Accessed December 6, 2015.

Centers for Disease Control and Prevention (CDC): *Frequently asked questions: about surgical site infections*, 2012a, http://www.cdc.gov/HAI/pdfs/ssi/SSI_tagged.pdf. Accessed December 7, 2015.

Centers for Disease Control and Prevention (CDC): Vital signs: binge drinking prevalence, frequency, and intensity among adults—United States, 2010, *MMWR Morb Mortal Wkly Rep* 61(1):14, 2012b.

Centers for Disease Control and Prevention (CDC): *Adult obesity facts*, 2015a, CDC, http://www.cdc.gov/obesity/data/adult.html. Accessed December 7, 2015.

Centers for Disease Control and Prevention (CDC): *Childhood obesity facts*, 2015b, CDC, http://www.cdc.gov/obesity/data/childhood.html. Accessed December 7, 2015.

Centers for Medicare and Medicaid Services (CMS): *Adverse events in hospitals: public disclosure of information about events*, Washington, DC, 2010, Office of Inspector General, http://oig.hhs.gov/oei/reports/oei-06-09-00360.pdf. Accessed December 7, 2015.

Chapin JW, Geibel J: *Malignant hyperthermia*, 2015, http://emedicine.medscape.com/article/2231150-overview#a2. Accessed December 7, 2015.

Clayton JL: Special needs of older adults undergoing surgery, *AORN J* 87(3):557, 2008.

Cleveland Clinic: *Pulse and your target heart rate*, 2015, http://my.clevelandclinic.org/services/heart/prevention/exercise/pulse-target-heart-rate. Accessed December 7, 2015.

Cleveland Clinic: *Diseases and conditions: latex allergy*, 2014, http://my.clevelandclinic.org/health/diseases_conditions/hic_Latex_Allergy. Accessed December 7, 2015.

Costantini R, et al: Controlling pain in the post-operative setting, *MA Int J Clin Pharmacol Ther* 49(2):116, 2011.

Davis S: Incentive spirometry after abdominal surgery, *Nurs Times* 108(26):22, 2012.

Dunham M: Caring for patients undergoing bariatric surgery, *Nursing* 43(10):44, 2013.

Edelman CL, Mandle CL: *Health promotion throughout the lifespan*, ed 8, St Louis, 2014, Mosby.

Fetzer SJ: Postoperative nausea and vomiting. In Schick L, Windle PE, editors: *PeriAnesthesia nursing core curriculum: preprocedure, phase I and phase II PACU nursing*, ed 3, St Louis, 2015, Elsevier.

Fink JB: Forced expiratory technique, directed cough and autogenic drainage, *Respir Care* 52(9):1210, 2007.

Galanti GA: *Caring for patients from different cultures*, ed 4, Philadelphia, 2008, University of Pennsylvania Press.

Hart SR, et al: Unintended perioperative hypothermia, *Ochsner J* 11(3):259, 2011.

Johns CD, et al: Malignant hyperthermia: a crisis response plan, *OR Manager* 28(6):18, 2012.

Kotthoff-Burrell E: Perioperative assessment of the older adult, *Try This Best Pract Nurs Care Older Adults* (SP6):1, 2012.

Lee S, et al: The effectiveness of a perioperative smoking cessation program: a randomized clinical trial, *Anesth Analg* 117(3):605, 2013.

Lehne RA: *Lehne's pharmacology for nursing care*, ed 9, St Louis, 2016.

Lewis S, et al: *Medical-surgical nursing: assessment and management of clinical problems*, ed 9, St Louis, 2014, Mosby.

Malignant Hyperthermia Association of the United States: *Managing an MH crisis*, 2015, http://www.mhaus.org/healthcare-professionals/managing-a-crisis. Accessed December 7, 2015.

Massey RL: Return of bowel sounds indicating an end of postoperative ileus: is it time to cease this long-standing nursing tradition?, *Medsurg Nurs* 21(3):146, 2012.

McCaffrey R: Make PONV prevention a priority, *OR Nurse* 1(2):39, 2007.

Meiner SE: *Gerontologic nursing*, ed 5, St Louis, 2015, Mosby.

National Quality Forum (NQF): *National voluntary consensus standards for public reporting of patient safety event information: a consensus report*, Washington, DC, 2010, NQF.

Nelson JM, Carrington JM: Transitioning the older adult in the ambulatory care setting, *AORN J* 94(4):348, 2011.

Operating Room Nurses Association of Canada (ORNAC): *Our philosophy*, 2015, https://ornac.ca/en/about-us/our-philosophy. Accessed November 30, 2015.

Pruitt B: Help your patient combat postoperative atelectasis, *Nursing* 36(5):64, 2006.

Reitman E, Flood P: Anaesthetic considerations for non-obstetric surgery during pregnancy, *Br J Anaesth* 107(Suppl 1):i72, 2011.

Rothrock JC: *Alexander's care of the patient in surgery*, ed 15, St Louis, 2015, Mosby.

Sifain A, Papadakos PJ: Pump lungs: the conundrum of cardiopulmonary bypass, *Can J Respir Ther* 47(3):29, 2011.

Stuart RH, et al: Unintended perioperative hypothermia, *Oschner J* 11(3):259, 2011.

Tamura-Lis W: Teach-Back for quality education and patient safety, *Urol Nurs* 33(6):267, 2013.

The Joint Commission (TJC): *Advancing effective communication, cultural competence, and patient-and-family-centered care: a roadmap for hospitals*, 2014, http://www.jointcommission.org/topics/health_equity.aspx. Accessed December 7, 2015.

The Joint Commission (TJC): *Accountability measure list*, 2015, http://www.jointcommission.org/assets/1/18/ACCOUNTABILITYMEASURESList_2014_May2015.pdf. Accessed December 7, 2015.

The Joint Commission (TJC): *2016 National Patient Safety Goals*, Oakbrook Terrace, IL, 2016, The Commission. Available at http://www.jointcommission.org/standards_information/npsgs.aspx. Accessed November 2015.

Williams B: Supporting self-care of patients following general abdominal surgery, *J Clin Nurs* 17(5):584, 2008.

RESEARCH REFERENCES

Alanazi AA: Reducing anxiety in preoperative patients: a systematic review, *Br J Nurs* 23(7):387, 2014.

Askarpour ST, et al: Study of the effect of early feeding, chewing gums, and laxative on ileus in patients who underwent open cholecystectomy, *Internet J Surg* 22(2):2010.

Awad S, Lobo DN: What's new in perioperative nutritional support? *Curr Opin Anesthesiol* 24(3):339, 2011.

Bulfone G, et al: A longitudinal study of the incidence of pressure sores and the associated risks and strategies adopted in Italian operating theatres, *J Perioper Pract* 22(2):50, 2012.

Chung F, et al: Predictive performance of the STOP-BANG score for identifying obstructive sleep apnea in obese patients, *Obes Surg* 23(12):2050, 2013.

Douketis JD, et al: Perioperative management of antithrombotic therapy: antithrombotic therapy and prevention of thrombosis, ed 9, American College of Chest Physicians Evidence-Based Clinical Practice Guidelines, *Chest* 141(Suppl 2):e326S, 2012.

Dumville JC, et al: Preoperative skin antiseptics for preventing surgical wound infections after clean surgery, *Cochrane Database Syst Rev* (3):CD003949, 2013.

Fearon KC, Luff R: The nutritional management of surgical patients: enhanced recovery after surgery, *Proc Nutr Soc* 62(4):807, 2003.

Gärtner R, et al: Recovery at the postanaesthetic care unit after breast cancer surgery, *Dan Med Bull* 57(2):A4137, 2010.

Giakoumidakis K, et al: Effects of intensive glycemic control on outcomes of cardiac surgery, *Heart Lung* 42(2):146, 2013.

Goodnough LT, et al: Detection, evaluation, and management of preoperative anaemia in the elective orthopaedic surgical patient: NATA guidelines, *Br J Anaesth* 106(1):13, 2011.

Gould ML, et al: Prevention of VTE in nonorthopedic surgical patients: antithrombotic therapy and prevention of thrombosis, ed 9, American College of Chest Physicians Evidence-Based Clinical Practice Guidelines, *Chest* 141(Suppl 2):e227S, 2012.

Grawe JS, et al: Impact of preoperative patient education on postoperative pain in consideration of the individual coping style, *Der Schmerz* 24(6):575, 2010.

Haufler K, Harrington M: Using nurse-to-patient telephone calls to reduce day-of-surgery cancellations, *AORN J* 94(1):19, 2011.

Hazem ESM, Mokbel EM: Postoperative analgesia after major abdominal surgery: fentanyl-bupivacaine patient–controlled epidural analgesia versus fentanyl patient–controlled intravenous analgesia, *Egyptian J Anesth* 30(4):393, 2014.

Jang SY, et al: First flatus time and xerostomia associated with gum-chewing after liver resection, *J Clin Nurs* 21(15):2188, 2012.

Kapoor R, et al: Comparison of two instruments for assessing risk of postoperative nausea and vomiting, *Am J Health Syst Pharm* 65(5):448, 2008.

Kehlet H, Wilmore DW: Evidence-based surgical care and the evolution of fast-track surgery, *Ann Surg* 248(2):189, 2008.

Kobelt P, et al: Evaluation of a standardized sedation assessment for opioid administration in the postanesthesia care unit, *Pain Manag Nurs* 15(3):672, 2014.

Kovac A: Update on the management of postoperative nausea and vomiting, *Drugs* 73(14):1525, 2013.

Kwon S, et al: Importance of perioperative glycemic control in general surgery: a report from the Surgical Care and Outcomes Assessment Program, *Ann Surg* 257(1):8, 2013.

Landis EM: Micro-injection studies of capillary blood pressure in human skin, *Heart* 15:209, 1930.

Lipshutz AKM, Gropper MA: Perioperative glycemic control an evidence-based review, *Anesthesiology* 110:408, 2009.

Liu CK, Fielding RA: Exercise as an intervention for frailty, *Clin Geriatr Med* 27(1):101, 2011.

Lockhart EM, et al: Obstructive sleep apnea screening and postoperative mortality in a large surgical cohort, *Sleep Med* 14(5):407, 2013.

Madsen D, et al: Listening to bowel sounds: an evidence-based practice project, *Am J Nurs* 105(12):40, 2005.

Marwah S, et al: Role of gum chewing on the duration of postoperative ileus following ileostomy closure done for typhoid ileal perforation: a prospective randomized trial, *Saudi J Gastroenterol* 18(2):111, 2012.

Mira JJ, et al: Predictors of patient satisfaction in surgery, *Surgery* 145(5):536, 2009.

National Institute for Health and Care Excellence (NICE): *Venous thromboembolism: reducing the risk for patients in hospital,* 2010, http://www.nice.org.uk/guidance/cg92/chapter/1-recommendations. Accessed December 7, 2015.

Olrich T, et al: Hourly rounding: a replication study, *Medsurg Nurs* 21(1):23, 2012.

Paice J, et al: Efficacy and safety of scheduled dosing of opioid analgesics: a quality improvement study, *J Pain* 6(10):639, 2005.

Partridge JSL, et al: Frailty in the older surgical patient: a review, *Age Ageing* 41(2):142, 2012.

Petrovic MA, et al: Pilot implementation of a perioperative protocol to guide operating room–to–intensive care unit patient hand-offs, *J Cardiothorac Vasc Anesth* 26(1):11, 2012.

Ronco M, et al: Patient education outcomes in surgery: a systematic review from 2004-2010, *Int J Evid Based Healthc* 10(4):309, 2012.

Seamon MJ, et al: The effects of intraoperative hypothermia on surgical site infection: an analysis of 524 trauma laparotomies, *Ann Surg* 255(4):789, 2012.

Simpson L, et al: High prevalence of undiagnosed obstructive sleep apnoea in the general population and methods for screening for representative controls, *Sleep Breath* 17(3):967, 2013.

Tocher JM: Expectations and experiences of open abdominal aortic aneurysm repair patients: a mixed methods study, *J Clin Nurs* 23(3/4):421, 2014.

Williams S, et al: Dynamic measurement of human capillary blood pressure, *Clin Sci (Lond)* 74(5):507, 1988.

Willson M, et al: Nursing interventions to decrease the risk of catheter-associated urinary tract infection. Part 2: Staff education, monitoring and care techniques, *J Wound Ostomy Cont Nurs* 36(2):137, 2009.

GLOSSARY

A

abduction Movement of a limb away from the body.

abrasion Scraping or rubbing away of epidermis; may result in localized bleeding and later weeping of serous fluid.

absorption Passage of drug molecules into the blood. Factors influencing drug absorption include route of administration, ability of the drug to dissolve, and conditions at the site of absorption.

acceptance Fifth stage of Kübler-Ross's stages of grief and dying. An individual comes to terms with a loss rather than submitting to resignation and hopelessness.

accessory muscles Muscles in the thoracic cage that assist with respiration.

accommodation Process of responding to the environment through new activity, thinking, and changing the existing schema or developing a new schema to deal with the new information. For example, a toddler whose parent consistently corrects him when he calls a horse a "doggie" accommodates and forms a new schema for horses.

accountability State of being answerable for one's actions—a nurse answers to himself or herself, the patient, the profession, the employing institution such as a hospital, and society for the effectiveness of nursing care performed.

accreditation Process whereby a professional association or nongovernmental agency grants recognition to a school or institution for demonstrated ability to meet predetermined criteria.

acculturation Process of adapting to and adopting a new culture.

acne Inflammatory, papulopustular skin eruption, usually occurring on the face, neck, shoulders, and upper back.

acromegaly Chronic metabolic condition caused by overproduction of growth hormone and characterized by gradual, marked enlargement and elongation of bones of the face, jaw, and extremities.

active listening Listening attentively with the whole person—mind, body, and spirit. It includes listening for main and supportive ideas; acknowledging and responding; giving appropriate feedback; and paying attention to the other person's total communication, including the content, intent, and feelings expressed.

active range-of-motion (ROM) exercise Exercise to the joint by the patient while doing activities of daily living or during joint assessment.

active strategies of health promotion Activities that depend on the patient's motivation to adopt a specific health program.

active transport Movement of materials across the cell membrane from lesser concentration to greater concentration by enzymes and energy that allows the cell to admit larger molecules than would otherwise be possible.

activities of daily living (ADLs) Activities usually performed in the course of a normal day in the patient's life such as eating, dressing, bathing, brushing the teeth, or grooming.

activity tolerance Kind or amount of exercise or work that a person is able to perform.

actual loss Loss of an object, person, body part or function, or emotion that is overt and easily identifiable.

acuity recording Mechanism by which entries describing patient care activities are made over a 24-hour period. The activities are then translated into a rating score, or acuity score, that allows for a comparison of patients who vary by severity of illness.

acute care Pattern of health care in which a patient is treated for an acute episode of illness, for the sequelae of an accident or other trauma, or during recovery from surgery.

acute illness Illness characterized by symptoms that are of relatively short duration, are usually severe, and affect the functioning of the patient in all dimensions.

adduction Movement of a limb toward the body.

adolescence Period in development between the onset of puberty and adulthood. It usually begins between 11 and 13 years of age.

adult day care centers Facility for the supervised care of older adults; provides activities such as meals and socialization during specified day hours.

advanced practice registered nurse (APRN) Generally the most independently functioning nurse. An APRN has a master's degree in nursing, advanced education in pathophysiology, pharmacology, and physical assessment; and certification and expertise in a specialized area of practice.

advanced sleep phase syndrome Common in older adults; a disturbance in sleep manifested by early waking in the morning with an inability to get back to sleep. It is thought that this syndrome is caused by advancing of the circadian rhythm of the body.

adventitious sounds Abnormal lung sounds heard with auscultation.

adverse effect Harmful or unintended effect of a medication, diagnostic test, or therapeutic intervention.

adverse reaction Any harmful, unintended effect of a medication, diagnostic test, or therapeutic intervention.

advocacy Process whereby a nurse objectively provides patients with the information they need to make decisions and supports the patients in whatever decisions they make.

afebrile Without fever.

affective learning Acquisition of behaviors involved in expressing feelings about attitudes, appreciation, and values.

afterload Resistance to left ventricular ejection; the work the heart must overcome to fully eject blood from the left ventricle.

age-related macular degeneration Progressive disorder in which the macula (the specialized portion of the retina responsible for central vision) degenerates as a result of aging and loses its ability to function efficiently. First signs include blurring of reading matter, distortion or loss of central vision, sensitivity to glare, and distortion of objects.

agnostic Individual who believes that any ultimate reality is unknown or unknowable.

airborne precautions Safeguards designed to reduce the risk of transmission of infectious agents through the air that a person breathes.

alarm reaction Mobilization of the defense mechanisms of the body and mind to cope with a stressor; the initial stage of the general adaptation syndrome.

aldosterone Mineralocorticoid steroid hormone produced by the adrenal cortex with action in the renal tubule to regulate sodium and potassium balance in the blood.

allergic reactions Unfavorable physiological response to an allergen to which a person has previously been exposed and has developed antibodies.

alopecia Partial or complete loss of hair; baldness.

Alzheimer's disease Disease of the brain parenchyma that causes a gradual and progressive decline in cognitive functioning.

AMBULARM Device used for the patient who climbs out of bed unassisted and is in danger of falling. This device is worn on the leg and signals when the leg is in a dependent position such as over the side rail or on the floor.

amino acid Organic compound of one or more basic groups and one or more carboxyl groups. Amino acids are the building blocks that construct proteins and the end products of protein digestion.

anabolism Constructive metabolism characterized by conversion of simple substances into more complex compounds of living matter.

analgesic Relieving pain; drug that relieves pain.

analogies Resemblances made between things otherwise unlike.

anaphylactic reactions Hypersensitive condition induced by contact with certain antigens.

aneurysm Localized dilations of the wall of a blood vessel; usually caused by atherosclerosis, hypertension, or a congenital weakness in a vessel wall.

anger Second stage of Kübler-Ross's stages of grief and dying. During this stage an individual resists loss by expressing extreme displeasure, indignation, or hostility.

angiotensin Polypeptide occurring in the blood, causing vasoconstriction, increased blood pressure, and the release of aldosterone from the adrenal cortex.

anion gap Difference between the concentrations of serum cations and anions; determined by measuring the concentrations of sodium cations and chloride and bicarbonate anions.

anions Negatively charged electrolytes.

anthropometric measurements Body measures of height, weight, and skinfolds to evaluate muscle atrophy.

anthropometry Measurement of various body parts to determine nutritional and caloric status, muscular development, brain growth, and other parameters.

antibodies Immunoglobulins essential to the immune system that are produced by lymphoid tissue in response to bacteria, viruses, or other antigens.

anticipatory grief Grief response in which the person begins the grieving process before an actual loss.

antidiuretic hormone (ADH) Hormone that decreases the production of urine by increasing the resorption of water by the renal tubules. ADH is secreted by cells of the hypothalamus and stored in the posterior lobe of the pituitary gland.

antiembolic stockings Elasticized stockings that prevent formation of emboli and thrombi, especially after surgery or during bed rest.

antigen Substance, usually a protein, that causes the formation of an antibody and reacts specifically with that antibody.

antipyretic Substance or procedure that reduces fever.

anxiolytics Drugs used primarily to treat episodes of anxiety.

aphasia Abnormal neurological condition in which language function is defective or absent; related to injury to speech center in cerebral cortex, causing receptive or expressive aphasia.

apical pulse Heartbeat as listened to with the bell or diaphragm of a stethoscope placed on the apex of the heart.

apnea Absence of respirations for a period of time.

apothecary system System of measurement. The basic unit of weight is a grain. Weights derived from the grain are the gram, ounce, and pound. The basic measure for fluid is the minim. The fluidram, fluid ounce, pint, quart, and gallon are measures derived from the minim.

approximate To come close together, as in the edges of a wound.

arcus senilis Opaque ring, gray to white in color, that surrounds the periphery of the cornea. The condition is caused by deposits of fat granules in the cornea. Occurs primarily in older adults.

asepsis Absence of germs or microorganisms.

aseptic technique Any health care procedure in which added precautions are used to prevent contamination of a person, object, or area by microorganisms.

assault Unlawful threat to bring about harmful or offensive contact with another.

assertive communication Type of communication based on a philosophy of protecting individual rights and responsibilities. It includes the ability to be self-directive in acting to accomplish goals and advocate for others.

assessment First step of the nursing process. Activities required in the first step are data collection, validation, sorting, and documentation. The purpose is to gather information for health problem identification.

assimilation To become absorbed into another culture and adopt its characteristics.

assisted living Residential living facilities in which each resident has his or her own room and shares dining and social activity areas.

associative play Form of play in which a group of children participates in similar or identical activities without formal organization, direction, interaction, or goals.

atelectasis Collapse of alveoli, preventing the normal respiratory exchange of oxygen and carbon dioxide.

atheist Individual who does not believe in the existence of God.

atherosclerosis Common arterial disorder characterized by yellowish plaques of cholesterol, lipids, and cellular debris in the inner layers of the walls of the large- and medium-size arteries.

atrioventricular (AV) node Part of the cardiac conduction system located on the floor of the right atrium; receives electrical impulses from the atrium and transmits them to the bundle of His.

atrophied Wasted or reduced size or physiological activity of a part of the body caused by disease or other influences.

attachment Initial psychosocial relationship that develops between parents and the neonate.

attentional set Internal state of the learner that allows focusing and comprehension.

auditory Related to or experienced through hearing.

auscultation Method of physical examination; listening to the sounds produced by the body, usually with a stethoscope.

auscultatory gap Disappearance of sound when obtaining a blood pressure; typically occurs between the first and second Korotkoff sounds.

authority Right to act in areas in which an individual has been given and accepts responsibility.

autologous transfusion Procedure in which blood is removed from a donor and stored for a variable period before it is returned to the donor's own circulation.

autonomy Ability or tendency to function independently.

B

back-channeling Active listening technique that prompts a respondent to continue telling a story or describing a situation. Involves use of phrases such as "Go on," "Uh huh," and "Tell me more."

bacteriuria Presence of bacteria in the urine.

balance Position in which the person's center of gravity is correctly positioned so falling does not occur.

bandages Available in rolls of various widths and materials, including gauze, elasticized knit, elastic webbing, flannel, and muslin. Gauze bandages are lightweight and inexpensive, mold easily around contours of the body, and permit air circulation to underlying skin to prevent maceration. Elastic bandages conform well to body parts but can also be used to exert pressure over a body part.

bargaining Third stage of Kübler-Ross's stages of grief and dying. A person postpones the reality of a loss by attempting to make deals in a subtle or overt manner with others or with a higher being.

baridi Condition among the Bena people of Tanzania attributed to disrespectful behavior within the family or transgression of cultural taboos. The person experiences physical and psychological symptoms and is usually treated by a traditional healer, who has the person make a public admission or an apology or who treats the person with herbal remedies.

basal cell carcinoma Malignant epithelial cell tumor that begins as a papule and enlarges peripherally, developing a central crater that erodes, crusts, and bleeds. Metastasis is rare.

basal metabolic rate (BMR) Amount of energy used in a unit of time by a fasting, resting subject to maintain vital functions.

battery Legal term for touching another's body without consent.

bed boards Boards placed under the mattress of a bed that provide extra support to the mattress surface.

bed rest Placement of the patient in bed for therapeutic reasons for a prescribed period.

benchmarking Identifying best practices and comparing them to current organizational practices to improve performance. This process helps to support the claims of quality care delivery by the institution.

beneficence Doing good or actively promoting doing good; one of the four principles of the ethical theory of deontology.

benign breast disease (fibrocystic) Benign condition characterized by lumpy, painful breasts and sometimes nipple discharge. Symptoms are more apparent before the menstrual period. Known to be a risk factor for breast cancer.

bereavement Response to loss through death; a subjective experience that a person suffers after losing a person with whom there has been a significant relationship.

biases and prejudices Beliefs and attitudes associating negative permanent characteristics to people who are perceived as different from oneself.

bi-level positive airway pressure (BiPAP) Ventilatory support used to treat patients with obstructive sleep apnea, patients with congestive heart failure, and preterm infants with underdeveloped lungs.

bilineally Kinship that extends to both the mother's and father's sides of the family.

binders Bandages made of large pieces of material to fit specific body parts.

bioethics Branch of ethics within the field of health care.

biological clock Cyclical nature of body function. Functions controlled from within the body are synchronized with environmental factors; same meaning as biorhythm.

biological half-life Time it takes for the body to lower the amount of unchanged medication by half.
biotransformation Chemical changes that a substance undergoes in the body such as by the action of enzymes.
blanchable hyperemia Redness of the skin caused by dilation of the superficial capillaries. When pressure is applied to the skin, the area blanches, or turns a lighter color.
body image Peoples' subjective concept of their physical appearance.
body mechanics Coordinated efforts of the musculoskeletal and nervous systems to maintain proper balance, posture, and body alignment.
bone resorption Destruction of bone cells and release of calcium into the blood.
borborygmi Audible abdominal sounds produced by hyperactive intestinal peristalsis.
botanica Place that sells religious and herbal remedies.
bradycardia Slower-than-normal heart rate; heart contracts fewer than 60 times/min.
bradypnea Abnormally slow rate of breathing.
bronchospasm Excessive and prolonged contraction of the smooth muscle of the bronchi and bronchioles, resulting in an acute narrowing and obstruction of the respiratory airway.
bruit Abnormal sound or murmur heard while auscultating an organ, gland, or artery.
buccal Of or pertaining to the inside of the cheek or the gum next to the cheek.
buccal cavity Consists of the lips surrounding the opening of the mouth, the cheeks running along the side walls of the cavity, the tongue and its muscles, and the hard and soft palate.
buffer Substance or group of substances that can absorb or release hydrogen ions to correct an acid-base imbalance.
bundle of His Part of the cardiac conduction system that arises from the distal portion of the atrioventricular (AV) node and extends across the AV groove to the top of the intraventricular septum, where it divides into right and left bundle branches.

C

cachexia Malnutrition marked by weakness and emaciation, usually associated with severe illness.
capitation Payment mechanism in which a provider (e.g., health care network) receives a fixed amount of payment per enrollee.
capnography Also known as end titled CO_2 monitoring, it provides instant information about how effectively CO_2 is eliminated by the pulmonary system, how effectively it is transported through the vascular system, and how effectively CO_2 is produced by cellular metabolism. Capnography is measured near the end of exhalation.
carbohydrates Dietary classification of foods comprising sugars, starches, cellulose, and gum.
carbon monoxide Colorless, odorless, poisonous gas produced by the combustion of carbon or organic fuels.
cardiac index Adequacy of the cardiac output for an individual. It takes into account the body surface area (BSA) of the patient.
cardiac output (CO) Volume of blood expelled by the ventricles of the heart, equal to the amount of blood ejected at each beat multiplied by the number of beats in the period of time used for computation (usually 1 minute).
cardiopulmonary rehabilitation Actively assisting the patient with achieving and maintaining an optimal level of health through controlled physical exercise, nutrition counseling, relaxation and stress management techniques, prescribed medications and oxygen, and compliance.
cardiopulmonary resuscitation (CPR) Basic emergency procedures for life support consisting of artificial respiration and manual external cardiac massage.
care To feel concern for or interest in one who has sorrow or difficulties.
caring Universal phenomenon that influences the way we think, feel, and behave in relation to one another.
carriers People or animals who harbor and spread an organism that causes disease in others but do not become ill themselves.
case management Organized system for delivering health care to an individual patient or group of patients across an episode of illness and/or a continuum of care; includes assessment and development of a plan of care, coordination of all services, referral, and follow-up; usually assigned to one professional.
case management plan Multidisciplinary model for documenting patient care that usually includes plans for problems, key interventions, and expected outcomes for patients with a specific disease or condition.
catabolism Breakdown of body tissue into simpler substances.
cataplexy Condition characterized by sudden muscular weakness and loss of muscle tone.
cataracts Abnormal progressive condition of the lens of the eye characterized by loss of transparency.
cathartics Drugs that act to promote bowel evacuation.
catheterization Introduction of a catheter into a body cavity or organ to inject or remove fluid.
cations Positively charged electrolytes.
center of gravity Midpoint or center of the weight of a body or object.
centigrade Denotes temperature scale in which 0° is the freezing point of water and 100° is the boiling point of water at sea level; also called Celsius.
cerumen Yellowish or brownish waxy secretion produced by sweat glands in the external ear.
chancres Skin lesions or venereal sores (usually primary syphilis) that begin at the site of infection as papules and develop into red, bloodless, painless ulcers with a scooped-out appearance.
change-of-shift report Report that occurs between two scheduled nursing work shifts. Nurses communicate information about their assigned patients to nurses working on the next shift of duty.
channel Method used in the teaching-learning process to present content: visual, auditory, taste, smell. In the communication process a method used to transmit a message: visual, auditory, touch.
charting by exception (CBE) Charting methodology in which data are entered only when there is an exception from that which is normal or expected; reduces time spent documenting in charting. It is a shorthand method for documenting normal findings and routine care.
chest percussion Striking the chest wall with a cupped hand to promote mobilization and drainage of pulmonary secretions.
chest physiotherapy (CPT) Group of therapies used to mobilize pulmonary secretions for expectoration.
chest tube Catheter inserted through the thorax into the chest cavity for removing air or fluid; used after chest or heart surgery or pneumothorax.
Cheyne-Stokes respiration Occurs when there is decreased blood flow or injury to the brainstem.
chronic illness Illness that persists over a long time and affects physical, emotional, intellectual, social, and spiritual functioning.
circadian rhythm Repetition of certain physiological phenomena within a 24-hour cycle.
circular transactional communication process Communication model that enhances the linear communication by enabling the sender and receiver to view perceptions, attitudes, and potential reactions of others via a mental picture. This is a continuous and interactive activity.
circulating nurse Assistant to the scrub nurse and surgeon whose role is to provide necessary supplies; dispose of soiled instruments and supplies; and keep an accurate count of instruments, needles, and sponges used.
civil law Statutes concerned with protecting a person's rights.
climacteric Physiological, developmental change that occurs in the male reproductive system between the ages of 45 and 60.
clinical criteria Objective or subjective signs and symptoms, clusters of signs and symptoms, or risk factors.
clinical decision making Problem-solving approach that nurses use to define patient problems and select appropriate treatment.
clinical-decision support systems Computerized programs used within the health care setting to support decision-making.
Clinical Information System (CIS) A computer-based system that collects, stores, and manipulates data to allow health care providers to make informed decisions about patient care.
closed-ended question Form of question that limits a respondent's answer to one or two words.
clubbing Bulging of the tissues at the nail base caused by insufficient oxygenation at the periphery, resulting from conditions such as chronic emphysema and congenital heart disease.

code of ethics Formal statement that delineates a profession's guidelines for ethical behavior. A code of ethics sets standards or expectations for the professional to achieve.

cognitive learning Acquisition of intellectual skills that encompass behaviors such as thinking, understanding, and evaluating.

collaborative interventions Therapies that require the knowledge, skill, and expertise of multiple health care professionals.

collaborative problem Physiological complication that requires the nurse to use nursing- and health care provider–prescribed interventions to maximize patient outcomes.

colloid osmotic pressure Abnormal condition of the kidney caused by the pressure of concentrations of large particles such as protein molecules that will pass through a membrane.

colon Portion of the large intestine from the cecum to the rectum.

colonization Presence and multiplication of microorganisms without tissue invasion or damage.

comforting Acts toward another individual that display both an emotional and physical calm. The use of touch, establishing presence, the therapeutic use of silence, and the skillful and gentle performance of a procedure are examples of comforting nursing measures.

common law One source for law that is created by judicial decisions as opposed to those created by legislative bodies (statutory law).

communicable disease Any disease that can be transmitted from one person or animal to another by direct or indirect contact or by vectors.

communication Ongoing, dynamic series of events that involves the transmission of meaning from sender to receiver.

community health nursing Nursing approach that combines knowledge from the public health sciences with professional nursing theories to safeguard and improve the health of populations in the community.

community-based nursing Acute and chronic care of individuals and families to strengthen their capacity for self-care and promote independence in decision making.

comorbidity A chronic, long term condition existing simultaneously with and usually independently of another medical condition.

compassion The feeling that arises when a person is confronted with another's suffering and feels motivated to relieve that suffering. Compassion shows kindness, caring, and a willingness to help others.

competence Specific range of skills necessary to perform a task.

complete bed bath Bath in which the entire body of a patient is washed in bed.

compress Soft pad of gauze or cloth used to apply heat, cold, or medications to the surface of a body part.

computer-based patient record Comprehensive computerized system used by all health care practitioners to permanently store information pertaining to a patient's health status, clinical problems, and functional abilities.

concentration Relative content of a component within a substance or solution.

concentration gradient Gradient that exists across a membrane, separating a high concentration of a particular ion from a low concentration of the same ion.

concept map Care-planning tool that assists in critical thinking and forming associations between a patient's nursing diagnoses and interventions.

confianza Trust.

confidentiality Act of keeping information private or secret; in health care the nurse only shares information about a patient with other nurses or health care providers who need to know private information about a patient to provide care for him or her; information can only be shared with the patient's consent.

conjunctivitis Highly contagious eye infection. The crusty drainage that collects on eyelid margins can easily spread from one eye to the other.

connectedness Having close spiritual relationships with oneself, others, and God or another spiritual being.

connotative meaning Shade or interpretation of the meaning of a word influenced by the thoughts, feelings, or ideas that people have about the word.

conscious sedation Administration of central nervous system–depressant drugs and/or analgesics to provide analgesia, relieve anxiety, and/or provide amnesia during surgical, diagnostic, or interventional procedures.

constipation Condition characterized by difficulty in passing stool or an infrequent passage of hard stool.

consultation Process in which the help of a specialist is sought to identify ways to handle problems in patient management or in planning and implementing programs.

contact precautions Safeguards designed to reduce the risk of transmission of epidemiologically important microorganisms by direct or indirect contact.

continent urinary diversion (CUR) Surgical diversion of the drainage of urine from a diseased or dysfunctional bladder. Patient uses a catheter to drain the pouch.

continuous positive airway pressure (CPAP) Ventilatory support used to treat patients with obstructive sleep apnea, patients with congestive heart failure, and preterm infants with under developed lungs.

convalescence Period of recovery after an illness, injury, or surgery.

coping Making an effort to manage psychological stress.

core temperature Temperature of deep structures of the body.

cough Sudden, audible expulsion of air from the lungs. The person breathes in, the glottis is partially closed, and the accessory muscles of expiration contract to expel the air forcibly.

counseling Problem-solving method used to help patients recognize and manage stress and enhance interpersonal relationships. It helps patients examine alternatives and decide which choices are most helpful and appropriate.

crackles Fine bubbling sounds heard on auscultation of the lung; produced by air entering distal airways and alveoli, which contain serous secretions.

crime Act that violates a law and that may include criminal intent.

criminal law Concerned with acts that threaten society but may involve only an individual.

crisis Transition for better or worse in the course of a disease, usually indicated by a marked change in the intensity of signs and symptoms.

crisis intervention Use of therapeutic techniques directed toward helping a patient resolve a particular and immediate problem.

critical pathways Tools used in managed care that incorporate the treatment interventions of caregivers from all disciplines who normally care for a patient. Designed for a specific care type, a pathway is used to manage the care of a patient throughout a projected length of stay.

critical period of development Specific phase or period when the presence of a function or reasoning has its greatest effect on a specific aspect of development.

critical thinking Active, purposeful, organized, cognitive process used to carefully examine one's thinking and the thinking of other individuals.

crutch gait Gait achieved by a person using crutches.

cue Information that a nurse acquires through hearing, visual observations, touch, and smell.

cultural and linguistic competence Set of congruent behaviors, attitudes, and policies that come together in a system or agency or among professionals that enables effective work in cross-cultural situations.

cultural assessment Systematic and comprehensive examination of the cultural care values, beliefs, and practices of individuals, families, and communities.

cultural awareness Gaining in-depth awareness of one's own background, stereotypes, biases, prejudices, and assumptions about other people.

cultural care accommodation or negotiation Adapting or negotiating with the patient/families to achieve beneficial or satisfying health outcomes.

cultural care preservation or maintenance Retaining and/or preserving relevant care values so patients are able to maintain their well-being, recover from illness, or face handicaps and/or death.

cultural care repatterning or restructuring Reordering, changing, or greatly modifying a patient's/family's customs for a new, different, and beneficial health care pattern.

cultural competence Process in which the health care professional continually strives to achieve the ability and availability to work effectively with individuals, families, and communities.

cultural encounters Engaging in cross-cultural interactions; refining intercultural communication skills; gaining in-depth understanding of others and avoiding stereotypes; and managing cultural conflict.

cultural imposition Using one's own values and customs as an absolute guide in interpreting behaviors.

cultural knowledge Obtaining knowledge of other cultures; gaining sensitivity to, respect for, and appreciation of differences.

cultural pain Feeling that a patient has after a health care worker disregards the patient's valued way of life.

cultural skills Communication, cultural assessment, and culturally competent care.

culturally congruent care Care that fits people's valued life patterns and sets of meanings generated from the people themselves. Sometimes this differs from the professionals' perspective on care.

culturally ignorant or blind Uneducated about other cultures.

culture Integrated patterns of human behavior that include the language, thoughts, communications, actions, customs, beliefs, values, and institutions of racial, ethnic, religious, or social groups.

culture care theory Leininger's theory that emphasizes culturally congruent care.

culture-bound syndromes Illnesses restricted to a particular culture or group because of its psychosocial characteristics.

culturological nursing assessment Systematic and comprehensive examination of the cultural care values, beliefs, and practices of individuals, families, and communities.

cutaneous stimulation Stimulation of a person's skin to prevent or reduce pain perception. A massage, warm bath, hot and cold therapies, and transcutaneous electrical nerve stimulation are some ways to reduce pain perception.

cyanosis Bluish discoloration of the skin and mucous membranes caused by an excess of deoxygenated hemoglobin in the blood or a structural defect in the hemoglobin molecule.

D

DAR (data, action, patient response) Format used in focus charting for recording patient information.

data analysis Logical examination of and professional judgment about patient assessment data; used in the diagnostic process to derive a nursing diagnosis.

data cluster Set of signs or symptoms that are grouped together in logical order.

database Store or bank of information, especially in a form that can be processed by computer.

debridement Removal of dead tissue from a wound.

decentralized management Organizational philosophy that brings decisions down to the level of the staff. Individuals best informed about a problem or issue participate in the decision-making process.

decision making Process involving critical appraisal of information that results from recognizing a problem and ends with generating, testing, and evaluating a conclusion. Comes at the end of critical thinking.

deconditioning Physiological change following a period of inactivity, bed rest or sedentary lifestyle. It results in functional losses in such areas as mental status, degree of continence and ability to accomplish activities of daily living.

defecation Passage of feces from the digestive tract through the rectum.

defendant Individual or organization against whom legal charges are brought in a court of law.

defining characteristics The observable assessment cues that cluster as manifestations of a problem focused or health promotion nursing diagnosis.

dehiscence Separation of the edges of a wound, revealing underlying tissues.

dehydration Excessive loss of water from the body tissues accompanied by a disturbance of body electrolytes.

delegation Process of assigning another member of the health care team to be responsible for aspects of patient care (e.g., assigning nurse assistants to bathe a patient).

delirium Acute state of confusion that is potentially reversible and often has a physical cause.

dementia Generalized impairment of intellectual functioning that interferes with social and occupational functioning.

denial Unconscious refusal to admit an unacceptable idea.

denotative meaning Meaning of a word shared by individuals who use a common language. The word *baseball* has the same meaning for all individuals who speak English, but the word *code* primarily denotes cardiac arrest to health care providers.

dental caries Abnormal destructive condition in a tooth caused by a complex interaction of food, especially starches and sugars, with bacteria that form dental plaque.

deontology Traditional theory of ethics that proposes to define actions as right or wrong based on the characteristics of fidelity to promises, truthfulness, and justice. The conventional use of ethical terms such as *justice, autonomy, beneficence,* and *nonmaleficence* constitutes the practice of deontology.

depression (1) Reduction in happiness and well-being that contributes to physical and social limitations and complicates the treatment of concomitant medical conditions. It is usually reversible with treatment. (2) Fourth stage of Kübler-Ross's stages of grief and dying. In this stage the person realizes the full impact and significance of the loss.

dermis Sensitive vascular layer of the skin directly below the epidermis; composed of collagenous and elastic fibrous connective tissues that give the dermis strength and elasticity.

determinants of health Many variables that influence the health status of individuals or communities.

detoxify To remove the toxic quality of a substance. The liver acts to detoxify chemicals in drug compounds.

development Qualitative or observable aspects of the progressive changes that one makes in adapting to the environment.

developmental crises Crises associated with normal and expected phases of growth and development (e.g., the response to menopause); same as maturational crises.

diabetic retinopathy Disorder of retinal blood vessels. Pathological changes secondary to increased pressure in the blood vessels of the retina result in decreased vision or vision loss caused by hemorrhage and macular edema.

diagnosis-related group (DRG) Group of patients classified to establish a mechanism for health care reimbursement based on length of stay. Classification is based on the following variables: primary and secondary diagnosis, co-morbidities, primary and secondary procedures, and age.

diagnostic process Mental steps (data clustering and analysis, problem identification) that follow assessment and lead directly to the formulation of a diagnosis.

diagnostic reasoning Process that enables an observer to assign meaning to and classify phenomena in clinical situations by integrating observations and critical thinking.

diaphoresis Secretion of sweat, especially profuse secretion associated with an elevated body temperature, physical exertion, or emotional stress.

diaphragmatic breathing Respiration in which the abdomen moves out while the diaphragm descends on inspiration.

diarrhea Increase in the number of stools and the passage of liquid, unformed feces.

diastolic Pertaining to diastole, or the blood pressure at the instant of maximum cardiac relaxation.

dietary reference intake (DRI) Information on each vitamin or mineral to reflect a range of minimum-to-maximum amounts that avert deficiency or toxicity.

diffusion Movement of molecules from an area of high concentration to one of lower concentration.

digestion Breakdown of nutrients by chewing, churning, mixing with fluid, and chemical reactions.

direct care interventions Treatments performed through interaction with the patient. For example, a patient may require medication administration, insertion of an intravenous infusion, or counseling during a time of grief.

discharge planning Activities directed toward identifying future proposed therapy and the need for additional resources before and after returning home.

discrimination Prejudicial outlook, action, or treatment.

disease Malfunctioning or maladaptation of biological or psychological processes.

disinfection Process of destroying all pathogenic organisms except spores.

disorganization and despair One of Bowlby's four phases of mourning in which an individual endlessly examines how and why the loss occurred.

distress Damaging stress; one of the two types of stress identified by Selye.

disuse osteoporosis Reductions in skeletal mass routinely accompanying immobility or paralysis.

diuresis Increased rate of formation and excretion of urine.

documentation Written entry into the patient's medical record of all pertinent information about him or her. These entries validate the patient's problems and care and exist as a legal record.

dominant culture Customs, values, beliefs, traditions, and social and religious views held by a group of people that prevail over another secondary culture.

dorsiflexion Flexion toward the back.

drainage evacuators Convenient portable units that connect to tubular drains lying within a wound bed and exert a safe, constant, low-pressure vacuum to remove and collect drainage.

droplet precautions Safeguards designed to reduce the risk of droplet transmission of infectious agents.

dysmenorrhea Painful menstruation.

dysphagia Difficulty swallowing; commonly associated with obstructive or motor disorders of the esophagus.

dyspnea Sensation of shortness of breath.

dysrhythmia Deviation from the normal pattern of the heartbeat.

dysuria Painful urination resulting from bacterial infection of the bladder and obstructive conditions of the urethra.

E

ecchymosis Discoloration of the skin or bruise caused by leakage of blood into subcutaneous tissues as a result of trauma to underlying tissues.

ectropion Eversion of the eyelid that exposes the conjunctival membrane and part of the eyeball.

edema Abnormal accumulation of fluid in interstitial spaces of tissues.

egocentric Developmental characteristic wherein a toddler is only able to assume the view of his or her own activities and needs.

electrocardiogram (ECG) Graphic record of the electrical activity of the myocardium.

electrolyte Element or compound that, when melted or dissolved in water or other solvent, dissociates into ions and can carry an electrical current.

electronic health record An electronic record of patient health information generated whenever a patient accesses medical care in any health care delivery setting.

electronic infusion device Piece of medical equipment that delivers intravenous fluids at a prescribed rate through an intravenous catheter.

electronic medical record Part of the electronic health record that contains patient data gathered in a health care setting at a specific time and place.

embolism Abnormal condition in which a blood clot (embolus) travels through the bloodstream and becomes lodged in a blood vessel.

emerging adulthood The time from adolescence to the young adult when responsibilities of a stable job, marriage and parenthood begin. It includes five features: the age of identity exploration; the age of instability, the age of self-focus, the age of feeling in between and the age of possibilities.

emotional intelligence Assessment and communication technique used to better understand and perceive emotions of themselves. This assists in building a therapeutic relationship.

empathy Understanding and acceptance of a person's feelings and the ability to sense the person's private world.

empowered Gave legal authority to or enabled an individual or group; promoted self-actualization of an individual or group.

endogenous infections Infections produced within a cell or organism.

endorphins Hormones that act on the mind such as morphine and opiates and produce a sense of well-being and reducing pain.

endotracheal tube Short-term artificial airways to administer mechanical ventilation, relieve upper airway obstruction, protect against aspiration, or clear secretions.

enema Procedure involving introduction of a solution into the rectum for cleansing or therapeutic purposes.

enteral nutrition (EN) Provision of nutrients through the gastrointestinal tract when the patient cannot ingest, chew, or swallow food but can digest and absorb nutrients.

entropion Condition in which the eyelid turns inward toward the eye.

environment All of the many factors (e.g., physical and psychological) that influence or affect the life and survival of a person.

epidermis Outer layer of the skin that has several thin layers in different stages of maturation; shields and protects the underlying tissues from water loss, mechanical or chemical injury, and penetration by disease-causing microorganisms.

epidural infusion Type of nerve block anesthesia in which an anesthetic is intermittently or continuously injected into the lumbosacral region of the spinal cord.

erythema Redness or inflammation of the skin or mucous membranes that is a result of dilation and congestion of superficial capillaries; sunburn is an example.

eschar Thick layer of dead, dry tissue that covers a pressure ulcer or thermal burn. It may be allowed to be sloughed off naturally, or it may need to be surgically removed.

ethical dilemma Dilemma existing when the right thing to do is not clear. Resolution requires the negotiation of differing values among those involved in the dilemma.

ethical principles Set of guidelines for the expectations a profession and the standards of behavior for its members.

ethics Principles or standards that govern proper conduct.

ethics of care Delivery of health care based on ethical principles and standards of care.

ethnicity Shared identity related to social and cultural heritage such as values, language, geographical space, and racial characteristics.

ethnocentrism Tendency to hold one's own way of life as superior to that of others.

ethnohistory Significant historical experiences of a particular group.

etiology Study of all factors that may be involved in the development of a disease.

eupnea Normal respirations that are quiet, effortless, and rhythmical.

eustress Stress that protects health; one of the two types of stress identified by Selye.

evaluation Determination of the extent to which established patient goals have been achieved.

evidence-based knowledge Knowledge that is derived from the integration of best research, clinical expertise, and patient values.

evidence-based practice Use of current best evidence from nursing research, clinical expertise, practice trends, and patient preferences to guide nursing decisions about care provided to patients.

evisceration Protrusion of visceral organs through a surgical wound.

exacerbations Increases in the gravity of a disease or disorder as marked by greater intensity in signs or symptoms.

excessive daytime sleepiness Extreme fatigue felt during the day. Signs of this include falling asleep at inappropriate times such as while eating, talking, or driving. May indicate a sleep disorder.

excoriation Injury to the surface of the skin caused by abrasion.

exhaustion stage Phase that occurs when the body can no longer resist the stress (i.e., when the energy necessary to maintain adaptation is depleted).

exogenous infection Infection originating outside an organ or part.

exostosis Abnormal benign growth on the surface of a bone.

expected outcomes Expected conditions of a patient at the end of therapy or a disease process, including the degree of wellness and the need for continuing care, medications, support, counseling, or education.

extended care facility Institution devoted to providing medical, nursing, or custodial care for an individual over a prolonged period such as during the course of a chronic disease or the rehabilitation phase after an acute illness.

extension Movement by certain joints that increases the angle between two adjoining bones.

extracellular fluid (ECF) Portion of body fluids composed of the interstitial fluid and blood plasma.

exudate Fluid, cells, or other substances that have been discharged from cells or blood vessels slowly through small pores or breaks in cell membranes.

F

face-saving Way of speaking or acting that preserves dignity.

Fahrenheit Denotes temperature scale in which 32° is the freezing point of water and 212° is the boiling point of water at sea level.

faith Set of beliefs and a way of relating to self, others, and a Supreme Being.

fajita Cotton binder used on a newborn's abdomen among Hispanics and Filipinos to prevent gas and umbilical hernia.

family Group of interacting individuals composing a basic unit of society.

family as context Nursing perspective in which the family is viewed as a unit of interacting members having attributes, functions, and goals separate from those of the individual family members.

family caregiving A family process that occurs in response to an illness and encompasses multiple cognitive, behavioral, and interpersonal processes.

family diversity Unique needs and characteristics of each member in a family.

family durability System of support for a family that includes immediate and extended family members.

family forms Patterns of people considered by family members to be included in the family.

family functioning Processes families use to achieve their goals.

family hardiness Internal strengths and durability of the family unit; characterized by a sense of control over the outcome of life events and hardships, a view of change as beneficial and growth-producing, and an active rather than passive orientation in responding to stressful life events.

family health Determined by the effectiveness of the family's structure, the processes that the family uses to meet its goals, and internal and external forces.

family as patient Nursing approach that takes into consideration the effect of one intervention on all members of a family.

family resiliency Family's ability to cope with expected and unexpected stressors.

family structure Based on organization (i.e., ongoing membership) of the family and the pattern of relationships.

farmacia Place to obtain prescribed medications.

febrile Pertaining to or characterized by an elevated body temperature.

fecal impaction Accumulation of hardened fecal material in the rectum or sigmoid colon.

fecal incontinence Inability to control passage of feces and gas from the anus.

fecal occult blood test (FOBT) Measures microscopic amounts of blood in the feces.

feces Waste or excrement from the gastrointestinal tract.

feedback Process in which the output of a given system is returned to the system.

felony Crime of a serious nature that carries a penalty of imprisonment or death.

feminist ethics Ethical approach that focuses on the nature of relationships to guide participants in making difficult decisions, especially relationships in which power is unequal or in which a point of view has become ignored or invisible.

fever Elevation in the hypothalamic set point so body temperature is regulated at a higher level.

fictive Nonblood kin; considered family in some collective cultures.

fidelity Agreement to keep a promise.

fight-or-flight response Total physiological response to stress that occurs during the alarm reaction stage of the general adaptation syndrome. Massive changes in all body systems prepare a human being to choose to flee or remain and fight the stressor.

filtration Straining of fluid through a membrane.

fistula Abnormal passage from an internal organ to the surface of the body or between two internal organs.

flashback Recollection so strong that the individual thinks that he or she is actually experiencing the trauma again or seeing it unfold before his or her eyes.

flatus Intestinal gas.

flora Microorganisms that live on or within a body to compete with disease-producing microorganisms and provide a natural immunity against certain infections.

flow sheets Documents on which frequent observations or specific measurements are recorded.

fluctuance Soft, boggy feeling when tissue is palpated; usually a sign of tissue infection.

fluid volume deficit (FVD) Fluid and electrolyte disorder caused by failure of bodily homeostatic mechanisms to regulate the retention and excretion of body fluids. The condition is characterized by decreased output of urine, high specific gravity of urine, output of urine that is greater than the intake of fluid in the body, hemoconcentration, and increased serum levels of sodium.

fluid volume excess (FVE) Fluid and electrolyte disorder characterized by an increase in fluid retention and edema, resulting from failure of bodily homeostatic mechanisms to regulate the retention and excretion of body fluids.

focus charting Charting methodology for structuring progress notes according to the focus of the note (e.g., symptoms and nursing diagnosis). Each note includes data, actions, and patient response.

focused cultural assessment Method of evaluating a patient's ethnohistory, biocultural history, social organization, and religious and spiritual beliefs to find issues that are most relevant to the problem at hand.

food poisoning Toxic processes resulting from the ingestion of a food contaminated by toxic substances or bacteria-containing toxins.

food security All members of a household have access to sufficient, safe, nutritious food to maintain a healthy lifestyle.

foot boots Soft, foot-shaped devices designed to reduce the risk of footdrop by maintaining the foot in dorsiflexion.

footdrop Abnormal neuromuscular condition of the lower leg and foot characterized by an inability to dorsiflex, or evert, the foot.

friction Effects of rubbing or the resistance that a moving body meets from the surface on which it moves; a force that occurs in a direction to oppose movement.

functional health illiteracy Inability of an individual to obtain, interpret, and understand basic information about health.

functional health patterns Method for organizing assessment data based on the level of patient function in specific areas (e.g., mobility).

functional nursing Method of patient care delivery in which each staff member is assigned a task that is completed for all patients on the unit.

future orientation Time dimension emphasized by dominant American culture. It is characterized by direct communication and is focused on task achievement, whereas past orientation communication is circular and indirect and is focused on group harmony.

G

gait Manner or style of walking, including rhythm, cadence, and speed.

gastrostomy feeding tube Insertion of a feeding tube through a stoma into the stomach to provide enteral nutrition.

general adaptation syndrome (GAS) Generalized defense response of the body to stress; consists of three stages: alarm, resistance, and exhaustion.

general anesthesia Intravenous or inhaled medications that cause the patient to lose all sensation and consciousness.

genomics Describes the study of all the genes in a person and interactions of those genes with one another and with that person's environment.

geriatrics Branch of health care dealing with the physiology and psychology of aging and the diagnosis and treatment of diseases affecting older adults.

gerontology Study of all aspects of the aging process and its consequences.

gingivae Gums of the mouth; mucous membrane with supporting fibrous tissue that overlies the crowns of unerupted teeth and encircles the necks of teeth that have erupted.

glaucoma Abnormal condition of elevated pressure within an eye caused by obstruction of the outflow of aqueous humor. If untreated, it often results in peripheral visual loss, decreased visual acuity with difficulty adapting to darkness, and a halo effect around lights.

globalization Worldwide scope or application.

glomerulus Cluster or collection of capillary vessels within the kidney involved in the initial formation of urine.

gluconeogenesis Formation of glucose or glycogen from substances that are not carbohydrates such as protein or lipid.

glucose Primary fuel for the body; needed to carry out major physiological functions.

glycogen Polysaccharide that is the major carbohydrate stored in animal cells.

glycogenesis Process for storing glucose in the form of glycogen in the liver.

goals Desired results of nursing actions set realistically by the nurse and patient as part of the planning stage of the nursing process.

Good Samaritan laws Legislation enacted in some states to protect health care professionals from liability in rendering emergency aid unless there is proven willful wrong or gross negligence.

graduated measuring container Receptacle for volume measurement.

granny midwives Amateur health practitioners that assist in labor and delivery.

granulation tissue Soft, pink, fleshy projections of tissue that form during the healing process in a wound not healing by primary intention.

graphic record Charting mechanism that allows for the recording of vital signs and weight in such a manner that caregivers can quickly note changes in the patient's status.

grief Form of sorrow involving the person's thoughts, feelings, and behaviors that occurs as a response to an actual or perceived loss.

grieving process Sequence of affective, cognitive, and physiological states through which the person responds to and finally accepts an irretrievable loss.

grounded Connection between the electric circuit and the ground, which becomes part of the circuit.

growth Measurable or quantitative aspect of an individual's increase in physical dimensions as a result of an increase in number of cells. Indicators of growth include changes in height, weight, and sexual characteristics.

guided imagery Method of pain control in which the patient creates a mental image, concentrates on that image, and gradually becomes less aware of pain.

gustatory Pertaining to the sense of taste.

H

halal Foods permissible for Muslims to eat.

hand rolls Rolls of cloth that keep the thumb slightly adducted and in opposition to the fingers.

hand-wrist splints Splints individually molded for the patient to maintain proper alignment of the thumb, slight adduction of the wrist, and slight dorsiflexion.

haram Foods prohibited by Muslim religious standards.

health Dynamic state in which individuals adapt to their internal and external environments so there is a state of physical, emotional, intellectual, social, and spiritual well-being.

health belief model Conceptual framework that describes a person's health behavior as an expression of his or her health beliefs.

health beliefs Patient's personal beliefs about levels of wellness that can motivate or impede participation in changing risk factors, participating in care, and selecting care options.

health care–acquired infection Infection that was not present or incubating at the time of admission to a health care setting.

health care problems Any conditions or dysfunctions that the patient experiences as a result of illness or treatment of an illness.

health disparities Preventable differences in the burden of disease, injury, violence, or opportunities to achieve optimal health that are experienced by socially and economically disadvantaged populations.

health informatics Application of computer and information science in all basic and applied biomedical sciences to facilitate the acquisition, processing, interpretation, optimal use, and communication of health-related data.

health literacy Patients' reading and mathematics skills, comprehension, ability to make health-related decisions, and successful functioning as a consumer of health care.

health promotion Activities such as routine exercise and good nutrition that help patients maintain or enhance their present level of health and reduce their risk of developing certain diseases.

health promotion model Defines health as a positive, dynamic state, not merely the absence of disease. The health promotion model emphasizes well-being, personal fulfillment, and self-actualization rather than reaction to the threat of illness.

health status Description of health of an individual or community.

heat exhaustion Abnormal condition caused by depletion of body fluid and electrolytes resulting from exposure to intense heat or the inability to acclimatize to heat.

heat stroke Continued exposure to extreme heat that raises the core body temperature to 40.5° C (105° F) or higher.

hematemesis Vomiting of blood, indicating upper gastrointestinal bleeding.

hematoma Collection of blood trapped in the tissues of the skin or an organ.

hematuria Abnormal presence of blood in the urine.

hemolysis Breakdown of red blood cells and release of hemoglobin that may occur after administration of hypotonic intravenous solutions, causing swelling and rupture of erythrocytes.

hemoptysis Coughing up blood from the respiratory tract.

hemorrhoids Permanent dilation and engorgement of veins within the lining of the rectum.

hemostasis Termination of bleeding by mechanical or chemical means or the coagulation process of the body.

hemothorax Accumulation of blood and fluid in the pleural cavity between the parietal and visceral pleurae.

hernia Protrusion of an organ through an abnormal opening in the muscle wall of the cavity that surrounds it.

hilots Amateur health practitioners that assist in labor and delivery among Filipinos.

holistic Of or pertaining to the whole; considering all factors.

holistic health Comprehensive view of the person as a biopsychosocial and spiritual being.

home care Health service provided in the patient's place of residence to promote, maintain, or restore health or minimize the effects of illness and disability.

homeostasis State of relative constancy in the internal environment of the body; maintained naturally by physiological adaptive mechanisms.

hope Confident but uncertain expectation of achieving a future goal.

hospice System of family-centered care designed to help terminally ill people be comfortable and maintain a satisfactory lifestyle throughout the terminal phase of their illness.

Hoyer lift Mechanical device that uses a canvas sling to easily lift dependent patients for transfer.

humidification Process of adding water to gas.

humor Coping strategy based on an individual's cognitive appraisal of a stimulus that results in behavior such as smiling, laughing, or feelings of amusement that lessen emotional distress.

hydrocephalus Abnormal accumulation of cerebrospinal fluid in the ventricles of the brain.

hydrostatic pressure Pressure caused by a liquid.

hyperactive/overactive bladder Common bladder complaint that occurs more frequently with aging and includes the symptoms of urgency, frequency, nocturia, and urge incontinence.

hypercalcemia Greater-than-normal amount of calcium in the blood.

hypercapnia Greater-than-normal amounts of carbon dioxide in the blood; also called hypercarbia.

hyperextension Position of maximal extension of a joint.

hyperglycemia Elevated serum glucose levels.

hypertension Disorder characterized by an elevated blood pressure persistently exceeding 120/80 mm Hg.

hyperthermia Situation in which body temperature exceeds the set point.

hypertonic Situation in which one solution has a greater concentration of solute than another; therefore the first solution exerts greater osmotic pressure.

hypertonicity Excessive tension of the arterial walls or muscles.

hyperventilation Respiratory rate in excess of that required to maintain normal carbon dioxide levels in the body tissues.

hypnotics Class of drug that causes insensibility to pain and induces sleep.

hypostatic pneumonia Pneumonia that results from fluid accumulation as a result of inactivity.

hypotension Abnormal lowering of blood pressure that is inadequate for normal perfusion and oxygenation of tissues.

hypothermia Abnormal lowering of body temperature below 35° C, or 95° F, usually caused by prolonged exposure to cold.

hypotonic Situation in which one solution has a smaller concentration of solute than another; therefore the first solution exerts less osmotic pressure.

hypotonicity Reduced tension of the arterial walls or muscles.

hypoventilation Respiratory rate insufficient to prevent carbon dioxide retention.

hypovolemia Abnormally low circulating blood volume.

hypoxemia Arterial blood oxygen level less than 60 mm Hg; low oxygen level in the blood.

hypoxia Inadequate cellular oxygenation that may result from a deficiency in the delivery or use of oxygen at the cellular level.

I

identity Component of self-concept characterized by one's persisting consciousness of being oneself, separate and distinct from others.

idiosyncratic reaction Individual sensitivity to effects of a drug caused by inherited or other bodily constitution factors.

illness (1) Abnormal process in which any aspect of a person's functioning is diminished or impaired compared with his or her previous condition. (2) The personal, interpersonal, and cultural reaction to disease.

illness behavior Ways in which people monitor their bodies, define and interpret their symptoms, take remedial actions, and use the health care system.

illness prevention Health education programs or activities directed toward protecting patients from threats or potential threats to health and minimizing risk factors.

immobility Inability to move about freely; caused by any condition in which movement is impaired or therapeutically restricted.

immunity Quality of being insusceptible to or unaffected by a particular disease or condition.

immunization Process by which resistance to an infectious disease is induced or augmented.

implementation Initiation and completion of the nursing actions necessary to help the patient achieve health care goals.

impression management Ability to interpret others' behavior within their own context of meanings and behave in a culturally congruent way to achieve desired outcomes of communication.

incentive spirometry Method of encouraging voluntary deep breathing by providing visual feedback to patients of the inspiratory volume they have achieved.

incident rates Rate of new cases of a disease in a specified population over a defined period of time.

incident report Confidential document that describes any patient accident while the person is on the premises of a health care agency. (See occurrence report.)

independent practice association (IPA) Managed care organization that contracts with physicians or health care providers who usually are members of groups and whose practices include fee-for-service and capitated patients.

indirect care interventions Treatments performed away from the patient but on behalf of the patient or group of patients.

induration Hardening of a tissue, particularly the skin, because of edema or inflammation.

infection Invasion of the body by pathogenic microorganisms that reproduce and multiply.

inference (1) Judgment or interpretation of informational cues. (2) Taking one proposition as a given and guessing that another proposition follows.

infiltration Dislodging an intravenous catheter or needle from a vein into the subcutaneous space.

inflammation Protective response of body tissues to irritation or injury.

informed consent Process of obtaining permission from a patient to perform a specific test or procedure after describing all risks, side effects, and benefits.

infusion pump Device that delivers a measured amount of fluid over a period of time.

infusions Introduction of fluid into the vein, giving intravenous fluid over time.

inhalation Method of medication delivery through the patient's respiratory tract. The respiratory tract provides a large surface area for drug absorption. Inhalation can be through the nasal or oral route.

injections Parenteral administration of medication; four major sites of injection: subcutaneous, intramuscular, intravenous, and intradermal.

insensible water loss Water loss that is continuous and not perceived by the person.

insomnia Condition characterized by chronic inability to sleep or remain asleep through the night.

inspection Method of physical examination by which the patient is visually systematically examined for appearance, structure, function, and behavior.

instillation To cause to enter drop by drop or very slowly.

institutional ethics committee Interdisciplinary committee that discusses and processes ethical dilemmas that arise within a health care institution.

instrumental activities of daily living (IADLs) Activities necessary for independence in society beyond eating, grooming, transferring, and toileting; include such skills as shopping, preparing meals, banking, and taking medications.

integrated delivery network (IDN) Set of providers and services organized to deliver a coordinated continuum of care to the population of patients served at a capitated cost.

interpersonal communication Exchange of information between two persons or among persons in a small group.

interstitial fluid Fluid that fills the spaces between most of the cells of the body and provides a substantial portion of the liquid environment of the body.

interview Organized, systematic conversation with the patient designed to obtain pertinent health-related subjective information.

intracellular fluid Liquid within the cell membrane.

intradermal (ID) Injection given between layers of the skin into the dermis. Injections are given at a 5- to 15-degree angle.

intramuscular (IM) Injections given into muscle tissue. The intramuscular route provides a fast rate of absorption that is related to the greater vascularity of the muscle. Injections are given at a 90-degree angle.

intraocular Method of medication delivery that involves inserting a medication disk similar to a contact lens into the patient's eye.

intrapersonal communication Communication that occurs within an individual (i.e., people "talk with themselves" silently or form an idea in their own mind).

intravascular fluid Fluid circulating within blood vessels of the body.

intravenous Injection directly into the bloodstream. Action of the drug begins immediately when given intravenously.

intravenous fat emulsions Soybean- or safflower oil–based solutions that are isotonic and may be infused with amino acid and dextrose solution through a central or peripheral line.

intubation Insertion of a breathing tube through the mouth or nose into the trachea to ensure a patent airway.

intuition Inner sensing that something is so.

irrigation Process of washing out a body cavity or wounded area with a stream of fluid.

ischemia Decreased blood supply to a body part such as skin tissue or to an organ such as the heart.

isolation Separation of a seriously ill patient from others to prevent the spread of an infection or protect the patient from irritating environmental factors.

isometric exercises Activities that involve muscle tension without muscle shortening, do not have any beneficial effect on preventing orthostatic hypotension, but may improve activity tolerance.

isotonic Situation in which two solutions have the same concentration of solute; therefore both solutions exert the same osmotic pressure.

J

jaundice Yellow discoloration of the skin, mucous membranes, and sclera caused by greater-than-normal amounts of bilirubin in the blood.

jejunostomy tube Hollow tube inserted into the jejunum through the abdominal wall for administration of liquefied foods to patients who have a high risk of aspiration.

joint contracture Abnormality that may result in permanent condition of a joint; is characterized by flexion and fixation; and is caused by disuse, atrophy, and shortening of muscle fibers and surrounding joint tissues.

joints Connections between bones; classified according to structure and degree of mobility.

judgment Ability to form an opinion or draw sound conclusions.

justice Ethical standard of fairness.

K

Kardex Trade name for card-filing system that allows quick reference to the particular need of the patient for certain aspects of nursing care.

karma Asian Indian belief that attributes mental illness to past deeds in one's previous life.

knowing the patient An in-depth knowledge of the patient's patterns of responses; fosters skilled clinical decision making.

Korotkoff sound Sound heard during the taking of blood pressure using a sphygmomanometer and stethoscope.

Kussmaul respiration Increase in both rate and depth of respirations.

kyphosis Exaggeration of the posterior curvature of the thoracic spine.

L

la cuarantena Period of rest and restricted physical activity after childbirth that usually lasts 40 days.

laceration Torn, jagged wound.

language Code that conveys specific meaning as words are combined.

laryngospasm Sudden uncontrolled contraction of the laryngeal muscles, which in turn decreases airway size.

lateral violence Hostile, aggressive, and harmful verbal and nonverbal behavior by a nurse to another nurse via attitudes, actions, words, or behaviors. This behavior includes criticizing, intimidations, blaming, fighting, public humiliation, isolating, withholding assistance, or undermining efforts in completing assignments. This leaves the nurse feeling bullied, inadequate and powerless.

law Rule, standard, or principle that states a fact or relationship between factors.

laxatives Drugs that act to promote bowel evacuation.

learning Acquisition of new knowledge and skills as a result of reinforcement, practice, and experience.

learning objective Written statement that describes the behavior that a teacher expects from an individual after a learning activity.

left-sided heart failure Abnormal condition characterized by impaired functioning of the left ventricle caused by elevated pressures and pulmonary congestion.

leukoplakia Thick, white patches observed on oral mucous membranes.

licensed practical nurse (LPN) Also known as the licensed vocational nurse (LVN) or in Canada, registered nurse's assistant (RNA); trained in basic nursing skills and the provision of direct patient care.

licensed vocational nurse (LVN) The LVN is the same as a licensed practical nurse (LPN), an individual trained in the United States in basic nursing techniques and direct patient care who practices under the supervision of a registered nurse. The LVN is licensed by a board after completing what is usually a 12-month educational program and passing a licensure examination. In Canada an LVN is called a certified nursing assistant.

lipids Compounds that are insoluble in water but soluble in organic solvents.

lipogenesis Process during which fatty acids are synthesized.

living wills Instruments by which a dying person makes wishes known.

local anesthesia Loss of sensation at the desired site of action.

logroll Maneuver used to turn a reclining patient from one side to the other or completely over without moving the spinal column out of alignment.

lordosis Increased lumbar curvature.

M

maceration Softening and breaking down of skin from prolonged exposure to moisture.

mal de ojo Evil eye.

malignant hyperthermia Autosomal-dominant trait characterized by often fatal hyperthermia in affected people exposed to certain anesthetic agents.

malpractice Injurious or unprofessional actions that harm another.

malpractice insurance Type of insurance to protect the health care professional. In case of a malpractice claim, the insurance pays the award to the plaintiff.

managed care Health care system in which there is administrative control over primary health care services. Redundant facilities and services are eliminated, and costs are reduced. Preventive care and health education are emphasized.

Maslow's hierarchy of needs Model developed by Abram Maslow that is used to explain human motivation.

matrilineal Kinship that is limited to only the mother's side.

maturation Genetically determined biological plan for growth and development. Physical growth and motor development are a function of maturation.

maturational loss Loss, usually of an aspect of self, resulting from the normal changes of growth and development.

Medicaid State medical assistance to people with low incomes, based on Title XIX of the Social Security Act. States receive matching federal funds to provide medical care and services to people meeting categorical and income requirements.

medical asepsis Procedures used to reduce the number of microorganisms and prevent their spread.

medical diagnosis Formal statement of the disease entity or illness made by the physician or health care provider.

medical record Patient's chart; a legal document.

Medicare Federally funded national health insurance program in the United States for people over 65 years of age. The program is administered in two parts. Part A provides basic protection against costs of medical, surgical, and psychiatric hospital care. Part B is a voluntary medical insurance program financed in part from federal funds and in part from premiums contributed by people enrolled in the program.

medication abuse Maladaptive pattern of recurrent medication use.

medication allergy Adverse reaction such as rash, chills, or gastrointestinal disturbances to a medication. Once a drug allergy occurs, the patient can no longer receive that particular medication.

medication dependence Maladaptive pattern of medication use in the following patterns: using excessive amounts of the medication, increased activities directed toward obtaining the medication, or withdrawal from professional or recreational activities.

medication error Any event that could cause or lead to a patient's receiving inappropriate drug therapy or failing to receive appropriate drug therapy.

medication interaction Response that occurs when one drug modifies the action of another drug. The interaction can potentiate or diminish the actions of another drug; or it may alter the way a drug is metabolized, absorbed, or excreted.

melanoma Group of malignant neoplasms, primarily of the skin, that are composed of melanocytes. Common in fair-skinned people having light-colored eyes and those who have been sunburned.

melena Abnormal black, sticky stool containing digested blood that is indicative of gastrointestinal bleeding.

menarche Onset of a girl's first menstruation.

Ménière's disease Chronic disease of the inner ear characterized by recurrent episodes of vertigo; progressive sensorineural hearing loss, which may be bilateral; and tinnitus.

menopause Physiological cessation of ovulation and menstruation that typically occurs during middle adulthood in women.

message Information sent or expressed by sender in the communication process.

metabolic acidosis Abnormal condition of high hydrogen ion concentration in the extracellular fluid caused by either a primary increase in hydrogen ions or a decrease in bicarbonate.

metabolic alkalosis Abnormal condition characterized by the significant loss of acid from the body or increased levels of bicarbonate.

metabolism Aggregate of all chemical processes that take place in living organisms and result in growth, generation of energy, elimination of wastes, and other functions concerned with the distribution of nutrients in the blood after digestion.

metacommunication Dependent not only on what is said but also on the relationship to the other person involved in the interaction. It is a message that conveys the sender's attitude toward self and the message and the attitudes, feelings, and intentions toward the listener.

metastasize Spread of tumor cells to distant parts of the body from a primary site (e.g., lung, breast, or bowel).

metered-dose inhaler (MDI) Device designed to deliver a measured dose of an inhalation drug.

metric system Logically organized decimal system of measurement; metric units can easily be converted and computed through simple multiplication and division. Each basic unit of measurement is organized into units of 10.

microorganisms Microscopic entities such as bacteria, viruses, and fungi that are capable of carrying on living processes.

micturition Urination; act of passing or expelling urine voluntarily through the urethra.

milliequivalent per liter (mEq/L) Number of grams of a specific electrolyte dissolved in 1 L of plasma.

mind mapping Graphic approach to represent the connections between concepts and ideas (e.g., nursing diagnoses) that are related to a central subject (e.g., the patient's health problems).

mindfulness A moment-to-moment present awareness with an attitude on non-judgment, acceptance, and openness. Mindfulness meditative practices are effective in reducing psychological and physical symptoms or perceptions of stress.

minerals Inorganic elements essential to the body because of their role as catalysts in biochemical reactions.

minimum data set (MDS) Required by the Omnibus Budget Reconciliation Act of 1987, the MDS is a uniform data set established by the Department of Health and Human Services. It serves as the framework for any state-specified assessment instruments used to develop a written and comprehensive plan of care for newly admitted residents of nursing facilities.

misdemeanor Lesser crime than a felony; the penalty is usually a fine or imprisonment for less than 1 year.

mobility Person's ability to move about freely.

moderate sedation/analgesia/conscious sedation Administration of central nervous system depressant drugs and/or analgesics to provide analgesia, relieve anxiety, and/or provide amnesia during surgical, diagnostic, or interventional procedures. Routinely used for diagnostic or therapeutic procedures that do not require complete anesthesia but simply a decreased level of consciousness.

monosaturated fatty acid Fatty acid in which some of the carbon atoms in the hydrocarbon chain are joined by double or triple bonds. Monounsaturated fatty acids have only one double or triple bond per molecule and are found as components of fats in such foods as fowls, almonds, pecans, cashew nuts, peanuts, and olive oil.

morals Personal conviction that something is absolutely right or wrong in all situations.

motivation Internal impulse that causes a person to take action.

motivational interviewing Interview technique used to identify patient's thoughts, beliefs, fears and current health care behavior with the aim of helping them to identify improved self-care behaviors.

mourning Process of grieving.

murmurs Blowing or whooshing sounds created by changes in blood flow through the heart or abnormalities in valve closure.

muscle tone Normal state of balanced muscle tension.

myocardial contractility Measure of stretch of the cardiac muscle fiber. It can also affect stroke volume and cardiac output. Poor contraction decreases the amount of blood ejected by the ventricles during each contraction.

myocardial infarction Necrosis of a portion of cardiac muscle caused by obstruction in a coronary artery.

myocardial ischemia Condition that results when the supply of blood to the myocardium from the coronary arteries is insufficient to meet the oxygen demands of the organ.

N

NANDA International North American Nursing Diagnosis Association organized in 1973. It formally identifies, develops, and classifies nursing diagnoses.

narcolepsy Syndrome involving sudden sleep attacks that a person cannot inhibit. Uncontrollable desire to sleep may occur several times during a day.

nasogastric (NG) tube Tube passed into the stomach through the nose to empty the stomach of its contents or deliver medication and/or nourishment.

nebulization Process of adding moisture to inspired air by the adding water droplets.

necessary losses Losses that every person experiences.

necrotic Of or pertaining to the death of tissue in response to disease or injury.

negative health behaviors Practices actually or potentially harmful to health such as smoking, drug or alcohol abuse, poor diet, and refusal to take necessary medications.

negative nitrogen balance Condition occurring when the body excretes more nitrogen than it takes in.

negligence Careless act of omission or commission that results in injury to another.

neonate Stage of life from birth to 1 month of age.

nephrons Structural and functional units of the kidney containing renal glomeruli and tubules.

neurotransmitter Chemical that transfers the electrical impulse from the nerve fiber to the muscle fiber.

nociceptors Somatic and visceral free nerve endings of thinly myelinated and unmyelinated fibers. They usually react to tissue injury but may also be excited by endogenous chemical substances.

nocturia Urination at night; can be a symptom of renal disease or may occur in persons who drink excessive amounts of fluids before bedtime.

nonblanchable hyperemia Redness of the skin caused by dilation of the superficial capillaries. The redness persists when pressure is applied to the area, indicating tissue damage.

noninvasive positive-pressure ventilation (NPPV) Used to prevent using invasive artificial airways (endotracheal [ET] tube or tracheostomy) in patients with acute respiratory failure, cardiogenic pulmonary edema, or exacerbation of chronic obstructive pulmonary disease. It has also been used following extubation of an ET tube.

nonmaleficence Fundamental ethical agreement to do no harm. Closely related to the ethical standard of beneficence.

nonrapid eye movement (NREM) sleep Sleep that occurs during the first four stages of normal sleep.

nonshivering thermogenesis Occurs primarily in neonates. Because neonates cannot shiver, a limited amount of vascular brown adipose tissue present at birth can be metabolized for heat production.

nonverbal communication Communication using expressions, gestures, body posture, and positioning rather than words.

normal sinus rhythm (NSR) The wave pattern on an electrocardiogram that indicates normal conduction of an electrical impulse through the myocardium.

numbing One of Bowlby's four phases of mourning. It is characterized by the lack of feeling or feeling stunned by the loss; may last a few days or many weeks.

Nurse Practice Acts Statutes enacted by the legislature of any of the states or the appropriate officers of the districts or possessions that describe and define the scope of nursing practice.

nurse-initiated interventions Response of the nurse to the patient's health care needs and nursing diagnoses. This type of intervention is an autonomous action based on scientific rationale that is executed to benefit the patient in a predicted way related to the nursing diagnosis and patient-centered goals.

Nursing Clinical Information System (NCIS) A system that incorporates the principles of nursing informatics to support the work that nurses do by facilitating documentation of nursing process activities and offering resources for managing nursing care delivery.

nursing diagnosis Formal statement of an actual or potential health problem that nurses can legally and independently treat; the second step of the nursing process, during which the patient's actual and potential unhealthy responses to an illness or condition are identified.

nursing health history Data collected about a patient's present level of wellness, changes in life patterns, sociocultural role, and mental and emotional reactions to illness.

nursing intervention Any treatment based on clinical judgment and knowledge that a nurse performs to enhance patient outcomes.

Nursing Outcomes Classification A systematic organization of nurse sensitive outcomes into groups or categories based upon similarities, dissimilarities, and relationships among the outcomes.

nursing process Systematic problem-solving method by which nurses individualize care for each patient. The five steps of the nursing process are assessment, diagnosis, planning, implementation, and evaluation.

nursing-sensitive outcomes Outcomes that are within the scope of nursing practice; consequences or effects of nursing interventions that result in changes in the patient's symptoms, functional status, safety, psychological distress, or costs.

nurturant Behavior that involves caring for or fostering the well-being of another individual.

nutrients Foods that contain elements necessary for body function, including water, carbohydrates, proteins, fats, vitamins, and minerals.

O

obesity Abnormal increase in the proportion of fat cells, mainly in the viscera and subcutaneous tissues of the body.

objective data Information that can be observed by others; free of feelings, perceptions, prejudices.

occurrence report Confidential document that describes any patient accident while the person is on the premises of a health care agency. (See incident report.)

olfactory Pertaining to the sense of smell.

oncotic pressure Total influence of the protein on the osmotic activity of plasma fluid.

Open-ended question Form of question that prompts a respondent to answer in more than one or two words.

operating bed Table for surgery.

operating room (1) Room in a health care facility in which surgical procedures requiring anesthesia are performed. (2) Informal: a suite of rooms or an area in a health care facility in which patients are prepared for surgery, undergo surgical procedures, and recover from the anesthetic procedures required for the surgery.

ophthalmic Drugs given into the eye in the form of either eye drops or ointments.

ophthalmoscope Instrument used to illuminate the structures of the eye to examine the fundus, which includes the retina, choroid, optic nerve disc, macula, fovea centralis, and retinal vessels.

opioid Drug substance derived from opium or produced synthetically that alters perception of pain and that, with repeated use, may result in physical and psychological dependence (narcotic).

oral hygiene Condition or practice of maintaining the tissues and structures of the mouth.

orthopnea Abnormal condition in which a person must sit or stand to breathe comfortably.

orthostatic hypotension Abnormally low blood pressure occurring when a person stands.

osmolality Concentration or osmotic pressure of a solution expressed in osmoles or milliosmoles per kilogram of water.

osmolarity Osmotic pressure of a solution expressed in osmoles or milliosmoles per kilogram of the solution.

osmoreceptors Neurons in the hypothalamus that are sensitive to the fluid concentration in the blood plasma and regulate the secretion of antidiuretic hormone.

osmosis Movement of a pure solvent through a semipermeable membrane from a solution with a lower solute concentration to one with a higher solute concentration.

osmotic pressure Drawing power for water, which depends on the number of molecules in the solution.

osteoporosis Disorder characterized by abnormal rarefaction of bone, occurring most frequently in postmenopausal women, sedentary or immobilized individuals, and patients on long-term steroid therapy.

ostomy Surgical procedure in which an opening is made into the abdominal wall to allow the passage of intestinal contents from the bowel (colostomy) or urine from the bladder (urostomy).

otoscope Instrument with a special ear speculum used to examine the deeper structures of the external and middle ear.

ototoxic Having a harmful effect on the eighth cranial (auditory) nerve or the organs of hearing and balance.

outcome Condition of a patient at the end of treatment, including the degree of wellness and the need for continuing care, medication, support, counseling, or education.

outliers Patients with extended lengths of stay beyond allowable inpatient days or costs.

outpatient Patient who has not been admitted to a hospital but receives treatments in a clinic or facility associated with the hospital.

oxygen desaturation A decrease in oxygen concentration in the blood resulting from any condition that affects the exchange of carbon dioxide and oxygen.

oxygen saturation Amount of hemoglobin fully saturated with oxygen, given as a percent value.

oxygen therapy Procedure in which oxygen is administered to a patient to relieve or prevent hypoxia.

P

pain Subjective, unpleasant sensation caused by noxious stimulation of sensory nerve endings.

palliative care Level of care that is designed to relieve or reduce intensity of uncomfortable symptoms but not to produce a cure. Palliative care relies on comfort measures and use of alternative therapies to help individuals become more at peace during end of life.

pallor Unnatural paleness or absence of color in the skin.

palpation Method of physical examination whereby the fingers or hands of the examiner are applied to the patient's body to feel body parts underlying the skin.

palpitations Bounding or racing of the heart associated with normal emotions or a heart disorder.

Papanicolaou (Pap) smear Painless screening test for cervical cancer. Specimens are taken of squamous and columnar cells of the cervix.

parallel play Form of play among a group of children, primarily toddlers, in which each one engages in an independent activity that is similar to but not influenced by or shared with the others.

paralytic ileus Usually temporary paralysis of intestinal wall that may occur after abdominal surgery or peritoneal injury and that causes cessation of peristalsis; leads to abdominal distention and symptoms of obstruction.

parenteral administration Giving medication by a route other than the gastrointestinal tract.

parenteral nutrition (PN) Administration of a nutritional solution into the vascular system.

parteras Lay midwives.

partial bed bath Bath in which body parts that might cause the patient discomfort if left unbathed (i.e., face, hands, axillary areas, back, and perineum) are washed in bed.

passive range-of-motion (PROM) exercises Range of movement through which a joint is moved with assistance.

passive strategies of health promotion Activities that involve the patient as the recipient of actions by health care professionals.

pathogenicity Ability of a pathogenic agent to produce a disease.

pathogens Microorganisms capable of producing disease.

pathological fractures Fractures resulting from weakened bone tissue; frequently caused by osteoporosis or neoplasms.

patient-centered care Concept to improve work efficiency by changing the way that patient care is delivered.

patient-and-family-centered care Model of nursing care in which mutual partnerships between the patient, family and health care team are formed to plan, implement and evaluate the nursing and health care delivered.

patient-controlled analgesia (PCA) Drug delivery system that allows patients to self-administer analgesic medications on demand.

patrilineal, patrilineally Kinship that is limited to only the father's side.

pay for performance Quality improvement program that rewards excellence through financial incentives to motivate change to achieve measurable improvements and improve patient care quality and safety.

perceived loss Loss that is less obvious to the individual experiencing it. Although easily overlooked or misunderstood, a perceived loss results in the same grief process as an actual loss.

perception Peoples' mental image or concept of elements in their environment, including information gained through the senses.

percussion Method of physical examination whereby the location, size, and density of a body part is determined by the tone obtained from the striking of short, sharp taps of the fingers.

perfusion (1) Passage of a fluid through a specific organ or an area of the body. (2) Therapeutic measure whereby a drug intended for an isolated part of the body is introduced via the bloodstream. (3) Relates to the ability of the cardiovascular system to pump oxygenated blood to the tissues and return deoxygenated blood to the lungs.

perineal care Procedure prescribed for cleaning the genital and anal areas as part of the daily bath or after various obstetrical and gynecological procedures.
perioperative nursing Refers to the role of the operating room nurse during the preoperative, intraoperative, and postoperative phases of surgery.
peripherally inserted central catheter (PICC) Alternative intravenous access when the patient requires intermediate-length venous access greater than 7 days to 3 months. Intravenous access is achieved by inserting a catheter into a central vein by way of a peripheral vein.
peristalsis Rhythmical contractions of the intestine that propel gastric contents through the length of the gastrointestinal tract.
peritonitis Inflammation of the peritoneum produced by bacteria or irritating substances introduced into the abdominal cavity by a penetrating wound or perforation of an organ in the gastrointestinal or reproductive tract.
PERRLA Acronym for "pupils equal, round, reactive to light, accommodation"; the acronym is recorded in the physical examination if eye and pupil assessments are normal.
personalismo Personalistic.
petechiae Tiny purple or red spots that appear on skin as minute hemorrhages within dermal layers.
pharmacokinetics Study of how drugs enter the body, reach their site of action, are metabolized, and exit from the body.
phlebitis Inflammation of a vein.
physician-initiated interventions Based on the physician's response to a medical diagnosis, the nurse responds to his or her written orders.
PIE note Problem-oriented medical record; the four interdisciplinary sections are the database, problem list, care plan, and progress notes.
placebos Dosage form that contains no pharmacologically active ingredients but may relieve pain through psychological effects.
plaintiff Individual who files formal charges against an individual or organization for a legal offense.
planning Process of designing interventions to achieve the goals and outcomes of health care delivery.
plantar flexion Toe-down motion of the foot at the ankle.
pleural friction rub Adventitious lung sound caused by inflamed parietal and visceral pleura rubbing together on inspiration.
pneumothorax Collection of air or gas in the pleural space.
point of maximal impulse (PMI) Point where the heartbeat can most easily be palpated through the chest wall. This is usually the fourth intercostal space at the midclavicular line.
point of view Way of looking at issues that reflects an individual's culture and societal influences.
poison Any substance that impairs health or destroys life when ingested, inhaled, or absorbed by the body in relatively small amounts.
poison control center One of a network of facilities that provides information regarding all aspects of poisoning or intoxication, maintains records of their occurrence, and refers patients to treatment centers.
polypharmacy Use of a number of different drugs by a patient who may have one or several health problems.
polyunsaturated fatty acid Fatty acid that has two or more carbon double bonds.
population Collection of individuals who have in common one or more personal or environmental characteristics.
positive health behaviors Activities related to maintaining, attaining, or regaining good health and preventing illness. Common positive health behaviors include immunizations, proper sleep patterns, adequate exercise, and nutrition.
postanesthesia care unit (PACU) Area adjoining the operating room to which surgical patients are taken while still under anesthesia.
postmortem care Care of a patient's body after death.
postural drainage Use of positioning along with percussion and vibration to drain secretions from specific segments of the lungs and bronchi into the trachea.
postural hypotension Abnormally low blood pressure occurring when an individual assumes the standing posture; also called orthostatic hypotension.
posture Position of the body in relation to the surrounding space.
power of attorney for health care Person designated by the patient to make health care decisions for the patient if the patient becomes unable to make his or her own decisions.
preadolescence Transitional developmental stage that occurs between childhood and adolescence.
preanesthesia care unit Area outside the operating room where preoperative preparations are completed.
preload Volume of blood in the ventricles at the end of diastole, immediately before ventricular contraction.
preoperative teaching Instruction regarding a patient's anticipated surgery and recovery that is given before surgery. Instruction includes, but is not limited to, dietary and activity restrictions, anticipated assessment activities, postoperative procedures, and pain-relief measures.
presbycusis Hearing loss associated with aging. It usually involves both a loss of hearing sensitivity and a reduction in the clarity of speech.
presbyopia Gradual decline in ability of the lens to accommodate or focus on close objects; reduces ability to see near objects clearly. This condition commonly develops with advancing age.
prescriptions Written directions for a therapeutic agent (e.g., medication, drugs).
presence Deep physical, psychological, and spiritual connection or engagement between a nurse and patient.
present time orientation Time dimension that focuses on what is happening here and now. Communication patterns are circular, and this time orientation is in conflict with the dominant organizational norm in health care that emphasizes punctuality and adherence to appointments.
pressure ulcer Inflammation, sore, or ulcer in the skin over a bony prominence.
presurgical care unit (PSCU) Area outside the operating room where preoperative preparations are completed.
preventive nursing actions Nursing actions directed toward preventing illness and promoting health to avoid the need for primary, secondary, or tertiary health care.
primary appraisal Evaluating an event for its personal meaning related to stress.
primary care First contact in a given episode of illness that leads to a decision regarding a course of action to resolve the health problem.
primary health care Combination of primary and public health care that is accessible to individuals and families in a community and provided at an affordable cost.
primary intention Primary union of the edges of a wound, progressing to complete scar formation without granulation.
primary nursing Method of nursing practice in which the patient's care is managed for the duration by one nurse who directs and coordinates other nurses and health care personnel. When on duty, the primary nurse cares for the patient directly.
primary prevention First contact in a given episode of illness that leads to a decision regarding a course of action to prevent worsening of the health problem.
problem focused diagnosis A clinical judgment concerning an undesirable human response to a health condition/life process that exists in an individual, family or community.
problem identification One of the steps of the diagnostic process in which the patient's health care problem is recognized as a result of data analysis based on professional knowledge and experience.
problem solving Methodical, systematic approach to explore conditions and develop solutions, including analysis of data, determination of causative factors, and selection of appropriate actions to reverse or eliminate the problem.
problem-oriented medical record (POMR) Method of recording data about the health status of a patient that fosters a collaborative problem-solving approach by all members of the health care team.
productive cough Sudden expulsion of air from the lungs that effectively removes sputum from the respiratory tract and helps clear the airways.
professional standards review organization (PSRO) Focuses on evaluation of nursing care provided in a health care setting. The quality, effectiveness, and appropriateness of nursing care for the patient are the focus of evaluation.
prone Position of the patient lying face down.
proprioception Ability of the body to sense its position and movement in space.
prospective payment system (PPS) Payment mechanism for reimbursing hospitals for

inpatient health care services in which a predetermined rate is set for treatment of specific illnesses.

prostaglandins Potent hormonelike substances that act in exceedingly low doses on target organs. They can be used to treat asthma and gastric hyperacidity.

proteins Any of a large group of naturally occurring, complex, organic nitrogenous compounds. Each is composed of large combinations of amino acids containing the elements carbon; hydrogen; nitrogen; oxygen; usually sulfur; and occasionally phosphorus, iron, iodine, or other essential constituents of living cells. Protein is the major source of building material for muscles, blood, skin, hair, nails, and the internal organs.

proteinuria Presence in the urine of abnormally large quantities of protein, usually albumin. Persistent proteinuria is usually a sign of renal disease or renal complications of another disease, hypertension, or heart failure.

protocol Written and approved plan specifying the procedures to be followed during an assessment or in providing treatment.

pruritus Symptom of itching; an uncomfortable sensation leading to the urge to scratch.

psychomotor learning Acquisition of ability to perform motor skills.

ptosis Abnormal condition of one or both upper eyelids in which the eyelid droops; caused by weakness of the levator muscle or paralysis of the third cranial nerve.

puberty Developmental period of emotional and physical changes, including the development of secondary sex characteristics and the onset of menstruation and ejaculation.

public health nursing Nursing specialty that requires the nurse to care for the needs of populations or groups.

public communication Interaction of one individual with large groups of people.

pulmonary hygiene More frequent turning, deep breathing, coughing, use of incentive spirometry, and chest physical therapy (PT) if ordered.

pulse deficit Condition that exists when the radial pulse is less than the ventricular rate as auscultated at the apex or seen on an electrocardiogram. The condition indicates a lack of peripheral perfusion for some of the heart contractions.

pulse pressure Difference between the systolic and diastolic pressures, normally 30 to 40 mm Hg.

Purkinje network Complex network of muscle fibers that spread through the right and left ventricles of the heart and carry the impulses that contract those chambers almost simultaneously.

pursed-lip breathing Deep inspiration followed by prolonged expiration through pursed lips.

pyrexia Abnormal elevation of the temperature of the body above 37° C (98.6° F) because of disease; same as fever.

pyrogens Substances that cause a rise in body temperature, as in the case of bacterial toxins.

Q

QSEN The Quality and Safety in the Education of Nurses (QSEN) initiative is the commitment of nursing to the competencies outlined in the Institute of Medicine report related to nursing education. QSEN encompasses six competencies: patient-centered care, teamwork, collaboration, evidence-based practice, quality improvement, and safety.

quality improvement Monitoring and evaluation of processes and outcomes in health care or any other business to identify opportunities for improvement.

quality indicator Quantitative measure of an important aspect of care that determines whether quality of service conforms to requirements or standards of care.

R

race Common biological characteristics shared by a group of people.

Ramadan Religious observance held during the ninth month of the Islamic calendar year. It involves fasting from sunrise to sunset.

range of motion (ROM) Range of movement of a joint from maximum extension to maximum flexion as measured in degrees of a circle.

rapid eye movement (REM) sleep Stage of sleep in which dreaming and rapid eye movements are prominent; important for mental restoration.

reaction Component of the pain experience that may include both physiological responses such as in the general adaptation syndrome and behavioral responses.

reality orientation Therapeutic modality for restoring an individual's sense of the present.

receiver Person to whom message is sent during the communication process.

reception Neurophysiological components of the pain experience in which nervous system receptors receive painful stimuli and transmit them through peripheral nerves to the spinal cord and brain.

record Written form of communication that permanently documents information relevant to health care management.

recovery Period of time immediately following surgery when the patient is closely observed for effects of anesthesia, changes in vital signs, and bleeding. The area is usually in the postanesthesia care unit.

referent Factor that motivates a person to communicate with another individual.

reflection Process of thinking back or recalling an event to discover the meaning and purpose of that event. Useful in critical thinking.

refractive error Defect in the ability of the lens of the eye to focus light such as occurs in nearsightedness and farsightedness.

regional anesthesia Loss of sensation in an area of the body supplied by sensory nerve pathways.

registered nurse (RN) In the United States a nurse who has completed a course of study at a state-approved, accredited school of nursing and has passed the National Council Licensure Examination (NCLEX-RN).

regression Return to an earlier developmental stage or behavior.

regulatory agencies Local, state, provincial, or national agencies that inspect and certify health care agencies as meeting specified standards. These agencies can also determine the amount of reimbursement for health care delivered.

rehabilitation Restoration of an individual to normal or near-normal function after a physical or mental illness, injury, or chemical addiction.

reinforcement Provision of a contingent response to a learner's behavior that increases the probability of recurrence of the behavior.

related factor Any condition or event that accompanies or is linked with the patient's health care problem.

relaxation Act of being relaxed or less tense.

reminiscence Recalling the past to assign new meaning to past experiences.

remissions Partial or complete disappearances of the clinical and subjective characteristics of chronic or malignant disease; remission may be spontaneous or the result of therapy.

renal calculi Calcium stones in the renal pelvis.

renin Proteolytic enzyme produced by and stored in the juxtaglomerular apparatus that surrounds each arteriole as it enters a glomerulus. The enzyme affects the blood pressure by catalyzing the change of angiotensinogen to angiotensin, a strong repressor.

reorganization Last phase of Bowlby's phases of mourning. During this phase, which sometimes requires a year or more, the person begins to accept unaccustomed roles, acquire new skills, and build new relationships.

reports Transfer of information from the nurses on one shift to the nurses on the following shift. Report may also be given by one of the members of the nursing team to another health care provider (e.g., a physician or therapist).

reservoir Place where microorganisms survive, multiply, and await transfer to a susceptible host.

residual urine Volume of urine remaining in the bladder after a normal voiding; the bladder normally is almost completely empty after micturition.

resistance stage Third stage of the stress response, when the person attempts to adapt to the stressor. The body stabilizes; hormone levels stabilize; and heart rate, blood pressure, and cardiac output return to normal.

resource utilization group (RUG) Method of classification for health care reimbursement for long-term care facilities.

respeto Respectful.

respiration Exchange of oxygen and carbon dioxide during cellular metabolism.

respiratory acidosis Abnormal condition characterized by increased arterial carbon dioxide concentration, excess carbonic acid, and increased hydrogen ion concentration.

respiratory alkalosis Abnormal condition characterized by decreased arterial carbon dioxide concentration and hydrogen ion concentration.

respite care Short-term health services to dependent older adults either in their home or in an institutional setting.

responsibility Carrying out duties associated with a particular role.

restorative care Health care settings and services in which patients who are recovering from illness or disability receive rehabilitation and supportive care.

restraint Device to aid in the immobilization of a patient or patient's extremity.

return demonstration Demonstration after the patient has first observed the teacher and then practiced the skill in mock or real situations.

rhonchi Abnormal lung sound auscultated when the patient's airways are obstructed with thick secretions.

right-sided heart failure Abnormal condition that results from impaired functioning of the right ventricle; characterized by venous congestion in the systemic circulation.

risk factor Any internal or external variable that makes a person or group more vulnerable to illness or an unhealthy event.

risk management Function of hospital or other health facility administration that is directed toward identification, evaluation, and correction of potential risks that could lead to injury of patients, staff members, or visitors and result in property loss or damage.

risk nursing diagnosis A clinical judgment concerning the vulnerability of an individual, family, group or community for developing an undesirable human response to health conditions/life processes.

role performance Way in which a person views his or her ability to carry out significant roles.

root cause analysis Process of data collection and analysis that aids in finding the real cause of the problem and working on dealing with it rather than just dealing with its effects.

S

Sabbath From sundown on Friday to sundown on Saturday, this religious observance is a day of rest and worship for Jews and some Christian sects.

sandbags Sand-filled plastic tubes that can be shaped to body contours. They can immobilize an extremity or maintain body alignment.

saturated fatty acid Fatty acid in which each carbon in the chain has an attached hydrogen atom.

scientific method Codified sequence of steps used in the formulation, testing, evaluation, and reporting of scientific ideas.

scientific rationale Reason why a specific nursing action was chosen based on supporting literature.

scoliosis Lateral spinal curvature.

scrub nurse Registered nurse or operating room technician who assists surgeons during operations.

secondary appraisal Evaluating one's possible coping strategies when confronted with a stressor.

secondary intention Wound closure in which the edges are separated; granulation tissue develops to fill the gap; and, finally, epithelium grows in over the granulation, producing a larger scar than results with primary intention.

secondary prevention Level of preventive medicine that focuses on early diagnosis, use of referral services, and rapid initiation of treatment to stop the progress of disease processes.

sedatives Medications that produce a calming effect by decreasing functional activity, diminishing irritability, and allaying excitement.

segmentation Alternating contraction and relaxation of gastrointestinal mucosa.

self-concept Complex, dynamic integration of conscious and unconscious feelings, attitudes, and perceptions about one's identity, physical being, worth, and roles; how a person perceives and defines self.

self-esteem Feeling of self-worth characterized by feelings of achievement, adequacy, self-confidence, and usefulness.

self-transcendence Sense of authentically connecting to one's inner self.

sender Person who initiates interpersonal communication by conveying a message.

sensible water loss Loss of fluid from the body through the secretory activity of the sweat glands and the exhalation of humidified air from the lungs.

sensory deficits Defects in the function of one or more of the senses, resulting in visual, auditory, or olfactory impairments.

sensory deprivation State in which stimulation to one or more of the senses is lacking, resulting in impaired sensory perception.

sensory overload State in which stimulation to one or more of the senses is so excessive that the brain disregards or does not meaningfully respond to stimuli.

sequential compression stockings Plastic stockings attached to an air pump that inflates and deflates the stockings, applying intermittent pressure sequentially from the ankle to the knee.

serum half-life Time needed for excretion processes to lower the serum drug concentration by half.

sexual dysfunction Inability or difficulty in sexual functioning caused by physiological or psychological factors or both.

sexual orientation Clear, persistent erotic preference for a person of one sex or the other.

sexuality "A function of the total personality … concerned with the biological, psychological, sociological, spiritual and culture variables of life …" (Sex Information and Education Council of the United States, 1980).

sexually transmitted infection Infectious process spread through sexual contact, including oral, genital, or anal sexual activity.

shear Force exerted against the skin while the skin remains stationary and the bony structures move.

side effect Any reaction or consequence that results from medication or therapy.

side rails Bars positioned along the sides of the length of the bed or stretcher to reduce the patient's risk of falling.

simpatia Friendly.

sinoatrial (SA) node Called the *pacemaker of the heart* because the origin of the normal heartbeat begins at the SA node. The SA node is in the right atrium next to the entrance of the superior vena cava.

situational crisis Unexpected crisis that arises suddenly in response to an external event or a conflict concerning a specific circumstance.

situational loss Loss of a person, thing, or quality resulting from a change in a life situation, including changes related to illness, body image, environment, and death.

sitz bath Bath in which only the hips or buttocks are immersed in fluid.

skilled nursing facility Institution or part of an institution that meets criteria for accreditation established by the sections of the Social Security Act that determine the basis for Medicaid and Medicare reimbursement for skilled nursing care, including rehabilitation and various medical and nursing procedures.

sleep State marked by reduced consciousness, diminished activity of the skeletal muscles, and depressed metabolism.

sleep apnea Cessation of breathing for a time during sleep.

sleep deprivation Condition resulting from a decrease in the amount, quality, and consistency of sleep.

SOAP note Progress note that focuses on a single patient problem and includes subjective and objective data, analysis, and planning; most often used in the problem-oriented medical record (POMR).

social determinants of health Factors that contribute to a person's current state of health. These factors may be biological, socioeconomic, psychosocial, behavioral, or social in nature.

socializing Interacting with friends or other people; communicating with others to form relationships and help people feel relaxed.

solute Substance dissolved in a solution.

solution Mixture of one or more substances dissolved in another substance. The molecules of each of the substances disperse homogeneously and do not change chemically. A solution may be a liquid, gas, or solid.

solvent Any liquid in which another substance can be dissolved.

source record Organization of a patient's chart so each discipline (e.g., nursing, medicine, social work, or respiratory therapy) has a separate section in which to record data. Unlike POMR, the information is not organized by patient problems. The advantage of a source record is that caregivers can easily locate the proper section of the record in which to make entries.

sphygmomanometer Device for measuring the arterial blood pressure that consists of an arm or leg cuff with an air bladder connected to a tube, a bulb for pumping air into the bladder, and a gauge for indicating the amount of air pressure being exerted against the artery.

spiritual distress State of being out of harmony with a system of beliefs, a Supreme Being, or God.

spiritual well-being Individual's spirituality that enables a person to love, have faith and hope, seek meaning in life, and nurture relationships with others.

spirituality Spiritual dimension of a person, including the relationship with humanity, nature, and a supreme being.

standard of care Minimum level of care accepted to ensure high-quality care to patients. Standards of care define the types of therapies typically administered to patients with defined problems or needs.

standard precautions Guidelines recommended by the Centers for Disease Control and Prevention (CDC) to reduce risk of transmission of bloodborne and other pathogens in hospitals.

standardized care plans Written care plans used for groups of patients who have similar health care problems.

standing order Written and approved documents containing rules, policies, procedures, regulations, and orders for the conduct of patient care in various stipulated clinical settings.

statutory law Of or related to laws enacted by a legislative branch of the government.

stenosis Abnormal condition characterized by the constriction or narrowing of an opening or passageway in a body structure.

stereotypes Generalizations that are made about individuals without further assessment.

sterilization (1) Rendering a person unable to produce children; accomplished by surgical, chemical, or other means. (2) A technique for destroying microorganisms using heat, water, chemicals, or gases.

stoma Artificially created opening between a body cavity and the surface of the body (e.g., a colostomy formed from a portion of the colon pulled through the abdominal wall).

stress Physiological or psychological tension that threatens homeostasis or a person's psychological equilibrium.

stressor Any event, situation, or other stimulus encountered in a person's external or internal environment that necessitates change or adaptation by the person.

striae Streaks or linear scars that result from rapid development of tension in the skin.

stroke volume (SV) Amount of blood ejected by the ventricles with each contraction. It can be affected by the amount of blood in the left ventricle at the end of diastole (preload), the resistance to left ventricular ejection (afterload), and myocardial contractility.

subacute care Level of medical specialty care provided to patients who need a greater intensity of care than that provided in a skilled nursing facility but who do not require acute care.

subcultures Various ethnic, religious, and other groups with distinct characteristics from the dominant culture.

subcutaneous (sub-Q) Injection given into the connective tissue under the dermis. The subcutaneous tissue absorbs drugs more slowly than those injected into muscle. Injections are usually given at a 45-degree angle.

subjective data Information gathered from patient statements; the patient's feelings and perceptions. Not verifiable by another except by inference.

sublingual Route of medication administration in which the medication is placed underneath the patient's tongue.

Sunrise Model A model developed by Leininger that aids the health care practitioner in designing care decisions and actions in a culturally congruent fashion.

supine Position of the patient in which the patient is resting on his or her back.

suprainfection Secondary infection usually caused by an opportunistic pathogen.

suprapubic catheter Catheter surgically inserted through abdomen into bladder.

surfactant Chemical produced in the lungs to maintain the surface tension of the alveoli and keep them from collapsing.

surgical asepsis Procedures used to eliminate any microorganisms from an area. Also called *sterile technique*.

sympathy Concern, sorrow, or pity felt by the nurse for the patient. Sympathy is a subjective look at another person's world that prevents a clear perspective of all sides of the issues confronting that person.

synapse Region surrounding the point of contact between two neurons or between a neuron and an effector organ.

syncope Brief lapse in consciousness caused by transient cerebral hypoxia.

synergistic effect Effect resulting from two drugs acting synergistically. The effect of the two drugs combined is greater than the effect that would be expected if the individual effects of the two drugs acting alone were added together.

systolic Pertaining to or resulting from ventricular contraction.

T

tachycardia Rapid regular heart rate ranging between 100 and 150 beats/min.

tachypnea Abnormally rapid rate of breathing.

tactile Relating to the sense of touch.

tactile fremitus Tremulous vibration of the chest wall during breathing that is palpable on physical examination.

teaching Implementation method used to present correct principles, procedures, and techniques of health care; to inform patients about their health status; and to refer patients and family to appropriate health or social resources in the community.

team nursing Decentralized system in which the care of a patient is distributed among the members of a team. The charge nurse delegates authority to a team leader, who must be a professional nurse.

teratogens Chemical or physiological agents that may produce adverse effects in the embryo or fetus.

tertiary prevention Activities directed toward rehabilitation rather than diagnosis and treatment.

therapeutic communication Process in which the nurse consciously influences a patient or helps the patient to a better understanding through verbal and/or nonverbal communication.

therapeutic effect Desired benefit of a medication, treatment, or procedure.

thermoregulation Internal control of body temperature.

threshold Point at which a person first perceives a painful stimulus as being painful.

thrill Continuous palpable sensation like the purring of a cat.

thrombus Accumulation of platelets, fibrin, clotting factors, and the cellular elements of the blood attached to the interior wall of a vein or artery, sometimes occluding the lumen of the vessel.

tinnitus Ringing heard in one or both ears.

tissue ischemia Point at which tissues receive insufficient oxygen and perfusion.

tolerance Point at which a person is not willing to accept pain of greater severity or duration.

tort Act that causes injury for which the injured party can bring civil action.

total patient care Nursing delivery of care model originally developed during Florence Nightingale's time. In the model a registered nurse (RN) is responsible for all aspects of care for one or more patients. The RN works directly with the patient, family, physician or health care provider, and health care team members. The model typically has a shift-based focus.

touch To come in contact with another person, often conveying caring, emotional support, encouragement, or tenderness.

toxic effect Effect of a medication that results in an adverse response.

tracheostomy Procedure whereby a surgical incision is made into the trachea and a short artificial airway (a tracheostomy tube) is inserted.

transcendence The belief that there is a force outside of and greater than the person that exists beyond the material world.

transcultural Concept of care extending across cultures that distinguishes nursing from other health disciplines.

transcultural nursing Distinct discipline developed by Leininger that focuses on the comparative study of cultures to understand similarities and differences among groups of people.

transcutaneous electrical nerve stimulation (TENS) Technique in which a battery-powered device blocks pain impulses from reaching the spinal cord by delivering weak electrical impulses directly to the surface of the skin.

transdermal disk Medication delivery device in which the medication is saturated on a wafer-like disk, which is affixed to the patient's skin. This method ensures that the patient receives a continuous level of medication.

transfer report Verbal exchange of information between caregivers when a patient is moved from one nursing unit or health care setting to another. The report includes information necessary to maintain a consistent level of care from one setting to another.
transformational leadership A leadership style that focuses on change and innovation through effective communication and team building. Engagement, empowerment, and accountability are critical to team effectiveness.
transfusion reaction Systemic response by the body to the administration of blood incompatible with that of the recipient.
trapeze bar Metal triangular-shaped bar that can be suspended over a patient's bed from an overhanging frame; permits patients to move up and down in bed while in traction or some other encumbrance.
trimester Referring to one of the three phases of pregnancy.
trochanter roll Rolled towel support placed against the hips and upper leg to prevent external rotation of the legs.
trough The lowest serum concentration of a medication before the next medication dose is administered.
turgor Normal resiliency of the skin caused by the outward pressure of the cells and interstitial fluid.

U

unsaturated fatty acid Fatty acid in which an unequal number of hydrogen atoms are attached and the carbon atoms attach to one another with a double bond.
ureterostomy Diversion of urine away from a diseased or defective bladder through an artificial opening in the skin.
urge incontinence A type of urinary incontinence that results from sudden, involuntary contraction of the muscles of the urinary bladder, resulting in an urge to urinate.
urinal Receptacle for collecting urine.
urinary diversion Surgical diversion of the drainage of urine such as a ureterostomy.
urinary incontinence Inability to control urination.
urinary reflux Abnormal, backward flow of urine.
urinary retention Retention of urine in the bladder; condition frequently caused by a temporary loss of muscle function.
urine hat Receptacle for collecting urine that fits toilet.
urometer Device for measuring frequent and small amounts of urine from an indwelling urinary catheter system.
urosepsis Organisms in the bloodstream.
utilitarianism Ethic that proposes that the value of something is determined by its usefulness. The greatest good for the greatest number of people constitutes the guiding principle for action in a utilitarian model of ethics.
utilization review (UR) committees Physician-supervised committees to review admissions, diagnostic testing, and treatments provided by physicians or health care providers to patients.

V

validation Act of confirming, verifying, or corroborating the accuracy of assessment data or the appropriateness of the care plan.
Valsalva maneuver Any forced expiratory effort against a closed airway such as when an individual holds his or her breath and tightens his or her muscles in a concerted, strenuous effort to move a heavy object or change positions in bed.
value Personal belief about the worth of a given idea or behavior.
valvular heart disease Acquired or congenital disorder of a cardiac valve characterized by stenosis and obstructed blood flow or valvular degeneration and regurgitation of blood.
variances Unexpected event that occurs during patient care and that is different from CareMap predictions. Variances or exceptions are interventions or outcomes that are not achieved as anticipated. Variance may be positive or negative.
variant Differing from a set standard.
vascular access devices Catheters, cannulas, or infusion ports designed for long-term, repeated access to the vascular system.
vasoconstriction Narrowing of the lumen of any blood vessel, especially the arterioles and the veins in the blood reservoirs of the skin and abdominal viscera.
vasodilation Increase in the diameter of a blood vessel caused by inhibition of its vasoconstrictor nerves or stimulation of dilator nerves.
venipuncture Technique in which a vein is punctured transcutaneously by a sharp rigid stylet (e.g., a butterfly needle), a cannula (e.g., an angiocatheter that contains a flexible plastic catheter), or a needle attached to a syringe.
ventilation Respiratory process by which gases are moved into and out of the lungs.
verbal communication Sending of messages from one individual to another or to a group of individuals through the spoken word.
vertigo Sensation of dizziness or spinning.
vibration Fine, shaking pressure applied by hands to the chest wall only during exhalation.
virulence Ability of an organism to rapidly produce disease.
visual Related to or experienced through vision.
vital signs Temperature, pulse, respirations, and blood pressure.
vitamins Organic compounds essential in small quantities for normal physiological and metabolic functioning of the body. With few exceptions, vitamins cannot be synthesized by the body and must be obtained from the diet or dietary supplements.
voiding Process of urinating.
vulnerable populations Collection of individuals who are more likely to develop health problems as a result of excess risks, limits in access to health care services, or being dependent on others for care.

W

wellness Dynamic state of health in which an individual progresses toward a higher level of functioning, achieving an optimum balance between internal and external environments.
wellness education Activities that teach people how to care for themselves in a healthy manner.
wellness nursing diagnosis Clinical judgment about an individual, group, or community in transition from a specific level of wellness to a higher level of wellness.
wheezes, wheezing Adventitious lung sounds caused by a severely narrowed bronchus.
work redesign Formal process used to analyze the work of a certain work group and change the actual structure of the jobs performed.
worldview Cognitive stance or perspective about phenomena characteristic of a particular cultural group.
wound culture Specimen collected from a wound to determine the specific organism that is causing an infectious process.

Y

yearning and searching Second phase of Bowlby's phases of mourning. It is characterized by emotional outbursts of tearful sobbing and acute distress.

Z

Z-track injection Technique for injecting irritating preparations into muscle without tracking residual medication through sensitive tissues.

INDEX

b indicates boxes, *f* indicates illustrations, and *t* indicates tables.

SPECIAL FEATURES

Evidence-Based Practice

Patient Teaching

Concept Maps